Oxford Textbook of Palliative Medicine

Third Edition

Edited by

Derek Doyle OBE

Formerly Medical Director/Consultant in Palliative Medicine, St Columba's Hospice, Edinburgh, UK

Geoffrey Hanks

Professor of Palliative Medicine, University of Bristol, Bristol Haematology and Oncology Centre, Bristol, UK

Nathan I Cherny

Director, Cancer Pain and Palliative Medicine, Department of Medical Oncology and Palliative Medicine, Share Zedek Medical Center, Jerusalem, Israel

and

Sir Kenneth Calman

Vice-Chancellor and Warden, University of Durham, Durham, UK

OXFORD
UNIVERSITY PRESS

OXFORD
UNIVERSITY PRESS

Great Clarendon Street, Oxford OX2 6DP

Oxford University Press is a department of the University of Oxford.
It furthers the University's objective of excellence in research, scholarship,
and education by publishing worldwide in

Oxford New York

Auckland Bangkok Buenos Aires Cape Town Chennai
Dar es Salaam Delhi Hong Kong Istanbul Karachi Kolkata
Kuala Lumpur Madrid Melbourne Mexico City Mumbai Nairobi
São Paulo Shanghai Taipei Tokyo Toronto

Oxford is a registered trade mark of Oxford University Press
in the UK and in certain other countries

Published in the United States
by Oxford University Press Inc., New York

First edition published 1993
First published in paperback 1995
Second edition published 1998
Reprinted 1998
Second edition published in paperback 1999
Reprinted 2001, 2003
Third edition published 2004

British Library Cataloguing in Publication Data

Data available

ISBN 0 19 851098 5

10 9 8 7 6 5 4 3 2 1

Typeset by Newgen Imaging Systems (P) Ltd, Chennai, India
Printed in Italy
on acid-free paper by Lego Print

Oxford Textbook of

Palliative Medicine

Indexer Newgen Imaging Systems (P) Ltd
Production Manager Kate Martin
Design Manager Andrew Meaden
Typographer Jonathan Coleclough
Publisher Catherine Barnes

Summary of contents

Contents

Preface to the third edition

We continue to be delighted with the success of this textbook and grateful for the many comments and suggestions sent to us by colleagues round the world. In the few years since the last edition was published many new palliative care services have been established, Palliative Medicine has been recognized as a specialty in more countries, and everywhere this textbook has come to be recognized as the definitive text on a fast-developing subject.

Our editorial team has changed. Our sense of loss when Neil MacDonald had to retire from the team was, to some extent, eased when he agreed to write several chapters and when we found not one, but two distinguished colleagues to replace him. Neither needs much introduction. Nathan Cherny, an Australian–trained physician works in Jerusalem, but is equally well known and respected in the United States where he pursued his studies in Memorial Sloan Kettering Cancer Center in New York. Sir Kenneth Calman, now Vice Chancellor of Durham University, England was previously the first professor of oncology in the University of Glasgow and instrumental in establishing palliative care services in that city before becoming, in turn, the Chief Medical Officer, Scotland and Chief Medical Officer, England.

We introduced many changes and innovations into the second edition and in this, the third edition, we have made even more changes—many of them suggested by readers. In many respects this is a new book; so comprehensive are the changes. There are new chapters devoted to palliative medicine in the context of care of the elderly and intensive care. A chapter is devoted to complementary and alternative medicine in relation to patients receiving palliative care, and a whole section to the contributions to palliative medicine of allied health professionals as they are now termed.

Increasingly is it being recognized that the principles of palliative medicine are applicable in the care of people with non-malignant conditions. Reflecting that we have introduced chapters on non-malignant respiratory disease, non-malignant neurological disease, cardiac disease, dietary and nutritional problems, while many other sections from previous editions have been totally rewritten, often by new authors whom we have been delighted to welcome to this work.

So important do we regard education and training in our subject that this section has also been rewritten and the opportunity taken to introduce new ideas and new technologies such as internet learning and video conferencing. Readers will not be surprised to see lists of recommended websites, and references to websites.

We feel privileged to have worked with contributors from so many countries including Australia, Canada, China, Germany, India, Israel, Italy, Norway, Sweden, and the United States. All exceedingly busy, they have willingly written for our textbook and shared their wealth of knowledge and clinical experience. Our especial thanks, however, must go to our secretaries, Debbie Ashby in Bristol and Judith Sunter in Durham, to our professional colleagues, to Catherine Barnes and all at Oxford University Press, and to Mukesh of Newgen Imaging.

As with previous editions we dedicate this textbook to suffering patients around the world and to our colleagues who care for them.

Derek Doyle
Geoffrey Hanks
Nathan I. Cherny
Kenneth Calman
September 2003

Preface to the second edition

When the first edition of this textbook was published in 1993 we were honoured to receive many appreciative reviews: several of them raised points to consider in a second edition and offered most constructive suggestions. We have been able to add comments from colleagues all over the world, to all of whom we express our appreciation. Our publishers have persuaded us to produce a new edition into which we can incorporate the many points raised.

Several people commented that the textbook appeared to be exclusively for doctors, yet palliative care, as is so frequently stated in the text, is team caring, interprofessional in fact rather than multiprofessional. We make no apology for it being a *medical textbook* for that is exactly what we intended and explained in the Preface to the first edition. We continue to see a need for a medical reference book whilst fully respecting and appreciating the roles of colleagues in other professions. In the same way we feel the title is right in referring to *palliative medicine* rather than palliative care or hospice care but readers will notice that throughout the text, wherever team collaboration is mentioned, the word used is *care* rather than *medicine*, and the much-loved word *hospice* is used when that is the title of a particular unit or service.

Another important comment was that the first edition appeared to focus on malignant disease although the principles of palliative medicine are said to apply to all diseases. In particular, some colleagues asked why a section had not been devoted exclusively to palliation in the geriatric population. The first comment has been addressed in this new edition by requesting all our contributors to demonstrate the relevance of palliative medicine across the clinical spectrum, where necessary highlighting special areas and issues for attention. We sought the opinion of specialist geriatricians and in the light of their comments have decided not to devote a special chapter to their patients.

What we *have* done is to introduce completely new chapters and make the book bigger and even more comprehensive. The increasingly important contribution of interventional radiology has been recognized with a full chapter, as have the subjects of audit and the economics of palliative medicine, and AIDS in children. A new chapter is devoted to pruritus and sweating, another to pain assessment, and yet another to pharmacological aspects of palliative medicine.

The section on cultural issues was appreciated by many readers and in this new edition it has been expanded with the additions of chapters on the cultures of sub-Saharan Africa, China and Japan, and Australian indigenous peoples, reflecting the worldwide spread and appropriateness of palliative medicine. A new team of authors has written the ethics section and, in recognition of the ethical issues in caring for children, a new chapter has been introduced on ethical issues in paediatric palliative medicine. Even when chapter titles have not been changed readers will find that many alterations have been made in the text, much new material added, and many new references cited, reflecting the considerable advances in this specialty in a very few years.

We pay tribute to those contributors to the first edition who so graciously agreed to stand down and hand over the baton to other authorities, and welcome our many new colleagues. To them all we express very sincere thanks for all the time, work, and endless patience they have so generously shared with us.

We have enjoyed working with our friends in Oxford University Press and make no apology for singling out Dr Irene Butcher whose skills, patience, and wisdom seem to us to be limitless. Finally, but with great sincerity, we acknowledge our immeasureable debt to our assistants, secretaries, and colleagues who in diverse ways made this new edition possible.

Derek Doyle
Geoffrey W.C. Hanks
Neil MacDonald
October 1997

Preface to the second edition

Preface to the first edition

We offer this new textbook as our contribution to modern palliative medicine. Our readers deserve some explanation about its contents and our fellow contributors our *unqualified* appreciation and respect.

Until quite recently terminal care, as it used to be called, consisted of little more than 'tender loving care' married to pain and symptom control using basic drugs skilfully prescribed. Some argued that there was little else to it and certainly not sufficient to merit a major textbook. We felt differently as, clearly, do many others who have made the subject their life's work. We were conscious of how much can be done, how much there is to learn, and how little we ourselves knew. Equally we were aware of how much our colleagues in related disciplines and specialties could share with us, how much valuable research had been done and how much remains to be done. Hence this textbook. Our aim has been to produce as comprehensive a book as possible, with a body of knowledge based on sound research as well as extensive clinical experience. To some extent we believe we have succeeded. Readers will note differing opinions, each firmly held by those with that level of experience and authority. We have made no attempt to reconcile all such differences for they are important. They demonstrate where dogmatism may be inappropriate and where further studies are still needed. Having said that, we have been impressed with the unanimity demonstrated in most areas and the professional open-mindedness and humility displayed by our contributors.

On many more occasions than might have been expected, we have been reminded what a strong scientific base palliative medicine is built on. Little of what has been written is merely anecdotal, valuable as that can be. Much has been studied and researched, forming the basis of this textbook.

Inevitably some will criticize the book as too much related to, and reflecting, 'Westernized' medical practice without due attention to the needs of the 'palliative care Third World'. Throughout, we have never ignored the needs of those having to work with limited resources but have tried to demonstrate not only what can be done in the medically-sophisticated world but also by colleagues less fortunate than ourselves. Treatment regimens include basic principles as well as sophisticated techniques, always emphasizing the totality of care, and the roles and needs not only of other professionals but also the relatives. We are deeply conscious that, while for a few, palliative medicine is the final stage of years of sophisticated therapeutic management, for millions of others all they can ever hope for is that its benefits will eventually become available to them and their families.

Clearly it would be impossible to detail each drug, each with as many different proprietary names, for every country where this book may be read. Rather we have chosen to use generic names.

Palliative medicine impinges on and frequently overlaps with many other medical specialties. Gone are the days when a patient receiving palliative care never again had further investigations or benefited from the advice of surgeons and oncologists. We have tried to demonstrate the contributions of other specialists by inviting them to share their knowledge and their contributions with us and have been honoured by their unstinting willingness to do so. Technical details of their work would have been out of place in such a textbook but readers will appreciate how they too can contribute to the complex kaleidoscope which confronts us and challenges us in palliative medicine.

In the same way in which we have encouraged these coauthors to share their wisdom in their own way, so too have we not attempted to impose a consistency of style on their writing but left them to express their thoughts and share their deeply-held feelings in their own inimitable way. We believe that this has enriched the book.

To our contributors we offer our profound thanks and respect. Few have worked alone; most have been assisted by many others, perhaps unnamed in this book, and by clinician colleagues who have acted for them when their writing took up days and weeks of precious time. To them all, named and unnamed, we extend our appreciation. They have all borne with our demands and our criticisms with unfailing patience making us appreciate what sensitive, understanding clinicians they must be.

Traditionally all authors and editors close with a grateful tribute to their publishers. In our case we would go further. We could never have dared to expect such patience with our shortcomings, such guidance when we so often called for it, and such genuine interest in, and enthusiasm for, our subject and this book. We are deeply grateful. We feel particularly privileged to have worked with Dr Irene Butcher who was an unfailing source of encouragement, support, and advice. No editors could have been better served.

Our secretaries deserve a special mention. Irene Turnbull (Edinburgh), Felicity Fleetwood (London), and Sheila Parr and Patricia McDonald (Edmonton) have given unstintingly of their skills, time, and loyalty, and to each we offer our unqualified thanks.

We dedicate this textbook to the colleagues with whom we work, those who have taught and inspired us and, most of all, to those we serve, our patients and their families.

Derek Doyle
Geoffrey W.C. Hanks
Neil MacDonald
1993

Foreword

Cicely M. Saunders, OM, DBE

President and Founder, St Christopher's Hospice, London, UK

But I have promises to keep, and miles to go before I sleep.
Robert Frost

The above quotation reminds us of all that people can achieve during the last phase of life. This textbook, now into another edition in response to demand, covers ground much wider than just a systematic approach to symptom control but is concerned with the whole impact of persistent disease upon a person and the whole family. Its historical development was summed up by Wall in 1986:

> Up to the 19th century, most medical care related to the amelioration of symptoms while the natural history of the disease took its course toward recovery or death. By 1900, doctors and patients alike had turned to a search for root cause and ultimate cure. In the course of this new direction, symptoms were placed on one side as sign posts along a highway which was being driven toward the intended destination. Therapy directed at the sign posts was denigrated and dismissed as merely symptomatic. By the second half of this century, a reaction set in as seen by such remarkable developments as the hospice movement. The immediate origins of misery and suffering need immediate attention while the long-term search for basic cure proceeds. The old methods of care and caring had to be rediscovered and the best of modern medicine had to be turned to the task of new study and therapy specifically directed at pain.[1]

Such pain is not merely physical. By 1964 it was noted that the single word *pain* could refer to 'total pain' with mental distress and social and spiritual problems, with patients making such statements as, 'it seemed that all of me is wrong'.[2]

Approaches to death and dying reveal much about the attitude of the society as a whole towards the individuals who go through it. The development of ideas of what constitutes a good death can even be traced to prehistory. Funeral rites can be dated back 50 000 years, and from this time show how early men laid down their dead in grief and in some hope of a continued existence.[3] Gentles traces the way funeral rites have become less and less elaborate and comparatively less costly over the millennia in proportion to the wealth of society.[4] But there seems to be more to it than that. The fantastic wealth of Egyptian funerals and the expenditure of time and human effort on such memorials as the pyramids were concentrated on the Pharaohs who in some sense personified the longings for immortality of the rest of the populace. Attitudes to death reflect attitudes to religion and community.

Aries reviewed Western attitudes towards death from the Middle Ages to the present.[5] At the beginning of the period he describes 'tamed death', when the dying person was sure of his role in preparing for the end according to ritual or custom (ref. 5, pp. 2–9). He was himself the centre of the stage, hopeful, if all was done in order, of a safe passage to the next world. Aries compares this with Solzhenitsyn's description of the death of the simple people of the country who 'departed easily, as if they were just moving into a new house'.[6] Similarly, Aries points out, the cemeteries of the early Middle Ages were open and public places and 'the living were as familiar with the dead as they were familiarised with the idea of their own death' (ref. 5, p. 25).

Gradually, during the Middle Ages subtle modifications gave a dramatic and personal meaning to this traditional familiarity. An increasing emphasis on the Last Judgement and the displacing of this to the end of each life, with all its concentration on feelings of sin and failure, together with a macabre interest in physical decomposition, gave a more personal, threatening focus. One's own death, and an urge somehow to maintain identity despite the loss of all material attachments, took the place of the familiar resignation to the collective destiny of the species (ref. 5, pp. 27–52). The individual has his/her particular place in the Christian Gospel (e.g. the search for the one lost sheep to join the ninety and nine safe in the fold) but the emphasis grew more urgent with the Renaissance.

Aries traces in the exaggeration of mourning that developed in the nineteenth century, a new fear, not so much of the death of the self as the death of another—the origin of the cult of tombs and cemeteries as we know them. This development was sharply brought to an end in many places in the twentieth century by a process far more abrupt than any so far summarized, surely related to the carnage of the War of 1914. From now on we see a process by which death becomes, as Aries puts it, 'shameful and forbidden', something to be hidden from those around.

The increasing tendency not to tell the dying person the truth of his/her condition, the likelihood of dying in hospital, often alone, rather than at home, and the inability of the society to allow any display of emotions in public, all made death an outlaw, a forbidden subject. We have not found our way to come to terms with our mortality, and each person, each family, with little help from ritual, or tradition, or from those around, has somehow to find a way to come to terms with and grow from loss. The old acceptance of destiny has disappeared and a new sense of outrage that modern advances cannot finally halt the inevitable makes caring for the dying and for their families demanding and often difficult, but perhaps all the more rewarding as truth becomes more openly discussed.

The present volume, looking at the whole field of the multidisciplinary speciality of palliative medicine, addresses aspects of this problem and, importantly, shows how appropriate treatment before a patient can rightly be termed 'dying' can make a radical difference to the last span of life and to the way the family lives afterwards.

The early hospices

A considerable part of this new and positive attitude, with its new range of possibilities, stems from the attitudes and skills of the modern hospice. An ancient word, although not originally concerned with dying, it has some connotations that introduce interesting comparisons with the aims of a modern hospice and palliative care teams. The Latin word *hospes* first meant 'stranger'. By late classical times, the word had changed and denoted a host, while *hospitalis* meant friendly—the welcome to the stranger. From it was derived hospitality and thence many words used today—hospital, hostel, hostelry, hotel—and hospice. Another noun was derived—*hospitium*, originally the warm feeling between host and guest, and later the place where this feeling was experienced. The Greek version was *xenodochium* and by the fourth century came the first of many Christian institutions under both names, arising first in the Byzantine area[7] and later spreading to Rome and finally throughout Europe as hospice or hospital.[8] They were based on the Christian command 'As you did it to one of the least of these my brethren, you did it to me' (Matt. 25, v. 40). This was a radically different approach from the Hippocratic tradition in which a doctor did not treat the incurably sick or terminally ill. It was thought unethical to treat a patient with a deadly disease, for in so doing the doctor risked paying the penalty awaiting those mortals who challenged nature and the gods.[9]

These hospices welcomed pilgrims, often very battered and perhaps dying, and gradually came the connotation of sickness as Christians set out not only to welcome strangers and give food and drink, but also to care for the sick. As hospices developed along the pilgrim routes, local people in need undoubtedly came for help and were not sent away. Hospices lasted throughout the Middle Ages, but most came to a rather abrupt end with the Reformation. The state of the incurable and dying, no longer the honoured guests but often consigned to Poor Law or equivalent institutions, could be desperate. An example of how the Church's concern for the sick and poor was missed is illustrated by a petition to Henry VIII from the Lord Mayor and citizens of London. They implored the King to re-found the priory of St Bartholomew in Smithfield and that of St Thomas across London Bridge in Southwark 'for the ayde and comfort of the poore sikke, blynde, aged and impotent persones, beying not able to helpe themselffs, nor hauyning any place certeyn whereyn they may be lodged, cherysshed and refressed tyll they be cured and holpen of theyre dyseases and sycknesse'.[10]

The modern hospice movement

As has been pointed out, the medieval hospice was not primarily associated with dying people, and over the centuries it had come to welcome an impossible mix of patients along with travellers and pilgrims, orphans, and the destitute, with varying degrees of segregation. Such cure as could be attained was a primary aim, but with comparatively little to offer many must have died, being cared for to the end with much emphasis on spiritual comfort.

The first use so far discovered of the word 'hospice' solely for care of the dying was by Mme Jeanne Garnier in Lyons, France, in 1842, who founded several such hospices or *Calvaires*. There was no connection with the Irish Sisters of Charity who opened Our Lady's Hospice in Dublin in 1879 and St Joseph's Hospice in East London in 1905, both for incurable and dying patients, but Calvary Hospital in New York (1899) drew its inspiration from this source. Three Protestant Homes had been opened in London by the time St Joseph's welcomed patients. These were the Friedensheim Home of Rest (later St Columba's Hospital) in 1885, the Hostel of God (later Trinity Hospice) in 1891, and St Luke's Home for the Dying Poor in 1893. Several small catholic, protestant, and Jewish homes were founded under different titles in the turn of the nineteenth and twentieth centuries in the USA and Australia. The author's 7 years from 1948 as a volunteer nurse in St Luke's, by then named Hospital, and the reading of its many complete and lively annual reports by Dr Howard Barrett, its founder, were a major influence in the early planning of St Christopher's Hospice.

These reports are full of individual stories of carefully observed people. Here we are not meeting 'the dying' but people, often part of destitute families. In 1909 Dr Barrett wrote:

> We do not think or speak of our inmates as 'cases'. We realize that each one is a human microcosm, with its own characteristics, its own aggregate of joys and sorrows, hopes and fears, its own life history, intensely interesting to itself and some small surrounding circle. Very often it is confided to some of us.

None of these homes had much impact upon general care for dying people.[11]

There was also much to learn from the Marie Curie Memorial Foundation. In 1952 it published a report detailing a great deal of suffering among patients dying of cancer at home.[12] Their response in supplying home nurses and in opening a series of cancer-care homes marked another important milestone in terminal care. But above all, the author's 7 years in clinical care at St Joseph's listening to patients, introducing records, and monitoring the results of the development of pain and symptom control first seen in St Luke's as the regular administration of oral opioids were crucial. Patients' comments and conditions revealed the need for appropriate treatments, for care in their own homes to supplement the existing community services, and for family support both before and after bereavement. Above all, the need for research and education in what was eventually to become a new speciality was revealed through much reading and many visits during those years.

The opening of St Christopher's in 1967 as the first research and teaching hospice that included home care, family support throughout illness and bereavement follow up, led to several different systems of offering care. This began to be termed the Hospice Movement in North America, where patterns other than free-standing inpatient units were first developed. Similar systems arose not long afterwards in the United Kingdom. In 1974, The Connecticut Hospice began offering home care with a medical and professional team leading many volunteers, without its own back-up beds. In New York, a consulting team began working throughout St Luke's Hospital during the same year. In early 1975, Mount opened the Palliative Care Service in Royal Victoria Hospital, Montreal. The founders of all these teams had spent sabbatical periods of study and experience at St Christopher's Hospice. These developments demonstrated that hospice care did not have to be limited to a separate building, but that the new attitudes and skills could be practised in a variety of settings. Since those early days, a world-wide spread has shown that the basic principles can be interpreted in widely differing cultures and with few resources other than the family values of the developing world.[13]

The Montreal Unit was not the first such use of the word palliative, although apparently there was no connection. In 1890, Dr Herbert Snow, Surgeon to the Cancer Hospital, Brompton, London, published a book on 'The Palliative Treatment of Incurable Cancer, with an Appendix on the Use of the Opium Pipe'.[14] He also published an article in the British Medical Journal on 'Opium and cocaine in the Treatment of cancerous disease.'[15] The Cancer Hospital (now the Royal Marsden Hospital) was next door to the Brompton Hospital for Diseases of the Chest. Perhaps the pharmacists were in touch when the latter hospital produced the Brompton Cocktail in the early 1930s with its main ingredients of morphine or diamorphine and cocaine. Its regular four-hourly usage in St Luke's Hospital can be traced back to 1935, through the memories of a former matron. The Cancer Hospital was committed to patients with advanced disease. In 1909 Dr Horder was allocated 19 beds for such patients and in 1964 a ward was re-opened with 16 beds in Dr Horder's name. No record of what happened in the interim period can be found.

New tools for relief

All the new teams set out first to establish the control of the distress that had led to their patients' referral. For this they had many new tools on which to depend due to the work and discoveries of the 1950s, including new psychotropic drugs, phenothiazines, antidepressants and anxiolytics, synthetic steroids, and nonsteroidal anti-inflammatory drugs. New analgesics were also available, although even now none has so far replaced the well-tried opioids. Rather, it has been a continuing challenge to understand their actions, and to compare and test different routines, compositions, and methods of administration. At the same time, reports came from new pain clinics, and work concerning better understanding of family dynamics and bereavement was undertaken at the Tavistock Centre for Human Relations. Developments in both cancer chemotherapy and intensive care units also had their impact in both contrast and continuity with the work of the new teams. A detailed study of 102 matched patients by Hinton[16] on 'The physical and mental distress of the dying' documented the need to address problems largely ignored by the main thrust of medical development in general hospitals at that time. A short, but comprehensive, nationwide study by Hughes showed the woeful gap in adequate care of dying people.[17] Even earlier, in 1945, four social workers in Boston revealed some of the inadequacies in end of life care in a series of 200 patients.[18]

During the 1960s Kubler-Ross began her series of interviews with patients talking about dying in a large general hospital in Chicago. Her book 'On Death and Dying'[19] had a major impact on the public and on many professionals, and undoubtedly prepared the ground for the growth of hospice home-care teams in the United States. It also had an impact in other countries, although the original impetus, summarized above, came from more traditional sources, developing 'in the interstices of the NHS'.[20]

At about the same time Parkes began publishing his studies of bereavement. His approach to the whole family had a major influence on the planning and early development of St Christopher's and, from there on, the whole movement. He was to carry out much of the early evaluation of hospice work.[21]

The influences that came together include barely remembered influences. Most important is the impact of the many hundreds of patients whose notes were summarized, whose conversations were tape-recorded, and whose memories remain. They were the real founders of the hospice movement. Workers in clinical pain research were encountered and studied in researching the hospice foundation. Contacts with pain clinics were also developed.

There are, of course, other sources of the whole spectrum of palliative medicine as it is brought together in this book. The most important element that links the early teams and the present widely developing branch of medicine is an awareness of the many needs of a person and his family as they grapple with all the demands and challenges introduced by the inexorable progress of a disease that has outstripped the possibilities of cure. Although the early foundations took such subtitles as 'for the dying', the new teams had early on established, as their main objective, the quality of life until death. The message was: 'You matter because you are you, and you matter until the last moment of your life. We will do all we can, not only to help you die peacefully, but also to live until you die'.[22] These words together with the concept of total pain—a combination of physical, psychological, social, and spiritual elements—were built into St Christopher's and from thence into the modern hospice movement.

St Christopher's Hospice brought together these elements to set up this work, to demonstrate and evaluate its practice, and to encourage others to consider similar work in their different ways and settings. This had all been discussed in detail with the Ministry of Health, and in 1966 a research and development grant was awarded to set up a home-care service (established in 1969), to conduct a comparative study of oral morphine and diamorphine (begun the same year), and to perform an evaluation of local services and the effect that the presence of the Hospice would have upon them (from 1967). Research and rigour in developing clinical practice and education were built in from the beginning.

It was important to emphasize that what was being developed was not a soft option that would only be termed 'care', but a more appropriate treatment for people with advanced disease and for their families. The main focus on malignant disease enabled the workers to concentrate on a limited range of symptoms and social and emotional problems and to produce a number of studies and publications, first from St Christopher's and soon from other centres such as Montreal and later Oxford, Southampton, and elsewhere. The present volume makes clear how widely these challenges are now recognized and tackled.

If there had not been a great amount of distress documented, among others, by the Marie Curie Memorial Foundation in the home and by Hinton in hospital and felt deeply by all who could remember a sadly unrelieved death in their family or among their acquaintances, there would not have been the spread of interest and action, first in the United Kingdom and then in North America, Europe, Australia, Southern Africa, and many countries throughout the world. If there had not been continued contact with both fundamental scientists and clinicians occupied in research in pain and with many workers in other specialties, there would have been no sound basis of practice to share and to become one of the roots of the whole development of the spectrum of palliative medicine as presented in this textbook with all the updates and additions of this new edition.

Challenges and principles

A chapter on 'Terminal care' in the *Oxford Textbook of Medicine*[23] was reviewed as 'a characteristic mixture of tough clinical science and compassion'.[24] All the work of the professional team—the increasingly skilled symptom control, the supportive nursing, the social and pastoral works, the home care, and the mobilization of community resources—enable people to live until they die, at their own maximum potential, performing to the limit of their physical activity and mental capacity, with control and independence wherever possible. If they are recognized as unique and are helped to live as part of their families and in other relationships, they can still reach out to their hopes and expectations and to what has deepest meaning for them and end their lives with a sense of completion. The family, so often the caring team, will share this.

Awareness of what 'quality of life' means to people now demands full consideration of both the nature of their suffering and the appropriateness of various possible treatments and settings in their particular circumstances. Alertness to any remission of their disease or disability should accompany the optimum control of all the manifestations of an inexorable advance.

Patients should end their lives in the place most appropriate to them and to their families, and where possible, have choices in the matter. Some insight into the serious nature of their disease by the patient will help towards realistic decisions. Continuity of care can be maintained in the midst of change if there is effective care as presented anew by the contributors to this textbook.

When a person is dying the family find themselves in a crisis situation, with the joys and regrets of the past, the demands of the present, and the fears of the future, all brought into stark focus. Help may be needed to deal with guilt, depression, and family discord, and in this time of crisis there is the possibility of resolving old problems and finding reconciliations that greatly strengthen the family. If this time is to be fully used, there needs to be some degree of shared awareness of the true situation. Truth needs to be available (though not pressured) so that the family can travel together. In general, sharing is more creative than deception. The often-surprising potential for personal and family growth at this stage is one of the strongest objections most hospice workers raise for the legalization of a deliberately hastened death or for an automatic policy of 'shielding' a patient from the truth. No one should have information forced upon them, but any continuing communication with a patient is likely to open up the subject sooner or later. The doctor who overcomes his own fears of the subject will learn how, and when, and what to tell.

At times the work will cause pain and bewilderment to all members of the staff. If they do not have the opportunity of sharing their strain and questions, they are likely to leave this field or find a method of hiding behind a professional mask. Those who commit themselves to remaining near the suffering of dependence and parting find that they are impelled to develop a basic philosophy, part individual and part corporate. This grows out of the work undertaken together as members find that they each have to search, often painfully, for some meaning in the most adverse circumstances and gain enough freedom from their own anxieties to listen to another's questions of distress.

Most of the early homes and hospices were Christian in origin, their workers believing that if they continued faithfully with the work to which they felt called, help would reach their patients from God who had Himself died and risen again. Some of the traditional ways of expressing this faith are being interpreted afresh today, but there are also many people entering this field who do not have such a commitment, or who belong to other faiths or none.

Now that palliative care is spreading worldwide it has still, according to the definition of the World Health Organization[25] kept a concern for the spiritual needs of its patients and their families. The whole approach has been based on the understanding that a person is an indivisible entity, a physical and a spiritual being. The search for meaning, for something on which to trust, may be expressed in many ways, direct and indirect, in metaphor or in silence, in gesture or in symbol or, perhaps most of all, in healing relationships and in a new experience of creativity. Those who work in palliative care may have to realize that they too are being challenged to face this dimension for themselves. Many, both helper and patient, live in a secularized society and have no religious language. Some will, of course, still be in touch with their roots in this area and find a familiar practice, liturgy, or sacrament to help their need. Others, however, will not, and insensitive suggestions in this field will be unwelcome. However, if we can come together not only in our professional capacity but also in our common, vulnerable humanity, there may be no need of words on our part, only of respect and concerned listening. For those who do not wish to share their deepest concerns, care is given in a way that can reach the most hidden places. Feelings of fear and guilt may seem inconsolable but many of us have sensed that an inner journey has taken place and that a person nearing the end of their life has found peace. Important relationships may be developed or reconciled at this time and a new sense of self developed.

A human as well as a professional basis has a fundamental bearing on the way that the work is done, and everyone meeting these patients and their families is challenged to have some awareness of this dimension. Their search for meaning can create a climate in which patients and families can reach out trustingly towards what they see as true and find acceptance of what is happening to them.

The values that the hospice movement tried to establish, alongside its commitment to excellence in practice, have shown that there are ways of seeking for 'good death' today. Its 'holistic' approach has been built into the whole spectrum of palliative medicine and is presented anew by the contributors to this textbook.

The hospice movement and the specialty of palliative care that has grown out of it, reaffirms the importance of a person's life and relationships. Focused research, attention to details, and a developing expertise has aimed to avoid the isolation that many have suffered, often increased by inappropriate interventions. If people know they are respected as part of the human family (and here the developing countries have much to teach us all), the ending of life can be a final fulfillment of all that has gone before. As the modern hospice began by listening to patients, let one patient have the last word: 'Loneliness is not so much a matter of being alone as of not belonging'.[(26)]

References

1. **Wall, P.D.** (1986). Editorial: 25 volumes of pain. *Pain* **25**, 1–4.
2. **Saunders, C.** (1964). The symptomatic treatment of incurable cancer. *Prescribers Journal* **4** (4), 68–73.
3. **Eisley, L.** *The Firmament of Time.* London: Gollancz, 1961, p. 113.
4. **Gentles, I.** *Care for the Dying and the Bereaved.* Toronto: Anglican Book Centre, 1982, pp. 121–32.
5. **Aries, P.** *Western Attitudes towards Death from the Middle Ages to the Present.* Open Forum Series. London: Marion Boyars, 1976.
6. **Solzhenitsyn, A.** *Cancer Ward.* London: Bodley Head, 1968, p. 115.
7. **Miller, T.S.** *The Birth of the Hospital in the Byzantine Empire.* Baltimore: Johns Hopkins Press, 1985.
8. **Phipps, W.E.** (1988). The origin of hospices/hospitals. *Death Studies* **12**, 91–9.
9. **Lord Walton.** *Method in Medicine. The Harveian Oration of 1990.* London: Royal College of Physicians, 1991.
10. **Clark-Kennedy, A.E.** *London Pride: The Story of a Voluntary Hospital.* London: Hutchinson Benham, 1979.
11. **Humphreys, C.** (2001). Waiting for the last summons: the establishment of the first hospices in England. *Mortality* **6** (2), 146–66.
12. **Marie Curie Memorial Foundation.** *Report on a National Survey Concerning Patients Nursed at Home.* London: Marie Curie Memorial Foundation, 1952.
13. **Saunders, C. and Kastenbaum, R.** *Hospice on the International Scene.* New York: Springer, 1997.
14. **Snow, H.** *The Palliative Treatment of Incurable Cancer, with an Appendix on the Use of the Opium-Pipe.* London: J. & A. Churchill, 1890.
15. **Snow, H.** (1896). Opium and cocaine in the treatment of cancerous disease. *British Medical Journal* **2**, 718–19.
16. **Hinton, J.M.** (1963). The physical and mental distress of the dying. *Quarterly Journal of Medicine* **32**, 1–21.
17. **Glyn Hughes, H.L.** *Peace at the Last.* Gulbenkian Foundation, 1960.
18. **Abrams, R.** et al. (1945). Terminal care in cancer. A study of two hundred patients attending Boston Clinics. *New England Journal of Medicine* **232** (25), 719–27.
19. **Kubler-Ross, E.** *On death and Dying.* Toronto: Macmillan, 1969.
20. **Clark, D.C.** (1999). Cradled to the grave? Terminal care in the United Kingdom 1948–67. *Mortality* **4** (3), 225–47.
21. **Seale, C.H.** (1989). What happens in hospices: a review of research evidence. *Social Science and Medicine* **28**, 551–9.
22. **Saunders, C.** (1976). Care of the dying—the problem of euthanasia (2) *Nursing Times* **72** (27), 1049–52.
23. **Saunders, C.M.** (1983). Terminal care. In *Oxford Textbook of Medicine* Section 28 (ed. D.J. Weatherall, J.G.G. Ledingham, and D.A. Warrell), pp. 1–28. Oxford: Oxford University Press.
24. **Launer, J.** (1983). Overcoming prejudice. *British Medical Journal* **286**, 1029.
25. **World Health Organisation.** *Cancer Pain Relief and Palliative Care*, 1990, pp. 11–12.
26. **Holden, T.** Patiently speaking. In *Nursing Times*, 12 June 1980, pp. 1035–6.

Contributors

Andy Adam Professor of Interventional Radiology, Department of Radiology, St Thomas' Hospital, London, UK
8.1.5 Interventional radiology

Julia M. Addington-Hall Professor, Department of Palliative Care and Policy, GKT School of Medicine, King's College, London, UK
2.2 The epidemiology of death and symptoms

Linda Armstrong Hon. Research Fellow, Department of Speech and Language Sciences, Queen Margaret University College, Edinburgh, UK
15.5 The contribution of speech and language therapy to palliative medicine

Caroline Badger Research Fellow—Systematic Reviews, Royal College of Nursing, RCN Institute, London, UK
8.9.3 Lymphoedema

Greg Bailly Chief Resident, Department of Urology, Dalhousie University, Nova Scotia, Canada
8.10 Genito-urinary problems in palliative medicine

Vincent G. Bain Associate Professor, Department of Gastroenterology, University of Alberta, Edmonton, Canada
8.3.5 Jaundice, ascites, and hepatic encephalopathy

Claudia Bausewein Attending Physician, Interdisciplinary Palliative Care Unit, Munich University Hospital—Grosshadern, Munich, Germany
8.15 Brain tumours

Steven Bayles Assistant Professor, Vanderbilt-Bill Wilkerson Center for Otolaryngology and Communication Sciences, Nashville, TN, USA
8.11 Head and neck cancer

Michaela Bercovitch Palliative Care Physician, The Hospice, Sheba Medical Centre, Tel Aviv, Israel
8.2.8 Transcutaneous electrical nerve stimulation (TENS)

Cheryl R. Billante Adjunct Assistant Professor of Otolaryngology, Vanderbilt Voice Center, Nashville, TN, USA
8.11 Head and neck cancer

Gian Domenico Borasio Chief Attending Physician, Interdisciplinary Palliative Care Unit and Department of Neurology, Munich University Hospital—Grosshadern, Munich, Germany
8.15 Brain tumours
10.6 Palliative medicine in non-malignant neurological disorders

Mark Bower Consultant Medical Oncologist, Chelsea and Westminster Hospital, London, UK
8.13 Endocrine and metabolic complications of advanced cancer

Jo Bray Director, The Diana Princess of Wales Memorial Trust, The Royal Marsden Hospital, London, UK
15.1 The contribution of occupational therapy to palliative medicine

William Breitbart Chief of Psychiatry Service, Department of Psychiatry and Behavioural Sciences, Memorial Sloan Kettering Cancer Center, New York, USA
8.2.10 Psychological and psychiatric interventions in pain control
8.17 Psychiatric symptoms in palliative medicine

Stephen C. Brown Pain Program Director, Department of Anaesthesia, The Hospital for Sick Children, Toronto, Canada
9.1 Pain control

Eduardo Bruera Professor and Chief of Service, Department of Pain Control and Palliative Care, University of Texas, MD Anderson Cancer Center, USA
8.4.4 Pharmacological interventions in cachexia and anorexia
8.5 Fatigue and asthenia

Graham Buckley Chief Executive, NHS Education for Scotland, Edinburgh, UK
3.4 Educating for professional competence in palliative medicine

Sir Kenneth Calman Vice Chancellor and Warden, University of Durham, Durham, UK
1 Introduction
3.1 Introduction
4.3 Communication with the public, politicians, and the media
20.1 Introduction

Augusto Caraceni Consultant Neurologist, Rehabilitation and Palliative Care, Istituto Nazionale dei Tumori, Milan, Italy
8.14 Neurological problems in advanced cancer

Rev. Joseph P. Cassidy Principal, St Chad's College, University of Durham, Durham, UK
11 Cultural and spiritual aspects of palliative medicine

Barrie R. Cassileth Professor and Chief of Service, Integrative Medicine Service, Memorial Sloan Kettering Cancer Center, New York, USA
16 Complementary therapies in palliative medicine

Fiona Cathcart Senior Clinical Psychologist, St Columba's Hospice, Edinburgh, UK
15.8 The contribution of clinical psychology to palliative medicine

Kin-Sang Chan Chief of Service and Consultant, Pulmonary and Palliative Care Unit, Haven of Hope Hospital, Kowloon, Hong Kong
8.8 Palliative medicine in malignant respiratory diseases

Sir Cyril Chantler Emeritus Professor, University of London/Chairman, Great Ormond Street Hospital for Children, London, UK
3.5 Palliative medicine and children: ethical and legal issues

Nathan I. Cherny Director, Cancer Pain and Palliative Medicine, Department of Medical Oncology and Palliative Medicine, Share Zedek Medical Center, Jerusalem, Israel
1 Introduction
2.1 The problem of suffering
8.2.3 Opioid analgesic therapy
8.2.7 Neurosurgical approaches in palliative medicine

Harvey Max Chochinov Professor, Department of Psychiatry, University of Manitoba, Winnipeg, Canada
8.17 Psychiatric symptoms in palliative medicine

Nicholas Christakis Professor, Department of Health Care Policy, Harvard Medical School, Boston, USA
2.4 Predicting survival in patients with advanced disease

David Clark Professor, Institute for Health Research, Lancaster University, Lancaster, UK
21 Palliative medicine—a global perspective

Anthony Cmelak Assistant Professor, Department of Radiation Oncology, Vanderbilt-Ingram Cancer Center, Nashville, TN, USA
8.11 Head and neck cancer

Simon Cohen Consultant Physician, Department of Medicine, Bloomsbury Institute of Intensive Care, London, UK
10.8 Palliative medicine in intensive care

John J. Collins Head, Pain and Palliative Care Services, Children's Hospital, Westmead, Sydney, Australia
9.2 Symptom control in life-threatening illness

Jill Cooper Head Occupational Therapist, Department of Occupational Therapy, The Royal Marsden Hospital, London, UK
15.1 The contribution of occupational therapy to palliative medicine

Michael J. Cousins Professor, Department of Anaesthesia and Pain Management, Royal North Shore Hospital, Sydney, Australia
8.2.6 Anaesthetic techniques for pain control

Sarah Cox Consultant in Palliative Care, Chelsea and Westminster Hospital, London, UK
8.13 Endocrine and metabolic complications of advanced cancer

Nessa Coyle Director, Supportive Care Program, Department of Neurology, Memorial Sloan Kettering Cancer Center, New York, USA
5.3 Qualitative research

Isobel Davidson Senior Lecturer, Department of Dietetics and Nutrition, Queen Margaret University College, Edinburgh, UK
8.4.3 Dietary and nutritional aspects of palliative medicine
15.3 The contribution of the dietician and nutritionist to palliative medicine

Andrew N. Davies McAlpine Macmillan Consultant Senior Lecturer in Palliative Medicine, University of Bristol Department of Palliative Medicine, Bristol Haematology and Oncology Centre, Bristol, UK
7 Principles of drug use in palliative medicine

Betty Davies Professor, Family Health Care Nursing, UCSF School of Nursing, San Francisco, USA
9.5 Special consideration for children in palliative medicine
9.6 Bereavement issues and staff support

Rev. Douglas J. Davies Department of Theology, University of Durham, Durham, UK
11 Cultural and spiritual aspects of palliative medicine

Franco De Conno Director, Rehabilitation and Palliative Care, Istituto Nazionale Dei Tumori, Milan, Italy
8.12 Mouth care

Carol Dealey Research Fellow, Research Development Team, University Hospital Birmingham NHS Trust, Queen Elizabeth Hospital, Birmingham, UK
8.9.2 Nursing aspects

Ellie Dowling Speech-Language Pathologist, Vanderbilt-Bill Wilkerson Center for Otolaryngology and Communication Sciences, Nashville TN, USA
8.11 Head and neck cancer

Robin Downie Professor of Moral Philosophy, University of Glasgow, Glasgow, UK
3.3 Truth-telling and consent

Derek Doyle, OBE Formerly Medical Director/Consultant in Palliative Medicine, St Columba's Hospice, Edinburgh, UK
1 Introduction
17.1 Palliative medicine in the home
18 The terminal phase

Len Doyal Professor of Ethics, The Royal London Hospital NHS Trust, London, UK
3.5 Palliative medicine and children: ethical and legal issues

Luke Doyle Senior Physiotherapist, Calvary Hospital, Kogorah & nbsp, Sydney, Australia
15.4 The contribution of physiotherapy to palliative medicine

Francis G. Dunn Consultant Cardiologist/Clinical Director, Cardio-Thoracic Directorate, Stobhill NHS Trust, Glasgow, UK
10.5 Palliative medicine for patients with end-stage heart disease

Mark Emberton Senior Lecturer in Oncological Urology, Institute of Urology, London, UK
8.1.3 Surgical palliation

Robin L. Fainsinger Director, Palliative Care Program, Royal Alexandra Hospital, Edmonton, Canada
8.4.2 Clinical assessment and decision-making in cachexia and anorexia

Marie Fallon Consultant in Palliative Medicine/Senior Lecturer, Department of Oncology and Palliative Care, Western General Hospital NHS Trust, Edinburgh, UK
8.2.3 Opioid analgesic therapy
10.1 Introduction

Lesley Fallowfield Professor of Psycho-Oncology, Psychosocial Oncology Group, School of Biological Sciences, University of Sussex, Brighton, UK
4.1 Communication with the patient and family in palliative medicine

Betty R. Ferrell Associate Research Scientist, City of Hope National Medical Center, Duarte, California, USA
12.2 Emotional problems in the family

Helen Fielding Principal Clinical Pharmacist, Fairmile Marie Curie Centre, Edinburgh, UK
15.9 The contribution of the clinical pharmacist to palliative medicine

Jacqueline Filshie Consultant Anaesthetist, Royal Marsden Hospital, London, UK
8.2.9 Acupuncture

Baroness Ilora Finlay of Llandaff Professor of Palliative Medicine, University of Wales College of Medicine, Velindre NHS Trust, Cardiff, UK
20.2 Training family physicians

Sarah Fisher Senior Physiotherapist, The Beacon Community Cancer and Palliative Care Centre, Guildford, UK
15.4 The contribution of physiotherapy to palliative medicine

Kathleen M. Foley Professor, Department of Neurology, Memorial Sloan Kettering Cancer Center, New York, USA
8.2.2 Acute and chronic cancer pain syndromes

Karen Forbes Consultant and Macmillan Senior Lecturer in Palliative Medicine, Department of Palliative Medicine, Bristol Haematology and Oncology Centre, Bristol, UK
8.2.11 Difficult pain problems: an integrated approach

Carl Johan Fürst Medical Director, Palliative Care Unit, Stockholms Sjukhem Foundation, Associate Professor Oncology, Karolinska Institute, Stockholm, Sweden
18 The terminal phase

Charles S.B. Galasko Professor of Orthopaedic Surgery, Hope Hospital, Salford, UK
8.1.4 Orthopaedic principles and management

Paul Glare Consultant in Palliative Medicine, Royal Prince Alfred Hospital, Sydney, Australia
2.4 Predicting survival in patients with advanced disease
10.2 AIDS in adults

Ann Goldman Consultant in Paediatric Palliative Medicine, Great Ormond Street Hospital for Children, London, UK
3.5 Palliative medicine and children: ethical and legal issues

Gilbert R. Gonzales Attending Physician, Pain and Palliative Care Service, Memorial Sloan Kettering Cancer Center, New York, USA
8.2.1 Pathophysiology of pain in cancer and other terminal diseases

Patricia Grocott Research Fellow, Florence Nightingale School of Nursing and Midwifery, King's College London, London, UK
8.9.2 Nursing aspects

Geoffrey Hanks Professor of Palliative Medicine, University of Bristol, Bristol Haematology and Oncology Centre, Bristol, UK
1 Introduction
5.2 Research in palliative care: getting started
7 Principles of drug use in palliative medicine
8.2.3 Opioid analgesic therapy
8.2.11 Difficult pain problems: an integrated approach

Samuel J. Hassenbusch Associate Professor, Department of Neurosurgery, MD Anderson Medical Center, Houston, USA
8.2.7 Neurosurgical approaches in palliative medicine

Anne P. Hemingway Professor of Diagnostic Radiology, Department of Imaging, Hammersmith Hospital, London, UK
8.1.5 Interventional radiology

Irene J. Higginson Department of Palliative Care and Policy, King's College London, London, UK
2.2 The epidemiology of death and symptoms
6.2 Clinical and organizational audit in palliative medicine

Katherine Hopkins Consultant Physician, Palliative Care Team, Royal Free Hospital, London, UK
14 Rehabilitation in palliative medicine

Peter J. Hoskin Consultant Clinical Oncologist, Mount Vernon Centre for Cancer Treatment, Middlesex, UK
8.1.2 Radiotherapy in symptom management

Andrew M. Hoy Consultant in Palliative Medicine/Medical Director, Princess Alice Hospice, Esher, UK
20.3 Training specialists in palliative medicine

Jane M. Ingham Director, Palliative Care Programme and Associate Professor of Medicine, Georgetown University Medical Center, Washington DC, USA
6.1 The measurement of pain and other symptoms

David Jeffrey Consultant in Palliative Medicine, 3 Counties Cancer Centre, Cheltenham, UK
4.2 Communication with professionals

Stein Kaasa Professor of Palliative Medicine, University Hospital of Trondheim, Trondheim, Norway
5.2 Research in palliative care: getting started
6.3 Quality of life in palliative medicine—principles and practice

Menelaos Karanikolas Assistant Professor of Anesthesiology, Pain Management Center, Washington University School of Medicine, St Louis, USA
8.2.6 Anaesthetic techniques for pain control

Krikor Kichian Consultant Physician, Department of Gastroenterology, University of Alberta, Edmonton, Canada
8.3.5 Jaundice, ascites, and hepatic encephalopathy

Deborah Kirklin Head of Medical Humanities Unit, University College London, London, UK
20.5 The role of the humanities in palliative medicine

David W. Kissane Professor, Centre for Palliative Care, Department of Medicine, University of Melbourne, Victoria, Australia
5.5 Research into psychosocial issues
19 Bereavement

Linda J. Kristjanson Professor of Palliative Care, Edith Cowen University, Churchlands, Australia
5.3 Qualitative research

Vic Larcher Consultant Paediatrician, The Royal London Hospital NHS Trust, London, UK
3.5 Palliative medicine and children: ethical and legal issues

Richard M. Leach Consultant Chest Physician, Guys and St Thomas' Hospital Trust, St Thomas' Hospital, London, UK
10.4 Palliative medicine and non-malignant, end-stage respiratory disease

S. Lawrence Librach Professor of Pain Control and Palliative Care, University of Toronto, Mount Sinai Hospital, Toronto, Canada
17.2 Palliative care in the home: North America

J. Norelle Lickiss, AO Professor and Director, Sydney Institute of Palliative Medicine, Royal Prince Alfred Hospital, Sydney, Australia
2.5 The interdisciplinary team

Jon Håvard Loge Professor, Department of Behavioural Sciences in Medicine, University of Oslo and Consultant at the Centre for Palliative Medicine, Ullevaal University Hospital, Oslo, Norway
6.3 Quality of life in palliative medicine—principles and practice

Charles L. Loprinzi Specialist Medical Oncologist, Mayo Clinic, Minnesota, USA
8.7 Pruritus and sweating in palliative medicine

David Lussier Fellow, Department of Pain Medicine and Palliative Care, Beth Israel Medical Centre, New York, USA
8.2.5 Adjuvant analgesics in pain management
8.2.11 Difficult pain problems: an integrated approach

Alison MacDonald Senior Lecturer, Department of Speech and Language Sciences, Queen Margaret University College, Edinburgh, UK
15.5 The contribution of speech and language therapy to palliative medicine

Neil MacDonald, CM Division of Palliative Medicine, Department of Oncology, University of Montreal, Quebec, Canada
2.3 Palliative medicine and modern cancer care
3.2 Confidentiality
3.6 Ethical issues in palliative care research

Peter Maguire Consultant Psychiatrist/Senior Lecturer, Cancer Research Psychological Medicine Group, Manchester, UK
20.4 Learning counselling

Kathryn A. Mannix Consultant in Palliative Medicine, Newcastle Marie Curie Centre, Newcastle upon Tyne, UK
8.3.1 Palliation of nausea and vomiting

Cinzia Martini Physician, Neurology Unit, Rehabilitation and Palliative Care, Istituto Nazionale dei Tumori, Milan, Italy
8.14 Neurological problems in advanced cancer

Mitchell B. Max Director, Clinical Trials Unit, Pain and Neurosensory Mechanisms Branch, National Institute of Dental Research, Bethesda, MD, USA
5.4 Clinical trials of treatments for pain

Alan Maynard Professor, Department of Health Economics, University of York, Heslington, UK
2.6 Economics-based palliative medicine

Dorothy McArthur Principal Clinical Pharmacist, St Columba's Hospice, Edinburgh, UK
15.9 The contribution of the clinical pharmacist to palliative medicine

Jenny McClure Clinical Specialist in HIV/Palliative Care, Department of Physiotherapy, Edenhall Marie Curie Centre, London, UK
15.4 The contribution of physiotherapy to palliative medicine

Andrew D. McGavigan Clinical Research Fellow, Cardio-Respiratory Directorate, Stobhill Hospital, Glasgow, UK
10.5 Palliative medicine for patients with end-stage heart disease

Patricia A. McGrath Director, Pediatric Pain Program, Child Health Research Institute, Ontario, Canada
9.1 Pain control

Malcolm McIllmurray Professor, Department of Medical Oncology, Royal Lancaster Infirmary, Lancaster, UK
8.1.1 Palliative medicine and the treatment of cancer

Henry J. McQuay Professor of Pain Relief, University of Oxford, Pain Research Unit, The Churchill Hospital, Oxford, UK
5.1 The principles of evidence-based medicine
8.2.4 Non-opioid analgesics

Diane E. Meier Professor of Geriatrics and Palliative Care, Mount Sinai Hospital, New York, USA
10.7 Palliative medicine and care of the elderly

Sebastiano Mercadante Consultant in Pain and Palliative Care, Pain Relief and Palliative Care Unit, La Maddelena Cancer Center, Palermo, Italy
8.3.4 Pathophysiology and management of malignant bowel obstruction

Anna Monias Fellow, Department of Geriatrics and Palliative Care, Mount Sinai Hospital, New York, USA
10.7 Palliative medicine and care of the elderly

Barbara Monroe Chief Executive, St Christopher's Hospice, London, UK
13 Social work in palliative medicine

Andrew Moore Director of Research, Pain Research Unit, The Churchill Hospital, Oxford, UK
5.1 The principles of evidence-based medicine
8.2.4 Non-opioid analgesics

Peter S. Mortimer Professor and Consultant Dermatologist, Skin Department, St George's Hospital, London, UK
8.9.1 Medical aspects
8.9.3 Lymphoedema

Timothy Mould Consultant Gynaecological Oncologist, Department of Gynaecological Oncology, University College London Hospitals, London, UK
8.1.3 Surgical palliation

Barbara A. Murphy Associate Professor, Vanderbilt-Ingram Cancer Center, Nashville TN, USA
8.11 Head and neck cancer

Hans Neuenschwander Specialist Oncologist, FMH Medicina Interna Specialita Oncologia, Switzerland
8.5 Fatigue and asthenia

Simon R. Noble Specialist Registrar in Palliative Medicine, All Wales Training Programme, Velindre Hospital, Wales, UK
20.2 Training family physicians

Richard W. Norman Professor, Department of Urology, Dalhousie University, Halifax, Canada
8.10 Genito-urinary problems in palliative medicine

Clare O'Callaghan Principal Music Therapist, Social Work Department, Peter MacCallum Cancer Centre, Melbourne, Australia
15.2 The contribution of music therapy to palliative medicine

James M. Oleske François-Xavier Bagnoud Professor of Pediatrics, UMDNJ/New Jersey Medical School, Newark, USA
10.3 Palliative medicine for children and adolescents with HIV/AIDS

Stacy Orloff Bereavement Counsellor, The Hospice of the Florida Suncoast, USA
9.6 Bereavement issues and staff support

Joan T. Panke Executive Director, DC Partnership to Improve End-of-Life Care, Washington DC, USA
12.2 Emotional problems in the family

Steven D. Passik Director, Symptom Management and Palliative Care Program, Markey Cancer Center, Associate Professor of Medicine and Behavioral Science, University of Kentucky, Kentucky, USA
8.2.10 Psychological and psychiatric interventions in pain control
8.17 Psychiatric symptoms in palliative medicine

Ugo Pastorino Consultant Surgeon, Department of Thoracic Surgery, European Institute of Oncology, Milan, Italy
8.1.3 Surgical palliation

David Payne Assistant Attending Psychologist, Psychiatry Service, Memorial Sloan Kettering Cancer Center, New York, USA
8.2.10 Psychological and psychiatric interventions in pain control

Rich Payne Chief, Pain and Palliative Care Department, Memorial Sloan Kettering Cancer Center, New York, USA
8.2.1 Pathophysiology of pain in cancer and other terminal diseases

Ian C. Pearson Specialist Registrar in Dermatology, Skin Department, St George's Hospital, London, UK
8.9.1 Medical aspects

Jose Pereira Professor of Palliative Medicine, Department of Oncology, University of Calgary, Alberta, Canada
8.4.2 Clinical assessment and decision-making in cachexia and anorexia

Carolyn Pitceathly Research Associate, Cancer Research Psychological Medicine Group, The Christie Hospital, Manchester, UK
20.4 Learning counselling

Mark R. Pittelkow Associate Professor of Dermatology, The Mayo Clinic, Minnesota, USA
8.7 Pruritus and sweating in palliative medicine

M. Lois Pollock Co-ordinator, Social Work/Community Work, Aged Services, Jewish Care, Sydney, Australia
2.5 The interdisciplinary team

Russell K. Portenoy Chairman, Department of Pain and Palliative Medicine, Beth Israel Hospital, New York, USA
5.4 Clinical trials of treatments for pain
6.1 The measurement of pain and other symptoms
8.2.5 Adjuvant analgesics in pain management
8.2.11 Difficult pain problems: an integrated approach

Thomas J. Prendergast Associate Professor of Medicine and Anaesthesiology, Section of Pulmonary and Critical Care Medicine (3D), Dartmouth-Hitchcock Medical Center, Lebanon, USA
10.8 Palliative medicine in intensive care

Fiona Randall Consultant in Palliative Medicine, Christchurch Hospital, Christchurch, UK
3.3 Truth-telling and consent

Claud Regnard Consultant in Palliative Medicine, St Oswald's Hospice, Newcastle upon Tyne, UK
8.3.2 Dysphagia, dyspepsia, and hiccup
20.6 Internet and IT learning

Rosemary Richardson Senior Lecturer, Department of Dietetics and Nutrition, Queen Margaret University College, Edinburgh, UK
8.4.3 Dietary and nutritional aspects of palliative medicine
15.3 The contribution of the dietician and nutritionist to palliative medicine

Carla Ripamonti Consultant in Medical Oncology and Clinical Pharmacology, Rehabilitation and Palliative Care, Istituto Nazionale dei Tumori, Milan, Italy
8.3.4 Pathophysiology and management of malignant bowel obstruction
8.12 Mouth care

Margaret Robbins Research Fellow, University of Bristol, Department of Palliative Medicine, Bristol Haematology and Oncology Centre, Bristol, UK
5.2 Research in palliative care: getting started

Clive J.C. Roberts Clinical Dean of Bristol Medical School & Consultant Senior Lecturer in Clinical Pharmacology and Therapeutics, Department of Medicine, Bristol Royal Infirmary, Bristol, UK
7 Principles of drug use in palliative medicine

Angela Rogers Research Fellow, Department of Palliative Care and Policy, Guys, King's and St Thomas' School of Medicine, King's College, London, UK
10.6 Palliative medicine in non-malignant neurological disorders

David J. Roy, OC, Director of the Center for Bioethics, Clinical Research Institute, Montreal, Canada
3.7 Euthanasia and withholding treatment

Tarun Sabharwal Consultant Interventional Radiologist, Department of Radiology, St Thomas's Hospital, London, UK
8.1.5 Interventional radiology

Richard Sainsbury Senior Lecturer in Surgery, Royal Free and University College London Medical School, London, UK
8.1.3 Surgical palliation

Mave Salter Clinical Nurse Specialist/Stoma Therapist, Community Liaison, Surrey, UK
15.7 The contribution of stoma therapy to palliative medicine

Robert B. Santulli Associate Professor of Psychiatry, Dartmouth-Hitchcock Sleep Disorders Center, Dartmouth Medical Center, Lebanon, USA
8.16 Sleep in palliative care

Michael J. Sateia Associate Professor of Psychiatry & Director, Dartmouth-Hitchcock Sleep Disorders Center, Dartmouth Medical School, Lebanon, USA
8.16 Sleep in palliative care

Cicely M. Saunders, OM, DBE, President and Founder, St Christopher's Hospice, London, UK
Foreword

Alberto Sbanotto Physician, Department of Neurology, Istituto Nazionale dei Tumori, Milan, Italy
8.12 Mouth care

Karon Scharpen-von-Heussen Consultant in Palliative Medicine, Edenhall Marie Curie Centre, London, UK
14 Rehabilitation in palliative medicine

Glenn Schulman Physician, Integrative Medicine Service, Memorial Sloan Kettering Cancer Center, New York, USA
16 Complementary therapies in palliative medicine

Michael M.K. Sham Consultant in Palliative Care and Chest Medicine, Nam Long Hospital, Hong Kong
8.8 Palliative medicine in malignant respiratory diseases

Fabio Simonetti Physician, Neurology Unit, Rehabilitation and Palliative Care, Istituto Nazionale dei Tumori, Milan, Italy
8.14 Neurological problems in advanced cancer

Ann Smyth Director of Training for Psychology Services, NHS Education for Scotland, Edinburgh, UK
3.4 Educating for professional competence in palliative medicine

Michael M. Stevens Senior Staff Specialist and Head, Oncology Unit, The Children's Hospital, Westmead, Sydney, Australia
9.3 Psychological adaptation of the dying child
9.4 Care of the dying child and adolescent: family adjustment and support

Jan Stjernswärd International Director, WHO Collaborating Centre and Oxford International Centre for Palliative Care, Churchill Hospital, Oxford, UK
21 Palliative medicine—a global perspective

Florian Strasser Assistant Professor, Department of Oncology and Palliative Medicine, Kantonsspital, St Gallen, Switzerland
8.4.1 Pathophysiology of the anorexia/cachexia syndrome

Annette F. Street Senior Lecturer, School of Nursing and Midwifery, La Trobe University, Australia
5.5 Research into psychosocial issues

Lizabeth H. Sumner Director of Pediatric Program, Project Director, National Alliance for Children with Life-Threatening Conditions, San Diego Hospice, San Diego, USA
9.5 Special consideration for children in palliative medicine

Robert A. Swarm Chief, Pain Management Center, Washington University School of Medicine, Washington, USA
8.2.6 Anaesthetic techniques for pain control

Catherine Sweeney Research Officer/Medical Tutor, Marymount Hospice, Cork, Republic of Ireland
8.4.4 Pharmacological interventions in cachexia and anorexia
8.5 Fatigue and asthenia

Nigel Sykes Medical Director, St Christopher's Hospice, Sydenham, London, UK
8.3.3 Constipation and diarrhoea

John W. Thompson Hon. Physician and Honorary Consultant in Medical Studies, St Oswald's Hospice, Newcastle-upon-Tyne, UK
8.2.9 Acupuncture

Anne Berit Thorsen Associate Consultant in Palliative Care, Palliative Care Unit, Haven of Hope Hospital, Hong Kong
8.8 Palliative medicine in malignant respiratory diseases

Adrian J. Tookman Consultant in Palliative Medicine/Medical Director, Edenhall Marie Curie Centre, London, UK
14 Rehabilitation in palliative medicine

Doris M.W. Tse Chief of Service, Department of Medicine and Geriatrics, Caritas Medical Centre, Hong Kong
8.8 Palliative medicine in malignant respiratory diseases

Kristen S. Turner Palliative Medicine Specialist, Sydney Institute of Palliative Medicine, Sydney, Australia
2.5 The interdisciplinary team

A. Robert Turner Professor, Department of Oncology, Cross Cancer Institute, Northern Alberta Cancer Program, Alberta, Canada
8.6 Clinical management of anaemia, cytopenias, and thrombosis in palliative medicine

Mary L.S. Vachon Consultant Clinical Psychologist, Psychotherapy & Consulting Inc, Toronto, Canada
12.1 The emotional problems of the patient in palliative medicine
12.3 The stress of professional caregivers

Carolynne Vaizey Consultant Surgeon, GI Unit, The Middlesex Hospital, London, UK
8.1.3 Surgical palliation

Vittorio Ventafridda Scientific Director, Fondazione Floriani, Milan, Italy
8.12 Mouth care

Raymond Voltz Professor, Department of Neurology, University of Munich, Munich, Germany
8.15 Brain tumours
10.6 Palliative medicine in non-malignant neurological disorders

Alexander Waller Medical Director, The Hospice, Sheba Medical Center, Tel Aviv, Israel
8.2.8 Transcutaneous electrical nerve stimulation (TENS)

Charles Weijer Associate Professor, Department of Bioethics, Dalhousie University School of Medicine, Halifax, Canada
3.6 Ethical issues in palliative care research

Philip Wiffen Coordinating Editor Cochrane Pain and Supportive Care Group, Pain Research Unit, The Churchill Hospital, Oxford, UK
5.1 The principles of evidence-based medicine

Michèle Wood Art Therapist/Senior Lecturer, Edenhall Marie Curie Centre, London, UK
15.6 The contribution of art therapy to palliative medicine

Roger Woodruff Director of Palliative Care, Austin and Repatriation Medical Centre, Heidelberg, Victoria, Australia
10.2 AIDS in adults

Ram Yogev Medical Director, Pediatric and Maternal HIV Infection, Division of Infectious Diseases, Children's Memorial Hospital, Chicago, USA
10.3 Palliative medicine for children and adolescents with HIV/AIDS

1 Introduction

Derek Doyle, Geoffrey Hanks, Nathan I. Cherny, and Kenneth Calman

Much has happened since we wrote the Introduction to the first edition of this textbook little more than a decade ago. In it we tried to define palliative medicine, to answer some of the questions being asked about it, and to outline the challenge of bringing modern palliative care to the many in need of it around the world. Even then we sensed a growing interest in it and hoped that this textbook would contribute to the setting of standards and the development of palliative medicine.

Today, as we prepare this third Introduction, there are over 8000 palliative care services worldwide, admittedly mainly in the developed world but with an encouraging number starting in the developing world. From a mere handful there are now hundreds of hospital palliative care teams. There are now many professorial chairs in Palliative Medicine, the subject is being taught in more medical schools, and several of the major textbooks on medicine, geriatrics, family medicine, and oncology include chapters on it. It is even occasionally mentioned in scientific papers on other aspects of medicine, though in our view not as frequently as it deserves to be.

However, there is no reason for triumphalism. For every person who receives good palliative care there must be hundreds or even thousands who need it and have no access to it. It remains a gamble whether or not they are offered it even in the affluent countries of the West.

Countless young doctors still qualify with no training whatsoever in it. However, the picture is not as bleak as it might at first appear. Increasingly, doctors are recognizing inadequacies in their knowledge and clinical skills, resulting in considerable demand worldwide for high-quality education in palliative medicine.

Perhaps one reason for satisfaction is that important questions are increasingly being asked about palliative medicine. When should it be started? Who might benefit from it? How should it be provided and by whom? Is anything to be gained by it having specialty status as is currently the case in the United Kingdom, Australasia, Hong Kong, Taiwan, and Romania? Can it really be taught or are the skills needed for it inherited rather than acquired? Does it have a big enough knowledge base to merit all the attention being paid to it with a textbook such as this?

To begin to address such questions it seems prudent, as in the first two editions of this textbook, to start with definitions.

What is palliative medicine?

We shall use the definition prepared and adopted in the United Kingdom in 1987 when palliative medicine was accorded specialist status:

Palliative Medicine is the study and management of patients with active, progressive, far-advanced disease, for whom the prognosis is limited and the focus of care is the quality of life.

By intention, this definition is for doctors. By common assent, when other clinicians such as nurses, occupational- or physiotherapists, or pastoral care workers, are involved we refer to palliative *care* rather than palliative medicine because such care is almost always multi-professional, or interdisciplinary—to use the more appropriate word though both terms are used interchangeably in this textbook. This book, however, has been prepared to address the needs of doctors, though naturally we hope some of its contents will interest and assist other colleagues who refer to it.

For all the criticisms levelled at this definition it has many merits. It emphasizes that it is a subject worthy of study, and therefore by implication, of research. Later in this section we shall look at education and training, as well as at research. Many chapters are devoted to these in this book.

The definition refers to 'active disease' thereby excluding such things as post-traumatic syndromes, the disability which can result from cerebrovascular accidents, and several chronic conditions which, whilst undoubtedly incapacitating and distressing, may run a course of many years before they ever become life-threatening.

The inclusion of the word 'progressive' emphasizes the clinical basis for the definition because we are now able to measure disease progression better than ever before. It may be by simple clinical examination and assessment or by straight X-rays. It may require the sophistication of CT scans, magnetic resonance imaging (MRI), or biochemical or tumour markers. Palliative medicine, according to this definition, is for those whose underlying illness is now progressing inexorably, though as a result of some palliative interventions remission may still be achieved.

Some critics have questioned whether there needs to be mention of 'far-advanced' when, later in the definition, it is said that palliative medicine is for people with a limited prognosis. However, its inclusion excludes those with an illness which is certainly progressing, and will eventually prove fatal though that time may be some considerable time off—a reminder, if any was needed, of the chronicity of many fatal illnesses. We shall return to this topic of when to commence palliative medicine later in this section.

Probably the most important feature of the definition, however, is its bold assertion that the focus of palliative medicine is on the quality of life. Predictably similar claims would be made by most medical specialties, but only within recent memory have attempts been made to define the quality of life or devise tools for its measurement. More often the focus of medical care has appeared to be on cure or, failing that, on life-preservation or prolongation. Palliative medicine is not about curing. Nor does it ever set out to prolong life (any more than it sets out to abbreviate it), though many patients receiving palliative care seem to outlive the prognoses given by their doctors. The focus is on the quality of life—something which some would regard as an oxymoron. How can one speak of quality of life for people confronting death? The fact is that quality of life is something frequently spoken about by the patients themselves, something they seem more aware of and concerned about than most of us would expect, were we not working in palliative medicine. It is a concept, a goal that receives much mention in this book.

It will be noticed that no mention is made of the nature of the patient's illness. It has traditionally been regarded as the final care appropriate for those dying from malignant disease though within the last 20 years or so more and more patients with motor neurone disease (AML) have received palliative care.

A valid criticism of the definition is that it makes no explicit mention of relatives, though concern for them is perhaps implicit. There is no question that palliative medicine is concerned with their needs and welfare as well as those of the patients, and in particular is sensitive to bereavement in its many manifestations. The needs of relatives and friends receive much attention in this book.

When should palliative care start?

To address this question we have to look at something which has received much attention since the first edition of this book was prepared a decade or so ago.

Many of those who recognized the need for skilled and compassionate care of the terminally ill and made every effort to practise palliative care in their daily work expressed reservations about palliative medicine being regarded as a specialty. They pointed out that its principles were those many doctors try to follow in everything they do, whether or not their patients suffer from a mortal illness, whether their prognosis is long or short. Some family physicians reminded us that almost all their work is palliative, whether it is for cardiac, respiratory, or degenerative conditions, for cancer, or for chronic illnesses. At the same time many agreed that there comes a time, usually in the terminal phase of an illness but not exclusively then, when such major problems arise that the help of a specialist is much appreciated, as is the existence of an inpatient unit to which they can refer such patients for skilled palliation. The more this was debated the more was it acknowledged that there can be equally challenging problems of pain, coping, accepting the diagnosis, and being nursed at home much earlier in the illness, long before it could be described as terminal. On such occasions the help of a specialist might assist but not if it implied to the patient that death was imminent. Yet another input to this debate was that of surgeons and oncologists who reminded us that some of their contributions to patient care are never intended to cure but are essentially palliative. This did not qualify them to be termed palliative medicine specialists nor did they want that title.

Out of this debate have come three concepts.

- The *principles of palliative care* are integral and intrinsic to all good clinical care whatever the nature or the stage of a patient's illness. To differentiate this care from specialist palliative care some have recommended that it be known as *non-specialist or general palliative care.*
- *Palliative procedures and techniques* have an important role to play in achieving pain and symptom relief. They include the formation of ostomies, the insertion of stents, paracenteses, orthopaedic procedures such as hip replacement and spinal stabilization, the insertion of spinal catheters, radiotherapy, and many cancer chemotherapy regimens.
- *Specialist palliative medicine* focuses on patients with active, progressive, and far-advanced illness and a limited prognosis, but can make important contributions to the care of patients at earlier stages in their illness. As a 'specialty', whether officially recognized as such or not, it also has responsibility for research, education, and setting professional standards in the discipline.

These should help us to answer the question on when palliative care should start. The answer is that *non-specialist palliative care, that is to say palliative care provided by the patient's general practitioner or family physician employing the principles of palliative care, starts at the time of diagnosis and continues until death, whatever the underlying pathology.* Every person has the right to expect relief from suffering, whatever its nature, whether or not its cause can be eradicated. Every person has a right to expect their doctors to be concerned with the quality of their life.

This has important implications. It reminds us that life prolongation is not the ultimate goal of medical care, deeply gratifying as it can be when it is possible. All care should be patient-centred rather than pathology-centred, profoundly important as it is that the doctor be familiar with the pathology and its manifestations and complexity. Because palliative care is holistic care—equally concerned with physical, psychosocial, and spiritual aspects of each patient—all care should be holistic. Clearly, this does not imply that every physician, surgeon, radiation oncologist, and psychologist with whom they come in contact must attempt to solve every such problem, even if they were trained and competent to do so. It does, however, mean that they must never lose sight of the fact that everyone has different dimensions in their life. This has implications for our professional education and training as we shall discuss shortly.

It might be thought there is no problem about the use of palliative procedures and techniques and when they are appropriate. However, experience has shown that sometimes they are resorted to when a less-invasive treatment is equally appropriate and available. Some have performed subtotal hepatectomies in the final week of life to relieve the pain of malignant secondaries when the patient had never been given a trial of opioids. Other patients have had epidural catheters inserted before being offered oral opioids. Some patients have been given what has been curiously called 'placebo chemotherapy' rather than being told truthfully that no further chemotherapy is appropriate for them. Of course, the opposite is sometimes true. Some frail patients are left in considerable pain from their pancreatic carcinoma when a coeliac plexus block earlier in their illness might have been highly effective. Others suffer the anguish of rectal discharge and incontinence when a resection of the rectum at the time of diagnosis could have prevented it. The use of palliative procedures also raises ethical issues: issues of resource allocation, of ascertaining what the patient regards as quality of life, of ensuring that anything done to the patient is beneficial and not either futile or harmful in the short or long term. Much emphasis is provided in this book to such ethical issues.

The moral of this is clear. There needs to be collaboration and co-operation among medical colleagues from start to finish of a patient's care. In many of the health care systems in the world today, patients are referred from one doctor to another when each has done all within his/her power and skill. Rather than risk upsetting the patient or appearing to leave them to their fate, each doctor either holds on to them for as long as possible or continues to see them long after he or she has nothing further to offer. For many doctors, calling in a specialist in palliative medicine is seen as a defeat, an admission that they have reached the end of their therapeutic options. A group of cardiologists in the United Kingdom was asked when they would consider referring patients to a specialist palliative care service. The answer was 'when we have no more drugs to offer'. It is interesting that when asked if they took into account how long was left for the patient they said that it was usually a month or so before the patient's death. Examination of patient records showed that it was more usually 6 months before death. In a series of interviews neurologists were asked the same question, when would they start palliative care. Many said palliative care should start at the time of diagnosis in the case of patients with primary or secondary cerebral malignancies, variant CJD, and motor neurone disease. Several observed that few neurological conditions are curable and, though they seldom used the word, most of their work was essentially palliative in nature and many of the units in which they work are ill-suited and ill-staffed for inpatient care of mortally ill patients.

We are still left with the question of when to start specialist palliative care. Our definition should be adequate. Unlike non-specialist palliative care which is appropriate from the day of diagnosis, specialist palliative care is usually only needed *when the problems of the patient are either so numerous, so severe, so difficult to relieve, or so unusual* that a team with expert and specialist skills needs to be called in. A key member of such a team will be a palliative medicine specialist. This is a scenario familiar to all family physicians. They can manage most conditions without resorting to specialists or experts. Every now and then they come across something outside their knowledge or experience. Far from being a defeat or a disgrace, their training and skill enable them to identify the specialist best qualified to help their patient, and such expert help is invoked. The same principle applies to where such specialist care should be given. Provided it is thought that the patient is receiving the best care possible then he or she can remain where they are—home, general hospital, or nursing home. When specialist care skills are needed, consideration needs to be given to a transfer to a hospice or specialist palliative care unit.

What patients should receive specialist palliative care?

It has just been said that *all* patients have a right to receive palliative care, whether it is generalist or specialist. It should not depend on their pathology any more than it should be affected by their colour, their religion, their culture, their financial means, or their social class.

Traditionally it has been seen as exclusively for cancer patients, only recently being widened to accept patients suffering from motor neurone disease and AIDS. There would seem to be no clinical or ethical reason why it should not be available to all patients, whatever their pathology.

However, some have argued that existing services can hardly cope with the number of cancer patients being referred to them. They fear that admitting other patients will be too much for their limited resources, but recent work in the United Kingdom has shown that a unit prepared to admit non-cancer patients seldom has more than 15–20 per cent of them under its care at any one time, even though cancer only accounts for 25 per cent of deaths and cardiovascular disease 55 per cent of deaths in the Western world. Others have pointed out that to be able to give the same quality of care to patients with cardiac, respiratory, endocrine, and neurological conditions would require radical changes in the training of both palliative care doctors and nurses.

The acceptance of palliative care being appropriate from the time of diagnosis and equally applicable to all pathologies may appear to some as though palliative care is becoming 'care of the chronically ill', something that was never intended. It could easily result in the medical profession being divided into 'curers' and 'carers'. This would be wrong. All doctors are carers. All doctors are committed to relieving suffering, wherever and whenever they encounter it in the course of their work.

A frequently expressed criticism of the first two editions of this book was that the focus was almost exclusively on malignant disease. This has been addressed in this edition. There are now major sections on non-malignant conditions, written with the needs of palliative medicine doctors and family physicians in mind though, hopefully, they will also interest and be of value to colleagues working in those non-malignant disease specialties. Where not otherwise stated readers can assume that the general principles enunciated in this book apply, whatever the pathology.

We are committed to seeing the principles of palliative care, and all the knowledge which has come from specialist palliative care, being made available to all who suffer, whatever the nature of their illness.

Who can practice palliative medicine?

This question has been answered in what has been discussed earlier. It is the responsibility of every doctor to employ the principles of palliative medicine in their work. Whether or not they feel confident and competent to do so is another matter. That will largely depend on their professional education and training and on something else not yet mentioned—their access to specialist palliative medicine physicians (or at least those practising it full time). The educational role and potential of such specialists cannot be exaggerated.

Debate continues in many countries about whether or not it is necessary to have specialists in this subject. Countries which have gone down the road of specializing believe that it has given palliative care a much higher professional and public profile, has made a significant educational and academic impact, and has raised the standard of palliative care across the spectrum. Some go further and believe it has made politicians and health service planners more aware of the needs of patients with end-stage disease and of their obligation to address those needs.

The opponents of specializing fear that it might lead to elitism, to a schism between family medicine and palliative medicine, and to an exaggerated focus on end of life issues to the detriment of continuing and supportive care throughout life. We do not share this fear.

Does palliative medicine have universal relevance?

This question has also been answered in what has been discussed earlier. It would be morally unacceptable if it was available exclusively to certain geographical, ethnic, or social groups, or to those articulate enough to ask for it or wealthy enough to pay for it.

However, it might be argued that in some parts of the world there is a greater urgency to develop palliative care than in others. Some might question the ethics of having the levels of primary, secondary, and tertiary care currently available in most developed countries, though not also providing high-quality palliative care. Of course, in some developing countries there may be little or no primary care. Hospitals may be few in number, under-staffed, under-resourced, and ill-equipped. There may be few, if any, specialists or facilities where they can practice their skills. There are countries where there are no radiotherapy units, where many drugs, and particularly cancer chemotherapy, cannot be afforded, and where opioids are unobtainable for one reason or another. In such countries there is no possibility whatsoever of curing an illness, little possibility of bringing about even a modest remission in many progressive conditions, and all that people can hope for—and their basic right—is that simple, effective, and efficient means may be found to ease their suffering. Few things can be more important in the world than that palliative care becomes available worldwide as a matter of greatest urgency.

It might be argued that this is a political issue, not a medical one. Presumably, all would agree that the most effective thing that can be done in developing countries is to ensure safe water and provide access to basic health care facilities. We agree but would argue that it is a responsibility of doctors worldwide to keep politicians informed about not only such health promotion and disease prevention, but also health care priorities, one of which is undoubtedly palliative care. At the same time, doctors have a responsibility to research their work, to be conscious of the financial implications of all they do, and to advise politicians responsibly. It is for this reason that so much emphasis has been given in this book to research issues and to the economics of palliative care provision. One of the lessons learnt in the developed world is that public opinion can and does influence politicians, when well presented. We are said to live in a consumer-driven society and few would deny that palliative care is a consumer-centred subject. When the general public, supported by their doctors, argue for more dignified and compassionate care for the terminally ill, politicians have been shown to be receptive and responsive.

It is to be expected, and indeed welcomed, that in different countries innovative new models for the provision of palliative care will be tried. No matter how successful and acceptable the models developed in the West have proved to be, the models of care provision must be appropriate for each community receiving it rather than be a clone of one tried in the West. Self-evident as this may be, there are still places in the developing world trying to reproduce services they have seen first hand in the West and doctors going abroad from the West, energetically promoting such models. In time one hopes that the developed countries will be willing to learn from their younger colleagues in developing countries how to provide the best care more economically and appropriately than at present.

Education and training in palliative medicine

Most doctors are dedicated to easing the suffering of their patients even though they may not glorify this aspect of their work with the name of palliative medicine. Many studies have demonstrated that doctors are conscious of the palliative needs of their patients and are keen to provide good care. However, many studies have also shown that they lack both the confidence and competence in palliative care, and have until now had little or no training in it.

Worldwide experience seems to confirm that one of the strengths of palliative care, and one of the lessons others might learn from it, is the value of team work. Presumably, most clinicians will claim that they all work closely with colleagues from other disciplines, sharing skills, supporting each other, all working towards agreed goals. Those experienced in palliative care would go further. They would claim that effective palliative care can only be provided by a team—another major and very complex issue addressed in this book.

As this book will demonstrate, there is more to palliative medicine than 'tender loving care', a high level of sympathy, and time and inclination to sit by the bedside holding a patient's hand. Palliative medicine has a large and growing knowledge base. It calls for heightened skills in communicating (including listening) and an educated understanding of the training and skills of colleagues in other disciplines and professions. It may surprise some readers that a section of this book is devoted to professions allied to medicine. It has not been written for *their* benefit but so that doctors practising palliative medicine may know better what each of these professions has to offer as part of the clinical team.

Another section in the book, also written to educate and inform palliative medicine doctors, is on Complementary Medicines in relation to palliative care. Predictably some will be surprised, even dismayed, that such a book includes this section. Presumably no one will deny that in the West more people try complementary medicines than most doctors would care to admit, that many studies have shown that palliative care nurses have expressed such interest in aromatherapy that thousands have undertaken training in it, and that the general public, rightly or wrongly, seem to expect hospices to offer such therapies. Colleagues in China and the Far East tell us that close on 100 per cent of their patients have tried, or are still taking, traditional herbal remedies when they come to palliative care. We believe we have a responsibility to know more about complementary medicine and its place in palliative medicine. If it interests our patients sufficiently for them to resort to it we must learn more about it whilst endeavouring to enhance our skills in orthodox medicine.

Many writers take great pains to remind us that palliative medicine is more than an exercise in clinical pharmacology and that palliative medicine physicians should be more than symptomatologists. We wholeheartedly concur. Experience has shown many of us that freeing a patient from pain does not necessarily restore happiness to them or give them an inner peace. The answer to fear is seldom an anxiolytic, any more than an anti-depressant is a cure for sadness. The diagnostic challenges and the complexities of pharmacological manipulation will be fully explored in the pages which follow, but even then we may not have encapsulated what lies at the heart of palliative medicine. The task is not an easy one.

It has been said that palliative medicine is concerned with three things—the quality of life, the value of life, and the meaning of life. The quality of life is, by general assent, intimately related to freedom from pain, fear, and other distressing symptoms. It is bound up with our relationship with loved ones and with those who care for us, and is affected by the quality of that care and its focus on personal dignity. In our modern society it is often said that life seems to have less value than used to be the case. Value seems often to be measured in terms of a person's economic potential in society weighed against the financial burden of caring for them when they are ill, frail, or dying. Often, little thought seems to be given to what they have contributed and probably still are contributing to the society in which they live. How often terminally ill people tell you that they wonder if they are of any further use to anyone, if they are still needed, or if society would be better off without them. They are, in their own way, looking not at the quality of life but the value of life. The meaning of life brings us into the realm of the existential or what has come to be termed spirituality, something that most would agree is not the same as religion. Is it possible for any doctor to care for a terminally ill person and not be asked, and also to wonder, why Man must suffer?

We mention all this because it has led some to question whether doctors can be taught palliative medicine. Some have suggested that palliative medicine calls for attitudes and skills that are inherent. They claim that a doctor either possesses them or does not. They would argue that teaching the skills of clinical pharmacology is one thing, teaching philosophy, existentialism, and spirituality is something different. Perhaps they are right when they say that what is most needed in doctors is a change in attitude towards their patients, their needs, and their care. Can attitudinal changes be achieved through a book such as this? We believe they can. This is more than an educational challenge that is addressed in the section devoted to education and training. It is a thread which will be found woven into every page of the book we now offer to our friends and colleagues around the world.

2

The challenge of palliative medicine

2 The challenge of palliative medicine

2.1 The problem of suffering

Nathan I. Cherny

Despite the advances in modern medicine, many illnesses continue to evade cure. Chronic progressive incurable illness is a major cause of disability, distress, suffering, and, ultimately, death. This is true for many causes of cancer, progressive neurologic disorders, AIDS, and other disorders of vital organs. Progressive chronic diseases of this ilk are most common in late adulthood and old age, but they occur in all ages.

When cure is not possible, as often it is not, the relief of suffering is the cardinal goal of medicine. Recognition of this axiom is at the heart of the philosophy, science, and practice of palliative medicine.

Understanding suffering

For the patient with incurable illnesses, such as cancer, the goals of care may be stated as the alleviation of suffering, the optimization of quality of life until death ensues, and the provision of comfort in death.[1–3] Persistent suffering that is inadequately relieved (or the anticipation of this situation) undermines, for the sufferer, the value of life. Without hope that this situation will be relieved, patients, their families, and professional health care providers may see elective death by suicide, euthanasia, or assisted suicide as their only alternatives. The truth of the perception that patients need to be killed or assisted to kill themselves to be adequately relieved of suffering depends upon the adequacy of the available measures to relieve suffering. The essence of the controversy is the problem of suffering.

The alleviation of suffering is universally acknowledged as a cardinal goal of medical care.[1,4–10]

The ability to formulate a response to the challenge of suffering requires a clinically relevant understanding of the nature of the problem.[3,10–15] Paradoxically, however, the medical literature on the nature of suffering is sparse. Cassell described suffering as arising from a threat to the integrity of the person, and elucidated multiple factors that may contribute to that threat.[16,17] He asserts, however, that the nature of suffering precludes the development of a clinical taxonomy, and that the ability to recognize suffering is an acquired skill.[17] Cicely Saunders has described a model of suffering as 'Total Pain'. Although this model does not define the nature of the problem, it does outline some of the various physical, psychological, emotional, existential, and social factors that contribute to the experience.[18] Some authors have suggested that there remains a need for a definition of suffering that is clinically relevant and a paradigm of cancer-related suffering that acknowledges the interrelated distress of the patient, the family, and the health care providers as they face a terminal disease.[2,10–12,19,20]

Defining suffering

In the cancer setting, clinical and psychosocial research has helped define the scope and prevalence of distresses experienced by patients, their families, and their attending health care professionals, and has highlighted the complex interrelations between these groups. Based on a review of this research, a new definition of suffering and a taxonomy of factors that may contribute to the experience was proposed.[21] In this model, suffering is described as an aversive experience characterized by the perception of personal distress that is generated by adverse factors that undermine quality of life.[21] The defining characteristics of suffering include: (a) the presence of perceptual capacity (sentience), (b) the fact that the factors undermining quality of life are appraised as distressing, and (c) the fact that the experience is aversive. According to this definition, suffering is a phenomenon of conscious human existence, the intensity of which is determined by the number and severity of the factors diminishing from quality of life, the processes of appraisal, and perception. Each of these variables is amenable to therapeutic interventions.

The triangular model of suffering

The encounter with terminal illness is a potential cause of great distress to patients, their families, and the professional caregivers attending them. Among patients with advanced cancer, for instance, at least two-thirds of patients with advanced cancer have significant pain[22–25] and numerous other physical symptoms that can equally diminish the patient's quality of life.[22,26–29] Furthermore, many patients endure enormous psychological distress,[30–34] and in some cases, form an existential perspective that, even without pain or other physical symptoms, continued life is without meaning.[35–37] For the families and loved ones of patients there is, likewise, great distress in this process: anticipated loss, standing witness to the physical and emotional distress of the patient, and bearing the burdens of care.[38–40] Finally, professional caregivers may potentially be stressed by the suffering which they witness and which challenges their clinical and emotional resources.[41–44]

According to this model, the suffering of each of these three groups is inextricably interrelated such that the perceived distress of any one of these three groups may amplify the distress of others (Fig. 1).

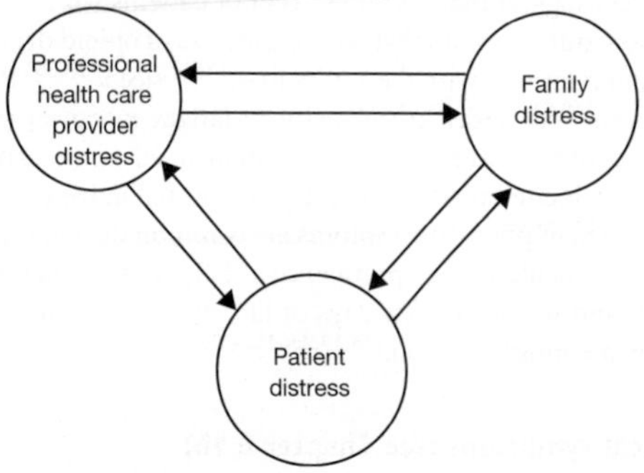

Fig. 1 The interrelationship between the distress of the patient, their family, and the health care providers.

Suffering and personal growth

The potential for personal development and net positive gain in overcoming situations of adversity and suffering is widely recognized. This potential, however, is predicated on the ability to cope with the prevailing problems and challenges. It is the phenomenon of coping that generates the potential for growth and reward.[45,46] Coping does not occur if the demands of the situation are overwhelming (distinct from merely being appraised as overwhelming). For example, the patient with inadequately relieved pain, shortness of breath, or vomiting may be absolutely unable to address issues related to his offspring and spouse. The spouse and offspring who are overwhelmed by problems of daily care requirements may be absolutely unable to appreciate time with the patient. Suffering in chronic debilitating illness cannot be eliminated, but if adequate relief is achieved then coping and growth can occur. By understanding and addressing the factors that may potentially overwhelm the patient, family, and health care providers, the necessary preconditions for coping and growth are established.

Relieving suffering: a right

It is widely held that terminally ill patients have a right to adequate relief of uncontrolled suffering. Indeed, the World Health Organization asserts that the relief of pain and other symptoms is a right of the patient with advanced and incurable cancer[47] and the right to the adequate provision of palliative care for the terminally ill has been ratified by the American Medical Association, Academy of Psychosomatic Medicine, American Academy of Hospice and Palliative Medicine, American Board of Hospice and Palliative Medicine, American College of Chest Physicians, American Pain Society, and the National Kidney Foundation.[48]

The corollary of this right is the responsibility of caregivers to ensure that adequate provisions are made for relief. The formulation of a therapeutic response requires an understanding of the phenomenon of suffering and the factors that contribute to it. Failure to appreciate, or to effectively address, the full diversity of contributing factors may confound effective therapeutic strategies.

Cancer as a model of suffering and terminal illness

The interrelated elements of suffering in terminal illness is well illustrated by an evaluation of distress among cancer patients, their families, and the caring health care providers.

Patient distress

Physical symptoms (see Section 8)

Prevalence data suggest that 70–90 per cent of patients with advanced disease will have significant pain that requires the use of opioid drugs.[24,49–56] Persistent pain interferes with the ability to eat,[57] sleep,[58,59] think, interact with others,[60,61] and is correlated with fatigue in cancer patients.[62] The prevalence of symptoms other than pain in an advanced cancer patient have been well documented in the hospice and palliative care literature: multiple concurrent physical symptoms are common during the last weeks of life, with a particularly high prevalence of fatigue and generalized weakness[22,26–29] and in the last few days of life, dyspnoea, delirium, nausea, and vomiting are most common.[18,19,23–25,36,38]

Psychological symptoms (see Chapter 8.16)

Psychiatric problems occur in greater than 60 per cent of patients with far-advanced cancer;[63,64] the most common problems are adjustment disorders, depression, anxiety, and delirium.[63,64] All four of these symptoms may contribute to the development of suicidal thoughts, and indeed, psychiatric disorders are present in the vast majority cancer patients who are suicidal.[65] Assessment of suicidal cancer patients at the Memorial Sloan-Kettering Cancer Center by the Psychiatry Service diagnosed one-third with major depression, 20 per cent with a delirium, and 50 per cent with an adjustment disorder with anxious and depressed features at the time of evaluation.[65]

Factors that adversely influence the prevalence and severity of psychological distress are: the presence of advanced disease, distressing physical symptoms (especially pain),[61,66–68] disability, unresolved previous experiences of loss or separation,[66,69,70] feelings of frustration and hopelessness,[66] a lack of perceived support from at least one loved person,[69] strained interpersonal relationships,[69] controlling personality trait,[71,72] difficulties in adapting to the illness and its implications,[71,73] economic concerns, impaired cognitive abilities,[66,74] and unsatisfactory communication regarding illness or treatment (particularly where there has been the precipitous disclosure of poor prognosis without allowance for a process of adjustment and assimilation of information).[75,76] Uncontrolled pain is an important precipitant of psychological distress and is a suicide risk factor. In a large prospective study of psychological symptoms in cancer patients,[67] the prevalence of cancer-related pain was 39 per cent in those who had a psychiatric diagnosis and only 19 per cent in those without such a diagnosis. Indeed, it has been observed that psychiatric symptoms commonly resolve with adequate pain relief.[68]

Existential distress (see Chapters 8.16 and 11)

Common existential issues for patients with advanced cancer include hopelessness, futility, meaninglessness, disappointment, remorse, death anxiety, and disruption of personal identity.[16,36,77–79] Existential distresses may be related to past, present, or future concerns. Current personal integrity, the sense of who one is as a person, can be disrupted by changes in body image, somatic, intellectual, social, and professional functions, and in perceived attractiveness as a person and as a sexual partner.[16,37] For some patients retrospection can trigger profound disappointment (from unfulfilled aspirations or a depreciation of the value of previous achievements) or remorse from unresolved guilt.[16,37,78] If life is perceived to offer, at best, comfort in the setting of fading potency or, at worst, ongoing physical and emotional distress as days pass slowly until death, anticipation of the future may be associated with feelings of hopelessness, futility, or meaninglessness such that the patient sees no value in continuing to live.[32,37,78–82] Death anxiety is common among cancer patients; surveys have shown that 50–80 per cent of terminally ill patients have concerns or troubling thoughts about death, and that only a minority achieve an untroubled acceptance of death.[37,83,84] Together, these symptoms have been labelled a 'demoralization syndrome'.[85]

Although these existential issues are sometimes referred to as 'spiritual',[86–90] they appear to be universal, and independent of religion and religious practice.[36,78]

Family/social distress

The perception by the patient of the distress of family, friends, and health care providers, can further amplify the patient's distress,[74,91] and thus contribute to the nihilistic conclusion that ongoing existence only constitutes a perpetuation of the burden to self and to others.

Family distress (see Chapters 9.4, 12.1, and 12.2)

The development of advanced cancer in a family member impacts upon the entire family.[74,92–96] The challenges confronting the family: to acknowledge the ending of life as they have known it, and to define a new way of constructively living out their final days together as best possible, engender great stresses.[96] Among the contributing factors to the ensuing distress are empathic suffering with the distress of the patient, grief and bereavement, role changes, and the physical, financial, and psychological sequelae of the burdens of care.[74,92–96] Furthermore, the family carers of cancer patients have been shown to constitute a vulnerable population. In one study almost a quarter of the family caregivers for the terminally ill had chronic health problems themselves;[97] other studies have highlighted the further detriment to health incurred by family carers.[98] A very high prevalence of anxiety and adjustment difficulties have also been identified among family members, the severity of which is often as great as that of the patients' themselves.[74,99]

Psychosocial factors

A review of the data on the impact of cancer on the family members identified 11 major issues for family members: emotional strain, physical demands, uncertainty, fear that the patient will die, alteration in roles and lifestyles, financial concerns, ways to comfort the patient, perceived inadequacy of care services, existential concerns, sexuality, and non-convergent needs among family members.[100] These issues can be profoundly influenced by the trajectory of the illness.[74] For example, a long illness characterized by a remitting and relapsing course may produce persistent anxiety and uncertainty, which can produce severe emotional fatigue. To resolve those feelings, family members may, in some circumstances, hope for the patient's rapid demise. In contrast, when the time from diagnosis to impending death has been short, there may be little opportunity for family members to come to terms with the presence of life-threatening illness, let alone impending death.

Grief

In most cases, the pre-terminal phase of the cancer experience is associated with a period of anticipatory grieving[101] in which the family undergoes a transition associated with the patient's 'fading away'.[96] In one study[96] the onset of this transition was generally heralded by a deterioration in the patient's condition that challenged ongoing denial. The most heralding events were unrecoverable weakness, loss of independence in ambulation and personal care, and loss of mental clarity. These events are distressing in that they constitute losses, diminish hope for recovery, and focus attention on the inevitability of the patient's demise.

Caregiver burden

Although most patients die in the hospital setting, most of the care prior to dying is carried out at home by the family members with the support of health care professionals. The care of a terminally ill family member greatly strains the physical, emotional, and psychological resources of the family unit and its individual members.[74,102–104] Home care often involves participation in personal hygiene needs, administration of medication by non-invasive or invasive routes, attention to nutritional needs, psychological support, and emergency management of such problems as pain, dyspnoea, or bleeding.[105–107] The heavy physical work of transferring a weak or immobile patient, and attending to other needs (such as laundering or cleaning), is often further compounded by exhaustion due to sleep deprivation as a result of anxious thoughts or patient care needs. For many this is a new experience, and the uncertainties about the dying process and the ability to cope with the problems that lie ahead may become a focus for anxiety or ruminative thoughts.[105–107]

Financial distress

Financial distress has been under-appreciated and is often neglected in routine care.[108] Studies comparing the relative costs of home- and hospital-based terminal care[109,110] have neglected the financial and social costs to the family.[111–113] In the National Hospice Study, 26 per cent of primary care takers either left their work or lost their jobs, and 60 per cent reported a significant reduction in income due to either absenteeism or a change in work arrangements.[114] Permanent loss of employment occurred most frequently among those who could least afford it: older women and low-income families.[114] The costs of caring for a family member can leave the surviving family with severely compromised resources. This distress is often exacerbated by inadequate insurance coverage.[115]

Caregiver conflicts

The caregiver may experience profound conflict in this situation: conflict between the desire to provide adequate relief of distressing symptoms while, at the same time, wanting to preserve their loved one's alertness and to avoid hastening death[98] and conflict between the duty to care for a loved-one and to care for oneself, and one's other responsibilities.[116]

Family needs

The needs of the families of patients with advanced cancer have been surveyed by several researchers.[106,117–122] The prompt and effective relief of patient symptoms is a major priority for family members, as are the needs for education in the comfort care of the patient, and for physician and nursing availabilities.[106,117–120,123,124] The need for communication from health care providers that is honest, direct, and compassionate, in which family concerns and opinions are heard and valued, and that conveys information that can help in patient care has been commonly reported.[117–119,125,126] Material supports, such as a hospital bed, and professional supports in the framework of family meetings are similarly valued.[117] Commonly unmet needs include the need to receive assurance of the patient's comfort, to be informed of the patient's condition, to ventilate emotions, to receive comfort and support from family members, and to receive acceptance, support, and comfort from health care professionals.[121,122,126–128]

Risk identification

The endurability of the burdens of care is an important consideration in long-term care planning; the family members' current and future welfare is an important consideration when care demands are great and supportive resources for home care are limited.[116] In a large retrospective survey 22 per cent of families of terminally ill patients were unable or unwilling to provide personal or medical care.[129]

The identification of populations at particularly high risk for early intervention is facilitated by an assessment of stressors, particular family needs, and the resources available to the family. Family groups which have been identified to be at particular risk include the families of older males with lung cancer and the families of young women with cervix cancer,[130] family systems that alternated between emotional distress and open conflict,[129] and the families of patients who are poorly adjusted to their illness and condition.[129] In contrast, the attributes identified to facilitate effective function include: the ability to work cohesively, prior successful experience in handling stress, a substantial and flexible repertoire of coping strategies, family stability, financial security, the availability of outside supports to which the family is receptive, and a readiness to view this difficult period as potentially growth-producing.[131]

Health care professional distress (see Chapter 12.3)

Stressors

Health care professionals may experience distress due to the constant exposure to suffering, loss, and grief that they are expected to be able to ease or relieve.[44,132,133] Among the stressors experienced by professionals working in this field are: patients who experience high morbidity and mortality, high work pressure, frequent life and death decisions (which sometimes occur in ambiguous circumstances), high consumer expectations, interstaff conflict, severe patient dependency, debilitation, or disfigurement, severe emotional distress among patients and their families, and issues relating to suffering and distress caused by the treatments themselves.[44] Stresses that are specific to the cancer setting include the uncertainty and fear associated with the disease, the high prevalence of side-effects from cancer treatments, the palliative rather than curative nature of most interventions, the difficulties of therapeutic decision-making (particularly in the setting of progressive disease or treatment associated with high risk of death), difficulties in confronting patient and family reactions while continuing to treat the patient, and difficulties in communicating with others outside the workplace about the stresses to which they are exposed.[134]

Physician distress

In a survey of 598 oncologists,[135] 56 per cent reported some degree of burnout. Burnout was experienced variably as frustration and a sense of failure (56 per cent), depression (34 per cent), disinterest (20 per cent), and boredom (18 per cent). Of those affected, it adversely impacted on their personal and social lives (85 per cent) and on their professional lives (50 per cent). Major contributing factors were insufficient personal or vacation time (57 per cent), continuous exposure to fatal illness (53 per cent), and frustration due to limited therapeutic success (45 per cent). While almost half the respondents felt that this experience was intrinsic to the nature of the work, the prevalence of burnout was related to the proportion of time spent in direct patient care.

A study of 393 cancer clinicians in the United Kingdom found that burnout was more prevalent among radiotherapists than among medical oncologists and palliative care specialists.[136] Burnout was associated with the stress of feeling overload, dealing with treatment toxicity/errors, deriving little satisfaction from professional status/esteem, high stress and low satisfaction from dealing with patients, and from a perceived lack of resources. Insufficient training in communication and management skills were identified as impotant stressors.[136]

In a survey of 81 French general practitioners,[137] 86 per cent endorsed the assertion that encounters with death were a cause of physician suffering. The major causes of physician suffering were the end of the doctor–patient relationship (58 per cent), feelings of uselessness (55 per cent) and failure (38 per cent), increased awareness of their own mortality (49 per cent), and the presence of 'questions without answers' (31 per cent). The most commonly reported feelings that were experienced by these physicians at the bedside of the dying patient were sadness (94 per cent), helplessness (89 per cent), failure (61 per cent), disappointment (59 per cent), and loneliness (51 per cent). Anecdotal reports attest to a significant prevalence of stress among trainees in cancer medicine, particularly in dealing with end-of-life issues.[107–109]

Nursing distress

Studies of nurses working in palliative care have yielded mixed results, whereas an international study evaluating stress levels and coping mechanisms among professionals who work with illness and death found that palliative care and hospice workers had less stress and better coping than those in other fields.[138] Despite that, the potential for exhaustion and burnout is well described.[138,139] Major sources of stress include perceived deficiencies in symptom control, deep emotional involvement in work, dealing with young patients, dealing with the emotional needs of distressed relatives, and conflict with the participating physicians over the goals of care.[140–142]

Developing a clinical strategy for the relief of distress and the control of suffering

An effective approach to the alleviation of suffering for patients with incurable or terminal illness is predicated upon careful case assessment, identification of care needs, formulation of a multidisciplinary therapeutic intervention to address those needs, and the provision of ongoing monitoring with readiness to re-evaluate the care plan as problems arise or needs change.

Assessment

An appreciation of the full diversity of factors that may contribute to suffering underscores the need for a methodical approach to the assessment of each individual case. The objectives of the assessment are to identify current problems that are a source of distress to each of the parties, to assess their care needs, and to evaluate the adequacy of the available resources. This evaluation must incorporate: medical variables in the patient, family, and available community medical system; psychological variables in the patient, family, and psychosocial community supports; and social and financial variables in the patient and family. Since both the patient and the family are part of the unit of care, assessment requires discussion with both. The clinician must maintain a clinical posture that affirms relief of suffering as the central goal of therapy, and which encourages open and effective communication about perceived problems.

Patient assessment

The prevalence of poorly controlled pain and other physical symptoms, and the impact of these factors on the lives of all involved, emphasize the importance of addressing these issues at the earliest opportunity. The early establishment of good symptom control conveys concern, builds the trust of patients and their families, and facilitates the ability to address other important issues.

Patient variables that must be assessed include the disease status, expected disease progression, present functional level, symptoms, current therapies, and anticipated future problems. Of particular importance is the patient's level of function, reflecting his or her mobility (e.g. fully bedbound or fully mobile without any aid), ability to communicate (from severe, as with brain tumours, to minimal impairment), ability to perform activities of daily living, bowel and bladder functions (from incontinence to full self-care), and level of alertness (from coma to full alertness). The use of validated pain and symptom assessment instruments can provide a format for communication between the patient and health care professionals and can also be used to monitor the adequacy of therapy.

It is important to ascertain the patient and the family's understanding of the nature and extent of the illness and their expectations of treatment and outcome. As part of this process, the clinician must develop an understanding of the patient's prioritization of the sometimes conflicting goals of care: optimization of comfort, function (interactional function in particular), and duration of survival.

Family assessment

Family assessment should encompass medical variables, psychosocial concerns, and the adequacy and availability of supports. Concurrent medical problems in a family member, particularly a primary caregiver, need to be evaluated since the viability of the home care plan may depend upon the family member's ability to participate in care. Evaluation of the willingness and ability of home carers to provide home care, and the availability of supports are essential. Since the ability of families to cope with home care is largely determined by the nature of the available home care supports, the family assessment must include an assessment of available health care professional and community supports.

It is important to ascertain the family's understanding of the nature and extent of the patient's illness and their expectations of treatment and outcome. Discrepancies between what is known and understood by the patient and the family should be identified, and the reasons for these discrepancies should be carefully explored. Knowledge deficits may have been deliberately maintained: the family or patient not wanting information overload, the patient protecting the family from knowledge of poor prognosis, or the family protecting the patient from the impact of such information. This part of the assessment requires a non-judgemental posture and sensitivity to psychological and cultural factors that may influence the transmission of information.

Health care professional assessment

Evaluation of the professional caregiver supports usually requires greater detail than that which can be provided by the patient and family alone. To effectively plan for ongoing care, the clinical coordinator must understand the limitations of the involved health care professionals (knowledge, experience, and availability for home care), their difficulties in coping with the situation, and their perceived needs to improve the care outcome. As previously described, the coping of professional caregivers maybe severely strained by issues pertaining to communication, conflict with the patient, family or colleagues, perceived therapeutic failure, excessive workload or emotional strain, and difficult therapeutic or ethical decisions.

Family meetings

A common source of distress for patient, family, and professional carers occurs when there is a lack of coordination in the desired goals of patient care. The goals of care are often complex, but can generally be grouped into three broad categories: (i) prolonging survival, (ii) optimizing comfort, and (iii) optimizing function. The relative priority of these goals provides an essential context for therapeutic decision-making. The prioritization of these goals is a dynamic phenomenon which changes with the evolution of the disease: whereas the optimization of comfort, function, and survival may share equal priority during the phase of ambulatory palliation, the provision of comfort usually assumes overriding priority as death approaches. When patients equally prioritize optimal comfort and function, the therapeutic intent is to achieve an adequate degree of relief without compromising cognitive and physical functions. When comfort is the overriding goal of care, the overriding intent is to achieve relief. In the latter circumstance, there is a willingness to continue therapies that may impair function or even foreshorten life expectancy.

Family meetings, with relevant members of the professional health care team, provide a useful format for discussing the needs of all parties involved, clarifying care goals, sharing and exploring concerns, and developing a therapeutic plan that adequately addresses those needs. The participants should be determined on an individual case basis. Since the family is an appropriate unit of care, and its members have a right to confidentiality, it may be appropriate, on occasion, to meet without the participation of the patient, to address their concerns and needs. Meetings with the participation of all persons who are involved can open communication, improve coordination in the formulation of a care plan, and facilitate better personal coping for each of the individuals involved.

Formulation and implementation of a care plan

The assessment of the patient and their family will identify specific care needs to be addressed, as well as the strengths and weakness' of available resources. The formulation of a flexible care plan aimed at reducing suffering must address the spectrum of problems that have been identified, using the coordinated skills of a range of health care providers.

Coordination of the many participants in this sort of multidisciplinary care requires an identified leader for each case. This role is usually filled by either a physician or a nurse, and the specific person may change in the course of an illness as the predominant care needs change. For example, with the progression of the cancer from a diagnostic stage to a palliative stage, the responsibility may shift sequentially from a surgeon, to a medical oncologist, and finally, to a home care nurse. The coordinator, or case manager, is responsible for monitoring the degree to which care needs are being met, and for facilitating change when necessary. Similarly the well-being and function of the health care professionals must be monitored, ensuring the availability of appropriate manpower and expertise to effectively manage the prevailing problems. For security and safety in the event of a clinical crisis, it is essential that the patient and family have access to a contact person with 24-h availability. This model represents a family-centred, multidisciplinary, collaborative approach among physicians, nurses, social workers, other therapists, and community supports.

Conclusion

An understanding of the nature of suffering and the factors that contribute to it are essential to the task of palliative medicine. Suffering is a complex human experience which requires evaluation in order to construct an effective therapeutic response that is appropriate to presenting problems. An effective approach incorporates careful case assessment, identification of care needs, formulation of a multidisciplinary therapeutic intervention to address those needs, and the provision of ongoing monitoring with readiness to re-evaluate the care plan as problems arise or needs change.

References

1. **Wanzer, S.H.** et al. (1989). The physician's responsibility toward hopelessly ill patients. A second look. *New England Journal of Medicine* **320** (13), 844–9.
2. **van Hooft, S.** (1998). Suffering and the goals of medicine. *Medical Health Care and Philosophy* **1** (2), 125–31.
3. **Byock, I.R.** (1996). The nature of suffering and the nature of opportunity at the end of life. *Clinical Geriatric Medicine* **12** (2), 237–52.
4. **Roy, D.J.** (1991). Relief of suffering: the doctor's mandate (editorial). *Journal of Palliative Care* **7** (4), 3–4.
5. **Angell, M.** (1982). The quality of mercy (editorial). *New England Journal of Medicine* **306** (2), 98–9 (the above reports in MacintoshPCUNIX TextHTML format).
6. **American Medical Association** (1996). Good care of the dying patient. Council on Scientific Affairs, American Medical Association. *Journal of the American Medical Association* **275** (6), 474–8.
7. **American Nurses Association Center for Ethics and Human Rights Task Force on the Nurse's Role in End-of-life Decisions.** *Compendium of Position Statements on the Nurse's Role in End-of-life Decisions.* ANA Publications, 1992, pp. 1–13.
8. **President's Commission for the Study of Ethical Problems in Medical and Biomedical and Behavioral Research.** *Deciding to Forgo Life Sustaining Treatment: Ethical and Legal Issues in Treatment Decisions.* Washington DC: US Government Printing Office, 1983.
9. **Rich, B.A.** (2001). Physicians' legal duty to relieve suffering. *Western Journal of Medicine* **175** (3), 151–2.
10. **Roy, D.J.** (1993). Biology and meaning in suffering. *Journal of Palliative Care* **9** (2), 3–4.
11. **Burge, F.** (1992). The epidemiology of palliative care in cancer. *Journal of Palliative Care* **8** (1), 18–23.
12. **Van Eys, J.** (1991). The ethics of palliative care. *Journal of Palliative Care* **7** (3), 27–32.
13. **Van Eys, J.** *Therapeutic Interventions for Suffering: Professional and Institutional Perspectives.* New York: NLN Publishers, 1992 (15–2461), pp. 115–26.
14. **Churchill, L.R.** (1991). Why we need a theory of suffering, and lots of other theories as well: commentary. *Journal of Clinical Ethics* **2** (2), 95–7.
15. **Copp, L.A.** (1974). Pain and suffering. The spectrum of suffering. *American Journal of Nursing* **74** (3), 491–5.
16. **Cassell, E.J.** (1982). The nature of suffering and the goals of medicine. *New England Journal of Medicine* **306** (11), 639–45.
17. **Cassell, E.J.** (1991). Recognizing suffering. *Hastings Centential Reports* **21** (3), 24–31.
18. **Saunders, C.** (1984). The philosophy of terminal care. In *The Management of Terminal Malignant Disease* (ed. C. Saunders), pp. 232–41. Baltimore MD: Arnold Publishers.
19. **Williams, J.R.** (1991). When suffering is unbearable: physicians, assisted suicide, and euthanasia. *Journal of Palliative Care* **7** (2), 47–9.
20. **Dantz, B.** (1999). Commentary: who defines suffering? *Journal of Pain and Symptom Management* **17** (4), 302.
21. **Cherny, N.I., Coyle, N., and Foley, K.M.** (1994). Suffering in the advanced cancer patient: a definition and taxonomy. *Journal of Palliative Care* **10** (2), 57–70.
22. **Conill, C.** et al. (1997). Symptom prevalence in the last week of life. *Journal of Pain and Symptom Management* **14** (6), 328–31.
23. **Vainio, A. and Auvinen, A.** (1996). Prevalence of symptoms among patients with advanced cancer: an international collaborative study. Symptom Prevalence Group. *Journal of Pain and Symptom Management* **12** (1), 3–10.
24. **Portenoy, R.K.** et al. (1994). The Memorial Symptom Assessment Scale: an instrument for the evaluation of symptom prevalence, characteristics and distress. *European Journal of Cancer* **30A** (9), 1326–36.

25. **Grond, S.** et al. (1994). Prevalence and pattern of symptoms in patients with cancer pain: a prospective evaluation of 1635 cancer patients referred to a pain clinic. *Journal of Pain and Symptom Management* **9** (6), 372–82.
26. **Kutner, J.S., Kassner, C.T., and Nowels, D.E.** (2001). Symptom burden at the end of life: hospice providers' perceptions. *Journal of Pain and Symptom Management* **21** (6), 473–80.
27. **Chang, V.T.** et al. (2000). Symptom and quality of life survey of medical oncology patients at a veterans affairs medical center: a role for symptom assessment. *Cancer* **88** (5), 1175–83.
28. **Mercadante, S., Casuccio, A., and Fulfaro, F.** (2000). The course of symptom frequency and intensity in advanced cancer patients followed at home. *Journal of Pain and Symptom Management* **20** (2), 104–12.
29. **Portenoy, R.K.** et al. (1994). Symptom prevalence, characteristics and distress in a cancer population. *Quality of Life Research* **3** (3), 183–9.
30. **Massie, M.J. and Holland, J.C.** (1990). Depression and the cancer patient. *Journal of Clinical Psychiatry*, **51** (Suppl.), 12–17, (discussion, 18–19).
31. **Massie, M.J., Gagnon, P., and Holland, J.C.** (1994). Depression and suicide in patients with cancer. *Journal of Pain and Symptom Management* **9** (5), 325–40.
32. **Breitbart, W.** et al. (2000). Depression, hopelessness, and desire for hastened death in terminally ill patients with cancer. *Journal of the American Medical Association* **284** (22), 2907–11.
33. **Morasso, G.** et al. (1999). Psychological and symptom distress in terminal cancer patients with met and unmet needs. *Journal of Pain and Symptom Management* **17** (6), 402–9.
34. **Bottomley, A.** (1998). Depression in cancer patients: a literature review. *European Journal of Cancer Care (England)* **7** (3), 181–91.
35. **Yalom, I.D.** (1980). Meaninglessness and psychotherapy. In *Existential Psychotherapy*, pp. 461–86. New York: Basic Books.
36. **Kissane, D.W.** (2000). Psychospiritual and existential distress. The challenge for palliative care. *Australian Family Physician* **29** (11), 1022–5.
37. **Bolmsjo, I.** (2000). Existential issues in palliative care—interviews with cancer patients. *Journal of Palliative Care* **16** (2), 20–4.
38. **Weitzner, M.A., McMillan, S.C., and Jacobsen, P.B.** (1999). Family caregiver quality of life: differences between curative and palliative cancer treatment settings. *Journal of Pain and Symptom Management* **17** (6), 418–28.
39. **Kinsella, G.** et al. (1998). A review of the measurement of caregiver and family burden in palliative care. *Journal of Palliative Care* **14** (2), 37–45.
40. **Blanchard, C.G., Albrecht, T.L., and Ruckdeschel, J.C.** (1997). The crisis of cancer: psychological impact on family caregivers. *Oncology (Huntington)* **11** (2), 189–94 (discussion, 196, 201–2).
41. **Grunfeld, E.** et al. (2000). Cancer care workers in Ontario: prevalence of burnout, job stress and job satisfaction. *Canadian Medical Association Journal* **163** (2), 166–9.
42. **Vachon, M.L.** (1999). Reflections on the history of occupational stress in hospice/palliative care. *Hospice Journal* **14** (3–4), 229–46.
43. **Astudillo, W. and Mendinueta, C.** (1996). Exhaustion syndrome in palliative care (see comments). *Support Care in Cancer* **4** (6), 408–15.
44. **Kash, K.M.** et al. (2000). Stress and burnout in oncology. *Oncology (Huntington)* **14** (11), 1621–33 (discussion, 1633–4, 1636–7).
45. **Lazarus, R.S.** (1985). The psychology of stress and coping. *Issues in Mental Health and Nursing* **7** (1–4), 399–418.
46. **Folkman, S.** et al. (1986). Appraisal, coping, health status, and psychological symptoms. *Journal of Personal and Social Psychology* **50** (3), 571–9.
47. **World Health Organization.** *Cancer Pain Relief* 2nd edn. Geneva: World Health Organization, 1996, p. 63.
48. **Cassel, C.K. and Foley, K.M.** (1999). Principles for care of patients at the end of life: an emerging consensus among the specialties of medicine. In *Milbank Memorial Fund Reports,* p. 32. MY: Milbank Memorial Fund.
49. **Cleeland, C.S.** et al. (1994). Pain and its treatment in outpatients with metastatic cancer. *New England Journal of Medicine* **330** (9), 592–6.
50. **Larue, F.** et al. (1995). Multicentre study of cancer pain and its treatment in France. *British Medical Journal* **310** (6986), 1034–7.
51. **Kelsen, D.P.** et al. (1995). Pain and depression in patients with newly diagnosed pancreas cancer. *Journal of Clinical Oncology* **13** (3), 748–55.
52. **Portenoy, R.K.** et al. (1994). Pain in ovarian cancer patients. Prevalence, characteristics, and associated symptoms. *Cancer* **74** (3), 907–15.
53. **Portenoy, R.K.** et al. (1992). Pain in ambulatory patients with lung or colon cancer. Prevalence, characteristics, and effect. *Cancer* **70** (6), 1616–24.
54. **Tay, W.K., Shaw, R.J., and Goh, C.R.** (1994). A survey of symptoms in hospice patients in Singapore. *Annals of the Academy of Medicine, Singapore* **23** (2), 191–6.
55. **Brescia, F.J.** et al. (1992). Pain, opioid use, and survival in hospitalized patients with advanced cancer. *Journal of Clinical Oncology* **10** (1), 149–55.
56. **Donnelly, S. and Walsh, D.** (1995). The symptoms of advanced cancer. *Seminars in Oncology* **22** (2 Suppl. 3), 67–72.
57. **Feuz, A. and Rapin, C.H.** (1994). An observational study of the role of pain control and food adaptation of elderly patients with terminal cancer. *Journal of the American Dietetics Association* **94** (7), 767–70.
58. **Thorpe, D.M.** (1993). The incidence of sleep disturbance in cancer patients with pain. In *7th World Congress on Pain: Abstracts,* abstract 451. Seattle WA: IASP Publication.
59. **Cleeland, C.S.** et al. (1996). Dimensions of the impact of cancer pain in a four country sample: new information from multidimensional scaling. *Pain* **67** (2–3), 267–73.
60. **Ferrell, B.R.** (1995). The impact of pain on quality of life. A decade of research. *Nursing Clinics of North America* **30** (4), 609–24.
61. **Massie, M.J. and Holland, J.C.** (1992). The cancer patient with pain: psychiatric complications and their management. *Journal of Pain and Symptom Management* **7** (2), 99–109.
62. **Burrows, M., Dibble, S.L., and Miaskowski, C.** (1998). Differences in outcomes among patients experiencing different types of cancer-related pain. *Oncology Nursing Forum* **25** (4), 735–41.
63. **Breitbart, W. and Jacobsen, P.B.** (1996). Psychiatric symptom management in terminal care. *Clinical Geriatric Medicine* **12** (2), 329–47.
64. **Breitbart, W.** et al. (1995). Neuropsychiatric syndromes and psychological symptoms in patients with advanced cancer. *Journal of Pain and Symptom Management* **10** (2), 131–41.
65. **Breitbart, W.** (1988). Suicide in cancer patients. *Scandinavian Journal of Social Medicine* **16** (3), 149–53.
66. **Nordin, K.** et al. (2001). Predicting anxiety and depression among cancer patients: a clinical model. *European Journal of Cancer* **37** (3), 376–84.
67. **Derogatis, L.R.** et al. (1983). The prevalence of psychiatric disorders among cancer patients. *Journal of the American Medical Association* **249** (6), 751–7.
68. **Breitbart, W.** (1990). Cancer pain and suicide. In *Second International Congress on Cancer Pain* (ed. K.M. Foley, J.J. Bonica, and V. Ventafridda), pp. 399–412. New York: Raven Press.
69. **Stedeford, A.** (1984). Psychological aspects of the management of terminal cancer. *Comprehensive Therapy* **10** (1), 35–40.
70. **Vachon, M.L.** (1987). Unresolved grief in persons with cancer referred for psychotherapy. *Psychiatric Clinics of North America* **10** (3), 467–86.
71. **Farberow, N.L., Schneiderman, E.S., and Leonard, C.V.** (1963). Suicide among general medical and surgical hospital patients with malignant neoplasms. *Medical Bulletin* **9**. Washington DC: US Veterans Administration.
72. **Watson, M.** et al. (1990). Locus of control and adjustment to cancer. *Psychology Reports* **66** (1), 39–48.
73. **Bredart, A.** et al. (1999). Psychological distress in cancer patients attending the European Institute of Oncology in Milan. *Oncology* **57** (4), 297–302.
74. **Vachon, M.L.** (1998). Psychosocial needs of patients and families. *Journal of Palliative Care* **14** (3), 49–56.
75. **Mager, W.M. and Andrykowski, M.A.** (2002). Communication in the cancer 'bad news' consultation: patient perceptions and psychological adjustment. *Psychooncology* **11** (1), 35–46.
76. **Ellis, P.M. and Tattersall, M.H.** (1999). How should doctors communicate the diagnosis of cancer to patients? *Annals of Medicine* **31** (5), 336–41.
77. **Moberg, D.O. and Brusek, P.M.** (1978). Spiritual well-being: a neglected subject in quality of life research. *Social Indicators Research* **5**, 303–23.
78. **Yalom, I.D.** *Existential Psychotherapy*. New York: Basic Books, 1980, p. 523.
79. **Ellis, J.B. and Smith, P.C.** (1991). Spiritual well-being, social desirability and reasons for living: is there a connection? *International Journal of Social Psychiatry* **37** (1), 57–63.
80. **Breitbart, W. and Rosenfeld, B.D.** (1999). Physician-assisted suicide: the influence of psychosocial issues. *Cancer Control* **6** (2), 146–61.

81. **Chochinov, H.M.** et al. (1999). Will to live in the terminally ill. *Lancet* **354** (9181), 816–19.
82. **Chochinov, H.M.** et al. (1995). Desire for death in the terminally ill. *American Journal of Psychiatry* **152** (8), 1185–91.
83. **Neubauer, B.J. and Lai, J.Y.** (1988). Death anxiety and attitudes toward hospice care. *Psychology Reports* **63** (1), 195–8.
84. **Stedeford, A.** (1981). Couples facing death. I-Psychosocial aspects. *British Medical Journal (Clinical Research and Education)* **283** (6298), 1033–6.
85. **Kissane, D.W., Clarke, D.M., and Street, A.F.** (2001). Demoralization syndrome—a relevant psychiatric diagnosis for palliative care. *Journal of Palliative Care* **17** (1), 12–21.
86. **World Health Organization.** *Cancer Pain Relief and Palliative Care.* Geneva: World Health Organization, 1990.
87. **Purdy, W.A.** (2002). Spiritual discernment in palliative care. *Journal of Palliative Medicine* **5** (1), 139–41.
88. **Kuuppelomaki, M.** (2001). Spiritual support for terminally ill patients: nursing staff assessments. *Journal of Clinical Nursing* **10** (5), 660–70.
89. **Storey, P.** (2001). Spiritual care at the end of life. *Texas Medicine* **97** (8), 56–9.
90. **Krizek, T.J.** (2001). Spiritual dimensions of surgical palliative care. *Surgical Oncology Clinics of North America* **10** (1), 39–55.
91. **Orr, R.D., Paris, J.J., and Siegler, M.** (1991). Caring for the terminally ill: resolving conflicting objectives between patient, physician, family, and institution. *Journal of Family Practitioners* **33** (5), 500–4.
92. **Heath, S.** (1996). Childhood cancer—a family crisis. 1. The impact of diagnosis. *British Journal of Nursing* **5** (12), 744–8.
93. **Heath, S.** (1996). Childhood cancer—a family crisis. 2. Coping with diagnosis. *British Journal of Nursing* **5** (13), 790–3.
94. **Kristjanson, L.J. and Ashcroft, T.** (1994). The family's cancer journey: a literature review. *Cancer Nursing* **17** (1), 1–17.
95. **Lewis, F.M.** (1993). Psychosocial transitions and the family's work in adjusting to cancer. *Seminars in Oncology Nursing* **9** (2), 127–9.
96. **Davies, B., Reimer, J.C., and Martens, N.** (1990). Families in supportive care—Part I. The transition of fading away: the nature of the transition. *Journal of Palliative Care* **6** (3), 12–20.
97. **West, S.R.** et al. (1986). A retrospective study of patients with cancer in their terminal year. *New Zealand Medical Journal* **99** (798), 197–200.
98. **Schachter, S.** (1992). Quality of life for families in the management of home care patients with advanced cancer. *Journal of Palliative Care* **8** (3), 61–6.
99. **Siegel, K.** et al. (1996). Depressive distress among the spouses of terminally ill cancer patients. *Cancer Practice* **4** (1), 25–30.
100. **Lewis, F.** (1986). The impact of cancer on the family: a critical analysis of the research literature. *Patient Education and Counselling* **8**, 269–89.
101. **Kissane, D.W., McKenzie, D.P., and Bloch, S.** (1997). Family coping and bereavement outcome. *Palliative Medicine* **11** (3), 191–201.
102. **Hinds, C.** (1985). The needs of families who care for patients with cancer at home: are we meeting them? *Journal of Advances in Nursing* **10** (6), 575–81.
103. **Ekberg, J.Y., Griffith, N., and Foxall, M.J.** (1986). Spouse burnout syndrome. *Journal of Advances in Nursing* **11** (2), 161–5.
104. **Hull, M.M.** (1989). Family needs and supportive nursing behaviors during terminal cancer: a review. *Oncology Nursing Forum* **16** (6), 787–92.
105. **Ferrell, B.R.** et al. (1992). Home care: maintaining quality of life for patient and family. *Oncology (Huntington)* **6** (2 Suppl.), 136–40.
106. **Ferrell, B.R.** et al. (1991). Pain as a metaphor for illness. Part II. Family caregivers' management of pain. *Oncology Nursing Forum* **18** (8), 1315–21.
107. **Addington-Hall, J.** et al. (1995). Symptom control, communication with health professionals, and hospital care of stroke patients in the last year of life as reported by surviving family, friends, and officials. *Stroke* **26** (12), 2242–8.
108. **Jones, R.V., Hansford, J., and Fiske, J.** (1993). Death from cancer at home: the carers' perspective. *British Medical Journal* **306** (6872), 249–51.
109. **Ventafridda, V.** et al. (1989). Comparison of home and hospital care of advanced cancer patients. *Tumorigenesis* **75** (6), 619–25.
110. **Beck-Friis, B., Norberg, H., and Strang, P.** (1991). Cost analysis and ethical aspects of hospital-based home-care for terminal cancer patients. *Scandinavian Journal of Primary Health Care* **9** (4), 259–64.
111. **Bloom, B.S., Knorr, R.S., and Evans, A.E.** (1985). The epidemiology of disease expenses. The costs of caring for children with cancer. *Journal of the American Medical Association* **253** (16), 2393–7.
112. **Bodkin, C.M., Pigott, T.J., and Mann, J.R.** (1982). Financial burden of childhood cancer. *British Medical Journal (Clinical Research and Education)* **284** (6328), 1542–4.
113. **Lansky, S.B.** et al. (1979). Childhood cancer: nonmedical costs of the illness. *Cancer* **43** (1), 403–8.
114. **Muurinen, J.M.** (1986). The economics of informal care. Labor market effects in the National Hospice Study. *Medical Care* **24** (11), 1007–17.
115. **Glajchen, M.** (1994). Psychosocial consequences of inadequate health insurance for patients with cancer. *Cancer Practice* **2** (2), 115–20.
116. **Callahan, D.** (1988). Families as caregivers: the limits of morality. *Archives of Physical and Medical Rehabilitation* **69** (5), 323–8.
117. **Kristjanson, L.J.** (1989). Quality of terminal care: salient indicators identified by families. *Journal of Palliative Care* **5** (1), 21–30.
118. **Kristjanson, L.J., Atwood, J., and Degner, L.F.** (1995). Validity and reliability of the family inventory of needs (FIN): measuring the care needs of families of advanced cancer patients. *Journal of Nursing Measures* **3** (2), 109–26.
119. **Kristjanson, L.J.** et al. (1997). Family members' care expectations, care perceptions, and satisfaction with advanced cancer care: results of a multi-site pilot study. *Journal of Palliative Care* **13** (4), 5–13.
120. **Ferrell, B.R.** et al. (1991). Pain as a metaphor for illness. Part I. Impact of cancer pain on family caregivers. *Oncology Nursing Forum* **18** (8), 1303–9.
121. **Milberg, A. and Strang, P.** (2000). Met and unmet needs in hospital-based home care: qualitative evaluation through open-ended questions. *Palliative Medicine* **14** (6), 533–4.
122. **Soothill, K.** et al. (2001). The significant unmet needs of cancer patients: probing psychosocial concerns. *Support Care in Cancer* **9** (8), 597–605.
123. **Ferrell, B.R.** et al. (1995). The impact of cancer pain education on family caregivers of elderly patients. *Oncology Nursing Forum* **22** (8), 1211–18.
124. **Grobe, M.E., Ahmann, D.L., and Ilstrup, D.M.** (1982). Needs assessment for advanced cancer patients and their families. *Oncology Nursing Forum* **9** (4), 26–30.
125. **Wright, K. and Dyck, S.** (1984). Needs of the grieving spouse in a hospital setting. *Nursing Research* **6**, 371–4.
126. **Field, D.** et al. (1992). Care and information received by lay carers of terminally ill patients at the Lancestershire Hospice. *Palliative Medicine* **6**, 237–42.
127. **Hinds, C.** (1985). The needs of families who care for patients with cancer at home: are we meeting them? *Journal of Advances in Nursing* **10** (6), 575–81.
128. **Tolle, S.W.** et al. (2000). Family reports of barriers to optimal care of the dying. *Nursing Research* **49** (6), 310–17.
129. **Wellisch, D.** et al. (1989). An evaluation of psychosocial problems of the homebound cancer patient: relationship of patient adjustment to family problems. *Journal of Psychosocial Oncology* **7**, 55–76.
130. **Wellisch, D.** et al. (1983). Evaluation of psychosocial problems of the homebound cancer patient: the relationship of disease and the socioeconomic variables of patients to family problems. *Journal of Psychosocial Oncology* **1**, 1–15.
131. **Quinn, W. and Herndon, A.** (1986). The family ecology of cancer. *Journal of Psychosocial Oncology* **4**, 45–59.
132. **Mount, B.M.** (1986). Dealing with our losses. *Journal of Clinical Oncology* **4** (7), 1127–34.
133. **Billings, J.** (1985). On being a reluctant physician—strains and rewards in caring for the dying at home. In *Outpatient Management of Advanced Cancer* (ed. J. Billings), pp. 309–18. Philadelphia PA: Lippincott.
134. **Barni, S.** et al. (1996). Oncostress: evaluation of burnout in Lombardy. *Tumorigenesis* **82** (1), 85–92.
135. **Whippen, D.A. and Canellos, G.P.** (1991). Burnout syndrome in the practice of oncology: results of a random survey of 1000 oncologists (see comments). *Journal of Clinical Oncology* **9** (10), 1916–20.
136. **Ramirez, A.J.** et al. (1995). Burnout and psychiatric disorder among cancer clinicians. *British Journal of Cancer* **71** (6), 1263–9.
137. **Schaerer, R.** (1993). Suffering of the doctor linked with the death of patients. *Palliative Medicine* **7**, 27–37.

138. **Vachon, M.L.** (1995). Staff stress in hospice/palliative care: a review. *Palliative Medicine* **9** (2), 91–122.
139. **Astudillo, W. and Mendinueta, C.** (1996). Exhaustion syndrome in palliative care. *Support Care in Cancer* **4** (6), 408–15.
140. **Harris, R., Bond, M., and Turnbull, R.** (1990). Nursing stress and stress reduction in palliative care. *Palliative Medicine* **4**, 191–6.
141. **Wilkes, L.M. and Beale, B.** (2001). Palliative care at home: stress for nurses in urban and rural New South Wales, Australia. *International Journal of Nursing Practice* **7** (5), 306–13.
142. **Newton, J. and Waters, V.** (2001). Community palliative care clinical nurse specialists' descriptions of stress in their work. *International Journal of Palliative Nursing* **7** (11), 531–40.

2.2 The epidemiology of death and symptoms

Irene J. Higginson and Julia M. Addington-Hall

What is epidemiology?

Epidemiology is the study of the distribution and determinants of disease in defined populations.[1,2] It describes groups of patients or whole populations and their different characteristics. In addition to using raw numbers, epidemiology calculates proportions and rates, so that we can know how common a condition occurs within the denominator (total) population. Epidemiological information is used to plan and evaluate strategies to prevent illness or future problems and as a guide to the management of patients in whom disease has already developed.

Traditionally, epidemiology has used information about deaths to calculate numbers of deaths and mortality rates. These may be standardized by age and gender, so that the types and cause of death can be compared in different areas. Crude information on the numbers of deaths is also useful to determine how many patients and families might need care. Both these types of information are useful in planning palliative and end of life care. This is described in detail in the section on the epidemiology of death.

In a parallel way we can consider symptoms. The same epidemiological methods are used as for a disease. Thus, we can study how often a symptom, for example, fatigue, pain, constipation, breathlessness, or depression, occurs in different groups of people, and why. This is helpful in better understanding the relevance of each symptom in a specific disease, in studying its cause and what is associated with this cause and in developing and testing strategies to improve the management of symptoms.[2]

Before we consider the epidemiology of death and the symptoms, it is useful to review the main definitions.

Main epidemiological definitions

Incidence and prevalence are the classical ways used to describe how common a disease, symptom, or problem are in a population. These are often used incorrectly in palliative care reports. Further understanding the relationship between incidence and prevalence can help to place epidemiological information into better context for needs assessment.

Incidence quantifies the number of new diseases or symptoms that develop in a population at risk during a given period of time (e.g. new symptoms such as new instances of pain or fatigue). Incidence is quantified as a rate:

$$\text{incidence} = \frac{\text{number of new symptoms during a given period of time}}{\text{total population (or person-time) at risk}}$$

Incidence provides an estimate of the probability (or risk) that a patient will develop the symptom (or disease if that is being considered) during the given period of time.[2]

For diseases which occur once and are invariably fatal (e.g. most lung cancers or motor neurone disease), incidence rates are very similar to death (or mortality) rates. The latter can then be used to estimate the former.

Prevalence quantifies the proportion of a given population with a symptom (e.g. fatigue) or a disease (e.g. lung cancer) at a designated time. When the term is used without qualification of a time period it is usually the point prevalence. For example, the proportion of patients with fatigue at a given point in time. Note that, although the term 'prevalence rate' is used for prevalence, prevalence is a proportion, not a rate.

$$\text{prevalence} = \frac{\text{number of patients with the problem}}{\text{total population}} \text{ at a designed time}$$

The period prevalence refers to the proportion of a given population with a problem (e.g. fatigue, or if a disease is being considered, cancer or motor neurone disease) at any time during a specified period (old and new cases). Period prevalence can refer to the proportion with a problem at any time in one year (annual prevalence) or at any time in their life (lifetime prevalence).

The longer the time period used to calculate the period prevalence, the greater the prevalence is likely to be. For example, if we ask a group of Masters Programme students if they have had fatigue in the last 3 days, many will respond negatively (unless it is examination time). However, if we ask the same group if they have had fatigue in the past year, then we are likely to find that a greater number will say they have had fatigue. Thus the time period used when asking questions about symptoms will strongly influence the result, and any questions that ask about prevalence in the past year will give higher levels than questions that ask about a shorter time period.

Incidence and prevalence are closely related. Prevalence (the proportion of a population with a disease or symptom at a designated time) depends on both the incidence (the rate of new disease or symptom during a period of time) and the duration of the disease or symptom. A disease or symptom with a long duration will have a high probability to be counted at that designated time when prevalence is estimated.[2]

Epidemiology of death

Mortality statistics provides information on the number of deaths each year, their cause and location, how these are related to demographic characteristics such as age, occupation, and place of birth, and changes over time in, for example, life expectancy and causes of death. They are important for health policy and planning, in general, and are an useful source of information for those responsible for planning and providing palliative care services. Their usefulness depends on two assumptions, the first that the data is reliable and valid and the second that palliative care need is directly related to cause of death.

Reliability and validity of mortality statistics

In developed countries much effort is taken to ensure that mortality statistics are reliable and valid: all deaths are registered, the cause of death is coded according to rules specified by the World Health Organization (WHO), using the International Classification of Diseases (ICD), and is often automated to reduce coder error, and systems of quality checks and validation exist to ensure the highest achievable quality of data.[3] Nevertheless, there remain sources of bias.

Information on the decedent's socio-demographic characteristics are provided by the person who registers the death, who may not know the correct information. For example, age may be inaccurately recorded in death certificates in the United States, with a systematic under-reporting but with too many deaths reported at 95 years or older.[4] Race and origin may also be inaccurately reported.[5]

Completing a death certificate requires doctors to give the condition or the sequence of conditions that led directly to the death, as well as any associated conditions that contributed to the death but were not part of the sequence. Many thousands of doctors write death certificates, and the quality is therefore bound to be inconsistent, given the variations in doctors' training in death certification, their habits, and their knowledge. Errors are common: a Canadian study reported that a third of the death certificates completed in a teaching hospital contained a major error.[6] Whether a consequence of error or a lack of knowledge about the patient by the certifying doctor, mortality from dementia is under-estimated[7] whilst mortality from coronary heart disease may be over-estimated.[8]

Mortality statistics as indicators of need for palliative care

The use of mortality statistics to establish need for palliative care assumes that the causes of death likely to be indicative of such need can be identified in these statistics, and that the data are accurate. This may be a reasonable assumption in cancer, at least amongst younger people (cancer may be under-reported in the very elderly[9]). Outside of cancer, the use of mortality statistics is more problematic. As outlined above, for example, mortality statistics under-estimate the prevalence of dementia, and will lead to an under-estimate of need if used to plan palliative care services. In addition, there is growing evidence that people with severe heart failure have palliative care needs.[10] When they die, however, their deaths will usually be attributed to the underlying cause of the heart failure, rather than to the heart failure per se. Mortality statistics will be of little use in establishing the need for palliative care amongst these patients.

Mortality statistics alone are not sufficient to estimate palliative care needs, even in cancer. To give a complete picture of population-level need, they need to be combined with information from prospective studies of quality of life and of functional decline in the last weeks and months of life.[11] Although not complete, particularly at the level of individual cancers, much is now known about the pattern of decline in cancers and about the epidemiology of symptoms and other problems. These can be combined with mortality statistics to assess need. The evidence for palliative care needs amongst people dying from heart failure or chronic obstructive pulmonary disease (COPD) is less well-established and it is therefore difficult to use it to estimate need at the population level. A minority of deaths from heart failure follow the cancer trajectory of rapid decline. Most patients will experience gradual and unpredictable decline and/or die suddenly.[12] Accurate information on the proportions falling into each group is, however, unknown, as is the relationship between dying trajectory and the patient's quality of life. Even if all deaths from heart failure were identifiable from mortality statistics, in the absence of better epidemiological data on the last months of life this would still shed little light on palliative care needs in heart failure.

Death certification requires doctors to indicate the condition or sequence of conditions that led directly to death, as well as any associated conditions that contributed to death. Mortality statistics are based on the underlying cause of death coded according to WHO guidelines from these data. They do not necessarily provide complete information on all the medical conditions the patient had. This is a particular issue for older people, who are likely to have had a number of co-morbidities and in whom indeed it may be difficult to establish any one cause of death. Palliative care is concerned with the whole person and their holistic needs. Again, mortality statistics will not give a complete picture of these.

In summary, mortality statistics can give useful information on the likely levels of need for palliative care at a population level, particularly when combined with the findings of epidemiological studies of the prevalence of symptoms and other problems amongst patients and families. Mortality statistics are a starting point, at least in indicating the total number of people who die. They are currently most useful in establishing the need for palliative care amongst cancer patients. But outside of cancer or among older people[13] these will be subject to errors. Mortality information needs to be adjusted by results from prospective and retrospective studies, by estimates of the types of illness a person may have had, and by likely errors in coding.

Epidemiology of dying in England and Wales

Despite these limitations, a basic understanding of the epidemiology of dying is important for the information it provides (albeit imperfectly) on population-level need for palliative care, and because it raises questions about whether these services are provided in a way that is fair and equitable or whether there are groups who are currently under-served by palliative care. Knowing trends in, for example, the cause of death can also be important in planning future palliative care provision.

Death registration data from England and Wales are used in this section to illustrate causes of death in developed countries, and their relationship to age, gender, ethnicity, and place of death. People in these countries no longer die in large numbers from infectious illnesses, usually rapidly and with little warning. Instead, they survive to succumb eventually to the new killers: cancer and chronic diseases such as CHD and chronic lung diseases. This contrasts to developing countries, where infections including AIDS/HIV remain important causes of death. However, mortality rates in many developing countries are declining with a consequent rapid growth in the number of older people and in the proportion of deaths from chronic diseases: the WHO have projected that by 2020 three-quarters of all deaths in developing countries could be age-related, with CHD, cancer, and diabetes becoming important causes of death.[13] The patterns of mortality reported below will therefore become increasingly common across the world in the next decades.

Who dies?

In the year 2000, 530 870 people aged 15 or above died in England and Wales (Table 1). Just over a thousand in every 100 000 people die each year—1 per cent of the population. Most people live until old age. Sixteen per cent of the deaths in 2000 occurred between the ages of 15 and 64, 19 per cent between 65 and 74, 33 per cent between 75 and 84, and 31 per cent at the age of 85 or above. Men, on an average, die earlier than women do. Women aged 60 in 1997 had a life expectancy of 22.7 years, and men 18.9 years. In 2000, 62 per cent of people who died between the ages of 15 and 64 were men, compared with 41 per cent of those who died at the age of 75 or above. Twenty-one per cent of men who died in 2000 in England and Wales were aged between 15 and 64, compared with 12 per cent of women. Conversely, 73 per cent of women died at the age of 75 or above, compared with only 55 per cent of men.

In the United Kingdom, as in other developed countries, there is a social class gradient in mortality.[14] For example, one study found that men in manual occupations were twice as likely to die before the age of 65 over a 20-year follow-up period as their contemporaries working in non-manual occupations. This appears to be related to differences in wealth and associated standing in the society rather than to absolute levels of poverty.[15]

In 1991 people from non-white ethnic groups made up 5.9 per cent of the United Kingdom population.[16] Ethnicity is related to social

Table 1 Deaths of people aged 15 or over in England and Wales in 2000, by age and sex[a]

Age (years)	Deaths in each age-group (%)		Deaths within gender category (%)		Total deaths (%)
	Men	Women	Men	Women	
15–44	65	35	4.7	2.3	3.4
45–64	61	39	16.3	9.5	12.8
65–74	59	41	24.0	15.2	19.4
75+	41	59	55.0	73.0	64.4
No. of deaths			252 825	278 045	530 870

[a] Office of National Statistics, DH2, No. 27, The Stationery Office, London, 2001.

Table 2 Variations in selected causes of death by age in England and Wales in 2000

ICD 9	Diagnosis	Deaths in each age-group (%)				Total no. of deaths	Deaths (%)
		15–64	65–74	75–84	85+		
140–208	Malignant neoplasms	37.5	35.9	24.0	13.3	132 420	24.9
290, 797	Presenile and senile organic psychotic conditions; senility—no mention of psychosis	0.06	0.4	2.1	9.4	19 631	3.7
390–459	Diseases of the circulatory system	27.4	38.7	43	41.1	207 089	39
410–414	Ischaemic heart disease	17.4	23.5	22.8	17.8	108 415	20.4
430–438	Stroke	4.6	7.1	10.9	13.3	52 478	9.9
460–519	Diseases of the respiratory system	6.7	13.3	18.4	24	92 253	17.4
490–496	Chronic obstructive pulmonary disease and allied conditions	3.2	6.4	6.2	3.4	25 559	4.8
480–486	Pneumonia	3.3	5.4	10.3	17.9	56 242	10.5
800–999	Injury and poisoning	11.7	1.4	1.3	1.7	16 122	3
No. of deaths		86 301	102 767	176 436	165 366	530 870	

deprivation, and thus to an increased risk of premature death. In addition, mass migration into the United Kingdom began in the late 1940s, and minority ethnic groups include increasing numbers of older people. In 1999, there were nearly 250 000 people aged 60 years or above from these groups in the United Kingdom, and this number is expected to increase rapidly in the next two decades.(17) Given the relationship between increased age and death the number of deaths in the United Kingdom from these groups will also increase. Hospices and specialist palliative care services will increasingly need to ensure that their services are acceptable to and appropriate for people from minority groups.(18)

Of what?

The major causes of death in England and Wales are listed in Table 2, together with the number of people who died from each cause in 2000. Infectious diseases were the main cause of death 100 years ago. These declined, particularly during the first half of the last century, and diseases of the circulatory system (including heart disease and stroke) then became more prominent. These have also been in decline as a cause of mortality, although they remain the leading cause of death, accounting for 39 per cent of deaths in 2000. With these reductions in mortality, the proportion of deaths due to cancer has increased. In 2000 cancer accounted for 25 per cent of deaths.

The proportion of deaths attributable to cancer declines with age, from 38 per cent of deaths between the ages of 15 and 64 to 12 per cent of deaths in the oldest age-group. As indicated above, cancer may be under-diagnosed in the very elderly, but it is still likely that the incidence decreases with age. It is the leading cause of death in the youngest age-group, and comes a close second to diseases of the circulatory system in the 65–74 age-group. Nevertheless, it kills nearly as many people aged over 75 as under it (63 134 versus 69 286). Lung cancer is the leading cancer type, responsible for 22 per cent of all cancer deaths (Table 3). In men, lung cancer accounts for 21 per cent of deaths, followed by prostrate cancer (13 per cent), and colorectal cancer (11 per cent). In women, the three leading cancers in terms of mortality are breast cancer (18 per cent), lung cancer (17 per cent), and colorectal cancer (11 per cent). Lung cancer mortality rates in women continue to rise, whilst mortality from some other cancers—notably breast cancer—are falling in response to improved treatments and earlier detection.(16)

Injuries and poisoning show the same pattern as cancer in that there is an inverse relationship between the proportion of deaths attributed to these causes and age-group. In contrast, the proportion of deaths due to dementia increases sharply with age from less than 1 per cent of deaths in the youngest age-group compared with nearly 10 per cent in the oldest (itself an under-estimation(7)).

Circulatory diseases as a whole increase in importance with age, but this is largely due to an increase in the proportion of deaths due to stroke (from 5 per cent to 13 per cent). The proportion of deaths attributable to heart disease remains fairly stable across the age-groups. The incidence of heart failure is increasing as the population ages, and it has a poor prognosis. Its importance as a cause of death is not reflected here because, as discussed above, most heart failure deaths are attributed to the underlying cause of the heart failure.

Some causes of death affect relatively few people but are important in palliative care (i) because of the distress they cause and (ii) because there is a long trajectory of illness (compared with cancer), increasing the prevalence of symptoms and problems (see section on incidence and prevalence). A good example is motor neurone disease, which was the underlying cause

Table 3 Variation by age in selected site of cancer in 2000 death registrations in England and Wales[a]

ICD 9 code	Malignant neoplasm site	Total no.	Cancer deaths (%)	Cancers in age-group (%)			
				15–64	65–74	75–84	85+
150	Oesophagus	6061	4.6	4.6	4.5	4.6	4.4
151	Stomach	5779	4.4	3.1	4.6	4.7	5.4
153–154	Colon, rectum, rectosigmoid junction, and anus	14235	10.7	8.8	10.4	11.4	13.1
162–163	Trachea, bronchus, lung, and pleura	29555	22.3	20.1	27.4	23.2	13.8
174	Female breast	11363	8.6	13.3	6	6.5	9.8
179–184	Female reproductive organ	6787	5	7	5	4.3	4.4
185–187	Male reproductive organ	8458	6.4	2	5.5	8.5	10.4
188–189	Bladder/kidney	7132	5.3	4.3	5.3	5.8	6.4
200–208	Lymphatic and haematopoietic tissue	9764	7.4	8.2	7.1	7.1	7.0
No. of deaths		132421		32378	36901	42755	20379

[a] From Office of National Statistics, DH2, no. 27.

Table 4 Place of death for all deaths in England and Wales in 1999, by age

	Total no.	Cancer deaths (%)	Cancers in age-group (%)			
			15–64	65–74	75–84	85+
Psychiatric hospitals	3807	0.7	0.2	0.05	0.8	1.0
Hospices[a]	23 045	4.2	7.9	6.6	3.7	1.2
NHS hospitals and communal establishments for care of the sick (including NHS nursing homes)	297 677	54	52.8	58	58	47.8
Non-NHS hospitals and communal establishments for care of sick (including private nursing homes)	59 392	10.8	2.4	4.6	10.3	19.7
Other communal establishments	46 081	8.4	0.7	2.0	6.6	18.4
House	107 538	19.5	29	25.8	18.9	11.2
Other private homes and other places	13 376	2.4	6.9	2.5	1.8	0.8
Total	550 916	100				

[a] NHS hospices excluded.

of 1163 deaths in England and Wales in 2000. Many hospices and specialist palliative care services provided care for at least some of these patients in their last months and weeks of life. AIDS/HIV is another now-rare cause of death in the United Kingdom associated with distressing physical, psychological, and spiritual problems. In 2000, 181 people died from this, a decline since 1996, as a result of highly active antiretroviral drugs (although growing evidence of drug resistance suggests that the mortality rate may again increase in this country). Again, palliative care services have responded to the needs of some of these patients. However, there are still many who, for diverse reasons, continue to die from HIV/AIDS and need palliative care.(19) Worldwide this number is predicted to increase, such that HIV/AIDS will become the ninth most common cause of death in 2020.(10)

There are other causes of death which are not currently served by palliative care, at least in the United Kingdom, but for which there is growing evidence of unmet needs at the end of life.(10) These include chronic respiratory diseases and chronic liver disease. The former killed 25 559 people in 2000, 64 per cent of whom were aged 75 or above. In contrast, only 4768 people died from cirrhosis and chronic liver disease, 69 per cent of whom died before the age of 65. The number of affected patients is likely to grow over the next two decades, due to the increased prevalence of hepatitis C infection. The palliative care needs of these patients have received little attention.

Where do people die?

In 1999, 54 per cent of deaths in England and Wales took place in NHS hospitals (and other NHS establishments for care of the sick, including NHS nursing homes). One in five (19.5 per cent) took place at home, and 11 per cent in 'non-NHS hospitals and communal establishments for care of the sick', a category which includes private nursing homes; 4 per cent took place in hospices, an under-estimation as the 12 or so NHS hospices are included in the NHS hospital category. The proportion of deaths in NHS hospitals declines in the oldest age-group, whilst that in 'other communal establishment' (including residential homes for the elderly) increases in this age-group. The proportion of deaths in a hospice or at home has an inverse relationship with age, whilst deaths in non-NHS hospitals and communal establishments increase with age (Table 4). This presumably reflects on the use of private nursing homes, but these data are not currently coded in a way that makes it possible to identify nursing home deaths.

Table 5 Deaths of cancer patients in hospice and palliative care centres in 1999 by age in England and Wales[a]

Age at death (years)	No. of cancer deaths	Cancer deaths (%)	No. of hospice deaths[b]	Hospice deaths (%)
15–44	3891	2.9	804	3.6
45–64	29 095	21.4	5881	26.6
65–74	38518	28.4	6969	31.5
75–84	43718	32.2	6573	29.7
85+	20611	15.2	1879	8.5
Total no. of deaths	135833		22106	

[a] The 12 NHS hospices are not included. It is estimated that hospice deaths in 1998 were therefore under-estimated by about 1700.

[b] Deaths from causes other than cancer are excluded. For 22 106 out of 23 045 hospice deaths the underlying cause of death was cancer (95.9 %).

The proportion of cancer patients who die in NHS hospitals has fallen since 1985 from 58 to 47.3 per cent, whilst the proportion of home deaths seems to be rising slightly following falls in the early 1990s.[(20)] Cancer patients living in less-affluent areas are less likely to die at home than people in more affluent areas.[(21)] The proportion dying at home decreases with age[(22)] as does the proportion dying in a hospice (Table 5). Place of death varies between ethnic groups. People born in the Caribbean are less likely to die at home than people born in the United Kingdom, whilst migrants from the Indian sub-continent are more likely to do so.[(23)]

The trajectory of dying

Some people die suddenly, with no warning, no preceding illness, and no time for care. Figures on the proportion of deaths which follow this trajectory are difficult to obtain. Two nationally representative surveys of people who died in England and Wales estimated that one in 10 deaths[(24,25)] could be categorized in this way. In contrast, other people die after a period of terminal illness, where it is recognized by health professionals—and usually by patients and families—that the patient has an incurable condition which will result in their death. As discussed above, this type of dying trajectory has been particularly associated with cancer. Neurological conditions such as motor neurone disease also fit into this category. Hospices and specialist palliative care services have developed in the past 30 years to advance understanding of how to care for these patients and to directly provide care for some.

Others die from chronic conditions such as chronic heart failure and COPD. These have mortality rates similar to those of some cancers[(26,27)] but only a minority of patients, if any, show the relatively predictable trajectory of decline associated with terminal cancer. Instead, patients may die suddenly—particularly those with heart failure. For the remainder, their dying trajectory is characterized by unpredictable periods of deterioration followed by periods of stability and even recovery. They are not usually seen as terminal illnesses, and it can be very difficult to distinguish a terminal episode from previous severe episodes from which the patient has recovered. Their clinical course is characterized by uncertainty, both for patients and families and for health professionals. There is growing recognition that these patients may benefit from palliative care, but further work is needed to identify their needs and, in particular, to identify the best way to offer these patients palliative care support.[(10)]

Epidemiology of symptoms

Information about the epidemiology of symptoms is important for the care of patients.[(28)] Symptoms are a prerequisite to making diagnoses; the identification and treatment of symptoms is an essential part of medical and nursing training. Understanding how common symptoms are and what factors affect them help doctors and nurses to develop their clinical abilities. The prevalence of symptoms contributes to determining the patients' needs in terms of symptom control, and therefore provision of services. Measuring symptom changes over time is used to assess whether treatments are effective.

For example, epidemiological research into fatigue can:

- describe frequency and severity of fatigue at different stages of disease or in different groups of patients,
- categorize different types of fatigue,
- describe the different factors associated with increased fatigue,
- develop predictive indicators of those people most likely to experience fatigue, and
- compare the outcomes of different treatments.

Robust measurement is vital for all of these uses—whether a study reports how common the symptom is, what factors are associated with it, or attempts to determine how effective a treatment is by considering changes in the symptom over time.

This section reviews the difficulties in measuring symptom prevalence, some of the common symptom assessment systems that are used to assess symptom prevalence, and some of the data on the prevalence of symptoms in different patient groups.

Problems with the information

Studies to date show a wide variation in the reported prevalence of even very common symptoms in cancer or in other conditions. For example, the prevalence of pain varies greatly between different studies, even in cancer.[(29,30)] Other symptoms can vary even more. Three main factors influence this.

Firstly, variation in the design of prevalence studies (e.g. different patient groups, including the different abilities of some patients to complete questionnaires, different ways of recruiting subjects, different time periods—from 1 day to 1 year). As the disease progresses the prevalence of many symptoms, for example, pain and breathlessness, increases. Therefore, studies of patients entering an inpatient hospice are likely to be different from patients referred to an outpatient clinic. This makes generalization of different health care settings or different patient groups difficult.[(31)]

Secondly, there are difficulties in assessing the presence or absence of the symptom. No one 'gold standard' assessment system exists, and patient, family, and staff assessments can vary. There are only modest correlations between these different assessors, although it is likely that family members report some symptoms more frequently than do patients, and staff report them slightly less so.[(32–34)] In some circumstances symptom assessments can be poor.[(35)]

This variation is exacerbated by the different ways of grading symptom severity, for example, using visual analogue scales, Likert-type scales or others.

Table 6 Four alternative interactions between two concurrent symptoms

Symptoms are due to the same pathological process
One symptom is a consequence of the pathological process of the other
One symptom is a side effect of the treatment of the other
Symptoms are unrelated in aetiology

The way the question is understood by the respondent is also important. For example, some patients asked if they have pain will respond positively, because they are receiving analgesics, and some others may say no because they do not want to take analgesics.[36] But asking how much the pain is *affecting* them, or how well it is controlled, will give a different picture. This situation is more difficult for symptoms that may be interpreted differently by different assessors, or those that may be overlooked by some patients, families, or professionals. For example, depression may be difficult to detect—professionals may fail to detect it and patients may not wish or be able to acknowledge its presence.[37] Fatigue, although now accepted as very common in progressive illness, has a long history of being overlooked because it was seen as inevitable, and consequently professionals did not ask about it and patients did not volunteer information about it.

Thirdly, there are difficulties in defining the type of symptom.[38] The symptom may be chronic, or acute, or a combination, have different pathophysiologies (e.g. neuropathic or nociceptive pain), and have different causes, either as a direct or an indirect result of the patient's main illness, as a side-effect of treatment, or due to another cause entirely[39,40] (see Table 6). In progressive illness symptoms are multiple and interact with each other (Tables 6 and 7).[41] So, for example, lack of sleep may be a direct result of pain, diarrhoea, or another symptom; a dry mouth may be a result of dehydration, a side-effect of opioids or tricyclics, a mouth infection, or poor mouth care.

Table 7, adapted from a review of gastrointestinal symptom prevalence by Potter and Higginson,[28] illustrates the variation in time period, measures, and, even simply, the number of symptoms included in different reports of the prevalence of symptoms. The different approaches will have led to very different results. Over time more systematic approaches, rather than just a review of patient charts, have been used. Appraising the way the symptom is detected and measured is essential when reviewing any study that assesses symptom prevalence (very few studies assess symptom incidence, see section on definitions).

Because of these problems in assessing symptom prevalence, tables that report the prevalence of symptoms in cancer patients, or those with other conditions, must be interpreted with caution, especially when data from different studies are combined. The reported prevalence will be different simply because of the different methods and patient groups used in the studies.

Application of epidemiological data to assess need for care

If data is required to estimate the numbers of patients likely to need care, for example, in an epidemiologically based needs assessment for a district,[11] then it is probably sensible to try to use an assessment based on a complete population—for example, a random sample of people who died in that area. This allows generalization to that local population. For the purposes of service planning, it is probably better to use period prevalence estimates, considering fairly long periods of several months. This will ensure that the more rare episodes of symptoms will be included. But this will not provide information on how long each symptom episode lasted, nor any information about changing severity.

Such information can be useful in giving a broad indication of how many people, in the time period considered, are likely to need care or treatment for that symptom. Based on this, estimates of the need for palliative care have been developed and used in several countries.[11] Table 8 reproduces information from the London (England) Regional Strategy for Palliative Care,[42] which provided estimates of the numbers of patients in broad categories who could need palliative care, based on the numbers of people likely to be experiencing symptoms.

One drawback of collecting information about a representative sample is that the best way of finding that representative sample is through complete population data sets, such as registers of death (mortality) or diseases. Too often disease registers are incomplete or not sufficiently up to date to allow prospective studies. Thus, retrospective studies are conducted, usually taking information from surveys of bereaved family members identified through death registrations. While these sacrifice some validity in terms of measurement, they have the advantage of providing a complete sample, at least of younger people who died—the most elderly often do not have family members who were close enough to give information.

However, this method may be problematic in the future because of changes in data protection legislation. Acquiring a representative sample is also dependent on a sufficiently high response rate. The new data protection law in the United Kingdom, has stipulated that researchers may not write to bereaved relatives directly, using a sample drawn by the Office of National Statistics (ONS). Instead individuals are approached by ONS and only if they respond positively will their details be forwarded to researchers who then contact them. This extra stage, and the requirement that respondents have to 'opt in' to the study, rather than 'opt out', is likely to reduce the response rate. The long-term effect will be that need assessments will be less reliable and health care planning weakened by this change in the law.

Symptom assessment systems

To help establish more robust ways of assessing symptoms, measurement tools have been tested and used in different patient groups. These have often been validated against a clinician's assessment (common in the validation of scales to assess depression), the physical condition of the patient, or an existing scale that is somehow considered to be better. There is often no 'absolute' test of a symptom, and the patient's description of how much it is affecting or distressing them is often the most important, although note that some symptoms are not so easily volunteered by patients, especially psychological or potentially embarrassing ones.

Table 9 reviews some of the different range of standardized measures for prospectively assessing symptoms.[43] All of these measures have been tested and found to have some degree of validity and reliability and are worth considering, rather than attempting to devise a new measure.[44,45] They also have the advantage of allowing comparison between studies, or even possibly meta-analysis of data sets, because the same information has been used. They avoid the problems found in Table 7, of variations even in the numbers of symptoms assessed. For those interested in single symptoms, there are also measurement tools for these, such as for depression,[37] pain,[46,47] or gastrointestinal.[28]

Prevalence of symptoms in progressive illness

All studies, of all conditions, show that in progressive illnesses symptoms are common and multiple. Table 10 reviews two multi-centre data sets.[48,49] Both analyses are flawed because of variations between settings in the way the data was collected, and because in the case of Kutner et al. there was a heavy reliance on staff assessment of symptoms. A wide range of prevalence of symptoms were reported among palliative care patients, although some common patterns emerged. First, patients had multiple symptoms. Second, pain, fatigue (weakness or lack of energy), and anorexia (loss of appetite) were very common, but the patterns of other symptoms are almost as varied as in Table 7 as it is in different studies. What is lacking in this field is good longitudinal studies using validated standard measures, examining symptom incidence and prevalence over time, and the factors associated with greater or lesser symptoms.

Table 7 Examples of different symptom studies involving at least 100 palliative care patients. Adapted from Potter and Higginson[28]

Author	Sample size	Study details	Outcome measures	Notes
Twycross, 1986	6677	Cancer patients referred to palliative care team (PCT)	Data collected from medical notes 1975–1984	Six symptoms recorded Data quoted in text, not published in journal
Watchel, 1988	1119	Terminally ill cancer patients receiving hospice care	Two-weekly questionnaire Spitzer QOL	Eight symptoms recorded Patient or proxy Period prevalence: 2 weeks
Reuben, 1988	1592	Terminally ill cancer patients Expected prognosis less than 6 months	Two-weekly questionnaire KPS scale	14 symptoms recorded Patient or proxy Period prevalence: 2 weeks
Mcillmurray, 1989	256	Cancer patients admitted for terminal care to a hospice	Questionnaire on admission then weekly until death or discharge	Three symptoms recorded Patient or proxy
Lichter, 1990	200	All patients in hospice Last 48 h of life	Questionnaire	13 symptoms recorded Patient or proxy
Ventafridda, 1990	120	Cancer patients referred to hospice home care team Assessment of symptoms requiring sedation	Review of medical notes	Four symptoms that needed sedation
Brescia, 1990	1103	Cancer patients admitted to oncology hospital and dying within 6 months of admission	Review of medical records	Six symptoms recorded
Dunphy, 1990	547	Cancer patients referred to PCT	Review of medical records	Seven symptoms recorded Patient or proxy
Seale, 1991	800 216 cancer	Carers of patients who died in 1987	Questionnaire	23 symptoms recorded Only proxy (bereaved family member or relative)
Faisinger, 1991	100	Cancer patients in last week of life in hospice	Multiple VASs	Eight symptoms recorded Patient or proxy
Curtis, 1991	100	Cancer patients referred to hospital PCT	Questionnaire Severity scale	30 symptoms recorded Patient only?
Krech, 1992	100	Lung cancer patients referred to PCT	Questionnaire Severity scale	30 symptoms recorded Patient only?
Sebastian, 1993	312	All cancer patients attending oncology OPD	Questionnaire	Nine symptoms recorded Patient only
Grond, 1994	1635	Cancer patients referred to pain clinic	Questionnaire Activity on VRS	15 symptoms recorded Patient or proxy
Addington-Hall, 1995	2074	Carers of cancer patients who died in United Kingdom in 1990	Questionnaire Severity scale	16 symptoms recorded Period prevalence: last year and last week of life All proxy
Donnelly, 1995	1000	Cancer patients referred to PCT. Last week of life?	Questionnaire Severity scale	20 symptoms recorded Period prevalence: 1 week Patient or proxy
Ellershaw, 1995	125	Cancer patients referred to hospital PCT	PACA McCorkle symptom distress scale	Eight symptoms recorded Patient only
Vainio, 1996	1640	Cancer patients referred to PCT	Questionnaire Severity scale	Nine symptoms recorded Patient only
Conill, 1997	176	Cancer patients referred to PCT in last week of life	Questionnaire	18 symptoms recorded Period prevalence: 1 week Patient only?
Ng, 1998	100 59 cancer	Cancer and non-cancer admissions to hospital PCT	Questionnaire	16 symptoms recorded Patient or proxy
Schuitt, 1998	151	All patients attending oncology OPD	Questionnaire Symptom distress scale	Nine symptoms recorded Patient only Data collected on general population
Edmonds, 1998	352 324 cancer	All patients referred to hospital PCT	Modified STAS Repeated measure every 2 weeks until death	11 symptoms reported Period prevalence: 2 weeks Proxy only

Table 8 Extract from London (England) Regional Strategy for Palliative Care (Higginson, 2000)[42]

London Region: the population

London Region includes the largest city in the United Kingdom with a population in inner and outer London of almost 7 million in 1997, 14% of the population of England. There are areas of high deprivation and poorer health status (approximately 2 million people), as well as areas of relative affluence (approximately 2.3 million people). In the 1991 census, 80% of the population classified themselves as White, 8% Black, 10% Asian, and 2% other. At a borough level the proportion of people from Black or minority ethnic groups ranges from 4 to 45%. Over the next 10 years the White population of London is expected to decrease, and all other ethnic groups will increase.

There are 16 health districts within the boundaries of the new London Region, formed in 1998, with populations ranging from 249 437 (Hillingdon) to 737 066 (Lambeth, Southwark, and Lewisham). The health of the population of London is broadly similar to the rest of England, although it is substantially worse for people aged under 65 years: the all cause standardized mortality ratio for 1989–1994 was 96, that for those aged under 65 is 104. Spending on health services in 1994–1995 was £3.3 billion (compared with 13.9 billion for the rest of England).

The London Region: incidence of people needing palliative care

The incidence of patients that need palliative care can be estimated from the number of deaths due to common conditions that might require palliative care.

In 1995, in London Region, there were 64 609 deaths: 24% from cancer, 41% from diseases of the circulatory system, 18% from diseases of the respiratory system, 4% from diseases of the neurological system, 4% from diseases of the digestive system, 1% from diseases of the genitourinary system, 4% from external injury and poisoning, and 9% from others. The NHS Executive guidance on the needs assessment of palliative care[a] groups those conditions requiring palliative care as follows:

- *Progressive cancers:* the main categories are cancers of lung, trachea, bronchus, gastrointestine, genitourinary, female breast, ear, nose and throat, lymphatic, leukaemia and haemopoetic, brain, and other cancers, including those which present with metastasis and where the primary cancer is not known.
- *Progressive non-malignant diseases, which can have a palliative period:* these include diseases of the circulatory system (most commonly heart diseases, such as chronic heart failure, and cerebrovascular diseases, such as stroke), diseases of the respiratory system (most commonly chronic obstructive pulmonary disease), disease of the nervous system and sense organs (most commonly motor neurone disease, multiple sclerosis, ALS), dementia, and AIDS/HIV.
- *Children's terminal illnesses, and hereditary diseases, including degenerative disorders such as muscular dystrophy and cystic fibrosis:* this last group is beyond the scope of this report and needs separate consideration.

This suggests that almost 60 000 people each year died from conditions that had a progressive period, as above, and would benefit from good symptom management and palliative care.

The London Region: prevalence of problems in the last year of life

To help to estimate the need for palliative care, it is useful to examine the likely prevalence of problems. This is based on estimates of the prevalence of problems in the last year of life, drawn from research among random samples of patients who died. Details of the calculation are provided in the Epidemiologically-Based Needs Assessment for Palliative and Terminal Care.

These estimates suggest that in the London Region there are, each year, 13 300 cancer patients who experience pain that requires treatment in the last year of life, 8000 who experience nausea and/or vomiting, 7400 who experience trouble breathing or breathlessness. Many other symptoms are also present. Table 9 shows the estimates for each health district. Note that one patient will have several symptoms.

Among patients who have conditions other than cancer, estimates suggest that in the London Region each year 30 200 experience pain that requires treatment in the last year of life, 12 200 experience nausea and/or vomiting, 22 100 experience trouble breathing or breathlessness. As for cancer patients, many other symptoms are also present. As for cancer patients, one patient will have several symptoms. However, the total number of patients with symptoms is roughly double that of cancer patients.

[a] Higginson, I.J. (1997). Health care needs assessment: palliative and terminal care. In *Health Care Needs Assessment* 2nd Series (ed. A. Stevens and J. Raftery). Oxford: Radcliffe Medical Press.

Conclusions and recommendations for future work

Although they have limitations, epidemiological mortality data are useful in planning and providing palliative care. Both current data and likely future trends are useful. Most people in developed countries—particularly women and the more affluent—can now expect to live until they are in their 70s or 80s. Their deaths will be ageing-related and due to chronic and disabling diseases such as cancer, stroke, heart failure, and respiratory diseases. If the current relationships between advanced age and institutional care continue to hold, nursing and residential homes will become increasingly important and the proportion of deaths in these settings will rise. Palliative care will therefore increasingly need to address the needs of older people, including the oldest of olds. It will also need to address the needs of members of minority ethnic groups, particularly in the United Kingdom, as the first generation of post-war migrants age. Although the ageing of the population is likely to be central to the future of development of palliative care, as it will be to health care in general, it is important not to overlook the needs of the one in six who die before reaching retirement age, two-fifths of whom will die from cancer. Current trends in mortality suggest that deaths from chronic liver disease may become more common, particularly in this age-group. Understanding the epidemiology of the dying will help hospices and palliative care services ensure that they meet the needs of those currently dying, as well as enable them to plan for the future.

Symptom epidemiology helps us to better understand symptoms, how they come about, what factors affect them, and which patient-groups have those symptoms. This information can help to anticipate problems and plan care for individual patients. In education, clinical staff need to know how often they are likely to encounter a symptom and what its likely causes are. Symptom epidemiological data can help to direct assessments of health care need, for planning services, and to indicate how many services are needed. Further, symptom measurement information can direct research and audit. We need to measure symptom prevalence to learn how effective treatments are.

But knowledge is limited because of variations in assessment methods, in populations studied, and because of a reliance on cross-sectional, rather than on longitudinal studies. Further, some groups have been little studied. In the future, work should concentrate on:

- measuring symptoms, factors associated with them, and interactions in longitudinal populations as well as in cross-sectional studies;

Table 9 Examples of some multi-dimensional measures used to assess symptoms in prospective palliative care studies, that can give more systematic information about symptoms. Adapted from Higginson and Bruera[43]

Name of measure	Number of items and domains covered	Validity	Time	Administration
An initial assessment of suffering	43 (patient); mood, symptoms, fears and family worries, knowledge and involvement, support	Correlates with Spitzer Quality of Life Index physical health groups	Not known	Patient completion or by professional interview
Edmonton Symptom Assessment Schedule—ESAS	9 (patient); pain, activity, nausea, depression, anxiety, drowsiness, appetite, well-being, shortness of breath	Correlates with STAS (except for activity)	Few minutes	Patient completion or with nurse assistance
European Organisation for Research on Treatment of Cancer—EORTC QLQ-C30	30 (patient); 9 multi-item scales including 5 functional, 3 symptom scales, and a global quality of life scale	Inter-scale correlation, correlates with clinical status	11–12 min	Patient completion
The McGill Quality of Life Questionnaire—MQOL	17 (patient); physical symptoms, psychological symptoms, outlook on life and meaningful existence	Correlates with Spitzer Quality of Life Index and single item index	Not known	Patient completion
The McMaster Quality of Life Scale—MQLS	32 (patient); physical symptoms, functional status, social functioning, emotional status, cognition, sleep and rest, energy and vitality, general life satisfaction, meaning of life	Correlates with Spitzer Quality of Life Index	Patients 3–30 min, staff under 3 min, families approximately 3 min	Patient, family, or staff completion
Rotterdam Symptom Checklist—RSCL	34 (patient); physical and psychosocial symptoms	Inter-scale correlation for psychological dimension, less for physical distress items	8 min	Patient completion
Extended versions of the Support Team Assessment Schedule—E-STAS	17 (patient and carer); pain and symptom control, and other psychological and social outcomes. Extended versions (called E-STAS) examine wide range of symptoms, including breathlessness, nausea, vomiting, constipation, cough	Correlates with patient's and families ratings and with HRCA-QL, correlates with original STAS	2–5 min, depending on number of symptoms included	Professional completion
Symptom Distress Scale—SDS	13 (patient); nausea, mood, loss of appetite, insomnia, pain, mobility, fatigue, bowel pattern, concentration and appearance	Correlates with global Quality of Life measures	Not known	Patient completion in the presence of an interviewer

Table 10 Results from two multi-centre analysis of symptom prevalence of patients with progressive illness

Study	Population no. and type of sites, no. of patients, and conditions if given	How symptoms are assessed	Prevalence of common symptoms (%)
Kutner et al., 2001	16 hospices, $n = 348$, 55% cancer (14% cardiac failure, 12% neurological, 11% respiratory, 16% other)	Memorial symptom assessment scale (staff assessed) recorded in cross-sectional sample of patients in care of hospice teams	Lack of energy, 83; pain, 76; lack of appetite, 63; feeling drowsy, 61; sad, 51; short of breath, 48; agitation, 48; worrying, 43; cough, 42; nervous, 42; constipation, 39; irritability, 38; swelling of arms and legs, 36; difficulty sleeping, 35; weight loss, 35; dry mouth, 34 (plus 16 other symptoms with prevalences ranging 3–30)
Vainio et al., 1996	7 hospice or palliative care services, $n = 1840$, all cancer	Range of standardized and non-standardized measures, only 8 symptoms recorded assessed at referral to the units, in some instances by staff and sometimes by patients	Pain, 57; weakness, 51; weight loss, 39; anorexia, 30; constipation, 23; nausea, 21; dyspnoea, 19; insomnia, 9; confusion, 8

- using and improving the standardized measurement tools and assessment systems; and
- exploring symptom prevalence in some of the more-neglected disease groups (e.g. those with dementia) and communities, such as those of different ethnic groups.

References

1. **Ebrahim, S.** (1996). Principles of epidemiology in old age. In *Epidemiology in Old Age* (ed. S. Ebrahim and A. Kalache), pp. 12–21. London: BMJ.
2. **Higginson, I.J. and Costantini, M.** (2002). Epidemiological methods in studies of symptoms in advanced disease. In *Interactive Textbook on Clinical*

Symptoms Research (ed. M. Max and J. Lynn). New York: National Institutes of Health.

3. **Office of National Statistics**. *Mortality Statistics: General (Series DH1).* London: Office of National Statistics, DH1, no. 32, 1999.
4. **Preston, S.H., Elo, I.T., Rosenwaike, I., and Hill, M.** (1996). African-American mortality at older ages: results of a matching study. *Demography* **33**, 193–209.
5. **Rosenberg, H.M., Maurer, J.D., Sorlie, P.D., Johnson, N.J., MacDorman, M.F., Hoyert, D.L., Spitler, J.F., and Scott, C.** (1999). Quality of death rates by race and Hispanic origin: a summary of current research. *Vital & Health Statistics* Series 2, September 1–13.
6. **Myers, K.A. and Farquhar, D.R.** (1998). Improving the accuracy of death certification. *Canadian Medical Association Journal* **158**, 1317–23.
7. **Ganguli, M. and Rodriguez, E.G.** (1999). Reporting of dementia on death certificates: a community study. *Journal of the American Geriatric Society* **47**, 842–9.
8. **Coady, S.A., Sorlie, P.D., Cooper, L.S., Folsom, A.R., Rosamond, W.D., and Conwill, D.E.** (2001). Validation of death certificate diagnosis for CHD: the Atherosclerosis Risk in Communities (ARIC) study. *Journal of Clinical Epidemiology* **54**, 40–50.
9. **Stanta, G., Campagner, L., Cavallieri, F., and Giarelli, L.** (1997). Cancer of the oldest old. What we have learned from autopsy studies. *Clinics in Geriatric Medicine* **13**, 55–68.
10. **Addington-Hall, J.M. and Higginson, I.J.** *Palliative Care for Non-cancer Patients.* Oxford: Oxford University Press, 2001.
11. **Higginson, I.J.** (1997). Health care needs assessment: palliative and terminal care. In *Health Care Needs Assessment* 2nd Series (ed. A Stevens and J. Raftery). Oxford: Radcliffe Medical Press, 1997.
12. **Teno, J.M.** (2001). Quality of life and quality indicators for end of life cancer care: hope for the best, yet prepare for the worst. In *Improving Palliative Care for Cancer* (ed. K.M. Foley and H. Gelband), pp. 96–131. Washington DC: National Academy Press.
13. **World Health Organization**. *Population Ageing—A Public Health Challenge.* Fact sheet No 135, Geneva: World Health Organization, 1998.
14. **Davey-Smith, G., Hart, C., Blane, D., Gillis, C., and Hawthorne, V.** (1997). Lifetime socioeconomic position and mortality: prospective observational study. *British Medical Journal* **314**, 547.
15. **Wilkinson, R.** (1997). Socioeconomic determinants of health: health inequalities or absolute material standards? *British Medical Journal* **314**, 591.
16. **Office of National Statistics**. *Data from 1991 Census on Ethnic Composition of UK.* London: Office of National Statistics, 2002.
17. **Evandrou, M.** (2000). Ethnic inequalities in health in later life. *Health Statistics Quarterly* **8**, 20–9.
18. **Koffman, J. and Higginson, I.J.** (2001). Accounts of carers' satisfaction with health care at the end of life: a comparison of first generation black Caribbeans and white patients with advanced disease. *Palliative Medicine* **15**, 345.
19. **Higginson, I.J. and O'Neill, J.** (2001). Conclusions and recommendations: palliative care in the age of HIV and AIDS, report of the meeting. *Journal of the Royal Society for Medicine* **94**, 428.
20. **Higginson, I.J., Astin, P., and Dolan, S.** (1998). Where do cancer patients die? Ten-year trends in the place of death of cancer patients in England. *Palliative Medicine* **12**, 353–63.
21. **Higginson, I.J., Astin, P., Dolan, S., and Jarman, B.** (1999). Do social factors affect place of death? Analysis of 10 years data in England. *Journal of Public Health Medicine* **21**, 22–8.
22. **Quinn, M. and Bubb, P.** (2000). Cancer trends in England and Wales, 1950–1999. *Health Statistics Quarterly* **8**, 5–19.
23. **Hearn, J. and Higginson, I.J.** (1997). Variations in place of death amongst minority ethnic groups. *Proceedings of the European Association of Palliative Care Conference.*
24. **Cartwright, A., Hockey, J., and Anderson, J.L.** *Life Before Death.* London: Routledge & Kegan Paul, 1973.
25. **Cartwright, A.** (1987). Changes in life and care in the year before death 1969–1987. *Journal of Public Health and Medicine* **13**, 81–7.
26. **Cowie, M.R.** et al. (2000). Survival of patients with a new diagnosis of heart failure: a population-based study. *Heart* **83**, 505–10.
27. **Connor, A.F.** et al. (1996). Outcomes following acute exacerbation of severe chronic obstructive lung disease. *American Journal of Respiratory Critical Care and Medicine* **154**, 959–67.
28. **Potter, J. and Higginson, I.J.** (2002). Frequency and severity of gastrointestinal symptoms in advanced cancer. In *Gastro-Intestinal Symptoms* (ed. E. Bruera and C. Ripamonte), pp. 1–15. Oxford: Oxford University Press.
29. **Bonica, J.J.** (1990). Evolution and current status of pain programs. *Journal of Pain and Symptom Management* **5**, 368–74.
30. **Higginson, I.J. and Edmonds, P.** (2000). Effectiveness and efficiency in the management of cancer pain: current dilemmas in clinical practice. In *The Effective Management of Cancer Pain* (ed. R. Hillier, I. Finlay, J. Welsh, and A. Miles), pp. 3–14. London: Aesculapius Medical Press.
31. **Grond, S., Zech, D., Diefenbach, C., and Bischoff, A.** (1994). Prevalence and pattern of symptoms in patients with cancer pain: a prospective evaluation of 1635 cancer patients referred to a pain clinic. *Journal of Pain and Symptom Management* **9**, 372–82.
32. **Hinton, J.** (1996). How reliable are relatives' retrospective reports of terminal illness? Patients and relatives' accounts compared. *Social Science and Medicine* **43**, 1229–36.
33. **Butters, E., Higginson, I., George, R., and McCarthy, M.** (1993). Palliative care for people with HIV/AIDS: views of patients, carers and providers. *AIDS Care* **5**, 105–16.
34. **Higginson, I.J. and McCarthy, M.** (1993). Validity of the support team assessment schedule: do staffs' ratings reflect those made by patients or their families? *Palliative Medicine* **7**, 219–28.
35. **Sengstaken, E.A. and King, S.A.** (1993). The problems of pain and its detection among geriatric nursing home residents. *Journal of the American Geriatric Society* **41**, 541–4.
36. **Weiss, S.C., Emanuel, L.L., Fairclough, D.L., and Emanuel, E.J.** (2001). Understanding the experience of pain in terminally ill patients. *Lancet* **357**, 1311–15.
37. **Hotopf, M., Chidgey, J., Addington-Hall, J., and Lan Ly, K.** (2002). Depression in advanced disease: a systematic review. Part 1. Prevalence and case finding. *Palliative Medicine* **16**, 81–97.
38. **Foley, K.M. and Gelband, H.** *Improving Palliative Care for Cancer. Summary and Recommendations.* National Cancer Policy Board Institute of Medicine and National Research Council. Washington DC: National Academy Press, 2001.
39. **Bookbinder, M.** et al. (1996). Implementing national standards for cancer pain management: program model and evaluation. *Journal of Pain and Symptom Management* **12**, 334–47.
40. **Portenoy, R.K.** (1996). Opioid therapy for chronic nonmalignant pain: a review of the critical issues. *Journal of Pain and Symptom Management* **11**, 203–17.
41. **Ingham, J. and Portenoy, R.** (2002). Approaches to the assessment of symptoms. In *Cachexia—Anorexia in Cancer Patients* (ed. E. Bruera and I.J. Higginson), pp. 158–71. Oxford: Oxford University Press.
42. **Higginson, I.J.** *Palliative Care for Londoners: A Report Commissioned by the London Regional Health Authority.* London: Department of Palliative Care and Policy, 2000.
43. **Higginson, I.J. and Bruera, E.** (2001). Care of patients who are dying, and their families. In *Oxford Textbook of Oncology* (ed. R.L. Souhami, I. Tannock, P. Hohenberger, and J.-C. Horiot), pp. 1103–20. Oxford: Oxford University Press.
44. **Hearn, J. and Higginson, I.J.** (1997). Outcome measures in palliative care for advanced cancer patients: a review. *Journal of Public Health and Medicine* **19**, 193–9.
45. **Higginson, I.J.** *Outcome Measures in Palliative Care.* ISBN 1 898915 06 7. London: National Council for Hospice and Specialist Palliative Care Services, 1995.
46. **Walsh, T.D.** (1984). Measurement of chronic pain in advanced cancer. In *Pain Proc Joint Meeting Europ Chapters, Int Assoc for the Study of Pain Abano Terme 15–21 May 1983* (ed. R. Rizzi and M. Visentin), pp. 253–6. Padua: Piccin/Butterworths.
47. **Wilkie, D.J., Lovejoy, N., Dodd, M., and Tesler, M.D.** (1990). Cancer pain intensity measurement: Concurrent validity of three tools: Finger dynamometer, pain intensity number scale, visual analogue scale. *Hospice Journal* **6**, 1–13.

48. Vainio, A. and Auvinen, A. (1996). Symptom prevalence group. Prevalence of symptoms among patients with advanced cancer: an international collaborative study. *Journal of Pain and Symptom Management* 12, 3–10.
49. Kutner, J.S., Kassner, C.T., and Nowels, D.E. (2001). Symptom burden at the end of life: hospice providers perceptions. *Journal of Pain and Symptom Management* 21, 473–80.

2.3 Palliative medicine and modern cancer care

Neil MacDonald

It is innately human to comfort and provide care to those suffering from cancer, particularly those close to death. Yet what seems self-evident at an individual, personal level has, by and large, not guided policy at the level of institutions in this country.

Kathleen Foley[1]

Introduction

As in other areas of medicine and surgery, the scientific advances of the nineteenth and twentieth centuries led oncologists to adopt a biological model of disease. Cancer came to be regarded as a disease of organ dysfunction rather than an illness—an illness with psychological and spiritual dimensions embracing both the patient and the patient's family and community.

The public never fully accepted the biological model of cancer. To most non-physicians in every culture, cancer is regarded as an illness with panoramic social and psychological ramifications rather than as simply an organ-based disease. The community reaction to the biological model of cancer provides a continuing strong impetus for the palliative care movement.

Progress in the surgical management of cancer was rapid in the first half of the twentieth century. In the 1950s the availability of megavoltage radiotherapy units increased the capacity for cure of localized cancers. Following the introduction of alkylating agents and the first antimetabolite, amethopterin, in 1945–1950, progress in cancer chemotherapy led to the organization of a third cancer treatment speciality, medical oncology.

Cancer therapy was initially based on the concept that tumours were homogenous entities which proceeded in orderly fashion from local growth to lymph node involvement and subsequent haematological dissemination. Cancer was thought to consist of aberrant tissue that acted like a foreign invader and thus could be repulsed like other external threats such as bacteria. Indeed, the treatment of cancer is often expressed in military terms. A 'war' on cancer was declared and patients 'battled' with cancer. The 'war' however, resembled the First World War, with initial rapid progress followed by a pattern reminiscent of the trench warfare of 1914–1918. Similar to the optimism of Marshall Haig and his colleagues, oncologists thought that 'the millennium may soon be upon us' and hoped that a few more drugs or forms of radiation energy would bring about the cure of advanced cancer.

Unfortunately, current research on cell and molecular biology discounts this possibility. In 2001, cancer is recognized as a disorder involving cells with often multiple genetic errors which enable them to escape normal control systems and to rapidly develop cytotoxic drug resistance. Cancer may not be a distinct entity; under the rubric 'Cancer' multiple distinct forms probably exist.[2] Even within a specific cancer, because of the propensity for cancer cells to alter their genetic apparatus, cancer tissue is soon composed of multiple populations of cells with different responses to growth factors and anticancer therapy.[3] Cancer cure rates now lies in the range of 50 per cent in the industrialized countries, but in developing countries cure remains an uncommon event.

Our understanding of cancer continues to improve, allowing the introduction of more rational biologic therapies. Research on tumour angiogenesis, genetic aberrations, and other aspects of molecular biology may ultimately result in uniformly available curative treatment, but this remains to be determined. In any event, the tortuous process of moving from the laboratory to the bedside and providing cost-effective therapies is likely, in the best of circumstances, to evolve over several years.

Age standardized cancer incidence and mortality rates are either stable or slightly decreasing in some industrialized nations.[4,5] Because of success in preventing death from infectious diseases and, in the Western world, from cardiovascular disease, a shift in the mean age of population is occurring. Overall cancer incidence rises with age. Consequently, a global increase in patients with cancer is anticipated. In developing countries, most patients will continue to present with advanced ultimately fatal disease.

In the face of these expectations, artificial lines drawn between disease modifying therapy and palliative care are inappropriate. Since this chapter appeared in the second edition, throughout the Western world one notes multiple reports, replete with recommendations, on the status of palliative care. These publications emanating from august academic or government bodies, clearly outline the extent of suffering encountered by patients with advanced cancer and the lack of a proportionate response from those responsible for cure at all levels. They commonly conclude with a ringing endorsement for change. While one's cynical side notes the continuing misalignment of need and response, in the author's opinion there has been a sea change in the interest of the cancer establishment in palliative care research, education, and care. The more enlightened cancer centres are assuming a mantle of leadership and taking steps to nurture integrated systems of cancer care wherein the principles of palliative care can be applied throughout the course of illness in concert with traditional treatment of malignant disease. The demonstrated success of these programmes should ultimately convince laggard philistines to offer support for palliative care in keeping with its importance. This chapter will consider the rationale for a comprehensive cancer control system incorporating palliative care.

Relations between cancer centres and palliative care programmes

There are four phases of cancer prevention:

1. prevention of the disease (public education and policy),
2. prevention of advanced disease (early diagnostic programmes),
3. prevention of death (anticancer treatment), and
4. prevention of suffering.[6]

The four phases are often not co-ordinated within a cancer control programme. Until recently cancer centres have concentrated on the first three phases, which stimulated the development of the palliative care movement to deal with the fourth phase.

Cancer centre interest in palliative medicine

Although most cancer patients will die of their disease, studies on the aetiology and treatment of their symptoms have not received a high priority within cancer centres. Research studies accurately assess survival and objective tumour response, but the effect of cancer therapies on pain, other physical symptoms, and on psychosocial parameters is seldom reported to this day.

For example, the *Journal of Clinical Oncology* during 1986 and 1987 published 24 phase II–phase III studies on the chemotherapeutic response of advanced carcinoma of the oesophagus, stomach, colon, pancreas, and non-small-cell lung cancer. These tumours, then and now, are poorly responsive to chemotherapy and, even in responders, prolongation of life is modest.

Because major changes in cure rates or survival could not be expected for patients with these poor response tumours, it is logical to expect that investigators would have concentrated on the impact of chemotherapy on the symptoms of these patients. Each article provided an assessment of tumour response and drug toxicity; none of them reported on the effect of chemotherapy on pain.[7]

While psychologists and quality of life committees have become associated with a number of the major cooperative chemotherapy groups, and national drug regulatory bodies often require quality of life data, the pattern is changing slowly. Information on quality of life and symptom control was contained in only two of the 10 comparable reports of the 1986–1987 survey published in the *Journal of Clinical Oncology* between January and June 2001. Symptoms are seemingly regarded as problems of a second order of importance. For example, pain, dyspnoea, fatigue, and cachexia–anorexia are commonly present in patients with advanced cancer. Aside from cancer pain, these symptoms are poorly understood and ineffectually treated, but promising new approaches are emerging from laboratory studies. And yet, out of 3127 abstracts offered for presentation of the 2001 meeting at the American Society of Oncology, the index lists only 44 studies concerned with these common problems. In contrast, an old, generally ineffectual, chemotherapy agent, 5 F.U., was featured in 129 studies.[8] Proportionately, abstract submissions covering issues of importance in palliative care actually appear to be decreasing.[9]

Palliative medicine reaction—anticancer therapy

Because of the failure of disease-modifying therapy to help advanced cancer patients in many instances, palliative medicine physicians and nurses may deride the use of these therapies in situations where they may be helpful. They may overestimate the toxicities associated with chemotherapy used in a palliative setting and regard oncologists as automatons, enslaved by the icon of tumour response, without reference to the usefulness of a response for the patient. Conversely, oncologists may sometimes think that palliative care colleagues are simply addressing 'soft' issues at the end of life, while downplaying the intellectual rigour and complexities involved in controlling patient suffering. A state of 'two solitudes' may come into existence wherein both groups fail to consult each other adequately, and fail to arrive at an obvious conclusion: that both groups should work as team members pooling their skills, to assist patients and families throughout the full course of illness.

Reluctance to encourage integration of palliative care with other aspects of cancer care is encountered from leaders in both spheres. Both groups may feel that linkage will result in distortion of objectives and dilution of resources. Oncologists may say that we already look after all the needs of cancer patients (although we have not measured their degree of suffering as rigorously as we have measured the size of their tumour nodules and may overestimate our symptom control skills). Alternatively, palliative medicine physicians may state that the oncologists, while mastering symptom control techniques (and that is all for the good), may miss the heart of the matter, and fail to introduce the 'warm envelope' of care that characterizes palliative care at its best. Moreover, they may believe that the complexity of the problem is such that, with the best of will, those whose primary interest lies in screening, tumour biology, or pharmacology, will never have the time and energy to address the needs of dying patients and their families. Although most of their patients have cancer, palliative medicine physicians may also be concerned that too close a tie with cancer programmes will blunt their efforts to provide palliative care for other dying patients.

The above professional issues may confuse the community as patients and their families should reasonably expect continuity of care throughout their illness and are puzzled when jurisdictional priorities and barriers require them to take a zigzag path to obtain appropriate care. When this exists, patients and families caught in the centre will suffer.

Integration of palliative medicine in a cancer control programme

Palliative care as an exercise in prevention

Palliative care has traditionally concentrated on the last days of life; a time when pain, other symptoms, and psychosocial distress are often prominent and difficult to control. A seemingly never ending pattern of reaction to new crises is often present. Would the task be easier if patients had received good palliative care throughout their trajectory of illness?

Prevention is the cornerstone of excellent medical practice, early recognition of a problem may prevent a disaster or alleviate its full flowering. It is reasonable to assume that cancer centres imbued with the philosophy of palliative care will be more likely to prevent long-term patient distress by integrating excellent palliative care and antitumour therapy earlier in the course of illness. They will more likely achieve this end if the cancer centre has established close contact with a palliative care group or has included a palliative care division or department within their own organization.

Most cancer centres throughout the world have not acted on this logical proposition. It is gratifying to note, however, that the United Kingdom Policy Framework for Commissioning Cancer Services[10] recommends both the formation of palliative care programmes within cancer centres and their coordination with community palliative care. The report strongly endorses the concept of palliative care as a preventive exercise. 'Palliative care is required for many patients early in the course of their disease, sometimes from the time of diagnosis. It should not be associated only with terminal care. The palliative care team should integrate in a seamless way with all cancer treatment services to provide the best possible quality of life for the patient and their family.' The WHO also recognizes the wisdom of linking palliative care with other aspects of cancer care, and regards it as an exercise in prevention.[11]

Evidence exists that early identification of causes of suffering improves patient–family quality of life. Vachon and others report that poorly handled transfer of information and recognition of anxiety at the time of diagnosis translates into increased problems later in the course of illness. Studies on pain demonstrate the plasticity of afferent sensory pain pathways when exposed to unrelated chronic stimulation.[12] Pain thresholds are lowered, previously uninvolved neuronal systems transmit pain messages, and the relief of pain requires larger doses of analgesics and co-analgesics. Confusional states are common at the end of life. Dr Bruera and his colleagues correlate a reduction in delirium with the introduction of preventive measures including routine assessments, maintenance of hydration, and opioid rotation.[13]

Studies in basic science laboratories support the concept that 'pain can kill'[14] as can emotional stress.[15,16] The cachexia–anorexia syndrome will also directly cause death if a critical state of malnutrition is reached.[17,18]

Less clearly established is the thesis that poor symptom control may influence the course of human illness. Cancer symptoms represent a body defense mechanism gone awry. Virtually all acute symptoms have a role in protecting the body from threat or injury. For example, nausea and vomiting have their place in protecting us from ingestion of harmful substances and pain will cause us to withdraw from a real or potential source of injury. As stated in another forum,[19] 'when the symptom switch is left on, the stress reaction engendered is not helpful and may cause great harm. For example, symptoms associated with advanced cancer may arise from a stew of cytokines surrounding the tumour, joined in unholy purpose with tumour products, causing adverse activation of the neuro-endocrine immune system, with concomitant devastating effect on quality of life and patient comfort'. Chronic stimulation of these systems can stimulate tumour growth and adversely influence treatment.[20]

Is there human evidence that poor symptom management not only affects quantity but quality of life? Reflecting the state of palliative care research, a large differential is noted between laboratory studies relevant to this point and the paucity of related patient studies.[21,22] The weight and logic of animal symptom studies do dictate, however, that symptom control research should receive priority not only because of the potential effect on suffering, but also because symptom control may go hand in hand with disease control.

If one accepts this thesis, it is clear that cancer centres must adopt major changes in their *modus operandi.* The application of impeccable symptom control from disease onset means that palliative care colleagues within a cancer centre will become essential focal points for education, clinical research, and assisting in the care of patients with particularly difficult problems. Palliative care skills, however, will need to be demonstrated by all oncologists and other physicians responsible for the care of patients with advanced chronic illness, as palliative care physicians see only a small proportion of cancer patients early in their course.[23] These patients are advised by oncologists and primary care physicians. Consequently, a radical change in physician education and attitude must take place.[24]

Palliative medicine—interface with oncology

Cancer centres and palliative care units can learn from each other to their mutual benefit and that of the people they serve.[25] Cancer centres will recognize more clearly that:

1. *Continuity of care is important.* Patients should not be exposed to constantly changing flotillas of doctors and nurses. A specific physician–nursing team should be recognized by the patient and family as their primary source of support within the centre.

In some jurisdictions, the patient may not have contact with a family practitioner skilled in palliative medicine. The cancer centre should not discharge the patient into a void for palliative care by the family doctor without assurance that community resources are in place to assist the patient and family. Oncologists, palliative care groups and family practice programmes must establish these interfaces.

2. *Pain and other symptoms can be assessed in a formal manner.* Assessment dictates that we ask about the presence of problems. When asked, patients and families will bring forward information which otherwise could be passed over in a busy clinic.[26]

There is current evidence that oncologists may underestimate their patients' pain and home–family concerns. Slevin et al.[27] compared quality of life assessments, finding a wide variation. Even Karnofsky ratings (a measure of physical status) showed low correlations between patient–physician pairs. In another study on prostate cancer,[28] one-quarter of severely disabled patients were judged by their physicians to be either asymptomatic or only slightly limited. Obtaining information on pain, other symptoms, and psychosocial distress is assisted through the use of patient-oriented assessment forms and assessments by other health professionals.

3. *Pain and other symptoms can be relieved* but, as in other areas of oncology, rigorous attention to detail, including protocols for patient–family teaching are required.

4. *Hierarchy of problems.* At any time, the hierarchy of problems may vary considerably, among family, patient, and medical attendants.[29] The last may be most concerned with drug toxicity or drug doses; the family may have financial concerns uppermost, including the loss of income caused by prolonged waiting in an outpatient department; while the patient may be primarily upset by unrelieved pain and anxiety. A palliative care approach will elicit patient–family concerns and recognize their primacy.

5. *Home care.* The home is the focal point for palliative care and therapies are designed to be suitable for home use. Palliative care teams have established special techniques to allow previously hospital-bound patients to return home. Examples are the use of pump-delivered subcutaneous medications, epidural analgesic regimens, and, most importantly, regular assessment and follow-up by palliative care nurses in the home. Close integration between cancer centres and palliative care home care teams, keeps people at home, enhances the patients' lives and improves the efficient operation of the cancer centre (Section 17.1).

6. *Joint clinics.* Patients constantly report that waiting in impersonal hospital clinics to see yet another new consultant is a very enervating experience. A cancer centre with a palliative care group can coordinate patient visits so that the antitumour therapy decisions are reached in concert with plans for home care management of pain and other symptoms. The patient will appreciate the obvious evidence of a team approach to problems.

In turn, palliative care groups will learn from their close contact with cancer centres. Lessons to be learned include:

1. *Self-criticism.* The messianic aspects of palliative care should be complemented by critical review of existing dogma. Cancer centres will question unsubstantiated claims of therapeutic success and subject their therapies to tests of efficacy. Adoption of their approach will strengthen both the academic and the resource bases of palliative care. The *British Medical Journal* editorialized, 'evidence based medicine is a phrase that is currently familiar to only a few doctors, but we will all know it by the millennium'.[30] Several recent publications[31,32] contain an analysis of the evidence backing current pain management practice. While sound studies support approaches using opioids and NSAIDs, adjuvant drug therapy and non-pharmaceutical pain interventions are commonly based on modest evidence. One's recent encounters with health administrators and pharmacy committees indicate that hard data are needed to balance their bottom-line financial concerns. Evidence-based studies will not only improve clinical care, but will also influence and guide policy makers responsible for setting health care priorities.

2. *Emphasis on quality research.* Cancer centres thrive on clinical trials, and oncologists have established common classification systems and multi-institutional groups, enabling them to carry out first-rate clinical research. The cancer centres include basic science workers whose presence can result in a flow of research ideas from laboratory to the clinics.

The oncology cooperative model for conducting multi-centre research could be copied with profit by palliative care groups. In contrast to oncology, internationally established criteria for definition and assessment of symptoms do not exist. Therefore, most palliative care research studies enrol small numbers of patients whose characteristics may not be clear to other investigators. If tumour biologists can be involved in symptom control research, they will produce the needed information on the pathophysiology of currently uncontrolled symptoms, such as asthenia. Tumour biologists are located in cancer centres and may become interested in problems of importance to palliative medicine through regular contact with palliative medicine physicians.

3. *Resources.* Cancer centres tend to be relatively well supported by their communities and government institutions (a crass but important concept).

4. *Enhanced access to palliative anticancer therapy.* The need for quick and easy access to interventional procedures or palliative radiotherapy is sometimes unpredictable and can be facilitated if palliative care physicians work together with oncologists on a day-to-day basis. Moreover, the technical resources and consultant base of a cancer centre are often needed to resolve difficult symptom problems. A clinical example follows:

Mrs L., with metastatic breast cancer and leptomeningeal involvement, was receiving excellent care in her home community. She was on regular opioids which controlled her pain and allowed her to continue her life as a mother and a community leader. The pain in her left hip became severe, and her family physician steadily increased her dose of opioids, to the point where she was still in severe pain, but stuporous. X-rays of her bones did not suggest that she had any recent damage. Nothing else acute seemed to have happened. She was afebrile, and her white count had not changed, nor had her haemoglobin dropped. This lady needed the services of an acute care hospital and, when she was transferred to such a hospital, CT scans and ultrasounds of her pelvis revealed that she had a pelvic abscess. She had been on steroids, which may have dampened the usual signs of infection. The abscess cavity was drained, the patient was placed on antibiotics, and she returned home in good pain control, alert on her previous dose of opioids.[33]

Mrs L. illustrates the benefits arising from continued interaction between community-based palliative care and a sophisticated cancer centre. On occasion 'high tech' approaches are required to alleviate suffering.

During the next decade, cancer centres will increasingly recognize their responsibility for balancing the phases of cancer prevention and should welcome the incorporation of palliative medicine within their organizations. They have recognized the need for sub-speciality development in various fields of oncology, and it is reasonable that they should also develop programmes designed to address the palliative needs of cancer patients and their families and to conduct research and teaching in this special field.

The comprehensive cancer programme concept

Patients with newly diagnosed inoperable carcinomas, including those arising in the colon, pancreas, kidney, and lung (non-small-cell variety) have a fatal illness which predictably will end their lives, often within a few months to a year. They do not have the time to embark on a probable futile course of chemotherapy which will further exacerbate the cachexia problem that may accompany their diagnosis then only at a late stage of disease transferring to a palliative care programme.

It is logical that they should be treated in a fully comprehensive fashion at diagnosis. A comprehensive cancer care programme is based on the concept that organ system, cellular, molecular, and psychosocial aberrations are interdependent. Physicians within such a programme recognize the influence on the illness and therapeutic response of the patient's emotional status (autonomic nervous system changes), pain (generalized stress reaction), nutrition (metabolic abnormalities, muscle proteolysis, cytokine, and tumour-factor-mediated muscle proteolysis), and functional status (ability to exercise). A comprehensive cancer care programme will incorporate each of these themes.[34] For a patient with cancer of the pancreas, this may include:

- cancer chemotherapy—preferably in a trial setting,
- nutritional counselling and an opportunity to participate in programmes addressing the cachexia–anorexia syndrome—preferably in a trial setting,
- skilled interventional access including stents (both ductal and intestinal) and coeliac plexus blocks carried out by experienced people,
- assessment of psychological factors and use of antidepressants if indicated, and
- access to rehabilitation programmes geared to strengthen and maintain muscle function and to manage fatigue through a combination of exercise and pharmacologic approaches.

Similar comprehensive programmes re-tailored to match the anticipated cancer course can be introduced for patients with other predictably fatal cancers at diagnosis. The successful operation of a comprehensive programme is dependent upon a degree of interdisciplinary cooperation, which remains alien in most large centres. Moreover, the programme is dependent upon a major change in mind set on the part of all participants; for example, a medical oncologist may not think that physiotherapy and a nutritional clinical trial could turn out to be useful components of overall patient care. Studies on comprehensive approaches are modest indeed in comparison to the wealth of single-minded chemotherapy trials that continue to flood the oncology literature.

Ethical considerations at the interface

Do cancer centres have a moral responsibility to ensure that cancer patients in the region they serve have access to impeccable palliative care? Institutions, like the professionals who staff them, have ethical duties.[35] These considerations must influence their role in a community, in concert with all the other factors that shape an institution's mission. It is common practice for cancer centres to formally publish their mission and goals and, in so doing, to clearly state the areas of cancer care for which they will accept responsibility. Centres, however, often have a mandated role to serve as a focal point for comprehensive cancer care in a region. Even in the absence of a formal mandate, their presence strongly influences the overall arrangements for cancer care.

Commonly, a cancer centre may define itself as a centre for tertiary patient care, focusing on the application of complex technological approaches to treatment, and on the organization and conduct of clinical trials. Indeed, most cancer centres have a strong academic component, and the physicians working in these centres are expected to carry out clinical research.

A cancer centre may define its mission in a manner which does not call upon it to assume responsibilities for all four phases of a comprehensive cancer control programme. If so, the centre must reconcile its role as an institution with specific priorities addressing the needs of a measured number of patients in its catchment area, and its role as a component of a comprehensive cancer programme within which all patients are entitled to equal consideration. Wearing the latter mantle, the centre has a responsibility to guarantee continuity of care for cancer patients. The onus is on the cancer centre to either develop a comprehensive palliative care service or to use its influence and resources to ensure that a fully coordinated autonomous community programme is in place.

For example, the emphasis in cancer centres in clinical trials must not damage the prospects of those patients who, for whatever reason, do not enter a trial, or who subsequently discontinue participation in research protocols. Often, poor performance status will disenfranchise a patient for consideration in a trial, or advancing disease will cause them to be dropped from continued care within a clinical trial setting. As the limited time of the clinicians within the cancer centre may be primarily taken up with clinical trial activities, could a clinical trial impact negatively on the care of many patients not enrolled in the trial? This scenario could develop in centres where arrangements for formal interaction with community palliative care services are not in place, with consequent discharge of patients into a void.

The financial stringencies observed in every land can have a deleterious effect on cancer centre–palliative care interactions. Reimbursement increasingly relates to dictated norms; financial penalties are associated with deviations from these parameters. Dying often does not adhere to administrative fiats. As a result, patients with advanced disease who, nevertheless, need the technical skills of a cancer centre, may not be welcome. Factors diminishing the access of dying patients to hospitals may particularly affect the poor, who are less likely to have means enhancing home care[36] and who may have greater levels of distress.[37]

A single-minded emphasis on 'the bottom line' may not only be ethically problematic, but may also prove to be a bad business decision. A Harvard Business Review study illustrated the perils associated with cost-cutting (in industries outside the health field) without due regard to maintenance of ethical standards.[38] The study provided examples of companies with an exclusive focus on cost-cutting, with resultant drop in staff morale, customer satisfaction, and further financial losses, in contrast to other companies who thrived through balancing resource allocation with ethical reflection.

Callahan has stated 'No moral impulse seems more deeply embedded than the need to relieve suffering … it has become a foundation stone for the practice of medicine, and it is at the core of the social and welfare programmes of all civilized nations'.[39] If this tenet is applied to the organization of cancer control programmes, palliative care will thrive in a state of equipoise with other aspects of cancer care.

Will this newly recognized responsibility of cancer centres damage the existing palliative care movement; a movement which has recruited thousands of theologians, social workers, trained volunteers, family practitioners, and others who have no ties with cancer programmes? The inclusion of palliative medicine as just another part of a large hospital programme would be a mistake, leading to a loss of the platform of community interest which has nourished palliative care. When the question is asked, the community gives the needs of dying patients a high priority.[40]

Community support can be harnessed through creating parallel structures, such as Palliative Care Community Councils, with volunteer community members who will monitor the development of palliative care in a town or region and foster community–government education exercises. In some jurisdictions, these councils could assume funding and supervisory responsibilities. The advancement of palliative medicine at the community hospital level will extend the arm of palliative care towards people with other chronic ultimately fatal, disorders, while the skills of palliative care physicians can be employed in concert with others to help assist people with chronic non-fatal illnesses.(41)

An essential tenet of palliative care organizations is the establishment of broad community understanding and support. If this is present, then a programme web with strong filaments connecting cancer centre palliative care groups, community hospitals (where palliative inpatient units may be located), community volunteer groups, and dedicated home care programmes servicing all hospitals can be developed. As in all areas of human endeavour, ultimately, the success of an integrated community programme depends on the maturity and goodwill of the participants. If they are willing to lower institutional barriers and cherish cooperative activity rather than insularity, palliative care will thrive in all parts of the community, including the cancer centre.

References

1. **Foley, K.M.** (2001). Preface. In *Improving Palliative Care for Cancer—Summary and Recommendations* (ed. K.M. Foley and H. Gelband), p. ix. Institute of Medicine and National Research Council. Washington DC: National Academy Press.
2. **Schein, P.S.** (2001). The case for a new national program for the development of cancer therapeutics. *Journal of Clinical Oncology* **19** (12), 3142–53.
3. **Fidler, I.J.** (2001). Angiogenic heterogeneity: regulation of neoplastic angiogenesis by the organ microenvironment. *Journal of the National Cancer Institute* **93** (14), 1040–1.
4. **National Cancer Institute of Canada.** *Canadian Cancer Statistics 2001.* Toronto, Canada, 2001.
5. **Howe, H.L., Wingo, P.A., Thun, M.J., Ries, L.A.G., Rosenberg, H.M., Feigal, E.G., and Edwards, B.K.** (2001). Annual report to the nation on the status of cancer (1973 through 1998), featuring cancers with recent increasing trends. *Journal of the National Cancer Institute* **93** (11), 824.
6. **MacDonald, N.** (1991). Palliative care—the fourth phase of cancer prevention. *Cancer Detection and Prevention* **15**, 3253–5.
7. **MacDonald, N.** (1989). The role of medical oncology in cancer pain control. In *Advances in Pain Research and Therapy* Vol. 11 (ed. C.S. Hill, Jr. and W.S. Fields). New York: Raven Press.
8. **Grunberg, S.M.**, ed. *Thirty-Seventh Annual Meeting of the American Society of Clinical Oncology. Program/Proceedings.* Baltimore: Lippincott Williams & Wilkins, 2001.
9. **Sweeney, C., Beattie-Palmer, L., Palmer, J.L., and Bruera, E.** (2001). Changing patterns of symptom control and palliative care paper presentations at the Annual Meeting of the American Society of Clinical Oncology. *Journal of Clinical Oncology* **19/14**, 3438–9.
10. **Calman Report/Recommendations.** *A Policy Framework for Commissioning Cancer Services.* Calman Report/Recommendations for Cancer Services. Consultative Document. London: Her Majesty's Stationery Office, 1994.
11. **World Health Organization** (2002). Pain relief and palliative care. In *National Cancer Control Programmes. Policies and Managerial Guidelines* 2nd edn. Geneva: World Health Organization.
12. **Coderre, T.J., Katz, J., Vaccarino, A.L., and Melzack, R.** (1993). Contribution of central neuroplasticity to pathological pain: review of clinical and experimental evidence. *Pain* **52**, 259–85.
13. **Bruera, E.** et al. (1995). Changing pattern of agitated impaired mental status in patients with advanced cancer: association with cognitive monitoring, hydration and opioid rotation. *Journal of Pain and Symptom Management* **10**, 287–91.
14. **Liebeskind, J.C.** (1991). Pain can kill. *Pain* **44**, 3–4.
15. **Wulsin, L.R.** (2000). Does depression kill? *Archives of Internal Medicine* **160**, 1731–2.
16. **Schulz, R., Beach, S.R., Ives, D.G., Martire, L.M., Ariyo, A.A., and Kop, W.J.** (2000). Association between depression and mortality in older adults: the Cardiovascular Health Study. *Archives of Internal Medicine* **160**, 1761–8.
17. **Tisdale, M.** (1997). Cancer cachexia. *Journal of the National Cancer Institute* **89** (23), 1763–73.
18. **Warren, S.** (1932). The immediate causes of death in cancer. *American Journal of Medical Sciences* **184**, 610–15.
19. **MacDonald, N.** (2002). Re-defining symptom management. *Journal of Palliative Medicine* **5** (2), 301–4.
20. **Balkwill, F. and Mantovani, A.** (2001). Inflammation and cancer: back to Virchow? *Lancet* **357**, 539–45.
21. **Lillemoe, K.D.** (1998). Palliative care therapy for pancreatic cancer. *Surgical Oncology Clinics of North America* **7** (1), 199–216.
22. **Gogos, C.A., Ginopoulos, P., Salsa, B., Apostolidou, E., Zoumbos, N.C., and Kalfarentzos, F.** (1998). Dietary omega-3 polyunsaturated fatty acids plus vitamin E restore immunodeficiency and prolong survival for severely ill patients with generalized malignancy: a randomized control trial. *Cancer* **82** (2), 395–402.
23. **MacDonald, N.** et al. (1997). A Canadian survey of issues in cancer pain management. *Journal of Pain and Symptom Management* **14** (6), 332–42.
24. **Abrahm, J.L.** (1999). The oncologist's expanding role. *Cancer* **85** (8), 1645–8.
25. **MacDonald, N.** (1991). Cure and care: interaction between cancer centres and palliative care units. In *Recent Results in Cancer Research* Vol. 121 (ed. H.J. Senn and A. Glaus), pp. 399–407. Berlin: Springer.
26. **Rhodes, D.J., Koshy, R.C., Waterfield, W.C., Wu, A.W., and Grossman, S.A.** (2001). Feasibility of quantitative pain assessment in outpatient oncology practice. *Journal of Clinical Oncology* **19** (2), 501–8.
27. **Slevin, M.L., Plant, H., Lynch, D., Drinkwater, J., and Gregory, W.M.** (1988). Who should measure quality of life, the doctor or the patient? *British Journal of Cancer* **57**, 109–12.
28. **Fossa, S.D.** et al. (1990). Quality of life and treatment of hormone resistant prostatic cancer. *European Journal of Cancer* **26** (11–12), 1133–6.
29. **Grobe, M.E., Ahmann, D.L., and Ilstrup, D.N.** (1982). Assessment of needs of terminal cancer patients. *Oncology Nursing Forum* **9**, 26–30.
30. **Morrison, I. and Smith, R.** (1994). The future of medicine. *British Medical Journal* **309** (6962), 1099–100.
31. **US Department of Health and Human Services.** *Management of Cancer Pain. Clinical Practice Guideline Number 9.* US Department of Health and Human Services, Public Health Service, Agency for Health Care Policy and Research, 1994, pp. 221–5.
32. **The Steering Committee on Clinical Practice Guidelines for the Care and Treatment of Breast Cancer** (1998). The management of chronic pain in patients with breast cancer. *Canadian Medical Association Journal* **158** (3 Suppl.), S71–81.
33. **Mackey, J.R., Birchell, I., and MacDonald, N.** (1995). Occult infection as a cause of hip pain in a patient with metastatic breast cancer. *Journal of Pain and Symptom Management* **10** (5), 1–4.
34. **MacDonald, N., Ayoub, J.P., Barkun, A., Dalzell, M.A., Gagnon, B., and Rosenberg, L.** (2000). Carcinoma of the pancreas—an integrated programme. *Cancer Strategy* **2**, 17–24.
35. **Reiser, S.J.** (1994). The ethical life of health care organizations. *Hastings Center Report* **24** (6), 28–35.
36. **Higginson, I., Webb, D., and Lessof, L.** (1994). Reducing hospital beds for patients with advanced cancer. *Lancet* **344**, 409.
37. **Cleeland, C.S.** et al. (1994). Pain and its treatment in outpatients with metastatic cancer. *New England Journal of Medicine* **330** (9), 392–6.
38. **Paine, L.S.** (1994). Managing for organizational integrity. *Harvard Business Review* March–April, 106–17.
39. **Callahan, D.** *The Troubled Dream of Life: In Search of a Peaceful Death.* New York: Simon & Schuster, 1993, p. 94.
40. **Hadorn, D.C.** (1991). The Oregon priority-setting exercise: quality of life and public policy. *Hastings Center Report* **21** (May–June Suppl.), 11–16.
41. **Addington-Hall, J.M. and Higginson, I.J.**, ed. *Palliative Care for Non-Cancer Patients.* New York: Oxford University Press, 2001.

2.4 Predicting survival in patients with advanced disease

Paul Glare and Nicholas Christakis

Introduction

Why the renewed interest in the importance of prognosis in palliative medicine?

The three great clinical skills in medicine are diagnosis, treatment, and prognosis. Prior to the turn of the twentieth century, prognosis was much more prominent than it is today. For example, the nineteenth century physician was esteemed if he could diagnose pneumonia, and in the absence of effective treatment, predict whether a patient was likely to succumb to the illness. As effective therapies for many previously fatal illnesses were discovered during the first half of the twentieth century, prognosis gave way to treatment as the core clinical skill accompanying diagnosis; increasingly successful therapies made details of the natural history of illness progression seem less relevant to the clinician.(1)

The rise of palliative medicine as the study of specialized care for patients with incurable illnesses has set the scene for a renaissance of prognostication as a clinical skill. But unlike the nineteenth century, where prognosis often involved acute illness in young adults, in palliative medicine, prognosis frequently relates to chronic progressive and ultimately fatal diseases and co-morbidities in the elderly. The reasons for prognostication in incurable disease that have been put forward are therefore not to predict recovery but:

- to provide patients and their families with information about what the future is likely to hold so that they can set their goals, priorities, and expectations of care;(2–6)
- to help patients develop insight into their dying;(5)
- to assist clinicians in their decision-making;(7)
- to compare like patients with regard to outcomes;(8)
- to establish patients' eligibility for care programmes, including timely referral to hospice programmes;(7,9)
- to establish patients' eligibility for clinical trials;
- for policy making with respect to appropriate resource utilization and allocation of support services, for example, frequency of contacts if home care is proposed; and(5–7)
- to provide a common language for health care professionals involved in end of life care.

It is apparent that some of the foregoing items are more relevant before referral to palliative care services while others are more relevant after referral.

Prognosis in 'terminal' disease

Prognosis is a generic term related to predicting any health outcome. When it is related to a potentially life-threatening illness such as cancer, it is closely related to diagnosis, in that the same clinical and pathological factors which are used to make a diagnosis are also relevant to the prognosis. Most of the literature dealing with prognosis in cancer concerns factors that influence the probability of cure. For example, in the case of early breast cancer, tumour size and grade, oestrogen receptor status, age, menopausal status, and axillary lymph node involvement are used to stage the disease and these have prognostic import with respect to standard oncological outcomes that include, but are not restricted to, survival: the length of time until disease recurrence, median survival, and the percentage of cases still alive at standard oncological time points, such as 5 and 10 years. Different treatments are also compared with respect to their impact on survival: for example, after their initial surgery and radiotherapy, post-menopausal women with breast cancer and positive nodes have less local recurrence and a 10.9 per cent reduction in the probability of dying at 10 years if they are given adjuvant hormone therapy with tamoxifen.(10)

In patients with incurable advanced cancer, the diagnostic, pathological, and treatment differences that determine survival in early stage disease are typically less relevant. Moreover, because this is a very heterogeneous group of patients with respect to tumour type, these factors are replaced by different clinical and treatment factors which are not related to the principal diagnosis but to broader syndromic manifestations of terminal illness: physical dependency, the anorexia–cachexia syndrome, lymphopaenia, poor quality of life, and so on. Nevertheless, some patients with incurable cancer can be on the brink of death while others are relatively healthy and have months or even years to live.

In other eventually fatal illnesses, like COPD and cardiac failure, disease-specific factors like arterial blood gas levels and left ventricular function are more relevant to prognosis. Non-specific factors like symptoms (e.g. dyspnoea at rest), functional level, and quality of life are still very relevant nevertheless.

Different death trajectories

A fundamental issue affecting the prediction of survival is the possibility of prototypal death trajectories (Fig. 1).(11,12) The extent to which such hypothesized prototypal death trajectories actually occur is not fully understood at present, nor is it clear what fraction of patients with each of several different kinds of illness show each of these, or other possible, trajectories.

Nevertheless, it is clear that there is little role for palliative care in sudden death, other than to offer bereavement follow-up (Trajectory a). The prototypal cancer death involves a relatively predictable decline in health status over a period of weeks or months (Trajectory b). This is the bailiwick of palliative care and the pattern of deterioration for which traditional palliative care services such as hospices are best designed. This inexorable decline occurs because the cancer–cachexia syndrome seems to be the final common pathway of most solid tumours.(13) While the causes of death in cancer patients are quite diverse and often ultimately result from acute, potentially reversible problems with variable outcomes, such as infection,(14) in most cases the underlying tumour precipitates the cause of death (with anorexia–cachexia syndrome and coma as the final common pathway—see section on symptoms).

In chronic progressive illnesses other than cancer, different death trajectories may apply and two main ones have been described. One is the

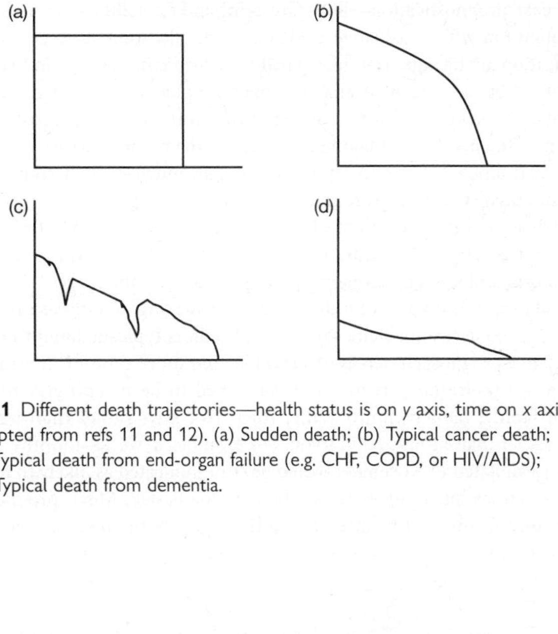

Fig. 1 Different death trajectories—health status is on *y* axis, time on *x* axis (adapted from refs 11 and 12). (a) Sudden death; (b) Typical cancer death; (c) Typical death from end-organ failure (e.g. CHF, COPD, or HIV/AIDS); (d) Typical death from dementia.

slow decline punctuated by acute crises from which the individual recovers to—or close to—the prior health state until the final crisis occurs that cannot be, or is not, treated (Trajectory c). The AIDS-related death and most end-organ failure deaths [e.g. chronic obstructive pulmonary disease (COPD) and congestive heart failure (CHF)] are typical of this pattern. The other is long-term languishing in a very poor health state culminating in death at some unpredictable time following no obvious event, typical of the post-stroke or Alzheimer's death (Trajectory d). Such possible differences in death trajectory may make the role of palliative care harder to define in non-cancer diagnoses.

Some authors have tried to make a distinction between advanced cancer (when disease is widespread but there is still some realistic hope of controlling it, if not curing it) and terminal cancer (when disease is widespread and there is no realistic way of controlling it) and to thereby determine the length of the so-called 'terminal phase'. The following durations of the terminal phase have been calculated:

Author	Country	Year	Survival (days)	
			Mean	Median
McCusker[4]	United States	1984	94	45
Vigano[15]	Canada	2000	175	107
Llobera[16]	Spain	2001	99	59

Thus it can be seen that the median duration of the terminal phase of cancer is around 2–4 months.

Different cultural aspects of prognostication at the end of life

The importance that physicians place on predicting survival at the end of life will be strongly influenced by socio-cultural factors. In his book, the *Nature of Suffering*, Cassell reminds us that in Hippocrates' day, the physician who was a good prognosticator was most highly esteemed amongst his colleagues.[17] By contrast, many religious traditions insist that only God or Allah knows the hour of an individual's death.

In liberal, pluralist Western societies physicians are generally willing to discuss the prognosis, along with the diagnosis and treatment, of a life-threatening illness. In many non-English speaking cultures, such discussions have traditionally been avoided, although this situation may be gradually changing.

The traditional palliative medicine approach to prognostication

In the past, prognostication—both foreseeing and foretelling—has received little attention within palliative medicine. Typically, some aspects of prognostication are brought out during palliative medicine training in Britain, the United States, and Australia. The main emphasis of training is good clinical decision-making in the context of far-advanced disease. Most stress is given to the necessity of taking into account the natural history of eventually fatal illnesses (without ever being taught much explicit content of that) and predicting the future consequences of a therapeutic act/omission, rather than predicting length of survival. Nevertheless, it is generally recognized that patients and (more often) families would sometimes ask for a prognosis, and it is a fundamental principle that the patient's goals, priorities, and expectations are what drives decision-making, not disease-related issues. The palliative medicine trainee in Britain is typically taught not to formulate a prognosis in terms of a specific amount of time,[18] but rather to offer a timeframe that has been supposed to be meaningful to the patient/family: namely, hours rather than days, days rather than weeks, weeks rather than months, and so on. For example, a 'weeks–months' prognosis formulated in November would be communicated as 'likely to make it to Christmas but unlikely to still be here for Easter'. Much prognostic importance is attached to interpreting how quickly the disease seems to have been progressing. A similar pattern has been documented in the United States.[19]

In terms of disclosing the prognosis, trainees are explicitly and implicitly taught to only disclose the formulated prognosis when it is requested and then to give a frank disclosure.[19] Much is made of the prognostic accuracy of the experienced nursing staff in the hospice unit regarding when an imminently dying patient would finally die, and the phenomenon that individuals very close to death would 'hang on' until they achieved closure. There is some suggestion that patients can indeed postpone death until symbolically meaningful occasions.[20]

In the Department of Palliative Care at Royal Prince Alfred Hospital, Sydney, Australia, the proforma that was developed for the patient database asked the registrar/fellow completing the form to give a temporal estimate of the expected survival. This is expressed in terms of a time interval: less than 1 week (representing hours–days), 1–4 weeks (days–weeks), 4–12 weeks (weeks–months), or greater than 12 weeks (months–years). There was never any training in how to formulate these temporal estimates or any evaluation of the accuracy of these formulations, although recently this has been considered in a preliminary way.[21] Nor was it clear what the time was meant to represent. Was it the actual time this individual would live? Or the worse case scenario? Or the median survival of other patients like this? Or the 90 per cent survival of other patients like this? Or something else? In the United States, many hospices formally require admission paperwork to indicate expected survival but this is typically limited to checking a box that the patient has 'less than 6 months' to live. And again, the meaning of this statement has not been made clear, although physicians are very inaccurate.[2]

Deconstructing prognostication: foreseeing versus foretelling

There are two fundamental aspects to the clinical skill of prognostication. The first is foreseeing, that is, formulating the prediction. The second is foretelling, that is, communicating the prediction to the patient. Both foreseeing and foretelling can be studied and improved upon.[22]

Formulating a prognosis in the patient with advanced cancer

Prognostication is not restricted to predicting survival. Prognostication simply means predicting an outcome. In its strictest sense, it refers to 'the relative probabilities that the patient will develop each of the alternative outcomes of the natural history of his/her disease',[23] and so is amenable to sophisticated statistical analysis. In the case of kidney stones, for example, there are prognoses for spontaneous passage, need for surgery, response to other treatments, pain, and recurrence. In the case of cancer, there are prognoses for cure, restoration of function, recurrence, and response to therapy, pain, other symptoms, and death. In the case of palliative care, which is primarily concerned with eventually fatal illnesses, time to death is the key outcome of interest.

There are various ways the practicing clinician can rationally formulate a prognosis. One can rely on one's own experience, but this depends on having seen a lot of similar cases, having a reliable memory, and remaining dispassionate in one's assessments. One can consult an 'expert' in the field but this is not always feasible and is subject to the expert's own biases. One can consult a textbook, but as mentioned above, modern textbooks contain little or no information about the relative probabilities of outcomes of interest. One can employ validated, published algorithms of variable ease of use.[24–26] Finally one can do an electronic search of the medical literature, but again there have been few studies or systematic reviews done to date, although this is changing for survival prediction, especially in patients with advanced cancer.[27]

As with all research, the quality of the methodology of prognostic studies and the way it is reported has improved enormously over the past

Table 1 Characteristics of well-designed studies to evaluate the association of prognostic factors with survival[81]

There is a well-defined study population
An inception cohort design is used
The prognostic factors selected for study are appropriate and clearly defined
The sample size is adequate for the study to have sufficient statistical power
The end point is clearly defined
There is completeness of follow-up
The data analysis is appropriate to test the association between the study factors and survival, using the appropriate statistical tests
There is a measure of agreement between the predicted and actual survival
The definition of accuracy is explicit and appropriate

20 years. Several authors have attempted to review the literature on prognostication in patients with terminal illness and each has commented on the methodological weaknesses—and difficulties interpreting—the studies, especially the older ones.[3,27,28] Well-designed studies to evaluate the association of prognostic factors with survival need the characteristics shown in Table 1.

Clinical predictions of survival

The classic paper on clinicians' estimation of survival (CES) in terminal cancer was published in the British Medical Journal in 1972. (It is perhaps the ultimate irony that, according to the footnote at the end of the BMJ paper, the Parkes study was planned and initiated by the late Dr Ronald Welldon shortly before his own unexpected death in 1969.) In that study, patients with a cancer diagnosis admitted to St Christopher's Hospice for 'terminal care' were studied.[29] Referring doctors (GPs or hospital staff) at the time of referral made predictions of individuals' duration of survival (in weeks). Hospice medical and nursing staff also made predictions at the time of admission. Although most patients died within 12 weeks, the predictions of survival showed little relation to actual length of survival. Moreover, greater than 80 per cent of the erroneous predictions were in the overly optimistic direction (often out by a factor of 2 or more).

Subsequently there have been close to a dozen studies of CES in advanced cancer with varying types of predictions by doctors and other health care professionals of varying experience in terminal care.[2,5,6,15,16,30–37] The diversity of study designs used makes it hard to be certain how accurate clinical predictions are. Most series used so-called *temporal* predictions of survival, expressed in terms of the actual time to be lived by the individual patient, as an ordinal variable (i.e. actual number of days or, more usually, weeks) and these are the least accurate and generally overly optimistic (see Table 2).

Other studies have expressed survival duration as a probability, asking the estimator to state the probability that the patient would survive to a certain time point (e.g. what are the chances that the patient survive 2 months or less, 6 months or more, a year or more?). Others have asked the estimators to provide upper and lower estimates of survival, or to give the smallest interval that would include 90 per cent of deaths of similar patients. Still others have asked estimators to put patients into temporal groups. These last studies hint that physicians may be less prone to error if prognosis is elicited this way.[5,15,30,33,34,36] For example, when asked to decide if individual patients had more or less than a year to live, doctors and nurses assigned more than 1000 hospitalized cancer patients to the correct survival category in more than 75 per cent of cases, and were as likely to over-estimate as under-estimate survival.[33] In another study, two physicians had an accuracy of 60 per cent in predicting whether hospice patients would survive 4 weeks or not.[34] Table 3 provides some illustrative ways that prognoses might be elicited from estimators, with answers that are denominated in different units. The inaccuracy of temporal prognostication has been confirmed in our own systematic review of these studies which is evaluating more than 1500 temporal prediction-actual survival dyads.[38] The heterogeneity of the studies is high, making formal meta-analysis impossible but the pooled results show that CES consistently over-estimates survival, by 45 per cent in general. CES were correct to within 1 week of actual survival (AS) in only 25 per cent cases, and over-estimated AS by at least 4 weeks in 27 per cent. There was increasing variability in AS as CES increases. Nevertheless, although the level of agreement between CES and AS was low (weighed kappa 0.36), they were highly correlated, with $R^2 = 0.51$ for log transformations of both (Fig. 2).

Aside from the issue of whether different ways of eliciting prognoses are more or less accurate, there are other questions to ask about CES:

- *Are repeated estimates more accurate?* In the original Parkes study, doctors were actually less accurate a week later. Subsequently, several investigators have found that doctors' ensuing predictions on the same patients correlate more strongly with survival than their initial ones.[5,37,39]
- *Is there a 'horizon effect'?* Prognosis has a dynamic quality and may change (becoming more or less certain) as time passes. Whether CES are more accurate in those patients who are closer to dying has only been studied to a limited extent. In one study where patients had a median survival of 15 weeks, physicians were most likely to be correct (positive predictive value 74 per cent) when predicting a short survival (<2 months), but they only predicted this in a small number (31 per cent) of the patients who actually survived less than 2 months.[15] Data from a study of more than 500 terminally ill patients (median survival 24 days) referred to hospices in Chicago, IL, in whom their own physicians were asked to make prognostic estimates, suggest that the extent of prognostic error varied depending on both observed and predicted survival, as shown in Table 8.[2] Because physicians were in general so optimistic in their estimates, the longer the *observed* survival, the lower the error. Conversely, the longer the *predicted* survival, the greater the error.
- *Does discipline make a difference?* In the Parkes paper, no significant differences were found between the accuracy of predictions made at referral by GPs, by hospital doctors, by hospice doctors on the day of admission, or by ward sisters and senior nurses at the same time. Several subsequent studies have mostly found no differences in the prognostic abilities of health care workers from different disciplines, although the numbers of prognosticators were usually small.[2,5,15,16,32] One recent British study found that while doctors were the best initial predictors, nurse auxiliaries became very accurate in the last few days of life ($r = 0.98$), presumably because of the amount of time they spend with the patient.[37]
- *Does experience make a difference?* Table 1 suggests that doctors working in the terminal care field have improved their powers of survival estimation over the past 20 years. In one study, the correlation between CES by palliative care specialists and AS increased with clinician experience, and as a group these prognosticators made errors (using the Parkes criterion, i.e. actual survival = predicted survival ± 100 per cent) in only 30 per cent cases, although most errors were still overly optimistic.[6] In the Chicago hospice study, only 20 per cent of the doctors' predictions were accurate (predicted survival = actual survival ± 33 per cent), 63 per cent were overly optimistic (predicted survival > actual survival + 33 per cent), and 17 per cent were overly pessimistic (predicted survival < actual survival − 33 per cent).[2] Multivariate modelling showed that most types of doctors are prone to error in most types of patients, although the greater the experience of the doctor the greater their prognostic accuracy. However, the stronger the doctor–patient relationship, the lower their prognostic accuracy. This suggests that the dispassionate, experienced physician is likely to be the most accurate prognosticator and raises the concept of seeking a 'second opinion' when a definitive prognosis is required.

Despite the inaccuracy of CES, it seems to be an important prognostic factor as it has been retained as an independent predictor of survival on multivariate analysis of a range of possible prognostic variables by several different investigators.[24,40] CES seems to depend more on the individual

Table 2 Association of clinicians' estimates of survival and actual survival in 12 studies

Author, country	Year	Prognosticator/s	Type of prediction	*n*	Median predicted survival (weeks)	Median actual survival (weeks)	Predictions that were accurate (%)	Predictions that were over-optimistic (%)
Parkes, United Kingdom	1972	Hospice doctors	Actual survival (weeks)	74	4.5	~3	8	66
Scotto, United States	1972	Oncologists	Actual survival (months)	178	NS	NS	NS	52
Evans, United Kingdom	1985	Terminal care support team	Upper and lower limits (days)	45	NA	~7	54	37
Heyse-Moore, United Kingdom	1987	Referring doctor	Actual survival (weeks)	50	8	2	4	88
Forster, United States	1988	University oncologist	Interval of likely death (weeks–months)	101	NA	3.5	NS	1[a]
Addington-Hall, United Kingdom	1990	Doctors and nurses	Live more or less than 1 year	1128	NA	17.5	75–83	12
Bruera, Canada	1992	Hospice physicians	Live more or less than 4 weeks	47	NA	4 (mean)	60	26–34
Maltoni, Italy	1994	Palliative care MD	Actual survival (weeks)	100	6	5	15	63
McKillop, Canada	1997	Attending physicians	Likely survival (months)	39	NA	~52	75	NS
Oxenham, United Kingdom	1998	Palliative care senior registrars	Date of death	30	NS	2.5	NS	NS
Vigano, Canada	1999	Oncologists	Actual survival (weeks–months)	233	15.3	14.5	52	NS
Christakis, United States	2000	GPs, internists, oncologists	Actual survival (weeks–months)	468	18	3.5	20	63
Llobera, Spain	2000	Oncologists, GPs	NS	200	NS	7.5	22–27	55–63

[a] 'seriously' over-optimistic, according to authors.

Notes: NA = not applicable, NS = not stated.

Table 3 Ways that prognoses might be elicited, with answers denominated in different units

'What is your best estimate of how long this patient has to live?'
'What is your best estimate of this patient's per cent chance of surviving for 7/30/90/180/360 days or more?'
'Of 100 such patients, how long would it typically be before 20/50/80 died?'
'How likely is this patient to live for 7/30/90/180/360 days or more?'
'Into which of the following categories is the patient's survival most likely to fall: 0–7, 8–30, 31–90, 91–180, or 181–365 days?'

perceptions of the person making the prediction rather than on 'common observations' (although it has been shown to correlate positively with performance status). Given that experienced physicians are more accurate prognosticators, it seems logical to ask if the prognosticators were willing to verbalize the thinking behind their estimates of life expectancy, this might provide useful insights into consideration and valuation of select clinical and social information.[41] A useful paradigm for conceptualizing prognostication, based on the ideas of MacKillop,[28] is shown in Fig. 3.

Performance status

Since CES does not seem to be very accurate, other ways of predicting survival duration in terminal cancer have been investigated. Various factors have been associated with survival, including demographics (age, gender, marital status), tumour-associated factors (primary site, histology, stage), performance status, symptoms, and psychological well being: almost 150 different variables that have been evaluated for their ability to predict survival.[27,42,43] Of all of them, performance status has been studied the most extensively and consistently shows an association with survival duration (see Table 4).

Ever since the development of the Karnofsky performance status (KPS) scale in the 1940s to assess the effects of chemotherapy on functional level, performance status has been recognized as a predictor of oncological outcomes, including survival (see Table 5). The first study to evaluate clinical variables as predictors of survival in advanced cancer evaluated the KPS scale. In that study, the authors primarily aimed to comprehensively establish the statistical properties of the KPS scale; in order to demonstrate its validity, the association of KPS scale score with other clinical variables including duration of survival was evaluated.[44] In a rehabilitation programme 152 cancer patients who had a predicted survival in the 3–12 months range were evaluated; 104 died during the follow-up period and it was found that that a poor performance status (KPS score <50) was associated with a short survival (although one patient with KPS score <50 survived beyond 6 months). While those with a better KPS score generally lived longer, the corollary was not true. A good KPS score (>50) did not guarantee a long survival in this population, the KPS score rapidly dropped in the final 2 months of life. Many other authors have subsequently confirmed this association between KPS score and survival in advanced cancer.[5,6,13,16,27,45]

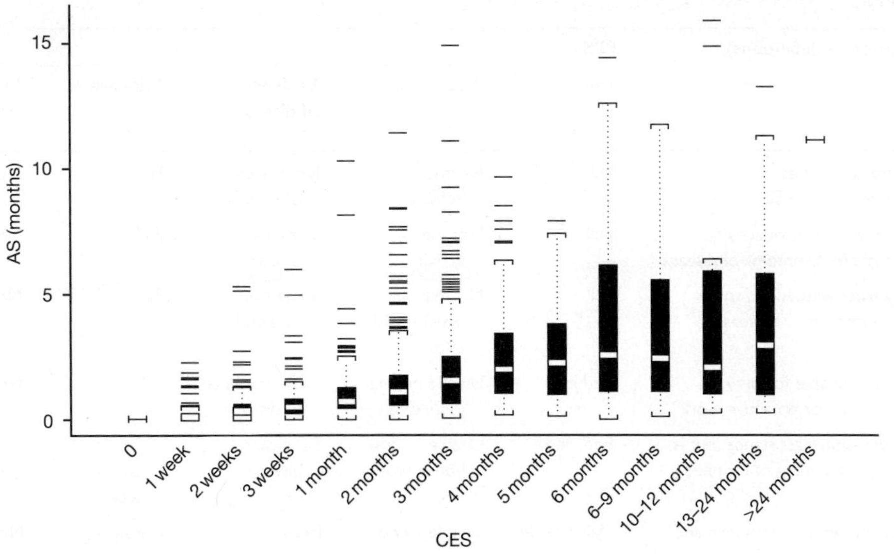

Fig. 2 Association between clinical prediction of survival and actual survival.(38) This is a plot of the differences between CES and AS. The boxes indicate the interquartile range (IQR) of AS, expressed in months. The middle bar is the median survival for the group. The whiskers are drawn to 1.5 times the IQR, which would represent the 99.65 percentile if the data were normally distributed (which they are not). Points beyond are drawn individually. It can be observed that when CES exceeds 6 months there is no predictive value in this measure. When CES is 6 months or less, AS equals or exceeds this estimate in no more than one in four patients. Thus the clinician's estimate is generally optimistic. The figure also demonstrates the increasing variability in AS as CES increases and the skewed distribution of AS, given the CES.

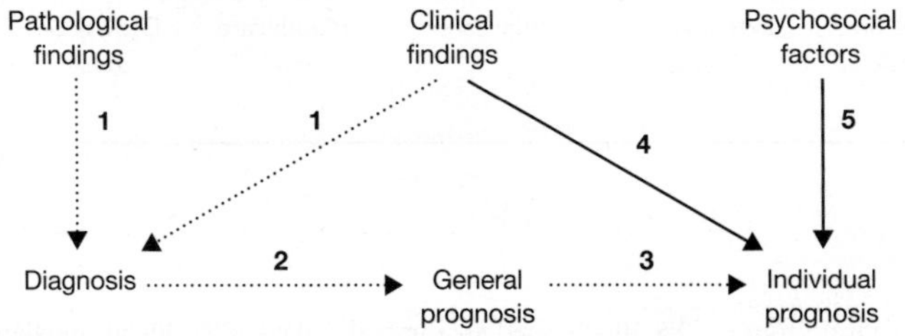

Fig. 3 Formulating a prognosis (adapted from ref. 27). Clinicopathological findings such as tumour histology, grade, and site/number of metastases lead to the diagnosis of the individual's disease. **1**, there is a general prognosis associated with this diagnosis, induced from the clinician's experience of previous patients with the same disease (expressed as 5-year survival rate, median survival, etc.); **2**, this general prognosis is then attributed to the individual patient; **3**, but needs to be modified according to other clinical findings such as performance status, symptoms, metabolic problems; **4**, and quality of life scores or other psychosocial variables; **5**, in patients with far-advanced/terminal cancer, factors **4** and **5** (solid lines) seem to be more important than **1**, **2**, or **3** (broken lines).

The National Hospice Study undertaken in the United States in the early 1980s involved over 1000 patients referred to hospice programmes, with an overall median survival of 37 days.(45) It found that the KPS score accounted for only a small amount of the variability in survival, but that it was highly statistically significant. In general, each increase in KPS level (e.g. from 10 to 20) added approximately 2 weeks to the remaining life span in this study. Furthermore, the KPS scores were used to group patients into survival risk classes (KPS score 10–20: median survival 2 weeks; KPS score 30–40: 7 weeks; KPS score ≥50: 12 weeks). Others have also shown that the KPS score can be used to stratify terminally ill patients for survival risk.(6)

It is unclear whether performance status is a better prognostic indicator than CES as neither has much positive predicative value for individual survival to a certain time point. One group found that the KPS score was more strongly correlated with survival than CES made at the initial visit,(5) while others came to the opposite conclusion (Maltoni, 1994). The latter study

Table 4 The extent to which various clinical variables appear to be predicative of survival in patients with far-advanced cancer(40)

Variable	Number of positive studies[a]	Total number of evaluating studies	Strength of association
Poor performance status	14	14	Definite
Anorexia	8	9	Definite
CES	7	7	Definite
Cognitive failure	7	8	Definite
Dyspnoea	7	8	Definite
Dry mouth	5	6	Definite
Weight loss	4	5	Definite
Dysphagia	4	5	Definite
Primary site	5	10	Possibly yes
Pain	5	10	Possibly yes
Serum albumin	3	4	Possibly yes
Tachycardia	3	4	Possibly yes
Gender (male)	3	11	Possibly yes
Marital status	2	5	Probably not
Nausea	2	5	Probably not
Age	2	9	Probably not
Fever	1	4	Probably not
Anaemia	0	4	Probably not

[a] Positive on either univariate or multivariate analysis.

showed that the CES and KPS score were closely correlated ($r^2 = 0.37$). In other words, 37 per cent of the variation in the survival estimates was accounted for by changes in the performance status. It is possible that the greater accuracy of the survival estimates made by experienced clinicians

Table 5 KPS score and PPS

Percentage of normal performance status	KPS (Karnofsky definitions)	PPS					
		Ambulation	Activity level	Evidence of disease	Self-care	Intake level	Conscious
100	Normal, no complaints, no evidence of disease	Full	Normal activity	No evidence of disease	Full	Normal	Full
90	Able to carry on normal activity, minor signs or symptoms of disease	Full	Normal activity	Some evidence of disease	Full	Normal	Full
80	Normal activity with effort, some signs or symptoms of disease	Full	Normal activity with effort	Some evidence of disease	Full	Normal or reduced	Full
70	Cares for self, unable to carry on normal activity or do active work	Reduced	Unable normal job/work	Some evidence of disease	Full	Normal or reduced	Full
60	Requires occasional assistance, but is able to care for most of his needs	Reduced	Unable hobby/ house work	Significant disease	Occasional assistance necessary	Normal or reduced	Full or confusion
50	Requires considerable assistance and frequent medical care	Mainly sit/lie	Unable to do any work	Extensive disease	Considerable assistance necessary	Normal or reduced	Full or drowsy or confusion
40	Disabled, requires special care and assistance	Mainly in bed	Unable to do any work	Extensive disease	Mainly assistance	Normal or reduced	Full or drowsy or confusion
30	Severely disabled, hospitalization is indicated although death not imminent	Totally bed bound	Unable to do any work	Extensive disease	Total care	Reduced	Full or drowsy or confusion
20	Very sick, hospitalization necessary, active supportive treatment necessary	Totally bed bound	Unable to do any work	Extensive disease	Total care	Minimal sips	Full or drowsy or confusion
10	Moribund, fatal process progressing rapidly	Totally bed bound	Unable to do any work	Extensive disease	Total care	Mouth care only	Drowsy or coma
0	Dead	Dead					

compared with inexperienced ones is that they have learnt to take performance status into account when prognosticating, although this remains to be proven. Other investigators have confirmed this strong association between KPS score and CES, to the point that performance status dropped out of their survival models.(16,46) One problem with the KPS score is that, like other clinical scales, it is scored with varying degrees of inter-rated reliability. This improves with training and care is need when scoring it.(45) Patient-rated KPS scores provide independent prognostic information in addition to physician-rated KPS score.(13)

Other performance status ratings have not been investigated as extensively as the KPS score has. The ECOG scale has been shown to be predictive of survival in both advanced cancer(13) and terminal cancer.(47) ADL scores have also been associated with survival of cancer patients.(48) More recently, the Palliative Performance Scale (PPS), a modification of the KPS, has been developed by home hospice nurses in Canada as a new tool for measuring physical status in patients referred to palliative care services (see Table 5).(49) Initial testing of PPS showed that performance status in terminal cancer could be used for predicting various outcomes, including short-term survival. For example, patients admitted to a hospice unit with a PPS score of 10 all died in the unit, with an average survival of 1.9 days, while 56 per cent of those with a PPS score of 40 on admission died in the unit, with an average survival of 10 days. Full validation of the PPS is awaited, especially regarding whether it is more reliable than KPS score. Very similar results have been obtained with PPS for inpatients admitted to an Australian palliative care unit.(50) A Japanese group has shown that PPS scores are highly correlated with KPS scores (Spearman's $\rho = 0.94$) and tend to stratify patients admitted to a palliative care unit, who had an overall median survival of approximately 1 month, into three homogenous survival groups (PPS 10–20, median survival 6 days; PPS 30–50, median survival 41 days, and PPS 60–70, median survival 108 days).(51)

Symptoms

The onset of various symptoms has also been associated with poor survival in patients with far-advanced cancer. Classic work on this topic was first published by Alvin Feinstein in the mid-1960s, wherein it was argued that symptoms are a more robust indicator of cancer progression and hence prognosis than alternative pathology-based systems.(42) Following on from the findings in the early 1980s that performance status, while strongly associated with survival, did not have sufficient predictive accuracy to guide clinical decision-making in individual cases,(44,45) data from the National Hospice Study of patients after referral to hospice was used to determine whether symptom profile would supplement the accuracy of KPS score in accurately predicting survival.(52) This study showed that five of 14 symptoms evaluated were predictive of survival, namely, anorexia, weight loss, xerostomia, dysphagia, and dyspnoea. These symptoms supplemented prognostic information provided by performance status, especially for patients with better performance status. For example, patients with a KPS score greater than 50 and none of the five key symptoms had a median survival of approximately 6 months and a small (10 per cent) chance of living for 1.5 years; on the other hand, patients with similar performance status and all five symptoms had a median survival of only 2 months and a 10 per cent chance of living for 9 months. In patients with poor performance status, the results were as follows: patients with KPS score 10–20 with no symptoms have a median survival of 8 weeks while those with all the symptoms had a median survival of only 2 weeks.

The best association between survival and symptoms is for the symptoms associated with the anorexia–cachexia syndrome, namely, anorexia and weight loss (see Table 2). Generalized debility and weakness may be the terminal syndrome or pathway, prompting some to call cachexia the 'final common pathway' in patients dying from cancer.[13,53–55] While some studies have not found the symptom of anorexia per se to retain independent prognostic importance on multivariate analysis, other nutritional indices have inevitably been included in the regression models (e.g. weight loss, decreased serum albumin).

Subsequent to the National Hospice Study, several other authors have found dyspnoea to be a survival predictor.[7,24,47,56,57] There is also strong evidence for cognitive failure/confusion as a predictor of a poor survival in far-advanced cancer. A small study of patients admitted to a Canadian PCU was one of the first to explore the link between cognitive failure and poor survival. Patients with a mini-mental state examination score of less than 24, weight loss, and dysphagia had an increased risk of surviving for less than 4 weeks.[34] Somewhat surprisingly, neither anorexia nor dyspnoea was predictive of a short survival in that study. A number of others since,[16,35,56,58] but not all[47] have confirmed this finding.

Somewhat surprisingly, pain is not usually considered to be predictive of poor survival,[34,52] even though it is well known that pain increases in frequency and severity as cancer progresses. However, episodes of severe, uncontrollable ('unendurable') pain and breathlessness have been reported to be more common in the last few weeks of life.[59] Treatment with opioids does not have any impact on survival rate according to several groups of investigators.[47,60]

Quality of life

The relationship between symptoms and survival may be broadened to include the prognostic implications of measures of 'quality of life', in part because symptom distress scores have been recommended as a quality of life measure. A Canadian study of 434 patients with cancer who were within the first 6 months of diagnosis and had a median survival after enrollment of 300 days found that Symptom Distress Scores (SDS) were highly correlated with survival ($r = -0.49$).[61] In this study, fatigue, insomnia, frequent pain, and 'outlook' (sic) were the symptoms most commonly given high distress scores, but not anorexia (notably, weight loss, dysphagia, and dry mouth are not included in the SDS). Similar to performance status, low symptom distress scores did not guarantee long-term survival, but patients with high symptom distress all virtually had short survival times. There were significant differences in levels of symptom distress according to disease site.

A study of patients with hepatic metastases from colorectal cancer specifically showed that the physical symptom subscale score of the Rotterdam Symptom Checklist was the sole quality of life indicator (QOL) predicting survival.[62] In another study—of cancer patients with a median survival in excess of 2 years—a number of quality of life instruments were evaluated; on multivariate analysis, the physical symptom subscale score of the Memorial Symptom Assessment Scale—which averages the frequency, severity, and distress associated with 12 prevalent symptoms—was the only quality of life measure to independently predict reduced survival.[63]

The role of psychological factors in cancer survival has been controversial for more than two decades. A well-known study of over 350 newly diagnosed cancer patients conducted in the 1980s by Cassileth et al. found that 'the inherent biology of the disease [cancer] alone determines the prognosis',[64] and others have confirmed this finding more recently.[65] On the other hand, equally well-known studies like those by Greer and co-workers have identified psychosocial aspects of cancer survivors, such as the 'fighting spirit'.[66–68] Qualitative research of terminally ill cancer patients who were exceptionally long survivors showed that they adopted an 'active coping stance', characterized by: (i) belief in recovery, (ii) positive intentionality, (iii) a meaningful relationship with one doctor, (iv) an intense desire to stay alive.[69] Subsequently, a recent prospective study of psychosocial issues and breast cancer survival by Greer and colleagues found a significantly increased risk of death from all causes by 5 years in women with a high scores for depression and helplessness/hopelessness but there were no significant results found for fighting spirit.[70]

The relationship between survival and patient-related quality of life has been examined for advanced cancer in the oncology literature, and there is some evidence of an association. A significant association has been reported between patient-rated well being and survival time in women receiving treatment for advanced breast cancer,[71] and patient's perception of well being, measured by the Functional Living Index-Cancer (FLIC) instrument (a patient self-rated, cancer-specific QOL questionnaire) is more important in predicting survival in advanced lung cancer than other predictors like KPS score or weight loss.[72] Patients with high FLIC scores lived twice as long (6 months) as those with low scores (3 months). In patients with metastatic melanoma, various measures of QOL (Spitzer QLI, VAS for mood, appetite, and global QOL) have also been shown to be independent predictors of survival, along with KPS score and liver secondaries.[73]

More recently, global QOL scores measured using the EORTC QLQ C30 has been shown to be a strong prognostic indicator in patients with inoperable lung cancer, along with weight loss.[46] In the univariate analysis, a number of QOL subscales, symptoms (anorexia, fatigue, and dyspnoea), and performance status were significant, but dropped out in the multivariate analysis. Shadbolt has found that the global health status item at the beginning of the SF-36 is the best predictor of survival in patients with advanced, but not terminal, cancer.[74]

QOL has not been looked into much in patients with far-advanced disease after referral to hospice/palliative care services. Furthermore, measuring QOL in patients with terminal cancer is fraught with difficulties: (i) the usual QOL definitions and tools are not very applicable in dying patients, (ii) short survival and poor cognitive function makes QOL data difficult to collect, and (iii) the use of ratings by proxies has only limited value.[75]

Nevertheless, there has been some attempt to examine this question. The Spitzer Quality of Life Index (SQLI) has been evaluated for its ability to reduce prognostic uncertainty.[33] In patients estimated to live less than 1 year, there was a trend for those with a low SQLI score to be more likely to die within 6 months than those with a high SQLI. However, the individual patients' scores were not strong predictors of 6-month survival. For example, while 86 per cent of patients who died within 6 months had an SQLI score of less than 7, 65 per cent of those with an SQLI less than 7 were still alive at 6 months.

A validated Italian QOL questionnaire designed for use in hospice/palliative care, the Therapeutic Impact Questionnaire (TIQ), uses four-point Likert scales to rate four major components of QOL—physical symptoms, function, psychological state, and family and social relationships. Global well being is also evaluated. Of all the data provided by TIQ, only the patient-rated perception of cognitive function and global well being showed independent prognostic value. Patients had median survivals of 137, 50, and 17 days for impairment of neither, one, or both scales, respectively.[58]

The association between QOL and survival raises the same issues as with any other statistical association: causality, that is, does the patient's QOL actively influence the natural history of the disease and therefore the survival, or is the QOL merely a reflection of the severity of the illness, progressing inexorably towards death? This issue has been controversial for more than two decades, and needs well-designed clinical trials of interventions that improve quality of life to answer it. Other non-medical factors that influence survival include marital status and socioeconomic status. Marital status has been shown to modify the effect of QOL on survival in cancer patients.[72]

Biological parameters

It is well established that biological parameters are associated with survival of patients with early-stage cancer undergoing treatment. This observation includes both complex biological parameters, such as pathological grade and tumour receptor status, and simple biological parameters such as sodium, albumin, and lymphocyte levels.[76] For example, it has been recognized for 20 years that hyponatraemia is a predictor of a poor outcome in lung cancer, and this was the first biological variable to be evaluated with respect to far-advanced cancer.[32]

Interest in biological parameters has gradually increased over the past 10 years. An Australian study in the early 1990s found a single biological parameter—elevated serum bilirubin—to be one of only four diverse clinical parameters that were predictive of survival on admission to a palliative care unit.[47] An Italian group has done the first large multicentre study of simple biological factors in far-advanced cancer.[77] They collected blood and urine in 530 patients from 22 palliative care centres who had a median survival of 32 days. They looked at various haematological and hepatic synthetic parameters, parameters that they hypothesized to be relevant. Specifically, they evaluated haemoglobin, white blood cell (WBC) count, and differential percentages (but not platelets), transport iron, transferrin, pseudocholinesterase, serum albumin, and proteinuria. They did not evaluate serum electrolytes, liver function tests, or serum calcium, all of which have been found to be important in other, smaller series. Most patients had abnormal values, except for the neutrophil, basophil, monocyte, and eosinophil percentages. Univariate analysis of survival found that the following were all associated with reduced survival: high total WBC, high neutrophil percentage, low lymphocyte percentage, low serum pseudocholinesterase, low serum albumin, and elevated proteinuria. On multivariate analysis, only high total WBC and low lymphocyte percentage retained independent prognostic significance.

Other parameters that have been evaluated include low serum albumin—for which the evidence is conflicting[40,47]—and elevations of serum alkaline phosphatase, lactate dehydrogenase, and C-reactive protein.

Prognostic scores/models

From all of the foregoing, it appears that there is the potential to combine various simple clinical and laboratory factors which are easily evaluated and measured in terminally ill cancer patients to provide physicians with accurate information about prognosis of the type '*x* per cent chance of surviving *y* days'. However, the concept of group probabilities—statistical relations between disease factors and outcomes—verges on anathema to many professionals within palliative care. The philosophical basis of palliative care focuses on understanding the patient as a person, the uniqueness of their suffering, and the clinician's personal interaction with the patient and their family, carefully avoiding anything that dehumanises the individual.

Nevertheless, although individuals exhibit unique features, clinicians cannot avoid making predictions about outcomes. Research commencing within the field of clinical psychology has shown that in general actuarial (statistical) methods are superior to clinical judgement in predicting human behaviour and other outcomes.[78] Actuarial judgement uses empirically established relationships between data and the condition or event of interest. Throughout clinical medicine, simple scoring systems, such as the Glasgow Coma Scale and the Killip Class of myocardial infarction, have proved useful. In cancer medicine, both physiological and psychological factors have been investigated for their ability to compare the accuracy of estimation of survival time. The parameters used for predicting 5-year survival rates in patients with earlier stages of cancer, such as primary site, stage of disease, clinical presentation and history, number of metastases, and location of metastases are generally not useful for predicting survival time as death approaches (see Fig. 3). Instead, several attempts have been made to combine one or more of the factors known to predict survival in the terminally ill (performance status, symptoms, quality of life, biological parameters) into a parsimonious mathematical model that can be used at the bedside to improve CES. The fact that actuarial judgement is more accurate than clinical judgement in advanced cancer is undoubtedly related to the fact that the underlying tumour precipitates the cause of death in the majority of cases making the final common pathway of the anorexia–cachexia syndrome so predictable (i.e. Trajectory B), and it has been recognized since the 1980s that poor performance status, nutritional symptoms like anorexia and weight loss, and the associated metabolic derangement constitute a 'terminal cancer syndrome'.[53,79]

Attempts to develop prognostic models for advanced cancer have been based on similar models in early-stage cancer where, for example, 61 biological variables were assessed for their prognostic value prior to commencement of chemotherapy in 400 patients with small-cell lung cancer.[75] Multiple regression analysis revealed that only tumour stage, KPS score, and four biochemical variables (serum sodium, bicarbonate, alkaline phosphatase, and lactate dehydrogenase levels) were important. Combining these six factors into a simple scoring system—the so-called 'Manchester Index'—the authors were able to accurately distinguish patients belonging to three different prognostic groups, the best of which contained all long-term survivors whereas the bad prognostic group contained no patient surviving greater than 1 year.

In patients with far-advanced cancer, many studies have developed multiple regression models to determine the association between prognostic factors and survival, but few have tested the predictive accuracy of their final models, a key step in prognostic model building.[80–82] Some of the better-developed ones are discussed in greater detail here.

National hospice study life table[52]

Using data from the US National Hospice Study of hospice referrals in the 1980s, these investigators looked at combining performance status—in this case KPS score—and symptoms. As mentioned previously, a poor KPS score (<50) is associated with poor survival, although better performance status (KPS score ≥ 50) does not guarantee good survival. Using these data and statistical modelling, the investigators found that the presence or absence of certain key symptoms was able to differentiate the patients with better performance who had short and long prognoses. Five out of 14 symptoms collected in the data set were identified as being predictive of poor survival: anorexia, weight loss, dysphagia, dry mouth, and dyspnoea. In patients with KPS scores greater than or equal to 50 and none of these symptoms, the median survival was 6 months; if all the symptoms were present it was only 6 weeks. If some were present, the prognosis was intermediate and depended on which of the combination were present. On the other hand, for patients with a very poor performance status (KPS score 10–20), symptoms were less important: if none were present, the median survival was 6 weeks; if all the symptoms were present it was 2 weeks. What makes this study particularly important is that the data from this analysis are presented in the form of a life table that can be easily read off by the clinician at the bedside. For example, a patient with a KPS score 30–40 and anorexia, weight loss, and dry mouth has a median survival of 59 days and a 10 per cent chance of still being alive in 258 days. Although internally validated on the source data set, these predictions are yet to be externally validated.

Australian study[47]

The Australian study of patients with far-advanced cancer requiring inpatient care used various clinical and physiological variables to predict survival. Multivariate analysis of 19 variables identified four that were independently prognostic: poor performance status (ECOG), hyperbilirubinaemia, hypotension, and, need for hospice admission at first clinic visit.

Patients were then categorized into 16 groups depending on which combination of these factors was present, and then these groupings were used to stratify patients into three survival groups: less than 1 month, 1–3 months, or greater than 3 months. The positive predictive value of the 16 groups for the stratification was low, ranging from 0.41 to 0.79 (median 0.5).

SUPPORT study[25]

This study was set up to identify deficiencies in the care of patients with eventually fatal illnesses (only some of whom had cancer) and who were hospitalized, making it difficult to compare with the other data about terminal cancer. Nevertheless, this study is relevant because it aimed to use accurate prognostic information as the cornerstone of improved decision-making about end of life care in hospitals. Based on the APACHE system for prognostication in critically ill patients in ICU's, individuals' clinical and physiological parameters were utilized in a complex algorithm that was computer generated and gave a probability for the hospitalized patient being alive in 2 and 6 months' time.(25) While the mathematical model is complex and not suitable for routine use by the clinician at the bedside and the information provided (chance of being alive in 6 months) is relevant to only a small minority of cancer patients referred to hospice/palliative care, it shows that application of epidemiological methodology has the potential to provide the clinician with very accurate prognostic data.

Palliative Prognostic (PaP) score(24)

The Italian group who have identified elevated white cell count and low lymphocyte percentage as predictive of a poor survival have looked at combining these laboratory values with other parameters to develop a simple model for predicting survival that is useful for the palliative care/hospice clinician. As a result of multivariate analysis of more than 30 parameters, performance status, symptoms, and the haematological parameters are included with the CES in the final mathematical model. Points are allocated for each of these factors, and these subscores are then summed to give a final score, known as the Palliative Prognostic (PaP) score which predicts for short-term survival, as shown in Table 6.

In developing the PaP score system, the investigators found that this model is highly predictive of short-term survival and is able to split a heterogeneous sample of patients with far-advanced cancer (median survival around 30 days) into three groups, that is, those with a high (>70 per cent), intermediate (30–70 per cent), and low (<30 per cent) chance of still being alive in 30 days. The range of PaP scores, readily calculable at the bedside at the time of first contact with the patient, is 0–17.5, higher scores representing worse survival. Cut points of 5.5 and 11 for the three groups (i.e. 0–5.5 for the high-probability group, 6–11 for the intermediate, and 11.5–17.5 for the low-probability group) have been identified.

The PaP score has been subsequently validated by the investigators in almost 500 Italian patients, the overwhelming majority of whom were being visited by community care teams,(60) and independently in 100 hospitalized terminally ill patients in Australia.(83) The PaP score continues to be developed and a new version incorporating cognitive failure has been proposed by the investigators.

Table 6 How to compute PaP score(24)

	Partial score
Dyspnoea	
No	0
Yes	1
Anorexia	
No	0
Yes	1.5
Karnofsky performance status	
≥30	0
10–20	2.5
Clinician's estimate of survival (weeks)	
>12	0
11–12	2
7–10	2.5
5–6	4.5
3–4	6
1–2	8.5
Total white cell count	
≤8.5	0
8.6–11.0	0.5
>11	1.5
Lymphocyte percentage	
20–40	0
12–19.9	1
<12	2.5
Risk groups	*Total score*
A (30 day survival probability >70%)	0–5.5
B (30 day survival probability 30–70%)	5.6–11
C (30 day survival probability <30%)	11.5–17.5

Simple Indicator (Japan)(56)

Performance status and symptoms are combined to form a Simple Indicator to predict short-term survival in terminally ill cancer patients.(56) The Simple Indicator dichotomizes heterogeneous groups of patients according to whether or not they will live for more than 3 weeks or more than 6 weeks. The indicator performed well in the hands of its originators, having a high level of accuracy for both time points (84 and 76 per cent, respectively). It is unclear how the authors actually use the indicator to distinguish between the two groups: the indicators in both groups are a PaP Scale (see section on performance status) score of 10–20, dyspnoea at rest and delirium, with oedema being an additional risk factor for 6-week survival but not for 3-week survival.

GBU Index(84)

Over the past 10 years, the North Central Cancer Treatment Group of the United States has also identified performance status and nutritional factors as being predictive of short-term survival in patients enrolled in chemotherapy trials. Recently, this group has reported the 'GBU' (i.e. good, bad, or uncertain) Index which, like the Australian model and the Simple Indicator, uses combinations of four factors to stratify patients into three prognostic groups (good, bad, or uncertain chance of surviving 1 year). The GBU Index is most useful in patients with performance status scores ECOG 0–1. Like the Manchester Index, GBU has little relevance to the palliative care population, but it helps to further this interesting concept.

Formulating a prognosis in diseases other than cancer

Even more so than cancer, prognosis is critical to the discussion of terminal care in patients with various eventually fatal illnesses such as CHF, COPD, and Alzheimer's disease.(85–88) In the United States, such patients must have a prognosis of less than 6 months 'if the disease follows its usual course' to meet referral criteria to hospice programmes. In other countries, accurate prognostic information is important for the many other reasons identified in the introduction section.

However, formulating a prognosis in these illnesses may be more complicated than it is in cancer because of the difference in the death trajectories. Many of these illnesses may have precipitous declines that may not be reversible due to acute exacerbations [Fig. 1(c)]. As a result, the risk of dying can fluctuate wildly, soaring during acute exacerbations of illness and receding if the process can be stabilized.(89) For example, ER physicians identified 17 per cent of patients admitted for acute exacerbations of heart failure as having less than 10 per cent chance of surviving 90 days, when in fact 67 per cent did not survive.(90) The CES for hypothetical COPD patients with respiratory failure revealed marked variability in estimates.(91)

Nevertheless, there are some similarities with advanced cancer in terms of how one formulates a prognosis in the patient who is terminally ill with a non-cancer diagnosis. Firstly, the 'McKillop' model of prognostication

(Fig. 3) presumably remains relevant: pathology, clinical features, and environmental factors all contribute to the one general and individual prognoses as they do in cancer.[21] Secondly, performance status seems to be a useful global measure of survival in both types of conditions. Thirdly, the emotional and mental status of the patient and family influence the length of survival. Fourthly, the rate of disease progression is important in both the rate of hospitalization and the rate of development of new complications, especially in non-cancer diagnoses.

There are general and specific indicators of the terminal stage of non-cancer diagnoses.[85,92,93] The general ones are impaired performance status and impaired nutritional status. As for cancer, impaired performance status plays an important role in prognostication; it has been shown to predict mortality in the elderly in several studies,[94] and is the basis for the current (United States) National Hospice Organization (NHO) guidelines on prognostication in non-cancer illnesses.[95] Nutritional status is also significant: patients who experience a greater than 10 per cent weight loss over 6 months have been shown to have an increased risk of dying. Decreased serum albumin is also associated with mortality, especially if it is less than 25 g/dl.[96] When impaired performance status and impaired nutritional status occur together, they are highly predictive of short-term mortality.

Unfortunately, in the SUPPORT study, predictions of having less than 6-month survival in the subset of patients with CHF, COPD, and chronic liver disease (CLD) but without malignancy, multi-organ system failure, or acute respiratory failure were very inaccurate.[97] Not only were 70 per cent of individuals who were identified as being expected to die in 6 months still alive at the end of that period, but 54 per cent of those not expected to die in the period did so. Most strikingly, 41 per cent of patients given less than 10 per cent chance of surviving 6 months survived beyond this time frame. Even in the last 2–3 days of life, patients with CHF and COPD were given an 80 and 50 per cent chance of surviving 6 months, respectively.

With regard to individual disease indicators, the following specific predictors have been identified.

- *CHF:* age greater than 64 years, New York Heart Association (NYHA) Class, left ventricular ejection fraction less than 20 per cent, dilated cardiomyopathy, uncontrolled arrhythmias, systolic hypotension, and chest X-ray signs of left heart failure are all associated with poor short-term survival. The NHO criteria for a prognosis of less than 6 months are: (i) NYHA Class IV (chest pain and/or breathless at rest/minimal exertion) and (ii) already optimally treated with diuretics and vasodilators.
- *COPD:* advanced age, forced expiratory volume at 1 s (FEV_1) of less than 30 per cent, and pulmonary hypertension with cor pulmonale/right heart failure are poor prognostic signs. The NHO criteria include: (i) dyspnoeic at rest, (ii) on 24-h home oxygen with pO_2 less than 50 mm Hg and/or pCO_2 more than 55 mm Hg, and (iii) documented evidence of cor pulmonale.
- *Alzheimer's disease:* functional status appears to be the main predictor of survival. The onset of inability to walk unaided indicates entering the final phase of the illness. In one study, 30 per cent patients with dementia who were greater than 90 years of age and referred to a United States hospice programme were alive 3 years later.[98] NHO criteria include: (i) advanced disease (unable to walk independently and/or hold a meaningful conversation) and (ii) onset of medical complications (e.g. aspiration pneumonia, UTI, decubitus ulcers).
- *NHO criteria* are also available for HIV/AIDS, CLD, renal failure, stroke, coma, and motor neurone disease.

Few prognostic models have been developed for predicting survival in terminal non-cancer illnesses. The HELP study developed a nomogram for accurately estimating the length of life in the hospitalized elderly (>80 years of age) using a limited amount of clinical information, but has not been widely validated.[25] Gender, duration of illness, age at onset, Mini-Mental State Examination score, and extrapyramidal or psychotic features have been combined in a validated model that predict time to nursing home placement or death for patients with Alzheimer's disease.[99]

Communicating a prognosis

While foreseeing is the formulation of a prognosis by a clinician, foretelling is the specialized form of doctor–patient communication of a prognosis. The issue here is not merely whether and how physicians formulate prognosis, but also whether and how they might communicate them. Predicting survival in patients with far-advanced cancer and communicating the prognosis can be seen to have much in common with other forms of 'breaking bad news' in patients with a life-threatening illness.

Why communicate the formulated prognosis to the patient?

In the last 30 years, there has been a sea change in attitudes regarding disclosure of information to patients with cancer. It is now expected that the oncologist would have an open and frank discussion with the patient at the time of initial diagnosis about all aspects of the disease, including what the future holds, especially in terms of what can be expected from treatment.

Despite this openness, it is unclear what patients want in terms of prognostic information. Physicians in turn often regard it as taboo to talk about the length of time remaining for a patient perceived to be in the terminal stage of their illness. The reasons for this are multifactorial. Firstly, we still live in a death-denying society. Secondly, doctors' prognoses are notoriously inaccurate and many doctors are not confident about their prognosis-formulating skills—the popular culture is full of stories of patients 'beating the odds'.[100] Thirdly, it is dramatic and unpleasant for the doctor to forecast that the patient's death is imminent—not only does the doctor have to admit that medicine as an institution and they as an individual physician have 'failed', but they also will be apprehensive about how the patient will react to the prognosis and how they will react if the patient becomes very emotional. Furthermore, physicians are poorly prepared for the tasks of formulating and communicating prognosis, with medical schools, textbooks, and journals all tending to neglect prognostication.[19]

Physicians cope with the stress of having to formulate or communicate prognoses by adopting certain 'norms' of behaviour regarding prognostication (Table 7):

Foretelling an accurate prognosis is important because there is data that patients who are optimistic about their outlook will demand more aggressive life-sustaining treatment than those who are pessimistic about their outlook. If this optimism is unrealistic, this could have bad consequences for the patient if the aggressive life-sustaining treatment that they demand is futile and overly-burdensome for them. Moreover, most studies show that most patients want and need prognostic information in order to make the best possible clinical and personal decisions.[101] If this optimism is discordant with what the physician foresees as the prognosis, then there are a number of possible explanations for the discrepancy:

- the doctor has not given the patient a diagnosis/prognosis;
- the doctor has, but the patient is in denial;
- the doctor has, but the patient has misinterpreted what the doctor has said; and

Table 7 Norms of prognostication[19]

Do not make predictions
Keep what predictions you make to yourself
Do not communicate predictions to patients unless asked
Do not be specific
Do not be extreme
Be optimistic

- the doctor has said something vague or more optimistic than what he believes.

One study sought to shed light on these possibilities.(102) It involved asking physicians to formulate prognoses in specific patients of theirs and then asking them to state what they would communicate to these patients if the patients insisted on being told their prognosis. As mentioned previously, the formulated prognosis (median 75 days) was overly optimistic by a factor of 3 (median actual survival 26 days) (Table 8). They found that the doctors would give a frank disclosure of their prognosis to 37 per cent, not offer any prognosis to 23 per cent of patients, and offer a discrepant prognosis in 40 per cent, with the majority (70 per cent) of the discrepant prognoses in the over-optimistic direction. The authors' conclusion is that many patients are thus 'twice removed' from the reality of their outlook, because not only is the prognosis not formulated accurately but also the prognosis is then often communicated even more optimistically, a point illustrated by Fig. 4. This may help to explain the discrepancy between doctors and patient's perspective on their illness. The authors also examined various patient, prognostic, and physician characteristics to see if they correlated with the different categories of disclosure type.

Table 8 Physicians' overestimates of patient survival, by observed and predicted survival(2)

Duration of survival (days)	% overestimate in survival (mean)	*N*
Observed		
1–30	795	251
31–90	288	130
91–180	136	49
>180	71	38
Overall	526	468
Predicted		
1–30	192	150
31–90	382	144
91–180	501	119
>180	1872	55
Overall	526	468

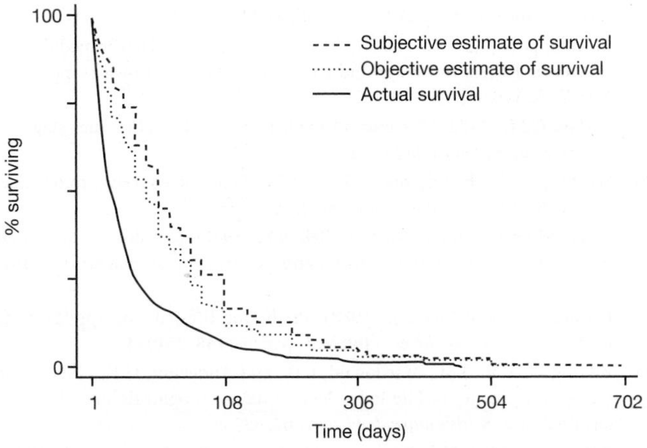

Fig. 4 Relationship between subjective, objective, and actual survival.(102) The graph illustrates the differences between actual survival, formulated 'objective' survival (told to the investigators), and communicated 'subjective' survival (that would be told to patients) in 300 terminally ill cancer patients. The median actual survival was 24 days, the median objective prognosis was 75 days, and the median survival disclosed to the patient was 90 days. *Source:* Lamont and Christakis, 2001.

Why might the physician want to disclose a prognosis that is more optimistic than what they believe it to be? Other work has identified the phenomenon of the 'self-fulfilling prophecy' in the psychology of the physician, and the possibility that giving an overly-optimistic prognosis to the patient will produce a better outcome than would have otherwise happened—and vice versa for a pessimistic prognosis. There is other data to support the view that doctors believe in the self-fulfilling prophecy and that being hopeful/optimistic produces better outcomes.(103) Because of the clear importance of maintaining hope in oncology, the task of foretelling an accurate prognosis to a patient with terminal cancer may be a greater challenge than accurately foreseeing it.

The first three norms listed above relate to the 'when' of prognosticating. Most patients with an eventually fatal illness are interested in some discussion about their preferences for end of life care and a meaningful discussion can only take place if the patient has a realistic understanding of where they are situated in the trajectory of their illness. It is well documented that there is a discrepancy between what physicians and patients understand about the goals of treatment and what the future holds throughout the spectrum of the cancer illness, and this has been documented in the terminal phase as well.

How to communicate the formulated prognosis to the patient

While we have clarified what prognostic information the physician should try to provide in terms of significant content and scientific authority, the best process for conveying the prognosis remains problematic. In fact, it has been called the 'next communication frontier for oncology'.(104) There seem to be a number of preconditions to be fulfilled. Firstly, the doctor has to be willing to disclose the prognosis truthfully, and as we have already stated, the norms of medical practice counteract this. Secondly, a single conversation may not be sufficient: an open, supportive, and ongoing dialogue may often be required. Thirdly, development of communication aids such as question prompt sheets for patients/families or tools for illustrating concepts like probabilities that are difficult to simply explain need to be explored.

Communicating the prognosis—especially when it is unfavourable—is best seen as the prototype of breaking bad news. Thus, the doctor needs to be truthful, accurate, empathetic, and still try to foster hope. The rules for breaking bad news in other contexts should be followed: the doctor begins by ensuring the setting is as optimal as possible (i.e. privacy, sitting, partner), then ascertain how much information the patient wants, then ascertain what they already know, then deliver the news accordingly. The doctor should check that the patient has understood, then arrange to return subsequently to check that it has been understood, answer any more questions, and ensure the patient is coping.

Conclusion

Prognostication remains a controversial topic in palliative care. In the past 20 years, much research has been undertaken to identify ways of improving the accuracy and precision of clinicians' estimates. While we are now in a better position to give the patient '*x* per cent chance of surviving for *y* weeks/months', predictions that are precise enough to drive treatment plans remain elusive. Furthermore, models that predict survival should be thought of like any diagnostic test, that is, they should not be interpreted in isolation but as a way of improving the pre-test probability of survival, which is based on clinical judgement.

Clinical judgement alone may be sufficient if the issue is acknowledging that there is a probability of dying from an illness in the foreseeable future. The SUPPORT study showed that patients will change their planning behaviour once they understand that the chance of surviving beyond 6 months is small.

What ultimately may be needed is not so much an accurate prediction of time but an acknowledgement of the possibility of dying, communicated carefully by the compassionate and skillful physician.

Summary

- Prognostication is important in end of life care.
- The precision of the survival estimate depends on the reason for prognosticating.
- Doctors (and other health care professionals) are not very accurate when making temporal estimates in individual patients, although this may be improving.
- Experience improves prognostication accuracy, but this is modified by the closeness of the doctor–patient relationship.
- Probabilistic predictions are more accurate.
- The clinical estimate of survival is a powerful independent prognostic indicator.
- In general, patients with a poor performance status live for shorter periods than those who are more functional.
- Symptoms like anorexia, breathlessness, and confusion are important predictors that an individual is rapidly approaching the end of life.
- QOL scores may be more powerful than KPS scores or symptom reports in predicting survival.
- Simple, reliable, and valid prognostic models that combine these factors have been developed and can be readily used at the bedside of terminally ill cancer patients.
- Predicating survival in patients dying of diseases other than cancer is much harder.
- Communicating survival predictions is an important part of cancer care.

References

1. **Christakis, N.A.** (1997). The ellipsis of prognosis in modern medical thought. *Social Science and Medicine* **44**, 301–5.
2. **Christakis, N.A. and Lamont, E.B.** (2000). Extent and determinants of error in doctors' prognoses in terminally ill patients: prospective cohort study. *British Medical Journal* **320**, 469–72.
3. **Den Daas, N.** (1995). Estimating length of survival in end-stage cancer: a review of the literature. *Journal of Pain and Symptom Management* **10**, 548–55.
4. **McCusker, J.** (1984). The terminal period of cancer: definition and descriptive epidemiology. *Journal of Chronic Diseases* **37**, 377–85.
5. **Evans, C. and McCarthy, M.** (1985). Prognostic uncertainty in terminal care: can the KPS help? *Lancet* **1** (8439), 1204–6.
6. **Maltoni, M.** et al. (1994). Clinical prediction of survival is more accurate than the Karnofsky performance status in estimating life span of terminally ill cancer patients. *European Journal of Cancer* **30A** (6), 764–6.
7. **Hardy, J.R., Turner, R., Saunders, M.A., and A'Hern, R.** (1994). Prediction of survival in a hospital-based continuing care unit. *European Journal of Cancer* **30A**, 284–8.
8. **Justice, A.C.** *The Development, Validation, and Evaluation of Prognostic Systems: An Application to the Acquired Immunodeficiency Syndrome (AIDS)*. Ann Arbor MI: University Microfilms, 1996.
9. **Smith, J.L.** (2000). Commentary. Why do doctors overestimate? *British Medical Journal* **320**, 472–3.
10. **Early Breast Cancer Trialists' Collaborative Group** (1998). Tamoxifen for early breast cancer: an overview of the randomised trials. *Lancet* **351**, 1451–67.
11. **Field, M.J. and Cassel, C.K.**, ed. *Approaching Death: Improving Care at the End of Life/Committee on Care at the End of Life.* Washington DC: National Academy Press, Division of Health Care Services, Institute of Medicine, 1997.
12. **Lynn, J.** (2001). Helping patients who may die soon and their families. The role of hospice and other services. *Journal of the American Medical Association* **285**, 925–32.
13. **Loprinzi, C.L.** et al. (1994). Prospective evaluation of prognostic variables from patient completed questionnaires. *Journal of Clinical Oncology* **12**, 601–7.
14. **Inagaki, J., Rodriguez, V., and Bodey, G.P.** (1974). Causes of death in cancer patients. *Cancer* **33**, 568–73.
15. **Vigano, A., Dorgan, M., Bruera, E., and Suarez-Almazor, M.E.** (1999). The relative accuracy of the clinical estimation of the duration of life for patients with end of life cancer. *Cancer* **86**, 170–6.
16. **Llobera, J., Esteva, M., Rifa, J., Benito, E., Terrasa, J., Rojas, C., Pons, O., Catalan, G., and Avella, A.** (2000). Terminal cancer, duration and prediction of survival time. *European Journal of Cancer* **36** (16), 2036–43.
17. **Cassell, E.** *The Nature of Suffering.* New York: Oxford University Press, 1991.
18. **Rich, A.** (1999). How long have I got?—Prognostication and palliative care. *European Journal of Palliative Care* **6**, 179–82.
19. **Christakis, N.A.** *Death Foretold.* Chicago IL: University of Chicago Press, 1999.
20. **Phillips, D.P. and Smith, D.G.** (1990). Postponement of death until symbolically meaningful occasions. *Journal of the American Medical Association* **263**, 1947–51.
21. **Chye, R.** *Predicting Prognosis in Palliative Care—A Five Year Retrospective Analysis (abstract).* Annual Scientific Meeting, Royal Australasian College of Physicians, Sydney, Australia, May 13–16, 2001.
22. **Lamont, E.B. and Christakis, N.A.** (1999). Some elements of prognosis in terminal cancer. *Oncology* **13**, 1165–70.
23. **Sackett, D., Haynes, R.B., Guyatt, G.H., and Tugwell, P.** *Clinical Epidemiology: A Basic Science for Clinical Medicine* 2nd edn. Boston MA: Little Brown and Co., 1991.
24. **Pirovano, M.** et al. and an Italian Multicentre Study Group on Palliative Care (1999). A new palliative prognostic score: a first step for the staging of terminally ill cancer patients. *Journal of Pain and Symptom Management* **17**, 231–9.
25. **Knaus, W.A.** et al. (1995). The SUPPORT prognostic model: objective estimates of survival for seriously ill hospitalised adults. *Annals of Internal Medicine* **122**, 191–203.
26. **Teno, J.M.** et al. (2000). Prediction of survival for older hospitalized patients: the HELP survival model. *Journal of the American Geriatric Society* **48**, S16–24.
27. **Vigano, A., Dorgan, M., Buckingham, J., Bruera, E., and Suarez-Almazor, M.E.** (2000). Survival prediction in terminal cancer patients: a systematic review of the literature. *Palliative Medicine* **14**, 363–74.
28. **Mackillop, W.J.** (2001). The importance of prognosis in cancer medicine. In *Prognostic Factors in Cancer* 2nd edn. (ed. M. Gospodarowicz), pp. 3–14. New York: Wiley-Liss.
29. **Parkes, C.M.** (1972). Accuracy of predictions of survival in later stages of cancer. *British Medical Journal* **2**, 29–31.
30. **Scotto, J. and Schneiderman, M.A.** (1972). Predicting survival in terminal cancer. *British Medical Journal* **4** (831), 50.
31. **Heyse-Moore, L.H. and Johnson-Bell, V.E.** (1987). Can doctors accurately predict the life expectancy of patients with terminal cancer? *Palliative Medicine* **1**, 165–6.
32. **Forster, L.E. and Lynn, J.** (1988). Predicting lifespan for applicants to inpatient hospice. *Archives of Internal Medicine* **148**, 2540–3.
33. **Addington-Hall, J.M., Macdonald, L.D., and Anderson, H.R.** (1990). Can the Spitzer Quality of Life Index help to reduce prognostic uncertainty in terminal care. *British Journal of Cancer* **62**, 695–9.
34. **Bruera, E., Miller, M.J., Kuehn, N., MacEachern, T., and Hanson, J.** (1992). Estimate of survival of patients admitted to a palliative care unit: a prospective study. *Journal of Pain and Symptom Management* **7**, 82–6.
35. **Maltoni, M.** et al. (1995). Prediction of survival of patients terminally ill with cancer. Results of an Italian multicenter study. *Cancer* **75**, 2613–22.
36. **Mackillop, W.J. and Quirt, C.F.** (1997). Measuring the accuracy of prognostic judgements in oncology. *Journal of Clinical Epidemiology* **50**, 21–9.

37. **Oxenham, D. and Cornbleet, M.A.** (1998). Accuracy of prediction of survival by different professional groups in a hospice. *Palliative Medicine* **12**, 117–18.

38. **Glare, P., Jones, M., Virik, K., Hudson, M., Eychmuller, S., Christakis, N., and Simes, J.** Meta-analysis of predicted survival for terminally ill cancer patients (in preparation).

39. **Poses, R.M., Bekes, C., Copare, F.J., and Scott, W.E.** (1990). What difference do two days make? The inertia of physicians' sequential prognostic udgments for critically ill patients. *Medical Decision Making* **10**, 6–14.

40. **Vigano, A., Bruera, E., Jhangri, G.S., Newman, S.C., Fields, A.L., and Suarez-Almazor, M.E.** (2000). Clinical survival predictors in patients with advanced cancer. *Archives of Internal Medicine* **160**, 861–8.

41. **Perlman, R.A.** (1988). Inaccurate predictions of life expectancy. Dilemmas and opportunities. *Archives of Internal Medicine* **148**, 2538–9.

42. **Feinstein, A.R.** (1966). Symptoms as an index of biological behaviour and prognosis in human cancer. *Nature* **209**, 241–5.

43. **Justice, A.C., Covinsky, K.E., and Berlin, J.A.** (1999). Assessing the generalizability of prognostic information. *Annals of Internal Medicine* **130** (6), 515–24.

44. **Yates, J.W., Chalmer, B., and McKegney, P.** (1980). Evaluation of patients with advanced cancer using the Karnofsky Performance Status. *Cancer* **45**, 2220–4.

45. **Mor, V., Laliberte, L., Morris, J.N., and Wiemann, M.** (1984). The Karnofsky Performance Status scale. An examination of its reliability and validity in a research setting. *Cancer* **53**, 2002–7.

46. **Langendyk, H., Aaronson, N.K., de Jong, J.M.A., ten Velde, G.P.M., Muller, M.J., and Wouters, M.** (2000). The prognostic impact of quality of life assessed with the EORTCQLQ C30 in inoperable non-small cell lung carcinoma treated with radiotherapy. *Radiotherapy in Oncology* **55**, 19–25.

47. **Rosenthal, M.A., Gebski, V.J., Kefford, R.F., and Stuart-Harris, R.C.** (1993). Prediction of life expectancy in hospice patients: identification of novel prognostic factors. *Palliative Medicine* **7**, 199–204.

48. **Bennett, M. and Ryall, N.** (2000). Using the modified Barthel index to estimate survival in cancer patients in hospice: observational study. *British Medical Journal* **321** (7273), 1381–2.

49. **Anderson, F., Downing, G.M., Hill, J., Casorso, L., and Lerch, N.** (1996). Palliative Performance Scale (PPS): a new tool. *Journal of Palliative Care* **12** (1), 5–11.

50. **Virik, K. and Glare, P.** (2002). Validation of the Palliative Performance Scale for inpatients admitted to a palliative care unit in Sydney, Australia (letter). *Journal of Pain and Symptom Management* **23** (6), 455–7.

51. **Morita, T., Tsunoda, J., Inoue, S., and Chihara, S.** (1999). Validity of the Palliative Performance Scale from a survival perspective. *Journal of Pain and Symptom Management* **18**, 2–3.

52. **Reuben, D.B., Mor, V., and Hiris, J.** (1988). Clinical symptoms and length of survival in patients with terminal cancer. *Archives of Internal Medicine* **148**, 1586–91.

53. **Wachtel, T., Masterson, S.A., Reuben, D., Goldberg, R., and Mor, V.** (1989). The end stage cancer patient: terminal common pathway. *Hospice Journal* **4** (4), 43–80.

54. **Ma, G. and Alexander, H.R.** (1998). Prevalence and pathophysiology of cancer cachexia. In *Topics in Palliative Care* Vol. 2 (ed. E. Bruera and R.K. Portenoy), pp. 91–129. New York: Oxford University Press.

55. **Vigano, A., Dorgan, M., Bruera, E., and Suarez-Almazor, M.E.** (1999). Terminal cancer syndrome: myth or reality. *Journal of Palliative Care* **15** (4), 32–9.

56. **Morita, T., Tsunoda, J., Inoue, S., and Chihara, S.** (1999). Survival prediction of terminally ill cancer patients by clinical symptoms: development of a simple indicator. *Japanese Journal of Clinical Oncology* **29** (3), 156–9.

57. **Escalante, C.P.** et al. (2000). Identifying risk factors for imminent death for cancer patients with acute dyspnea. *Journal of Pain and Symptom Management* **20**, 318–25.

58. **Tamburini, M., Brunelli, C., Rosso, S., and Ventafridda, V.** (1996). Prognostic value of quality of life scores in terminal cancer patients. *Journal of Pain and Symptom Management* **11**, 32–41.

59. **Ventafridda, V., Ripamonti, C., Tamburini, M., Cassileth, R.B., and De Conno, F.** (1990). Unendurable symptoms as prognostic indicators of impending death in terminal cancer patients. *European Journal of Cancer* **26**, 1000–1.

60. **Maltoni, M.** et al. and an Italian Multicentre Study Group on Palliative Care (1999). Successful validation of the Palliative Prognostic Score in terminally ill cancer patients. *Journal of Pain and Symptom Management* **17**, 240–7.

61. **Degner, L.F. and Sloan, A.** (1995). Symptom distress in newly diagnosed ambulatory cancer patients and as a predictor of survival in lung cancer patients. *Journal of Pain and Symptom Management* **10**, 423–31.

62. **Earlam, S., Glover, C., Fordy, C., Burke, D., and Allen-Mersh, T.G.** (1996). Relation between tumour size, quality of life, and survival in patients with colorectal liver metastases. *Journal of Clinical Oncology* **14** (1), 171–5.

63. **Chang, V.T., Thaler, H.T., Ployak, T.A., Kornblith, A.B., Lepore, J.M., and Portenoy, R.K.** (1998). Quality of life and survival. The role of multidimensional symptom assessment. *Cancer* **83**, 173–9.

64. **Cassileth, B.R.** et al. (1985). Psychosocial correlates of survival in advanced malignant disease? *New England Journal of Medicine* **312**, 1551–5.

65. **Ringdal, G.I., Götestam, K.G., Kaasa, S., Kvinnsland, S., and Ringdal, K.** (1996). Prognostic factors and survival in a heterogeneous sample of cancer patients. *British Journal of Cancer* **73**, 1594–9.

66. **Greer, H.S., Morris, T., and Pettingale, K.W.** (1979). Psychological response to breast cancer: effect on outcome. *Lancet* **2** (8146), 785–7.

67. **Pettingale, K.W., Morris, T., Greer, S., and Haybittle, J.L.** (1985). Mental attitudes to cancer: an individual prognostic factor. *Lancet* **i**, 750.

68. **Spiegel, D., Bloom, J.R., Kraemer, H.C., and Gottheil, E.** (1989). Effect of psychosocial treatment on survival of patients with metastatic breast cancer. *Lancet* **ii**, 888–91.

69. **Roud, P.C.** (1987). Psychosocial variables associated with the exceptional survival of patients with advanced malignant diseases. *Journal of National Medical Association* **79**, 97–102.

70. **Watson, M., Haviland, J.S., Greer, S., Davidson, J., and Bliss, J.M.** (1999). Influence of psychological response on survival in breast cancer: a population-based cohort study. *Lancet* **354** (9187), 1331–6.

71. **Coates, A.** et al. (1992). Prognostic value of quality of life scores during chemotherapy for advanced breast cancer. *Journal of Clinical Oncology* **10**, 1833–8.

72. **Ganz, P.A., Lee, J.J., and Siau, J.** (1991). Quality of life assessment: an independent prognostic variable for survival in lung cancer. *Cancer* **67**, 3131–5.

73. **Coates, A.** et al. (1993). Prognostic value of QOL scores in a trial of chemotherapy with or without interferon in patients with metastatic malignant melanoma. *European Journal of Cancer* **29A**, 1731–4.

74. **Shadbolt, B., Barresi, J., and Craft, P.** (2002). Self-related health as a predictor of survival among patients with advanced cancer. *Journal of Clinical Oncology* **20**, 2514–9.

75. **Paci, E.** et al. (2001). Quality of life assessment and outcome of palliative care. *Journal of Pain and Symptom Management* **21** (3), 179–88.

76. **Cerny, T., Blair, V., Anderson, H., Bramwell, V., and Thatcher, N.** (1987). Pre-treatment prognostic factors and scoring system in 407 small-cell lung cancer patients. *International Journal of Cancer* **39**, 146–9.

77. **Maltoni, M.** et al. and an Italian Multicentre Study Group on Palliative Care (1997). Biological indices predictive of survival in 519 Italian terminally ill cancer patients. *Journal of Pain and Symptom Management* **13**, 1–9.

78. **Dawes, R.M., Faust, D., and Meehl, P.E.** (1989). Clinical versus actuarial judgement. *Science* **243**, 1668–74.

79. **Schonwetter, R.S., Teasdale, T.A., and Storey, P.** (1989). The terminal cancer syndrome (letter). *Archives of Internal Medicine* **149**, 965–6.

80. **Steyerberg, E.W. and Harrell, F.J.** (2002). Statistical models for prognostication. In *Symptom Research: Methods and Opportunities* (ed. M.B. Max and J. Lynn) (http://symptomresearch.nih.gov, accessed May 16th, 2002).

81. **Koss, N. and Feinstein, A.R.** (1971). Computer-aided prognosis. II. Development of a prognostic algorithm. *Archives of Internal Medicine* **127** (3), 448–59.

82. **Altman, D.G.** (2001). Systematic reviews of studies of prognostic variables. *British Medical Journal* **323**, 224–8.

83. **Glare, P. and Virik, K.** (2001). Independent validation of Palliative Prognostic Score in terminally ill cancer patients in the acute care setting in Australia. *Journal of Pain and Symptom Management* **22**, 891–8.

84. **Sloan, J.A.** et al. (2001). A simple stratification factor prognostic for survival in advanced cancer: the Good/Bad/Uncertain Index. *Journal of Clinical Oncology* **19**, 3539–46.

85. **Fries, J.F. and Ehrlich, G.B.** *Prognosis: Contemporary Outcomes of Disease.* Bowie MD: Charles Press, 1981.

86. **Kapoor, A.S. and Singh, B.N.**, ed. *Prognosis and Risk Assessment in Cardiovascular Disease.* New York: Churchill Livingstone, 1993.

87. **McKellar, D.P.** et al. *Prognosis and outcomes in surgical disease.* St Louis MO: Quality Medical Publishing, 1998.

88. **Schonwetter, R.S. and Jani, C.R.** (2000). Survival estimation in non-cancer patients with advanced disease. In *Topics in Palliative Care* Vol. 4 (ed. E. Bruera and R.K. Portenoy), pp. 55–74. Oxford: Oxford University Press.

89. **Finucane, T.E.** (1999). How gravely ill becomes dying?. A key to end-of-life care (editorial). *Journal of the American Medical Association* **282**, 1670–2.

90. **Poses, R.M.** et al. (1997). Physicians' survival predictions for patients with acute congestive heart failure. *Archives of Internal Medicine* **157**, 1001–7.

91. **Perlman, R.A.** (1987). Variability in physician estimates of survival for acute respiratory failure in chronic obstructive pulmonary disease. *Chest* **91**, 515–21.

92. **Von Gunten, C.F. and Twaddle, M.L.** (1996). Terminal care for noncancer patients. *Clinics in Geriatric Medicine* **12** (2), 349–58.

93. **Stuart, B.** (1999). Advanced cancer and comorbid conditions: prognosis and treatment. *Cancer Control* **6** (2), 168–74.

94. **Reuben, D.B., Rubenstein, L.V., Hirsch, S.H., and Hays, R.D.** (1992). Value of functional status as a predictor of mortality: results of a prospective study. *American Journal of Medicine* **93**, 663–9.

95. **Standards and Accreditation Committee, Medical Guidelines Taskforce of the National Hospice Organization.** *Medical Guidelines for Determining Prognosis in Selected Non-cancer Disease* 2nd edn. Arlington VA: National Hospice Organisation, 1996.

96. **Corti, M.C., Guralnik, J., Salive, M.E., and Sorkin, J.D.** (1994). Serum albumin level and physical disability as predictors of mortality in older persons. *Journal of the American Medical Association* **272**, 1036–42.

97. **Fox, E., Landrum-McNiff, K., Zhong, Z., Dawson, N.V., Wu, A.W., and Lynn, J.** (for the SUPPORT Investigators) (1999). Evaluation of prognostic criteria for determining hospice eligibility in patients with advanced lung, heart and liver disease. *Journal of the American Medical Association* **282**, 1638–45.

98. **Aguero-Torres** et al. (1998). Prognostic factors in very old demented adults: a seven-year follow-up from a population-based survey in Stockholm. *Journal of the American Geriatric Society* **46**, 444–52.

99. **Stern, Y.** et al. (1997). Predicting time to nursing home care and death in individuals with Alzheimer's disease. *Journal of the American Medical Association* **277**, 806–12.

100. **Gould, S.J.** (1998). The median is not the message. In *Narrative Based Medicine* (ed. T. Greenhalgh and B. Hurwitz). London: BMJ Books. www.cancerguide.org/median_not_msg.html.

101. **Weeks, J.C.** et al. (1998). Relationship between cancer patients' predictions of prognosis and their treatment preferences. *Journal of the American Medical Association* **279**, 1709–14.

102. **Lamont, E.B. and Christakis, N.A.** (2001). Prognostic disclosure to patients with cancer near the end of life. *Annals of Internal Medicine* **134**, 1096–115.

103. **Del Vecchio Good, M.J., Munakata, T., Kobayashi, Y., Mattingly, C., and Good, B.J.** (1994). Oncology and narrative time. *Social Science and Medicine* **38** (6), 855–62.

104. **Siminoff, L.A.** (1992). Improving communication with cancer patients. *Oncology (Huntington)* **6** (10), 83–7 (discussion 87–9).

2.5 The interdisciplinary team

J. Norelle Lickiss, Kristen S. Turner, and M. Lois Pollock

Introduction

A team is a strategy to achieve a goal, a means to an end. Team efforts centred on facilitating human flourishing in the face of eventually fatal illness, and especially in the face of approaching death, need clearly articulated goals, reformulated as often as necessary, in the light of changing circumstances and ethical dimensions. The increasing complexity of the tasks involved in palliative care as demonstrated in this book, and in the practice of palliative medicine as an ingredient of care, calls for a recognition of the increasing complexity (and multiplicity) of teams involved in the care of even one patient and his/her significant others.

The following scenarios may indicate the variability of the tasks and the challenges for interdisciplinary teams called to supplement the efforts of the core of any team: the patient and his or her closest associates. The questions may be asked of every case: What needs are obvious? At what points in the story? And what teams were involved in this patient's care?

1. A young village woman with locally advanced cancer of cervix, is brought by her husband to a city hospital in a developing country. She has severe pain in the left side of her pelvis, extending down the left thigh and into her calf. She can neither walk without pain nor sleep. The gynaecologist and the clinic provided her with paracetamol tablets. The hospital permits three injections of morphine in the post-operative period, but no morphine is permitted for medical use in other circumstances. There is no oral morphine. There are small supplies of codeine. Radiotherapy is available, with a 2-month waiting list: the cost of radiotherapy is equivalent to one quarter of her family's annual income. The woman has three small children in the village. There is a nurse at the village aid post, and arrangements are made for this patient to be taken home for care until radiotherapy can be commenced.

2. A village-based man, aged 40, father of five children, is found in a base hospital in a developing country to have advanced hepatocellular cancer. The family is advised to take him home to care for him until he dies, with the help of a nurse at a village aid post.

3. A professional man, 45, had melanoma excised from his upper back, in a major surgical referral centre in a university hospital. Two years later, he had a lump in the axilla (proven recurrence) excised and had local radiotherapy. Within 3 months, whilst remaining well and active he developed pain in the sacral region, worse on walking and he went to his local hospital. A fracture was noted on fifth lumbar vertebra, and he was transferred to the university hospital. Within the next few days pain had began to radiate down the anterior and lateral thigh, and although neurological tests were normal, he noted slight loss of power in right leg especially hip flexion and constipation for several days. A palliative medicine consultant recommended change in the analgesic regime and MRI, which demonstrated a mass near the cauda equina. Radiotherapy was begun that evening. The patient was emotionally shattered by the unequivocal evidence of metastatic melanoma. He does not wish his wife to be told that he has incurable and eventually fatal melanoma. A trial of chemotherapy (investigative) will be undertaken.

4. A woman in her 80s was sent down from a rural area, for surgery in a city hospital for presumed disc protrusion. Adenocarcinoma was found at the site: there was no obvious primary cancer. She became septic in the post-operative period, with delirium. A decision was made (with involvement of her daughter) for comfort care, with if possible,

transfer back to the country hospital under the care of general practitioner, (with the assistance of the hospital based palliative nurse consultant). She died before transfer was possible.

5. A professional woman in her early 60s, with considerable previous morbidity (including bilateral breast cancer 10 years previously), remained active in an artistic profession but noted rapidly progressive weakness over some months. Eventually, after extensive investigations at a tertiary institution, a diagnosis of motor neurone disease was made. She took legal steps to ensure that life-prolonging measures such as PEG feeding (in the face of increasing difficulty with swallowing) were not to be undertaken. She was transferred for care to a private hospital under the care of a palliative medicine specialist, with planned transfer to a specialist palliative care hospital if appropriate.
6. A woman in her 40s has slowly (over several years) progressing ovarian cancer despite extensive therapy, including debulking surgery twice, and several courses of chemotherapy. She is being cared for at home by a general practitioner with the assistance of a home care team and is socially active. She has experienced bouts of infection in the huge tumour mass, and again requires hospitalization for intensive antibiotic therapy, under the care of the palliative medicine specialist. She has recently noted depression and describes feeling fragile during the recent admission: earlier in her life she has experienced major depression. A liaison psychiatrist in consultation advises antidepressants. She hopes to return home, and wishes to be in a hospice for the last few days of her life.
7. A man with extensive head and neck cancer (currently admitted to a teaching hospital), with now well-relieved pain, refuses radiotherapy, or PEG feeding, and wants to be allowed to die. He has no one to care for him at home, but says he has a daughter, not seen for 30 years, in another city.
8. A woman aged 50 with glioblastoma is a single mother with an intellectually impaired son, a daughter involved in IV heroin use (both living with her), and a son in gaol for robbery. Her former partner was a violent alcohol abuser and has contact with her daughter. She can no longer care for her family, and her general practitioner advises that home care is no longer feasible, and she needs institutional care.
9. A woman in her 60s was found to have extensive recurrent cancer of her cervix: she had been previously treated with radiotherapy and had no signs of disease for 5 years. The tumour did not respond to chemotherapy, and she developed severe renal failure due to ureteric obstruction. Ureteric stents were inserted—with good result. Three months later she became severely dyspnoeic, with pulmonary metastases, pleural effusion, and possible pulmonary embolus. She wanted to be allowed to die, but her husband wanted 'everything to be done to save my wife'.

These cases, drawn from current practice, are merely an indication of the diverse spectrum of situations encountered. It is evident that the tasks in caring for patients with eventually fatal illness, and especially as death approaches, vary with:

1. the characteristics of the individual patient (age, gender, environment, personal history, cultural and biological inheritance, and the point in the illness saga);
2. prevailing needs and priorities of the patient and his/her family or significant others;
3. the context of care (place, economic, and cultural context);
4. resources (personal and non-personal) available, as well as required; notably, the skills and other competence needed;
5. agreed reasonable and appropriate goals.

The structure, and even more obviously, the function, and longevity of interdisciplinary teams relate to the varying tasks. Professionals in specialist palliative care services will necessarily have varying interfaces with professionals based in other services. Interdisciplinary teams will form, and reform, and change like the patterns in a kaleidoscope in the changing scenarios in health care systems—but what unifies the whole enterprise is the patient whose story is the common thread. All are at the service of this patient's well-being—as perceived by the patient in relation to his/her close associates. Such close associates, charged with assisting the patient, may include one trusted professional who is there throughout much of the story (be it years, months, weeks, or days), if he or she is fortunate, such as the family doctor, or an oncologist, or a palliative medicine practitioner, or a nurse practitioner, or a social worker or a pastoral care person—or person with legal status holding durable power of attorney.

Tasks

Tasks involved in palliative care may include the following of particular relevance to the practice of palliative medicine (by whoever exercises this responsibility):

1. diagnosis of progression or recurrence of disease—and appropriate communication of such information;
2. formulation of treatment plans for the disease and/or for symptoms, with due regard to ethical dimensions of the scenario;
3. implementing, monitoring, and formulation of new plans;
4. recognition of the dying phase ('the diagnosis of dying');
5. comprehensive personal care, support, recognition of suffering, alleviation of distress, restructuring of hope;
6. facilitating remote or proximate preparation for death;
7. professional support of family/carers, and especially including any involved children.

These tasks will be undertaken in most communities worldwide with little reference to specialist palliative care services. For example, an oncologist with a comprehensive view of cancer care, and familiarity with contemporary palliative medicine, and appropriate professional colleagues may well carry out such tasks. Specialists in immunology, respiratory medicine, cardiology, nephrology, in conjunction with general practitioners, regularly supervise the palliative care of the large numbers of patients with relevant progressive diseases. Specialist palliative care services (which may include trained, supported, and supervised volunteers) may efficiently supplement such mainstream health care services—or in some countries, may play a more prominent role, especially where the resources for antidisease therapy are limited (e.g. in HIV/AIDS), and good symptom relief, support and comprehensive care, however meagre the resources, becomes the keystone to the edifice of care. In many under-resourced communities the only help available may be non-professional carers, hopefully with some educational and personal support, even at a distance.

Prerequisites for good team work in interdisciplinary teams

Whatever the composition of teams, there are some fundamental prerequisites for effective and efficient teamwork:

- consensus and clarity regarding goal/objectives/strategies;
- recognition of the specific personal contribution of each team member;
- competence of each team member in his or her own discipline and understanding and respect for the competence and role of each other team member and procedures;
- clear definition of tasks and responsibility/accountability and means for communication within the teams;
- competent leadership appropriate to the structure and function of the team and the task(s) at hand (and leadership may vary with tasks);

- procedures for evaluating the effectiveness and quality of team efforts;
- bereavement care of staff as appropriate;
- recognition of the contribution of patients in furthering professional understanding.

All of these elements are interlinked, but for convenience may be considered separately—since each is complex, sometimes fraught with difficulties, and needs to be understood, and examined by all as part of the professional preparation for team participation.

Consensus and clarity regarding goals/objectives/strategies

If the goals/objectives and strategies are not agreed, tension within a team is inevitable. There may be diverse points of view with regard to matters such as patient priorities, or the balance to be struck in the face of competing demands or competing ethical principles. However, consensus must be reached, sometimes in a situation of considerable emotional tension.

It is useful to define precisely what are the differences of perspective or fact or opinion held by different team members. Sometimes the issues are matters of information: members of the team may not have complete information about, for example, the extent of a tumour, options remaining for antidisease therapy, unfortunate experiences with specific therapies in the past, or facts about family structure or function which need to be clear to all.

At other times the issues are philosophical, or ethical in the broad sense: for example, the value for personal development and growth of the last phase of life, as against a view that truncation of this phase to ensure unconsciousness or death even as soon as possible. Such matters require a sound anthropology(1) and point to necessary features of education for end-of-life care. It is an exercise of wisdom to balance respect for autonomy, commitment to beneficence, and to avoiding maleficence, with awareness of the demands of personal and social justice. There may be differences of opinion based in perceived legal difficulties: it is the responsibilities of educators to ensure that the legal dimensions of the practice of palliative medicine with respect to the location (country, state) of practice are understood and respected, and implemented.

In the process of reaching consensus there may be need to pause, while information is clarified, and team members have an opportunity to reflect on the situation—for a limited time (hours or days), and then communicate again. In most instances, consensus is readily achieved, but in the interface situation, where personnel from several hospital services are necessarily involved, as a team, for some hours, days or weeks, agreement needs to be carefully achieved and nurtured, with changes in focus, as time goes on, also agreed. The care of patients with progressive, eventual fatal disease, and especially near to death in acute hospitals, is receiving more attention and close scrutiny (see Chapter 2.2). Striving for continuity of care in such a context, where patients may move sometimes several times between hospitals, and between hospitals and community (home, hostel, or nursing home) requires efficient team work across several boundaries; extending for months, even years in the case of patients with relapsing, or partially controlled, but eventually fatal chronic conditions.

Continuity of care across the hospital–community interface is usually more easily achieved by having structures and procedures in place for discharge planning. A case manager—someone (or delegate) available to patient and family on a continuous basis—may be the wisest approach, where feasible. Where a patient moves within various elements of a palliative care service, communication is facilitated ideally by the possession of a core of attitudes and competence nurtured during education in palliative medicine, palliative nursing or palliative care centred social work. The goals and objectives as well as strategies should in such instances be readily understood as well as communicated. In other circumstances, much work is needed to communicate and ensure understanding of the goals of care and strategies being used.

Recognition of the specific personal contribution of each team member, and the allocation of tasks

In some settings (e.g. acute hospital settings), ad hoc team members may hardly know each other as persons—although their disciplines are readily understood (e.g. intensivist, cardiologist, etc). In other circumstances, especially within a comprehensive palliative care service with hospice/hospital/community components, one's team members become personally familiar. In either circumstance, but especially in the latter, there needs to be sensitive awareness to what a team member-as-person brings to the team (in addition to his or her professional competence). In brief, he or she will bring a specific personal style, his/her unique personal history, or an inheritance (biological and cultural) which will influence the rest, and he or she will usually have his or her own support system and personal network, outside the work situation. The person who must draw virtually all his/her personal sustenance from palliative care—or the one who uses other persons (patients or team members) as means to personal ends—are potentially hazardous for team work in palliative care. Self-awareness is essential, and opportunities for consideration of such matters, and the processes of personal growth and development need to be built into the educational process.

Competence of each team member in his or her own discipline

Interdisciplinary teams should not involve blurring the boundaries between disciplines: there may instead be a heightened need for specialized competence appropriate to the task. Doctors need to be good doctors, nurses to be good nurses, social workers to be good social workers and so on, but each should understand the capacities, as well as the limitations of the other disciplines. Responsibility and accountability of components of a group task can be then assigned, and boundaries clarified. Such a mosaic is a basis for integrated effort, not fragmentation.

Competent and appropriate leadership

A leader motivates, guides, and facilitates the activity of a team and takes overall responsibility for setting directions and planning strategies to achieve them, but acts in collaboration with team members. The principle of subsidiarity applies to the team: members should be facilitated to make decisions and exercise their highest capacities with individual accountability, but the leader must take overall responsibility for the direction struck and the quality of the total effort, and to be accountable for the well being of the team members in so far as work effort contributes, or detracts from this. The leader needs to recognize burdens too heavy for a team member to bear, or the team member who takes on unreasonable and worse, unauthorized care burdens, the team member who works incessantly maybe because there is no life outside work, or the team member who is 'burned out'(see Chapter 12.3). The leader does have a responsibility for the care of the team, whilst not at all taking away the responsibility of each individual for his or her own care.

Situations of tragedy may arise in the course of work devoted to the care of patients in the closing phase of life. A sense of tragedy may be compounded by the personal experience of the professional, and it is essential for professionals not to internalize the distress of their patients. Patients dying in despair, seriously at odds with the self, others, all that is, and hurting those who would care, or with horrific diseases causing disfigurement, and profound suffering (quite apart from symptoms difficult to relieve): patients can cause much distress in carers.

Research with respect to the suffering of doctors at the death of patients has prompted the following words which need to be borne in mind with reference to all team members.

> There is a last point to make about the doctor's suffering: suffering cannot be restricted to a list of feelings, causes, reactions and coping strategies . . . Human suffering does not amount to a physical or moral pain or to a difficulty. Suffering is something like crossing a sea, traversing a mountain or a desert; it is an experience,

painful indeed, in which the person will become more oneself and will discover oneself; it is an experience in which a person will experience evil, and yet, at the same time, will be led to discover and express the deepest meaning of one's life. This is true also for the suffering of the doctor.[2]

Procedures for evaluating the effectiveness and quality of team efforts

Evaluation of palliative care has rapidly evolving methodology (see Chapters 6.2 and 6.3). In addition to any systematic collection of patient/family data undertaken in the course of care, some process is needed for a team, as a team, to reflect on the experience of care, and any need to modify practice.

In an atmosphere of 'no fault', just a search for what may be regarded as 'bad outcomes' (just as a car manufacturer wants to find faulty cars) it is possible to have an experience of evaluation, directed at quality improvement. The 'bad outcomes' to be noted need to be agreed in advance, deaths without dignity according to agreed criteria, poor symptom relief, presentation to emergency department of a hospital, etc. and varied according to prevailing circumstances.[3] Whether or not this occurred in patients with whom a consultative service is in contact (or for whom a service is responsible), and the team then considers whether or not this occurrence was available—and if so, what could be done better in the future. Such a procedure assists in team building, in support in debriefing after traumatic stress to some extent, in sharing unavoidable or avoidable failure, and in immediate planning and implementation of new procedures.

The prerequisites in general for good team work in interdisciplinary teams have been demonstrated in a remarkable manner in the care of patients with HIV/AIDS. In particular, there has been recognition of the unique contributions of patients with AIDS, especially gay men with AIDS, in advancing medical science, in determining the appropriate shape of care systems, including emphasis on self-support.[4] There is pressing need for the innovations achieved in relation to HIV/AIDS to be extended into other areas of patient care.

Bereavement care of staff—as appropriate

The processes of bereavement may need to be facilitated not only for family and friends but also staff (see Chapters 12.2, 12.3, and 19). Bereavement overload, or disenfranchised grief, are both risks of professionals involved in palliative care. Post-traumatic stress disorder (PTSD) must also be recognized as a hazard, and appropriate debriefing procedures are essential for all staff.

Difficulties in team work

Attention to matters thus far considered may minimize problems in teams. However, problems can and do arise because of our shared humanity. Within teams grounded in specialist palliative care services where interpersonal relations are necessarily frequent and persistent over considerable periods of time, problems may arise with negative impact not only on team members, but on patient care. Conflict and demoralization need recognition. Conflict and/or demoralization in an interdisciplinary team may be provoked by poorly defined roles, deficiencies in communication, ineffective leadership, personality factors, scarcity of resources, poorly managed change, or events casting doubt on fundamental ideals or principles.

Conflict should usually be resolved peripherally—at the level at which the conflict is occurring—with minimal involvement of other persons. Where this is not possible, the existence of the conflict needs to be brought to the notice of the team leader, who may judge that a more senior administrator or facilitator may need to be involved. Such procedures should be rarely needed, but when truly needed, may be essential. Conflict between interfacing teams, if jeopardizing patient care, needs also to be addressed. Fundamentally, the conflict needs to be admitted, the shape of it articulated, the difference in perception of fact or of judgement clarified at the same time as common ground is sought as a basis for consensus. In most conflicts arising in teams (or between teams) comprised of conscientious staff, agreement should be achievable with respect to goals/objectives, and the precise areas of disagreement—and on the fundamentals of approaches to resolve the conflict by agreed solutions to be tried and evaluated.

Demoralization may accompany, result from, or reinforce conflict. The demoralization syndrome in patients is increasingly recognized. Demoralization in a team may be expressed in absenteeism, apathy, resistance to change, or deep sadness. A team may be wounded by poor leadership, or unreasonable burdens, but loss of vision, or loss of belief that the objectives are worth striving for, or utterly unachievable, requires recognition and attention. The team leader may need assistance from an outside resource to assist in rebuilding the team. Re-examining the foundations is a good start—such as, belief in the value of each person (however vulnerable and wounded), and in the potential of professional competence to enhance life, even at its close. Without a vision, the people perish—and so does a team. The philosopher Ernest Bloch, noted that a distinguishing feature of a leader is 'at midnight to be confident of the dawn'. Whoever is designated leader—whether by appointment, or consensus may need at times to recall such words.

Stresses to be faced by interdisciplinary teams involved in palliative care in the future

The burden humanity bears is in many ways, increasing, not only an increase in morbidity because of sheer force of numbers, but related to increases in mass disasters. Palliative care in circumstances of massive civil disaster is a challenge to teamwork of the highest order, and guidance is available.[5]

In other more conventional circumstances, two significant issues emerge, requiring consideration.

Increasing complexity in the needs of the patients to be cared for

Antidisease treatments are constantly evolving. Disease which were in recent memory regarded as inevitably and often rapidly fatal, are now seen as often or even usually controllable for some time (e.g. HIV/AIDS) or curable (e.g. childhood leukaemia).

The extensive inquiry in end-of-life care in the United States[6] has led to the recommendation that the principles of palliative care (with or without involvement of specialist palliative care services) should be in place from the time of diagnosis of eventually fatal illness with the emergence of the preferred 'mixed management model'. Such a concept enlarges considerably the scope of inquiry into teams and their roles in the care of patients in the closing phase of life, be it years, months, weeks, or days. It also has implications with reference to education and research.[7]

The earlier that patients are seen in their disease trajectory—by any professionals—and especially by specialists in palliative medicine, the more adequate the knowledge needed of options for antidisease treatment. Woe betide a palliative medicine practitioner, at least in an industrialized nation, who does not understand that some diseases may mimic cancer, that many patients with advanced cancers mandate serious consideration of chemotherapy, or that patients with advanced cardiac failure or neurological disease, or respiratory failure should experience adequate trials of appropriate therapy. Evidence-based medicine (EBM) must be taken into account when appraising whether or not a patient referred for assistance has had an adequate trial of antidisease therapy. Personal knowledge of EBM will always be limited, but communication is essential with relevant colleagues perceived then as team members in the search for knowledge as part of the task of patient care.

Patients become more complex with increasing complexity of evidence-based antidisease treatment capable of disease control, for a time at least.

Such a change affects the psyche also—for the patient is almost inevitably on a roller coaster with changing hopes, bouts of despair, the burden of an information load (significance of tumour markers, CT results, and so on) capable of deflecting energy from the task of living life to the full in a situation of probable time limitation. Furthermore, patients with diseases other than HIV/AIDS and their carers, are becoming more informed with respect to their diseases, and can be expected to play a far more significant role in the future in the evaluation, and in the evolution of systems of comprehensive care.

No patient can live without hope—but it is the task of team members sometimes to assist the patient (and family) on focusing hope on what will not fail: personal worth and dimensions of personal achievement, the fidelity of carers and so on, rather than on strategies which are means, not ends (such as blood counts, X-rays and other images, markers, or new drugs). The focus of hope will change, and team members require sensitivity to the implications of such change. Such a task—the support of patients on roller coasters—requires that each team member has a sound personal philosophy and an adequate view of the human condition and of human possibility. The team as a whole needs to have an understanding of what is being done to assist an individual patient—what is being said, and what is being hoped for, and the possibility of realizing that hope.

Increasing complexity and diversity of the context in which care is given

Care is needed wherever needy patients are located: good palliative care is not context bound, but strategies vary in different contexts: palliative care offered in an intensive care unit, or in an emergency department, or in a nursing home requires teamwork appropriate to the circumstance, and open to new approaches, and new complexities.

Obvious considerations are the diversities of location within the health system, changes in family structure and function, and in communities, and increasing cultural diversity: all these have implications for teams, so does extreme poverty. But there are other considerations quite central to the practice of palliative medicine and palliative care.

The history of the word 'hospice' has been outlined by many: hospice designed first a place (of safety on a journey) then a programme, then a philosophy. It has become useful to consider a person—a professional committed to palliative care—as a hospice—a place of safety. There is stress on the patient as guest in such a place: a challenge for hospitals and professions in all contexts.

Should an interdisciplinary team, which may include volunteers, regard itself as a team and its member individually as guests and the patient host? Issues such as avoiding the overloading of patients with unnecessary and uninvited professionals become more clear. It is the patient who should invite the professional. It is the professional who should behave as guest.

Privacy issues also become more clear. It is the patient who owns all clinical information—any other with access should recognize that it is by delegation of the patient, not by right. This concept is being embodied in law in several countries. There is rarely justification for private information concerning a patient to be divulged to team members in person or in writing either without the consent of the patient or in a situation where such consent would be unlikely to be given. What could not be said, of a personal nature, in the presence of a patient, should not normally be shared with a team unless the well being of the patient, family or the team are clearly at stake. The issue of confidentiality in patient care requires re-examination in connection with interdisciplinary team work, so that the values in which team work is rooted, fundamentally doing good (beneficence), aiding human flourishing, is carried out by the guest professionals in a manner appropriate to and acceptable to the patient, the team's host.

Interconnectedness of individuals needs to be fostered in the twenty-first century as old certainties become more fragile or even pass away and grand narratives may fail. Teams involved in the care of the frail and most vulnerable in society have the opportunity to demonstrate fundamental human solidarity and even as such to be bringers of hope.

References

1. **ten Have, H.** (1998). Images of man in philosophy of medicine. *Advances in Bioethics* 4, 173–93.
2. **Schaerer, R.** (1993). Suffering of the doctor linked with the death of patients. *Palliative Medicine* 7 (Suppl. 1), 27–37.
3. **Glare, P.A. and Lickiss, J.N.** (1992). Quality assurance in palliative care. *Medical Journal of Australia* **157**, 572.
4. **Woodruff, R. and Glare, P.** (2004). AIDS in adults. In *Oxford Textbook of Palliative Medicine*, 3rd edn. (ed. D. Doyle, N.I. Cherny, K. Calman, and G. Hanks), pp. 847–80. Oxford: Oxford University Press.
5. **International Working Group on Death, Dying and Bereavement.** Guidelines for Civil Disaster (in press).
6. **Field, M.J. and Cassel, K.**, ed. *Approaching Death: Improving Care at the End of Life.* Washington Institute of Medicine, National Academy Press, 1997, p. 85.
7. **Glare, P.A. and Virik, K.** (2001). Can we do better in end-of-life care? The mixed management model and palliative care. *Medical Journal of Australia* **175**, 530–3.

2.6 Economics-based palliative medicine

Alan Maynard

Introduction

Economists are often known as 'the dismal scientists' who produce doom-laden forecasts about topics such as unemployment, inflation, and economic growth. Health economists, a sub-species of the main tribe, tend to emphasize that there are only two things that are certain in life: death and taxes!

However, whilst death and taxes are unavoidable, they are not immutable. Life can be enhanced by health care investments, which not only can delay death but also improve patient well-being by repairing, stabilizing and controlling physical, social, and psychological quality of life. Furthermore, death can be humane and given dignity if resources are used carefully. In reality, then, health economics is a cheerful trade, concerned with postponing death and disability and reducing taxes by ensuring, in state-run health care systems like the United Kingdom National Health Service (NHS), that resource use is efficient and the tax burden on householders in minimized.

The pursuit of goals such as these by health economists is, inevitably, a collaborative enterprise. Everywhere, the dominant influence on resource allocation in health care is the physician. Medical practitioners are generally trained in the Hippocratic tradition, with an individualistic perspective. The Hippocratic oath involves, inter alia, an undertaking by the physician to:

> use my power to help the sick to the best of my ability and judgement; I will abstain from harming or wronging any man(1)

Modern medicine, like the society in which it operates, pays little attention to death.(2) Montaigne argued we 'should be ever booted and spurred and ready to depart'. Nowadays death, particularly if 'premature', is seen as a failure rather than something for which we should be prepared. An essential part of that preparation is an evidence base that is freely available for use by all. Such an evidence base might include how best to provide death education as well as how to palliate pain and distress in the closing period of life. The role of the medical professions in this latter activity is considerable.

The physician's ability to benefit his patient depends on the evidence he has available to determine which therapies improve the length and quality of life of which patients and to what extent. Cochrane[3] and others[4] challenged their medical colleagues with the assertion and evidence that many interventions had little or no scientific evidence as to their effect (hope-fully beneficial!) on the patient.

One effect of this criticism and questioning of the evidence based on the effectiveness of clinical interventions was the development of the evidence-based medicine (EBM) movement. David Sackett was a leading advocate of EBM. An American doctor who worked in Canada (McMaster University) and the United Kingdom (Oxford), Sackett asserted:

> Doctors practising evidence-based medicine will identify and apply the most efficacious interventions to maximise the quality and quantity of life for individual patients; this may raise rather than lower the cost of their care.[5]

The EBM approach has been challenged as an incomplete method for determining which patients should be treated.[6] This challenge is based on the economic concept of opportunity cost, or the value of what is given up (in terms of health gain) when one patient is treated and another is inevitably denied treatment. The economic perspective emphasizes measurement of the cost effectiveness of competing interventions, not just clinical effectiveness or whether a treatment 'works'. This is the new EBM, where the initials stand for economics-based medicine. With the new EBM, the policy focus is maximizing improvements in population health from a given, fixed budget by targeting treatments on the basis of their relative cost effectiveness.

Increasingly, the economic approach is likely to dominate choices about health care investment. The new EBM has to be understood, applied and utilized in palliative care as in all other areas of health and social care. Without understanding and applying techniques of economic evaluation, investment in palliative care may be fragmented and inadequate, leaving patients and their carers in avoidable disability, distress, and pain.

Why use the new EBM? (see Chapter 5.1)

Why is there a need for the new EBM? Always and everywhere resources are scarce. Whether in the case of the individual, the clinical team, the hospital, the hospice, or the NHS, resources are limited, and difficult choices have to be made as to who will be left in what degree of pain and discomfort and who, in extremis, will be left to die, hopefully in humane and well-cared-for circumstances. This problem is not new:

> who shall live and who shall die, who shall fulfil his days and shall die before his time
>
> Yom Kippur (Day of Atonement) Prayer Book

Traditionally, medicine has addressed such rationing issues with the old-style EBM: evidence-based medicine.[5] This approach emphasized the individual ethic inherent in the Hippocratic Oath and the consequent necessity to demonstrably 'do good' to the patient. To meet this requirement, physicians needed to know which interventions were clinically effective. Armed with information about 'what worked' in the medical armoury, the role of physicians was to treat the patient to the best of their ability until, in the limit, the benefits of care were zero. This individual perspective is of great appeal to patients and is part of the basis of patient–physician trust, with doctors acting as independent agents, doing their best for the patient in their care.

Whilst this approach to the deployment of scarce resources in health has dominated much of twentieth century medicine, it is incomplete. Paradoxically, at least in the initial stages, this was the prevailing perspective in the development of the Cochrane Collaboration, which informed old-style EBM. Yet Archie Cochrane, the physician after whom the network was named, clearly articulated the need to deploy resources on the basis of new-style EBM (or economics-based medicine). Thirty years ago he wrote:

> Allocation of funds and facilities are nearly always based on the opinions of senior consultants but, more and more requests for additional facilities will have to be based on detailed arguments with 'hard evidence' as to the gain to be expected from the patients' angle and the cost. Few can possibly object to this. (p. 82)[3]

Despite this clear advocacy of resource allocation in health care being based on the relative costs and benefits of competing patient interventions, the medical paradigm (old-style EBM) has continued to dominate health policy. This focus on clinical effectiveness is not wrong, but it is incomplete.

An illustration of this problem is:

(i) Therapy A produces 5 years of good quality life (or quality adjusted life years: QALYs) and therapy B produces 10 QALYs. (The QALY is a composite measure of health outcomes in which time in a health state is weighted by its quality. The weights assigned are between 1, best possible health, and 0, dead.)

(ii) The clinician and the individual patient would prefer therapy B, which gives the greatest benefit and is more clinically effective.

(iii) If therapy A costs £1000 and therapy B £7000, A produces a QALY at an average cost of £200, whilst therapy B's average cost per QALY is £700. Therapy B produces 5 more QALYs than therapy A, at an additional cost of £6000, making the incremental cost of QALY B £1200.

(iv) Whilst therapy B is clinically effective, therapy A is also clinically effective, though less so than therapy B, but more cost effective.

(v) If the total budget available in this therapeutic area is £700 000, investing in B produces 1000 QALYs, whilst investment in therapy A produces 3500 QALYs.

(vi) If the social goal is the allocation of resources to maximize improvements in population health from a given budget, the adoption of a more cost effective intervention (A) ensures achievement of this goal.

To illustrate how such considerations are no longer academic but central to the rationing of health care resources, it is useful to examine the United Kingdom regulatory agency, the National Institute for Clinical Excellence (NICE). When it was established, its Chairman, Professor Michael Rawlins, argued that NICE's function was not to ration resources, but to advise decision makers.[7] However, the subsequent behaviour of the Appraisal Committee of NICE contradicts Professor Rawlins' intentions.[8] In the 2001 annual report of NICE, it was acknowledged that the Appraisal Committee had consistently approved for NHS use, new technologies with a cost of below £30 000 per QALY. Beta-interferon for multiple sclerosis, the recent drug technology rejected by NICE in its initial decision, had cost-QALY characteristics of £40 000 and upwards.[9]

A mechanism similar to NICE, the Pharmaceutical Benefits programme, was initiated in Australia is 1993 and uses economic evidence to determine which new drugs are reimbursed is the Government's Medicare programme. Economic evidence is increasingly being used in other parts of the European Union (e.g. Finland, the Netherlands, and Spain) to inform decisions about the use of new technologies, especially pharmaceuticals.

The worldwide movement involving the adoption of the new EBM as advocated by Cochrane 30 years ago, will radically transform the way in which scarce health care resources are managed. Increasingly, palliative care managers, both clinical and non-clinical, will be challenged and purchasers will demand evidence that the investment in services offered to the dying are more cost effective than competing interventions such as the new drugs approved by NICE, as well as procedures such as hip replacements, coronary artery by-pass grafts, and renal analysis. Whilst this process will be gradual, it seems both inevitable and sensible for society's resources to be used in ways consistent with public policy goals.

What is involved in the new EBM?

EBM consists of the systematic evaluation of the costs and benefits of alternative ways of spending scarce health care resources. At its simplest,

Table 1 Types of economic evaluation

Type of evaluation	Cost measurement (£)	Outcome measurement	Outcome valuation
Costing studies	Yes	No	None
Cost minimization analysis (CMA)	Yes	No	None
Cost effectiveness analysis (CEA)	Yes	Yes	Specific, condition specific
Cost benefit analysis (CBA)	Yes	Yes	Monetary (£)
Cost utility analysis (CUA)	Yes	Yes	Generic (e.g. QALY)

economics is about valuing what is given up when a patient is treated (the opportunity cost of the value of alternative ways of using resources) and what is gained (the benefit, in terms of changes in the length and quality of life for the patients and their carers). The different types of economic evaluation are summarized in Table 1.

The costing of diseases is not proper economic evaluation (as no comparator is involved) but included here as a warning. Valuations of the cost of asthma, diabetes, and alcohol abuse are common in the literature, but tell decision-makers nothing about the clinical or economic effectiveness of competing interventions. Diseases may be costly with no efficient or effective treatment. Mere estimation of their cost is not a reason for investing in treatment in such areas!

Cost minimization analysis (CMA) involves the costing of two alternative interventions in a therapeutic area whilst assuming the outcomes are identical. The latter assumption is very strong and unrealistic as interventions usually have very different effects on patients. These techniques (costing and CMA) are of limited use for informing rationing choices.

Cost effectiveness analysis (CEA) was developed by the United States Pentagon in the Korean War. They used 'body count' as the 'outcome' measure and investigated the costs of alternative methods (e.g. artillery, napalm, and infantry) of killing their enemies! In health care, the outcome measure is usually condition specific (e.g. lives saved by renal dialysis and millimetre of mercury score decreased by hypertension treatment). CEA identifies the costs of the alternative and the condition-specific benefits. CEA is, as a consequence, useful in informing choices about interventions within a therapeutic area (e.g. renal dialysis or renal transplantation) but not for informing choices between therapeutic areas (e.g. renal or cardiac interventions).

Application of CEA in palliative care can, for instance, compare the use of chemotherapy and the use of best-available supportive care (BASC). If the end-point measure used in such an evaluation is, for example, 2- and 3-month survival, chemotherapy may give the best effect at the highest cost. However, this narrow focus (survival duration) gives no information to decision-makers about the comparative quality of survival.

Cost benefit analysis (CBA) is a term often used by the uninitiated as being the same as economic evaluation. The latter is a generic term, whilst CBA is a specific type of economic evaluation. It involves the identification of the costs and benefits of the alternatives and their valuation in a common denominator—money. Valuation of the control of pain is difficult enough, but the translation of such pain measures into monetary equivalents is even more difficult. Various techniques can be used to elicit the values people place on complex medical benefits: for example, the willingness to pay approach and the use of discrete choice analysis.

Cost utility analysis (CUA) involves the costing of the alternatives and the valuation of benefits in terms of the generic measure (e.g. QALYs). The use of generic measure means that this type of analysis can be used to inform choices within and between therapeutic categories. It is this approach that has been used by NICE. An example of its use in palliative care is a Canadian paper,[10] which compared two chemotherapy regimes and BASC. The latter had the lowest cost per QALY ($23 368) and the cost per QALY of the chemotherapy options exceeded $40 000.

Guidelines for economic evaluation

Guidelines or checklists to facilitate the practice of economic evaluation have been available for over 25 years (e.g. see Williams' checklist in Appendix 1[11]). The economic evaluation literature is complex and esoteric in some respects. A guide to this literature is offered in Appendix 2.

There are seven fundamental steps in economic evaluation in health care:

(i) identification of the study question,

(ii) identification of the alternatives to be appraised,

(iii) identification, measurement, and valuation of all the relevant costs,

(iv) identification, measurement, and valuation of all the relevant benefits,

(v) adjustment of costs and benefits to take account of their timing (discounting) and uncertainty,

(vi) undertaking of sensitivity analysis, and

(vii) identification and agreement of the decision rule (considerations of efficiency and equity).

These steps will now be elaborated in the context of palliative care. Palliative care has been defined by the WHO as 'the active total care of patients whose disease is not responsive to curative treatment. Control of pain, of other symptoms and of psychological, social and spiritual problems is paramount. The goal of palliative care is achievement of the best possible quality of life for patients and their families.'[12] Like many WHO definitions, this is vague, well intentioned, and totally isolated from new EBM considerations.

According to the United States Institute of Medicine (IOM), four basic elements are required for the care of the dying: understanding the physical, psychological, spiritual, and practical dimensions of care-giving; identifying and communication diagnosis and prognosis; establishing goals and plans; and fitting palliative and other care to these goals.[13] As with the WHO definition, the IOM's basic elements are useful but incomplete, tending to underplay the need to evaluate the relative costs and benefits of care to ensure that it is cost effective.

The literature on palliative medicine increasingly recognizes the incomplete nature of the evidence about the clinical effectiveness of care options.[14] There is relatively little literature reporting economic evaluations in palliative care, although several authors have identified the need for such analyses.[15–18] Economic evaluation in this area offers some challenges.

Identification of the study question

Whilst advocacy of economic evaluation of palliative care may be easy, identifying and agreeing upon the study question is often difficult and contentious. For instance, Hearn and Higginson[19] carried out a systematic review of specialist palliative care teams and their effects on outcomes for cancer patients. They identified 18 studies, some of which were randomized control studies (in many cases the randomization methods were not reported) and others used different quasi-experimental methods. They concluded that there was some evidence that specialist care did provide better outcomes for cancer patients.

Their review demonstrates the strengths and weaknesses of the study question. Whilst specialist teams give apparent benefits, the heterogeneity in the nature of the specialist teams and the weak costing, rather than proper economic evaluation, makes it difficult to identify the causes and the costs of the improved outcomes produced by the different specialist teams.

Identification of the alternatives to be appraised

Economic evaluation, like clinical evaluation, is about the comparison of the characteristics of alternative ways of delivering care to a patient with a particular diagnosis. Inappropriate selection of a comparator can produce biased estimates in the evaluation. Some regulatory authorities, which require economic evaluation to inform their reimbursement decisions, set out clearly the choice of comparator, for example, the 'usual' current treatment or the cheapest alternative treatment. Careless, or 'strategic' selection of a comparator can corrupt the evidence base. For instance, it is not clear whether it was careless or strategic when one team investigating the therapeutic characteristics of a new antipsychotic compared it with a very high dose of the usual treatment, haloperidol.[20] This made the new product look very 'attractive'.

Identification, measurement, and valuation of all relevant costs

The distinctions between identification, measurement, and valuation are important and the authors of studies should be explicit about which costs get fully appraised and which are omitted (and why) during the course of a study. In many study areas, and palliative care is one, costs are imposed on the patient, the carer agencies (public and private), and carers (e.g. relatives and friends).

Identification, measurement, and valuation of all relevant benefits

Once again, benefits may accrue to patients and their carers. In palliative care, the goal may not be so much enhancing the length of life but ensuring the quality of the remaining weeks or months is controlled (e.g. in terms of pain) and is of the best possible quality. Authors advocating the increased use of economic evaluation in palliative care typically point to the area of benefit measurement as being one of the most difficult.[15–18] Practitioners in the subject area use a range of different specific quality of life instruments and there is concern, not only about the lack of consensus as to which of these is best for measuring particular end points, but also about the sensitivity of generic quality of life measures, such as short form 36 (SF36) and the Euro-qol (EQ5D). Systematic exploration of the relative attributes of both specific (e.g. pain control instruments) and generic quality of life measures (which evaluate physical, social, and psychological well being in simple and succinct ways) should be a priority in future evaluation work in palliative medicine.

In all estimations of benefits, the result is influenced by the selection of the end-point. Survival is often emphasized as the end-point in many cancer trials, but for patients, quality of life is crucial. Combining such end-points into, for instance, estimates of QALYs can be important but remains a rather crude science.

Adjustments for timing and uncertainty

Whilst much palliative medicine is short term and intense in the last weeks of life, some interventions may be over a longer time period. For such interventions and much of the rest of health care, these time horizons need to be dealt with carefully in economic evaluation.

If you are offered the choice between £1000 now or £1000 in 1 year, generally you will prefer £1000 now. If you are offered the choice of repaying a debt of £1000 now or in a year's time, you will likely prefer the latter. This is what is called time preference. When costs and benefits occur over time, it is usual to adjust their value, a process called discounting, to take account of time preference. Similarly, adjustments may be made if elements of the costs and benefits have varying degrees of uncertainty associated with them. Adjustments to take account of a range of probabilities can be made.

Sensitivity analysis

As in clinical evaluation, the results of any appraisal should be subjected to sensitivity analysis. Variations in the values of elements of the costs and benefits streams should be applied to determine the robustness of the study results.

Agreeing the decision rule

The construction of the study results should ensure the production of data relevant to the decision-makers' rules about the prioritization of investments in patient care. Increasingly, as evidenced by the work of NICE in the United Kingdom, this means that cost–QALY estimates should be generated so that the ranking of the technology in some 'league table' can be identified. Alternative decision rules and elaboration of the procedures can be found in the standard textbooks about economic evaluation.[21,22]

Making difficult decisions

Rationing is ubiquitous. It is nonsense to debate whether there is rationing in health care. The issue is not 'if' but 'how' it is practised. Rationing in health care occurs 'when someone is denied (or simply not offered) an intervention that everyone agrees would do them some good and which they would like to have'.[23] This simple definition emphasizes that denial of care, even when it is clinically effective (but not cost effective), should be expected in all health care systems which seek to use scarce resources efficiently. Thus, beta-interferon benefits are relatively small and because the cost of an annual course of this drug is high (and three times that in Australia), the intervention is not cost effective—as NICE has pointed out.

Another important aspect of this definition concerns therapies the patient 'would like to have'. Often the attributes of alternative therapies are not well defined, let alone shared with patients and carers. Better evaluation, both clinical and economic, could be used to inform patients more fully. There is now good evidence (e.g. from experimentation comparing well-informed patient decisions with surgeon-led decisions in prostate care) that patients choose far more conservatively than medical practitioners. 'Commando surgery' in head and neck cancer may be regretted by ill-informed patients struggling for marginal additions to survival with 'tolerable' quality of life.

Efficacy and equity

The new EBM approach emphasizes the goal of efficiency, though the society shows by its public choices that this is not the only policy consideration. The investments made to enhance the survival of low birth weight babies are inefficient: they produce, at high cost, survivors who often exhibit high degrees of intellectual and physical disabilities. However, the society continues to invest in low birth weight and other marginal babies because of the apparent high value it places on 'new, young' life. These choices imply that the society is prepared to pay more for a QALY in this area, than it is to buy a QALY for mature adults.

This 'equity' consideration has been elaborated in a number of different ways. For instance, Williams[24] has put forward the 'fair innings' argument in which he (now in his mid-70s) advocates discrimination against the elderly (who have had a fair innings) in favour of, for instance, the young disabled (who have not had a good innings). A consequence of adopting such a rule would be that hip replacements for the elderly (a cost-effective intervention) might be delayed to fund beta-interferon for young multiple sclerosis sufferers (an inefficient intervention).

An alternative argument might be that discrimination and the use of inefficient interventions might be socially preferred not only at birth but also at death. We might, then, weight QALYs generated from investment in the care of the dying to reflect a higher social valuation than care for a hernia repair for a middle-aged adult. Such weighting would reflect the society's desire for people to have a good death.

Such propositions raise major issues of how equity weights should be determined and by whom. Any such weighting is a decision to give up greater health gains by treating patients efficiently, and to achieve fewer health gains by treating patients inefficiently. Such choices should be explicit and those who make them should be publicly accountable (unlike at present!). 'Efficiency rules OK!' is the implicit value inherent in economics. However, as many practitioners of the cheerful science have emphasized, distributional or equity considerations are a fact of political life which need to be built into resource allocation or rationing decisions. To ignore equity and preach efficiency alone is a dangerous game. But equally, to preach clinical effectiveness ignoring efficiency and equity issues, as many physicians and other health professionals do, is a disservice to both patients and their carers.

Making treatment and care choices within palliative care and between palliative care and the numerous other health areas is little more than an unevaluated social experiment at present. This leads to inefficient medical practices and depriving patients of care from which they would benefit. In future, the criteria used to determine such difficult choices should be explicit and socially agreed upon so that all involved can be accountable.

Conclusion

Practitioners are delivering care packages that have not been evaluated from the clinical, let alone economic perspective (new EBM). As in all areas of medicine, there is some relevant evidence to inform intervention choices but more knowledge is needed to inform the allocation or rationing of resources in palliative care.[14] The tradition of medicine, to believe that good is being done to patients at least cost in the absence of evidence, has to be replaced by scepticism which can only be displaced by the best scientific knowledge.

Social experimentation based on beliefs and unsubstantiated assertions is inefficient and unethical. Patients in their last weeks and months of life can, and often do, face a lottery determined by the presence or absence of local leadership and the provision of care. With better measurement of the economic attributes of palliative care, existing funding can be better defended and new funding acquired if such investments are demonstrably cost effective. If they are not cost effective and the resources could generate greater health benefits to patients elsewhere in the health care system, it is sensible (i.e. efficient) to deprive palliative care of funding. Playing Oliver and demanding 'more' will no longer serve the interests of patients in any part of the health care system.

To return to the beginning, Benjamin Franklin declared in 1789 'in this world nothing can be said to be certain, except death and taxes'. Researchers, advocates, and providers in palliative care need to adopt the new EBM perspective to ensure that death is delayed and of good quality and that taxes are minimized. Any other action would be a folly.

Appendix 1

Williams' checklist for economic evaluation

1. What precisely is the question that the study was trying to answer?
2. What is the question that it has actually answered?
3. What are the assumed objectives of the activity studied?
4. By what measures are these represented?
5. How are they weighted?
6. Do they enable us to tell whether the objectives are being attained?
7. What range of options was considered?
8. What other options might there have been?
9. Were they rejected, or not considered, for good reasons?
10. Would their inclusions have been likely to change the results?
11. Is anyone likely to be affected who has not been considered in the analysis?
12. If so, why are they excluded?
13. Does the notion of cost go wider or deeper than the expenditure of the agency concerned?
14. If not, is it clear that these expenditures cover all the resources used and accurately represent their value if released for other uses?
15. If so, is the line drawn so as to include all potential beneficiaries and losers and are the resources costed at their value in their best alternative use?
16. Is the differential timing of the items in the streams of benefits and costs suitably taken care of (e.g. by discounting and, if so, at what rate)?
17. Where there is uncertainty, or known margins of error, is it made clear how sensitive the outcome is to these elements?
18. Are the results, on balance, good enough for the job in hand?
19. Has anyone else done better?

He remarked in conclusion: 'The last two have been added because I do not want to be accused of advocating a counsel of perfection. Decisions do have to be made and will continue to be made on the basis of imperfect knowledge. But I am anxious to ensure that we know how little we know when we do what we have to do.'

Appendix 2

A guide to the literature on economic evaluation

1. For practitioners and researchers who have little experience of the economics literature, some initial reading should include:
   a. Jefferson, T., Dermichi, V., and Mugford, M. *Elementary Economic Evaluation in Health Care* 2nd edn. London: BMJ Publishing, 2000.
   b. Williams.[11]
2. The standard text books in economic evaluation are:
   a. Gold et al.[22] which is American in its orientation.
   b. Drummond, M.F.[21] which is British–Canadian in its orientation.
3. An invaluable aid to an understanding of these economic techniques is to see how guideline criteria can be used to 'take apart' and review some of the existing literature. Examples of this are:
   a. Drummond, M.F. *Studies in Economic Appraisal of Health Care.* Oxford: Oxford University Press, 1981.
   b. NHS Economic Evaluation Database: this can be accessed through both the NHS Centre for Reviews and Dissemination at the University of York and the Cochrane Collaboration. This database is updated each month. Users can directly access individual records as well as the general website (http://nhscrd.york.ac.uk/nhsdhp.htm). Readers of this database will find that most of the palliative care studies listed are not regarded as economic evaluations but as limited cost studies. All proper economic evaluations are critically appraised on this website in a way similar to Drummond's book of case studies (3a. above).

References

1. **Lloyd, G.E.R.**, ed. *Hippocratic Writings.* Harmondsworth: Penguin Books, 1983.
2. **Smith, R.** (2000). A good death. *British Medical Journal* **320**, 129–30.
3. **Cochrane, A.L.** *Effectiveness and Efficiency: Random Reflections on Health Services.* London: Nuffield Provincial Hospitals Trust, 1972.
4. **Bunker, J., Barnes, B., and Mosteller, F.**, ed. *Costs, Risks and Benefits of Surgery.* New York: Oxford University Press, 1977.
5. **Sackett, D.L., Rosenberg, W.M.C., Muir Gray, J.A., Haynes, R.B., and Richardson, W.S.** (1996). Evidence based medicine: what it is and what it isn't. *British Journal of Medicine* **213**, 71–2.
6. **Maynard, A.** (1977). Evidence based medicine: an incomplete method for informing treatment choices. *Lancet* **349**, 126–8.
7. **Rawlins, M.** (1999). In pursuit of quality: the national institute for clinical excellence. *Lancet* **353**, 1079–82.
8. **Timmins, N.** *Drugs and the NHS's £30000 question.* Financial Times, August 10th, 2001, p. 17.
9. **National Institute for Clinical Excellence.** *Appraisal of Beta Interferon/ Glatiramer for Multiple Sclerosis Provisional Appraisal Determination.* August 2001. Available at http://www.nice.org.uk/
10. **Kennedy, W.** et al. (1995). Cost utility of chemotherapy and best supportive care in non-small cell lung cancer. *PharmacoEconomics* **8**, 316–23.
11. **Williams, A.** (1974). The cost–benefit approach. *British Medical Bulletin* **30** (3), 252–6.
12. **World Health Organization.** *WHO Definition of Palliative Care,* www.who.int/hiv/topics/palliative/PalliativeCare/en, 1990.
13. **Institute of Medicine.** *Approaching Death: Improving the End of Life.* Washington DC: National Academy of Sciences, 1997.
14. **Higginson, I.J.** (1999). Evidence based palliative care. *British Medical Journal* **319**, 462–3.
15. **Normand, C.** (1996). Economics and evaluation of palliative care. *Palliative Medicine* **10**, 3–4.
16. **Watkins-Bruner, D.** (1998). Cost effectiveness and palliative care: seminars on oncology. *Nursing* **14** (2), 164–7.
17. **Bruera, E. and Suarez-Almozor, M.** (1998). Cost effectiveness in palliative care. *Palliative Medicine* **12**, 315–16.
18. **Higginson, I. and Edmonds, P.** (1999). Services, costs and appropriate outcomes in end of life care. *Annals of Oncology* **10**, 135–6.
19. **Hearn, J. and Higginson, I.** (1997). Do specialist palliative care teams improve outcomes for cancer patients? A systematic literature review. *Palliative Medicine* **12**, 317–32.
20. **Geddes, J., Freemantle, N., Harrison, P., and Bebbington, P.** (2000). Atypical antipsychotics in the treatment of schizophrenia: systematic overview and meta-regression analysis. *British Medical Journal* **321**, 1371–6.
21. **Drummond, M.F., O'Brien, B., Stoddart, G.L., and Torrance, G.W.** *Methods for the Economic Evaluation of Health Care Programmes* 2nd edn. Oxford: Oxford University Press, 1997.
22. **Gold, M., Siegel, J.E., Russell, L.B., and Weinstein, M.C.**, ed. *Cost Effectiveness in Health and Medicare.* New York: Oxford University Press, 1996.
23. **Williams A.** Personal communication, 1998.
24. **Williams, A.** (1997). Rationing health care by age: the case for. *British Medical Journal* **314**, 820–2.

3

Ethical issues

3 Ethical issues

3.1 Introduction

Kenneth Calman

It might be asked why it is relevant to have a chapter on ethics in a textbook of palliative medicine. The reason should be clear, in that much of the reasoning behind making decisions with patients on how best to manage the complexity of the problems requires that judgements are made. Such judgements are based on values held by the patient, the family, and the doctor. There may well be differences in views, and almost always there will be uncertainty. It is this uncertainty which makes the whole field so difficult and one in which legitimate differences of opinion can occur.

The purpose of having an ethical view of palliative care

The purpose of this chapter is to assist the professional to be able to analyse a clinical issue from an ethical point of view, and indeed to be able to identify an ethical issue in the first place. It will also introduce a range of concepts which are helpful in understanding ethical issues, and allow a comparison to be made between the person's own values and those of others. It should also encourage a logical approach and the ability to marshal arguments in favour of one's own position and understand that others may have different views. In essence, it is about understanding one's own values and how they compare with those of others.

This chapter is designed to set the scene for the more detailed sections which follow in subsequent chapters.

Developing an ethical framework

A discussion of ethical issues in palliative care usually revolves around a series of values held by all participants, which influence the clinical decision-making process. This will always include the patient's values and almost always those of the family. The way we consider our own values is generally around a framework of concepts, some of which may even be mutually incompatible. The framework may be based on duties, rights, or a series of principles such as autonomy, and it is the balance between such principles which determines the outcome of the decision-making.

The framework adopted by any individual (patient, family member, or professional) may vary on these factors (duties, right, and principles) alone. However, if one adds into this differences in social, cultural, and spiritual aspects of life, then the possibilities become much more complex. From this brief discussion certain conclusions can be drawn.

- There are many different ways in which framework for ethical decision-making can be constructed.
- These variations are relevant to making decisions which will almost always be in the face of uncertainty, and thus judgements will be required.
- Because of this there is ample scope for disagreement on what to do.
- There can be no right or wrong approach, just differences between different value bases held by individuals.

These brief conclusions raise other issues such as what to do when there is a disagreement, and how such disagreements should be dealt with, and these will be discussed later.

Where do values come from?

If values are so important how are our own values formed, and where do they come from? There are a whole series of ways some of which, and for each individual, may be more important than others. These might include;

- *Upbringing and parental values.* These can be important in terms of early religious experiences, attitudes to discipline and the context of the family. Political influences and attitudes may also be established in this process.
- *Schooling is the next major factor.* The role of the teacher, school values, and subjects taught also influence our thinking.
- *Religious background may be critical in setting values.* Different religions have different ways of looking at issues and even within a single religious group there may be considerable variation in views. For example, within the Christian religion views on end of life decisions and abortion vary considerably.
- *Peer pressure.* This can be very important in setting values as the need to conform, and not have views which would be outside the context of the group, which may be seen as abnormal. This pressure occurs not only in the context of school but also at work and at play.
- *Role models.* We all have role models, people we look up to and admire, and whose values we espouse. For professionals these can be crucial. The 'hidden' agenda in medicine is very powerful. Doctors, and others, learn from the attitudes and behaviour of seniors. It is difficult to underestimate the importance of this, especially if there are differences of views in the clinical team. For patients the comments of friends and loved ones, those who play a significant part in their lives, are very relevant indeed.
- *Professional education and experience.* As medical students and postgraduate staff learn more about the possibilities in palliative care, and lack of them, for the management of symptoms, or improving quality of life, so views can change. Meeting and helping a particular patient can have a profound effect, both positive and negative.
- *The media.* Debates in the media, for example, about end of life issues, can influence public opinion and those of patients and their families. The discussions may be informative, but are sometimes unrealistic and can raise expectations about possible outcomes.

- *Learning about ethics.* Part of being a professional is being concerned with ethical issues. It is necessary therefore to take time to learn about the concepts which are relevant and to be able to justify one's own position. Ethics may be learned in a variety of ways: through courses, reading, and by testing experience against the concepts. It should be clear, however, that having an ethical approach to palliative care is not about a 1-week lecture course, it is about attitudes and values which occur in everyday practice. It is an ongoing process and a part of continuing professional development.
- *Codes of ethics.* In some cases the values which are seen to be important have been codified and written down. The most famous of these is the Hippocratic Oath, which sets out some of the ethical principles which the doctor should follow. There are many others, including the Helsinki Declaration and the Declaration of Human Rights. These provide useful checks and prompts for those practising palliative medicine.

Such influences, and there are many others, shape our feelings and our values and it is these which are tested at times of uncertainty. They guide us in what to do in difficult circumstances. This leads to a discussion on the concepts and principles, which we collectively call our values.

Some key concepts

The following section sets out some of the key concepts which may be relevant in building up a personal ethical framework. It draws from a variety of different sources over several millennia, and the reader is advised to consult the reading list at the end of this chapter for further information and greater detail.

- *A duty to alleviate suffering.* This is an obvious concept, but like all such concepts not as simple as it seems. Of course we should alleviate suffering, but at what cost, either clinical or financial? How far should we go to alleviate suffering? Would this include active euthanasia? What if the symptom is difficult to alleviate and we fail? Have we failed in our duty?
- *Respect for persons.* Once again, this is an obvious concept to consider. It is important that we consider the individual and their dignity in the palliative care setting. How we communicate, how we show respect and courtesy, all matter. This also means respecting the wishes of patients and their values, even if they differ from our own, and this can be a source of conflict. Respect for persons is associated with the concept of confidentiality. This sets out the right of the patient to have information about them, or their condition, kept within a limited number of members of the team, and in some instances by only one of them. It is a very important principle and one which can be easily breached as teams become larger and access to information easier.
- *Autonomy.* This is a concept, related to respect. It states that each individual has a right to make decisions about his/her own life and as a sentient human being is capable of so doing. It is difficult to disagree with this concept but it can, like so many other issues, raise problems. These include how far we should bend to patient's wishes, and whether we should at anytime refuse to do what the patient wants. Such issues need to be thought through and would include the patients asking for a particular treatment which might not be available, or is too expensive, or one's own ethical framework is at odds with the patient's decision. A key part of autonomy is the ability of the patient to consent to treatment or care. Their wishes should be respected and they have a right to refuse treatment offered whether or not it makes sense to the doctor.
- *Non-maleficence.* This at first sight seems entirely appropriate. We should not do anything which may cause a potential harm to the patient. Once again how this works in practice is more difficult. Much of what we do, for example, in cancer treatment is potentially harmful, and the benefit might not always be clear. The dictum, *primum non nocere*—first do no harm—can be difficult to live up to.
- *Beneficence.* This implies that we should always do the best for our patients. Difficult to disagree with. However, it also implies that we as individual professionals have the skills and expertise to deal with the problem, and the wisdom to refer the patient to someone else if we already have not. There is a major ethical issue here in the professional competence of the doctor and this is discussed in greater detail in Chapter 3.4 and Section 20.
- *Utility.* This is an important concept in developing our framework of ethics. In short, it makes the point that the basis for care should be for the greatest good of the greatest number. We should do what we can to alleviate the suffering of the majority. This has obvious difficulties faced with an individual patient who might fall outside of the category of 'greatest number' for whatever reason, but when resources are limited, and that includes our time, how do we rationalize this concept?
- *Justice.* This implies fairness for all and equity and equality of care. Clearly this is impossible to achieve in all instances. Even in the field of palliative care it is obvious that patients with cancer have a greater chance of being looked after by a palliative care service than a patient with cardiac and respiratory disease. Is this right and fair?
- *Human rights.* A good case can be made for using a rights-based approach. This begins by defining what such rights are and how they can be enforced. The right to life, the right to respect, the right to education, are all part of this approach.

This brief review does no more than indicate some of the concepts that form part of the development of a framework of ethics which help each of us to make difficult decisions in the face of uncertainty.

Some example of conflicts

The principles listed above are often in conflict with each other, and the following examples give some indication of the complexities involved. Here are a few clinical examples to put these principles in context.

- *The right to life.* This is a fundamental principle with which few would disagree. However, in end of life situations how far should we go to keep life going? Should no expense be spared even if this means that others cannot have a service provided, either through a funding shortage or lack of clinical time? This has especial difficulty in the case of children where emotional issues are raised and these are fully discussed in Chapter 3.5.
- *Autonomy.* The patient has a right to his or her own views, but what happens if we disagree? Suppose the patient wants us to 'end it all' and asks for euthanasia as an active process and that this is against our own values? The concept of autonomy suggests that the wishes should be enacted, but it is impossible for us to do so.
- *Telling the truth.* It would be natural to tell the truth to patients about their illness and the possible treatment. Several different scenarios present themselves, however. The first is when a relative approaches the doctor and asks that the patient is not told of the diagnosis or the prognosis. The second is the converse where the patient does not wish the family to know, but what if this is an infectious disease (HIV infection) or a genetic disorder which might be transmitted to a member of the family?
- *Issues of research.* There are many ways in which conflicts may arise in research projects and these are dealt with in detail in Chapter 3.6. One familiar example, particular to nursing staff engaged in observational research, is when the procedure being studied is being performed badly. Does one intervene and correct the process, and hence destroy the research work, or leave the situation and potentially harm the patient?

Making decisions

At the end of the day it is our values that are of assistance in making decisions. The issue of uncertainty and the need for judgement have already been alluded to. The section looks at some of the components of the decision-making process.

- First, what is the evidence available about the patient, the possible symptom, and how can it best be controlled? What treatments are available, including non-pharmacological methods?

- What is the usual outcome of the process? Would the treatment be better carried out elsewhere? Are all the skills and expertise required available?
- What are the views of the patient? Are they the same as that of the family and the physician?
- If the views are different, can you see a way of supporting the wishes of the patient, or do you disagree?
- Has the patient been given all the information and have they consented to the possible intervention?

Going through this process (or something similar to it) can sometimes identify ways of reconciling differences of view or identify new ways of approaching the problem. It is part of good medical practice and is not a new method.

A key part of the whole process is the issue of trust between the patient and the doctor. Such trust takes time to build and can be lost rapidly. The old proverb 'trust comes on foot and goes on horse back' feels true. How can this trust be developed? It will require getting to know the patient, being honest, and always keeping promises. Explaining the procedures, what will happen, who will be there, and what their roles will be is very much part of this. Trust means allowing someone to do something one would not normally let them do. It means giving up some autonomy. An example might help to illustrate some of these issues. Suppose you are going out for the evening and you ask a 20-year old to look after your two children aged 5 and 7. You trust the person, though you know that something untoward may happen. You know that if it does it will not be deliberate. The baby sitter has the interest of the children at heart. The same concept applies to patients. If they trust the doctor, then they give up some of their own control and give it to the doctor whom they know will not do anything deliberately harmful and will always be doing it in the best interests of the patient. The patient knows that they will be kept fully informed and that their views will be respected at all times.

The reason this concept is so important is that in the management of uncertainty there will always be unknowns. It will not always be possible to give all of the information because the nature of the problem may be unknown. Trust bridges the gap and allows the patient to have the most appropriate course of action. Martin Buber in his book 'I and Thou' sets this out rather differently, but with the same outcome. He makes the point that some relationships are 'I and You' ones. There is respect but there is also a professional distance between the patient and the doctor. Some of the relationships however, are 'I and Thou' ones which are much closer, there is real trust, there is a 'sharing of hearts', and the depth of the relationship is considerable. Trust is part of this and those who work regularly in the palliative care field will recognize such relationships. Trust is a fundamental part of the patient–doctor relationship.

Dealing with disagreements (see Chapters 17.1 and 20.4)

So far there has been an assumption that everyone will agree with the outcome of the decision-making process. As the examples discussed above make clear, this is not always the case and the problem is what to do in such circumstances. There are three possible scenarios.

1. *The patient and the doctor disagree.* It is not difficult to see how such differences can come about. Poor communication, lack of trust, and differences in values, all contribute. The real issue is what to do about it? This is a situation where the doctor must not be proud and must show humility. The patient is generally right. There should be an open referral to another professional who may look at the situation from a different perspective and with a different value base. Such referrals should be made early in the process before resentment and anger build up.
2. *The patient and the family disagree.* This is a particularly tragic problem, when at a time when the family should be supportive and positive, there are family disagreements, tension, and difficulty in communicating. It requires a skilled professional to help the family come together and make the most of the remaining life of the patient.
3. *Inter-professional disputes.* These are common and the result of professional education and the building of values. Disagreements can be a positive and learning experience for all. The problem arises when one member of the staff has values which are different from the others' and after discussion there is no meeting of minds. This can often occur when a new member joins the team and challenges the values of others. What should be done in this instance? There can be an agreement to differ and that the group view, or that of the senior professional, prevails. The learning experience following the outcome of the decision can be very important. This may not be sufficient, however, and the member of staff still disagrees. Under these circumstances, where the ethical principles of the doctor may be compromised, it is often useful to talk the problem over with a senior colleague. It may be that the practice is unethical in the views of others and this must be shared. In extreme circumstances, the views of the individual may be so incompatible with that of the team that the staff member has to resign.

Working in other cultures

A particular subset of the differences in values which may occur relates to working in different cultures, religious faiths, or social systems. Here, the differences may be very significant and the doctor may have to accept the views of the different culture, no matter how difficult it may seem. We can learn from others and their views, while challenging, may be just as relevant, they are to the individuals concerned. It is necessary for doctors and others to familiarize themselves with such differences and to be sensitive to the range of values that may be presented to them.

Research ethics review committees

All research to be carried out should be reviewed by an independent research ethics committee. These are set up in different ways but have as their primary function the interests of the patient and their protection. They can comment and ask questions of the research workers and ensure that patients are not disadvantaged and that the research meets ethical standards. These too may vary from country to country and from culture to culture. They are an essential safeguard for patients.

Role of the humanities

In an earlier section of the chapter, reference was made to learning about ethics and the range of methods available. One of these, covered in Chapter 20.5, is the use of the humanities, and in particular, literature. The use of novels, plays, and poems to illustrate difficult ethical issues and their complexity, can be very powerful mechanisms in assisting in the understanding of very difficult clinical problems.

Further reading

American Medical Association. *Codes of Medical Ethics*, 1994.

Beauchamp, T.L. and Childress, J.F. *Principles of Biomedical Ethics* 5th edn. Oxford: Oxford University Press, 2001.

British Medical Association. *The Medical Profession and Human Rights.* London: Zed Books Ltd, 2001.

Buber, M. *I and Thou.* Edinburgh: T.T. Clark, 1958.

Downie, R.S. and Calman, K.C. *Healthy Respect* 2nd edn. Oxford: Oxford University Press, 1994.

Downie, R.S. and Macnaughton, J. *Clinical Judgement. Evidence in Practice.* Oxford: Oxford Medical Publications, 2000.

Boyd, K.M., Higgs, R., and Pinching, A.J., ed. *The New Dictionary of Medical Ethics.* London: BMJ Publishing Group, 1997.

Fulford, K.W.M., Dickenson, D.L., and Murray, T., ed. *Healthcare Ethics and Human Values.* Oxford: Blackwell Publishing, 2002.

3.2 Confidentiality

Neil MacDonald

> What I may see or hear in the course of the treatment or even outside of the treatment in regard to the life of men, which on no account one must spread abroad, I will keep to myself holding such things shameful to be spoken about.
>
> Oath of Hippocrates

Not all of the dictums in the ancient oath of Hippocrates have stood the test of time. He was an antiabortionist who would restrict medical practice to 'brothers in male lineage'. The concept of risk versus benefit for patients was not familiar to him, as Hippocrates abjures the use of any 'deadly' drug in treatment, and he may have been unduly paternalistic in his approach to patients—the oath says nothing about providing patients with information, or respecting patient autonomy.

Amongst the Hippocratic principles, the statement on confidentiality remains fresh and topical. Nevertheless, modern societal mores challenge the bedrock principles of a physician's individual responsibility for a patient, including respect for 'what I may see or hear in the course of treatment or even outside of treatment in regard to the life of men'. Current codes of medical practice regard a physician's respect for patient confidentiality as a fundamental tenet, but one shaded by societal expectations. For example, The Canadian Medical Association Code of Ethics states:

> Respect the patient's right to confidentiality except when this right conflicts with your responsibility to the law, or when the maintenance of confidentiality would result in a significant risk of substantial harm to others or to the patient if the patient is incompetent; in such cases, take all reasonable steps to inform the patient that confidentiality will be breached.
>
> When acting on behalf of a third party, take reasonable steps to ensure that the patient understands the nature and extent of your responsibility to the third party.
>
> Upon a patient's request, provide the patient or third party with a copy of his or her medical record, unless there is a compelling reason to believe that information contained in the record will result in substantial harm to the patient or others.

They do, however, often spell out scenarios where physicians may break the seal of confidentiality even if not bound to do so by the law.

Physicians should refrain from disclosure of patient information, even after the death of a patient, but exceptions are permitted:

1. with patient consent;
2. for legal demand;
3. when judged to be in the patient's interest—that is, family discussions on occasion;
4. for registration of illnesses;
5. to protect society.

The law echoes societal views and anticipates that patients regard their communications with physicians as privileged, and expect that these communications will not be revealed to others without consent. The physician may breach this compact only if it is clearly to the patient's benefit (generally, in situations where the patient may not be competent), where the duties to protect society outweigh patient privilege (e.g. where a psychiatrist may know about forthcoming events whereby the patient may harm others[(1)]) or where the law demands that a physician breach the vow of confidentiality. In general, physicians do not enjoy the same level of respect for privileged communication enjoyed by their legal brethren.[(2,3)] Absolute privilege is an aspect of lawyer–client interaction, as the law believes that it could not properly function if this rule were not in place. Arguably, the significance of trust in medical communications can be viewed in a similar light, but it is clearly not regarded by the law as absolute; the protection for patient/physician discourse varies from place to place.

Modern medical ethical principles and western trends of thought value highly the principle of autonomy. Central to a respect for personal autonomy, is the concept that the privacy of individuals must be respected.*

Fidelity and trust are essential characteristics of a physician's covenant with sick and vulnerable people seeking treatment, care, and healing. For this relationship to work, doctors need information from patients as much as patients seek information from doctors. There is a difference, though. To give their professional advice and counsel, and to guide their treatment prescriptions, doctors often require kinds of information about the body and biography of sick people, information patients would not normally be willing to share with anyone else.

The duty to protect confidentiality binds not only the physician primarily in charge of a patient's treatment and care. That duty extends to all other members of a clinical care team who need access to a patient's medical chart if they are to make their special contribution to a patient's care. It is misguided to consider their access to a patient's medical records as a break of confidentiality. It may happen, however, that patients may entrust to a doctor or nurse confidences of a particularly personal nature that should not be written down in the medical record. Decisions in this matter call for sound judgement and open discussion with patients.

Confidentiality in research

Participants in research may be harmed psychologically, socially, or even financially if their privacy is invaded or if information about them, including their participation in certain kinds of research, is not kept confidential. There is now heightened sensitivity to the critical importance of safeguards for privacy and confidentiality, particularly in surveillance studies and in research on conditions that are socially stigmatizing and likely to render people susceptible to various kinds of discrimination. The HIV epidemic, for instance, has occasioned the development of detailed guidelines and of ingenious coding methods for electronic data storage to protect privacy and confidentiality in the research setting.

Information sheets accompanying consent forms for participants in clinical research should routinely state that rights to privacy and to confidentiality of information will be respected in clinical trials. The World Medical Association Declaration of Helsinki states that every precaution should be taken to respect the privacy of research subjects. The Code of Federal Regulations of the United States requires, for Institutional Review Board approval of research with human subjects, that there are adequate provisions to protect the privacy of subjects and to maintain the confidentiality of data.

The requirements for adequate protection of privacy and confidentiality will vary in keeping with the nature of the research, the disease or condition under study, and the laws of each country. Where shields do not exist in law, researchers may be restricted with regard to the extent of protection of confidentiality they can guarantee research subjects. Clinical studies involving follow-up of patients after closure of the study also require that attention be given to the protection of privacy. Research subjects should be alerted to the possibility of future contact and they should give free and informed consent to any follow-up plan.[(4)]

It is reasonable for purposes of medical audit and epidemiologic surveys that records be accessed by responsible colleagues. Ordinarily, specific patient consent for this type of work is not required, although an official custodian of the records must review requests and provide access only if scientific standards and strict confidentiality are assured.

Perhaps the public's greatest concern relevant to the privacy of health information relates to 'macro-issues' such as the intrusion of modern

* Ethical considerations require a strict interpretation of the use of words and symbols. In this discussion, the term 'privacy' is taken to mean 'the right of an individual to limit access by others to some aspect of the person' (Gostin, L.O. et al. (1993). Privacy and security of personal information in a new health care system. *Journal of the American Medical Association* **270**, 2487–93). 'Confidentiality' is defined as a form of informational privacy characterized by a special relationship, such as the physician–patient relationship. Personal information obtained in the course of that relationship should not be revealed to others unless the patient is first made aware and consents to its disclosure.

techniques of communication into the health field, with the potential for broad access to individual health data by a wide range of agencies and individuals.[5] The participation by many professionals and volunteers in the therapy of patients, the demands by a host of agencies for patient information, and the ready electronic recording and transfer of this information challenge the maintenance of the ancient dictum of strict confidentiality.

It is now possible to embed all of our health information on a plastic 'smart card'. This advance is helpful to us, as our health profiles will follow us as we make our way through increasingly complex health care systems. The risks are obvious—this information could be available to people with less-than-charitable interest in us. Access to information about us by alien agencies is a clear and evident risk which has been discussed in a number of publications and editorials on both sides of the Atlantic.[6–10]

Common issues in confidentiality

In this section we will consider ethical issues in confidentiality which palliative care colleagues may encounter on a daily basis. We will limit further discussion to the problem of balancing the interpretation of psychosocial information for patient good and the casual distribution of privileged patient information with consequent loss of respect and dignity. Three scenarios, based on actual experiences, with details changed to preserve confidentiality, will illustrate the issues which arise.

Case 1

Case 1 (Box 1) is an account where secret information from a family, of a nature which any of us would regard as privileged, is disclosed by a medical consultant. Several issues arise.

- When we are provided with private information about a patient, can we share secret information with others while withholding it from the patient?
- A medical chart is a public record. Does not our duty to protect patient privacy require us to preclude the publication of implicitly private matters in a public record?
- Information changes the way we think about a patient. As information may be inaccurate and cause us to adopt attitudes or policies inimical to a patient, questions of dignity aside, is it not our duty to reconcile our information with the patient's account?

Box 1 Privileged information disclosed by a medical consultant

Medical consultation

To: Psychiatry

Reason for request: 'Drug addiction' (Pt. has metastatic chondrosarcoma with severe chronic pain syndrome due to invasion of a knee joint).

Consultative note

Thank you. 35 year old male with metastatic chondrosarcoma. In pain and using up to 100 codeine plus acetaminophen tablets a week. Wife feels he is addicted—sleeps most of the day, no ambition. Pt. doesn't think his medications are a concern, but he is worried about things—bills are piling up—he has a family to support—fights constantly with his wife. The pain in his knee is severe (average 8/10 on pain scale). Any movement makes it worse; the patient cannot weight-bear. He is severely anhedonic—no appetite for food or zest for life. He can't concentrate on any task and can't 'get it together' to do anything. No interest in sex for months according to his wife. He knows he is depressed, but denies suicidal thoughts. However, he told his wife he might shoot self if things got worse (he has the means to do so).

Social history

Unhappy childhood; history of dysphoric family with spousal abuse. Wife states still in love, but she can't cope with his physical problems and moods. She feels like leaving him sometimes (he doesn't know this).

On social assistance—financially strapped.

(Physical examination and recommendations regarding pain management, family counselling and antidepressants follow).

Public record

An institutional medical chart may be read by scores of people. Seigler, describing the chart access of a woman entering hospital for a routine cholecystectomy, notes that in excess of 80 people (physicians, students, volunteers, administrators, maintenance staff, and other health professionals) may read the record.[11] A colleague who has worked in hospitals for 30 years has stated 'If I must be hospitalized, I'll react like a military prisoner and give them only my name, occupation, and Medicare number!' His circumspect view may be extreme, albeit based on disturbing observations over time. However, maintaining due respect for the public nature of a medical record should temper both the nature of matters discussed, and the language chosen to relate those matters. The consult note (Box 1) disregards these principles. The ward staff are given details about the patient's mental state, sexuality, and family life; details which in some instances are not known by the patient.

When private information on a patient is received from others, the burden is on the physician to justify withholding this material from a patient. However, this general moral principle must be wisely interpreted in the individual situation—will feedback to the patient cause alienation and family strife, as it almost certainly would in this case?[12] What is the value and accuracy of hearsay information? Physicians traditionally are repositories of patient secrets, both those relayed by patients and by friends and family. We may conclude that, while openness remains the ideal, we are free to use this information as we deem appropriate to further the patient's good, including remaining silent both in print and in conversation.

Case 2

You have been asked to see Mrs C.H., a 38-year-old woman with advanced metastatic breast cancer, primarily to bone, with consequent generalized pain. Her pain control, previously good, is now inadequate, despite therapy with regularly increasing doses of opioids, spot radiation therapy, and a recent trial of a biphosphonate. The ward nurses report increasing mood swings, with periods of obvious sadness and weeping.

After a period of hesitant conversation in which Mrs C.H. appears reluctant to discuss psychosocial issues which may contribute to her suffering, she suddenly states: 'You would have pain, too, if your husband was playing around with your best friend'. She then reports that she had previously partnered her husband in a small business. As she was no longer able to work with him, she encouraged a friend to take her place. The staff had previously noted that Mrs C.H. was often visited by her husband, accompanied by this friend. Following further discussion, it seems to you that the depth of anguish created for Mrs C.H. by this situation is indeed a major contributor to her deteriorating physical and psychological status.

Shortly after this interview, you are participating in the weekly palliative care team review of all patients on the unit. How should you contribute to the discussion on Mrs C.H.?

Team discussion

Working as a team requires periodic meetings to discuss patient problems. Nevertheless, the salutary goal of working together to assist patients and families may adversely affect privacy and patient-family dignity. It is a privilege to share a family's most intimate secrets. If we are to help a family to the fullest extent, it is sometimes necessary that we are able to share this information with colleagues in our interdisciplinary team. Team discussions of patient-family problems, however, have a potentially serious negative component. Hearsay information on marital infidelities, spousal abuse, sexual performance, and other subjects usually regarded as inherently of a confidential nature, may be bandied about, sometimes in a humorous vein. Transmission of information on our Case 2 patient without her specific permission violates universally held principles of timeless importance. Revelations of this nature before a group represent a fundamental attack on patient-family dignity, while unsubstantiated information may influence the reaction of hospital staff to a patient or family member.

Are we so professional that accounts of peccadilloes and moral failings will not influence unfavourably our degree of involvement and patient concern? The saintly amongst us may not be unduly swayed; for the rest, it is best that the physicians not test the charity and understanding of health care colleagues sharing patient responsibilities through unhelpful revelations.

While communication of patient information with hospital teams is essential for patient well-being, physicians and nurses should remember that when we pass on information we are acting as if we have implied consent from the patient. We should get the patient's specific permission to pass on to specifically designated members of a health care team material which an ordinary person would judge to be sensitive.

In Case 2, it may be important for certain members of the palliative care team to know about Mrs C.H.'s suspicions, as they are contributing to her suffering and may be incorrect. Counselling will help. Quite certainly, Mrs C.H.'s permission to share this information should be sought. She may give the permission willingly, and she may want and need to speak to certain members of the team about her sadness and distress. She may also have her own personal reasons for restricting disclosure only to certain team members in whom she has a high degree of trust. As the case evolved, Mr C.H. was probably not unfaithful; the corticosteroids may have contributed to Mrs C.H.'s paranoia.

Case 3

You are standing within the confines of the ward station, discussing with a colleague the paranoid delusions of a delirious patient. Your eye is drawn to the nearby elevator where a startled visitor, not associated with the patient in question, has obviously overheard your discussions. He appears shocked, and you wonder if the visitor may believe that you were discussing his loved one. With a sense of remorse, you once again resolve not to discuss patient information in other than a fully secure environment.

Probably all of us have violated the tenets of confidentiality in a scene similar to the above. Discussion of patient information in public elevators and cafeterias is an obvious avoidable problem. However, few hospitals are built with adequate provisions for private space. A particular problem still emerges from the 'Grand Ward Round', wherein senior staff, residents, students, and nursing colleagues parade around from bed to bed, discussing patient issues. This scenario has been associated with offenses to patient dignity in a variety of guises. The patient may be referred to in the third person as people hover around the bed, while personal information is bandied about amongst both the members of the ward-walk and the patients and visitors currently in the room at that time.

Efficiency of operation does not take precedence over the fundamental ethical responsibilities of physicians to honour patient privacy. The ward-walk must be so tailored as to ensure that the common violations which were the product of our training are not accepted as a standard which will be followed by future generations of physicians.

Professional confidentiality

Physicians regard maintenance of confidentiality as a cardinal imperative. This virtue is manifest not only in respect to their patients, but also to their colleagues. Guarding patient confidentiality is a straightforward ethical proposition, albeit constantly threatened by administrative and third party pressures. Professional confidentiality, however, does present a series of problematic ethical issues. Sissela Bok[13] states that 'confidentiality, like all secrecy, can then cover up for and in turn lead to a great deal of error, injury, pathology and abuse'. These issues may more commonly arise when maintenance of confidentiality is used as a shield to protect colleagues or to honour demands placed upon physicians by third parties which if not honoured may result in personal loss. Examples include:

- *Covenants to maintain confidentiality of research results.* It is reasonable that confidentiality should be respected in research sponsored by pharmaceutical firms as undue release of trial background information and details may damage a firm's prospects. Balanced against the duty of a physician to a sponsoring firm or agency, is the overriding duty to ensure that patients are not harmed. For example, recently a Canadian physician was threatened with a suit by a pharmaceutical firm for releasing trial information at a meeting and subsequently publishing this material. In so doing, she broke a confidentiality clause contained in her contract.

  Pharmaceutical firms must not include absolute bonds of confidentiality in their contracts, nor can physicians agree to these strictures. Acquiescence not only violates academic integrity but could result in patient harm. Pharmaceutical firms and their principal investigators involved in institutional trials may rightfully expect that confidentiality will be maintained throughout the course of a trial until established end-points are reached, scientific analysis is carried out, and the trial data is ready for presentation and publication. It is unethical for participants to violate this expectation unless, in conscience, they are in possession of data which suggests that continuation is harmful to prospective enrollees. Under these circumstances, they should discuss their concerns with the sponsors and other investigators. If honest doubt exists with respect to investigator views, trial confidentiality should be maintained. If, however, the investigator is not in doubt that maintenance of trial confidentiality will harm others, the investigator must speak out. Investigators must also be free to publish the results of completed trials within a reasonable period of trial completion, regardless of sponsor interests; absolute gag clauses in sponsor-investigator clinical trial contracts are not ethical.

- *Physician benefits with potential influence on therapy.* On occasion, physicians have benefited from restricting patient services and profited by adopting certain pharmaceutical regimes. Patients must be informed about physician financial arrangements which can impact on their care; this principle is straightforward.

  Regardless of disclosure, should physicians engage in such practices under any circumstances? Decisions on this issue must satisfy the ethical dictate calling upon physicians to ensure that patient well-being trumps pecuniary gain when the two interests are in conflict.

- *Physician opinions—other professionals.* It is usually in a patient's best interest that physicians demonstrate respect for their colleagues and do not bandy about unsubstantiated comments which might damage patient confidence in another professional.

  Tolerance of the occasional error by an otherwise competent individual is both humane and ethical providing that arrangements are in place for regular review of practice and adoption of corrective measures. Patients or families should be told about the error and its consequences by the professional who made the error.

What to do in the face of an established pattern of incompetent behaviour?—or if patient error with correctable consequences is not acknowledged? Reports of notable cover-ups within the law, medicine, the clergy, and the military are frequently fodder for the media. An ethical dilemma does not exist when a pattern of inadequate care is present. Rather, it is clearly an imperative that mechanisms are in place to change people and systems responsible for substandard activity. Easier said than done, one may say because of the inherent inertia of long-established programmes and the sometimes misplaced but nevertheless compassionate regard for failing colleagues. Nevertheless, in these circumstances the responsibility of those who have supervisory responsibility for our practice is clear.

On occasion, palliative care physicians working with cancer patients may sharply differ with their oncology colleagues with respect to aggressive use of therapy in seemingly futile situations. These are complex issues as such decisions on chemotherapy depend heavily on informed patient judgement, interest of the patient in taking part in experimental therapy, and the sometime demands of patients and families to receive toxic treatments even though a very slim opportunity for any degree of success is present. Do ethical considerations with respect to physician financial reward?; the continuing application of chemotherapy as a facile but harmful means of keeping communication lines open?; or a slavish adherence to research protocol therapy sometimes play a role? Perhaps, on occasion, but such assumptions are often wrong and cannot be acted upon in the absence of evidence.

As in other areas of complex care, the onus is on palliative care physicians to present their ideas clearly and rationally to colleagues who share care in anticipation that, within professional ranks, a sensible joint recommendation for patients will emerge. Again, an outcome which is readily expressed on paper but often taxing to apply in clinical practice, particularly if a palliative care programme is not involved early in the patient's course. Nevertheless, the failure of communication, albeit difficult and awkward, between professional colleagues should not be tolerated if the consequences are misguided harmful decisions on therapy.

References

1. **Quinn, K.M.** (1984). The impact of Tarasoff on clinical practice. *Behavioural Sciences and the Law* **2**, 319–29.
2. **Hoffman, B.** (1992). Disclosure of medical information without consent: the patient's right to confidentiality. *Health Law in Canada* **13**, 156–9.
3. **Marshall, M.** (1992). Case comment: R.V. Gruenke. *Health Law in Canada* **12**, 112–14.
4. **Tri-Council Working Group**. *Code of Conduct for Research Involving Humans.* Ottawa: Minister of Supply and Services Canada, 1996.
5. **Lewis, Harris and Associates.** *Weston AF Health Information Privacy Survey.* Atlanta GA: Equifax Inc., 1993.
6. **Marr, P.** (1994). Maintaining patient confidentiality in an electronic world. *International Journal of Bio-Medical Computing* **35** (Suppl. 1), 213–17.
7. **Gostin, L.O.** et al. (1993). Privacy and security of personal information in a new health care system. *Journal of the American Medical Association* **270**, 2487–93.
8. **Anderson, R.** (1995). NHS-wide networking and patient confidentiality. *British Medical Journal* **311**, 5–6.
9. Editorial (1989). The selling of patients' data. *Lancet* **ii**, 1078.
10. **Black, D.** (1992). Personal health records. *Journal of Medical Ethics* **18**, 5–6.
11. **Siegler, M.** (1982). Confidentiality in medicine—a decrepit concept. *New England Journal of Medicine* **307**, 1518–21.
12. **Burnum, J.F.** (1991). Secrets about patients. *New England Journal of Medicine* **324**, 1130–3.
13. **Sissela Bok.** *Secrets: On the Ethics of Concealment and Revelation.* New York: Vintage Books, 1984, p. 123.

3.3 Truth-telling and consent

Robin Downie and Fiona Randall

The importance of truth-telling

Honesty, of which a disposition to tell the truth is a central aspect, is one of the most valued of all moral characteristics. As the poet Robert Burns says:

> An honest man's the noblest work of God.[1]

It is not difficult to understand why this should be so. First, human beings are essentially language-users, and language-use presupposes that we can expect that people will at least usually try to tell the truth in communication. If they don't, communication will break down. Second, human beings are not self-sufficient; they have constant need for the help of others. Human beings therefore need to rely on each other and reliability presupposes truth-telling in the statement of intentions, the giving of information, advice, and so on. Third, truth-telling is important in human relationships, although few human relationships could survive the whole truth and nothing but the truth all of the time! This last point becomes especially important, as we shall see, when we move specifically to the professional–patient relationship. In general terms then, a very high moral value is placed on truth-telling in everyday life. Is that also the case in medical practice?

Truth-telling in palliative care

It has not always been the case, for the reason that traditionally doctors did not see it as part of their medical aim to pass on information, or to enable patients to plan their futures, or to establish authentic relationships.[2] Rather, they saw their role as that of alleviating suffering and prolonging life where possible, and regarded truth-telling as not at the top of that agenda. To put it another way, whereas truth-telling might be central to ordinary human relationships, the professional–patient relationship was regarded as a special one in which the centrality of truth-telling was less obvious. And of course, if there is no obligation to tell the truth (and no ethical code mentions such an obligation), then life becomes a little easier for the doctor, who can avoid the obligation to confront the patient with distressing information.

Times have changed, however, and the traditional position is no longer acceptable to the public or to the majority of doctors. In the present climate the stress is on openness, or 'transparency', in all relationships, including professional ones. In the professional–patient relationship, there is an emphasis on trust. Of course, it might be argued that the patient trusts the professional to relieve suffering, not to tell the truth. But in the professional–patient relationship trust cannot be compartmentalized in this way. A trusting professional–patient relationship requires openness about what can and cannot be achieved.[3,4]

But that position still leaves a number of problems which require more detailed discussion in a medical context, for the professional–patient relationship is a special one. This is especially the case in palliative care for three reasons.

First, the patients in palliative care are approaching the ends of their lives, so information to be communicated will inevitably be distressing or at least sad. So, even if we agree that we must tell the truth there remain important questions about how much of the truth should be told, how it should be told, and when it should be told.[5] Second, the patients will typically be weak and frail and sometimes confused. Hence, special consideration is necessary to ensure that the information which is provided is also understood. Third, the WHO definition of palliative care gives relatives a central place in the remit—the aim of palliative care is the best possible quality of life for patients and their families—so there are special problems of how much to tell relatives and how that should be done.[6] The problems of truth-telling cannot be divorced from those of confidentiality.

How much truth?

There are two approaches that can be taken to the question of how much of the truth should be told to patients in palliative care. First, there is the position that patients must be told all the information they can comprehend, and second the position that the professional's task is limited to giving only that amount of information that patients indicate they want.[7,8]

The first proposal can clearly have adverse outcomes, for it means that patients will be given a large amount of bad news, including information about likely ways in which they will die. Even if information of this kind is delivered in the best possible manner it may have the result that patients will be unnecessarily traumatized. This is especially unjustifiable when we remember that much of the information may turn out in the end to be irrelevant.

The second proposal is that professionals should answer patients' questions truthfully but always literally and should not go beyond what the patient is asking. This approach has the advantage that patients can gain knowledge at a pace which enables them to assimilate it. But there are drawbacks.

First, it can be used by the professional as a way of avoiding the responsibility for deciding what aspects of the truth should be told. The professional may be fully aware that the patient's questions may not be leading to the crux of the matter, either because the patient does not know what to ask or is afraid to ask the hard question. Perhaps the duty of the professional is to assist the patient in confronting the truth which he suspects but does not quite know how to ask.

Second, even if a patient has indicated that he/she does not wish to hear bad news, it may still be the duty of the professional to provide a limited amount of this bad news to prevent further harm. For example, if a patient with carcinoma of the breast and also neck pain is found to have metastases in the cervical spine, with a risk of cord compression and quadriplegia, then a hard collar should be worn and the patient told to avoid falls, etc. In this situation the patient has to be given the bad news of cervical metastases in order to adjust lifestyle patterns to minimize the risk of very serious harm of quadriplegia.

Of course, it might be argued that if the patient gives signs that bad news is emphatically not wanted then the professional should not give it—and just hope that the adverse consequences will not happen. But this seems an abdication of responsibility. The other possibility in this situation is to ask permission of the patient to make the best decisions on their behalf without full explanation. The professional can then give advice on lifestyle, etc. without unwanted explanations as to their necessity. If the patient seems resistant to a full explanation this may be the best solution.

The professional should never tell lies to the patient, but there may be circumstances in which the professional should be 'economical with the truth', as is sometimes said in political circles. For example, a very ill patient may ask if he has 2 years to live. The professional may have good reason for thinking that 4 weeks is a more likely survival time, but saying this might be unnecessarily harsh. The professional might reasonably reply that survival for 2 years is very unlikely, rather than that it is impossible. This is far from being the whole truth, but it is truth, tempered with kindness. The conclusion seems to be that the professional should always tell the truth, but how much of the truth to tell should be based partly on the patient's wishes, and partly on a harms/benefits calculus.[9,10]

Perhaps a balanced view is provided in *Harry Potter and the Philosopher's Stone:* 'The truth', Dumbledore sighed. 'It is a beautiful and terrible thing, and should therefore be treated with great caution. However, I shall answer your questions unless I have a very good reason not to, in which case I beg you'll forgive me. I shall not, of course, lie' (p. 216).[11]

Patients and relatives

To whom should the truth be told? The obvious answer is 'the patient'. In practice, the situation in palliative care is not so simple, partly because, as we have seen, the WHO definition builds in care of relatives as part of the remit, and partly because in palliative care the patients are weak and the relatives are concerned and protective. The relatives therefore often express a wish to be in control of the flow of information. And of course professionals may be happy to go along with this because it can be easier to discuss matters with relatives than with patients.

But this situation is at variance with all codes of ethics, which stress patient confidentiality. We must therefore try to square off what tends to be the practice of palliative care, and what may be the custom in some cultures,[7,12,13] with the requirements of codes of ethics. The only way to do this is to ensure that the competent patient gives permission for relatives to be informed. Indeed, with the permission of the patient it can be very helpful if the patient is given explanations in the presence of relatives who may later be able to discuss the information and ask further questions.

Some relatives may wish to go further than this, however, to control the flow of information to the competent patient, or indeed to attempt to prevent any kind of bad news being given to the patient. This situation is one which professionals must resist. In the United Kingdom, at least, relatives have no moral or legal right to control the information which is given to patients. This is easily said, but dealing with angry relatives can require great tact and courage. Nevertheless, it is a professional responsibility to put the patient first.

The situation becomes more complicated when the patient is confused and not competent to make decisions or to assimilate information. In England the legal position is that relatives have no legal right to make decisions on behalf of incompetent, adult patients; decision-making power remains with the doctor. Nevertheless, it is clearly a matter of good practice to involve the relatives as much as possible.

There is another sort of situation in which the relatives should be given information, and that is the one in which the relatives are going to be involved as carers. Acting as a carer in a humane and efficient way, without damage either to the patient or to the carer, requires that information be provided.

How much information should members of the professional team be given? Obviously, they must be given enough to enable them to carry out their professional duties. Sometimes, however, a patient may confide in a team member something of a private and personal nature. Does this need to be shared with the team? If the professional concerned is sure that the information is relevant to the care of the patient then permission should be asked of the patient to share it with other professionals on a 'need to know' basis.

Truth-telling and treatment decisions

We have so far been discussing truth-telling mainly in connection with diagnosis and prognosis. Slightly different issues arise over truth-telling in the context of treatment decisions. These problems will be discussed further in the context of obtaining consent for treatment, but here we should note that the truth should be told in a manner which enables the patient to understand what is going to happen.

For example, there may be a palliative chemotherapy treatment which has a 40 per cent chance of causing some disease regression, with a 70 per cent chance of distressing side-effects, and a 10 per cent chance of life-threatening infection as a result of bone-marrow suppression. Now these facts may be presented to patients in several ways, all of which consist entirely of true statements. But some ways of putting the facts will encourage the patient to accept the treatment and some ways may encourage the patient to decline. Honesty requires that the harms and risks should be presented in various ways, to try to ensure that the patient really does understand the harms and benefits involved.

Truth-telling and communication skills (see Chapter 4.1)

Sometimes 'communication skills' are referred to in this kind of context, as if they answered all difficulties. But there are various problems with communication skills in this context.[14]

The first is that they are associated with 'breaking bad news' and therefore the emphasis tends to be on proceeding slowly, with compassion, and so on. No doubt such a manner of communication is important in palliative care, but it is also important in the context of treatment decisions that the emphasis should be on what is said. For example, in the type of case mentioned above it is important that the patient is told not just that the treatment proposed carries a 'reasonable' chance of response with some side-effects and a low chance of infection, but also that the treatment has a 60 per cent chance (greater than even) of doing no good at all whilst carrying a 70 per cent chance of causing distressing side-effects and a 10 per cent chance of a life-threatening infection. Both ways of putting the issues consist of true statements but both are necessary if the patient is to understand what the proposed treatment involves.

It might be said that communication skills will enable us to put the issues to the patient in the 'best possible way'. But what does that mean?

This takes us to the second difficulty with 'communication skills'. They are a means to an end, but what is the end? Is the end to persuade or manipulate the patient into accepting the treatment which the professional believes to be in the best interests of the patient, or is it to enable the patient to understand the situation so that he/she can make an informed choice? The easy answer, especially in palliative care, is that the patient supported by relatives must make the choice. But in practice this is not always easy to accept if the patient is choosing in what the professional considers to be an irrational manner. We cannot resolve this here, but stress in this context that truth cannot be dissolved into communication skills.

Truth-telling and consent

We have said that one of the purposes of truthful communication between health care professionals and patients is to enable patients to make an informed choice as to whether to accept or reject the proposed health care options. The process by which patients make this choice has come to be known as 'obtaining consent'. In more formal terms, consent is the granting to someone of permission to do what he would not otherwise have the right to do. Let us discuss this.[7,15–17]

In the course of providing health care it is necessary to examine patients, carry out investigations, and provide treatment. Each of these acts has a direct effect on the patient, on his or her body and mind. Given that we believe that people should have the right to determine what is done to their bodies, then so long as the patient can make those choices consent is necessary for the provision of health care. It is especially important in palliative care to note that consent is also required before pursuing treatment or interventions, including 'counselling', aimed at alleviating mental distress or suffering.

In the ensuing discussion, in order to avoid tedious repetition, we have used 'treatment' as a generic term to encompass examination and investigation as well as drug and other treatment measures aimed at enhancing physical or mental well being. In the first part of the discussion we have assumed that the patient is competent to give consent. The abilities necessary to be competent are described later.

Consent, agreement, demand, and joint decision-making

Once the professional has offered the treatments (together with the necessary information which we discuss below) the patient has the right to choose which treatment he or she will accept and which he or she will refuse. By consenting the patient is doing more than simply agreeing to a treatment. Consent involves exercising a right. The idea of consent as mere acquiescence or agreement is too weak a notion.

It is sometimes suggested that consent entails a right to demand a certain investigation or treatment. But consent as a 'right to demand' is too strong a notion. In order to explain why this is so it is necessary to consider the moral positions of the patient and professional in their relationship, and also to reflect on the nature of what can be achieved in health care, particularly in the context of terminal illness.

In palliative care it is often the case that treatments to prolong life may be associated with a low probability of success and with significant harms and risks, and so it is a matter of judgement for health care professionals as to which treatments they consider have a reasonable prospect of conferring net benefit. Treatments to alleviate suffering may also be associated with harms and risks, though these are usually less severe.

Now some patients may be willing to accept major harms and risks for the sake of a low probability of prolonging life for a short time. Sometimes they may also be willing to accept significant harms and risks for the sake of possible relief of suffering. Because of this fact it is sometimes suggested that the duty of the health care professional is to offer, and be willing to provide, every technically possible investigation and treatment and to let the patient decide on the management plan. In other words, it is suggested that the patient has the right to demand that a particular management plan be followed, even if the professional considers that in the specific clinical circumstances it is very likely to result in overall harm to the patient.

This is a misleading and consumerist model of the relationship between the health care professional and patient, and it is a misleading and invalid interpretation of the concept of consent. The patient's right to consent to a treatment is not a right to demand any treatment. The patient does not have unilateral power to determine the treatment plan. Professional integrity must be defended against patient consumerism. Professionals are moral agents and cannot be expected to provide a treatment which would cause overall harm.[7]

Given that the professional can refuse to provide a particular investigation or treatment, and the patient can refuse to accept any investigation or treatment, it is clear that the process of deciding on a management plan, of 'obtaining consent', must require joint decision-making. The patient and the professional each has a power of veto. During the consent process they need to reach agreement about the best course of action for the patient.

This process of discussion, of description of the details of benefits, harms, and risks in the particular clinical situation, of exploration of the patient's wishes and goals, is absolutely essential to the aim of providing the health care treatment that is best for the particular patient. Consent seen in this way as a continuous process of joint decision-making is the ethical basis of palliative care.

Consent and competence

In order to be able to make health care choices patients require certain abilities. If they possess these abilities they are said to be competent, or to have capacity, to give informed consent. Adult patients are presumed to be competent unless proved otherwise. In palliative care there are often circumstances in which the patient is incompetent to give consent, for example, because of confusion, diminution of consciousness, or dementia. Where there is any doubt about the patient's competence, it is the responsibility of the health care professionals to assess it and to judge whether or not the patient is capable of making the treatment choice.

Competence is decision-specific. The question is whether the patient can make the particular health care decision, not whether he or she can make any other decision, such as what to have for breakfast or what to write in a last will and testament. Patients may be competent to make some simple decisions, but they may be unable to make those that involve complex choices.

Assessing competence can be surprisingly difficult, but it is a crucial judgement.[18] When patients are incompetent, other people must try to make the best possible decisions on their behalf. We discuss this situation briefly below. Competence requires possession of all of the following five abilities:

1. the ability to understand the necessary facts and probabilities,
2. the ability to retain this information so as to deliberate on it,
3. the ability to make a voluntary, uncoerced choice,
4. the ability to make a reasoned choice, and
5. the ability to communicate that choice.

It follows from the above list that there are two basic capacities required for competence: the capacity to receive and understand information, and the capacity to make reasoned voluntary choices. We shall examine both requirements.

Receiving and understanding information

Many treatment choices require the patient to be able to understand, retain, and deliberate on a large amount of unfamiliar information. In order to make a treatment choice the patient needs to know the following:

1. the diagnosis of the illness and its prognosis untreated;
2. the nature, magnitude, and likelihood of the benefits of treatment; and
3. the nature, magnitude, and likelihood of the harms and risks of treatment.

For example, if a patient with an inoperable malignant oesophageal stricture is asked whether he wants a stent inserted to improve worsening dysphagia, he needs to know that he has cancer of the oesophagus, that he may become completely unable to swallow, and that the illness is terminal, with some guide as to the time scales involved. He then needs to know about the possible benefits of the stent in terms of prolonging life and improving his comfort. This information includes whether stent insertion is likely to be successful, how much it will improve his swallowing, how long its effect may last, and whether it will make him more comfortable. He needs to know about the harms and risks of stent insertion, which include pain after the procedure and the (small but serious) risk of perforation of the oesophagus.

The patient in this example needs to be able to retain this information, deliberate on it, make a reasoned and voluntary choice, and then communicate that choice to the doctor who will perform the stent insertion. As is often the case in palliative care, this treatment choice requires the patient to be in possession of a large amount of information, much of which is unpleasant.

Not surprisingly, it sometimes happens that patients indicate that they do not want this information, but instead would prefer to agree to a treatment plan proposed by the professional team. In this situation the patient is making a positive choice to hand over much of the decision-making responsibility to the professionals. But the doctors and nurses may find it extremely difficult to know what would be best for the particular patient, especially where there is a fine balance between the potential benefit and the harms and risks.

When patients indicate they do not want to make an adequately informed choice the health care professionals are left in a morally difficult position. It is our view that it is a right, not a duty, to give informed consent to treatment. In other words, patients do not have to give informed consent as a condition of receiving treatment. They should be allowed the option of being offered that treatment which the health care team feel is best in the particular circumstances, and then the patient can accept or refuse the treatment offered. As we have argued, accepting or refusing is distinct from giving consent, as that term has come to be used in health care.

An exception to this general rule occurs where benefit, harm, and risk are finely balanced. This would be the case in the above example if the insertion of the stent was expected to be technically difficult and risky and the patient already had liver metastases, but the dysphagia was rapidly worsening. In this situation the professionals concerned might ask the patient about his goals at this point in the illness, and about the things which now mattered most in his life. Armed with this information they would be in a slightly better position to offer the best treatment plan. However, if they felt that they simply could not make the best choice without more specific guidance from the patient, then they might insist that he should know some crucial information and give some indication of his wishes. It is reasonable to refuse to provide a treatment which has significant harms and risks and limited benefits unless the patient gives adequately informed consent.

The process of joint decision-making, as we have described, does require the health care professionals to make some judgements.[19] They must decide what care options to offer, judge whether the patient is competent, and also judge what information is necessary in the circumstances for adequately informed consent. Such professional decisions cannot be determined by guidelines removed from the actual case.

Nevertheless, we can conclude that where benefit is small or statistically unlikely and the harms and risks are significant, a high standard of disclosure of information is required for adequately informed consent, and that it is reasonable for health care professionals to decline to provide that treatment unless the competent patient gives consent in the full sense.

Voluntary choice

In order to be morally and legally valid, consent must be freely given. Patients must not be coerced by health care professionals, and the latter must accept the competent patient's refusal of treatment following consideration of the necessary information. Rational and balanced presentation of the benefits, harms, and risks of treatment is necessary, whereas an unbalanced presentation of the facts or coercion are not acceptable.

Unfortunately, patients may be subject to coercion by their relatives, particularly where those relatives want the patient to accept life-prolonging treatment. It also happens that relatives may want unpleasant information withheld from the patient, and occasionally they may request that the professionals either omit crucial information or deliberately mislead the patient. In such circumstances it is clear that the rights of the competent patient, and the duties of the health care professionals to the patient, override the wishes of the relatives.

It is often difficult for professionals in the field of palliative care to uphold the rights and interests of patients when there is conflict with the wishes and interests of their relatives. This occurs because of the idea, in this area of health care, that the professionals have duties to benefit the relatives. It is our view that, if there are any duties to benefit relatives, those duties should not override our duties to patients and our obligations to respect and uphold their rights.

Incompetent patients and advance statements

When adult patients are incompetent, and when children are too young to be able to consent to treatment, health care decisions are made for them by others. Laws which govern this process vary from country to country. Generally, parents can consent to or refuse treatment on behalf of their children, but the situation becomes much more complex where the children have some ability to comprehend the decision.

It is essential that professionals have adequate knowledge of the laws of their own country. For example, in the United Kingdom the law dictates that if the adult patient is incompetent then no-one can consent to or refuse treatment on the patient's behalf, and it is the moral and legal responsibility of the health care team to make care decisions based on their assessment of the patient's best interests. In so doing they must take into account whatever can be known of what the patient's wishes might have been in the circumstances, and the relatives should be asked to help in this endeavour.

Competent patients sometimes make written or verbal 'advance statements' about their wishes regarding treatment if they become incompetent to make decisions themselves. An advance refusal of treatment is binding on professionals if the refusal was competently made and if the circumstances which have arisen are believed to be those to which the refusal was intended to apply. However, a patient cannot, via an advance statement, require that a particular treatment be given. The health care team has a duty not to give harmful treatments to incompetent patients, in the same way as they have a duty not to harm competent patients. The laws regarding advance statements vary from country to country.[20]

The ethical issues surrounding consent to research in palliative care are discussed in Chapter 3.6.

Justifying the need for consent

The most obvious moral justifications for consent are respect for the patient's autonomy and the goal of achieving the best possible health care management for the particular patient. But the whole process of decision-making also fosters trust in the relationship, and promotes public and social values, such as the value of each human being even when very ill and dependant on others for care. The pursuit of informed consent helps to avoid patients being victims of fraud or duress, and protects patients taking part in research.

The moral justifications for obtaining informed consent are based on the necessity of preserving the essential nature of the patient–professional relationship, and there are wider social benefits to be gained by upholding the rights and duties of both the patient and the professional in that relationship.

References

1. **Burns, R.** (1786). The Cotter's Saturday Night. In *Longer Scottish Poems* Vol. 2 (ed. D. Crawford, D. Hewitt, and A. Law), pp. 216–21. Edinburgh: Scottish Academic Press.
2. **Krisman-Scott, M.A.** (2000). An historical analysis of disclosure of terminal status. *Journal of Nursing Scholarship* **32** (1), 47–52.
3. **Kim, M.K. and Alvi, A.** (1999). Breaking the bad news of cancer: the patient's perspective. *Laryngoscope* **109** (7 pt 1), 1064–7.
4. **Anderlik, M.R.** et al. (2000). Revisiting the truth-telling debate: a study of disclosure practices at a major cancer center. *Journal of Clinical Ethics* **11** (3), 251–9.
5. **Ellis, P.M. and Tattershall, M.H.** (1999). How should doctors communicate the diagnosis of cancer to patients? *Annals of Medicine* **31** (5), 336–41.
6. **World Health Organization.** *Cancer, Pain Relief and Palliative Care.* Report of a WHO Expert Committee, Technical Report Series no. 804. Geneva: World Health Organization, 1990.
7. **Randall, F. and Downie, R.S.** *Palliative Care Ethics* 2nd edn. Oxford: Oxford University Press, 1999.
8. **Girgis, A. and Sanson-Fisher, R.W.** (1998). Breaking bad news: current best advice for clinicians. *Behavioural Medicine* **24** (2), 53–9.
9. **Brusamolino, E. and Surbone, A.** (1997). Telling the truth to the patient with cancer. A cross-cultural dialogue. *Annals of the New York Academy of Science* **809**, 411–21.
10. **Campbell, E.M. and Sanson-Fisher, R.W.** (1998). Breaking bad news. 3. Encouraging the adoption of best practice. *Behavioural Medicine* **24** (2), 73–80.
11. **Rowling, J.K.** *Harry Potter and the Philosopher's Stone.* London: Bloomsbury, 1997.
12. **Chiu, T.Y.** et al. (2000). Ethical dilemmas in palliative care: a study in Taiwan. *Journal of Medical Ethics* **26** (5), 353–7.
13. **Gordon, D.R. and Paci, E.** (1997). Disclosure practices and cultural narratives: understanding concealment and silence around cancer in Tuscany, Italy. *Social Science and Medicine* **44** (10), 1433–52.
14. **Jenkins, V.L.** et al. (2001). Information needs of patients with cancer: results from a large study in UK cancer centres. *British Journal of Cancer* **84** (1), 48–51.
15. **Mason, J.K. and McCall Smith, R.A.** *Law and Medical Ethics* 4th edn. London: Butterworths, 1994, pp. 218–37.
16. **Montgomery, J.** *Health Care Law.* Oxford: Oxford University Press, 1997, pp. 227–48.
17. **Jonsen, A.R.** *The Birth of Bioethics.* Oxford: Oxford University Press, 1998, pp. 353–8.
18. **British Medical Association and the Law Society.** *Assessment of Mental Capacity: Guidance for Doctors and Lawyers.* London: British Medical Association, 1995.
19. **Downie, R.S. and Macnaughton, J.** *Clinical Judgement: Evidence in Practice.* Oxford: Oxford University Press, 2000.
20. **British Medical Association.** *Advance Statements.* London: British Medical Association, 1995.

Further reading

The following books give the official British medical consensus on the topics covered in the chapter:

British Medical Association. *Medical Ethics Today: Its Practice and Philosophy,* London: BMJ Publishing Group, 1998.

British Medical Association. *The Older Person: Consent and Care.* London: BMJ Publishing Group, 1995.

British Medical Association. *Rights and Responsibilities of Doctors.* London: BMJ Publishing Group, 1992.

British Medical Association. *Advance Statements.* London: BMJ Publishing Group, 1995.

British Medical Association. *Assessment of Mental Capacity: Guidance for Doctors and Lawyers.* London: British Medical Association, 1995.

Department of Health. *Reference Guide to Consent for Examination or Treatment.* London: Department of Health, 2001.

General Medical Council. *Seeking Patients' Consent.* London: General Medical Council, 1998.

The following book analyses and defends the role of judgement in medical decision-making:

Downie, R.S. and Macnaughton, R.J. *Clinical Judgement: Evidence in Practice.* Oxford: Oxford University Press, 2000.

The following books, provide balanced accounts of truth-telling in health care:

Higgs, R. (1985). On telling patients the truth. In *Moral Dilemmas in Modern Medicine* (ed. M. Lockwood), pp. 187–202. Oxford: Oxford University Press.

Randall, F. and Downie, R.S. *Palliative Care Ethics: A Companion for all Specialties.* Oxford: Oxford University Press, 1999, pp. 128–9 (see also pp. 140–1, 133–40).

The following books discuss the ethical aspects of consent:

Jonsen, A.R. *The Birth of Bioethics.* Oxford: Oxford University Press, 1998, pp. 353–8.

Kuczewski, M.G. and Pinkus, R.L.B. *An Ethics Casebook for Hospitals.* Washington DC: Georgetown University Press, 1999, pp. 1–27.

Kushner, T.K. and Thomasma, D.C. *Ward Ethics.* Cambridge: Cambridge University Press, 2001, pp. 18–25.

Randall, F. and Downie, R.S. *Palliative Care Ethics: A Companion for all Specialties* 2nd edn. Oxford: Oxford University Press, 1999, Chapters 2, 10, 11.

The following books discuss legal perspectives on consent:

Mason, J.K. and McCall Smith, R.A. *Law and Medical Ethics* 4th edn. London: Butterworths, 1994, Chapter 10.

Montgomery, J. *Health Care Law.* Oxford: Oxford University Press, 1997, pp. 227–48 (see also Chapter 10).

3.4 Educating for professional competence in palliative medicine

Graham Buckley and Ann Smyth

> The most unethical thing a practising doctor can do is to let his competence fall away[1]

Introduction

As succinctly stated by Sir Douglas Black for doctors, individual ethical responsibility is at the heart of clinical competence for all who care for the sick. In this chapter we describe the quality assurance processes designed to identify and eliminate poor performance and incompetence. These do not alter the ethical imperative for the doctor (and other clinicians), since 'to practice competently is primarily a charge on his own conscience'.[1] How to acquire and maintain clinical skills is an educational question. This chapter consequently largely addresses training issues and does so in the context of the ethical basis of clinical practice.

Professional competence is a deceptively simple label to describe the complex set of attributes and behaviours required of health professionals who are caring for people with incurable illnesses. There is an extensive literature on the desired competencies as defined by educational and professional groups.[2–5] A better starting point is to explore what patients and their families look for in their professional carers.[6] Although this literature base is less extensive it is consistent in defining good practitioners as trusted people who will listen, respond, and act together to optimize patient care and make the end of life as creative, as dignified, and as comfortable as possible. To achieve this requires a synthesis of humanist, technical, and behavioural attributes that we can, in our better moments, identify with professionalism. These attributes have been dissected, arranged, and rearranged in a variety of ways by different professional associations, organizations, and staff groups. There is much commonality in these frameworks, covering the key components of communication skills, symptom management (in particular, pain control), and effective team working. Frameworks are of value in the design of educational curriculae and in assessing the acquisition of these competencies. Separating out the different components of professional practice in this way should not undermine the importance of synthesizing these attributes to ensure that patients receive care that is effective and appropriate to them as individuals in their unique personal, social, and cultural context.

Training in palliative care is clearly of major importance in its own right. Recognition of this has led to significant increases in the time devoted to palliative care in the basic training of doctors and nurses over the past 10 years.[7] In parallel to this development has been the recognition that learning how to provide palliative care can be a powerful, central, and integrating subject for the whole of the curriculum. This is because palliative care raises major biomedical, ethical, communication, social, and personal learning challenges.

In exploring these challenges a generic framework is used here as the model for exploring how competencies can be acquired, deployed, and assessed for the benefit of patients.

A framework of competencies

Competency- or outcome-based education is in the ascendancy in current thinking about the training of health professionals. Critics from the liberal arts tradition are concerned that an exclusive focus on educational outcomes may replace education with mechanistic training. Authors such as McKernan[8] see education as a journey of exploration and discovery in which the outcome cannot be pre-determined. However, the educational debate is in some sense artificially polarized. Among the desired outcomes of the education of health professionals is the need to acquire the skills to challenge prevailing orthodoxy and the intelligence to reflect on practice so that the whole of one's professional career becomes a journey of exploration and discovery.

Brown University Medical School[9] was one of the first to adopt a systematic approach to the definition of outcome-based training and to translate these outcomes into learning plans and assessment strategies designed to integrate competency domains. Building on the work at Brown University, the five Scottish Medical Schools have collaborated in producing their framework, The Scottish Doctor.[10] This is presented here because it is generic and has the potential to be applied to all health professions and all phases of learning.

Translating these generic learning outcomes into specific competencies for different professional groups at different stages in their training is the task of professional bodies, educational providers, employers, and statutory bodies. The detailed make up of these competencies is defined in this textbook. For example, within the emotional intelligence of the generic framework, awareness of psychosocial issues in the context of palliative care requires practitioners to be sensitive to how patients approaching the end of life understand and wish to be supported during a final illness. It can be seen that this competence is not discrete. The links with ethical understanding and with communication skills are obvious. It is, therefore, not surprising that formulations of the competencies needed for good palliative care are usually stated as higher order or meta-competencies. An Australian approach has been to describe these meta-competencies for physicians in terms of a journey through care (adapted from ref. 2):

- Managing entry into palliative care
  - Establish relationship with patient and care giver
  - Identify range and type of problems
- Develop management plan with interdisciplinary team
  - Contribute medical perspective to developing team approach to management
- Review, monitor, and update management plan with interdisciplinary team
  - Monitor medical component of the management plan
- Manage terminal phase and bereavement
  - Redefine and communicate changing problems and priorities with patients, care givers, and interdisciplinary team
- Actively support other members of interdisciplinary team

A more traditional formulation of competencies was constructed through the American Board of Internal Medicine End-of-Life Patient Care Project:

Components	Examples of competencies
Medical knowledge	Assessment of pain and other symptoms
Interviewing and counselling skills	Giving bad news
Team approach	Enhancing ability of team members to fulfil professional responsibilities
Symptom and pain control assessment and management	Awareness and use of treatment guidelines
Professionalism	Confidentiality
Humanistic qualities	Compassion
Medical ethics	Conflicts of interest Surrogate decision making

It is beyond the scope of this chapter to define a complete educational curriculum for training in palliative care. The outlines set out above indicate the broad scope of such a curriculum in terms of competencies. The next question to be considered in planning a training programme is the choice of educational strategy. This requires a basic understanding of the theoretical basis of different educational techniques.

Educational theories relevant to training for palliative care

Kaufman et al.[11] have helpfully summarized the educational strategies and theories that can support practice in the education of health professionals: social cognitive theory, reflective learning, transformative learning, self-directed learning, and experiential learning. There is overlap and concordance between the theories and each adopts the principles of adult learning[12] which can be summarized as:

- a safe learning environment in which challenge is balanced by support;
- learners involved in shaping learning processes and in the context of formal educational interventions;
- learners encouraged to identify their own learning needs and objectives;
- learners actively involved in exploring learning resources and devising strategies to meet their objectives;
- constructive individual feedback on performance and progression forming a central feature of the educational process; and
- learners helped to evaluate their own learning.

The value of the different theoretical perspectives is in the information they give to the complex educational task of creating a fully rounded practitioner.

Social learning. The key concept in social learning or social cognitive theory as it is sometimes termed, is the powerful impact of interaction between the learner and the totality of the environment in determining learning. The prior knowledge, motivation, values, and attitudes held by the learner interact with hidden as well as the explicit and formal elements of an educational programme. The observed behaviours of teachers as positive or negative role models are part of this hidden curriculum. Personal reflection will reveal how significantly these aspects of a learning experience influence engagement with the subject.

Reflective learning is the most seductive of these theories for doctors who tend to feel comfortable within the logical positivism of the biological sciences. Schön[13] built on the positivist paradigm to argue that practitioners have to test and revise their theoretical constructs through reflection in and on practice. He examined the behaviour of practitioners across a range of professions. High quality was associated with individuals who constantly question their performance and who use the unexpected to test and modify their constructs of illness patterns and therapeutics. Encouraging these professional behaviours is seen as a central part of training viewed from this theoretical perspective. Educational programmes can utilize this perspective by incorporating strategies, such as portfolio learning as a practical tool, to gather evidence of practice and facilitate reflection.

Transformative learning theory is similar to social learning in defining learning as a social process of constructing and internalizing new meanings of one's experience as a guide to action. However, it focuses not on the incremental elaboration of existing constructs but looks at what is necessary to radically alter them. How can existing but faulty assumptions, beliefs, feelings, and interpretations be challenged? In the context of training for palliative care is this necessary? It can be argued that this is the key educational task in the culturally and emotionally charged arena of caring for the dying. For this reformist educational agenda, the educator needs to be a co-learner and provocateur. This is one of the strongest theoretical arguments in support of small-group learning. Peers can challenge, in a supportive environment, the beliefs and behaviours of each other to achieve radical change.

Self-directed learning is not so much a theory as an aspiration with moral overtones. It builds on humanist traditions of personal development and the technical evidence of the effectiveness that flows from encouraging learners to control their own education. As such it embodies the key principles of adult learning.

Experiential learning emphasizes the centrality of learning in an environment that links concrete experiences with conceptual models. This linkage is important even in childhood as judged by the work of Piaget. Kolb[14] defines the environment in terms of feeling, thinking, watching, and doing. Learning is seen to be enhanced by engaging with all four modalities.

Desirable features of educational programmes

As can be gathered from the above resumé of relevant educational concepts there is a rich theoretical basis on which to build a curriculum for training in palliative care. The fact that there is no single dominant theory or model leaves room for flexibility. Constructing a curriculum is not like using a recipe book to bake a cake. Local needs, tradition, and resources legitimately colour approaches to training. The professional background, extent of prior knowledge, and current clinical responsibility will also legitimately influence the design of the curriculum. Understanding the theoretical basis and principles of learning offers a framework against which to gauge the potential value of an educational strategy or event. For example, portfolio learning may be ineffective unless it is placed within a process of feedback from mentors so that active reflection on practice is encouraged.

From the consideration of educational principles, theories, and evidence base it is possible to advocate a number of features for successful training programmes:

(i) early experience of palliative care and continuing contact throughout the training period;

(ii) guided reflection on clinical practice and personal development throughout the training period;

(iii) explicit definition of the expected outcome of the training programme in terms of a competency framework;

(iv) an assessment strategy derived from the definitions of educational outcomes;

(v) opportunities for participation in peer group learning or other mechanisms capable of combining personal support with challenge of beliefs and attitudes; and

(vi) encouragement of critical self-appraisal through clinical audit.

Good examples of mapping the acquisition of competencies into this educational approach come from nursing. The framework by Collquhoun and Dougan[4] is of particular value in that it identifies the gradation of competencies required of nurses fulfilling different roles within a health care system.

Designing a curriculum

From the general set of competencies outlined above and the theoretical models described it is possible to construct a specific curriculum for a defined group of learners utilizing available resources. Having established 'what' is to be learned the key questions to be addressed by teachers and learners in developing the curriculum are 'when?' and 'how?'.

When

Boyd[15] has advocated a basic temporal sequence for acquiring competence in breaking bad news:

- awareness of the issues,
- elaboration in context,
- integration into overall array of skills, and
- application.

This approach can be generalized to other learning outcomes in palliative care and offers a helpful guide to curriculum planning. Guidance from expert groups such as the United States National Consensus Conference on Medical Education for Care Near the End of Life[16] are also of value in constructing the different stages of a curriculum. As an example, for the early years of the undergraduate medical curriculum they identify the following outcomes:

1. Understanding the psychological, sociologic, cultural, and spiritual aspects of death and dying:

   (a) suffering

Table 1 The learning outcomes for a competent and reflective practitioner, based on the three-circle model

A. What the doctor is able to do—'doing the right thing', Technical intelligence

1 **Clinical skills**	2 **Practical procedures**	3 **Patient investigations**	4 **Patient managements**	5 **Health promotion and disease preventions**	6 **Communication**	7 **Appropriate information handling skills**
❑ History ❑ Physical examination ❑ Interpretation of findings ❑ Formulation of action plan to characterize problem and reach a diagnosis	❑ Cardiology ❑ Dermatology ❑ Endocrinology ❑ Gastroenterology ❑ Haematology ❑ Musculo-skeletal ❑ Nervous system ❑ Ophthalmology ❑ Otolaryngology ❑ Renal/urology ❑ Reproduction ❑ Respiratory ❑ Surgery ❑ General	❑ General principles ❑ Clinical ❑ Imaging ❑ Biochemical medicine ❑ Haematology ❑ Immunology ❑ Microbiology ❑ Pathology ❑ Genetics	❑ General principles ❑ Drugs ❑ Surgery ❑ Psychological ❑ Physiotherapy ❑ Radiotherapy ❑ Social ❑ Nutrition ❑ Emergency medicine ❑ Acute care ❑ Chronic care ❑ Rehabilitation ❑ Alternative therapies ❑ Patient referral	❑ Recognition of causes of threats to health and individual at risk ❑ Implementation where appropriate of basics of prevention ❑ Collaboration with other health professionals in health promotion and disease prevention	❑ With patient ❑ With relatives ❑ With colleagues ❑ With agencies ❑ With media/press ❑ Teaching ❑ Managing ❑ Patient advocate ❑ Mediation and negotiation ❑ By telephone ❑ In writing	❑ Patient records ❑ Accessing data sources ❑ Use of computers ❑ Implementation of professional guidelines ❑ Personal records (log books, portfolios)

B. How the doctor approaches their practice—'doing the thing right'			C. The doctor as a professional—'the right person doing it'	
Intellectual intelligence	**Emotional intelligence**	**Analytical and creative intelligence**	**Personal intelligence**	
8 **Understanding of social, basic and clinical sciences, and underlying principles**	9 **Appropriate attitudes, ethical understanding, and legal responsibilities**	10 **Appropriate decision making skills, and clinical reasoning and judgement**	11 **Role of the doctor within the health service**	12 **Personal development**
❑ Normal structure and function ❑ Normal behaviour ❑ The life cycle ❑ Pathophysiology ❑ Psychosocial model of illness ❑ Pharmacology and clinical pharmacology ❑ Public health medicine ❑ Epidemiology ❑ Preventative medicine and health prevention ❑ Education ❑ Health economics	❑ Attitudes ❑ Understanding of ethical principles ❑ Ethical standards ❑ Legal responsibilities ❑ Human rights issues ❑ Respect for colleagues ❑ Medicine in multicultural societies ❑ Awareness of psychosocial issues ❑ Awareness of economic issues ❑ Acceptance of responsibility to contribute to advance of medicine ❑ Appropriate attitude to professional institution and health service bodies	❑ Clinical reasoning ❑ Evidence-based medicine ❑ Critical thinking ❑ Research method ❑ Statistical understanding ❑ Creativity/resourcefulness ❑ Coping with uncertainty ❑ Prioritization	❑ Understanding of health care systems ❑ Understanding of clinical responsibilities and role of doctor ❑ Acceptance of code of conduct and required personal attributes ❑ Appreciation of doctor as researcher ❑ Appreciation of doctor as mentor or teacher ❑ Appreciation of doctor as manager including quality control ❑ Appreciation of doctor as member of multiprofessional team and of roles of other health care professionals	❑ Self-learner ❑ Self-awareness • enquires into own competence • emotional awareness • self-confidence ❑ Self-regulation • self-care • self-control • adaptability to change • personal time management ❑ Motivation • achievement drive • commitment • initiative ❑ Career choice

Notes: Harden et al.[18] see also AMEE Education Guide No. 14, Outcome-based education.

(b) loss

(c) bereavement

(d) ritual and meaning at the end of life

2. Develop basic interviewing and communication skills essential to end of life care:

(a) how to listen to the impact of illness on life

(b) how to explore hope, hopelessness, and fear

(c) how to discuss loss and grief

3. Understand the pathophysiology and management of common symptoms at the end of life:

(a) pain

(b) shortness of breath

(c) dehydration

(d) depression

4. Identify significant points of consensus and controversy in the ethical aspects of end of life care:

(a) withholding/withdrawing treatment, assisted suicide, and euthanasia

(b) pain management

(c) allocation of resources and access to high-quality palliative care

(d) non-abandonment of patients

5. Improve their ability to reflect self-critically on their personal and professional experiences around death and loss:

(a) death in their personal experience

(b) views of the afterlife

(c) the goals of medicine

(d) the role of the doctor and the health care team in caring for the dying

How

Integration of these competencies into a general curriculum can be achieved through curriculum mapping.[17] This can be achieved most readily by using a generic framework such as the Scottish Doctor[9] (Table 1) model and listing the desirable competencies alongside those for other complex and important clinical responsibilities, such as the management of pregnancy. The degree of overlap in areas other than specific knowledge bases will be seen to be considerable. This allows the programme designer to develop generic attributes such as interviewing skills by selection of patients and problems across a broad range of clinical scenarios and developing these skills by introducing greater complexity over time.

Spiral curriculum

The above describes the basic concept of the spiral curriculum.[18] For both generic and clinical training and programmes specifically targeted on palliative care, the aim in a spiral curriculum is to provide learners with a taste of the full range of clinical challenges in the first cycle of the course. This raises awareness of fundamental issues and provides an overall framework for the learners and makes it possible for them to identify gaps and weaknesses that they can address in subsequent cycles.

The following is a guide to the content of the first cycle of a spiral curriculum for training in palliative care:

- develop awareness and understanding of the psychological, social, cultural, and spiritual aspects of death and dying;
- begin in a supportive environment to explore the self-knowledge of the learner around their own beliefs and emotions in relation to death and dying;
- develop basic communication skills and how to conduct interviews which are emotionally charged;
- on the basis of increasing knowledge of psychology pathophysiology and pharmacology start to understand the management of common symptoms at the end of life; and
- from a general understanding of underlying principles begin to understand significant points of consensus and controversy in the ethical aspects of palliative care, for example, resource allocation, euthanasia, personal and professional boundaries.

Synthesis

From the above it will be clear that a range of educational strategies are required in the training programme. Conventional lectures and study guides can deal with the factual elements of the curriculum. The emotional intelligence required of professionals in clinical practice, particularly in palliative care, requires a participative approach to learning. From the psychology and education literature it is clear that facilitated small-group learning is a powerful way for learners to examine and modify beliefs and understanding of themselves and others. The power of this technique places a strong moral obligation on the teachers and institutions to make this experience beneficial to all the participants. Within a supportive group, techniques such as role play allow learners to develop skills of interviewing within a safe environment as well as of addressing key ethical issues and exploring values and beliefs. Following Boyd's framework, a spiral curriculum will present increasing complexity of clinical challenge and utilize progressively the actual experience of the learner in observing and then contributing to the provision of palliative care.

With notable exceptions, the planned and structured education for health professionals almost completely evaporates on entry to career posts. This may be the moment of maximum personal and professional challenge as full responsibility for patient care is assumed. Maladaptive behaviours and responses to the demands of caring for people at the end of life may originate at this time leading in some cases to burn out and drug or alcohol misuse. A number of initiatives have tackled this problem in generic and targeted ways.[19] It is increasingly recognized that health professionals who carry continuing responsibilities for people at the end of life need to understand their own needs for support, have ready access to help, and be part of a professional environment which builds in support as a normal part of the therapeutic community. A crucial dimension of professional competence, particularly in palliative care, is this ability to monitor all aspects of one's performance.

Poor performance and incompetence

In this chapter we concentrate on the educational frameworks and strategies required to help health professionals become competent. A wide range of professional and regulatory bodies accredit the attainment of clinical competence. Traditional reliance on initial professional qualifications as guarantors of continuing competence has been undermined by a series of high-profile disciplinary and legal cases in the United Kingdom and elsewhere. These have revealed in stark fashion the gap, for some practitioners, between their ability to attain acceptable standards in test conditions and their performance to these standards in day-to-day care of patients.

The need to assure the public of the continuing competence and satisfactory performance of health professionals, has led to the introduction of professional re-certification and clinical audit. The difference between the assessment of competence and measurement of performance can be likened to the difference between *in vitro* and *in vivo* research.

In vitro or competency assessment takes place in a regulated and defined context to ensure reliability in judging the attainment of explicit standards of knowledge and skills. Although attempts are made to incorporate attitudinal measures into these assessments the difficulty in making them reliable means that these components rarely influence pass/fail decisions in high-stake professional examinations. In contrast *in vivo* or performance assessments take place in the real complex world of clinical practice. Values, interpersonal relationships, team working, and other personal attributes play a crucial part in determining whether technical competence leads to effective performance. There are of course factors beyond the control of the individual that impact on performance. The literature on clinical error and medical mishaps provides evidence of the crucial importance of good systems of care. Error is rarely only due to the behaviour of an individual clinician.

The key issue is how can we assure patients that they are receiving good standards of care. Two related approaches are being pursued in many different countries. The first is to require health professionals to demonstrate their continuing competence in order to maintain their professional certification. Early initiatives in nursing in Australia[(19)] relied on evidence of participation in formal and informal continuing education. Licensing bodies, employers, and governments acting on behalf of patients are now seeking to go beyond this educational proxy for competence by examining the performance of clinicians. Norcini[(20)] has documented the difficulties encountered in the United States in devising rigorous and fair assessments that rely on patient outcome measures. Such measures are now used routinely to provide performance profiles but case mix differences and problems in attributing outcomes to individuals in a team setting limit their use in re-certification.

From the perspective of the patient it is the standard of overall care that matters. This shifts the focus from individual professional competence to the performance of teams. Clinical audit is the second and more important of the ways of assuring the public about standards of care. Health care organizations in many parts of the world are implementing clinical audit in a systematic fashion. One good example comes from Scotland. The Clinical Standards Board as part of the National Health Service has published the set of standards they will use in reviewing the performance of units providing specialist care.[(21)] The standards cover areas such as: access to care, range of skills available to patients, the programmes of continuing education for staff members, effectiveness of communication to other care providers including the families of patients, specialist interventions for symptom control, and patients' preferred place of death being sensitively ascertained and responded to. For each area a statement of the standard is published together with the evidence base or rationale behind it, the detailed criteria that will be used to judge achievement of the standard, and the specific data that will be collected. Using the terminology of Donabedian, the standards relate to structure and process rather than to outcome, but in palliative care this makes sense.

The title for this section invites negativity and the burgeoning industry of quality assurance in health care potentially adds to the stress of committed practitioners. The challenge to achieve high standards of care needs to be balanced by support. Just as the maintenance of competence is the ethical responsibility of the individual clinicians, the support provided by employers to sustain doctors, nurses, and others in the intellectually and emotionally challenging field of palliative care is also an ethical issue.

Re-certification and quality audit programmes therefore need to be designed to stimulate and support clinical teams. Celebration of good practice needs to feature the identification of areas where performance can improve. Early experience of the involvement of patients in the performance review processes of the General Medical Council suggests that they achieve this balanced approach more easily than professionally qualified assessors do.

References

1. **Black, D.** (2001). A bottom line in medical ethics. *Clinical Medicine* **1** (6), 455–6.
2. **Yuen, K.** et al. (1998). Educating doctors in palliative medicine: development of a competency-based training program. *Journal of Palliative Care* **14** (3), 79–82.
3. **Blank, L.L.** (1995). Defining and evaluating physician competence in end-of-life patient care. *Western Journal of Medicine* **163**, 297–301.
4. **Colquhoun, M. and Dougan, H.** (1997). Performance standards: ensuring that the specialist nurse in palliative care is special. *Palliative Medicine* **11**, 381–7.
5. **American Board of Internal Medicine.** *Caring for the Dying: Identification and Promotion of Physician Competency.* Philadelphia PA: ABIM, 1996.
6. **Block, S. and Billings, J.A.** (1998) Nurturing humanism through teaching palliative care. *Academic Medica* **7**, 764–5.
7. **Field, M.J. and Cassel, C.K.**, ed. *Approaching Death: Improved Care at the End of Life. Report from the Institute of Medicine Committee on Care at the End of Life.* Washington DC: National Academy Press, 1997.
8. **McKernan, J.** (1993). Perspectives and Imperatives: some limitations of outcome-based education. *Journal of Curriculum and Supervision* **8** (4), 343–53.
9. **Smith, R.S. and Dollase, R.** *AMEE Education Guide No. 14.* Association for the Study of Medical Education in Europe, Dundee, AMEE 1999.
10. **Harden, R.M., Crosby, J.R., Davis, M.H., and Friedman, M.** (1999). From competency to meta-competency: a model for the specification of learning outcomes. *Medical Teacher* **21** (6), 546–52.
11. **Kaufman, D.M., Mann, K.V., and Jennett, P.A.** *Teaching and Learning in Medical Education: How Theory can Inform Practice.* ASME Education Booklet. Association for the Study of Medical Education, Edinburgh, ASME 2000.
12. **Knowles, M.S.** *The Modern Practice of Adult Education: From Pedagogy to Andragogy* 2nd edn. New York: Cambridge Books, 1980.
13. **Schön, D.A.** *The Reflective Practitioner: How Professionals Think in Action.* New York: Basic Books, 1983.
14. **Kolb, D.A.** *Experiential Learning: Experience as the Source of Learning and Development.* Eaglewood Cliffs NJ: Prentice Hall, 1984.
15. **Boyd, K.M.** (1994). Helping future doctors learn how to break bad news. *Medical Teacher* **16** (4), 297–301.
16. **Barnard, D.** et al. (1999). Preparing the ground: contributions of the pre-clinical years to medical education for care near the end of life. *Academia Medica* **74** (5), 499–505.
17. **Harden, R.M.** *Curriculum Mapping: A Tool for Transparent and Authentic Teaching and Learning.* AMEE Education Guide No 21. Association for the Study of Medical Education in Europe, Dundee, AMEE 2001.
18. **Harden, R.M. and Stamper, N.** (1999). What is spiral curriculum? *Medical Teacher* **21** (2), 141–3.
19. **Newble, D., Paget, N., and McLaren, B.** (1999). Revalidation in Australia and New Zealand: approach of the Royal Australasian College of Physicians. *British Medical Journal* **319**, 1185–8.
20. **Norcini, J.J.** (1999). Re-certification in the United States. *British Medical Journal* **319**, 1183–5.
21. *Specialist Palliative Care Draft Standards.* Clinical Standards Board for Scotland, Edinburgh, 2001.

3.5 Palliative medicine and children: ethical and legal issues

Len Doyal, Ann Goldman, Vic Larcher, and Cyril Chantler

The impending death of a child poses practical, intellectual, and emotional challenges for the child, their family, and professionals alike. One of the roles of good palliative care is to respond to these challenges. However, a prerequisite to the effective provision of palliative care is the acceptance by all concerned of a change in the goal of treatment from cure to palliation. Of course, some aspects of palliative care will accompany attempts to cure, especially when the overall prognosis remains in doubt. Decisions to change the goals of care mean, in effect, that there are circumstances when it is no longer morally or legally acceptable or necessary to initiate or to continue to provide life-sustaining treatment.

The purpose of this chapter is to explore the moral and legal arguments concerning the provision of palliative care when a decision has been made not to prolong life. It will outline the ethico-legal basis of such decisions as they apply to a variety of situations in childhood terminal illness. Finally, suggestions about the management of conflict will be provided, along with procedural mechanisms for dealing with the moral indeterminacy that may accompany the decision-making progress. While the focus of legal analysis will be on law within the United Kingdom, similar principles and reasoning will apply to other national legal jurisdictions.

Background

Both technological advances and improved public health have contributed to falling death rates in infants and children. Survival rates for extremely premature babies have increased, cure of childhood leukaemia is the rule rather than the exception and patients with chronic diseases such as cystic fibrosis have an increased life expectancy. Many paediatricians do not have significant experience of death in childhood, and the context in which such deaths occur is extremely variable. Acute deaths may occur in neonates who sustain brain haemorrhage or in victims of accidents. The process of dying may be more protracted (e.g. relapsed leukaemia) while other children may face a slow decline as a result of a naturally shortened life span (e.g. those with severe psychomotor disability).

Responses of children, parents, and professionals are as variable as the circumstances that provoke them. Some parents may want active treatment, directed at prolonging life, continued to the very moment of death. Others, seeing the pain and suffering of their child and perhaps uncertain whether they have the strength and will to support him or her, may wish for a speedy and peaceful death. There may be a sense of loss of future potential, feelings of anger, bewilderment, betrayal, and desolation at the cruel hand that fate has dealt, coupled with a sense of injustice and perhaps depression. Professionals, confronted with such situations may share many of the feelings of the child and their family and may be unsure as to how they are to fulfil their duty to protect life and health. Given the assumed potential for growth and development that children have, it is perhaps not surprising that paediatricians frequently give their patients more chances to recover from their illness than adults might receive. As a consequence some children may receive treatments that carry greater burdens with less chances of success than those used for adults.

It is in these circumstances that palliative care assumes great importance. If health can be defined as the absence of physical and mental disabilities that otherwise would be caused by disease then it is clear that the intention to use palliative care is entirely consistent with the duty to restore health. It achieves this by attempting to relieve both pain and suffering, promoting the development of the child's emotional and cognitive abilities, and enabling the child to sustain his or her capabilities for as long as possible. In short, the aim of good palliative care is to maximize the child's potential, while acknowledging the constraints imposed by their illness. Such care also involves supporting parents and professional carers in their duties and responsibilities to the child in the face of the suffering imposed by terminal illness. Seen in these terms palliative care involves far more than provision of effective pain relief and has many positive attributes, which apply throughout a terminal illness.

However, the decision to opt for palliative care instead of potentially curative treatment also poses intellectual and emotional problems for all concerned, because it involves changing the goals of care. Inherent in this process is the decision both not to provide or to withdraw life-sustaining treatment (NPWLST) and its timing. It is therefore essential to consider the circumstances, in the context of the child's illness, when it is felt that life-sustaining treatment is no longer morally or legally justified. A prerequisite for such decision-making is the availability of palliative care which is crucial in optimizing the comfort and dignity of patients and supporting carers. Almost inevitably those who provide palliative care will be involved in the decision-making process.

Although there may be certain circumstances that are relatively straight forward—for example, the management of a child who is actually dying, decisions not to try to prolong life can provoke self-doubt in professionals and conflict with parents. This is especially so in situations where death is not imminent but there are serious moral questions about sustaining life, even though it may be technically possible to do so. It is therefore important that those who undertake palliative care have a good understanding of the ethical and legal principles that underpin such decisions and which may enable them to negotiate the potential minefields of dilemmas and uncertainties that may exist. This understanding is necessary so that the basis on which decisions are made can be sensitively communicated with the child (if possible) and their parents in a constructive and open fashion. Practitioners in palliative care rightly emphasize the importance of the qualities of sympathy, empathy, good communication, and team work in the management of terminal illness. The exhibition of these qualities depends on the clarity of moral and legal reasoning of those involved; provision of such clarity is also a goal of this chapter.

Moral arguments about not prolonging life

The first duty of clinical care is to respect the life and health of patients to an acceptable standard.[1] Individuals whose lives are at risk and can be saved, or who are suffering from illness that can be cured or effectively managed, should receive appropriate medical help. For clinicians to breach this duty of care is a potentially serious offence, which may entail professional censure or exclusion and legal, possibly criminal, culpability. For example, if clinicians do nothing to save the lives of patients whose death is foreseeable, then they may be prosecuted for murder as the result of such inaction. This is because they will have knowingly and deliberately acted in direct contravention of their duty of care.[2]

However, despite these caveats, it is also the case that in some circumstances, clinicians are not only professionally and legally allowed to make decisions NPWLST where it is clear that death is likely to result, but also do so with considerable frequency.[3,4] How can this be reconciled with their general duty of care and the potentially punitive consequences of not abiding by it? Morally, the argument is clear. In most circumstances, protecting and saving the lives of patients is in their best interests, because medical treatment can benefit them. This is why making a decision NPWLST cannot simply be morally justified by statements to the effect that 'nature should be allowed to take its course' or 'it would be better not to try too hard' to sustain a patient's life. Therefore, given the duty to protect life, there can be only one coherent justification for not doing so—that for some reason, to do so is not in the patient's best interests.

The moral justification for non-treatment decisions inevitably relates to circumstances where it is no longer clear that patients' objective interests as humans are best served by prolonging their lives.[5] It is in this context that the benefits and burdens of medical treatment will be evaluated. Unless continued life is in the best interest of patients, further life-prolonging treatment can have no benefit and cannot be worth the burden. The crucial moral question then becomes: when is it more in the interest of a patient to die than to continue to live? Generally speaking, this will be when the patient is permanently unable—or is no longer so able—to engage minimally, and with some sense of sustained self-awareness and well being, in any of the activities that uniquely characterize human life.[5,6] Such inability may occur in a range of circumstances:

- Patients may be so close to death and in such a physically and emotionally weakened state that they are no longer able to initiate any coherent action.

- Patients may be so brain damaged that they have minimal capacities to reason, to choose, to plan ahead, and thus to interact intentionally with others. It is through such interaction that individuals continue to expand their understanding of themselves, of other humans, and of the rest of the world.

Inability aside, patients may have all of the characteristic human attributes and self-awareness and be fully capable of interaction with others. However, they may themselves decide that, because of the physical and emotional impact of their terminal illness, life does not have enough sustained meaning for them to wish to continue it. They may judge the provision or continuation of life-prolonging treatment as a burden that is no longer in their best interest.

In all these circumstances clinicians may decide that it is morally and professionally unacceptable to strive to prolong the lives of patients by medical means.[1] Against the background of poor quality of life and prospects for anything resembling a minimally fulfilled human life, the ratio of benefit to burden of treatment can no longer warrant further life-prolonging medical intervention.[6] To ignore this fact on the grounds of the 'sanctity of life' is clearly just as much a breach of the duty of care as not clinically intervening when it is in the patients best interests.[7,8]

Despite these arguments, decisions NPWLST would be morally unacceptable if they in any way added to the suffering or indignity of the patients concerned. As has been noted, terminally ill patients who are candidates for such decisions will have often already benefited from palliative care focused on the relief of physical and psychological pain and discomfort. Terminal illness that culminates in a decision NPWLST can take place abruptly (e.g. as the result of an accident) or can occur over a long period.[9] To this extent, palliative care should not in itself be identified with non-treatment decisions. Rather, such care underlines the importance of the moral obligation to minimize the suffering of terminally ill patients, even after it has been agreed that life-sustaining medical treatment is of no further benefit to them. The knowledge that pain and other forms of suffering can be effectively managed can also be of great help to relatives and professional carers who recognize and feel the moral enormity of deciding that a patient should be allowed to die without further medical intervention.[10,11]

The legality of decisions not to provide or sustain life-prolonging treatment

Until recently, clinicians who allowed patients to die as a result of decisions NPWLST did so within a legal environment that was potentially punitive. Prior to 1989, the only legal precedent for such decisions in the United Kingdom was a ruling by Lord Justice Templeman. In Re B (81) he suggested that if infants—and therefore all people—had lives that were 'demonstrably awful' it might be appropriate to allow them to die without medical intervention.[12] Templeman was unclear about the precise clinical meaning of this phrase, although it was clear contextually that he envisaged a level of brain damage and disability more extreme than Down's Syndrome. Until the law was further clarified, therefore, clinicians who made non-treatment decisions exposed themselves to criminal charges, including murder.

The situation changed dramatically during the 1990s, with a series of legal cases concerning severely damaged infants. Again, these cases had consequences for all patients and their outcome established the legality of non-treatment decisions in specific circumstances and the criteria by which such decisions could be made. These criteria directly reflect the moral arguments already outlined, in terms of their focus on best interests.

- Re C (89).[13] This infant was *imminently and irreversibly close to death* as a result of hydrocephalus and cerebral malformation.
- Re J (90).[14] Here, the baby was not close to death but was so brain damaged that he would *never be able to engage in any form of self-directed activity*. The baby had probable severe spastic quadriplegia, deafness, blindness, and very little intellectual potential or capacity to feel pain.
- Re J (92).[15] The child in this case was also not close to death but had severe brain damage as a consequence of microcephaly with severe cerebral palsy. The clinical decision to NPWLST was legally upheld against the wishes of the child's mother. It established that clinicians *cannot be forced to administer life-sustaining treatments that they believe are not in the best interests of patients with very severe brain damage, even when the patients are children and parents insist that treatment continues.*
- Airedale NHS Trust v Bland (93).[16] As the result of severe injury, Tony Bland (an adult) was in a persistent vegetative state for over 2 years. It was held that further medical treatment would not be of any benefit to him and could be withdrawn.
- Re R (96).[17] In this case, it was held that the non-provision of life-sustaining antibiotic therapy and cardio-pulmonary resuscitation was acceptable for an adult with very severe brain damage.

These cases provided clinical substance to what Templeman had earlier meant by a 'demonstrably awful' life and they continue to influence professional and legal thinking about non-treatment decisions. In effect, they legalize what can be called passive euthanasia within the United Kingdom.[18] However, it is inconceivable that these cases would have been decided as they were without the availability of effective palliative care, since they were concerned with minimizing the long-term suffering of patients through decisions NPWLST. This would be impossible without such care. However, it is equally clear that the judges in question did not reduce the potential interest of patients in staying alive to just the successful management of their physical or emotional discomfort. Ultimately, their judgement to legalize decisions NPWLST was essentially moral in character, as it must be in other national legal jurisdictions where similar principles prevail.

Paediatric guidelines for non-provision and withdrawal of life-sustaining treatment

In 1997, these moral and legal arguments concerning NPWLST decisions were accepted and further developed by the Royal College of Paediatrics and Child Health (RCPCH).[19] In some cases involving children, such decisions—although traumatic—may not be too difficult for professional and parental carers (e.g. when the child is a terminally ill infant with no prospect of a future life). In others, they will raise more problems (e.g. when the terminally ill child has a fully developed personality and, on the face of it, everything to live for but no opportunity to do so).

The RCPCH guidelines address all of these different prospects and state that withholding or withdrawing curative medical treatment might be considered when:

1. The child has been appropriately diagnosed as brain dead.
2. The child has been appropriately diagnosed to be in a permanent vegetative state (PVS).
3. The situation is one of 'no chance' where death is only being marginally delayed, without significant alleviation of suffering.
4. There is 'no purpose' in keeping the child alive because of a dramatic and unacceptable degree of physical or mental impairment, such that it would be unreasonable to expect him or her to tolerate it. Either because of age or the severity of brain damage, the child will never be able to participate in 'decisions regarding treatment or its withdrawal'.
5. The child's future life will be 'unbearable'. In the face of 'progressive and irreversible' illness the child and/or the family believe that further treatment is more than the child can endure with any acceptable degree of human fulfilment. Such children may or may not be mentally impaired. If they are for whatever reason, the impact of such impairment on the child must be considered.

Legally, the first criterion has been long established and the second was confirmed by Airedale NHS Trust v Bland (93). The third criterion is based on Re C (89) and the fourth on Re J (90) and Re J (92), at least to the extent that it is meant to pertain to very severe brain damage. The fifth criterion is legally more complicated, as will be shown.

Since brain death and PVS are clinically well understood, the focus here will be on the last three criteria. Each can be illustrated as follows:[20]

- *No chance.* These are cases where there is a consensus that further clinical intervention will be futile—will not achieve the goal of significant prolongation of life. An example might be a child of 18 months who presents with meningo-coccal septicaemia, but who, despite intensive care, develops multiple organ failure.
- *No purpose.* Here, brain damage is so extensive that the child will develop or will regress to only minimal self-awareness and capacity for self-directed activity or interaction with others. Thus a 3-month-old girl resuscitated at birth (weight 480 g) might require immediate ventilation and neonatal intensive care followed by further ventilation, high doses of steroids, no significant improvement in lung function, and the occurrence of severe intraventricular haemorrhages in the brain with a high probability of severe mental disability. This may occur in any stage of childhood depending on the type of illness concerned (e.g. Tay–Sachs, Battens, and other incurable genetic diseases associated with childhood).
- *Unbearable.* Such cases entail the necessity for repeated, dramatic, and potentially traumatic clinical interventions whose burden is deemed by parents, professional carers, and perhaps the children themselves, as being too great in light of the potential benefit. A case would be a 10-year-old boy with renal failure, with dysmorphic kidneys, moderately severe learning difficulties, but with a degree of physical independence, an attractive personality, and much love from parents and siblings. After extensive discussion with the clinical team, his school, the parents of other similarly affected children, social workers, and a chaplain, his parents decided that dialysis should not begin. Similar clinical cases may involve children who are mature enough to decide to refuse such clinical intervention themselves where their decision is supported by the family and clinical team. An example might be the child with advanced lung disease as a result of cystic fibrosis who refuses heart–lung transplantation.

With the first three criteria (i.e. brain death, PVS, and futile intervention) parental views and demands for treatment do not confer legal obligations—as Re J (92) confirms. Yet while the child is and should be the focus of the paediatric duty of care, it is equally clear that some further moral duty is owed to the parents. Their distress and concern are themselves forms of suffering that deserve support and guidance.[10] Clinical teams, especially those providing palliative care, inevitably bear the brunt of the responsibility to provide both. They must delicately negotiate with parents, helping them to understand the nature of their child's condition, prognosis, and why the NPWLST is believed to be in the child's best interest. If done sensitively and with appropriate communication skills, such counselling can often lead to successful outcomes both for the child and the parent, however ambiguous the word 'success' must be in this context.

However, this may be impossible. For example, parents may insist on the continuation of medical intervention that will neither significantly sustain life nor confer clinical benefit (e.g. in brain stem death or PVS). Here, the clinical team must affirm their belief that the interests of the child will not be served by further active treatment, and that it is their professional duty not to provide it.[21] While courts in the United Kingdom have made it clear that they will support such clinical judgments, this picture becomes more complex in other legal national jurisdictions, where parents are deemed to have more authority. Generally, parents who reject the advice of the clinical team and wish for life-sustaining treatment to continue should:

- be counselled with respect and dignity;
- be advised that they may wish to go to court to obtain judicial intervention in their favour, but informed that this is unlikely to be the outcome;
- be told how to go about this and, where practical, helped to do so;
- be supported sympathetically with regard to the clinical and moral reasons for non-treatment; and
- not be engaged in adversarial conflict and debate.

These issues will often emerge in the broader context of discussions about on-going palliative care, and those responsible for such care may be actively involved in these sensitive negotiations.

The chronically deteriorating immature child

The fourth and fifth criteria of the RCPCH guidelines raise moral and legal issues more contentious than the first three.[22] Using them to justify decisions NPWLST should therefore be approached with caution. The fourth criterion of 'no purpose' suggests that non-treatment may be acceptable in children with a small degree of cognitive function—enough, say, for minimal levels of self-directed activity and social interaction—but who also have overwhelming physical disability. There is imprecision about the nature and type of physical or mental impairment envisaged. However, this criterion expressly refers to the fact that maintaining the life of such a child would have 'no purpose'. This suggests that the brunt of the dramatic impairment is meant to be primarily neurological in the context of a very short life expectancy—at whatever point in the child's life that this is revealed. Clinical examples of this kind have already been outlined.

This emphasis on severe neurological damage does not apply to the fifth criterion of 'unbearable' because this partly encompasses children who are capable of clear but limited cognitive and emotional development. The maturity of such children may be compromised by disability, by age, or by the effect of illness. On the one hand, through invasive treatment, their lives may be sustainable in the short to long-term, perhaps even through adolescence and beyond. On the other hand, their personal experience of life under these circumstances may be terrible.

Such children may be able to experience and conceptualize bewilderment and despair about their physical disabilities and their consequent inability to achieve whatever goals they are capable of setting for themselves. They are therefore well outside the 'no purpose' criterion. But it is precisely this increased but limited level of awareness and understanding—and the sadness and frustration that may go with it—that can make the point of continued life-sustaining treatment and continued life itself so questionable for them, their parents, and professional carers. Such children may indeed reach a state where the prospect of further invasive and disruptive life-prolonging treatment is more than those who love and care for them believe that they can bear.

Clinical conditions relevant to decisions of this kind NPWLST include respiratory, cardiac, or kidney diseases that are incurable and rapidly degenerative. Equally important are childhood cancers where unpleasant treatment has been repeated, and where further treatment may extend life but with an increasingly uncertain therapeutic outcome. In these circumstances, some parents may believe that their children have such limited potential for human fulfilment that further treatment to preserve life is no longer in the child's best interest. Conversely, other parents may take the opposite view and believe that they can and should provide maximum support for their child, to continue to try to optimize their potential for as long as possible.[23]

It should now be clear why the fifth RCPCH criterion differs from the others. Cognitive impairment may vary in children in this category but case law only refers to the most dramatic forms of such impairment. Yet in the circumstances that have been described, it may well be that continued life is not in the best interests of children who lack the maturity to make such a judgment for themselves and whose disabilities are worsening with no hope of significant improvement. If the health care team is convinced that this is so then it is highly unlikely that a decision NPWLST will lead to any suggestion of legal impropriety—provided that parents also agree.

A problem might arise if the team believes that life-sustaining treatment should be withdrawn and the parents disagree. Here, the wishes of the parents should be respected—unless there is some reason to believe that they are practically incapable of providing the support and resources required to optimize their child's personal potential. In the face of further dispute, a judicial ruling should be obtained.

This analysis leads to what some may regard as a disquieting conclusion. Children, with the same clinical condition, will in one situation (parental support) have their lives sustained, while in another situation (the withdrawal of parental support) will have their lives foreshortened.[5] The moral justification for this is that, since there is some indeterminacy about the child's cognitive, emotional, and physical potentials, it would be wrong to force the beliefs of the clinical team on parents who disagreed. After all, it is the parents and not the team who will have to live with either committing themselves to caring for their child or with the knowledge that they morally participated in a decision that foreshortened their child's life.

In either circumstance, effective palliative care becomes essential. In the case of the young child for whom parents and clinicians agree that continued life has become too unbearable, NPWLST—which might include any item on the 'therapeutic menu'—might not bring about immediate death. However, if such withdrawal is clinically managed, palliative measures should ensure:

- minimal suffering and discomfort for the child,
- maximal support for parents though sensitive and constructive communication,
- provision of relevant information so that parental decisions can be as informed as possible,
- maximum intimate contact with the child if death will occur in hospital, and
- measures that will optimize the potential success of the bereavement process.

Similarly, if the decision is to continue to sustain the child's life, then the inevitability of further deterioration will necessitate palliative measures designed to optimize physical and emotional functions and to minimize discomfort. Support for the parents entails the provision of appropriate information and practical help to assist them to ensure that their child will sustain the best quality of life possible.

Respect for the autonomy of the chronically deteriorating mature child

It can be seen that a paediatrician's duty of care demands acting in the best interests of their immature patients and that this may lead to NPWLST decisions. However, paediatricians also have another duty of care. This is to respect the autonomy of their patients—their moral right to make informed and reasoned choices about their illnesses and treatments.

Terminally ill children may develop high levels of maturity before they die. Although their life expectancy may be brief and their degrees of autonomy may vary considerably, these young people may have much that they wish to try to accomplish. The combination of life-sustaining intervention with effective palliative care is essential in assisting them to this end. To this extent, the second duty of care will be consistent with the first. Most children will want to optimize their life expectancy and the quality of their life just as much as will their parents and clinicians. As a result, they will wish to co-operate with their clinical management. Such partnership in care can be enormously rewarding for all concerned, despite the circumstances in which it occurs.

A minority of children may choose not to co-operate with or simply to refuse the provision of life-prolonging care. For whatever reason, and irrespective or whatever potential benefits that good clinical and palliative care may offer, they may decide that they do not wish to continue to live with the burden that their illness imposes. Here, the duty to protect life and health comes into direct conflict with the duty to respect autonomy—to the degree that such children may be said to possess it.

The importance of respecting the autonomy of children

Respect for the autonomy of children is of particular importance. If the dignity of adults is abused through denying them informed choice, their capacity to return to some state of normality will probably be preserved. This is because their cognitive and emotional foundations for individual personality and personal identity are well developed. The opposite holds, however, for children. They are in the process of developing their personalities and learn through their interactive relationships with adults. Their personal identities are forged around experiencing themselves as the kinds of persons who are deemed by adults to do some things well and others not so well. Their emotional confidence and health will very much depend on their self-satisfaction with these dynamic and evolving achievements.[24]

Hence, lack of respect for a child's autonomy can severely undermine both intellectual skills and emotional confidence in ways that can be irretrievable. This is why disrespect of children can be so damaging to their future potential as persons and why it can be so psychologically traumatic for them when it occurs. Yet equally, children must be protected in circumstances where they are at risk and not able to protect themselves. Finding this balance can be complex in the clinical care of children.[25]

Younger children may lack sufficient autonomy to be able to consent to or refuse medical treatment. This does not mean that it is unnecessary to consult them about their thoughts and feelings concerning their illness and its treatment. Such consultation is mandated by the United Nations Convention on the Rights of the Child and nationally in the United Kingdom by the Children Act.[26,27] Thus the beliefs of an immature child with a chronically deteriorating terminal illness must be taken into account in any medical decisions made about them, even when these beliefs are ultimately rejected. Here, the balance between respect and protection weighs in favour of the latter. On the other hand, if the child is autonomous or mature enough to conform to the same criteria of competence as an adult the balance is in favour of respecting autonomy. In such circumstances, their right to refuse medical treatment should be respected because they are competent.

Adults are competent to consent to and refuse treatment, including life-sustaining treatment provided they have the capacity:[28]

- to understand relevant information about treatment proposals and the consequences of refusing them,
- to remember the most important aspects of this information,
- to reason or deliberate about the any clinical choices that are proposed, and
- to believe that information communicated applies to the patient who is given it and, for example, is not being made up in order to deceive or harm.

Therefore, adults may be competent and still make choices about their medical care that clinicians deem irrational and dangerous. Provided that they are competent, the choice of such patients to embark upon a course of non-treatment that will, in effect, kill them should be respected. It is important to note that competence is essentially task-oriented and context-dependent. An adult may be incompetent to do or understand many things and still be competent to understand, remember, deliberate about, and believe basic clinical information to make crucial choices about their care.

The right of the competent child to refuse life-sustaining treatment

Why should competent children be regarded as any different? After all, if treatment is in their best interests and they consent to it then no further moral reason (e.g. further parental consent) is required to proceed. But what if they refuse? It is a great injustice to force unwanted treatment on such a child simply because of his/her age, when they can be shown to be competent using adult criteria.[8] Not only may such intervention lead to the same loss of dignity that it does with adults, the loss may be compounded because competent children may be less physically and socially able to resist whatever force is administered.

It is now widely accepted that competent children who refuse treatment that can be postponed without loss of life or serious injury should have their decision respected.[29] Not to do so may generate anger and hostility towards health professionals, placing the young person at potential risk of serious harm through their rejecting future clinical help when it is needed. Equally, a competent child who understands that death will result from the refusal of treatment will weigh up their choice against the background of their experience of their illness and its treatment. Forced or coerced treatment can only add to this desperate feeling of helplessness and indignity. It may reach the stage where it can be argued to be analogous to a form of torture—no matter how well intentioned.[30]

Forcing unwanted treatment on competent young people who refuse it is, therefore, immoral. Depending on the jurisdiction, however, the law does not necessarily agree. In England, two further important cases in the early 1990s judged that age rather than competence should determine whether young people should have the same right to refuse treatment which was felt to be in their best interests.[31,32] As a result, English law accepts that although a competent young person may consent to such medical treatment they cannot refuse it until they are 18. Conversely, Scottish law makes no distinction between the right of a competent young person to agree or to refuse such treatment, with no apparent disastrous consequences.[33]

Procedural rules for children who refuse treatment

The only coherent justification for not giving a competent young person the right to refuse life-sustaining treatment is procedural rather than a matter of moral principle. It is reasonable to argue that it is difficult to determine whether young persons are competent to make such important decisions about their health care and its impact on their family. Life and death mistakes cannot be corrected. This underlines the importance of having clinical procedures in place to assess a child's competence to make specific decisions irrespective of their age.[34]

If such procedures determine that a child is competent, then the right of choice should be with the child and no one else, although they may choose to share decision-making with others, or even delegate it to them. For example, a very young person suffering from leukaemia may competently decide that they do not wish to have any more chemotherapy and understand that the result will be that they may not live for very long. As with adults, their autonomy should be respected and should trump the duty of clinicians and/or parents to protect their life and health. This should be the case irrespective of age or the understandable desire to guard the interests of children in ways that are perceived to be their best interests.

Conflict between such young people and parents—or between clinicians and parents—may arise under these circumstances.[35] Clinicians may continue to question the competence of such young people, even when all the appropriate procedural steps have been taken to verify it. The stakes may just seem too high.[7] Of course, where such steps have not been taken (e.g. interviews with the duty social worker and consultant paediatric psychiatrist) the primary task is to help the child to understand their importance and in such a way that maximizes their feeling of being treated with respect and dignity. If appropriate procedural steps do confirm the competence of such children, it is the duty of their clinician to counsel the parents—and if necessary seek counselling themselves—about the terrible consequences of continuing to force life on a child for whom it has lost meaning.[36] Of course, the need for sensitivity, patience, and compassion in discussions and debates of these kinds—if they are not to degenerate into angry incomprehension—cannot be overestimated. It is precisely in these contexts that the skills and insights associated with paediatric palliative care will prove invaluable.[9]

Consequences for palliative care

Good palliative care has an important role to play in the duty to respect autonomy of children. Although children may be terminally ill they may still want to get things done—and as competently as possible! Some children will engage in a variety of activities at home or in hospital with no clear understanding of the closeness of their death. Others will have varying amounts of understanding but will also be keen to be as active as possible. Competent children who have a full understanding of their terminal prognosis will want to do many of the things that characterize adults in such circumstances—to see and converse with people, to make some record of their experiences, to make what they believe to be important choices about a variety of matters ... to reflect on their life and what it has meant to them. To be unable to do things of this kind properly because of inadequate pain relief and other support can be as harrowing as the pain and suffering themselves.

Pain and other forms of suffering may be detrimental to the exercise of competent choice. Effective palliative care can enable children to express their desires in a way that influences their clinical management. This may include a desire no longer to accept life-sustaining treatment. If such children believe that they have been able to make their views clear and that they have been listened to, this will help enormously in their ability to face their illness and its consequences. Whether or not their desires are achieved, they can at least know that they were treated with respect and dignity. For children at the very end of their lives, such feelings and beliefs will be the ones with which they die. If their death is peaceful and pain-free this is surely a testament to the moral worth of good palliative care.

Conclusion: palliative care and moral indeterminacy

For the purposes of exposition it has been necessary to analyse many issues as though they were more or less straightforward. In fact, this is far from the truth. It is one thing to observe that coherent moral and legal principles dictate the boundaries of good paediatric practice. It is another thing believe that in practice these principles will be interpreted in the same ways. They will not! Paediatricians, parents, and children will all, at times, disagree about what the correct interpretation should be.[37,38]

As regards non-treatment issues, these disagreements will be fuelled by a variety of conflicting values about, among others:

- the sanctity of life,
- the most appropriate circumstances in which to foreshorten life through the NPWLST,
- what constitutes competence in a young person who refuses life-prolonging treatment,
- the amount of coercion that is acceptable in forcing treatment on semi-competent children, and
- how much duty is owed to protecting the well being of parents—for example, by preserving life longer than is in a child's best interests or through not supporting a competent refusal of life-saving treatment.

It would be foolish to pretend that in such cases of moral and, perhaps, legal indeterminacy, definitively correct solutions can or will be found.

In the face of such uncertainty, it is essential that the discussions about how to proceed should take place in a form which optimizes the rationality of decision-making.[39] These decisions may be a compromise, one not completely satisfying to any of the participants. It will be important, therefore, that all participants believe that the decision emerged from a rigorous and fair discussion. Given the fraught emotions that often face ethico-legal indeterminacy in paediatric decisions about the end of life, this belief should help to strengthen the realization that certainty is sometimes more than anyone can expect.

More specifically, procedural fairness dictates that relevant discussions concerning non-treatment issues are organized so that the voices of key participants are heard and respected. Thus the traditional power of the senior personnel in the clinical team must be suspended and no single person or interest group should be allowed to dominate communication and debate. For this to be a practical reality, patients and parents involved in such discussions may need to be represented by advocates who can help them to articulate their beliefs and concerns. If they are present within the hospital, clinical ethics committees or ethics consultants may also be of help, to the degree that their advice is perceived to be objective and independent.[40]

However such ethico-legal uncertainty is procedurally approached, the most important factor in its successful resolution will be the transparency of the care and concern of the paediatric staff. Of particular importance will be their ability to reach out to patients and parents—without this necessarily entailing agreement with what they decide.[41] This is hardly surprising. Most experienced practitioners know that it is this process that constitutes good medicine. Those who specialize in palliative care will have particular skills and experience in facilitating good communication and education about the material factors surrounding terminal care and death—most of them experience, in discussing with parents, the delicate balance between their concern for the interests of their children and the necessary emotional hardship brought upon them by their child's illness.[9–11] This experience can and should inform all aspects of the management of the moral indeterminacy that can surround decisions relating to NPWLST. Indeed, without the wisdom and reassurance that such experience can provide children, parents, and professional carers, the burden of such decisions would be even more intolerable.

Acknowledgement

Many thanks to Professor Lesley Doyal for her advice and support.

References

1. **Chantler, C. and Doyal, L.** (2000). Medical ethics: the duties of care in principle and practice. In *Clinical Negligence* (ed. M. Powers and N. Harris), pp. 549–72. London: Butterworths.
2. **Kennedy, I. and Grubb, A.** *Medical Law.* London: Butterworths, 2000.
3. **van der Wal, M.E., Renfurm, L.N., van Vught, A.J., and Gemke, R.J.B.J.** (1999). Circumstances of dying in hospitalised children. *Intensive Care Medicine* **158**, 560–5.
4. **Balfour-Lynn, I.M. and Tasker, R.C.** (1996). At the coalface—medical ethics in practice. Futility and death in paediatric medical intensive care. *Journal of Medical Ethics* **22**, 279–81.
5. **Doyal, L.** (1998). When life may be too precious: the severely damaged neonate. *Seminars in Neonatology* **3** (4), 297–382.
6. **British Medical Association.** *Withholding and Withdrawing Life-prolonging Medical Treatment.* London: BMJ Books, 1999, pp. 1–12.
7. **Kenny, N.P. and Frager, G.** (1996). Refractory symptoms and terminal sedation of children: ethical issues and practical management. *Journal of Palliative Care* **12** (3), 1996.
8. **Levetown, M.** (1996). Ethical aspects of pediatric palliative care. *Journal of Palliative Care* **12**, 35–9.
9. **Association for Children with Life-Threatening or Terminal Conditions and their Families.** *A Guide to the Development of Children's Palliative Care Services.* London: Royal College of Paediatrics and Child Health, 1997.
10. **Trapp, A.** (1998). Support for the family. In *Care of the Dying Child* (ed. A. Goldman), pp. 76–92. Oxford: Oxford University Press.
11. **Stein, A. and Woolley, H.** Caring for the carers. In *Care of the Dying Child* (ed. A. Goldman), pp. 164–82. Oxford: Oxford University Press.
12. Re B (1981) 1 WLR 1421.
13. Re C (1989) 2 All ER 782.
14. Re J (1990) 6 BMLR 25.
15. Re J (1992) 9 BMLR 10.
16. Airedale NHS Trust v Bland (1993) 1 All ER 821.
17. Re R (1996) 2 FLR 99.
18. **Montgomery, J.** *Health Care Law.* Oxford: Oxford University Press, 2002, pp. 437–9.
19. **Royal College of Paediatrics and Child Health.** *Withholding or Withdrawing Life Saving Treatment in Children: A Framework for Practice.* London: Royal College of Paediatrics and Child Health, 1997.
20. **Goldman, A., Burne, R., and Rees, P.** (1998). Different illnesses and the problems they cause. In *Care of the Dying Child* (ed. A. Goldman), pp. 14–42. Oxford: Oxford University Press.
21. **Jecker, N.S. and Schneiderman, L.J.** (1995). When families request that 'everything possible' be done. *Journal of Medicine and Philosophy* **20**, 145–63.
22. **Doyal, L. and Larcher, V.** (2000). Drafting guidelines for the withholding or withdrawing of life sustaining treatment in critically ill children and neonates. *Archive of Diseases of Childhood. Fetal and Neonatal Edition* **83**, F60–3.
23. **Pinkerton, J.A.V.** et al. (1997). Parental rights at the birth of a near-viable infant: conflicting perspectives. *American Journal of Obstetrics and Gynaecology* **177**, 283–8.
24. **Doyal, L. and Gough, I.** *A Theory of Human Need.* London: Macmillan, 1991.
25. **Kurtz, Z.** (1995). Do children's rights to health care in the UK ensure their best interests? *Journal of the Royal College of Physicians of London* **29**, 508–16.
26. **General Assembly of the United Nations.** *Convention on the Rights of the Child 1989.* London: The Stationary Office, 1996.
27. Children Act 1989, s.1(3)(a).
28. Re C (1994) 1 All ER 819 (FD).
29. **British Medical Association.** *Consent, Rights and Choices in Health Care for Children and Young People.* London: BMJ Books, 2001.
30. **Doyal, L.** (1998). Can medicine be torture? In *Childhood Abused* (ed. G. Van Bueren), pp. 155–74. Ashgate: Aldershott.
31. Re R (1991) 4 All ER 177.
32. Re W (1992) 4 All ER 627.
33. Reference to Scottish Law.
34. **Dixon-Woods, M., Young, B., and Heney, D.** (1999). Partnerships with children. *British Medical Journal* **319**, 778–80.
35. **Doyal, L. and Henning, P.** (1994). Stopping treatment for end-stage renal failure: the rights of children and adolescents. *Paediatric Nephrology* **7**, 768–71.
36. **Dorner, S.** (1976). Adolescents with spina bifida: how they see their situation. *Archives of Diseases in Childhood* **51**, 439–44.
37. **Randolph, A.G., Zollo, M.B., Egger, M.J., Guyatt, G.H., Nelson, R.M., and Stidham, G.L.** (1999). Variability in physician opinion on limiting pediatric life support. *Pediatrics* **103** (4), e46.
38. **Farsides, C.C.S.** (1998). Autonomy and its implications for palliative care: a northern European perspective. *Palliative Medicine* **12**, 147–51.
39. **Doyal, L.** (1990). Medical ethics and moral indeterminacy. *Journal of Law and Society* **17**, 1–16.
40. **Doyal, L.** (2001). Clinical ethics committees and the formulation of health care policy. *Journal of Medical Ethics* **27** (Suppl. II), 44–9.
41. **Gillis, J.** (1997). When lifesaving treatment in children is not the answer. *British Medical Journal* **315**, 1246.

3.6 Ethical issues in palliative care research

Neil MacDonald and Charles Weijer

Introduction

In the past the term 'palliative care' has been synonymous with care of persons near the end of life. As reflected in this third edition the term palliative care is now more expansive; clearly patients with predictably fatal illnesses should have the principles of palliative care applied to assist them from the point of diagnosis. Moreover, these principles will also benefit patients with severe but potentially curable illnesses such as those receiving an arduous course of treatment for cancer. The general principles of research ethics cover palliative care research which engages patients who are not expected to die in the near future. This chapter will consider ethical issues which arise when persons are in the last days, weeks, or months of their lives.

In the past, persons near the end of life were enrolled in palliative care programmes after all avenues of interventional therapy to arrest the basic disease were explored. Usually, research opportunities were not open to them, as few hospice/palliative care groups were involved in clinical studies. While many factors have limited palliative care research,[1] at the core lies an ethical concern that patients are uniquely vulnerable at the end of their lives. Consequently, much of our work in palliative care is anecdotally based as the field has attracted relatively few research scientists or support.

This situation is unsatisfactory, as, similar to any other field, palliative care programmes must develop on a research base. Palliative care will suffer if our organizational arrangements and therapies are not backed up by sound research.

Relevance of palliative care research

From a patient and family viewpoint, early access to research advances benefit participants in successful clinical trials; even those who did not receive the 'winning' therapy in a randomized trial tend to do better than similar patients treated off study.[2–5] The concept that research participation results in patient exploitation must be balanced by a recognition that clinical trials may offer both a societal and a personal benefit. On the face of it, shielding dying patients from the cares of the world, including research decisions, makes eminent sense. However, the coin has two sides. Shielding implies the control of information, with consequent reduced access to options, negation of autonomy, and the loss of dignity inherent in choosing one's destiny. 'Comfort care' may simply translate into the application of traditional inadequate therapies.

Global relevance

Recent publications have stressed the importance of prioritizing both research and health care initiatives according to their relevance to large human populations, opportunity for proceeding from basic studies to clinical application, and ease of implementation and evaluation.[6,7] If such guidelines were applied, palliative care research would surely flourish.

Chronic non-infectious disorders (notably cancer and cardiovascular disease) will soon be the major global cause of death in both developing and technically advanced nations. Because of cost and distribution problems, many Western cancer research initiatives are not relevant in the impoverished countries of the world. Thus, the gap between have- and have-not countries will widen in the twenty-first century with the advent of new therapies. A reasonable proportion of research resources should be directed towards new therapies which have global relevance. Many of the initiatives of research interest in palliative care today are not expensive and may be more readily accessed in all global health care systems.

Magnitude of potential benefit from palliative care research

Aside from pain, the current status of symptom research is not satisfactory. For example, cachexia–anorexia and fatigue are the most common problems afflicting advanced cancer patients.[8,9] It is ironic that there is so little research on this devastating problem, the principal reason for patient loss of independence, when one considers the growing evidence that the syndrome is due to a long-term, useless activation of inflammatory cytokine systems, perhaps compounded by production of proteolytic substances by tumours.[10,11] Both aetiologic factors are potentially subject to safe intervention, as demonstrated by a number of animal and human studies.[12–14]

The pathophysiologic basis of symptoms is similar across disorders. Presumably, an intervention enabling a cancer patient to obtain pain relief or to improve appetite and muscle mass will also benefit patients with other chronic illnesses and similar problems. Therefore, research on problems associated with end-stage disease of any type may have a striking multiplier effect.

In addition to symptom research, as reflected in the 1998 ASCO statement on end of life care,[15] research on access to care, the impact of funding mechanisms on end of life issues, the needs of families who are increasingly beset by the obligation of home care, and bereavement issues, are fields of research clearly worthy of current emphasis.

Evidence-based medicine

'Evidence-based medicine' will increasingly influence policy-makers responsible for the prioritization of health programmes. While this approach is welcome, as it calls upon us to think critically about our therapies, it could increase the emphasis on research areas where 'evidence' is easily obtained, and funding, often from pharmaceutical firms, is readily available (e.g. cancer chemotherapy). Palliative care patients will be disadvantaged if research in the field is thwarted, and the lack of research is then used as a reason for failing to support palliative care initiatives.[16] Promising areas of palliative care research include cheap and commercially unprofitable approaches, such as studies on off-patent medications and inexpensive opioids (e.g. methadone). Special assistance from public granting bodies will be required for palliative care research studying therapies where demonstration of success will have public benefit, without substantial commercial gain.

Ethical distinctiveness of research in palliative care

While the principles which govern the moral conduct of research in other situations are pertinent to the participation of end of life patients in research trials, a number of unique factors amplify the ethical issues posed by research involving dying patients.

Purpose—Palliative care research is usually designed to improve the patient's quality of life or to determine factors which impact on patient–family well being. Trial interventions usually have a low risk of causing harm while the benefit of participation in a successful trial may be rapidly realized. In this respect, palliative care research stands in contrast to Phase I drug trials whose primary objective is a biologic endpoint (agent tolerance and safety, and secondarily, efficacy may also be considered).

Competence—Patients engaged in research must understand their options after receiving relevant information, and must be able to both use that information to reach a decision and clearly communicate that decision.[17] The competence of patients to give informed consent is a particular concern at the end of life. The incidence of dementia and delirium is increased[18,19] while, without formal testing, defects in cognitive function may be masked.[20] Bruera reports that 13 of 67 patients otherwise judged eligible to participate in a research study were found to have Folstein Mini-Mental Status examinations of less than 24/30: these patients appeared to be mentally competent in clinical assessments, were able to read and sign a consent form, but probably could not offer valid informed consent.

Personal goals—At any time, the uniqueness of individuals and the need to ensure that their goals are consonant with those of the investigators is important. Using cancer as an example, earlier in the trajectory of illness, it is more likely that these goals will be fully shared—that is, both parties are primarily interested in curing the illness or in a meaningful prolongation of life. Towards the end of life, when a curative therapeutic trial is no longer possible, the aims of investigators, patients, and families may be quite different or, indeed, in conflict. These differences may affect a variety of research processes, including mutual agreement on research objectives, obtaining informed consent, trial design (e.g. parallel versus crossover designs), changes in design as the study proceeds, and trial termination.

Clinical instability—Patients with advanced illness are subject to a barrage of constantly changing physical and psychosocial problems. At any time, patients may average 8–11 symptoms, occurring against a background of co-morbidity from other chronic illnesses.[21] Each problem may demand its own therapeutic approach, and many of the drugs employed will result in the addition of other agents to balance the adverse effects of the first drugs. As a result, polypharmacy may reign, and a patient with constantly changing patterns of illness may also suffer from iatrogenic problems, further compounding the patient's fragile status. Aside from the impact of the patient's unstable condition on research results, the patient may not be able to complete the research trial.

Age—Aged patients are often excluded from participation in clinical trials.[22,23] Aside from AIDS patients, the majority of patients dying with advanced chronic illness are elderly. The role of an older person in a research trial is compounded by all of the issues raised in the above sections. Nevertheless, many research programmes are not particularly germane to the needs of the aged.

Performance status—Investigators either preclude enrollment of patients with limited performance status or choose not to approach them. As one consequence, information on the effects of anticancer therapy on symptom status is limited. While the risk of inducing harm out of proportion to benefit wisely influences decisions to exclude some patients, a misguided application of this principle could reduce interest in designing trials of gentler therapy particularly germane to the problems of patients with more advanced illness.

Site—Location should not a priori disqualify a patient or family from research participation. The development of palliative care and hospice facilities independent of association with academic centres, is a major factor which has limited clinical and health services research. Progressively, links are now established between academia and community programmes. The staff of many hospices, however, may feel uncomfortable about the intrusion of research, not only because of staff time and patient vulnerability issues but also as they may lack training in the conduct of clinical research. The lack of staff familiarity with the process of clinical research may sharply limit access. The world of clinical research has its own language and increasingly complex processes for support, administration, and review. How can already stressed, overworked hospice professionals embrace these new intrusions on their lives and the lives of their patients?

Casarett et al.[24] have recently published a policy paper of the National Hospice Organization (United States) clearly articulating problems involved in hospice research and providing a series of cogent recommendations which, if adopted, can resolve some of the problems outlined above. The paper stresses the need for staff education on the conduct of research while emphasizing that the review process [primarily involving so-called 'Institutional Review Boards' (IRB) in the United States] must be clearly and efficiently articulated. Anecdotally, Canadian palliative care colleagues have experienced a few problems with IRB review. These bodies, often familiar with far more dangerous complex cancer chemotherapy protocols, sometimes seem to freeze when approached with protocols involving dying patients. Not only do hospice staff, patients, and families require tutoring on research ethics and process, IRB members also require education to assist them with review of symptom control and other issues in end of life care.

Non-patient ethical issues—the concept of trial hierarchy

Opportunities for patients to take part in symptom control clinical trials should increase, as many compounds which may relieve suffering are now available for study. Access to these trials, however, is problematic for a number of reasons:

- Often contact points (e.g. family physicians and oncologists) are not familiar with the trials.
- Contact points may be aware of the trials but their mind set is directed towards chemotherapy trials to the exclusion of other approaches to managing a patient's problems.
- Contact points are familiar with symptom control trials but their patient also qualifies for a chemotherapy trial. The pharmaceutical firm sponsoring the chemotherapy trial will usually include an exclusion clause which forbids participation of the patient in alternate trials, a clause sanctioned by the ICH 'Good Clinical Practice Guidelines'. This sounds reasonable, after all, as a successful symptom control trial may affect the results of the chemotherapy trial, while double trial participation may increase patient burden. Nevertheless, the patient may be denied an opportunity to participate in a programme of potential benefit because of the chemotherapy imperative. Thus an ethical dilemma arises.

Clinical trial ethics are problematic if a chemotherapy trial is favoured over a symptom control trial because of added financial reward associated with a pharmaceutical firm trial, or if the patient is enrolled on a chemotherapy trial in some part because a full range of alternative therapies, including access to a symptom control trial, was not discussed with the patient. The ethical dilemma is resolved if patients with advanced cancer considering palliative chemotherapy trials, which are unlikely to alter survival in a meaningful way, are fully informed of alternative approaches, including participation in symptom control trials. With respect to the potential enticement of financial gain for the investigators or their departments, the primary ethical rule that physicians, at all circumstances, must value patient well being above other considerations, should ensure that money does not influence judgement. One hopes that this is not a naïve statement.

Risk—Relevant to any discussion on vulnerability is the degree of risk which patients and families may be asked to assume. Physicians have an obligation to assess the vulnerability of these prospective research subjects to adverse effects of study participation, and to exclude those susceptible to enhanced risk.[25] Beyond this, American regulations limit the degree of risk to which various groups of research subjects may be exposed. In any setting, research interventions must meet the expectations of clinical equipoise; that is, there must exist honest, professional disagreement in the community of expert practitioners as to the preferred treatment (vi).[26,27]

Often a research protocol will require that patients undergo additional investigation purely for scientific reasons. In considering these interventions, the concept of 'minimal risk' comes into play. This concept may be interpreted as follows: 'minimal risk means that the probability and magnitude of harm or discomfort anticipated in the research are not greater in and of themselves than those ordinarily encountered in daily life or during the performance of routine physical or psychological examinations or tests' (45 Code of Federal Regulations 46.102(i)).

The degree of risk encountered in daily life varies from person to person; a high base line risk is inherent in the day-to-day life of a fighter pilot, or a patient with advanced disease, compared with a healthy sedentary office worker. While one must be extremely careful to avoid burdening palliative care patients and families with non-therapeutic initiatives, investigative studies if linked with necessary diagnostic tests (e.g. linking a study on 'molecular epidemiology' of cachexia–anorexia with routine blood draws) should be encouraged. Patients and families are frequently interviewed in the normal course of events by health professionals; a limited expansion of these discussions in the psychosocial realm which involves research questionnaires or interviews may be ethically acceptable if careful attention is given to the added burden placed upon the patient or family member.

The question of vulnerability

Is palliative care research ethically proscribed because of inherent vulnerability of involved patients and families? An absolutist view is held by some who believe that palliative care patients and families are so vulnerable that they should never be invited to participate in a study, even with their informed consent. 'To research at all in to the needs and experiences of this client group could be said to be an affront to the dignity of those people who are terminally ill, and an expression of profound disrespect for the emotional and physical state of such patients.'[28] Those who hold this view seemingly believe that patients in palliative care are characterized primarily by their status as 'dying'—already in an ante chamber separate from the rest of us.

The absolutist view has emotional appeal, but it is not, however, a fully articulated position. What does 'vulnerability' mean? In what ways are persons at the end of life vulnerable? If, indeed, some persons at the end of life are deemed to be vulnerable, does it follow that research on them ought to be prohibited?

The word vulnerability is often used in an inexact fashion. Levine defining vulnerability states: 'In general, we identify as vulnerable those who are relatively (or absolutely) incapable of protecting their own interests. More formally, they have insufficient power prowess intelligence resources strength or other needed attributes to protect their own interest through negotiations for informed consent'.[29]

He cautions 'it should be understood that each person, when measured against the highest standards of capability, is relatively vulnerable. We are all dependent upon someone or something and susceptible to temptation ... it is easy to identify too many persons as vulnerable'.[29]

The Common Rule (United States) directs review boards to be 'particularly cognizant of the special problems of research involved in vulnerable populations such as children, prisoners, pregnant women, mentally disabled persons or economically or educationally disadvantaged persons'. The very diversity of the list suggests the complexity of the vulnerability concept which must encompass differing degrees of vulnerability. Even in groups where vulnerability would seem to have clear lines of demarcation, such as that involved in prisoners and the incompetent, research is not proscribed; rather, additional protections are now in place or have been proposed.[30]

Persons at the end of life may be vulnerable for a variety of reasons including:

- increased risk of adverse effects associated with experimental treatment;
- inability to make an informed choice temporarily, intermittently, or permanently;
- undue dependence upon others;
- unrealistic expectations because of desperate straits in which they find themselves with consequent willingness to take part in trials with very low probability of success (a problem more likely to confront participants in Phase I chemotherapy trials).

Patients with advanced ultimately fatal disease can fall into any or all of the above categories. They are ill, exhausted, often depressed, and because of these factors perhaps more susceptible to proposals which are not in their best interests. Varying degrees of cognitive failure may be present.

While the inherent degree of vulnerability of the dying magnifies the requirement for their protection, it does not follow that research participation must be prohibited. Vulnerable persons may be included in research if two general conditions are fulfilled:

- Research bears direct relevance to their medical condition and carries the opportunity of medical benefit to those enrolled or the opportunity to advance knowledge for the class of patients to which they belong.
- Recognizing the risk of enhanced vulnerability, dedicated safeguards should be in place.

Case study* CG, a 68-year-old businessman was referred to the palliative care unit of a teaching hospital with non-small-cell lung cancer, widely metastatic to liver and bone. Pain was rapidly controlled using an opioid and a non-steroidal anti-inflammatory drug. The patient had a variety of gastro-intestinal complaints, but no evidence of tumour involvement of the GI tract. Nausea and constipation were rapidly controlled. The patient, however, who had a recent history of a loss of 10 kg in weight over a 2-month period remained with a poor appetite, early satiety, and severe fatigue. CG required assistance for even limited ambulation because of generalized weakness. He had a moderate anaemia, a low albumen content, and a very high C-reactive protein content. CG's physicians concluded that he had the cachexia–anorexia syndrome. CG received nutritional counselling, and an attempt was made to provide him with nutritious foods which he previously enjoyed. The family wanted him to receive Omega-3 fatty acids in capsule form, which the professional staff endorsed. They advised the family on what is thought to be the optimal dose of an Omega-3 preparation.

CG is a candidate for a current research study on cachexia–anorexia: a randomized, double-blind, placebo-controlled trial of thalidomide. He gives informed consent for participation in the study. Several members of the palliative care team, including nurses and two physicians, do not agree with palliative care research of any kind. Can a study such as the thalidomide study be justified for CG or other patients in his situation? Do current methods for obtaining informed consent reliably indicate mental competence and adequately protect patients in studies such as these?

CG is already receiving seven medications. There is limited data on how thalidomide may interact with any of these. Should CG be exposed to unknown risk of drug interaction? The study investigator is a member of the palliative care team. Does this create an unacceptable conflict of interest?

* This is a composite case based on author experience.

Questioning research in palliative care

The physician and nurses in the above scenario might express the following concerns to justify their antiresearch stance:[31]

- Clinical researchers, whether using quantitative or qualitative strategies, risk treating subjects merely as a means to the research end, thus contravening the central palliative care tenet that considers the patient and family member and their needs as ends in themselves. Palliative care physicians and nurses state that they aim to support the goals and aspirations of patient and family, rather than enlisting their support in fulfilling the researchers' goals.
- In safeguarding the well being of the research subject, the depersonalization implicit in the impersonal nature of the experimental method may introduce unavoidable role conflict as the investigator acts as agent for both patient well being and study completion.
- Informed consent is problematic because the stability and duration of consent are uncertain, and may be influenced by events emerging in the course of the study. Thus 'informed consent' at the outset can, at best, be simply consent to commence.
- Participant observation in palliative care research may be burdened by an intrinsic power differential between researcher and subject. Typically when we speak of consent to research participation, we assume that physician and patient are on a 'level playing field': information is exchanged, risks are described, and the patients can decide for themselves whether to participate. But, of course, seriously ill people are not on a level playing field with health professionals, particularly those who are responsible for both care and research.
- Palliative care patients may be particularly vulnerable to the close attention of the researcher in qualitative studies and to a deepening relationship with this researcher as the study progresses. Role blurring may become an additional problem which may interfere with withdrawal from the study. Is the researcher perceived to be a friend? nurse? or researcher? The researcher must be adequately trained and supervised to identify and manage the transference and counter-transference that are likely to occur. Are adequate safeguards built into the termination of the relationship.
- The effects of each of the drugs received by CG are well known when used as single agents. We do not know the outcome of adding thalidomide to a complex drug regime in a malnourished person. In our ignorant state we should not ask CG to accept additional risk.
- The whole research process remains value laden by virtue of the selective availability of research funding which supports issues dictated by cultural or economic preoccupations.

In support of palliative care research

In rebutting an article decrying the conduct of palliative care research, a group of physicians engaged in palliative care research state: '… the suggestion that others have the right to deprive them (i.e. patients) of making their own decisions regarding whether they wish to participate in clinical research is paternalistic, demeaning and disrespectful. The frailty of the very ill does not preclude autonomous decision making, participating in society, giving to others or finding purpose and meaning. The personhood, integrity and sanctity of all individuals must be equally respected'.[31] The ethical argument for of research in palliative care emerges from the following considerations.

Acceptability in principle

Research wherein the patient is the 'means to the end' is not, prima facie, unethical. If this were the case, a moral imperative against all clinical research would exist. Moreover, the 'means, end' language may misrepresent the real relationship existing between researchers and participant patients. The collaboration of each requires a unique contribution of each to the research venture. In that collaboration, it is difficult to say that either the researcher or the participating patient is a means to the attainment of the other's end. Both should strive towards the same end. This breaks down when researchers manipulate patients, fail to respect their dignity, and reduce them to merely means.

Independent of patient benefit, research may advance the pool of human knowledge and the investigator's prestige and career. These research outcomes are not inherently odious; they only become so if they represent the prime purpose of research with participatory patient interests as secondary goals.

Purpose is a key issue in ethical discussions. While the investigator's main purpose may be to produce generalizable knowledge, secondary benefits potentially accruing to the patient, to other patients, or to the investigator, are ethically acceptable ends.

Informed consent

Truly informed consent, if freely offered, may resolve ethical issues arising in this situation. The concept of patient autonomy supports the potential involvement of patients in research that may not be of immediate benefit to themselves. It remains a noble gesture to 'shake one's fist at the inevitable' and to make a contribution to the common good. The sense of purpose, sometimes lost in the course of suffering from a chronic illness, may be enhanced even from one's bed, if a continuing contribution to the community may be offered. The noble nature of man is demeaned if research is simply conceived as a utilitarian effort.

However, analyses of patients participating in some Phase I trials tells us that many patients participate in these studies primarily in the hope of personal benefit.[32] Did they not understand the study explanation? Was it properly carried out? Did they choose to see only what they wished to see? We don't know, but their responses raise the concern that 'informed consent' may be reduced to a medical oxymoron.[33] In the final analysis, the patient's protection must lie in the physician's observation of the Helsinki dictum—'the interest of science and society should never take precedence over the well-being of the subject'.

This issue represents a tangible application of the cardinal principles of medical ethics. These principles are sterile if not applied within a compassionate environment by wise, charitable, and moral investigators.

Placebo use in research

Placebo use is regarded by some as controversial in palliative care research. Recent guidelines on research in palliative care[34] state: 'Giving a placebo is not just if there is a therapy known to be more effective than a placebo. Therefore, placebo-controlled double blind trials are unlikely to be ethical'. This view presupposes that a treatment is known to be effective before study. If this is so, then a placebo trial is obviously unethical, regardless of the phase in the trajectory of the patient's illness in which it is conducted. Placebo trials are ethical at all stages of illness *providing that placebos do not replace standard efficacious therapy, and providing that patients know and understand that they may be receiving a placebo.*

As stated in the 'Tri-Council Policy Statement for the Ethical Conduct of Research Involving Humans' (MRC, NSERC, SSHRC), 'a placebo may be used as the control treatment in a clinical trial in the following circumstances:

(a) there is no standard treatment;

(b) standard therapy has been shown to be no better than placebo;

(c) evidence has arisen creating substantial doubt regarding the net therapeutic advantage of standard therapy;

(d) effective treatment is not available to patients due to cost constraints or short supply (this may only be applied when background conditions of justice prevail within the health care system in question; for example, a placebo-controlled trial is not permissible when effective but costly treatment is made available to the rich but remains unavailable to the poor and uninsured);

(e) in a population of patients who are refractory to standard treatment and for whom no standard second line treatment exists;

(f) testing add-on treatment to standard therapy when all subjects in the trial receive all treatments that would normally be described, or;

(g) patients have obtained an informed refusal of standard therapy for a minor condition for which patients commonly refuse treatment, and when withholding such therapy will not lead to undue suffering or the possibility of irreversible harm of any magnitude.'

When placebo use is considered, an evaluation of the rationale for foregoing 'standard therapy' will need to be rigourously carried out.

If placebo research is approved, the investigators must ensure that patients, family members, or legally designated third parties are fully informed that a therapy may be withheld or withdrawn, to be replaced by a placebo, and fully informed of any consequences which may predictably occur following the withholding or withdrawal of the therapy.

Must a patient always have the right to the active agent? This issue has surfaced in many AIDS trials, albeit primarily with respect to therapies used in early or mid-disease trajectory.

This issue is negated in research trials involving '*n* of *1*' or short-span crossover designs. These are particularly useful approaches for palliative care research, although inherent design problems such as carryover effects and the constantly changing clinical setting may limit study interpretation. Moreover, regulatory agencies prefer randomized placebo studies.[35]

The concept of clinical equipoise

Participation in a clinical trial can never be justified if it results in less-than-optimal care. However, many 'standard' approaches in palliative care may not have proven efficacy, may not confer patient benefit and, under certain circumstances, may be harmful. For example, corticosteroids, in certain doses at certain stages of illness, appear to be helpful in increasing appetite, patient weight, and possibly even energy levels, with low risk of toxicity. However, at higher doses over time, toxicity may be a problem. A blind assumption from early trials that corticosteroids or progestational agents are helpful in all circumstances would result in erroneous and harmful practice.

There is a consensus that at the beginning of an RCT comparing two or more treatments, an honest null hypothesis must exist.[36] In other words, uncertainty must exist as to the relative merits of the treatments being tested in the trial.[37] Some authors have argued that this means the treatments in a trial must be precisely balanced—referred to as 'theoretical equipoise'—that is, no empirical grounding for a preference for one treatment over another in a trial can exist.[38] As Freedman has pointed out, this understanding of equipoise is all too fragile: the fate of a single patient in an RCT could throw the balance in favour of one treatment or the other, thus requiring that the trial be stopped.[39] Freedman has persuasively argued for a different understanding of equipoise, termed 'clinical equipoise'. Clinical equipoise exists when there is 'an honest, professional disagreement among expert clinicians about the preferred treatment'.[39]

> At the start of the trial, there must be a state of clinical equipoise regarding the merits of the regimens to be tested, and the trial must be designed in such a way as to make it reasonable to expect that, if it is successfully concluded, clinical equipoise will be disturbed. In other words, the results of a successful trial should be convincing enough to resolve the dispute among clinicians.[39]

The question hinges on the analysis of equipoise. If, in the physician's opinion, equipoise is not absolute, this view should be shared with the patient. Even if equipoise does exist, patients must receive an explanation of what this means. If there is no scientifically relevant difference between two treatments under study, there may be a personally relevant difference for the patient. Subsequent decisions in practice will depend on other factors such as cost and drug access.

Double agents?

Yes, a physician or nurse conducting clinical research is acting as a double agent. While this situation can induce an ethical dilemma, it does not, de facto, place one in an unethical stance. Increasingly, we are called upon to act as double agents, with responsibilities not only to our patients, but to their families, our colleagues, departments and institutions, medical faculties and, most problematic of all, the state (or, in the United States, private insurance agencies or Health Management Organizations). Moreover, in our private lives, we must constantly address the balance between responsibilities to our own families and the patients we serve.

While one must often accept double agency status, the ethical problems therein arising may be resolved if priorities are set so that, as has been the tradition in medical practice throughout the ages, patient well being is maintained as a physician's top priority.

This problem is not unique to research settings. Indeed, although not receiving proportionate attention, it may be of greater concern in the non-research setting.[40,41] Currently, clinical research protocols must be accompanied by carefully constructed informed consent documents which should, prior to their introduction, be reviewed by uninvolved physicians, scientists, and members of the lay community. While patient comprehension of these forms and the purposes of research is often poor,[42] this may reflect a more general ethical problem in patient communication. If patient understanding of their illness and the purpose of the clinical research trial is often not clear, what happens in the course of day-to-day care outside a research setting?

The data on cognitive impairment at the end of life are sufficient in the authors' opinion to dictate the routine use of a screening tool, such as the Folstein Mini-Mental Status test. While not an absolute litmus test, an abnormal test result should raise serious questions about patient capability to provide informed consent.

As in other research areas, informed consent may need to be repeatedly renegotiated during the course of a study. It is not a blanket permit. This is necessary to provide patients with updated information which may alter study equipoise. It is of particular importance in palliative care research, since patient cognition, health status, and degree of vulnerability may change, with consequent re-setting of the terms for informed consent.

The community as partners in research

Clemenceau, noting the singularly unimaginative approach of his military to World War I battle strategy, stated 'War is too important to be left in the hands of the generals'. A similar sentiment may apply to the dearth of research interest in the problems of dying patients. The 2001 American Society of Clinical Oncology abstracts contain 12 times as many studies on an old chemotherapeutic agent, 5FU, as there are on cachexia–anorexia and fatigue.

In order to make clinical trials at the end of life more responsive to the needs of patients, greater involvement of patients and their families in the design and conduct of cancer research is clearly needed.[43] Clinical science inevitably involves value-laden decisions. Currently these decisions appear to be weighted heavily towards seemingly repetitive interventional trials, with consequent reduced emphasis on psychosocial and symptom control issues. The balance will be heavily influenced by the traditional interests of academic oncology, buttressed by the availability of support from the pharmaceutical industry. Is this balance logical, and does it reflect the expectations of the community? Possibly not—the answer will be more clearly apparent when we involve patients and patient communities, not only in the ethical review of trials (a practice now well established), but also in the planning and conduct of research. The AIDS community has achieved this, to a certain extent. With respect to cancer, the concerned community may be less clearly defined. However, as cancer affects between one in three and one in four members of the community, there is an abundance of thoughtful, well-informed people whose families have been touched by cancer, and who could be drawn upon to help in this process.

Towards resolving the case dilemma

The issues surrounding CG's care and possible involvement in research generated considerable debate and, indeed, strife amongst the members of the ward team. The following steps could be taken to resolve the dilemma presented:

1. A workshop on ethical issues in palliative care research was organized, with wide participation by staff members.
2. A Folstein Mini-Mental Status examination could be carried out, with CG's permission. He scores 27/30. Subsequently, as a supplement to the standard informed consent process, the physician and nurse with primary responsibilities discuss some of the troublesome issues that could arise following CG's participation in two research trials.

As a result joint agreement can be achieved with CG, his family (whose advice he had sought), the primary involved physicians and nurses, and the clinical investigators, that his involvement in a thalidomide trial, with the problematic issues that could arise through adding yet another medication with multiple adverse effects, could create a polypharmaceutical stew, with potential risks judged to out-balance potential benefits.

Limiting factors in palliative care research (MacDonald, N. (1993). Priorities in education and research in palliative care. *Palliative Medicine* **7** (Suppl. 1), 65–76.)

Aside from ethical issues, research involving dying patients presents formidable logistic, funding, demographic, and academic barriers (outlined below). Consequently, few investigators are currently attracted to this area of endeavour.

Specific suggestions to enhance ethical conduct of palliative care research

As stated earlier, adherence to published ethical guidelines for the conduct of research should, by and large, encompass most of the concerns which may arise in a palliative care setting. Nevertheless, it may be helpful to emphasize a few issues in order to support the confidence and interest of palliative care staff and patients in the research process. These include:

A. Patient enrollment

1. Potential research participants in palliative care research should be advised to discuss their participation in a research trial with close family members and/or confidants.

Palliative care stresses that families represent the fundamental unit of care. In keeping with this principle, family members, as defined by the patient, should be involved in discussions on the decision to participate in a research programme. They should also be kept informed of clinical trial progress.

Commonly, family members will share research burdens (e.g. research-related clinic visits, medication arrangements); it is reasonable that their input is recognized and honoured.

2. Researchers should not automatically exclude potential research participants on the basis of age, frailty, mental or physical disability, locale of care, or the nature of their health insurance.

The published ethical regulations and guidelines governing clinical research in both the United States and Canada are silent on the issue of involving dying patients in research. The Canadian Tri-Council Policy Statement clearly stresses the application of the principle of just distribution in determining exclusion criteria. 'Members of society should neither bear an unfair share of the direct burdens of participating in research nor should they be unfairly excluded from the potential benefits of research participation.'[44] As in other aspects of life, it is never ethically acceptable to stigmatize or stereotype an individual's rights because of a perceived attribute.

3. Patients in palliative care units should have standardized tests of cognitive function prior to requests for participation in research.

Patients in a palliative care setting are at particular risk of developing a confusional state. Contributing factors include age, polypharmacy, institutional setting, the common occurrence of dehydration, infection, and hypoxia, and direct damage to the central nervous system induced by the underlying chronic disorder. Often, cognitive impairment may not be obvious to health professionals or family members, as people can mask the worrisome signs of loss of mental function. Such patients may only offer obvious signs of an anxiety state or depression.

Adequate comprehension of the study at onset and continued understanding enabling participants to withdraw by choice are fundamental components of ethical research. When cognition is problematic, competency assessment and monitoring are essential components of palliative care research for reasons stated earlier in the text.

4. Patients with advanced, ultimately fatal chronic illnesses should be encouraged to complete a comprehensive advance directive, including their views on participation in research, early in the trajectory of illness.

While it is advisable for all of us to complete advance directives, those with an illness which may predictably end their lives after a period of disability should receive particular encouragement.

5. Incompetent patients may be considered for participation in research if the research is of potential direct benefit to them and does not expose them to more-than-minimal risk. Under these circumstances, the informed consent of the patient's representative will be required. Authorized representatives may be legally mandated individuals or family members recognized by the professional staff as sharing responsibility for family care. While, ethically, such family members should be able to influence patient care of both a research and non-research nature, in some jurisdictions only legally authorized individuals may be able to participate in research decisions.

These recommendations are consonant with published ethical research codes. The concept of minimal risk, however, bears closer examination. What is minimal risk for a delirious patient in the last days of life, whose authorized representative and family members could be asked to consider enrolling their loved one in a study of a new antipsychotic known to be both safe and efficacious in the management of schizophrenia? We believe that a proportionate approach to judging the ethical aspects of research participation should be employed. Therefore, it may be acceptable to study new agents in end of life delirium as the bar for 'minimal risk' is considerably raised for these patient, and agents not previously studied in delirium, but clearly demonstrated to be safely used in patients with other forms of psychosis, may hold an acceptable benefit–risk ratio for the patient and family.

B. Design

1. Protocols should be so written as to encourage understanding and participation by members of the palliative care team working with the patient-participant.

Palliative care is a multidisciplinary activity. The design and conduct of palliative care research studies should reflect this basic principle.

2. Trial methodology must emphasize maintenance of patient comfort and dignity through routine inclusion of assessments of the factors which contribute to this goal.

Recognition and alleviation of suffering is the *raison d'être* for palliative care. This goal must be reflected in the planning and conduct of clinical trials. Tangible expressions of this concept include the routine use of symptom control and quality of life assessments in longitudinal clinical trials.

3. Community members with palliative care experience should be involved in the decisions on which research is to be conducted and in the formulation of a research plan.

Palliative care programmes may tangibly apply the above guideline through enlistment of their volunteers to participate in Research Committees. Most sophisticated palliative care programmes include volunteers, many of whom have past experiences with palliative care as involved family members.

C. Conduct

1. For studies which involve more-than-minimal risk, tests of cognitive status should be repeated at regular intervals, not to exceed 4 weeks.

2. Patients may become incompetent after enrollment in a research project. Continued participation should be dependent upon demonstration of continued patient benefit while on the experimental therapy and clear evidence that the therapy is not responsible for the development of incompetence.

3. If an incompetent research participant becomes competent in the course of the research project, continuing participation should only occur after the participant has directly provided informed consent.

D. Publication

1. Upon completion of a research project, consideration should be given to circulation of the study results amongst family members of research participants, the palliative care volunteer group, and any community members with an interest in palliative care.

The above guideline is advanced as a technique for both fulfilling an obligation to honour the participation of those who enrolled in the studies and to improve the appreciation and interest of the community in palliative care research. Decisions on circulation of research information are dependent on the primary obligation to the community involved.

CG may conclude that, while it might be somewhat tiring, he would actually enjoy participating in a music therapy study which can be successfully carried out.

The thalidomide trial proceeds with enrollment of patients, with a better performance status and a probable longer stable period of illness, who could logically receive thalidomide or placebo, without the potential risks and study contamination introduced by using it in a patient with predictably only a few weeks to live and at high risk from unpredictable polypharmacy.

Not everyone would agree with the ultimate steps taken—debate continues in the representative palliative care ward.

Acknowledgement

The authors wish to thank the Soros Foundation—Project on Death in America for their support.

References

1. **MacDonald, N.** (1995). Suffering and dying in cancer patients. *Western Journal of Medicine* **163** (3), 278–86.
2. **Slevin, M.** et al. (1995). Volunteers or victims: patients' view of randomized cancer trials. *British Journal of Cancer* **71**, 1270–4.
3. **Weijer, C., Freedman, B., Fuks, A., Robbins, J., Shapiro, S., and Skrutkowska, M.** (1996). What difference does it make to be treated in a clinical trial? *Clinical and Investigative Medicine* **19**, 179–83.
4. **Meadows, A.T., Kramer, S., Hopson, R., Lustbader, E., Jarrett, P., and Evans, A.E.** (1983). Survival in childhood acute lymphangitic leukemia: effect of protocol and place of treatment. *Cancer Investigation* **1**, 49–85.
5. **Davis, S.** et al. (1995). Participants in clinical trials for resected non small cell lung cancer have improved survival compared with non-participants in such trials. *Cancer* **56** (7), 1710–18.
6. **Council on Ethical and Judicial Affairs, American Medical Association.** Ethical issues in managed care. (Council report) (1995). *Journal & the American Medical Association* **273** (4), 330–5.
7. **Bennett, K., Tugwell, P., Sackett, D., and Haynes, B.** (1990). Relative risks, benefits and costs of intervention. In *Tropical and Geographical Medicine* 2nd edn. (ed. K.S. Warren, A.S.F. Adel, and A. Mahmoud), pp. 205–28. New York: McGraw-Hill.
8. **Donnelly, S., Walsh, D., and Rybicki, L.** (1995). The symptoms of advanced cancer: identification of clinical and research priorities by assessment of prevalence and severity. *Journal of Palliative Care* **11** (1), 27–32.
9. **Dunlop, R.** (1996). Clinical epidemiology of cancer cachexia. In *Cachexia–Anorexia in Cancer Patients* (ed. E. Bruera and I. Higginson), pp. 76–82. New York: Oxford University Press.
10. **Lecker, S.H., Solomon, V., Mitch, W.E., and Goldberg, A.L.** (1999). Muscle protein breakdown and the critical role of the ubiquitin-proteasome pathway in normal and disease states. *Journal of Nutrition* **129**, 227S–37S.
11. **Todorov, P., Cariuk, P., McDevitt, T., Coles, B., Fearon, K., and Tisdale, M.** (1996). Characterization of a cancer cachectic factor. *Nature* **379** (6567), 739–42.
12. **Tisdale, M.J. and Beck, S.A.** (1991). Inhibition of tumour-induced lypolysis *in vitro* and cachexia and tumour growth *in vivo* by eicosapentanoic acid. *Biochemical Pharmacology* **41**, 103.
13. **Gogos, C.A., Ginopoulos, P., Salsa, B., Apostolidou, E., Zoumbos, N.C., and Kalfarentzos, F.** (1998). Dietary omega-3 polyunsaturated fatty acids plus vitamin E restore immunodeficiency and prolong survival for severely ill patients with generalized malignancy: a randomized control trial. *Cancer* **82** (2), 395–402.
14. **Barber, M.D.** et al. (1999). An oral nutritional supplement enriched with fish oil reverses weight-loss in patients with pancreatic cancer. *British Journal of Cancer* **8** (1), 80–6.
15. (1998). Cancer care during the last phase of life. (Adopted on 20 February 1997 by the American Society of Clinical Oncology) *Journal of Clinical Oncology* **16** (5), 1986–96.
16. **MacDonald, N.** (1998). Palliative care: an essential component of cancer Control. *Canadian Medical Association Journal* **158** (13), 1709–16.
17. **Appelbaum, P.S. and Grisso, T.** (1988). Assessing patients' capacities to consent to treatment. *The New England Journal of Medicine* **319** (25), 1635–88.
18. **Bruera, E., Franco, J.J., Maltoni, M., Watanabe, S., and Suarez-Almazor, M.** (1995). Changing pattern of agitated impaired mental status in patients with advanced cancer: association with cognitive monitoring, hydration, and opiate rotation. *Journal of Pain and Symptom Management* **10** (4), 287–91.
19. **Massie, M.J., Holland, J.C., and Glass, E.** (1983). Delirium in terminally ill cancer patients. *American Journal of Psychiatry* **140**, 1048–50.
20. **Bruera, E., Spachynski, K., MacEachern, T., and Hanson, J.** (1993). Cognitive failure in cancer patients in clinical trials (Letter). *Lancet* **341**, 247–8.
21. **Portenoy, R.K.** et al. (1994). Symptom prevalence, characteristics and distress in a cancer population. *Quality of Life Research* **3** (3), 183–9.
22. **Kennedy, B.J.** (1991). Needed: clinical trials for older patients. *Journal of Clinical Oncology* **9** (5), 718–20.
23. **Fuks, A., Weijer, C., Freedman, B., Shapiro, S., Skrutkowski, M., and Riaz, A.** (1997). A study in contrasts: eligibility criteria in a twenty-year sample of NSABP and POG clinical trials. *Journal of Clinical Epidemiology* **51**, 69–79.
24. **Casarett, D., Ferrell, B., Kirschling, J., Levetown, M., Merriman, M.P., Ramey, M., and Silverman, P.** (2001). NHPCO task force statement on the ethics of hospice participation in research. *Journal of Palliative Medicine* **4** (4), 441–9.
25. **Weijer, C. and Fuks, A.** (1994). The duty to exclude: excluding people at undue risk from research. *Clinical and Investigative Medicine* **17**, 115–22.
26. **Freedman, B.** (1987). Equipoise and the ethics of research. *New England Journal of Medicine* **317**, 141–5.
27. **Freedman, B., Fuks, A., and Weijer, C.** (1992). Demarcating research and treatment: a systematic approach for the analysis of the ethics of clinical research. *Clinical Research* **40**, 653–60.
28. **de Raeve, L.** (1994). Ethical issues in palliative care research. *Palliative Medicine* **8**, 298–305.
29. **Levine, R.J.** *Ethics and Regulation of Clinical Research.* New Haven: Yale University Press, 1988, pp. 187–90.
30. **US National Bioethics Advisory Commission.** *Research Involving Persons With Mental Disorders that may Affect Decision Making Capacity.* Washington DC: US Government Printing Office, 1998 (45 CFR 46.305).
31. **Mount, B.M., Cohen, R., MacDonald, N., Bruera, E., and Dudgeon, D.** (1995). Ethical issues in palliative care research revisited. *Palliative Medicine* **9**, 165–70.
32. **Kodish, E., Stocking, C., Ratain, M.J., Kohrman, A., and Siegler, M.** (1992). Ethical issues in phase I oncology research: a comparison of investigators and institutional review board chairpersons. *Journal of Clinical Oncology* **10**, 1810–16.
33. **Raghavan, D.** (1991). Clinician surrogates and equipoise: an analogy to lawyers who represent themselves? *European Journal of Cancer* **27** (9), 1072–4.
34. **The National Council for Hospice and Specialist Palliative Care Services.** *Guidelines on Research in Palliative Care*, London, 1995.
35. **Elliott, C. and Weijer, C.** (1995). Cruel and unusual treatment. *Saturday Night.* December, 31–4.
36. **Levine, R.J.** *Ethics and Regulation of Clinical Research.* New Haven: Yale University Press, 1988, pp. 187–90.
37. **Fried, C.** *Medical Experimentation: Personal Integrity and Social Policy.* Amsterdam: North Holland Publishing, 1974.
38. **Shaw, L.W. and Chalmers, T.C.** (1970). Ethics in cooperative clinical trials. *Annals of the New York Academy of Sciences* **169**, 487–95.
39. **Freedman, B.** (1987). Equipoise and the ethics of clinical research. *The New England Journal of Medicine* **317** (3), 141–5.
40. **Annas, G.J.** (1994). Informed consent, cancer, and truth in prognosis. *The New England Journal of Medicine* **330** (3), 223–5.
41. **MacDonald, N.** (1992). Quality of life in clinical and research ethics. *Journal of Palliative Care* **8** (3), 46–51.
42. **Williams, C.J. and Zwitter, M.** (1994). Informed consent in European multi centre randomised clinical trials—are patients really informed? *European Journal of Cancer* **30A** (7), 907–10.
43. **Weijer, C.** (1995). Our bodies, our science. *The Sciences.* May/June, 41–5.
44. **Tri-Council Statement.** *Ethical Conduct for Research Involving Humans. Section 5.* Canada: Public Works and Government Services, 1998.

3.7 Euthanasia and withholding treatment

David J. Roy

Introduction

Ethical issues in palliative medicine and palliative care arise with particular intensity, although not exclusively, at the bedsides of gravely ill and dying people. There would be no issues to resolve if there were no uncertainties and conflicts about what clinically should and should not be done in the care of patients afflicted with advanced and irreversible disease. The issues are ethical because they centre upon beliefs about how human beings should live and die, about the values individuals and groups should uphold, and about which values may be sacrificed when all values at stake in a specific situation cannot be honoured and maintained. The issues are also ethical because they centre on the purposes and responsibilities of the medical and nursing professions as well as upon the relationships of law to medical and nursing practice.

This chapter's consideration of withholding or withdrawing life-prolonging treatment and of euthanasia opens with a brief discussion of clinical ethics, the primary perspective of the entire chapter. Of course, what happens at the bedsides of sick and dying people happens also within hospitals and health care institutions, and these are societal institutions. So the ethical issues raised by the withholding of life-prolonging treatment and by euthanasia and physician-assisted suicide could be analysed and discussed by focusing attention on the ethics of a health care institution, or on the ethics of the medical and nursing professions, or more broadly, on the public ethics of a given society. However, the choice taken here is to consider withholding treatment and euthanasia primarily from the perspective of clinical ethics, a specialization of ethics that is not to be identified with, although it inevitably intersects with, the ethics of an institution, of a profession, of a religion, or of the public ethics of a society.[1]

Clinical ethics

People in Western societies today clash profoundly on two levels: on the level of their cultural beliefs, within which people define the goals of life and the meaning of death; and on their hierarchies of value against which people decide which values may be sacrificed and which values must be maintained at all costs. In this context, ethics requires a shift from a divergent to a convergent method and mode of thought. The required shift is from the task of constructing arguments in support of diverse value systems to the work of constructing practical judgments about what must be done, what should be prohibited, and what can be tolerated in the care of very sick people. The shift from theoretical to practical reasoning in ethics is needed to reach the decisions that often have to be made quite rapidly at the bedside of the sick and the dying. This is the shift required to extricate clinical ethics and the ethics of palliative medicine from the deadlock of interminable discourse about matters upon which people are likely never to agree.[2]

The starting point of clinical ethics, as also of clinical practice, is the consideration of patients in their full particularity, what Charles Fried has called the principle of personal care.[3] The complete palliative physician holds together two seemingly incompatible excellences: sensitivity to signals of the patient's body and receptivity to the messages of a life in crisis—at the crossroads or at the terminus of a personal history.

The clinical goals to be pursued for each patient, and the requirements of clinical care, inevitably change along the continuum of disease. While diseases vary considerably both as to rate and as to continuity of evolution, the evolution of disease is also always unique to each individual patient. It is the nature of a patient's response to treatment plans that indicates when the times arrive to down-regulate intensive life-prolonging care and up-regulate palliative care. The shift is rarely abrupt or of the on–off, binary kind of change. Moreover, certain interventions, such as radiotherapy or surgery, may serve curative clinical goals for some patients and palliative goals for others. Along this continuum of evolving disease and correspondingly changing clinical goals, moments are reached when it is clinically, ethically, and legally justifiable to withhold or to discontinue clinical treatments, such as resuscitation procedures, respiratory support, dialysis, antibiotics, chemotherapy, surgery, and assisted hydration and nutrition; the discontinuance of this last-mentioned intervention being still very controversial.

The kinds of decisions that have to be taken *for* and *with* gravely ill and dying persons are not purely technical. These decisions become an intrinsic component of the event of dying. Depending on the content of these decisions, and on the way they are made, some people will have the chance to die well, masters of their dying, not alone and not lonely. Others may die before their time, without a chance to live their dying through. Others may die too late, reduced to biological systems that have to be tended. Some may die uninformed and unenlightened, caught trying to play 'scene two' when life's drama is in fact about to close. Still others may die, who could have lived.

Decisions having such consequences demand that comprehensive attention be given to patients in their full particularity; that attention is focused on the unique biology, clinical condition, needs, desires, life plans, hopes, sufferings, strengths, vulnerabilities, and limitations of *this* particular person *now*. Decisions of this kind, and they are the primary outcome of clinical ethics in palliative medicine, cannot be deduced from any one principle or set of principles. These decisions result rather from a process of highly practical reasoning. The method of clinical ethics in palliative medicine is inductive. It works by passing the existing principles of the philosophical and religious moral traditions through the grid of particular personal and clinical histories to learn gradually what these principles command, prohibit, or tolerate. This knowledge is not all worked out in advance, completed, and awaiting to be applied. The clinical ethical order within these principles is, to use an expression of David Bohm, an implicate order.[4] An implicate order cannot be made explicit as a whole. It is manifested slowly and only partially as it is worked out in the case-by-case practical judgments reached at the bedsides of utterly unique persons as their disease advances and their biographies come to a close.

Withholding or withdrawing therapy

A contemporary consensus

Although saving lives always has been, and will ever remain, a primary goal of clinical practice, the initiation and continuation of intensive life-prolonging procedures may result in little more than a stretching out of the dying curve, or in the extension of an unbearable and unrelentingly miserable life. Over the last 20 years or so, patients, families, nurses, doctors, and people from all walks of life have been asking whether extension of life to the bitter biological end is the right thing to do, particularly when the sick and the dying find the physical, emotional, and personal costs of such treatment to be hardly bearable. A trend has developed over more than two decades, and its direction is away from an ethic of prolonging life at all costs towards an ethic emphasizing the quality of life and of dying over the duration of life taken as an absolute value. This trend, as evidenced in a line of court cases and in a voluminous literature in medicine, nursing, ethics, and law, is against the tethering of people with advanced, irreversible illness to life-prolonging treatments and technologies, particularly when the underlying disease is progressing and cannot be halted; and when the life extended is only marginally bearable or definitely miserable.[5–16]

This consensus regarding withholding or withdrawing life-prolonging treatments has crystallized around seven basic considerations.

First, decisions about withholding or discontinuing life-sustaining treatments cannot be made adequately on the basis of a pre-determination that some treatments are *extraordinary* and others are *ordinary*.[7,17,18] The real clinical–ethical issue is whether any treatment, be it technically simple or complex, be it an instrument of basic or of advanced life support, is in keeping with the current clinical goals for each individual patient. For this reason, the distinction between extraordinary and ordinary means has given way to the more meaningful distinction between proportionate and non-proportionate treatments.[19,20]

Second, the proportionate/non-proportionate distinction implies that there are *no intrinsic moral or ethical imperatives attached to different categories of treatment*, such as cardiopulmonary resuscitation, ventilatory support, dialysis, medication such as vasopressors, antibiotics, and insulin, and the provision of assisted nutrition and hydration. Decisions to use, to forego, or to discontinue any of these and other kinds of treatment should be taken as a function of, and not in isolation from, the clinical goals of the total treatment plan for each patient.

Third, binary thinking that would set *sacredness of life* in opposition to *quality of life*, so that respect of the one would require abandonment of the other, is not the way to reach ethically sound clinical decisions.

Fourth, *quality of life* decisions are inescapable in clinical practice because physicians and clinical teams are ethically and professionally obligated to gauge the consequences of their work on the bodies and lives of the people they are professionally presuming to help. Yet, the quality of human life varies from person to person, and, indeed, varies for each person across the ages of the life cycle. The ethical danger in 'quality of life' decisions is that some lives may be judged as not worth living because they will never match up to some inflexible notions or scales, inevitably culturally conditioned, of what worthwhile human living means. Thinking of quality of life in absolute rather than in relative terms risks the mistake of ignoring that a meaningful human life is possible even far-out from the centers of biological, psychological, and intellectual normalcy.

Fifth, an ethical danger also lurks within any absolute emphasis on the *sacredness of life*. Since the introduction of powerful life-prolonging technologies in hospitals, people have feared being technologically tethered to the biologically living relic of the persons they once were, and can never be again. They have feared being clinically forced into the extension of a life now irreversibly damaged by disease, depleted of energy, and intolerant of enjoyment. In such and similar circumstances, it is now widely recognized as being ethically erroneous to read the sacredness of life principle as compelling absolute persistence in extending life by all means and at all costs, right up to the moment when a patient's biology has utterly lost all capacity to respond. To insist on the contrary would be equivalent to insisting that a sick person's biology is more sacred than their person.

Sixth, the emphasis in the contemporary consensus, at least within the countries and culture of the West, is on shared decision-making between physician and patient, with the patient holding primacy of power to decide. This emphasis comes to expression, to cite one example, in an amendment to the Criminal Code of Canada, proposed some years ago by the then existing, and now disbanded, Law Reform Commission of Canada. The amendment was designed to prohibit any relevant paragraph of the code from being interpreted as requiring a physician 'to continue to administer or to undertake medical treatment against the expressed wishes of the person for whom such treatment is intended'.[21]

Seventh, it would be a mistake to read the contemporary emphasis on self-determination as implying that there is no place in the contemporary consensus for withholding or discontinuing life-prolonging treatment when patients can no longer express their will and never expressed any thought about these matters before falling gravely ill. There is general agreement that incompetent patients have the same rights as competent patients.[22,23] There is also general agreement that doctors and clinical teams should not be bound by law to administer treatments that are therapeutically useless and not in the patient's best interests.[23,24]

Physicians, clinical teams, and family members do not, of course, always agree on what are the best interests of irreversibly ill or dying persons. Moreover, some family members, when speaking with doctors about discontinuing life-prolonging treatments, may not have the best interests of a dying person as their decisive priority. These situations, as will be considered below, may provoke intensely difficult scenes at the bedside.

The contemporary clinical-ethical consensus about withholding or discontinuing life-prolonging treatments may simply fail to operate when there is no continuing communication among doctors, nurses, patients, and families; when doctors and nurses are not educated to attend both to the body and to the biography of patients; and when the organization of care in hospitals promotes the unreflective use of technology rather than the careful mastery of technology in the service of the patients' goals and aspirations.[25] When these failures occur, a technologically and bureaucratically dominated system tends to take charge, and that system may not know when or how to stop life-extending treatments, in great part because that system is not in intimate contact with the sick and dying people it is meant to serve.[26]

The consensus in practice: principles and cases

The method of clinical ethics in palliative medicine, outlined in the section on clinical ethics, will now be exemplified in a series of considerations of when and why it is ethically justified to withhold or to discontinue life-extending therapy. These considerations refer to the principles most frequently invoked when decisions about treatment have to be made with or for the dying. Specific real cases, greatly modified to protect confidentiality, are described to illustrate how principles have to be interpreted in the light of individual patient histories if they are to offer any practical guidance at the bedside.

When patients refuse treatment

If confusion, the undue influence of other persons, and pathologic depression can be excluded, many hold to the principle that 'the will of the patient, not the health of the patient, should be the supreme law' governing decisions about initiating or discontinuing life-prolongation measures.[27] A classic expression of the principle of self-determination is Justice Benjamin Cardozo's 1914 statement: 'Every human being of adult years and sound mind has a right to determine what shall be done with his own body'.[28] In the same vein, the Law Reform Commission of Canada has proposed an amendment to the Criminal Code of Canada to prohibit any relevant paragraph of the code from being interpreted as requiring a physician 'to continue to administer or to undertake medical treatment against the expressed wishes of the person for whom such treatment is intended'.[21]

This clear and reasonable principle may conflict sharply with strongly held clinical perceptions and certain dominant values in our culture. People increasingly give public support to patient autonomy and to the value of self-determination against the potential abuse of medical technology. However, it is not always easy to live according to the same categories in which we think. People can generally agree on the justification of abandoning life-prolonging procedures when a patient's loss of consciousness is irreversible. Many, however, experience a strong visceral opposition to discontinuing or withholding life-prolongation treatment—whether this be respiratory support, chemotherapy, or total parenteral nutrition—from an intelligent, conscious, and lucid patient.

This spontaneous opposition may be reinforced by bonds to the patient forged during the earlier fight for life. Decisive and distressed family members may also intensify the difficulty of respecting a patient's refusal of life support. Moreover, although the principle of autonomy or of self-determination may be easy to state, it is often very difficult to ascertain whether some patients who are speaking coherently are not perhaps so dominated by a particular state of mind, such as a depression, that they really are unable to make decisions on their own behalf.

Case study Several years ago, a 27-year-old woman entered a hospital with leukaemia. She had been abandoned by her parents shortly after her birth, and subsequently lived in one foster home after another. Through adolescence she lived a wild sex and drug life and came to despise herself at the age of 19. At this time she met a couple who had never had children, and they offered her a room in their home. She gradually became their own child in fact, if not by law, and this young woman, highly intelligent, went on to finish her schooling, her university undergraduate studies, and had dreams of becoming an architect.

Her leukaemia was diagnosed at this point in her life. A young physician was very supportive, assuring this young woman that effective treatments were available, and that she had every chance of pursuing her professional dream. When he outlined the treatment plan, the young woman agreed to everything except the blood transfusions. She could not accept transfusions she said, because her new parents' Jehovah's Witness faith had become her own. She didn't want to die but could not accept a treatment that for her was tantamount to betrayal of her faith, and to a betrayal of the parents and extended family who had given her a new life.

The physician opposed her refusal, insisted that she was not going to enter the cemetery because of some silly belief, and that she was totally wrong in refusing a treatment, when that refusal was, in his view, equal to a choice of death. When he threatened to force treatment on the young woman, the relationship broke down, and another, older physician entered the scene. He spoke to the younger physician, reminding him of their shared religious beliefs, some of which were looked upon as bizarre and even foolish by some of their very bright and competent colleagues. The older physician said 'It's not for us to judge her faith but to make sure she is really speaking her own mind and is not being pressured by others.'

It became quite clear over several considerations that this young woman was quite thoroughly independent, was not being pressured by family or friends, and held the Jehovah's Witness belief as her very own. Her refusal of transfusions was then respected by the entire clinical team, with the young physician maintaining a very reluctant silence.

After the young woman's death and funeral, that reluctant silence exploded in rage directed against the older physician who had orchestrated respect for the young woman's decision. The young physician's accusation? 'If it were not for you and your ethics, doctor, she'd be at the university now, and probably dancing on Saturday. Now she's dead, and you seduced me into betraying my basic mission as a doctor, which is to save life. I could have saved hers.' The older physician's response? 'Do you think it is your mission to save life at all costs? Even at the cost of crushing a patient's liberty? If you do, you're wrong. At times liberty is a value higher than health or even life.'

This one case illustrates how difficult it can be at times to respect an instance of human freedom that is highly conscious of itself, superbly capable of self-expression, and articulating itself in a choice that affronts a dominant value or moral persuasion. This case also illustrates how the whole biography of this young patient, not only her clinical condition and the treatments available, entered into the deliberation required to reach a clinical decision. Many, but not all, would argue that the decision reached in this case, matched the full particularity of this young woman. For that reason, it was the right decision. However, if principles can be generalized, specific clinical-ethical decisions cannot.

Case study The clinical circumstances of the following case are quite different from those of the young woman with leukaemia, just discussed. This woman, 53 years old, entered a hospital in a state of renal failure. She was accompanied by her husband and her adult daughter. The physician explained to the woman that she would have to start dialysis, but she refused, stating that it was time for her 'to go into the arms of God'. Over lengthy conversations that afternoon, the woman's refusal of dialysis was persistent, and her refusal was strongly supported by her husband and daughter. She appeared lucid and coherent, but fatigued and withdrawn. She insisted on leaving the hospital and returning to her village many miles away, to be cared for by her doctor there, and basically to let nature take its course.

Her son, however, arrived at the hospital late in the afternoon, before her departure, and explained that his mother had been depressed over the last 10 years and had never, in his opinion, been adequately diagnosed or treated. Supported by her son, and against her protests and those of her husband and daughter, the doctor had the woman admitted to hospital and dialysis was started. The woman also received psychiatric attention. Over months she improved and changed her mind thoroughly about the dialysis, with which she collaborated enthusiastically, and about wanting to live. As she gradually rediscovered her former better self, she took up activities and re-established friendships she had long abandoned. Her husband and daughter changed too, recognizing in her the woman they had once loved but who, over years of depression, had become for them a constant source of stress and even a symbol of death.

It was not immediately obvious to the doctor, even after a lengthy conversation that afternoon, that this woman's depression, not her genuine self, was refusing treatment and seeking death. This case illustrates a situation in which respect for a patient's self-determination requires clinical opposition to a patient's and to her family's refusal of treatment.

When burdens are not proportionate to benefits

The principle of proportionality, succinctly stated, affirms that life-prolonging treatments are contraindicated when they cause more suffering than benefit.(27) This principle also comes to expression in the Canadian Law Reform Commission's recommendation that the Criminal Code should not bind physicians to administer therapeutically useless treatments or treatments that conflict with a patient's best interests.(21) Other position papers have also cited this principle or its equivalent.(8,23) The Vatican Declaration on Euthanasia proposes that it is ethically justifiable to discontinue the use of life-prolonging techniques 'where the results fall short of expectations'. Direct appeal is made to the principle of proportionality when this document observes that patient, family, and staff may judge that 'the techniques applied impose on the patient strain or suffering out of proportion with the benefits which he or she may gain from such techniques'.(19)

It was on the basis of a proportionality judgment that the court supported a mother's and grandmother's refusal of additional chemotherapy treatment for Carole Couture-Jacquet's saccrococcygeal teratoma. This little girl, under 5 years old, had already suffered greatly from the side-effects of previous chemotherapeutic regimens. The suffering included constant nausea, loss of at least 50 per cent of kidney function, and a significant diminishing of hearing function. Physicians estimated that a renewed chemotherapy regimen had a 10–20 per cent chance of arresting the advance of Carole's cancer.

The Quebec Court of Appeal did not find the mother's and grandmother's refusal of additional chemotherapy for Carole to be unreasonable. That refusal, rather, was seen as based on reasonable proportionality judgment that the low probability of success did not justify submitting Carole to more of the intolerable suffering she had already endured.(29)

Case study A 42-year-old man, severely handicapped intellectually, and with multiple metastases to the brain, presented his two sisters and a clinical team with a choice initially found by all involved to be most difficult. The treatments available at the time would probably prolong this man's life for a period of 6 months to 1 year beyond the time he could be expected to live without treatment. Yet these treatments required the patient's collaboration, and he could not collaborate. He didn't understand what doctors and nurses and hospitals were, and had no concept whatsoever of disease, treatment, and side-effects. He was a powerfully built person and still capable of quite devastating resistance to anyone he thought threatening or harmful. He also had lovely hair, and prized this personal characteristic above everything. He would spend hours grooming himself and admiring himself in the mirror, and would glow when complimented about his hair.

How, his sisters and physician asked, would he react to the hair loss and other side-effects of his treatment? Would he resist treatment if he made the connection between his hair loss and what doctors were doing to him? Would it not be better for our brother, the sisters asked, if he could have a relatively comfortable 8 months of life rather than 11 months or so of life filled with losses, complications of daily living, and misery he could never understand? This is how the sisters and the clinical team came to understand the choice they had to make for this man, and they judged aggressive antitumour treatment as being out of keeping with what this patient could tolerate, as likely to cause this man harm out of all proportion to the good it would bring him.

When treatments are bound to fail

Although several guidelines have stated that patients are not obliged to undergo, and physicians are not obliged to offer, begin, or continue treatments that are futile,[5,30] there is continuing confusion and controversy about the meaning and usefulness of futility as an indicator for the withholding or withdrawal of treatments.[31–39]

In this section, the futility of an intervention is to be judged in terms of the clinical goals for each individual patient. The central question is: will the intervention benefit the patient as a whole? Antibiotics will clear up a pneumonia in a patient locked into a persistent state of unawareness. That *effect* can be achieved. Because this effect can be achieved, some physicians believe antibiotic therapy *in this situation* is not futile, and hence obligatory. However, what is the goal of treatment for a patient who will never regain consciousness? If the clinical goal of this treatment is to return the patient to even a minimum of intellectual and relational capacity, then this treatment for patients in this state is indeed futile and non-obligatory, for those patients will never return to consciousness and awareness.

It is essential to distinguish and even separate two components in the concept of futility: the component of physiological effect and the component of benefit.[40] Some treatments are futile because they cannot produce a desired physiological effect for a particular patient or a particular category of patients. For example, the probability of chemotherapeutically halting a metastatic process may, on the basis of clinical trial results or on the basis of accumulated clinical experience, be nil or so low as to constitute the rare and unpredictable exception.

Other treatments may be futile because they are useless in attaining the clinical goals of care, even if they can have the effect of prolonging biological life. If the goal of clinical treatment is to restore a patient to a measure of independent life, then treatments are futile if they only prolong a dying process, or preserve the patient in a permanent state of unconsciousness, or tether the patient indefinitely to life-support machines in an intensive care unit.[41]

Consideration of each individual patient in his or her body and biography, the total patient, is the key to proper use of futility as a criterion for withholding or discontinuing advanced or even basic life support. Prolonging a dying process may be justifiable if the patient and family need that extra time to achieve important personal goals.

Case study One man in an irreversible and advanced stage of leukaemia returned to a hospital time and again for blood transfusions. Some members of the clinical team accused others of excessive agressivity in their treatment of this man. They came to think differently, though, on the day the man returned to hospital one last time, this time to die. He explained that, though he knew the treatments would never cure him, they at least gave him the time to complete the porch he was building around the house for his wife. In a quite different situation, a physician aggressively maintained life support for a severely brain damaged teenager so that the mother and father could synchronize their schedules of grief. The father, unrealistically expecting his son's return to conscious life, was accusing his more realistic wife of abandoning hope, of abandoning their son. The marriage and the equilibrium of the surviving 9-year-old brother were in danger. The physician, a neurologist, worked carefully and sensitively with the father who, 5 months later, came to the hospital with his wife and son. He apologized to his wife in the presence of the doctor and both husband and wife requested that no further efforts whatsoever be continued to prolong the biological shell of their child. Efforts to prolong the life of a non-salvageable child can be justified, within reasonable limits, if they contribute to the healing of an endangered family life.

Treatments of the most varied sorts are means to ends and the futility of treatments in clinical practice should be judged in terms of how likely it is that any given treatment will obtain the current clinical goals for this patient now.

When being alive is no longer meaningful

Some people, perhaps many, believe that survival in a state of persistent unawareness is not meaningful human existence and may indeed be a fate worse than death.[51] Useful studies and reviews[42–45] discuss the clinical characteristics of persistent vegetative state and the basis for its diagnosis. Our concern in this section is to discuss how far physicians may ethically go in allowing patients in states of persistent unawareness to die. Is there an ethically defensible distinction between advanced life-support measures that may be discontinued and basic support measures, such as assisted nutrition and hydration, that ethically must be continued?

As mentioned earlier in this section, and as bears repeating, medical, ethical, and even legal consensus[46–49] is growing in support of the view that there are no intrinsic moral differences between categories of treatment, such as CPR, ventilatory support, medications, and the provision of nutrition and hydration by artificial means. Decisions to start or discontinue assisted nutrition and hydration, as all other treatment decisions, should be taken as a function of, and not in isolation from, the goals of the total treatment plan for each patient.[50] This question, however, remains controversial.[51–55]

The ethically critical question regarding assisted nutrition and hydration of children and adults in persistent vegetative state is not: 'Are we justified in *dis*continuing such treatment?' but rather: 'What justification is there for *continuing* this treatment?' This latter question is based upon the assumption that every medical and surgical intervention into the body of a patient has to be justified. A range of invasive procedures in emergency and intensive care units are normally justified by the likelihood of curing the patient, stabilizing the patient, or restoring the patient to a level of meaningful life.

When physicians reliably diagnose that a patient is in a state of persistent unawareness, and that the patient's emergence from that state is impossible or overwhelmingly unlikely, there is little justification for continuing assisted nutrition and hydration. These procedures, as one mother expressed it, 'are only preventing my son from completing his death'.

If assisted nutrition and hydration may be essential measures in the palliative care of some dying patients,[56] this is rarely the case for patients, adults, or children, in deep and irreversible coma.[57] Relatives, and some physicians and nurses, may be very opposed to discontinuing assisted hydration and nutrition for a patient in a state of persistent unawareness because they believe and fear that the patient will suffer the pain and discomforts of hunger and thirst. This is unlikely if the diagnosis of persistent vegetative state is correct. A person in this state is, by definition, unable to perceive a wide range of stimuli, and the brain functions required to permit self-perceived affective response to stimuli have been destroyed.[58] At least one other working group agrees that the neurological mechanisms needed for the experience of pain and suffering are no longer operating in vegetative state patients, and that feeding does not benefit these patients.[59] If decisions have been taken to discontinue assisted hydration and nutrition, good nursing care and oral hygiene will assure the patient's bodily dignity until death occurs.

When the evolution of the disease is uncertain

The evolution of the patient's clinical course usually indicates when the time has arrived to discontinue life-sustaining treatment and to allow a patient to die. However, time *is not always* on the physician's or the patient's side. The conscious, alert, and ventilator-dependent patient certainly presents one of the greatest and most difficult challenges to clinicians and family in deciding when to stop support that could prolong life indefinitely in an intensive care unit.[60] The term 'entrapment' has been used to describe this situation that may occur more frequently in spinal cord injury and neuromuscular disease than in other clinical conditions.[61] Entrapment may also occur outside the context of respiratory support, for example, in clinical situations marked by a slowly cascading series of organ failures and infections.

There is no one single ethical protocol that can cover these situations. The following considerations, however, offer a direction for difficult decisions. First, there is no clinical or moral obligation for physicians and family to adhere to a treadmill of increasing therapy and diminishing returns for a patient who will, in all probability, never be freed from a regimen of intensive care. Second, there is no ethical difference, and it is also increasingly recognized that there is no legal difference, between not starting and stopping life-prolonging treatment.[62,63] Third, the purpose of resuscitation, respiratory support, and other emergency and intensive care measures is to return a person in acute collapse to some reasonable measure of normal human life. Intensive care treatment has reached its limits when its only result is to entrap a patient into permanent bondage and residency in an intensive care unit. Intensive care has reached its limits, and may be stopped, when it can do little more than totally tie the patient's time and energy to the procedures of survival.[36,64] Fourth, it is not always possible, but it sometimes happens that patients are able to understand their predicament and are able also to help family and physicians with the difficult decisions that have to be made.

Case study A 10-year-old boy, neurologically damaged but cognitively unimpaired after an automobile accident, had already suffered several episodes of respiratory failure and would continue to do so indefinitely. This little boy, while still on respirator after his last respiratory arrest, clearly told his parents and doctor that he wanted to go home and was altogether too fatigued by the whole process to ever want to be resuscitated again. Nancy, B., a 25-year-old woman in Québec, afflicted with extensive muscular atrophy resulting from Guillain-Barré syndrome, initiated the discussion and deliberation that eventually elicited Superior Court agreement with her request to stop the respirator on which she would be dependent for breath and life for the rest of her life.[65,66]

When families clash with physicians

Decisions about life-prolonging treatments involve a complex interplay of clinical facts and probabilities and personal values. They are not purely medical in nature. Physicians, on the basis of their knowledge and experience, carry prime responsibility for ascertaining a patient's condition and prognosis, and for assessing the clinical efficacy, benefits, and risks of alternative treatments. Patients and families, on the other hand, have a need and a right to receive from physicians clear and comprehensive clinical information so that they can decide which of alternative available treatments, or whether only palliative treatment, is in their own or their family member's best interests.

When patients are unconscious, confused, or otherwise unable to participate in decisions about their care, physicians inevitably have to share these decisions with parents, close family members, close friends of the patient, or with the patient's guardian, as the case may be.

The principle of proximity states that loved ones who have lived years with a gravely ill and dying person are normally best situated to interpret what is in that patient's best interests and to defend those interests. To act responsibly on behalf of a dying loved one, family members need the same clinical information that the patients themselves would require.

When shared decision-making works well, neither physician nor family members take the final decision alone. They carry responsibility for that decision together. However, shared decision-making may, on occasion, break down totally. The causes of such breakdowns are usually complex, and may in some situations be due to some physicians insensitivity to, and lack of understanding of, a particular patient and family. Some physicians may also be relatively uncommunicative or may be seeking to impose their moral views on the patient or family. Since case descriptions of breakdowns in shared decision-making would require at least a chapter, attention may be best focused here on situations where families are trying, as it were, to play doctor.

The impending death of a central figure in a family can provoke multiple shifts in the relationship of the family members, one to all and all to each. The relationship of power and leadership among family members may undergo rapid change right at the bedside, and precisely on the issue of what is to be done for a dying relative.

Case study A large family led by one of the sons demanded that all antibiotics and all other supportive treatments be stopped so that their mother could die in peace. Extensive discussions between the clinical team and four consultants had the greatest difficulty in bringing the family to understand that the patient was going through a normal post-operative course after repair of an abdominal aorta. The patient's situation was indeed most grave, and prognosis was most guarded, but it was still too early, 10 days after the operation, to say that this woman would not recover and was dying. The family finally opposed the dominant and dominating son and agreed to the continuation of all treatments so that their mother's body would have time to 'have its say'.

This family, however, was most unstable. Within 3 days of the clinical discussion that ended with the family's acceptance of life-supporting treatment, the family arrived in full numbers, led by the son, and demanded of the physician in charge that all treatments be stopped. The physician was overwhelmed, and complied. They thought their mother would die within a few hours. When their mother was still alive 2 days later, the family panicked and asked that treatment of the post-operative infections be started again. It was too late, though. Septicaemia had spread and a woman died who might have lived.

Families who try to play doctor need to be gently and firmly opposed, while all efforts continue to achieve common understanding between the family and clinical team. This opposition may be particularly important when family members are insisting on maximal aggression treatment of a dying patient. Physicians and hospitals, unfortunately, can be fearful, fearful of bad publicity, fearful of legal entanglements, and they can fail for these reasons to oppose unreasonable family demands that are damaging to dying patients.

Case study Such an event occurred when a niece demanded on behalf of her 82-year-old aunt, who was in the terminal phase of advanced cancer, that dialyses be started when her aunt's kidneys failed. The niece also threatened legal proceedings if she suspected her aunt died more rapidly than expected due to heavy administration of analgesics. This elderly patient's dying was prolonged because of hospital and physician acquiescence to the niece's demands, and this patient's pain was inadequately medicated because of the niece's threats.

When advance directives cause ethical dilemmas

Advance care planning is a strategy to ensure that the norm of consent is still operative and respected where sick persons are no longer able to discuss their treatment options with physicians and thereby exercise control over the course of their care. Planning in advance may typically include written directives indicating who a person would want to make treatment decisions on his or her behalf, and specifying also what kinds of treatment one would or would not want in certain states of illness.[67–73]

It is illusory, however, to think that advanced directives or living wills will prevent all clinical-ethical uncertainties and conflicts. People themselves may change, and may change their minds and attitudes towards certain states of illness, between the time they write their advance directives and when the occasion arrives for their implementation. Proxy decision-makers, appointed in advance, may be uncertain as to whether the sick person, now unconscious or otherwise incompetent, really is in the clinical situation described in the advance directives as requiring non-initiation or discontinuance of certain kinds of treatment. It may also happen that people, in their advanced directives, have requested life-prolonging interventions that now, in their current specific clinical condition, are totally unrealistic.

Quite different situations can occur within which advance directives create an ethical dilemma for clinicians, and possibly also for family members.

Case study Such an event occurred in an emergency unit when a woman arrived in ambulance accompanied by the ambulance physician and her two sons. This 67-year-old woman had a long history of rheumatoid arthritis and had taken an overdose of barbiturates. Finding their mother unconscious, the sons called the ambulance. However, they also arrived with two documents, signed by their mother and stating clearly that she intended to end her life when her arthritis reached a stage that no longer permitted her to live independently and in her own apartment. One document was a living will or advance directives text, signed 6 months earlier, and naming her sister as the person who should speak and decide for her when she was no longer able to do so herself. The second document was signed the day before the woman took the overdose. That document specified that the woman intended to end her life, that no resuscitation should be attempted, and that she would sue in the event that she were to be successfully resuscitated.

The physician in the emergency service telephoned the sister and she, along with the woman's two sons, insisted that this woman should not be resuscitated.

This woman did not have a medical record in the hospital where she was brought by ambulance, and the physician felt extremely uneasy about not resuscitating a suicide victim about whom he has so little medical information. Should this woman, despite her clear advance directives, be resuscitated, only to be left in the situation of having to try suicide all over again? Was this woman suffering from a treatable depression? Had this woman really received optimal treatment for her arthritis? In the face of all these unknowns, and with only minutes to spare, the emergency room physician decided not to attempt resuscitation, and the woman died shortly after that decision was taken.

This situation provoked intense controversy within the hospital and it was impossible to achieve consensus in several discussions that followed upon his event.[74]

When anguish or pain are overwhelming

Whether heavy sedation of patients prior to their deaths, sometimes called terminal sedation,[75,76] is ever ethically justifiable remains controversial. The controversy, in part, is about what happens to people who are dying from advanced cancer. Some claim and others deny that there is a crescendo of pain and suffering in the final days of dying from cancer, a crescendo admitting of relief only through heavy sedation and the induction of sleep prior to death.[77–79] This controversy is about events and numbers, and it can only be resolved by additional research.

The use of heavy sedation to control pain and other causes of suffering is ethically controversial not least because one class of sedatives, the barbiturates, are frequently used to administer capital punishment, for euthanasia, and for suicide.[80–82] Some who can ethically accept the use of heavy sedation to manage refractory pain and refractory symptoms such as dyspnoea and agitated delirium may be ethically very uncertain about the use of sedation to control severe and persistent anxiety, depression, and existential distress.[83,84]

Pain and symptoms are said to be refractory when they 'cannot be adequately controlled despite aggressive efforts to identify a tolerable therapy that does not compromise consciousness'.[85] The ethical evaluation of heavy sedation, including the use of barbiturates for the control of refractory symptoms, largely depends on the clinical goals and intentions of patients, families, and clinicians. There should be no ethical objection to the use of heavy sedation when this is the only effective measure available to bring patients relief from agonies that torment their bodies and minds. The choice of which sedative to use, and in what doses, and by which route of administration remains a matter of clinical assessment and clinical judgment in palliative medicine. Attention should be given to the fact that clinical strategies for managing refractory existential suffering and severe anxiety in the dying are perhaps less well established than for the management of pain and physical symptoms.[85] Moreover, existential suffering and anxiety may not be constant, and may wax and wane over time.

The determination that suffering of the mind is refractory requires 'repeated assessment by a knowledgeable clinician who has established a relationship with the patient and his or her family'. If anxiety, depression, and existential suffering resist all consciousness-preserving methods of control, then the use of heavy sedation may be ethically justifiable.[80,86–88] Relief from crushing agonies is for some, and perhaps for many dying patients, a higher value than the maintenance of consciousness.

Although some may find the difference between euthanasia and induction of deep sleep or heavy drowsiness to be thin and logically uncompelling,[89,90] the distinction, despite this perception, is clinically, ethically, and legally real and essential. Some people do need to sleep before they die, and conflicts of perception regarding the ethereality versus the reality of the distinction between sedation and euthanasia[91–93] should never be allowed to frustrate fulfillment of that need.

Euthanasia

There are excellent surveys, covering the period from the 1870s to the present, of how people have thought, acted, and legislated regarding euthanasia.[94–98] Physicians of various medical specialties, nurses, and the general public have been polled over the last several years to ascertain attitudes and practices towards euthanasia.[99–113] Various associations and working groups have issued positions on the matter[114–122] and philosophers, theologians, ethicists, lawyers, physicians, and nurses have, over the last decade, analysed, defended, and criticized the many reasons and arguments put forth to justify or reject the legalization of euthanasia or its ethical acceptability.[123–133]

A comprehensive review of this voluminous reflection would far exceed the space of a chapter, let alone a subsection of a chapter, on ethics in palliative medicine, and might even distract from the purpose of this chapter's discussion of euthanasia. That purpose is to stimulate those involved in the practice of palliative medicine to formulate reasoned responses to two crucial questions; crucial because they affect in a major way how palliative medicine will be understood, practiced, and supported. The first question is whether euthanasia can ever be ethically acceptable or tolerable within palliative medicine. The second question is whether euthanasia should be decriminalized, legalized, or declared to be an excusable exception, under some regulatory scheme or other, to homicide laws. In this section we centre attention on the second of these two questions.

These two questions are quite distinct[134,135] although there is a tendency to collapse the second question about the status of euthanasia by law to the status of euthanasia in the clinical ethics of palliative medicine. Some would propose that if euthanasia can reasonably be thought to be ethically acceptable, or at least ethically tolerable as the lesser of evils in some circumstances, then euthanasia should be permitted by law. *The central argument of this chapter is that euthanasia, even if it may be ethically tolerable in some circumstances, should not be decriminalized, nor legalized, nor legally excused under some regulatory scheme of conditions that would uphold the legal prohibition of euthanasia in principle.*

Euthanasia: a definition and distinctions

To facilitate discussion of this section's central question, we first propose a working definition of euthanasia and then distinguish euthanasia, so defined, from acts of foregoing or discontinuing life-prolonging treatments as well as from the use of various analgesics or sedatives to relieve the dying from pain, symptoms, or overwhelming distress.

A definition

People have been thinking, writing, and proposing legislation about euthanasia for a long time, but the discussion is bedeviled by the many different and conflicting understandings of what euthanasia means. If what is said is not what is meant, then many things that should be done may remain undone, and what should not be done may be championed as the only right thing to do.

A large measure of confusion could be removed from discussions about the ethical acceptability of euthanasia or about its legalization, if the term were taken to mean: *the deliberate and painless termination of life of a person afflicted with an incurable and progressive disease leading inexorably to death.* Euthanasia in this chapter means the administration of death to the dying.

Euthanasia should not be confused with cessation of treatment

A central element in the controversy over euthanasia is the fact that some people acknowledge, and others deny, that there is an ethically relevant distinction between euthanasia and withholding or discontinuing life-prolonging treatments.[136,137] This chapter emphasizes that this distinction is clinically, ethically, and legally essential, logically defensible, and should be sustained.[138–141]

The distinction rests on the assumption that doctors do not possess, nor should they be given, unlimited authority to intervene into the bodies and lives of sick and dying people. Such unlimited authority over the life of another human being is what doctors assume or are given by the dying themselves or by others when they administer euthanasia, defined above, as the administration of death. Such unlimited authority is also what doctors exercise when they insist on continuing life-prolonging treatments that have reached the limit of any good they can do for the dying but have not reached the limit of the suffering they can intensify. To discontinue life-prolonging treatments when these can no longer restore health, function, or consciousness is to recognize the limits of a physician's authority and power over a human life. To discontinue life-prolonging treatments in these circumstances is to allow a dying person to die. This is not the administration of death and it is not euthanasia.

However, the distinction between euthanasia and cessation of life-prolonging treatments, and the reservation of the term euthanasia for the act of administrating death, does not mean that all acts of withholding or withdrawing life-prolonging treatments are ethically or legally justifiable acts of allowing people to die. Withholding life-prolonging treatments from persons who need not die or who are not ready to die may be deeply reprehensible ethically and possibly even legally criminal. But acts of withholding or discontinuing life-sustaining treatments should be ethically evaluated on their own merits and should not be confused with euthanasia.

Administering pain control is not the administration of death

One of the essential elements of dying with dignity is freedom from pain, and the various kinds of bodily and mental fatigue and distress, that can dominate consciousness and leave no psychic space free for the personally important things people want to think, say, and do before they die. Constant, wracking, and mind-twisting pain separates dying persons from themselves and from their loved ones. That pain combined with other kinds of relentless biological and psychic stress can drive the dying from coping, control, and integration to chaos and hopelessness.[142,143]

Patients have a right to request, and doctors have an obligation of fidelity to the dying to employ, every *proportionate* means available to relieve the suffering and agony provoked by relentless pain and symptoms distress. Administering medications in combinations, dosages, and frequencies needed to relieve effectively the suffering of the dying is logically, clinically, and ethically totally different from the act of administering death. These two acts differ both as to end and as to means. The goal of palliative medicine is emancipation, the freeing of the dying person's consciousness from the domination of pain. The goal of euthanasia is death.

It is in part because of a failure to grasp the essential distinction between euthanasia and the palliative control of pain and symptoms that some doctors, unreasonably fearful of legal liability for hastening death, have gone just so far, and not far enough, in their use of medications to give patients the relief they need and request. Patients should never have to beg for relief because of doctors' unenlightened fears. And it is indeed foolish to deny patients relief from suffering because of unsubstantiatable fears and concerns that effective relief of pain will shorten life.[144,145] A dying patient receiving frequent medication for pain and symptom control will eventually die after receiving a dosage of medication. It is a fallacy to conclude that the medication and not the last surge of the underlying disease caused the patient's death.

The legalization of euthanasia: key events

Euthanasia has been practiced in the Netherlands for many years, particularly since the Dutch Supreme Court declaration in 1984 that euthanasia would be legally excusable if physicians found themselves to be in a conflict of duties. In such a conflict a physician would face the dilemma: respect the Dutch Penal Code's prohibition of euthanasia or respect a patient's request for euthanasia as a release from suffering. However, voluntary euthanasia is now decriminalized or legalized (both terms having been used in the literature) in the Netherlands. Members of Parliament voted in November 2000 to approve legislation to decriminalize voluntary euthanasia and the Dutch Senate voted 46 votes to 28 for approval on 10 April 2001. Voluntary euthanasia is no longer a criminal offence if doctors fulfill requirements similar to those proposed by the Royal Dutch Medical Association in 1984. A physician still has to notify the municipal coroner of an act of euthanasia and the coroner forwards both the physician's notification and written report to one of the regional review committees established in 1998. These committees now have the power to decide whether a physician has performed euthanasia in keeping with the legislated requirements and to close the case or send it on to the prosecutor.[146–148]

In North America, pressure is growing to legalize assisted euthanasia. In November 1991, voters in Washington State took part in a referendum on death with dignity, which included a provision to legalize euthanasia. Despite public opinion polls that showed a two-thirds majority in favour of voluntary euthanasia, the proposal was defeated by 54 per cent of voters. A similar proposal was defeated by California voters in November 1992, by an almost identical margin.

In 1996, two United States Appeal Courts ruled against the ban of certain states against physician-assisted death. On 6 March 1996, the Ninth Circuit Court of Appeals, exercising jurisdiction over the State of Washington and eight other states, ruled that terminally ill patients have the right to seek a doctor's aid to hasten death. The ruling applies to terminally ill adults, who have 'a strong liberty interest in choosing a dignified and humane death rather than being reduced at the end'.[149] On 2 April 1996, the Second Circuit Court of Appeals, which covers the states of New York, Vermont, and Connecticut, ruled that the state of New York's ban on physician-assisted suicide or euthanasia was unconstitutional. The Court expressed the view that: 'Physicians do not fulfill the role of "killer" by prescribing drugs to hasten death any more than they do by disconnecting life-support systems.'[150] Moreover, prohibitions of physician-assisted euthanasia or suicide, in the view of this Court 'are not rationally related to any legitimate state interest'. That interest, the Court stated, 'lessens as the potential for life diminishes. And what business is it of the state to require the continuation of agony when the result is imminent and inevitable?'[150]

On 8 November 1994, Oregon voters approved the Death with Dignity Act.[151] A legal injunction that delayed implementation of the act was lifted in October 1997 and a measure to repeal the Death with Dignity Act was rejected by Oregon voters in November 1997. That act allows a terminally ill patient to request in writing a prescription for medication to end life. This law specifically prohibits physicians from performing euthanasia, but allows them to assist patients by prescribing medications patients can use to advance their own deaths. Physicians are also required to report to the Oregon Health Division all prescriptions for lethal medications. In February 2001, the Oregon Health Division reviewed 3 years of physician-assisted suicide practice under the Death with Dignity Act.[152]

The practice of physician-assisted suicide in Oregon is being attacked by the United States Attorney General, John Ashcroft, who believes the Oregon Death with Dignity Act violates the federal Controlled Substances Act. In his ruling of 6 November 2001, the Attorney General instructed the Drug Enforcement Administration to take action against physicians who would have prescribed lethal medications after 9 November 2001, the effective date of the ruling.[153,154] The Oregon Department of Justice mounted a legal challenge to this ruling and United States District Judge Robert E. Jones, on

20 November 2001, extended a restraining order on the Ashcroft ruling for up to 5 months. The Death with Dignity Act will remain in force until Judge Jones issues his final ruling, expected in the Spring of 2002, on Oregon's challenge to the Ashcroft ruling.[155,156]

In Canada, the Supreme Court, in September 1993, ruled against a British Columbia woman's request for physician-assisted euthanasia. Sue Rodriguez was dying of amyotrophic lateral sclerosis, a motor neuron disease. The Supreme Court judges were split 5–4 in their ruling that the Criminal Code's prohibition of assisted suicide or euthanasia does not violate the Canadian Charter of Rights and Freedoms.

Australia's Northern Territory legalized voluntary euthanasia when it passed its Rights of the Terminally Ill Act on 25 May 1995. Physicians are specifically prohibited from administering or assisting euthanasia if there are effective palliative care options available for the relief of a patient's pain and suffering.[157] This Act was reversed by the Australian Federal Parliament in March 1997.[158]

Reasoning in favour of legalizing euthanasia

The strongest arguments advanced to support the legalization of euthanasia are usually complex combinations of statements of fact, of principle, of logic, and of belief.

As to *statements of fact*, those requesting that euthanasia be decriminalized, legalized, or legally excused under some regulatory scheme emphasize the current limits of palliative medicine. Euthanasia, it is claimed, is often the only effective means of relieving dying patients from intense suffering. Although palliative medicine and palliative care have over the last three decades made remarkable progress, it is still quite true, as a *Lancet* editorial on the Dr Nigel Cox case observed, that there is a long way to go before it becomes possible to promise that no terminal state is so bad that it cannot be palliatively controlled, with dignity maintained by the coordinated administration of medications and other forms of treatment and care.[159] Moreover, it is also a matter of fact, documented in a number of studies, that currently effective methods of palliative medicine are so frequently neither mastered nor used by clinical teams, that patients continue to die miserably.[160–162] It is also quite true that access to expert palliative medicine and care remains extremely limited in most countries of the world.[163–166]

At this point *statements of principle* lock into the argument. There is the *principle of compassion*. Over 25 years ago, A.B. Downing, in advocating the legalization of euthanasia, emphasized that we shall probably never be able to eliminate totally from human experience the suffering that is both hard to bear and hard to behold. He buttressed this observation with the words of the former Dean of St Paul's Cathedral, the Very Reverend W.R. Matthews, who stated: 'It seems to be an incontrovertible proposition that, when we are confronted with suffering that is wholly destructive in its consequences and, so far as we can see, could have no beneficial result, there is a *prima facie* duty to bring it to an end'.[167] Because palliative medicine and care are neither universally effective nor universally available, and probably never will be, compassion requires that euthanasia be legally available to patients when no other effective means of relief are at hand.

A second *statement of principle* in the prolegalization argument would limit the administration of legalized euthanasia to those who are suffering consciously and who voluntarily request the hastening of their deaths. Only those should receive euthanasia, who, with full knowledge of their condition, stably request death, unpressured by others and unconstrained by depression. This is an appeal to the principle of autonomy and self-determination. The combination of the principle of compassion with the principle of self-determination leads to the ethical conclusion that it would be wrong not to honour patients' informed, lucid, free, and stable requests for rapid and painless death, as their chosen way of release from suffering they find unbearable. Physicians should be authorized to administer euthanasia to suffering patients, who want to advance their death but cannot do so themselves for lack of knowledge, ability, or both. Given the primacy of individual liberty among the values Western societies hold dear, the burden of proof should be on those who would legally restrict the liberty of competent adults to request and receive euthanasia.

The prolegalization argument evolves with an appeal to *statements of logic*. If we ethically and legally allow doctors to withhold or to discontinue life-prolonging treatments, fully aware that patients will die as a result, then there is no logically compelling reason to treat voluntary euthanasia differently. There is no compelling ethical reason to reject the legalization of euthanasia, since discontinuance of life-sustaining treatments is already widely accepted, clinically, ethically, and legally, and there is no ethical difference between death resulting from the withdrawal of life-prolonging treatment and death resulting from euthanasia. In fact, so the logic presses, it would be more compassionate to deliver death rapidly and painlessly to those who request it than to force them, by our euthanasia inaction, to stumble through a perhaps lengthy dying until they collapse, exhausted, into death. The United States Federal Second Circuit Court of Appeal's ruling, on 2 April 1996, that the State of New York's ban on doctor-assisted suicide should be struck down invoked the logic of 'no-difference' when the court stated: 'Physicians do not fulfill the role of "killer" by prescribing drugs to hasten death any more than they do by disconnecting life-support systems'.[150]

Nearly all proposals for the legalization of euthanasia admit the necessity of procedures and safeguards to prevent potential abuses of euthanasia. If not legalized, euthanasia, it is believed, will be practiced clandestinely, and without adequate legal supervision and control, abuses will likely occur. However, it is also believed, practicable, effective, and enforceable safeguards, which will not bureaucratically complicate that last days of those asking for euthanasia, are designable, Moreover, it is also believed, these safeguards will prevent most categories of abuse, if not every possible instance of abuse within any given category.

What would constitute an abuse of euthanasia? The most frequently cited examples refer to various categories of non-voluntary euthanasia: the administration of euthanasia to patients who have been submitted to pressure and manipulation; to persons who have not consented, or who cannot consent, to the advancing of their deaths.

At this point a *decisive statement of belief* enters into the prolegalization argument. One may grant, for the sake of argument, that safeguards and regulations may be effective in preventing abuse, but they will be so only so long as certain acts of euthanasia continue to be seen as an abuse. The statement of belief is that a society, our society, will never come to perceive euthanasia as an act of compassion for the comatose, for those in persistent vegetative state, for those in prolonged states of senile dementia, for persons afflicted with persistent, difficult-to-treat depression, or for persons afflicted with other forms of chronic mental or physical disability.

The Cartesian assumption that clarity, order, and pre-established procedure will govern the practice of euthanasia, and will do so successfully, floats in abstraction above the real world in which euthanasia will be practiced. This is a world of infinitely complex interactions, across society as a whole, among patients, doctors, nurses, families, hospital managers, health care budget planners, politicians, and conflicting moral groups who, such is the human condition, so often fall far short of the ideal agents these euthanasia proposals would require. Indeed, whether clear legal guidelines translate into adequate social control of euthanasia and whether euthanasia in practice brings about the peaceful death for which it is desired and designed is open to question and is being questioned.[168–172]

Why euthanasia should not be legalized

There is a valid distinction between ethically justifying or tolerating an individual act of euthanasia and ethically defending a regulatory policy or law authorizing a wide range of acts of euthanasia.[134] We accept this distinction and now turn to a summary of the reasons why euthanasia should not be legalized.

Opposition to the legalization of euthanasia is not only a matter of theoretical reasoning and argument. In its most decisive phase, that opposition is also a matter of practical judgment. A change in the law prohibiting euthanasia would represent a profound societal change, and a most significant departure from the accumulated wisdom of generations of human beings, who have thought it essential to circumscribe the administration of death with clear and stable restrictions. It is the cumulative impact of the high questionability, if not illusions, of so many of the assumptions of those favouring legalization of euthanasia that militates decisively against any legal change that would grant doctors, or any other persons, authority to administer death to the dying. The questionable or illusory assumptions are as follows.

Regarding voluntariness

It is highly questionable that any society will be able to uphold the voluntary character of euthanasia once euthanasia becomes a legally and socially acceptable option. Voluntary means freedom from coercion, pressure, undue inducement, and psychological and emotional manipulation. There is no law permitting voluntary euthanasia that could, even if implemented via complex procedures, protect conscious and vulnerable people against subtle manipulation to request socially acceptable administered death when they would rather live and be cherished.

Attention should be given to the fears many have of being a burden on others when they are very old or very sick and dependent. This fear was cited as one of the two most common reasons people in the United States put forth in support of legalizing euthanasia, the other reason being a fear of dying a painful death.[134,173] The decision of two United States Federal appeal courts to lift bans on euthanasia has provoked the observation: 'People who are sick already feel that they are a financial and emotional burden to their families and to society. … Now society is telling them, "You have an option. You have the right to die." For them, this translates easily into an obligation to die'.[174]

Regarding extension of euthanasia to those who cannot consent

Those who propose legalization of euthanasia usually claim, but not always, that only voluntary euthanasia should be legally permitted. The assumption is that after legalization of voluntary euthanasia, societies in the Western world would be enduringly willing and able to withstand pressure for an extension of euthanasia to those who never were able, or to those who have irreversibly lost the ability, to request or to consent to the termination of their lives.

There are good reasons to believe this assumption is illusory. There are many persons in hospitals, chronic care wards, and nursing homes across the land whose lives, by standards external to themselves and in the eyes of others, are hardly worth living. Many of these persons retain little more than the ability to sense and experience biological pain and comfort, gentleness of care, pleasing sound, human presence, and warmth. Some can hardly experience even these things, but their relatively strong bodies still cling to life.

It is naive to imagine that social barriers against non-voluntary euthanasia would not crumble in a society that legalizes voluntary euthanasia on the basis of compassion. Should compassion not also extend to those who, in the eyes of others, are suffering the indignity of profound mental and physical handicaps, even if they are suffering no pain, but who cannot request euthanasia?

This naivety is reinforced when one adverts to the fact that insistence on *voluntary* euthanasia was for some proponents of euthanasia in the Netherlands little more than a strategic move towards a much more expanded administration of euthanasia.[175] The 1985 report of the Netherlands State Commission on Euthanasia accepted euthanasia for comatose patients upon family request when such patients continued to live despite discontinuance of life-prolonging treatments. Moreover, the 1994 Dutch law on notification procedures for euthanasia included a notification procedure for euthanasia when persons, such as handicapped newborn children or comatose patients, cannot request or consent to the termination of their lives.[176] Some physicians in the Netherlands do not even consider such terminations of life to be euthanasia because they consider that euthanasia, by definition, has to be voluntary. Some would consider the rapid and painless termination of life in these circumstances to be little more than normal medical practice.[177]

Regarding the necessity of euthanasia

The case for legalizing euthanasia appeals to compassion. Euthanasia, it is claimed, should be legalized because it is inhumane to allow people to continue suffering when they request release by the painless termination of life. The assumptions behind this claim are that patients frequently suffer agony from pain that is uncontrollable; and that administration of death is the only effective release from suffering that arises, not from unmanageable pain, but from the human condition.

The first illusion in this assumption is that euthanasia or physician-assisted suicide will faultlessly deliver patients a tranquil death as the release from suffering that they desire and are requesting. A recent study has found that complications, such as myoclonus and vomiting, occurred in 7 per cent of cases of assisted suicide in the Netherlands. Problems with completion of assisted suicide, such as a longer-than-expected time to death, failure to induce coma, or induction of coma followed by awakening of the patient, occurred in 16 per cent of cases of assisted suicide. In the practice of euthanasia in the Netherlands, complications occurred in 3 per cent and problems with completion occurred in 6 per cent of cases. The authors comment that unexpected events can be traumatic.[178]

The second illusion in this assumption is the notion that doctors and nurses have generally mastered the state-of-the-art knowledge and skills that bring about an adequate management of pain and symptoms. But they have not. Where the binary logic, dying with pain or euthanasia, still holds true, the most reasonable solution would require widespread *education of doctors and nurses in the methods of palliative medicine and palliative care.* Legalization of euthanasia is an unjustifiable substitute for such education.[179]

Regarding the ability of doctors to communicate with the dying

Should legal authorizations to administer death, to practice euthanasia, be given to doctors, some of whom may very well not know how to listen to and to talk to suffering and dying patients? Is it not illusory to think that doctors generally are masters of the sensitive art of communication with the dying?[180–182]

That art is both difficult and complex. It is difficult because the care of dying people, who may also be suffering intensely, may provoke feelings of hopelessness, helplessness, failure, or demoralization within a doctor.[183,184] It may be difficult for a doctor when experiencing these feelings to avoid reinforcing in patients a sense of helplessness and of diminished self-worth coming to expression in a patient's demand for death. The art of communication with suffering and dying persons is also complex because the interaction between doctor and dying patient shapes and limits what each hears from and says to the other.[185] 'The patient's request for euthanasia may be more than just a reflection of the patient's individual despair; it may be an indication that others have despaired of the patient or have been perceived by the patient as having experienced such despair.'[186]

The existence of legalized euthanasia or physician-assisted suicide may also perilously simplify communication between physicians and dying patients, particularly when these conversations centre on a dying patient's request for death. If some psychiatric observers are correct in reporting that the legal availability of euthanasia as a medical option is resulting in physicians' loss of knowledge about how to deal with suicidal thoughts in the gravely ill,[187] physician–patient conversations that would thoroughly explore the origin and meaning of the suicidal ideation, and that would also help a patient discover her adaptive and coping strengths, may simply never occur.

It would be unwise to give doctors legal authorization to administer death when some physicians are insensitive to the psychological complexity of their conversations with dying patients. There should be no move to decriminalize or legalize euthanasia or physician-assisted suicide until we have mounted a credible and sustained effort to train doctors in the skills, including the communicative skills, required for a professional care of the dying.

Regarding the stability of societal compassion

The illusion to be mentioned here, the most dangerous of all, docks in the bay of well-meaning simplicity, the simplicity of assuming that a society permitting voluntary euthanasia and tolerating non-voluntary euthanasia could remain committed to high standards of care for vulnerable, poor, and marginalized people. The simplicity, and the naivety, consists in the narrow focus on the particular situation in which one person, a physician, wants to do good for another person, a patient requesting release from unbearable suffering. It is naive to imagine that a policy and a law permitting euthanasia will not lead to insensitive, inhumane, and intolerable abuse simply because those who designed the law were governed by pure motives and noble purposes.[188]

This narrow and naive focus of attention is blind to what Loren Graham, writing about eugenics and genetics in Russia and Germany during the 1920s, has called 'second-order' links between changing values and the uses a society can make of a science or a policy. Second-order links are difficult to see. They depend upon existing, and changing, political and social situations, and upon the persuasiveness of current, and emerging, philosophies and ideologies, however flawed these may be.[189] A societal acceptance of euthanasia or physician-assisted suicide, and the consequences of these practices on the compassionate care of vulnerable and dying people, are influenced by a society's economic situation, by its health care system, and by its management of health care technology.[190,191] The abuses which a law permitting euthanasia could come to serve depend upon second-order links between such a law and currently latent, or later emergent, ideologies of human insensitivity.

Regarding the costs of care

It is illusory to imagine that second-order links are not now being forged between social-economic stresses and a future law that would permit voluntary euthanasia and possibly tolerate non-voluntary euthanasia. The constraints and strains on our health care budgets, and our much vaunted universal health care systems, are growing in intensity. As many have observed, medical and hospital costs rise steeply with increasing age. In these circumstances, could socially and legally acceptable euthanasia not come to seem altogether too socially convenient? Could euthanasia then not come to be seen as a tolerable substitute for spending limited resources to develop and expand programmes of palliative care tailored for patients with cancer, HIV disease, amyotrophic lateral sclerosis, and other destructive and mortal diseases?

The danger in economically tough times is that we may easily slip into a triage mentality and adopt for everyday life the principles of exception that are tolerable only in extreme emergency situations. In such situations, where resources are just not immediately at hand to treat all who are sick or injured, treatment begins with those who are most severely ill or injured but who are salvageable, then moves on to those who are in lesser danger of dying, and finally is given last of all to those who cannot be saved, to the dying. This approach becomes particularly threatening to the humanitarian values and ethic of a society when it is put forth as necessary not only in crises of short duration, but as a matter of course. That the dying should come last when resources are distributed is reflected in a statement of the United States Court of Appeals for New York State in the Court's decision to strike down the New York State ban on euthanasia. The Court said: 'Surely the state's interest lessens as the potential for life diminishes'.[150] Those who believe that palliative care should be one of the first of the services to be cut when health care and hospital budgets are drastically slashed should stop and reflect upon the consequences of extending to everyday life the principles of triage that apply to emergency situations. Charles Fried has warned: 'It is when emergencies become usual that we are threatened with moral disintegration, dehumanization'.[192]

There is reason for concern that legalized euthanasia could come to be an expression of moral disintegration and of dehumanization of which we would never have thought ourselves capable.

Caution in reasoning against the legalization of euthanasia

In this chapter, opposition to the legalization of euthanasia is presented as a matter of practical and prudential judgment. Each of the reasons advanced in the preceding subsection against changing laws currently prohibiting the administration of death to the dying is open to question, and has been questioned in one publication or another written by those who believe and argue that healers should be legally authorized to administer euthanasia in response to voluntary requests of competent patients suffering from a terminal illness.[193–195] In our judgment, the reasons put forward to promote 'a carefully designed social experiment with legalized, voluntary euthanasia'[195] are, both when taken individually and when taken together as an argument, too naive and too insensitive to the complexities, and to the extremes of moral views in pluralistic modern societies to justify such a radical departure, as euthanasia would be, from long-standing legal interdictions on the administration of death.

This chapter's opposition to the legalization of euthanasia recognizes the difference between *reasonable* and *effective* distinctions.[196] The distinction between voluntary euthanasia on the one hand and non-voluntary or pressured euthanasia on the other is intellectually clear and ethically significant. The concern and practical judgment of this chapter is that it will probably be very difficult effectively to maintain this distinction in practice. Will societal attitudes towards non-voluntary euthanasia change and become more benign as people become more and more accustomed to various extensions and modifications of voluntary euthanasia?

An event in the world of art may suggest what could happen in the world of ethics. Bernard Williams cites Nelson Goodman's explanation of how increasingly incompetent forgeries by van Meegeren came to be accepted as genuine Vermeers.[196,197] What process was at work that could so distort the faculties of aesthetic perception and judgment? It was a process of incremental adaptation to incrementally poor forgeries. Only when the latest and poorest of the forgeries were compared, not to preceding and somewhat better forgeries, but to the original Vermeers, did the poverty of the fakery become strikingly clear.

The chapter's judgment that voluntary euthanasia as a compassionate release from suffering should not be legalized includes the concern that a process similar to that at work with the van Meegeren forgeries may come to distort ethical perceptions and evaluations of extensions of euthanasia to those who are neither dying nor able to consent. This concern is not purely speculative. The tolerance, if not the desire, for non-voluntary euthanasia in the Netherlands,[198] the 1994 legal authorization of a notification procedure for non-voluntary euthanasia in the Netherlands, and the Dutch Supreme Court's decision in June 1995 not to penalize psychiatrist Dr Boudewijn Chabot for assisting the suicide of a woman suffering from grief and depression[199] are all events that give justifiable cause to pause and to wonder how far enlightened societies at the beginning of this century will be prepared to go in extending the putative benefits of compassionate euthanasia.

Position statement

At the beginning of this century, the signs in Western societies of overt discrimination, of latent racism, of utilitarian insensitivity to vulnerable people, and of tendencies to devaluate human beings[200] are too prominent to justify insouciant attitudes regarding the legalization of euthanasia. The law prohibiting euthanasia, even voluntary euthanasia, should be maintained.

Those who favour legalization of voluntary euthanasia believe it to be utterly unproved and quite unlikely that legalization of euthanasia will provoke a societal slide down the slippery slope to intolerable abuses. Admittedly, such a slide is not certain. The issue is whether we should try this social experiment. This chapter argues that we should not.

Of course, there is no law, not even a law prohibiting euthanasia, that can cover the infinite variety of human situations or the infinite variety of unique human suffering. Maintaining a law against euthanasia will require of all of us the kind of common sense that knows when such a law should not be applied, or not applied in all its force.

Conclusion

At the close of this chapter we draw attention to the distinction between *ethics within palliative care* and *the ethic within which palliative care operates.*

This chapter has been about *ethics within palliative care.* The bedside of the dying has centred the chapter's discussions about resolving value conflicts and uncertainties, about how to make and justify the myriad decisions required of the dying, of families and of doctors, nurses, and other professionals on behalf of the dying. The clinical goal of palliative medicine underlying the discussion of ethical issues encompasses the coordination of knowledge, skills, reflection, and compassion to allow us, at the end of our days, to die as Philip Aries[201] outlines:

> Death must simply become the discreet but dignified exit of a peaceful person from a helpful society. A death without pain or suffering, and ultimately without fear.

But what of those who do not find their way into this ideal place? What of those who die alone, abandoned in their final plight? Any answer to this question confronts the *ethic within which palliative care operates.* That ethic encompasses a vision and the reach of humanity beyond the bedside. It is an ethic of action.

In his novel *The Death of Virgil,* Hermann Brock has the poet considering a decision to destroy his manuscript of the Aeneid.[202] Why? Because Brock sees Virgil coming to realize that the beauty and truth of language are inadequate to cope with human suffering. A poetry more immediate that that of words is needed: a poetry of action.[203]

Like such a poetry, the ethic within which palliative care operates needs to be an ethic of action, an ethic that mobilizes and links governments, institutions, programmes, services, persons, and resources to form a tissue of effective bonds of compassion, an ethic based on the vision that no one is a stranger to us among those who anguish and suffer as they face loss and death.

References

1. **Roy, D.J., Williams, J.R., and Dickens, B.M.** *Bioethics in Canada.* Scarbourough, Ontario: Prentice-Hall, 1994, pp. 27–60.
2. **Toulmin, S.** (1981). The tyranny of principles. *Hastings Center Report* **11**, 31–9.
3. **Fried, C.** *Medical Experimentation. Personal Integrity and Social Policy.* Amsterdam: North-Holland Publishing Company, 1974, pp. 101–5.
4. **Bohm, D.** *Wholeness and the Implicate Order.* London: Routledge and Kegan Paul, 1980.
5. **The Hastings Center.** *Guidelines on the Termination of Life-Sustaining Treatment and the Care of the Dying.* Briarcliff Manor, NY: The Hastings Center, 1987.
6. **The Appleton International Conference** (1992). Developing guidelines for decisions to forego life-prolonging medical treatment. *Journal of Medical Ethics* **18** (Suppl.), 3–23 (John M. Stanley, Guest Editor).
7. **President's Commission for the Study of Ethical Problems in Medicine and Biomedical and Behavioral Research.** *Deciding to Forego Life-Sustaining Treatment. Ethical, Medical, and Legal Issues in Treatment Decisions.* Washington DC: US Government Printing Office, 1983.
8. **National Council for Hospice and Specialist Palliative Care Services.** *Key Ethical Issues in Palliative Care: Evidence to House of Lords Select Committee on Medical Ethics* Occasional Paper 3. London: National Council for Hospice and Special Palliative Care Services, July 1993.
9. **Council on Ethical and Judicial Affairs, American Medical Association** (1992). Decisions near the end of life. *Journal of the American Medical Association* **267**, 2229–33.
10. **Sherlock, R.** (1982). For everything there is a season; the right to die in the United States. *Brigham Young University Law Review* **3**, 545–616.
11. **Gostin, L.** (1986). A right to choose death: the judicial trilogy of Brophy, Bouvia, and Conroy. *Law, Medicine & Health Care* **14**, 198–202.
12. **Meisel, A.** *The Right to Die.* New York: John Wiley & Sons, 1989.
13. **Ruark J.E., Raffin, T.A., and the Stanford University Medical Center Committee on Ethics** (1988). Initiating and withdrawing life support. *New England Journal of Medicine* **318**, 25–30.
14. **Buchanan, A.E. and Brock, D.** *Deciding for Others: The Ethics of Surrogate Decisionmaking.* London: Cambridge University Press, 1989.
15. **Wanzer, S.** et al. (1989). The physician's responsibility toward hopelessly ill patients: a second look. *New England Journal of Medicine* **244**, 1846–53.
16. **Solomon, M.Z.** et al. (1993). Decisions near the end of life: professional views on life-sustaining treatments. *American Journal of Public Health* **83**, 14–23.
17. **McCartney, J.T.** (1980). The development of the doctrine of ordinary and extraordinary means of preserving life in Catholic moral theology before the Karen Quinlan case. *Linacre Quarterly* **47**, 215–24.
18. **McCormick, R.A.** *How Brave a New World? Dilemmas in Bioethics.* New York: Doubleday & Company, 1981.
19. **Sacred Congregation for the Doctrine of the Faith** (1980). *Declaration on Euthanasia* **10** (10), 154–7. Rome: Origins.
20. **Panicola, M.** (2001). Catholic teaching on prolonging life: setting the record straight. *Hastings Center Report* **31** (6), 14–25, (see also p. 4, 9).
21. **Law Reform Commission of Canada.** *Euthanasia, Aiding Suicide and Cessation of Treatment.* Report #20. Ottawa: Minister of Supply and Services Canada, 1983, p. 32.
22. **Meisel, A.** (1993). The legal consensus about forgoing life-sustaining treatment: its status and prospects. *Kennedy Institute of Ethics Journal* **2**, 309–45.
23. **Paris, J. and Reardon, F.E.** (1991). Moral, ethical, and legal issues in the intensive care unit. *Journal of Intensive Care Medicine* **6**, 175–95 (see also p. 191).
24. **Task Force on Ethics of the Society of Critical Care Medicine** (1990). Consensus report on the ethics of foregoing life-sustaining treatments in the critically ill. *Critical Care Medicine* **18**, 1435–9.
25. **Feinstein, A.R.** (1983). An additional basic science for clinical medicine: IV. The development of clinimetrics. *Annals of Internal Medicine* **99**, 848.
26. **Lo, B.** (1995). Improving care near the end of life. Why is it so hard? *Journal of the American Medical Association* **274**, 1634–6.
27. **Cassem, N.** (1980). When illness is judged irreversible: imperative and elective treatments. *Man & Medicine* **5**, 154–66.
28. **Faden, R., Beauchamp, T.L., and King, N.M.P.** *A History and Theory of Informed Consent.* Oxford: Oxford University Press, 1986, p. 123.
29. **Carole Couture-Jacquet, C.** (1986). The Montreal Children's Hospital [1986]. *R.J.Q.* 1221–8 (Cour d'Appel).
30. **Stanley, J.M., ed.** (1992). The Appleton International Conference. Developing guidelines for decisions to forego life-prolonging medical treatment. *Journal of Medical Ethics* **18** (Suppl.), 3–23.
31. **Veatch, R.M. and Spicer, C.M.** (1992). Medically futile care: the role of the physician in setting limits. *American Journal of Law & Medicine* **18**, 15–36.
32. **Truog, R.D., Brett, A.S., and Frader, J.** (1992). The problem with futility. *New England Journal of Medicine* **326**, 1560–4.
33. **Heft, P.R., Siegler, M., and Lantos, J.** (2000). The rise and fall of the futility movement. *New England Journal of Medicine* **343**, 293–6.
34. **Council on Ethical and Judicial Affairs, American Medical Association** (1999). Medical futility in end-of-life care. Report of the Council on Ethical and Judicial Affairs. *Journal of the American Medical Association* **281** (10), 937–41.
35. **Brody, H.** (1998). Bringing clarity to the futility debate: don't use the wrong cases. *Cambridge Quarterly of Health Care Ethics* **7**, 269–73.
36. **Schneiderman, L.J.** (1998). Commentary. Bringing clarity to the futility debate: are the cases wrong? *Cambridge Quarterly of Health Care Ethics* **7**, 273–8.
37. **Trotter, G.** (1999). Response to 'Bringing clarity to the futility debate: don't use the wrong cases' by Brody, H. and 'Commentary. Bringing clarity to the futility debate: are the cases wrong?' by Schneiderman, L.J. (*C.Q.* Vol. 7, No. 3). Mediating disputes about medical futility. *Cambridge Quarterly of Health Care Ethics* **8**, 527–37.
38. **Schneiderman, L.J. and Capron, A.M.** (2000). How can hospital futility policies contribute to establishing standards of practice? *Cambridge Quarterly of Health Care Ethics* **9**, 524–31.
39. **Dunphy, K.** (2000). Futilitarianism: knowing how much is enough in end-of-life care. *Palliative Medicine* **14**, 313–22.
40. **Schneiderman, L.J.** et al. (1990). Medical futility: its meaning and ethical implications. *Annals of Internal Medicine* **112**, 949–54.
41. **Feinberg, W.M. and Ferry, P.C.** (1984). A fate worse than death. The persistent vegetative state in childhood. *American Journal of Diseases of Children* **138**, 128–30.

42. **Munstat, T.L.** et al. (1989). Guidelines on the vegetative state: commentary on the American Academy of Neurology Statement. *Neurology* **39**, 123–4.
43. **American Neurological Association Committee on Ethical Affairs** (1993). Persistent vegetative state: report of the American Neurological Association Committee on Ethical Affairs. *Annals of Neurology* **33**, 386–90.
44. **Tresch, D.D.** et al. (1991). Clinical characteristics of patients in the persistent vegetative state. *Archives of Internal Medicine* **151**, 930–2.
45. **Working Group, Royal College of Physicians** (1996). The permanent vegetative state. Review by a Working Group convened by the Royal College of Physicians and endorsed by the Conference of Medical Royal Colleges and their Faculties of the United Kingdom. *Journal of the Royal College of Physicians of London* **30**, 119–21.
46. **Steinbrook, R. and Lo, B.** (1988). Artificial feeding—solid ground, not a slippery slope. *New England Journal of Medicine* **318** (5), 286–90.
47. **Cantor, N.L.** (1989). The permanently unconscious patient, non-feeding and euthanasia. *American Journal of Law & Medicine* **15**, 381–437.
48. **Lynn, J.**, ed. *By No Extraordinary Means*. Bloomington IN: Indiana University Press, 1986.
49. **Pollock, S.G.** (1988–89). Life and death decisions; who makes them and by what standards? *Rutgers Law Review* **41**, 505–40.
50. **Bernat, J.L.** et al. (1993). Patient refusal of hydration and nutrition. *Archives of Internal Medicine* **153**, 2723–7.
51. **Kamisar, Y.** (1989). Dilemma over the night that ends all nights; right to die, or license to kill? *New Jersey Law Journal* **124** (21), 7.
52. **Gillick, M.R.** (2000). Rethinking the role of tube feeding in patients with advanced dementia. *New England Journal of Medicine* **342**, 206–10.
53. **Wade, D.T.** (2001). Ethical issues in diagnosis and management of patients in the permanent vegetative state. *British Medical Journal* **322**, 352–4.
54. **Hildebrand, A.J.** (2000). Masked intentions: the masquerade of killing thoughts used to justify dehydrating and starving people in a 'persistent vegetative state' and people with other profound neurological impairments. *Issues in Law & Medicine* **16**, 143–65.
55. **Gillon, R.** (1999). End-of-life decisions. *Journal of Medical Ethics* **25**, 435–6.
56. **MacDonald, N. and Fainsinger, R.** (1996). Indications and ethical considerations in the hydration of patients with advanced cancer. In *Cachexia–Anorexia in Cancer Patients* (ed. E. Bruera and I. Higgins), vol. 7, pp. 94–109. Oxford: Oxford University Press <http://www.growthhouse.org/books/bruera2.htm>
57. **Lynn, J. and Childress, J.F.** (1983). Must patients always be given food and water? *Hastings Center Report* **13** (5), 17–21.
58. **Council of Scientific Affairs and Council on Ethical and Judicial Affairs** (1990). Persistent vegetative state and the decision to withdraw or withhold life support. *Journal of the American Medical Association* **263**, 426–30.
59. **Institute of Medical Ethics Working Party on the Ethics of Prolonging Life and Assisting Death** (1991). Withdrawal of life-support from patients in a persistent vegetative state. *Lancet* **337**, 96–8.
60. **Gillis, J.** et al. (1989). Ventilator-dependent children. *Medical Journal of Australia* **150**, 10–14.
61. **Gillis, J. and Kilham, H.** (1990). Entrapment. *Critical Care Medicine* **18**, 897.
62. **Smedera, N.** et al. (1990). Withholding and withdrawal of life support from the critically ill. *New England Journal of Medicine* **322**, 309–15.
63. **NIH Workshop** (1986). Withholding and withdrawing mechanical ventilation. *American Review of Respiratory Disease* **134**, 1327–30.
64. **McCormick, R.A.** (1975). A proposal for 'quality of life' criteria for sustaining life. *Hospital Progress* **56**, 76–9.
65. **Roy, D.J.** Decision offers Nancy B. a measure of dignity. Life-support technology not sole solution. *The Financial Post* 8 January 1992, p. 10.
66. **Roy, D.J.** Respecter le désir et la dignité de Nancy B. *Le Devoir* 2 December 1991, Vol. 1, p. 4.
67. **Singer, P.A., Robertson, G., and Roy, D.J.** (1999). Advance care planning. In *Bioethics at the Bedside: A Clinician's Guide* (ed. P.A. Singer), pp. 39–46. The Clinical Basics Series. Ottawa: Canadian Medical Association.
68. **Emanuel, L.L. and Emanuel, E.J.** (1989). The medical directive: a new comprehensive advance care document. *Journal of the American Medical Association* **261**, 3288–93.
69. **Hackler, C., Moseley, R., and Vawter, D.** *Advance Directives in Medicine*. New York: Praeger, 1989.
70. **Singer, P.A.** et al. (1992). Advance directives: are they an advance? *Canadian Medical Association Journal* **146**, 127–34.
71. **Silverman, H.J., Vinicky, J.K., and Gasner, M.R.** (1992). Advance directives: implications for critical care. *Critical Care Medicine* **20**, 1027–31.
72. **Ditto, P.H.** et al. (2001). Advance directives as acts of communication. A randomized controlled trial. *Archives of Internal Medicine* **161**, 421–30.
73. **Coppola, K.M.** et al. (2001). Accuracy of primary care and hospital-based physicians' predictions of elderly outpatients' treatment preferences with or without advance directives. *Archives of Internal Medicine* **161**, 431–40.
74. **Désaulniers, P.** (1994). L'éthique clinique à l'urgence: réfléchir contre la montre. In *Collection Panétius—Archives de l'éthique clinique. 1. Au chevet du malade: analyse de cas à travers les spécialités médicales* (ed. D.J. Ray, C.H. Rapin, and M.R. Morisstte), pp. 99–101. Montréal: Centre de bioéthique, Institut de recherches cliniques de Montréal.
75. **Cowan, J.D. and Walsh, D.** (2001). Terminal sedation in palliative medicine—definition and review of the literature. *Supportive Care in Cancer* **9** (16), 403–7.
76. **Chater, S.** et al. (1998). Sedation for intractable distress in the dying—a survey of experts. *Palliative Medicine* **12**, 255–69.
77. **Ventafridda, V.** et al. (1990). Symptom prevalence and control during cancer patients' last days of life. *Journal of Palliative Care* **6** (3), 7–11.
78. **Mount, B.** (1990). A final crescendo of pain? *Journal of Palliative Care* **6** (3), 5–6.
79. **Roy, D.J.** (1990). Need they sleep before they die? *Journal of Palliative Care* **6** (3), 3–4.
80. **Truog, R.D., Berde, C.B., Mitchell, C., and Grier, H.E.** (1992). Barbiturates in the care of the terminally ill. *New England Journal of Medicine* **327**, 1678–81.
81. **Bedau, H.A.**, ed. *The Death Penalty in America* 3rd edn. New York: Oxford University Press, 1982, pp. 17–18.
82. **Quill, T.E.** (1991). Death and dignity: a case of individualized decision-making. *New England Journal of Medicine* **324**, 691–4.
83. **Sholl, J.G.** (1993). Barbiturates in the care of the terminally ill (Letter). *New England Journal of Medicine* **328** (18), 1350.
84. **Donnelly, S., Nelson, K., and Walsh, T.D.** (1993). Barbiturates in the care of the terminally ill (Letter). *New England Journal of Medicine* **328** (18), 1350–1.
85. **Cherny, N.I. and Portenoy, R.K.** (1994). Sedation in the management of refractory symptoms; guidelines for evaluation and treatment. *Journal of Palliative Care* **10** (2), 31–8.
86. **Cherny, N., Coyle, N., and Foley, K.M.** (1994). The treatment of suffering when patients request elective death. *Journal of Palliative Care* **10** (2), 71–9.
87. **Saunders, C.** (1984). Pain and impending death. In *Textbook of Pain* (ed. P. Wall, and R. Melzack), pp. 477–8. New York: Churchill Livingstone.
88. **Mount, B. and Hamilton, P.** (1994). When palliative care fails to control suffering. *Journal of Palliative Care* **10** (2), 24–6.
89. **Scott, M.** (1944). Commentaries. When palliative care fails to control suffering. *Journal of Palliative Care* **10** (2), 30.
90. **Gauthier, C.C.** (2001). Active voluntary euthanasia, terminal sedation, and assisted suicide. *The Journal of Clinical Ethics* **12** (1), 43–50.
91. **Morita, T.** et al. (1999). Do hospice clinicians sedate patients intending to hasten death? *Journal of Palliative Care* **15** (3), 20–3.
92. **Loewy, E.H.** (2001). Terminal sedation, self-starvation, and orchestrating the end of life. *Archives of Internal Medicine* **161**, 329–32.
93. **Smith II G.P.** (1998). Terminal sedation as palliative care: revalidating a right to a good death. *Cambridge Quarterly of Health Care Ethics* **7**, 382–7.
94. **Emanuel, E.J.** (1994). Euthanasia. Historical, ethical, and empirical perspectives. *Archives of Internal Medicine* **154**, 1890–901.
95. **Van Der Sluis, I.** (1979). The movement for euthanasia 1875–1975. *Janus* **66**, 131–71.
96. **Gruman, G.J.** (1973). An historical introduction to ideas about voluntary euthanasia; with a bibliographic survey and guide for interdisciplinary studies. *OMEGA* **4**, 87–138.
97. **Silving, H.** (1954). Euthanasia: a study in comparative criminal law. *University of Pennsylvania Law Review* **103**, 350–89.
98. **Portnoy, R.K.**, ed. (1991). Special issue on medical ethics: physician-assisted suicide and euthanasia. *Journal of Pain and Symptom Management* **6**, 279–339.

99. **Davis, A.J.** et al. (1993). An international perspective of active euthanasia: attitudes of nurses in seven countries. *International Journal of Nursing Studies* **30**, 301–10.
100. **Ward, B.J. and Tate, P.A.** (1994). Attitudes among NHS doctors to requests for euthanasia. *British Medical Journal* **308**, 1332–4.
101. **Shapiro, R.S.** et al. (1994). Willingness to perform euthanasia. A survey of physician attitudes. *Archives of Internal Medicine* **154**, 575–84.
102. **Paume, P. and O'Malley, E.** (1994). Euthanasia: attitudes and practices of medical practitioners. *Medical Journal of Austria* **161**, 137–44.
103. **Kinsella, T.D. and Verhoef, M.J.** (1993). Alberta euthanasia survey. 1. Physicians' opinions about the morality and legalization of active euthanasia. *Canadian Medical Association Journal* **148**, 1921–6.
104. **Verhoef, M.J. and Kinsella, T.D.** (1993). Alberta euthanasia survey. 2. Physicians' opinions about the acceptance of active euthanasia as a medical act and the reporting of such practice. *Canadian Medical Association Journal* **148**, 1929–33.
105. **Stevens, C.A. and Hassan, R.** (1994). Management of death, dying and euthanasia: attitudes and practices of medical practitioners in South Australia. *Journal of Medical Ethics* **20**, 41–6.
106. **Meier, D.E.** et al. (1998). A national survey of physician-assisted suicide and euthanasia in the United States. *New England Journal of Medicine* **338**, 1193–201.
107. **Shah, N.** et al. (1998). National survey of UK psychiatrists' attitudes to euthanasia. *Lancet* **352**, 1360.
108. **Willems, D.L.** et al. (2000). Attitudes and practices concerning the end of life. A comparison between physicians from the United States and from the Netherlands. *Archives of Internal Medicine* **160**, 63–8.
109. **Valverius, E., Nilstun, T., and Nilsson, B.** (2000). Palliative care, assisted suicide and euthanasia: nationwide questionnaire to Swedish physicians. *Palliative Medicine* **14**, 141–8.
110. **Emanuel, E.J., Fairclough, D.L., and Emanuel, L.L.** (2000). Attitudes and desires related to euthanasia and physician-assisted suicide among terminally ill patients and their caregivers. *Journal of the Medical American Association* **284**, 2460–8.
111. **Grassi, L.** et al. (2000). Medical students' opinions of euthanasia and physician-assisted suicide in Italy. *Archives of Internal Medicine* **160**, 1226–2227.
112. **Warner, T.D.** et al. (2001). Uncertainty and opposition of medical students toward assisted death practices. *Journal of Pain and Symptom Management* **22**, 657–67.
113. **Asai, A.** et al. (2001). Doctors' and nurses' attitudes towards and experiences of voluntary euthanasia: survey of members of the Japanese Association of Palliative Medicine. *Journal of Medical Ethics* **27**, 324–30.
114. **British Medical Association.** *Euthanasia.* London: BMA, 1988.
115. **The American Geriatrics Society Ethics Committee** (1995). Physician-assisted suicide and voluntary active euthanasia. *Journal of the American Geriatrics Society* **43**, 579–80.
116. **Institute of Medical Ethics Working Party on the Ethics of Prolonging Life and Assisting Death** (1990). Assisted death. *Lancet* **336**, 610–13.
117. **House of Lords Select Committee on Medical Ethics.** *Report.* London: H.M. Stationery Office, 1994.
118. **Canadian Medical Association** (1995). CMA policy summary. Physician-assisted death. *Canadian Medical Association Journal* **152**, 248A–B.
119. **The Senate of Canada, Special Senate Committee on Euthanasia and Assisted Suicide.** *Of Life and Death. Report of the Special Senate Committee on Euthanasia and Assisted Suicide.* Ottawa: Minister of Supply and Services Canada, 1995.
120. **Académie Suisse des Sciences Médicales** (1995). Directives médico-éthiques sur l'accompagnement médical des patients en fin de vie ou souffrant de troubles cérébraux extrêmes. *Bulletin des Médecins Suisses* **29** (30), 1226–8.
121. **Sahm, S.W.** (2000). Palliative care versus euthanasia. The German position: the German General Medicine Council's principles for medicine care of the terminally ill. *Journal of Medicine and Philosophy* **25**, 195–219.
122. **Snyder, L. and Sulmasy, D.P.** (2001). Physician-assisted suicide. *Annals of Internal Medicine* **135**, 209–16.
123. **Gillett, G.** (1998). Euthanasia, letting die and the pause. *Journal of Medical Ethics* **14**, 61–8.
124. **Brock, D.W.** (1992). Voluntary active euthanasia. *Hastings Center Report* **22** (2), 10–22.
125. **Callahan, D.** (1992). When self-determination runs amok. *Hastings Center Report* **22** (2), 52–5.
126. **Miller, F.G. and Fletcher, J.C.** (1993). The case for legalized euthanasia. *Perspectives in Biology and Medicine* **36** (2), 159–76.
127. **Kamisar, Y.** (1995). Against assisted suicide—even a very limited form. *University of Detroit Mercy Law Review* **72**, 735–69.
128. **Keown, T.**, ed. *Euthanasia Examined. Ethical, Clinical and Legal Perspectives.* London: Cambridge University Press, 1995.
129. **Dworkin, R.** et al. Assisted suicide: the philosophers' brief. *New York Review of Books* 27 March 1997, pp. 41–7.
130. **Dubois, J.M.** (1999). Physician-assisted suicide and public virtue: a reply to the liberty thesis of 'The Philosophers' Brief'. *Issues en Law & Medicine* **15**, 159–79.
131. **Beauchamp, T.L.** (1999). The medical ethics of physician-assisted suicide. *Journal of Medical Ethics* **25**, 437–9.
132. **Fraser, S.I. and Walters, J.W.** (2000). Death—whose decision? Euthanasia and the terminally ill. *Journal of Medical Ethics* **26**, 121–5.
133. **Doyal, L. and Doyal, L.** (2001). Why active euthanasia and physician-assisted suicide should be legalised. *British Medical Journal* **323**, 1079–80.
134. **Truog, R.D. and Berde, C.B.** (1993). Pain, euthanasia, and anesthesiologists. *Anesthesiology* **78**, 353–60.
135. **Brock, D.W.** (1992). Euthanasia. *The Yale Journal of Biology and Medicine* **65**, 121–9.
136. **Rachels, J.** (1995). Active and passive euthanasia. *New England Journal of Medicine* **292**, 78–80.
137. **Gillon, R.** (1988). Euthanasia, withholding life-prolonging treatment, and moral differences between killing and letting die. *Journal of Medical Ethics* **14**, 115–17.
138. **Callahan, D.** (1989). Can we return death to disease? (Suppl. Mercy, Murder & Morality: Perspectives on Euthanasia). *Hastings Center Report* **19** (1), 4–6.
139. **The New York State Task Force on Life and the Law.** *When Death is Sought: Assisted Suicide and Euthanasia in the Medical Context.* New York: The New York State Task Force on Life and the Law, 1994.
140. **Larson, E.J.** (1995). Seeking compassion in dying: the Washington State law against assisted suicide. *Seattle University of Law Review* **18**, 509, 517.
141. **Scofield, G.R.** (1995). Exposing some myths about physician-assisted suicide. *Seattle University of Law Review* **18**, 473, 481.
142. **Chapman, C.R. and Gavrin, J.** (1993). Suffering and its relationship to pain. *Journal of Palliative Care* **9** (2), 5–13.
143. **Liebeskind, J.C.** (1991). Editorial. Pain can kill. *Pain* **44**, 3–4.
144. **Trowell, H.** *The Unfinished Debate on Euthanasia.* London: SCM Press Ltd, 1973, p. 83.
145. **Smith, R.S.** (1993). Ethical issues surrounding cancer pain. In *Current and Emerging Issues in Cancer Pain: Research and Practice* (ed. C.R. Chapman and K.M. Foley), pp. 385–92. New York: Raven Press.
146. **Sheldon, T.** (2001). Holland decriminalises voluntary euthanasia. *British Medical Journal* **322**, 947.
147. **Weber, W.** (2001). Netherlands legalise euthanasia. *Lancet* **357**, 1189.
148. **Wise, J.** (2001). Netherlands, first country to legalize euthanasia. *Bulletin of the World Health Organization* **79** (6), 580.
149. United States Court of Appeals for the Ninth Circuit, Compassion in Dying, a Washington non-profit corporation. Jane Roe; John Doe; James Poe; Harold Gluchsberg, M.D., v. State of Washington; Christine Gregoire, Attorney General of Washington. 6 March 1996 : 14.
150. United States Court of Appeals for the Second Circuit, Timothy Quill, M.D., Samuel C. Klagskrun, M.D., and Howard A. Grossman, M.D. v. Denaris C. Vacco, Attorney General of the State of New York, George E. Palaki, Governor of the State of New York, Robert M. Morgenthau, District Attorney of New York County. 2 April 1996 : 12.
151. **Annas, G.J.** (1994). Death by prescription. The Oregon initiative. *New England Journal of Medicine* **331**, 1240–3.
152. **Department of Human Services, Oregon Health Division, Center for Disease, Prevention, and Epidemiology.** *Oregon's Death with Dignity*

Act: Three Years of Legalized Physician-Assisted Suicide. Portland OR: Department of Human Services, Oregon Health Division, 2001.

153. **Ashcroft J.** (Attorney General). *Dispensing of Controlled Substances to Assist Suicide.* Washington DC: Department of Justice, Office of the Attorney General 9 November 2001 (http://www.deadiversion.usdoj.gov/fed_regs/notices/2001/fr1109.htm).
154. **McLellan, F.** (2001). US government undercuts Oregon's assisted-suicide law. *Lancet* **358**, 1788.
155. **State of Oregon Department of Justice**. *Attorney General Hardy Myers to take Legal Action to Protect Oregon's Physician-Assisted Suicide Law.* Media Releases, 6 November 2001 (http://www.doj.state.or.us/releases/rel110701.htm).
156. **McCall, W.** *Oregon's Physician-Assisted Suicide Law gets Another Temporary Reprieve.* The Associated Press, 20 November 2001 (http://www.worldrtd.org/OregonReprieve.html).
157. **Ryan, C.J. and Kaye, M.** (1996). Euthanasia in Australia—The Northern Territory Rights of the Terminally Ill Act. *New England Journal of Medicine* **334**, 326–8.
158. **Fleming, J.I.** (2000). Death, dying, and euthanasia: Australia versus the Northern Territory. *Issues in Law & Medicine* **15**, 291–305.
159. Editorial (1992). The final autonomy. *Lancet* **340**, 757–8.
160. **The SUPPORT Principal Investigators** (1995). A controlled trial to improve care for seriously ill hospitalized patients: the study to understand prognoses and preferences for outcomes and risks of treatments (SUPPORT). *Journal of the American Medical Association* **274** (20), 1591–8.
161. **Cleeland, C.S.** et al. (1994). Pain and its treatment in outpatients with metastatic cancer. *New England Journal of Medicine* **330**, 592–6.
162. **Foley, K.M.** (1991). The relationship of pain and symptom management to patient requests for physician-assisted suicide. *Journal of Pain and Symptom Management* **6**, 289–97.
163. **Stjernsward, J.** et al. (1994). Opioid availability in Latin America: the Declaration of Florianoloplis. *Journal of Palliative Care* **10** (4), 11–14.
164. **Vainio, A.** (1995). Treatment of terminal cancer pain in France: a questionnaire study. *Pain* **62**, 155–62.
165. **Rhymes, J.** (1990). Hospice care in America. *Journal of the American Medical Association* **264**, 369–72.
166. **Wank, R.** et al. (1993). Country reports: status of cancer pain and palliative care in Argentina, Australia, Canada, China, Columbia, Costa Rica, Egypt, France, Germany, Greece, Hungary, India, Indonesia, Japan, Papua New Guina, Phillipines, Singapore, Thailand, United States, and Vietnam. *Journal of Pain and Symptom Management* **8** (6), 385–442.
167. **Downing, A.B.**, ed. *Euthanasia and the Right to Death.* London: Peter Owen, 1969, p. 23.
168. **Cohen-Almagor, R.** (2001). An outsider's view of Dutch euthanasia policy and practice. *Issues in Law & Medicine* **17** (1), 35–68.
169. **Cohen-Almagor, R.** (2001). 'Culture of death' in the Netherlands: Dutch perspectives. *Issues in Law & Medicine* **17** (2), 167–79.
170. **Jochemsen, H. and Keown, J.** (1999). Voluntary euthanasia under control? Further empirical evidence from the Netherlands. *Journal of Medical Ethics* **25**, 16–21.
171. **Gunning, K.F.** (2000). Die Euthanasie in Holland ausser Kontrolle. Kritischer Bericht eines holländischen Arztes. *Der Internist* **6**, M144–6.
172. **Horton, R.** (2001). Euthanasia and assisted suicide: what does the Dutch vote mean? *Lancet* **357**, 1221–2.
173. **Blondin, R.J., Szalay, U.S., and Knox, R.A.** (1992). Should physicians aid their patients in dying? *Journal of the American Medical Association* **267**, 2658–62.
174. **Fein, E.B.** Will the right to suicide become an obligation? *The New York Times*, 7 April 1996, p. 24.
175. **de Watcher, M.A.M.** (1992). Euthanasia in the Netherlands. *Hastings Center Report* **22** (2), 29.
176. **Schwartz, R.L.** (1995). Euthanasia and assisted suicide in the Netherlands. *Cambridge Quarterly of Healthcare Ethics* **4**, 117–18.
177. **ten Have HAMJ and Welie JVM.** (1992). Euthanasia: normal medical practice? *Hastings Center Report* **22** (2), 34–8.
178. **Groenewoud, J.H.** et al. (2000). Clinical problems with the performance of euthanasia and physician-assisted suicide in the Netherlands. *New England Journal of Medicine* **342**, 551–6.
179. **Emanuel, E.J.** (2001). Euthanasia: where the Netherlands leads will the world follow? *British Medical Journal* **322**, 1376–7.
180. **Annas, G.J.** (1993). Physician-assisted suicide: Michigan's temporary solution. *New England Journal of Medicine* **328**, 1573.
181. **Ramirez, A.J.** et al. (1995). Burnout and psychiatric disorder among cancer clinicians. *British Journal of Cancer* **71** (6), 1263–9.
182. **Ramirez, A.J.** et al. (1996). Mental health of hospital consultants: the effects of stress and satisfaction at work. *Lancet* **347**, 724–8.
183. **Cherny, N.I.** et al. (1994). Suffering in the advanced cancer patient: a definition and taxonomy. *Journal of Palliative Care* **10** (2), 57–70.
184. **Cherny, N.I.** et al. (1994). The treatment of suffering when patients request elective death. *Journal of Palliative Care* **10** (2), 71–9.
185. **Modestin, J.** (1987). Countertransference reactions contributing to completed suicide. *British Journal of Medical Psychology* **60**, 379–85.
186. **Varghese, F.T. and Kelly, B.** (2001). Countertransference and assisted suicide. *Issues in Law & Medicine* **16** (3), 252.
187. **Hamilton, N.G. and Hamilton, C.A.** (2000). Therapeutic response to assisted suicide request. *Issues in Law & Medicine* **16** (2), 167–76.
188. **Fairbairn, G.J.** (1988). Kuhse, Singer and slippery slopes. *Journal of Medical Ethics* **14**, 132–4.
189. **Graham, L.R.** (1977). Political ideology and genetic theory: Russia and Germany in the 1920's. *Hastings Center Report* **7** (5), 30–9.
190. **Rizzo, R.F.** (2000). Physician-assisted suicide in the United States: the underlying factors in technology, health care and palliative medicine. Part One. *Theoretical Medicine* **21**, 277–89.
191. **Rizzo, R.F.** (2000). Physician-assisted suicide in the United States: confronting legal and medical reasoning. Part Two. *Theoretical Medicine* **21**, 291–304.
192. **Fried, C.** (1975). Rights and health care—beyond equity and efficiency. *New England Journal of Medicine* **293**, 245.
193. **Quill, T.E., Cassel, C.K., and Meier, D.** (1992). Care of the hopelessly ill. Proposed criteria for physician assisted suicide. *New England Journal of Medicine* **327**, 1380–4.
194. **Brody, H.** (1992). Assisted death—a compassionate response to a medical failure. *New England Journal of Medicine* **327**, 1384–8.
195. **Miller, T.G. and Fletcher, J.C.** (1993). The case for legalized euthanasia. *Perspectives in Biology and Medicine* **36** (2), 159–76 (see also p. 168).
196. **Williams, B.** (1985) Which slopes are slippery? In *Moral Dilemmas in Modern Medicine* (ed. M. Lockwood), pp. 126–37. Oxford: Oxford University Press.
197. **Goodman, N.** *Languages of Art—an Approach to a Theory of Symbols.* Indianapolis In: Hackett Publishing Co., 1976, pp. 110–11.
198. **Hendin, H.** (1994). Seduced by death: doctors, patients, and the Dutch care. *Issues in Law & Medicine* **10**, 123–68.
199. **CQ Interview** (1995). Arlene Judith Kotzko and Dr Boudewijn Chabot discuss assisted suicide in the absence of somatic illness. *Cambridge Quarterly of Health Care Ethics* **4**, 239–49.
200. **Woollacot, M.** Paying the price for insecurity. *The Manchester Guardian Weekly*, 28 August 1994, p. 25.
201. **Ariès, P.** *L'Homme devant la mort.* Paris: Éditions du Seuil, 1977, p. 608.
202. **Broch, H.** *The Death of Virgil.* San Francisco: North Point Press, 1983.
203. **Steiner, G.** (1982). The hollow miracle. In *Language and Silence. Essays on Language, Literature, and the Inhuman* (ed. G. Steiner), p. 103. New York: Atheneum.

4

Communication and palliative medicine

4 Communication and palliative medicine

4.1 Communication with the patient and family in palliative medicine

Lesley Fallowfield

Introduction

> I think the best physician is the one who has the providence to tell to the patients according to his knowledge the present situation, what has happened before, and what is going to happen in the future (Hippocrates)

Talking about sad, bad, and difficult things is a fundamental and an inevitable part of the health care professional's (HCPs) work, but one in which few have received sufficient help or training.[1,2] In an endeavour to shield patients from uncomfortable and distressing facts, doctors and nurses frequently censor their information giving in the mistaken belief that what someone does not know does not harm them. This misguided albeit well-intentioned assumption is made at all stages of the disease trajectory. Less-than-honest disclosure is apparent when a patient first reports suspicious symptoms, at confirmation of the diagnosis, when the putative therapeutic benefits of treatment are discussed, at recurrence or relapse, and towards the end of life. Most attempts by doctors to protect patients from the reality of their situation often creates further problems for patients, their relatives, and their friends. Furthermore, it can lead to inconsistent messages being given by other members of the multidisciplinary team. Economy with the truth often leads to conspiracies of silence that usually build up to a heightened state of fear, anxiety, and confusion, rather than one of calmness and equanimity. The kinds of ambiguous or deliberately misleading messages received by patients may afford them short-term benefits while things continue to go well, but it has unfortunate long-term consequences. A patient with a shortened or uncertain future needs time and scope to reorganize and adapt their life towards the attainment of achievable goals. Realistic hopes and aspirations can only be generated from honest disclosure. In this chapter evidence from research studies will be provided showing that although communicating the truth can be painful, deceit may well provoke greater problems. Some suggestions will also be made about practical ways to communicate about difficult issues in palliative care.

Good palliative care presents substantial clinical, nursing, communication, and emotional challenges for all HCPs. If accomplished well, palliative care can also offer tangible, satisfying, professional and personal benefits. It might well be assumed that a speciality dealing with the care of dying people would appeal to those who possess not only good clinical and communication skills but also attitudes and beliefs compatible with an openness towards honest disclosure and truth-telling. Although the skills required for the provision of physical care may be excellent, effective communication is often less well honed. Questionable approaches towards honest disclosure may be the consequence of poor training or may represent unawareness of the impact that dishonesty has on patients; it may also demonstrate genuine differences in cultural expectations. For example, Bruera et al.[3], conducted an interesting postal survey which examined the attitudes and beliefs of palliative care specialists towards communication with the terminally ill. Respondents were based in French-speaking Europe, South America (Argentina and Brazil), and Canada. Every clinician said that they would like to be told the truth about their own terminal illness. However, only 93 per cent of Canadian physicians, 26 per cent of European clinicians, and 18 per cent of South American clinicians thought that the majority of their patients would wish to know ($P = 0.001$). Similar attitudes prevailed when clinicians were asked to estimate how many relatives would want patients to know about the terminal nature of their illness. Clearly what clinicians *think* that their patients want and what the patients and their families *actually* want is often very different. The evidence for really substantial cultural differences regarding patients' actual rather than assumed information needs about prognosis is in fact rather thin or inconclusive. For example, well-conducted studies by Fielding and Hung in Hong Kong[4] challenge the notion that Asian patients with cancer and their families want less information than their Western counterparts. A vital clinical point to make is that HCPs should make concerted efforts to base their communication on an individual's expressed preference, whatever their cultural background, and not make assumptions about the needs of different ethnic groups.

Information needs of patients and their families

It is of course important to determine the information needs of patients if people are to be able to give informed consent and make educated decisions. Their future management might include further treatment options or participation in Phase I trials, but people cannot contribute to these decisions if they lack the necessary information. Truthful communication about the future is also vital if patients are to be permitted the dignity of deciding how to spend their remaining time. Unfortunately doctors worldwide seriously underestimate not only the information needs of their patients[4,5] but also their preferences about decision making.[6] Some patients express a desire for more limited information at different timepoints during the course of their disease,[7] but they represent the minority. Research conducted in the United Kingdom by Jenkins et al.[8] with a large heterogeneous sample of 2331 patients with cancer showed that 2027 (87 per cent) wanted all possible information, be that good or bad news.

Some doctors would argue that honest disclosure is reasonable in patients for whom cure is a realistic prospect but that when the outlook is bleak then they are less likely to provide full information. Results from a recent extension to the study by Jenkins et al.[9] make this position untenable. The study has now recruited 2809 patients, 1032 of whom were being treated palliatively. The general information preferences of palliatively

Table 1 Specific information preferences of patients with cancer

	Absolutely need/ would like to have (%)		Do not want (%)	
	Palliative	Non-palliative	Palliative	Non-palliative
Specific name of the illness	87	91	13	9
Whether or not it is cancer	98	98	2	2
Week-by-week progress	90	93	10	7
Chances of cure	93	97	7	3
All possible treatments	94	95	6	5
All possible side effects	97	97	3	3
How treatment works	91	93	9	7

treated patients were compared with those of patients receiving potentially curative treatment or who were in remission. Irrespective of treatment intent, the overwhelming majority of patients expressed a preference for the doctor to give as much information as possible, be that good or bad news. Slightly more of the palliatively treated patients (7.3 per cent) than the non-palliative group (3.9 per cent) wanted additional information only if it was good news ($P < 0.001$) although the numbers of patients overall who endorsed this option were very small 144/2809. Little difference was found when the more specific information needs of palliative and non-palliative groups were compared (see Table 1), although there were some interesting sex differences. In general, women wanted more information than men for most items ($P < 0.01$), although both men and women had an equal need to know whether or not it was cancer and what the chances of cure were. Among the palliatively treated patients the sex differences disappeared, with the majority of men and women wanting the same sorts of information apart from the chances of cure, where again more women than men wanted this information ($P = 0.021$).

The effect of age was also examined; in general younger patients under 65 years wanted more information than those over 65 ($P < 0.01$) apart from knowing their chances of cure, where needs were the same irrespective of age. Among the palliatively treated patients, more younger people wished to know about the specific name of the cancer they had, what all possible treatments were, and how any treatments worked ($P < 0.01$).

Appraisal of these results suggests that the intuitive censoring of information that many doctors engage in on the grounds that patients prefer not to know is unfounded. Patients may feel isolated and scared that nothing can or will be done to help them if doctors fail to give adequate information about test results, potential ways of managing symptom, and the true therapeutic aim of different treatments. Precisely at a time when the majority of people are most in need of truthful communication and support, when they have changing thoughts and feelings and need to make important decisions, a conspiracy of silence may envelop them, and the resulting anxiety and tension may hinder adjustment. In the words of Charles Fletcher '*No news is not good news, it is an invitation to fear*'.[10]

Practical ways to help

Assuming that HCPs accept the ethical imperative that they should at all times aim for supportive, honest disclosure, what other aids are there to assist patients and their families with the assimilation of difficult information?

Audiotapes

Many now recognize the utility of providing cancer patients with tape-recordings of their consultations as an aid to improving recall and satisfaction.[11] One group of researchers suggested that although audiotapes helped retention of information it did not reliably reduce psychological distress and could be unhelpful to some patients with a poor prognosis.[12] A more recently reported RCT examined the efficacy of an audiotaped recording of the consultation with a palliative care team in addition to written information for 60 patients with advanced disease.[13] The audiocassette with written information significantly improved overall satisfaction with the clinic and recalling of information given during the consultation. Patients also expressed a high level of satisfaction with the tape which was also valued by family members and friends.

Written material

Although verbal communication should be the primary method for transfer of information for patient education, written materials are useful adjuncts for some patients and their families. Patients can drown under a sea of paper, however, and may need guidance seeking out the most appropriate aids for them, in particular, information about reliable websites. Excellent materials in the form of booklets and leaflets are available from CancerBACUP in the United Kingdom and from their website. For individual HCPs and organizations wishing to produce more locally relevant informational aids, the Centre for Health Information Quality (ChiQ) has a useful set of guides for developing readable information using a tool known as DISCERN.[14] The King's Fund in London also has an excellent guide called the practicalities of producing patient information (POPPI)[15] developed with help from CHiQ and the Plain English Forum.

Prompt sheets

Some researchers have investigated the utility of prompt sheets for patients before they see the doctor in an attempt to facilitate greater participation and asking of questions.[16,17] There are some concerns that this merely increases the numbers of questions asked without necessarily helping patients to discuss those topics of most concern and relevance to them. Nevertheless, prompt sheets are a cheap and easy intervention in a palliative setting where patients and families may not know what to ask or be too frightened to ask without prompting. They are certainly worthy of more research, in particular, harnessing the input of patients and families themselves who may be in a better position than HCPs to highlight the types of questions they wished that they had asked.

Decision-making preferences of patients in palliative care

As we have seen, patients want considerably more information than is often provided to enable them to understand the logic behind treatment recommendations made by HCPs, but how involved do they wish to be in decision-making? Desire for more information and actual participation in decision-making are not one and the same thing.[18,19] Certainly, in the non-palliative setting there is a large body of evidence suggesting that for women newly diagnosed with breast cancer many wished to assume a more passive role in decision-making than a general population sample or women with benign breast disease, who tended to prefer more active or collaborative roles.[20–22] Importantly, this work has also revealed how poor doctors are at recognizing which patients desire active or more passive roles.[5] In another study of 78 patients in a palliative setting, the concordance between clinicians' perceptions of their patients' preferences and patients' actual perceptions showed that only 38 per cent of the cases matched. The clinicians tended to underestimate patients' desire for more shared decision-making. Patients' age or sex had no influence on the accuracy of prediction.[6] As doctors manifestly lack the skills to identify patient preferences accurately, it would seem sensible for a clinic nurse to assess this prospectively prior to the patient meeting with the doctor. Card sort techniques such as those described by Degner and Sloan are an effective means of ensuring that patient preferences are met.[20] One cautionary note, however, is that preferences may well change over time as disease progresses, thus decision-making preferences need to be checked regularly as the coping strategies employed by patients are more dynamic and adaptive than is sometimes thought.

Emotional impact on doctors and nurses

There is a body of evidence suggesting that a reluctance to give bad and sad news probably reflects the difficulty that the doctor experiences conveying this type of information as much as a desire to protect patients from the distress such knowledge provokes.[1,23] Some of the reasons doctors and nurses have problems with this area can be seen in Table 2.

Inadequate skills

In the course of a professional career spanning may be 40 years, an oncologist in the United Kingdom is likely to conduct around 150–200 000 interviews with patients and their families. Thus communication is a core clinical skill, yet one in which few doctors have received much useful training.[24] Many are aware that this lack of training contributes to their own stress and burnout.[25,26] The good news is that properly structured, intensive communication skills courses employing cognitive, behavioural and affective components have been shown in a randomized trial to significantly improve cancer doctors' skills in clinics.[27] Following the course, doctors adopted a more patient-centred approach, used more open-ended questioning, displayed more empathy, responded more appropriately to patients' cues, and used fewer leading questions. Furthermore, they also changed their attitudes and beliefs about the importance of communicating in this way which led to the transfer of these skills into clinics.[28]

Nurses experience similar communication difficulties as doctors do and complain about inadequate training. Few, like the doctors involved in cancer care, have received much useful formal training in basic interviewing, assessment, and counselling skills. Some find their position even more stressful when patients are given conflicting information about the diagnosis by doctors in the care team.[29] Research looking at the skills of hospice nurses revealed a disturbing level of blocking behaviours, especially when patients needed to talk about psychological concerns.[30,31] Nurses also appear to benefit from further communication skills training courses in terms of improved attitudes,[32] confidence, and skills.[29,33]

Table 2 Some reasons for doctors' problems

Inadequate skills due to poor training
Fear of provoking emotional distress
Not knowing how to handle an emotional outburst
Worries about containing one's own emotions
Fear of being blamed by patients and relatives for failure
Over identification with certain patients
Having to confront one's own fears about death

Fear of provoking distress and handling emotion

Breaking bad news and talking about advanced disease and death will invariably provoke some emotional response from patients and whoever else is present. Most HCPs fear extreme expression of emotion and tears although some report withdrawn, stunned silence even more challenging to deal with.[1] Some doctors assume that the nursing staff are more capable than they are in this type of situation and are therefore the best people to leave distressed patients and relatives with following a difficult interview. However, dealing with emotional reactions was perceived as the most difficult communication challenge for 46 per cent of senior oncology nurses.[29] Learning how to manage the expression of emotion by others and in ourselves is of paramount importance if HCPs are to be honest but supportive bearers of bad news.

Containing one's own emotions

Becoming emotionally close to patients is inevitable for many of us working within the so-called caring professionals and has a cost. Worries about becoming upset ourselves often inhibits expression of ordinary kindness and compassion towards a distressed patient. It is not always wrong to display some emotion, in some situations it has been shown to be of value. Grieving parents just told about the death of a child appreciated those who looked moved or who shed a tear with them.[34] Nevertheless, many doctors invest considerable energy cultivating a posture of cool detachment on the grounds that it represents the more professional type of response expected of doctors. Unfortunately patients and relatives can view this detached attitude as evasive, cold, and unsympathetic, occurring at just the time that they are in much need of empathy and support. Whilst no one would be helped by an hysterical, weeping nurse or doctor, I have yet to hear of a complaint that the doctor looked too concerned and tearful whereas reports of cold indifference are frequently heard.

Being blamed for failure, over-identification, and confronting one's own death fears

In most Western cultures there is an inclination 'to deny death altogether and celebrate new forms of technology designed to forestall death'.[35] Not only lay population but also doctors themselves often harbour quite unrealistic expectations about the therapeutic benefits of modern medicine, consequently anything other than cure can feel like failure. Some HCPs retreat from truthful disclosure if treatment has been less successful than was hoped; it is as though they still lived in ancient times when the bearer of the bad news that a battle had been lost would be executed. Younger, less-experienced doctors and nurses need opportunities to talk about these feelings in addition to being given training in how to deal with patients and families who react to bad news with anger and aggression, trying to find someone to blame.

Sometimes people who have difficulty accepting the inevitability of death engage in 'doing something behaviours'. For a family this might involve dragging the hapless patient around the world in a quest to find a miracle cure. Doctors may continue with a treatment regimen that has very little prospect of alleviating symptoms or enhancing survival. As fanciful as this might seem it is a phenomenon in which the patient becomes a kind of 'talisman' for the doctor. It is a means of defying death by keeping people alive.[36] These types of problems can influence the openness of communication in sometimes quite subtle ways and may be more obvious to an observer than to the doctor. Hoping against hope that things might just have a better outcome is more likely when the doctor identifies with the patient or the relatives. Awareness of how these issues influence and affect our communication is important.

Worldwide most palliative care is provided by many different HCPs many of whom may not be palliative care specialists. Surgeons, medical and radiation oncologists, haematologists, chest physicians, dermatologists, and others will all see patients for whom curative treatment is not a feasibility, and many of these clinicians feel neither confident nor competent when communicating with patients seen as 'therapeutic failures'. Sadly unless the cure rates for most of the common solid tumours increases considerably, a majority of oncologists will spend the bulk of their clinical careers discussing palliation with patients and their families. Thus knowing how to pace and tailor communication about difficult issues appropriately should be a prerequisite for anyone working in the field of cancer. But in palliation few find this an easy or even satisfying task.

As part of a randomized trial of a communication skills training,[9,27] clinicians were asked to rate on a visual analogue scale, their satisfaction with their consultations immediately after patients had left the room. Mean satisfaction following 1039 palliative care consultations was significantly lower ($P < 0.0001$) than that following the 1768 consultations about active curative treatment or remission.

During previous communication skills courses[24] informing patients about the withdrawal of active, curative treatment and discussing palliation instead was seen as a major source of stress for senior clinicians in cancer medicine. Participants self-rated their confidence on a 10 cm visual analogue scale to items such as 'telling patients that you are replacing active therapy with symptomatic care only'. Mean rating was 5.76 cm and low when compared with, for example, 'telling patients they have a recurrence' (6.62 cm) or 'discussing side effects of treatment' (7.28 cm). The doctor's unease is often picked up leading to further anxiety, distress, and feelings of abandonment by patients.

Doctors' styles of communication

Doctors do have very different communication styles; some are helpful, others merely exacerbate their patients' difficulties. Brewin outlined three ways of breaking bad news to patients.[37] The first was a blunt and insensitive approach based on an assumption that people would be upset however they were told. The second was to appear kind and sad, but fail to provide support, encouragement, or to express any optimism. The third way was to adopt an understanding, positive, flexible, reassuring, and empathic approach, one that few doctors receive much formal help or training to develop.

Patients' views about their doctors when discussing the transition from curative to palliative care were investigated in an interesting Swedish study. Six categories of doctor were identified from a qualitative analysis of semi-structured interviews: the inexperienced messenger, the emotionally burdened, the rough and ready expert, the benevolent but tactless expert, the distanced doctor, and the empathic professional. The patients stressed how much their ability to cope with the information depended on their relationship with the doctor.[38] As doctors acknowledge so many personal difficulties and barriers when communicating within this area, there is a clear need for improved training opportunities. Unless taught a patient-centred, biopsychosocial approach of relating to and talking with patients, doctors may be oblivious to the impact that their communication has on patients or feel helpless when trying to be appropriately supportive and to lessen the blow of bad news.

Effects of minimization or ambiguity

If doctors are uncomfortable with handling transitions they may minimize the significance of test results or the true therapeutic aims of treatment, thus denying patients opportunities to make plans and utilize whatever time is left. Examples of this captured on audiotape and videotape in our research include the following examples: a patient with multiple myeloma who had benefited from only a few months remission following high dose chemotherapy, bone marrow transplantation, and maintenance interferon became very upset when told that tests confirmed relapse. In response to the patients' manifest distress the doctor said 'there's only a small amount of Bence-Jones protein in your urine'. Thus implying that things were not really too bad. We have also heard several doctors talking about 'a few hot spots on bone scans', the significance of which was lost on patients when interviewed by us later. At times communication is so ambiguous, oblique, or incomplete that patients are ill-prepared for the future and adjustment is impaired.[39] The following quotes reveal unfortunate examples of this. In the first a woman with metastatic breast cancer reported that her doctor had said, 'Take the tamoxifen, that'll hold it ... it's quite simple to have your lung drained'. She then commented that they had talked of only 'evidence of secondaries in the lung', which she presumed meant that things were 'hopefully not too bad'. She died 9 weeks after this interview from her lung metastases.[40]

The next example shows the interaction between a doctor and an elderly man with lung cancer before his expected third cycle of chemotherapy:

Doctor: As you may remember when we first started this chemotherapy we told you that we would check your blood and X-rays before each cycle. I have looked at your tests today and there are signs that things are progressing so we do not think that you should have anymore chemotherapy.

Patient: Oh! So what happens now then?

Doctor: Well we just want you to come and see us if you develop any further problems with the breathing and we'll treat those symptoms.

Patient: Right then, well thank you very much doctor.

Immediately after this consultation the patient was asked by a researcher what he remembered, he said, 'well it's good news really ... the doctor thinks things are progressing so I don't need anymore chemo and to just come back if my breathing starts up again ... getting breathless you know'.

This scenario illustrates another problem, to add to the difficulty many have even discussing palliation, that is the ambiguity of the language that is used. Words and phrases such as 'things are progressing' or 'positive' and 'negative' nodes have the opposite meanings when used in a lay rather than medical context. It is so important to check exactly what patients have understood before the consultation ends, as studies reveal that there are often major discrepancies between what doctors think they have said and what the patient has actually heard or understood.[41] This calls into question the veracity of any consent given for treatment.

Consultations were tape-recorded in a recently published report from Australia in which 118 patients with incurable cancer were seeing one of nine oncologists for a first consultation about their disease.[42] Although the majority (84.7 per cent) were told about the aim of chemotherapy, 25.4 per cent were not explicitly told their cancer was incurable, and 42.4 per cent were not told their likely prognosis. Alternatives to embarking on anticancer therapy were only presented to 44.1 per cent, and only 36.4 per cent were told about side effects likely to impinge on quality of life. Choices about management were not offered to 69.3 per cent, and patient understanding was checked in only 10.2 per cent of consultations. Greater information disclosure was not related to anxiety but greater participation in decision-making was. It is interesting to speculate whether or not the decisional conflict and anxiety experienced by some patients was due to incomplete understanding about treatment. People cannot make decisions if they lack vital information about the available options.

Despite doctors' genuine lack of awareness that sometimes they have seriously misled or confused patients, others admit to using misleading and euphemistic terminology and justify this with arguments that patients do not really want to know the truth when things are bad. The data regarding patient information preferences described earlier point to the fallacy of this position. Finally whatever verbal communication takes place there is a necessity to ensure the congruency of this with any non-verbal communication. Appropriate facial expressions and affect are needed to reinforce the intended message.

Unwillingness to discuss prognosis

We have already seen examples of less-than-honest disclosure but problems for patients and their families are compounded further by doctors' reluctance to prognosticate; they rarely initiate discussions about prognosis and are often evasive even if the patient is brave enough to ask. No one would deny that this is a tricky topic as many cancers do have uncertain outcomes making prediction difficult. Doctors may feel so insecure and lacking in confidence when predicting how long someone might live that they try to avoid doing it at all. Failure to talk about such important issues arises for more complex reasons than mere uncertainty and inaccuracy about the likely course of the disease. Many studies have been reported in which doctors ability to predict survival of patients with cancer was examined. In one of the earliest,[43] using a liberal interpretation of prediction accuracy, that is no more than twice and no less than half the actual duration of survival, 53 per cent of predictions were wrong. For the majority of these inaccuracies (90 per cent) the direction of error was for an optimistic rather than a pessimistic prediction, showing a propensity for overestimation rather than for underestimation of survival.

Many more recent publications have substantiated Parkes original studies showing that things have not changed much despite better diagnostic tools, so we need to look for other reasons for this.[44–46] Several references have already been made in this chapter to the fact that over identification with patients can have negative effects. Research also shows that the better the doctor knows the patient in terms of the length and intensity of their contact, the more likely the doctor is to overestimate survival.[47] Doctors may need to hope against hope that things are better than they really are and this becomes more evident if the doctor has built up a close relationship with the patient. This also provides a partial explanation as to why doctors may promote further toxic treatment regimens for patients that have very little prospect of benefit, rather than have an honest discussion about supportive care.

Extending further the arguments first expressed by Hippocrates,[48] Lamont and Christakis[49] have described how patients may unwittingly become 'twice removed' from the truth about their illness. Disclosure of prognosis is conceptualized as comprising two distinct elements, those of foreseeing and foretelling. Foreseeing can be defined as the unexpressed cognitive estimate or prediction that a doctor may make about a patient's likely survival, which we know is inclined to be optimistic. Foretelling is the communication about this with a patient which we know may be liable to conscious and accidental ambiguity or deliberate evasion. So the 'twice removed patient' can end up with a wildly inaccurate estimation of their likely survival and consequently are unable to prepare appropriately for the future.

Effect on patients of truth about prognosis

'Rare are the cases where making or offering a carefully considered and framed prognosis results in choices that are harmful to the patient.... As a result of a failure to prognosticate, let alone prognosticate accurately, patients may die deaths they deplore in locations they despise. They may seek noxious chemotherapy rather than good palliative care, enrol in clinical trials of experimental therapy that offer more benefit to the researchers than to themselves, or reassure loved ones that it is not yet time to pay a visit only to lapse into a coma before there is time to say goodbye.' [47]

An argument is frequently made that most patients should not be told the truth about their prognosis as they will lose hope, become overwhelmed with an immobilizing depression, and not enjoy whatever time is left. Little hard evidence exists to support this position; in fact it is more likely that misguided evasion or frank dishonesty may add considerably to a patient's distress and prolong the necessary adjustment process. Most of the patients referred to one psychotherapist for anxiety management and adjustment disorders, had not been given honest information about their cancer in the first place.[50] Likewise of 101 patients with inoperable tumours, highest drug use, anxiety, and depression were found in those *not* told the truth of their condition.[51] As Simpson has asserted 'Hope is based on knowledge, not ignorance.' and that 'what remains unspoken is unspeakable'.[52] If potentially distressing disclosures to patients are avoided then we give patients no opportunities to reveal their own fears and worries. This can leave them in anxiety-ridden isolation, convinced that the most unspeakably horrible fate awaits them. The uninformed patient may construct a scenario that bears little relationship to their likely demise.

Dealing with the misinformed patient

The palliative care team can find themselves dealing with a great deal of hostility and anger from patients and families who feel that they were never given honest information by HCPs involved earlier on in their care. They may feel that the choices and decisions that were made about therapeutic options were based on inaccurate or overoptimistic advice. The patient who feels very strongly that they were misled is unlikely to trust the new team members trying to offer reassurances about symptomatic care. Considerable investment in relationship-building skills is needed if the patient and relatives are going to develop the important degree of trust that will ease the physical and emotional pains that lie ahead. Discussion about why different outcomes to those hoped for have arisen is important and can sometimes be enough to correct some of the misunderstandings. However, familiarity with the official complaints procedure for the really angry person might be needed. Above all, recognition that the anger might be justified and that it may be the only way that some people have of expressing their distress and disappointment is required. Accurate documentation in hospital records about who said what to whom and when is obviously useful as are satisfactory communication channels with the multidisciplinary team in order to provide feedback to others about what has happened and to perhaps avoid such situations in the future.

Anxiety and depression

Although avoidance of communication about advanced disease does not protect patients from experiencing considerable psychological distress, palliative patients certainly do have significantly higher psychological morbidity than other patients with curable cancer.[53] It is a sorry fact that much of this often goes unrecognized and therefore untreated. In the United Kingdom 2850 patients were given the General Health Questionnaire (GHQ12) and 837 (36.4 per cent) had scores suggestive of psychological morbidity.

The 1046 palliative patients were more likely than other patients to have high GHQ scores ($P < 0.0001$). The ability of the clinicians to detect this probable morbidity was low overall but there were some interesting differences. The clinicians true positive (sensitivity) rates were higher for their palliative patients than for their other patients. Unfortunately their specificity (true negative) rates were lower and misclassification rates greater. At least 408/1046 palliative patients were either thought to have significant psychological morbidity when they did not, or were thought to be psychologically well when they needed some extra help. One interpretation of these findings is that doctors nihilistically assume that people with incurable disease will be psychologically distressed. Doctors then lack the communication skills to determine how patients are coping. Unfortunately there was very little evidence of psychosocial probing during consultations which might permit more accurate assessment and referral on to appropriate support services.

Palliation should include treatment and amelioration of all symptoms including psychological ones. There is increasing evidence from well-conducted trials that psychosocial interventions are effective with adult cancer patients.[54] Assuming that the institutions where patients are being treated have access to psychological services, it is vital that clinicians are trained in basic skills to determine which patients need help. Screening patients with validated questionnaires prior to seeing the doctor might improve detection rates.

Communication needs of the family

The most important source of psychological and physical support for most patients is likely to be a family member. Encouraging a good therapeutic alliance with partners and carers is therefore vital. Many HCPs find communicating with dying or seriously ill patients less stressful than that with relatives who can appear threatening, obstructive, and hard to deal with. However, much of the difficulty can be managed or at least understood if one steps back a pace and considers the enormous strain and stress that carers have to shoulder. Some family members can look more ill and care-worn than their dying relative as a result of the increased pressures, new roles, and expectations placed upon them.

Most HCPs will at some stage have to cope with families who wish them to conceal the truth from their dying relative on the grounds that they would not be able to take it and would suffer unnecessarily. This is always hard to manage but families need help understanding that there is little or no convincing evidence supporting the contention that terminally ill patients who have not been told the truth of their situation die happily in blissful ignorance. A dying person witnesses their deteriorating body, fatigue, and reduction in ability to function.

Concealment of the truth is rarely achievable as relatives, friends, and HCPs find it hard not to give out non-verbal clues as to what is happening. The hollow cheerfulness and feigned optimism about quite unrealistic future goals are excruciating to witness, as are the anxious and stressed expressions on faces of people trying to maintain a lie. Particularly upsetting is watching families, who have not been gently helped to confront reality, locked into stilted discussions about trivia or frozen in silence. In Lawrence Goldie's words, 'couples instead of drawing closer together wither in each other's arms'.[55] Facilitating opportunities for partners to discuss death with each other demands tact and skill and there may occasionally be exceptional circumstances where it might not be appropriate but these exceptions are rare. Collusion with relatives of dying patients in an attempt to sustain the myth of immortality is an abrogation of our responsibility to assist patients through the stages that might be needed for people to achieve a calm acceptance and more serene and dignified death. Additionally the inability to talk through death leaves much 'unfinished business' which relatives can bitterly regret later.

Just as families may wish to stop their loved ones from learning the sad fact that they are dying, occasionally patients themselves may ask that their relatives are not told the truth. This is a tricky situation as from an ethical standpoint, if conscious, the patient does have the right of confidentiality. Family dynamics can be hard to understand but the legal next of kin may not actually be the person from whom the patient has derived most support during their life. As well as 'protecting' relatives from the hurtful news of impending death, a desire to withhold this information can be the last defiant and punitive act left to a person. The only real suggestion that can be offered in such circumstances, although this is not based on any empirical evidence, is to try and find out why the patient feels so reluctant to share the knowledge about impending death with their relative. It might help to point out that a failure to reveal the truth and to discuss the subject with relatives might mean that the patient's wishes about such things as funeral service, burial, or wishes about their estate and will are not handled appropriately. Also it might prevent reconciliation of old enmities. The services of a family therapist, social worker, or clinical psychologist might be invaluable.

Conclusion

Honest communication is surely an ethical imperative for the truly caring clinician. Patients need to plan and make decisions about the place of their death, put their affairs in order, say good-byes or forgive old adversaries, and be protected from embarking on futile therapies. All HCPs who work within an oncology or palliative care setting experience occasions when tough and distressing issues need to be discussed. Their behaviour and communication of caring and competence at this time have a major influence on the ability of patients and families to assimilate the news, consider options, and adapt and adjust to what lies ahead. Even if the news is gloomy the right touch, look, and supportive kind word always makes a difference. We know the effects that poor communication exerts but need to recognize that if patients are to receive optimal care then the training needs and emotional support required by HCPs cannot be ignored.

References

1. **Fallowfield, L.J.** (1993). Giving sad and bad news. *Lancet* **341**, 476–8.
2. **Maguire, P.** (1999). Improving communication with cancer patients. *European Journal of Cancer* **35** (14), 2058–65.
3. **Bruera, E., Neumann, C.M., Mazzocato, C., Stiefel, F., and Sala, R.** (2000). Attitudes and beliefs of palliative care physicians regarding communication with terminally ill cancer patients. *Palliative Medicine* **14** (4), 287–98.
4. **Fielding, R.G. and Hung, J.** (1996). Preferences for information and involvement in decisions during cancer care among a Hong Kong Chinese population. *Psychooncology* **5**, 321–9.
5. **Degner, L.F.** et al. (1997). Information needs and decisional preferences in women with breast cancer. *Journal of the American Medical Association* **277** (18), 1485–92.
6. **Bruera, E., Sweeney, C., Calder, K., Palmer, L., and Benisch-Tolley, S.** (2001). Patient preferences versus physician perceptions of treatment decisions in cancer care. *Journal of Clinical Oncology* **19** (11), 2883–5.
7. **Leydon, G.M.** et al. (2000). Faith, hope, and charity: an in-depth interview study of cancer patients' information needs and information-seeking behavior. *British Medical Journal* **173** (1), 26–31.
8. **Jenkins, V., Fallowfield, L., and Saul, J.** (2001). Information needs of patients with cancer: results from a large study in UK cancer centres. *British Journal of Cancer* **84** (1), 48–51.
9. **Fallowfield, L.J., Jenkins, V.A., and Beveridge, H.A.** (2002). Truth may hurt but deceit hurts more: communication in palliative care. *Palliative Medicine* **16**, 297–303.
10. **Fletcher, C.** (1980). Listening and talking to patients. *British Medical Journal* **281**, 994.
11. **Scott, J.T., Entwistle, V.E., Sowden, A.J., and Watt, I.** (1999). Recordings or summaries of consultations for people with cancer (Cochrane review). *The Cochrane Library* **4**, 1–49.
12. **McHugh, P.** et al. (1995). The efficacy of audiotapes in promoting psychological wellbeing in cancer patients: a randomised, controlled trial. *British Journal of Cancer* **71**, 388–92.
13. **Bruera, E., Pituskin, E., Calder, K., Neumann, C.M., and Hanson, J.** (1999). The addition of an audiocassette recording of a consultation to written recommendations for patients with advanced cancer: a randomized, controlled trial. *Cancer* **86** (11), 2420–5.
14. **Charnock, D., Shepperd, S., Needham, G., and Gann, R.** (1999). DISCERN: an instrument for judging the quality of written consumer health information on treatment choices. *Journal of Epidemiology and Community Health* **53** (2), 105–11.
15. **Duman, M. and Farell, C.** *The Practicalities of Producing Patient Information—The POPPI Guide*. London: The King's Fund, 2000.
16. **Butow, P.N., Dunn, S.M., Tattershall, M.H.N., and Jones, Q.J.** (1994). Patient participation in the cancer consultation: evaluation of a question prompt sheet. *Annals of Oncology* **5**, 199.
17. **Brown, R.F., Butow, P.N., Dunn, S.M., and Tattersall, M.H.** (2001). Promoting patient participation and shortening cancer consultations: a randomised trial. *British Journal of Cancer* **85** (9), 1273–9.
18. **Sutherland, H.J., Llewellyn-Thomas, H.A., Lockwood, G.A., Tritchler, D.L., and Till, J.E.** (1989). Cancer patients: their desire for information and participation in treatment decisions. *Journal of the Royal Society of Medicine* **82**, 260–3.
19. **Fallowfield, L.** (2001). Participation of patients in decisions about treatment for cancer. *British Medical Journal* **323** (7322), 1144.
20. **Degner, L.F. and Sloan, J.A.** (1992). Decision-making during serious ilness: what role do patients really want to play? *Journal of Clinical Epidemiology* **45** (9), 941–50.
21. **Luker, K.A., Beaver, K., Leinster, S.J., Owens, R.G., Degner, L.F., and Sloan, J.A.** (1995). The information needs of women newly diagnosed with breast cancer. *Journal of Advances in Nursing* **22** (1), 134–41.

22. **Beaver, K., Luker, K.A., Owens, R.G., Leinster, S.J., Degner, L.F., and Sloan, J.A.** (1996). Treatment decision making in women newly diagnosed with breast cancer. *Cancer Nursing* **19** (1), 8–19.
23. **Buckman, R.** (1984). Breaking bad news: why is it still so difficult? *British Medical Journal (Clinical Research Edition)* **288** (6430), 1597–9.
24. **Fallowfield, L.J., Lipkin, M., and Hall, A.** (1998). Teaching senior oncologists communication skills: results from phase 1 of a comprehensive longitudinal program in the UK. *Journal of Clinical Oncology* **16**, 1961–8.
25. **Fallowfield, L.J.** (1995). Can we improve the professional and personal fulfilment of doctors in cancer medicine? *British Journal of Cancer* **71**, 1132–3.
26. **Ramirez, A.J.** et al. (1995). Burnout and psychiatric disorder among cancer clinicians. *British Journal of Cancer* **71** (6), 1263–9.
27. **Fallowfield, L., Jenkins, V., Farewell, V., Saul, J., Duffy, A., and Eves, B.** (2002). Efficacy of a Cancer Research UK communication skills model: a randomised controlled trial. *Lancet* **359**, 650–6.
28. **Jenkins, V. and Fallowfield, L.** (2002). Can communication skills training alter physicians? Beliefs and behavior in clinics? *Journal of Clinical Oncology* **20** (3), 765–9.
29. **Fallowfield, L., Saul, J., and Gilligan, B.** (2001). Teaching senior nurses how to teach communication skills in oncology. *Cancer Nursing* **24** (3), 185–91.
30. **Booth, K., Maguire, P.M., Butterworth, T., and Hillier, V.F.** (1996). Perceived professional support and the use of blocking behaviours by hospice nurses. *Journal of Advanced Nursing* **24** (3), 522–7.
31. **Heaven, C.M. and Maguire, P.** (1997). Disclosure of concerns by hospice patients and their identification by nurses. *Palliative Medicine* **11** (4), 283–90.
32. **Razavi, D., Delvaux, N., Marchal, S., Bredart, A., Farvacques, C., and Paesmans, M.** (1993). The effects of a 24 hour psychological training programe on attitudes, communication skills and occupational stress in oncology: a randomised study. *European Journal of Cancer* **29A** (13), 1858–63.
33. **Wilkinson, S., Bailey, K., Aldridge, J., and Roberts, A.** (1999). A longitudinal evaluation of a communication skills programme. *Palliative Medicine* **13** (4), 341–8.
34. **Finlay, I. and Dallimore, D.** (1991). Your child is dead. *British Medical Journal* **302** (6791), 1524–5.
35. **Annas, G.J.** (1994). Informed consent, cancer, and truth in prognosis. *New England Journal of Medicine* **330** (3), 223–5.
36. **Trillin, A.S.** (1981). Of dragons and garden peas: a cancer patient talks to doctors. *New England Journal of Medicine* **304** (12), 699–701.
37. **Brewin, T.B.** (1991). Three ways of giving bad news. *Lancet* **337**, 1207–9.
38. **Friedrichsen, M.J., Strang, P.M., and Carlsson, M.E.** (2000). Breaking bad news in the transition from curative to palliative cancer care—patient's view of the doctor giving the information. *Support Care in Cancer* **8** (6), 472–8.
39. **Dunn, S.M., Patterson, P.U., Butow, P.N., Smartt, H.H., McCarthy, W.H., and Tattersall, M.H.** (1993). Cancer by another name: a randomized trial of the effects of euphemism and uncertainty in communicating with cancer patients. *Journal Clinical Oncology* **11** (5), 989–96.
40. **Hall, A., Fallowfield, L.J., and A'Hern, R.P.** (1996). When breast cancer recurs: a 3-year prospective study of psychological morbidity. *The Breast Journal* **2** (3), 197–203.
41. **Quirt, C.F.** et al. (1997). Do doctors know when their patients don't? A survey of doctor–patient communication in lung cancer. *Lung Cancer* **18** (1), 1–20.
42. **Gattellari, M., Voigt, K.J., Butow, P.N., and Tattersall, M.H.** (2002). When the treatment goal is not cure: are cancer patients equipped to make informed decisions? *Journal Clinical Oncology* **20** (2), 503–13.
43. **Parkes, C.M.** (1972). Accuracy of predictions of survival in later stages of cancer. *British Medical Journal* **2** (5804), 29–31.
44. **Muers, M.F., Shevlin, P., and Brown, J.** (1996). Prognosis in lung cancer: physicians' opinions compared with outcome and a predictive model. *Thorax* **51** (9), 894–902.
45. **Mackillop, W.J. and Quirt, C.F.** (1997). Measuring the accuracy of prognostic judgments in oncology. *Journal of Clinical Epidemiology* **50** (1), 21–9.
46. **Christakis, N.A. and Lamont, E.B.** (2000). Extent and determinants of error in doctors' prognoses in terminally ill patients: prospective cohort study. *British Medical Journal* **320** (7233), 469–72.
47. **Christakis, N.A.** *Death Foretold.* Chicago IL: University of Chicago Press, 1999.
48. **Hippocrates** (1978). Prognosis. In *Hippocratic Writings* (ed. G.E.R. Lloyd), pp. 170–85. London: Penguin Books.
49. **Lamont, E.B. and Christakis, N.A.** (1999). Some elements of prognosis in terminal cancer. *Oncology (Huntington)* **13** (8), 1165–70 (discussion 1172–4, 1179–80).
50. **Stedford, A.** *Facing Death.* London: Heinemann, 1984.
51. **Gerle, B., Lunden, G., and Sandblom, P.** (1960). The patient with inoperable cancer from the psychiatric and social standpoints. *Cancer* **13**, 1206–17.
52. **Simpson, M.A.** (1982). Therapeutic uses of truth. In *The Dying Patient* (ed. E. Wilkes), pp. 255–62. Lancaster: MYP Press.
53. **Fallowfield, L., Ratcliffe, D., Jenkins, V., and Saul, J.** (2001). Psychological morbidity and its recognition by doctors in patients with cancer. *British Journal of Cancer* **84** (8), 1011–15.
54. **Meyer, T.J. and Mark, M.M.** (1995). Effects of psychosocial interventions with adult cancer patient: a meta analysis of randomised experiments. *Health Psychology* **14**, 101–8.
55. **Goldie, L.** (1982). The ethics of telling the patient. *Journal of Medical Ethics* **8**, 128–33.

4.2 Communication with professionals

David Jeffrey

Introduction

Patients with advanced life-threatening diseases which are no longer curable, have a variety of complex physical, psychosocial, and spiritual needs. No single individual can meet all these needs. However, an effective multidisciplinary team can deliver a high standard of palliative care.[1,2] The number of health care professionals involved in the team and the importance of their ability to work collaboratively, increases with the complexity of the patient's needs.[3] A high quality of patient care and family support depends on sharing of information, good communication, and joint decision-making among the different professionals.

In the past there has been an emphasis on improving communication between health care professionals and patients, but, communication between health care professionals is often poor.[4–6] Poor communication is not only a waste of time but also a threat to patient care and a source of staff stress.[7] It is now appropriate to review communication issues among the many professionals involved in the patient's care.

Barriers to effective interprofessional communication

The Calman–Hine report, on cancer services in the United Kingdom, emphasized the importance of good communication among those caring for cancer patients.[8] For communication between health care professionals to be effective a number of potential barriers need to be considered:

- Palliative care is provided in a number of settings, for example, home, community hospital, nursing home, hospice, and hospital.
- Specialist palliative care teams often work at the interface between curative and palliative care.

- Specialist palliative care teams need to liaise among teams of differing health care professionals, voluntary, and statutory agencies.
- Maintaining patient confidentiality in multidisciplinary teams may be difficult.
- Health care professionals tend to work autonomously.

A multidisciplinary team which is not communicating effectively will be prone to interprofessional and intraprofessional rivalries, strife, and delayed decision-making.[9]

Problems of interprofessional communication can be illustrated in the context of the journey of a patient with advanced cancer. It should be remembered that the principles of specialist palliative care and the importance of effective communication among professionals are as relevant in the care of patients with life-threatening non-malignant disease as in cancer care. This chapter will follow the patient, family, and carers through referral, assessment, care, discharge, death, and bereavement. The central role of communication in maintaining effective professional relationships which foster a high standard of care is emphasized. Differing communication behaviours are analysed and ways of improving communication among professionals are discussed.

The patient's journey

Once cancer is diagnosed the world is filled with uncertainty for the patient and family. Good communication among all health professionals is vital to ensure they receive a comprehensive service which involves as little misunderstanding as possible.[10] Two differing clinical approaches to the same patient highlight how communication among professionals can affect the patient's quality of life.[11]

A non-collaborative approach

A 45-year-old woman with advanced ovarian cancer and multiple liver metastases was admitted to hospital. The surgeon told her that her disease was now advanced and was inoperable. He referred her to an oncologist, who felt she would not benefit from further chemotherapy. She was discharged from hospital, and referred back to her general practitioner and district nurse. She became withdrawn and took to her bed where she died, 3 weeks later.

A collaborative approach

In this scenario, the surgeon requested a joint assessment by an oncologist and a specialist palliative care nurse. During this joint assessment, the patient revealed that she was worried: she feared she would be in pain and she did not think her husband would cope on his own. The specialist nurse addressed each of the patient's concerns and advised her on the resources which were available. The patient was relieved to hear that her symptom control would be regularly monitored by her general practitioner and district nurse and that a community specialist palliative care nurse could also be involved to support both her and her husband. She felt confident about her discharge home and died at home peacefully 3 weeks later. Three months after her death her husband accepted bereavement support offered by the community specialist palliative care nurse.

These two approaches illustrate the differing quality of life which a patient with advanced cancer may experience as a result of differing communications among the health care professionals. In both situations the patient died 3 weeks following discharge from hospital. In the first approach, although the patient's physical symptoms were well controlled, there was neglect of her psychosocial concerns. The opportunity was lost for the patient to resolve unfinished emotional business and her husband received no bereavement support. In contrast, in the second approach, the patient had the same short survival but was able to come to terms with her fears and to be involved in planning support for her husband. The non-collaborative model adopts a problem-based approach, whilst the collaborative model anticipates problems.[11]

It is now appropriate to examine the problems encountered in interprofessional communication at the various stages of the patient's journey.

Interprofessional communication problems

Referral

The point at which the health care professional, either in the community or in hospital, refers to specialist palliative care can present challenges.[12,13] An audit of palliative care at home in part of the United Kingdom showed services were frequently involved too late and provision of information was often lacking or patchy.[14] Referrers often give the relevant medical details but less information on the social, psychological, or spiritual aspects of the patient's history.[15] Delayed referral to specialist services may result in patients receiving inadequate palliative care.

The reasons for delayed referral may be based on:

- lack of knowledge among patients and health care professionals of the role of the palliative care team, and of their skills and expertise;
- a sense of vulnerability and guilt among the primary carers that problems have not been resolved;
- a desire to protect a professional boundary, the 'my patient' syndrome, where the professional feels that he/she can cope with all the patient's needs; and
- a wish to protect patients from distress, since referral to specialist palliative care usually involves addressing the fact that the underlying disease is no longer curable.

Some doctors still mistakenly believe that specialist palliative care is confined to the terminal phase of the illness, when the patient is obviously dying. If patients are only referred at the terminal stage of their illness then this belief will be reinforced both among professionals and the public. The doctor or nurse may fear the reaction of the patient when palliative care is mentioned, and so delay referral to avoid this potentially distressing discussion.

Referral may be delayed if the doctor or nurse feels that they can respond to all the patient's needs. They may be unaware of the skills and expertise of the specialist palliative care team, particularly if such teams do not have clear referral criteria. Some professionals have reservations that too many people will be involved in the patient's care and delay referral to preserve the patient's privacy.

Interdisciplinary assessment

The quality of interdisciplinary teamwork is dependent upon a complex process of sharing: the different professionals have to consider clinical, emotional, and social assessments of the patient and family. Communicating these assessments is an essential element of effective interdisciplinary care.

There may be problems in communicating the results of assessments from hospital to the community. Outpatients may not return to see their general practitioner but telephone requesting a prescription suggested by the hospital specialist. The general practitioner may not have received the hospital letter and may spend time tracing the hospital specialist to find out what she has suggested. In a qualitative study of referral and reply letters among oncologists, surgeons, and general practitioners, oncologists wanted information about the patient's medical status and involvement of other doctors. The referring surgeons and general practitioners identified delays in receiving the consultant's reply and reported insufficient detail in their letters. They wanted information regarding the proposed treatment, expected outcomes, and psychological concerns; however, these items were often omitted.[16] General practitioners valued easy access to specialists and a rapid response to requests.[16] The transition between curative to palliative care can be a time of uncertainty for patients and professionals; for example, referral to an oncologist may in itself lead a patient to believe that further active treatments are available.[13]

Confidentiality

Communication of patient information within and among hospital, hospice, and primary care teams is essential for patient well being. Professionals may act as if they have implied consent to share patient information. However, a health care professional has a duty not to divulge information about a patient to a third party without the explicit consent of the patient. Without a requirement for confidentiality it would be impossible to build a trusting relationship with the patient. On the other hand, if interdisciplinary teamwork is to be effective then information about the patient has to be shared amongst members of the team. It is necessary to explain to the patient that you are a member of a team and request permission to share information with other professionals. Different levels of information about the patient can be shared with other professionals on a 'need to know' basis, in order to benefit the patient.[12] If information is judged to be highly sensitive, the patient's permission should be sought, to pass on information to designated members of the team.

Continuity of care

Continuity of care is one of the essential components of high-standard palliative care. With the changes in organization of primary care in the United Kingdom, involving the use of out-of-hours co-operatives and less emphasis on home visiting, continuity of care becomes more difficult to provide. Doctors may blame their colleagues for failing to keep them informed of changes occurring in the patient's illness. The diversity that gives the interdisciplinary team its potential for effectiveness can also make the team vulnerable if there is insufficient communication.[17] All team members have a role; the challenge is how to achieve information exchange. During team communication and delegation there is a risk of distortion of the message.

The goals of care may not be clear; there may be a tension between curing and caring. If consensus is not reached as to the aim of care, then team members may be pulling in different directions, so patients and carers receive mixed messages, which only heighten uncertainty and distress. Situations where pain has been difficult to manage may be a barrier to communication, professionals may be reluctant to discuss what they perceive as a failure in their management. General practitioners may lose touch with patients who are being followed up in hospital clinics and feel marginalized in their care.[13]

Discharge planning

There is an increasing trend of rapid turnover of inpatients in National Health Service hospitals in the United Kingdom; so newly discharged patients are dependant on carefully planned care in the community. The provision of such co-coordinated care requires effective communication across the hospital community interface.[18] However, gaps in care cause patients frustration when they are transferred from specialist to primary care. General practitioners do not want to give a conflicting message to that of the hospital team, or be ignorant of facts when facing patients and relatives. Anecdotal evidence exists of interprofessional rivalries, and of poor communication among health care professionals.[19,20] With the emergence of palliative care specialists, some family doctors feel their expertise has declined and their competence undermined.[21] Consequently there may be reluctance for them to seek help.

Terminal care and bereavement support

There are a number of ethical dilemmas which may arise at the end of a patient's life. Examples include requests for euthanasia, issues surrounding withdrawal of nutrition and hydration, 'do not attempt resuscitation' orders, and advance directives. Ethical dilemmas do not have easy answers; it is often difficult to reach a moral consensus in the team.

Interprofessional communication may break down following the death of the patient. In one study, when deaths occurred in hospital the general practitioner was informed within 24 h in only 16 per cent of cases.[22] Failure to inform the primary care team can lead to the embarrassing error of a member of the team visiting the patient's home in ignorance of the death, or to a lack of provision of bereavement support to the family.

Organizational problems

Health care systems suffer enormous inefficiency because of a poor communication infrastructure.[23] During times of stress, effective communication is threatened.[24] Organizational change is a feature of modern health care and is unsettling to the professionals. In a survey of hospital admissions, it was found that communication problems were the most common cause of preventable disability or death.[25]

Despite the importance of communication in the provision and organization of health care there has been little research of communication systems and what work has been done is driven largely by technology rather than by understanding of clinical needs.[23]

Although, doctors and nurses may prefer face to face communication, they risk contributing to an interruptive workplace culture: doctors may generate twice as many interruptions via the telephone and paging system as they receive.[23] We need to be aware that interruption may have psychological costs: diversion of attention, forgetfulness, errors, and rescheduling of work plans.[23] For example, doctors may carry out a series of calls to book an investigation: eight telephone calls and one pager request over 54 minutes to arrange a CT scan.[23] The doctor in this example, was involved in following a trail of telephone numbers, speaking to a variety of radiology administrative staff, radiographers, and radiologists before he could complete the scan booking.[23] Doctors rarely considered the effect that a telephone call or pager would have on the other party, selfishly valuing the completion of their own tasks over that of their colleagues.[23]

Hospital palliative care teams may experience difficulties in integrating the collaborative approach into hospital practice.[11] Historically, doctors have had total authority and nurses carried out their orders. These outdated models of care have been replaced by collaborative teamwork in which professional boundaries are blurred and access to the patient is shared depending on the individual's need. However, such working practices take time to develop and where there is role conflict it can cause stress amongst the health care professionals.

Communication and stress

Unsatisfactory communication lies at the heart of many of the stresses experienced by professionals working in palliative care. Complaints from patients may be generated by a criticism of one professional by another. Much of palliative care is uncertain; decisions have to be made with inadequate information, or where advice from colleagues is conflicting. Arranging admission of a patient to hospital may be stressful for general practitioners.[13]

Many of the stresses reported by professionals when caring for the dying were not directly as a result of working with the patient or the family but arose from difficulties with colleagues and institutional hierarchies: perhaps where there was rivalry for patients or the blocking of patient referral.[26] Health care professionals are at risk of being overwhelmed by the quantity of information available to them.

Improving interprofessional communication

In order for communication to be effective there must be opportunities to meet, exchange information, plan interventions, and take shared responsibility for the patient's care. This section seeks to explore ways in which we can address the problems highlighted during the patient's journey.

Referral

The initiation of a team approach often depends on the doctor's recognition of the need for an interdisciplinary approach to care.[1] The general practitioner is in an ideal position to both initiate the team approach and to share knowledge and insights with other members of the team.[1] The primary team caring for the patient, whether in the community or the hospital, should be adopting the palliative care approach.

This approach involves good communication among general practitioners, community nurses, between hospital staff. The communication among these professionals forms the lynch pin of palliative care provision. However, the needs of some patients and families will exceed the resources of these teams and further support will be required from a specialist palliative care service. The patients and families need to be fully aware and in agreement with referral to the specialist palliative care team. This means that the referring doctor or nurse needs a clear understanding of the role of the palliative care team and is comfortable about discussing issues which the patient may raise at the time of this referral. The patient may ask 'Am I going to die?' or perhaps 'Am I going to get better?'

It is perhaps unusual that in specialist palliative care, teams accept referrals from a variety of health care professionals, professions allied to medicine, patients, and carers. It is essential that the specialist team liaises with the medical team managing the patient and that the primary team has the full knowledge and agreement that the specialist palliative care team should be involved. It is a privilege for a specialist team to be invited to share care. They should be aware that the primary referring professional may feel threatened or guilty that pain or symptoms have not been controlled.[27]

Most patients trust their general practitioners, which facilitates the introduction of other health care professionals into their care.[1] The decision to refer should be based on whether the quality of life of patients with advanced disease could be improved. Appropriate referral to a specialist team should be made whenever a health care professional reaches the limits of their own skills. We need to keep up-to-date with the work of our colleagues. If we are unaware of their skills and expertise then we may fail to make appropriate referrals. The introduction of clinical governance has placed more emphasis on being sure that patients receive the right care in the right setting and at the right time.

Palliative care teams have developed referral criteria and eligibility criteria to clarify the process of referral.[28] For instance, the 'Leeds eligibility criteria' emphasize that to be eligible for specialist palliative care the patient should meet three key criteria:[28]

1. progressive and advanced disease,
2. the patient has an extraordinary level of need, and
3. following referral the patient to be assessed by a specialist palliative care service.

It is preferable that a letter or an entry in the medical notes requesting a specialist palliative care assessment should confirm verbal referrals; the reason for referral and the degree of urgency should also be specified. The specialist palliative care team needs to communicate their hours of availability and their standard of response. The referring doctor should provide the relevant information about the patient's history, current condition, drug therapy, management plan, and any particular concerns they may have.[29]

Interdisciplinary assessment

General practitioners need to encourage multiprofessional primary care team working as well as enlisting the skills and knowledge of the specialist palliative care team.[30] The professional relationship between general practitioners and specialists is better than the literature and anecdotal evidence might suggest.[31]

Referrals to the specialist palliative care team are discussed in an interdisciplinary team meeting. These meetings are essential to plan the highest standards of care. They also provide an opportunity for education and to facilitate continuity of care. Effective communication between nurses and doctors is enhanced by the formation of good interpersonal relationships in a friendly supportive atmosphere.[32] The ability of nurses to communicate informally results in them being able to express their intuitions regarding their patient's condition, without fear of being ridiculed by their medical colleagues.[32] It is part of good clinical practice to ensure that everyone is given an opportunity or chance to express their views. Nurses are closer to patients, so doctors need to listen to their views before making decisions. Sharing of ideas within the team takes time; managers need to acknowledge the value of collaborative practice in palliative care and accept that time is necessary for such communication.

The specialist palliative care team assessment of the patient should be shared with the primary referring team: the patients progress, medication, level of awareness, and needs of the family should be discussed. Joint working among different professions can be facilitated in a number of practical ways; palliative care posts exist which work across hospital and community situations.[33] Role blurring is an inevitable feature of interprofessional teamwork as the individuals making up the team depend on each other. This interdependence can result in either a competitive or a collaborative relationship.[11]

Continuity of care

It is in the patient's best interest for one doctor, usually a general practitioner, to be fully informed and responsible for continuity of the patient's medical care. The nursing care can similarly be best co-coordinated by the district nurse, although on occasions it may be appropriate for another member of the team to be designated the key worker. Decision-making procedures should be clear and known and communication regular and routine. There is a need for regular meetings between the doctor and nurse to hand over details of the patient's progress, drug changes, and any important communications between the professional and the patient or family. In all communications, whether among doctors, among doctors and nurses, or among nurses, it is reassuring to patients and family to hear that details are being passed among them.[12,21]

Practical issues to address at such meetings are:[34]

- what information does my colleague need?
- what is the management plan?
- is everyone clear about his or her responsibilities?
- how should we communicate again?

Record keeping

Documentation is an important part of interprofessional communication which guides practice, provides information, and forms a measure of the quality of care.[35] The district nursing record which remains with the patient can be a helpful mechanism for communication between primary and specialist services.[8] Patient-held records may also be useful when moving from one setting to another, creating better continuity and improving interprofessional communication.[10,35] Integrated care pathways are a new initiative which act as guidelines and multidisciplinary case records, facilitating interprofessional communication in their preparation, implementation, and review.[36]

The oncology–palliative care interface

Specialist palliative care has become integrated with cancer care and co-ordinates with community care.[8] Good communication at the oncology–palliative care interface, in the form of joint assessments and parallel clinics, ensures that patients receive expert pain and symptom control and psychosocial care. At the same time they are also able to retain easy access to palliative anticancer treatments such as chemotherapy or radiotherapy.

Advocacy

Advocacy implies pleading or representing the case of another person to a higher authority.[37] In the past, advocacy in health care has tended to be considered as a nursing issue. In an ideal world advocacy would be redundant; anyone close to the patient can act as an advocate.[38] It is critical that there is trust and flexibility among team members so that when advocacy issues arise, the team accepts this as a way of considering the patient's interest and not as personal criticism of an individual team member.

Discharge planning

General practitioners and district nurses are the key professionals responsible for medical and nursing care at home; they should be the first professionals consulted when planning a discharge from hospital.[12] This is also a good time to anticipate which other members of the team should be involved in care, such as occupational therapists, physiotherapists, and social workers. It is vital that the primary care team should have detailed information: they need to know the diagnosis, prognosis, aims of care, drug treatments, and details of what information has been given to the patient, on the day of discharge from hospital. The social worker is generally responsible for co-ordinating the package of care at home. This involves integrating home care assistance, the primary care team, specialist palliative care, and non-professional voluntary support. Good communication is essential if these various agencies are to be co-coordinated to provide care to meet the assessed needs of the patient and family.

Discharge letters from hospital should reach the general practitioner on the day of discharge and detail diagnosis, drug management, the patient's and families understanding, future care plans, and details of other agencies involved.[19] Such information may be supplemented by talking to the general practitioner or district nurse on the telephone or communication by fax. In this way, general practitioners and district nurses are not left ignorant of the patient's medical details when facing patients and relatives on their return home.[19]

Terminal care and bereavement support

Communication within the team ensures co-coordinated care which respects the patients' need for privacy. Whilst the general practitioner and district nurse are the key professionals when the patient is dying at home, it is important to remember that the specialist palliative care team is available for advice and help. Indeed some services offer 24 h advice to professionals. Good communication among the professionals can maximize therapeutic effectiveness and create an environment in which the patient and family can feel a sense of security.[1] When there has been a difficult death arrangements can be made to review the case in a discussion facilitated by one of the specialist team.

There needs to be an efficient means of notifying the general practitioner and the primary care team of the patient's death. The team need to identify an appropriate key worker who will be responsible for offering the family bereavement support and arranges a follow up bereavement visit 3–6 months after death to assess how the person is coping.[12] It is helpful to make a record of the death in the bereaved's notes.

Communication, conflict, and stress

Doctors, nurses, and other members of the team need clear ways of communicating. Mutual respect and trust among team members leads to their corporate and individual skills being employed in an optimal way. It is never helpful to be critical of colleagues in front of patients or relatives; such behaviour only serves to reduce the patient's confidence in the team. Professionals should monitor signs of stress in their colleagues and offer support when it is needed. It is sometimes easier to identify a stressed colleague than to intervene to help and support. Professionals should extend the support that they give to patients, to each other. Palliative care is filled with uncertainty; professionals need to be able to acknowledge this uncertainty and to share their concerns with colleagues. Ethical dilemmas can cause team stress, calling a family meeting or case conference to debate the issues can be a constructive way of helping to reach a team consensus.

When conflict occurs it should be acknowledged and resolved. In resolving conflict, it is vital to retain the self-respect of other individuals and to focus on specific patient-centred issues. One must resist scape-goating or blaming individuals. Clinical supervision, mentoring, and peer appraisal can be methods of supporting and encouraging colleagues. Time spent building bridges or 'networking' is rarely wasted.

Communication facilities

Team members need instruction in appropriate use of communication facilities. Voice-mail, e-mail, and mobile communication can improve support, but there is a need to reassure staff that their messages have been acted on.[23] Health care professionals need to think about the consequences of communication action with regard to their colleagues and to reflect on the use of resources and alternative approaches. There is a need for dialogue between disciplines to teach health care professionals how to design, evaluate, and set up efficient communication systems. Joint consultations may be facilitated by tele-conferencing through sound and video links without clinicians having to leave their usual work place.[39] The internet may unite practices and hospitals to reduce paperwork, speeding up access to results, hospital referral, and discharge letters through e-mail.[40]

Education and clinical audit

Ideas of multiprofessional and interprofessional education are central to the development of the new National Health Service in the United Kingdom. Learning in a clinical as well as a classroom setting may hold the key.[41] A major objective of interprofessional education is fostering of mutual respect.

Common training programmes in communication skills also challenge working practices.[42] While updates of clinical knowledge for individual doctors remain important, other learning is needed including strategies for multidisciplinary and multiprofessional working.[3]

It could be argued that by the time doctors and nurses have undergone professional training their views are so entrenched that they may be unwilling to develop a true appreciation of each other's roles, putting the team approach at risk. Perhaps teaching doctors and nurses together would allow some of these barriers to be removed through an opportunity for communication.[40,42] Recent reforms in health provision in the United Kingdom place an emphasis on collaborative working in health, social, and voluntary sectors.[43]

Clinical audit is another mechanism for improving interprofessional communication and is an integral part of clinical governance. The General Medical Council of the United Kingdom issued guidance on maintaining good medical practice which indicated that one of the key tests of a good team is that the members can be 'open and honest about professional performance' both together and separately. This requires a willingness to engage directly across professional boundaries that have long been impermeable.[44]

Conclusions

Collaborative practice involves good communication, an understanding of each other's roles, and trusting interpersonal relationships. Collaborative models of care are complex but this may be because they mirror the complexity of human suffering.[45] Professionals in hospital and the community need to maintain clear channels of communication, to acknowledge uncertainty, and to try to reach a consensus with the patient rather than perceiving one discipline as being critical of another. Patients and families will benefit if physicians are aware both of their own abilities and limitations and are willing to enlist the skills of others. A collaborative coordinated approach is particularly important as the disease progresses and the patient becomes frailer and the needs of the patient and family become more pronounced. As the number of professionals involved in the care increases, communication is essential to maintain maximized therapeutic effects, minimize confusion, and facilitate a coherent system of care. A team of reliable professionals who are communicating well with each other provides patients with a sense of security, consistency, and comfort. Such collaborative practice is essential if we are to have any chance of meeting the needs of patients and their families.

References

1. **Ingham, J.M. and Coyle, N.** (1997). Teamwork in end of life care: a nurse–physician perspective on introducing physicians to palliative care concepts. In *New Themes in Palliative Care* (ed. D. Clark, J. Hockley, and S. Ahmedzai), pp. 255–74. Buckingham: Open University Press.
2. **Lockhart-Wood, K.** (2001). Nurse–doctor collaboration in cancer pain management. *International Journal of Palliative Nursing* **7**, 6–16.
3. **Headrick, L.A., Wilcock, P.M., and Batalden, P.B.** (1998). Interprofessional working and continuing medical education. *British Medical Journal* **316**, 771–4.
4. **NHS Centre for Reviews. University of York** (2000). Informing, communicating and sharing decisions with people who have cancer. *Effective Health Care* **6**, 1–8.
5. **Charles, C., Gafni, A., and Whelan, T.** (2000). How to improve communications between doctors and patients. *British Medical Journal* **320**, 1220–1.
6. **Gosbee, J.** (1998). Communications among health professionals. *British Medical Journal* **316**, 642.
7. **Salter, R., Brettle, P., and Hobbs, F.D.R.** (1998). Poor communication puts patients at risk. *British Medical Journal* **317**, 279.
8. **Calman, K. and Hine, D.** *A Policy Framework for Commissioning Cancer Services.* London: Department of Health, 1995.
9. **Fottrell, E.** (1990). Multidisciplinary functioning: will it still be of use? *British Journal of Hospital Medicine* **43**, 253.
10. **McGann, C.** (1998). Communications in cancer care: introducing patient held records. *International Journal of Palliative Nursing* **4**, 222–9.
11. **Coyle, N.** (1997). Interdisciplinary collaboration in hospital palliative care: chimera or goal? *Palliative Medicine* **11**, 265–6.
12. **Doyle, D. and Jeffrey, D.** *Palliative Care in the Home.* Oxford: Oxford University Press, 2000.
13. **Jeffrey, D.** *Cancer from Cure to Care.* Manchester: Hochland & Hochland, 2000.
14. **Miller, D.G., Carroll, D., Grimshaw, J., and Watt, B.** (1998). Palliative care at home: an audit of cancer deaths in Grampian region. *British Journal of General Practice* **48**, 1299–302.
15. **Massorotto, A., Carter, H., MacLeod, R., and Donaldson, N.** (2000). Hospital referrals to a hospice: timing of referrals, referrers expectation, and the nature of referral information. *Journal of Palliative Care* **16**, 22–9.
16. **McConnell, D., Burton, P.N., and Tattersall, M.H.** (1999). Improving the letters we write; an exploration of doctor–doctor communications in cancer care. *British Journal of Cancer* **80**, 427–37.
17. **Mystakidou, K.** (2001). Interdisciplinary working: a Greek perspective. *Palliative Medicine* **15**, 67–8.
18. **Closs, S.J.** (1997). Discharge communications between hospital and community health care staff: a selective review. *Health, Social Care and Community* **5**, 181–97.
19. **Black, O.J.** (1996). Supportive and shared care. In *Cancer Care in the Community* (ed. B. Hancock), pp. 117–29. Oxford: Radcliffe Medical Press.
20. **White, F.** (1996). A review of palliative care in the community and the need for specialist services. *Journal of Cancer Care* **5** (4), 83–90.
21. **Hill, A.** (1998). Multiprofessional teamwork in hospital palliative care teams. *International Journal of Palliative Nursing* **4**, 214–21.
22. **Quinn, R. and Joyce, K.** (2000). How do general practitioners learn of their patient's death? *Irish Medical Journal* **93**, 282–3.
23. **Coiera, E. and Tombs, V.** (1998). Communication behaviour in a hospital setting: an observational study. *British Medical Journal* **316**, 673–6.
24. **Cooper, J.** *Stepping into Palliative Care.* Oxford: Radcliffe Medical Press, 2000, pp. 189–96.
25. 1995. 14 000 preventable deaths in Australian hospitals. *British Medical Journal* **310**, 1487.
26. **Vachon, M.L.S.** (1995). Staff stress in hospice/palliative care: a review. *Palliative Medicine* **9**, 91–122.
27. **Smith, R.** (1996). What clinical information do doctors need? *British Medical Journal* **313**, 1062–8.
28. **Bennett, M., Adam, J., Alison, D., Hicks, F., and Stockton, M.** (2000). Leeds eligibility criteria for specialist palliative care services. *Palliative Medicine* **14**, 157–8.
29. **General Medical Council.** *Good Medical Practice.* London: GMC, 2001.
30. **Peppiatt, R.** (1998). Palliative terminal care. *British Journal of General Practice* **48**, 1297–8.
31. **Marshall, M.N.** (1998). How well do general practitioners and hospital consultants work together? A qualitative study of co-operation and conflict within the medical profession. *British Journal of General Practice* **48**, 1379–82.
32. **Mackay, L.** *Conflicts in Care, Medicine and Nursing.* London: Chapman & Hall, 1993.
33. **Chilver, K.** (2001). Joint working, joint roles: streamlining patient care. *European Journal of Palliative Care* **8**, 112–14.
34. **Buckman, R.** (1998). Communication in palliative care: a practical guide. In *Oxford Textbook of Palliative Medicine* 2nd edn. (ed. D. Doyle, G.W.C. Hanks, and N. MacDonald), pp. 153–4. Oxford: Oxford University Press.
35. **Anderson, E.E.** (2000). Professional practice issues surrounding record keeping in district nursing practice. *British Journal of Community Nursing* **5**, 352–6.
36. **Ellershaw, J.** et al. (1997). Developing an integrated care pathway for the dying patient. *European Journal of Palliative Care* **4**, 203–7.
37. **Webb, P.** *Ethical Issues in Palliative Care.* Oxford: Radcliffe Medical Press, 2000.
38. **Randall, F. and Downie, R.S.** *Palliative Care Ethics. A Good Companion.* Oxford: Oxford University Press, 1999.
39. **Harrison, R., Clayton, W., and Wallace, P.** (1996). Can telemedicine be used to improve communications between primary and secondary care? *British Medical Journal* **313**, 1377–80.
40. **Willmot, M. and Sullivan, F.** (2000). NHS net in Scottish primary care. Lessons for the future. *British Medical Journal* **321**, 878–81.
41. **Finch, J.** (2000). Interprofessional education and team working: a view from the education providers. *British Medical Journal* **321**, 1138–40.
42. **Keogh, K., Jeffrey, D., and Flanagan, S.** (1999). The Palliative Care Education Group for Gloucestershire (PEGG): an integrated model of multidisciplinary education in palliative care. *European Journal of Cancer Care* **8**, 44–7.
43. **Department of Health.** *The NHS Plan: A Plan for Investment, A Plan for Reform.* London: Department of Health, 2000.
44. **General Medical Council.** *Guidance on Maintaining Good Medical Practice.* London: General Medical Council, 1998.
45. **Lorenz, A.D., Mauksch, L.B., and Gawinski, B.A.** (1999). Models of collaboration. *Primary Care* **26**, 401–10.

4.3 Communication with the public, politicians, and the media

Kenneth Calman

Introduction

It might well be asked why a chapter on such an issue should appear in this textbook, which is essentially concerned with issues of care, quality of life, ethical and research issues, and the delivery of a service. The answer lies precisely in that statement. Each of these areas is of direct relevance to the public (who might need the service), to politicians (who may be funding the service), and the media (who will be reporting on the service). A glance through almost any newspaper in almost any country will show how much news and political noise can be made over issues in palliative care.

Three brief examples will illustrate the kind of issues which need to be addressed:

End of life issues. Euthanasia is a subject which is not only the province of professionals, but the public at large. The public and politicians want to know what the issues are, what discussions are taking place at the moment, what is happening in other countries, and how can their views be heard?

Resource allocation. Almost every health system is currently looking to see how palliative care can be developed and funded. It is an emotional issue and attracts publicity. Campaigns can be readily mounted to build a hospice, raise money for a post or educational purposes, and for many other reasons. But why should palliative care be funded at the expense of other services? How can the case be made to those who make the decisions?

Quality of care. One of the commonest complaints against health professionals is that of poor communication. Not surprisingly this becomes particularly relevant in those circumstances when patients die in inappropriate circumstances and the family are unhappy.

Add to these examples other high profile issues in the press at any time, and the justification for some thinking about the topic becomes clearer. There are many more examples which could have been used; however, these should suffice to show the importance of the topic. The danger is that without thought and preparation, the doctor, the speciality, or the palliative care service may be misunderstood and under these circumstances it is much more difficult to get on top of the agenda. Better to be ahead of the game than trying to recover from a public relations disaster.

The purpose of these processes is to build up trust between the doctor and the palliative care service and the media, politicians, and the public. Trust is a key part of the process and takes time to build up and very easy to lose. The remainder of this chapter deals with the issues which arise when clinical interests in palliative care interface with the public, politicians, and the media.

The purpose of communication

The communication of an issue around palliative care to the public or the media has several different functions. First it might be to inform the public of the scope of palliative care or give the details of a new service or treatment which is available. Second it may be to raise the profile of the speciality or a particular service in order that funding might be approved or donations granted. It might be to assist in the patient or the public making choices, either about the services available or to raise an ethical issue such as euthanasia or other end of life issues. It might also be to encourage professional staff to consider palliative care as a career and see it as an opportunity for personal development. From the political point of view it will partly be to raise awareness of the subject and allow opportunities to meet and talk to politicians about the ways in which palliative care can be of benefit to a wide range of people.

Part of the problem is that the response to any issue can be reactive or proactive; in so many instances it is the former—responding to a news item rather than setting the news. Both of course are relevant and can be very valuable but in reactive mode the story line is usually set and it may be difficult to change it. It is generally someone else's agenda.

Taking the lead and thus shaping the agenda sounds the right thing to do, but it can be very difficult. The media may not be interested, they tend to like 'bad news' stories where there is conflict and death, where there is controversy, or where patient lives have been put at risk. 'Good news' stories are much more difficult to get into the press though local media, print, and television are often looking for news. What often matters, with deadlines to be met, is to have a full press release available so that it can be used without much editing.

Each palliative care service must therefore hold the contact numbers of key media personnel and local politicians and invite them on a regular basis to visit the facility, meet staff, and if appropriate, patients. Such visits build up trust and a working atmosphere, which, if problems arise can allow them to be handled more readily. This inevitably takes time and in the short term there may be nothing to show for the effort. However, if the media and the public are aware of what palliative care is, and what can be offered, then they are more likely to be responsive if something new comes on the scene or a problem arises.

Communication with the public is also about providing information about health and illness, and in the palliative care setting, about death and dying. These latter two topics are still taboo in many places and the palliative care service, through a carefully developed communication strategy, can bring such topics into the public consciousness. They can help in the debate and discussion, pose questions and begin to give some of the answers, and deal with fears and misconceptions about such issues. They can help to form attitudes and ensure that when problems do arise then they know where they might get help. The provision of information is one of the services which can be provided. The use of leaflets, audio tapes, and videos can assist in this process. Notices and posters in local shops or pharmacies can be another way of disseminating information. Local seminars with other professional groups, with the public, and with the media may be another way of doing this. It is not an easy area to discuss and requires careful and sensitive writing and producing. However, if the public, the media, and the politicians can learn more and their attitudes change then a great deal will have been gained.

Mechanisms of communication

Communication with the public, the media, and the politicians is not a simple matter. However, there are some principles which have been found to be useful in assisting the process.

- Be clear about the message and consider the language used very carefully. Is it understandable? Is too much jargon used? Is there a single clear message? It is sometimes useful to use a non-medical colleague to check the press statement. If it is not understandable by them, then it will not be by the public.
- Have you considered all those who might be affected by the message? Could some of the key players be involved in the process in order that they are supportive when the message is released? For example, if a new service is being launched, local health providers and professionals might like to know this and be prepared to support the new venture rather than oppose it, a possible occurrence, if they have not been involved.
- Check out any possible financial implications. What does it cost? How will it be funded? Will this take resource away from other services?
- Make sure that you have prepared a 'question and answer' brief for the person who will be in the lead. In particular, highlight any controversial areas, or areas into which an interviewer may lead. For example, though the press launch may be to set out a new pain unit, the discussion might all be about euthanasia. Consider all aspects. Preparation is everything.
- Make sure you are aware of any related stories in the press which you might be asked about, and whether or not a particular politician has a special interest in some aspect of palliative care. Background information is critical if you are not to be caught out.
- Decide early on who will be in the lead, and that individual should be involved in the process from the beginning, not brought in at the end.
- Where relevant, hard copy information should be made available for interested parties to take away and use.
- Where appropriate, have internal meetings of key external stakeholders to ensure that there are no surprises for them.
- Finally, after the event, a full de-briefing should be held to work through any of the problems and improve the presentation next time.

Some organizations find it helpful to use a checklist which is developed over the years and which fits the organization and the subject matter. Such checklists include key contacts and access to legal advice where required. Difficult issues usually occur on Friday nights when people have left the service. Make sure you are prepared. One way of doing this is to take the next public incident and ask whether your organization could tackle it, and how. Ensure that you have available telephone numbers of staff and key personnel. There may be a rapid need to check the data, inform or meet key stakeholders, prepare a well-understood message free from jargon, and identify the individual to present the information. Audio-visual aids may be required and these should be prepared early.

Dealing with the public and the media are now regular occurrences for many palliative care services. It is worth considering staff training specifically for this purpose. It can increase confidence and ensure that important aspects of the process are not missed. This is also relevant to National Organizations and Speciality Groups. There is merit, on a regional or national basis, having a list of specialists who can be available to deal with specific issues. Once again, media training for this group is likely to be helpful. Remember that in press releases it is useful to have them checked for 'reading age' (a technique to establish its readability) and by a lay person for its comprehension and avoidance of jargon.

Dealing with an urgent issue

The description given above is concerned mainly with the situation in which there is a clear need to speak to the press or politicians, and which can be planned and prepared for. The alternative situation which has to be dealt with is where a problem arises and which needs immediate action, or which is a source of questioning by the public or the media. Such situations might include the use of a new and controversial treatment, an increased number of unexpected deaths, a major complaint against the hospice for poor care, a disgruntled relative (perhaps with good cause), a controversial statement made by a member of staff on an issue relevant to palliative care which might or might not have been misinterpreted, and many others.

In these situations there is much less time to prepare, and the work done before hand on the checklist—who should speak, contact numbers, etc.—will become very useful. In such situations, however, it is often clear that there has been a problem and that it might have been present for some time. This is often called the anticipatory phase of the response to an unexpected risk. Part of the function of the senior management in the hospice is to be alert to possible problems (risks), to identify them, and where possible deal with them as early as can be. Looking back, the problem may even have been detected early but no one took action. In the public presentation of the problem, whatever it is, one of the first questions usually asked is, why was this not detected earlier? Who was responsible for this, and why was no action taken? Answers to these will be needed at the press conference. Think through all possible questions and have a mock press conference with your staff who think of the difficult questions. The time to have media training is before this incident occurs.

The process during the second phase of communication of an urgent issue is similar to that described earlier, but some aspects need emphasizing.

- A key contact list is essential.
- If other players are involved, or might have a view (e.g. the community nursing service, a pharmaceutical company, the local medical group, or health authority) then it is generally wise to inform then and meet them.
- The message needs to be clear, and potential questions need to be identified and answered. Hard copies of the press release should be available and checked for any errors and for language.
- Nothing should be held back or concealed and if the information is not known or available then this should be made public. It can be noted that more information will be made available as it becomes known.
- It is often helpful to enlist the views of outsiders who can put the issue into perspective and allay public fears, if there may be some. Such individuals and other key groups should, if possible, be at the press conference to answer questions.
- When issues like this arise, the media should not be avoided or dismissed. If they have no comment or copy to use they will make it up or use other people's views. Provide them with something to take away and use.
- If you have a website then it can be used to provide updated information. Refer to it in the press briefing.
- The language used in the presentation has to be very carefully considered. The choice of words can be crucial and this is not a task which can be done without very careful presentation or rehearsal in many instances. Making comments in the press is not a trivial task as words and phrases can be so easily misconstrued.
- As before, the evaluation of the outcome is critical and should help to inform any other problems in the future. It is often assumed that this will be a one off and will never happen again. This is not likely to be true. Such events will continue to occur and the palliative care service needs to be able to respond.

Such communication issues are common to many different palliative care organizations and it might be useful for a local, regional, or national grouping to get together and share experience of these issues.

Media training

In a palliative care service which has regular contact with the media and the public it may be of value to have senior people trained in media skills. This allows the individual to think through some of the issues and have professional advice on presentation and on how to raise difficult issues. There are many agencies in most countries which can provide such a service. It allows confidence to be built up so that the doctor is less frightened of the media and politicians, and faces them without feeling threatened. This is of course easier if the doctor has already met the individuals and begun the process of engagement.

Evaluating the outcome—how do we know if we have been successful?

This is the final phase of the response and the one which is often neglected. Once the dust has settled and the press has gone home, what has been learned? It is easy to say that this is a one off, that it couldn't possibly happen again, but it might. Could the processes be tightened up? Have the basic problems been dealt with? Has a regular process of audit been set up to ensure that any further problems will be identified at the earliest possible time? If the hospice, service, or clinician is to learn from past experiences then this needs to be built into the thinking and the culture of the organization.

Interacting with politicians

Politicians, both local and national, can be of great value to a palliative care service. It is important, therefore, that efforts are made to get to know them and to ensure that they understand the work of the care service. They can be great allies. In particular, they may be of help in the following ways.

Public policy. Politicians have an important responsibility in public policy and in setting a national framework for action. They do this through the democratic process in parliament, senate, or congress. They can influence public opinion, and are influenced by it. Issues such as the use of cannabis or in the ending of life are just some of the policy issues they may deal with. They make laws and have the ability to change the way in which a service operates or is funded. They can therefore shape a palliative care service for a whole nation, and provide the resource. They will need assistance in this and are likely to turn to advisors for specialist advice. While ministers or senior politicians will generally make the running, local parliamentarians will have significant input.

Parliamentary processes. In addition to the functions described above there are other important areas to consider. There are select committees which investigate particular issues, and there are specialist parliamentary groups whose members focus on such topics as palliative care. They are usually 'All Party Associations' and thus generally free from party politics. Such groups are an important source of input into decision making. As 'Lobbying' groups they are important source of advocacy for patients and for the services they require.

International issues. There are many international bodies which have interests in palliative care and other relevant issues such as ethics. These include the World Health Organization, medical and professional organizations, and regional groupings such as the European Union and the Council of Europe. There are many others across the world and they are a useful source of information and expertise.

Conclusion

Dealing with the media is a professional task. It requires care, planning. It is a process which has been thought out and worked on with sufficient energy at a very high level in the palliative care team. Working with politicians can be very rewarding and can influence decisions about the future of the speciality. Invitations to meet senior people should be accepted with alacrity. Eating for my hospice is an occupational hazard.

Further reading

Bennett, P. and Calman, K.C. *Risk Communication and Public Health.* Oxford: Oxford University Press, 1999.

5

Research in palliative medicine

5 Research in palliative medicine

5.1 The principles of evidence-based medicine

Henry J. McQuay, Andrew Moore, and Philip Wiffen

What constitutes evidence?

Finding and using the best available evidence should be part of our professional lives. Archie Cochrane said in 1979 'It is surely a great criticism of our profession that we have not organized a critical summary, by specialty or subspecialty, adapted periodically, of all relevant randomized controlled trials'. We have been slow to grasp this nettle.

There are several interlinked strands:

- finding the evidence;
- appraising the evidence;
- making the evidence (doing trials or systematic reviews);
- using the evidence.

The focus in this chapter is on randomized trials and systematic reviews of existing trials. Systematic reviews and large randomized trials constitute the most reliable sources of evidence we can muster (Table 1). Put simply, they are the best chance we have to determine what is true. We discuss how to find trials, and how to appraise their quality. Further on there is advice on how to appraise the quality of systematic reviews themselves.

Table 1 Type and strength of efficacy evidence[1] (Oxford CEBM levels of evidence; May 2001)

Level	Therapy/prevention, aetiology/harm
1a	SR (with homogeneity) of RCTs
1b	Individual RCT (with narrow CI)
1c	All or none
2a	SR (with homogeneity) of cohort studies
2b	Individual cohort study (including low quality RCT; e.g. <80% follow-up)
2c	'Outcomes' research: ecological studies
3a	SR (with homogeneity) of case-control studies
3b	Individual case-control study
4	Case-series (and poor quality cohort and case-control studies)
5	Expert opinion without explicit critical appraisal, or based on physiology, bench research, or 'first principles'

http://cebm.jr2.ox.ac.uk/docs/levels.html

Evidence-based medicine

The strident debate between the proponents and the opponents of evidence-based medicine (EBM) has led slowly to clearer thoughts. A current definition of EBM is that it is the conscientious, explicit, and judicious use of current best evidence in making decisions about the care of individual patients.[2] The practice of EBM requires the integration of individual clinical expertise with the best available external clinical evidence from systematic research. Decisions that affect the care of patients should be taken with *due weight* accorded to *all* valid, relevant information. There are many factors as well as the results of randomized controlled trials (RCTs) which may weigh heavily in both clinical and policy decisions, such as patient preferences and resources, and these must contribute to decisions about the care of patients (*due weight*). Valid, relevant evidence should be considered alongside these other factors in the decision-making process. No one sort of evidence should necessarily be the determining factor in a decision. *All* implies that there should be an active search for that valid, relevant information and that an assessment should be made of the accuracy of the information and the applicability of the evidence to the decision in question, that is, information should be appraised. EBM is thus what most health care professionals have been trying to practice all their working lives.

What is changing is that there is an increasing number of well-conducted RCTs and systematic reviews, and that there is a political pressure, both from those receiving care and from those who pay for it, to support our treatment choices with high quality evidence. That should not be too irksome, given that professionally we would all wish to do the best for our patients. What happens is that the evidence supports some interventions and suggests that others are considerably less effective than some of us believe. This should not make us paranoid. Precisely the same message has emerged in the other areas of medicine which have received similar attention. What is clear is that very often the quality of the trials of invasive interventions is much lower than the quality of drug trials. The onus must be on us to do bigger and better trials if we wish to continue using some of these techniques.

Evidence-based medicine and palliative care

Palliative care has the same generic problems found in other therapeutic areas, but also has some which are specific to palliative care. One generic problem is the narrative review. The traditional narrative review, an overview of part or all of the speciality, often written by a key opinion leader, has a number of features which leave it open to bias. The author may select just her papers, or those of her friends, and ignore those of her competitors. This bias in the selection of the literature may not always be easy to identify, and obviously can produce a biased conclusion. The bias may be compounded by an absence of rigour in criteria for including papers, that is, not only has the author used just her own papers, but she has included some high-quality work and some of low quality. Data may not have been extracted in a logical way. The systematic review should prevent the problems of a narrative review, because the way in which the literature is searched is transparent, and so are the inclusion and exclusion criteria. The way in which data are extracted should also be crystal clear, so that the reader could repeat the search, find the papers, rule individual papers in or out, and extract the data. The reader might not reach the same conclusion as the original author, but at least the starting point is the same, which is unlikely to be the case with the narrative review.

A second problem is that not all the interventions which are made in palliative care are easy to study with the gold standard randomized trial. The methods for compiling credible systematic reviews described below require credible component trials. If a topic, a particular intervention, has resisted study with high quality trials, then it may be impossible to produce a credible review. A further level of complexity is when we want to know if a particular package of interventions is better than another package—home care versus hospital care for instance. The absence of good study methods for packages of care is obvious from parallel work in other therapeutic areas, intensive care and cognitive behavioural therapy are two examples. Until we have good study methods for individual trials it will remain difficult to draw strong evidence-based conclusions about service delivery and packages of care.

A third problem in palliative care is that trials are notoriously difficult to conduct, compared for instance with acute pain. Some, but not all, of the interventions in palliative care will have been studied in other settings, such as chronic non-malignant pain. The question then arises of the legitimacy of extrapolating high quality evidence derived in other therapeutic areas. The corollary is 'Is it necessary to trial an intervention in palliative care when it has been shown to work well elsewhere?'. The pragmatic answer is that this has to be context dependent. An intervention which is safe and effective for neuropathic pain in chronic non-malignant pain will likely work well in palliative care, but may of course have additional problems in sicker patients or with different drug–drug interactions.

Where do you get the evidence?

Evidence which is both relevant and valid is necessary for effective care. The RCT is the most reliable way to estimate the effect of an intervention. The principle of randomization is simple. Patients in a randomized trial have the same probability of receiving any of the interventions being compared. Randomization abolishes selection bias because it prevents investigators influencing who has which intervention. Randomization also helps to ensure that other factors, such as age or sex distribution, are equivalent for the different treatment groups. Inadequate randomization, or inadequate concealment of randomization, lead to exaggeration of therapeutic effect.[3]

To produce valid reviews of evidence, the reviews need to be systematic, and to be systematic, qualitative, or quantitative, they need to include all relevant RCTs. Identifying all the relevant trials is a 'fundamental challenge'[4] which is easily underestimated.

The first obstacle faced by any reviewer is finding out how many eligible RCTs exist. Commonly the total is unknown. Usually only for newer interventions are reviewers likely to be sure that they have found all the RCTs. Otherwise the only way to find how many RCTs there are would be to scan every record in each of the available bibliographic databases, to search by hand all non-indexed journals, theses, proceedings, and textbooks, to search the reference lists of all the reports found, and to ask investigators of previous RCTs for other published or unpublished information.[5] In practice, constrained by time and cost, reviewers have to compromise, and then hope that what they have found is a representative sample of the unknown total population of trials. The more comprehensive the searching the more trials will be found, and any conclusions will then be stronger. Comprehensive searches can be very time consuming and costly, so again this emphasizes the necessary compromise, where the target is the highest possible yield for given resources.

Retrieval bias is the failure to identify reports which could have affected the results of a systematic review or meta-analysis.[6] This failure may be because trials are still ongoing, or completed but unpublished (publication bias) or because although published the search did not find them. Trying to identify unpublished trials by asking researchers had a very low yield,[7] and was not cheap. Registers of ongoing and completed trials are another way to find unpublished data, but such registers are rare.

Developing a citation database for a review

This process has three phases: definition of inclusion criteria, identification of reports, and information management. The example used is for a wide search for all analgesic interventions.[8] For a particular intervention, the reviewer would follow the same path but narrow the inclusion criteria.

Inclusion criteria

A report was regarded as eligible if the following criteria were fulfilled:

- Allocation to the intervention was described as randomized (no precise description of the method of randomization was required) or as double-blind or as both, or if it was suggested that the interventions were given at random and/or under double-blind conditions, and
- Analgesic interventions with pain or adverse effects as outcomes, and/or any intervention using pain as an outcome measure, were compared.
- Reports were excluded which investigated analgesic effectiveness during (as opposed to after) diagnostic or surgical procedures.

Identification of reports

Since we developed our original process,[8] electronic searching is much easier, and we use a range of databases, MEDLINE, EMBASE, the Cochrane Library, CINAHL, and PSYCHLIT as part of our standard operating procedures. The citations to the identified reports are downloaded, and stored in a reference management program. Each downloaded citation is checked on screen for definite eligibility, probable eligibility or ineligibility and coded accordingly. Hard copies of eligible and probable reports are obtained, and if necessary are translated, and eligibility is then confirmed.

Hand searching of journals

Some topics may by their nature be published in journals which are not indexed by the major databases, and these journals may need to be searched by hand to find relevant studies. These reports, either missed by MEDLINE indexing, or in non-indexed journals, are then added to the citation database if perusal of the hard copy confirms that they are indeed eligible.

Conclusions

The importance of basing systematic reviews on the highest quality evidence (randomized trials) is obvious from our experience in the pain field,[9] and from the experience of others. This means that very considerable time and effort has to be spent to gather all the relevant material for each review.

The process outlined here is a laborious task, made easier now because citations of known RCTs have been added to the Cochrane Library, so that others do not have to repeat the hand-searching process. For topics that are not mainstream the hand-searching process will still have to be done.

Judging the quality of trials

Once you have found all the reports of the trials relevant to your question there is another stage in the process. This stage is first to confirm that these reports meet certain *quality standards* and second that, even though a report may pass those quality standards, whether the trial is *valid*.

Imagine a situation where you found 40 reports of trials on your question. You then discover that 20 of the reports say that the intervention is terrific, and 20 conclude that it should never be used. Delving deeper you find that the 20 'negative' reports score highly on your quality standards scale. The 20 'positive' reports score poorly for quality. What then will you conclude? Without a quality scale you would vote for the intervention. With the quality scale you would vote against.

The quality scale should include measures of bias. Bias is the simplest explanation why poor-quality reports give more positive conclusions than high-quality reports. The quality standards which you require cannot be absolute, because for some clinical questions there may not be any RCTs. Setting RCTs as a minimum absolute standard would therefore be inappropriate for all the questions we might want to answer. In the pain world, however, there are two reasons for setting this high standard, and requiring trials to be randomized. The first reason is that we do have, particularly for drug interventions, quite a number of RCTs. The second is that we would argue that it is even more important to stress the minimum quality standards of randomization and double-blinding when the outcome measures are subjective.

Developing and validating a quality scale

What makes a trial worthy of the label 'high quality'? Quality could refer to the clinical relevance of the study, to the likelihood of biased results, to the appropriateness of the statistical analysis, to the presentation of the data, or to the ethical implications of the intervention or to the literary style of the manuscript. We think that quality must primarily indicate the likelihood that the study design reduced bias. Only by avoiding bias is it possible to estimate the effect of a given intervention with any confidence.

The simple scale (Tables 2 and 3) which we developed,[(10)] and which is now used widely, was designed to assess the likelihood of the trial design to generate unbiased results and approach the 'therapeutic truth'. Other trial characteristics such as clinical relevance of the question addressed, data analysis and presentation, literary quality of the report, or ethical implications of the study are not included in our definition.

Table 2 Scale (3 point) to measure the likelihood of bias in pain research reports

This is not the same as being asked to review a paper. It should not take more than 10 min to score a report and there are no right or wrong answers

Please read the article and try to answer the following questions (see attached instructions):

1. Was the study described as randomized (this includes the use of words such as randomly, random, and randomization)?
2. Was the study described as double-blind?
3. Was there a description of withdrawals and drop outs?

Scoring the items

Give a score of 1 point for each 'yes' and 0 points for each 'no'. There are no in-between marks:

Give 1 additional point if:	On question 1, the method of randomization was described *and* it was *appropriate* (table of random numbers, computer generated, coin tossing, etc.)
and/or:	If on question 2 the method of double-blinding was described *and* it was *appropriate* (identical placebo, active placebo, dummy, etc.)
Deduct 1 point if:	On question 1, the method of randomization was described *and* it was *inappropriate* (patients were allocated alternatively, or according to date of birth, hospital number, etc.)
and/or:	On question 2 the study was described as double-blind but the method of blinding was *inappropriate* (e.g. comparison of tablet versus injection with no double dummy)

Table 3 Advice on using the scale

1. Randomization:
If the word randomized or any other related words such as random, randomly, or randomization are used in the report, but the method of randomization is not described, give a positive score to this item. A randomization method will be regarded as appropriate if it allowed each patient to have the same chance of receiving each treatment and the investigators could not predict which treatment was next. Therefore, methods of allocation using date of birth, date of admission, hospital numbers, or alternation should not be regarded as appropriate

2. Double-blinding:
A study must be regarded as double-blind if the word double-blind is used (even without description of the method) or if it is implied that neither the caregiver nor the patient could identify the treatment being assessed

3. Withdrawals and drop outs:
Patients who were included in the study but did not complete the observation period or who were not included in the analysis must be described. The number *and* the reasons for withdrawal must be stated. If there are no withdrawals, it should be stated in the article. If there is no statement on withdrawals, this item must be given a negative score (0 points)

Comments on the scale

The 3-point scale is simple, short, valid, and reliable. Our results suggest that even without clinical or research experience users should be able to score the quality of research reports consistently. Chalmers et al. suggested many years ago that the quality of clinical reports should be assessed blind.[(11)] We found that such blinded assessment produced significantly lower scores. This may be very important if absolute cut-off scores are imposed by systematic reviewers, and if quality scores are used to weight the results of primary studies in subsequent meta-analysis.[(12,13)] The results of open evaluations are good enough for busy readers. The improved reliability with blind testing is of more relevance to journal editors for manuscript selection and to systematic reviewers. Quality scales without clinimetric evaluation have already been used in pain work to support the conclusions of systematic reviews.[(14–16)]

None of the items is specific to pain studies. The three items are very similar to the components of a scale used extensively to assess the effectiveness of interventions during pregnancy and childbirth,[(17)] and also appear in most other scales. Control of selection bias and rater bias is obviously crucial to quality.

Selection bias is best controlled by allocating patients at random to the different study groups. Each patient should have the same probability of being included in each comparison group, and the allocation should be concealed until after the patient has given consent to take part. Methods of allocation based on alternation, date of birth, or hospital record number cannot be regarded as random. Failure to secure proper randomization increases the likelihood that potential participants in a 'randomized' study will be admitted to the study selectively because of prior knowledge of the group to which they would be allocated or excluded selectively before formal admission in the study.[(18)] Ideal methods of randomization are those in which individuals with no direct relationship to the study participants are in charge of the allocation (e.g. allocation by telephone from a central coordinating office, concealed from the investigators). Appropriate simpler alternatives are coin tossing, tables of random numbers, and numbers generated by computers, but at higher risk of selective selection.

All these methods are regarded as appropriate for the purposes of our scale, although we are aware that selective selection is still possible even if the group allocation is concealed until after consent has been obtained. We rate the randomization method as inappropriate if the potential participants did not have the same chance of being included in any of the comparison groups (methods based on date of birth, hospital number, or alternation).

Even with excellent randomization selection bias may still be introduced if biased and selective withdrawal and drop outs occur after the allocations have been made.[19] This is why an adequate description of withdrawals and drop outs is included in the scale. With that information it is possible to analyse on an intention-to-treat basis (all those randomized whether or not they were exposed to the study interventions[20]).

Rater bias can be minimized by blinding the person receiving the intervention, the individual administering it, the investigator measuring the outcome, and the analyst. Blinding can be tested by asking the study patients and the researchers which intervention they had. This is not often done. The usual 'best' level of blinding is blinding of the study subject and those making the observations (double-blinding). Double-blinding is often achieved by using control interventions with similar physical characteristics to those of the intervention under evaluation, or by the use of dummies when two or more interventions have to be given by different routes. Sometimes, however, one of the interventions may produce effects which make blinding very difficult to sustain. Then the use of active placebos or active controls may decrease the likelihood of rater bias. All these precautions are relatively easy to achieve in drug studies. In non-drug studies testing under blind conditions is either difficult or inappropriate (e.g. surgical procedures) or impossible (e.g. acupuncture or TENS). The risk of rater bias limits the confidence with which conclusions can be reached. We know that studies which are not double-blind risk an average exaggeration of treatment effect of 17 per cent.[3]

Validity of trials

A study may of course be both randomized and double-blind, and describe withdrawals and drop outs in copious detail (so scoring well on this quality scale) and yet be invalid. Two examples from the pain world illustrate this point. One is from the injection of morphine into the knee joint to reduce pain after arthroscopy.[21] In some trials, this injection was made after the operation without knowledge of whether or not the patients had enough pain for the intervention to make a difference. If they had just mild pain rather than moderate or severe pain it is quite possible that the success ascribed in that trial to the intervention was actually due to the fact that they did not have any pain to begin with. The second example comes from attempts to show the efficacy of pre-emptive analgesia, where comparisons were made at multiple time points after surgery between patients receiving analgesia before pain and the group who received the same analgesia after the pain had started. A statistical difference at one of eight time points is then held up as proof that giving the analgesia before the pain is successful, when at the other seven points there was no difference. These are criticisms of the validity of the trials, and including these trials uncritically in a review will affect the conclusions. A third example is a review which proclaimed that fewer patients would die after major surgery if they had regional plus general anaesthesia.[22] The statistical significance which led the authors to this potentially important conclusion came from a number of small trials with 30 per cent mortality rates, rates so high as to make one question the validity of the trials.

How can these pitfalls be avoided? We attempted to build a checklist of validity checks,[23] hoping this would be a generic solution across all therapeutic areas. In reality, while some of the items are generic some are specific to the field, so that the reader, the author and the reviewer must all be aware of the potential problems.

Judging the quality of reviews

As professionals we want to use the best treatments and, as patients, to be given them. Knowing that an intervention works (or does not work) is fundamental to clinical decision-making. When is the evidence strong enough to justify changing practice? Some of the decisions we make are based on individual studies, often on small numbers of patients, which, given the random play of chance, may lead to incorrect decisions. Systematic reviews and large randomized trials constitute the most reliable sources of evidence we can muster (Table 1).[1] Systematic reviews identify and review all the relevant studies, and are more likely to give a reliable answer. They use explicit methods and quality standards to reduce bias. Their results are the closest we are likely to get to the truth in the absence of satisfactorily large randomized trials.

The questions a systematic review should answer for us are:

- How well does an intervention work (compared with placebo, no treatment, or other interventions in current use)?
- Is it safe?
- Will it work and be safe for the patients in our practice?

Clinicians need to be able to synthesize their knowledge of a particular patient in their practice, their experience and expertise, and the best external evidence from systematic review. They can then be confident that they are doing their best. But the product of systematic review and particularly meta-analysis—often some sort of statistical output—is often not interpretable or usable in day-to-day clinical practice. A common currency to help make the best treatment decision for a particular patient is what is needed. We believe that this common currency is the number-needed-to-treat (NNT). The choice of analgesic for both professional and patient will be made on the balance between efficacy and risk, where the risk may be adverse effect or drug interaction with other drugs which the patient is taking.

Quality control

Systematic reviews of inadequate quality may be worse than none, because faulty decisions may be made with unjustified confidence. Quality control in the systematic review process, from literature searching onwards, is vital. How to judge the quality of a systematic review is encapsulated in the questions:[24]

- Were the question(s) and methods stated clearly?
- Were the search methods used to locate relevant studies comprehensive?
- Were explicit methods used to determine which articles to include in the review?
- Was the methodological quality of the primary studies assessed?
- Were the selection and assessment of the primary studies reproducible and free from bias?
- Were differences in individual study results explained adequately?
- Were the results of the primary studies combined appropriately?
- Were the reviewers' conclusions supported by the data cited?

When systematic reviews of the same topic use data from different numbers of papers, reasons should be sought. Reviews can use criteria that exclude information important to individual clinicians, or may be too lax by including studies with inadequate trial design. The defence against either mistake is to read the inclusion and exclusion criteria critically to see if they make sense in your clinical circumstance.

Outcome measures chosen for data extraction should also be sensible. Usually this is not a problem, but again it is a part of the methods that needs to be read carefully to see if you agree with the outcome measure extracted. The reviewer may have used all that is available, and any problems were due to the original trials, but it is a determinant of the clinical utility of the review.

Therapeutic interventions: which study designs are admissible?

For a systematic review of therapeutic efficacy, the gold standard is that eligible studies should be RCTs to exclude selection bias. If trials are not randomized, estimates of treatment effect may be exaggerated by up to 40 per cent.[3] In a systematic review of transcutaneous electrical nerve stimulation (TENS) in post-operative pain, 17 reports on 786 patients could be regarded unequivocally as RCTs in acute post-operative pain. Fifteen of these 17 RCTs demonstrated no benefit of TENS over placebo. Nineteen reports had pain outcomes but were not RCTs; in 17 of these 19, TENS was considered by their authors to have had a positive analgesic effect.[9] When appropriate, and particularly with subjective outcomes, the gold standard for an efficacy systematic review is studies that are both randomized and double-blind (to exclude observer bias). The therapeutic effect may be exaggerated by up to 20 per cent in trials with deficient blinding.[3]

Databases can provide records of many patients were or were not taking a particular medicine. They may record how well the patient or the health care professional thought the medicine worked. Conclusions about the efficacy of the treatment made from databases are however necessarily subject to the selection bias and the observer bias which the randomized trial, and the systematic review which uses randomized trials to derive its efficacy estimate, are designed to minimize. Estimates or treatment efficacy from database data are therefore likely to be overestimates.[3] The purist argument has to be that efficacy estimates derived from databases are likely to be of poor quality, subject to bias, and confounded by other influences, such as the medical condition itself and by other drugs.

Not all data can be combined in a meta-analysis: qualitative systematic reviews

It is often not possible or sensible to combine (pool) data, resulting in a qualitative rather than a quantitative systematic review. Combining data is not possible if there is no quantitative information in the component trials of the review. Combining data may not be sensible if trials used different clinical outcomes or followed the patients for different lengths of time. Combining continuous rather than dichotomous data may be difficult. Even if trials measure and present dichotomous data, how many patients did or did not achieve a specified outcome, if the trials are otherwise of poor quality[10] it may not be sensible to combine the data.

Making decisions from qualitative systematic reviews

Making decisions about whether or not a therapy works from such a qualitative systematic review may look easy. In the example above, 15 of the 17 RCTs of TENS in acute pain showed no benefit compared with control. The thinking clinician will realize that TENS in acute pain is not an effective analgesic. The problem with this simple vote counting, counting how many trials showed benefit and how many did not, is that it may mislead. It ignores the sample size of the constituent studies, the magnitude of the effect in the studies and the validity of their design even though they were randomized.[23]

Evaluating efficacy

Combining data: quantitative systematic reviews

There are also two parts to the 'does it work?' question: how does it compare with placebo and how does it compare with other therapies. Whichever comparison is being considered, the three stages of examining a review are a L'Abbé plot, statistical testing (odds ratio or relative risk), and a clinical significance measure such as NNT.

L'Abbé plots[25]

A first stage for evaluating therapies is to look at a simple scatter plot, which can yield a surprisingly comprehensive qualitative view of the data. Even if the review does not show the data in this way it can be done from information on individual trials presented in the review tables. Figure 1 contains data from an updated systematic review of single dose paracetamol in acute pain. Each point on the graph is the result of a single trial, the size of each point being proportional to the size of each trial, and what happens with paracetamol (experimental event rate [EER]) is plotted against the event rate with placebo (control event rate [CER]).

Trials in which the experimental treatment proves better than the control (EER > CER) will be in the upper left of the plot, between the *y*-axis and the line of equality. Paracetamol was better than placebo in all the trials; although the plot does not say how much better. If experimental was no better than control then the point would fall on the line of equality (EER = CER), and if control was better than experimental then the point would be in the lower right of the plot, between the *x*-axis and the line of equality (EER < CER).

Visual inspection gives a quick and easy indication of the level of agreement among trials. Heterogeneity is often assumed to be due to variation in the EER—the effect of the intervention. Figure 1 shows that variation in the CER can also be a source of heterogeneity, even though the controls were all matched placebos in relatively homogeneous acute pain conditions with single dose treatment.

L'Abbé plots have several benefits and the simple visual presentation is easy to assimilate. They make us think about the reasons why there can be such wide variation in (especially) placebo responses, and about other factors in the overall package of care that can contribute to effectiveness. They explain the need for placebo controls if ethical issues about future trials arise. They keep us sceptical about overly good or bad results for an intervention in a single trial where the major influence may be how good or bad was the response with placebo.

Variation in control (placebo) response rates Variation in CER is not unusual. Similar variation was seen in trials of antiemetics in post-operative vomiting,[26] and in six trials of prophylactic natural surfactant for preterm

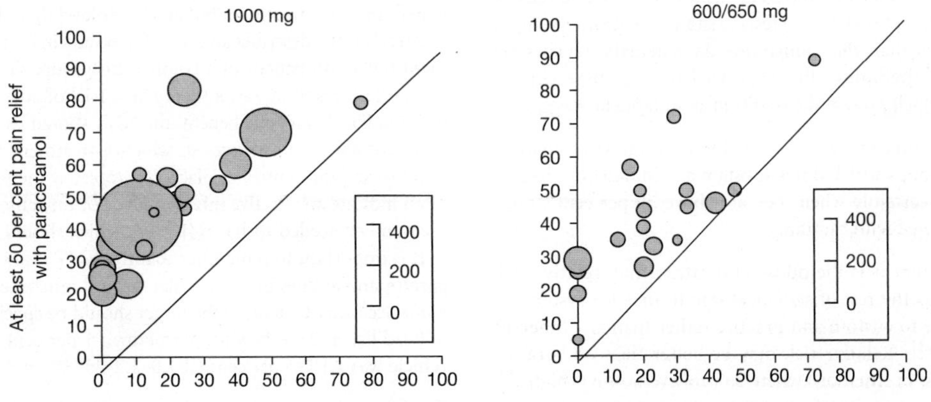

Fig. 1 L'Abbé plot of EER (% >50% relief on treatment) against CER (% >50% relief on placebo) for RCTs of paracetamol 1000 and 600/650 mg.

infants, the CER for bronchopulmonary dysplasia was 24–69 per cent.[27] Such variation would not be expected in other circumstances, like use of antimicrobials. Rates of eradication of *Helicobacter pylori* with short-term use of ulcer healing drugs were 0–17 per cent in 11 RCTs (with 10 of 11 below 10 per cent).[28]

The reason for large variations in event rates with placebo may have something to do with trial design and population. The overwhelming reason for large variations in placebo rates in pain studies (and probably studies in other clinical conditions) is the relatively small group sizes in trials. Group sizes are chosen to produce statistical significance through power calculations—for pain studies, the usual size is 30–40 patients for a 30 per cent difference between placebo and active analgesic. An individual patient can have no pain relief or 100 per cent pain relief. Random selection of patients can therefore produce groups with low placebo response rate or high placebo response rate, or somewhere in between. Mathematical modelling based on individual patient data shows that while group sizes of up to 50 patients are likely to show a statistical difference 80–90 per cent of the time, to generate a close approximation to the 'true' clinical impact of a therapy requires as many as 500 patients per group (or more than 1000 patients in a trial).[29] Credible NNTs for analgesics need data from 500 patients.

The lessons are that information from individual trials of small size should be treated with circumspection in pain and probably other therapeutic areas, and that variation in outcomes seen in trials of small size is probably artefactual.

Heterogeneity Clinicians making decisions on the basis of systematic reviews need to be confident that apples are not being compared with oranges. The L'Abbé plot is a qualitative defence against this problem. While statistical testing ostensibly provides a quantitative way of checking for heterogeneity, the tests lack power,[30] so that while a test positive for heterogeneity suggests mixed fruits are being compared, a negative test does not provide complete reassurance that there is no heterogeneity. Heterogeneity will also appear to occur because of variations in control and experimental event rates due to the random play of chance in trials of small size. Generally, trials of fewer than 10 patients per group should be omitted from systematic reviews,[25] but considerable variability will occur in group sizes below 50 patients. The crucial issues are whether the trials are clinically homogeneous and sufficiently large.

Indirect versus direct comparisons What clinicians really need are the results of direct comparisons of the different interventions, so called head-to-head comparisons. These are rarely available, and what we have to work with are comparisons of each of the interventions with placebo. Indeed, at present we have no method to use the data from the direct comparisons of efficacy. The methods illustrated here tell us how fast each competitor runs against the clock, rather than who crosses the line first in a head-to-head challenge.

Statistical significance

When it is legitimate and feasible to combine data, the odds ratio and relative risk (or benefit) are the accepted statistical tests to show that the intervention works significantly better than the comparator. As systematic reviews are used more to compare therapies, clinicians need to grip these clinical epidemiological tools, which present the results in an unfamiliar way.

Odds ratios The odds ratio can give a distorted impression when analyses are conducted on subgroups which differ substantially in baseline risk.[31] Where CERs are high (certainly when they are above 50 per cent), odds ratios should be interpreted with caution.

Relative risk The fact that it is the odds ratio rather than relative risk reduction that is used as the test of statistical significance for systematic reviews seems to be due to custom and practice rather than any inherent intellectual advantage.[31] Relative risk may be better than odds ratios because it is more robust in situations where control event rate is high.[32] With event rates above 10 per cent relative risk produces more conservative figures.[33] There is still considerable uncertainty and disagreement amongst statisticians and reviewers as to whether odds ratios or relative risk should be used. Importantly odds ratios should be interpreted with caution when events occur commonly—as in treatments—and odds ratio may overestimate the benefits of an effect when event rates are above 50 per cent. They are likely to be superseded by relative risk because it is more robust in situations where event rates are high.[2,31]

How well does the intervention work? Clinical significance

While odds ratios and relative risks can show that an intervention works compared with control they are of limited help in telling clinicians how well the intervention works—the size of the effect or its clinical significance.

Effect size One method of estimating the amount of benefit, the effect size is to use the standardized mean difference.[34] The advantages of this approach are that it can be used to compare the efficacy of different interventions measured on continuous rather than dichotomous scales, and even using different outcome measures. The *z*-score output is in standard deviation units, and therefore is scale-free. The (major) disadvantage of effect size is that it is not intuitive for clinicians.

Number-needed-to-treat The NNT is the number of people who have to be treated for one to achieve the specified level of benefit. This concept is proving to be a very effective alternative as the measure of clinical significance from quantitative systematic reviews. It has the crucial advantage of applicability to clinical practice, and shows the effort required to achieve a particular therapeutic target.

Technically, the NNT is the reciprocal of the absolute risk reduction, and is given by the equation

$$\mathrm{NNT} = \frac{1}{(\mathrm{IMP}_{\mathrm{act}}/\mathrm{TOT}_{\mathrm{act}}) - (\mathrm{IMP}_{\mathrm{con}}/\mathrm{TOT}_{\mathrm{con}})}$$

where $\mathrm{IMP}_{\mathrm{act}}$ is the number of patients given active treatment achieving the target, $\mathrm{TOT}_{\mathrm{act}}$, the total number of patients given the active treatment, $\mathrm{IMP}_{\mathrm{con}}$, the number of patients given a control treatment achieving the target, and $\mathrm{TOT}_{\mathrm{con}}$, the total number of patients given the control treatment.

Advantage The advantage of the NNT is that it is clinically intuitive, showing how many patients need to be treated for one to benefit. It is treatment specific. It describes the difference between active treatment and control. The level of benefit or threshold used to calculate NNT can be varied, but the NNT is likely to be relatively unchanged because changing threshold changes results for both active and control. The threshold used for the single dose analgesic data (see Fig. 2) was 50 per cent pain relief. This is a difficult target for analgesics, and, in cancer pain, patients feel a treatment is beneficial if it produces 30 per cent relief.[35] What is judged worthwhile relief may vary with the clinical context, but in terms of the NNT calculation the choice of threshold makes little impact on the relative efficacy of the different treatments, because the results for the control will improve if the threshold is lowered, and deteriorate at a higher threshold. Some patients will of course benefit from the treatment but at a lower level than the threshold.

An NNT of 1 describes an event that occurs in every patient given the treatment but in no patient in a comparator group. This could be described as the 'perfect' result in, say, a therapeutic trial of an antibiotic compared with placebo. For therapeutic benefit, the NNT should be as close as possible to 1; there are few circumstances in which a treatment is close to 100 per cent effective and the control or placebo completely ineffective, so NNTs of 2 or 3 often indicate an effective intervention. For unwanted effects, NNT becomes the number-needed-to-harm (NNH), which should be as large as possible.

It is important to remember that the NNT is always relative to the comparator and applies to a particular clinical outcome. The duration of treatment necessary to achieve the target should be specified. The NNT for cure of head lice at 2 weeks with permethrin 1 per cent compared with control vehicle was 1.1 (95 per cent CI 1.0–1.2).[36,37]

Confidence intervals The confidence intervals of the NNT are an indication that 19 times out of 20 the 'true' value will be in the specified range. If there

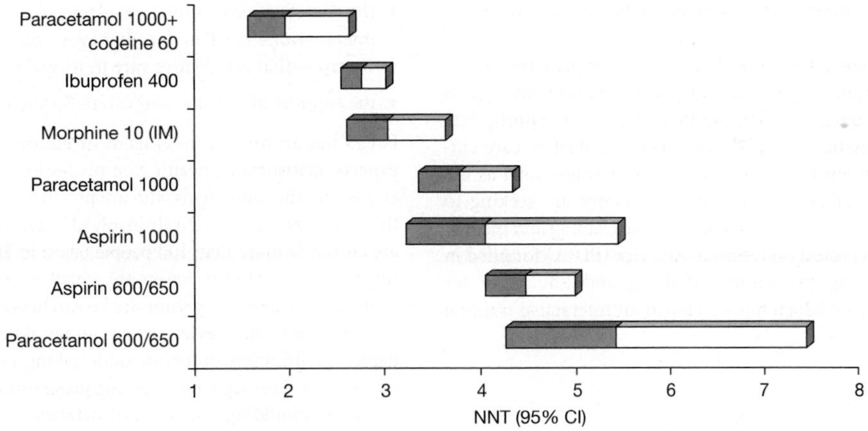

Fig. 2 NNT for 50% pain relief in post-operative pain (single dose). NNT point estimate is at the junction of the grey and white bar segments. Grey bar segment is the lower 95% confidence interval, white is the upper.

is inadequate or conflicting data then the NNT may not have finite confidence intervals, and the statistical tests (odds ratio or relative risk) will not be statistically significant. An NNT with an infinite confidence interval may still have clinical value as a benchmark, but should be treated cautiously until further data permits finite confidence intervals.

Disadvantages The disadvantage of the NNT approach—apparent from the formula—is that it needs dichotomous data. Continuous data can be converted to dichotomous for acute pain studies so that NNTs may be calculated, by deriving a relationship between the two from individual patient data.[38] Because of the way it is calculated, NNT will also be sensitive to trials with high CERs. As CER rises, the potential for treatment specific improvement decreases: higher (and apparently less effective) NNTs result. So, as with any summary measure from a quantitative systematic review, NNT needs to be treated with caution, and comparisons can only be made confidently if the pooled trials do not show major variation in their CERs.

Evaluating safety

Estimating the risk of harm is a critical part of clinical decisions. Systematic reviews should report adverse events as well as efficacy, and consider the issue of rare but important adverse events. Large RCTs apart, most trials study limited patient numbers. New medicines may be launched after trials on 1500 patients,[39] missing these rare but important adverse events. The rule of three is important here. If a particular serious event does not occur in 1500 patients given the treatment, we can be 95 per cent confident that the chance of it occurring is at most 3/1500.[40]

Much the same rules apply to harm as to efficacy, but with some important differences, the rules of admissible evidence and the NNH rather than NNT. The absence of information on adverse effects in systematic reviews reduces their usefulness.

Rules of evidence

The gold standard of evidence for harm—as for efficacy—is the RCT. The problem is that in the relatively small number of patients studied in RCTs rare serious harm may not be spotted. Therefore, study architectures of lower intrinsic quality may be admissible for an adverse effect systematic review. An extreme example is that observer blinding is superfluous if the outcome is death. Such rare and serious harm cannot and should not be dismissed just because it is reported in a case report rather than in an RCT. The 'process rules' in this area have yet to be determined.

Number-needed-to-harm

For adverse effects reported in RCTs, NNH may be calculated in the same way as NNT. When there is low incidence it is likely that point estimates alone will emerge (infinite confidence intervals). Major harm may be defined in a set of RCTs as intervention-related study withdrawal, and be calculated from those numbers. Precise estimates of major harm will require much wider literature searches to trawl for case reports or series. Minor harm may similarly be defined in a set of RCTs as reported adverse effects. The utility of these reports is because they are reported simply as present or absent, with no indication of severity or importance to the patient.

Conclusion: using NNT and NNH to evaluate analgesics

In the ideal world you will have three numbers for each intervention, an NNT for benefit and NNHs for minor and major harm. The thrust of this chapter is that these methods can be used to show the effectiveness or otherwise of a range of interventions, and if effective, to use the NNT as a benchmark of just how effective a particular intervention is. This then becomes the yardstick against which alternative interventions, each with its NNT for benefit, NNH for minor harm and NNH for major harm should be judged, and is the pivot for the clinical decision on whether or not to use the intervention for an individual patient. Figure 2 ranks the analgesics by their efficacy estimate; clinical choice might be to prescribe or take a safer although marginally less effective drug.

To provide robust recommendations on choice of analgesic, prescription or over-the-counter, requires evidence of the highest quality. These methods can deliver high quality efficacy estimates if there are randomized trials of adequate size and quality, but not if the trials are deficient in number, size or quality. Safety estimates are more difficult, not least because the data from which they are derived come commonly from study designs which are not randomized and hence more subject to bias.

Extrapolation to palliative care

More than 15 000 RCTs have been identified in the general area of pain and a few hundred systematic reviews exist.[41] The palliative care seam is much thinner with some 1200 RCTs identified, about half of which deal with palliative chemotherapy. There are just a handful of systematic reviews to inform practice. Systematic reviews by definition rely on RCTs as the raw material. EBM has highlighted many gaps in its pursuit of answers and this is equally true in palliative medicine. There are signs of a positive move to higher quality research but this depends on funding, academic recognition, high-quality journals, and greater coordination and collaboration between palliative care centres.[42] The US Institute of Medicine publication *Approaching Death—Improving Care at the End of Life*[43] states 'Important gaps in scientific knowledge about the end of life need serious attention from researchers', and 'current knowledge and understanding are insufficient to guide and support the consistent practice of evidence-based medicine at the end of life'.

There is an increasing voice for promoting research in palliative medicine,(44) against a background where some considered research among this group of patients to be unethical. The limited amount of appropriate research itself limits the chances of improvements in a palliative care culture which relies primarily on clinical experience.(44) Groups such as the European Association of Palliative Care research network are seeking to change this.(45) Other developments seeking to improve training and incorporate evidence include the Project on Death in America (PDIA) founded in 1994 aimed at transforming the culture of dying and Education for Physicians on end-of-life care which has developed an interactive training programme.(46)

The Cochrane Pain, Palliative Care and Supportive Care Collaborative Review Group (PaPaS)

The Cochrane Collaboration(47) is an international not-for-profit organization that aims to 'prepare, maintain and disseminate *systematic reviews* of the effects of health care'. It has come about as a product of several concerns and developments:

- an awareness of the huge volume of medicine related literature and a lack of any coordinated analysis of this;
- the emergence of EBM concepts which have grown to embrace the whole of healthcare and health care practitioners;
- the availability and potential of the Internet. This has enabled a global research community to develop and thrive in a collaborative fashion.

Systematic reviews undertaken by the Cochrane Collaboration are published in *The Cochrane Library*(48) which is available by subscription as a CD-ROM (issued quarterly) or on-line via the Internet. The published reviews include a full publication containing the background and methods, a detailed analysis with graphical displays where appropriate, an abstract and 100-word synopsis.

As well as Cochrane systematic reviews, other health care databases are included in *The Cochrane Library:*

- the Cochrane Controlled Trials Register (a bibliographic database of controlled trials)—this contains some 300 000 references to RCTs that have been identified by the Collaboration;
- the Database of Abstracts of Reviews of Effectiveness (DARE) (structured abstracts of over 2000 systematic reviews which have been critically appraised by reviewers at the NHS Centre for Reviews and Dissemination in York and by other people, e.g. from the American College of Physicians' Journal Club and the journal *Evidence-Based Medicine*);
- the Cochrane Methodology Register (a bibliography of articles on the science of research synthesis).

Collaborative Review Groups (CRGs) comprise an international multidisciplinary group from around the world who share an interest in developing and maintaining systematic reviews relevant to a particular health area. Groups are coordinated by an editorial team who edit and assemble completed reviews for inclusion in *The Cochrane Library*. Each group is organized around a small team of coordinating editor and review group coordinator who are responsible for managing the group and for the quality of its output. There are currently 50 CRGs based in a number of countries, each addressing a particular health care area. The Pain, Palliative and Supportive Care Group (PaPaS)(49) is one such group and has its editorial base at the Pain Research Unit, Oxford, UK. PaPaS aims to generate evidence about the effectiveness of health care treatments relevant to:

- the prevention and treatment of pain;
- the relief of symptoms resulting from both the disease process, interventions used in the management of the disease, and symptom control—that is palliative care in its widest sense;
- the support of patients and carers through the disease process.

PaPaS has an international team of editors and peer reviewers—clinical experts, statisticians, health care professionals, consumers—who support and advise the individuals who are preparing systematic reviews. As regards the reviewers who are actively involved in preparing systematic reviews, there are currently more than 100 people based in 18 countries that are contributing to reviews. Most reviewers are practitioners who are researching a review topic in their own time; some are researchers who have obtained funding to work full-time on a review, or are undertaking a review as part of a higher degree qualification, others are undertaking a review as the research element of their specialist registrars training programme in palliative medicine.

PaPaS is building a specialized database of all known RCTs and clinical controlled trials related to pain, palliative and supportive care—irrespective of language of publication. This database is used as a resource by reviewers to identify trials for possible inclusion in systematic reviews.

In the first 4 years of operation, PaPaS has published 26 research protocols and 17 completed reviews in the Cochrane Library; there are a further 50 reviews in progress.

Some examples from the palliative care field include:

- benzodiazepines for insomnia in palliative care;
- calcitonin for bone pain and complications secondary to bone metastases;
- drug treatments for anxiety in palliative care;
- drug treatments for delirium in palliative care;
- interventions for supporting adults and children through bereavement;
- interventions for the management of constipation in cancer patients;
- interventions for the management of skin (and mucous membranes) before, during, and after radiation therapy;
- ketamine as an adjuvant to opioids for cancer pain;
- metoclopramide for chemotherapy-induced nausea and vomiting;
- pharmacological and psychological interventions for low mood in palliative care patients;
- radionucleotides for bone pain and complications secondary to bone metastases;
- supportive care for symptom relief in patients with gastrointestinal cancer;
- acupuncture for chemotherapy-induced nausea or vomiting among cancer patients;
- bisphosphonates for pain secondary to bone metastases;
- cannabinoids for chemotherapy-induced nausea and vomiting;
- cannabinoids for pain management;
- dexamethasone for the treatment of emesis induced by cytotoxic drugs;
- feeding regimes for bone marrow transplant patients;
- hydromorphone for pain relief;
- massage and aromatherapy massage for symptom relief in patients with cancer;
- megestrol for cancer cachexia;
- opioids for the palliation of breathlessness in terminal illness;
- pleurodesis for malignant pleural effusions;
- psychotherapeutic treatments for the management of chronic pain in children;
- reflexology for symptom relief in patients with cancer.

Table 4 shows the number of journals identified by the PaPaS group as containing trials relevant to palliative care, the spread of languages and the

Table 4 Identified journals in palliative care

Number of journals	31
Languages	6 (2 Asian)
Indexed in MEDLINE	6
Indexed in EmBASE	3 (2 unique)
Hand-searched by PaPaS	11

fact that many are not indexed in MEDLINE or EmBASE. Clearly, there is still a lot to do.

Conclusions

If there is a theme to this chapter on evidence-based medicine and palliative care, it is that we know how to provide robust evidence about the efficacy of interventions. To provide that evidence we need high-quality trials. We should not shy away from doing high-quality trials in palliative care just because they are difficult. At the same time we need to acknowledge that the methodology is not adequate yet to design quality studies of the ways in which we deliver care, either packages of care or the context in which they are delivered. The finite necessities are the fact that we know how to do some (relatively simple) trials and reviews. The infinite luxuries are all the questions to which we do not yet have the answers.

References

1. **Oxford Centre for Evidence-based Medicine.** Levels of Evidence and Grades of Recommendations (Web page). Available at http://cebm.jr2.ox.ac.uk/docs/levels.html. (Accessed 30 January 2002.)
2. **Sackett, D., Richardson, W.S., Rosenberg, W., and Haynes, B.** *Evidence Based Medicine.* London: Churchill Livingstone, 1996.
3. **Schulz, K.F., Chalmers, I., Hayes, R.J., and Altman, D.G.** (1995). Empirical evidence of bias: dimensions of methodological quality associated with estimates of treatment effects in controlled trials. *Journal of the American Medical Association* **273**, 408–12.
4. **Chalmers, I., Dickersin, K., and Chalmers, T.** (1992). Getting to grips with Archie Cochrane's agenda. *British Medical Journal* **305**, 786–7.
5. **Jadad, A.R. and McQuay, H.J.** (1993). A high-yield strategy to identify randomized controlled trials for systematic reviews. *Online Journal of Current Clinical Trials* (Serial Online) Doc No. 33; 3973 words, 39 paragraphs, 5 tables.
6. **Simes, R.J.** (1987). Confronting publication bias: a cohort design for meta-analysis. *Statistics in Medicine* **6**, 11–29.
7. **Hetherington, J., Dickerson, K., Chalmers, I., and Meinert, C.** (1989). Retrospective and prospective identification of unpublished controlled trials: lessons from a survey of obstetricians and pediatricians. *Pediatrics* **84**, 374–80.
8. **Jadad, A.R., Carroll, D., Moore, A., and McQuay, H.** (1996). Developing a database of published reports of randomised clinical trials in pain research. *Pain* **66**, 239–46.
9. **Carroll, D., Tramer, M., McQuay, H., Nye, B., and Moore, A.** (1996). Randomization is important in studies with pain outcomes: systematic review of transcutaneous electrical nerve stimulation in acute postoperative pain. *British Journal of Anaesthesia* **77** (6), 798–803.
10. **Jadad, A.R.** et al. (1996). Assessing the quality of reports of randomized clinical trials: is blinding necessary? *Controlled Clinical Trials* **17**, 1–12.
11. **Chalmers, T.C.** et al. (1981). A method for assessing the quality of a randomized control trial. *Controlled Clinical Trials* **2**, 31–49.
12. **Fleiss, J.L. and Gross, A.J.** (1991). Meta-analysis in epidemiology, with special reference to studies of the association between exposure to environmental tobacco smoke and lung cancer: a critique. *Journal of Clinical Epidemiology* **44**, 127–39.
13. **Nurmohamed, M.T.** et al. (1992). Low molecular-weight heparin versus standard heparin in general and orthopaedic surgery: a meta-analysis. *Lancet* **340**, 152–6.
14. **ter Riet, G., Kleijnen, J., and Knipschild, P.** (1990). Acupuncture and chronic pain: a criteria-based meta-analysis. *Journal of Clinical Epidemiology* **43** (11), 1191–9.
15. **Koes, B.W., Bouter, L.M., Beckerman, H., van, d.H.G., and Knipschild, P.G.** (1991). Physiotherapy exercises and back pain: a blinded review (see comments). *British Medical Journal* **302** (6792), 1572–6.
16. **Koes, B.W., Assendelft, W.J., van, d.H.G., Bouter, L.M., and Knipschild, P.G.** (1991). Spinal manipulation and mobilisation for back and neck pain: a blinded review (see comments). *British Medical Journal* **303** (6813), 1298–303.
17. **Chalmers, I., Hetherington, J., Elbourne, D., Keirse, M.J.N.C., and Enkin, M.** (1989). Materials and methods used in synthesizing evidence to evaluate the effects of care during pregnancy and childbirth. In *Effective Care in Pregnancy and Childbirth* (ed. I. Chalmers, M. Enkin, and M.J.N.C. Keirse), pp. 38–65. Oxford: Oxford University Press.
18. **Chalmers, I.** (1989). Evaluating the effects of care during pregnancy and childbirth. In *Effective Care in Pregnancy and Childbirth* (ed. I. Chalmers, M. Enkin, and M.J.N.C. Keirse), pp. 1–37. Oxford: Oxford University Press.
19. **Sackett, D.L. and Gent, M.** (1979). Controversy in counting and attributing events in clinical trials. *New England Journal of Medicine* **301**, 1410–12.
20. **Peto, R.** et al. (1976). Design and analysis of randomised clinical trials requiring prolonged observation of each patient. 1. Introduction and design. *British Journal of Cancer* **34**, 585–612.
21. **Kalso, E., Tramer, M., Carroll, D., McQuay, H., and Moore, R.A.** (1997). Pain relief from intra-articular morphine after knee surgery: a qualitative systematic review. *Pain* **71**, 642–51.
22. **Rodgers, A.** et al. (2000). Reduction of postoperative mortality and morbidity with epidural or spinal anaesthesia: results from overview of randomised trials. *British Medical Journal* **321** (7275), 1493.
23. **Smith, L.A., Oldman, A.D., McQuay, H.J., and Moore, R.A.** (2000). Tearing apart quality and validity in systematic reviews: an example from acupuncture trials in chronic neck and back pain. *Pain* **86**, 119–32.
24. **Oxman, A.D. and Guyatt, G.H.** (1988). Guidelines for reading literature reviews. *Canadian Medical Association Journal* **138**, 697–703.
25. **L'Abbé, K.A., Detsky, A.S., and O'Rourke, K.** (1987). Meta-analysis in clinical research. *Annals of Internal Medicine* **107**, 224–33.
26. **Tramer, M., Moore, A., and McQuay, H.** (1995). Prevention of vomiting after paediatric strabismus surgery: a systematic review using the numbers-needed-to-treat method. *British Journal of Anaesthesia* **75** (5), 556–61.
27. **Soll, J.C. and McQueen, M.C.** (1992). Respiratory distress syndrome. In *Effective Care of the Newborn Infant* (ed. J.C. Sinclair and M.E. Bracken), Chapter 15, p. 333. Oxford: Oxford University Press.
28. **Moore, R.A.** *Helicobacter pylori* and peptic ulcer. A systematic review of effectiveness and an overview of the economic benefits of implementing that which is known to be effective (Web page), 1995: Available at http://www.jr2.ox.ac.uk/Bandolier/bandopubs/hpyl/hpall.html.
29. **Moore, R.A., Gavaghan, D., Tramer, M.R., Collins, S.L., and McQuay, H.J.** (1998). Size is everything—large amounts of information are needed to overcome random effects in estimating direction and magnitude of treatment effects. *Pain* **78** (3), 209–16.
30. **Gavaghan, D.J., Moore, R.A., and McQuay, H.J.** (2000). An evaluation of homogeneity tests in meta-analyses in pain using simulations of individual patient data. *Pain* **85**, 415–24.
31. **Sinclair, J.C. and Bracken, M.B.** (1994). Clinically useful measures of effect in binary analyses of randomized trials. *Journal of Clinical Epidemiology* **47** (8), 881–9.
32. **Sackett, D.L., Deeks, J.J., and Altman, D.G.** (1996). Down with odds ratios! *Evidence-Based Medicine* **1**, 164–6.
33. **Deeks, J.** (1996). What the heck's an odds ratio? *Bandolier* **3** (3), 6–7.
34. **Glass, G.V.** (1976). Primary, secondary, and meta-analysis of research. *Education Research* **5**, 3–8.
35. **Farrar, J.T., Portenoy, R.K., Berlin, J.A., Kinman, J.L., and Strom, B.L.** (2000). Defining the clinically important difference in pain outcome measures. *Pain* **88** (3), 287–94.

36. **Van der Stichele, R.H., Dezeure, E.M., and Bogaert, M.G.** (1995). Systematic review of clinical efficacy of topical treatments for head lice. *British Medical Journal* **311**, 604–8.

37. **Moore, R.A., McQuay, H., and Gray, M.** *Bandolier—The First 20 Issues.* Oxford: Bandolier, 1995.

38. **Moore, A., McQuay, H., and Gavaghan, D.** (1996). Deriving dichotomous outcome measures from continuous data in randomised controlled trials of analgesics. *Pain* **66**, 229–37.

39. **Moore, T.J.** *Deadly Medicine.* New York: Simon & Schuster, 1995.

40. **Eypasch, E., Lefering, R., Kum, C.K., and Troidl, H.** (1995). Probability of adverse events that have not yet occurred: a statistical reminder. *British Medical Journal* **311**, 619–20.

41. **Systematic reviews on pain topics** (Web page). Available at http://www.jr2.ox.ac.uk/Bandolier/painres/MApain.html. (Accessed 15 March 2002.)

42. **Bruera, E.** (1998). Research into symptoms other than pain. In *Oxford Textbook of Palliative Medicine* 2nd edn, Section T.3. (ed. D. Doyle, G. Hanks, and N. MacDonald), Oxford: Oxford University Press.

43. **Field, M.J.C.C.** *Approaching Death: Improving Care at the End of Life.* Washington DC: National Academy Press, 1997.

44. **Kaasa, S. and De Conno, F.** (2001). Palliative care research. *European Journal of Cancer* **37** (Suppl. 8), S153–9.

45. **EAPC—European Association of Palliative Care** (Web page). Available at www.eapcnet.org/home.html. (Accessed 20 February 2002.)

46. **EPEC. Education for Physicians on end of life care** (Web page). 31 January 2002. Available at www.epec.net.

47. **Cochrane. The Cochrane Collaboration** (Web page). Available at www.cochrane.org. (Accessed 20 February 2002.)

48. **Cochrane Library. The Cochrane Library** (Web page). Available at www.update-software.com/Cochrane/default.HTM. (Accessed 20 February 2002.)

49. **PaPaS—Pain, Palliative and Supportive Care Group, Cochrane Collaboration** (Web page). Available at www.jr2.ox.ac.uk/cochrane. (Accessed 20 February 2002.)

5.2 Research in palliative care: getting started

Geoffrey Hanks, Stein Kaasa, and Margaret Robbins

> Ignorance has risks, but they are largely unseen and unnoticed. Gaining knowledge has risks which are noticed, but largely unpredictable, and it is very costly (though less so than prolonged ignorance). It focuses blame, whereas ignorance dispels it. So, maintaining ignorance often seems more attractive than gaining knowledge.
>
> Duncan Vere[1]

Introduction

We make no apology for opening this chapter again with the words of Professor Duncan Vere, Professor of Clinical Pharmacology & Therapeutics at the London Hospital, and a research adviser at St Christopher's Hospice in the early days of modern palliative care. Research in palliative care remains in the doldrums in spite of apparent wide recognition of its importance amongst palliative care practitioners and the continued development of new clinical services across the world. These developments are not being driven by research findings. We do not have data that tell us what is the most cost-effective model of service delivery of palliative care, or, in fact, can we answer the more basic question of what models are *effective.* There remain large areas of clinical practice in palliative care that are based on clinical experience rather than high-quality evidence, and this applies even to core activities such as the control of pain. There is an urgent need to establish a more substantial evidence base, because this is a cross-cutting area of health care that is relevant to many other specialties and disciplines.

A report on cancer research in the United Kingdom from the recently established National Cancer Research Institute (NCRI) highlights the fact that one of the most poorly funded areas in the combined research portfolios of the major cancer research funding organizations in the United Kingdom is palliative care.[2] This has prompted the NCRI to set up a strategic review group to analyse the background and reasons for the relatively poor state of palliative care research and make proposals for remedying this situation. This is not a problem unique to the United Kingdom: analysis of research outputs in terms of publications and potential impact suggests that this relative paucity of research activity is a worldwide phenomenon. In this chapter, we explore some of the reasons for this, give some advice about practical aspects of undertaking research in palliative care, and also suggest some possible ways to progress in the future. Other chapters in this section discuss in more detail evidence-based medicine and qualitative research in palliative care.

Research in palliative care: the beginning

Modern palliative care has its origins in the opening of St Christopher's Hospice in London in 1967. St Christopher's was different from other long-established hospices and homes for the terminally ill because its aim was to integrate 'a scientific programme concerned with the discriminating use of drugs with the tender loving care'[3] provided within these other institutions. From the outset, research was a priority and the studies in pain control by Twycross[4] and in the evaluation of hospice care by Murray-Parkes[5] had a considerable impact on the development of the specialty and widespread influence outside it. Since that time, much has been achieved and there have been many advances that are described throughout this book. However, that initial urgency and enthusiasm to gain a basic understanding of the physiology and pharmacology of the dying/severely ill patient and to evaluate rigorously the care that was provided and the treatment that was given has not grown and matured. As palliative care has developed into the mainstream of health care, research, paradoxically, has tended to take a back seat. Indeed, there is still a widespread view that scientifically rigorous clinical research is incompatible with the basic tenets of palliative care: 'few people associate hospices with science-based medicine'.[6] Yet, as in any other field of health care, practitioners have an obligation to provide the best possible treatment and care to patients at the end of their lives. The only way to ensure that high standards are established and maintained is through an understanding of the pathophysiological processes involved in patients with advanced disease and by evaluating the treatments that are employed using the most robust methodology that can be applied. Research is essential in order to be confident that current practice is best practice. However, there is a need now for strategic investment in researchers, facilities, and infrastructure to give some substance to the often articulated exhortations for more research in palliative care.

Obstacles to research in palliative care

Research has not yet become embedded in the culture of palliative care. The issues of the primacy of the individual and whole person care versus the 'greatest happiness of the greatest number' are brought sharply into focus in palliative care. The physician's obligation to keep the patient's interest paramount is a fundamental precept of medical practice and is given great emphasis in palliative care. However, the physician has another obligation, which is to promote the acquisition of scientific knowledge. These obligations constitute a real conflict and raise difficult ethical dilemmas. In daily clinical practice, patient care seems always 'to win' over research when time is limited. Other members of the team will face similar dilemmas and this may be particularly acute for non-medical practitioners who are not so constrained by the biomedical model of health and ill-health and may be unsympathetic to research that is focused only or predominantly in this direction. Thus, there is a need to change the culture of palliative care so that research is seen as an integral and essential part of the discipline, and also to be eclectic in the approach to research and the choice of methodologies that are employed.

There are problems in attracting high-quality researchers into palliative care. This is partly a consequence of the uncertain career structures and a relative lack of training opportunities (which reflects the lack of funds and investment). There are very few academic departments and fewer still that have sufficient core funding to allow the development of blue sky research programmes. Substantial investment in departments that have the critical mass and facilities to allow high-quality research to be undertaken would take research in palliative care a quantum leap forward. But no such investment is on the horizon and palliative care researchers need to compete with other disciplines who have decades of tradition in performing research. 'Comfort care' research is always likely to be less attractive to grant awarding bodies than molecular genetics. However, it is increasingly apparent that molecular biology may be a fertile area for exploring research questions of direct relevance to palliative care practice. Translational research is one of the priority areas for palliative care: academic departments of palliative care may need to broaden their base to include laboratory scientists as well as social anthropologists, ethicists, and clinicians.

Palliative medicine has been a recognized speciality in the United Kingdom for 15 years but it remains the case that physicians may reach consultant status (attending, specialist) with very little experience of research. Even if they do have experience and are interested in doing research the clinical pressures and lack of infrastructure support may make it impossible for them to engage in worthwhile studies. The situation in other countries in Europe and in the United States has been similar though new initiatives to establish academic departments and research networks are now emerging in many parts of the world and in some training programmes in palliative medicine it is necessary to undertake and publish a research project. Research is a mandatory part of the training programme in the Nordic Curriculum in Palliative Medicine and in the United Kingdom may take up 1 year of the 4-year higher specialist training. There is a need to encourage specialist trainees to take time out to do research. It is vital that we consolidate what has been achieved already and do not lose key posts as the first generation of palliative care researchers approach retirement. At the same time new training and substantive posts for researchers are needed together with the right sort of support for them.

National and international organizations in palliative care have a key role to play. The European Association for Palliative Care has led the way by establishing a Research Network and one of its initial studies, a cross-sectional survey of palliative care in Europe, has demonstrated the great potential of palliative care research networks to work in a coherent and collaborative fashion.(7) Few individual services are able to complete good clinical studies in a reasonable period of time because of small numbers. The future for palliative care research lies with networks be they local, regional, national, or international.

The ethics of research in palliative care (see also Chapter 3.6)

Much progress in medicine is achieved through advances in basic science, but it also depends on clinical research, which, by definition, means research involving patients. Serendipity continues to play a role in advancing knowledge as does astute clinical observation. But none of these mechanisms can be relied on to ensure progress; human experimentation based on the scientific method is essential for medicine to continue to advance. This argument applies to palliative care as it does to any other area of medicine.

The Declaration of Helsinki, drawn up by the World Medical Association in 1964 (and amended in 1975 and 1983) was a response to the need for a code of ethics on human experimentation that would be applicable to all countries and all situations where human subjects were involved in research.(8) The code acknowledges the need for guidance for physician investigators caught in the conflict between the patient's own best interests and the necessity to advance knowledge for the benefit of society as a whole.

The Declaration of Helsinki is generally accepted as an ethical code of practice for clinical research and its principles are applicable to palliative medicine. It is important that clinical research is seen to conform to these principles and that all research projects are scrutinized by independent assessors to ensure that this is the case. This function is usually under-taken by a local Research Ethics Committee and now in many countries there is a comprehensive network of local and multicentre research ethics committees.

Research governance

In recent years, there has been a trend towards increasingly explicit guidelines and regulations relating to research involving patients. In the United Kingdom, these guidelines are described under the heading of 'research governance'. Research can involve an element of risk regarding both the return on investment and the safety and well-being of participants. The research governance guidelines are designed to minimize risk and improve research performance and they provide a useful framework, particularly for those new to research, which has general applicability and is not only relevant in the United Kingdom.

Research governance is 'the means by which we ensure high scientific, ethical, and financial standards for the conduct of research and involves transparent decision-making processes, clear allocation of responsibilities, and robust monitoring arrangements'. The research governance framework for health and social care in the United Kingdom encompasses five domains. These are ethics (the dignity, rights, safety, and well-being of participants); science (the quality and appropriateness of research); information (the requirements for free access to research information); health, safety, and employment (of participants and research and other staff); and finance and intellectual property. The background and details of the Research Governance Framework are available at: www.doh.gov.uk/research/RD3/nhsrandd/researchgovernance.htm.

Controlled clinical trials and informed consent in palliative medicine

Austin Bradford Hill set out the ethical precepts for randomized controlled trials (RCTs) in his Marc Daniels Lecture at the Royal College of Physicians in 1963.(9) In the United States, Henry Beecher had a similar influence on the development of ethical guidelines for clinical research,(10) and the subject has been debated in many places since. It is not appropriate to discuss this subject in detail here but the reader is referred to these reviews as they make two important points. The first is that the prospective RCT is the most efficient, scientific way of evaluating a new treatment or of comparing alternative treatments, but the second is that it is not the only way of ensuring the advance of reliable knowledge.

Controlled clinical trials are necessary in palliative medicine, and the usual guidelines and ethical principles will apply. Some points need particular emphasis in the palliative care setting. Patients are invariably at a low ebb physically and many are elderly and frail; most have a multitude of physical and emotional and perhaps social and spiritual problems. When they come to the palliative care unit or team many of these problems will be dealt with, and some, particularly the psychosocial issues, may receive attention for the first time. The supportive environment in palliative care may make patients particularly keen to give something back to the carers, to show their gratitude for the care they are receiving. All of these factors make patients particularly vulnerable when they are asked to participate in any sort of research project, for many will feel almost an obligation to accede to such a request. Researchers in palliative care must be on their guard not to take advantage of this situation.

In palliative care, cognitive impairment and often frank confusion is a problem encountered in many patients; when this is obvious they will be excluded from consideration for entry to a study. However, often the impairment is mild or variable. Such patients need careful assessment, and, wherever there is any doubt that the patient is able to understand what is being asked of him, he or she should not be considered for inclusion.

There is a fine balance that needs to be achieved here. The special vulnerability of patients receiving palliative care dictates the need for special handling in obtaining consent to participate in research but at the same time the researcher must not go out of his or her way to talk the patient out of wanting to take part.

Evidence-based palliative care (see Chapter 5.1)

The principles of evidence-based medicine underpin our day-to-day clinical practice. Evidence-based medicine 'is the conscientious, explicit, and judicious use of current best evidence in making decisions about the care of individual patients. The practice of evidence-based medicine means integrating individual clinical expertise with the best available external clinical evidence from systematic research'.

Evidence-based medicine is not a new idea. It has always been implicit that clinical practice should be based on the best possible evidence. However, what was relatively new 10 years ago was the widespread recognition that this is not happening. The evolution of current thinking about evidence-based medicine is described in Chapter 5.1.

Evidence-based medicine is about finding ways in which to bridge the gap between the huge amount of published data and clinical practice, and encompasses a number of strategies. One of these has been the development of scientific methods (systematic reviews and meta-analyses) to combine data from a number of different randomized studies of the same or similar treatments in any particular condition. Systematic reviews differ from other types of review in that they adhere to a strict scientific design in order to make them more comprehensive, to minimize the chance of bias, and so ensure their reliability.

Taken at face value, it seems reasonable to assume that the data from several studies that have been combined according to agreed scientific methodology should be more meaningful than the evidence from single studies. This is not universally accepted and there is no doubt that the methodology and application of these techniques must continue to be looked at critically. However, systematic reviews and meta-analyses are powerful tools in aggregating and evaluating large amounts of data and have become an important area of research activity in palliative medicine. One function they serve is to highlight research questions and thus contribute to the research agenda by careful and comprehensive review of the available evidence. A regular quarterly update from the Cochrane Pain, Palliative and Supportive Care Group (PaPaS) is published in the journal *Palliative Medicine* and will alert readers to reviews currently in progress or planned.

Evidence-based medicine and the future of palliative care

Evidence-based medicine has already had a major impact on the development of health care in a time of ever increasing demands but limited resources. It is likely that resource allocation will increasingly be based on evidence not just of efficacy but of cost-effectiveness. Where proof of efficacy is lacking, funds will not be provided by government or other health care agencies. This has particular implications for palliative care because it is an area where such research-based evidence is sparse. There are many activities within palliative care that are not amenable to investigation by randomized controlled studies. But, as noted above, the RCT is not the only valid method of ensuring advances in knowledge. The recent focus on evidence-based medicine makes all the more urgent the investment in palliative care research.

The scope of research in palliative care

One of the challenges in palliative care research is setting boundaries around the field. Because the subject and event of dying and death is at the centre of practitioners' concerns, it can be tempting to include all dimensions of scholarship related to 'death' within the field of interest. Death, as one of the major rites of passage for individuals, families, and societies, attracts research on its many ramifications, manifestations, and meanings in everyday life. The cultural context in which people present themselves as patients, come to approach death, and are cared for through their dying, is open to wide and varied interpretations drawn from historical, sociological, anthropological, theological, philosophical, and psychological perspectives; each with its own research traditions. Understanding the significance of death as a rite of passage as well as a biological or medical event is important for the skills of the practitioner when faced with communication challenges with dying patients and their families, and so the field of palliative care research could be immense. Practically, however, the field is generally focused on a narrower range of interests, of immediate concern, and relevance to practitioners and planners.

The principal questions that face palliative care professionals are those of clinical effectiveness and acceptability, service efficiency and organization, and meeting changing needs in the population. These are basic questions concerned with *what* palliative care practitioners do, and *how* they do it. The research skills to answer these questions are commonly drawn from the traditions of clinical research (medical, nursing, and allied health professional), health services research, and also epidemiology.

Epidemiological research

Descriptive epidemiology seeks to describe the prevalence and incidence of conditions within defined populations. Assessing the need for palliative care in different sectors of the population is clearly important for informing the process of service development and planning. In relation to palliative care, epidemiological research has been hampered by an absence of clearly defining population indicators linked to levels of clinical need, as well as changing perceptions within the profession of palliative care as to the appropriate 'catchment population'. The extended application of palliative care from its original main constituency of terminally ill cancer patients, to patients with any life-limiting illness, from point of diagnosis onwards, poses problems of classification. The majority of health service utilization data and measures of morbidity and mortality are based on disease categories. These do not give an indication of symptom burden or dependency levels, and thus little indication of the need for different forms of palliative care.

Clinical research

Traditionally, clinical research tends to focus on biochemical, microbiological, and physiological processes and the effect of pharmacological and other therapeutic agents. In palliative care, this focus is much broader because of the complexity of advanced disease and the high prevalence of psychological and existential distress. Clinical trials are based on an experimental approach and will often use outcomes from the laboratory derived from body samples (blood, tissue) or images (X-rays or scans) as well as patient responses recorded by questionnaire or structured interview. It is at the level of clinical research that trial-based research methodologies are most effective and applicable. The need for access to skilled technicians and laboratory facilities will tend to limit research capacity in clinical research for researchers working in non-academic or community settings.

Health services research

Research that is not strictly epidemiological or clinical can be categorized into the wider area named health services research. This kind of research is primarily focused on the evaluation of the organization and delivery of health care. Frequently, the research is applied to particular problems faced by policy-makers, managers, practitioners, and patients, and can range from questions of cost and effectiveness, policy formulation and implementation, the evaluation of new technologies, through to patient and public preferences and perceptions. Research approaches include those that underpin the social sciences as well as the more experimentally based approaches of the natural sciences. Much of the multidisciplinary research carried out in palliative care is focused on questions of innovation and organization in services, and assessing the need for and access to different types of intervention.

Wider humanistic research

The contribution of other disciplines and research traditions to the body of research in palliative care is well recognized and valued. Concern with the ethical, moral, spiritual, and philosophical dimensions of care for the dying and bereaved from all perspectives informs a body of scholarship, which broadens out the focus of research that can be relevant to palliative care practitioners. However, lack of familiarity with disciplinary roots and epistemological theory can make the contributions from the social sciences and humanities impenetrable to practitioners schooled in the natural sciences.

Clinical and health services research: practical considerations

There are particular difficulties associated with clinical research in palliative care, in addition to the ethical constraints described above. The patient population from which potential trial candidates are taken is characterized by old age, multisystem disease, generally severe illness with many symptoms, a progressive clinical condition, and limited survival time. In addition, polypharmacy is the rule, and environmental and psychological factors have a variable but potentially very great influence on physical well-being. Prospective randomized controlled studies are thus particularly difficult to carry out, because there are major problems in accrual of patients to trials, attrition, and missing data.[11–14]

The choice of trial design for prospective studies will be much influenced by these characteristics of the patient population. Endpoints or outcomes are also difficult to define. Outcome measures are not generally based on hard data such as biochemical indices or survival, which are relatively easy to quantify, but on changes in symptoms and quality of life, which are much more difficult to measure. The choice of trial design and measurements will be influenced also by the need to ensure that all procedures are designed to place the least possible additional burden on patients.

Defining the patient population

A particularly complex issue is the definition of a palliative care patient population. The lack of strict criteria for defining the patient population is a threat to both the internal and external validity of research in palliative care. In this context, internal validity can be understood as the ability to define the cohort of patients included in a given study. For example, if the true patient population is more heterogeneous than the one defined, the heterogeneity might obscure, even obliterate the positive effect of a particular intervention. External validity is about the representativeness of the sample. In clinical practice research data might be inappropriately applied if the precise characteristics of the population included in a particular research project are not accurately described. Research methods are generally predicated on the comparison of one population with another; studies of effectiveness are only meaningful when one treatment is set against another within similar or homogeneous populations. Palliative care populations are difficult to standardize, however, since referral to a palliative care team is made for a wide variety of reasons, most of which will be patient generated, but will also include reasons that involve the patient's family and professional carers, and the facilities available to the patient. Prognosis on referral is one way of categorizing patients, which is generally a matter of clinical judgement and use of dependency scores, while time from referral to death is another way; but this is only possible retrospectively. Another possibility is symptom burden, which is in most cohorts closely related to expected survival.[15–17]

Methodology

The evaluation of the effectiveness of treatments in palliative care has either not been undertaken at all or has been conducted using poor or inadequate research methodology. This was also the case in clinical medicine generally until the late 1960s and early 1970s. Only in recent years has it become evident that properly designed and well-conducted clinical trials are needed in palliative care as much as in any other area of medicine. Most of the published studies of the effectiveness of treatments in palliative care have been related to pain and quite often the patients included have been at an early stage of their disease. Whether the results of these studies can be extrapolated to palliative care patients is open to question.

A clinical trial is any investigation that follows the principles of a scientific experiment allowing for the evaluation of the clinical effect of an intervention in a valid and reliable way. The term 'clinical trial' is not synonymous with 'randomized controlled trial' (RCT). A clinical trial in the broadest sense of the term may mean any kind of planned experiment in patients, ranging from open descriptive studies to RCTs. The trial design will be determined by the research question.

Drawing on the experience of drug development, clinical trials are usually described in three (or four) phases. This three/four-stage process could also provide a model for research in palliative care in that it describes a sequential process requiring different experimental designs at different stages.

The choice of an appropriate study design will depend on what is already known about the particular question to be investigated. With the recent emphasis on evidence-based medicine there has been much discussion of the need for RCTs and of the fact that the RCT is the 'gold standard' and the most robust method for evaluating new treatments. However, many research questions do not need to be answered in an RCT. Furthermore, when attempting to design a randomized study, a lack of sufficient descriptive data may make it difficult to decide upon a study design and on appropriate outcomes or to perform a valid sample size calculation. This is commonly the case in palliative care research. The choice of trial design is crucial and in this process collaboration between experts is essential. This is the stage at which a project group should be established, at the very beginning of the planning process of a study.

In palliative care, a pilot study (or simply a non-systematic observation of a particular intervention) could be described as 'phase I'. Such a non-systematic study is not a rigorous research experiment but is the first step in the research plan. Thus, before embarking on an RCT it is necessary to go through a process analogous to phase I and II drug studies. This step-by-step approach highlights the fact that clinical research is a time-consuming process. Researchers and clinicians should not expect too many answers from each study.

Guidelines and books[18,19] on clinical trial methodology are widely available. The objectives and design of a study will be driven by the research question(s) and the resources available. This is not just about funding but also about academic and clinical resources and the availability of sufficient patients. A common problem in clinical research (not by any means unique to palliative care) is that investigators invariably and substantially overestimate the number of patients they are likely to see who would be suitable for a particular study. Changes in treatment policies might influence the availability of patients for a particular study even more if the entry criteria are based on previous policy.

A general criticism of palliative care research is that too many small studies are performed with an open non-comparative design, and thus the impact of the results in terms of changing practice will be limited. For example, in a recent systematic review of ketamine in cancer-related pain, the reviewers found 32 case series but only two RCTs of good quality (and these involved a total of only 20 patients). This makes it impossible to draw firm conclusions about the efficacy of ketamine.[20]

How to plan a clinical trial

The planning process of any clinical study often starts with new encouraging data from the laboratory or, probably more often in palliative care, from chance or non-systematic observations in the clinic. Aside from the need to collect together background information, the planning process involves a series of basic steps, which will need to be considered to provide the framework for the study (Table 1).

Usually, one will start with a literature review to see what is known about an intervention and the target condition or symptom. If the review indicates that a formal study is necessary or worthwhile, a research question or hypothesis should be formulated and this will determine the aim of the study.

A common mistake in clinical research is to bring too many ideas together and try to answer too many questions at the same time. Many studies are too complex with many research questions that cannot be answered with a limited number of patients.

Explicit definition of the aim of the study is crucial. Many clinical research projects are undertaken without a clear and concise aim, and the consequence is a lack of precision in the subsequent steps of the planning process and ultimately a poor study or one that is impossible to complete. The aim should be written in clear and understandable language and ideally it should be easily understood by a lay person. It should be formulated in a brief way in one or two sentences. It is often expressed as a general question and this is broken down into specific research questions or hypotheses.

The research questions will determine the patient population to be studied. There are several factors to take into consideration such as 'which group of patients will best give an answer to these questions?' For example, if a study was designed to examine patients' attitudes towards euthanasia and physician-assisted suicide in palliative care, the researchers would need to decide whether to ask the patient directly. In similar studies, patients themselves have not been asked, but the questions have been put to proxies or the general public. If the researchers decide to ask the patients, they must then decide how to select patients (in this example perhaps 'not too ill, but not too far away from being confronted with death and dying'). The patient sample must also be representative of the population of patients to whom the results will be applied. In other words, if a select subgroup of the general population is recruited to a study, the usefulness and applicability of the results (the external validity or generalizability) will be compromised.

In studies evaluating the effect of adjuvant chemotherapy in breast cancer or combination therapy for HIV, the primary outcomes are easy to select; for example, tumour response or survival time.[21] However, in recent years in oncology trials criticisms have been made about limiting the outcomes to survival or cure and not taking account of late side-effects of the treatment. During the last decade, for example, several studies have described the high prevalence of subjective side-effects, such as fatigue, in Hodgkin's disease survivors.[22] These experiences emphasize that selection of outcomes, even in curative treatment studies, might be less straightforward than it at first appears. In palliative care the number of outcomes can easily get out of hand, because of the complexity of the patient population and studies have been reported with 10–20 and even more outcome measures. This multiplicity of outcomes is further driven by the multidimensionality of the concept of health-related quality of life and the range of scales and single items used in these measures.[23,24] It is important not to fall into this trap. In general, one or two primary outcomes and perhaps two to three secondary outcomes are the most that should be included.

All of these issues should be thoroughly discussed by the researchers and the involved clinicians together with the larger study group before the research protocol can be finalized.

Table 1 The evolution of a research project in palliative care

Describe clearly the clinical problem or observations that prompted the idea for a study
Discuss the relevance and validity of the observations with clinical colleagues
Carry out a comprehensive review of the literature to find out what is already known about the topic
Formulate a research question or two or three questions. These will define the aim of the study
Define the patient population
Decide on the appropriate study design
Decide on the outcomes to be measured
With these decisions made, write the protocol

Randomization and blinding

The concept of random allocation of patients when comparing different treatments (or any other interventions) is important in the design of a clinical experiment. The purpose of randomization is to reduce selection bias. Non-randomized trials have a tendency to overestimate the effect of treatment. Randomization also provides a basis for use of standard methods of statistical analysis. When a new treatment is introduced enthusiastic clinicians and researchers tend to overestimate its beneficial effects. For example in the early open studies of cisplatin in the treatment of non-small cell lung cancer, the response rate was double that found in later randomized studies.[25] The same tendency is also seen when using historical controls as a comparison group or when using other quasi-experimental designs.

In palliative care, randomized studies are particularly difficult to undertake and complete. Therefore, other types of studies might be important to consider and might be preferable. Caution needs to be exercised in the analysis and in the interpretation of data from non-randomized studies. Other designs may be appropriate and may represent a slightly less robust option than an RCT but still produce persuasive data. For example, in the evaluation of palliative care programmes, cluster randomized designs have been used.[26]

Unblinded trials also overestimate the effect of treatment. Blinding may be difficult to achieve and needs to be thought about early in the planning process, particularly it if involves the manufacture of placebo formulations or other manufacturing processes to conceal the identity of treatments. Palliative care researchers should consult with statisticians and clinical trial methodologists early in the planning process of the study, and preferably include these advisors in the project group. There are useful texts on clinical trial methodology,[18] study design,[27] an introduction to statistics,[28] and more comprehensive textbooks on medical statistics.[29] Such texts provide basic background reading for researchers.

Statistical considerations

The project group will need to consult with a statistician, or preferably include a statistician, early in the process of designing the study. The statistician should have continuing input through the project. Medical statisticians have skills and expertise in several areas of clinical research, that is, study design, sample size estimation, and in the analysis of the data. One essential step in the planning process of any clinical study is to decide how many patients will be needed to get a valid result.

The purpose of this 'sample size' calculation is to ensure that the study is large enough to detect a clinically important difference should one exist, or exclude the possibility of such a difference should none be detected. In order to estimate the sample size the statistician will want to know how small a difference in the main outcome measures it is important to be able to detect in terms of clinical significance. For example, the number of patients treated with a new opioid, reaching a Numerical Rating Scale (NRS) score below three within 2 weeks of the initiation of treatment. In comparative studies of pain relief, the mean value of the NRS is often used as a primary outcome. The clinicians need to specify how small a difference between groups will be considered to be of clinical significance (e.g. 2 on a 0–11 NRS scale). It would also be helpful to have information about what could be expected to happen in the control group (mean and standard deviation) and this information may be derived from a pilot study or from published literature. The required number of patients is calculated according to how confident one wants to be about detecting a difference between interventions if one exists (the power of the study).

The protocol

A study cannot exist for long as an idea in researchers' minds and a few hastily written notes and memos. It has to be formalized into a protocol, which acts as the 'blue print' of the project. The protocol evolves through a series of stages to become a comprehensive document detailing the 'why', 'when', and 'how' of the study. In its final form, the protocol will describe the background to the study and its scientific relevance, the rationale behind the chosen study design, and a description of the organizational and ethical dimensions. Importantly, the protocol will include a detailed description of how the study will be carried out, from the methods of patient selection and recruitment, the procedures of data collection and handling, through to the plans for analysis. Every step along the way needs to be considered, as well as the procedures to be followed in the case of deviations. Every study will encounter unexpected consequences and unpredictable effects. In this sense, the protocol may well be added to at various points during the study to take account of unforeseen circumstances (commonly called 'protocol deviations'). Table 2 outlines a typical structure of a protocol for a clinical study.

The process of developing a rough draft of a study protocol through to a stage where all aspects of the study have been considered and piloted is a major research effort on its own. In theory, it means that short of actually carrying out the study, everything that could be done has been done. In practice, researchers who skimp on the protocol and associated development work will often find themselves faced with untenable or 'un-doable' research studies.

Access to patients

A major challenge in palliative care research involving relatively large numbers of patients is in identifying the patient population and gaining access to them. When research involves selected patients in a clinic, or on a ward, identifying those appropriate for research may not be problematic, especially if the clinician involved is carrying out the research. However, for non-clinical researchers, or for clinical researchers wanting to recruit patients from settings other than their own, identification and access are crucial aspects of patient recruitment. In these situations, co-operation will be needed from the other health care professionals caring for the patients. To gain access to patients may require lengthy negotiation, involving presentations at clinical meetings, permission from professional bodies, as well as a strategy for communication and keeping the research project uppermost in clinicians' minds.

It can be useful to develop information sheets, specific for each professional concerned, early on in the stages of introducing a project to those who are affected. Thinking through likely questions and their answers can help to take the project off the drawing board and ground it in the reality of clinical life. Colleagues and peers will be concerned that the research is well designed and addresses a clinically important question. Justifying the purpose and value of a research project to one's peers is particularly critical in relation to palliative care research where non-palliative care colleagues may question the probity of carrying out research with this patient group. There are probably few palliative care researchers who have not, at some time, had their research intentions questioned. In addition, it will be important to listen to colleagues' concerns and offer flexibility in the carrying out of the research. Colleagues will be particularly resistant to participating in anything that involves more paperwork or disruptions to routines. The effort and time involved in securing access to patients from professional colleagues should not be underestimated.

Table 2 Writing the protocol: the headings

1. Introduction
    - Current state of knowledge and literature review
    - Reasons for study
    - Specific aspect of problem to be investigated
2. Aim(s) and objectives
3. Methods
    - *Design of investigation*
    - Observational or experimental
    - Descriptive or analytical
    - Prospective (cohort)
    - Retrospective (case–control)
    - Control group
    - Schedule with justification of design chosen
    - *Definitions*
    - Diagnostic criteria
    - Definition of terms
    - *Populations*
    - Identification
    - Sampling
    - Inclusion and exclusion criteria
    - Randomization (where appropriate)
    - Losses and refusals
    - *Data*
    - Study variables and extraneous variables
    - Sources of data
        - Pre-existing records
        - Interview/examination
        - Postal survey
    - Design of survey documents
        - Questionnaire
        - Interview schedules
        - Data abstraction forms
    - *Ethical and funding issues*
    - Discussion where appropriate
    - *Analysis*
    - Indicate how each question in the objectives is to be answered
    - Tabulations to be prepared and how
    - Statistical tests to be used
    - Sample size calculation where appropriate
4. Timetable and programming of the work
    - Including time to develop and pilot questionnaires if necessary
5. Appendices
    - Patient information sheet
    - Patient consent form
    - Information sheets for
        - GP
        - Patient's consultant
        - Nursing staff
        - Carers
        - As appropriate
    - Data collection forms
    - Questionnaires
        - Designed for study
        - Validated, for example,
            - McGill Pain Questionnaire
            - HADS
            - EORTC $QLQC_{30}$

Reproduced with permission from University of Bristol MSc in Palliative Medicine Handbook, 2003 (ed. K. Forbes and A. Davies).

It is also important to feed back to practitioners who have been involved in the research through facilitating access to patients, or providing information, at the end of the research. Knowing what the findings are and what importance they hold for future service configurations helps make the research a collaborative experience, and can be an element in service development and change where that is indicated. This affirms the stakeholder role, which professional carers hold in the research process.

Significant others to the patient—non-professional carers

Care at the end of life embraces not only the patient, but also those close to him or her. Supporting family carers in their caring role is important in relieving some of the practical difficulties and burdens that are encountered during protracted periods of high dependency care in the home, as well as addressing the psychological distress that is associated with the loss of a close relative. Research similarly involves not only the patient but also those close to the patient in a caring role. Research interest may take several forms; it may focus on the long-term health of those who survive the patient (bereavement studies), but as frequently, it may focus on how patients and their home carers cope with the illness together, and the perceptions of the home carers of the professional care received by the patient. Even when research is solely concerned with patient-based indicators, those close to the patient are important in the research process by acting as intermediaries. Home or family carers can take on a number of roles in relation to patients' involvement in research and each role needs to be appreciated by the research team.

Gatekeepers/protectors

Family members adopting a caring role also act as 'gatekeepers' to the patients. This is likely to be increasingly critical as the patient's stamina declines, when dependency increases, and when the patient himself/herself has delegated certain aspects of decision-making to a trusted family carer. When patients are approached for recruitment to a research study it is generally advisable, therefore, to approach whoever appears to be most in contact with the patient (in hospital or at home). Research can appear threatening to those who are striving to care for the patient; primarily they may worry about the research tiring and distracting the patient, and about questions upsetting the patient—either by providing too much information or opening up areas of contemplation that may further disturb the patient. When time is perceived to be short, carers may well resent the attention of the patient being taken by people outside of the family. How family carers weigh up the benefits of participating in a research study (short-term benefits of additional monitoring and attention and long-term benefits to society) against the costs to the patient (and themselves) of time commitments and possibly extra upset will be pivotal in the recruitment process.

The family carer's role as gatekeeper is often regarded negatively by researchers, as one of the barriers to achieving adequate sample sizes. While researchers regard adult patients as autonomous, self-determining individuals who can decide for themselves whether they want to participate in research, the vulnerability of some palliative care patients can make this problematic. The tensions between dealing with a patient as a family member rather than as simply an individual are all too apparent. Participation in research is an intervention in itself (patients are not 'passive subjects') with consequences that cannot be wholly predicted, however meticulously procedures are followed. Family carers can be more aware of this than researchers since to them the patient is not one 'number' amongst many; he or she is a spouse, parent, sibling, or child. Being involved in research can involve the wider family context, and so the extended boundaries of the palliative care patient need to be appreciated by researchers, with procedures in place to inform and include family members.

Interpreters, substitutes, and advocates

When patients have difficulty communicating their thoughts and feelings, family members may take on the role of interpreter and substitute (proxy). Interpretation can be needed for both speech and language difficulties (translation). In the face of cognitive impairment, the views of family carers may be used as a substitute for the patients' views. A number of studies have investigated the validity of proxy ratings, concluding that proxies tend to underestimate the severity of certain symptoms (pain and depression) but that in the absence of patient-derived data, proxy data are valuable.

A role that sits between gatekeeper and interpreter is that of advocate. The extent to which family carers take on this role varies with their own confidence and the situations within which they find themselves. Researchers should be aware that advocacy can work in different ways; at times making sure that the best interests of the patient are promoted, at others, following an agenda that is not the patient's but that of the family member. This is another reason for extreme sensitivity to be exercised by the research team.

Significant others to the patient—professional carers

Professional carers can likewise act as gatekeepers, interpreters, substitutes, and advocates, with all the cautions outlined above. Similarly, they are also a subject of great interest in their own right from the point of view of service/practitioner efficiency and effectiveness, and understanding the process of delivering high-quality palliative care. There is a growing body of research on the training and educational needs of practitioners, the dynamics of interprofessional and multidisciplinary team working, and management processes to preserve and enhance occupational health.

Finance and management

There are many sources of funding that are relevant to palliative care but securing funds for research in this area is a competitive exercise as it is in any area of health care. As indicated at the beginning of this chapter, palliative care research is a relatively neglected area as far as the major funders of cancer research are concerned. The great majority of patients currently being treated by palliative care services are patients with cancer so this means that funding for studies in non-cancer patients is in even shorter supply. However, the climate is changing and this is happening in many different parts of the world. It is not possible here to give detailed information about funding sources since these will vary from country to country. This sort of information is obviously of considerable relevance to future researchers and it is one area where the scientific journals in palliative care could play a useful role.

Finance for individual projects

The length of time between securing finance for a project and actually starting data collection is always underestimated. This period can be divided into two main phases: the time before project funds are actually drawn upon, when research staff are being recruited and when a considerable amount of planning and groundwork is being carried out. The second phase is when the funds are being disbursed and piloting work is being undertaken. It is crucial that as much work as possible is carried out in the first phase, even though the work is essentially not funded. Efficient management of time and resources from the very start of a project are obviously key factors in its successful running.

Project group

All research projects benefit from being exposed to a group of people who have experience in the subject under research and who are interested in the project. This is particularly important for large studies. The role of a project group can vary along a spectrum of responsibilities that range from being highly involved in the administration and day-to-day concerns of the project, to being relatively distant, and receiving information about the project on a regular though infrequent basis. The value of project groups are as follows:

1. they can provide peer review to the research project, thus validating the research in the eyes of external sponsors and host institutions;
2. they can provide research experience and expertise, especially during the early stages of a project;
3. they can provide contacts and entry to otherwise hard to access sectors;
4. they can provide moral support and encouragement during the course of the project;

5. they can act as a sounding board, and also participate in the understanding and analysis of data;
6. they can help to disseminate the findings of the research and have a wider view of its relevance to policy and practice.

Depending on the size of the project, it can sometimes be helpful to institute a steering group of key stakeholders who are sympathetic to the research but who do not have much time to devote to it, and a management group of people who are accessible regularly and become close to the project and data collection, and who report back to the steering group.

The staffing and management of major research projects will tend to be as follows:

1. the researcher(s) conducting the research and collecting data on a day-to-day basis;
2. a group of researchers (including all or some of those listed in point 1) who monitor the progress of the study on a regular basis and who provide support, advice, and suggestions, and act as a sounding board;
3. a wider group of interested parties who may (or may not) be formally constituted as a steering group.

At an early stage, agreement needs to be reached about decision-making (research and finance), supervision, and mentoring.

Piloting the study and study procedures

Research studies do not start off as fully formed projects. Indeed, it is impossible to anticipate all the challenges that a study will face at the planning stage. The word 'pilot' derives from the job of steering a boat on its course and the metaphor of guiding a ship through uncertain and troubled waters is an apt one. Without preliminary studies, it is difficult to steer the course of a large project. Pilot work is important for testing all aspects of research design, from the face validity and acceptability of data collection procedures, to the workability of allocation schedules, and administration tasks. Dealing with the questions and issues raised by pilot studies can be demanding at a stage when there is impatience to start the main study, not least due to the pressure on obtaining funds for research and the need to work to deadlines. However, learning the lessons from pilot work can be critical to the success of the project. For researchers working alone, the use of a research journal can encourage a reflective attitude to the pilot work, and help to refine the research design. For researchers in a team, frequent meetings at this stage, with records made of the discussions and decisions will again help to re-define and re-model the research into a workable proposition. Re-writing the protocol with the findings of the pilot work is important for the auditing of the research project.

Administration and paperwork

It will be readily appreciated that a research study will quickly develop different strands of paperwork, reflecting the different administrative tasks:

1. Background work relating to the development of the study, reviews of the scientific literature, and any position papers and early proposals.
2. Paperwork relating to the funding and approval of the study (sponsors, ethics committees, other professional and regulatory bodies).
3. Correspondence and paperwork relating to the formation of the steering and project group(s), together with the minutes and agendas of each formally convened meeting.
4. A record of the protocol as it develops through successive drafts.
5. Sources of information targeted at specific sectors of the study population: information sheets for patients and their professional and non-professional carers, information posters for hospital or hospice wards or other settings, information in local media about the study.
6. Paperwork used for collecting data, ranging from consent forms, case record forms, to questionnaires and data abstraction forms. This might also include letters or cards sent by the research team to patients and carers after data collection to thank them for their participation, as well as any correspondence from the study population regarding the research, including letters of complaint or inquiry. Restricting access to this kind of documentation is central to preserving patient confidentiality (lockable rooms or filing cabinets).
7. A developing account of the way the study is progressing. Most projects benefit from regular review, although this will depend on its size and timescale. Even in the absence of interim analysis, it can be the important to monitor recruitment rates, protocol deviations, and any other problems with the management of the project. This can also be an opportunity for informal reflections on the study, particularly from the point of view of the day-to-day researcher(s).
8. Paperwork relating to data preparation and data analysis, including any conventions used in coding data, and where the data are held and in what form. This aspect of project administration is most important for the understanding and interpretation of data in analysis.
9. Finally, the project will be written up as a report in various formats for various audiences, and it is important to keep records of the drafts as they develop and become finalized.

Efficient administration is essential in two quite common scenarios. One is where a project is required to audit its activities and give an account of the funds that have been used, and the procedures that have been followed. This can happen as a result of a rolling programme of research audit within an institution or sector, or can happen as a result of a special investigation, triggered by a number of different concerns (perhaps unrelated to the study). Another more common scenario is where researchers move away from the project before its conclusion, which may seriously affect the smooth running of a study, but the effect can be minimized by comprehensive paperwork. Again, the role of a project group is critical to the orientation of a new researcher, mid-study, with the dangers of keeping decision-making and discussion to too small a group all too evident.

Good clinical practice

Good clinical practice or GCP relates to drug trials and evolved from FDA guidelines (the Food and Drug Administration in the United States) but are now applicable worldwide. GCP regulations were designed to ensure that reliable, verifiable, and retrievable data are obtained in a drug trial and have become essential to the drug development process. GCP guidelines explicitly outline the investigators' responsibilities: for example, in obtaining ethical approval for the study; ensuring that all patients entered into the study have given written informed consent; and in conducting the study and completing the case record forms according to the protocol. In addition, the investigator must report all adverse events; keep records of the dispensing and return of all study drugs; file all documentation in the investigators site file; and set aside time for discussion during visits of the study monitor and the quality assurance auditor.

GCP applies to all trials on medicinal products in human beings. Usually, such studies are being carried out under the sponsorship of a commercial company and the details will be monitored by the clinical research associates employed by the company. However, clinical researchers will need to familiarize themselves with these requirements because they need to be strictly adhered to. In the European Union (EU) new legislation is currently going through a process of consultation as a prelude to implementation of an EU Directive 2001/20/EC on Good Clinical Practice in Clinical Trials. The new law will significantly extend the scope of GCP to cover all clinical trials of medicinal products, including trials not directly supported by pharmaceutical companies and phase I healthy volunteer studies. One major change in the new regulations is that breach of the obligations contained in them may be in some circumstances a criminal offence. There are major implications in the proposals for Research Ethics Committees and (in the United Kingdom) for the Research Governance Framework for Health and Social Care. Again these regulations will have wide-ranging influence outside of the United Kingdom. More detailed information is available on the EU Commission website 'http://pharmacos.eudra.org/' and on the Department of Health website 'www.doh.gov.uk/clinicaltrialsconsult.index.htm'.

Supporting researchers and the clinical team (keeping it going)

The initial rush of enthusiasm for a project is difficult to sustain over time without conscious management of the research team. Studies can get into difficulty quite quickly when unexpected problems start to shake the confidence of the supporting clinical teams or the front-line researchers. Encountering slow patient recruitment or high dropout rates, for example, can be disillusioning and de-motivating. However, a project that is conceived as a collaborative venture, where support from others is openly valued, and where there is a commitment to teamwork, is likely to develop mechanisms for keeping the study going. Attention needs to be focused on the individual needs and group dynamics of the research team, as well as the wider group of staff who are involved in facilitating the study. Morale and support for the study can be promoted in a number of ways:

1. For clinical staff, provision of regular feedback and direct contact with the study team to answer queries and address any concerns is desirable. This is also important considering the high turnover of clinical staff; new staff will need to be identified and inducted especially during a long-running study. Busy clinical staff anyway will also tend to forget about studies, and so an important aspect of regular contact is to remind them that the study is still running.
2. Within the research team, time should be set aside for team-building activities (e.g. away days and social events), and to help prevent 'burn-out', the provision of mentoring, co-counselling, or de-briefing should be considered.

Databases and data management

Considerable thought needs to be devoted to the system of recording and holding data early in the planning of a research study. The success of subsequent analysis will depend on the quality of the data, its reliability, and completeness. Most research data will be held in an electronic database, which is basically a way of holding, organizing, and indexing the records transferred from data-capture forms (generally paper-based but can be electronic given the use of lap-top computers or palm-held devices). Many databases are used for more than their 'filing system' capacities. Records can be sorted and selected for basic ordering and counting purposes, and data held in a database can be accessed by other software packages for administrative tasks such as bulk mailings, other correspondence, and automated updates. Because of the individual characteristics and requirements of each study, a certain amount of customization of the database package used is generally necessary.

Within a research study it is important to manage the data, by attending to three crucial processes:

1. how data gets onto the database;
2. how the database is maintained;
3. how data are used for analysis and report formation.

Questions of sufficient computer hardware and software should be addressed in the early stages of a study, and adequate funds made available. In addition, information and computer technology (ICT) orientation and on-going training should be available for all researchers engaged on the project who are either responsible for data input, or who require access to the data. The process of inputting data during the study should be piloted for 'user-friendliness'. This would cover efficiency and ease of input, taking care not to make the process over-burdensome. The requirements of the analysis need to be borne in mind in order to avoid excessive (and costly) data recording.

However diligent researchers are in the recording and inputting of data, mistakes happen, especially when people are rushed, tired, or distracted. Accuracy of data input can be built into data-entry protocols, but it cannot always be programmed for. Regular checks of the data can show up gross inaccuracies and perhaps consistent mistakes, which becomes an important part of data management and the subsequent integrity of the data. Checking as the study progresses can also mean that omissions can be followed-up quickly, rather than being left to the end when it becomes a more time-consuming task. The way that data are coded and entered needs to be written up in a manual that should sit alongside the database, allowing other researchers to understand and access the database.

The security and protection of the database is also an important aspect of data management. First, there is the necessity of adhering to national and international data protection and patient confidentiality requirements. This may determine or limit some of the data items that are actually held on the database, and may also require special consent from the research subjects. Second, the database needs to be held securely, possibly by restricting physical access to it (access to computers, servers), and protecting it through the use of passwords. In addition, back-up discs of the database, which are needed in the event of computer problems, also need to be protected.

Ease of export of data to supporting software packages is clearly an important aspect of the analysis and report-writing stage of a study and warrants careful consideration of the options available, together with the adequacy of training and on-going support for the life of the study. How the data will be used for analysis will depend partly upon *who* will be responsible for this, and this should be planned for at the earliest stages of the study. A statistical analysis will involve collaboration with a statistician and the data should be held in such a way that it is easily manipulated into files for use by a variety of statistical packages. Analysis of qualitative data also requires planning of the way textual data are collected and recorded. The CAQDAS (Computer Assisted Qualitative Data Analysis Software) Project, funded by the UK Economic and Social Research Council, provides practical support, training, and information in the use of a range of software programmes that have been designed to assist qualitative data analysis. This can be accessed through their website, www.caqdas.soc.surrey.ac.uk.

Finally, questions of archiving study data and pooling or sharing data with other studies should be considered. Studies finish and researchers move on, so having a known repository for study data can be important for future researchers. More value can also be derived from a study when data are shared with other researchers working in the national or international context. The importance of this in palliative care research is particularly apt, given the many difficulties in recruiting large numbers of research participants.

Analysing and interpreting the data and presenting and publishing the results

The analysis of the data should be straightforward if all of the preceding steps have been properly adhered to and an adequate number of subjects have been recruited. The statistical methods to be used will already have been decided and the data will have been 'cleaned' and stored in files in a database that allows easy manipulation in statistical software packages. Recruitment and attrition are major problems in palliative care research as has been discussed earlier and missing data need careful attention and handling, but all of these problems will have been anticipated and ways of managing them agreed. As the numbers start taking shape towards one conclusion or another there is a sense of excitement and anticipation that they will add up to a meaningful advance in knowledge.

The next step will be to present the data to colleagues and at scientific meetings to begin the process of peer review. Usually, the first public presentation of the data will be at a scientific meeting such as the biennial Congress of the European Association for Palliative Care. Some practical advice about getting abstracts accepted, whether for poster presentation or oral communication, is outlined in Table 3.

Submitting a paper for publication

Much research is undertaken and completed and even presented at a scientific meeting but is never published in a peer-reviewed journal. There may be many reasons for this and it is not possible briefly to discuss them all here. However, Table 4 gives some advice about submitting papers for publication.

Table 3 Submitting abstracts for free communications at research meetings

Find out the final date for submission as early as possible
Read the instructions to authors carefully and follow them precisely
Decide whether the data are best presented as a poster or as an oral communication. Oral communications typically are allocated 10 min plus 5 min for questions. The larger the meeting paradoxically the smaller the likely audience (because there are usually many parallel sessions in large meetings)
Follow the usual structure of Introduction, Aims, Patients/Subjects, Methods, Results, Conclusions, unless instructions say otherwise
Write impeccable English (or other language if appropriate) with accurate terminology and good grammar
Do not exceed the word allowance
Scientific committees look for originality and interest, topicality, and sound methodology. They need some reassurance that you will have data to present (i.e. that the study has actually started or is in progress) so try to avoid submitting an abstract with no data at all
Posters need to be eye-catching and succinct. However interesting the topic, poor presentation and endless detail in small print will deter people from reading it

Table 4 Submitting a paper for publication

Decide which journal to go for. Are the data relevant to a general journal (*New England Journal of Medicine, Lancet, BMJ*) or a specialist journal (*Cancer, Journal of Clinical Oncology, Palliative Medicine*)? The general journals are much more difficult to be published in
Aim high (but appropriately so) because sometimes you will catch an editor's interest and with the leading journals you will usually get a very rapid response if the paper is rejected (one of the authors had experience of acknowledgement of receipt of a paper within a week of posting, and a letter of rejection 24 h later)
Do not be too discouraged by rejection but try to learn from it. Usually authors will get some feedback explaining why the paper has been rejected. This should enable them to improve the paper before submitting it to another journal
Before submission to any journal, study the Instructions to Authors and abide by them strictly particularly in terms of length, style, and references
In general, it is not worth arguing with editors if they have made it clear that they do not wish to publish your paper. However, if you believe the comments of referees or editors are unreasonable or just erroneous it is perfectly legitimate to challenge them. Occasionally the editor may change his mind
Similarly, if your paper is accepted but the referees or editors suggest changes that you are not happy with, respond and explain why you feel the changes are not justified
After publication make sure you read the journal (even if it is not one you regularly take) so that you can respond to any correspondence about your paper

Conclusions

Research in palliative care is essential for maintaining standards and advancing knowledge and improving practice. It is challenging, some-times frustrating, sometimes daunting but always exciting and rewarding when a study is successfully completed whether the outcome is positive or negative. We hope that this chapter will help those who are new to research to begin some research, and complete it, thus contributing to improving outcomes for patients with advanced disease, which is ultimately the aim of this endeavour.

References

1. **Vere, D.** (1981). Controlled clinical trials: the current ethical debate. *Journal of the Royal Society of Medicine* **74**, 85–7.
2. **National Cancer Research Institute**. *Strategic Analysis 2002*. London: National Cancer Research Institute.
3. **Saunders, C.** (1978). Hospice care. *American Journal of Medicine* **65**, 76–8.
4. **Twycross, R.G.** (1977). Choice of strong analgesic in terminal cancer: diamorphine or morphine? *Pain* **3**, 93–104.
5. **Murray-Parkes, C.** (1985). Terminal care: home, hospital or hospice? *Lancet* **i**, 155–7.
6. **Hanks, G.W.** (1985). The care of advanced cancer patients. In *Medical Perspectives in Cancer Research* (ed. A.J.S. Davis and P.S. Rudland), pp. 263–72. Chichester: Ellis Horwood.
7. **Blumhuber, H., Kaasa, S., and De Conno, F.** (2002). The European Association for Palliative Care. *Journal of Pain and Symptom Management* **24**, 124–7.
8. **Anonymous** (1964). Human experimentation: code of ethics of the World Medical Association. *British Medical Journal* **2**, 177.
9. **Bradford-Hill, A.** (1963). Medical ethics and controlled trials. *British Medical Journal* **ii**, 1043–9.
10. **Beecher, H.K.** (1966). Ethics and clinical research. *New England Journal of Medicine* **274**, 1354–60.
11. **McWhinney, I.R., Bass, M.J., and Donner, A.** (1994). Evaluation of a palliative care service: problems and pitfalls. *British Medical Journal* **309**, 1340–2.
12. **Rinck, G.C., van den Bos, G.A.M., Kleijnen, J., de Haes, H.J., Schade, E., and Veenhof, C.H.** (1997). Methodologic issues in effectiveness research on palliative cancer care: a systematic review. *Journal of Clinical Oncology* **15**, 1697–707.
13. **Hanks, G.W.** et al. (2002). The imPaCT study: a randomised controlled trial to evaluate a hospital palliative care team. *British Journal of Cancer* **87**, 733–9.
14. **Kaasa, S. and Loge, J.H.** (2003). Quality of life in palliative care: principles and practice. *Palliative Medicine* **17**, 11–20.
15. **Kaasa, S., Mastekaasa, A., and Lund, E.** (1989). Prognostic factors for patients with inoperable non-small cell lung cancer, limited disease. *Radiotherapy and Oncology* **15**, 235–42.
16. **Maltoni, M., Pirovano, M., Scarpi, E., Marinari, M., Indelli, M., Arnoldi, E., Gallucci, M., Frontini, L., Piva, L., and Amadori, D.** (1995). Prediction of survival of patients terminally ill with cancer. Results from an Italian Prospective Multicentric Study. *Cancer* **75**, 2613–22.
17. **Vigano, A., Bruera, E., Jhangri, G.S., Newman, S.C., Fields, A.L., and Suarez-Almazor, M.E.** (2000). Clinical survival predictors in patients with advanced cancer. *Archives of Internal Medicine* **160**, 861–8.
18. **Pocock, S.J.** *Clinical Trials: A Practical Approach* 1st edn Chichester: John Wiley & Sons.
19. **Karlberg, J. and Tsang, K.** *Introduction to Clinical Trials*, Merck Sharp & Dohme (Asia) Ltd. Clinicals Trials Centre, Faculty of Medicine, The University of Hong Kong, 1998.
20. **Bell, R., Eccleston, C., and Kalso, E.** (2003). Ketamine as an adjuvant to opioids for cancer pain. *Cochrane Database Systems Review* **1**, CD003351.
21. **Early Breast Cancer Trialists' Group** (1998). Tamoxifen for early breast cancer: an overview of the randomized trials. *Lancet* **351**, 1451–67.
22. **Loge, J.H., Foss Abrahamsen, A., Ekeberg, O., and Kaasa, S.** (1999). Hodgkin's disease survivors more fatigued than the general population. *Journal of Clinical Oncology* **17**, 253–61.
23. **Aaronson, N.K.** et al. (1993). The European Organisation for Research and Treatment of Cancer QLQ-C30: a quality of life instrument for use in international clinical trials in oncology. *Journal of the National Cancer Institute* **85**, 365–76.
24. **Cohen, S.R., Mount, B.M., Strobel, M.G., and Bui, F.** (1995). The McGill quality of life questionnaire: a measure of quality of life appropriate for people with advanced disease: a preliminary study of validity and acceptability. *Palliative Medicine* **9**, 207–19.
25. **Kaasa, S., Thorud, E., Host, H., Lien, H.H., Lund, E., and Sjolie, I.** A randomized study evaluating radiotherapy versus chemotherapy in patients

with inoperable non-small cell lung cancer. *Radiotherapy and Oncology* **11**, 7–13.

26. **Jordhoy, M.S.** et al. (2000). A palliative care intervention and death at home: a cluster randomised trial. *Lancet* **356**, 888–93.
27. **Rothman, K.J. and Greenland, S.** *Modern Epidemiology*, 2nd edn. London: Lippincott Williams & Wilkins 1998.
28. **Rosner, B.** *Fundamentals of Biostatistics* 5th edn., Pacific Grove: Duxbury Press, 1999.
29. **Altman, D.G.** *Practical Statistics for Medical Research.* London: Chapman & Hall/CRC, 1991.

5.3 Qualitative research

Linda J. Kristjanson and Nessa Coyle

How do we undertake research in palliative care that addresses the range of complex questions that face clinicians in a way that is scientifically credible and ethically sensitive? In some instances, quantitative research methods are the most appropriate means of addressing certain research questions. However, not everything in health care or, more specifically, palliative care can be understood by or reduced to numbers. In other instances, therefore, qualitative methods are the best or only approaches to achieve scientific resolution for the evaluation of certain research problems. And in some cases, qualitative methods in combination with quantitative approaches are indicated. Researchers should be able to use both types of methods.

In both palliative care and qualitative research, there is an emphasis on understanding individual experiences that may not fit into established categories of knowledge. There is recognition that each person's perspective is unique, complex, and multifaceted. Personal experience is valued as a means of determining what is relevant to care and research. The varying ways people perceive and interpret their experiences as they construct meaning are respected. Both researcher and caregivers strive to create an atmosphere of trust and mutual respect, to suspend pre-determined beliefs, and to embrace the ambiguity of multiple realities inherent in this approach to knowing the patient's world.

In this chapter, we will explore how qualitative methods can help to address palliative care research questions, starting from the premise that the nature of the clinical research question is the most valuable guide to determining the methodology to be used. We will provide an overview of qualitative research 'scaffolding', discuss three of the most commonly used qualitative methods, outlining differences amongst these methods with examples of their application in palliative care. We will then outline the challenging research issues that palliative care clinicians and researchers face when embarking upon qualitative studies with palliative care populations. We will conclude by identifying ways in which palliative care research can be served by qualitative methods and will offer recommendations for palliative care research using qualitative methods.

What is qualitative research?

The term 'qualitative research' encompasses a wide domain of methods and research practices that have certain common characteristics. The most defining characteristic is that the approach to inquiry is not dependent upon statistical procedures of quantification. Qualitative research recognizes that the values researchers hold influence the types of research questions. Qualitative research seeks meaning and understandings about processes and phenomena, with attention to narratives, personal experiences, and language.[1] The differences between quantitative and qualitative methods are not simply idiosyncrasies of research techniques. Rather, the underpinning philosophical orientations or paradigms that inform the methods are divergent and merit discussion.

Paradigms and ways of knowing

Kuhn[2] first described the term 'paradigm' in relation to traditions of science. Kuhn argued that each scientific community has its own way of viewing what constitutes a scientific problem and consequently determines the appropriate manner in which the problems should be addressed. He used the term 'paradigm' to denote a collective view of what constitutes the nature of the world. He suggested that the set of values arising from this worldview guided the investigator in the type of research question asked and in the subsequent method that allow these questions to be best answered.

Quantitative researchers generally rely on a positivistic approach to science and knowledge development. Positivism refers to a belief that all sciences, including social science, can be scientific in the same way as the physical sciences, such as physics or chemistry.[3] Research undertaken using most quantitative research methods assumes that only observed, objective phenomenon and positive facts are worthy of attention. Positivists usually prefer to measure things using structured questions and by constructing scales that can be analysed with statistics.

Qualitative researchers ground their reasoning and methods in an inductive, interpretive approach to science and understanding. The interpretative, qualitative paradigm of the social sciences acknowledges the inherent value-laden nature of inquiry, seeking to acknowledge the ability of human beings to interpret their world and to give meaning to their subjective experiences.[1]

A simple comparison of quantitative and qualitative approaches is offered by LeCompte and Preissle,[4] who succinctly stated, 'deductive researchers hope to find data to match a theory; inductive researchers hope to find a theory that explains their data' (p. 42).

Despite these apparent differences, it is becoming increasingly common for health-related research to use a mix of methods, depending upon the nature of the research question and the scope of the study aims.

The qualitative research question?

Research questions best informed by qualitative methods often begin with questions such as 'how', 'what', 'who', and 'why'. In several types of qualitative approaches, there is an assumption that the researcher may not know the real or relevant research question until he/she is immersed in the field situation. Broad, open-ended research questions are quite acceptable, with anticipation that the research question will be refined or modified as the study proceeds. No matter how the research question is stated, the amount of time allocated for conducting the study must fit the scope of the research problem and the realities of the field situation. Data used to answer these questions are based upon interviews or extended periods of observation or document review. Key features include: capturing the individual's point of view, examining aspects of everyday life, and ensuring that the ensuing descriptions are full of detail. The depth of qualitative research makes it difficult to reproduce or replicate in the exact same form. The nature of the methods means that the interaction between the researcher and participant may not be something that another researcher could attain in the same depth, detail, or scope. When a person tells their story to someone, the story is rarely told in exactly the same manner. However, the general themes, issues, concerns, and perceptions should endure—and it is this level of consistency that would be explored in subsequent studies.

Qualitative research scaffolding

There are a number of methods within the domain of qualitative research. We will discuss three of the most commonly used methods—*ethnography, phenomenology*, and *grounded theory*. Each of these approaches has arisen from a different parent discipline, has somewhat different aims/outcomes and may use similar data collection methods, but employ different analysis techniques. Differences amongst these three methods are briefly summarized in Table 1.

The researcher should be guided by the research question and the overall aim of the study to determine which qualitative method is most appropriate. However, in examining the recent qualitative research in the field, it is apparent that rigid adherence to one particular procedure is not common. A description of each method and an example of palliative care research undertaken using each of these methods is briefly summarized below.

Ethnography

Ethnography is a methodology that incorporates a variety of theoretical traditions. However, it is more closely associated with anthropological research than with sociology. Ethnography focuses on the culture of a group, the webs and patterns of meaning that make up a culture and that guide and make sense of people's actions.[3] Ethnography focuses on discovering the cultural frameworks, analysing their structure and content, and using this as a basis for explanation of particular social phenomena. Ethnography is distinct as an approach in that it attempts to interpret and present findings from a cultural perspective. Ethnography searches out the patterns of meaning and emotions that make up culture and how these make sense of actions in everyday life. At the heart of ethnography is good or 'thick' description, typically obtained through an immersion in the everyday life of the group or a given social setting.

Morales[5] used an ethnographic methodology to study the meaning of touch to hospitalized Puerto Ricans with cancer. Eight cancer patients receiving care in a 12-bed oncology research unit in Puerto Rico participated. Data gathering methods included participant observation and several interviews during 1-month period. Participant observation is a valuable data collection method that follows the anthropologist's research model, in which the study of people in their natural settings is undertaken using a toolkit of observation technique, with the researcher becoming immersed in the setting to a greater or lesser degree (Spradley, 1980).[6] The researcher who observes human beings cannot escape, having to participate in some fashion in the experience and actions of those he/she observes. Through this type of participatory interaction, the researcher is able to see things from the people's perspectives and hence to have a deeper understanding of the people that he/she is learning from.[3] Issues of the risk of a 'Hawthorne effect' that are a concern in quantitative methods are not relevant in this type of research. In qualitative research, the researcher *is the instrument of data collection*, through use of observation, field notes, and interviews. No claim is made that the interviewer is separate from the data collection tool or process. However, it is essential that qualitative research reports include details of whether researchers are insiders or outsiders to the setting, and the relevant, existing assumption they bring to the study. Use of this technique also requires an extended period of observation so that the early influence of the observer or interviewer lessens and those observed return to their usual practices and behaviours.

Content analysis was then used to identify patterns of behaviour and meaning. Analysis of field notes and interview was undertaken to search for domains. Theme analysis was used in the search for the relationships among domains. Themes are recurrent patterns in the data that are used to connect domains. Domains are categories of meaning that refer to specific social or cultural scenes or observations.[7] In the analysis of the patient interviews, two types of touch (i.e. domains) were identified: procedural and affective. The predominant theme about perceptions of nurses' touch was that of conveying confidence (this is the recurrent pattern when examining different domains or types of touch). Confidence was related to the patient's increase in positive expectation as much as the possibility of recovery from the cancer illness. Two domains (sub-components of the theme) emerged within the confidence theme: enhancement of the patient's coping abilities and a message of acceptance of the patient as a person during their illness experience. Use of ethnographic methods for this type of study was most appropriate and provided the researcher with an opportunity to construct culturally relevant knowledge.

Phenomenology

Phenomenologists study situations in the everyday world from the viewpoint of the experiencing person. In contrast to the emphasis on culture that is characteristic of ethnographers, phenomenology emphasizes the individual's construction of 'life-world'.[8] The life-world includes taken-for-granted assumptions about everyday life, such as what clothes should be worn, the way to greet someone who is dying, and how to manage embarrassing moments during personal care. The aim is to determine the meaning of an experience for the people who have had the experience and are able to provide a comprehensive description of it. Further, use of phenomenology specifies that people's actions should be explained with reference to their conscious intentions, and with references to the types or categories of understandings that people develop.

Tarzian[9] used phenomenology to study nurses' experiences of caring for dying patients who have 'air hunger'. Ten hospice, long-term care, oncology, or emergency medicine nurses who cared for air-hungry dying patients were recruited. Interviews with two family members who witnessed their dying spouses suffer from air hunger were also used to complement the nurses' accounts. Three themes were identified and provided a framework for a new vision of 'doing everything' for a dying person who suffers from air hunger. These themes included *the patient's look—panic* that beckoned them to respond, a sense of *surrendering and sharing control*, and *fine-tuning dying*. Nurses described ways they responded to relieve a patient's air hunger, including being prepared before air hunger occurs, calming patients and families, medicating patients, improvising care, attending to family members' needs, and drawing distinctions between

Table 1 Qualitative approaches, parent discipline, aim, and methods

Qualitative approach	Parent discipline	Aim	Data collection techniques	Analysis methods
Ethnography	Anthropology	To understand a phenomenon from using a cultural perspective	Interviews Participant observation Document reviews	Language as unit of analysis Search for customs, practices, mores, and norms
Phenomenology	Philosophy	To understand the lived experience of an individual or group of individuals	Interviews Focus group interviews	Search for meanings, essences, lived experiences, stories, and narratives
Ground theory	Sociology	To understand a psycho-social or social process	Interviews Focus groups Participant observation	Search for common themes, sub-themes, and categories Identify contexts, contrasts, co-variates, consequence

palliating and killing. When air hunger occurs in people who are close to death, it often triggers increasing panic and breathlessness. As one home hospice nurse stated, 'He died with his eyes wide open, just gasping for breath, clearly panicked. And I just felt so bad for his wife and daughter who were at his bedside. And I felt after that, I don't ever want this to happen again to anybody' (ref. 9, p. 2).

This study focussed on a research question that has previously been only tangentially addressed in prior empirical work. No prior studies were found regarding the experience of air hunger when death is imminent. The ethical and practical obstacles of this type of study are notable. However, use of the phenomenological approach allowed the researcher to undertake this inquiry in a sensitive, systematic, and in-depth manner that resulted in articulation of new knowledge.

Grounded theory

Grounded theory methods are based upon the argument that theory can be built up through careful observation of the social world. A grounded theory is one that is inductively derived from the study of the phenomenon it represents. That is, it is discovered, developed, and provisionally verified through systematic data collection and analysis of data pertaining to that phenomenon.[10] The methods have their roots in symbolic interactionism founded within American sociological writings. Symbolic interactionism is an analytic framework that argues that human beings construct action on the basis of the meanings of the objects they encounter. This research tradition studies the importance of meanings and symptoms to help understand human behaviour. Symbolic interactionists examine how people make sense of their experiences through a common set of symbols, emphasizing that these symbols are developed and find meaning through shared interactions. Through a process of role-taking, a person imagines how they themselves appear to others, thus becoming a symbolic object to them.

At the heart of grounded theory are two specific techniques, theoretical sampling and thematic analysis. Theoretical sampling involves a process where the representativeness of concepts, not representativeness of persons, is crucial. The aim is not simply to generalize the findings to the broader population, but to construct a theoretical explanation by specifying the conditions and processes that give rise to variations in a phenomenon. The units of analysis are concepts. Thematic analysis is used and involves a process of coding, sorting, and organizing data.

Davies[11] used grounded theory methods to examine the long-term outcomes of adolescent sibling bereavement. She conducted a series of intensive, semi-structured interviews with 12 adults who, in their early adolescence, lost a sibling. This study resulted in the development of a theoretical scheme that captured the reactions and consequences of this experience. Long-term outcomes included psychological growth, a sense of feeling different, and withdrawal from peers. Sibling who withdrew from their peers at a time when peer relationships are critical to completing developmental tasks suffered long-term feelings of sadness and loneliness.

Use of grounded theory methods was appropriate for this study question as it allowed the researcher to identify a psychosocial process, describe and theorize about the meaning and response to a traumatic life event that occurs within a complex social and developmental context. The techniques used by Davies, the reporting methods documented, and the contributions of this work to understanding long-term effects of adolescent bereavement are notable and could not have been achieved using other research methods.

These are only three of the more commonly reported methodologies in qualitative research that may be helpful in addressing research questions in the area of palliative care. The reader may wish to pursue additional literature that describes these methods in greater depth or other types of qualitative methods (e.g. participatory action research, feminist analysis, critical theory, narrative analysis).[3,12–14] Although presented as separate methods, these approaches need not be followed rigidly. Rather, it is important to apply methods with integrity, clear accounts, and a constructive critique of one's own approaches. This said, the notion of rigour in qualitative research methods warrants discussion.

Rigour in qualitative research

One of the major issues related to use of qualitative research methods is the problem of how to appraise the rigour and merits of qualitative methods. The methods of assessing reliability and validity of quantitative methods do not apply and are inappropriate for judging qualitative methods. The qualitative research community holds differing viewpoints on the type of criteria, the need for criteria, and the extent to which an agreed upon set of criteria for judging qualitative research should be expected. Notwithstanding the debates amongst qualitative researchers regarding the best criteria for evaluating qualitative methods, the researcher faced with a need to justify his/her methods, explain the merits of the proposal to a funding body, or report findings in a transparent and credible manner must rely on some criteria.

Miles and Huberman,[15] drawing principally on the work of Guba and Lincoln,[16–18] have listed five criteria that researchers should apply to try to ensure that the qualitative research process is followed and emerging findings are trustworthy. These criteria are *credibility, transferability, dependability, confirmability,* and *authenticity*.

Credibility is enhanced when researchers describe and document their experience as researchers. Self-reflection on the part of the researcher is essential. One way of increasing self-reflection is to keep a journal in which the content and process of interactions are noted, including reactions to various events. This is precisely the aim of a field journal. A journal becomes the record to these relationships and provides material for reflection. Another way of establishing credibility is by consulting participants themselves and asking them to read and discuss the construction derived from the analysis. This technique is referred to as member checking.

Transferability refers to the extent to which the findings from a study might be applied to another situation. Guba and Lincoln[17] suggest that transferability is dependent upon the degree of similarity between two situations or contexts. The authors use the term 'fittingness' to help determine the degree of similarity between two contexts. The original context must be described adequately so that a reader can make a judgement regarding transferability. According to Sandelowski,[19] a study meets the criterion of fittingness when its findings can 'fit' into contexts outside the study situation and when its audience views its findings as meaningful and applicable in terms of their own experiences.

Dependability refers to the consistency of the data. Auditability is the criterion for rigour when dealing with the consistency of data. According to Sandelowski,[19] a study and its findings can be audited when another researcher can clearly follow the decision trail used by the investigator in the study. In addition, another researcher could arrive at the same or comparable, but not contradictory, conclusions given the researcher's data, perspective, and situation.

Confirmability is concerned with assuring that data, interpretations, and outcome inquires are rooted in contexts and persons apart from the evaluation and not simply a figment of the evaluator's imagination. Confirmability requires one to show the way in which interpretations have been arrived at via the inquiry.[20] This requires that data (constructions, assertions, facts, etc.) can be tracked to their sources, and that the logic used to assemble the interpretations into structurally coherent and corroborating wholes is both explicit and implicit in the narrative or a case study. Thus, both the raw products and the processes used to compress them are available to be inspected and confirmed by an outside reviewer of the study. One of the techniques to assess confirmability of a study is a confirmability audit. Guba and Lincoln indicate that confirmability is established when credibility, transferability, and dependability are achieved.

Authenticity is the fifth criterion added later by Guba and Lincoln[21] to acknowledge that multiple constructed realities lie at the heart of the constructivist paradigm. Authenticity is demonstrated if researchers can show that they have represented a range of different realities (fairness in representing and reporting findings). Research should also develop more sophisticated understandings of a phenomenon being studied (ontological authenticity), be shown to have helped members appreciate the viewpoints of people other than themselves (educative authenticity), have stimulated some form of action (catalytic authenticity), and have empowered members to act (tactical authenticity).

Processes and techniques to enhance trustworthiness

In quantitative methods, the terms reliability and validity are used to assess the rigour of the methods used. In qualitative research, the term trustworthiness is appropriate and refers to the extent to which the researcher has addressed five criteria (dependability, authenticity, transferability, credibility, and confirmability). A number of processes to achieve these criteria have been specified and are outlined here. These include use of triangulation, an audit trail, peer debriefing, prolonged engagement, member checking, and techniques to enhance reflexivity. Each of these is described in Table 2.

The researcher endeavouring to demonstrate the trustworthiness of study findings will employ these techniques and processes as is appropriate to the method chosen. The overall trustworthiness of a study is always negotiable and open-ended, not being a matter of final proof whereby readers are compelled to accept an account.

Research issues and pitfalls

Palliative care research can be especially challenging to undertake given the vulnerability of the populations to be studied, the quickly changing nature of the patient's illness, and the complexities of the phenomena to be studied. Three particular issues that merit discussion from the perspective of qualitative methods are outlined here: methodological challenges, the range of palliative care populations to be studied, and medical and social complexities of palliative care.

Methodological challenges

Clinicians and researchers who embark upon palliative care research do so in a field that is fraught with challenges. Participant dying patients often have unpredictable illness trajectories that make longitudinal studies almost impossible. They are frequently distressed by symptoms and their competence affected by the high doses of drugs needed to relieve symptoms. Family members are also under pressure from changes in family dynamics, preparatory grief, and a desire to protect their loved one from any added burden. Health-care professionals have complex workloads, not only in the care of patients and families but also in the building and maintenance of their teams. Because palliative care is a relatively new area of health care, there are often difficulties in finding data collection tools that are proven to be valid and reliable in this field. Often, research methods are dependent on large numbers of relatively homogeneous subjects, whereas in palliative care, we have small numbers of potential participants, each experiencing their illness uniquely, scattered through many organizations. Problems of attrition in palliative care research are well documented(24,25) and use of randomized clinical trials may also pose challenges.

These challenges may prompt use of qualitative methods, which may assist in circumventing some of the difficulties outlined. For example, use of a qualitative design may allow the researcher to examine variations within an illness trajectory more closely. A more personal approach afforded by qualitative methods may facilitate patient participation and decrease the magnitude of attrition. Use of qualitative techniques may elicit information that would not otherwise be retrieved through surveys or paper-and-pencil questionnaires and may provide the basis for development of instruments that are more precise and appropriate for use in palliative care.

Use of qualitative methods may also present practical challenges of how to manage large amounts of complex data and the need to master qualitative data management systems (e.g. NU.DIST, IN.VITRO). These data management software programs are particularly helpful in handling large amounts of data, quickly confirming coding decisions, facilitating re-coding of data, and enhancing the transparency of the data coding and analysis process. However, time must be allowed to learn how to use these software packages so that they serve as a useful tool. It is also important to remember that these packages are only meant to manage the data; the analysis still remains the intellectual responsibility of the researcher.

It may be also difficult for qualitative researchers to know how to reduce the rich, in depth stories that they hear from patients into categories and themes in such a way that retains the poignancy and context of the patient's experience. The intellectual prowess required to hold detail, context, variations, and similarities in one's mind at the same time whilst reviewing and analysing the data cannot be over-stated. The qualitative analysis process might be likened to the action of a high-powered camera lens. The researcher must be able to move close to the data (zoom in) and then move back to the broader context (pan the scene) with flexibility, consistency, and clarity. This analytic technique is a particular skill required for high-quality qualitative research, which may be particularly challenging to learn without experienced research consultation.

The qualitative researcher must also be alert to a potential blurring of boundaries between research and therapy. The intent of the qualitative research interview process is not to develop a therapeutic relationship with the patient or problem-solving therapy for the patient. The intent is to describe a phenomenon or experience that the patient is fully informed of for the purpose of the research. This is not to say that participation in a qualitative interview may not be 'therapeutic'. Many participants describe the research interview as 'invigorating' and helpful. However, the primary aim of qualitative research interviews it not to offer therapy. This distinction has important ethical and methodological implications that the researcher must bear in mind. A researcher, who identifies that the participant may be requiring therapeutic support, must be alert to the need for referral (with the participant's permission) to clinicians or health professionals who may offer this assistance. Researchers should not confuse their role by taking on this role themselves.

Range of palliative care populations

Palliative care populations reach far beyond individuals living with cancer and their families. The needs of those with non-cancer diagnosis, elderly patients receiving care in aged care facilities, and those receiving other approaches to care (e.g. acute care, alternative therapies) in parallel with palliative care may be best studied using qualitative methods. Individuals from non-dominant cultural groups, those in lower socioeconomic groups, children requiring palliative care support, and those in rural and remote communities might all benefit from qualitative research approaches.

Individuals with non-cancer diagnoses

Palliative care is appropriate for patients with neurodegenerative disorders, those with end-stage cardiac or renal failure, persons living with AIDS, and children with various health conditions. To date, few studies have been undertaken to examine the palliative care needs of these populations. Use of phenomenology to understand the meaning of these illness trajectories or studies employing grounded theory techniques may reveal useful social and psychosocial processes relevant to palliative care of these groups.

Elderly individuals

Predictions for the year 2025 confirm an ageing population, with more people worldwide dying from chronic or progressive illnesses rather than acute conditions.(26) Therefore, it is quite imaginable that an array of palliative care services will be required to meet the range of needs of individuals who might benefit from palliative care. To date, little empirical work has been reported on the palliative care needs of the elderly. Qualitative methods may help to elucidate care processes, expressions of symptomatology, and issues of family caring that are unique to this population.

Table 2 Processes, definitions, and approaches to enhancing trustworthiness in qualitative studies

Processes	Definitions	Approaches/variations	Methodological challenges in relation to palliative care
Triangulation	Use of multiple methods within one study[13]	Data triangulation Investigator triangulation Theory triangulation Methods triangulation	Patients and family members may have difficulty participating if multiple methods are used due to fatigue
Prolonged engagement and persistent observation	Sufficient involvement must occur to ensure that data collected are relevant and complete[21]	Extended time in the field Repeated visits to data collection site/participants Rapport of researcher in study context	Persistent observation may be difficult because of unpredictable illness trajectories and changes in cognitive status of patients
Peer debriefing	Practice of involving a peer at various steps of the research process, especially in analysis phase[21]	Multiple researchers for data collection and coding Peer-review panels to discuss challenge data collection steps, analysis process, and researchers' reflections	Researcher(s) may have limited access to colleagues who can serve as research peers. Palliative care clinicians may be available, but may not be able to serve in this role because of confidentiality requirements of research
Member-checking	Verification with participants that what they said has been interpreted with the meaning they ascribed[17]	Formal Informal Individuals Groups Intermittent or final	Patient's cognitive status changes or meaning of the experience changes over time making member-checking unsuitable. Patients may die before member checks occur
Audit trails	Process of research is documented in a way that can be tracked[22]	Maintenance of audit trail notes, decision points, and coding notes	Usually feasible. Volume of detailed, complex notes must be well organized for management of data analysis
Reflexivity techniques	Ways investigators use to document personal reflections on the research process, which are used in the analysis enhance transparency and construction of meanings[23]	Field notes Journals Memos	Usually feasible. Time consuming and emotionally demanding given the type of research undertaken and the sensitive nature of the work; however, is essential due to the above

Individuals receiving palliative care concurrently with other types of services

Palliative care services function adjacent to existing health-care services and must be well linked with other areas of the health-care system to ensure that services are coordinated and well sequenced. This interface requires that research methods and approaches take into consideration patient care needs at earlier phases of an illness trajectory or the needs of patients who may be receiving concurrent active treatments. Qualitative methods may be helpful in examining these types of interactions, illness journeys, and treatment narratives. These approaches may elucidate hypotheses or theoretical postulates concerning the effects of earlier phases of an illness on palliative care. Although health professionals may easily discern differences between palliative care and acute care treatment, patients and families may not make this distinction as crisply. Therefore, 'following' patients from one type of care service/setting to another may be helpful in understanding questions about the transition to palliative care, the history of symptomatology, and the meaning of illness experiences.

Individuals from non-dominant cultural and lower socioeconomic groups

There is also evidence that individuals in minority groups are under-served by current palliative care models. There has been little research undertaken to understand the health and caring perspectives of different cultural groups. Yet, there is a pressing need for this type of empirically based knowledge, because cultural responses to death and dying may take on increased importance once the biomedical interventions have failed to cure. It is often at this stage of illness that patients and families turn to more culturally familiar and comforting beliefs and practices. Some reports also indicate that patients in socially deprived areas have limited access to palliative care. A family's social and cultural background may influence relationship with health-care professionals, access to care, and the carer roles assumed. It is clear that ethnographic methods may offer particular advantages in addressing these types of research questions, providing knowledge that takes into account the social and cultural context and meanings of illness from these perspectives.

Paediatric patients

The development of palliative care services for adults has not been paralleled in paediatrics. It is not that death is less common amongst children than adults. The dying child has been avoided in the literature and in practice, perhaps for emotionally charged reasons. According to Frager,[27] the provision of paediatric palliative care is patchy and inconsistent. One of the reasons may be that many of the diseases are rare and the children suffering from these diseases are distributed over a broad geographic area. Most deaths are due to uncontrollable malignant disease following unsuccessful attempts at curative treatment, and although cure rates for cancer have increased markedly in recent years, nearly one-third of childhood malignancies result in death. However, paediatric palliative care needs extend beyond cancer diagnoses and may be appropriate for a range of progressive, life-threatening illnesses (e.g. neurodegenerative and metabolic disorders, organ failure).

Qualitative methods allow investigations with smaller populations such as the paediatric population, and may provide a useful foundation for examining sensitive topics with these vulnerable patients. The methods of qualitative research are generally less intrusive (e.g. participant observation, play interviews, use of drawings) and are more context sensitive than many quantitative methods, allowing ethically sound and developmentally appropriate approaches to paediatric research.

Individuals in rural and remote communities

Health-care providers in rural and remote communities confront additional challenges associated with delivery of palliative care. They must serve as 'advanced generalists' to a wide range of patients with various health concerns with the expectation that they are able to respond equally well to these problems. Difficulties of isolation, lack of resources, and added emotional pressures associated with long-term patient–health professional relationships may challenge care providers further. The need for responsive models of palliative care appropriate to the needs of these communities is pressing. However, the issue of sample size and geographic dispersion can again be difficult. It is also important that the interventions tested and approaches to care evaluated are appropriate to the community and the social context in which they will be applied. In many instances, use of qualitative methods (e.g. ethnography, action research, grounded theory methods) are particularly useful in obtaining relevant data from a rural community and ensuring that the results obtained will be positively received and implemented.

Ethical research issues specific to the field

Palliative care research usually involves vulnerable patients, family members, and health care professionals. The vulnerability of patients and families in palliative care settings often means that quantitative methods using batteries of data collection tools are unsuitable.

Qualitative research approaches may in these situations be ideal methods for providing rich insights into what might otherwise be hidden areas of practice. However, patients may sometimes feel obligated to participate in research, as gratitude for the care they are receiving. Therefore, palliative care researchers (regardless of the methods chosen) must take special precautions to ensure that some distance is created in the research process between participants and their carers, to ensure that participants are not dependent on care from the researchers. Researchers must also ensure that consenting procedures are clear, open, and honest in their assessment of benefit to the patient. Participants must also be given clear opportunities to withdraw from the project. Often, this requires the researcher to be especially sensitive to signs from potential participants that they do not wish to be involved any more. Therefore, consenting procedures should be dynamic, in this way, so that there is a process of revisiting consent and renegotiation of participation.

There are also a number of consistent reports that indicate that patients and family carers who participate in qualitative studies do not report feeling burdened from their involvement. In contrast, they report feeling affirmed by the opportunity to contribute their experiences to others, may see their involvement as a type of testimony and last contribution that they offer the wider community, and may gain insights from having an opportunity to reflect on their experiences. Some participants report feeling invigorated by this participation. It seems important, therefore, to consider the potential positive benefits that occur through use of qualitative research in a palliative care context.

Summary

Qualitative research is an area of basic scientific inquiry, the fundamental description of mechanisms, processes, structures, and phenomenon. This basic research is needed in the area of palliative care to build clinical interventions and more effective clinical programmes.

Some of the benefits or advantages of qualitative methods include: an ability to examine situations in depth with open-ended questions, the capacity to explore complex questions, and a research approach that is flexible enough for application to a wide range of patients.

Yedida and MacGregor[28] illustrate the potential for depth and breadth in qualitative research through an ethnographic study designed to identify dominant themes characterizing patients' perspectives on death during the last months of life. The seven motifs they identified that characterized these perspectives were: struggle (living and dying are difficult), dissonance (dying is not living), endurance (triumph of inner strength), coping (finding a new balance), incorporation (belief system accommodates death), quest (seeking meaning kin death), and volatile (unresolved and unresigned). Yedidia and MacGregor found that the patients ($n = 30$, with a mean of 4.2 interviews per patient) showed a strong capacity for coherence, integrating their responses to dying with broader motifs in their life stories. The richness of this type of data and its implications for palliative care are only possible to elicit through a qualitative research approach.

References

1. **Berglund, C.A.**, ed. *Health Research.* South Melbourne, Victoria: Oxford University Press, 2001.
2. **Kuhn, T.** *The Structure of Scientific Revolutions.* Chicago: University of Chicago Press, 1970.
3. **Rice, P.L. and Ezzy, D.** *Qualitative Research Methods: A Health Focus.* South Melbourne, Victoria: Oxford University Press, 1999.
4. **LeCompte, M. and Preissle, J.** *Ethnography and Qualitative Design in Educational Research,* 2nd edn. San Diego CA: Academic Press Inc., 1993.
5. **Morales, E.** (1994). Meaning of touch to hospitalised Puerto Ricans with cancer. *Cancer Nursing* **17**, 464–9.
6. **Spradley, J.P.** *Participant Observation.* New York: Holt, Rinchart & Winston, 1980.
7. **Gillis, A. and Jackson, W.** *Research for Nurses: Methods and Interpretation.* Philadelphia: FA Davis Company, 2002.
8. **van Manen, M.** *Researching Lined Experience: Human Science for an Action Sensitive Pedagogy.* New York: State University of New York, 1990, pp. 30–3.
9. **Tarzian, A.J.** (2000). Caring for dying patients who have air hunger. *Journal of Nursing Scholarship* **32**, 137–43.
10. **Strauss, A. and Corbin, J.** *Basics of Qualitative Research: Grounded Theory Procedures and Techniques.* Newbury Park CA: Sage Publications Inc., 1990.
11. **Davies, B.** (1991). Long-term outcomes of adolescent sibling bereavement. *Journal of Adolescent Research* **6**, 83–96.
12. **Clough, P.** *Feminist Thought.* Oxford: Blackwell, 1994.
13. **Denzin, N. and Lincoln, Y.**, ed. *Handbook of Qualitative Research.* Thousand Oaks CA: Sage Publications, 2000.
14. **Whyte, W.F.**, ed. *Participatory Action Research.* Newbury Park CA: Sage Publications, 1991.
15. **Miles, M.B. and Huberman, A.M.** (1994). Data management and analysis methods. In *Handbook of Qualitative Research* (ed. N. Denzin and Y. Lincoln), pp. 428–44. Thousand Oaks CA: Sage Publications.
16. **Guba, E.G. and Lincoln, Y.S.** *Naturalistic Inquiry.* Beverly Hills CA: Sage, 1981.
17. **Guba, E.G. and Lincoln, Y.S.** *Fourth Generation Evaluation.* Newbury Park CA: Sage Publications, 1989.
18. **Lincoln, Y.S. and Guba, E.G.** *Naturalistic Inquiry.* Beverly Hills CA: Sage, 1985.
19. **Sandelowski, M.** (1986). The problem of rigor in qualitative research. *Advances in Nursing Science* **8**, 27.
20. **Koch, T.** (1994). Establishing rigour in qualitative research: the decision trail. *Journal of Advanced Nursing* **19**, 976–86.
21. **Guba, E.G. and Lincoln, Y.S.** (1994). Competing paradigms in qualitative research. In *Handbook of Qualitative Research* (ed. N. Denzin and Y. Linkcon), pp. 105–17. Thousand Oaks CA: Sage Publications.
22. **Silverman, M., Ricci, E., and Gunter, M.** (1990). Strategies for increasing the rigor of qualitative methods in evaluation of health care programs. *Evaluation Review* **14**, 57–74.
23. **Grbich, C.** *Qualitative Research in Health: An Introduction.* St Leonards NSW: Allen & Unwin, 1999.
24. **Bruera, E.** (1994). Ethical issues in palliative care research. *Journal of Palliative Care* **10**, 7–9.
25. **Kristjanson, L.J., Hanson, E.J., and Balneaves, L.G.** (1994). Research with palliative care populations: ethical issues. *Journal of Palliative Care* **10**, 10–15.
26. **Davis, R., Wagner, E.H., and Groves, T.** (1999). Managing chronic disease. *British Medical Journal* **318**, 1090–1.
27. **Frager, G.** (1996). Pediatric palliative care: building the model, bridging the gaps. *Journal of Palliative Care* **12**, 9–12.
28. **Yedida, M. and MacGregor, B.** (2001). Confronting the prospect of dying: reports of terminally ill patients. *Journal of Pain and Symptom Management* **22** (4), 807–19.

5.4 Clinical trials of treatments for pain

Mitchell B. Max and Russell K. Portenoy

Introduction

The development of a scientific basis for symptom treatment is an imperative for the field of palliative care. Several historical circumstances make pain research an area of particular promise. First, a range of new treatments have been made possible by advances in both neuroscience and therapeutic technology. Examples include the development of selective agonists and antagonists of neural receptors mediating pain and analgesia, and the development of novel methods of analgesic administration, such as spinal, transdermal, or patient-controlled analgesic infusions. Second, the scientific foundation for research into pain therapy has already been established. Thousands of clinical trials have shown that simple measures of pain relief can reliably quantify analgesic efficacy. Third, there are great opportunities for methodological innovation, including multidose drug comparisons, assessment of treatment toxicity and quality of life, and controlled studies of spinal opiate infusions or neurolytic procedures.

This chapter is written for the palliative care clinician who plans to conduct controlled clinical trials of treatments for pain. In this brief review, no attempt will be made to be comprehensive; for example, biostatistical issues, such as sample size calculation, sequential analysis methods, and specific statistical tests, are left to other works. Rather, several of the key issues in designing a clinical analgesic trial will be discussed in some depth: formulating the research question, choosing treatments and controls in a way that will maximize the chance for a meaningful positive or negative result, and tailoring the most efficient study procedures for a particular situation (e.g. patient selection, the choice between parallel or crossover design, and the choice of outcome measures). To complement this chapter, the beginning investigator may wish to refer to longer works on analgesic study design,[1–3] monographs on clinical trials methods in general,[4–6] pain assessment,[7–9] and biostatistics.[10,11] An interactive, research case-based presentation of this material and research on other symptoms is available at http://symptomresearch.nih.gov.[12]

Clarifying the question to be studied

Clinical trials in palliative medicine might examine any of a wide variety of pain relief interventions, including treatments aimed at the lesion causing pain, new analgesic drugs or routes of drug administration, neuroablative procedures, cognitive treatments for pain, and efforts to improve physicians' prescribing practices. Each type of investigation requires numerous design choices. For most of these interventions, there have been few or no clinical trials, and it is not possible to give specific rules for their design. Nonetheless, there are several general questions common to all studies that may help the investigator to focus limited resources on the crucial issues.

What shortcomings of conventional treatments is the proposed treatment intended to correct?

The outcome measures and overall design of the study should focus on the components of this particular clinical dilemma. For example, the most common dose-limiting side-effects of opioids are sedation and nausea. In studies of adjuvant drugs intended to specifically augment opioid analgesia, these side effects must be carefully quantitated, and the treatments, controls, and outcome measures be sufficient to prove that the addition of the adjuvant not only increases analgesia, but causes less sedation and nausea than an equianalgesic dose of the opioid alone. Such data are lacking on adjuvants in current use[13] (Chapter 8.2.3).

Is the study primarily intended to elucidate a biological principle, or to guide the clinician's empirical choice of treatment in that particular patient population?

Schwartz and Lellouch[14,15] distinguish between two different purposes of clinical trials, which they call 'explanatory' and 'pragmatic'. An 'explanatory' approach seeks to elucidate a biological principle. The study population is considered to be a model from which one may learn principles of analgesic pharmacology or pain physiology—principles that are likely to shed light on a variety of clinical problems. For example, the 'analgesic equivalency tables' that guide opioid prescribing in a variety of conditions are largely based on studies in cancer patients.[1,2] A 'pragmatic' approach, in contrast, focuses on the question, 'What is the better treatment in the *particular clinical circumstances* of the patients in the study?'

As an illustration of how these approaches to design differ, consider a hypothetical analgesic that animal studies had shown to be effective in models of visceral pain. Looking first at patient selection, a palliative care researcher oriented towards the explanatory approach might select only a small subset of cancer patients in whom there was unequivocal radiological proof of hollow viscera involvement, while the pragmatic clinical researcher might open the study to patients with ill-defined abdominal pain. An explanatory approach would try to maximize the therapeutic response by selecting a high dose and monitoring patients frequently; the pragmatically oriented investigator might choose an intermediate dose and provide the looser supervision common in clinical practice. An explanatory approach will usually mandate a placebo, because even small amounts of pain relief over the placebo response may provide information about the mechanisms of visceral pain transmission and relief. A pragmatic approach, in contrast, generally compares the new treatment to the best treatment in clinical use. Placebo comparisons may still be desirable in such studies, particularly when there is no significant difference between the study drug and standard control (see below), but detection of a small therapeutic effect is of less interest.

The dichotomous explanatory/pragmatic schema is an oversimplification, of course. The investigator usually wishes to address both theoretical *and* practical concerns. This distinction may, however, offer a useful perspective for making design choices in complex cases.

How can previous clinical experience with the proposed treatment guide the design of a controlled trial?

Retrospective or prospective surveys of clinical experience can provide insights into the nature and variety of therapeutic and adverse effects produced by a treatment, and thereby help determine the methods for future controlled studies. Among other factors, surveys can suggest the major sources of variability in the response to an intervention. For example, a survey of approximately 700 cancer patients treated with non-steroidal anti-inflammatory drugs suggested that pain relief was greater in patients with bony or other somatic lesions than in those with nerve lesions.[16]

Surveys may also enable the investigator to estimate the time-course of response. In a controlled trial, treatment periods should be long enough so that patients will approach maximal response, unless a significant incidence of drop outs or spontaneous change in the disease over that length of time mandates a compromise on study duration. This will help to maximize the power of the study to detect treatment differences. In some cases, survey data must be supplemented by prospective open-label pilot studies. For analgesic drug treatments, survey data or prospective dose-ranging studies will suggest a maximum safe dose for initial studies and may suggest a range of doses or blood levels that will produce analgesia.[17] Such pilot studies can also provide variance estimates for the major outcome measures, which are needed to choose the sample size.[4] The use of surveys and non-randomized controlled trials are discussed further in other articles.[18,19]

Choice of treatments and controls

A clear-cut positive *or* negative result of a clinical trial is often useful to other researchers, and ultimately, to patients. Unfortunately, many clinical studies turn out to be inconclusive (and often unpublishable) because of poor selection of control groups. During the 40-year history of analgesic clinical trials, a distinct logic has evolved regarding the choice of controls and the interpretation of clinical trials. This framework, illustrated in Fig. 1(a)–(h), is now widely applied in determining the validity of single-dose analgesic trials.[20,21]

Interpreting analgesic studies: test drug, placebo, and positive control

Although the simplest of the classic designs consists of two treatments—the test medication and a placebo—most modern single-dose trials also include a standard analgesic 'positive control'. In single-dose trials, common positive controls include morphine, aspirin, or ibuprofen.

To demonstrate the value of these controls, consider a hypothetical study comparing the putative analgesic drug X to a morphine 'positive control' and a placebo (Fig. 1(a)). Using summed pain relief scores as the measure of analgesia, drug X tended to be slightly but not statistically significantly more effective than morphine, and both drug X and morphine were statistically superior to placebo. The conclusions are straightforward: drug X is an effective analgesic, and the study methods were sufficiently sensitive to distinguish morphine from placebo.

The omission of a positive control does not fatally flaw the study if drug X is superior to placebo (Fig. 1(b)), although one cannot be certain about the strength of the effect. The positive control serves as a yardstick against which to compare the magnitude of the analgesia produced by drug X. In pain syndromes for which there is no accepted positive control—for example, some types of neuropathic pain—the comparison of test drug to placebo must suffice. Should drug X fail to produce more analgesia than the placebo, however, the omission of the positive control will render the study uninterpretable (Fig. 1(c)). One cannot reliably conclude that drug X is ineffective in this condition. Perhaps the drug is truly analgesic in patients with this condition, but the study methods were too insensitive to observe this effect. This could happen because patients were too stressed by the clinical setting to respond to medication, the pain questionnaires were insensitive, the procedures of the nurse-observer were variable or confusing, or merely because of random variation. If a morphine positive control were included and shown superior to both placebo and drug X (Fig. 1(d)), this would validate the study methodology and indicate that drug X was not analgesic in this population. Alternatively, if morphine produced no more analgesia than drug X and the placebo (Fig. 1(e)), one could conclude that the study methods were inadequate to show the effects of even a strong analgesic.

What are the consequences of omitting the *placebo* and comparing drug X only to a standard analgesic? As in the previous case, this omission is less damaging when the assay shows a difference between the two treatments. The data in Fig. 1(f) suggest that drug X is an effective analgesic in this population, although the proportion of analgesia attributable to the placebo effect cannot be determined for either drug X or morphine. If the responses to drug X and standard analgesic were similar, however (Fig. 1(g)), interpretation would be troublesome. The data might reflect either that drug X and morphine were both effective analgesics, or that neither was effective and there was a large placebo effect.[22]

If the use of a placebo group is difficult, an alternative approach is to use a second dose level of the standard analgesic. Figure 1(h) shows that morphine 12 mg surpassed morphine 6 mg, demonstrating the sensitivity of the study methods, and implying that the effects of both drug X and morphine 12 mg were not merely placebo effects.

In addition to doses of a test drug, a standard analgesic, and a placebo, most analgesic studies include additional treatment groups or controls that are chosen to further elucidate the major research question. For example, when evaluating a range of doses of test analgesic, one might add additional

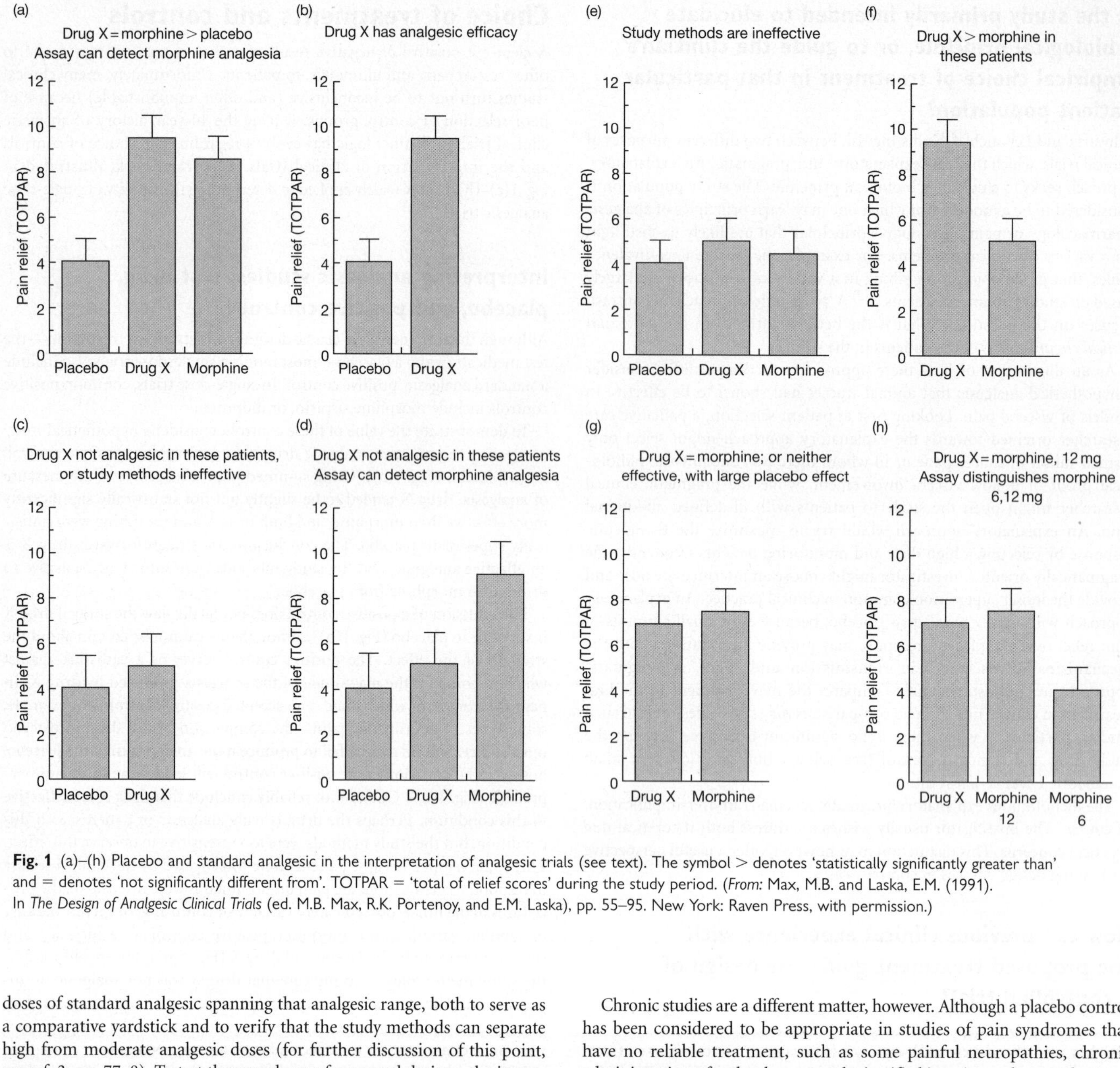

Fig. 1 (a)–(h) Placebo and standard analgesic in the interpretation of analgesic trials (see text). The symbol > denotes 'statistically significantly greater than' and = denotes 'not significantly different from'. TOTPAR = 'total of relief scores' during the study period. (*From:* Max, M.B. and Laska, E.M. (1991). In *The Design of Analgesic Clinical Trials* (ed. M.B. Max, R.K. Portenoy, and E.M. Laska), pp. 55–95. New York: Raven Press, with permission.)

doses of standard analgesic spanning that analgesic range, both to serve as a comparative yardstick and to verify that the study methods can separate high from moderate analgesic doses (for further discussion of this point, see ref. 3, pp. 77–8). To test the soundness of proposed designs, the investigator may wish to graph the possible outcomes as in Fig. 1(a)–(h). If the conclusion, given a particular outcome is ambiguous, it may be wise to consider additional treatment groups that would distinguish among the alternative explanations. The addition of treatment or control groups is costly, however. One must either recruit more patients or reduce the size of each treatment group, lessening the statistical power of the comparisons. In many cases, particularly where negative results will not be of great interest, researchers may choose to omit controls whose main value is to clarify the interpretation of the negative result.

Placebo and positive controls in chronic palliative care studies

In single-dose analgesic studies in cancer pain, there are rarely ethical objections to the use of placebos, because patients understand that they can terminate the study and take additional analgesic at any time. In actual practice, many patients experience some placebo analgesia, and most tolerate the study for the 1–2 h needed to evaluate the response to the placebo.

Chronic studies are a different matter, however. Although a placebo control has been considered to be appropriate in studies of pain syndromes that have no reliable treatment, such as some painful neuropathies, chronic administration of a placebo cannot be justified in pain syndromes that generally respond to therapy, such as most cancer pain syndromes. Moreover, attrition rates under such circumstances are likely to be high; for example, in a placebo-controlled drug trial in cancer patients,[23] 90 per cent of the placebo group withdrew on the first day. The same problem exists for studies of discrete interventions, for example, coeliac block, that require a prolonged observation period after the treatment.

In these situations, therefore, the only feasible way to conduct placebo-controlled studies may be to give both placebo and active treatment groups access to a standard analgesic 'rescue' dose. An example of a chronic placebo-controlled study of ibuprofen for metastatic bone pain is shown in Fig. 2. Stambaugh and Drew[24] enrolled a group of inpatients whose bone pain required at least four daily doses of an oxycodone/acetaminophen (oxy/APAP) combination. Strong parenteral opioids were also given for severe breakthrough pain, but patients requiring more than one injection daily were dropped from the study. For the first 7 days of the study, no intervention took place; the daily dose of oxy/APAP was monitored, and patients assessed pain intensity and relief once a day. On days 8–14, half the patients received ibuprofen 600 mg po four times daily, and the other half

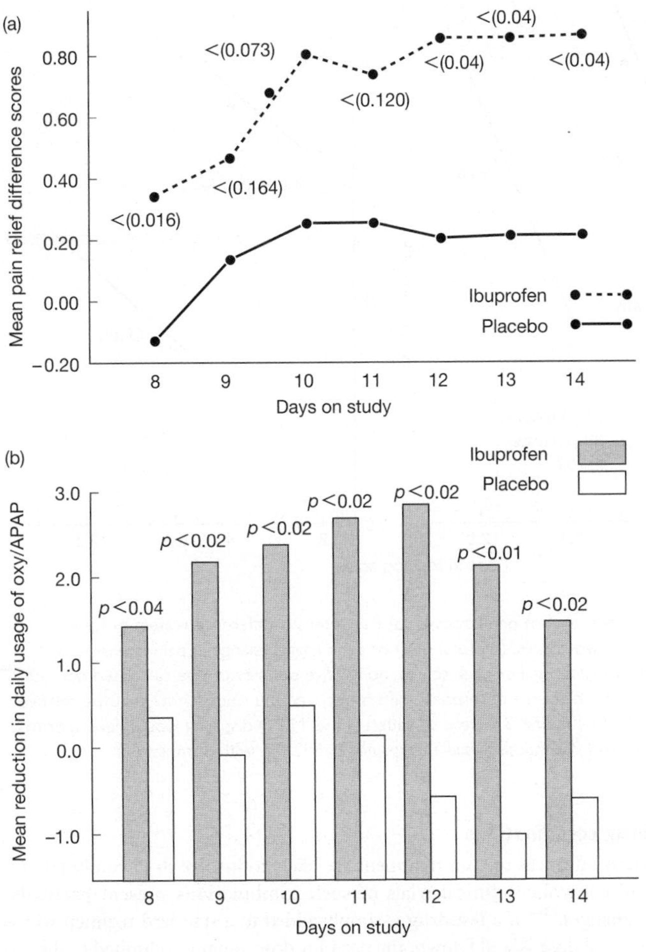

Fig. 2 (a) Comparison of mean pain relief differences of ibuprofen, 600 mg four times per day versus placebo, both in combination with oxy/APAP as needed. Values in parentheses represent *p* values of ibuprofen versus placebo. Day 8 was the first day ibuprofen or placebo were added, after 7 days of baseline observations of pain and oxy/APAP consumption. (b) Alterations of oxy/APAP use after the addition of ibuprofen or placebo. Mean reduction scores were determined by comparing oxy/APAP use on Days 6 and 7 with means for each of Days 8–14. For each day, oxy/APAP use was reduced by the addition of ibuprofen. (*From:* Stambaugh, J.E. and Drew, J. (1988). *Clinical Pharmacology and Therapeutics* **44**, 665–9, with permission.)

received placebo. Figure 2 shows that pain relief was better with ibuprofen than placebo, and that the ibuprofen-treated group reduced their oxy/APAP consumption relative to the placebo group. This example illustrates how use of the background or rescue analgesic becomes another important outcome measure. Similar strategies have been used to study the analgesic effects of sustained-release morphine in cancer patients[25–27] and many types of interventions in postoperative pain.[28,29]

In these designs, the rescue analgesic may be given by any of a variety of routes, including oral, intramuscular, or intravenous (commonly by patient-controlled analgesic devices). Both pain report and rescue analgesic consumption should be examined as primary outcome measures. Although some investigators have used the the amount of rescue drug consumed as the only outcome measure, many patients may not change their analgesic demands enough to completely offset any change in pain (as in Fig. 2 and refs 27 and 28). In addition, the reduction of analgesic consumption alone is not a compelling clinical advantage, unless pain or analgesic side effects can also be shown to be reduced. An analytic method has been proposed that integrates pain score and rescue analgesic consumption into a single summary variable.[30]

In repeated-dose studies just as in single-dose studies, positive controls or multiple levels of the test drug may also be used to answer the research question.[31,32] As with the placebo-controlled studies discussed above, provisions must generally be made for a rescue analgesic treatment of some sort. In addition, the protocol should allow for lowering doses of the test drug or standard analgesic should drug toxicity occur.

Designing the appropriate control interventions may also be a challenge for non-pharmacological treatments. Control or sham interventions are possible with diverse treatments such as cognitive pain control techniques or acupuncture, but they are often open to criticism.[33] With more invasive methods such as neuroablative procedures, placebo or sham procedures are generally considered inappropriate.

Comments on several specialized design problems

Dose-ranging studies

Knowledge of a drug's dose–response curve guides its use in clinical practice. This relationship is clarified through studies that compare the effects produced by a range of doses. The dose range to be examined in these trials may be chosen on the basis of Phase I toxicity studies, which indicate an upper limit, or by prior clinical experience. Methods for examining the dose–response relationship is an area of current research interest,[34–36] although there has been little work with chronic analgesic therapies.

A few general points can be made about dose-ranging. First, doses should be chosen over a wide range of levels. For dose ranges that may be of clinical interest, several levels of a standard analgesic control are also often desirable, allowing a direct comparison of adverse effects for the test and standard treatment at levels producing equal analgesia. Second, efforts to estimate the optimal therapeutic range are often assisted by the analysis of blood levels of drug or active metabolites, particularly in the case of drugs whose pharmacokinetics have great variability.[17] Third, to draw firm conclusions about dose–response curves, it is important that several different dosing schemes be specified prospectively; these may include parallel group designs, crossover studies[34] (see below), or studies using several different ascending dose-titration schedules.[37]

Relative potency studies

One of the most useful tools in guiding the dosing of opioid analgesics has been the class of designs called relative potency bioassays.[38] Relative potency bioassays consist of a comparison of two or more doses of a test drug with two or more doses of a standard (Fig. 3). A placebo may not be necessary in such trials, because the demonstration of a statistically significant positive slope for the dose–response curves establishes assay sensitivity. A placebo is necessary, however, if one wishes to estimate the lowest dose at which analgesic efficacy might be detected.

There are several advantages in expressing the outcome of a study or group of studies[39,40] in terms of relative potency. First, such estimates allow clinicians to tailor the dosing of a new drug to the individual patient, based on the specific dose of the standard usually used by that patient. Second, this method eliminates the problem of expressing a drug's effect in units on an arbitrary analgesic scale, measurements whose absolute size may vary with the patient population, study methods, and placebo effect. Finally, relative potency studies allow one to test whether a new analgesic or drug combination is superior to the standard in terms of toxicity as well as efficacy; the relative intensity of adverse effects can be estimated for the two treatments at doses providing the same analgesia.[13,41]

There are also pitfalls in interpreting relative potency assays. If the dose–response curves of the test and standard drugs are not linear and parallel, or the doses chosen are not in the same analgesic range, the calculated relative potency may be incorrect or meaningless. In addition, if the drugs to be compared have different kinetics, the relative potency may vary greatly depending upon whether the peak pain relief or the summed scores over

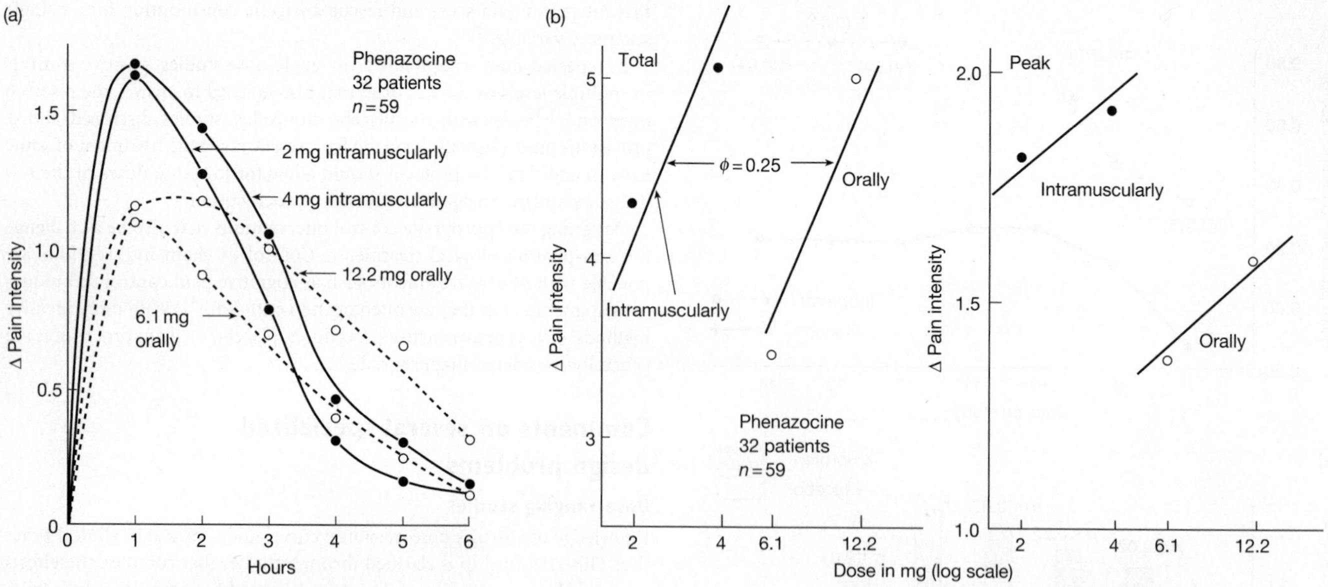

Fig. 3 Four-point relative potency study comparing intramuscular (filled circles) and oral (open circles) phenazocine. (a) Pain intensity difference (category scale) is plotted against time (left). Note the difference between the time-course of analgesia for the two routes. (b) Total (left) or peak (right) change in pain intensity are plotted against dose. For total scores, oral phenazocine is one-fourth as potent as intramuscular drug. For peak scores, no relative potency can be calculated because there was no overlap between the level of response seen with the two routes. Because the time-course of response differs between the routes, note that the relative potency calculated for total scores will change according to the length of the study; e.g., if only the first 3 h were considered, the IM/PO disparity would have appeared even greater. (*From:* Beaver, W.T., Wallenstein, S.L., Houde, R.W., and Rogers, A. (1968). *Clinical Pharmacology and Therapeutics* **9**, 582–97, with permission.)

time are used. For example, using summed scores over time will favour a drug with longer duration (Fig. 3, left).

In addition, relative potency estimates derived from single-dose studies may not be sufficient to predict chronic dosing requirements, particularly when the pharmacokinetics of the treatments and their active metabolites differ. For example, the slowly metabolized analgesic methadone is equipotent to morphine as a single parenteral dose, but observations in cancer patients being converted from chronic treatment with one drug to the other suggest methadone is more than 10 times more potent.[42] Additional repeated-dose relative potency studies of the common opioid analgesics are needed to provide a better basis for clinical treatment. One must be wary of several potential biases. If relative potency estimates are based on unidirectional shifts from opioid A to opioid B, the relative effectiveness of opioid B might be underestimated if opioid tolerance develops or if the underlying disease progresses in a way that tends to increase pain. One can avoid this bias by running the conversion in both directions.[12,43,44]

Studies to assess whether two treatments are equivalent

A common error in study design is to assume that the demonstration of no significant difference between two analgesics proves that they are equivalent.[45] The error in this reasoning is illustrated by the following example: In a controlled trial, cancer patients received either intramuscular morphine, 10 mg, or intramuscular morphine, 5 mg, *plus* a peptide shown to potentiate opioid analgesia in animals. In the clinical trial, similar pain relief scores were observed for the two treatments, and the investigator concluded that the peptide doubled the analgesic effects of morphine. The data do not support this; without controls such as morphine, 5 mg alone, or placebo, there was no demonstration that the study methods would have been sensitive enough to detect a true difference between analgesics (Fig. 1(g)). Even if both morphine, 10 mg, and morphine, 5 mg + peptide had surpassed a control group, a convincing demonstration of equivalence would require demonstrating that the 95 per cent confidence interval for the difference between the two treatments was also small.[46–48] This generally requires a much larger sample size than is needed to distinguish an active treatment from placebo.[45]

Drug combinations

Many advances in pain treatment are likely to involve drug combinations, and controlled clinical trials of such combinations present particular challenges.[49] If a test drug is simply added to a standard regimen whose optimal dose is well known, the need for dose-ranging is limited to the test drug.[50] Should uncertainty exist about the dose of each component, however, a rather complex study may be needed.[51] For example, one might determine dose–response curves for each component alone and for several dose ratios of the combination (current work is reviewed in refs 12, 20, 49, and 52–54).

Parallel versus crossover designs

In a parallel group (also termed 'completely randomized') design, each patient receives a single treatment. In a crossover design, each patient receives some (incomplete block) or all (complete block) of the treatments being studied.

There are several obvious advantages to crossover designs. Analgesic studies often require large sample sizes because detection of a drug effect must compete with so many other causes of variation in pain report: the subject's painful lesion, tolerance to opioid medications, psychological makeup, previous pain experience, age, race, weight, interaction with the study personnel, etc. Much of this between patient variation can be eliminated by using a crossover design, in which treatment comparisons are largely or entirely within the same patient.[55–60] Because of this reduction in variance, and because each patient is used several times, crossover studies usually have greater statistical power for a given sample size than parallel group designs.[49] This is an important practical advantage, particularly when studies are performed in a single center. Crossover designs have been used frequently in studies of cancer pain.[1,61]

Such advantages notwithstanding, there may be problems with the use of crossover designs in palliative care settings. First, change in the painful lesions over time may introduce great variability into patient responses, thereby undermining the major potential advantage of the crossover design. This necessitates that the total duration of the crossover study be short enough to ensure such within-patient variation will be less than the variation already existing between the patients enrolled. The changes in the underlying disease, as well as logistical factors and voluntary withdrawals, usually cause a higher dropout rate in crossover than in parallel group studies. Although the greater power of the crossover approach may compensate for a higher dropout rate, reviewers may doubt the general applicability of the results of a study completed by a minority of the patients entered.

Another major concern with crossover studies is the possibility of bias produced by unequal 'carryover effects'. Carryover effects are changes in the efficacy of treatments resulting from treatments given in earlier periods; they may be mediated by persistence of drug or metabolites, changes in brain or peripheral tissues caused by the treatment, or behavioural or psychological factors. The major problem with carryover effects occurs with the two-treatment, two-period design ('2 × 2'; Table 1, left). Results may be difficult to interpret whenever the treatment effect differs for the two periods. In this event, one cannot distinguish with any certainty whether this is due to a carryover effect (persistence of a pharmacological or psychological effect of the first treatment into the second period), a 'treatment × period interaction' (the passage of time affects the relative efficacy of the treatments; e.g. by the second period, patients who initially received placebo might be too discouraged to respond to any subsequent treatment), or a difference between the groups of patients assigned the two different orders of treatment. For this reason, regulatory agencies have been particularly reluctant to rely upon data from such designs.

Fortunately, these statistical difficulties are largely limited to the 2 × 2 case. If the investigator adds several other treatment sequences (Table 1, Alternative #1) or a third treatment period (Alternative #2, 3) unbiased estimates of treatment effects are possible even in the presence of various types of carryover effects.[58–60,62] For studies involving three or more treatments, there are a variety of designs that allow these effects to be distinguished.[58,63] Thus, although the relative brevity and simplicity of the 2 × 2 design may make it attractive for single-centre pilot studies and for situations in which previous experience suggests that there is no significant carryover effect, the need to estimate treatment effects with greater certainty will usually recommend the use of alternative designs.

A variant of the crossover design, the 'enriched enrolment' design, may be useful in studying treatments to which only a minority of patients respond.[64,65] If the results are not statistically significant in a conventional clinical trial, one cannot retrospectively point at the responders and claim that the treatment accounted for their relief. One can, however, enter them into a second prospective trial, or a series of comparisons between treatment and placebo. If the results of the second trial considered alone are statistically significant, this suggests that the patients' initial response was not just due to chance. While statistically defensible, enriched enrollment designs are open to the criticism that prior exposure to the treatment may defeat the double-blind procedure (particularly with treatments that have distinctive side effects), and sometimes result in spurious positive results.

Parallel study designs are preferable when there are strong concerns about carryover effects or when the natural history of the pain syndrome makes disease-related changes in pain likely during the period required for a crossover study. Between-patient variability is the major problem posed by parallel group designs, and several approaches have been suggested to mitigate its impact.[66] For example, baseline pain scores may be subtracted from the treatment scores to yield pain intensity difference scores, or they may be treated as a covariate. This often eliminates a large part of the variance, thereby increasing the power of treatment comparisons. In single-dose analgesic drug trials, the baseline has generally been determined under 'no treatment conditions', but as discussed above, a standard pain treatment regimen will generally be needed in palliative care contexts.

The investigator should also make an effort to balance the treatment groups for variables that predict response, whenever these predictors are known or suspected.[67] If one wishes to examine response in specific subgroups, assignments must also be balanced appropriately. Groups can be balanced using stratification or various techniques of adaptive randomization.[4,6] In studies with sample sizes typical of single-centre trials, 20–40 patients per group, these methods can significantly increase the power of a study if the prognostic variables are well chosen and the statistical methods take the balancing method into account.[66] If stratification is not feasible, post hoc covariate analyses or other statistical techniques may be an acceptable substitute if the variables in question are distributed fairly evenly among the treatment groups.

Table 1 Some alternative designs for two-treatment cross-over studies

Standard 2 × 2	Alternative 1	Alternative 2	Alternative 3
A–B	A–B	A–B–B	A–B–B
B–A	B–A	B–A–A	B–A–A
	A–A		A–B–A
	B–B		B–A–B

Selecting the patient sample

Many characteristics of the patients may influence the outcome of analgesic studies (Table 2). Depending upon the purpose of the study (see above), investigators may either choose to define the population narrowly for a number of factors, or may open the study to a broad group of patients. Narrow criteria bring certain benefits—potentially lower variance in outcome measures, and as discussed above, more solid grounding for 'explanatory' conclusions. On the other hand, multiple rigorous entry criteria

Table 2 Factors that contribute to the heterogeneity of the population suffering from cancer pain

Pain-related factors	Pain characteristics
	Intensity and duration of chronic pain
	Pain intensity at study onset
	Quality
	Temporal pattern
	Precipitants
	Pain mechanisms and site of lesion
	Prior therapy
	Duration and extent of prior analgesic use
	Efficacy of previous analgesics
	Prior adverse effects from analgesics
Patient-related factors	Demographics
	Psychological factors
	Affective disorders
	Other psychiatric disorders
	Behavioural disturbances
	Cognitions, expectations, and fears
	Intellectual capacity
	Degree of placebo response
	Other historical factors
	History of chronic pain
	History of substance abuse
	History of psychiatric disorder
Disease-related factors	Related to neoplasm
	Type of tumour
	Extent of disease
	Previous antineoplastic therapy
	Ongoing antineoplastic therapy
	Other pathological processes
	Major organ dysfunction
	Number and severity of other symptoms
	Other treatments
	Concurrent use of centrally acting drugs
	Use of drugs that may be coanalgesic

may slow patient accrual, or introduce selection biases that may limit the generalizability of the results. For example, the decision to exclude elderly cancer patients from a trial may reduce the risk of adverse effects, but will also limit the value of the efficacy and safety data for treating older patients.

Factors related to the pain

In selecting patients for cancer pain studies, particular attention should be paid to pain mechanisms, temporal characteristics, baseline pain intensity, and prior opioid intake.[68]

It is reasonable to assume that pain mechanisms may not be uniform among pains arising from different tissues, and that these differences may affect responses to particular treatments. Although pain mechanisms may sometimes be directly assessed using techniques such as stimulation or blockade of particular nerve fiber populations, this will rarely be practical in palliative care clinical trials. Pain mechanisms may be imputed from knowledge of the involved tissues, and from the patient's pain report. Therefore it is important that researchers characterize patients by the site of pain-producing lesions during enrollment into the study, and by the quality and temporal characteristics of the pain. Current studies at Memorial Sloan-Kettering Cancer Center use the following categories: *Somatic pain* denotes pain arising from bone, joint, muscle, skin, or connective tissue, which is usually aching or throbbing in quality and well localized. For some purposes, investigators may wish to consider particular subclasses, such as bone pain. *Visceral pain* can be sub-divided into a relatively well-localized and aching pain associated with tumor involvement of organ capsules and the poorly localized, usually intermittent cramping associated with obstruction of a hollow viscus. These two sub-types should be distinguished in analgesic studies. *Neuropathic pain* is most commonly burning or stabbing in quality, is often associated with a sense of distortion of the body part or light-touch evoked discomfort, and is accompanied by evidence of appropriately localized injury to the peripheral or central nervous system.

Although many pains in patients with cancer are relatively steady, some patients have intermittent transient pains, such as the so-called 'incident pains' that are triggered by movement. The analgesic efficacy of any therapeutic modality may be difficult to assess when these pains are frequent and severe. In some studies, it may be reasonable for the investigator to exclude patients in whom they are particularly prominent, whereas in other studies, it may be useful to consider quantitating the frequency and intensity of these pains as an additional outcome measure.

Baseline pain intensity and consumption of analgesic drugs prior to the study (including type and dose of drug, duration of treatment, and time of last dose) must also be recorded as potentially important covariates.[69–71] In the case of opioids, the latter factor may operate, at least in part, through the influence of tolerance. Variability in prior opioid consumption may greatly increase the variation in response to the test doses of the experimental opioids. This possibility is usually addressed during the study through the use of appropriate selection critieria (e.g. a designated range of prior opioid consumption) or by stratification by previous drug intake. Alternatively, variable degrees of tolerance within the study sample can potentially be managed by flexibility in the test doses used during the study; if the relative potency of the test drug and baseline drug is known, doses of the study drug can be determined as a proportion of the patient's prior opioid exposure, rather than as a fixed milligram amount.

Factors related to the patient

A large number of patient characteristics (Table 2) must also be considered in the selection of appropriate candidates for study. In those patients who participate in the study, these characteristics may become important covariates to evaluate vis-a-vis the analgesic response. In some fields, notably psychopharmacology, it is customary practice to try to identify particular patients as 'placebo responders' during a single-blind treatment with placebo during a run-in period before the study. Patients are then excluded from the study. This has not been the tradition in analgesic studies because single-dose trials in the early 1950s suggested that most patients will sometimes report decrease of pain with placebo. However, this issue has not been rigorously examined in repeated dose analgesic studies. Some of the controversies about trying to characterize and exclude placebo responders are reviewed in ref. 72.

Factors related to the disease

The medical condition of the patient must be carefully considered in the selection process. Major organ failure, including pulmonary or renal insufficiency, cardiac or liver disease, or encephalopathy, may increase the risks to the patient of participation in the study, potentially undermine data collection, or bias patients towards rating treatments as unacceptable even if they relieve pain. Mild degrees of delirium or dementia are common in cancer patients[73] and may impair the patient's ability to discriminate effects.

Outcome measures

Pain and pain relief

Most of the clinical analgesic trials in the literature have used category scales and visual analogue scales (VAS), such as those shown in Fig. 4.[74] In single-dose analgesic comparisons, patients are asked to complete these scales at regular intervals and derived measures such as peak relief (or reduction in pain intensity score) and summed relief scores are used as outcome measures.[20] In these studies, relief category scales and VAS for pain intensity and relief appear more somewhat more sensitive than pain category scales in detecting drug treatment effects.[75,76]

In chronic studies, researchers have generally used category scales, VAS, or the McGill Pain Questionnaire (MPQ)[77] to assess pain. A measure developed specifically for the cancer patient, the Brief Pain Inventory (BPI) combines a 0–10 rating of pain intensity with assessments of mood, pain-related interference with common daily activities, and sleep.[78] Studies to compare these tools in palliative care settings are needed.[79]

Many investigators prefer to use pain intensity rather than pain relief scales in chronic studies because they allow the patient to directly estimate the pain. Any assessment of pain relief, in contrast, requires a comparison with the memory of baseline pain, which may be difficult in studies of long duration. Although single-dose studies have suggested that the pain intensity VAS may be more sensitive than the pain intensity category scale,[75] the VAS may be confusing to some elderly patients and those with a poor grasp of English. A study in which only written instructions were given found that 11 per cent of chronic pain patients failed to complete the VAS, while all used the category scale correctly.[80] Some of these failures can be prevented by careful instruction of the patient.[81,82]

Pain intensity category scale (4-point)		Pain relief category scale (5-point)	
Severe	3	Complete	4
Moderate	2	Lots	3
Mild	1	Moderate	2
None	0	Slight	1
		None	0

LEAST possible pain	Visual analogue scale, pain intensity	WORST possible pain
NO relief of pain	Visual analogue scale, pain relief	COMPLETE relief of pain

Fig. 4 Examples of standard category and VAS used to assess pain and pain relief in analgesic studies. (Adapted from: Fishman, B., Pasternak, S., Wallenstein, S.L., Houde, R.W., Holland, J., and Foley, K.M. (1987). *Cancer* **60**, 1151–8, with permission.)

The MPQ has been extensively validated as a multidimensional pain scale for acute and chronic pain conditions.[83] Its disadvantages are that it takes about 5 minutes to complete, compared to seconds for VAS and category scales, requires a rich vocabulary, and confuses some patients.[78,84] In a study of cancer patients, an Italian version of the MPQ was shown to reflect only one dimension, which appeared to be most closely related to pain intensity.[85] If this finding generalizes within the cancer population, it would suggest that the potential value of multidimensional assessment is not realized in cancer pain. A pain intensity rating is more simply acquired using a briefer scale, such as the VAS.

The first large studies to directly compare the sensitivity of the commonly used pain scales in detecting treatment effects were carried out by Bellamy et al.[86,87] in studies of anti-inflammatory treatment in patients with osteoarthritis and rheumatoid arthritis. They found that a 0–10 numerical scale and 100 mm VAS were equally sensitive, but considerably larger sample sizes would have required to reach significance with the standard four-point pain intensity category scale or the MPQ. Because of the occasional confusion provoked by the more abstract VAS, we consider the 0–10 numerical scale best for chronic studies. Additional analyses of this scale have been done by Farrar et al.,[88] who suggest that a reduction of about 30 per cent in the average intensity of this scale over a 2-month trial is the best 'cut-point' to suggest that the response is clinically meaningful to the patient.

An important issue in the conduct of analgesic trials is the frequency of pain assessment. Many chronic studies have used single ratings before and after treatments, even though many types of cancer-related pain fluctuate over hours or days. Because single retrospective ratings covering a long period may be strongly affected by the pain level over the past day or two, treatment effects determined using the mean of frequent ratings over a long period (e.g. daily or several times daily) may be more robust;[89] there will still be random fluctuations, but they will tend to average out over the study period. Although the possibility of missing data is compounded by the request for frequent pain measurement, the successful completion of studies that incorporated nightly[90] or multiple daily pain measures[27] suggests that this degree of patient burden is not excessive for most ambulatory populations. Frequent and prospective pain evaluation is particularly important if separate pains (e.g. steady pain and incident pains) or various characteristics of the pain are to be assessed independently. This type of evaluation can yield data that may be relevant to pain mechanisms or to the clinical utility of an intervention.

Analgesic use

As discussed above, most chronic studies of cancer pain require the use of a background analgesic regimen and/or the provision of rescue doses, the need for which can be used as an ancillary measure of analgesic efficacy. Before the study begins, it is often advisable to revise patients' analgesic regimen to a standard set of treatments—for example, an aspirin-like agent and an appropriate dose of morphine. This may make the population more homogeneous and enhance the sensitivity of the study. Whatever the method for adjusting analgesic maintenance or rescue doses, it is important that procedures for making decisions are as uniform as is practical, particularly between clinicians or study sites. As discussed above, the efficacy of a standard opioid rescue dose may vary with the degree of prior opioid tolerance.

A recent controlled study[90] evaluated the analgesic outcome associated with a new chemotherapy for pancreas cancer using change in pain and analgesic consumption as two of the primary outcome measures. To accomplish this, a standardized opioid regiment was implemented during a 'run-in' period. This regimen incorporated a baseline opioid and a rescue dose. During the study period that followed, patients were randomly assigned to receive one of two chemotherapeutic drugs. Each patient received multiple treatment cycles over a period of many months. The treating oncologist made whatever adjustments in the opioid regimen that were needed to retain optimal pain control during this lengthy period. At the end of the study, both pain scores and analgesic consumption differed significantly between the two study groups. The standardization of the analgesic regimen in this design presumably reduced the within-group variability, and may have increased the likelihood that these significant group differences would be found.

Drug side-effects

Numerous checklists have been devised to survey adverse effects during drug trials.[91] The more extensive of these[92,93] assess a variety of characteristics for each adverse event, including severity, relationship to the drug, temporal charactistics (timing after a dose, duration and pattern during the day), contributing factors, course, and action taken to counteract the effect. Symptoms can be listed a priori or can be recorded as observed by the investigator. Each characteristic can be quantitated with scales of various complexity. For example, the likelihood of a relationship between the adverse event and the study drug in clinical drug trials has been recorded on a categorical scale (none, remote, possible, probable, definite) according to the presence or absence of specific features;[94] these may include a reasonable temporal relationship, foreknowledge that such an event may occur with the specific drug, improvement following discontinuation of the drug, and reappearance of the effect following repeated exposure. If appropriate, specific instruments can be used to assess one or more side effects, such as nausea[95] or cognitive impairment.[96] A simpler approach assesses the intensity of a symptom on a VAS adapted for the purpose; this has been accomplished successfully with sedation, for example.[97]

The detailed assessment of adverse events can add considerably to the time and effort required for the evaluation of the study intervention. The degree to which the various characteristics are pursued should be determined by the overall goals of the study. The evaluation of a new type of analgesic drug, for example, may warrant this effort, whereas such detail may be appropriately neglected in lieu of other assessments in studies of accepted opioids, for which the side effect spectrum is well appreciated.

In studies comparing a placebo to a putative therapeutic drug that also produces side effects, patients' perception of side-effects may increase their expectation of benefit, and lead to a false positive result.[98,99] While there is no consensus about how to deal with this potential bias, suggestions have included the use of 'active placebos' that mimic the side-effects of the test drug, use of questionnaires to assess whether patients and staff can see through the blind,[100] or simpler measures such as the careful recording of side-effects or the use of multiple dose levels of the test drug. In the latter case, the finding of a positive dose–response relationship above the level where side effects begin suggests a specific analgesic effect.

Mood, function, and global assessments

The effects of pain treatment on mood, function, and other dimensions of the quality of life are essential measures for chronic pain studies in palliative care settings. Measurement of these outcomes is discussed in Chapters 5.5 and 6.3 of this volume.

Because a treatment may relieve pain, but produce side-effects or worsen symptoms associated with the underlying disease, it is valuable to have the patient make an overall rating of treatment acceptability. In parallel designs, a category scale can be used (e.g. 'How satisfied have you been with the treatment you received during the study?': not at all, slightly, moderately, a great deal, completely). In crossover trials, patients may be asked to compare one intervention to the other ('Did you prefer treatment A, treatment B, or have no preference?'). All studies can incorporate a query about the future use of a treatment ('Would you be willing to continue treatment with this intervention?').

Conclusion

This brief chapter has sought to identify key issues in designing controlled trials of pain relief in palliative care settings. Practical difficulties of research in this patient group are great, but aided by patience, frequent consultations with a statistician and other pain researchers, and a familiarity with the principles of pain research outlined here, palliative care clinicians have the opportunity shape a new research tradition.

References

1. **Houde, R.W., Wallenstein, S.L., and Beaver, W.T.** (1966). Evaluation of analgesics in patients with cancer pain. In *Clinical Pharmacology, Section 6, International Encyclopedia of Pharmacology and Therapeutics* (ed. L. Lasagna), pp. 59–97. New York: Pergamon Press.
2. **Houde, R.W., Wallenstein, S.L., and Beaver, W.T.** (1965). Clinical measurement of pain. In *Analgesics* (ed. G. de Stevens), pp. 75–122. New York: Academic Press.
3. **Max, M.B., Portenoy, R.K., and Laska, E.M.**, ed. *The Design of Analgesic Clinical Trials.* New York: Raven Press, 1991.
4. **Friedman, L.M., Furberg, C.D., and DeMets, D.L.** *Fundamentals of Clinical Trials*, 2nd edn. Littleton MA: PSG Publishing Company, 1985.
5. **Pocock, S.J.** *Clinical Trials: A Practical Approach.* Chichester UK: John Wiley & Sons, 1983.
6. **Meinert, C.L.** *Clinical Trials: Design, Conduct, and Analysis.* New York: Oxford University Press, 1986, pp. 71–89.
7. **Chapman, C.R. and Loeser, J.D.**, ed. *Issues in Pain Measurement.* New York: Raven Press, 1989.
8. **Price, D.D.** *Psychological Mechanisms of Pain and Analgesia.* Seattle WA: IASP Press, 1999.
9. **Turk, D.C. and Melzack, R.**, ed. *Handbook of Pain Assessment.* New York: Guilford Press, 1992.
10. **Bailar, J.C., III and Mosteller, F.** *Medical Uses of Statistics.* Waltham MA: NEJM Books, 1986.
11. **Pocock, S.J.** (1977). Group sequential methods in the design and analysis of clinical trials. *Biometrika* **64**, 191–9.
12. **Max, M.B. and Lynn, J.**, ed. *Interactive Textbook of Symptom Research.* Bethesda MD: National Institute of Dental and Craniofacial Research, 2002. URL: http://symptomresearch.nih.gov.
13. **Max, M.B.** (1994). Challenges in the design of clinical trials of drug combinations. In *Proceedings of the VII World Congress on Pain* (ed G.F. Gebhart, D.L. Hammond, and T.S. Jensen), pp. 569–86. Seattle WA: IASP Publications.
14. **Schwartz, D. and Lellouch, J.** (1967). Explanatory and pragmatic attitudes in therapeutic trials. *Journal of Chronic Diseases* **20**, 637–48.
15. **Schwartz, D., Flamant, R., and Lellouch, J.** *Clinical Trials* (Transl. M.J.R. Healy). London: Academic Press, 1980.
16. **Ventafridda, V., Fochi, C., De Conno, F., and Sganzerla, E.** (1980). Use of nonsteroidal anti-inflammatory drugs in the treatment of pain in cancer. *British Journal of Clinical Pharmacology* **10**, S343–6.
17. **Inturrisi, C.E. and Colburn, W.A.** (1986). Application of pharmacokinetic–pharmacodynamic modeling to analgesia. In *Opioid Analgesics in the Management of Clinical Pain* (ed K.M. Foley and C.E. Inturrisi), pp. 441–52. New York: Raven Press.
18. **Feinstein, A.R.** (1983). An additional basic science for clinical medicine: II. The limitations of randomized trials. *Annals of Internal Medicine* **99**, 544–50.
19. **Portenoy, R.K.** (1991). Cancer pain: general design issues. In *The Design of Analgesic Clinical Trials* (ed. M.B. Max, R.K. Portenoy, and E.M. Laska), pp. 233–95. New York: Raven Press.
20. **Max, M.B. and Laska, E.M.** (1991). Single-dose analgesic comparisons. In *The Design of Analgesic Clinical Trials* (ed. M.B. Max, R.K. Portenoy, and E.M. Laska), pp. 55–95. New York: Raven Press.
21. **Food and Drug Administration.** *Guideline for the Clinical Evaluation of Analgesic Drugs.* Rockville MD: US Department of Health and Human Services, 1992.
22. **Turner, J.A., Deyo, R.A., Loeser, J.D., Von Korff, M., and Fordyce, W.E.** (1994). The importance of placebo effects in pain treatment and research. *Journal of the American Medical Association* **271**, 1609–14.
23. **Stambaugh, J.E. and McAdams, J.** (1987). Comparison of intramuscular dezocine with buorphanol and placebo in chronic cancer pain: a method to evaluate analgesia after both single and repeated doses. *Clinical Pharmacology and Therapeutics* **42**, 210–19.
24. **Stambaugh, J.E. and Drew, J.** (1988). The combination of ibuprofen and oxycodone/acetaminophen in the management of chronic cancer pain. *Clinical Pharmacology and Therapeutics* **44**, 665–9.
25. **Savarese, J.J., Thomas, G.B., Homesley, H., and Hill, C.S.** (1988). Rescue factor: a design for evaluating long-acting analgesics. *Clinical Pharmacology and Therapeutics* **43**, 376–80.
26. **Cundiff, D.** et al. (1989). Evaluation of a cancer pain model for the testing of long-acting analgesics. *Cancer* **63**, 2355–9.
27. **Portenoy, R.K., Maldonado, M., Fitzmartin, R., Kaiko, R., and Kanner, R.** (1989). Controlled-release morphine sulfate: analgesic efficacy and side effects of a 100 mg tablet in cancer pain patients. *Cancer* **63**, 2284–8.
28. **Lehmann, K.A.** (1991). Patient-controlled intravenous analgesia for postoperative pain relief. In *The Design of Analgesic Clinical Trials* (ed. M.B. Max, R.K. Portenoy, and E.M. Laska), pp. 481–506. New York: Raven Press.
29. **VadeBoncouer, T.R., Riegler, F.X., Gautt, R.S., and Weinberg, G.L.** (1989). A randomized double-blind comparison of the efficacy of interpleural bupivicaine and saline on morphine requirements and pulmonary function after cholecystectomy. *Anesthesiology* **71**, 339–43.
30. **Silverman, D.G., O'Connor, T.Z., and Brull, S.J.** (1993). Integrated assessment of pain scores and rescue morphine use during studies of analgesic efficacy. *Anesthesia and Analgesia* **77**, 168–70.
31. **Max, M.B.** (1994). Divergent traditions in analgesic clinical trials. *Clinical Pharmacology and Therapeutics* **56**, 237–41.
32. **Jadad, A.R., Carroll, D., Glynn, C.J., Moore, R.A., and McQuay, H.J.** (1992). Morphine responsiveness of chronic pain: double-blind randomized crossover study with patient-controlled analgesia. *Lancet* **339**, 1367–71.
33. **Chapman, C.R. and Donaldson, G.W.** (1991). Issues in designing trials of nonpharmacological treatments for pain. In *The Design of Analgesic Clinical Trials* (ed. M.B. Max, R.K. Portenoy, and E.M. Laska), pp. 699–711. New York: Raven Press.
34. **McQuay, H.J., Carroll, D., and Glynn, C.J.** (1993). Dose–response for analgesic effect of amitriptyline in chronic pain. *Anaesthesia* **48**, 281–5.
35. **Sheiner, L.B., Beal, S.L., and Sambol, N.C.** (1989). Study designs for dose-ranging. *Clinical Pharmacology and Therapeutics* **46**, 63–77.
36. **Temple, R.** (1989). Dose–response and registration of new drugs. In *Dose–Response Relationships in Clinical Pharmacology* (ed. L. Lasagna, S. Erill, and C.A. Naranjo), pp. 147–70. Amsterdam: Elsevier.
37. **Bolognese, J.A.** (1983). A Monte Carlo comparison of three up-and-down designs for dose ranging. *Controlled Clinical Trials* **4**, 187–96.
38. **Laska, E.M. and Meisner, M.J.** (1987). Statistical methods and applications of bioassay. *Annual Review of Pharmacology and Toxicology* **27**, 385–97.
39. **Beaver, W.T., Wallenstein, S.L., Houde, R.W., and Rogers, A.** (1968). A clinical comparison of the effects of oral and intramuscular administration of analgesics: pentazocine and phenazocine. *Clinical Pharmacology and Therapeutics* **9**, 582–97.
40. **Laska, E.M., Sunshine, A., Mueller, F., Elvers, W.B., Siegel, C., and Rubin, A.** (1984). Caffeine as an analgesic adjuvant. *Journal of the American Medical Association* **251**, 1711–18.
41. **Belville, J.W., Forrest, W.H., Elashoff, J., and Laska, E.** (1968). Evaluating side effects of analgesics in a cooperative clinical study. *Clinical Pharmacology and Therapeutics* **9**, 303–13.
42. **Lawlor, P.G., Turner, K.S., Hanson, J., and Bruera, E.D.** (1998). Dose ratio between morphine and methadone in patients with cancer pain: a retrospective study. *Cancer* **82**, 1167–73.
43. **Heiskanen, T. and Kalso, E.** (1997). Controlled-release oxycodone and morphine in cancer related pain. *Pain* **73**, 37–45.
44. **Max, M.B.** et al. *Principles of Analgesic Use in the Treatment of Acute Pain and Cancer Pain*, 4th edn. Skokie IL: American Pain Society, 1987, 1989, 1992, 1999.
45. **Temple, R.** (1982). Government viewpoint of clinical trials. *Drug Information Journal* **16**, 10–17.
46. **Detsky, A.S. and Sackett, D.L.** (1985). When was a 'negative' clinical trial big enough? How many patients you needed depends on what you found. *Archives of Internal Medicine* **145**, 709–12.
47. **Makuch, R.W. and Johnson, M.F.** (1986). Some issues in the design and interpretation of 'negative' clinical studies. *Archives of Internal Medicine* **146**, 986–9.

48. **Makuch, R. and Johnson, M.** (1989). Issues in planning and interpreting active control equivalence studies. *Journal of Clinical Epidemiology* **42**, 503–11.

49. **Beaver, W.T.** (1984). Combination analgesics. *American Journal of Medicine* September 10 Suppl., 38–53.

50. **Lavigne, G.J., Hargreaves, K.M., Schmidt, E.A., and Dionne, R.A.** (1989). Proglumide potentiates morphine analgesia for acute surgical pain. *Clinical Pharmacology and Therapeutics* **45**, 666–73.

51. **Levine, J.D. and Gordon, N.C.** (1988). Synergism between the analgesic actions of morphine and pentazocine. *Pain* **33**, 369–72.

52. **Carter, W.H., Jr. and Carchman, R.A.** (1988). Mathematical and biostatistical methods for designing and analyzing complex chemical interactions. *Fundamentals of Applied Toxicology* **10**, 590–5.

53. **Plummer, J.L. and Short, T.G.** (1990). Statistical modelling of the effects of drug combinations. *Journal of Pharmacological Methods* **23**, 297–309.

54. **Brunden, M.N., Vidmar, T.J., and McKean, J.W.** *Drug Interactions and Lethality Analysis.* Boca Raton FL: CRC Press, 1988.

55. **James, K.E., Forrest, W.H., and Rose, R.L.** (1985). Crossover and non-crossover designs in four-point parallel line analgesic assays. *Clinical Pharmacology and Therapeutics* **37**, 242–52.

56. **Louis, T.A., Lavori, P.W., Bailar, J.C., and Polansky, M.** (1984). Crossover and self-controlled designs in clinical research. *New England Journal of Medicine* **310**, 24–31.

57. **Brown, B.W., Jr.** (1980). The crossover experiment for clinical trials. *Biometrics* **36**, 69–79.

58. **Jones, B. and Kenward, M.G.** *Design and Analysis of Cross-over Trials.* London: Chapman and Hall, 1989.

59. **Ratkowsky, Da., Evans, M.A., and Alldredge, J.R.** *Cross-over Experiments: Design, Analysis, and Application.* New York: Marcel Dekker, 1993.

60. **Senn, S.** *Cross-over Trials in Clinical Research.* Chichester UK: John Wiley, 1993.

61. **Bruera, E.** (1991). Cancer pain: chronic studies of adjuvants to opioid analgesics. In *The Design of Analgesic Clinical Trials* (ed. M.B. Max, R.K. Portenoy, and E.M. Laska), pp. 267–81. New York: Raven Press.

62. **Laska, E.M., Meisner, M., and Kushner, H.B.** (1983). Optimal crossover designs in the presence of carryover effects. *Biometrics* **39**, 1087–91.

63. **Cochran, W.G. and Cox, G.M.** *Experimental Designs*, 2nd edn. New York: John Wiley & Sons, 1957.

64. **Byas-Smith, M.G., Max, M.B., Muir, J., and Kingman, A.** (1995). Transdermal clonidine compared to placebo in painful diabetic neuropathy using a two-stage 'enriched enrollment' design. *Pain* **60**, 267–74.

65. **Sang, C.N., Booher, S., Gilron, I., Parada, S., and Max, M.B.** (2002). A randomized, placebo-controlled trial of dextromethorphan and memantine in painful diabetic neuropathy and postherpetic neuralgia. *Anaesthesiology* **96**(5), 1053–61

66. **Lavori, P.W., Louis, T.A., Bailar, J.C., and Polansky, M.** (1983). Designs for experiments—parallel comparisons of treatment. *New England Journal of Medicine* **309**, 1291–8.

67. **Kaiko, R.F., Wallenstein, S.L., Rogers, A.G., and Houde, R.W.** (1983). Sources of variation in analgesic responses in cancer patients with chronic pain receiving morphine. *Pain* **15**, 191–200.

68. **Bruera, E., MacMillan, K., Hanson, J., and MacDonald, R.N.** (1989). The Edmonton staging system for cancer pain: preliminary report. *Pain* **37**, 203–10.

69. **Thaler, H.T.** (1991). Outcome measures and the effect of covariates. In *The Design of Analgesic Clinical Trials* (ed. M.B. Max, R.K. Portenoy, and E.M. Laska), pp. 106–11. New York: Raven Press.

70. **Wallenstein, S.L.** et al. (1990). Clinical analgesic assay of repeated and single doses of heroin and hydromorphone. *Pain* **41**, 5–14.

71. **Portenoy, R.K., Payne, D., and Jacobsen, P.** (1999). Breakthrough pain: characteristics and impact in patients with cancer pain. *Pain* **81**, 129–34.

72. **Max, M.B.** (2002). Small clinical trials. In *Principles and Practice of Clinical Research* (ed. J.I. Gallin), pp. 207–24. New York: Academic Press.

73. **Silberfarb, P.M. and Oxman, T.E.** (1988). The effects of cancer therapies on the central nervous system. In *Psychiatric Aspects of Cancer* (ed. R.J. Goldberg), pp. 13–25. Basel: Karger.

74. **Fishman, B., Pasternak, S., Wallenstein, S.L., Houde, R.W., Holland, J., and Foley, K.M.** (1987). The Memorial pain assessment card: a valid instrument for the evaluation of cancer pain. *Cancer* **60**, 1151–8.

75. **Littman, G.S., Walker, B.R., and Schneider, B.E.** (1985). Reassessment of verbal and visual analog ratings in analgesic studies. *Clinical Pharmacology and Therapeutics* **38**, 16–23.

76. **Sriwatanakul, K., Lasagna, L., and Cox, C.** (1983). Evaluation of current clinical trial methodology in analgesimetry based on experts' opinions and analysis of several analgesic studies. *Clinical Pharmacology and Therapeutics* **34**, 277–83.

77. **Melzack, R.** (1975). The McGill Pain Questionnaire: major properties and scoring methods. *Pain* **1**, 277–99.

78. **Daut, R.L., Cleeland, C.S., and Flannery, R.C.** (1983). Development of the Wisconsin Brief Pain Questionnaire to assess pain in cancer and other diseases. *Pain* **17**, 197–210.

79. **Bradley, L.A. and Lindblom, U.** (1989). Do different types of chronic pain require different measurement technologies? In *Issues in Pain Measurement* (ed. C.R. Chapman and J.D. Loeser), pp. 445–54. New York: Raven Press.

80. **Kremer, E., Atkinson, J.H., and Ignelzi, R.J.** (1981). Measurement of pain: patient preference does not confound pain measurement. *Pain* **10**, 241–8.

81. **Scott, J. and Huskisson, E.C.** (1976). Graphic representation of pain. *Pain* **2**, 175–84.

82. **Sriwatanakul, K., Kelvie, W., Lasagna, L., Calimlim, J.F., Weis, O.F., and Mehta, G.** (1983). Studies with different types of visual analog scales for measurement of pain. *Clinical Pharmacology and Therapeutics* **34**, 234–9.

83. **Melzack, R., Katz, J., and Jeans, M.E.** (1985). The role of compensation in chronic pain: analysis using a new method of scoring the McGill Pain Questionnaire. *Pain* **23**, 101–12.

84. **Chapman, C.R., Casey, K.L., Dubner, R., Foley, K.M., Gracely, R.H., and Reading, A.E.** (1985). Pain measurement: an overview. *Pain* **22**, 1–32.

85. **De Conno, F.** et al. (1994). Pain measurement in cancer patients: a comparison of six methods. *Pain* **57**, 161–6.

86. **Bellamy, N., Campbell, J., and Syrotuik, J.** (1999). Comparative study of self-rating pain scales in rheumatoid arthritis patients. *Current Medical Research and Opinion* **15**, 121–7.

87. **Bellamy, N., Campbell, J., and Syrotuik, J.** (1999). Comparative study of self-rating pain scales in osteoarthritis patients. *Current Medical Research and Opinion* **15**, 113–19.

88. **Farrar, J.T., Young, J.P., Jr., LaMoreaux, L., Werth, J.L., and Poole, R.M.** (2001). Clinical importance of changes in chronic pain intensity measured on an 11-point numerical pain rating scale. *Pain* **94**, 149–58.

89. **Jensen, M.P. and McFarland, C.A.** (1993). Increasing the reliability and validity of pain intensity measurement in chronic pain patients. *Pain* **55**, 195–203.

90. **Burris, H.A., III, Moore, M.J., Anderson, J., Green, M.R., Rothenberg, M.L., Modiano, M.R., Cripps, M.C., Portenoy, R.K., Storniolo, A.M., Tarassoff, P., Nelson, R., Dorr, F.A., Stephens, C.D., and Von Moff, D.D.** (1997). Improvement in survival and clinical benefit with gemcitabine as first-line therapy for patients with advanced pancreas: a randomized trial. *Journal of Clinical Oncology* **15**, 2403–13.

91. **Koeppen, D., Mohr, R., and Streichenwien, W.** (1989). Assessment of adverse drug events during the clinical investigation of a new drug. *Pharmacopsychiatry* **22**, 93–8.

92. **Guy, W., ed.** *ECDEU Assessment Manual for Psychopharmacology (DOTES: Dosage Record and Treatment Emergent Symptom Scale).* Rockville MD: National Institute of Mental Health, 1976, pp. 223–44.

93. **Levine, J. and Schooler, N., ed.** *Systematic Assessment for Treatment Emergent Events (SAFTEE-GI).* Rockville MD: National Institute of Mental Health, 1983.

94. **Karch, F.E. and Lasagna, L.** (1975). Adverse drug reactions. *Journal of the American Medical Association* **234**, 1236–41.

95. **Morrow, G.R.** (1984). The assessment of nausea and vomiting. *Cancer* **53**, 2267–80.

96. **Bruera, E., Macmillan, K., Hanson, J., and MacDonald, R.N.** (1989). The cognitive effects of the administration of narcotic analgesics in patients with cancer pain. *Pain* **39**, 13–16.

97. **Inturrisi, C.E., Portenoy, R.K., Max, M.B., Colburn, W.A., and Foley, K.M.** (1990). Pharmacokinetic–pharmacodynamic relationships of methadone infusions in patients with cancer pain. *Clinical Pharmacology and Therapeutics* **47**, 565–77.

98. **Greenberg, R.P. and Fisher, S.** (1994). Seeing through the double-masked design: a commentary. *Controlled Clinical Trials* **15**, 244–6.

99. **Max, M.B.** (1991). Neuropathic pain. In *The Design of Analgesic Clinical Trials* (ed. M.B. Max, R.K. Portenoy, and E.M. Laska), pp. 193–202. *Advances in Pain Research and Therapeutics* Vol. 18. New York: Raven Press.

100. **Moscucci, M., Byrne, L., Weintraub, M., and Cox, C.** (1987). Blinding, unblinding, and the placebo effect: an analysis of patients' guesses of treatment assignment in a double-blind trial. *Clinical Pharmacology and Therapeutics* **41**, 259–65.

5.5 Research into psychosocial issues

David W. Kissane and Annette F. Street

Psychosocial research needs to be conducted in accordance with the core values and principles of palliative care. Patient- and family-centred care acknowledges the unique experience of each person and their family members. Key values include respect for the dignity of all, advocacy on behalf of their expressed wishes, and equity in access to services. In response, psychosocial researchers seek not only the most effective interventions, but are also concerned with the meaning such treatments have for patient and family.

In this chapter, we want to highlight the scope of psychosocial questions and interests by drawing on a number of different methods that have formed the basis of psychosocial research. In doing so we have made choices. We have not covered all the possible research methods for the investigation of topics of concern in palliative care. Many of these methods are covered in detail in other chapters in this section on research. Rather, our focus has been on highlighting formative and current research, delineating the problems involved in conducting research with dying people, and making some suggestions about where future psychosocial research should be directed. A feature of the chapter is a section analysing the various instruments in use in psychosocial research. Sometimes, researchers are unaware of the potential range of validated questionnaires that can aid psychosocial research. Similarly, we have analysed a range of computer-assisted qualitative analysis programs. This chapter will serve as a most useful resource.

The scope of psychosocial research in palliative medicine

Research activity can be grouped into broad domains or themes of inquiry. Many interesting questions and controversies arise in each domain. These are listed in Box 1.

Box 1 Domains of psychosocial research in palliative medicine

- Communication studies: breaking bad news, discussing prognosis and dying
- Coping and adaptation to change
- Cultural issues including those of indigenous peoples
- Dying process
- Ethics of end-of-life care
- Family studies: carers, family support
- Grief and bereavement
- Interventions: psychotherapy, pharmacological, physical
- Lived experience of illness: impact on self, the body, dignity, and burden on others
- Paediatric aspects of adaptation, coping, and care
- Psychiatric disorders: anxiety, depression, delirium, etc.
- Sexuality and intimacy
- Quality of life
- Social issues: relationships, recreation, work, and living arrangements
- Suffering, existential and spiritual distress

The choice of research issue is commonly determined by awareness of unmet needs, concern about the standard of care, or a desire to improve the outcome of treatment. We illustrate pertinent issues about a number of these domains as we discuss relevant methodology and return to the challenges for the future at the end of this chapter.

Literature review and meta-analysis

A comprehensive literature review is a *sine qua non* as many ideas have been considered before. Exploring the boundaries of knowledge necessitates firstly identifying what is known, what aspects remain unclear, and thinking through where the benefits of further study will lie. A formal literature search is thus crucial before the hypothesis is generated or aims and objectives of the study are delineated.

While the history of any construct and its application is of interest, the recent emphasis on a clinical approach that is evidence-based strives to avoid mistakes that are derived from the slavish adherence to tradition and dogmatic assumptions without true evidence of outcome benefits. To ensure that one is not drawn into the perpetuation of such myths by the biased selection of previously published research, a systematic approach to literature review is encouraged. This incorporates conceptualization of the relevant issues and selection of appropriate key words and search bases (e.g. MEDLINE, PsycInfo, CINAL, Proquest 5000), methodological review of the techniques that generated any data, and an integrative review of its meaning and significance.

Few systematic reviews of psychosocial palliative care topics have been conducted. In an examination of the impact of specialist palliative care on quality of life for patients, Salisbury and Bosanquet[1] argued that there was little good-quality evidence upon which to base any conclusions; most palliative care standards and models are based on opinion without systematic scientific support. However, a systematic review of survival prediction in terminal care provides a recent example.[2]

Meta-analyses provide level I evidence for the efficacy of treatment regimens and these also exist in psychooncology. For instance, there is incontrovertible evidence from these about the effectiveness of psychoeducational[3] and psychotherapeutic[4] interventions in cancer care. Setting standards about methodology prior to examining studies is a key requirement of study selection for these meta-analytic techniques.

Concept and construct development

The building up of a theory provides a conceptual framework on which further observations can be based and ultimately delivers an empirical basis for the development of interventions. The qualitative approach to construct development begins in grounded theory, while quantitative methodology creates instruments to measure constructs, which in turn need to be carefully validated and demonstrated to have reliability for recurrent use.

Instrument development

The commonly used rating scales used in psychosocial research in palliative medicine have been summarized in Tables 1–9. Instruments that measure distress, mood states, coping, quality of life, support, and family functioning tend to be well validated, while measures of spirituality, dignity, and existential domains warrant further work.

Rating scales can be used for screening, diagnosis, measurement of severity and change—attention needs to be paid to the purpose for which any instrument was designed and its reliability and validity in that role. In choosing an instrument, the researcher needs to consider what they seek to measure and for what purpose. For instance, sensitivity of scales to detect small changes will vary, sometimes at the expense of specificity, and the scales' practicality and brevity will often be important when considered for use with palliative patients.

Grounded theory

Glaser and Strauss[47,48] initially developed grounded theory to examine the practices, behaviours, beliefs, and attitudes of individuals in their natural setting. Their seminal works *Awareness of Dying* and *Time for Dying* challenged the notion that knowledge can only be generated through the testing of *a priori* theories about dying. Instead, they demonstrated that when a subject is not well theorized, as was the situation with death and dying at that time, information could be collected concerning the actions, interactions, and social processes to generate theory from the ground up. They demonstrated how relationships with the dying are structured around key awareness concepts that guide communication and action.

Chamanz[49] exemplified a landmark study using grounded theory in which the loss of self was seen as a fundamental form of suffering in cancer patients and the chronically ill. Morse,[50] a nurse anthropologist, provided a further example in identifying important palliative care concepts such as 'enduring', 'uncertainty', 'suffering', and 'hope', and then examining their interrelationships. Similarly, as few studies had dealt with the mental survival of patients with advanced cancer, grounded theory was used to explore the concept of protection and hope in those patients with malignant gliomas.[51]

Case studies and narratives

Clinical case reports

Clinical reports of individual patients have always served an important function in highlighting relevant issues of presentation, diagnosis, or management. One example was a series of patients who sought euthanasia under the Northern Territory of Australia's Rights of the Terminally Ill legislation, which operated for 9 months in 1996.[52] These cases exemplified non-recognition of depression, a poor standard of medical care, and disagreement over the terminal status of patients, highlighting the defective gate-keeper roles set up by the legislation. Building up collections of case reports points to the need for cohort and longitudinal studies as observational evidence is mounted. The corresponding narrative inquiry of the qualitative approach brings an equally in-depth appraisal as the detailed clinical case account.

Narrative inquiry

Narratives constructed from research interviews mirror the social life of the person, with language forming the major cultural resource that participants draw on jointly to create meaning.[53] A particular 'narrative self' is constituted through the story, occasioned by the presence of a listener who brings his/her own set of historically and theoretically framed questions and comments to the encounter. The seminal work of Kleinman[54] on illness narratives and Frank's[55] writings on the wounded storyteller have shaped a narrative tradition designed to offer explanatory models of the world of people experiencing life-limiting illnesses. Recent nursing work has developed individual and group narratives to explore close nurse–patient relationships in palliative care.[56]

Ethnography

Ethnography as a research technique developed in medical anthropology and is the in-depth study of people and their culture. Palliative care facilities have been studied through ethnography in order to expose the taken-for-granted assumptions, discourses, norms, values, rituals, and traditions that structure care relationships. Formative ethnographies[57–59] explored the understanding of emotional labour involved in care for the dying and the 'good death' experience.

In a fascinating recent ethnography, Lawton[60] explored the dying process in relation to the management of the difficult symptoms of the 'unbound body', the perceived loss of personhood, and the 'social death'. She spent five months in a hospice day care centre and 10 months in an in-patient hospice.

Table 1 Self-report instruments measuring distress

Instrument name	Item number and response style	Factor structure	Reliability	Validity	Comments on utility
General Health Questionnaire (GHQ)[5]	12-item briefest, response 0/1; also 60-, 30-, 28-item scales	1. Somatic 2. Anxiety 3. Social function 4. Depression	Cronbach's $\alpha = 0.93$	Extensively validated in community and hospital patients	For GHQ-28, a score >9 indicates probability of caseness for distress. GHQ-12 is also a useful brief screen
Brief Symptom Inventory (BSI)[6]	53 items, 4-point Likert response	Nine symptom factors and 3 global scales	Subscale internal consistency 0.71–0.85	Predictive validity evident from over 1000 studies	Excellent screening tool derived from the Hopkins Symptom Checklist-90. Also shortened to the BSI-18 incorporating anxiety, depression, and somatization scales
Impact of Events Scale (IES)[7]	15 items, 4-point response	1. Intrusion 2. Avoidance	$\alpha = 0.92$	Well validated	Records subjective distress associated with a current situational event. Widely used in cancer patients

Table 2 Self-report instruments measuring depression

Instrument name	Item number and response style	Factor structure	Reliability	Validity	Comments on utility
Beck Depression Inventory (BDI)[8]	21 items, 4-point response	1. Cognitions 2. Somatic symptoms	$\alpha = 0.86$	Well validated, correlations with clinical ratings of depression >0.60	Over 40 years use; uses 13 cognitive items in palliative medicine
Center for Epidemiological Studies (CES-D)[9,10]	20 items, 4-point response	1. Cognitive 2. Somatic	Satisfactory	Concurrent validity: 60% RDC major and 71% minor depression	Much used in epidemiological studies
Brief Zung (Brief ZSDS)[11]	11 items after removing 9 somatic items	Cognitive scale	$\alpha = 0.84$	Correlates well with longer scale ($r = 0.92$)	Cognitive version well regarded in medically ill
Hospital Anxiety & Depression Scale (HAD)[12,13]	14 items, 4-point response	1. Anxiety 2. Depression	Satisfactory	Correlation of 0.69 with Clinical Anxiety Scale and 0.81 with Montgomery–Asberg Depression	Face validity of depression based only on cheerfulness and joy. Anxiety subscale useful
Profile of Mood States (POMS)[14]	65 items, 5-point response	6 factors	α varies between 0.84 and 0.95; test–retest between 0.65 and 0.74	Well validated in cancer studies	Useful change measure for RCTs
Affects Balance Scale (ABS)[15]	40 items, 5-point response	8 factors: 4 positive and 4 negative affect states	Satisfactory	Well validated in cancer studies	Useful change measure; better capture of positive affects

Table 3 Self-report instruments measuring anxiety

Instrument name	Item number and response style	Factor structure	Reliability	Validity	Comments on utility
Death Anxiety Scale (DAS)[16,17]	15 items, true–false	1 factor	Test–retest 0.83; $\alpha = 0.76$	Well validated	Reveals preoccupation with and anxiety about death
HAD anxiety subscale[13]	7 items	1 factor	Satisfactory	Well validated	Useful
State-Trait Anxiety Inventory (STAI)[18]	40 items, 4-point response	1. State 2. Trait	Test–retest 0.65–0.86; $\alpha > 0.90$	Good concurrent validity	Separates situational from personality-based responses

In order to blend in, she also took on the role of volunteer. This raised ethical questions about the information she received in this capacity rather than as a researcher. Likewise, the notion of informed consent that was gained on the patient's entry to the facility could not necessarily be considered to cover the entirety of their experience, with some staff expressing disquiet at her attendance at meetings. Yet, the ethnographic method enabled her to make a sustained examination of the dying process in UK hospice settings and to write about those elements of care that are not made explicit.

Cohort and longitudinal studies

Observational studies may be either retrospective or prospective. In the former, past events are studied through case notes or by interview. They may be limited by incomplete recording or biased recall, but are inexpensive and serve as a useful beginning. In contrast, prospective studies eliminate the bias of memory and permit examination of a number of associations, but may be limited by the availability of suitable subjects for recruitment within a reasonable time frame. In addition, subjects may be lost to follow-up.

Cross-sectional studies

Cross-sectional studies are both observational and descriptive, typically being used to measure the prevalence of a symptom or illness. They can be further used to identify clinical associations, well exemplified by the study of the 'desire for death' by Chochinov and colleagues in 200 Canadian hospice inpatients, which was found to be genuine and persistent in 8.5 per cent and significantly associated with depressive disorder, isolation from family, and pain.[61]

Case–control studies

The case–control study is used generally to test an aetiological hypothesis, by comparing a group with a disease or specific treatment, matched with controls. The methodological challenge is in the selection criteria for the cases to ensure that they are a representative sample and similarly the variables on which matching is achieved, and whether this is by random community selection or paired match. For instance, studies of men with prostate cancer have shown global quality of life to be equivalent to

Table 4 Self-report measures of cognitive attitudes and coping

Instrument name	Item number and response style	Factor structure	Reliability	Validity	Comments on utility
Ways of Coping Questionnaire (WCQ)[19]	31 items	1. Problem-solving 2. Avoidance 3. Social support	α between 0.75 and 0.9	Well validated	Based on classic Lazarus and Folkman model
Life Orientation Test (LOT)[20]	8 items, 4-point response	1. Optimism	Satisfactory test–retest and internal consistency	Good convergent and discriminant validity	Useful dispositional measure of expectations about outcomes; correlates with longer survival
General Coping Strategies Scale (COPE)[21]	15 items, 5-point response	1. Active 2. Distraction 3. Avoidant	Satisfactory	Satisfactory	Measures frequency of use of a series of problem-focused and emotion-focused strategies
Mental Adjustment to Cancer Scale (MAC)[22]	40 items, 4-point response	1. Fighting spirit 2. Anxious preoccupation 3. Fatalism 4. Helpless/hopeless 5. Avoidance	Cronbach's α between 0.65 and 0.84	Kappa = 0.72 against clinical evaluation	Factor structure alters with different cultural attitudes; translated into several languages
Mini-MAC[23]	29 items, 4-point response	5 factors as above, strengthening of cognitive avoidance	α between 0.62 and 0.88	Concurrent validity against HAD	Retains 16 original items, better avoidance scale

Table 5 Self-report measures of social adjustment, support, and family functioning

Instrument name	Item number and response style	Factor structure	Reliability	Validity	Comments on utility
Modified Social Adjustment Scale (SAS-M)[24]	42 items, 5-point response	1. Work 2. Household 3. Social and leisure 4. Extended family 5. Children 6. Family 7. Marital	Satisfactory	Pearson $r = 0.72$ for clinical interview	Useful change measure for monitoring social adjustment during interventions
Psychosocial Adjustment to Illness Scale (PAIS)[25]	46 items, 4-point response	1. Health care 2. Work 3. Domestic 4. Sexual 5. Extended family 6. Social and leisure 7. Distress	α between 0.62 and 0.93; inter-rater reliabilities between 0.56 and 0.86	Satisfactory convergent validity; also predictive	Useful in the medically ill including cancer patients
Interpersonal Support Evaluation List (ISEL)[26]	40 items, true–false	1. Instrumental aid 2. Perception of support 3. Self-esteem 4. Sense of belonging	α between 0.73 and 0.85	Well validated	Helpful appraisal of perceptions of social support
Brief Social Provisions Scale (BSCS)[27]	9 items	1. Social integration 2. Reassurance of worth	α between 0.71 and 0.66	Satisfactory	Assesses perception of interpersonal support
Family Environment Scale (FES-Short form)[28]	40 items, true/false response	10 factors; 3 forming Family Relationship Index are most relevant: cohesion, conflict, and expressiveness	α values vary between 0.61 and 0.78; test–retest between 0.68 and 0.86 over 2 months	Good criterion and predictive validity	Relationship factors form a useful screening tool to identify dysfunctional families
Family Assessment Device (FAD)[29]	Full-scale 60 items; 12-item general function scale; 4 points	Full scale has 6 factors	α between 0.72 and 0.92; test–retest between 0.66 and 0.76	Good concurrent validity	Useful measure of family functioning

Table 6 Self-report measures of quality of life

Instrument name	Item number and response style	Factor structure	Reliability	Validity	Comments on utility
McGill Quality of Life (McGillQOL)[30]	16 items, 10-point response based on experience of last 2 days	1. Somatic 2. Well being 3. Psychological 4. Social support 5. Existential	Cronbach's α between 0.62 and 0.83	Convergent validity against other QOL scales in cancer and HIV	Meaning, goals, and worth are usefully captured by existential subscale
Functional Assessment of Cancer Therapy (FACT-G)[31]	27 items	1. Physical 2. Functional 3. Social 4. Emotional	Cronbach α between 0.72 and 0.85	Satisfactory	Well used in cancer patients
Functional Living Index for Cancer (FLIC)[32]	22 items, 7-point response	1. Physical 2. Social 3. Emotional	Satisfactory	Satisfactory	Useful, well-used measure
European EORTC QLQ-C30[33]	30 items; yes/no and 4-point responses	1. Physical 2. Role 3. Social 4. Cognitive 5. Emotional 6. Symptom severity	Internal consistency between 0.59 and 0.85	Satisfactory	Developed for chemotherapy trials; has specific modules for specific cancer types
Medical Outcomes Study (SF-36)[34]	36 items	8 factors	α between 0.65 and 0.89	Satisfactory	A general health survey used in community samples
Symptom Distress Scale (SDS)[35]	13 items	Symptom severity	$\alpha = 0.84$	Good predictive validity	High scores reflect poor symptom control
Karnofsky Performance Scale Status (KPS)[36]	1 item	Physical function	Satisfactory	Satisfactory	Useful proxy for QOL

Table 7 Self-report measures of religiosity and spirituality

Instrument name	Item number and response style	Factor structure	Reliability	Validity	Comments on utility
Spiritual wellbeing of FACIT-Sp[37,38]	12 items	1. Meaning/peace 2. Faith	α between 0.81 and 0.88	Satisfactory	Meaning and religious conviction are useful constructs
Systems of Beliefs Inventory (SBI-15)[39]	15 items	1. Beliefs and practices 2. Social support from a faith community	Satisfactory	Satisfactory	Addresses religion and support but not existential issues
Royal Free Spirituality Scale[40]	20 items, specific responses and 10-point linear analogue scale	1. Spiritual scale 2. Philosophical scale	α between 0.81 and 0.60; test–retest 0.67–1.0	Satisfactory	Applicable to a range of faiths and public religions
Religious Orientation Scale (ROS)[41]	24 items	1. Intrinsic religiousness 2. Extrinsic practices	Satisfactory	Satisfactory	Intrinsic scale predicts psychological health; extrinsic predicts maladaptiveness

Table 8 Measures used in paediatric studies

Instrument name	Item number and response style	Factor structure	Reliability	Validity	Comments on utility
Child Behaviour Checklist (CBCL)[42]	Parental report	1. Competency in school, social, and activity domains 2. Internalizing and externalizing behaviours	Satisfactory	Satisfactory	Normative data are available
Children's Depression Inventory (CDI)[43]	27-item self-report; reading age	1. Negative mood 2. Interpersonal 3. Ineffectiveness 4. Anhedonia 5. Self-esteem	Satisfactory; well used by adolescents	Satisfactory	Raw scores are converted into age- and gender-specific *T*-scores; normative data are available

Table 9 Self-report measures of caregiver burden

Instrument name	Item number and response style	Factor structure	Reliability	Validity	Comments on utility
Caregiver Level of Burden Scale (CLBS)[44]	29 items	1. Health 2. Psychological well-being 3. Social life 4. Finances 5. Relationship with impaired person	Internal consistency of 0.86	Satisfactory	Useful appraisal of caregiver's capacity to cope
Instrumental Activities of Daily Living (IADL)[45]	Charts specific tasks	1. Communication 2. Finances 3. Food preparation 4. Home maintenance 5. Medication assistance	Internal consistency of 0.91	Satisfactory	Monitors caregiver's role
Caregiver Reaction Assessment (CRA)[46]	24 items, 5-point response	1. Caregiver's esteem 2. Family support 3. Finances 4. Impact on schedule 5. Health	Cronbach's α 0.80–0.90	Concurrent validity with CES-D; satisfactory construct validity	Developed with cancer carers (mean age 59) as well as elderly carers of Alzheimers and physically ill patients

community samples of similarly aged men, but urinary incontinence, impotence, and bowel symptoms to be causally related to the treatments these men have received.[62]

Cohort studies

Cohort studies are both observational and analytical in prospectively following groups of patients with key differences to assess outcome. They provide valuable information on the nature of a relationship and whether there is a causal association. Thus, the King's College cohort of women with breast cancer were followed across 15 years of illness to determine the influence of coping style on survival.[63] Women who were fatalistic, overly anxious, or hopeless/helpless in their cognitions died earlier than those using positive avoidance or fighting spirit. Time available for follow-up is an obvious limitation in palliative medicine.

Cross-sectional, case–control, and cohort studies using quantitative techniques are paralleled by phenomenological, interview, and focus group methods in qualitative research.

Phenomenology

Phenomenology aims to describe the 'lived experience' of the particular situation and is derived from an existential, philosophical approach. It explores the everyday life of the person in great detail to understand how they generate meaning. Life experiences, such as living with bowel cancer, contain both the physical experience and an inner consciousness of what bowel cancer means based on their past, the images it conjures up, and how they perceive the experience.

Phenomenological research has explored the perception of hope in oncological palliative care from the perspective of nurses.[64,65] Likewise, MacLeod[66] interviewed doctors to examine the unique aspects of their experience of patients' deaths, along with identification of significant shared patterns.

A limitation of such studies is that although they are very useful in assisting people to understand the meaning of experiences, their philosophical approach does not directly inform practical outcomes or therapeutic interventions.

Discourse analysis

Recognition of the social construction of daily life has led to research that deconstructs taken-for-granted assumptions in medical practice. Armstrong's[67,68] early work deconstructed the relationships between nurses and patients, explored the patient's view of the dying process and how silence and truth are constructed in palliative care. Seale[69] deconstructed the issues around dying and bereavement to show the effects of social understandings on medical and community practices. The constructions of dignity and euthanasia in end-of-life care were analysed to show the psychosocial aspects of patient's understandings that sit against professional interpretations.[70]

Qualitative interviews and focus group studies

Alongside qualitative studies described by a particular theoretical position are some studies that are merely described as 'qualitative research'. These studies invariably adopt some of the strategies of the major approaches but do not attempt to develop a concept or theory, describe phenomena or experiences of a cultural group, or deconstruct the effects of practices, relationships, and structures. Rather, their focus is on providing contextual and explanatory analysis of certain topics. Such studies are usually designed for one of three reasons: to find out enough information about a new area to develop a survey tool or intervention; to explain the meaning of results from controlled studies, for example, contextual information to illustrate why compliance is problematic; and to use a mixed method approach in response to the growing awareness of the value of complementary research.

Leading qualitative researchers have argued against the number of small projects that are independent and not directed at establishing a programmatic approach to the development of knowledge. In response, research programmes are emerging with larger samples and interrelated research questions. For instance, a study by Kuuppelomäki[71] interviewed 32 patients, 13 family members, 13 doctors, and 13 nurses from a variety of settings to explore their conceptions and beliefs about death as part of a larger study that examined suffering and death.

Controlled clinical trials

Preventive or therapeutic interventions are generally tested through controlled studies such as the randomized controlled trial (RCT), which could be double blinded, placebo-controlled, or cross-over in design. The methodological assumption that needs to be proven is that the groups are in every way equal before the treatment is delivered. The likelihood of a chance difference being observed is reduced by prior declaration of the primary

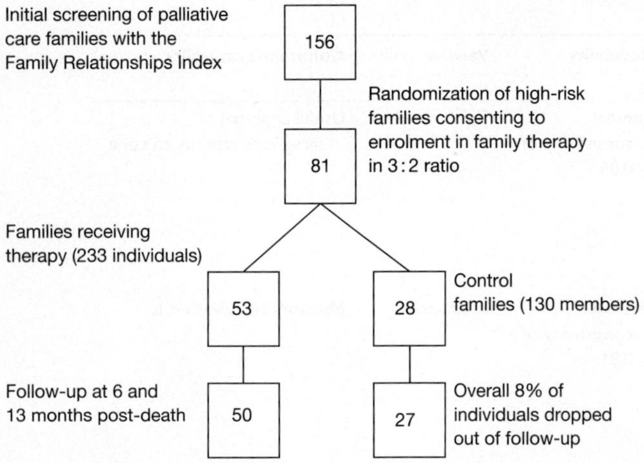

Fig. 1 Typical design of randomized controlled trials (RCTs) used in psychosocial research in palliative medicine. In this example, an RCT study of Family Focused Grief Therapy is given.[73] Variations could include use of screening, stratification when randomizing, number of arms used, and length of longitudinal follow-up with differing frequency of outcome measure points.

outcome, use of a sample size with adequate power to determine a sufficient difference, and significance testing.

Randomization needs to be performed independently of the therapists, and stratification by known prognostic factors is worthwhile in cancer studies. In multicentre trials, pre-stratification of patients by centre is standard practice because of the likelihood that prognoses will differ between centres and to minimize the awkwardness of any within-centre imbalance.

The place of controlled trials has been much debated in palliative medicine, yet they are vital when outcome is examined as the endpoint. Pharmacological trials, for instance, demonstrating the efficacy of antidepressants, provide the obvious example of double blind RCTs.[72] The study of Family Focused Grief Therapy during palliative care and bereavement (see Fig. 1) delivered to 'high-risk' families selected by screening and thereafter randomized to intervention or control is another example of a carefully designed and methodologically sound study, this time a psychotherapeutic intervention.[73] Analysis based on 'intention to treat' principles incorporates the acceptance or otherwise of any planned intervention (including withdrawals because of side-effects) into the final analysis of benefits.

Methodological difficulties experienced in controlled trials include patient refusers and withdrawals, undeclared confounding treatments, dose variations and fidelity of the treatment applied, defaults in interim assessments, and deaths prior to outcome measurements. Despite such inherent challenges, the quality of evidence achieved necessitates greater utilization of these designs in future research in palliative medicine.

Power analyses to assist choice of sample size are vital to avoid the unethical conduct of worthless research. In controlled trials in which we wish to demonstrate a 15 per cent difference in response between study arms, tradition usually accepts a 5 per cent risk (or one in 20 chance) of a falsely positive finding being determined by chance (a type I error). Similarly, the sensitivity of a false negative result (type II error) is usually set to be at least 0.80, so that there is a chance of one in five or less of missing an important difference between treatments. However, effect size also has an important influence on power, the larger the effect the more probable it is that positive results will be detected. As the sample size increases, the precision of the estimate of the difference between treatments increases—this can be reflected in 95 per cent confidence limits whose interval will typically decrease as the sample size rises.

Mixed qualitative quantitative methodology

Increasingly, psychosocial research is being designed utilizing a combined methodology approach. An excellent recent example of this is found in a study of coping during illness with HIV.[74] In setting out to identify the predictors of coping outcome, Folkman and colleagues began a longitudinal study in 1990 with a cohort of 253 carers of gay men dying from AIDS during the era before triple therapies became available. The design involved bimonthly assessment over 2 years, during which two-thirds became bereaved. The researchers candidly admitted their intention to focus on negative affects, but were struck by the interviewees' desire to share positive experiences. Indeed, with the exception of the period around death, positive affects were as frequent as negatives.

This qualitative observation led the researchers to question the adaptational significance of positive affect and to ask what kinds of coping processes sustained it? After controlling for social support, optimism, ways of coping, and health, they found that perception of meaning in life accounted for a significant variance in positive affects but not depressive symptoms. Analysis of 106 narratives revealed that meaning-centred coping increased self-worth, sense of resilience, wisdom, and a perspective that no longer feared death. Moreover, a task- and role-oriented approach to instrumental care provision promoted a sense of mastery, which also maintained positive affect. The importance of meaning-based coping emerged to expand the earlier theory of coping (problem- or emotion-focused processes that regulate distress).

Without incorporating the qualitative dimension into what otherwise looked like a solidly designed quantitative study, it seems unlikely that insight into this important third method of appraisal in coping (meaning-based, generating positive affects) would have been recognized. Coping strategies was also the focus of another recent mixed method study of caregivers that followed stages of coping through diagnosis to bereavement.[75]

A problem with many multimethod approaches is the minimal level of skill and expertise demonstrated in the 'themes' derived from low-level qualitative work. The assumption that 'anyone can do qualitative research but only experts can do quantitative research' is evident in many conference presentations on palliative care or psychooncology research. There is no sense of the 'aha' experience, that nod of recognition, or the impetus to think differently that good qualitative research brings to the reading/listening audience. Development of expertise is equally important for both qualitative and quantitative research and collaboration between such researchers generates a powerful armamentarium.

Characterization of psychological outcome can be through both form and content. Quantitative studies mostly emphasize the content through measurement of specific dimensions, which can be compared to controls over time, but usually at specific points. Qualitative studies add insight into form, with recognition of the pattern of change in outcome over time. Then, repeated measures analysis, with attention to the slope and variability of change using qualitative techniques, enriches understanding of the evaluation process.

Computer-assisted qualitative data analysis software

Computers have become an integral part of the repertoire of tools for qualitative analysis.[76] There are a number of packages available from the relative simple text retrievers that are useful to sort and manage data into categories of information, to the highly sophisticated new-generation multi-media capacities of NVivo. It is important to understand what capabilities are needed for the research process before deciding on a software package.

The features of commonly used packages are listed in Table 10.

Table 10 Computer-assisted qualitative data analysis software

Type of software	Function	Products
Text retrievers	Recover data pertaining to a category using keywords	Matamorph The Text Collector Word Cruncher ZyINDEX Sona Professional
Code-and-retrieve packages	Divide texts into segments, attach codes to segments, find and display segments with a given code or combination of codes	HyperQual Kwalitan QUALPRO The ETHNOGRAPH
Code-based theory building	Code-and-retrieve, develop more abstract, formal classifications, query patterns or display networks of coding, and search for combinations of coding and text, link to statistics packages, and test propositions	WinMAX NUD*IST (N5) HyperRESEARCH AQUAD Ethno QCA Atlas/ti for Windows
Interpretive–iterative	Theory-building capacities not dependent on coding—integrate coding with qualitative linking, shaping and modelling, iterative searching, and reviewing of interpretation	NVivo

Methodological difficulties in psychosocial research in palliative medicine

Psychosocial researchers encounter significant specific difficulties in conducting research with dying people.[77,78] The recruitment of patients, attainment of an adequate sample size,[79] attrition rates, and the variability of the patient's condition[80] create problems for researchers internationally. Employment of trained data managers, adoption of several recruitment methods, and use of well thought out inclusion criteria does assist sampling problems.[79] Moreover, ethical debates exist regarding the impact of research on patients at the end of their lives,[81] the withholding of treatment in controlled trials,[82] and the informed consent process when delirium is present.[83] Extensive interviews and use of batteries of questionnaires can be stressful and intrusive at a vulnerable and potentially poignant time in the life-cycle.[84]

In contrast, Frank[55] reminds us that sharing a heroic account of the life lived is often part of the process of coming to terms with its impending closure. Likewise, Doyle and colleagues cite the tremendous benefits derived from studies of the subcutaneous use of the opioids.[85] Furthermore, only seeking a carer's perspective does not provide a reliable picture of the patient's needs.[86] Despite the challenges involved in such psychosocial research, its value is beyond question and critical to our endeavours to improve the care of the dying.

Outcomes in psychosocial research and future directions

The clinical significance or utility of each study merits careful reflection so that standards of care are steadily improved. Quality assurance programmes have highlighted the importance of the feedback loop, which leads to altered practice, innovation, and change.[45] This should be a cyclical activity.

For palliative medicine to grow as a discipline, its research activity must be scholarly and generate the needed evidence that informs purposeful clinical activity. Psychosocial research is a cardinal component of such endeavours. It needs to grow through well thought out national and international collaborations, utilizing integrated methodologies of the highest standards. For too long, clinicians have defensively avoided good science through flawed claims about the unsuitability of palliative patients for research. Fortunately, the specialty is maturing and recognizes the imperative for its future of excellence in research studies.

Psychosocial research in the future needs to embrace RCTs to establish a sound evidence base for its practice. Examples of needed pharmacological trials include the comparison of benzodiazepines with the newer major tranquilizers for patients with delirium and comparison of newer antidepressants (e.g. venlafaxine and mirtazapine) with amitriptyline in the management of neuropathic pain. Further, RCTs are needed of psychotherapies, particularly meaning-centred therapies, to treat existential and spiritual distress. Interpersonal psychotherapy is one manualized and standardized intervention waiting to be applied in palliative care—its emphasis on grief, transitions, roles, and relationships makes it particularly suitable with this population. Interventions need to be both patient- and family-centred.

Suffering remains a cardinal domain for future research activity. Observational studies using mixed methodologies are needed to explore demoralization, dignity, shame, and unworthy dying, incorporating the experience of patients, families and carers, doctors and nurses, and all related support staff to build a complete gestalt of the many intersecting influences on outcome. Over the next decade, such a body of work should guide future intervention studies aimed at further improving the standard of psychosocial care.

Communication studies have developed in oncology over the past decade but remain a vital research domain for palliative medicine. Discussion of prognosis and preparation for death are some of the most challenging conversations, yet there is a corresponding dearth of systematic research to guide the approach that clinicians take. Promotion of adaptive coping and maintenance of hope alongside acceptance of the reality of impending death constitute a fundamental feature of the effective communication needed in palliative medicine. There is much research here still to be grappled with.

Research into decision-making and informed consent in end-of-life care is also needed to provide empirical evidence to inform the otherwise theoretical ethical debate that abounds globally. There is still much to learn about the complexities of influence and competence of patients to make choices in vulnerable settings.

There are many important questions needing to be addressed. Researchers need to utilize a variety of methods to answer them. Mixed-method, observational studies, and RCTs are crucial approaches needing to be used in psychosocial research in the future. Moreover, an urgent requirement in many countries of the world is the training of dedicated researchers who can then address many of these problems. Without solid education and experience, the pitfalls appear formidable; skill development in research methodology is crucial to respond to the many challenges emerging in this young discipline.

References

1. **Salisbury, C. and Bosanquet, N.** (1999). The impact of different models of specialist palliative care on patient's quality of life: a systematic review of the literature. *Palliative Medicine* **13**, 3–17.
2. **Vigano, A., Dorgan, M., Buckingham, J., Bruero, E., and Suarez-Almazor, M.** (2000). Survival prediction in terminal cancer patients: a systematic review of the medical literature. *Palliative Medicine* **14**, 363–74.
3. **Devine, E. and Westlake, S.** (1995). The effects of psychoeducational care provided to adults with cancer: meta-analysis of 116 studies. *Oncology Nursing Forum* **22**, 1369–81.
4. **Meyer, T. and Mark, M.** (1995). Effects of psychosocial interventions with adult cancer patients: a meta-analysis of randomised experiments. *Health Psychology* **14**, 101–8.
5. **Goldberg, D.** *The Detection of Psychiatric Illness by Questionnaire.* London: Oxford University Press, 1972.
6. **Derogatis, L.** *Brief Symptom Inventory (BSI) Administration, Scoring and Manual.* Minneapolis: National Computer Systems, 1994.
7. **Horowitz, M., Wilner, N., and Alvarez, W.** (1979). Impact of event scale: a measure of subjective distress. *Psychosomatic Medicine* **41**, 209–18.
8. **Beck, A., Steer, R., and Garbin, M.** (1988). Psychometric properties of the Beck Depresion Inventory: twenty-five years of evaluation. *Clinical Psychology Review* **8**, 77–100.
9. **Radloff, L.** (1977). The CES-D scale: a self-report depression scale for research in the general population. *Applied Psychological Measures* **1**, 385–401.
10. **Roberts, R. and Vernon, S.** (1983). The center for epidemiologic studies depression scale: its use in a community sample. *American Journal of Psychiatry* **140**, 41–6.
11. **Dugan, W., McDonald, M., Passik, S., Rosenfeld, B., Theobald, D., and Edgerton, S.** (1998). Use of the Zung Self-Rating Depression Scale in cancer patients: feasibility as a screening tool. *Psycho-Oncology* **7**, 483–93.
12. **Zigmond, A. and Snaith, R.** (1983).The hospital anxiety and depression scale. *Acta Psychiatrica Scandinavica* **67**, 361–70.
13. **Snaith, R. and Taylor, C.** (1985). Rating scales for depression and anxiety: a current perspective. *British Journal of Clinical Pharmacology* **19**, 17S–20S.
14. **McNair, D., Lorr, M., and Droppleman, L.** *Profile of Mood States (Manual).* San Diego: Edits/Educational & Industrial Testing Service, 1992.
15. **Derogatis, L.** *The Affects Balance Scale: a Preliminary Guide to Administration, Scoring & Application.* Towson: Clinical Psychometric Research Inc., 1992.
16. **Templer, D.** (1970). The construction and validation of a death anxiety scale. *Journal of General Psychology* **82**, 165–77.
17. **Lonetto, R. and Templer, D.** *Death Anxiety.* New York: Hemisphere, 1986.
18. **Spielberger, C.** (1975). Anxiety-State-Trait-Process. In *Stress and Anxiety* (ed. C. Spielberger and I. Sarasen), pp. 115–43. New York: Halsted Press.
19. **Lazarus, R. and Folkman, S.** *Stress, Appraisal and Coping.* New York: Springer, 1984.
20. **Scheier, M. and Carver, C.** (1985). Optimism, coping and health: assessment and implications of generalized outcome expectancies. *Health Psychology* **4**, 219–47.
21. **Weisman, A. and Worden, J.** (1976). The existential plight in cancer: significance of the first 100 days. *International Journal of Psychiatry in Medicine* **7**, 1–15.
22. **Watson, M., Greer, S., and Bliss, J.** *Mental Adjustment to Cancer Scale User's Manual.* Sutton, Surrey: Cancer Research Campaign Medical Research Group, Royal Marsden Hospital, 1989.
23. **Watson, M., Law, M., dos Santos, M., Greer, S., Baruch, J., and Bliss, J.** (1994). The Mini-MAC: further development of the mental adjustment to cancer scale. *Journal of Psychosocial Oncology* **12**, 33–46.
24. **Cooper, P., Osborn, M., Gath, D., and Feggetter, G.** (1982). Evaluation of a modified self-report measure of social adjustment. *British Journal of Psychiatry* **141**, 68–76.
25. **Derogatis, L.** (1986). The psychosocial adjustment to illness scale (PAIS). *Journal of Psychosomatic Research* **30**, 77–91.
26. **Cohen, S., Mermelstein, R., Kamarck, T., and Hoberman, H.** (1985). Measuring the functional components of social support. In *Social Support: Theory, Research and Applications* (ed. I. Sarasen and B. Sarason), pp. 73–94. New York: Wiley.
27. **Cutrona, C. and Russel, D.** (1987). The provisions of social relationships and adaptation to stress. *Advances in Personal Relations* **1**, 37–67.
28. **Moos, R. and Moos, B.** *Family Environment Scale Manual.* Palo Alto CA: Consulting Psychologists Press, 1981.
29. **Epstein, N., Baldwin, L., and Bishop, D.** (1983). The McMaster Family Assessment Device. *Journal of Marital and Family Therapy* **9**, 171–80.
30. **Cohen, S., Mount, B., Bruera, E., Provost, M., Rowe, J., and Tong, K.** (1997). Validity of the McGill Quality of Life Questionnaire in the palliative care setting: a multi-centre Canadian study demonstrating the importance of the existential domain. *Palliative Medicine* **11**, 3–20.
31. **Cella, D.** *Manual of the Functional Assessment of Chronic Illness Therapy (FACIT Scales)—Version 4.* Evanston IL: Center on Outcomes, Research and Education (CORE), Evanston Northwestern Healthcare and Northwestern University, 1997.
32. **Schipper, H., Clinch, J., McMurray, A., and Levitt, M.** (1984). Measuring the quality of life of cancer patients: the Functional Living Index—Cancer: development and validation. *Journal of Clinical Oncology* **2**, 472–83.
33. **Aaronson, N., Ahmedsai, S., and Bergman, B.** (1993). The European organization for research and treatment of cancer QLQ-C30: a quality-of-life instrument for use in international clinical trials in oncology. *Journal of National Cancer Institute* **85**, 365–76.
34. **Ware, J., Snow, K., Kosinski, M., and Gandek, B.** *SF-36 Health Survey: Manual and Interpretation Guide.* Boston: The Health Institute New England Medical Center, 1993.
35. **McCorkle, R. and Young, K.** (1978). Development of a symptom distress scale. *Cancer Nursing* **1**, 373–8.
36. **Karnofsky, D. and Burchenal, J.** (1949). Clinical evaluation of chemotherapeutic agents in cancer. In *Evaluation of Chemotherapeutic Agents* (ed. C. Macleod), pp. 191–205. New York: Columbia Press.
37. **Fitchett, G., Peterman, A., and Cella, D.** Spiritual beliefs and quality of life in cancer and HIV patients. *Proceedings of Annual meeting of the Society for the Scientific Study of Religion and the Religious Research Association*, 9 November 1996, Nashville, TN.
38. **Brady, M., Peterman, A., Fitchett, G., Mo, M., and Cella, D.** (1999). A case for including spirituality in quality of life measurement in oncology. *Psycho-Oncology* **8**, 417–28.
39. **Holland, J. et al.** (1998). A brief spiritual beliefs inventory for use in quality of life research in life-threatening illness. *Journal of Psychosocial Oncology* **7**, 460–9.
40. **King, M., Speck, P., and Thomas, A.** (1995). The Royal Free Interview for religious and spiritual beliefs: development and standardization. *Psychological Medicine* **25**, 1125–34.
41. **Donahue, M.** (1985). Intrinsic and extrinsic religiousness: review and meta-analysis. *Journal of Personality and Social Psychology* **48**, 400–19.
42. **Achenbach, T.** *Manual of the Child Behavior Checklist/4–18 and 1991 Profile.* Burlington VT: University of Vermont, 1991.
43. **Kovacs, M.** *Children's Depression Inventory Manual.* North Tonawanda NY: Multi-Health Systems, 1992.
44. **Zarit, S., Reever, K., and Bach-Peterson, J.** (1980). Relatives of the impaired elderly: correlates of feeling the burden. *The Gerontologist* **20**, 649–55.
45. **Lawton, M.** (1971). The functional assessment of elderly people. *Journal of American Geriatric Society* **19**, 465–80.
46. **Given, C.W., Given, B., Stommel, M., Collins, C., King, S., and Franklin, S.** (1992). The Caregiver Reaction Assessment (CRA) for caregivers to person

with chronic physical and mental impairment. *Research in Nursing and Health* **15**, 271–83.
47. **Glaser, B.G. and Strauss, A.L.** *Awareness of Dying*. Chicago: Aldine, 1965.
48. **Glaser, B.G. and Strauss, A.L.** *Time for Dying*. Chicago: Aldine, 1968.
49. **Charmaz, K.** (1983). Loss of self: a fundamental form of suffering in the chronically ill. *Sociology of Health and Illness* **5**, 168–95.
50. **Morse, J. and Penrod, J.** (1999). Linking concepts of enduring uncertainty, suffering and hope. *Image: Journal of Nursing Scholarship* **31**, 145–50.
51. **Salander, P., Bergenheim, T., and Henriksson, R.** (1996).The creation of protection and hope in patients with malignant brain tumours. *Social Science and Medicine* **42**, 985–96.
52. **Kissane, D., Street, A., and Nitschke, P.** (1998). Seven deaths in Darwin: case studies under the Rights of the Terminally Ill Act, Northern Territory, Australia. *Lancet* **352**, 1097–102.
53. **Charmaz, K.** Stories of suffering: subjective tales and research narratives. *Qualitative Health Research: Keynote Address from the Fourth Qualitative Health Research Conference*, Vol. 9, 1999, pp. 362–82.
54. **Kleinman, A.** *The Illness Narratives: Suffering, Healing and the Human Condition*. New York: Basic Books, 1988.
55. **Frank, A.W.** *The Wounded Storyteller*. Chicago: University of Chicago Press, 1995.
56. **Aranda, S. and Street, A.** (2001). From individual to group: use of narratives in a participatory research process. *Journal of Advanced Nursing* **33**, 791–7.
57. **McNamara, B., Waddell, C., and Colvin, M.** (1994). The institutionalization of the good death. *Social Science and Medicine* **39**, 1501–8.
58. **McNamara, B., Waddell, C., and Colvin, M.** (1995). Threats to the good death: the cultural context of stress and coping among hospice nurses. *Sociology of Health and Illness* **17**, 222–44.
59. **James, N. and Field, D.** (1992). The routinization of hospice: charisma and bureaucratization. *Social Science and Medicine* **34**, 1363–75.
60. **Lawton, J.** *The Dying Process: Patient's Experiences of Palliative Care*. London: Routledge, 2000.
61. **Chochinov, H.** et al. (1995). Desire for death in the terminally ill. *American Journal of Psychiatry* **152**, 1185–91.
62. **Litwin, M.** et al. (1995). Quality-of-life outcomes in men treated for prostate cancer. *Journal of the American Medical Association* **273**, 129–35.
63. **Greer, S., Morris, T., Pettingale, K., and Haybrittle, J.** (1990). Psychological responses to breast cancer and 15 year outcome. *Lancet* **i**, 49–50.
64. **Benzein, E. and Saveman, B.** (1998). Nurses' perception of hope in patients with cancer: a palliative care perspective. *Cancer Nursing* **21**, 10–16.
65. **Benzein, E., Borberg, A., and Saveman, B.** (2001). The meaning of the lived experience of hope in patients with cancer in palliative home care. *Palliative Medicine* **15**, 117–26.
66. **MacLeod, R.D.** (2001). On reflection: doctors learning to care for people who are dying. *Social Science and Medicine* **52**, 1719–27.
67. **Armstrong, D.** (1984). The patient's view. *Social Science and Medicine* **18**, 737–44.
68. **Armstrong, D.** (1987). Silence and truth in death and dying. *Social Science and Medicine* **24**, 651–7.
69. **Seale, C.** *Constructing Death: The Sociology of Dying and Bereavement*. Cambridge: Cambridge University Press, 1998.
70. **Street, A.F. and Kissane, D.W.** (2001). Constructions of dignity in end-of-life care. *Journal of Palliative Care* **17**, 93–101.
71. **Kuuppelomäki, M.** (2000). Cancer patients', family members' and professional helpers conceptions and beliefs concerning death. *European Journal of Oncology Nursing* **4**, 39–47.
72. **Holland, J., Romano, S., Heiligenstein, J., Tepner, R., and Wilson, M.** (1998). A controlled trial of fluoxetine and desipramine in depressed women with advanced cancer. *Psycho-Oncology* **7**, 291–300.
73. **Kissane, D.W. and Bloch, S.** *Family Focused Grief Therapy*. Buckingham: Open University Press, 2002.
74. **Folkman, S.** (2001). Revised coping theory and the process of bereavement. In *Handbook of Bereavement Research. Consequences, Coping, and Care* (ed. M. Stroebe, R. Hansson, W. Stroebe, and H. Schut), pp. 563–84. Washington DC: American Psychological Association.
75. **Grbich, C., Parker, D., and Maddocks, I.** (2001). The emotions and coping strategies of caregivers of family members with a terminal cancer. *Journal of Palliative Care* **17**, 30–6.
76. **Fielding, N.** (2001) Computer applications in qualitative research. In *Handbook of Ethnography* (ed. P. Atkinson, A. Coffey, S. Delamont, J. Lofland, and L. Lofland), pp. 453–67. London: Sage.
77. **Field, D., Clark, D., Corner, J., and Davis, C.**, ed. *Researching Palliative Care*. Buckingham: Open University Press, 2001.
78. **Glare, P.** (1999). Trials in palliative care. *Cancer Forum* **23**, 147–8.
79. **Jordhoy, M.** (1999). Challenges in palliative care research: recruitment and attrition and compliance: experience from a randomized controlled trial. *Palliative Medicine* **13**, 299–310.
80. **Kirkham, S. and Abel, J.** (1997). Placebo-controlled trials in palliative care: the argument against. *Palliative Medicine* **11**, 489–92.
81. **de Raeve, L.** (1994). Ethical issues in palliative care research. *Palliative Medicine* **8**, 298–305.
82. **Corner, J.** (1996). Is there a research paradigm for palliative care? *Palliative Medicine* **10**, 201–8.
83. **Karim, K.** Conducting research involving palliative patients. In *Nursing-Standard* (NURS-STAND), September 27–October 3, 2000; **15** (2), 34–6 (28 refs).
84. **Atkinson, P. and Silverman, D.** (1997). Kundera's immortality: the interview society and invention of the self. *Qualitative Inquiry* **3**, 304–25.
85. **Doyle, D., Hanks, G.W.C., and MacDonald, N.** Introduction. In *Oxford Textbook of Palliative Medicine*, 2nd edn. Oxford: Oxford University Press, 1999.
86. **Seale, C. and Kelly, M.** (1997). A comparison of hospice and hospital care for people who die: views of the surviving spouse. *Palliative Medicine* **11**, 93–100.

Further reading

Cresswell, J.W. *Qualitative Inquiry and Research design*. Thousand Oaks CA: Sage Publications, 1998. Useful qualitative methodological text with comparisons of methods in different approaches.

Freeman, C. and Tyrer, P., ed. *Research Methods in Psychiatry*, 2nd edn. London: Royal College of Psychiatrists, 1995. Useful guide for the beginner to psychosocial research.

Field, D., Clark, D., Corner, J., and David, C., ed. *Researching Palliative Care*. Buckingham: Open University Press, 2001. An illustrative compilation of palliative care studies.

Higginson, I., ed. *Clinical Audit in Palliative Care*. Oxford: Radcliffe Medical Press, 1993. A basic primer of quality assurance that incorporates the psychosocial.

Sederer, L.I. and Dickey, B., ed. *Outcomes Assessment in Clinical Practice*. Baltimore: Williams & Wilkins, 1996. A useful resource into clinical outcomes assessment.

6

Patient evaluation and outcome measures

6 Patient evaluation and outcome measures

6.1 The measurement of pain and other symptoms

Jane M. Ingham and Russell K. Portenoy

Introduction

Medical intervention aims to eliminate disease, mitigate disease effect, and maximize quality of life. As clinicians endeavour to fulfil these goals, symptoms present both diagnostic clues and therapeutic challenges. For patients, the disease experience is inextricably linked to symptoms and the distress they produce. Distress, in turn, is influenced by diverse psychosocial and cultural factors. The assessment of symptoms and symptom distress is, therefore, a vital aspect of clinical care, particularly in advanced and incurable illnesses for which the primary goals of care may relate to comfort and quality of life (QOL).

Ideally, the management of symptoms should be guided by a comprehensive assessment that incorporates an understanding of the multidimensional nature of symptoms and quality of life. Symptom measurement is a part of symptom assessment and should similarly reflect the complexity of patient perceptions. This complexity can be addressed by reviewing: (a) the principles of symptom assessment and measurement; (b) the clinical and research applications of these principles; (c) the measurement instruments for several common symptoms; and (d) the challenges in the application of symptom measures in the palliative care setting.

Principles of symptom assessment and measurement

Symptoms—a general definition

The study of symptoms has been hampered to some degree by a lack of consistency in terminology. The Oxford Dictionary defines symptom as 'a physical or mental phenomena, circumstance or change of condition arising from and accompanying a disorder and constituting evidence for it . . . specifically a *subjective* indicator perceptible to the patient and as opposed to an *objective* one (cf. sign)'.[1] Thus, symptoms are inherently subjective. They are perceptions, usually conveyed by language. Symptom measurement attempts to quantify aspects of these perceptions in a manner that is valid and reliable.

This definition also highlights the distinction between symptoms, signs, and pathological processes or diagnoses. Usually, a disease process causes a spectrum of symptoms, each of which may clarify the disease process and diagnosis. Symptoms are subjective physical and psychological phenomena that arise from pathological states or disorders and should never be viewed as diagnoses. Signs are clinical observations, the observation of which contributes to the process that allows a clinician to formulate a diagnosis. For example, a patient may report 'confusion'—a symptom in this instance—and the clinician may note 'signs' including poor concentration and evidence of memory loss. After eliciting a history the clinician may ascertain the 'diagnosis' which in this instance may be dementia or delirium. The existence of confusion, however, should not be used synonymously with either the diagnosis of delirium or dementia, or with any of the other disease processes with which this symptom may be associated. Further 'confusion' should not be used as a 'diagnosis' as there are a number of conditions with which it may be associated.

Defining specific symptoms

Although languages are made rich by the many nuances that are applied to words that describe human perceptions, the measurement of these perceptions is made more challenging by these nuances. The complexity of measurement is compounded when the words used to label symptoms, such as 'pain' or 'fatigue', have a plethora of meanings for patients and a wide range of implications in the medical setting.

In contrast to the generally accepted definition for 'pain' and the development of a taxonomy for the study of this symptom,[2] no such definition or taxonomy has evolved to clarify other symptoms. For example, the measurement of 'fatigue', 'confusion', and even 'breathlessness', is complicated by the absence of specific definitions and the range of implications associated with each. Fatigue may be interpreted by some patients as sleepiness and by others as muscle weakness. The word 'confusion' may be used to refer to impaired concentration, disorganized thinking, forgetfulness, or even hallucinations. A study that investigated the descriptors used by patients with dyspnoea found that 8 per cent answered 'no' to the statement 'I feel breathless' despite answering 'yes' for numerous other descriptors that are applied to dyspnoea.[3] Dyspnoea certainly provides an illustration of the fact that an understanding of the language used describe symptoms is crucial, both in the clinical setting to interpret distress and in the research setting with instrument development. Recent work has demonstrated that the descriptors of breathlessness used by healthy individuals reflect distinct and separable cognitive constructs that are not simply dependent on the presence of an underlying pathophysiology or on a specific disease condition.[4,5] That stated, however, it was demonstrated in the same population that distinct qualities of breathlessness appear to relate to different physiologic mechanisms underlying respiratory discomfort.[4,5]

To further illustrate the complexity of the linguistics involved with this issue, another study explored QOL in a population of cancer patients and found that there was instrument-to-instrument variation in the prevalence of identical symptoms (Table 1).[6–9] In addition, items that appeared to assess similar experiences, such as 'anxiety' and 'nervousness', had differing prevalence rates. These data indicate that symptom assessment and measurement is dependent on the clarity of meanings attached to symptom descriptors. The variability of these meanings justifies the need for formal validation of symptom assessment instruments.

Subjectivity in assessment and measurement

Because symptoms are inherently subjective, patient self-report must be the primary source of information.[10–16] Numerous studies have demonstrated

Table 1 Prevalence of selected symptoms by instrument

Symptom	ESAS[a] (%) n = 233	FACT[b] (%) n = 238	MSAS[c] (%) n = 232
Pain	57	61	58
Nausea	29	23	24
Depression	40	—	—
Sadness	—	42	29
Anxiety	63	—	—
Nervous feeling	—	46	37

Adapted from published data in Chang, V.T., Hwang, S.S., and Feuerman, M. (2000). Validation of the Edmonton Symptom Assessment Scale. *Cancer* **88** (9), 2164–71.

[a] Edmonton Symptom Assessment Scale.

[b] Functional Assessment of Cancer Therapy Scale.

[c] Memorial Symptom Assessment Scale.

that observer and patient assessments are not highly correlated, and that the accuracy of a clinician's assessment cannot be assumed.[10–14] For example, a low correlation has been demonstrated between patients' visual analogue scores (VAS) for pain and those of health care providers.[10] Clinician accuracy has been demonstrated to be especially poor even in settings where clinicians are assessing patients with the most severe pain, suggesting that inferences about subjective states may be most uncertain at a level of patient distress that is most clinically relevant. A study that concurrently assessed patients and their spouse caregivers found that, although the caregivers agreed with patients on objective measures with observable referents (e.g. ability to dress independently), they disagreed with subjective aspects of patient functioning (e.g. depression, fear of future, and confidence in treatment).[11] Another study revealed that retrospective assessments by bereaved family members did not accurately depict patient symptoms at the end of life.[12]

The optimal approach to symptom assessment and measurement must incorporate patient ratings of subjective experiences. In some cases, objective signs can be monitored to complement subjective data, but this information cannot substitute for self-report. For example, dyspnoea measurement may be complemented by measurement of oxygen saturation or blood gases. Nausea measurement may be supplemented by assessment of the frequency of emesis, and pain measurement may be clarified by functional assessment.

In some populations, such as demented or obtunded patients or preverbal children, it may not be possible to obtain or interpret patient self-reports. Although family members and staff may be useful proxies for clinical and research purposes, these data must be interpreted cautiously. This latter approach to data collection has been effective in some studies of symptoms and quality of life towards the end of life.[17–23] Nonetheless, to facilitate accurate interpretation of data, investigators should always acknowledge the source of the data and describe the self-report and proxy data separately, if both are acquired.[24]

Symptoms as measurable multidimensional experiences

Symptoms are multidimensional experiences that may be evaluated in terms of their specific characteristics and impact (Table 2). The impact of symptoms may be described in relation to spheres of functioning; any variety of family, social, financial, spiritual, and existential issues; or various global constructs such as overall symptom distress or QOL.[25–28]

Symptom characteristics

Although surveys of symptoms have often assessed prevalence, or prevalence and a single descriptor (usually severity), a more detailed assessment of the characteristics of specific symptoms is often valuable. This may appear to be self-evident in the clinical setting, where history taking frequently

Table 2 The measurable aspects of symptoms

Specific dimensions	Frequency Severity Distress
Symptom impact on specific factors	Other physical and psychological symptoms or diagnoses Function Family, social, financial, spiritual, and existential resources and concerns
Symptom impact on global constructs	Global symptom distress Health-related quality of life

incorporates the assessment of the frequency, severity, and distress associated with each symptom. Assessment of these characteristics has not, however, been extensively applied in the research setting.

The variability of symptom characteristics has been described repeatedly.[8,25–27,29–32] For example, a study of 215 patients with prostate, colon, breast, or ovarian cancer described variations in the frequency, severity and distress (the degree to which they considered the symptom to be bothersome) associated with 32 physical and psychological symptoms.[25] Some of the symptoms were reported to be frequent or severe, but not highly bothersome or distressing, suggesting that the mere report of a symptom does not imply that it is burdensome or in need of treatment. Similar variability in the characteristics of symptoms has been demonstrated in the paediatric setting.[30]

Symptom impact

The impact of symptoms can be evaluated in terms of many phenomena. In the setting of advanced medical disease, the presence of multiple symptoms and other adverse influences on QOL can complicate efforts to define the impact of a particular symptom.

Pain provides a useful example of this complexity. Pain may induce depression, exacerbate anxiety, interfere with the ability to interact socially, impair physical performance, prevent the patient from working, and decrease family income. These secondary effects can be specifically measured. The Brief Pain Inventory (BPI), for example, contains a validated subscale that assesses pain-related interference with function, mood, and enjoyment of life.[33] Surveys in the cancer population have shown that the relationship between pain severity and interference with function is non-linear and characterized by a disproportionate impairment in function above a pain severity rating of 4 on a 10-point scale.[34,35] This finding has been demonstrated to be consistent across four cultures and may ultimately be useful in research to quantify target ranges of pain severity and better assess the effectiveness of pain treatment strategies.[35]

The complexity of symptom impact is reflected in the many options available to measure it. Depending on the goals of measurement, symptom impact may be illuminated by the evaluation of other physical or psychological symptoms, patient function, global symptom distress, or other domains of QOL.

Symptoms and global constructs

Several studies have explored the utility of the construct 'global symptom distress' as an indicator of overall symptom burden in the cancer population.[8,28,31,36] Brief measures have been validated to measure this construct (see below).[28,31] The development of these brief measures demonstrates that unidimensional assessment of a small group of highly prevalent physical and psychological symptoms can validly indicate global symptom distress, which correlates with both a relatively poor QOL and impairment of performance status.[25,31] Although multidimensional assessment probably has a greater potential for clarifying the impact of symptoms on QOL,[8] the use of a brief measure, requiring limited evaluation time, can provide clinically relevant information with minimal effort.

The multidimensional construct of QOL reflects the broad influence of many positive and negative factors on perceived well-being.[24,37–44] Physical and psychological symptoms contribute to QOL, but are merely elements within a complex set of factors that increase or temper distress, or enhance well-being. This complexity is particularly apparent in the setting of advanced medical disease, which is characterized by numerous physical and psychological symptoms[25,26,30,31,45–54] and a diverse range of physical, emotional, social, ethical, and spiritual phenomena. Each of the latter concerns has the potential to independently influence QOL, and to augment or lessen the distress associated with specific symptoms.

Figure 1 illustrates the impact that a pathophysiological process and various modifying factors may have on the perception of symptom-associated distress and overall QOL. Assessment of these complex interactions may be facilitated by the use of valid multidimensional measures of QOL (see Chapter 6.3).

Multidimensional measurement of symptoms may provide the most information about the interactions between symptoms and QOL. For example, a recent study of symptoms in patients with cancer provided empirical evidence that information relating to the impact of symptoms on QOL was maximized by concurrent measurement of 'symptom distress' and either frequency or intensity.[8] Of the three dimensions assessed, distress was the most informative. These data suggest that distress, or if possible, distress and another dimension, should be assessed if the goal of the evaluation is to clarify the interaction between symptoms and QOL. Further validation of this concept has been undertaken in a recent study, which explored the role of measurement of each of 32 symptoms with respect to distress (for physical symptoms) or frequency (for psychological symptoms) alone.[31]

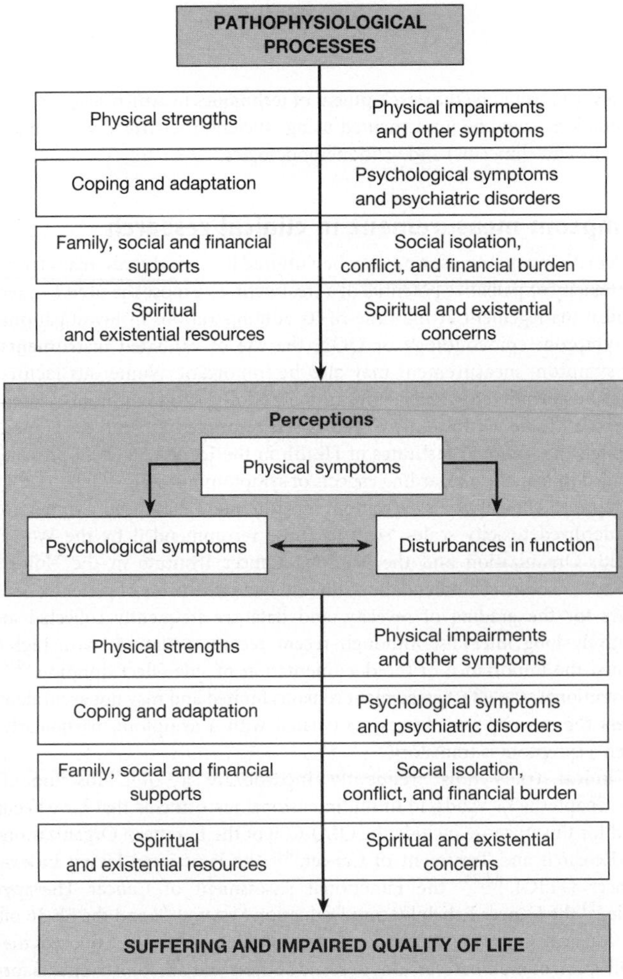

Fig. 1 Interactions between pain, symptoms, and quality of life.

Symptom assessment and measurement over time

Symptoms usually change over time. Characteristics may change or the symptom itself may remit or recur. Clinically, this observation is usually addressed through repeated assessments throughout the course of disease. In the research setting, and particularly in clinical trials, the challenge of symptom measurement is to capture the relevant concerns as they evolve, using measures that are simple and brief enough to both limit patient burden and encourage compliance.[55,56]

Numerous factors influence the changes in symptom prevalence and characteristics. Even problems that remain static, such as aphonia following laryngectomy, may be perceived differently as the disease, or the availability of treatment, changes or the consequences on function or psychosocial status evolve. Although such symptoms may continue to be described by the patient as severe, the associated distress and impact on QOL may increase or decrease. These observations suggest that longitudinal measurement of multiple symptom dimensions may be essential to accurately characterize the long-term impact of symptoms, interventions, or disease-related processes on QOL.

Clinical and research applications

Historically, symptom measurement has been used in clinical investigations to determine the positive and negative impact of disease-oriented therapies or palliative treatments. Although symptom measurement could potentially have clinical utility as a part of the routine monitoring of cancer patients in treatment settings,[10,16,57–60] it has rarely been applied in this way. More recently however some investigators have been exploring the utility of the routine use of patient-rated QOL and successfully applied this using computer-based methodology in the clinical setting.[61–66]

Symptom measurement in routine clinical management

The effective implementation of therapeutic strategies is contingent on comprehensive symptom assessment. The clinical approach to symptom assessment, which has been well described in basic medical textbooks and in specialized reviews, requires a detailed evaluation of symptom characteristics, pathogenesis, and impact (Table 3).[67–70] Although rarely used, instruments for structured history taking and for assessment of patient needs have been developed.[71–73]

Symptom measurement is one aspect of comprehensive evaluation, but the routine clinical application of symptom measures, particularly for symptoms other than pain, has not been systematically explored. This is unfortunate given the possibility of increased awareness of symptom-related distress and improved outcomes associated with careful, ongoing monitoring.[60] Systematic pain measurement may improve the understanding of health professionals of the pain status of individual hospitalized patients.[74] In a cancer centre, regular measurement has been incorporated into a continuous quality improvement strategy and preliminary data suggest that nurse's knowledge and attitudes about pain, and patient satisfaction with pain management, have improved subsequently.[59,75] In the latter study, pain measurement was facilitated by the addition of a pain scale to the bedside chart. An example of such a chart is seen in Fig. 2. Recent guidelines from the Agency for Health Care Policy and Research[16] and the American Pain Society[58] have recommended the regular use of pain rating scales to assess pain severity and relief in all patients who commence or change treatments. These recommendations also suggest that clinicians teach those patients who are at risk for experiencing pain, and their family members, to use assessment tools in the home to promote continuity of pain management in all settings.

Table 3 Clinical symptom assessment

Medical history	Psychosocial issues	Current medications
Diagnosis Chronology Therapeutic interventions including operative procedures, chemo- and radiotherapy Patient's knowledge of current extent of disease *Assessment* Review of systems For each symptom: chronology and frequency severity degree of distress impact on function other clinical characteristics impact of each symptom on other symptoms patient perception of aetiology prior treatment modalities and their efficacy other factors that alleviate or modulate distress associated with specific symptoms e.g. coping strategies and supports *Physical examination*	Family history Social resources Impact of disease and symptoms on patient and family *Global symptom impact* Global symptom distress impact of overall symptom distress on quality of life Impact of symptoms on quality of life: physical condition psychological status social interactions Factors that modulate global symptom distress e.g. coping strategies and family supports *Assess available laboratory and imaging data*	*Pathophysiology* For each symptom: inferred pathophysiology relationship to other symptoms differing pathophysiologies same pathophysiology causal pathology induced by another symptom causal factor is treatment directed at another symptom

Adapted from Ingham and Portenoy (1996), ref. 69.

The experience with pain measurement in the clinical setting could be expanded to the measurement of other symptoms. Symptom checklists, which have been developed to explore the spectrum of common physical and psychological symptoms in particular disease states, may be useful in symptom detection. Unfortunately, these simple, face-valid instruments have notable limitations, which include the lack of adequate validation and the inability to address more than one symptom dimension.[6,76–79] Face validity, by which is meant the intuitive assumption of validity based on the appearance of the items, is less than adequate in the research setting. In the routine clinical setting, where the scale is complemented by a full clinical evaluation, extensive validation of an instrument may not be needed. Recent studies have yielded new validated measures that supersede these simple checklists for research purposes (see below).[8,25,28,36,80,81] Although the application of the newer, more comprehensive measures has not been explored outside the research setting, some of the simple checklists have been used in routine clinical practice in palliative care units.[6,77] As discussed above, some investigators have utilized QOL measures in the clinic setting using computer-based touch screen methodology.[62–66] In addition to focusing staff attention on symptom assessment, such measures may be used as a means of reviewing the quality of patient care and ascertaining situation-specific barriers to symptom control.[6,51,82,83]

In the clinical setting, comprehensive symptom assessment should also query the impact of symptoms on global symptom distress and other quality of life concerns. Although instruments exist for the evaluation of global distress[8,25,28,36] and QOL,[7,44,84–87] the use of this type of instrument also has not been adopted in routine patient care.

Recently, a number of organizations, including those that accredit hospital organizations and national bodies such as the National Comprehensive Cancer Network (NCCN) in the United States, have recommended the implementation of routine detection methods for symptoms, in particular for pain, and the use of clinical practice guidelines for the treatment of distress and various symptoms.[88–90] To date, there is not a widely accepted methodology for the implementation of these recommendations in the clinical setting. Increasingly it is becoming apparent that a useful contribution to this field would be the development of techniques by which such recommendations could be implemented using efficient, user-friendly (for both patients and clinicians) and valid methodologies.

Symptom measurement in clinical research

Systematic symptom assessment, when utilized in clinical trials, may clarify the toxicity or palliative potential of a treatment, or expose the need to alter clinical management at the time of its administration. In investigations of symptom epidemiology or QOL, the use of validated instruments for symptom measurement may also be important. Numerous factors must be considered when planning methodology for symptom-related research (Table 4). Recently a web-based resource has been developed through the National Institutes of Health in the United States to provide detailed information regarding aspects of symptom research.[91]

In most clinical trials, symptom measurement has been limited to standardized toxicity scales, such as those recommended by the World Health Organization and the National Cancer Institute in the United States.[76] These recommendations do not mandate the use of patient-rated scales for the grading of severity, and data are frequently collected at relatively long intervals. Although recent recommendations have highlighted the importance of the documentation of side-effect duration,[92] conventional side-effect assessment remains limited and may not accurately assess the severity and distress associated with a symptom, particularly when a symptom is transitory.

Clinical trials now frequently incorporate a QOL instrument (see Chapter 6.3). Validated multidimensional instruments that have been used for this purpose include the QLQ-C30 of the European Organization for Research and Treatment of Cancer,[44] the Functional Living Index-Cancer (FLIC),[84,85] the Functional Assessment of Cancer Therapy Scale,[7] the Cancer Rehabilitation Evaluation System,[86] and the SF-36 of the Medical Outcome Study.[87] Recent studies have also explored the application of modified versions of some of these and other instruments for QOL assessment in populations with symptomatic HIV infection and other illnesses.[93–97]

INSTRUCTIONS: Record numbers, letters or symbols for appropriate measure		
TIME:		
Temp.		
BLOOD PRESSURE	Lying	
	Sitting	
	Standing	
Pulse		
Respirations		
Pulse Ox–O_2 Sat %		
FIO_2		
Blood glucose		
TIME:		
PAIN ASSESSMENT	Pain scale: 0–10 (none–most intense)	
	Key: Descriptors B = Burning A = Aching S = Shooting T = Throbbing ST = Stabbing ✗ = No Change — Site	
	Intervention N = None PCA = Pump MED = Medication COM = Comfort measures ★ = see note — Description	
	Intervention	
	Reassessment Time 30° p IV 60° p PO	
	Reassess with Pain Scale	

Fig. 2 Georgetown University Hospital observation chart. Patients are asked if there is pain 'right now' and if so to rate it on a scale where 0 = no pain and 10 = the worst pain. The hospital's policy and forms support a regular approach to assessment in which the pain score is documented, the character of the pain charted and an assessment of any intervention administered for the pain undertaken within a 30–60 min time frame of the assessment and detection of pain. 'Interventions' include medications and an array of non-pharmacological 'comfort' measures including, for example, repositioning. Reproduced with permission of Georgetown University Hospital. Copyright: MedStar–Georgetown Medical Center, Inc.

Table 4 Methodological considerations for symptom measurement in research settings

Patient-related factors	Factors related to investigator goals and resources	Instrument-related factors
Patient's ability to provide consent and comprehend instruments	*Study aims and method*	*Validity and reliability*
Age-related factors	Which symptoms and dimensions of symptoms need to be assessed?	Validity of instrument for assessment of symptom in general and in particular population
Cognitive state	When should symptoms be assessed?	Ability of instrument to assess the dimensions and impact of symptom
Cultural and language barriers	What methodological controls are needed?	
Patient's descriptors for symptom	*Data management and statistical analysis*	*Clinical utility and appropriateness*
Presence of other symptoms	Available resources for data collection and analysis	Capacity of instrument to assess hypothesis
Patient's willingness to participate in data collection		Instrument complexity and respondent burden
Patient reluctance to participate in investigation or to report specific symptom		

All of these recently developed, validated, multidimensional measures of health-related QOL assess a selected group of prevalent symptoms, including pain, fatigue, and anxiety.[7,44,84,86] Although this information may be clinically meaningful and sufficient for many purposes, these instruments cannot fully clarify the prevalence rates or characteristics of the diverse array of physical and psychological symptoms experienced by patients. O'Brien, Chang, Cella and colleagues have recently explored the feasibility of computer-assisted, immediate QOL monitoring in lung cancer in the setting of a clinical trial. Using this approach, physicians were provided with a graph of patient's QOL scores across the FACT-L subscales and symptom domains, as a means of emphasizing important patient concerns. The success of this type of 'real-time' assessment has suggested the role of such assessments in clinical trials but has also highlighted their potential utility in the clinic setting.[98]

Although a detailed assessment of symptoms may not be required in some studies, large clinical trials or epidemiological surveys may benefit from measurement of a broad spectrum of physical or psychological symptoms. This can be accomplished by the concurrent use of a QOL instrument and an instrument that is specially designed to measure symptoms. Alternatively, a more 'tailored' approach can be used in which a screening instrument is combined with some specific supplemental measures that capture information relevant to the disease or clinical setting. The recent development of multidimensional QOL instruments with disease- or treatment-specific modules derives from this perspective.[7,38,39,44] Depending on the purpose of the assessment, the aims of the research, the anticipated outcomes and toxicities, and the resources of the investigator, tailoring can be focused on specific assessment of a single symptom or phenomenon, multiple symptoms, or of related disease- and treatment-specific issues (e.g. performance status or psychological function).[7,38,39,44,56]

The utility of this 'tailored' approach to symptom and QOL assessment was demonstrated in a recent study, which explored the importance of specific pain assessments during routine QOL evaluation.[56] This phase II trial of paclitaxel and recombinant human granulocyte-colony stimulating factor for breast cancer, previously observed clinical observations had suggested that frequent short-lived episodes of pain were likely to occur during this treatment regimen. To capture this information, supplemental pain measurements were included with QOL measures. The assessment revealed a marked disparity between the pain data obtained during a routine QOL assessment performed at 3-week intervals and those acquired through the supplemental pain evaluation obtained twice weekly. In contrast to the interval assessment, which revealed a marked decline in median pain scores, the supplemental assessment demonstrated transient acute and severe pains in almost half the patients. Clearly, such a tailored approach to measurement may be important in clarifying the usefulness of a therapy in symptom palliation, altering clinical management at the time of treatment or determining the long-term effects of therapy on well-being. This study also illustrates the need, in all settings, for careful consideration of the optimal timing of evaluations.

Finally, in relation to 'measurement' in clinical research, consideration must not only be given to the utility of an instrument to measure a subjective effect but also to whether a reasonable presumption can be made about the extent to which a change in the measured score reflects a 'clinically relevant' change in symptom severity or distress. Statistical significance, particularly in tests of group averages, may or may not indicate that the difference is meaningful in the clinical sense. For example, a clinical trial of an analgesic with a large sample size may show that the group receiving treatment A had an average change in a pain score of 1.0 on a 0–10 scale, whereas the group that received treatment B had an average change of 1.8. This difference may be statistically significant but clinically irrelevant. Moreover, this difference reflects average scores and may hide the fact that some patients had very large changes after a treatment, whereas some changed not at all.

The studies needed to clarify clinically relevant measurements are scant and much research is needed in this area. A variety of approaches to interpreting change have been proposed.[91,99] Rather than group averages, it may be more meaningful to use categorical measures that make intuitive sense clinically. Using pain to illustrate, the investigator can, for example, compare the number of patients who achieve pain relief greater than 50 per cent, the number of patients who must be treated to yield one patient who attains at least 50 per cent relief (known as Number Needed to Treat, or NNT),[100] or the number of treatment days on which pain control was good.[101] New analyses of data from large pain studies suggests that change scores of 2 or more on 0–10 scale, or a 30 per cent change on an analogue scale reflects clinically meaningful change; the investigator could therefore compare the number of patients who achieve one of these criteria. An analysis of the BPI suggested specific scores that could be interpreted as 'mild', 'moderate', or 'severe' pain.[102] A comparison of the number of patients who change from one category to another yields similar information. In the same manner, it may be possible to combine variables into an index of 'clinical benefit'. One group, for example, have suggested that changes in three variables (reduction in pain by 50 per cent, weight gain of 5 per cent, and improvement in KPS of 20 per cent) along with duration of improvement (4 weeks) may be suggestive of 'clinical significance'.[103–105] Of note, the Cochrane reviews have taken a systematic review approach to assessing the impact of symptom-related therapies through the use of meta-analyses.[106]

There continue to be many issues to be resolved through future studies.[99] Is an improvement of 50 per cent in a pain score of 2 to 1 on an 11-point numeric scale as clinically significant as a change from 9 to 4.5? Can clinical significance of a therapy be evaluated without controlling for side-effects, and if not, how should these be measured and indexed? In the complex palliative care setting, can the clinical relevance of a single symptom be truly explored when most patients experience multiple distressing symptoms concurrently? These issues must be considered when interpreting the measurement of any symptom in clinical reports and further research hopefully will clarify methods for measuring and interpreting meaningful data.

Validated instruments for symptom assessment

Instrument selection for symptom measurement must be guided by an understanding of the goals of assessment and the practicality, applicability, and acceptability of the instrument, or instruments, in the particular patient population. Careful consideration must be given to the burden imposed on patients, clinicians, and investigators by the use of each instrument. Measurement strategies that are simple and brief may limit patient burden and encourage compliance. The effort to achieve this, however, should not preclude the assessment needed to capture complex symptom-related concerns or QOL. If the information is salient and would not be assessed otherwise, the increased burden may be warranted.

Instruments for the measurement of multiple symptoms

Historically, the spectrum of common physical and psychological symptoms has, most frequently, been explored using simple, face-valid measures, often in the form of symptom checklists.[6,51,76,77] Recent studies have resulted in the development of new, validated measures that may supersede these simple checklists, particularly in the assessment of multiple symptoms.

Memorial Symptom Assessment Scale (MSAS):[8,25] The MSAS is a validated, patient-rated measure that provides multidimensional information about a diverse group of common symptoms (Fig. 3). This instrument characterizes 32 physical and psychological symptoms in terms of intensity, frequency and distress. The MSAS provides a Global Distress Index (MSAS-GDI), a 10-item subscale that reflects global symptom distress, and separate subscales that measure physical (MSAS-PHYS) and psychological (MSAS-PSYCH) symptom distress, respectively. The MSAS may be a useful measure in a variety of research settings. Further studies are needed to establish its reliability and validity with repeated administration, assess its utility as an outcome measure in cancer clinical trials, and confirm its value in patients with various types of cancer and disease states. Recently, Chang et al. have developed and validated 'short-form' of this instrument (MSAS-SF).[31] Work is ongoing by the same group on the validation of a further 'condensed' version of this same instrument. These latter instruments, being short and easily administered, are likely to prove useful in the clinic setting and their utility in this arena is currently being explored. Recently Collins et al. have validated a paediatric version of the MSAS (see below—Special populations).[30]

MEMORIAL SYMPTOM ASSESSMENT SCALE

NAME: DATE:

SECTION 1:

INSTRUCTIONS: We have listed 24 symptoms below. Read each one carefully. If you have had the symptom during this past week, let us know how OFTEN you had it, how SEVERE it was usually and how much it DISTRESSED OR BOTHERED you by circling the appropriate number. If you DID NOT HAVE the symptom, make an "X" in the box marked "DID NOT HAVE"

DURING THE PAST WEEK, Did you have any of the following symptoms?	DID NOT HAVE	IF YES, How OFTEN did you have it?				IF YES, How SEVERE was it usually?				IF YES, How much did it DISTRESS or BOTHER you?				
		Rarely	Occas-ionally	Frequ-ently	Almost cons-tantly	Slight	Moder-ate	Severe	Very severe	Not at all	A little bit	Some-what	Quite a bit	Very much
Difficulty concentrating		1	2	3	4	1	2	3	4	0	1	2	3	4
Pain		1	2	3	4	1	2	3	4	0	1	2	3	4
Lack of energy		1	2	3	4	1	2	3	4	0	1	2	3	4
Cough		1	2	3	4	1	2	3	4	0	1	2	3	4
Feeling nervous		1	2	3	4	1	2	3	4	0	1	2	3	4
Dry mouth		1	2	3	4	1	2	3	4	0	1	2	3	4
Nausea		1	2	3	4	1	2	3	4	0	1	2	3	4
Feeling drowsy		1	2	3	4	1	2	3	4	0	1	2	3	4
Numbness/tingling in hands/feet		1	2	3	4	1	2	3	4	0	1	2	3	4
Difficulty sleeping		1	2	3	4	1	2	3	4	0	1	2	3	4
Feeling bloated		1	2	3	4	1	2	3	4	0	1	2	3	4
Problems with urination		1	2	3	4	1	2	3	4	0	1	2	3	4

Continued on other side............

DURING THE PAST WEEK, Did you have any of the following symptoms?	DID NOT HAVE	IF YES, How OFTEN did you have it?				IF YES, How SEVERE was it usually?				IF YES, How much did it DISTRESS or BOTHER you?				
		Rarely	Occas-ionally	Frequ-ently	Almost cons-tantly	Slight	Moder-ate	Severe	Very severe	Not at all	A little bit	Some-what	Quite a bit	Very much
Vomiting		1	2	3	4	1	2	3	4	0	1	2	3	4
Shortness of breath		1	2	3	4	1	2	3	4	0	1	2	3	4
Diarrhea		1	2	3	4	1	2	3	4	0	1	2	3	4
Feeling sad		1	2	3	4	1	2	3	4	0	1	2	3	4
Sweats		1	2	3	4	1	2	3	4	0	1	2	3	4
Worrying		1	2	3	4	1	2	3	4	0	1	2	3	4
Problems with sexual interest or activity		1	2	3	4	1	2	3	4	0	1	2	3	4
Itching		1	2	3	4	1	2	3	4	0	1	2	3	4
Lack of appetite		1	2	3	4	1	2	3	4	0	1	2	3	4
Dizziness		1	2	3	4	1	2	3	4	0	1	2	3	4
Difficulty swallowing		1	2	3	4	1	2	3	4	0	1	2	3	4
Feeling irritable		1	2	3	4	1	2	3	4	0	1	2	3	4

Continued on next page............

Fig. 3 Continued.

SECTION 2:

INSTRUCTIONS: We have listed 8 symptoms below. Read each one carefully. If you have had the symptom during this past week, let us know how SEVERE it was usually and how much it DISTRESSED OR BOTHERED you by circling the appropriate number. If you DID NOT HAVE the symptom, make an "X" in the box marked "DID NOT HAVE".

DURING THE PAST WEEK, Did you have any of the following symptoms?	DID NOT HAVE	IF YES, How SEVERE was it usually?				IF YES, How much did it DISTRESS or BOTHER you?				
		Slight	Moderate	Severe	Very severe	Not at all	A little bit	Somewhat	Quite a bit	Very much
Mouth sores		1	2	3	4	0	1	2	3	4
Change in the way food tastes		1	2	3	4	0	1	2	3	4
Weight loss		1	2	3	4	0	1	2	3	4
Hair loss		1	2	3	4	0	1	2	3	4
Constipation		1	2	3	4	0	1	2	3	4
Swelling of arms of legs		1	2	3	4	0	1	2	3	4
"I don't look like myself"		1	2	3	4	0	1	2	3	4
Changes in skin		1	2	3	4	0	1	2	3	4

** IF YOU HAD ANY OTHER SYMPTOMS DURING THE PAST WEEK, PLEASE LIST BELOW AND INDICATE HOW MUCH THE SYMPTOM HAS DISTRESSED OR BOTHERED YOU.

OTHER:	0	1	2	3	4
OTHER:	0	1	2	3	4
OTHER:	0	1	2	3	4

Fig. 3 Revised version of the Memorial Symptom Assessment Scale.[8] Reprinted from *European Journal of Cancer* **V60**, Portenoy, R.K. et al. The Memorial Symptom Assessment Scale: an instrument for the evaluation of symptom prevalence, characteristics and distress, pp. 1151–8. Copyright (1994), with permission from Elsevier.

The Edmonton Symptom Assessment System (ESAS):[6] The ESAS evaluates eight symptoms on VAS's and has been extensively used in palliative care research. The validity and reliability of this instrument has recently been explored and in advanced cancer it is apparent that the ESAS is a valid instrument.[9] Of note, in the validation study undertaken by Chang et al. test–retest validity was better at 2 days than at 1 week and the ESAS 'distress' score appeared to reflect physical well being. Certainly, this instrument's convenience, applicability in patients with far-advanced disease, and ease of use seem advantageous.

Rotterdam Symptom Checklist (RSCL):[80,81] The RSCL is a validated patient-rated measure that evaluates a spectrum of common symptoms in terms of patient-rated distress. Thirty physical and psychological symptoms are included and an additional eight items specifically attempt to define the impact of symptoms on physical activity and function. The RSCL provides quantitative information about global symptom distress and subscales that distinguish physical and psychological symptom distress. This instrument does not address the issue of multidimensional assessment and no information is provided about potentially relevant dimensions, such as intensity or frequency. Some symptoms that may be common in advanced disease, such as change in taste and appearance, are not evaluated. Although there are questions about pain in the head, back, abdomen, and mouth, there is no general pain item.

Symptom Distress Scale (SDS):[28,36] The SDS is a 13-item patient-rated scale that evaluates 11 symptoms, nine physical and two psychological, in terms of frequency, intensity, or distress. Responses are answered on a 5-point Likert scale ranging from 1 (no distress) to 5 (extreme distress). Although the SDS provides only limited information about specific symptoms, it is a valid and useful measure of global symptom distress. The potential utility of this score has been further demonstrated in a study of lung cancer patients in which the symptom distress score was a significant predictor of survival.[107]

Instruments for the measurement of specific symptoms

Although numerous instruments have been validated for the assessment of some symptoms,[91] such as pain and depression, there is a paucity of similar instruments for other symptoms that are prevalent in advanced disease, such as anorexia, dry mouth, or change in appearance. Moreover, many symptom-specific instruments have been validated in specific populations and may not be valid in others. For example, dyspnoea measurement has been developed in the disciplines of pulmonary medicine and cardio-logy,[4,5,108–113] and, there is little information specifically derived in the oncology setting.[114–116] To illustrate the range of options available and the practical issues that may be important in selecting an instrument, the following discussion focuses on measures for four common symptoms—pain, impaired cognition, dyspnoea, and fatigue. For further detail about specific symptoms, readers are referred to specific chapters in this text and to the recently developed web-based resource that focuses on symptom research.[91]

Instruments for the assessment of pain

Unidimensional scales of intensity or relief, including visual analogue, numerical, and categorical scales, have been the traditional focus of pain measurement. Multidimensional instruments, which provide a more comprehensive evaluation of pain and its impact, comprise the McGill Pain

Questionnaire (MPQ)[117–119] and an instrument that has been extensively validated in the cancer population, the BPI.[33]

The Memorial Pain Assessment Card (MPAC)[120] is a brief, validated measure that uses VAS's to characterize pain intensity, pain relief and mood, and an 8-point verbal rating scale (VRS) to further characterize pain intensity (Fig. 4). The mood scale, correlates with measures of overall psychological distress, depression, and anxiety, and is considered to be a valid measure of global psychological distress. Although this instrument provides limited information, its brevity, simplicity, and reliability are attractive and it has been used in many analgesic trials.

The BPI[33] is a self-administered, easily understood measure that provides information about pain history, intensity, location and quality (Fig. 5). Numeric scales (Range 0–10) indicate the intensity of pain in general, at its worst, at its least, and right now. A percentage scale quantifies relief from current therapies. A body figure allows localization of the pain. Seven questions evaluate the degree to which pain interferes with function, mood, and enjoyment of life. The BPI has now been translated into several languages.

The MPQ[117–119] is a self-administered questionnaire that evaluates the sensory, affective, and evaluative dimensions of pain and provides global scores and subscale scores for each of these dimensions. The scores are derived from the adjectival pain descriptors selected by the patient. A 5-point verbal categorical scale characterizes the intensity of pain and a pain drawing localizes the pain. Additional information is collected about the impact of medications and other therapies. This instrument does not assess the impact of pain on function. To date, the predominant application of the MPQ has been in the assessment of chronic, non-malignant pain and the utility of the subscale scores has not been demonstrated for cancer pain.[121]

Instruments for the assessment of impaired cognition

Instruments have been developed to specifically identify cognitive impairment and others have been developed to determine the likelihood that the impairment can be ascribed to a specific diagnosis, such as delirium.

Screening tests for cognitive impairment include the Mini Mental Status Exam[122] and the Blessed Orientation-Memory-Concentration Test.[123] These tools are sensitive indicators of impairment,[83,124,125] but are not specific for the diagnosis of delirium or dementia. Further assessment with either a clinical interview or the administration of another validated instrument, is necessary to clarify the diagnosis of the cause of cognitive impairment. Electroencephalography or brain imaging studies may supplement the clinical assessment and assist in the clarifying of the diagnosis.

The instruments used to diagnose delirium provide an example of instruments that specifically assess a specific 'diagnosis' to further describe the nature of a clinical state of confusion. Delirium is common in hospitalized cancer patients[53,54,83] and in the medically ill elderly.[126–128] It is also highly prevalent in those with chronic illness who are nearing the end of life,[83,129–131] and recent evidence suggests that this syndrome is highly distressing for patients, and their family and professional caregivers.[132] The instruments for delirium assessment have been extensively reviewed by Smith et al.,[133] and although the clinical psychiatric interview using the criteria outlined by the American Psychiatric Association in the Diagnostic and Statistical Manual (DSM) IV[134] remains the 'gold standard' for the diagnosis of delirium several instruments are available that facilitate the diagnosis. These include the Confusion Assessment Method,[135] the Delirium Symptom Interview,[136] and the Delirium Rating Scale (DRS).[137] These instruments, which were developed based on the earlier criteria outlined in the DSM III[138] or DSM III-R,[139] use an interview format to clarify the characteristics of the cognitive impairment. Either a score above a cut-off point or an algorithm documents the presence or absence of delirium. Although none of these measures have been adequately validated as a measure of delirium severity, they may be useful in providing a method for the monitoring of patients predisposed to delirium or receiving treatment for this condition.

Recently, Breitbart et al. have developed the Memorial Delirium Assessment Scale (MDAS).[140] The MDAS is a 10-item instrument that quantifies the severity of symptoms that are found in delirium and is based on criteria that are included in both the DSM III-R and the DSM IV. Scores from the MDAS and DRS have been shown in one study to be significantly correlated and, in the same study the scores on both also correlated with a global clinical judgment of delirium severity.[141] The MDAS is intended for repeated administrations over a short time period and this new instrument may prove to be useful for capturing short-term fluctuations in delirium.[142] This instrument has now been translated into Italian and Japanese,[141,143] and a recent report described the use of the MDAS, along with other symptom assessment instruments, for routine detection of symptoms in a French-speaking palliative care setting.[144]

Instruments for the assessment of fatigue

Fatigue is among the most prevalent symptoms reported by patients with advanced illness, including cancer. Despite this, unlike exists for pain, there is no generally accepted definition of fatigue.[2] The experience is frequently characterized by a spectrum that includes muscular weakness, lethargy, sleepiness, mood disturbance (particularly depression), cognitive

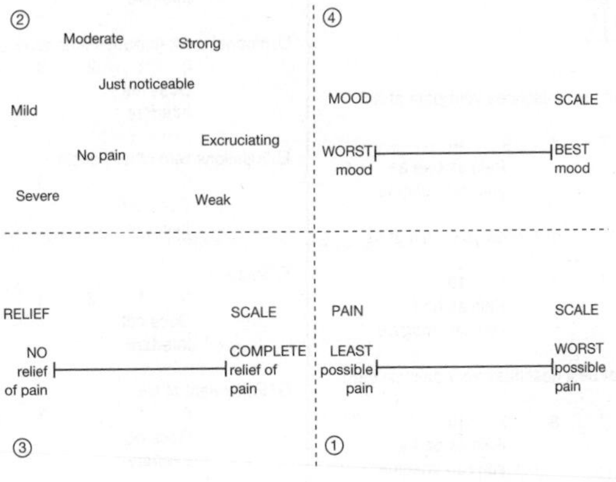

Fig. 4 The Memorial Pain Assessment Card. *Cancer* **60**(5), 1987, pp. 1151–8. Copyright © (1987) American Cancer Society. Reprinted by permission of Wiley-Liss, Inc., a subsidiary of John Wiley & Sons, Inc.

Brief Pain Inventory

Date: ___/___/___

Name: ____________ ____________ ____________
Last First Middle Initial

Phone: (___) ____________ Sex: ☐ Female ☐ Male

Date of Birth: ___/___/___

1) Marital Status (at present)
1. ☐ Single 3. ☐ Widowed
2. ☐ Married 4. ☐ Separated/Divorced

2) Education (Circle only the highest grade or degree completed)
Grade 0 1 2 3 4 5 6 7 8 9
10 11 12 13 14 15 16 M.A./M.S.
Professional degree (please specify) ____________

3) Current occupation ____________
(specify titles; if you are not working, tell us your previous occupation)

4) Spouse's Occupation ____________

5) Which of the following best describes your current job status?
☐ 1. Employed outside the home, full-time
☐ 2. Employed outside the home, part-time
☐ 3. Homemaker
☐ 4. Retired
☐ 5. Unemployed
☐ 6. Other

6) How long has it been since you first learned your diagnosis? _____ months

7) Have you ever had pain due to your present disease?
1. ☐ Yes 2. ☐ No 3. ☐ Uncertain

8) When you first received your diagnosis, was pain one of your symptoms?
1. ☐ Yes 2. ☐ No 3. ☐ Uncertain

9) Have you had surgery in the past month? 1. ☐ Yes 2. ☐ No

10) Throughout our lives, most of us have had pain from time to time (such as minor headaches, sprains, and toothaches). Have you had pain **other** than these everyday kinds of pain during the **last week**? 1. ☐ Yes 2. ☐ No

IF YOU ANSWERED YES TO THE LAST QUESTION, PLEASE GO ON TO QUESTION 11 AND FINISH THIS QUESTIONNAIRE. IF NO, YOU ARE FINISHED WITH THE QUESTIONNAIRE. THANK YOU.

11) On the diagram, shade in the areas where you feel pain. Put an X on the area that hurts the most.

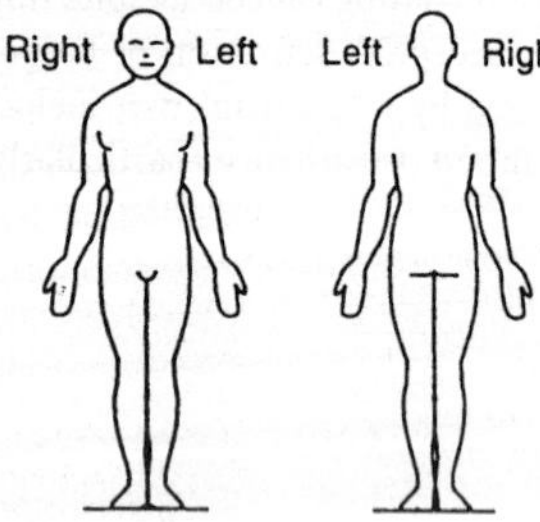

12) Please rate your pain by circling the one number that best describes your pain at its **worst** in the last week.
0 1 2 3 4 5 6 7 8 9 10
No Pain — Pain as bad as you can imagine

13) Please rate your pain by circling the one number that best describes your pain at its **least** in the last week.
0 1 2 3 4 5 6 7 8 9 10
No Pain — Pain as bad as you can imagine

14) Please rate your pain by circling the one number that best describes your pain on the **average**.
0 1 2 3 4 5 6 7 8 9 10
No Pain — Pain as bad as you can imagine

15) Please rate your pain by circling the one number that tells how much pain you have **right now**.
0 1 2 3 4 5 6 7 8 9 10
No Pain — Pain as bad as you can imagine

16) What kinds of things make your pain feel better (for example, head, medicine, rest)?
____

17) What kinds of things make your pain worse (for example, walking, standing, lifting)?
____

18) What treatments or medications are you receiving for your pain?
____

19) In the last week, how much relief have pain treatments or medications provided? Please circle the one percentage that most shows how much relief you have received.
0% 10% 20% 30% 40% 50% 60% 70% 80% 90% 100%
No Relief — Complete Relief

20) If you take pain medication, how many hours does it take before the pain returns?
☐ 1. Pain medication doesn't help at all
☐ 2. One hour
☐ 3. Two hours
☐ 4. Three hours
☐ 5. Four hours
☐ 6. Five to twelve hours
☐ 7. More than twelve hours
☐ 8. I do not take pain medication

21) Circle the appropriate answer for each item.
I believe my pain is due to:
☐ Yes ☐ No 1. The effects of treatment (for example, medication, surgery, radiation, prosthetic device).
☐ Yes ☐ No 2. My primary disease (meaning the disease currently being treated and evaluated).
☐ Yes ☐ No 3. A medical condition unrelated to primary disease (for example, arthritis).

22) For each of the following words, check yes or no if that adjective applies to your pain.

Aching	☐ Yes	☐ No	Exhausting	☐ Yes	☐ No
Throbbing	☐ Yes	☐ No	Tiring	☐ Yes	☐ No
Shooting	☐ Yes	☐ No	Penetrating	☐ Yes	☐ No
Stabbing	☐ Yes	☐ No	Nagging	☐ Yes	☐ No
Gnawing	☐ Yes	☐ No	Numb	☐ Yes	☐ No
Sharp	☐ Yes	☐ No	Miserable	☐ Yes	☐ No
Tender	☐ Yes	☐ No	Unbearable	☐ Yes	☐ No
Burning	☐ Yes	☐ No			

23) Circle the one number that describes how, during the past week, **pain has interfered** with your:

A. General Activity
0 1 2 3 4 5 6 7 8 9 10
Does not Interfere — Completely interferes

B. Mood
0 1 2 3 4 5 6 7 8 9 10
Does not Interfere — Completely interferes

C. Walking ability
0 1 2 3 4 5 6 7 8 9 10
Does not Interfere — Completely interferes

D. Normal work (includes both work outside the home and housework)
0 1 2 3 4 5 6 7 8 9 10
Does not Interfere — Completely interferes

E. Relations with other people
0 1 2 3 4 5 6 7 8 9 10
Does not Interfere — Completely interferes

F. Sleep
0 1 2 3 4 5 6 7 8 9 10
Does not Interfere — Completely interferes

G. Enjoyment of life
0 1 2 3 4 5 6 7 8 9 10
Does not Interfere — Completely interferes

Pain Research Group, Department of Neurology, University of Wisconsin-Madison

Fig. 5 Brief pain inventory. Reproduced with permission from Charles Cleeland, PhD.[33]

disturbances (such as difficulty concentrating), and others. Depending on the purpose of the assessment, the measurement of fatigue may need to attempt to capture this spectrum of disturbances.[145–148] Thus, fatigue provides an interesting example of the 'spectrum' of measurement that is feasible for a symptom.

Although unidimensional scales have been used, a thorough assessment of fatigue evaluates the temporal dimensions of the symptom, its physical and psychological components, and its associated distress. That stated clinicians and investigators may have differing goals in assessment—aiming to capture severity, quality, impact, or phenomena conceptually related to fatigue.[149–151] Unidimensional fatigue scales include single-item scales and those that are incorporated into symptom checklists and other validated symptom assessment instruments.[28,81,149,152,153] The latter includes the fatigue subscale of the Profile of Mood States (POMS)[154] and a measure created from the EORTC QLQ-C30 as a three-item subscale for fatigue (Were you tired?, Have you felt weak?, Did you need a rest?—each categorized on a 4-point verbal rating scale).[155] Scales developed in the industrial setting have also been applied to clinical assessment.[147,156–160]

Several multidimensional scales have been validated in the medically ill. These are detailed in Table 5.[149,161–169] As an example, the 41-item Piper Fatigue Self Report Scale (PFS) addresses the severity, distress, and impact of fatigue, and can be administered as either a series of VAS's or as numeric scales.[161,162] This scale was developed to assess the multiple dimensions of fatigue in patients receiving radiation therapy and has demonstrated excellent reliability and moderate construct validity in this population. Another example is the Visual Analogue Scale-Fatigue (VAS-F)—an 18-item, multidimensional patient-rated instrument. This instrument has been validated in a population with sleep disorders and has demonstrated high internal consistency and significant correlations with the POMS fatigue subscale and a sleepiness scale.[163] The VAS-F has not been widely used in populations with advanced medical disease, but may prove useful because of its comparative brevity.

Recent discussion in the literature has also focused on the potential and value associated with the measurement of assessing various symptoms and problems that may be 'associated' with fatigue.[149,150] For example, in a series of studies evaluating psychostimulants in patients receiving opioids, investigators used a VAS to assess 'drowsiness' and other scales to evaluate cognitive status.[170–173] As an 'objective' outcome some investigators have linked the assessment of fatigue interventions with measures of exercise capacity.[174,175] Others have evaluated sleep, and sleep efficiency in the setting of fatigue. The latter leads into an area that could relate to the impact of fatigue, or alternately could be a 'cause' of fatigue. In this category it has been proposed that when measuring fatigue in certain settings it may be appropriate to measure aspects related to potential aetiologies and co-morbidities. The latter may include measurement of symptoms, sleep, psychological distress, metabolic parameters, and other factors.[149]

Fatigue, in a similar manner to pain, cognitive impairment and indeed any symptom that is very distressing, may itself impose limitations on assessment. In the setting of fatigue, the length of the multidimensional fatigue assessment instruments may be problematic in populations with advanced disease and/or severe fatigue. In the initial validation study of the PFS, for example, 24 per cent of patients experienced difficulties in responding to the scales and almost half the patients approached for the study refused to participate. This problem compounds the challenges posed by the lack of a widely accepted definition, the complexity of the dimensions that constitute the symptom and the paucity of instruments that are both validated and accepted. Ongoing research will hopefully clarify some of these problems and guide the development of assessment instruments.

Table 5 Multidimensional fatigue questionnaires

Piper Fatigue Scale (Piper et al., 1998)
Lee Fatigue Scale (Lee et al., 1991)
Fatigue Assessment Questionnaire (Glaus, 1996)
Functional Assessment of Cancer Therapy—Anaemia/Fatigue (Yellen et al., 1997)
Brief Fatigue Inventory (Mendoza et al., 1999)
Cancer Fatigue Scale (Okuyama et al., 2000)
Schwartz Cancer Fatigue Scale (Schwartz, 1998)
Multidimensional Fatigue Inventory (Smets et al., 1995)

Reproduced from Portenoy, R.K. (2001). Fatigue. In *Interactive Clinical Research Textbook* Chapter 9 (ed. M. Max and J. Lynn). National Institute of Dental and Craniofacial Research. Available online on http://www.symptomresearch.com

Instruments for the assessment of dyspnoea

The instruments for the measurement of dyspnoea have, for the most part, been developed in the setting of chronic pulmonary and cardiac conditions. Like other symptoms, numerous aspects and dimensions of dyspnoea can be assessed.[176] These include antecedents, or physiologic and psychogenic factors that precede the onset of the symptom; environmental or personal characteristics that mediate dyspnoea; subjective responses and reactions to dyspnoea; and consequences or outcomes of dyspnoea.[111,176] Instruments may assess one or more of these dimensions.

To clarify the appropriateness of the language employed in dyspnoea assessment, the descriptors used by patients have been explored using adjectival checklists.[3,177,178] These studies indicate that patients use a variety of descriptors for dyspnoea and those particular descriptors, or clusters of descriptors, vary in relation to specific lung pathologies. For example, a study of patients with a spectrum of chronic lung diseases, including emphysema-bronchitis, asthma, restrictive lung disease, and vascular lung disease, demonstrated that although most patients endorsed the descriptor 'I feel short of breath', those with asthma were more likely than others to describe 'chest tightness'.[177] As mentioned above, the work of Mahler et al., in an outpatient population with seven different conditions demonstrated that each diagnosis was associated with a unique set of clusters (e.g. asthma with 'work/effort' and 'tight', interstitial lung disease with 'work/effort' and 'rapid' breathing).[4] The 'work/effort' cluster was common for all diagnoses. These investigators suggested that the use of a questionnaire containing descriptors of breathlessness might help to establish a specific diagnosis and to identify mechanisms whereby a specific intervention relieves dyspnoea. These disease-specific characteristics emphasize the importance of selecting instruments for dyspnoea measurement that have been validated in the appropriate disease population.

VASs are the most commonly utilized measures for the assessment of dyspnoea in patients with advanced disease. VASs generally have good within-subject reproducibility, particularly when dyspnoea is assessed repeatedly in a single session using a standard exercise task to induce dyspnoea.[108,179,180] The VAS has been found to be less reliable when the same exercise task is repeated at longer intervals, such as 2 weeks.[181] In addition, considerable between-subject variation has been demonstrated[182] and, in some individuals, VAS scores are insensitive and poorly reproducible.

Verbal categorical scales and numerical scales have also been used to assess dyspnoea.[109,110,178,183] The modified Borg scale is an example of a commonly used categorical scale.[184,185] This scale, which has been validated in healthy individuals and in patients with chronic non-malignant pulmonary disease, rates the patient's perception of their dyspnoea in relation to a perceived level of exertion. For example, the dyspnoea is rated as equating with exertion that is 'very, very weak', 'very, very strong', and varying degrees in between.

The measurement of dyspnoea, unlike that of many other symptoms, frequently involves the administration of an instrument with a dyspnoea-producing task, usually standardized or graded exercise. Indeed, although the commonly used dyspnoea measures, such as VASs and the Borg scale,[184,185] have been shown to be reliable and valid measures of dyspnoea when assessment is linked to such an exercise task, the validity and reliability of these measures have only rarely been evaluated *without* such a stress.[114,186,187] In addition, the work to date suggests the VAS is *not* appropriate for comparing dyspnoea in different patients as there are no standard principles that allow the scales to be used consistently by different subjects.(176)

It is clear that the reliability of dyspnoea assessment can be improved by the use standardized exercise task and thus consideration must be given in assessment to the type of task and timing of assessment that is appropriate in a given setting. One approach involves the assessment of each subject's ability to reproduce a dyspnoea score on the VAS in response to a standard degree of exertion.(179) Other investigators have attempted to use a standardized exercise to 'calibrate' the VAS with respect to each subjects quantity and quality of breathlessness.(109,110) In such a 'calibrated' scale, the upper end of the VAS is 'anchored' to the dyspnoea associated with a specific strenuous exercise.(109) The dyspnoea at the moment that the exercise is terminated is defined as the maximum point on the VAS. This has been shown to have utility in detecting clinically significant changes in pulmonary rehabilitation of patients with chronic obstructive pulmonary disease.(180)

In addition to enhancing the reliability of the assessment, an approach that incorporates an exercise task allows the assessment of therapeutic interventions that may have little impact on baseline dyspnoea but substantial effect on exercise-induced dyspnoea. When assessing dyspnoea in a population with advanced disease, it is important to define a standardized exercise that is not limited by other symptoms or disabilities. For example, in some populations, the use of short walk or treadmill exercise may be limited by pain or fatigue, whereas repetitive arm or leg lifting exercises may be feasible.

Other instruments assess the consequences of dyspnoea in relation to limitations on function. Although useful in the patient suffering from breathlessness as a single symptom, these instruments, which include the Modified Medical Research Council Dyspnoea Scale,(188) the American Thoracic Society Five Level Scale of Breathlessness,(189) the Baseline Dyspnoea Index,(190) and the Transition Dyspnoea Index,(190) have obvious limitations when function is limited by other symptoms such as pain or fatigue. That stated however, especially in patients with dyspnoea as their primary symptom in the setting of cardio-pulmonary disease and even in those with other symptoms, it has been suggested that in many settings it is most appropriate to measure the effects on activities of daily living for 'benchmarking' patient progress(191) and that instruments that quantify function and health-related quality of life have great utility for documenting outcomes (although these may be limited as to documenting treatment responsiveness for specific clinical interventions).(191,192)

Challenges in palliative medicine

There are significant challenges in bringing systematic symptom measurement to the very ill palliative care population. These include both attitudinal and conceptual barriers to the use of such measures, practical barriers, and barriers that are specific to special populations.

Conceptual and attitudinal barriers to the use of symptom measures

Conceptual and attitudinal barriers to the use of health status measures in patient care and clinical trials(193) are likely to be relevant in the palliative care setting. These include skepticism about the validity and importance of self-rated health measures, preferences for physiologic outcomes or death rates, unfamiliarity of health care providers with the scoring of measures, and a paucity of direct comparisons among instruments.

Education of health professionals about measurement techniques should be viewed as a priority in efforts aimed at eliminating barriers and improving symptom management. In a recent survey of physicians providing care for patients with cancer, 76 per cent stated that the single most important barrier to adequate pain management was poor pain assessment.(194) In another survey, less than one-half of patients with pain had a staff member ask about pain or note pain in their record during the 72-h period after their admission to the hospital.(195) The routine use of symptom assessment measures in clinical practice may be useful in approaching these difficulties.(60) Recent directives by accreditation organizations, such as the Joint Commission for the Accreditation of Hospital Organizations in the United States—mandating that hospitals and nursing facilities assess pain routinely—have intensified the focus on symptom assessment in 'routine' patient care settings.

Practical barriers that occur in patients with advanced disease

The absence of valid measures for the assessment of many common symptoms represents a major methodologic barrier to improving symptom measurement. As a result, many studies have used checklists to measure symptom prevalence without reference to symptom distress and impact. New, validated measures that assess symptom characteristics are clearly preferable and many of these have been discussed above. There remains an ongoing need for the development of instruments for the specific assessment of the less common symptoms.

Some symptoms are difficult to measure or, in themselves, compromise the assessment of subjective concerns. The high prevalence of delirium and fatigue in patients with advanced disease is a potential barrier to the completion of subjective measures, and severe distress—from any cause—is likely to be an impediment to comprehensive assessment, at least in the immediate setting of severe distress. Studies have suggested that the prevalence of delirium in hospitalized medical and surgical patients is approximately 10 per cent.(127,196) A higher prevalence, ranging to 50 per cent in some studies, exists in some inpatient populations, including the elderly and patients in the post-operative period.(126,127) The prevalence of delirium in hospitalized cancer patients ranges from 8 to 40 per cent.(53,54,83) A consistently higher prevalence, up to 85 per cent, has been found in studies of cancer populations with very advanced disease, particularly those in the last week of life.(83,131,197)

Cognitive impairment may preclude accurate measurement of subjective data. The difficulty that some cognitively intact individuals experience in completing VASs(109,198–200) is likely to be increased among the cognitively impaired. It has been suggested that studies should incorporate a methodology for assessing an individual's ability to consistently use measurement instruments, such as the VAS, and consideration should be given to eliminating patients who are unable to reliably use the instrument from studies designed to assess the specific interventions.(109)

In the clinical setting, it is crucial to assess pain and other causes of distress in the cognitively impaired and to develop a methodology by which a patient's distress and the impact of interventions can be assessed over time. Recent studies involving cognitively impaired elderly patients have demonstrated that many of these patients can report pain.(201,202) Those with mild to moderate cognitive impairment usually can respond to a self-report instrument.(201,202) To reduce the under-reporting of pain,(201) it is important to teach patients how to use the scales and to repeat enquiries about pain.(203,204) For non-verbal patients with severe cognitive impairment, pain assessment must rely on behavioural scales. These scales have drawbacks and should not be used if self-report is possible. Behaviour can reflect distress caused by problems other than pain, and severe dementia can 'blunt' physical responses and lead to an underestimate of distress. Although these behavioural measures can be useful in clinical assessment, the extent to which they can validly measure change over time has not been adequately explored.(205–207) This area is deserving of more study.

As an illustration of the use of a behavioural tool, Kavoch et al. developed an 'Assessment of Discomfort in Dementia Protocol' as a systematic method for addressing both physical pain and distress in patients with severe dementia.(207) This protocol uses the response to 'as needed' analgesics as a part of the assessment process. As noted, the goal of this approach is to measure 'discomfort', another proxy for pain, in those with severe cognitive impairment.

Fatigue is also an extremely prevalent concern in patients with advanced disease. Fatigue is the most common symptom in populations with advanced cancer, occurring with a prevalence of 40–70 per cent,[25,26,45–47,50,208] and although the impact of fatigue on the ability of patients to complete assessment measures has not been specifically empirically evaluated, it is an important theoretical concern.

A further methodologic difficulty relates to the measurement of symptoms in patients experiencing multiple symptoms concurrently. In a study of patients with prostate, colon, breast, or ovarian cancer the median number of symptoms per patient was 11.5 and the range was 0–25.[25] The development of instruments for the measurement of global symptom distress has provided a method by which the impact of multiple symptoms can be explored.[8,25,28,36]

The priorities of the patient and family may be another barrier to systematic symptom assessment in the palliative care setting. Patients may be unwilling to participate in clinical studies or provide information that requires the use of complex, time-consuming instruments. One survey demonstrated that patients in a palliative care unit gradually reduced their compliance with twice daily VAS measures for pain, activity, nausea, drowsiness, appetite, sensation of well-being, depression and anxiety, as their disease progressed.[51] In contrast to the day of admission, when 69 per cent of the VASs were completed by the patient and 28 per cent by the nurse, only 8 per cent of the measures were completed by the patient on the day of death.

The willingness or ability of patients with advanced medical disease to participate in symptom studies has not been studied. Clearly, this willingness will vary with the characteristics of the patient, family, disease, and study methodology. It is reassuring to note that several surveys of symptoms and QOL in patients with advanced medical illness suggest that relatively good compliance is possible. Of 1427 consecutive outpatients with recurrent or metastatic cancer who were asked to participate in a study using the BPI, only 119 patients (8.3 per cent) did not participate; of these, 68 (4.7 per cent) refused, 34 (2.4 per cent) were too ill to participate, and 17 (1.2 per cent) were unable to comprehend or complete the forms.[209] In another study of 308 patients with advanced, symptomatic HIV disease, 67 per cent participated, 15 per cent refused, and the remaining 18 per cent could not be enrolled for 'logistic' reasons.[210] The group who participated provided self-report data despite severe symptoms (mean symptom number 11) and a low performance status (41 per cent limited in self-care activities).

Concern about the response of medically ill patients to sensitive questions at a time when they are experiencing numerous physical, psychological, and emotional stressors has also not been addressed in the literature. Evidence exists, however, that sensitive areas of concern can be assessed. For example, in a survey of patients with cancer who were expected to die within a year, patients were asked to participate in interviews at biweekly or monthly intervals to discuss issues regarding their preferred place of death.[211] Of 98 patients approached, 84 (86 per cent) agreed to be interviewed, of whom 70 (83 per cent) died during the study. Clearly willingness to participate in such studies and to answer sensitive questions will be influenced by many factors including, among others, cultural preferences.

In summary, the concerns that cognitive impairment may interfere with subjective reporting, and that fatigue and/or symptom burden may limit patient ability or willingness to provide subjective data, have important implications for clinical practice and research methodology in the palliative care population. Clinically, these issues impact on the approach to assessing patient concerns. In the research setting, these issues emphasize the importance of selection criteria, documentation of cognitive status, and recording of reasons for refusal or inability to participate in data collection.

Special populations

Symptom measurement is particularly challenging in several subpopulations. These include the paediatric population, the imminently dying, those patients whose language or culture differs from that of the health care professionals involved in their care, and the cognitively impaired. Approaches to the symptom assessment and measurement in the cognitively impaired have been discussed above.

In the paediatric literature, symptom assessment has predominantly focused on procedural pain.[212–215] There has been little attention directed towards the assessment of chronic pain or other symptoms that occur in the setting of chronic illness. Procedural pain has been evaluated with self-report VASs and 'faces' scales,[216–221] and observational scales such as the Observational Scale of Behavioral Distress[222] and the Procedure Behavior Checklist.[218] These measures quantify the occurrence, intensity, and range of a child's pain during procedures. Although a behavioural observation scale for assessment of tumour-related pain in children aged 2–6 years has been developed,[223] the 17 items in the scale lack operational definitions and demonstrated poor inter-rater reliability. Other scales have been used for the assessment of chemotherapy-related nausea and vomiting,[224,225] including VASs and 'face' scales for frequency, severity, and distress, but these have not been extensively validated. The MSAS has recently been adapted for use for the measurement of multiple symptoms in the population aged 10–18 years.[30] This instrument can provide multidimensional information about symptoms experienced by children. Its use to date has been for research in the paediatric population with cancer.

The difficulties encountered in the assessment of the imminently dying population have led both clinicians and investigators to rely on observer-rated data despite concerns about the validity of this approach. This area interfaces closely with that discussed above related to cognitive impairment. The prevalence of cognitive impairment varies by disease and general rules cannot be proffered. For example, only 15 per cent of 16 000 decedents in the National Mortality Followback Survey had 'trouble understanding where he or she was during the last few hours or days'.[226] Although some surveys have described cancer patients with advanced disease as commonly being *unable* to communicate for significant periods of time towards the end of life,[51,129,130,227,228] a recent survey of 102 inpatient and homecare cancer deaths found that significant numbers (over 50 per cent) of patients were able to interact up to 12 h before death but by the hour before death few (less than 10 per cent) were communicative.[229] Thus, in the majority of those who die the major deterioration in mental status only occurs in the days immediately prior to death. Although this issue poses significant methodological challenges for the assessment of distress in the imminently dying and similar issues apply to those that were discussed above in the section addressing cognitive impairment, it is apparent that oftentimes assessment of the subjective experience is a feasible goal even in the imminently dying.

Significant problems relating to symptom assessment and measurement also may be encountered in patients whose culture and language differ from the professionals involved in their care.[230] Without meticulous attention to skilled translation, the nuances of the language used to describe symptoms may obscure meaning across cultures. Only a few instruments have been shown to be reliable and valid across cultures and languages,[141,231,232] and translation and validation of other symptom measures is needed. In the clinical setting, health care professionals may need to develop simple, face-valid symptom measures to overcome language barriers. A discussion among the clinician, the patient and an interpreter can facilitate the construction of a simple, two-language verbal rating scale to keep by the bedside. To assist a patient who is being cared for in the setting of cultural or language barriers with communication of symptom-related issues, the symptoms on these face-valid rating scales should take into account the current concerns of the patient and anticipated concerns given the patient's clinical problems. To monitor the level of distress and impact of interventions, such scales should, at a minimum, address both symptom intensity and relief. This approach is important to ensure that symptom distress can be minimized at all times, particularly when interpreters are not freely available.

Conclusion

Systematic symptom assessment is a foundation of clinical practice and research. Instruments for the measurement of symptoms have been developed and may facilitate this process. Quantification of symptoms may be able to improve symptom management and further the goal of enhanced QOL. Clinicians and investigators should become familiar with these instruments and develop methods for their use in routine clinical practice, the research environment, and the palliative care setting.

References

1. **Brown, L., ed.** *The New Shorter Oxford English Dictionary*. Oxford: Clarendon Press, 1993.
2. **IASP, Subcommittee on Taxonomy** (1980). Pain terms: a list with definitions and notes on usage. *Pain* **8**, 249–52.
3. **Elliott, M.W.** et al. (1991). The language of breathlessness. Use of verbal descriptors by patients with cardiopulmonary disease. *American Review of Respiratory Diseases* **144** (4), 826–32.
4. **Mahler, D.A.** et al. (1996). Descriptors of breathlessness in cardiorespiratory diseases. *American Journal of Respiratory and Critical Care Medicine* **154** (5), 1357–63.
5. **Harver, A.** et al. (2000). Descriptors of breathlessness in healthy individuals: distinct and separable constructs. *Chest* **118** (3), 679–90.
6. **Bruera, E.** et al. (1991). The Edmonton Symptom Assessment System (ESAS): a simple method for the assessment of palliative care patients. *Journal of Palliative Care* **7** (2), 6–9.
7. **Cella, D.F.** et al. (1993). The Functional Assessment of Cancer Therapy scale: development and validation of the general measure. *Journal of Clinical Oncology* **11** (3), 570–9.
8. **Portenoy, R.K.** et al. (1994). The Memorial Symptom Assessment Scale: an instrument for the evaluation of symptom prevalence, characteristics and distress. *European Journal of Cancer* **30A** (9), 1326–36, Elsevier Science Limited.
9. **Chang, V.T., Hwang, S.S., and Feuerman, M.** (2000). Validation of the Edmonton Symptom Assessment Scale. *Cancer* **88** (9), 2164–71.
10. **Grossman, S.A.** et al. (1991). Correlation of patient and caregiver ratings of cancer pain. *Journal of Pain and Symptom Management* **6** (2), 53–7.
11. **Clipp, E.C. and George, L.K.** (1992). Patients with cancer and their spouse caregivers. Perceptions of the illness experience. *Cancer* **69** (4), 1074–9.
12. **Higginson, I., Priest, P., and McCarthy, M.** (1994). Are bereaved family members a valid proxy for a patient's assessment of dying? *Social Science & Medicine* **38** (4), 553–7.
13. **Slevin, M.L.** et al. (1988). Who should measure quality of life, the doctor or the patient? *British Journal of Cancer* **57**, 109.
14. **Kahn, S.B., Houts, P.S., and Harding, S.P.** (1992). Quality of life and patients with cancer: a comparative study of patient versus physician perceptions and its implications for cancer education. *Journal of Cancer Education* **7**, 241.
15. **Osoba, D.** (1994). Lessons learned from measuring health-related quality of life in oncology. *Journal of Clinical Oncology* **12**, 608.
16. **Jacox, A.** et al. *Management of Cancer Pain. Clinical Practice Guideline*. No. 9. US Department of Health and Human Services, Public Health Service, Agency for Health Care Policy and Research, 1994.
17. **Greer, D.S.** et al. (1986). An alternative in terminal care: results of the National Hospice Study. *Journal of Chronic Diseases* **39** (1), 9–26.
18. **Morris, J.N.** et al. (1986). Last days: a study of the quality of life of terminally ill cancer patients. *Journal of Chronic Diseases* **39** (1), 47–62.
19. **Reuben, D.B. and Mor, V.** (1986). Dyspnea in terminally ill cancer patients. *Chest* **89** (2), 234–6.
20. **Mor, V.** (1987). Cancer patients' quality of life over the disease course: lessons from the real world. *Journal of Chronic Diseases* **40**, 535–44.
21. **Mor, V. and Masterson-Allen, S.** (1990). A comparison of hospice versus conventional care of the terminally ill cancer patient. *Oncology (Huntington)* **4** (7), 85–91 (discussion 94, 96).
22. **Higginson, I.J. and McCarthy, M.** (1994). A comparison of two measures of quality of life: their sensitivity and validity for patients with advanced cancer. *Palliative Medicine* **8** (4), 282–90.
23. **The Support Study Investigators** (1995). A controlled trial to improve care for seriously ill hospitalized patients: SUPPORT. *Journal of the American Medical Association* **274**, 1591–8.
24. **Aaronson, N.K.** (1990). Quality of life research in cancer clinical trials: a need for common rules and language. *Oncology* **4** (5), 59–66.
25. **Portenoy, R.K.** et al. (1994). Symptom prevalence, characteristics and distress in a cancer population. *Quality of Life Research* **3** (3), 183–9.
26. **Dunlop, G.M.** (1989). A study of the relative frequency and importance of gastrointestinal symptoms and weakness in patients with far advanced cancer. *Palliative Medicine* **4**, 37–43.
27. **Welch, J.M., Barlow, D., and Richardson, P.H.** (1991). Symptoms of HIV disease. *Palliative Medicine* **5**, 46–51.
28. **McCorkle, R. and Young, K.** (1978). Development of a symptom distress scale. *Cancer Nursing* **1**, 373–8.
29. **Portenoy, R.K. and Hagen, N.A.** (1990). Breakthrough pain: definition, prevalence and characteristics (see comments). *Pain* **41** (3), 273–81.
30. **Collins, J.J.** et al. (2000). The measurement of symptoms in children with cancer. *Journal of Pain and Symptom Management* **19** (5), 363–77.
31. **Chang, V.T.** et al. (2000). The memorial symptom assessment scale short form (MSAS-SF). *Cancer* **89** (5), 1162–71.
32. **Chang, V.T.** et al. (2000). Symptom and quality of life survey of medical oncology patients at a veterans affairs medical center: a role for symptom assessment. *Cancer* **88** (5), 1175–83.
33. **Daut, R.L., Cleeland, C.S., and Flanery, R.C.** (1983). Development of the Wisconsin Brief Pain Questionnaire to assess pain in cancer and other diseases. *Pain* **17** (2), 197–210.
34. **Daut, R.L. and Cleeland, C.S.** (1982). The prevalence and severity of pain in cancer. *Cancer* **50** (9), 1913–18.
35. **Serlin, R.C.** et al. (1995). When is cancer pain mild, moderate or severe? Grading pain severity by its interference with function. *Pain* **61** (2), 277–84.
36. **McCorkle, R. and Quint-Benoliel, J.** (1983). Symptom distress, current concerns and mood disturbance after diagnosis of a life-threatening disease. *Social Science & Medicine* **17** (7), 431–8.
37. **Till, J.E.** (1994). Measuring quality of life: apparent benefits, potential concerns. *Canadian Journal of Oncology* **4** (1), 243–8.
38. **Aaronson, N.K., Bullinger, M., and Ahmedzai, S.** (1988). A modular approach to quality of life assessment in cancer clinical trials. In *Recent Results in Cancer Research* (ed. H. Scheurlen, R. Kay, and M. Baum), p. 231. Berlin: Springer-Verlag.
39. **Moinpour, C.M.** et al. (1989). Quality of life end points in cancer clinical trials: review and recommendations. *Journal of the National Cancer Institute* **81** (7), 485–95.
40. **Moinpour, C.M.** et al. (1990). Quality of life assessment in Southwest Oncology Group trials. *Oncology* **4** (5), 79–84.
41. **Cella, D.F. and Tulsky, D.S.** (1990). Measuring quality of life today: methodological aspects. *Oncology* **4** (5), 29–38.
42. **Aaronson, N.K.** (1991). Methodologic issues in assessing the quality of life of cancer patients. *Cancer* **67** (Suppl. 3), 844–50.
43. **Nayfield, S.G.** et al. (1992). Report from a National Cancer Institute (USA) workshop on quality of life assessment in cancer clinical trials. *Quality of Life Research* **1** (3), 203–10.
44. **Aaronson, N.K.** et al. (1993). The European Organization for Research and Treatment of Cancer QLQ-C30: a quality-of-life instrument for use in international clinical trials in oncology. *Journal of National Cancer Institute* **85** (5), 365–76.
45. **Curtis, E.B., Krech, R., and Walsh, T.D.** (1991). Common symptoms in patients with advanced cancer. *Journal of Palliative Care* **7** (2), 25–9.
46. **Coyle, N.** et al. (1990). Character of terminal illness in the advanced cancer patient: pain and other symptoms during the last four weeks of life. *Journal of Pain and Symptom Management* **5** (2), 83–93.
47. **Dunphy, K.P. and Amesbury, B.D.W.** (1990). A comparison of hospice and homecare patients: patterns of referral, patient characteristics and predictors on place of death. *Palliative Medicine* **4**, 105–11.
48. **Brescia, F.J.** et al. (1990). Hospitalized advanced cancer patients: a profile. *Journal of Pain and Symptom Management* **5** (4), 221–7.
49. **Grosvenor, M., Bulcavage, L., and Chlebowski, R.T.** (1989). Symptoms potentially influencing weight loss in a cancer population. Correlations with primary site, nutritional status, and chemotherapy administration. *Cancer* **63** (2), 330–4.

50. **Ventafridda, V.** et al. (1990). Quality-of-life assessment during a palliative care programme. *Annals of Oncology* **1** (6), 415–20.

51. **Fainsinger, R.** et al. (1991). Symptom control during the last week of life on a palliative care unit. *Journal of Palliative Care* **7** (1), 5–11.

52. **Reuben, D.B., Mor, V., and Hiris, J.** (1988). Clinical symptoms and length of survival in patients with terminal cancer. *Archives of Internal Medicine* **148** (7), 1586–91.

53. **Levine, P.M., Silberfarb, P.M., and Lipowski, Z.J.** (1978). Mental disorders in cancer patients: a study of 100 psychiatric referrals. *Cancer* **42** (3), 1385–91.

54. **Derogatis, L.R.** et al. (1983). The prevalence of psychiatric disorders among cancer patients. *Journal of the American Medical Association* **249** (6), 751–7.

55. **Guyatt, G.H.** et al. (1987). Quality of life in patients with chronic airflow limitation. *British Journal of Diseases of the Chest* **81** (1), 45–54.

56. **Ingham, J.** et al. (1996). An exploratory study of frequent pain measurement in a cancer clinical trial. *Quality of Life Research* **5** (5), 503–7.

57. **Jacox, A., Carr, D.B., and Payne, R.** (1994). New clinical-practice guidelines for the management of pain in patients with cancer. *New England Journal of Medicine* **330** (9), 651–5.

58. **Max, M.** (1990). American Pain Society quality assurance standards for relief of acute pain and cancer pain. In *Proceedings VI World Congress on Pain* (ed. M.R. Bond, J.E. Charlton, and C.J. Woolf), pp. 185–9. Amsterdam: Elsevier.

59. **Bookbinder, M., Coyle, N., Kiss, M., Goldstein, M.L., Holritz, K., Thaler, H., Gianella, A., Derby, S., Brown, M., Racolin, A., Ho, M.N., and Portenoy, R.K.** (1996). Implementing national standards for cancer pain management: program model and evaluation. Journal of Pain and Symptom Management **12** (6), 334–47.

60. **Foley, K.M.** (1995). Pain relief into practice: rhetoric without reform. *Journal of Clinical Oncology* **13** (9), 2149–51.

61. **Morris, J., Perez, D., and McNoe, B.** (1998). The use of quality of life data in clinical practice. *Quality of Life Research* **7** (1), 85–91.

62. **Velikova, G.** et al. (1999). Automated collection of quality-of-life data: a comparison of paper and computer touch-screen questionnaires. *Journal of Clinical Oncology* **17** (3), 998–1007.

63. **Carlson, L.E.** et al. (2001). Computerized quality-of-life screening in a cancer pain clinic. *Journal of Palliative Care* **17** (1), 46–52.

64. **Taenzer, P.** et al. (2000). Impact of computerized quality of life screening on physician behaviour and patient satisfaction in lung cancer outpatients. *Psycho-oncology* **9** (3), 203–13.

65. **Cull, A.** et al. (2001). Validating automated screening for psychological distress by means of computer touchscreens for use in routine oncology practice. *British Journal of Cancer* **85** (12), 1842–9.

66. **Velikova, G.** et al. (2002). Computer-based quality of life questionnaires may contribute to doctor–patient interactions in oncology. *British Journal of Cancer* **86** (1), 51–9.

67. **Foley, K.M.** (1993). Pain assessment and cancer pain syndromes. In *Oxford Textbook of Palliative Medicine* (ed. D. Doyle, G. Hanks, and N. Macdonald), pp. 148–65. Oxford: Oxford University Press.

68. **Cherny, N.I. and Portenoy, R.K.** (1994). Cancer pain: principles of assessment and syndromes. In *Textbook of Pain* (ed. P.D. Wall and R. Melzack), pp. 787–823. Edinburgh: Churchill Livingstone.

69. **Ingham, J.M. and Portenoy, R.K.** (1996). Symptom assessment. In *Hematology/Oncology Clinics of North America* (ed. N.I. Cherny and K.M. Foley), pp. 21–40. Philadelphia PA: WB Saunders.

70. **Sui, A.L., Reuben, D.B., and Moore, A.A.** (1994). Comprehensive geriatric assessment. In *Principles of Geriatric Medicine and Gerontology* (ed. W.R. Hazzard et al.), pp. 203–11. New York: McGraw-Hill.

71. **Pecoraro, R.E.** et al. (1979). Validity and reliability of a self-administered health history questionnaire. *Public Health Reports* **94**, 231–8.

72. **Brodman, K.** et al. (1949). The Cornell Medical Index, an adjunct to medical interview. *Journal of the American Medical Association* **140**, 530–4.

73. **Coyle, N.** et al. (1996). Development and validation of a patient needs assessment tool (PNAT) for oncology clinicians. *Cancer Nursing* **19** (2), 81–92.

74. **Au, E.** et al. (1994). Regular use of a verbal pain scale improves the understanding of oncology inpatient intensity. *Journal of Clinical Oncology* **12** (12), 2751–5.

75. **Bookbinder, M.** et al. (2003). Implementing national standards for cancer pain management: program model and evaluation. *Oncology Nursing Forum* (in press).

76. **Miller, A.B.** et al. (1981). Reporting results of cancer treatment. *Cancer* **47**, 207–14.

77. **Donnelly, S. and Walsh, D.** (1995). The symptoms of advanced cancer. *Seminars in Oncology* **22** (No. 2, Suppl. 3), 67–72.

78. **Burgess, A.P., Irving, G., and Riccio, M.** (1993). The reliability and validity of a symptom checklist for use in HIV infection: a preliminary analysis. *International Journal of STD and AIDS* **4**, 333–8.

79. **Osoba, D.** (1993). Self-rating symptom checklists: a simple method for recording and evaluating symptom control in oncology. *Cancer Treatment Reviews* **19** (Suppl. A), 43–51.

80. **de Haes, J.C.J.M.** et al. (1987). Evaluation of the quality of life of patients with advanced ovarian cancer treated with combination chemotherapy. In *The Quality of Life of Cancer Patients* (ed. N.K. Aaronson and J. Beckman), pp. 217–25. New York: Raven Press.

81. **de Haes, J.C.J.M., van Kippenberg, F.C.E., and Neijt, J.P.** (1990). Measuring psychological and physical distress in cancer patients: structure and application of the Rotterdam Symptom Checklist. *British Journal of Cancer* **62**, 1034–8.

82. **Bruera, E.** et al. (1990). Palliative care in a cancer center: results in 1984 versus 1987. *Journal of Pain and Symptom Management* **5** (1), 1–5.

83. **Stiefel, F., Fainsinger, R., and Bruera, E.** (1992). Acute confusional states in patients with advanced cancer. *Journal of Pain and Symptom Management* **7** (2), 94–8.

84. **Schipper, H.** et al. (1984). Measuring the quality of life of cancer patients: The Functional Living Index-Cancer: development and validation. *Journal of Clinical Oncology* **2** (5), 472–83.

85. **Morrow, G.R., Lindke, J., and Black, P.** (1992). Measurement of quality of life in patients: psychometric analyses of the Functional Living Index-Cancer (FLIC). *Quality of Life Research* **1**, 287–96.

86. **Ganz, P.A.** et al. (1992). The CARES: a generic measure of health related quality of life for patients with cancer. *Quality of Life Research* **1**, 19–29.

87. **Stewart, A.L., Hays, R.D., and Ware, J.E.** (1988). The MOS short-form general health survey: reliability and validity in a patient population. *Medical Care* **26**, 724–35.

88. **Holland, J.C.** (1997). Preliminary guidelines for the treatment of distress. *Oncology (Huntington)* **11** (11A), 109–14 (discussion 115–17).

89. **Mock, V.** et al. (2000). NCCN Practice Guidelines for cancer-related fatigue. *Oncology (Huntington)* **14** (11A), 151–61.

90. **Payne, R.** (1998). Practice guidelines for cancer pain therapy. Issues pertinent to the revision of national guidelines. *Oncology (Huntington)* **12** (11A), 169–75.

91. **Max, M. and Lynn, J.** *Interactive Clinical Research Textbook*. National Institute of Dental and Craniofacial Research, 2001.

92. **Creekmore, S.P., Urba, W.J., and Longo, D.L.** (1991). Principles of the clinical evaluation of biological agents. In *Biologic Therapy of Cancer* (ed. V.T. Devita, S. Hellmen, and S.A. Rosenberg), pp. 67–86. Philadelphia PA: Lippincott Co.

93. **Kaplan, R.M.** et al. (1989). The Quality of Well-Being Scale: applications in AIDS, cystic fibrosis, and arthritis. *Medical Care* **27**, 35–49.

94. **Wu, A.W.** et al. (1991). A health status questionnaire using 30 items from the Medical Outcomes Study. *Medical Care* **29** (8), 786–98.

95. **Wachtel, T.** et al. (1992). Quality of life in persons with human immunodeficiency virus infection: measurement by the Medical Outcomes Study instrument (see comments). *Annals of Internal Medicine* **116** (2), 129–37.

96. **Cleary, P.D.** et al. (1993). Health-related quality of life in persons with acquired immune deficiency syndrome. *Medical Care* **31** (7), 569–80.

97. **Bozzette, S.A.** et al. (1994). A Perceived Health Index for use in persons with advanced HIV disease: derivation, reliability and validity. *Medical Care* **32** (7), 716–31.

98. **O'Brien, P.** et al. (2001). Feasibility of computer-assisted, immediate quality of life (QOL) monitoring in lung cancer. In *Proceedings of ASCO*

Vol. 20, abstract 1865. Program Proceedings American Society of Clinical Oncology. 37th Annual Meeting. Published by the American Society of Clinical Oncology, produced and printed by Lippincott, Williams and Wilkins, Philadelphia.

99. **Chang, V. and Ingham, J.M.** (2003). Symptom control: a review. *Cancer Investigations* (in press).
100. **Cook, R.J. and Sackett, D.L.** (1995). The number needed to treat: a clinically useful measure of treatment effect. *British Medical Journal* **310**, 452–4.
101. **Zech, D.F.** et al. (1995). Validation of World Health Organization Guidelines for cancer pain relief: a 10-year prospective study. *Pain* **63**, 65–76.
102. **Serlin, R.C.** et al. (1995). When is cancer pain mild, moderate or severe? Grading pain severity by its interference with function. *Pain* **61** (2), 277–84.
103. **Rothenberg, M.L.** et al. (1996). A rationale for expanding the endpoints for clinical trials in advanced pancreatic carcinoma. *Cancer* **78** (3 Suppl.), 627–32.
104. **Rothenberg, M.L.** et al. (1996). A phase II trial of gemcitabine in patients with 5-FU-refractory pancreas cancer (see comments). *Annals of Oncology* **7** (4), 347–53.
105. **Burris, H.A., III** et al. (1997). Improvements in survival and clinical benefit with gemcitabine as first-line therapy for patients with advanced pancreas cancer: a randomized trial. *Journal of Clinical Oncology* **15** (6), 2403–13.
106. Bandolier Library. Palliative and Supportive Care. http://www.jr2.ox.ac.uk/bandolier/booth/booths/pall.html. Last accessed May 9, 2003.
107. **Kukull, W.A., McCorkle, R., and Driever, M.** (1986). Symptom distress, psychosocial variables and survival from lung cancer. *Journal of Psychosocial Oncology* **4**, 91–104.
108. **Stark, R.D., Gambles, S.A., and Lewis, J.A.** (1981). Methods to assess breathlessness in healthy subjects: a critical evaluation and application to analyse the acute effects of diazepam and promethazine on breathlessness induced by exercise or by exposure to raised levels of carbon dioxide. *Clinical Science* **61** (4), 429–39.
109. **Stark, R.D.** (1988). Dyspnoea: assessment and pharmacological manipulation. *European Respiratory Journal* **1** (3), 280–7.
110. **Cockcroft, A., Adams, L., and Guz, A.** (1989). Assessment of breathlessness. *Quarterly Journal of Medicine* **72** (268), 669–76.
111. **McCord, M. and Cronin, S.D.** (1992). Operationalizing dyspnea: focus on measurement. *Heart & Lung* **21** (2), 167–79.
112. **Eakin, E.G., Kaplan, R.M., and Ries, A.L.** (1993). Measurement of dyspnoea in chronic obstructive pulmonary disease. *Quality of Life Research* **2** (3), 181–91.
113. **Mahler, D.A. and Harver, A.** (2000). Do you speak the language of dyspnea? *Chest* **117** (4), 928–9.
114. **Brown, M.L.** et al. (1986). Lung cancer and dyspnea: the patient's perception. *Oncology Nursing Forum* **13** (5), 19–23.
115. **Bruera, E.** et al. (1993). Effects of oxygen on dyspnoea in hypoxaemic terminal-cancer patients. *Lancet* **342** (8862), 13–14.
116. **Roberts, D.K., Thorne, S.E., and Pearson, C.** (1993). The experience of dyspnea in late-stage cancer. Patients' and nurses' perspectives. *Cancer Nursing* **16** (4), 310–20.
117. **Melzack, R.** (1975). The McGill pain questionnaire: major properties and scoring methods. *Pain* **1**, 277–99.
118. **Graham, C.** et al. (1980). Use of the McGill Pain Questionnaire in the assessment of cancer pain: replicability and consistency. *Pain* **8**, 377–87.
119. **Melzack, R.** (1987). The short-form McGill Pain Questionnaire. *Pain* **30**, 191–7.
120. **Fishman, B.** et al. (1987). The Memorial Pain Assessment Card. A valid instrument for the evaluation of cancer pain. *Cancer* **60** (5), 1151–8.
121. **DeConno, F.** et al. (1994). Pain measurement in cancer patients: a comparison of six methods. *Pain* **57**, 161–6.
122. **Folstein, M.F., Folstein, S.E., and McHugh, P.R.** (1975). Mini-mental state. *Journal of Psychiatric Research* **12**, 189–98.
123. **Katzman, R.** et al. (1983). Validation of a short orientation–memory–concentration test of cognitive impairment. *American Journal of Psychiatry* **140** (6), 734–9.
124. **Bruera, E.** et al. (1992). Cognitive failure in patients with terminal cancer: a prospective study. *Journal of Pain and Symptom Management* **7** (4), 192–5.
125. **Fainsinger, R.L., Tapper, M., and Bruera, E.** (1993). A perspective on the management of delirium in terminally ill patients on a palliative care unit. *Journal of Palliative Care* **9** (3), 4–8.
126. **Lipowski, Z.J.** (1987). Delirium (acute confusional states). *Journal of the American Medical Association* **258** (13), 1789–92.
127. **Levkoff, S.E.** et al. (1992). Delirium. The occurrence and persistence of symptoms among elderly hospitalized patients. *Archives of Internal Medicine* **152** (2), 334–40.
128. **Breitbart, W. and Strout, D.** (2000). Delirium in the terminally ill. *Clinics in Geriatric Medicine* **16** (2), 357–72.
129. **Exton-Smith, A.N.** (1961). Terminal illness in the aged. *Lancet* **2**, 305–8.
130. **Witzel, L.** (1975). Behavior of the dying patient. *British Medical Journal* **2**, 81–2.
131. **Massie, M.J., Holland, J., and Glass, E.** (1983). Delirium in terminally ill cancer patients. *American Journal of Psychiatry* **140** (8), 1048–50.
132. **Breitbart, W., Gibson, C., and Tremblay, A.** (2002). The delirium experience: delirium recall and delirium-related distress in hospitalized patients with cancer, their spouses/caregivers, and their nurses. *Psychosomatics* **43** (3), 183–94.
133. **Smith, M.J., Breitbart, W.S., and Platt, M.M.** (1995). A critique of instruments and methods to detect, diagnose, and rate delirium. *Journal of Pain and Symptom Management* **10** (1), 35–77.
134. **American Psychiatric Association**. *Diagnostic and Statistical Manual of Mental Disorders* 4th edn. Washington DC: American Psychiatric Association, 1994.
135. **Inouye, S.K.** et al. (1990). Clarifying confusion: the confusion assessment method. *Annals of Internal Medicine* **113**, 941–8.
136. **Albert, M.S.** et al. (1992). The delirium symptom interview: an interview for the detection of delirium symptoms in hospitalized patients. *Journal of Geriatric Psychiatry and Neurology* **5** (1), 14–21.
137. **Trzepacz, P.T., Baker, R.W., and Greenhouse, J.** (1988). A symptom rating scale for delirium. *Psychiatry Research* **23**, 89–97.
138. **American Psychiatric Association**. *Diagnostic and Statistical Manual of Mental Disorders* 3rd edn. Washington DC: American Psychiatric Association, 1980.
139. **American Psychiatric Association**. *Diagnostic and Statistical Manual of Mental Disorders* 3rd, revised edn. Washington DC: American Psychiatric Association, 1987.
140. **Breitbart, W.** et al. (1997). The Memorial Delirium Assessment Scale (see comments). *Journal of Pain and Symptom Management* **13** (3), 128–37.
141. **Grassi, L.** et al. (2001). Assessing delirium in cancer patients: the Italian versions of the Delirium Rating Scale and the Memorial Delirium Assessment Scale. *Journal of Pain and Symptom Management* **21** (1), 59–68.
142. **Breitbart, W., Tremblay, A., and Gibson, C.** (2002). An open trial of olanzapine for the treatment of delirium in hospitalized cancer patients. *Psychosomatics* **43** (3), 175–82.
143. **Matsuoka, Y.** et al. (2001). Clinical utility and validation of the Japanese version of Memorial Delirium Assessment Scale in a psychogeriatric inpatient setting. *General Hospital Psychiatry* **23** (1), 36–40.
144. **Mancini, I.** et al. (2002). Supportive and palliative care: experience at the Institut Jules Bordet. *Supportive Care in Cancer* **10** (1), 3–7.
145. **Irvine, D.M.** et al. (1991). A critical appraisal of the literature investigating fatigue in the individual with cancer. *Cancer Nursing* **14** (4), 188–99.
146. **Smets, E.M.** et al. (1993). Fatigue in cancer patients. *British Journal of Cancer* **68** (2), 220–4.
147. **Glaus, A.** (1993). Assessment of fatigue in cancer and non-cancer patients and in healthy individuals. *Supportive Care in Cancer* **1**, 305–15.
148. **Winningham, M.L.** et al. (1994). Fatigue and the cancer experience: the state of the knowledge. *Oncology Nursing Forum* **21** (1), 23–34.
149. **Portenoy, R.K.** (2001). Fatigue. In *Interactive Clinical Research Textbook* Chapter 9 (ed. M. Max and J. Lynn), National Institute of Dental and Craniofacial Research. http://www.symptomresearch.com/. Produced by the

US Department of Health and Human Services, National Institute of Dental and Craniofacial Research, Bethesda, MD.

150. **Richardson, A.** (1998). Measuring fatigue in patients with cancer. *Supportive Care in Cancer* **6** (2), 94–100.

151. **Ream, E. and Richardson, A.** (1999). From theory to practice: designing interventions to reduce fatigue in patients with cancer. *Oncology Nursing Forum* **26** (8), 1295–303 (quiz 1304–5).

152. **McNair, D., Lorr, M., and Deoppleman, L.F.** *Profile of Mood States Manual.* San Deigo CA: Educational and Industrial Testing Service, 1971.

153. **Brunier, G. and Graydon, J.** (1996). A comparison of two methods of measuring fatigue in patients on chronic haemodialysis: visual analogue versus Likert scale. *International Journal of Nursing Studies* **33** (3), 338–48.

154. **Cella, D.F.** et al. (1987). A brief POMS measure of distress for cancer patients. *Journal of Chronic Diseases* **40** (10), 939–42.

155. **Aaronson, N.K.** et al. (1993). The European Organization for Research and Treatment of Cancer QLQ-C30: a quality-of-life instrument for use in international clinical trials in oncology. *Journal of the National Cancer Institute* **85** (5), 365–76.

156. **Pearson, P.G. and Byars, G.E.** The Development and Validation of a Check List Measuring Subjective Fatigue. Randolf AFB TX: School of Aviation, USAF, 1956.

157. **Yoshitake, H.** (1971). Relations between the symptoms and feelings of fatigue. *Ergonomics* **14**, 175–96.

158. **Haylock, P.J. and Hart, L.K.** (1979). Fatigue in patients receiving localized radiation. *Cancer Nursing* **2** (12), 461–7.

159. **Kogi, K. and Saito, Y.** (1971). Assessment criteria for mental fatigue. A factor-analytic study of phase discrimination in mental fatigue. *Ergonomics* **14** (1), 119–27.

160. **Kobashi-Schoot, J.A.M.** et al. (1985). Assessment of malaise in cancer patients treated with radiotherapy. *Cancer Nursing* **8** (6), 306–13.

161. **Piper, B.F.** et al. (1989). The development of an instrument to measure the subjective dimension of fatigue. In *Key Aspects of Comfort. Management of Pain, Fatigue and Nausea* (ed. S.G. Funk et al.), pp. 199–208. New York: Springer Publishing Company.

162. **Piper, B.F.** et al. (1998). The revised Piper Fatigue Scale: psychometric evaluation in women with breast cancer. *Oncology Nursing Forum* **25** (4), 677–84.

163. **Lee, K.A., Hicks, G., and Nino-Murcia, G.** (1991). Validity and reliability of a scale to assess fatigue. *Psychiatry Research* **36**, 291–8.

164. **Glaus, A.** (1998). Fatigue in patients with cancer. Analysis and assessment. *Recent Results in Cancer Research* **145**, I–XI, 1–172.

165. **Yellen, S.B.** et al. (1997). Measuring fatigue and other anemia-related symptoms with the Functional Assessment of Cancer Therapy (FACT) measurement system. *Journal of Pain and Symptom Management* **13** (2), 63–74.

166. **Mendoza, T.R.** et al. (1999). The rapid assessment of fatigue severity in cancer patients: use of the Brief Fatigue Inventory. *Cancer* **85** (5), 1186–96.

167. **Okuyama, T.** et al. (2000). Development and validation of the cancer fatigue scale: a brief, three-dimensional, self-rating scale for assessment of fatigue in cancer patients. *Journal of Pain and Symptom Management* **19** (1), 5–14.

168. **Schwartz, A.L.** (1998). The Schwartz Cancer Fatigue Scale: testing reliability and validity. *Oncology Nursing Forum* **25** (4), 711–17.

169. **Smets, E.M.** et al. (1995). The Multidimensional Fatigue Inventory (MFI) psychometric qualities of an instrument to assess fatigue. *Journal of Psychosomatic Research* **39** (3), 315–25.

170. **Bruera, E.** et al. (1987). Methylphenidate associated with narcotics for the treatment of cancer pain. *Cancer Treatment Reports* **71** (1), 67–70.

171. **Bruera, E.** et al. (1989). Use of methylphenidate as an adjuvant to narcotic analgesics in patients with advanced cancer. *Journal of Pain and Symptom Management* **4** (1), 3–6.

172. **Bruera, E.** et al. (1992). The use of methylphenidate in patients with incident cancer pain receiving regular opiates. A preliminary report. *Pain* **50** (1), 75–7.

173. **Bruera, E.** et al. (1992). Neuropsychological effects of methylphenidate in patients receiving a continuous infusion of narcotics for cancer pain. *Pain* **48** (2), 163–6.

174. **Mock, V.** et al. (1997). Effects of exercise on fatigue, physical functioning, and emotional distress during radiation therapy for breast cancer. *Oncology Nursing Forum* **24** (6), 991–1000.

175. **Larson, J.L.** et al. (1996). Reliability and validity of the 12-minute distance walk in patients with chronic obstructive pulmonary disease. *Nursing Research* **45** (4), 203–10.

176. **Dudgeon, D.** (2002). Multidimensional assessment of dyspnea. In *Issues in Palliative Care Research* (ed. R. Portenoy and E. Bruera), pp. 83–96. New York: Oxford University Press.

177. **Janson-Bjerklie, S., Carrieri, V.K., and Hudes, M.** (1985). The sensations of dyspnea. *Nursing Research* **35** (3), 154–9.

178. **Simon, P.M.** et al. (1989). Distinguishable sensations of breathlessness induced in normal volunteers. *American Review of Respiratory Diseases* **140**, 1021–7.

179. **O'Neill, P.A.** et al. (1986). The effect of indomethacin on breathlessness in patients with diffuse parenchymal disease of the lung. *British Journal of Diseases of the Chest* **80** (1), 72–9.

180. **de Torres, J.P.** et al. (2002). Power of outcome measurements to detect clinically significant changes in pulmonary rehabilitation of patients with COPD. *Chest* **121** (4), 1092–8.

181. **Wilson, R.C. and Jones, P.W.** (1989). A comparison of the visual analogue scale and modified Borg scale for the measurement of dyspnea during exercise. *Clinical Science* **76**, 277–82.

182. **Stark, R.D.** et al. (1983). Effects of codeine on the respiratory responses to exercise in healthy subjects. *British Journal of Clinical Pharmacology* **15** (3), 355–9.

183. **Eakin, E.G., Kaplan, R.M., and Ries, A.L.** (1993). Measurement of dyspnea in chronic obstructive pulmonary disease. *Quality of Life Research* **2**, 181–91.

184. **Borg, G.** (1970). Perceived exertion as an indicator of somatic stress. *Scandinavian Journal of Rehabilitation Medicine* **2–3**, 92–8.

185. **Borg, G.** (1982). Psychophysical bases of perceived exertion. *Medicine and Science in Sports and Exercise* **14** (5), 377–81.

186. **Gift, A.G.** (1989). Clinical measurement of dyspnea. *Dimensions of Critical Care Nursing* **8**, 210–16.

187. **Dhand, R., Kalra, S., and Malik, S.K.** (1988). Use of visual analogue scales for assessment of the severity of asthma. *Respiration* **54** (4), 255–62.

188. **Research Council Committee on the Aetiology of Chronic Bronchitis** (1960). Standardized questionnaires on respiratory symptoms. *British Medical Journal* **2**, 1665.

189. **Thoracic Society** (1978). Recommended respiratory disease questionnaires for use with adults and children in epidemiological research. *American Review of Respiratory Diseases* **118**, 7–53.

190. **Mahler, D.** et al. (1984). The measurement of dyspnea: contents, interobserver agreement, and physiologic correlates of two new clinical indexes. *Chest* **85**, 751–8.

191. **Cullen, D.L. and Rodak, B.** (2002). Clinical utility of measures of breathlessness. *Respiratory Care* **47** (9), 986–93.

192. **Mahler, D.A.** (2000). How should health-related quality of life be assessed in patients with COPD? *Chest* **117** (Suppl. 2), 54S–7S.

193. **Deyo, R.A. and Patrick, D.L.** (1989). Barriers to the use of health status measures in clinical investigation, patient care, and policy research. *Medical Care* **27** (Suppl. 3), S254–68.

194. **VonRoenn, J.H.** et al. (1993). Physician attitudes and practice in cancer pain management: a survey from the Eastern Cooperative Oncology Group. *Annals of Internal Medicine* **119**, 121–6.

195. **Donovan, M., Dillon, P., and McGuire, L.** (1987). The incidence and characteristics of pain in a sample of medical–surgical outpatients. *Pain* **30**, 69–87.

196. **Lipowski, Z.J.** *Delirium: Acute Confusional States.* New York: Oxford University Press, 1990.

197. **Lawlor, P.G.** et al. (2000). Occurrence, causes, and outcome of delirium in patients with advanced cancer: a prospective study. *Archives of Internal Medicine* **160** (6), 786–94.

198. **Stark, R.D., Gambles, S.A., and Chatterjee, S.S.** (1982). An exercise test to assess clinical dyspnoea: estimation of reproducibility and sensitivity. *British Journal of Diseases of the Chest* **76** (3), 269–78.

199. **Ganz, P.A.** et al. (1988). Estimating the quality of life in a clincal trial of patients with metastatic lung cancer using the Karnofsky Performance Status and the Functional Living Index-Cancer. *Cancer* **61**, 849.

200. **Selby, P. and Robertson, B.** (1987). Measurement of quality of life in patients with cancer. *Cancer Surveys* **6**, 521–43.

201. **Parmelee, P.A., Smith, B., and Katz, I.R.** (1993). Pain complaints and cognitive status among elderly institution residents. *Journal of the American Geriatric Society* **41** (5), 517–22.

202. **Ferrell, B.A., Ferrell, B.R., and Rivera, L.** (1995). Pain in cognitively impaired nursing home patients. *Journal of Pain and Symptom Management* **10** (8), 591–8.

203. **McCaffery, M. and Pasero, C.**, ed. *Pain Clinical Manual.* Mosby Inc., 2nd edn., 1999.

204. **Sengstaken, E.A. and King, S.A.** (1993). The problems of pain and its detection among geriatric nursing home residents. *Journal of the American Geriatric Society* **41** (5), 541–4.

205. **Baker, A.** et al. (1996). Chronic pain management in cognitively impaired patients: a preliminary research project. *Perspectives* **20** (2), 4–8.

206. **Simons, W. and Malabar, R.** (1995). Assessing pain in elderly patients who cannot respond verbally. *Journal of Advanced Nursing* **22** (4), 663–9.

207. **Kovach, C.R.** et al. (2002). The assessment of discomfort in dementia protocol. *Pain Management Nursing* **3** (1), 16–27.

208. **McCarthy, M.** (1990). Hospice patients: a pilot study in 12 services. *Palliative Medicine* **4**, 93–104.

209. **Cleeland, C.S.** et al. (1994). Pain and its treatment in outpatients with metastatic cancer. *New England Journal of Medicine* **330**, 592–6.

210. **Cunningham, W.E.** et al. (1995). Comparison of health-related quality of life in clinical trial and nonclinical trial human immunodeficiency virus-infected cohorts. *Medical Care* **33** (4), AS15–25.

211. **Townsend, J.** et al. (1990). Terminal cancer care and patients' preference for place of death: a prospective study. *British Medical Journal* **301** (6749), 415–17.

212. **Karoly, P.** (1991). Assessment of pediatric pain. In *Children in Pain: Clinical and Research Issues from a Developmental Perspective* (ed. J.P. Bush and S.W. Harkins), pp. 59–82. New York: Springer-Verlag.

213. **Manne, S.L. and Andersen, B.L.** (1991). Pain and pain-related distress in children with cancer. In *Children in Pain: Clinical and Research Issues from a Developmental Perspective* (ed. J.P. Bush and S.W. Harkins), pp. 337–72. New York: Springer-Verlag.

214. **Matthews, J.R., McGrath, P.J., and Pigeon, H.** (1993). Assessment and measurement of pain in children. In *Pain in Infants, Children and Adolescents* (ed. N.L. Schechter, C.B. Berde, and M. Yaster). Baltimore MD: Williams and Wilkins.

215. **Gaffney, A., McGrath, F., and Dick, B.** (2003). Measuring pain in children: Developmental and instrument issues. In *Pain in Infants, Children and Adolescents* (ed. N.L. Schechter, C.B. Berde, and M. Yaster), pp. 128–41. Philadelphia: Lippincott Williams and Wilkins.

216. **Jay, S.** et al. (1987). Cognitive–behavioral and pharmacologic interventions for childrens' distress during painful medical procedures. *Journal of Consulting and Clinical Psychology* **55**, 860–5.

217. **Katz, E., Kellerman, J., and Ellenberg, L.** (1987). Hypnosis in the reduction of acute pain and distress in children with cancer. *Journal of Pediatric Psychology* **12**, 379–94.

218. **LeBaron, S. and Zeltzer, L.K.** (1984). Assessment of pain and anxiety in children and adolescents by self-reports, and a behavior checklist. *Journal of Consulting and Clinical Psychology* **52** (5), 729–38.

219. **Kuttner, L., Bowman, M., and Teasdale, M.** (1988). Psychological treatment of distress, pain and anxiety for children with cancer. *Developmental and Behavioral Pediatrics* **9**, 374–81.

220. **Manne, S.** et al. (1990). Behavioral intervention to reduce child and parent distress during venipuncture. *Journal of Consulting and Clinical Psychology* **58**, 565–72.

221. **Jay, S. and Elliott, C.** (1984). Behavioral observation scales for measuring childrens' distress: the effects of increased methodological rigor. *Journal of Consulting and Clinical Psychology* **52**, 1106–7.

222. **Elliott, C., Jay, S., and Woody, P.** (1987). An observational scale for measuring childrens' distress during medical procedures. *Journal of Pediatric Psychology* **12**, 543–51.

223. **Gauvain-Piquard, A.** et al. (1987). Pain in children aged 2–6 years: a new observational rating scale elaborated in a pediatric oncology unit—a preliminary report. *Pain* **31**, 177–88.

224. **Zeltzer, L.K.** et al. (1988). Can children understand and use a rating scale to quantify somatic symptoms? Assessment of nausea and vomiting as a model. *Journal of Consulting and Clinical Psychology* **56** (5), 567–72.

225. **Tye, V.L.** et al. (1993). Chemotherapy induced nausea and emesis in pediatric cancer patients: external validity of child and parent emesis ratings. *Developmental and Behavioral Pediatrics* **14** (4), 236–41.

226. **Seeman, I.** (1992). National Mortality Followback Survey: 1986 Summary, United States National Center for Health Statistics. *Vital and Health Statistics* **20** (19).

227. **Saunders, C.** (1984). Pain and impending death. In *Textbook of Pain* (ed. P. Wall and R. Melzack), pp. 472–8. New York: Churchill Livingstone.

228. **Hinton, J.M.** (1963). The physical and mental distress of the dying. *Quarterly Journal of Medicine* **32** (125), 1–21.

229. **Ingham, J.M.** et al. (1994). Pain and distress in cancer patients during the dying process. American Pain Society Abstracts, No. 94623, November.

230. **Waxler-Morrison, N., Anderson, J.M., and Richardson, E.**, ed. *Cross Cultural Caring: A Handbook for Health Professionals in Western Canada.* University of BC Press, 1990.

231. **Cleeland, C.S. and Ryan, K.M.** (1994). Pain assessment: global use of the Brief Pain Inventory. *Annals of the Academy of Medicine Singapore* **23** (2), 129–38.

232. **Cleeland, C.S.** et al. (1988). Multidimensional measurement of cancer pain: comparisons of US and Vietnamese patients. *Journal of Pain and Symptom Management* **3** (1), 23–7.

6.2 Clinical and organizational audit in palliative medicine

Irene J. Higginson

Quality of care: a worldwide concern?

Throughout the world there is a growing emphasis on ensuring quality and value for money in health care. Higher public expectations and the move towards quality service in many public and private companies have all heightened the desire to introduce quality assurance, audit, and evaluation into clinical care.[1,2] In response, clinicians, managers, and governments have sought to standardize clinical practice to that which is the 'best' possible practice, or which is proven to be the most effective and efficient.[1] Although many terms in the quality dictionary are new, many of the ideas, such as clinical review, are not. The history of quality assessment and audit can be traced back as far as 1700 BC in Egypt when King Hammurabi, introduced penalties, sometimes quite drastic, for different degrees of what was deemed as 'surgical incompetence' (although it is not clear who judged this incompetence). In 1518, the Charter of the Royal College of Physicians included: 'to uphold the standards of medicine both for their own honour and public benefit'. The General Nursing Council (GNC) was established in

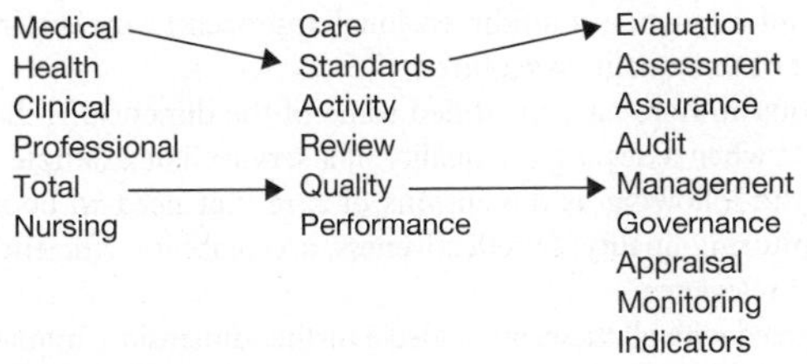

Fig. 1 Different approaches. Audit by any other name: combine terms from the table below.

1919 to 'monitor nurses' practice and conduct'. Florence Nightingale was one of the first clinicians to insist on measuring the outcome of care for her patients, to evaluate treatment.[3] Grand rounds, postgraduate lectures, and clinical presentations already contributed to the review of medical and nursing performance. However, the new emphasis on audit and quality improvement and governance has brought four main differences:

- explicit criteria for good practice should be applied by all clinicians rather than those in exemplary centres;
- all patients in care and all centres should be included in quality monitoring rather than a few 'interesting' cases;
- patients and families will have information about care to empower them to seek the best care;
- funding or accreditation may be withheld from those units which do not comply with quality standards or which are found to be ineffective or inefficient.[4]

References in the medical and nursing literature to quality assurance and clinical audit began in the late 1970s. They continue to increase in number, although the terms have changes over time (see Fig. 1), and most recently terms such as continuous quality improvement, and clinical governance have begun to emerge.

Why assess quality or audit palliative care: benefits and costs?

Palliative care arose out of a desire to improve the quality of care for patients with advancing disease and their families. This was based on evidence that care for people with progressive illness, and at death, was poor.[5,6] The newness of the field coupled with scepticism or reluctance to support this form of care often resulted in many of the early evaluations of palliative services which compared hospice, home, and hospital care.[7–14] Therefore, palliative care often led the way in developing ways to examine the quality of care and sought to influence those working in oncology and other professions.[15] However, there was no cause for complacency. These evaluations were limited to a few exemplary centres.[15]

Since then, palliative care has grown rapidly such that there are services in over 90 countries of the world. With this growth have emerged, many different tools and measures of the quality of palliative care and for audit, and their use is becoming more common.[16–18] Further, there is now evidence demonstrating the effectiveness of palliative care and hospice services, based on empirical studies in different sites and systematic literature reviews.[19,20] But one major criticism of the evidence reviews is the lack of comparison of different models of care.[21–23] Practice still varies from one country to another, from one part of a country to another, and from one service to another, even in simple aspects such as staffing levels and mix within a hospice or home care team, the catchment populations, the operational policies, and the throughput.[24,25] Even today, we need to know which models of care work best and for which types of problems palliative care is most effective. Those providing and those who resource palliative care services need to know which interventions and in what combination work best, for what kinds of patients and families, and in which type of localities. Research is important in discovering some of these aspects, but equally audit or quality assessment, is important to identify what works best, for whom and when.

Hospices and palliative care services bring new therapies, such as new treatments for symptoms, support and counselling services, or complementary therapies. However, new therapies and approaches must be evaluated and audited, to determine if and for whom these are useful. Otherwise hospices' resources and the patient's time will be wasted. There is a great danger in concentrating on only current concerns without reviewing previous failings and using those findings to plan improved care in the future.

Antipathy to quality assessment and audit is based on various arguments such as:

- There is no problem since palliative care is of a high quality (I once heard of a chief executive of a hospice who said that there was no need to measure the quality of care, because she 'knew that their care was good').
- Palliative care is self-auditing, because staff spend time with patients and families.
- The outcomes of palliative care cannot be measured—they are too complicated or intangible.
- Measuring more simple outcomes of palliative care, such as pain or symptom control, is not enough and until we can measure everything audit should not be attempted.
- Resources, information, and time are not available.
- Audit looks back at practice which has gone, not the problems which lie ahead.

None of these arguments can be supported by evidence. Numerous audits and quality assessments of palliative care have helped to improve care. Audit has had major impact in the development of hospice and palliative care in much of Europe, Canada, and Australia. The results have been used in the following ways:[2,16,17,26–37]

- In assisting the development of local and regional palliative care programmes.
- In providing outcomes information that has allowed the programme leaders to argue for increased funding.
- In demonstrating the effectiveness of different interventions and allowed for an increase in patient referrals.
- In reviewing the quality of care and identifying ways to improve it for patients and families in the future.
- In identifying components where care is less effective, allowing services to be better targeted and identifying patients who should be referred earlier in the future.
- Systematic assessments of patients and families have helped to ensure that:
  - aspects of care were not overlooked;
  - communication between patients and families and professionals and also within the team improved;
  - there is a more holistic approach to care; and
  - new staff were better integrated, giving them a clear understanding of what to assess.
- In helping to establish referral criteria and develop ways to predict those patients and families who may run in to more difficulties and thereby should be referred earlier.

Audit is important for education and training, because the structured review allows analysis, comparison, and evaluation of individual performance; it promotes adherence to local clinical policies and offers opportunity for publication of results. Educational programmes can be constructed to meet the demonstrated needs of individuals or groups.

Increasingly, audit, clinical governance, or quality review are required for the recognition of training posts and for the revalidation of doctors. Royal

Colleges and Faculties increasingly seek evidence of formally organized review and could withdraw recognition from departments that do not provide this.

Audit is important for those who resource palliative care, such as commissioners, primary care trusts, health care insurance agencies, because it provides tangible evidence that the service is seeking the most effective use of existing clinical resources and aims to improve the quality of care. This is increasingly important when competing for health care contracts.[38] Requirements for audit and the implementation of research findings may well be included in such contracts.[2]

Some examples of the costs of *not* auditing are as important as the benefits of auditing.[2,16] These include:

- Extra inappropriate treatment, which wastes the patients' and families' time and resources on such treatment, as well as wasting staff time and resources. Such resources could be used elsewhere where they may be more effective.
- Uncontrolled symptoms may cause admission to hospice or hospital, or delay discharge. Most significantly this causes suffering to the patient, family, and staff.
- There may be extra inappropriate services, for example, unnecessary outpatient attendance.

However, quality assessment and audit takes time and resources. These should not be underestimated. Indeed it may be impossible to undertake audit if a service is struggling, with insufficient numbers of staff to give even basic care such as washing and administering drugs. Perhaps the audit here is to show simply that the service cannot even measure and assess a patient's needs properly. Indeed, simple assessments, such as whether follow-up occurs, can be useful in assessing practice.[39] The resources needed for audit and quality assessment can include:

- Time from all staff to prepare for audit, to agree the standards or topic, and to review the findings.
- Time from some staff to carry out the audit and to analyse its results and document the findings and any recommendations.
- Commitment from *all* staff, managers, nurses, doctors, etc. to consider the results and act upon them.
- Resources to pay for the staff time involved, plus any other analytical or computing support needed.

The costs of audit mean that it is important to ensure that the audit itself is as effective as possible. What is the purpose of collected audit data if the changes are not acted on? Mechanisms to review the audit and to ensure it is effective are discussed in a later section.

Computers are not necessary for audit. They can help if they are used to streamline the information collected and if they include ready prepared programmes to make the analysis easy. A number of computer programs have been specifically designed for recording clinical data for palliative care and other services. The audit measures can be included within these programs, and increasingly application in clinical practice is aided by staff using hand-held computers, or even patients completing information.[17] However, if the audit is small or in its early stages, too rigid use of computers by inexperienced staff can be a hindrance, because the need to update the computer delays the evolution of the audit.

What do we mean by quality?

Quality, as defined in many dictionaries, pertains to 'degree of excellence' or 'general excellence'. But what constitutes excellence in the context of a service, who defines it, and what components should be addressed. For example, should 'excellence' be limited to clinical skills, or should it encompass broader aspects, such as whether the service reaches all those in need? Surely, when measuring quality of a service all the features and characteristics that bear on its ability to satisfy the stated or implied needs of the users of that service should be assessed. Quality in health care is a multidimensional concept, and as such, a multidimensional approach to measurement and assessment of that quality is required.[40]

Numerous authors have identified some of the dimensions that should be included when assessing the quality of a service. For example, Maxwell identifies the following as dimensions of care that need to be measured when monitoring quality:[41] effectiveness, acceptability, efficiency, access, equity, and relevance.

Black agreed with all these, but added a further dimension: humanity,[42] a dimension which would be particularly important for palliative care services.

So how do we determine whether we are offering a good quality service if we have to consider all these dimensions? One method of assessing and ensuring service quality, is to conduct a programme of review and improvement of the service, and this process is what clinical audit, quality assurance and improvement is concerned with.

How do we assess the quality of palliative care?

Donabedian[40] and others[16] have translated the assessment of the quality of health care into:

1. *Structure/or inputs:* resources in terms of manpower, equipment, and money.
2. *Process:* how the resources are used (such as domiciliary visits, beds, clinics, drugs, or treatments given).
3. *Output:* productivity or throughput (such as rates of clinic attendance or discharge, inpatient throughput—the number of patients admitted over a given period of time).
4. *Outcome:* change in health status or quality of life that can be attributed to health care.

This model is built on manufacturing industry and, despite limitations discussed below, it has value, in that it defines the steps in which health and social care are delivered.

Structural aspects influence the process of care so that its quality can be either diminished or enhanced. Similarly changes in the process of care, including variations in its quality, will influence the output, and in turn the effect of care on health status and outcomes. Thus, there is a functional relationship between these in that:

structure →process → output → outcome.[16,40]

Structure is easiest to measure because its elements are the most stable and identifiable. However, it is an indirect measure of the quality of care and its value depends on the nature of its influence on care. Structure is relevant to quality in that it increases or decreases the probability of a good performance. Process and output are closer to changes in the health status of individuals. Their advantage is that they measure the most immediately discernible attributes of care activities. However, they are only valuable as a measure once the elements of process are known to have a clear relationship with the desired changes in health status.[50] Outcome reflects the true change in health status, and thus is the most relevant for patients and society. However, it is difficult to eliminate other causes for change, such as prior care or external events. A useful approach is to focus on the difference between the desired outcome and the actual outcome. Services can then identify whether or not their goals are being achieved and investigate any failings.

Organizational audits usually assess the structure and process of care, whereas clinical audits often measure the process and outcome of care. Although structure is easiest to measure it is furthest from influencing change in the patient and family. Outcome is most difficult to measure but is of direct relevance to the patient and family. Standards of structure or process are most useful when these are of proven effectiveness, or if there is an overwhelming consensus that these are desirable. Structure, process, and outcome measures which have been either used or advocated to assess palliative care are shown in Table 1.

Table 1 Aspects of care that could be measured to assess structure, process, output, or outcome in palliative care

Type of measure	Examples
Structure	Values or aims of the service
	Financial resources
	Home care/hospital/hospice services
	Day hospice places
	Number of staff or services per cancer patient in the population
	Staffing mix, grades
	Number of staff per patient
	Drugs and equipment available
	Building design
	Physical environment—for example, safety, pleasantness of surroundings
Process	Number of visits
	Number of admissions
	Procedures followed
	Documentation
	Time taken in a visit
	Policies and procedures for staff training and working
	Mechanism for handling complaints and the documentation of this
	Adherence to ethical and legal codes
	Staff support given
Output	Rate of discharge
	Number of completed consultant episodes
	Throughput
	Rate of equipment given out
	Drugs given
	Well coordinated care—telephone communication etc.
	Supply of medicines after discharge
	Completed patient management plans
	Early arrival of discharge information to GP
	Satisfaction of professionals referring to the service
Outcome	Reduction in distressing symptoms
	Improved mental health of patient and carer
	Patient and carer satisfaction
	Satisfied with place of care
	Open and honest communication as the patient wishes
	Resolved communication, fears, grief, anger
	Resolved need to plan future events—for example, funeral or meetings
	Good use of remaining time
	Any spiritual problems resolved or fulfilment
	Reduced carer strain
	Improved carer health
	Resolved grief after death (if appropriate)

More recently, Stewart et al.,[43] have extended the model, sub-dividing the 'structure' elements into: (i) personal and social environment of the patient and family; and (ii) the structural aspects of care, such as resources, staffing, buildings, etc. They also sub-divided the outcomes into: (a) satisfaction; and (b) quality and length of life. These sub-divisions are consistent with the earlier model of Donabedian,[40] and those proposed for palliative care audit in the United Kingdom.[16] However, Stewart et al.'s differentiation of the personal and social environment is a useful demonstration of how audit results may be different because of different settings, or with a different 'case-mix' where patients and families have differing conditions or problems.

A rose by any other name would smell as sweet: the evolving terms—audit, quality improvement, governance?

Over the last 20 years it has been interesting to observe how different terms have come in and out of vogue to describe the evolving approaches to assessing and ensuring the quality of health care. There are also differences between countries. Somewhat disappointingly, the literature in one country tends to ignore audit and quality improvement initiatives in another, thereby reducing the chance to learn. In the United Kingdom and many other European countries, clinical audit (as opposed to financial audit, concerned only with financial matters), became the initial term of choice. Later, this was accompanied by quality assurance (which tended to include a programme of several audits, all working together). Such a programme was similar to the development of total (or continuous) quality improvement in the United States and many other countries, which incorporated a cycle called Plan, Do, Study, Act.[2,43]

There are various terms. Indeed, combining the one term from each of column 1, 2 and in some instances 3, in Fig. 1, will provide examples of the terms available. In that way we can form the terms clinical audit, clinical governance, total quality assessment, and so on. Some of the widely accepted definitions are shown in Table 2.

Common/basic concepts, which are essential, and common to all types of audit or quality review, are:

- that assessment is systematic;
- that there is a cycle where care is monitored, the results reviewed and there is a change to improve practice;
- standards of care are set, either locally or nationally;
- that the cycle is then repeated;

Figure 2 shows one cycle; most approaches are consistent with this. For the remaining part of the chapter, for simplicity, the word audit will be used, to incorporate the different approaches. Through the cycle, audit aims to improve care for patients and families by assessing whether we are doing the right thing well. Therefore, we have to: first, know what we are trying to achieve, second, have a way of observing practice to assess whether we achieve the goals or standards and third, change practice to improve care. Standards for the delivery of care are agreed. Then practice is observed and compared with the standards. This often demonstrates successes, but also failings and need for change. The results are then fed back and examined, so that new or modified standards can be set. The audit cycle is then repeated anew. The cycle can be entered at any point—for example, it is possible to begin by observing practice and acting on the results, and then proceed to setting standards.

Some common distinctions

Clinical audit

Clinical audit is the systematic critical analysis of the quality of clinical care including the procedures used for diagnosis and treatment, the use of resources and the resulting outcome and quality of life for the patient.[16]

Early forms of audit involved only single professions—for example, medical or nursing audit (Table 2). However, it is now widely accepted that audit in palliative care should be multiprofessional, to reflect the multiprofessional nature of care. Clinical audit is like medical and nursing audit but involves all professionals and volunteers, rather than only doctors or nurses.

The audit can be prospective, where the standards and measures are agreed at the start and are recorded on patients and families during their care, or retrospective, which looks back at the care of patients using either the clinical notes and extracting the information or by asking families.

Organizational audit

The Kings Fund Centre in London originally described organizational audit as the developmental and voluntary stage towards accreditation.[44]

Table 2 Common definitions: audit and quality assurance

Term	Definition
Medical audit	The systematic critical analysis of the quality of medical care including the procedures used for diagnosis and treatment, the use of resources, and the resulting outcome and quality of life of the patient[5]
Clinical audit	The systematic critical analysis of the quality of clinical care including the procedures used for diagnosis and treatment, the use of resources, and the resulting outcome and quality of life of the patient Clinical audit is like medical audit but involves all professionals and volunteers rather than only doctors
Nursing audit	The methods by nurses compare their actual practice against pre-agreed guidelines and identify areas for improving their care
Prospective audit	The standards and measures are recorded on patients and their families during their care
Retrospective audit	This looks back at the care of patients who have been discharged or have died, and the standards are applied to the information available from case notes or by asking families about the care after the patient has died
Quality assurance	The definition of standards, the measurement of their achievement and the mechanisms to improve performance The quality assurance cycle is as for medical audit or clinical audit. However, quality assurance implies a planned programme involving the whole unit or health services. Clinical or medical audit is usually described as one part of a quality assurance programme

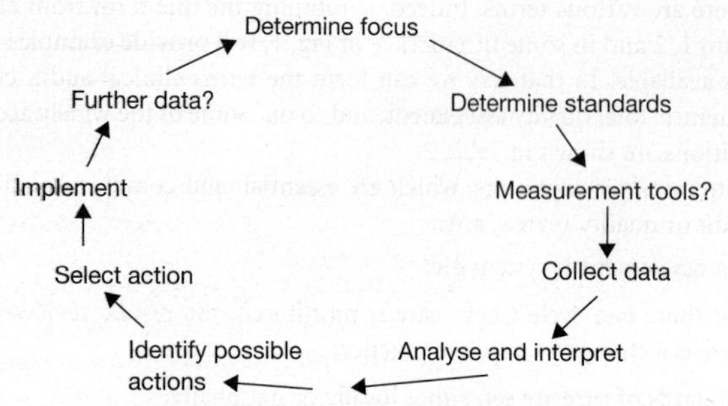

Fig. 2 Cycles of quality assurance, performance measurement, and audit.

Accreditation schemes exist in many countries and usually operate nationally. For example, Royal Colleges inspect training posts and agree where doctors can be trained. In the United Kingdom, there are two main country-wide systems of organization audit. The King's Fund Centre, London, developed a project initially called 'Accreditation UK' and later called 'Organizational Audit',[44] which worked voluntarily with NHS and private hospitals to agree a lengthy document of standards. The programme reviews acute general hospitals against published standards, and more recently extended its work to primary care. Following from this a palliative care organizational audit was developed. Various regions have developed their own organizational audits, for example, the Yorkshire Peer Review system or audits in the North West of the United Kingdom.[45]

These organizational standards were developed because of evidence of organizational variation, which limits the quality of care. These included administrative delays, uncoordinated care, poor environment or sign-posting, poor staff training, etc. Organizational standards need to be straight forward enough to be monitored by an external surveyor.

Organizational audit and accreditation are usually developed in three stages:

1. Developing organizational standards of the systems and process of care.
2. Implementation of the standards by the hospices, hospitals, or units included.
3. Evaluation of compliance with the standards, usually by external surveyors or auditors, sometimes called peer review.

The first stage, developing standards, can often be quite lengthy, because the standards need to be agreed and written in clear, non-ambiguous language, and then tested to determine if the standards can distinguish between good and sub-optimal practice. If the standards are able to detect only the poorest practice, then they could have the effect of reducing standards to just above this level, because units will not need to strive higher. Units with higher standards, which are not recognized as having higher standards, may appear to have higher costs for the same level of practice as units with just acceptable standards.

Quality assurance and total quality management programmes

Although there are various definitions for quality assurance, a widely accepted one is the 'definition of standards, the measurement of their achievement, and the mechanisms to improve performance'. Thus, the cycle is as clinical audit. Clinical audit lies within the frame of quality assurance: clinical audit being the review of the quality of local clinical practice on a regular basis, for example through internal 'peer review' by practising clinicians.

Total quality management is a term which has recently entered the jargon in quality in health care and its definition is included for completeness. It has been defined as a strategy to get an organization working to its maximum effectiveness and efficiency. It has been facilitated by closer working relationships been clinicians and managers[1] and builds on the other definitions, but switches the focus from quality practised within professionals to quality within the whole organization. Thus, clinical audit would lie within a total quality management programme. It also introduces the concept of managing the quality process, such as cataloguing reports of local quality initiatives[1] and using managers to ensure that improvements in quality occur.

Clinical governance

Clinical governance is a framework to ensure that all NHS organizations have proper processes for monitoring and improving clinical quality (and care). It aims to safeguard high standards of care and create a working environment where excellence can flourish. It examines what doctors, nurses, and other professionals do, seeking to support and value staff. This, in addition to clinical audit, and quality initiatives across the organization, focuses attention also on training, continued professional development and competency to practice of staff. It seeks to ensure and develop the practice of all clinicians. Clinical governance is of greater concern in modern medicine than ever in the past because of the rapid pace of developments in clinical practice, available diagnostic investigations and treatments, especially those with potentially dangerous effects if not carried out properly. Many health care services are already required to establish clinical governance, and in the future in many countries doctors will have to have been reviewed through such programmes to be re-validated to practice.[4,5]

Who carries out audit and what is measured?

The different approaches to audit and the assessment of quality can be categorized according to two axes: first, who carries out the audit—the local clinicians, managers, or external organization; and second, whether the audit considered the care of an individual or a few patients, or the whole organization or population. Common forms of audit according to these two axes—internal versus external and individual versus organization/population—are shown in Fig. 3. The type of appropriate audit is determined by the setting. It is extremely difficult for those resourcing services or for external bodies to assess the clinical quality of care. Instead, they are more likely to rely on organizational or environmental standards or, when

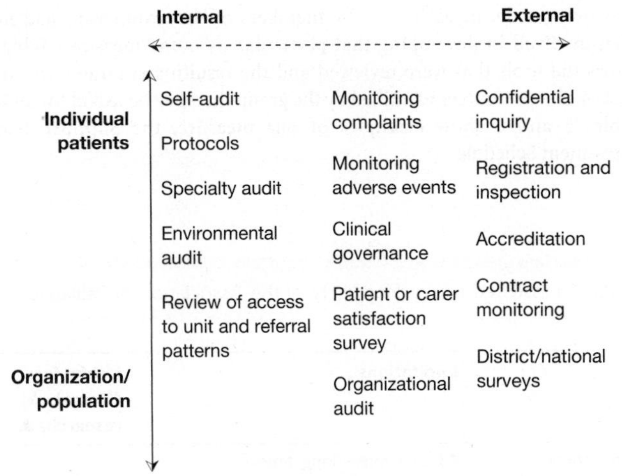

Fig. 3 Range of activities possible within audit.

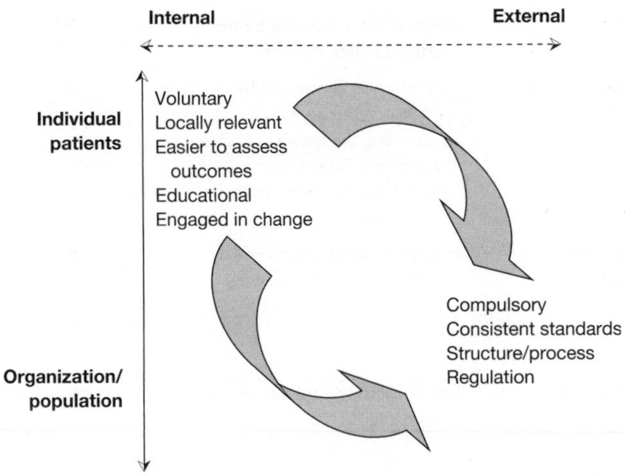

Fig. 4 Effect of activities within audit.

determining whether the professionals are employing proven high quality treatments, examine staff-mix and whether a clinical audit programme is in place. Thus those audits that are more orientated towards internal and individual assessment are more likely to be educational and voluntary. Those audits concerned with organizational aspects and undertaken by external experts or by inspection are more likely to be mandatory and funding or accreditation may depend on their outcome (see Fig. 4).

Applying audit to palliative care

The next section reviews the steps in audit, when it is applied to palliative care.

Know what we are trying to achieve: goals or standards

The definitions of palliative care and palliative medicine (see Chapter 20 of the textbook) provide good guidance on the goals of palliative care, which might be measured in audit. These include aspects of pain and symptom control, improving the quality of life for the patient, relieving fears and anxiety, and caring for the family members or carers. Therefore, in analysing the goals or standards of care, many have audited their effectiveness in controlling symptoms, such as pain or dyspnoea, their effect on a patient's quality of life or psychological well-being, or the patient's or family members' satisfaction with care, or has suggested indicators of these aspects.[2,28,31–33,35,46–58]

There are other aspects which might be included. Various work has examined the features of 'a good or appropriate' death,[59] building on Weisman's definition of 'appropriate death' as 'an absence of suffering, preservation of important relationships, an interval for anticipatory grief, relief of remaining conflicts, belief in timeliness, exercise of feasible option in activities, and consistency with physical limitations, all within the scope of one's ego ideal'.[60] Kellehear described the features of a modern 'good death' as 'awareness of dying, social adjustments and personal preparations, public preparations (legal, financial, religious, funeral, medical), work or activities reduced, and farewells'.[61] Singer et al. identified five domains of quality end-of-life care: receiving adequate pain and symptom management, avoiding inappropriate prolongation of dying, achieving a sense of control, relieving burden, and strengthening relationships with loved ones.[62] Payne also assessed different perspectives.[63] These definitions might suggest audit of aspects of patient and family awareness of the illness or their planning of personal and public preparations, and such aspects have been included in some measures, such as the Support Team Assessment Schedule.[64]

In many countries, the role of palliative care in supporting, advising, and educating other professions is stressed[19,20] (see also other chapters). Family practitioners have identified educational needs for symptom control and patient and family support.[65–73] Therefore, another form of audit could examine the educational and supportive role of palliative care services.

Poor communication is a frequent cause of stress for patients and families.[74–80] Doctors and nurses need to communicate well with patients and their families rather than withdrawing or appearing hurried or abrupt in their manner. Communication is needed between professional staff caring for the patient and family member, to ensure liaison and to prevent duplication or delay. These aspects are also goals suitable for audit.

Total pain has been described as including physical, emotional, social, and spiritual components. Although the earlier discussions have covered the emotional and physical aspects of palliative care, it is also important to consider audit of the spiritual and social aspects. Spiritual audit might consider whether patients are able to raise aspects of spiritual concern to them and find a mechanism to relieve problems or whether patients are in any form of spiritual crisis. Social aspects might include whether the patient and family have sufficient practical and financial support to remain at home.

There are also simple goals, such as preferred place of death, or meeting other patient or family preferences, or access of certain patient groups (such as those from ethnic minorities, or non-cancer conditions)[81] that might be suitable for audit. One problem with this though, is that these goals may not reflect the wishes of all patients. For example, although around 70 per cent of patients would prefer to die at home, increasingly patients choose hospice as a second choice, wishes are very individual, are little understood in some sections of society and are altered by experience.[82] Thus this indicator, like other process indicators, needs to be reviewed cautiously.

How can these goals be turned into standards? Any goal or standard which is set must be measurable, sufficiently challenging but achievable. It would be unrealistic to set a goal or standard that all patients would be free from pain, but it would be reasonable to set a goal of what proportion of patients' pains might be controlled and in what circumstances pain might be uncontrolled. A baseline could be established from current practice. Standards of action when pain is uncontrolled could be audited.

Have a way of assessing and re-assessing the quality of care

For all of the above aspects, measurement tools or indicators are needed. There are now a number of these available in palliative care, which have been validated to different degrees. The Association for Palliative Medicine of the United Kingdom established a working party to review these and subsequently published a WHICH TOOL GUIDE.[83] The group carried out a MEDLINE search to identify potential measures and to check whether they had been used in more than one centre. Then the group provided a preliminary guide as to whether they would recommend the tools in research or clinical audit of palliative care. In order to avoid conflicts of interest, the decision on awarding a research 'triangle' or clinical 'star' was made, in each case, by members of the group who had not been involved in developing that particular outcome measure. Table 3 shows the tools that were reviewed and the resulting commentary, and Table 4 other resources identified by the group that may be useful for audit. Tables 5 and 6 show examples of one measure, the Support Team Assessment Schedule.

Table 3 Review of measures and indicators that could potentially be used in audit. As assessed by working party of the Association of Palliative Medicine, UK[a]

Measure, scale, or tool	Used in ...	Strengths	Limitations	Useful for: Clinical, ☆; research, ▲
An initial assessment of suffering[89]	Acute hospitals, advanced cancer	Can be used either by patient or a trained nurse interview	43 questions—long, time to complete not known	
Cambridge Palliative Audit Schedule[90] CAMPAS	Developed from STAS for use in primary care to assess palliative care	Developed for primary care team members, useful for recording assessments and monitoring care	Not very widely tested or validated	
Edmonton Functional Assessment Tool[91]	Inpatients in palliative care units	Simple to use—10 items, mainly function	Function alone may not be the patient's chief concern	☆
Edmonton Symptom Assessment Scale[92]	Inpatient setting	Quick and can be used either by patient or with nurse assistance	Potential bias introduced by change in the person recording the answers as care continues. Patient may have concerns other than symptoms	☆
European Organisation for Research into Treatment of Cancer (EORTC)-QLQ C30[93,94]	Developed for chemotherapeutic cancer trials—lung cancer patients; work of palliative module underway	Reliable and valid in research settings, broad ranging	Functional questions may cause distress if asked repeatedly	▲
Functional Assessment of Cancer Therapies[95,96] (FACT)	General cancer settings in US, especially research studies—has a palliative module	Major validation programme	Use in palliative care not yet widely reported	▲
Hebrew Rehabilitation Centre for Aged, Quality of Life Index[97] (HRCA-QL)	Adapted from the Spitzer Quality of Life Index, used in the National Hospice Study, in inpatient, home care, and conventional care—inelderly populations	Short and quick	Has not been re-validated and lacks responsiveness in advanced disease, completed by professionals	
Linear pain or comfort rating scales	Forms basis of many assessment tools—for example, post-surgical pain management evaluation	A patient-centred approach, simple, relatively quick	Pain relief alone may not be patient's chief concern. Need to look more widely, in some visual analogue scales are hard to use	☆▲
McGill Quality of Life Questionnaire[98–100]	Advanced cancer and HIV patients at home or inpatient palliative care unit	Includes an existential domain, as well as symptoms and psychological issues	Has not been widely tested in UK settings	▲
Magnet—single outcome that pulls together all related individual outcomes[83]	Of whole palliative care service	Easy to understand and adapt locally, simple, and relatively easy to use	Not validated or tested widely, depends upon what outcome is chosen as the magnet	
Measure your own medical outcome profile[101] (MYMOP)	Used for rating effect of complementary therapies and in chronic bronchitis	Allows patient to identify the symptoms of greatest importance to them and monitor impact of care/intervention on these	Patients need to be guided in its use	
Palliative Care Assessment[102] (PACA)	Hospital palliative care team and outpatient	Short and relatively simple to use	Professional completion	☆

Table 3 Continued

Measure, scale, or tool	**Used in ...**	**Strengths**	**Limitations**	**Useful for: Clinical, ☆; research, ▲**
Palliative Care Core Standards[103] (PCCS)	Inpatient hospice	Comprehensive tool, covering structure, process, education and training	Lengthy—expected to take 10 min to complete	
Palliative Care Outcome Scale[104–106] (POS)	Used in inpatient hospice, day care, hospital support team, home care, and primary care	Simple and short—has patient completion and staff completion component; tested for validity and reliability, has items for individual patient generation	May not be sufficiently detailed; some aspects require further testing	☆▲
Proportion who die at home[107,108]	Used by health authorities to monitor overall care	Quick and easy to measure and aggregate. Easy to make comparisons	Home death may not have been patient choice. May be distorted by lack of appropriate inpatient provision	
Proportion who die in their place of choice	Used by some palliative home care and primary care teams	Reflects patient choice and individual wishes	Difficult to get information in some circumstances, choice may change over time	
Proportion of final weeks spent at home	A proxy measure that can give some indication of the availability of community support services	Quick and easy to measure and aggregate. Clear operational definitions allow valid comparisons between districts	May be distorted by lack of appropriate inpatient provision	
Rotterdam Symptom Checklist[109]	Use in inpatient palliative care setting	Short; validity tested in cancer trials	Reports of use in palliative care mixed	▲
Spitzer Quality of Life Index[110]	Used as basis for comparison with McGill Quality of Life Scale	Short and quick	Has not been validated in palliative care and lacks responsiveness in advanced disease, completed by professionals	
Support Team Assessment Schedule[47,64,111,112] (STAS)	Used by community palliative care teams, hospital teams, day care, inpatient units, and hospital at home services	A wide-ranging checklist looking at clinical and communication issues; available in other languages and has been modified with additional specific items	Teams need to actively use this questioning each section, not just ticking boxes; professional completion	☆▲
Symptom Distress Scale[113]	Life-threatening cancer and heart disease	Some validation; looks at symptoms and mood in relation to quality of life	Patient completion in presence of interviewer	
Schedule for the Evaluation of Individual Quality of Life[114] (SEIQoL)	Inpatient palliative care	Patient centred, the patient identifies the important areas	Can be complex and time consuming	☆▲
Views Of Informal Cares, Experience and Services[106,115–118] (VOICES)	Population based, views of bereaved carer or person who knew most about the patient's last year of life	Includes carers, and most persons irrespective of the service received, developed from questionnaire used since 1967, postal	Carers may not represent the patient's views, and are not available for some. May not get good response from minority groups	▲

[a] The criteria for assessment were: research—used in more that one centre for research in palliative care; relevant to palliative care goals; clinical—used in more than one centre for clinical practice in palliative care; relevant to palliative care goals; short and easy to use.

Most of the measures described here audit a series of key indicators, for example, pain, symptoms, and patient needs. An alternative is to audit one single symptom or problem, for example, constipation, communication, or access to care. This is called topic review. Other approaches are also possible, although seldom used. Table 7 reviews these.

Organizational audits and peer review systems have tended to develop indicators that can be used in inspections of services, and concentrate on the structure and process of care, such as:

- *Service values*—a statement of service values and objectives related to the palliative care service guides the organization and delivery of high quality care.
- *Organization and management*—the palliative care service or organization is managed efficiently to ensure patients and families receive suitable and effective multidisciplinary care.
- *Organizational and operational policy*—organizational and operational policies reflect current knowledge and principles and are consistent with the requirements of statutory bodies, purchasing authorities, and service objectives.
- *Physical environment for care*—the physical environment is safe and accommodates individual and shared needs.
- *Self-determination and climate for care*—the caring environment for patients and families is conducive to independence, self-esteem, and participation in daily life.
- *Direct patient and family care*—professional staff manage to ensure that patient and family needs are assessed, planned, implemented, and evaluated on an individual basis.

Table 4 Other useful resources for audit and evaluation noted by the Working Party of the Association for Palliative Medicine

PEPSI COLA Checklist developed in primary care for palliative care needs of dying patients; includes needs/support matrix[83]
Compass A 'clinical value' compass that identifies the balance between functional health status, satisfaction against need, total costs, and clinical outcomes[119]
Review by Hearn and Higginson A published review of outcome measures in palliative care for advanced cancer patients[120]
Care of the Dying Pathway Provides a flowsheet which outlines the expected course of patient's care during last 48 h of life[121]
'Evaluating Palliative Care/Evidence-based Palliative Care' (a) *Evaluating Palliative Care* by Margaret Robbins—includes outcome indicators that can be used to evaluate palliative care from a patient, carer, staff, and service perspective[122] (b) *Evidence-based palliative care* by Huda Abu-Saad, includes review of evidence and chapter discussing ways to measure outcomes[123]
Examples of websites on quality of life measures and related indicators www.chcr.brown.edu www.picker.org www.hospicecare.com www.atsqol.org
Minimum Data Set (collected in UK and other countries) and other activity statistics Allows comparison between local data and regional/national data; its usefulness depends on reliability and accuracy of data, especially in the way data is collected

Table 5 Example of items in the Support Team Assessment Schedule[16,64]

Patient and family items
Pain control
Symptom control
Patient anxiety
Family anxiety
Patient insight
Family insight
Spiritual
Planning
Predictability
Communication between patient and family
Service items
Practical aid
Financial
Wasted time
Communication from professionals to patient and family
Communication between professionals
Professional anxiety
Advising professionals

Table 6 Definition and ratings of Support Team Assessment Schedule item 'pain control'[16]

Pain control = Effect of his/her pain on the patient

Rating	Definition
0	None
1	Occasional or grumbling single pain. Patient is not bothered to be rid of symptom
2	Moderate distress, occasional bad days, pain limits some activity possible within extent of disease
3	Severe pain present often. Activities and concentration markedly affected by pain
4	Severe and continuous overwhelming pain. Unable to think of other matters

- *Multidisciplinary working and team work*—a range of skills is available to meet service goals, and specific contributions are identified and integrated.
- *Staffing and skill mix*—good employment practices are in place and staffing levels are systematically determined in order to meet service needs.
- *Education, training, and staff development*—staff have access to education and training programmes, which reflect the different levels of activity and practice necessary to meet service goals, provide appropriate care and respond to change.
- *Staff support*—staff support systems are in place as an integral part of the organization and a healthy working environment is promoted, which recognizes the possible physical and emotional effects of work on staff.
- *Ethics and law*—there is guidance and support for staff to comply with statutory requirements and use a systematic approach to decision-making where ethical and legal status issues are involved.

Tables 8 and 9 show an example of how one of these aspects, interdisciplinary working, is assessed. Consistent with the model in Figs 3 and 4, the emphasis is on documentary evidence.

Change practice to ensure that any deficiencies are corrected

This stage closes the audit loop in the cycle.[2,16] Any weaknesses in practice need to be considered and discussed with the whole team to determine what changes might be appropriate. This may involve a review of the literature or consulting with other individuals to determine whether they have solutions to particular problems. For example, in London we identified that our control of dyspnoea in the last weeks of life was not reaching our targets: this was the most severe symptom in patients.[84] To decide what change was needed we had to consult chest physicians, physiotherapists, and other colleagues about what treatment might be appropriate in the home, review the literature on effective treatment, and examine the possible causes of dyspnoea. This led us to substantially change our practice and it also has probably led to further research into the management of dyspnoea.

In larger specialist palliative care services, difficulties in implementing the change have been described.[36,85] These include:

Table 7 Types of audit: an appraisal of their uses in palliative care

Key indicators
These can be based on the structure or process of care, as in organizational audit or can be based on clinical indicators, such as in clinical audit. In organizational audit the indicators are reviewed by inspection, in clinical audit they are reviewed by the clinical team (see Figs 3 and 4)
Routinely collected data, such as throughput, visits, or re-admission rates can be used in some areas of health care, but in palliative care these may not be appropriate and the clinical record may have to be amended to include relevant items. In clinical audit a few key indicators are chosen and recorded prospectively and examined after a period of care. In organizational audit or peer review, the survey team ask for information about the indicators and then seek evidence of these. In clinical audit—measure such as those shown in Table 3 are used
Topic review
A topic is chosen and reviewed prospectively or retrospectively. Although the latter often reveals inadequacies in the clinical records it is often valuable in providing a baseline for later comparison. Examples of topics are: medical records and letters, referral or admission procedures, control of a particular symptom, prescribing practice, or the diagnostic procedures used
Random case review
Here notes are selected at random and critically reviewed by doctors not involved in that person's care. This method may lose direction if the aims and criteria for quality are not clear. One way to focus the audit is to develop a previously agreed checklist for use in the critical review. The method can be linked with key indicators—a random sample of notes are examined for the key indicators
Patient or family satisfaction
The simplest method is to analyse patient and family complaints. However, in palliative care patients may die before they are able to complain. Surveys of patients' or families' views may be included in the overall quality improvement plan of a hospice or hospital, see Table 3 for examples of how this may be used
Adverse patient events
This systematically identifies events during a patient's treatment which may indicate some lapse in the quality of care. Patients' clinical records are reviewed retrospectively by a health professional or a ward clerk for examples of agreed adverse events. This method is of value in specialities such as surgery, where adverse events (e.g. death or post-operative infection) are usually recorded in the patients' records. However, in palliative care the method is awkward, because adverse palliative events are more difficult to identify routinely and may not be included in the patient's records unless these are standardized

Table 8 Example of criteria used in organizational audit and peer review systems

Interdisciplinary working and teamwork
Criteria
1. Systems exist for referral to the therapy professions, social workers, and ministers of religion
2. Mechanisms exist for liaison within and between disciplines, including volunteers, to ensure continuity of care
3. Staff demonstrate awareness of differing roles, relationships, and responsibilities
4. Mechanisms exist for monitoring the performance of the multidisciplinary team
5. There are systems to inform patients and families of the range of skills and services available
6. There are arrangements for liaison and cooperation between patients and families and health care agencies

Table 9 Evidence to be considered from the standard on interdisciplinary team work, used in organizational audits and peer review

Interdisciplinary working and teamwork
For Criterion 1—Do systems exist for referral to the therapy professions, social workers/counsellors, ministers of religion, complementary therapists, dieticians, interpreters, and other specialist medical or nursing services (i.e. ostomy nurse, psychiatrist)?
Documents
Referral forms
Response time statistics
Discussion
How is liaison maintained?
How are referrals made?
How quickly are referrals met?
Do these staff have post-qualification specialist training?
Observation
Observe referrals and team relationship

1. Inadequate cascading of the information from those present at the audit meetings to other staff.
2. Difficulties in ensuring that those with hands-on patient contact but at the end of the cascade, such as auxiliary nurses, feel ownership of any changes and therefore are willing to take part in them.
3. Difficulties if the main communicator is a resistor to change. Many health care professionals have inane conservatism to resist the change of long-cherished views. This may be partly from fear of their deficits being revealed.[86–88]

Continuing education is important to achieve change.[36,85] It can be targeted to ensure that those to be educated feel part of the teaching or learning process. One mechanism, which Finlay has described, asks the full team of nurses to evolve policy themselves with the facilitator of the tutor.[86]

Audit in developing countries—is it appropriate?

As palliative medicine evolves globally, one question emerges, is audit relevant in developing as well as developed countries? The currently available measurement and audit systems may be of limited use in countries with scarce resources such as India, Africa, South America, and Eastern Europe. Programmes in these countries have relatively few health care professionals, and these have varied levels of training.[37] In addition, some patients and families have high levels of illiteracy making self-completion of assessment forms impossible. The burden of illness and symptom distress in patients dying of AIDS, tuberculosis, malaria, and even the cancer-related syndromes in some of these programmes is different, just as belief systems vary, and therefore the tools may need to adjust to the main symptom problems in these patients.[37]

On the other hand, the basic principles of documenting the results of our interventions and using them to guide our future direction are not different in these regions. It can be argued that the limited resources make it even more imperative to ensure that as the programmes evolve they are capable of serving the largest possible number of patients and families in the most effective possible way. Audit is one way to minimize the risk of failure, and to learn, at an early stage, about potential problems and to identify success.[37]

However, the development is not without challenges, as many programmes in developing countries have limited access to resources and technology to successfully incorporate audit. Higginson and Bruera recently proposed a way to establish audit in developing countries, through collaboration between local programmes with specific needs and those with audit experience and methodological skills.[37]

Conclusions

Audit approaches and methods are now well advanced in palliative care, especially in clinical audit. We have a choice of possible and already tried methods and measures which we can adapt for our own needs, rather than having to undertake much of the development ourselves. Practical measures for clinical audit include the Support Team Assessment Schedule, the new shorter Palliative Outcome Scale, which is under development and the Edmonton Symptom Assessment Scale (which have either been validated or are being tested for this), and topic audits. Clinical audits which use satisfaction surveys or surveys after bereavement are probably more costly, but are still possible. Apart from completing the audit cycle, clinical audit can look to developing clinical protocols for treatment, or algorithms to predict patient problems and the need for specialized care. Organizational audit and peer review is also now well established, and different systems are available.

Audit, or the various alternative terms that describe this assessment of the quality of care, is here to stay, and is now widely accepted. But it requires resources, and so it must be sure to benefit patients and families, be kept as simple and efficient as possible, and have a strong educational component. Further work is needed to evaluate the impact of different audit approaches and methods on improving care, so that we know which approach is most cost-effective. In addition, there is a need to develop and test methods of audit in developing countries. If palliative care approaches extend backwards to include patients earlier in care, rather than those just near to death then the audit could become a means for clinical dialogue and education between specialties. Palliative medicine could take the lead in encouraging this, promoting methods among their medical and surgical colleagues and presenting their own results.

References

1. **Shaw, C.D.** (1993). Quality assurance in the United Kingdom. *Quality Assurance in Health Care* **5**, 107–18.
2. **Lynn, J.** (2001). Reforming care through continuous quality improvement. In *Palliative Care for Non-Cancer Patients* (ed. J.M. Addington-Hall and I.J. Higginson), pp. 210–16. Oxford: Oxford University Press.
3. **Rosser, R.M.** (1985). A history of the development of health indices. In *Measuring the Social Benefits of Medicine* (ed. G.T. Smith), London: Office of Health Economics.
4. **Shaw, C.D.** *Medical Audit. A Hospital Handbook.* London: King's Fund Centre, 1989.
5. **Buckingham, R.W., Lack, S.A., Mount, B.M., Maclean, L.D., and Collings, J.T.** (1976). Living with dying: use of the technique of participant observation. *Canadian Medical Association* **115**, 1211–15.
6. **Cartwright, A., Hockey, J., and Anderson, J.L.** *Life Before Death.* London: Routledge & Kegan Paul, 1973.
7. **Parkes, C.M.** (1979). Terminal care evaluation of in-patient service at St Christopher's Hospice: Part 1. *Postgraduate Medical Journal* **55**, 517–25.
8. **Parkes, C.M.** (1979). Terminal care: evaluation of in-patient services at St Christopher's Hospice: Part 2—self assessment of effects of the service on surviving spouses. *Postgraduate Medical Journal* **55**, 523–7.
9. **Parkes, C.M.** (1980). Terminal care: evaluation of an advisory domiciliary service at St Christopher's Hospice. *Postgraduate Medical Journal* **56**, 685–9.
10. **Barzelai, L.P.** (1981). Evaluation of a home based hospice. *Journal of Family Practice* **12**, 241–5.
11. **Brooks, C.H. and Smyth-Starvch, K.** (1984). Hospice home care cost savings to third party insurers. *Medical Care* **22**, 691.
12. **Kane, R.L., Klein, S.J., Bernstein, L., Rothenberg, R., and Wales, J.** (1985). Hospice role in alleviating the emotional stress of terminal patients and their families. *Medical Care* **23**, 189–97.
13. **Mor, V., Morris, J.N., Hiris, J., and Sherwood, S.** (1988). The effects of hospice care on where patients die. In *The Hospice Experiment* (ed. V. Mor, D.S. Greer, and R. Kastenbaum), pp. 133–46. Baltimore MD: Johns Hopkins University Press.
14. **Ward, A.W.M.** (1976). The impact of a special unit for terminal care. *Social Science and Medicine* **10**, 373–6.
15. **Higginson, I.J.** (1993). Palliative care: a review of past changes and future trends. *Journal of Public Health Medicine* **15**, 3–8.
16. **Higginson, I.J.** *Clinical Audit in Palliative Care.* Oxford: Radcliffe, 1993.
17. **Higginson, I.J. and Carr, A.J.** (2001). Measuring quality of life: using quality of life measures in the clinical setting. *British Medical Journal* **322**, 1297–300.
18. **Ingleton, C. and Faulkner, A.** (1995). Quality assurance in palliative care—a review of the literature. *Journal of Cancer Care* **4**, 49–55.
19. **Higginson, I.J.** et al. (2002). Do hospital based palliative care teams improve outcomes for patients or families at the end of life. *Journal of Pain and Symptom Management* **23**, 96–106.
20. **Higginson, I.J., Finlay, I.G., Goodwin, D.M., Cook, A.M., Edwards, A.G.K., Hood, K., Douglas, H.-R., and Normand, C.E.** The role of palliative care teams: a systematic review of their effectiveness and cost-effectiveness. *Final Report to the Welsh Office for Research and Development.* London: Department of Palliative Care and Policy, 2001.
21. **Hearn, J. and Higginson, I.J.** (1998). Do specialist palliative care teams improve outcomes for cancer patients? A systematic literature review. *Palliative Medicine* **12**, 317–32.
22. **Higginson, I.J.** (1999). Evidence based palliative care—there is some evidence and there needs to be more. *British Medical Journal* **319**, 462–3.
23. **Salisbury, C.** et al. (1999). The impact of different models of specialist palliative care on patient's quality of life: a systematic literature review. *Palliative Medicine* **13**, 3–17.
24. **Bosanquet, N.** (1999). Background and patterns of use of service. In *Providing a Palliative Care Service: Towards an Evidence Base* (ed. N. Bosanquet and C. Salisbury), pp. 8–10, 33–42. Oxford: Oxford University Press.
25. **Eve, A. and Higginson, I.J.** (2000). Minimum dataset activity for hospice and hospital palliative care services in the UK 1997–98. *Palliative Medicine* **14**, 395–404.
26. **Higginson, I.J., Hearn, J., and Webb, D.** (1996). Audit in palliative care: does practice change? *European Journal of Cancer Care England* **5**, 233–6.
27. **Higginson, I.J.** (1994). Clinical audit and organizational audit in palliative care. *Cancer Surveys* **21**, 233–45.
28. **Blyth, A.C.** (1990). Audit of terminal care in a general practice. *British Medical Journal* **300**, 983–6.
29. **Butters, E., Higginson, I., George, R., and McCarthy, M.** (1993). Palliative care for people with HIV/AIDS: views of patients, carers and providers. *AIDS Care* **5**, 105–16.
30. **Finlay, I., Wilkinson, C., and Gibbs, C.** (1992). Planning palliative care services. *Health Trends* **24**, 139–41.
31. **Glickman, M.** Making palliative care better: quality improvement, multiprofessional audit and standards. Occasional Paper 12. London: National Council for Hospice & Specialist Palliative Care Services, 1997.
32. **Ingleton, C. and Faulkner, A.** (1993). Quality assurance. Audit in palliative care: a senior nurse perspective. *Nursing Standards* **7**, 8–9.
33. **Lloyd Williams, M.** (1996). An audit of palliative care in dementia. *European Journal of Cancer Care England* **5**, 53–5.
34. **McKee, C.M., Lauglo, M., and Lessof, L.** (1989). Medical audit: a review. *Journal of the Royal Society of Medicine* **82**, 474–8.
35. **Rogers, M.** Palliative care audit in primary care report: Anglia Clinical Audit and Effectiveness Team. Cambridge: Institute of Public Health, 1996.

36. **Hayes, A.** (1993). Audit experience: assessing staff's views. In *Clinical Audit in Palliative Care* (ed. I.J. Higginson), pp. 138–43. Oxford: Radcliffe Medical Press.
37. **Higginson, I.J. and Bruera, E.** (2002). Do we need palliative care audit in developing countries? *Palliative Medicine* **16**, 546–7.
38. **Clark, D., Neale, B., and Heather, P.** (1995). Contracting for palliative care. *Social Science and Medicine* **40**, 1193–202.
39. **Bromberg, M.H. and Higginson, I.** (1996). Bereavement follow-up: what do palliative support teams actually do? *Journal of Palliative Care* **12**, 12–17.
40. **Donabedian, A.** (1980). The definition of quality and approaches to its assessment. In *Explorations in Quality Assessment and Monitoring* Vol. 1 (ed. A. Donabedian), Michigan: Health Administration Press.
41. **Maxwell, R.** (1992). Dimensions of quality revisited: from thought to action. *Quality in Health Care* **1**, 171–7.
42. **Black, N.** (1990). Quality assurance of medical care. *Journal of Public Health Medicine* **12**, 97–104.
43. **Stewart, A.L., Teno, J.M., Patrick, D.L., and Lynn, J.** (1999). The concept of quality of life of dying persons in the context of health care. *Journal of Pain and Symptom Management* **17**, 93–108.
44. **King's Fund Centre.** *Organisational Audit (Accreditation UK): Standards for an Acute Hospital.* London: King's Fund Centre, 1990.
45. **Working Party of Clinical Governance of the Quality and Clinical Governance Committee.** *Clinical Governance and Quality Approaches in Palliative Care.* London: National Council for Hospice and Specialist Palliative Care, 2002.
46. **Bullen, M.** (1995). The role of the specialist nurse in palliative care. *Professional Nursing* **10**, 755–6.
47. **Butters, E., Higginson, I., George, R., Smits, A., and McCarthy, M.** (1992). Assessing the symptoms, anxiety and practical needs of HIV/AIDS patients receiving palliative care. *Quality of Life Research* **1**, 47–51.
48. **Finlay, I.G. and Dunlop, R.** (1994). Quality of life assessment in palliative care. *Annals of Oncology* **5**, 13–18.
49. **Kristjanson, L.J.** (1989). Quality of terminal care: salient indicators identified by families. *Journal of Palliative Care* **5**, 21–30.
50. **Vachon, M.L., Kristjanson, L.J., and Higginson, I.** (1995). Psychosocial issues in palliative care: the patient, the family, and the process and outcome of care. *Journal of Pain and Symptom Management* **10** (2), 142–50.
51. **Haidet, P.** et al. (1998). Outcomes, preferences for resuscitation, and physician–patient communication among patients with metastatic colorectal cancer. SUPPORT Investigators. Study to Understand Prognoses and Preferences for Outcomes and Risks of Treatments. *American Journal of Medicine* **105**, 222–9.
52. **Higginson, I.J. and Bruera, E.** (2001). Care of patients who are dying, and their families. In *Oxford Textbook of Oncology* (ed. R.L. Souhami, I. Tannock, P. Hohenberger, and J.-C. Horiot), pp. 1103–20. Oxford: Oxford University Press.
53. **Higginson, I.J.** *Health Care Needs Assessment: Palliative and Terminal Care.* Oxford: Radcliffe Medical Press, 1997.
54. **Harper, R., Ward, A., Westlake, L., and Williams, B.T.** Good practice in terminal care: some standards and guidelines for hospital inpatient units and day hospices. Sheffield: University of Sheffield, 1988.
55. **Ingleton, C. and Faulkner, A.** (1993). Audit issues in palliative care: the perspective of senior nurses. *Journal of Cancer Care* **2**, 201–6.
56. **Latimer, E.** (1991). Auditing the hospital care of dying patients. *Journal of Palliative Care* **7**, 12–17.
57. **Lunt, B.** (1983). Goal-setting in terminal care: a method for recording treatment aims and priorit. *Journal of Advanced Nursing* **8**, 495–505.
58. **Teno, J.M.** (2001). Quality of life and quality indicators for end of life cancer care: hope for the best, yet prepare for the worst. In *Improving Palliative Care for Cancer* (ed. K.M. Foley and H. Gelband), pp. 96–131. Washington DC: National Academy Press.
59. **Emanuel, E.J. and Emanuel, L.L.** (1998). The promise of a good death. *Lancet* **351** (Suppl. 2), SII21–9.
60. **Weisman, A.D.** (1988). Appropriate death and the hospice program. *Hospice Journal* **4**, 65–77.
61. **Kellehear, A.** *Dying of Cancer. The Final Year of Life.* London: Harwood, 1990.
62. **Singer, P.A., Martin, D.K., and Kerner, M.** (1999). Quality end-of-life care: patients' perspectives. *Journal of the American Medical Association* **281**, 163–8.
63. **Payne, S., Smith, P., and Dean, S.** (1999). Identifying the concerns of informal carers in palliative care. *Palliative Medicine* **13**, 37–44.
64. **Higginson, I.J. and McCarthy, M.** (1993). Validity of the support team assessment schedule: do staffs' ratings reflect those made by patients or their families? *Palliative Medicine* **7**, 219–28.
65. **Cartwright, A.** *The Role of the General Practitioners in Caring for People in the Last Year of Their Lives.* London: King Edward's Hospital Fund for London, 1990.
66. **Copperman, H.** (1988). Domiciliary hospice care: a survey of general practitioners. *Journal of the Royal College of General Practitioners* **38**, 411–13.
67. **Doyle, D.** (1982). Domiciliary terminal care: demands on statutory services. *Journal of the Royal College of General Practitioners* **32**, 285–91.
68. **Edgar, I. and Bytheway, A.** (1988). Information exchange: the hospice nurse and the community nurse. *Nursing Times* **84**, 42–4.
69. **Finlay, I.** (1992). Care of the dying in general practice. *British Medical Journal* **291**, 179–81.
70. **Grande, G.E. and Todd, C.F.** *Care Needs at Home during Terminal Illness: GPs', Patients' and Relatives' Views.* Cambridge: Department of Public Health, 1993.
71. **Grande, G.E., Todd, C., Barclay, S.I.G., and Doyle, J.H.** (1996). What terminally ill patients value in the support provided by GPs, district and Macmillan nurses. *International Journal of Palliative Nursing* **2** (3), 138–43.
72. **Hjortdahl, P. and Laerum, E.** (1992). Continuity of care in general practice: effect on patient satisfaction. *British Medical Journal* **304**, 1287–90.
73. **Jones, R.V.H.** (1993). Teams and terminal cancer care at home: do patients and carers benefit? *Journal of Interprofessional Care* **7**, 239–45.
74. **Todd, C.J. and Still, A.W.** (1984). Communication between general practitioners and patients dying at home. *Social Science Medicine* **18**, 667–72.
75. **Addington-Hall, J.M., Lay, M., Altmann, D., and McCarthy, M.** (1995). Symptom control, communication with health professionals, and hospital care of stroke patients in the last year of life as reported by surviving family, friends, and officials. *Stroke* **26**, 2242–8.
76. **Baile, W.F., Glober, G.A., Lenzi, R., Beale, E.A., and Kudelka, A.P.** (1999). Discussing disease progression and end-of-life decisions. *Oncology (Huntingt)* **13**, 1021–31.
77. **Buckman, R.** (1998). Communication in palliative care: a practical guide. In *Oxford Textbook of Palliative Medicine* (ed. D. Doyle, G.W.C. Hanks, and N. MacDonald), pp. 141–56. Oxford: Oxford University Press.
78. **Buckman, R.** *I don't Know What to Say: How to Help and Support Someone Who is Dying.* London: Papermac, 1988.
79. **Fallowfield, L.** (1993). Giving sad and bad news. *Lancet* **341**, 476–8.
80. **Faulkner, A., Webb, P., and Maguire, P.** (1991). Communication and counseling skills: educating health professionals working in cancer and palliative care. *Patient Education and Counseling* **18**, 3–7.
81. **Koffman, J. and Higginson, I.J.** (2001). Accounts of carers' satisfaction with health care at the end of life: a comparison of first generation black Caribbeans and white patients with advanced disease. *Palliative Medicine* **15**, 345.
82. **Higginson, I.J. and Sen-Gupta, G.J.A.** (2000). Place of care in advanced cancer: a qualitative systematic literature review of patient preferences. *Journal of Palliative Medicine* **3**, 287–300.
83. **Clinical Effectiveness Working Group, Higginson, I.J., Campion-Smith, C., Miller, M., Thomas, K., and Wee, B.** *The Which Tool Guide?* Southampton: Association for Palliative Medicine, UK, 2002.
84. **Higginson, I.J. and McCarthy, M.** (1989). Measuring symptoms in terminal cancer: are pain and dyspnoea controlled? *Journal of the Royal Society of Medicine* **82**, 264–7.
85. **McKee, E.** (1993). Audit experience: a nurse manager in home care. In *Clinical Audit in Palliative Care* (ed. I.J. Higginson), pp. 128–37. Oxford: Radcliffe Medical Press.
86. **Finlay, I.** (1993). Audit experience: views of a hospice director. In *Clinical Audit in Palliative Care* (ed. I.J. Higginson), pp. 144–57. Oxford: Radcliffe Medical Press.

87. **Finlay, I. and Fowell, A.** (2000). A good death: care pathways in Wales aims to improve care of dying patients. *British Medical Journal* **320**, 1205.

88. **McQuillan, R., Finlay, I., Branch, C., Roberts, D., and Spencer, M.** (1996). Improving analgesic prescribing in a general teaching hospital. *Journal of Pain and Symptom Management* **11**, 172–80.

89. **MacAdam, D.B. and Smith, M.** (1987). An initial assessment of suffering in terminal illness. *Palliative Medicine* **1**, 34–47.

90. **Rogers, M.S., Barclay, S.I., and Todd, C.J.** (2002). Developing the Cambridge palliative audit schedule (CAMPAS): a palliative care audit for primary health care teams. *British Journal of General Practice* **48**, 1224–7.

91. **Kaasa, T., Loomis, J., Gillis, K., Bruera, E., and Hanson, J.** (1997). The Edmonton Functional Assessment Tool: preliminary development and evalu-ation for use in palliative care. *Journal of Pain and Symptom Management* **13**, 10–19.

92. **Bruera, E.** et al. (1991). The Edmonton Symptom Assessment System (ESAS): a simple method for the assessment of palliative care patients. *Journal of Palliative Care* **7**, 6–9.

93. **Aaronson, N.K.** et al. (1993). The European Organisation for Research and Treatment of Cancer QLQ-C30: a quality-of-life instrument for use in international clinical trials in oncology. *Journal of the National Cancer Institute* **85**, 365–76.

94. **Aaronson, N.K., Bullinger, M., and Ahmedzai, C.** (1988). A modular approach to quality-of-life assessment in cancer clinical trials. *Recent Results in Cancer Research* **111**, 231–49.

95. **Cella, D.F. and Tulsky, D.S.** (1990). Measuring quality of life today: methodological aspects. *Oncology* **4**, 29–37.

96. **Brady, M.J. and Cella, D.** (1999). Assessing the quality of life in palliative care. *Cancer Treatment and Research* **100**, 203–16.

97. **Morris, J.N.** et al. (1986). Last days: a study of the quality of life of terminally ill cancer patients. *Journal of Chronic Diseases* **39**, 47–56.

98. **Cohen, S.R., Mount, B.M., Tomas, J.J.N., and Mount, L.F.** (1996). Existential well-being is an important determinant of quality of life: Evidence from the McGill Quality of Life Questionnaire. *Cancer* **77**, 576–86.

99. **Cohen, S.R., Mount, B.M., Strobel, M.G., and Bui, F.** (1995). The McGill Quality of Life Questionnaire: a measure of quality of life appropriate for people with advanced disease. A preliminary study of validity and acceptability. *Palliative Medicine* **9**, 207–19.

100. **Cohen, S.R., Mount, B.M., Bruera, E., Provost, M., Rowe, J., and Tong, K.** (1997). Validity of the McGill Quality of Life Questionnaire in the palliative care setting: a multi-centre Canadian study demonstrating the importance of the existential domain. *Palliative Medicine* **11**, 3–20.

101. **Patterson, C.** (1996). Measuring outcomes in primary care: a patient generated measure, MYMOP, compared with the SF-36 health survey. *British Medical Journal* **312**, 1016–20.

102. **Ellershaw, J.E., Peat, S.J., and Boys, L.C.** (1995). Assessing the effectiveness of a hospital palliative care team. *Palliative Medicine* **9**, 145–52.

103. **Trent Hospice Audit Group.** *Palliative Care Core Standards: A Multidisciplinary Approach.* Trent Hospice Audit. Derby: Nightingale Macmillan Continuing Care Unit, 1992.

104. **Hearn, J. and Higginson, I.J.** (1999). Development and validation of a core outcome measure for palliative care: the palliative care outcome scale. *Quality in Health Care* **8**, 219–27.

105. **Aspinal, F., Hughes, R., Higginson, I.J., Thompson, M., and Dunckley, M.** *The Palliative Outcome Scale: User Guide.* London: Department of Palliative Care and Policy, 2002.

106. **Hughes, R., Higginson, I.J., Addington-Hall, J.M., Aspinal, F., Thompson, M., and Dunckley, M.** (2001). Project to impROve Management Of Terminal illnEss (PROMOTE). *Journal of Interprofessional Care* **15**, 398–9.

107. **Higginson, I.J., Astin, P., Dolan, S., and Jarman, B.** (1999). Do social factors affect place of death? Analysis of 10 years data in England. *Journal of Public Health Medicine* **21**, 22–8.

108. **Higginson, I.J., Astin, P., and Dolan, S.** (1998). Where do cancer patients die? Ten-year trends in the place of death of cancer patients in England. *Palliative Medicine* **12**, 353–63.

109. **de Haes, J.C.J.M. and van Knippenberg, F.C.E.** (1990). Measuring psychological and physical distress in cancer patients: structure and application of the Rotterdam symptom checklist. *British Journal of Cancer* **62**, 1034–8.

110. **Spitzer, W.O.** et al. (1981). Measuring the quality of life of cancer patients: a concise QL-index for use by physicians. *Journal of Chronic Disease* **34**, 585–9.

111. **Higginson, I.J. and McCarthy, M.** (1994). A comparison of two measures of quality of life: their sensitivity and validity for patients with advanced cancer. *Palliative Medicine* **8**, 282–90.

112. **Higginson, I.J.** *Audit Methods: A Community Schedule.* Oxford: Radcliffe, 1993.

113. **McCorkle, R. and Young, K.** (1978). Development of a symptom distress scale. *Cancer Nursing* **101**, 373–8.

114. **Joyce, C.R.B., McGee, H.M., and O'Boyle, C.A.** *Individual Quality of Life. Approaches to Conceptualisation and Assessment.* Amsterdam: Harwood Academic Publishers, 1999.

115. **Addington-Hall, J. and Kalra, L.** (2001). Measuring quality of life: who should measure quality of life? *British Medical Journal* **322**, 1417–20.

116. **Addington-Hall, J.M., Walker, L., Jones, C., Karlsen, S., and McCarthy, M.** (1998). Development of a questionnaire to measure satisfaction with services received in the year before death. *Journal of Epidemiology and Community Health* **52**, 802–7.

117. **Addington-Hall, J.M. and McCarthy, M.** (1995). Regional study of care for the dying: methods and sample characteristics. *Palliative Medicine* **9**, 27–35.

118. **Edmonds, P.M., Karlsen, S., and Addington-Hall, J.M.** (2000). Palliative care needs of hospital in-patients. *Palliative Medicine* **14**, 227–8.

119. **Nelson, E.C.** et al. (1996). Improving health care. Part 1: The Clinical Value Compass. *Joint Commission Journal on Quality Improvement* **22**, 243–58.

120. **Hearn, J. and Higginson, I.J.** (1997). Outcome measures in palliative care for advanced cancer patients: a review. *Journal of Public Health Medicine* **19**, 193–9.

121. **Ellershaw, J., Murphy, D., Foster, A., Shea, T., and Overill, S.** (1997). Developing an integrated care pathway for the dying patient. *European Journal of Palliative Care* **4**, 203–7.

122. **Robbins, M.** *Evaluating Palliative Care: Establishing the Evidence Base.* Oxford: Oxford University Press, 1998.

123. **Abu-Saad, H.** *Evidence-Based Palliative Care.* London: Blackwell Science, 2001.

6.3 Quality of life in palliative medicine—principles and practice

Stein Kaasa and Jon Håvard Loge

Introduction

Quality of life (QOL) is a central concept in palliative care. It is not a new idea, one of the main goals of the health care system in ancient Greece was to improve patients' QOL.[1] The assessment tools and the medical interventions they had in hand were limited, but still they probably achieved an improvement in patients QOL by their interventions. The term 'QOL' was not established as a distinct entity, but rather as a general term, 'everything in life taken into consideration'.

Most people will agree that the ultimate goal for a society is to achieve an optimal QOL for the population. However, the means by which this is achieved through the political process differ. A communist from Russia, a

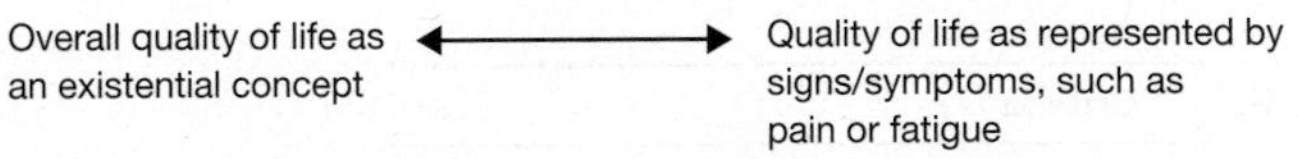

Fig. 1 Quality of life as a continuum from existentiality to single symptoms.

socialist from Poland, a social democrat from Norway, and a Republican from Texas would probably strongly disagree about which political strategies one should choose in order to improve the general QOL in society.

In a sociological context QOL is described in theories of measures of human welfare (defined as level of education, economic and industrial growth). In studies from the 1950s it was found that an economic improvement did not necessarily result in greater level of happiness, lower levels of worries, or a better outlook.(2) It was recognized that there was need for alternative indicators of social welfare in addition to the economic and material indicators currently used. As a result subjective indicators of human welfare were developed. A different terminology is used by different groups to describe the phenomenon. Some use the term subjective social indicators, others indicators of general well being or of QOL.(3,4) The common denominator was that the measures were of a subjective nature and the information was collected by means of interviews or questionnaires.

The overall goal in health care has always been and will always be to improve patients' QOL. Despite the more widespread use of the term as a theoretical concept and empirically, no precise common definition exist. However, in order to simplify the discussion, one may target two general approaches in the understanding of the concept. QOL, as a broad concept encompasses 'how is your life, everything taken in consideration' and QOL as a more distinct health-oriented concept focuses on some specific aspect of health or health care, such as symptom control and physical function. These are not mutually exclusive concepts, but rather a continuum of issues between two extremes allowing an intuitive flexibility in defining QOL in terms of established phenomenon or as a single sign or symptom, as illustrated in Fig. 1.

Overall QOL

In a sociological, psychological, and medical context, QOL has been defined as a broad concept. As described above, these definitions connect psychological, mental, and spiritual domains of a person's life. In the process of finding indicators of these various abstract phenomena satisfaction, happiness, morale, and positive and negative effects have been put forward as important components of the QOL concept. In some of the literature there is an emphasis on normality, viewing QOL as fulfillment of life and the possibilities to live a normal life, while others focus more on mental capacity, to think clearly, to see, to love and be loved, to make decisions for oneself, to maintain contact with family and friends, to live at home, and/or to be physically active. The ability to make individual decisions has also been emphasized as an important aspect of QOL, including the capacity of the individual to realize his life, and the perception of personal meaning.

According to these definitions QOL is strongly linked to normality, including normal function or that a minimum of human needs are met. Such a minimum of needs were also described by Maslow,(5) which is often refered to as 'Maslow's needs hierarchy', consisting of biological needs, needs for close relationships, needs for meaningful occupation, and need for change. This concept has further been elaborated in a QOL context viewing QOL as the level of a person's activity, the ability to relate to others, self-esteem, and a basic mood of happiness.(6)

The theoretical concept of normality and biological fulfilment is challenged empirically in that many patients with major physical and/or psychological limitations, may report a high degree of global QOL.(7) These empirical findings fit well with another theory, the so-called Gap Theory of Calman.(8) He described QOL as an inverse relationship to the difference between an individual's expectations and their perception of the given situation, 'the smaller the gap the better quality of life'. According to this gap theory, as illustrated in Fig. 2, a change in QOL from T0 to T1 can be caused by changes in both expectations and experience, case A and B report the same QOL at T0 and T1; however, the underlying causes of the change from T0 to T1 is different in the two individuals.

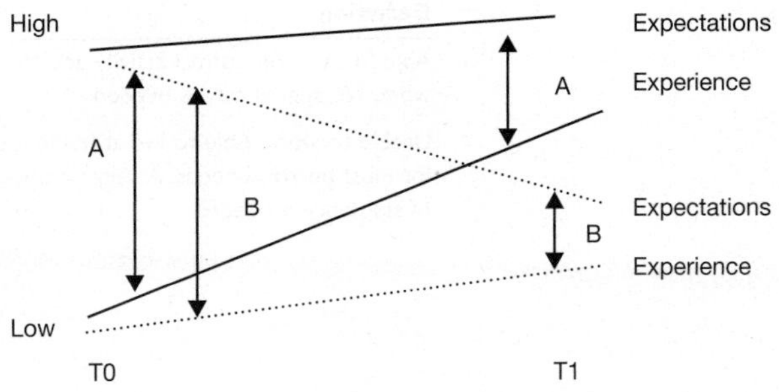

Fig. 2 Quality of life as the gap between expectations and experience.

QOL in medicine

In health care research QOL encompasses a range of components, which are measurable and related to health, disease, illness, and medical interventions. In health care, as well as in life in general, QOL means different things to different people and takes on different meanings according to the illness, experience, support, etc. Furthermore, a professional's focus may also influence the perception of QOL. For example, a medical oncologist may rate tumour response after delivering combination chemotherapy to a patient with a non-Hodgkin's lymphoma as the most important achievement to improve QOL, while a nurse may focus on patients' ability to deal with daily activities. For a physician in palliative medicine improvement of QOL for one patient may mean pain control, and for another to establish necessary social support. In the context of clinical trials one is rarely interested in QOL as a global concept, but rather as a focused outcome caused by the intervention in question, such as improved pain control during night time by delivery of slow-release morphine at bedtime or reduced dyspnoea after chest irradiation for a patient with lung cancer. Despite the ongoing discussion about how to define QOL most researchers and clinicians agree that QOL in palliative medicine is related to symptom control, physical function, psychological well being, and meaning and fulfilment (existential and spiritual issues). This multidimensional health-oriented concept has been named by many clinicians and researchers as health-related quality of life (HRQOL).(9–13)

The WHO definition of health captured already in 1947—the multidimensionality of health: 'Health is not only the absence of infirmity and disease, but also a state of complete physical, mental and social well-being'.(14) In many aspects this definition has been identified by several researchers as the beginning of a new era in the approach to health care. Historically, another important step in the same direction was described by Karnofsky in 1948. He evaluated the palliative effect of nitrogen mustard on various malignant tumours by means of subjective improvement, objective improvement, and performance status.(15) Performance status was defined according to specific criteria, which have become widely used and known as the Karnofsky performance status scale (Table 1). This simple scale has been shown to be significant predictor of survival in patients with metastatic disease, as have measurers of HRQOL.(16–19)

During the 1970s standardized questionnaires were developed in co-operative groups and in university settings. 'Linear analogue self-assessment scales' (LASA) were used to capture the QOL of specific cancer groups, such as breast-cancer patients. These measures included a variety of subjective domains, such as well being, mood, anxiety, activity, pain, and

Table 1 Performance status

Definition	%	Criteria
Able to carry on normal activity and to work. No special care is needed	100	Normal; no complaints; no evidence of disease
Unable to work. Able to live at home, care for most personal needs. A varying amount of assistance is needed	90	Able to carry on normal activity; minor signs or symptoms of disease
	80	Normal activity with effort; some signs or symptoms of disease
	70	Cares for self; unable to carry on normal activity or to do active work
	60	Requires occasional assistance; but is able to care for most of his needs
	50	Requires considerable assistance and frequent medical care
Unable to care for self. Requires equivalent of institutional or hospital care. Disease may be progressing rapidly	40	Disabled; requires special care and assistance
	30	Severely disabled; hospitalization is indicated although death not imminent
	20	Very sick; hospitalization necessary; active supportive treatment necessary
	10	Moribund; fatal processes progressing rapidly
	0	Dead

Table 2 No of papers indexed in Medline under the keyword 'Quality of Life' 1961–2000

1961–65	1966–70	1971–75	1976–80	1981–85	1986–90	1991–95	1996–2000
0	8	180	1159	1881	4541	9464	12 749

social activity.[9,10] Others developed measures of health status in order to capture patient's general perception of health, some examples are the Sickness Impact Profile,[11] Nottingham Health Profile,[20] SF-36,[21,22], and more physically oriented scales such as the Barthel Index.[12] Other measures, which also are classified as QOL measures focus primarily on psychological domains, such as the General Health Questionnaire (GHQ)[13] and Profile of Mood States.[23]

At the same time similar development of measures were seen within the area of pain assessment based upon the International Association for the Study of Pain's (IASP) definition of pain. IASP defined pain as 'an unpleasant sensory and emotional experience associated with actual or potential tissue damage, or described in terms of such damage'.[24] This definition is conceptually very similar to most definitions of QOL—both rely on patients self-report, and the questionnaire methodology is most commonly used. Previously pain measurement had involved a standardized external stimulus, such as radiant heat, which were used to obtain a psychophysiological standard against which to measure clinical pain. A 'language of pain' was developed, which is well illustrated by the McGill pain questionnaire (MPQ).[25] More simple tools were also used to assess pain intensity, such as verbal rating scales (VRS), numerical rating scales (NRS), and visual analogue scales (VAS).[26]

Most of the HRQOL and pain measures are built upon a questionnaire concept, more or less well suited for palliative care patients. For severely ill patients assessment by means of interview may be more appropriate. Interviews are flexible and provide detailed information, but are expensive and time-consuming to perform. Further, their usefulness is often limited in multicentre trials where HRQOL is often assessed at several time points.[27] Therefore assessment by use of questionnaires has become the most commonly used approach. The questionnaires are often in paper format, but questionnaires can be administered in an electronic format.[28]

The enormous increase in publications indexed under the subject heading 'QOL in Medline' reflects the increased focus on the patients' QOL during the last 30–35 years (Table 2). The rapidly increasing number of papers and newly developed questionnaires are a reminder of the ambiguity of the concept QOL.

A textbook published in 1996 included more than 200 different measures of QOL.[29] Many of these questionnaires have not been developed based upon explicit definitions and operationalizations of the phenomena they are supposed to measure. Different wordings of the same phenomena across different questionnaires exemplified by fatigue versus vitality and psychological functioning versus mental health underline the lack of precision, not only on the level of single items and scales, but also in communication about each concept.

In palliative care

The goals of palliative care are acknowledged to include the domain of HRQOL as well as spirituality, loss/grief, family involvement, and coping. Many of the most common HRQOL tools have been thought inadequate by researchers in palliative care. They have been criticized for being too narrow by only including physical, psychological, and social aspects of a patient's life. Thus outcome measures require questions that reflect the specific goals of palliative care,[30] such as improving the QOL before death, controlling symptoms and supporting the family (Table 3). It has been proposed that meaning should also be included, as well as purpose, spirituality, and grief.[31–33]

During end-stage disease patients will often not be able to complete HRQOL instruments and proxies will be the only possible source of collection of information, either by means of interviews (open, semi-structured, or structured) or questionnaires.

One possible strategy is to let the health care provider or the family member complete the instrument. However, many studies have shown that the assessment of health care providers or family members differs from the response obtained from the patients. In some conditions observers seems to overestimate the psychological burden, while pain and other symptoms are often underestimated.

In summary, HRQOL is of subjective nature and the patient is the primary source of information. It is a dynamic phenomenon, probably with varying dimension in focus, depending upon individual factors, disease factors, symptomatology, coping ability, closeness to death, etc. By reviewing the definition of the concept it is clear that the content is highly

Table 3 HRQOL measurement in palliative care

Content of measures—dimensions
◆ Symptoms
◆ Physical function
◆ Emotional function
◆ Existential issues (spirituality)
Proxy ratings
◆ Health care providers
◆ Family members
Quality of life
◆ Patient and family assessment?

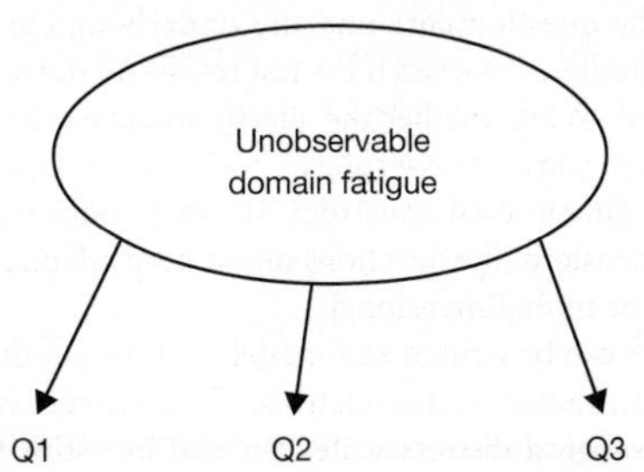

Fig. 3 Items/questions.

influenced by setting, that is, the severity of physical symptoms, general health, spirituality, coping, existentially, etc. However, there is a general agreement to at least include symptomatology, physical, psychological, and social domains into the measures, although in many circumstances existential and spiritual domains also seem appropriate to include.

Measurement theory

HRQOL is regarded as an 'underlying concept', which is abstract, not directly observable, individual, and multidimensional. The experience from clinical practice can be used to better understand the practicalities related to measurement theory. In a clinical interview, specific questions are asked in order to gain knowledge about the phenomena in question. In order to communicate about an abstract phenomenon, one needs to agree upon a definition of the concept, how to explore the concept, and how to summarize the findings. In other words, an accurate description of a subjective phenomenon depends upon how the concept is defined, how data is collected, processed, and communicated.

It is well documented that reliable and valid information is best collected by standardized procedures, such as clinical interview and examination, which include standardized data collection, documentation routines, interpretation, and communication in patients' records and orally to colleagues.

For example, fatigue is generally agreed to be an important domain in the concept of HRQOL in palliative care, and a set of items or questions often based upon not only first hand clinical experience but also existing measures that might be derived.

Theoretically, as illustrated in Fig. 3, the three questions Q1, Q2, and Q3 should all contribute to measure the level of fatigue in palliative care patients. The number of items needed to measure a given concept as precisely as possible depends upon factors such as the complexity of the phenomenon in question and the level of reliability needed. The reliability will improve by increasing the number of items, according to common measurement theory.

Validity and reliability

Reliability is linked to the reproducibility of a measure, such as a lab test, an X-ray, or a QOL measure. The basic idea is that under different circumstances the underlying concept is constant and the measure captures the concept across the variations in context. In more technical terms reliability is an estimate of the degree of random error of any given instrument. There are a number of ways in which reliability is estimated in QOL research. The most common procedure is to estimate the internal consistency of a unidimensional score. The assumption by estimating the internal consistency of a set of items is that all of the items address the same underlying dimension. The estimate will represent the average correlations among all of the items in the measure. Cronbach alpha is often used to calculate the correlations.[34] Stability or reproducibility is another estimate of reliability. One might ask about the degree of agreement between observers (interobserver reliability), observation on the same patients on two different occasions (test–retest reliability), and so forth.

Validity refers to whether the test measures what it is intended to measure. If there is an established instrument which measures the underlying phenomenon, say for example anxiety, this instrument can be used as the gold standard. By comparing the new instrument with the old, estimates of validity can be calculated. However, the situation is often that no gold standard exists, which means that indirect methods must be used in order to establish the validity of the new instrument. The approach of construct validity is often used, which is based upon a theory of a given construct, for example, physical function or fatigue. Validity in this context is defined as the extent to which a method measures the underlying construct in question.[35] The validity is not a 'fixed' property of an instrument, and may change when the context and study population vary between studies. The terminology of validity testing can be confusing. Most authors, however, agree that there are three basic types of validity: content, criterion, and construct validity (the three C's).

Content validity

'Content validity'—or the related 'face validity'—refers to the extent to which the scale looks reasonable. The face validity indicates whether, on the face of it, the instrument appears to be assessing the desired qualities, while the content validity is a judgement of whether the questionnaire samples all the relevant and important dimensions we are interested in. There are no empirical ways of testing this; the judgement is usually based on a review and consensus by an expert panel of health care workers and/or patients.

Criterion validity

Criterion validity is the correlation of a scale with some other measure of the dimensions under study, ideally a gold standard. It is usually divided into concurrent and predictive validity.

Concurrent validity is established by comparing a new method with the old way of assessment, with both assessments performed at the same time. In laboratory medicine a criterion or a standard is often used to calibrate a new instrument. Since there is no established gold standard for measuring cancer patients' QOL, quite often new scales are compared with old ones, which might have suboptimal validity. Another approach is to use indirect methods of comparisons, such as observer- or interview-based ratings. This can introduce difficulties in the interpretation of the results. If an expected association between, for example, a questionnaire and an observer-rated instrument is not confirmed, it is difficult to tell whether the questionnaire, or the observer-rated instrument, or both, have low validity. Predictive validity is a measure of the extent to which the questionnaire can predict an event or a test result in the future. The results from a screening instrument for psychological distress could, for example, be compared with the level of psychiatric morbidity assessed by a clinical interview at a later point in time.

Construct validity

Construct validity relates to the extent to which the instrument assesses an unobservable, hypothetical construct we are interested in, such as pain, body image, or anxiety. Evaluation of smaller construct validity is an ongoing process where the questionnaire and the underlying construct must be tested in various studies. However, if the test results do not support our hypotheses, it is difficult to tell whether the questionnaire has low construct validity or whether the construct is wrong or both. Pain, for example, could be defined as a unidimensional construct. If a pain questionnaire seems to assess several dimensions, the questions might need adaptation or the construct of pain may be multidimensional.

Hypothesized constructs can be written as a model, and the goodness of fit can be examined by confirmatory factor analyses. The construct validity of scales, such as a psychological distress scale, can also be estimated by comparing results between extreme groups such as patients with or without anxiety and depression in a clinical interview. By testing the convergent validity and discriminant validity, the correlations between the new instrument and other methods are reviewed. A high correlation is expected with scales assessing similar constructs like other psychological distress scales (convergent validity), and low correlation with instruments assessing other constructs such as physical function (discriminant validity).

Patient population

Patient population in palliative care and compliance with QOL assessment tools

There are several issues one must take into account when assessing HRQOL in palliative care. Patients are sick and disabled. Valid and reliable data may therefore be difficult to collect, particularly in the later stages of life. Patients often have several symptoms at the same time and physical symptoms may give rise to psychological problems (and *vice versa*). These relationships in palliative care in general and specifically in end of life care, have been discussed and addressed empirically.

What is a palliative care population?

A palliative care population is not a well-defined group of patients. In some programmes most patients are dying, while in others the majority of the patients have a longer life expectancy. In discussing the use of methodology to collect HRQOL data, the patient population in question should be specified. Several indicators might be used to describe the population, such as expected survival, type of tumour-directed treatment, do not resuscitate (DNR) status, symptom burden, and type of oncological treatment. Most patients in palliative oncological trials who receive chemotherapy have a performance status above 60–70 and consequently an expected survival of more than 6 months with large variations depending upon the primary diagnosis. A second category of patients are those admitted to a palliative care programme, either as in-patients or as out-patients, but not imminently dying often with an average survival of 1–3 months. And the third category may be the imminently dying patients with a Karnofsky performance status of 30–40 and lower. This latter category can be divided into a group of cognitively intact and cognitively impaired patients (Table 4).

The content of the assessment tools, the total length of instrument, and the use of proxy raters are some of the important issues to consider in relation to the patient population being investigated.

Compliance and patient population

Missing data is a potential source of selection bias in cancer research and quality assurance programme.[36] The missing data are not random—patients in poorest health, with shortest life expectancy are the noncompliers.[37] When data are missing for some patients, basic questions arise as to whether the patients with missing data differ from those with complete datasets. In order to evaluate the scientific report and to compare

Table 4 Patient population in palliative care. A suggestion of classification

	Expected survival	Karnofsky
Primary palliation	>6 months	60–70
Early palliation	2–3 months	50–60
Late palliation	<1 month	30–40
Immediately dying	<1–2 weeks	≤10

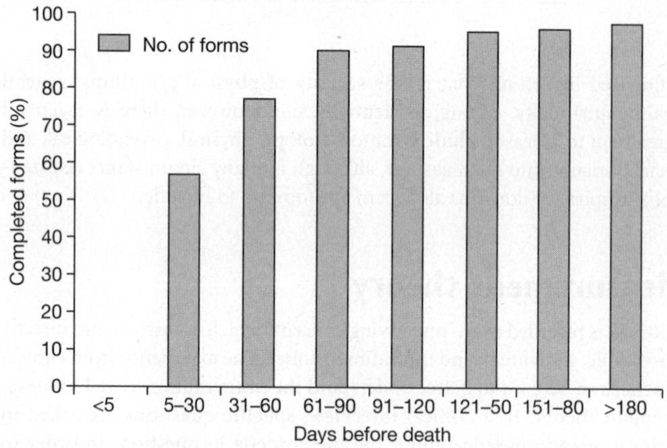

Fig. 4 Number of HRQOL forms completed in proportion to those distributed within various time frames prior to patients' death.

cohorts between studies a standard reporting system of compliance, including all available information, should be required. Compliance is often defined as the number of questionnaires completed as a proportion of the number expected. The issue of compliance is described in greater detail in textbooks[38] and in the statistical literature.[39] In this chapter some issues relating to compliance in palliative care will be discussed.

When patients become increasingly ill with progressive disease, they will find it difficult to complete questionnaires. Acceptable compliance can be achieved with HRQOL questionnaires in palliative care, though several patients will need assistance to complete the measures. During end of life care, the last 1–2 months of the patient's life, more patients will need help to complete the assessment tools due to cognitive impairment, severe symptom distress, and/or emotional burdens, and consequently compliance decreases substantially if help is not provided,[40] (Fig. 4). Patients who are nearly dying will experience many distressing symptoms, and if they are excluded from not just research but also quality assurance and in evaluating clinical practice, there is a potential of lack of systematic treatment procedures for this fragile population.[41]

Proxy ratings

Proxies may be considered as an alternative or complementary source of information, especially during end of life care.[42] However, there has been a general negative attitude towards the use of proxy rating in the HRQOL literature because it has been repetitively argued that assessment directly from the patient is the most valid way of collecting subjective data.

Review articles[43,44] and commentaries[45,46] have been written on the topic of caregivers and significant others as raters. Most of the published articles, which address this issue, relate to general cancer populations or those in 'early palliation'. The studies have been criticized because of small sample sizes, major limitations in methodology, and use of unstandardized

Table 5 Limitations of proxy ratings

A better understanding of when and why proxy ratings and patients ratings differ
Simpler and shorter assessment tools
Instruments with known psychometric properties, a clinically understandable measure, and directly comparable to a patient ratings

ad hoc instruments. The findings of the published studies are not totally consistent; however they can be summarized as follows:

- Health care providers tend to overestimate patients' anxiety, depression, and general psychological distress.
- Agreement between health care providers and patients' ratings was better in the absence of distress than in the presence of distress.
- Pain and other symptoms seem to be underestimated.
- Proxy rating seems to be more accurate when the domains are concrete and observable.

There are several unanswered questions related to the use of proxy raters (Table 5): the limitation of proxy data, the content of proxy rating instruments, and the development of a common measure.

Even with these limitations caregivers or health care providers can be recommended as proxy raters and it is probably best to use one of the short validated tools in order to compare data between studies and allow for familiarity of measures for the clinicians. The COOP/WONCA chart,(47) Edmonton Symptom Assessment Schedule (ESAS),(48) or EORTC QOLQ C-30(49) are examples of such instruments. Another alternative is the SF-8,(50) which has not been validated in palliative care populations. This instrument has the advantage that it can be scored on the same measures as the SF-36 scales and its summary measures.(21)

However, before proxy ratings can be recommended outside a methodological research setting in palliative care, measurement tools and report systems need to be further developed into a user-friendly format and the strengths and limitations of proxy ratings need to be addressed.

Questionnaires

The rapidily increasing number of questionnaires available makes it a challenge to choose the right measure. The first step in the selection procedure is to specify the aims of the project or clinical problems in question and to compare these with the content of the questionnaire. It is generally recommended to assess HRQOL with multidimensional instruments because such measures are more comprehensive than unidimensional scales.(51) The HRQOL measures are commonly divided into generic, disease-specific, and domain-specific. The generic measures are not specific to any population or disease. They are therefore applicable for subjects with more than one condition, and they make comparisons across populations and conditions possible. The disease-specific measures are developed for specific groups of patients, for example, the EORTC-QLQ-C30 and the FACT(49,52) or instruments specifically developed for palliative care. Most of the instruments include various aspects of functioning such as physical, role, and social functioning, and subjective appraisal of symptoms and well being.(53) Most recent generic and disease-specific instruments also assess positive health; that is, good health and well being and not merely the absence of problems.(54) The domain-specific instruments assess specific domains within the overall concept of HRQOL, such as fatigue, pain, or psychological distress. Assessments of QOL will often include combinations of generic, disease-specific, and domain-specific instruments based upon the specific purpose of the study. For example, if one wants to compare the effects of single fraction irradiation with multiple fractions in a population with painful bone metastasis, a disease-specific questionnaire such as the EORTC-QLQ-C30 in combination with domain-specific questionnaires of measurement of pain might be relevant. The number of questionnaires must fit the purpose of the assessment, but must also be balanced against the burden upon the respondents and the costs of the data collection. The increased amount of information gained by including domain-specific measures is not always obvious and is clearly dependent on the psychometric properties, the content, and the sensitivity of the instruments. For example, if a fatigue instrument does not have better measurement qualities than the fatigue scale within a generic or disease-specific instrument, it is probably best not to be included because of the increased burden to the patient.

Comparative data on various instruments measuring the same constructs are relatively scarce. The researcher might be best off by choosing instruments that are commonly used and found relevant within similar populations and settings. By choosing commonly used instruments, one's finding can more easily be evaluated in a broader perspective. The psychometric properties of an instrument might vary across populations, therefore applying a questionnaire for the first time within a 'new population', generally requires retesting of the psychometric properties of the instrument.

A good example of this phenomenon is the assessment of depression. Measures of depression have been developed for psychiatric populations, such as The Beck Depression Inventory and Hamilton's Depression Scale.(55,56) They include several somatic depressive symptoms, such as fatigue, weight loss, and sleeping difficulties, which confound the assessment of depression in somatically ill patients.(57) The use of these instruments in a palliative care population without testing the measurement properties in this group of patients might overestimate the prevalence of 'depressive symptomatology' caused by the disease itself and not by a depressive condition.

In the following some commonly used instruments are briefly discussed. This does not imply that these instruments are superior to other available instruments.

Generic instruments

The first instruments were published in the 1970s and 1980s, such as the Sickness Impact Profile (SIP)(58) and the Nottingham Health Profile.(20) For a more detailed description we refer to other reviews.(29,54,59) The first generation of instruments was generally lengthy and time-consuming to complete.

SF-36

The Short Form 36 (SF-36) is a typical second-generation instrument, developed from a larger questionnaire.(21) Eight concepts that were not specific to any disease, age, population, or treatment group were chosen to measure health conceptualized in two main dimensions: physical and mental health (Table 6). The instrument should satisfy minimum psychometric standards necessary for group comparisons. The psychometric properties are generally very good with Cronbachs alphas in the range 0.80–0.93.(22) The instrument is available in two versions: a standard version with a timeframe of 4 weeks and an acute version with a timeframe of 1 week. The SF-36 has been translated into more than 40 languages, and considerable effort has been made for international harmonization of the instrument and collection of normative data through the IQOLA-project.(60,61)

The SF-36 physical and mental component summary scales capture about 85 per cent of the reliable variance in the instrument.(62) On this background it was decided that a questionnaire with fewer items could be constructed. Twelve items from the SF-36 were therefore selected and the instrument labelled the SF-12,(63) and later the even shorter SF-8.(50) The SF-12 reproduces the eight-scale profile of the SF-36. It yields less-precise scores, as would be expected for single- and two-item scales.

WHOQOL

The WHO has developed the WHO quality of life assessment instrument (WHOQOL).(64) The instrument was developed, according to a standardized protocol, simultaneously in several languages and cultures at 15 international centres.(65) The original instrument encompasses five domains measured by 100 items: physical health, psychological health, level of independence, social relationship, spirituality, and environment. Each domain includes several facets, in total 24. Each facet contains four items, and the last four items measure overall QOL and general health. The validity of the instrument is not fully documented. Because of the limitations posed upon

Table 6 Some commonly used generic and disease-specific HRQOL-questionnaires

Name	Type	Domains	No. of items	First publ.	Ref.
WHOQOL	Generic	Physical Psychological Independence Social relations Environment Spirituality Overall QOL	100	1993	
WHOQOL-BREF	Generic	Physical Psychological Social relations Environment	26	1998	
SF-36	Generic	Health transition General health Bodily pain Physical function Role function, physical Role function, emotional Vitality Mental health Social function	36	1992	
SF-12	Generic	Physical Mental	12	1996	
SF-8			8	1999?	
EORTC QLQ C-30	Disease-specific (cancer)	Physical Cognitive Emotional Social +8 symptoms	30	1993	
FACT-G	Disease-specific (cancer)	Physical Social/family Emotional Functional	27	1993	

the use of the instrument's length, a 26-item abbreviated scale has been published, primarily for use in epidemiological studies.[66]

Disease-specific measures

EORTC QOL-C30

The development of the cancer-specific questionnaires, the EORTC QLQ-C30 (European Organization for Research and Treatment of Cancer) started in 1980, and the first 30-item version was finalized in 1993.[49] Modified versions have been published and the group recommends version 3.0 of the questionnaire.[67] The questionnaire covers five functional scales (physical, role, cognitive, emotional, and social), general QOL, three symptom scales, (fatigue, pain, and nausea and vomiting) and six single items. The single items assess common symptoms in cancer patients such as dyspnoea, loss of appetite, insomnia, constipation, and diarrhoea. Two items ask for overall evaluation of health and QOL. These two items have seven response choices, all the other items have four response choices. The scores for each functional scale, symptom scale, and single item are transformed to scales with a possible range of scores from 0 to 100. For the functional scales, a higher score means higher level of functioning while for the symptom scales/items, a higher score means a higher level of symptoms.

The timeframe for the assessment is 1 week, which may be of particular relevance in clinical trials. The instrument is copyrighted. The questionnaire is translated and validated in 38 languages and has been used in more than 1500 studies worldwide. The instrument has good psychometric properties including test–retest reliability.[68,69] This is an important characteristic of the instrument because it was originally developed for use in clinical trials. The instrument has also been used for other purposes such as studying the communication between patient and physician.[70]

The so-called modular approach adopted by the EORTC QOL Group infers that the core questionnaire can be supplemented with additional questionnaires designed for specific cancer sites.[71] These include disease-specific supplements for lung cancer (LC13),[72] breast cancer (BR23),[73] and head and neck cancer (H&N35).[74] Phase III modules that are available include modules for bladder cancer, brain cancer, colorectal cancer, gastric cancer, multiple myeloma, ophthalmic cancer, pancreatic cancer, prostate cancer, and satisfaction with care. The modules that are presently being field-tested are the oesophageal and ovarian modules. At present, no specific module for palliative care exists. Updates on the latest development of the EORTC questionnaires are found in the website[67] www.eortc.be/home/qol/eortc.

FACT-G

The Functional Assessment of Cancer—General Version (the FACT-G) is part of a measurement system called Functional Assessment of Chronic Illness Therapy (FACIT) intended for use in chronic diseases. The FACT-G was first published in 1993 and includes 27 items arranged in subscales covering four dimensions: physical well being, social/family well being, emotional well being, and functional well being.[52] Each of the items has five response alternatives and scores for each scale are sums of subscale scores; a total score is also provided. In the latest versions of FACIT the subjects are asked to rate the impact of each domain of overall QOL. The timeframe is 1 week, and the psychometric properties are reported as comparable to the EORTC QLQ-C30.[52] There seems to be a tendency for the FACT-G to be used more frequently in the United States than in Europe, while the EORTC QLQ-C30 is used primarily in Europe.

The FACIT measurement system has also adopted a modular approach with cancer-specific, symptom-specific, and treatment-specific subscales. This includes, among others, two instruments for measurement of anaemia and fatigue.[75] For an update on the complete FACIT measurement system refer to the study group's website[76] www.facit.org/facit_questionnair.htm.

Domain-specific measures

Generic or disease-specific instruments might not be sensitive enough for detection of differences in HRQOL. Questionnaires, also called domain-specific instruments, have been designed to assess specific symptoms, such as pain, fatigue, and anxiety. In some instances these types of instruments might be preferable to use. Numerous instruments are available, and for a more comprehensive description we refer to relevant textbooks.[29,59] For example, in a study of patients with advanced prostate cancer, the EORTC QLQ-C30 fatigue scale did not detect variations in fatigue over time whereas two fatigue-specific instruments captured group differences.[77] This finding may be related to the so-called floor and ceiling effects. A ceiling effect occurs when a high proportion of the total respondents grade themselves as having the maximum score and a floor effect is an excessive use of the minimum values of the scales.

Anxious and depressive symptoms

Domain-specific instruments for measurement of anxiety and depression are generally old and many researchers and clinicians will regard them as first-generation instruments. For example, the Hospital Anxiety and Depression Scale (the HADS) was constructed in 1983, but it has relatively recently been recommended for use in oncology and in palliative care.[78–80] Other commonly used instruments for measurement of depression such as the Beck Depression Inventory (BDI) and Hamilton Depression Scale (HDS) were first published as early as the 1960s.[55,56]

For instruments measuring anxiety and depression in palliative care it is important to examine for somatic items (fatigue, weight-loss, loss of appetite, etc.). Such symptoms are valid symptoms of anxious and depressive conditions in psychiatric and healthy populations, and they are included in the present diagnostic criteria for these disorders.[81] However, these symptoms are not valid to measure anxiety and depression in palliative care because they may only reflect the underlying somatic disease. For example, five of the 21 items in the BDI are of a somatic nature. In spite of the relatively extensive research literature addressing this methodological challenge, many published papers do not pay attention to the consequences of including somatic items in assessments of anxiety and depression in the physically ill. HADS is one of the most frequently used instrument for measuring anxious (seven items) and depressive symptoms (seven items) in oncology and palliative medicine. Five of the items constituting the depression subscale are about anhedonia, one item is about mood, and one is about retardation. HADS is therefore affected by somatic status to a higher degree than stated by the constructors and assumed by many users. Further, anhedonia is probably influenced by somatic condition to a much higher extent than previously recognized. It has been demonstrated that a total score, including both the anxiety and depression subscales, is a better predictor of major depression in palliative care patients than scores on the depressive subscale.[82] This partly reflects the fact that recent progress in the measurement of depressive symptoms and in the diagnosis of depression among severely ill patients is not integrated in the HADS.

Fatigue

Fatigue is the most frequent symptom in palliative care and is experienced by nearly all patients with advanced disease.[83,84] In palliative care, as opposed to healthy populations, fatigue only weakly correlates with psychological distress and probably reflects the subjective experience of being ill.[84]

Instruments specifically designed for measuring fatigue were first published in the late 1980s. At present several instruments are available[85,86] and most of these should be classified as first-generation instruments.

Most researchers agree that fatigue is a multidimensional phenomenon, but the number and types of dimensions is debated. All present fatigue-measures include physical fatigue, which corresponds to the subjective feeling of being exhausted and lacking energy. A short (11 items) fatigue instrument, Fatigue Questionnaire (FQ), measures fatigue in two dimensions: physical and mental fatigue.[87] Mental fatigue is about the subjective experience of being mentally exhausted, and the items are about concentration, memory, and speech. The FQ has good and stable psychometric properties across quite different populations, but the wording of the response categories is problematic in palliative care because they ask about a comparison with what is usual. For cancer patients with active disease for several years, such a comparison might be confusing.

Pain

Pain is the second most prevalent symptom in palliative care, and for the majority of patients it is the most distressing symptom. It is well documented that pain is underdiagnosed and often undertreated when diagnosed.[88] Pain is also the main target for pharmacological interventions during palliative care. In general, pain is included as single items or as separate subscales in all existing generic and disease-specific instruments. It is also important to underscore that pain is a complicated and controversial area for assessment, although some of the problems are reflecting general challenges for HRQOL assessments. For example, to what extent shall a pain assessment include assessment of physical and emotional distress caused by pain? How shall pain be measured in patients receiving analgesics? How to deal with pain thresholds which vary between individuals and with each individual's access to support? What about differentiating between specific types of pain? How to measure specific cancer pains such as break-through pain?

Domain-specific tools for measurement of pain, such as the (MPQ), measure pain as a multidimensional phenomenon, but it is rather extensive and thereby often difficult to apply in debilitated palliative care patients.[89] A shorter version of this instrument has been developed and validated.[90] Others, for example, the Brief Pain Inventory (BPI),[91] measure the impact of pain upon physical functioning in addition to measuring pain intensity. There is reason to question whether functional consequences of pain can be validly separated from functional limitations due to other factors.[92] This point is of particular relevance in palliative care because of the complexity of the disease process, functional limitations, and the appearance of several symptoms at the same time.

In most situations, pain intensity is the main target for pain measurements. Additional aspects such as variation in pain over time, pain triggered by physical activity or break-through pain might be of relevance in many situations. In such cases, available instruments must be evaluated for their properties in measuring these aspects of the pain experience.

Use of single items

The use of single items either as self-constructed items or as items borrowed from a complete instrument is generally not recommended. The validity of self-constructed items is generally uncertain and moving an item from its context might affect the responses. However, if one wants to measure, for example, sleep, very few instruments include item(s) on this important aspect of health and disease. Instead of constructing single items, it is preferable to use items that have been developed and validated as part of multidimensional questionnaires. The EORTC QLQ C-30 includes one item about problems with sleeping.[49] This item measures the subjective experience of having sleeping difficulties but does not describe them in detail, difficulty in getting off to sleep, frequent wakening, early wakening or hypo-/hypersomnia. Given the importance of sleep for many patients and the high prevalence of sleep disturbances in palliative care, improved instruments for assessing sleep are required.

Cognitive impairment

Cognitive impairment as part of dementia, amnestic disorder, or delirium is prevalent in palliative care.[93] Among patients with terminal cancers, 20–40 per cent develop delirium or other neuropsychiatric conditions.[94]

We are not aware of any HRQOL studies in cancer patients, which have discussed their results in relation to possible cognitive impairment among the subjects. Cognitive impairment affects completion rate, data quality, and possibly the validity of HRQOL studies in palliative care.

Interviews conducted by health care providers by means of specific interview guides and observation are the most appropriate methods for the detection of cognitive impairment. The subjective experience of cognitive impairment is weakly related to neuropsychiatric disturbances but much stronger to psychological distress.[95] Consequently, the cognitive functioning scale within HRQOL questionnaires might measure mental fatigue rather than cognitive functioning. The most commonly used interview-based instruments in assessments of cognitive impairment in palliative care is the Mini Mental State Examination (MMSE) and the Memorial Delirium Assessment Scale (MDAS).[96,97] Physicians or other health professionals can administer these measures without specific preparation although it is wise to compare first-time performances with more experienced personnel as part of the introduction routines into a research project or clinical practice. The MDAS is a brief, reliable tool for assessing delirium severity, while the MMSE is designed for diagnosing cognitive impairment irrespective of the cause or neuropsychiatric diagnosis. For the MMSE it has been demonstrated that the score of 12 selected items scored binomially is equally efficient as the sum score of all the 20 items in identifying cognitive impairment in elderly patients.[98] However, more research is needed before such an abbreviated version can be recommended.

Palliative care-specific

A short-form individual quality of life questionnaire (SEIQOL)

During the last decade several HRQOL instruments have been developed and validated within palliative care. A short summary of some of these scales will be described. The schedule for the evaluation of individual QOL (SEIQOL) was developed in order to let the patient assess QOL from an individual perspective without imposing a predetermined set of items to respond to. It was designed specifically to assess three questions: what areas of life are important, how is the individual doing in each of these areas, and what is the importance of the area?[99]

The SEIQOL is a complex measure and its use in routine clinical practice may prove impractical. An abbreviated form has been developed recently, the SEIQOL-direct weighting (SEIQOL-DW)[100] and validated in a population of advanced cancer patients.[101] One limitation in the study was the high number of exclusions of terminally ill patients. It was concluded that the SEIQOL-DW seems most appropriate for routine clinical settings, while the original SEIQOL is more suitable for in-depth exploration of QOL.

Therapy impact questionnaire (TIQ)

Therapy impact questionnaire (TIQ) is a 36-item questionnaire assessing both disease and therapy impact, and divided into four dimensions—physical symptoms, functional status, emotional and cognitive domains, and social interaction.[102]

The questionnaire has been validated in Italy in a population with advanced cancer. To our knowledge the questionnaire is not extensively used outside Italy.

McGill quality of life questionnaire (MQOL)

MQOL is a 17-item questionnaire derived from patient interviews, literature review, and existing instruments.[103] The instrument was designed in response to the criticism that existing HRQOL instruments developed for cancer patients in general lacked questions on existential concerns.[104] The instrument consists of five distinct subscales: physical well being, physical symptoms, psychological symptoms, existential well being, and support (or relationships).[31,105] The questionnaire was validated in a multicentre study with patients recruited from palliative care services and later in a combined population consisting of oncology out-patients and palliative care services.[106] MQOL has recently been validated cross-culturally in a Hong Kong Chinese population and found to be cross-culturally robust.[107] The reliability was found to be satisfactory for use on a group level, but not on an individual level. The MQOL is shown to be responsive to detect changes between good and bad days.

The Missoula-VITAS quality of life index

The subjective experience of an individual living with the interpersonal, psychological and existential, or spiritual challenges accompanying advanced disease was used as the basic definition when this instrument was developed, focusing on the terminal phase of life.[32] The instrument is composed of 25 items and the content is based upon a literature review, formal interview of hospice professionals, patients, and their family members. It has been validated in a hospice setting. It covers five domains: symptoms, function, interpersonal, well being, and spirituality. Most questions are of a global nature, including the assessment of symptoms. The instrument seems most suitable for use in the planning of care and probably in quality control. The validity of the questionnaire needs to be explored in greater detail.

The life evaluation questionnaire (LEQ)

The LEQ is a 45-item questionnaire developed to evaluate aspects of life that are relevant to patients with incurable cancer and that are not measured by established questionnaires.[108] The content is based upon in-depth interviews with patients and carers. The instrument consists of five main domains, freedom versus restrictions, appreciation of life, contentment, resentment, and social interaction.

McMaster quality of life scale (MQLS)

This measure was developed to assess QOL from the palliative care patients' perspective.[109] It is a 32-item questionnaire measuring physical, emotional, social, and spiritual domains. Each domain is subdivided into scales with low (0.09) to moderate high (0.79) internal consistency. Each item is rated on a seven-point NRS. A parallel form is used for family and staff ratings. The interater reliability was satisfactory within the patient population, while the agreement between patient and family ($r = 0.64$) and patient and staff ($r = 0.50$) was moderate.

HRQOL—during end of life care or for the dying

Research on QOL for the dying patient is sparse—probably related to several factors, such as a lack of focus on dying patients and the dying process in general ('the battle is lost—why bother with it'). Furthermore, the dying patient is vulnerable and the ethics related to the research is debatable.

There are several methodological challenges related to HRQOL assessment in the dying, including the rapid change in most biological processes and loss of cognition, which is highly relevant to the ability to collect subjective data. As previously pointed out, there are major problems with compliance in this subpopulation with the use of traditional HRQOL questionnaires (Table 7). In most palliative care programmes the aim is to support the family to care for the dying at home in addition to providing specialist professional care. Consequently the team is caring for the patient in a family network. In end of life care 12 important domains of physicians have been identified by patients; acceptability and continuity, team co-ordination and communication, communication with patients, patient education, inclusion and recognition of family, competence, pain and symptom management, emotional control, personalization, attention to patient values, respect and humanity, and support for patient decision making.[110]

Another group involved in the development of assessment tools for patients with life limiting illness, reached similar conclusions: the outcome

Table 7 Palliative care-specific HRQOL questionnaires

Name	Domains	No. of items	Ref.
SEIQOL	Self-determined		
TIQ	Physical Functional Emotional Cognitive	36	
MRQOL	Physical well being Physical symptoms Psychological symptoms Existential well being Support	17	
Missoula-VITAS	Symptoms Function Interpersonal Well being Transcendence	25	
LEQ	Freedom versus restriction Appreciation of life Contentment Resentment Social interaction	45	

Table 8 Quality at the end of life

Important domains
Singer:[112]
Symptom management
Avoiding inappropriate prolongation of dying
Achieving sense of control
Relieving burden
Strengthening of relationship between loved ones

should be patient focused and family centred, clinical meaningful, administratively manageable, and psychometrically sound.[111]

QOL assessment is by definition subjective in nature. In the dying patient, who is cognitively impaired, 'subjective data' needs to be collected by observers.

There is a lack of validated instruments specifically designed for dying patients; however, there is a growing literature addressing measurement issues for this patient population, focusing on the development of a conceptual framework.[112,113]

In summary one may say that the patient-focused assessment recommended is very similar to the strategy developed earlier in the disease trajectory, focusing on symptom control and how to relieve patient burden. However, during end of life care spiritual and existential issues need to be addressed in greater detail in addition to family members' perception of quality of care (Table 8).

Family satisfaction, HRQOL, grief, and other domains may be used as an outcome of quality of death. A variety of instruments have been used in the published studies to examine different aspects and models of care,[114–117] and no consensus on content or on type of instruments seems to be arrived upon. In several studies a general high level of satisfaction with care has been observed and only minor differences between various palliative care programmes, which may indicate a poor ability of the existing instruments to discriminate between groups when measuring satisfaction with care and HRQOL.[118–123]

How to measure HRQOL during end of life care?

The complexity, length, and content of the existing HRQOL instruments seem inappropriate for use during the dying process. Shorter and simpler instruments are needed here. To our knowledge there is no single instrument widely used for this purpose, but simple NRS have been developed. The ESAS is a short 10-item instrument[124] and has been used extensively in several scientific reports by the Edmonton group.[125] Other symptom assessment schedules are also used, such as the Memorial Symptom Assessment Scale Short Form (MSAS-SF), which is one of the several alternatives for symptom assessment. However, there is a lack of consensus on how to measure HRQOL in the dying patient. New, shorter and more comprehensive instruments need to be developed, which ideally could be completed by both the patient and proxy raters in sequence.

Analysis and interpretation of data

Clinical significance

What is the clinical relevance of a summary score or a single item when comparing groups of patients or individuals? This is one basic question to ask both in daily clinical practice, in interpreting clinical research, and in sample size calculation in the planning process of a clinical trial. The clinical significance is related to the importance of the symptoms or the sign.

In pain assessment a numerical rating scale ranging from 0 to 10 is often used as a simple unidimensional outcome. When discussing the clinical significance of a pain score, two important questions need to be answered: what is a relevant cut off point in order to classify the pain score in need of intervention? What is the minimum improvement on a pain measure, say on a 0–10 scale in a randomized trial, comparing two different pain medications in order to consider the difference to be of clinical importance?

Change in any clinical variable, independent of the nature of the variable, that is, physiological (blood pressure), psychological (anxiety), and performance (physical ability), needs to be interpretated in a clinical framework. It is not a methodological or statistical question whether a change of 20 on a scale from 0 to 100 is of clinical significance. In order to be able to make a valid judgement on the magnitude of a measure in order to regard it as 'clinically significant', the clinician needs at least to understand the nature of the measure, including insight into the content of the composite score, the clinical meaning of the measure, and how it relates to individual patients. The discussion on clinical significance is not unique to QOL assessment. Similar discussions arise, for example, in interpreting the clinical significance of blood pressure medication, in interpreting the reduction of tumour size in oncology caused by chemotherapy, and in the importance of change in median survival in patients with non-small-cell lung cancer admitted to a randomized chemotherapy trial.

These are some of the general problems. A more specific problem related to palliative care is the interpretation of change in several QOL estimates in the same study (Table 9). The outcome is by nature multidimensional, the estimate is often based on a summary score of several questions, and a common metric does not apply between scales and domains (i.e. is 40 on a pain measure similar in symptom burden to 40 on a nausea measure?). In palliative care where most patients are living with a progressive disease, improvement in overall condition cannot be expected, thus the 'improvement' expected on a single or a multiple measure may actually be merely a 'slow down' or stabilization of symptom burden. The complexity of human biology may cause an increase in intensity in one symptom when another symptom is relieved. Furthermore, most patients have a mosaic of symptoms, which often needs broad interventions, and consequently one specific outcome may be difficult to identify.

Multidimensionality

The strength of the HRQOL concept is its multidimensionality; however, during analysis (see later) and in the interpretation of the outcomes, the multidimensionality is a problem. Based upon a careful clinical consideration, it is recommended to identify the primary outcomes, that is, the domains of most importance, before the study is launched. Outcomes should be limited to two or three and the remaining data from the HRQOL questionnaire must be considered as additional information, and should not be used as an indicator for change of practice.

Table 9 Problems related to outcome interpretation

Multidimensionality	Generic
Content of the measure	Generic
No common metric	Generic
Heterogenic intervention	Palliative care-specific
Multiple problems (symptoms)	Palliative care-specific
Progressive disease	Palliative care-specific

Content of the measure

Measures may consist of multiple questions. Before any questionnaire is applied in the study, the researcher and the clinician need to investigate in detail the content of each scale. The content is the basis for a clinical understanding of the score. Without an intuitive understanding of the measure, a valid judgement of the final estimate is difficult. The use of several HRQOL methods reduces the chances for an intuitive understanding of the outcomes. Therefore, the number of methods should be kept to a minimum both for clinical monitoring and for clinical research.

The lack of a common measure between scales within the same instrument is a problem. How much this phenomenon also influences the size of what is a clinical significant change in the instrument is still an unresolved question.

In a recent systematic review on HRQOL in palliative care no clear pattern was found in how various researchers address this issue.[126] In some reports a group mean change of 10 on a 0–100 scale has been proposed as a clinically significant difference.[127] Others have said that half a standard deviation is a clinically significant difference, which is close to 10 on a 0–100 scale.

Data presentation

HRQOL has become mandatory in many cancer clinical trials, and in palliative medicine HRQOL domains are the primary outcome in most studies.

A careful evaluation of the aims of the study is crucial in the planning process in order to be able to identify the primary outcomes. For example, in a study of the effects of cardiocentesis for pericardial effusions in patients with advanced cancer, it is reasonable to consider pain, physical functioning, and dyspnoea as the primary outcomes and not changes on ultrasound or X-ray. The design of the study and the choice of explanatory and primary outcome variables are the main determinants in choosing the appropriate analysis strategy. The design and the variables should reflect the aims of the study, so the analytical strategy is, in large part determined before the actual analysis starts.

No one wants to end up in a situation in which an important explanatory variable has not been included in the data collection although many probably have. This implies that the data analyses should have been planned far before the study was initiated, and ideally all tables (not the numbers) should have been constructed during the planning process of the study. Clear hypotheses will definitely make this work easier and will reduce the possibilities for the researcher ending up in endless searches for significant *P*-values.

Still, many studies must be conducted without the possibility to perform confirmatory tests of predefined hypotheses, for example, prevalence studies. Neither can one single study support a whole series of hypotheses. It is therefore sensible to limit the number of confirmatory hypotheses, and much of the analytical process therefore has to be exploratory (i.e. suggested by the data). In the latter situation it is possible to test specific hypotheses suggested by the data, but then the *P*-values should be used as guidelines and treated carefully.

If the limit for statistical significance is set at 0.05, then each 20th analysis will by chance reach statistical significance. Typically this occurs in univariate tests in prospective studies, where at a particular time-point a subscale demonstrates statistically significant differences between groups. This can seriously inflate the type-I (false positive) error rate. Irrespective of the possible clinical consequences, this problem makes it difficult for the researcher to distinguish between true and false positive differences. There are several possible ways in which to handle this problem, although none of them are ideal and the literature does not suggest one specific strategy. Common sense and careful consideration will always be the basis of analysis and interpretation. Possible solutions are suggested in other reviews and papers.[38,128,129] In the planning phase of a study, the problem can best be solved by stating clearly which scales within the battery of HRQOL assessments, are defined as the primary outcomes (e.g. pain and fatigue). These variables will then be in the focus of the analysis and correction for multiplicity of endpoints might perhaps be unnecessary. For the rest of the scales the number of analyses should be reduced as much as possible, and some type of correction for the multiplicity of endpoints, either by Bonferroni correction and similar methods or by the use of more conservative *P*-values (e.g. $P < 0.01$). The interpretation of the latter analyses should reflect that the analyses are hypothesis generating and the results indicate a need for confirmation in later studies.

Several strategies have been proposed for solving the problem of non-random missing data. Imputation of missing data is not any problem if the data are missing by random. It is also a preferable strategy if the missing data are not-random, for example, related to disease status or subsequent death. However, before imputation is performed, careful analyses of patterns for missing data are necessary to identify the bias in the existing data. Missing scores in prospective studies may be imputed by carrying the last value forward. Imputation of missing items within multi-item scales can be achieved by calculating person-specific means for the items within the scale that has been filled in. For missing single items no good strategy exists. Instruments such as the SF-36 and the EORTC QLQ C-30 include algorithms for imputation of missing data.[130,131] Although exclusion of all subjects with missing data definitely introduces a bias, imputation of missing values without prior examination of possible patterns for missing data is not recommended. For more detailed descriptions of other aspects of analyses of HRQOL data we refer to textbooks in medical statistics and HRQOL assessments.[29,38]

There is at present increasing focus upon a transparent presentation of research data, and we strongly advise the presentation of data in accordance with the predefined aims of the study. The CONSORT statement includes 21 items that should be presented in a paper. The essence is that the researchers shall provide enough information about the study so the reader can judge the reliability of the results.[132] In the situation described above, it is correct to tell the reader how the study was designed, and that the main findings were carried out as predefined secondary endpoints.

A related challenge is the treatment of criteria for statistical significance, because most HRQOL measurements include multiple endpoints and this may lead to the so-called multisignificance problem. It is generally recommended to include all assessments in the presentation, but this may lead to data overload in the paper. This requires careful consideration and some pragmatism, but the presentation of the data shall always reflect the original protocol. In many instances the authors therefore end up with several endpoints, and in most cases it is therefore correct to perform some sort of adjustment for the multiplicity of endpoints, as mentioned previously.

A detailed checklist for presentation of HRQOL studies has been presented.[133] In general, this guideline is in accordance with the general rules for writing a paper. However, there are some specific points to notice for HRQOL studies apart from the points commented upon above.

Relatively few HRQOL studies examine specific hypotheses since observational studies are by far the commonest type of study. Accordingly, the rationale for selection of HRQOL instruments should be presented. The population should be described in terms of those variables that can affect the outcome variables. These include interalia age, gender, ethnicity, educational status, functional status, timing of the assessments, compliance, data completeness, and attrition due to death.[134] In palliative care, functional status and time to death are variables that strongly influence the results of the measurements.[135]

Computer-adaptive testing

Several reports indicate that doctors and health professionals both in general oncology and in palliative care do not recognize subjective symptoms in their patients.[136–138] These findings may be related to the fact that measurement of HRQOL has not become an integral part of clinical practice. There are probably several explanations to these shortcomings, such as the content of the measures, that is, many of the scales may not have enough clinical relevance, clinicians do not believe in the importance of assessing subjective experience and/or the impracticalities in using comprehensive measures in daily clinical practice. These comprehensive measures may be difficult to interpret and not easily accessible in the clinical decision-making process. Furthermore, HRQOL instruments display Cronbach alphas ranging from 0.80 to 0.90, which is not high enough for individual assessments.

The distribution of HRQOL questionnaires in paper format has until now been the standard administration form although some recent studies have administered the HRQOL instruments as computer-based touch-screen programmes with promising results.[28,139] The existing measures are a compromise between shortness and precision, shortness as a consequence of the paper and pencil format and lack of precision because of the shortness of the questionnaire. A patient's functional capacity must be covered by relatively few items, and subjects with functional capacity at one extreme say best possible function must answer rather irrelevant items covering the opposite extreme of the functional range. For example, a person responding that he is barely able to walk 50 m will obviously find an item about the ability to walk 2 miles irrelevant. The result is that the existing measures are somewhat imprecise and display rather large standard deviations. The latter implies that the number of participants must be high to achieve sufficient power in clinical trials. Most instruments also display 'floor- and ceiling-effects', which implies that a substantial number of the respondents tend towards the minimum or maximum scores of the scale, meaning that group differences will not be possible to detect. Another challenge and possible obstacle for taking full advantage of the existing measures is the interpretation of the scores. For all published multidimensional instruments, a score of 50 on a 0–100 scale is not comparable with a numerically identical score on another scale, which is exemplified empirically in that a change in score does not relate linearly to an external criteria.[140]

In palliative care measurement of symptoms may also be restricted by the patients' limited physical capacity, and even relatively short instruments are often too demanding to fill in for many patients.[141] Instruments that yield valid and reliable results with the smallest possible effort for the patients are therefore urgently needed. Instruments that are suitable both for individual assessments (i.e. diagnosis and monitoring of individual patients) and for research have, therefore, obvious advantages for the clinicians, the patients, and the researchers. Ideally, measures of subjective symptoms should be precise, easy to administer, and be filled in with the smallest possible effort by the doctor and the patient.

Modern psychometric methods like the Rasch models and the Item Response Theory (IRT) have great potential to achieve precise and efficient measurement of subjective symptoms at individual patient level.[142,143] The basic idea of these methods is that a particular response to a particular item depends on the type of item (item difficulty) and on the underlying (latent) health construct. Both item difficulty and the respondent's ability are measured on the same scale or ruler. Combining IRT with a computer algorithm allows individualized selection of items to provide the most precise information for the particular patient and to score all items on a common scale. On the basis of the answer to the first question, the computer will select a new question, and in the next step the computer will select a new question based on the answer to the second question and so forth until a preset level of precision is reached. This approach can be illustrated by measurement of depression. It is demonstrated that a single question: 'Are you depressed?' is a good predictor of depression in patients with advanced cancer.[144] Assessment of depression within the IRT system could start with such a question. The next questions would then build on the answers to the first, and one will consequently achieve a precise estimation of the level of depression.

CAT methodology uses a computer interface for the patient (or a computerized interview/clinician report) that is tailored to the unique ability level of the patient. The basic notion of an adapted test is to mimic what an experienced clinician would do. A clinician learns most when he/she directs questions at the patient's approximate level of proficiency. Administering functional items that are either too easy or too hard provides little information. An adaptive test first asks questions in the middle of the ability range, and then directs questions to an appropriate level based on the patient's responses, without asking unnecessary questions. This allows for fewer items to be administered (individual respondent, interview, or clinical judgement) while gaining precise information regarding an individual's placement along a continuum of functional ability. CAT applications require a large set of items in any one functional or symptom area (item pools), items that consistently scale along a dimension of low to high functional proficiency, and rules guiding starting, stopping, and scoring procedures.[142]

The psychometric methods that make it possible to calibrate questionnaire items on a standard metric ('ruler') also yield the algorithms necessary to run the 'engine' that powers CAT assessments. These statistical models tell how likely it is that a person at each level of health will choose each response to each survey question. This logic is reversed to estimate the probability of each health score from a particular pattern of item responses. The resulting likelihood function makes it possible to estimate each person's score, along with a person-specific confidence interval.

Doctors or nurses can administer the CAT assessments. Alternatively the patients can respond directly on the computer. The computerized form will allow for more flexible ways of administering the tool, including downloading from the Internet, administration by proxies, and the employment of hand-held devices. Scores will be computed immediately and in digital form. This entire development process was strongly suggested in a recent paper in the British Medical Journal.[144] The latter will make integration with other clinical parameters easier, as patient records generally are more often stored in computerized form.

At present this approach to measurements of subjective symptoms and functioning has not moved outside the research laboratories although the first practical tests have been performed with success in migraine patients.[142]

Summary

QOL is described both as a multidimensional and a unidimensional concept. Multidimensional measures consist of items covering physical, psychological, and social aspects of life. These types of measures are also often called HRQOL measures. In palliative care these types of measures have been criticized for being too limited in not covering the existential and spiritual issues well enough.

A series of measures for use in health care in general (generic instruments), and for use in specific diagnostic groups, such as cancer (cancer-specific) and palliative care (palliative care-specific), have been developed and validated. A third category of instruments are the domain-specific measures. They are developed for assessing specific symptoms or signs, such as pain, fatigue, depression, anxiety, physical function, and spirituality.

Most instruments are developed for use in research and may not be suited for use in daily clinical practice. However, in the future one may expect to have instruments which are computer based and suitable for use in both clinical practice and in research. In the meantime a reasonable strategy is to choose one of the commonly used HRQOL instruments for use in research. The content of the questionnaire needs to be carefully reviewed to ensure that it fits the research questions addressed in each specific project.

References

1. **Aristotle** 384–322BC *Nichomachean Ethics*, Book 1 (Iv). H. Rackham, 1926 (transl.)
2. **Bradburn, N.** *The Structure of Psychological Well-Being*. Chicago IL: Aldine, 1969.
3. **Andrews, F. and Withey, S.** *Social Indicators of Well-Being: Americans' Perceptions of Life Quality*. New York: Plenum, 1976.

4. **Campbell, A., Converse, P., and Rodgers, W.** *The Quality of Life Perceptions, Evaluations, Satisfactions.* New York: Russel Sage Foundation, 1976.
5. **Maslow, A.** *Motivation and Personality.* New York: Harper, 1970.
6. **Naess, S.** *Quality of Life Research. Concepts, Methods and Applications.* Oslo: Institute of Applied Social Research, 1987.
7. **Hjermstad, M., Holte, H., Evensen, S., Fayers, P., and Kaasa, S.** (1999). Do patients who are treated with stem cell transplantation have a health-related quality of life comparable to the general population after 1 year? *Bone Marrow Transplant* **24**, 911–18.
8. **Calman, K.C.** (1984). Quality of life in cancer patients—an hypothesis. *Journal of Medical Ethics* **10**, 124–7.
9. **Priestman, T. and Baum, M.** (1976). Evaluation of quality of life in patients receiving treatment for advanced breast cancer. *Lancet* **1**, 899–901.
10. **Coates, A., Dillenbeck, C., and McNeil, D.** (1983). Linear analogue self-assessment (LASA) in evaluation of apects of the quality of life of cancer patients receiving therapy. *European Journal of Cancer and Clinical Oncology* **19**, 1633–7.
11. **Bergner, M., Bobbitt, R., Carter, W., and Gilson, B.** (1981). The sickness impact profile: development and final revision of a health status measure. *Medical Care* **19**, 787–805.
12. **Wade, D. and Qollin, C.** (1988). The Barthel ADL index: a standard measure of physical disability. *International Disability Studies* **10**, 64–7.
13. **Goldberg, D. and Williams, P.** *A User's Guide to the General Health Questionnaire.* The NFER-NELSON Publishing Company Ltd., 1988.
14. **World Health Organization.** *The First Ten Years of the World Health Organization.* Geneva: World Health Organizations, 1958.
15. **Karnofsky, D.A., Abelmann, W.H., Craver, L.F., and Burchenal, J.H.** (1948). The use of the nitrogen mustrads in the palliative treatment of carcinoma. *Cancer* 634–56.
16. **Coates, A., Porzsolt, F., and Osoba, D.** (1997). Quality of life in oncology practice: prognostic value of EORTC QLQ-C30 scores in patients with advanced malignancy. *European Journal of Cancer* **33**, 1025–30.
17. **Maltoni, M., Pirovano, M., Scarpi, E., Marinari, M., Indelli, M., Arnoldi, E., Gallucci, M., Frontini, L., Piva, L., and Amadori, D.** (1995). Prediction of survival of patients terminally ill with cancer. Results of an Italian prospective multicentric study. *Cancer* **75**, 2613–22.
18. **Lagakos, S.W.** (1983). Prognostic factors for patients with inoperable lung cancer. In *Lung Cancer Clinical Diagnosis and Treatment* (ed. M.J. Straus). New York: Grune and Stratton.
19. **Kaasa, S., Mastekaasa, A., and Lund, E.** (1989). Prognostic factors for patients with inoperable non-small cell lung cancer, limited disease. The importance of patients' subjective experience of disease and psychosocial well-being. *Radiotherapy in Oncology* **15**, 235–42.
20. **Hunt, S.M. and McEwen, J.** (1980). The development of a subjective health indicator. *Sociology of Health & Illness* **2**, 231–46.
21. **Ware, J.E. Jr. and Sherbourne, C.D.** (1992). The MOS 36-item short-form health survey (SF-36). I. Conceptual framework and item selection. *Medical Care* **30**, 473–83.
22. **Ware, J.E. Jr.** (1996). The SF-36 health survey. In *Quality of Life and Pharmaeconomics in Clinical Trials* (ed. B. Spilker). Philadelphia PA: Lippincott-Raven.
23. **McNair, D., Lord, M., and Droppleman, L.** *EITS Manual for the Profile of Mood States.* San Diego CA: Educational Testing Service, 1971.
24. **IASP Task Force on Taxonomy.** *Classification of Chronic Pain* 2nd edn. Seattle WA: IASP Press, 1994, pp. 209–14.
25. **Melzack, R. and Torgerson, W.S.** (1971). On the language of pain. *Anesthesiology* **34**, 50–9.
26. **Jensen, M.P., Karoly, P., and Braver, S.** (1986). The measurement of clinical pain intensity: a comparison of six methods. *Pain* **27**, 117–26.
27. **Kaasa, S.** (1992). Measurement of quality of life in clinical trials. *Oncology* **49**, 289–94.
28. **Velikova, G., Wright, E.P., Smith, A.B., Cull, A., Gould, A., Forman, D., Perren, T., Stead, M., Brown, J., and Selby, P.J.** (1999). Automated collection of quality-of-life data: a comparison of paper and computer touch-screen questionnaires. *Journal of Clinical Oncology* **17**, 998–1007.
29. **Spilker, B.** *Quality of Life and Pharmaeconomics in Clinical Trials.* Philadelphia PA: Lippincott-Raven, 1996.
30. **Hearn, J. and Higginson, I.J.** (1997). Outcome measures in palliative care for advanced cancer patients: a review. *Journal of Public Health and Medicine* **19**, 193–9.
31. **Cohen, S. and Myhr, G.** (1992). Quality of life in terminal ilness: defining and measuring subjective well-being in the dying. *Journal of Palliative Care* **8**, 40–5.
32. **Byock, I.R. and Merriman, M.P.** (1998). Measuring quality of life for patients with terminal illness: the Missoula-VITAS quality of life index. *Palliative Medicine* **12**, 231–44.
33. **Waldron, D., O'Boyle, C.A., Kearney, M., Moriarty, M., and Carney, D.** (1999). Quality-of-life measurement in advanced cancer: assessing the individual. *Journal of Clinical Oncology* **17**, 3603–11.
34. **Chronbach, L.** (1951). Coefficient alpha and the internal structure of tests. *Psychometrica* **16**, 297–334.
35. **Streiner, D. and Norman, G.** (1989) Validity. In *Health Measurement Scales: A Practical Guide to Their Development and Use.* (ed. D. Streiner and G. Norman). Oxford: Oxford University Press.
36. **Bernhard, J., Cella, D.F., Coates, A.S., Fallowfield, L., Ganz, P.A., Moinpour, C.M., Mosconi, P., Osoba, D., Simes, J., and Hurny, C.** (1998). Missing quality of life data in cancer clinical trials: serious problems and challenges. *Statistics in Medicine* **17**, 517–32.
37. **Anderson, H., Hopwood, P., Stephens, R.J., Thatcher, N., Cottier, B., Nicholson, M., Milroy, R., Maughan, T.S., Falk, S.J., Bond, M.G., Burt, P.A., Connolly, C.K., McIllmurray, M.B., and Carmichael, J.** (2000). Gemcitabine plus best supportive care (BSC) vs BSC in inoperable non-small cell lung cancer—a randomized trial with quality of life as the primary outcome. UK NSCLC Gemcitabine Group. Non-small cell lung cancer. *British Journal of Cancer* **83**, 447–53.
38. **Fayers, P. and Machin, D.** *Quality of life—Assessment, Analysis and Interpretation.* New York: Wiley, 2000.
39. **Colton, T., Johnson, A., and Machin, D.** *Statistics in Medicine.* New York: Wiley, 1998, pp. 517–796.
40. **Jordhoy, M.S., Kaasa, S., Fayers, P., Ovreness, T., Underland, G., and Ahlner-Elmqvist, M.** (1999). Challenges in palliative care research; recruitment, attrition and compliance: experience from a randomized controlled trial. *Palliative Medicine* **13**, 299–310.
41. **Sneeuw, K.C., Aaronson, N.K., Sprangers, M.A., Detmar, S.B., Wever, L.D., and Schornagel, J.H.** (1997). Value of caregiver ratings in evaluating the quality of life of patients with cancer. *Journal of Clinical Oncology* **15**, 1206–17.
42. **Brunelli, C., Costantini, M., Di Giulio, P., Gallucci, M., Fusco, F., Miccinesi, G., Paci, E., Peruselli, C., Morino, P., Piazza, M., Tamburini, M., and Toscani, F.** (1998). Quality-of-life evaluation: when do terminal cancer patients and health-care providers agree? *Journal of Pain and Symptom Management* **15**, 151–8.
43. **Higginson, I., Priest, P., and McCarthy, M.** (1994). Are bereaved family members a valid proxy for a patient's assessment of dying? *Society for Science and Medicine* **38**, 553–7.
44. **Sprangers, M.A. and Aaronson, N.K.** (1992). The role of health care providers and significant others in evaluating the quality of life of patients with chronic disease: a review. *Journal of Clinical Epidemiology* **45**, 743–60.
45. **Lampic, C. and Sjoden, P.O.** (2000). Patient and staff perceptions of cancer patients' psychological concerns and needs. *Acta Oncologia* **39**, 9–22.
46. **Sprangers, M.A. and Sneeuw, K.C.** (2000). Are healthcare providers adequate raters of patients' quality of life—perhaps more than we think? *Acta Oncologia* **39**, 5–8.
47. **Van Weel, C.** (1993). Functional status in primary care: COOP/WONCA charts. *Disability and Rehabilitation* **15**, 96–101.
48. **Bruera, E., Kuehn, N., Miller, M., Selmser, P., and Macmillan, K.** (2002). The Edmonton Symptom Assessment System (ESAS): a simple method. *Incomplete.*
49. **Aaronson, N.K. et al.** (1993). The European organization for research and treatment of cancer QLQ-C30: a quality-of-life instrument for use in international clinical trials in oncology. *Journal of National Cancer Institute* **85**, 365–76.
50. **Ware, J.E., Kosinski, M., Dewey, J., and Gandek, B.** How to Score and Interpret Single-Item Health Status Measures: A Manual for Users of the SF-8 Health Survey. Lincoln RI: Quality Metric Incorporated, 2001.
51. **Osoba, D.** (1994). Lessons learned from measuring health-related quality of life in oncology. *Journal of Clinical Oncology* **12**, 608–16.
52. **Cella, D.F., Tulsky, D.S., Gray, G., Sarafian, B., Linn, E., Bonomi, A., Silberman, M., Yellen, S.B., Winicour, P., and Brannon, J.** (1993). The functional assessment of cancer therapy scale: development and validation of the general measure. *Journal of Clinical Oncology* **11**, 570–9.

53. **Muldoon, M., Barger, S., Flory, J., and Manuck, S.** (1998). What are quality of life measurements measuring? *British Medical Journal* **316**, 542–5.

54. **Ware, J.E. Jr.** (1995). The status of health assessment. *Annual Review of Public Health* **16**, 327–54.

55. **Beck, A., Ward, C., Mendelson, M., Mock, J., and Erbaugh, J.** (1961). An inventory for measuring depression. *Archives of General Psychiatry* **4**, 561–71.

56. **Hamilton, M.** (1960). A rating scale for depression. *Journal of Neurology, Neurosurgery and Psychiatry* **23**, 56–62.

57. **Massie, M. and Popkin, M.** (1998). Depressive disorders. *Psycho-Oncology.*

58. **Bergner, M., Bobbitt, R.A., Kressel, S., Pollard, W.E., Gilson, B.S., and Morris, J.R.** (1976). The sickness impact profile: conceptual formulation and methodology for the development of a health status measure. *International Journal of Health Services* **6**, 393–415.

59. **Bowling, A.** *Measuring Disease.* Philadelphia PA: Open University Press, 1995.

60. **Aaronson, N.K., Acquadro, C., Alonso, J., Apolone, G., Bucquet, D., Bullinger, M., Bungay, K., Fukuhara, S., Gandek, B., and Keller, S.** (1992). International quality of life assessment (IQOLA) Project. *Quality of Life Research* **1**, 349–51.

61. **Wagner, A.K., Gandek, B., Aaronson, N.K., Acquadro, C., Alonso, J., Apolone, G., Bullinger, M., Bjorner, J., Fukuhara, S., Kaasa, S., Leplege, A., Sullivan, M., Wood-Dauphinee, S., and Ware, J.E. Jr.** (1998). Cross-cultural comparisons of the content of SF-36 translations across 10 countries: results from the IQOLA Project. International quality of life assessment. *Journal of Clinical Epidemiology* **51**, 925–32.

62. **McHorney, C.A., Ware, J.E. Jr., and Raczek, A.E.** (1993). The MOS 36-item short-form health survey (SF-36): II. Psychometric and clinical tests of validity in measuring physical and mental health constructs. *Medical Care* **31**, 247–63.

63. **Ware, J. Jr., Kosinski, M., and Keller, S.D.** (1996). A 12-item short-form health survey: construction of scales and preliminary tests of reliability and validity. *Medical Care* **34**, 220–33.

64. **Study protocol for the World Health Organization project to develop a Quality of Life Assessment Instrument (WHOQOL)** (1993). *Quality of Life Research* **2**, 153–9.

65. **Szabo, S.** (1996). The World Health Organization Quality of Life (WHO-QOL) assessment instrument. In *Quality of Life and Pharmaeconomics in Clinical Trials* (ed. B. Spilker). Philadelphia PA: Lippincott-Raven, 1996.

66. **Development of the World Health Organization WHOQOL-BREF Quality of Life Assessment. The WHOQOL group** (1998). *Psychology in Medicine* **28**, 551–8.

67. http://www.eortc.be, 2002.

68. **Bjordal, K. and Kaasa, S.** (1992). Psychometric validation of the EORTC core quality of life questionnaire, 30-item version and a diagnosis-specific module for head and neck cancer patients. *Acta Oncologia* **31**, 311–21.

69. **Hjermstad, M.J., Fossa, S.D., Bjordal, K., and Kaasa, S.** (1995). Test/retest study of the European organization for research and treatment of cancer core quality-of-life questionnaire. *Journal of Clinical Oncology* **13**, 1249–54.

70. **Detmar, S.B., Aaronson, N.K., Wever, L.D., Muller, M., and Schornagel, J.H.** (2000). How are you feeling? Who wants to know? Patients' and oncologists' preferences for discussing health-related quality-of-life issues. *Journal of Clinical Oncology* **18**, 3295–301.

71. **Aaronson, N.K.** (1994). The EORTC modular approach to quality of life assessment in oncology. *International Journal of Mental Health* **23**, 75–96.

72. **Bergman, B., Aaronson, N.K., Ahmedzai, S., Kaasa, S., and Sullivan, M.** (1994). The EORTC QLQ-LC13: a modular supplement to the EORTC core quality of life questionnaire (QLQ-C30) for use in lung cancer clinical trials. EORTC study group on quality of life. *European Journal of Cancer* **30A**, 635–42.

73. **Bjordal, K., Ahlner-Elmqvist, M., Tollesson, E., Jensen, A.B., Razavi, D., Maher, E.J., and Kaasa, S.** (1994). Development of a European Organization for Research and Treatment of Cancer (EORTC) questionnaire module to be used in quality of life assessments in head and neck cancer patients. EORTC quality of life study group. *Acta Oncologia* **33**, 879–85.

74. **Sprangers, M.A., Cull, A., Bjordal, K., Groenvold, M., and Aaronson, N.K.** (1993). The European organization for research and treatment of cancer. Approach to quality of life assessment: guidelines for developing questionnaire modules. EORTC study group on quality of life. *Quality of Life Research* **2**, 287–95.

75. **Cella, D.** (1997). The functional assessment of cancer therapy-anemia (FACT-An) scale: a new tool for the assessment of outcomes in cancer anemia and fatigue. *Seminars in Hematology* **34**, 13–19.

76. http://www.facit.org/facit questionnaire.htm, 2002.

77. **Stone, P., Hardy, J., Huddart, R., A'Hern, R., and Richards, M.** (2002). Fatigue in patients with prostate cancer receiving hormone therapy. *European Journal of Cancer* **36**, 1134–41.

78. **Zigmond, A. and Snaith, R.** (1983). The hospital anxiety and depression scale. *Acta Psychiatrica Scandinavica* **67**, 361–70.

79. **Maguire, P. and Selby, P.** (1989). Assessing quality of life in cancer patients. *British Journal of Cancer* **60**, 437–40.

80. **Barraclough, J.** (1997). ABC of palliative care. Depression, anxiety, and confusion. (Review). *British Medical Journal* **315**, 1365–8.

81. **American Pshychiatric Association DSM-IV.** *Diagnostic and Statistical Manual of Mental Disorders.* Washington DC: APA, 1994.

82. **Le Fevre, P., Devereux, J., Smith, S., Lawrie, S.M., and Cornbleet, M.** (1999). Screening for psychiatric illness in the palliative care inpatient setting: a comparison between the hospital anxiety and depression scale and the general health questionnaire-12. *Palliative Medicine* **13**, 399–407.

83. **Coyle, N., Adelhardt, J., Foley, K.M., and Portenoy, R.K.** (1990). Character of terminal illness in the advanced cancer patient: pain and other symptoms during the last four weeks of life. *Journal of Pain and Symptom Management* **5**, 83–93.

84. **Stone, P., Hardy, J., Broadley, K., Tookman, A.J., Kurowska, A., and A'Hern, R.** (1999). Fatigue in advanced cancer: a prospective controlled cross-sectional study. *British Journal of Cancer* **79**, 1479–86.

85. **Loge, J.H. and Kaasa, S.** (1998). Fatigue and cancer—prevalence, correlates and measurement. *Progress in Palliative Care* **6**, 43–7.

86. **Stone, P., Richards, M., and Hardy, J.** (1998). Fatigue in patients with cancer. *European Journal of Cancer* **34**, 1670–6.

87. **Chalder, T., Berelowitz, G., Pawlikowska, T., Watts, L., Wessely, S., Wright, D., and Wallace, E.P.** (1993). Development of a fatigue scale. *Journal of Psychosomotor Research* **37**, 147–53.

88. **Grond, S., Zech, D., Diefenbach, C., Radbruch, L., and Lehmann, K.A.** (1996). Assessment of cancer pain: a prospective evaluation in 2266 cancer patients referred to a pain service. *Pain* **64**, 107–14.

89. **Melzack, R.** (1975). The McGill pain questionnaire: major properties and scoring methods. *Pain* **1**, 277–99.

90. **Melzack, R.** (1987). The short-form McGill pain questionnaire. *Pain* **30**, 191–7.

91. **Daut, R.L., Cleeland, C.S., and Flanery, R.C.** (1983). Development of the Wisconsin brief pain questionnaire to assess pain in cancer and other diseases. *Pain* **17**, 197–210.

92. **Radbruch, L., Loick, G., Kiencke, P., Lindena, G., Sabatowski, R., Grond, S., Lehmann, K.A., and Cleeland, C.S.** (1999). Validation of the German version of the brief pain inventory. *Journal of Pain and Symptom Management* **18**, 180–7.

93. **Robinson, J.** (1999). Cognitive assessment of palliative care patients. *Progress in Palliative Care* **7**, 291–8.

94. **Pereira, J., Hanson, J., and Bruera, E.** (1997). The frequency and clinical course of cognitive impairment in patients with terminal cancer. *Cancer* **79**, 835–42.

95. **Cull, A., Hay, C., Love, S.B., Mackie, M., Smets, E., and Stewart, M.** (1996). What do cancer patients mean when they complain of concentration and memory problems? *British Journal of Cancer* **74**, 1674–9.

96. **Folstein, M.F., Folstein, S.E., and McHugh, P.R.** (1975). 'Mini-Mental State'. A practical method for grading the cognitive state of patients for the clinician. *Journal of Psychiatric Research* **12**, 189–98.

97. **Breitbart, W., Rosenfeld, B., Roth, A., Smith, M.J., Cohen, K., and Passik, S.** (1997). The Memorial Delirium Assessment Scale. *Journal of Pain and Symptom Management* **13**, 128–37.

98. **Braekhus, A., Laake, K., and Engedal, K.** (1992). The Mini-Mental State examination: identifying the most efficient variables for detecting cognitive impairment in the elderly. *Journal of the American Geriatric Society* **40**, 1139–45.

99. **O'Boyle, C.A.** (1994). The schedule for the evaluation of individual quality of life. *International Journal of Mental Health* **23**, 3–23.

100. **Hickey, A.M., Bury, G., O'Boyle, C.A., Bradley, F., O'Kelly, F.D., and Shannon, W.** (1996). A new short form individual quality of life measure

(SEIQoL-DW): application in a cohort of individuals with HIV/AIDS. *British Medical Journal* **313**, 29–33.

101. **Waldron, D., O'Boyle, C.A., Kearney, M., Moriarty, M., and Carney, D.** (1999). Quality-of-life measurement in advanced cancer: assessing the individual. *Journal of Clinical Oncology* **17**, 3603–11.
102. **Tamburini, M., Rosso, S., Gamba, A., Mencaglia, E., De Conno, F., and Ventafridda, V.** (1992). A therapy impact questionnaire for quality-of-life assessment in advanced cancer research. *Annals of Oncology* **3**, 565–70.
103. **Cohen, S.R., Mount, B.M., Strobel, M.G., and Bui, F.** (1995). The McGill quality of life questionnaire: a measure of quality of life appropriate for people with advanced disease. A preliminary study of validity and acceptability. *Palliative Medicine* **9**, 207–19.
104. **Cohen, S.R., Mount, B.M., and MacDonald, N.** (1996). Defining quality of life. *European Journal of Cancer* **32A**, 753–4.
105. **Cohen, S.R., Mount, B.M., Bruera, E., Provost, M., Rowe, J., and Tong, K.** (1997). Validity of the McGill quality of life questionnaire in the palliative care setting: a multi-centre Canadian study demonstrating the importance of the existential domain. *Palliative Medicine* **11**, 3–20.
106. **Cohen, S.R. and Mount, B.M.** (2000). Living with cancer: 'Good' days and 'Bad' days—what produces them. *American Cancer Society* 1854–65.
107. **Lo, R.S., Woo, J., Zhoc, K.C., Li, C.Y., Yeo, W., Johnson, P., Mak, Y., and Lee, J.** (2001). Cross-cultural validation of the McGill quality of life questionnaire in Hong Kong Chinese. *Palliative Medicine* **15**, 387–97.
108. **Salmon, P., Manzi, F., and Valori, R.M.** (1996). Measuring the meaning of life for patients with incurable cancer: the life evaluation questionnaire (LEQ). *European Journal of Cancer* **32A**, 755–60.
109. **Sterkenburg, C.** (1996). A reliability and validity study of the McMaster quality of life scale (MQOLS) for a palliative population. *Journal of Palliative Care* **12**, 18–25.
110. **Randall Curtis, J., Marjorie, M., Wenrich, D., Carline, J., Shannon, S., Amrozy, D., and Ramsey, P.** (2001). Understanding physicians' skills at providing end-of-life care. *Journal of General Internal Medicine* **16**, 41–9.
111. **Teno, J.M., Byock, I., and Field, M.J.** (1999). Research agenda for developing measures to examine quality of care and quality of life of patients diagnosed with life-limiting illness. *Journal of Pain and Symptom Management* **17**, 75–82.
112. **Singer, P.A., Martin, D.K., and Kelner, M.** (1999). Quality end-of-life care: patients' perspectives. *Journal of the American Medical Association* **281**, 163–8.
113. **Stewart, A.L., Teno, J., Patrick, D.L., and Lynn, J.** (1999). The concept of quality of life of dying persons in the context of health care. *Journal of Pain and Symptom Management* **17**, 93–108.
114. **Rinck, G.C., van den Bos, G.A., Kleijnen, J., de Haes, H.J., Schade, E., and Veenhof, C.H.** (1997). Methodologic issues in effectiveness research on palliative cancer care: a systematic review. *Journal of Clinical Oncology* **15**, 1697–707.
115. **Hearn, J. and Higginson, I.J.** (1998). Do specialist palliative care teams improve outcomes for cancer patients? A systematic literature review. *Palliative Medicine* **12**, 317–32.
116. **Smeenk, W. et al.** (1998). Effectiveness of home care programmes for patients with incurable cancer on their quality of life and time spent in hospital: systematic review. *British Medical Journal* **16**, 1939–44.
117. **Salisbury, C., Bosanquet, N., Wilkinson, E.K., Franks, P.J., Kite, S., Lorentzon, M., and Naysmith, A.** (1999). The Impact of different models of specialist palliative care on patients' quality of life: a systematic literature review. *Palliative Medicine* **13**, 3–17.
118. **Kane, R.L., Wales, J., Bernstein, L., Leibowitz, A., and Kaplan, S.** (1984). A randomised controlled trial of hospice care. *Lancet* **1**, 890–4.
119. **Zimmer, J.G., Groth-Juncker, A., and McCusker, J.** (1985). A randomized controlled study of a home health care team. *American Journal of Public Health* **75**, 134–41.
120. **Addington-Hall, J. et al.** (1992). Randomised controlled trial of effects of coordinating care for teminally ill cancer patients. *British Medical Journal* **305**, 1317–22.
121. **Hughes, S.L., Cummings, J., Weaver, F., Manheim, L., Braun, B., and Conrad, K.** (1992). A randomized trial of the cost effectiveness of VA hospital-based home care for the terminally ill. *Health Service Research* **26**, 801–17.
122. **Jordhoy, M.S., Fayers, P., Saltnes, T., Ahlner-Elmqvist, M., Jannert, M., and Kaasa, S.** (2000). A palliative-care intervention and death at home: a cluster randomised trial. *Lancet* **356**, 888–93.
123. **Jordhoy, M.S., Fayers, P., Loge, J.H., Ahlner-Elmqvist, M., and Kaasa, S.** (2001). Quality of life in palliative cancer care: results from a cluster randomized trial. *Journal of Clinical Oncology* **19**, 3884–94.
124. **Bruera, E., Kuehn, N., Miller, M.J., Selmser, P., and Macmillan, K.** (1991). The Edmonton symptom assessment system (ESAS): a simple method for the assessment of palliative care patients. *Journal of Palliative Care* **7**, 6–9.
125. **Chang, V.T., Hwang, S.S., Feuerman, M., Kasimis, B.S., and Thaler, H.T.** (2000). The Memorial Symptom Assessment Scale Short Form (MSAS-SF). *Cancer* **89**, 1162–71.
126. **Kaasa, S. and Loge, J.H.** (2002). Quality of life assessment in palliative care. *Lancet* **3**, 175–82.
127. **Hjermstad, M.J., Evensen, S.A., Kvaloy, S.O., Fayers, P.M., and Kaasa, S.** (1999). Health-related quality of life 1 year after allogeneic or autologous stem-cell transplantation: a prospective study. *Journal of Clinical Oncology* **17**, 706–18.
128. **Altman, D.** *Practical Statistics for Medical Research.* London: Chapman & Hall, 1991.
129. **Fairclough, D. and Gelber, R.** (1996). Quality of life: statistical issues and analysis. In *Quality of Life and Pharmaeconomics in Clinical Trials* (ed. B. Spilker). Philadelphia PA: Lippincott-Raven, 1996.
130. **Wade, M., Darling, H., Grossman, J., McNerney, W., Tarlov, A., and Ware, J.E.** *How to Score the SF-36 Health Survey 2.* Boston MA: Medical Outcomes Trust, 1994.
131. **Fayers, P., Aaronson, N., Bjordal, K., and Sullivan, M.** *EORTC QLQ-C30. Scoring Manual.* Brussels: Quality of life Unit, EORTC Data Center, 1995.
132. **Begg, C., Cho, M., Eastwood, S., Horton, R., Moher, D., Olkin, I., Pitkin, R., Rennie, D., Schulz, K.F., Simel, D., and Stroup, D.F.** (1996). Improving the quality of reporting of randomized controlled trials. The CONSORT statement. *Journal of the American Medical Association* **276**, 637–9.
133. **Staquet, M., Berzon, R., Osoba, D., and Machin, D.** (1996). Guidelines for reporting results of quality of life assessments in clinical trials. *Quality of Life Research* **5**, 496–502.
134. **Hjermstad, M.J., Fayers, P.M., Bjordal, K., and Kaasa, S.** (1998). Health-related quality of life in the general Norwegian population assessed by the European organization for research and treatment of cancer core quality-of-life questionnaire: the QLQ − C30 (+3). *Journal of Clinical Oncology* **16**, 1188–96.
135. **Osoba, D., Rodrigues, G., Myles, J., Zee, B., and Pater, J.** (1998). Interpreting the significance of changes in health-related quality-of- life scores. *Journal of Clinical Oncology* **16**, 139–44.
136. **Cull, A., Stewart, M., and Altman, D.G.** (1995). Assessment of and intervention for psychosocial problems in routine oncology practice. *British Journal of Cancer* **72**, 229–35.
137. **Passik, S.D., Dugan, W., McDonald, M.V., Rosenfeld, B., Theobald, D.E., and Edgerton, S.** (1998). Oncologists' recognition of depression in their patients with cancer. *Journal of Clinical Oncology* **16**, 1594–600.
138. **Shuster, J.L. Jr., Breitbart, W., and Chochinov, H.M.** (1999). Psychiatric aspects of excellent end-of-life care. Ad hoc committee on end-of-life care. The Academy of Psychosomatic Medicine. *Psychosomatics* **40**, 1–4.
139. **Velikova, G., Stark, D., and Selby, P.** (1999). Quality of life instruments in oncology. *European Journal of Cancer* **35**, 1571–80.
140. **Ware, J.E. and Keller, S.D.** (1996). Interpreting general health measures. In *Quality of Life and Pharmaeconomics in Clinical Trials* (ed. B. Spilker). Philadelphia PA: Lippincott-Raven, 1996.
141. **Urch, C.E., Chamberlain, J., and Field, G.** (1998). The drawback of the hospital anxiety and depression scale in the assessment of depression in hospice inpatients. *Palliative Medicine* **12**, 395–6.
142. **Ware, J.E., Bjorner, J.B., and Kosinski, M.** (2000). Practical implications of item response theory and computerized adaptive testing: a brief summary of ongoing studies of widely used headache impact scales. *Medical Care* **38**, 1173–82.
143. **Lord, F.** *Applications of Item Response Theory to Practical Testing Problems.* Hillsdale NJ: Erlbaum Associates, 1980.
144. **Higginson, I.J. and Carr, A.J.** (2001). Measuring quality of life: using quality of life measures in the clinical setting. *British Medical Journal* **322**, 1297–300.

7

Principles of drug use in palliative medicine

7 Principles of drug use in palliative medicine

Geoffrey Hanks, Clive J.C. Roberts, and Andrew N. Davies

The control of distressing symptoms is central to the practice of palliative medicine. It is the foundation of 'whole patient' care in that it is not possible to deal with psychological, social, or spiritual concerns if patients have uncontrolled physical symptoms. The management of these symptoms is largely based on drug treatment, which means that effective symptom control requires some understanding of clinical pharmacology. The purpose of this chapter is to describe those principles of clinical pharmacology that are relevant to day-to-day palliative medicine practice.

Symptom management is unfortunately not a simple exercise of targeting a particular symptom with a specific drug. Patients with advanced disease are a vulnerable population and it is necessary to recognize that environmental and psychological factors have a variable but potentially very great influence on physical well-being. The response to drug treatment may be sometimes unpredictable for these reasons.

One hazard for palliative medicine physicians that has been a recent focus of attention is the use of drugs for unlicensed indications or by unlicensed routes of administration which is common in pain and symptom management. Fifteen per cent of all prescriptions, affecting up to two-thirds of inpatients in specialist palliative care units (in the United Kingdom), may fall into this category.(1,2) This highlights the obligation of prescribers to clearly understand the principles of drug use that should guide their practice and the specific limitations of whatever data are available.

There are other complicating factors in this patient population. The patients are predominantly elderly with many concurrent symptomatic problems and often with multisystem dysfunction. Polypharmacy is almost invariable and the potential for drug interactions and modified or abnormal responses to drugs is considerable. Iatrogenic problems are commonplace in that prescription of one symptomatic remedy—for example, an opioid analgesic—will invariably cause other symptoms, in this case constipation, drowsiness, and possibly nausea and dry mouth. A laxative, antiemetic, psychostimulant, and artificial saliva may all be added to the treatment regimen as a result. The skill of the palliative medicine physician is to deal effectively with each symptom without imposing a greater burden on the patient because of intolerable, unwanted drug effects or too complex a drug regimen. The principles of effective symptom control need always to be kept in mind: make a diagnosis of the underlying mechanism or cause of each symptom, individualize the treatment, and keep it simple.

Clinical pharmacology

Clinical pharmacology may be broadly divided into pharmacokinetics ('what the body does to the drug') and pharmacodynamics ('what the drug does to the body'). It is often assumed that these are theoretical and rather esoteric disciplines that do not have much direct 'clinical' relevance. As we shall demonstrate, this assumption is wrong. For example, palliative care patients commonly require parenteral administration of drugs at some stage of their illness, and disordered handling of drugs by the body as a result of disease is common. Drugs are often used in special formulations, either involving modified release of orally administered agents or novel forms designed for administration by other routes. These are everyday clinical situations that cannot be properly managed without some pharmacokinetic knowledge.

Pharmacodynamics is about drug action in man and, like pharmacokinetics, its measurement has become highly sophisticated; for example, in the use of imaging techniques to monitor biochemical changes in target organs such as the brain. However, one of the challenges of drug use in palliative care is that outcome measures are often not easy to define and measure. In palliative care, drugs are not being used to cure disease but to improve comfort. Subjective symptoms such as pain, nausea, or depression are less easy to quantify than biochemical changes in the brain or even tumour size, serum calcium, or haemoglobin concentrations. Yet, these are common targets for drug treatment in palliative medicine. Knowledge of the basic modes of action of drugs will underpin the logical selection and use of the most appropriate remedies for these symptoms.

Pharmacokinetics

Pharmacokinetics is often arbitrarily described under the headings of absorption, distribution, metabolism, and excretion of drugs. A number of other terms are used to describe the way in which the body handles drugs. These terms can be defined and modelled mathematically. However, the practising clinician should not be put off by the complex mathematical formulae that are often applied to the subject. A broad understanding of the physiological, pharmacological, and pathophysiological factors that influence the ultimate concentration of a drug in the blood and eventually at its site of action is invaluable and does not need an understanding of complex mathematics.

This section will define commonly used kinetic terms and identify, where possible, factors contributing to the variability of each. In order to illustrate the terminology, some pharmacokinetic parameters for frequently used drugs will be described at the end of each section.

Half-life ($t_{1/2}$)

This is perhaps the most well known and commonly used pharmacokinetic parameter. It is a measure of the rate at which a particular process takes place. For example, the elimination half-life is a measure of the time taken for half the drug in the body to be removed. However, the process is often complex. For example, the decay in drug concentration following intravenous administration may comprise several exponentials, representing movement of drug inwards and outwards of body compartments and also the elimination of the drug from the body. It is generally the elimination half-life that correlates most closely with the duration of action of the drug, though this is not always the case. Technical difficulties in defining a drug's half-life (e.g. complex assay procedures) may account for variation in quoted figures.

The elimination half-life is a dependent variable—dependent on volume of distribution and clearance. In the simplest kinetic model, half-life ($t_{1/2}$) equals volume of distribution (V_d) multiplied by a constant (k) divided by clearance (Cl):

$$t_{1/2} = k\,\frac{V_d}{\mathrm{Cl}}.$$

What this means is that half-life is prolonged as distribution volume increases and clearance reduces. These terms are defined below.

Drugs with a long half-life may accumulate over a prolonged period of time and build up to toxic levels. For example, this may happen with methadone, which on regular dosing has a half-life of 20–40 h.[3]

The elimination half-life of benzodiazepine hypnotics to some extent predicts the potential of each drug to cause residual or hangover effects the next day. Temazepam ($t_{1/2}$ 8–10 h) and triazolam ($t_{1/2}$ 2–3 h) are much less likely to cause daytime drowsiness than flurazepam (which has an active metabolite desalkylflurazepam with a $t_{1/2}$ of 2–4 days).

Apparent volume of distribution (V_d)

This term is defined as the volume into which all the drug in the body would need to be distributed to achieve the blood concentration. For drugs that are taken up into fat stores or muscle, the volume may be many times body size. Thus, it is not a real volume that can be described in anatomical terms but a mathematical concept that is a convenient way of expressing how a drug is distributed in the body. This is why it is termed 'apparent'. Similarly, a 'compartment' does not have an anatomical equivalent but is a theoretical space (often shown diagramatically as a box).

The volume of distribution is important as a determinant of half-life and is also of theoretical importance in the calculation of a loading dose where one is needed. Alteration in body composition and in the physicochemical environment of the body causes changes in distribution volume. Such changes for individual drugs in specific conditions may be quite difficult to predict. However, emaciation may reduce the distribution volume of many centrally acting agents and lead to an enhanced effect after single doses. If a drug is normally highly bound to plasma protein, distribution volume may increase when plasma proteins are reduced because more drug is available for tissue-binding sites. However, because the proportion of active (unbound) drug is increased, a lower plasma concentration of drug will produce a given therapeutic effect. Thus, the net result is that the effects of these changes will tend to cancel each other out.

Digoxin is rapidly and extensively taken up by body tissues, particularly skeletal and cardiac muscle and in a 70-kg man has a volume of distribution of some 490 l. In contrast, morphine, which is relatively hydrophilic and little taken up in tissue stores, has a volume of distribution of 140 l. In both of these examples the 'apparent' volume of distribution is greater than the size of the body.

Clearance

This is the volume of blood that is completely cleared of the drug in a unit of time. It, therefore, most closely reflects the efficiency of the elimination process. It is a major determinant of half-life and of the steady state drug concentration. This is because at steady state the amount of blood being cleared in the interval between doses will contain an amount of drug equivalent to the dose (assuming 100 per cent bioavailability). The two major organs of elimination are the liver and the kidney, both of which are susceptible to pharmacological and pathophysiological sources of variability. Clearance can be measured experimentally by plotting blood concentrations of the drug after a dose has been administered. Clearance (Cl) can then be calculated as

$$\mathrm{Cl} = \frac{\text{dose}}{\text{area under the plasma concentration/time curve}}.$$

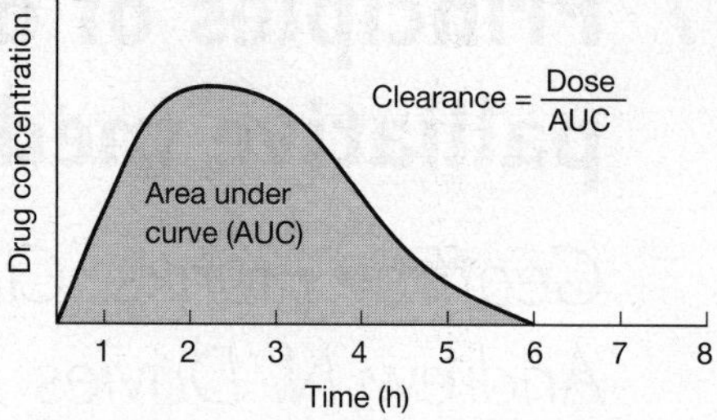

Fig. 1 Plasma concentrations of a typical drug after oral administration. The shaded area is the 'area under the curve' of plasma concentration versus time and can be calculated mathematically, and from this can be derived the clearance.

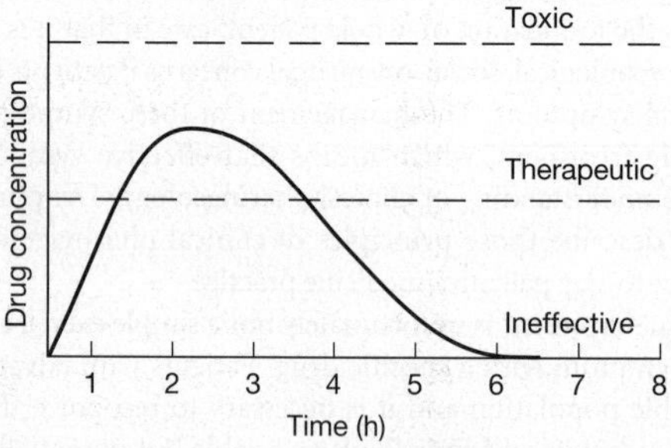

Fig. 2 Plasma concentrations of a typical drug after oral administration of a single dose. The aim in chronic dosing is to maintain plasma concentrations within the therapeutic range.

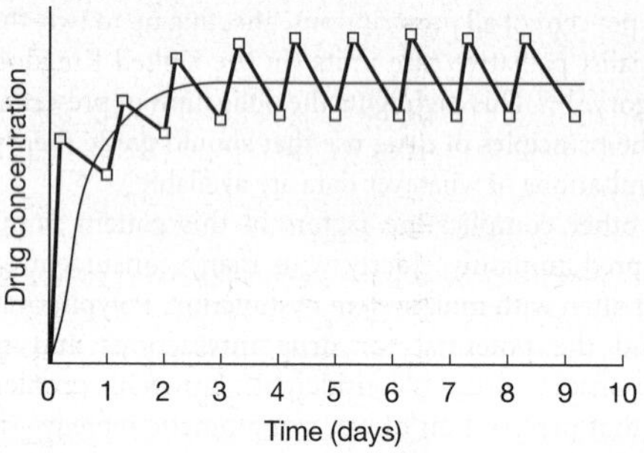

Fig. 3 Steady state plasma concentration of a short-acting drug showing peaks and troughs after each dose.

This is illustrated in Fig. 1.

Most drugs are cleared from the bloodstream either by metabolism in the liver or by excretion by the kidney, or by a combination of both. Total blood clearance determines steady state concentration and is the sum of all clearance mechanisms. Whilst it is often claimed that if one organ of elimination is compromised by disease the other can compensate by allowing increased excretion of the drug, this does not prevent a rise in drug level in the body, which is determined by total clearance.

Steady state plasma concentration (C_{ss})

The aim of any dosing regimen in an individual patient is to achieve a concentration of drug in the blood that is not so high as to produce adverse effects but high enough to give the intended effect (Fig. 2). This concentration can never be completely steady as peaks will occur at the point of maximum drug absorption after administration and troughs occur immediately before each dose (Fig. 3). Steady state is said to have been achieved when all trough and all peak concentrations do not vary. The degree of swing between peak and trough is determined by the drug's elimination half-life and the frequency of drug administration. For instance, where a drug has a short half-life and the difference between peak concentration and trough concentration is small, then dosing should be frequent. The actual steady state concentrations achieved in any patient are dependent on the dose administered, the bioavailability of the drug in that patient, and the clearance of the drug from the blood in that patient.

It is a common misconception that steady state drug concentration is dependent on the size of the body. In fact, the volume into which the drug is distributed plays no part. The reason why smaller people and children often require reduced doses is because they have smaller organs of elimination and therefore lower clearance rates. This is pertinent in the context of palliative care where it cannot be predicted that a patient whose body is wasted may need to be given a smaller dose. The elimination process itself may be unimpaired.

Time to reach steady state plasma concentration

Whilst the actual concentration of drug in the blood is independent of its half-life, the time it takes to reach that level is entirely and solely dependent on this parameter. As a rough guide, if a drug is given to a patient in constant dosage at a constant time interval, it takes about four half-lives to reach 95 per cent of the steady state plasma concentration. This applies only to drugs whose elimination is governed by 'first-order kinetics'. Fortunately, this comprises the vast majority of drugs, with phenytoin being the notable exception. During a first-order process a constant proportion of remaining drug is eliminated in a unit of time. Indeed, that is why the term half-life can be applied—that is, half the drug in the body is removed in the half-life interval.

A first-order process is independent of the concentration of drug; the proportion eliminated is the same per unit of time whilst the actual amount of drug eliminated increases. A zero-order process is dependent on concentration and the amount eliminated per unit of time is fixed. Phenytoin is initially metabolized according to first-order kinetics but the enzyme system responsible has limited capacity. Once this system is 'saturated', metabolism of phenytoin continues as a zero-order process.

It is clear, therefore, that for a first-order process the amount of drug in the body must build up until the amount of drug being eliminated during the dose interval equates with the dose. Because the time to reach steady state depends on half-life, when this is very long it may be necessary to give a loading dose initially and then to follow with a reduced maintenance dose.

The elimination half-life ($t_{1/2}$) of morphine is 2–4 h. Thus, when morphine is administered at regular 4-hourly intervals steady state will be 95 per cent achieved after 16 h or so. In contrast, the half-life of digoxin is about 2 days so that it would take at least 8–10 days to achieve steady state. It is usual to give a loading dose of digoxin and then maintain patients on a single daily dose.

Bioavailability

This is the percentage of administered drug that gains access unchanged to the systemic circulation. It is of most clinical relevance after oral administration. It can be measured in individual patients by comparing the area under the plasma concentration time curves after oral and after parenteral administration allowing for any difference in the dose administered and assuming no change in the rate of elimination. Many factors may contribute to a reduction of bioavailability below 100 per cent. Variation in the pharmaceutical formulation of drugs such as digoxin and phenytoin may account for significant differences in bioavailability and the extent of drug absorption may be susceptible to changes in gastrointestinal function.

More important, however, is the extent of presystemic (or 'first pass') metabolism (Fig. 4). Once absorbed from the gastrointestinal tract, all drugs must pass via the portal venous system through the liver. If within that organ there is an avid system of enzymes for metabolizing the particular drug, then a percentage will be biotransformed before passing through the liver to the systemic circulation. For some drugs, the amount extracted during one pass through the liver (extraction ratio) may be as high as 80 per cent, giving an oral bioavailability of only 20 per cent. The steady state blood concentration of such drugs after oral administration may exhibit high variability; minor changes in the extraction ratio will be reflected by large percentage changes in bioavailability. Thus, interactions with other drugs that induce or inhibit hepatic enzymes or changes in hepatic function due to disease may have a profound effect on such drug levels after oral administration but relatively little effect when the drug is given parenterally. In patients with chronic liver disease or hepatic metastases, blood may be 'shunted' from portal to systemic vessels. The drug may thus by-pass hepatic enzymes, the presystemic metabolism will be reduced, and the bioavailability may be considerably increased. Consequently, very much higher levels of drug may build up after oral administration if the enhanced bioavailability is not taken into account. The effect of presystemic metabolism on drug bioavailability must also be taken into account when calculating oral doses during conversion from parenteral regimens. The bioavailability of some drugs may also be reduced by intraluminal degradation in the gastrointestinal tract or metabolism by enzymes within the intestinal wall.

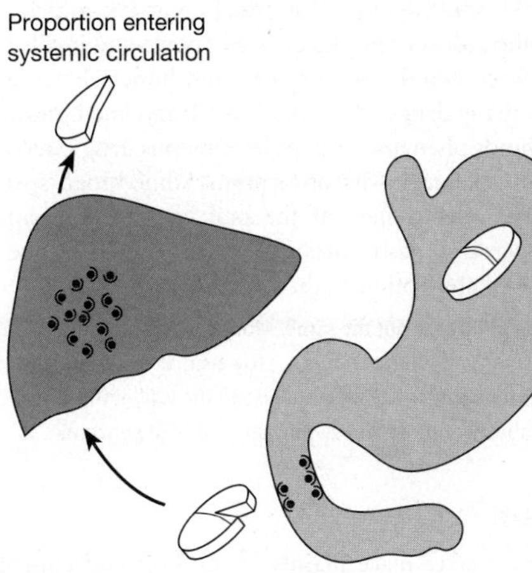

Fig. 4 'First pass' metabolism may take place in the liver (and sometimes also in the intestinal mucosa) before the absorbed drug enters the systemic circulation.

Drug absorption

The absorption of drugs is mainly a passive process along a concentration gradient across a lipid cell membrane. As long as the drug is in solution and has a degree of lipid solubility, there is sufficient surface area for diffusion, and the drug remains in contact with the absorptive areas for long enough, problems should not arise.

Most drugs are absorbed where the greatest surface area is available; that is, in the small bowel. A reduced rate of absorption may, therefore, occur if there is a delay in emptying of the stomach. This might arise as part of a pathological process or result from pharmacological agents that slow gastric motility, such as drugs with anticholinergic effects or opioid analgesics.

Drugs must have the physicochemical characteristics to facilitate dissolution in the gut and once presented to the vast surface area of the small bowel their potential for full absorption should be easily achieved. Only the most severe of structural gastrointestinal disease will cause problems.

Many drugs are now formulated as controlled release preparations. For them to achieve their expected absorptive profile they may need to remain in the small bowel for a prolonged length of time. Such formulations have usually only been tested under ideal conditions in healthy volunteers. For the patient with gastrointestinal hurry who takes a controlled release drug there is a risk that it will be propelled past the absorptive zone of the gut before all of the drug has been released and this will result in therapeutic failure.

Within the gut there is some potential for drug interaction, which results in reduced bioavailability. Most examples are well known and involve loose chemical binding between two drugs within the gut lumen. For example, cholestyramine binds many drugs, iron salts and tetracycline bind to each other, and sucralfate binds phenytoin. Other less obvious drug interactions may occur involving interference with absorption. Some broad-spectrum antibiotics decrease the effectiveness of the oral contraceptive and the mechanism may be increased gastrointestinal transit caused by the antibiotic, leading to reduced absorption of the contraceptive.

Absorption and bioavailability are not the same. Morphine, for example, is more or less completely absorbed (i.e. 100 per cent). However, it undergoes extensive presystemic metabolism, mainly in the liver but also in the wall of the gastrointestinal tract. The bioavailability of morphine is thus about 20–30 per cent.

Drug metabolism

Drug biotransformation takes place mainly in the liver and contributes both to the rate of elimination of drug and to its bioavailability. The rate at which the metabolic process proceeds usually determines the clearance, but where the removal is particularly avid (high extraction ratio) the rate of delivery of drug to the liver rather than the rate of metabolism may determine clearance (flow-dependent kinetics). For such drugs if liver blood flow is markedly reduced, drug accumulation will result.

The biochemical processes of drug metabolism are complex. Two phases of metabolism are usually described involving initially oxidation or hydrolysis (phase I) followed by conjugation (phase II), but this concept can be misleading. All of the reactions involve the production of products that are more polar and, therefore, more water soluble and amenable to excretion by the kidney. The so-called phase II reactions may take place in some circumstances without prior phase I. Phase I reactions involve oxidation, reduction, hydrolysis, hydration, dethioacetylation, and isomerization. Such reactions may prepare the drug molecule for a phase II reaction by producing or uncovering a chemically reactive group which then forms the substrate for a phase II reaction.

Of the phase I reactions, oxidation involving the 'mixed-function oxidase system' is the most important and its behaviour is best understood. This system of enzymes is based in hepatic microsomes and requires molecular oxygen, NADPH and cytochrome P450, and NADPH–cytochrome P450 reductase. Amongst the reactions catalysed by the mixed-function oxidase system are aromatic hydroxylation, aliphatic hydroxylation, epoxidation, *N*-dealkylation, *O*-dealkylation, oxidative deamination, *N*-oxidation, *S*-oxidation, and alcohol oxidation. Not all oxidative processes are carried out by this system; alcohol dehydrogenation is performed by a non-microsomally located enzyme that is responsible for the major pathway for alcohol detoxification (in non-enzyme induced subjects).

Phase II reactions mostly involve conjugation: glucuronidation, glycosylation, sulfation, methylation, and acetylation or conjugation with glutathione or with certain amino acids.

The intricacies of drug metabolism may appear irrelevant to clinicians but an appreciation of the complexity of the process is necessary in developing a scientific approach to dose management.

Pharmacodynamics

Drugs produce their effects on the body by combining with receptors, by modifying enzyme processes, or by a direct chemical or physical action.

Receptors, agonists, and antagonists

Receptors are specialized areas of the cell membrane that are highly specific for certain drug or hormone molecules. A drug that combines with a receptor to 'activate' it is called an agonist and this terminology initially derived from the actions of hormones and neurotransmitters. The term refers to a drug that binds to cell receptors to induce changes in the cell that stimulate physiological activity. Some drugs can combine with receptors without initiating any change in cell function. Such drugs are called antagonists because they interfere with the action of agonists by blocking the receptor sites ('competitive antagonists'). Non-competitive antagonists do not compete for the same receptor as the agonist but block the effect of the agonist in some other way.

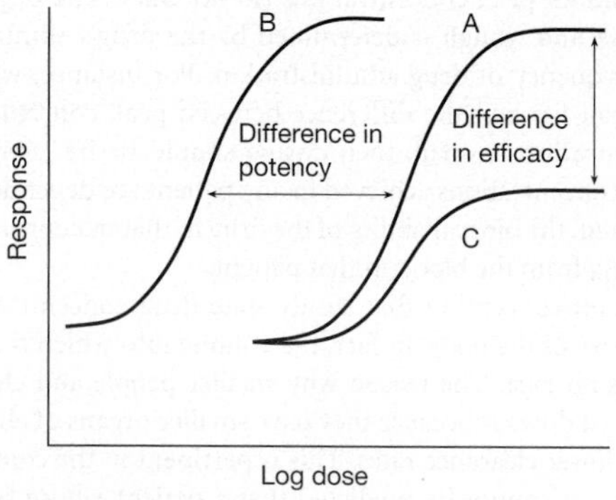

Fig. 5 Log dose–response curves for two full agonist drugs A and B, and a partial agonist C. Drug B is more potent than drug A but no more effective. Drug A is more effective than drug C but has similar potency.

A partial agonist is a drug with low intrinsic activity (efficacy) so that its dose–response curve exhibits a ceiling effect at less than the maximal effect produced by a full agonist. The difference between a partial agonist and a full agonist is, thus, a difference in efficacy (Fig. 5). This should not be confused with potency, which is a measure of the amount of drug required to produce a given effect, and is a measure also of affinity for receptors; the more potent a drug, the greater its affinity for receptors. Thus, a drug may be a partial agonist (less effective) but still more potent than a full agonist. This is the case with buprenorphine, which has limited efficacy compared with morphine but greater potency (0.3 mg intramuscular buprenorphine ≡ 10 mg intramuscular morphine).[4] However, because it is more potent it has greater affinity for μ opioid receptors and can displace morphine from them. In this way, it can act as an 'antagonist' of morphine by reducing the overall μ opioid effect (see Chapter 8.2.3). Buprenorphine is, therefore, sometimes classified as an 'agonist antagonist'. Other opioid analgesics, such as pentazocine, are also classified as 'agonist antagonists' but have a different profile. These drugs have both agonist and antagonist effects at receptors, but at different receptors (see below).

There are similar examples in other therapeutic areas, and they are likely to increase as new receptors and receptor subtypes are identified. For example, metoclopramide has been long regarded primarily as a dopamine receptor blocker, which it is at low doses. At high doses metoclopramide blocks (antagonizes) $5HT_3$ receptors and is a much more effective antiemetic. Metoclopramide also has a prokinetic effect on the upper gastrointestinal tract and this is mediated through an agonist effect at $5HT_4$ receptors, leading to an enhancement of the effects of acetylcholine release in the gut. Metoclopramide is, thus, both an agonist and an antagonist at different serotonin receptors.

Morphine is an agonist at μ opioid receptors. Buprenorphine is a partial agonist at μ receptors and can in certain circumstances reverse ('antagonize') the effects of morphine. Pentazocine is a weak competitive antagonist at μ receptors (so may also antagonize the effects of morphine but by a different mechanism) and is a partial agonist at a different type of opioid receptor, κ. Naloxone is an antagonist at the μ opioid receptor and will block the effects of μ agonists and partial agonists (but with varying efficiency).

Drugs that alter enzyme activity

Non-steroidal anti-inflammatory drugs block the effect of the enzyme cyclo-oxygenase and thereby interfere with the synthesis of prostaglandins; this is believed to be the basis for their anti-inflammatory activity. Monoamine oxidase inhibitor antidepressants interfere with the degradation of monoamine neurotransmitters, thus, enhancing their effect in central synapses; angiotensin-converting-enzyme inhibitors block the conversion of angiotensin I to angiotensin II by inhibiting the relevant enzyme and are effective in the treatment of hypertension and cardiac failure. Thus, drugs affecting enzyme processes may have diverse therapeutic applications but many of them share in common the fact that they are inhibitors of enzyme actions.

Drugs that have a direct chemical or physical action

Antacids are an example of drugs with a direct chemical action. They are bases that neutralize gastric acid. Drugs with a physical mode of action include the bulk laxatives such as ispaghula husk. While the mode of action of such drugs seems far less complex than that of drugs that interact with receptors, the same attention to detail in their use and individualized approach are necessary to maximize the benefits and reduce potential adverse effects.

Tolerance, drug dependence, and drug resistance

Tolerance

Tolerance refers to the phenomenon of decreasing response to a drug, as a consequence of its continued use. It is manifest by a shift to the right in the dose–response curve: an increased dose is required to achieve a similar effect (Fig. 6). In contrast, sensitization refers to the phenomenon of increasing response to a drug, as a consequence of its continued use. It is manifest by a shift to the left in the dose–response curve: a decreased dose is required to achieve a similar effect (Fig. 6). Sensitization is a relatively uncommon phenomenon.

Tolerance may be due to:

- An alteration in the pharmacokinetic profile of a drug (pharmacokinetic tolerance). For example, tolerance to barbiturates has been linked to induction of hepatic microsomal enzymes, which results in an increased metabolism of the barbiturate.
- Or an alteration in the pharmacodynamic profile of the drug (pharmacodynamic tolerance). Tolerance to opioids has been linked to uncoupling of opioid/G protein receptor complexes, which results in a decreased effect of the opioid.

Tolerance occurs at a variable time after initiation of the drug. Moreover, it may occur to some, or all, of the effects of the drug. For example, tolerance

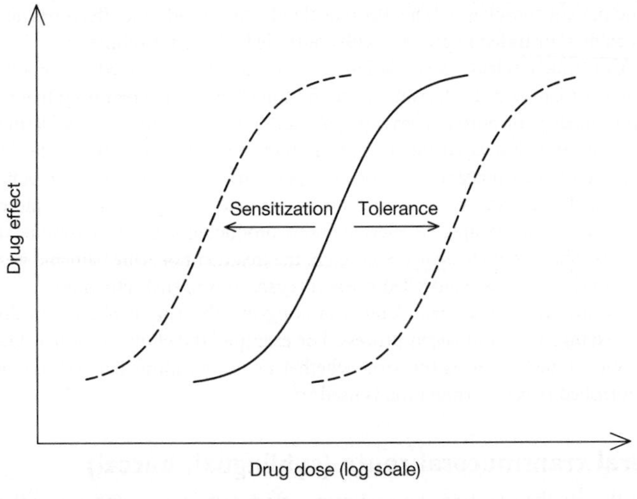

Fig. 6 Graphical representation of drug tolerance and sensitization.

to the analgesic effects of opioids is uncommon in clinical practice. Indeed, increases in opioid requirements are invariably related to progression of disease, rather than to development of tolerance.[5] However, tolerance to some of the adverse effects of opioid drugs is common in clinical practice. Thus, sedation and nausea and vomiting usually settle within a few days, or a week or two.

Cross-tolerance refers to a decreased response to a drug, as a consequence of the use of a similar drug (similar structure, similar function). It may occur to some, or all of the effects of the drugs. The extent of cross-tolerance between opioid drugs is very variable. The practice of opioid switching relies on incomplete cross-tolerance between opioids. Thus, opioid switching will only be successful if cross-tolerance to the analgesic effects is less than cross-tolerance to the adverse effects.[6]

Drug dependence

In pharmacological terms, drug dependence has been divided into two types:[7]

- *Psychological dependence*—characterized by a compulsion to continue to take the drug. This is a pathological response to the drug.
- *Physical dependence*—characterized by a withdrawal syndrome if the drug is not taken (or if an antagonist drug is taken). This is a normal physiological response to the drug.

The relationship between the two types of drug dependence is variable: patients may develop psychological dependence only, or physical dependence, or a combination of psychological and physical dependence. For example, patients receiving opioids for cancer pain rarely develop psychological dependence, although they often develop physical dependence to the opioid.[8] In contrast, opioid drug abusers invariably develop a combination of psychological and physical dependence.

Psychological dependence is associated with a positive (perceived) effect from taking the drug. Drugs that produce a rapid effect are more likely to induce psychological dependence than drugs that produce a delayed effect. For example, a drug given intravenously is more likely to induce psychological dependence than the same drug given orally. The positive effects of the drug are often reinforced by the rituals associated with drug taking, and also by the environment used for drug taking. Indeed, the treatment of psychological dependence involves measures aimed at reducing these reinforcing factors.[7]

Physical dependence is associated with a negative effect from not taking the drug (i.e. with a withdrawal syndrome). The features of the withdrawal syndrome are usually the opposite to the features of the drug's acute effect. The treatment of physical dependence involves trying to reduce the impact of this reinforcing factor.[7] A variety of different 'detoxification' regimens have been used, including gradual reduction of the original drug, gradual reduction of a substitute drug, and symptomatic treatment of the withdrawal syndrome. Many patients require a combination of different strategies in order to overcome their drug dependence.

Drug resistance

Resistance refers to the phenomenon of lack of responsiveness to a drug. The expression is primarily applied to antimicrobial and cytotoxic drugs, but could equally be applied to other classes of drug.

Drug resistance has been sub-classified into: (a) primary or intrinsic resistance—this type of resistance develops de novo; (b) secondary or acquired resistance—this type of resistance develops after exposure to the drug. Drug resistance may involve a single drug, may involve several drugs from the same class (cross-resistance), or several drugs from different classes (also described as cross-resistance). Cross-resistance is invariably due to a common molecular mechanism.

Drug resistance is primarily related to the genetic profile of the cell. Resistance may occur in response to spontaneous mutation, or, in the case of antimicrobial agents, to transfer of genetic material (involving plasmids, bacteriophages, or other mechanisms). The molecular mechanisms

Table 1 Molecular mechanisms of drug resistance

Molecular mechanisms of drug resistance	Specific example
Drug inactivated	Resistance to penicillin may result from the production of β-lactamase
Drug prevented from entering into the cell	Melphalan resistance has been linked to deactivation of various active transport systems (e.g. system L)
Drug prevented from remaining in the cell	Fluconazole resistance has been linked to activation of various active transport systems (e.g. major facilitator efflux pump)
Pro-drug not activated	Resistance to 5-fluorouracil may result from the abnormalities of several enzymes in its metabolic pathway
Alteration of drug 'target'	Amphotericin resistance has been linked to alteration of cell membrane
Overproduction of drug 'target'	Methotrexate resistance has been linked to overproduction of dihydrofolate reductase
Effect of drug counteracted	Resistance to cisplatin may result from repair of damaged DNA

underlying drug resistance are shown in Table 1. Continuing drug usage encourages the development of resistance by suppressing the growth of sensitive cells and, thereby, encouraging the growth of resistant cells.

Antimicrobial drug resistance has become a major clinical problem. Indeed, the Standing Medical Advisory Committee Sub-Group on Antimicrobial Resistance (UK) has used the expression 'looking into the abyss' to describe the current situation.[9] Antimicrobial drug resistance involves not only antibacterial agents, but also antifungal and antiviral agents. Infections caused by resistant organisms generally result in increased morbidity, increased mortality, and increased use of resources.[9]

There is relatively little information about the impact of antimicrobial resistance in palliative medicine. However, a study from the United Kingdom reported that methicillin-resistant *Staphylococcus aureus* (MRSA) infections in hospices were, indeed, associated with increased morbidity (physical and psychological), and increased use of resources.[10] Moreover, this study reported that MRSA infections resulted in major operational problems for the relevant hospices (secondary to infection-control measures).

Antimicrobial drugs should generally only be prescribed for cases of proven infection, and not for prophylaxis of infection. Narrow spectrum drugs should be employed, and these should be prescribed in relatively high doses, for relatively short courses.[9] Other strategies that are relevant include the use of appropriate infection-control measures (e.g. hand washing).

Cytotoxic drug resistance is a perennial clinical problem.[11] Many tumours are primarily resistant, whilst many other tumours become secondarily resistant.

Routes of administration of drugs in palliative care

A variety of different routes of drug administration are used in palliative care. The choice of route will depend on a combination of patient, drug, and organizational factors (availability of drug formulation, financial resources, human resources). Moreover, the choice of route will often vary over the course of the patient's illness.

Oral route

The oral route is the main route of administration of drugs in palliative care. The advantages of this route are that it is simple, non-invasive, and acceptable to patients. Moreover, the majority of drugs used in palliative care are available in oral forms, and, often, in different oral formulations (liquid, solid). The disadvantages of this route are that there are numerous factors that can affect the absorption and bioavailability of the drug.

Modified release formulations for oral administration

There are two theoretical benefits of sustained or controlled release oral preparations. They are either to prolong the absorption time and thereby

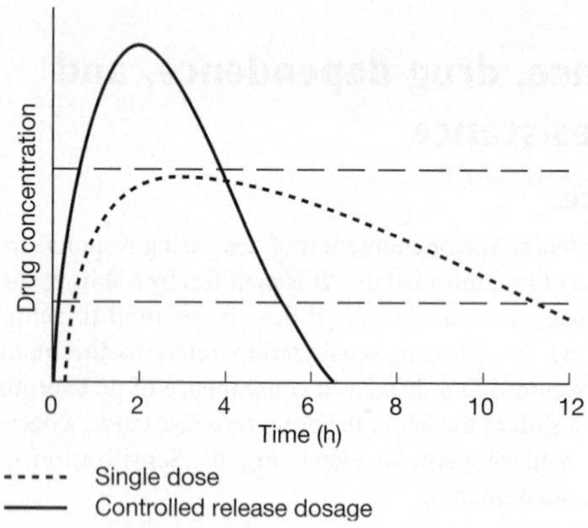

Fig. 7 Typical plasma concentration profile for an immediate release and controlled release formulation of the same drug.

extend the overall duration of action of a short-acting drug (Fig. 7) or to attenuate peak plasma concentrations of a drug where such peak concentrations could be associated with adverse effects. The commonest example in palliative medicine is controlled release morphine. Morphine is a short-acting drug with a duration of analgesia of about 4 h, so in order to maintain control of chronic pain it has to be given six times a day. Controlled release morphine tablets have a 12- or 24-h duration of effect. Reduction in the frequency of dosing has important benefits in terms of patient acceptance and patient compliance. The theoretical reduction in adverse effects has not been demonstrated in practice with controlled release morphine.

Controlled release formulations are, in general, designed for maintenance treatment. The plasma concentration profile is different from that of an immediate or normal release preparation in that the time to peak plasma concentration is delayed and the peak is attenuated. This has implications for the use of such preparations. For example, some drugs need to be rapidly absorbed and have a relatively short duration of action if they are to achieve their intended therapeutic effect without producing significant unwanted effects. This applies to analgesics used in the treatment of acute pain and it is inappropriate to use controlled release preparations in such situations.

Controlled release formulations prolong the absorption phase, but do not change the elimination process. For example, the elimination half-life of morphine (2–4 h) is the same whether or not an immediate release or controlled release formulation is used.[12]

Oral transmucosal route (sublingual, buccal)

In theory, the oral transmucosal route offers certain advantages over the oral route, particularly increased speed of drug absorption, and increased drug bioavailability (for drugs that undergo 'first pass' hepatic metabolism). However, in practice, the oral transmucosal route is limited by the lack of suitable drug formulations, and by the prevalence of salivary gland dysfunction. Recently, there has been interest in the use of this route to treat breakthrough pain,[13] and also to treat epileptic seizures.[14]

Nasogastric/enteral feeding tubes

The decision to use this route is dependent on a number of factors, including the availability of a suitable formulation of the drug, the compatibility of the drug and enteral feed, and various practical issues (the position of the feeding tube and the size of the feeding tube).[15]

Ideally, liquid drug formulations should be used with feeding tubes. However, solid drug formulations can be used, though it is necessary to dissolve them in water, or crush and suspend them in water (see below). Occasionally, parenteral drug formulations are used in place of oral formulations. The appropriateness of crushing solid drug formulations, and of using parenteral formulations, should be verified with a reliable source of drug information.

In general, modified-release formulations should not be crushed, since this can affect their physical characteristics and as a result alter their pharmacokinetic profile (usually resulting in an increased rate of absorption—'dose dumping'). Dose dumping may result in decreased efficacy, and decreased tolerability to the extent of serious drug toxicity. In general, enteric-coated tablets should also not be crushed (unless the end of the feeding tube is situated beyond the stomach).

Drugs should always be administered separately from the enteral feed and the feeding tube should be flushed with water before, and after, the drug is given. Similarly, drugs should always be administered separately and the tube should be flushed before, and after, each drug is given. In the case of drugs that do not interact with food/enteral feed, the feed can be stopped immediately before, and can be restarted immediately after, the drug has been administered.

Rectal route

The rectal route remains an important route of administration of drugs in palliative care. Its main advantage is that it is simple (and does not require additional equipment). Indeed, non-professional carers can be taught to administer drugs via this route. Its main disadvantage is that it is not acceptable to many patients and may be inconvenient for very ill patients. A variety of drugs can be given rectally: some are formulated specifically for rectal use, whilst others are given as oral or parenteral formulations.

The absorption of drugs from the rectum can be very variable: absorption is limited by the small surface area, the presence of faeces, defaecation, and involuntary expulsion of the drug. Drugs given rectally are subject to some 'first pass' hepatic metabolism: the venous drainage of the lower and middle part of the rectum is the inferior vena cava, whilst the venous drainage of the upper part of the rectum is the portal vein (there are significant anastomoses between these two venous systems).

It has been recommended that drugs are inserted one finger-length into the rectum, and, if the rectum is dry, that 10 ml of warm water is co-administered (to ensure dissolution).[16] Alcohol/glycol-containing formulations should be avoided, since these substances can cause rectal irritation.

Subcutaneous route

The subcutaneous route is the most commonly used parenteral route in palliative care. The advantages of the subcutaneous route are that it is simple, and acceptable to patients. Subcutaneous injections are less painful than intramuscular injections. Moreover, a subcutaneous cannula can be inserted, which allows repeated administration of intermittent boluses of drugs, or administration of continuous infusions of drugs (and reduces the need for repeated puncture of the skin). A number of drugs may be given subcutaneously, although in most cases they are not licensed for this route of administration.

Subcutaneous infusions can be given via conventional infusion devices, or, more commonly, via small, battery-powered, syringe drivers. A recent survey from the United Kingdom reported that a variety of different combinations of drugs were being given by continuous infusion.[17] However, the stability/compatibility of many of these combinations is not known. (The compatibility of drug combinations is dependent on a number of factors, including the types of drugs, the concentrations of drugs, the diluent, and other factors such as temperature and UV light.) A database of compatible drug combinations is now available on the Internet (http://www.pallmed.net/). Generally, infusions should contain as few drugs as possible. Indeed, most experts recommend that infusions should contain no more than three drugs. It should be noted that the absence of precipitation within a drug mixture is not synonymous with compatibility between the drugs in that mixture.[18]

Intermittent subcutaneous bolus injections of drugs are usually rapidly absorbed, which makes this route suitable for the emergency treatment of symptoms. Continuous infusions produce stable blood levels of drugs, which make this route suitable for the background treatment of symptoms. However, the absorption of drugs may be affected if the cutaneous blood flow is compromised in any way. Drugs given via the subcutaneous route, and via other parenteral routes, are not susceptible to 'first pass' hepatic metabolism. Indeed, drugs given via the subcutaneous route tend to have a high bioavailability (generally near 100 per cent).

Intramuscular route

The intramuscular route is used infrequently in palliative care: it is generally used in circumstances where the subcutaneous route is contraindicated, such as when the drug is irritant to the skin, when the drug is of large volume, and when the cutaneous blood supply is compromised.

Intravenous route

The intravenous route is also used infrequently in palliative care: it is generally used in emergency situations to obtain a rapid response, and in circumstances where the other parenteral routes are contraindicated, such as where there is a bleeding diathesis and when the peripheral blood supply is compromised. However, if a patient has an indwelling central venous catheter, it would seem appropriate to use the intravenous route rather than the other parenteral routes.

Dermal route

Drugs are usually applied to the skin in order to achieve a local effect. For example, parenteral formulations of diamorphine and morphine (in suitable bases) have been used to treat localized pain secondary to non-malignant ulceration, tumour infiltration, and tumour fungation.[19] However, drugs can also be applied to the skin in order to achieve a systemic effect. For example, specific transdermal formulations of fentanyl and buprenorphine have been developed to treat chronic pain.

Few drugs are reliably absorbed through the skin. Absorption is limited by the physical characteristics of the epidermis and is increased if the epidermis is damaged or destroyed. The absorption of drugs is also dependent on cutaneous hydration (poor hydration leads to decreased absorption), and cutaneous blood flow (poor blood flow leads to decreased absorption). Drugs that are absorbed through the skin are not susceptible to 'first pass' hepatic metabolism.

Pulmonary route

In palliative care, the pulmonary route is primarily used to administer drugs to the lungs. Drugs are administered in the form of either a fine powder or an aerosol, and are administered via an inhaler (± a holding chamber/'spacer') or a nebulizer. The addition of a holding chamber improves the efficiency of inhalers. A recent systematic review concluded that bronchodilators administered via an inhaler and holding chamber were as effective as bronchodilators administered via a nebulizer in acute asthma.[20]

The pulmonary route of administration of drugs is discussed in more detail in Chapter 8.8.

Spinal route

The spinal route refers to administration of drugs either into the epidural space ('epidural'/'extradural'), or into the subarachnoid space ('intrathecal'/ 'subarachnoid').

The spinal route of administration of drugs is discussed in detail in Chapter 8.2.6.

Other routes

Other routes of administration that have been used in palliative care include intranasal, intracavity, and regional application of drugs. The intranasal route can be used to deliver drugs systemically, as well as to deliver drugs locally. Indeed, the role of intranasal opioids in the treatment of breakthrough pain (akin to the use of the oral transmucosal route) is currently being investigated.[21] There have been several reports of the successful use of intracavity local anaesthetics for localized pain: local anaesthetic administered into the pleural cavity have been used to manage chest wall pain,[22] whilst local anaesthetic administered into the joint space has been used to manage bone pain secondary to a pathological fracture.[23] Similarly, there have been several reports of the successful use of regional (perineural) application of local anaesthetics for neuropathic pain.[24]

Variability in drug response

Wide variability in the rates of drug metabolism occurs between individuals as a result of genetic factors, pathological processes, concurrent medication, and ageing, and creates the major obstacle to matching dose to patients' requirements.

Both pharmacokinetic and pharmacodynamic factors may be responsible for therapeutic failure or adverse effects and the mechanism of each may relate to drug interaction, disease, genetics, or the effect of old age. The study of variability in drug response encompasses the whole of the science of clinical pharmacology. In this section, we will merely highlight important principles and provide examples most relevant to palliative medicine.

Pharmacogenetics

Wide interindividual variation in the rates of metabolism of drugs has been observed for many years and a combination of genetic and environmental factors is assumed to be responsible. Our understanding of the influence of genetic factors is increasing rapidly with the advent of modern molecular biological techniques. For example, the rate of elimination of isoniazid within populations has been recognized to have a bimodal distribution.[25] This drug is *N*-acetylated and it is well known now that the rate of drug acetylation is under the control of two autosomal alleles, R for fast acetylation and r for slow (R being dominant and r recessive).[26] 'Fast acetylators' of isoniazid may be more susceptible to hepatic damage caused by the drug and at the same time may be at risk of under dosage with other agents which are acetylated.[27]

The high incidence of the recessive trait, which determines slow acetylation, may indicate a selective advantage for slow acetylators, which is not related to drug metabolism. There is variation in the proportion of fast and slow acetylators in different populations and ethnic groups. In most European groups, about 40 per cent are fast acetylators and in the United States 45 per cent, but 80–90 per cent of Asian populations and nearly 100 per cent of Canadian Eskimos are fast acetylators.[28] Numerous drugs are metabolized by acetylation and the effects of genetic polymorphism have not been studied for all. Hydralazine, some sulfonamides, and some benzodiazepines are worthy of mention but within the field of palliative medicine, where in general dose can be titrated to patients' needs, there do not appear to be significant clinical implications of this phenomenon.

A genetic component to drug oxidation was first documented when rates of metabolism of antipyrine were shown to have a greater degree of concordance in identical twins than in fraternal twins.[29] This was difficult to interpret because of the singular lack of any observed correlation in the rates of oxidation of different drugs between individuals. However, it was subsequently demonstrated that people who were slow oxidizers of debrisoquine were also slow metabolizers of other drugs such as sparteine, phenformin, phenytoin, metoprolol, nortriptyline, and others.[30] We now know that the enzyme system involved, cytochrome P450, can be classified into a number of subfamilies each of which is probably under genetic and environmental control. The most widely studied is the debrisoquine 4-hydroxylation phenotype, which is under the control of cytochrome P450 2D6. About 90 per cent of the population are extensive metabolizers of debrisoquine and family studies have indicated that this is a dominant trait.[31,32] Using kinetic tests it has been shown that different racial groups exhibit different proportions of poor and extensive metabolizers. Egyptians show the lowest incidence of debrisoquine poor metabolizer status (about 1 per cent), whereas West Africans show the highest (about 13 per cent), and Caucasians have an intermediate incidence. CYP2D6 is involved in the methylation of codeine and failures of this drug to produce analgesia have been attributed to the inability to metabolize codeine to the active moiety—morphine. There is evidence of genetic control in the metabolism of mephenytoin in which another isoform of cytochrome P450 is involved (2C9). About 3 per cent of Caucasians and 18 per cent of Japanese are poor metabolizers of mephenytoin.[33] CYP1A2, responsible for the metabolism of theophylline amongst many other drugs, is easily induced by alcohol and flavonoids found in the diet, especially cruciferous vegetables and polycyclic aromatic hydrocarbons found in barbecued food. The variation between genetically determined poor and extensive metabolism is wide and it is important, therefore, that the doses of susceptible drugs should be very carefully managed.

There are, of course, pharmacodynamic examples of genetic variation in drug response. These include resistance to the effects of warfarin due to increased sensitivity to vitamin K, haemolysis in patients with glucose-6-phosphate dehydrogenase deficiency in response to drugs such as sulfonamides or nitrofurantoin, and flushing in response to alcohol in patients taking chlorpropamide.[34]

Disease states

A myriad of conditions, both acute and chronic, can affect the response to drugs by both pharmacokinetic and pharmacodynamic mechanisms. From the pharmacokinetic viewpoint, diseases of the two most important organs of elimination, the kidney and the liver, are most important.

Excretion of drugs by the kidney depends either upon filtration of drug unbound to plasma protein at the glomerulus or upon the active transport systems that secrete drug at the renal tubule. In reality, the reduction in the renal clearance of any drug closely follows renal function as measured by creatinine clearance. The consequences of renal disease, therefore, depend upon the extent to which renal clearance contributes to total drug clearance and how critical drug concentration is in terms of toxicity. Information about the need for dose adjustment in patients with renal impairment is usually readily available in prescribing information sources.

A more complex situation exists for hepatically metabolized drugs. The relevance to palliative medicine is much greater because centrally active drugs tend to be those requiring metabolism simply because they are lipid soluble—a necessary property for penetration into the brain. The metabolic process converts them into more polar, water-soluble metabolites. The liver is also much more commonly affected in malignant disease, not least because it is a common site for metastases.

In chronic liver disease, there exist intrahepatic and extrahepatic anastomoses ('shunts') between the portal and systemic circulation. This means that drugs that normally have a low bioavailability because of presystemic metabolism in the liver can by-pass that metabolic process and may achieve a greatly increased oral bioavailability. This has been shown to occur with pentazocine, pethidine,[35] and chlormethiazole[36] (and many other drugs not used in palliative medicine) and may be expected to occur with methadone,[37] metoclopramide,[38] and others. Reduced metabolite formation of several drugs in the absence of a reduction in systemic clearance in patients with hepatic metastases suggests that such shunting can also take place within tumour deposits inside the liver.[39] This has great implications for oral dosing in malignant disease of drugs with normally low bioavailability.

In chronic liver disease, the total mass of functioning hepatocytes is reduced. It is not surprising that drug metabolism is generally impaired. However, normal interindividual variation in drug metabolism rates is so wide that the effect of the disease may only be evident when severe. The level of serum albumin has been shown to correlate as closely as any parameter to the degree of pharmacokinetic disturbance.[40]

The situation is further complicated by an apparent differential effect on the enzyme system involved. Thus, glucuronidation seems to be relatively protected from the effects of liver disease compared to oxidation and demethylation and there is also evidence of a differential effect on the subfamilies of cytochrome P450.[39]

Hepatic drug metabolizing capacity is not just susceptible to local effects within that organ but widespread pathophysiological changes may affect drug clearance rates. Acute febrile illnesses and endocrine abnormalities may impair drug metabolism.

Some drugs rely on conversion within the liver to their active moiety, for example, prednisone, methylprednisone, and many of the angiotensin converting enzyme inhibitors. This may render some drugs less effective than others in the presence of liver disease and influence the choice of drug in this situation.[39]

In malignant disease of the liver, there appears to be no overall loss of functional hepatocytes so that systemic clearance is usually unimpaired.[41] Some more detailed studies of cytochrome P450 subfamilies are now emerging. It has been shown that CYP1A2 and CYP2E1 are decreased in cirrhosis but not in hepatocellular carcinoma,[42] and there is evidence that P450s of the 2C subfamily may actually be upregulated (i.e. have increased activity) in patients with carcinoma.[43]

Not only renal and hepatic failure but also other organ failures can cause changes in distribution volume either through reducing plasma proteins to which drugs bind or through a qualitative change in the binding sites. Tissue binding may also be affected and the changes in body composition in relation to organ failure and cachexia may be expected to change a drug's distribution volume according to whether they are distributed mainly in water or in lipid tissue. Although poorly studied, the kinetic profile of many drugs is likely to be abnormal in the presence of advanced malignant disease.

In disease states pharmacodynamic mechanisms may cause altered response. Increased sensitivity to centrally acting agents and those acting on the cardiovascular system is common. Particular care is needed when both pharmacodynamic and pharmacokinetic changes are potentially occurring in the same patient, for example, when using drugs with sedating properties in patients with hepatic impairment or respiratory insufficiency.

Ageing

Much of what has been said in respect of disease processes can be applied to the elderly, for after the age of about 65 years there is a gradual decline in renal and hepatic function. Body composition changes so that there is an increase in lipid in relation to total body weight and plasma albumin gradually declines. However, it should be emphasized that the changes in pharmacokinetics are quite small and are only detectable in group studies. The most notable change associated with ageing is an increase in variability so that no assumptions can be made about reduced doses being required and titration of dose to patients' requirements is just more difficult in the aged.

Well studied and of great interest is the effect of the ageing process on hepatic drug metabolism. Total hepatic mass decreases with age and much of the documented decline in drug metabolizing capacity can be attributed to the sheer reduction in total functional hepatocyte mass.[44] It appeared from studies with antipyrine and other agents that it was only microsomally located enzyme systems that decline in activity with age but the results of studies are inconsistent[45] and it has been estimated that only 3 per cent of total variance in drug metabolic rate could be attributed to ageing.[46] A further source of debate is the response of the cytochrome P450 system to enzyme inhibitors and inducers with the obvious implications for drug interaction. There appears little doubt that cimetidine, and presumably other enzyme inhibitors, have a similar effect in the elderly compared to the young.[47] Earlier studies had suggested that microsomal enzymes in the elderly were incapable of being induced[48] (see below) but this suggestion is now completely refuted[45,49] and it is clear that elderly patients are at risk of drug interaction through these mechanisms in the same way as the young.

Reduced cardiovascular and other homeostatic mechanisms and reduced central nervous system function in the aged make this group susceptible to excessive effects from diuretics, blood pressure lowering agents, and central nervous system depressants. The prescription of prochlorperazine for the symptom of dizziness illustrates the potential hazards. The dizziness is usually due to age-related postural hypotension. However, the α-adrenergic blocking properties of the phenothiazine cause vasodilation and worsen the symptom, the dopamine receptor blocking effect precipitates parkinsonism, and the sedating effect causes intellectual impairment!

Drug interaction

Patients who develop terminal illnesses may already be receiving drugs for a variety of conditions. Some may still be required but others may not be necessary but may be continued because of the adverse impact of discontinuing them. If drugs to relieve symptoms are added, this creates an enormous potential for drug interaction. Interaction is adverse if it causes therapeutic failure or toxicity from any one drug. It may be regarded, therefore, as simply another source of variability in drug response. Remembering all the possible drug interactions is virtually impossible, so frequent consultation with prescribing information is important. However, a knowledge of the underlying mechanisms of drug interaction can put the prescriber on guard.

In broad terms, drug interactions are either pharmacokinetic or pharmacodynamic. Kinetic interaction results in a change in the total body exposure to the drug reflected in a change in blood concentration. The effect is entirely predictable from that change. However, the existence of a pharmacokinetic interaction can not be easily predicted—every drug has to be studied before its potential for kinetic interaction can be recognized.

The site of pharmacodynamic interaction is the receptor and so it follows that the consequences of such interaction are common to pharmacological groupings of drugs and are, therefore, to some extent predictable from a working knowledge of each drug group.

Kinetic interaction arises through alteration in rate and extent of absorption, changes in metabolism (both presystemic and elimination), changes in distribution, and in renal excretion. Drugs such as metoclopramide, anticholinergics,[50] and opioid analgesics,[51] which alter the rate of gastric emptying, will affect the speed of absorption of other agents. Again, the resultant effects may not be easily predictable. It is of interest, for example, that food increases the bioavailability of morphine[52] and metoclopramide increases morphine's rate of absorption and sedative effects.[53] Some drugs bind others in the gastrointestinal tract and affect their bioavailability. Certain antacid preparations, iron salts, and cholestyramine are the worst offenders and care is necessary in the use of these drugs concurrently with others.

Of least importance are interactions through changes in distribution. This is because, as we have seen, volume of distribution is not a determinant of steady state concentration although an acute change could cause a temporary effect. In the past, much was made of interactions between drugs as a result of plasma protein binding displacement but this is actually rarely a problem. Even if a drug is very heavily bound to protein, displacement will result in only a temporary rise in the free (unbound) fraction because of immediate compensatory mechanisms. There will be wider distribution throughout the distribution volume and the first-order nature of the elimination process results in increased removal of drug. Most clinically significant interactions previously ascribed to protein binding displacement have now been explained by enzyme inhibition.[54]

Drug interaction resulting from changes in the rate of metabolism by the liver will result in both changes in bioavailability (for those drugs with significant 'first pass' effect) and decreased clearance. Steady state concentrations of drug may be profoundly affected. A number of drugs (particularly the barbiturates, carbamazepine, phenytoin, and rifampicin) are capable of inducing the mixed function oxidase and glucuronidase enzyme systems in the liver. The process involves hypertrophy of the endoplasmic reticulum and takes some weeks to be fully achieved. There is a myriad of substrates for this interaction, amongst them warfarin, corticosteroids, the oral contraceptive, and anticonvulsant drugs. Serum methadone levels can be reduced by the concurrent use of carbamazepine, phenobarbitone, and phenytoin[55] and by rifampicin.[56] The oestrogen component of the oral contraceptive has been shown to double the clearance of morphine by induction of glucuronyl transferase, suggesting the need for increased doses in patients on oestrogens.[57] Important to the care of patients with malignancy is the trebling in plasma clearance of dexamethasone, which can occur in patients receiving concurrently phenytoin, phenobarbitone, or rifampicin, or presumably other enzyme inducers, leading to a reduced bioavailability and shortened half-life.[58]

Our understanding of the process of inhibition of the mixed function oxidase system by drugs has increased dramatically in recent years with the identification of the subfamilies of cytochrome P450. Previously, there was no explanation as to why one drug might reduce the clearance of a second but not that of a third. It is now clear that some drugs inhibit specific subfamilies whilst others, such as cimetidine, are capable of inhibiting all forms of cytochrome P450. That is why cimetidine causes interaction with so many other agents. Cimetidine has been reported to precipitate apnoea in patients taking methadone[59] and to have had a similar effect in a patient taking morphine,[60] but others have found only a small and insignificant effect on morphine kinetics.[61] Other H2 receptor blocking drugs have no enzyme inhibitory effect and the proton pump inhibitor omeprazole has a modest and rather unpredictable effect.

Clomipramine and amitriptyline increase the bioavailability and reduce the clearance of morphine and enhance the analgesic effect. The mechanism seems to be both kinetic, through enzyme inhibition, and pharmacodynamic, through the antidepressants' analgesic effects.[62] Enzyme inhibition tends to occur rapidly so that the full effect is seen after four or five of the newly prolonged half-lives. The list of drugs that cause interaction through enzyme inhibition is long but non-steroidal anti-inflammatory drugs, especially azapropazone,[63] and some of the opioid analgesics, such as dextropropoxyphene,[64] are implicated.

Interactions between drugs and foods through hepatic enzyme induction and inhibition are now recognized. Flavonoids in cabbage and broccoli, etc., may induce some cytochrome P450 sub-families whereas a component of grapefruit juice can inhibit them. These interactions may reach clinical significance where these foodstuffs are being taken in large quantity.

The most important drug interactions in the kidney involve competition between agents for active tubular secretion. This process is used by organic acids and the most frequent 'interactors' are the loop diuretics and some non-steroidal anti-inflammatory drugs. The renal excretion of methotrexate may be inhibited by some non-steroidal anti-inflammatory drugs through this mechanism.[65] Although renal excretion of some drugs is pH dependent, and this can be useful in the management of poisonings, it has in general minor implications in normal therapeutics. There are a few exceptions; for example, methadone's renal clearance is considerably enhanced by concurrent use of urinary acidifiers such as acetazolamide.[66]

Of pharmacodynamic interactions, those of greatest import in palliative medicine involve intracerebral mechanisms. Drugs that cause sedation also have the potential to cause confusion. Not only can central nervous system depressants summate in their action but if the ionic or metabolic environment is deranged by other drugs, such as diuretics, the problem may be compounded. It is of interest that certain benzodiazepines have been shown to oppose the respiratory depressant action of some opioid analgesics[67] whilst increasing the drowsiness associated with others without affecting kinetics.[68] Phenothiazines increase the risk of respiratory depression, sedation, and hypotension.[69]

Polypharmacy

Polypharmacy is endemic in palliative medicine. A recent survey of 385 patients 3 weeks after referral to a palliative care service found that the median number of drugs per patient was five, with a maximum of 11.[70] These numbers are similar to those reported in other elderly patient populations, particularly those admitted to hospital with drug-induced illness.[71] There are several causes of polypharmacy[72] and in palliative medicine some justification. Patients with advanced cancer invariably suffer several symptoms, many of which will be amenable to drug therapy. This may justify the use of combinations of drugs but the overriding principle here must be to avoid unnecessary duplicate prescribing that may occur with significant frequency even in leading specialist centres[70] and to be aware of potential consequences of multiple drug use. Clearly, the more drugs employed at any one time the greater the likelihood of drug interaction. Sometimes, such interaction will be unpredictable, but often adverse consequences of polypharmacy may be both predictable and avoidable. Increasingly, there is a move towards the production of clinical guidelines and drug formularies that should have the effect of improving prescribing habits and encouraging the use of the simplest effective remedies.

Apart from avoiding duplicate prescribing of similar drugs, there are other important principles of good practice that will reduce the tendency towards polypharmacy. The drug regimen should be regularly reviewed and potentially redundant treatments identified. It is always easier to continue treatments particularly if they are not causing any obvious problems, and often patients are reluctant to give up old friends. Both patient and physician need to be persuaded of the benefit of stopping drugs. Adverse effects of one symptomatic remedy may be self-limiting, both in terms of severity and duration, so that any additional treatment introduced to deal with them may be continued unnecessarily. Nausea associated with morphine, for example, is usually an initiation side-effect, if it occurs at all, and may need specific treatment only for a few days; similarly drowsiness, which will usually not require any additional drug intervention. Trials of therapy for specific symptoms should be encouraged and the treatment changed if ineffective rather than continued in conjunction with a new drug.

Use of drugs for unlicensed indications

Legislation regarding the manufacture, marketing, and medical use of therapeutic drugs varies throughout the world. Pharmaceutical companies can only market drugs that have an appropriate marketing authorization (aka product licence). Moreover, pharmaceutical companies can only market drugs within the specific criteria laid out in the marketing authorization (indications for use, patient populations, formulations of the drug, dosages of the drug). In contrast, doctors are permitted to prescribe drugs beyond the specific criteria laid out in the marketing authorization. This practice is known as 'off licence', or 'unlicensed' use of drugs.

The use of unlicensed drugs is common in palliative medicine as noted at the beginning of the chapter. Observational studies from two inpatient units in the United Kingdom reported that ~15 per cent of all prescribed drugs were being used for an unlicensed indication,[1,2] and that 12 per cent of all prescribed drugs were being given via an unlicensed route (i.e. subcutaneously).[2] Indeed, in the study by Todd et al., 68 per cent of the patients were prescribed at least one drug for an indication outside of its marketing authorization (Todd, personal communication).

The use of unlicensed drugs has implications for clinical governance, and medical litigation. Thus, the decision to use an unlicensed drug should be influenced by the:

1. benefit–risk ratio for the patient;
2. strength of evidence for the use of the drug;

Table 2 Selected Internet sources of drug information

Website address	Website content
http://www.druginfozone.org/	Generic website for information about all aspects of clinical pharmacology (UK Medicines Information, NHS, UK)
http://www.bnf.org/	British National Formulary online
http://www.emc.vhn.net/	Association of British Pharmaceutical Industry (ABPI) Medicines Compendium online
http://www.palliativedrugs.com/	Palliative Care Formulary online
http://www.pallmed.net/	Generic website with syringe driver drug compatibility database
http://nccam.nih.gov/	Generic website for information on complementary medicines (National Center for Complementary and Alternative Medicine, National Institute of Health, USA)
http://fda.gov/orphan/index.htm	Generic website for information on orphan drugs (Food and Drug Administration, USA)

3. availability of alternative pharmacological therapies;
4. availability of alternative non-pharmacological therapies;
5. practice of other palliative medicine physicians.

It has been recommended that consent should be obtained before starting the drug, that the reasons for prescribing the drug are recorded in the clinical notes, and that these reasons are conveyed to other members of the health care team.(73) However, a recent survey suggested that it was not routine practice to obtain consent before starting an unlicensed drug in the United Kingdom:(74) the reasons given for this state of affairs included the impracticality of obtaining consent, and the potential distress to patients/carers of obtaining consent.

Sources of drug information

There are a number of different sources of information on the drugs used in palliative medicine, including conventional educational resources (journals, textbooks), national pharmacopoeias, drug information units, drug regulatory authorities, and pharmaceutical companies.

Many sources of information are generic in nature, and provide limited information specifically about the uses of drugs in palliative medicine. However, some sources are specific, such as the Palliative Care Formulary.(75) The Palliative Care Formulary is modelled on the British National Formulary and it provides similar information (formulations, cautions, side-effects), with additional information about the uses of the drug (indications, regimens, references) in palliative medicine.

An increasingly important source of information is the World Wide Web. The Internet has a number of advantages, especially ease of access, but also a number of disadvantages, particularly the lack of peer review of information.(76) The Health On the Net Foundation (Switzerland) was set up in response to the latter problem: it provides impartial information about the quality of health care websites; it also produces a voluntary code of conduct for the developers of health care websites (see Table 2).

There are an ever-increasing number of drug resources on the Internet. Indeed, the use of generic search engines often leads to 'information overload', as a result of the indiscriminate identification of vast numbers of websites. Table 2 gives a list of some useful drug resources on the Internet: these websites are maintained by respected organizations, are freely accessible to health care professionals, and have links to other relevant websites.

Clinical pharmacists can also be useful sources of drug information (see Chapter 15.9). A study from Australia reported that a clinical pharmacist identified potential problems with the drug regimen of 13 per cent of hospice inpatients, and that changes in the drug regimen resulted in improvements in care in the majority of instances.(77) The problems identified included inappropriate drug dose, inappropriate drug frequency, and potential drug interactions; the problems were predominantly related to drugs being used for general medical indications, rather than for palliative care indications.

Conclusions

The skilful use of drugs to palliate symptoms is essential to the practice of palliative medicine. Individualization of drug and dose and simplicity are the watchwords whatever type of treatment is being used. An understanding of the principles outlined in this chapter should facilitate day-to-day management of clinical problems, improve the risk–benefit ratio of drugs used in symptom control, and ultimately contribute to improving the quality of life of patients with advanced disease.

References

1. **Atkinson, C.V. and Kirkham, S.R.** (1999). Unlicensed uses for medication in a palliative care unit. *Palliative Medicine* **13**, 145–52.
2. **Todd, J. and Davies, A.** (1999). Use of unlicensed medication in palliative medicine. *Palliative Medicine* **13**, 446.
3. **Ettinger, D.S., Vitale, P.J., and Trump, D.L.** (1979). Important clinical pharmacologic considerations in the use of methadone in cancer patients. *Cancer Treatment Reports* **63**, 457–9.
4. **Bullingham, R.E.S., McQuay, H., Dwyer, D., Allen, M.C., and Moore, R.A.** (1981). Sublingual buprenorphine used post-operatively: clinical observations and preliminary pharmacokinetic analysis. *British Journal of Clinical Pharmacology* **12**, 117–22.
5. **Collin, E., Poulain, P., Gauvain-Piquard, A., Petit, G., and Pichard-Leandri, E.** (1993). Is disease progression the major factor in morphine 'tolerance' in cancer pain treatment? *Pain* **55**, 319–26.
6. **Fallon, M.** (1997). Opioid rotation: does it have a role? *Palliative Medicine* **11**, 177–8.
7. **Littleton, J.** (1997). Drug dependence and drugs of abuse. In *Integrated Pharmacology* (ed. C.P. Page, M.J. Curtis, M.C. Sutter, M.J.A. Walker, and B.B. Hoffman), pp. 539–51. London: Mosby.
8. **Kanne, R.M. and Foley, K.** (1981). Patterns of narcotic use in a cancer pain clinic. *Annals of New York Academy of Science* **362**, 161–72.
9. **Standing Medical Advisory Committee Sub-Group on Antimicrobial Resistance.** *The Path of Least Resistance*. London: Department of Health, 1998.
10. **Prentice, W., Dunlop, R., Armes, P.J., Cunningham, D.E., Lucas, C., and Todd, J.** (1998). Methicillin-resistant *Staphylococcus aureus* infection in palliative care. *Palliative Medicine* **12**, 443–9.
11. **Souhami, R.L., Tannock, I., Hohenberger, P., and Horiot, J.C.**, ed. *Oxford Textbook of Oncology* 2nd edn. Oxford: Oxford University Press, 2002.
12. **Savarese, J., Goldenheim, P.D., Thomas, G.B., and Kaiko, R.F.** (1986). Steady-state pharmacokinetics of controlled release oral morphine sulphate in healthy subjects. *Clinical Pharmacokinetics* **11**, 505–10.

13. **Farrar, J.T., Cleary, J., Rauck, R., Busch, M., and Nordbrock, E.** (1998). Oral transmucosal fentanyl citrate: randomized, double-blinded, placebo-controlled trial for treatment of breakthrough pain in cancer patients. *Journal of National Cancer Institute* **90**, 611–16.
14. **Scott, R.C., Besag, F.M., and Neville, B.G.** (1999). Buccal midazolam and rectal diazepam for treatment of prolonged seizures in childhood and adolescence: a randomised trial. *Lancet* **353**, 623–6.
15. **Gilbar, P.J.** (1999). A guide to enteral drug administration in palliative care. *Journal of Pain and Symptom Management* **17**, 197–207.
16. **Warren, D.E.** (1996). Practical use of rectal medications in palliative care. *Journal of Pain and Symptom Management* **11**, 378–87.
17. **O'Doherty, C.A., Hall, E.J., Schofield, L., and Zeppetella, G.** (2001). Drugs and syringe drivers: a survey of adult specialist palliative care practice in the United Kingdom and Eire. *Palliative Medicine* **15**, 149–54.
18. **Grassby, P.F. and Hutchings, L.** (1997). Drug combinations in syringe drivers: the compatibility and stability of diamorphine with cyclizine and haloperidol. *Palliative Medicine* **11**, 217–24.
19. **Krajnik, M., Zylicz, Z., Finlay, I., Luczak, J., and van Sorge, A.A.** (1999). Potential uses of topical opioids in palliative care—report of 6 cases. *Pain* **80**, 121–5.
20. **Cates, C.J. and Rowe, B.H.** (2001). Holding chambers versus nebulisers for beta-agonist treatment of acute asthma (Cochrane Review). In *The Cochrane Library* Issue 4. Oxford: Update Software.
21. **Zeppetella, G.** (2000). An assessment of the safety, efficacy, and acceptability of intranasal fentanyl citrate in the management of cancer-related breakthrough pain: a pilot study. *Journal of Pain and Symptom Management* **20**, 253–8.
22. **Amesbury, B., O'Riordan, J., and Dolin, S.** (1999). The use of interpleural analgesia using bupivacaine for pain relief in advanced cancer. *Palliative Medicine* **13**, 153–8.
23. **Shabat, S., Stern, A., Kollender, Y., and Nyska, M.** (2001). Continuous intra-articular patient-controlled analgesia in a cancer patient with a pathological hip fracture. A case report. *Acta Orthopaedica Belgica* **67**, 304–6.
24. **Wang, M.Y., Teitelbaum, G.P., Loskota, W.J., Eng, D., Albuquerque, F., and Gruen, J.P.** (2000). Brachial plexus catheter reservoir for the treatment of upper-extremity cancer pain: technical case report. *Neurosurgery* **46**, 1009–12.
25. **Evans, D.A.P., Manley, K.A., and McKusick, V.A.** (1960). Genetic control of isoniazid metabolism in man. *British Medical Journal* **ii**, 485.
26. **Sim, E. and Hickman, D.** (1991). Polymorphism in human *N*-acetyltransferase—the case for the missing allele. *Trends in Pharmacological Science* **12**, 1211–13.
27. **Ellard, G.A. and Gammon, P.T.** (1977). Acetylator phenotyping of tuberculosis patients using matrix isoniazid on sulphadimidine and its prognostic significance for treatment with several intermittent isoniazid-containing regimens. *British Journal of Clinical Pharmacology* **4**, 5–14.
28. **Lunde, P.K.M., Frislid, K., and Hansteen, V.** (1977). Disease and acetylation polymorphism. *Clinical Pharmacokinetics* **2**, 182.
29. **Vesell, E.S.** (1975). Pharmacogenetics. *Biochemical Pharmacology* **24**, 445–50.
30 **Steiner, E., Iselius, L., Alvan, G., Lindstein, J., and Sjoqvist, F.** (1985). A family study of genetic and environmental factors determining polymorphic hydroxylation of debrisoquine in man. *Clinical Pharmacology and Therapeutics* **38**, 394–401.
31. **Eichelbaum, M. and Gross, A.S.** (1990). The genetic polymorphism of debrisoquine/sparteine metabolism—clinical aspects. *Clinical Pharmacology and Therapeutics* **46**, 377–94.
32. **Gonzalez, F.J. and Meyer, U.A.** (1991). Molecular genetics of the debrisoquine/sparteine polymorphism. *Clinical Pharmacology and Therapeutics* **50**, 233–8.
33. **Gibson, G.G. and Skett, P.** *Introduction to Drug Metabolism* 2nd edn. Glasgow: Blackie Academic and Professional, 1994.
34. **Anonymous** (1999). Pharmacogenetics. In *A Textbook of Clinical Pharmacology* 4th edn. (ed. J.M. Ritter, L.D. Lewis, and T.G.K. Mant), pp. 108–18. London: Arnold.
35. **Pond, S.M., Tong, T., Benowitz, N.L., and Jacob, P.** (1980). Enhanced bioavailability of pethidine and pentazocine in patients with cirrhosis of the liver. *Australian and New Zealand Journal of Medicine* **10**, 515.
36. **Pentikainen, P.J., Neuvonen, P.J., and Jostell, K.G.** (1980). Pharmacokinetics of chlormethiazole in healthy volunteers and patients with cirrhosis of the liver. *European Journal of Pharmacology* **17**, 275.
37. **Inturrusi, C.E. and Verebely, K.** (1972). Disposition of methadone in man after a single oral dose. *Clinical Pharmacology and Therapeutics* **13**, 923–30.
38. **Bateman, D.N.** (1983). Clinical pharmacokinetics of metoclopramide. *Clinical Pharmacokinetics* **8**, 523–9.
39. **Morgan, D.J. and McLean, A.J.** (1995). Clinical pharmacokinetic and pharmacodynamic considerations in patients with liver disease. *Clinical Pharmacokinetics* **29**, 370–91.
40. **Homeida, M., Jackson, L., and Roberts, C.J.C.** (1978). Decreased first pass metabolism of labetalol in chronic liver disease. *British Medical Journal* **2**, 1048.
41. **Robertz-Vaupel, G.M. et al.** (1992). Disposition of antipyrine inpatients with extensive metastatic liver disease. *European Journal of Clinical Pharmacology* **42**, 465–9.
42. **Guengerich, F.P. and Turvy, C.G.** (1991). Comparison of levels of several human microsomal cytochrome P450 enzymes and epoxide hydrolase in normal and disease states using immunochemical analysis of surgical liver samples. *Journal of Pharmacology and Experimental Therapeutics* **256**, 1189–91.
43. **Murray, M.** (1992). P450 enzymes: inhibition mechanisms, genetic regulation and effects of liver disease. *Clinical Pharmacokinetics* **23**, 132–46.
44. **Swift, C.G., Homeida, M., Halliwell, M., and Roberts, C.J.C.** (1985). Antipyrine disposition and liver size in the elderly. *European Journal of Clinical Pharmacology* **20**, 119–28.
45. **Durnas, C., Loi, C.M., and Cusack, B.J.** (1990). Hepatic drug metabolism and aging. *Clinical Pharmacokinetics* **19**, 359–89.
46. **Vestal, R.E. et al.** (1975). Antipyrine metabolism in man: influence of age, alcohol, caffeine and smoking. *Clinical Pharmacology and Therapeutics* **18**, 425–32.
47. **Feely, J., Pareira, I., Guy, E., and Hockings, N.** (1984). Factors affecting the response to inhibition of drug metabolism by cimetidine—dose response and sensitivity of elderly and induced subjects. *British Journal of Clinical Pharmacology* **17**, 77–81.
48. **Salem, S.A.M., Rajjayabun, P., Shepherd, A.M.M., and Stevenson, I.H.** (1978). Reduced induction of drug metabolism in the elderly. *Age and Ageing* **7**, 68–73.
49. **Pearson, M.W. and Roberts, C.J.C.** (1984). Drug induction of hepatic enzymes in the elderly. *Age and Ageing* **13**, 313–16.
50. **Nimmo, J., Heading, R.C., Tothill, P., and Prescott, L.F.** (1973). Pharmacological modification of gastric emptying: effects of propantheline and metoclopramide on paracetamol absorption. *British Medical Journal* **1**, 587–9.
51. **Nimmo, W.S., Heading, R.C., Wilson, J., Tothill, P., and Prescott, L.F.** (1975). Inhibition of gastric emptying and drug absorption by narcotic analgesics. *British Journal of Clinical Pharmacology* **2**, 509–13.
52. **Gourlay, G.K., Plummer, J.L., Cherry, D.A., Foate, J.A., and Cousins, M.J.** (1989). Influence of a high fat meal on the absorption of morphine from oral solutions. *Clinical Pharmacology and Therapeutics* **46**, 463–8.
53. **Manara, A.R., Shelley, M.P., Quinn, K., and Park, G.R.** (1988). The effect of metoclopramide on the absorption of oral controlled release morphine. *British Journal of Clinical Pharmacology* **25**, 518–21.
54. **Kristensen, M.B.** (1983). Drug interaction and clinical pharmacokinetics. In *Handbook of Clinical Pharmacokinetics* (ed. M. Gibaldi and L. Prescott) pp. 242–64. Auckland: ADIS Health Science Press.
55. **Bell, J., Seves, V., Bowren, P., Lewis, J., and Batey, R.** (1988). The use of serum methadone levels in patients receiving methadone maintenance. *Clinical Pharmacology and Therapeutics* **43**, 623–9.
56. **Bending, M.R. and Skacel, P.O.** (1977). Rifampicin and methadone withdrawal. *Lancet* **i**, 1211.
57. **Watson, K.J.R., Ghabrial, H., Mashford, M.L., Harman, P.J., Breen, K.J., and Desmond, P.V.** (1986). The oral contraceptive pill increases morphine clearance but does not increase hepatic blood flow. *Gastroenterology* **90**, 1779.
58. **Anonymous** (1991). Dexamethasone. In *Therapeutic Drugs* (ed. C. Dollery et al.), pp. D44–50. Edinburgh: Churchill Livingstone.

59. **Dawson, G.W. and Vestal, R.E.** (1984). Cimetidine inhibits the *in vitro* *N*-demethylation of methadone. *Research Communications in Chemical Pathology and Pharmacology* **46**, 301–4.

60. **Fine, A. and Churchill, D.N.** (1981). Potential lethal interaction of cimetidine and morphine. *Canadian Medical Association Journal* **124**, 1434.

61. **Lam, A.M. and Clement, J.L.** (1984). Effect of cimetidine pre-medication on morphine-induced ventilatory depression. *Canadian Anaesthetic Society Journal* **31**, 36–43.

62. **Ventafridda, V., Ripamonti, C., De Conno, F., Bianchi, M., Pazzuconi, F., and Panereai, A.E.** (1987). Antidepressants increase bioavailability of morphine in cancer patients. *Lancet* **i**, 1204.

63. **Roberts, C.J.C., Daneshmend, T.K., Macfarlane, D., and Dieppe, P.A.** (1981). Anti-convulsant intoxication precipitated by azapropazone. *Postgraduate Medical Journal* **57**, 191.

64. **Orme, M. and Breckenridge, A.** (1976). Warfarin and distalgesic interaction. *British Medical Journal* **i**, 200.

65. **Daly, H.M., Scott, G.L., Boyle, J., and Roberts, C.J.C.** (1986). Methotrexate toxicity precipitated by azapropazone. *British Journal of Dermatology* **114**, 733–5.

66. **Bellward, G.D., Warren, D.M., Howald, W., Axelson, J.E., and Abbott, P.S.** (1977). Methadone maintenance: effect of urinary pH on renal clearance in chronic high and low doses. *Clinical Pharmacology and Therapeutics* **22**, 92–9.

67. **McDonald, C.F., Thomson, S.A., Scott, N.C., Scott, W., Grant, I.W.B., and Crompton, G.K.** (1986). Benzodiazepine–opiate antagonism—a problem in intensive care therapy. *Intensive Care Medicine* **12**, 39–42.

68. **Pond, S.M., Benowitz, N.L., Jacob, P., and Rigod, J.** (1982). Lack of effect of diazepam on methadone metabolism in methadone-maintained addicts. *Clinical Pharmacology and Therapeutics* **31**, 139–43.

69. **Grothe, D.R., Ereshefsky, L., Jann, M.W., and Fidone, G.S.** (1986). Clinical implication of the neuroleptic–opioid interaction. *Drug Intelligence in Clinical Pharmacology* **20**, 75–7.

70. **Twycross, R.G., Bergl, S., John, S., and Lewis, K.** (1994). Monitoring drug use in palliative care. *Palliative Medicine* **8**, 137–43.

71. **Colt, A.G. and Shapiro, A.P.** (1989). Drug induced illness as a cause for admission to a community hospital. *Journal of the American Geriatric Society* **37**, 323–6.

72. **Kroenke, K.** (1985). Polypharmacy. Causes, consequences, and cure. *The American Journal of Medicine* **79**, 149–52.

73. **Ferner, R.E.** (1996). Prescribing licensed medicines for unlicensed indications. *Prescribers' Journal* **36**, 73–8.

74. **Pavis, H. and Wilcock, A.** (2001). Prescribing of drugs for use outside their licence in palliative care: survey of specialists in the United Kingdom. *British Medical Journal* **323**, 484–5.

75. **Twycross, R., Wilcock, A., and Thorp, S.** *Palliative Care Formulary. PCF 1*. Oxford: Radcliffe Medical Press, 1998.

76. **Pereira, J. and Bruera, E.** (1998). The Internet as a resource for palliative care and hospice: a review and proposals. *Journal of Pain and Symptom Management* **16**, 59–68.

77. **Lucas, C., Glare, P.A., and Sykes, J.V.** (1997). Contribution of a liaison clinical pharmacist to an inpatient palliative care unit. *Palliative Medicine* **11**, 209–16.

66. Wood, S.M., Mahaffey, M.J., Smith, P., and Read, J. (1992). Local effect of [illegible] acetate, [illegible] [illegible] and [illegible]. Journal of Pharmacology and Therapeutics, [illegible].
67. Gardner, D.M., Shulman, K.I., Walker, S.E., and Tailor, S.A. (1996). [illegible] of the [illegible] interaction. Journal of Clinical Psychiatry, 57, [illegible].
68. Twycross, R.G., Bergl, S., John, S., and Lewis, K. (1990). Monitoring drug use in palliative care. Palliative Medicine, 4, 27–34.
69. Oh, [illegible] and Shapiro, A.P. (1979). [illegible] and [illegible] in a community hospital. Journal of the American Geriatric Society, 27, [illegible].
70. Lincoln, K. (1987). [illegible] Causes, [illegible]. American Journal of Medicine, 79, 149–52.
71. Farrer, K. (1988). [illegible] hospital [illegible]. Journal of Pharmacy, 16, 61–5.
72. Evans, H. and Wilcock, A. (2000). [illegible] drug use in the United Kingdom. British Medical Journal, 320, [illegible].
73. Twycross, R., Wilcock, A., and Thorp, S. Palliative care formulary (PCF). Radcliffe Medical Press, 1998.
74. Pereira, J. and Bruera, E. (1998). The [illegible] in palliative medicine: a review. Journal of Pain and Symptom Management, 10, [illegible].
75. Gilbar, P., Wood, R.S., and Sykes, P.P. (1999). Contribution of a hospital pharmacist to [illegible] care. Palliative Medicine, 13, [illegible].
76. Drummer, O.H. and Wood, R.H. (1993). [illegible]. Journal of Medicine, 46, [illegible].
77. Hine, M. and Copeland, [illegible] (1981). [illegible] interactions of [illegible]. Journal of [illegible], 131, [illegible].
78. Lam, J.M. and Garland, D.J. (1991). [illegible] of [illegible] on [illegible] in the [illegible]. [illegible].
79. [illegible], V., Ripamonti, C., De Conno, F., Bianchi, M., Panerai, A.E., and Parolaro, A.E. (1998). [illegible] bioavailability of [illegible]. Lancet, [illegible].
80. Jacob, D., Gleeson, D., Montgomery, D., and Moore, D.A. (1991). [illegible] intoxication precipitated by [illegible]. Palliative Medicine, 5, 161.
81. [illegible] and Brackenridge, A.R. (1988). [illegible]. British Medical Journal, 1, 101.
82. Daly, R.M., Scott, E.L., Ralph, L., and Roberts, C.J.C. (1996). [illegible] by [illegible]. British Journal of [illegible], [illegible].
83. [illegible], [illegible], Wesson, D.M., Howard, W., [illegible], and Ahlgren, E.S. (1997). [illegible] in [illegible]. Journal of Clinical Pharmacology, 37, [illegible].
84. McDonald, C.J., Thomson, N.A., Smith, N., Smith, W., Cloud, A.M.K., and [illegible], K. (1998). [illegible] on the [illegible]. Journal of Palliative Care, 12, 7[illegible].

8 Symptom management

8 Symptom management

8.1 Disease modifying management

8.1.1 Palliative medicine and the treatment of cancer

Malcolm McIllmurray

The optimal management of cancer requires a multidisciplinary team approach in which palliative care physicians and surgical, radiation, and medical oncologists play an important part. Patients may experience physical, emotional, psychological, and spiritual distress at any time during the course of the illness, and involving palliative care physicians from diagnosis ensures that patients are referred for specialist palliative care when they need it. However, so that they are fully integrated members of the multidisciplinary team, palliative care physicians should understand the respective roles of the oncologists in the team and know about the cancers which they treat and the expectations and side effects of their treatments. In addition, this knowledge should ensure that palliative care physicians are able to recognize patients in their care who might benefit from cancer treatment and refer them to an appropriate oncologist.

This chapter describes the medical treatment of cancer which is provided by the medical oncologist in the multidisciplinary team. In some countries this role is shared between medical and radiation oncologists. Emphasis is placed on the treatment of advanced and incurable cancer because palliative care physicians are more likely to be involved in that clinical setting although patients with early and curable cancer may also need their expertise.

Background

Cancer is a disease which is derived from the mutation of a single cell. The mutation is the result of defects in the genes associated with the cell cycle and the cell signalling pathways which control cell replication and cell death. The defects can be inherited, occur by chance, or be acquired by exposure to certain viruses or carcinogens. The mutated cell (the cancer phenotype) has various characteristics which include the ability:

- to avoid apoptosis (programmed cell death),
- to resist the normal ageing process,
- to replicate outside normal controlling mechanisms,
- to produce chemicals which dissolve surrounding connective tissue (matrix metalloproteinases),
- to stimulate a microvascular blood supply (angiogenesis),
- to invade and disseminate to other parts of the body (metastatic spread), and
- to overcome or paralyse the immune system.

Cell signalling pathways begin with cell surface receptors which, when activated, initiate a cascade of molecular events that transfer instructions from outside the cell to the cell nucleus. Over-expression of receptors, which are activated by growth factors and which instruct the cell to divide, is also a feature of the cancer phenotype.

An understanding of the relationship between a cancer cell and its environment and of the cellular changes which produce these various biological effects has given rise to the treatment of some cancers with hormones or hormone-blocking drugs (hormone therapy) and with other receptor or protein-modifying agents (biological therapy). However, the gold standard for the medical treatment of cancer is the use of cytotoxic drugs (chemotherapy) whose effects do not depend on the genetic differences that distinguish cancer cells from their normal counterparts. This chapter considers the use of these three types of treatment in a palliative care setting and gives the reader an understanding of the principles which underlie their use. Prescribing details are omitted because this is the responsibility of the oncologist and not of the palliative care physician.

Chemotherapy in palliative care

The mode of action of cytotoxic drugs

Cells divide in an orderly sequence known as the cell cycle (Fig. 1) in which DNA synthesis (S phase) is followed by mitosis (M phase) with gaps between these two events (G1 and G2) during which DNA copy defects are identified and corrected or the cell is programmed to die (apoptosis). Cells can leave the cell cycle and remain in a resting phase (G0) until they re-enter the cycle in response to an appropriate stimulus.

Cytotoxic drugs target cells during cell division in the cell cycle. However, some drugs only kill cells if they happen to be in a particular phase of the

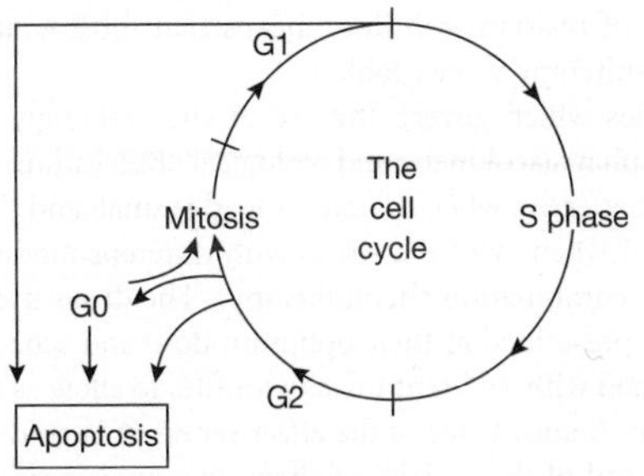

Fig. 1 The cell cycle.

cycle when the drug is administered (phase-specific drugs). Prolonging the time during which a cancer is exposed to a phase-specific drug will increase the number of cells killed because dividing cells cycle at random and all dividing cells must pass through that phase of the cycle for maximum cytotoxic effect. Other drugs kill cells in cycle in whatever phase of division the cells have reached when the drug is administered (cycle-specific drugs) and the number of cells killed is related to the administered dose of the drug rather than to the exposure time. The distinction between phase-specific and cycle-specific drugs is useful when it comes to selecting drugs and doses for combination regimens because, for example, it makes sense to avoid administering two drugs together which are specific for the same phase of the cell cycle; and when two cycle-specific drugs are administered together, the doses of each must be reduced to avoid severe toxic side effects.

Cytotoxic drugs can also be classified according to their pharmacological effects on the biological events which take place during the cell cycle as follows.

Antimetabolites interfere with the incorporation of nucleic acid bases into the DNA molecule. Their activity is greatest in the S phase of the cell cycle. Examples are 5-fluorouracil, fludarabine, methotrexate, and gemcitabine.

Alkylating drugs typically form linkages between the strands of DNA which prevent them from separating during the M phase of the cell cycle, but they also have other biochemical effects and are cycle-specific rather than phase-specific. Examples are cyclophosphamide, ifosfamide, chlorambucil, and melphalan. Other drugs with alkylating activity include the platinum compounds, cisplatin, and carboplatin.

Antitumour antibiotics act through a number of different mechanisms but typically interfere with the binding of base-pair molecules and prevent the separation of the DNA strands during the M phase of the cell cycle. Some drugs are phase-specific, such as bleomycin, and others are cycle-specific, such as doxorubicin and epirubicin.

Plant alkaloids are derived from natural sources. They are phase-specific and are either mitotic spindle inhibitors, such as vincristine, vinblastine, and the taxanes, paclitaxel and docetaxel, or topoisomerase inhibitors, such as topotecan, irinotecan, and etoposide.

The effect of cytotoxic drugs on cancer cells

The factors that determine the greater damage inflicted by cytotoxic drugs on cancer tissues compared to normal tissues are related to two important observations. Firstly, the proportionate cell kill following treatment is generally greater in cancer tissues than in normal tissues because cytotoxic drugs only affect dividing cells and the proportion of dividing cells (the growth fraction) is generally higher in cancer tissues than in normal tissues. Secondly after cytotoxic damage, the processes of repair are more efficient in normal tissues than in cancer tissues. Therefore if treatment is given intermittently and the time between treatments is just enough to allow normal tissues to recover, there is a gradual reduction in the population of cancer cells whilst the normal cell population is maintained. In theory it should be possible to eliminate all cancer cells if treatment is continued for long enough but, in practice it is rare for cancers to be cured in this way. As cancers grow they outstrip their own blood supply, which reduces drug penetration, and they contain an increasing number of mutant cell lines some of which are sensitive to cytotoxic drugs and others which are not. The continued growth of resistant cell lines means that most cancers cannot be cured by chemotherapy alone (Table 1).

The principles which govern the use of chemotherapy in cancers are based on these pharmacokinetic and biological observations. Thus, chemotherapy is most effective when the cancer load is small and the growth fraction is high and when cytotoxic drugs with different modes of action are given together (combination chemotherapy). The drugs used in combination should be prescribed at their optimum dose and schedule and drugs should be selected with different toxicity profiles to allow as wide a range of dose as possible. A knowledge of the effectiveness of chemotherapy in each type of cancer and of the toxicity of chemotherapy is necessary to inform the discussion which must take place between the patient and oncologist about the decision to treat.

Table 1 Response of cancers to chemotherapy and hormone therapy

Cancers which can be cured by chemotherapy (including patients with advanced disease)
Germ cell
Chorioncarcinoma
Non-Hodgkin lymphoma (high-grade)
Hodgkin's lymphoma
Acute lymphoblastic leukaemia
Cancers which can be cured by induction,[a] or adjuvant chemotherapy[b] and/or hormone therapy[c]
Breast[a,b,c]
Non-small cell lung (local advanced)[a]
Colon[b]
Osteosarcoma[b]
Cancers in which survival may be prolonged by chemotherapy[a] and/or hormone therapy[b] in patients with advanced disease
Breast[a,b]
Non-Hodgkin lymphoma (low-grade)[a]
Colon[a]
Myeloma[a]
Prostate[b]
Small cell lung[a]
Bladder[a]
Ovary[a]
Rectum[a]
Endometrium[b]
Acute myeloid lukaemia[a]
Cancers which may respond to chemotherapy for advanced disease with little effect on survival but with possible quality of life benefits
Non-small cell lung
Cervix
Melanoma
Oesophagus
Pancreas
Stomach
Glioma
Head/neck
Soft tissue sarcoma
Cancers which are resistant to chemotherapy
Renal
Mesothelioma
Prostate
Endometrium

The effectiveness of chemotherapy

The process whereby drugs move from the laboratory to clinical practice is painstakingly slow. Extensive animal testing establishes cytotoxic efficacy and safety and is followed by three phases of clinical trials involving patients. These are designed to determine the optimum dose and schedule and the toxicity profile of the drug (phase I trials), the response of different cancers to the drug (phase II trials), and the clinical benefits, either alone or in combination with other cytotoxic drugs, in the cancers which respond (phase III trials). Informed consent for treatment is mandatory for all patients recruited into clinical trials.

Clinical decisions are based on the outcome of phase III trials. A phase III trial usually takes the form of a randomized controlled trial (RCT) in which the new drug, either alone or in combination, is compared to standard treatment which may be supportive care only. Patients selected for RCTs must meet eligibility criteria which are clearly defined so that both treatment groups are comparable. Stratification may be necessary to control for the patient and cancer characteristics which are known to affect the outcome. Differences between treatment groups are usually small and large numbers of patients are needed to detect a significant effect of a new drug. Many phase III trials are not large enough to detect small differences and it is necessary to combine the data from all published trials of a particular treatment for a particular cancer to obtain proof of effectiveness. This is called a meta-analysis and is a method of evaluating new drugs and combinations in common cancers.

The effectiveness of chemotherapy in treating patients with cancer is assessed by the effect it has on:

- the survival time from commencement of treatment;
- the time from commencement of treatment to cancer progression;
- the cancer response rate which is the proportion of treated patients whose cancer either becomes undetectable (complete remission) or reduces in size by at least 50 per cent (partial remission) or stays the same size (stable disease) or continues to grow during treatment (progressive disease); and
- the quality of life.

Quality of life measurements have become very important in the evaluation of cytotoxic drugs since it was shown that the quality of life of cancer patients can be improved by chemotherapy despite the associated toxicity and without there necessarily being any improvement in survival time.[1,2]

The toxicity of chemotherapy

The normal tissues which are most vulnerable to the effects of chemotherapy are those which are in a constant state of regeneration and repair. It can be predicted therefore that the commonest toxicities will arise from the effects on the bone marrow, gastrointestinal tract, and skin. Other toxicities such as the effects on kidneys, nervous system, lungs, and heart are less predictable and much less common.

Bone marrow

Erythrocytes, neutrophils, and platelets are produced by haemopoeitic stem cells in the bone marrow. Their production rate is such that new cell formation keeps pace with cell losses; in the normal steady state about 5 per cent of stem cells are undergoing cell division (in cell cycle) at any one time. These dividing stem cells are vulnerable to the effects of cytotoxic drugs. A fall in the number of circulating neutrophils which follows a course of chemotherapy will take several days to appear because the life span of a mature neutrophil is about 10 days. For erythrocytes the period is much longer, about 120 days, and for platelets about 5 days. Low erythrocyte counts (anaemia) and low platelet counts (thrombocytopenia) can be corrected by transfusion if necessary or, in the case of the erythrocyte by the administration of erythropoietin, the naturally occurring erythrocyte stem-cell growth factor; these effects are rarely life-threatening.

By contrast, a low neutrophil count exposes a patient to the risks of serious and sometimes fatal infection. This is especially dangerous for there is no symptom which will alert a patient to a falling neutrophil count and it may only be brought to their attention when infection is established. Thus in any chemotherapy service, there must be clear instructions to patients about recognizing the symptoms and signs of infection and fast-tracking them through the health care services so that the combination of a low neutrophil count and a fever is identified and treated without delay. Such patients must be regarded as acute medical emergencies and they require immediate admission to hospital. After obtaining samples of body fluids and secretions for culture, treatment with broad-spectrum potent antibiotics given intravenously must be initiated and continued until positive specimen cultures suggest more specific treatment or until the fever has abated and the body temperature has been normal for at least 48 h. If the fever persists and the neutrophil count remains low ($<1.5 \times 10^6/\text{mm}^3$), neutrophil recovery should be stimulated by the administration of a granulocyte stem-cell growth factor (GCSF) but this is not usually necessary.

Gastrointestinal tract

The mucosal lining of the gastrointestinal tract is being shed and replaced continuously, and the clinical effects of cytotoxic drugs on the mucosal stem cells in cycle is seen within days of treatment. These include nausea, vomiting, mucositis, and diarrhoea. There is considerable variation in the severity of these symptoms amongst individuals and amongst different cytotoxic drugs but the symptoms can be so severe that admission to hospital may be necessary for parenteral hydration and alimentation.

There are other causes for the nausea and vomiting associated with cytotoxic drugs which involve 5HT3 and dopamine receptors found peripherally and in the central nervous system. Symptoms can occur acutely (within 24 h of chemotherapy) or be delayed (from 48 h onwards) and can be abolished or diminished by the administration of 5HT3 receptor-blocking drugs, such as ondansetron and granisetron, an hour or so before chemotherapy is given and orally for several days thereafter if necessary. Dexamethasone given orally or by intravenous injection has a similar antiemetic effect and recent evidence suggests that it may be more effective. The combination of a 5HT3 blocking drug with dexamethasone appears to have important advantages over either given alone.[3] The mechanism of action of dexamethasone is not known. These drugs have largely replaced metoclopramide, a drug which blocks dopamine receptors in the medulla of the brain (and has a variety of other receptor effects). Although effective as an antiemetic the doses needed were frequently associated with extrapyramidal side effects. Short-acting benzodiazepines such as lorazepam can be useful adjuncts to antiemetic therapy in patients where anxiety is a factor. With some cytotoxic drugs their potential for causing vomiting is so low that no prophylactic treatment is necessary although it is a sensible precaution to give an oral antiemetic such as domperidone an hour or so before chemotherapy is given.

Delayed nausea and vomiting can be prevented by oral medication such as domperidone, dexamethasone in reducing doses, and ondansetron taken by mouth for between 5 and 10 days depending on the severity of the symptoms. There may be a psychological component to these symptoms and the phenomenon of anticipatory vomiting where patients vomit at the thought of treatment or at the sight or smell of the hospital, is well described and can be alleviated by behavioural therapy such as hypnosis.

Diarrhoea as a toxic effect of cytotoxic drugs is rarely severe and is usually self-limiting. Preventative measures are not necessary and constipating drugs can be taken as required should it arise. There are exceptions, however. For example, the diarrhoea from irinotecan, a cytotoxic drug commonly used in the treatment of colorectal cancer, can be so severe that serious dehydration is a real possibility. With sensible precautions, such as subcutaneous atropine with treatment and the use of potent constipating drugs if symptoms arise, treatment with irinotecan has become safe and manageable.

Mucositis, an inflammation of the mucous membranes of the mouth, tongue, pharynx, and sometimes extending into the oesophagus, can vary from slight redness to severe ulceration which can make eating and drinking impossible. The combination of severe mucositis and a low neutrophil count is dangerous because the inflamed mucous membrane can be a portal of entry for bacteria into the systemic circulation. Mucositis settles in time and the discomfort can be relieved by local anaesthetics such as benzydamine hydrochloride as a mouthwash or spray. If mucositis is severe and prolonged, patients may need admission to hospital and strong analgesics may be required until the symptoms have resolved. Oral and oesophageal candidiasis which is common in these patients can be indistinguishable in appearance from drug-induced mucositis. It is prudent to culture the inflamed mucosa and treat with antifungal agents where there is doubt.

Skin

Surprisingly skin rashes are uncommon with cytotoxic drugs. Photosensitivity, urticaria, hyperpigmentation, and dermatitis have been described. The worst effects are those associated with the hair and nails. Hair thinning or total hair loss is predictable with certain drugs and it can be seen soon after the first course of chemotherapy. Various techniques for cooling the scalp have been developed to prevent hair loss but they are not wholly satisfactory and are not in general use. The hair loss is not permanent and hair can grow again before chemotherapy has been completed.

The nail changes can result in horizontal ridges of the nails, each ridge marking a course of treatment, or in complete avulsion of the nail bed. There are no effective preventative measures and eventually these changes will grow out. The hand/foot syndrome is a curious skin reaction associated with 5-fluorouracil especially with treatment by continuous infusion. It is a painful, erythematous desquamation with fissuring of the palms of the hands and soles of the feet which recovers if the drug is withdrawn.

Kidneys

Renal damage from cytotoxic drugs is most often associated with the platinum derivatives, particularly cisplatin. This is a dose-related effect and because the blood level is itself related to renal function, it is essential that renal function is determined before each course of chemotherapy is prescribed and an adjustment made to the dose as appropriate. Drugs that cause renal toxicity should not be administered unless the creatinine clearance is greater than 40 ml/min. Toxic damage can be permanent.

Nervous system

An altered mental state has been associated with methotrexate, ifosfamide, and other cytotoxic drugs giving rise to confusion, depression, and drowsiness. Cerebellar disturbance can occur with 5-fluorouracil and seizures have been described with vincristine, cisplatin, and ifosfamide. A peripheral neuropathy is more common and can occur with the vinca alkaloids, platinum drugs, the taxanes, and etoposide. Symptoms include numbness and parasthesiae and if the autonomic nerves are involved, colicky abdominal pain and constipation. The platinum drugs in high doses cause nerve deafness but this is rarely seen at recommended dose levels. If it does occur recovery is slow and damage may be permanent.

Lungs

Cytotoxic drugs such as bleomycin, methotrexate, and cyclophosphamide are well-documented causes of lung toxicity. It is more likely with concomitant chest radiotherapy. Symptoms include cough and breathlessness and may occur acutely or be delayed for many years after treatment. The radiological changes in the lungs can be difficult to distinguish from pulmonary oedema, lymphangitis carcinomatosa, and infection. Transbronchial lung biopsy may be required to establish the diagnosis.

Heart

Cardiotoxicity is a feature of the anthracycline drugs, particularly the parent compound doxorubicin. At total cumulative doses not exceeding 450 mg/m^2 the incidence of cardiomyopathy is 2 per cent; this rises to 7 per cent at 550 mg/m^2, 15 per cent at 600 mg/m^2, and 40 per cent at 700 mg/m^2. The clinical features are those of congestive cardiac failure which typically appears 30–60 days after the last dose. The response to diuretic therapy, digoxin, and ACE inhibitors is disappointing and patients may die. Cardiac ischaemia can be caused by 5-fluorouracil resulting in arrhythmias, angina, hypotension, and congestive cardiac failure. Patients at risk are the elderly with pre-existing cardiac disease and previous mediastinal radiotherapy.

A list of cytotoxic drugs commonly used in palliative chemotherapy schedules with common toxicities is shown in Table 2.

To treat or not to treat

The goal of palliative chemotherapy is cancer control, with the expectation of prolonged survival and improved quality of life, including the relief or prevention of symptoms, rather than cure. It is preferable that patients participate in the treatment decision and chemotherapy should not be given without the patient's informed consent. Treatment decisions are based on a consideration of the balance between the benefits expected and the toxicity and risks of chemotherapy which are different for each patient. Sometimes improved quality of life is the only expected benefit and indication for treatment. Patients can share in the decision only if they are given the relevant information. The fear that imparting this information to patients with incurable cancer might leave them bereft and in a state of despair has proved unfounded.[4,5] Indeed patients are eager for information and want to be involved in decisions about treatment.[6] They want to know the duration of treatment and the effect it may have on their working capacity and lifestyle, as well as information about their disease, the treatment options, the possible outcomes, and the toxicity of treatment.

Table 2 Common toxicity profiles of commonly used cytotoxic drugs

Drug	Toxicity			
	Bone marrow	Hair loss	Vomiting	Other
Anti-metabolites				
5-Fluorouracil	+++[a]		+	M D
Methotrexate	++			N M
Gemcitabine	+		+	L
Alkylating drugs				
Cyclophosphamide	+++	+++	++	L B M
Melphalan	++			
Cisplatin	++	+	+++	N K
Carboplatin	+++		+	
Antitumour antibiotics				
Doxorubicin	+++	+++	++	H D
Epirubicin	+++	+++	++	
Bleomycin		++	+	L M
Plant alkaloids				
Vincristine	+	++	+	N C
Vinblastine	+++	+	+	N C
Vinorelbine	+++	+	+	N C
Paclitaxel	++	+++	+	N H
Docetaxel	++	+++	++	N
Irinotecan	++	+	+	D
Topotecan	+++	++	+	
Etoposide	++	+	+	N

[a] Key: +, mild; ++, moderate; +++, severe; M, mucositis; D, diarrhoea; C, constipation; N, neuropathy; B, bladder; K, kidney; H, heart; L, lung.

Table 3 Performance status scales

Karnofsky scale		ECOG[a]/WHO scale	
No complaints; no evidence of disease	100	0	Normal activity No restrictions
Able to carry on normal activity; minor signs or symptoms of disease	90	1	Restricted but ambulatory; able to carry out light work
Some signs or symptoms of disease; Normal activity with effort	80		
Cares for self; unable to carry on normal activity or to do active work	70	2	Ambulatory and self-caring but unable to carry out light work; up more than 50% of waking hours
Requires occasional assistance but is able to care for personal needs	60		
Requires considerable assistance and frequent medical care	50	3	Limited self-care; symptomatic, confined to bed or chair more than 50% of waking hours
Disabled; requires special care and assistance	40	4	Completely disabled; totally confined to bed; may need hospitalization
Severely disabled; hospitalization indicated although death not imminent	30	5	Dead
Very sick; hospitalization necessary; requires active supportive treatment	20		
Moribund; fatal processes progressing rapidly	10		
Dead	0		

[a] ECOG, Eastern Cooperative Oncology Group.

The medical assessment of each patient should include a detailed history and examination with bidirectional measurements of any palpable masses. Histological diagnosis and staging investigations are essential. A blood count, and kidney and liver function tests are important baseline tests. Physical fitness is graded according to validated performance status scales as shown in Table 3. These are used for defining eligibility for clinical drug trials and for recording changes in physical fitness over time.

The decision to treat or not to treat is made when the oncologist can interpret these findings and place the patient's situation into a clinical context. The histological diagnosis and staging investigations will determine the chemotherapy options, if any, which are based on response, survival, and quality of life data from previous controlled clinical trials. Comorbid conditions, blood tests, age, and performance status may affect the decision to treat or the choice of drugs and indicate the need for any dose modifications. For example, chemotherapy is usually only appropriate for patients with a performance status score of 60 or above (Karnofsky scale) because they need to be reasonably physically robust to cope with the toxicity of treatment. An exception, however, may be a patient whose cancer can be cured by chemotherapy, when the additional risks associated with the treatment because of their poor physical condition, may be worth taking. In presenting this information to patients medical jargon should be avoided and understanding can be increased by the use of information leaflets, diagrams, and taped recordings of the consultation. Careful thought should be given to the way in which information is presented because this may affect the patient's choice of a treatment option; for example, outcome can be expressed as the chance of survival rather than the probability of death. Some patients find it helpful to meet other similar patients or to obtain a second opinion or to access a nurse counsellor. Chemotherapy involves a commitment to repeated hospital visits, venepunctures, cannulations, investigations, and assessments and to a risk of hospital admissions and death. It should not be taken lightly. Some patients with treatable cancer prefer to allow the disease to run its course without intervention and this view should always be respected. Some patients with untreatable cancer may ask to be treated with chemotherapy but this can only be justified in the context of phase I or phase II clinical trials and any pressure to administer speculative treatments should be resisted.

The timing of chemotherapy

Typically chemotherapy is given to patients when there is demonstrable metastatic spread but it may be given to treat local disease when surgery or radiotherapy are either not possible or are inappropriate. Occasionally chemotherapy is given before surgery or radiotherapy (neo-adjuvant or induction chemotherapy) to reduce the size of a cancer so that surgery or radiotherapy can be done more easily. Chemotherapy may be given after surgery (adjuvant chemotherapy) in the absence of demonstrable disease to reduce the chance of systemic relapse in patients with micrometastases. This approach has been shown to increase the 5- and 10-year survival rates in early-stage breast[7] and colon[8] cancer.

The administration of chemotherapy

Chemotherapy is usually administered by intravenous injection or infusion although, increasingly, oral formulations of cytotoxic drugs are being developed. Most chemotherapy regimens dictate that the drugs are given intermittently with 3–4 weeks between each course of treatment to allow time for normal tissues to recover. There is evidence that some chemotherapy may be better tolerated and as effective when given more frequently, say weekly in smaller doses[9] and the optimal scheduling of chemotherapy is under continuous review. A course of chemotherapy should not be administered unless the neutrophil count is greater than $1.5 \times 10^6/\text{mm}^3$ and any drug-induced gastrointestinal symptoms have settled. Dose reductions or the addition of GCSF should be considered for subsequent courses of chemotherapy after a life-threatening toxic episode.

Multiple courses of chemotherapy means repeated venepunctures and cannulations. Cytotoxic drugs are irritants and local phlebitis is common. Venous access can be a problem unless a permanent access line is established. This is necessary anyway for continuous infusional treatment. There are various devices for securing permanent venous access. They involve the insertion of a long polymerized silicone rubber (Silastic) catheter into the right atrium. The catheter may be single, double, or triple lumen and some devices include a subcutaneous implantable injection port so that the whole system is concealed beneath the skin. Intravenous fluid, drugs, and blood can be administered and blood samples can be taken through the catheter. Catheter-related deaths are rare but infection and thrombosis can occur and a pneumothorax can complicate the insertion procedure. Reasons for early withdrawal of the catheter include persistent fever and jugular or superior vena caval thrombosis.

Intra-arterial chemotherapy is occasionally considered for the treatment of localized cancer in the limbs, head and neck, and liver. Its use is experimental and confined to specialized units. Similarly installation of cytotoxic drugs into the abdominal cavity is being evaluated for the treatment of ovarian cancer.

Chemotherapy should be administered in specialized units by staff who are properly trained and under the supervision of cancer specialists (oncologists). There should be procedures for preparing and administering treatment which protect the staff from skin and aerosol contamination and for dealing with drug spillage and extravasation.

The monitoring of chemotherapy

Patients on chemotherapy require regular assessment and it is normal practice to record symptoms, toxicity, and response before each course of treatment. The methods for monitoring response depend on the cancer type and the sites of disease and include repeated measurements of palpable masses, or masses identified radiologically or with scanning techniques, and serum tumour markers. Tumour markers are substances, usually proteins, that are produced by cancers and can be detected and quantified in the blood or urine. The serum tumour markers commonly used in clinical practice for monitoring as well as for diagnosis and detecting recurrence are shown in Table 4. It is not necessary to repeat the radiological investigations each time but a formal review of the disease status should be carried out after no more than three courses of treatment have been given. Chemotherapy should be withdrawn if there is evidence of progressive disease or if there are other compelling clinical reasons for doing so. Only by treating the patient and monitoring the response can the sensitivity of the cancer to chemotherapy be determined. There are, as yet, no predictive tests as there are, for example, for antibiotics in the treatment of infection.

The number of courses of chemotherapy and the duration of continuous infusional chemotherapy is not fixed. Much depends on the regimen, the

Table 4 Serum tumour markers which are used in clinical practice

Marker	Cancer
Carcinoembryonic antigen	Colorectal, breast, lung (small cell)
CA 125	Ovary
CA 15-3	Breast
CA 19-9	Pancreas
Prostate specific antigen	Prostate
Lactic dehydrogenase	Lymphoma, lung (small cell)
Alpha fetoprotein	Germ cell, hepatoma
Human chorionic gonadotrophin	Germ cell Chorioncarcinoma
Thyrocalcitonin	Thyroid (medullary)
Monoclonal immunoglobulin	Myeloma, lymphoma

toxicity, the patient's condition and the disease status. Some cytotoxic drugs have cumulative toxicities and maximum recommended doses should not be exceeded. Clearly if toxicity is minimal and the patient's condition is improved by treatment it is reasonable to continue until there is evidence of disease progression. However, the tolerability of some regimens is such that a maximum of 4–6 courses, or for continuous infusional chemotherapy, a maximum period of 6 months, is recommended. Patients whose cancer is resistant to one chemotherapy regimen can be treated with another. Similarly, different regimens can be given to patients with relapsed disease, although response rates become progressively less.

There are many questions about cancer chemotherapy which remain largely unanswered, such as the optimal combination of cytotoxic drugs and the optimal scheduling , timing, and duration of treatment to give the highest response with the lowest toxicity for each type of cancer. These issues can only be resolved by RCTs. It is the ambition of oncologists that as many patients as possible be treated in the context of an RCT.

Hormone therapy in palliative care

The mode of action of hormones and hormone therapy

Hormones are polypeptides produced by the endocrine system which influence metabolic processes throughout the body. The effects are mediated either directly by binding with specific cell surface receptors or indirectly by stimulating or inhibiting the local production of cell growth factors. Some cancers contain cells which require particular hormones to proliferate (hormone-dependent) and these are the cancers that are amenable to hormone therapy (Table 1). The therapy either blocks the binding of hormones to receptors or reduces the circulating and cellular concentrations of the hormone. The cancers most susceptible to this approach are breast cancer and prostate cancer.

Breast cancer

Hormone-dependent breast cancer cells proliferate under the influence of oestrogen. Oestrogen is produced mainly by the ovaries in pre-menopausal women and from the conversion of androgens mainly from the adrenal glands in post-menopausal women. Androgens are converted into oestrogen by aromatase, an enzyme found in peripheral sites such as adipose tissue, skin, muscle, and liver, and in up to 70 per cent of breast cancers.[10] Oestrogen production can be reduced by surgical intervention (oophorectomy, adrenalectomy, hypophysectomy), radiation of the ovaries, or by gonadotrophin-releasing hormone analogues all of which have the same effect in pre-menopausal women. Aromatase inhibition is used in post-menopausal women and this can be achieved by the administration of steroidal androgen analogues such as exemestane which inactivate the enzyme irreversibly or by non-steroidal drugs such as anastrozole and letrozole which are less specific and reversible and whose inhibitory effects depend on the continued presence of the drug. Both types of aromatase inhibitors reduce circulating oestrogen to nearly undetectable levels in post-menopausal women but the steroidal drugs may be more effective and responses are seen in patients who have progressed on treatment with non-steroidal drugs. The side effects of oestrogen depletion include hot flushes, sweats, and osteoporosis.

Antioestrogens such as tamoxifen bind to oestrogen receptors and their clinical effects in breast cancer are largely confined to patients with oestrogen-receptor-positive disease. Tamoxifen has other pharmacological effects and can act as an agonist when oestrogen concentrations are low. Newer drugs which are purely competitive inhibitors are being introduced into clinical practice.[11] The agonist activity of tamoxifen is thought to explain the small increased incidence of endometrial cancer in patients taking it for many years. Other side effects include hot flushes, thromboembolism, and corneal and retinal deposits. Any serious effects are rare, however, and tamoxifen is a remarkably well-tolerated drug.

Progestational drugs such as medroxyprogesterone acetate are used to treat hormone-dependent breast cancer and response rates are similar to that of tamoxifen. The mechanism of action is unknown but they may interfere with binding to progesterone and oestrogen receptors and with aromatization. Side effects include weight gain, vaginal bleeding, and thromboembolism.

Prostate cancer

Hormone-dependent prostate cancer cells proliferate under the influence of androgens. Most androgen activity comes from testosterone, which is produced in the testes. Secretion is regulated by luteinizing hormone (LH) from the pituitary gland which in turn is regulated by luteinizing hormone-releasing hormone (LHRH) from the hypothalamus. Other androgens are synthesized in the adrenal glands and are converted peripherally to testo-sterone. Their secretion is regulated by adrenocorticotrophic hormone (ACTH). Testosterone is metabolized to dihydro-testosterone (DHT) which drives cell proliferation and DHT receptors are found in hormone-dependent prostate cancer cells.

Testosterone production can be reduced by surgical intervention (castration) or by drugs which inhibit LH secretion (oestrogens, cyproterone acetate, and LHRH agonists, such as goserelin and leuprolide acetate), ACTH secretion (glucocorticoids), and steroid synthesis (ketoconazole). Oestrogens are no longer used alone in the treatment of prostate cancer because of cardiovascular side effects, although in combination with nitrogen mustard (estramustine) they may have a place in second-line treatment. The LHRH agonists produce an initial rise in serum testosterone concentration followed by a fall to castration levels. The rise can produce a tumour 'flare' and a temporary worsening of symptoms which can be blocked by a peripheral antiandrogen drug such as cyproterone acetate or flutamide. Side effects include loss of potency and hot flushes. The advantages of castration compared to LHRH agonists are the rapidity of the effect, cost effectiveness, and the elimination of compliance as an issue. However, there are psychological consequences which make it an unacceptable option for some patients.

Glucocorticoids and ketononazole have modest effects on serum testosterone levels and their side effects have limited their use in the treatment of prostate cancer.

Non-steroidal antiandrogens such as flutamide bind to DHT receptors in prostate cancer cells. The steroidal antiandrogen cyproterone acetate is less effective as a binding agent but has progestational activity and suppresses LH secretion as well. Total androgen blockade can be achieved by combining testosterone deprivation with an antiandrogen. Both flutamide and cyproterone acetate can cause serious liver toxicity and liver function tests must be monitored.

Miscellaneous cancers

Hormone-dependent endometrial cancer is regulated by an interaction between circulating oestrogen and progesterones. Cancer regression is seen in up to 30 per cent of patients during treatment with progestational drugs such as medroxyprogesterone acetate and megestrol acetate, and response rates are higher in progesterone-receptor-positive, well-differentiated cancers.

Some ovarian cancers express oestrogen and progesterone receptors, some malignant melanomas express oestrogen receptors, some renal cancers express progesterone receptors, and some pancreas cancers express androgen receptors but it is doubtful if hormone therapy has any part to play in the management of these cancers.

Biological agents in palliative care

Biological agents to treat cancer have been developed from an understanding of the molecular changes which characterize the cancer phenotype and of the effects cancer cells have on their immediate surroundings and on host defence mechanisms. This is an evolving science and the reader is given an insight into some of the new targets for anticancer treatments and examples of agents which are being introduced into clinical practice.

Growth factor receptors and tyrosine kinases

Cell signalling pathways are the means by which cells receive the instruction to proliferate or to die. They begin with the activation of surface receptors which cause messages to cascade through the cytoplasm to the nucleus and to the cell cycle. Any of the genes which code for the proteins involved in these processes (proto-oncogenes) may be abnormally expressed in a cancer cell (known then as an oncogene) and can result in either a continuous drive to cell proliferation or escape from apoptosis. Oncogenes and their protein products are potential targets for anticancer treatment. One of the pathways includes epidermal growth factor receptors (EGFRs) and a family of enzymes the tyrosine kinases, which transfer the information from activated cell surface receptors into the cytoplasm. These receptors and enzymes are over-expressed in a number of epithelial cancers, (cancer of the breast, ovary, pancreas, stomach, colon, rectum, and non-small cell lung cancer) and probably have a part to play in their pathogenesis.[12] Several treatment strategies for targeting EGFR-expressing cancers are being pursued. These include anti-EGFR monoclonal antibodies and tyrosine kinase inhibitors which block the transfer of signals in different ways.

Trastuzumab (herceptin) is a humanized monoclonal antibody (one in which specific regions of a murine antibody are inserted into the framework of a generic human IgG antibody) that binds to the EGFR-related receptor HER2 which is over-expressed in 30 per cent of breast cancers, where it is associated with a poor prognosis.[13] A number of studies have demonstrated the efficacy of trastuzumab in HER2-positive metastatic breast cancer either alone[14] or in combination with chemotherapy.[15] Similar studies are being conducted with trastuzumab in the other epithelial cancers which over-express HER2.[16]

Imatinide (glivec) is a small molecule that inhibits a particular tyrosine kinase which is the protein product of the bcr-abl oncogene. This oncogene is expressed as a result of a chromosome translocation and the fusion of the bcr gene on chromosome 22 with the abl gene on chromosome 9, and is the genetic abnormality that characterizes chronic myeloid leukaemia (the Philadelphia chromosome). The continuous production of the bcr-abl tyrosine kinase is thought to drive cell proliferation. Imatinide produces complete haematological responses in most patients in the chronic and accelerated phases of the disease.[17] In addition to improving symptoms and prolonging survival, it is possible that imatinide, either alone or in combination with conventional treatment, will cure patients with chronic myeloid leukaemia.

The cell cycle

When the signal to proliferate reaches the cell nucleus, replication begins. The orderly progression of the cell cycle is initiated and controlled by cyclins and cyclin-dependent kinases (CDKs). Cyclins are over-expressed in a number of different cancers and together with CDKs are targets for therapeutic intervention.[18]

Normally, if damaged DNA is detected during cell replication, the cell cycle is arrested at the G1/S and G2/M interfaces (known as check points) whilst the damage is repaired. If repair is not possible, the cell is triggered into apoptosis (Fig. 1). In this way mutations in proto-oncogenes which might lead to a cancer phenotype may be eliminated. The check points are controlled by protein products of genes known as tumour suppressor genes which have the effect of slowing or blocking progression through the cell cycle by inhibiting the formation of cyclin complexes. If tumour suppressor genes are inactivated, abnormal genetic material passes on to successive generations of the original cell. Inactivation of one tumour suppressor gene in particular, known as P53, is critical in carcinogenesis. Mutations are found in 50 per cent of cancers. The technology exists to transfer non-mutated P53 DNA into cancer cells, to raise antibodies against mutated P53 protein, and to produce vaccines that kill cells containing mutated P53[19]—three more ways of treating cancer if theoretical possibilities can be translated into clinical practice.

Matrix metalloproteinases and angiogenesis

As a cancer grows, the surrounding connective tissue matrix is reorganized through the release of metalloproteinase enzymes. This process facilitates invasion and spread of cancer cells and is an important step in allowing the migration of endothelial cells which lead to new blood vessel formation (angiogenesis). Angiogenesis is controlled by stimulatory and inhibitory molecules released by cancer cells and by cells contained within the connective tissue. The stimulatory molecules include fibroblast growth factor, vascular endothelial growth factor (VEGF), platelet-derived growth factor, and various matrix metalloproteinases. The inhibitory molecules include interferon and angiostatin. The balance between the two determines the micro-environment and influences the growth characteristics of the cancer and its potential for metastatic spread. These discoveries provide a number of possibilities for treating cancer by inhibiting angiogenesis and the reorganization of the connective tissue stroma. Matrix metalloproteinase inhibitors, VEGF receptor inhibitors, interferon alpha, endogenous angiostation, and drugs such as thalidomide which have antiangiogenic properties are all being evaluated in clinical trials. Thalidomide has anticancer activity in multiple myeloma.[20]

Host defence mechanisms

Sometimes cancer cells express or secrete tumour-associated or tumour-specific proteins which provoke an immune response. The response includes the release of cytokines by macrophages and lymphoid cells which activate cytotoxic T lymphocytes and natural killer cells and the production of antibodies by B lymphocytes which activate antibody-dependent cell-mediated cytotoxicity. The reasons why the immune system fails to eliminate these cancer cells are unclear but enhancing the response through immunological manipulation can have anticancer effects and different methods of doing this are being evaluated in clinical practice.

Although it is not a tumour antigen as such, the CD20 antigen is a cell surface protein which characterizes the B lymphocyte. Large numbers of B lymphocytes are produced and accumulate in some forms of low-grade non-Hodgkin lymphoma. Rituximab is a humanized monoclonal antibody raised against the CD20 antigen and is a new approach to the treatment of this disease.[21]

Treatment strategies

In this section, the treatment strategies of certain cancers are outlined. Breast cancer, lung cancer, and colorectal cancer are selected because they are common, their clinical course is often protracted, and together they account for a large part of the workload of a palliative care physician. Myeloma is selected because patients are often symptomatic at the outset and may present first to a palliative care physician and it is important to recognize that myeloma responds well to medical treatment. Carcinoma from an unknown primary source (CUP) is selected because these patients present doctors with difficult diagnostic and management decisions and may be referred to palliative care physicians without a full oncology assessment. The reader is referred to textbooks of cancer medicine for information about the medical treatment of the other cancers listed in Table 1.

Response rates and survival data are given as an indication of the effectiveness of treatment but an improvement in quality of life measures may be the main expected benefit and these details are not given here. It is worth stating that an improvement in median survival of say 3 months may seem small to the reader but it may be very significant to a patient whose life-expectancy is only 6 months.[22] Certainly patients view small gains from treatment as being much more worthwhile than do the prescribing doctors.[23]

Breast cancer

The management of metastatic breast cancer depends on the site or sites of disease, whether the disease is local or systemic, and if systemic whether it is life-threatening (involving liver or lung) or not (involving bone or soft tissue). Other important factors include the patient's menopausal status, performance status, and physical symptoms, and the cancer's oestrogen, progesterone, and HER2 receptor status. The choice of treatment and the expected outcomes are as follows.

Hormone therapy[24]

Hormone therapy is only considered for patients with oestrogen- and/or progesterone-receptor-positive breast cancer. It is preferred to chemotherapy because the administration is easier, side effects are fewer, and responses are more durable. However, it is used only if the patient is not symptomatic and the situation is not life-threatening because the response to hormone therapy is slow and a failure to respond in these circumstances would not adversely effect the patient's comfort or survival. Otherwise chemotherapy is used first and is followed by hormone therapy. In pre-menopausal patients, hormone therapy includes any of the surgical, radiation, and medical techniques to remove or prevent oestrogen production, and anti-oestrogens such as tamoxifen. Tamoxifen, anastrozole, exemestane, and progesterones are used in post-menopausal patients.

Most patients do not present with metastatic disease and will have been treated previously for early-stage breast cancer with adjuvant hormone therapy. If relapse occurs within 1 year of primary treatment, the disease is likely to be hormone-resistant and chemotherapy is recommended. If relapse occurs after 1 year of primary treatment, with say tamoxifen, or within 1 year of stopping it, the next line of hormone therapy, with say anastrozole, should be used. Otherwise tamoxifen is used again. Whilst a cancer continues to demonstrate hormone sensitivity, the different hormones can be used in sequence for each episode of relapse. Sometimes stopping hormone therapy for disease progression is followed by regression of the cancer. In contrast, the administration of hormone therapy may produce a temporary exacerbation of symptoms known as a tumour flare which may result in hypercalcaemia in patients with metastatic bone disease.

The overall response to first-line hormone therapy is between 30 and 40 per cent, although it can be as high as 60 per cent in patients with non-visceral disease and a long disease-free interval, factors which predict a good response. Response rates of 25 per cent and between 10 and 15 per cent are seen with second- and third-line hormone therapy, respectively. Responses may last for several years.

Chemotherapy[25]

In addition to its use for life-threatening disease, chemotherapy is recommended for patients with metastatic breast cancer which is oestrogen-receptor-negative or which is refractory or becomes resistant to hormone therapy. HER2-positive disease (between 20 and 30 per cent of all patients) may also be an indication for chemotherapy because it is associated with hormone resistance in breast cancer which is also oestrogen-receptor-positive. There is also an increased rate of cancer growth, an enhanced rate of metastases, a shorter disease-free interval, and a reduced overall survival in these patients.

Chemotherapy regimens have changed over the years as new drugs and combinations are introduced into clinical practice. First-line chemotherapy for metastatic disease is either one or a combination of two or three of any of the following: cyclophosphamide, methotrexate, 5-fluorouracil, doxorubicin, and epirubicin, avoiding any drugs that were used previously as adjuvant treatment. Second- and third-line chemotherapy is either one or a combination of any of the same drugs, together with vinorelbine, docetaxel, and paclitaxel avoiding drugs that were used as first-line treatment.

Overall response rates to first-line treatment are between 40 and 60 per cent which includes between 10 and 20 per cent complete responses. The median duration of the response is between 6 and 10 months. Response rates of 25 per cent or less are seen with second- and third-line chemotherapy. High-dose chemotherapy with GCSF to hasten bone marrow recovery has not shown a survival benefit and is not recommended.[26]

Biological agents

Phase II trials have demonstrated the efficacy of trastuzumab in patients with HER2-positive disease and early phase III data have shown improvement in response rates, median time to progression, and survival when trastuzumab is added to first-line chemotherapy in metastatic breast cancer.[15] The combination of trastuzumab and an anthracycline should be used with caution for increased cardiac toxicity has been reported when they are given together.

Other treatments

The bone is the commonest site for metastases in breast cancer and may be the only site of spread for several years. Metastatic bone disease can give rise to serious morbidity, including pathological fractures, hypercalcaemia, and spinal cord compression, especially when the metastases are associated with increased osteoclastic activity and osteolysis. Bisphosphonates inhibit osteoclastic activation. They control hypercalcaemia and reduce the frequency of fractures and the severity of bone pain.[27] They may also reduce the incidence of bone metastases, but this has not been confirmed,[28] and there is no evidence of an increase in survival. Patients with metastatic bone disease and osteolysis should be treated with bisphosphonates indefinitely.

Lung cancer[29]

The management of lung cancer depends on the histological subtype, either small cell or non-small cell (includes squamous, adenocarcinoma, and large cell cancers), the stage of the disease, and the performance status of the patient.

Small cell lung cancer (20 per cent)

Metastatic spread occurs early in the natural history of the disease. It may be associated with inappropriate antidiuretic hormone secretion, ectopic ACTH secretion, and a myasthaenic syndrome. The median survival of untreated patients is about 2 months. Prognostic factors include the performance status, the stage of disease (either limited to one hemithorax, 30 per cent, or beyond this limit, 70 per cent, and called extensive disease), and serum sodium and lactic dehydrogenase concentrations. Patients with limited disease, a good performance status, and normal biochemistry respond well to systemic chemotherapy. The standard regimen is a combination of either cisplatin or carboplatin and etoposide. The response rate is between 80 and 95 per cent and the median survival is 20 months. Between 50 and 60 per cent are complete responders and a proportion of these patients (between 10 and 20 per cent) are long-term survivors provided they have prophylactic cranial[30] and mediastinal radiation[31] therapy as well.

Patients with extensive disease and poor prognostic factors may also respond to chemotherapy.[32] Regimens which include vincristine, doxorubicin, etoposide, or cyclophosphamide are used in these patients because they are better tolerated than platinum-based regimens. The response rate is about 40 per cent but there are few complete responders. The median survival is between 7 and 10 months. Few patients live beyond 2 years.

The prognosis for patients after relapse is poor. There is no standard second-line chemotherapy regimen but the taxanes and the newer topoisomerase inhibitors (topotecan and irinotecan) are being studied and look promising.

Non-small cell lung cancer[33] (80 per cent)

Where possible, non-small cell lung cancer is treated by surgical resection which results in a 5-year survival rate of about 60 per cent in patients with early-stage disease. An additional benefit from adjuvant chemotherapy has not yet been established. Induction chemotherapy in locally advanced disease can sometimes convert an unresectable cancer to one which is resectable. Response rates of 75 per cent and resection rates of 60 per cent have been reported with up to 25 per cent of patients alive and in remission after 5 years. However, patients in these studies were carefully selected by age, performance status, and medical history and the results may not be widely applicable. Patients with locally advanced unresectable non-small cell lung cancer (30 per cent) are treated by induction chemotherapy followed by radiotherapy which increases median and 2-year survival compared to radiotherapy alone.[34]

About 50 per cent of patient's with non-small cell lung cancer present with evidence of metastatic spread. The median survival for these patients is about 6 months and there is no prospect of cure. Several randomized trials have shown the benefit of chemotherapy in good performance status patients compared to supportive care alone.[35] There is an overall increase of 3 months in median survival and an increase from 30 to 40 per cent in the numbers of patients alive at 1 year. More importantly, there is an improvement in a range of quality of life measures, including the relief of physical symptoms, if chemotherapy is used.[1] Cisplatin or docetaxel combined with vinorelbine or gemcitabine give the highest response and survival rates. Any of these drugs not used as first-line chemotherapy can be used to treat relapsed disease.

Table 5 Immunochemical markers in common use

Marker	Cancer
Cytokeratin	Carcinoma
Vimentin	Sarcoma
Common leucocyte antigen	Lymphoma
S100	Malignant melanoma
Prostate-specific antigen	Prostate
Oestrogen receptor	Breast
Alpha fetoprotein Human chorionic gonadotrophin Placental alkaline phosphatase	Germ cell
Chromogranin	Neuroendocrine

Colorectal cancer

About 60 per cent of patients with colorectal cancer have metastatic disease either at presentation or after surgical resection and adjuvant chemotherapy. The liver and lungs are the commonest sites of involvement. Until recently, chemotherapy with 5-fluorouracil modulated by the concomitant administration of folinic acid was the standard regimen giving a response rate of 30 per cent and a median survival of between 12 and 14 months, 6 months more than supportive care alone. However, the combination of these two drugs with irinotecan has increased the response rate to nearly 50 per cent and the median survival to 17 months and has become the new gold standard regimen.[36] Other new active drugs, oxaliplatin[37] (a platinum derivative) and capecitabine[38] (an orally administered precurser of 5-fluorouracil) are being evaluated in phase II and III trials. A novel approach with a monoclonal antibody targeting a cell surface glycoprotein which is preferentially expressed on adenocarcinomas is also being evaluated in these patients.[39]

Myeloma[40]

Multiple myeloma is a cancer of bone marrow plasma cells. A monoclonal protein (paraprotein) secreted by the cancer is found in the serum in 80 per cent of patients and free immunoglobulin light chains are often found in the urine. In 20 per cent of patients light chains only are produced by the cancer. Symptoms include bone pain (60 per cent), and the symptoms associated with anaemia, hypercalcaemia, infection, and renal failure. Standard medical treatment is chemotherapy with melphalan and prednisolone which gives a response rate (greater than 50 per cent reduction in the paraprotein concentration) of 50 per cent. Maintenance chemotherapy is ineffective. More aggressive chemotherapy with vincristine, doxorubicin, and dexamethasone is appropriate for patients with a good performance status and gives a response rate of between 60 and 80 per cent.[41] Patients under 60 years who have chemosensitive myeloma may go on to high-dose therapy supported by peripheral blood or bone marrow stem cell transplantation.[42] This increases the median survival from 2 years to 5 years. Thalidomide gives responses in 30 per cent of patients whose myeloma is resistant to chemotherapy.[20] Other treatments include bisphosphonates which reduce bone pain, hypercalcaemia, and the frequency of pathological bone fractures;[43] blood transfusions or erythropoietin for anaemia; and plasmaphoresis for the hyperviscosity syndrome.

Carcinoma of unknown primary (CUP)[44]

About 3 per cent of cancers present with metastatic spread and the primary cancer cannot be found despite careful clinical examination and screening X-rays, CT scans, and mammography. The management of these patients is difficult because the tissue of origin of the cancer is an important factor in determining a treatment plan. In these circumstances treatment decisions are based on additional information derived from immunochemical staining of tissue samples (Table 5) and serum tumour marker studies (Table 4) and from the distribution of the metastases which may indicate the most likely source of the cancer.

The distribution of histological subtypes in CUPs is adenocarcinoma (60 per cent), squamous cancer (5 per cent), and poorly/undifferentiated cancer (35 per cent). About two-thirds of the primary cancers can be found at autopsy and their distribution gives an indication of the range of primary sites which can present as a CUP. The commonest sites for an adenocarcinoma are lung, pancreas, stomach, and prostate; for a squamous cancer are head and neck, oesophagus, skin and lung; and for an undifferentiated cancer are lymphoma, germ cell, melanoma, and neuroendocrine. It is essential to identify germ cell tumours and lymphomas because these cancers may be curable (Table 1). Similarly patients with prostate cancer may have prolonged survival with hormone treatment. If the primary cancer remains unknown after a thorough evaluation, chemotherapy may be offered to patients with a good performance status with regimens which reflect the most likely source of the cancer.[45] Alternatively vincristine, doxorubicin, and cyclophosphamide in combination give a response rate of 20 per cent.[46] The median survival of these patients is only 6 months and only 20 per cent live beyond 1 year.

Future directions

Further progress in the medical treatment of cancer may come from new cytotoxic drug development or modifying the schedules and combinations of the cytotoxic drugs already in use. However, this is likely to produce small incremental gains rather than a dramatic revolution in treatment outcomes. Real hope for the future comes from the increasingly detailed understanding of the molecular changes which characterize the cancer phenotype and from the innovative ways of correcting and combating them. Treatments which target some of these changes are already being used in clinical practice and have been described (trastuzumab, rituximab, and imatinide). Many more like them are being developed and evaluated.[47] Furthermore it is now possible to inactivate oncogenes and their products, to restore the function of damaged proto-oncogenes and tumour-suppressor genes, and to target cells containing particular gene defects with cytotoxic agents, giving rise to further possibilities for specific cancer treatments in the future.

It can be predicted that these biological therapies will be most effective when they are given early in the disease process because of better drug penetration and fewer cell mutations when the cancer load is small. Thus, unless or until molecular techniques for earlier diagnosis and more sensitive screening become a reality, the need for conventional debulking procedures (surgery, radiotherapy, chemotherapy) will remain.

References

1. **Anderson, H.** et al. (2000). Gemcitabine plus best supportive care (BSC) versus BSC in inoperable non-small-cell lung cancer—a randomised trial with quality of life as the primary outcome. *Bristol Journal of Cancer* **83**, 447–53.
2. **Thatcher, N.** et al. (1995). Symptomatic benefit from gemcitabine and other chemotherapy in advanced non-small cell lung cancer: changes in performance status and tumour-related symptoms. *Anti-Cancer Drugs* **6** (Suppl. 6), 39–48.
3. **Ioannidis, J.P.A., Hesketh, P.J., and Lau, J.** (2000). Contribution of dexamethasone to control of chemotherapy-induced nausea and vomiting: a meta-analysis of randomised controlled trials. *Journal of Clinical Oncology* **18**, 3409–22.
4. **Fallowfield, L., Ford, S., and Lewis, S.** (1994). Information preferences of patients with cancer. *Lancet* **344**, 1576.
5. **Ajaj, A., Singh, M.P., and Abdullah, A.J.J.** (2001). Should elderly patients be told they have cancer? Questionnaire survey of older people. *British Medical Journal* **323**, 1160.
6. **Meredith, C.** et al. (1996). Information needs of cancer patients in West Scotland: cross-sectional survey of patients' views. *British Medical Journal* **313**, 724–6.
7. **Early Breast Cancer Trialist 5 Collaborative Group** (1992). Systemic treatment of early breast cancer by hormonal, cytotoxic or immune therapy. 133 randomised trials involving 31 000 recurrences and 24 000 deaths among 75 000 women. *Lancet* **339**, 71–85.
8. **Midgley, R.S.J. and Kerr, D.J.** (2000). ABC of colorectal cancer: adjuvant therapy. *British Medical Journal* **321**, 1208–11.
9. **Seidman, A.D.** et al. (1998). Dose-dense therapy with weekly 1-hour paclitaxel infusions in the treatment of metastatic breast cancer. *Journal of Clinical Oncology* **16**, 3353–61.
10. **Millar, W.R.** (1990). Endocrine treatment for breast cancers: biological, rationale and current progress. *Journal of Steroid Biochemistry and Molecular Biology* **37**, 467–80.
11. **Howell, A. and Dowsett, M.** (1997). Recent advances in endocrine therapy of breast cancer. *British Medical Journal* **315**, 863–6.
12. **Salomon, D.S.** et al. (1995). Epidermal growth factor-related peptides and their receptors in human malignancies. *Critical Reviews in Oncology and Haematology* **19**, 183–232.
13. **Klijn, J.G.** et al. (1992). The clinical significance of epidermal growth factor receptor in human breast cancer: a review of 5232 patients. *Endocrine Review* **13**, 3–17.
14. **Cobleigh, M.A.** et al. (1999). Multinational study of the efficacy and safety of humanized anti—HER2 monoclonal antibody in women who have HER2—overexpressing metastatic breast cancer that has progressed after chemotherapy for metastatic disease. *Journal of Clinical Oncology* **17**, 2639–48.
15. **Slamon, D.J.** et al. (2001). Use of chemotherapy plus a monoclonal antibody against HER2 for metastatic breast cancer that overexpresses HER2. *New England Journal of Medicine* **344**, 783–92.
16. **Scholl, S., Beuzeboc, P., and Pouillart, P.** (2001). Targeting HER2 in other tumour types. *Annals of Oncology* **12** (Suppl. 1), 81–7.
17. **Mughal, T.I. and Goldman, J.M.** (2001). Chronic myeloid leukaemia: STI 571 magnifies the therapeutic dilemma. *European Journal of Cancer* **37**, 561–8.
18. **Sausville, E.A.** (1999). Cyclin-dependent kinases: novel targets for cancer treatment. *Thirty-fifth Annual Meeting of the American Society of Clinical Oncology: Educational Book*, 9–21. The American Society of Clinical Oncology. Baltimore MD: Lippincott Williams and Wilkins.
19. **Harris, C.C.** (1996). Structure and function of the P53 tumour suppressor gene: clues for rational cancer therapeutic strategies. *Journal of the National Cancer Institute* **88**, 1442–55.
20. **Singhal, S.** et al. (1999). Antitumour activity of thalidomide in refractory myeloma. *New England Journal of Medicine* **341**, 1565–71.
21. **McLaughlin, P.** et al. (1998). Rituximab chimeric anti-CD20 monoclonal antibody therapy for relapsed indolent lymphoma: half of patients respond to a four-dose treatment programme. *Journal of Clinical Oncology* **16**, 2825–33.
22. **Silvestri, G., Pritchard, R., and Welch, H.G.** (1998). Preferences for chemotherapy in patients with advanced non-small-cell lung cancer: descriptive study based on scripted interviews. *British Medical Journal* **317**, 771–5.
23. **Slevin, M.L.** et al. (1990). Attitudes to chemotherapy: comparing views of patients with cancer with those of doctors, nurses and general public. *British Medical Journal* **300**, 1458–60.
24. **Goldhirsch, A. and Gelber, R.D.** (1996). Endocrine therapies of breast cancer. *Seminars in Oncology* **23**, 494–505.
25. **Fossati, R.** et al. (1998). Cytotoxic and hormonal treatment for metastatic breast cancer: a systematic review of published randomised trials involving 35 510 women. *Journal of Clinical Oncology* **16**, 3439–60.
26. **Pusztai, L. and Hortobagyi, G.N.** (1998). Discouraging news for high-dose chemotherapy in high-risk breast cancer. *Lancet* **352**, 501–2.
27. **van Holten-Verzantvoort, A.T.** et al. (1993). Palliative bone treatment in patients with bone metastases from breast cancer. *Journal of Clinical Oncology* **11**, 491–8.
28. **Kanis, J.A.** et al. (1996). Clodronate decreases the frequency of skeletal metastases with breast cancer. *Bone* **19**, 663–7.
29. **Hoffman, P.C., Mauer, A.M., and Vokes, E.E.** (2000). Lung cancer. *Lancet* **355**, 479–85.
30. **Auperin, A.** et al. (1999). Prophylactic cranial irradiation for patients with small-cell lung cancer in complete remission. *New England Journal of Medicine* **341**, 476–84.
31. **Perry, M.L.** et al. (1987). Chemotherapy with or without radiation therapy in limited small-cell carcinoma of the lung. *New England Journal of Medicine* **316**, 912–18.
32. **Chute, J.P.** et al. (1999). Twenty years of phase III trials for patients with extensive stage small-cell lung cancer. Perceptible progress. *Journal of Clinical Oncology* **17**, 1794–1801.
33. **Carney, D.N. and Hansen, H.H.** (2000). Non-small-cell lung cancer—stalemate or progress? *New England Journal of Medicine* **343**, 1261–2.
34. **Pritchard, R.S. and Anthony, S.P.** (1996). Chemotherapy plus radiotherapy compared with radiotherapy alone in the treatment of locally advanced, unresectable, non-small cell lung cancer: a meta-analysis. *Annals of Internal Medicine* **125**, 723–9.
35. **Non-Small Cell Lung Cancer Collaborative Group** (1995). Chemotherapy in non-small cell lung cancer: a meta-analysis using updated data on individual patients from 52 randomised clinical trials. *British Medical Journal* **311**, 899–908.
36. **Douillard, J.Y.** et al. (2000). Irinotecan combined with fluorouracil compared with fluorouracil alone as first-line treatment for metastatic colorectal cancer: a multicentre randomised trial. *Lancet* **355**, 1041–7.
37. **Mainfrault-Goebel, F.** et al. (1999). High dose oxaliplatin with the simplified 48 h bi-monthly leucovorin and 5-fluorouracil regimen in pre-treated metastatic colorectal cancer. *Proceedings of the American Society of Clinical Oncology* **18**, 898.
38. **Twelves, C.** et al. (1999). A phase III trial of capecitabine in previously untreated advanced/metastatic colorectal cancer. *Proceedings of the American Society of Clinical Oncology* **18**, 1010.
39. **Ragnhammar, P.** et al. (1993). The therapeutic use of the unconjugated monoclonal antibody 17-1A in combination with GM-CSF in the treatment of colorectal carcinoma. *Medical Oncology and Tumour Pharmacology* **10**, 61–70.
40. **Samson, D. and Singer, C.** (2001). Multiple myeloma, *Journal of the Royal College of Physicians of London* **1**, 365–70.
41. **Samson, D.** et al. (1989). Infusion of vincristine and doxorubicin with oral dexamethasone as first-line therapy for multiple myeloma. *Lancet* **2**, 882–5.
42. **Attal, M.** et al. (1996). A prospective randomised trial of autologous bone marrow transplantation and chemotherapy for multiple myeloma. *New England Journal of Medicine* **335**, 91–7.
43. **Berenson, J.R.** et al. (1996). Efficacy of pamidronate in reducing skeletal events in patients with advanced multiple myeloma. *New England Journal of Medicine* **334**, 488–93.
44. **Le Chevalier** et al. (1988). Early metastatic cancer of unknown origin at presentation. A clinical study of 302 consecutive autopsied patients. *Archives of Internal Medicine* **148**, 2035–9.

45. **Mainsworth, J.D. and Greco, F.A.** (1993). Treatment of patients with cancer of an unknown primary site. *New England Journal of Medicine* **329**, 257–63.

46. **Anderson, H.** et al. (1983). VAC chemotherapy for metastatic carcinoma from unknown primary site. *European Journal of Cancer* **19**, 49–52.

47. **Schnipper, L.E. and Strom, T.B.** (2001). A magic bullet for cancer—how near and how far? *New England Journal of Medicine* **345**, 283–4.

Further reading

Ross, D.W. *Introduction to Oncogenes and Molecular Cancer Medicine.* New York: Springer, 1998.

Casciato, D.A. and Lowitz, B.B. *Manual of Clinical Oncology* 3rd edn. New York: Little, Brown and Company, 1995.

Skeel, R.T. and Lachant, N.A. *Handbook of Cancer Chemotherapy* 4th edn. New York: Little, Brown and Company, 1995.

Souhami, R.L. et al. *Oxford Textbook of Oncology* 2nd edn. Oxford: Oxford University Press, 2001.

8.1.2 Radiotherapy in symptom management

Peter J. Hoskin

Introduction

The majority of cancer patients will require radiation therapy at some time in the course of their disease, with many having several treatment episodes; over half of all radiation treatments are given with palliative intent for control of local symptoms. Radiotherapy has a major role in symptom control where this is due to localized tumour effect but in this setting has no influence over the natural history of the tumour outside the irradiated area.

General principles of radiotherapy

Radiobiology

Radiotherapy is treatment with ionizing radiation which causes damage to cellular DNA. The most frequently used forms of ionizing radiation in clinical practice are X-rays produced from an X-ray machine or linear accelerator and gamma rays produced from a radioactive source. Some radioisotopes in clinical use also release beta particles which have a similar effect. Other radiation types such as neutrons and protons remain in experimental use in some parts of the world but are not relevant to palliative treatment. The results of radiation passing through a living cell are to cause both direct and indirect damage to the reproductive material of the cell. Direct damage results in base deletions and single and double strand breaks in the DNA chain. Indirect damage, which is probably the major component of the radiation effect, is a result of the interaction of radiation with water molecules in the cell releasing toxic free radicals. Normal cells have a large capacity to repair most of this 'sub-lethal' radiation damage but this is often deficient in transformed malignant cells and these differences in repair capacity may partly account for the variations seen in radiosensitivity. The mechanism of cell death after radiation exposure may be either reproductive failure due to DNA damage or apoptosis through its impact on the cell regulatory mechanisms.

The response of cells to radiation is affected by many factors including oxygenation (hypoxic cells are relatively radioresistant), the number of cells actively dividing (cells in certain phases of the cell cycle are more sensitive than others; non-cycling cells are relatively radioresistant), and the rate of repopulation within the tumour. These parameters of repair, reoxygenation, repopulation, and redistribution within the cell cycle, are the fundamental influences on the cellular response to radiation. They are relevant to the response of tumours in clinical practice and directly influence the way in which radiation is delivered to maximize tumour cell kill whilst minimizing normal tissue damage.

Palliative compared to radical radiotherapy

The aim of radical radiotherapy is to cure local tumour by the complete eradication of tumour cells with minimum associated long-term normal tissue damage; the aim of palliative radiotherapy is to control local symptoms with minimum associated acute radiation reaction.

These two very different aims result in different philosophies in the delivery of radiation. To minimise normal tissue damage small doses built up over a lengthy period are required and hence many patients will require treatment on a daily basis. There is conflict, however, between minimizing normal tissue damage and maximizing tumour control which in general requires high doses close to or beyond those which surrounding normal tissues will tolerate. Radiation schedules shown to improve tumour control may involve *acceleration* in which the dose is given two or three times a day over a much shorter period to reduce the opportunities for tumour repopulation during the course of treatment or *hyperfractionation* in which the treatment is given over the same period but in two or three much smaller doses per day than when delivered as a single daily dose. This considerable investment in time by the patient can be readily justified where cure is the aim, but for patients with a survival of only a few weeks or months where a treatment period of 6–8 weeks would be a major proportion of their remaining life span simpler, more pragmatic schedules are more appropriate provided they are effective in their aim of achieving local symptom control. In general symptom control does not require complete eradication of a tumour mass and indeed in some scenarios, for example, metastatic bone pain, symptom response appears independent of tumour shrinkage.

It is also important to realize that a large proportion of cells, between 60 and 80 per cent of the total, will be killed by the first one or two radiation exposures from a course of treatment. In radical treatment the challenge is to eradicate the remainder whilst in palliative treatment this initial effect may be more than adequate for long-term symptom control. Thus most palliative treatments can be delivered in one or two treatments and rarely is it necessary to extend a course of treatment beyond 1 week. The delivery of short low dose schedules will also result in less troublesome acute reactions and a very low risk of late damage to normal tissues within the expected life span of the patient.

Clinical radiation delivery

The aim of radiotherapy in clinical practice is to deliver an effective dose of radiation with minimal side effects in an environment which the patient finds comfortable and friendly. Unfortunately some of the constraints of radiation delivery may impinge upon these latter aims, for example, the need to immobilize the patient in a fixed position, the use of hard wooden flat couches, and the need for staff to leave the patient isolated whilst radiation delivery is taking place.

The most common type of radiotherapy is external beam irradiation. The different modes of external beam radiation are shown in Table 1. In a modern radiotherapy unit most radiotherapy will be given using an X-ray beam from a linear accelerator or, for more superficial lesions, electron beams from a linear accelerator or orthovoltage X-rays. Figure 1 shows patient being prepared for treatment on a modern linear accelerator. Ionizing radiation can also be delivered by the application of a radioactive source into or around the tumour site. This is known as brachytherapy and examples of this are shown in Table 2. Radiation is damaging to normal

Table 1 Types of external beam radiotherapy

	Energy	Source	Depth of penetration	Clinical use
Superficial X-rays	50–150 kV	X-ray tube	5–10 mm	Surface skin tumours
Orthovoltage X-rays	250–500 kV	X-ray tube	15–30 mm	Surface tumours Superficial bones e.g. ribs, sacrum
Electrons	4–20 MeV	Linear accelerator	15–70 mm	Surface tumours Superficial bones e.g. ribs, sacrum Lymph nodes
Megavoltage X-rays	4–25 MV	Linear accelerator	3–20 cm	Main source of radiation beams for sites other than above
Gamma rays	2.5 MV	Cobalt source	5–10 cm	All sites except superficial skin

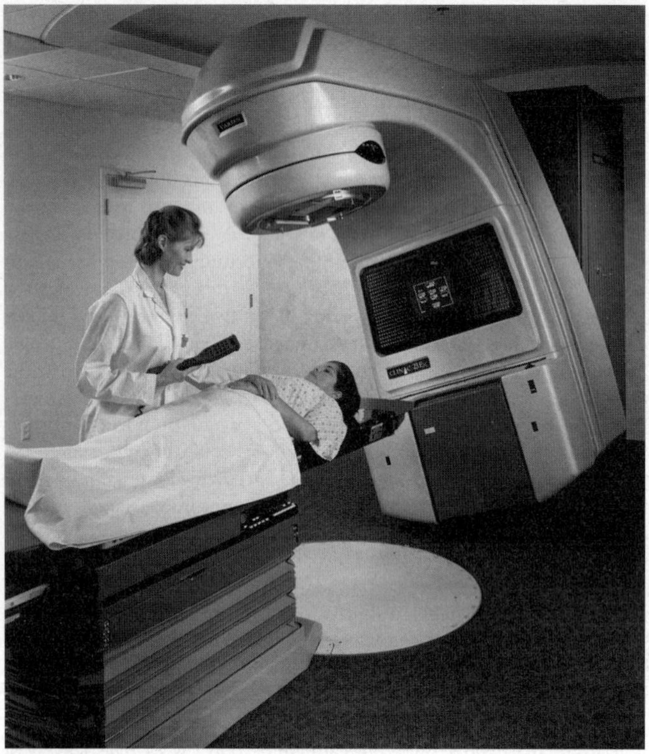

Clinac® Accelerators: Clinac 23EX with MLC-120 and PortalVision™

Fig. 1 Treatment with a modern linear accelerator (Courtesy of Varian Medical, United Kingdom).

tissues and it is therefore important to ensure that it is directed as accurately as possible to the area requiring treatment whilst minimizing the amount of sensitive normal tissue within the treated area. For superficial lesions which are visible or palpable the area to be localized can be easily defined on clinical examination but deep-seated tumours require radiographic localization using a treatment simulator. In many common palliative scenarios such as bone metastases or a primary lung tumour plain X-ray images are sufficient for localization. A treatment simulator will be used which is an X-ray machine identical to the therapy machine in its geometric specifications and movement but which differs by emitting a diagnostic X-ray beam producing an image of the proposed therapeutic beam. For more deep-seated tumours localization can be enhanced by coupling the simulator process with CT scanning which is of particular value in sites such as the bladder, prostate, and pancreas. In addition to accurate localization it is vital that if an area is to be treated more than once in a course of treatment the beam position relative to the patient can be accurately reproduced from day to day. This is ensured by both careful measurement and documentation of the beam position within indelible marking of accurately defined skin entry points on the patient. It may also be necessary to immobilize the patient when treating an area where small movements can result in the beam passing through critical structures, for example, around the eye. The patient may be immobilized using simple techniques such as sandbags, or for more complex treatments a plastic shell using an individualized face mask may be necessary.

A linear accelerator produces high energy radiation at a rate of around 1 Gy/min which means that most treatments even using large single fractions in the palliative setting will last for only a few minutes. There are no accompanying symptoms during radiation exposure provided the patient is comfortable at the outset. It is important to facilitate patient compliance with the procedure to ensure that they can co-operate in achieving the required position and in lying still during treatment. This may require the judicious administration of analgesia or anxiolytic drugs prior to treatment for those having significant pain or other symptoms.

Table 2 Isotope use in brachytherapy

Intra-cavitary	Caesium Cobalt Iridium	Intra-uterine Intra-vaginal Endo-oesophageal Endobronchial Endorectal
Interstitial	Iridium	Tongue, floor of mouth Buccal mucosa Breast Anal canal Vulva/vagina
Surface (mould)	Iridium	Skin Penis

Side effects of radiotherapy

The side effects of radiotherapy are categorized into two groups based on their timing relative to the radiation exposure. Acute effects will be seen during and may persist for several weeks after radiotherapy. Late effects are rarely seen before 9 months after treatment but there is then an ongoing risk for many years, if not forever, that they may appear. They are therefore two distinct events with different aetiologies.

The common clinical manifestations of acute and late radiation toxicity are shown in Table 3.

Acute toxicity represents loss of surface epithelial cells resulting in skin erythema or desquamation, mucositis, oesophagitis, cystitis, or gastrointestinal irritation. Repair of the denuded surface with new epithelial cells occurs once treatment is completed provided that the underlying stem cell population has not been damaged irreparably. Recovery usually occurs within a period of a few days or weeks from treatment. On rare occasions,

Table 3 Acute and late effects of radiation

Site	Acute effect	Late effect[a]
Skin	Erythema Desquamation	Atrophy, fibrosis Telangectasia Necrosis
Gastrointestinal tract	Nausea, anorexia Vomiting Diarrhoea	Stricture Telangiectasia, bleeding Perforation Malabsorption Chronic enteritis, colitis, proctitis
Bladder	Sterile cystitis	Reduced volume Telangiectasia, bleeding Urethral or ureteric stricture Fistula
Oral cavity Pharynx	Mucositis Dry mouth Taste loss	Mucosal atrophy Telangiectasia, bleeding Dental caries Mandibular necrosis
Lung	Pneumonitis	Fibrosis
Central nervous system	Transient demyelination (Lhermitte's sign) Local oedema	Myelitis Necrosis
Eye	Keratitis	Cataract Entropion or ectropion Dry eye

[a] In most patients only minor late effects are seen. These are minimized by reducing the dose of radiation delivered to sensitive structures with the treated region to known safe 'tolerance' doses. Late effects are not expected after palliative radiotherapy.

however, there may be persistent damage, termed 'consequential damage' seen particularly in vulnerable sites such as the back or the lower leg where skin healing appears less efficient. Poor healing after radiotherapy may also be seen where there is secondary infection or trauma and it is these events which can predispose to the rare occurrence of radionecrosis.

Late radiation damage is the major cause of treatment related loss of function and even mortality in patients receiving radical treatment. Its major cause is vascular damage with pathological changes of progressive endarteritis obliterans resulting in progressive closure of small blood vessels. The clinical manifestations of this may be relatively minor such as the commonly observed appearance of skin atrophy or telangiectasia on the skin or mucosal surfaces where radiation was delivered. More serious consequences due to tissue breakdown may, however, occasionally be seen. Common sites are within the pelvis where the bowel or bladder may be damaged resulting in fibrosis and bowel perforation or fistula formation between the bladder, bowel, or vagina. In the central nervous system because of its very limited ability to repair damage catastrophic necrosis will occur if dose limits are exceeded. For every tissue a 'tolerance dose' is defined up to which late normal tissue damage is not expected in the 'normal' population. One of the reasons for the complex planning systems which have evolved for radiation delivery is the strenuous effort required to avoid exceeding these doses whilst delivering effective doses to nearby tumour. Unfortunately there are genetically predisposed individuals to radiation damage where even a conventional tolerance dose may result in late damage.

Management of radiation side effects

Acute side effects may still occur, even after relatively low dose palliative radiation. Management requires no more than relief of symptoms whilst allowing the affected area to heal.

Mild skin reactions require no active treatment. Local skin irritation can be relieved by application of aqueous or 1 per cent hydrocortisone cream.

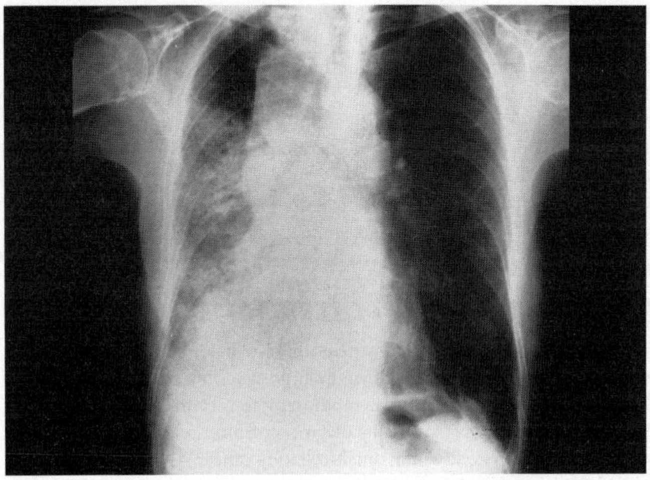

Fig. 2 Interstitial pneumonitis in the right mid and lower zones on chest radiograph after palliative irradiation for carcinoma of the bronchus.

Desquamation will rarely if ever be seen after palliative doses. The use of topical preparations such as gentian violet is to be discouraged and talcum powder and proprietary creams containing metallic salts should be avoided at all costs during treatment as these can enhance the reaction. Starch powder as found in proprietary baby powders may be helpful in keeping the surrounding skin dry and comfortable.

Nausea during irradiation to the abdomen or pelvis will usually respond to simple anti-emetic therapy such as metoclopramide 10 mg 6–8 hourly or where more severe ondansetron 8 mg twice daily. Where anti-emetics are ineffective, a small dose of steroid such as prednisolone 10–30 mg daily may be valuable.

Radiation-induced acute diarrhoea usually responds to dietary advice—avoiding fruit and other fibre-containing foods—and where required loperamide taken with each loose stool or codeine phosphate on a regular basis three to four times daily.

Radiation cystitis may be more difficult to control with no satisfactory local treatment. The use of an alpha blocker such as tamsulosin may be effective where there is severe bladder spasm and potassium citrate or cranberry juice are time-honoured remedies which may be of supportive value. Where there is significant dysuria or strangury then systemic analgesics are also of value.

Oropharyngeal mucositis occurs within the radiation field when treating the head and neck region. It is important to maintain a high level of oral hygiene using regular chlorhexidine mouthwashes and prophylactic anti-candidal preparations with nystatin suspension or clotrimazole gel. Local relief of pain may be achieved using soluble aspirin or benzydamine mouthwashes. Radical high dose treatment to the oral cavity, particularly where the salivary glands are included in the treatment volume, can result in troublesome mouth dryness, loss of taste, and predispose to major dental caries and osteo-radionecrosis of the jaw. For this reason formal dental assessment pre-treatment and meticulous dental hygiene using fluoride dental gel, both during radiotherapy and thereafter, is important in these patients. However, where simple low dose palliative treatment is to be given, for example, to a metastasis in the mandible, then such measures are not required. Throughout the oral cavity and pharyngeal tract, symptoms will be made worse in those patients who smoke or take spirits and where possible these should be avoided during treatment. If severe, typically during radical treatment, enteral feeding using a nasogastric fine bore tube or more commonly a percutaneous gastrostomy, may be required to provide nutritional support through treatment.

Pneumonitis may be seen even after palliative treatment to the lungs. This will present with a dry cough and dyspnoea up to 4 months after treatment and has a classical appearance on chest X-ray shown in Fig. 2, with patchy shadowing conforming to the geometry of the radiation field. A 2- to 3-week course of systemic steroids with antibiotics for secondary infection is recommended but continuing symptoms and late radiation fibrosis may well ensue.

Finally it is important to anticipate probable acute side effects, explain their likelihood to the patient, and encourage the prophylactic use of anti-emetics, anti-diarrhoeal drugs, and mouthwashes. The patient should also be reassured that these are temporary events which will resolve following completion of radiotherapy.

Combined modality treatment

There is increasing use of radiochemotherapy in radical treatments with many sites now having been shown in large randomized phase III trials to benefit from the addition of chemotherapy to a radical course of radiotherapy. This includes treatments of cancers from the oesophagus,(1) anal canal,(2) uterine cervix,(3) non-small-cell lung cancer,(4) and head and neck region.(5) In these settings the chemotherapy is given with radiation to enhance the effect of radiotherapy rather than achieving a systemic cell kill effect. There are other instances, however, where chemotherapy may be given before (neo-adjuvant) or, more commonly, after (adjuvant) radiotherapy to provide early control of micro-metastasis whilst the radiotherapy obtains local control of the more bulky primary site. Examples are seen in the modern management of breast cancer, small-cell lung cancer, colorectal cancer, and lymphoma. Few if any of these treatments, however, fall readily within the scope of palliative medicine.

Specific indications for radiotherapy and symptom control

Radiotherapy is effective for many symptoms where their basis is local tumour interference with normal tissue structures through either pressure or infiltration. A simple classification and examples of these areas is shown in Table 4.

Table 4 Indications for radiotherapy in symptom palliation

Symptom	Cause
Pain	
Bone pain	Bone metastases
Visceral pain	Soft tissue metastases
Neuropathic pain	Bone metastases
	Soft tissue primary or metastases
	Intrinsic tumour in nerve tissue
Local pressure	
Spinal canal compression	Extradural metastases
	Bone metastases
Cranial nerve palsies	Skull base bone metastases
	Meningeal metastases
	Intrinsic brain tumour
Obstruction	
Bronchus	Intrinsic bronchial tumour
	Extrinsic lymphadenopathy
Oesophagus	Intrinsic bronchial tumour
	Extrinsic lymphadenopathy
Superior vena cava	Primary mediastinal tumour
	Primary lung or oesophageal tumour
	Metastatic mediastinal lymphadenopathy
Hydrocephalus	Malignant meningitis
	Primary or metastatic brain tumour
Limb swelling	Metastatic lymphadenopathy
Bleeding	
Haemoptysis	Primary bronchial tumour
	Metastatic bronchial or lung tumour
Haematuria	Primary tumour in kidney, ureter, bladder, prostate
Vaginal bleeding	Primary tumours of vagina, cervix or uterus
	Metastases in vagina
Rectal bleeding	Primary anal or colorectal tumours

Bone metastases

Radiotherapy may be indicated for bone metastases because of bone pain, pathological fracture, or pressure on nerves.

Bone pain

Radiotherapy is highly effective in the treatment of local metastatic bone pain. The majority of patients with bone metastases survive for less than one year and radiotherapy will achieve pain control over this period for the majority of patients. With short median predicted survival times a simple short treatment schedule is most appropriate and for the majority of situations a single treatment delivering a dose of 8 Gy is adequate. The results from a large randomized trial evaluating this are shown in Fig. 3 with a probability of pain relief at 3, 6, and 12 months after treatment of around 80 per cent.(6) Whilst there is now considerable data in the literature supporting the use of single doses in this setting some patients will receive a more protracted fractionated course of treatment delivering 20–30 Gy over 1–2 weeks which is preferred by some centres where there is concern over possible fracture or nerve compression.

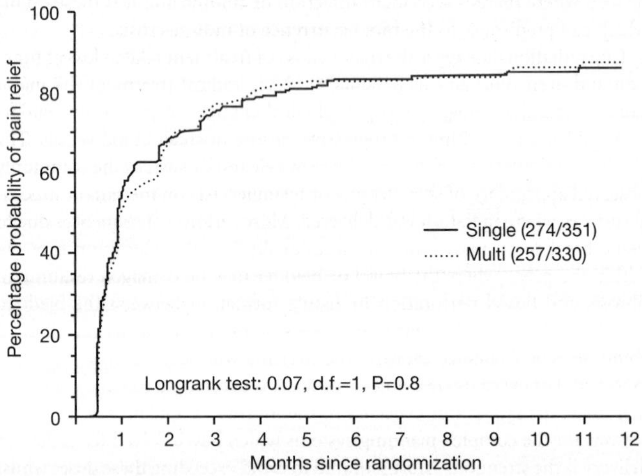

Fig. 3 Probability of pain relief after single or multiple fraction treatments for metastatic bone pain (from United Kingdom Bone Pain Trial Working Party, 1999;(6) reproduced with permission).

The treatment techniques for bone metastasis are simple. Superficial bones such as the clavicle, ribs, and sacrum may be treated with a direct field using orthovoltage X-rays or electrons and other sites will be treated using a linear accelerator or cobalt beam. Under optimal conditions the site will be localized using a treatment simulator based on clinical examination and radiographic or bone scan evidence of metastatic disease. It is particularly important to document carefully the field margin since most patients will have multiple sites of metastasis and further treatment with the potential for overlap of fields may be required. This is of particular concern in the spine where metastasis at several levels may require sequential treatment. Overlap of fields in the spine can result in overdosage to the spinal cord with the risk of subsequent radiation myelitis and irreversible neurological deterioration developing within 6–9 months from treatment. For patients with a short prognosis this may not be relevant and a positive decision to accept an overlap may be made, with the full knowledge of the patient, where it is considered that benefit from treatment in the short term outweighs any theoretical hazard of later myelitis; in others, however, where the expected prognois is greater than 6 months the risks may be an issue.

Many patients have multiple sites of disease with pain that is often not well localized but presents as a diffuse symptom affecting multiple sites. Such patients should be considered for wide field radiotherapy or radioisotope therapy.

Wide field radiotherapy delivers treatment to an area which may include up to half the body as described above using doses of 6 Gy to the upper half-body, where the lungs limit higher doses, or 8 Gy to the lower half-body. Again no advantage for higher doses has been seen, although a recent large randomized trial has recommended 8 Gy in two fractions as the optimum dose.[7] Inevitably wide field treatment is associated with greater toxicity than local field irradiation with around two-thirds of patients having gastrointestinal symptoms of nausea, vomiting, or diarrhoea and the majority of a period of bone marrow suppression following treatment. This may result in some patients requiring blood transfusions but rarely is severe enough to cause clinically relevant neutropenia or thrombocytopenia. Spontaneous recovery is to be expected and indeed sequential treatment of upper and lower half-bodies is possible given a 4-to 6-week gap for marrow recovery. The most serious consequence of upper hemibody irradiation is the development of radiation pneumonitis, usually avoided by limiting the dose to 6 Gy after correction for the increased transmission of the X-ray beam through the lungs. Where the occasional case does occur it is invariably progressive and fatal. Despite this hemibody irradiation is a valuable tool for the treatment of widespread bone pain and response rates are consistently around 80 per cent maintained in the majority of patients until their death.[7,8]

When accurate prospective assessments of pain have been used to monitor the response to the local irradiation of painful bone metastasis an increasing incidence pain relief is seen for several weeks from the time of treatment and whilst around half of patients will respond achieving pain relief within the first 2–4 weeks others may yet experience improved pain 6–8 weeks after treatment. The timing of response varies between local radiotherapy to an isolated bone metastasis and wide field hemibody radiotherapy. Rapid responses are often seen after wide field radiotherapy and this contrast is illustrated in Fig. 4. Timing of response is important in considering whether alternative treatments or reirradiation should be considered. Re-irradiation should certainly be considered where pain returns after a previous good response but may also be of value where the initial response is unsatisfactory. The probability of response after re-treatment

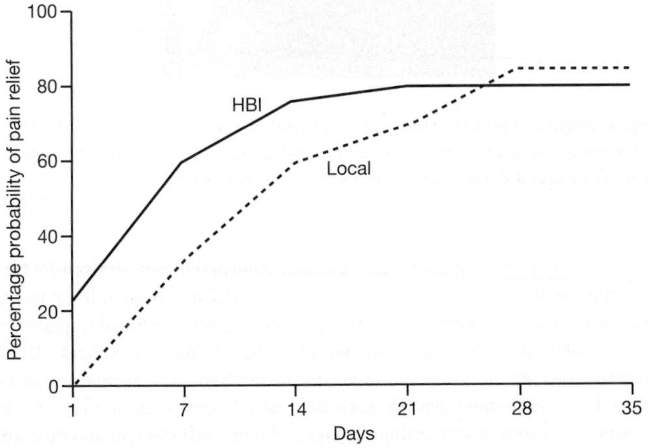

Fig. 4 Comparison of onset of pain relief following hemibody irradiation (HBI) and local irradiation for bone pain (after Salazar et al. 1986,[8] reproduced with permission).

is around 80 per cent, similar to that after primary treatment and is not always predicted by the initial response.[9]

Radioisotope treatment is an alternative means of delivering radiation to multiple sites of bone metastasis. It uses systemic administration of a radioactive isotope which is then selectively concentrated at sites of bone metastasis. This may be because of tumour-specific isotope concentration as in differentiated thyroid cancer concentrating radio-iodine, or bone-specific localization exploiting the uptake of phosphate and calcium at sites of remineralization. The isotopes used deliver their radiation dose by the release of beta particles with a short range of only a few millimetres thereby concentrating their dose within the immediate area of uptake.

In the specific case of differentiated thyroid cancer, using radio-iodine, published series reported disappointingly low response rate in terms of bone pain relief after radio-iodine, and external beam therapy is considered better for painful bone metastasis in this setting.[10]

Isotopes exploiting remineralization include phosphorus and strontium[11] which are concentrated in the same way as calcium and samarium[12] and rhenium which are localised by chelation with a phosphonate compound (Sm-EDMP and Re-HDMP). Strontium and samarium are the two isotopes most readily available in commercial formulations for clinical use. Prostate cancer has been used as the model for the development of this treatment having typically a florid osteoblastic remineralisation response. Both isotopes are highly effective in achieving pain relief with very few side effects; best results are probably achieved in patients relatively early in their natural history with good performance status, serum PSA less than 100 μg/l, and haemoglobin greater than 10 g/dl.[13] Both are given as a single outpatient intravenous injection considerably simplifying administration for the patient, and radiation hazards are few provided the patient does not have urinary incontinence. Transient bone marrow depression may be seen but is rarely of clinical significance and less than that seen with hemibody radiotherapy; however, severe bone marrow depression is a contraindication to the use of these agents. Using similar parameters to those for chemotherapy, that is, a neutrophil count less than 1.5×10^9/l and a platelet count less than 50×10^9/l would make their use hazardous. Since the substances are cleared by renal excretion the other relative contra-indication is renal impairment. In addition to prostate cancer their efficacy has been demonstrated in other primary sites in particular breast cancer and the main barrier to the more widespread application of radioisotope therapy in metastatic bone pain is the substantial cost associated with their use.

The mechanism by which radiation achieves pain control is not clear. Tumour cells are undoubtedly killed even after small single doses of radiation which result in pain relief but other factors may be important. Evidence suggesting that tumour shrinkage itself may not be necessary include the observation that rapid pain relief may be seen within 24 h of treatment particularly after hemibody irradiation (Fig. 4), that no relationship has been shown between the response in terms of pain relief and different histological types of tumour correlating with variations in radiosensitivity, and that no clear dose response effect above 8 Gy has been shown for the onset or duration of pain relief. This implies that local effects upon the hose tissue possibly affecting the release of pain-mediating humeral agents and osteoblast/osteoclast interaction are important co-factors in achieving and maintaining pain relief. Further evidence to support this hypothesis comes from the efficacy of bisphosphonates, the potent osteoclast inhibitors, in metastatic bone pain relief and the demonstration that changes in biochemical markers of osteoclast activity occur following radiotherapy to bone pain which can predict for response.[14]

Prophylactic radiotherapy to bone metastases

There has been considerable interest in the role of radiation preventing the development and subsequent morbidity from bone metastasis. Inadvertent irradiation of certain sites such as the thoracic spine when a breast is irradiated has been shown to reduce the instance of subsequent metastatic events in bones in this area. More recently the value of hemibody irradiation at the time of presentation of localized bone pain has been evaluated and a reduction in subsequent episodes of bone pain demonstrated.[15] Similarly the use of radioactive strontium has been explored when bone metastases first present and this also has been shown to reduce or delay the need for further treatment for bone pain.[16] The gains are relatively modest, hemibody irradiation resulting in a 16 per cent reduction in requirements for additional local radiotherapy and strontium delaying the median time to further radiotherapy for a site of bone pain by 15 weeks.

It is likely also that bisphosphonates will have an increasing role in both the primary treatment and prophylaxis of bone metastases particularly in breast and prostatic cancer. The relative roles of radiotherapy and bisphosphonates and the interaction between them in the overall management of bone metastases have yet to be clearly defined.

Pathological fracture

Pathological fracture at a site of bone metastasis may occur spontaneously or as a result of minor trauma particularly in weight-bearing bones. Surgical internal fixation is the preferred management in long bones but there will be situations including vertebral collapse and fractures of the rib and girdle bones where surgery is not feasible and other scenarios where a patient has advanced disease and poor performance status where surgery is inappropriate. In these cases local irradiation remains a valuable palliative tool both to achieve local pain relief and to enable bone healing. When the object of treatment is pain relief alone a single dose of 8 Gy is adequate treatment and following irradiation around two-thirds of patients with pathological fracture will achieve pain relief. There are no comparative data defining the optimal dose to achieve bone healing after pathological fracture. Remineralization is reported in one-third of patients after doses of 40–50 Gy delivered in 4–5 weeks but is also seen after lower doses of only 20 Gy in 2 weeks. In practice most patients will receive courses delivering 20–30 Gy in 5–10 fractions over 1–2 weeks.

Radiotherapy may also be indicated post-operatively following internal fixation to prevent further progression of the remaining metastatic tumour and enable healing of the bone around the prosthesis. There is, however, little published data to support this common practice although non-randomized data suggest better functional recovery when radiotherapy is given.[17] Conventionally fields covering the entire length of the prosthesis or intra-medullary nail are used because of the perceived risk of dissemination through the marrow cavity by the operative procedure. Patients with widespread metastatic disease and limited survival whose pain is controlled post-operatively gain little benefit from post-operative radiotherapy and this should be deferred unless local pain develops.

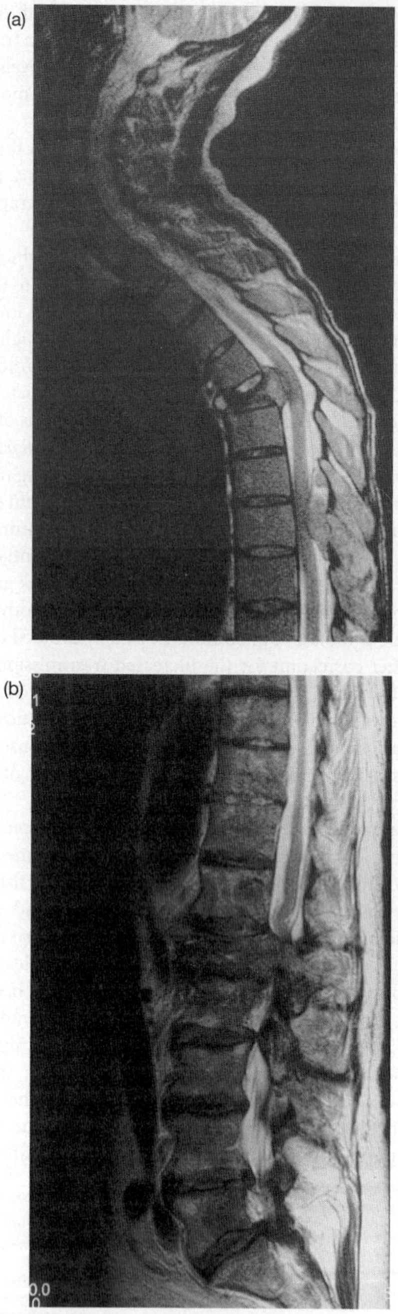

Fig. 5 Magnetic resonance scans of spinal cord compression demonstrating (a) areas of extradural metastases with in addition an area of vertebral collapse and (b) vertebral bone involvement causing cord compression.

Neurological symptoms

Spinal cord and cauda equina compression

Spinal cord or cauda equina compression with loss of function of limbs and loss of sphincter control is catastrophic It occurs because of tumour compression of neurological tissue in the spinal canal. The initial events are predominantly vascular with venous engorgement and oedema followed by mechanical compression with ultimately irreversible damage to the nervous tissue. Magnetic resonance imaging (MRI) of spinal cord compression has shown around one-quarter of these cases to be due to direct encroachment of the spinal canal by tumour arising in a vertebral body with the remainder attributable to blood borne extradural or intra-dural metastasis[18] as demonstrated in Fig. 5. Approximately 70 per cent of cases involve thoracic cord, 20 per cent the lumbosacral region, and 10 per cent the cervical cord.

Early diagnosis is essential in this condition and the major determinant of outcome independent of treatment. It should be considered and excluded in any patient presenting with sensory or motor changes in the limbs or urinary symptoms, in particular where there is associated backache or known vertebral metastasis. Urgent imaging of the spinal canal using MRI as the method of choice is mandatory even where recent investigations have shown no evidence of metastatic disease. Alternative but less satisfactory imaging methods of the spinal canal where MRI is unavailable or in the occasional patient where it is contra-indicated because of metal implants or a pacemaker, include spinal myelography and CT imaging. Where MRI is negative and the picture is of cauda equina involvement a lumbar puncture should be performed having excluded raised intra-cranial pressure, to exclude carcinomatous meningitis. Figure 5 demonstrates spinal cord compression from direct invasion of a bone metastasis (a) and extradural tumour metastasis (b).

Histological diagnosis is essential before embarking upon definitive treatment. In many patients there will already be an underlying diagnosis of metastatic malignancy but in one series 48 per cent of patients presenting with spinal cord compression had no previous history of malignant disease.[19] The commonest sites for spinal cord compression are breast, lung, and prostate, each accounting for around 20 per cent of patients in most series. Most other primary sites have also been associated with spinal canal involvement, the next two commonest being kidney and lymphoma. Where a patient with known metastatic disease presents with spinal cord compression it is usually reasonable to assume that this will be the same disease process unless there are atypical features to suggest a second primary. In most cases where a histological diagnosis is not available a CT guided fine needle aspirate cytology specimen or needle biopsy will be sufficient.[20]

Both radiotherapy and decompressive surgery are effective in the initial management of spinal cord compression. Whilst no randomized comparison of the two modalities of treatment with sufficient numbers to provide a true comparison has been undertaken, no advantage of surgery over radiotherapy has been demonstrated in published series where patients have a previously confirmed diagnosis of malignant disease and no evidence of vertebral collapse. A non-randomized comparison has suggested that better pain relief is seen after radiotherapy or where radiotherapy is given post-operatively.[21] Initial management for most patients should include high dose steroids and local irradiation to the spinal site. Certain histological types of tumour should be considered for primary chemotherapy rather than for radiotherapy or for surgery. These include lymphoma and small-cell lung cancer. Patients with these tumours relapsing with spinal canal compression after previous chemotherapy, however, will be best treated initially with radiotherapy, second line chemotherapy being much less certain to achieve a response in this critical situation.

The radiation technique in most cases is simple using a single posterior field to encompass the vertebral level and a suitable margin. With accurate localization using MR one vertebral body or 3 cm above and below the area of cord compression is adequate. Problems may arise where there are multiple sites of compression, particularly if anatomically distant, and in some patients more than one radiation field may be required to cover, for example, sites in the high thoracic and lumbar region. Where there is a large para-vertebral mass more complex planning may be necessary to ensure complete coverage. Two or three angled fields to cover the tumour volume taking care to avoid sensitive para-vertebral structures, in particular the kidneys in the lower thoracic and upper lumbar regions, may be needed.

Most patients with good performance status will receive fractionated courses of treatment delivering 20–30 Gy in 5–10 fractions. Recovery after paraplegia that has been established for more than 24 h is not to be expected and in these patients single doses of 8–10 Gy are often given for pain relief without any expectation of neurological recovery. In other selected cases, particularly those with a localized potentially curable tumour such as a solitary plasmacytoma, higher doses of up to 40 or 50 Gy over 3–5 weeks may be delivered.

In patients who have extensive vertebral collapse with intrusion into the spinal canal radiotherapy is of little value in re-establishing neurological function. It is in this group of patients that surgery has its main application with the use of anterior spinal surgery involving resection and spinal stabilization. This represents a more invasive procedure than radiotherapy with significant operative morbidity and even mortality but results in series of selected patients are superior to either laminectomy or radiotherapy alone, with between 62 and 83 per cent of patients being able to walk following anterior surgery and pain relief being achieved in 71 per cent.[22,23] Many of these patients, however, have poor general condition as shown by a 30 per cent mortality in one series of 26 consecutive patients operated on for pain or neurological deficits, and careful selection of patients for surgical referral is therefore required.[23] Surgery should also be considered for relapse after or progression during radiotherapy and in some cases where there is localized involvement of the spinal canal by tumour conventionally regarded as 'radioresistant', for example, soft tissue sarcoma.

The outcome of treatment depends primarily upon the speed of diagnosis and neurological status at initiation of treatment. When patients present ambulatory, 79 per cent are still ambulant following radiotherapy treatment; in contrast of those presenting with para-paresis only 42 per cent become ambulant and 20–25 per cent will suffer significant neurological deterioration during treatment by radiotherapy alone. Where pain relief is the goal of treatment, radiotherapy will achieve this in over three-quarters of patients compared with only one-third of patients following laminectomy. Histology may influence outcome, patients with myeloma and lymphoma having a better outcome than those with breast cancer, who in turn respond better than those with lung or kidney primary tumours.

In patients with a sufficiently long survival, recurrence of symptoms may occur from tumour regrowth or development of other sites in the spine. Previously irradiated sites may be subject to reirradiation but a lower dose given in smaller fraction sizes will be used, for example, 20 Gy in 10 daily fractions to avoid incurring radiation damage to the cord. In these circumstances where the tumour is localized surgical decompression should be considered.

Since the outcome of treatment is best when diagnosis is made very early there would be considerable advantages in predicting those patients at risk of spinal cord compression and treating them prophylactically. It is possible using MRI to detect metastasis in vertebral bodies at very early stages of development and minor encroachment into the spinal canal which is often clinically asymptomatic and not detectable on plain radiographs. Other predictors for spinal canal compression reported in small-cell lung cancer are local back pain associated with positive bone scan in the spine or cerebral metastasis with a positive bone scan. These situations are associated with cord compression in 36 and 25 per cent, respectively.[24] There is some evidence from the use of bisphosphonates that prophylactic treatment of sub-clinical bone metastasis can reduce spinal complications and similar observations have been made using early antiandrogen treatment in prostate cancer. In some centres there is an aggressive policy of prophylactic irradiation for spinal metastasis on this basis.

The most important issues in the management of spinal cord compression remain a high awareness of condition and a low threshold for investigating relatively minor symptoms, particularly in patients with known vertebral metastasis or disease in the nervous system.

Brain metastasis

Up to 10 per cent of all cancers metastasize to the brain, the most common primary sites being the lung and breast; approximately one-third of these will be solitary deposits. Disability from brain metastasis is disproportionate to the bulk of the tumour with a very small deposit on the motor cortex having catastrophic results for the patient whilst a deposit of similar size would have little effect in the lung or liver. In general therefore active treatment of brain metastases as soon as they have presented is indicated although in some patients their impact will be such that performance status of the patient is already very poor and treatment non-contributory. Confirmation of the diagnosis is obtained using CT or MR scanning. Initial management usually includes the use of steroids to reduce and control raised intra-cranial pressure and where symptoms are due to oedema rather than tumour infiltration some initial improvement in neurological deficit is often seen. There is, however, also evidence that high dose steroids in this setting contribute significantly to morbidity and total doses of 4–8 mg dexamethasone daily may be adequate.

Radiotherapy is well established as an effective palliative treatment for cerebral metastasis. Overall headache, motor and sensory loss, and confusion will respond to treatment in around 80 per cent of selected patients with a complete response of between 35 and 55 per cent.[25] However, the median survival after irradiation for brain metastasis is less than 6 months reflecting the fact that brain metastasis often heralds widespread advanced metastatic disease with the majority of patients dying from the combined effect of distant metastasis rather than progressive disease in the brain alone. Twenty per cent of patients who embark upon a course of radiotherapy for brain metastases fail to complete the course and this argues for careful selection in determining which patients may benefit from radiotherapy. In particular those with multiple metastases outside the central nervous system and those with poor performance status with rapidly progressive disease are most likely to succumb within the period of treatment. Factors influencing survival after radiation are shown in Table 5.

As with any other symptomatic metastatic disease it is important to have an underlying histological diagnosis. In general whilst it is preferable to diagnose a site other than the brain, where a solitary metastasis is present or if this is the first manifestation of malignancy there may be no alternative.

Further management will then depend upon the general condition of the patient, underlying primary site, and the distribution of the brain metastases. A simple algorithm is shown in Fig. 6.[26]

Treatment techniques for multiple brain metastases are simple using lateral fields from each side (parallel opposed fields) covering the entire intracranial contents. A series of randomized trials have shown no benefit for doses greater than 20–30 Gy in 1–2 weeks[25] and more recent trials have shown that 12 Gy in two fractions is equivalent to 30 Gy in 10 fractions for symptom control with a small but clinically not significant improvement in survival of 7 days in the 30 Gy arm.[27] This difference was greater in a sub-group of good prognosis patients and the longer schedule may therefore be selected for this group, but for patients with advanced disease and only moderate performance status a simple two fraction schedule is to be recommended.

There is usually little acute toxicity from a short palliative course of whole brain radiotherapy for multiple brain metastasis but an unfortunate and unavoidable effect is complete alopecia. Hair regrowth will occur within a period of 2–3 months but for many patients this is a particularly distressing and on occasions unacceptable cost of treatment. Mild scalp erythema may also occur particularly around the external pinnae and most patients will continue steroids through treatment; transient rises in intracranial pressure having been reported which can be troublesome if pressure is already raised when treatment starts. It is also important, following completion of cranial irradiation, to reduce and if possible discontinue the steroids in order to minimize long-term side effects provided there is no neurological deterioration whilst doing so.

The majority of patients with multiple cerebral metastases will die from widespread metastatic disease outside the central nervous system but around a quarter will suffer persistent or recurrent symptomatic cerebral metastasis. Steroids may achieve short-term control of symptoms but significant side effects may occur. Re-treatment following a dose of 20–30 Gy carries a risk of radiation damage to the brain and there is often reluctance to consider reirradiation for recurrent disease. Without treatment, however, progressive morbidity and ultimately death from brain metastasis will occur and neurological sequelae from radiation damage may take many months if not years to be manifest. On this basis therefore low dose re-treatment delivering a further 20–30 Gy in 2–3 weeks may be beneficial for selected patients who have a good initial response to treatment.

Solitary metastases usually reflect a more favourable prognosis and in selected patients with no detectable systemic disease elsewhere surgical removal gives good local and long-term control. Post-operative radiotherapy is usually recommended on the basis of two randomized trials showing a statistically significant reduction in brain recurrence, but because of a high incidence of death from progressive systemic disease there was no impact on overall survival. However, a third larger trial has failed to confirm this advantage for post-operative radiotherapy.[26] Localized high dose radiotherapy using radiosurgery is an alternative to surgical excision. There has been no formal comparison between the two but where surgery is limited by the site of metastasis and proximity to functionally critical structures it may be considered as an alternative. This uses either a dedicated multi-source cobalt unit (gamma knife) or a stereotactic multiple-arc radiotherapy technique from a linear accelerator. The role of whole brain radiotherapy in addition to radiosurgery, analogous to the use of post-operative radiotherapy, remains uncertain but this is also recommended in some centres. Similarly there is no consensus on radiation doses in this setting but radiosurgery is typically delivered as single doses of 15–20 Gy. Unfortunately, despite surgery or radiosurgery achieving local control, most patients still ultimately succumb to the effects of distant metastasis

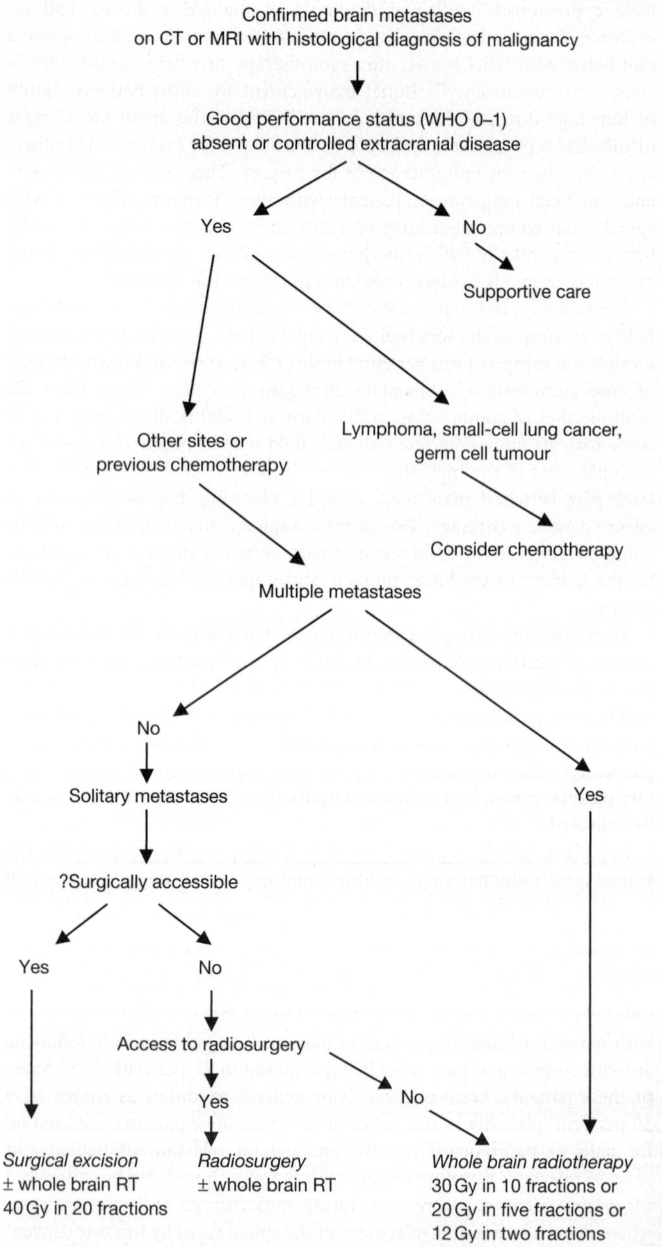

Fig. 6 Algorithm for the management of brain metastases (derived from Hoskin and Brada[26]).

Table 5 Prognostic factors influencing survival after irradiation of brain metastases

Increased survival	Decreased survival
Brain first site of relapse	Multiple lobes involved
Brain sole site of relapse	Meningeal disease
Long disease-free interval prior to brain relapse	
Primary site in brain	
Performance status 0/1	
Age <60 years	

and careful selection and screening is required before embarking upon aggressive local therapy of this type.

Primary brain tumours

Primary brain tumours (including low grade I or II astrocytoma, oligondendroglioma, ependymoma, and meningioma) will in most cases be treated by surgery, radiotherapy, or both with curative intent. However, high grade astrocytomas (grade III or IV) are extremely malignant incurable tumours with, if untreated, a prognosis of only a few months. Palliative radiotherapy may be of value in this situation for selected patients with good performance status and the best results are seen in those aged under 60 with no neurological deficits who present with fits. High dose treatment delivering 60 Gy in 30 fractions over 6 weeks has been shown to be superior to 45 Gy in 20 fractions over 4 weeks in this group[28] and the role of adjuvant chemotherapy in this setting remains under investigation. Despite this only 10 per cent of patients with high grade astrocytoma will be alive 2 years after treatment and a significant number will fail to benefit from this high dose treatment schedule. In these patients where symptoms are progressive short pragmatic schedules delivering doses of 20–30 Gy may be considered.[29] For those aged over 60 years presenting with major neurological deficits and poor performance status radiotherapy generally has little benefit.

Malignant meningitis

Diffuse meningeal carcinomatosis is generally a pre-terminal event with a median survival of only a few weeks if untreated. It commonly presents with multiple spinal root symptoms and signs and multiple cranial nerve palsies. Raised intra-cranial pressure may occur resulting in headache and other symptoms. Common primary sites associated with malignant meningitis are carcinoma of the breast and lung. Central nervous system relapse of leukaemia also typically presents with malignant meningitis.

Intensive treatment may be indicated where there is a treatable underlying malignancy. In the case of acute leukaemia and lymphoma sustained remissions may be achieved by the use of intra-thecal chemotherapy using methotrexate and cytosine arabinoside often combined with craniospinal irradiation (radiotherapy to the entire brain and spinal cord) or cranial irradiation alone. Such treatment is no small undertaking and may be associated with morbidity due to bone marrow depression and nausea, vomiting, and alopecia from the radiotherapy. In children there are also the associated issues of impaired spinal growth and intellectual development after radiotherapy to the spine and brain, respectively. Furthermore it is unfortunately the case that despite initial remission, central nervous system relapse of lymphoma or leukaemia is generally associated with a poor overall prognosis and subsequent relapse with death often occurs within a few months.

The outlook for carcinomatous meningitis from solid tumours, however, is even worse and whilst untreated the median survival is only a few weeks even intensive therapy with intrathecal chemotherapy and craniospinal irradiation will extend this to no more than a few months, much of which may be taken up with treatment.[30] On this basis judicious local irradiation to specific sites causing symptoms such as the skull base when cranial nerves are involved or the segments of the spinal cord related to nerve root symptoms, delivering a dose of 20 Gy in five fractions offers a more pragmatic approach, achieving effective palliation whilst minimizing the morbidity and duration of treatment in a universally fatal condition.

Cranial nerve palsies

Cranial nerve symptoms and signs due to metastatic cancer may arise from intrinsic metastasis in the brain stem and mid brain, infiltration of the leptomeninges, compression by extra-dural deposits, or bone involvement in the skull base. The management of intrinsic metastasis and leptomeningeal metastasis has been discussed above; results of whole brain irradiation for cranial nerve deficits due to cerebral metastasis show an overall response rate of 78 per cent and a complete response rate of 42 per cent.[25] Local irradiation of the skull base is of value where diffuse bone involvement has resulted in cranial nerve compression and symptomatic improvement is reported in between 50 and 78 per cent of patients maintained until death in around 80 per cent. In general patients with skull base metastasis, representing metastatic bone disease, will have a better prognosis than those with intrinsic central nervous system metastases, their median survival being between 10 and 20 months.[31,32]

Peripheral nerve symptoms

Involvement of peripheral nerves will typically result in nerve root pain and loss of motor function in the distribution of that nerve. This may be due to compression of the nerve by tumour at any point from the spinal root canal to its peripheral receptors. Cauda equina compression from spinal canal tumour has been discussed in the section above. Outside the spinal canal symptoms may arise because of direct tumour compression and infiltration particularly in the brachial plexus from apical lung tumours or metastatic lymph nodes and at the lumbosacral plexus from pelvic tumours of the bowel, bladder, ovary, or uterus. Lumbosacral neuropathic pain will respond to palliative doses of radiotherapy with complete pain relief within 1 month reported in 85–100 per cent of patients.[33] Pelvic irradiation for pain relief for recurrent colorectal cancer is successful in up to 80 per cent of patients with no difference detected between a 3-week course of treatment delivering 45 Gy and a single dose of 10 Gy.[34] Treatment to apical lung tumours or axillary recurrence of breast cancer causing upper limb pain due to brachial plexus neuropathy is reported to be successful in up to 77 per cent of patients using typical doses of 20–30 Gy in 1–2 weeks.[35]

Choroidal and orbital metastasis

Metastases to the eye are unusual but may cause distressing symptoms of proptosis, pain, and visual disturbance. The most common intra-occular site is the choroid where over 50 per cent of metastases arise from primary breast cancer, 30 per cent from lung cancer, and around 25 per cent are bilateral. The diagnosis is made on fundoscopy or slit lamp examination. Untreated there is progressive deterioration and ultimately loss of vision. Local treatment with radiotherapy delivering doses of 30–40 Gy in 2–4 weeks is reported to achieve stabilization and improvement of vision in 70–85 per cent of patients.[36] Metastasis at other intra-orbital sites are less common and may arise not only from blood-borne secondary spread but also as a result of direct invasion from other head and neck sites, in particular the nasopharynx, nasal cavity, and sinuses. Palliative local irradiation is again of value in preventing and relieving local symptoms from pressure and infiltration.

Radiotherapy to the eye and orbit requires meticulous attention to technique, avoiding as far as possible direct irradiation of the cornea which can result in painful keratitis. Radiation cataracts may be induced after only small doses of 5–10 Gy to the lens of the eye and wherever possible, therefore, this should also be shielded. In the context of palliative treatment, however, it is important to bear in mind that radiation cataracts may take many years to evolve and should not be considered a reason for avoiding radiation to the orbit where indicated.

Cerebral lymphoma

Primary lymphoma of the central nervous system is a rare extranodal site for non-Hodgkins lymphoma but has increased in incidence considerably in recent years due to its association with HIV infection when it is often a manifestation of advanced, late stage disease. It may cause headache, fits, cranial nerve palsies, or other focal neurological signs. Initial treatment with steroids will often achieve good symptom palliation and some regression. Whole brain radiotherapy has an important role both in the primary treatment when 'radical' doses of 40–50 Gy may be given[37] and also in palliation when a typical dose is 30 Gy in 10 fractions over 2 weeks. In the HIV setting good palliation can be achieved, with death then ensuing from opportunist infection rather than from progressive lymphoma; in the immunocompetent sporadic cases more intensive treatment, often in combination with chemotherapy, results in a median survival of 10–18 months.[38]

Obstructive symptoms

Mediastinal compression and superior vena cava obstruction

The syndrome of superior vena cava obstruction (SVCO) may arise due to occlusion by extrinsic compression, intraluminal thrombosis, or direct invasion of the vessel wall. The majority of cases are due to malignant tumour within the mediastinum but other rare causes which should be excluded include aortic aneurysm, chronic mediastinitis, trauma, or thrombosis following central venous catheterization. Approximately 3 per cent of patients with carcinoma of the bronchus and 8 per cent of those with lymphoma will develop SVCO and of the patients who present with this syndrome 75 per cent will have primary bronchial carcinomas (40 per cent of which will be small-cell lung cancer) and 15 per cent will have mediastinal lymphoma.

The clinical effects arise as a result of increased venous pressure above the site of obstruction. The extent to which this produces symptoms will depend on the efficiency of collateral vessels (particularly the internal mammary vessels, pulmonary veins, and the thoracic and vertebral venous plexuses) which may bypass the obstruction. Because of this obstruction above the azygos vein will have less effect than obstruction below this level. A wide variety of presenting symptoms may result, including headaches, somnolence, and dizziness, together with the effects of oedema and pressure within the mediastinum causing dysphagia, dyspnoea, cough, or hoarseness; more rarely convulsions may result from cerebral hypertension. Examination may reveal fixed engorgement of arm and neck veins with visible dilatation of superficial skin veins, cyanosis, and facial oedema. Management requires both alleviation of symptoms and shrinkage of intra-thoracic tumour to relieve the obstruction. SVCO, whilst potentially a hazardous condition, rarely needs emergency treatment and it is more important to have a full and accurate assessment of the underlying disease together with a histological diagnosis in order that correct effective therapy may be instigated. Presentation with SVCO is not a contra-indication to radical curative treatment in patients where this is appropriate, for example, mediastinal Hodgkin's disease. It is important not to compromise the management of these patients by inappropriate emergency treatment. A policy of delayed treatment until definitive tissue diagnosis can be achieved has been evaluated in a large review of 1986 patients presenting with SVCO which found only one death directly attributable to venous obstruction which occurred as a result of inhalation from an epistaxis.[39]

The first approach to management therefore should always be to obtain a histological diagnosis and to fully stage the patient so that those patients eligible for radical treatment, and those for whom chemotherapy as the primary treatment will be more appropriate than radiotherapy, can be identified. Whilst there are theoretical problems in performing a biopsy within a region of raised venous pressure, with an increased risk of haemorrhage, in practice bronchoscopy, mediastinoscopy, or lymph node biopsy are performed without major complications and should be undertaken unless there is life-threatening large airways obstruction. Patients presenting with acute symptoms should be considered for initial bronchoscopy and stenting as the most appropriate primary treatment and similarly for severe venous occlusion the insertion of an SVC stent will be more immediately successful than radiotherapy or chemotherapy. During the acute phase of investigation steroids may also be of value in high doses, such as dexamethasone 12–16 mg daily although there is no good objective data to support this practice. Once a tissue diagnosis has been confirmed and where indicated and feasible a stent has been placed, definitive treatment with chemotherapy or radiotherapy should be instigated.

On the basis of a histological diagnosis those patients with chemosensitive tumours, in particular small-cell lung cancer, Hodgkin's disease, non-Hodgkin's lymphoma, and germ cell tumours, can be identified and treated with primary chemotherapy. For the remainder, the majority of whom will have non-small-cell lung cancer, radiotherapy to the mediastinum covering the tumour mass and adjacent lymph nodes areas where appropriate is indicated. This may present technical difficulties in patients with impaired respiratory function if they are unable to lie flat for treatment and on occasions it may be necessary to compromise on technique treating the patient sitting up until symptoms improve. In the palliative setting it is usual to deliver doses of 20–30 Gy in 1–2 weeks but where the primary tumour is localized and radical treatment would otherwise be indicated a radical course of radiotherapy or chemoradiation should not be denied the patient.

Symptomatic relief following irradiation for SVCO is reported in 50–95 per cent of patients within the first two weeks of treatment. The survival of patients presenting with SVCO is determined by their underlying disease rather than the syndrome itself with the exception of the relatively rare instance of large airway obstruction or cerebral oedema when urgent treatment is required. There is data to suggest treatment has little effect upon the obstruction to blood flow in the SVC which persists in three-quarters of patients. This implies that the development of collaterals is most important in achieving the observed clinical improvement rather than the physical release of compression from the SVC.[39]

Lung collapse secondary to bronchial obstruction

Complete bronchial occlusion will lead to collapse of lung distal to that site. Obstruction may occur due to extrinsic compression by mediastinal lymph nodes secondary to bronchial or other epithelial cancers or lymphoma. A more common cause is intrinsic carcinoma of the bronchus. When obstruction occurs rapidly, acute dyspnoea with associated cough due to the secondary lung collapse will be the presenting symptom. Treatment is aimed at restoring the patency of the bronchus. For intrinsic tumours this may be best achieved by local treatment such as cryotherapy or laser therapy via a bronchoscope. For extrinsic tumours appropriate radiotherapy or in the case of chemosensitive tumours chemotherapy is indicated. As with SVCO, presentation with bronchial obstruction does not preclude radical treatment in those patients where that would be appropriate, for example, lymphoma, limited disease small-cell lung cancer, or localized non-small-cell lung cancer. Lymphoma and small-cell lung cancer will be best treated with primary chemotherapy. Localized non-small-cell lung cancer will benefit from radical doses of radiotherapy given either as an accelerated schedule such as CHART (continuous hyperfractionated accelerated radiotherapy) or within a chemoradiation programme.[40] For poor performance status patients and those with distant metastasis palliative radiotherapy is indicated. In these patients a single dose of 10 Gy has been shown to be as effective as more prolonged schedules in large randomized trials being equivalent in terms of both symptom control and survival, with a reduced risk of acute morbidity.[41,42] There is an intermediate group of good performance status patients with advanced tumours who may have a small but significant survival advantage from higher dose radiotherapy. A randomized trial comparing a schedule of 39 Gy in 13 fractions with 17 Gy in two fractions found a median improvement in survival of 54 days in favour of the higher dose and a 1-year survival of 36 per cent after 13 fractions compared to 31 per cent after two fractions, which was statistically significant.[43]

An alternative method of delivering radiotherapy in the bronchial lumen is using the technique of endobronchial irradiation. This may be particularly appropriate for patients relapsing after previous external beam irradiation. It is performed as a day case requiring fibreoptic bronchoscopy during which a fine plastic catheter is passed through the suction channel of the bronchoscope and under direct vision left to lie alongside the tumour-bearing region of bronchus, shown in Fig. 7. This area is irradiated using brachytherapy via a high dose rate afterloading machine which passes a radioactive source, iridium 192, along the catheter to dwell within the area bearing tumour where treatment is required. This technique can be combined with either laser therapy or cryotherapy to restore the lumen where there is complete bronchial obstruction. Endobronchial brachytherapy has now been compared in a randomized controlled trial with external beam radiotherapy.[44] No difference in survival or symptom control scores for cough, haemoptysis, shortness of breath, or hoarseness was seen but external beam radiotherapy was found to be superior for symptoms of chest pain, anorexia, tiredness, and nausea. In contrast less

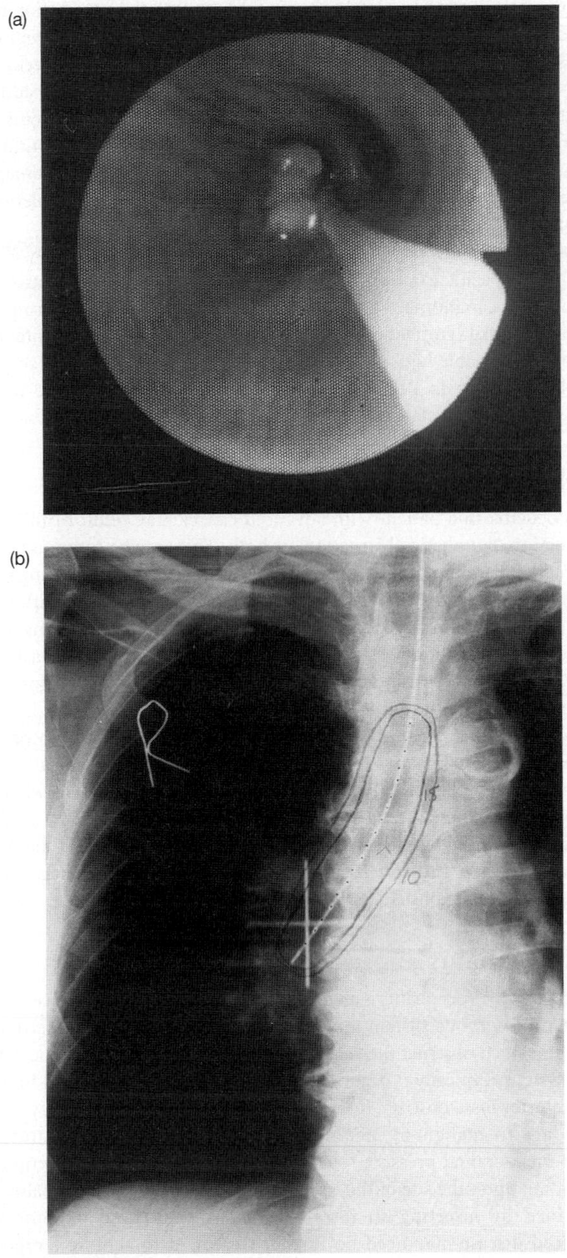

Fig. 7 Endobronchial brachytherapy demonstrating (a) passage of treatment catheter under direct vision at bronchoscopy and (b) subsequent radiograph to verify position prior to treatment.

dysphagia was found in patients receiving endobronchial brachytherapy. The standard dose is 15 Gy at 1 cm and the major advantage of brachytherapy is that it can be given as a single procedure often possible as an outpatient day case.

It is also important to recognize that chemotherapy has an increasing place in the management of inoperable lung cancer and many patients will benefit from both chemotherapy and radiotherapy in this setting.[40]

Dysphagia

Pain and difficulty in swallowing is a common symptom in patients with advanced cancer within the mediastinum. This may be due to intrinsic tumour arising from the wall of the oesophagus, hypopharynx (piriform fossa, post-cricoid region, and posterior pharyngeal wall), and stomach. Alternatively there may be extrinsic compression from mediastinal lymph nodes or tumours in the thymus, thyroid gland, or adjacent bronchus. Post mortem data shows that around 80 per cent of patients presenting with dysphagia have intrinsic tumour within the oesophagus and in one study multiple levels of obstruction were seen in almost a quarter of these patients.[45] Local symptoms may be alleviated with analgesia and anticholingergic drugs to reduce secretion while nutrition can be maintained by a fine bore nasogastric tube or percutaneous gastrostomy. Where there is widespread metastatic disease in poor performance patients more active treatment may be inappropriate and unsuccessful. In selected patients, however, with good performance status and limited disease surgical intervention with either radical resection or if not appropriate laser resection or stenting should be considered and has the advantage of rapid symptom relief if successful. There is, however, a significant morbidity and procedure-related mortality associated with these approaches and external beam irradiation should also be considered as a means of relieving dysphagia both for intrinsic tumour obstruction and for where there is extrinsic compression. A typical radiation field for this is shown in Fig. 8, the usual dose delivered to such an area being 20–30 Gy in 1–2 weeks with re-established swallowing reported in over 80 per cent of patients maintained for a mean duration of 6 months.[46] The disadvantage of radiotherapy in this setting, however, is that relief is not immediate, may take several weeks to occur, and there may initially be a period of enhanced dysphagia because of acute oesophagitis. This should be managed with simple topical medication such as soluble aspirin in a viscous muscilage.

There is some evidence that higher doses of radiotherapy delivering 50 Gy in 5 weeks or more may give a higher and more durable response rate and this should be considered for patients who have good performance status and limited disease, in whom a longer prognosis may be expected.[47] Where radical treatment using radiotherapy is used, chemoradiation has been shown to be superior to radiotherapy alone using concomitant cisplatin and 5FU during the course of radiotherapy.[1]

An alternative technique is endo-oesophageal radiotherapy which is similar to that of endobronchial brachytherapy. A tube is passed through the area of oesophageal constriction and a radioactive source passed along the tube shown in Fig. 8. A small diameter high dose afterloading source will pass readily through a fine catheter which itself fits inside a nasogastric tube and the procedure can be undertaken as an outpatient. The nasogastric tube is passed with local anaesthetic followed by X-ray verification of its position and delivery of the treatment which typically takes only a few minutes. Used alone sustained improvement in swallowing is reported in 54 per cent of patients.[48] This technique has also been used in an attempt to achieve high local doses in combination with external beam radiotherapy for radical treatment. Randomized trials suggest there may be an advantage to this approach and one series of 171 patients reports improved swallowing for three or more months in 90 per cent of patients with 56 per cent achieving complete restoration of normal swallowing.[49] The role of this approach within chemoradiation schedules is currently under investigation.

In addition to acute toxicity there may be later changes which develop within the life span of patients with advanced disease. Of these, oesophageal stricture is the most common late complication reported in 35 per cent of cases receiving combined external beam and brachytherapy.[49] In contrast, after short palliative doses of 20–30 Gy, stricture is unusual in the absence of tumour recurrence. After palliative doses of radiotherapy other more severe complications such as perforation and fistula are also unusual unless related to tumour progression.

Urinary tract obstruction

Urinary tract obstruction may arise because of obstruction of the renal pelvis, ureter, bladder, or urethra at any point. This may be due to both benign and malignant conditions, and the most satisfactory means of re-establishing renal drainage is a surgical procedure to bypass the obstruction using a nephrostomy, ureteric stents, or transurethral resection of an intrinsic urethral tumour.

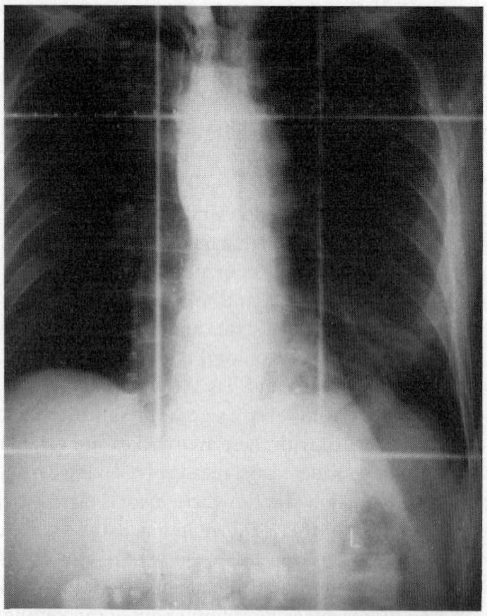

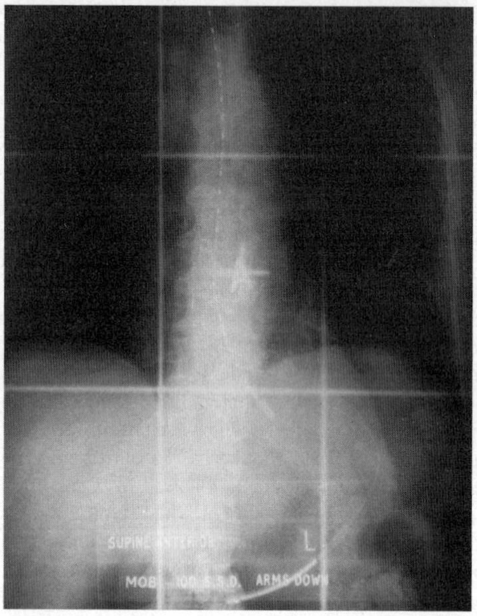

Fig. 8 Palliative radiation field for external beam treatment of oesophageal cancer causing dysphagia. (a) Retreatment in this patient was possible using the endoluminal technique (b) with the catheter containing dummy sources shown in position at the time of swallowing contrast material to demonstrate the site of obstruction.

The role of radiotherapy in relieving urinary tract infection is restricted to those patients in whom surgery is either technically not possible or otherwise inappropriate, but it is also important to consider radiotherapy following immediate relief of obstruction to treat the underlying cause. Common clinical scenarios include locally advanced cancer of the cervix, bladder, or prostate, or recurrence of colorectal tumour. It is important to ascertain the primary site of the tumour and in the setting of para-aortic lymphadenopathy obtain histological confirmation since in some instances, for example, lymphoma and germ cell tumour primary chemotherapy with curative intent will be appropriate. Radiotherapy for the underlying tumour should be based on the merits of the tumour and radical treatment not denied the patient. Conventionally primary tumours of the cervix, prostate, or bladder causing urinary tract obstruction in the absence of lymph node or distant metastasis will be treated with high radiation doses to achieve tumour shrinkage and re-establish urinary flow with the expectation that a proportion of patients will have long-term disease control or even cure. Doses of 50–55 Gy in 20 daily fractions or 60–65 Gy in 6–6$\frac{1}{2}$ weeks with intra-cavitary brachytherapy being given for cervical cancers in addition to external beam treatment will be necessary. One series of patients with carcinoma of the prostate presenting with urinary retention found that radiotherapy alone was sufficient to restore normal urinary drainage in 84 per cent with a mean time to catheter removal from completion of radiotherapy of 10 weeks.[(50)]

In some instances intra-luminal or interstitial radiotherapy may also be possible, a specific example being that of a sub-urethral metastasis from endometrial carcinoma. This is a recognized pattern of spread from submucosal vaginal lymphatic invasion to the urethra meatus. An interstitial implant will enable high dose local treatment to be delivered. Techniques are also available to deliver intra-luminal brachytherapy to the urethra where recurrent prostate cancer or bladder base tumours are troublesome.

Limb oedema

Limb oedema in a patient with advanced cancer may result from venous obstruction, lymphatic obstruction, or both. This may be compounded by general debility, immobility, and poor nutrition with accompanying hypoalbuminaemia. In a proportion of patients, particularly those with upper limb oedema due to carcinoma of the breast, post-radiation changes may have caused lymphatic obstruction; ipsilateral arm oedema is seen in over 30 per cent of patients undergoing both axillary surgery and radiotherapy to the axilla for breast cancer.

Local radiotherapy may be of value in the treatment of limb oedema where enlarged malignant axillary, inguinal, or pelvic nodes are the cause of obstruction. The best results are obtained with early treatment when the circulatory obstruction can be reversed. Relatively low doses of 20–30 Gy in 1–2 weeks are used taking care to preserve, wherever possible, a channel of unirradiated skin and soft tissue through which lymph drainage can be maintained despite post-radiation changes.

Hydrocephalus

Obstructive hydrocephalus is an uncommon manifestation of cancer within the central nervous system and may result from primary or secondary tumours which obstruct the cerebrospinal fluid at any point in the ventricular system. Typically it occurs when tumours of either the mid brain or the posterior fossa obstruct the aqueduct or fourth ventricle; it may also be secondary to malignant meningitis. Patients present with features of raised intra-cranial pressure together with focal neurological symptoms, depending upon the site of the tumour. Rapid relief of hydrocephalus may be gained by inserting an intra-ventricular shunt and patients with advanced disease may need no further treatment to achieve temporary symptom control. Where surgery is not feasible or where there are multiple intra-cerebral lesions palliative radiotherapy should be given in the same way as discussed for the management of brain metastasis in the previous section.

Advanced primary central nervous system tumours of the mid brain and posterior fossa are also treated by radiotherapy usually delivering doses of 50–55 Gy given over 6–7 weeks.

Haemorrhage

Haemoptysis

Haemoptysis is a common symptom of bronchial carcinoma occurring in around 50 per cent of patients at presentation. It may also accompany pulmonary metastasis and is distressing for the patient although rarely of haemodynamic significance. It is life-threatening only when a major vein or bronchial artery is eroded and then usually beyond all treatment. Haemoptysis is otherwise an indication for local radiotherapy and control rates of up to 80 per cent are reported with palliative doses using either external beam treatment or endobronchial brachytherapy as discussed above. The randomized trials show that a single dose of 10 Gy external beam is as effective as other more prolonged schedules with less acute morbidity.(41)

It is important to remember that haemoptysis is a presenting symptom of bronchial carcinoma and is not in itself a contra-indication to radical treatment in patients having localized disease which can be radically resected or encompassed in a high dose radiation volume. Screening for this possibility should always occur prior to embarking upon palliative irradiation. Patients with non-small-cell lung cancer having stage I or II disease, that is, without involvement of mediastinal lymph nodes, should all be considered for surgery or high dose radiotherapy using either accelerated schedules such as CHART or chemoradiation.(40) Patients with good performance status and stage III disease, that is mediastinal node involvement, may also in selected cases benefit from high dose radiotherapy. Patients with small-cell lung cancer will usually be selected for primary chemotherapy but in the face of advanced extensive disease palliative radiotherapy for symptoms such as haemoptysis is highly effective using the same techniques as those used for non-small-cell lung cancer.

The management of haemoptysis due to pulmonary metastasis is more difficult. Local irradiation is only of value where a specific site of haemorrhage can be identified or where there is only a solitary metastasis. Bronchoscopic confirmation of the origin of bleeding is therefore needed where there are multiple metastasis; arbitrary irradiation of the particular area of metastatic disease is not to be recommended although low dose whole lung irradiation delivering a dose of 25 Gy in 20 fractions over 4 weeks has been used in the past for widespread metastasis from radiosensitive tumours such as Ewing's sarcoma or Wilms' tumour. In general, however, chemotherapy or hormone therapy is the preferred treatment in this setting and only when this has failed should palliative irradiation be explored.

There is no proven advantage in terms of survival for treating the asymptomatic patient with inoperable lung cancer but some evidence suggests that tumours greater than 10 cm in diameter, whether primary or metastatic, carry a significant risk of haemorrhage and it has been suggested that such lesions should receive prophylactic treatment.

Haematuria

Haematuria may be related to bleeding from primary or metastatic disease at any site along the urinary tract from the renal pelvis to the urethra. Thus before embarking upon palliative treatment careful localization of the site of bleeding, including intravenous urography, CT scanning, or cystoscopy is vital. Haematuria in patients with advanced cancer is usually caused by bleeding from a local bladder tumour which may be primary or secondary to local infiltration of an advanced rectal or uterine carcinoma. Other common causes are advanced renal cell carcinoma and urethral infiltration by carcinoma of the prostate. Other causes that may be relevant to the cancer patient are infective cystitis, chemical cystitis associated with certain chemotherapy agents such as cyclophosphamide or ifosfamide, bladder telangiectasia as a late change following high dose radiotherapy to the bladder or as a rare manifestation of thrombocytopenia, or a blood coagulation defect.

The main role of radiotherapy in this setting is to achieve haemostasis in patients with inoperable or recurrent tumours. Haematuria may settle with conservative measures such as bladder irrigation, administration of antifibrinolytic drugs such as tranexamic acid, and cystoscopic diathermy. Where this fails modest doses of irradiation delivered to a small volume encompassing the site of haemorrhage will often be successful.

In advanced muscle invasive bladder cancer a large randomized trial comparing 35 Gy in 10 fractions with 21 Gy given in three fractions on alternate days over 1 week has shown equivalent symptomatic improvement of bladder related symptoms with no excess toxicity from the shorter 21 Gy schedule.(51) Haematuria was found to be improved in 50 per cent of patients at completion of treatment and in 63 per cent at 3 months after treatment. Careful localization of bladder tumours is important using a cystogram or CT scan. In poor performance status patients single doses of 8–10 Gy may be equally effective and 17 Gy in two fractions has also been reported as a useful schedule in this setting with a 59 per cent response rate for haematuria.(52)

As with other sites haematuria may be the presentation of a potentially curable primary bladder or prostatic carcinoma and full assessment of the patient both in terms of their tumour and general status is important before deciding upon palliative treatment. For advanced tumours of the bladder radical radiotherapy is appropriate delivering doses of 55 Gy in 4 weeks or 60–65 Gy in $6–6\frac{1}{2}$ weeks. Radical radiotherapy to the prostate gland will deliver doses of 65–70 Gy in $6\frac{1}{2}–7$ weeks with some centres now using dose escalation to even higher doses. Again, however, palliative schedules using single doses or 21 Gy in three fractions to the prostate for local symptoms is effective in the patient where palliation is the aim of treatment.

Haematuria due to locally advanced inoperable renal carcinoma may also benefit from local irradiation where a nephrectomy is not possible. The tolerance of the normal kidney to radiation is low, and even with modest palliative doses it is to be expected that the kidney bearing the tumour will be damaged with loss of function. It is therefore important to ensure that renal function from the contra-lateral kidney is normal before treatment. Doses of 10 Gy as a single dose, 21 Gy in three fractions over 1 week, or 20–30 Gy over 1–2 weeks have all been used in this setting; there is little published data on the expected response rate.

Treatment of the bladder or prostate may result in diarrhoea because of the inevitable inclusion of some of the rectum in the treatment volume. In the MRC randomized trial of palliative radiotherapy in bladder cancer there was a 5 per cent incidence of mild diarrhoea not requiring medication and a 2 per cent incidence of moderate diarrhoea requiring medication for control.(51) Treatment of the kidney may include stomach or small bowel resulting in nausea, vomiting, and diarrhoea. Careful explanation and reassurance about these side effects together with ready availability of anti-diarrhoeal agents and anti-emetics is an important part of management.

Uterine and vaginal bleeding

Tumours of the uterus, including endometrial and cervical cancer and uterine sarcomas, frequently present with abnormal vaginal bleeding. This is rarely excessive and readily managed conservatively before embarking upon definitive treatment. Occasionally major haemorrhage may be the presenting feature of a uterine tumour requiring urgent resuscitation and vaginal packing before urgent treatment is instigated. Haemorrhage in patients with advanced and metastatic cancer may be due to recurrent or locally advanced tumours of the cervix or uterus, local infiltration from advanced cancers of the bladder or rectum, or metastatic mucosal deposits along the vaginal wall typical of the pattern of spread from endometrial cancer. Haemorrhagic mucosal deposits are also a particular feature of vulval or vaginal melanoma.

Radiotherapy is of value in obtaining definitive control of bleeding using either external beam irradiation or intra-cavitary treatment as appropriate. Where vaginal bleeding represents the primary presentation of advanced cervical cancer, radical radiotherapy is often appropriate delivering external beam treatment to a dose of around 50 Gy in 5 weeks followed by intra-cavitary treatment to the cervix and para-cervical tissues. Similarly where locally advanced bladder, rectal, or uterine tumours are the cause and previous radiotherapy has not been given palliative pelvic doses are effective using a schedule of 21 Gy in three fractions or 20–30 Gy over 1–2 weeks. Where previous radiotherapy has been given to the pelvis further low doses can often be considered and these can be effective in obtaining haemostasis although there may be risks of additional late bowel damage associated with this. These decisions must be balanced between the severity of symptoms and the anticipated life expectancy of the patient. Where thought appropriate single doses of 8 Gy or short courses of up to 20 Gy in five fractions are effective.

Where bleeding is from small volume disease, such as nodules of the vaginal vault or along the vaginal mucosa, intra-cavitary treatment may be

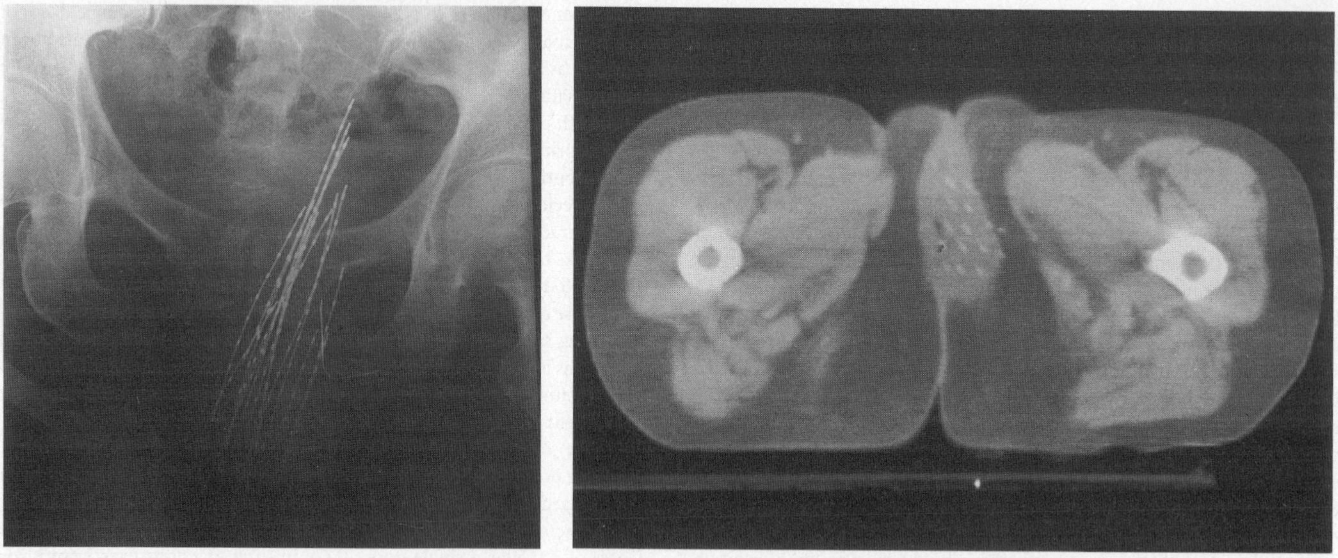

Fig. 9 X-ray and CT planning scans demonstrating positions of brachytherapy catheters containing dummy sources after implantation of a larger symptomatic fungating vulval tumour. After verification and calculation of the radioactive loadings required, treatment is given by afterloading using an iridium source passed down the catheters shown here.

preferable. Vaginal sources in the form of either ovoids or a vaginal tube can be introduced directly into the vagina and used to carry a radiation source in the form of caesium or iridium which whilst in position within the applicator will deliver local radiation to its surface along the vaginal wall. The use of intra-cavitary brachytherapy in this way enables a high surface dose to be given to the mucosa but with a rapid fall off in dose away from the source so that critical structures such as bladder and rectum are relatively spared from the radiation dose. This may be of value in patients who have previously received radiotherapy to the pelvis but is also highly effective in otherwise untreated patients. This form of treatment does, however, have limitations in being able to treat only a depth of 5–10 mm. For larger recurrent tumours around the vulva and vaginal region and in the peri-urethral tissues an interstitial implant may be necessary. Whilst more demanding for the patient requiring a general anaesthetic and either radioactive needles or afterloading radioactive tubes to be placed through the tumour area, as shown in Fig. 9, it enables high dose treatment to be delivered locally within the tumour even where previous radiotherapy has been given to the pelvis and may provide highly effective palliation from an otherwise very difficult situation of progressive tumour in the vulvo-vaginal tissues.

Gastrointestinal haemorrhage

Symptomatic gastrointestinal haemorrhage may arise from either the upper or lower gastrointestinal tract resulting in haematemesis, melaena, or rectal bleeding. The underlying tumour may be a primary neoplasm arising within the gastrointestinal tract, most commonly from the stomach, large bowel, or rectum, or as a result of direct invasion by locally advanced tumour in adjacent structures such as the uterus, bladder, or prostate invading the rectum. Blood-borne metastasis to the bowel are rare but metastatic malignant melanoma is a recognized cause of haemorrhagic deposits within the small bowel wall and Kaposi's sarcoma, seen with HIV infection, may cause a similar problem.

As in other sites local radiotherapy in modest doses to a site of haemorrhage within the bowel will often achieve effective and durable control of bleeding. In the lower bowel tumours in the rectum and colon are usually readily identified and localized within a treatment volume. Treatment of the stomach may be more difficult both because it can be a relatively mobile structure and also because the sensitivity of surrounding tissues, in particular liver, small bowel, and kidneys, limits tolerance and the dose that can be delivered safely. Localization of tumours within the small bowel can be difficult because of its mobility and radiation to the stomach and small bowel can have considerable associated morbidity with nausea, vomiting, and diarrhoea.

The most common scenario will be recurrent tumours of the rectum or sigmoid colon, particularly at the site of an anastomosis where a primary has been previously resected. External beam radiotherapy for bleeding from recurrent colorectal cancer has been reported to achieve an overall response rate of 85 per cent with complete control of bleeding in 63 per cent of patients following a dose of 30–35 Gy in 10 fractions over 2 weeks.[53] An alternative approach is again to use intra-luminal brachytherapy similar to the technique used for vaginal bleeding, passing a tube into the rectum through which a radioactive source can be placed to deliver a high surface dose to the rectal mucosa and associated tumour area. This approach has the advantage of being delivered as a single outpatient procedure when high dose rate afterloading brachytherapy is used, the actual technique being little different to a sigmoidoscopic examination. It is, however, limited to accessible tumours in the lower sigmoid colon, rectum, and anal canal.

Chest wall and other skin lesions

Locoregional recurrence remains a significant problem in patients with breast cancer occurring in 7–10 per cent of those with early disease and up to 40 per cent of those presenting with advanced local disease. Post-operative irradiation at the time of primary treatment significantly reduces the likelihood of locoregional relapse but despite this a number of patients with recurrent metastatic breast cancer will also have progressive loco-regional tumour on the chest wall which will fungate and bleed.

Where total mastectomy is possible this may be the best procedure to surgically clear recurrent tumour on the chest wall. In many cases, however, the tumour will be fixed and inoperable with multiple satellite nodules across the chest, often involving the contra-lateral breast or extending laterally across the mid axillary line on to the back. In general, chemotherapy will be the most appropriate initial treatment but often such disease will recur and not remain chemosensitive. Where no previous radiotherapy has been given and there is no evidence of distant metastasis, high dose local irradiation may be appropriate delivering doses of up to 60 Gy in 6 weeks. In patients with distant metastasis and a poor prognosis shorter schedules of 10 Gy in one fraction or 20–30 Gy in 1–2 weeks may be more appropriate. Often it is not possible to encompass the entire extent of clinically detectable disease and in these circumstances those causing greatest symptoms may be targeted.

Where there has been recurrence despite previous irradiation further radiotherapy may be possible to a limited area of symptomatic tumour since the risks of skin necrosis are negligible compared with the effects of progressive fungating tumour within the skin. Superficial X-ray treatment or low energy electrons to fungating or bleeding chest wall nodules is often highly effective and a single dose of 8–10 Gy or a longer course delivering 20–30 Gy over 1–2 weeks is commonly used. More complex techniques using a surface mould in which radioactive sources are placed over the involved area or interstitial brachytherapy in which large tumour masses are implanted with radioactive needles or afterloading applicator tubes can also be considered.

Skin nodules may also be a manifestation of primary tumours in other sites and once established may fungate and bleed. These will, by definition, reflect blood-borne metastasis and therefore radical treatment is usually inappropriate but local treatment to symptomatic nodules is of value. Techniques and doses similar to those discussed above for recurrent breast cancer will be employed.

Primary skin tumours may also present with locally advanced inoperable disease. Bleeding and fungation are likely to become major problems in the management of these patients and local radiotherapy is of value in their control. In the absence of metastasis, and in the case of basal cell carcinoma which does not metastasize, high radical doses may be considered using appropriate techniques with either electrons of appropriate energy to treat to the depth of the tumour or tangential X-ray beams to cover the tumour volume. Doses of 60 Gy in 6 weeks or equivalent are given to large tumours where this is appropriate in the light of the patient's general performance status. For patients with poor performance status or metastatic disease shorter courses delivering doses of 20–30 Gy in 1–2 weeks may be considered and will be effective in achieving growth delay and stopping haemorrhage. Melanoma characteristically presents with haemorrhagic tumours and may in more advanced cases result in multiple skin nodules. Local radiotherapy delivering higher doses of 30 Gy in five to six fractions treating twice weekly is often used with good effect.[54]

Other local tumour effects

Fungation

Fungation of a superficial tumour mass is a distressing feature of locally advanced cancer. It is seen most commonly in chest wall recurrence after breast carcinoma and with metastatic lymph nodes in the neck or groin. Local irradiation is most valuable in the prevention of fungation at a time when the overlying skin is intact. A palliative course of treatment delivering 20–30 Gy in 1–2 weeks will usually delay growth within a tumour mass sufficient to prevent fungation. In certain instances where local tumour is the sole manifestation of malignancy, higher doses may be appropriate. The most common scenario of this type is the presence of a cervical lymph node containing squamous carcinoma from the head and neck region or inguinal lymph nodes with squamous carcinoma from the perineal region. Occasionally large lymph nodes may present without an obvious underlying primary tumour. Radical radiotherapy to malignant nodes from an unknown primary in the neck can achieve long-term control in this setting with overall 5 year survival figures of 20–30 per cent in selected series.[55]

Once fungation has occurred successful treatment is more difficult but alongside nursing care and administration of analgesics and antibiotics, local irradiation may still be of value in reducing the underlying tumour bulk, arresting surface haemorrhage, and drying the surface as the process of healing is allowed to commence. This will make nursing care simpler and relieve the patient from the distress of local haemorrhage.

Kaposi's sarcoma

Kaposi's sarcoma is now most commonly seen as a feature of HIV infection and is the most common AIDS-related malignancy. It may also be seen in sporadic cases when it typically presents in the skin of the lower limbs in European men. Multiple skin lesions are usual but extracutaneous disease is also common affecting the oral cavity and gastrointestinal tract. The characteristic purplish raised plaques may bleed and ulcerate. In contrast to other soft tissue sarcomas Kaposi's is markedly radiosensitive and small doses of irradiation will result in complete regression of lesions in up to 70 per cent of patients.[56] There is good evidence that single doses are as effective as more prolonged schedules and superficial irradiation delivering 8 Gy to symptomatic sites is recommended.

Liver metastases

In most instances the presence of liver metastasis heralds the terminal phases of advanced cancer. Clinical symptoms will include anorexia, malaise, and weight loss alongside local pain and discomfort from hepatic enlargement and stretching of the liver capsule. Pain may be acute where there is rapid expansion of the liver or haemorrhage into a metastasis. Local radiotherapy may be of value particularly in those patients with good performance status and normal bilirubin and where the primary site is other than stomach or pancreas.[57] If the primary tumour is chemosensitive this is usually the first line of approach and where there are solitary metastases, resection should be considered. For other patients, however, palliative low dose radiotherapy may provide valuable relief of symptoms. Two prospective randomized trials have demonstrated relief of hepatic pain in 80 per cent of patients with complete relief in 55 per cent and improvements in nausea, vomiting, fever, and night sweats in 45 per cent.[57,58]

The liver has limited tolerance to radiation and so hepatic radiotherapy may be associated with side effects and when doses greater than 30 Gy are given there is a risk of inducing radiation hepatitis. Toxicity is related not only to dose but also the volume of liver included in the treatment volume and unless there is diffuse infiltration of the entire organ, uninvolved liver should be excluded from the radiation volume. With doses of 30 Gy delivered in 2–3 weeks relatively mild self-limiting toxicity is reported with lethargy and nausea being the predominant symptoms.

Splenomegaly

Symptomatic splenomegaly from malignant disease is usually associated with haematological malignancies, in particular, chronic granulocytic leukaemia and certain types of non-Hodgkin's lymphoma. It is also a feature of myelodysplasia. Surgical removal of the spleen is the preferred management but in advanced disease or in patients with poor performance status this may not be appropriate and local irradiation is an effective means of palliation. Symptoms due to local bulk (causing pain and discomfort) and hypersplenism (causing consumption of red cells and platelets) benefit from treatment. Pain relief is reported in over 90 per cent of patients and durable size reduction in 60 per cent.[59] The spleen containing lymphoma or leukaemia is extremely sensitive to radiation and high doses should be avoided as these may precipitate pancytopenia and rapid tumour lysis. Single doses of 1 Gy or less delivered at weekly intervals are recommended to a total dose of between 3 and 10 Gy with weekly assessment before each treatment to evaluate the effect on the peripheral blood count and the degree of splenic shrinkage. Even at these low doses precautions should be taken against the effects of rapid tumour lysis ensuring the patient is well hydrated and giving allopurinol to prevent hyperuricaemia.

Hypercalaemia

Hypercalaemia complicates the clinical course of around 10 per cent of all patients with malignant disease, particularly those with common epithelial tumours such as breast and lung cancer. Whilst it frequently occurs in patients with widespread metastatic disease no clear correlation with the extent of bone metastasis is usually demonstrated and it is thought that many cases arise due to the production of chemical agents promoting osteoclastic reabsorption of bone, in particular parathyroid hormone-related protein. The initial management of a patient with hypercalcaemia secondary to advanced cancer includes rehydration, diuresis, and bisphosphonates. However, whilst the initial reduction of serum calcium is usually achieved, rebound hypercalcaemia frequently follows, requiring further intensive treatment, and often a refractory phase is entered after several episodes. Where a potential source of the chemical agent can be identified, such as locally advanced endobronchial carcinoma, local irradiation to reduce its production and enable stabilization of blood calcium levels may be of value. Standard palliative doses are usually delivered as described above and whilst anecdotally a valuable treatment in this setting no published data is available for accurate estimates of response.

Paraneoplastic phenomena

Certain conditions may be seen in patients with malignancy which are not directly related to the process of tumour growth, invasion and metastasis but are nonetheless associated with the malignant process. Their severity often mirrors the extent of the associated tumour.

The most common association is with primary carcinoma of the bronchus when neoplastic symptoms arise in around 2 per cent of patients and include neuropathies, myopathies, myasthenia (the Eaton–Lambert syndrome), and cutaneous manifestations such as acanthosis nigricans, erythema gyratum, or hairy man syndrome. It is probable that these symptoms reflect secretion of a humeral agent possibly an auto-antibody. The paraendocrine syndromes are associated with ectopic production of ACTH, ADH, human chorionic gonadotrophin, 5 hydroxytryptamine, or thyroid stimulating hormone, as well as those mentioned above in the context of hypercalcaemia. Where there is an identifiable local tumour and where surgical excision is not possible or appropriate, local irradiation may result in improvement and resolution of the paraneoplastic symptoms as the tumour regresses. In advanced disease only palliative doses may be appropriate but in localized disease the presence of a paraneoplastic syndrome should not exclude consideration of radical treatment. As with hypercalcaemia there is no good data on precise response rates to treatment in this setting.

Conclusion

Local irradiation is a valuable treatment for palliation of local symptoms with consistently high response rates in the relief and control of bone pain, neurological symptoms, obstructive symptoms, and haemorrhage. Short treatments and simple techniques can minimize disruption and acute morbidity for the patient with advanced cancer whilst enabling control of symptoms.

References

1. **Herskovic, A.** et al. (1992). Combined chemotherapy and radiotherapy compared with radiotherapy alone in patients with cancer of the esophagus. *New England Journal of Medicine* **24**, 1593–8.
2. **Ryan, D.P., Compton, C.C., and Mayer, R.J.** (2000). Carcinoma of the anal canal. *New England Journal of Medicine* **342**, 792–800.
3. **Thomas, G.M.** (1999). Improved treatment for cervical cancer—concurrent chemotherapy and radiotherapy. *New England Journal of Medicine* **340**, 1198–9.
4. **Komakil, R.** et al. (2000). Sequential vs. concurrent and radiation therapy for inoperable non-small cell lung cancer (NSCLC): analysis of failures in a Phase III Study (RTOG 9410). *International Journal of Radiation Oncology Biology Physics* **48** (Suppl.), 5.
5. **Munro, A.J.** (1995). An overview of randomised controlled trials of adjuvant chemotherapy in head and neck cancer. *British Journal of Cancer* **71**, 83–91.
6. **Bone Pain Trial Working Party** (1999). 8 Gy single fraction radiotherapy for the treatment of metastatic skeletal pain: randomised comparison with a multifraction schedule over 12 months of patient follow-up. *Radiotherapy and Oncology* **52**, 111–21.
7. **Salazar, O.M.** et al. (2001). Fractionated half-body irradiation (HBI) for the rapid palliation of widespread, symptomatic, metastatic bone disease: a randomized phase III trial of the International Atomic Energy Agency (IAEA). *International Journal of Radiation Oncology Biology Physics* **50**, 765–75.
8. **Salazar, O.M.** et al. (1986). Single dose hemibody irradiation in palliation of multiple bone metastases from solid tumours. *Cancer* **58**, 29–36.
9. **Mithal, N., Needham, P.R., and Hoskin, P.J.** (1994). Retreatment with radiotherapy for painful bone metastases. *International Journal of Radiation Oncology Biology Physics* **29**, 1011–14.
10. **Brown, A.P.** et al. (1984). Radioiodine treatment of metastatic thyroid carcinoma: The Royal Marsden Hospital experience. *British Journal of Radiology* **57**, 323–7.
11. **Hoskin, P.J.** (1994). Strontium. In *Therapeutic Drugs* (Suppl. 2) (ed. C. Dollery), pp. 223–7. Edinburgh: Churchill Livingstone.
12. **Serafini, A.N.** et al. (1998). Palliation of pain associated with metastatic bone cancer using Samarium-153 Lexidronam: a double-blind placebo-controlled clinical trial. *Journal of Clinical Oncology* **16**, 1574–81.
13. **Windsor, P.M.** (2001). Predictors of response to strontium-89 (Metastron) in skeletal metastases from prostate cancer. *Clinical Oncology* **13**, 219–27.
14. **Hoskin, P.J., Stratford, M.R.I., and Folkes, L.K.** (2000). Effect of local radiotherapy for bone pain on urinary markers of osteoclast activity. *Lancet* **355**, 1428–9.
15. **Poulter, C.** et al. (1992). A phase III study of whether the addition of single dose hemibody irradiation to standard fractionated local field irradiation is more effective than local field irradiation alone in the treatment of symptomatic osseous metastases. *International Journal of Radiation Oncology Biology Physics* **23**, 74–8.
16. **Porter** et al. (1993). Results of a randomised Phase III trial to evaluate the efficacy of strontium-89 adjuvant to local field external beam irradiation in the management of endocrine-resistant metastatic prostate cancer. *International Journal of Radiation Oncology Biology Physics* **25**, 805–13.
17. **Townsend, P.W.** et al. (1995). Role of postoperative radiation therapy after stabilization of fractures caused by metastatic disease. *International Journal of Radiation Oncology Biology Physics* **31**, 43–9.
18. **Pigott, K., Baddeley, H., and Maher, E.J.** (1994). Pattern of disease in spinal cord compression on MRI scan and implications for treatment. *Clinical Oncology* **6**, 7–10.
19. **Shaw, M.D.M., Rose, J.E., and Patterson, A.** (1980). Metastatic extradural malignancy of the spine. *Acta Neurochirurgica* **52**, 113–20.
20. **Findlay, G.F.G.** (1988). The role of needle biopsy in the management of cervical metastases. *British Journal of Neurosurgery* **2**, 479–84.
21. **Findlay, G.F.G.** (1984). Adverse effects of the management of malignant spinal cord compression. *Journal of Neurology, Neurosurgery and Psychiatry* **47**, 761–8.
22. **Siegal, T. and Siegal, T.** (1985). Surgical decompression of anterior and posterior malignant epidural tumours compressing the spinal cord: a prospective study. *Neurosurgery* **17**, 424–32.
23. **Moore, A.J. and Uttley, D.** (1989). Anterior decompression and stabilisation of the spine in malignant disease. *Neurosurgery* **24**, 713–17.
24. **Goldman, J.M.** et al. (1989). Spinal cord compression in small cell lung cancer: a retrospective study of 610 patients. *British Journal of Cancer* **59**, 591–3.
25. **Borgelt, B.** et al. (1982). The palliation of brain metastases: final results of the first two studies by the Radiation Therapy Oncology Group. *International Journal of Radiation Oncology Biology Physics* **6**, 1–9.
26. **Hoskin, P.J. and Brada, M. (on behalf of the participants of the Second Workshop on Palliative Radiotherapy and Symptom Control, London)** (2000). *Clinical Oncology* **13**, 91–4.
27. **Priestman, T.J.** et al. (1996). Final results of the Royal College of Radiologists' trial comparing two different radiotherapy schedules in the treatment of cerebral metastases. *Clinical Oncology* **8**, 308–15.
28. **Bleehan, N.** et al. (1991). A Medical Research Council trial of two radiotherapy doses in the treatment of grades 3 and 4 astrocytoma. *British Journal of Cancer* **64**, 769–74.

29. **Thomas, R.** et al. (1994). Hypofractionated radiotherapy as a palliative treatment in poor prognosis patients with high grade glioma. *Radiotherapy and Oncology* **33**, 113–16.
30. **Wasserstrom, W.R., Glass, J.P., and Posner, J.B.** (1982). Diagnosis and treatment of leptomeningeal metastases from solid tumours. *Cancer* **49**, 759–72.
31. **Vikram, B. and Chu, F.** (1979). Radiation therapy to metastases to the base of the skull. *Radiology* **130**, 465–8.
32. **Hall, S., Buzdar, A., and Blumenschein, G.** (1983). Cranial nerve palsies in metastatic breast cancer due to osseous metastases without intercranial involvement. *Cancer* **52**, 180–4.
33. **Russi, E.G.** et al. Palliative radiotherapy in lumbosacral carcinomatous neuropathy. *Radiotherapy and Oncology* **26**, 172–3.
34. **James, R.D.** et al. Prognostic factors in locally recurrent rectal carcinoma treated by radiotherapy. *British Journal of Surgery* **70**, 469–72.
35. **Ampil, F.L.** (1985). Radiotherapy for carcinomatous brachial plexus plexopathy. *Cancer* **56**, 2185–8.
36. **Dobrowsky, W.** (1988). Treatment of choroidal metastases. *British Journal of Radiology* **61**, 140–2.
37. **Laperriere, N.J.** et al. (1997). Primary lymphoma of brain: results of management of a modern cohort with radiation therapy. *Radiotherapy and Oncology* **43**, 247–52.
38. **Denton, A.S. and Spittle, M.F.** (1995). Leukaemia and lymphoma. *Current Medical Literature, The Royal Society of Medicine* **3**, 35–41.
39. **Ahman, F.R.** (1984). A reassessment of the clinical implications of the superior vena caval syndrome. *Journal of Clinical Oncology* **2**, 961–8.
40. **Timothy, A.R.** et al. (2001). Radiotherapy for inoperable lung cancer. *Clinical Oncology* **13**, 86–7.
41. **MRC Lung Cancer Working Party** (1991). Inoperable non-small cell lung cancer (NSCLC): a Medical Research Council randomised trial of palliative radiotherapy with two fractions or ten fractions. *British Journal of Cancer* **63**, 265–70.
42. **MRC Lung Cancer Working Party** (1992). A Medical Research Council (MRC) randomised trial of palliative radiotherapy with two fractions or a single fraction in patients with inoperable non-small cell lung cancer (NSCLC) and poor performance status. *British Journal of Cancer* **65**, 934–41.
43. **MRC Lung Cancer Working Party** (1996). Randomized trial of palliative two-fraction versus more intensive 13-fraction radiotherapy for patients with inoperable non-small cell lung cancer and good performance status. *Clinical Oncology* **8**, 167–75.
44. **Stout, R.** et al. (2000). Clinical and quality of life outcomes in the first United Kingdom randomized trial of endobronchial brachytherapy (intraluminal radiotherapy) versus external beam radiotherapy in the palliative treatment of inoperable non-small cell lung cancer. *Radiotherapy and Oncology* **56**, 323–7.
45. **Sykes, N.P., Baines, M., and Carter, R.L.** (1998). Clinical and pathological study of dysphagia conservatively managed in patients with advanced malignant disease. *Lancet* **ii**, 726–8.
46. **Wara, M.** et al. (1976). Palliation for carcinoma of the oesophagus. *Radiology* **121**, 717–20.
47. **Leslie, M.D.** et al. (1992). The role of radiotherapy in carcinoma of the thoracic oesophagus: an audit of the Mount Vernon experience 1980–1989. *Clinical Oncology* **4**, 114–18.
48. **Brewster, A.E.** et al. (1995). Intraluminal brachytherapy using the highdose rate microselectron in the palliation of carcinoma of the oesophagus. *Clinical Oncology* **7**, 102–5.
49. **Flores, A.D.** et al. (1990). The impact of new radiotherapy modalities in the surgical management of cancer of the oesophagus and cardia. In *Brachytherapy HDR and LDR* (ed. A.A. Martinez, C.G. Orton, and R.F. Mould), pp. 27–43. Columbia: Nucletron.
50. **Wells, P.** et al. (1996). The effect of radiotherapy on urethral obstruction from carcinoma of the prostate. *British Journal of Urology* **78**, 752–5.
51. **Duchesne, G.M.** et al. (2000). A randomized trial of hypofractionated schedules of palliative radiotherapy in the management of bladder carcinoma: results of Medical Research Council Trial BA09. *International Journal of Radiation Oncology Biology Physics* **47**, 379–88.
52. **Srinivasan, V., Brown, C.H., and Turner, A.G.** (1994). A comparison of two radiotherapy regimes for the treatment of symptoms from advanced bladder cancer. *Clinical Oncology* **6**, 11–13.
53. **Taylor, R.E., Kerr, G.R., and Arnott, S.J.** (1987). External beam radiotherapy for rectal adenocarcinoma. *British Journal of Surgery* **74**, 455–9.
54. **Overgaard, J.** (1986). The role of radiotherapy in recurrent and metastatic malignant melanoma: a clinical radiobiological study. *International Journal of Radiation Oncology Biology Physics* **12**, 867–72.
55. **Fletcher, G.H.** (1990). Controversial views in the management of cervical metastases. *International Journal of Radiation Oncology Biology Physics* **19**, 1101–2.
56. **Munro, A.J. and Stewart, J.S.W.** (1989). Aids: incidence and management of malignant disease. *Radiotherapy and Oncology* **14**, 121–31.
57. **Leibel, S.A.** et al. (1987). A comparison of misonidazole sensitised radiation therapy to radiation therapy alone for the palliation of hepatic metastases: results of a Radiation Therapy Oncology Group randomised study. *International Journal of Radiation Oncology Biology Physics* **13**, 1057–64.
58. **Borgelt, B.B.** et al. (1981). The palliation of hepatic metastases: results of the Radiation Therapy Oncology Group pilot study. *International Journal of Radiation Oncology Biology Physics* **7**, 587–91.
59. **Paulino, A.C. and Reddy, S.P.** (1996). Splenic irradiation in the palliation of patients with lymphoproliferative and myeloproliferative disorders. *American Journal of Hospice and Palliative Care* **13**, 32–5.

8.1.3 Surgical palliation

Richard Sainsbury, Carolynne Vaizey, Ugo Pastorino, Timothy Mould, and Mark Emberton

General introduction

The incidence of cancer continues to rise as the population increases and ages. The mortality from cancer has shown a mixed picture with some instances where the mortality has decreased (female breast cancer in the white population) and others where it has remained depressingly constant such as in carcinoma of the pancreas. What has changed is the way that patients with cancer are cared for. Earlier diagnosis, multidisciplinary team management, the use of appropriate therapies, and the avoidance of treatments unlikely to prove successful, coupled with the involvement of specialist nurses and the palliative care team have all contributed to a form of care that was the exception a decade ago.

The role of the surgeon has changed since this chapter was first written. Surgical specialization is a double-edged sword. There are undoubted benefits to the patient with an established diagnosis when looked after by a surgical expert but for the patient who has yet to achieve a diagnosis the demise of an experienced general surgeon may lead to delay and unnecessary investigations.

The surgeon used to have a key role in the diagnostic process but the interventional radiologist who will undertake a guided percutaneous biopsy increasingly supplants him. The radiologist may also be involved in the process of palliation, again by diagnosis of recurrence, or in the therapeutic arena as in the placement of stents or the percutaneous blocks of various nervous plexii.

Is all lost for the surgeon? Not yet. The enclosed contributions make clear that the judicious use of surgery has a major role in the management of patients with advanced disease. Surgeons are involved with the initial evaluation and management of the patient prior to disease recurrence, they are often the first doctor to detect recurrence then have a role in staging and further local control. They have specific skills in the management of discharge and haemorrhage and some forms of pain are best controlled by surgical fixation rather than increasing analgesia. Finally reconstruction and rehabilitation may well be needed as part of palliation and certainly require surgical skills.

The disappointment of medical oncology in providing long-term local control in the majority of solid tumours means that adequate surgery is still required even if a tumour is downstaged. Surgical involvement at the outset will often determine operability and potential curability. Joint assessment of complex patients is essential and the establishment of multidisciplinary teams has been one of the major advances in recent years. It is easier to provide a multidisciplinary team when one works in a cancer centre with access to neurosurgeons, orthopaedic surgeons, plastic surgeons, and specialist tumour site-specific surgeons. It may be harder to reproduce this range of expertise in the district hospital and patients may need to be referred into the centre for such care. This should not be seen as a failure by the local treating team and good centre/district communication should allow patients to move easily between the two with a return to the local team for ongoing care.

Breast cancer

The incidence of breast cancer continues to rise and although the mortality has fallen in the United Kingdom and in the white population of America it still remains a significant problem. In a population of patients taken from a Cancer Registry where the effect of delay in diagnosis was being examined it was found that 9 per cent of patients still presented with advanced disease (i.e. with surgically unresectable disease or with symptomatic bone or liver metastases). Given that there are 32 000 new cases of breast cancer a year in the United Kingdom (and probably a million worldwide) this represents a significant number of people in whom the management from the outset will be palliative rather than curative. The acceptance of core biopsy as an accurate diagnostic tool and the ability to obtain tissue for oestrogen receptor analysis means that many of these patients no longer require formal open surgery.

Downstaging of advanced disease

Depending on the rapidity of presentation and the hormone receptor status, a choice between endocrine therapy and chemotherapy as the primary treatment may be made. The newer third generation aromatase inhibitors such as letrozole, anastrozole, and examestane seem to achieve better responses than tamoxifen both in terms of overall response and speed of onset. There is also some evidence that they may work better when there are low levels of oestrogen receptors present. If the patient is pre-menopausal then ovarian ablation can be undertaken by surgery, radiotherapy or, more commonly now, with luteinizing hormone releasing hormone (LHRH) superagonists such as goseralin or leuprolide. Having rendered the patient post-menopausal the chance of endocrine response is higher. It is assumed that the combination of an LHRH agonist with an aromatase inhibitor will be beneficial and anecdotally this appears to be true although there are, as yet, no reported randomized controlled trials in the advanced setting to confirm this.

If the patient responds to an endocrine manipulation for a worthwhile time then a second or third line endocrine agent should be tried and we have all seen occasional patients with prolonged control of advanced disease by multiple endocrine manipulations.

If the patient is endocrine unresponsive or hormone receptor negative then chemotherapy will be used. Off trial the FEC regimen (5-FU, epirubicin, and cyclophosphamide) is currently popular and the taxanes and trazumatab (a monoclonal antibody to the Her-2 receptor) have yet to become first-line agents. Newer agents currently under trial will further extend the options available. If the patient achieves a satisfactory response then surgery to help control local disease should be carried out. This may take the form of a local resection or mastectomy with or without reconstruction. Radiotherapy is usually indicated for this group of patients and this normally follows surgery although in the case of an inflammatory cancer (which has responded to chemotherapy) the radiotherapy is often given prior to surgery. The prognosis for patients with inflammatory cancer has improved dramatically with modern management—at one time the prognosis was universally fatal whereas now with modern chemotherapy, radiotherapy, and surgery 60–70 per cent will survive to 5 years.

Achievement of local control is required even if the patient presents with disseminated disease. It is much less common nowadays to see patients with recurrent chest wall disease. This is because appropriate primary surgery with radiotherapy have been used more often. There are, however, worrying trends for inappropriate primary therapy being undertaken in some centres with failure to adhere to the principles of good local control. Examples include primary medical therapy with no completion surgery or radiotherapy after initial 'response'.

Occasionally, recurrent chest wall disease occurs in the absence of dissemination. After careful staging it may be appropriate to consider a major resection. This may include the breast, underlying muscle and chest wall. One site for such recurrences is the internal mammary chain of lymph nodes. This is being seen more commonly as they are no longer irradiated in order to protect the coronary vasculature. Such a recurrence may present as pain or a vague mass which is seen on CT scan to permeate between the ribs.

Depending on the defect created a number of techniques are available to reconstruct the defect. If the chest wall remains stable then a simple myocutaneous flap[1] may be sufficient. If stability is needed then a microvascular free bone graft may be required.[2] Additional tissue to provide cover can be brought up from the abdomen by means of an omental flap.[3] Skin grafting can be used on top of the omentum to provide skin cover.[4] The previous use of radiotherapy may render the tissues less tolerant and may limit the options available. Knowledge of the previous radiotherapy fields is often useful in planning a major operation. Such major surgery requires a multidisciplinary approach with surgical oncologist, plastic surgeon, thoracic or cardiac surgeon, and suitable post-operative care.

Reconstruction

It was once suggested that patients who underwent breast conservation had a better psychological outcome but it was subsequently shown that patients who were treated by clinicians who gave them choice fared better and that the diagnosis of cancer, per se, was a bigger threat than the type of surgery undertaken. For patients with advanced disease, be it a large primary tumour or recurrent chest wall disease, resection with or without reconstruction often improves quality of life. It adds little to overall survival but may control further local recurrence. Reconstruction of the breast or cover of a large defect may be required. There are various techniques available from simple insertion of a prosthesis to complicated flap procedures. The choice depends on the size of the defect and whether or not radiotherapy has been or is about to be used. The cosmetic outcome is less satisfactory if radiotherapy is used when a prosthesis has been inserted. This is because a significant capsular contracture can occur. Sometimes a period of tissue expansion is needed prior to insertion of a prosthesis in order to create enough space and some ptosis. Flaps may be raised from a number of sources—the commonest being the latissimus dorsi flap which may include both muscle and skin. A transverse rectus abdominis myocutaneous (TRAM) flap involves movement of the lower abdominal skin and fat with some muscle. This can either be swung on a pedicle or used as a free flap with microvascular anastomosis of the inferior epigastric vessels to the internal mammary vessels. There are variations of this type of flap but all require specialist skills and are time consuming. These are major operations with risks of failure of the anastomosis and loss of the flap and problems with the donor site. The patient needs to be counselled as to these risks. Attention is often needed to the contralateral breast, which may require a mastopexy or reduction in order to achieve symmetry.

Cancer of the gastrointestinal tract

Malignant tumours of the gastrointestinal tract account for around 40 000 deaths a year in England and Wales—nearly 30 per cent of all deaths from malignancy. Many patients have advanced disease at presentation and survival figures for those regarded as ostensibly curable suggest many of them already have disseminated disease. While surgery undoubtedly cures patients with minimally invasive tumours, its contribution lies chiefly in symptom relief and local disease control.

The principal symptoms of gastrointestinal malignancy are obstruction of a hollow conduit, pain due to tumour infiltration, and blood loss—either acute or chronic. The most effective way to relieve them is to excise the primary tumour completely, even in some cases, when metastases are unequivocally present. If this is technically feasible, there may be little practical difference between curative and palliative procedures. When complete excision is impossible, or when associated risks are unacceptably high, symptoms from obstruction can still be relieved by surgical bypass or decompression or by establishing a channel through the tumour by endoscopic means. Unless the primary tumour is removed, however, symptoms of obstruction may recur and those caused by other pathological processes, such as bleeding, may become more prominent. Some symptoms, like the pain of malignant infiltration, may not be alleviated by surgery at all; other symptoms may relate to metastatic disseminated disease rather than the primary tumour itself. In these circumstances, surgical intervention of any kind may be inappropriate.

With the recent introduction of disease-specific quality of life assessments to study outcome of palliative procedures for gastrointestinal cancer[5,6] further insight into the patient's perception of the benefits or harms of treatments will be gained. It is to be hoped that studies using these tools will lead to the further optimization of palliative treatments in the future.

Carcinoma of the oesophagus

Oesophageal cancer is the cause of 2 per cent of cancer deaths in the United Kingdom each year. Adenocarcinoma has a rapidly rising incidence and now accounts for most oesophageal tumours. Treatment is seldom curative and median survival after diagnosis is 10 months with only 10 per cent of patients surviving for 5 years.[7] Most clinicians agree palliation is the most important aspect of management. Surgical excision is only possible in about a third of cases but there is recent evidence that neoadjuvant chemotherapy may improve resectability. Resectability is assessed on pre-operative investigations including ultrasound and computerized tomographic scanning. The recent introduction of endoscopic ultrasound has provided an investigatory tool which is superior to CT scanning for the assessment of T staging. The use of positron emission tomography (PET) to detect occult metastases is currently under investigation. Despite a fall in the operative mortality rate to about 5–10 per cent, largely due to improved anaesthesia and post-operative care, complications of resection are still common. Retrospective studies suggest that surgical excision may offer better palliation than radical radiotherapy but this may simply reflect the selection of less advanced cases for surgery. The most that can be concluded from uncontrolled studies is that the best results of surgery are achieved by experienced teams in carefully selected cases.

Patients fall broadly into two groups—those without evidence of advanced disease who are fit for surgery or those who have advanced disease or are unfit or surgery. Patients in the first group are best served by resection as this affords the chance of a cure or the most sustained palliation from dysphagia. Tumours at the gastro-oesophageal junction are approached through a left thoracoabdominal or thoracic incision with incision of the diaphragm. More proximal tumours require the two-stage Ivor–Lewis approach using a right thoracotomy following mobilization of the stomach at laparotomy. Some surgeons favour a three-stage procedure to achieve an adequate resection margin, with an anastomosis in the neck through a third stage cervical incision.

In the technique of transhiatal oesophagectomy the oesophagus is removed through cervical and abdominal incisions without opening the chest. Proponents of this approach claim there are less pulmonary complications but there is little evidence to support a reduction in morbidity or mortality and the procedure does not achieve adequate clearance in advanced disease. Endoscopic ultrasonography may assist selection for this procedure and the introduction of minimally invasive techniques now makes it possible to mobilize the thoracic oesophagus under direct vision. The stomach is the most popular organ for oesophageal replacement; the colon and small bowel are alternatives and free jejunal grafts have been used to replace the cervical oesophagus with encouraging results.

There are a number of treatment methods available for those patients who are not suitable for resection. Radical radiotherapy has an increasing place in the treatment of patients with inoperable disease.

Several studies have shown a promising response to radiotherapy and combination chemotherapy with cisplatinum-based regimens in patients with advanced disease. There are early data to suggest that patients with advanced local disease may do well with radical radiotherapy or chemoradiotherapy.

Relief of dysphagia

For those patients who are not suitable for resection, a permanent gastrostomy is hardly ever justifiable. Palliative radiotherapy, like oesophageal dilatation, provides only temporary symptomatic relief with over 60 per cent of patients experiencing recurrent dysphagia. Bypass procedures are associated with a particularly high operative mortality rate (at least 30 per cent) and should probably be reserved for tumours that prove unresectable at operation contrary to expectation.

Oesophageal intubation is the standard way of relieving symptoms in patients with unresectable tumours or malignant tracheo-oesophageal fistulas. Previously, intubation was achieved using reinforced silicone or latex tubes either by traction at open operation or by pulsion through an endoscope. These tubes usually have a funnelled upper end and an additional distal flange, to prevent upward displacement. Migration, however, still occurs in up to a third of cases. Additionally the serious complication of perforation occurs in 10 per cent and mortality is 3–10 per cent.[8] The lower complication rates and decreased length of hospital stay[9,10] offset the marked increase in cost of the now favoured self-expanding stents when compared to the rigid tubes. Metal stents are placed endoscopically (Fig. 1) and have the advantage of a small delivery system. The procedure can be performed under conscious sedation and 90 per cent of patients are able to tolerate a semi-solid or a normal diet following insertion. However, they may not be as good as initially thought with increasing reports of patients experiencing discomfort and even pain after insertion. Late complications occur in up to 50 per cent of those treated and repeated endoscopic interventions may be necessary to enhance the patient's quality of life.

Many patients with oesophageal tubes require a semi-solid diet. Steak, unless minced and fresh bread are particularly liable to stick. Blockage may resolve spontaneously and can be encouraged to do so by administering

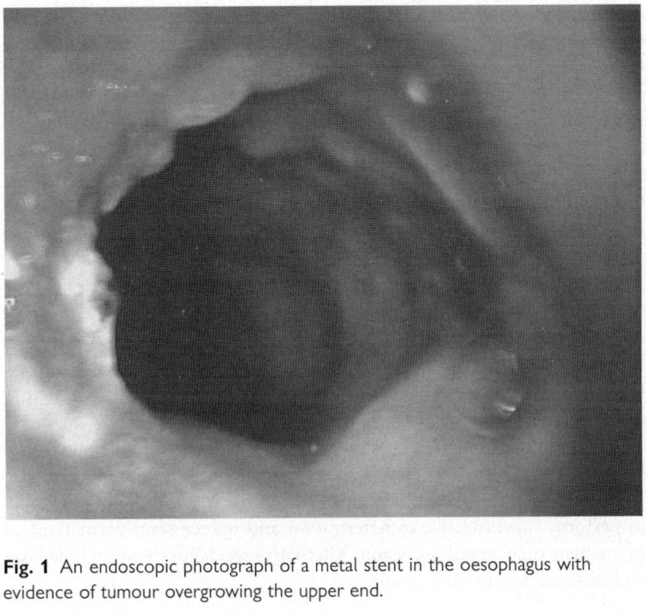

Fig. 1 An endoscopic photograph of a metal stent in the oesophagus with evidence of tumour overgrowing the upper end.

fizzy drinks. If not, a nasogastric tube should be passed to try to dislodge the bolus before resorting to endoscopy.

Neodymium yittrium–aluminium-garnet (Nd:YAG) laser therapy is an alternative to intubation and can also be undertaken without general anaesthesia. It is only suitable for exophytic tumours which account for two-thirds of oesophageal tumours. The laser is used to burrow through the tumour on successive occasions or to photocoagulate the majority of the tumour at one session after preliminary dilatation. Dysphagia is relieved in over 90 per cent of cases, after a median of two treatments, and one-half of patients can take a normal diet. The complication rate is low. More than 50 per cent of patients require further courses of treatment, sometimes after only a few weeks; additional external beam radiotherapy significantly reduces the need for frequent treatments. Brachytherapy post-laser treatment can prolong relief of dysphagia for up to 5 months without the need to resort to a stent.

Another development is the introduction of photodynamic therapy (PDT) which uses light energy to produce destruction of tissues that have been pre-treated with photosensitizing drugs. This technique has been shown to be similar in outcome to laser treatments; accidental oesophageal perforation is less likely with PDT and, as healing apparently occurs by tissue regeneration rather than by fibrosis, strictures are supposed to develop less frequently. The disadvantage of this approach is prolonged photosensitivity which can last for up to 3 months.

Control of fistulas or treatment of perforation of tumours

These complications occur in 5 per cent of patients. Endoscopic methods can be used to treat most complications including perforations—stents can often be placed over the site of the tear, in a similar manner in which they are used to treat a tracheo-oesophageal fistula.

Treatment of bleeding

Significant bleeding is a rare complication of oesophageal cancers. Argon plasma coagulation (APC) is the treatment of choice although at the moment there is a lack of published evidence. It produces a superficial thermodestructive effect on tissues and this is suited, not only to use for coagulation of bleeding areas of tumour, but also to destruction of small tumour nodules, or control of tumour overgrowth over the ends of a stent. Similar results, although at much lower cost have been reported using absolute alcohol given by injection endoscopically,[11] and an increasing number of small studies report the value of combining tumour destruction with intubation.[12]

Carcinoma of the stomach

About 16 000 people die from gastric cancer in the United Kingdom every year. Most patients present with advanced disease with less than a third being suitable for curative resection. Several retrospective studies have shown that patients with incurable gastric cancer have better symptomatic relief and a longer life expectancy after resection than after bypass procedures or with no treatment at all. While the results may simply reflect a selection bias, there is little doubt that symptoms due to mechanical obstruction or haemorrhage are relieved more successfully by resection (80–85 per cent) than by procedures that leave the tumour in place such as a gastroenterostomy (30–80 per cent).

The operative mortality rate of palliative resection is related to the type of operation performed. Figures vary widely but within the last decade operative mortality rates have fallen: figures of 4–8 per cent are now quoted for total gastrectomy. Although this operation can be followed by severe nutritional deficiencies, the majority of patients have a good or satisfactory quality of life after surgery.

Bleeding, in the emergency setting, in unfit patients or in the absence of symptoms of obstruction, may be best treated by embolization techniques. Refinement of technique and materials has enhanced the radiologist's ability to perform superselective catheterization and induce semi-permanent or permanent small vessel occlusion. Alternative modalities may include laser and external beam radiotherapy.

The less common complication of perforation of a gastric cancer may occur in a previously undiagnosed patient. As this is often associated with advanced disease it is accepted that a simple closure with biopsy may be performed. Emergency resection offers good palliation, albeit with an increased mortality, although long-term survival is not enhanced.[13]

There is currently great interest in the use of pre-operative combination chemotherapy for patients with advanced gastric cancer. Response rates of 70 per cent, with complete remission in just over 10 per cent, have been obtained with epirubicin–cisplatinum–fluorouracil in patients with advanced disease enabling some of them (50 per cent) to proceed to surgery and successful resection. A trial of pre-operative chemoradiotherapy prior to the resection of gastric cancer resulted in significant pathological responses in the majority of patients and this may enhance resection rates in the future.[14]

For patients with unresectable tumours options are limited. Tumours confined to the cardia can be treated by intubation or laser therapy, as described for cancer of the oesophagus, although there is an increased incidence of tube dislodgement. There are now reports of relief of obstructing gastric outlet tumours using self-expanding metal stents.[15] Simple bypass of antral tumours offers temporary relief from vomiting but gastric emptying can be unsatisfactory and the Devine antral exclusion operation may be preferable.

Malignant obstructive jaundice

The majority of pancreatobiliary carcinomas are too far advanced at presentation and are not amenable to surgical resection for cure. Most patients with carcinoma of the pancreas present with obstructive jaundice. Relief of biliary obstruction results in a prolonged and more comfortable survival, free of distressing pruritis. Duodenal obstruction and pain are the other major considerations in the palliation of pancreatic or biliary tumours. With the development of endoscopic techniques for the relief of jaundice and, with the improvement in pre-operative assessment of operability the role of palliative surgery has declined sharply. Data on palliative resection is limited but anecdotal reports suggest a better quality of life following resection and less pain in the terminal stages than with more conservative therapies. Although mortality rates for resection should now be below 5 per cent, morbidity rates remain high. Palliative resection may, however, be performed in cases where the tumour is found to be infiltrating at a point in the operation which is considered to be past the 'point of no return'.

When a patient is found to be unsuitable for resection prior to the 'point of no return' a bypass operation can be accomplished by anastomosis of the duodenum or jejunum to the gall bladder or common bile duct. When the cystic duct is occluded by tumour, the jejunum is joined to the hepatic duct by means of a Roux loop. Cholecystojejunostomy is an easy procedure to perform but there is sufficient evidence that this is associated with an unacceptable complication rate particularly recurrent jaundice and cholangitis to discourage its use.[16,17] Most surgeons perform a choledochoduodenostomy or a more complex choledochojejunostomy with Roux-en-Y. The former procedure has the advantage of simplicity and maintenance of easy endoscopic access if there is recurrent jaundice.

Duodenal obstruction occurs in 5 per cent of patients at presentation and in a further 15–30 per cent within 12 months. Most surgeons, therefore, perform a gastrojejunostomy at the same time as the biliary bypass, the addition of which is not associated with a greater mortality rate or a longer recovery period. With a biliary bypass alone 17 per cent of patients will get symptoms from duodenal obstruction by 8.5 months.[17] Laparoscopic techniques are used by enthusiasts for staging in equivocal cases and there are now techniques developed for both biliary and gastric bypasses.

Advanced tumours of the distal bile duct and ampulla are treated in the same way as pancreatic carcinoma. Those of the gall bladder carry an extremely poor prognosis. Unresectable tumours of the proximal biliary tree were historically managed by surgical bypass but are now palliated with endoscopic or percutaneous stenting. The bypass was achieved by joining a Roux loop to the intrahepatic biliary tree. This was found by incising the bridge of tissue joining the quadrate and left lobes to expose the left hepatic duct, as described by Hepp and Couinaud in 1956, or by following the round ligament into the umbilical fissure as described by Soupault and Couinaud in 1957.

Percutaneous transhepatic or endoscopically placed endoprostheses are associated with a lower mortality rate and fewer early complications than surgical bypass and the majority of cases with malignant jaundice are now treated with stenting techniques.

Until recently, endoscopic biliary stenting was performed with Teflon, polyethylene, or polyurethrane endoprostheses and had similar results to percutaneous stenting and surgical bypass. The mortality rate was less than that reported for surgical bypass and recovery was quicker, but occlusion of the stent occurred within a few months. The newer self-expanding metal stents have larger diameters and occlusion is therefore less common. A further major advantage is that they can be used in the duodenum to treat obstruction. However, they are expensive and very difficult to remove. As a general rule, patients who are expected to survive less than 3 months are suitable for a 'plastic' stent; those with a longer survival or those needing duodenal stenting should have a self-expanding metal stent.

Bypass and stenting procedures both fail to address the symptom of pain associated with tumour infiltration. Current treatment of intractable pain that fails to respond to adequate doses of opioid analgesia is usually either a percutaneous splanchnic block or a thoracoscopic splanchnicectomy. Persistent pain may also respond to external beam radiotherapy. Percutaneous chemical splanchnic blocks involve the percutaneous injection of the coeliac plexus with 40 ml of 5 per cent phenol or 20 ml of 50 per cent alcohol under fluoroscopic or computed tomography guidance. In specialist centres endoscopic ultrasound-guided coeliac plexus block has been shown to have a similar efficacy to the percutaneous approach and theoretically this technique should have a lower complication rate. Thoracoscopic splanchnicectomy can also be performed with a low complication rate with the nerve being readily identifiable beneath the pleura.

Small bowel tumours

Malignant tumours of the small intestine are uncommon. As a rule they can be resected or bypassed with little difficulty.

Colorectal cancer

Colorectal cancer is the second commonest cause of cancer death in the United Kingdom, where an estimated 27 000 new cases occur each year. There is a 37 per cent 5-year survival, which has improved little in recent years. In 10–15 per cent of patients, death occurs from locoregional disease progression; the remaining 50 per cent die from disseminated disease, particularly involving the liver. Palliation of colorectal cancer may therefore be considered as control of local or control of disseminated disease.

Local disease

About 20 per cent of patients present with locally advanced disease with involvement of adjacent viscera. However, only about 5 per cent are not amenable to primary surgical resection. Complete surgical excision is the only effective treatment for locally advanced colorectal cancer, and offers a chance of cure that is comparable to similar stage disease that has not invaded adjacent tissues. Future management may be simplified by the use of staple guns which 'mark' the site of an anastomosis and further clips can be used to mark where tumour appears macroscopically close to the resection margins.

The most useful pre-operative test for assessment of extent of local invasion of colonic cancer is CT scanning, now usually performed as pneumocolography. Tumours of the rectum may be assessed using CT scanning, magnetic resonance imaging (MRI), or endorectal ultrasound. The traditional assessment of tumour fixity by rectal examination, usually performed under anaesthesia, suggests extramural involvement with 60 per cent accuracy in palpable rectal tumours. Pre-operative irradiation of locally advanced disease, in the rectum, can downstage the tumour and allow resection, some operative specimens showing no residual evidence of local disease.

Despite modern imaging surgeons are still sometimes faced with intra-operative decisions about resectability. Bypass surgery including the formation of a stoma relieves symptoms of obstruction but has no effect on symptoms of bleeding, mucous discharge, tenesmus, or on the pain of infiltration. In some cases, however, the decision to perform a resection can be associated with a high morbidity and even a high mortality. Excision of adjacent structures including the abdominal wall is usually feasible; proximity of major vessels particularly the pelvic veins or infiltration of the retroperitoneum may indicate irresectability. A so-called trial of dissection should be made with care as a point of no return can be reached all too quickly with the onset of bleeding or with perforation of the bowel.

Recurrent disease after primary resection occurs solely at the site of tumour excision in 30 per cent of cases but is associated with distant metastases in 70 per cent of cases of local recurrence. Abdominal and pelvic CT scanning provide the most comprehensive assessment of the site and extent of local recurrence. Sacral MRI can be useful where there is unexplained pelvic pain, which is usually due to sacral nerve involvement with recurrent disease after rectal cancer excision.

Surgical excision of local recurrence helps symptom control in about 10 per cent of cases and should be considered in appropriately fit patients with limited disease. Endoscopic evidence of recurrence is usually revealed to represent the 'tip of the iceberg' when the area is imaged with CT or MRI. Localized small bowel obstruction can be relieved with intestinal bypass, but this is rarely helpful when there are multiple areas of hold up requiring multiple bypasses. When the diagnosis of multiple areas of obstruction can be made before laparotomy, for example, from a follow through study or abdominal CT scan, the patient is probably better managed by non-operative measures.

Ileostomies should be as distal as possible to ensure maximum small bowel absorption, and avoidance of the need to provide fluid and electrolyte supplementation. A loop ileostomy can often be performed through a trephine incision and in some cases, where the patient is frail, this can be done under local anaesthesia. The use of tube caecostomies should be a last resort,[18] as even with a Foley-type catheter with a balloon and anchoring sutures faecal leakage can occur and in the absence of complications they do not represent a long-term solution.

Distal colonic or rectal obstruction can be relieved by a defunctioning colostomy proximal to the site of obstruction. Rectal or distal colonic obstruction can also be relieved by endoluminal stenting or laser resection but these do not help to control pelvic pain. Control of pain and bleeding can be achieved by irradiation of areas of local recurrence but this is better used where obstruction has first been resolved by one of the methods mentioned above. Insertion of self-expanding endoluminal stents for obstruction of the left colon is performed via an endoscopy using fluoroscopy to confirm positioning.[19] These stents (Fig. 2) can also be used to relieve obstruction and allow adequate bowel preparation prior to definitive surgery.

The use of major surgery such as exenteration with or without sacral resection is an option in the fit patient with the prospective of long-term palliation of symptoms. This type of surgery requires both physical and mental strength on the part of the patient and should be reserved for motivated individuals and performed by a multidisciplinary team.[20] However, the worst scenario that can be imagined for a patient is the uncontrolled external growth of rectal or perineal recurrence and avoidance of this may involve a lowering of surgical thresholds.

Disseminated disease

For many patients with metastatic disease at presentation, resection of the primary tumour will afford the best palliation. However, there are some frail patients with advanced metastatic disease and an absence of symptoms relating to their primary tumour in whom surgical intervention is inappropriate. Judgement of the sequence of events leading to death may be necessary in the decision whether or not to operate and this is not always a

(a)
(b)

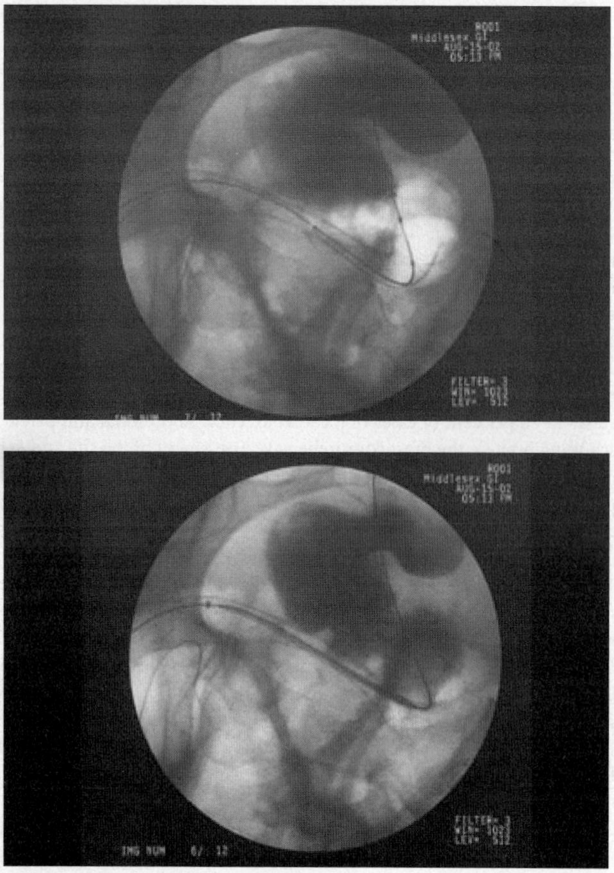

Fig. 2 (a) A screening X-ray taken during the placement of an expanding metal stent into the sigmoid colon of a patient with a malignant stricture. (b) A screening X-ray taken of a second stent being passed through the first stent to extend the length of stenting.

simple assessment. In the presence of irresectable metastatic disease there is a place for limited resections, or more minimally invasive surgery using laparoscopic or laparoscopically assisted techniques.(21)

The commonest site of metastasis in colorectal cancer is the liver which is involved in about 80 per cent of patients with disseminated disease. It is thought that secondary metastasis from the liver to other sites is the main source of general dissemination. Uncontrolled liver metastases produce pain, abdominal distension, jaundice, and inferior vena cava obstruction. The only proven curative treatment for colorectal metastases is surgical resection, which is technically feasible in about 20 per cent of affected patients. The operative mortality should be less than 4 per cent and the 5-year survival approaches 30 per cent. There is some variability in criteria for suitability for metastasis resection among surgeons but most would prefer to operate on patients with fewer than four metastases, confined to one lobe of the liver, not adjacent to major vessels and with no evidence of residual disease elsewhere after the primary resection.

Recurrent disease develops within the liver in 25 per cent and elsewhere in 50 per cent of patients who have previously undergone liver metastasis resection. The majority of liver metastasis patients cannot be helped by resection. Although chemotherapy can be used to downstage liver metastases so that they become resectable this can render the liver more friable and prone to haemorrhage.

Theoretically, there are advantages to the administration of chemotherapy directly into the hepatic artery, so reducing systemic exposure. However, there is the counter argument that other parts of the body should be exposed to reduce the number of metastases that occur elsewhere. Despite good response rates there has been little demonstrable effect on survival to date. Although the fully implantable pump systems reduce mechanical problems to a minimum there is still the small chance of liver toxicity.

Ablation techniques, usually performed percutaneously under imaging are beginning to show promising results. As with most new developments these treatments were initially confined to those patients who were unsuitable for any other treatments. Freezing and laser, and more recently, radiofrequency ablation techniques have been developed. Randomized controlled trials comparing ablation with surgery will be difficult to establish, however, while many surgeons retain their belief that surgery is the optimal treatment. Radiofrequency ablation produces heat by ionic agitation. Cooled tip electrodes and high-powered generators have improved the efficacy of this therapy. It has the advantage of ease of ablation of a normal rim of tissue around the tumour.(22) It is possible to perform ablation therapy in the operating theatre when metastases are difficult to image and combined surgical and ablation techniques may be used to eradicate disease in cases which are somewhat too advanced for surgery alone.

Rarely, resection of an isolated lung metastasis can produce long-term survival but the development of lung, bone or brain metastases usually indicates that the disease is incurable. The pain of bone metastases can usually be controlled by irradiation, and prophylactic bone fixation may be required for metastases affecting long bones. For brain metastases cerebral irradiation plus high dose corticosteroids can reduce intracerebral pressure and delay neurological deterioration.

Since most patients with colorectal carcinoma are not cured, it could be argued that the majority of patients receive palliative treatment. Careful judgement is required in deciding the correct mixture of radical surgery, radiotherapy, and chemotherapy to produce the best chance of prolonged, high-quality survival.

Lung cancer

Bronchogenic carcinoma is a major cause of mortality world-wide and the survival rate has not improved significantly in the last 20 years. Over 150 000 new cases of lung cancer are diagnosed in Europe every year but less than 10 per cent are cured even with the best standards of medical treatment. With the exception of a few patients whose small cell lung cancers may be eradicated by chemotherapy and radiotherapy, the majority of patients with lung cancer can only be cured by complete surgical resection. Unfortunately, the proportion of primary lung cancers amenable to curative surgery is only 10 per cent in the United Kingdom, compared to 20–30 per cent in the United States. In the vast majority of cases, surgery is not feasible because of the tumour extent (local spread or distant metastases) or the poor general condition of the patient.

In large retrospective series, there are virtually no long-term survivors after resection of T4 or bulky N2-N3 disease. Induction chemotherapy or chemoradiotherapy is reported to improve the proportion of patients with advanced non-small cell lung cancer (NSCLC) (stage IIIA-B) suitable for resection, resulting in a higher 5-year survival than historical series (18 versus 9 per cent). However, in those with bulky N2 disease the long-term survival after induction chemotherapy was only 4 per cent.

Due to the poor surgical and medical curability of lung tumours, the role of palliative treatment has increased. Only in very rare instances can surgery be usefully combined with other treatment modalities to prolong the survival of patients who otherwise have no chance of cure. Recent technological progress in developing new surgical instruments and minimally invasive techniques have improved the results of palliative treatment. Video-assisted bronchoscopy and thoracoscopy now enable the surgeon to perform complex endobronchial and intrathoracic procedures with greater accuracy and safety, without the need for open thoracotomy, and new synthetic materials provide more flexible and durable bronchial stents and other endoprostheses.

Locally advanced or metastatic lung cancer

In the management of primary lung cancer, major surgery is rarely justified for palliation alone. Incomplete or debulking surgery does not influence the patient's life expectancy or improve quality of life. A few long-term survivors can be identified after incomplete resection followed by post-operative radiotherapy, but similar results can be achieved with radiotherapy alone.

To describe complete resection as 'palliative' is misleading, as typical symptoms such as cough, dyspnoea, or chest pain are likely to be worse after surgery than they were before. Radiotherapy with or without chemotherapy is preferable to incomplete resection in patients with locally advanced lung cancer, and symptoms of bronchial obstruction and haemoptysis are better treated by endoscopic resection and/or brachytherapy. Even in the presence of the paraneoplastic syndromes, durable control of hormone related symptoms is only achieved by complete excision of the disease.

Lung abscess or acute sepsis are rare indications for partial resection, and even experienced thoracic surgeons have only anecdotal cases. Salvage resection is sometimes indicated for acute life-threatening complications such as the massive necrosis of heavily irradiated lung parenchyma.

Lung resection in the presence of cytological positive pleural effusion is associated with a mean survival of 3–6 months. A similar survival time can be anticipated after resection of T4 tumours invading mediastinal structures such as the superior vena cava, aorta, myocardium, or oesophagus.

Patients presenting with operable lung cancer and a solitary distant metastasis may benefit from resection of both tumour foci. The probability of long-term survival after resection of a brain metastasis and the lung primary is between 10 and 20 per cent at 5 years, with no significant difference in survival between patients with synchronous and metachronous presentation of the brain lesion. Resection of the brain metastasis plus brain irradiation is better than radiotherapy alone in terms of median survival and quality of life. Long-term survivors have also been reported after resection of isolated adrenal metastases.

It is more difficult to assess the prognosis after resection of synchronous intrapulmonary metastases as they are virtually indistinguishable from multiple primary cancers. Clinically, concurrent lung lesions should be considered as independent primary tumours and treated with curative intent whenever possible.

Airway obstruction

Obstruction of the trachea and main bronchi, with severe dyspnoea and stridor, is an infrequent but serious complication of lung cancer, leading to life-threatening respiratory distress. Occasionally patients with a localized endoluminal tumour may be candidates for curative resection.

In the majority of cases, however, obstruction results from compression of the airway due to metastatic involvement of mediastinal nodes at the carina or in the paratracheal chain. Such metastatic spread is common in lung cancer and other extrathoracic malignancies such as breast cancer and lymphoma. Extraluminal compression may be associated with an intraluminal component in lung cancer cases. Palliative therapy is usually best provided by external irradiation. In an emergency, however, or if relapse occurs after external irradiation or prior resection, the surgeon may be involved.

If the chief component of airway obstruction is endoluminal, endoscopic resection provides immediate and safe relief of symptoms. This is achieved by various techniques including simple 'core out', Nd: YAG laser photocoagulation, cryotherapy, or diathermy resection. Whilst laser photocoagulation was originally applied through the fibreoptic bronchoscope under local anaesthesia, the use of a rigid bronchoscope and Sanders Venturi ventilation under general anaesthesia offers a number of definite advantages and has now become the accepted approach. Using the rigid bronchoscope it is now possible to maintain adequate ventilation during the whole procedure even when there is significant bleeding, and haemostasis can be secured at the end of resection. Other modalities can be applied at the same time, such as the insertion of an endobronchial stent. The results of endoscopic disobliteration may be consolidated by giving high-dose intraluminal radiotherapy within a few days of endoscopic resection.

Where the major component of obstruction is extrinsic compression (resistant or recurrent disease after external irradiation) the insertion of an endobronchial stent can relieve symptoms, and is especially useful in an emergency.

Initial experience of tracheobronchial stenting was based on the Montgomery T tube or T–Y tube, inserted through a tracheostomy incision under bronchoscopic control. This procedure remains a valid option for high tracheal obstructions, being easily managed and tolerated by the patient, even for long periods. A further advance has been the development of fully endobronchial silicone stents, manufactured from T tubes at the time of endoscopy, or commercially available in various shapes. Silicone stents can be easily removed if obstruction is relieved by further irradiation (external or endobronchial) and reinserted in case of relapse.

Expandable wire stents have been used as an alternative to silicone, to provide a larger internal lumen and to avoid displacement (Fig. 3). However, tumour ingrowth is a problem and covered expanding devices have now been developed.

(a)
(b)

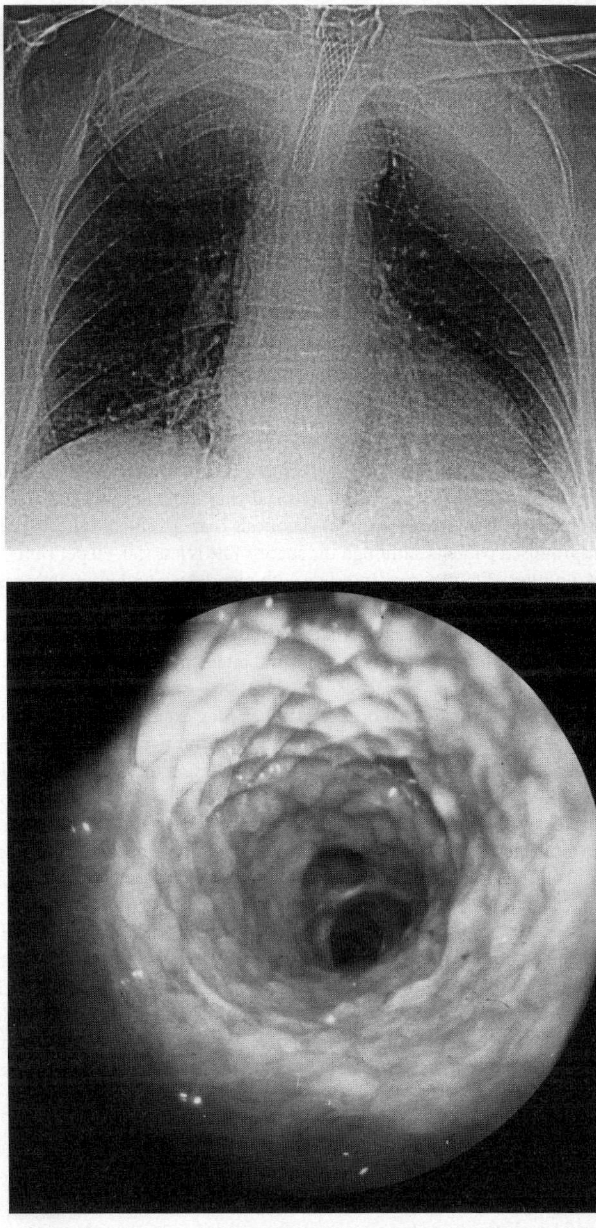

Fig. 3 Wallstent prosthesis, radiological (a) and endoscopic (b) appearance.

Table 1 Endoscopic techniques in the palliation of malignant airways obstruction

Endoscopic techniques		Advantages versus disadvantages
Disobliteration	Nd:YAG laser	Effective/costly
	Diathermy	Effective/not widely available
	Cryotherapy	Effective/repeated application required
Brachytherapy	Iridium afterload	Tolerable in previous irradiation, day case treatment/not widely available
Silicone stents	T or T/Y tubes	Cheap, stable/tracheostomy required
	Endobronchial stents	Cheap/can displace
Metal stents	Gianturco	Expandable/tumour ingrowth
	Wallstent	Thin wall/tumour ingrowth
	Covered	High internal versus external ratio

Thus, a combination of therapies can now be applied to treat the intraluminal as well as extrinsic component of the obstruction (Table 1) at a single endoscopic procedure. In our experience, diathermy resection is an effective and safe way of relieving intraluminal obstruction at less financial cost than laser resection, and can be combined with silicone stent insertion if there is an extraluminal component to the obstruction. Multiple sequential bronchoscopies are often required to reassess the disease, resect endobronchial recurrence, and/or reposition the stent. Although the median survival of these patients is 5–6 months, occasional long-term survivors have been reported.

Pleural effusion (see also Chapter 8.7)

The aim of palliation is to achieve as complete an expansion of the lung as possible, preferably with permanent pleurodesis to prevent recurrence. Surgical pleurodesis by talc poudrage at thoracoscopy or thoracotomy is the most effective technique, achieving permanent control in over 90 per cent of cases. Medical pleurodesis with intercostal chest drainage and intrapleural instillation of tetracycline or other chemicals is an acceptable alternative in compromised patients, although the success rate is less (50–60 per cent).

A number of factors may interfere with pleurodesis and ultimately result in clinical failure. They include: incomplete drainage of the effusion; an ineffective agent; insufficient contact between agent and pleural surface due to adhesion or fibrin from previous pleural interventions; and failed apposition of the two pleural surfaces.

Surgical pleurodesis cannot succeed when lung expansion is restricted by a malignant or benign cortex as apposition of the two pleural surfaces is essential. In patients in whom the lung will not expand sufficiently to allow apposition, the insertion of a pleuroperitoneal shunt may be effective. Video-assisted thoracoscopy is the best way to assess the results and it is then possible to proceed to talc pleurodesis or insertion of a pleuroperitoneal shunt. Both procedures provide reliable long-term control of effusion, without the need for repeated readmission and pleural aspiration.

In our experience of 180 patients treated with either talc pleurodesis or pleuroperitoneal Denver shunt at the Royal Brompton Hospital, effective palliation was achieved in over 95 per cent of patients. In the whole series, there was no intraoperative mortality but a few patients (5 per cent) died within the first month due to respiratory or multiorgan failure related to their advanced malignant disease. Median survival was 5 months (range 1–53). These results justify the early surgical referral of any patient with good performance status and recurrent malignant effusion.

The cause of dyspnoea in these patients is often complex and multifactorial. It may result from chest wall restriction due to previous surgery or radiotherapy, or infiltration by recurrent breast cancer. There may be bronchial obstruction due to metastatic nodal disease, lymphangitis, and pulmonary fibrosis secondary to radiotherapy or airway obstruction. Pleural effusion may be the only correctable component, but it can be difficult to assess its contribution to the dyspnoea prior to treatment.

Tumour recurrence along the track of a chest drain or pleuroperitoneal shunt has been occasionally observed in patients with malignant effusions. It seldom causes significant symptoms but radiotherapy may be required to control pain and discourage local progression.

Pericardial effusion

Surgery is often required for patients with malignant pericardial involvement where constriction or effusion causes cardiac tamponade. Pericardiectomy relieves constriction and pericardial fenestration provides effective and continued drainage for effusion. Survival after pericardiectomy for malignant constriction is dismal and surgery is not justified for tumours with a poor prognosis such as lung cancer. Fenestration is possible via thoracotomy or video-assisted thoracoscopy. The subxiphoid approach has been reported to be a safer alternative for pericardial fenestration than the intrathoracic procedure. Other techniques have been used, such as percutaneous balloon pericardiotomy or pericardioperitoneal shunt.

Superior vena cava obstruction

Major surgery has no role in the palliation of superior vena cava syndrome due to advanced lung cancer. Resection and reconstruction of the superior vena cava or innominate vein with polytetrafluoroethylene grafts is only justified for cases of primary germ cell tumours of the mediastinum or invasive thymoma, for whom surgery aims at cure or long-term survival. For other malignancies including lung cancer, chemotherapy and/or radiotherapy offers better palliation than surgery.

The recent development of intravascular stenting techniques provides new possibilities for managing persistent or recurrent superior vena cava obstruction (see Section 8). The percutaneous transvenous insertion of expandable wire stents, with or without prior balloon dilatation, can be a safe and effective alternative to conventional therapy.

Chest wall invasion and Pancoast syndrome

Chest wall resection for locally advanced lung cancer yields excellent results, providing tumour excision is macroscopically and microscopically complete and mediastinal node involvement excluded. The 5-year survival is approximately 50 per cent for T3N0 and 30 per cent for T3N1.

The development of safe techniques for chest wall reconstruction, including polypropylene mesh (Marlex), methyl methacrylate composite prosthesis, and soft tissue reconstruction using myocutaneous flaps, has expanded the role of surgery in this field. Extensive chest wall resections, including total sternectomy, can now be performed with a low operative mortality in selected cases.

Such major surgery is only justified by an intention to cure. There is no symptomatic or survival benefit after incomplete resection and such cases are best treated by radiotherapy alone. Palliative surgery is often advocated in superior sulcus or Pancoast tumours but there is little evidence that incomplete resection in these circumstances affords better control of chest pain than radiotherapy alone. Median survival after incomplete resection of Pancoast tumours is less than 1 year, with 10–15 per cent of patients surviving 3 years and none alive at 5 years. In the unique experience of Memorial Sloan Kettering, where post-operative brachytherapy has been regularly used as an adjuvant treatment for patients undergoing resection of superior sulcus tumours, 9 per cent of patients survived 5 years after incomplete resection. However, there was no difference in survival between these patients and those who did not undergo resection, and median survival after surgery was only 11 months.

Radiotherapy remains the principal treatment for symptomatic bone metastases. Rib or sternal resection may be sometimes be advised if relapse occurs after radiotherapy and the patient's life expectancy is otherwise reasonable, or if there are no other sites of disease and the primary tumour is controlled.

Dysphagia

In patients with locally advanced lung cancer, oesophageal obstruction may occur as a result of mediastinal lymphadenopathy or direct extension of the primary tumour (at the level of the carina or left main bronchus). Occasionally, tumour spread may be associated with a broncho-oesophageal fistula, which more commonly follows radiotherapy.

Radiation can relieve dysphagia, but local relapse is frequent and recurrent dysphagia may require further management.

The insertion of an endoprosthesis often provides adequate palliation. As discussed above, the use of self-expanding stents has now generally replaced older reinforced silicone or latex tubes.

Oesophageal bypass is inadvisable for oesophageal obstruction from primary lung cancer but may be required in patients with tracheo-oesophageal fistula who otherwise have a favourable prognosis and a good performance status.

Conclusion

The thoracic surgeon has a valuable role in the palliation of some manifestations of advanced intrathoracic disease. Survival is usually measured in months but some patients will benefit for years.

Gynaecological malignancy

Six thousand and five hundred women die from gynaecological cancer per year. Four thousand of these deaths are from ovarian cancer, 1200 from cervix cancer, 800 from endometrial cancer, and 350 from vulval cancer. In the palliative care of these women, surgical intervention may be useful in alleviating the symptoms of a number of problems. The symptoms that commonly come under review for treatment with surgical techniques are bowel obstruction, fistulas, bleeding, discharge, and odour.

Bowel obstruction

Bowel obstruction can occur in any tumour with intra-abdominal spread. Seventy-five per cent of women with ovarian cancers present with stage III disease where it is already spread within the abdomen. Although stage III ovarian cancer may be put into complete remission with a treatment combination of surgery and chemotherapy, it is common for it to reoccur within the abdominal cavity. This tends to occur on the surfaces of the intra-abdominal organs. The tumour deposits then cause adhesions and strictures which result in bowel obstruction. Intra-abdominal metastases leading to bowel obstruction can also occur with advanced endometrial, cervical, and rarely, vulval cancer.

The role of surgery in malignant bowel obstruction due to advanced gynaecological cancer remains controversial. Most of the research evidence is retrospective and comes to varying conclusions ranging from a significant role for surgery to no role at all. In the vast majority of retrospective reviews quality of life post-surgery is rarely measured or reported. In the palliative context of surgery, quality of life is the most important factor. These issues are summarized in an excellent systematic review published recently.[23]

When a woman presents with bowel obstruction due to advanced gynaecological cancer, initial conservative measures of intravenous fluids plus nasogastric tube and aspiration should be initiated. As the onset of obstruction in these cases tends to be an insidious process, with perforation rarely a complication, urgent surgical intervention is not usually required. Thus, there should be time for the woman to be reviewed by a multidisciplinary team. This multidisciplinary team should include a gynaecological oncology surgeon, a chemotherapy specialist, and a palliative care specialist. The following factors should then be assessed:

1. The chemotherapy options and the likely prognosis.
2. Whether the obstruction is likely to be at a single site or if multiple sites of obstruction due to widespread intra-abdominal disease are expected.
3. The patient's performance status and expected quality of life.
4. The patient's wishes and symptoms.

The first assessment is to decide the likely prognosis of the patient. In the case of ovarian cancer, the most important prognostic factor is the previous chemotherapy that has been used, and whether further chemotherapeutic options exist. If chemotherapy options remain, surgical treatment of the obstruction should be considered early, while serum albumin remains high. If all the therapeutic options have been used, then the obstruction probably represents an end stage event in the disease history and surgery to relieve the obstruction is unlikely to prolong life significantly.

From the surgical point of view it is important to assess whether the obstruction is likely to be at a single site, or whether there are multiple sites of obstruction due to widespread intra-abdominal disease. It is possible to relieve the obstruction in 80–100 per cent of cases.[24] If a single site of obstruction is found, the obstructed bowel may be excised or bypassed. However, if there is multiple site disease the obstruction may only be relieved by a high ileostomy or even a jejunostomy. A high output stoma of this type may significantly reduce the patient's quality of life.

An assessment of the patient's general condition including pre-obstruction performance status is important in order to determine whether the patient is likely to recover from the surgical insult of the surgery, and what quality of life they may be expected to attain following surgery.

These factors should be considered together with the patient's wishes. The patient should be fully informed in an open manner as to the likely prognosis and the likely chances of surgery succeeding. They also need to be told of the high possibility of a stoma being necessary following surgery. These issues should be discussed with the gynaecological and palliative care clinical nurse specialists. In the face of poor prognosis and widespread intra-abdominal disease, the presence of the palliative care team at the consultation allows the option of non-surgical treatment to be fully discussed. If the non-surgical route is taken, then effective control of symptoms can often be achieved by the skilful use of drugs, usually delivered by continuous subcutaneous infusion. The patient can usually be managed without a nasogastric tube or other invasive procedures (see Chapter 8.3.4).

Fistulas

Advanced cervical cancer is the most common cause for a fistula in gynaecological malignancies. Pelvic radiotherapy may compound the effect of malignant disease to cause fistulas. The fistula may be vesico-vaginal or recto-vaginal. A combination of both types of fistula is not uncommon. A multidisciplinary team including a gynaecological oncologist, palliative care specialist, incontinence nurse, and gynaecological oncology clinical nurse specialist should assess the patient. Patients with a poor prognosis and poor mobility are best treated with conservative measures. This is particularly the case with a vesico-vaginal fistula. Urine loss can be dealt with by the use of incontinence pads. The continence clinical nurse specialist and the gynaecological oncology clinical nurse specialist have a major role in managing this distressing problem. If the patient has a good performance status and their prognosis allows significant time, then a urinary diversion should be performed. The simplest urinary diversion with the least chance of complication and morbidity should be offered. This is generally an ileal conduit. More complicated continent diversions are generally not appropriate in this situation, but again this depends on the life expectancy of the patient and the patient's wishes.

Recto-vaginal fistulas are often less acceptable to patients than urinary fistulas. The discomfort and odour from faecal discharge makes the patient more likely to request a bowel diversion rather than deal with the problem with incontinence pads. The simplest bowel diversion is indicated in these cases, although this can be complicated by the presence of widespread intra-abdominal disease.

There are occasions when continent fistula repairs are appropriate. Short-term repair of vaginal fistulas is possible using a three-layer colpocleisis technique. This procedure obliterates the vagina using a graft from either the gracilis or the fat pad of the labia majora to provide healthy tissue in the middle of two layers of vaginal skin. It can be used for both recto-vaginal and vesico-vaginal fistulas. In patients who have a vesico-vaginal fistula, a fenestration is made through to the rectum to allow drainage of urine into the rectum and the patient evacuates both urine and faeces through the anus.

Haemorrhage, discharge, and local fungation

Haemorrhage is most commonly caused by recurrent cervical or endometrial carcinoma at the top of the vaginal vault. It may be appropriate to treat tumours which cause recurrent haemorrhage by surgical means. Often the surgical procedures can be extensive and careful discussion between the multidisciplinary team and the patient must occur. If haemorrhage is occuring from recurrent tumour at the top of the vagina, surgical excision of the tumour may require an exenterative procedure. This is generally inappropriate for a patient in palliative care. Surgical ligation of the internal iliac vessels may reduce haemorrhage, but this would require a laparotomy. Other techniques which are less invasive and cause less morbidity must be considered first. Chemotherapy and particularly small doses of radiotherapy may be effective in stopping haemorrhage. Interventional radiology to embolize the main feeding artery is becoming more common and can be extremely effective in these cases.

Discharge can come from a tumour at the top of the vagina or from locally fungating vulval tumours. Initial efforts to control the odour and discharge will involve the use of metronidazole to reduce the infective processes. Washing with povidone iodine solutions may help in some circumstances. Charcoal dressings can be used to prevent odour.

For locally fungating tumours on the vulva, surgical excision can be considered. This would generally be considered if radiotherapy or chemoradiotherapy treatment had failed. Surgical excision in this scenario may require a myocutaneous graft to cover the defect. This would bring in fresh blood supply to the area to ensure that healing is as quick as possible. Gracilis or vertical rectus abdominus grafts are the most commonly used. If the tumour involves the external urethra, 1 cm of urethra can be excised without loss of continence. If the tumour extends along the anterior vaginal wall, the entire urethra may need to be excised. An ileal conduit may be fashioned, but if the patient is frail and life expectancy is not long, then a simpler procedure may be desired. In this case, the bladder base can be sutured after excision of the urethra and a permanent suprapubic catheter placed.

Palliative urological surgery

The malignancies that most commonly require palliative intervention from the urological team are (in descending order) prostate cancer, urothelial tumours of the bladder, renal cell tumours, and urothelial tumours of the renal collecting systems and ureters. Men with penile and testicular cancer will occasionally require some form of intervention but this will be an uncommon occurrence because of the relatively low prevalence of these tumours.

The symptoms that most commonly require palliation are not specific to any of the malignancies described above. All the tumours mentioned can result in haematuria, retention, obstruction, infection, and fistula formation though they do so with different propensities. As the surgical principles involved in relieving an individual of these symptoms are not specific to the underlying tumour it makes sense to structure this section by the presenting complaints and to describe the specific examples where management is determined by the tumour itself rather than the complication it has caused. We will limit ourselves to surgical interventions alone and therefore will neither refer to hormonal manipulation nor to chemo- or radiotherapy unless administration of these adjuvant therapies requires a surgical operation in order to render them effective.

Bleeding

Haematuria is the most common symptom in patients with locally advanced or metastatic urological malignancy. It results in problems for the patient for three reasons. First, it is distressing. Second, if prolonged it can result in anaemia or hypovolaemia. Third, if there is sufficient blood in the urine clots will form. These can cause obstruction to the ureters and result in painful clot colic. Clots, if sufficiently large, can also obstruct the bladder outlet and result in acute urinary retention. It is self-evident that clot retention of urine could result directly from bleeding from a renal tumour, transitional cell carcinoma anywhere along the urinary tract, or indeed from prostate cancer extending into the trigone of the bladder. As well as arising directly from tumour invasion, haematuria in advanced malignancy might occur as a result of previous radiotherapy, most commonly to the bladder or to the prostate. Management is the same irrespective of the cause.

Making the diagnosis

Ultrasound of the urinary tract and/or IVU in addition to cystoscopy will confirm the diagnosis in almost all cases and, importantly, exclude obstruction of the upper tracts due to clot formation. Very rarely bleeding will be intermittent and remain elusive. This might require spiral CT scanning of the upper tracts or ureteroscopy.[25] Very rarely, angiography will be required to diagnose the site of bleeding and in order to arrest it by embolization.[26]

Management

Acute retention due to clots in the bladder requires catheterization with a large three-way irrigating catheter. Regular washouts of the bladder might be required until a system of bladder irrigation can be established. Clots in the bladder will block the catheter intermittently, resulting in pain and 'by passing' of the catheter during bladder contractions. On rare occasions clearance of the clots will not be possible with a catheter alone and a washout of the bladder will have to be done under general anaesthetic with a cystoscope incorporating Elick's clot evacuators or some similar device. Identifying the site of bleeding during an acute episode is usually futile. If control can be achieved either conservatively or via catheter irrigation it is usually best to defer cystoscopy or imaging until the bleeding has settled. Once this has happened it is usually possible to visualize the site of bleeding if it is of lower urinary tract origin (carcinoma or the bladder or prostate) and to deal with it by fulguration, vaporization, or resection. If the bleeding is diffuse (such as that which arises from radiation or chemotherapy associated cystitis) then systemic or topical treatments might be considered. These are usually tried empirically in the following order (to limit toxicity): epsilon amino caproic acid administered orally, intravesical alum, formalin, silver nitrate, and phenol. If diffuse bleeding persists and is life-threatening, the following have been tried: internal iliac artery embolization, hyperbaric oxygen, percutaneous urinary diversion, and cystectomy as a last resort. The number of available treatment options, none of which have been subjected to controlled trials should alert the reader that diffuse bleeding from the bladder is both a rare event and can be difficult to treat. A thoughtful review by Crew et al.[27] provides an algorithm that places emphasis on a conservative approach.

Clot retention in the bladder will arise quite frequently from bleeding coming from a renal cell tumour or a urothelial carcinoma of the ureter or renal collecting system. Again often all that is required is complete evacuation of the clots within the bladder and irrigation of the bladder via a three-way urethral catheter. Severe recurrent or life-threatening haemorrhage is controlled by angiographic embolization or in exceptional circumstances by nephrectomy or nephro-ureterectomy.

Retention

The most common form of urinary retention occurring in patients with advanced urological malignancy is retention that arises as a result of clots obstructing the bladder outlet. The management of this condition has been described above.

Less commonly, obstruction of the bladder outlet can occur as a result of local tumour extension. Growth of a prostate or bladder carcinoma can make it impossible for the bladder to empty. Prior radiotherapy can contribute to this problem by stiffening the bladder neck, prostate and external sphincter resulting in a voiding dysfunction.

Making the diagnosis

The diagnosis will be made from the history. Sudden acute retention of urine resulting in clear urine on catheterization will be easily dealt with. The more insidious presentation of incomplete bladder emptying accompanied by urinary incontinence may take longer to become recognized. The history should lead the clinician to the problem that can be confirmed either by ultrasound or by catheterization.

Occasionally, urethral catheterization will not be possible and a suprapubic puncture will be required, though this should be resisted in the presence of a bladder carcinoma as a troublesome malignant fistula may result.

Management

In some cases, a catheter may seem the best option if life expectancy is short. In the medium to long-term, catheters usually cause problems because of encrustation, blockage or infection. Endoscopic resection of the tumour is the most commonly undertaken intervention. It is frequently undertaken for local progression of prostate cancers and can result in a re-establishment of normal or near normal voiding. In this situation men need to be warned of two things. First, that if successful the intervention may need to be repeated as blockage may recur. Second, that if the tumour extends into the distal (voluntary) sphincter, relieving a proximal obstruction will result in a decrease in outlet resistance and sometimes result in total incontinence because of a non-functioning sphincter. If this does occur it is usually managed by a long-term catheter or in certain selected cases with an artificial urinary sphincter.

The role of self-expanding stents in lower urinary tract obstruction is being explored, largely as a result of the favourable reports in ureteric obstruction (see below). At present there is limited experience and resection remains the mainstay of treatment. Palliative cystectomy is available if repeat resections fail or if the bladder becomes so dysfunctional (small and scarred or unstable) as to make the patient's life a misery.

Obstruction (of the ureter)

Obstruction of the ureter can result from three broad categories of tumour. First are those that have their origin outside the ureter. These can arise from direct invasion from a colonic tumour or by compression resulting from a lymph node that could be arising from a metastatic renal cell or testicular tumour. Second are those that arise from the ureter itself. These are mainly transitional cell tumours. Third are those that cause obstruction within the lumen of the ureter. This occurs most commonly as a result of clots but on rare occasions a pedunculated tumour of the renal pelvis may extend into the ureter and cause obstruction and hydronephrosis.

Making the diagnosis

Sometimes advanced malignancy can obstruct a ureter slowly and quietly. It is not unusual to undertake a bone scan as part of the staging of a man with advanced prostate cancer and reveal an asymptomatic unilateral hydronephrosis and hydroureter. Most clinicians after consultation with the patient would probably elect not to treat this type of obstruction unless relief of that obstruction would contribute significantly to the patient's overall renal function. It used to be advised (and indeed was advocated in a previous edition of this book) that relief of obstruction should be avoided 'as death from renal failure appears more peaceful than death from uncontrolled malignancy'. This may well be the case but when the options of intervention versus non-intervention are presented to the patient together with their relative harms and benefits it is rare to find a patient who chooses not to be treated.

Management

If treatment is contemplated it should be as minimally invasive as possible. As a first option placement of a retrograde ureteric stent using cystoscopy and fluoroscopy seems reasonable though it does require a general anaesthetic. One of the benefits of this approach is that, if successfully placed, it requires no puncture and no external drainage device. Modern ureteric stents can be left in place for about 6 months. Some patients tolerate them very well, others seem to report considerable bladder irritation, recurrent infections, and loin pain on voiding (though this usually gets better with time). Stents can also block, encrust or migrate, though if changed according to the manufacturers instructions these complications are rare.

Sometimes placement of a retrograde stent is not possible. If the tumour obscures the ureteric orifice within the bladder then the stent will need to be placed from above, in an antegrade manner using a percutaneous puncture. It is customary to leave a nephrostomy for a day or two prior to placing a guide wire across the stricture and guiding a stent through it and down into the bladder. Very occasionally, a so-called 'rendezvous' procedure is required. A guide wire is inserted down to the malignant stricture in an antegrade manner. At the same time, the operator will resect in the region of the tip of the guide wire using fluoroscopy. Eventually, the guide wire is seen and pulled through the tumour into the bladder. Once this is done, a stent can be placed over the guide wire, across the stricture and into the bladder.

One of the problems that occur with traditional plastic stents in the presence of malignancy is blockage. Plastic stents are of small calibre and can be compressed or infiltrated by tumour. This has led a number of investigators to experiment with materials other than plastic in order to obtain long-term relief of malignant obstruction. Although a number of different types have been tried with mixed success, most of the interest rests with new generation thermo-expandable stents.[28] These prostheses have the advantage that they can be introduced into a small lumen in their unexpanded state and then expanded using warm irrigation. Their construction (like a tightly coiled spring) prevents tumour entering the lumen. Because of their metal alloy construction they are unlikely to be compressed by tumour. Moreover, if they fail they can be removed with relative ease.

It is unusual these days to have to resort to major open surgery in order to relieve obstruction. On rare occasions, such as obstruction complicated by frequent infections requiring hospitalization, operations such as nephrectomy or various forms of diversion might be contemplated.

Fistulas

Malignant urinary fistulas rarely heal, particularly so if complicated by prior radiotherapy. They can make life intolerable for the patient and nursing nearly impossible as the patient will be constantly wet. The most common ones include vesico-vaginal, vesico-colic, prostato-rectal, and uretero-enteric in addition to the various cutaneous fistulas. In the presence of extensive pelvic malignancy urinary diversion may be the only option. If life expectancy is limited then this may be achieved by nephrostomy alone. In other situations diversion with an ileal conduit or ureterostomies may be more appropriate. It would be rare to contemplate a primary repair with tissue interposition in a person with advanced malignancy.

References

1. **Taylor, M.E.** (2002). Breast cancer: chest wall recurrences. *Current Treatment Options in Oncology* **3** (2), 175–7.
2. **Cordeiro, P.O., Santamaria, E., and Hidalgo, D.** (2001). The role of microsurgery in reconstruction of oncologic chest wall defects. *Plastic and Reconstructive Surgery* **108** (7), 1924–30.
3. **Henderson, M.A., Burt, J.D., Jenner, D., Crookes, P., and Bennett, R.C.** (2001). Radical surgery with omental flap for uncontrolled locally recurrent breast cancer. *Australian and New Zealand Journal of Surgery* **71** (11), 675–9.
4. **Sato, M., Tanaka, F., and Wada, H.** (2002). Treatment of necrotic infection on the anterior chest wall secondary to mastectomy and postoperative radiotherapy by the application of omentum and mesh skin grafting: report of a case. *Surgery Today* **32** (3), 261–3.
5. **Blazeby, J.M., Alderson, D., and Farndon, J.R.** (2000). Quality of life in patients with oesophageal cancer. *Recent Results in Cancer Research* **155**, 193–204.

6. Schmier, J., Elixhauser, A., and Halpern, M.T. (1999). Health-related quality of life evaluations of gastric and pancreatic cancer. *Hepatogastroenterology* **46**, 1998–2004.
7. Bancewicz, J. (1999). Palliation in oesophageal neoplasia. *Annals of the Royal College of Surgeons of England* **81**, 382–6.
8. Khulusi, S. and Morris, T. (2000). Endoscopic palliation of gastrointestinal malignancy. *European Journal of Gastroenterology and Hepatology* **12**, 397–402.
9. Davies, N., Thomas, H.G., and Eyre-Brook, I.A. (1998). Palliation of dysphagia from inoperable oesophageal carcinoma using Aitkinson tubes or self-expanding metal stents. *Annals of the Royal College of Surgeons of England* **80**, 394–7.
10. Siersema, P.D., Hop, W.C., Dees, J., Tilanus, H.W., and van Blankenstein, M. (1998). Coated self-expanding metal stents versus latex prostheses for esophagogastric cancer with special reference to prior radiation and chemotherapy: a controlled, prospective study. *Gastrointestinal Endoscopy* **47**, 113–20.
11. Carazzone, A., Bonavina, L., Segalin, A., Ceriani, C., and Peracchia, A. (1999). Endoscopic palliation of oesophageal cancer: results of a prospective comparison of Nd:YAG laser and ethanol injection. *European Journal of Surgery* **165**, 351–6.
12. Kubba, A.K. and Krasner, N. (2000). An update in the palliative management of malignant dysphagia. *European Journal of Surgical Oncology* **26**, 116–29.
13. Rice, D., Geller, A., Bender, C.E., Gostout, C.J., and Donohue, J.H. (2000). Surgical and interventional palliative treatment of upper gastrointestinal malignancies. *European Journal of Gastroenterology and Hepatology* **12**, 403–8.
14. Lowy, A.M., Feig, B.W., Janjan, N., Rich, T.A., Pisters, P.W., Ajani, J.A., and Mansfield, P.F. (2001). A pilot study of preoperative chemoradiotherapy for resectable gastric cancer. *Annals of Surgical Oncology* **8**, 519–24.
15. Wai, C.T., Ho, K.Y., Yeoh, K.G., and Lim, S.G. (2001). Palliation of malignant gastric outlet obstruction caused by gastric cancer with self-expanding metal stents. *Surgical Laparoscopy, Endoscopy & Percutaneous Techniques* **11**, 161–4.
16. Sarfeh, I.J., Rypins, E.B., Jakowatz, J.G., and Juler, G.L. (1988). A prospective, randomized clinical investigation of cholecystenterostomy and choledochoenterostomy. *American Journal of Surgery* **155**, 411–14.
17. Watanapa, P. and Williamson, R.C.N. (1992). Surgical palliation for pancreatic cancer: developments during the past two decades. *British Journal of Surgery* **79**, 8–20.
18. Sagar, P.M. and Pemberton, J.H. (2000). Surgical palliation of colorectal cancer. *European Journal of Gastroenterology and Hepatology* **12**, 409–13.
19. Law, W.L., Chu, K.W., Ho, J.W., Tung, H.M., Law, S.Y., and Cu, K.M. (2000). Self-expanding metallic stent in the treatment of colonic obstruction caused by advanced malignancies. *Diseases of the Colon and Rectum* **43**, 1522–7.
20. Sardi, A., Bolton, J.S., Hicks, T.C., and Skenderis, B.S. (1994). Total pelvic exenteration with or without sacral resection in patients with recurrent colorectal cancer. *Southern Medical Journal* **87**, 363–9.
21. Milsom, J.W., Kim, S.H., Hammerhofer, K.A., and Fazio, V.W. (2000). Laparoscopic colorectal cancer surgery for palliation. *Diseases of the Rectum and Colon* **43**, 1512–16.
22. Taylor, I. and Gillams, A.R. (2000). Colorectal metastases: alternatives to resection. *Journal of the Royal Society of Medicine* **93**, 576–9.
23. Feuer, D.J. et al. (1999). Systematic review of surgery in malignant bowel obstruction in advanced gynaecological and gastrointestinal cancer. *Gynaecologic Oncology* **75**, 313–22.
24. Rubin, S.C. et al. (1988). Palliative surgery for intestinal obstruction in advanced ovarian cancer. *Gynecologic Oncology* **34**, 16–19.
25. Bagley, D.H. and Smith, A.D., ed. (1995). Treatment of haematuria. In *Controversies in Endourology* (ed. D. Arthur and A.D. Smith), Chapter 14, pp. 220–5. Philadelphia PA: WB Saunders.
26. Mitty, H.A. and Goldman, H. (1974). Angiography in unilateral bleeding with a negative urogram. *American Journal of Radiology* **121**, 508–17.
27. Crew, J.P., Jephcott, C.R., and Reynard, J.M. (2001). Radiation induced haemorrhagic cystitis. *European Urology* **40**, 111–23.
28. Kulkarni, R.P. and Bellamy, E.A. (1999). A new thermo-expandable shape memory nickel–titanium alloy stent for the management of ureteric strictures. *British Journal of Urology International* **83**, 755–9.

8.1.4 Orthopaedic principles and management

Charles S.B. Galasko

Palliate is defined in the *Concise Oxford Dictionary* as 'alleviate (disease) without curing'. This applies to much of orthopaedic surgery but a detailed description of all types of orthopaedic palliative care is beyond the scope of this book.

Orthopaedic surgeons are involved in the treatment of patients with incurable diseases such as rheumatoid arthritis, cerebral palsy, muscular dystrophy, and other neuromuscular disorders such as Paget's disease and skeletal dysplasias.

Rheumatoid arthritis is best treated by a multi-disciplinary team which includes rheumatologists, physiotherapists, occupational therapists, and orthopaedic surgeons. Operations such as total hip replacement and total knee replacement are highly successful in relieving pain and restoring function but do not affect the underlying disorder. Surgery, however, is not without its complications and the artificial joints will not last forever.

Many of the patients with neuromuscular disorders develop secondary deformities as a result of muscle imbalance, unequal growth of abnormal muscle and normal underlying bone resulting in progressive shortening of the muscle during growth, and the effect of gravity where the underlying muscles are extremely weak. Surgery may be required to restore plantigrade feet to aid mobility, correct contractures at other sites, and treat painful subluxing or dislocated hips. One of the most significant secondary deformities is progressive scoliosis in patients with Duchenne muscular dystrophy and other neuromuscular conditions where the child is wheelchair bound. In these patients progressive scoliosis is associated with progressive pelvic obliquity which interferes with sitting balance, leads to sitting discomfort, and may eventually make sitting impossible because of the pain secondary to gross pelvic obliquity. Surgical correction of the scoliosis and spinal fusion is a major operation. In these patients the aim of surgery is to restore sitting balance and prevent the progression of the scoliosis and pelvic obliquity thus maintaining comfortable sitting. Foot deformity may affect the gait of patients who otherwise would be independently mobile and dislocation of the hip secondary to muscle imbalance may be painful and affect sitting balance.

The orthopaedic surgeon can do much to improve the quality of life of patients with neuromuscular disease by trying to prevent the secondary development of deformities and the surgical correction of the deformities should they occur.[1,2]

Metabolic bone disease (including Paget's disease of bone, osteoporosis, and osteomalacia) is extremely common. Paget's disease of bone may be associated with secondary arthritis, particularly of the hip, and stress fracture. Osteoporosis predisposes to fractures, most commonly in the proximal femur, distal radius, and spine. The management of osteoporotic fractures forms a major component of the work of orthopaedic surgeons. This is likely to increase and it is anticipated that the number of osteoporotic fractures will at least double by 2020. In many instances the underlying metabolic disease can be treated medically. The orthopaedic surgeon can do much to improve the quality of life of these patients by treating the complications of these disorders, for example, by joint replacement in patients with Paget's disease and secondary osteoarthritis of the hip, prophylactic stabilization of a pagetoid bone with impending fracture, internal fixation of pagetoid stress fractures and osteoporotic fractures, and replacement arthroplasty of some osteoporotic fractures.

The prevalence of degenerative disorders of the musculoskeletal system will increase in an ageing population. These disorders cannot be cured but there is much that the orthopaedic surgeon can do to improve the quality of life of patients with disabling degenerative disorders of their musculoskeletal system.

Although less common than the above, the orthopaedic surgeon is also involved in the palliative care of patients with malignant disease. It is this aspect of palliative orthopaedics that will be discussed in greater detail in this chapter. With improvements in oncology, patients with malignant disease are living longer and the management of their secondary skeletal disease is becoming more important in their overall care.

Primary bone tumours

The treatment depends on the extent of the neoplasm. If it is localized the emphasis is on radical resection and chemotherapy (the type of resection depending on the type, site, and local dissemination of the tumour) in an attempt to obtain a cure and, in the appendicular skeleton maintain the limb. If the tumour has disseminated or is inoperable, the treatment is palliative.

Skeletal metastases

The principles of treatment are:

1. pain relief,
2. preservation/restoration of skeletal integrity,
3. preservation/restoration of function, and
4. elimination or prevention of neurologic compromise.

The main role of the orthopaedic surgeon in the treatment of metastatic bone disease is in the treatment of the complications of skeletal metastases.

Pain is the commonest form of presentation of skeletal metastases and occurs in two-thirds of patients with radiographically detectable lesions;[3] the pain may develop before the lesion becomes detectable on radiographs. Unless a further complication arises, the orthopaedic surgeon is not usually involved in the treatment of painful skeletal metastases but he may be involved in their diagnosis as patients with bone pain are frequently referred initially to an orthopaedic surgeon. Magnetic resonance imaging is the most sensitive method of detecting early metastases, especially in the spine, but skeletal scintigraphy is still probably the investigation of choice in assessing the degree of skeletal dissemination.

A variety of modalities of treatment are available for the management of non complicated skeletal metastases and the associated pain, including analgesics, non steroidal anti-inflammatory drugs, endocrine therapy, radiotherapy, chemotherapy, and systemic radionuclide therapy (e.g. using phosphorus-32, strontium-89, samarium-153, rhenium-186, and tin-117m).

Bone pain may be the presenting feature of hypercalcaemia and an increase in bone pain was the commonest symptom of this condition in at least one series.[4]

Bisphosphonates are being increasingly used in the management of skeletal metastases, particularly in mammary cancer and myeloma (see below). They may also be useful in the treatment of painful skeletal metastasis due to hormone refractory prostatic cancer.[5] Tumour growth is dependent on angiogenesis. Multiple strategies for therapeutic angiosuppression are currently under investigation. These include matrix metalloproteinase inhibitors, endothelial cell proliferative inhibitors, and antivascular endothelial growth factor.[6]

The orthopaedic surgeon is usually not involved in the treatment of the painful uncomplicated lesion although he may have made the diagnosis but becomes involved when one of the following complications arise.

1. impending fracture,
2. pathological fracture,
3. spinal instability, and
4. spinal cord or cauda equina compression.

Impending fracture

Large lytic metastases are evident on plain radiographs and usually present with pain. By the time a large, lytic metastasis has developed there is considerable disruption and the cortex of the affected bone has been involved. The mechanism of pain in these lesions is not fully understood but may be associated with infractions of the surrounding bone or stretching of the periosteum by growing tumour.[7] The risk of fracture is high. Fidler[8] reported a fracture incidence of 3.7 per cent when 25–50 per cent of the cortex was involved, 61 per cent when the degree of cortical involvement ranged between 50 and 75 per cent, and 79 per cent if more than 75 per cent of the cortex was involved.

Mirels[9] proposed a scoring system for diagnosing impending fractures. His scoring system was based on the site of the metastasis, the severity of pain, the radiographic appearance of the lesion, and the size of the lesion. The most serious prognostic signs were lesions in the peritrochanteric region, pain sufficiently severe to interfere with function, lytic lesions, and lesions that involved more than two-thirds of the bone. Hipp et al.[10] thought that routine radiographs and computer tomography (CT) scans were unreliable in predicting pathological fracture but that new methods, which applied engineering principles to the analysis of quantitative CT, may provide a more objective guideline for determining the treatment strategy for each patient. Menck et al.[11] suggested that the indications for prophylactic internal fixation for femoral metastases were a ratio of $\geqslant 0.60$ between the width of the metastasis and the diameter of the bone, axial cortical destruction in the femoral neck $\geqslant 13$ mm and in other parts of the femur $\geqslant 30$ mm, or cortical destruction of the circumference $\geqslant 50$ per cent.

Although most fractures are associated with large, lytic metastases, they can also occur in other types of metastases. There are basically three types of bone destruction consequent upon skeletal metastases.[12,13]

Geographic

These are large solitary, well-defined lytic areas, more than 1 cm in diameter and usually with a sharply demarcated edge (Fig. 1).

'Moth-eaten'

These are multiple, smaller, lytic metastases (2–5 mm) which may coalesce to form larger confluent areas. The margins are usually ill defined.

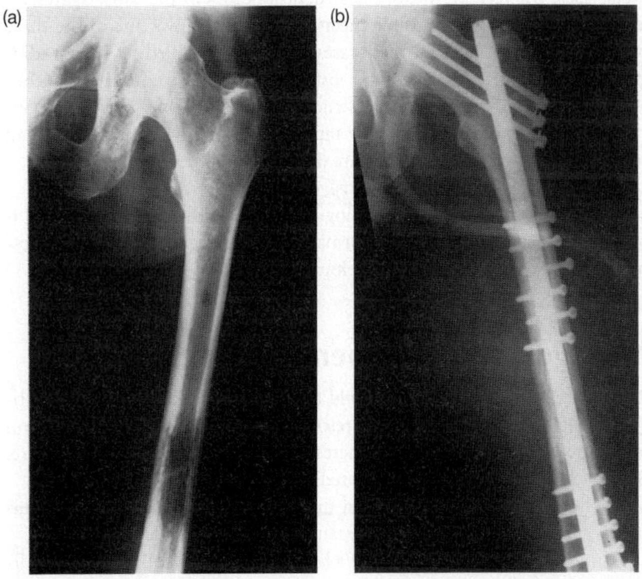

Fig. 1 (a) Patient with a large 'Geographic' metastasis in the mid shaft of the femur. There is a further metastasis in the proximal femur. Prophylatic stabilization of the femur is indicated, but it is essential that all the lesions in the affected bone should be stabilized. (b) Stabilization of the femur using an interlocking nail and stabilizing the entire bone. The lesion in the mid femoral shaft has been curetted out and the defect filled with methyl methacrylate.

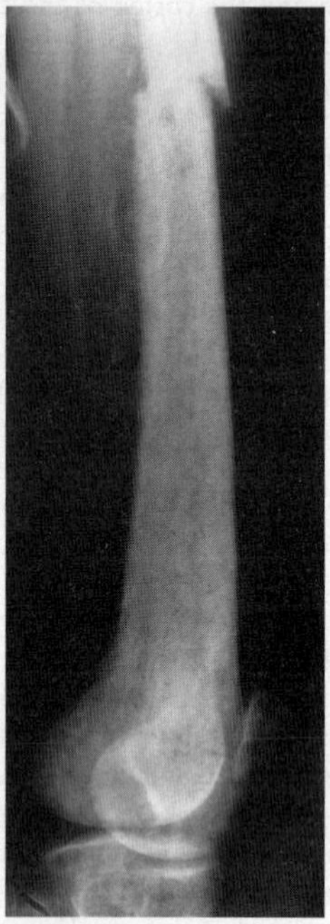

Fig. 2 Patient with multiple 'permeative' metastases. The entire femur was riddled with these tiny lesions. He has developed a pathological fracture through the shaft of the femur.

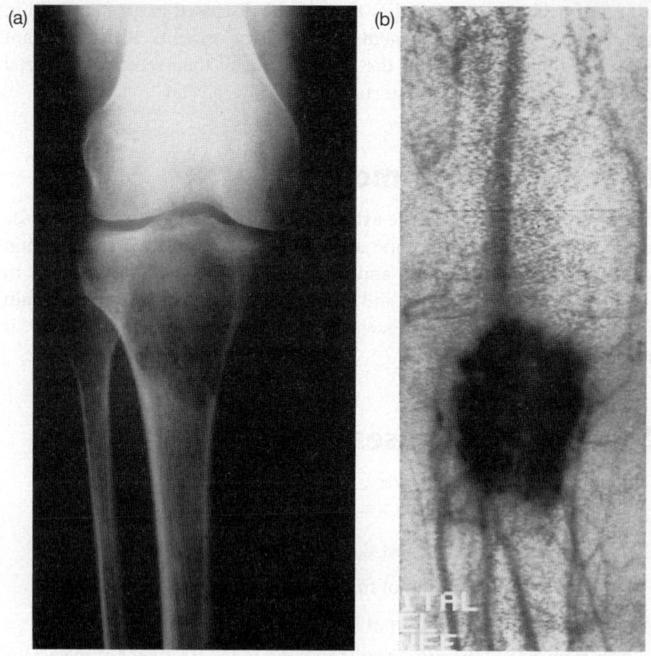

Fig. 3 (a) Patient with isolated metastasis from renal carcinoma in proximal tibia. (b) Arteriogram. The lesion is extremely vascular.

Permeative

These are multiple, tiny, lytic areas (usually 1 mm or less) seen principly in cortical bone (Fig. 2). The bone is weakened and such lesions predisposed to pathological fracture, even though a large lytic metastases cannot be seen on the radiographs.

Geographic destruction is usually found in the slowest developing metastases, whereas permeative destruction occurs in the most aggressive lesions. A patient with multiple metastases usually shows one of the three principle patterns. Skeletal metastases are often classified by their radiographic appearance as osteolytic, osteoblastic, or mixed although they almost invariably induce bone destruction and new bone formation concurrently except in myeloma, very rapidly enlarging lytic metastases, and solid deposits from leukaemia where the lesion may be purely lytic.[14]

Osteoblastic lesions have a low risk of fracture.

Weight bearing pain is a physiological test of structural integrity and is probably caused by excessive deformation in the region of the bone destruction. It often precedes the development of a pathological fracture.

Management of impending fractures

Radiotherapy relieves pain but could temporarily weaken the bone, probably due to the associated transient resorption. Should this occur, irradiation of a large lytic metastasis could increase the risk of pathological fracture. Biopsy of the metastasis may also predispose to fracture.

Bisphosphonates play no role in the management of large, lytic metastases. They may be useful in the treatment of other smaller metastases.

Primary internal stabilization of a large lytic deposit, followed by irradiation, has certain advantages. It is easier to fix the bone whilst it is still intact; the rehabilitation and convalescence are much shorter and easier. Prior to internal stabilization the general fitness of the patient must be assessed, the presence of malignant hypercalcaemia excluded, and the extent of the dissemination of the tumour evaluated. Resection and prosthetic replacement of an isolated skeletal metastasis, with no other evidence of dissemination, must be considered, particularly if the patient has renal carcinoma. Other factors to take into consideration include the prognosis and the medical condition of the patient. Patients who are near death (survival of 2–4 weeks) are poor candidates for surgery. Patients with breast and prosthetic carcinoma have the best overall prognosis; those with lung cancer have the worst.

Large, lytic metastases, particularly if secondary to renal carcinoma, may be very vascular, and surgery may be associated with torrential haemorrhage. Such lesions may require pre-operative arteriography (Fig. 3) and, if necessary, embolization prior to surgery.[15,16]

Where feasible, closed intramedullary nailing is preferred, with interlocking screws to provide additional stability (Fig. 2). If indicated, a biopsy specimen can be taken using bronchial forceps or through a separate incision.

Intramedullary nailing may not provide adequate stabilization for large metastases at the end of long bones and, in some sites, replacement arthroplasty may be indicated. Care must be taken to avoid producing a fracture when positioning the patient or whilst stabilizing the lesion.

It is essential that the internal stabilization of the lesion provides sufficient strength to allow unsupported use of the limb, including weight bearing in the lower limb. If the implant is not likely to provide this, the stabilization should be supplemented with methyl methacrylate cement. In this case, the tumour is removed, the cavity filled with methyl methacrylate, and the implant fixed across the methyl methacrylate whilst it is still soft, in addition to bridging normal bone above and below the lesion.

Irradiation is an essential part of treatment to inhibit further tumour growth since the latter will result in progressive bone destruction and resultant loosening of the stabilization with increased risk of fracture. Post-operative irradiation is preferred to pre-operative irradiation as the latter may pre-dispose to problems with wound healing and wound breakdown. Post-operative irradiation is usually postponed for 10–14 days following surgery. The sutures are usually left in for a minimum of 3 weeks. Metal staples should not be used to close the skin nor should zinc oxide dressings be applied as they may affect the post-operative radiotherapy.

There is some evidence to suggest that the incorporation of chemotherapeutic agents in the methyl methacrylate may inhibit local tumour growth.[17] Depending on the primary lesion the patient may also require endocrine therapy or chemotherapy and bisphosphonates may be helpful in controlling other small metastases.

Internal fixation carries the theoretical risk of disseminating tumour cells but there is no evidence that internal fixation causes increased tumour spread, even in the same bone or beyond. Furthermore, there is no evidence that the combined effect of surgical intervention and general anaesthesia has affected the overall prognosis in these patients. On the contrary, there is some evidence to suggest that internal stabilization of these lesions is associated with a lower incidence of pulmonary metastases.[18] Intramedullary reaming is associated with embolization of marrowfat and other constituents of the bone marrow. This may result in acute systemic hypertension, pulmonary hypertension, oxygen desaturation, and occasionally cardiac arrest. This is a well-recognized complication associated with reaming and pressurization of the femoral canal in procedures such as hip arthroplasty and intramedullary fixation of femoral fractures. It may also occur following intramedullary nail fixation of femoral metastases.[19]

It is important that, prior to treatment, scintigrams and radiographs are obtained of the entire length of the affected bone so that any other metastases, which may subsequently develop into a pathological fracture, are stabilized and are included in the radiotherapy field (Fig. 1). A pathological fracture at the edge of an implant, particularly if the implant has been fixed with methyl methacrylate, is more difficult to treat than if there was no implant in the bone. Furthermore, it is difficult to irradiate a metastasis if part of the lesion has been included in a previous field.

In general terms, patients with skeletal metastases have a better prognosis and a longer survival than patients with visceral metastases and it is important that the stabilization outlives the patient. Patients who only have skeletal metastases may have a lengthy survival but suffer considerable morbidity from cancer mediated bone destruction. Dürr et al.[20] found that solitary bone involvement and more than 12 months latency between the diagnosis of renal cell carcinoma and the detection of bone metastases were the two independent factors with a significant prognostic value. Patients who fulfilled these criteria had a 5-year survival of 54 per cent, patients who fulfilled one criterion had a 5-year survival of 17 per cent, and those with no positive factor had a 5-year survival of 0 per cent.

Skeletal metastases occur commonly and it is essential to diagnose them early if the patient is to receive optimum treatment. The diagnosis of the lesion should include not only the site of the lesion and the degree and site of dissemination but also the presence of any complications, the extent of soft tissue involvement particularly with spinal metastases, and the vascularity of the lesion. Magnetic resonance imaging is the most sensitive method of detecting early metastases in the spine but skeletal scintigraphy is probably still the investigation of choice in detecting skeletal metastases elsewhere and particularly in assessing the degree of dissemination. The advantages of skeletal scintigraphy are its high sensitivity and the ability to examine the entire skeleton. The disadvantage is its low specifity. CT scanning does not have a primary role in the diagnosis of skeletal metastases but is extremely useful in the confirmation of isolated lesions. The advantages are the axial images, the ability to reconstruct in any plane, good tissue contrast, and excellent resolution. The disadvantages are the irradiation, single scanning plane, limited areas that can be examined, and implant artefact. Magnetic resonance imaging is the method of choice for examining the spine. The advantages are the excellent contrast, the ability to image in any plane, the possibility of imaging a relatively large area, and the demonstration of the soft tissues. It may demonstrate the relation of the lesion to other structures. The bone cortex is not as well visualized as with CT scanning and the presence of metal implants including surgical clips may preclude its use. Biochemical bone markers play no role in the diagnosis of skeletal metastases but may be helpful in assessing the response to treatment.[21] If there is any doubt about the diagnosis, a biopsy should be taken before definitive surgery. Nailing of an isolated lesion of a long bone which subsequently proves to be a primary bone tumour is a disaster, spreading tumour cells throughout the marrow cavity and often precluding limb salvage surgery.

Appropriate surgical management of skeletal metastases is cost effective, especially if previously immobile patients can mobilize and dependent patients become able to care for themselves.

Pathological fractures

Although virtually every malignant tumour can metastasize to bone and may be associated with a pathological fracture, mammary carcinoma is responsible for approximately 50 per cent (Table 1); the other tumours that commonly metastasize to bone are prostatic, lung, and renal cancers. Multiple myeloma is the second commonest cause of a malignant pathological fracture.

The commonest site of pathological fracture is in the femur (Table 2) but virtually any long bone is at risk. It is probable that the majority of tumour emboli which develop into skeletal metastases are carried there via Batson's vertebral plexus[22,23] which would explain why some tumours appear to metastasize preferentially to bone and would also explain the sites of skeletal metastases and pathological fracture. The development of a pathological fracture is not necessarily a terminal event. With improvements in chemotherapy and endocrine therapy the average survival has increased during the past two decades. The survival is related to the primary tumour. Virtually no patient with bronchial carcinoma has survived, following a pathological fracture, for more than 6 months[24–26] whereas the mean survival for patients with prostatic carcinoma is in excess of 2 years and many patients with mammary carcinoma have lived for several years after a pathological fracture has been suitably treated.

There are three aspects to the treatment of pathological fractures.

1. The orthopaedic management,
2. localized irradiation, and
3. the treatment of the causative tumour.

The orthopaedic management will be discussed in this chapter.

Table 1 Pathological fractures

Primary tumour	Number of patients	Number of fractures
Breast	105	120
Lung	25	26
Prostate	22	23
Kidney	8	8
Rectum	6	6
Stomach	4	4
Bladder	3	3
Melanoma	2	2
Uterus	2	2
Thyroid	1	1
Colon	1	1
Oesophagus	1	1
Bile duct	1	1
Cervix	1	1
Penis	1	1
Squamous cell	1	1
Lymphoma	4	5
Leukaemia	6	6
Myeloma	25	35
Not known	5	5
Total	224	252

Table 2 Pathological fractures

Site		Number
Pelvis		3
Femur	Transcervical	60
	Intertrochanteric	26
	Subtrochanteric	29
	Shaft	41
	Distal	10
Humerus	Proximal	20
	Shaft	50
	Distal	3
Tibia	Proximal	2
	Shaft	1
Radius	Shaft	2
Ulna	Shaft	1
Clavicle		3
Mandible		1
Total		252

Localized irradiation is an essential part of treatment in an attempt to control the underlying tumour and prevent further osteolysis with resultant loosening of the implant. It can be delayed until the wound has healed but this is not essential. The implant does not appear to affect the irradiation providing orthovoltage is not used, because of dose enhancement in the immediate vicinity of the metal and the shielding of tumour cells in the shadow of the implant.

As with impending fractures, the evaluation of a patient with a pathological fracture includes an assessment of the general fitness of the patient, the degree of dissemination of the tumour, the primary tumour, and the presence of other complications. In addition to a careful clinical examination, the evaluation includes appropriate blood tests, radiographs, skeletal scintigraphy, and magnetic resonance imaging of the affected bone. If the primary lesion is not known or if there is any uncertainty about the origin of a pathological fracture, a biopsy of the lesion is essential. This can be carried out at the time of surgical stabilization.

Orthopaedic management of pathological fractures

The orthopaedic management depends on the site and type of fracture as well as the general condition of the patient. Patients who are terminal, with a life expectancy of only 2–4 weeks should be made comfortable but should not be subjected to major surgery. The pain relief gained by orthopaedic intervention, in the vast majority of patients, warrants surgery in patients whose life expectancy is more than 4 weeks and who are fit for the procedure. Clohisy et al.[27] attempted to evaluate the effect of surgery for impending fractures and pathological fractures using SF36. They found that the heterogeneous nature of the patients undergoing surgical treatment, the potential for very poor health status prior to surgery, low patient enrolment, and high attrition through death made it very difficult to study these patients. High attrition and adjuvant treatment with radiation or chemotherapy made it impractical to draw firm conclusions about the effect of surgical treatment on the overall quality of life but they found a trend towards improvement in selected health status measures for both physical and mental health. Analysis of patient-rated health-status scores as predictors of survival indicated that improvement in these scores 6 weeks following surgery was associated with an increased survival.

Pathological transcervical femoral fractures do not unite, irrespective of the method of treatment[24] probably due to the effect of irradiation on an area where fractures are associated with impaired vascularity. This failure to unite is irrespective of the degree of displacement. Replacement arthroplasty gives the best results. The type of arthroplasty depends on the degree of tumour involvement. If there are no metastases in the acetabulum, proximal femoral endoprosthetic replacement may be all that is required but generally total hip replacement is preferred, particularly if the patient has a reasonable life expectancy. The endoprosthesis should be fixed with methyl methacrylate cement and should be long enough to stabilize other metastases in the affected femur. If the acetabulum is involved, total replacement arthroplasty is required. The type of pelvic reconstruction depends on the amount of bone destruction. Where it is limited, the tumour is curetted from the acetabulum and a conventional total hip replacement arthroplasty is carried out, the defect being filled with methyl methacrylate. If there is more extensive involvement of the acetabulum, reconstruction may be required at the time of arthroplasty.[28] Scintigrams or magnetic resonance images should be obtained of the rest of the femur prior to surgery. If there are more distant metastases, these should be stabilized at the time of replacement arthroplasty, a long stemmed femoral component being used. If there are lesions distal to the stem of the prosthesis, additional stabilization of the distal femur may be required. At the time of surgery intralesional curettage of the lesion is carried out and the defect filled with methyl methacrylate.

Unstable pathological fractures of the pelvis requiring surgical intervention are uncommon and usually occur in the periacetabular area. Harrington[28] has classified these fractures according to the location and extent of the tumour or radiation lysis.

Class I: The lateral cortices and superior and medial acetabular walls are structurally intact. Conventional fixation of the acetabular component of a total hip arthroplasty is usually successful.

Class II: The medial wall is deficient. This requires a reconstructive technique that transfers the stress of weight bearing away from the deficient wall and onto the intact acetabular rim. Some form of protrusion shell is required.

Class III: The lateral cortices and the medial and superior acetabular walls are deficient. These require constructive techniques that transmit load bearing stresses into structurally intact bone in the upper ilium and adjacent to the sacro–iliac joint. Harrington[29] used Steinmann pins, a protrusion shell, and an acetabular component of a total hip replacement with methyl methacrylate to reconstruct such fractures whereas others use specially constructed modular prostheses with a pelvic saddle prosthesis. The durability of reconstruction for periacetabular metastases requires appropriate use of acetabular mesh, Steinmann pins, acetabular reinforcement rings, a long stemmed femoral prosthesis, and methyl methacrylate cement. A protrusio cup may be needed. The combination of an allograft combined with a prosthesis to form an allograft–prosthetic composite is another alternative but this carries a higher risk of infection, in addition to non-union, and most authors avoid this in the management of metastatic fractures.

Patients who have acetabular metastases that are refractory to radiation and chemotherapy have a short life expectancy. Surgical reconstruction generally provides satisfactory short-term palliation, is sufficiently durable to exceed the life expectancy of the patients, and is associated with an improvement in the patient's quality of life.[30,31]

Nilsson et al.[32] reported the outcome of reconstruction, using the Harrington technique, in 32 patients with advanced periacetabular metastatic destruction. The median survival was 11 months; 13 patients lived for a year or more. At follow-up after 1 year, 10 of the 13 were free of pain at rest and weight-bearing, six were walking with and seven without support and 11 lived outside a health care facility. Kunisada and Choong[33] found that all 37 patients who underwent total hip arthroplasty with pelvic reconstruction for metastatic periacetabular tumour showed improvements in hip pain, analgesic use, ambulation, and mobility post-operatively.

Percutaneous injection of methylmethacrylate has also been suggested for the management of acetabular metastases. Weill et al.[93] reported on 18 patients with painful acetabular malignancies; 17 patients had metastases and one had multi-focal bone sarcoma. In four patients (22 per cent) there was total improvement, seven (39 per cent) gained 'clear improvement', four (22 per cent) obtained moderate improvement, in one (6 per cent) there was no improvement, and in two (11 per cent) their symptoms worsened in keeping with a cement leak in contact with the sciatic nerve and towards to joint. They concluded that percutaneous injection of acrylic surgical cement was a minimally invasive and low cost procedure that provided immediate and long-term pain relief of acetabular metastases in some patients.

It is sometimes impossible to stabilize a pathological fracture of the proximal humerus because of the lack of bony support proximal to the fracture. This may also apply to pathological fractures at other ends of long bones. Under these circumstances prosthetic replacement should also be considered.

The indications for endoprosthetic replacement in the management of skeletal metastases are:

1. resection of a solitary metastasis, usually secondary to renal carcinoma, with the aim of achieving a wide margin of healthy tissue around the tumour;
2. transcervical femoral fractures;
3. some metastases or pathological fractures involving the epiphysis or metaphysis of long bones, where other forms of treatment are not practical; and
4. some failures of previous fixation.

Most intertrochanteric femoral fractures are probably best treated by internal fixation, prosthetic replacement being reserved for those patients where extensive destruction of the proximal femur precludes effective internal fixation. Diaphyseal fractures are probably best fixed with an interlocking nail whereas fractures of the intertrochanteric region and supracondylar region may be best treated by implants specifically designed for these sites. Unreamed intramedullary nails have also been used for impending and pathological femoral fractures.[34]

Unlike transcervical femoral fractures, the majority of pathological fractures involving the rest of the femur or tibia are best treated with internal fixation, usually supplemented with methyl methacrylate[35,36] even though this may interfere with callus formation. Internal fixation provides definite advantages over external support. It gives the patient greater and much more rapid relief of pain; it is associated with easier nursing, more comfortable turning of the patient and prevention of pressure sores; it allows much earlier mobilization of the patient and discharge from hospital. It is also thought to increase the prospect of union. As with impending fractures, it is essential that the stabilization allows weight bearing. Methyl methacrylate will not compensate for inadequate mechanical instability due to a poorly positioned implant or the use of an inadequate implant. As indicated above, the method of fixation must also stabilize other metastases in the involved bone to avoid the risk of subsequent fracture adjacent to the implant.

Internal fixation of humeral pathological fractures has also been shown to be of benefit, in that it provides the patient with much greater mobility, earlier use of the limb, and more rapid and greater relief of pain although the advantages over conservative treatment are not as marked as with pathological fractures of the lower limb.[37] McCormack et al.[38] suggested that a functional brace was indicated if the patient had a limited life expectancy but for those patients expected to survive for more than 3 months, internal fixation was the method of choice to ensure pain relief, restoration of function, and avoid later refracture. Some fractures of the distal humerus might be best treated in a cast brace because of the complexity of internal stabilization, with radiotherapy. The type of stabilization depends on the site of fracture and includes the Russell–Taylor humeral nail,[39] or Ender nails.[40] Harrington[29] advised two Rush rods supplemented by intramedullary methyl methacrylate for supracondylar humeral fractures. In most cases intramedullary fixation is preferable to plating and interlocking nailing is indicated for diaphysial fractures.

The principle of fixation of a pathological fracture is different from that of a traumatic fracture. In the latter instance the aim of surgery is to fix the bone in as optimum a position as possible, with minimum dissection of the soft tissues to encourage healing by bone. In many instances this may require protected weight bearing for some weeks. With pathological fractures, secondary to metastatic cancer, one cannot reliably depend on bone healing and in a patient with a limited life expectancy, optimum palliation requires unrestricted use of the limb following surgical stabilization. Fractures of the humeral shaft treated by internal fixation and post-operative radiotherapy may heal rapidly with exuberant callus.

Multiple fractures

Some patients present with several pathological fractures and each must be treated on its merits. This may require the stabilization of several fractures.

Fracture through an isolated metastasis

Occasionally patients present with an isolated skeletal metastasis. They usually present with pain, may present with an impending fracture, and occasionally with a pathological fracture. The commonest primary is renal carcinoma and, provided there is no other evidence of dissemination of the tumour, resection of the lesion should be considered, usually in the form of local resection and prosthetic replacement, including intercalary replacement of the diaphysis. It is easier to excise and replace a metastasis than one that has already fractured. The haematoma consequent upon the latter may cause widespread dissemination of tumour, which may make it impossible to carry out a local resection with adequate margins.

Baloch et al.[41] evaluated the results of excision of a solitary bony metastasis from renal cell carcinoma in 25 patients. Two patients underwent excision only, five had an amputation, and 18 had excision with endoprosthetic replacement. One, three, and five year cumulative survival rates were 88, 54, and 13 per cent, respectively. Of the 25 patients, 10 remained free from disease at a mean follow-up of 42 months and 15 developed further metastases at a mean of 17.4 months. One patient suffered a local recurrence which was treated by further excision. The 5-year survival, in these patients, from the time of nephrectomy was 45 per cent. They recommended radical excision of the solitary bony metastasis in renal cell carcinoma, both for control of local disease and because of the prospect of long-term survival in some patients.

Post-operative irradiation

Local irradiation does not interfere with fracture healing, providing the fracture is adequately immobilized.[25,42] The optimum time for irradiation is after surgery has been carried out. Pre-operative irradiation makes the tissues more friable. Ideally, post-operative irradiation should wait until the wound has settled down. It is not necessary to wait until the sutures have been removed but the sutures should be retained for 3–4 weeks in patients who have undergone surgery for metastatic cancer. Under these circumstances, the radiotherapy can be given at about 12–14 days post-operatively.

Townsend et al.[43] estimated the probability of achieving normal use of the extremity following internal stabilization was 53 per cent for patients who had had post-operative radiation versus 11.5 per cent for patients who underwent surgery alone ($P < 0.01$).

Spinal instability

Back pain is a frequent symptom of disseminated carcinoma and in 10 per cent is due to spinal instability.[44] Carcinoma of the breast is the commonest primary tumour associated with spinal instability, followed by myeloma (Table 3). However, any tumour can metastasize to the spine and can cause sufficient destruction to render the spine unstable. Spinal instability can cause excruciating pain which is mechanical in nature. In its severe form the patient is only comfortable when lying absolutely still. Any movement, including log rolling by two or three trained nurses is associated with agonizing pain and the patient may not be able to sit, stand, or walk because of

Table 3 Type of primary tumour in patients who had spinal instability secondary to tumour-induced osteolysis

Primary tumour	Number of patients
Breast	40[a]
Multiple myeloma	10
Kidney	6
Lung	4
Prostate	4
Melanoma	2
Cervix	2
Bladder	1
Colon	1
Uterus	1
Ovary	1
Stomach	1
Vagina	1
Parotid	1
Lymphoma	1
Chordoma	1
Chondrosarcoma	1
Histiocytoma	1
Unknown	1
Total	80

[a] One patient underwent lumbar stabilization 22 months after a successful dorsal spinal stabilization.

Table 4 Results of spinal stabilization in 80 patients with spinal instability secondary to tumour-induced bone destruction

Result	Percentage of patients
Complete relief of pain	89
Partial relief of pain	5
Failure of implant ± infection	5
Paraplegia but pain controlled	1
Death due to septicaemia	1

the pain, even with the use of a spinal orthosis. In the milder form, the patient may be relatively free from pain when wearing a rigid spinal orthosis but any movement of the back, for example, turning in bed, sitting, or standing may be impossible without support. Plain radiographs show destruction of bone with vertebral collapse of a greater or lesser degree. It is unusual to see a discreet fracture. Nevertheless spinal instability should be considered the equivalent of a pathological fracture in an appendicular bone because the pain is due to the instability and not due to the metastasis. Radiotherapy or chemotherapy will not alleviate the pain. Like pathological fractures of the long bones, stabilization is required for pain relief. The spine can be stabilized from either an anterior or a posterior approach, the decision depending on the site and the extent of the lesion(s). Vascular metastatic lesions necessitate pre-operative embolization, particularly if anterior stabilization is being considered.(16,45) This is particularly relevant with regard to metastases from renal carcinoma but other tumours may also be very hyperaemic. Spinal metastases usually initially involve the vertebral body and if the unstable segment is limited to one or possibly two adjacent vertebrae anterior resection of the lesion together with vertebral replacement using a cage filled either with bone graft or methyl methacrylate, and stabilization with a Kaneda device is indicated whereas, if the lesion is more extensive or there are two areas of instability posterior stabilization is required, modern spinal implants having the flexibility of being fixed with intrapedicular screws, hooks, and/or wires. When the lumbar spine is stabilized the rod is contoured to provide a lumbar lordosis and when the thoracic spine is stabilized the rod is contoured to provide a dorsal kyphosis. If posterior fixation is inadequate for stabilization of the spine in patients with metastatic lesions in the fourth and fifth lumbar vertebrae a combined anterior and posterior stabilization procedure might be necessary.

The spine can be stabilized by either a posterior or anterior approach. We have previously reported on 80 patients with spinal instability secondary to metastatic disease (Table 4).(46) Of these 70 were treated with posterior stabilization, five by anterior stabilization, and five by combined anterior and posterior stabilization. With the exception of the first patient, all patients were investigated to determine whether there was any tumour within the spinal canal and if there was, the spinal cord or cauda equina (depending on the level of the lesion) was decompressed at the time of stabilization. Magnetic resonance imaging is the investigation of choice to determine whether there is any extension of the tumour into the canal.

Seventy-one (89 per cent) of the 80 patients had complete relief of pain (Table 4) and four patients (5 per cent) had partial relief. In five patients treatment failed. One patient died of septicaemia after a wound infection. Another patient developed a deep infection requiring removal of the implant. Two patients in whom we had used Harrington rods and hooks had loosening of the implant. This instrumentation was the best available at that time, but now has been superseded by a variety of other implants with better fixation. Since the new implants have become available and have been used, we have not had a further case of loosening. The fifth patient had complete relief of pain but paraplegia developed as a result of an extradural bleed despite removal of the clot. He had received anticoagulants for the treatment of an intercurrent illness. Pre-operative radiation therapy predisposed to infection.

The first patient in this series had multiple myeloma and had been treated with chemotherapy and radiation therapy. Although his tumour was successfully treated, he was unable to sit up or walk and was confined to bed because of excruciating back pain. Even log rolling by two trained nurses was painful. At the time that he was evaluated, the only device that was available to stabilize the spine was the Harrington rod. His thoracic spine was stabilized with two Harrington rods and the hooks were cemented in situ with methyl methacrylate. Even though one hook loosened, the patient had total relief of pain to the extent that he could walk and could return home. Eight months later, he was re-admitted to the hospital with clinical signs of cord compression. The implant had to be removed at the time of decompression of the spinal cord. As indicated above it is now routine practice to evaluate the spinal canal and, if there is any tumour in the canal, irrespective of whether the patient has neurological symptoms or not, the spinal cord or cauda equina, depending on the level of involvement, is decompressed at the time of stabilization. In the initial years of our series, the spinal canal was evaluated with myelography; subsequently, it was evaluated with myelography combined with CT; and, currently, magnetic resonance imaging is used. The decompression is carried out prior to stabilization. Once the decompression has been carried out the spine is stabilized irrespective of whether the patient has neurological signs or symptoms.

Anterior decompression and stabilization is now carried out more frequently. In the next 44 patients referred with spinal instability, 25 underwent anterior decompression and stabilization, 15 underwent posterior decompression and stabilization, two underwent combined anterior and posterior stabilization with decompression, and in two patients the disease was too advanced for surgery to be considered. One patient with breast carcinoma underwent anterior decompression and stabilization but her tumour did not respond to treatment and 7 months later she required posterior decompression and stabilization for neural compression.

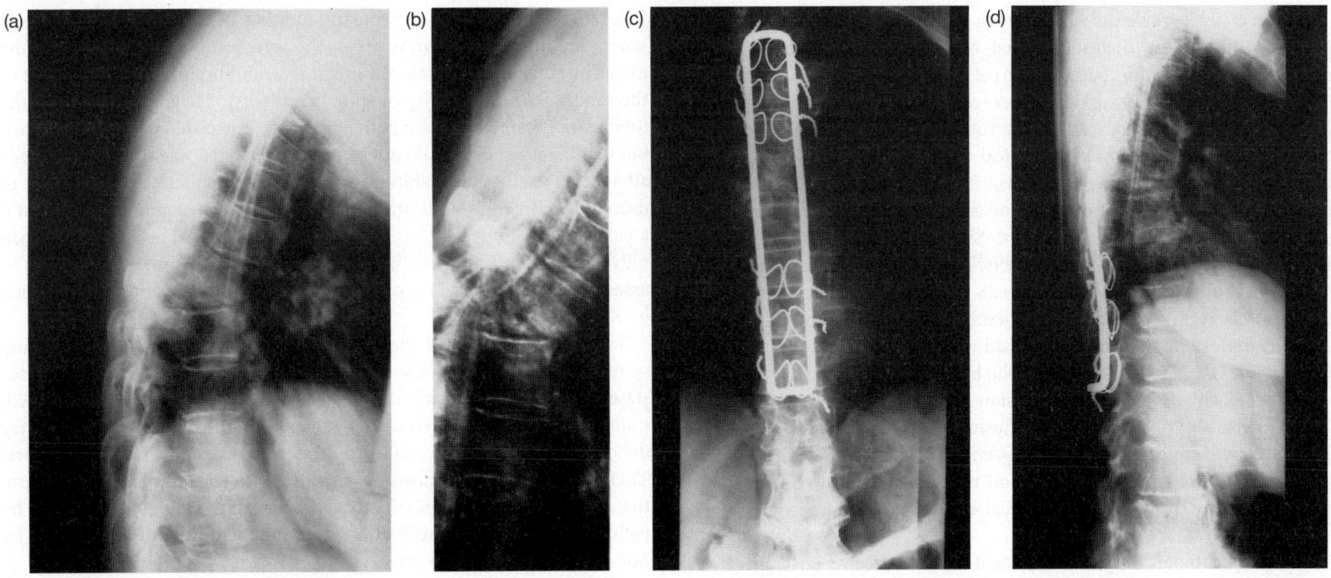

Fig. 4 Patient with mammary carcinoma. (a) Lateral radiograph of the spine, showing complete collapse of the dorsal vertebra with spinal instability. (b) Myelogram. There is compression of the spinal cord at the level of the lesion. In addition to the agonising back pain the patient also had marked weakness affecting both lower limbs. (c) and (d) Antero-posterior and lateral radiographs following posterior decompression of the spine, stabilization with a Hartshill rectangle, and correction of the kyphus. The patient obtained complete relief of pain and regained full neurological function.

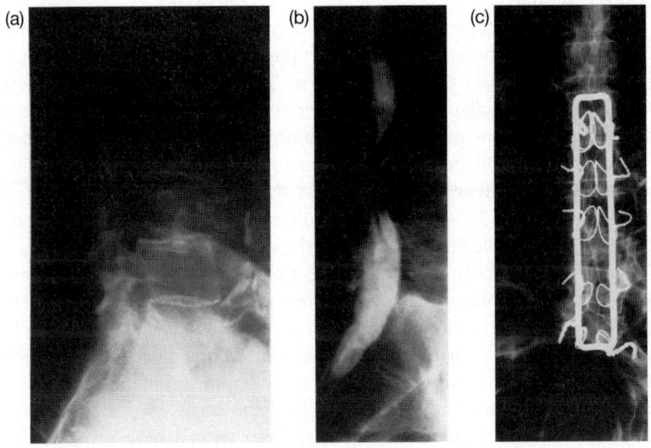

Fig. 5 Patient with mammary carcinoma who presented with excrutiating pain due to spinal instability. Clinical examination revealed significant weakness affecting both lower limbs. (a) Lateral radiographs showing destruction of L4 with spinal instability. (b) Myelogram. Extradural tumour is compressing the cauda equina. (c) The patient was treated with posterior decompression and stabilization using a Hartshill rectangle. She obtained complete relief of pain and made a full neurological recovery.

Thirty-four of the 80 patients in our first series[46] showed some clinical evidence of compression of their spinal cord or cauda equina, usually weakness of the lower limbs severe enough to affect walking or standing (Figs 4 and 5). These patients were treated by decompression at the time of stabilization.[46] Twenty-three of the 34 (68 per cent) obtained major recovery of neurological function, sufficient to allow them to walk without orthoses and restoration of bladder function where it had been compromised. It must be emphasized that these patients presented primarily with pain due to spinal instability. In two of these patients cord compression recurred 10 and 14 months after decompression.

Others have reported similar results. Onimus et al.[48] reported the results of operative intervention in 100 patients with spinal metastases. Anterior stabilization was carried out in 58 patients, posterior stabilization in 33, and combined anterior and posterior stabilization in nine. Pre-operatively, 96 patients had vertebral pain and 43 had radicular pain. Walking was impossible for 50 patients, either due to neural compression or due to pain caused by the spinal instability. Thirty-five (70 per cent) of the 50 patients were able to walk after decompression and stabilization. Of the 38 patients with a neurological deficit pre-operatively, 30 had a decrease of the deficit post-operatively. Sixty-two patients completely stopped using analgesics after the operation. Overall, there was clinical improvement in 80 of the 100 patients.

Weigel et al.[49] retrospectively assessed 86 surgical interventions in 76 consecutive patients with symptomatic spinal metastases. Back pain and/or radicular pain was present in all patients before surgery and in 76 per cent of patients it was severe. Sixty per cent of patients obtained marked pain relief following surgery and 29 per cent moderate improvement. In 11 per cent there was no change. No patients reported worsening of pain. The relief of pain was permanent, returning only in patients who developed local tumour recurrence or new metastatic spinal disease. The mean post-operative survival was 13.1 months, the highest survival rates being seen in patients with multiple myeloma and breast carcinoma with very poor survival in patients with lung carcinoma (2.1 months) and melanoma (1.5 months). Survival in patients with these tumours was significantly shorter than the overall survival of the other 64 patients ($P < 0.0001$). In 45 instances there was a neurological deficit. Improvement was observed in 58 per cent. They found that 19 per cent of the operations were associated with complications.

Hatrick et al.[50] evaluated 42 patients who underwent surgery for metastatic disease of the spine. Post-operatively, pain improved in 38 (90 per cent), the neurological deficit in 20 of the 29 patients with a deficit (69 per cent), and the ambulatory ability in 25 of the 32 patients (78 per cent) with very restricted mobility.

Jackson et al.[51] reviewed the results in 79 patients who underwent 107 spinal operations for metastatic renal cell carcinoma. Indications for surgery included disabling pain [94 (88 per cent) of 107 procedures] and/or neurological dysfunction [55 (51 per cent) of 107 procedures]. The anatomical location and extent of the tumour determined the choice of anterior, posterior, or combined surgical approach. Internal fixation was carried out in all but three patients. Pre-operative embolization was required in approximately one-half of the patients. The median post-operative survival was 12.3 months. Significant pain reduction was achieved in 84 (89 per cent) of the 94 cases presenting with disabling pain. Neurological improvement was seen in 36 (65 per cent) of the 55 patients.

Ghogawala et al.[52] found that patients who had radiation before surgical decompression and stabilization had a three fold greater wound complication rate ($P < 0.05$) than patients who had surgery followed by radiation.

Endoscopically assisted decompression of metastatic thoracic tumours has also been described.[53] His conclusion was that endoscopic-assisted decompression could reduce morbidity, and may aid surgery by improving the surgeon's vision providing light and magnification as well as a more direct view. This author has no personal experience of thoroscopic vertebrectomy.

As with pathological fractures, patients should receive post-operative irradiation. There are occasions, however, when the patient has received the maximum tolerable dose pre-operatively and further radiotherapy would put the cord at risk of developing transverse myelitis. The underlying tumour may require treatment by endocrine therapy or chemotherapy and bisphosphonates may be indicated for other small skeletal metastases demonstrated in the pre-operative investigations. These patients require pre-operative evaluation in the same way as patients with impending or pathological fractures.

McPhee et al.[47] found that pre-operative protein depletion and perioperative administration of corticosteroids were risk factors for wound infection in patients undergoing surgery for spinal metastases.

Instability of the cervical spine is uncommon compared with involvement of the dorsal or lumbar spine but does occur (Fig. 6). The principles of treatment are the same—namely, spinal stabilization (with decompression if there is any evidence of cord compression) followed by localized irradiation (if feasible) and endocrine therapy, chemotherapy, and/or bisphosphonate therapy. Minor degrees of cervical instability can be controlled by a collar. However, if this does not control the pain, surgical stabilization is indicated. Several methods of stabilization have been used, including bone-grafting, posterior stabilization, anterior resection and stabilization, and anterior replacement.

Tokuhashi et al.[54] have developed an assessment system for the prognosis of metastatic spinal tumours. Their system employs six parameters: the general condition of the patient, the number of extra spinal bone metastases, the number of metastases in the vertebral body, metastases to the major internal organs (lungs, liver, kidneys, and brain), the primary site of the cancer, and the severity of spinal cord palsy. They concluded that the total score obtained for each patient could be correlated with the prognosis but that the prognosis could not be predicted from a single parameter. They advised an excisional operation, using extensive curettage at the time of decompression and stabilization in the patients with a good prognosis and a palliative procedure in those with a poor prognosis. The latter was aimed only at securing support with no or only partial resection of the lesion. To assess the general condition of the patient they used the criteria established by Karnofsky (1967).[55]

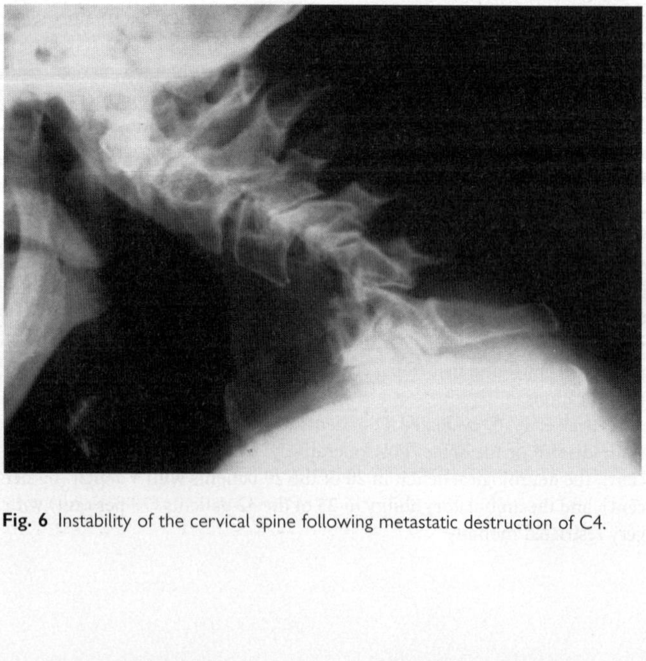

Fig. 6 Instability of the cervical spine following metastatic destruction of C4.

Tomita et al.[64] based their surgical strategy on a prognostic scoring system which used the grade of malignancy, visceral metastases (no metastases, treatable, untreatable), and skeletal metastases (solitary or isolated, multiple). Their surgical strategy was based on the prognostic score. They divided their patients into four groups depending on the prognostic score. Those with the best prognosis were treated with wide or marginal excision, the next group by marginal intralesional excision, the third group by palliative surgery with stabilization, and those with the worst prognosis by non-operative supportive care.

The mean survival time in the first group was 38.2 months, in the second group was 21.5 months, and in those treated by palliative surgery and stabilization was 10.1 months. The mean survival time of patients treated with terminal care was 5.3 months. It is this author's view that if a patient is in excruciating pain spinal stabilization is warranted even if the survival is no more than a few weeks.

Enkaoua et al.[56] assessed the utility of the Tokuhashi score and felt that it was successful as a prognostic tool except that patients with metastases from renal cancer did better than those with metastases from an unknown primary tumour.

As with appendicular lesions, the question arises as to whether impending vertebral collapse can be assessed and prophylactic stabilization carried out. Taneichi et al.[57] have attempted to do so. They suggested that there was a significant risk of collapse of thoracic vertebrae if there was 50–60 per cent tumour involvement of the vertebral body with no destruction of other structures or 25–30 per cent involvement of the vertebral body with costovertebral joint destruction and, in the thoracolumbar and lumbar spine if there was 35–40 per cent involvement of the vertebral body or 20–25 per cent of the vertebral body with pedicle destruction.

Percutaneous vertebroplasty is being used increasingly to treat patients with painful compression fractures from osteoporosis, osteolytic metastases, and multiple myeloma. The technique consists of percutaneous needle placement into the vertebral body followed by the injection of radio-opaque methyl methacrylate under radiographic guidance, resulting in reduction of pain and strengthening of the bone. Most of the cases reported where skeletal metastases have been treated have involved the thoracic or lumbar spine[61,62] but the cervical spine can also undergo vertebroplasty.[58]

It is this author's view that vertebroplasty is still experimental. There are no long follow-up studies, there is a significant risk that the presence of cement in the vertebral bodies will lead to further osteoporosis and collapse of the surrounding bone and, depending on the integrity of the cortex, the cement may be injected into the spinal canal causing damage to the spinal cord or cauda equina. Preoperative magnetic resonance scanning of patients with spinal instability frequently shows tumour within the spinal canal suggesting that if the methyl methacrylate was injected into the tumour deposit, some of it would escape into the spinal canal potentially putting the spinal cord or cauda equina at risk. Good short-term results in patients with osteoporotic compression fractures have been reported by Heini et al.[59] Lieberman et al.[60] used an inflatable bone tamp together with the methyl methacrylate in an attempt to restore vertebral height but reported cement extravasation in several instances. Most of the studies have also included only a small number of patients with a limited follow-up. There have been no randomized, controlled studies comparing vertebroplasty with standard medical therapy for osteoporosis. Significant complications are probably less than 10 per cent and have included increased pain, radiculopathies, spinal cord compression, pulmonary embolism, infection, and rib fractures.[63] Cement leakage, where reported, is common, ranging from 30 to 67 per cent but in osteoporosis did not generally lead to clinical complications.[63] They noted that cement leakage leading to radiculopathy or spinal cord injury was more common after treatment of metastases or myeloma than for osteoporotic fractures. Despite the number of articles published on this procedure, few have clearly defined the outcome measures and virtually none have provided a long-term follow-up in terms of the clinical indications, expected complications, and inherent risks. What happens with time?

Standard barium-impregnated methyl methacrylate is not sufficiently radio-opaque to be adequately and safely visualized fluoroscopically during injection. The addition of either sterile tantalum or tungsten to the methyl methacrylate greatly enhances its visibility and minimizes the risk of the cement extravasating beyond the confines of the vertebral cortices.

Compression of the spinal cord or cauda equina

Schaberg and Gainor[65] reported that cord compression occurred in 20 per cent of patients with vertebral metastases and Constans et al.[66] thought it likely that 5–10 per cent of patients developed symptomatic neurological manifestations of their metastases. Kramer[67] estimated that spinal cord compression occurred in up to 5 per cent of patients with malignancy. Compression of the spinal cord or corda equina may occur in association with spinal instability (where the treatment of choice is spinal stabilization, decompression, and post-operative radiotherapy) or in isolation. In the latter circumstance the choice of treatment (surgical decompression and stabilization, radiotherapy, and steroids) depends on the duration, severity, and rapidity of onset of the symptoms. Pain is almost invariable and persisting and increasing back pain may herald spinal cord compression. Pain is frequently localized to the site of disease and is probably caused by stimulation of pain receptors in the longitudinal ligaments, dura, or periosteum as the tumour expands. Radicular pain is less common. It is important to be aware of the possible significance of localized spinal or radicular pain. Nevertheless, by the time treatment is started up to 50 per cent of patients will no longer be able to walk and 10–30 per cent will be paraplegic.[68,69] Other symptoms include weakness, disturbance of gait, paraesthesia, urinary hesitancy or precipitancy, and constipation or spurious diarrhoea. The sequence of events is often pain, motor dysfunction, paraesthesia, and sensory loss. Pinprick and deep pain sensation may be retained until late. Results depend heavily on the neurological status of the patient at the time of starting treatment and it is important, therefore, to make the diagnosis urgently. The assessment of the patient is as described for patients with spinal instability, except that the investigations may have to be carried out as an emergency, outside normal working hours. Ideally, the investigation should only be carried out in a centre where immediate surgical decompression with stabilization is available.

When indicated, surgical decompression is urgent. It is indicated in patients with recent onset of symptoms, particularly a developing paraplegia or urinary retention of less than 24 h duration; a block, shown on the preoperative magnetic resonance image to be localized to no more than two or three segments; and in a patient with a life expectancy of at least 6–8 weeks. Once a paraplegia has been established for some days or urinary retention has been present for more than 30 h, surgical decompression with stabilization is often associated with some return of sensation and pain relief but not with useful recovery of bladder or motor function. Under these circumstances, irradiation is indicated as is the case with a more extensive block. However, occasionally anterior decompression and stabilization may be associated with major neurological recovery in patients with long-standing neurological disturbances, providing the onset of the symptoms has been gradual. In general terms, patients with a gradual onset of neurological disturbances do better than patients who have developed paraplegia and urinary retention extremely rapidly.

Because of the risk of subsequent instability, the spine must be stabilized at the time of decompression.[70–73] The decompression can be carried out anteriorly or posteriorly but it is essential that decompression is associated with stabilization to avoid the development of progressive kyphosis which may produce further compression of the spinal cord and neurological impairment. Laminectomy alone is contraindicated. Laminar removal and replacement has been described.[74]

It has previously been suggested that treatment, whether surgical or nonsurgical, should be combined with a short course of high dosage corticosteroids in order to minimize the oedema. Recently, the efficacy of steroids has been questioned, but in view of the devastating nature of this complication, it is the author's view that steroids should be used until they are shown to have no value in the treatment of this complication. Dexamethasone is usually used. If surgical decompression is undertaken post-operative radiotherapy should be given if feasible.

Laminectomy, on its own, is contraindicated. It may destabilize the spine, cause spinal instability, or lead to progressive kyphosis with stretching of the spinal cord resulting in further damage. Unfortunately, many of the articles comparing surgery with radiotherapy have compared inadequate surgery (namely laminectomy alone) with radiotherapy and it is not surprising, therefore, that they found that radiotherapy combined with steroids was at least as effective as laminectomy.[75–77] Surgical management of spinal cord or cauda equina compression is decompression (either anteriorly or posteriorly) combined with stabilization.

McBroom[78] recommended that the choice of treatment of spinal cord compression, without deformity or instability, depended on severity and speed of progression of the neurological symptoms and the radiosensitivity of the tumour. Patients with minor neurological symptoms that had been slow in onset responded favourably to irradiation, irrespective of tumour type. Dense paraparesis or rapid neurological deterioration were poor prognostic indicators, irrespective of the treatment. Under these circumstances the only chance of achieving a functional recovery lay in rapid decompression of the spinal cord. If the tumour was radiosensitive, irradiation could affect cord compression as quickly as surgery. Radio-resistant tumours are slow to respond and require urgent surgical decompression. Radiotherapy will not be as effective in symptomatic patients with progressive kyphotic spinal deformity or spinal instability. These patients require decompression and stabilization. Cowap et al.[79] evaluated 166 patients who presented to a cancer centre with malignant spinal cord compression proved by magnetic resonance imaging. The majority of patients (92 per cent) were treated with radiotherapy. Changes in functional capability over time were assessed using performance and neurological status. Over the course of treatment there was no significant change in either performance or neurological status. The median survival from confirmation of diagnosis was 82 days but survival was significantly better for those presenting with good functional status.

Prevention of bone lysis

The main role of the orthopaedic surgeon, in the palliation of patients with skeletal metastases, is in the treatment of the complications of these lesions. These complications are usually caused by bone lysis resulting in impending fracture, pathological fracture, and spinal instability. The aim of treatment, in the future, must be to prevent this progressive bone destruction. Endocrine therapy and chemotherapy may be effective in some patients. The tumour induced osteolysis is mediated by osteoclasts, the osteoclasts being stimulated by cytokines and growth factors secreted by the tumour.[80] Some of these factors may also affect the cell adhesion molecules. For example, Evans et al.[81] have shown that myeloma inhibits the normal osteoblastic response to bone destruction, this action being mediated by factors secreted by the tumour and which affect the ability of the osteoblast to adhere to the bone surface. Adhesion molecules may also explain why certain tumours metastasize to specific sites—this may be because the tumour cells have the capacity to bind selectively to those organs.

If it is not possible to destroy the cancer cells, the treatment of choice for skeletal metastases may be to inhibit the secondary bone resorption which subsequently occurs and which is responsible for much of the morbidity associated with skeletal metastases. Bisphosphonates inhibit osteoclast bone resorption. They are useful in the management of small lesions but have not yet been shown to be of benefit in large, lytic lesions that are likely to develop into a pathological fracture or spinal instability. It may be that with the development and use of these agents tumour induced bone osteolysis will be minimized and the complications that require orthopaedic intervention avoided.

Tumours only grow if they develop their own blood supply. This is dependent on local angiogenetic factors and another possibility of controlling tumour growth is by the use of anti-angiogenic drugs.

Non-metastatic orthopaedic conditions in patients with malignant disease

Patients with malignant disease may develop benign disorders of the skeleton which mimic metastases. These must be differentiated from metastatic disease and should be treated on their merits. Like any individual, a patient with a cancer may sustain a traumatic fracture. If the patient has a past history of malignancy and there is no evidence of dissemination, a biopsy should be taken from the fracture. In some instances, this may be the first manifestation of recurrence of the disease, even though there has been a long disease-free interval. The development of a non-pathological fracture may subsequently be associated with dissemination of the cancer.

Galasko and Sylvester[44] found that a benign lesion was responsible for the back pain that developed in 11 of 31 consecutive patients with an underlying malignant disease. Benign conditions included spondylolisthesis, prolapsed disc, degenerative spondylosis, pyogenic infection, and chronic back strain. The author has treated four patients with a history of malignant disease and who had a prolapsed intervertebral disc confirmed by radiological imaging. In one patient the symptoms settled with conservative management; three patients required excision of the prolapsed disc. In three patients (including the patient who responded to conservative treatment) there was no evidence of metastatic disease and none of the patients developed metastatic disease during 2 years follow-up, whereas the fourth patient had disseminated carcinoma. Nevertheless, it was felt that surgical excision was warranted in view of her severe symptoms, to improve the quality of her remaining life. This patient was alive and asymptomatic 1 year later.

Painful osteoarthritis and other orthopaedic conditions may occur in patients with malignancy and in some patients may be secondary to avascular necrosis of the femoral or humeral head as a result of irradiation or steroid treatment. If symptoms warrant it, joint replacement arthroplasty is indicated, even in the presence of dissemination carcimona.[82]

Failure of education

Although orthopaedic surgery can do much to improve the quality of life of patients with metastatic cancer, many suitable patients are not being referred. Galasko et al.[83] analyzed the records of 1412 women who were diagnosed with and treated for breast cancer in 31 hospitals. Of these 963 had complete records which were used for the analysis.

The results are shown in Table 5. All the patients who developed a pathological fracture of femur were referred for an orthopaedic appointment. Only four out of nine patients with a pathological fracture of their humerus were referred for an orthopaedic opinion. It is possible that surgery may not have been the optimum form of providing palliative care in all the other five patients but it is likely that it would have been the optimum form of treatment in many of them. Of the six patients who developed neurological

Table 5 Referral of patients who had complications from skeletal metastases

Complication	Total[a]	Referred to orthopaedic surgeon	Operative treatment	Non-operative treatment
Pathological fracture of femur	22	22 (100%)	19	3
Pathological fracture of humerus	9	4	2	7
Neurological compression	6	2	1	5
Spinal instability	51	6 (12%)	0	51

[a] The values represent the number of patients.

compression only two were referred for an orthopaedic opinion. More worrying is that only six (12 per cent) of the 51 women who developed spinal instability were referred for an orthopaedic opinion. An analysis of textbooks revealed that only two of nine oncological textbooks and one of 12 textbooks on breast cancer mentioned spinal instability secondary to metastatic disease of the spine.

The British Medical Journal, in a review article on myeloma[84] published a radiograph which was suggestive of spinal instability.[85,86] The caption to the radiograph was 'Bone pain from mechanical effects of myeloma damage (as in spine shown here) often necessitates long-term treatment with strong analgesia despite response to chemotherapy'. The reader might ask why the editor accepted this article, which made no mention of operative stabilization of the spine despite the publication, for more than 15 years, of reports on the need for stabilization and its efficacy.

In 'ABC of Breast Diseases', neither spinal instability nor spinal stabilization for metastatic cancer of the spine was mentioned.[87,88] However, it was stated that 'cord compression is not usually amenable to surgery' and that 'patients with isolated metastases causing cord compression who are fit can be treated by emergency laminectomy' even though, as indicated above, laminectomy should not be carried out in a patient who has metastatic disease of the spine unless the procedure is combined with stabilization.

O'Donoghue et al.[89,90] reported similar results. They evaluated 269 consecutive patients with breast cancer who had been seen in an internationally known breast unit. They found that patients who had a pathological fracture did better after operative intervention with adjunctive therapy than did those who had non-operative treatment alone. Forty-seven women had a total of 82 instances of structural bone destruction, 52 (63 per cent) of which involved the spine and 11 of which were associated with cord compression. The average duration of symptom-free survival was 39 weeks in the group that had been treated operatively for spinal structural bone destruction compared with 11 weeks in the group treated non-operatively. The average duration of overall survival was 22 and nine months, respectively ($P < 0.05$ for both comparisons). They concluded that clinical review by an orthopaedic surgeon would have been appropriate in 89 per cent of the instances but was sought in only 46 per cent and that operative intervention was feasible in 65 per cent but was carried out in only 31 per cent.

Domchek et al.[91] evaluated 718 women with metastatic breast cancer. During the study period 7.8 per cent had a pathological fracture, 9.7 per cent required surgical intervention to bone, 40.8 per cent underwent radiation therapy to bone, and 8.5 per cent developed spinal cord compression. The true incidence of these complications is higher in that they noted that some of their patients developed these complications after the end of the study period.

A 'Bone Metastases Clinic' has been established at the Toronto–Sunnybrook Regional Cancer Centre whose staffing includes Radiation Oncologists and

Orthopaedic Surgeons. With very few exceptions, only patients with pathological fractures or those with impending fractures of the long bone are booked into the clinic.[92] What is required are bone pain clinics for patients who have metastatic cancer based in large orthopaedic departments. Then, if a patient required operative intervention for a complication secondary to skeletal metastases, it would be carried out by the appropriate orthopaedic surgeon in that department. Treatment based on the site of involvement would include spinal stabilization with or without decompression by the spinal surgeon, proximal femoral replacement with or without acetabular reconstruction by the hip surgeon, fixation of pathological fractures by the trauma surgeon, and so on. The development of such clinics would do much to improve the quality of life of patients who have skeletal metastases.

Conclusions

The development of an impending fracture, pathological fracture, spinal instability, or spinal cord/cauda equina compression in patients with metastatic cancer is not necessarily a terminal event. These lesions are associated with severe pain. The aims of treatment are to alleviate pain, restore mobility and the use of the affected limb or spine, prevent neurological compression, or restore neurological function.

In the vast majority of impending and pathological fractures this is best achieved by internal stabilization or replacement arthroplasty. The type of stabilization depends on the site of the lesion. If the stabilization is not adequate to provide unsupported use of the limb, which includes weight bearing in a lower limb long bone it should be supplemented by methyl methacrylate. Post-operative radiotherapy is an essential part of the treatment. The causative tumour should be treated by endocrine therapy or chemotherapy as indicated and other small skeletal metastases, treated by bisphosphonates particularly in breast cancer and multiple myeloma.

Before treating the lesion, the patient must be carefully evaluated to determine the degree of dissemination of the cancer and particularly any other areas of involvement in the affected bone as this may influence the type of surgery and the radiotherapy field. Optimum treatment of these lesions may require major surgery which should not be carried out if a patient is terminal. The aim of treatment is to palliate the symptoms and improve the patients' quality of life. Orthopaedic treatment does not affect the life expectancy. Irrespective of whether surgical reconstruction is possible, the patient should always be made comfortable, kept comfortable and allowed to die with dignity.

Contraindications to surgery include a terminally ill patient, a high risk of fixation failure due to the extent of bone destruction, or the presence of infection.

The same principles apply to the management of spinal instability and neural compression. The former requires stabilization, with decompression as necessary, supplemented by post-operative radiotherapy (if feasible), chemotherapy, or endocrine therapy and bisphosphonates if indicated. The latter requires decompression combined with stabilization, post-operative radiotherapy and chemotherapy or endocrine therapy and bisphosphonates. In patients with metastatic cancer of their spine, spinal decompression must always be supplemented by spinal stabilization to prevent progressive collapse of the spine resulting in kyphosis and stretching of the spinal cord.

Although orthopaedic surgery has much to offer in the palliation of patients with complications from skeletal metastases, the minority of patients with these spinal disorders are being referred for treatment. Better education of oncologists and cancer surgeons is required.

It is hoped that improved understanding of the underlying pathophysiological changes that occur when tumour invades bone may lead to effective osteoclast inhibiting drugs, which may obviate the development of large lytic metastases in the future. The treatment of primary malignant tumours depends on the extent of the tumour but frequently the emphasis of treatment is on radical resection and chemotherapy.

References

1. **Galasko, C.S.B.** *Neuromuscular Problems in Orthopaedics.* Oxford: Blackwell Scientific Publications, 1987.
2. **Galasko, C.S.B.** (1994). The orthopaedic management of neuromuscular disease. In *Disorders of Voluntary Muscle* (ed. J. Walton, G. Karpati, and D. Hilton-Jones), pp. 851–77. Edinburgh: Churchill-Livingstone.
3. **Galasko, C.S.B.** (1972). Skeletal metastases and mammary cancer. *Annals of the Royal College of Surgeons of England* **50**, 3–28.
4. **Galasko, C.S.B. and Burn, J.I.** (1971). Hypercalcaemia in patients with advanced mammary cancer. *British Medical Journal* **3**, 573–7.
5. **Heidenreich, A., Hofmann, R., and Engelman, U.H.** (2001). The use of bisphosphonates for the palliative treatment of painful bone metastasis due to hormone refractory prostate cancer. *Journal of Urology* **165**, 136–40.
6. **Brem, S.** (1999). Angiogenesis and cancer control: from concept to therapeutic trial. *Cancer Control* **6**, 436–58.
7. **Garrett, I.R.** (1993). Bone destruction in cancer. *Seminars in Oncology* **20**, 4–9.
8. **Fidler, M.** (1981). Incidence of fracture through metastases in long bones. *Acta Orthopaedica Scandinavia* **52**, 623–7.
9. **Mirels, H.** (1989). Metastatic disease in long bones: proposed scoring system for diagnosing impending pathologic fractures. *Clinical Orthopaedics and Related Research* **249**, 256–64.
10. **Hipp, J.A., Springfield, D.S., and Hayes, W.C.** (1995). Predicting pathologic fracture risk in the management of metastatic bone defects. *Clinical Orthopaedics and Related Research* **312**, 120–35.
11. **Menck, H., Schulze, S., and Larsen, E.** (1988). Metastasis size in pathologic femoral fracture. *Acta Orthopaedica Scandinavia* **59**, 151–4.
12. **Lodwick, G.S.** (1964). Reactive response to local injury in bone. *Radiological Clinics of North America* **2**, 209–19.
13. **Lodwick, G.S.** (1965). A systematic approach to the roentgen diagnosis of bone tumours. In *Tumours of Bone and Soft Tissue*, pp. 49–68. Chicago: Year Book Publishers.
14. **Galasko, C.S.B.** (1982). Mechanisms of lytic and blastic metastatic disease of bone. *Clinical Orthopaedics and Related Research* **169**, 20–7.
15. **Roscoe, M.W.** et al. (1989). Preoperative embolization in the treatment of osseous metastases from renal cell carcinoma. *Clinical Orthopaedics and Related Research* **238**, 302–7.
16. **Olerud, C.** et al. (1993). Embolization of spinal metastases reduces peroperative blood loss. Twenty-one patients operated on for renal cell carcinoma. *Acta Orthopaedica Scandinavia* **64**, 9–12.
17. **Wang, H.M.** et al. (1996). The effect of methotrexate loaded bone cement on local destruction by the VX_2 tumour. *Journal of Bone and Joint Surgery* **78B**, 14–47.
18. **Bouma, W.H., Mulder, J.H., and Hop, W.C.J.** (1983). The influence of intramedullary nailing upon the development of metastases in the treatment of an impending pathological fracture: an experimental study. *Clinical and Experimental Metastasis* **1**, 205–12.
19. **Barwood, S.A.** et al. (2000). The incidence of acute cardiorespiratory and vascular dysfunction following intramedullary nail fixation of femoral metastasis. *Acta Orthopaedica Scandinavia* **71**, 147–52.
20. **Dürr, H.R.** et al. (1999). Surgical treatment of osseous metastasis in patients with renal cell carcinoma. *Clinical Orthopaedics and Related Research* **367**, 283–90.
21. **Galasko, C.S.B.** (1995). Diagnosis of skeletal metastases and assessment of response to treatment. *Clinical Orthopaedics and Related Research* **312**, 64–75.
22. **Batson, O.V.** (1940). The function of the vertebral veins and their role in the spread of metastasis. *Annals of Surgery* **112**, 138–49.
23. **Batson, O.V.** (1942). The role of the vertebral veins in metastatic processes. *Annals of Internal Medicine* **16**, 38–45.
24. **Galasko, C.S.B.** (1974). Pathological fractures secondary to metastatic cancer. *Journal of the Royal College of Surgeons of Edinburgh* **19**, 351–62.
25. **Gainor, B.J. and Buchert, P.** (1983). Fracture healing in metastatic bone disease. *Clinical Orthopaedics and Related Research* **178**, 297–302.

26. **Harrington, K.D.** (1988). Anterior decompression and stabilisation of the spine as a treatment for vertebral collapse and spinal cord compression from metastatic malignancy. *Clinical Orthopaedics and Related Research* **233**, 177–97.

27. **Clohisy, D.R.** et al. (2000). Evaluation of the feasibility of and results of measuring health-status changes in patients undergoing surgical treatment for skeletal metastases. *Journal of Orthopaedic Research* **18**, 1–9.

28. **Harrington, K.D.** (1981). The management of acetabular insufficiency secondary to metastatic malignant disease. *Journal of Bone and Joint Surgery* **63A**, 653–64.

29. **Harrington, K.D.** (1995). Orthopaedic management of extremity and pelvic lesions. *Clinical Orthopaedics and Related Research* **312**, 136–47.

30. **Giurea, A.** et al. (1997). The benefits of surgery in the treatment of pelvic metastases. *International Orthopaedics (SICOT)* **21**, 343–8.

31. **Marco, R.A.** et al. (2000). Functional and oncological outcomes of acetabular reconstruction for the treatment of metastatic disease. *Journal of Bone and Joint Surgery* **82-A**, 642–51.

32. **Nilsson, J.** et al. (2000). The Harrington reconstruction for advanced periacetabular metastatic destruction. *Acta Orthopaedica Scandinavia* **71**, 591–6.

33. **Kunisada, T. and Choong, P.F.** (2000). Major reconstruction for peri-acetabular metastasis. Early implications and outcome following surgical treatment in 40 hips. *Acta Orthopaedica Scandinavia* **71**, 585–600.

34. **Giannoudis, P.V.** et al. (1999). Unreamed intramedullary nailing for pathological femoral fractures. Good results in 30 patients. *Acta Orthopaedica Scandinavia* **70**, 29–32.

35. **Harrington, K.D.** et al. (1972). The use of methylmethacrylate as an adjunct in the internal fixation of malignant neoplastic fractures. *Journal of Bone and Joint Surgery* **54A**, 1665–76.

36. **Yablon, I.G. and Paul, G.R.** (1976). The augmentive use of methylmethacrylate in the management of pathologic fractures. *Surgery, Gynecology and Obstetrics* **143**, 177–83.

37. **Galasko, C.S.B.** (1980). The management of skeletal metastases. *Journal of the Royal College of Surgeons of Edinburgh* **25**, 143–61.

38. **McCormack, R.R. Jr., Glass, D.B., and Lane, J.M.** (1985). Functional case bracing of metastatic humeral shaft lesion. *Orthopedic Transactions* **9**, 50–1.

39. **Ikpeme, J.O.** (1994). Intramedullary interlocking nailing for humeral fractures: experiences with the Russell-Taylor humeral nail. *Injury* **25**, 447–55.

40. **Hyder, N. and Wray, C.C.** (1993). Treatment of pathological fractures of the humerus with Ender nails. *Journal of the Royal College of Surgeons of Edinburgh* **38**, 370–2.

41. **Baloch, K.G.** et al. (2000). Radical surgery for the solitary bony metastasis from renal cell carcinoma. *Journal of Bone and Joint Surgery* **82-B**, 62–7.

42. **Bonarigo, B.C. and Rubin, P.** (1967). Non-union of pathologic fractures after radiation therapy. *Radiology* **88**, 889–98.

43. **Townsend, P.W.** et al. (1994). Impact of post-operative radiation therapy and other perioperative factors on outcome after orthopaedic stabilization of impending or pathologic fractures due to metastatic disease. *Journal of Clinical Oncology* **12**, 2345–50.

44. **Galasko, C.S.B. and Sylvester, B.S.** (1978). Back pain in patients treated for malignant tumours. *Clinical Oncology* **4**, 273–83.

45. **Gellad, F.E.** et al. (1990). Vascular metastatic lesions of the spine; preoperative embolization. *Radiology* **176**, 683–6.

46. **Galasko, C.S.B.** (1999). Spinal instability secondary to metastatic cancer. In *Lumbar Segmental Instability* (ed. M. Szpalski, R. Gunzburg, and M.H. Pope), pp. 85–90. Philadelphia: Lippincott Williams and Wilkins.

47. **McPhee, I.B., Williams, R.P., and Swanson, C.E.** (1998). Factors influencing wound healing after surgery for metastatic disease of the spine. *Spine* **23**, 726–32.

48. **Onimus, M., Papin, P., and Gangloff, S.** (1996). Results of surgical treatment of spinal thoracic and lumbar metastases. *European Spine Journal* **5**, 407–11.

49. **Weigel, B.** et al. (1999). Surgical management of symptomatic spinal metastases. Postoperative outcome and quality of life. *Spine* **24**, 2240–6.

50. **Hatrick, N.C.** et al. (2000). The surgical treatment of metastatic disease of the spine. *Radiotherapy and Oncology* **56**, 335–9.

51. **Jackson, R.J., Gokaslan, Z.L., and Loh, S-C.A.** (2000). Metastatic renal cell carcinoma of the spine: surgical treatment and results. *Journal of Neurosurgery* (Spine 1) **94**, 18–24.

52. **Ghogawala, Z., Mansfield, F.L., and Borges, L.F.** (2001). Spinal radiation before surgical decompression adversely affects outcomes of surgery for symptomatic metastatic spinal cord compression. *Spine* **26**, 818–24.

53. **McLain, R.F.** (1998). Endoscopically assisted decompression for metastatic thoracic neoplasms. Spine **23**, 1130–5.

54. **Tokuhashi, Y.** (1990). Scoring system for the preoperative evaluation of metastatic spine tumour prognosis. *Spine* **15**, 1110–13.

55. **Karnofsky, D.A.** (1967). Clinical evaluation of anticancer drugs: cancer chemotherapy. *GANN Monograph* **2**, 223–31.

56. **Enkaoua, E.A.** et al. (1997). Vertebral metastases. A critical appreciation of the preoperative prognostic Tokuhashi score in a series of 71 cases. *Spine* **22**, 2293–8.

57. **Taneichi, H.** et al. (1997). Risk factors and probability of vertebral body collapse in metastases of the thoracic and lumbar spine. Spine **22**, 239–45.

58. **Tong, F.C.** et al. (2000). Transoral approach to cervical vertebroplasty for multiple myeloma. *American Journal of Roentgenology* **175**, 1322–4.

59. **Heini, P.F., Wälchli, B., and Berkmann, U.** (2000). Percutaneous transpedicular vertebroplasty with PMMA: operative technique and early results. A prospective study for the treatment of osteoporotic compression fractures. *European Spine Journal* **9**, 445–50.

60. **Lieberman, I.H.** et al. (2001). Initial outcome and efficacy of 'kyphoplasty' in the treatment of painful osteoporotic vertebral compression fractures. *Spine* **26**, 1631–8.

61. **Cotten, A.** et al. (1996). Percutaneous vertebroplasty for osteolytic metastases and myeloma: effects of the percentage of lesion filling and the leakage of methyl methacrylate at clinical follow-up. *Radiology* **200**, 525–30.

62. **Weill, A.** et al. (1996). Spinal metastases: indications for and results of percutaneous injection of acrylic surgical cement. *Radiology* **199**, 241–7.

63. **Garfin, S.R., Yuan, H.A., and Reiley, M.A.** (2001). Kyphoplasty and vertebroplasty for the treatment of painful osteoporotic compression fractures. *Spine* **26**, 1511–15.

64. **Tomita, K.** et al. (2001). Surgical strategy for spinal metastases. *Spine* **26**, 298–306.

65. **Schaberg, J. and Gainor, B.J.** (1985). A profile of metastatic carcinoma of the spine. *Spine* **10**, 19–20.

66. **Constans, J.P.** et al. (1983). Spinal metastases with neurological manifestations. Review of 600 cases. *Journal of Neurosurgery* **59**, 111–18.

67. **Kramer, J.** (1992). Spinal cord compression in malignancy. *Palliative Medicine* **6**, 202–11.

68. **Shaw M.D.M., Rose, J.E., and Paterson, A.** (1980). Metastatic extradural malignancy of the spine. *Acta Neurochirurgica* **52**, 113–20.

69. **Shapiro, W.R. and Posner, J.B.** (1983). Medical versus surgical treatment of metastatic spinal cord tumours. In *Controversies in Neurology* (ed. R.A. Thompson and J.R. Green), pp. 57–65. New York: Raven Press.

70. **DeWald, R.L.** et al. (1985). Reconstructive spinal surgery as palliation for metastatic malignancies of the spine. *Spine* **10**, 21–6.

71. **Johnson, J.R., Leatherman, K.D., and Holt, R.T.** (1983). Anterior decompression of the spinal cord for neurological deficit. *Spine* **8**, 396–405.

72. **Kostuik, J.P.** (1983). Anterior spinal cord decompression for lesions of the thoracic and lumbar spine, techniques, new methods of internal fixation, results. *Spine* **8**, 512–31.

73. **Siegal, T. and Siegal, T.** (1985). Vertebral body resection for epidural compression by malignant tumours. *Journal of Bone and Joint Surgery* **67A**, 375–82.

74 **Fidler, M.W. and Bongartz, E.B.** (1988). Laminar removal and replacement: a technique for the removal of epidural tumour. *Spine* **13**, 218–20.

75 **Findlay, G.F.G.** (1984). Adverse effects of the management of malignant spinal cord compression. *Journal of Neurology, Neurosurgery and Psychiatry* **47**, 761–8.

76. **Cobb, C.A.III., Leavens, M.E., and Eckles, N.** (1977). Indications for non-operative treatment of spinal cord compression due to breast cancer. *Journal of Neurosurgery* **47**, 653–8.

77. **Gilbert, R.W., Kim, J.H., and Posner, J.B.** (1978). Epidural spinal cord compression from metastatic tumour: diagnosis and treatment. *Annals of Neurology* **3**, 40–51.

78. **McBroom, R.** (1988). Radiation or surgery for metastatic disease of the spine. *Royal Society of Medicine Current Medical Literature—Orthopaedics* **1**, 97–101.
79. **Cowap, J., Hardy, J.R., and A'Hern, R.** (2000). Outcome of malignant spinal cord compression at a cancer centre: implications for palliative care services. *Journal of Pain and Symptom Management* **19**, 257–64.
80. **Galasko, C.S.B.** (1976). Mechanisms of bone destruction in the development of skeletal metastasis. *Nature* **263**, 507–8.
81. **Evans, C.E.** et al. (1992). Myeloma affects both the growth and function of human osteoblast-like cells. *Clinical and Experimental Metastasis* **10**, 33–8.
82. **Galasko, C.S.B.** *Skeletal Metastases.* London: Butterworths, 1986.
83. **Galasko, C.S.B., Norris, H.E., and Crank, S.** (2000). Spinal instability secondary to metastatic cancer. Current concepts review. *Journal of Bone and Joint Surgery* **82-A**, 570–6.
84. **Singer, C.R.** (1997). ABC of clinical haematology. Multiple myeloma and related conditions. *British Medical Journal* **314**, 960–3.
85. **Galasko, C.S.B.** (1997). Multiple myeloma. Surgical stabilisation often provides good pain relief. *British Medical Journal* **315**, 186.
86. **Krikler, S.J.** (1997). Multiple myeloma. Surgery is often more effective than analgesia for mechanical pain. *British Medical Journal* **315**, 186.
87. **Leonard, R.C., Roger, A., and Dixon, J.M.** (1994). ABC of breast diseases. Metastatic breast cancer. *British Medical Journal* **309**, 1501–4.
88. **Leonard, R.C.F., Roger, A., and Dixon, J.M.** (1995). Metastatic breast cancer. In *ABC of Breast Diseases* (ed. J.M. Dixon), London: British Medical Publishing Group.
89. **O'Donoghue, D.S., Howell, A., and Walls, J.** (1997). Implications of fracture in breast cancer bone metastases. *Journal of Bone and Joint Surgery* **79-B** (Suppl. i), 97.
90. **O'Donoghue, D.S., Howell, A., and Walls, J.** (1997). Orthopaedic management of structurally significant bone destruction in breast cancer bone metastases. *Journal of Bone and Joint Surgery* **79-B** (Suppl. i), 98.
91. **Domchek, S.M.** et al. (2000). Predictors of skeletal complications in patients with metastatic breast carcinoma. *Cancer* **89**, 363–8.
92. **Andersson, L.** et al. (1999). The ultimate one-stop for cancer patients with bone metastasis: new combined bone metastasis clinic. *Canadian Oncology and Nursing Journal* **9**, 103–4.
93. **Weill, A., Kobaiter, H., and Chiras, J.** (1998). Acetabulum malignancies: technique and impact on pain of percutaneous injection of acrylic surgical cement. *European Radiology* **8**, 123–9.

8.1.5 Interventional radiology

Tarun Sabharwal, Anne P. Hemingway, and Andy Adam

One of the most significant medical discoveries was that of X-rays by Roentgen in November 1895. Exactly a century later, the discipline of radiology would be unrecognizable to the early pioneers. Conventional radiographic techniques have been joined by other modalities, including computerized tomography, nuclear medicine, ultrasound, and magnetic resonance imaging. Added to all these diagnostic modalities has been the discipline of interventional radiology.[1,2] The emergence of this specialty has been made possible by enormous technological advances in relation to catheter and instrument design and manufacture, imaging systems, and radiological expertise. Interventional radiological procedures have virtually replaced several more invasive and hazardous surgical alternatives. Other interventional techniques offer completely new therapeutic options. Some diagnostic radiological procedures are frequently followed by therapeutic manoeuvres. For example, percutaneous antegrade pyelography, performed to delineate the site and nature of renal obstruction, is usually followed immediately by the placement of a nephrostomy drainage catheter.[3] Purely diagnostic procedures, such as percutaneous biopsy, will not be discussed in any detail, as they are largely inappropriate for the patient with a known terminal or neoplastic process receiving palliative care.

All interventional procedures carry some risk, which is related to the underlying condition, the nature of the procedure, and the experience of the radiologist. Therefore, it is important in patients with advanced malignant disease receiving palliative care to contemplate only those procedures that will alleviate symptoms, and in which the potential benefits outweigh the risks.

Interventional radiology can make a significant contribution to the palliation of patients with irresectable malignant tumours, as many of the procedures can relieve symptoms without the need for general anaesthesia, a prolonged stay in hospital, or the discomfort associated with recovery from a surgical operation. The vast majority of procedures are performed using local anaesthesia and mild sedation. The emphasis in this chapter is on the indications, contraindications, and likely outcomes, rather than on detailed technical descriptions.

Therapeutic interventional radiological procedures

A summary of procedures that may be useful in patients undergoing palliative care is shown in Table 1.

Percutaneous puncture and drainage procedures

Utilizing fluoroscopy, ultrasound, or computerized tomography it is possible to image and drain obstructed renal and biliary systems, cysts, abscesses, and effusions.

Renal tract[4]

Antegrade pyelography and percutaneous nephrostomy are used in the management of a variety of situations, including malignant obstruction of the urinary tract, haemorrhagic cystitis secondary to chemotherapy (where it is desirable to divert the urine to 'rest' the bladder), and in patients with recto-vaginal or recto-vesical fistula caused by pelvic malignancy. Diversion of urinary flow may assist in healing of the fistulas, ease nursing problems, and allow patients to become 'dry' (Fig. 1).

Table 1 Interventional radiological procedures

Procedure	Examples of indications
Drainage	Malignant obstruction of renal and biliary tract, pleural effusions, ascites
Dilation/stenting	Malignant gastrointestinal, biliary, ureteric and airway obstruction, superior or inferior vena caval obstruction, etc.
Feeding	Venous access—Hickman lines peripherally-inserted central catheter (PICC) lines Percutaneous gastrostomy
Extraction	Retrieval or resiting of venous lines
Infusion	Regional, selective infusion of chemotherapeutic agents
Embolization	Hormone producing metastases, primary hepatocellular carcinoma, skeletal metastases, etc.
Neurolysis	Coeliac ganglion in pancreatic cancer
Vertebroplasty	Vertebral metastasis, osteoporosis
Tumour ablation	Liver, renal, bony, and soft tissue tumours

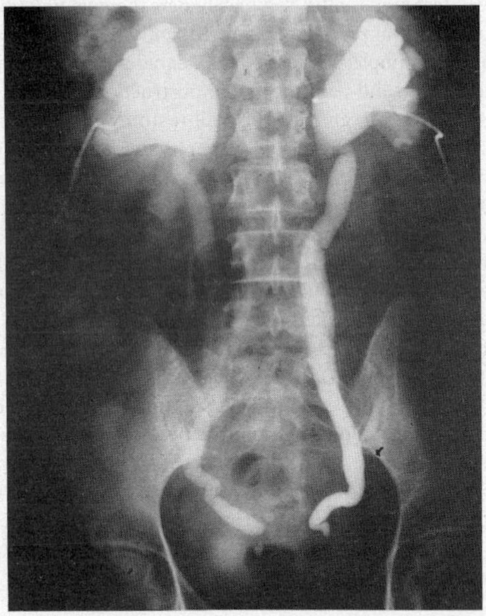

Fig. 1 Percutaneous renal drainage.

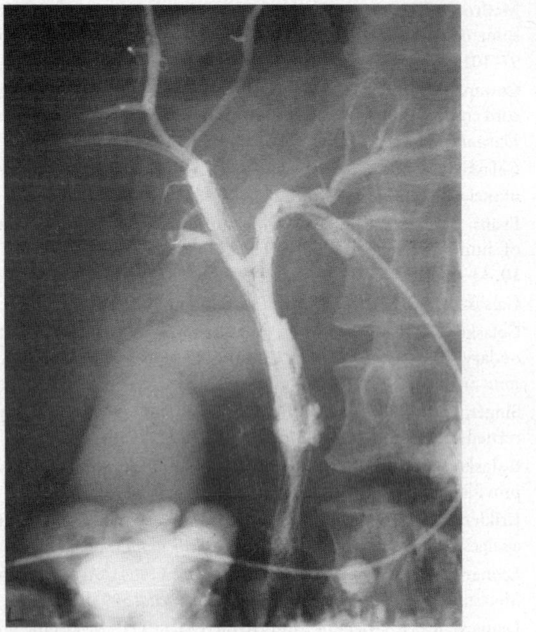

Fig. 2 Percutaneous biliary drainage.

The pelvicalyceal system is initially punctured with a fine gauge needle through which radiographic contrast medium is instilled to determine the level of obstruction. Urine can be aspirated for microbiological and cytological examinations. Percutaneous nephrostomy entails the insertion into the collecting system of a pigtail configuration catheter with multiple, large side-holes. If drainage is to be of short duration, an external bag may be satisfactory; however, if long-term drainage is required and if it is possible to cross the area of obstruction, an internal stent is preferred,[5] as it allows the patient to be free of 'bags'. It is noteworthy that, in most cases, it is possible to manipulate a catheter across an area of apparently complete obstruction. Although a contrast study may indicate total obstruction, a hydrophilic guide wire can usually be advanced through the 'obstruction', as it finds the (very narrow) lumen and follows it. The balloon catheter can then be advanced over the guide wire to dilate the stricture and restore patency before a stent is inserted.

In patients with pelvic malignancy and fistulas to the perineum it may prove necessary to combine nephrostomy with ureteric embolization using steel coils or segments of gelatine sponge to prevent any urine reaching the skin of the perineum.[6] A catheter can be manipulated into the ureter and embolic materials, such as steel coils and sterile sponge, can be injected to occlude the ureter.

Biliary tract

Ultrasound is used to determine the site of malignant biliary tract obstruction, following which percutaneous transhepatic cholangiography is performed. An external drain is inserted into the dilated biliary system to allow decompression and is usually followed immediately by insertion of an internal–external drain or an endoprosthesis (Fig. 2). Stents may be inserted endoscopically for lesions affecting the low common bile duct or percutaneously in patients with lesions at the hilum of the liver. Self-expandable metallic endoprostheses can be inserted using relatively small introducing catheters and yet they achieve a large internal diameter when released across the obstructing lesion.

The commonest form of occlusion of plastic biliary endoprostheses is bile encrustation, the occurrence of which is inversely proportional to the calibre of the stent. As self-expandable metallic stents have a much larger internal lumen than plastic endoprostheses, they are much less prone to occlusion due to encrustation of bile. However, they can become blocked by tumour growing through the mesh of the stent (ingrowth) or extending above or below the endoprosthesis (overgrowth). The overall failure rate of plastic stents is in the region of 30–40 per cent, whereas that of metallic stents is 10–15 per cent. The frequency of cholangitis is approximately 30 per cent in patients with plastic stents and approximately 10 per cent in patients with metallic endoprostheses. Occluded plastic stents can be replaced using a variety of endoscopic or percutaneous techniques. Occluded metallic endoprostheses cannot be removed but their patency can be restored by the introduction of a second device inserted coaxially within the first. Unless life expectancy is very short, it is well worth considering restoring the patency of an occluded stent, as this can greatly improve the patient's quality of life.[7,8]

Malignant pleural effusions

Most patients with a malignant pleural effusion (MPE) will have symptoms referable to it. While effusions due to lymphoma, small-cell lung cancer, and germ cell tumours may recede with systemic therapy, the remainder usually require local, palliative treatment. The most common aetiologies are lung cancer, breast cancer, lymphoma, ovarian cancer, and gastric cancer. Patients with MPE have a mean life-expectancy of only 6–12 months. A patient who presents with an MPE should first have a diagnostic and therapeutic thoracocentesis. This can be done under ultrasound guidance. It is important to assess for symptom improvement and the ability of the lung to re-expand. The fluid will re-accumulate in almost all patients, at which time local treatment is needed. This typically consists of tube thoracostomy, usually followed by instillation of a sclerosing agent (doxycycline, bleomycin, or talc) to chemically induce pleurodesis.[9] A tunnelled pleural catheter (Denver Biomaterials, Inc., Golden, CO) is also available for those patients who are ineligible or fail sclerotherapy. This is a 66-cm long 15.5 French soft silicone catheter with a polyester cuff to promote fibrosis to the subcutaneous tissue and multiple side-holes to enhance drainage. A valve in its hub is opened only when a dilator is passed through it. This prevents inadvertent entry of air or leakage of fluid. The drainage system consists of a vacuum bottle with a pre-connected tube that has a dilator at its end to pass into the hub of the catheter. Drainage will typically take no longer than 15 min and should be performed at least every other day. In the outpatient setting, this can be done by a visiting nurse, family members, or the patient.

Abscess drainage[10]

Percutaneous puncture of an abscess cavity under ultrasound guidance, computerized tomography, or magnetic resonance imaging and aspiration of contents for bacteriological analysis can be followed by insertion of a drainage catheter. It is possible to instil antibiotics into the cavity and percutaneous drainage may be effective either as the definitive treatment or as a temporary measure until the appropriate surgery can be undertaken.

Dilatation techniques[2]

Dilatation procedures are most commonly employed for the treatment of non-malignant conditions in the vascular tree (percutaneous transluminal angioplasty). However, these techniques can also be applied to benign and malignant stenoses and occlusions in other systems, including the gastrointestinal tract, and the renal and biliary systems.

Gastrointestinal tract

Within the gastrointestinal tract, fluoroscopically-guided balloon dilatation has proved to be a particularly useful technique. Dilatation alone is unlikely to be effective in malignant strictures and should be followed by some form of stenting.

Oesophagus

The main indication for oesophageal stenting is the alleviation of dysphagia in patients with irresectable oesophageal cancer. Rigid plastic tubes inserted endoscopically have been used for several years. More recently, self-expandable metallic endoprostheses have become available.[11] Such stents are usually covered with plastic in order to prevent ingrowth of tumour through the wall of the stent. They can be introduced using fluoroscopic guidance under light sedation, unlike rigid plastic tubes that are too large to be inserted without the use of general anaesthesia in many patients. Placement of a metallic stent across a tight stricture produces a virtually immediate and substantial improvement in swallowing. A commonly used device is the Ultraflex stent (Boston Scientific Corp., USA), which consists of a woven Nitinol mesh, and is available in covered and uncovered forms. The procedure can be performed rapidly, on an outpatient basis if necessary. The quality of swallowing can be graded from 0 for normal swallowing to 4 for complete dysphagia. The mean dysphagia score of patients with oesophageal carcinoma treated with self-expandable metallic endoprostheses is 1.[12] Most patients treated with rigid plastic tubes have a dysphagia score greater than 2, and the majority can manage only a liquid or semi-liquid diet. A prospective randomized comparison has shown that although metallic stents are more expensive than rigid plastic tubes, they are cost-effective, because they minimize the rate of complications and reduce the length of hospital stay.[13]

Other palliative options for relieving dysphagia in patients with oesophageal cancer include surgery, radiotherapy, chemotherapy, brachytherapy, and endoscopic laser therapy. Metallic stents relieve dysphagia better than endoscopic laser therapy does, which should be reserved for special cases, such as exophytic tumours.[12] Stent insertion is a straightforward procedure with negligible mortality and low morbidity, and seldom needs to be repeated in the majority of patients.

Plastic-covered stents are also very useful in the management of malignant oesophageal fistulas. Unlike fistulas associated with benign diseases, which may heal with conservative therapy, fistulas associated with malignant lesions do not heal spontaneously. Without definitive treatment, most patients succumb to malnutrition and thoracic sepsis within weeks. Radiological insertion of a covered metallic stent can result in immediate sealing of the fistula and the patient can drink fluids a few hours after the procedure, resuming a normal diet on the following day[11] (Fig. 3).

Gastroduodenal and colorectal

Self-expanding metallic stents are playing an increasingly important role in the treatment of gastroduodenal obstruction and acute colonic obstruction.[14,15] Patients with these conditions are often elderly and frail with dehydration and electrolyte imbalance. Self-expanding stents offer a non-surgical therapeutic alternative that rapidly relieves the obstruction and improves their clinical condition, with a high success rate and low morbidity.

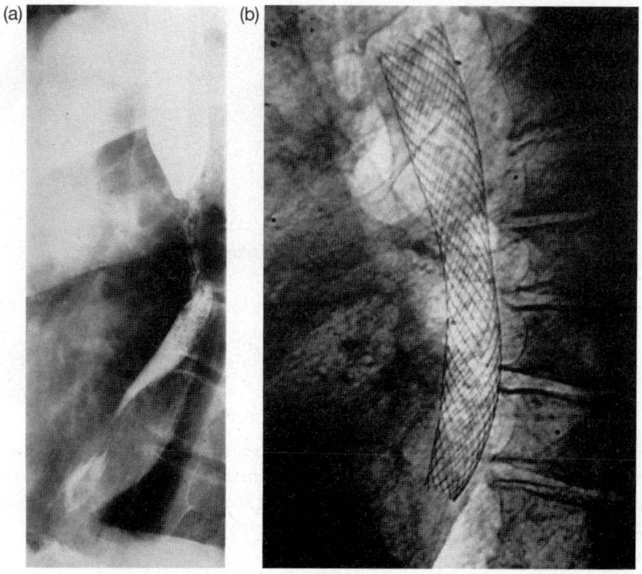

Fig. 3 Oesophageal stenting.

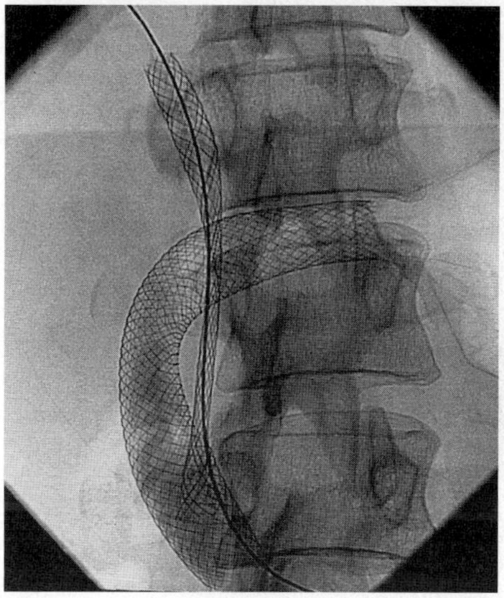

Fig. 4 Concurrent percutaneous biliary (wallstent) and gastroduodenal (enteral) stent in patient with inoperable pancreatic cancer.

Currently the 22-mm 'Enteral' Wallstent (Schneider, Bulach, Switzerland) seems the most suitable stent because of its high longitudinal flexibility, adequate self-expanding force, and small diameter introducer system (Fig. 4).

Percutaneous puncture and decompression of the caecum (in cases of distal obstruction) and for afferent loop obstruction have been described.[16]

Tracheobronchial

Self-expandable metallic stents can be inserted in the trachea or main bronchi of patients with irresectable tracheobronchial malignancy to restore patency of the airways and prevent collapse and/or infection of the lung distal to a malignant stenosis.[17] This procedure is best carried out under general anaesthesia, as a combined effort between an interventional radiologist and a bronchoscopist. Bronchoscopic visualization is used to

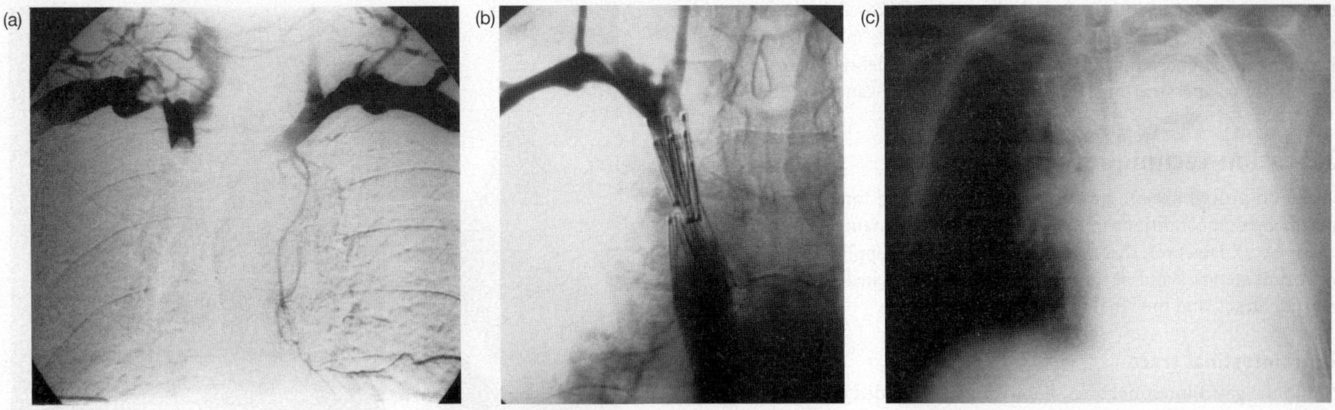

Fig. 5 Superior vena caval stenting. (a) Superior venocavogram reveals extensive thrombosis and narrowing of the superior vena cava by tumour. (b) Following selective thrombolysis, metallic stents have been placed across the compressed area which was initially dilated with a balloon. A repeat venogram confirms patency of the superior vena cava. (c) A chest radiograph shows the stents in place and the extensive tumour affecting the left hemithorax and mediastinum. The patient's symptoms showed immediate improvement and had completely resolved by 24 h.

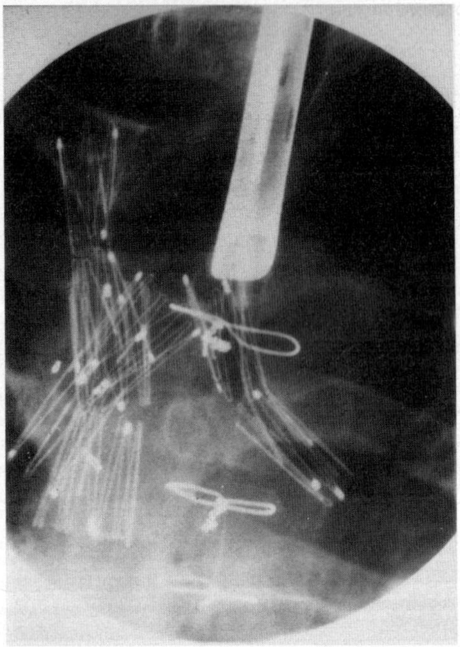

Fig. 6 Tracheal and superior vena cava stenting. Double bronchial stents and superior vena cava stents in a patient with myasthenia gravis with compression following surgery and radiotherapy. (Reproduced with kind permission from I.D. Irving and R. Dick.)

determine the position of the stricture, the limits of which are marked with a radio-opaque marker. The stricture is then dilated under fluoroscopic guidance. Following dilatation, a self-expandable metallic stent (such as a Wallstent endoprosthesis) is released across the stricture, again under fluoroscopic guidance. This can result in significant symptomatic improvement and prevent infection and abscess formation beyond an obstructing lesion. There are few indications for inserting metallic stents in benign disease of the airways. However, successful palliation in a case of irresectable benign disease has been reported.(18) Placement of plastic-covered metallic stents in the trachea is an effective method of managing tracheo-oesophageal fistulae unsuitable for treatment with covered oesophageal stents.(19)

Venous obstruction

The superior vena cava syndrome often represents as a very distressing pre-terminal event in patients with thoracic malignancy. It is most commonly related to mediastinal neoplasia, particularly primary and secondary lung tumours and lymphoma. The obstruction, which can be partial or complete, can be caused by caval compression and/or invasion by tumour and is frequently complicated by venous thrombosis.

Superior venocavography delineates the site and extent of the obstruction. If extensive thrombosis is present, selective intravenous thrombolysis with a catheter placed within the thrombus is undertaken under local anaesthesia. Percutaneous transfemoral dilatation of the narrowed superior vena cava is followed by the insertion of a self-expandable metallic endoprosthesis. Flow is restored immediately, providing excellent and immediate palliation of symptoms(20) (Fig. 5). This procedure can be performed prior to, in conjunction with, or after therapy, including radiotherapy or chemotherapy (Fig. 6). Malignant involvement of the inferior vena cava can be managed in a similar fashion. All patients with malignant superior or inferior vena caval obstruction should be considered for this relatively straightforward and usually successful procedure, which can readily improve their quality of life.

Percutaneous insertion of an inferior vena cava filter is indicated in patients with recurrent pulmonary embolism refractory to or unsuitable for treatment with anticoagulation therapy and in those patients with free-floating thrombus in the inferior vena cava.(21)

Feeding techniques

Venous access

Central venous access may be essential in some patients with terminal disease for feeding and the delivery of medication, particularly analgesia. A variety of long-term venous access systems (e.g. tunnelled central venous catheters, peripherally inserted central catheters (PICCs), and venous ports), have been developed for insertion under fluoroscopic and ultrasound guidance.(22,23) The procedure is now usually performed in the radiology department under local anaesthesia and strict asepsis.(24) The main advantage over the surgical venous cut-down technique is that performing the procedure under fluoroscopic guidance ensures that the tip of the catheter is always in the correct position and virtually eliminates the need for repositioning the catheter at a later date. The procedure is rapid, well tolerated by the patient, and associated with high success and low complication rates.(25) In our experience, it is virtually always possible to gain venous access using interventional radiological methods. The rate of occurrence of pneumothorax when using a subclavian approach is approximately 1 per cent. This complication is very rare when access is gained via the internal jugular vein. The long-term complications of occlusion and infection of the catheter are not significantly different from those observed when a surgical method of venous access is used. The traditional surgical method of placement without imaging guidance is associated with a misplacement rate of approximately 6 per cent, whereas this complication does not occur when catheter placement is performed under imaging guidance.

Percutaneous gastrostomy

Nutritional support is commonly required in patients with end-stage disease. This sometime raises difficult questions particularly in relation to parental nutrition (see Chapter 8.4.3). Enteral feed is generally a simpler option and can be accomplished by the insertion of gastrostomy tubes. The insertion of a feeding gastrostomy tube either under fluoroscopic or endoscopic guidance and local anaesthesia can significantly improve the patient's well being and ease of management, often avoiding the need for uncomfortable psychologically distressing nasogastric tubes and intravenous lines. A gastrostomy tube can be readily managed in the home environment by the patient's family and carers as well as by nursing staff.[26]

Gastro-jejunostomy tubes are preferable when there is gastric outlet obstruction or in cases of gastro-oesophageal reflux.

Extraction techniques[2,27]

Developments in intravenous feeding therapy and monitoring techniques have led to a vast increase in the number of indwelling venous cannulas and catheters. Unfortunately, these occasionally break or become disconnected and a part or all of the catheter is 'lost' within the venous system.[28] It is important to retrieve these intravascular foreign bodies as they not only perforate vascular structures and cause dysrhythmias but also act as a seat of infection, particularly in immunosuppressed patients. Surgical retrieval of catheter fragments is hazardous (and sometimes impractical), necessitating a thoracotomy. It is almost invariably possible to retrieve these catheter fragments, which usually lodge within the right side of the heart or the pulmonary arteries, percutaneously under fluoroscopic guidance. Detailed descriptions of all the retrieval techniques available are beyond the scope of this chapter but any interventional radiologist offering a comprehensive vascular service is well advised to become acquainted with the various methods and have the necessary equipment available.[29]

The ability to snare or 'catch' the end of a catheter can also be of value when the tip of an indwelling central venous catheter has become displaced into the jugular vein. It is usually possible to 'pull' such a catheter back into a correct position using a percutaneous vascular approach under local anaesthesia.

Infusion

The ability to site vascular catheters in virtually any area of the body in either the venous or arterial system has enabled the radiologist/clinician to deliver a variety of chemotherapeutic agents directly to the site of disease. Cytotoxic agents, thrombolytic agents, and analgesics can be delivered safely and effectively by this method, if required.

Vascular embolization[2]

The deliberate occlusion of arteries and/or veins by the injection of embolic agents through selectively placed catheters, is one of the major therapeutic applications of interventional radiology in the patient with neoplastic disease. This technique has been employed in the management of severe and disabling symptoms from a very wide variety of tumours throughout the body. Embolization, which usually involves a percutaneous technique with local anaesthesia, offers an attractive alternative to surgery under general anaesthesia and, in some situations, is the only therapeutic option available. A wide variety of embolic agents are available.[30] The broad categories of substances used include particulate emboli (Spongostan; polyvinyl alcohol—Ivalon), mechanical emboli (balloons, steel coils), and liquids (50 per cent dextrose, absolute alcohol, lipiodol). The appropriate agent or combination of agents depends on the lesion to be treated and its site (with particular reference to adjacent vulnerable vascular structures).

Embolization can be used definitively to treat benign conditions and pre-operatively to assist effective, safe surgery, but in many cases it is used palliatively to alleviate distressing symptoms (Fig. 7).

Palliative embolization

Embolization can be used to control pain, haemorrhage, and hormone production as well as to reduce tumour bulk. The technique may be used as the primary mode of treatment in inoperable malignancy and embolization of metastatic deposits has, in some situations, been shown to extend survival times in advanced disease.[31] Tumours in all sites have been treated in this fashion (liver, kidney, bone, lung, soft tissues, nervous system, and

(a)

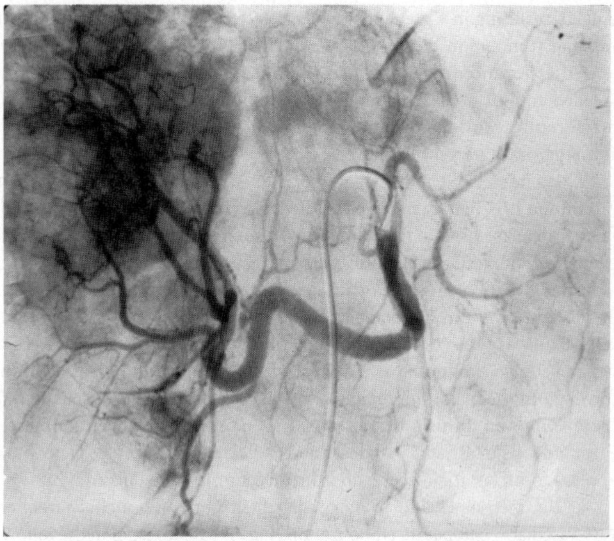

(b)

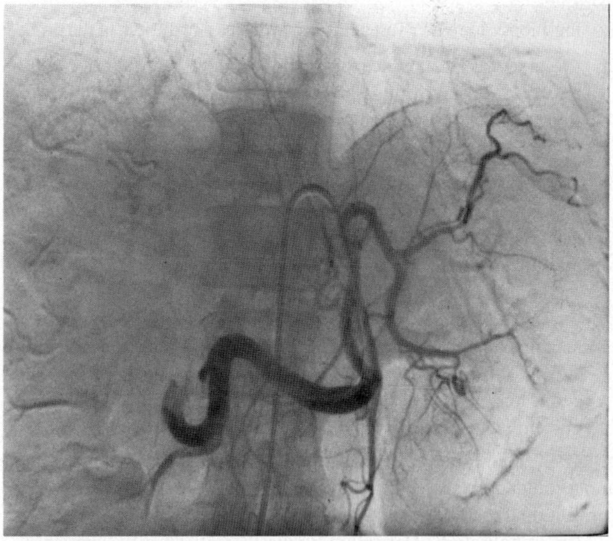

Fig. 7 Hepatic embolization for metastatic carcinoid tumour. (a) The arterial parenchymal phase shows hepatic enlargement and reveals multiple tumour deposits. (b) Post-embolization arteriogram shows that the arterial supply has been obliterated. The patient's symptoms (flushing and diarrhoea) were dramatically alleviated by this procedure.

gastrointestinal tract). Hormone secreting neoplasms such as metastatic APUD cell tumours show the greatest therapeutic response to arterial embolization. The APUD cell systems are widespread in the body and are concerned with the production and release of polypeptides and proteins with hormonal activity. Carcinoid tumours of the appendix and ileum are examples of the APUD cell system in the gastrointestinal tract. Appropriate pharmacological blockade is necessary during the embolization to avoid the effects of a dramatic outpouring of hormone as the tumour is deprived of its blood supply. The beneficial effects of embolization may become apparent within a matter of hours. In embolization procedures it is important that adequate premedication is given prior to the procedure, including broad-spectrum antibiotics. In many situations, for example, liver and bone, it is necessary to continue antibiotics for 10 days after the procedure to prevent sepsis developing in the devascularized tissue.

A significant advance in tumour embolization has been the development of chemoembolization.(32) In this technique embolic materials are mixed with chemotherapeutic drugs; the emboli cause ischaemia of the tumour cells and by increasing the transit time through the tumour vascular bed, the contact time between the cytotoxic agent and the neoplastic cells is prolonged, resulting in a greater therapeutic effect. It has been discovered that vascular tumours in the liver have a particular affinity for lipiodol injected into the hepatic artery. The possibility of tagging cytotoxic agents or labelled monoclonal antibodies to the lipiodol is under investigation in many centres worldwide. Some preliminary results, for example, in primary hepatoma, are very encouraging.(33,34)

In patients with cirrhosis of the liver complicated by hepatocellular carcinoma it is best to avoid arterial embolization because it may lead to further deterioration in liver function. In such patients percutaneous injection of alcohol into the tumour under ultrasound guidance has been shown to lead to a significant increase in life expectancy. Unfortunately, the results of this procedure in patients with multiple hepatic metastases are not as satisfactory as those obtained in hepatocellular carcinoma. This is because hepatocellular carcinoma is a very vascular tumour and alcohol diffuses throughout the mass, whereas most metastases are not very vascular so that there is uneven diffusion of alcohol and many cells survive the injection. Percutaneous treatment with laser and radiofrequency probes is now being applied to metastatic disease, and the initial results are encouraging.

Skeletal metastases and primary malignant bone tumours are frequently very vascular. Therapeutic embolization (Fig. 8) can be useful in the following situations:

1. Pre-biopsy, to reduce vascularity, thus decreasing the risk of the procedure.
2. Pre-operatively, to reduce tumour bulk and vascularity prior to tumour resection. This technique has proved valuable prior to limb preservation surgery for malignant or for potentially malignant lesions such as osteoclastoma and osteogenic sarcoma.
3. For palliation of inoperable neoplasms, to reduce pain and tumour bulk. The commonest embolization materials are sterile absorbable gelatine sponge and steel coils. Occasionally, liquid emboli, such as absolute alcohol and iso-butyl-2-cyanocrylate, are used. Cyanoacrylate sets quickly after coming into contact with human tissue and can be difficult to handle. It is important not to embolize outside the target area and measures must be taken to avoid the adhesive incorporating the tip of the delivery catheter into the embolic plug. Various types of resins and polymers with more controllable setting characteristics are currently being developed.

Embolization can result in occlusion of vessels uninvolved by malignancy and should be reserved for patients who have not responded to more conventional therapy.

After embolization of large tumour masses, patients may experience some discomfort and pain and they may have a fever for a few days accompanied by a feeling of malaise and an elevated white cell count. This combination of signs and symptoms has been called the *post-embolization syndrome*, and is an indicator of the presence of necrotic tissue. Sustained pyrexia should alert the clinician to the possibility of abscess formation and blood cultures plus regional ultrasound should be performed. Elevated serum C-reactive protein can also provide a useful indication that infection may be present.(35)

Neurolysis

Some patients with malignant conditions develop intractable pain, which can be relieved by injection of alcohol. For example, certain patients with carcinoma of the pancreas experience severe pain which may be relieved by coeliac plexus block. In these patients the coeliac ganglion may be ablated safely by injecting alcohol under computerized tomography guidance.

Percutaneous vertebroplasty

Percutaneous vertebroplasty involves injection of bone cement into a cervical, thoracic, or lumbar vertebral body for the relief of pain and the strengthening of bone. This procedure is being used for patients with lytic lesions due to bone metastases, aggressive haemangiomas, or multiple myeloma, and for the relief of intractable debilitating pain resulting from osteoporotic vertebral collapse. Up to 80 per cent of patients with pain unresponsive to conventional medical treatment experience a significant degree of pain relief, and few serious complications have been reported.(36,37)

The choice between vertebroplasty, surgery, radiation therapy, and medical treatment depends upon a number of factors, including the local and general extent of the disease, the spinal level involved, and the patient's general state of health, life expectancy and neurological condition.

Percutaneous vertebroplasty is usually performed under local anaesthesia combined with sedation, and may be carried out as an outpatient procedure or may require a short hospital stay. Computerized tomography and/or fluoroscopic guidance is used. The patient lies in the prone position, and a large bore (10–15 gauge) needle is placed into the vertebral body. Acrylic bone cement, usually methyl methacrylate, mixed with contrast medium, is then injected into the affected vertebra. This material is viscous to minimize leakage into adjacent structures or blood vessels. The procedure usually takes 1–2 h. Non-steroidal anti-inflammatory drugs can be used for 2–4 days after vertebroplasty to minimize the inflammatory reaction to the acrylic compound. Pain relief is expected within 24 h of the procedure (Fig. 9).

Gene therapy

One of the more exciting recent developments and research areas in medicine is gene therapy. The underlying principle is to identify and clone a gene, and then insert it into a vector capable of directing expression in mammalian tissues. The principle aim at present is to treat genetic deficiencies and malignant diseases refractory to conventional therapies. The delivery systems involved include retroviral vectors, adenoviral vectors, and cationic liposomes, along with strategies that involve ultrasound, computerized tomography, and transcatheter angiographic gene delivery. Examples of genes being evaluated in current trials include oncogenes, tumour suppressor genes, suicide genes, and antiangiogenesis factors.(38)

Percutaneous tumour ablation

Until recently, the alternatives to surgical treatment of malignancy have been limited to radiotherapy and chemotherapy. Recurrent malignancy in areas of previous radiation therapy, localized metastatic disease, and primary neoplasms in patients who are poor surgical candidates can, in many instances, be problematic for conventional therapy. However, the outlook for some patients who might otherwise be left to systemic chemotherapy or supportive care may be helped largely in part by new innovative image-guided therapies. Percutaneous techniques of local tumour ablation may be categorized into three major groups: injection (ethanol, acetic acid, hot saline), heating (radiofrequency,(39) electrocautery, interstitial laser therapy, microwave coagulation therapy, high-intensity focused ultrasound), and freezing (cryotherapy). Advantages of the ablative therapies compared to surgical resection include reduced morbidity and mortality, low cost, suitability for real-time image guidance, and the ability to perform procedures

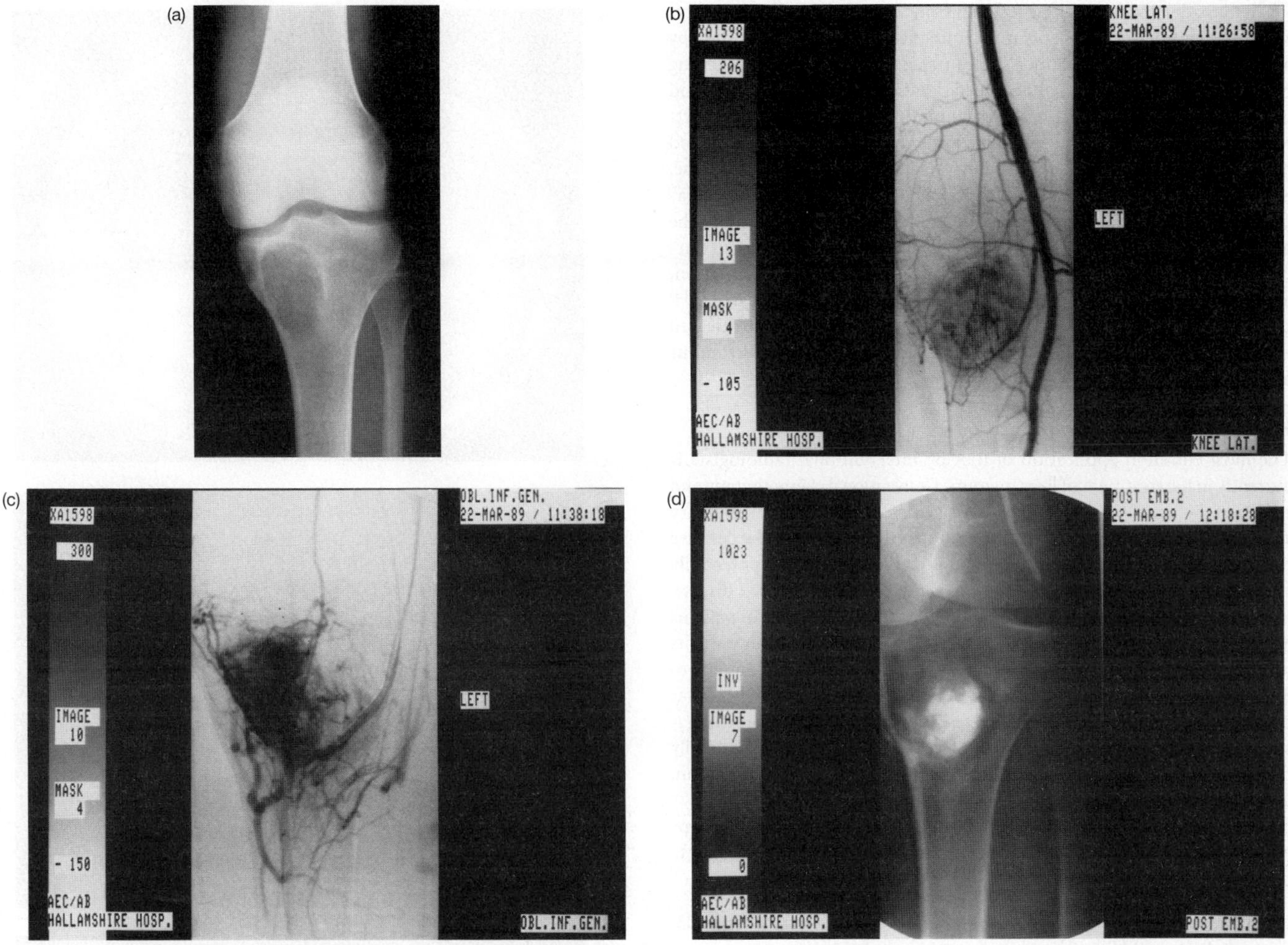

Fig. 8 Embolization of a painful skeletal metastasis from a primary renal carcinoma in a 55-year-old man. (a) Anteroposterior radiograph of the left knee shows a large lytic metastasis in the upper tibia in a patient with a known renal malignancy. (b) A femoral arteriogram (lateral) shows hypervascularity in the region of the metastasis. (c) The main vessel supplying this region was selectively catheterized. Fine particulate embolic material suspended in contrast medium and hypertonic dextrose was injected selectively into the vessels supplying the tumour. (d) Post-embolization radiograph shows stagnant contrast and embolic agent within the tumour. The patient experienced some increased pain for 24 h controlled with opioid analgesics. After this period his symptoms were significantly alleviated.

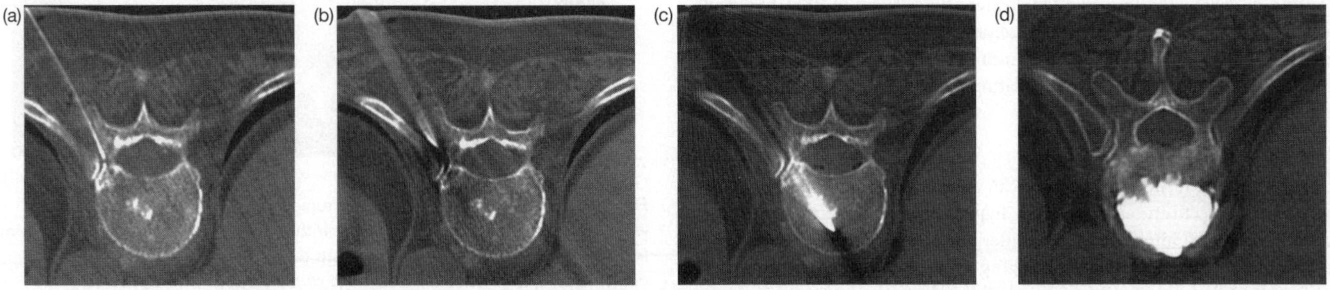

Fig. 9 Percutaneous vertebroplasty. Fluoroscopic images. (a) 22G spinal needle in situ for local anaesthetic injection. (b) 11G vertebroplasty needle has been percutaneously positioned with tip in vertebral body using computerized tomography and fluoroscopic guidance. (c) Careful injection of cement through needle. (d) Post-cement injection. (Films reproduced with kind permission from Prof A. Gangi.)

on an outpatient basis. All these techniques induce cell death by coagulative necrosis. Current developments in radiofrequency ablation (RFA) therapy are allowing treatment of larger size tumours (3–5 cm) and this exciting new technique has already demonstrated significant benefits for cancer and palliative care patients. RFA has been found to be effective for the short-term local control of painful soft tissue tumours in multiple locations, and may temporarily decrease or obviate the need of opioids in palliative care. Successful cases of RFA have been performed for painful bone metastases.(40) Other examples of the role of RFA in palliative care include the treatment of uncontrolled haematuria in patients with renal cell carcinoma,(41) and relief of distressing symptoms of bowel obstruction, abdominal distension, and pain from a large pancreatic metastatic mass (42) (Fig. 10). Better methods of imaging guidance and more sophisticated equipment are likely to increase the importance of percutaneous tumour ablation in the future.

Percutaneous liver tumour ablation

The most common application of RFA by interventional radiologists is currently in the treatment of liver tumours. Conventional chemotherapy and radiation therapy are ineffective for management of primary or secondary malignant hepatic tumours. Hepatic resection is the mainstay in the curative management of hepatic malignancies and is considered the only potentially curative therapy for these tumours. However, because of advanced disease, unfavourable location, or poor clinical condition, only a minority of patients are eligible for surgical resection. Actuarial survivals achieved in patients undergoing resection for hepatocellular carcinoma range from 55 to 80 per cent at 1 year and from 25 to 50 per cent at 5 years.(43) Similar outcomes have been achieved with the resection of colorectal hepatic metastases. These poor results have led to the development of multiple minimally invasive forms of therapy. These include intra-arterial chemoembolization, injection of ethanol, and interstitial laser, microwave, or RFA.

Of these the most widely used are percutaneous ethanol injection for hepatocellular carcinoma and thermal ablation methods for hepatic metastases.

Percutaneous ethanol injection therapy

Percutaneous ethanol injection therapy (PEIT) was first described in 1983. Since that time PEIT has been used extensively for treatment of unresectable hepatocellular carcinoma.(44) There is no absolute limitation to the size or number of lesions treated. However, as tumour size increases, homogeneity of ethanol diffusion diminishes at the periphery, increasing the probability that residual viable tumour cells will persist at the margin of the lesion following therapy. The limitation of diffusion radius and homogeneity is particularly relevant to metastases that have a firmer consistency than hepatocellular carcinoma, making them more resistant to ethanol diffusion at any size. The frequent need for multiple treatment sessions for each lesion, and the limited injection volume tolerated in a single session, place practical limitations on the number of lesions treated. For these reasons, as well as the documented greater effectiveness of PEIT for small, solitary tumours, many restrict the use of PEIT to nodular lesions 3 cm or less in diameter and three or fewer in number. However, PEIT is sometimes used in conjunction with thermal ablation in an effort to increase the area of tumour destruction.

Thermal ablation

Lesional heating techniques such as RFA and interstitial laser photocoagulation (ILP) effect tumour necrosis by hyperthermia. RF electrodes or laser fibres are inserted into the tumour under ultrasound, computerized tomography, or magnetic resonance imaging guidance. They generate intralesional heat by local hyperthermia which has been shown to cause almost immediate coagulation necrosis at temperatures of 50°C or greater, and to have a preferential cytotoxic effect on tumour cells at temperatures between 41 and 45°C. The time required to achieve a cytotoxic effect at these lower temperatures ranges from 15 min at 45°C to 240 min at 41°C, with the time doubling for each degree drop in temperature.(45) ILP produces thermal coagulation by conversion of absorbed light energy into heat.(46)

(a)

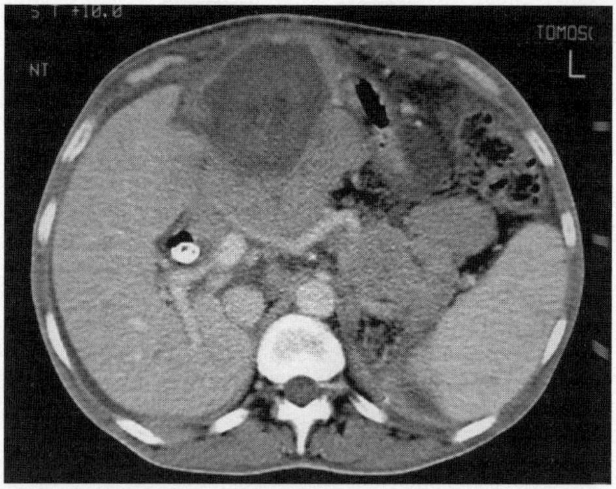

(b)

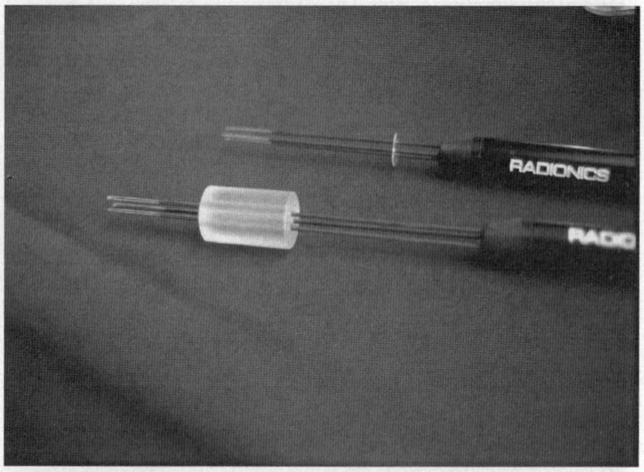

(c)

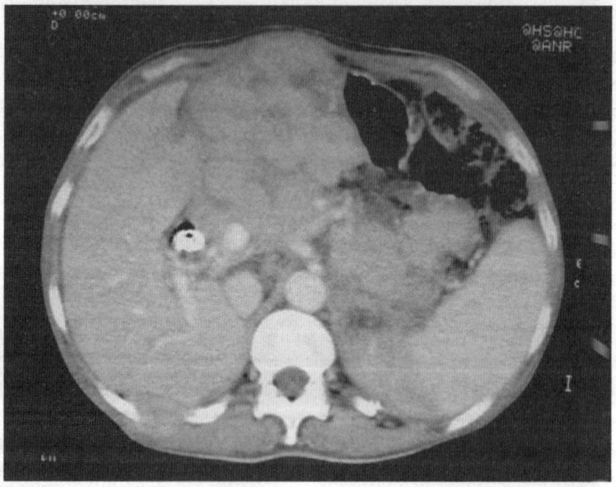

Fig. 10 RFA of a pancreatic secondary tumour. Patient had inoperable disease with metastatic melanoma and suffered with symptoms of severe abdominal pain and bowel obstruction. (a) Computerized tomography scan of abdomen demonstrating large tumour in the head of the pancreas thought to be responsible for current symptoms. (b) Radionics triple cooled RF probe that was used for percutaneous RFA therapy. (c) Follow-up computerized tomography scan (1 week later) showed a low attenuation area within the tumour mass that represents necrosis; the pancreatic tumour lesion is smaller and there was now less mass effect. Patient's symptoms were significantly alleviated.

In RFA, alternating current induces ionic agitation, which results in frictional heat production within the tissue. The size and shape of the necrotic lesion produced by RF has been shown to be a function of the probe gauge, length of the exposed probe tip, temperature along the exposed electrode, and duration of therapy. Lesion diameter increases with local temperature up to 90°C and reaches a maximum of 1.6 cm for a single probe. Strategies aimed at increasing the volume of tissue coagulation include the use of multi-probe electrodes and saline enhancement.[47] Cooling the electrode with saline during the ablation procedure prevents charring of the liver and reduces the impedance of the tissues adjacent to the electrode. In turn, this permits dissemination of heat further out into the tumour and increases the area of coagulation. The procedure is tolerated well and causes either no or only slight and transient abnormalities of liver function tests. Serious complications are rare and consist mainly of intraperitoneal haemorrhage and liver abscess formation.

The goal in RF thermal ablation is to kill the target tumour as well as a 5–10-mm circumferential cuff of normal hepatic parenchyma. Tumours smaller than 3 cm are easily encompassed by the 3-cm spread of heat from a triple RF electrode. However, we usually perform two overlapping ablations for tumours of this size. Tumours 3–4 cm in diameter require approximately six overlapping ablations, either during the same session or in two separate sessions. It is best to adopt a systematic approach using overlapping 'thermal cylinders' of coagulation. A cylinder is created around the tract of the electrode from the deepest to the most superficial portions of the tumour. Each ablation is overlapped by 50 per cent. Therefore, more than 12 ablations are required for tumours larger than 4 cm in maximum diameter.

The follow-up of patients after all forms of percutaneous tumour ablation includes a combination of imaging, tumour marker assay, and selected use of fine needle aspiration biopsy. It is useful to follow serial levels of alpha-fetoprotein or carcino-embryonic antigen, in the case of hepatocellular carcinoma or metastatic disease, respectively, only when the serum levels of these markers are elevated prior to the initiation of therapy. The immediate goal of imaging is to assess whether complete necrosis has been achieved. Ultrasound does not usually provide useful information, as the echogenicity of fibrosis and neoplastic tissue overlap. Contrast enhanced-magnetic resonance imaging and contrast enhanced-computerized tomography are capable of demonstrating remaining viable tumour requiring treatment. However, in difficult cases, PET scanning may provide additional information.

Several clinical series using different methods of RFA have been reported. The results appear to be promising, showing a 40 per cent 5-year survival rate and 52–67 per cent complete ablation rate. RF thermal ablation is a quick, relatively safe, and highly effective technique for bulking primary and secondary malignant hepatic tumours. Also, it holds great promise as a technique for local tumour eradication. However, it is difficult to create an adequate tumour-free margin around tumours and failure to do so results in incomplete ablations and tumour recurrence. There are two factors responsible for this difficulty: (i) the differential blood flow that exists between tumours and normal hepatic parenchyma, and (ii) difficulty in accurate placement of the RF electrode.

RF thermal ablation has many potential advantages over existing therapies. It is far more effective for debulking tumours than is radiation therapy or systemic chemotherapy. Unlike surgical resection or cryosurgery, it is minimally invasive and can be repeated as necessary to treat new tumours. It has far fewer complications than chemoembolization. Lastly, it has two major advantages compared to percutaneous ethanol ablation: it can be used to treat primary and secondary malignant hepatic tumours, and it requires fewer sessions to treat hepatocellular carcinoma.

Conclusions

This chapter was not intended to be an exhaustive list of every procedure that can be performed but to give an overall impression of the vast range of interventional techniques available. The patient undergoing palliative care should not be subjected to any unnecessary procedures or instrumentation. However, there are many readily performed, well tolerated, and safe interventional procedures which can significantly alleviate distressing symptoms, improve the quality of remaining life, and ease the nursing burden. Further detailed information can be obtained from the many reviews, journals, and books on the subject, some of which are included in the reference list.

References

1. **Athanasoulis, C.A.** et al. *Interventional Radiology.* Philadelphia PA: WB Saunders, 1981.
2. **Allison, D.J., Wallace, S., and Machan, L.S.** (1992). Interventional radiology. In *Diagnostic Radiology: An Anglo-American Textbook of Organ Imaging* 3rd edn. (ed. R.G. Grainger and D.J. Allison), pp. 2483–550. Edinburgh: Churchill Livingstone.
3. **Wallace, S. and Charanangavej, C.** (1987). Interventional radiology in renal neoplasms. *Seminars in Roentgenology* **22**, 303.
4. **Pfister, R.C., Yoder, I.C., and Newhouse, J.H.** (1981). Percutaneous uroradiologic procedures. *Seminars in Roentgenology* **16**, 62–71.
5. **Pingoud, E.G.** et al. (1980). Percutaneous antegrade bilateral ureteral dilation and stent placement for internal drainage. *Radiology* **134**, 780.
6. **Dick, R.A., Adam, A., and Allison, D.J.** (1992). Interventional techniques in the hepatobiliary system. In *Diagnostic Radiology: An Anglo-American Textbook of Organ Imaging* 3rd edn. (ed. R.G. Grainger and D.J. Allison), pp. 1235–58. Edinburgh: Churchill Livingstone.
7. **Adam, A.** et al. (1991). Self-expandable stainless steel endoprostheses for treatment of malignant bile duct obstruction. *American Journal of Roentgenology* **156**, 321–5.
8. **Davids, P.H.P.** et al. (1992). Randomized trial of self-expanding metal stents versus polyethylene stents for distal malignant biliary obstruction. *Lancet* **340**, 1488–92.
9. **Patz, E.F.** et al. (1996). Ambulatory sclerotherapy for malignant pleural effusions. *Radiology* **199** (1), 133–5.
10. **Gerzof, S.G., Spira, R., and Robins, A.H.** (1981). Percutaneous abscess drainage. *Seminars in Roentgenology* **16**, 62–71.
11. **Watkinson, A.F.** et al. (1995). Oesophageal carcinoma: initial results of palliative treatment with covered self-expanding endoprostheses. *Radiology* **195**, 821–71.
12. **Adam, A.** et al. (1997). Palliation of inoperable esophageal carcinoma: a prospective randomised trial of laser therapy and stent placement. *Radiology* **202**, 344–8
13. **Knyrim, K.** et al. (1993). A controlled trail of an expansile metal stent for palliation of oesophageal obstruction due to inoperable cancer. *New England Journal of Medicine* **329**, 1302–3.
14. **De Baere, T.** et al. (1997). Self-expanding metallic stents as palliative treatment of malignant gastro-duodenal stenosis. *American Journal of Radiology* **169**, 1079–83.
15. **Mainar, A.** et al. (1996). Colorectal obstruction: treatment with metallic stents. *Radiology* **198**, 761–4.
16. **Casola, J.** et al. (1986). Percutaneous cecostomy for decompression of the massively distended cecum. *Radiology* **158**, 793–4.
17. **Hatrick, A., Sabharwal, T., and Adam, A.** (2001). Tracheobronchial stents. *Seminars in Interventional Radiology* **18**, no. 3.
18. **Davitt, S.** et al. (2002). Tracheobronchial stent insertions in the management of major airway obstruction in a patient with Hunter syndrome (type II mucopolysaccharidosis). *European Radiology* **12**, 458–62.
19. **Morgan, R.** et al. (1997). Malignant esophageal fistulas and perforations: management with plastic-covered metallic endoprostheses. *Radiology* **204**, 527–32.
20. **Irving, J.D.** et al. (1992). Gianturco self-expanding stents: clinical experience in the vena cava and large veins. *Cardiovascular and Interventional Radiology* **15**, 351–5.
21. **Becker, D.M., Philibrick, J.T., and Selby, J.B.** (1992). Inferior vena cava filters: indications, safety, effectiveness. *Archives of Internal Medicine* **152**, 1985–94.
22. **Robertson, L.J., Mauro, M.A., and Jacques, P.F.** (1989). Radiologic placement of Hickman catheters. *Radiology* **170**, 1007–9.

23. **Parkinson, R.** et al. (1998). Establishing an ultrasound guided peripherally inserted central catheter (PICC) insertion service. *Clinical Radiology* **53** (1), 33–6.
24. **Adam, A.** (1995). Insertion of long term central venous catheters: time for a new look. *British Medical Journal* **311**, 341–2.
25. **Page, A.C.** et al. (1990). The insertion of chronic indwelling central venous catheters (Hickman lines) in interventional radiology suites. *Clinical Radiology* **10**, 105–9.
26. **Bell, S.D.** et al. (1995). Percutaneous gastrostomy and gastrojejunostomy: additional experience in 519 procedures. *Radiology* **194**, 817–20.
27. **Rossi, P.** (1982). Percutaneous removal of intravascular foreign bodies. In *Interventional Radiology* (ed. R.A. Wilkins and M. Viamonte), pp. 359–69. Oxford: Blackwell Scientific Publications.
28. **Gibson, R.N.** et al. (1985). Major complications of central venous catheterization. A report of five cases and brief review of the literature. *Clinical Radiology* **36**, 204–8.
29. **Belli, A.M. and Hemingway, A.P.** (1993). Retrieval of intravascular foreign bodies. In *Interventional Radiology in the Peripheral Vascular System* Vol. 4. (ed. A.M. Belli), pp. 88–92. London: Edward Arnold.
30. **Hemingway, A.P.** (1986). Materials for embolization. *Radiology Now*, 63–4.
31. **Chuang, V.P. and Wallace, S.** (1987). Hepatic artery embolization in the treatment of hepatic neoplasms. *Radiology* **140**, 51–8.
32. **Kato, L.** et al. (1981). Arterial chemoembolization with microencapsulated anticancer drug. *Journal of the American Medical Association* **245**, 1123–7.
33. **Takayasu, K.** et al. (1987). Hepatocellular carcinoma: treatments with intra-arterial iodized oil with and without chemotherapeutic agents. *Radiology* **162**, 345–51.
34. **Kobayashi, H.** et al. (1987). Intra-arterial injection of adriamycin/mitomycin C lipiodol suspension in liver metastases. *Acta Radiologica* **28**, 275–80.
35. **Hemingway, A.P. and Allison, D.J.** (1986). Complications of embolization: analysis of 410 procedures. *Radiology* **166**, 669–72.
36. **Gangi, A.** et al. (1999). Computed tomography (CT) and fluoroscopy-guided vertebroplasty: results and complications in 187 patients. *Seminars in Interventional Radiology* **16**, 137–42.
37. **Cotton, A.** et al. (1998). Percutaneous vertebroplasty: state of the art. *Radiographics* **18**, 311–23.
38. **Voss, S.D. and Kruskal. J.B.** (1998). Gene therapy: a primer for radiologists. *Radiographics* **18**, 1343–72.
39. **Solbiata, L.** et al. (1997). Percutaneous US-guided RF tissue ablation of liver metastases: long-term follow-up. *Radiology* **202**, 195–203.
40. **Dupuy, D.E.** et al. (1998). Percutaneous radiofrequency ablation of osseous metastatic disease. *Radiology* **202** (Suppl.), 146.
41. **McGovern, F.J.** et al. (1999). Radiofrequency ablation of renal cell carcinoma via image guided needle electrodes. *Journal of Urology* **161**, 599–600.
42. **Sabharwal, T. and Adam, A.** Radiofrequency ablation treatment for the palliation of large secondary pancreatic mass. *Eurorad Database* (case no. 678).
43. **Nagorney, D.M.** et al. (1989). Primary hepatic malignancy: surgical management and determinants of survival. *Surgery* **106**, 740–9.
44. **Castells, A.** et al. (1993). Treatment of small hepatocellular carcinoma in cirrhotic patients: a cohort study comparing surgical resection and percutaneous ethanol injection. *Hepatology* **18** (5), 1121–6.
45. **Dickson, A. and Calderwood, S.** (1983). Thermosensitivity of neoplastic tissues *in vivo*. In *Hyperthermia in Cancer Therapy* (ed. F.K. Storm), pp. 63–141. Boston MA: GK Hall Medical Publishers.
46. **Livraghi, T.** et al. (1997). Saline-enhanced radiofrequency tissue ablation in the treatment of liver metastases. *Radiology* **202**, 205–10.
47. **Steger, A.** et al. (1992). Multiple-fibre low-power interstitial laser hyperthermia: studies in normal liver. *British Journal of Surgery* **79**, 139–45.

8.2 The management of pain

8.2.1 Pathophysiology of pain in cancer and other terminal diseases

Rich Payne and Gilbert R. Gonzales

Pathophysiology of pain: inferences from clinical syndromes

Recent advances in the understanding of fundamental neurobiological mechanisms of nociception have provided insights into the evaluation and treatment of clinical pain.(1) Pain caused by cancer and other medical illnesses may be caused by direct effects of the disease (e.g. tumour infiltration of pain sensitive structures in cancer, infarction of tissue in sickle cell anaemia) or by the treatment associated with the disease, which injures visceral, musculoskeletal, and nervous tissue. For example, surgery, chemotherapy, and radiation therapy, which are necessary to treat cancer are all associated with potentially painful sequelae.(2)

Acute pain serves the purpose of alerting the organism to the presence of harmful (or potentially harmful) stimuli in the internal or external environment. Acute pain may be repetitive in circumstances in which recurrent and/or progressive tissue injury is experienced. This is typically the case when pain accompanies medical disorders such as cancer, sickle cell disease, haemophilia, multiple sclerosis, etc. Although these conditions cause pain extended over a period of time, and are often referred to as chronically painful conditions, they should be distinguished from the chronic 'pain state'. The latter term is usually used in the context of patients who report pain on a long-term basis, with no apparent tissue injury component or at least no apparent evidence of persistent nociceptor activation. Pain in this setting serves no known useful biological purpose. The psychological counterparts to the chronic pain state include depression, anxiety, and other affective states, and are key to understanding the disability associated with this condition.(3)

It is therefore important to recognize that chronic pain is not merely a temporal extension of acute pain. New data emerging from studies evaluating the central modulation of nociception indicate that a major distinction between acute and chronic pain may be found in the differences in central neural responses induced by the chronic afferent neural impulses of nociceptor activity.(3) Changes in central neural processing induced by these impulses activate *N*-methyl-D-aspartate (NMDA) receptors, and other biochemical and physiological processes, which may allow a persistent pain sensation to occur in the presence of diminishing nociceptive activity, in the absence of such activity, or to normally non-painful activity such as touch (see below).

Much recent experimental evidence suggests that acute persistent pain (such as that induced by experimental arthritis production in animals) may promote biochemical, physiological, and pharmacological changes in the peripheral and central nervous systems, which may promote the continuation of pain.(4) These data are detailed in the sections below dealing with inflammatory and neuropathic pain models. Although acute pain may be associated with profound psychological reactions such as anxiety and fear, and may also be accompanied by activation of the sympathetic nervous system, many of these physiological and psychological reactions become habituated as pain persists. Adaptation of sympathetic activity and the development of chronic vegetative signs, including a decrease in appetite, malaise, sleep disturbances, irritability, and reduced activity, characterize chronic pain.

Traditionally, the cancer patient has served as a model for acute and chronic pain in man, and several broad 'physiological' types of pain have been distinguished: somatic, visceral, and neuropathic, and perhaps even sympathetically maintained pain. Somatic or nociceptive pain occurs as a result of activation of nociceptors in cutaneous and deep musculoskeletal tissues. This pain is typically well localized and may be felt in superficial

Table 1 'Physiological' pain categories

Type of pain	Examples	Putative mechanisms
Nociceptive	Arthritis, fracture, bone metastasis, cellulitis	Activation of nociceptors
Visceral	Pancreatitis, peptic ulcer, myocardial infarction	Activation of nociceptors
Neuropathic	Herpes zoster, neuropathy, post-stroke pain, trigeminal neuralgia	Ectopic discharges within nervous system, spontaneous activity in nerves, neuroma formation, others
Complex regional pain syndromes[a]	Persistent focal pain following trauma with or without evidence of sympathetic involvement	Sensitization of spinal neurones, ephaptic transmission, others

[a] See Stanton-Hicks et al.[12]

cutaneous or deeper musculoskeletal structures. Examples of somatic pain include bone metastasis, post-surgical incisional pain, and pain accompanying myofascial or musculoskeletal inflammation or spasm (Table 1).

Visceral pain is also common in the cancer patient and results from infiltration, compression, distension, or stretching of thoracic and abdominal viscera (e.g. liver metastasis and pancreatic cancer). This type of pain is poorly localized, often described as 'deep, squeezing' and 'pressure', and may be associated with nausea, vomiting, and diaphoresis, particularly when acute. Visceral pain is often referred to cutaneous sites that may be remote from the site of the lesion (e.g. shoulder pain with diaphragmatic irritation). Tenderness and pain on touching the referred cutaneous site may occur.[5]

Neuropathic pain results from injury to the peripheral and/or central nervous systems.[6] Pain resulting from lesions to the peripheral nerves (especially those which are traumatic in origin and which partially or completely interrupt afferent sensory transmission between the peripheral and central nervous systems) has sometimes been termed 'deafferentation' pain. Pain resulting from injury to the spinal cord or brain, especially pain complicating strokes, is usually termed 'central pain'. The terms 'deafferentation' and 'central' pain are forms of neuropathic pain and are often used to denote pain following injury or dysfunction to peripheral or central neural structures, respectively.

In the cancer patient, neuropathic pain most commonly occurs as a consequence of tumour compression or infiltration of peripheral nerves, nerve roots, or the spinal cord. In addition, surgical trauma, chemical, or radiation-induced injury to peripheral nerves or the spinal cord from cancer therapies may also result in this type of pain. Examples of common neuropathic pains include metastatic or radiation-induced brachial or lumbosacral plexopathies, epidural spinal cord and/or cauda equina compression, postherpetic neuralgia, and painful vincristine, cisplatin, or paclitaxel neuropathy. Pain resulting from neural injury is often severe and is different in quality as compared to somatic or visceral pain. It is typically described as a constant dull ache, often with a pressure or 'vice-like' quality; superimposed paroxysms of burning and/or electrical shock-like sensations are common. These paroxysms of pain may be associated with spontaneous and ectopic activity in the peripheral[7] and central nervous systems.[8]

Although much is now known about the biochemical and neurophysiological processes associated with activation of nociceptors, a complete understanding of the pathophysiology of pain in specific patients is seldom possible. Although different physiological mechanisms of pain frequently coexist in patients with advanced cancer and other chronic medical illnesses, their recognition often has direct diagnostic and therapeutic implications.[1] This is particularly true for neuropathic pain. For example, the presence of paroxysmal or lancinating pain may indicate the appearance of spontaneous action potential propagation, and usually leads the clinician to suspect a neuropathic aetiology, even in the absence of compelling evidence for neural injury. Anticonvulsant medications that inhibit these discharges (such as phenytoin, carbamazepine, valproic acid, gabapentin, or clonazepam) may successfully manage this lancinating pain when traditional analgesics such as opioids or non-steroidal anti-inflammatory analgesics have failed. On the other hand, continuous burning dysaesthetic pains, which commonly accompany toxic metabolic polyneuropathies (e.g. diabetic neuropathy), may respond better to tricyclic antidepressants than to either anticonvulsants or opioids. Although the mechanisms by which the dysaesthesias are generated are not well understood, the clinician can make important treatment decisions based on the quality of the pain, which is likely to reflect differences in the pathophysiology of different forms of neuropathic pain.

Injury to nervous tissue may activate nociceptive systems and produce pain without stimulating nociceptors. Pain that occurs as a result of neurological injury is often qualitatively different from somatic or visceral pain, which results from activation of nociceptors in the setting of a normal nervous system. Given the different mechanisms and quality of neuropathic pain, it is not surprising that this pain may respond to drugs such as anticonvulsants, which are not useful in somatic or visceral pain.

The sympathetic nervous system may be involved in these pain states (particularly acute visceral and neuropathic pain), although its role is poorly understood.[9] Evidence for the involvement of the sympathetic nervous system in pain include:

1. the improvement of some forms of pain with sympathetic nerve blocks or with adrenergic blocking drugs such as propranolol and phenoxybenzamine;
2. increase in pain with sympathetic stimulation in some patients with causalgia and other complex regional pain syndromes;
3. animal studies of peripheral nerve injury that show the development of new α-adrenergic receptors and the sensitivity of regenerating nerve sprouts to systematic or locally applied catecholamines and sympathetic nerve blocks.[10]

However, the primary role of the sympathetic nervous system in chronic pain states has been challenged recently.[11] A recent review of this subject suggested that a new term, 'complex regional pain syndrome' be used rather than 'reflex sympathetic dystrophy' or 'sympathetically maintained pain' to avoid any inferences regarding mechanisms of sympathetic involvement in these pain states that are not conclusively determined.[12]

Nociceptors and peripheral nerve physiology

Sensory receptors that are preferentially sensitive to noxious (tissue damaging) or potentially noxious stimuli are prevalent in skin, bone, muscle, connective tissues, thoracic, abdominal, and pelvic viscera.[13] The free nerve endings that transduce these noxious stimuli conduct electrical discharges to the spinal cord utilizing two types of nerve fibres, A*- and C-fibres. A*-fibres are thinly myelinated, about 2.5 μm thick, and conduct action potentials at a rate of 5 m/s or less. Activation of these fibres by electrical stimulation is typically associated with sharp, stinging painful sensations. C-fibres are unmyelinated, about 0.3 μm thick, and conduct action potentials at a rate of 2 m/s or less. Patterns of electrical activity in C-fibres evoked by noxious stimuli are often associated with vaguely localized pain of a 'dull' and 'burning' quality. In human cutaneous peripheral nerves 10 per cent of all myelinated fibres carry nociceptive information, and more than 90 per cent of all unmyelinated fibres are nociceptive (Figs 1 and 2).[14]

Cutaneous nociceptors and hyperalgesia

Cutaneous nociceptors are defined morphologically by their appearance in light and electron microscopy, and physiologically by their patterns of response to mechanical, thermal, and chemical cutaneous stimuli.[15] On this basis, nociceptors have been classified as A* mechanical nociceptors,

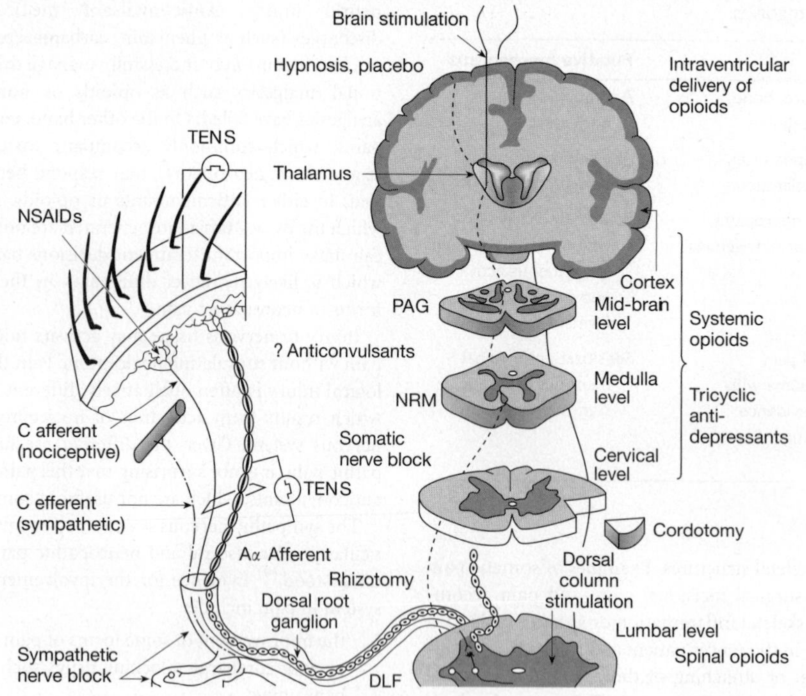

Fig. 1 Diagram of ascending and descending neural pathways involved in nociception.

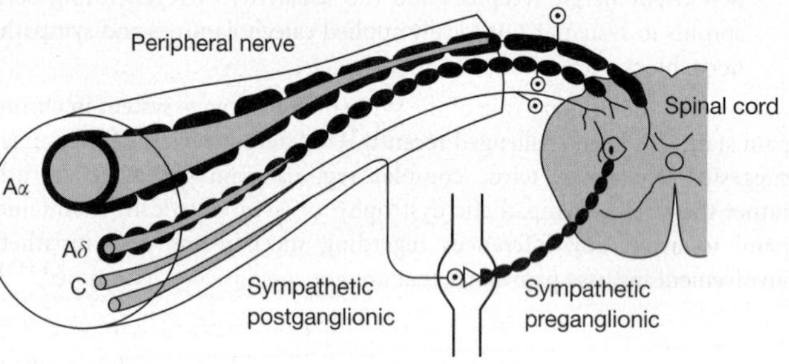

Fig. 2 Diagram of peripheral nerve mosaic 'cables'.

C-polymodal nociceptors, and silent or sleeping nociceptors, the latter being discovered only recently.[16] The silent nociceptor is mechanically insensitive and is only active when tissue is injured. Several research strategies have been used to correlate verbal reports of pain with patterns of electrical activity in these units. For example, one can correlate pain responses to laser heat applied to human skin (in which nerve fibre activity cannot be measured easily) with recordings from afferent C-fibres in the primate stimulated by the identical stimulus.[17] Using this paradigm, it has been demonstrated that human judgements of pain following a brief laser burn injury to the skin (i.e. defined as primary hyperalgesia) were most closely matched by increased responses in A* rather than C-afferent fibres. This demonstrates that burning pain and hyperpathia are not exclusively mediated by unmyelinated C-fibre units as had been previously thought (Fig. 3).[17]

Another strategy used to investigate more directly the relationship between peripheral nerve activity in man and unpleasant or painful sensations involves the use of microneurography.[18] This technique allows the stimulation and recording from single afferent or efferent fibres in peripheral nerves of conscious patients or volunteers, and also allows the correlation of electrical activity in afferent nociceptive fibres with verbal reports of pain. Microneurographic techniques have shown that activation of a single myelinated nociceptor is sufficient to cause pain, and direct electrical stimulation of unmyelinated nociceptors to discharge frequencies greater than 1.5/s is associated with a dull, burning, or aching pain.[14] Microneurographic recordings have confirmed that positive symptoms and signs of peripheral nerve disease such as Tinel's sign, Lhermitte's symptom, or positive straight leg raising in S_1 root compression are associated with spontaneous activity in peripheral nerves. Paraesthesias are represented by ectopic paroxysmal activity and high-frequency (>220 Hz) discharges in peripheral nerves as observed in microneurographic recordings.[19]

Nociceptors are not spontaneously active but may show sensitization, particularly after thermal injury to the skin.[17] Sensitization is manifested as:

1. decreased threshold of activation after injury;
2. increased intensity of a response to a noxious injury;
3. the emergence of spontaneous activity.

Sensitization of nociceptors may occur within minutes after a thermal injury and may last for hours. Sensitization of nociceptors produces the clinical phenomenon of hyperalgesia, defined as an increased response to a stimulus that is normally painful.

Sensitization of nociceptors may be mediated by efferent sympathetic activity (see below) as well as by chemical substances that are liberated by tissue injury and inflammation—potassium, adenosine triphosphate, bradykinin and prostaglandins, tachykinins, and other peptides.[20,21]

Nociceptor sensitization is the physiological correlate of primary hyperalgesia, which occurs after tissue injury, and is a mechanism of persistent pain in man. Secondary hyperalgesia results from central nervous system changes induced by tissue injury and nociceptor sensitization. The clinical expression of secondary hyperalgesia includes expansion of the zone of cutaneous hyperalgesia outside of the area of initial injury. This phenomenon is caused by hyperexcitability or 'central sensitization' of the second-order neurones in the spinal cord, upon which the nociceptive afferents terminate. Central sensitization is mediated by a complex set of biochemical and physiological events in which NMDA receptors play an important role.[22]

Central sensitization is dependent on NMDA receptor activation.[22] The amino acid glutamate binds postsynaptically to the NMDA receptor.

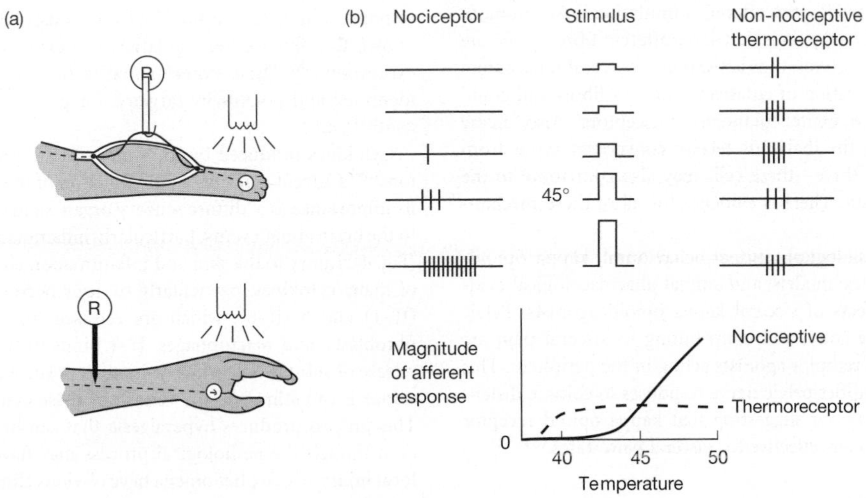

Fig. 3 Graph of a nociceptor versus a simple thermoreceptor.

When coupled with glutamate, the NMDA receptor is activated and functions as a divalent cation channel regulator, admitting Ca^{2+} and Mg^{2+} cations into the cell. Glutamate and NMDA receptors are found in high concentration in the dorsal horn of the spinal cord. Glutamate depolarized spinal cord neurones when applied iontophoretically and is known to be released from spinal cord preparations following electrical stimulation or noxious chemical stimulation *in vivo*. Blockade of NMDA receptors by drugs such as ketamine, dextrophan, phencyclidine, and MK-801 reduces windup (e.g. progressive increase in the number of spikes evoked by a single stimulus in response to repeated stimulation of peripheral C-fibres) to C-fibre stimulation, and can also prevent or terminate central sensitization once it has begun. Spinal administration of non-steroidal anti-inflammatory drugs block the hyperalgesia produced by formalin injection into the hind paw in animal models of pain, indicating that prostaglandins are important to the central as well as peripheral anti-inflammatory actions of this group of analgesics.[(23)] Hyperalgesia seen in inflammatory pain can arise through inflammatory mediators and these mediators can sensitize dorsal horn neurons through signalling pathways including protein kinase A, protein kinase C, and others.[(24)]

A second type of excitatory amino acid receptor, α-amino-3-hydroxy-5-methyl-4-isoxazoleproprionic acid (AMPA), has also been implicated in analgesia. This receptor admits Na^+ and K^+ when activated; blockade of AMPA receptors by selective antagonists such as CNQX (cyano-7-nitro-quinoxaline-2,3-dione) appears to be antinociceptive in animals. Thus, pharmacological agents which are very selective antagonists at NMDA and AMPA receptors hold great promise for future development as analgesics.

Synthesis of a great body of recent work on central nervous system modulation of nociception has shown that the NMDA receptor modulation has many clinical implications. It is apparent that several pre- and post-synaptic systems converge to provide a complex network of interactions that may contribute to the persistence of pain, even in the absence of ongoing nociceptive stimulation. Better understanding of these systems has major implications for:

1. explaining the persistent or chronic pain in the absence of ongoing nociception;
2. new opportunities for analgesic drug development;
3. opportunities for pre-emptive analgesia to prevent hyperalgesia and chronic pain.

The synthesis of nitric oxide, a gaseous neurotransmitter, is accomplished by activation of the enzyme nitrous oxide synthetase. This enzyme is activated by Ca^{2+}; the calcium gains access to the cell via activation of A receptors, which is a calcium channel ionophore. Nitric oxide is an excitatory neurotransmitter, and as a gas can diffuse across the synaptic cleft to induce retrograde effects such as release of glutamate and other neurotransmitters. It also appears to interact with adjacent neurones and glia. Thus, the synthesis of nitric oxide has important, widespread ramifications.[(25,26)] There are also findings that show that changes in tetrodotoxin (TTX)-sensitive and TTX-resistant sodium channels in nerve injury result in neuropathic pain that may lead to the development of subtype-specific Na^+ channel blockers.[(27)]

Visceral and bone nociceptors and deep pain

Bone pain from metastatic disease is perhaps the most common cause of pain in advanced cancer. Tumour metastasis to bone is associated with bone destruction and new bone formation and prostaglandins are important in this.[(28)] Myelinated and unmyelinated afferent fibres exist in bone and are in highest density in the periosteum; prostaglandins E_1 and E_2 are known to sensitize nociceptors and produce hyperalgesia.[(29)]

Deep pain originating from bone and visceral structures in the thoracic, abdominal, and pelvic cavities is, in fact, more common than cutaneous pain. Although much less well studied than their cutaneous counterparts, muscle and visceral nociceptors do exist in almost all organs studied thus far and appear to have different physiological properties than do cutaneous nociceptors, including the property of referred pain.[(5)] When normal human viscera are cut or otherwise manipulated, pain is usually not elicited, thus, unlike their cutaneous counterparts, visceral nociceptors appear to have a different function for the organism than as a simple 'acute warning system' for the presence of harmful tissue damaging stimuli. The type of stimuli that are sufficient to cause visceral pain include such things as chemical or mechanical irritation of the mucosal and serosal surfaces or torsion, traction, and distension of the mesentery or a hollow viscus. It has been emphasized recently that visceral nociceptors have a wide range of responsiveness, and so-called 'silent' nociceptors may be recruited in the presence of inflammation.[(5)]

Visceral pain has a deep (rather than superficial) and aching quality, is poorly localized, and often referred to a cutaneous point (which may be tender). Common examples of referred pain in cancer patients include back pain and paraspinal muscle tenderness that occurs with pancreatic and endometrial cancer, right shoulder pain that occurs with hepatoma or liver metastasis, and abdominal or leg pain, occurring in prostatic cancer. The mechanism of referred pain is not fully understood, but may be related to convergence of cutaneous and visceral sensory input onto common spinothalamic tract cells in the spinal cord.[(30)] It is hypothesized that pain is referred to the skin because the brain 'misinterprets' the source of the input, since cutaneous non-nociceptive afferent stimulation is so common. Another explanation for referred pain is that some afferent fibres innervate both somatic and visceral structures, thus activation of visceral nociceptors would cause antidromic activation of cutaneous sensory fibres and could release algesic substances to excite cutaneous nociceptors. Also, many spinothalamic tract cells in the thalamus receive convergent input from skin, muscle, viscera, or all three—these cells may also contribute to the phenomenon of referred pain. There is evidence for all of these mechanisms for referred pain.[30]

There is now electrophysiological, animal behavioural, kappa opioid-deficient gene targeting mouse models, and animal pharmacological evidence of the attenuating effects of visceral kappa opioid agonists. Pelvic nerve fibres innervating the colon and contributing to visceral pain are modulated by kappa opioid receptor agonists acting in the periphery. This opioid receptor subtype modifies pelvic nerve responses to colonic distension as well as animal behaviour suggesting that kappa opioid receptor agonists could be therapeutically effective for visceral pain states.[31–34]

Inflammatory pain models

Nociceptors exist in periarticular joint surfaces and much recent work has reported on the time course and physiology of 'the response of' these nociceptors to experimentally induced arthritis. The inflammatory reaction is often induced by direct injection of Freund's adjuvant or another immunogen (i.e. carrageenan, yeast extract, formalin, etc.) into a joint or foot pad, and is associated with pain-related behaviours (e.g. limping, guarding of the limb, circling, etc.) in the animal. As discussed below, inflammation also exposes opioid receptors on peripheral nerves and causes the migration of immune cells that have opioid receptors on their surface.

These inflammatory pain models thus offer an alternative to the more traditional, static and acute models (e.g. tail flick) that are dependent on reflex spinal activity rather than more highly organized animal behaviours, and thus allow one to study pain states that may more closely reproduce human conditions. For example, the ability to produce persistent pain states in animals using inflammatory models has demonstrated that peripheral noxious stimulation could induce gene expression in central nervous system neurons.[35] Thus, it has been demonstrated that unilateral inflammatory pain that may induce expression of a proto-oncogene resulting in opioid gene expression for dynorphin ipsilateral to the side of the inflammatory lesion.[36] In addition, the proto-oncogene *c-fos* mRNA may act as a messenger molecule in signal transduction systems of preproencephalin and preprodynorphin, which then may regulate the production of the endogenous opioids methionine, leucine encephalin, and dynorphin in response to noxious stimuli.[37] Exogenously administered opioids are also known to influence the regulation and expression of opioid peptide gene expression.[38] These experimental techniques allow activated cells to be identified and potentially targeted for pharmacological manip-ulation to control pain.

Cytokines produced by immune cells are potent activators of nociceptors.[39] Current concepts of the function of the immune system emphasize its importance as a 'diffuse sensory organ' signalling important information to the brain about events, particularly inflammatory events, in the periphery (Fig. 4). Injury to the skin and inflammation changes cause the elaboration of many cytokines, particularly tumour necrosis factor and interleukin 1 (IL-1) and 6 (IL-6), which are released from mast cells, keratinocytes, fibroblasts, and macrophages. IL-1 binds to the peripheral nerve causing release of substance P, which initiates a positive feedback loop because substance P can stimulate the release of these cytokines from immune cells. This process produces hyperalgesia that can be diffuse in its distribution, even though the pathological process may have been initiated from very focal injury. These phenomena have obvious clinical relevance. For example, specific antagonists of IL-1 have been shown to block hyperalgesia in the rat,[39] thereby pointing to the possibilities of new analgesic agents.

The newest class of non-steroidal anti-inflammatory drug (NSAID), the cycloxygenase-2 (COX-2) inhibitors, blocks the COX-2 enzyme, and controls the production of prostaglandin from arachidonic acid that is released from cell membranes at the time of injury. COX-2 is involved in inflammation production whereas COX-1 is responsible for gastric irritation and other activities. The COX-2 inhibitors have apparent reduced GI toxicity. Newer COX-2 inhibitors, besides rofecoxib and celecoxib, can be expected to be available to treat inflammatory pain.

Peripheral opioid effects

It is now apparent that opioids have peripheral antinociceptive and anti-inflammatory effects.[40] Peripheral opioid receptors of the μ (morphine-preferring), δ (encephalin-preferring), and κ (dynorphin-preferring) subtypes appear to be located on primary afferents, especially C-fibre afferents. One can demonstrate antinociceptive effects of opioids that are administered topically to peripheral tissues at sites of inflammation and the excitability of the afferent fibre is reduced. The release of substance P is also inhibited.[41]

Peripheral opioid effects can be observed within minutes of an inflammatory response but are not observed in the absence of inflammation.[42] The relatively brief time course needed for expression of peripheral analgesic effects and binding studies suggest that these opioid receptors are pre-existing on peripheral nerves and are not dependent on *de novo*

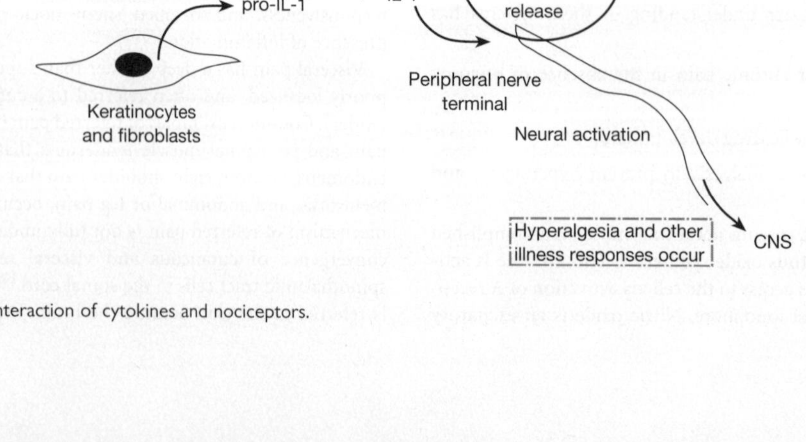

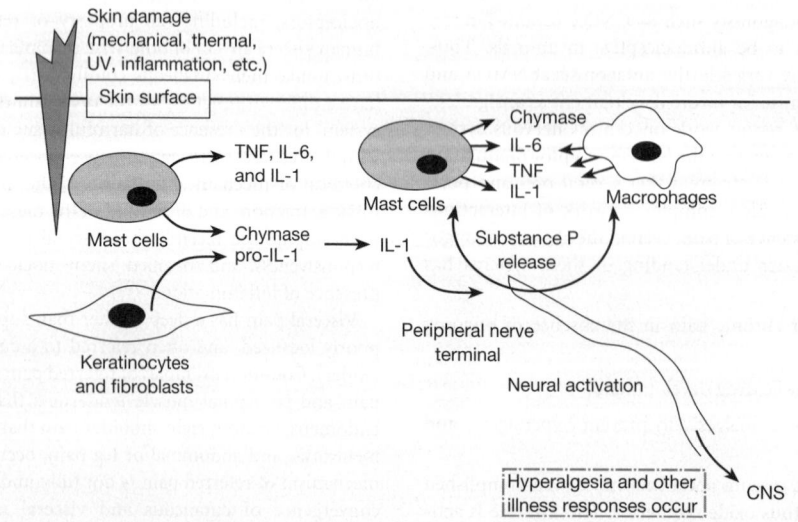

Fig. 4 Cartoon illustrating the interaction of cytokines and nociceptors.

synthesis. It appears that inflammation may disrupt the perineurium and expose the receptors.(43)

Several human studies have demonstrated analgesia to intra-articular injection of morphine for the treatment of postoperative pain.(44) In fact, intra-articular injection is more effective than perineural injection of morphine. The observation that opioid receptors are transported from the cell body in the dorsal root ganglion down the peripheral nerve axon to the terminal during inflammatory injury may explain this observation, since axonal receptors appear to be in transit and probably less functional.(42)

Opioid receptors are also present on immunocompetent cells that migrate to inflamed tissue.(45) Local application of opioids which are polar and which do not cross the blood–brain barrier would be advantageous in order to avoid adverse central nervous system effects such as sedation, nausea, respiratory depression, and mental clouding, and require direct investigation in inflammatory pain states in man.

Animal models of neuropathic pain and bone pain

Several models of neuropathic pain have been described.(46–49) These models have been helpful in dissection of the physiological pharmacological mechanisms of neuropathic pain. The chronic constriction model of Bennett and Xie is of particular interest because it produces unilateral spontaneous pain within 4 days of tying a loose ligature around the rat sciatic nerve. In addition to pain behaviours that are inferred by the guarding of the extremity, hyperalgesia and allodynia to sensory testing, a temperature abnormality in the nerve-injured limb also occurs. Thus, this animal model of neuropathic pain appears to mimic many important clinical findings that are seen in peripheral nerve injury in man. Recent quantitative neuropathological analysis of the nerve injury indicates that, initially, oedema produces a fourfold increase in the fascicular area; later, myelinated fibres are decreased to less than 0.5 per cent of their control values by day 14 after injury.(50) Unmyelinated fibres decrease in the first 5 days, but increase thereafter secondary to nerve fibre sprouting. Macrophage invasion occurs over time. It appears that Wallerian degeneration and macrophage activation are important peripheral components of hyperalgesia.

Although peripheral nerve injuries can be produced and quantified in these animal models, it is apparent that there are important changes occurring in the central nervous system as a consequence of the nerve lesions, and the ubiquitous NMDA receptors and the excitatory amino acid glutamate have been implicated in these changes. For example, one can demonstrate the presence of 'dark neurones' in the spinal cords ipsilateral to nerve injury, which are thought to be caused by NMDA-mediated excitotoxicity.(51) Blockade of NMDA receptors may reduce this cytotoxicity by decreasing spontaneous discharges in the peripheral nerve following injury.(52) In addition, the thermal hyperalgesia that occurs after the nerve injury is mediated by nitric oxide.(53)

A bone cancer pain animal model has revealed that a unique set of neurochemical changes occur in the spinal cord ipsilateral to the bone destruction and periosteal invasion. In one model, spinal cord astrocytic hypertrophy without neuronal loss and expression of dynorphin and internalization of the substance P receptor were seen. These and other changes were correlated with the extent of tumour growth and bone destruction(54,55) (Fig. 5).

Dorsal horn circuitry and the spinothalamic tracts

Afferent fibres from nociceptors enter the spinal cord laterally in the dorsal root and ascend or descend one to two segments in Lissauer's tract to synapse in the dorsal horn. The dorsal horn consists of six laminas with lamina I, the marginal zone, being the most dorsal. Lamina II and III together comprise the substantia gelatinosa, which is an important site of integration of nociceptive and non-nociceptive input into the spinal cord (Fig. 6).(56) However, as much as 30 per cent of afferent fibres are also known to enter through the ventral root; this is an explanation for the failure of dorsal rhizotomy to relieve pain permanently.(57)

Dorsal horn neurones receiving input from primary afferent fibres can have two types of responses: (1) nociceptive-specific and (2) wide dynamic

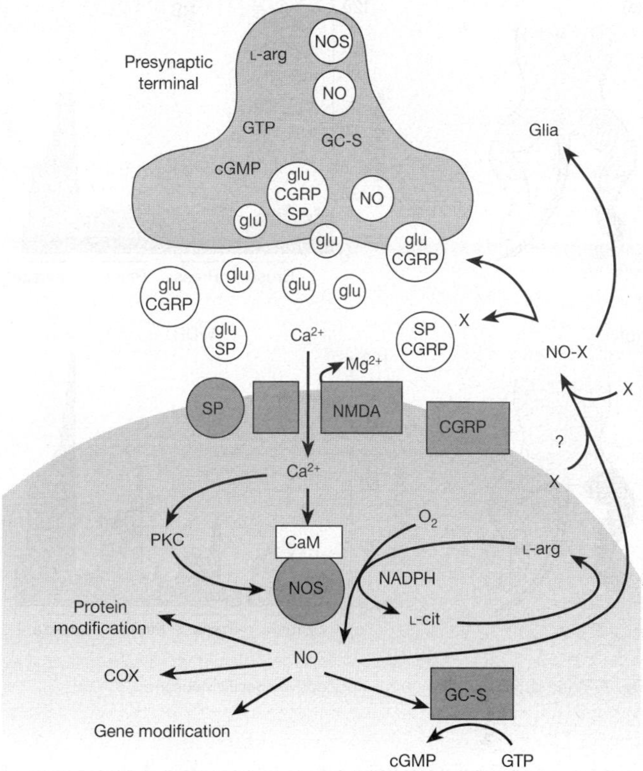

Fig. 5 Factors such as prostaglandin E, growth factors, cytokines and parathyroid hormone-related protein are secreted by malignant cells. These factors affect bone formation directly or indirectly. (See Rubens and Coleman.(55))

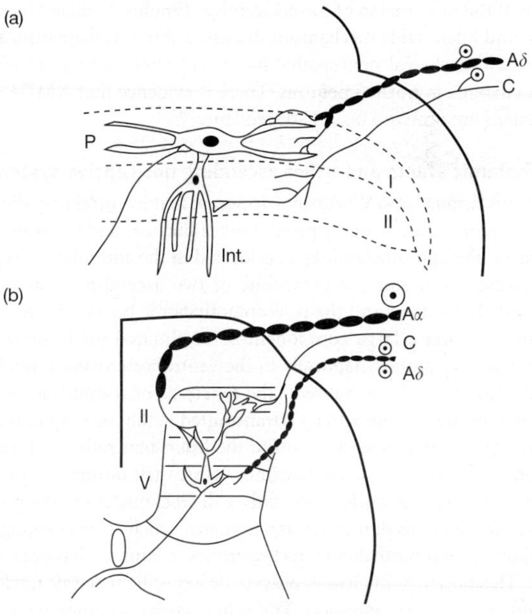

Fig. 6 Dorsal horn circuitry.

range (Fig. 7).(13) Similar responses can also be observed in thalamic and cortical cells receiving projections from the spinothalamic tract. Both types of neuronal responses appear important in pain perception. The wide dynamic range neurone responds to innocuous and noxious stimuli of

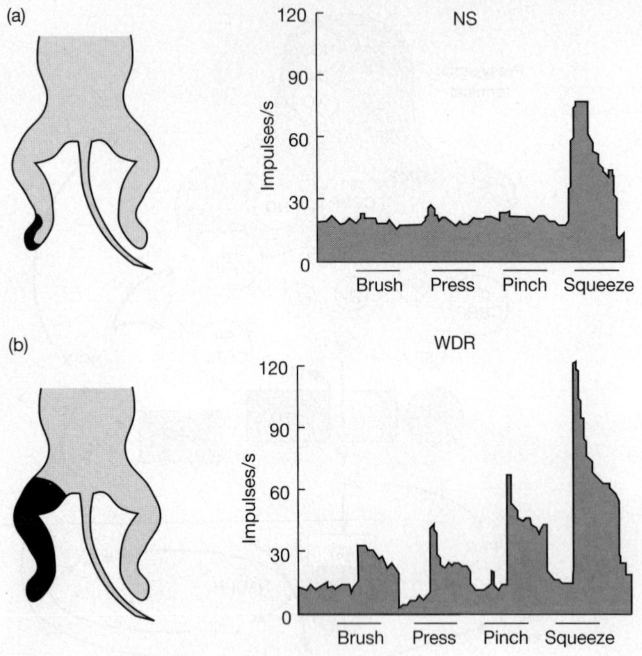

Fig. 7 Wide dynamic range versus nociceptive-specific neurones.

many types and increases its firing pattern in proportion to the intensity of the stimulus. These neurones probably provide the central nervous system with information relative to the quality of the perceived painful stimulus. The nociceptive-specific neurone responds only to intense noxious stimulation; they probably signal the central nervous system with respect to the presence or absence of tissue damaging stimuli. The dorsal horn is the site of much of the modulation of the nociceptive stimulus mediated by opioid, NMDA, and nitric oxide mechanisms discussed above. Gabapentin, a medication used in clinical neuropathic pain conditions, appears to enhance NMDA currents in normal neurons. There is evidence that NMDA receptor channels are protein kinase C-dependent.[(58)]

Spinothalamic tracts and other ascending nociceptive systems

Axons from lamina I and V neurones decussate in the central grey the spinal cord and become the ascending projections of the neo- and paleospinothalamic tracts. The spinothalamic tract is located in the anterolateral segment of the spinal cord, and is a composite of two ascending systems—the neospinothalamic tract and the paleospinothalamic tracts. The neospinothalamic tract has a large component of myelinated nociceptive fibres (A*) that project monosynaptically to the ventroposterolateral nucleus of the thalamus. These fibres subserve the functions of stimulus localization and pain intensity. C-fibre activity is transmitted in the paleo-spinothalamic tract with projections branching off to the brainstem reticular formation and to the medial regions of the thalamus before their ultimate termination in ventroposterolateral nucleus. Recently, a distinct nucleus in the posterior thalamus in the brains of monkey and humans, which receives topographic projections from spinothalamic tract neurones in lamina I has been identified.[(59)] This posterior nucleus appears to be a specific thalamic nucleus for pain and temperature sensation. The ventrobasilar complex (ventroposterolateral nucleus, ventroposteromedial thalamic nucleus) axons project to the parietal somatosensory cortex. The medial thalamic nuclear group projects to the striatum and cerebral cortex.

Several other ascending spinal tracts have been identified including the spinohypothalamic tract, spinoreticular tract, spinopontoamygdala tract, and the dorsal column tract.[(60)] The spinoreticular tract, which projects to the brainstem reticular formation, and the spinocervicothalamic tract ascend in the ipsilateral dorsolateral quadrant and travel with the spinothalamic tract in the medial lemniscus. Dorsal column fibres transmit both proprioceptive and nociceptive information and ascend in the ipsilateral medial lemniscus to the thalamus.[(61)] In fact, recent neurophysiological and neuroanatomical studies also indicate a convergence of somatic and visceral afferent information in this tract.[(62)] The multiple ascending non-spinothalamic tracts may be responsible for the recurrence of painful symptoms following ablative procedures such as cordotomy.

The composition of the spinothalamic tracts suggests functional diversity.[(63)] The neospinothalamic tract probably subserves the sensory-discriminatory aspects of pain perception (stimulus localization and intensity). The phylogenetically older paleospinothalamic tract appears to subserve the arousal, emotional, and affective/suffering components of pain. In addition to receiving inputs from the paleospinothalamic tracts, the intralaminar nuclear complex of the thalamus also receives afferents from the cerebellum and projects efferent fibres to the striatum. This suggests that this system is also important in mediating the inevitable reflex withdrawal responses that accompany the reaction to unexpected painful stimuli.[(63)]

The trigeminal subnucleus caudalis (spinal trigeminal nucleus) and adjacent reticular formation are the equivalent of the spinal dorsal horn, and modulate nociceptive information entering the nervous system from head and neck structures. This nucleus has a similar laminar structure and afferent synaptic connections as the spinal dorsal horn. Descending fibres in the spinal trigeminal tract convey pain, thermal, and tactile information from the ipsilateral face, forehead, and mucous membranes of the nose and mouth. The spinal trigeminal nucleus appears to be the only part of the trigeminal complex uniquely concerned with pain and thermal sensation. It has a laminated structure and neurons within laminas I and V and the adjacent reticular formation encodes nociceptive information in the same manner as do spinal dorsal horn neurones. Second-order neurones cross to the other side of the brainstem and ascend in the contralateral medial lemniscus, eventually terminating in the ventroposteromedial thalamic nucleus.[(63)]

A newly described midline posterior column pathway, which mediates the perception of visceral pain in pelvic and abdominal structures, can be ablated with punctate midline myelotomy for the relief of visceral cancer pain.[(64)] Significant pain relief has been reported with minimal neurological sequeli using punctuate midline myelotomy. This technique may provide an alternative method for treating cancer-associated visceral pain, especially in patients with pain refractory to opioids or where side-effects preclude using opioids and non-invasive adjuvants.

Cerebral cortex and pain

Lesions of the cerebral cortex that are large and destroy the somatosensory area have been reported to produce minimal or no pain, while small and highly localized cortical lesions outside of this area can be associated with increased pain perception. Clinically, it is clear that cortical lesions can produce central pain and cortical stimulation rarely has been demonstrated to produce pain.[(65)] The primary somatosensory cortex receives projections from ventroposterolateral and ventroposteromedial thalamic nuclei—areas which receive heavy input from nociceptive systems. A syndrome of 'asymbolia for pain' has been described, which is associated with lesions of the insular cortex.[(66)] These patients have normal thresholds to experimental cutaneous pain stimuli contralateral to the insular lesion, but do not generate emotional responses to the stimuli and appear not to perceive the stimuli as noxious.

A lesion anywhere in the first-, second-, or third-order neurones of the spinothalamic and thalamocortical projections may result in central pain symptoms. Thus, lesions affecting the spinal cord, brainstem, and cortex may impact on critical thalamic functions to induce central pain.[(67)] For example, a report of central pain complicating a toxoplasmosis abscess in the internal capsule and thalamus indicates the range of pathologies that can cause this syndrome.[(68)] However, mass lesions such as primary or metastatic tumours involving the brainstem, thalamus, and cortex only very rarely produce pain of this type. Brain tumours may be associated with headache when accompanied by increased intracranial pressure, but this is not considered to be central pain. Hypoalgesia (i.e. reduced appreciation of painful stimuli such as pinprick) is a common accompaniment of central pain, and in the case of ischaemic thalamic injury decreased temperature sensation of the affected area is an almost invariable accompaniment.[67]

The loss of inhibitory influences on excitatory pathways has been proposed to be the mechanism for the initiation of central pain. Lhermitte proposed that the thalamus acts as a gating mechanism on sensory fibres along the route to the cortex.[69] Electrophysiological studies in animal models suggest that removal of inhibition exerted by the neospinotha-lamic system (lateral thalamus) on the paleospinothalamic system (medial thalamus) might be important in the aetiology of some cases of central pain.[67] Although the lateral thalamus is often destroyed in cases of thalamic pain, it is difficult to assign a single thalamic structure as the only centre for initiation of all cases of central pain.

Endogenous pain suppression pathways and the neuropharmacology of nociception

Neuroanatomical pathways that arise in the brainstem and descend to the spinal cord function to modulate activity in the ascending nociceptive pathways (Fig. 1).[70] One such pathway begins in the periaqueductal grey of the midbrain and descends to the nucleus raphe magnus in the medulla. From the nucleus raphe magnus there is a projection to the dorsal horn of the spinal cord via the dorsal longitudinal fasciculus. This pathway terminates in laminas I, II, and IV of the spinal cord to modulate afferent nociceptive impulses. A second, more laterally placed descending pathway, starting in the nucleus reticularis paragigantocellularis in the pons, projects to the dorsal horn via the dorsal longitudinal fasciculus. Electrical stimulation or microinjection of morphine into these brainstem and/or spinal cord sites produces analgesia in the absence of motor, sensory, or autonomic blockade.

Serotonin and noradrenaline are putative neurotransmitters in these brainstem endogenous pain suppression pathways in animals and man, and drugs that affect their pharmacological actions may have analgesic activity. For example, tricyclic antidepressant compounds, such as amitriptyline, block the presynaptic uptake of both chemicals, thus augmenting their postsynaptic actions in the descending pain suppression pathways. The actions of both noradrenaline and serotonin appear to be important for analgesia, since antagonists of these amines partially block analgesia.[71] However, noradrenaline appears to be the more important of the two neurotransmitters in the mediation of analgesia because relative 'pure' serotonin reuptake inhibitors, such as zimelidine, appear not to be as effective as amitriptyline,[72] and relatively 'pure' noradrenaline reuptake blocks such as desipramine have demonstrated analgesic actions in randomized controlled clinical trials in postherpetic neuralgia.[73] Drugs such as clonidine, which are α_2-agonists at adrenergic receptors in the spinal cord, produce analgesia when delivered directly into the spinal epidural space.[74]

Amitriptyline has analgesic properties independent of its antidepressant effects and has been used for the management of many painful conditions, including, postherpetic neuralgia and painful diabetic neuropathy. Amitriptyline may also augment the effects of morphine analgesia in animals.[75] It is postulated that activation of these descending systems by opioid medications, such as morphine, or by endogenous substances, such as serotonin, methionine and leucine encephalin, or dynorphin, leads to the release of putative neurotransmitter agents such as serotonin, which then modulate the activity of ascending spinothalamic pathways. For example, it has been reported recently that an important action of morphine is to activate 'off cells' in the brainstem, which then inhibit phasic electrical activity in the descending systems, thereby permitting ascending transmission of nociceptive stimuli (Fig. 8).[70] Also, it has been suggested that activation of this descending control system by the action of endogenous opioids such as ∃-endorphin and encephalon may account for the phenomenon of placebo

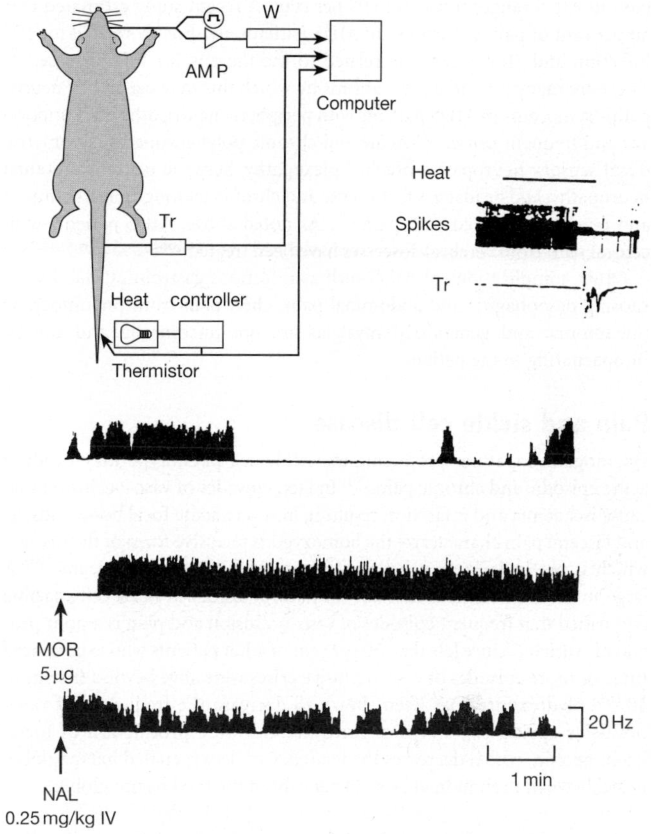

Fig. 8 On–off cells and morphine analgesia.

and acupuncture analgesia.[70] However, the reversibility of these phenomena by naloxone and the true role of endogenous opioid systems in their production is still in doubt.

Acute and chronic pain in medical disorders

Many chronic, incapacitating, and/or ultimately fatal disease processes may be accompanied by severe pain, especially in their terminal phases. Cancer is the most obvious and widely discussed condition, but AIDS, multiple sclerosis, central pain following stroke, and musculoskeletal pain secondary to joint immobility, and arthritis complicating neurodegenerative dementing illnesses such as Parkinson's disease, amyotrophic lateral sclerosis, and Alzheimer's disease are but a few other examples of this problem. In addition, birth defects attendant to prematurity and birth-related trauma, which produce catastrophic neurological deficits that lead to disability and death, may be associated with pain in the neonate which is particularly problematic to assess and treat. This is so because the physiology of nociception in the developing nervous system has only been investigated recently, and the assessment of pain in preverbal children is difficult.[76] The following section highlights specific examples of pain in these clinical conditions that are likely to be encountered by physicians involved in palliative care of terminally ill patients.

Painful conditions complicating HIV infection and AIDS

Pain is now recognized as a significant problem in patients with acquired immunodeficiency syndrome (AIDS).[77] Statistics on the prevalence of pain in AIDS ranges from 30 to 97 per cent. A recent study estimated that 50 per cent of pain syndromes in AIDS patients are directly related to HIV infection and 30 per cent are related to the therapy for HIV disease.(77) There are many potential mechanisms by which this may occur, but neuropathic symptoms in AIDS patients with peripheral neuropathy is an important and frequent cause.(78) Acute and chronic polyneuropathy, symmetric distal sensory neuropathy, brachial plexopathy, herpetic neuralgia, cranial neuropathy, and headaches from acute and chronic meningitis are common and may be associated with pain.(79) As noted above, AIDS patients with central pain from cerebral abscesses have been treated.(68)

Other complications of AIDS such as infectious gastrointestinal disease causing oesophagitis and abdominal pain, chest pain from pneumocystic pneumonia, and generalized myalgias are not uncommon and can be incapacitating to the patient.

Pain and sickle cell disease

Haemoglobinopathies producing the sickle cell phenotype may produce acute episodic and chronic pain.(80) In fact, episodes of vaso-occlusion that cause ischaemia and infarction resulting in severe acute focal bone, muscle, and visceral pain characterize the homozygous recessive form of the disease, which is particularly prevalent in Africans and African-Americans.(80) A large study undertaken to describe the natural history of sickle cell anaemia confirmed that frequent episodes of vaso-occlusion and pain is a poor prognostic variable, since less than 50 per cent of adult patients who experienced three or more episodes of vaso-occlusive crises were alive beyond the age of 40.(81) Hydroxyurea has been shown to decrease the frequency of vaso-occlusive episodes.(82) Hydroxyurea increases the production of foetal haemoglobin, which decreases the tendency of deoxygenated haemoglobin to sickle when present in at least 20 per cent of the total haemoglobin.

Pain syndromes in multiple sclerosis

It is generally accepted that pain in patients with multiple sclerosis is common. As much as 55–82 per cent of multiple sclerosis patients have pain complaints.(83) A possible pathophysiological mechanism of pain in multiple sclerosis includes ectopic spontaneous discharges in central demyelinated axons. This has been proposed to be the cause of paroxysmal pain in conditions such as trigeminal neuralgia complicating multiple sclerosis. The pain associated with optic neuritis and periorbital pain with eye movement has been suggested to be due to traction on the meninges that envelops the swollen optic nerve.(84) Extremity pain, especially with a dysaesthetic component and painful electric shock-like sensations (i.e. L'hermitte's sign associated with neck flexion) is thought to be due to posterior column demyelination and ephaptic conduction of impulses (i.e. cross-excitation of nerves by shunting of current between fibres in close apposition). Other causes of extremity pain and low back pain in multiple sclerosis have been attributed to musculoskeletal abnormalities, which become secondarily irritated or develop spasm as a result of abnormal gait and posturing because of the neurological abnormalities.

Cerebrovascular disease

As much as 1–2 per cent of stroke patients may develop central post-stroke pain. Decreased temperature sensation on the affected side may be an absolute accompaniment in these patients.(67) The onset of pain may be delayed for several years after the stroke, and the pain may be superficial or deep. The pain is often severe in intensity and may be accompanied by hyperalgesia and allodynia. Paroxysms of severe pain may occur and may be elicited by emotional episodes and movement. Another common cause of pain in the hemiplegic post-stroke patient is mechanical shoulder pain unrelated to the central injury.(67)

Spinal cord injury

Central pain may occur from a traumatic injury at any level of the spinal cord. Central pain usually occurs in the area of spinal cord or root somatosensory deficit.(84) If the nerve root is injured, neuropathic pain in a radicular distribution may add to the central pain of spinal cord origin. The pathophysiology of central pain caused by a spinal cord lesion is not known and not everyone with similar lesions develops pain. The traumatic spinal cord lesions that have been reported to cause central pain include: traumatic hemisection of the cord, traumatic haematomyelia of the cervical cord, post-traumatic vascular lesions, and syringomyelia. High-dose corticosteroids administered within hours of the injury may ameliorate acute pain and aid recovery of neurological function.(85)

Pain in Parkinson's disease

Pain sensations are more common than the medical profession gives credit to in the Parkinson's disease patient.(86) Sensory symptoms that are painful in Parkinson's disease can be classified as musculoskeletal, neuropathic, pain associated with dystonic and akathisia movements, and non-localizing burning-type pain described as 'Central pain'.(86) The site of nervous system dysfunction that leads to the pain symptoms in Parkinson's patients has been postulated to be the basal ganglia or the release of sensory centres from extrapyramidal influence.(87,88)

Pathophysiology of pain in special circumstances

Pain in the infant or preverbal child

Although this is not a common circumstance in palliative medicine, the assessment and treatment of pain in the very young child poses significant challenges. However, it is now clear that in the human foetus the neuroanatomic pathways necessary for pain perception are developed, and analysis of the behavioural and physiological responses to putatively painful stimuli suggest that the human neonate can, indeed, perceive pain.(89) The available evidence suggests that analgesic and anaesthetic agents should be used in procedures and operations that are known to be painful in older individuals or when the infant is responding in a way that is consistent with discomfort. Unique issues with respect to the pharmacokinetic and pharmacodynamic responses to analgesic and anaesthetic agents in this age group in comparison to older individuals is beyond the scope of this chapter; however, this is also under intense study.

Pain in the elderly and demented patient

Chronic pain in patients over the age of 65 has been reported to occur in 20 per cent of people in this age group.(90) Patients in this age group have been considered to have a greater sensitivity to medications with sedative effects such as opioids, tricyclic antidepressants, anticonvulsants, and benzodiazepines. Body fluid volume decreases with age and this may affect the distribution and concentration of drugs such as morphine in the elderly patient.(91)

Acute confusional states may occur with many medications, especially in the patient with abnormal baseline cortical function, that is, the demented individual. Adverse effects of the opioids that may be enhanced in the elderly include constipation, hypotension, and, with certain opioids such as pethidine, the accumulation of toxic metabolites (especially in the setting of renal dysfunction), which may cause convulsions, myoclonic jerks, hallucinations, agitation, and psychotomimetic effects. There is also an increased risk of drug interactions. In general, opioids and other drugs with short plasma half-lives (e.g. morphine, hydromorphone, or oxycodone) should be used in elderly patients, as opposed to those with longer plasma half-lives (e.g. methadone or levorphanol), as there is less likelihood of accumulation with repetitive dosing and therefore less chance to cause confusion.

Summary

There have been major advances in our understanding of fundamental neurobiological processes involved in nociception. The increased understanding offers the opportunity for new therapeutic agents to treat pain in patients in all stages of diseases, including terminal illnesses. Evaluation of the pathophysiological mechanisms of pain in specific patient populations may also improve our ability to target treatment strategies for optimal outcomes.

References

1. **Payne, R.** (1989). Cancer pain—anatomy, physiology and pharmacology. *Cancer* **63**, 2266–74.
2. **Foley, K.M.** (1986). Pain syndromes in patients with cancer. In *Contemporary Neurology Series: Pain Management: Theory and Practice* Vol. 48 (ed. R.K. Portenoy and R.M. Kanner), p. 215. Philadelphia: FA Davis.
3. **Cleeland, C.S. and Syrjala, K.L.** (1992). How to assess cancer pain. In *Handbook of Pain Assessment* (ed. D.C. Turk and R. Melzack), pp. 360–87. New York: Guilford Press.
4. **Woolf, C.S.** (1990). Central mechanisms of acute pain. In *Proceedings of the IVth World Congress on Pain*, pp. 25–34. Amsterdam: Elsevier.
5. **Cevero, F. and Morrison, J.F.B.**, ed. *Visceral Sensation*. Amsterdam: Elsevier Science, 1986.
6. **Elliott, K. and Foley, K.M.** (1989). Neurologic pain syndromes in patients with cancer. *Neurologic Clinics* **7**, 333–60.
7. **Wall, P. and Glutnic, M.** (1974). Ongoing activity in peripheral nerves: the physiology and pharmacology of impulses originating from a neuroma. *Experimental Neurology* **43**, 580–93.
8. **Albe-Fessard, D.G. and Lombard, M.C.** (1983). Use of an animal model to evaluate the origin of and protection against deafferentation pain. In *Advances in Pain Research and Therapy* Vol. 5 (ed. J.J. Bonica, U.L.F. Lindblom, and A. Iggo), pp. 691–738. New York: Raven Press.
9. **Nathan, O.W.** (1983). Pain and the sympathetic nervous system. *Journal of Autonomic Nervous System* **7**, 363–70.
10. **Bennett, G.J.** (1993). An animal model of neuropathic pain: a review. *Muscle and Nerve* **16**, 1040–8.
11. **Verdago, R.J. and Ochoa, J.L.** (1994). Sympathetically maintained pain I. Phentolamine block questions the concept. *Neurology* **44**, 1003–10.
12. **Stanton-Hicks, M., Janis, W., Hassenbusch, S., Haddox, J.D., Boas, R., and Wilson, P.** (1995). Reflex sympathetic dystrophy: changing concepts and taxonomy. *Pain* **63**, 127–33.
13. **Willis, W.D.** *The Pain System: The Neural Basis of Nociceptive Transmission in the Mammalian Nervous System*. Basle: S Karger, 1985.
14. **Torebjork, H.E. and Hallin, R.G.** (1974). Identification of afferent C units in intact human skin nerves. *Brain Research* **67**, 387–403.
15. **Burgess, P.R. and Perl, E.R.** (1973). Cutaneous mechanoreceptors and nociceptors. In *Handbook of Sensory Physiology, Vol. II: Somatosensory System* (ed. A. Iggo), pp. 29–78. Berlin: Springer-Verlag.
16. **Schmidt, R., Schmelz, M., Forer, C., Ringkamp, M., and Torbejork, E.** (1995). Novel classes of responsive and unresponsive C-nociceptors in human skin. *Journal of Neuroscience* **15**, 333–41.
17. **Raja, S., Meyer, R.A., and Campbell, J.N.** (1990). Hyperalgesia and sensitization of primary afferent fibers. In *Pain Syndromes in Neurology* (ed. H.D. Fields), pp. 19–45. London: Butterworth.
18. **Burke, D.** (1993). Microneurography: impulse conduction and parasthesia. *Muscle and Nerve* **16**, 1025–32.
19. **Torebjork, H.E. and Ochoa, J.L.** (1980). Specific sensations evoked by activity in single identified sensory units in man. *Acta Physiologica Scandinavica* **110**, 445–7.
20. **Levine, J.D., Fields, H.L., and Basbaum, A.I.** (1993). Peptides and the primary afferent nociceptor. *Journal of Neuroscience* **13**, 2273–86.
21. **Walker, K., Perkins, M., and Dray, A.** (1995). Kinins and kinin receptors in the nervous system. *Neurochemistry International* **26L**, 1–16.
22. **Gordh, T., Kaarlsten, R., and Kristensen, J.** (1995). Intervention with spinal NMDA, adenosine, and NO systems for pain modulation. *Annals of Medicine* **27**, 229–34.
23. **Malmberg, A.B. and Yaksh, T.L.** (1992). Hyperalgesia mediated by spinal glutamate or substance P receptor blocked by spinal cyclooxygenase inhibition. *Science* **257**, 1276–9.
24. **Aley, K.** et al. (2001) Nociceptor sensitization by extracellular signal-regulated kinases. *Journal of Neuroscience* **21**, 6933–9.
25. **Bredt, D.S. and Snyder, S.H.** (1994). Nitric oxide: a physiologic messenger molecule. *Annual Review of Biochemistry* **63**, 175–95.
26. **Meller, S.T., Pechman, P.S., Gebhart, G.F., and Maves, T.J.** (1992). Nitric oxide mediates the thermal hyperalgesia produced in a model of neuropathic pain in the rat. *Neuroscience* **50**, 7–10.
27. **Mao, J. and Chen, L.L.** (2000). Systemic lidocaine for neuropathic pain relief. *Pain* **87**, 7–17.
28. **Galasko, C.S.B.** (1976). Mechanisms of bone destruction in the development of skeletal metastasis. *Nature* **263**, 507–10.
29. **Ferreira, S.H., Nakamura, M., and Castro, M.S.A.** (1978). The hyperalgesic effects of prostacyclin and protaglandin E2. *Prostaglandins* **16**, 31–7.
30. **Milne, R.J.** et al. (1981). Convergence of cutaneous and pelvic visceral nociceptive inputs onto primate spinothalamic neurons. *Pain* **11**, 163–81.
31. **Burton, M.D. and Gebhart, G.F.** (1998) Effects of kappa-opioid receptor agonists on responses to colorectal distension in rats with and without acute colonic inflammation. *Pharmacology and Experimental Therapeutics* **285**, 707–15.
32. **Black, D. and Trevethick, M.** (1998) The kappa opioid receptor is associated with the perception of visceral pain. *Gut* **43**, 312–13.
33. **Gebhart, G.F.** (2000). J.J. Bonica Lecture—2000: Physiology, pathophysiology, and pharmacology of visceral pain. *Regional Anesthesia and Pain Medicine* **25**, 632–8.
34. **Friese, N.** et al. (1997) Reversal by kappa-agonists of peritoneal irritation-induced ileus and visceral pain in rats. *Life Sciences* **60**, 625–34.
35. **Hunt, S.P., Pini, A., and Evan, G.** (1987). Induction of c-fos like protein in spinal cord neurons following sensory stimulation. *Nature* **328**, 632–4.
36. **Iadorola, J.J., Douglass, J., Civelli, O., and Naranjo, J.R.** (1988). Differential activation of spinal cord dynorphin and enkephalin neurons during hyperalgesia: evidence using cDNA hybridization. *Brain Research* **455**, 205–12.
37. **Draisci, G. and Iadarola, M.** (1989). Temporal analysis of increases in c-fos, preprodynorphin and preproenkephalin in mRNAs in rat spinal cord. *Molecular Brain Research* **6**, 31–7.
38. **Crosby, G., Chaar, M., and Uhl, G.R.** (1990). Subarachnoid morphine alters opiate peptide gene expression. *Pain* (Suppl. 5), S455.
39. **Watkins, L.R., Maier, S.F., and Goehler, L.E.** (1995). Immune activation: the role of pro-inflammatory cytokines in inflammation, illness responses and pathological pain states. *Pain* **63**, 289–302.
40. **Stein, C.** (1995). The control of pain in peripheral tissues by opioids. *New England Journal of Medicine* **332**, 1685–90.
41. **Stein, C., Millan, M.J., Shippenberg, T.S., Peter, K, and Herz, A.** (1989). Peripheral opioid receptors mediating antinociception in inflammation. Evidence for involvement of mu, delta and kappa receptors. *Journal of Pharmacology and Experimental Therapy* **248**, 1269–75.
42. **Stein, C., Schafer, M., and Hassan, A.H.S.** (1995). Peripheral opioid receptors. *Annals of Medicine* **27**, 219–21.
43. **Antonijevic, I., Mousa, S.A., Schafer, M., and Stein, C.** (1995). Perineural defect and peripheral opioid analgesia in inflammation. *Journal of Neuroscience* **15**, 165–72.
44. **Stein, C.** et al. (1991). Analgesic effect of intraarticular morphine after arthroscopic knee surgery. *New England Journal of Medicine* **325**, 1123–6.
45. **Sibinga, N.E.S. and Goldstein, A.** (1988). Opioid peptide and opioid receptors in cells of the immune system. *Annual Review of Immunology* **6**, 219–49.
46. **Wall, P.D., Devor, M., Inbal, R., Scadding, J.W., Schonfeld, D., Seltzer, Z., and Tomkiewicz, M.M.** (1979). Autotomy following peripheral nerve lesions: experimental anesthesia dolorosa. *Pain* **7**, 103–9.
47. **Bennett, G.J. and Xie, Y.K.** (1988). A peripheral mononeuropathy in the rat that produces disorders of pain sensation like those seen in man. *Pain* **33**, 87–107.
48. **Kim, S.H. and Chung, J.M.** (1992). An experimental model for peripheral neuropathy produced by segmental spinal nerve litigation in the rat. *Pain* **50**, 355–63.
49. **Seltzer, Z., Dubner, R., and Shir, Y.** (1990). A novel behavioral model of neuropathic pain disorders produced by partial sciatic nerve injury. *Pain* **43**, 205–18.
50. **Sommer, C., Lalonde, A., Heckman, H.M., Rodriguez, M., and Myers, R.R.** (1995). Quantitative neuropathology of a focal nerve injury causing hyperalgesia. *Journal of Neuropathology and Experimental Neurology* **54**, 635–43.

51. **Sugiomoto, T., Bennett, G.J., and Kajander, K.C.** (1990). Transynaptic degeneration in the superficial dorsal horn after sciatic nerve injury: effects of a chronic construction injury, transection and strychnine. *Pain* **42**, 205–13.
52. **Tal, M. and Bennett, G.J.** (1993). Dextrorphan relieves neuropathic heat-evoked hyperalgesia. *Neuroscience Letters* **151**, 107–10.
53. **Meller, S.T., Penchman, P.S., Gebhart, G.F., and Maves, T.J.** (1992). Nitric oxide mediates the thermal hyperalgesia produced in a model of neuropathic pain in the rat. *Neuroscience* **50**, 7–10.
54. **Schwei, M.J.** et al. (1999). Neurochemical and cellular re-organization of the spinal cord in a murine model of bone cancer pain. *Journal of Neuroscience* **19**, 10886–97.
55. **Rubens, R.D. and Coleman, R.E.** (1995) Bone metastases. In *Clinical Oncology* (ed. M.D. Abeloff, J.O. Armitage, A.S. Lichter et al.), pp. 643–8. New York NY: Churchill Livingstone.
56. **Cervero, F. and Iggo, A.** (1980). The substantia gelatinosa of the spinal cord. A critical review. *Brain* **103**, 717–22.
57. **Coggeshall, R.E.** (1979). Afferent fibers in the ventral root. *Neurosurgery* **4**, 443–8.
58. **Gu, Y. and Huang, L.Y.** (2001). Gabapentin actions on *N*-methyl-D-aspartate receptor channels are protein kinase C-dependent. *Pain* **93**, 85–92.
59. **Craig, D.D., Bushnell, M.C., Zhang, E.-T., and Blomqvist, A.** (1994). A thalamic nucleus specific for pain and temperature sensation. *Nature* **372**, 770–3.
60. **Giesler, G.J., Katter, J.T., and Dado, R.J.** (1994). Direct spinal pathways to the limbic system for nociceptive information. *Trends in Neuroscience* **17**, 244–50.
61. **Besson, J.M. and Chaouch, A.** (1987). Peripheral and spinal mechanisms of nociception. *Physiological Review* **67**, 67–185.
62. **Berkley, K.J. and Hubscher, C.H.** (1995). Are there separate central nervous system pathways for touch and pain? *Nature Medicine* **1**, 766–73.
63. **Mehler, W.R., Feferman, M.E., and Nanta, W.J.H.** (1960). Ascending axon degeneration following anterolateral cordotomy: an experimental study in the monkey. *Brain* **83**, 718–50.
64. **Nauta, H.J., Hewitt, E., Westlund, K.N., and Willis, W.D. Jr.** (1997) Surgical interruption of a midline dorsal column visceral pain pathway. Case report and review of the literature. *Journal of Neurosurgery* **86** (3), 538–42.
65. **Penfield, W. and Boldrey, E.** (1937). Somatic motor and sensory representation in the cerebral cortex of man as studied by electrical stimulation. *Brain* **60**, 389–443.
66. **Bertheier, M., Startstein, S., and Leiguarda, R.** (1988). Asymbolia for pain: a sensory-limbic disconnection syndrome. *Annals of Neurology* **24**, 41–9.
67. **Casey, K.L.** *Pain and the Central Nervous System Disease: The Central Pain Syndromes*. New York: Raven Press, 1991.
68. **Gonzales, G.R., Herskovitz, S., Rosenblum, M., Kanner, R., Foley, K.M., Portenoy, R., and Brown, A.** (1990). Clinicopathologic correlation of Dejerine–Roussy syndrome (DRS) caused by CNS toxoplasmosis in patients with AIDS. *Neurology* **40** (Suppl. 1), 117, 437.
69. **Lhermitte, J.** (1933). Physiologie des ganglions centraux. Les corps stries. La couche optique. Les formations sous-thalamiques. In *Traite de Physiologice Normale et Pathologique* Vol. 9 (ed. B.J. Roger), pp. 357–402. Paris: Masson.
70. **Fields, H.L. and Besson, J.M.**, ed. (1986). Pain modulation. *Progress in Brain Research* **77**.
71. **Taiwo, Y.O., Fabian, H., Pazoles, C.J., and Fields, H.L.** (1985). Potentiation of MS anti-nociception by monoamine reuptake inhibitors in rat spinal cord. *Pain* **21**, 329–37.
72. **Watson, C.P.N. and Evans, R.J.** (1985). A comparative trial of amitriptyline and zimelidine in post-herpetic neuralgia. *Pain* **23**, 387–94.
73. **Kishore, K.R., Max, M.B., Schafer, S.C., Ganghan, M.A., Smoller, B., Gracey, R.H., and Dubner, R** (1990). Desipramine relieves postherpetic neuralgia. *Clinical and Pharmacological Therapy* **47**, 305–12.
74. **Eisenach, J.C., DuPen, S., Dubois, M., Miguel, R., Allin, D., and Payne, R.** (1995) and the Epidural Clonidine Study Group. Epidural clonidine analgesia for intractable cancer pain. *Pain* **61**, 391–9.
75. **Botney, M. and Fields, H.L.** (1983). Amitriptyline potentiates morphine analgesia by a direct action on the central nervous system. *Annals of Neurology* **13**, 160–4.
76. **Anand, K.J.S. and Hickey, P.R.** (1987). Pain and its effects in the human neonate and fetus. *New England Journal of Medicine* **317**, 1321–9.
77. **Breitbart, W. and Patt, R.** (1995). Pain management in patients with AIDS. *Annals of Hematology–Oncology* **2**, 391–9.
78. **Lipton, S.A.** (1994). HIV-related neuronal injury. Potential therapeutic intervention with calcium channel antagonists and NMDA antagonists. *Molecular Neurobiology* **8**, 181–96.
79. **Britton, C.B. and Miller, J.R.** (1984). Neurologic complications in acquired immunodeficiency syndrome (AIDS). *Neurologic Clinics* **2**, 315.
80. **Patt, R.B. and Payne, R.** (1995). Management of pain. In *Williams' Textbook of Hematology* (ed. B.S. Collier and T.S. Kipps), pp. 203–8. London: McGraw-Hill.
81. **Platt, O.S., Branbilla, D.J., and Rosse, W.F.** (1994). Mortality in sickle cell disease. Life expectancy and risk factors for early death. *New England Journal of Medicine* **330**, 1639–44.
82. **Charche, S.** et al. (1995). Effect of hydroxyurea on the frequency of painful crises in sickle cell anemia. *New England Journal of Medicine* **332**, 1317–22.
83. **Moulin, D.E.** (1989). Pain in multiple sclerosis. *Neurologic Clinics* **7**, 321–31.
84. **Tasker, R.R.** (1990). Pain resulting from central nervous system pathology (central pain). In *The Management of Pain* 2nd edn. (ed. J.J. Bonica), pp. 267–83. Philadelphia: Lea and Febiger.
85. **Akdemir, H. and Pasaoglu, A.** (1992). Histopathology of experimental spinal cord trauma. Comparison of treatment with TRH, naloxone and dexamethasone. *Research in Experimental Medicine* **192**, 177–83.
86. **Ford, B.** (1998). Pain in Parkinson's disease. *Clinical Neuroscience* **5**, 63–72.
87. **Snider, S.R., Fahn, S., Isgreen, W.P., and Cote, L.J.** (1976). Primary sensory symptoms in parkinsonism. *Neurology* **26**, 423–9.
88. **Chudler, E.H. and Dong, W.K.** (1995). The role of the basal ganglia in nociception and pain. *Pain* **60**, 3–38.
89. **Owen, J.A.** et al. (1983). Age related morphine kinetics. *Clinical Pharmacology and Therapy* **34**, 364–8.
90. **Crook, J., Hideout, E., and Brown, G.** (1984). The prevalence of pain complaints in a general population. *Pain* **18**, 299–314.
91. **Payne, R. and Pasternak, G.** (1990). Pain and pain management. In *Geriatric Medicine* 2nd edn. (ed. C.K. Cassel, D.E. Riesenberg, L.B. Sorenson, and J.R. Walsh), pp. 585–606. New York: Springer-Verlag.

8.2.2 Acute and chronic cancer pain syndromes

Kathleen M. Foley

Adequate assessment is the critical first step to define a treatment strategy for patients with pain. The major goal of an assessment strategy is to use the most appropriate diagnostic and therapeutic approaches to define the cause of the pain and to direct its treatment. Advances in our understanding of the pathophysiology of cancer pain, coupled with the availability of validated pain measurement tools, facilitates such an assessment. Identification and categorization of a wide range of distinct and characteristic pain syndromes provide the clinical basis for choosing specific therapeutic strategies.

Prevalence data indicates that there are currently about 25 million people living with cancer worldwide. Numerous studies have demonstrated that the prevalence of pain increases with progression of disease and that the intensity, type and location of pain varies according to the primary site of cancer, extent of disease, progression, and the treatments employed.[1–3] Several countrywide studies have reported comparable epidemiologic data suggesting consistent prevalence rates of 30–40 per cent of patients in active therapy reporting pain and 70–90 per cent of patients with advanced disease reporting pain.[4–6] In a US survey of 1308 oncology outpatients treated by the Eastern Cooperative Oncology Group, 67 per cent reported recent pain, with 36 per cent describing pain severe enough to impair function.[7] In a similar study undertaken in France, 69 per cent of the cancer patients surveyed rated their worst pain to be at a level that impaired their ability to function.[8]

Studies have also looked at the global impact of pain in cancer patients. Uncontrolled pain precludes a satisfactory quality of life. Persistent pain markedly interferes with activities of daily living and social interaction. The impact of pain on mood and psychological functioning is complex, but numerous studies point to the increased risk of anxiety, depression, and suicidal ideation.[9,10] In a study of ambulatory patients with recurrent or metastatic lung or colon cancer, as many as 90 per cent experienced pain more than 25 per cent of the time.[11] More than one-half of the patients reported that pain interfered moderately or more with general activity and work. More than one-half of patients reported moderate or greater pain interference with sleep, mood, and enjoyment in life. In short, pain is prevalent among well-functioning ambulatory patients and substantially compromises function in about one-half of the patients that experience it.

In a study to validate the Memorial Symptom Assessment Scale, Portenoy et al. reported pain was present in 63 per cent of 246 randomly selected inpatients and outpatients undergoing active treatment for prostrate, colon, breast, or ovarian cancers, and was rated moderate to severe by 43 per cent of respondents.[12] In surveys of patients admitted to palliative care or hospice services, pain was inadequately relieved in 64–80 per cent of patients at the time of intake.[6,13] In a survey combining epidemiologic and ethnographic data, 2266 cancer patients who were referred to an anaesthesiology-based pain service were prospectively evaluated.[3] On referral, 98 per cent of patients suffered pain, with the average pain intensity on the day prior to admission rated as severe or worse by 70 per cent of the patients, despite 92 per cent of patients having been previously treated with analgesics or co-analgesics. These various studies point out the wide variation in assessing prevalence of pain in various populations of patients with cancer; however, they also point to the fact that cancer pain is a major problem and significantly impacts quality of life.

There are numerous ways to categorize the types of pain that occur in patients with cancer. These include definitions based on the neurophysiologic mechanisms of pain, its temporal aspects, its intensity, the categories of patients with pain, and on the specific pain syndromes that occur in such patients. These categories have practical value because they capture the multidimensional aspects of pain. Although this chapter will focus on the specific pain syndromes that occur in patients with cancer, a brief discussion of these categorical aspects is useful.

Neurophysiologic mechanisms of pain

Three types of pain—somatic, visceral and neuropathic—have been described based on neurophysiologic mechanisms. These are reviewed in Chapter 8.2. Pain may also be defined on a temporal basis. It is well recognized that cancer patients have both acute and chronic pain. This division is based on our increased understanding of pain mechanisms and on the recognition that the central modulation for these types of pain states may be different and that the clinical management of, and response to, treatment is different.

Temporal patterns of pain

Acute pain

Acute pain is categorized by a well-defined temporal pain onset generally associated with subjective and objective physical signs and with hyperactivity of the autonomic nervous system. These signs provide the health care professional with objective evidence that substantiates the patient's complaint of pain. Acute pain is usually self-limited and responds to treatment with analgesic drug therapy and treatment of its precipitating cause.

Acute pain can be further sub-divided into sub-acute and intermittent or episodic types. Sub-acute pain describes pain that comes on over several days, often with increasing intensity, and represents a pattern of progressive pain symptomatology. Episodic pain refers to pain that occurs during confined periods of time, on a regular or irregular basis. Intermittent pain is used to describe episodic pain. All of the pains in this category of acute pain usually have associated autonomic hyperactivity.

Chronic pain

In contrast, chronic pain is defined as pain that persists for more than 3 months, often with a less well-defined temporal onset. Adaptation of the autonomic nervous system occurs and patients with chronic pain lack the objective signs common to the patient with acute pain. Chronic pain is associated with significant changes in personality, lifestyle, and functional ability. Such patients require a management approach that encompasses not only treatment of the cause of the pain, but also treatment of its complications that have ensued in their functional status, social lives, and personalities.[14] Treatment of chronic pain is especially challenging because it requires careful assessment of not only the intensity of pain, but the degree of psychological distress as well.

Breakthrough pain

More recently, a language using more specific terms to define and convey pain that occurs in cancer patients with both acute and chronic pain states has been implemented. Baseline pain is defined as the pain reported by patients as the average pain intensity experienced for 12 h or more during a 24-h period. Breakthrough pain is characterized by a transient increase in pain to greater than moderate intensity occurring on a baseline pain of moderate intensity or less.[15]

Breakthrough pain has a diversity of characteristics. In some patients, it characterizes pain onset or marked worsening of pain, at the end of the dosing interval of the regularly scheduled analgesic. In other patients, it is caused by an action of the patient and referred to as incident pain. In some patients, incident pains have a non-volitional precipitate, such as flatulence. The majority of breakthrough pains are usually thought to be associated with a known malignant cause, but a small percentage may be unrelated to either the cancer or its treatment.

Pain intensity

Pain may also be defined on the basis of intensity, and there is an extensive literature in the use of words to describe pain intensity. However, it is well recognized that there are limitations in a unidimensional concept of pain. Specific categorical scales of pain intensity have been used, in which patients are asked to describe their pain as mild, moderate, severe, or excruciating. Visual analogue scales have also been used. These are often a 10-cm line anchored on either end by two points—'no pain' or 'worse possible pain'—and the patient is asked to mark on the line the intensity of their pain. Numerical scales are also commonly used, asking patients to rate their pain from a number 1 ('no pain') to a 10 ('worse possible pain'). These different scales used to capture a patient's experience have now been validated.

Pain intensity assessment must be appropriate to the patient under study; for example, in children the measurement of pain intensity includes various age-specific methods that again have been validated. Symptom measurement, including the measurement of pain, is discussed in much greater detail in Chapter 6.1.

Pain setting

Pain can also be defined by the setting in which it occurs: for example, post-operative pain and procedural pain. Post-operative pain, procedural pain, and traumatic pain all occur in patients with cancer and are usually described as acute pain in which there is an identifiable cause and associated therapy.

Special groups of patients with pain

Pain can also be described by the special group of patients in which it occurs, such as pain in children, in the elderly, and in the mentally incompetent. It is beyond the scope of this chapter to define these different groups except to acknowledge that they represent aspects of the cancer patient population and that the specific aspects of age, gender, cognitive state, and ethnicity may have some impact on both the assessment and the therapeutic perspective taken to manage them.

Types of patients with pain

A series of specific types of patients with pain have been described in the cancer population (Table 1). Group I comprises patients with acute cancer-related pain. A sub-group of this category includes patients in whom pain is the major symptom related to the diagnosis of cancer. For this group, pain has a special meaning as the harbinger of their illness. The occurrence of pain during the course of the illness or after successful therapy has the immediate implication of recurrent disease. Determination of the cause of the pain may present a diagnostic problem, but effective treatment of the cause, for example, radiation therapy for bone metastases, is usually possible and associated with dramatic pain relief in the majority of patients.

The second sub-group of Group I include patients who have acute pain associated with their cancer therapy, for example, pain after surgery or secondary to the acute effects of chemotherapy. The cause of the pain is readily identified and its course is predictable and self-limiting. Such patients endure such pain for promise of a successful outcome. This is most readily observable in patients undergoing bone marrow transplant, who commonly under-medicate themselves for oral mucositis pain.

Group II consists of patients with chronic cancer related pain with difficult diagnostic and therapeutic problems. The group can be sub-divided into patients with chronic pain associated with tumour progression, and those with chronic pain related to cancer treatment. Both sub-groups have pain that has persisted for more than 3 months. In patients with chronic pain associated with the progression of disease, such as those with carcinoma of the pancreas, the pain escalates in intensity and combinations of antitumour therapy, analgesic drug therapy, and anaesthetic blocks and behavioural approaches to pain control are all attempted with varying degrees of success.[16] Psychological factors may play an important role in this patient population in whom palliative anticancer therapy may be of little value and is physically debilitating. A sense of hopelessness and fear of impending death may add to and exaggerate the pain, which then contributes to the overall suffering of the patient.[17] Identification of both the pain and the suffering component is essential for the provision of adequate therapy. It is for this group of patients that Cicely Saunders has used the phrase 'total pain' to describe the aetiologic components other than a noxious physical stimulus, including emotional, social, bureaucratic, financial, and spiritual pain.[18] Those caring for this group of patients must be concerned with all aspects of distress and discomfort if the experience of physical pain is to be alleviated. The chronicity of the pain is associated with a series of psychological signs—disturbances in sleep, reduction in appetite, impaired concentration, and irritability—and with the clinical signs and symptoms mimicking a depressive disorder.

Table 1 Types of patients with cancer pain

Group I—Patients with acute cancer-related pain
Associated with the diagnosis of cancer
Associated with the cancer therapy (surgery, chemotherapy, and radiation therapy)
Group II—Patients with chronic cancer-related pain
Associated with cancer progression
Associated with cancer therapy (surgery, chemotherapy, and radiation therapy)
Group III—Patients with pre-existing chronic pain and cancer-related pain
Group IV—Patients with a history of drug addiction and cancer-related pain
Actively involved in illicit drug use
In methadone maintenance programme
With a history of drug abuse
Group V—Dying patients with cancer-related pain

Patients with chronic pain associated with cancer therapy usually require treatment directed at the symptoms, not the cause. Treatment of the pain is often limited by the lack of available methods to remove the cause of the pain. This group of patients closely parallels those in the general population with chronic intractable pain. Identification of the group of patients is imperative because recognition of the cause of the pain as independent of the cancer markedly alters the patients' therapy, prognosis, and psychological state. All approaches intended to maintain the functional state should be employed. For example, post-mastectomy pain occurring in a patient following a simple mastectomy is a commonly described treatment-related cancer pain syndromes.[19] The persistent neuropathic pain often interferes with the patient's quality of life and is a constant reminder to the patient of their breast cancer diagnosis and surgical management. In patients with treatment related pain syndromes, approaches other than drug therapy may often provide effective alternatives to pain management. This group of patients is increasing in size and accounts for up to 25 per cent of patients referred to the Memorial Sloan-Kettering Cancer Pain Clinic.[20]

Group III includes patients with a history of chronic non-malignant pain who have cancer and associated pain. Psychological factors play an important part in this group of patients whose psychological and functional status is already compromised. They are at risk for further functional incapacity and escalating chronic pain. However, their history should not be used in a punitive way to minimize their complaints. Identification of this group of patients as a high-risk group helps to improve their psychological assessment and intervention.

Group IV includes patients with a history of drug addiction who have a cancer-related pain.[21] Three sub-groups can be identified: one, patients actively involved in illicit drug use and drug-seeking behaviour; two, those receiving methadone in a methadone maintenance programme; and three, those who have not used drugs in several years. Under-treatment with analgesic drugs occurs most commonly in this Group IV population of patients. Assessment of reported pain by physicians and nurses is coloured by the fact that pain symptoms are confused with drug-seeking behaviour. Attention to the medical and psychological needs of these patients requires individual assessment and consultation with experts in drug-related problems. The first sub-group represents a major management problem, straining the most tolerant of medical care systems. Pain in the other two sub-groups is readily managed with the recognition that the psychological stresses consequent to the pain in cancer may place the patient at high risk for recidivism.

Group V includes dying patients with pain. In this group, diagnostic and therapeutic consideration should be directed at maintaining the comfort of the patient.[22,23] Issues of hopelessness and of death and dying become prominent and a suffering component of the illness must be addressed. Inadequate control of pain exacerbates the suffering and demoralizes both the family and the medical personnel, who feel that they have failed in treating the patient's pain at a time when adequate treatment may have mattered most. Rapid escalation of analgesic drug therapy and attempts to ameliorate the psychological symptoms should be employed. The risk/benefit ratios associated with analgesic approaches become less of an issue, as the goal of pain therapy is the comfort of the patient. A clear understanding of the common associated symptoms that occur in this population of patients and the use of approaches that actively search out and provide appropriate symptom control are particularly important in this group of patients. The use of end-of-life care pathways, the potential use for sedation to control intractable symptoms, and the comprehensive attention and impeccable attention in management of the wide variety of symptoms in dying patients can dramatically improve their care.

Clinical assessment of pain

Certain general principles should be adhered to when evaluating all cancer patients who complain of pain (Table 2). Lack of attention to these general principles is the major cause of misdiagnosis of a specific pain syndrome.

Believe the patient's complaint of pain

Critical to the management of the patient with cancer pain is the establishment of a trusting relationship with the physician. The complaint of pain is a symptom, not a diagnosis. Pain perception is not simply a function of the amount of physical injury sustained by the patient, but is a complex state determined by multiple factors. It is important to remember that the diagnosis of a specific pain syndrome and a complete understanding of the psychological state of the patient are not always made on the initial evaluation. In fact, it may take several weeks to define its nature because of the lack of radiological or pathological verification. It may take a similar period to comprehend fully the psychological makeup of the individual patient. There are numerous examples in the assessment of patients with pain and cancer that point out the limitations of the diagnostic procedures. It is not uncommon for patients with tumour infiltration of the brachial plexus with either lung or breast cancer to have pain for several weeks or months prior to the onset of objective radiologic and neurologic findings.(24,25) Similarly, it is not uncommon for patients with recurrent ovarian cancer to have new defined pain syndromes as the first and only sign of their progressive disease.(26) A comprehensive evaluation involves taking a careful history, performing a detailed medical, neurological, and psychological evaluation, developing a series of diagnosis-related hypotheses, and ordering the appropriate diagnostic studies.

Table 2 Clinical assessment of pain

1.	Believe the patient's complaint of pain
2.	Take a careful history of the pain complaint to place it temporally in the patient's cancer history
3.	Assess the characteristics of each pain, including its site, its pattern of referral, its aggravating and relieving factors and its impact on activities of daily living and quality of life
4.	Clarify the temporal aspects of the pain; acute, sub-acute, chronic, baseline, intermittent, breakthrough, or incident
5.	List and prioritize each pain complaint
6.	Evaluate the response to previous and current analgesic and antitumour therapies
7.	Evaluate the psychological state of the patient
8.	Ask if the patient has a past history of alcohol or drug dependence
9.	Perform a careful medical and neurological examination
10.	Order and personally review the appropriate diagnostic procedures
11.	Treat the patient's pain to facilitate the necessary workup
12.	Design the diagnostic and therapeutic approach to suit the individual
13.	Provide continuity of care from evaluation to treatment, to ensure patient compliance and to reduce patient anxiety
14.	Reassess the patient's response to pain therapy
15.	Discuss advance care planning with the patient and the family

Take a careful history of the pain complaint

This should include the patient's description of:

1. the site of the pain;
2. quality of pain;
3. exacerbating and relieving factors;
4. its temporal pattern;
5. its exact onset;
6. the associated symptoms and signs;
7. interference with activities of daily living;
8. impact on the patient's psychological state;
9. response to previous and current analgesic therapies.

Multiple pain complaints are common in patients with advanced disease and need to be ordered in terms of priority and classification.

Evaluate the psychological state of the patient

It is imperative to clarify the patient's current level of anxiety and depression and to learn whether he/she experienced such feelings before this illness. Knowing whether the patient has had psychiatric care can help to clarify the patient's psychological risk for decompensation during this acute stressful situation of a new or recurrent diagnosis of cancer.

Does a patient have a history or family history of acute or chronic pain? Information on how he/she handled previous painful events may provide insights into whether the patient has demonstrated chronic illness behaviour. A personal or family history of alcohol or drug dependence may explain why the patient may be fearful or refuses to take opioid drugs. Has the patient seen someone die a painful death? From our experience, patients who have had such an experience are particularly fearful of their own death and have serious concerns about their ability to receive adequate care.

Since each patient has his or her own understanding about the meaning of pain, it is useful to have the patient elaborate this meaning. Do they think it represents recurrent tumour or are they convinced that it is simply a non-malignant pain syndrome? There is good evidence to suggest that when patients have a clear understanding of the meaning of their pain as representing recurrent tumour, they have increased psychological distress.

The importance of identifying psychological factors is supported by a variety of studies, which have focused on the impact of suffering in patients with pain.(17) Taxonomy of suffering has been described and the interface between pain and suffering is discussed in Chapters 8.2.10 and 8.17. There are a series of psychiatric syndromes that have been described in patients with cancer.(9) Awareness of the common psychiatric syndromes when evaluating the pain complaint may expand the physician's understanding of such a complaint.

Although it is critical to know as much as possible about each individual patient with pain, such information may not be readily available on the first interview, and in some instances may never be available because of the lack of intellectual competence on the part of the patient to define clearly these various components of their pain complaint. It is also necessary to verify the history from a family member who may provide information that the patient is unable or unwilling to provide; the family member may be more objective in assessing the disability of the patient who underreports his symptoms. Similarly, in a patient who is a poor historian, the family members may be able to provide essential information that may alter the diagnostic approach. All attempts should be made to compile a careful history and to define the medical, neurological, and psychological profile.

It is also critical, as the patient focuses on issues of quality of life, to ask the patient to define what he/she would do if the pain were intractable or intolerable. Does he have suicidal thoughts or a pact with a family member? Does he have a family history of suicide? Has he made previous suicide attempts? Does he have drugs reserved for such an event, or a gun in the house that he might use if he feels desperate? Such questions may allow patients to discuss openly their enormous fears of death and the need to take matters into their own hands rather than trust the health care professional to provide them with adequate control of their intractable pain or significant suffering. Such open discussion can allow the treating physician better to define for patients their options for care and reassure patients of his commitment to their care. Patients will rarely offer this information unless requested by physicians. Therefore, it is critical that a repertoire of specific questions be developed that can be integrated readily into the initial history taking by the physician. At the same time, it is important to ask patients questions about their advance directives, such as who is the their health care proxy and how they have viewed the use and application of their advance directives.(27)

Perform a careful medical and neurological examination

The medical and neurologic examination helps to provide the necessary data to substantiate the history. Knowledge of referral patterns of pain in the common cancer pain syndromes can direct the examination. The characteristics of pain in breast cancer patients with brachial plexopathy is so specific that they can help to define the diagnosis of tumour infiltration of the brachial plexus from radiation fibrosis of the brachial plexus.(24) Similarly, the commonly described post-mastectomy pain syndrome in women following surgical procedures on the breast—from lumpectomy to mastectomy—is readily separable from pain due to tumour infiltration.(19) The physical and neurologic exam also allows one to inspect visually and palpate the site of pain, and to look for the associated physical and neurological signs that might help to define the nature of the pain symptom.

Defining the degree of motor or sensory changes can help identify the specific site in the nervous system that may be involved. Similarly, in patients with sensory loss, the presence of allodynia and hyperesthesia and changes in thermal sensation can further define the nature of the sensory problem. Moreover, the degree of muscle spasm, gait instability, and impaired coordination can only be assessed following such a full examination.

Order and personally review the appropriate diagnostic studies

Diagnostic studies confirm the clinical diagnosis and define the site and extent of tumour infiltration in those patients with metastatic disease. Computerized trans-axial tomography (CT) and magnetic resonance imaging (MRI) represent the most useful diagnostic procedures in evaluating patients with cancer pain. The CT scan provides a detailed visualization of bone and soft tissue in a two-dimensional view and is most useful in defining early bony changes. CT is also useful in directing needle placement for biopsies and for anaesthetic procedures such as coeliac plexus block. More recently, the combination of CT with positron emission tomography (PET) has allowed for the detection of very small tumours that are not easily defined on CT scan only. MRI is particularly useful in evaluating vertebral involvement in epidural spinal cord compression as well as in parenchymal brain metastases, but has recently been extended to be most useful in evaluating the presence of diffuse lymph nodes in patients with breast and abdominal cancer. Along with the use of these major radiologic diagnostic techniques, there are a host of procedures including ultrasonography, radio-labelled tumour markers, and isotope scanning devices, as well as traditional bone scans based on radio-isotope uptake of abnormal areas in bone or soft tissue that can aid in assessing tumour recurrence.

The critical rule in using these techniques appropriately is that negative studies do not necessarily rule out a tumour aetiology for the cause of the pain. For example, numerous studies demonstrate that, for example, a negative bone scan does not rule out bony metastatic disease. Therefore, the physician, when ordering the necessary diagnostic procedures, should review them personally with the radiologist to correlate any pathological changes with the site of the pain, and should repeat these studies over time if the patient's pain complaint persists or neurological or physical signs develop.

Evaluation of the extent of metastatic disease may help to discern the relationship of the pain complaint to possible recurrent disease; for example, the post-mastectomy pain syndrome that occurs secondary to the interruption of the intercostobrachial nerve is, in our experience, never causally related with recurrent disease.(19) In contrast, in patients with carcinoma of the lung, the presence of recurrent disease is often associated with the appearance of a late post-thoracotomy pain syndrome.(28) The use of tumour markers, of which there are now a wide variety, can be very helpful in identifying that the new pain complaint may in fact represent a metastatic disease. These include the CEA antigen, CA125, CA15-2, prostrate specific antigen (PSA), and a new host of antigens that serve as indirect markers of recurrent tumour.

Treat the pain to facilitate the appropriate workup

No patient should be evaluated inadequately because of a significant pain problem. Early management of the pain while investigating the source will markedly improve the patient's ability to participate in the necessary diagnostic procedures. During the initial evaluation of the pain complaint, the use of a wide range of methods of pain control including anaesthetic and neurosurgical approaches, should be considered: for example, the temporary use of local anaesthetics via an epidural catheter to manage sacral pain or the use of a percutaneous cordotomy in a patient with unilateral pain below the waist from a lumbosacral plexopathy.(29) These approaches should not be considered for use only when all else fails, but should be an integral part of the assessment of the patient with pain.

Reassess the patient's response to therapy

Continual reassessment of the response of the patient's pain complaint to the prescribed therapy provides the best method to validate that the initial diagnosis is correct. However, in those patients in whom the effective therapy is less than predicted or in whom exacerbation occurs, reassessment of the treatment approach or the search for a new cause should be considered. An example is the patient with epidural spinal cord compression who develops a second block proximal to the one being irradiated, with neurological signs mimicking those of the original block.

Design the diagnostic and therapeutic approach to suit the individual

The evaluation of the patient must be closely allied to the patient's level of function, ability to participate in a diagnostic workup, willingness to undergo the necessary diagnostic approaches, objective evidence that treatment approaches may be beneficial, and the patient's life expectancy. Careful judgement should be employed in the use of diagnostic approaches that will have a direct impact on the choice of the therapeutic strategy or answer a specific question. The random use of diagnostic procedures in this group of patients is inappropriate, and may have an adverse effect on the quality of life for such patients. Open discussion with the patient about the need for assessment as well as the therapeutic options is critical to allow the necessary dialogue that will allow the patient to be part of the decision making process. In some patients, diagnostic procedures may be inappropriate because they simply confirm the existence of disease for which there are no treatments available or for which the treatments are major surgical procedures that would be inappropriate in, for example, a dying patient. Patient refusal of evaluation or treatment must be respected when the physician has fully explained the options to the patient and is convinced that the patient has an accurate understanding of the potential consequences of no further workup or treatment.

In a variety of studies, it has been demonstrated that new pathologies are commonly identified through a comprehensive assessment offering the opportunity for new therapeutic approaches, as well as pain management approaches, in managing the patient's symptoms.(30)

Discuss advance directives with the patient and the family

Lastly, it is critical in developing approaches for pain management that there be an open discussion about advance care planning so that the physician has a clear understanding of the patient's goal for therapy. The physician must have unconditional positive regard for the patient, placing the control of symptoms of pain and treatment of the patient's psychological distress in highest regard.[31] Knowledge of the patient's decisions about resuscitation, living wills, health care proxies, and symptom management should he/she become incompetent improves the physician's ability to care for the patient with advanced disease appropriately and humanely. Discussions related to the sedative effects of opioid therapy should help clarify the patient's perspective on their cognitive status during the course of their pain management. The discussion should include patient input on whether they would accept being sleepy as a consequence of pain therapy if their pain could not be controlled with them awake and cognitively intact.[23]

Cancer pain syndromes

Cancer pain has also been classified according to a series of common pain syndromes and their pathophysiologic mechanisms. The pain syndromes that occur commonly in patients with cancer have been evaluated in both inpatient and outpatient settings and have been divided into three major categories: (a) The first and foremost cause of pain in patients with cancer is that associated with direct tumour involvement. This accounted for 78 per cent of pain problems in a survey of the Memorial Sloan-Kettering Cancer Center inpatient population and for 62 per cent of the problem in an outpatient survey.[20] Metastatic bone disease, hollow viscous involvement, and nerve compression or infiltration are the most common causes of pain from direct tumour involvement. (b) The second group of pain syndromes are those associated with cancer therapy. This group accounts for approximately 19 per cent of pain problems in an inpatient population and 25 per cent of problems in an outpatient population. It includes pain that occurs in the course, or as a result, of surgery, chemotherapy, or radiation therapy. (c) A third category of pain syndromes includes those unrelated to the cancer or the cancer therapy. Approximately 3 per cent of inpatients have pain unrelated to their cancer or their cancer therapy, and this figure increases to 10 per cent when an outpatient population is surveyed.

These data reflect information about the prevalence of pain symptoms in adults with pain and cancer. Several other authors have noted comparable figures and have demonstrated that direct cancer involvement is the major cause of pain in cancer patients. Studies of an inpatient population of children with cancer demonstrated that one-third of children in active therapy and two-thirds with advanced disease have significant pain. Of interest, in children in active therapy, the major cause of pain is procedure-related pain, in contrast to tumour-related pain[20] (see Chapter 9.1).

In this section, a series of acute and chronic pain syndromes are described. The wide variety of syndromes has also been categorized as acute or chronic, as neurological, as tumour-specific, and as site-specific. A detailed description of all of the extant pain syndromes is beyond the scope of this chapter. Tables 3 and 4 list some of the more common clinical syndromes and incorporate previous classifications described by Foley et al., Cherny et al., and numerous other investigators.[16,20,28,32–36]

Acute pain syndromes associated with cancer

There are a series of well-described cancer-related acute pain syndromes that occur most commonly due to diagnostic or therapeutic interventions. Effective treatment directed at the cause is the common approach for management.

Table 3 Cancer-related acute pain syndromes[33]

Acute pain associated with diagnostic and therapeutic interventions

- Acute pain associated with diagnostic intervention
  - Lumbar puncture headache
  - Arterial or venous blood sampling
  - Bone marrow biopsy
  - Lumbar puncture
  - Colonoscopy
  - Myelography
  - Percutaneous biopsy
  - Thoracocentesis
- Acute post-operative pain
- Acute pain caused by other therapeutic interventions
  - Pleurodesis
  - Tumour embolization
  - Suprapubic catheterization
  - Intercostal catheter
  - Nephrostomy insertion
- Acute pain associated with analgesic techniques
  - Injection pain
  - Opioid headache
  - Spinal opioid hyperalgesia syndrome
  - Epidural injection pain

Acute pain associated with anticancer therapies

- Acute pain associated with chemotherapy infusion techniques
  - Intravenous infusion pain
    - Venous spasm
    - Chemical phlebitis
    - Vesicant extravasation
    - Anthracycline associated flare reaction
  - Hepatic artery infusion pain
  - Intraperitoneal chemotherapy abdominal pain
- Acute pain associated with chemotherapy toxicity
  - Mucositis
  - Corticosteroid-induced perineal discomfort
  - Steroid pseudorheumatism
  - Painful peripheral neuropathy
  - Headache
    - Intrathecal methotrexate meningitic syndrome
    - L-asparaginase associated dural sinuses thrombosis
    - Trans-retinoic acid headache
  - Diffuse bone pain
    - Trans-retinoic acid
    - Colony-stimulating factors
  - 5-flurouracil-induced anginal chest pain
  - Post-chemotherapy gynaecomastia
- Acute pain associated with hormonal therapy
  - Luteinizing hormone releasing factor tumour flare in prostate cancer
  - Hormone-induced pain flare in breast cancer
- Acute pain associated with immunotherapy
  - Interferon-induced acute pain
- Acute pain associated with radiotherapy
  - Incident pain associated with positioning
  - Oropharyngeal mucositis
  - Acute radiation enteritis and proctocolitis
  - Early onset brachial plexopathy
  - Sub-acute radiation myelopathy

Acute pain associated with infection

- Acute herpes zoster and post-herpetic neuralgia

Acute pain associated with diagnostic interventions

Common acute pain syndromes include: pain following bone marrow aspiration, thoracentesis, and post-lumbar puncture headache. Post-lumbar

Table 4 Cancer-related chronic pain syndromes

Bone pain syndromes
- Multiple bony metastases
- Pain syndromes of the bony pelvis and hip
  - Hip joint syndrome
- Pain syndromes associated with base of skull metastases
  - Orbital syndrome
  - Parasellar syndrome
  - Middle cranial fossa syndrome
  - Jugular foramen syndrome
  - Occipital condyle syndrome
  - Clivus syndrome
  - Sphenoid sinus syndrome
  - Odontoid fracture and atlantoaxial destruction
- Back pain and epidural spinal cord compression

Visceral pain syndromes from tumour infiltration
- Pain syndrome associated with pancreatic cancer
- Pain syndrome associated with ovarian cancer
- Pain syndrome associated with colorectal cancer
- Hepatic distention syndrome
- Midline retropentoreal syndrome
- Chronic intestinal obstruction
- Peritoneal carcinomatosis
- Malignant peritoneal pain
- Ureteric obstruction

Pain syndromes associated with tumour infiltration of nerves
- Tumour infiltration of the peripheral nerve
- Painful peripheral neuropathy
  - Sensory neuropathy
  - Sensorimotor neuropathy
- Tumour infiltration of the cervical plexus
- Tumour infiltration of the brachial plexus
- Tumour infiltration of the lumbar plexus
- Tumour infiltration of the meninges (leptomeningeal metastases)

Chronic pain syndromes associated with cancer therapy
- Post-chemotherapy pain syndromes
  - Chronic painful peripheral neuropathy
  - Avascular necrosis of femoral or humeral head
  - Plexopathy associated with intra-arterial infusion
  - Gynaecomastia with hormonal therapy for prostate cancer
- Post-surgical pain syndromes
  - Post-mastectomy pain syndrome
  - Post-radical neck dissection pain
  - Post-thoracotomy pain
  - Post-operative frozen shoulder
  - Phantom pain syndromes
    - Phantom limb pain
    - Phantom breast pain
    - Phantom anus pain
    - Phantom bladder pain
  - Stump pain
  - Post-surgical pelvic floor myalgia
- Chronic post-radiation pain syndromes
- Radiation-induced peripheral nerve tumour
- Radiation-induced brachial and lumbosacral plexopathies
- Chronic radiation myelopathy
- Chronic radiation enteritis and proctitis
- Burning perineum syndrome
- Osteoradionecrosis

puncture headache is an acute pain syndrome, which is typically precipitated by assuming an upright posture.[37,38] The incidence of headache is related to the calibre of the lumbar puncture needle and to the amount of cerebrospinal fluid removed. Persistent lumbar puncture headache is thought to be related to continuous cerebrospinal fluid leak, with reduced cerebrospinal fluid volume and traction on the meninges secondary to the loss of volume. It usually occurs hours to several days following the procedure and is most commonly described as a dull pain, usually with associated neck and shoulder pain. Persistent headache may necessitate application of an epidural blood patch, but assuming a recumbent position will dramatically relieve the pain.[38]

Acute pain associated with invasive therapeutic interventions

These include the pain associated with tumour embolization, chemical pleurodesis, and the most common acute pain, post-operative pain. Each of these pain syndromes have a known aetiology and are associated with transient pain which slowly improves, for example, with post-operative pain, in a matter of several days to 1 week.

Similarly, there are acute pain syndromes associated with analgesic techniques ranging from the pain following injection by either the intramuscular, or subcutaneous route or the pain induced in certain patients sensitive to histamine release. Opioid-induced headache is a rare complication of opioid drug therapy and appears to occur in a selective population of patients. Switching from morphine to drugs with less histamine release such as oxymorphone or fentanyl can often obviate this acute pain syndrome.[29] Spinal opioid hyperalgesia is a rare pain syndrome that occurs in patients following either epidural or intrathecal injections of high doses of opioids. It is typically characterized by hyperaesthesia and diffuse pain in the perineal, buttock or bilateral legs and may include segmental myoclonus, and priapism. The use of naloxone or a benzodiazepine has been reported anecdotally to provide relief. Reduction in drug by the removal of drug from the cerebrospinal fluid is associated with dramatic pain relief.[39]

Acute pain associated with cancer therapy

Acute pain syndromes associated with chemotherapy

Intravenous infusion pain

Four intravenous infusion-related pain syndromes have been described: venospasm, chemical phlebitis, vesicant extravasation, and anthracycline-associated flare.[40,41]

Hepatic artery infusion pain

Hepatic arterial infusion for patients with hepatic metastasis may be associated with a diffuse abdominal pain syndrome.[42] The pain is usually self-limiting and stops with discontinuation of the infusion. In rare instances, continuous infusions may be associated with a persistent pain syndrome. Some studies report that reduction in the infusion to a lower dose may ameliorate the syndrome.[43]

Intraperitoneal chemotherapy pain

Approximately 25 per cent of patients receiving intraperitoneal chemotherapy reported transient mild abdominal pain associated with a sensation of fullness and bloating. Another 25 per cent report moderate or severe pain necessitating opioid analgesia or discontinuation of the therapy.[44] The differential diagnosis of moderate to severe pain is either chemical peritonitis or infection. Certain drugs such as mitoxantrone and doxorubicin can produce chemical peritonitis. In those patients who develop fever and leukocytosis, an infectious peritonitis must be ruled out.[45,46]

Acute pain associated with chemotherapy toxicity

Severe mucositis is the most common consequence of chemotherapy and/or radiotherapy. Grading systems for the severity of mucositis have been developed and its treatment usually requires the use of both local and systemic analgesic therapies. Superinfection with fungal or viral microorganisms is common and careful attention to such infections is necessary to prevent systemic sepsis.[47]

Corticosteroid-induced perineal burning

This pain syndrome is characterized by transient burning sensation in the perineum following the rapid intravenous infusion of doses of dexamethasone. This transient pain lasts through the infusion time only and is usually associated with the use of large doses of dexamethasone in the range of 20–100 mg per intravenous bolus.[28]

Steroid-pseudorheumatism

This is another pain syndrome associated with the use of corticosteroids. It manifests as diffuse arthralgia and myalgia with muscle and joint tenderness following withdrawal from steroids. The symptoms occur with rapid or slow withdrawal, and may occur in patients who have been taking corticosteroids for long or short periods of time. The pathogenesis of this syndrome is poorly understood, but it has been speculated that steroid withdrawal may sensitize joint and muscle mechanoreceptors and nociceptors. Treatment consists of re-instituting steroids at a higher dose and withdrawing them more slowly.[48]

Painful neuropathy or mono-neuropathy

A variety of chemotherapeutic agents may produce a toxic peripheral neuropathy. The syndrome is manifest by painful paraesthesia and hyperreflexia, and less frequently, by motor and sensory loss or autonomic dysfunction. The drugs most commonly associated with peripheral neuropathy are the vinca alkaloids, especially vincristine, cisplatin, and procarbazine, and, more rarely, misonidazole and hexamethylmelamine. Dysaesthesias and paraesthesia occur in up to 100 per cent of patients treated with vinca alkaloids.[49] The painful sensations in patients with neuropathy are usually localized to the hands and feet, burning in quality, and frequently exacerbated by cutaneous stimulation of the distal extremities. Many patients complain of a significant hyperaesthesia and may develop associate autonomic changes. In patients with severe peripheral neuropathy and significant autonomic changes, sympathetic blocks may be indicated.

In patients receiving intra-arterial infusion of a chemotherapeutic agent, such as cisplatin, into the iliac artery, the therapy may result in a lumbosacral plexopathy or mono-neuropathy. In this syndrome, patients develop symptoms within 48 h of the procedure, characterized by the acute onset of pain, weakness, and paraesthesia in the distribution of the lumbosacral plexus. This syndrome is thought to be due to small vessel damage and infarction of the plexus or nerve at the site of injection. The prognosis for neurological recovery has not been fully established. Such patients have a pain syndrome of a neuropathic type, characterized by burning dysaesthetic pain in the leg, in an area with both motor and sensory dysfunction.

Chemotherapy-induced headache

An acute meningitic syndrome can occur in 5–50 per cent of patients treated for leukaemia or leptomeningeal metastases with intrathecal methotrexate. Headache is the prominent symptom and may be associated with vomiting, nuchal rigidity, fever, irritability, and lethargy.[50] The symptoms usually begin within hours following the treatment and persist for several days. The cerebrospinal fluid examination reveals a pleocytosis, which may mimic bacterial meningitis. Patients at risk for the development of this syndrome include those who have received multiple intra-thecal injections and those patients undergoing treatment for proven leptomeningeal metastases. A second syndrome associated with headache following chemotherapy administration is L-asparaginase-induced thrombosis of the cerebral veins or dural sinuses.[51] This occurs in upwards of 1–2 per cent of patients receiving this treatment as a result of the depletion of asparagine, which leads to the reduction of plasma proteins involved in coagulation and fibrinolysis. Headache followed by seizures, hemiparesis, delirium, vomiting, or cranial nerve palsies may occur. The diagnosis is established by gradient-echo sequences on MRI scan or by angiography. A third chemotherapeutic agent trans-retinoic acid therapy which is used in the treatment of acute promyelocytic leukaemia (APML) can cause a transient severe headache.[52] The mechanism may be related to pseudo-tumour induced by hypervitaminosis A.

Diffuse bone pain of acute onset

Acute bone pain is another common adverse effect of trans-retinoic acid therapy in patients with APML. The pain is generalized, variable in intensity, and closely associated with a transient neutrophilia.[53] A similar pain syndrome occurs following the administration of colony-stimulating factors.[54] The aetiology at the present time remains unclear.

5-Fluorouracil-induced anginal chest pain

5-Flourouracil (5-FU) in continuous infusion may be associated with the development of ischaemic chest pain.[55] Coronary vasospasm is the underlying mechanism and studies with continuous ambulatory electrocardiograph (ECG) monitoring of patients demonstrate a near threefold increase in ischaemic episodes over pre-treatment recordings. These ECG changes were more common among patients with known coronary artery disease.

Post-chemotherapy gynaecomastia

Painful gynaecomastia can occur as a delayed complication of chemotherapy.[56] It occurs most commonly in testicular cancer and resolves spontaneously. It is thought to be secondary to cytotoxic-induced disturbance of androgen secretion and it needs to be differentiated from tumour-related gynaecomastia, which may herald early recurrence of a testicular tumour.

Acute pain associated with hormonal therapy

Luteinizing hormone releasing factor (HRF) hormonal therapy

Initiation of LHRF hormonal therapy in patients with prostate cancer can produce a transient flare in pain symptoms in 5–25 per cent of patients.[57] Exacerbation of bone pain or urinary retention are the most common associated symptoms. This syndrome occurs typically within the first week of therapy lasting upwards of 1–3 weeks. Co-administration of an androgen antagonist at the start of LHRF agonist therapy can prevent this tumour flare from occurring.

Hormone-induced pain flare in breast cancer

Various hormonal therapies for the treatment of metastatic breast cancer can precipitate a sudden onset of diffuse musculoskeletal pain, commencing within hours to weeks of initiation of therapy. Erythema around cutaneous lesions changes in liver function studies and hypercalcaemia are other manifestations of this hormone-induced tumour flare. The underlying mechanism is not understood.

Acute pain associated with immunotherapy

Interferon (IFN)-induced acute pain

Patients treated with IFN may experience an acute syndrome consisting of fever, chills, myalgia, arthralgia, and headache that often begins shortly after initial dosing and improves with continuous administration of the drug.[58] The severity of symptoms is related to the type of IFN, route of administration, schedule, and doses.

Acute pain associated with radiotherapy

Oral pharyngeal mucositis, stomatitis and/or pharyngitis are radiotherapy induced-acute pain syndromes involving the oral mucosa. They occur with doses above 1000 cgy.[58]

These occur following radiation therapy to the head and neck region and are associated with inflammation and ulceration of mucous membranes. Acute cystitis, proctitis, and vaginitis can also similarly occur with local radiation therapy to the perineal region. These syndromes occur several days to a week after the initiation of radiation therapy and may take several weeks to clear. The prevalence of these syndromes varies. There is data to suggest the following abdominal and pelvic radiotherapy, 50 per cent of patients may develop an acute radiation proctocolitis associated with rectal pain, tenesmus, diarrhoea, and mucus discharge and bleeding.

A sub-acute radiation myelopathy may also occur and an Lhermitte sign has been reported as an early acute pain syndrome in patients receiving radiation therapy to an area that includes the cervical or thoracic spinal cord.[50] It is most frequently observed after radiation therapy for head and neck cancers and Hodgkin's disease. It is characterized by a painful shock-like sensation in the neck precipitated by neck flexion. Such pains radiate down the spine and into one or more extremities. This syndrome usually begins weeks to months after the completion of radiotherapy and typically resolves within a 3–6 month period.

Acute pain associated with an infection

Cancer patients have a high incidence of viral infection most commonly associated with the varicella virus and the clinical syndrome of acute herpetic neuralgia. Acute herpes zoster is characterized by the onset of pain or itch followed by the development of a dermatome rash occurring in the trigeminal distribution or in the cervical, thoracic, or lumbar region. Pain is initially dull and aching, progresses to continuous and is often associated with an acute lancinating component. Post-herpetic neuralgia is the term used to describe pain persisting beyond the clearance of the skin lesions. Aggressive therapy with antiviral medications within 72 h of the eruptions has been demonstrated to reduce the prevalence of chronic pain syndromes secondary to this viral infection. In some instances, acute herpes zoster may appear in an area overlying a malignancy and it occurs twice as frequently in previously irradiated dermatomes as in non-irradiated areas[59,60] (see Chapter 8.9.1).

Chronic pain syndromes associated with tumour infiltration

This category includes those syndromes associated with the common sites for tumour invasion of bone, hollow viscus, and nerve.

Bone pain syndromes

Bone tumours, either primary or metastatic, are the most common causes of pain in patients, with cancer. Tumour involvement of bone produces pain in one of two ways: by direct involvement of the bone and activation of nociceptors locally; or by compression of the adjacent nerves, soft tissues, or vascular structures. Bone pain is reviewed in detail in Chapters 8.1.2 and 8.1.4. There are a range of bone pain syndromes, which are associated with the common sites of bony involvement including proximal long bones, vertebrae, and skull. For example, both the hip and pelvis are common sites of metastatic involvement. The weight-bearing function of these structures essential for normal ambulation contributes to the propensity of disease at these sites to cause incident pain with ambulation. The bone pain syndromes associated with neurological signs and symptoms are also briefly reviewed here as they occur commonly and early diagnosis can prevent serious neurologic compromise.[28]

Hip joint syndrome

Tumour involvement of the acetabulum or head of the femur typically produces localized hip pain, which is aggravated by weight bearing and movement of the hip. The pain may radiate to the knee or medial thigh and occasionally this may be the only site of pain. Medial extension of acetabular tumour can involve the lumbosacral plexus as it travels through the pelvic sidewall. Bone scans, CT, and MRI are the common diagnostic approaches to assess pain symptomatology involving the hip. The value of both CT and MRI is that they can demonstrate the extent of adjacent soft tissue involvement (Fig. 1). An MRI scan seems to be more sensitive to early changes within the hip joint itself.

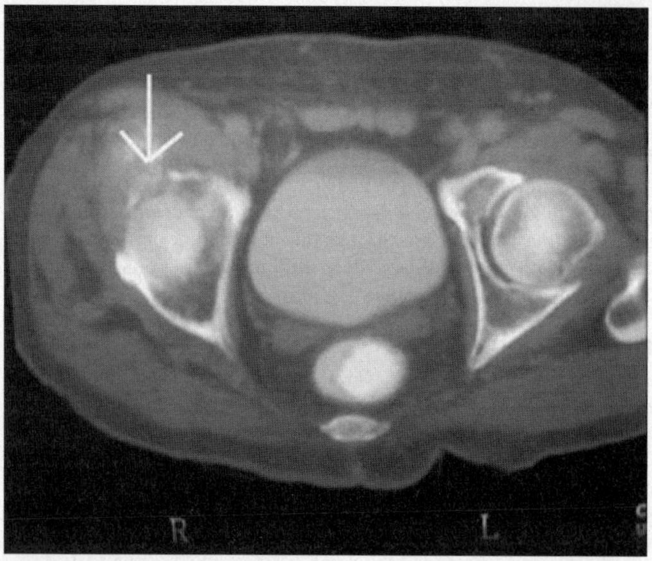

Fig. 1 CT of the pelvis demonstrating lytic metastasis in the anterior column of the right acetabulum.

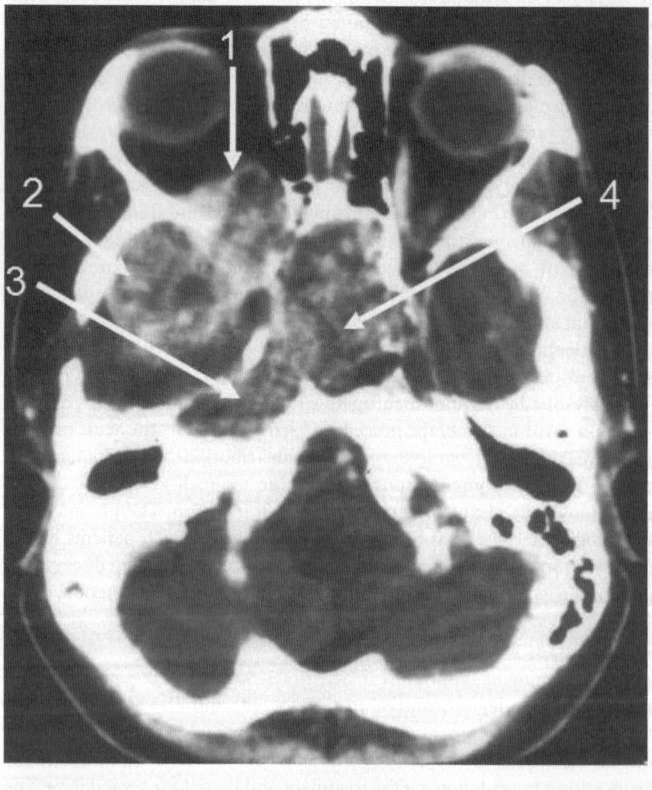

Fig. 2 CT scan of the base of skull demonstrating extensive metastases involving: (1) posterior orbit; (2) middle cranial fossa; (3) clivus; (4) sphenoid sinuses.

Pain syndromes associated with skull metastases

At least five clinical syndromes associated with metastases to the base of skull have been identified. These can occur with any tumour but are more commonly seen with breast cancer, prostate cancer, and less commonly lung and colorectal cancer. They maybe directly associated with nasopharyngeal tumours and they appear to be often diagnosed late in the course of illness.[61] They are best imaged by CT or MRI axial tomography (Fig. 2).

The orbital syndrome

The first symptom of this syndrome is progressive continuous pain in the supraorbital area of the affected eye. Blurred vision is followed by double vision. Examination reveals proptosis of the involved eye and external ophthalmoplegia. There maybe decreased sensation in the ophthalmic division of the trigeminal nerve or a palpable orbital tumour.

The parasellar syndrome

Parasellar syndrome presents as unilateral, supraorbital, and frontal headache in up to 83 per cent of patients and as diplopia without proptosis. Some patients may have an associated ocular paresis or papilledema.

Middle fossa syndrome

Most patients with a middle fossa syndrome present with numbness, paraesthesias, or pain referred to the second or third divisions of the trigeminal nerve. Over one-half of the patients experience a dull ache in the cheek or jaw. Pain similar to trigeminal neuralgia but without trigger points has been reported as a presentation. Sensory symptoms in the trigeminal distribution precede other symptoms by weeks or months. Diplopia, headache, dysarthria, and dysphasia can then develop. Headache occurs in up to 28 per cent of patients with a middle fossa syndrome; examination reveals sensory loss in the trigeminal nerve distribution in most patients, as well as signs of weakness in the pterygoids and masseter muscles, signs of abducens palsy and other ocular palsies.

Jugular foramen syndrome

The presenting syndrome in patients with a jugular foramen syndrome is hoarseness or dysphasia. Two patients had glossopharyngeal neuralgia and one of whom presented with glossopharyngeal neuralgia and syncope. Other patients have had unilateral pain behind the ear. The neurologic signs include unilateral weakness of the palate, vocal cord, and sternocleido mastoid and trapezius, and tongue muscles.

Occipital condyle syndrome

The presentation of this syndrome is with severe unilateral occipital pain worsened with neck flexion and associated with stiffness of the neck. Examination reveals tenderness to palpation over the occipital area and cranial nerve XII paralysis. Some patients may have weakness of the sternocleidomastoid muscle and dysarthria.

Clivus metastases

Presentation of this lesion is often with a vertex headache, which is exacerbated by neck flexion. Typically, there is involvement of the lower cranial nerves with evidence of their weakness and the signs maybe bilateral.

Sphenoid sinus metastases

Sphenoid sinus metastases often present with bifrontal headache radiating to the temples and intermittent retro orbital pain that may be associated with nasal congestion and diplopia. Examination may reveal the presence of unilateral or bilateral sixth nerve paresis.

Odontoid fractures

This lesion may simulate a base of skull metastases. The pain radiates over the posterior aspect of the skull to the vertex and is exacerbated by neck movement, particularly flexion. Fractures of the odontoid process are usually secondary to destruction of the atlas. Pathologic fracture may result in secondary subluxation and spinal cord or brainstem compression. Pain is the earliest symptom and neurologic signs of progressive sensory, motor, and autonomic dysfunction in the upper extremities may be observed.

Back pain and epidural spinal cord compression

Tumour infiltration of the vertebrae is one of the most common causes of pain in patients with cancer and is seen with the majority of tumours especially breast, lung, and prostate cancer. One of the most serious neurological complications of vertebral body metastases is the development of epidural spinal cord compression[50,62,63] (see also Chapter 8.14). In fact, most examples of epidural spinal cord compression (ESCC) are caused by metastases to the vertebral body that then spreads to the epidural space. Pain from vertebral body destruction usually precedes neurologic signs of epidural spinal cord compression by a prolonged period. Because the outcome of therapy for ESCC is dependent on early diagnosis, back pain must be considered a serious complaint whose misdiagnosis may lead to irreversible paraplegia or quadriplegia. Severe back pain is the initial symptom in greater than 95 per cent of patients with ESCC. However, it may also be the only neurologic sign despite a complete or near complete epidural block in 10 per cent of patients. The pain may be local, radicular, referred, or funicular. Local pain over the involved vertebral body, which results from involvement of the vertebral periosteum, is dull and exacerbated by recumbency (Table 5).

Radicular pain from compressed or damaged nerve roots is usually unilateral in the cervical and lumbosacral regions and bilateral in the thorax, where it is experienced as a tight band across the chest or abdomen. Referred pain in the midscapular region or in both shoulders may accompany cervicothoracic epidural disease, and bilateral sacroiliac and iliac crest pain may be observed with L-1 vertebral compression. Funicular pain is uncommon and presumably results from compression of the sensory tracts in the spinal cord. It usually occurs some distance below the site of the compression and is typically described as a hot or cold pain in a poorly localized non-dermatomal distribution.

The patient may develop neurological signs and symptoms including weakness, sensory loss, autonomic dysfunction, and reflex abnormalities. Weakness may be segmental owing to nerve root damage or pyramidal in distribution if the spinal cord is injured. Sensory abnormalities include ascending paraesthesias, a sensory loss, or complete loss of all sensory modalities below the dermatomal level in paraplegic patients. The upper level of sensory findings may correspond to the location of the epidural tumour or be below it by many segments. Bladder and bowel dysfunction is rarely the presenting symptom but may appear after sensory symptoms

Table 5 Clinical features suggestive of ESCC and cauda equina compression

Clinical features	Notes
Rapid progression of back pain	Ominous occurrence
Radicular pain	Can be intermittent in cervical and lumbosacral regions Usually bilateral in the thorax Exacerbated by recumbency, cough, sneeze, or valsalva
Weakness	Segmental: suggestive of radiculopathy Lumbosacral multisegmental: suggestive of cauda equina compression Pyramidal distribution: suggestive of spinal cord compression Variable rate of progression After development of weakness, 30% develop paraplegia within 7 days
Sensory abnormalities	May also begin segmentally May ultimately evolve into a sensory level Upper level of sensory findings may correspond to the location of the epidural tumour
Bladder and bowel dysfunction	Generally occurs late Early symptoms of conus medullaris or cauda equina lesion
Musculoskeletal features	Scoliosis Asymmetrical wasting of paravertebral musculature Gibbus (palpable step) in the dorsal spine Spinal tenderness to percussion

have developed. The exception to this generalization occurs with compression of the conus medullaris, which presents with acute urinary retention and constipation without preceding motor or sensory symptoms.

Reflex abnormalities from spinal cord involvement include absence of superficial cutaneous reflexes, increases in deep cutaneous and deep tendon reflexes at or below the level of compression and extensor plantar responses. Asymmetric flaccid motor weakness and sensory loss with absent lower limb reflexes characterize cauda equina compression. Conus medullaris lesions may present with a rapidly progressive symmetric perineal pain followed by early autonomic dysfunction and saddle sensory loss and motor weakness. Ataxia without pain maybe the initial presentation of epidural compression in 1 per cent of patients; this finding is presumably due to early involvement of the spinocerebellar tract.

In patients with back pain and a normal neurologic examination, the presence of a greater than 50 per cent collapse of the vertebral body on plain X-rays (Fig. 3) is associated with an 87 per cent chance of ESCC. Back pain in patients with normal plain radiograph requires further workup including a definitive study with MRI scanning. At the current time, MRI scans (Fig. 4) are the diagnostic procedures of choice but for those patients who are unable or unwilling to tolerate an MRI scan, the use of CT scanning with or without myelography (Fig. 5) are the other appropriate procedures of choice.

Critical to the care of the patient with back pain and impending neurological compromise is the use of appropriate diagnostic studies and treatment with steroids and radiation therapy. In some instances, surgery through either an anterior or posterior approach is appropriate to make the necessary diagnosis in those patients who have an unknown cancer or in patients who have been previously irradiated to the site for whom radiation therapy is no longer an option. Combinations of steroids, surgery, and radiation therapy and the choice of these approaches must be tailored to the individual needs of the patient. But at the current time, standard therapy is a short course of corticosteroids with focal radiotherapy.

Visceral pain syndromes

Pain from tumour invasion of a hollow viscus, with or without pleural or peritoneal involvement, is the second most common cause of pain in patients with cancer. These syndromes are addressed in some of the other chapters, for example, those related to symptom control and intestinal obstruction.[63–67] A brief consideration of the pain syndrome associated with pancreatic and ovarian cancer are mentioned for their unique aspects.[16,35,36]

Pain associated with pancreatic cancer

Pain associated with pancreatic cancer (see also Chapter 8.2.2) is associated with a variety of pain syndromes that have been referred to as both acute and chronic. From the available data, less than 10 per cent of patients when diagnosed with pancreatic cancer have tumours confined to the pancreas alone; 40 per cent have locally advanced tumours involving lymph nodes and peri pancreatic tissue and more than 50 per cent have visceral metastatic disease.[64] The most frequent metastatic sites include regional lymph

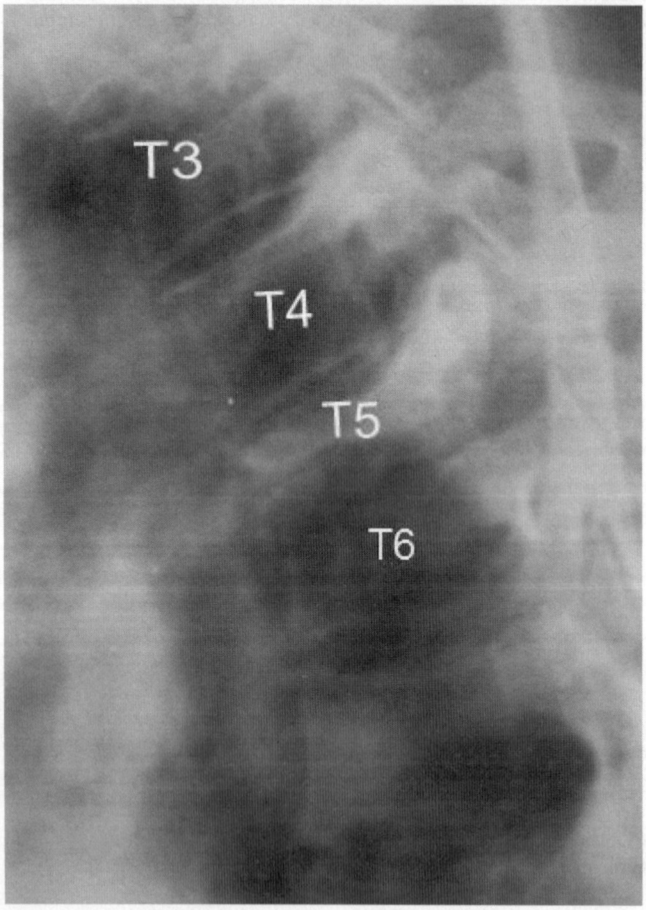

Fig. 3 Lateral spine X-ray demonstrating collapse of the T5 vertebral body.

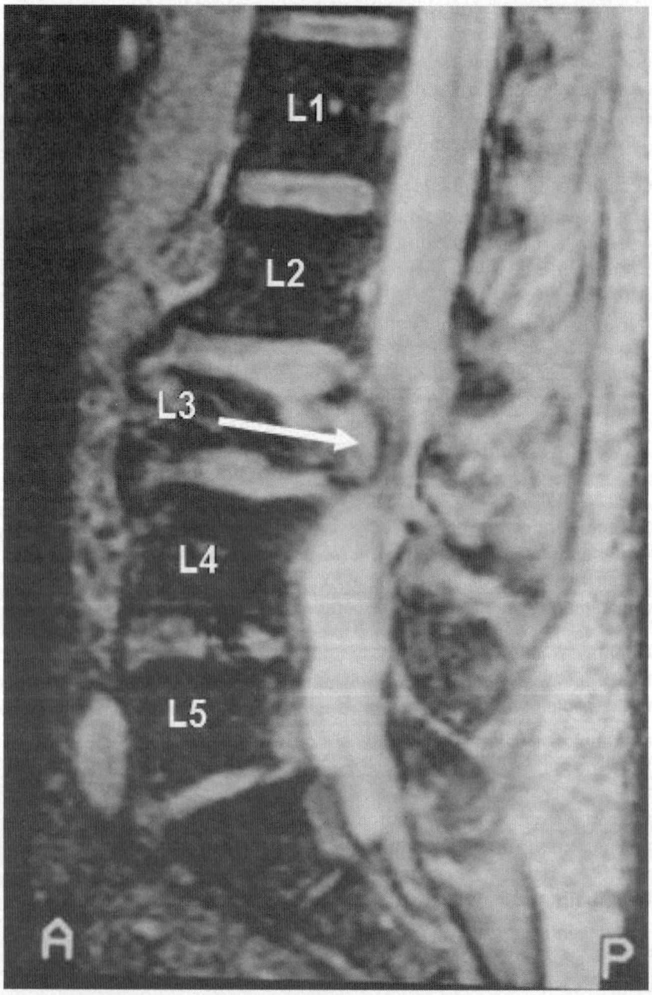

Fig. 4 Saggital MRI scan demonstrating compression of the thecal sac by a collapsed L3 vertebral body with posterior displacement.

(a)
(b)
(c)

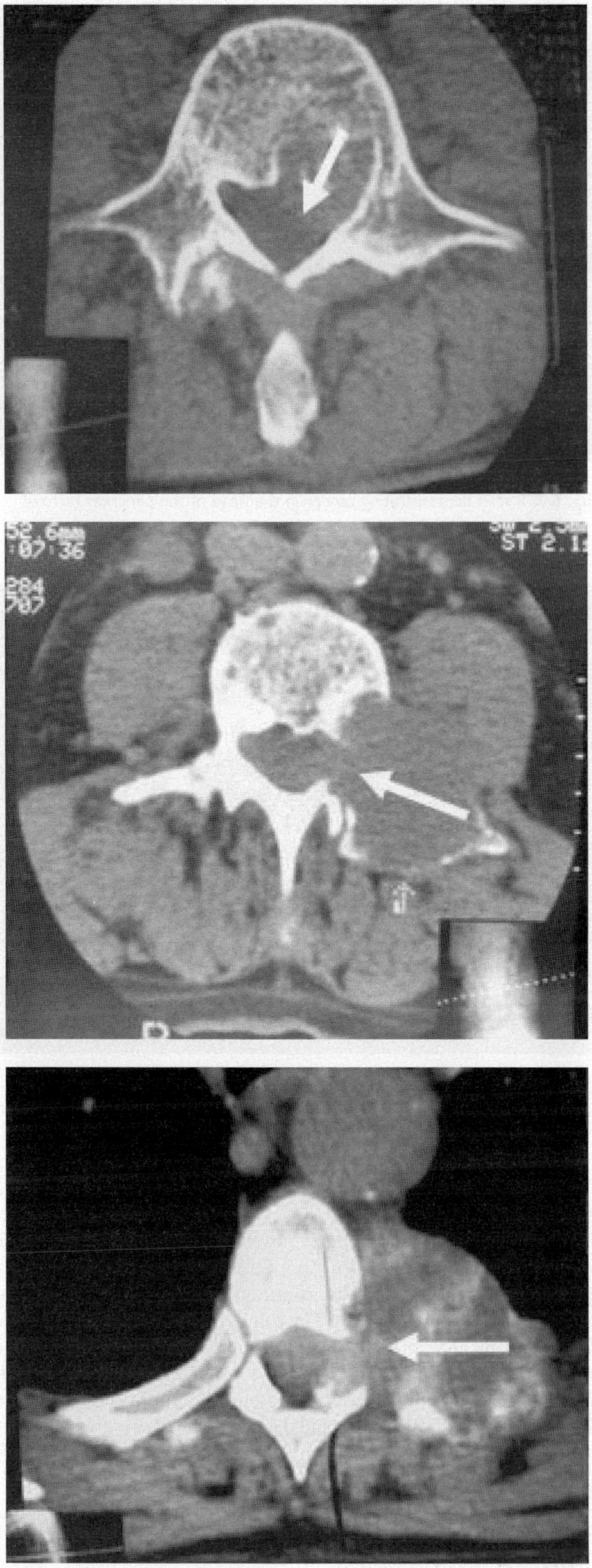

Fig. 5 CT images of ESCC: (a) metastasis in vertebral body encroaching directly into the spinal canal; (b) metastasis in transverse processes extending into the canal via the intervertebral foramen; (c) paravertebral tumour (from rib) encroaching via the intervertebral canal.

nodes, liver, peritoneum, and abdominal viscera. At the time of presentation the type of pain and its pattern are closely associated with the site of tumour within the pancreas. For example, tumours in the head of the pancreas produce biliary obstruction, a painless jaundice, with subsequent abdominal obstruction. Seventy-two per cent of patients with tumour in the head of the pancreas will have pain, in contrast to 87 per cent with tumour occurring in the body or the tail of pancreas. In the latter group, studies have suggested that pain occurs late in the course of the disease and results from gastric and retroperitoneal invasion. Metastases to the liver, to the peritoneum which results in ascites, to the retroperitoneal nodes to vascular structures and to the epidural space are the major sites of involvement for the development of intractable pain in pancreatic cancer.

Patterns of referred pancreatic pain have been studied by electrical stimulation of the head, body and tail of the pancreas following insertion of corresponding electrodes during elective surgery.(65) Pain originating from stimulation in the head of the pancreas localizes to the epigastrium and right of midline and is mediated by the right splanchnic nerves through the right thoracic sympathetic ganglia over the 6th–12th thoracic nerves. Blockade of these pathways by local anaesthetics is associated with relief of pain. Pain from stimulation of the body of the pancreas localizes to the mid epigastrium is mediated by the right splenic nerves and thoracic sympathetic ganglia bilaterally and can be relieved by bilateral blockade of these afferent pathways. Pain from stimulation of the tail of the pancreas is localized to the left epigastrium and left posterior intercostal space is mediated by the left splenic nerves and sympathetic ganglia from the sixth thoracic to the first lumbar nerve and can be alleviated by interruption of these pathways. The complexity of the innervation of the pancreas by somatic and visceral nerves points out the multiplicity of the nature of pain in this disease. Table 6 outlines a series of pain syndromes that have been identified in pancreatic cancer, including those associated with direct tumour infiltration and those associated with therapeutic interventions.(66)

Pain associated with ovarian cancer

In a study of the prevalence of pain in patients with ovarian cancer, 62 per cent of patients reported that pain preceded their diagnosis or their recurrence of disease.(26) Pain often readily disappears with antineoplastic therapy, either chemotherapy or surgery. Seventy-four per cent of patients reported that pain was located in the abdomen or pelvis with 15 per cent describing

Table 6 Pain syndromes in pancreatic cancer(66)

Tumour in the head of the pancreas
Tumour in the head of the pancreas with small bowel compression and/or obstruction
Tumour in the head of the pancreas with bilary obstruction
Tumour in the body or tail of the pancreas
Tumour in the body or tail of the pancreas with gastric compression or invasion
Tumour in the peripancreatic nodes with perineural splanchnic invasion
Tumour in the peripancreatic nodes with paraspinal or epidural extension
Tumour compression of portal vessels
Tumour compression of portal vessels with nerve compression
Tumour invasion of the peritoneum
Tumour invasion of the peritoneum with large bowel obstruction
Tumour invasion of the peritoneum with ascites
Tumour invasion of liver
Pain related to cancer therapy for pancreatic cancer
Acute post-operative pain
Chronic post-surgical diversion pain
Post-biliary shunt pain
Post-gastrostomy pain
Post-jejunostomy pain
Chronic post-cholecystectomy syndrome

the site as lower back, rectum, or genital area. Seventy-five per cent of patients described the pain as sharp and aching or cramping and two-thirds of those reported had an intermittent or prominent fluctuating component. Of particular interest, the prevalence of pain was similar to prevalence rates in populations with other solid tumours. Up to 30–50 per cent had pain during active antineoplastic therapy and as high as 80 per cent had pain associated with far advanced disease. Up to two-thirds of patients in one study described a highly stereotyped pain syndrome that usually disappeared after antineoplastic therapy of any type. This observation suggested that there is a clinically identifiable pain syndrome that may well herald the recurrence of disease.[26]

In short, pain symptomatology in patients with ovarian cancer is common and appears to be closely related to the presence of disease or as an early sign of recurrence suggesting that the onset of a new pain or recurrence over the previous pain should be an important sign to indicate the need for further diagnostic studies to evaluate the presence of new or metastatic disease.

Hepatic distention syndrome

Gross hepatomegaly or expanding intrahepatic metastasis may produce pain in the right subcostal region and occasionally in the right mid back or flank. The pain may be referred to the right neck or shoulder or in the region of the right scapula. The pain is typically described as dull and aching and maybe exacerbated by movement, pressure on the abdomen, and deep inspiration. It is commonly associated with anorexia and nausea. The pain originates from stretching of the hepatic capsule or from distention or compression of vessels in the biliary tract. Appropriate imaging of the liver and retroperitoneal space can determine the aetiology of the pain and steroids maybe effective in treating tumour-induced hepatic distention.[35]

Midline retroperitoneal syndrome

Tumour infiltration of the pancreas or lymph node enlargement in the paravertebral and retroperitoneal spaces are the most common causes of pain referred to the posterior abdominal wall and bilateral flank region. The pain may also be referred anteriorly to the epigastrium. It is commonly dull and boring in character exacerbated by lying down and improved by sitting. Ultrasound along with either CT or MRI scanning of the abdomen are the diagnostic procedures of choice (Fig. 6). This syndrome needs to be differentiated from ESCC which shares characteristic pain features with retroperitoneal tumour invasion and is common as tumour extends into local vertebrae and the epidural space.

Chronic intestinal obstruction

Diffusive abdominal pain is a common complication of chronic gastrointestinal obstruction.[35] These syndromes and their treatment are discussed in Chapter 8.3.4.

Peritoneal carcinomatosis

This syndrome occurs most commonly associated with colonic and ovarian cancer and is commonly associated with peritoneal inflammation, malignant adhesions and ascites.[35] CT scanning with contrast may demonstrate evidence of bowel infiltration and peritoneal nodules (Fig. 7).

Malignant peritoneal pain

Tumours of the gastrointestinal, genitourinary, and reproductive tract are commonly associated with perineal pain.[36] The pain is often characterized as constant and aching, aggravated by sitting or standing and maybe associated with tenesmus or bladder spasms. Characteristically, the tumour may spread by perineal invasion or by compression and infiltration of the musculature of the deep pelvis. CT and MRI scanning can provide an appropriate diagnosis, but many patients commonly complain of pain for long periods of time before radiologic documentation of new or recurrent tumour. In this setting, the use of tumour markers can sometimes be used to document the progression of disease without radiologic documentation.

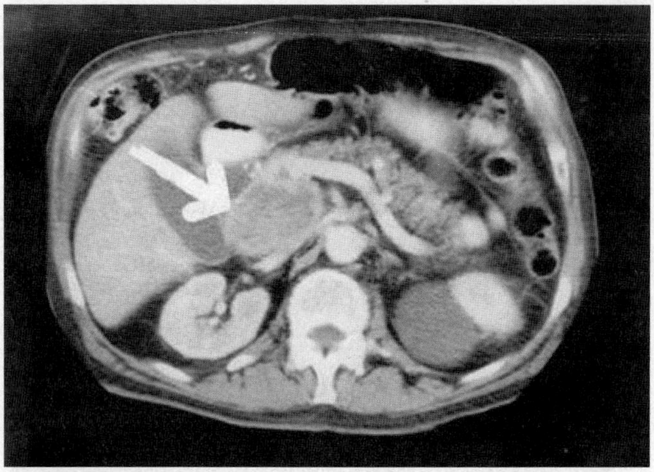

Fig. 6 CT scan demonstrating cancer in the head of the pancreas (arrow).

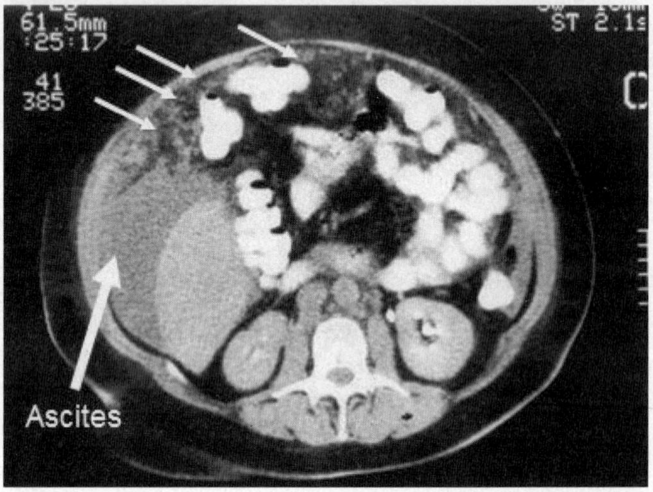

Fig. 7 CT demonstrating peritoneal carcinomatosis (small arrows) with associated ascites.

Ureteric obstruction

Tumour infiltration paravertebrally as well as within the pelvis is commonly associated with ureteric obstruction. Gastrointestinal, genitourinary, and gynaecologic cancers are most commonly associated with progressive obstruction of the ureters.[36,67] The pain is commonly unilateral radiating from the flank anteriorly to the groin region and exacerbated by standing and partially relieved by sitting. In some instances the pain maybe associated with acute spasms. The use of ultrasound, CT, or MRI can demonstrate the presence of hydronephrosis and define the site of compression. Ureteral stints can often dramatically improve this unilateral pain syndrome (see Chapter 8.1.5).

Pain syndromes associated with tumour infiltration of nerves

Tumour infiltration of nerve is the third most common cause of pain in cancer patients. They are briefly reviewed. Tables 3 and 4 list the common acute and chronic pain syndromes evaluated by an inpatient and outpatient pain consultation service and by a supportive care programme in comprehensive cancer centre.[20,35,68]

Tumour infiltration of the peripheral nerve

Constant burning pain with hyperaesthesia and dysaesthesia in the area of sensory loss is the usual clinical presentation. Tumour compression of peripheral nerve proximately occurs most commonly and is associated with paravertebral or retroperitoneal tumour. The pain is radicular and unilateral, and a careful sensory examination can often delineate the site of nerve compression. Metastatic tumour in the rib often produces intercostal nerve involvement.

Painful peripheral neuropathies

Painful peripheral neuropathies have multiple causes including nutritional deficiencies (B-1 and B-12), metabolic (diabetes and renal and hepatic dysfunction) abnormalities, neurotoxic effects of chemotherapy (vincristine and cisplatinum), direct invasion by tumour, and rarely, paraneoplastic syndromes. This latter cause for painful peripheral neuropathy is important as such remote effects commonly present as the initial manifestation of an underlying malignancy. Their course is usually independent of the primary tumour except for the neuropathy associated with myeloma.[50,69]

Sensory neuropathy

In this disorder, pain is a presenting complaint and is usually characterized by tingling sensations in the extremities, burning paraesthesias, sensory ataxia with marked impairment of joint position sense and occasional lancinating or lightening pains. These sensory symptoms result from an inflammatory process involving the dorsal root ganglia and are often part of a more general condition effecting the limbic lobe, brainstem, and spinal cord. The course of this dorsal root ganglionitis is independent of the primary tumour and does not appear to improve with treatment of the underlying malignancy. It is usually associated with small cell carcinoma of the lung and occasionally with carcinomas of the breast, ovary, and colon.

Sensorimotor neuropathy

Sensorimotor peripheral neuropathy is associated with a spectrum of findings ranging from dysaesthesias and sensory loss to extensive muscle waisting and weakness. This disorder rarely presents as a Guillian Barré syndrome.[70] The peripheral neuropathy associated with multiple myeloma is an example. Clinically evident peripheral neuropathy occurs in 13–14 per cent of patients with multiple myeloma and electrophysiologic evidence can be found in 40 per cent of patients. A progressive, painful neuropathy in a middle-aged man requires a search for multiple myeloma. The neuropathy precedes detection of the myeloma in 80 per cent of patients. Several sub-types can be identified including a small fibre amyloid neuropathy and a neuropathy associated with osteosclerotic myeloma. Multiple aetiologies for the myeloma-associated neuropathy have been proposed.

Tumour infiltration of the cervical plexus

The upper four cervical ventralrami join to form the cervical plexus. The plexus lies close to the upper four ventralrami between the deep and anterior lateral muscles of the neck and is covered by the sternocleidomastoid muscle. Damage to the plexus may present as aching pain the preauricular and postauricular region and the anterior neck. This injury may be due to a primary head and neck malignancy, metastases to the cervical lymph nodes or nerve damage following surgery on the neck. A Horner's syndrome maybe present if the superior cervical ganglion is involved. Because of overlap of innervations of the face and neck region from cranial nerves V, VII, VIIII, X, pain from a cervical plexopathy may commonly present as a facial pain syndrome.

Tumour infiltration of the brachial plexus

Tumour infiltration of the brachial plexus results from the contiguous relationship of the plexus to draining lymph nodes and occurs commonly in patients with lymphoma, breast, and lung cancer. In patients with lung cancer, the syndrome is often referred to as the superior pulmonary sulcus or Pancoast syndrome and results from tumour infiltration of the lower brachial plexus. In this patient population, this syndrome is characterized by pain radiating to the ipsilateral shoulder, posterior aspect of the arm and elbow and a C8–T1 distribution. Typically, the neurologic symptoms of pain and paraesthesias occur in the fourth and fifth fingers and may precede objective clinical signs for several weeks to months. These paraesthesias progress to numbness and weakness in a C-7, C-8, T-1 distribution. The supraclavicular and axillary regions maybe normal. The presence of a Horner's syndrome suggests involvement of the paravertebral space.[25]

In patients with breast cancer, the syndrome is often quite comparable to that occurring in patients with Pancoast syndrome.[24,71] For the most part, pain is the most common symptom and precedes neurologic signs or symptoms for up to 9 months. The pain's distribution depends on the site of plexus involvement. Eight-five per cent of patients with tumour infiltration present with pain, which is moderate to severe, beginning in the shoulder girdle and radiating to the elbow, medial side of the forearm and fourth and fifth fingers. In some patients, pain is localized to the posterior aspect of the arm or to the elbow. Some patients complain of a burning or freezing sensation and hypersensitivity of the skin along the ulnar aspect of the arm. This distribution of pain is consistent with involvement of the lower plexus. In some patients, pain is restricted to either the shoulder girdle or tips of the finger, either the index finger or thumb. In these patients infiltration of the upper plexus (C-5–6) often in the supraclavicular fossa is the site of nerve compression. By the time of diagnosis of a brachial plexus lesion, 98 per cent of patients have pain that is most often reported as severe. Paraesthesias occur as a presenting symptom in approximately 15 per cent of patients. The clinical signs include focal weakness, atrophy and sensory changes in the distribution of the C-7, C-8, and T-1 roots. This occurs in more than 75 per cent of patients. Twenty-five per cent of patients in one series presented with whole plexus weakness. Electrodiagnostic studies may be useful and may reveal fibrillation potentials and positive waves characteristic of denervation in the distribution of the brachial plexus. Radiographic studies such as computed tomography (Fig. 8) and magnetic resonance imaging with contrast are the definitive studies.

Tumour infiltration of the plexus must be distinguished from a radiation-induced reversible brachial plexopathy or radiation injury to the plexus or an acute aschemic brachial plexopathy. However, the clinical presentation of pain and the progression of neurologic deficit, particularly in a patient with evidence of active disease, should strongly suggest the diagnosis of tumour infiltration and lead to further diagnostic studies (see Chapter 8.1.5).

Tumour infiltration of the lumbar plexus

Lumbosacral plexopathy is one of the more disabling complications of pelvic tumours because both leg weakness and incapacitating pain immobilize the

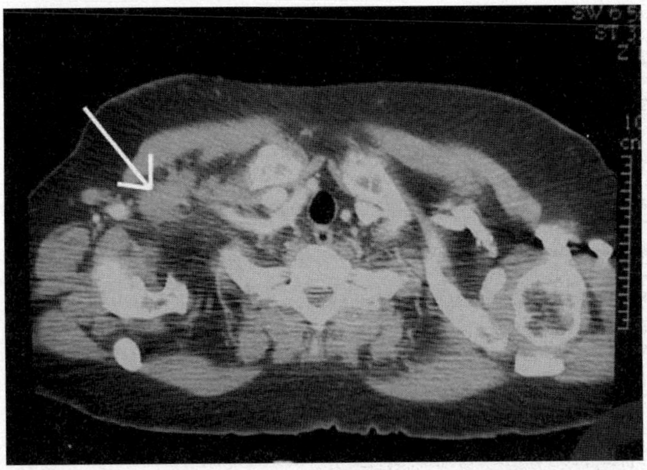

Fig. 8 CT scan demonstrating tumour mass (arrow) compressing right brachial plexus.

patient, leading to secondary infection, and venous thrombosis. In studies of patients with documented pelvic tumour by CT or biopsy, three clinical syndromes have been delineated. Pain is the most common clinical symptom in patients, with up to 70 per cent of patients having the insidious onset of pelvic or radicular leg pain, followed weeks to months later by sensory symptoms and eventually weakness. The quintet of leg pain, weakness, oedema, rectal mass, and hydronephrosis suggests plexopathy due to cancer. These syndromes can be divided into three groups including: (a) a lower lumbosacral plexopathy, which was the most common occurring from tumour infiltration of L-4 through S-1; (b) an upper plexopathy, characterized by tumour infiltration of L-1 through L-4 occurring in up to 31 per cent of patients; and (c) a pan plexopathy from L-1 to S-3 occurring in 18 per cent of patients.

Each of these clinical syndromes of lumbosacral plexopathy can be distinguished by their associated motor, sensory, and reflex abnormalities; all are associated with pain, with a characteristic pattern directly related to their site of involvement. For example, in patients with an upper plexopathy, the tumours are posterior-medially placed in the paravertabral gutter and extend into the true pelvis. In those patients with tumour extending above the pelvic rim, complaints of lumbar and flank pain are common. In lower plexopathy patients, tumours are posteriorly placed in the true pelvis and erode the sacrum. Posterior radicular leg pain is most common in this group of patients. But of note, patients also complain of flank, groin, and anterior thigh pain. Table 7 delineates the symptoms and signs by level of plexus involvement in a prospective population of patients studied for lumbosacral plexopathy.[67]

Leptomeningeal metastases

Leptomeningeal metastases result from diffuse multifocal involvement of the sub-arachnoid space by metastatic tumour. This disorder presents with symptoms and signs of structural disease involving the neuroaxis at more than one anatomic site. Neurologic signs are often more prominent and widespread than the symptoms alone. They may include cerebral, cranial nerve, and spinal cord symptoms and signs. Headache and radicular pain in the low back and buttock are the common pain symptoms. Headache appears to be one of the most common presenting complaints. It is often severe, intractable, and associated with nausea, vomiting, and nuchal rigidity. The headache may be associated with changes in mental status including lethargy, confusion, or loss of memory. In some instances, seizures may be the first sign of leptomeningeal involvement. Up to one-third of patients may present with cranial nerve symptoms characterized by double vision, hearing loss, facial numbness, or decreased vision. Both atypical facial pain resembling cluster headache as well as glossopharyngeal neuralgia with syncope have been reported. Back and radicular pain, weakness and paraesthesias in the lower extremities, and bowel or bladder dysfunction have also been reported, with more than half of patients having spinal cord and nerve root involvement upon examination.

A natural history of leptomeningeal metastases is one of progressive neurologic dysfunction at multiple sites. The diagnosis is confirmed through the use of MRI scans with contrast (Fig. 9) and a direct analysis of the cerebrospinal fluid following lumbar puncture.[50,71]

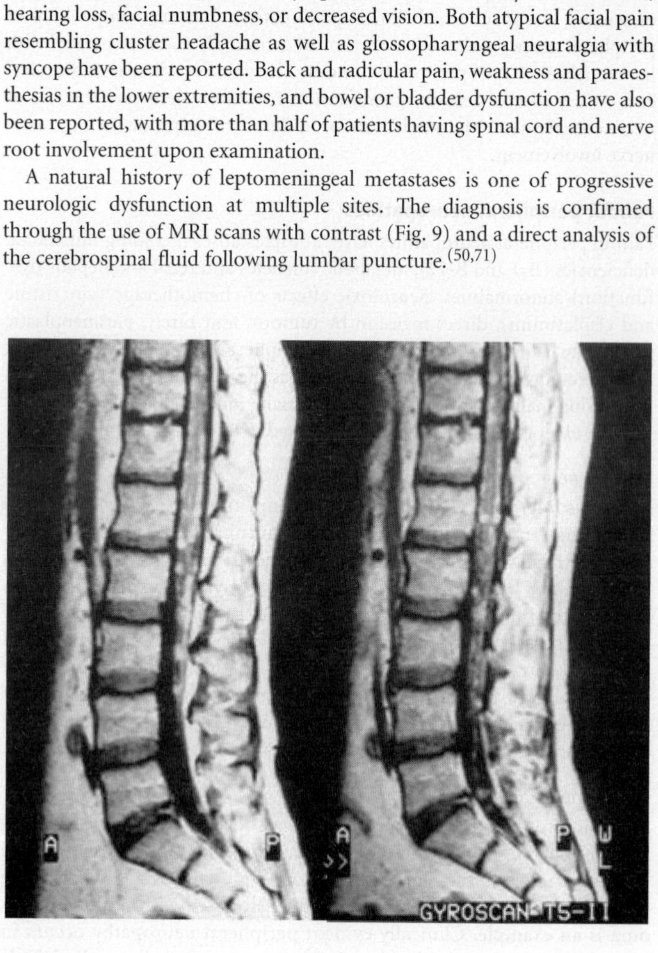

Fig. 9 Sagittal MRI of the spine with gadolinium contrast demonstrating multiple enhancing tumour deposits characteristic of leptomeningeal metastases.

Table 7 Symptoms and signs by level of plexus involvement. Prospective patients ($n = 34$)[67]

Clinical level	Upper	Lower	Pain
Number of patients	12	16	6
Most common tumour	Colorectal	Sarcoma	Genitourinary
Pain distribution			
Local	Lower abdomen	Buttock, perineum	Lumbosacral
Radicular	Anterolateral thigh	Posterolateral thigh, leg	Variable
Referred	Flank, iliac crest	Hip and ankle	Variable
Numbness/paraesthesias	Anterior thigh	Perineum, thigh, sole	Anterior thigh, leg, foot
Motor and reflex changes	L2–L4	L5–S1	L2–S2
Sensory loss	Anterolateral thigh	Posterior thigh, sole	Esp. anterior thigh, leg
Tenderness	Lumbar	Sciatic notch, sacrum	Lumbosacral
Positive SLRT[a]			
Direct	6/12	8/16	5/6
Reverse	2/12	8/16	5/6
Leg oedema	5/12	6/16	5/6
Rectal mass	3/12	8/16	0/6
Sphincter weakness	0/12	8/16	0/6

[a] Straight leg raising test.

Chronic pain syndromes associated with cancer therapy

Post-surgical pain syndromes

In assessing a patient with a post-surgical pain syndrome, knowledge of the exact time of onset of the syndrome is critical to help differentiate it from recurrent tumour. Post-surgical syndromes are characterized by either persistent pain following a surgical procedure or recurrent pain after the initial surgical pain has cleared. A series of post-surgical pain syndromes have been identified in cancer patients undergoing common surgical procedures.

Post-mastectomy pain syndrome

Four to 10 per cent of women who undergo any surgical procedure on the breast, from lumpectomy to radical mastectomy, are at risk to develop this syndrome. The pain can occur immediately, several days following the procedure, or as late as 6 months following the surgery.[19,28,72] Pain is characterized by a constricting, burning sensation localized to the posterior arm, axilla, and anterior chest wall in the area of sensory loss. It is aggravated by arm movement and relieved by immobilization. Patients often develop a frozen shoulder because they posture the arm in a flexed position, close to the chest wall to reduce the pain associated with movement. In the majority of patients, a trigger point in the axilla or anterior chest wall can often be palpated and corresponds to the site of a traumatic neuroma. Following a series of anatomical studies, the aetiology of post-mastectomy pain is believed to be a neuroma originating from the intercostobrachial nerve, a cutaneous sensory branch of T1–T2. The nature of the pain and the clinical symptoms should distinguish it readily from tumour infiltration of the brachial plexus. There is marked anatomical variation in the size and distribution of the intercostobrachial nerve, accounting for its variable appearance in patients undergoing mastectomy. The syndrome appears to occur more commonly in patients who have had post-operative complications at the time of their breast surgery, such as local haematoma, infection, or problems in wound closure. Those patients who demonstrated an increased risk for the development of keloids may also be at risk for this syndrome. The neuropathic quality of the pain is often reported by patients as dysaesthetic and hyperaesthetic, and, on examination, a significant degree of allodynia may be demonstrated. In those patients complaining of a tight constricting sensation, breast reconstruction does not alter this phenomenon. Management of this pain syndrome includes physical therapy, local trigger point injections, sympathetic blocks, topical application of capsaicin, and, in isolated cases, surgical exploration of the area of traumatic neuroma.

Post-radical neck dissection pain

This pain results from injury to the cervical nerves and cervical plexus at the time of surgery. A sensation of tightness with burning dysaesthesias in the area of sensory loss are the characteristic symptoms. Patients typically report acute lancinating pain in the area of sensory loss. They may also complain of a second type of pain, resulting from the musculoskeletal imbalance that occurs in the shoulder following surgical removal of neck muscles, similar to the droopy shoulder syndrome. Thoracic outlet symptoms and signs of suprascapular nerve entrapment can occur.[73,74] Selective weakness and wasting of the supraspinatus muslces, with or without aching discomfort in the shoulder, are the characteristic clinical signs and symptoms. Escalating pain in this group of patients may signify recurrent tumour or soft-tissue infection. The latter is often difficult to diagnose in tissue damaged by radiation and surgery. Empirical treatment with antibiotics in patients with head and neck tumours and escalating pain has been reported to be associated with dramatic resolution of symptoms.[75] The diagnostic approach to these patients depends upon repeated CT scans through the area of pain, and frequent head and neck examinations to rule out the presence of recurrent tumour. The treatment of patients with post-radical neck dissection pain includes physical therapy, trigger point injections, and appropriate bracing of the shoulder and back, as well as pharmacological approaches.

Post-thoracotomy pain

This pain is typically characterized as an aching and burning sensation in the distribution of the thoracotomy incision, often associated with sensory loss and occasionally with autonomic changes. Patients complain of exquisite point tenderness at the most medical and apical points of the scar. The pain results from traction or disruption of the intercostal nerve following surgery on the chest wall. The intercostal neurovascular bundle (vein, artery, and nerve) courses along a groove in the inferior border of the rib. Traction on the ribs and rib resection are the common causes of nerve injury during a surgical procedure of the chest. Studies by Kanner, in a series of 126 patients undergoing thoracotomy at the Memorial Sloan-Kettering Cancer Center, have defined the pattern of pain following thoracotomy.[76] Kanner identified three groups of patients: Group I consisted of patients with immediate post-operative pain that diminished by 2 months after surgery. When pain recurred in this group of patients, in all cases the pain was due to recurrence of tumour. In Group II, in whom pain persisted following the thoracotomy and then increased during the follow-up period, local recurrences of disease and infection were the most common causes of increasing pain. Group III had stable or decreasing pain, which gradually resolved over an 8-month period, although recurrence of the tumour was noted. Late post-thoracotomy pain, which characterized patients in Groups I and II, was due to recurrent or persistent tumour or infection. Thus, the persistence of pain for more than 8 months, the recurrence of pain after initial improvement, and the persistent escalating pain during the post-operative recovery all suggest recurrent tumour and, less commonly, infection as aetiological factors in this pain symptomatology. This is in contrast to patients with post-mastectomy pain, where both a recurrent tumour and infection are rarely, if ever, associated with escalating pain symptomatology. Chest radiographs are insufficient to evaluate recurrent chest disease, and a CT scan through the chest, with bone and soft-tissue windows, is the diagnostic procedure of choice. The CT scan is also necessary prior to the consideration of an intercostal nerve block in the management of pain in these syndromes. If pain management is inadequate or patients are not actively rehabilitated following surgery, a frozen shoulder and a secondary reflex sympathetic dystrophy involving the arm may develop.

Phantom limb and stump pain

Pain following surgical amputation of a limb is of two types: pain in the phantom limb and stump pain. Preamputation limb pain influences the development of phantom pain.

Phantom limb pain

The incidence of phantom pain is significantly lower in patients with short-lasting preamputation pain and in patients who do not have pain in the limb the day before the amputation.[76,77] After amputation, phantom limb pain may initially magnify and then slowly fade over time. The pain has a paroxysmal burning or shooting quality and may be associated with bothersome paraesthesias. The phantom often assumes painful and unusual postures and telescopes as it approaches the stump with time. Pre-operative lumbar epidural blockade significantly reduces the incidence of phantom limb pain in the first years after the amputation, and pre-operative analgesic control appears to be the treatment of choice as multiple medical therapies, including antidepressants, opioids, anticonvulsants, sympathetic blockade, and transcutaneous electrical nerve stimulation (TENS), have met with limited success once the pain is well established (see Chapter 8.2.8).

Stump pain

Stump pain occurs at the site of the surgical scar several months to years following amputation. It results from the development of a traumatic neuroma at the site of the nerve section. The pain is characterized by burning dysaesthesias, which are often exacerbated by movement and blocked by the injection of a local anaesthetic. Careful assessment of the patient with pain will help distinguish stump pain from phantom pain. Stump pain is treated by identifying the trigger-point site and treating it locally, readjusting the prosthesis, and using drugs to suppress neuronal firing, such as anticonvulsants and antidepressants. Recurrence of pain in a phantom limb is an ominous sign, and should alert the physician to reassess the patient for proximal recurrence of tumour. We have evaluated several patients who began to complain of phantom leg pain several years after leg resection for primary tumours of bone. The pain proved to be the first symptom of recurrent disease in the pelvis following below-the-knee or above-the-knee amputation.[28]

Other phantom pain syndromes

Several phantom pain syndromes have been described following surgical procedures.[78,79] These include phantom breast pain following mastectomy, which occurs in 15–30 per cent of patients and appears to occur most commonly in those patients who report pre-operative pain. The pain tends to start in the region of the nipple and spread to the entire breast. Boas has reported a phantom anus syndrome occurring in 15 per cent of patients who undergo abdominal perineal resection of the rectum. This pain syndrome may occur in the early post-operative period or after a latency of months to years. Of note, late onset pain is almost always associated with tumour recurrence.[79]

Post-radiation pain syndromes

Pain occurring as a complication of radiation therapy is less common than post-chemotherapy and metastatic pain syndromes.[50] Pain occurs following damage to a peripheral nerve or the spinal cord, either as a result of changes in the microvasculature of the connective tissue surrounding the peripheral nerve, from fibrosis and chronic inflammation in connective tissues, or from demyelination and focal necrosis of white and grey matter in the spinal cord. These syndromes occur late in the course of a patient's illness and the differential diagnosis always includes recurrent tumour. In all instances, pain is a component of the syndrome, but usually it is not as prominent a complaint as when the syndrome is associated with recurrent tumour.

Radiation fibrosis of the brachial plexus

Pain in the distribution of the brachial plexus following radiation therapy is due to fibrosis of surrounding connective tissue and secondary nerve injury.[24,71,72,80] Pain occurs in only 18 per cent of patients at the time of presentation. Radiation changes in the skin, lymphoedema, and weakness in the C5, C6 distribution typically occurs. This disorder may begin as early as 6 months or as late as 20 years after the radiation therapy. The neurological deficits are relentlessly progressive and ultimately result in a useless, often oedematous limb. In contrast to malignant infiltration, electromyogram studies show myokymic discharges. The CT scan usually demonstrates diffuse infiltration that cannot be distinguished from tumour infiltration. The MRI scan demonstrates diffuse soft-tissue changes that do not enhance with gadolinium. A careful history, knowledge of the radiation ports and total dose of radiation therapy, and a clear assessment of the patient's extent of disease, coupled with radiological and electrodiagnostic studies can help in making the diagnosis.

Radiation fibrosis of the lumbosacral plexus

Radiation fibrosis of the lumbosacral plexus is rare, but may present from 1 to 30 years following radiation treatment.[28,50] The use of intracavitary radium implants with pelvis radiation for carcinoma of the cervix may be an additional risk factor. Presenting symptoms include weakness of the legs, associated with sensory symptoms and numbness and paraesthesias. Pain occurs in only 10 per cent of patients. Symptoms and signs are usually bilateral upon presentation, and weakness commences distally in the L5, S1 segments and slowly progresses. Radiation necrosis of the pelvic bone commonly accompanies this disorder and can help in furthering the diagnosis.

Radiation myelopathy

Pain may be an early symptom and is localized in the area of spinal cord damage. It is characterized as a typical central pain, burning in quality, associated with pain and temperature loss. This particular pain is often refractory to therapy and associated with significant motor and sensory neurological findings. MRI scan may demonstrate an area of hypointensity in the spinal cord. The etiology is thought to be changes in both the vascular supply and myelin in the spinal cord.[28,50]

Radiation-induced peripheral nerve tumours

Malignant peripheral nerve tumours and secondary primary tumours in a previously irradiated site may occur and present as a painful, expanding mass in a patient with a history of previously treated cancer. Patients with neurofibromatosis have an increased risk of developing malignant peripheral nerve tumours following radiation therapy.[80] The diagnosis maybe difficult in a patient presumed cured of his/her underlying malignancy who presents with progressive pain, with or without a palpable mass in the plexus. The use of MRI scan can be helpful, particularly if there is evidence of gadolinium enhancement, but often the diagnosis is made by surgical exploration and pathological confirmation.

References

1. **Ahles, T.A., Ruckdeschel, J.C., and Blanchard, E.B.** (1984). Cancer-related pain: prevalence in an outpatient setting as a function of stage of disease and type of cancer. *Journal of Psychosomatic Research* **28**, 115–19.
2. **Banning, A., Sjogren, P., and Henriksen, H.** (1991). Pain causes in 200 patients referred to a multidisciplinary cancer pain clinic. *Pain* **45**, 45–8.
3. **Grond, S., Zech, D., Diefenbach, C., Radbruch, L., and Lehmann, K.** (1996). Assessment of cancer pain: a prospective evaluation in 2266 cancer patients referred to a pain service. *Pain* **64**, 107–14.
4. **Larue, F., Colleau, S.M., Brasseur, L., and Cleeland, C.S.** (1995). Multicentre study of cancer pain and its treatment in France. *British Medical Journal* **310**, 1034–7.
5. **Greenwald, H.P., Bonica, J.J., and Bergner, M.** (1987). The prevalence of pain in four cancers. *Cancer* **60**, 2563–9.
6. **Zenz, M., Zenz, T., Tryba, M., and Strumpf, M.** (1995). Severe undertreatment of cancer pain: a 3 year survey of the German situation. *Journal of Pain and Symptom Management* **10**, 187–91.
7. **Von Roenn, J.H., Cleeland, C.S., Gonin, R., Hatfield, A., and Pandya, K.J.** (1993). Physicians' attitudes and practice in cancer pain management: a survey from the Eastern Cooperative Oncology Group. *Annals of Internal Medicine* **119**, 121–6.
8. **Larue, F., Colleau, S.M., Fontaine, A., and Brasseur, L.** (1995). Oncologists and primary care physicians attitudes towards pain control and morphine prescribing in France. *Cancer* **76**, 2375–82.
9. **Breitbart, W., Chochinov, H.M., and Passik, S.** (1998). Psychiatric aspects of palliative care. In *Oxford Textbook of Palliative Medicine* 2nd edn. (ed. D. Doyle, G.W. Hanks, and N. MacDonald), pp. 933–56. Oxford: Oxford University Press.
10. **Chochinov, H.M., Wilson, K.G., Enns, M., and Lander, S.** (1997). Are you despressed? Screening for depression in the terminally ill. *American Journal of Psychiatry* **154**, 674–6.
11. **Portenoy, R.K.** et al. (1992). Pain in ambulatory patients with lung or colon cancer: prevalence, characteristics and impact. *Cancer* **70**, 616–24.
12. **Portenoy, R.K.** et al. (1994). The Memorial Symptom Assessment Scale: an instrument for the evaluation of symptom prevalence, characteristics and distress. *European Journal of Clinical Oncology* **30**, 1326–36.
13. **Morris, J.N.** et al. (1986). The effects of treatment settings and patient characteristics on pain in terminal cancer patients: a report from the National Hospice Study. *Journal of Chronic Diseases* **39**, 27–35.
14. **Turk, D.C. and Meichenbaum, D.H.** (1989). A cognitive behavioral approach to pain management. In *Textbook of Pain* (ed. P.D. Wall and R. Melzack). Oxford: Oxford University Press.

15. **Portenoy, R.K. and Hagen, N.A.** (1990). Breakthrough pain: definition, prevalence and characteristics. *Pain* **41**, 273–82.
16. **Salzburg, D. and Foley, K.M.** (1989). The management of pancreatic cancer pain. In *Surgical Clinics of North America* (ed. H. Reber), pp. 629–50. Philadelphia PA: WB Saunders.
17. **Cherny, N.I., Coyle, N., and Foley, K.M.** (1994b). Suffering in the advanced cancer patient. Part I: a definition and taxonomy. *Journal of Palliative Care* **10** (2), 57–70.
18. **Saunders, C.** *The Management of Terminal Illness.* London: Edward Arnold, 1967.
19. **Granek, I., Ashikari, R., and Foley, K.M.** (1983). Postmastectomy pain syndrome: clinical and anatomic correlates. *Proceedings of the American Society of Clinical Oncology* **3**, 122.
20. **Foley, K.M.** (1979). Pain syndromes in patients with cancer. In *Advances in Pain Research and Therapy* Vol. 2. *International Symposium on Pain in Advanced Cancer* (ed. J.J. Bonica and V. Ventafridda), pp. 59–76. New York: Raven Press.
21. **Passik, S.D., Kirsh, K.L., and Portenoy, R.** (1999). Understanding aberrant drug-taking behavior. Addiction redefined for palliative care and pain management settings. *Principles and Practices of Supportive Oncology* **2** (Suppl. 2), 29–54.
22. **Foley, K.M.** (1999). A 44-year-old woman with severe pain at the end of life. *Journal of the American Medical Association* **281** (20), 1937–45.
23. **Foley, K.M. and Cherny, N.I.** (1996). Guidelines for the care of the dying. In *Hematology/Oncology Clinics of North America* (ed. N.I. Cherny and K.M. Foley), pp. 261–86. Philadelphia PA: WB Saunders.
24. **Kori, S.H., Foley, K.M., and Posner, J.B.** (1981). Brachial plexus lesions in patients with cancer: clinical findings in 100 cases. *Neurology* **31**, 45–50.
25. **Kanner, R.M., Martini, N., and Foley, K.M.** (1982). Incidence of pain and other clinical manifestations of superior pulmonary sulcus tumour (Pancoast's tumours). In *Advances in Pain Research and Therapy* Vol. 4 (ed. J.J. Bonica and V. Ventafridda), pp. 27–38. New York: Raven Press.
26. **Portenoy, R.K.** et al. (1994). Pain in ovarian cancer patients: prevalence, characteristics, and associated symptoms. *Cancer* **74**, 907–15.
27. **Emanuel, L.L., Danis, M., Pearlman, R.A., and Singer, P.A.** (1995). Advance care planning as a process: structuring the discussions in practice. *Journal of American Geriatrics Society* **43**, 440–6.
28. **Elliott, K. and Foley, K.M.** (1989). Neurologic pain syndromes in patients with cancer. *Neurologic Clinics* **7**, 333–60.
29. **Carver, A.C. and Foley, K.M.** Management of cancer pain. In *Cancer Medicine* 6th edn. (ed. D. Kufe et al.). Ontario, Canada: BC Decker, Inc., (2003).
30. **Gonzalez, G.R., Elliott, K.J., Portenoy, R.K., and Foley, K.M.** (1991). Impact of a comprehensive evaluation in the management of cancer pain. *Pain* **47**, 141–4.
31. **Cassell, E.J.** (1982). The nature of suffering and the goals of medicine. *New England Journal of Medicine* **306**, 639–45.
32. **Foley, K.M.** (1987). Pain syndromes in patients with cancer. In *Medical Clinics in North America* Vol. 71 (ed. K.M. Foley and R. Payne), pp. 169–84. Philadelphia PA: WB Saunders.
33. **Cherny, N. and Portenoy, R.K.** (1994). Cancer pain: principles of assessment and syndromes. In *Textbook of Pain* (ed. P.D. Wall and R. Melzack), pp. 787–823. Edinburgh: Churchill Livingstone.
34. **Portenoy, R.K.** (1992). Cancer pain: pathophysiology and syndromes. *Lancet* **339**, 1026–31.
35. **Cherny, N. and Foley, K.M.** (1994). Colorectal and anal cancer pain: pathophysiology, assessment, syndromes and management. In *Cancer of the Colon, Rectum, and Anus* (ed. A.M. Cohen, S.J. Winawer, M.A. Friedman, and L.L. Gunderson), pp. 1075–117. New York: McGraw-Hill.
36. **Stillman, M.J.** (1990). Perineal pain: diagnosis and management, with particular attention to perineal pain of cancer. In *Advances in Pain Research and Therapy* Vol. 16 (ed. K.M. Foley, J.J. Bonica, and V. Ventafridda), pp. 359–78. Second International Congress on Cancer Pain. New York: Raven Press.
37. **Raskin, N.H.** (1990). Lumbar puncture headache: a review. *Headache* **30**, 197–200.
38. **Heide, W. and Diener, H.C.** (1990). Epidural blood patch reduces the incidence of post lumbar puncture headache. *Headache* **30**, 280–1.
39. **Stillman, M.J., Moulin, D.E., and Foley, K.M.** (1987). Paradoxical pain following high-dose spinal morphine. *Pain* (Suppl. 4), S389. Fifth World Congress on Pain, IASP.
40. **Molloy, H.S., Seipp, C.A., and Duffey, P.** (1989). Administration of cancer treatments: practical guide for physicians and oncology nurses. In *Cancer: Principles and Practice of Oncology* 3rd edn. (ed. V.T. DeVita, S. Hellman, and S.A. Rosenberg), pp. 2369–402. Philadelphia PA: Lippincott.
41. **Curran, C.F., Luce, J.K., and Page, J.A.** (1990). Doxorubicin-associated flare reactions. *Oncology Nurses Forum* **17**, 387–9.
42. **Kemeny, N., Cohen, A., Bertino, J., Sigerson, E.R., Botet, J., and Oderman, P.** (1990). Continuous intrahepatic infusion of floxuridine and leucovorin through an implantable pump for the treatment of hepatic metastases from colorectal carcinoma. *Cancer* **65**, 2446–50.
43. **Botet, J.F., Watson, R.C., Kemeny, N., Daly, J.M., and Yeh, S.** (1985). Cholangitis complicating intraarterial chemotherapy in liver metastasis. *Radiology* **156**, 335–7.
44. **Almadrones, L. and Yerys, C.** (1990). Problems associated with the administration of intraperitoneal therapy using the Port-A-Cath system. *Oncology Nurses Forum* **17**, 75–80.
45. **Fitsch, E., Sevelda, P., Schmidl, S., and Salzer, H.** (1990). First experiences with intraperitoneal chemotherapy in ovarian cancer. *European Journal of Gynaecological Oncology* **11**, 19–22.
46. **Markman, M., Howell, S.B., Lucas, W.E., Pfeifle, C.E., and Green, M.R.** (1984). Combination intraperitoneal chemotherapy with cisplatin, cytarabine, and doxorubicin for refractory ovarian carcinoma and other malignancies principally confined to the peritoneal cavity. *Journal of Clinical Oncology* **2**, 1321–6.
47. **Chapko, M.K., Syrjala, K.L., Schilter. L., Cummings, C., and Sullivan, K.M.** (1990). Chemoradiotherapy toxicity during bone marrow transplantion: time course and variation in pain and nausea. *Bone Marrow Transplantion* **4**, 181–6.
48. **Rotstein, J. and Good, R.A.** (1957). Steroid pseudorheumatism. *Archives of Internal Medicine* **99**, 545–55.
49. **Mollman, J.E.** et al. (1988). Cisplatin neuropathy: risk factors, prognosis and protection by WR-2721. *Cancer* **61**, 2192–5.
50. **Posner, J.** *Neurologic Complications of Cancer.* Philadelphia PA: FA Davis Company, 1995.
51. **Feinberg, W.M. and Swenson, M.R.** (1988). Cerebrovascular complications of L-asparaginase therapy. *Neurology* **38**, 127–33.
52. **Huang, M.E.** et al. (1998). Use of all-*trans* retinoic acid in the treatment of acute promyelocytic leukemia. *Blood* **72**, 567–72.
53. **Castaigne, S.** et al. (1990). All-*trans* retinoic acid as a differentiation therapy for acute promyelocytic leukemia. I. Clinical results. *Blood* **76**, 1704–9.
54. **Balmer, C.M.** (1991). Clinical use of biologic response modifiers in cancer treatment: an overview. Part II. Colony-stimulating factors and interleukin-2. *Dalian Institute of Chemical Physics* **25**, 490–8.
55. **Eskilsson, J. and Albertsson, M.** (1990). Failure of preventing 5-fluorouracil cardiotoxicity by prophylactic treatment with verapamil. *Acta Oncologica* **29**, 1001–3.
56. **Trump, D.L. and Anderson, S.A.** (1983). Painful gynecomastia following cytotoxic therapy for testis cancer: a potentially favorable prognostic sign? *Journal of Clinical Oncology* **1**, 416–20.
57. **Quesada, J.R., Talpaz, M., Rios, A., Kurzrock, R., and Gutterman, J.U.** (1986). Clinical toxicity of interferons in cancer patients: a review. *Journal of Clinical Oncology* **4**, 234–43.
58. **Rider, C.A.** (1990). Oral mucositis. A complication of radiotherapy. *New York State Dental Journal* **56**, 37–9.
59. **Segal, A.Z. and Rordorf, G.** (1996). Gabapentin as novel treatment for postherpetic neuralgia. *Neurology* **46** (4), 1175–6.
60. **Fields, H.L., Rowbotham, M., and Baron, R.** (1998). Postherpetic neuralgia: irrilable nociceptors and deafferentation. *Neurobiological Disease* **5**, 209–27.
61. **Greenberg, H.S.** et al. (1981). Metastases to the base of the skull: clinical findings in 43 patients. *Neurology* **31**, 530–8.
62. **Portenoy, R.K., Lipton, R.B., and Foley, K.M.** (1987). Back pain in the cancer patient: an algorithm for evaluation and management. *Neurology* **37** (1), 134–8.
63. **Clouston, P., DeAngelis, L., and Posner, J.B.** (1992). The spectrum of neurologic disease in patients with systemic cancer. *Annals of Neurology* **31**, 268–73.

64. Kelsen, D., Portenoy, R.K., Thaler, H., Niedzwiecki, D., Passik, S., Banks, W., Brennan, M., and Foley, K.M. (1995). Pain and depression in patients with newly diagnosed pancreas cancer. *Journal of Clinical Oncology* **13** (3), 748–55.
65. Briss, W.R. et al. (1950). Localization of referred pancreatic pain induced by electrical stimulation. *Gastroenterology* **16**, 317–23.
66. Foley, K.M. (1988). Pain syndromes and pharmacologic management of pancreatic cancer pain. *Journal of Pain and Symptom Management* **3** (4), 176–87.
67. Jaeckle, K.A., Young, D.F., and Foley, K.M. (1985). The natural history of lumbosacral plexopathy in cancer. *Neurology* **35** (1), 8–15.
68. Coyle, N. et al. (1990). Character of terminal illness in the advanced cancer patient: pain and other symptoms during the last four weeks of life. *Journal of Pain and Symptom Management* **5**, 83–93.
69. Davis, D. (1972). Myeloma neuropathy. *Archives of Neurology* **27**, 507–11.
70. Phanthumehinda, K. et al. (1988). Guillian Barré syndrome and optic neuropathy in acute leukemia. *Neurology* **38**, 1324–5.
71. DeAngelis, L.M., Rogers, L.A., and Foley, K.M. (2000). Leptomeningeal metastasis. In *Diseases of the Breast* 2nd edn. (ed. J.R. Harris, M.E. Lippman, M. Morrow, and C.K. Osborne), pp. 867–91. Philadelphia PA: Lippincott Williams & Wilkins.
72. Vecht, C.J. (1990). Arm pain in the patient with breast cancer. *Journal of Pain and Symptom Management* **5**, 109–17.
73. Cailliet, R. *Shoulder Pain*. Philadelphia PA: F.A. Davis, 1966.
74. Swift, T.R. and Nichols, F.T. (1984). The droopy shoulder syndrome. *Neurology* **34**, 212–15.
75. Bruera, E. and Macdonald, N. (1986). Intractable pain in patients with advanced head and neck tumours: a possible role of local infection. *Cancer Treatment Reports* **70**, 691–2.
76. Bressler, B., Cohen, S.J., and Magnussen, S. (1955). The problem of phantom breast and phantom pain. *Journal of Nervous and Mental Disorders* **123**, 181–7.
77. Frederiks, J.A.M. (1985). Phantom limb and phantom limb pain. In *Handbook of Clinical Neurology Vol. 1: Clinical Neuropsychology* (ed. J.A.M. Fredericks), pp. 395–404. New York: Elsevier Science.
78. Kroner, K., Krebs, B., Skov, J., and Jorgensen, H.S. (1989). Immediate and long-term phantom breast syndrome after mastectomy: incidence, clinical characteristic relationship to pre-mastectomy breast pain. *Pain* **36**, 327–35.
79. Boas, R.A. (1983). Phantom anus syndrome. In *Proceedings of the Third World Congress on Pain. Advances in Pain Research and Therapy* (ed. J.J. Bonica, U. Lindblom, and A. Iggo), pp. 947–51. New York: Raven Press.
80. Foley, K.M., Woodruff, J.M., and Ellis, F.T. (1980). Radiation-induced malignant and atypical peripheral nerve sheath tumours. *Archives of Neurology* **7**, 311–18.

8.2.3 Opioid analgesic therapy

Geoffrey Hanks, Nathan I. Cherny, and Marie Fallon

Introduction

Treatment with analgesic drugs is the mainstay of cancer pain management.[1,2] Although concurrent use of other approaches and interventions may be appropriate in many patients, and necessary in some, analgesic drugs are needed in almost every case. Drugs whose primary clinical action is the relief of pain are conventionally classified on the basis of their activity at opioid receptors as either opioid or non-opioid analgesics. A third class, adjuvant analgesics, are drugs with other primary indications that can be effective analgesics in specific circumstances. The major group of drugs used in cancer pain management are the opioid analgesics.

During the last 20 years there has been a dramatic increase in our knowledge of the sites and mechanism of action of the opioids. The development of analytical methods has also been of great importance in facilitating pharmacokinetic studies of the disposition and fate of opioids in patients. More recently advances in genomic research have indicated the potential importance of pharmacogenetic factors in the response to opioid analgesics.[3] These studies have begun to offer us a better understanding of some of the sources of variation between individuals in their response to opioids and to suggest ways of minimizing some of their adverse effects. Although there are gaps in our knowledge of opioid pharmacology, the rational and appropriate use of these drugs is based on the knowledge of their pharmacological properties derived from well-controlled clinical trials.

Terminology

In this chapter and throughout this text, we have adopted the following conventions in terminology.

Opiate is a specific term that is used to describe drugs derived from the juice of the opium poppy. For example, morphine is an opiate but methadone (a completely synthetic drug) is not.[4]

Opioid is a general term that includes naturally occurring, semi-synthetic, and synthetic drugs which produce their effects by combining with opioid receptors and are stereospecifically antagonized by naloxone. In this context we refer to opioid agonists, opioid antagonists, opioid peptides, and opioid receptors.

Narcotic is commonly used to describe morphine-like drugs and other drugs of abuse. The term is derived from the Greek *narke*, meaning numbness or torpor. Since this is an imprecise and pejorative term that is not useful in a pharmacological context, its use with reference to opioids is discouraged. The term narcotic is not used in this book.

Opioid receptors

Opioids are agonists at highly specific receptor sites, and there is general agreement on the existence of at least three types of opioid receptor: the morphine receptor μ (mu), the κ (kappa) receptor at which the prototype agonist is ketocyclazocine, and the enkephalin receptor δ (delta). A fourth receptor, σ (sigma), was originally included in this group. However, actions mediated through σ receptors are not reversed by naloxone so it is not a true opioid receptor. The μ receptors have been further sub-classified into two distinct sub-types ($\mu 1$ and $\mu 2$), as have the δ receptors ($\delta 1$ and $\delta 2$). Kappa receptors have been divided into $\kappa 1$, $\kappa 2$, and $\kappa 3$ sub-types. Recently, several of these receptors have been successfully cloned.

In animal models, some laboratories have cloned up to 10µ receptor sub-types.[5] However, the functional significance of these 'spliced variants' remains unclear at present

Table 1 shows the putative effects mediated by the three main opioid receptors.[6] This classification is based on the original description by Martin et al.[7] The effects presumed to be mediated at μ receptors have been defined as a result of both human and animal studies, while the effects mediated at κ receptors derive predominantly from animal models. κ receptors mediate analgesia that persists in animals made tolerant to δ agonists; κ agonists produce less respiratory depression and miosis than μ agonists. It is assumed that opioid receptors mediate the sedative and mental clouding effects of opioids, in addition to their other pharmacological actions.

Table 1 Responses mediated by activation of opioid receptors

Receptor	Response on activation
μ	Analgesia, respiratory depression, miosis, euphoria, reduced gastrointestinal motility
κ	Analgesia, dysphoria, psychotomimetic effects, miosis, respiratory depression
δ	Analgesia

Opioid receptors are found in several areas of the brain, particularly in the periaqueductal grey matter, and throughout the spinal cord. Supraspinal systems have been described for $\mu 1$, $\kappa 3$, and $\delta 2$ receptors, whereas $\mu 2$, $\kappa 1$, and $\delta 1$ receptors modulate pain at the spinal level.[8] Our understanding of the effect profiles of opioid receptors remains incomplete, as new advances make it clear that their disposition and structure are extremely complex.

The molecular pharmacology of opioids

Molecular biology techniques have enabled the primary amino acid sequence of the human μ, κ, and δ opioid receptors to be determined. The pharmacological and functional properties of the cloned receptors, the development of 'knockout' animals (which are deficient in a receptor or part of a receptor), and the manipulation and substitution of various amino acids in critical domains of the various opioid receptors are providing new information on receptor function and organization that will lead to an increased understanding of opioid neurotransmission at the molecular level and of the factors controlling the development of responses to opioid drugs.

The three opioid receptor genes, encoding mu (MOR), delta (DOR), and kappa (KOR) have been cloned. The binding affinities of a range of opioids to the μ-, κ-, and δ-opioid receptors and also to the cloned μ receptor have been examined in animals. The animal data indicate that while the commonly prescribed opioids (agonists and antagonists) bind preferentially to the μ receptor, they also interact with all three receptor types. Morphine and normorphine (a minor metabolite of morphine) show the greatest relative preference for the μ receptor. Methadone (which also has some NMDA-receptor blocking activity) shows significant binding to δ receptors, while buprenorphine, and to a lesser extent naloxone, avidly bind to all three receptor types. There is evidence (albeit inconsistent) that the d-enantiomer of methadone blocks the NMDA receptor. The binding affinity of buprenorphine to the μ receptor is much greater than that of naloxone, which explains why the latter only partially reverses buprenorphine toxicity.

Animal data also indicate that codeine and diamorphine have very poor binding to opioid receptors, which reinforces the possibility that both are prodrugs where the pharmacologically active species are morphine[9] and 6-monoacetyl morphine,[10] respectively. Oxycodone may also act through an active metabolite, though there are some data which suggest that this is not the case.[11]

Pethidine is considered to be a potent μ receptor agonist, but it does bind weakly to all three opioid receptors. Ketobemidone has a lower affinity for the μ receptor than does morphine, but it shows greater discrimination for this receptor compared to κ receptors. The binding of both of these opioids to the δ receptor is similar.[12]

The binding of morphine, methadone, buprenorphine, and naloxone to the cloned human μ receptor shows excellent congruence with the animal data.[13,14] Fentanyl shows a similar binding affinity, while codeine demonstrates greater binding affinity to the cloned human receptor. Thus, for these commonly administered opioids, there is no great variability in their affinity for the human μ receptor.

The clinical relevance of these data is that different opioids act in different ways. We are aware too from anecdotal clinical experience that there is considerable interindividual variability in response to each opioid and this reinforces our need to assess an individual's response to opioid analgesia carefully. It would be premature to extrapolate from laboratory data, which in many instances have not yet been replicated, to the clinic. However, these data increasingly inform the clinical use of these drugs and will be particularly relevant to new approachs to their use such as 'opioid switching'.

Agonists, antagonists, potency, and efficacy

Based on their interactions with the various receptor sub-types, opioid compounds can be divided into agonist, agonist–antagonist, and antagonist classes (Table 2).

Agonists

An agonist is a drug that has affinity for and binds to cell receptors to induce changes in the cell that stimulate physiological activity. The agonist opioid drugs have no clinically relevant ceiling effect to analgesia. As the dose is raised, analgesic effects increase in a log linear function, until either analgesia is achieved or dose-limiting adverse effects supervene. Efficacy is defined by the maximal response induced by administration of the active agent. In practice, this is determined by the degree of analgesia produced following dose escalation through a range limited by the development of adverse effects. Potency, in contrast, reflects the dose–response relationship. Potency is influenced by pharmacokinetic factors (i.e. how much of the drug enters the body systemic circulation and then reaches the receptors) and by affinity to drug receptors.

The concepts of efficacy and potency are illustrated in Fig. 1, which shows the dose–response curves for two drugs A and B. If the logarithm of dose is plotted against response an agonist will produce an S-shaped or sigmoid curve. The efficacy of the two drugs, defined by maximum response is the same. Drug A produces the same response as B but at a lower dose, and therefore is described as more potent.

Antagonist

Antagonist drugs have no intrinsic pharmacological action but can interfere with the action of an agonist. Competitive antagonists bind to the same receptor and compete for receptor sites, whereas non-competitive antagonists block the effects of the agonist in some other way.

Agonist–antagonist

The agonist–antagonist analgesics can, in turn, be subdivided into the mixed agonist–antagonists and the partial agonists, a distinction also based

Table 2 Classification of opioid analgesics into agonist, agonist–antagonist and antagonist classes

Agonists	*Partial agonists*
Morphine	Buprenorphine
Codeine	*Agonist–antagonists*
Oxycodone	Pentazocine
Dihydrocodeine	Butorphanol
Oxymorphone	Nalbuphine
Pethidine	Dezocine
Levorphanol	Meptazinol
Hydromorphone	*Antagonists*
Methadone	Naloxone
Fentanyl	Naltrexone
Dextropropoxyphene	
Diamorphine (heroin)	
Tramadol	
Phenazocine	
Dextromoramide	
Dipipanone	

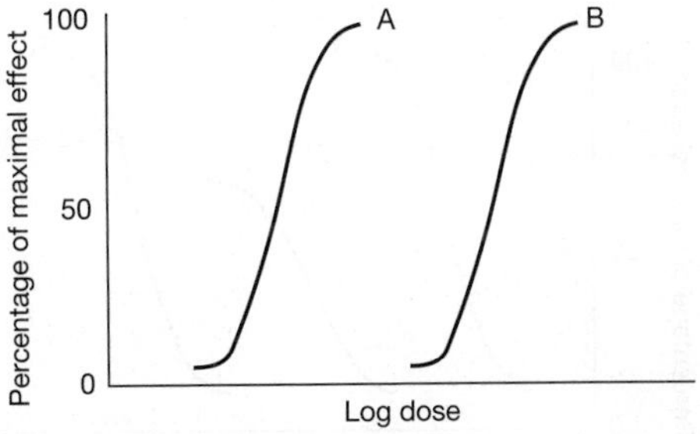

Fig. 1 Dose–response curves for two full opioid agonists (A and B) similar in efficacy but different in potency (A is more potent than B).

on specific patterns of drug–receptor interaction. Both the partial agonist and agonist–antagonist drugs have a ceiling effect for analgesia, and although they produce analgesia in the opioid-naive patient, in theory they can precipitate withdrawal in patients who are physically dependent on morphine-like drugs. For these reasons, they have been considered generally to have a limited role in the management of patients with cancer pain.

Mixed agonist–antagonists

The mixed agonist–antagonist drugs produce agonist effects at one receptor and antagonist effects at another. Pentazocine is the prototype agonist–antagonist: it has agonist effects at κ receptors and weak μ antagonist actions. Thus in addition to analgesia, pentazocine may produce κ-mediated psychotomimetic effects not seen with full or partial μ agonists. When a mixed agonist–antagonist is administered together with an agonist, the antagonist effect at the μ receptor can generate an acute withdrawal syndrome.

Partial agonists

A partial agonist has low intrinsic activity (efficacy) so that its dose–response curve exhibits a ceiling effect at less than the maximum effect produced by a full agonist. Buprenorphine is the main example of a partial agonist opioid. Increasing the dose of such a drug above its ceiling does not result in any further increase in response. This phenomenon is illustrated in Fig. 2 in which C is a partial agonist. C is more potent than B (in the lower part of the curve it will produce the same response at a lower dose), but is less effective than both A and B because of its ceiling effect.

When a partial agonist is administered together with an agonist, displacement of the agonist can cause a net reduction in pharmacological action which may be sufficient to generate an acute withdrawal syndrome. Whilst this is a theoretical possibility with morphine and buprenorphine, no such interaction has been reported. Similarly, it has been suggested that the effects of morphine may be blocked in a patient switched from buprenorphine, because of the prolonged action of buprenorphine and the assumption that it will 'antagonize' the effect of morphine. This has been one of the reasons why buprenorphine has not been in cancer pain management. However, the recent development of a transdermal formulation of buprenorphine may encourage its use in chronic cancer pain (and chronic non-cancer pain). An analgesic ceiling with buprenorphine is only reached at doses of 8–16 mg or more in 24 h.[15] When used in usual recommended doses (for example, two patches of 70 μg/h of transdermal buprenorphine, equivalent to 3–4 mg per 24 h) buprenorphine can be considered a full μ agonist since at these doses its effect will lie on the linear part of the dose–response curve.

Relative potency and equianalgesic doses

Relative potency is the ratio of the doses of two analgesics required to produce the same analgesic effect. By convention the relative potency of each of the commonly used opioids is based upon a comparison with 10 mg of parenteral morphine. Data from single- and repeated-dose studies in patients with acute or chronic pain have been used to develop an equianalgesic dose table (Table 3) that provides guidelines for dose selection when the drug or route of administration is changed. The information contained in the equianalgesic dose table does not represent standard doses, nor is it intended as an absolute guideline for dose selection. Many variables may influence the appropriate dose for an individual patient, including intensity of pain, prior opioid exposure in terms of drug, duration, and dose (and the degree of cross-tolerance that this confers), age, route of administration, level of consciousness, metabolic abnormalities (see below), and genetic polymorphism in the expression of relevant enzymes or receptors.

Dose–response relationship

As noted above, there is no ceiling to the analgesic effects of full agonist opioids. As the dose is raised, analgesic effects increase as a log linear function. In practice, the appearance of adverse effects, including confusion, sedation, nausea, vomiting, or respiratory depression, imposes a limit on the useful dose of an opioid agonist. Thus the efficacy of any particular drug in an individual patient will be determined by the degree of analgesia produced following dose escalation to intolerable and unmanageable side-effects.

The role of opioids in the management of cancer pain

Analgesic therapy with opioids, non-opioids, and adjuvant analgesics is developed for the individual patient through a process of continuous evaluation so that a favourable balance between pain relief and adverse pharmacological effects is maintained.

The analgesic ladder

An expert committee convened by the Cancer and Palliative Care Unit of the World Health Organization (WHO) proposed a structured approach to drug selection for cancer pain, which has become known as the 'WHO analgesic ladder'.[16] When combined with appropriate dosing guidelines, this approach is capable of providing adequate relief to 70–90 per cent of patients.[17–23] Emphasizing that the intensity of pain, rather than its specific aetiology, should be the prime consideration in analgesic selection, the approach advocates three basic steps (Fig. 3):

1. Patients with mild cancer-related pain should be treated with a non-opioid analgesic, which should be combined with adjuvant drugs

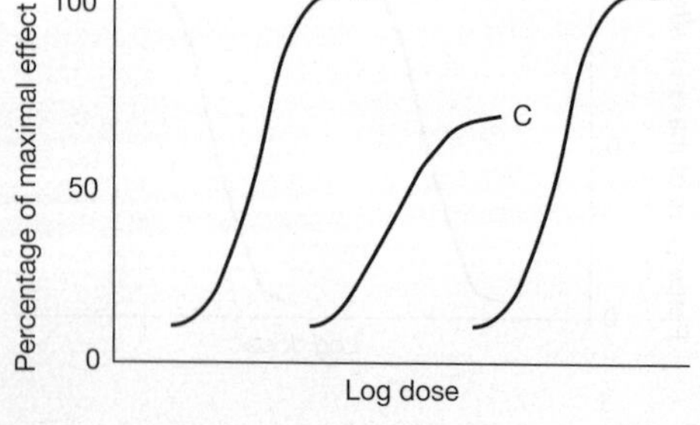

Fig. 2 Dose–response curves for two full opioid agonists (A and B) and a partial opioid agonist C.

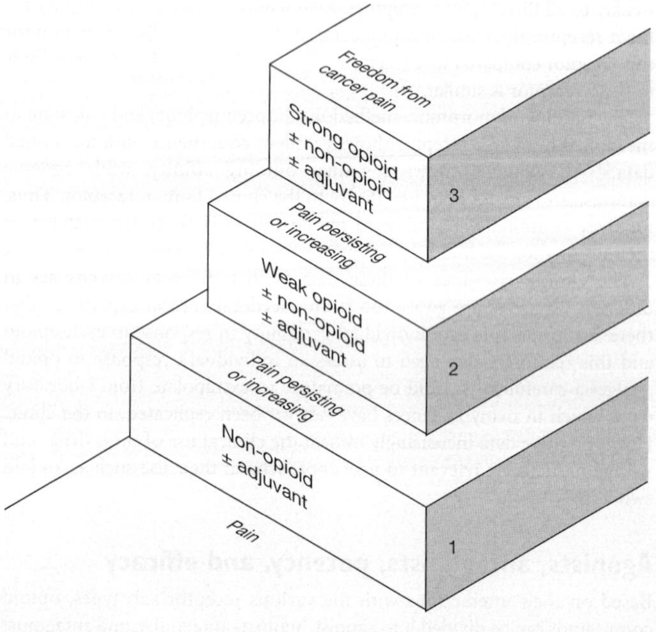

Fig. 3 The WHO three-step analgesic ladder. (Reproduced with permission from ref. 2.)

Table 3 Opioid analgesics (pure μ agonists) used for the treatment of chronic pain

Morphine-like agonists	Equi-analgesic doses[a]	Half-life (h)	Peak effect (h)	Duration (h)	Toxicity	Comments	Oral bioavailability (%)	Active metabolites
Morphine	10 s.c. 20–60 p.o.[b]	2–3 2–3	0.5–1 1.5–2	3–6 4–7	Constipation, nausea, sedation most common; respiratory depression rare in cancer patients	Standard comparison for opioids; multiple routes available	20–30	M6G
Sustained-release morphine	20–60 p.o.[b]	2–3	3–4	8–12		Twice daily administration	20–30	M6G
Sustained-release morphine	20–60 p.o.[b]	2–3	4–6	24		Once-a-day morphine approved in some countries	20–30	M6G
Hydromorphone	1.5 s.c. 7.5 p.o.	2–3 2–3	0.5–1 1–2	3–4 3–4	Same as morphine	Used for multiple routes	35–80	No
Oxycodone	20–30	2–3	1	3–6	Same as morphine	Combined with aspirin or paracetamol (acetaminophen), for moderate pain in USA; available orally without non-opioid for severe pain	60–90	Oxymorphone
Sustained-release oxycodone	20–30	2–3	3–4	8–12				Oxymorphone
Oxymorphone	1 s.c. 10 p.r.	— —	0.5–1 1.5–3	3–6 4–6	Same as morphine	No oral formulation		Glucuronides
Pethidine (meperidine)	75 s.c.	2–3	0.5–1	3–4	Same as morphine + CNS excitation; contraindicated in those on MAO inhibitors	Not used for cancer pain due to toxicity in higher doses and short half-life	30–60	Norpethidine
Diamorphine	5 s.c.	0.5	0.5–1	4–5	Same as morphine	Analgesic action due to metabolites, predominantly morphine; only available in some countries		Morphine
Levorphanol	2 s.c. 4 p.o.	12–16	0.5–1	4–6	Same as morphine	With long half-life, accumulation occurs after beginning or increasing dose		No
Methadone[c]	10 s.c. 20 p.o. *(see text)*	12–>150	0.5–1.5	4–8	Same as morphine	Risk of delayed toxicity due to accumulation; useful to start dosing on p.r.n. schedule	60–90	No
Codeine	130 s.c. 200 p.o.	2–3	1.5–2	3–6	Same as morphine	Usually combined with non-opioid	60–90	Morphine
Propoxyphene HCl (dextropropoxyphene)	—	12	1.5–2	3–6	Same as morphine plus seizures with overdose	Toxic metabolite accumulates but not significant at doses used clinically; usually combined with non-opioid	40	Norpropoxyphene

(Continued)

Table 3 Continued

Morphine-like agonists	Equi-analgesic doses[a]	Half-life (h)	Peak effect (h)	Duration (h)	Toxicity	Comments	Oral bioavailability (%)	Active metabolites
Propoxyphene napsylate (dextropropoxyphene)	—	12	1.5–2	3–6	Same as hydrochloride	Same as hydrochloride	40	Norpropoxyphene
Hydrocodone	—	2–4	0.5–1	3–4	Same as morphine	Only available combined with paracetamol; only available in some countries		Hydromorphone
Dihydrocodeine	—	2–4	0.5–1	3–4	Same as morphine	Only available combined with aspirin or paracetamol in some countries	20	Morphine
Fentanyl	—	3–12	—	—	Same as morphine	Can be administered as a continuous i.v. or s.c. infusion; based on clinical experience, 100 μg/h is roughly equianalgesic to morphine 4 mg/h i.v.	25/buccal <2/oral	No
Fentanyl transdermal system	—	13–22	—	48–72	Same as morphine	Based on clinical experience 100 μg/h is roughly equianalgesic to morphine 4 mg/h; recent study indicates a ratio of oral morphine: transdermal fentanyl of 100 : 1	90/transdermal	No

[a] Dose that provides analgesia equivalent to 10 mg i.m. morphine. These ratios are useful guidelines when switching drugs or routes of administration.

[b] Extensive survey data suggest that the relative potency of i.m. : p.o. or s.c. : p.o., morphine of 1 : 6 changes to 1 : 2–3 with chronic dosing.

[c] When switching from another opioid to methadone, the potency of methadone is much greater than indicated in this table.

if a specific indication for these exists. For example, a patient with mild to moderate arm pain caused by radiation-induced brachial plexopathy may benefit when a tricyclic antidepressant is added to paracetamol (acetaminophen).[24,25]

2. Patients who are relatively non-tolerant and present with moderate pain, or who fail to achieve adequate relief after a trial of a non-opioid analgesic, should be treated with an opioid conventionally used for mild to moderate pain (formerly known as a 'weak' opioid). This treatment is typically accomplished using a combination product containing a non-opioid (e.g. aspirin or paracetamol) and an opioid (such as codeine, oxycodone, or propoxyphene). This combination can also be coadministered with an adjuvant analgesic. The doses of these combination products can be increased until the maximum dose of the non-opioid analgesic is attained (e.g. 4000–6000 mg paracetamol); beyond this dose, the opioid contained in the combination product could be increased as a single agent, or the patient could be switched to an opioid conventionally used in step 3.
3. Patients who present with severe pain, or who fail to achieve adequate relief following appropriate administration of drugs on the second step of the analgesic ladder, should receive an opioid conventionally used for moderate to severe pain (formerly known as a 'strong' opioid). This group includes morphine, diamorphine, fentanyl, oxycodone, phenazocine, hydromorphone, methadone, levorphanol, and oxymorphone. These drugs may also be combined with a non-opioid analgesic or an adjuvant drug. Clearly, the boundary between opioids used in the second and third steps of the analgesic ladder is somewhat artificial since low doses of morphine or other opioids for severe pain can be less effective than high doses of codeine or propoxyphene.

According to these guidelines, a trial of opioid therapy should be given to all patients with pain of moderate or greater severity.

The evidence of the long-term efficacy of this approach and the evidence base underlying its recommendations has been the subject of criticism.[26] Several other developments have also contributed to a reevaluation of the WHO ladder. The introduction of low-dose formulations of opioid agonists traditionally used for severe pain, and of other agents such as tramadol has widened the repertoire of agents suitable for the management of moderate pain (step 2). Indeed, many authorities now advocate the use of the same opioid for all pains of moderate or greater intensity.[27–30]

Despite these reservations, the guiding principle that analgesic selection should be primarily determined by the severity of the pain remains sound, and continues to be widely endorsed.[1,27,31]

Opioid analgesics

The division of opioid agonists into 'weak' or 'strong' opioids, which was incorporated into the original analgesic ladder proposed by the WHO, was not based on fundamental differences in their pharmacology, but rather reflected the customary manner in which these drugs were used. In this chapter we will refer to opioids for mild to moderate pain and opioids for moderate to severe pain rather than 'weak' or 'strong' opioids. This terminology is now incorporated into the current version of the WHO analgesic ladder.

Opioids for mild to moderate pain

Codeine

Codeine (methylmorphine) is a naturally occurring opium alkaloid used as an analgesic, antitussive, and antidiarrhoeal agent (Fig. 4). Codeine is much less potent than morphine and produces its analgesic effects in part by binding to μ opioid receptors but with low affinity and, in part through biotransformation to morphine by cytochrome P-450 CYP2D6 (sparteine oxygenase) which exhibits genetic polymorphism. Approximately 7 per cent of Caucasians lack CYP2D6 activity (poor metabolizers) due to inheritance of two non-functional alleles and in these individuals codeine has a diminished analgesic effect.[32,33]

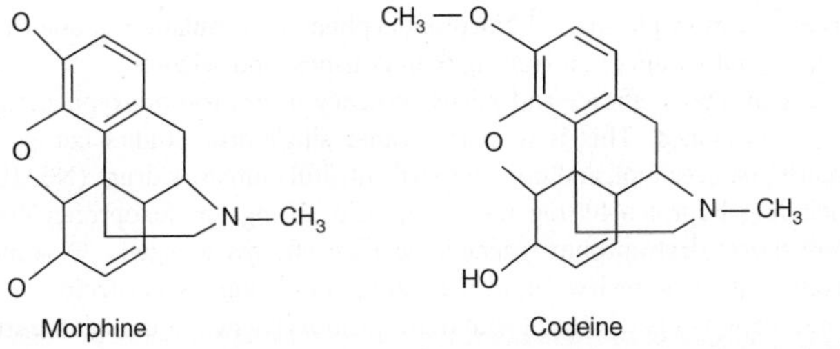

Fig. 4 The chemical structures of morphine and codeine.

Codeine phosphate is absorbed well from the gastrointestinal tract, but oral bioavailability varies considerably between individuals (from 12 to 84 per cent in one study[34]). The main metabolite is codeine-6-glucuronide, with much smaller amounts of norcodeine, morphine, and morphine 3- and 6-glucuronides also being produced.[35] The usual oral dose of codeine is 30–60 mg and its duration of action is 4–6 h.

Codeine is not generally given as a single agent when used orally as an analgesic, but is usually combined with a non-opioid and recent systematic reviews confirm that the combination of codeine and paracetamol is more effective that paracetamol alone.[36,37] A sustained-release formulation of codeine is available in some countries. When changing from regular administration of a codeine/non-opioid combination to morphine, patients receiving a total daily dose of 240–360 mg codeine are usually started on 60 mg morphine daily.

Dihydrocodeine

Dihydrocodeine is a semi-synthetic analogue of codeine that is used as an analgesic, antitussive, and antidiarrhoeal agent. When administered by mouth, dihydrocodeine is equianalgesic to codeine. However, when administed parenterally it is approximately twice as potent as codeine. This may be explained by the consistently poorer bioavailability of dihydrocodeine (20 per cent), which probably results from hepatic presystemic metabolism.[38]

The usual starting dose is 30 mg every 4–6 h (by mouth), and this may be increased to 60 mg. However, dihydrocodeine appears to have a narrower therapeutic index than codeine, with a high incidence of adverse effects at the 60-mg dose. A controlled-release formulation of dihydrocodeine is available in several countries.

There have been a number of reports of severe toxicity associated with dihydrocodeine in patients with impaired renal function.[39,40] The mechanism is not clear because of the limited data available on the pharmacokinetics of this drug, although it seems most likely that the cause is accumulation of active glucuronide metabolites, as occurs with morphine.

There is confusion about the relative analgesic potency of dihydrocodeine. It seems reasonable to assume that oral dihydrocodeine is roughly equipotent to oral codeine, and to use a similar conversion ratio when changing to morphine.

Dextropropoxyphene

Propoxyphene is a synthetic derivative of methadone, and its dextrorotatory stereoisomer dextropropoxyphene is responsible for its analgesic activity. Dextropropoxyphene is a μ agonist with low receptor affinity similar to that of codeine. It is readily absorbed from the gastrointestinal tract with peak serum levels about 2 h after administration. The mean elimination half-life is about 12 h, with steady state levels being reached after 3–4 days of regular administration every 6–8 h. The half-life may be very long (over 50 h) in elderly patients.[41]

Dextropropoxyphene undergoes extensive first-pass metabolism. Its principal metabolite is norpropoxyphene, which is active but penetrates the brain to a much lesser extent and has much weaker opioid effects. Norpropoxyphene has a longer half-life (about 23 h) than dextropropoxyphene itself and accumulates in plasma.[42] Norpropoxyphene accumulation is associated with excitatory effects, including tremulousness and seizures.

The analgesic efficacy and relative potency of dextropropoxyphene have been questioned. This is in part because single-dose studies comparing aspirin, paracetamol, and non-steroidal anti-inflammatory drugs (NSAIDs), including ibuprofen 400 mg, mefenamic acid 250 mg, and fenoprofen 50 mg, have shown dextropropoxyphene to be a less effective analgesic.[43] A more recent systematic review found that paracetamol alone is as effective as the combination of paracetamol with dextropropoxyphene,[44] though the studies included were again all single-dose studies. Single-dose studies may be misleading, as is the case with single-dose studies of oral morphine.

The extensive first-pass metabolism of dextropropoxyphene is dose dependent such that the systemic availability of the drug increases with increasing oral doses.[45] Thus, with regular administration, there is enhanced bioavailability and some degree of accumulation because of the long elimination half-lives of the parent drug and its main metabolite. Both dextropropoxyphene and norpropoxyphene reach plasma concentrations in the steady state which are five to seven times greater than those found after the first dose. There is therefore a pharmacokinetic basis for believing that repeated doses of dextropropoxyphene are likely to be more effective than single doses. The usual starting dose of morphine for patients receiving dextropropoxyphene–paracetamol combinations every 4–6 h (representing 260–390 mg of dextropropoxyphene daily) is 60 mg per day.

Toxicity of dextropropoxyphene

For a long time a combination of dextropropoxyphene and paracetamol was the most commonly prescribed analgesic in the United Kingdom and some Scandinavian countries, but it received much adverse publicity because of its lethal effects in overdose and fears about its addiction potential. Part of this concern was stimulated by its very widespread use. In addition to usual opioid adverse effects, propoxyphene may rarely induce a hepatotoxic reaction,[46] cardiac conduction disorder,[47] and potentially dangerous drug interactions have been reported when propoxyphene has been administered along with carbamazepine,[48] warfarin,[49] or alcohol.[50] At present, however, there is insufficient evidence to conclude that dextropropoxyphene is inherently more toxic than codeine or other opioids of similar efficacy, nor is there evidence that one is more effective than another.

Oxycodone

Oxycodone is a semi-synthetic congener of morphine, which has been on the market for 80 years but until recently was only available in formulations which effectively circumscribed its use. In the United States, it has been prescribed in low-dose combination products with a non-opioid for oral administration (usually 5 mg of oxycodone with either aspirin or paracetamol) and has traditionally been used as a step 2 analgesic. In the United Kingdom and some other countries only a rectal suppository and no oral formulations have been available, so that it has been used only for patients unable to take oral medication.[51] Oxycodone has been more widely used by mouth as a first line step 3 opioid in Scandinavia where it has also been widely used as a post-operative opioid.[52] Recently, oxycodone has been produced as a single agent in new oral formulations, both normal release and sustained release, which has substantially improved the convenience of administration. In many countries sustained release oxycodone is available in 5, 10, 20, 40, and 80 mg formulations with a corresponding range of normal release formulations. Oxycodone is increasingly used as a step 3 opioid,[53–55] though the low-dose formulations allow its use at step 2 also. Oxycodone probably provides the best example of the overlap in efficacy between opioids at steps 2 and 3.

Tramadol

Tramadol is a centrally acting analgesic which possesses opioid agonist properties and may also activate monoaminergic spinal inhibition of pain.[56] It has modest affinity with μ opioid receptors, with weak affinity to δ and κ receptors, and its analgesic effect is reversed by naloxone. Unlike other opioids, it also inhibits the uptake of noradrenaline and serotonin, and in an animal model systemically administered yohimbine or ritanserin blocks tramadol-induced analgesia,[56] suggesting that this effect contributes significantly to the drug's analgesic action.

Tramadol can be administered orally, rectally, intravenously, subcutaneously, or intramuscularly. In many countries, it is available in both normal- and sustained-release formulations. Parenterally, 50–150 mg of tramadol is equianalgesic to 5–15 mg morphine.[57] There are insufficient data for a reliable assessment of its oral to parenteral relative analgesic potency and estimates range from 1 : 4[58] to 1 : 10.[59]

Recent studies have demonstrated the efficacy of oral tramadol in the management of chronic cancer pain of moderate severity.[58–60] Few patients with severe pain are adequately managed by tramadol.[59,61] Tramadol has a similar side-effect profile to morphine, but may cause less constipation and respiratory depression at equianalgesic doses.

Opioids in combination with non-opioids

The second step of the analgesic ladder

By convention, formulations combining aspirin or paracetamol with a low dose of codeine, oxycodone, or propoxyphene have been recommended for pain of moderate intensity (step 2 of the analgesic ladder). This recommendation was pragmatic rather than evidence based. It reflected the concern that in many parts of the world it would be unacceptable to use morphine or other potent opioids for moderate pain.

Overall, these combination preparations have frequently proved to be relatively ineffective because the dose of opioid was too low (e.g. codeine 8 or 16 mg). Indeed, in the validation studies of the WHO ladder few patients using these agents maintained adequate relief for more than a few weeks.[17] Additionally, these formulations all have a short duration of effect and require patients to use repeated doses every 3–4 h to achieve continuous analgesia in the setting of chronic pain.

The most frequently employed step 2 analgesics in cancer pain are combination preparations containing 300–500 mg paracetamol with 30 mg codeine, 32.5 mg dextropropoxyphene, or 5 mg oxycodone. The combination of dextropropoxyphene with paracetamol (coproxamol in the United Kingdom) has theoretical disadvantages of pharmacokinetic incompatibility (dextropropoxyphene has a much longer elimination half-life than paracetamol) and accumulation of dextropropoxyphene and its active metabolite norpropoxyphene. However, neither problem appears to have any clinical consequence in practice and this combination remains widely used. Codeine and paracetamol are pharmacokinetically more compatible, and at present either combination would be an appropriate choice.

Recent studies comparing single doses of opioid/non-opioid combinations with various NSAIDs in post-operative pain have shown advantages for the latter in terms of greater efficacy and less adverse effects.[62–64] Chronic use of NSAIDs may negate any advantage in terms of unwanted effects, although at present there are no comparative data for chronic cancer pain. NSAIDs are increasingly employed as step 2 analgesics.

Given the limitations of the conventional approach many clinicians now use a variety of single agent opioid agonists, some previously designated as 'step 3' opioids, in an appropriate dose, for moderate pain. Over recent years, sustained-release formulations of oxycodone, tramadol and morphine in dose formulations appropriate for pain of moderate severity have become widely available and are now often used in this setting. This practice is supported by evidence of efficacy.[54,60,65]

The partial agonist opioid buprenorphine also may be used in this setting since it has recently become available in a transdermal formulation. Preliminary experience has been reported in the management of moderate cancer pain.[66] A low-dose formulation of transdermal fentanyl is also under development and is designed for use in patients who may be opioid naive. There are potential dangers in the earlier use of the most potent opioids, particularly when administered in long acting formulations and more clinical trial data are required to clarify some of the issues surrounding these trends in opioid prescribing.

Opioids for moderate to severe pain

Morphine-like agonists

The morphine-like agonist drugs (Table 2) are widely used to manage cancer pain. Although they may differ from morphine in quantitative characteristics they qualitatively mimic the pharmacological profile of morphine, including both desirable and undesirable effects. Controversy has developed over the choice of an opioid drug, in part because of the dearth of well-controlled studies comparing the efficacy and side-effects of these drugs during chronic administration, and in part because of the large amount of survey data and anecdotal reports supporting one drug over another.

Clinicians in most countries have some choice when selecting which opioid drug(s) to prescribe, but the options can vary from country to country.

Morphine is still considered to be the opioid drug of choice by many practitioners[30] and has occupied this place throughout recorded history. However, some of the other potent μ receptor agonists are gaining popularity for a variety of reasons. While greater choice is very important in analgesic therapy, it should not be forgotten that morphine is an excellent analgesic and maintains a key position and reference point for all opioids in our therapeutic armamentarium. Similarly, while there is theoretical evidence (on the basis of receptor binding profiles) that opioid combinations may give optimum analgesia with a more favourable side-effect profile, there is as yet no good clinical evidence to support such treatment strategies which are likely to be appropriate only in rare situations.

Morphine

Morphine is a potent μ-agonist drug that was first introduced into clinical use almost 200 years ago. It is the main naturally occurring alkaloid of opium derived from the poppy *Papaver somniferum* and is available for therapeutic use as the sulphate, hydrochloride, and tartrate. Recent evidence suggests that biosynthetic pathways for morphine exist in animal and human tissues such as liver, blood, and brain.[67] Its chemical structure is shown in Fig. 4. The WHO has placed oral morphine on the Essential Drug List, and preparations are available for oral, rectal, parenteral, and intraspinal administration.

Bioavailability

Morphine is available in four oral formulations: an elixir, a normal-release tablet, a modified-release tablet or capsule (of which there are now several preparations using different sustained-release mechanisms), and sustained-release suspensions. Absorption of morphine after oral administration occurs predominantly in the alkaline medium of the upper small bowel (morphine is a weak base) and is more or less complete. After oral administration, extensive presystemic elimination of the drug occurs predominantly in the liver. In healthy volunteers and cancer patients, the average bioavailability for oral morphine is 20–30 per cent.[68–70] Like all other pharmacokinetic parameters, bioavailability demonstrates marked inter-individual variability. In patients with normal renal function the plasma half-life (2–3 h) is somewhat shorter than the duration of analgesia (4–6 h). The pharmacokinetics remain linear with repetitive administration, and there does not appear to be autoinduction of biotransformation even following large chronic doses.[71]

Morphine is relatively hydrophilic and, when administered epidurally or intrathecally, it is not rapidly absorbed into the systemic circulation. This results in a long half-life in cerebrospinal fluid (90–120 min) and extensive rostral redistribution.[72]

Metabolism

About 90 per cent of morphine is converted into metabolites (Fig. 5), principally the glucuronide conjugates morphine-3-glucuronide (M3G) and morphine-6-glucuronide (M6G); minor metabolites include codeine, normorphine, and morphine ethereal sulfate. The liver appears to be the predominant site of metabolism in humans, although in animal models extrahepatic metabolism has been demonstrated in the small bowel and the proximal renal tubule of rodents. These sites may become important where liver function is impaired. M3G is the major metabolite and in recent years there has been some controversy about its possible role as an opioid antagonist or in mediating some of the adverse effects of morphine.

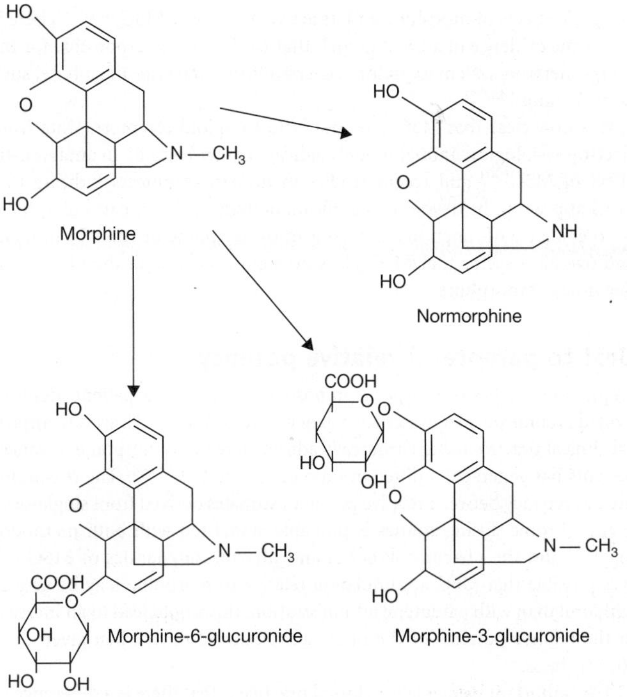

Fig. 5 The metabolites of morphine.

Morphine-6-glucuronide

M6G binds to opioid receptors[73] and produces potent opioid effects in animals[73–75] and humans.[73,76–78] M6G excretion by the kidney is directly related to creatinine clearance;[79] its elimination half-life is 2–3 h in patients with normal renal function (similar to that of morphine) but becomes progressively longer with deteriorating function, resulting in significant accumulation.[79] In patients with impaired renal function, M6G may accumulate in blood and cerebrospinal fluid,[80] and high concentrations of this metabolite have been associated with toxicity.[76,81] Although further studies are needed to clarify the clinical importance of M6G and other metabolites, the data available are sufficient to recommend caution when administering morphine to patients with renal impairment. Patients who are receiving regular morphine and develop acute renal failure in a previously stable situation (e.g. a rapidly developing obstructive uropathy in a patient with pelvic malignancy) may develop a sudden onset of signs and symptoms of opioid toxicity, necessitating temporary withdrawal of the morphine and subsequent dose reduction, and/or less frequent administration.

M6G is thought to be a potent analgesic and studies in acute post-operative pain are currently ongoing. It is not yet clear whether M6G will have fewer side-effects than morphine, though it has been suggested that M6G causes less respiratory depression.[82–84]

Morphine-3-glucuronide

For many years, it has been assumed that M3G is inert as is the case with most glucuronide metabolites.[85] Recent behavioural studies in rodents, however, suggested that M3G produces a functional antagonism of the analgesic effects of morphine and its active metabolite M6G.[86,87] There is also some evidence in animal models that M3G may be responsible for the central nervous system excitatory adverse effects seen with morphine, such as myoclonus.[88,89]

It is now clear that M3G does not bind to opioid receptors. Data from electrophysiological animal models indicate no evidence of an antagonistic effect of M3G[90] and recent studies in human volunteers indicate that M3G appears to be devoid of significant activity.[83,91] In particular, there is no evidence of functional antagonism of morphine or M6G in humans and overall it seems that M3G plays no significant role in the pharmacodynamics of morphine.

Oral to parenteral relative potency

Single-dose studies of morphine in post-operative cancer patients demonstrated an oral-to-intramuscular potency ratio of 1 : 6.[92] However, empirical clinical practice using chronically administered oral morphine in cancer patients has generated a different ratio of 1 : 3 or 1 : 2.[93,94] The reason for the discrepancy between relative potency estimates derived from single-dose versus chronic dosing studies is probably associated with both methodology[95] and the pharmacokinetics and pharmacodynamics of M6G.[93] It is possible that M6G accumulation relative to morphine may be greater with oral than with parenteral administration; this would lead to an increase in the relative potency of the orally administered drug when given on a chronic basis.

The important principle for clinical practice is that there is a difference in relative analgesic potency when the route of administration is changed, and that adjustment of dose is necessary in order to achieve an equivalent effect and to avoid either underdosing or toxicity. The usual practice when converting from oral morphine to subcutaneous morphine (or diamorphine) is to divide the oral dose by two or three.[30]

Parenteral morphine

The inorganic salts of morphine (morphine sulphate and morphine hydrochloride) have limited solubility. Standard formulations are available up to 20 mg/ml, and morphine can be constituted from lyophilized power up to 50 mg/ml. Morphine tartrate is substantially more soluble and, in some countries, is formulated in a concentration of 80 mg/ml.

Sustained-release morphine preparations

The development of modified-release morphine preparations has had a major impact on clinical practice. These preparations, which are usually administered on a 12-h schedule, provide a much more convenient means of administering oral morphine.[96] Several preparations are available worldwide with a range of dose formulations (10, 15, 30, 60, 100, and 200 mg depending on the country), allowing considerable flexibility in their use. Some preparations allow once-daily administration and sustained-release suspensions are also available.[97]

In contrast with morphine solution or normal-release tablets, where peak plasma concentrations are achieved within the first hour followed by a rapid decline and an elimination half-life of 2–4 h, sustained-release morphine typically achieves peak plasma concentrations 3–6 h after administration, the peak is attenuated, and plasma concentrations are sustained over a 12- or 24-h period.[98–100] The type and incidence of adverse effects with sustained-release morphine and normal-release oral morphine appear to be similar with the currently available formulations.

Although some clinicians advocate the use of sustained-release morphine when initiating morphine therapy in cancer patients, a normal-release preparation is generally recommended in the dose titration period.[30] Initial dose titration using sustained-release morphine is difficult because of the delay in achieving peak plasma concentrations, the attenuation of peak concentrations, and the long duration of action. In this situation, dose finding is performed more efficiently with a short-acting morphine preparation. Once the effective dose is identified using a normal-release formulation, this may be changed to a sustained-release preparation using a milligram-to-milligram conversion. For the same reasons, sustained-release morphine is not appropriate for the treatment of acute pain or 'breakthrough' pain. A normal-release morphine preparation should be provided to patients stabilized on sustained-release morphine to be used 'as required' for breakthrough pain.

Diamorphine (heroin)

Diamorphine (diacetylmorphine) is a semi-synthetic analogue of morphine and has a long tradition of use for cancer pain in the United Kingdom. It is only available for legal medicinal use in the United Kingdom and Canada.

Following oral administration of diamorphine, only morphine can be measured in the patient's blood. The use of oral diamorphine is an inefficient way of delivering morphine to the systemic circulation. There is no good basis to believe that there is any difference between these two drugs when given by mouth. Sublingual administration of diamorphine has been advocated by some but, as discussed below, this route is not appropriate for either morphine or diamorphine because of poor absorption.

It has been thought that diamorphine does not itself bind to the μ opioid receptor but must be biotransformed to 6-acetylmorphine and morphine to produce its analgesic effect.[101] However, recent studies with mor-knockout mice seem to indicate that it does not produce its effects through μ receptor binding and may have effects at other receptors.[102] This may explain some of the pharmacodynamic differences between morphine and diamorphine when given parenterally.

Since diamorphine is more soluble and lipophilic than morphine, it does have some advantages for parenteral administration. When administered by subcutaneous or intramuscular injection, diamorphine is approximately twice as potent as morphine. There are also differences between diamorphine and morphine administered by intravenous injection: diamorphine has a marginally quicker onset of action, produces greater sedation, and possibly less vomiting.[103] This may be explained by different receptor binding. The greater solubility of diamorphine (shared also with hydromorphone and morphine tartrate) is of particular advantage for patients who require large doses of subcutaneous opioids.

Methadone

Methadone is a synthetic opioid with an oral-to-parenteral potency ratio of 1 : 2 and an oral bioavailability greater than 85 per cent. In single-dose studies, methadone is only marginally more potent than morphine; however, with repeated administration it is several times more potent. Methadone has a very long plasma half-life, averaging approximately 24 h (with a range from 12 to over 150 h).[104,105] Whereas most patients can be well controlled on 8–12-h dosing, some patients require dosing at a 4–8-h interval to maintain analgesic effects.[106] Methadone may be a useful alternative to morphine, but its safe administration requires knowledge of its pharmacology and experience of its use.

After treatment is initiated or the dose is increased, plasma concentration rises over a prolonged period, and this may be associated with a delayed onset of side-effects. Consequently, patients must be followed closely until there is reasonable certainty that a steady state plasma concentration has been approached (approximately 1 week). Serious adverse effects can be avoided if the initial period of dosing is accomplished with 'as needed' administration.[107] When steady state has been achieved, scheduled dose frequency should be determined by the duration of analgesia following each dose.[108]

Oral and parenteral preparations of methadone are available. Subcutaneous infusion is possible[109] but caution is required since local skin toxicity may be a problem.[110]

The equianalgesic dose ratio of morphine to methadone has been a matter of confusion and controversy. Recent data from crossover studies with morphine and methadone and hydromorphone and methadone indicate that methadone is much more potent than previously described in literature, and that the ratio correlates with the total opioid dose administered before switching to methadone.[111] Among patients receiving low doses of morphine, the ratio is 4 : 1. In contrast, for patients receiving more than 300 mg of oral morphine (or parenteral equivalent) the ratio is approximately 10 : 1 or 12 : 1.[111]

Pethidine (meperidine)

Pethidine is a synthetic opioid with agonist effects similar to those of morphine but a profile of potential adverse effects that limits its utility as an analgesic for chronic cancer pain. Intramuscular pethidine 75 mg is equivalent to 10 mg of intramuscular morphine. Pethidine has an oral bioavailability of 40–60 per cent, and its oral-to-parenteral potency ratio is 1 : 4. It is more lipophilic than morphine, and produces a faster onset and shorter duration of analgesia of 2–3 h.

Pethidine is *N*-demethylated to norpethidine, which is an active metabolite that is twice as potent as a convulsant and half as potent as an analgesic compared with its parent compound. Accumulation of norpethidine after repetitive dosing of pethidine can result in central nervous system excitability characterized by subtle mood effects, tremors, multifocal myoclonus, and occasionally, seizures.[112,113] Naloxone does not reverse pethidine-induced seizures, and it is possible that its administration to patients receiving pethidine chronically could precipitate seizures by blocking the depressant action of pethidine and allowing the convulsant activity of norpethidine to become manifest.[114] If naloxone is necessary in this situation, it should be diluted and slowly titrated while appropriate seizure precautions are taken. Selective toxicity of pethidine can also occur following administration to patients receiving monoamine oxidase inhibitors. This combination may produce a syndrome characterized by hyperpyrexia, muscle rigidity, and seizures which may occasionally be fatal.[115] The pathophysiology of this syndrome is related to excess availability of serotonin at the $5HT_{1A}$-receptor in the central nervous system.

Although accumulation of norpethidine is most likely to affect patients with overt renal disease, toxicity is sometimes observed in patients with normal renal function. These potential adverse effects contraindicate pethidine for the management of chronic cancer pain. Given the availability of alternative drugs that lack these toxicities, its use in acute pain management is also not recommended.[117]

Hydromorphone

Hydromorphone is another morphine congener. It is five times more potent than morphine and can be administered by the oral, rectal, parenteral, and intraspinal routes. Its oral bioavailability varies from 35 to 80 per cent, and its oral-to-parenteral potency ratio is 1 : 5.[118] Its half-life is 1.5–3 h and it has a short duration of action. Although it is largely excreted unchanged by the kidney, it is partially metabolized in the liver to a 3-glucuronide, which is excreted by the kidneys.[118,119]

Its solubility, the availability of a high-concentration preparation (10 mg/ml), and high bioavailability by the subcutaneous route (78 per cent) make it particularly suitable for subcutaneous infusion.[120] In the United States, it is routinely available in oral, rectal, and injectable formulations, and a sustained-release oral formulation.[121] For patients who require very high opioid doses via the subcutaneous route, hydromorphone can be constituted in concentrations of up to 50 mg/ml from lyophilized powder. It has also been administered via the epidural and intrathecal routes to manage acute and chronic pain. Hydromorphone is hydrophilic and, when administered via the epidural route, its pharmacokinetic profile, including its long half-life and extensive rostral distribution in cerebrospinal fluid, is similar to that of morphine.[122]

The equianalgesic ratio of parenteral morphine to hydromorphone has become a matter of controversy; recent data suggests that for chronic dosing it is less than the traditionally quoted ratio of 1 : 7 and that it is probably closer to 1 : 4.[123,124]

Levorphanol

Levorphanol is a morphine congener with a long half-life (12–16 h).[125] It is five times more potent than morphine and has an oral-to-parenteral potency ratio of 1 : 2.[126] Like methadone, the discrepancy between plasma half-life (12–16 h) and duration of analgesia (4–6 h) may predispose to drug accumulation following the initiation of therapy or dose escalation. Although dose titration needs to be done carefully in the opioid-naive patient, problems with drug accumulation appear to be less than those produced by methadone.

In the United States, levorphanol is generally used as a second-line agent in patients with chronic pain who cannot tolerate morphine. The possibility that this drug may be particularly useful in morphine-tolerant patients has been proposed on the basis of its affinity for receptors $\kappa 3$ and δ that are presumably not involved in morphine analgesia.[127] It is no longer available in the United Kingdom or Canada.

Oxycodone

As previously described, oxycodone is a synthetic morphine congener that has a high oral bioavailability (60–90 per cent) and an analgesic potency 30–50 per cent greater than morphine.[128,129] Since the development of sustained release formulations in doses suitable for severe pain, it is now widely used for this indication. The sustained release formulation is available in a wide range of dose formulations (5, 10, 20, 40, and 80 mg)[55] and has a duration of action of 8–12 h. The sustained-release formulation achieves effective therapeutic levels within an hour[130] and appears to be suitable for dose titration.[131] Oxycodone pectinate is available in the United Kingdom as a 30-mg rectal suppository which has a delayed absorption and prolonged duration of effect.[51]

There has been confusion about the relative efficacy of oxycodone. Until recently, it has been viewed primarily as a 'step 2' opioid because it has for long been available in low dose in combination products with non-opioid analgesics. It seems clear that the relative potency of oxycodone has been underestimated in early clinical studies in which it appeared to be less potent than morphine. As indicated above more recent studies indicate that it is more potent, in a ratio of about 1.5 : 1.[128]

There remains uncertainty also about the role of its active metabolite oxymorphone in mediating the effects of oxycodone. However, current evidence suggests that the metabolites of oxycodone including oxymorphone do not contribute significantly to its pharmacological effects.[11]

Oxymorphone

Oxymorphone is a lipophilic congener of morphine. It is currently most widely used in suppository form, infrequently used parenterally on a chronic basis, and is not available orally. The injectable formulation is 10 times more potent than morphine.[132] A rectal formulation that is approximately equipotent with parenteral morphine is also available in the United States. The plasma half-life of oxymorphone is 1.2–2 h, and its duration of action is 3–5 h. It is less likely to produce histamine release than morphine,[133] and may be particularly useful for patients who develop itch in response to other opioids.[134] Oxymorphone is currently not available in the United Kingdom.

Fentanyl

Fentanyl is a semisynthetic opioid and is a highly selective μ agonist[135] that is about 80 times as potent as parenteral morphine in the non-tolerant acute pain patient. It is also extremely lipophilic and is extensively taken up into fatty tissue.[136] Its elimination half-life ranges from 3 to 12 h and is influenced by the duration of prior administration and the extent of fat sequestration. Fentanyl has been used mainly as an intravenous anaesthetic agent and continues to be used parenterally as a pre-medication for painful procedures and in continuous infusions. When used intravenously, fentanyl has a very short duration of action of 0.5–1 h. This is related to the rapid redistribution of the drug into body tissues rather than to hepatic and renal elimination.[137] The development of a transdermal system and an oral transmucosal formulation has broadened the clinical utility of fentanyl for the management of cancer pain.

Transdermal fentanyl

The low molecular weight and high lipid solubility of fentanyl facilitate absorption through the skin and a transdermal formulation that delivers 25, 50, 75, or 100 μg/h is widely available.[138–140] The transdermal system consists of a drug reservoir that is separated from the skin by a copolymer membrane that controls the rate of drug delivery to the skin surface. The drug is released at a nearly constant amount per unit time along a concentration gradient from the patch to the skin. After application of the transdermal system, serum fentanyl concentration increases gradually, usually levelling off after 12–24 h, and then remaining stable for a time before declining slowly. When the patch is removed, serum concentration falls 50 per cent in approximately 17 h (range 13–22 h).[141] The slow onset of effect after application and an equally slow decline in effect after removal are consistent with the development of a subcutaneous depot of drug that maintains the plasma concentration. There is significant interindividual variability in fentanyl bioavailability by this route and dose titration is necessary.[141] The dosing interval for each system is usually 72 h, but interindividual pharmacokinetic variability is large and some patients require a dosing interval of 48 h.[142]

Familiarity with the kinetics of the transdermal system is essential for optimal use. Since there is a delay of 8–12 h in achieving effective analgesia after initial application of the patch, it is necessary to provide alternative analgesia for this initial period. It is prudent to apply the patch in the early hours of the day so that the patient can be observed as blood levels rise over the ensuing 12 h to minimize the risk of overdosing during sleep. Significant concentrations of fentanyl can remain in the plasma for up to 24 h after removal of the patch because of delayed release from tissue and subcutaneous depots. Neither age nor patch location appears to affect fentanyl absorption from the transdermal system.[140] There is a potential for temperature-dependent increases in fentanyl release from the system associated with increased skin permeability in patients with fever, who should be monitored for opioid side-effects. Patients should also avoid exposing the patch to direct external heat.

Empirically, the indications for the transdermal route include intolerance of oral medication, poor compliance with oral medication, and occasionally the desire to provide a trial of fentanyl to patients who have reacted unfavourably to other opioids. However, there are a number of limitations. The delay in onset of analgesia and in the establishment of steady state blood levels require the liberal use of an alternative short-acting opioid (usually morphine) for breakthrough pain during the early treatment period. Because of its 3-day duration of action, transdermal fentanyl is generally unsuitable for patients with unstable pain, and if a patient's pain goes out of control management may be complicated because of the delay in re-establishing steady state. If dose reductions are required or discontinuation is indicated, the continuing absorption following patch removal must be taken into account. Poor patch adhesion may be a problem in some patients. Set against these considerations are the advantages in terms of convenience and compliance and there is high patient acceptability of this mode of administration. Additionally there are experimental and clinical data to suggest that transdermal fentanyl is associated with less constipation than morphine.[143,144]

Empirical observations suggest that a 100-μg/h fentanyl patch is approximately equianalgesic to 2–4 mg/h of intravenous morphine (or equivalent). The relative potency ratio that is applicable when converting patients from oral morphine to transdermal fentanyl has been the subject of some controversy, but the dosing recommendations of the manufacturer seem about right. The patch should be placed in an area where skin movement is limited, such as the upper anterior chest wall or either side of the midline on the back, preferably the lower back. Studies have shown that all areas of skin absorb the drug at roughly the same rate.[140] Since the adhesive strips on these patches are less than optimal, securing the patch with non-irritant tape is often necessary.

Transdermal fentanyl is best reserved for patients whose opioid requirements are stable[30] and in general it is likely to be a second-line choice. However, for suitable patients it works well and they like it.[145]

Oral transmucosal fentanyl citrate (OTFC)

An oral transmucosal formulation of fentanyl (which incorporates the drug in a hardened lozenge on a stick) that is absorbed across the buccal mucosa, has recently been introduced in many countries for the management of breakthrough pain. The lozenge is rubbed gently against the inside of the cheek until it has dissolved. The formulation is rapidly absorbed and achieves blood levels and time to peak effect that are comparable to parenterally administered fentanyl. Indeed, the time to onset of analgesia is 5–10 min[146–149] and studies in cancer patients suggest that it can provide rapid and very effective relief of breakthrough pain. Formulations incorporating 200, 400, 600, 800, and 1600 μg are available. The most common adverse effects associated with this formulation are somnolence, nausea, and dizziness. One interesting observation which has emerged from the clinical trials and clinical use is that the successful dose of OTFC cannot be predicted and is not directly related to the daily dose of regular opioids being received for background pain. This raises some questions about the current management of breakthrough pain with conventional formulations of oral or parenteral opioids (see Chapter 8.2.11). The use of OTFC is still relatively limited but initial experience has been good.

Other drugs

Phenazocine

Phenazocine is a synthetic opioid structurally related to morphine with strong binding to the σ receptor. One 5-mg tablet is equivalent to 25 mg of oral morphine, which means that there is less flexibility in its use. Phenazocine may be given sublingually, although administration by this route is usually avoided because of its bitter taste and variable absorption. In the United Kingdom, it was often used for patients who are unable to tolerate oral morphine, but it is now largely replaced by the more recently available alternative opioids such as oxycodone, fentanyl, and hydromorphone.

Dextromoramide

Dextromoramide is a μ agonist and is approximately twice as potent as morphine when taken by mouth. Few data on its pharmacokinetics are available because of difficulties in accurately assaying the drug, but in clinical practice in cancer pain it has a rapid onset of action but a shorter duration than morphine. Tolerance to dextromoramide seems to develop rapidly in humans and, although the duration of analgesia may initially be 2–4 h, with repeated administration this may be reduced to only 1 or 2 h. For this reason, it is unsuitable for maintenance treatment in chronic cancer pain, although it has been used successfully as a short-acting strong analgesic for breakthrough pain in some patients. It does not have any particular advantages over morphine used in this way, and in general the use of dextromoramide in chronic cancer pain is not recommended.

Dipipanone

Dipipanone is a diphenylpropylamine structurally related to both dextromoramide and methadone. As an analgesic, it is approximately half as potent as morphine, and in the United Kingdom it is only available in a combination tablet containing 10 mg dipipanone and 30 mg cyclizine. For many patients this results in excessive sedative and anticholinergic side-effects related to cyclizine when adequate analgesic doses are given, and thus it has only limited application in the management of chronic cancer pain.[150]

Agonist–antagonist opioid analgesics

The agonist–antagonist opioid analgesics are a heterogeneous group of drugs with moderate to strong analgesic activity, comparable with that of the agonist opioids such as codeine and morphine. The group includes drugs which act as an agonist or partial agonist at one receptor and as an antagonist at another (pentazocine, dezocine, butorphanol, nalbuphine)—'the mixed agonist–antagonists'—and drugs acting as a partial agonist at a single receptor (buprenorphine). These two groups of drugs can be also classified as nalorphine- or morphine-like. Meptazinol fits neither classification and occupies a separate category. The place of this group of drugs in chronic cancer pain has been limited.(151) However, the recent development of a transdermal formulation of buprenorphine may allow its more widespread use in both chronic cancer and non-cancer pain.

Mixed agonist–antagonist analgesics

The agonist–antagonists produce analgesia in the opioid-naive patient but may precipitate withdrawal in patients who are physically dependent on morphine-like drugs. Therefore, when used for chronic pain, they should be tried before repeated administration of a morphine-like agonist drug.

Pentazocine, butorphanol, and nalbuphine are μ antagonists and κ agonists or partial agonists. All three drugs are strong analgesics when given by injection: pentazocine is one-sixth to one-third as potent as morphine, nalbuphine is roughly equipotent with morphine, and butorphanol is 3.5–7 times as potent. The duration of analgesia is similar to that of morphine (3–4 h). Oral pentazocine is closer in analgesic efficacy to aspirin and paracetamol than the weak opioid analgesics, such as codeine. Neither nalbuphine nor butorphanol is available as an oral formulation, and butorphanol is no longer available in any form in the United Kingdom.

At usual therapeutic doses, nalbuphine and butorphanol have respiratory depressant effects equivalent to that of morphine (although the duration of such effects may be longer with butorphanol). Unlike morphine, there appears to be a ceiling to both the respiratory depression and the analgesic action.

All three drugs have a lower abuse potential than the agonist opioid analgesics such as morphine. However, all have been subject to abuse and misuse, and pentazocine (but not the others) is subject to controlled drug restrictions. In North America, the oral preparation of pentazocine is marketed in combination with naloxone (but is available without naloxone elsewhere).

Meptazinol is a synthetic hexahydroazepine derivative with opioid agonist and antagonist properties, but is unlike either the nalorphine-type agonist–antagonists or buprenorphine. Meptazinol has central cholinergic properties which may account at least in part for its analgesic effects. Receptor binding studies show it to be a specific μ1 agonist. Meptazinol is one-tenth as potent as morphine by intramuscular injection and has a duration of action of about 4 h. Some studies have shown adverse effects to be more frequent than with morphine, although respiratory depression and constipation appear to be less.

In therapeutic doses, the mixed agonists–antagonists may produce certain self-limiting psychotomimetic effects in some patients; pentazocine is the most common drug associated with these effects. These drugs play a very limited role in the management of chronic cancer pain because the incidence and severity of the psychotomimetic effects increase with dose escalation, and nalbuphine and butorphanol are only available for parenteral use.

A transnasal formulation of butorphanol is now on the market in the United States, but there is no reported experience of its use in the management of chronic cancer pain.

Partial agonist analgesics

Buprenorphine (Table 2) is a semi-synthetic derivative of thebaine and chemically closely related to the strong agonist etorphine. Buprenorphine is a true partial agonist at the μ receptor and exhibits a ceiling effect in dose response curves in various animal models. In some, a bell-shaped curve is seen, indicating that at doses above a certain level the pharmacological effect actually decreases with increasing dose.(152) Buprenorphine has until recently only been available by injection or for sublingual administration. A dose of 0.4 mg sublingually gives similar analgesia to 0.2–0.3 mg intramuscularly, with an onset of analgesia within 30–60 min of administration and a duration of 6–9 h.(153) In contrast, if taken orally, buprenorphine is a poor analgesic due to extensive presystemic elimination.(154) The long duration of analgesia with buprenorphine may be related to its affinity for the μ-opioid receptor and an unusually slow dissociation constant for the drug–receptor complex.

Buprenorphine has been in clinical use for more than 25 years and has been evaluated in a variety of acute pain models. Direct single dose comparisons with other analgesics such as morphine is complicated by its long duration of action, but results from a number of studies in post-operative pain suggest that single doses of 0.3 mg buprenorphine parenterally or 0.4 mg sublingually give equivalent analgesia to 10–15 mg intramuscular morphine. A ceiling effect for analgesia in humans has not been clearly demonstrated.

Buprenorphine produces typical opioid adverse effects. Overall the available data (which is limited) suggest that the incidence of common adverse effects compared with morphine is similar. Naloxone appears to be relatively ineffective in reversing opioid effects due to buprenorphine.(155) Co-administration of buprenorphine to patients receiving high doses of a morphine-like agonist may precipitate withdrawal symptoms.

Buprenorphine was introduced in high-dose sublingual tablet formulations in 1999 for the management of drug dependence. This potential use of the drug has long been recognized(156) and it has been suggested that there is less overdose risk compared with other opioids.(157)

Buprenorphine has been recently introduced in a patch for transdermal administration. The drug is incorporated in a polymer adhesive matrix (with no liquid reservoir). Three patch sizes are available delivering 35, 52.5, and 70 µg buprenorphine per hour, and each lasts for 3 days. Therapeutic plasma concentrations are achieved within 11–21 h and steady state between the second and third applications of the patch. At usual clinical doses of 3–4 mg per 24 h buprenorphine functions as a pure μ agonist.

Transdermal buprenorphine has been licensed for use in both cancer pain and non-cancer pain but clinical experience with this formulation is limited.

Principles of opioid administration

The effective clinical use of opioid drugs requires familiarity with the different drugs available, routes of administration, dosing guidelines, and potential adverse effects.

Indications

A trial of opioid therapy should be given to all patients with pain of moderate or greater severity, irrespective of the underlying pathophysiological mechanism. As discussed in Chapter 8.2.11, the suggestion that some forms of pain, such as neuropathic pain, are intrinsically refractory to opioid analgesia has been refuted by several studies that demonstrate that pain mechanisms do not accurately predict analgesic outcome from opioid therapy.(158) Given the variability of response, all opioid trials in the clinical setting should include dose titration until adequate analgesia occurs or intolerable adverse effects supervene. This approach will identify those responders who can gain substantial clinical benefit from opioid therapy.

Patients whose pain is not easily controlled with an opioid analgesic because of troublesome adverse effects may benefit from alternative strategies and these are discussed below.

Drug selection

The factors that influence opioid selection include pain intensity, pharmacokinetic considerations and available formulations, previous adverse effects, and the presence of co-existing disease.

Pain intensity

Patients who present with severe pain are usually treated with a 'step 3' opioid (morphine, hydromorphone, oxycodone, oxymorphone, fentanyl, methadone, or levorphanol). Patients with moderate pain are conventionally treated with a combination product containing paracetamol or aspirin plus a conventional step 2 opioid [codeine, dihydrocodeine, hydrocodone, oxycodone (low dose), and propoxyphene].

Pharmacokinetic considerations and type of formulation

Any of the available agonist opioids can be selected for the opioid-naive patient without major organ failure. Short-half-life opioids (morphine, hydromorphone, oxycodone, or oxymorphone) are generally favoured because they are easier to titrate than the long-half-life drugs, which require a longer period to approach steady state plasma concentrations. Among the short-half-life opioids, the range of available formulations often influences specific drug selection. For ambulatory patients who are able to tolerate oral opioids, morphine sulphate is generally preferred since it has a short half-life and is easy to titrate in its normal-release form; it is also available as sustained-release preparations that allow 12- and 24-h dosing intervals. The long-half-life opioids methadone and levorphanol are not usually considered for first-line therapy because they can be difficult to titrate and present challenging management problems if delayed toxicity develops as plasma concentrations gradually rise following dose increments. For the reasons previously described, the use of pethidine, dextromoramide, and dipipanone for the management of cancer pain is discouraged.

When the oral route of opioid administration is contraindicated, the available routes of administration may become an important consideration in opioid selection. Fentanyl and buprenorphine are available for administration by the transdermal route. Although most of the full agonist drugs are well absorbed by subcutaneous infusion, some (like morphine tartrate, hydromorphone, and diamorphine) are more suitable by virtue of their high solubility and low irritability. Methadone and fentanyl may produce significant local irritation when administered by the subcutaneous route. For cultural and aesthetic reasons, the subcutaneous route is often preferred to rectal administration. Subcutaneous infusion may be also preferable in patients at the end of life because it is less disruptive than using intermittent analgesic suppositories when nursing a sick patient.

Response to previous trials of opioid therapy

It is always important to review the response to previous trials of opioid therapy. If the current opioid is well tolerated, it is usually continued unless difficulties in dose titration occur or the required dose cannot be administered conventionally. If dose-limiting side-effects develop, a trial of an alternative opioid should be considered as discussed in the section on adverse effects.

Co-existing disease

Pharmacokinetic studies of pethidine, pentazocine, and propoxyphene have revealed that liver disease may decrease the clearance and increase the bioavailability and half-lives of these drugs.[159,160] These changes may result in above-normal plasma concentrations. Mild or moderate hepatic impairment has only a minor impact on morphine clearance;[161] however, advanced disease may be associated with reduced elimination.[162]

Patients with renal impairment may accumulate the active metabolites of propoxyphene (norpropoxyphene), pethidine (norpethidine), and morphine (M6G). Particular caution is required in the administration of these drugs to such patients.[76,79,163,164] Until more data are available, it may be wise to assume that other opioids with active metabolites may produce similar problems of toxicity in patients with impaired renal function.

Morphine remains the standard step 3 opioid analgesic against which others are measured and is the most widely available in a variety of oral formulations.[30] It has limitations; the systemic availability of morphine by the oral route is poor (20–30 per cent) and this contributes to the sometimes unpredictable onset of action and great interindividual variability in dose requirements and response. Active metabolites may contribute to toxicity particularly in patients with renal impairment.[164] Sometimes the pain does not respond well or completely to morphine, notably neuropathic pain. However, none of the alternatives to morphine has so far demonstrated advantages which would make it preferable in routine use as the first-line oral opioid for cancer pain. Morphine remains the standard but for reasons of familiarity, availability and cost rather than proven superiority.

Routes of administration

Opioids should be administered by the least invasive and safest route capable of providing adequate analgesia. In a survey of patients with advanced cancer, more than half required two or more routes of administration prior to death, and almost a quarter required three or more.[165]

Oral administration

The oral route of opioid administration remains the most important and appropriate in routine practice. Orally administered drugs have a slower onset of action, a delayed peak time, and a longer duration of effect compared with parenterally administered drugs. The time to peak effect depends on the drug and the nature of the formulation. For most normal-release oral formulations, peak effect is typically achieved within 60 min. The oral route of drug administration is inappropriate for patients who have impaired swallowing or gastrointestinal obstruction, and for some patients who require a rapid onset of analgesia. For patients who require very high doses, the inability to prescribe a manageable oral opioid regimen may be an indication for the use of a non-oral route.

When given orally, the opioids differ substantially with respect to their relative analgesic potency compared with parenteral administration. To some extent, this reflects differences in presystemic metabolism, that is, the degree to which they are inactivated as they are absorbed from the gastrointestinal tract and pass through the liver into the systemic circulation. As indicated in Table 3, morphine, diamorphine, pethidine, hydromorphone and oxymorphone, have ratios of oral to parenteral potency ranging from 1 : 3 to 1 : 12. Methadone, levorphanol, and oxycodone are subject to less presystemic elimination and also demonstrate a lower oral-to-parenteral potency ratio of at least 1 : 2. Failure to recognize these differences may result in a substantial reduction in analgesia when a change from parenteral to oral administration is attempted without upward titration of the dose, or toxic effects when changing in the opposite direction.

Rectal administration

The rectal route is a non-invasive alternative to parenteral routes for patients unable to use oral opioids. Rectal suppositories containing morphine, hydromorphone, oxymorphone, and oxycodone are available. The pharmacokinetics and bioavailability of drugs given rectally may differ from that of oral administration because of delayed or limited absorption and partial bypassing of presystemic hepatic metabolism. In practice, however, the potency of opioids administered rectally is approximately equal to that achieved by oral dosing.[166] In contrast with morphine, rectal oxycodone appears to have a delayed absorption and prolonged duration of action.

For many patients, the rectal route is not used because it is more convenient to convert directly to a subcutaneous infusion of opioid using a portable syringe driver or similar device.

Parenteral administration

Bolus injections

Parenteral routes of administration are considered for patients who have impaired swallowing or gastrointestinal obstruction, those who require a rapid onset of analgesia, and those who require very high doses that cannot be conveniently administered by other methods. Repeated parenteral bolus injections, which can be delivered by the intravenous, intramuscular, or subcutaneous routes, may be complicated by the occurrence of untoward 'bolus' effects (toxicity at peak concentration and/or pain breakthrough at the trough). Intravenous bolus provides the most rapid onset; the time to peak effect correlates with the lipid solubility of the opioid, ranging from 2 to 5 min for methadone and from 10 to 15 min for morphine. Although repetitive intramuscular injections are commonplace in some countries, they are painful and offer no pharmacokinetic advantage, and their use is not recommended.[30,31] Repeated bolus doses, if required, can be accomplished without frequent skin punctures by using an indwelling intravenous or subcutaneous infusion device. To deliver repeated subcutaneous injections, a 25–27 gauge 'butterfly' can be left under the skin for up to a week.[167] The discomfort associated with this technique is partially related to the volume to be injected; it can be minimized by the use of concentrated formulations.

Continuous infusions

Continuous infusions avoid the problems associated with the 'bolus effect' and can be administered intravenously or subcutaneously.[168,169] Continuous subcutaneous infusion using a portable battery-operated syringe driver or other similar device was originally devised to administer infusions of desferrioxamine to patients with thalassemia, but was subsequently used to deliver diamorphine to patients with advanced cancer who were unable to take oral drugs.[170] This technique is now well established in palliative care and is used to administer analgesics, antiemetics, anxiolytic sedatives, and dexamethasone.

Ambulatory infusion devices vary in complexity, cost, and ability to provide patient-controlled 'rescue doses' as an adjunct to a continuous basal infusion. A variety of devices have been employed, all designed to be lightweight and portable, and in one case disposable. Opioids suitable for continuous subcutaneous infusion must be soluble, well absorbed and non-irritant. Extensive experience has been reported with morphine, diamorphine, hydromorphone, fentanyl, and oxymorphone.[120,168,171] Methadone[110] and fentanyl appear to be relative irritants and are best avoided by this route.

Studies suggest that dosing with subcutaneous administration can proceed in a manner identical to continuous intravenous infusion: a post-operative study comparing patients who received an identical dose of morphine by either intravenous or subcutaneous infusion found no difference in blood levels,[172] and a controlled study of hydromorphone calculated a bioavailability of 78 per cent for the subcutaneous route and observed that analgesic outcome was identical during intravenous or subcutaneous infusion. To maintain the comfort of an infusion site, the subcutaneous infusion rate should not exceed 5 ml/h. Subcutaneous infusion has become the first choice when parenteral analgesia is required in palliative care patients.

Continuous intravenous infusion may be the most appropriate way of delivering an opioid for patients with a pre-existing implanted central line, when there is a need for infusion of a large volume of solution, or when using methadone. If continuous intravenous infusion must be continued on a long-term basis, a permanent central venous port is recommended.

Continuous infusions of drug combinations may be indicated when pain is accompanied by nausea, anxiety, or agitation. In such cases an antiemetic, neuroleptic, or anxiolytic may be combined with an opioid provided that it is non-irritant, miscible, and stable in combined solution. As noted later in the text, a variety of different combinations of drugs are commonly given by continuous infusion.[173] However, the stability/compatibility of many of these combinations is not known. The compatibility of drug combinations is dependent on a number of factors, including the types of drugs, the concentrations of drugs, the diluent and temperature, and UV light. A database of compatible drug combinations is now available on the internet (http://www.pallmed.net/). Generally infusions should contain as few drugs as possible, preferably no more than three. The absence of precipitation within a drug mixture is not synonymous with compatibility between the drugs in that mixture.[174]

Epidural, intrathecal, and intraventricular administration (see also Chapter 8.2.6)

The discovery of opioid receptors in the dorsal horn of the spinal cord led to the development of intraspinal opioid delivery techniques. In general, they provide a longer duration of analgesia at doses lower than required by systemic administration. The delivery of low opioid doses near the sites of action in the spinal cord may decrease supraspinally mediated adverse effects. Opioid selection for intraspinal delivery is influenced by several factors. Hydrophilic drugs, such as morphine and hydromorphone, have a prolonged half-life in cerebrospinal fluid and significant rostral redistribution.[175] Lipophilic opioids, such as fentanyl and sufentanil, have less rostral redistribution and therefore less prolonged adverse effects if these become a problem.

The addition of local anaesthetic such as bupivacaine to an epidural or intrathecal opioid has been demonstrated to improve analgesia without increasing toxicity.[176,177] Unlike in acute post-operative pain, where a large volume of low concentration local anaesthetic is used, in chronic cancer pain, a small volume of high concentration of local anaesthetic is preferred and can be mixed with an appropriate dose of a small volume of opioid.

The initial conversion of opioid dose from systemic subcutaneous diamorphine or morphine is:

- epidural—1/10 of systemic dose;
- intrathecal—1/10 of epidural dose.

Thus, if a patient were on 100 mg of subcutaneous morphine or diamorphine/day, the equivalent epidural dose would be 10 mg, and the equivalent intrathecal dose would be 1 mg/day.

The initial solution used for epidural infusion is usually:

- 9 ml 0.5 per cent bupivacaine;
- 150 μg clonidine;
- morphine or diamorphine dose according to individual patient requirements (as calculated above).

This gives a total volume of 10 ml infused over 24 h.

The initial solution used for intrathecal infusion is normally around 1/10 of the above, that is:

- 1 ml 0.5 per cent bupivacaine;
- 15 μg clonidine;
- morphine or diamorphine according to individual patient requirements.

Should there be a major problem with pump malfunction, and the whole dose is delivered as a bolus, this should *not* result in a major, life-threatening overdose.

There are no trials comparing the intrathecal and epidural routes in cancer pain. The epidural route is generally preferred because the techniques to accomplish long-term administration are simpler. A combined analysis of adverse effects observed in numerous trials of epidural or intrathecal administration suggests that the risks associated with these techniques are similar (see Chapter 8.2.6). The potential morbidity associated with these procedures emphasizes the need for a well-trained clinician and long-term monitoring.

Limited experience suggests that the administration of an opioid into the cerebral ventricles can provide long-term analgesia in selected patients. This technique has been used for patients with upper-body or head pain or with severe diffuse pain. Schedules have included both intermittent injection via an Ommaya reservoir and continual infusion using an implanted pump.

The indication for the spinal routes of administration of opioid analgesics in palliative care patients is discussed in more detail in Chapter 8.2.6.

Other routes and modes of administration

Transdermal

As previously described, fentanyl and buprenorphine are available in a transdermal formulation and their use is discussed above.

Sublingual

Sublingual absorption could potentially occur with any opioid, but bioavailability is very poor with drugs that are not highly lipophilic.[178,179] A sublingual preparation of buprenorphine is available in some countries, although not in the United States. Anecdotally, sublingual morphine has also been reported to be effective; given the poor sublingual absorption of this drug, this efficacy may be related in part to swallowing of the dose. Both fentanyl and methadone are well absorbed sublingually, but no preparations are currently available for clinical use. Thus the sublingual approach has limited value owing to the lack of true sublingual formulations, poor absorption of most drugs, and the inability to deliver high doses or to prevent swallowing of the dose. Sublingual administration of an injectable formulation is occasionally used in patients requiring low doses of opioids who temporarily lose the option of oral dosing. Sublingual administration of fentanyl and related drugs (alfentanyl) has also been reported to be effective in the management of breakthrough pain.[180] The injectable formulation is used and is much cheaper than the oral transmucosal formulation of fentanyl (OTFC). However, it is not really a practical option for patients who are still mobile and at home for whom OTFC may work well and is more convenient to use.

Oral transmucosal and nasal

The management of 'breakthrough' pain has been a topic of considerable recent interest[181] partly stimulated by the development of OTFC and other novel approaches to the administration of potent opioids. The nasal route may be effective for a number of opioids[182] and nasal diamorphine spray has been shown to provide effective pain relief for children and teenagers presenting to emergency departments in acute pain with clinical fractures.[183] This approach is also currently being investigated in adult cancer patients with troublesome acute episodic pain.

Topical

There are several case series and one very small randomized controlled trial (in press) that examine the role of topical morphine for local analgesia. The small amount of existing evidence seems to point to a role in some situations, for example, cutaneous ulcers or tumour with cutaneous inflammation. Doses of 10–40 mg of morphine are used in simple gel, saline soaks, or local anaesthetic gel.[184–186]

Changing the route of administration

As described above, when changing from the oral to parenteral routes, or vice versa, an adjustment in dose is required to avoid either toxic effects or a reduction in analgesia. The ratios of oral to parenteral relative potency given in Table 3 are estimates and should not be taken as precise figures but used as guidelines to achieve a roughly equianalgesic effect. There is considerable variation between patients, and upward or downward adjustment may then be required for individual patients. The slower onset of analgesia after oral administration often requires some adaptation on the part of a patient who is accustomed to the more rapid onset seen after parenteral opioid. In some patients, the problems associated with switching from the parenteral to the oral route of opioid administration may need to be minimized by slowly reducing the parenteral dose and increasing the oral dose over a 2–3-day period.

Usually, no dose adjustment is required when patients are switched from the subcutaneous to the intravenous route or vice versa.

Scheduling opioid administration

'Around-the-clock' dosing

To provide the patient with continuous relief by preventing the pain from recurring, patients with continuous or frequent pain are usually scheduled for 'around-the-clock' dosing. However, clinical vigilance is required in patients with no previous opioid exposure and those administered drugs with long half-lives. With methadone, for example, delayed toxicity may develop as plasma concentration rises slowly toward steady state levels.

Rescue doses

All patients who receive an around-the-clock opioid regimen should also be offered a 'rescue dose', that is, a supplemental dose given on an as-needed basis to treat pain that breaks through the regular schedule.[30] The integration of scheduled dosing with rescue doses provides a method for safe and rational stepwise dose escalation and is applicable to all routes of opioid administration. The rescue drug is typically identical to that administered on a continuous basis, with the exception of transdermal fentanyl and methadone; the use of an alternative short-half-life opioid is recommended for the rescue dose when these drugs are used. The frequency with which the rescue dose can be administered depends on the time to peak effect for the drug and the route of administration. Oral rescue doses can be offered up to every 60–90 min, and parenteral rescue doses can be offered up to every 15–30 min. Clinical experience suggests that the size of the rescue dose should be equivalent to one-sixth of the 24-h baseline dose, that is, the same as the 4-hourly dose of opioid. The magnitude of the rescue dose should be individualized and some patients with low baseline pain but severe exacerbations may require rescue doses that are substantially larger.

Scheduling with sustained-release formulations

Sustained-release formulations can reduce the inconvenience associated with around-the-clock administration. These formulations should not be used for rapid titration of the dose in patients with severe pain. Sustained-release oral morphine sulfate and oxycodone, and transdermal fentanyl are now widely used, and sustained-release formulations of codeine, tramadol, and hydromorphone have been introduced in various countries.

A normal-release formulation of a short-half-life opioid (usually the same drug) is generally used as the rescue medication. Sustained- and normal-release formulations of oral morphine are dose equivalent; switching from one to the other is done on a milligram-for-milligram basis after the daily dose requirement is identified using a normal-release formulation.

As-needed dosing

In some limited situations, an as-needed dosing regimen alone can be recommended. This type of dosing provides additional safety during the initiation of opioid therapy in the opioid-naive patient, particularly when rapid dose escalation is needed or a long-half-life drug is administered. This technique is strongly recommended when starting methadone therapy and for patients with acute renal failure.

Patient-controlled analgesia

Patient-controlled analgesia is a technique of parenteral drug administration in which the patient controls a pump that delivers bolus doses of an analgesic according to parameters set by the physician. Use of a patient-controlled analgesia device allows the patient to titrate the opioid dose carefully to his or her individual analgesic needs. Long-term patient-controlled analgesia in cancer patients is accomplished via subcutaneous or intravenous routes using an ambulatory infusion device.[187] The more technologically advanced of these devices have programmable variables, including infusion rate, rescue dose, and lock-out interval. The option for bolus dosing is typically used in conjunction with continuous opioid infusion. There is relatively little experience of patient-controlled analgesia in chronic cancer pain; it is a technique largely confined to the management of acute post-operative pain.

Dose selection and adjustment

Initial dose selection

A patient with severe pain that is not controlled with a step 2 opioid–non-opioid combination in full dose should begin one of the opioid agonists at a dose equivalent to 10 mg oral morphine sulphate every 4 h.

Dose titration

Inadequate pain relief should be addressed by gradual escalation of the opioid dose until adequate analgesia is reported or intolerable side-effects (that cannot be managed by simple interventions) supervene. Because analgesic response to opioids increases linearly with the logarithm of the dose, dose escalations of less than 30–50 per cent are not likely to improve analgesia significantly. Clinical experience indicates that a dose increment of this order of magnitude is safe and is large enough to observe a meaningful change in effects. In most cases, gradual dose escalation identifies a favourable balance between analgesia and side-effects which remains stable for a prolonged period. While doses can become extremely large during this process, the absolute dose is immaterial as long as the balance between analgesia and side-effects remains favourable. In a retrospective study of 100 patients with advanced cancer, the average daily opioid requirement was equivalent to 400–600 mg of intramuscular morphine, but approximately 10 per cent of patients required more than 2000 mg and one patient required over 30 000 mg every 24 h. Other centres have generally reported lower doses. A median dose of 60 mg/day in one centre[188] and 120 mg/day in another.[189]

A simple method of dose titration using oral morphine is to prescribe a dose of immediate-release morphine every 4 h and the same dose for rescue (for breakthrough pain).[30] The rescue dose can be given as often as required (e.g. every hour) and the total dose of morphine can be reviewed daily. The regular dose can then be adjusted according to how many rescue doses have been given.

Rate of dose titration

The severity of the pain should determine the rate of dose titration. Patients with very severe pain can be managed by repeated parenteral dosing every 15–30 min until pain is partially relieved when an oral dosing regimen should be started.

Tolerance

Patients vary greatly in the opioid dose required to manage their pain. The need for escalating doses is a complex phenomenon. Most patients reach a dose that remains constant for prolonged periods. When the need for dose escalation arises, any of a variety of distinct processes may be involved. Clinical experience suggests that true pharmacological tolerance is a much less common reason than disease progression or increasing psychological distress. Changes in the pharmacokinetics of an analgesic drug could also be implicated.

True pharmacological tolerance probably involves changes at the receptor level, and in this situation continued drug administration itself induces an attenuation of effect. Clinically, tolerance to the non-analgesic effects of opioids appears to occur commonly albeit at varying rates for different effects. For example, tolerance to respiratory depression, somnolence, and nausea generally develops rapidly, whereas tolerance to opioid-induced constipation develops very slowly, if at all. Tolerance to these opioid side-effects is not a clinical problem, and indeed is a desirable outcome that allows effective dose titration to proceed.

From the clinical perspective, the concern is that tolerance to the analgesic effect of the drug will develop and that this will necessitate rapid dose escalation which may continue until the drug is no longer useful. Induction of true analgesic tolerance which could compromise the utility of treatment can only be said to occur if a patient manifests a need for increasing opioid doses in the absence of other factors (e.g. progressive disease) that would be capable of explaining the increase in pain. Extensive clinical experience suggests that most patients who require an escalation in dose to manage increasing pain have demonstrable progression of disease.

This conclusion has two important implications: concern about tolerance should not impede the use of opioids early in the course of the disease, and worsening pain in a patient receiving a stable dose of opioid should not be attributed to tolerance but taken as presumptive evidence of disease progression or, less commonly, increasing psychological distress.

Opioid pharmacokinetic factors that may influence drug dosing

Hepatic and renal impairment

The impact of hepatic and renal impairment on opioid metabolism and excretion has been described previously. Neither hepatic nor renal dysfunction is a contra-indication to the use of opioid analgesics in cancer pain. Care is required, particularly in patients with renal impairment, but most situations can be managed without complex or exceptional measures. Opioids may exacerbate the central nervous system signs and symptoms in patients with severe hepatic or renal dysfunction. A high level of vigilance is required, and clinical signs and symptoms are more important than biochemical data in indicating appropriate intervention.

Drug interactions

The tricyclic antidepressants clomipramine and amitriptyline may increase plasma morphine levels as measured by an increase in bioavailability and the half-life of morphine in cancer patients.[190] The concurrent administration of drugs that induce the hepatic mixed function oxidase system can alter the disposition of certain opioids. The metabolism of pethidine is increased by phenobarbitone and phenytoin, and that of methadone is increased by phenytoin and rifampicin. Methadone has also been reported to induce its own metabolism.

The potential for additive side-effects and serious toxicity from drug combinations must be recognized. The sedative effect of an opioid may add to that produced by numerous other centrally acting drugs such as anxiolytics, neuroleptics, and antidepressants. Likewise, the constipating effects of opioids are probably worsened by drugs with anticholinergic effects. A severe adverse reaction, including excitation, hyperpyrexia, convulsions, and death, has been reported after the administration of pethidine to patients treated with a monoamine oxidase inhibitor.

Advanced age

It appears that all phases of pharmacokinetics are affected by the ageing process. Absorption may be influenced by decreases in gastric acid, intestinal blood flow, mucosal cell mass, and intestinal motility. The clearance of morphine, fentanyl, and nalbuphine is decreased in the elderly, and this age-related difference in pharmacokinetics may partially explain the greater sensitivity of older patients to therapeutic opioid doses compared with younger patients. Pharmacodynamic responses may also be altered in older patients. Increased receptor sensitivity and concurrent alterations in mental status may account in part for the increased response shown by elderly patients to opioid analgesics. In practice, reducing the dose or lengthening the time interval between doses for the elderly patient will minimize the development of serious adverse effects.

Children

The management of pain in children with opioid analgesics follows the same principles as described for the adult patient (see Chapter 9.1). The oral and intravenous routes are commonly used to avoid repetitive needle injections. Continuous subcutaneous infusion has also been used in the terminally ill child. Individualization of doses and titration to the needs of the child are essential.

Management of opioid adverse effects

Successful opioid therapy requires that the benefits of analgesia clearly outweigh treatment-related adverse effects. This requires understanding of adverse opioid effects and the strategies used to prevent and manage them are essential skills for all involved in cancer pain management.[191] The adverse effects that are frequently observed in patients receiving oral morphine and other opioids are summarized in Table 4. The most common are sedation, constipation, and nausea and vomiting, but there are other adverse effects including confusion, hallucinations, nightmares, urinary retention, multifocal myoclonus, dizziness, and dysphoria. The mechanisms that underlie these various adverse effects, even the most common, are only partly understood and, as discussed above, appear to depend upon a number of factors including age, extent of disease and organ dysfunction, concurrent administration of certain drugs, prior opioid exposure, and the route of drug administration. Studies comparing the adverse effects of one opioid analgesic with another in this population are lacking. Similarly, controlled studies comparing the adverse effects produced by the same opioid given by various routes of administration are also lacking.

As a general rule, caution is required when using opioids in patients in acute pain with impaired ventilation, bronchial asthma, or raised intracranial pressure; the same caveats do not usually limit dose titration in chronic cancer pain management.

Factors predictive of opioid adverse effects

Drug related

Overall, there is very little reproducible evidence suggesting that any one opioid agonist has a substantially better adverse effect profile than any other. Pethidine is not recommended in the management of chronic cancer pain because of concerns regarding its side-effect profile. Recent data from controlled studies indicate that the transdermal administration of fentanyl is associated with a lesser incidence of constipation than oral morphine.(145,192)

Route related

There is very limited evidence to suggest differences in adverse effects associated with specific routes of systemic administration. Compared to oral administration of morphine, small studies have demonstrated less nausea and vomiting with rectal(193) and subcutaneous administration.(194) As noted above, transdermal fentanyl appears to be associated with less constipation than oral morphine. It is not clear whether this is a route- or drug-related effect.

Table 4 Common opioid-induced adverse effects

Gastrointestinal	Nausea Vomiting Constipation
Autonomic	Xerostomia Urinary retention Postural hypotension
Central nervous system	Drowsiness Cognitive impairment Hallucinations Delirium Respiratory depression Myoclonus Seizure disorder Hyperalgesia
Cutaneous	Itch Sweating

Patient related

For reasons that are not well explained, there is striking interindividual variability in the sensitivity to adverse effects from morphine and other opioid drugs. Genetic variability may be at least part of the explanation in that it may influence both therapeutic and unwanted effects.

Some of this variability is related to co-morbidity. Ageing is associated with altered pharmakokinetics particularly characterized by diminished clearance and volume of distribution. This has been well described for morphine(195) and fentanyl.(196,197) In a study of morphine in chronic cancer pain, overall elderly patients required lower doses than their younger counterparts without exhibiting an enhanced risk for opioid induced adverse effects.(198) In patients with impaired renal function there is delayed clearance of the metabolite M6G.(199) Anecdotally, high concentrations of M6G have been associated with toxicity,(76,200,201) however, in a prospective study of patients with opioid-induced delirium or myoclonus no relationship to renal function was observed.(202)

Other patient-related factors that may enhance the risk of adverse effects include the co-administration of drugs which may have cumulative toxicity or other concurrent co-morbidity (Table 5).

Opioid initiation and dose escalation

Some adverse effects appear transiently, after the initiation of an opioid or after dose escalation and spontaneously abate. This phenomenon has been well demonstrated in a prospective study of morphine dose escalation and its effects on cognitive function.(203) This study demonstrated that cognitive impairment which was evident at the start of treatment with morphine or when the dose was increased commonly improved after 7 days. This phenomenon, though often described, has not been formally studied with other adverse effects.

There is substantial variability in the dose response of opioid adverse effects. A dose–response relationship is most commonly evident with central

Table 5 Co-morbidity that may mimic opioid-induced adverse effects

Cause		Adverse effects
Central nervous system	Cerebral metastases	Drowsiness, cognitive impairment, nausea, vomiting
	Leptomeningeal metastases	Drowsiness, cognitive impairment, nausea, vomiting
	Cerebrovascular event	Drowsiness, cognitive impairment
	Extradural haemorrhage	Drowsiness, cognitive impairment
Metabolic	Dehydration	Drowsiness, cognitive impairment
	Hypercalcaemia	Drowsiness, cognitive impairment, nausea, vomiting
	Hyponatraemia	Drowsiness, cognitive impairment
	Renal failure	Drowsiness, cognitive impairment, nausea, vomiting, myoclonus
	Liver failure	Drowsiness, cognitive impairment, nausea, vomiting, myoclonus
	Hypoxaemia	Drowsiness, cognitive impairment
Sepsis/infection		Drowsiness, cognitive impairment, nausea, vomiting
Mechanical	Bowel obstruction	Nausea, vomiting
Iatrogenic	Tricyclic antidepressants	Drowsiness, cognitive impairment, constipation
	Benzodiazepines	Drowsiness, cognitive impairment
	Antibiotics	Nausea and vomiting
	Vinca alkaloids	Constipation
	Flutamide	Constipation
	Corticosteroids	Agitated delirium
	Non-steroidal anti-inflammatory drugs	Nausea, drowsiness
	Chemotherapy	Nausea, vomiting, drowsiness, cognitive impairment
	Radiotherapy	Nausea, vomiting, drowsiness

nervous system effects of sedation, cognitive impairment, hallucinations, myoclonus, and respiratory depression. Even among these, however, there is very substantial interindividual variability Additionally, as tolerance develops to some effects, the spectrum of adverse effects changes over time. Commonly, patients who have had prolonged opioid exposure have a lesser tendency to develop sedation or respiratory depression, and the predominant central nervous system effects become the neuroexci-tatory ones of delirium and myoclonus. Gastrointestinal adverse effects generally have a weaker dose–response relationship. Some, like nausea and vomiting, are common with the initiation of therapy but are subsequently unpredictable with resolution among some patients and persistence among others. Constipation is virtually universal and demonstrates no consistent dose relationship.

Differential diagnosis

Adverse symptoms in patients taking opioids are not always caused by the opioid. Drug induced effects must be differentiated from other causes and from drug interactions (Table 2). Indeed, the appearance of a new adverse change in patient well-being that occurs in the setting of stable opioid dosing is rarely caused by the opioid, and an alternative explanation should be vigorously sought.

Strategies for management of opioid adverse effects

In general, four different approaches to the management of opioid adverse effects have been described:

1. dose reduction of systemic opioid;
2. specific therapy to reduce the adverse effect;
3. opioid switch (or rotation);
4. change in the route of administration.

Dose reduction of systemic opioid

Reducing the dose of administered opioid usually results in a reduction in dose-related adverse effects. When patients have well-controlled pain, gradual reduction in the opioid dose will often result in the resolution of dose-related adverse effects whilst preserving adequate pain relief.(204)

When opioid doses cannot be reduced without the loss of pain control, reduction in dose must be accompanied by the addition of an accompanying synergistic approach.

The addition of a non-opioid co-analgesic

The analgesia achieved from NSAIDs is additive and often synergistic with that achieved by opioids.(205–208)

The addition of an adjuvant analgesic that is appropriate to the pain syndrome and mechanism (see Chapter 8.2.5)

Adjuvant analgesics (see below) may be combined with primary analgesics to improve the outcome for patients who cannot otherwise attain an acceptable balance between pain relief and side-effects.(209) There is great interindividual variability in the response to all adjuvant analgesics and, for many only limited benefit. Many of the adjuvant analgesics have the potential to cause side-effects that may be additive to the opioid-induced adverse effects that are already problematic. In evaluating the utility of an adjuvant agent in a particular patient setting, one must consider the likelihood of benefit, the risk of adverse effects, the ease of administration, and patient convenience.

The application of a therapy targeting the cause of the pain

Specific antitumour therapies, such as radiotherapy, chemotherapy, or surgery targeting the cause of cancer related pain can provide substantial relief and thus reduce the need for opioid analgesia. Radiotherapy is of proven benefit in the treatment of painful bone metastases, epidural neoplasm and headache due to cerebral metastases (see Chapter 8.1.2). In other settings, there is a lack of well established supportive data, and the use of radiotherapy is largely anecdotal. Despite a paucity of evidence concerning the specific analgesic benefits of chemotherapy,(210,211) there is a strong clinical impression that tumour shrinkage is generally associated with relief of pain. Surgery may have a role in the relief of symptoms caused by specific problems, such as obstruction of a hollow viscus, unstable bony structures and compression of neural tissues (Chapters 8.1.3 and 8.1.4).

The application of a regional anaesthetic or neuroablative intervention (see Chapter 8.2.6)

The results of the WHO analgesic ladder validation studies suggest that 10–30 per cent of patients with cancer pain do not achieve a satisfactory balance between relief and side-effects using systemic pharmacotherapy alone without unacceptable drug toxicity. Anaesthetic and neurosurgical techniques may reduce or eliminate the requirement for systemically administered opioids to achieve adequate analgesia. In general, regional analgesic techniques such as intraspinal opioid and local anaesthetic administration or intrapleural local anaesthetic administration are usually considered first because they can achieve this end without compromising neurological integrity. Neurodestructive procedures, however, are valuable in a small subset of patients; and some of these procedures, such as coeliac plexus blockade in patients with pancreatic cancer, may have a favourable enough risk benefit ratio that early treatment is warranted.

Symptomatic therapy to reduce the adverse effects

Symptomatic drugs used to prevent or control opioid adverse effects are commonly employed. With few exceptions, the literature describing these approaches is anecdotal. Very few studies have prospectively evaluated efficacy and no studies have evaluated the toxicity of these approaches over the long term. In general, this approach involves the addition of a new medication, adding to medication burden and with the associated risks of additional or different adverse effects or drug interactions.

Opioid switch (or rotation)

It has long been observed anecdotally that patients who develop intolerable adverse effects with morphine while achieving inadequate analgesia may sometimes benefit from switching to an alternative oral opioid agonist.(212,213) In recent years, the practice has focused particularly on the problems of cognitive impairment and the possible relationship with toxic metabolites of morphine and other opioids. The frequency with which this is a problem and the suggested pathophysiology has been the subject of some controversy(214,215) and some have advocated multiple switches if the first change in drug does not achieve or maintain the desired effect.(216–219) Improvements in cognitive impairment, sedation, hallucinations, nausea, vomiting, and myoclonus have been commonly reported. This approach requires familiarity with a range of opioid agonists and with the use of equianalgesic tables to convert doses when switching between opioids. While this approach has the practical advantage of minimizing polypharmacy, outcomes are variable and unpredictable. When switching between opioids, even with prudent use of equianalgesic tables, patients are at risk for under-or-over dosing by virtue of individual sensitivities.

Dose adjustments when switching opioids

When patients are switched from one opioid analgesic to another, lack of attention to the drug-dependent differences in opioid dose may result in undermedication or overdose. In this setting familiarity with the use of the equianalgesic dose table (Table 3) is essential. For patients with good pain control, the starting dose of the new drug should be reduced to 50–75 per cent of the equianalgesic dose to account for incomplete cross-tolerance. However, if the patient had inadequate pain control on the previous opioid, a smaller dose reduction is used and the starting dose of the new drug can be usually 75–100 per cent of the equianalgesic dose. Clinical experience suggests that additional caution is needed when the change is to methadone; a reduction to 25–33 per cent of the equianalgesic dose is prudent. After any change from one opioid to another, patients must be monitored to assess the adequacy of analgesia and to detect the development of side-effects. Subsequent dose adjustments are usually necessary.

This information has been gained empirically but is based upon the concept that cross-tolerance is not complete among opioids and conforms to our recognition that the relative potency of some of the opioid analgesics may change with repetitive dosing, particularly those opioids with a long plasma half-life.

The biological basis for the observed interindividual variability in sensitivity to opioid analgesia and adverse effects is multifactorial. Preclinical studies show that opioids can act on different receptors or sub-type receptors[220] and individual receptor profiles may influence the analgesia as well as the side-effects. The genetic makeup of the individual plays an important role in analgesia for some opioids[221] and similar phenomena may contribute to variability in adverse effect sensitivity.

Change in the route of systemic administration

There is no good evidence that efficacy is dependent on route of administration: in general, morphine has equal efficacy if given in appropriate dosage by oral, parenteral, or spinal routes. However, there are limited data that indicate that some adverse side-effects among patients receiving oral morphine can be relieved by switching the route of admission to the subcutaneous route. In one small study, this phenomenon was reported for nausea and vomiting,[194] in another there was less constipation, drowsiness, and nausea.[222]

Initial management of the patient receiving opioids who presents with adverse effects

Among patients receiving opioid analgesic therapy, there are two key steps in the initial management of adverse effects. First, the clinician must distinguish between morphine adverse effects and co-morbidity or drug interactions, and deal with the latter appropriately. In patients with advanced cancer, side-effects due to drug combinations are common. The potential for additive side-effects and serious toxicity from drug combinations must be recognized. The sedative effect of an opioid may add to that produced by numerous other centrally acting drugs, such as anxiolytics, neuroleptics, and antidepressants.[223] Likewise, drugs with anticholinergic effects probably worsen the constipating effects of opioids.

If it seems that there is a true adverse effect of the opioid, consideration should be given to reducing the opioid dose. If the patient has good pain control, the morphine dose should be reduced by 25 per cent.

Gastrointestinal side-effects

The gastrointestinal adverse effects of opioids are common. In general, they are characterized by having a weak dose–response relationship.

Constipation

Constipation is the most common adverse effect of chronic opioid therapy.[224] Laxative medications should be routinely prescribed prophylactically to most patients.

Nausea and vomiting

Opioids may produce nausea and vomiting through both central and peripheral mechanisms. These drugs stimulate the medullary chemoreceptor trigger zone, increase vestibular sensitivity, and have effects on the gastrointestinal tract (including increased gastric antral tone, diminished motility, and delayed gastric emptying). With the initiation of opioid therapy, patients should be informed that nausea can occur and that it is usually transitory and controllable. Routine prophylactic administration of an antiemetic is not necessary, except in patients with a history of severe opioid-induced nausea and vomiting, but patients should have access to an antiemetic at the start of therapy if the need for one arises. Anecdotally, the use of prochlorperazine, metoclopromide, or haloperidol in low dose has usually been sufficient.

Central nervous system side-effects

The central nervous system side-effects of opioids are generally dose related. The specific pattern of central nervous system adverse effects is influenced by individual patient factors, duration of opioid exposure and dose.

Sedation

Initiation of opioid therapy or significant dose escalation commonly induces sedation that persists until tolerance to this effect develops, usually in days to weeks. It is useful to forewarn patients of this potential, and thereby reduce anxiety and encourage avoidance of activities, such as driving, that may be dangerous if sedation occurs.[225] Some patients have a persistent problem with sedation, particularly if other confounding factors exist. These factors include the use of other sedating drugs or co-existent diseases such as dementia, metabolic encephalopathy, or brain metastases. Both dextroamphetamine and methylphenidate have been used in the treatment of opioid-induced sedation.[226] Treatment with methylphenidate or dextroamphetamine is typically begun at 2.5–5 mg in the morning, which is repeated at midday if necessary to maintain effects until evening. Doses are then increased gradually if needed. Few patients require more than 40 mg per day in divided doses. This approach is relatively contra-indicated among patients with cardiac arrhythmias, agitated delirium, paranoid personality, and past amphetamine abuse.

Confusion and delirium

Mild cognitive impairment is common following the initiation of opioid therapy or dose increases. Similar to sedation, however, pure opioid-induced encephalopathy appears to be transient in most patients, persisting from days to a week or two. Although persistent confusion attributable to the opioid alone occurs, the aetiology of persistent delirium is usually related to the combined effect of the opioid and other contributing factors, including electrolyte disorders, neoplastic involvement of the central nervous system, sepsis, vital organ failure, and hypoxaemia.[226] A stepwise approach to management (Table 6) often culminates in a trial of a neuroleptic drug. Haloperidol in low doses (0.5–1.0 mg PO or 0.25–0.5 mg intravenously or intramuscularly) is most commonly recommended because of its efficacy and low incidence of cardiovascular and anticholinergic effects.

Respiratory depression

When sedation is used as a clinical indicator of central nervous system toxicity and appropriate steps are taken, respiratory depression is rare. When, however, it does occur it is always accompanied by other signs of central nervous system depression, including sedation and mental clouding. Respiratory compromise accompanied by tachypnoea and anxiety is never a primary opioid event.

With repeated opioid administration, tolerance appears to develop rapidly to the respiratory depressant effects of opioid drugs and consequently clinically important respiratory depression is a very rare event in the cancer patient whose opioid dose has been titrated against pain.

The ability to tolerate high doses of opioids is also related to the stimulus related effect of pain on respiration in a manner that is balanced against the

Table 6 A stepwise approach to the management of confusion and delirium

1. Discontinue non-essential centrally-acting medications
2. If analgesia is satisfactory, reduce opioid dose by 25%
3. Exclude sepsis or metabolic derangement
4. Exclude CNS involvement by tumour
5. If delirium persists, consider: —trial of neuroleptic (e.g. haloperidol) —change to an alternative opioid drug —a change in opioid route to an intraspinal route (± local anaesthetic) —a trial of other anaesthetic or neurosurgical options

depressant opioid effect. Opioid-induced respiratory depression can occur, however, if pain is suddenly eliminated (such as may occur following neurolytic procedures) and the opioid dose is not reduced.[227]

When respiratory depression occurs in patients on chronic opioid therapy, administration of the specific opioid antagonist, naloxone, usually improves ventilation. This is true even if the primary cause of the respiratory event was not the opioid itself, but rather, an intercurrent cardiac or pulmonary process. A response to naloxone, therefore, should not be taken as proof that the event was due to the opioid alone and an evaluation for these other processes should ensue.

Naloxone can precipitate a severe abstinence syndrome and should be administered only if strongly indicated. If the patient is bradypnoeic but readily arousable, and the peak plasma level of the last opioid dose has already been reached, the opioid should be withheld and the patient monitored until improved. If severe hypoventilation occurs (regardless of the associated factors that may be contributing to respiratory compromise), or the patient is bradypnoeic and unrousable, naloxone should be administered. To reduce the risk of severe withdrawal following a period of opioid administration, dilute naloxone (1 : 10) should be used in doses titrated to respiratory rate and level of consciousness. In the comatose patient, it may be prudent to place an endotracheal tube to prevent aspiration following administration of naloxone.

Multifocal myoclonus

All opioid analgesics can produce myoclonus. Mild and infrequent myoclonus is common. In occasional patients, however, myoclonus can be distressing or contribute to breakthrough pain that occurs with the involuntary movement. If the dose cannot be reduced due to persistent pain, consideration should be given to either switching to an alternative opioid[216] or to symptomatic treatment with a benzodiazepine (particularly clonazepam or midazolam), dantrolene or an anticonvulsant.[226]

Other effects

Urinary retention

Opioid analgesics increase smooth muscle tone and can occasionally cause bladder spasm or urinary retention (due to an increase in sphincter tone). This is an infrequent problem that is usually observed in elderly male patients. Tolerance can develop rapidly but catheterization may be necessary to manage transient problems.

Opioids and driving

The ability to continue driving is very important to maintaining the quality of life of many patients with advanced cancer. Many assume that they must stop driving whilst taking regular potent opioid analgesics, but this is not necessarily so. The usual advice to patients is that they should not drive or engage in other skilled activities such as operating machinery when they first start on morphine or a similar opioid, or when they increase the dose. However, once the initial sedative effects have resolved and both the patient and physician are confident that cognitive and psychomotor performance are no longer impaired, driving and other similar activities may restart.

This advice is based to a large extent on empirical experience and there have been few objective data to substantiate it. However, recent studies confirm, perhaps surprisingly, that morphine produces little measurable impairment of cognitive and psychomotor function,[228] particularly in patients receiving continuous treatment with stable doses.[229] In one study, which used a battery of performance tests designed specifically to assess functions related to driving ability, chronic morphine use was associated with slower reaction times, more mistakes, and a slowing in ability to process visual information and perform motor sequences, but these changes were not statistically significant compared with a control group of cancer patients not taking morphine.[225] These data support the clinical impression that stable doses of morphine are unlikely to cause substantial impairment of the psychomotor skills required for driving, and allow us to continue to advise patients to this effect.

'Allergy' and intolerance to morphine

Morphine and other opioids cause histamine release, and this is said to contribute to asthma or urticaria in allergic patients.[133,230,231] There is no published information on the incidence of this phenomenon and, in our experience, it is very rare.

However, it is not uncommon for patients to claim that they are 'allergic' to morphine. This usually means that they have had a bad experience with the drug but, on investigation, what they describe are its common side-effects. There is no doubt that most patients experience some adverse effects when they first start regular morphine treatment. Most commonly this is sedation, nausea, and, less often, vomiting. All patients must be warned about this and appropriate measures must be taken, as described above. If patients are not warned and experience unpleasant adverse effects they will be discouraged from continuing with the drug, and if they do not understand what is going on they may assume they that are 'allergic' to it.

The opioid-dependent patient: definitions and misconceptions

Addiction and substance abuse are social and medical problems of pandemic proportions which are associated with major social and human costs. Commonly, opioid drugs are the preferred substances of abuse. This association, combined with the principle of non-maleficence is the basis for concern regarding risk of addiction caused by the medical use of opioids. In recent years, the relationship between the medical use of opioids and the risk of addiction has been the focus of policy makers, medical sociologists, and pain clinicians. Overall, this body of research has demonstrated: (i) the risk of developing addictive behaviours or substance abuse as a consequence of the medical use of opioids is low; (ii) patient, family members, members of the health care professions, and regulators commonly overestimate the risk of addiction; (iii) patient, family members, members of the health care professions, and regulators often confuse physical dependence and addiction and; (iv) together, these concerns contribute substantially to physician reluctance to prescribe opioids and patient reluctance to use them.[232–234]

To understand these phenomena as they relate to opioid treatment of cancer pain, it is useful first to present a concept that might be called 'therapeutic dependence'. Patients who require a specific drug therapy to control a symptom or disease process are clearly dependent on the therapeutic efficacy of the drugs in question. Examples of this 'therapeutic dependence' include the requirements of patients with congestive cardiac failure for cardiotonic and diuretic medication or the reliance of insulin-dependent diabetics on insulin therapy. In these patients, undermedication or withdrawal of treatment would result in serious untoward consequences. Patients with chronic cancer pain have an analogous relationship to their analgesic therapy. This relationship may or may not be associated with the development of physical dependence, but is virtually never associated with addiction.

Psychological dependence and 'addiction'

The properties of the opioid analgesics that are most likely to lead to their being misused are effects mediated in the central nervous system. The term addiction refers to a psychological and behavioural syndrome characterized by a continued craving for an opioid drug to achieve a psychic effect (psychological dependence) and associated aberrant drug-related behaviours, such as compulsive drug-seeking, unsanctioned use or dose escalation, and use despite harm to self or others. Addiction should be suspected if patients demonstrate compulsive use, loss of control over drug use, and continuing use despite harm. The term addiction should not be used to describe physical dependence.

There is a common perception that opioid use, for any reason, is associated with a high risk of iatrogenic psychological dependence and that it is best avoided or minimized.[235] This bias is largely derived from experience with patients suffering from substance abuse disorder who use opioids in settings other than pain. Many health care professionals and laypersons fail to distinguish between patients with substance abuse disorder and psychologically well patients with pain, and consequently overestimate the risk of iatrogenic addiction. This skews evaluation of the therapeutic index of opioids, and impacts adversely on the likelihood of a clinician to prescribe opioids and on the patients' compliance with an opioid prescription.

Despite very extensive use of opioids in the management of acute pain and cancer pain, and a growing experience in the use of opioids in recurrent acute pain and chronic non-cancer pain, there have been relatively few studies that have specifically addressed the risk of iatrogenic addiction.

In the only reported prospective study among cancer patients treated with morphine, Schug et al. identified one case of substance abuse among 550 cancer patients who were treated for a total of 22 525 treatment days.[236] In a national survey of burn centres, no cases of addiction were identified among more than 10 000 patients who were administered opioids for pain.[237] The largest prospective study involved a mixed population of 11 882 patients treated with acute or chronic cancer pain in the hospital setting. In this study only four cases of addiction could be identified among patients with no history of addiction who received at least one dose of an opioid for strong pain.[238] Finally, among 2369 headache patients, most of whom had access to opioid therapy, only three cases of addiction were identified.[239]

Physical dependence

Physical dependence is the term used to describe the phenomenon of withdrawal when an opioid is abruptly discontinued or an opioid antagonist is administered.[240] The severity of withdrawal is a function of the dose and duration of administration of the opioid just discontinued (i.e. the patient's prior opioid exposure). The administration of an opioid antagonist to a physically dependent individual produces an immediate precipitation of the withdrawal syndrome. Patients who have received repeated doses of a morphine-like agonist to the point where they are physically dependent may experience an opioid withdrawal reaction when given a mixed agonist–antagonist. It can be shown that prior exposure to a morphine-like drug greatly increases a patient's sensitivity to the antagonist component of a mixed agonist–antagonist. Therefore, when used for chronic pain, the mixed agonist–antagonists should be tried before prolonged administration of a morphine-like agonist is initiated.

The abrupt discontinuation of an opioid analgesic in a patient with significant prior opioid experience will result in signs and symptoms characteristic of the opioid withdrawal or abstinence syndrome.[241] The onset of withdrawal is characterized by the patient's report of feelings of anxiety, nervousness and irritability, and alternating chills and hot flushes. A prominent withdrawal sign is 'wetness' including salivation, lacrimation, rhinorrhoea, sneezing, and sweating, as well as gooseflesh. At the peak intensity of withdrawal patients may experience nausea and vomiting, abdominal cramps, insomnia, and, rarely, multifocal myoclonus. The time course of the withdrawal syndrome is a function of the elimination half-life of the opioid on which the patient has become dependent. Abstinence symptoms generally appear within 6–12 h and reach a peak at 24–72 h following cessation of a short-half-life drug such as morphine, while onset may be delayed for 36–48 h with methadone, which has a long half-life. Therefore, it is important to emphasize that, even in a patient in whom pain has been completely relieved by a procedure (e.g. a cordotomy), it is necessary to decrease the opioid dose slowly to prevent withdrawal.

Experience indicates that the usual daily dose required to prevent withdrawal is equal to 75 per cent of the previous daily dose. Following this rule of thumb, doses can be gradually titrated down until the drug is discontinued.

'Pseudoaddiction'

Some cancer patients who continue to experience unrelieved pain manifest intense concern about opioid availability and drug-seeking behaviour that is reminiscent of addiction but ceases once pain is relieved, often through opioid dose escalation. This behaviour has been termed 'pseudoaddiction'.[242] Pain relief usually produced by dose escalation eliminates this aberrant behaviour and distinguishes the patient from the true addict. Misunderstanding of this phenomenon may lead the clinician inappropriately to stigmatize the patient with the label 'addict', which may compromise care and erode the doctor–patient relationship. In the setting of unrelieved pain, the request for increases in drug doses requires careful assessment, renewed efforts to manage pain, and avoidance of stigmatizing labels.

Management of cancer pain in patients with a history of drug abuse

Patients with a history of abuse of opioid analgesics may develop cancer and severe pain.[243,244] The management of such patients is, in principle, exactly the same as that outlined in this chapter. Our approach is to maintain such patients on oral medication if possible, even though they may require very much larger doses than normal. If parenteral medication is required, continuous subcutaneous infusion remains the mode of administration of choice.

For patients receiving therapy for drug abuse, with or without opioid maintenance therapy (e.g. methadone maintenance), it is essential that the issues relating to the use of opioid analgesics for pain management are discussed not only with the patient but also with his or her family and drug abuse counsellors, so that the patient's support group reaches a consensus on the utility and appropriateness of analgesic therapy. An open and supportive approach, and the use of concomitant psychotropic medication as appropriate, will aid the effective management of these patients.[244]

In managing such patients, clinicians should be aware of several common issues that may confound therapy. Mental clouding, either as an effect of disease progression or as an iatrogenic adverse effect, commonly raises concerns about the relapse or recurrence of psychological dependence. A request for escalation of their opioid dose may be generated by increased psychological stress rather than pain alone. Aberrant drug-seeking behaviour such as acquisition of opioids from multiple sources, 'loss' of prescribed drugs or prescriptions, unsanctioned dose escalation, and prescription fraud must be recognized as suggestive of true addiction and addressed openly as such. In all cases, one clinician should be identified as responsible for pain management, and these patients should be reviewed frequently.[244,245]

Conclusions

There have been many developments in our understanding of opioid pharmacology, particularly at a molecular level, in the 10 years since the first edition of this textbook. Genomic research promises further major advances in allowing us to understand many of the clinical dilemmas surrounding the use of these drugs in patients with pain. New formulations and increased availability of a wide range of drugs have resulted in much greater sophistication in their use. But the overarching advice remains the same. That optimal therapy for the cancer patient with pain depends on a comprehensive assessment of his or her pain, medical condition, and psychosocial status as well as an understanding of the clinical pharmacology of analgesic drugs. Cancer patients with pain vary greatly in their response to analgesics. Genetic, pharmacokinetic and pharmacodynamic factors, as well as psychological factors, will influence the effectiveness of an analgesic in an individual patient. Through a process of repeated evaluation and continuous review, analgesic therapy with opioids, non-opioids, and adjuvant analgesics is individualized so that a favourable balance between pain relief and adverse pharmacological effects is maintained.

References

1. **World Health Organization**. *Cancer Pain Relief* 2nd edn. Geneva: WHO, 1996.
2. **Portenoy, R.K. and Lesage, P.** (1999). Management of cancer pain. *Lancet* **353**, 1695–700.
3. **Lötsch, J.** et al. (2002). The polymorphism A118G of the human mu-opioid receptor gene decreases the pupil constrictory effect of morphine-6-glucuronide but not that of morphine. *Pharmacogenetics* **12**, 3–9.

4. **Hughes, J. and Kosterlitz, H.W.** (1983). Introduction (to opioid peptides). *British Medical Bulletin* **39**, 1–3.
5. **Pasternak, G.** (2001). The pharmacology of mu analgesics: from patients to genes. *Neuroscientist* **7**, 220–31.
6. **Reisine, T. and Pasternak, G.** (1996). Opioid analgesics and antagonists. In *Goodman and Gilman's Pharmacological Basis of Therapeutics* 9th edn (ed. J.G. Hardman, L.E. Limbird, P.B. Molinoff, R.W. Ruddon, and A.G. Gilman), pp. 521–55. New York: McGraw-Hill.
7. **Martin, W.R., Eades, C.G., Thompson, J.A., Huppler, R.E., and Gilbert, P.E.** (1976). The effects of morphine and nalorphine-like drugs in the non-dependent and morphine-dependent spinal dog. *Journal of Pharmacology and Experimental Therapeutics* **197**, 517–32.
8. **Pasternak, G.W.** (1993). Pharmacological mechanisms of opioid analgesics. *Clinical Neuropharmacology* **16**, 1–18.
9. **Sindrup, S.H.** et al. (1991). Codeine increases pain thresholds to copper vaper laser stimuli in extensive but not poor metabolisers of sparteine. *Clinical Pharmacology and Therapeutics* **49**, 686–93.
10. **Inturrisi, C.E.** et al. (1983). Evidence from opiate binding studies that heroin acts through its metabolites. *Life Sciences* **33**, 773–6.
11. **Heiskanen, T., Olkkola, K.T., and Kalso, K.** (1998). Effects of blocking CYP2D6 on the pharmacokinetics and pharmacodynamics of oxycodone. *Clinical Pharmacology and Therapeutics* **64**, 603–11.
12. **Christensen, C.B.** (1993). The opioid receptor binding profiles of ketobemidone and morphine. *Pharmacology and Toxicology* **73**, 344–5.
13. **Raynor, K.** et al. (1995). Characterization of the cloned human mu opioid receptor. *Journal of Pharmacology and Experimental Therapeutics* **272**, 423–8.
14. **Traynor, J.R.** (1996). The mu-opioid receptor. *Pain Reviews* **3**, 221–48.
15. **Johnson, R.E.** (1997). Review of US clinical trials of buprenorphine. *Research and Clinical Forums* **19**, 17–23.
16. **World Health Organization**. *Cancer Pain Relief.* Geneva: WHO, 1986.
17. **Ventafridda, V., Tamburini, M., Caraceni, A., DeConno, F., and Naldi, F.** (1987). A validation study of the WHO method for cancer pain relief. *Cancer* **59**, 851–6.
18. **Takeda, F.** (1990). Japan's WHO cancer pain relief program. In *Advances in Pain Research and Therapy* Vol. 16 (ed. K.M. Foley, J.J. Bonica, V. Ventafridda, and M.V. Callaway), pp. 475–83. New York: Raven Press.
19. **Walker, V.A.** et al. (1988). Evaluation of WHO analgesic guidelines for cancer pain in a hospital-based palliative care unit. *Journal of Pain and Symptom Management* **3**, 145–9.
20. **Goisis, A.** et al. (1989). Application of a WHO protocol on medical therapy for oncologic pain in an internal medicine hospital. *Tumori* **75**, 470–2.
21. **Schug, S.A.** et al. (1990). Cancer pain management according to WHO analgesic guidelines. *Journal of Pain and Symptom Management* **5**, 27–32.
22. **Zech, D.F.J., Grond, S., Lynch, J., Hertel, D., and Lehman, K.A.** (1995). Validation of World Health Organization guidelines for cancer pain relief. A 10-year prospective study. *Pain* **63**, 65–76.
23. **Mercadante, S.** (1999). Pain treatment and outcomes for patients with advanced cancer who receive follow-up care at home. *Cancer* **85**, 1849–58.
24. **McQuay, H.J. and Moore, R.A.** (1997). Antidepressants and chronic pain. *British Medical Journal* **314**, 763–4.
25. **Kalso, E.** et al. (1998). Systemic local-anaesthetic-type drugs in chronic pain: a systematic review. *European Journal of Pain* **2**, 3–14.
26. **Jadad, A.R. and Browman, G.P.** (1995). The WHO analgesic ladder for cancer pain management. *Journal of the American Medical Association* **274**, 1870–3.
27. **Benedetti, C.** et al. (2000). NCCN Practice Guidelines for cancer pain. *Oncology* **14**, 135–50.
28. **Cleary, J.F.** (2000). Cancer pain management. *Cancer Control* **7**, 120–31.
29. **Walsh, D.** (2000). Pharmacological management of cancer pain. *Seminars in Oncology* **27**, 45–63.
30. **Hanks, G.W.** et al. (2001). Morphine and alternative opioids in cancer pain: the EAPC recommendations. *British Journal of Cancer* **84**, 587–93.
31. **Agency for Health Care Policy and Research: Cancer Pain Management Panel.** *Management of Cancer Pain. Clinical Practice Guideline 9.* Washington DC: US Department of Health and Human Services, 1994.
32. **Sindrup, S.H. and Brosen, K.** (1995). The pharmacogenetics of codeine hypoalgesia. *Pharmacogenetics* **5**, 335–46.
33. **Poulsen, L.** et al. (1996). Codeine and morphine in extensive and poor metabolizers of sparteine: pharmacokinetics, analgesic effect and side effects. *European Journal of Clinical Pharmacology* **51**, 289–95.
34. **Persson, K., Hammarlund-Udenaes, M., Mortimer, O., and Rane, A.** (1992). The postoperative pharmacokinetics of codeine. *European Journal of Clinical Pharmacology* **42**, 663–6.
35. **Vree, T.B. and Verwey-van Wissen, C.P.** (1992). Pharmacokinetics and metabolism of codeine in humans. *Biopharmaceutics and Drug Disposition* **13**, 445–60.
36. **de Crean, A.J.M., Di Guiulio, G., Lampe-Schoenmaeckers, A.J.E.M., Kessels, A.G.H., and Kleijnen, J.** (1996). Analgesic efficacy and safety of paracetamol–codeine combinations versus paracetamol alone: a systematic review. *British Medical Journal* **313**, 321–5.
37. **Moore, A., Collins, S., Carroll, D., and McQuay, H.** (1997). Paracetamol with and without codeine in acute pain: a quantitative systematic review. *Pain* **70**, 193–201.
38. **Rowell, F.J., Seymour, R.A., and Rawlins, M.D.** (1983). Pharmacokinetics of intravenous and oral dihydrocodeine and its acid metabolites. *European Journal of Clinical Pharmacology* **25**, 419–24.
39. **Barnes, J.N. and Goodwin, F.J.** (1983). Dihydrocodeine narcosis in renal failure. *British Medical Journal* **286**, 438–9.
40. **Barnes, J.N., Williams, A.J., Tomson, M.J.F., Toseland, P.A., and Goodwin, F.J.** (1985). Dihydrocodeine in renal failure: further evidence for an important role of the kidney in the handling of opioid drugs. *British Medical Journal* **290**, 740–2.
41. **Crome, P., Gain, R., Ghurye, R., and Flanagan, R.J.** (1984). Pharmacokinetics of dextropropopoxyphene and nordextropropoxyphene in elderly hospital patients after single and multiple doses of Distalgesic. Preliminary analysis of results. *Human Toxicology* **3**, 41S–8S.
42. **Inturrisi, C.E., Colburn, W.A., Vereby, K., Dayton, H.E., Woody, G.E., and O'Brien, C.P.** (1982). Propoxyphene and norpropoxyphene kinetics after single and repeated doses of propoxyphene. *Clinical Pharmacology and Therapeutics* **31**, 157–67.
43. **Beaver, W.T.** (1984). Analgesic efficacy of dextropropoxyphene and dextropropoxyphene-containing combinations: a review. *Human Toxicology* **3**, 191S–220S.
44. **Li Wan Po, A. and Zhang, W.Y.** (1997). Systematic overview of co-proxamol to assess analgesic effects of addition of dextropropoxyphene to paracetamol. *British Medical Journal* **315**, 1565–71.
45. **Perrier, D. and Gibaldi, M.** (1972). Influence of first-pass effect on the systemic availability of propoxyphene. *Journal of Clinical Pharmacology* **12**, 449–52.
46. **Rosenberg, W.M.** et al. (1993). Dextropropoxyphene induced hepatotoxicity: a report of nine cases. *Journal of Hepatology* **19**, 470–4.
47. **Hantson, P.** et al. (1995). Adverse cardiac manifestations following dextropropoxyphene overdose: can naloxone be helpful? *Annals of Emergency Medicine* **25**, 263–6.
48. **Pippenger, C.E.** (1987). Clinically significant carbamazepine drug interactions: an overview. *Epilepsia* **28** (Suppl. 3), S71–6.
49. **Justice, J.L. and Kline, S.S.** (1988). Analgesics and warfarin. A case that brings up questions and cautions. *Postgraduate Medicine* **83**, 217–18, 220.
50. **Whittington, R.M.** (1984). Dextropropoxyphene deaths: coroner's report. *Human Toxicology* **3** (Suppl.), 175S–85S.
51. **Leow, K.P.** et al. (1995). Pharmacokinetics and pharmacodynamics of oxycodone when given intravenously and rectally to adult patients with cancer pain. *Anesthesia and Analgesia* **80**, 296–302.
52. **Kalso, E., Poyhia, R., Onnela, P., Linko, K., Tigerstedt, I., and Tammisto, T.** (1991). Intravenous morphine and oxycodone for pain after abdominal surgery. *Acta Anaesthesiologica Scandinavica* **35**, 642–6.
53. **Glare, P.A. and Walsh, T.D.** (1993). Dose-ranging study of oxycodone for chronic pain in advanced cancer. *Journal of Clinical Oncology* **11**, 973–8.
54. **Heiskanen, T. and Kalso, E.** (1997). Controlled-release oxycodone and morphine in cancer related pain. *Pain* **73**, 37–45.
55. **Hanks, G.W. and Hawkins, C.** (2000). Agreeing a gold standard in the management of cancer pain: the role of opioids. In *The Effective Management*

of Cancer Pain (ed. R. Hillier, I. Finlay, J. Welsh, and A. Miles), pp. 57–77. London: Aesculapius Medical Press.

56. **Raffa, R.B., Friderichs, E., Reimann, W., Shank, R.P., Codd, E.E., and Vaught, J.L.** (1992). Opioid and non-opioid components independently contribute to the mechanism of action of tramadol, an 'atypical' opioid analgesic. *Journal of Pharmacology and Experimental Therapeutics* **260**, 275–85.
57. **Lee, C.R.** et al. (1993). Tramadol. A preliminary review of its pharmacodynamic and pharmacokinetic properties, and therapeutic potential in acute and chronic pain states. *Drugs* **46**, 313–40.
58. **Wilder Smith, C.H., Schimke, J., Osterwalder, B., and Senn, H.J.** (1994). Oral tramadol, a mu-opioid agonist and monoamine reuptake-blocker, and morphine for strong cancer-related pain. *Annals of Oncology* **5**, 141–6.
59. **Grond, S.** et al. (1999). High-dose tramadol in comparison to low-dose morphine for cancer pain relief. *Journal of Pain and Symptom Management* **18**, 174–9.
60. **Petzke, F.** et al. (2001). Slow-release tramadol for treatment of chronic malignant pain—an open multicenter trial. *Supportive Care in Cancer* **9**, 48–54.
61. **Radbruch, L.** et al. (1996). A risk–benefit assessment of tramadol in the management of pain. *Drug Safety* **15**, 8–29.
62. **McEvoy, A.** et al. (1996). Comparison of diclofenac sodium and morphine sulphate for postoperative analgesia after day case inguinal hernia surgery. *Annals of the Royal College of Surgeons of England* **78**, 363–6.
63. **St Charles, C.S.** et al. (1997). A comparison of ibuprofen versus acetaminophen with codeine in the young tonsillectomy patient. *Otolaryngology—Head and Neck Surgery* **117**, 76–82.
64. **Innes, G.D.** et al. (1998). Ketorolac versus acetaminophen-codeine in the emergency department treatment of acute low back pain. *Journal of Emergency Medicine* **16**, 549–56.
65. **De Conno, F.** et al. (1991). A clinical study on the use of codeine, oxycodone, dextropropoxyphene, buprenorphine, and pentazocine in cancer pain. *Journal of Pain and Symptom Management* **6**, 423–7.
66. **Kopp, M.** (1994). Buprenorphine transdermal system (TTS) delivery rate 35 mcg/h in an open long-term study with chronic patients. In *3rd Congress of the European Federation of IASP Chapter* Nice, France. September 2000. Abstracts.
67. **Benyhe, S.** (1994). Morphine: new aspects in the study of an ancient compound. *Life Sciences* **55**, 969–79.
68. **Sawe, J., Dahlstrom, B., Paalzow, L., and Rane, A.** (1981). Morphine kinetics in cancer patients. *Clinical Pharmacology and Therapeutics* **30**, 629–35.
69. **Hoskin, P.J., Hanks, G.W., Aherne, G.W., Chapman, D., Littleton, P., and Filshie, J.** (1989). The bioavailability and pharmacokinetics of morphine after intravenous, oral and buccal administration in healthy volunteers. *British Journal of Clinical Pharmacology* **27**, 499–505.
70. **Gourlay, G.K., Plummer, J.L., Cherry, D.A., and Purser, T.** (1991). The reproducibility of bioavailability of oral morphine from solution under fed and fasted conditions. *Journal of Pain and Symptom Management* **6**, 431–6.
71. **Sawe, J., Svensson, J.O., and Rane, A.** (1983). Morphine metabolism in cancer patients on increasing oral doses—no evidence for autoinduction or dose dependence. *British Journal of Clinical Pharmacology* **16**, 85–93.
72. **Max, M.B., Inturrisi, C.E., Kaiko, R.F., Grabinski, P.Y., Li, C.H., and Foley, K.M.** (1985). Epidural and inthrathecal opiates: cerebrospinal fluid and plasma profiles in patients with chronic cancer pain. *Clinical Pharmacology and Therapeutics* **38**, 631–41.
73. **Paul, D., Standifer, K.M., Inturrisi, C.E., and Pasternak, G.W.** (1989). Pharmacological characterization of morphine-6-beta-glucuronide, a very potent morphine metabolite. *Journal of Pharmacology and Experimental Therapeutics* **251**, 477–83.
74. **Shimomura, K.** et al. (1971). Analgesic effect of morphine glucuronides. *Tohoku Journal of Experimental Medicine* **105**, 45–52.
75. **Pasternak, G.W., Bodnar, R.J., Clark, J.A., and Inturrisi, C.E.** (1987). Morphine-6-glucuronide, a potent mu agonist. *Life Sciences* **41**, 2845–9.
76. **Osborne, J.R., Joel, S.P., and Slevin, M.L.** (1986). Morphine intoxication in renal failure: the role of morphine-6-glucuronide. *British Medical Journal* **292**, 1548–9.
77. **Osborne, R., Thompson, P., Joel, S., Trew, D., Patel, N., and Slevin, M.L.** (1992). The analgesic activity of morphine-6-glucuronide. *British Journal of Clinical Pharmacology* **34**, 130–8.
78. **Portenoy, R.K., Thaler, H.T., Inturrisi, C.E., Friedlander-Klar, H., and Foley, K.M.** (1992). The metabolite, morphine-6-glucuronide, contributes to the analgesia produced by morphine infusion in pain patients with normal renal function. *Clinical Pharmacology and Therapeutics* **51**, 422–31.
79. **Portenoy, R.K.** et al. (1991). Plasma morphine and morphine-6-glucuronide during chronic morphine therapy for cancer pain: plasma profiles, steady state concentrations and the consequences of renal failure. *Pain* **47**, 13–19.
80. **D'Honneur, G., Gilton, A., Sandouk, P., Scherrmann, J.M., and Duvaldestin, P.** (1994). Plasma and cerebrospinal fluid concentrations of morphine and morphine glucuronides after oral morphine. The influence of renal failure. *Anesthesiology* **81**, 87–93.
81. **Lehmann, K.A. and Zech, D.** (1993). Morphine-6-glucuronide a pharmacologically active morphine metabolite: a review of the literature. *European Journal of Pain* **12**, 28–35.
82. **Peat, S.J., Hanna, M.H., Woodham, M., Knibb, A.A., and Ponte, J.** (1991). Morphine-6-glucuronide: effects on ventilation in normal volunteers. *Pain* **45**, 101–4.
83. **Penson, R.T., Joel, S.P., Bakhshi, K., Clark, S.J., Langford, R.M., and Slevin, M.L.** (2000). Randomised placebo-controlled trial of the activity of the morphine glucuronides. *Clinical Pharmacology and Therapeutics* **68**, 667–76.
84. **Penson, R.T., Joel, S.P., Roberts, M., Gloyne, A., Beckwith, S., and Slevin, M.L.** (2000). The bioavailability and pharmacokinetics of subcutaneous, nebulized and oral morphine-6-glucuronide. *British Journal of Clinical Pharmacology* **53**, 347–54.
85. **Hanks, G.W.** (1991). Morphine pharmacokinetics and analgesia after oral administration. *Postgraduate Medical Journal* **67** (Suppl. 2), S60–3.
86. **Smith, M.T., Watt, J.A., and Cramond, T.** (1990). Morphine-3-glucuronide—a potent antagonist of morphine analgesia. *Life Sciences* **47**, 579–85.
87. **Gong, Q.-L., Hedner, J., Bjorkman, R., and Hedner, T.** (1992). Morphine-3-glucuronide may functionally antagonise morphine-6-glucuronide induced antinociception and ventilatory depression in the rat. *Pain* **48**, 249–55.
88. **Yaksh, T.L. and Harty, G.J.** (1987). Pharmacology of the allodynia in rats evoked by high dose intrathecal morphine. *Journal of Pharmacology and Experimental Therapeutics* **244**, 501–7.
89. **Labella, F.S., Pinsky, C., and Havlicek, V.** (1979). Morphine derivatives with diminished opiate receptor potency show enhanced central excitatory activity. *Brain Research* **174**, 263–71.
90. **Hewett, K., Dickenson, A.H., and McQuay, H.J.** (1993). Lack of effect of morphine-3-glucuronide on the spinal antinociceptive action of morphine in the rat: an electrophysicological study. *Pain* **53**, 59–63.
91. **Penson, R.T., Joel, S.P., Clark, S., Gloyne, A., and Slevin, M.L.** (2001). Limited phase I study of morphine-3-glucuronide. *Journal of Pharmaceutical Sciences* **90**, 1810–16.
92. **Houde, R.W., Wallenstein, S., and Beaver, W.T.** (1965). Clinical measurement of pain. In *Analgesics* (ed. G. Stevens), pp. 75–122. New York: Academic Press.
93. **Hanks, G.W., Hoskin, P.J., Aherne, G.W., Turner, P., and Poulain, P.** (1987). Explanation for potency of repeated oral doses of morphine? *Lancet* **ii**, 723–5.
94. **Twycross, R.G.** (1988). The therapeutic equivalence of oral and subcutaneous/intramuscular morphine sulphate in cancer patients. *Journal of Palliative Care* **2**, 67–8.
95. **Kaiko, R.F.** (1986). Commentary: equianalgesic dose ratio of intramuscular/oral morphine, 1 : 6 versus 1 : 3. In *Advances in Pain Research and Therapy* Vol. 8 (ed. K.M. Foley and C.E. Inturrisi), pp. 87–93. New York: Raven Press.
96. **Hanks, G.W.** (1989). Controlled-release morphine (MST Contin) in advanced cancer: the European experience. *Cancer* **623**, 2378–82.
97. **Forman, W.B., Portenoy, R.K., Yanagihara, R.H., Hunt, C., Kush, R., and Shepard, K.** (1993). A novel morphine sulphate preparation: clinical trial of a controlled-release morphine suspension in cancer pain. *Palliative Medicine* **7**, 301–6.

98. **Savarese, J.J., Goldenheim, P.D., Thomas, G.B., and Kaiko, R.F.** (1986). Steady-state pharmacokinetics of controlled release oral morphine sulphate in healthy subjects. *Clinical Pharmacokinetics* **11**, 505–10.

99. **Poulain, P.** et al. (1988). Relative bioavailability of controlled release morphine tablets (MST Continus) in cancer patients. *British Journal of Anaesthesia* **61**, 569–74.

100. **Gourlay, G.K., Cherry, D.A., Onley, M.M., Tordoff, S.G., Conn, D.A., Hood, G.M., and Plummer, J.L.** (1997). Pharmacokinetics and pharmacodynamics of 24 hourly Kapanol compared to 12 hourly MST Contin in the treatment of severe cancer pain. *Pain* **69**, 295–302.

101. **Inturrisi, C.E., Max, M.B., Foley, K.M., Schultz, M., Shin, S.-U., and Houde, R.W.** (1984). The pharmacokinetics of heroin in patients with chronic pain. *New England Journal of Medicine* **210**, 1213–17.

102. **Pasternak, G.W. and Standifer, K.M.** (1995). Mapping of opioid receptors using antisense oligodeoxynucleotides: correlating their molecular biology and pharmacology. *Trends in Pharmacological Sciences* **16**, 334–50.

103. **Kaiko, R.F., Wallenstein, S.L., Rogers, A.G., Grabinski, P.Y., and Houde, R.W.** (1981). Analgesic and mood effects of heroin and morphine in cancer patients with postoperative pain. *New England Journal of Medicine* **304**, 1501–5.

104. **Ripamonti, C.** et al. (1997). An update on the clinical use of methadone for cancer pain. *Pain* **70**, 109–15.

105. **Davis, M.P. and Walsh, D.** (2001). Methadone for relief of cancer pain: a review of pharmacokinetics, pharmacodynamics, drug interactions and protocols of administration. *Supportive Care in Cancer* **9**, 73–83.

106. **Grochow, L., Sheidler, V., Grossman, S., Green, L., and Enterline, J.** (1989). Does intravenous methadone provide longer lasting analgesia than intravenous morphine? A randomized double-blind study. *Pain* **38**, 151–7.

107. **Sawe, J.** et al. (1981). Patient-controlled dose regimen of methadone for chronic cancer pain. *British Medical Journal* **282**, 771–3.

108. **Mercadante, S.** et al. (1996). Patient-controlled analgesia with oral methadone in cancer pain: preliminary report. *Annals of Oncology* **7**, 613–17.

109. **Mathew, P. and Storey, P.** (1999). Subcutaneous methadone in terminally ill patients: manageable local toxicity. *Journal of Pain and Symptom Management* **18**, 49–52.

110. **Bruera, E., Fainsinger, R., Moore, M., Thibault, R., Spoldi, E., and Ventafridda, V.** (1991). Local toxicity with subcutaneous methadone. Experience of two centers. *Pain* **45**, 141–5.

111. **Ripamonti, C.** et al. (1998). Equianalgesic dose/ratio between methadone and other opioid agonists in cancer pain: comparison of two clinical experiences. *Annals of Oncology* **9**, 79–83.

112. **Szeto, H.H., Inturrisi, C.E., Houde, R., Saal, R., Cheigh, J., and Reidenberg, M.M.** (1977). Accumulation of normeperidine an active metabolite of meperidine, in patients with renal failure or cancer. *Annals of Internal Medicine* **86**, 738–41.

113. **Eisendrath, S.J., Goldman, B., Douglas, J., Dimatteo, L., and Van, D.C.** (1987). Meperidine-induced delirium. *American Journal of Psychiatry* **144**, 1062–5.

114. **Umans, J.G. and Inturrisi, C.E.** (1982). Antinociceptive activity and toxicity of meperidine and normeperidine in mice. *Journal of Pharmacology and Experimental Therapeutics* **223**, 203–6.

115. **Sporer, K.A.** (1995). The serotonin syndrome. Implicated drugs, pathophysiology and management. *Drug Safety* **13**, 94–104.

116. **Kaiko, R.F.** et al. (1983). Central nervous system excitatory effects of meperidine in cancer patients. *Annals of Neurology* **13**, 180–5.

117. **Agency for Health Care Policy and Research: Acute Pain Management Panel.** *Acute Pain Management: Operative or Medical Procedures and Trauma.* Washington DC: US Department of Health and Human Services, 1992.

118. **Houde, R.W.** (1986). Clinical analgesic studies of hydromorphone. In *Advances in Pain Research and Therapy* Vol. 8 (ed. K.M. Foley and C.E. Inturrisi), pp. 129–36. New York: Raven Press.

119. **Sarhill, N.** et al. (2001). Hydromorphone: pharmacology and clinical applications in cancer patients. *Supportive Care in Cancer* **9**, 84–96.

120. **Moulin, D.E., Kreeft, J.H., Murray, P.N., and Bouquillon, A.I.** (1991). Comparison of continuous subcutaneous and intravenous hydromorphone infusions for management of cancer pain. *Lancet* **337**, 465–8.

121. **Hays, H.** et al. (1994). Comparative clinical efficacy and safety of immediate release and controlled release hydromorphone for chronic severe pain. *Cancer* **74**, 1808–16.

122. **Brose, W.G., Tanalian, D.L., Brodsky, J.B., Mark, J.B.D., and Cousins, M.J.** (1991). CSF and blood pharmacokinetics of hydromorphone and morphine following lumbar epidural administration. *Pain* **45**, 11–17.

123. **Collins, J.J.** et al. (1996). Patient-controlled analgesia for mucositis pain in children: a three- period crossover study comparing morphine and hydromorphone. *Journal of Pediatrics* **129**, 722–8.

124. **Lawlor, P.** et al. (1997). Dose ratio between morphine and hydromorphone in patients with cancer pain: a retrospective study. *Pain* **72**, 79–85.

125. **Dixon, R., Crews, T., Inturrisi, C.E., and Foley, K.M.** (1983). Levorphanol: pharmacokinetics and steady-state plasma concentrations in patients with pain. *Research Communications in Chemistry, Pathology and Pharmacology* **41**, 3–17.

126. **Wallenstein, S.L., Rogers, A.G., Kaiko, R.F., and Houde, R.W.** (1986). Clinical analgesic studies of levorphanol in acute and chronic cancer pain. In *Advances in Pain Research and Therapy* Vol 8 (ed. K.M. Foley and C.E. Inturrisi), pp. 211–15. New York: Raven Press.

127. **Moulin, D.E., Ling, G.S., and Pasternak, G.W.** (1988). Unidirectional cross tolerance between morphine and levorphanol in the rat. *Pain* **33**, 233–9.

128. **Kalso, E. and Vainio, A.** (1990). Morphine and oxycodone hydrochloride in the management of cancer pain. *Clinical Pharmacology and Therapeutics* **47**, 639–46.

129. **Poyhia, R., Vainio, A., and Kalso, E.** (1993). A review of oxycodone's clinical pharmacokinetics and pharmacodynamics. *Journal of Pain and Symptom Management* **8**, 63–7.

130. **Kaiko, R.F.** et al. (1996). Pharmacokinetic–pharmacodynamic relationships of controlled-release oxycodone. *Clinical Pharmacology and Therapeutics* **59**, 52–61.

131. **Salzman, R.T.** et al. (1999). Can a controlled-release oral dose form of oxycodone be used as readily as an immediate-release form for the purpose of titrating to stable pain control? *Journal of Pain and Symptom Management* **18**, 271–9.

132. **Eddy, N.B. and Lee, L.E.** (1959). The analgesic equivalence and relative side action liability of oxymorphone. *Journal of Pharmacology and Experimental Therapeutics* **125**, 116–21.

133. **Hermens, J.M., Hanifin, J.M., and Hirshman, C.A.** (1985). Comparison of histamine release in human skin mast cells by morphine, fentanyl and oxymorphone. *Anesthesiology* **62**, 124–9.

134. **Rogers, A.** (1991). Considering histamine release in prescribing opioid analgesics. *Journal of Pain and Symptom Management* **6**, 44–5.

135. **Yeadon, M. and Kitchen, I.** (1988). Comparative binding of mu and delta selective ligands in whole brain and pons/medulla homogenates from rat: affinity profiles of fentanyl derivatives. *Neuropharmacology* **27**, 345–8.

136. **Hess, R., Steibler, G., and Herz, A.** (1972). Pharmacokinetics of fentanyl in man and the rabbit. *European Journal of Clinical Pharmacology* **4**, 135–41.

137. **Mather, L.E.** (1983). Clinical pharmacokinetics of fentanyl and its newer derivatives. *Clinical Pharmacokinetics* **8**, 422–46.

138. **Lehmann, K.A. and Zech, D.** (1992). Transdermal fentanyl: clinical pharmacology. *Journal of Pain and Symptom Management* **7** (Suppl.), S8–16.

139. **Varvel, J.R., Shafer, S.L., Hwang, S.S., Coen, P.A., and Stanski, D.R.** (1989). Absorption characteristics of transdermally administered fentanyl. *Anesthesiology* **70**, 928–34.

140. **Southam, M.A.** (1995). Transdermal fentanyl therapy: system design, pharmacokinetics and efficacy. *Anti-Cancer Drugs* **6** (Suppl. 3), 26–34.

141. **Portenoy, R.K.** et al. (1993). Transdermal fentanyl for cancer pain: repeated dose pharmacokinetics. *Anesthesiology* **78**, 36–43.

142. **Jeal, W. and Benfield, P.** (1997). Transdermal fentanyl. A review of its pharmacological properties and therapeutic efficacy in pain control. *Drugs* **53**, 109–38.

143. **Megens, A., Artois, K., and Vermeire, J.** (1998). Comparison of the analgesic and intestinal effects of fentanyl and morphine in rats. *Journal of Pain and Symptom Management* **15**, 253–7.

144. **Haazen, L., Noorduin, H., and Megens, A.** (1999). The constipation-inducing potential of morphine and transdermal fentanyl. *European Journal of Pain* **3** (Suppl.), 9–15.

145. **Payne, R.** et al. (1998). Quality of life and cancer pain: satisfaction and side effects with transdermal fentanyl versus oral morphine. *Journal of Clinical Oncology* **16**, 1588–93.

146. **Fine, P.G.** et al. (1991). An open label study of oral transmucosal fentanyl citrate (OTFC) for the treatment of breakthrough cancer pain. *Pain* **45**, 149–53.

147. **Farrar, J.T.** et al. (1998). Oral transmucosal fentanyl citrate: randomized, double-blinded, placebo-controlled trial for treatment of breakthrough pain in cancer patients. *Journal of the National Cancer Institute* **90**, 611–16.

148. **Christie, J.M.** et al. (1998). Dose-titration, multicenter study of oral transmucosal fentanyl citrate for the treatment of breakthrough pain in cancer patients using transdermal fentanyl for persistent pain. *Journal of Clinical Oncology* **16**, 3238–45.

149. **Egan, T.D.** et al. (2000). Multiple dose pharmacokinetics of oral transmucosal fentanyl citrate in healthy volunteers. *Anesthesiology* **92**, 665–73.

150. **Faull, C., McKechnie, E., Riley, J., and Ahmedzai, S.** (1994). Experience with dipipanone elixir in the management of cancer related pain: case study. *Palliative Medicine* **8**, 63–5.

151. **Hoskin, P.J. and Hanks, G.W.** (1991). Opioid agonist antagonist drugs in acute and chronic pain states. *Drugs* **41**, 326–44.

152. **Rance, M.J.** (1979). Animal and molecular pharmacology of mixed agonist–antagonist analgesic drugs. *British Journal of Clinical Pharmacology* **7**, 281–6.

153. **Bullingham, R.E.S., McQuay, H.J., and Moore, R.A.** (1983). Clinical pharmacokinetics of narcotic agonist-antagonist drugs. *Clinical Pharmacology* **8**, 332–43.

154. **Bullingham, R.E.S., McQuay, H.J., Dwyer, D., Allen, M.C., and Moore, R.A.** (1981). Sublingual buprenorphine used post-operatively: clinical observations and preliminary pharmacokinetic analysis. *British Journal of Clinical Pharmacology* **12**, 117–22.

155. **Gal, T.J.** (1989). Naloxone reversal of buprenorphine-induced respiratory depression. *Clinical Pharmacology and Therapeutics* **45**, 6–71.

156. **Mello, N.K. and Mendelson, J.H.** (1980). Buprenorphine suppresses heroin use by heroin addicts. *Science* **207**, 657–9.

157. **Hammersley, R., Cassidy, M.T., and Oliver, J.** (1995). Drugs associated with drug related deaths in Edinburgh and Glasgow, November 1990–October 1992. *Addiction* **90**, 959–65.

158. **Portenoy, R.K., Foley, K.M., and Inturrisi, C.E.** (1990). The nature of opioid responsiveness and its implications for neuropathic pain: new hypotheses derived from studies of opioid infusions. *Pain* **43**, 273–86.

159. **Neal, E.A., Meffin, P.J., Gregory, P.B., and Blaschke, T.F.** (1979). Enhanced bioavailability and decreased clearance of analgesics in patients with cirrhosis. *Gastroenterology* **77**, 96–102.

160. **Giacomini, K.M., Giacomini, J.C., Gibson, T.P., and Levy, G.** (1980). Propoxyphene and norpropoxyphene plasma concentrations after oral propoxyphene in cirrhotic patients with and without surgically contructed portacaval shunt. *Clinical Pharmacology and Therapeutics* **28**, 417–24.

161. **Patwardhan, R.V.** et al. (1981). Normal metabolism of morphine in cirrhosis. *Gastroenterology* **81**, 1006–11.

162. **Hasselstrom, J., Eriksson, L.S., Persson, A., Rane, A., Svensson, J., and Sawe, J.** (1990). The metabolism and bioavailability of morphine in patients with severe liver cirrhosis. *British Journal of Clinical Pharmacology* **29**, 289–97.

163. **Chan, G.L. and Matzke, G.R.** (1987). Effects of renal insufficiency on the pharmacokinetics and pharmacodynamics of opioid analgesics. *Drug Intelligence in Clinical Pharmacology* **21**, 773–83.

164. **McQuay, H.J. and Moore, R.A.** (1997). Opioid problems, and morphine metabolism and excretion. In *Handbook of Experimental Pharmacology* (ed. A.H. Dickenson and J.-M. Besson), pp. 335–60. Berlin: Springer-Verlag.

165. **Coyle, N., Adelhardt, J., Foley, K.M., and Portenoy, R.K.** (1990). Character of terminal illness in the advanced cancer patient: pain and other symptoms during last four weeks of life. *Journal of Pain and Symptom Management* **5**, 83–9.

166. **Hanning, C.D.** (1990). The rectal absorption of opioids. In *Advances in Pain Research and Therapy* Vol. 14 (ed. C. Benedetti, C.R. Chapman, and G. Giron), pp. 259–69. New York: Raven Press.

167. **Coyle, N., Cherny, N.I., and Portenoy, R.K.** (1994). Subcutaneous opioid infusions in the home. *Oncology* **8**, 21–7.

168. **Oliver, D.J.** (1985). The use of the syringe driver in terminal care. *British Journal of Clinical Pharmacology* **20**, 515–16.

169. **Portenoy, R.K.** (1987). Continuous intravenous infusions of opioid drugs. *Medical Clinics of North America* **71**, 233–41.

170. **Russell, P.S.B.** (1979). Analgesia in terminal malignant disease. *British Medical Journal* **i**, 1561.

171. **Bruera, E., Brenneis, C., Michaud, M., MacMillan, K., Hanson, J., and MacDonald, R.N.** (1988). Patient-controlled subcutaneous hydromorphone versus continuous subcutaneous infusion for the treatment of cancer pain. *Journal of the National Cancer Institute* **80**, 1152–4.

172. **Waldmann, C.S., Eason, J.R., Rambohul, E., and Hanson, G.C.** (1984). Serum morphine levels. A comparison between continuous subcutaneous infusions and intravenous infusions in post-operative patients. *Anaesthesia* **39**, 768–71.

173. **O'Doherty, C.A., Hall, E.J., Schofield, L., and Zeppetella, G.** (2001). Drugs and syringe drivers: a survey of adult specialist palliative care practice in the United Kingdom and Eire. *Palliative Medicine* **15**, 149–54.

174. **Grassby, P.F. and Hutchings, L.** (1997). Drug combinations in syringe drivers: the compatibility and stability of diamorphine with cyclizine and haloperidol. *Palliative Medicine* **11**, 217–24.

175. **Moulin, D.E., Inturrisi, C.E., and Foley, K.M.** (1986). Epidural and intrathecal opioids: cerebrospinal fluid and plasma pharmacokinetics in cancer pain patients. In *Pain Research and Therapy* Vol. 8 (ed. K.M. Foley and C.E. Inturrisi), pp. 369–84. New York: Raven Press.

176. **Du Pen, S. and Williams, A.R.** (1992). Management of patients receiving combined epidural morphine and bupivacaine for the treatment of cancer pain. *Journal of Pain and Symptom Management* **7**, 125–7.

177. **Hogan, Q., Haddox, J.D., Abram, S., Weissman, D., Taylor, M.L., and Janjan, N.** (1991). Epidural opiates and local anesthetics for the management of cancer pain. *Pain* **46**, 271–9.

178. **Weinberg, D.S.** et al. (1988). Sublingual absorption of selected opioid analgesics. *Clinical Pharmacology and Therapeutics* **44**, 335–42.

179. **Ripamonti, C. and Bruera, E.** (1991). Rectal, buccal and sublingual narcotics for the management of cancer pain. *Journal of Palliative Care* **7**, 30–5.

180. **Zeppetella, G.** (2001). Sublingual fentanyl citrate for cancer-related breakthrough pain: a pilot study. *Palliative Medicine* **15**, 323–8.

181. **Mercadante, S.** et al. (2002). Episodic (breakthrough) pain. *Cancer* **94**, 832–9.

182. **Dale, O., Hjortkjaer, R., and Kharasch, E.D.** (2002). Nasal administration of opioids for pain management in adults. *Acta Anaesthesiologica Scandinavica* **46**, 759–70.

183. **Kendall, J.M., Reeves, B.C., and Latter, V.S.** (2001). Multicentre randomised controlled trial of nasal diamorphine for analgesia in children and teenagers with clinical fractures. *British Medical Journal* **322**, 261–5.

184. **Stein, C.** (1995). The control of pain in peripheral tissues by opioids. *New England Journal of Medicine* **332**, 1685–90.

185. **Back, I.N. and Finlay, I.** (1995). Analgesic effect of topical opioids on painful skin ulcers. *Journal of Pain and Symptom Management* **10**, 493.

186. **Krajnik, M.** et al. (1999). Potential uses of topical opioids in palliative care—reports of 6 cases. *Pain* **80**, 121–5.

187. **Citron, M.L., Kalra, J.M., Seltzer, V.L., Chen, S., Hoffman, M., and Walczak, M.B.** (1992). Patient-controlled analgesia for cancer pain: a long-term study of inpatient and outpatient use. *Cancer Investigation* **10**, 335–41.

188. **Walsh, T.D. and Cheater, F.M.** (1983). Use of morphine for cancer pain. *Pharmaceutical Journal* **231**, 525–8.

189. **Brooks, D.J., Gamble, W., and Ahmedzai, S.** (1995). A regional survey of opioid use by patients receiving specialist palliative care. *Palliative Medicine* **9**, 229–38.

190. **Ventafridda, V., Ripamonti, C., DeConno, F., Bianchi, M., Pazzuconi, F., and Panerai, A.E.** (1987). Antidepressants increase bioavailability of morphine in cancer patients. *Lancet* **i**, 1204.

191. **Cherny, N.** et al. (2001). Strategies to manage the adverse effects of oral morphine: an evidence-based report. *Journal of Clinical Oncology* **19**, 2542–54.

192. **Donner, B.** et al. (1996). Direct conversion from oral morphine to transdermal fentanyl: a multicenter study in patients with cancer pain. *Pain* **64**, 527–34.

193. **Babul, N., Provencher, L., Laberge, F., Harsanyi, Z., and Moulin, D.** (1998). Comparative efficacy and safety of controlled-release morphine suppositories and tablets in cancer pain. *Journal of Clinical Pharmacology* **38**, 74–81.

194. **McDonald, P.** et al. (1991). Regular subcutaneous bolus morphine via an indwelling cannula for pain from advanced cancer. *Palliative Medicine* **5**, 323–9.
195. **Baillie, S.P.** et al. (1989). Age and the pharmacokinetics of morphine. *Age and Ageing* **18**, 258–62.
196. **Bentley, J.B.** et al. (1982). Age and fentanyl pharmacokinetics. *Anesthesia and Analgesia* **61**, 968–71.
197. **Holdsworth, M.T.** et al. (1994). Transdermal fentanyl disposition in elderly subjects. *Gerontology* **40**, 32–7.
198. **Rapin, C.H.** (1989). The treatment of pain in the elderly patient. The use of oral morphine in the treatment of pain. *Journal of Palliative Care* **5**, 54–5.
199. **Osborne, R.** et al. (1993). The pharmacokinetics of morphine and morphine glucuronides in kidney failure. *Clinical Pharmacology and Therapeutics* **54**, 158–67.
200. **Hagen, N.A.** et al. (1991). Chronic nausea and morphine-6-glucuronide. *Journal of Pain and Symptom Management* **6**, 125–8.
201. **Sjogren, P.** et al. (1993). Myoclonic spasms during treatment with high doses of intravenous morphine in renal failure. *Acta Anaesthesiologica Scandinavica* **37**, 780–2.
202. **Tiseo, P.J.** et al. (1995). Morphine-6-glucuronide concentrations and opioid-related side effects: a survey in cancer patients. *Pain* **61**, 47–54.
203. **Bruera, E.** et al. (1989). The cognitive effects of the administration of narcotic analgesics in patients with cancer pain. *Pain* **39**, 13–16.
204. **Fallon, M.T. and O'Neill, W.M.** (1998). Substitution of another opioid for morphine. Opioid toxicity should be managed initially by decreasing the opioid dose. *British Medical Journal* **317**, 81.
205. **Sevarino, F.B.** et al. (1992). The efficacy of intramuscular ketorolac in combination with intravenous PCA morphine for postoperative pain relief. *Journal of Clinical Anesthesia* **4**, 285–8.
206. **Bjorkman, R.** et al. (1993). Morphine-sparing effect of diclofenac in cancer pain. *European Journal of Clinical Pharmacology* **44**, 1–5.
207. **Joishy, S.K. and Walsh, D.** (1998). The opioid-sparing effects of intravenous ketorolac as an adjuvant analgesic in cancer pain: application in bone metastases and the opioid bowel syndrome. *Journal of Pain and Symptom Management* **16**, 334–9.
208. **Minotti, V.** et al. (1998). Double-blind evaluation of short-term analgesic efficacy of orally administered diclofenac, diclofenac plus codeine, and diclofenac plus imipramine in chronic cancer pain. *Pain* **74**, 133–7.
209. **Portenoy, R.K.** (1996). Adjuvant analgesic agents. *Hematology/Oncology Clinics of North America* **10**, 103–19.
210. **Queisser, W.** (1984). Chemotherapy for the treatment of cancer pain. *Recent Results in Cancer Research* **89**, 171–7.
211. **Rubens, R.D.** et al. (1992). Appropriate chemotherapy for palliating advanced cancer. *British Medical Journal* **304**, 35–40.
212. **Twycross, R.G. and Lack, S.A.** *Symptom Control in Far-Advanced Cancer: Pain Relief.* London: Pitman Books, 1983.
213. **Hanks, G.W.** (1991). Opioid-responsive and opioid-non-responsive pain in cancer. *British Medical Bulletin* **47**, 718–31.
214. **de Stoutz, N.D.** et al. (1995). Opioid rotation for toxicity reduction in terminal cancer patients. *Journal of Pain and Symptom Management* **10**, 378–84.
215. **Fallon, M.** (1997). Opioid rotation: does it have a role? *Palliative Medicine* **11**, 177–8.
216. **Cherny, N.J.** et al. (1995). Opioid pharmacotherapy in the management of cancer pain: a survey of strategies used by pain physicians for the selection of analgesic drugs and routes of administration. *Cancer* **76**, 1283–93.
217. **Bruera, E.** et al. (1995). Changing pattern of agitated impaired mental status in patients with advanced cancer: association with cognitive monitoring, hydration, and opioid rotation. *Journal of Pain and Symptom Management* **10**, 287–91.
218. **Bruera, E.** et al. (1996). Opioid rotation in patients with cancer pain. A retrospective comparison of dose ratios between methadone, hydromorphone, and morphine. *Cancer* **78**, 852–7.
219. **Ashby, M.A.** et al. (1999). Opioid substitution to reduce adverse effects in cancer pain management. *Medical Journal of Australia* **170**, 68–71.
220. **Pasternak, G.W. and Standifer, K.M.** (1995). Mapping of opioid receptors using antisense oligodeoxynucleotides: correlating their molecular biology and pharmacology. *Trends in Pharmacological Sciences* **16**, 344–50.
221. **Brosen, K.** et al. (1993). Role of genetic polymorphism in psychopharmacology—an update. *Psychopharmacology Series* **10**, 199–211.
222. **Drexel, H.** et al. (1989). Treatment of severe cancer pain by low-dose continuous subcutaneous morphine. *Pain* **36**, 169–76.
223. **Pies, R.** (1996). Psychotropic medications and the oncology patient. *Cancer Practice* **4**, 164–6.
224. **Fallon, M. and O'Neill, B.** (1997). ABC of palliative care. Constipation and diarrhoea. *British Medical Journal* **315**, 1293–6.
225. **Vainio, A.** et al. (1995). Driving ability in cancer patients receiving long-term morphine analgesia. *Lancet* **346**, 667–70.
226. **Portenoy, R.K.** (1994). Management of common opioid side effects during long-term therapy of cancer pain. *Annals of the Academy of Medicine Singapore* **23**, 160–70.
227. **Hanks, G.W., Twycross, R.G., and Lloyd, J.W.** (1981). Unexpected complication of successful nerve block. Morphine-induced respiratory depression precipitated by removal of severe pain. *Anaesthesia* **36**, 37–9.
228. **O'Neill, W.M., Hanks, G.W., Simpson, P., Fallon, M.T., Jenkins, E., and Wesnes, K.** (2000). The cognitive and psychomotor effects of morphine in healthy subjects: a randomised controlled trial of repeated (four) oral doses of dextropropoxyphene, morphine, lorazepam and placebo. *Pain* **85**, 209–15.
229. **Zacny, J.P.** (1996). Should people taking opioids for medical reasons be allowed to work and drive? *Addiction* **91**, 1581–4.
230. **Warner, M.A.** et al. (1991). Narcotic-induced histamine release: a comparison of morphine, oxymorphone, and fentanyl infusions. *Journal of Cardiothoracic and Vascular Anesthesia* **5**, 481–4.
231. **Katcher, J. and Walsh, D.** (1999). Opioid-induced itching: morphine sulfate and hydromorphone hydrochloride. *Journal of Pain and Symptom Management* **17**, 70–2.
232. **McCaffery, M.** (1992). Pain control. Barriers to the use of available information. World Health Organization Expert Committee on Cancer Pain Relief and Active Supportive Care. *Cancer* **70** (Suppl. 5), 1438–49.
233. **Ward, S.E.** et al. (1993). Patient-related barriers to management of cancer pain. *Pain* **52**, 319–24.
234. **Mortimer, J.E. and Bartlett, N.L.** (1997). Assessment of knowledge about cancer pain management by physicians in training. *Journal of Pain and Symptom Management* **14**, 21–8.
235. **Sees, K.L. and Clark, H.W.** (1993). Opioid use in the treatment of chronic pain: assessment of addiction. *Journal of Pain and Symptom Management* **8**, 257–64.
236. **Schug, S.A.** et al. (1992). A long-term survey of morphine in cancer pain patients. *Journal of Pain and Symptom Management* **7**, 259–66.
237. **Perry, S. and Heidrich, G.** (1982). Management of pain during debridement: a survey of US burn units. *Pain* **13**, 267–80.
238. **Porter, J. and Jick, H.** (1980). Addiction rare in patients treated with narcotics. *New England Journal of Medicine* **302**, 123.
239. **Medina, J.L. and Diamond, S.** (1977). Drug dependency in patients with chronic headaches. *Headache* **17**, 12–14.
240. **Jasinski, D.R.** (1981). Opiate withdrawal syndrome: acute and protracted aspects. *Annals of the New York Academy of Sciences* **362**, 183–6.
241. **Rogers, A.G.** (1991). Prevention of the withdrawal syndrome in an opioid-dependent one-year-old child with decreasing pain. *Journal of Pain and Symptom Management* **6**, 129.
242. **Weissman, D.E. and Haddox, J.D.** (1989). Opioid pseudoaddiction—an iatrogenic syndrome. *Pain* **36**, 363–6.
243. **Passik, S.D.** et al. (1998). Substance abuse issues in cancer patients. Part 1: Prevalence and diagnosis. *Oncology (Huntington)* **12** (4), 517–21, 524.
244. **Passik, S.D.** et al. (1998). Substance abuse issues in cancer patients. Part 2: Evaluation and treatment. *Oncology (Huntington)* **12** (5), 729–34.
245. **Passik, S.D. and Theobald, D.E.** (2000). Managing addiction in advanced cancer patients. Why bother? *Journal of Pain and Symptom Management* **19**, 229–34.

8.2.4 Non-opioid analgesics

Henry J. McQuay and Andrew Moore

Non-opioid analgesics are fundamental to managing pain, both on and off prescription, and this is as true in palliative care as in other areas of medicine. Patients use them off-prescription to treat minor ailments, we prescribe them as part of the analgesic ladder, and we believe that they, or some of them, have a special role in bone pain. The optimal use of these drugs emphasizes that the phrase analgesic ladder is slightly misleading. Unlike on a real ladder, where the climber goes up or down the rungs, best pain relief may be obtained if all the rungs on the analgesic ladder are used simultaneously, in the sense that the non-opioid analgesics work through different mechanisms compared with the opioids, and the analgesia from one drug class adds to the analgesia provided by the other class. Hence, the importance of the non-opioid analgesics.

The development of the COX-2 non-steroidal anti-inflammatory drugs (NSAIDs) has given us a clearer picture of the mechanism of NSAID action, but we are still ignorant as to precisely where, and in some cases how, the non-opioid analgesics work. Aspirin after all was discovered in 1753 at Chipping Norton near Oxford, and preparations of willow have been used in herbal and folk medicine for thousands of years.

Beyond understanding where and how the non-opioid analgesics work the clinical questions about their pharmacology are intriguing. These drugs work as analgesics, but we need to know which is the most and which is the least effective, and whether different routes offer any efficacy advantage. The choice of drug to prescribe, given that they all work, has to take into account their relative safety. The safety issues include adverse effects at therapeutic dosage, gastrointestinal, cardiac and renal, the impact of the drugs on other diseases such as asthma, and drug–drug interactions with warfarin or prophylactic aspirin.

While the major focus of the chapter is on paracetamol and NSAIDs, both COX-1 and COX-2, there is also brief mention of dipyrone and nefopam.

Where and how do they work?

NSAIDs: COX-1 and COX-2

The classic explanation of how NSAIDs work was that they inhibited the enzyme cyclo-oxygenase (Fig. 1), decreasing prostaglandin synthesis, which in turn reduced the pain-sensitizing effect of the prostaglandins. The cyclo-oxygenase was believed to be expressed constitutively with constant levels in individual tissues. The increase in prostaglandin synthesis in inflammation was ascribed to increased release of precursor.(1) Two clues that this was an inadequate explanation were increased cyclo-oxygenase activity in inflammation and the ability of corticosteroids to block this increase (Fig. 1). A further conundrum was (and is) the analgesic efficacy of the drugs in conditions which did not involve inflammation.

The classic site of action, from the work of Vane in the 1970s, was thought to be peripheral, at the site of inflammation. A solely peripheral site of action, however, does not fit easily with the antipyretic effects, or aspirin's ability to produce tinnitus, which seem likely to be occurring centrally.

The research which followed the identification of two isoforms of cyclo-oxygenase, COX-1 and COX-2, has made some of the mechanisms of action clearer.(1) The two enzymes are very similar. Both are membrane-associated. Arachidonic acid released from neighbouring damaged membranes is converted by the enzymes into prostaglandins. The differences between the two enzymes are in their internal configuration, which dictates which drugs bind

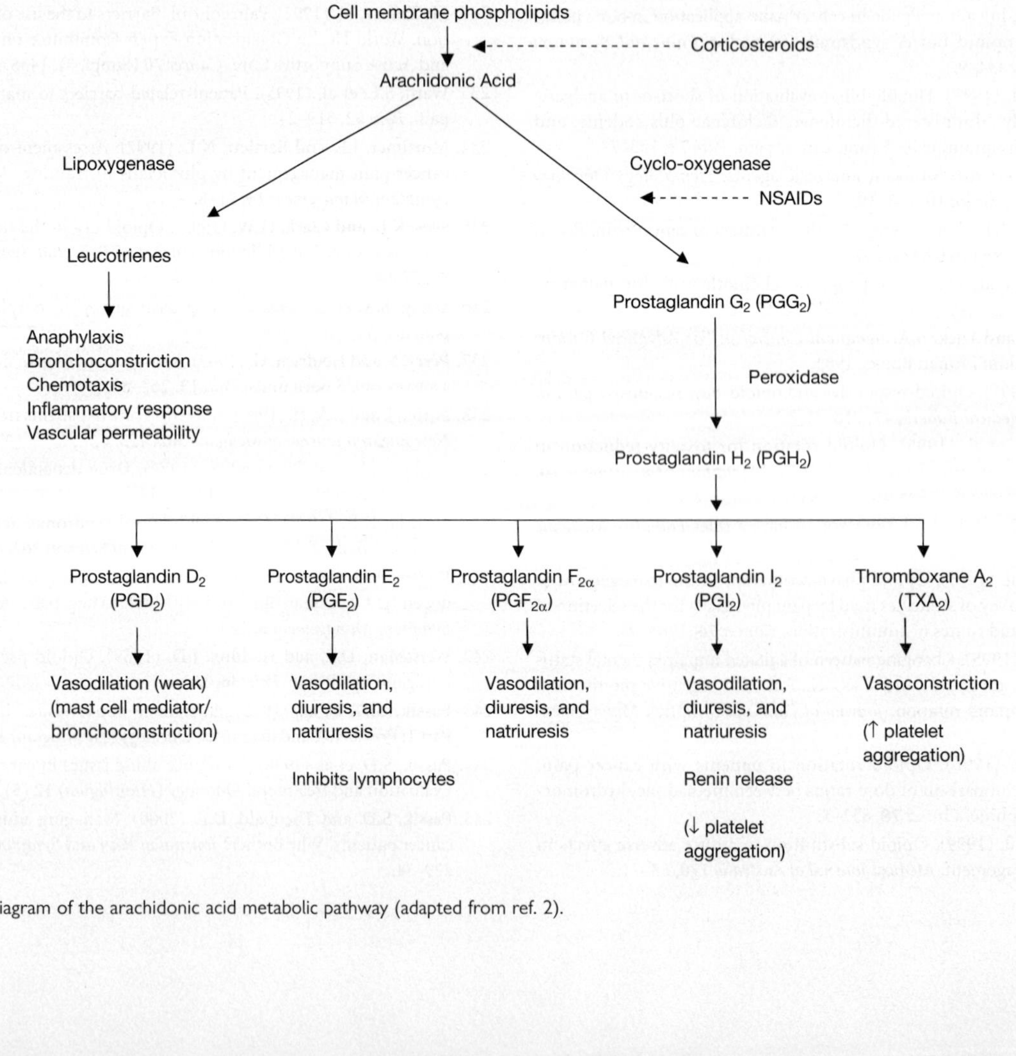

Fig. 1 Schematic diagram of the arachidonic acid metabolic pathway (adapted from ref. 2).

to each, in their distribution in different body tissues, and in their relative preponderance in normal conditions (constitutive) and in response to inflammation (induced). The broad distinction between the two systemic isoforms, COX-1 and COX-2, is that COX-1 is mainly expressed constitutively and gives rise to prostaglandins that mediate normal cellular processes, whereas COX-2 is generally considered to be an inducible enzyme, induced by inflammation and 'called up' to synthesize more prostanoids. COX-1, as the 'constitutive' isoform, is necessary for normal functions and is found in most cell types. COX-2, despite being the inducible isoform, is expressed constitutively (i.e. under normal conditions) in a number of tissues, which may include brain, testis, kidney, and lung.

It is because these prostanoids play a variety of important roles in the normal physiology and functioning of the gastrointestinal tract, the renal system, and the cardiovascular system that NSAID therapy, by inhibiting prostaglandin and thromboxane production, can interfere with prostaglandin-mediated maintenance of these systems, resulting in a range of potential adverse effects.

Enantiomeric *R* and *S* forms—potentially separating analgesia and anti-inflammatory actions

One of the clinical enigmas surrounding NSAIDs is the extent to which the analgesic and anti-inflammatory actions are separate. A further stage to this question is that if these two actions can be separated are they generated at the same sites or at different sites? The proprionic acid NSAIDs (-bufen, -profen, naproxen) are isomers, with the *S* enantiomer active and the *R* inactive. Naproxen is marketed in the *S* enantiomeric form, the others as racemates. Separation of the analgesic and anti-inflammatory actions has been shown with the *R* and *S* enantiomers of flurbiprofen. The *S* form has both anti-inflammatory and analgesic action. The *R* form blocks nociception but has little effect on PG formation and inflammation. In addition, while the *S* form is ulcerogenic the *R* form is said to have negligible effect. These findings do not seem to have had much clinical impact.

Paracetamol, dipyrone, and nefopam

Nobody knows precisely where paracetamol or dipyrone works. The standard explanation for paracetamol is that it acts as a cyclo-oxygenase inhibitor in the brain, explaining both its analgesic and its antipyretic actions. The lack of clinical anti-inflammatory activity may be because paracetamol is not active on peripheral cyclo-oxygenase. Similar comments are made for dipyrone. Nefopam, while undoubtedly an analgesic, is not an opioid and does not have NSAID-like activity. It is neither anti-inflammatory nor antipyretic, and, like paracetamol and dipyrone, its site of action is presumed to be in the central nervous system.

Clinical efficacy

How well does the intervention work?

Clinicians need to know how *well* the intervention works—the size of the effect or its clinical significance. Knowing only that an intervention works is much, much less helpful, especially when a range of similar interventions is available. The information on relative efficacy given here uses the number-needed-to-treat (NNT) as the measure of clinical significance, with data derived from quantitative systematic reviews. The NNT describes the *difference* between active treatment and control, and in the case of Figs 2 and 3 this is the difference between active drug and placebo in the proportion of patients who achieve at least 50 per cent pain relief over 6 h following a single postoperative dose of the drug. By deriving the NNT for different analgesics from comparisons with placebo the relative efficacy can be compared, and such 'league tables' (Fig. 2) are easy to understand. As more systematic reviews compile similar data on other analgesics, the league table can be extended, allowing drug comparison on a credible evidence-base. The league table is legitimate only because it uses information on similar patients with valid inclusion criteria (pain of moderate or severe intensity), similar measurement methods, similar outcomes, and a common comparator, placebo. While it can be argued that head-to-head comparison between analgesics would be better, the problem is that few such head-to-head comparisons exist, and randomized trials to detect small differences in efficacy between two analgesics would need to be massive to be able to detect differences in direction, let alone in the magnitude of the difference.

Oral non-opioids

Figure 2 shows the information (at least 400 patients at each dose) for oral single doses of the NSAIDs, diclofenac, ibuprofen, and aspirin, and for paracetamol, at the doses specified on the axis label. The data came from systematic reviews of randomized controlled trials of single doses in

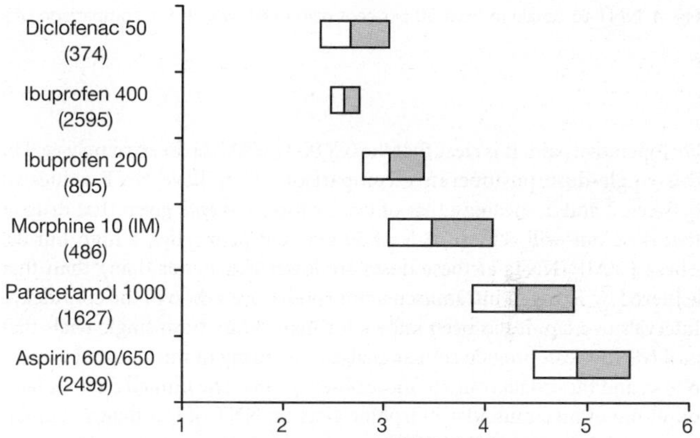

Fig. 2 Numbers-needed-to-treat (NNT) for 50% pain relief in postoperative pain (single dose). (NNT point estimate is at the junction of the grey and white bar segments. Grey bar segment is the lower 95% confidence interval, white is the upper. Number of patients given active drug shown in brackets on *y*-axis label.)

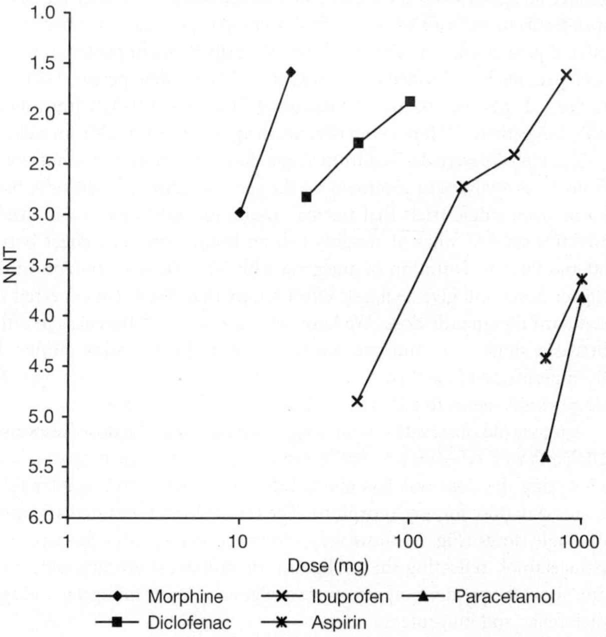

Fig. 3 Dose–response relationships for numbers-needed-to-treat (NNT) for 50% pain relief in postoperative pain (single dose).

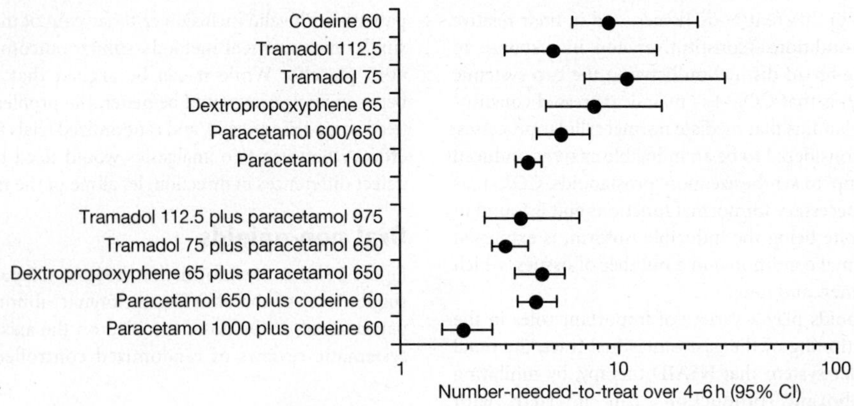

Fig. 4 NNT to obtain at least 50 per cent pain relief over 4–6 h: comparison of single-dose combination drugs and their components.

postoperative pain. It is clear that the (COX-1) NSAIDs do extremely well in this single-dose postoperative comparison. They have NNT values of between 2 and 3, meaning that of two or three patients given that drug at that dose one will achieve at least 50 per cent pain relief, a high hurdle. These NSAID NNTs at these doses are lower (i.e. better than) than that achieved by 10 mg of intramuscular morphine, even though the confidence intervals overlap. It has been known for many years from single trials that oral NSAIDs can provide similar analgesia to 10 mg of intramuscular morphine, and these data confirm those observations. The limited data we have on 20 mg of intramuscular morphine gives an NNT of less than 2. Similar conclusions about the relative efficacy of oral NSAIDs and 10 mg intramuscular morphine were reached in an earlier review.(3)

Aspirin 600/650 mg and paracetamol 1000 mg are significantly less effective than 10 mg intramuscular morphine. The point estimates of the NNT are higher, and there is no overlap of the confidence intervals. The original trial results of Houde and Wallenstein suggested milligram for milligram equianalgesic equivalence between aspirin and paracetamol in postoperative pain, and this is borne out by our results. There is no reason to expect any greater analgesia from the COX-2 inhibitors, which were after all designed specifically to reduce gastro-intestinal haemorrhage rather than because they offered greater efficacy. The NNT for rofecoxib 50 mg in postoperative pain (600 patients in published trials) is about 2.3 (J. Barden, personal communication). Dipyrone 500 mg oral has an NNT of 2.4 (1.9–3.2) from data on only 143 patients.(4) It too is an effective drug. We have no NNT for nefopam.

These NNTs were derived from single-dose pain studies. It is not possible from these analyses to comment on the speed of onset of analgesia, but we know from single trials that normal release formulations of the 'original' NSAIDs start to work at roughly half an hour, with peak effect between 60 and 90 min. Duration of analgesia with NSAIDs is a function of dose. Bigger doses will give analgesic effect longer than the 4–6 h expected from standard therapeutic dose. We know little about any differences in efficacy between single and multiple dosing. Most multiple dosing studies have been performed in arthritis, and the relative efficacy data shown here from single doses seems to tally well with the multiple dosing studies.

Another old observation from single trials was that the dose–response for analgesia with NSAIDs was 'flat', meaning that the increase in analgesia from increasing the dose was less marked than was seen with a similar relative increase in dose for, say, morphine. The results from the systematic reviews of single doses (Fig. 3) show very similar dose–responses for aspirin and paracetamol, reflecting the milligram for milligram efficacy equivalence, and show the greater potency, more analgesia at lower milligram dosage, of diclofenac and ibuprofen.

The largest doses of diclofenac and ibuprofen produce NNTs approaching 1, which is the theoretically perfect NNT. Dose is plotted in Fig. 3 as the logarithm, and this (visually) tends to minimize the difference in the slope of the dose–response curve between morphine and the non-opioid analgesics. This perhaps emphasizes the clinical perception of the ceiling to non-opioid analgesia. Rapid and effective control of an acute severe (nociceptive) pain is better achieved with opioid titration.

Analgesic efficacy of the non-opioid analgesics is improved by combination with weak opioids (Fig. 4).(5)

Combination of paracetamol 600/650 mg with codeine or dextropropoxyphene lowers (improves) the NNT of the combination to levels similar to that of 10 mg intramuscular morphine. At a practical clinical level, combinations of simple analgesics with opioids are considered effective, and are often used as one rung in the ladder of analgesic treatments for cancer. The central argument used against them is that a combination of A plus B is no better than A alone. Figure 4 illustrates that pooling information from individual trials can provide evidence to deal with this argument in a way that individual trials of conventional size cannot. Clearly, the combinations were better than the individual components alone, and the argument that a combination of A plus B is no better than A alone can be rebutted.

Other routes of administration

Topical

Surprising evidence that topical NSAIDs are effective in strains and sprains and in arthritic conditions came from a systematic review of 86 randomized controlled trials involving 10 160 patients.(6) Measures approximating at least half pain relief were used with analysis at 1 week for acute and 2 weeks for chronic conditions. In acute pain conditions placebo controlled trials had an NNT of 3.9 (3.4–4.4). Analysing by drugs (at least three trials) ketoprofen (NNT 2.6), felbinac (3.0), ibuprofen (3.5), and piroxicam (4.2) had significant efficacy. Benzydamine and indomethacin were not distinguished from placebo. In placebo controlled trials of chronic pain conditions, the NNT for topical NSAIDs was 3.1 (2.7–3.8). This analgesia was not due to rubbing a cream onto the painful area, because both placebo and the topical NSAID were applied in the same way. We do not understand the biology of the topical NSAIDs, but the limited comparisons of topical and oral formulations show that both work. Topical NSAIDs thus have a place in the armamentarium.

Injected and rectal

We do not have the same league table of relative analgesic efficacy for injected or rectal NSAIDs in postoperative or other acute pain states. The reason for this is that almost all trials of injected or rectal NSAIDs were conducted with the analgesic given where there was no pain—before the operation began, for instance. This was fashionable because of the (unsubstantiated) belief that if pain can be pre-empted then the need for analgesics postoperatively is reduced.

Injected NSAIDs, paracetamol (propacetamol), dipyrone, and nefopam are all effective analgesics, but it is difficult to establish if they are any more effective than their oral equivalents. Indeed, oral ketorolac 10 mg was equivalent to intramuscular ketorolac 30 mg in one review.[7] If oral and injected formulations are equally effective then the advantage of the injected formulations would be restricted to contexts where the patients cannot swallow, or, if injected formulation was faster in onset of action, to contexts where rapid analgesia was required. To prove that injected formulations are better than oral formulations requires that the same drug be compared at the same dose across the two routes. A systematic review[8] of 26 randomized controlled trials (2225 analysed patients), published between 1970 and 1996, which examined the difference in analgesic efficacy and adverse effects of NSAIDs given by different routes of administration, found few trials which included this necessary comparison.

Different doses of eight different NSAIDs (diclofenac, ibuprofen, indomethacin, ketoprofen, ketorolac, naproxen, piroxicam, tenoxicam), given by intravenous, intramuscular, intrawound, rectal, and oral route, were tested in 58 single-dose or multiple-dose comparisons. Fifteen trials compared the same drug by different routes. In nine of them (35 per cent of all trials) the same drug was compared at the same dose.

Five postoperative pain trials were valid direct comparisons comparing diclofenac or ketorolac across routes. In one trial, diclofenac 1 mg/kg injected intravenously at induction of anaesthesia led to significantly lower pain intensity scores 30 min after surgery than the same dose given intramuscularly at induction. In two other trials no difference was found between ketorolac 30 mg given either intravenously or intramuscularly at induction; both intramuscular and intravenous ketorolac 30 mg at induction led to significantly lower pain scores and less rescue analgesics at 90 min after surgery than the same dose taken orally, but 1 h before surgery. Group sizes in this trial were small (i.e. 14 patients per group) and no double-dummy design was used. Another trial with larger groups (50 patients per group), but again without a double-dummy design, reported less pain and rescue analgesics at discharge with diclofenac 75 mg intramuscularly compared with the same drug given orally but at a lower dose (50 mg). Yet another trial compared diclofenac 150 mg taken orally with 50 mg intramuscularly plus 100 mg orally. The drugs were given as a premedication using a double-dummy design, and group sizes were large (50 patients per group). No difference was found between the two forms of administration.

There were three valid direct comparisons in renal colic comparing dipyrone, diclofenac, and indomethacin given by different routes. In one trial pain relief was tested with dipyrone 1 or 2 g, and diclofenac 75 mg, given intramuscularly compared with intravenously. At 10 and 20 min after administration of the drugs the proportion of patients with at least 50 per cent improvement was significantly in favour of the intravenous route with each drug and dose. In the two other trials intravenous indomethacin 50 mg was compared with the same drug given rectally but double the dose. Despite there being only half the intravenous dose both trials reported significant improvement (less pain intensity, less rescue analgesics) with the intravenous route compared with the rectal. Again these differences were apparent only at 10 or 20 min.

A simple clinical conclusion is that we lack convincing evidence that the same dose of NSAID is any more effective when given by injection than when given at the same dose by mouth. One might then argue that it makes little sense to give that dose by injection instead of by mouth to a patient who can swallow.

Safety

NSAIDs can cause a number of minor adverse effects at recommended doses, but can also cause major adverse effects at recommended doses. At recommended doses paracetamol can also cause minor adverse effects, but no major adverse effects. It is only in overdose that paracetamol is dangerous, with the potential to cause hepatic failure. Dipyrone is not available in many countries because of concerns about agranulocytosis; controversy continues about the incidence of this problem. Dipyrone was (re)withdrawn from the market in Sweden recently after six cases in 10 000 patients were exposed. This is a much higher incidence than that encountered in other countries where the drug is used widely.

With the NSAIDs it is worth recalling the concept that the slope of the dose–response curve for analgesia may not be as steep as that for morphine (Fig. 3). The slope of the dose–response curves for adverse effects need not be the same as that for analgesia. If the slope for adverse effects is steeper than that for analgesia then dose increase to produce greater analgesia may produce proportionately greater increase in adverse effects.

NSAID safety in acute use

Major problems

In acute pain, the main concerns with NSAIDs are renal and coagulation problems. Acute renal failure can be precipitated in pre-existing heart or kidney disease, those on loop diuretics, or those who have lost more than 10 per cent of blood volume. NSAIDs cause significant lengthening (by about 30 per cent) of the bleeding time, usually still within the normal range. This can last for days with aspirin, but hours with non-aspirin NSAIDs. This raises the possibility that NSAIDs can cause significant increase in blood loss. A comparison of ketorolac, diclofenac, and ketoprofen in over 11 000 patients having major surgery, and given injected then oral doses of one of the three NSAIDs, gave a 1 per cent incidence of increased surgical site bleeding, a 0.1 per cent incidence of allergy, 0.1 per cent incidence of acute renal failure, and 0.04 per cent incidence of gastrointestinal bleeding.[9] There was no difference among the three NSAIDs. The problem with the paper is that we do not know what would happen in the absence of NSAIDs. These estimates are in a sense the worst case, and tell us what happens in the presence of NSAIDs, and confirm that the postoperative risk of acute renal failure with NSAIDs is greater than the risk of gastrointestinal bleeding.

Minor problems

Adverse effects from single-dose oral acute pain studies have been examined systematically for paracetamol, ibuprofen, and aspirin.[10] The common adverse effects like nausea, dizziness, or drowsiness were reported more often when diaries were used, and drowsiness was reported more often in dental rather than other pain models. The incidence of any adverse effect with any single dose of analgesic was low, but for paracetamol and ibuprofen, but not aspirin, was statistically greater than placebo. Gastric irritation was two to three times more common with aspirin rather than placebo, with a number needed to harm of 22 (95 per cent confidence interval 22–174).[11]

Other routes

For injected and rectal administration, commonly reported adverse effects independent of the route of administration were nausea, vomiting, dizziness, drowsiness, sedation, anxiety, dyspepsia, indigestion, and dry mouth.[8] Two studies reported bleeding time changes. In 12 patients with rheumatoid arthritis treated with indomethacin 100–150 mg orally and rectally, respectively, in a cross-over design for 2 weeks, endoscopically diagnosed gastric mucosal damage was independent of the route of administration.

Adverse effects related to the route of administration were most often reported for intramuscular and rectal regimens. Discomfort at the site of injection was the most frequent complaint in relation to intramuscular injections. After rectal administration, diarrhoea, rectal irritation, and non-retention of suppositories were reported.

For topical NSAIDs in both acute and chronic pain, local and systemic adverse events, and drug-related study withdrawal, had a low incidence and were no different from placebo.

NSAID safety in chronic use

Oral NSAIDs cause ulcers in some people. In some of those who have ulcers, some also have symptoms, which include bleeding ulcers. In some of those who have bleeding ulcers, the bleeding is sufficiently severe to result in hospital admission, and may cause death. The variables are drug and dose, duration of exposure, and patient characteristics. The total burden is large, with some 106 000 NSAID-related hospital admissions and 16 500 deaths in the United States every year.[12] Age and sex are the major risk factors for serious gastrointestinal complications with NSAIDs, though a history of previous ulcers and heart disease are also important. Of the different NSAIDs, some are implicated more than others, though case–control and cohort studies give somewhat different estimates. Both types of study indicate that ibuprofen is among the safest of the NSAIDs.

The size of the problem of gastrointestinal emergencies associated with oral NSAID use is large. Two recent UK studies, each on about 1 per cent of the UK population, indicate, first, that 1.9 per cent of NSAID users might be admitted to hospital each year with upper gastrointestinal emergencies,[13] and, second, that one episode of ulcer bleeding in the elderly will be expected for each 2823 prescriptions.[14] Another way of putting this is that if oral NSAIDs are taken for at least 2 months, the risk of an endoscopic ulcer is 1 in 5, of a symptomatic ulcer is about 1 in 70, of a bleeding ulcer is about 1 in 150, and of a death from a bleeding ulcer about 1 in 1300.[15] None of these risks is associated with topical NSAIDs, which have much lower plasma concentrations.

Gastrointestinal adverse effects

Epidemiological studies associating NSAID use and upper GI problems and published in the 1990s have been reviewed and the data pooled to give a much clearer picture of risks.[16] To be included studies had to be case–control or cohort studies on non-aspirin NSAIDs, with data on bleeding, perforation, or other serious upper gastrointestinal tract event resulting in hospital admission or referral to a specialist, and have data to calculate relative risk. Eighteen studies were found, all of which had specific definitions of exposure and outcome and similar ascertainment for comparison groups. All but two attempted to control for potential confounding factors, like age, sex, history of ulcer, or concomitant medicines.

The main results are summarized in Figs 5 and 6. Compared with non-users, NSAID users had a higher risk of upper GI bleed (UGIB) when they were current NSAID users and used a higher dose. The duration of use was unimportant, but different NSAIDs had different risks, with ibuprofen (especially doses below 2400 mg a day) being least harmful.

The effect of ulcer history and age is shown in Figs 7 and 8. People with a history of ulcer or with a previous bleed who took NSAIDs were at much greater risk than those with no history of ulcer who took NSAIDs. Older patients who took NSAIDs were at greater risk than those under 50 years of age who took NSAIDs. This is obviously highly relevant in palliative care.

The limited evidence available suggests that there are fewer dyspeptic symptoms with COX-2 inhibitors than with COX-1.[17]

Renal failure

NSAIDs can cause acute renal failure with chronic use, as they can with acute use. If renal function depends on prostaglandin 'overdrive', then taking NSAIDs which reduce the prostaglandin overdrive will impair function. The risk factors, as with acute NSAID use, include pre-existing heart or kidney disease, those on loop diuretics, or those who have lost more than 10 per cent of blood volume; palliative care patients are therefore often at risk. A recent estimate of the risk came from a study conducted among all members of the Tennessee Medicaid programme aged 65 years or more in 1987–1991 and enrolled for at least 1 year.[18] Those with first admission to hospital for acute renal failure (admission creatinine level of 180 μmol/L or more at admission) were the cases of community acquired acute renal failure. Controls were randomly selected for all persons in the study population. Exclusions were people with end-stage renal disease and those with hospital acquired acute renal failure. NSAID exposure was ascertained from prescriptions filled in the year before the index date.

There were 1799 cases with an annual incidence of community acquired acute renal failure of 4.5 admissions per 1000. The median hospital stay was 8 days. Thirty-six per cent died within 30 days. Forty-two per cent were classified as having new renal disease. The remainder were classified as having chronic renal failure with acute exacerbation based on a prior creatinine

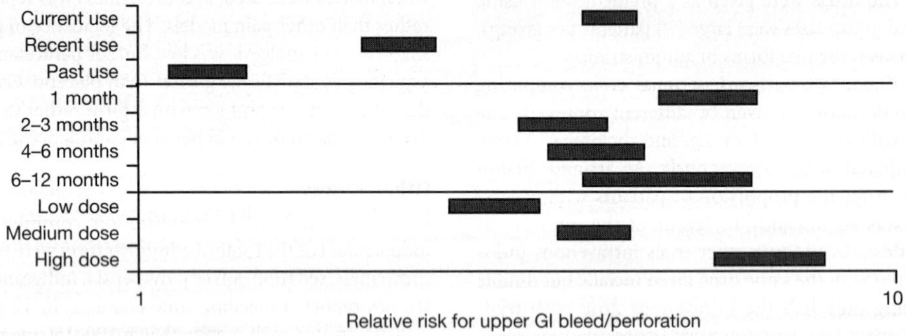

Fig. 5 Risk of upper GI bleed for NSAIDs users, compared with non-users. (Bars represent 95% CI of relative risk.)

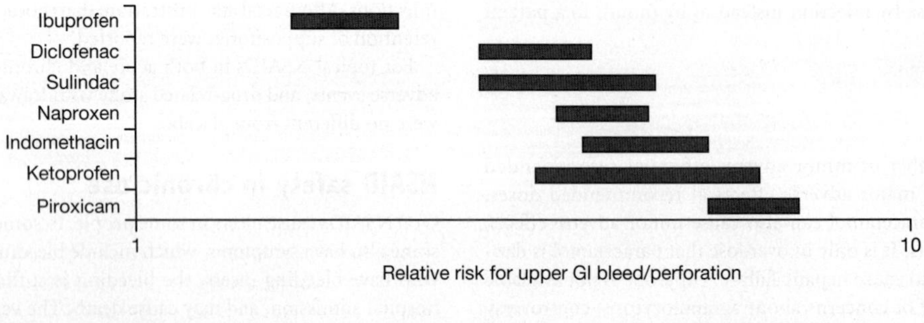

Fig. 6 Risk of upper GI bleed for particular NSAIDs, users compared with non-users. (Bars represent 95% CI of relative risk.)

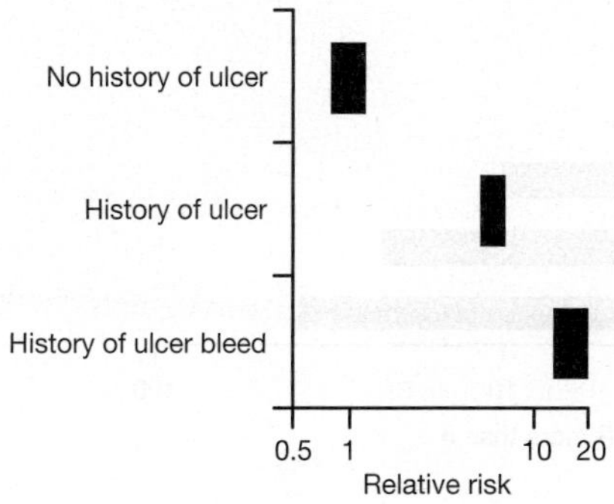

Fig. 7 Effect of history of ulcer in users of NSAIDs. (Bars represent 95% CI of relative risk.)

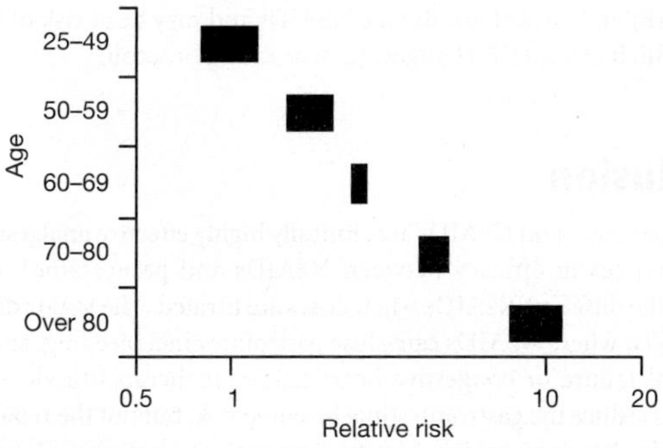

Fig. 8 Effect of age in users of NSAIDs. (Bars represent 95% CI of relative risk.)

level above 122 μmol/L, a documented history of chronic renal failure, or imaging studies compatible with chronic renal disease. There were 9899 controls. Controls were less likely to be nursing home residents or to be 85 years or older.

NSAID use was higher (18 per cent) in cases than in controls (11 per cent). For current NSAID use the odds ratio was 1.6 (95 per cent confidence interval 1.3–1.9). Those who had stopped using NSAIDs within the past 30 days had no increased risk of renal failure. For certain NSAIDs where there was sufficient information, ibuprofen and indomethacin, there was a dose response for risk. For individual NSAIDs, ibuprofen, piroxicam, fenoprofen, and indomethacin had the greatest increased risk, with odds ratios of about 2.

A previous detailed study, though on smaller numbers, indicated that previous renal disease, or gout, but particularly a combined history of gout plus previous renal disease were major risks for renal failure with NSAIDs.[19] Patients using NSAIDs with half-lives of 12 h or more in the previous week had particularly increased risk of renal failure.

There seems no biological reason why the risk of renal problems should be lower with COX-2 inhibitors than with the COX-1 NSAIDs.

Congestive heart failure

The third in the triad of major problems is congestive heart failure (CHF) in older people,[20] and this problem has had a much lower profile than gastrointestinal bleeding and renal failure. This low profile may have been inappropriate, because as many hospital admissions may result from NSAID induced congestive heart failure as for gastrointestinal bleeding.

A study at two hospitals in New South Wales (population about 450 000) enrolled as cases consecutive patients between 1993 and 1995 where the medical officer admitting the case and the attending physician agreed that the primary reason for admission was CHF.[20] Patients admitted for other reasons with incidental CHF were not included. Study nurses ensured that all included cases met Framingham criteria for CHF. Controls (target two per case) were patients of the same sex and within 5 years of age admitted to the same hospital, but with no clinical or radiological signs of CHF.

Table 1 NSAID use and history of heart disease: effect on risk of developing congestive heart failure

Heart disease	NSAID use	Odds ratio (95% CI)
No history	Non-user	1
No history	User	1.6 (0.7–3.7)
History	Non-user	2.5 (1.4–4.3)
History	User	26 (6–119)

There were 365 cases and 658 controls, with a mean age of 76 years. Most cases had moderate or severe CHF. Use of non-aspirin NSAIDs was 17 per cent in the cases in the week before admission, compared with 12 per cent in controls. The adjusted odds ratio was 2.1 (5 per cent confidence interval 1.2–3.3) for all cases, and 2.8 (1.5–5.1) for the 272 cases with first admission for CHF (Table 1).

CHF was far more likely in those patients with a prior history of heart disease, in which the odds ratio was 26 (5.8–119). Complicated statistical analysis confirmed the effect of pre-existing heart disease, and suggested that NSAIDs with longer half-lives (naproxen, piroxicam, and tenoxicam) had much higher risk than those with short half-lives (ibuprofen, diclofenac, for instance), though on small numbers in a subgroup analysis.

The importance of the NSAID precipitation of CHF was substantiated by a large study from Sweden.[21] Ecological line regression established an increased relative risk of 1.26 (1.23–1.28) between outpatient NSAID use and hospitalized heart failure.

Hypertensive effects of analgesics

NSAIDs raise blood pressure in some individuals, but with variable extent.[22] Hypertensive patients on NSAIDs are more susceptible to blood pressure increases than normotensives, and the mean increase in blood pressure was slightly higher in untreated hypertensive patients than in normotensive patients.[23] Hypertensive patients receiving antihypertensive therapy experienced a greater mean increase in supine blood pressure as a result of NSAID therapy than uncontrolled hypertensive patients (4.7 versus 1.8 mmHg), and blood pressure increases were greater in patients receiving β-blockers, than in those receiving vasodilators and diuretics.[23] In normotensive patients, hypertensive effects of conventional NSAIDs appear to be minimal.[23,24] COX-2 drugs probably have similar effects, but the information is still limited.[22]

Comment

These three major NSAID risks, gastrointestinal bleeding, renal failure, and congestive heart failure, are important in palliative care, particularly because increased age is such an important factor. Putting all this into the perspective of an average primary care grouping of 100 000,[25] then in this population (3500 over 65 taking NSAIDs) there would be 18 hospital admissions every year for upper gastrointestinal bleeding, 10 for acute renal failure, and 22 for congestive heart failure. The majority of the renal and heart failure cases would be in those aged 75 and over. For both renal failure and CHF, NSAIDs 'uncover' existing disease problems, and for both there are plausible mechanisms, dose–response relationships, and particular association with NSAIDs with longer half-lives.

What can be done to minimize these risks? The risk of gastrointestinal bleeding with COX-1 inhibitors may be reduced by co-administration of proton pump inhibitors or misoprostol. Gastrointestinal adverse effects limit the tolerability of misoprostol. For gastrointestinal bleeding the COX-2 inhibitors reduce but do not eliminate the risk. With rofecoxib, for instance, 50 mg daily resulted in 2.1 confirmed gastrointestinal events per

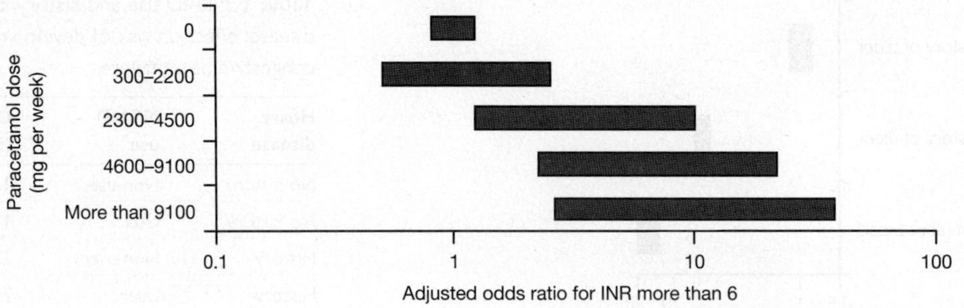

Fig. 9 Effect of paracetamol dose on risk of INR above 6.0.

100 patient-years compared with 4.5 per 100 patient-years on naproxen 500 mg twice daily (relative risk, 0.5; 95 per cent CI 0.3–0.6), with a median follow-up of 9 months.[26] The respective rates of complicated confirmed events (perforation, obstruction, and severe upper gastrointestinal bleeding) were 0.6 per 100 patient-years and 1.4 per 100 patient-years (relative risk, 0.4; 95 per cent CI 0.2–0.8). COX-2 inhibitors, however, do not reduce the risk of renal failure or of congestive heart failure, and for these risks there has to be a clinical balance between the analgesia provided by an NSAID, COX-1 or COX-2, and the risk of complication. Over half the patients in the CLASS study[27] of celecoxib versus COX-1 drugs in arthritis were on hypertensive treatment, a reminder of the awkward fact that the patients with pain will often be hypertensive and hence at risk. There is no evidence that the risk of congestive heart failure is higher with COX-2 than with COX-1, but for rofecoxib there is debate about thrombotic safety.[28] Equally there is no evidence that the risk of renal failure is higher with COX-2 than with COX-1. The three risks can only be minimized by sensible assessment and selection.

Contra-indications

A history of gastrointestinal bleeding, particularly in the past year, and co-administration of steroids which also increase the risk of gastrointestinal bleeding, are potential contra-indications to NSAID use, as would be the presence of moderate or severe renal problems. In mild renal dysfunction dose reduction and use of shorter half-life drugs may reduce risk.

Asthma and allergy

NSAIDs may make asthma worse, and NSAIDs should be avoided in any patient who has had exacerbation of asthma, or angioedema or urticaria or rhinitis while taking aspirin or any other NSAID. The advice to use paracetamol as the alternative in this circumstance seems sound. Recent publications claiming that paracetamol causes asthma appear to suffer from confounding by indication.[29] Asthmatics are told not to take NSAIDs but to take paracetamol. Therefore, many people taking paracetamol have asthma, but the paracetamol is not causal.

Drug interactions

Warfarin

In a case–control study of patients attending the anticoagulant therapy unit (2000 patients) over a single year, who had been on warfarin for at least 1 month, had a target INR of 2.0–3.0, but who had an INR greater than 6.0, paracetamol was a risk factor.[30] Taken mainly for acute pains, the more of it used in the week before the test, the greater the chance of a raised INR (Fig. 9). More than nine 500 mg tablets a week gave an odds ratio of 7, and more than 18 tablets a week an odds ratio of 10.

Clearly again there is a risk of confounding by indication, in that patients on warfarin are advised not to take NSAIDs and may be at risk of the other factors which cause INR changes, such as eating broccoli.

Conclusion

Simple analgesics and NSAIDs are clinically highly effective analgesics. There are differences in efficacy between NSAIDs and paracetamol, but little between the different NSAIDs when doses are titrated. The major differences are in safety, where NSAIDs can cause gastrointestinal bleeding, and precipitate renal failure or congestive heart failure at therapeutic dose. COX-2 inhibitors reduce the gastrointestinal bleeding risk, but not the renal or heart failure risks. Paracetamol is safe at therapeutic dose, but a little less effective. This balance between efficacy and safety is critical to optimal use of the drugs in all therapeutic areas; palliative care presents a particular challenge.

References

1. **Hawkey, C.J.** (1999). COX-2 inhibitors. *Lancet* **353**, 307–14.
2. **Whelton, A.** (2000). Renal and related cardiovascular effects of conventional and COX-2-specific NSAIDs and non-NSAID analgesics. *American Journal of Therapeutics* **7**, 63–74.
3. **Eisenberg, E., Berkey, C.S., Carr, D.B., Mosteller, F., and Chalmers, T.C.** (1994). Efficacy and safety of nonsteroidal antiinflammatory drugs for cancer pain: a meta-analysis. *Journal of Clinical Oncology* **12** (12), 2756–65.
4. **Edwards, J.E., Meseguer, F., Faura, C.C., Moore, R.A., and McQuay, H.J.** (2001). Single-dose dipyrone for acute postoperative pain (Cochrane Review). *Cochrane Database Systems Review* **3**, CD003227.
5. **Edwards, J., McQuay, H., and Moore, R.A.** (2002). Combination analgesic efficacy. Individual patient data meta-analysis of single-dose oral tramadol plus acetaminophen in acute postoperative pain. *Journal of Pain and Symptom Management* **23**, 121–30.
6. **Moore, R.A., Tramèr, M.R., Carroll, D., Wiffen, P.J., and McQuay, H.J.** (1998). Quantitive systematic review of topically-applied non-steroidal anti-inflammatory drugs. *British Medical Journal* **316**, 333–8.
7. **Smith, L.A., Carroll, D., Edwards, J.E., Moore, R.A., and McQuay, H.J.** (2000). Single dose ketorolac and pethidine in acute postoperative pain: a systematic review with meta-analysis. *British Journal of Anaesthesia* **84**, 48–58.
8. **Tramèr, M.R., Williams, J.E., Carroll, D., Wiffen, P.J., Moore, R.A, and McQuay, H.J.** (1998). Comparing analgesic efficacy of non-steroidal anti-inflammatory drugs given by different routes in acute and chronic pain: a qualitative systematic review. *Acta Anaesthesiologica Scandanavica* **42**, 71–9.
9. **Forrest, J.B.** et al. (2002). Ketorolac, diclofenac, and ketoprofen are equally safe for pain relief after major surgery. *British Journal of Anaesthesia* **88** (2), 227–33.
10. **Edwards, J.E., McQuay, H.J., Moore, R.A., and Collins, S.L.** (1999). Reporting of adverse effects in clinical trials should be improved. Lessons from acute postoperative pain. *Journal of Pain and Symptom Management* **81**, 289–97.

11. **Edwards, J.E.** et al. (2000). Single dose oral aspirin for acute pain. *Cochrane Database Systems Review* 2, CD002067.
12. **Singh, G.** (1998). Recent considerations in nonsteroidal anti-inflammatory drug gastropathy. *American Journal of Medicine* **105** (1B), 31S–8S.
13. **Moore, R.A. and Phillips, C.J.** (1999). Cost of NSAID adverse effects to the UK National Health Service. *Journal of Medical Economics* **2**, 45–55.
14. **Hawkey, C.J., Cullen, D.J., Greenwood, D.C., Wilson, J.V., and Logan, R.F.** (1997). Prescribing of nonsteroidal anti-inflammatory drugs in general practice: determinants and consequences. *Aliment Pharmacology and Therapeutics* **11**, 293–8.
15. **Tramer, M.R., Moore, R.A., Reynolds, D.J., and McQuay, H.J.** (2000). Quantitative estimation of rare adverse events which follow a biological progression: a new model applied to chronic NSAID use. *Pain* **85** (1–2), 169–82.
16. **Hernandez-Diaz, S. and Rodridguez, L.A.G.** (2000). Association between nonsteroidal anti-inflammatory drugs and upper gastrointestinal tract bleeding/perforation. *Archives of Internal Medicine* **160**, 2093–9.
17. **Watson, D.J.** et al. (2000). Gastrointestinal tolerability of the selective cyclooxygenase-2 (COX-2) inhibitor rofecoxib compared with nonselective COX-1 and COX-2 inhibitors in osteoarthritis. *Archives Internal Medicine* **160**, 2998–3003.
18. **Griffin, M.R., Yared, A., and Ray, W.A.** (2000). Nonsteroidal antiinflammatory drugs and acute renal failure in elderly persons. *American Journal of Epidemiology* **151** (5), 488–96.
19. **Henry, D.** et al. (1997). Consumption of non-steroidal anti-inflammatory drugs and the development of functional renal impairment in elderly subjects. Results of a case–control study. *British Journal of Clinical Pharmacology* **44**, 85–90.
20. **Page, J. and Henry, D.** (2000). Consumption of NSAIDs and the development of congestive heart failure in elderly patients. *Archives of Internal Medicine* **160**, 777–84.
21. **Merlo, J.** et al. (2001). Association of outpatient utilisation of non-steroidal anti-inflammatory drugs and hospitalised heart failure in the entire Swedish population. *European Journal of Clinical Pharmacology* **57**, 71–5
22. **Hillis, W.S.** (2002). Areas of emerging interest in analgesia: cardiovascular complications. *American Journal of Therapeutics.* **9** (3), 259–69.
23. **Johnson, A.G., Nguyen, T.V., and Day, R.O.** (1994). Do nonsteroidal anti-inflammatory drugs affect blood pressure? *Annals of Internal Medicine* **121**, 289–300.
24. **Pope, J.E., Anderson, J.J., and Felson, D.T.** (1993). A meta-analysis of the effects of nonsteroidal anti-inflammatory drugs on blood pressure. *Archives of Internal Medicine* **153**, 477–84.
25. **Blower, A.L.** et al. (1997). Emergency admissions for upper gastrointestinal disease and their relation to NSAID use. *Ailment Pharmacology and Therapeutics* **11**, 283–91.
26. **Bombardier, C.** et al. (2000). Comparison of upper gastrointestinal toxicity of rofecoxib and naproxen in patients with rheumatoid arthritis. *New England Journal of Medicine* **343** (21), 1520–8.
27. **Silverstein, F.E.** et al. (2000). Gastrointestinal toxicity with celecoxib versus nonsteroidal anti-inflammatory drugs for osteoarthritis and rheumatoid arthritis. The CLASS study: a randomised controlled trial. *Journal of the American Medical Association* **284** (10), 1247–55.
28. Food and Drug Administration. Cardiovascular safety of rofecoxib (Web Page). 2001; Available at http://www.fda.gov/ohrms/dockets/ac/01/briefing/3677b2_06_cardio.pdf. (Accessed 11 March 2002.)
29. **Signorello, L.B., McLaughlin, J.K., Lipworth, L., Friis, S., Sørensen, H.T., and Blot, W.J.** (2002). Confounding by indication in epidemiologic studies of commonly used analgesics. *American Journal of Therapeutics* **9** (3), 199–205.
30. **Hylek, E.M.** et al. (1998). Acetaminophen and other risk factors for excessive warfarin anticoagulation. *Journal of the American Medical Association* **279** (9), 657–62.

8.2.5 Adjuvant analgesics in pain management

David Lussier and Russell K. Portenoy

The term 'adjuvant analgesic' describes any drug that has a primary indication other than pain, but is analgesic in some painful conditions. In the palliative care literature, this term is often used synonymously with 'coanalgesic' to refer to a drug that is administered with a primary analgesic, usually an opioid, to enhance pain relief, treat pain that is refractory to the analgesic, or allow reduction of the analgesic dose for the purpose of limiting side-effects.

This terminology is widely accepted, but can be problematic. In the palliative care setting, adjuvant analgesics are a subset of a much larger group of 'adjuvant drugs', which are coadministered with analgesics for a variety of reasons. Adjuvant drugs may be administered to treat the side-effects produced by the analgesic or manage other symptoms associated with the pain. In this sense, laxatives and antiemetics are adjuvant drugs.

It may also be confusing to note that the term 'adjuvant' itself can be a misnomer. The adjuvant analgesics are often used alone—not as adjuvant to any other therapy. Indeed, this group includes some drugs that are non-specific, multipurpose analgesics and others that are commonly used in selected disorders as primary analgesics. This is particularly true in populations with chronic pain unrelated to cancer or other progressive medical diseases.

Given this imprecise terminology and the expanding use of adjuvant analgesics as non-traditional primary analgesics, it is important to understand the pharmacology of these drugs and their therapeutic role in varied patient populations. In this way, the use of the adjuvant analgesics can be optimized, both as 'add-on' therapy to an opioid regimen and as distinct, primary therapy in those painful disorders that are likely to demonstrate a good response.

General considerations

Several principles guide the administration of all adjuvant analgesics. These emphasize the importance of a comprehensive patient assessment and a broad foundation in analgesic pharmacotherapy.

Comprehensive assessment

The selection of a drug and optimal dosing regimen depends on a systematic assessment of the patient.[1,2] This assessment requires a careful history and review of records, physical examination, and appropriate laboratory and imaging studies. The information obtained includes the following:

1. characteristics of the pain, including severity, location, temporal features, quality, and syndrome;
2. aetiology of the pain and its relationship to the underlying disease;
3. inferences about the predominating type of pain pathophysiology, for example, nociceptive or neuropathic (see Chapter 8.2.1);
4. impact of pain on function and quality of life;
5. presence of associated factors (comorbidities), including physical and psychological symptoms, functional impairments, psychiatric disorder, family or social disruption, financial problems, and spiritual or religious concerns, and their effects on quality of life.

The need for systematic assessment continues during the course of therapy with an adjuvant analgesic. Over time, changes in pain, side-effects, or any of the broader quality of life concerns may impel a shift in therapeutic strategy. The use of adjuvant analgesics in the management of pain is a 'labour-intensive' endeavour, which requires frequent contact with the patient to ensure continuous, appropriate administration of the drug.

Positioning of treatment

Extensive experience in the cancer population indicates that the adjuvant analgesics are, as a group, less reliable analgesics than opioids. This characteristic may be determined by a smaller proportion of treated patients who respond adequately, a higher likelihood of troublesome side-effects, or a slower onset of analgesic effect for most drugs (perhaps due to the need to initiate therapy at low doses to avoid side-effects). For example, in contrast to survey data that demonstrate a favourable outcome within days for 70–90 per cent of cancer patients who receive opioid therapy,[3–17] studies of the tricyclic antidepressants show that these drugs require treatment for weeks to obtain optimal results and offer 50 per cent, or greater, relief to 50–75 per cent of patients with neuropathic pain.[18,19]

This observation suggests that most patients with moderate or severe pain related to serious medical illness who have no relative contraindications to opioid therapy should not receive an adjuvant analgesic until opioid therapy has been optimized. Although some clinicians attempt to improve patient response by initiating therapy with an opioid and an adjuvant analgesic concurrently, this approach increases the risk of additive toxicity. Unless another indication for an earlier trial exists (e.g. a comorbidity that may also respond to the drug, a history of problems with opioids, or a type of pain that may be particularly responsive to a specific adjuvant), the safest and most efficient approach usually involves the addition of an adjuvant analgesic to an opioid regimen that is yielding inadequate analgesia despite dose escalation to limiting side-effects. This positioning of the adjuvant analgesics must be understood in relation to the other options that exist in this situation (Table 1). In the absence of data from comparative clinical trials, the decision to use an adjuvant analgesic drug instead of an alternative therapy, such as a trial of spinally administered opioids or a nerve block, is usually a matter of clinical judgement.

The selection of a specific adjuvant analgesic may be suggested by the characteristics of the pain (see below) or, in some instances, by the existence of another symptom concurrent with pain that may be amenable to a non-analgesic effect of the drug. In many situations, multiple options exist and priorities for therapeutic trials must also be developed on the basis of a comprehensive assessment of the patient and best clinical judgement.

Pharmacological characteristics

To select and properly administer an adjuvant analgesic, the clinician must be familiar with the drug's actions, approved indications, unapproved indications accepted in medical practice, likely side-effects and potential serious adverse effects, usual time–action relationship, pharmacokinetics, specific dosing guidelines for pain, and interactions with other drugs. Very few of the adjuvant analgesics have been studied in the palliative care setting and the information used to develop dosing guidelines is usually extrapolated from other patient populations.

Table 1 Therapeutic options when opioid therapy regimen fails due to dose-limiting toxicity

Approach	Therapeutic options
Pharmacological techniques to reduce systemic opioid requirement	Use of adjuvant analgesics Use of spinal opioids
Identifying an opioid with a more favourable balance between analgesia and side-effects	Sequential opioid trials
Improving the tolerability of the opioid regimen to allow further dose escalation	More aggressive side-effect management (e.g. psychostimulants for opioid-induced somnolence)
Non-pharmacological techniques to reduce the systemic opioid requirement	Anaesthetic approaches Surgical approaches Rehabilitative approaches Psychological approaches

Caution is usually appropriate as adjuvant analgesics are used in a medically ill population. Low initial doses and gradual dose escalation may avoid early side-effects and identify dose-dependent analgesic effects that can be explored to optimize the balance between pain relief and adverse effects. The use of low initial doses and dose titration may delay the onset of analgesia, however, and patients must be forewarned of this possibility to improve adherence with the therapy.

Interindividual and intraindividual variability

There is great variability in the response to all adjuvant analgesics. Although specific patient characteristics, such as advanced age or coexistent major organ failure, may increase the likelihood of some (usually adverse) responses, it is nonetheless true that neither favourable effects nor specific side-effects can be reliably predicted in the individual patients. Additionally, there is remarkable intraindividual variability in the response to different drugs, including those within the same class. Implicit in both these observations is the potential utility of sequential trials of adjuvant analgesics. The process of sequential drug trials, like the use of low initial doses and dose titration, should be explained to the patient at the start of therapy to enhance adherence and reduce the distress that may occur as treatments fail.

Risks and benefits of polypharmacy

Adjuvant analgesics are typically administered to patients who are receiving several other drugs. Although this is widely regarded as appropriate, the potential for additive side-effects and unpredictable adverse effects must be anticipated by the practitioner whenever an adjuvant is added to an existing drug regimen. The decision to add, or continue, a therapy must be based on a careful assessment of outcomes and a clear understanding of the goals of care. If a treatment yields demonstrable benefit without serious risk, and without cumulative side-effects that otherwise impair function or quality of life, there is ample justification for continuing. Additional pain relief at the price of somnolence or mental clouding is not acceptable for patients whose goals include restoration of function, but may be completely appropriate for those who seek comfort as the only goal.

The risks of additive toxicity from polypharmacy derive from both pharmacokinetic and pharmacodynamic changes. For example, the addition of a tricyclic antidepressant to a morphine regimen may produce somnolence due to an increase in morphine plasma concentration[20] or a pharmacodynamic interaction independent of changes in drug concentration.

Adjuvant analgesics

The adjuvant analgesics comprise an extraordinarily diverse group of drug classes (Table 2). A generally useful, broad classification distinguishes

Table 2 Adjuvant analgesics: major classes

Antidepressants
Anticonvulsants
Local anaesthetics
Neuroleptics
N-Methyl-D-aspartate (NMDA) receptor blockers
Sympatholytics
Alpha-2 adrenergic agonists
Corticosteroids
Gamma aminobutyric acid (GABA) agonists
Muscle relaxants
Benzodiazepines
Osteoclast inhibitors
Radiopharmaceuticals

those that may be considered non-specific, multipurpose analgesics from those used for more specific indications. A review of the evidence supporting the analgesic efficacy of agents in each class provides the foundation for the development of clinical guidelines.

Multipurpose analgesics

The data supporting the analgesic efficacy of some drug classes derive from numerous studies of very diverse syndromes. The range of positive outcomes for these drugs suggests that they can be considered multipurpose analgesics, fundamentally similar in this respect to the opioid and non-opioid analgesics (Table 3). This designation is appropriate even if these drugs are used only for selected indications in the palliative care setting.

Antidepressant drugs

As reviewed elsewhere,[21–28] there is compelling evidence that the tricyclic antidepressants are analgesic in a variety of chronic pain syndromes. The efficacy of the tertiary amine compounds has been demonstrated in a large number of controlled and uncontrolled trials. Amitriptyline was effective in migraine and other types of headache,[29–36] arthritis,[37] chronic low back pain,[38] post-herpetic neuralgia,[39–42] fibromyalgia,[43–45] painful diabetic polyneuropathy,[18,46–48] central pain,[49] chronic facial pain,[50] cancer pain,[51] and psychogenic pain.[52] In contrast, two studies in populations with HIV-related peripheral neuropathy failed to show any benefit of amitriptyline treatment.[53,54] Imipramine was useful for arthritis,[55] headache,[33] painful diabetic neuropathy,[56–58] low back pain,[59] and idiopathic chest pain.[60] Doxepin relieved coexistent pain and depression,[61,62] headache,[35,63] and low back pain.[64] Topical doxepin applied to skin has been shown to decrease neuropathic pain in a controlled trial,[65] and a single-dose study suggested that oral topical doxepin can be effective in pain from radiation-induced mucositis.[66] Clomipramine was analgesic in various neuropathic pains and idiopathic pain[67–70] and dothiepin was effective in fibromyalgia and psychogenic pain.[71,72]

Analgesic efficacy has also been demonstrated for the secondary amine tricyclic antidepressants. In controlled trials, desipramine was analgesic in postherpetic neuralgia[19] and painful diabetic neuropathy.[46,70] Nortriptyline was effective in mixed neuropathic pains[67] and, combined with fluphenazine, in painful diabetic polyneuropathy.[73] For postherpetic neuralgia, it has been shown to be as effective as amitriptyline, with fewer intolerable side-effects.[42]

The non-tricyclic antidepressants also have been studied, with more equivocal results. The analgesic efficacy of the norepinephrine reuptake blocker maprotiline has been established in controlled comparisons against clomipramine in idiopathic pain[69] and against amitriptyline in postherpetic neuralgia.[40] It has also been shown to decrease the intensity of chronic low back pain[74] and pain due to peripheral neuropathy.[47] Although a trial of trazodone for dysaesthetic pains in patients with traumatic myelopathy did not demonstrate a favourable effect,[75] benefits were suggested in another controlled trial performed in patients with cancer pain.[51]

Although some studies have reported positive results with selective serotonin reuptake inhibitors (SSRIs), randomized controlled trials and clinical experience have yielded mixed outcomes.[26,46] Paroxetine has been shown to be effective in painful diabetic neuropathy,[76] where it relieves both steady and lancinating pain, but not in chronic low back pain.[74] Citalopram seems effective in painful diabetic neuropathy.[77] Zimelidine was found to be analgesic in a controlled trial of patients with mixed organic and psychogenic pain syndromes,[78] but was ineffective for postherpetic neuralgia in an open-label comparison against amitriptyline.[79] Limited evidence suggests that fluoxetine might have a role in the prophylaxis of chronic daily headache[80] and the treatment of fibromyalgia.[81,82] A controlled trial in patients with diabetic neuropathy, however, failed to demonstrate benefit from this drug.[46] In studies that directly compared SSRIs and tricyclic antidepressants, the SSRIs have been less effective as analgesics.[46,79] Other serotonin reuptake inhibitors (e.g. fluvoxamine, sertraline) have not been systematically studied as analgesics in patient populations.

Monoamine oxidase inhibitors have been evaluated in limited clinical settings. A controlled trial of phenelzine demonstrated analgesic efficacy in patients with atypical facial pain[83] and several favourable uncontrolled trials of phenelzine and tranylcypromine for treatment of migraine have also been reported, but these trials date from more than 30 years ago.[84]

Venlafaxine inhibits presynaptic reuptake of both serotonin and noradrenaline without the anticholinergic effects of the tricyclic antidepressants. Although evidence of analgesic efficacy is still very limited, the data are promising. The drug has been shown to increase experimental pain tolerance.[85] Case series support analgesic effects in painful diabetic neuropathy[86] and other types of neuropathic pain,[87,88] and in a randomized study, it relieved pain from polyneuropathy but was not as efficacious as imipramine.[89] Thus, the evidence suggests that venlafaxine is analgesic; like the SSRIs, however, its overall effectiveness probably is exceeded by the tricyclic antidepressants.

Bupropion is another promising second-generation non-tricyclic, which specifically inhibits neuronal norepinephrine reuptake and, less potently, dopamine reuptake. Case series suggest analgesic effects in chronic headache[90,91] and chronic low back pain.[92] More recently, an open-label trial[93] and a randomized study[94] reported substantial pain relief in patients with neuropathic pain. Bupropion has a low risk of somnolence and sexual dysfunction, side-effects that may be limiting with other antidepressants. Anecdotally, patients may report increased energy that appears to be unrelated to mood effects, which has led to empirical use for fatigue. These favourable characteristics suggest that a trial of bupropion as an adjuvant analgesic should be considered for selected patients.

Nefazodone also inhibits serotonin and norepinephrine reuptake. Unlike other antidepressants, it also has a direct postsynaptic serotonin antagonist effect. This drug has been reported to potentiate morphine analgesia in animals but there have been no controlled human trials confirming efficacy.[95] At this time, nefazodone usually is considered for a trial when other antidepressant analgesics have been ineffective and a drug with sedative effects may be beneficial.

Very few clinical trials have specifically evaluated the efficacy of antidepressants as analgesics for cancer pain. Nonetheless, partially controlled[51,96,97] and uncontrolled trials[98–100] generally confirm the analgesic potential of the tricyclic antidepressants in the cancer population. Other drugs have not been studied.

In summary, there is very substantial evidence that antidepressant drugs have analgesic effects in diverse types of chronic pain. Given the range of pain syndromes that are potentially responsive, it is appropriate to classify these drugs as non-specific, multipurpose analgesics. The strongest evidence of analgesic efficacy is found in the numerous controlled trials of the

Table 3 Non-specific multipurpose adjuvant analgesics

Class	Examples
Antidepressants	
Tricyclic antidepressants	Amitriptyline, nortriptyline, desipramine, doxepin, imipramine, clomipramine
Selective serotonin reuptake inhibitors	Paroxetine, citalopram, fluoxetine, sertraline, fluvoxamine
Noradrenaline serotonin reuptake inhibitors	Venlafaxine
Monoamine oxidase inhibitors	Phenelzine
Others	Maprotiline, bupropion, trazodone
Alpha-2-adrenergic agonists	Clonidine, tizanidine
Corticosteroids	Dexamethasone, prednisone, methylprednisolone
Neuroleptics	Methotrimeprazine

tertiary amine drugs, the best studied of which has been amitriptyline. Although less abundant data support the efficacy of the secondary amine tricyclic drugs, desipramine and nortriptyline have been carefully studied and have clear analgesic potential. Drugs with more selective actions at specific monoaminergic synapses are also analgesic. Among the nontricyclic drugs, paroxetine and maprotiline have established efficacy and there are limited supporting data for citalopram, venlafaxine, and bupropion. Given the relatively good side-effect profile of the SSRIs and other newer drugs,[26,101–105] there is particularly strong clinical interest in these antidepressants. In the next few years, the analgesic effect of these drugs should be assessed more precisely by randomized controlled trials.

Mechanism of action

Although effective treatment of concurrent depression can contribute to a favourable outcome from antidepressant therapy in patients with chronic pain, the analgesic effect of these drugs is not dependent on their antidepressant activity. Controlled studies have demonstrated that the usually effective analgesic dose is often lower than that required to treat depression, and the onset of analgesia typically occurs much sooner, usually within 1 week.[39,49,56,58,67,68,70,76] Moreover, non-depressed patients can experience analgesia and depressed patients can report pain relief without a change in mood.[18,19,46,49,59] Finally, single-dose studies of amitriptyline in animal models have demonstrated dose-dependent antinociception,[106–109] further suggesting an independent analgesic effect from these drugs.

Several hypotheses may be proposed to explain the analgesia produced by the antidepressants. The most widely accepted postulates that their ability to block the reuptake of monoamines increases activity in endogenous monoamine-mediated pain modulating pathways, the best characterized of which descend from the brainstem and use serotonin or norepinephrine as transmitters.[110–113] Interestingly, favourable clinical studies with drugs that have selective serotonergic or noradrenergic effects suggest that increased neurotransmitter availability in either pathway can yield analgesic effects.

Animal studies have also demonstrated that the acute antinociceptive effects produced by various classes of antidepressants can be partially blocked by the specific opioid antagonist, naloxone.[107–109,113,114] This finding suggests that activation of the opioid systems by these drugs could account for part of their analgesic effect. This activation seems to be both direct, through an interaction with the opioid receptor, and indirect through enhanced release of opioid peptides.[114]

When a tricyclic antidepressant is coadministered with an opioid, some of the benefit may relate to a pharmacokinetic interaction that results in higher opioid concentrations. Such an interaction has been demonstrated when clomipramine or amitriptyline is added to a morphine regimen.[20] Neither the importance of this mechanism in comparison to other effects on pain modulation, nor the degree to which this pharmacokinetic interaction occurs with other drugs is known.

The tricyclic antidepressants are not highly selective and they also interact with other types of receptors (e.g. acetylcholine and histamine) that may be important in the development of analgesia.[115–118] Further elucidation of these mechanisms awaits additional investigations using more selective drugs.

Adverse effects

Although serious adverse effects are uncommon at the doses of antidepressant usually administered for pain, such morbidity does occur and less serious side-effects are frequent.[101,102] Dose-related side-effects can occur even at low doses, particularly in patients who may be predisposed to adverse effects due to major organ dysfunction, use of multiple other drugs, or advanced age. Moreover, some patients who receive low doses of the tricyclic antidepressant actually attain relatively high plasma drug concentrations,[119] and this pharmacokinetic variability may also account for some cases of toxicity.

Among the antidepressants, the tricyclic drugs are most likely to produce side-effects, and the incidence of side-effects is highest with the tertiary amine drugs. The most serious adverse effect, cardiotoxicity, is very uncommon.[120] Patients who have significant heart disease, including conduction disorders, arrhythmia, or heart failure, should not be treated with a tricyclic. Due to their cardiac toxicity, overdose of a tricyclic can be lethal. Orthostatic hypotension is far more common than cardiac toxicity during treatment with a tricyclic antidepressant.[120] It is more likely in the elderly and, combined with the cognitive effects of these drugs, probably accounts for an increased risk of hip fracture in this population.[121] Patients who are predisposed to orthostasis, such as those with autonomic neuropathy, usually are considered better candidates for an antidepressant in an alternative class. The likelihood of cognitive side-effects, including somnolence, mental clouding, and, less commonly, delirium, is increased in the elderly and those with predisposing factors, such as dementia, brain metastases, prior cranial radiotherapy, or concurrent use of other centrally acting drugs.

Most of the minor side-effects produced by the tricyclic antidepressants are related to their anticholinergic properties. These include dry mouth, blurred vision, and constipation. These problems usually are tolerated or effectively managed. Rarely, more serious anticholinergic toxicity can occur, including precipitation of acute angle closure glaucoma, tachycardia, severe constipation, or urinary retention. Due to the risk of precipitating an attack, the tricyclics are contraindicated in those with a known history of a narrow anterior chamber of the eye or prior attacks of acute glaucoma. Eye pressures usually should be followed more closely when these drugs are given to patients with open-angle glaucoma. The likelihood of urinary retention can be reduced in male patients by inquiring about symptoms of prostatism prior to therapy.

The secondary amine tricyclic drugs, desipramine and nortriptyline, are less anticholinergic and, therefore, better tolerated than the tertiary amines, such as amitriptyline. They also are less likely to cause orthostatic hypotension, somnolence, and cognitive impairment. Nortriptyline has been shown to be as effective and better tolerated than amitriptyline in patients with postherpetic neuralgia.[42] Patients who are predisposed to the side-effects associated with the tricyclics, or who have distressing side-effects during a trial of a tertiary amine drug, should be considered for a trial of desipramine or nortriptyline.

The main advantage of the SSRIs is their more favourable side-effect profile.[26,122] The most common adverse events from SSRIs are nausea, headache, sedation, insomnia, weight gain, impaired memory, sweating, tremor, and sexual dysfunction.[123,124] Clinical experience and several case reports suggest that SSRIs can induce or worsen akathisia and parkinsonian symptoms,[125] but the evidence is conflicting.[126] Rapid discontinuation of SSRIs, especially the short-acting paroxetine, can cause a discontinuation syndrome characterized by both somatic (dizziness, light-headedness, nausea, fatigue, lethargy, sleep disturbances) and psychological (anxiety, agitation, crying, irritability) symptoms.[127,128] A gradual tapering should avoid these symptoms. Post-marketing surveillance has revealed that major adverse reactions to SSRIs are very uncommon.[123] Fatalities related to overdoses have only been reported with citalopram.[123]

Venlafaxine is usually well tolerated, in both its immediate-release and sustained-release formulations. The most frequent adverse events are nausea, dizziness, somnolence, insomnia, ejaculatory disturbances, sweating, and dry mouth.[129] A dose-related hypertension has also been reported, which warrants regular blood-pressure monitoring. As with the SSRIs, withdrawal symptoms have been reported following its abrupt discontinuation.[127]

The most common side-effects of bupropion are dry mouth, insomnia, nausea, headache, rash, and agitation/excitement.[130] It decreases seizure threshold, and is relatively contraindicated in patients with factors predisposing to seizures, such as sedative-hypnotic withdrawal states, coadministered drugs with seizure-lowering potential, and central nervous system pathology.[105,131,132] The main advantages of bupropion are the absence of sexual side-effects and its propensity to increase the energy level rather than causing lethargy, which can be very helpful in depressed or sedated patients.[105]

Pharmacology

The tricyclic antidepressants are metabolized by several isozymes of cytochrome P450. The tertiary amines are metabolized by CYP1A2 and CYP2C19, whereas the secondary amines are cleared by CYP2D6. There is large interindividual variation in these metabolic pathways. For example, the extensive metabolizers of desipramine and nortriptyline clear the drug up to seven times faster than poor metabolizers,[133] which require a 2-week period before achieving a steady state.[134]

Tricyclic antidepressants may be coadministered with SSRIs during treatment for depression or pain. There is an important drug interaction between these classes. SSRIs may produce a reduction in the clearance of the tricyclics and, therefore, result in a significantly higher plasma level.[135–138] This potential suggests that the tricyclic dose should be lowered initially when adding an SSRI.

Most SSRIs, especially paroxetine and fluoxetine, inhibit CYP2D6, which could produce interactions with other medications metabolized by this isozyme.[139] Clinically significant drug interactions with paroxetine seem to be limited, however.[140] As their effect on CYP2D6 is less, sertraline and citalopram are less likely to interact with other drugs.[139] Due to the presence of an active metabolite, fluoxetine has a much longer half-life than the other SSRIs and is more prone to drug–drug interactions.[138]

Venlafaxine also is highly metabolized by CYP2D6 and can interact with other drugs affected by this isozyme. Although unexpected adverse effects can occur with such drug combinations, the clinical significance of these interactions in practice appears to be limited. The dose of venlafaxine should be reduced in patients with several renal disease or cirrhosis, due to lower clearance. Dose adjustments are not required in the setting of advanced age alone.[129]

Like venlafaxine, the dose of bupropion should be reduced in patients with several renal or liver disease. Drug interactions are uncommon.[105]

Indications

The antidepressant drugs are multipurpose analgesics and potentially could be considered for the treatment of any chronic pain syndrome. The available evidence does not support their use as analgesics for acute pain,[141,142] despite the demonstrated efficacy of selected tricyclic antidepressants in animal models of acute nociception[106] and human experimental pain.[143]

As discussed previously, treatment with an adjuvant analgesic, such as an antidepressant drug, is usually considered in the palliative care setting when a favourable balance between analgesia and side-effects cannot be attained with an opioid. There are many potential reasons for a poor response to an opioid,[144] among which is a 'neuropathic' pathophysiology (see Chapter 8.2.1).[145,146] Given the established benefit of the antidepressants in patients with diverse types of neuropathic pains,[18,19,39,40,46,49,57,58,67,70,79] these drugs may be particularly valuable in painful conditions related to such mechanisms. Thus, the strongest indication for the use of an antidepressant as an adjuvant analgesic in palliative care occurs in the patient with neuropathic pain whose response to opioids has been inadequate.

There is great heterogeneity in the range of symptoms presented by patients with neuropathic pains. Conceivably, specific symptoms may indicate the existence of mechanisms that respond differently to drugs with varying modes of action. Although there has been little systematic investigation of this possibility, the clinical literature has guidelines, based on anecdotal observation, that reflect this perspective. For example, it is generally accepted that antidepressants are more useful for neuropathic pains characterized by continuous dysaesthesias, regardless of the specific syndrome, than pains described as lancinating (stabbing). This impression continues, notwithstanding controlled trials that have demonstrated the efficacy of amitriptyline and desipramine for continuous and lancinating dysaesthesias in patients who are experiencing both.[18,19] The latter data suggest that antidepressant trials may be considered for patients with predominating lancinating neuropathic pains who have failed other specific adjuvant analgesics (see below).

Early use of an adjuvant analgesic is also considered when pain is accompanied by a comorbid condition that may respond to a non-analgesic effect of the drug. Antidepressants are commonly used when pain is complicated by depression. The sedative tricyclic antidepressants are often added when pain is accompanied by insomnia, whereas the anxiolytic SSRIs can be useful in anxious patients and bupropion is more indicated in sedated or fatigued patients.

Dosing guidelines

Given the very extensive data supporting the analgesic efficacy of the tricyclic antidepressants, especially amitriptyline, it is reasonable to select one of these drugs as the first-line treatment for pain. Amitriptyline should be considered for a trial in relatively young patients who have limited factors predisposing to anticholinergic, sedative, or cardiovascular side-effects. Medically ill patients who are predisposed to these toxicities are better considered for an initial trial with a secondary amine drug, specifically desipramine or nortriptyline. If tricyclic antidepressants have not been tolerated, or are expected to yield problematic effects, trials of other, better-tolerated antidepressants, such as paroxetine, citalopram, venlafaxine, or bupropion, should be considered. Maprotiline is another option, but generally is sedating and may not be preferred on this basis.

It is now common practice to combine antidepressants in different classes as a strategy to address treatment-refractory depression. Anecdotally, the same approach may be useful when pain is the indication for these drugs. A combination of a tricyclic (amitriptyline) and an SSRI (fluoxetine) has been shown to be more effective than either drug alone in relieving pain from fibromyalgia.[82] In patients with medical illness, this approach usually is considered in the setting of severe neuropathic pain that has not responded to conservative pharmacotherapy. Typically, a tricyclic drug is combined with a non-tricyclic, or an SSRI (or venlafaxine) is combined with bupropion.

Anecdotal observation and very limited empirical data[40] suggest that there is substantial variability in the analgesic response to the different antidepressants. Failure of a drug due to inefficacy, therefore, might reasonably be followed by a trial of an alternative drug. There are no guidelines for drug selection during these sequential trials and the process usually proceeds by trial and error.

The starting dose of the tricyclic antidepressants should be low, 10 mg in the elderly or the medically ill, and 25 mg in younger patients. The initial dosing increments are usually the same size as the starting dose. Doses can be increased every few days. The usual effective dose range for amitriptyline or desipramine is 50–150 mg; some patients will benefit from doses below or above this range. Although most patients can be treated with a single night-time dose, some patients have less morning 'hangover' and some report less late-afternoon pain if doses are divided.

The SSRIs paroxetine and citalopram should be started at a daily dose of 20 mg in young patients or 10 mg in elderly or medically ill patients. They can be increased gradually up to the usually effective dose of 20–40 mg daily. Higher doses sometimes are more effective. Discontinuation of these drugs should be done gradually, to avoid withdrawal symptoms.

Venlafaxine can be started at 75 mg in young and 50 mg daily in elderly patients. The immediate-release formulation should be given in two divided doses, whereas the extended-release formulation can be given once a day. The dose can be increased as tolerated, up to a usual maximum dose of 225–375 mg/day. The only controlled trial on the use of venlafaxine as adjuvant analgesic used a daily dose of 225 mg/day[89] but good analgesic effects have been reported with doses as low as 75 mg/day.[86,87] The dose should be reduced by 25 per cent in mild-moderate renal function impairment and by 50 per cent in dialysis patients. If it is used for more than 6 weeks, the dose should be tapered over 2 weeks when discontinuing its use.

Treatment with bupropion may be initiated at a dose of 100–150 mg/day with the immediate-release formulation in two divided doses, or with the extended-release formulation once a day.[93,94] The maximum daily dose usually is 450 mg/day; to reduce concerns about peak concentration toxicity (specifically seizures), it is prudent to limit any single dose to 300 mg.

Given evidence of dose-dependent analgesic effects, at least for the tricyclic antidepressants,[18,58] it is reasonable to continue upward dose titration beyond the usual analgesic doses in patients who fail to achieve benefit and have no limiting side-effects. This course is clearly justified in patients with a coexistent depression, but should be considered even in patients without evidence of this disorder. There is currently no justification for increasing doses beyond the levels associated with antidepressant effects.

Although current data are insufficient to define concentration–effect models for antidepressant analgesia, it is useful to monitor plasma drug concentration during therapy, if feasible. In non-responders, low plasma drug concentration suggests either poor compliance or an unusually rapid metabolism; in the latter case, doses can be increased while repeatedly monitoring the plasma drug level. Likewise, non-responders whose plasma concentration is not very low, but is lower than the antidepressant range, should be considered for a trial of higher doses if side-effects are not a problem. For patients who are benefiting from therapy, plasma levels provide a baseline for comparison should pain recur in the future.

Changes in pain, mood, cognitive status, sleep pattern, and other clinical effects must be carefully monitored during dose escalation. There are limited, anecdotal observations that suggest the existence of a therapeutic window for analgesia during dose escalation with some tricyclic drugs. That is, it is possible that analgesic effects could decline as the dose is increased above some threshold and that dose reduction from this level could regain analgesia. This potential for a therapeutic window emphasizes the importance of careful monitoring during dose escalation.

A favourable analgesic effect is usually observed within a week after achieving an effective dosing level and, in some patients, maximal effect appears to evolve over days or weeks thereafter. This delay, combined with the many days required to increase the dose to a therapeutic level, may result in a prolonged period during which patients experience unsatisfactory effects from the therapy, and sometimes experience uncomfortable side-effects. Unless the patient is well informed about this potential, non-compliance is likely.

Corticosteroids

Corticosteroid drugs have many potential indications in the palliative care setting. Numerous studies have suggested that these drugs may improve appetite, nausea, malaise, and overall quality of life.[147–157] Although concern about toxicity has generally limited chronic use to patients with advanced disease and short life expectancies, there is a substantial anecdotal experience with both short-term and long-term administration for a variety of clinical problems, including pain.

Data from controlled trials and clinical series supports the classification of corticosteroids as multipurpose analgesics. Efficacy has been suggested in reflex sympathetic dystrophy, a type of neuropathic pain,[158] and diverse types of cancer pain, including bone pain, neuropathic pain from infiltration or compression of neural structures, headache due to increased intracranial pressure, arthralgia, and pain due to obstruction of a hollow viscus (e.g. bowel or ureter).[150,154,159–161]

Analgesic effects have been described for a variety of corticosteroids and a broad range of doses. A placebo-controlled trial in patients with far-advanced cancer demonstrated that relatively low doses of methylprednisolone (16 mg twice daily) were analgesic but that these effects waned over a 20-day evaluation period.[152] A survey of patients administered high doses of dexamethasone (96 mg/day for 2 weeks) for malignant epidural spinal cord compression observed pain relief in 64 per cent within hours of the initial dose.[159] A randomized trial confirmed that dexamethasone was profoundly analgesic in spinal cord compression but could not identify any difference between a high (100 mg) and low (10 mg) initial dose.[162] Symptoms related to bowel obstruction have been shown to respond to dexamethasone 8–60 mg/day[160,161] and methylprednisolone 30–50 mg/day.[150]

This accumulated experience establishes the analgesic potential of corticosteroid drugs in a variety of chronic pain syndromes. Differences among drugs have not been discerned, and there are no data by which to judge dose-response relationships, relative potencies among drugs, and long-term efficacy.

Mechanism of action

The mechanism of analgesia produced by corticosteroids is unknown. Any of several processes may be involved. Compression of pain-sensitive structures may be relieved by reduction of peritumoural oedema[163] or, in the case of steroid-responsive neoplasms, by shrinkage of tumour masses themselves.[164] Activation of nociceptors may be lessened by reduced tissue concentrations of some inflammatory mediators—specifically prostaglandins and leukotrienes. Aberrant electrical activity in damaged nerves may also be tempered by these agents.[165]

Adverse effects

Well-recognized adverse effects are associated with short- and long-term administration of corticosteroids, and with the withdrawal of these drugs following chronic use.[166,167] The risk of serious toxicity increases with the dose of the drug, the duration of therapy, and predisposing factors associated with the medical condition of the patient.

Although acute toxicity is possible, transitory corticosteroid therapy is usually well tolerated. The potential toxicities include adverse neuropsychological effects, hyperglycaemia, fluid retention (which can lead to hypertension or volume overload in predisposed patients), and gastrointestinal disturbances ranging from dyspepsia to frank ulceration. A study of a high-dose dexamethasone regimen for epidural spinal cord compression (96 mg intravenously, followed by 96 mg orally for 3 days, then a taper for 10 days) noted three cases of serious toxicity among the 27 patients randomized to the steroid therapy (11 per cent); one patient became hypomanic, one developed a confusional state, and one developed a perforated gastric ulcer.[168]

The neuropsychological toxicity associated with corticosteroid therapy ranges from delirium to relatively isolated changes in mood, cognitive functioning, or perception. Mood disturbances can themselves vary from euphoria to depression. In another study of patients who received a high-dose dexamethasone regimen for epidural spinal cord compression (100 mg followed by 24 mg every 6 h), the overall rate of psychiatric disorders was no greater than a comparison group, but there was a greater incidence of major depressive disorders and a trend toward a greater incidence of delirium in the steroid-treated group; those who received steroids also had more depressive and anxious symptomatology.[169] Although neuropsychological toxicity is usually observed early during treatment and when relatively high doses are administered, these adverse effects can complicate any steroid regimen at any time. There is no proven association with any specific drug and the occurrence of acute toxicity during one course of therapy does not predict a similar response during subsequent courses.

Chronic administration of a corticosteroid can produce a cushingoid habitus; changes in integument, subcutaneous tissues, and connective tissues; weight gain; hypertension; severe osteoporosis; myopathy; increased risk of infection; hyperglycaemia; gastrointestinal toxicity; and late neuropsychological effects.[166] Long-term treatment with relatively low doses is generally well tolerated, however, even among patients with advanced illness. A study of advanced cancer patients chronically administered prednisolone or dexamethasone at varying doses observed oropharyngeal candidiasis in approximately one-third of patients and oedema or cushingoid habitus in less than one-fifth; dyspepsia, weight gain, neuropsychological changes, and ecchymoses occurred in 5–10 per cent, and the incidence of other adverse effects, such as hyperglycaemia, myopathy, and osteoporosis, was even lower than this.[156]

Chronic administration of a corticosteroid approximately doubles the risk of peptic ulcer.[170] This risk is increased further by coadministration of a non-steroidal anti-inflammatory drug.[171] This potentiation of gastrointestinal toxicity relatively contraindicates the combined use of a corticosteroid and a non-steroidal anti-inflammatory drug in the palliative care setting. Steroid use also increases the risk of gastrointestinal perforation, even during short-term therapy.[172,173] This complication may be associated with constipation.[172]

Steroid withdrawal following chronic therapy can produce a syndrome of myalgia and arthralgia known as steroid 'pseudorheumatism'.[174] Withdrawal may also produce other symptoms, such as malaise, headache, and mood disturbance, or yield a flare of the symptoms for which steroid therapy had been initiated previously. Following a reduction to low doses, patients also may be at risk for disturbances associated with hypocortisolism, particularly during a period of intercurrent stress such as systemic infection. The symptoms associated with steroid withdrawal can occur with either dose reduction or discontinuation of therapy. In some cases, symptoms appear after a relatively modest decline in a relatively high baseline dose.

Escalation of the steroid dose can provide relief, and a slower, more gradual taper may avoid recurrence.

Pharmacology

Dexamethasone is metabolized by the hepatic isozyme CYP3A4.[139] It can increase the metabolism of other drugs metabolized by this subunit of the P450 system, including the tertiary tricyclics, methadone, carbamazepine, venlafaxine, and dextromethorphan. Phenytoin and nefazodone, which are inhibitors of CYP3A4, can theoretically increase the effect of dexamethasone but the clinical significance of this interaction remains unknown.[139]

Indications

Corticosteroids are used acutely in the management of epidural spinal cord compression, raised intracranial pressure, and superior vena cava syndrome. Pain may accompany each of these syndromes and symptomatic relief is one of the goals of therapy.

On the basis of anecdotal experience, corticosteroids are also administered for many other painful syndromes, including metastatic bone pain, neuropathic pain due to compression or infiltration of peripheral nerves or nerve plexus, painful lymphoedema, pain due to obstruction of a hollow viscus, and pain due to organ capsule distension. Like other adjuvant analgesics, corticosteroids are usually added to an opioid regimen following dose escalation to limiting toxicity. Patients who present with these pain syndromes commonly have other symptoms that could potentially be improved by steroid therapy, such as nausea or malaise, and corticosteroid therapy may be considered earlier if primarily indicated by these other symptoms.

Dosing guidelines

The relative risks and benefits of the various corticosteroids are unknown. In the United States, dexamethasone is usually selected, a choice that gains theoretical support from the relatively low mineralocorticoid effects of this drug. Prednisone and methylprednisolone have also been used.

On the basis of clinical experience, corticosteroids are usually administered either in a high- or a low-dose regimen. A high-dose regimen (e.g. dexamethasone 100 mg followed initially by 96 mg/day in divided doses) has been used for patients who experience an acute episode of very severe pain that cannot be promptly reduced with opioids, such as that associated with a rapidly worsening malignant plexopathy.[147] This regimen may also be appropriate when treating an oncological emergency that may be steroid-responsive, such as superior vena cava syndrome or epidural spinal cord compression. The dose can be tapered over weeks, concurrent with the initiation of other analgesic approaches such as radiotherapy.

A low-dose corticosteroid regimen (e.g. dexamethasone 1–2 mg once or twice daily) has been used for patients with advanced medical illness who continue to have pain despite optimal dosing of opioid drugs. In most cases, long-term therapy is planned. Although the risks associated with prolonged steroid use in this setting are more than balanced by the need for enhanced comfort, repeated assessments are required to ensure that benefits are sustained.[149] Ineffective regimens should be tapered and discontinued and, in all cases, the lowest dose that yields the desired results should be sought.

Alpha-2 adrenergic agonists

Classification of the alpha-2 adrenergic agonists as non-specific, multipurpose analgesics is supported by both animal and human studies. Strong antinociceptive effects in animals can be produced by clonidine, a partial agonist at the alpha-2 adrenergic receptor,[175–177] and by both medetomidine, a full alpha-2 agonist,[178] and dexmedetomidine, the active D-isomer of medetomidine.[179] These effects can be observed in a variety of experimental models, including models of neuropathic pain.[177,179] In humans, analgesic effects in diverse pain syndromes have been established in controlled studies of systemic dexmedetomidine,[180] and both systemic and intraspinal clonidine.[181–185] These and other reports suggest that clonidine can be beneficial in pain syndromes that may be relatively less opioid-responsive, including chronic headache, non-malignant neuropathic pains,[181,184–189] and some cancer pain syndromes (including neuropathic cancer-related pain).[182,190–193]

Two controlled trials have illuminated the role of clonidine as an analgesic. The first study used an 'enriched enrolment' design, in which an open-label phase was used to identify patients with painful diabetic polyneuropathy who might be potential clonidine responders; these patients were then tested in a controlled trial of transdermal clonidine.[181] This trial confirmed an earlier report[194] in demonstrating that less than one-fourth of patients are potential responders, and that those who do respond can experience analgesia that is both substantial and sustained.

The second study compared a 14-day epidural infusion of clonidine (30 μg/h) with an epidural placebo infusion in patients with cancer pain who were receiving titrated intraspinal opioids via epidural morphine patient-controlled analgesia.[182] Overall, clonidine reduced pain but not opioid consumption. Therapeutic success, defined as either reduced opioid requirement or pain reduction, occurred in 45 per cent of those who received clonidine and 21 per cent of those who received placebo. Remarkably, most of this difference in success rates was due to the response of patients with neuropathic pain; in this subgroup, success was achieved by 56 per cent of those who received clonidine and only 5 per cent of those who received placebo.

These data provide evidence that clonidine is a multipurpose analgesic that may be particularly useful in the management of neuropathic pain. Both systemic administration, by the oral or transdermal route, and epidural administration can yield favourable effects. Although a minority (less than one-fourth during systemic administration) are likely to respond, those that do can experience clinically meaningful effects.

Tizanidine is another centrally acting alpha-2 agonist and is commercially available in the United States as an antispasticity agent, with established efficacy in hypertonicity associated with multiple sclerosis,[195] acquired brain injury,[196] and spinal cord injury.[197] Its antinociceptive properties have been observed in animal studies[198,199] and a few open-label studies have revealed some analgesic effect in fibromyalgia[200] and chronic daily headache.[201] Although the evidence of analgesic efficacy is limited, the mechanism of this drug and a favourable clinical experience has supported its use as a multipurpose analgesic.

Mechanism of action

The mechanism of clonidine analgesia has not been established and is likely to be complex.[177] Noradrenergic receptors are clearly important in the modulation of nociceptive processing and it is possible that interaction with alpha-2 receptors in the spinal cord[179,202] or brainstem[203] activates endogenous systems that reduce nociceptive input to the central nervous system. Presumably, these systems may be relatively more or less involved in the processing of different types of noxious stimuli[177] or the development of different types of pain syndromes.

It is also possible that clonidine may produce analgesia in some cases through interference with the mechanisms that perpetuate so-called sympathetically maintained pain, a subtype of neuropathic pain.[188] Clonidine may reduce sympathetic tone and, in this way, ameliorate pains that are sustained, at least in part, by circulating catecholamines or efferent activity in the sympathetic nervous system.

The analgesic effect of tizanidine is also likely explained by its alpha-2-adrenergic properties.[204] A study in fibromyalgia patients also suggested that this drug dose-dependently changes substance P levels in cerebrospinal fluid, an effect with theoretical consequences on nociception.[200]

Adverse effects

In placebo-controlled trials, the most common adverse effects associated with systemic or epidural clonidine administration have been somnolence, hypotension (usually orthostatic), and dry mouth.[181,182] In patients without severe concurrent medical illness, the major toxicity produced by clonidine is usually somnolence. The potential for adverse effects, including serious hypotension, presumably is increased in the meically ill. The controlled trial of epidural clonidine in cancer pain demonstrated that the drug produced sustained hypotensive effects in almost one-half of the patients;[182] specifically, six of the 38 patients (16 per cent) who received clonidine experienced serious blood pressure changes associated with dizziness, hypotension, or rebound hypertension.

The most frequent side-effects associated with tizanidine are somnolence and dry mouth.[196] This drug has less affinity for the alpha-1 adrenergic receptor and, therefore, produces hypotension less often than clonidine.[204]

Pharmacology

Clonidine is metabolized by the liver to inactive metabolites, which are renally excreted. The drug interactions are minimal and mainly concern potentiation of the effects of other hypotensive medications.[205]

Indications

Like other multipurpose analgesics, clonidine and tizanidine can be considered for a therapeutic trial in any chronic pain state. In the medically ill, anecdotal experience has generally been limited to patients with opioid-refractory pain, typically neuropathic pains. Although the data in support of analgesic effects are better for clonidine, a trial of tizanidine may be favoured because of concern about hypotension. Both drugs are usually avoided in patients who are haemodynamically unstable, predisposed to serious hypotension (e.g. by autonomic neuropathy, intravascular volume depletion, or concurrent therapy with potent hypotensive agents), or markedly somnolent from other causes. Given limited experience with the adrenergic agonists in those with advanced illness, trials of these drugs are usually considered after other adjuvant analgesics, such as the antidepressants, oral local anaesthetics, and anticonvulsants, have failed.

Dosing guidelines

When administered systemically for pain, clonidine is typically initiated at a relatively low dose, 0.1 mg/day orally or one-half of a TTS-1 patch transdermally. Given its delivery characteristics, the transdermal system can be safely cut into pieces to change the dose.

Monitoring of both pain and adverse effects is necessary during gradual dose escalation. Neither dose-dependent effects nor the potential for a ceiling dose has been evaluated during systemic clonidine therapy. Consequently, gradual dose escalation should continue until significant side-effects occur or blood pressure declines to a degree that is worrisome. Anecdotally, some patients have benefited from relatively high doses (as high as 2 mg/day in rare cases), and it is reasonable to continue upward dose titration until dose-limiting toxicity is encountered.

Tizanidine is usually started with a dose of 2 mg at bedtime and can be gradually increased by 2 mg increments every few days. Most patients do not exceed a maximal dose of 24 mg daily. The dose is usually divided, but some patients benefit from a nighttime dose alone.

Neuroleptics

The demonstration of antinociceptive effects in animal models[206] and the favourable results of several controlled clinical trials in diverse pain syndromes[207–211] suggest that some neuroleptics might be considered non-specific, multipurpose analgesics. Nonetheless, there is relatively little evidence of analgesic activity for most neuroleptic compounds and their role as adjuvant analgesics is limited by this lack of definitive data and the potential for adverse effects.[212]

Controlled trials have yielded mixed results. The strongest evidence of analgesic efficacy has been acquired in studies of the phenothiazine, methotrimeprazine. Favourable studies of this drug have been conducted in patients with cancer pain,[208] other chronic pain states[207,209,213] (including some with neuropathic pain), and acute pain following surgery or myocardial infarction.[214] In these studies, the analgesic potency of methotrimeprazine 10–20 mg approximated morphine 10 mg in patients with little or no prior opioid exposure.

A controlled comparison of pimozide (4–12 mg/day) and carbamazepine in patients with trigeminal neuralgia demonstrated that pimozide has analgesic efficacy in this lancinating neuropathic pain syndrome.[211] Unfortunately, a very high incidence of disturbing side-effects, including physical and mental slowing, tremor, and parkinsonian symptoms, limited the value of this therapy. The analgesic efficacy of fluphenazine in headache was similarly suggested in a controlled, multiple dose (1 mg/day) study of 50 patients with chronic tension headache.[210]

The analgesic efficacy of neuroleptic drugs was not confirmed in other, single-dose controlled studies. These evaluated chlorpromazine,[215] promethazine,[216] and haloperidol[217] in varied pain models.

The possibility of neuroleptic-mediated analgesic effects has also been suggested in numerous anecdotal reports. Trifluoperazine, chlorprothixine, haloperidol, and fluphenazine have been administered for a variety of pain syndromes,[218–224] including chronic headache and neuropathic pains,[218,220] and various neuroleptics have been reported to be coanalgesic when added to another psychotropic or an opioid.[73,97,225] An opioid-sparing effect has been described in some,[97] but not all,[226] surveys of patients with cancer pain.

Olanzapine is a second-generation (atypical) antipsychotic agent. Case reports and case series have reported efficacy in aborting cluster headache[227] and relieving pain from fibromyalgia.[228] These data are, however, still minimal and further studies are required to confirm the analgesic effect of olanzapine or any other of the newer atypical antipsychotic agents.

Thus, the available data establish the analgesic potential of one neuroleptic, methotrimeprazine, and suggest that others may be similarly characterized. The evidence is limited, however, and some well-controlled studies have failed to confirm this effect.

Mechanism of action

The mechanism of neuroleptic analgesia is unknown, but may involve the effect of dopaminergic blockade on endogenous pain modulating systems. Dopamine receptors, specifically the D_2 subtype, are represented among the numerous pathways that subserve pain modulation.[229] Studies in animals have suggested that selective dopamine antagonists can potentiate morphine analgesia[206,230] and controlled clinical trials have demonstrated that metoclopramide, a relatively selective blocker of the D_2 receptor, is analgesic in humans.[231,232] This evidence, however, does not confirm that a dopaminergic mechanism underlies the analgesic effects of neuroleptic drugs, because all these drugs interact with other receptors that could potentially mediate analgesic effects.

Even metoclopramide has effects on another central nervous system receptor, specifically the 5-HT_3 serotonin receptor subtype, that could mediate analgesia.[233]

Adverse effects

Common side-effects of neuroleptic drugs include sedation, orthostatic dizziness, and anticholinergic effects. Some patients experience mental clouding or confusion. Phenothiazines, such as chlorpromazine and fluphenazine, are more likely to produce these effects than other subclasses, such as the butyrophenones (e.g. haloperidol). The sedation produced by the neuroleptics can be additive to other central nervous system depressants. Rare, idiosyncratic reactions include blood dyscrasias, dermatoses (including photosensitivity), and hepatic damage.

The possibility of extrapyramidal side-effects is perhaps the greatest concern in the clinical use of neuroleptic drugs. The incidence of these disorders varies with the drug, duration of therapy, and dose.[234] Compared to other neuroleptics, both fluphenazine and haloperidol are relatively more likely to produce these effects, whereas olanzapine is less likely to induce them.[235]

The most serious extrapyramidal reaction is the neuroleptic malignant syndrome, which is characterized by rigidity, autonomic instability, and encephalopathy.[236] Successful management requires prompt diagnosis, discontinuation of the neuroleptic, and intensive supportive measures. The use of dantrolene and bromocriptine has been suggested in severe cases.[236]

Some extrapyramidal effects tend to occur early in therapy. These include acute dystonic reactions (e.g. trismus, torticollis, and even opisthotonos), akathisia, and parkinsonism. The management of these complications usually involves discontinuation of the neuroleptic, with or without the administration of an anticholinergic drug, such as benztropine. Akathisia has also been managed anecdotally with a benzodiazepine.

Tardive syndromes, including dyskinesias and the less-common dystonias, occur late and may become intractable. Tardive dyskinesia is more common in the elderly and women. Although believed to be related to the quantity of the neuroleptic consumed, it has been observed even in those consuming low doses for a period of months. Treatment of a tardive dyskinesia syndrome usually requires tapering and then discontinuation of the drug. Rarely, tapering of the neuroleptic will be accompanied by the development of worsening dyskinesias (so-called 'withdrawal emergent dyskinesias'), which are usually transient. This phenomenon should not prevent a trial of a drug-free period.

Indications

In the palliative care setting, neuroleptics are used commonly in the management of delirium. Their specific use as analgesics has been limited by concerns about toxicity and the availability of alternative, safer drugs. Methotrimeprazine is difficult to obtain, but if available, may be useful in bedridden patients with advanced illness, who are experiencing pain associated with anxiety, restlessness, or nausea. For patients with advanced disease, the sedative, anxiolytic, and antiemetic effects of this drug can be highly favourable, and side-effects, such as orthostatic hypotension, are less of an issue.

The efficacy of pimozide in patients with trigeminal neuralgia[211] has suggested a role for this drug in the treatment of patients with refractory neuropathic pains characterized by a predominating lancinating or paroxysmal component. Given its side-effect liability, and the expanding pharmacologic options for neuropathic pain (see below), this drug is now rarely used. Other neuroleptics, such as haloperidol and fluphenazine, are sometimes considered for patients with various neuropathic pains that have not responded to opioids or preferred adjuvant analgesics (such as antidepressants), local anaesthetics, or anticonvulsants.

Dosing guidelines

With known dose-related toxicity and no confirmation of dose-dependent efficacy, the neuroleptics are prudently dosed to some arbitrary ceiling based on published reports, then discontinued if no analgesia ensues. For example, low initial doses of fluphenazine can be escalated to 1–2 mg three times daily, and the dose of haloperidol can be slowly increased to 2–5 mg two to three times a day.

Methotrimeprazine has been administered by intramuscular or subcutaneous bolus, by continuous subcutaneous infusion,[237] and brief intravenous infusion (administration over 20–30 min). Dosing usually begins with 5 mg every 6 h, or a comparable dose delivered by infusion, which is gradually increased as needed. Most patients will not require more than 20 mg every 6 h to gain desired effects.

Other adjuvant analgesics used for neuropathic pain

As noted previously, the focus on neuropathic pain as a target for the adjuvant analgesics in the palliative care setting derives from the observation that pains of this type may be relatively less responsive to opioid drugs than other pains.[144–146,238–241] A recent survey revealed that the appropriate use of both opioid and adjuvant analgesics can yield analgesic outcomes in cancer-related neuropathic pain that mirror those obtained during treatment of nociceptive or mixed pain syndromes.[17]

Inadequately relieved neuropathic pain is the usual indication for a trial of a multipurpose adjuvant analgesic. Indeed, the antidepressant analgesics are a first-line approach in this situation, and corticosteroids are considered early in the context of advanced illness. These drugs are complemented by many others that may be administered for the same indication (Table 4).

Oral and parenteral local anaesthetics

Numerous studies suggest that systemically administered local anaesthetics could be considered multipurpose analgesics. Nonetheless, a very large clinical experience has focused on the use of these drugs in the treatment of neuropathic pains. Analgesic trials have evaluated the local anaesthetics in both acute pain and various chronic pain syndromes.[242–244] Controlled trials[245–247] have demonstrated that a brief intravenous infusion of lignocaine (lidocaine) can relieve acute postoperative pain and pain due to burns. Surveys suggest benefit in a variety of chronic pains,[248–260] including arthritis,[255] musculoskeletal pains,[256] erythromelalgia,[260] vascular headache,[257] and migraine.[261] Randomized controlled studies have confirmed analgesic efficacy in central pain,[262,263] postherpetic neuralgia,[264] and painful diabetic neuropathy.[265] In contrast to this favourable experience, there also have been several negative studies of local anaesthetics in neuropathic cancer pain.[266–268]

Table 4 Adjuvant analgesics used for neuropathic pain

Class	Examples
First line	
Tricyclic antidepressants	See Table 3
Anticonvulsants	Gabapentin, topiramate, carbamazepine, phenytoin, valproate, oxcarbazepine, lamotrigine, levetiracetam, pregabalin
Non-tricyclic antidepressants	See Table 3
Other drugs	
Oral local anaesthetics	Mexiletine, tocainide, flecainide
Alpha-2 adrenergic agonists	Clonidine, tizanidine
N-Methyl-D-aspartate receptor antagonists	Dextromethorphan, ketamine
Topical agents	Capsaicin, lidocaine patch, EMLA
GABA agonists	Baclofen
Miscellaneous	Calcitonin

Prolonged relief of pain following a brief local anaesthetic infusion may be possible.[253] If pain recurs, long-term subcutaneous administration of lignocaine also has been used anecdotally to yield sustained relief of refractory neuropathic pain in cancer patients.[269]

Long-term systemic local anaesthetic therapy now is usually accomplished using an oral formulation. A survey of cancer patients suggested that flecainide can be effective in the treatment of pain due to tumour infiltration of nerves.[270] In controlled trials, tocainide was effective for trigeminal neuralgia[271] and mexiletine lessened the pain of diabetic neuropathy.[272,273] One randomized trial, however failed to observe benefit from mexiletine in HIV-related painful neuropathy.[274]

These data establish the analgesic potential of systemic local anaesthetic therapy. They suggest that diverse types of pain can potentially respond. Controlled trials have emphasized the value of this therapy in neuropathic pain, and this is the use that has been pursued in clinical practice.

Mechanism of action

Systemically administered local anaesthetics presumably alter the aberrant central processing of afferent stimuli that underlies some types of neuropathic pain. Animal studies reveal that intravenous lidocaine reduces hyperalgesia,[275–277] and a clinical trial observed an isolated effect on mechanical allodynia and hyperalgesia.[263]

It is well known that local anaesthetic drugs block sodium channels and thereby impose a non-depolarizing conduction block of the action potential.[278] A profound conduction block can be produced in peripheral axons following the local instillation of these drugs, a phenomenon exploited in regional anaesthesia. This type of peripheral effect, however, does not explain the analgesia produced by systemic administration of these drugs. Non-toxic systemic doses of local anaesthetics do not block the peripheral action potential, although amplitudes are decreased to a degree.[279]

Studies of experimental models have revealed that systemic administration of local anaesthetic drugs suppresses the activity of dorsal horn neurones that are activated by C fibre input,[280] as well as the spontaneous firing of neuromas and dorsal root ganglion cells.[281,282] Thus, systemic local anaesthetic drugs probably produce analgesic effects in neuropathic pain states through suppression of aberrant electrical activity or hypersensitivity in neural structures involved in the pathogenesis of the pain. These may include sensitized central neurones, neuroma associated with damaged peripheral axons, or both.

Adverse effects

The major dose-dependent toxicities associated with the local anaesthetics affect the central nervous system and the cardiovascular system. The central nervous system effects generally occur at a lower concentration than cardiac changes. Dizziness, perioral numbness and other paraesthesias, and tremor usually occur first; at higher plasma concentrations, progressive encephalopathy develops and seizures may occur.[278] There is a correlation between the local anaesthetic potency and the dose required to produce this central nervous system toxicity.[283]

Toxic concentrations of local anaesthetic drugs can produce cardiac conduction disturbances and myocardial depression.[278] The effect on the conduction system is first observed as prolongation of the PR interval and the QRS duration. At higher concentrations, bradycardia and other arrhythmias occur. If severe enough, the depression of myocardial contractility can result in pump failure. Similar to the central nervous system effects of these drugs, the likelihood of cardiovascular toxicity with relatively low doses is correlated with local anaesthetic potency.

Thus, all local anaesthetics share a spectrum of serious, dose-dependent adverse effects, the existence of which mandates caution in dose selection and titration. Although variability across drugs in the propensity to produce these effects may be clinically relevant, comparative trials of systemically administered local anaesthetic drugs have not been performed and clinical guidelines based on adverse effect data are largely inferential.

Long-term systemic treatment with a local anaesthetic is usually accomplished with one of the oral formulations; mexiletine, tocainide, or flecainide. In the United States, flecainide has not been used commonly due to an association with sudden death during a trial of therapy for patients immediately post-myocardial infarction.[284] Neither the general applicability of this risk of sudden death to other medical settings nor the degree to which it reflects a specific effect of flecainide is known. Nonetheless, flecainide does have relatively potent local anaesthetic effects and greater negative inotropic effects than the other oral local anaesthetics, and these pharmacological actions, combined with the association with sudden death, has tended to place it in a negative light as a therapy for chronic pain. In the absence of comparative safety data, it is reasonable to consider flecainide less preferred as a potential adjuvant analgesic than other oral local anaesthetics.

Troublesome side-effects occur commonly during therapy with mexiletine or tocainide and serious adverse effects also have been described.[285] A survey of patients administered tocainide for arrhythmia noted nausea in 34 per cent, dizziness in 31 per cent, light-headedness in 24 per cent, tremors in 22 per cent, palpitations in 17 per cent, vomiting in 16 per cent, and paraesthesias in 16 per cent.[286] Rare serious reactions include interstitial pneumonitis, severe encephalopathy, blood dyscrasia, hepatitis, and dermatological reactions;[285–288] of these, the pulmonary disorder appears to be most frequent.[285] Mexiletine often produces nausea and vomiting (diminished by ingesting the drug with food), tremor, dizziness, unsteadiness, and paraesthesias, which may induce discontinuation of dosing in up to 40 per cent of patients.[285,289] Serious side-effects, including liver damage and blood dyscrasias, are very rare, however.

Pharmacology

Lidocaine is metabolized by the liver and is a substrate of CYP3A4. It can, therefore, interact with other substrates and inhibitors of this isozyme. Its active metabolites can accumulate and cause neurological toxicity.[205]

Mexiletine is a substrate of CYP2D6 and an inhibitor or CYP1A2. Phenytoin can decrease mexiletine plasma concentrations, whereas SSRIs can increase it. Its half-life is increased in elderly and patients with liver or heart failure.[205]

Indications

Data from controlled trials and clinical experience suggest that any type of neuropathic pain can be considered a potential indication for systemic local anaesthetic therapy. A survey of patients treated with a brief lignocaine infusion found that neuropathic pains related to disorders of the peripheral nervous system are more likely to respond than pains related to a central nervous system lesion, but some patients with central pain do attain at least partial relief.[249] Both continuous and lancinating dysaesthesias can be ameliorated.[271,272]

The oral local anaesthetic drugs are usually considered for the long-term management of opioid-refractory neuropathic pain. There have been no comparative clinical trials to help define the appropriate use of these drugs in relation to the many other adjuvant analgesics that may be used for this indication. Based on the limited data available concerning long-term safety and efficacy, it is appropriate to position the local anaesthetics as second-line drugs for neuropathic pain. Specifically, a trial with an oral local anaesthetic usually is considered after antidepressant and anticonvulsant drugs have been tried (see below).[290]

The role of brief intravenous local anaesthetic infusions is even less well defined. Some patients experience immediate analgesia with this technique and favourable effects have been observed to continue for some period in a minority. Although one study showed that the response to an intravenous infusion of lidocaine is a good predictor of the response to oral mexiletine treatment,[291] this trial was limited by a very small sample size and the results should not be broadly generalized.

On the basis of clinical experience, a trial of a brief local anaesthetic infusion is sometimes implemented in patients with severe neuropathic pain that has not responded promptly to an opioid and requires immediate relief. This technique, therefore, may be a useful approach to the uncommon circumstance of 'crescendo' neuropathic pain.

Dosing guidelines

On the basis of the limited data available, mexiletine appears to be the oral local anaesthetic least likely to produce serious toxicity. Although intraindividual variability in the response to different drugs in this class has not been systematically assessed, such variability has been observed commonly with other drug classes and is likely to exist with the oral local anaesthetics as well. Thus, if mexiletine does not provide relief to a patient with severe neuropathic pain that has already proved refractory to opioids and other adjuvants, trials with tocainide or flecainide are justified.

There have been no controlled comparisons of the analgesic effects produced by brief intravenous infusions of the various parenteral anaesthetics. The published experience is greatest with procaine and lignocaine, and it is reasonable to consider these drugs first.

All local anaesthetic drugs must be used cautiously in patients with pre-existing heart disease. It is prudent to avoid this therapy in those patients with cardiac rhythm disturbances, those who are receiving anti-arrhythmic drugs, and those who have cardiac insufficiency. Patients who have significant heart disease should undergo cardiac evaluation before local anaesthetic therapy is administered.

Low initial doses and dose titration may reduce the likelihood of adverse effects. In the absence of contrary information, overall dosing levels should conform to those employed in the treatment of cardiac arrhythmias. For example, mexiletine should usually be started at 150 mg once or twice per day. This and subsequent doses are better tolerated when taken with food. If intolerable side-effects do not occur, the dose can be increased by a like amount every few days until the usual maximum dose of 300 mg three times per day is reached. Plasma drug concentrations, if available, can provide useful information as described previously for the tricyclic antidepressants.

There has been no systematic evaluation of the safety or efficacy of the combination of an oral local anaesthetic and other adjuvant drugs, such as a tricyclic antidepressant or anticonvulsant. Based on clinical experience, trials of such combinations, undertaken with close clinical monitoring, can be justified in patients with refractory neuropathic pain. If administration of the local anaesthetic has yielded meaningful partial analgesia, it should be continued as a trial while another drug is initiated. If there is a risk of drug interactions, or additive toxicities, dosing must be very cautious and monitoring must be intensified.

Dosing guidelines for local anaesthetics infusion are derived from the large clinical experience with this approach and a limited number of trials in patients with neuropathic pain. Lignocaine infusions have been administered at varying doses, typically within a range of 2–5 mg/kg infused over 20–30 min.[262] In the medically frail patient, it is prudent to start at the lower end of this range and provide repeated infusions at successively higher doses.

Anticonvulsant drugs

There is good evidence that the anticonvulsant drugs are useful in the management of neuropathic pains.[26,292,293] The older drugs, which have been used for decades, are now complemented by a rapidly increasing number of newer agents. Among the older drugs, evidence of efficacy is best for carbamazepine and phenytoin. The analgesic efficacy of carbamazepine has been established by controlled studies in patients with trigeminal neuralgia,[294–297] postherpetic neuralgia (in which an effect against lancinating but not continuous pains was demonstrated),[296] and painful diabetic neuropathy.[298] These data, along with uncontrolled trials in other types of neuropathic pain, suggest that carbamazepine has analgesic efficacy in lancinating neuropathic pain, regardless of the specific pathology that induces it.

In controlled trials, phenytoin was an effective analgesic for painful neuropathy in Fabry's disease[299] and painful diabetic neuropathy.[300] Surveys and case reports also suggested efficacy in other non-malignant neuropathic pains characterized by a prominent lancinating component, as well as in cancer pain.[301]

An expanding role for the anticonvulsants began with the advent of gabapentin. The analgesic efficacy of this drug has been established through randomized trials in populations with diabetic neuropathy[48,302,303] and postherpetic neuralgia.[304–306] Open label trials and surveys suggest its efficacy in complex regional pain syndrome,[307] HIV neuropathy,[308,309] neuropathic cancer pain,[310] and diverse pains from multiple sclerosis (paroxysmal pain,[311] trigeminal neuralgia,[312] painful nocturnal spasms[313]). One case report suggests possible use as a coanalgesic to relieve pain from wound dressing care.[314] Two studies comparing gabapentin and amitriptyline in diabetic neuropathy yielded conflicting results. In one trial, amitriptyline was more effective than gabapentin (difference not statistically significant) and the occurrence of adverse events was similar.[48] The other trial revealed gabapentin to be superior to amitriptyline in relieving pain and paraesthesias, and better tolerated.[303]

Due to its proven analgesic effect in several neuropathic pains, its good tolerability, and a paucity of drug–drug interactions, gabapentin has been recommended as a first-line agent for the treatment of neuropathic pain of diverse aetiologies.[16,292,293] This approach has largely been adopted in the medically ill, despite a lack of controlled trials in these populations. An open-label trial in patients with neuropathic cancer pain revealed gabapentin to be effective in reducing not only overall pain, shooting pain, and allodynia, but also burning pain.[310]

Lamotrigine has been shown in open-label trials to relieve pain from trigeminal neuralgia,[315,316] diabetic neuropathy,[317] and multiple sclerosis.[318] Randomized trials reported benefits in trigeminal neuralgia,[319] HIV neuropathy,[320] and central poststroke pain.[321] One study on diverse neuropathic pains, however, failed to observe any significant analgesia.[322] Only one case report suggested that lamotrigine could be beneficial in neuropathic cancer pain, providing pain relief and allowing a decrease of the opioid doses.[323]

The analgesic effect of topiramate also has been assessed in several studies. Two open-label trials observed benefit in diverse neuropathic pains[324,325] and randomized trials were positive in diabetic neuropathy[326] and migraine prevention.[327] In contrast, a recent randomized trial failed to observe any benefit in central pain.[328] Like gabapentin, pregabalin is a GABAergic compound. Recent studies confirm analgesic efficacy in pain from diabetic neuropathy,[329] postherpetic neuralgia,[330] and postoperative dental pain.[331]

Tiagabine is a GABA agonist and also has antinociceptive action in animal models.[332] In humans, it has only been studied in one small open-label trial, in which it was an effective treatment for diverse neuropathic pains.[333]

Felbamate has been used anecdotally to treat hemifacial spasm[334] and trigeminal neuralgia.[335] It has been associated with myelosuppression and hepatotoxicity. With many other options now available, it is very rarely considered for pain. Levetiracetam is antinociceptive in an animal model.[336] In a small open-label trial, adding levetiracetam following a poor response to gabapentin provided good or excellent relief in 60 per cent of patients.[337] Anecdotally, experience with this drug has been favourable and further trials are indicated. With support from animal studies,[338] zonisamide has been administered to patients with a variety of neuropathic pains, including complex regional pain syndrome.[339] It also has been used for the prevention of migraine headaches.[340] These limited data support a favourable clinical experience with this drug.

Oxcarbazepine is a metabolite of carbamazepine and has a similar spectrum of effects, with better tolerability.[341] Although the current evidence is limited to case series and open-label trials, it has been reported effective in diabetic neuropathy,[342] trigeminal neuralgia,[343] complex regional pain syndrome,[344] idiopathic neuropathic pain,[345] and other diverse neuropathic pains.[341,346] It has been effective in some patients who were refractory to carbamazepine[343] or gabapentin.[341,344] Placebo-controlled studies are currently under way to assess its efficacy in painful diabetic neuropathy.[342]

Several older anticonvulsants are widely used as analgesics for neuropathic pain despite limited data from clinical trials. There is a large clinical experience with both clonazepam[347,348] and valproate.[349,350] Clonazepam often is considered for an early trial if comorbid anxiety is a substantial problem. The role of valproate may change with the recent advent of a parenteral formulation, but this is yet to be determined.

In summary, selected anticonvulsant drugs may be effective for diverse types of neuropathic pain. Although the evidence is best for carbamazepine, the potential for adverse haematologic effects associated with this drug has limited its use in the medically ill patients. Gabapentin has become one of the first-line drugs for all types of neuropathic pain due to its proven efficacy and good tolerability. A number of the newer anticonvulsants appear very promising. There have been no comparative studies and experience in the treatment of cancer pain is limited.

Mechanism of action

The specific mechanisms of the analgesia produced by the anticonvulsant drugs are not known, but presumably relate to those actions underlying anticonvulsant effects. These include suppression of paroxysmal discharges and their spread from the site of origin, and reduction of neuronal hyperexcitability.[351] It can be postulated that the aberrant electrical activity that has been recorded from different levels of the neuraxis in experimental models of nerve injury [165,281,282,352–354] and in patients with chronic neuropathic pains[355–357] is the pathophysiological substrate for the experience of lancinating pains, and that the suppression of these discharges by anticonvulsant drugs results in analgesia.

Each drug has distinct mechanisms. Carbamazepine is an iminostilbene derivative chemically related to the tricyclic antidepressants. Analgesic effects could result from receptor interactions similar to those that characterize the latter drugs, or to more specific blockade of sodium and potassium channels. Oxcarbazepine has similar mechanisms. Phenytoin and lamotrigine are sodium channels blockers which also inhibit the presynaptic release of glutamate. The analgesic effect of valproic acid and topiramate presumably is mediated by sodium channels blockade and GABA enhancement. The mechanism of action of gabapentin is not completely understood. It is a GABA analogue but has no direct effects on GABA receptors. It increases overall GABA tone in the central nervous system and has other effects as well. Pregabalin is also a GABA analogue, with an agonistic effect on GABA receptors,[293] and tiagabine is a direct agonist of these receptors.

Adverse effects

Carbamazepine commonly causes sedation, dizziness, nausea, and unsteadiness. These effects can be minimized by low initial doses and gradual dose titration. The intensity diminishes in most patients maintained on the drug for several weeks. Of much greater concern is that carbamazepine causes leukopaenia and/or thrombocytopaenia in approximately 2 per cent of patients; aplastic anaemia is a rare complication.[358] Other rare adverse effects of carbamazepine include hepatic damage, hyponatraemia due to inappropriate secretion of antidiuretic hormone, and congestive heart failure.[359,360] Baseline liver and renal function tests should also be obtained prior to therapy.

Most of the common side-effects of phenytoin are dose-dependent. These include sedation or mental clouding, dizziness, unsteadiness, and diplopia.[361] These effects usually occur at plasma concentrations above the therapeutic range for seizure control. Occasional patients experience toxicity at lower concentrations. Ataxia, progressive encephalopathy, and even seizures can occur at toxic levels.[362] Of the idiosyncratic effects, the most serious are hepatotoxicity and exfoliative dermatitis. The occurrence of a maculopapular rash, which can be the harbinger of the more severe cutaneous reactions, should lead to discontinuation of the drug. A rare permanent cerebellar degeneration has been reported in patients with chronic phenytoin intoxication.[363]

At usual therapeutic doses, the side-effects of valproate are usually mild, consisting of sedation, nausea, tremor, and sometimes increased appetite. Hepatotoxicity, encephalopathy, dermatitis, alopecia, and a rare hyperammonaemia syndrome are among the reported idiosyncratic reactions.[364]

The newer anticonvulsant drugs, including gabapentin, lamotrigine, topiramate and oxcarbazepine, are generally associated with a favourable side-effect profile.[365–368] The most common side-effects are non-specific central nervous system complaints of somnolence, mental clouding, dizziness, fatigue, or unsteadiness. Gabapentin also may cause swelling. The most serious adverse effect associated with lamotrigine is an exfoliative rash, which occurs in approximately 0.3 per cent of treated patients. All types of rash, which affect more than 4 per cent of treated patients, are more likely to occur with high initial doses and in younger patients. For this reason, the drug should be started at a low initial dose (25–50 mg/day) and titrated over 1 month; patients younger than 15 years should not be treated in the usual circumstances. If any rash occurs, the drug must be stopped immediately.

Pharmacology

Carbamazepine is highly bound to proteins. It induces liver enzymes that are responsible for its metabolism and shortens its half-life with repetitive administrations.

Phenytoin also is highly bound to proteins. Its clearance is highly variable, dependent upon intrinsic hepatic function and dose administered. It is, therefore, helpful to monitor the serum levels in order to order the optimal dose. In order to get the active form of phenytoin, the level should be corrected depending on the albumin level.

Phenytoin is an inducer of the isozymes CYP2B6 and CYP3A, and is a substrate of CYP2C9.[205] It is well known for its numerous drug interactions. It increases clearance of other drugs metabolized by CYP3A4, including methadone, midazolam, and imipramine.[139] Patients receiving phenytoin and one of these drugs might, therefore, require a higher dose of the other medication. It also decreases serum concentrations or effectiveness of lamotrigine, warfarin, corticosteroids, cyclosporin, theophylline, rifampin, quinidine, mexiletine, dysopyramide, dopamine, and several muscle relaxants.[205] Via a competitive inhibition of the enzyme system, phenytoin levels are decreased by erythromycin and increased by fluoxetine and sertraline. Acute ingestion of alcohol decreases phenytoin levels and chronic administration increases that level. Interaction with valproic acid is complex and can cause both an increase and a decrease of the phenytoin level.[139]

Gabapentin is minimally protein bound and is excreted unchanged in the urine. It is not metabolized by the liver and has no known drug–drug interactions.[139,369] Due to a saturable absorption process in the gastrointestinal tract, its bioavailability varies from 60 per cent for a single 300-mg dose to 35 per cent for 1600 mg three times daily.[370] This declining oral bioavailability at higher doses may contribute to the ceiling effect observed clinically.

Lamotrigine undergoes both hepatic and renal metabolism and elimination. Its serum concentration is decreased by carbamazepine and phenytoin, and is increased by valproate. Topiramate is well-absorbed orally, has minimal protein binding and hepatic metabolism, and is excreted unchanged in the urine. Its serum concentration can be decreased by phenytoin, carbamazepine, and valproate.[205] Tiagabine is highly protein bound and undergoes significant hepatic metabolism, mainly by the CYP3A4 isozyme. Its half-life is decreased by coadministration of carbamazepine and phenytoin.[205] Like gabapentin, levetiracetam is not metabolized in the liver and has a low potential for drug interactions.[371] Oxcarbazepine has low protein binding and is mainly metabolized by non-inducible enzymes; its minimal metabolism by the cytochrome P450 diminishes its potential for drug interactions. It can nevertheless interact with some medications, including phenytoin and oral contraceptives.[372,373]

Indications

Anticonvulsant drugs are now widely considered for all types of neuropathic pain. Given a long tradition of use in syndromes characterized by lancinating and other episodic paroxysmal neuropathic pains, such as trigeminal neuralgia, one of these drugs usually is administered as the first-line strategy for neuropathic pains of this type. The treatment of lancinating or paroxysmal neuropathic pain may also be undertaken with other selected adjuvant analgesics. As noted previously, data from controlled studies indicate that the tricyclic antidepressants can ameliorate pain of this type,[18,19] but conventional practice continues to view these drugs as a second-line approach in patients with predominating lancinating dysaesthesias. Conventional practice at the present time supports early trials of either the anticonvulsants or the antidepressant analgesics (or in some settings, the corticosteroids) for neuropathic pain syndromes that do not have a predominating lancinating component. Among the anticonvulsants, gabapentin generally is now administered first due to its proven efficacy in different neuropathic pain syndromes and its good tolerability.[292,293] Other anticonvulsants usually are tried successively, with drugs selected empirically. Given its long history of use, carbamazepine may still be selected initially for trigeminal neuralgia.[374]

Dosing guidelines

Dosing guidelines employed in the treatment of seizures are typically extrapolated for the management of pain. When treating older patients or those with multiple medical illnesses, lower initial doses and more gradual upward dose titration are prudent to increase tolerability and compliance.

Low initial doses are appropriate for most anticonvulsants, but the administration of phenytoin often begins with the presumed therapeutic dose (e.g. 300 mg/day) or a prudent oral loading regimen (e.g. 500 mg twice, separated by hours). When low initial doses are used, dose escalation should ensue until favourable effects occur, intolerable side-effects supervene, or plasma drug concentration has reached some arbitrary level (customarily at the upper end of the therapeutic range for seizures).

Although gabapentin can be started at doses between 300 and 900 mg/day, it is usually prudent to begin at 100–300 mg at bedtime in elderly patients or those with advanced illness. The dose can be increased by an amount equal to the starting dose every few days. The effective dose range is very broad. Some patients report benefit at 300–600 mg/day, whereas others require more than 3600 mg/day. The usual effective dose range is 900–2700 mg/day in two to three divided doses. The dose can be increased as long as it is well tolerated and an increase provides further relief. The initial dose should be lowered and the tapering more gradual in patients with renal insufficiency.

Carbamazepine is usually started at 100–200 mg twice daily. The dose can be increased gradually at intervals of days to weeks depending on the clinical situation. The usual therapeutic dose is 600–1600 mg daily in two to four divided doses.

Lamotrigine should be started at a dose of 25–50 mg/day. The dose should be increased on a weekly or biweekly basis (weekly increments of

25 mg/day after starting at 25 mg, or an increase from 25 mg twice daily to 50 mg twice daily after 2 weeks on the lower dose). This approach to dosing reduces the risk of cutaneous hypersensitivity. After the dose reaches 100 mg/day, further increments can be performed more quickly, and in larger amounts. The usual effective dose is between 200 and 500 mg/day.

Topiramate can be initiated at 25 mg daily and titrated gradually up to 400 mg/day, in two divided doses. The usual effective dose range is 100–300 mg/day in two divided doses. Pregabalin has been shown effective at doses of 600 mg/day for patients with normal function and 300 mg/day for patients with mild to moderate renal insufficiency. Tiagabine should be initiated with a dose of 4 mg at bedtime and increased gradually. The maximum dose studied has been 12 mg/day, in three divided doses.(333) Levetiracetam can be initiated at 500–1000 mg/day, then gradually increased. In one study, the maximum tolerated dose was 1000 mg and a mean daily dose of 750 mg was effective.(337) Higher doses are used in the clinical setting. The initial daily dose of oxcarbazepine should be 75–150 mg twice daily; doses can be gradually increased to a usual maximum of 2400 mg/day in divided doses. Analgesia seems to be achieved with relatively low doses compared to those required for epilepsy, with a mean daily dose of 814 mg in one study.(342) Zonisamide is usually started at a dose of 100–200 mg/day. The usual effective dose range is yet unclear. Clinical trials started with administration of 100 mg every fourth night, with gradual increase up to 400 mg/day over several weeks.(339,340)

Baclofen

As noted previously, several non-anticonvulsant drugs have been used in the management of lancinating or paroxysmal neuropathic pains, including the neuroleptic pimozide,(211) systemically administered local anaesthetics, and the tricyclic antidepressants.(18,19) Baclofen is another alternative, a trial of which typically precedes these other therapies (Table 4).

Baclofen, an agonist at the gamma aminobutyric acid type B ($GABA_B$) receptor, has been conclusively demonstrated to have efficacy in trigeminal neuralgia(375) and is widely considered to be the second-line pharmacological approach in this condition, following anticonvulsants.(376) Other neuropathic pains characterized by an episodic lancinating or paroxysmal phenomenology have also been reported to respond to this drug.(377–379) Although there have been a few observations that suggest a broader analgesic potential,(380) baclofen is generally considered to have a relatively selective efficacy for lancinating or paroxysmal neuropathic pain. It usually is considered for a trial in other types of neuropathic pain only after a number of other trials have been ineffective.

The administration of baclofen for pain is undertaken in a manner similar to the use of the drug for its primary indication, spasticity. A starting dose of 5 mg two to three times per day is gradually escalated to the range 30–90 mg/day, and sometimes higher if side-effects do not occur. It is appropriate to continue dose escalation until pain is relieved or limiting side-effects occur. Doses may range well over 200 mg/day. The common side-effects (dizziness, somnolence, and gastrointestinal distress) are minimized by low starting doses and gradual dose escalation. The potential for a serious withdrawal syndrome, including delirium and seizure, exists with abrupt discontinuation following prolonged use;(381) doses should always be tapered before discontinuation of the drug.

N-Methyl-D-aspartate receptor blockers

Excitatory amino acids, such as glutamate and aspartate, are released by primary afferent neurons in response to noxious stimuli and are important in the central processing of the pain-related information. Interactions at the *N*-methyl-D-aspartate (NMDA) receptor are involved in the development of central nervous system changes that may underlie chronic pain and modulate opioid mechanisms—specifically tolerance.(382) Preclinical studies have established that the *N*-methyl-D-aspartate receptor is involved in the sensitization of central neurones following injury and the development of the 'wind-up' phenomenon, a change in the response of central neurones that has been associated with neuropathic pain.(383,384)

Antagonists at the *N*-methyl-D-aspartate receptor may offer another novel approach to the treatment of pain. Although there is evidence that such drugs may be multipurpose analgesics, which could potentially ameliorate acute pain(385,386) and diverse types of chronic pain,(387–392) the most intense interest has focused on their role as new therapies for neuropathic pain. The treatment of neuropathic pain may become an indication for the use of these drugs in the palliative care setting.

A variety of *N*-methyl-D-aspartate receptor antagonists are currently undergoing intensive investigation as potential analgesics. At the present time, there are three commercially available drugs in the United States, the antitussive dextromethorphan, the general anaesthetic ketamine, and the antiviral drug amantadine. These drugs have been shown to have analgesic effects in controlled studies of experimental pain.(393,394) Intravenous or subcutaneous ketamine has been shown to be effective in reducing pain from fibromyalgia(392) as well as diverse neuropathic pains,(395,396) including postherpetic neuralgia(397) and phantom limb pain.(398) Dextromethorphan relieves pain from diabetic neuropathy(399) and facial neuralgias(400) but clinical trials failed to show any benefit in postherpetic neuralgia.(399) A new compound containing morphine and dextromethorphan seems to be more effective than morphine alone in relieving chronic cancer and non-cancer pain.(401,402)

Dextromethorphan has been widely used for many years and is generally well tolerated. Its side-effects are dose-dependent; approximately one-third of patients report uncomfortable symptoms, including dysarthria, lightheadedness, nystagmus, gastrointestinal disturbances, at relatively high doses.(403) More serious but less common adverse events include memory loss, depression, dry mouth, unsteady gait, decreased coordination, and facial numbness.(403) A prudent starting dose is 45–60 mg/day, which can be gradually escalated until favourable effects occur, side-effects supervene, or a conventional maximal dose of 1 g is achieved.

Case reports,(404–407) case series,(408) open-label(409) and randomized trials(410,411) have reported effectiveness of ketamine in relieving cancer pain(403,406,408–411) or reducing opioid requirements.(410) A continuous infusion of ketamine is also used to induce sedation in the imminently dying.(412) Several different regimens have been recommended, including intravenous boluses (0.25–0.50 mg/kg),(404,411) continuous intravenous low- or high-dose infusion (up to 600 mg/day),(406) intravenous 'burst' doses (100–500 mg/day for 3–5 days),(409) subcutaneous infusions,(405,407) and oral doses (0.5 mg/kg tid).(408,410)

Clinicians who are experienced in the use of parenteral ketamine may, therefore, consider this option in patients with refractory pain. In the palliative care setting, this treatment may be useful, for example, in patients who have advanced disease and severe neuropathic pain that has not responded adequately to opioids and several adjuvant analgesics. The side-effect profile of ketamine, which includes delirium, nightmares, hallucinosis, and dysphoria, can be daunting, however, particularly in the medically frail. Nonetheless, given the low risk of serious toxicity when sub-anaesthetic doses are used, the risks may be justified when pain has been intractable to many routine approaches.

Typically, ketamine therapy for pain has been initiated at low doses given subcutaneously, such as 0.1–0.15 mg/kg by brief infusion or 0.1–0.15 mg/kg/h by continuous infusion. The dose can be gradually escalated, with close monitoring of pain and side-effects. Long-term therapy has been maintained using continuous subcutaneous infusion or repeated subcutaneous injections. Oral administration also has been used, but experience is more limited with this approach and the ratio of doses needed to maintain effects when converting from parenteral to oral dosing is uncertain.

Other NMDA antagonists also may be considered. Amantadine is a non-competitive NMDA antagonist and limited data suggest that it might reduce pain, allodynia, and hyperalgesia in chronic neuropathic pain(413) and surgical neuropathic cancer pain.(414) Although oral amantadine has been reported to be ineffective,(415) empirical trials sometimes are undertaken in refractory neuropathic pain. Common adverse events are nervousness, lightheadedness, concentration difficulty, depression, dizziness, and insomnia. Memantine, which like amantadine may be relatively well tolerated, also blocks the NMDA receptor and has been used for refractory neuropathic pain. These drugs deserve further studies to confirm efficacy and determine whether benefits outweigh the risk of toxicity in the medically ill.

The D-isomer of the opioid methadone also blocks the NMDA receptor.[416–418] In many countries, methadone is available as the racemic mixture, 50 per cent of which is the D-isomer. The contribution of this non-opioid molecule to the analgesia produced by methadone is uncertain,[419,420] but a growing clinical experience with this drug suggests that it plays a role. There are no data, however, to support the conclusion that methadone is better than other opioids for the treatment of neuropathic pain.

New *N*-methyl-D-aspartate receptor antagonists are in development and may ultimately prove useful for a variety of medical indications. Advances in this area have occurred rapidly and it is likely that the role of these agents in the management of pain will be much better defined within a few years.

Calcitonin

Calcitonin is an interesting drug that may have several pain-related indications in the palliative care setting. Its potential role in bone pain is discussed below. In recent years, evidence has accumulated that calcitonin may also have efficacy in neuropathic pain states. Favourable controlled trials have been reported in populations with complex regional pain syndrome[421] and acute phantom pain.[422] Although the mechanisms that may be responsible for these analgesic effects are unknown, these observations justify an empirical trial of calcitonin in refractory neuropathic pain of diverse types. The adverse effects and dosing guidelines are similar to those for use as coanalgesics in bone pain, described below.

Other drugs for sympathetically maintained pain

Sympathetically maintained pain is a form of neuropathic pain in which dysaesthesias are believed to be sustained through efferent activity in the sympathetic nervous system.[423] This type of pain is believed to occur most often in patients with a clinical syndrome consistent with complex regional pain syndrome, which is characterized by the occurrence of focal autonomic dysregulation (e.g. swelling, vasomotor disturbances, and sweating abnormalities), focal motor disturbances (e.g. tremor or dystonia), or trophic changes (e.g. focal osteoporosis, atrophy of skin or subcutaneous tissues, and changes in nail or hair growth) in the region of the pain. Sympathetic nerve blocks are an important diagnostic test, and if positive, a first-line of treatment. Drug therapy is usually considered if nerve blocks fail or are contraindicated.

Drug treatments for pain that is presumed to be sympathetically maintained may involve the non-specific use of any of the aforementioned classes of adjuvant analgesics, either multipurpose drugs or drugs used specifically for neuropathic pain. Alternatively, therapy may focus on trials of drugs that either influence sympathetic function or have been specifically studied in this condition, such as phenoxybenzamine, prazosin, guanethidine, propranolol, and nifedipine.[424]

Topical analgesics

Topical therapies for neuropathic pain have been used for those syndromes characterized by both a predominating peripheral mechanism and continuous dysaesthesia. Available topical therapies include capsaicin preparations, formulations containing aspirin or a non-steroidal anti-inflammatory drug, local anaesthetic, and tricyclic preparations.[425]

The potential value of topical capsaicin in both painful mononeuropathies and polyneuropathies has been suggested from surveys of patients with postherpetic neuralgia or postmastectomy pain[426–430] and controlled trials in populations with postherpetic neuralgia[431] and painful diabetic neuropathy.[432,433] Other controlled trials, which demonstrate that topical capsaicin may relieve the pain associated with osteoarthritis of the finger joints,[434] also suggest that some painful somatic disorders may be amenable to this therapy. The benefit of topical capsaicin in painful diabetic neuropathy and osteoarthritis, as well as one non-painful condition, psoriasis, was confirmed in a meta-analysis of available controlled trials.[435] One controlled trial in HIV-associated painful peripheral neuropathy failed to show any analgesic effect.[436] In cancer patients, capsaicin cream was effective in reducing neuropathic postsurgical pain (postmastectomy, postthoracotomy, postamputation).[437]

There is some preliminary evidence that much higher doses of capsaicin (7.5–10 per cent rather than 0.025–0.075 per cent currently used clinically) could allow greater relief from burning pain, which could persist for several months after a single capsaicin exposure.[438] Application of this high-concentration formula is accomplished using general or regional anaesthesia to reduce the acute pain. The safety and efficacy of this approach remains to be clarified in future studies.

Capsaicin cream 0.025–0.075 per cent must be applied to the painful area four times a day by rubbing it in until it vanishes. A trial of several weeks is needed to adequately judge effects. Hands must be washed thoroughly immediately after application. Many patients experience severe burning pain after the first applications, which usually gradually decreases over a few days if the cream is applied regularly. Some patients tolerate the cream better if application is preceded by application of a local anaesthetic or ingestion of an analgesic. A cream combining capsaicin with the tricyclic doxepin might also cause less burning pain.[439]

Capsaicin is the ingredient of the chilli pepper producing its pungent taste. When applied topically, it binds to the vanilloid (VRI) capsaicin receptor on the afferent membrane of the small, unmyelinated, polymodal C-fibres, thereby causing the depolarization of the nociceptors and release of substance P.[440] This initial release explains the increased burning pain felt with the first applications of capsaicin. Regular use eventually leads to depletion of substance P from the terminals of afferent C-fibres, potentially leading to a decreased pain perception. Prolonged use of capsaicin can also induce degeneration of epidermal nerve fibres, which may contribute to the analgesic effect.[441]

Numerous anti-inflammatory drugs have been investigated for topical use in populations with neuropathic pain, particularly postherpetic neuralgia, and results have generally been mixed. Although one small controlled trial demonstrated efficacy greater than placebo for topical aspirin, indomethacin, and diclofenac in patients with acute herpetic neuralgia or postherpetic neuralgia,[442] another controlled trial found no efficacy whatsoever for topical treatment with a benzydamine cream in a similar patient population.[443] Survey data are similarly conflicting.[425] These limited data suggest that the efficacy of topical anti-inflammatory drugs for neuropathic pain remains unproved.

Preliminary evidence indicates that local application of a cream containing the tricyclic doxepin can relieve neuropathic pain of diverse origins, to a similar extent as capsaicin.[439,444] It is still unclear whether this analgesic effect is mediated by peripheral adenosine receptors or there is a systemic absorption of doxepin.[439] Given the safety of this approach, a trial of a topical cream compounded with this tricyclic drug, or another drug in this class, is reasonable during the treatment of chronic neuropathic pain.

A commercially available mixture of local anaesthetics, which contains a 1 : 1 mixture of prilocaine and lignocaine, is capable of penetrating the skin and producing a dense local cutaneous anaesthesia. This product, known as eutectic mixture of local anaesthetics (EMLA®) is widely used to prevent the pain of needle puncture or incision, as well as from debridement of leg ulcers.[445] A limited study in patients with postherpetic neuralgia suggests its utility in the management of some chronic neuropathic pains.[446] Surveys of relatively high concentrations of topical lignocaine,[425,447] and a controlled trial of 5 per cent lignocaine gel,[448] have also been positive in patients with postherpetic neuralgia. There is a very remote risk of toxicity from systemic absorption of a topical local anaesthetic.[446,448] Careful monitoring is needed if the anesthetic is applied repeatedly to mucous membranes or open wounds.

Guidelines for a trial of topical local anaesthetic are ill defined. To create an area of dense sensory loss using the eutectic mixture of lignocaine and prilocaine, a relatively thick application must remain in contact with the skin under an occlusive dressing for at least 1 h. This mode of administration may be difficult if the painful area is large or adjacent to the face or a mobile region of the body. There is no evidence in populations with neuropathic pain that cutaneous anaesthesia is necessary to gain benefit from a topical local anaesthetic and, anecdotally, some patients seem to respond favourably to a thin application applied without a dressing. In the absence of any systematic evaluation of dosing techniques, the patient should be encouraged to try various modes of administration in an effort to identify a salutary approach. If possible, one of these trials should include an occlusive dressing of some type (ordinary plastic wrap can be used for large areas) and a duration of application of at least 1 h.

Topical application of local anaesthetics recently has been facilitated by the development of a lidocaine 5 per cent patch. There is evidence that the lidocaine patch reduces pain and allodynia from postherpetic neuralgia,(449,450) and it is now commonly used for this indication.(28) Evidence of its analgesic effect in other neuropathic conditions is still scarce,(451) but clinical experience has been positive. The patch can be used for several years with continued moderate or greater pain relief.(450) Although the patch was studied with use limited to 12 h per day, continuous application is common in the clinical setting. Multiple patches are often used. There are limited data that indicate a high level of safety with up to three patches for periods up to 24 h.(452–454) Application of more than three patches may be useful for some patients, but this approach should be accompanied by initial monitoring for local anesthetic toxicity. An adequate trial may require several weeks of observation. The most frequently reported adverse event is mild to moderate skin redness, rash, or irritation at the patch application site, which seems to be related to the vehicle rather than to lidocaine.(450)

Anticholinesterase drugs

Anecdotal reports have described the successful use of a variety of anticholinesterase drugs in patients with diverse types of neuropathic pain.(455,456) Physostigmine has also been reported to have favourable effects when combined with morphine during the treatment of acute pain.(457) The mechanism of the putative benefits produced by these drugs is not established and treatment is associated with the potential for serious adverse effects, such as bradycardia. A trial of one of these drugs should only be considered for medically stable patients with severe refractory pain.

Benzodiazepines for neuropathic pain

The evidence for benzodiazepine analgesia is limited and conflicting. Despite some positive studies with clonazepam and alprazolam(347,348) in the management of lancinating and cancer-related neuropathic pains, critical reviews of the current information about these drugs do not support the analgesic effects of benzodiazepines for neuropathic pain.(458,459) A trial of clonazepam can nevertheless still be justified in refractory neuropathic pain on the basis of anecdotal experience, especially in the case of the common coexistence of pain and anxiety.

Adjuvant analgesics used for bone pain

Bone pain is a common problem in the palliative care setting. Radiation therapy is usually considered when bone pain is focal and poorly controlled with an opioid, or is associated with a lesion that appears prone to fracture on radiographic examination. Anecdotally, multifocal bone pain has been observed to benefit from treatment with a non-steroidal anti-inflammatory drug or a corticosteroid.(460) Other adjuvant analgesics that are potentially useful in this setting include calcitonin, biphosphonate compounds, gallium nitrate, and selected radiopharmaceuticals (Table 5). There have been no comparative trials of these adjuvant analgesics for bone pain and the selection of one over another is usually based on convenience, patient preference, and the clinical setting.

Table 5 Adjuvant analgesics used for malignant bone pain[a]

Corticosteroids
Calcitonin
Bisphosphonates
Clodronate
Pamidronate
Radionuclides
Strontium-89 (^{89}Sr)
Rhenium-186 (^{186}Re)
Samarium-153 (^{153}Sm)
Gallium nitrate

[a] Anecdotal data suggest that non-steroidal anti-inflammatory drugs are also useful in bone pain.

Calcitonin

The use of calcitonin in the treatment of various neuropathic pains has been described previously.(421,422) Bone pain may be another indication for this compound in the palliative care setting.

Calcitonin provides significant analgesia in acute osteoporotic vertebral compression fractures,(461–464) allowing earlier mobilization.(464) Although not studied, benefits also may be seen in those with other types of lesions, such as pelvic fracture.

In cancer patients, calcitonin may relieve pain from bone metastasis.(465–468) The most frequent routes of administration are subcutaneous or intranasal. If subcutaneous boluses are used, they should be preceded by skin testing with 1 IU to screen for hypersensitivity reactions, especially in patients with a history of reactions to salmon or seafood. The optimal dose is not known. A trial may be initiated at a relatively low dose, then gradually increased to 200 IU, if tolerated, and sometimes higher. The intranasal formulation avoids the need for subcutaneous injections, facilitating the use of this drug in home care. It is administered once daily, with an initial dose of 200 IU in one nostril, alternating nostrils every day.(461–463,465) Although the potential for better efficacy with higher doses have not been studied, an inadequate response can be followed by a trial of two sprays per day (400 IU), and even more in some cases. Suppositories and continuous subcutaneous administration of calcitonin also have been reported to be effective.(464,466)

Apart from infrequent hypersensitivity reactions, the main side-effect of calcitonin is nausea. The likelihood and severity of this effect may be reduced by gradual escalation from a low starting dose. According to clinical experience, nausea usually subsides after a few days and is less frequent with the intranasal form. Periodic monitoring of calcium and phosphorus is prudent during treatment.

The mechanism of action of calcitonin is still unclear and may be mulifactorial. The drug can increase endorphin levels in the central nervous system(466) and possibly can interact with the serotonergic system.(469) Peripheral effects may involve an anti-inflammatory action or a direct effect on osteoclasts.(466,469)

Intrathecal calcitonin has also been suggested to produce analgesic effects,(470) presumably independent of its putative mechanism of action in bone pain. The long-term risks and benefits of this approach are not known and this approach should be considered experimental at the present time.

Biphosphonates

Bisphophonates are analogues of inorganic pyrophosphate that inhibit osteoclast activity and, consequently, reduce bone resorption in a variety of illnesses. As such, they are mainstay approaches in the treatment of osteoporosis, Paget's disease, and tumour-induced hypercalcaemia. Many surveys and several controlled trials have established the analgesic efficacy of these compounds, particularly pamidronate and clodronate.(471–476)

Although the analgesic effect of clodronate has been shown in studies of prostate cancer,(477) multiple myeloma,(478) and various neoplasms,(472,479,480) the data are not uniformly positive.(481) An intravenous dose of 600 mg weekly provides analgesia and decreases the use of analgesics.(472,476) The main advantage of clodronate over pamidronate is its good oral bioavailability, which avoids the need of an intravenous administration. An oral dose of 1600 mg daily resulted in moderate analgesic effect and seems to be the optimal dose.(476)

Pamidronate has been extensively studied in populations with bone metastases.[476] It has been proven to have good analgesic effect in several studies of breast cancer[482–484] and multiple myeloma.[485] Although different doses have been used, the usual recommendation calls for the administration of 60–90 mg intravenously every 3–4 weeks.[476] This dose benefits approximately 50 per cent of patients.[474] There are dose-dependent effects, and a poor response at 60 mg can be followed by a trial of 90 mg; if the patient tolerates 90 mg but gets only partial relief, a trial of 120 mg can be considered. The only significant adverse events observed are occasional hypocalcaemia and nausea. It is safe in patients with impaired renal function.

Among the other biphosphonates, etidronate has been studied in two trials and failed to demonstrate any significant analgesic effect.[486,487] The analgesic effects of alendronate, zolendrenate, and ibandronate have not been studied specifically. These drugs are very potent and are likely to be active in patients with bone metastases.

The biphosphonates may also reduce other skeletal morbidity. Recent studies indicate that zolendronate can reduce skeletal morbidity in patients with multiple myeloma and breast cancer patients.[488,489] Pamidronate 90 mg every 4 weeks reduces skeletal complications (pathological fractures, need for bone radiation or surgery, spinal cord compression, hypercalcaemia) in metastatic breast cancer[484] and multiple myeloma[485] patients. Women with recurrent breast cancer and no known metastases developed fewer bone metastases, hypercalcaemic episodes, vertebral deformities, and overall rate of morbid skeletal events when clodronate was added to antitumour therapy.[490] Although the latter study did not reveal a survival advantage from clodronate therapy, the results suggest that prophylactic biphosphonates therapy may influence the presentation of metastatic disease and, in turn, reduce the likelihood of adverse disease-related outcomes.

In summary, bisphosphonates have definite analgesic effects, and reduce skeletal morbidity in patients with bone metastases from breast cancer, prostate cancer, and multiple myeloma. These drugs presumably could benefit symptoms related to osteoblastic metastases from any tumor type. Data supporting these palliative effects are compelling for pamidronate and clodronate; with the exception of etidronate, a drug with relatively poor potency, other drugs have not been studied. Newer third-generation agents alendronate, ibandronate, and zolendronate, which are much more potent, could potentially provide analgesia with oral administration. Studies are needed to confirm these effects in populations with diverse tumour types. Apart from a need to monitor for hypocalcaemia, especially in patients with extensive metastases, side-effects are usually uncommon. Given current information, a trial of pamidronate, clodronate, or a potent oral agent could be justified in most patients with symptoms related to bone metastases. The dose–response relationship should be considered when administering these drugs. If a drug other than pamidronate or clodronate is used and symptoms do not improve, a trial of one of the established agents could be considered.

Radiopharmaceuticals

Radionuclides that are absorbed at areas of high bone turnover have been evaluated as potential therapies for metastatic bone disease.[491,492] The first radionuclide introduced into clinical practice was phosphorus-32 orthophosphate. Numerous series suggest that this drug can relieve bone pain in as many as 80 per cent of patients.[493] Bone marrow suppression is the major toxicity, and the desire for a compound with a better therapeutic index has spurred the development of several new radionuclides.

Many newer radionuclides have been advocated as potential therapies for bone pain.[491,492] Strontium chloride-89, rhenium-186 hydroxyethylenediphosphonic acid, and samarium-153 ethylene-diaminetetramethylenephosphonic acid have been most promising thus far. Surveys of patients with bone metastases from a variety of tumour types have provided strong evidence that these compounds can reduce bone pain without undue risk to bone marrow or other vital structures.[494–502]

Strontium-89, which is commercially available in the United States, has been most extensively evaluated as a treatment for bone pain. Favourable effects have been reported in numerous surveys[494–496] and confirmed in placebo-controlled trials.[503,504] The larger of these controlled trials evaluated strontium-89 as an adjunct to conventional radiotherapy in 126 patients with advanced prostate cancer; treatment reduced the need for both radiotherapy and analgesic drugs.[503] Strontium-89 has also been shown to compare favourably with hemibody irradiation in a randomized trial.[505]

Reviews of the extensive clinical experience with strontium-89 suggest that pain relief occurs in approximately 80 per cent of patients, 10 per cent of whom attain complete relief.[506,507] Initial clinical response occurs in 7–21 days and peak response may be delayed for a month or more. Approximately 5–10 per cent of patients experience a transitory pain flare immediately after treatment. The usual duration of benefit is 3–6 months, after which retreatment may regain a favourable effect. Following treatment, clinically significant leucopaenia or thrombocytopaenia occur in approximately 10 and 33 per cent of patients, respectively.[503] The nadir of bone marrow effects occurs 4–8 weeks after injection and usually undergoes at least partial return to baseline by 12 weeks.

In the absence of comparative trials, the profile of clinical effects produced by strontium-89 can help clarify its role in relation to the other strategies used for bone pain. Strontium-89 is only potentially effective in the treatment of pain due to osteoblastic bone lesions or lesions with an osteoblastic component. An osteoblastic component should be confirmed by positive bone scintigraphy before treatment with this drug. Given the delayed onset and peak effects, treatment should not be administered unless patients have a life expectancy of greater than 3 months. This delay also implies that treatment should not be considered as the sole approach for patients with severe pain.

Due to the potential for bone marrow toxicity, treatment with strontium-89 should not be considered unless adequate bone marrow reserve has been documented. In the case of strontium-89, this is usually considered to be a platelet count above 60 000 and a white blood cell count above 2400.[507] Patients who continue to be candidates for myelosuppressive chemotherapy should not be treated because the effects on bone marrow may worsen the toxicity of later cytotoxic therapy or limit the ability to rebound after therapy.

Other drugs for bone pain

Gallium nitrate is another osteoclast inhibitor that may be analgesic for multifocal malignant bone pain. Experience is currently limited to a series of cases.[508] Future studies are needed to clarify the value of this drug.

Anecdotal reports have suggested that L-dopa can ameliorate metastatic bone pain.[509] More recent experience, however, has been disappointing,[510,511] and the approach cannot be recommended for routine trials.

Adjuvant analgesics used for bowel obstruction

The management of symptoms associated with malignant bowel obstruction may be challenging.[512] If surgical decompression is not feasible, the need to control pain and other obstructive symptoms, including distension, nausea, and vomiting, becomes paramount. The use of opioids may be problematic due to dose-limiting toxicity (including gastrointestinal toxicity) or the intensity of breakthrough pains. Anecdotal reports suggest that anticholinergic drugs, the somatostatin analogue octreotide, and corticosteroids may be useful adjuvant analgesics in this setting. The use of these drugs may also ameliorate non-painful symptoms and minimize the number of patients who must be considered for chronic drainage using nasogastric or percutaneous catheters.

Anticholinergic drugs

Anticholinergic drugs could theoretically relieve the symptoms of bowel obstruction by reducing propulsive and non-propulsive gut motility and decreasing intraluminal secretions.

Some patients appear to benefit from the administration of hyoscine (scopolamine).[513,514] In some countries, hyoscine is only commercially available as the hydrobromide salt, which readily crosses the blood–brain barrier. Although this formulation can be delivered via a transdermal system, which simplifies treatment in patients with bowel obstruction, it is likely to be associated with a relatively higher incidence of central nervous system side-effects, such as somnolence and confusion, than an anticholinergic drug with less penetration through the blood–brain barrier. Two small series demonstrated that hyoscine butylbromide, which is less likely to pass the blood–brain barrier due to low lipid solubility, can be effective for obstructive symptoms, including pain.[515,516] Glycopyrrolate has a pharmacological profile similar to hyoscine butylbromide, but has not been systematically evaluated in a population with symptomatic bowel obstruction. In medically ill patients who are predisposed to central nervous system toxicity, a trial of one of the latter drugs may be warranted on theoretical grounds.

Octreotide

The somatostatin analogue octreotide inhibits the secretion of gastric, pancreatic, and intestinal secretions and reduces gastrointestinal motility. These effects probably underlie the analgesic effects that have been reported in case series of symptomatic treatment of bowel obstruction.[516] The benefits of these drugs may occur more rapidly than hyoscine.[517] Octreotide has also been used to manage severe diarrhoea due to enterocolic fistula, high output jejunostomies or ileostomies, or secretory tumours of the gastrointestinal tract.[518–520]

Octreotide has a good safety profile but is expensive. In some settings, however, the cost may be balanced by an excellent clinical response or the avoidance of the costs involved in the use of a gastrointestinal drainage procedure.

Corticosteroids

As discussed previously, the symptoms associated with bowel obstruction may improve with corticosteroid therapy. The mode of action is unclear and the most effective drug, dose, and dosing regimen are unknown. A broad range of doses have been described anecdotally. For example, dexamethasone has been used for this indication in a dose range of 8–60 mg/day[160,161] and methylprednisolone has been administered in a dose range of 30–50 mg/day.[150] One study even used a dose as high as 240 mg/day for 3 days, however, without showing any benefit compared to 40 mg/day.[521] The potential for complications during long-term therapy, including an increased risk of bowel perforation,[172,173] may limit this approach to patients with short life expectancies.

Adjuvant analgesics used for musculoskeletal pain

Although pains that originate from injury to muscle or connective tissue are prevalent in the medically ill,[522] there has been no systematic evaluation of analgesic therapies for this problem. In the management of acute traumatic sprains or strains in the non-medically ill, non-opioid and opioid analgesics are commonly supplemented by treatment with so-called muscle relaxant drugs or benzodiazepines. The role of the latter drugs for opioid-refractory musculoskeletal pains in populations with advanced medical illness remains ill defined.

Muscle relaxants

The so-called muscle relaxants include drugs in a variety of classes, all of which are marketed for the treatment of acute musculoskeletal pain. In the United States, this group includes drugs that are also administered as antihistamines (e.g. orphenadrine), tricyclic compounds structurally similar to the tricyclic antidepressants (e.g. cyclobenzaprine), and other types of drugs (e.g. carisoprodol, chlorzoxazone, metaxalone, and methocarbamol).

The efficacy of the muscle relaxant drugs in common musculoskeletal pains has been established in placebo-controlled studies.[523–526] Some studies have demonstrated analgesic effects that are superior to either aspirin or acetaminophen, and others have shown that the combination of a muscle relaxant and one of the latter drugs provides better analgesia than does aspirin or acetaminophen alone. There have been no controlled comparative trials or studies that have directly compared the efficacy and side-effect profiles of these drugs with either non-steroidal anti-inflammatory drugs or opioids.

Although muscle relaxant drugs can relieve musculoskeletal pains, these effects may not be specific and do not depend on relaxation of skeletal muscle. The label 'muscle relaxant' notwithstanding, there is actually no evidence that these drugs relax skeletal muscle in the clinical setting. They do inhibit polysynaptic myogenic reflexes in animal models, but the relationship between this action and analgesia is not known.

Thus, the muscle relaxant drugs are best viewed as alternatives to the anti-inflammatory drugs and opioids, which may be indicated in musculoskeletal pains because of the evidence of analgesic efficacy in these conditions. These drugs should not be administered in the mistaken belief that they relieve muscle spasm.

The muscle relaxant drugs are generally well tolerated, but have sedative effects that may be additive to other centrally acting drugs, including the opioids. Anecdotally, some patients report differences among drugs in analgesic efficacy or sedative side-effects, and it is reasonable to switch to an alternative drug if treatment is initially ineffective. Although the dose–response relationships of the muscle relaxant drugs have not been systematically explored, there are probably dose-dependent effects and the use of a low initial dose followed by gradual dose escalation can be recommended as a means to identify the most salutary balance between analgesia and side-effects. Experience with these drugs is too limited to pursue dose escalation beyond the usual recommended range.

If the muscle spasm is believed to be related to the pain, it may be justifiable to consider a trial of a drug with established effect on skeletal muscle. Treatment with diazepam or another benzodiazepine,[527] the alpha-2 adrenergic agonist tizanidine, or the $GABA_B$ agonist baclofen could be tried. A trial of one of the muscle relaxants might be considered, but not as a drug with specific efficacy, and the potential for side-effects and withdrawal phenomenon should elicit caution in selecting drugs of this class.[528]

Other adjuvant analgesics

Many other drugs have analgesic effects, but are not usually administered for pain in the palliative care setting. Some, such as the psychostimulants, are given for alternative indications; others have been disappointing in clinical practice or are yet too new to confirm safety and efficacy in the medically ill population.

Psychostimulants

There is substantial evidence that psychostimulant drugs have analgesic effects.[529] Controlled, single-dose studies have established the analgesic efficacy of dextroamphetamine in postoperative pain,[530] methylphenidate in pain associated with Parkinson's disease[531] or cancer,[532] and caffeine in headache, sore throat, and oral surgery pain.[533–536] Although pain is not considered a primary indication for these drugs, this potential for analgesic effects may influence the decision to recommend a trial in the medically ill.

Controlled trials of methylphenidate in the cancer population have established that this drug can reduce opioid-induced somnolence,[532,537,538] improve cognition,[539] treat depression,[540,541] and alleviate fatigue.[542] The management of central nervous system side-effects is an important issue, and, accordingly, the practical use of psychostimulants in the palliative care setting has focused on this indication, rather than the treatment of unrelieved pain.

Modafinil, a newer psychostimulant with a unique mechanism, has been used to alleviate somnolence in narcolepsy patients,[543] enhance antidepress-ant therapy,[544] and relieve fatigue in multiple sclerosis patients.[545] It is now also used to reduce opioid-induced somnolence in cancer patients.[546]

The psychostimulants are usually well tolerated. A survey of 50 patients treated with methylphenidate observed early toxicity in two patients (hallucinations and a paranoid reaction, respectively) and no late toxicity.[547] Anecdotal experience suggests that the other psychostimulants have a similarly favourable therapeutic index. The potential for tremulousness, anorexia and weight loss, insomnia, and tachycardia or hypertension should be recognized and monitored during therapy.

Treatment with methylphenidate or dextroamphetamine is typically begun at 2.5–5 mg in the morning and again at midday, if necessary, to keep the patient alert during the day and not interfere with sleep at night. The second is usually needed. Doses are increased gradually until efficacy is established. Although few patients require more than 40 mg/day in divided doses, occasional patients benefit from higher doses. Some patients require dose escalation later in the course of therapy. Modafinil is usually started at 100 mg/day and then increased. Maximal doses have not been defined.

Antihistamines

Controlled, single-dose studies have established that diphenhydramine, hydroxyzine, orphenadrine, phenyltoloxamine, and pyrilamine can have analgesic effects.(523,525,548–553) Favourable effects from antihistamine-containing proprietary pain relievers have also been observed.(554) These data suggest that antihistaminic drugs may be non-specific analgesics.

Although recent case reports reported some adjuvant analgesic efficacy from diphenydramine,(555) clinical experience has been disappointing. The reason for this disparity is not evident, but the failure to observe substantial analgesia from the addition of an antihistamine suggests that treatment should be considered only for patients who have indications other than pain. Hydroxyzine, for example, is sometimes administered to patients with pain complicated by anxiety, nausea, or itch in the hope that analgesia will be augmented while these other symptoms are relieved. The use of these agents must also be tempered by the potential for side-effects (e.g. somnolence) that add to those produced by other centrally acting drugs, including the opioids.

Cannabinoids

Cannabinoids have antinociceptive effects in animal models(556,557) and single-dose studies of intramuscular levonantradol in postoperative pain and oral delta-9-tetrahydrocannabinol in cancer pain demonstrated clear analgesic effects.(558,559) In the study of cancer pain, for example, 10 mg of delta-9-tetrahydrocannabinol was well tolerated and produced analgesic effects similar to 60 mg codeine, but a higher dose yielded severe side-effects in many patients.(558) Thus, the therapeutic window for this drug appears narrow and maximal efficacy at tolerable doses is limited. Various cannabinoids are now being studied for their potential medical effects. Given the involvement of central cannabinoid receptors in nociceptive processing, the possibility of clinically relevant analgesic effects from these drugs should be pursued in future studies.

Conclusions

Although the use of adjuvant analgesics in palliative care remains largely guided by anecdotal experience, controlled clinical trials have begun to provide a scientific rationale for many therapies. Future investigations of nociceptive processes and pain pathophysiology will undoubtedly lead to the development of novel drugs. For example, the adjuvant analgesics may one day include drugs that modulate peripheral nociceptive processes, such a substance P or bradykinin antagonists, or drugs that alter central processing by interacting with gangliosides or second messenger systems activated by excitatory amino acids. Although opioid drugs continue to be the major approach to the treatment of pain in the palliative care setting, adjuvant analgesics offer opportunities for improved outcomes in the substantial group of patients who cannot attain an acceptable balance between pain relief and side-effects.

References

1. **Cherny, N.I. and Portenoy, R.K.** (1999). Cancer pain: principles of assessment and syndromes. In *Textbook of Pain* 4th edn. (ed. P.D. Wall and R. Melzack), pp. 1017–64. London: Churchill Livingstone.
2. **Gonzales, G.R., Elliot, K.J., Portenoy, R.K., and Foley, K.M.** (1991). The impact of a comprehensive evaluation in the management of cancer pain. *Pain* (1990) **47**, 141–4.
3. **Jorgensen, L., Mortensen, M.-J., Jensen, N.-H., and Eriksen, J.** (1990). Treatment of cancer pain patients in a multidisciplinary pain clinic. *The Pain Clinic* **3**, 83–9.
4. **Moulin, D.E. and Foley, K.M.** (1990). Review of a hospital-based pain service. In *Advances in Pain Research and Therapy* Vol. 16 (ed. K.M. Foley, J.J. Bonica, and V. Ventafridda), pp. 413–27. Second International Congress on Cancer Pain. New York: Raven Press.
5. **Portenoy, R.K.** (1989). Cancer pain: epidemiology and syndromes. *Cancer* **63**, 2298–307.
6. **Schug, S.A., Zech, D., and Dorr, U.** (1990). Cancer pain management according to WHO analgesic guidelines. *Journal of Pain and Symptom Management* **5**, 27–32.
7. **Schug, S.A., Zech, D., Grond, S., Jung, H., Meurser, T, and Stobbe, B.** (1992). A long-term survey of morphine in cancer pain patients. *Journal of Pain and Symptom Management* **7**, 259–66.
8. **Takeda, F.** (1986). Results of field testing in Japan of the WHO draft interim guidelines on relief of cancer pain. *The Pain Clinic* **1**, 83–9.
9. **Toscani, F. and Carini, M.** (1989). The implementation of WHO guidelines for the treatment of advanced cancer pain at a district general hospital in Italy. *The Pain Clinic* **3**, 37–48.
10. **Ventafridda, V., Tamburini, M., and De Conno, F.** (1985). Comprehensive treatment in cancer pain. In *Advances in Pain Research and Therapy* Vol. 9 (ed. H.L. Fields, R. Dubner, and F. Cervero), pp. 617–28. Proceedings of the Fourth World Congress on Pain. New York: Raven Press.
11. **Ventafridda, V., Tamburini, M., Caraceni, A., De Conno, F, and Naldi, F.** (1987). A validation study of the WHO method for cancer pain relief. *Cancer* **59**, 850–6.
12. **Vijayaram, S., Bhargava, K., Ramamani, C.S., Heranjal, R., and Lobo, B.** (1989). Experience with oral morphine for cancer pain relief. *Journal of Pain and Symptom Management* **4**, 130–4.
13. **Walker, V.A., Hoskin, P.J., Hanks, G.W., and White, I.D.** (1988). Evaluation of WHO analgesic guidelines for cancer pain in a hospital-based palliative care unit. *Journal of Pain and Symptom Management* **3**, 145–9.
14. **World Health Organization.** *Cancer Pain Relief and Palliative Care.* Geneva: World Health Organization, 1990.
15. **Portenoy, R.K. and Lesage, P.** (1999). Management of cancer pain. *Lancet* **353**, 1695–700.
16. **Ripamonti, C. and Dickerson, E.D.** (2001). Strategies for the treatment of cancer pain in the new millennium. *Drugs* **61**, 955–77.
17. **Grond, S., Radbruch, L., Meuser, T., Sabatowki, R., Loick, G., and Lehmann, K.A.** (1999). Assessment and treatment of neuropathic cancer pain following WHO guidelines. *Pain* **79**, 15–20.
18. **Max, M.B., Culnane, M., Schafer, S.C., Gracely, R.H., Walther, D.J., Smoller, B., and Dubner, R.** (1987). Amitriptyline relieves diabetic neuropathy pain in patients with normal or depressed mood. *Neurology* **37**, 589–96.
19. **Kishore-Kumar, R., Max, M.B., Schafer, S.C., Gaughan, A.M., Smoller, B., Gracely, R.H., and Dubner, R.** (1990). Desipramine relieves postherpetic neuralgia. *Clinical Pharmacology and Therapeutics* **47**, 305–12.
20. **Ventafridda, V., Bianchi, M., Ripamonti, C., Sacerdote, P., De Conno, F., Zecca, E., and Panerai, A.E.** (1990). Studies on the effects of antidepressant drugs on the antinociceptive action of morphine and on plasma morphine in rat and man. *Pain* **43**, 155–62.
21. **Monks, R. and Merskey, H.** (1999). Psychotropic drugs. In *Textbook of Pain* 4th edn. (ed. P.D. Wall and R. Melzack), pp. 1155–86. London: Churchill Livingstone.
22. **Onghena, P. and Van Houdenhove, B.** (1992). Antidepressant-induced analgesia in chronic nonmalignant pain: a meta-analysis of 39 placebo-controlled studies. *Pain* **49**, 205–19.
23. **Watson, C.P.** (2000). The treatment of neuropathic pain: antidepressants and opioids. *Clinical Journal of Pain* **16** (2 Suppl.), S49–55.
24. **Ansari, A.** (2000). The efficacy of newer antidepressants in the treatment of chronic pain: a review of current literature. *Harvard Review of Psychiatry* **7**, 257–77.
25. **Salerno, S.N., Browning, R., and Jackson, J.L.** (2002). The effect of antidepressant treatment on chronic back pain: a meta-analysis. *Archives of Internal Medicine* **162**, 19–24.
26. **Collins, S.L., Moore, R.A., McQuay, H.J., and Wiffen, P.** (2000). Antidepressants and anticonvulsants for diabetic neuropathy and postherpetic neuralgia: a quantitative systematic review. *Journal of Pain and Symptom Management* **20**, 449–58.
27. **Sindrup, S.H. and Jensen, T.S.** (2000). Pharmacologic treatment of pain in polyneuropathy. *Neurology* **55**, 915–20.

28. **Kanazi, G.H., Johnson, R.W., and Dworkin, R.H.** (2000). Treatment of postherpetic neuralgia: an update. *Drugs* **59**, 1113–26.
29. **Gobel, H., Hamouz, V., Hansen, C., Heininger, K., Hirsche, S., Lindner, V., Heuss, D., and Soyka, D.** (1994). Chronic tension-type headache: amitriptyline reduces clinical headache duration and experimental pain sensitivity but does not alter pericranial muscle activity readings. *Pain* **59**, 241–50.
30. **Couch, J.R., Ziegler, D.K., and Hassanein, R.** (1976). Amitriptyline in the prophylaxis of migraine: effectiveness and relationship of antimigraine and antidepressant effects. *Neurology* **26**, 121–7.
31. **Diamond, S. and Baltes, B.J.** (1971). Chronic tension headache—treatment with amitriptyline—a double-blind study. *Headache* **11**, 110–16.
32. **Gomersall, J.D. and Stuart, A.** (1973). Amitriptyline in migraine prophylaxis. *Journal of Neurology, Neurosurgery and Psychiatry* **3C**, 684–90.
33. **Lance, J.W. and Curran, D.A.** (1964). Treatment of chronic tension headache. *Lancet* **1**, 1236–9.
34. **Indaco, A. and Carrieri, P.B.** (1988). Amitriptyline in the treatment of headache in patients with Parkinson's disease: a double-blind placebo-controlled study. *Neurology* **38**, 1720–2.
35. **Okasha, A., Ghaleb, A.A., and Sadek, A.** (1973). A double-blind trial for the clinical management of psychogenic headache. *British Journal of Psychiatry* **122**, 181–3.
36. **Descombes, S., Brefel-Courbon, C., Thalamas, C., Albucher, J.F., Rascol, O., Montastruc, J.L., and Senard, J.M.** (2001). Amitriptyline treatment in chronic drug-induced headache: a double-blind comparative pilot study. *Headache* **41**, 178–82.
37. **Frank, R.G., Kashani, J.H., Parker, J.C., Beck, N.C., Brownlee-Duffeck, M., Elliott, T.R., Haut, A.E., Atwood, C., Smith, E., and Kay, D.R.** (1988). Antidepressant analgesia in rheumatoid arthritis. *The Journal of Rheumatology* **15**, 1632–8.
38. **Ward, N.G.** (1986). Tricyclic antidepressants for chronic low back pain: mechanism of action and predictors of response. *Spine* **11**, 661–5.
39. **Watson, C.P.N., Evans, R.J., Reed, K., Merskey, H., Goldsmith, L., and Warsh, J.** (1982). Amitriptyline versus placebo in postherpetic neuralgia. *Neurology* **32**, 671–3.
40. **Watson, C.P.N., Chipman, M., Reed, K., Evans, R.J., and Birkett, N.** (1992). Amitriptyline versus maprotiline in postherpetic neuralgia: a randomized double-blind, crossover trial. *Pain* **48**, 29–36.
41. **Bowsher, D.** (1997). The effects of pre-emptive treatment of postherpetic neuralgia with amitriptyline: a randomized, double-blind, placebo-controlled trial. *Journal of Pain and Symptom Management* **13**, 327–31.
42. **Watson, C.P.N., Vernich, L., Chipman, M., and Reed, K.** (1998). Nortriptyline versus amitriptyline in post-herpetic neuralgia: a randomized trial. *Neurology* **51**, 1166–71.
43. **Carette, S., McCain, G.A., Bell, D.A., and Fam, A.G.** (1986). Evaluation of amitriptyline in primary fibrositis: a double-blind, placebo-controlled study. *Arthritis and Rheumatism* **29**, 655–9.
44. **Dinerman, H., Felsen, D., and Goldenberg, D.** (1985). A randomized clinical trial of naproxen and amitriptyline in primary fibromyalgia. *Arthritis and Rheumatism* **159** (Suppl.), 28–33.
45. **Carette, S.** et al. (1994). Comparison of amitriptyline, cyclobenzaprine, and placebo in the treatment of fibromyalgia: a randomized, double-blind clinical trial. *Arthritis and Rheumatism* **37**, 32–40.
46. **Max, M.B., Lynch, S.A., Muir, J., Shoaf, S.E., Smoller, B., and Dubner, R.** (1992). Effects of desipramine, amitriptyline, and fluoxetine on pain in diabetic neuropathy. *New England Journal of Medicine* **326**, 1250–6.
47. **Vrethem, M., Boivie, J., Arnqvist, H., Holmgren, H., Lindstrôm, T., and Thorell, L.H.** (1997). A comparison of amitriptyline and maprotiline in the treatment of painful polyneuropathy in diabetics and nondiabetics. *Clinical Journal of Pain* **13**, 313–23.
48. **Morello, C.M., Leckband, S.G., Stoner, C.P., Moorhouse, D.F., and Sahagian, G.A.** (1999). Randomized double-blind study comparing the efficacy of gabapentin with amitriptyline on diabetic peripheral neuropathy pain. *Archives of Internal Medicine* **159**, 1931–7.
49. **Leijon, G. and Boivie, J.** (1989). Central post-stroke pain: a controlled trial of amitriptyline and carbamazepine. *Pain* **36**, 27–36.
50. **Sharav, Y., Singer, E., Schmidt, E., Dionne, R.A., and Dubner, R.** (1987). The analgesic effect of amitriptyline on chronic facial pain. *Pain* **31**, 199–209.
51. **Ventafridda, V., Bonezzi, C., Caraceni, A., De Conno, F., Guarise, G., Ramella, G., Saita, L., Silvani, V., Tamburini, M., and Toscani, F.** (1987). Antidepressants for cancer pain and other painful syndromes with deafferentation component: comparison of amitriptyline and trazodone. *Italian Journal of Neurological Sciences* **8**, 579–87.
52. **Pilowsky, I., Hallett, E.C., Bassett, D.L., Thomas, P.G., and Penhall, R.K.** (1982). A controlled study of amitriptyline in the treatment of chronic pain. *Pain* **14**, 169–79.
53. **Kieburtz, K., Simpson, D., Yiannoutsos, C., Max, M.B., Hall, C.D., Ellis, R.J., Marra, C.M., McKendall, R., Singer, E., Dal Pan, G.J., Clifford, D.B., Tucker, T., and Cohen, B.** (1998). A randomized trial of amitriptyline and mexiletine for painful neuropathy in HIV infection. *Neurology* **51**, 1682–8.
54. **Shlay, J.C., Chaloner, K., Max, M.B., Flaws, B., Reichelderfer, P., Wentworth, D., Hillman, S., Brizz, B., and Cohn, D.L.** (1998). Acupuncture and amitriptyline for pain due to HIV-related peripheral neuropathy: a randomized controlled trial. *Journal of the American Medical Association* **280**, 1590–5.
55. **Glick, E.N. and Fowler, P.D.** (1979). Imipramine in chronic arthritis. *Pharmacology and Medicine* **1**, 94–6.
56. **Kvinesdal, B., Molin, J., Froland, A., and Gram, L.F.** (1984). Imipramine treatment of painful diabetic neuropathy. *Journal of the American Medical Association* **251**, 1727–30.
57. **Sindrup, S.H., Ejlertsen, B., Froland, A., Sindrup, E.H., Brosen, K., and Gram, L.F.** (1989). Imipramine treatment in diabetic neuropathy: relief of subjective symptoms without changes in peripheral and autonomic nerve function. *European Journal of Clinical Pharmacology* **37**, 151–3.
58. **Sindrup, S.H., Gram, L.F., Skjold, T., Froland, A., and Beck-Nielsen, H.** (1990). Concentration–response relationship in imipramine treatment of diabetic neuropathy symptoms. *Clinical Pharmacology and Therapeutics* **47**, 509–15.
59. **Alcoff, J., Jones, E., Rust, P., and Newman, R.** (1982). Controlled trial of imipramine for chronic low back pain. *Journal of Family Practice* **14**, 841–6.
60. **Cannon, R.O.** et al. (1994). Imipramine in patients with chest pain despite normal coronary angiograms. *New England Journal of Medicine* **330**, 1411–17.
61. **Ward, N.G., Bloom, V.L., and Friedel, R.P.** (1979). The effectiveness of tricyclic antidepressants in the treatment of coexisting pain and depression. *Pain* **7**, 331–41.
62. **Evans, W., Gensler, F., Blackwell, B., and Galbrecht, C.** (1973). The effects of antidepressant drugs on pain relief and mood in the chronically ill. *Psychosomatics* **14**, 214–19.
63. **Morland, T.J., Storli, O.V., and Mogstad, T.E.** (1979). Doxepin in the treatment of mixed vascular and tension headaches. *Headache* **19**, 382–3.
64. **Hameroff, S.R., Weiff, J.L., Lerman, J.C., Cork, R.C., Watts, K.S., Crago, B.R., Neuman, C.P., Womble, J.R., and Davis, T.P.** (1982). Doxepin effects on chronic pain, depression and plasma opioids. *Journal of Clinical Psychiatry* **43**, 22–7.
65. **McCleane, G.** (2000). Topical application of doxepin hydrochloride, capsaicin and a combination of both produces analgesia in chronic human neuropathic pain: a randomized, double-blind, placebo-controlled study. *British Journal of Clinical Pharmacology* **49**, 574–9.
66. **Epstein, J.B., Truelove, E.L., Oien, H., Allison, C., Le, N.D., and Epstein, M.S.** (2001). Oral topical doxepin rinse: analgesic effect in patients with oral mucosal pain due to cancer or cancer therapy. *Oral Oncology* **37**, 632–7.
67. **Panerai, A.E., Monza, G., Movillia, P., Bianchi, M., Francucci, B.M., and Tiengo, M.** (1990). A randomized, within-patient crossover, placebo-controlled trial on the efficacy and tolerability of the tricyclic antidepressants chlorimipramine and nortriptyline in central pain. *Acta Neurologica Scandinavica* **82**, 34–8.
68. **Langohr, H.D., Stohr, M., and Petruch, F.** (1982). An open and double-blind crossover study on the efficacy of clomipramine (Anafranil) in patients with painful mono- and polyneuropathies. *European Neurology* **21**, 309–17.
69. **Eberhard, G., von Knorring, L., Nilsson, H.L., Sundequist, U., Bjorling, G., Linder, H., Svard, K.O., and Tysk, L.** (1988), A double-blind randomized study of clomipramine versus maprotiline in patients with idiopathic pain syndromes. *Neuropsychobiology* **19**, 25–34.
70. **Sindrup, S.H., Gram, L.F., Skjold, T., Grodum, E., Brosen, K., and Beck-Nielsen, H.** (1990). Clomipramine versus desipramine versus placebo in the treatment of diabetic neuropathy symptoms. A double-blind cross-over study. *British Journal of Clinical Pharmacology* **30**, 683–91.

71. **Caruso, I., Sarzi Putini, P.C., Boccassini, L., Santandrea, S., Locati, M., Volpato, R., Montrone, F., Benvenuti, C., and Beretta, A.** (1987). Double-blind study of dothiepin versus placebo in the treatment of primary fibromyalgia syndrome. *Journal of International Medical Research* **15**, 154–7.
72. **Feinman, C., Harris, M., and Cawley, R.** (1984). Psychogenic facial pain: presentation and treatment. *British Medical Journal* **288**, 436–8.
73. **Gomez-Perez, F.J., Riell, J.A., Dies, H., Rodriguez-Rivera, J.G., Gonzalez-Barranco, J., and Lozano-Castaneda, O.** (1985). Nortriptyline and fluphenazine in the symptomatic treatment of diabetic neuropathy. A double-blind crossover study. *Pain* **23**, 395–400.
74. **Atkinson, J.H., Slater, M.A., Wahlgren, D.R., Williams, R.A., Zisook, S., Pruitt, S.D., Epping-Jordan, J.E., Patterson, T.L., Grant, I., Abramson, I., and Garfin, S.R.** (1999). Effects of noradrenergic and serotonergic antidepressants on chronic low back pain intensity. *Pain* **83**, 137–45.
75. **Davidoff, G., Guarracini, M., Roth, E., Sliwa, J., and Yarkony, G.** (1987). Trazodone hydrochloride in the treatment of dysesthetic pain in traumatic myelopathy: a randomized, double-blind, placebo-controlled study. *Pain* **29**, 151–61.
76. **Sindrup, S.H., Gram, L.F., Brosen, K., Eshoj, O., and Mogensen, E.F.** (1990). The selective serotonin reuptake inhibitor paroxetine is effective in the treatment of diabetic neuropathy symptoms. *Pain* **42**, 135–44.
77. **Sindrup, S.H., Bjerre, U., Dejgaard, A., Brojen, K., Aaes-Jorgensen, T., and Gram, L.F.** (1992). The selective serotonin reuptake inhibitor citalopram relieves the symptoms of diabetic neuropathy. *Clinical Pharmacology and Therapeutics* **52**, 547–52.
78. **Johansson, F. and von Knorring, L.** (1979). A double-blind controlled study of a serotonin uptake inhibitor (zimelidine) versus placebo in chronic pain patients. *Pain* **7**, 69–78.
79. **Watson, C.P.N. and Evans, R.J.** (1985). A comparative trial of amitriptyline and zimelidine in postherpetic neuralgia. *Pain* **23**, 387–94.
80. **Diamond, S. and Frietag, F.G.** (1989). The use of fluoxetine in the treatment of headache. *Clinical Journal of Pain* **5**, 200–1.
81. **Geller, S.A.** (1989). Treatment of fibrositis with fluoxetine hydrochloride (Prozac). *American Journal of Medicine* **87**, 594–5.
82. **Goldenberg, D., Mayskiy, M., Mossey, C., Ruthazer, R., and Schmid, C.** (1996). A randomized, double-blind crossover trial of fluoxetine and amitriptyline in the treatment of fibromyalgia. *Arthritis and Rheumatism* **39**, 1852–9.
83. **Lascelles, R.G.** (1966). Atypical facial pain and depression. *British Journal of Psychiatry* **122**, 651–9.
84. **Anthony, M. and Lance, J.W.** (1969). Monoamine oxidase inhibitors in the treatment of migraine. *Archives of Neurology* **21**, 263–8.
85. **Enggaard, T.P., Klitgaard, N.A., Gram, L.F., Arendt-Nielsen, L., and Sindrup, S.H.** (2001). Specific effect of venlafaxine on single and repetitive experimental painful stimuli in humans. *Clinical Pharmacology & Therapeutics* **69**, 245–51.
86. **Davis, J.L. and Smith, R.L.** (1999). Painful peripheral diabetic neuropathy treated with venlafaxine HCl extended release capsules. *Diabetes Care* **22**, 1909–10.
87. **Pernia, A., Mico, J.A., Calderon, E., and Torres, L.M.** (2000). Venlafaxine for the treatment of neuropathic pain. *Journal of Pain and Symptom Management* **19**, 408–9.
88. **Sumpton, J.E. and Moulin, D.E.** (2001). Treatment of neuropathic pain with venlafaxine. *Annals of Pharmacotherapy* **35**, 557–9.
89. **Sindrup, S.H., Bach, F.W., Madsen, C., and Jensen, T.S.** (2002). Venlafaxine compared to imipramine in painful polyneuropathy. *Journal of Pain* **3** (2 Suppl. 1), 42 (abstract 767).
90. **Goodman, J.F.** (1997). Treatment of headache with bupropion. *Headache* **37**, 256.
91. **Pinsker, W.** (1998). Treatment of headache with bupropion. *Headache* **38**, 58.
92. **Davidson, J.R.T. and France, R.D.** (1994). Bupropion in chronic low back pain. *Journal of Clinical Psychiatry* **55**, 362.
93. **Semenchuk, M.R. and Davis, B.** (2000). Efficacy of sustained-release bupropion in neuropathic pain: an open-label study. *Clinical Journal of Pain* **16**, 6–11.
94. **Semenchuk, M.R., Sherma, S., and Davis, B.** (2001). Double-blind, randomized trial of bupropion SR for the treatment of neuropathic pain. *Neurology* **57**, 1583–8.
95. **Pick, C.G., Paul, D., Eison, M.S., and Pasternak, G.W.** (1992). Potentiation of opioid analgesia by the antidepressant nefazodone. *European Journal of Pharmacology* **211**, 375–81.
96. **Walsh, T.D.** (1986). Controlled study of imipramine and morphine in chronic pain due to advanced cancer. *Proceedings of the American Society of Clinical Oncology* **5**, 237.
97. **Breivik, H. and Rennemo, F.** (1982). Clinical evaluation of combined treatment with methadone and psychotropic drugs in cancer patients. *Acta Anaesthetica Scandinavica* **74**, 135–40.
98. **Magni, G., Arsie, D., and DeLeo, D.** (1987). Antidepressants in the treatment of cancer pain: a survey in Italy. *Pain* **29**, 347–53.
99. **Hugues, A., Chauvergne, J., Lissilour, T., and Lagarde, C.** (1963). L'imipramine utilisee comme antalgique majeur en carcinologie: etude de 118 cas. *Presse Medicale* **71**, 1073–4.
100. **Bernard, A. and Scheuer, H.** (1972). Action de la clomipramine (Anafranil) sur la douleur des cancers en pathologie cervico-faciale. *Journal Francais d'Oto-rhino-laryngologie* **21**, 723–8.
101. **Cooper, G.L.** (1988). The safety of fluoxetine: an update. *British Journal of Psychiatry* **153** (Suppl. 3), 77–86.
102. **Boyer, W.F. and Blumhardt, C.L.** (1992). The safety profile of paroxetine. *Journal of Clinical Psychiatry* **53** (Suppl. 2), 61–6.
103. **Kerr, J.S., Fairweather, D.B., Mahendran, R., and Hindmarch, I.** (1992). The effects of paroxetine, alone and in combination with alcohol on psychomotor performance and cognitive function in the elderly. *International Clinical Psychopharmacology* **7**, 101–8.
104. **Preskorn, S.H.** (1995). Comparison of the tolerability of bupropion, fluoxetine, imipramine, nefazodone, paroxetine, and venlafaxine. *Journal of Clinical Psychiatry* **56** (Suppl. 6), S12–21.
105. **Settle, E.C.** (1998). Bupropion sustained release: side-effect profile. *Journal of Clinical Psychiatry* **59** (Suppl. 4), S32–6.
106. **Spiegel, K., Kalb, R., and Pasternak, G.W.** (1983). Analgesic activity of tricyclic antidepressants. *Annals of Neurology* **13**, 462–5.
107. **Biegon, A. and Samuel, D.** (1980). Interaction of tricyclic antidepressants with opiate receptors. *Biochemistry and Pharmacology* **29**, 460–2.
108. **Isenberg, K.E. and Cicero, T.J.** (1984). Possible involvement of opiate receptors in the pharmacological profiles of antidepressant compounds. *European Journal of Pharmacology* **103**, 57–63.
109. **De Felipe, M.C., de Ceballow, M.L., and Fuentes, J.A.** (1986). Hypoalgesia induced by antidepressants in mice: a case for opioids and serotonin. *European Journal of Pharmacology* **125**, 193–9.
110. **Besson, J.M. and Chaouch, A.** (1987). Peripheral and spinal mechanisms of nociception. *Physiological Reviews* **67**, 67–186.
111. **Basbaum, A.I. and Fields, H.L.** (1984). Endogenous pain control systems: brainstem spinal pathways and endorphin circuitry. *Annual Review of Neuroscience* **7**, 309–38.
112. **Yaksh, T.L.** (1979). Direct evidence that spinal serotonin and noradrenaline terminals mediate the spinal antinociceptive effects of morphine in the periaqueductal gray. *Brain Research* **160**, 180–5.
113. **Schreiber, S., Backer, M.M., and Pick, C.G.** (1999). The antinociceptive effect of venlafaxine in mice is mediated through opioid and adrenergic mechanisms. *Neuroscience Letters* **273**, 85–8.
114. **Gray, A.M., Spencer, P.S.J., and Sewell, R.D.E.** (1998). The involvement of the opioidergic system in the antinociceptive mechanism of action of antidepressant compounds. *British Journal of Pharmacology* **124**, 669–74.
115. **Richelson, E.** (1979). Tricyclic antidepressants and neurotransmitter receptors. *Psychiatric Annals* **9**, 186–94.
116. **Charney, D.S., Menkes, D.B., and Heninger, F.R.** (1989). Receptor sensitivity and the mechanism of action of antidepressant treatment. *Archives of General Psychiatry* **38**, 1160–80.
117. **Potter, W.Z., Scheinin, M., Golden, R.N., Rudorfer, M.V., Cowdry, R.W., Calil, H.M., Ross, R.J., and Linnoila, M.** (1985). Selective antidepressants and cerebrospinal fluid: lack of specificity in norepinephrine and serotonin metabolites. *Archives of General Psychiatry* **42**, 1171–7.
118. **Cross, J.A. and Horton, R.W.** (1988). Effects of chronic oral administration of the antidepressants, desmethylimipramine and zimelidine on rat cortical, GABA-B binding sites: a comparison with 5 HT2 binding site changes. *British Journal of Pharmacology* **93**, 331–6.

119. **Preskorn, S.H. and Irwin, H.A.** (1982). Toxicity of tricyclic antidepressants—kinetics, mechanism, intervention: a review. *Journal of Clinical Psychiatry* **43**, 151–6.

120. **Glassman, A.H. and Bigger, J.T.** (1981). Cardiovascular effects of therapeutic doses of tricyclic antidepressants. *Archives of General Psychiatry* **38**, 815–20.

121. **Ray, W.A., Griffin, M.R., Schaffner, W., Baugh, D.K., and Melton, L.J.** (1987). Psychotropic drug use and the risk of hip fracture. *New England Journal of Medicine* **316**, 363–9.

122. **Solai, L.K., Mulsant, B.H., and Pollock, B.G.** (2001). Selective serotonin reuptake inhibitors for late-life depression: a comparative review. *Drugs Aging* **18**, 355–68.

123. **Edwards, J.G. and Anderson, I.** (1999). Systematic review and guide to selection of selective serotonin reuptake inhibitors. *Drugs* **57**, 507–33.

124. **Masand, P.S. and Gupta, S.** (1999). Selective serotonin-reuptake inhibitors: an update. *Harvard Review of Psychiatry* **7**, 69–84.

125. **Leo, R.J.** (1996). Movement disorders associated with the serotonin selective reuptake inhibitors. *Journal of Clinical Psychiatry* **57**, 449–54.

126. **Ceravolo, R., Nuti, A., Piccinni, A., Dell'Agnello, G., Bellini, G., Gambaccini, G., Dell' Osso, L., Murri, L., and Bonuccelli, U.** (2000). Paroxetine in Parkinson's disease: effects on motor and depressive symptoms. *Neurology* **55**, 1216–18.

127. **Rosenbaum, J.F. and Zajecka, J.** (1997). Clinical management of antidepressant discontinuation. *Journal of Clinical Psychiatry* **58** (Suppl. 7), 37–40.

128. **Michelson, D., Fava, Amsterdam, J., Apter, J., Londborg, P., Tamura, R., and Tepner, R.G.** (2000). Interruption of selective serotonin reuptake inhibitor treatment. Double-blind, placebo-controlled trial. *British Journal of Psychiatry* **176**, 363–8.

129. **Kent, J.M.** (2000). SNaRIs, NaSSAs, and NaRIs: new agents for the treatment of depression. *Lancet* **355**, 911–18.

130. **Wooltorton, E.** (2002). Bupropion (Zyban, Wellbutrin SR) reports of deaths, seizures, serum sickness. *Canadian Medical Association Journal* **166**, 68.

131. **Dunner, D.L., Zisook, S., Billow, A.A., Batey, S.R., Johnston, A., and Ascher, J.A.** (1998). A prospective safety surveillance study for bupropion sustained-released in the treatment of depression. *Journal of Clinical Psychiatry* **59**, 366–73.

132. **Davidson, J.** (1989). Seizures and bupropion: a review. *Journal of Clinical Psychiatry* **50**, 256–61.

133. **Brosen, K., Otton, S.V., and Gram, L.F.** (1986). Imipramine demethylation and hydroxylation: impact of the sparteine oxidation phenotype. *Clinical Pharmacology and Therapeutics* **40**, 543–9.

134. **Nordin, C., Siwers, B., Benitez, J., and Bertilsson, L.** (1985). Plasma concentrations of nortriptyline and its 10-hydroxy metabolite in depressed patients: relationship to the debrisoquine hydroxylation metabolic ratio. *British Journal of Clinical Pharmacology* **19**, 832–5.

135. **Brosen, K., Hansen, J.G., Nielsen, K.K., Sindrup, S.H., and Gram, L.F.** (1993). Inhibition by paroxetine of desipramine metabolism in extensive but not in poor metabolizers of sparteine. *European Journal of Clinical Pharmacology* **44**, 349–55.

136. **Harvey, A. and Preskorn, S.H.** (1995). Interactions of serotonin reuptake inhibitors with tricyclic antidepressants. *Archives of General Psychiatry* **52**, 783–5.

137. **Vandel, S.** et al. (1992). Tricyclic antidepressant plasma levels after fluoxetine addition. *Neuropsychobiology* **25**, 202–7.

138. **De Vane, C.** (1994). Pharmacogenetics and drug metabolism of newer antidepressant agents. *Journal of Clinical Psychiatry* **55**, 38–45.

139. **Bernard, S.A. and Bruera, E.** (2000). Drug interactions in palliative care. *Journal of Clinical Oncology* **18**, 1780–99.

140. **Nemeroff, C.** (1994). The clinical pharmacology and use of paroxetine, a new selective serotonin reuptake inhibitor. *Pharmacotherapy* **14**, 127–38.

141. **Kerrick, J.M., Fine, P.G., Lipman, A.G., and Love, G.** (1993). Low-dose amitriptyline as an adjunct to opioids for postoperative orthopedic pain: a placebo-controlled trial. *Pain* **52**, 325–30.

142. **Gordon, N.C., Heller, P.H., Gear, R.W., and Levine, J.D.** (1994). Interactions between fluoxetine and opiate analgesia for postoperative dental pain. *Pain* **58**, 85–8.

143. **Poulsen, L., Arendt-Nielsen, L., Brosen, K., Nielsen, K.K., Gram, L.F., and Sindrup, S.H.** (1995). The hypoalgesic effect of imipramine in different human experimental pain models. *Pain* **60**, 287–93.

144. **Bruera, E., Schoeller, T., Wenk, R., MacEachern, T., Marcelino, S., Hanson, J., and Suarez-Almazor, M.** (1995). A prospective multi-center assessment of the Edmonton staging system for cancer pain. *Journal of Pain and Symptom Management* **10**, 348–55.

145. **Arner, S. and Meyerson, B.A.** (1988). Lack of analgesic effect of opioids on neuropathic and idiopathic forms of pain. *Pain* **33**, 11–23.

146. **Portenoy, R.K., Foley, K.M., and Inturrisi, C.E.** (1990). The nature of opioid responsiveness and its implications for neuropathic pain: new hypotheses derived from studies of opioid infusions. *Pain* **43**, 273–86.

147. **Ettinger, A.B. and Portenoy, R.K.** (1988). The use of corticosteroids in the treatment of symptoms associated with cancer. *Journal of Pain and Symptom Management* **3**, 99–103.

148. **Watanabe, S. and Bruera, E.** (1994). Corticosteroids as adjuvant analgesics. *Journal of Pain and Symptom Management* **9**, 442–5.

149. **Needham, P.R., Daley, A.G., and Lennard, R.F.** (1992). Steroids in advanced cancer: survey of current practice. *British Medical Journal* **305**, 999.

150. **Farr, W.C.** (1990). The use of corticosteroids for symptom management in terminally ill patients. *American Journal of Hospice Care* **7**, 41–6.

151. **Wilcox, J.C., Corr, J., Shaw, J., Richardson, M., and Calman, K.C.** (1984). Prednisolone as an appetite stimulant in patients with cancer. *British Medical Journal* **288**, 27.

152. **Bruera, E., Roca, E., Cedaro, L., Carraro, S., and Chacon, R.** (1985). Action of oral methylprednisolone in terminal cancer patients: a prospective randomized double-blind study. *Cancer Treatment Report* **69**, 751–4.

153. **Della Cuna, G.R., Pelligrini, A., and Piazzi, M.** (1989). Effect of methylprednisolone sodium succinate on quality of life in preterminal cancer patients. A placebo-controlled multicenter study. *European Journal of Clinical Oncology* **25**, 1817–21.

154. **Tannock, I., Gospodarowicz, M., Meakin, W., Panzarella, T., Stewart, L., and Rider, W.** (1989). Treatment of metastatic prostatic cancer with low-dose prednisone: evaluation of pain and quality of life as pragmatic indices of response. *Journal of Clinical Oncology* **7**, 590–7.

155. **Popiela, T., Lucchi, R., and Giongo, F.** (1989). Methylprednisolone as palliative therapy for female terminal cancer patients: the Methylprednisolone Female Preterminal Cancer Study Group. *European Journal of Cancer* **25**, 1823–9.

156. **Hanks, G.W., Trueman, T., and Twycross, R.G.** (1983). Corticosteroids in terminal cancer. *Postgraduate Medical Journal* **59**, 702–6.

157. **Mercadante, S., Fulfaro, F., and Casuccio, A.** (2001). The use of corticosteroids in home palliative care. *Supportive Care in Cancer* **9**, 386–9.

158. **Kozin, F., Ryan, L.M., Carerra, G.F., Soin, L.S., and Wortmann, R.L.** (1981). The reflex sympathetic dystrophy syndrome (RSDS). III. Scintigraphic studies, further evidence for the therapeutic efficacy of systemic corticosteroids, and proposed diagnostic criteria. *American Journal of Medicine* **70**, 23–9.

159. **Greenberg, H.S., Kim, J., and Posner, J.B.** (1980). Epidural spinal cord compression from metastatic tumor: results with a new treatment protocol. *Annals of Neurology* **8**, 361–6.

160. **Reid, D.B.** (1988). Palliative management of bowel obstruction. *Medical Journal of Australia* **148**, 54.

161. **Fainsinger, R.L., Spanchynski, K., Hanson, J., and Bruera, E.** (1994). Symptom control in terminally ill patients with malignant bowel obstruction. *Journal of Pain and Symptom Management* **9**, 12.

162. **Vecht, Ch.J., Haaxma-Reiche, H., van Putten, W.L.J., de Visser, M., Vries, E.P., and Twijnstra, A.** (1989). Initial bolus of conventional versus high-dose dexamethasone in metastatic spinal cord compression. *Neurology* **39**, 1255–7.

163. **Yamada, K., Ushio, Y., Hayakawa, T., Anita, N., Yamada, N., and Mogami, H.** (1983). Effects of methylprednisolone on peritumoral brain edema. *Journal of Neurosurgery* **59**, 612–19.

164. **Posner, J.B., Howieson, J., and Cvitkovic, E.** (1977). 'Disappearing' spinal cord compression: oncolytic effects of glucocorticoids (and other chemotherapeutic agents) on epidural metastases. *Annals of Neurology* **2**, 409–13.

165. **Devor, M., Govrin-Lippman, R., and Raber, P.** (1985). Corticosteroids reduce neuroma hyperexcitability. In *Advances in Pain Research and*

Therapy Vol. 9 (ed. H.L. Fields, R. Dubner, and F. Cervero), pp. 451–5. Proceedings of the Fourth World Congress on Pain. New York: Raven Press.

166. **Haynes, R.C.** (1990). Adrenocorticotrophic hormone: adrenocortical steroids and their synthetic analogs: inhibitors of the synthesis and actions of adrenocortical hormones. In *The Pharmacological Basis of Therapeutics* 8th edn. (ed. A.G. Gilman, T.W. Rall, A.S. Nies, and P. Taylor), pp. 1431–62. New York: Pergamon Press.
167. **Weissman, D., Dufer, D., Vogel, V., and Abeloff, M.D.** (1987). Corticosteroid toxicity in neuro-oncology patients. *Journal of Neurooncology* **5**, 125–8.
168. **Sorensen, P.S., Helweg-Larsen, S., Mouridsen, H., and Hansen, H.H.** (1994). Effect of high-dose dexamethasone in carcinomatous metastatic spinal cord compression treated by radiotherapy: a randomized trial. *European Journal of Cancer* **30A**, 22–7.
169. **Breitbart, W., Stiefel, F., Kornblith, A.B., and Pannulo, S.** (1993). Neuropsychiatric disturbance in cancer patients with epidural spinal cord compression receiving high dose corticosteroids: a prospective comparison study. *Psycho-Oncology* **2**, 233–45.
170. **Messer, J., Reitman, D., Sacks, H.S., Smith, H., and Chalmers, T.** (1983). Association of adrenocorticosteroid therapy and peptic ulcer disease. *New England Journal of Medicine* **309**, 21–4.
171. **Piper, J.M., Ray, W.A., Daugherty, J.R., and Griffin, M.R.** (1991). Corticosteroid use and peptic ulcer disease—role of nonsteroidal anti-inflammatory drugs. *Annals of Internal Medicine* **114**, 735–40.
172. **Fadul, C.E., Lemann, W., Thaler, H.T., and Posner, J.B.** (1988). Perforation of the gastrointestinal tract in patients receiving steroids for neurologic disease. *Neurology* **38**, 348–52.
173. **ReMine, S.G. and McIlrath, D.** (1980). Bowel perforation in steroid-treated patients. *Annals of Surgery* **192**, 581–6.
174. **Dixon, R.A. and Christy, N.P.** (1980). On the various forms of corticosteroid withdrawal syndrome. *American Journal of Medicine* **68**, 224–30.
175. **Eisenach, J.C., Dewan, D.M., Rose, J.C., and Angelo, J.M.** (1987). Epidural clonidine produces antinociception, but not hypotension in sheep. *Anesthesiology* **66**, 496–501.
176. **Yaksh, T.L. and Reddy, S.V.R.** (1981). Studies in the primate on the analgesic effects associated with intrathecal actions of opiates, alpha adrenergic agonists and baclofen. *Anesthesiology* **54**, 451–67.
177. **Kayser, V., Desmeules, J., and Guilbaud, G.** (1995). Systemic clonidine differentially modulates the abnormal reactions to mechanical and thermal stimuli in rats with peripheral mononeuropathy. *Pain* **60**, 275–85.
178. **Pertovaara, A., Kauppila, T., and Tukeva, T.** (1990). The effect of medetomidine, an alpha-2 adrenoceptor agent in various pain tests. *European Journal of Pharmacology* **179**, 323–8.
179. **Puke, M.J.C. and Wiesenfeld-Hallin, Z.** (1993). The differential effects of morphine and the alpha 2 adrenoceptor agonists clonidine and dexmedetomidine on the prevention and treatment of experimental neuropathic pain. *Anesthesia and Analgesia* **77**, 104–9.
180. **Aho, M.S., Erkola, O.A., Scheinin, H., Lehtinen, A.M., and Korttila, K.T.** (1991). Effect of intravenously administered dexmedetomidine on pain after laparoscopic tubal ligation. *Anesthesia and Analgesia* **73**, 112–18.
181. **Byas-Smith, M.G., Max, M.B., Muir, H., and Kingman, A.** (1995). Transdermal clonidine compared to placebo in painful diabetic neuropathy using a two-staged 'enriched enrollment' design. *Pain* **60**, 267–74.
182. **Eisenach, J.C., Du Pen, S., Dubois, M., Miguel, R., Allin, D., and the Epidural Clonidine Study Group** (1995). Epidural clonidine analgesia for intractable cancer pain. *Pain* **61**, 391–400.
183. **Carroll, D., Jadad, A., King, L., Wiffen, P., Glynn, C., and McQuay, H.** (1993). Single-dose, randomized, double-blind, double-dummy, cross-over comparison of extradural and i.v. clonidine in chronic pain. *British Journal of Anaesthesiology* **7**, 665–9.
184. **Max, M.B., Schafer, S.C., Culnane, M., Dubner, R., Gracely, R.H.** (1988). Association of pain relief with drug side effects in postherpetic neuralgia: a single dose study of clonidine, codeine, ibuprofen and placebo. *Clinical Pharmacology and Therapeutics* **43**, 363–71.
185. **Tan, Y.-M. and Croese, J.** (1986). Clonidine and diabetic patients with leg pains. *Annals of Internal Medicine* **105**, 633.
186. **Petros, A.J. and Wright, R.M.B.** (1987). Epidural and oral clonidine in domiciliary control of deafferentation pain. *Lancet* **1**, 1034.
187. **Zeigler, D., Lynch, S.A., Muir, J., Benjamin, J., and Max, M.B.** (1992). Transdermal clonidine versus placebo in painful diabetic neuropathy. *Pain* **48**, 403–8.
188. **Glynn, C.J., Teddy, P.J., Jamous, M.A., Moore, R.A., and Lloyd, J.W.** (1986). Role of spinal noradrenergic system in transmission of pain in patients with spinal cord injury. *Lancet* **2**, 1249–50.
189. **Rauck, R.L., Eisenach, J.C., Jackson, K., Young, L.D., and Southern, J.** (1993). Epidural clonidine treatment for refractory reflex sympathetic dystrophy. *Anesthesiology* **79**, 1163–9.
190. **Coombs, D.W., Saunders, R., Gaylor, M., LaChance, B., and Jensen, L.** (1984). Clinical trial of intrathecal clonidine for cancer pain. *Regional Anesthesia* **9**, 34–5.
191. **Coombs, D.W., Saunders, R.L., LaChance, D., Savage, S., Ragnarsson, T.S., and Jensen, L.E.** (1985). Intrathecal morphine tolerance: use of intrathecal clonidine, DADLE and intraventricular morphine. *Anesthesiology* **62**, 357–63.
192. **Coombs, D.W., Saunders, R.L., Fratkin, J.D., Jensen, L.E., and Murphy, C.A.** (1986). Continuous intrathecal hydromorphone and clonidine for intractable cancer pain. *Journal of Neurosurgery* **64**, 890–4.
193. **Tumber, P.S. and Fitzgibbon, D.R.** (1998). The control of severe cancer pain by continuous intrathecal infusion and patient controlled intrathecal analgesia with morphine, bupivacaine and clonidine. *Pain* **78**, 217–20.
194. **Shafar, J., Tallett, E.R., and Knowlson, P.A.** (1972). Evaluation of clonidine in prophylaxis of migraine. *Lancet* **1**, 403–7.
195. **Smith, C., Birnbaum, G., Carter, J.L., Greenstein, J., and Lublin, F.D.** (1994). Tizanidine treatment of spasticity caused by multiple sclerosis: results of a double-blind, placebo-controlled trial. US Tizanidine Study Group. *Neurology* **44** (Suppl. 9), S34–43.
196. **Meythaler, J.M., Guin-Renfroe, S., Johnson, A., and Brunner, R.M.** (2001). Prospective assessment of tizanidine for spasticity due to acquired brain injury. *Archives of Physical Medicine and Rehabilitation* **82**, 1155–63.
197. **Nance, P.W., Bugaresti, J., Shellenberger, K., Sheremata, W., and Martinez-Arizala, A.** (1994). Efficacy and safety of tizanidine in the treatment of spasticity in patients with spinal cord injury. North American Tizanidine Study Group. *Neurology* **44** (Suppl. 9), S44–52.
198. **Kameyama, T., Nabeshima, T., Matsuno, K., and Sugimoto, A.** (1986). Comparison of alpha-adrenoceptor involvement in the antinociceptive action of tizanidine and clonidine in the mouse. *European Journal of Pharmacology* **125**, 257–64.
199. **Davies, J. and Johnston, S.E.** (1984). Selective antinociceptive effects of tizanidine (DS 103–282), a centrally acting muscle relaxant, on dorsal horn neurones in the feline spinal cord. *British Journal of Pharmacology* **82**, 409–21.
200. **Russell, I., Michalek, J., Xiao, Y., Haynes, W., Vertiz, R., and Lawrence, R.** (2002). Cerebrospinal fluid substance P in fibromyalgia syndrome is reduced by tizanidine therapy. *Journal of Pain* 3 (2 Suppl. 1), 41 (abstract 761).
201. **Saper, J.R., Lake, A.E. III, Cantrell, D.T., Winner, P.K., and White, J.R.** (2002). Chronic daily headache prophylaxis with tizanidine: a double-blind, placebo-controlled, multicenter outcome study. *Headache* **42**, 470–82.
202. **Yaksh, T.L.** (1985). Pharmacology of spinal adrenergic systems which modulate spinal nociceptive processing. *Pharmacology Biochemistry and Behavior* **22**, 845–58.
203. **Sagen, J. and Proudfit, H.** (1985). Evidence for pain modulation by pre- and postsynaptic noradrenergic receptors in the medulla oblongata. *Brain Research* **331**, 285–93.
204. **Coward, D.M.** (1994). Tizanidine: neuropharmacology and mechanism of action. *Neurology* **44** (Suppl. 9), S6–11.
205. **Semla, T.P., Beizer, J.L., and Higbee, M.D.** *Geriatric Dosage Handbook* 4th edn. Hudson OH: Lexi-Comp, 1998, pp. 238–40.
206. **Yjritsy-Roy, J.A., Standish, S.M., and Terry, L.C.** (1989). Dopamine D-1 and D-2 receptor antagonists potentiate analgesic and motor effects of morphine. *Pharmacology Biochemistry and Behavior* **32**, 717–21.
207. **Bloomfield, S., Simard-Savoie, S., Bernier, J., and Tetreault, L.** (1964). Comparative analgesic activity of levomepromazine and morphine in patients with chronic pain. *Canadian Medical Association Journal* **90**, 1156–9.
208. **Beaver, W.T., Wallenstein, S., Houde, R.W., and Rogers, A.** (1966). A comparison of the analgesic effects of methotrimeprazine and morphine in patients with cancer. *Clinical Pharmacology and Therapeutics* **7**, 436–46.

209. **Lasagna, L. and DeKornfeld, T.J.** (1961). Methotrimeprazine, a new phenothiazine derivative with analgesic properties. *Journal of the American Medical Association* **178**, 887–90.

210. **Hakkarainen, H.** (1977). Fluphenazine for tension headache: double-blind study. *Headache* **17**, 216–18.

211. **Lechin, F. et al.** (1989). Pimozide therapy for trigeminal neuralgia. *Archives of Neurology* **9**, 960–2.

212. **Patt, R.B., Proper, G., and Reddy, S.** (1994). The neuroleptics as adjuvant analgesics. *Journal of Pain and Symptom Management* **9**, 446–53.

213. **Montilla, E., Frederick, W.S., and Cass, L.J.** (1963). Analgesic effects of methotrimeprazine and morphine. *Archives of Internal Medicine* **111**, 725–8.

214. **Davidson, O., Lindenberg, O., and Walsh, M.** (1979). Analgesic treatment with levomepromazine in acute myocardial infarction. *Acta Medica Scandinavica* **205**, 191–4.

215. **Houde, R.W. and Wallenstein, S.L.** (1966). Analgesic power of chlorpromazine alone and in combination with morphine. *Federation Proceedings* **14**, 353.

216. **Keats, A.S., Telford, J., and Kurosu, Y.** (1961). Potentiation of meperidine by promethazine. *Anesthesiology* **22**, 31–41.

217. **Judkins, K.C. and Harmer, M.** (1982). Haloperidol as an adjuvant analgesic in the management of postoperative pain. *Anaesthesia* **37**, 1118–20.

218. **Davis, J.L., Lewis, S.B., Gerich, J.E., Kaplan, R.A., Schultz, T.A., and Wallin, J.D.** (1977). Peripheral diabetic neuropathy treated with amitriptyline and fluphenazine. *Journal of the American Medical Association* **238**, 2291–2.

219. **Kocher, R.** (1976). Use of psychotropic drugs for the treatment of chronic severe pain. In *Advances in Pain Research and Therapy* Vol. 1 (ed. JJ. Bonica and D. Albe-Fessard), pp. 579–82. Raven Press: New York.

220. **Nathan, P.W.** (1978). Chlorprothixene (Taractan) in postherpetic neuralgia and other severe pains. *Pain* **5**, 367–71.

221. **Raft, D., Toomey, T., and Gregg, J.M.** (1979). Behavior modification and haloperidol in chronic facial pain. *Southern Medical Journal* **72**, 155–9.

222. **Schubert, D.S.P., Patterson, M.B., and Long, C.** (1983). Phenothiazine analgesics in a patient with psychotic symptoms. *Psychosomatics* **24**, 599–600.

223. **Daw, J.L. and Cohen-Cole, S.A.** (1981). Haloperidol analgesia. *Southern Medical Journal* **74**, 364–5.

224. **Merskey, H. and Hester, R.A.** (1976). The treatment of chronic pain with psychotropic drugs. *Postgraduate Medical Journal* **48**, 594–8.

225. **Weis, O., Sriwatanakul, K., and Weintraub, M.** (1982). Treatment of postherpetic neuralgia and acute herpetic pain with amitriptyline and perphenazine. *South African Medical Journal* **62**, 274–5.

226. **Hanks, G.W., Thomas, P.J., Trueman, T., and Weeks, E.** (1983). The myth of haloperidol potentiation. *Lancet* **2**, 523–4.

227. **Rosen, T.D.** (2001). Olanzapine as an abortive agent for cluster headache. *Headache* **41**, 813–16.

228. **Kiser, R.S., Cohen, H.M., Freedenfeld, R.N., Jewell, C., and Fuchs, P.N.** (2001). Olanzapine for the treatment of fibromyalgia symptoms. *Journal of Pain and Symptom Management* **22**, 704–8.

229. **Yaksh, T.L.** (1999). Central pharmacology of nociceptive transmission. In *Textbook of Pain* 4th edn. (ed. P.D. Wall and R. Melzack), pp. 253–308. London: Churchill Livingstone.

230. **Bodnar, R.J. and Nicotera, N.** (1982). Neuroleptic and analgesic interactions upon pain and activity measures. *Pharmacology, Biochemistry and Behavior* **16**, 411–16.

231. **Rosenblatt, W.H., Cioffi, A.M., Sinatra, R., Saberski, L.R., and Silverman, D.G.** (1991). Metoclopramide: an analgesic adjunct to patient-controlled analgesia. *Anesthesiology and Analgesia* **73**, 553–5.

232. **Kandler, D. and Lisander, B.** (1993). Analgesic action of metoclopramide in prosthetic hip surgery. *Acta Anaesthesiologica Scandinavica* **37**, 49–53.

233. **Moss, H.E. and Sanger, G.J.** (1990). The effects of granisetron, ICS 205-930 and ondansetron on the visceral pain reflex induced by duodenal distension. *British Journal of Pharmacology* **100**, 497–501.

234. **Baldessarini, R.J.** (1990). Drugs and the treatment of psychiatric disorders. In *The Pharmacological Basis of Therapeutics* 8th edn. (ed. A.G. Gilman, T.W. Rall, A.S. Nies, and P. Taylor), pp. 383–435. New York: Pergamon Press.

235. **Tardy, D., Baldessarini, R.J., and Tazari, F.I.** (2002). Effects of newer antipsychotics on extrapyramidal function. *CNS Drugs* **16**, 23–45.

236. **Caroff, S.N. and Mann, S.C.** (1993). Neuroleptic malignant syndrome. *Medical Clinics of North America* **77**, 185–202.

237. **Storey, P., Hill, H.H., St. Louis, R., and Tarver, E.E.** (1990). Subcutaneous infusions for control of cancer symptoms. *Journal of Pain and Symptom Management* **5**, 33–41.

238. **Cherny, N.I., Thaler, H.T., Friedlander-Klar, H., Lapin, J., Foley, K.M., Houde, R., and Portenoy, R.K.** (1994). Opioid responsiveness of cancer pain syndromes caused by neuropathic or nociceptive mechanisms. *Neurology* **44**, 857–61.

239. **Mercadante, S., Maddaloni, S., Roccella, S., and Salvaggio, L.** (1992). Predictive factors in advanced cancer pain treated only by analgesics. *Pain* **50**, 151–5.

240. **McQuay, H.J., Jadad, A.R., Carroll, D., Faura, C., Glynn, C.J., Moore, R.A., and Liu, Y.** (1992). Opioid sensitivity of chronic pain: a patient-controlled analgesia method. *Anaesthesia* **47**, 757–67.

241. **Jadad, A.R., Carroll, D., Glynn, C.J., Moore, R.A., and McQuay, H.J.** (1992). Morphine responsiveness of chronic pain: double-blind randomised crossover study with patient-controlled analgesia. *Lancet* **339**, 1367–71.

242. **Glazer, S. and Portenoy, R.K.** (1991). Systemic local anesthetics in pain control. *Journal of Pain and Symptom Management* **6**, 30–9.

243. **Backonja, M.** (1994). Local anesthetics as adjuvant analgesics. *Journal of Pain and Symptom Management* **9**, 491–9.

244. **Mao, J. and Chen, L.L.** (2000). Systemic lidocaine for neuropathic pain relief. *Pain* **87**, 7–17.

245. **Cassuto, J., Wallin, G., Hogstrom, S., Faxen, A., and Rimback, G.** (1985). Inhibition of postoperative pain by continuous low dose infusion of lidocaine. *Anesthesia and Analgesia* **64**, 971–4.

246. **Birch, K., Jorgensen, B., Chraemer-Jorgensen, B., and Kehlet, H.** (1987). Effect of i.v. lignocaine on pain and the endocrine metabolic responses after surgery. *British Journal of Anaesthesia* **59**, 721–4.

247. **Bartlett, E.E. and Hutaserani, O.** (1961). Xylocaine for the relief of post-operative pain. *Anesthesia and Analgesia* **40**, 296–304.

248. **Edwards, W.T., Habib, F., Burney, R.G., and Begin, G.** (1985). Intravenous lidocaine in the management of various chronic pain states. *Regional Anesthesia* **10**, 1–6.

249. **Galer, B.S., Miller, K.V., and Rowbotham, M.C.** (1993). Response to intravenous lidocaine infusion differs based on clinical diagnosis and site of nervous system injury. *Neurology* **43**, 1233–5.

250. **Petersen, P., Kastrup, J., Zeeburg, I., and Boysen, G.** (1986). Chronic pain treatment with intravenous lidocaine. *Neurology Research* **8**, 189–90.

251. **Petersen, P. and Kastrup, J.** (1987). Dercum's disease (adiposa dolorosa): treatment of severe pain with intravenous lidocaine. *Pain* **28**, 77–80.

252. **Juhlin, L.** (1986). Long-standing pain relief of adiposa dolorosa (Dercum's disease) after intravenous infusion of lidocaine. *Journal of the American Academy of Dermatology* **15**, 383–4.

253. **Atkinson, R.L.** (1982). Intravenous lidocaine for the treatment of intractable pain of adiposis dolorosa. *International Journal of Obstetrics* **6**, 351–7.

254. **Iwane, T., Masanori, M., Matsuki, M., Ito, Y., and Shimoji, K.** (1976). Management of intractable pain in adiposis dolorosa with intravenous administration of lidocaine. *Anesthesia and Analgesia* **55**, 257–9.

255. **Graubard, D.J., Kovacs, J., and Ritter, H.H.** (1948). The management of destructive arthritis of the hip by means of intravenous procaine. *Annals of Internal Medicine* **28**, 1106–16.

256. **Marton, R., Spitzer, N., and Steinbrocker, O.** (1949). Intravenous procaine as an analgesic and therapeutic procedure in painful, chronic neuromusculo-skeletal disorders. *Annals of Internal Medicine* **10**, 629–33.

257. **Rosner, S.** (1984). A simple method of treatment for acute headache. *Headache* **24**, 50.

258. **Arner, S., Lindblom, U., Meyerson, B.A., and Molnar, C.** (1990). Prolonged relief of neuralgia after regional anesthetic blocks: a call for further experimental and systemic clinical studies. *Pain* **43**, 287–97.

259. **Boas, R.A., Covino, B.G., and Shahnarian, A.** (1982). Analgesic responses to IV lignocaine. *British Journal of Anaesthesia* **54**, 501–5.

260. **Kuhnert, S.M., Phillips, W.J., and Davis, M.D.P.** (1999). Lidocaine and mexiletine therapy for erythromelalgia. *Archives of Dermatology* **135**, 1447–9.

261. **Maciewicz, R., Chung, R.Y., Strassman, A., Hochberg, F., and Moskowitz, M.** (1988). Relief of vascular headache with intravenous lidocaine: clinical observations and a proposed mechanism. *Clinical Journal of Pain* **4**, 11–16.

262. **Backonja, M. and Gombar, K.** (1992). Response of central pain syndromes to intravenous lidocaine. *Journal of Pain and Symptom Management* **7**, 172–8.

263. **Attal, N., Gaudé, V., Brasseur, L., Dupuy, M., Guirimand, F., Parker, F., and Bouhassira, D.** (2000). Intravenous lidocaine in central pain: a double-blind, placebo-controlled, psychophysical study. *Neurology* **54**, 564–74.

264. **Rowbotham, M.C., Reisner-Keller, L.A., and Fields, H.L.** (1991). Both intravenous lidocaine and morphine reduce the pain of postherpetic neuralgia. *Neurology* **41**, 1024–8.

265. **Kastrup, J., Petersen, P., Dejgard, A., Angelo, H.R., and Hilsted, J.** (1987). Intravenous lidocaine infusion—a new treatment for chronic painful diabetic neuropathy. *Pain* **28**, 69–75.

266. **Bruera, E., Ripamonti, C., Brenneis, C., MacMillan, K., and Hanson, J.** (1992). A randomized double-blind crossover trial of intravenous lidocaine in the treatment of neuropathic cancer pain. *Journal of Pain and Symptom Management* **7**, 138–40.

267. **Elleman, K., Sjogren, P., Banning, A., Jensen, T.S., Smith, T., and Geertsen, P.** (1989). Trial of intravenous lidocaine on painful neuropathy in cancer patients. *Clinical Journal of Pain* **5**, 291–4.

268. **Chong, S.F., Bretscher, M.E., Mailliard, J.A., Tschetter, L.K., Kimmel, D.W., Hatfield, A.K., and Loprinzi, C.L.** (1997). Pilot study evaluating local anesthetics administered systemically for treatment of pain in patients with advanced cancer. *Journal of Pain and Symptom Management* **13**, 112–17.

269. **Brose, W.G. and Cousins, M.J.** (1991). Subcutaneous lidocaine for treatment of neuropathic cancer pain. *Pain* **45**, 145–8.

270. **Dunlop, R., Davies, R.J., Hockley, J., and Turner, P.** (1989). Letter to the Editor. *Lancet* **1**, 420–1.

271. **Lindstrom, P. and Lindblom, U.** (1987). The analgesic effect of tocainide in trigeminal neuralgia. *Pain* **28**, 45–50.

272. **Dejgard, A., Petersen, P., and Kastrup, J.** (1988). Mexiletine for treatment of chronic painful diabetic neuropathy. *Lancet* **1**, 9–11.

273. **Oskarsson, P., Ljunggren, J.G., and Lins, P.E.** (1997). Efficacy and safety of mexiletine in the treatment of painful diabetic neuropathy. *Diabetes Care* **20**, 1594–7.

274. **Kieburtz, K., Simpson, D., Yiannoutsos, C., Max, M.B., Hall, C.D., Ellis, R.J., Marra, C.M., McKendall, R., Singer, E., Dal Pan, G.J., Clifford, D.B., Tucker, T., and Cohen, B.** (1998). A randomized trial of amitriptyline and mexiletine in HIV infection. *Neurology* **51**, 1682–8.

275. **Chaplan, S.R., Bach, F.W., Shafer, S.L., and Yaksh, T.L.** (1995). Prolonged alleviation of tactile allodynia by intravenous lidocaine in neuropathic rats. *Anesthesiology* **83**, 775–85.

276. **Abdi, S., Lee, D.H., and Chung, J.M.** (1998). The anti-allodynic effects of amytriptyline, gabapentin, and lidocaine in a rat model of neuropathic pain. *Anesthesia and Analgesia* **87**, 1360–6.

277. **Koppert, W., Ostermeier, N., Sittl, R., Weidner, C., and Schmelz, M.** (2000). Low-dose lidocaine reduces secondary hyperalgesia by a central mode of action. *Pain* **85**, 217–24.

278. **Covino, B.G.** (1993). Local anesthetics. In *Postoperative Pain Management* (ed. F.M. Ferrante and T.R. VadeBoncouer), pp. 211–53. New York: Churchill Livingstone.

279. **deJong, R.H. and Nace, R.** (1968). Nerve impulse conduction during intravenous lidocaine injection. *Anesthesiology* **29**, 22–8.

280. **Woolf, C.J. and Wiesenfeld-Halli, Z.** (1985). The systemic administration of local anesthetic produces a selective depression of C-afferent evoked activity in the spinal cord. *Pain* **23**, 361–74.

281. **Chabal, C., Russell, L.C., and Burchiel, K.J.** (1989). The effect of intravenous lidocaine, tocainide and mexiletine on spontaneously active fibers originating in rat sciatic neuromas. *Pain* **38**, 333–8.

282. **Devor, M., Wall, P.D., and Catalan, N.** (1992). Systemic lidocaine silences ectopic neuroma and DRG discharge without blocking nerve conduction. *Pain* **48**, 261–8.

283. **Liu, P.L., Feldman, H.S., Giasi, R., Patterson, M.K., and Covino, B.G.** (1983). Comparative CNS toxicity of lidocaine, etidocaine, bupivacaine, and tetracaine in awake dogs following rapid intravenous administration. *Anesthesia and Analgesia* **62**, 375.

284. **CAST (Cardiac Arrhythmia Suppression Trial) Investigators** (1989). Preliminary report: effect of encainide and flecainide on mortality in a randomized trial of arrhythmia suppression after acute myocardial infarction. *New England Journal of Medicine* **321**, 406–12.

285. **Kreeger, W. and Hammill, S.C.** (1987). New antiarrhythmic drugs: tocainide, mexiletine, flecainide, encainide and amiodarone. *Mayo Clinic Proceedings* **62**, 1033–50.

286. **Horn, H.R., Hadidian, Z., Johnson, J.L., Vasallo, H.G., Williams, J.H., and Young, M.D.** (1980). Safety evaluation of tocainide in an American emergency use program. *American Heart Journal* **100**, 1037–40.

287. **Vincent, F.M. and Vincent, T.** (1985). Tocainide encephalopathy. *Neurology* **35**, 1804–5.

288. **Stein, M.G., Demarco, T., Gamsu, G., Finkbeiner, W., and Golden, J.** (1988). Computed tomography: pathologic correlates in lung disease due to tocainide. *American Review of Respiratory Diseases* **137**, 458–60.

289. **Campbell, R.W.F.** (1987). Mexiletine. *New England Journal of Medicine* **316**, 29–34.

290. **Jarvis, B. and Coukell, A.J.** (1998). Mexiletine: a review of its therapeutic use in painful diabetic neuropathy. *Drugs* **56**, 691–707.

291. **Galer, B.S., Harle, J., and Rowbotham, M.C.** (1996). Response to intravenous lidocaine infusion predicts subsequent response to oral mexiletine: a prospective study. *Journal of Pain and Symptom Management* **12**, 161–7.

292. **Backonja, M.M.** (2000). Anticonvulsants (antineuropathics) for neuropathic pain syndromes. *Clinical Journal of Pain* **16**, S67–72.

293. **Tremont-Lukats, I.W., Megeff, C., and Backonja, M.M.** (2000). Anticonvulsants for neuropathic pain syndromes: mechanisms of action and place in therapy. *Drugs* **60**, 1029–52.

294. **Campbell, F.G., Graham, J.G., and Zilkha, K.J.** (1966). Clinical trial of carbamazepine (Tegretol) in trigeminal neuralgia. *Journal of Neurology, Neurosurgery and Psychiatry* **29**, 265–7.

295. **Rockliff, B.W. and Davis, E.H.** (1966). Controlled sequential trials of carbamazepine in trigeminal neuralgia. *Archives of Neurology* **15**, 129–36.

296. **Killian, J.M. and Fromm, G.H.** (1968). Carbamazepine in the treatment of neuralgia. Use and side effects. *Archives of Neurology* **19**, 129–36.

297. **Nicol, C.F.** (1969). A four year double-blind study of carbamazepine in facial pain. *Headache* **9**, 54–7.

298. **Rull, J.A., Quibrera, R., Gonzalez-Millan, H., and Lozano Castaneda, O.** (1969). Symptomatic treatment of peripheral diabetic neuropathy with carbamazepine (Tegretol): double-blind cross-over trial. *Diabetologia* **5**, 215–18.

299. **Lockman, L.A., Hunninghake, D.B., Drivit, W., and Desnick, R.J.** (1973). Relief of pain of Fabry's disease by diphenylhydantoin. *Neurology (Minneap)* **23**, 871–5.

300. **Chadda, V.S. and Mathur, M.S.** (1978). Double-blind study of the effects of diphenylhydantoin sodium in diabetic neuropathy. *Journal of the Association of Physicians of India* **26**, 403–6.

301. **Yajnik, S., Singh, G.P., Singh, G., and Kumar, M.** (1992). Phenytoin as a coanalgesic in cancer pain. *Journal of Pain and Symptom Management* **7**, 209–13.

302. **Backonja, M., Beydoun, A., Edwards, K.R., Schwartz, S.L., Fonseca, V., Hes, M., LaMoreaux, L., and Garofalo, E.** (1998). Gabapentin for the symptomatic treatment of painful neuropathy in patients with diabetes mellitus: a randomized controlled trial. *Journal of the American Medical Association* **280**, 1831–6.

303. **Dallocchio, C., Buffa, C., Mazzarello, P., and Chiroli, S.** (2000). Gabapentin versus amitriptyline in painful diabetic neuropathy: an open-label pilot study. *Journal of Pain and Symptom Management* **20**, 280–5.

304. **Rowbotham, M., Harden, N., Stacey, B., Bernstein, P., and Magnus-Miller, L.** (1998). Gabapentin for the treatment of postherpetic neuralgia: a randomized controlled trial. *Journal of the American Medical Association* **280**, 1837–42.

305. **Rice, A.S.C. and Maton, S.** (2001). Gabapentin in postherpetic neuralgia: a randomised, double blind, placebo controlled study. *Pain* **94**, 215–24.

306. **Rosenberg, J.M., Harrell, C., Ristic, H., Werner, R.A., and de Rosayro, A.M.** (1997). The effect of gabapentin on neuropathic pain. *Clinical Journal of Pain* **13**, 251–5.

307. **Mellick, G.A. and Mellick, L.B.** (1995). Gabapentin in the management of reflex sympathetic dystrophy. *Journal of Pain and Symptom Management* **10**, 265–6.

308. **Vadivelu, N. and Berger, J.** (1999). Neuropathic pain after anti-HIV gene therapy successfully treated with gabapentin. *Journal of Pain and Symptom Management* **17**, 155–6.

309. **La Spina, I., Porazzi, D., Maggiolo, F., Bottura, P., and Suter, F.** (2001). Gabapentin in painful HIV-related neuropathy: a report of 19 patients, preliminary observations. *European Journal of Neurology* **8**, 71–5.

310. **Caraceni, A., Zecca, E., Martini, C., and De Conno, F.** (1999). Gabapentin as an adjuvant to opioid analgesia for neuropathic cancer pain. *Journal of Pain and Symptom Management* **17**, 441–5.

311. **Solaro, C., Lunardi, G.L., Capello, E., Inglese, M., Messmer Uccelli, M., Uccelli, A., and Mancardi, G.L.** (1998). An open-label trial of gabapentin treatment of paroxysmal symptoms in multiple sclerosis patients. *Neurology* **51**, 609–11.

312. **Solaro, C., Messmer Uccelli, M., Uccelli, A., Leandri, M., and Mancardi, G.L.** (2000). Low-dose gabapentin combined with either lamotrigine or carbamazepine can be useful therapies for trigeminal neuralgia in multiple sclerosis. *European Neurology* **44**, 45–8.

313. **Solaro, C., Uccelli, M.M., Guglieri, P., Uccelli, A., and Mancardi, G.L.** (2000). Gabapentin is effective in treating nocturnal painful spasms in multiple sclerosis. *Multiple Sclerosis* **6**, 192–3.

314. **Devulder, J., Lambert, J., and Naeyaert, J.M.** (2001). Gabapentin for pain control in cancer patients's wound dressing care. *Journal of Pain and Symptom Management* **22**, 622–6.

315. **Canavero, S. and Bonicalzi, V.** (1997). Lamotrigine control of trigeminal neuralgia. *Journal of Neurology* **244**, 527–32.

316. **Lunardi, G., Leandri, M., Albano, C., Cultrera, S., Fracassi, M., Rubino, V., and Favale, E.** (1997). Clinical effectiveness of lamotrigine and plasma levels in essential and symptomatic trigeminal neuralgia. *Neurology* **48**, 1714–17.

317. **Eisenberg, E., Alon, N., Ishay, A., Daoud, D., and Yarnitsky, D.** (1998). Lamotrigine in the treatment of painful diabetic neuropathy. *European Journal of Neurology* **5**, 167–73.

318. **Cianchetti, C., Zuddas, A., Randazzo, A.P., Perra, L., and Marrosu, M.G.** (1999). Lamotrigine adjunctive therapy in painful phenomena in MS: preliminary observations. *Neurology* **53**, 433.

319. **Zakrzewska, J.M., Chaudhry, Z., Nurmikko, T.J., Patton, D.W., and Mullens, E.L.** (1997). Lamotrigine (Lamictal) in refractory trigeminal neuralgia: results from a double-blind placebo controlled crossover trial. *Pain* **73**, 223–30.

320. **Simpson, D.M., Olney, R., McArthur, J.C., Khan, A., Godbold, J., and Ebel-Frommer, K.** (2000). A placebo-controlled trial of lamotrigine for painful HIV-associated neuropathy. *Neurology* **54**, 2115–19.

321. **Vestergaard, K., Andersen, G., Gottrup, H., Kristensen, B.T., and Jensen, T.S.** (2001). Lamotrigine for central poststroke pain: a randomized controlled trial. *Neurology* **56**, 184–90.

322. **McCleane, G.** (1999). 200 mg daily of lamotrigine has no analgesic effect in neuropathic pain: a randomised, double-blind, placebo controlled trial. *Pain* **83**, 105–7.

323. **Devulder, J.E.R.** (2000). Lamotrigine in refractory cancer pain: a case report (letter). *Journal of Clinical Anesthesia* **12**, 574–5.

324. **Potter, D., Edwards, K.R., and Bennington, V.T.** (1999). Potential role of topiramate in relief of neuropathic pain (abstract). *Neurology* **50**, A255.

325. **Movva, V., Royal, M., Jenson, M., Ward, S., Bhakta, B., and Gunyea, I.** (2002). Efficacy of topiramate in neuropathic pain: retrospective trial in 61 patients. *Journal of Pain* **3** (2 Suppl. 1), 41 (abstract 761).

326. **Edwards, K.** et al. (2000). Efficacy and safety of topiramate in the treatment of painful diabetic neuropathy: a double-blind, placebo-controlled study (abstract). *Neurology* **54** (S3), A81.

327. **Storey, J.R., Calder, C.S., Hart, D.E., and Potter, D.L.** (2001). Topiramate in migraine prevention: a double-blind, placebo-controlled study. *Headache* **41**, 968–75.

328. **Canavero, S., Bonicalzi, V., and Paolotti, R.** (2002). Lack of effect of topiramate for central pain. *Neurology* **58**, 831–2.

329. **Iacobellis, D.** et al. (2000). A double blind placebo-controlled trial of pregabalin for the treatment of pain from diabetic peripheral neuropathy. *Neurology* **54** (Suppl. 3), A177 (abstract P03.049).

330. **Corbin, A.E., Young, J.P. Jr., LaMoreaux, L., Sharma, U., Garofalo, E.A., and Poole, R.M.** (2002). Pregabalin reduces pain in patients with postherpetic neuralgia: supportive data from SF-McGill Pain Questionnaire (SF-MPQ). *Journal of Pain* **3** (2 Suppl. 1), 47 (abstract 785).

331. **Hill, C.M., Balkenohl, M., Thomas, D.W., Walker, R., Mathe, H., and Murray, G.** (2001). Pregabalin in patients with postoperative dental pain. *European Journal of Pain* **5**, 119–24.

332. **Ipponi, A., Lamberti, C., Medica, A., Bartolini, A., and Malmberg-Aiello, P.** (1999). Tiagabine antinociception in rodents depends on GABA(B) receptor activation: parallel antinociception testing and medial thalamus GABA microdialysis. *European Journal of Pharmacology* **368**, 205–11.

333. **Jenson, M., Ward, S., Royal, M., Movva, V., Bhakta, B., and Gunyea, I.** (2002). Tiagabine is an effective treatment of neuropathic pain: a prospective, open-label trial. *Journal of Pain* **3** (2 Suppl. 1), 40 (abstract 757).

334. **Mellick, G.A.** (1995). Hemifacial spasm: successful treatment with felbamate. *Journal of Pain and Symptom Management* **10**, 392–5.

335. **Cheshire, W.P.** (1995). Felbamate relieved trigeminal neuralgia. *Clinical Journal of Pain* **11**, 139–42.

336. **Ardid, D., Lamberty, Y., Alloui, A., Coudore-Civiale, M.-A., and Eschaller, A.** (2001). Levetiracetam (Keppra), a new antiepileptic drug, is effective in neuropathic but not acute pain models in rats. *Neurology* **56** (Suppl. 3), A350.

337. **Ward, S., Jenson, M., Royal, M., Movva, V., Bhakta, B., and Gunyea, I.** (2002). Gabapentin and levetiracetam in combination for the treatment of neuropathic pain. *Journal of Pain* **3** (2 Suppl. 1), 38 (abstract 750).

338. **McCumber, D., Chen, K.S., Meyer, K.E., and Yaksh, T.L.** (2002). A study of zonisamide (Zonegran®) in the formalin model of nociception. *Journal of Pain* **3** (2 Suppl. 1), 29 (abstract 715).

339. **Wallace, M.S.** (2002). Zonisamide for complex regional pain syndrome. *Journal of Pain* **3** (2 Suppl. 1), 42 (abstract 764).

340. **Drake, M.E. Jr.** (2002). Zonisamide in the prophylaxis of migraine headache. *Journal of Pain* **3** (2 Suppl. 1), 39 (abstract 754).

341. **Ward, S., Royal, M.A., Jenson, M., Bhakta, B., Gunyea, I., and Movva, V.** (2002). An open-label trial of oxcarbazepine in patients with radiculopathy refractory to gabapentin. *Journal of Pain* **3** (2 Suppl. 1), 42 (abstract 765).

342. **Carrazana, E., Beydoun, A., Kobetz, S., and Constantine, S.** (2002). An open-label, prospective trial of oxcarbazepine for the treatment of painful diabetic neuropathy. *Journal of Pain* **3** (2 Suppl. 1), 38 (abstract 751).

343. **Zakrzewska, J.M. and Patsalos, P.N.** (1989). Oxcarbazepine: a new drug in the management of intractable trigeminal neuralgia. *Journal of Neurology, Neurosurgery and Psychiatry* **52**, 472–6.

344. **Royal, M.A., Jenson, M., Bhakta, B., Gunyea, I., Movva, V., and Ward, S.** (2002). An open-label trial of oxcarbazepine in patients with complex regional pain syndrome refractory to gabapentin. *Journal of Pain* **3** (2 Suppl. 1), 41 (abstract 763).

345. **Hamza, M. and Rowlingson, J.** (2002). Initial experience with oxcarbazepine in the treatment of idiopathic neuropathic pain. *Journal of Pain* **3** (2 Suppl. 1), 40 (abstract 756).

346. **Dreyer, M.D., Edwards, K.R., and Norton, J.A.** (2002). Oxcarbazepine: preliminary clinical experience in the treatment of neuropathic pain. *Journal of Pain* **3** (2 Suppl. 1), 39 (abstract 755).

347. **Caccia, M.R.** (1975). Clonazepam in facial neuralgia and cluster headache: clinical and electrophysiological study. *European Neurology* **13**, 560–3.

348. **Martin, G.** (1981). The management of pain following laminectomy for lumbar disc lesions. *Annals of the Royal College of Surgeons of England* **63**, 244–52.

349. **Peiris, J.B., Perera, G.L.S., Devendra, S.V., and Lionel, N.D.W.** (1980). Sodium valproate in trigeminal neuralgia. *Medical Journal of Australia* **2**, 278.

350. **Raftery, H.** (1979). The management of postherpetic pain using sodium valproate and amitriptyline. *Journal of the Irish Medical Association* **72**, 399–401.

351. **Weinberger, J., Nicklas, W.J., and Berl, S.** (1976). Mechanism of action of anticonvulsants. *Neurology (Minneap)* **26**, 162–73.

352. **Devor, M. and Seltzer, Z.** (1999). Pathophysiology of damaged nerves in relation to chronic pain. In *Textbook of Pain* 4th edn. (ed. P.A Wall and R. Melzack), pp. 129–64. London: Churchill Livingstone.

353. **Albe-Fessard, D. and Lombard, M.C.** (1982). Use of an animal model to evaluate the origin of deafferentation pain and protection against it In *Advances in Pain Research and Therapy* Vol. 5 (ed. J.J. Bonica, U. Lindblom, and A. Iggo), pp. 691–700. New York: Raven Press.

354. **Guilbaud, G., Benoist, J.M., Levante, A., Gautron, M., and Willer, J.C.** (1992). Primary somatosensory cortex in rats with pain-related behaviours due to a peripheral mononeuropathy after moderate ligation of one sciatic nerve: neuronal responsivity to somatic stimulation. *Experimental Brain Research* **92**, 227–45.

355. **Lenz, F.A., Kwan, H.C., Dostrovsky, J.O., and Tasker, R.R.** (1989). Characteristics of the bursting pattern of action potentials that occurs in the thalamus of patients with central pain. *Brain Research* **496**, 357–60.

356. **Nystrom, B. and Hagbarth, K.E.** (1981). Microelectrode recordings from transected nerves in amputees in phantom limb pain. *Neuroscience Letter* **27**, 211–16.

357. **Loeser, J.D., Ward, A.A., and White, L.E.** (1968). Chronic deafferentation of human spinal cord neurons. *Journal of Neurosurgery* **29**, 48–50.

358. **Hart, R.G. and Easton, J.D.** (1982). Carbamazepine and hematological monitoring. *Annals of Neurology* **11**, 309–16.

359. **Van Amelsvoort, T., Bakshi, R., Devaux, C.B., and Schwabe, S.** (1994). Hyponatremia associated with carbamazepine and oxcarbazepine therapy: a review. *Epilepsia* **35**, 181–8.

360. **Terrence, C.F. and Fromm, G.H.** (1980). Congestive heart failure during carbamazepine therapy. *Annals of Neurology* **8**, 200–1.

361. **Ramsey, R.E., Wilder, B.J., Berger, J.R., and Bruni, J.** (1983). A double-blind study comparing carbamazepine and phenytoin as initial seizure therapy in adults. *Neurology* **33**, 904–10.

362. **Troupin, A. and Ojemann, L.M.** (1975). Paradoxical intoxication: a complication of anticonvulsant administration. *Epilepsia* **16**, 753–8.

363. **Ghatak, N.R., Santoso, R.A., and McKinney, W.M.** (1976). Cerebellar degeneration following long-term phenytoin therapy. *Neurology* **26**, 818–24.

364. **Schmidt, D.** (1984). Adverse effects of valproate. *Epilepsia* **25**, 44S–9S.

365. **Goa, K.L. and Sorkin, E.M.** (1993). Gabapentin: a review of its pharmacological properties and clinical potential in epilepsy. *Drugs* **46**, 409–27.

366. **Faught, E., Sachdeo, R.C., Remler, M.P., Chayasirisobhon, S., Iragui-Madoz, V.J., Ramsay, R.E., Sutula, T.P., Kanner, A., Harner, R.N., and Kuzniecky, R.** (1993). Felbamate monotherapy for partial-onset seizures: an active control trial. *Neurology* **43**, 688–92.

367. **Matsuo, F., Bergen, D., Faught, E., Messenheimer, J.A., Dren, A.T., Rudd, G.D., and Lineberry, C.G.** (1993). Placebo-controlled study of the efficacy and safety of lamotrigine in patient with partial seizures. *Neurology* **43**, 2284–91.

368. **Messenheimer, J., Ramsay, R.E., Willmore, L.J., Leroy, R.F., Zielinski, J.J., Mattson, R., Pellock, J.M., Valakas, A.M., Womble, G., and Risner, M.** (1994). Lamotrigine therapy for partial seizures: a multicenter, placebo-controlled, double-blind, cross-over trial. *Epilepsia* **35**, 113–21.

369. **Hemstreet, B. and Lapointe, M.** (2001). Evidence for the use of gabapentin in the treatment of diabetic peripheral neuropathy. *Clinical Therapeutics* **23**, 520–31.

370. **Perucca, E.** (1999). The clinical pharmacokinetics of the new antiepileptic drugs. *Epilepsia* **40** (Suppl. 9), S7–13.

371. **Hovinga, C.A.** (2001). Levetiracetam: a novel antiepileptic drug. *Pharmacotherapy* **21**, 1375–88.

372. **Wellington, K. and Goa, K.L.** (2001). Oxcarbazepine: an update of its efficacy in the management of epilepsy. *CNS Drugs* **15**, 137–63.

373. **Kalis, M.M. and Huff, N.A.** (2001). Oxcarbazepine, an antiepileptic agent. *Clinical Therapeutics* **23**, 680–700.

374. **Sindrup, S.H. and Jensen, T.S.** (2002). Pharmacotherapy of trigeminal neuralgia. *Clinical Journal of Pain* **18**, 22–7.

375. **Fromm, G.H., Terrence, C.F., and Chattha, A.S.** (1984). Baclofen in the treatment of trigeminal neuralgia: double-blind study and long-term follow-up. *Annals of Neurology* **15**, 240–4.

376. **Fromm, G.H.** (1994). Baclofen as an adjuvant analgesic. *Journal of Pain and Symptom Management* **9**, 500–9.

377. **Ringel, R.A. and Roy, E.P.** (1987). Glossopharyngeal neuralgia: successful treatment with baclofen. *Annals of Neurology* **21**, 14–15.

378. **Fromm, G.H., Graff-Radford, S.B., Terrence, C.F., and Sweet, W.H.** (1990). Pretrigeminal neuralgia. *Neurology* **40**, 1493–5.

379. **Terrence, C.F., Fromm, G.H., and Tenicela, R.** (1985). Baclofen as an analgesic in chronic peripheral nerve disease. *European Neurology* **24**, 380–5.

380. **Corli, O., Roma, G., Bacchini, M., Battagliarin, G., Di Piazza, D., Brambilla, C., and Grossi, E.** (1984). Double-blind placebo-controlled trial of baclofen, alone and in combination, in patients undergoing voluntary abortion. *Clinical Therapeutics* **6**, 800–7.

381. **Kofler, M. and Leis, A.A.** (1992). Prolonged seizure activity after baclofen withdrawn. *Neurology* **42**, 697.

382. **Mao, J., Price, D.D., and Mayer, D.J.** (1995). Experimental mononeuropathy reduces the antinociceptive effects of morphine: implications for common intracellular mechanisms involved in morphine tolerance and neuropathic pain. *Pain* **61**, 353–4.

383. **Woolf, C.J. and Thompson, S.W.N.** (1991). The induction and maintenance of central sensitization is dependent on *N*-methyl-D-aspartic acid receptor activation: implications for the treatment of post-injury pain hypersensitivity states. *Pain* **44**, 293–9.

384. **Dickenson, A.H. and Sullivan, A.F.** (1987). Evidence for a role of the NMDA receptor in the frequency dependent potentiation of deep dorsal horn nociceptive neurons following C fibre stimulation. *Neuropharmacology* **26**, 1235–8.

385. **Jahangir, S.M., Islam, F., and Aziz, L.** (1993). Ketamine infusion for post-operative analgesia in asthmatics: a comparison with intermittent meperidine. *Anesthesia and Analgesia* **76**, 45–9.

386. **Ilkjaer, S., Bach, L.F., Nielsen, P.A., Wernberg, M., and Dahl, J.B.** (2000). Effect of preoperative oral dextromethorphan on immediate and late postoperative pain and hyperalgesia after total abdominal hysterectomy. *Pain* **86**, 19–24.

387. **Mathisen, L.C., Skjelbred, P., Skoglund, L.A., and Oye, I.** (1995). Effect of ketamine, an NMDA receptor inhibitor, in acute and chronic orofacial pain. *Pain* **61**, 215–20.

388. **Cherry, D.A., Plummer, J.L., Gourlay, G.K., Coates, K.R., and Odgers, C.L.** (1995). Ketamine as an adjunct to morphine in the treatment of pain. *Pain* **62**, 119–21.

389. **Persson, J., Axelsson, G., Hallin, R.G., and Gustafsson, L.L.** (1995). Beneficial effects of ketamine in a chronic pain state with allodynia, possibly due to central sensitization. *Pain* **60**, 217–22.

390. **Stannard, C.F. and Porter, G.E.** (1993). Ketamine hydrochloride in the treatment of phantom limb pain. *Pain* **54**, 227–30.

391. **Hewitt, D.J.** (2000). The use of NMDA-receptor antagonists in the treatment of chronic pain. *Clinical Journal of Pain* **16**, S73–9.

392. **Graven-Nielsen, T., Aspegren Kendall, S., Henriksson, K.G., Bengtsson, M., Sörensen, J., Johnson, A., Gerdle, B., and Arendt-Nielsen, L.** (2000). Ketamine reduces muscle pain, temporal summation, and referred pain in fibromyalgia patients. *Pain* **85**, 483–91.

393. **Price, D.D., Mao, J., Frenk, H., and Mayer, D.J.** (1994). The *N*-methyl-D-aspartate antagonist dextromethorphan selectively reduces temporal summation of second pain in man. *Pain* **59**, 165–74.

394. **Park, K.M., Max, M.B., Robinovitz, E., Gracely, R.H., and Bennett, G.J.** (1994). Effects of intravenous ketamine and alfentanil on hyperalgesia induced by intradermal capsaicin. In *Proceedings of the 7th World Congress on Pain* (ed. G.F. Gebhardt, D.L. Hammond, and T.S. Jensen), pp. 647–55. Seattle: IASP Press.

395. **Backonja, A., Arndt, G., Gombar, K.A., Check, B., and Zimmermann, M.** (1994). Response of chronic neuropathic pain syndromes to ketamine: a preliminary study. *Pain* **56**, 51–7.

396. **Felsby, S., Nielsen, J., Arendt-Nielsen, L., and Jensen, T.S.** (1996). NMDA receptor blockade in chronic neuropathic pain: a comparison of ketamine and magnesium chloride. *Pain* **64**, 283–91.

397. **Eide, K., Stubhaug, A., Oye, I., and Breivik, H.** (1995). Continuous subcutaneous administration of the *N*-methyl-D-aspartic acid (NMDA) receptor antagonist ketamine in the treatment of post-herpetic neuralgia. *Pain* **61**, 221–8.

398. **Nikolajsen, L., Hansen, C.L., Nielsen, J., Keller, J., Arendt-Nielsen, L., and Jensen, T.S.** (1996). The effect of ketamine on phantom pain: a central neuropathic disorder maintained by peripheral input. *Pain* **67**, 69–77.

399. **Nelson, K.A., Park, K.M., Robinovitz, E., Tsigos, C., and Max, M.B.** (1997). High-dose oral dextromethorphan versus placebo in painful diabetic neuropathy and postherpetic neuralgia. *Neurology* **48**, 1212–18.

400. **Gilron, I., Booher, S.L., Rowan, J.S., Smoller, B., and Max, M.B.** (2000). A randomized, controlled trial of high-dose dextromethorphan in facial neuralgias. *Neurology* **55**, 964–71.

401. **Katz, N.P.** (2000). MorphiDex® (MS:DM) double-blind, multiple-dose studies in chronic pain patients. *Journal of Pain and Symptom Management* **19**, S37–41.

402. **Chevlen, E.** (2000). Morphine with dextromethorphan: conversion from other opioid analgesics. *Journal of Pain and Symptom Management* **19**, S42–9.

403. **Fisher, K., Coderre, T.J., and Hagen, N.A.** (2000). Targeting the *N*-methyl-D-aspartate receptor for chronic pain management: preclinical animal studies, recent clinical experience and future research directions. *Journal of Pain and Symptom Management* **20**, 358–73.

404. **Fine, P.G.** (1999). Low-dose ketamine in the management of opioid non-responsive terminal cancer pain. *Journal of Pain and Symptom Management* **17**, 296–300.

405. **Lloyd-Williams, M.** (2000). Ketamine for cancer pain. *Journal of Pain and Symptom Management* **19**, 79–80.

406. **Tarumi, Y., Watanabe, S., Bruera, E., and Ishitani, K.** (2000). High-dose ketamine in the management of cancer-related neuropathic pain. *Journal of Pain and Symptom Management* **19**, 405–7.

407. **Bell, R.F.** (1999). Low-dose subcutaneous ketamine infusion and morphine tolerance. *Pain* **83**, 101–3.

408. **Kannan, T.R., Saxena, A., Bhatnagar, S., and Barry, A.** (2002). Oral ketamine as an adjuvant to oral morphine for neuropathic pain in cancer patients. *Journal of Pain and Symptom Management* **23**, 60–5.

409. **Jackson, K., Ashby, M., Martin, P., Pisasale, M., Brumley, D., and Hayes, B.** (2001). 'Burst' ketamine for refractory cancer pain: an open-label audit of 39 patients. *Journal of Pain and Symptom Management* **22**, 834–42.

410. **Lauretti, G.R., Lima, I.C.P.R., Reis, M.P., Prado, W.A., and Pereira, N.L.** (1999). Oral ketamine and transdermal nitroglycerin as analgesic adjuvants to oral morphine therapy for cancer pain management. *Anesthesiology* **90**, 1528–33.

411. **Mercadante, S., Arcuri, E., Tirelli, W., and Casuccio, A.** (2000). Analgesic effect of intravenous ketamine in cancer patients on morphine therapy: a randomized, controlled, double-blind, crossover, double-dose study. *Journal of Pain and Symptom Management* **20**, 246–52.

412. **Berger, J.M., Ryan, A., Vadivelu, N., Merriam, P., Rever, L., and Harrison, P.** (2000). Ketamine–fentanyl–midazolam infusion for the control of symptoms in terminal life care. *American Journal of Hospice & Palliative Care* **17**, 127–32.

413. **Eisenberg, E. and Pud, D.** (1998). Can patients with chronic neuropathic pain be cured by acute administration of the NMDA receptor antagonist amantadine? *Pain* **74**, 337–9.

414. **Pud, D., Eisenberg, E., Spitzer, A., Adler, R., Fried, G., and Yarnitsky, D.** (1998). The NMDA receptor antagonist amantadine reduces surgical neuropathic pain in cancer patients: a double blind, randomized, placebo-controlled trial. *Pain* **75**, 349–54.

415. **Taira, T.** (1998). Comments on Eisenberg and Pud. *Pain* **74**, 337–9; *Pain* **78**, 221–6.

416. **Gorman, A.L., Elliott, K.J., and Inturrisi, C.E.** (1997). The D- and L-isomers of methadone bind to the non-competitive site on the *N*-methyl-D-aspartate (NMDA) receptor in rat forebrain and spinal cord. *Neuroscience Letter* **223**, 5–8.

417. **Davis, A.M. and Inturrisi, C.E.** (1999). D-methadone blocks morphine tolerance and *N*-methyl-D-aspartate-induced hyperalgesia. *Journal of Pharmacology and Experimental Therapeutics* **289**, 1048–53.

418. **Shimoyama, N., Shimoyama, M., Elliott, K.J., and Inturrisi, C.E.** (1997). D-Methadone is antinociceptive in the rate formalin test. *Journal of Pharmacology and Experimental Therapeutics* **283**, 648–52.

419. **Carpenter, K.J., Chapman, V., and Dickenson, A.H.** (2000). Neuronal inhibitory effects of methadone are predominantly opioid receptor mediated in the rat spinal cord *in vivo*. *European Journal of Pain* **4**, 19–26.

420. **Chizh, B.A., Schlutz, H., Scheede, M., and Englberger, W.** (2000). The *N*-methyl-D-aspartate antagonistic and opioid components of D-methadone antinociception in the rat spinal cord. *Neuroscience Letter* **296**, 117–20.

421. **Gobelet, C., Waldburger, M., and Meier, J.L.** (1992). The effect of adding calcitonin to physical treatment on reflex sympathetic dystrophy. *Pain* **48**, 171–5.

422. **Jaeger, H. and Maier, C.** (1992). Calcitonin in phantom limb pain: a double blind study. *Pain* **48**, 21–7.

423. **Backonja, M.** (1994). Reflex sympathetic dystrophy/sympathetically-maintained pain/causalgia: the syndrome of neuropathic pain with dysautonomia. *Seminars in Neurology* **14**, 263–71.

424. **Perez, R.S.G.M., Kwakkel, G., Zuurmond, W.W.A., and de Lange, J.J.** (2001). Treatment of reflex sympathetic dystrophy (CRPS type 1): a research synthesis of 21 randomized clinical trials. *Journal of Pain and Symptom Management* **21**, 511–26.

425. **Rowbotham, M.C.** (1994). Topical analgesic agents. In *Pharmacological Approaches to the Treatment of Chronic Pain: New Concepts and Critical Issues* (ed. H.L. Fields and J.C. Liebeskind), pp. 211–29. Seattle: IASP Press.

426. **Bernstein, J.E., Bickers, R.R., Dahl, M.V., and Roshal, J.Y.** (1987). Treatment of chronic postherpetic neuralgia with topical capsaicin. A preliminary study. *Journal of the American Academy of Dermatology* **17**, 93–6.

427. **Watson, C.P.N., Evans, R.J., and Watt, V.R.** (1988). Postherpetic neuralgia and topical capsaicin. *Pain* **33**, 333–40.

428. **Watson, C.P.N., Evans, R.J., and Watt, V.R.** (1989). The post-mastectomy pain syndrome and the effect of topical capsaicin. *Pain* **38**, 177–86.

429. **Watson, C.P.N. and Evans, R.J.** (1992). The postmastectomy pain syndrome and topical capsaicin: a randomized trial. *Pain* **51**, 375–9.

430. **Fusco, B.M. and Alessandri, M.** (1992). Analgesic effect of capsaicin in idiopathic trigeminal neuralgia. *Anesthesia and Analgesia* **74**, 375–7.

431. **Watson, C.P.N., Tyler, K.L., Bickers, D.R., Millikan, L.E., Smith, S., and Coleman, E.** (1993). A randomized vehicle-controlled trial of topical capsaicin in the treatment of postherpetic neuralgia. *Clinical Therapeutics* **15**, 510–26.

432. **Tandan, R., Lewis, G.A., Krusinski, P.B., Badger, G.B., and Fries, T.J.** (1992). Topical capsaicin in painful diabetic neuropathy. Controlled study with long-term follow-up. *Diabetes Care* **15**, 8–14.

433. **Capsaicin Study Group** (1991). Treatment of painful diabetic neuropathy with topical capsaicin. A multicenter, double-blind, vehicle-controlled study. *Archives of Internal Medicine* **151**, 2225–9.

434. **McCarthy, G.M. and McCarty, D.J.** (1992). Effect of topical capsaicin in the therapy of painful osteoarthritis of the hands. *Journal of Rheumatology* **19**, 604–7.

435. **Zhang, W.Y. and Li Wan Po, A.** (1994). The effectiveness of topically applied capsaicin: a meta-analysis. *European Journal of Clinical Pharmacology* **46**, 517–22.

436. **Paice, J.A., Ferrans, C.E., Lashley, F.R., Shott, S., Vizgirda, V., and Pitrak, D.** (2000). Topical capsaicin in the management of HIV-associated peripheral neuropathy. *Journal of Pain and Symptom Management* **19**, 45–52.

437. **Ellison, N., Loprinzi, C.L., Kugler, J., Hatfield, A.K., Miser, A., Sloan, J.A., Wender, D.B., Rowland, K.M., Molina, R., Cascino, T.L., Vukov, A.M., Dhaliwal, H.S., and Ghosh, C.** (1997). Phase III placebo-controlled trial of capsaicin cream in the management of surgical neuropathic pain in cancer patients. *Journal of Clinical Oncology* **15**, 2974–80.

438. **Robbins, W.R., Staats, P.S., Levine, J., Fields, H.L., Allen, R.W., Campbell, J.N., and Pappagallo, M.** (1998). Treatment of intractable pain with topical large-dose capsaicin: preliminary report. *Anesthesia and Analgesia* **86**, 579–83.

439. **McCleane, G.** (2000). Topical application of doxepin hydrochloride, capsaicin and a combination of both produces analgesia in chronic human neuropathic pain: a randomized, double-blind, placebo-controlled study. *Journal of Clinical Pharmacology* **49**, 574–9.

440. **Robbins, W.** (2000). Clinical applications of capsaicinoids. *Clinical Journal of Pain* **16**, S86–9.

441. **Nolano, M., Simone, D.A., Wendelschafer-Crabb, G., Johnson, T., Hazen, E., and Kennedy, W.R.** (1999). Topical capsaicin in humans: parallel loss of epidermal nerve fibers and pain sensation. *Pain* **81**, 135–45.

442. **DeBenedittis, G., Besana, F., and Lorenzettit, A.** (1992). A new topical treatment for acute herpetic neuralgia and postherpetic neuralgia: the aspirin/diethyl ether mixture. An open-label study plus a double-blind controlled clinical trial. *Pain* **48**, 383–90.

443. **McQuay, H.J., Carroll, D., Moxon, A., Glynn, C.J., and Moore, R.A.** (1990). Benzydamine cream for the treatment of postherpetic neuralgia: minimum duration of treatment periods in a cross-over trial. *Pain* **40**, 131–5.

444. **McCleane, G.J.** (2000). Topical doxepin hydrochloride reduces neuropathic pain: a randomised, double-blind, placebo-conrolled study. *The Pain Clinic* **2**, 47–50.

445. **Lok, C.** et al. (1999). EMLA cream as a topical anesthetic for the repeated mechanical debridement of venous leg ulcers: a double-blind, placebo-controlled study. *Journal of the American Academy of Dermatology* **40**, 208–13.

446. **Stow, P.J., Glynn, C.J., and Minor, B.** (1989). EMLA cream in the treatment of post herpetic neuralgia: efficacy and pharmacokinetic profile. *Pain* **39**, 301–5.

447. **Rowbotham, M.C. and Fields, H.L.** (1989). Topical lidocaine reduces pain in postherpetic neuralgia. *Pain* **38**, 297–302.

448. **Rowbotham, M.C., Davies, P.S., and Fields, H.L.** (1995). Topical lidocaine gel relieves postherpetic neuralgia. *Annals of Neurology* **37**, 246–53.

449. **Rowbotham, M.C., Davies, P.S., and Galer, B.S.** (1996). Lidocaine patch: double-blind controlled study of a new treatment for post-herpetic neuralgia. *Pain* **65**, 39–44.

450. **Galer, B.S., Rowbotham, M.C., and Perander, J.** (1999). Topical lidocaine patch relieves postherpetic neuralgia more effectively than a vehicle topical patch: results of an enriched enrollment study. *Pain* **80**, 533–8.

451. **Devers, A. and Galer, B.S.** (2000). Topical lidocaine patch relieves a variety of neuropathic pain conditions: an open-label pilot study. *Clinical Journal of Pain* **16**, 205–8.

452. **Gammaitoni, A.R. and Davis, M.W.** (2002). Pharmacokinetics and tolerability of lidocaine patch 5 percent with extended dosing. *Annals of Pharmacotherapy* **36**, 236–40.

453. **Gammaitoni, A.R., Alvarez, N.A., and Galer, B.S.** (2002). Pharmacokinetics and safety of continuously applied lidocaine patches 5%. *American Journal of Health-System Pharmacy* **59**, 2215–20.

454. **Comer, A.M. and Lamb, H.M.** (2000). Lidocaine patch 5 per cent. *Drugs* **59**, 245–9.

455. **Schott, G.D. and Loh, L.** (1984). Anticholinesterase drugs in the treatment of chronic pain. *Pain* **20**, 201–6.

456. **Hampf, G., Bowsher, D., and Nurmikko, T.** (1989). Distigmine and amitriptyline in the treatment of chronic pain. *Anesthesia Progress* **36**, 58–62.

457. **Weinstock, M., Davidson, J.T., Rosin, A.J., and Schnieden, H.** (1982). Effect of physostigmine on morphine-induced postoperative pain and somnolence. *British Journal of Anaesthesia* **54**, 429–34.

458. **Dellemijn, P.L.I. and Fields, H.L.** (1994). Do benzodiazepines have a role in chronic pain management. *Pain* **57**, 137–52.

459. **Reddy, S. and Patt, R.B.** (1994). The benzodiazepines as adjuvant analgesics. *Journal of Pain and Symptom Management* **9**, 510–14.

460. **Payne, R.** (1989). Pharmacologic management of bone pain in the cancer patient. *Clinical Journal of Pain* **5**, S43–50.

461. **Punn, K.K. and Chan, M.B.** (1989). Analgesic effect of intranasal salmon calcitonin in the treatment of osteoporotic vertebral fractures. *Clinical Therapeutics* **11**, 205–9.

462. **Pontiroli, A.E., Pajetta, E., Scaglia, L., Rubinacci, A., Resmini, G., Arrigoni, M., and Pozza, G.** (1994). Analgesic effect of intranasal and intramuscular salmon calcitonin in post-menopausal osteoporosis: a double-blind, double-placebo study. *Aging* **6**, 459–63.

463. **Lyritis, G.P., Paspati, I., Karachalios, T., Ioakimidis, D., Skarantavos, G., and Lyritis, P.G.** (1997). Pain relief from nasal salmon calcitonin in osteoporotic vertebral crush fractures: a double-blind, placebo-controlled clinical study. *Acta Orthopedica Scandinavica* **61**, 10–15.

464. **Lyritis, G.P., Ioannidis, G.V., Karachalios, T., Roidis, N., Kataxaki, E., Papaioannou, N., Kaloudis, J., and Galanos, A.** (1999). Analgesic effect of salmon calcitonin suppositories in patients with acute pain due to recent osteoporotic vertebral crush fractures: a prospective double-blind, randomized, placebo-controlled clinical study. *Clinical Journal of Pain* **15**, 284–9.

465. **Szanto, J., Ady, N., and Jozsef, S.** (1992). Pain killing with calcitonin nasal spray in patients with malignant tumors. *Oncology* **49**, 180–2.

466. **Mystakidou, J., Befon, S., Hondros, J., Kouskouni, E., and Vlahos, L.** (1999). Continuous subcutaneous administration of high-dose salmon calcitonin in bone metastasis: pain control and beta-endorphin plasma levels. *Journal of Pain and Symptom Management* **18**, 323–30.

467. **Hindley, A.C., Hill, A.B., Leyland, M.J., and Wiles, A.E.** (1982). A double-blind controlled trial of salmon calcitonin in pain due to malignancy. *Cancer Chemotherapy Pharmacology* **9**, 71–4.

468. **Roth, A. and Kolaric, K.** (1986). Analgesic activity of calcitonin in patient with painful osteolytic metastases of breast cancer: results of a controlled randomized study. *Oncology* **43**, 283–7.

469. **Ormazabal, M.J., Goicoechea, C., Sanchez, E., and Martin, M.I.** (2001). Salmon calcitonin potentiates the analgesia induced by antidepressants. *Pharmacology, Biochemistry and Behavior* **68**, 125–33.

470. **Fraioli, F.** et al. (1984). Calcitonin and analgesia. In *Advances in Pain Research and Therapy* Vol. 7 (ed. C. Benedetti, C.R. Chapman, and G. Moricca), pp. 37–50. New York: Raven Press.

471. **Paterson, A.H.G., Powles, T.J., Kanis, J.A., McCloskey, E., Hanson, J., and Ashley, S.** (1993). Double-blind controlled trial of oral clodronate in patients with bone metastases from breast cancer. *Journal of Clinical Oncology* **11**, 59–65.

472. **Ernst, D.S., MacDonald, R.N., Paterson, A.H.G., Jensen, J., Brasher, P., and Bruera, E.** (1992). A double blind, cross-over trial of IV clodronate in metastatic bone pain. *Journal of Pain and Symptom Management* **7**, 4–11.

473. **Thiebaud, D., Leyvraz, S., von Fliedner, V., Perey, L., Cornu, P., Thiebaud, S., and Burckhardt, P.** (1991). Treatment of bone metastases from breast cancer and myeloma with pamidronate. *European Journal of Cancer* **27**, 37–41.

474. **Glover, D., Lipton, A., Keller, A., Miller, A.A., Browning, S., Fram, R.J., George, S., Zelenakas, K., Macerata, R.S., and Seaman, J.J.** (1994). Intravenous pamidronate disodium treatment of bone metastases in patients with breast cancer. *Cancer* **74**, 2949–55.

475. **Body, J.J.** (1999). Bisphosphonates for metastatic bone pain. *Supportive Care in Cancer* **7**, 1–3.

476. **Fulfaro, F., Casuccio, A., Ticozzi, C., and Ripamonti, C.** (1998). The role of bisphosphonates in the treatment of painful metastatic bone disease: a review of phase III trials. *Pain* **78**, 157–69.

477. **Adami, S. and Mian, M.** (1989). Clodronate therapy of metastatic bone disease in patients with prostatic carcinoma. *Cancer Research* **116**, 67–72.

478. **McCloskey, E.V., MacLennan, I.C.M., Kanis, J.A., MacLennan, I.C., and Drayson, M.T.** (2001). Effect of clodronate on progression of skeletal disease in multiple myelomatosis. *British Journal of Haematology* **113**, 1035–43.

479. **Robertson, A.G., Reed, N.S., and Ralston, S.H.** (1995). Effect of oral clodronate on metastatic bone pain: a double-blind, placebo-controlled study. *Journal of Clinical Oncology* **13**, 2427–30.

480. **Ernst, D.S., Brasher, P., Hagen, N., Paterson, A.H.G., MacDonald, N., and Bruera, E.** (1997). A randomized, controlled trial of intravenous clodronate in patients with metastatic bone disease and pain. *Journal of Pain and Symptom Management* **13**, 319–26.

481. **Lahtinen, R., Laasko, M., Palva, I., Virkkunen, P., and Elomaa, I.** (1992). Randomized placebo-controlled multicentre trial of clodronate in multiple myeloma. *Lancet* **340**, 1049–52.

482. **Van Holten-Verzantvoort, A.T.M., Kroon, H.M., Bijvoet, O.L., Cleton, F.J., Beex, L.V., Blijham, J., Hermans, J., Neijt, J.P., Papapoulos, S.E., and Sleebom, H.P.** (1993). Palliative pamidronate treatment in patients with bone metastases from breast cancer. *Journal of Clinical Oncology* **11**, 491–8.

483. **Lipton, A., Glover, D., Harvey, H., Grabelsky, S., Zelenakas, K., Macerata, R., and Seaman, J.** (1994). Pamidronate in the treatment of bone metastases: results of 2 dose-ranging trials in patients with breast or prostate cancer. *Annals of Oncology* **5** (Suppl. 7), S31–5.

484. **Hortobagyi, G.N., Theriault, R.L., Porter, L., Blayney, D., Lipton, A., Sinoff, C., Wheeler, H., Simeone, J.F., Seaman, J., and Knight, R.D.** (1996). Efficacy of pamidronate in reducing skeletal complications in patients with breast cancer and lytic bone metastases. *New England Journal of Medicine* **335**, 1785–91.

485. **Berenson, J.R., Lichtenstein, A., Porter, L., Dimopoulos, M.A., Bordoni, R., George, S., Lipton, A., Keller, A., Ballester, O., Kovacs, M.J., Blacklock, H.A., Bell, R., Simeone, J., Reitsma, D.J., Heffernan, M., Seaman, J., and Knight, R.D.** (1996). Efficacy of pamidronate in reducing skeletal events in patients with advanced multiple myeloma. *New England Journal of Medicine* **334**, 488–93.

486. **Belch, A.R., Bergsagel, D.E., Wilson, K., O'Reilly, S., Wilson, J., Sutton, D., Pater, J., Johnston, D., and Zee, B.** (1991). Effect of daily etidronate on the osteolysis of multiple myeloma. *Journal of Clinical Oncology* **9**, 1397–402.

487. **Smith, J.A.** (1989). Palliation of painful bone metastases from prostate cancer using sodium etidronate: results of a randomized, prospective, double-blind, placebo-controlled study. *Journal of Urology* **141**, 85–7.
488. **Berenson, J.R.** (2001). Zoledronic acid in cancer patients with bone metastases: results of Phase I and II trials. *Seminars in Oncology* **28** (2 Suppl. 6), 25–34.
489. **Berenson, J.R., Rosen, L.S., Howell, A., Porter, L., Coleman, R.E., Morley, W., Dreicer, R., Kuross, S.A., Lipton, A., and Seaman, J.J.** (2001). Zoledronic acid reduces skeletal-related events in patients with osteolytic metastases. *Cancer* **91**, 1191–200.
490. **Kanis, J.A., Powles, T., Paterson, A.H., McCloskey, E.V., and Ashley, S.** (1996). Clodronate decreases the frequency of skeletal metastases in women with breast cancer. *Bone* **19**, 663–7.
491. **Holmes, R.A.** (1993). Radiopharmaceuticals in clinical trials. *Seminars in Oncology* **20**, 22–6.
492. **Serafini, A.N.** (1994). Current status of systemic intravenous radiopharmaceuticals for the treatment of painful metastatic bone disease. *International Journal of Radiation Oncology and Biological Physics* **30**, 1187–94.
493. **Silberstein, E.B.** (1993). The treatment of painful osseous metastases with phosphorus-32-labeled phosphates. *Seminars in Oncology* **20**, 10–21.
494. **Laing, A.H., Ackery, D.M., Bayly, R.J., Buchanan, R.B., Lewington, V.J., McEwan, A.J., Macleod, P.M., and Zivanovic, M.A.** (1991). Strontium-89 chloride for pain palliation in prostatic skeletal malignancy. *British Journal of Radiology* **64**, 816–22.
495. **Robinson, R.G.** et al. (1987). Treatment of metastatic bone pain with strontium-89. *Nuclear Medicine Biology* **14**, 219–22.
496. **Silberstein, E.B. and Williams, C.** (1985). Strontium-89 therapy for the pain of osseous metastases. *Journal of Nuclear Medicine* **26**, 345–8.
497. **Maxon, H.R.** et al. (1988). Initial experience with 186-Re(Sn)-HEDP in the treatment of painful skeletal metastases. *Journal of Nuclear Medicine* **29**, 776.
498. **Turner, J.H. and Claringbold, P.G.** (1991). A phase II study of treatment of painful multifocal skeletal metastases with single and repeated dose samarium-153 ethylenediaminetetramethylene phosphonate. *European Journal of Cancer* **27**, 1084–6.
499. **Maxon, H.R.** et al. (1992). Rhenium-186 hydroxyethylidene diphosphonate for the treatment of painful osseous metastases. *Seminars in Nuclear Medicine* **22**, 33–40.
500. **Turner, J.H., Claringbold, P.G., Hetherington, E.L., Sorby, P., and Martindale, A.A.** (1989). A phase I study of samarium-153 ethylenediamenetramethylene phosphonate therapy for disseminated skeletal metastases. *Journal of Clinical Oncology* **7**, 1926–31.
501. **Farhanghi, M., Holmes, R.A., Volkert, W.A., Logan, K.W., and Singh, A.** (1992). Samarium-153-EDTMP: pharmacolkinetic, toxicity and pain response using an escalating dose schedule in treatment of metastatic bone pain. *Journal of Nuclear Medicine* **33**, 1451–8.
502. **Holmes, P.A.** (1992). [153Sm]EDTMP: a potential therapy for bone cancer pain. *Seminars in Nuclear Medicine* **22**, 41–5.
503. **Porter, A.T.** et al. (1993). Results of a randomized phase-III trial to evaluate the efficacy of strontium-89 adjuvant to local field external beam irradiation in the management of endocrine resistant metastatic prostate cancer. *International Journal of Radiation, Oncology, and Biologic Physics* **25**, 805–13.
504. **Lewington, V.J., McEwan, A.J., Ackery, D.M., Bayly, R.J., Keeling, D.H., Macleod, P.M., Porter, A.T., and Zivanovic, M.A.** (1991). A prospective, randomized double-blind cross-over study to examine the efficacy of strontium-89 in pain palliation in patients with advanced prostate cancer metastatic to bone. *European Journal of Cancer* **27**, 954–8.
505. **Quilty, P.M., Kirk, D., Bolger, J.J., Dearnaley, D.P., Lewington, V.J., Mason, M.D., Reed, N.S., Russell, J.M., and Yardley, J.** (1994). A comparison of the palliative effects of strontium-89 and external beam radiotherapy in metastatic prostate cancer. *Radiotherapy and Oncology* **31**, 33–40.
506. **Robinson, R.G., Preston, D.F., Baxter, K.G., Dusing, R.W., and Spicer, J.A.** (1993). Clinical experience with strontium-89 in prostatic and breast cancer patients. *Seminars in Oncology* **20**, 44–8.
507. **Robinson, R.G., Preston, D.F., Schiefelbein, M., and Baster, K.G.** (1995). Strontium-89 therapy for the palliation of pain due to osseous metastases. *Journal of the American Medical Association* **274**, 420–4.
508. **Warrell, R.P., Lovett, D., Dilmanian, F.A., Schneider, R., and Heelan, R.T.** (1993). Low-dose gallium nitrate for prevention of osteolysis in myeloma: results of a pilot randomized study. *Journal of Clinical Oncology* **11**, 2443–50.
509. **Minton, J.P.** (1974). The response of breast cancer patients with bone pain to L-dopa. *Cancer* **33**, 358–63.
510. **Hanks, G.W.** (1988). The pharmacological treatment of bone pain. *Cancer Surveys* **7**, 87–101.
511. **Sjolin, S. and Trykker, H.** (1985). Unsuccessful treatment of severe pain from bone metastases with Sinemet 25/100. *New England Journal of Medicine* **302**, 650–1.
512. **Ripamonti, C.** (1994). Management of bowel obstruction in advanced cancer patients. *Journal of Pain and Symptom Management* **9**, 193–200.
513. **Baines, M., Oliver, D.J., and Carter, R.L.** (1985). Medical management of intestinal obstruction in patients with advanced malignant disease: a clinical and pathological study. *Lancet* **2**, 990–3.
514. **Ventafridda, V., Ripamonti, C., Caraceni, A., Spoldi, E., Messina, L., and De Conno, F.** (1990). The management of inoperable gastrointestinal obstruction in terminal cancer patients. *Tumori* **76**, 389–93.
515. **De Conno, F., Caraceni, A., Zecca, E., Spoldi, E., and Ventafridda, V.** (1991). Continuous subcutaneous infusion of hyoscine butylbromide reduces secretions in patients with gastrointestinal obstruction. *Journal of Pain and Symptom Management* **6**, 484–6.
516. **Ripamonti, C., Mercadante, S., Groff, L., Zecca, E., De Conno, F., and Casuccio, A.** (2000). Role of octreotide, scopolamine butylbromide, and hydration in symptom control of patients with inoperable bowel obstruction and nasogastric tubes: a prospective randomized trial. *Journal of Pain and Symptom Management* **19**, 23–34.
517. **Mercadante, S., Ripamonti, C., Casuccio, A., Zecca, E., and Groff, L.** (2000). Comparison of octreotide and hyoscine butylbromide in controlling gastrointestinal symptoms due to malignant inoperable bowel obstruction. *Supportive Care in Cancer* **8**, 188–91.
518. **Mercadante, S.** (1992). Treatment of diarrhea due to enterocolic fistula with octreotide in a terminal cancer patient. *Palliative Medicine* **6**, 257–9.
519. **Mulvihill, S., Pappas, T.N., Passaro, E., and Debas, H.T.** (1986). The use of somatostatin and its analogues. *Surgery* **100**, 467–76.
520. **Ladefoged, K., Christensen, K.C., Hegnhoj, J., and Jarnum, S.** (1989). Effect of a long acting somatostatin analogue SMS 201-995 on jejunostomy effluents in patients with severe short bowel syndrome. *Gut* **30**, 943–9.
521. **Laval, G., Girardier, J., Lassaunière, J.M., Leduc, B., Haond, C., and Schaerer, R.** (2000). The use of steroids in the management of inoperable intestinal obstruction in terminal cancer patients: do they remove the obstruction? *Palliative Medicine* **14**, 3–10.
522. **Twycross, R.G. and Fairfield, S.** (1982). Pain in far-advanced cancer. *Pain* **14**, 303–10.
523. **Batterman, R.C.** (1965). Methodology of analgesic evaluation: experience with orphenadrine citrate compound. *Current Therapeutic Research* **7**, 639–47.
524. **Bercel, N.A.** (1977). Cyclobenzaprine in the treatment of skeletal muscle spasm in osteoarthritis of the cervical and lumbar spine. *Current Therapeutic Research* **22**, 462–8.
525. **Birkeland, I.W. and Clawson, D.K.** (1958). Drug combinations with orphenadrine for pain relief associated with muscle spasm. *Clinical Pharmacology and Therapeutics* **9**, 639–46.
526. **Gold, R.H.** (1978). Treatment of low back pain syndrome with oral orphenadrine citrate. *Current Therapeutic Research* **23**, 271–6.
527. **Tseng, T.C. and Wang, S.C.** (1971). Locus of action of centrally-acting muscle relaxants, diazepam and tybamate. *Journal of Pharmacology and Experimental Therapeutics* **178**, 350–60.
528. **Littrell, R.A., Hayes, L.R., and Stillner, V.** (1993). Carisoprodol (Soma): a new and cautious perspective on an old agent. *Southern Medical Journal* **86**, 753–6.
529. **Dalal, S. and Melzack, R.** (1998). Potentiation of opioid analgesia by psychostimulant drugs: a review. *Journal of Pain and Symptom Management* **16**, 245–53.
530. **Forrest, W.H., Brown, B.W., Brown, C.R., Defalque, R., Gold, M., Gordon, H.E., James, K.E., Katz, J., Mahler, D.L., Schroff, P., and Teutsch, G.**

(1977). Dextroamphetamine with morphine for the treatment of postoperative pain. *New England Journal of Medicine* **296**, 712–15.

531. **Cantello, R., Aguggia, M., Gilli, M., Delsedime, M., Riccio, A., Rainero, I., and Mutani, R.** (1988). Analgesic action of methylphenidate on parkinsonian sensory symptoms. Mechanisms and pathophysiological implications. *Archives of Neurology* **45**, 973–6.
532. **Bruera, E., Chadwich, S., Brenneis, C., Hanson, J., and MacDonald, R.N.** (1987). Methylphenidate associated with narcotics for the treatment of cancer pain. *Cancer Treatment Report* **71**, 67–70.
533. **Sawynok, J.** (1995). Pharmacological rationale for the clinical use of caffeine. *Drugs* **49**, 37–50.
534. **Schachtel, B.P., Fillingim, J.M., Lane, A.C., Thoden, W.R., and Baybutt, R.I.** (1991). Caffeine as an analgesic adjuvant: a double-blind study comparing aspirin with caffeine to aspirin and placebo in patients with severe sore throat. *Archives of Internal Medicine* **151**, 733–7.
535. **Laska, E.M., Sunshine, A., Mueller, F., Elvers, W.B., Siegel, C., and Rubin, A.** (1984). Caffeine as an analgesic adjuvant. *Journal of the American Medical Association* **251**, 1711–18.
536. **Forbes, J.A., Beaver, W.T., Jones, K.F., Kehm, C.J., Smith, W.K., Gongloff, C.M., Zeleznock, J.R., and Smith, J.W.** (1991). Effect of caffeine on ibuprofen analgesia in postoperative oral surgery pain. *Clinical Pharmacology and Therapeutics* **49**, 674–84.
537. **Wilwerding, M.B., Loprinzi, C.L., Mailliard, J.A., O'Fallon, J.R., Miser, A.W., van Haelst, C., Barton, D.L., Foley, J.F., and Athmann, L.M.** (1995). A randomized, crossover evaluation of methylphenidate in cancer patients receiving strong narcotics. *Supportive Care in Cancer* **3**, 135–8.
538. **Yee, J.D. and Berde, C.B.** (1994). Dextroamphetamine or methyphenidate as adjuvants to opioid analgesia for adolescents with cancer. *Journal of Pain and Symptom Management* **9**, 122–5.
539. **Bruera, E., Miller, M.J., Macmillan, K., and Kuehn, N.** (1992). Neuropsychological effects of methylphenidate in patients receiving a continuous infusion of narcotics for cancer pain. *Pain* **48**, 163–6.
540. **Fernandez, F.** et al. (1987). Methylphenidate for depressive disorders in cancer patients: an alternative to standard antidepressants. *Psychosomatics* **28**, 455–61.
541. **Macleod, A.D.** (1998). Methylphenidate in terminal depression. *Journal of Pain and Symptom Management* **16**, 193–8.
542. **Sarhill, N., Walsh, D., Nelson, K.A., Homsi, J., LeGrand, S., and Davis, M.P.** (2001). Methylphenidate for fatigue in advanced cancer: a prospective open-label pilot study. *American Journal of Hospice and Palliative Care* **18**, 187–92.
543. **US Modafinil in Narcolepsy Multicenter Study Group** (2000). Randomized trial of modafinil as a treatment for the excessive daytime somnolence of narcolepsy. *Neurology* **54**, 1166–75.
544. **Menza, M.A., Kaufman, K.R., and Castellanos, A.** (2000). Modafinil augmentation of antidepressant treatment in depression. *Journal of Clinical Psychiatry* **61**, 378–81.
545. **Rammohan, K.W., Rosenberg, J.H., Lynn, D.J., Blumenfeld, A.M., Pollak, C.P., and Nagaraja, H.N.** (2002). Efficacy and safety of modafinil (Provigil) for the treatment of fatigue in multiple sclerosis: a two centre phase 2 study. *Journal of Neurology, Neurosurgery and Psychiatry* **72**, 179–83.
546. **Cox, J.M. and Pappagallo, M.** (2001). Modafinil: a gift to portmanteau. *American Journal of Hospice and Palliative Care* **18**, 408–10.
547. **Bruera, E., Brenneis, C., Paterson, A.H., and MacDonald, R.N.** (1989). Use of methylphenidate as an adjuvant to narcotic analgesics in patients with advanced cancer. *Journal of Pain and Symptom Management* **4**, 3–6.
548. **Campos, V.M. and Solis, E.L.** (1980). The analgesic and hypothermic effects of nefopam, morphine, aspirin, diphenhydramine and placebo. *Journal of Clinical Pharmacology* **20**, 42–9.
549. **Hupert, C., Yacoub, M., and Turgeon, L.R.** (1980). Effect of hydroxyzine on morphine analgesia for the treatment of postoperative pain. *Anesthesia and Analgesia* **59**, 690–6.
550. **Stambaugh, J.E. and Lance, C.** (1983). Analgesic efficacy and pharmacokinetic evaluation of meperidine and hydroxyzine, alone and in combination. *Cancer Investigation* **1**, 111–17.
551. **Beaver, W.T. and Feise, G.** (1976). Comparison of the analgesic effect of morphine, hydroxyzine and their combination in patients with postoperative pain. In *Advances in Pain Research and Therapy* Vol. 1 (ed. J.J. Bonica), pp. 553–7. New York: Raven Press.
552. **Sunshine, A., Zighelboim, I., De Castro, A., Sorrentino, J.V., Smith, D.S., Bartizek, R.D., and Olson, N.Z.** (1989). Augmentation of acetaminophen analgesia by the antihistamine phenyltoloxamine. *The Journal of Clinical Pharmacology* **29**, 660–4.
553. **McColl, J.D. and Durkin, W.** (1982). The effect of pyrilamine on relief of symptoms of the premenstrual syndrome (PMS) and primary dysmenorrhea. *Federation Proceedings* **41**, 5572.
554. **Gilbert, M.M.** (1976). The efficacy of percogesic in relief of musculoskeletal pain associated with anxiety. *Psychosomatics* **17**, 190–3.
555. **Santiago-Palma, J., Fischberg, D., Kornick, C., Khjainova, N., and Gonzales, G.** (2001). Diphenhydramine as an analgesic adjuvant in refractory cancer pain. *Journal of Pain and Symptom Management* **22**, 699–703.
556. **Wilson, R.S., May, E.L., Martin, B.R., and Dewey, W.L.** (1976). 9-nor-9-Hydroxyhexahydrocannabinols. Synthesis, some behavioral and analgesic properties, and comparison with the tetrahydrocannabinols. *Journal of Medicinal Chemistry* **19**, 1165–7.
557. **Chesher, G.B., Dahl, C.J., Everingham, M., Jackson, D.M., Marchant-Williams, H., and Starmer, G.A.** (1973). The effect of cannabinoids on intestinal motility and their antinociceptive effect in mice. *British Journal of Pharmacology* **49**, 588–94.
558. **Noyes, R., Brunk, S.F., Avery, D.H., and Canter, A.** (1976). The analgesic properties of delta-9-tetrahydrocannabinol and codeine. *Clinical Pharmacology and Therapeutics* **18**, 84–9.
559. **Jain, A.K., Ryan, J.R., McMahon, F.G., and Smith, G.** (1981). Evaluation of intramuscular levonantradol and placebo in acute postoperative pain. *Journal of Clinical Pharmacology* **21**, 320S–6S.

8.2.6 Anaesthetic techniques for pain control

Robert A. Swarm, Menelaos Karanikolas, and Michael J. Cousins

Introduction

Fortunately, for the sake of persons with pain, health-care professionals today are generally more sophisticated in analgesic therapy than 10 or 20 years ago. As exemplified by the widespread use of the World Health Organization's algorithm[1] for analgesics in cancer pain, pain control now receives far more attention than ever before. However, some persons with pain will not have adequate pain control from systemic medications, whether due to the characteristics of a particular pain syndrome, analgesic-related adverse effects, or tolerance. For these clinical settings, various interventional therapies are available, many of which are adapted from operating-room anaesthetic techniques. Anaesthetic pain management techniques range from local anaesthetic or neurolytic neural blockade to the regional administration of pharmacologic agents that modify neuronal transmission, and also include newer techniques such as radiofrequency ablation. These techniques are important in the palliative care of persons with advanced disease when pain is not adequately controlled with systemic analgesics.

The role of anaesthetic techniques in palliative medicine

Systemic analgesics are the cornerstone of pharmacologic therapy for pain, and opioids are the principal agents for management of severe pain.[1,2]

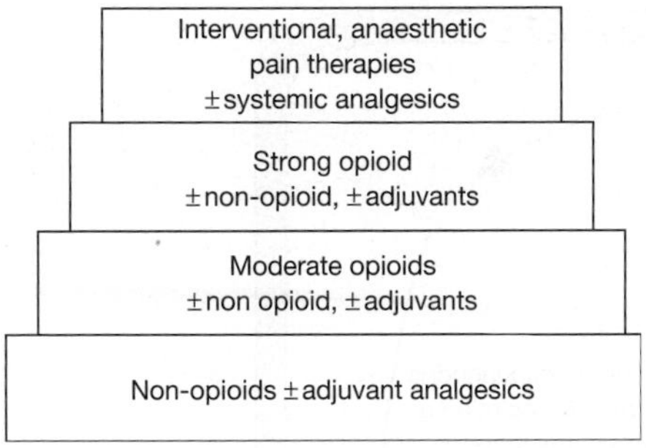

Fig. 1 Four-step analgesic ladder for stratified use of analgesic therapies.

Despite the proven efficacy of systemic analgesics, 2[3] to 10 per cent[4] of persons with advanced disease still experience severe pain. For them, the analgesic algorithm must be extended beyond systemic medications to include interventional, anaesthetic techniques of pain control (Fig. 1). The emphasis on pharmacologic and interventional therapies in this discussion presumes appropriate utilization of non-pharmacologic and psychosocial pain management strategies.[2]

Numerous disease and patient factors may limit the effectiveness of systemic analgesics.[5,6] Neuropathic pain may be less responsive to opioid analgesics than other types of pain; many resistant cancer pain syndromes include a component of neuropathic pain from compression or invasion of nervous tissue by tumour (e.g. brachial plexopathy in Pancoast tumours). Sharp, severe somatic pain, as with pathologic fracture or wound debridement, may be so intense as to surpass the efficacy of systemic 'analgesic' therapies and require more potent 'anaesthetic' therapies to block nociceptive transmission. Pain that fluctuates markedly in intensity (e.g. pain exacerbation with weight bearing, movement, etc.) is difficult to control, since a dose of opioid sufficient to control pain at peak intensity may be excessive when pain subsides. Patients' susceptibility to analgesic adverse effects varies widely, but there are rare individuals who are intolerant of opioids despite optimal use of strategies to manage nausea, constipation, and/or mental clouding. Patients with risk factors for ineffective pain control from systemic analgesics should be identified early so that interventional pain therapies can be given timely consideration.

Although the remarkable advances in our understanding of the neurobiology of pain in recent years have not yet resulted in widespread use of new pain therapies, there is increasing awareness of the limitations of conventional analgesic therapies. Currently available systemic analgesics do not effectively block mechanisms of peripheral and central nervous system (CNS) sensitization. To the contrary, there are many similarities between the hyperalgesic state produced by opioid tolerance and that of nerve injury.[7,8] Animal models indicate that *N*-methyl-D-aspartate (NMDA)-receptor mediated facilitation, and loss of inhibitory regulation, enhance pain signal transmission in both nerve injury and opioid tolerance. Persistent stimulation of spinal pain neurones results in activation of NMDA-receptor calcium channels and a marked increase in intracellular calcium, which activates protein kinase C (PKC). Persistent agonist effect at opioid receptors also activates PKC. Once activated, PKC alters NMDA-receptor calcium channels (to facilitate further calcium entry into the neurone) and opioid-receptor proteins. These changes facilitate nociceptive transmission and decrease analgesic efficacy of opioids. Persistent elevation of intracellular calcium also leads to activation of nitric oxide synthase and production of nitric oxide, which appears to be an essential factor in excitotoxic loss of spinal dorsal horn inhibitory interneurones. Either nerve injury or opioid tolerance appears to be sufficient for PKC and NO synthase activation and initiation of mechanisms of CNS sensitization (Fig. 2). In short,

1. pathophysiologic changes associated with nerve injury result in analgesic resistance to opioids; and
2. tolerance results from opioid-induced alterations in CNS function and structure similar to those seen in neuropathic pain.[7]

It has long been recognized that opioids are not ideal analgesics, but the concept that chronic opioid administration could facilitate pain signalling is of great clinical concern. Furthermore, a clinical syndrome of opioid toxicity has been described in the setting of advanced disease, severe pain, and pronounced opioid tolerance.[9] In such cases, escalating doses of opioid caused hyperalgesia and myoclonus, rather than improved analgesia. Opioid toxicity has been described after systemic[9] as well as spinal[10] administration of high-dose opioid.

To date, clinical pharmacologic strategies to block the development of tolerance are limited. Administration of NMDA-receptor antagonists with opioids limits tolerance in experimental animals, but the clinical efficacy of this strategy is uncertain. Clinical use of available NMDA-receptor antagonists, such as ketamine, is often limited by significant adverse effects.[11] Opioid rotation, or simple dose reduction, may be of real benefit in management of opioid toxicity. In difficult situations of uncontrolled pain due to tolerance and/or neuropathic causes, subcutaneous infusion of ketamine or lidocaine[12] may be invaluable (see below).

Opioid-tolerance-induced hyperalgesia and opioid-toxicity syndromes are reasons to consider anaesthetic techniques for control of pain. Local anaesthetic and neurolytic conduction blockade may limit nociceptive input, facilitation of pain transmission, and hyperalgesia. Spinal administration of opioid and non-opioid analgesics may result in enhanced pain control, even in the presence of significant opioid tolerance.[8,13,14] To the extent that anaesthetic techniques allow reduction in opioid dose, tolerance and opioid toxicity may be reduced or avoided.

The use of anaesthetic techniques for pain control does not preclude use of systemic analgesics or other pain therapies. Combinations of systemic and interventional techniques may include:

1. agents directed at peripheral pain receptors (anti-inflammatory drugs, topical agents);
2. techniques blocking axonal transmission (local anaesthetic or neurolytic conduction blockade);
3. sympathetic nervous system (local anaesthetic or neurolytic) blockade;
4. agents to decrease CNS reception and transmission of pain signals (systemic, spinal, or intraventricular opioids and/or other agents).

Anaesthetic techniques also may be used to help patients tolerate painful diagnostic or therapeutic procedures. For example, epidural blockade may be utilized to control pain and facilitate patient positioning for radiographic imaging, radiation therapy, or procedures such as neurolytic coeliac plexus block.

The pain management anaesthetist in palliative medicine

In the last decade, there has been considerable expansion of interventional, anaesthetic pain management techniques. New techniques, such as radiofrequency neural ablation techniques and intramuscular injection of botulinum toxin, have become widely used, whereas other procedures commonly carried out in the past (i.e. subarachnoid neurolytic block, neurolytic coeliac plexus block) are used less frequently. Pain management (pain medicine) has become a recognized area of subspecialization for anaesthetists. By extension of their basic knowledge and skills in surgical anaesthesia, anaesthetists with pain management training and expertise make unique contributions to palliative care. In addition to interventional analgesic techniques, anaesthetic pain management practice includes careful patient follow-up to ensure optimal care. Pain management anaesthetists have wide-ranging experience in the use of opioid and non-opioid analgesics, sedatives, antiemetics, and other drugs useful in palliative care. Not all pain in patients with cancer is directly related to the cancer, and in addition to cancer pain management expertise, pain management anaesthetists have broad experience in the management of pain in acute and non-cancer chronic pain settings. Beyond specific skills and expertise, successful incorporation of anaesthetic techniques into

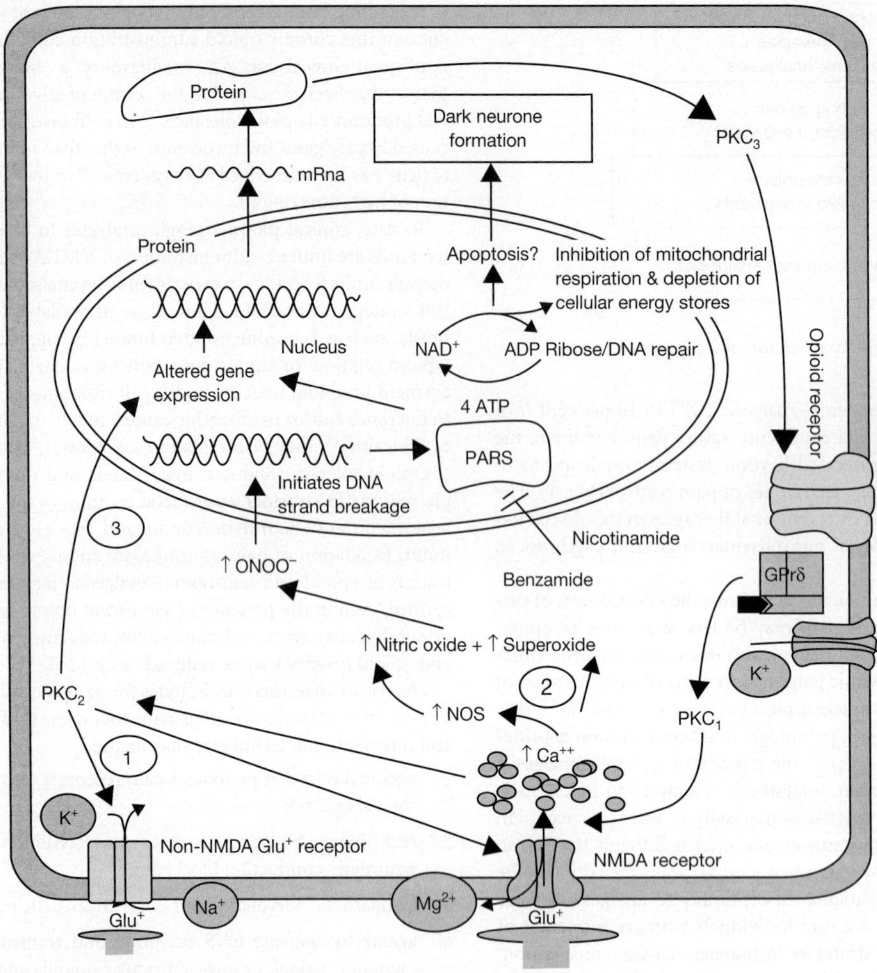

Fig. 2 A proposed model for the excitotoxic formation of dark neurones in the dorsal horn of the spinal cord from peripheral nerve injury or repeated morphine administration. Excessive excitation of the NMDA receptor and subsequent influx of Ca^{2+} occurs either directly by glutamate release from primary afferent input (nerve injury model) or indirectly by activation of μ-opioid receptors (repeated opioid administration). Activation of the μ-opioid receptor results in indirect NMDA receptor activation by initiating a second-messenger PKC translocation to the membrane. This PKC translocation activates the NMDA receptor by removal of the Mg^{2+} blockade. The removal of the Mg^{2+} blockade from the NMDA receptor allows an increased influx of Ca^{2+}. The influx of Ca^{2+}, via direct or indirect activation of the NMDA receptor, has several effects. It activates either a separate pool of PKC (PKC_2) or much greater amounts of the original pool of PKC_1. This second pool of PKC may be translocated directly to the membrane, modifying various excitatory amino acid or other receptors. It also may function as a transcription factor, resulting in the production of more PKC (PKC_3), which can result in uncoupling of the μ-opioid receptor from its associated G protein. Another effect of the influx of Ca^{2+} is that it activates NO synthase, which increases the production of NO. In addition, the influx of Ca^{2+} results in the production of superoxide from mitochondria. The simultaneous generation of these two molecules favours the production of peroxynitrite ($ONOO^-$), a very potent initiator of DNA strand breakage, which, in turn, initiates the production of the nuclear repair enzymes, PARS [poly (ADP-ribose) synthetase]. Pronounced activation of PARS can result in cell dysfunction and eventually cell death because of inhibition of mitochondrial respiration and depletion of cellular energy stores, which in turn may lead to the formation of dark neurones, perhaps by way of programmed cell death. PKC_x, various pools of protein kinase C; GPro, heterotrimeric guanine nucleotide binding protein; NOS, nitric oxide synthase. From Mayer, D.J. et al.[7]

palliative care requires careful planning so that appropriate therapies will be identified and made available in a timely fashion.

Techniques for pain control: the central nervous system

Spinal analgesia

When pain from cancer or advanced disease cannot be controlled with systemic analgesics, the spinal administration of analgesics is the most commonly used anaesthetic pain management therapy. In this context, 'spinal' includes both epidural and subarachnoid (or intrathecal) routes of administration (Table 1). Morphine is the most frequently used spinal analgesic for the management of chronic pain, but hydromorphone or fentanyl is also used. When spinal opioid alone proves inadequate, it is increasingly common to combine non-opioid analgesics, especially local anaesthetics (bupivacaine, ropivacaine) and/or α_2-adrenergic agonists (clonidine), with an opioid for spinal administration.

The rationale for spinal administration of analgesics is to provide more direct delivery of drug (e.g. morphine or clonidine) to relevant spinal receptors compared to systemic administration. The indications for spinal analgesics in palliative care and cancer pain management are:

1. pain not controlled with systemic analgesics;
2. unacceptable adverse effects from systemic analgesics, even if pain control is adequate.

Table 1 Administration sites for spinal analgesia

Spinal	All routes of administration near or within the spinal meninges ('spinal anaesthesia' is generally used to indicate subarachnoid administration of local anaesthetic)
Epidural	Immediately outside the dura mater, within the vertebral spinal canal
Intrathecal	Inside the thecal sac or dura mater. Intrathecal is often used synonymously with subarachnoid, but anatomically also includes the subdural space
Subdural	Between the dura mater and arachnoid mater
Subarachnoid	Inside the arachnoid mater. This space contains the cerebrospinal fluid

Spinal administration of analgesics is a potent therapy, but it must be used with skill and caution in order to minimize adverse outcomes. The keys to successful use of spinal analgesics are appropriate patient selection, meticulous attention to the technical details of spinal catheter system placement and maintenance, and careful analgesic dose adjustment. Some spinal analgesics used in clinical practice are not 'approved' for spinal administration. For example, morphine (epidural and subarachnoid), clonidine (epidural), and baclofen (subarachnoid) are the only drugs approved for chronic spinal administration by the US Food and Drug Administration. Using 'non-approved' spinal analgesics requires independently compounded 'custom' preparations, which may or may not be produced with the same high standards as commercially prepared pharmaceuticals.[15] Even with 'approved' analgesics, it should not be assumed that non-standard drug preparations, doses, or multiple-drug combinations will be void of significant neurotoxicity.[13,14] Humans should not be subjected to spinal analgesic therapies that have not undergone reasonable pre-clinical evaluation for neurotoxicity.

Spinal opioid administration

Although a relatively recent development, spinal opioid administration has an established role in management of severe pain. Soon after the first clinical reports in 1979, the application of spinal opioids quickly spread and is now used in various settings of acute pain, non-cancer chronic pain, and cancer-related pain.[8] Clinical experience has shown that with careful patient selection and dose adjustment, adverse effects from spinal opioids generally can be anticipated and managed; spinal opioid monotherapy has been recently reviewed with respect to the basic science and clinical practice.[16] Opioid tolerance and pain resistant to spinal opioid therapy are often managed with the co-administration of non-opioid spinal analgesics. In the future, spinal opioids and novel non-opioid drugs will likely play an important role in pain management as a mainstay of diverse analgesic therapies; combination spinal analgesia is the subject of a current systematic review.[17]

Spinal action of opioids

Spinal opioid administration enables the clinician to deliver opioid to the opioid receptors located within the dorsal horns of the spinal grey matter. These opioid receptors are one of many receptor types thought to modulate pain transmission in the spinal cord. Opioid binding to spinal receptors inhibits synaptic transmission between the primary afferent nociceptors and the second-order spinal neurones. By their presence on both the pre-synaptic (peripheral afferent nociceptor) and post-synaptic (second-order spinal neurone) nerve terminals, spinal opioid receptors are strategically positioned to inhibit nociceptive transmission.

Following lumbar spinal opioid administration, studies in humans have documented spinal CSF opioid concentrations far in excess of blood or plasma opioid concentrations. The time course of analgesia following epidural opioid administration correlates with spinal CSF opioid concentration rather than blood or plasma opioid concentrations.[8] Spinal administration is an effective way to deliver opioids to the spinal dorsal horns to decrease nociceptive transmission: clinically, this may result in enhanced analgesia.

Pharmacokinetic model of spinal opioids

There is considerable variation in the pharmacokinetics of different opioids when administered spinally, apparently related to differences in lipid solubility.[8,18] Following epidural administration, opioid must cross the dura, spread within the CSF, and penetrate into the spinal cord to reach spinal opioid receptors. Vascular uptake and absorption into nearby tissues reduces the quantity of drug available to reach opioid receptors. Pharmacokinetic considerations indicate that morphine has favourable characteristics for chronic spinal administration. Morphine is hydrophilic and, under physiological conditions, is highly ionized. The movement of the non-ionized moiety of morphine across the dura, as well as in and out of the spinal cord, is a slow process effected by small concentration gradients (Fig. 3). From the CSF, hydrophilic morphine moves slowly into the lipid-rich spinal cord. Morphine reaching spinal receptors has a long-lasting effect, as egress from the spinal cord is inhibited by the prolonged presence of morphine in the CSF.[8] Hydromorphone is very similar to morphine with regard to CSF pharmacokinetics following spinal administration.[19]

After epidural administration of a less-ionized, lipophilic opioid such as fentanyl, a greater proportion of the drug as compared with morphine will be present as a lipid-soluble moiety. This results in more rapid transfer of the drug across the dura, as well as in and out of the spinal cord. From the CSF, lipophilic opioid passes readily into the lipid-rich spinal cord, resulting in a rapid onset of analgesia. Egress from spinal receptors is enhanced by rapid systemic redistribution of opioid due to vascular uptake and by binding to various tissue sites. This model explains the rapid onset, short duration of analgesia, and limited cephalad migration of lipophilic opioids such as fentanyl.[18]

By comparison with morphine, sufentanil has a higher efficacy in that it need occupy a smaller fraction of opioid receptors to produce a comparable effect. Use of such high-efficacy agonists may reduce tolerance and increase the potency of spinal analgesia. Perhaps due to its relatively high cost, sufentanil is not widely used for chronic spinal administration; however, it is a second-choice agent when tolerance or insufficient effect limits spinal morphine analgesia.[6]

With subarachnoid administration, opioid is not subject to initial uptake by the epidural vasculature and epidural tissue binding sites, so subarachnoid doses of morphine are generally 10 per cent of doses required for epidural administration. There is a decrease in the time to onset of analgesia and a prolongation of effect following bolus subarachnoid, as compared with epidural, morphine administration.[8]

Following epidural or subarachnoid administration, morphine migrates from the spinal level of injection, due to the CSF circulation, to other spinal segments, and to supraspinal or brain structures. This extends the level of analgesia and increases the utility of spinal morphine in chronic pain. Unless CSF circulation is blocked[20,21] (e.g. tumour, congenital malformation, or arachnoiditis), spinal morphine need not be administered at the spinal segmental level of the pain. Hydromorphone, although somewhat more lipophilic than morphine, appears to be pharmacokinetically similar to spinal morphine,[19] especially with regard to the degree of cervical migration in CSF following lumbar administration.

Adverse effects of spinal opioids

The adverse effects and complications associated with spinal opioids are a result of the pharmacology of spinal opioids, or a consequence of the devices and techniques employed to deliver the opioids spinally (see technical considerations below). The most common adverse effects of spinal opioids are those of opioid therapy in general (Fig. 4). Fortunately, respiratory depression, nausea and vomiting, dysphoria, urinary retention, and

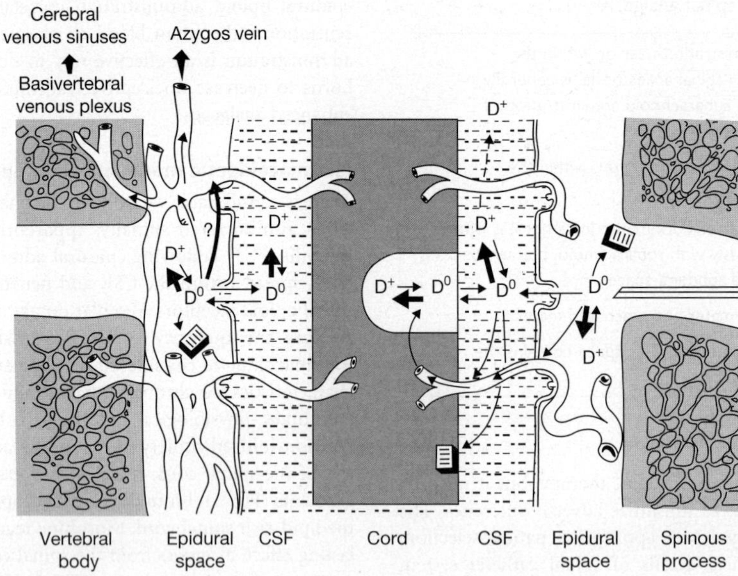

Fig. 3 Pharmacokinetic model of spinal opioid administration. An epidural needle (right) is shown delivering a hydrophilic opioid, such as morphine, to the epidural space. Within the epidural space, cerebrospinal fluid (CSF), and spinal cord equilibria of D^0 (non-ionized moiety of drug) and D^+ (ionized, hydrophilic moiety) are shown. Non-specific lipid binding sites are indicated by the shaded squares. The role of spinal arteries, in proximity to arachnoid granulations, in drug delivery is speculative. Epidural veins are the major point of clearance of epidural drugs. (Reproduced with permission from Cousins, M.J. and Bridenbaugh, P.O., ed. *Neural Blockade in Clinical Anesthesia and Management of Pain*, 3rd edn. Philadelphia: J.B. Lippincott, 1998.)

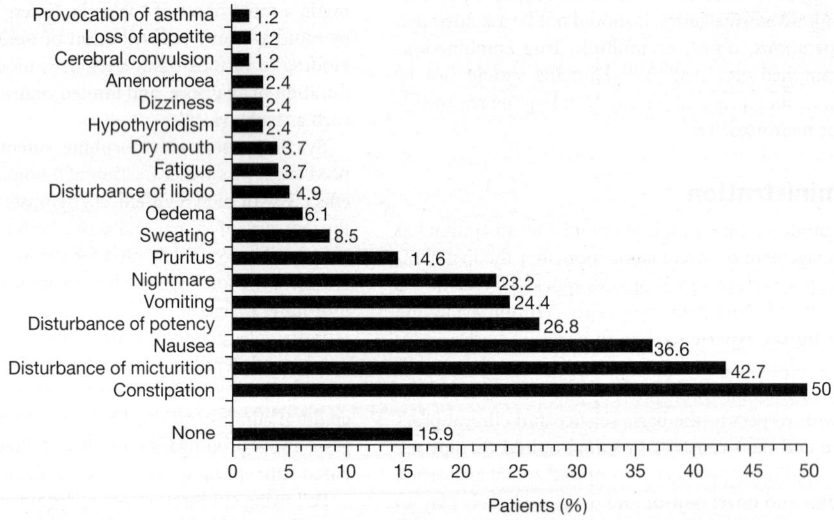

Fig. 4 Frequency of common adverse effects of chronic subarachnoid opioid therapy. (Reproduced with permission from Winkelmüller, M. and Winkelmüller, W. (1996). Long-term effects of continuous intrathecal opioid treatment in chronic pain of nonmalignant etiology. *Journal of Neurosurgery* **85**, 458–67.)

pruritus are not common following the spinal administration of opioids to patients with pain in palliative care. Such patients usually have been treated chronically with systemic opioids, and have developed some tolerance to opioid adverse effects. Therefore, these adverse effects are usually self-limiting or can be successfully managed by adjustment of the opioid dose. While opioid dose is being adjusted, these adverse effects may be managed with small doses of naloxone, often without reversal of opioid analgesia. In this setting, naloxone is best administered initially as an intravenous loading dose, given in 10–40 μg increments, followed by intravenous infusion of approximately 1–5 μg/kg h, titrated to effect. Constipation is a problem with both spinal and opioid systemic administration, which should be anticipated and managed.

Cephalad migration of morphine within the CSF appears to explain the delayed respiratory depression (onset 3–20 h) that can occur following spinal morphine administration in opioid-naive patients.[8] Clinically significant respiratory depression from spinal opioid is particularly rare in patients previously treated chronically with systemic opioids. Thus, with appropriate patient selection and careful dose titration, there appears to be a very low risk of respiratory depression with the use of spinal opioids as typically employed in palliative care.

Endocrine abnormalities, sweating, and peripheral oedema are adverse effects associated with chronic opioid therapy, whether given by systemic or spinal routes of administration. In one study of spinal opioid for non-malignant pain,[22] most male and all female patients developed hypogonadotropic hypogonadism, 15 per cent developed central hypocorticism, and 15 per cent developed adult growth hormone deficiency syndrome as indicated by deficient growth hormone response to insulin-induced hypoglycaemia. In a subgroup of patients with sexual dysfunction, hormone replacement therapy resulted in significant improvement.[22] Opioid-induced sweating, perhaps related to modest changes in basal body temperature regulation,[23] is not more prevalent (in the authors' experience) among patients receiving spinal as compared to systemic opioid. Peripheral oedema affects 6.1 per cent of people receiving long-term spinal opioid.[22] As with peripheral oedema associated with systemic opioids, oedema associated with spinal opioids appears related to an antidiuretic effect of opioids[23] and is usually managed with diuretics.

As with systemic opioid,[9] toxicity from very high doses of spinal opioid may be associated with myoclonus and hyperalgesia.[10] This syndrome of opioid-induced hyperalgesia should be suspected when individuals on high-dose opioid (e.g. subarachnoid morphine greater than 20 mg/day) develop generalized hyperalgesia, especially if associated with myoclonus.[24] Opioid toxicity may be managed with opioid rotation or dose reduction, perhaps with addition of non-opioid spinal analgesics.

Upon initiation of spinal opioid therapy, patients previously treated with systemic opioids may experience opioid withdrawal, if systemic opioid is suddenly ceased. Withdrawal symptoms may also develop if chronic epidural opioid is replaced with subarachnoid opioid. Withdrawal symptoms in these settings are readily managed with tapering doses of systemic opioid, while continuing to provide analgesia with spinal opioid. A useful strategy is to take advantage of the NMDA, as well as opioid actions of methadone. This allows the use of approximately 20 per cent of the morphine equivalent dose of methadone, facilitating systemic opioid tapering.

Non-opioid spinal analgesics

Local anaesthetics

When spinal opioids do not provide adequate analgesia, spinal local anaesthetic may be indicated.[13,14,25] In addition to the obvious, immediate analgesic effect of neuraxial conduction blockade, decreasing the nociceptive input to the spinal dorsal horns may decrease spinal sensitization. Reduction in opioid dose may limit the development of tolerance.[26] Bupivacaine is by far the most commonly used local anaesthetic for long-term spinal administration. It is not clear that ropivacaine offers advantage over bupivacaine when used for chronic pain. Chronic spinal lidocaine and tetracaine[13] are increasingly avoided due to concern for neurotoxicity.

Low-dose epidural local anaesthetic administration[8,27] can generally achieve good analgesia without significant motor or sensory impairment. This blockade of pain, rather than sensory or motor function, may be more readily obtained with epidural than subarachnoid local anaesthetic use, and is one of the main advantages of the epidural route of administration. Subarachnoid local anaesthetic administration may also provide good analgesic effect, without significant normal sensory or motor block, if doses are low (less than 30 mg bupivacaine per day). Long-term subarachnoid local anaesthetic, alone or with spinal opioid, has been successfully used to control otherwise intractable pain in a variety of clinical settings.[25,28,29]

In extreme cases, pain may not be relieved with spinal analgesics. In non-ambulatory, terminal patients with intractable lower back or lower extremity pain, continuous spinal anaesthesia, with dense sensory and motor block from intentional infusion of high doses of subarachnoid local anaesthetic (greater than 2 mg/h bupivacaine), may provide pain relief.[30]

Clonidine

In the past decade, clonidine has become well accepted as a second-line spinal analgesic[14] for use in chronic, severe pain not adequately controlled with spinal opioid. Systemic clonidine also has analgesic efficacy, but spinal clonidine is more potent.[8] The analgesic efficacy of spinal clonidine has been demonstrated in human, prospective, randomized trials in experimental pain,[31] cancer pain,[32] and spinal cord injury pain.[33] The analgesic effect of spinal clonidine appears to be mediated by the inhibitory effects of α_2-adrenergic receptors on spinal nociceptive transmission (Fig. 5).

In the United States, epidural clonidine is approved by the Food and Drug Administration for the control of cancer pain. Spinal clonidine has

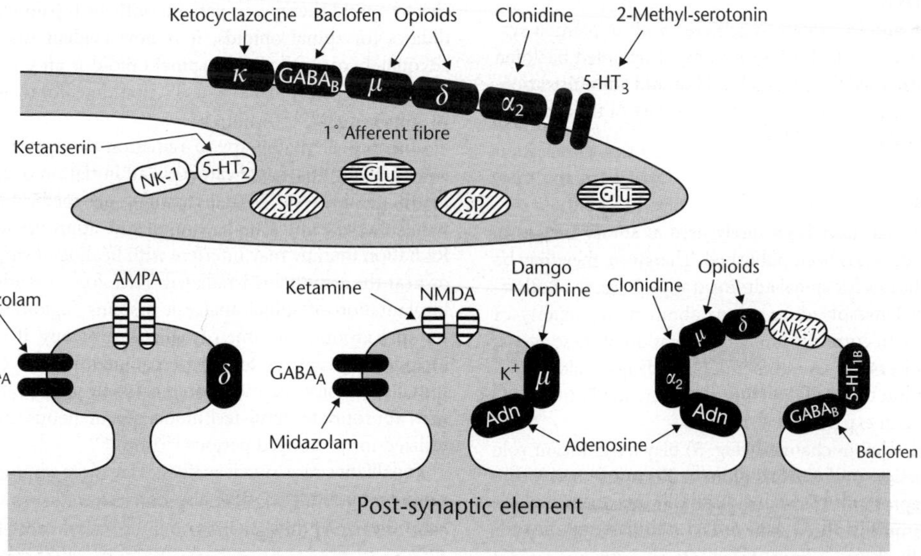

Fig. 5 Summary of neurotransmission from primary afferent sensory fibres to second-order spinal neurones (post-synaptic element) in the spinal dorsal horns. Neurotransmitters (open circles) include the excitatory amino-acid transmitters (i.e. glutamine = Glu) and neurokinins (i.e. substance P = SP). Activation of post-synaptic, excitatory amino-acid receptors (classified by their response to *N*-methyl-D-aspartate (NMDA) and α-amino-3-hydroxy-5-methyl-4-isoxazoleproprionic acid (AMPA)), as well as neurokinin receptors (NK-1), results in depolarization of the post-synaptic membrane. Excitatory receptors (open ovals) are also located pre-synaptically, where activation results in enhanced transmitter release (5-HT$_2$ = excitatory serotonin receptors). Activation of inhibitory receptors (filled ovals), located both pre- and post-synaptically, decreases the release and effectiveness of transmitters (κ, μ, δ, opioid; GABA, γ-aminobutyric acid; 5-HTβ, inhibitory serotonin receptor; α_2, α_2-adrenergic; Adn, adenosine). The drugs shown affect pain transmission, at least experimentally, and are believed to be active at the sites indicated (arrows). (Reproduced with permission from Cousins, M.J. and Bridenbaugh, P.O., ed. *Neural Blockade in Clinical Anesthesia and Management of Pain*, 3rd edn. Philadelphia: J.B. Lippincott, 1998.)

not been reported to cause neurotoxicity. The adverse effects of spinal clonidine, including hypotension, bradycardia, and sedation, are dose-related and generally manageable. Given its safety and efficacy, spinal clonidine is likely to remain an important spinal analgesic, often administered with opioid and/or local anaesthetic,[34] especially in clinical situations involving neuropathic pain.

Subarachnoid baclofen for spasticity and pain

The clinical management of severe spasticity, from upper motor neurone lesions, can be challenging.[35] Oral baclofen, a GABA analogue, can be successful in treating spasticity. Baclofen binding at (pre-synaptic) $GABA_B$ receptors on afferent neurones inhibits calcium influx into pre-synaptic terminals, suppressing release of excitatory neurotransmitters. This results in inhibition of spinal motor reflexes, clinically observed as reduced spasticity. Benzodiazepines, dantrolene, tizanidine, and spinal opioids[36] are also used in the management of spasticity, but oral baclofen has generally been found to be more effective and better tolerated. With higher doses of oral baclofen, sedation and other adverse effects may limit patient tolerance.

Subarachnoid baclofen is useful[35,37] in patients with severe spasticity unresponsive to, or with intolerable adverse effects from, oral baclofen. Subarachnoid administration results in significantly higher CSF concentrations than oral administration, even though subarachnoid doses are 100–1000 times lower. Human studies, with several year follow-up, indicate that subarachnoid baclofen is well tolerated[38] and no significant neurotoxicity has been identified. Baclofen also appears to have a role as a spinal analgesic when musculoskeletal pain is related to spasticity[39] and/or in settings of neuropathic pain.[40,41] Baclofen may well have significant utility as a second-line spinal analgesic, either alone or in combination with opioid.

The effectiveness of subarachnoid baclofen for control of spasticity is generally evaluated in each patient with a test dose before proceeding with chronic administration. Finding the appropriate dose is critical and may require adjustment: too little drug could lead to the erroneous conclusion of ineffectiveness, while an excessive dose may cause generalized muscle weakness or hypotonia. Accidental overdose may result in respiratory arrest through generalized weakness and/or CNS depression, but with appropriate support, including temporary mechanical ventilation, no long-term complications have been reported.

Chronic spinal baclofen administration is achieved with implanted systems, typically a computer-controlled infusion pump. Implanted baclofen pumps are the same as those used for subarachnoid opioid administration. Although highly reliable, the cost and technical complexity of these pumps is considerable (see technical considerations below).

Other spinal analgesics

Ketamine and midazolam each have been rarely used as spinal analgesics and some clinical efficacy data has been published. Therefore, they may be considered 'fourth-line' choices for spinal administration in cases of otherwise intractable pain.[14] Unresolved questions about neurotoxicity of spinal ketamine or midazolam currently limit consideration of these agents to the setting of terminal disease.[42] A number of other drugs could also be useful as spinal analgesics, but the available clinical data are too limited and, therefore, these agents remain experimental.[8,13,16]

NMDA-receptor-linked calcium channels (Fig. 5) play a significant role in spinal neural transmission and sensitization.[7] Ketamine and other experimental NMDA-receptor antagonists are potent analgesics in settings of hyperalgesia. Spinal ketamine has been shown to have analgesic efficacy,[43] although it has generally been administered along with an opioid (co-analgesic). Psychotropic adverse effects may limit utility of spinal ketamine.[44] Vacuolization of spinal neurones in an animal trial[42] and marked neurological deficit in a clinical case report[45] indicate the potential for neurotoxicity from subarachnoid ketamine.

γ-Aminobutyric acid (GABA) is an amino-acid neurotransmitter that inhibits synaptic transmission in the spinal dorsal horn through activation of inhibitory GABA receptors (Fig. 5). Benzodiazepines modulate GABA-mediated inhibition of neuronal transmission in the spinal cord by modifying the binding of agonists to $GABA_A$ receptors. Midazolam enhances the binding of GABA to (inhibitory) $GABA_A$ receptors and thereby inhibits neuronal transmission. Case reports indicate that spinal midazolam has analgesic efficacy; however, potential toxicity of midazolam itself and also toxicity of available midazolam preparations remains a concern.[13,42]

Palliative care indications for spinal analgesics

Spinal analgesics have been used most commonly for severe, cancer pain, but may also be used for palliation of intractable, non-cancer pain. The general indications for the use of spinal analgesics in palliative care are:

1. pain not controlled with systemic analgesics;
2. unacceptable adverse effects from systemic analgesics, even if pain control is adequate.

In both indications, it is assumed that prior analgesic trials included appropriate adjuvant drugs, in combination with adequate opioid.

In the management of both cancer and non-cancer pain, the nature of the underlying disease(s) and the character of the pain are important factors when considering spinal analgesic therapy. In cancer pain, the best response to spinal opioids is obtained in patients with deep, constant somatic pain. Other types of cancer pain are variably responsive, including cutaneous pain, intermittent somatic pain (pathologic fracture), intermittent visceral pain (intestinal obstruction), and coexistent cancer-related and non-cancer pain. Patients with extreme opioid tolerance (i.e. uncontrolled pain despite opioid doses over 1000 mg intravenous morphine per day) are unlikely to have good pain control with spinal opioid alone, and will likely require co-administration of non-opioid spinal analgesic(s). If the benefit of spinal analgesics is uncertain, a trial of spinal analgesic therapy through a temporary percutaneous catheter is recommended before implantation of a permanent delivery system. Limited life expectancy is a factor in selecting between spinal administration systems, but should not deter consideration of spinal analgesia.

Patients with severe, intractable pain not responsive to systemic analgesics may have a significant component of neuropathic pain. In the past, it was felt that 'central', neuropathic, or deafferentation pains were not responsive to opioid therapy, so patients with such pain were not considered candidates for spinal opioids. It is now evident that neuropathic pain not adequately controlled with spinal opioid is an indication for the addition of a non-opioid spinal analgesic (clonidine, local anaesthetic, or baclofen), to spinal opioid.

Ongoing chemotherapy or radiation therapy is not a contra-indication to placement of a spinal catheter and initiation of spinal analgesic therapy. Adequate analgesia, perhaps with spinal medications, may help patients with otherwise intractable pain tolerate appropriate antitumour therapies. Radiation therapy may interfere with healing of surgical wounds located in or near the areas being irradiated. Therefore, it is advisable to avoid surgical implantation of spinal analgesic systems (epidural ports, spinal infusion pumps) around the time of radiation therapy, if radiation portals would include surgical sites. Simple percutaneous spinal catheters may be used if spinal analgesics and radiation therapy need to be initiated simultaneously; with appropriate sterile technique, percutaneous spinal catheters have been utilized for prolonged periods.[25,28,29,46]

In palliative care, spinal analgesics are most commonly used for intractable cancer pain, but they have also been used for intractable non-cancer pain and other symptoms:

1. severe, inoperable peripheral vascular disease with ischaemic rest pain;
2. vertebral compression fractures and stress rib fractures (vertebroplasty may be a better option for pain due to vertebral compression fractures, especially with single-level fractures without severe spinal stenosis);
3. intractable, inoperable myocardial ischaemic pain and limited exercise tolerance;[29,47]
4. muscle spasticity due to CNS lesions[36] (intrathecal baclofen may be more effective[35]);

5. spinal cord injury pain;[33]
6. other conditions including neuropathic pain,[48,49] and intractable back pain,[48,50] including inoperable spinal stenosis.

Although spinal analgesics are potent, it is not realistic to expect elimination of pain. Patients selected for spinal analgesic therapies generally have severe pain problems, resistant to usual (systemic) analgesic therapies. Case series of patients with cancer[28] and non-cancer pain[48,50] indicate that 50–87 per cent of carefully selected patients received significant relief from spinal analgesic therapy.

Contraindications for spinal opioid therapy are similar to those for any regional anaesthetic technique, with a few additional concerns due to the chronicity of spinal analgesic use. Bleeding diathesis would increase the risk of spinal haematoma and neurologic deficit from spinal cord or nerve root compression. Septicaemia is a contraindication, due to the risk of infection of the spinal delivery system. Local, cutaneous infection is a contraindication if a site for implantation of the spinal catheter system, free of infection, cannot be found. Patients with immune suppression may be at higher risk of infection, but this is only a relative contraindication and must be evaluated for each patient.

The presence of epidural or spinal metastasis deserves special consideration. Spinal metastasis might be considered a contra-indication for spinal anaesthetic or analgesic techniques, yet patients with such lesions may have severe pain and, therefore, need spinal analgesia. The concern is that trauma to a friable tumour mass during catheterization could result in haemorrhage, epidural haematoma, and neural compression. Severe spinal stenosis, including that caused by tumour, also increases the risk of neural injury with neuraxial needle placement. To avoid such trauma, catheters should be inserted away from spinal metastases, perhaps under fluroscopy. Furthermore, the potential for eventual obstruction of CSF circulation, by an expanding tumour, should encourage the placement of catheters cephalad to known (or suspected) epidural or spinal metastases.[20,21,51]

Technical considerations and complications in spinal drug administration

Various technical considerations are important to the successful application of long-term spinal analgesic therapy. Long-term spinal analgesia requires catheter access to the subarachnoid or epidural space: the catheter may be a simple, percutaneous catheter for intermittent injection or part of a totally implanted, computer-controlled infusion pump system.[8,52] No single system is appropriate for all clinical settings, and any spinal system may be associated with complications such as infection, catheter dislodgement, or other technical failure, which must be properly assessed and managed. Before initiating spinal analgesia for long-term use, it is essential to ensure that appropriate nursing and social support will be available to assist with management of the patient and maintenance of the spinal administration system.

A percutaneous epidural catheter, as may be used for epidural anaesthesia or acute pain, is the simplest means of providing long-term analgesia. Epidural catheters are widely available, inexpensive, and may be used for days to weeks; however, even with careful technique, there is a risk of epidural infection and abscess. For longer-term use, *implanted epidural catheters* (epidural Port-A-Cath, Deltec; Du Pen catheters, Bard) are less likely to become dislodged and may have a lower infection rate.[46,53] The routine use of bacterial filters (0.2 μm) may help decrease the risk of infection,[46] but epidural abscess remains a concern.[54]

The long-term efficacy of epidural analgesia may be limited by epidural fibrosis, that is, formation of scar tissue around the catheter, within the epidural space.[55,56] Epidural fibrosis is a variable process, but may develop within 2 weeks of epidural catheter placement. Fibrosis limits the spread of analgesic solution, resulting in pain on injection and/or loss of analgesic effect. Management of epidural fibrosis requires repositioning the epidural catheter or replacing it with a subarachnoid catheter.

Percutaneous subarachnoid catheters have been used in palliative care of terminally ill persons with increasing frequency in recent years. The concern of infection and meningitis appears to be reasonably managed by the use of bacterial filters (0.2 μm) and a sterile technique that strictly minimizes the changing of external infusion pump reservoirs and tubing.[25,46,57] Advantages of subarachnoid analgesia are its efficiency and potency, which may translate into improved pain control with lower drug cost. Subarachnoid analgesics in widespread clinical use include opioid (e.g. morphine, hydromorphone), local anaesthetic (typically bupivacaine), clonidine, and baclofen.

Spinal analgesia can be provided with intermittent bolus dose administration (e.g. with needle and syringe via epidural Port-A-Cath[58]), but is typically delivered via infusion pump. Continuous infusion is necessary for administration of non-opioid spinal analgesics, and use of a closed system minimizes opportunities for infection. For long-term use, *implanted infusion pumps* for subarachnoid administration of analgesics have the lowest risk of infection and a low rate of technical complication.[59] Implanted pumps have the highest initial cost among all spinal administration systems, but appear to be cost-effective in the long run (several months to years) due to relatively low drug and maintenance costs.

An important limitation of implanted pumps is the small volume of the medication reservoir, which makes the use of commercial preparations of bupivacaine and/or clonidine impractical. Therefore, it is necessary to use solutions custom-made by a compounding pharmacist. Use of non-standard solutions is a potential source of neurotoxic contaminants or infection, but is done with increasing frequency worldwide.[13,14] Only preservative-free solutions should be used for spinal administration.

Adequate skilled nursing assistance and/or regular physician evaluation is essential for spinal analgesia to be successful. Implanted infusion pumps have the advantage that once implanted and adjusted, they only require refill every few weeks, but refills require physician or skilled nursing personnel. Percutaneous catheters or implanted injection portal systems with or without external infusion pumps may be managed by patients and/or family members, but generally require periodic nursing support. It is possible to initiate and maintain percutaneous subarachnoid analgesia in the home of terminally ill, homebound patients,[28] if physician home visits can be arranged. Follow-up can be accomplished through office evaluations, home visits, or institutionalization, depending on other aspects of patient care.[52,57] Hospital, home health service, and governmental nursing regulations concerning spinal administration systems vary widely. The impact of such local regulations on patient care must be anticipated and understood before initiating spinal analgesic therapy.

Infections of spinal catheter systems are among the most concerning problems associated with long-term spinal analgesia (Table 2). Infections are usually localized to the catheter insertion or implantation site, and cultures of any purulent drainage, followed by antibiotics, are necessary.[46,57] Epidural abscess and meningitis are rare, but must be treated aggressively, as they may result in permanent neurological deficit or death. In principle, epidural systems should be removed as part of the management of epidural abscess, yet the catheter may temporarily serve as a drainage conduit for the epidural space.[46] In rare cases, antibiotics may be delivered via the epidural catheter,[46] but if infection does not rapidly improve, the catheter should still be removed.[62] Meningitis, associated with subarachnoid catheter systems, should be treated with intravenous antibiotics as well as antibiotics delivered via the subarachnoid catheter system (Only antibiotics such as vancomycin, which are suitable for subarachnoid administration, should be administered through the implanted spinal catheter.). If the infection does not rapidly clear with antibiotics, the subarachnoid catheter system should be removed.[57,60,63]

Malfunctions in spinal catheter systems can result in the deterioration of previously satisfactory analgesia (Table 2). Loss of analgesia may be gradual (e.g. epidural fibrosis) or abrupt (e.g. infusion pump malfunction). Patients may report uncontrolled pain and/or symptoms of opioid withdrawal. Accurate function of infusion devices, implanted or external, must be verified. Epidurography or myelography may be used to verify spinal

Table 2 Evaluation and management of spinal catheter complications

Catheter system	Symptoms	Complication	Prevention	Evaluation	Management
Epidural	Back pain Paraesthesias on injection Loss of analgesic effect No signs of infection	Epidural fibrosis[56]	Unknown	Epidurography	Replace epidural or insert subarachnoid catheter
	Back and extremity pain Weakness Sensory abnormalities Fever, leukocytosis	Epidural infection or abscess[46]	Sterile technique, bacterial filters[46]	Catheter aspirate for gram stain, culture; spine MRI	Catheter aspiration for decompression Intravenous antibiotics Remove catheter
Epidural or subarachnoid	Loss of analgesic effect Opioid withdrawal	Catheter dislodgement or disconnection	Implanted rather than percutaneous system Subarachnoid catheter anchored to fascia	Plain radiographs with contrast injection via catheter	Revise or replace catheter
		Pump malfunction	Pump maintenance Utilize low volume and low battery alarm	Pump analysis Technical support from manufacturer	Revise or replace pump
	Erythema, tenderness at catheter insertion point or incision site	Infection at catheter insertion site	Sterile technique Catheter care	Culture: catheter exit site and, catheter aspirate	Antibiotics Local site care Remove catheter system if no rapid improvement
Subarachnoid	Meningeal irritation Severe headache Cervical stiffness Photophobia, fever	Meningitis[60]	Sterile technique[25] Bacterial filters for pump refill or on percutaneous catheters	Catheter aspirate (CSF) for cell count, gram stain, glucose, culture	Subarachnoid and systemic antibiotics Remove catheter system if no rapid improvement
	Spinal cord compression Paraesthesias Weakness	Subarachnoid granuloma[61]	Unknown Perhaps avoid excessive doses, concentrations of spinal opioid	Spine imaging: CT myelogram or MRI	Surgical resection of granuloma

spread of contrast injected through spinal catheters. It is essential to use non-ionic radiographic contrast suitable for myelography for all spinal (epidural and subarachnoid) contrast injections. Plain radiographs may be used to evaluate the structural integrity of spinal delivery systems.

Although the formation of scar tissue surrounding chronic epidural catheters ('epidural fibrosis') is fairly common, scarring around subarachnoid catheters is rare. Animal studies[64] suggest that chronic subarachnoid catheters may be associated with demyelination and other spinal cord abnormalities, but broad clinical experience (including histopathologic review[65]) indicates that subarachnoid-catheter-associated neural injury is rare in humans. Subarachnoid catheters used for baclofen administration have not been associated with inflammatory reactions. Subarachnoid catheters for spinal analgesics are associated with a small risk of catheter-tip granulomas, which can present as profound weakness or sensory abnormality indicating spinal cord compromise. In one case series, few patients actually presented with thoracic back pain, although many patients had experienced a prior period of severe thoracic back pain (perhaps an early sign of spinal inflammation) before other neurologic deficit was evident.[61] Spine MRI is the preferred imaging technique in this setting (patients with implanted spinal pumps *can* undergo MRI), but CT myelography is a reasonable alternative. After surgical resection of granuloma, complete or partial neurologic recovery can be expected in most cases, but there is a risk of permanent neurological deficit. High concentrations and high daily doses of opioid may be risk factors for spinal granulomas, but available data do not indicate what concentrations or doses are safe. These rare granulomas should not discourage the use of necessary spinal analgesic therapies in palliative care, but should encourage careful follow-up, so that appropriate interventions can be undertaken promptly.

Management of pain when spinal analgesia systems malfunction may be difficult since, generally, inadequate analgesia from systemic medications will have been the indication for the initiation of spinal analgesia. Nonetheless, such patients will require systemic analgesics for pain relief and prevention of opioid withdrawal. If an epidural catheter has malfunctioned due to epidural fibrosis, it is likely that the patient's pain can be managed equally well with systemic opioid at the same dose. This is because epidural fibrosis would have prevented spinal absorption, and the medication given would have been absorbed systemically. On the other hand, if the epidural system had been functioning well and opioid had been efficiently delivered to spinal receptors, systemic opioid doses equal to prior epidural doses will likely be insufficient for pain control, but will at least prevent opioid withdrawal. Therefore, if epidural systems malfunction, it is reasonable to use the prior epidural dose of opioid as the initial dose for systemic administration, with subsequent dose titration as needed.

Subarachnoid morphine doses are approximately 10 per cent of epidural doses and as low as 1 per cent of systemic (parenteral) doses, but these estimations are just starting points for titration of analgesics. These estimates must be used cautiously to prevent significant under- or over-dosing of patients (Table 3). When spinal local anaesthetic had been previously

Table 3 Equivalent morphine dose by administration route

Administration route	Morphine dose (approximate) (mg)	Dosing interval (h)
Oral	300	4
Intravenous	100	4
Epidural	10	6–8
Subarachnoid	1	12–24

Doses are approximate and must be applied to individual patients with caution. These ratios do not apply to other opioids. Conversion factors used to estimate equipotent doses for systemic administration of various opioids should not be used to predict equipotency of opioid doses for spinal administration due to variations in spinal pharmacokinetics.

added due to lack of efficacy of spinal opioid alone, it is unlikely that systemic opioid will provide reasonable analgesia should the spinal delivery system fail: additional anaesthetic or neurosurgical techniques for pain management will likely be necessary if the spinal system cannot be repaired/revised. An intravenous or subcutaneous infusion of a non-opioid analgesic (lidocaine, 50–100 mg/h, or ketamine, 10–20 mg/h) may be utilized to temporarily control otherwise intractable pain not responsive to opioids,[12] while other measures are initiated. If systemic ketamine is utilized, a benzodiazepine should also be administered to control possible dysphoric hallucinations.

Intracerebroventricular opioid administration

Catheter techniques similar to those used for spinal opioid administration have also been used to provide analgesia through the administration of opioid directly into the cerebral ventricles. There are several case series describing severe, intractable cancer pain in which intracerebroventricular opioid therapy provided good to excellent analgesia, in the majority of patients, with acceptable adverse effects.[66–68] Indications for intracerebroventricular opioid therapy include intractable pain (usually cancer-related pain) resistant to systemic opioid and adjuvant therapy in patients who also have one or more of the following indications:

1. inadequate analgesia through less complicated techniques;
2. inaccessible spinal epidural and subarachnoid spaces;
3. known spinal obstruction to the circulation of CSF; and/or
4. intractable head and neck pain.

Neurolytic blockade of the central nervous system

General consideration for neurolytic blockade

In general, neurolytic blocks are suitable for patients with short life expectancy and well-localized intractable pain.[69] Neurolytic blockade is less effective with widespread and/or deafferentation (neuropathic) pain. Somatic neurolytic blocks may, in fact, cause sufficient denervation to result in deafferentation pain, but incomplete neural destruction by neurolytic block may also produce a neuralgic type of pain. Deafferentation pain may be a sequela in as much as 14–30 per cent of patients undergoing peripheral neurolytic block, but is less common (1–3 per cent) after subarachnoid neurolysis. Neuropathic pain following neurolysis is most appropriately treated with transcutaneous electrical nerve stimulation, centrally acting analgesics, or spinal cord stimulation, rather than with further attempts at neurolysis.[69,70]

A local anaesthetic block may be of prognostic value, regarding both the degree of pain relief and potential complications from a proposed neurolytic block.[69] However, local anaesthetic blocks are not entirely predictive of the results of neurolytic block: systemically absorbed local anaesthetic, analgesic, and sedative medications given during the procedure, local anaesthetic spread to adjacent neural structures, neural plasticity, and placebo response may all contribute to a misleading temporary success from local anaesthetic blocks.[71] In terminally ill patients with severe pain, the combination of a prognostic local anaesthetic block, followed by neurolysis, may exceed the patient's willingness or ability to undergo procedures. In such terminal situations, it may be reasonable to proceed directly with neurolysis.

Phenol and ethyl alcohol (ethanol) are the neurolytic agents most frequently used in neural blockade.[72] Phenol has local anaesthetic as well as neurolytic effects, resulting in nearly painless injection. Doses of phenol, typically 6–10 per cent solution, should be limited to 1–10 ml for peripheral or sympathetic blocks, or 1–3 ml for subarachnoid injection. Excessive systemic doses or accidental intravascular injection of phenol may cause convulsions, followed by CNS depression, or even cardiovascular collapse. In contrast, ethanol is associated with few significant adverse effects from systemic absorption—at least with doses typically used in neurolytic blockade. There are few comparative data on which to base a choice of neurolytic agent. Prior to considering neurolytic blockade, it is important to accurately determine the aetiology of the pain. If possible, radiographic evaluation should be carried out to determine the extent of spinal tumour spread when considering neuraxial neurolysis: distortion of the epidural or subarachnoid spaces by tumour may lead to unpredictable, unacceptable spread of neurolytic solution.

Subarachnoid neurolytic blockade

The subarachnoid injection of a neurolytic agent is an effective analgesic technique, but should be restricted to patients with advanced malignancy and pain limited to a few spinal segments. The aim is to produce a chemical posterior rhizotomy, thereby interrupting the pain pathways from the affected area. Subarachnoid neurolytic blocks are best used for bilateral saddle (perineal) pain in patients with colostomy and permanent bladder catheter, or in relatively localized (unilateral) somatic pain of the chest wall or trunk[69] and should be avoided when the pain is widespread or of undiagnosed aetiology. Particular care must be taken to avoid increasing the patient's disability through motor weakness, incontinence, sexual dysfunction, or loss of position sense.

Interpretation of data on subarachnoid neurolytic blockade is limited by the variability of patient inclusion criteria, duration of follow-up, and techniques used to measure patient response, as well as the generally progressive nature of the underlying disease. In skilled hands, the results of phenol and alcohol subarachnoid block are probably similar (Table 4). Some patients may obtain relief for up to 6–12 months.[69] With appropriate patient selection and meticulous technique, complication rates seem to be in the range of 1–14 per cent, which may be acceptable for some patients. For example, if a bladder catheter is already in use, bladder incontinence may be of no consequence, whereas ambulatory patients will almost never accept incontinence even if pain relief by alternative methods is inferior. Subarachnoid neurolytic blocks are used less frequently now than in prior decades, likely reflecting more sophisticated use of systemic and other spinal analgesic therapies and increased awareness of potential complications.[70,79] Nonetheless, carefully performed subarachnoid neurolysis, in well-selected patients, continues to have a small but significant role in palliative care,[80,81] especially in settings where spinal analgesics are contraindicated or not available.

Standard techniques of neuraxial neurolysis may be insufficient in rare, extreme cases of lower body and/or lower extremity pain, for example, in bed-bound, terminally ill patients with significant nerve root or spinal cord tumour involvement. In such situations, chemical transection of the spinal cord at the upper lumbar or lower thoracic dermatomal level may be a reasonable alternative to terminal sedation or continuous spinal anaesthesia. This intervention is rarely used, but may offer high-quality relief of otherwise intractable pain and/or spasticity, in the appropriate setting.[69]

Table 4 Results of subarachnoid block with alcohol

Authors	Percentage results			
	Number of cases	Good	Fair	Poor
Dogliotti[73]	150	50	25	16
Greenhill[74]	>100	60	10	30
Hay[75]	252	46	32	22
Kuzucu et al.[76]	322	58.2	26.1	15.7
Combined series, Drechsel[77]	1908	60	21	19

Data from original articles and ref. 78.

'Good' means complete relief of pain for more than 1 month; 'fair' means complete relief of pain for less than 1 month, or reduction of pain for more than 1 month; 'poor' means relief for several days or no relief.

Epidural neurolytic blockade

Pain within the cervical dermatomes may be difficult to treat safely with subarachnoid neurolytic block, due to the rapid dilution of neurolytic solution by the faster CSF circulation in the neck. In addition, CSF flow may cause neurolytic solution to spread in an undesirable manner to adjacent neural structures. Therefore, epidural neurolysis may have an advantage over subarachnoid neurolysis in cervical and upper thoracic areas as solutions are placed outside the CSF-containing subarachnoid space. Epidural neurolysis may also be used at lower thoracic (for upper abdominal pain) and lumbar levels.(69) Epidural neurolytic techniques are rarely used, and are generally considered second-line therapies behind spinal analgesic therapies, in most clinical settings.

Spinal neurolysis for spasticity

Although most problems of spasticity may be managed medically, or with spinal baclofen, there is a role for subarachnoid neurolytic blockade in the palliative management of intractable spasticity.(69,82,83) Subarachnoid neurolysis for spasticity should only be considered in patients with no functional use of the lower extremities and severe, intractable spasticity. In such patients, spasticity may interfere with routine nursing and hygiene manoeuvres, and flaccid paralysis resulting from neurolytic blockade may be desirable.

Spinal cord stimulation

In spinal cord stimulation (SCS), electrodes are implanted in the epidural space, overlying the posterior aspect of the spinal cord, at a spinal level corresponding to the site of pain (e.g. T_{10} vertebral level for low back and lower lumbar pain). Electrical stimulation is provided by an implanted battery-pulse generator, or an external battery-pulse generator electromagnetically linked to the implanted electrodes.(84,85) Appropriately adjusted SCS is perceived by the patient as mild, tingling paraesthesias in the area of pain, which may be associated with significant pain relief. SCS analgesia is felt to result from interruption of nociceptive afferents through activation of endogenous inhibitory systems within the CNS; however, the analgesic mechanism of SCS has not been fully elucidated.

The main drawbacks to SCS include high cost and difficulty predicting which patients will gain lasting benefits. The hardware for SCS systems costs US$10 000–20 000, not including hospital costs and professional fees. Implantation of a permanent SCS system is preceded by a temporary trial of SCS, which adds to the cost, but helps to determine its potential benefit. Even after a successful trial, only 20–80 per cent of patients experience long-term analgesia from SCS.(84) Analgesic failures may be due to technical difficulties, placebo response during initial trial, development of tolerance to SCS, or progression of underlying pathology. If programmable arrays of multiple electrodes are used, the loss of effect may be overcome by using alternate combinations of electrodes. SCS has been used for many conditions, including chronic back and/or leg pain following lumbar spine surgery, intractable angina,(84) and various neuropathic conditions including complex regional pain syndrome (CRPS) and post-herpetic neuralgia. There is only one controlled trial comparing SCS with other therapies in CRPS, which reports efficacy in some patients with this condition.(86)

SCS can also be used in the management of severe extremity pain in patients with inoperable peripheral vascular disease. In animals, SCS improved microvascular blood flow, comparable to the improvement seen after surgical sympathectomy.(87) Prospective, randomized trials in inoperable peripheral vascular disease indicate that SCS is associated with improved pain control and/or a reduction in use of systemic analgesics.(88,89) It is less clear whether SCS reduces the extent of amputations. Although clinical reports of SCS are promising, there has been no comparison of SCS with neurolytic lumbar sympathetic block in inoperable peripheral vascular disease (see below).

The controversies and uncertainties of its use notwithstanding, SCS is an analgesic therapy that is successfully utilized in a number of settings, generally after inadequate response to systemic analgesics. SCS is a minimally invasive but expensive anaesthetic technique worthy of consideration when the palliation of appropriate symptoms has been resistant to other measures.

Techniques for pain control: the peripheral nervous system

Local anaesthetic blockade

Local anaesthetic blockade of peripheral nerves is useful in the management of severe somatic pain, such as pain from pathological fracture. Block techniques, perhaps with modification to include placement of a catheter for continuous infusion or repeated boluses of local anaesthetic, can be of considerable analgesic benefit.(90) Such techniques may be used temporarily to help patients tolerate other therapy or treatments (surgery for fracture stabilization, radiation therapy, or neurolytic block), or may serve as the primary analgesic therapy. Such use of catheters may be complicated by catheter-associated infection, local anaesthetic toxicity, catheter displacement, or other technical problems. As a result, these techniques are typically used as a temporary measure or for terminally ill patients. Examples of successful pain relief with continuous block are brachial plexus block for extremity pain,(91,92) suprascapular nerve block for shoulder pain,(93) and sciatic and femoral nerve block for lower extremity pain.(91)

Neurolytic blockade

Neurolytic blockade of peripheral nerves can be beneficial for patients with limited life expectancy who have severe somatic pain that is well characterized and localized. Somatic neurolytic blocks generally last up to 6 months, and are most appropriately viewed as complements to, rather than replacements for, systemic opioids and other pain therapies. Neuritis or deafferentation neuralgia may develop weeks to months following somatic neurolytic blockade in up to 30 per cent of patients, and the post-neurolysis pain may be worse than the original pain. Because of the limited duration of effect and the significant incidence of neuritis, neurolytic blocks are reserved for patients whose life expectancy is less than 6 months. Somatic neurolytic blockade should be avoided in patients where anticipated loss of innervated muscle function would add to morbidity. Alcohol and phenol are the agents most commonly used, but when life expectancy exceeds several months, cryoanalgesia or radiofrequency ablation is preferable, as the incidence of post-neurolysis neuropathic pain is lower.(69)

Recent improvements in pharmacologic management of pain, and the development of spinal analgesic therapies, have narrowed the indications for neurolytic blockade, so there are few patients for whom these procedures are yet indicated. For example, neurolytic intercostal nerve blocks or neurolytic paravertebral blocks may be used for management of intractable chest wall pain, as from chest wall invasion from pleural-based tumour. Generally, such pain problems are now managed with spinal analgesics, with neurolytic blocks reserved for those with contra-indication for spinal analgesics and a very short life expectancy. Before proceeding with neurolysis it is recommended that diagnostic local anaesthetic blocks be used to 'map' the nerves providing innervation to the pain area. Diagnostic/prognostic blocks are of particular importance in identifying which sacral nerve exerts a dominant effect on bladder tone, in order to avoid urinary incontinence after sacral neurolysis. The incidence of inadequate analgesia and neuralgia may be lessened by meticulous technique, perhaps using fluoroscopic guidance or nerve stimulator.(69)

Neurolytic blocks are used in palliative care not only for the management of pain, but also for the control of spasticity in patients with CNS disease. Neurolytic blockade of peripheral nerves(94,95) can result in considerable reduction of spasticity, but is reserved for situations where subarachnoid baclofen is ineffective or not indicated. Neurolytic pudendal nerve block also has been used successfully for the treatment of external sphincter hypertonicity in patients with spinal cord injury.(96) Compared to neuraxial neurolysis, peripheral nerve neurolysis may allow for more selective destruction, and this may be important in continent, ambulatory patients. The risk of neuralgia following peripheral neurolysis for control of spasticity is a concern that largely limits use of these techniques to palliative care.

Neurolytic trigeminal ganglion blockade

In the past, injection of the trigeminal (Gasserian) ganglion with alcohol or glycerol(69) was widely used in the management of trigeminal neuralgia, but this has largely been superseded by medical treatment with carbamazepine and other methods, such as surgical rhizotomy and radiofrequency gangliolysis.(85) The current role of trigeminal neurolysis in the management of cancer-related pain is unclear. Studies comparing trigeminal neurolysis with spinal analgesic therapies or other therapies for management of intractable facial pain of malignant origin have not been published, but in clinical practice, spinal analgesics and even intraventricular opioids are now used more commonly than neurolytic injection techniques.

Cryoanalgesia and radiofrequency lesioning

Radiofrequency lesioning

Radiofrequency ablation (RF) is the destruction of neural tissue with heat generated within tissue by a high-frequency electrical current.(69,97) As RF lesions are more predictable than chemical lesions, RF is now used for a variety of pain conditions.(85) However, as with other neuroablative techniques, pain relief is often accompanied by numbness, and there is a risk of dysaesthesias and motor weakness.

RF has been used for various procedures including ablation of the trigeminal ganglion; cervical, thoracic, and lumbar facet denervation; sacroiliac joint denervation; dorsal root ganglion ablation; and lesioning of the sympathetic chain at different levels (stellate, thoracic, and lumbar sympathetic ganglia). There are a few prospective studies on the use of RF for back pain with encouraging results,(98) but the long-term effects are unknown. There is, however, convincing data on the use of RF for trigeminal neuralgia.(85) A study of over 1000 patients showed that 95 per cent of patients had significant improvement of paroxysmal pain after trigeminal ganglion RF.(99) As trigeminal ganglion RF has approximately 35 per cent morbidity(99) and a low risk of mortality,(100) it is best reserved for patients who do not respond to, or cannot tolerate, medications.

A recent development is the use of pulsed RF (PRF), as an alternative to conventional RF. PRF consists of a train of short-duration, high-voltage, high-frequency pulses, whereby the maximal electrode temperature stays below 42°C, and analgesia can be achieved without nerve tissue damage. The mechanism of analgesia with PRF is not known, but animal data suggest it may be due to activation of pain-processing neurones in the dorsal horn of the spinal cord.(101) PRF has been reported to be effective in neuropathic (lumbar radiculopathy and chest wall) pain.(102) If further clinical experience confirms these anecdotal findings, PRF could be a very useful procedure for many chronic, debilitating neuropathic pain conditions. However, until more data are available, PRF is best reserved for patients who fail conventional pain therapies.

Cryoanalgesia

Cryoanalgesia is the destruction of neural tissue, by the application of extreme cold, to produce pain relief. The cryo needle is chilled to −50 to −70°C by the rapid expansion of carbon dioxide or nitrous oxide gas within the needle tip, and the low temperature produces variable degrees of nerve injury. The goal of cryoanalgesia is to induce loss of axonal continuity (axonotmesis) while preserving the architecture of the endo, peri, and ecto-neurium. Cryolesions cause wallerian axonal degeneration and breakup of the myelin sheath, followed by regeneration that starts from the proximal stump and advances distally. Although the risk of neuritis or dysaesthesia is lower than with other neuroablative techniques,(69) neuralgia can still occur;(103) therefore, cryoablation must be used with caution. Cryoanalgesia has been used mostly for post-thoracotomy pain, but its use has also been reported for various chronic pain problems. Cryoanalgesia may have a role in palliative care for the treatment of pain and spasticity: it may be applied to intercostal nerves for pain from rib fractures and has been used for palliation of hip adductor spasticity and obturator neuralgia.(104) The role of cryoanalgesia for the treatment of spasticity deserves further investigation.

Techniques for pain control: the sympathetic nervous system

Depending on the aetiology of pain, interruption of sympathetic nerves may have significant analgesic effect. The sympathetic chain and ganglia not only receive the efferent sympathetic fibres from the CNS, but are traversed (without synapse) by the visceral afferent nociceptive fibres. In various clinical settings, sympathetic block techniques may be used as follows:

1. blockade of afferent visceral nociceptive fibres may reduce or eliminate visceral pain;
2. sympathetic block may provide relief of ischaemic pain, produce cutaneous vasodilatation, and facilitate the healing of chronic ulceration as in inoperable peripheral vascular disease;
3. blockade of sympathetic (afferent) fibres may interrupt the interaction between nociceptive neurones and the sympathetic nervous system that appears to contribute to some cases of neuropathic pain.

The sympathetic nervous system appears to be variably involved in some clinical neuropathic pain problems, as well as animal models of nerve-injury pain.(105) Under normal conditions, nociceptors do not respond to sympathetic nervous system activity or administration of adrenergic agonists. After neural injury, however, sympathetic activation can result in enhanced nociceptor activity. Axotomized primary sensory afferents develop functional adrenoceptors and can be excited by sympathetic stimulation. Sprouting of sympathetic neurones, to envelop dorsal root ganglion neuronal cell bodies, has been demonstrated in experimental animals following nerve injury.(106) Although the functional significance of these sympathetic neuronal sprouts is uncertain, it has been postulated that such abnormal anatomic connections between sympathetic nervous fibres and primary afferent neurones may be part of the pathophysiology of some types of neuropathic pain.(107) In neuropathic pain, interruption of the sympathetic nervous system innervation to the area of pain may be of analgesic utility (Table 5).

Local anaesthetic sympathetic blockade

Local anaesthetic sympathetic blockade can be useful in some cases of neuropathic pain, renal colic, or ischaemic crises in Raynaud's disease or other obliterative arteriopathies.(108) Local anaesthetic sympathetic blockade is ineffective in treating established post-herpetic neuralgia,(108) but may be very useful in the management of pain from acute herpes zoster or subacute (less than 2-month duration) post-herpetic neuralgia. The role of sympathetic blockade in prevention of post-herpetic neuralgia is less clear. The incidence of post-herpetic neuralgia has been reported to be reduced in patients treated early with local anaesthetic sympathetic blockade,(112) but other studies have failed to show benefit.(113)

Temporary (local anaesthetic) sympathetic blockade may have value in predicting the response to neurolytic sympathetic block, but the response should be interpreted with caution. A number of factors, including systemic effect of absorbed local anaesthetic, concurrent somatic nerve block, patient expectations, and placebo response can make interpretation of the effects of local anaesthetic blockade problematic.(71)

Neurolytic sympathetic blockade

In the setting of advanced malignancy, neurolytic sympathetic blocks are used for the management of abdominal (coeliac plexus block), pelvic (superior hypogastric plexus block), and perineal (ganglion impar block) pain of visceral origin (Table 5). Neurolytic stellate ganglion block is infrequently carried out due to the proximity of, and potential for damage to, somatic nerves, vascular structures, and the brain stem.(69) Patients with mixed somatic and visceral pain, perhaps due to tumour invasion of somatic structures or distant metastases, may experience incomplete relief following sympathetic blockade. In some patients, however, even partial relief through neurolytic sympathetic blockade may improve overall pain control and allow reduction of opioid dose and opioid-related side effects.

Table 5 Types of neurolytic sympathetic block by location and clinical indication

Location	Clinical use	Results
Stellate ganglion block[a]	Angina, inoperable coronary artery disease Upper extremity pain Complex regional pain syndrome Peripheral vascular disease Raynaud's disease Brachial plexus infiltration by tumour Herpes zoster Phantom pain	Local anaesthetic block: variable, depending on pain condition Neurolytic block: unknown
Coeliac plexus block[b]	Visceral pain from Pancreatic cancer Other upper abdominal tumours	Partial to complete pain relief in 90% of patients alive after 3 months[109] Results similar for pancreatic cancer and other abdominal malignancies[109]
Lumbar sympathetic block[b]	Kidney pain (including 'phantom kidney pain') Intractable lower extremity pain Inoperable peripheral vascular disease Chronic painful leg ulceration Complex regional pain syndrome Phantom pain Herpes zoster Diabetic neuropathy Testicular pain	Variable, depending on pain condition Peripheral vascular disease: 50–80% of patients experience partial or complete relief of pain at rest[108,110]
Superior hypogastric plexus block[b]	Pelvic visceral pain from gynaecological, colorectal, or genitourinary cancer	Long-lasting relief in 72% of patients with positive response to diagnostic block[111]
Ganglion impar block[b]	Intractable perineal pain	Complete or significant relief in all patients[69]

[a] Neurolysis of the stellate ganglion is controversial, due to risk of complications. In some cases, persistent relief can be achieved from a series of local anaesthetic blocks.[69]

[b] Some clinicians do a local anaesthetic block before proceeding with neurolytic block to assess the effect of neurolysis.

Neurolytic coeliac plexus block

Pancreatic cancer pain is often described as relentless mid-epigastric pain radiating to the back.[69] Severe pain is a presenting symptom in only 10 per cent of pancreatic cancers,[114] but the incidence and severity of pain increases with disease progression. Neurolytic coeliac plexus block (NCPB) has been thoroughly studied and is known to be very effective for the relief of upper abdominal or back pain from pancreatic or other abdominal malignancies. With NCPB, good to excellent pain relief can be achieved in 85–90 per cent of patients[69,115] and pain relief persists until the time of death in 70–90 per cent of patients.

In a prospective randomized trial of patients with pancreatic cancer, NCPB provided equivalent pain relief with fewer adverse effects, compared to systemic analgesics.[116] Clinically, this information is useful in helping clinicians to select those individuals who may benefit from NCPB. Of course, if patients have good pain control with few and acceptable adverse effects related to systemic analgesics, there may be no further consideration given to NCPB. On the other hand, if patients have inadequate pain control, or they have significant adverse effects from medications, NCPB is a good pain management strategy. In the setting of unresectable pancreatic cancer, NCPB may be selected at any time, especially if pain is not well controlled with systemic analgesics.

In another prospective controlled trial, patients with unresectable pancreatic cancer were randomized to receive intraoperative neurolytic coeliac plexus block or placebo block. Among patients with significant preoperative pain, those receiving neurolytic coeliac plexus block had significantly longer survival than those treated with placebo.[117,118] Pending further investigation, it is unclear whether the improved survival is related to optimized pain control or some other effect of NCPB; however, the survival benefit appears to be another indication for NCPB in the setting of unresectable pancreatic cancer.

Following NCPB, 44 per cent of patients have diarrhoea (due to increased gastrointestinal motility) and 63 per cent have orthostatic hypotension. These symptoms are expected consequences of the interruption of the sympathetic innervation to the abdominal viscera, and are usually transient. In most patients NCPB can be done on an outpatient basis, but frail patients or those living long distances from the hospital/facility in which the block will be performed may be best served by overnight observation following NCPB for management of anticipated consequences of NCPB. Patients may rarely need oral ephedrine (30 mg three times daily) to control orthostatic hypotension or oral opioid to control diarrhoea. In patients previously treated with opioids, modest diarrhoea may be a welcome change, compared to opioid-related constipation.

Major, catastrophic complications can also occur after NCPB. A survey of 2730 patients treated with NCPB[119] found four cases of paraplegia, for an incidence of 1 : 683. There have also been several case reports concerning paraplegia following celiac plexus block. It is postulated that paraplegia is the result of vascular injury, perhaps due to vasospasm of the artery of Adamkiewicz, resulting in ischaemic injury to the spinal cord. Other serious complications include aortic dissection,[120] generalized seizures, or circulatory arrest.[69] Radiographic imaging for needle placement is recommended, although serious complications can still occur. Fluoroscopy is widely available and is used in many centres. CT may be advisable when there is known or suspected distortion of normal anatomy (such as in patients with massive ascites, organomegaly, or large pleural effusions), if a previous NCPB has been ineffective, or in young children.[121] Ultrasonography appears to be a reasonable alternative when the anterior approach is used.[122] It is unclear whether or not the risk of paralysis is affected by the technique used or the type of imaging.[123,124] A new approach for coeliac plexus block has been described via a transluminal endoscopic (gastroscopic) biopsy needle under endoscopic ultrasound guidance.[122] This technique may have utility,[125] especially when anatomic abnormalities preclude traditional approaches.[69] Pending further investigation, however, it is prudent to assume that all techniques of NCPB are associated with some risk of serious adverse effect. Paralysis after NCPB has even been described after open, intra-operative block.[126]

NCPB is sometimes used for chronic, non-cancer abdominal pain; however, except in terminal palliative care, this is controversial due to the limited duration of analgesia and the risk of complications.

Neurolytic lumbar sympathetic block

The most common indication for neurolytic lumbar sympathetic block (NLSB) is intractable lower extremity pain from ischaemia in patients with inoperable peripheral vascular disease. NLSB has been shown to increase cutaneous blood flow, reduce ischaemic rest pain, and enhance healing of chronic ischaemic ulceration.[110,127] It is also useful for neuropathic lower extremity pain. Less common indications are visceral pain from lower abdominal and pelvic structures, such as renal pain, testicular pain, and tenesmus.[108]

Lumbar sympathectomy can be done percutaneously with NLSB or surgically, with comparable results. With either approach, the majority of patients with peripheral vascular disease experience partial or complete relief of pain at rest, and the mean duration of effect is approximately 6 months. Compared to surgical sympathectomy, percutaneous NLSB is less invasive; has lower morbidity, mortality, and cost; and can easily be repeated.[127] Lumbar sympathectomy with radiofrequency has also been described, but seems inferior to NLSB.[128,129] The risk of serious complications from NLSB is low; however, it is recommended that radiographic imaging be used to verify appropriate needle placement and spread of neurolytic solution.

Neurolytic superior hypogastric plexus block

Neurolytic superior hypogastric plexus block has been shown to be safe and effective for pain control in patients with pelvic visceral pain from gynaecologic, colorectal, or genitourinary cancer.[111] Patients with pelvic pain from tumour invasion of the pelvic wall may have incomplete relief after superior hypogastric plexus block, because such pain likely has a significant somatic component that is unlikely to respond to sympathetic blockade. Extensive retroperitoneal disease, when present, may interfere with the spread of neurolytic agent and contribute to poor results. In patients with predominantly visceral pelvic pain, however, this technique may be very helpful. For very severe pain, or in cases involving significant somatic pain, spinal analgesics would seem to be a preferable analgesic technique; however, comparative data are not available.

Neurolytic ganglion impar block

The ganglion impar (also known as ganglion of Walther) is the terminal sympathetic ganglion of the paravertebral sympathetic chain and is located in the retroperitoneal space at the level of the sacrococcygeal junction. Neurolytic blockade of the ganglion impar may be used for the relief of intractable rectal or perineal pain, but available data are limited. Described techniques involve insertion of a needle through the anococcygeal ligament[69] or sacrococcygeal ligament.[130]

Miscellaneous anaesthetic techniques

Trigger point injections

Myofascial pain syndromes (MPS) are a common cause of pain that can involve any skeletal muscle. MPS may be the primary cause of pain or may be secondary to other pathology (i.e. disc herniation, vertebral compression fracture). MPS may complicate cancer-related pain, or be present as one cause of 'non-cancer-related pain' in cancer patients. As MPS are common, clinicians involved in palliative care need to be able to recognize and treat MPS.

Appropriate diagnosis of MPS requires careful physical examination for muscular 'trigger points' (TPs): a hyperirritable spot in skeletal muscle that is associated with a hypersensitive nodule that may be palpable. The TP is painful on compression and can cause characteristic referred pain and autonomic phenomena.[131] The aetiology of MPS is not fully known. TPs seem to arise from tissues affected by injury, which therefore become prone to further injury. Each new injury may result in additional TPs.[132] Cycles of sustained muscle contraction, impaired metabolic activity, and ischaemia may result in local sensitization of nociceptors and receptive field changes and account for the characteristic, complex patterns of referred pain that complicate MPS.[133]

Management of MPS depends on the severity and chronicity of pain. Injection of local anaesthetic or normal saline into TPs is often adequate to provide pain relief. For persistent pain, TP injections and other therapies (i.e. dry needling, vasocoolants, acupuncture, spray and stretch, analgesics)[132] need to be combined with removal of underlying or perpetuating factors (i.e. physical therapy for postural or muscular abnormalities, orthotic devices for structural abnormalities). When an underlying cause is present, such as disk disease or nerve root compression, treatment of resulting MPS is more likely to be successful if the underlying problem is directly addressed.

Botulinum toxin injections

Botulinum toxin (BTX) is a potent neurotoxin produced by the bacterium *Clostridium botulinum*, and is one important cause of food poisoning. The bacterium produces seven distinct toxins,[134] designated A, B, C, D, E, F, and G, all of which are potent neuroparalytic agents. There are at least two commercial preparations of BTX A complex for clinical use (Botox, Allergan; Dysport, Ipsen), and one preparation of BTX B complex (Myobloc in United States and Neurobloc in Europe, both by Elan). These BTX products have different doses, efficacy, and safety profiles, and therefore should not be considered as interchangeable generic equivalents.[134] BTX acts by irreversibly inhibiting the release of acetylcholine at the neuromuscular junction,[135] blocking neurotransmission, but after a few months, the neuromuscular junction is re-established. The effects of BTX start approximately 1 week after injection and last 3–4 months,[136] before regeneration of the neuromuscular junction occurs. Local injection of BTX results in a localized chemodenervation and the loss or reduction of neuronal activity at the target organ (e.g. muscle, glands), with minimal risk of systemic adverse effects.[134]

BTX has been used to treat disorders characterized by pathologically increased muscle activity,[137] such as spasticity, movement disorders, and chronic myofascial pain.[137,138] Patients who may benefit from BTX include those with hemiparesis after stroke, traumatic brain injury, multiple sclerosis, and paraparesis with focal spasticity. As typically used, BTX is well tolerated and safe, and no cases of permanent organ damage have been reported.[137] Reversible adverse effects include temporary bladder paresis, mild dysphagia, disabling muscle weakness, and even transient tetraparesis.[136] Repetitive injections may produce neutralizing antibodies, which render future use of BTX ineffective. Because of this concern, there should be an interval of at least 12 weeks between injections.[139]

The role of BTX in palliative care has not been well defined, but there are potential applications. BTX may be beneficial for patients with spasticity and may result in functional improvement by selectively weakening muscles involved in debilitating spasm. Specific benefits from BTX for spasticity include:[140]

1. improved motor function (ability to stand and walk, improved upper-extremity movement);
2. easier care of adults with spasticity (personal hygiene in patients with adductor spasticity, self-care, and dressing in patients with arm spasticity).

In addition, BTX can be beneficial for patients with chronic myofascial pain syndromes, such as those often associated with tension headaches, migraine, cervical pain, and low back pain.

Adjunctive physical therapy is very important if the benefits of BTX are to be maximized.[141] The high cost of the toxin is a significant factor that may limit the use of BTX in palliative care.

Interpleural analgesia

Interpleural (or intrapleural) analgesia (IPA) involving administration of local anaesthetics into the pleural space was first described for acute post-thoracotomy pain. IPA can be used to control pain from metastatic disease to the neck, arms, chest, brachial plexus, thorax, or abdomen,[142] and also to manage pain from acute pancreatitis,[143] acute herpes zoster, and post-herpetic neuralgia.[144] The proposed mechanism of IPA is diffusion of local anaesthetic through the pleura to block the intercostal nerves, thoracic sympathetic chain, splanchnic nerves, and brachial plexus.[145] In addition, the absorbed local anaesthetic may provide a systemic analgesic effect. Complications associated with IPA are pneumothorax in 2 per cent of patients, systemic toxicity from local anaesthetic (1.3 per cent), pleural effusion (0.4 per cent), pleural infection (0.4 per cent), and catheter rupture (0.1 per cent). Migration of the catheter into the lung has also been reported.[146]

IPA may be used for several weeks to months, with techniques similar to those used for chronic epidural access, including simple percutaneous catheters and subcutaneously implanted injection portals. IPA may be useful for control of both acute and chronic pain, but its relative merits, compared to spinal analgesia, are not defined.

Topical agents

Various medications have been used topically in an attempt to provide analgesia. Topical *lidocaine* seems to be effective in *post-herpetic neuralgia*[147] and other cases of neuropathic pain with significant mechano-allodynia. Pain during *dressing changes of open wounds* is difficult to control. In the authors' experience, 30–60 ml of 0.5–1 per cent lidocaine, simply sprayed over open wounds is safe and, if left in the wound for at least 5 min, is a very useful adjunct to systemic analgesics. This is most effective if applied to the old dressing, just before the final layer is removed. If 'wet-to-dry' dressing changes are needed for wound debridement, the local anaesthetic can be sprayed onto the wound surface after the old dressing is removed. Such topical application of local anaesthetic solution, or application of a local anaesthetic-soaked gauze pad for several minutes, also provides some degree of relief for superficial wound cleaning or debridement. More extensive wound debridement will require other regional or general anaesthetic techniques.

Oral topical doxepin (tricyclic antidepressant) has been reported in a single-dose case series to be effective for pain from oral mucositis secondary to radiation therapy or chemotherapy.[148] *Viscous lidocaine* (2 per cent) may also be invaluable in management of oral mucositis or oral herpes zoster.

Topical application of morphine to open wounds has been reported to be an effective analgesic therapy.[149,150] In these recent studies, morphine has been compounded into an aqueous gel used for wound care (e.g. IntraSite gel).[150] Opioid receptors, located on the peripheral terminals of primary afferent nociceptors, modulate nociceptive neural transmission.[151] In the setting of tissue inflammation, peripheral opioid receptors appear to be up-regulated, and are likely activated by endogenous opioids produced by peripheral immune cells. More clinical data are needed to evaluate the effects of topical morphine on wound healing and pain control. If the findings of these anecdotal reports are confirmed in future studies, the topical use of morphine for wound pain could be an important development.

Recent advances and future direction

The need for improved pain management techniques is clear: uncontrolled pain is a maleficent force that has significant adverse effects. In some cases, it appears that 'pain can kill'.[152] At the same time, opioid analgesics, the mainstay of analgesic therapy, are imperfect drugs associated with several adverse effects and opioid-tolerance-induced hyperalgesia. Clinical pain is not just simple nociception, but hyperalgesia with sensitization due to tissue injury/inflammation, nerve injury, and/or opioid tolerance. Fortunately, extensive research in recent years has yielded new insight into the pathophysiology of pain so that the translation of new anti-hyperalgesic therapies into clinical practice may become a reality.

The relationship between pain, analgesic therapies, and the medical consequences of unrelieved pain is the subject of ongoing research, but it is clear that chronic pain is never 'benign'. Severe physiologic stress, including unrelieved pain, can result in immune system suppression.[152] In experimental animals, post-operative pain appears to be a significant component of surgery-induced decrease in host resistance to tumour metastasis.[153] Clinical studies[154,155] have suggested similar surgery-induced immune suppression. Uncontrolled pain is also a risk factor for anxiety and depression, but in turn, anxiety and depression are risk factors for morbidity and mortality, perhaps also mediated by immune dysfunction.[156]

Analgesic therapies decreased the impact of surgery on host tumour resistance in animals;[153] however, a complicating issue is the finding that systemic morphine itself has some suppressant effect on immune function.[157] Spinal analgesics may have less effect on immune function than systemic morphine.[155,158] The importance of research in this area is evidenced by findings that neurolytic coeliac plexus block is associated with decreased pain, elevated mood, and improved survival in persons with pancreatic cancer pain.[117,118] In a recent randomized trial for refractory cancer pain, spinal analgesics were found to be associated with improved pain control and decreased analgesic toxicity, but also improved survival, compared to comprehensive medical management.[159] These data emphasize that, due to the consequences of uncontrolled pain, optimized pain control is an integral component of good medical care.

Recent research points the way towards new spinal analgesics for neuropathic pain and/or to address opioid tolerance.

- *Neurotrophins* are polypeptides that regulate nerve growth, differentiation, and function. After nerve injury, many of the changes in affected peripheral neurones are modulated by neurotrophins. Ectopic, spontaneous electrical activity in large Aβ neurones, which appears to be an essential component of mechano-allodynia, is related to neurotrophin-regulated abnormal density and distribution of sodium-channel subtypes on damaged neurons.[160] In animals, application of an exogenous neurotrophin prevented this abnormality in sodium channel regulation and decreased mechano-allodynia.[161]
- Neurotrophins also appear to regulate the CNS synapses of peripheral neurones. After nerve injury, there is reorganization of the central terminals of Aβ neurones, which develop new synapses with spinal cord neurones in pain pathways. Formation of these new synapses, which apparently contribute to development of mechano-allodynia, is regulated by Neurotrophin-3 (NT-3). In animals, subarachnoid administration of NT-3 antisense oligonucleotide attenuated the formation of new abnormal synapses, and limited development of mechano-allodynia.[162]

These lines of research, focusing on neuropathic pain and the effects of different neurotrophins, suggest that subarachnoid administration of pharmacologic agents with selected neurotrophin-like actions could be useful for neuropathic pain.

- *Adenosine and adenosine analogues* have been found to modulate pain transmission, apparently due to effects at spinal adenosine receptors (Fig. 5). Limited clinical studies have shown that adenosine has prolonged analgesic effect after subarachnoid administration,[163,164] but data on analgesic effects of systemic adenosine are inconclusive.[165,166] Initial evaluations of subarachnoid adenosine have not identified significant neurotoxicity or other adverse effects.[167] Therefore, adenosine or adenosine analogues may become useful spinal analgesics for neuropathic pain.
- *Opioid tolerance (hyperalgesia)* is the major limitation to successful use of chronic opioid therapy. Substance P is a known neurotransmitter in nociceptive pathways, but recent research has demonstrated that substance P also modulates the analgesic efficacy of opioid. Co-administration of substance P with low-dose morphine markedly

enhanced its analgesic effect. Subsequent animal research demonstrated that a *chimeric peptide* (ESP7), sharing amino acid sequences from substance P and endogenous opioid (endomorphin) tetrapeptides, has significant analgesic efficacy following subarachnoid administration. Most notably, tolerance to the analgesic effect did not develop with longer-term administration.[168] In another study, subarachnoid administration of a similar chimeric peptide (ESP6) with morphine prevented the development of analgesic tolerance to morphine.[169] Development of agents that limit tolerance to subarachnoid opioid could greatly enhance the utility of spinal analgesics.

- *Conotoxins* are extremely potent agents, some of that are specific for calcium channels in neurones that are associated with the NMDA receptor. Early examples (i.e. SNX-111) proved to be effective analgesics for neuropathic pain, but were found to have a very narrow therapeutic window.[170] A new, promising agent, AM336, is currently in clinical trials.

Current pain research continues to present clinicians with new understanding of familiar pain problems and new opportunities for improving analgesic therapies. Although rare pain problems cannot be adequately controlled with current therapies, the vast majority of patients in palliative care need not wait for future therapies to have adequate pain control. A large, diverse array of systemic, and interventional, anaesthetic pain therapies is currently available. The management of most current analgesic failures must only await the consistent application of pain management strategies already available.

References

1. **World Health Organization.** *Cancer Pain Relief and Palliative Care: Report of a WHO Expert Committee.* Technical Report Series. Geneva: World Health Organization, 1990, p. 804.
2. **Jacox, A.** et al. *Management of Cancer Pain. Clinical Practice Guideline No. 9.* Rockville: Agency for Health Care Policy and Research, US Department of Health and Human Services, 1994.
3. **Mercadante, S.** (1999). Pain treatment and outcomes for patients with advanced cancer who receive follow-up care at home. *Cancer* **85**, 1849–58.
4. **Cherny, N.I., Arbit, E., and Jain, S.** (1996). Invasive techniques in the management of cancer pain. *Hematology/Oncology Clinics of North America* **10**, 121–37.
5. **Mercadante, S. and Portenoy, R.K.** (2001). Opioid poorly-responsive cancer pain. Part 1: Clinical considerations. *Journal of Pain and Symptom Management* **21**, 144–50.
6. **Mercadante, S. and Portenoy, R.K.** (2001). Opioid poorly-responsive cancer pain. Part 2: basic mechanisms that could shift dose response for analgesia. *Journal of Pain and Symptom Management* **21**, 255–64.
7. **Mayer, D.J.** et al. (1999). Cellular mechanisms of neuropathic pain, morphine tolerance, and their interactions. *Proceedings of the National Academy of Sciences of the United States of America* **96**, 7731–6.
8. **Carr, D.B. and Cousins, M.J.** (1998). Spinal route of analgesia: opioids and future options. In *Neural Blockade in Clinical Anesthesia and Management of Pain* 3rd edn. (ed. M.J. Cousins and P.O. Bridenbaugh), pp. 915–83. Philadelphia: Lippincott-Raven.
9. **Bruera, E. and Pereira, J.** (1998). Recent developments in palliative cancer care. *Acta Oncologica* **37**, 749–57.
10. **De Conno, F.** et al. (1991). Hyperalgesia and myoclonus with intrathecal infusion of high-dose morphine. *Pain* **47**, 337–9.
11. **Mercadante, S.** et al. (2000). Analgesic effect of intravenous ketamine in cancer patients on morphine therapy: a randomized, controlled, double-blind, crossover, double-dose study. *Journal of Pain and Symptom Management* **20**, 246–52.
12. **Brose, W.G. and Cousins, M.J.** (1991). Subcutaneous lidocaine for treatment of neuropathic cancer pain. *Pain* **45**, 145–8.
13. **Bennett, G.** et al. (2000). Evidence-based review of the literature on intrathecal delivery of pain medication. *Journal of Pain and Symptom Management* **20**, S12–36.
14. **Bennett, G.** et al. (2000). Clinical guidelines for intraspinal infusion: report of an expert panel. PolyAnalgesic Consensus Conference 2000. *Journal of Pain and Symptom Management* **20**, S37–43.
15. **Jones, T.F.** et al. (2002). Neurologic complications including paralysis after a medication error involving implanted intrathecal catheters. *American Journal of Medicine* **112**, 31–6.
16. **Dougherty, P.M. and Staats, P.S.** (1999). Intrathecal drug therapy for chronic pain: from basic science to clinical practice. *Anesthesiology* **91**, 1891–918.
17. **Walker, S.M.** et al. (2002). Combination spinal analgesic chemotherapy: a systematic review. *Anesthesia & Analgesia* **95**, 674–715.
18. **Gourlay, G.K.** et al. (1989). Pharmacokinetics of fentanyl in lumbar and cervical CSF following lumbar epidural and intravenous administration. *Pain* **38**, 253–9.
19. **Brose, W.G.** et al. (1991). CSF and blood pharmacokinetics of hydromorphone and morphine following lumbar epidural administration. *Pain* **45**, 11–15.
20. **Rathmell, J.P., Roland, T., and DuPen, S.L.** (2000). Management of pain associated with metastatic epidural spinal cord compression: use of imaging studies in planning epidural therapy. *Regional Anesthesia and Pain Medicine* **25**, 113–16.
21. **Cherry, D.A., Gourlay, G.K., and Cousins, M.J.** (1986). Epidural mass associated with lack of efficacy of epidural morphine and undetectable CSF morphine concentrations. *Pain* **25**, 69–73.
22. **Winkelmuller, M. and Winkelmuller, W.** (1996). Long-term effects of continuous intrathecal opioid treatment in chronic pain of nonmalignant etiology. *Journal of Neurosurgery* **85**, 458–67.
23. **Reisine, T. and Pasternak, G.** (1996). Opioid analgesics and antagonists. In *Goodman & Gilman's The Pharmacologic Basis of Therapeutics* 9th edn. (ed. J.G. Hardman, L.E. Limbird, P.B. Molinoff, and R.W. Ruddon), pp. 521–55. New York: McGraw-Hill.
24. **Portenoy, R.K. and Savage, S.R.** (1997). Clinical realities and economic considerations: special therapeutic issues in intrathecal therapy—tolerance and addiction. *Journal of Pain and Symptom Management* **14**, S27–35.
25. **van Dongen, R.T., Crul, B.J., and De Bock, M.** (1993). Long-term intrathecal infusion of morphine and morphine/bupivacaine mixtures in the treatment of cancer pain: a retrospective analysis of 51 cases. *Pain* **55**, 119–23.
26. **van Dongen, R.T., Crul, B.J., and van Egmond, J.** (1999). Intrathecal coadministration of bupivacaine diminishes morphine dose progression during long-term intrathecal infusion in cancer patients. *Clinical Journal of Pain* **15**, 166–72.
27. **Du Pen, S.L.** et al. (1992). Chronic epidural bupivacaine-opioid infusion in intractable cancer pain. *Pain* **49**, 293–300.
28. **Mercadante, S.** (1994). Intrathecal morphine and bupivacaine in advanced cancer pain patients implanted at home. *Journal of Pain and Symptom Management* **9**, 201–7.
29. **Dahm, P.** et al. (1998). High thoracic/low cervical, long-term intrathecal (i.t.) infusion of bupivacaine alleviates 'refractory' pain in patients with unstable angina pectoris. Report of 2 cases. *Acta Anaesthesiologica Scandinavica* **42**, 1010–17.
30. **Berde, C.B.** et al. (1990). Subarachnoid bupivacaine analgesia for seven months for a patient with a spinal cord tumor. *Anesthesiology* **72**, 1094–6.
31. **Eisenach, J.C., Hood, D.D., and Curry, R.** (1998). Intrathecal, but not intravenous, clonidine reduces experimental thermal or capsaicin-induced pain and hyperalgesia in normal volunteers. *Anesthesia & Analgesia* **87**, 591–6.
32. **Eisenach, J.C.** et al. (1995). Epidural clonidine analgesia for intractable cancer pain. The Epidural Clonidine Study Group. *Pain* **61**, 391–9.
33. **Siddall, P.J.** et al. (2000). The efficacy of intrathecal morphine and clonidine in the treatment of pain after spinal cord injury. *Anesthesia & Analgesia* **91**, 1493–8.
34. **Tumber, P.S. and Fitzgibbon, D.R.** (1998). The control of severe cancer pain by continuous intrathecal infusion and patient controlled intrathecal analgesia with morphine, bupivacaine and clonidine. *Pain* **78**, 217–20.
35. **Burchiel, K.J. and Hsu, F.P.** (2001). Pain and spasticity after spinal cord injury: mechanisms and treatment. *Spine* **26**, S146–60.

36. **Chabal, C., Jacobson, L., and Terman, G.** (1992). Intrathecal fentanyl alleviates spasticity in the presence of tolerance to intrathecal baclofen. *Anesthesiology* **76**, 312–14.
37. **Penn, R.D.** et al. (1989). Intrathecal baclofen for severe spinal spasticity. *New England Journal of Medicine* **320**, 1517–21.
38. **Coffey, J.R.** et al. (1993). Intrathecal baclofen for intractable spasticity of spinal origin: results of a long-term multicenter study. *Journal of Neurosurgery* **78**, 226–32.
39. **Loubser, P.G. and Akman, N.M.** (1996). Effects of intrathecal baclofen on chronic spinal cord injury pain. *Journal of Pain and Symptom Management* **12**, 241–7.
40. **Zuniga, R.E., Schlicht, C.R., and Abram, S.E.** (2000). Intrathecal baclofen is analgesic in patients with chronic pain. *Anesthesiology* **92**, 876–80.
41. **Becker, R.** et al. (2000). Continuous intrathecal baclofen infusion in the management of central deafferentation pain. *Journal of Pain and Symptom Management* **20**, 313–15.
42. **Hodgson, P.S.** et al. (1999). The neurotoxicity of drugs given intrathecally (spinal). *Anesthesia & Analgesia* **88**, 797–809.
43. **Sator-Katzenschlager, S.** et al. (2001). The long-term antinociceptive effect of intrathecal S(+)-ketamine in a patient with established morphine tolerance. *Anesthesia & Analgesia* **93**, 1032.
44. **Stotz, M., Oehen, H.P., and Gerber, H.** (1999). Histological findings after long-term infusion of intrathecal ketamine for chronic pain: a case report. *Journal of Pain and Symptom Management* **18**, 223–8.
45. **Karpinski, N.** et al. (1997). Subpial vacuolar myelopathy after intrathecal ketamine: report of a case. *Pain* **73**, 103–5.
46. **Du Pen, S.** (1999). Complications of neuraxial infusion in cancer patients. *Oncology (Huntington)* **13**, 45–51.
47. **Blomberg, S.G.** (1994). Long-term home self-treatment with high thoracic epidural anesthesia in patients with severe coronary artery disease. *Anesthesia & Analgesia* **79**, 413–21.
48. **Anderson, V.C. and Burchiel, K.J.** (1999). A prospective study of long-term intrathecal morphine in the management of chronic nonmalignant pain. *Neurosurgery* **44**, 289–300.
49. **Hassenbusch, S.J.** et al. (1995). Long-term intraspinal infusions of opioids in the treatment of neuropathic pain. *Journal of Pain and Symptom Management* **10**, 527–43.
50. **Kumar, K., Kelly, M., and Pirlot, T.** (2001). Continuous intrathecal morphine treatment for chronic pain of nonmalignant etiology: long-term benefits and efficacy. *Surgical Neurology* **55**, 79–86.
51. **Appelgren, L.** et al. (1997). Spinal epidural metastasis: implications for spinal analgesia to treat 'refractory' cancer pain. *Journal of Pain and Symptom Management* **13**, 25–42.
52. **Ferrante, F.M.** (1999). Neuraxial infusion in the management of cancer pain. *Oncology (Huntington)* **13**, 30–6.
53. **de Jong, P.C. and Kansen, P.J.** (1994). A comparison of epidural catheters with or without subcutaneous injection ports for treatment of cancer pain. *Anesthesia & Analgesia* **78**, 94–100.
54. **Smitt, P.S.** et al. (1998). Outcome and complications of epidural analgesia in patients with chronic cancer pain. *Cancer* **83**, 2015–22.
55. **Coombs, D.W.** et al. (1985). Neuropathologic lesions and CSF morphine concentrations during chronic continuous intraspinal morphine infusion. A clinical and post-mortem study. *Pain* **22**, 337–51.
56. **Cherry, D.A. and Gourlay, G.K.** (1992). CT contrast evidence of injectate encapsulation after long-term epidural administration. *Pain* **49**, 369–71.
57. **Mercadante, S.** (1999). Problems of long-term spinal opioid treatment in advanced cancer patients. *Pain* **79**, 1–13.
58. **Gourlay, G.K.** et al. (1991). Comparison of intermittent bolus with continuous infusion of epidural morphine in the treatment of severe cancer pain. *Pain* **47**, 135–40.
59. **Hassenbusch, S.J.** et al. (1997). Clinical realities and economic considerations: economics of intrathecal therapy. *Journal of Pain and Symptom Management* **14**, S36–48.
60. **Bennett, M.I., Tai, Y.M., and Symonds, J.M.** (1994). Staphylococcal meningitis following synchromed intrathecal pump implant: a case report. *Pain* **56**, 243–4.
61. **Coffey, R.J. and Burchiel, K.** (2002). Inflammatory mass lesions associated with intrathecal drug infusion catheters: report and observations on 41 patients. *Neurosurgery* **50**, 78–86.
62. **van Diejen, D., Driessen, J.J., and Kaanders, J.H.** (1987). Spinal cord compression during chronic epidural morphine administration in a cancer patient. *Anaesthesia* **42**, 1201–3.
63. **Samuel, M., Finnerty, G.T., and Rudge, P.** (1994). Intrathecal baclofen pump infection treated by adjunct intrareservoir antibiotic instillation. *Journal of Neurology, Neurosurgery and Psychiatry* **57**, 1146–7.
64. **Yaksh, T.L., Noueihed, R.Y., and Durant, P.A.** (1986). Studies of the pharmacology and pathology of intrathecally administered 4-anilinopiperidine analogues and morphine in the rat and cat. *Anesthesiology* **64**, 54–66.
65. **Sjoberg, M.** et al. (1992). Neuropathologic findings after long-term intrathecal infusion of morphine and bupivacaine for pain treatment in cancer patients. *Anesthesiology* **76**, 173–86.
66. **Lazorthes, Y.R., Sallerin, B.A., and Verdie, J.C.** (1995). Intracerebroventricular administration of morphine for control of irreducible cancer pain. *Neurosurgery* **37**, 422–8.
67. **Karavelis, A.** et al. (1996). Intraventricular administration of morphine for control of intractable cancer pain in 90 patients. *Neurosurgery* **39**, 57–61.
68. **Ballantyne, J.C.** et al. (1996). Comparative efficacy of epidural, subarachnoid, and intracerebroventricular opioids in patients with pain due to cancer. *Regional Anesthesia* **21**, 542–56.
69. **Patt, R.B. and Cousins, M.J.** (1998). Techniques for neurolytic neural blockade. In *Neural Blockade in Clinical Anesthesia and Management of Pain* 3rd edn. (ed. M.J. Cousins and P.O. Bridenbaugh), pp. 1007–61. Philadelphia: Lippincott-Raven.
70. **Charlton, J.E. and Macrae, W.A.** (1998). Complications of neurolytic neural blockade. In *Neural Blockade in Clinical Anesthesia and Management of Pain* 3rd edn. (ed. M.J. Cousins and P.O. Bridenbough), pp. 663–72. Philadelphia: Lippincott-Raven.
71. **Hogan, Q.H. and Abram, S.E.** (1997). Neural blockade for diagnosis and prognosis: a review. *Anesthesiology* **86**, 216–41.
72. **Myers, R.R.** (1998). Neuropathology of neurolytic agents. In *Neural Blockade in Clinical Anesthesia and Management of Pain* 3rd edn. (ed. M.J. Cousins and P.O. Bridenbaugh), pp. 985–1006. Philadelphia: Lippincott-Raven.
73. **Dogliotti, A.M.** (1931). Traitement des syndrome douloureux de la peripheric par l'alcoolisation subarachnoidienne des racines posterieurs a leur emergencede las moelle epiniere. *Presse Medicale* **39**, 1249.
74. **Greenhill, J.P.** (1947). Sympathectomy and intra-spinal alcohol injections for relief of pelvic pain. *British Medical Journal* **2**, 859.
75. **Hay, R.C.** (1962). Subarachnoid alcohol block in control of intractable pain: report of 252 patients. *Anesthesia & Analgesia* **41**, 12.
76. **Kuzucu, E.Y., Derrick, W.S., and Wilber, S.A.** (1966). Control of intractable pain with subarachnoid alcohol block. *Journal of the American Medical Association* **195**, 541–4.
77. **Drechsel, U.** (1984). Treatment of cancer pain with neurolytic agents. *Recent Results in Cancer Research* **89**, 137–47.
78. **Swerdlow, M.** (1989). Intrathecal and extradural block in pain relief. In *Relief of Intractable Pain* 4th edn. (ed. M. Swerdlow and J.E. Charlton), pp. 223–57. Amsterdam: Elsevier.
79. **McGarvey, M.L.** et al. (2000). Irreversible spinal cord injury as a complication of subarachnoid ethanol neurolysis. *Neurology* **54**, 1522–4.
80. **Nagaro, T.** et al. (1994). Percutaneous cervical cordotomy and subarachnoid phenol block using fluoroscopy in pain control of costopleural syndrome. *Pain* **58**, 325–30.
81. **Rodriguez-Bigas, M.** et al. (1991). Intrathecal phenol rhizotomy for management of pain in recurrent unresectable carcinoma of the rectum. *Surgery, Gynecology and Obstetrics* **173**, 41–4.
82. **Scott, B.A.** et al. (1985). Intrathecal phenol and glycerin in metrizamide for treatment of intractable spasms in paraplegia. Case report. *Journal of Neurosurgery* **63**, 125–7.
83. **Asensi, V.** et al. (1999). Successful intrathecal ethanol block for intractable spasticity of AIDS- related progressive multifocal leukoencephalopathy. *Spinal Cord* **37**, 450–2.

84. **Muir, A. and Molloy, A.R.** (1997). Neuraxial implants for pain control. *International Anesthesiology Clinics* **35**, 171–96.

85. **Tasker, R.R.** (1998). Neurostimulation and percutaneous neural destructive techniques. In *Neural Blockade in Clinical Anesthesia and Management of Pain* 3rd edn. (ed. M.J. Cousins and P.O. Bridenbaugh), pp. 1063–111. Philadelphia: Lippincott-Raven.

86. **Kemler, M.A.** et al. (2000). Spinal cord stimulation in patients with chronic reflex sympathetic dystrophy. *New England Journal of Medicine* **343**, 618–24.

87. **Linderoth, B., Gunasekera, L., and Meyerson, B.A.** (1991). Effects of sympathectomy on skin and muscle microcirculation during dorsal column stimulation: animal studies. *Neurosurgery* **29**, 874–9.

88. **Jivegard, L.E.** et al. (1995). Effects of spinal cord stimulation (SCS) in patients with inoperable severe lower limb ischaemia: a prospective randomised controlled study. *European Journal of Vascular and Endovascular Surgery* **9**, 421–5.

89. **Klomp, H.M.** et al. (1999). Spinal-cord stimulation in critical limb ischaemia: a randomised trial. ESES Study Group. *Lancet* **353**, 1040–4.

90. **Vranken, J.H.** et al. (2001). Continuous brachial plexus block at the cervical level using a posterior approach in the management of neuropathic cancer pain. *Regional Anesthesia and Pain Medicine* **26**, 572–5.

91. **Fischer, H.B.** et al. (1996). Peripheral nerve catheterization in the management of terminal cancer pain. *Regional Anesthesia* **21**, 482–5.

92. **Aguilar, J.L.** et al. (1995). Long-term brachial plexus anesthesia using a subcutaneous implantable injection system. Case report. *Regional Anesthesia* **20**, 242–5.

93. **Mercadante, S., Sapio, M., and Villari, P.** (1995). Suprascapular nerve block by catheter for breakthrough shoulder cancer pain. *Regional Anesthesia* **20**, 343–6.

94. **Viel, E.J.** et al. (2002). Neurolytic blockade of the obturator nerve for intractable spasticity of adductor thigh muscles. *European Journal of Pain* **6**, 97–104.

95. **Chua, K.S. and Kong, K.H.** (2001). Clinical and functional outcome after alcohol neurolysis of the tibial nerve for ankle-foot spasticity. *Brain Injury* **15**, 733–9.

96. **Ko, H.Y. and Kim, K.T.** (1997). Treatment of external urethral sphincter hypertonicity by pudendal nerve block using phenol solution in patients with spinal cord injury. *Spinal Cord* **35**, 690–3.

97. **Kline, M.T. and Yin, W.** (2001). Radiofrequency techniques in clinical practice. In *Interventional Pain Management* 2nd edn. (ed. S.D. Waldman), pp. 243–93. Philadelphia: Saunders.

98. **Geurts, J.W.** et al. (2001). Efficacy of radiofrequency procedures for the treatment of spinal pain: a systematic review of randomized clinical trials. *Regional Anesthesia and Pain Medicine* **26**, 394–400.

99. **Broggi, G.** et al. (1990). Long-term results of percutaneous retrogasserian thermorhizotomy for essential trigeminal neuralgia—considerations in 1000 consecutive patients. *Neurosurgery* **26**, 783–7.

100. **Gocer, A.I.** et al. (1997). Fatal complication of the percutaneous radiofrequency trigeminal rhizotomy. *Acta Neurochirurgica (Wien)* **139**, 373–4.

101. **Higuchi, Y.** et al. (2002). Exposure of the dorsal root ganglion in rats to pulsed radiofrequency currents activates dorsal horn lamina I and II neurons. *Neurosurgery* **50**, 850–5.

102. **Munglani, R.** (1999). The longer term effect of pulsed radiofrequency for neuropathic pain. *Pain* **80**, 437–9.

103. **Conacher, I.D. Locke, T., and Hilton, C.** (1986). Neuralgia after cryoanalgesia for thoracotomy. *Lancet* **1**, 277.

104. **Kim, P.S. and Ferrante, F.M.** (1998). Cryoanalgesia: a novel treatment for hip adductor spasticity and obturator neuralgia. *Anesthesiology* **89**, 534–6.

105. **Baron, R., Levine, J.D., and Fields, H.L.** (1999). Causalgia and reflex sympathetic dystrophy: does the sympathetic nervous system contribute to the generation of pain? *Muscle & Nerve* **22**, 678–95.

106. **McLachlan, E.M.** et al. (1993). Peripheral nerve injury triggers noradrenergic sprouting within dorsal root ganglia. *Nature* **363**, 543–6.

107. **Siddall, P.J. and Cousins, M.J.** (1998). Introduction to pain mechanisms: implications for neural blockade. In *Neural Blockade in Clinical Anesthesia and Management of Pain* 3rd edn. (ed. M.J. Cousins and P.O. Bridenbaugh), pp. 675–99. Philadelphia: Lippincott-Raven.

108. **Breivik, H., Cousins, M.J., and Lofstrom, B.J.** (1998). Sympathetic neural blockade of upper and lower extremity. In *Neural Blockade in Clinical Anesthesia and Management of Pain* 3rd edn. (ed. M.J. Cousins and P.O. Bridenbaugh), pp. 411–45. Philadelphia: Lippincott-Raven.

109. **Eisenberg, E., Carr, D.B., and Chalmers, T.C.** (1995). Neurolytic celiac plexus block for treatment of cancer pain: a meta-analysis. *Anesthesia & Analgesia* **80**, 290–5.

110. **Alexander, J.P.** (1994). Chemical lumbar sympathectomy in patients with severe lower limb ischaemia. *Ulster Medical Journal* **63**, 137–43.

111. **Plancarte, R.** et al. (1997). Neurolytic superior hypogastric plexus block for chronic pelvic pain associated with cancer. *Regional Anesthesia* **22**, 562–8.

112. **Winnie, A.P. and Hartwell, P.W.** (1993). Relationship between time of treatment of acute herpes zoster with sympathetic blockade and prevention of post-herpetic neuralgia: clinical support for a new theory of the mechanism by which sympathetic blockade provides therapeutic benefit. *Regional Anesthesia* **18**, 277–82.

113. **Yanagida, H., Suwa, K., and Corssen, G.** (1987). No prophylactic effect of early sympathetic blockade on postherpetic neuralgia. *Anesthesiology* **66**, 73–6.

114. **Andren-Sandberg, A.** et al. (1999). Pain management of pancreatic cancer. *Annals of Oncology* **10** (Suppl. 4), 265–8.

115. **Mercadante, S. and Nicosia, F.** (1998). Celiac plexus block: a reappraisal. *Regional Anesthesia and Pain Medicine* **23**, 37–48.

116. **Mercadante, S.** (1993). Celiac plexus block versus analgesics in pancreatic cancer pain. *Pain* **52**, 187–92.

117. **Lillemoe, K.D.** et al. (1993). Chemical splanchnicectomy in patients with unresectable pancreatic cancer. A prospective randomized trial. *Annals of Surgery* **217**, 447–55.

118. **Staats, P.S.** et al. (2002). The effects of alcohol celiac plexus block, pain, and mood on longevity in patients with unresectable pancreatic cancer: a double-blinded, randomized, placebo-controlled study. *Pain Medicine* **2**, 28–34.

119. **Davies, D.D.** (1993). Incidence of major complications of neurolytic coeliac plexus block. *Journal of the Royal Society of Medicine* **86**, 264–6.

120. **Kaplan, R., Schiff-Keren, B., and Alt, E.** (1995). Aortic dissection as a complication of celiac plexus block. *Anesthesiology* **83**, 632–5.

121. **Tanelian, D. and Cousins, M.J.** (1989). Celiac plexus block following high-dose opiates for chronic noncancer pain in a four-year-old child. *Journal of Pain and Symptom Management* **4**, 82–5.

122. **Abedi, M. and Zfass, A.M.** (2001). Endoscopic ultrasound-guided (neurolytic) celiac plexus block. *Journal of Clinical Gastroenterology* **32**, 390–3.

123. **Rathmell, J.P., Gallant, J.M., and Brown, D.L.** (2000). Computed tomography and the anatomy of celiac plexus block. *Regional Anesthesia and Pain Medicine* **25**, 411–16.

124. **Moore, D.C.** (2001). Despite waffling and minimaxing, computed tomography is optimal when performing a neurolytic celiac plexus block. *Regional Anesthesia and Pain Medicine* **26**, 285–7.

125. **Wiersema, M.J., Wong, G.Y., and Croghan, G.A.** (2001). Endoscopic technique with ultrasound imaging for neurolytic celiac plexus block. *Regional Anesthesia and Pain Medicine* **26**, 159–63.

126. **Abdalla, E.K. and Schell, S.R.** (1999). Paraplegia following intraoperative celiac plexus injection. *Journal of Gastrointestinal Surgery* **3**, 668–71.

127. **Walsh, J.A.** et al. (1985). Blood flow, sympathetic activity and pain relief following lumbar sympathetic blockade or surgical sympathectomy. *Anaesthesia and Intensive Care* **13**, 18–24.

128. **Rocco, A.G.** (1995). Radiofrequency lumbar sympatholysis. The evolution of a technique for managing sympathetically maintained pain. *Regional Anesthesia* **20**, 3–12.

129. **Haynsworth, R.F., Jr. and Noe, C.E.** (1991). Percutaneous lumbar sympathectomy: a comparison of radiofrequency denervation versus phenol neurolysis. *Anesthesiology* **74**, 459–63.

130. **Wemm, K., Jr. and Saberski, L.** (1995). Modified approach to block the ganglion impar (ganglion of Walther). *Regional Anesthesia* **20**, 544–5.

131. **Simons, D.G., Travell, J.G., and Simons, L.S.** (1999). *Myofascial Pain and Dysfunction: The Trigger Point Manual.* Baltimore: Williams & Wilkins.

132. **Sola, A.E.** (1999). Upper extremity pain. In *Textbook of Pain* 4th edn. (ed. P.D. Wall and R. Melzack), pp. 559–78. Edinburgh: Churchill Livingstone.

133. **Mense, S.** (1993). Nociception from skeletal muscle in relation to clinical muscle pain. *Pain* **54**, 241–89.

134. **Aoki, K.R.** (2001). Pharmacology and immunology of botulinum toxin serotypes. *Journal of Neurology* **248** (Suppl. 1), 3–10.

135. **Wheeler, A.H., Goolkasian, P., and Gretz, S.S.** (2001). Botulinum toxin A for the treatment of chronic neck pain. *Pain* **94**, 255–60.
136. **Hesse, S.** et al. (2001). Botulinum toxin A treatment of adult upper and lower limb spasticity. *Drugs and Aging* **18**, 255–62.
137. **Gobel, H.** et al. (2001). Evidence-based medicine: botulinum toxin A in migraine and tension-type headache. *Journal of Neurology* **248** (Suppl. 1), 34–8.
138. **Foster, L.** et al. (2001). Botulinum toxin A and chronic low back pain: a randomized, double-blind study. *Neurology* **56**, 1290–3.
139. **Jankovic, J. and Brin, M.F.** (1991). Therapeutic uses of botulinum toxin. *New England Journal of Medicine* **324**, 1186–94.
140. **Reichel, G.** (2001). Botulinum toxin for treatment of spasticity in adults. *Journal of Neurology* **248** (Suppl. 1), 25–7.
141. **Porta, M.** (2000). A comparative trial of botulinum toxin type A and methyl-prednisolone for the treatment of myofascial pain syndrome and pain from chronic muscle spasm. *Pain* **85**, 101–5.
142. **Myers, D.P.** et al. (1993). Interpleural analgesia for the treatment of severe cancer pain in terminally ill patients. *Journal of Pain and Symptom Management* **8**, 505–10.
143. **Reiestad, F.** et al. (1989). Successful treatment of chronic-pancreatitis pain with interpleural analgesia. *Canadian Journal of Anaesthesia—Journal Canadien D Anesthesie* **36**, 713–16.
144. **Reiestad, F.** et al. (1990). Interpleural analgesia in the treatment of severe thoracic postherpetic neuralgia. *Regional Anesthesia* **15**, 113–17.
145. **Amesbury, B., O'Riordan, J., and Dolin, S.** (1999). The use of interpleural analgesia using bupivacaine for pain relief in advanced cancer. *Palliative Medicine* **13**, 153–8.
146. **Harrison, P., Kent, E.A., and Lema, M.J.** (1993). Interpleural analgesia: its use, and a complication, in a quadriplegic patient with chronic benign pain. *Journal of Pain and Symptom Management* **8**, 238–41.
147. **Rowbotham, M.C.** et al. (1996). Lidocaine patch: double-blind controlled study of a new treatment method for post-herpetic neuralgia. *Pain* **65**, 39–44.
148. **Epstein, J.B.** et al. (2001). Oral topical doxepin rinse: analgesic effect in patients with oral mucosal pain due to cancer or cancer therapy. *Oral Oncology* **37**, 632–7.
149. **Krajnik, M.** et al. (1999). Potential uses of topical opioids in palliative care—report of 6 cases. *Pain* **80**, 121–5.
150. **Twillman, R.K.** et al. (1999). Treatment of painful skin ulcers with topical opioids. *Journal of Pain and Symptom Management* **17**, 288–92.
151. **Stein, C.** (1995). The control of pain in peripheral tissue by opioids. *New England Journal of Medicine* **332**, 1685–90.
152. **Liebeskind, J.C.** (1991). Pain can kill. *Pain* **44**, 3–4.
153. **Page, G.G., Blakely, W.P., and Ben Eliyahu, S.** (2001). Evidence that postoperative pain is a mediator of the tumor-promoting effects of surgery in rats. *Pain* **90**, 191–9.
154. **Logan, H.L.** et al. (2001). Pain and immunologic response to root canal treatment and subsequent health outcomes. *Psychosomatic Medicine* **63**, 453–62.
155. **Page, G.G.** (2002). Analgesia administration attenuates surgery-induced tumor promotion. *Regional Anesthesia and Pain Medicine* **27**, 197–9.
156. **Kiecolt-Glaser, J.K.** et al. (2002). Emotions, morbidity, and mortality: new perspectives from psychoneuroimmunology. *Annual Review of Psychology* **53**, 83–107.
157. **Roy, S. and Loh, H.H.** (1996). Effects of opioids on the immune system. *Neurochemical Research* **21**, 1375–86.
158. **Hamra, J.G. and Yaksh, T.L.** (1996). Equianalgesic doses of subcutaneous but not intrathecal morphine alter phenotypic expression of cell surface markers and mitogen-induced proliferation in rat lymphocytes. *Anesthesiology* **85**, 355–65.
159. **Smith, T.J.** et al. (2002). Randomized clinical trial of an implantable drug delivery system compared to comprehensive medical management for refractory cancer pain: impact on pain, drug related toxicity and survival. *Journal of Clinical Oncology* **20**, 4040–9.
160. **Kocsis, J. and Devor, M.** (2000). Altered excitability of large-diameter cutaneous afferents following nerve injury: consequences for chronic pain. In *Proceedings of the 9th World Congress on Pain* (ed. M. Devor, M.C. Rowbotham, and Z. Wiesenfeld-Hallin), pp. 119–35. Seattle: IASP Press.
161. **Boucher, T.J.** et al. (2000). Potent analgesic effects of GDNF in neuropathic pain states. *Science* **290**, 124–7.
162. **White, D.M.** (2000). Neurotrophin-3 antisense oligonucleotide attenuates nerve injury-induced Abeta-fibre sprouting. *Brain Research* **885**, 79–86.
163. **Eisenach, J.C., Hood, D.D., and Curry, R.** (2002). Preliminary efficacy assessment of intrathecal injection of an American formulation of adenosine in humans. *Anesthesiology* **96**, 29–34.
164. **Belfrage, M.** et al. (1999). The safety and efficacy of intrathecal adenosine in patients with chronic neuropathic pain. *Anesthesia & Analgesia* **89**, 136–42.
165. **Dirks, J.** et al. (2001). Effect of systemic adenosine on pain and secondary hyperalgesia associated with the heat/capsaicin sensitization model in healthy volunteers. *Regional Anesthesia and Pain Medicine* **26**, 414–19.
166. **Gyllenhammar, E. and Nordfors, L.O.** (2001). Systemic adenosine infusions alleviated neuropathic pain. *Pain* **94**, 121–2.
167. **Eisenach, J.C., Hood, D.D., and Curry, R.** (2002). Phase I safety assessment of intrathecal injection of an American formulation of adenosine in humans. *Anesthesiology* **96**, 24–8.
168. **Foran, S.E.** et al. (2000). A substance P-opioid chimeric peptide as a unique nontolerance-forming analgesic. *Proceedings of the National Academy of Sciences of the United States of America* **97**, 7621–6.
169. **Foran, S.E.** et al. (2000). Inhibition of morphine tolerance development by a substance P-opioid peptide chimera. *Journal of Pharmacology and Experimental Therapeutics* **295**, 1142–8.
170. **Penn, R.D. and Paice, J.A.** (2000). Adverse effects associated with the intrathecal administration of ziconotide. *Pain* **85**, 291–6.

8.2.7 Neurosurgical approaches in palliative medicine

Samuel J. Hassenbusch and Nathan I. Cherny

It is estimated that 10 per cent or more of cancer patients do not receive adequate relief with pharmacological treatment options, often troubled by dose-limiting side-effects such as nausea or cognitive dysfunction.[1] The relative roles of ablative and augmentative procedures are still unclear in neurosurgical pain management (Fig. 1). Many of the ablative procedures have been available for 40–50 years yet, in many situations, have been replaced by newer augmentative procedures over the past 10 years.

Pain relief from ablative procedures may be of a shorter duration than that resulting from augmentative techniques (e.g. stimulation or spinal infusion), and may be accompanied by deafferentation pain.[2] As with long-term spinal infusions of morphine, it remains unclear whether delayed recurrence of pain represents extension of the underlying tumour to new anatomic areas or late failure of the procedure.[3,4] More recently, however, older techniques for intracranial ablative procedures have been updated. With the use of improved stereotactic equipment and guidance by computerized tomography (CT) and magnetic resonance imaging (MR), the accuracy of intracranial procedures has been improved and the need for ventriculography largely eliminated. The procedures can be performed under local anaesthesia, perhaps with intravenous sedation, and require only a twist drill hole, rather than a burr hole or a craniotomy.

Patients generally must have severe pain that is not relieved adequately by systemic medications or simple neurolytic procedures. Though some of the procedures, such as thalamotomy and cingulotomy often have been used for pain of non-cancer causes, these operations are most beneficial for cancer patients. In addition to logistical issues, choice of a specific operation also needs to take into consideration the type of pain, severity, location, and the primary cause of the painful sensation.

Consideration of invasive approaches requires a word of caution. Interpretation of data regarding the use of alternative analgesic approaches

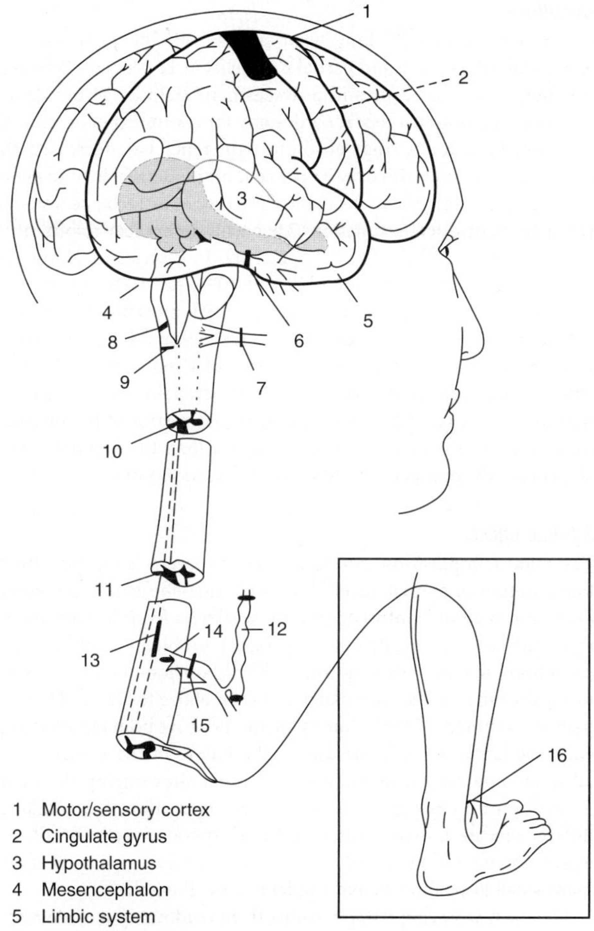

Fig. 1 Overview of anatomic sites for pain procedures in the central nervous system. (*From:* Raj, P.P. *Practical Management of Pain*. St Louis MO: Mosby, Inc., 2000, p. 793.)

and extrapolation to the presenting clinical problem require care. The literature is characterized by the lack of uniformity in patient selection, inadequate reporting of previous analgesic therapies, inconsistencies in outcome evaluation and paucity of long-term follow-up. Furthermore, reported outcomes in the literature may not predict the outcomes of a procedure performed on a medically ill patient by a physician who has more limited experience with the techniques involved.

When indicated, the use of invasive and neurodestructive procedures should be based on an evaluation of the likelihood and duration of analgesic benefit, the immediate and long-term risks, the likely duration of survival, the availability of local expertise, and the anticipated length of hospitalization.

For most pain syndromes, there exists a range of techniques that may theoretically be applied. In choosing between a range of procedures the following principles are salient:[5]

1. Ablative procedures are deferred as long as pain relief is obtainable by non-ablative modalities.
2. The procedure most likely to be effective should be selected. If there is a choice, however, the one with the fewest and least serious adverse effects is preferred.
3. In progressive stages of cancer, pain is likely to be multifocal and a procedure aimed at a single locus of pain, even if completed flawlessly, is unlikely to yield complete relief of pain until death. A realistic and sound goal is a lasting decrease in pain to a level that is manageable by pharmacotherapy with minimal side-effects.
4. Since there is a learning curve with all of the procedures, performance by a physician who is experienced in the specific intervention may improve the likelihood of a successful outcome.

Techniques

Though neurosurgical approaches to lesion placement are fairly standardized, the requisite tools have changed as technology has progressed. Ablative procedures using open surgical techniques or techniques guided by air or contrast ventriculography have been superceded by closed operations using stereotaxis under ventriculogram, CT, or MRI guidance. These newer approaches also increase the surgeon's ability to correct for individual patient variation in anatomy.[6] For example, using MRI, the actual trajectory for the electrode placement can be planned in relation to other brain structures.

Since no method is entirely exact, a variety of intraoperative procedures are often used to confirm lesion placement.[7] Such techniques include the use of intraoperative testing of the area without causing permanent damage; low-frequency stimulation that aids determination of the function of the region surrounding the target; and single-unit microelectrode recording to ensure preservation of critical structures in the area.[7]

Radiosurgery, for example, using the Gamma Knife, is increasingly employed to create ablative lesions for treatment of chronic pain.[8,9] Targets in the thalamus and the anterior limb of the internal capsule have been frequently reported.[8,10,11] The radiosurgical technique for these pain-relieving lesions uses a similar technique to that for focused radiation (radiosurgery) of a brain tumour. Although radiosurgery is non-invasive to the brain, it remains unclear to what extent the lesions become smaller over time and thus what degree of pain relief can be expected at various time points after the radiation exposure.

Description of specific procedures

The following procedures either are currently being practised or, based upon past reports, offer significant efficacy of relief with minimal morbidity. As seen from the descriptions that follow, some of these procedures treat specific pain areas such as the head or legs while others treat more generalized areas of pain. The various approaches have been divided into ablative and augmentative techniques and listed within each group beginning with the most commonly used technique first.

Ablative procedures

Cordotomy

Anatomy

The aim of the operation is to disrupt the spinothalamic tract just below where it enters the medulla. However, the mechanism of action for this procedure has been suggested to affect more than just C-fibres because pain relief coincides with a lessened sensation of pinching skin and temperature cooling.[12]

Indication

Cordotomy is most effective for unilateral pain that does not approach the midline.[13,14] Greatest experience has been reported with pain in the pelvis and lower limbs.[13,14] Substantial analgesia has also been reported with unilateral chest and upper limb pain.[13,15]

Technique

In the percutaneous method, X-ray fluoroscopy is used to position a radiofrequency electrode needle at the level of the C1–2 interspace in the lateral spinothalamic tract as determined by the area of pain[16] (Fig. 2(a) and (b)). CT guidance allows for better visualization and more accurate insertion of the electrodes into the spine.[15] A cordotomy needle puncture is made in the side of the neck contralateral to the site of pain with the aid of a questioning stimulation in which the patient is asked about sensory changes and twitching. The open surgical technique for cordotomy is similar to the percutaneous method except that it is often carried out with the patient seated in an upright position. In this procedure, the anterolateral surface of the spinal cord is viewed and an avascular area is found for the incision. The blade projects 6 mm through the cervical area and 4–5 mm in the thoracic area, and then cuts ventrally in order to transect the ventral quadrant but spare the medial funiculus. The open operation is not generally preferred because of the greater risks it entails in comparison with the percutaneous procedure.

A patient's case must be exactly suited to the procedure in order for pain relief to be successfully achieved. Proper preoperative respiratory/pulmonary function is critical because mortality is almost always related to respiratory problems.

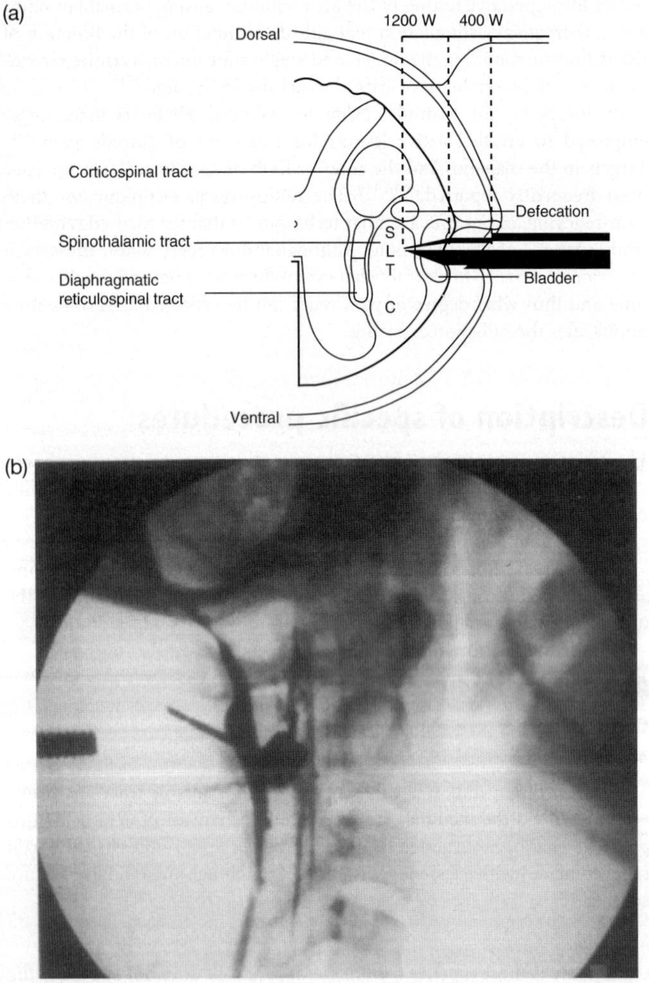

Fig. 2 (a) Drawing of placement of electrode in the posterolateral section of the spinothalamic tract for percutaneous cordotomy using CT-guidance. (b) Lateral cervical spine X-ray fluoroscopy showing positioning of the cordotomy electrode anterior to the dentate ligament, which is outlined with injected contrast. (*From:* North, R.B. and Levy, R.M. *Neurosurgical Management of Pain*. New York: Springer-Verlag, 1997, p. 206(a), 203(b).)

Outcomes

In one large series,[14] long-term success with no pain was found in 33 per cent of patients, and partial pain relief in 12 per cent. Persistent pain was noted in 6 per cent and a dysaesthetic pain in 34 per cent, while 2.6 per cent required a repeat cordotomy for continued pain relief. Others, however, have found that absolute pain relief has decreased through post-operative time with only 37 per cent having satisfactory analgesia after 5–10 years.[17] Complications in the Tasker series included persistent paresis (2 per cent), bladder dysfunction (2 per cent), temporary respiratory failure (0.5 per cent), and death (0.5 per cent). In a series of 273 patients in Brisbane[13] treated between 1979 and 1991, satisfactory pain relief was achieved in 89 per cent of patients. First-week mortality was 3.3 per cent. Both of the two long-term survivors (8 and 5 years) have remained free of their original pain. In Nagaro et al.'s series of 45 patients,[18] 73 per cent of patients undergoing cordotomy developed new pains. The majority of these were mirror pains and a small minority was rostral to the original pain. In most cases, the new pain was less severe than the original pain and in 20 per cent the new pain resolved over weeks to months.

Adverse effects

The main complication during and after surgery is the possible loss of the sensation of temperature.[19] Possible side-effects of the percutaneous operation include contralateral limb weakness from lesioning too deep, transient Horner's syndrome, respiratory problems, and burning post-cordotomy dysaesthetic syndromes.[12,13] Post-lesional dysaesthesias and new pain either in the contralateral limb or above the level of the previous pain are common.[18,20,21] Some patients also have been reported to experience low levels of analgesia due to the failure of the surgery or lack of adequate anatomical localization of target sites during the operation. A small group has experienced new pain formation in a similar and/or different location, while others did not experience relief at all. In other words, the operation is fairly successful in achieving pain relief although many small impediments may hinder success along the way.

The most worrying complications from cordotomy include respiratory dysfunction and sleep apnoea. Respiratory dysfunction is the most significant complication from high percutaneous cervical cordotomy. High cervical cordotomy may result in disruption of the reticulospinal tract and lead to significant pulmonary compromise. Patients undergoing high unilateral percutaneous cordotomy are at risk for respiratory decompensation with concomitant pulmonary disease contralateral to the side of the cordotomy. Pre-operative pulmonary function tests are useful in predicting which of these patients may be affected. Lung disease per se is not a contraindication; indeed cordotomy has been successfully achieved in many patients with mesothelioma.[13,15,22]

Bilateral high cervical cordotomy has a higher risk of causing respiratory decompensation than the unilateral procedure and is associated with an additional risk of sleep apnoea. While forced vital capacity and maximum expiratory flow rate were not adversely affected following unilateral high percutaneous cordotomy, both values were significantly reduced following the bilateral procedure. Sleep apnoea has been reported in 0–18 per cent of cases following bilateral cordotomy. Patients appear to have normal respirations while awake because they maintain voluntary control which is mediated by the intact corticospinal tracts. Bilateral reticulospinal tract lesions cause a loss of autonomic respiratory drive when the patient falls asleep. Additionally, these lesions may result in a decreased response to hypercarbia as a stimulus to breathe. This scenario leads to sleep apnoea, or 'Ondine's curse'. Sleep apnoea generally develops within 5 days of the procedure but may occur at any time, often without warning. This condition is often self-limiting but patients may require interim ventilatory support. There is a high mortality from unrecognized sleep apnoea.

Other less severe adverse outcomes include hemiparesis or ataxia due to involvement of the corticospinal tracts. This is usually a transient finding occurring in 5–31 per cent of cases, but decreasing to less than 3 per cent long-term following both unilateral and bilateral cordotomy. While pre-existing bladder dysfunction may worsen following unilateral cordotomy; it is very common after bilateral cordotomy such that many patients require permanent catheterization.

Midline myelotomy

Anatomy

Myelotomy involves section of midline fibres posterior to the central canal of the spinal cord. The lesions are usually created at the lower thoracic spinal cord level although Gildenberg and others also have reported lesions at C1.[23] The procedure can be performed with mechanical ablation, radiofrequency techniques, or carbon dioxide laser.[24]

A commissural myelotomy on the spinal cord aims to interrupt all decussating second-order spinothalamic fibres that are contributing to pain perception on both sides of the body through the posterior commissure of the spinal cord. Two methods are presently available for patients: open and closed. The open operation requires an incision in the spinal cord down the exact midline between the two gracilis tracts and then continued ventrally until the posterior half of the cord is completely divided (Fig. 3). This transection disconnects the two sides of the posterior half of the spinal cord so that they are now independent of each other and can no longer communicate dorsally. The closed operation involves placement of a radiofrequency electrode between the two gracilis tracts using CT guidance.

Neurophysiology

There is evidence for a tract in the anterior part of the medial borders of the posterior columns mediating both pelvic and more proximal epigastric visceral pain.[25–27] Research conducted with laboratory animals has shown that lesions in the dorsal column reduce responses to noxious colorectal pain stimulation by 60–80 per cent, compared with the 20 per cent reduction that results from lesioning the ventral posterolateral nucleus of the thalamus.[28,29] Orthograde and retrograde tracers have shown the presence of a post-synaptic pathway (separate from the spinothalamic tract) that ascends in the gray matter around the central canal to the nucleus gracilis.[30] From there, nociceptive stimuli are relayed to the ventral posterolateral nucleus of the thalamus using the medial lemniscus.[30]

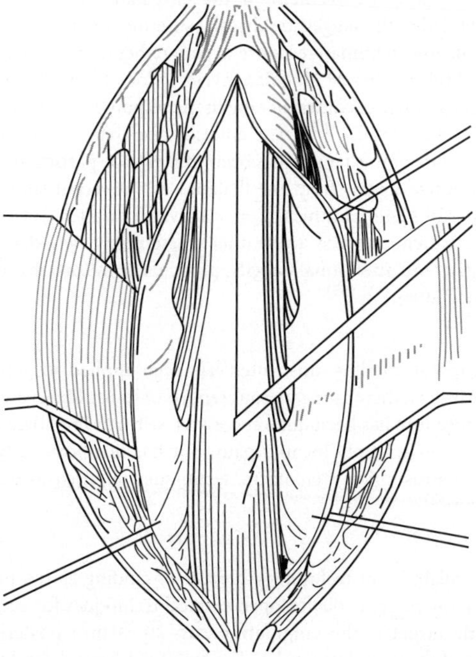

Fig. 3 Illustration of open exposure of posterior thoracic spinal cord and incision to create a plane between posterior columns down to the level of the central canal. Area of typical pain relief is shown. (*From:* Bonica, J.J., ed. *The Management of Pain*. Philadelphia: Lea & Febiger, 1990, p. 2074).

Indications

This procedure is particularly effective for visceral lower body pain in cancer patients where other procedures are inapplicable or unsuccessful.

Outcomes

Overall the experience with this technique is limited. The percentage of patients reporting moderate-to-marked pain relief has been approximately 70 per cent with only rare complications or side-effects noted. A study of cancer patients with visceral pain has confirmed that punctate midline myelotomy of the mid-thoracic spinal cord can reduce visceral pain and use of opioids without changes in sensation or motor function.[30] In general, analgesia from hyperpathia and background pain has been obtained without sensory loss but with preserved ability to localize and discriminate between sharp and dull stimuli.[23,31]

Hypophysectomy

Neurophysiology

The mechanism by which lesions of the pituitary gland bring pain relief is unclear, although it is generally agreed that neither the limbic system nor areas controlling affective responses are manipulated. A postulated hormonal mechanism involves changes in a humoural substance in the cerebrospinal fluid or hormonal changes via a direct neural mechanism.[32] Contrary to this proposal, it has been noted that pain relief occurs almost immediately without any regard for tumour regression. Relief can also occur in the thalamic pain regions and hormonally unresponsive tumours on a scale that could not be inferred given the degree of pituitary ablation experienced.[32–42] Still, very small amounts of tumour regression cannot be discounted.[33]

Modalities used to perform a hypophysectomy lend credence to the hypothalamic mechanism theory. A possible relation to the pain relief properties of the posteromedial hypothalamus can be observed, although the morphological effects of hypophysectomy, regardless of the technique used to create the lesions, centre in the anterior hypothalamus, specifically in the supraoptic and paraventricular nuclei.[43,44] Information suggesting the particularly strong impact that pituitary ablations have on the paraventricular nucleus coupled with knowledge of anatomical connections between this area and antinociceptive regions of the brain suggests the role of endogenous neurotransmitters. It has been observed, however, that naloxone does not reverse pain relief as it does with opioid-based relief. Although plasma concentrations of beta-endorphin were elevated in one study, no changes have been found in cerebrospinal fluid concentrations of metenkephalin or beta-endorphin.

Techniques

Techniques for open surgery on the area include the transcranial hypophysectomy and the open microsurgical hypophysectomy.[32] As technology has improved stereotactic methods, percutaneous stereotactic lesions are being created using alcohol, radiofrequency thermal techniques, cryotherapy, or interstitial placement of radioactive seeds.[36,45,46] The success of focused radiation therapy (e.g. Gamma Knife) on pituitary tumours has led to the use of this non-invasive modality to create similar lesions for pain relief.[10]

Of the various techniques for hypophysectomy, stereotactic instillation of alcohol into the pituitary gland is one of the best-described and most common techniques at this time. Alcohol has been shown to pass to the floor of the third ventricle, hypophyseal portal vessels, and the hypothalamus.[44] The use of stereotaxy for chemical hypophysectomy enables an injection of alcohol volumes between 1 and 5 ml. Better results have been achieved using alcohol volumes extending to the upper volumes of this range that are clearly greater than the volume of the sella.[44]

Indications

Hypophysectomy is occasionally considered for patients with severe cancer pain from diffuse areas of involvement from tumours such as metastatic breast or prostate carcinoma, regardless of receptor status. It can also be effective for other hormonally unresponsive tumours.[44]

Outcomes

In two different series of more than 100 patients each, chemical hypophysectomy appeared to provide significant pain relief. Excellent pain relief was reported in 45–65 per cent of all patients and 75–85 per cent of patients ceased using opioids. The mean post-operative survival time was 5 months, while the mean length of pain relief appeared to be 3 months. This length of pain relief was accomplished with one additional alcohol injection in 25–30 per cent of patients and with two additional injections in another 3–9 per cent.[44,47,48] Of the patients treated with alcohol injections, those suffering from breast or prostate carcinoma (50–75 per cent of patients) appeared to have slightly better pain relief than those with other types of tumours.[44] Approximately 25 per cent of patients had at least one significant exacerbation of pain after the procedure while one-third of these patients had more than one exacerbation.[44]

Adverse effects

Common complications included hormonal deficiency, such as diabetes insipidus, in 5–20 per cent of patients, cerebrospinal fluid leak in 1–10 per cent of patients, and ocular nerve palsy or temporal field visual loss in 2–10 per cent of patients.[44] Most of these changes were temporary. Other problems associated with the procedure on a far less frequent basis were meningitis in 0.5–1 per cent of patients, hypothalamic changes, headaches, and carotid artery damage in approximately 0.5 per cent of patients.[44] Despite a reported 2–5 per cent mortality rate, it seems likely that these numbers have been significantly lowered with the adoption of newer percutaneous and stereotactic methods.[10,44]

Thalamotomy

Neurophysiology

The thalamus is the termination site of the spinothalamic tract (lateral nucleus and central lateral nucleus of the medial thalamus), the pathway responsible for transmitting information about pain and temperature from the body to higher areas in the brain.[9] The lateral thalamus seems to be principally involved with sensory discrimination aspects of pain, while the medial thalamic nuclei are more involved in affective responses.[9] Using the effectiveness of pallidal lesions as corroborating evidence, investigators reasoned that lesions of their thalamic projections in the ventrolateral nucleus of the thalamus would also be effective.[49]

Indications

Thalamotomy is generally considered for intermittent shooting and hyperpathic or allodynic pain and not considered very effective for steady, burning or dysaesthetic components of central or deafferentation pain.[49] Despite its development for non-cancer pain, thalamotomy can be highly effective for and has been reported in the treatment of neuropathic cancer pain.[11,49,50] Advances in human stereotaxic procedures have led to resurgence in use of the thalamotomy.

Anatomy

Various thalamic sites have been targeted; these include the basal thalamus, medial thalamus, and dorsomedian thalamus affecting extralemniscal fibres, and thalamic projections terminating in the intralaminar nucleus, centromedianum nucleus, and the frontal lobe.[11,50] One of the most effective sites appears to be the inferior posteromedial thalamus, containing the intralaminar, centromedianum, and parafascicularis nuclei, all of which might affect the paleospinothalamic tract.[51] More recent literature has proposed that the medial thalamus is related to the spinoreticular tract, the descending pathway responsible for conducting impulses to many of the motor neurons.[9] Ablations of the lateral thalamus, particularly the ventrocaudal parvocellular nucleus, attempt to destroy the pain-receiving nucleus itself. Some authors have suggested that combination lesions, such as centromedianum and parafasicularis lesions with dorsomedial nucleus or the thalamic pulvinar lesions, might provide better long-term results.[51]

Techniques

Currently, a thalamotomy includes the use of stereotactic methods, frame imaging, referencing, target location(s) selection, and careful introduction of the probe so that sensitive motor structures remain intact.[49] These operative steps are followed by physiological testing to confirm the site.[49] The interactive nature of these tests requires the use of local anaesthesia to ensure patient cooperation. The testing site according to Tasker[49] should be approximately in the 15-mm sagittal plane or the tactile representation of the contralateral manual digits.

Outcomes

Both medial and lateral lesions of the thalamus are moderately effective (approximately 60 per cent pain relief) in dealing with cancer pain, but lateral thalamotomy carries with it higher rates of complication, nearly 32 per cent.[9] In treatment of nociceptive pain, thalamotomy has been reported to produce transient loss of all contralateral sensory modalities after the operation and also pseudoparesis in many of the cases studied by Tasker. The patients seemed to lose the appreciation of position and vibration sense due to the lesions in the ventrocaudal nucleus.[49] Pain relief is often unsustained and pain often recurs after 6–12 months.

Complications

Complications with these approaches are common;[9] they include paresis, cognitive disorders, infection and mortality (although rare in nociceptive pain cases), seizures and speech disturbance. Though lesions do not seem to affect cognitive ability, studies have shown that left-sided lesions affect language and the dominance of the right ear in listening exercises (right ear advantage).[9] Due to this limitted efficacy and the significant risks, some authorities have suggested that thalamic intraoperative testing stimulation should be carried out before considering the creation of a lesion.[49]

Cingulotomy

Neuroanatomy

This approach involves bilateral lesioning of a central white matter pathway that connects the frontal lobes with limbic structures, which modulate emotionality. Although its exact role in pain transmission is unclear, the anterior cingulate cortex incorporates motor, affective, memory and nociceptive functions, accounting for the various pathways connecting this area with the basal ganglia, frontal sub-sytems, and lateral frontal and parietal regions.[52,53] The involvement of the cingulate gyrus in emotional processes has led to the suggestion that the anterior cingulate cortex is most notable for its role in human response to pain rather than sensitivity to pain stimuli.[53] Still, studies of cingulate gyrus lesions in laboratory animals have shown a reduction contralaterally in the response to pain, particularly noxious thermal stimuli.[52,54] The anterior cingulate cortex, particularly the posterior side of this region, has been shown to be particularly responsive to nociceptive signals from the thalamus.[54] A recent study indicates that the anterior section of this region is activated by attention-demanding tasks. Some patients studied a year after cingulotomy were determined to have executive and attentional deficits, particularly in the areas of focused and sustained attention.[53]

Indications

While a cingulotomy has most often has been applied to patients with affective disorders, there are numerous reports of its use for severe pain control. The procedure has been quite successful with cancer patients suffering from diffuse or multiply located pain, but has not been fully adopted because of neurosurgical stereotactic techniques required to perform the operation.[52,55]

Techniques

With the availability of technology capable of guiding closed procedures, there is not any present role for open surgical techniques for cingulotomy. The specific target is the cingulate gyrus, 20–30 mm posterior to the anterior tip of the lateral ventricles. The target is 1.5 mm lateral to midline and 15 mm superior to the roof of the lateral ventricles.[56] (Fig. 4(a)). The radiofrequency method is used more commonly, with each lesion being created at 75°C for 60–90 s. The result is a cylindrical lesion approximately 10–20 mm long and 5–7 mm in diameter, centred in each cingulate gyrus (Fig. 4(b)).

(a)
(b)

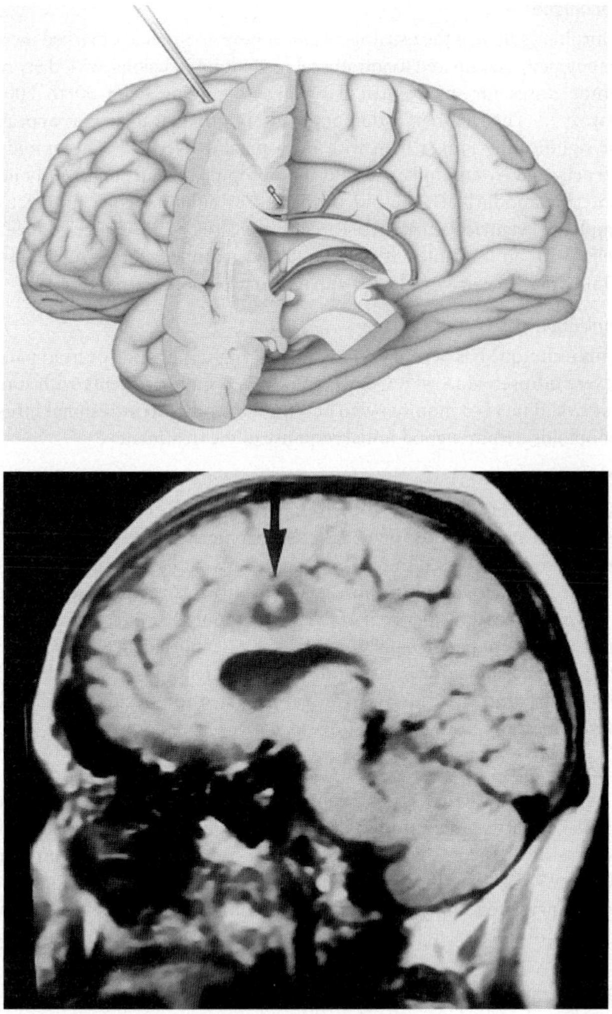

Fig. 4 (a) Placement of cingulotomy electrode through cortex so that the exposed electrode is located in the left cingulate gyrus near the distal portion of the anterior cerebral arteries (closed arrow) and lateral ventricles (open arrow). (b) Post-cingulotomy MRI (sagittal view) showing resultant cylindrical lesion in the cingulate gyrus (arrow). (*From:* Arbit, E., ed. *Management of Cancer-Related Pain.* Mount Kisco NY: Futura Publishing Company, Inc., 1993, p. 303.)

Outcomes

In the many reports of patients undergoing cingulotomy, as many as 30 per cent of these patients were treated for severe chronic pain. Approximately 51 per cent of these patients who were treated with intractable cancer pain had moderate, marked, or complete pain relief that lasted at least 3 months after the procedure. Like many ablative procedures, cingulotomy is more effective for patients with a shorter survival time.[55,57]

Complications

The main complications resulting from cingulotomy using old ventriculogram-guided techniques included controllable seizures (9 per cent incidence), transient mania (6 per cent incidence), decreased memory (3 per cent incidence), hemiplegia from intracerebral haematoma (0.3 per cent incidence), and a low, but measurable mortality rate (0.9 per cent).[56] In neuropsychiatric examination, some patients demonstarted difficulties in copying complex figures, performing two tapping tests, and successfully completing memory components of an organized serial learning test.[53] Present evidence suggests that changes in attention due to cingulate gyrus lesions do not significantly affect daily functioning and social behaviour for patients with severe cancer pain.

Trigeminal tractotomy

Neuroanatomy

The discovery that lesions in the descending trigeminal tract affected pain and temperature without diminishing touch sensation led to the study of this area and the adjacent nucleate caudalis as a target site for the ablative treatment of trigeminal neuralgia. The caudalis nucleate lies on the surface of the medulla posterior to the dorsal spinocerebellar tract, lateral to the fasciculus cuneatus, and inferior to the restiform body. It appears to act as a relay station for pain and temperature transmission from cranial nerves II, V, IX, and X so that destruction of its oral pole decreases neuron hyperexcitability and severs the ascending multisynaptic pathways for pain.[58]

Indications

Trigeminal tractotomy can be used for treatment of patients with unilateral head and neck cancer and with intractable pain in the distribution of the trigeminal nerve. Newer research indicates that, because the trigeminal, glossopharyngeal, and vagal nerves all meet at the spinobulbar juncture, ablative therapy in this region can also be used to treat vagoglossopharyngeal and geniculate neuralgias.

Techniques

Both percutaneous and open surgical techniques have been described for this operation. A percutaneous technique has been reported with needle penetration at the C1-foramen magnum area under stereotactic guidance.[59] Use of CT technology in particular allows direct visualization of the target and generates measurements of the spinal cord that are patient-specific.[60] An electrode with a 0.5–0.6 mm diameter is angled 30° cephalad and placed in the spinal cord, 6 mm lateral to the midline, to a depth of 4 mm. Under local anaesthesia, electrical stimulation at 50 Hz should provide facial response to low voltage. Stimulation will be felt in contralateral body areas via the spinothalamic tract if placement is too ventral, while placement that is too dorsal will be felt in ipsilateral areas via the fasciulus cuneatus.

When using an open approach, extension of the lesion to include part of both the spinothalamic tract and the fasciculus is recommended for mouth coverage. The open tractotomy is often combined with other nerve and/or root sections in the same area.

Results

Limited published reports of the results of this procedure, either with open or percutaneous techniques, suggest that about 75–85 per cent of patients with head and neck cancer have good pain relief.[61] Post-operative sensory changes in the area of the pain accompanied by limited relief have been documented as well. Duration of efficacy appears to be months rather than years after the procedure.

Complications

In some cases, pain associated with the percutaneous operation may result in termination of the procedure before completion. Temporary complications consist of changes in ipsilateral arm coordination, contralateral leg sensation, and ipsilateral arm (rarely leg) proprioception. Less frequent complications include Horner's syndrome, dysarthria, gait changes, and hiccoughs.

Mesencephalotomy (mesencephalic tractotomy)

Neurophysiology

Mesencephalic tractotomy aims to disrupt the mesencephalic spinothalamic tract (STT) and the spinoreticular tract (SRT).[9] By disrupting the junction of the STT and the SRT, the lesions on the mesencephalon disrupt two nociceptive pathways.[9]

Indication

Stereotactic mesencephalic tractotomy is an option in the management of cancer pain of the contralateral face, neck, or shoulder.

Technique

After fixing a stereotactic base ring to the patient's head, a localizer is fixed to the base ring and a series of MRI scan images is obtained. These images are exported to a computer workstation which is used to derive the stereotactic target coordinates and probe trajectory. The patient is then taken to the operating room. Under local anaesthesia, a frontal burr hole is created, and a stereotactic aiming arc is fixed to the base ring and used to guide a stimulating/lesioning probe to the mesencephalic lateral spinothalamic tract. Proper probe position is verified by stimulation. This usually produces a warm or cool sensation on the opposite side of the body. A radiofrequency lesion is then created which should produce contralateral thermanalgesia.

Outcomes

Mesencephalic tractotomy has been reported to provide significant pain relief in greater than 80 per cent of cancer patients on both short- and long-term (2–4 years) follow-ups.[9] The longest duration of pain relief in cancer patients is in the extremities while pain in the chest and abdomen do not respond adequately.[62] Pain relief usually lasts for at least 6 months.

Complications

The major side-effect appears to be difficulties with ocular movement and binocular vision with mortality rates varying from 1 to 7 per cent.[62–64] Post-operative dysaesthesia has been reported in studies of the medial lemniscus after large mesencephalic lesions in all different types of patients.[64]

Pulvinotomy

General

Pulvinotomy appears to be ideally suited to the treatment of intractable cancer pain whose symptoms are similar to those indicated for cingulotomy, particularly in patients with survival times up to 18 months.[65]

Neuroanatomy

Although the precise mechanisms for pain relief have not yet been ascertained, research indicates that the oral and medial parts of the pulvinar are involved in pain appreciation.[66] Electrophysiologic studies in cats have demonstrated that the pulvinar is involved in an indirect route for afferent stimuli.[67] From the pulvinar, afferent transmission connections have been traced to the temporal lobe and, from there, to the posterior sensory cortex.[68]

Technique

Pulvinar ablation is generally achieved using CT- or MRI-guided stereotaxis and radiofrequency ablation. Typically, lesion placement is in the medial area or in both the medial and lateral areas of pulvinar. Bilateral pulvinar ablation is more effective than ablation of the contralateral pulvinar alone.[65,69]

Results

Moderate to excellent pain relief has been reported in as many as 25 per cent of patients for periods ranging from 1 to 2.5 years.[68,70] When the lesions are extended backward to involve the pulvinar, the lesions, especially in the anterior pulvinar, have been found to be more effective than the centrum medianum thalamotomy.[68] Pre-existing pain is most affected by this operation and there is no reported loss of somatic sensation after the procedure.[51]

Complications

Analysis of patients after pulvinotomy has shown no apparent change in cognitive functions, although temporary changes in behaviour, such as tendencies towards childishness, excessive excitability, and euphoria, have all been observed.[70,71]

Augmentative procedures

Intraventricular infusion of opioid

The intraventricular infusion of opioids is one of the best-known intracranial augmentative procedures. It is normally among the last resort options for a patient's treatment.

Technique

Morphine sulfate is the usual agent and appears to provide a marked increase in potency as compared to intrathecal or epidural infusions, with daily morphine doses for intraventricular delivery ranging from 50 to 700 μg/day.[72–75] The length of action of the intraventricular injections appears to be significantly longer than with intraspinal delivery.[76] The opioid can be delivered by an implanted infusion pump placed subcutaneously in the anterior abdominal wall and connected by subcutaneous tubing to an implanted ventricular catheter. Patients may also be able to receive adequate relief with an implanted ventricular catheter connected to a subcutaneous Ommaya reservoir-type device with one to two injections per day.[77]

Indication

This technique has been used for patients with upper body or head pain, or severe diffuse pain.[72,74] Occasionally, it is used for patients with limited survival time (1–3 months) who develop a tolerance to intraspinal infusion of opioids despite a good initial response to the treatment.

Results

Karavelis et al.[72] reported their experience with 90 patients. All were started on an initial dose of 0.25 mg of morphine sulfate per 24 h which was progressively increased in 0.25-mg increments until optimal analgesia was attained. A daily morphine dose of up to 1 mg was adequate to achieve an analgesic effect in 77 per cent of the patients; only 10 per cent achieved less than 50 per cent pain relief. Lazorthes et al.[73] reported on 82 patients: with 95 per cent achieving satisfactory relief. Patients were started on 0.1–0.3 mg/day and the dose was gradually titrated to effect. The final doses were a mean of 2.5 mg (range, 0.10–60 mg).

Complications

The safety and side-effects of the intraventricular injections or infusions are similar to intraspinal infusions with the exception of the increased risk of respiratory depression noted in the first 3 days of the intraventricular delivery.[75,77] The most frequent side-effect is nausea/vomiting[72] and infusion-related complications such as colonized reservoirs, ventricular catheter dislodgement, catheters blockage, and meningitis.[74]

Deep brain stimulation

Neuroanatomy

The body's pain mechanisms are mediated by substances known as beta-endorphins, which are produced by certain brain cells. These beta-endorphins act to inhibit pain by their influence on two areas of the brain called the periventricular grey matter and the periaqueductal grey matter. Deep brain stimulation involves the implantation of electrodes to stimulate periventricular and periaqueductal grey matter.[78]

Technique

During this procedure, an electrode implant is carried out by placing the patient under local anaesthesia while a burr hole is made 3 cm from the midline in the coronal structure. These burr holes are made easily with CT- and MRI-guided stereotaxis because the technology enables accurate placement of the stimulating electrodes. For this operation, the initial targets are either the periventricular grey/periaqueductal grey (PVG/PAG) area, the ventral posterior lateral thalamus, or the internal capsule.[79] Stimulation of the PVG/PAG is best suited to nociceptive pain, while stimulation of areas in and around the thalamus (i.e. medial lemniscus ventralis basalis nucleus, internal capsule) is thought to work better for neuropathic pain.[79] The small size of thalamic targets as well as the numbness that may result from implantation have led some surgeons to prefer the internal capsule to the lateral thalamus.[79]

Many surgeons place electrodes temporarily in both areas and allow the patient to choose the location that best alleviates pain; others rely on intra-operative stimulation to determine placement. After 4 days, routine tests of the apparatus determine the frequencies that generate pain relief. Several days to 3 months after implantation, a radiofrequency-receiving device can be attached so that the patient can freely use the device.

Indications

Deep brain stimulation is rarely used in the management of cancer pain. It may be considered for patients with a good performance status who have pain that is refractory to systemic and regional analgesia and ablative procedures. This includes pain from diffuse bone metastases, midline or bilateral pain (especially of the lower body), brachial or lumbosacral plexopathy, and recurrent pain from head and neck cancer.[80]

Results

In a series of 31 patients with cancer pain who were treated with deep brain stimulation, 87 per cent of the patients experienced satisfactory relief with 55 per cent of these experiencing lasting relief until death.[80] In a trial of 68 patients over 15 years, 78 per cent underwent internalization of their devices and 79 per cent reported long-term relief.[79]

Complications

Complications are generally unavoidable because they are greatly influenced by the placement of the deep brain stimulator electrode. They occur less frequently when the electrode is placed in the PVG region than when it is placed in the PAG. The most reported complication in the Kumar study resulted from hardware malfunction, although 20–25 per cent of patients involved in the study reported the development of migraine-type headaches.

Summary

The neurosurgical options for treating intractable cancer pain are many. Advances in technology, particularly in the area of MRI guidance, have greatly improved the accuracy and ease of application of the intracranial techniques.

Over the past decade, the technology for and use of spinal procedures has remained fairly constant and as a result, information is still not complete concerning the best application of many of these procedures. Most certainly, it should be emphasized that these techniques are applied only to the small subset of patients with severe pain since many of the non-interventional options will suffice for pain that is minimal or mild in severity.

Selection of a specific technique can be based upon expected survival time of the cancer patient, pain location, and/or preference towards ablative or augmentative options. Despite the praise heaped by different clinical groups upon individual methods, information regarding the best modalities of treatment for specific pain syndromes is still lacking. This might be an indication that technology has outpaced our knowledge of the most effective application for each procedure. As knowledge of the efficacy of different various pain therapies grows, the role of each of these neurosurgical procedures in the overall management of cancer patients experiencing severe pain hopefully will be clarified.

References

1. **World Health Organization**. *Cancer Pain Relief* 2nd edn. Geneva: World Health Organization, 1996.
2. **Tasker, R.R.** (1987). The problem of deafferentation pain in the management of the patient with cancer. *Journal of Palliative Care* **2** (2), 8–12.
3. **Hassenbusch, S.J., Stanton-Hicks, M.S., and Walsh, J.** (1993). Opioid responsiveness with long-term intraspinal infusion of narcotic in nociceptive and neuropathic pain (Meeting abstract). *Proceedings of the Annual Meeting of the American Society for Clinical Oncology* **12**.
4. **Yaksh, T.L. and Onofrio, B.M.** (1987). Retrospective consideration of the doses of morphine given intrathecally by chronic infusion in 163 patients by 19 physicians. *Pain* **31** (2), 211–23.
5. **Cherny, N.I., Arbit, E., and Jain, S.** (1996). Invasive techniques in the management of cancer pain. *Hematology/Oncology Clinics of North America* **10** (1), 121–37.
6. **Hassenbusch, S.J.** (1995). Surgical management of cancer pain. *Neurosurgery Clinics of North America* **6** (1), 127–34.
7. **Holtzheimer, P.E. III, Roberts, D.W., and Darcey, T.M.** (1999). Magnetic resonance imaging versus computed tomography for target localization in functional stereotactic neurosurgery. *Neurosurgery* **45** (2), 290–7; discussion 297–8.
8. **Brisman, R., Khandji, A.G., and Mooij, R.B.** (2002). Trigeminal nerve–blood vessel relationship as revealed by high-resolution magnetic resonance imaging and its effect on pain relief after Gamma Knife radiosurgery for trigeminal neuralgia. *Neurosurgery* **50** (6), 1261–6, discussion 1266–7.
9. **Davis, K.D., Lozano, A.M., Tasker, R.R., and Dostrovsky, J.O.** (1998). Brain targets for pain control. *Stereotactic and Functional Neurosurgery* **71** (4), 173–9.
10. **Sloan, P.A., Hodes, J., and John, W.** (1996). Radiosurgical pituitary ablation for cancer pain. *Journal of Palliative Care* **12** (2), 51–3.
11. **Young, R.F., Jacques, D.S., Rand, R.W., and Copcutt, B.R.** (1994). Medial thalamotomy with the Leksell Gamma Knife for treatment of chronic pain. *Acta Neurochirurgica Supplement (Wien)* **62**, 105–10.
12. **Lahuerta, J., Bowsher, D., Lipton, S., and Buxton, P.H.** (1994). Percutaneous cervical cordotomy: a review of 181 operations on 146 patients with a study on the location of 'pain fibers' in the C-2 spinal cord segment of 29 cases. *Journal of Neurosurgery* **80** (6), 975–85.
13. **Stuart, G. and Cramond, T.** (1993). Role of percutaneous cervical cordotomy for pain of malignant origin. *Medical Journal of Australia* **158** (10), 667–70.
14. **Tasker, R.R.** (1988). Percutaneous cordotomy: the lateral high cervical technique. In *Operative Neurosurgical Techniques: Indications, Methods, and Results* (ed. H.H. Schmidek), pp. 1191–1205. New York: Grune & Stratton.
15. **Kanpolat, Y., Savas, A., Ucar, T., and Torun, F.** (2002). CT-guided percutaneous selective cordotomy for treatment of intractable pain in patients with malignant pleural mesothelioma. *Acta Neurochirurgica (Wien)* **144** (6), 595–9.
16. **Gildenberg, P.L.** (1976). Percutaneous cervical cordotomy. *Applied Neurophysiology* **39** (2), 97–113.
17. **Rosomoff, H.L. and Loeser, J.D.** (1990). Neurosurgical operations on the spinal cord. In *The Management of Pain* (ed. J.J. Bonica), pp. 2067–81. Philadelphia: Lea & Febiger.
18. **Nagaro, T., Adachi, N., Tabo, E., Kimura, S., Arai, T., and Dote, K.** (2001). New pain following cordotomy: clinical features, mechanisms, and clinical importance. *Journal of Neurosurgery* **95** (3), 425–31.
19. **Friehs, G.M., Schrottner, O., and Pendl, G.** (1995). Evidence for segregated pain and temperature conduction within the spinothalamic tract. *Journal of Neurosurgery* **83** (1), 8–12 (see comments).
20. **Nagaro, T., Amakawa, K., Arai, T., and Ochi, G.** (1993). Ipsilateral referral of pain following cordotomy. *Pain* **55** (2), 275–6.
21. **Nagaro, T., Amakawa, K., Kimura, S., and Arai, T.** (1993). Reference of pain following percutaneous cervical cordotomy. *Pain* **53** (2), 205–11.
22. **Jackson, M.B., Pounder, D., Price, C., Matthews, A.W., and Neville, E.** (1999). Percutaneous cervical cordotomy for the control of pain in patients with pleural mesothelioma. *Thorax* **54** (3), 238–41.
23. **Gildenberg, P.L.** (2001). Myelotomy through the years. *Stereotactic and Functional Neurosurgery* **77** (1–4), 169–71.
24. **Fink, R.A.** (1984). Neurosurgical treatment of nonmalignant intractable rectal pain: microsurgical commissural myelotomy with the carbon dioxide laser. *Neurosurgery* **14** (1), 64–5.
25. **Al-Chaer, E.D. and Traub, R.J.** (2002). Biological basis of visceral pain: recent developments. *Pain* **96** (3), 221–5.
26. **Al-Chaer, E.D., Lawand, N.B., Westlund, K.N., and Willis, W.D.** (1996). Pelvic visceral input into the nucleus gracilis is largely mediated by the postsynaptic dorsal column pathway. *Journal of Neurophysiology* **76** (4), 2675–90.
27. **Al-Chaer, E.D., Lawand, N.B., Westlund, K.N., and Willis, W.D.** (1996). Visceral nociceptive input into the ventral posterolateral nucleus of the thalamus: a new function for the dorsal column pathway. *Journal of Neurophysiology* **76** (4), 2661–74.
28. **Willis, W.D. Jr. and Westlund, K.N.** (2001). The role of the dorsal column pathway in visceral nociception. *Current Pain and Headache Reports* **5** (1), 20–6.

29. **Willis, W.D., Al-Chaer, E.D., Quast, M.J., and Westlund, K.N.** (1999). A visceral pain pathway in the dorsal column of the spinal cord. *Proceedings of the National Academy of Sciences USA* **96** (14), 7675–9.
30. **Nauta, H.J.** et al. (2000). Punctate midline myelotomy for the relief of visceral cancer pain. *Journal of Neurosurgery* **92** (Suppl. 2), 125–30.
31. **Becker, R., Gatscher, S., Sure, U., and Bertalanffy, H.** (2002). The punctate midline myelotomy concept for visceral cancer pain control—case report and review of the literature. *Acta Neurochirurgica Supplement* **79**, 77–8.
32. **Tindall, G.T., Nixon, D.W., Christy, J.H., and Neill, J.D.** (1977). Pain relief in metastatic cancer other than breast and prostate gland following trans-sphenoidal hypophysectomy. A preliminary report. *Journal of Neurosurgery* **47** (5), 659–62.
33. **Levin, A.B. and Ramirez, L.L.** (1984). Treatment of cancer pain with hypophysectomy: surgical and chemical. *Advances in Pain Research and Therapy* **7** (631), 631–45.
34. **Katz, J. and Levin, A.B.** (1977). Treatment of diffuse metastatic cancer pain by instillation of alcohol into the sella turcica. *Anesthesiology* **46** (2), 115–21.
35. **Carbonin, G.** (1978). Hypophysectomy and pain relief in cancer. *Journal of Neurosurgery* **48** (4), 666–7.
36. **Gye, R.S., Stanworth, P.A., Stewart, J.A., and Adams, C.B.** (1979). Cryohypophysectomy for bone pain of metastatic breast cancer. *Pain* **6** (2), 201–6.
37. **Fitzpatrick, J.M., Gardiner, R.A., Williams, J.P., Riddle, P.R., and O'Donoghue, E.P.** (1980). Pituitary ablation in the relief of pain in advanced prostatic carcinoma. *British Journal of Urology* **52** (4), 301–4.
38. **Levin, A.B., Katz, J., Benson, R.C., and Jones, A.G.** (1980). Treatment of pain of diffuse metastatic cancer by stereotactic chemical hypophysectomy: long term results and observations on mechanism of action. *Neurosurgery* **6** (3), 258–62.
39. **Sonntag, V.K.** (1981). Trans-sphenoidal hypophysectomy for intractable cancer pain. *Arizona Medicine* **38** (1), 23–5.
40. **Duthie, A.M., Ingham, V., Dell, A.E., and Dennett, J.E.** (1983). Pituitary cryoablation. The results of treatment using a transphenoidal cryoprobe. *Anaesthesia* **38** (5), 448–51.
41. **Cook, P.R., Campbell, F.N., and Puddy, B.R.** (1984). Pituitary alcohol injection for cancer pain. Use in a district general hospital. *Anaesthesia* **39** (6), 540–5.
42. **Ramirez, L.F. and Levin, A.B.** (1984). Pain relief after hypophysectomy. *Neurosurgery* **14** (4), 499–504.
43. **Takeda, F.** et al. (1983). Alterations of hypothalamopituitary interaction and pain threshold following pituitary neuroadenolysis—a clinical investigation of the mechanism of cancer pain relief. *Neurologia Medico-Chirurgica (Tokyo)* **23** (7), 551–60.
44. **Levin, A.B.** (1993). Hypophysectomy in the treatment of cancer pain. In *Management of Cancer-Related Pain* (ed. E. Arbit), pp. 281–95. Mt Kisco: Futura.
45. **Corssen, G., Holcomb, M.C., Moustapha, I., Langford, K., Vitek, J.J., and Ceballos, R.** (1977). Alcohol-induced adenolysis of the pituitary gland: a new approach to control of intractable cancer pain. *Anesthesia and Analgesia* **56** (3), 414–21.
46. **Fitzpatrick, J.M., Gardiner, R.A., Williams, J.P., Riddle, P.R., and Ep, O.D.** (1980). Pituitary ablation in the relief of pain in advanced prostatic carcinoma. *British Journal of Urology* **52** (4), 301–4.
47. **Miles, J.** (1979). Chemical hypophysectomy. *Advances in Pain Research and Therapy* **2**, 373–80.
48. **Madrid, J.L.** (1979). Chemical hypophysectomy. *Advances in Pain Research and Therapy* **2**, 381–91.
49. **Tasker, R.R.** (1990). Thalamotomy. *Neurosurgery Clinics of North America* **1** (4), 841–64.
50. **Whittle, I.R. and Jenkinson, J.L.** (1995). CT-guided stereotactic antero-medial pulvinotomy and centromedian-parafascicular thalamotomy for intractable malignant pain. *British Journal of Neurosurgery* **9** (2), 195–200.
51. **Sweet, W.H.** (1980). Central mechanisms of chronic pain (neuralgias and certain other neurogenic pain). *Research Publication—Association for Research in Nervous and Mental Disease* **58**, 287–303.
52. **Wong, E.T.** et al. (1997). Palliation of intractable cancer pain by MRI-guided cingulotomy. *Clinical Journal of Pain* **13** (3), 260–3.
53. **Cohen, R.A., Kaplan, R.F., Moser, D.J., Jenkins, M.A., and Wilkinson, H.** (1999). Impairments of attention after cingulotomy. *Neurology* **53** (4), 819–24.
54. **Davis, K.D.** et al. (2000). Activation of the anterior cingulate cortex by thalamic stimulation in patients with chronic pain: a positron emission tomography study. *Journal of Neurosurgery* **92** (1), 64–9.
55. **Hassenbusch, S.J., Pillay, P.K., and Barnett, G.H.** (1990). Radiofrequency cingulotomy for intractable cancer pain using stereotaxis guided by magnetic resonance imaging. *Neurosurgery* **27** (2), 220–3.
56. **Ballantine, H.T. Jr., Bouckoms, A.J., Thomas, E.K., and Giriunas, I.E.** (1987). Treatment of psychiatric illness by stereotactic cingulotomy. *Biological Psychiatry* **22** (7), 807–19.
57. **Pillay, P.K. and Hassenbusch, S.J.** (1992). Bilateral MRI-guided stereotactic cingulotomy for intractable pain. *Stereotactic and Functional Neurosurgery* **59** (1–4), 33–8.
58. **Kanpolat, Y., Deda, H., Akyar, S., and Caglar, S.** (1990). CT-guided pain procedures. *Neurochirurgie* **36** (6), 394–8.
59. **Schvarcz, J.R.** (1978). Spinal cord stereotactic techniques re trigeminal nucleotomy and extralemniscal myelotomy. *Applied Neurophysiology* **41** (1–4), 99–112.
60. **Kanpolat, Y., Savas, A., Batay, F., and Sinav, A.** (1998). Computed tomography-guided trigeminal tractotomy–nucleotomy in the management of vago-glossopharyngeal and geniculate neuralgias. *Neurosurgery* **43** (3), 484–9; discussion 490.
61. **Kanpolat, Y., Caglar, S., Akyar, S., and Temiz, C.** (1995). CT-guided pain procedures for intractable pain in malignancy. *Acta Neurochirurgica Supplement (Wien)* **64** (88), 88–91.
62. **Frank, F., Fabrizi, A.P., and Gaist, G.** (1989). Stereotactic mesencephalic tractotomy in the treatment of chronic cancer pain. *Acta Neurochirurgica (Wien)* **99** (12), 38–40.
63. **Shieff, C. and Nashold, B.S. Jr.** (1987). Stereotactic mesencephalic tractotomy for the relief of thalamic pain. *British Journal of Neurosurgery* **1** (3), 305–10.
64. **Shieff, C. and Nashold, B.S. Jr.** (1990). Stereotactic mesencephalotomy. *Neurosurgery Clinics of North America* **1** (4), 825–39.
65. **Yoshii, N.** et al. (1982). Comparative study between size of lesioned area and operative effects after pulvinotomy. *Applied Neurophysiology* **45** (4/5), 492–7.
66. **Strenge, H.** (1978). The functional significance of the pulvinar thalmi (author's translation). *Fortschritter der Neurologie-Psychiatrie Grenzgeb* **46** (9), 491–507.
67. **Tekian, A. and Afifi, A.K.** (1981). *Efferent connections of the pulvinar nucleus in the cat. Journal of Anatomy* **132** (Pt 2), 249–65.
68. **Laitinen, L.** (1977). Anterior pulvinotomy in the treatment of intractable pain. *Acta Neurochirurgica (Wien)* (Suppl. 24), 223–5.
69. **Yoshii, N. and Fukuda, S.** (1979). Effects of unilateral and bilateral invasion of thalamic pulvinar for pain relief. *Tohoku Journal of Experimental Medicine* **127** (1), 81–4.
70. **Yoshii, N., Mizokami, T., Ushikubo, T., Kuramitsu, T., and Fukuda, S.** (1980). Long-term follow-up study after pulvinotomy for intractable pain. *Applied Neurophysiology* **43** (3–5), 128–32.
71. **Yoshii, N. and Fukuda, S.** (1976). Several clinical aspects of thalamic pulvinotomy. *Applied Neurophysiology* **39** (34), 162–4.
72. **Karavelis, A., Foroglou, G., Selviaridis, P., and Fountzilas, G.** (1996). Intraventricular administration of morphine for control of intractable cancer pain in 90 patients. *Neurosurgery* **39** (1), 57–61.
73. **Lazorthes, Y.R., Sallerin, B.A., and Verdie, J.C.** (1995). Intracerebroventricular administration of morphine for control of irreducible cancer pain. *Neurosurgery* **37** (3), 422–8; discussion 428–9.
74. **Cramond, T. and Stuart, G.** (1993). Intraventricular morphine for intractable pain of advanced cancer. *Journal of Pain and Symptom Management* **8** (7), 465–73.
75. **Dennis, G.C. and DeWitty, R.L.** (1990). Long-term intraventricular infusion of morphine for intractable pain in cancer of the head and neck. *Neurosurgery* **26** (3), 404–7; discussion 407–8.

76. **Ballantyne, J.C., Carr, D.B., Berkey, C.S., Chalmers, T.C., and Mosteller, F.** (1996). Comparative efficacy of epidural, subarachnoid, and intracerebroventricular opioids in patients with pain due to cancer. *Regional Anesthesia* **21** (6), 542–56.
77. **Brazenor, G.A.** (1987). Long term intrathecal administration of morphine: a comparison of bolus injection via reservoir with continuous infusion by implanted pump. *Neurosurgery* **21** (4), 484–91.
78. **Boivie, J. and Meyerson, B.A.** (1982). A correlative anatomical and clinical study of pain suppression by deep brain stimulation. *Pain* **13** (2), 113–26.
79. **Kumar, K., Toth, C., and Nath, R.K.** (1997). Deep brain stimulation for intractable pain: a 15-year experience. *Neurosurgery* **40** (4), 736–46; discussion 746–7.
80. **Young, R.F.** (1993). Electrical stimulation of the brain for the treatment of intractable cancer pain. In *Management of Cancer-Related Pain* (ed. E. Arbit), pp. 257–69. Mt Kisco: Futura.

8.2.8 Transcutaneous electrical nerve stimulation (TENS)

Michaela Bercovitch and Alexander Waller

Transcutaneous electrical nerve stimulation (TENS) is a way of controlling pain through the 'gate' theory, where it is believed, selective electrical stimulation of certain nerve fibres block signals carrying pain impulses to the brain. It is usually administered by physiotherapists, upon referral by a physician. However, it is also employed directly by some physicians and in some hospital settings. Though it is commonly employed, and advocated by enthusiasts, firm evidence supporting its efficacy is scant.

The historic use of electricity to relieve pain

Pain has always been part of the human experience, and humans have always endeavoured to alleviate it.[1] One of the earliest records of pain relief, from Fifth Dynasty in Egypt (2500 BC), depicts the use of *Malapterurus electricus*, a fish with electrical properties, to relieve pain. Electricity as treatment for pain was also found during the Hippocratic era (400 BC).

The first written record of treating pain with electricity was attributed to Scribonius Largus (AD 46).[2] In 1759, John Wesely[3] described the use of electrotherapy for pain of sciatica, headache, gout, and kidney stones. Two centuries later, Sarlandiere used the effect of electrical stimulus on acupuncture points in treating pain of rheumatism, gout, neuralgia, and migraine headaches.[4] During the eighteenth and nineteenth centuries, galvanic sources were also used to relieve pain. In the twentieth century, electroanalgesia therapy became very popular, and was applied, in such diverse situations as dental extraction, labour pain, or amputation.[5,6]

Theoretic basis of TENS analgesia

Pain is defined as a sensory and emotional experience associated with total or partial tissue damage, or described in terms of such damage.[7] To better understand the mechanism of pain relief with TENS, a short description of pain mechanisms is useful.

The anatomy of pain transmission is described in Fig. 1.

The 'gate control theory', proposed in 1965 by Melzack and Wall, emphasized the modulation of inputs in the spinal dorsal horn and the dynamic role of the brain in processing pain.[8] The proposed mechanism of pain transmission is based on the existence of a 'barrier' between A-delta fibres and C fibres that project to the substantia gelatinosa of dorsal horn and synapses with the first central transmission cell—T-cell. The T-cell receives the impulses from peripheral fibres and activates the response and perception system. According to this theory, high-level stimulation of A-delta fibres have an inhibitory influence effectively 'closing the gate', of the T-cells of the ascending spinothalamic tract. Opening the gate is a result of high levels of activity from the C fibres producing excitation of T-cells and of biophysical mechanisms that lead to the perception of pain (Fig. 2).

Based on the gate control theory, it was postulated that using a low-level electrical stimulus will preferentially activate larger A-delta fibres. These fibres have a relatively low electrical threshold and may subsequently activate the small inhibitory interneurons of the substantia gelatinosa to effectively reduce the small fibre nociceptive input.[9]

In 1968, Melzack and Casey introduced a new concept to the basic gate theory—'the central control trigger'. According to this theory, dorsal column

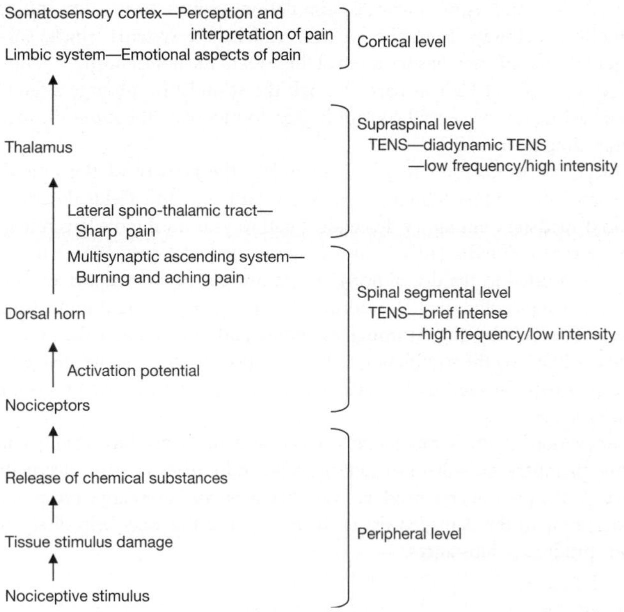

Fig. 1 The anatomy of pain transmission.

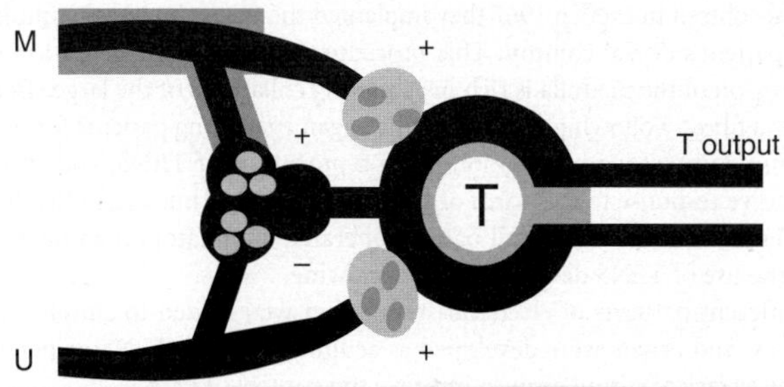

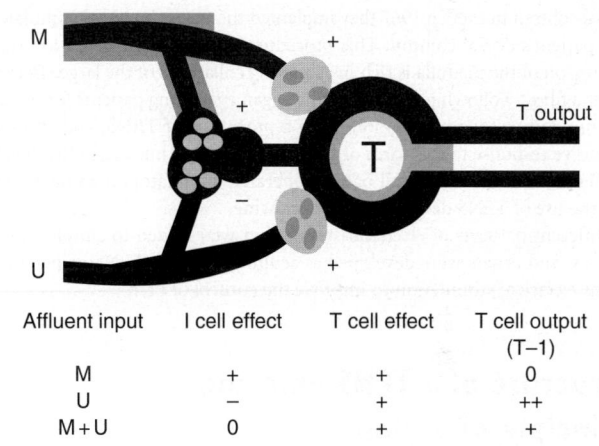

Affluent input	I cell effect	T cell effect	T cell output (T–1)
M	+	+	0
U	–	+	++
M+U	0	+	+

Fig. 2 Schematic diagram of the components of the 'Gate' in the dorsal horn of spinal cord.

stimulation and spinothalamic stimulation may activate descending inhibitory pathways from the reticular and limbic systems which, subsequently, modify the sensory input at the level of the dorsal horn.[10] Thus, TENS may act, at least in part, through the stimulation of large afferent fibres acting on the central control trigger, to modulate the input through descending pathways.

Electrical stimulation may also modulate the activity of the opioid-mediated descending inhibitory pathways. Basbaum and Fields described opioid-mediated inhibitory descending pathways from the nucleus reticularis gigantocellularis (RGC) through periaquaductal grey (PAG) nuclei are transmitted to the dorsal horn via the nucleus raphe magnus and the nucleus magnocellularis.[11] According to this theory, afferent input from small fibres is transmitted through ascending pathways to the thalamus and nucleus RGC. By the stimulation of PAG it is possible to generate analgesia, and it is hypothesized that TENS may act by excitation of the brainstem nuclei.

Activation of the sympathetic nervous system to produce changes in tissue chemistry is another mechanism proposed for relieving pain. Electricity used on the painful area produces vasodilatation via cholinergic receptors. Blood flow to the damaged tissues increases, and this may help dissipate pain-producing substances.

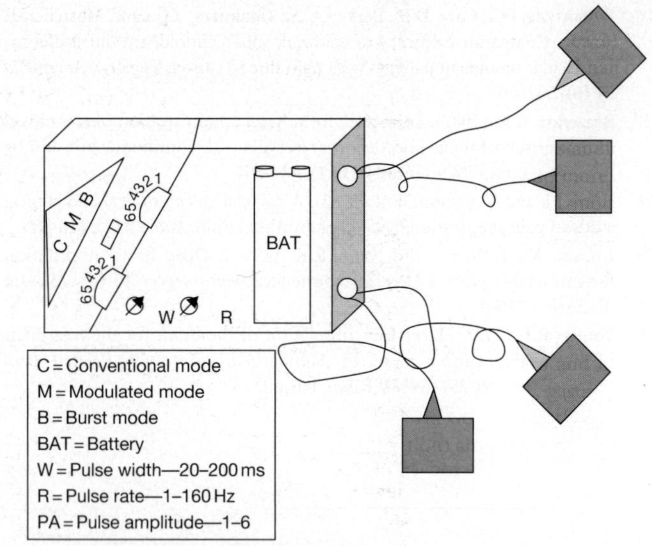

Fig. 3 Transcutaneous electrical stimulation system.

Early development of TENS

Two years after the gate theory was published, Shealy and his colleagues tried, and succeeded, to manage intractable back pain by stimulating the dorsal column in cats. In 1967 they implanted the first spinal cord stimulator in a patient's dorsal column. This procedure takes into consideration that this region of the medulla is rich in ascending collaterals of the large efferent A-delta fibres. Following this success, he began evaluating patients for dorsal column stimulator implantation using a prototype of TENS, and showed a positive response to this form of pain reduction.[9] Thus began the development of TENS, with small battery-operated stimulators manufactured, and the use of TENS devices spread worldwide.

Different patterns of electrical stimulation were added to simple TENS devices, and others were developed as acupuncture-like TENS or percutaneous electrical stimulation to improve the control of pain.

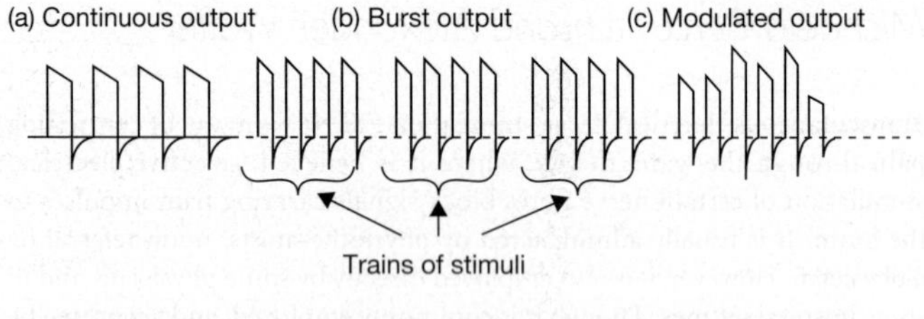

Fig. 4 Illustration of (a) continuous, (b) burst, and (c) modulated types of output available on most TENS units. (Adapted with permission from publisher. Walsh, D.M. (1997). TENS modes available. In *TENS Clinical Applications and Related Theory* 1st edn., p. 38. Edinburgh: Churchill Livingstone.)

Structure of a TENS unit and principle of action

A simple TENS unit consists of a hand-held, battery-operated, electrical pulse generator and electrodes (Fig. 3). The common commercial apparatus has three different pulse patterns: continuous, pulsed (burst), and modulated (ramped). These provide a cyclic variation of pulse duration, frequency, or amplitude that may offer the patient more comfort.

Electrotherapeutic devices used for pain treatment may be low frequency (LF)—1–4 Hz or high frequency (HF)—120–150 Hz. Some brands use low-frequency, high-intensity currents via electrodes applied to the skin over an 'acupuncture point', thus producing 'acupuncture-like TENS'.

Since the 1980s, a large number of such electrical stimulators have been developed, and with them, a variety of techniques for chronic and even acute pain management. TENS models range from single-channel devices to multichannel ones, with the single and dual models being battery operated (V battery). The multichannel unit requires an electrical outlet connection.

The type of TENS unit individualized to suit the patients prevailing condition. Mobile patients use a small single- or dual-channel units (e.g. Unitouch® or the British Tenscare), which are as small as 5.5 cm and weigh 60 g, and which are equipped with clips which attach them to clothing. These units are less powerful, and are recommended for chronic pain such as arthritis. Most TENS apparatus today are constructed to offer variable intensity, pulse duration, and frequency.[12] Moreover, they offer a choice as to type of output: continuous, burst, or modulation (Fig. 4).

Types of TENS administration

Conventional TENS

The conventional apparatus contains electrodes made of electroconductive material (carbon-filled vinyl sheets). Electrodes are applied to designated areas on the skin called dermatomal points. These 'dermatomal points' are areas that receive their nerve supply from a specified spinal nerve. Activation of the TENS unit results in transmission of electrical pulses in the selected dermatomal nerves.

There are four categories of anatomical sites to which the electrodes can be applied:

1. Close to the painful area. This stimulates the afferent sensory nerves that lead from the spinal cord to the painful area.[13–15]
2. Over a peripheral nerve with cutaneous distribution in the painful area (e.g. radial nerve, ulnar nerve, peroneal nerve). In these cases, the electrodes should be placed along the more superficial course of the nerve.[16] This approach has been reported in the management of peripheral nerve injury and peripheral neuropathy.[17–19]
3. Spinal nerve routes. Placing the electrodes paraspinally for stimulating the appropriate roots of spinal nerves which supply a specific dermatomal or myotomal painful area.[20]
4. Motor or trigger point placement. For stimulation of a specific group of skeletal muscles, tendons, joints, ligaments, periosteum.[21,22]

Acupuncture-like TENS

This technique employs a low-frequency, high-intensity stimulus administered to 'acupuncture points' over the skin, without using needles (see Chapter 8.2.9). The stimulus produces paraesthesia and muscle contraction. It is hypothesized[23] that it acts via the descending inhibitory pain pathways. The onset of analgesia is delayed, and lasts longer than using conventional TENS.[23]

Percutaneous electrical nerve stimulation (PENS)

PENS involves the use of electrically stimulated acupuncture needles at 'acupuncture points' or at 'dermatomal points'. In a small anecdotal series, PENS has been reported to have an analgesic effect in cancer patients with bone metastases. In this case, the electrode needles are placed in the soft tissue and muscle surrounding bones, thus bypassing the resistance of the cutaneous barrier and delivering the electrical stimulus closer to nerve endings located in the soft tissue, muscles and periosteum of the involved dermatomes.[24] Ahmed et al. report that two of three patients with bone pain who used PENS reported benefits from this technique.[25] Two patients with bone metastases reported significant pain relief, with a decreased need for analgesic drugs.

Efficacy of TENS therapy

The efficacy of TENS remains controversial. Beyond anecdotes and testimonies, there is very little data to support its utility in cancer pain. At best, it is advocated as an adjuvant approach to routine therapy,[26] at worst it is an ineffectual therapy, no more effective than placebos.[27]

The recent literature on TENS is sparse and anecdotal; it provides little substantive support for the effectiveness of this technique. In 1996, Khor et al. described a 39-year-old man with intractable metastatic femoral bone pain who received adjuvant therapy with TENS in addition to opioids.[28] In a survey of 20 patients with head and neck cancers, Chiarini et al. found that 60 per cent may have benefited from TENS, but only when the pain intensity is moderate or low.[29] As described above, Ahmed et al. reported their experience with percutaneous electrical stimulation in management of three patients with metastatic bone.[25] Finally, in a survey of analgesic techniques used in a sample of 593 cancer patients, 13 per cent received TENS as supportive therapy to systemic analgesia for nociceptive (1 per cent), neuropathic (6 per cent), and mixed (6 per cent) cancer pain.[30]

While there is no good evidence of efficacy for chronic pain, some of the alternative long-term analgesic approaches often involve either similarly limited efficacy or serious adverse effects. At least, TENS is unlikely to cause harm. If it is to be considered, TENS therapy should be undertaken with a realistic expectation of the results, and only continued after demonstrating a beneficial effect in that particular patient.

Administration of TENS

The treating physician will select the appropriate device based on the patient's needs and on availability. Stimulation sites are selected as described above (Fig. 5).

Selection of TENS parameters

After the optimal site has been found, the next step is to determine the best combination TENS electrical stimulation parameters to provide significant pain relief.

The output current of the TENS electrodes are characterized by:

- Frequency—the rate of change or the number of pulses delivered per second (measured in Hz).
- Amplitude (intensity)—the magnitude of current (measured in mA) and voltage (measured in V) applied by the TENS unit.
- Pulse duration (width)—measured in microseconds.
- Continuity—generated continuously or in bursts (trains of pulses or single pulses).
- Modulation—frequency, pulse duration, and amplitude change periodically.
- Current flow direction.

The TENS 'work modes' are combinations of these parameters. Common work modes include 'High frequency continuous' (50–200 Hz), low frequency continuous (1–4 Hz), 'high frequency bursts' in which the unit delivers brief bursts of high-frequency stimulation at a low frequency, that is, 2 Hz. The election of the most appropriate work mode is largely empirical.

Frequency

The signal frequency for conventional TENS is in the range of 50–200 Hz. This gives the optimum presynaptic inhibition through the gate mechanism.[31] Theoretically, high-frequency TENS is used to stimulate the large A-delta nerve fibres (which feature fast conduction rates and short refractory periods) and low frequencies are used to stimulate A-delta and C fibres (which have slower conduction rates and longer refractory periods, lower-frequency pulses should be used). A study conducted by Gopalkrishnan and Sulka[32] indicated a significant relief of primary and secondary heat and mechanical hyperalgesia when using high-frequency TENS signals.

Intensity

The conventional TENS uses low-intensity signals. In practice, intensity is adaptively set to a value that best fits the patient needs. While applying an incremental intensity TENS stimulus, the patient will be asked to report his/her sense of it. 'Vibration', 'tapping', 'buzzing', are terms usually used by the patient in relation with low-intensity stimulation. In general, the intensity should be set just below the pain threshold (when the patient reports discomfort) so that paraesthesias are felt in the painful region. Sometimes discomfort appears after a variable time interval from starting the treatment. Therefore, the patient's condition should be checked after about 10 min.

Current flow direction, pulse duration, and continuity

In some TENS units, the current flow between the TENS electrodes may be constant or change in a periodical or pulsed manner. Direct current (DC) describes a current constantly flowing in one direction, alternating current (AC) flows continuously but periodically changes its direction and pulsed current is periodic rather than constant. Pulsed current may be monophasic with current flows in one direction or biphasic with two phases of opposite flowing current.

Modulation

The periodical change in amplitude, frequency, or duration may have a positive effect on patient's comfort and treatment efficiency. Some TENS units offer a continuous change programme that is said to overcome the nerve fibre adjustment to the stimulus, maintaining its 'alertness' to the treatment.[33]

Guidelines for the application of TENS

1. Explain the technique to the patient.
2. Clean skin and hair and dry well.
3. Fix the electrode to the site of pain using hydrogel pads.
4. Assess the patient's sensation after 5 min and then again after 10 min of treatment and re-adapt the stimulus frequency and amplitude until pain threshold is reached such that the patient feels sensation of paraesthesias in the painful region.
5. Reassess the pain 30 min after beginning of treatment; if there is no analgesic effect, re-evaluate placement of the electrodes.

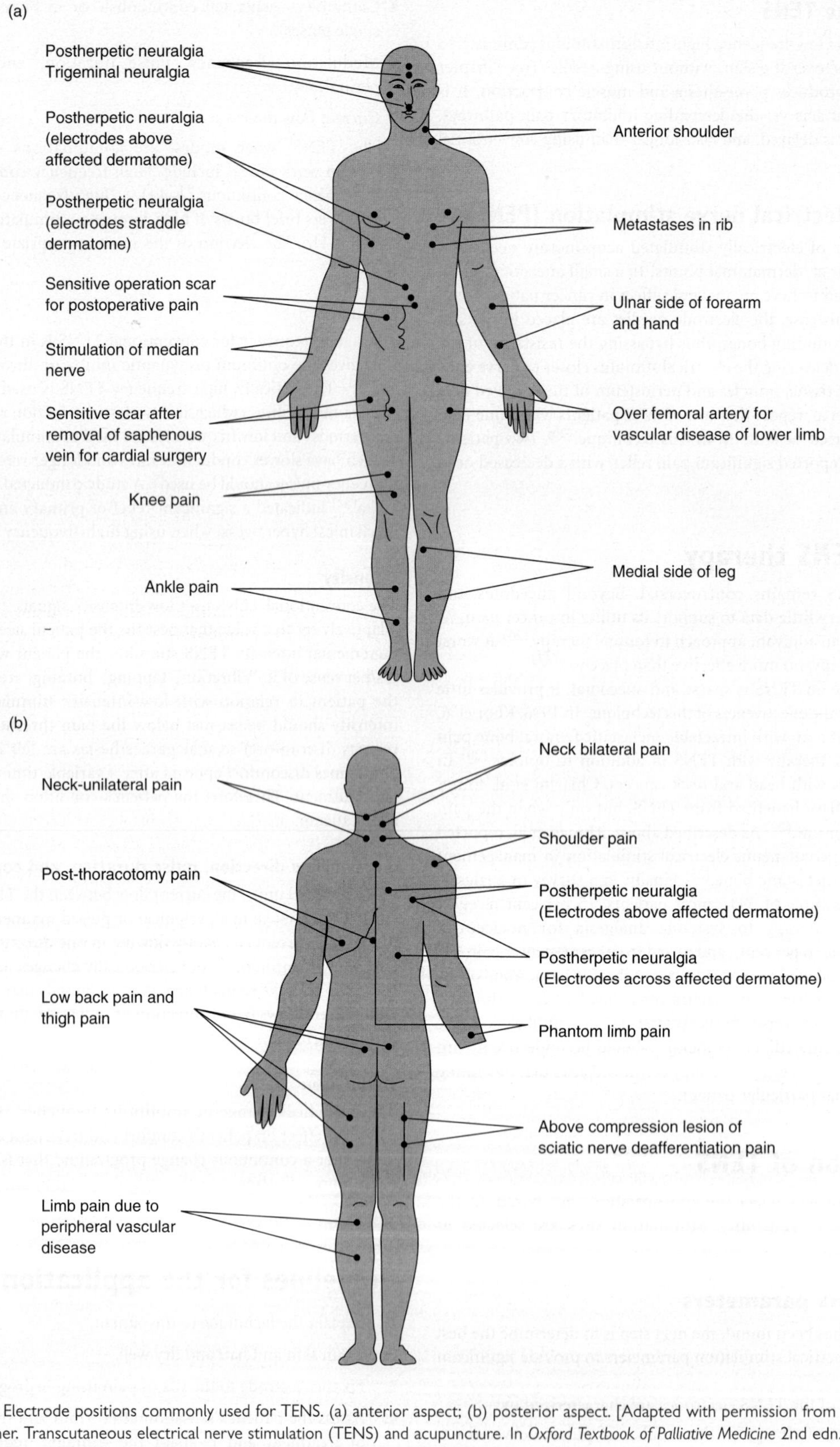

Fig. 5 Electrode positions commonly used for TENS. (a) anterior aspect; (b) posterior aspect. [Adapted with permission from publisher. Transcutaneous electrical nerve stimulation (TENS) and acupuncture. In *Oxford Textbook of Palliative Medicine* 2nd edn. (ed. D. Doyle, G.W.S. Hanks, and N. MacDonald), p. 423. Oxford University Press, 1998.]

6. If satisfactory analgesia is obtained, establish duration of daily treatment period for a trial of therapy.
7. Observe the appearance of the skin throughout treatment.

Once a successful strategy is identified this treatment should be followed by a trial of therapy at home. If the response to the treatment is favourable, patients should then rent or purchase their own unit. TENS treatments may be used as long as it is effective. In some settings, it is used on a fixed schedule, that is, for 10–60 min three times per day. Other patients may use it on an 'as needed' basis.

Pain indications

Indications

There is no evidence-based indication for the use of TENS in cancer patients. Given the lack of data, it is reasonable to consider a trial of therapy in patients who have achieved suboptimal outcomes from other evidence-based approaches. There is no data to indicate higher or lower likelihood of effect for different pain syndromes or mechanisms.

Contraindications

TENS has minimal side-effects and there are few contraindications. Documented contra-indications include:

1. severe allodynia;
2. incompetent patient;
3. cardiac pacemakers;
4. allergic reactions of the skin to the tape or electrode gel;
5. patients suffering from epilepsy;
6. during driving or operating machinery;
7. during pregnancy.

Additionally, electrodes placement on the anterior aspect of the neck, over the carotid sinuses, and eyes is contraindicated.

The use of TENS for other indications

Since the early 1900s, use of electroanalgesia has undergone a long sequence of changes. Initially used only for pain management, TENS has also come to be used for its non-analgesic effects.

Chemotherapy-induced nausea and vomiting

Beginning in 1989, the late Professor John Dundee demonstrated that electrical stimulation of the P6 acupuncture point has an antiemetic effect.[34] In 1991, McMillan et al. investigated the antiemetic effect of TENS applied to the P6 acupuncture point in addition to ondansetron in a group of 16 cancer patients receiving chemotherapy. Results showed significantly less nausea and vomiting when TENS was added to the antiemetic drugs.[35] In the same year, Dundee and colleagues compared the use of TENS and acupuncture as adjuvant treatment before cytotoxic treatment. They found benefits with TENS application in 77 per cent of administrations, with best results of 2-hourly self-administrated treatments of 15 Hz TENS.[34] Furthermore, in 1999, *Cancer Nursing* published a randomized double blind study by Pearl et al. that demonstrated once again the use of a miniaturized portable TENS as an adjuvant to standard antiemetic therapy for control of nausea and vomiting induced by cisplatin-based chemotherapy in 42 gynaecology patients.[36]

Lymphoedema

In 1995, Waller and Bercovitch used TENS for pain control in a patient after mastectomy for breast cancer who presented with painful lymphoedema. A considerable reduction in the degree of lymphoedema was observed after 2 days of systematic application. Two subsequent studies demonstrated the effectiveness of TENS application on lymphoedematous limbs (arms and legs). In 1996, they applied TENS for the relief of facial pitting oedema of one patient, using one channel and two electrodes. After 24 h there was a substantial reduction in the facial oedema. Further methodological research is needed.[37]

Wound healing—ulcers

Another interesting TENS application may be its use for healing ulcers. In 1983, Kaada reported the application of TENS in 10 patients with chronic leg and sacral ulcers. The ulcers, of various aetiology were resistant to standard treatment. By application of low-frequency bursts delivered at 2-Hz frequency, the authors reported successful healing in eight patients after few weeks of treatment.[38] Kaada's further studies showed clearly that electrical stimulation can be used to increase peripheral circulation and in this way to promote wound healing.

Conclusions

Accumulated anecdotal evidence suggests that TENS may have a role in relieving pain in general and cancer pain in particular. There is, however little substantiated evidence to support this belief. Given the potential for patient benefit and its low intrinsic morbidity it can be adopted as a trial therapy for patients with chronic pain. When it is considered, TENS therapy should be undertaken with a realistic expectation of the results, and only continued after demonstrating a beneficial effect in that particular patient.

References

1. **Meryl, R.G.** (2000). Electrotherapy in rehabilitation. In *TENS for Management of Pain and Sensory Pathology*, pp. 149–96. Philadelphia PA: FA Davis Company.
2. **Schonoch, W.** Die rezept sammlung des Scribonius. Jena: Baken Museum of Electricity in Life. Minneapolis MN, 1912–13.
3. **Wesley, J.** *The Desideratum: Or Electricity Made Plain and Useful.* London: W. Flexney, 1760.
4. **Sarlandiere, J.B.** *Memoires sur l'electro-puncture.* Paris: Delaumay, 1825.
5. **Burton, C.** (1975). Dorsal column stimulation: optimization of application. *Surgical Neurology* **4**, 169–77.
6. **Burton, C. and Maurer, D.D.** (1997). An assessment of the efficacy of physical therapy and physical modalities for the control of chronic musculo-skeletal pain. *Pain* **71**, 5–23.
7. **Merskey**, et al. (1979). Lecture delivered at the IASP Convention. *Proceedings of IASP.*
8. **Melzack, R.** (1993). Past, present and future pain. *Canadian Journal of Experimental Psychology* **47**, 615–29.
9. **Shealy, C.N., Mortimer, J.T., and Reswich, J.B.** (1967). Electrical inhibition of pain by stimulation of the dorsal column: preliminary clinical reports. *Anesthesia and Analgesia*, 45–8.
10. **Melzack, R. and Casey, K.L.** (1968). Sensory motivational and central control determinants of pain. In *The Skin Senses* (ed. D.R. Kenshalo), Springfield IL: Charles C Thomas.
11. **Basbaum, A.I. and Fields, H.L.** (1978). Endogenous pain control mechanisms: review and hypothesis. *Annual Journal of Neurology* **4**, 451.
12. **Stux, G. and Pomeranz, B.** *Basics of Acupuncture* 3rd edn. Berlin: Spinger-Verlag, 1995.
13. **Ebersold, M.** et al. (1976). Transcutaneous electrical nerve stimulation for treatment of chronic pain: A preliminary report. *Surgical Neurology* **4**, 96.
14. **Linzer, M. and Long, D.M.** (1976). Transcutaneous neural stimulation for relief of pain. IEEE *Transactions in Biomedical Engineering* **23**, 341.
15. **Loesor, J.D., Black, R.G., and Christman, A.** (1975). A relief of pain by transcutaneous stimulation. *Journal of Neurosurgery* **42**, 308.
16. **Berlandt, S.R.** (1984). Method of determining optimal stimulation sites for transcutaneous nerve stimulation. *Physical Therapy* **64**, 924.

17. **Picaza, J.A.** et al. (1975). Pain supression by peripheral stimulation. Part I. Observation with transcutaneous stimuli. *Surgical Neurology* **4**, 105.
18. **Sweet, W.H. and Wepsic, J.G.** (1968). Treatment of chronic pain by stimulation of primary afferent neuron. *Transactions of the American Neurological Association* **93**, 103.
19. **Mannheimer, J.S.** (1978). Electrode placements for transcutaneous electrical nerve stimulation. *Physical Therapy* **58**, 1455.
20. **Melzack, R., Stillwell, D.M., and Fox, E.J.** (1977). Trigger points and accupuncture points for pain: correlations and implications. *Pain* **3**, 3–23.
21. **Laitinen, J.** (1976). Accupuncture and transcutaneous electrical stimulation in the treatment of chronic sacrolumbalgia and ischialgia. *American Journal of Chinese Medicine* **4** (2), 169–75.
22. **Walsh, D.M.** *TENS Physiological Principles and Stimulation Parameters. The Clinical Application of TENS and Related Theory.* Edinbrugh: Churchill Livingstone, 1997, pp. 25–40.
23. **Paul, F.W., Philips, J., Thimoty, B.S., Proctor, J., Williams, B.A., and Craig, F.** (1999). *Bulletin of the American Pain Society* **9**.
24. **Wall, P.D. and Sweet, W.H.** (1967). Temporary abolition of pain in man. *Science* **155**, 108–9.
25. **Ahmed, H.E., Craig, W.F., White, P.F., and Mubber, P.** (1998). Percutaneous electrical nerve stimulation (PENS) a complementary therapy for the management of pain secondary to bone metastasis. *The Clinical Journal of Pain* **14**, 320–3.
26. **Lewis, B., Lewis, D., and Cumming, G.** (1994). The comparative analgesic efficacy of transcutaneous electrical nerve stimulation and a non-steroidal anti-inflammatory drug for pain osteoarthritis. *British Journal of Rheumatology* **33**, 455–60.
27. **Grond, S., Radbruch, L., Meusner, T., Sabatowsky, R., Loick, G., and Lehmann, K.A.** (1999). Assessment of treatment of neuropathic cancer pain following WHO guidelines. *Pain* **79** (1), 15–20.
28. **Khor, K.E. and Dittor, J.N.** (1996). Femoral nerve blockade in the multidisciplinary management of intractable localized pain due to metastatic tumor. A case report. *Journal of Pain and Symptom Management* **11** (1), 56–7.
29. **Chiarini, L., Stacca, R., Bertoldi, C., Malagnino, F., Pollastri, G., and Narni, F.** (1997). Management of facial pain resulting from cancer in oral and maxillofacial surgery. *Minerva Stomatologica* **46** (1/2), 27–38.
30. **Ghoname, E.A., Craig, W.F., White, P.F., Ahmed, H.E., Hamza, M.A., Gjraj, N.M., Vakharia, A.S., and Nohr, D.** (1999). The effect of stimulus frequency on the back pain. *Anesthesia and Analgesia* **88**, 841–6.
31. **Han, J.S., Chen, X.H., Sun, S.L., Xu, X.J., Yuan, Y., Yan, S.C., Hao, J.X., and Terenius, L.** (1991). Effect of low and high frequency TENS on met-enkephalin-org-phe and dynorphin A immunoreactivity in human lumbar CSF. *Pain* **47**, 295–8.
32. **Gopalkrishnan, P. and Sulka, K.A.** (2000). Effect of varying frequency, intensity and pulse duration of TENS on primary hyperalgesia in inflamed rats. *Archives of Physical Medicine and Rehabilitation.*
33. **Johnson, M.I., Ashton, C.H., Bousfeld, D.R., and Thompson, J.W.** (1991). Analgesic effects of different pulse patterns of transcutaneous electrical nerve stimulation on cold-induced pain in normal subjects. *Journal of Psychosomatic Research* **35** (2/3), 313–21.
34. **Dundee, J.W., Ghaly, R.G., Bill, K.M., Chestnutt, W.T., Fitzpatrick, K.T.J., and Lynas, A.G.A.** (1989). Effect of stimulation of the P-6 anti-emetic point on post operative nausea and vomiting. *British Journal of Anaesthesia* **63**, 612–18.
35. **McMillan, C., Dundee, J.W., and Abraham, W.P.** (1991). Enhancement of the antiemetic action of ondasetron by transcutaneous electrical stimulation of the P6 anti-emetic point in patients having highly anti-emetic citotoxic drugs. *British Journal of Cancer* **64**, 971–2.
36. **Pearl, M.L., Fisher, M., McCauley, D.L., Valea, F.A., and Chalas, E.** (1999). Transcutaneous electrical nerve stimulation as an adjunct for controlling chemotherapy induced nausea and vomiting in gynecologic oncology patients. *Cancer Nursing* **22** (4), 307–11.
37. **Waller, A. and Bercovitch, M.** *Treatment of lymphoedema with TENS. Lymphoedema.* Oxford: Radcliffe Medical Press, 2000, pp. 27–184.
38. **Kaada, B.** (1983). Promoted healing of chronic ulceration by transcutaneous nerve stimulation (TNS). *Vasa* **12**, 262–9.

8.2.9 Acupuncture

Jacqueline Filshie and John W. Thompson

Introduction

Medical historians and anthropologists have described numerous ways in which painful conditions have been managed by sensory modulation.(1) One common feature in such folklore techniques such as cupping, scarification, cauterization, and acupuncture is that a painful stimulus is applied to abolish the pain.

The exact timing of the origin of acupuncture is unclear(2) with reports that it may have been as early as the 21st century BC(3) with stone needles or 'Bian Shi' and bone needles being used. One of the earliest and most elegantly written texts about this ancient Chinese system of healing was *The Yellow Emperor's Classic of Internal Medicine.*(4) The Yellow Emperor or Huang Ti was thought to reign about 260 BC. He wanted the secrets of Medicine to be passed to his sons and his grandsons and the records to be made known to posterity. *Celestial Lancets* by Lu and Needham(5) provide the reader with a colourful description of historical and traditional Chinese acupuncture. More recently in 1991, Ötzi, the European ice man, was discovered in the Alps, having been preserved for 5200 years.(6) Imaging revealed widespread arthritis of the spine and lower legs and many of the 47 tattoos found on his body corresponded with acupuncture points currently used for arthritis. The asymmetrical location of the points and the fact that they were on areas normally covered by clothing are thought to represent therapeutic skin piercing rather than having ornamental significance.

Traditional Eastern style acupuncture involves a sophisticated and elaborate system of diagnosis based on 'energy flow' round the body, with subsequent selection of acupuncture points for stimulation by the insertion of fine needles in order to effect a 'cure'. Western practitioners use acupuncture following orthodox Western diagnosis by history, examination, and special investigations initially and use either a traditional form of acupuncture or a simplified neurophysiologically based method of point selection.

As covered elsewhere in the book, complementary and alternative medicine (CAM) has enjoyed unprecedented popularity in recent years. The reasons that patients access CAM therapies have been explored.(7,8) Many turn to it for help on account of the lack of a reliable cure for cancer and palliation of many of its symptoms in orthodox medicine. The perception that CAM represents gentle and more natural therapies is appealing, also the need for self-empowerment both emotionally and physically. The attitudes of medical, nursing, and allied health professionals to CAM is evolving. A survey of 141 health-care professionals in Ontario, working with cancer patients, identified acupuncture/acupressure as the first choice out of 19 non-pharmacological therapies about which they would like to learn more.(9) Acupuncture has an increasing role in the treatment of cancer pain and symptom management. In many Western pain clinics acupuncture has become a standard complementary form of treatment in addition to orthodox treatment methods.(10,11)

Techniques of acupuncture

The techniques employed by an individual acupuncturist vary enormously, not only on the selection of acupuncture points but also on the mode and length of stimulation (Table 1).

Traditional Chinese acupuncture

The traditional Chinese view included appreciation of the intimate relationship between man and his environment, much like Taoist philosophy. Historically, the Chinese described a circulation of vital energy Qi or Chi. Qi circulates in the body in deep channels and along meridians. Meridians are invisible lines joining a series of acupuncture points on the surface of the body. There are 12 paired, two unpaired, and several extra

Table 1 Techniques of acupuncture

Traditional Chinese acupuncture	'Qi' or energetic system with flow of vital energy Yin and Yang need to be balanced in health Pulse and tongue diagnosis and several laws utilized for traditional diagnosis 'De Qi' or needling sensation elicited with vigorous stimulation up to 30 min ± moxibustion
Western acupuncture	Manual acupuncture Minimal stimulation up to 20 min Maximal stimulation intermittently up to 20 min Electroacupuncture 2–4 Hz low frequency 50–200 Hz high frequency
Acupuncture analgesia	Vigorous manual stimulation or electroacupuncture Used for operations in China now as sole anaesthetic in <6% operations
Acupressure	No needles—less effective than needling
Auricular acupuncture	Needles inserted in tender regions or 'recipe' points
Ryodoraku	Reduced skin impedance treated electrically
Laser therapy	No needles—advantage paediatrics (not strictly acupuncture)
Veterinary	± electroacupuncture Unlikely to be a placebo!

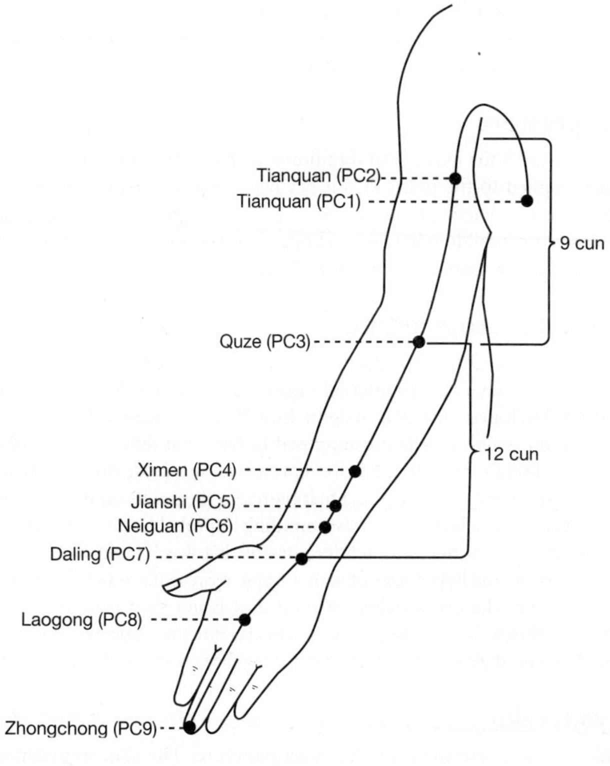

Fig. 1 The 'pericardium' meridian, in traditional Chinese acupuncture.

meridians. After taking a history, and a complex tongue and pulse diagnosis at both radial arteries, disease can be subtly diagnosed in 12 distant 'organs'. The validity of the pulse diagnosis has been seriously questioned in recent years.[12] The meridians and their associated 'organs', for example, spleen, kidney, and pericardium have no objective corresponding connections.

The Yellow Emperor believed that forces of opposite polarities were present in nature, Yin and Yang, negative and positive, dark and light, feminine and masculine. The Qi circulates round the body along the meridians to nourish both Yin and Yang components of internal organs in the following sequence: the lungs, large intestine, stomach, spleen, heart, small intestine, bladder, kidneys, pericardium (circulation), triple warmer (metabolism), gallbladder, and liver (Fig. 1).

Numerous 'laws' of acupuncture also help guide the traditional acupuncturist to make the correct diagnosis, including the law of the 'five elements'. Using these laws, points are selected and can be 'tonified' or 'sedated' if a deficiency or excess were found in any meridian. Chosen acupuncture points are manually stimulated with a needle until the patient feels a sensation of De Qi, a feeling of aching, numbness, tingling, heaviness, and fullness. Intriguingly, a very small percentage of patients, less than 1 per cent, experience a propagated sensation from the needle point which often follows the pathway of a meridian.[13] However, there is as yet no convincing evidence for the existence of meridians.

Needles are often stimulated thermally in addition to insertion and manipulation, usually by combustion of the pith of Artemesia Japonica (moxa) applied to the end of the needle or above acupuncture points. This is termed moxibustion. Many acupuncture points are somewhat tender to palpation in health and many more become tender in disease states. These points appear commonly in 'recipes' for treatment of various conditions.

It is not surprising that a rather seemingly bizarre system of diagnosis and treatment arose when one realizes that the study of formal anatomy only became possible in China in the early 20th century. Further history and philosophical background is available elsewhere.[2,3,5,14,15]

Medical acupuncture

Western-trained doctors rely on orthodox history taking, examination, and special investigations as deemed necessary before making a diagnosis. Such abstract concepts as Qi and Yin and Yang are relatively unacceptable to many western-trained doctors and have contributed to the scepticism with which many still view acupuncture. However, if the balance of Yin and Yang represents autonomic balance, and circulation of Qi, the circulation of oxygen, blood, and lymph, etc., the system can appear quite sophisticated and in some ways way ahead of the formal study of physiology.

Recent neuropharmacological and neurophysiological advances have given acupuncture a sound scientific basis and far more clinical credibility.[16] Acupuncture's actions are blocked by pre-treatment with injection of local anaesthetic.[17–19] It releases β-endorphin,[20,21] met-enkephalin, and dynorphins, which work on mu, delta, and kappa (MOR, DOR, and KOR) opioid receptors.[22,23] It releases serotonin with both analgesic and mood-enhancing properties.[22] Oxytocin is released, which is anxiolytic and analgesic.[24] It releases endogenous steroids[25] and has widespread autonomic effects.[26,27] Acupuncture is thought to up-regulate endogenous opioid gene production[28] (Zieglgänsberger 2002, personal communication), which in part explains why 'top-ups' are required to maintain the gene expression in a 'switched on' mode.

Acupuncture releases multiple endogenous substances that no single drug treatment could attempt to mimic. For further information, see the Neurophysiology section at the end of this chapter.

As further evidence accumulates, it seems likely that acupuncture works through neurophysiological modulation of multiple endogenous homeostatic mechanisms and less likely to work on energetic principles, or in a metaphysical way.

Clinical approaches

A pragmatic approach is more often taken with a mixture of segmental points appropriate to the disordered segment, trigger points, tender points, plus selected traditional 'strong' points. Trigger points are hyperirritable loci in taut bands of muscle that are painful on compression and can elicit a characteristic jump sign plus or minus a twitch response and may be accompanied by autonomic changes.[29] Referral patterns of discomfort often resemble the meridian lines and it is possible that the meridian theory developed as observations

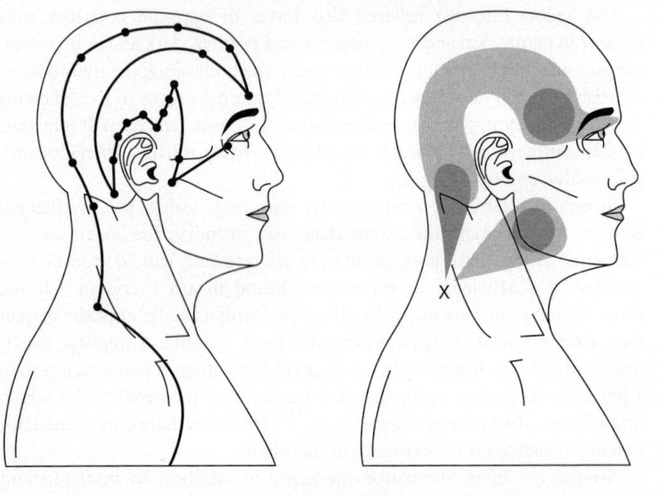

Fig. 2 This figure shows the close correlation between the referral pattern from a trigger point in upper trapezius and the path of the gallbladder meridian. The trigger point is anatomically co-incident with the acupuncture point GB21. From *Acupuncture—A Scientific Appraisal* by Ernst and White. Reprinted by permission of Elsevier Ltd.

of the referral pattern from trigger points or the coalescence of several trigger point patterns (see Fig. 2).[30,31] Needling trigger points can be most successful to treat pain of myofascial origin, which is very common in many cancer patients and also patients with musculoskeletal problems in primary care. Trigger points are exacerbated by a psychological stressor[32] and acupuncture is a particularly efficient way of deactivating them.[33]

Some use minimal stimulation from 5 secs up to 20 min and do not attempt to elicit De Qi. Some use more vigorous manual stimulation of the needles from seconds to many minutes. It has been noticed that some patients are more sensitive to acupuncture than others, so-called 'strong reactors', and require shorter gentle treatments.[34]

Patients in the main are treated somewhat empirically and treatment intensified or reduced on a trial and error basis, depending on individual progress. The treatment schedules are usually weekly for 6 weeks or twice weekly for 3 weeks with 'top-ups' at increasing intervals of 2 weeks, 3 weeks, etc., depending on the patient and their response, and how advanced the disease is in the patient.

A wide variety of techniques are both available and effective. These range from a Traditional Chinese approach on the one hand, in which point selection utilizes many historic laws and principles,[35,36] to the other extreme, in which many respected Western practitioners frankly do not believe in the special properties associated with formal Eastern acupuncture points, and who teach a simplified yet effective system of needling.[34,37,38]

Electroacupuncture (EA)

Electroacupuncture was first established as a substitute for the manual vigorous stimulation required for perioperative acupuncture or Acupuncture Analgesia.[39] An electric current is applied through the skin via the needles to stimulate chosen points. This is a stronger stimulus than transcutaneous electrical nerve stimulation (TENS), as the stimulus is transmitted through the skin via needles. Low-frequency electroacupuncture, 2–4 Hz, is more likely to stimulate the release of enkephalins and cortisol whereas high-frequency, 50–200 Hz, releases serotonin (5-HT) and dynorphin. Electroacupuncture is most frequently used for the treatment of acute pain and difficult pain problems such as fibromyalgia.[40]

Acupuncture analgesia

Acupuncture performed in a vigorous manner plus or minus electrical stimulation can raise pain tolerance to both experimental and surgically induced pain.[41–43] Acupuncture analgesia was introduced in 1958 and became popular in China for perioperative analgesia for many years. There were dramatic reports and video clips of patients having major surgery, for example, pneumonectomy, with only acupuncture as analgesia. The personal experience of James Reston, a journalist in the party accompanying President Nixon to China in 1973 and who benefited from acupuncture analgesia following an appendicectomy, was instrumental in the dissemination of knowledge about acupuncture in the West.

Numerous publications describe the use of acupuncture analgesia.[39] The lengthy induction time, coupled with inadequate analgesia in many cases, requiring opioid supplementation, understandably diminished its popularity. It is currently used, alone, for less than 6 per cent of operations in China. Nevertheless, it has had proven benefit as an adjunct to modern anaesthesia in diminishing postoperative analgesic requirements[44] and can enhance the quality of recovery with reduced morbidity.

Laser therapy

The use of external laser probes to deliver stimulation at acupuncture points is gaining acceptance,[45] although it remains controversial.[46] The mechanisms of action, particularly its effects on peripheral nerves, are uncertain and it may be misleading to include it with acupuncture. It is often described as 'laser acupuncture' but it is not strictly acupuncture because no needles are involved. One Cochrane review of laser therapy for osteoarthritis was equivocal, where wide variation in methods made assessment difficult.[47] Another review on short-term relief of pain and morning stiffness in patients with rheumatoid arthritis was positive.[48] Optimal parameters for treatment have yet to be elucidated. From an experimental point of view, laser therapy lends itself to testing with double blind trial methodology. There are anecdotal reports that laser therapy reduces mucositis following bone marrow transplantation, but no formal studies as yet.

Laser therapy, as it is painless, is more acceptable to paediatric patients, needle phobic patients, and veterinary subjects.

Acupressure

Acupressure is the massage of traditional acupuncture points. For example, when applied to the point PC6 it has been shown to reduce nausea and vomiting associated with chemotherapy.[49] Massage called 'Tuina' is used extensively on children in China. Though helpful, acupressure is believed to be less effective than acupuncture with needles.

Auricular acupuncture

In traditional Chinese acupuncture, the ear is deemed to be closely connected by channels to internal organs. In the 1950s, Nogier in France further developed auricular acupuncture[50] and suggested that different parts of the external helix are supposed to represent different parts of the body, as though the external helix represented an upside down foetus. By treating those areas on the pinna that represent the points on the body with pain, it could be alleviated. Whilst sounding improbable, one study showed some effect when needling tender sites in this way.[51] Further study is needed to test the hypothesis of somatotopic representation of the body on the ear. Since the ear is richly innervated, it is not surprising that strong sensory stimulation has far reaching effects. But the importance of point specificity on the ear has been challenged for the treatment of addictions.[52]

Ryodoraku

This is a Japanese form of electroacupuncture. The skin impedance is measured and if abnormal can be altered electrically.[53] Ryodoraku acupuncture points have been found in areas of skin containing sweat glands.

Veterinary acupuncture

Acupuncture and electroacupuncture are being used increasingly for domestic, farm, and racing animals.[54,55] The effectiveness of treatment in animals lends credence to the view that acupuncture is more than merely an elaborate placebo.

Equipment

Numerous wall charts and models are available, which depict traditional acupuncture points for accurate localization purposes. Acupuncture needles are usually made of surgical stainless steel and are disposable or reusable. Quality control of sterilization techniques is variable, so it should be mandatory to use disposable needles. The size, length, and gauges of needles vary according to practitioner preferences. Many use a plastic introducing guide tube to facilitate a quick and relatively painless insertion.

There is an enormous selection of electrical and laser equipment available. It is beyond the scope of this book to include this topic in any depth, so the reader is advised to consult standard textbooks and suppliers for further details.

Indications

In China, acupuncture is first-line treatment for hundreds of minor and major complaints,[35] and there is an increasing base of evidence accumulating on its use in the Western literature.[36,56,57] It is steadily gaining popularity in the West because of its perceived success in treating a host of common ailments, in many cases obviating the need for medication or at least reducing the dosage of drugs and the risk of side effects.

Selected topics have been chosen for their relevance to palliative medicine. The quality of some referenced articles is rather variable but this is not surprising as it is only comparatively recently that acupuncture has been the focus of serious observational work followed by randomized controlled trials.

Clinical research

Efficacy, safety, and cost-effectiveness need to be examined objectively in acupuncture, as they are in all aspects of modern healthcare. The results of clinical trials of acupuncture have been conflicting and this has been partly due to the complex issues surrounding the methodology of acupuncture trials. The generally accepted method of testing the efficacy of a new treatment is to subject it to a randomized, double blind, controlled trial. Randomization should not be a problem in any study. Blinding the therapist is difficult but not impossible. However blinding of the patient, independent observer, and statistician involved in the study should be feasible. The choice of a control is more problematic. Many studies have employed needling of non-traditional acupuncture points as the control treatment, but this procedure is now known to produce neurophysiological effects and is thus not truly inactive. Conversely, non-needling placebos may not be sufficiently credible. Recently, 'placebo needles' have been devised with retractable handles that do not penetrate the skin, operating on the 'stage dagger' principle. Even this sham control forcibly touches the skin and can cause some degree of sensory stimulation. Acupuncture needling was found to be superior to this sham control in one recent RCT on rotator cuff problems.[58] Trials that compare acupuncture with best standard treatment are also acceptable.

Acupuncture is a minimally invasive form of treatment and undoubtedly causes a strong placebo or non-specific effect. Placebo analgesia works in part via stimulation of endogenous opioids,[59] as does acupuncture, so it is quite testing to delineate one effect from the other. Thomas et al.[60] showed superiority of deep, superficial needling and diazepam over a placebo diazepam tablet for neck pain measured with VAS scores, but all four treatments improved the affective, emotional component of pain. Key research challenges remain for acupuncture.

Systematic reviews

Some of the early systematic reviews on acupuncture for pain control were inconclusive,[61,62] as they were based on pooled heterogeneous data with very flawed methodology. A more recent review examining much of the same evidence,[63] was similarly inconclusive, but did show limited evidence of the superiority of acupuncture treatment compared with untreated patients on a waiting list.

Significant positive evidence, based on systematic reviews, is available for the use of acupuncture in the control of nausea and vomiting, particularly post-operative nausea and vomiting,[64] for dental pain,[65] for headache,[66] for fibromyalgia,[67] and electroacupuncture for experimental pain.[42]

Acupuncture treatment for back pain is controversial with both a positive review[68] and a negative review[69] resulting from the authors' differing approaches to trial assessment. Addressing divergent conclusions, Cummings[70] has critically appraised the quality and validity in one systematic review of acupuncture for back pain, clearly demonstrating a lack of consistency and rigour in this review, which may account for the conflicting results. Inconclusive evidence exists for asthma, stroke, and neck pain, and negative evidence for weight loss and smoking cessation, although results of the latter are no worse than nicotine patches. Some feel any effects in aiding nicotine withdrawal may be useful in the short term.

Pain

Acupuncture has been found to help a wide variety of pain conditions with between 40 and over 80 per cent symptomatic improvement in primary care.[71–73] The shorter the duration of the problem, the better the response. Old age and multiple illnesses reduce the benefit. Ross[74] has recently shown the dramatic reduction in referrals from primary to secondary care, by extensively integrating its use in primary care. Other cost savings have been found by Christensen[75] and Lindall.[76]

Cancer pain and symptom control

The following sections discuss the use of acupuncture to treat acute post-operative pain in cancer patients and also chronic or intractable pain associated with cancer and its treatment.

Acute pain

Many aspects of acupuncture analgesia have been reviewed by White in 1998.[39] As already mentioned in the acupuncture analgesia section, acupuncture is much less frequently used as a sole anaesthetic because it is time consuming, requires lengthy counselling and a 20-min induction period before surgery. It does not give adequate muscle relaxation for abdominal surgery or mechanical ventilation. Only about 10 per cent of the population achieve sufficient analgesia to remain comfortable during surgery and awareness can be a problem.

The significant percentage of non-responders makes acupuncture analgesia risky as an alternative to general anaesthesia. Acupuncture as an adjuvant to anaesthesia is a different matter, decreasing analgesic requirement per- and post-operatively and improving post-operative recovery characteristics. Poulain showed this in 1997 in a series of 250 cancer patients having gynaecological surgery for cancer.[77] In a second study, not yet submitted for publication, Poulain blinded both the patient and the anaesthetic team, by having a second anaesthetic team give acupuncture or dummy acupuncture with no needles after induction and then the first team continued the surgery. The first anaesthetic team showed enhanced analgesia, and the independent observers showed enhanced post-operative recovery in the acupuncture group.

Aldridge[78] has recently shown a reduction in nausea and vomiting post-operatively compared with ondansetron in a series of 40 breast cancer patients and reduced post-operative pain.

The optimal choice of dose, points, timing of treatment pre-, per-, and post-operatively/combination, duration of needling, mode of stimulation, EA or manual are yet to be defined.

Cancer pain and cancer-related pain

The failure of pharmacological means alone to control pain has led many to use non-drug treatments including acupuncture and TENS. The pain can be caused by either primary or metastatic cancer, its treatment or be unrelated, and often due to a combination. It may include nociceptive or neuropathic components, or both. Acupuncture can improve pain control sufficiently to permit a decrease in dosage and side-effects of analgesics and co-analgesics. Acupuncture can help patients who are excessively sensitive to normal doses of analgesics as well as those who have pain despite appropriate titration of analgesics and co-analgesics.[79,80] It can also be relaxing for patients particularly distressed by anger or denial or who have difficulty in coming to terms with their disease (Filshie, unpublished observation).

The treatments are time consuming with treatment times often between 10 and 20 min, with six treatments planned in the initial course. This time is valuable for both the acupuncture itself and the therapeutic consultation. In clinical practice, results of treatment are undoubtedly due to the combination of the specific effects of the treatment and the opportunity for reflective listening and support given to the patient at a very crucial time in their lives.

At the first visit, gentle stimulation is given to assess whether the patient is a 'strong responder' or not. Then the treatment is subsequently tailored to the individual response. Appropriate segmental points are often chosen, plus trigger points and strong analgesic points, which may or may not be extrasegmental, for example, LI4. Figure 3(a) shows a combination of paravertebral segmental points and trigger points used for a patient with neck pain. The traditional point Large Intestine 4 or LI4 (Fig. 3(b)) is also often used, which has been shown to raise the pain threshold in numerous experimental studies.[42] The paravertebral points C7, T1, and T2 are particularly useful for pains and vascular problems in the head and neck, arm, and breast regions, and the paravertebral points L1–L5 for pain, with or without vascular problems, in the abdomen, low back, and lower leg (Fig. 3(c)). Sacral paravertebral points can be added for perineal pain.

Bowsher et al. in 1973 included a brief section by Mann[81] on eight cancer patients who obtained short-lived relief of 3–72 hours and a sense of relaxation and increased mental alertness. Wen[82] used several EA sessions a day reducing to one or two per day in a series of 29 patients whose pain was inadequately controlled in advanced disease and who were suffering from side-effects of opioids. Though time consuming, analgesia improved significantly and pain medication was significantly reduced.

Following the successful use in a series of 80 patients with advanced cancer-related pain, two summaries of extensive retrospective audits were published on 339 patients.[79,80] This group had a heterogeneous collection of symptoms, which had failed to respond to conventional treatment in a cancer hospital where clinicians are familiar with analgesics and co-analgesics. Fifty-two and 56 per cent, respectively, of patients obtained worthwhile analgesia after three weekly treatments to enable it to be a useful outpatient-based treatment.[79,80] An initial course of six treatments is followed by others given at increasing intervals. A further 30 and 22 per cent (respectively), often with late-stage disease, had only short-lived analgesia for 2 days or less.[79,80] The more advanced the disease, the shorter the response to treatment. Many patients had a significant improvement in mobility. Treatment-related pain such as post-surgical syndromes or post-irradiation pain often responded better and for longer. Muscle spasm, bladder spasm, and vascular problems were also helped significantly. Aung[83] describes similar results in an audit of 344 patients where a traditional approach was employed combined with Qi Gong, special breathing exercises and, in some cases, meditation. Leng, after his first year of acupuncture practice in a hospice, reported similar results.[84] A further audit of 89 patients for pain and xerostomia in particular showed similar results with 86 per cent of patients considering it 'very important' to continue to provide an acupuncture service.[85]

Another pain audit and detailed psychological profile in 67 patients with breast cancer and related pain showed a statistically significant drop in average pain, worst pain, interference with lifestyle, distress, pain behaviour, and depression after 1 month of weekly acupuncture treatments.[86] This improvement in symptoms and depression scores may be important because a high score for depression has been linked to a significantly decreased chance of survival.[87] Another study of patients in the 2-week period following breast surgery with axillary dissection showed improvement in pain and increased arm abduction compared with a control group having no acupuncture.[88]

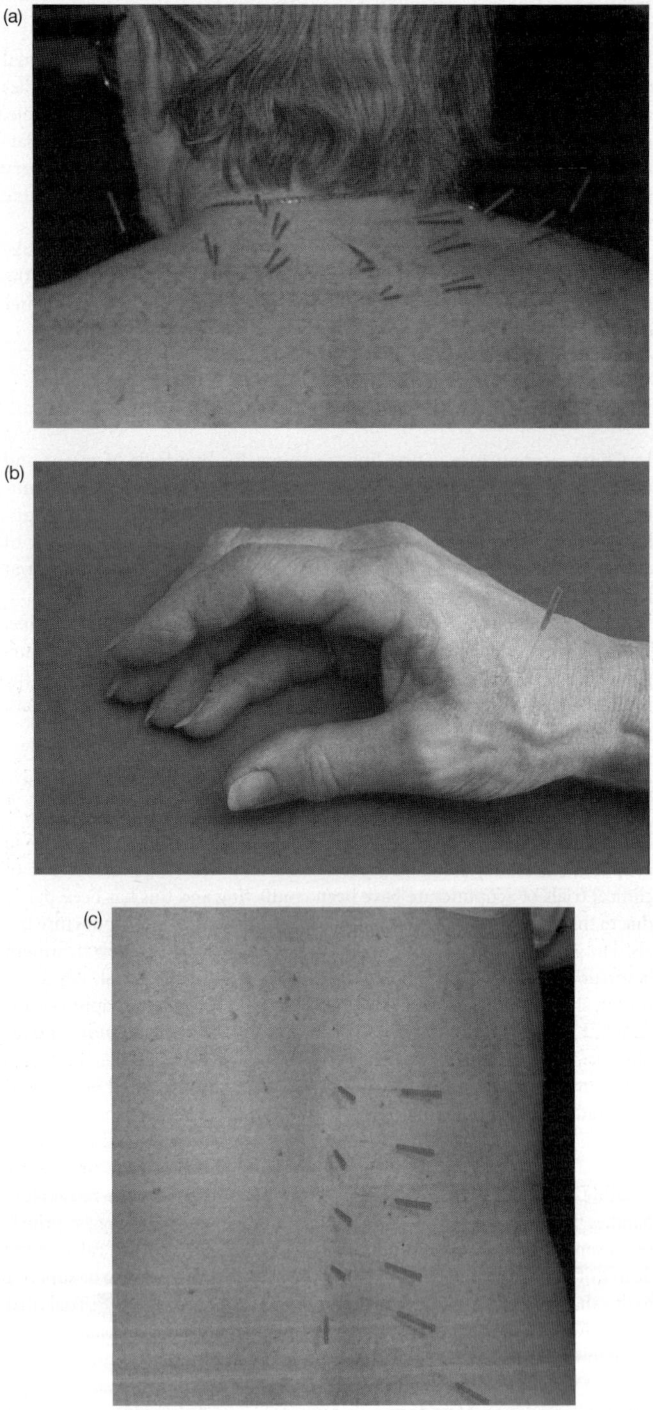

Fig. 3 (a) A combination of segmental and trigger points for a patient with neck pain. (b) The traditional acupuncture point Large Intestine 4 (LI4), which raises the pain threshold. (c) Segmental acupuncture in a patient with low back pain.

Phantom limb pain

Acupuncture can both elicit phantom limb pain (PLP), phantom limb sensation, and stump pain as well as alleviate pain.[89,90] In those patients who have a cold stump, the paravertebral sympathetic blocking points may help to give sympathetic blockade. Mirror sites are usually treated on the remaining limb together with needling of paravertebral and strong 'traditional points'. Pain relief can be instant and dramatic in selected patients, but as with many other forms of treatment for this condition, the majority are not necessarily helped and only short case series are described.(91)

Auriculoacupuncture for cancer pain

Dillon and Lucas(92) treated 28 hospice patients, including five with motor neurone disease, and found a statistically significant improvement in pain over a 4-week period. In another pilot series of 20 patients with various cancers, auriculoacupuncture produced a statistically significant reduction in pain intensity.(93)

Percutaneous electrical nerve stimulation (PENS)

PENS is reported as a 'novel treatment' but is simply electroacupuncture (EA) under a new title! Cummings(94) has reviewed the literature and found nothing to distinguish it from EA and no substantial justification to call it 'novel'. One anecdotal report claims that PENS helped two out of three patients when combined with periosteal needling.(95)

Acupuncture and TENS

TENS can often be used as a backup for acupuncture, if the acupuncture effect wears off between outpatient visits. The therapies are not necessarily interchangeable, some patients responding to acupuncture alone and others to TENS.

Tolerance

It is interesting to note that cancer patients with advanced disease need multiple treatments, two to eight weekly in general pain control. This is in marked contrast with patients with non-malignant disease who cope well with increasing intervals between treatments. Some patients, in addition, exhibit a reduced response to acupuncture with time. In fact, almost an inverse relationship was noted between tumour size and longevity of acupuncture response.(79,80) The larger the tumour burden, or the more active the disease, the shorter the beneficial effect of acupuncture. Advanced disease may have accounted for up to 30 per cent who only exhibited short-lived pain relief of 2 days or less in the two studies. Sudden tolerance occurring in a patient who had previously been acupuncture responsive was considered to be a sinister sign. Tolerance in such a patient was the reason for the patient to be immediately referred back to the oncologists for further investigation, as 17 out of 27 such patients had developed further metastases. Not only that, if metastatic disease was found and treated successfully by chemotherapy or radiotherapy, the patient could revert back to being acupuncture responsive again. Tolerance has been described in animal models when the opioid antagonists angiotensin 2(96) and CCK(97) were released with prolonged electroacupuncture. It is possible that patients with cancer have an increased or maximal output of endogenous opioids, which would prevent them from gaining an optimal response when treated.

Methods of overcoming acupuncture tolerance in late-stage disease include increasing the frequency of treatments or the use of semipermanent needles for the patients to massage and so help sustain the stimulation. Wen(82) used multiple acupuncture treatments daily in terminal patients to good effect such that the patients could reduce opioid medication and its attendant side-effects. Semipermanent needles have also been used to prolong analgesia and improve pain and symptom control in patients with advanced cancer.

Shortness of breath

In a randomized controlled trial of patients with chronic obstructive pulmonary disease (COPD), the traditional Chinese acupuncture-treated group showed significant benefit in subjective breathlessness and 6-min walking distance.(98) Objective measures of lung function were unchanged in both the treated and control groups.

The observation that acupuncture gave subjective improvement in shortness of breath in patients with advanced cancer in a pain clinic led to a pilot study. The short-term effects of acupuncture were studied in 20 patients with advanced cancer-related dyspnoea at rest where the symptom was directly related to primary or secondary malignancy.(99) Two sternal needles (Fig. 4(a)) and two traditional acupuncture points (LI4) (Fig. 3(b)) were used. Outcome measures showed significant improvement in VAS subjective scores of breathlessness, relaxation, and anxiety at 90 min. There was also an objective significant reduction in the respiratory rate that was sustained for the treatment period. Seventy per cent (14/20) of the patients reported marked symptomatic benefit from treatment. Eight of these patients elected to have two indwelling studs inserted onto the sternal points in an attempt to prolong the response (Fig. 4(b)). A clear plastic dressing was used to secure the needles. This gave patients control by enabling them to massage the studs during breathless 'panic attacks' or prior to any even trivial exercise. All eight reported varying degrees of benefit lasting up to 2 weeks. It was successful in patients who had failed to respond to multiple treatments for shortness of breath including steroids, opioids, various nebulizers, and oxygen. The two sternal semipermanent needles are now used in palliative care units in the United Kingdom and are named 'ASAD' points—or Anxiety, Sickness, and Dyspnoea points. They can remain in

(a)

(b)

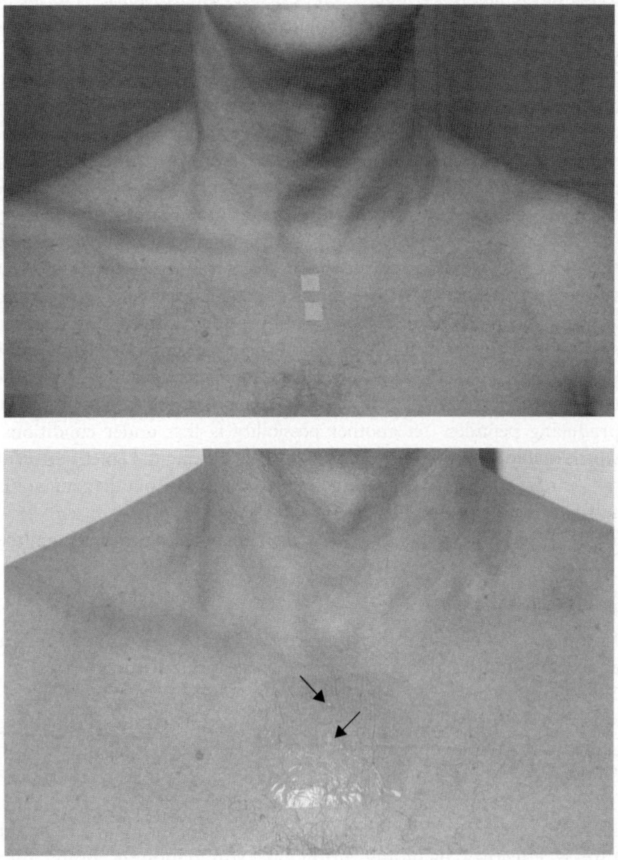

Fig. 4 (a) Two needles inserted at the top of the sternum for treatment of dyspnoea. (b) Two indwelling acupuncture needles shown by the arrows at ASAD points are covered by a clear plastic dressing which can be massaged to give relief in panic attacks or prior to activity.

place for up to 4 weeks at a time covered by a clear plastic dressing. Further prospective studies are in progress and the use of studs for COPD is also under evaluation.[100] Acupressure has also been used to assist pulmonary rehabilitation in patients with COPD.[101]

The mechanisms of action of acupuncture for dyspnoea remain speculative, but the sedative and central actions of endogenous opioid peptide release may be contributory. Acupuncture also has widespread effects on autonomic function, which, in turn, have a major influence on the respiratory system.

Nausea and vomiting

The late Professor John Dundee conducted numerous studies on acupuncture using a single needle placed at the point PC6 on the pericardium meridian (Fig. 1). He found PC6 a clinically useful anti-emetic treatment in postoperative nausea and vomiting, morning sickness, and as an additional anti-emetic for patients having chemotherapy. McMillan has summarized his findings.[102] Transcutaneous electrical nerve stimulation (TENS) has also been used with some success[103,104] to increase the scope of treatment. A systematic review by Vickers showed acupuncture for nausea and vomiting to be superior to a control group in 23 out of 33 randomized controlled trials. One recent high-quality randomized controlled trial has shown the benefit of acupuncture in nausea and vomiting associated with high-dose chemotherapy for breast cancer.[105]

In late-stage palliative care, nausea and vomiting is often multifactorial with possibly, opioids, electrolyte imbalance, anorexia, gastrointestinal symptoms, and dehydration contributing to the cause. In these cases, it may be necessary to add strong gastrointestinal points such as CV12, ST25, and ST36. Indwelling ASAD points can be helpful on occasions. As to the possible mechanisms of action of acupuncture for nausea and vomiting, there is, as yet, no clear-cut explanation.

Acupuncture is infrequently a cause of nausea and vomiting, which may be due simply to release of opioid peptides. When the provocative agent is a cytotoxic drug for example, it may have excited vomiting through some indirect mechanism involving activation of nerve pathways depending upon such transmitters as 5-hydroxytryptamine, dopamine, or opioid peptides (or possibly all three). Under these circumstances, the release of opioid peptides by acupuncture may switch on various inhibitory pathways that block the emetic pathway to the chemoreceptor trigger zone and/or the vomiting centre. An alternative explanation is that there may be significant antagonistic interaction between opioid peptides released by acupuncture such that when one group is present in high concentration (thus causing the emetic effect) the release of other opioid peptides (by acupuncture treatment) may release peptides that act as antagonists to the emetic-producing peptides. Yet another possibility is that under conditions in which opioid peptide concentration is high (causing the emetic effect) the anti-emetic effect of acupuncture is due to the release of other antagonistic substances such as, for example, CCK.[106]

Any effects of acupuncture on the cannabinoid receptors remain untested.

Xerostomia

Several studies have shown acupuncture to help xerostomia of different aetiology. Blom et al.[107] performed a randomized controlled trial on 38 patients with xerostomia following radiotherapy, using classical versus superficial acupuncture. Both groups showed a significant increase in salivary flow. In those patients who had had all the salivary gland irradiated, 50 per cent in both groups had increased flow rates at a 1-year follow-up. Thus, the superficial acupuncture was an active treatment. Lundeberg[27] discusses several studies and describes the mechanisms by which acupuncture is effective, including autonomic stimulation of both volume (parasympathetic) and viscosity (sympathetic) stimulation and release of the vasodilator calcitonin gene-related peptide (C-GRP), which also increases salivary secretion.

Fifty per cent of patients with xerostomia after radiotherapy for head and neck cancer, who were refractory to pilocarpine, benefited from acupuncture.[108] Acupuncture was found useful in patients in late-stage palliative care for xerostomia, dysphagia, and articulation.[109] Therefore, acupuncture may have a significant role in palliation of this unpleasant symptom in palliative care.

Vascular problems

Vascular problems may be helped by acupuncture. One anecdotal report describes two radionecrotic ulcers (which usually do not heal) but which healed completely using acupuncture.[110] Chronic ulcers have been healed by acupuncture, for example, those due to venous stasis. Lundeberg[27] has reviewed many of the effects of acupuncture on vascular problems, including angina, hypertension, and ischaemic skin flaps, and showed sympathetic blockade by acupuncture in certain circumstances.

Stroke

In a randomized controlled trial of 78 patients treated within l0 days of a severe stroke, the group receiving acupuncture (sensory stimulation) twice a week for l0 weeks recovered faster and spent less time in hospital.[111] Motor function, balance, activities of daily living (ADL), and quality of life were measured up to 12 months after stroke onset. In addition, rehabilitation costs for hospital and nursing care were reduced by US$26 000 per patient in the treatment group. The acupuncture group had enhanced recovery of postural function 2 years after the lesion and treatment.[112] A systematic review on the effectiveness of acupuncture for stroke subsequently showed six out of nine trials to be positive, but they concluded that there was no compelling evidence of effectiveness in stroke rehabilitation as two of the higher-quality studies were negative.[113]

Cancer-related hot flushes

Wyon et al.[114] demonstrated that acupuncture could decrease hot flushes in the natural climacteric. Tamoxifen-induced hot flushes contribute to 10 per cent of patients discontinuing therapy. Acupuncture has been found to reduce hot flushes.[115] Semipermanent needles were inserted at the point SP6 in severe cases who failed to respond to four weekly treatments.[116] Patients were advised to change the studs every 7–10 days. Clear plastic dressings secure the studs in each case and 'Do It Yourself' (DIY) kits are given to selected patients with clear instructions for cleansing, insertion, and safe disposal. (See Cautions and Contraindications for the insertion of semi-permanent needles.) Acupuncture has also helped to control vasomotor symptoms in men due to treatment of prostrate cancer.[117]

Miscellaneous

Acupuncture has helped dysphagia due to oesophageal obstruction,[118] intractable hiccup,[119,120] radiation rectitis following radiotherapy for carcinoma of the cervix,[121] experimentally induced itch,[122] and uraemic pruritus.[123]

AIDS

Greene et al.[124] showed that 48 per cent of 1016 HIV-infected participants used needle acupuncture to treat their symptoms. The majority of patients use complementary medicine to augment conventional therapy.[125] Individualized acupuncture treatment was helpful for treatment of sleep disturbance.[126] Increased sleep disturbance can contribute to cognitive dysfunction, though pain reduction from acupuncture may have contributed to the success. One large randomized controlled trial comparing acupuncture with amitriptyline and placebo failed to show any benefit of acupuncture or amitriptyline over placebo for peripheral neuropathy.[127] Possible infection with AIDS emphasizes the need to use disposable needles, as patients may not know their diagnosis, or fail to reveal it when seeking advice.

Immunological considerations

There is some limited evidence, mainly from studies in experimental animals, to suggest that acupuncture produces immunomodulating effects, similar to moderate exercise.[27,128,129] Much further study is required before recommending acupuncture wholeheartedly for immuno-enhancing effects, which may be beneficial alongside conventional treatment. The optimal points, dose, treatment frequency, and many other parameters would need to be identified first.

Anxiety and depression

Though not formally tested, the upper sternal 'ASAD' (Fig. 4(b)) points are used in the United Kingdom extensively for control of anxiety. Particularly anxious patients can give themselves a burst of anxiolysis by gently massaging the studs for 1–2 min. This can give the added benefit of a sense of control over this distressing symptom. Acupuncture was found to be equally as helpful as tricyclic drugs in depression in some studies.[130,131]

Complications and contraindications

Complications

Lazarou et al.[132] estimated that drugs are between the fourth and sixth commonest cause of death in the United State of America. By contrast, acupuncture is a safe method of treatment with low side-effects so that only 300 life-threatening episodes were found during a 30-year retrospective study.[133] More recently, Peuker and Grönemeyer reviewed rare but serious complications of acupuncture due to trauma,[134] as did Walsh, for infectious complications.[135]

Acupuncture's adverse effects have been classified into four groups:[134]

- delayed or missed diagnosis of the condition treated;
- negative reactions, for example, syncope, vertigo, and sweating;
- bacterial and viral infections (hepatitis B, C, and HIV);
- trauma of tissues and organs.

The safety aspects of acupuncture in palliative care have recently been reviewed.[136] Acupuncture can mask cancer and disease progression, for example, the pain of bone metastases. The disease must therefore be monitored continuously by both the oncology and palliative care teams. Furthermore, acupuncture treatment should be given by (or closely supervised by) a physician who has full knowledge about the stage and clinical condition of the patient.

Minor adverse events

Minor adverse effects include post-needling pain, bleeding, bruising, and sleepiness. Two recent prospective studies on 32 000 and 34 000 general acupuncture treatments concluded that there is a 14 per 10 000 and 13 per 10 000 chance, respectively, of a significant minor adverse event such as a forgotten needle or fainting following treatment.[137,138] Concordance between the studies was remarkably high, reporting, respectively, a low incidence of bleeding and bruising 3 and 2.9 per cent; pain 1 and 1.2 per cent; and aggravation of symptoms 1 and 2.8 per cent. The strengths and limitations of the studies were discussed frankly.

Cancer patients appear to be more sensitive to acupuncture than other patients and may become excessively sleepy during the treatment so that it is advisable to arrange for nursing assistance when treating these patients. Cachectic patients should be given superficial needling with particular care.

Infection due to the use of inadequately sterilized needles is also a major hazard. Disposable needles are the best way to reduce the risks and should be compulsory. Bacterial infection, including bacterial endocarditis, has been described,[139] and the most serious viral infections including hepatitis B.[140–142] It is unbelievable that clinics still exist both in the East and West where inadequate sterilization techniques continue to be used. For the safety of both patients and acupuncturists, it should be mandatory for all needles to be of the single use disposable type.

Although rare, serious anatomical damage to most organs and structures have been reported, including lungs (unilateral and bilateral pneumothorax), heart, liver, spleen, kidney, vessels, and nerves.[134] Some traditional Chinese textbooks include diagrams with alarmingly deep needling techniques which are more likely to cause damage, as is the failure to know basic anatomy. Some complications are life-threatening and arrhythmias and cardiac arrests have been reported with at least nine deaths. Burns from moxibustion and faulty electrical apparatus have also been described.

Table 2 Contraindications and cautions

Do not treat around unstable spine—could potentially lead to spinal cord injury or transection
Do not directly needle superficial tumour nodules or ulceration
Do not needle lymphoedematous limb
Do not needle if blood clotting is seriously impaired
Do not directly needle too close to or into a prosthesis
Do not needle intracranial deficits on skull or directly over spine following spinal surgery
Do not use electroacupuncture in a patient with a pacemaker
Cancer patients can be more sensitive to acupuncture and nursing assistance is recommended for each case
Needle only very superficially in cachectic patients
If tolerance occurs—it may represent progressive disease and full investigations of tumour status may be required
Cautions for semipermanent needles
Avoid in patients with heart valvular disease, post-heart transplant, or with a pacemaker
Caution in immunocompromised patients secondary to any cause including chemotherapy and radiotherapy and ITU
Severe immunosuppression
Post-splenectomy
Avoid in patients with known hepatitis B or C as risk from needle stick injury if they accidentally 'fall out' 'Strong reactors'
Caution in patients with keloid scars

Semipermanent needles are now used extensively to prolong the effects of acupuncture for treatment of cancer related pain, dyspnoea, anxiety, and hot flushes, so that their possible contraindications and cautions should be considered, as summarized in Table 2.[143]

Needles which 'fall out' can represent a sharps hazard and it is not always clear what happens to the needles after they have fallen out.[92,93] When DIY needle kits are given to a patient for self-treatment of symptoms, for example, hot flushes, these should include clear instructions on how to clean the skin and to use the needles; and a sharps box should be supplied so that the needles can be disposed of safely and where and when to return the box to hospital.

An unusual complication in one patient with rheumatoid arthritis and thyroid cancer was due to indwelling gold needles, which caused artifacts in the Bone I^{131} scan, similar to metastases.[144]

Any patient in whom acupuncture produces persistently short-lived relief merits further investigation in case this indicates disease progression.

Patients should not be given unrealistic expectations about the likely benefits of acupuncture (or any other complementary and alternative treatment). Inappropriate advice and counselling, which project guilt on to them over the cause of their cancer, are particularly harmful in this most vulnerable population.

Finally, many patients receiving acupuncture for pain describe *positive* side-effects,[138,145] with coincidental improvement of a wide variety of other conditions including hay fever, migraine, dumping syndrome, psoriasis, prostatism, and many more. This is a contrast of welcome side-effects!

Contraindications

Acupuncture needling is contraindicated in the area of an unstable spine due to metastatic disease, acute injury, or osteomyelitis in a patient with good neurological function below that level. It is safe to treat mild degenerative conditions, osteoporosis, or areas of old injury. There is the serious theoretical danger of removal of the protective muscle spasm around the unstable area, with ensuing danger of further compression or transection.[80] TENS is a useful alternative for local pain relief in these cases. However, acupuncture given to points in the legs of a patient has relieved excruciating hyperpathia, associated with vertebral metastasis and cord compression, and helped the pain disappear for up to 2 weeks per treatment. The mechanism may be similar to the use of regional sympathetic blockade in a limb to relieve central pain states.[110]

It is inadvisable to needle superficial sites of tumour growth and the affected limbs of a patient with moderate to severe lymphoedema. In practice, extremely gentle treatment with a 36-g needle does not seem to be problematic in an area of very mild lymphoedema for pain conditions.

Grossly abnormal clotting function is a contraindication and particularly if a patient bruises spontaneously. Superficial needling in patients with a platelet count above 20 000 may be permissible as with patients with a prolonged prothrombin time, within reason. It is contraindicated to use *electro*acupuncture in patients with a pacemaker, and many practitioners beware of treating patients with strong points or near the low back and abdomen during pregnancy to avoid inducing a miscarriage.

It should go without saying not to needle into or directly over a prosthesis, for example, breast implant, or directly over an intracranial deficit.

Neuroanatomy and neuropharmacology of acupuncture

During the past two decades considerable progress has been made with the study of the neuroanatomy and neuropharmacology of nociceptive systems including the possible mechanisms of both acupuncture and TENS. Figure 5 shows a diagram of the neuroanatomical and neuropharmacological basis of pain and the way in which this is modified by acupuncture and also by TENS. The diagram is based on the writings of Duggan and Foong,[146] Bowsher,[147,148] Han and Terenius,[22] Le Bars et al.,[149] Fields and Basbaum,[150] Jones et al.,[151] and Dickenson.[152] So-called 'first', 'rapid', or 'aversive' pain is due to the activation of small myelinated A delta fibres whereas 'second', 'slow', or 'tissue damage' pain is due to activation of mostly unmyelinated C fibres with activation of some A delta fibres.[147]

There are four conditions to be considered:

1. *Pathways for tissue damage pain:* peripheral polymodal nociceptor afferents (C) are activated as the result of, for example, a painful scar (as depicted in Fig. 5). The C fibre afferents terminate in the Substantia Gelatinosa (SG) (lamina II) where their axon terminals release the fast excitatory transmitters glutamate (GLU) and calcitonin gene related peptide (CGRP), and the slow excitatory transmitters Substance P (SP) or Vasoactive Intestinal Peptide (VIP), according to whether these arise from skin or viscera, respectively. The SG indirectlyexcitesTransmission cells (T) deep in the spinal grey matter whose axons form the spinoreticular tract and which constitutes one component of the crossed anterolateral funiculus which ascends to the brain. The spinoreticular tract sends collaterals to the hypothalamus (triggering autonomic responses to pain) and then synapses in the thalamus. In the latter it excites other neurones which are distributed widely over the cerebral cortex including the frontal cortex and also the limbic system, which give rise to the conscious sensation and emotional experience of tissue-damage (second) pain.
2. *Segmental acupuncture:* high threshold mechanoreceptors connected to small myelinated primary afferents (A delta) are activated by acupuncture. One central branch of the A delta afferent excites the inhibitory enkephalinergic interneuron (on the borders of laminae I and II), releasing enkephalin (Enk) which produces post-synaptic block of the SG cell. This prevents the onward transmission of noxiously generated information. This mechanism would explain segmental acupuncture.
3. *Extra-segmental acupuncture:* Waldeyer cells (W) in lamina I of the spinal grey matter are excited by acupuncture via another central branch of A delta primary afferents. The axons of the Waldeyer cells constitute another component (spinothalamic tract) of the crossed anterolateral funiculus and convey pin-prick information to consciousness through the ventral posterolateral nucleus of the thalamus and thence to the somatosensory cortex (where there is somatotopic representation). Collaterals excite the periaqueductal grey (PAG) which in its turn projects to the nucleus Raphe Magnus (nRM) situated in the midline of the lower brainstem reticular formation.

   Serotinergic (5HT) and adrenergic (Nad) axons of nRM cells descend through the dorsolateral funiculus of the spinal cord to synapse eventually with the cells described above and so block the onward transmission of noxiously generated information in the same manner as does segmental acupuncture. However, this descending inhibitory pathway gives off these connections *at all levels of the spinal cord* thereby explaining the extra-segmental effect of acupuncture.
4. *TENS*: By contrast with acupuncture, electrical stimulation excites A beta afferents connected to tactile receptors. After entering the spinal cord, these afferents ultimately ascend in the dorsal columns. However, at spinal cord level these A beta afferent fibres give collaterals which synapse with short interneurons, the endings of which end in proximity to the terminations of the C fibres as the latter synapse with SG cells. These interneurons release gamma-amino butyric acid (GABA) which causes presynaptic blockade of the C afferents thereby preventing them from exciting the SG cells and so blocking the onward transmission of nociceptive information. The elegant demonstration by Garrison and Foreman[153] that TENS decreases the activity of spontaneous and noxiously evoked dorsal horn cells is in accord with this explanation.

Duration of analgesia

A striking and puzzling difference between analgesia produced by acupuncture and TENS is the duration of pain relief. Whereas TENS usually produces analgesia for minutes or hours, acupuncture can, and often does, produce analgesia for weeks. The mechanisms discussed previously cannot account for the prolonged analgesia commonly seen after acupuncture and so some additional mechanisms must be involved. One suggested by Professor Jisheng Han of Beijing Medical University postulates that acupuncture sets up a so-called Meso-Limbic Loop of Analgesia[154] formed by the PAG, the nucleus Accumbens and the Habenula. Han and his colleagues have suggested that acupuncture may set in motion this particular loop of neuronal activity which, whilst it is in motion, blocks the upward transmission of nociceptive impulses from the spinal cord to the thalamus and cortex. In support of this hypothesis, Han and his colleagues[155] have shown that acupuncture analgesia can be blocked by injecting naloxone into any one of the main neuronal stations on the loop. It seems unlikely that naloxone would have this effect unless these areas operate as a loop and are thus interdependent in this way.

Presumably, once the loop has been set in motion it takes some time to slow down and it is during this time that analgesia occurs and so explains its prolonged effect. It is an exciting and novel concept but it remains to be substantiated by further experiments. The sustained effects of acupuncture may be due to up-regulation in analgesic gene expression and 'top-ups' are required to maintain the analgesic genes in a 'switched-on' mode.[28] Most recently, Sandkühler[156] has proposed a cellular mechanism in the spinal dorsal horn that may underlie the long-lasting analgesia that follows electroacupuncture, or *deliberately painful* TENS (intense TENS), of sufficient strength to stimulate Aδ nerve fibres.

Acupuncture, neurotransmitters, and clinical effects

There is now strong evidence that many of the analgesic (and other) effects of acupuncture are due to the action it has on various neurotransmitter

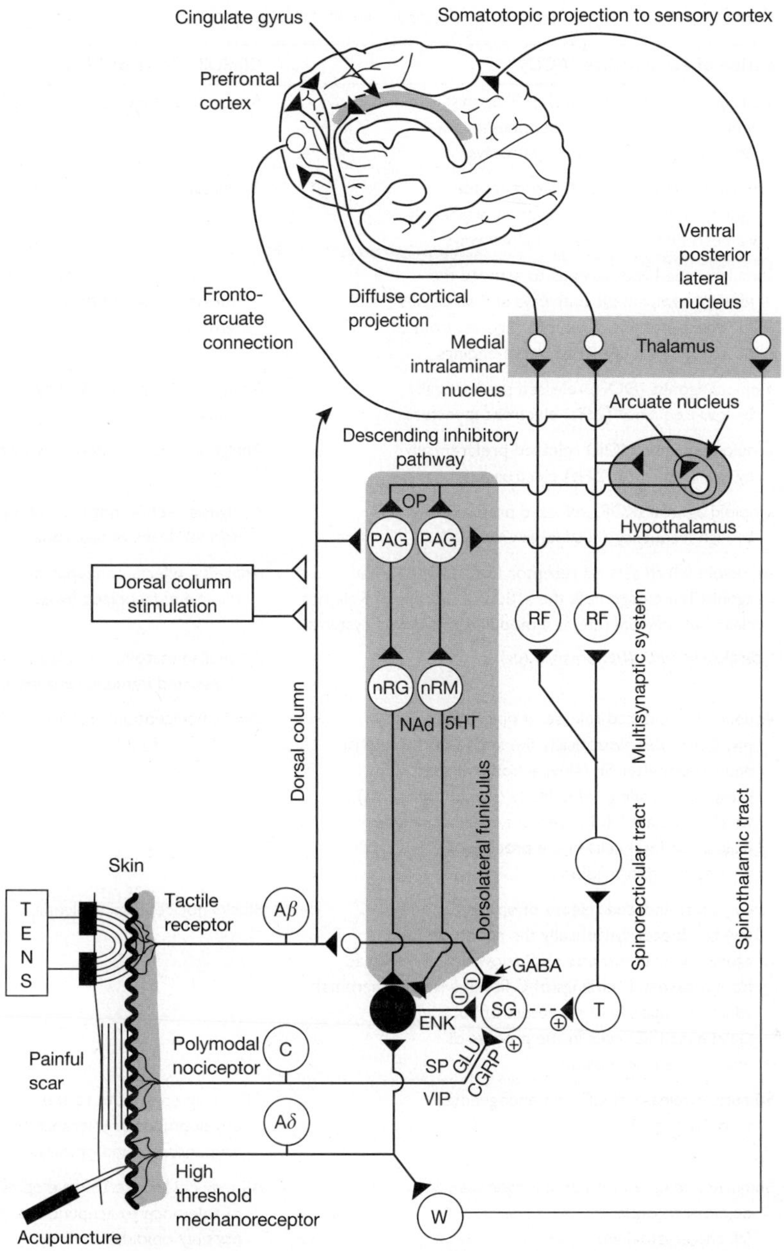

Fig. 5 Diagram to show neuronal circuits involved in acupuncture and TENS analgesia. The afferent pathways involved in transmitting nociceptive information from a painful scar to the higher centres via the dorsal horn, the ascending tracts, and the thalamus are shown. The connections to the descending inhibitory pathways which descend in the dorsolateral funiculus are also shown. The connections to the hypothalamus are indicated. Abbreviations: Aβ, C and Aδ represent the posterior root ganglion cells of Aβ, C, and Aδ fibres, respectively; CGRP = calcitonin gene related peptide; ENK = enkephalinergic neuron; GABA = γ-amino-butyric acid; GLU = glutamate; 5HT = 5-hydroxytryptamine, serotonin; Nad = noradrenaline = norepinephrine; nRG = nucleus raphé gigantocellularis; nRM = nucleus raphé magnus; OP = opioid peptides; PAG = periaqueductal grey; RF = reticular formation; SG = cell in the substantia gelatinosa; SP = substance P; T = transmission cell; VIP = vasoactive intestinal polypeptide; W = Waldeyer cell; + stimulant effect; − inhibitory effect.

systems (see Table 3). When acupuncture is used in palliative care, it is important to keep in mind the possible mechanisms that may or may not operate in an individual patient because this may have important implications for the best regimen to be used. For example, in patients with advanced cancer, the frequency of acupuncture therapy required to maintain analgesia often needs to be increased beyond that used in patients without cancer. It is likely that this is the result of neurotransmitter and immune systems (see Table 3) that are operating at reduced efficiency. This may well account for the different responses observed within and between patients and needs to be anticipated.

Epilogue

Acupuncture is not only of importance in its own right, but also because it has acted as a powerful catalyst in the study of the neurophysiology and neuropharmacology of pain. Acupuncture continues to help lead to a better understanding of the mechanism of pain and analgesia and also to the development of better analgesic agents. Acupuncture has an increasing role in the palliation of non-pain syndromes. While some of the mechanisms of action for these remain uncertain, the success in using a non-drug treatment with minimal side-effects is surely appealing for symptom management in palliative care.

Table 3 Clinical effects produced by the action of acupuncture on neurotransmitters (see also Fig. 5)

Neurotransmitter system	Action of acupuncture (ACU)	Clinical effects of ACU	Refs
5-Hydroxytryptamine (5HT), serotonin	Stimulates the release of this 5HT agonist which acts centrally and peripherally via descending pain inhibitory pathways	Analgesia and elevation of mood	Han and Terenius, 1982[22]
Noradrenaline (Nad), norepinephrine	Stimulates the release of this α receptor agonist which acts centrally and peripherally via descending pain inhibitory pathways	Analgesia	Han and Terenius, 1982[22]
Noradrenaline as transmitter in sympathetic nervous system	Stimulates the hypothalamus to activate the efferent sympathetic pathways and so causes the release of this α receptor agonist from postganglionic adrenergic nerve endings	Circulatory and metabolic effects; normalizes blood flow and skin temperature	Ernst and Lee, 1985;[26] Lundeberg, 1999[27]
met-Enkephalin	δ opioid agonist (DOR) released preferentially by low-frequency (2 Hz) electroacupuncture	Analgesia. Action blocked by naloxone	Han and Sun, 1990;[157] Han et al., 1991[23]
β-Endorphin	μ opioid agonist (MOR) released preferentially by low-frequency (2 Hz) electroacupuncture	Analgesia. Action blocked by naloxone	Han and Sun, 1990;[157] Han et al., 1991[23]
Dynorphin A & B	κ opioid agonist (KOR) released preferentially by high-frequency (100 Hz) EA	Analgesia. Action not blocked by normal doses of naloxone	Han and Sun, 1990;[157] Han et al., 1991[23]
Orphanin OFQ, nociceptin	An opioid which acts on receptor LC132/ORL1 as an agonist but antagonizes the action of morphine. Role not clear, but may operate as a modulator of opioid systems	Analgesic effects of acupuncture may be antagonized by orphanin	Tian et al., 1997[158]
Adrenocorticotrophic hormone (ACTH)	Co-released with β-endorphin (*qv*)	Anti-inflammatory, modulates stress, and immune responses	Roth et al., 1997[25]
Substance P (SP)	Acupuncture-induced release of opioid peptides (*qv*) block post-synaptically the action of the agonist neurotransmitter SP (slow action) released from presynaptic endings of C fibres (somatic afferents) which stimulate NK1 receptors of Substantia Gelatinosa (SG) cells in the process of nociceptive transmission	Blocks nociception; analgesia	Han, 1984;[159] Dickenson, 1996[152]
Vasoactive intestinal peptide (VIP)	Acupuncture-induced release of opioid peptides (*qv*) block post-synaptically the action of the agonist neurotransmitter VIP (slow action) released from presynaptic endings of C fibres (visceral afferents) which stimulate NK1 receptors of Substantia Gelatinosa (SG) cells in the process of nociceptive transmission	Blocks nociception; analgesia	Dickenson, 1996[152]
Cholecystokinin (CCK)	Stimulates release of CCK an endogenous opioid antagonist	CCK may contribute to the development of tolerance to acupuncture (and opioids)	Zhou et al., 1993[160]
Angiotensin II (AII)	Stimulates release of AII an endogenous opioid antagonist (cf. cholecystokinin)	AII may contribute to development of tolerance to acupuncture (and possibly opioids)	Wang and Han, 1990[161]
Calcitonin gene related peptide (CGRP)	Acupuncture-induced release of opioid peptides (*qv*) block post-synaptically this excitatory neurotransmitter released from presynaptic endings of C fibres during nociceptive transmission	Blocks nociception. CGRP is also released peripherally where it plays an important role as a powerful vasodilator	Dickenson, 1996;[152] Lundeberg, 1999[27]
Nerve growth factor (NGF)	Acupuncture may release NGF which increases production of CGRP and VIP	CGRP and VIP influence sensory and autonomic activity	Lundeberg, 1999[27]
Oxytocin	Releases oxytocin from posterior pituitary gland	Analgesia and sedation	Uvnäs-Moberg et al., 1993[24]
γ-Amino butyric acid (GABA)	TENS releases the inhibitory neurotransmitter GABA from endings of gabaergic neurons. Produces presynaptic inhibition of C fibre endings thereby blocking nociceptive transmission	Segmental analgesia	Garrison and Foreman, 1994[153]
Glutamate (GLU)	Acupuncture-induced release of opioid peptides (*qv*) block post-synaptically this excitatory neurotransmitter (fast action) released from presynaptic endings of C fibres during nociceptive transmission	Blocks nociception; analgesia	Dickenson, 1996[152]

Table 3 Continued

Neurotransmitter system	Action of acupuncture (ACU)	Clinical effects of ACU	Refs
Aspartate (ASP)	Acupuncture-induced release of opioid peptides (*qv*) block post-synaptically this excitatory neurotransmitter (fast action) released from presynaptic endings of C fibres during nociceptive transmission	Blocks nociception; analgesia	Dickenson, 1996[152]
Pre-prometenkephalin, pre-prodynorphin (opioid precursors)	Electroacupuncture (EA) modulates mRNA molecules coding for opioid precursors. EA 2 Hz induces the expression of prepromentenkephalin and EA 100 Hz induces the expression of preprodynorphin. Thus, EA may increase the distribution and amount of opioid peptides	This may be one of the mechanisms by which acupuncture induces analgesia of long duration	Guo et al., 1996[28]

Acknowledgements

The authors wish to acknowledge, with grateful thanks, the dedication, secretarial skills, and long suffering efforts of Mrs Jane Brooks during the preparation of this chapter.

References

1. **Melzack, R.** (1994). Folk medicine and the sensory modulation of pain. In *Textbook of Pain* (ed. R. Melzack and P.D. Wall), pp. 1209–17. Edinburgh: Churchill Livingstone.
2. **Beyens, F.** (1998). Reinterpretation of traditional concepts in acupuncture. In *Medical Acupuncture: A Western Scientific Approach* (ed. J. Filshie and A. White), pp. 391–407. Edinburgh: Churchill Livingstone.
3. **Ma, K.W.** (1992). The roots and development of Chinese acupuncture: from prehistory to early 20th century. *Acupuncture in Medicine* **10** (Suppl.), 92–9.
4. **Veith, I.** *The Yellow Emperor's Classic of Internal Medicine.* Berkeley: University of California Press, 1972.
5. **Lu, G.D. and Needham, J.** *Celestial Lancets, a History and Rationale of Acupuncture and Moxa.* Cambridge: Cambridge University Press, 1980.
6. **Dorfer, L.** et al. (1999). A medical report from the stone age? *Lancet* **354** (9183), 1023–5.
7. **Cassileth, B.R. and Brown, H.** (1988). Unorthodox cancer medicine. *CA: A Cancer Journal for Clinicians* **38** (3), 176–86.
8. **Cassileth, B.R. and Chapman, C.C.** (1996). Alternative cancer medicine: a ten-year update. *Cancer Investigation* **14** (4), 396–404.
9. **Sellick, S.M. and Zaza, C.** (1998). Critical review of 5 nonpharmacologic strategies for managing cancer pain. *Cancer Prevention and Control* **2** (1), 7–14.
10. **Woollam, C.H. and Jackson, A.O.** (1998). Acupuncture in the management of chronic pain. *Anaesthesia* **53** (6), 593–5.
11. **Clinical Standards Advisory Group (CSAG).** Services for Patients with Pain, 2000.
12. **Vincent, C.A.** (1992). Acupuncture research: why do it? *Complementary Medical Research* **6** (1), 21–4.
13. **Macdonald, A.J.** (1989). Acupuncture analgesia and therapy. In *Textbook of Pain* (ed. R. Melzack and P.D. Wall), pp. 906–19. Edinburgh: Churchill Livingstone.
14. **Ma, K.W.** (2000). Acupuncture: its place in the history of Chinese medicine. *Acupuncture in Medicine* **18** (2), 88–99.
15. **Mann, F.** *Acupuncture: The Ancient Chinese Art of Healing.* London: Heinemann, 1972.
16. **Ashton, H., Ebenezer, I., Golding, J.F., and Thompson, J.W.** (1984). Effects of acupuncture and transcutaneous electrical nerve stimulation on cold-induced pain in normal subjects. *Journal of Psychosomatic Research* **28** (4), 301–8.
17. **Chiang, C.-Y., Chang, C.-T., Chu, H.-L., and Yang, L.-F.** (1973). Peripheral afferent pathway for acupuncture analgesia. *Scientica Sinica* **16**, 210–17.
18. **Research Group of Acupuncture Anaesthesia** (1973). Effect of acupuncture on pain threshold of human skin. *Chinese Medical Journal* **3**, 151–7.
19. **Dundee, J.W. and Ghaly, G.** (1991). Local anesthesia blocks the antiemetic action of P6 acupuncture. *Clinical Pharmacology and Therapeutics* **50**, 78–80.
20. **Sjolund, B., Terenius, L., and Eriksson, M.** (1977). Increased cerebrospinal fluid levels of endorphins after electroacupuncture. *Acta Physiologica Scandinavica* **100** (3), 382–4.
21. **Clement-Jones, V., McLoughlin, L., Tomlin, S., Besser, G.M., Rees, L.H., and Wen, H.L.** (1980). Increased beta-endorphin but not met-enkephalin levels in human cerebrospinal fluid after acupuncture for recurrent pain. *Lancet* **2** (8201), 946–9.
22. **Han, J.S. and Terenius, L.** (1982). Neurochemical basis of acupuncture analgesia. *Annual Review of Pharmacology and Toxicology* **22**, 193–220.
23. **Han, J.S.** et al. (1991). Effect of low- and high-frequency TENS on Met-enkephalin-Arg-Phe and dynorphin A immunoreactivity in human lumbar CSF. *Pain* **47** (3), 295–8.
24. **Uvnäs-Moberg, K., Bruzelius, G., Alster, P., and Lundeberg, T.** (1993). The antinociceptive effect of non-noxious sensory stimulation is mediated partly through oxytocinergic mechanisms. *Acta Physiologica Scandinavica* **149** (2), 199–204.
25. **Roth, L.U., Maret-Maric, A., and Adler, R.H.** (1997). Acupuncture points have subjective (needling sensation) and objective (serum cortisol increase) specificity. *Acupuncture in Medicine* **15** (1), 2–5.
26. **Ernst, M. and Lee, M.H.** (1985). Sympathetic vasomotor changes induced by manual and electrical acupuncture of the Hoku point visualized by thermography. *Pain* **21** (1), 25–33.
27. **Lundeberg, T.** (1999). Effects of sensory stimulation (acupuncture) on circulatory and immune systems. In *Acupuncture: A Scientific Appraisal* (ed. E. Ernst and A. White), pp. 93–106. Oxford: Butterworth-Heinemann.
28. **Guo, H.F., Tian, J., Wang, X., Fang, Y., Hou, Y., and Han, J.** (1996). Brain substrates activated by electroacupuncture of different frequencies (I): comparative study on the expression of oncogene c-fos and genes coding for three opioid peptides. *Brain Research. Molecular Brain Research* **43** (1–2), 157–66.
29. **Travell, J.G. and Simons, D.G.** *Myofascial Pain and Dysfunction. The Trigger Point Manual.* Baltimore: Williams and Wilkins; 1983.
30. **Filshie, J. and Cummings, M.** (1999). Western medical acupuncture. In *Acupuncture: A Scientific Appraisal* (ed. E. Ernst and A. White), pp. 31–59. Oxford: Butterworth-Heinemann.
31. **Melzack, R., Stillwell, D.M., and Fox, E.J.** (1977). Trigger points and acupuncture points for pain: correlations and implications. *Pain* **3** (1), 3–23.
32. **McNulty, W.H., Gevirtz, R.N., Hubbard, D.R., and Berkoff, G.M.** (1994). Needle electromyographic evaluation of trigger point response to a psychological stressor. *Psychophysiology* **31** (3), 313–16.
33. **Baldry, P.E.** *Myofascial Pain and Fibromyalgia Syndromes.* Edinburgh: Churchill Livingstone, 2001.
34. **Mann F.** *Reinventing Acupuncture.* London: Butterworth Heinemann, 2000.
35. *Essentials of Chinese Acupuncture.* Beijing: Foreign Languages Press, 1980.
36. **Stux, G. and Hammerschlag, R.** *Scientific Basis of Acupuncture.* Berlin: Springer-Verlag, 2000.
37. **Baldry, P.E.** *Acupuncture, Trigger Points and Musculo-Skeletal Pain.* Edinburgh: Churchill Livingstone, 1993.

38. **Campbell, A.** *Acupuncture in Practice.* London: Butterworth Heinemann, 2001.
39. **White, A.** (1998). Electroacupuncture and acupuncture analgesia. In *Medical Acupuncture: A Western Scientific Approach* (ed. J. Filshie and A. White), pp. 153–75. Edinburgh: Churchill Livingstone.
40. **Deluze, C., Bosia, L., Zirbs, A., Chantraine, A., and Vischer, T.L.** (1992). Electroacupuncture in fibromyalgia: results of a controlled trial. *British Medical Journal* **305** (6864), 1249–52.
41. **Brockhaus, A. and Elger, C.E.** (1990). Hypalgesic efficacy of acupuncture on experimental pain in man. Comparison of laser acupuncture and needle acupuncture. *Pain* **43**, 181–5.
42. **White, A.** (1999). Neurophysiology of acupuncture analgesia. In *Acupuncture: A Scientific Appraisal* (ed. E. Ernst and A. White), pp. 60–92. Oxford: Butterworth-Heinemann.
43. **Price, D.D., Rafii, A., Watkins, L.R., and Buckingham, B.** (1984). A psychophysical analysis of acupuncture analgesia. *Pain* **19** (1), 27–42.
44. **Christensen, P.A., Noreng, M., Andersen, P.E., and Nielsen, J.W.** (1989). Electroacupuncture and postoperative pain. *British Journal of Anaesthesia* **62** (3), 258–62.
45. **Pontinen, P.J.** *Lower Level Laser Therapy as a Medical Treatment Modality: A Manual for Physicians, Dentists, Physiotherapists and Veterinary Surgeons.* Tampere: Art Upo Ltd, 1992.
46. **Baldry, P.** Laser Therapy. In *Medical Acupuncture: A Western Scientific Approach* (ed. J. Filshie and A. White), pp. 193–201. Edinburgh: Churchill Livingstone.
47. **Brosseau, L., Welch, V., Wells, G., deBie, R., Gam, A., Harman, K., Morin, M., Shea, B., and Tugwell, P.** Low Level Laser Therapy (Classes I, II & III) for Treating Osteoarthritis (Cochrane Review). *The Cochrane Library* (1), 2002. Oxford, Update Software.
48. **Brosseau, L., Welch, V., Wells, G., deBie, R., Gam, A., Harman, K., Morin, M., Shea, B., and Tugwell, P.** Low Level Laser Therapy (Classes I, II & III) for Treating Rheumatoid Arthritis (Cochrane Review). *The Cochrane Library* (1), 2002. Oxford, Update Software.
49. **Price, H., Lewith, G., and Williams, C.** (1991). Acupressure as an antiemetic in cancer chemotherapy. *Complementary Medical Research* **5**, 93–4.
50. **Nogier, P.F.M.** *Treatise of Auriculotherapy.* France: Maisonneuve, 1972.
51. **Oleson, T.D., Kroening, R.J., and Bresler, D.E.** (1980). An experimental evaluation of auricular diagnosis: the somatotopic mapping of musculoskeletal pain at ear acupuncture points. *Pain* **8**, 217–29.
52. **Lewith, G. and Vincent, C.A.** (1998). The clinical evaluation of acupuncture. In *Medical Acupuncture: A Western Scientific Approach* (ed. J. Filshie and A. White), pp. 205–24. Edinburgh: Churchill Livingstone.
53. **Nakatari, Y., Yamashita, K.** *Ryodoraku Acupuncture.* Ryodoraku Research Institute Ltd, 1977.
54. **Klide, A.M. and Shin, H.K.** *Veterinary Acupuncture.* Pennsylvania: Pennsylvania Press, 1986.
55. **Schoen, A.** *Veterinary Acupuncture, Ancient Art of Modern Medicine.* New York: Mosby, 1994.
56. **Filshie, J. and White, A.**, ed. *Medical Acupuncture: A Western Scientific Approach.* Edinburgh: Churchill Livingstone, 1998.
57. **Ernst, E. and White, A.**, ed. *Acupuncture: A Scientific Appraisal.* Oxford: Butterworth-Heinemann, 1999.
58. **Kleinhenz, J., Streitberger, K., Windeler, J., Gussbacher, A., Mavridis, G., and Martin, E.** (1999). Randomised clinical trial comparing the effects of acupuncture and a newly designed placebo needle in rotator cuff tendinitis. *Pain* **83** (2), 235–41.
59. **ter Riet, G., de Craen, A.J., de Boer, A., and Kessels, A.G.** (1998). Is placebo analgesia mediated by endogenous opioids? A systematic review. *Pain* **76** (3), 273–5.
60. **Thomas, M., Eriksson, S.V., and Lundeberg, T.** (1991). A comparative study of diazepam and acupuncture in patients with osteoarthritis pain: a placebo controlled study. *American Journal of Chinese Medicine* **19**, 95–100.
61. **Patel, M., Gutzwiller, F., Paccaud, F., and Marazzi, A.** (1989). A meta-analysis of acupuncture for chronic pain. *International Journal of Epidemiology* **18** (4), 900–6.
62. **ter Riet, G., Kleijnen, J., and Knipschild, P.** (1990). Acupuncture and chronic pain: a criteria-based meta-analysis. *Journal of Clinical Epidemiology* **43** (11), 1191–9.
63. **Ezzo, J., Berman, B., Hadhazy, V.A., Jadad, A.R., Lao, L., and Singh, B.B.** (2000). Is acupuncture effective for the treatment of chronic pain? A systematic review. *Pain* **86** (3), 217–25.
64. **Vickers, A.J.** (1996). Can acupuncture have specific effects on health? A systematic review of acupuncture antiemesis trials. *Journal of the Royal Society of Medicine* **89**, 303–11.
65. **Ernst, E. and Pittler, M.H.** (1998). The effectiveness of acupuncture in treating acute dental pain: a systematic review. *British Dental Journal* **184** (9), 443–7.
66. **Melchart, D.** et al. (1999). Acupuncture for recurrent headaches: a systematic review of randomized controlled trials. *Cephalalgia* **19** (9), 779–86.
67. **Berman, B., Ezzo, J., Hadhazy, V., and Swyers, J.P.** (1999). Is acupuncture effective in the treatment of fibromyalgia? *Journal of Family Practice* **48**, 213–18.
68. **Ernst, E. and White, A.R.** (1998). Acupuncture for back pain: a meta-analysis of randomized controlled trials. *Archives of Internal Medicine* **158** (20), 2235–41.
69. **Smith, L.A., Oldman, A.D., McQuay, H.J., and Moore, R.A.** (2000). Teasing apart quality and validity in systematic reviews: an example from acupuncture trials in chronic neck and back pain. *Pain* **86** (1–2), 119–32.
70. **Cummings, M.** (2000). Teasing apart the quality and validity in systematic reviews of acupuncture. *Acupuncture in Medicine* **18** (2), 104–7.
71. **Cummings, M.** (1996). Audit in acupuncture practice: a computerised audit of acupuncture in two populations: civilian and forces. *Acupuncture in Medicine* **14** (1), 37–9.
72. **Stellon, A.** (2001). An audit of acupuncture in a single-handed general practice over one year. *Acupuncture in Medicine* **19** (1), 36–42.
73. **Freedman, J.** (2002). An audit of 500 acupuncture patients in general practice. *Acupuncture in Medicine* **20** (1), 30–4.
74. **Ross, J.** (2001). An audit of the impact of introducing microacupuncture into primary care. *Acupuncture in Medicine* **19** (1), 43–5.
75. **Christensen, B.V., Iuhl, I.U., Vilbek, H., Bulow, H.H., Dreijer, N.C., and Rasmussen, H.F.** (1992). Acupuncture treatment of severe knee osteoarthrosis. A long-term study. *Acta Anaesthesiologica Scandinavica* **36** (6), 519–25.
76. **Lindall, S.** (1999). Is acupuncture for pain relief in general practice cost-effective? *Acupuncture in Medicine* **17** (2), 97–100.
77. **Poulain, P., Pichard Leandri, E., Laplanche, A., Montange, F., Bouzy, J., and Truffa-Bachi, J.** (1997). Electroacupuncture analgesia in major abdominal and pelvic surgery: a randomised study. *Acupuncture in Medicine* **XV** (1), 10–13.
78. **Aldridge, S.** Acupuncture helps breast cancer patients (abstract). *American Society of Anaesthesiologists Annual Scientific Session*, 2001.
79. **Filshie, J. and Redman, D.** (1985). Acupuncture and malignant pain problems. *European Journal Surgical Oncology* **11** (4), 389–94.
80. **Filshie, J.** (1990). Acupuncture for malignant pain. *Acupuncture in Medicine* **8** (2), 38–9.
81. **Bowsher, D., Mumford, J., Lipton, S., and Miles, J.** (1973). Treatment of intractable pain by acupuncture. *Lancet* **2**, 57–60.
82. **Wen, H.L.** (1977). Cancer pain treated with acupuncture and electrical stimulation. *Modern Medicine in Asia* **13** (2), 12–16.
83. **Aung, S.** (1994). The clinical use of acupuncture in oncology: symptom control. *Acupuncture in Medicine* **12** (1), 37–40.
84. **Leng, G.** (1999). A year of acupuncture in palliative care. *Palliative Medicine* **13**, 163–4.
85. **Johnstone, P.A.S., Polston, G.R., Niemtzow, R.C., and Martin, P.J.** (2002). Integration of acupuncture into the oncology clinic. *Palliative Medicine* **16**, 235–9.
86. **Filshie, J., Scase, A., Ashley, S., and Hood, J.** A study of the acupuncture effects on pain, anxiety and depression in patients with breast cancer (abstract). *Pain Society Meeting*, 1997.
87. **Watson, M., Haviland, J.S., Greer, S., Davidson, J., and Bliss, J.M.** (1999). Influence of psychological response on survival in breast cancer: a population-based cohort study. *Lancet* **354**, 1331–6.
88. **He, J.P., Friedrich, M., Ertan, A.K., Muller, K., and Schmidt, W.** (1999). Pain-relief and movement improvement by acupuncture after ablation and axillary lymphadenectomy in patients with mammary cancer. *Clinical Experimental Obstetrics and Gynecology* **26** (2), 81–4.

89. **Xue, C.C.** (1986). Acupuncture induced phantom limb and meridian phenomenon in acquired and congenital amputees. A suggestion of the use of acupuncture as a method for investigation of phantom limb. *Chinese Medical Journal (English)* **99** (3), 247–52.
90. **Monga, T.N. and Jaksic, T.** (1981). Acupuncture in phantom limb pain. *Archives of Physical Medicine and Rehabilitation* **62** (5), 229–31.
91. **Filshie, J. and Cummings, M.** Acupuncture. *Management of Phantom Limb Pain—The First International Consensus Meeting, Oxford University*, 2000.
92. **Dillon, M. and Lucas, C.F.** (1999). Auricular stud acupuncture in palliative care patients: an initial report. *Palliative Medicine* **13** (3), 253–4.
93. **Alimi, D., Rubino, C., Leandri, E.P., and Brule, S.F.** (2000). Analgesic effects of auricular acupuncture for cancer pain. *Journal of Pain and Symptom Management* **19** (2), 81–2.
94. **Cummings, M.** (2001). Percutaneous electrical nerve stimulation—electroacupuncture by another name? A comparative review. *Acupuncture in Medicine* **19** (1), 32–5.
95. **Ahmed, H.E., Craig, W.F., White, P.F., and Huber, P.** (1998). Percutaneous electrical nerve stimulation (PENS): a complementary therapy for the management of pain secondary to bony metastasis. *Clinical Journal of Pain* **14** (4), 320–3.
96. **Wang, K. and Han, J.S.** (1990). Accelerated synthesis and release of angiotensin II in the rat brain during electroacupuncture tolerance. *Science in China* **B33** (6), 686–93.
97. **Zhou, Y., Sun, Y.H., Shen, J.M., and Han, J.S.** (1993). Increased release of immunoreactive CCK-8 by electroacupuncture and enhancement of electroacupuncture analgesia by CCK-B antagonist in rat spinal cord. *Neuropeptides* **24** (3), 139–44.
98. **Jobst, K.** et al. (1986). Controlled trial of acupuncture for disabling breathlessness. *Lancet* **2** (8521–22), 1416–19.
99. **Filshie, J., Penn, K., Ashley, S., and Davis, C.L.** (1996). Acupuncture for the relief of cancer-related breathlessness. *Palliative Medicine* **10** (2), 145–50.
100. **Davis, C.L., Lewith, G.T., Broomfield, J., and Prescott, P.** (2001). A pilot project to assess the methodological issues involved in evaluating acupuncture as a treatment for disabling breathlessness. *Journal of Alternative and Complementary Medicine* **7** (6), 633–9.
101. **Maa, S.-H., Gauthier, D., and Turner, M.** (1997). Acupressure as an adjunct to a pulmonary rehabilitation program. *Journal of Cadiopulmonary Rehabilitation* **17**, 268–76.
102. **McMillan, C.M.** (1998). Acupuncture for nausea and vomiting. In *Medical Acupuncture: A Western Scientific Approach* (ed. J. Filshie and A. White), pp. 295–317. Edinburgh: Churchill Livingstone.
103. **McMillan, C.M. and Dundee, J.W.** (1991). The role of transcutaneous electrical stimulation of Neiguan antiemetic acupuncture point in controlling sickness after cancer chemotherapy. *Physiotherapy* **77**, 499–502.
104. **McMillan, C.M., Dundee, J.W., and Abram, W.P.** (1991). Enhancement of the antiemetic action of Ondansetron by transcutaneous electrical stimulation of the P6 antiemetic points in patients having highly emetic cytotoxic drugs. *British Journal of Cancer* **64**, 971–2.
105. **Shen, J.** et al. (2000). Electroacupuncture for control of myeloablative chemotherapy-induced emesis: A randomized controlled trial. *Journal of the American Medical Association* **284** (21), 2755–61.
106. **Wang, X.J., Wang, X.H., and Han, J.S.** (1990). Cholecystokinin octapeptide antagonized opioid analgesia mediated by mu- and kappa-but not delta-receptors in the spinal cord of the rat. *Brain Research* **523** (1), 5–10.
107. **Blom, M., Dawidson, I., Fernberg, J.O., Johnson, G., and Angmar-Mansson, B.** (1996). Acupuncture treatment of patients with radiation-induced xerostomia. *European Journal of Cancer. Part B, Oral Oncology* **32B** (3), 182–90.
108. **Johnstone, P.A.S., Peng, Y.P., May, B.C., Inouye, W.S., and Niemtzow, R.C.** (2001). Acupuncture for pilocarpine-resistant xerostomia following radiotherapy for head and neck malignancies. *International Journal of Radiation Oncology, Biology, Physics* **50** (2), 353–7.
109. **Rydholm, M. and Strang, P.** (1999). Acupuncture for patients in hospital-based home care suffering from xerostomia. *Journal of Palliative Care* **15** (4), 20–3.
110. **Loh, L., Nathan, P.W., and Schott, G.D.** (1981). Pain due to lesions of central nervous system removed by sympathetic block. *British Medical Journal* **282**, 1026–8.
111. **Johansson, K., Lindgren, I., Widner, H., Wiklund, I., and Johansson, B.B.** (1993). Can sensory stimulation improve the functional outcome in stroke patients? *Neurology* **43** (11), 2189–92.
112. **Magnusson, M., Johansson, K., and Johansson, B.B.** (1994). Sensory stimulation promotes normalization of postural control after stroke. *Stroke* **25** (6), 1176–80.
113. **Park, J., Hopwood, V., White, A.R., and Ernst, E.** (2001). Effectiveness of acupuncture for stroke: a systematic review. *Journal of Neurology* **248** (7), 558–63.
114. **Wyon, Y., Lindgren, R., Lundeberg, T., and Hammar, M.** (1995). Effects of acupuncture on climacteric vasomotor symptoms, quality of life, and urinary excretion of neuropeptides among post menopausal women. *Menopause* **2** (1), 3–12.
115. **Cumins, S.M. and Brunt, A.M.** (2000). Does acupuncture influence the vasomotor symptoms experienced by breast cancer patients taking tamoxifen? *Acupuncture in Medicine* **18** (1), 28.
116. **Towlerton, G., Filshie, J., O'Brien, M., and Duncan, A.** (1999). Acupuncture in the control of vasomotor symptoms caused by tamoxifen (letter). *Palliative Medicine* **13** (5), 445.
117. **Hammar, M., Frisk, J., Grimas, O., Hook, M., Spetz, A.-C., and Wyon, Y.** (1999). Acupuncture treatment of vasomotor symptoms in men with prostatic carcinoma: a pilot study. *The Journal of Urology* **161**, 853–6.
118. **Ruzhen, F.** (1984). Relief of oesophageal carcinomatous obstruction by acupuncture. *Journal of Traditional Chinese Medicine* **4** (1), 3–4.
119. **Liansheng, Y.** (1988). Treatment of persistent hiccupping with electro-acupuncture at 'hiccup-relieving' point. *Journal of Traditional Chinese Medicine* **8** (1), 29–30.
120. **Wong, S.K.A.** (1983). Treatment of hiccough by acupuncture—a report of two cases. *Medical Journal of Malaysia* **38** (1), 80–1.
121. **Zhang, Z.U.** (1987). Effect of acupuncture on 44 cases of radiation rectitis following radiation therapy for carcinoma of the cervix uteri. *Journal of Traditional Chinese Medicine* **7** (2), 139–40.
122. **Lundeberg, T., Bondesson, L., and Thomas, M.** (1987). Effect of acupuncture on experimentally induced itch. *British Journal of Dermatology* **117** (6), 771–7.
123. **Duo, L.J.** (1987). Electrical needle therapy of uremic pruritus. *Nephron* **47** (3), 179–83.
124. **Greene, K.B., Berger, J., Reeves, C., Moffat, A., Standish, L.J., and Calabrese, C.** (1999). Most frequently used alternative and complementary therapies and activities by participants in the AMCOA study. *Journal of the Association of Nurses in AIDS Care* **10** (3), 60–73.
125. **Standish, L.J.** et al. (2001). Alternative medicine use in HIV-positive men and women: demographics, utilization patterns and health status. *AIDS Care* **13** (2), 197–208.
126. **Phillips, K.D. and Skelton, W.D.** (2001). Effects of individualized acupuncture on sleep quality in HIV disease. *Journal of the Association of Nurses in AIDS Care* **12** (1), 27–39.
127. **Shlay, C.J.** et al. (1998). Acupuncture and amitriptyline for pain due to HIV-related peripheral neuropathy. *Journal of the American Medical Association* **280**, 1590–5.
128. **Jonsdottir, I.H.** (1999). Physical exercise, acupuncture and immune function. *Acupuncture in Medicine* **17** (1), 50–3.
129. **Gollub, R.L., Hui, K.K., and Stefano, G.B.** (1999). Acupuncture: pain management coupled to immune stimulation. *Zhongguo Yao Li Xue Bao* **20** (9), 769–77.
130. **Hechun, L., Yunkui, J., and Li, Z.** (1985). Electro-acupuncture versus amitriptyline in the treatment of depressive state. *Journal of Traditional Chinese Medicine* **5** (1), 3–8.
131. **Han, J.S.** (1986). Electroacupuncture: an alternative to antidepressants for treating affective diseases? *International Journal of Neuroscience* **29** (1–2), 79–92.
132. **Lazarou, J., Pomeranz, B.H., and Corey, P.N.** (1998). Incidence of adverse drug reactions in hospitalized patients: a meta-analysis of prospective studies. *Journal of the American Medical Association* **279** (15), 1200–5.
133. **Rampes, H. and James, R.** (1995). Complications of acupuncture. *Acupuncture in Medicine* **13** (1), 26–33.
134. **Peuker, E. and Grönemeyer, D.** (2001). Rare but serious complications of acupuncture: traumatic lesions. *Acupuncture in Medicine* **19** (2), 103–8.

135. **Walsh, B.** (2001). Control of infection in acupuncture. *Acupuncture in Medicine* **19** (2), 109–11.

136. **Filshie, J.** (2001). Safety aspects of acupuncture in palliative care. *Acupuncture in Medicine* **19** (2), 117–22.

137. **White, A., Hayhoe, S., Hart, A., and Ernst, E.** (2001). Survey of adverse events following acupuncture (SAFA): a prospective study of 32 000 consultations. *Acupuncture in Medicine* **19** (2), 84–92.

138. **MacPherson, H., Thomas, K., Walters, S., and Fitter, M.** (2001). A prospective survey of adverse events and treatment reactions following 34 000 consultations with professional acupuncturists. *Acupuncture in Medicine* **19** (2), 93–102.

139. **Spelman, D.W., Weinmann, A., and Spicer, W.J.** (1993). Endocarditis following skin procedures. *Journal of Infection* **26**, 185–9.

140. **Kent, G.P., Brondum, J., Keenlyside, R.A., LaFazia, L.M., and Scott, H.D.** (1988). A large outbreak of acupuncture-associated hepatitis B. *American Journal Epidemiology* **127** (3), 591–8.

141. **Slater, P.E.** et al. (1988). An acupuncture-associated outbreak of hepatitis B in Jerusalem. *European Journal of Epidemiology* **4** (3), 322–5.

142. (1998). CDSC. Outbreak of Hepatitis B associated with autohaemotherapy: update. *Communicable Disease Report, CDR Weekly* **8** (13), 113.

143. **Filshie, J.** (2000). Acupuncture in palliative care. *European Journal of Palliative Care* **7** (2), 41–4.

144. **Otsuka, N.** et al. (1990). Iodine-131 uptake in a patient with thyroid cancer and rheumatoid arthritis during acupuncture treatment. *Clinical Nuclear Medicine* **15**, 29–31.

145. **Odsberg, A., Schill, U., and Haker, E.** (2001). Acupuncture treatment: side effects and complications reported by Swedish physiotherapists. *Complementary Therapies in Medicine* **9** (1), 17–20.

146. **Duggan, A.W. and Foong, F.W.** (1985). Bicuculline and spinal inhibition produced by dorsal column stimulation in the cat. *Pain* **22**, 249–59.

147. **Bowsher, D.** (1985). Sensory mechanisms. In Frederiks, J.A.M. (ed.) *Clinical Neuropsychology* 45, 227–44. In *Handbook of Clinical Neurology* (ed. P.J. Vinken, G.W. Bruyn, and H.L. Klawans) **1** (45). Amsterdam: Elsevier.

148. **Bowsher, D.** (1987). The physiology of acupuncture. *Journal of the Intractable Pain Society of Great Britain and Ireland* **5**, 15–18.

149. **Le Bars, D., Dickenson, A.H., and Besson, J.M.** (1979). Diffuse noxious inhibitory controls (DNIC). II Lack of effect on non-convergent neurones, supraspinal involvement and theoretical implications. *Pain* **6**, 305–27.

150. **Fields, H.L. and Basbaum, A.L.** (1994). Central nervous system mechanisms of pain modulation. In *Textbook of Pain* 3rd edn (ed. P.D. Wall and R. Melzack), Chapter 12. Edinburgh: Churchill Livingstone.

151. **Jones, A.K.P.** et al. (1991). Cortical and subcortical localisation of response to pain in man using positron emission tomography. *Proceedings of the Royal Society of London, Series B* **244**, 39–44.

152. **Dickenson, A.H.** (1996). Pain mechanisms and pain syndromes. In *Pain 1996—an updated review* (ed. J.N. Campbell), pp. 113–21. Seattle: International Association for the Study of Pain.

153. **Garrison, D.W. and Foreman, R.D.** (1994). Decreased activity of spontaneous and noxiously evoked dorsal horn cells during transcutaneous electrical nerve stimulation (TENS). *Pain* **58**, 309–15.

154. **Han, J.S., Yu, L.C., and Shi, Y.S.** (1986). A Mesolimbic loop of analgesia. III A neuronal pathway from nucleus accumbens to periaquaductal grey. *Asian Pacific Journal of Pharmacology* **1**, 7–22.

155. **Zhou, Z.F., Du, M.Y., Wu, W.Y., Jiang, Y., and Han, J.S.** (1981). Effects of intracerebral microinjection of naloxone on acupuncture and morphine analgesia in the rabbit. *Scientia Sinica* **24**, 1166–78.

156. **Sandkühler, J.** (2000). Long-lasting analgesia following TENS and acupuncture: spinal mechanisms beyond gate control. In Proc. 9th World Congress on Pain, *Progress in Pain Research ands Management* Vol. 16 (ed. M. Devor, N.C. Rowbotham, and Z. Wiesenfeld-Hallin), pp. 359–69. International Association for the Study of Pain, Seattle.

157. **Han, J.S. and Sun, S.** (1990). Differential release of enkephalin and dynorphin by low and high frequencies electroacupuncture in the central nervous system. *Acupuncture: The Scientific International Journal (New York)* **1** (1), 19–27.

158. **Tian, J.** et al. (1997). Involvement of endogenous orphanin FQ in electroacupuncture-induced analgesia. *Neuroreport* **8**, 497–500.

159. **Han, J.S.** (1984). Progress in the pharmacological studies of acupuncture analgesia. *9th International Congress of Pharmacology* (ed. S.W. Paton et al.), London, Macmillan Proceedings, Vol. 1.

160. **Zhou, Y.** et al. (1993). Increased release of immunoreactive CCK-8 by electroacupuncture and enhancement of electroacupuncture analgesia by CCK-B antagonist in rat spinal cord. *Neuropeptides* **24**, 139–44.

161. **Wang, K. and Han, J.S.** (1990). Accelerated synthesis and release of angiotensin II in the rat brain during electroacupuncture tolerance. *Science in China (B)* **33**, 686–93.

8.2.10 Psychological and psychiatric interventions in pain control

William Breitbart, David Payne, and Steven D. Passik

Introduction

Effective management of pain in patients with advanced cancer or AIDS requires a multidisciplinary approach, enlisting expertise from a wide variety of clinical specialties including neurology, neurosurgery, anaesthesiology, and rehabilitation medicine.[1–3] The utilization of psychiatric interventions in the treatment of cancer and AIDS patients with pain and psychological distress has now also become an integral part of such a comprehensive approach.[4–6]

The scope of the problem

Prevalence of pain in cancer and AIDS

Pain is a common problem for cancer patients, with approximately 70 per cent of patients experiencing severe pain at some time in the course of their illness.[2] It has been suggested that nearly 75 per cent of patients with advanced cancer have pain[7] and that 25 per cent of cancer patients die in severe pain.[8] There is considerable variability in the prevalence of pain amongst different types of cancer. For example, approximately 5 per cent of leukaemia patients experience pain during the course of their illness as compared to 50–75 per cent of patients with tumours of the lung, gastrointestinal tract, or genitourinary system. Patients with cancers of the bone or cervix have been found to have the highest prevalence of pain, with as much as 85 per cent of patients experiencing significant pain during the course of their illness.[1] Yet, despite its prevalence, studies have shown that pain is frequently under-diagnosed and inadequately treated.[8,9] It is important to remember that pain is frequently only one of several symptoms present in cancer patients. In addition to pain, patients were found, in a survey of symptoms, to suffer from an average of three additional troubling physical symptoms.[10] With disease progression, the number of distressing physical symptoms also increases so that patients with advanced disease report a median of 11 symptoms.[11] Consequently, a global evaluation of the symptom burden allows for a more complete understanding of the impact of pain for the cancer patient.

Pain is a significant and often neglected problem in patients with AIDS. Estimates of the prevalence of pain in AIDS generally range from 30 to 90 per cent, with prevalence of pain increasing as the disease progresses.[12]

The incidence of disturbing pain in AIDS is as high as 88 per cent and 69 per cent of the patients suffered from pain that resulted in moderate to severe impairment in activities of daily living.[13] A retrospective chart review of hospitalized patients with AIDS revealed that over 50 per cent of patients required treatment for pain; with pain being the presenting complaint in 30 per cent (second only to fever).[14] In their study, chest pain occurred in 22 per cent, headache in 13 per cent, oral cavity pain in 11 per cent, abdominal pain in 9 per cent, and peripheral neuropathy in 6 per cent. A second retrospective review of pain in an AIDS population reported abdominal pain, peripheral neuropathy, and Kaposi's sarcoma as the three most frequent pain problems, which affected 15 per cent of patients.[15] Other reviews report that between 5 and 30 per cent of AIDS patients have painful peripheral neuropathy.[16–18] In a hospice setting, Schofferman and Brody[19] described pain in patients with far advanced AIDS. Fifty-three per cent of patients surveyed had pain, most commonly peripheral neuropathy, abdominal pain, headache, and Kaposi's sarcoma (skin pain). In an ambulatory AIDS population, 43 per cent of patients reported pain of at least 2 weeks duration.[20] Painful neuropathy accounted for 50 per cent of pain diagnoses and lower extremity pain related to Kaposi's sarcoma was found in 45 per cent. While pains of a neuropathic nature are an important clinical problem that has attracted a great deal of attention, the evolving literature on AIDS pain syndromes suggests that pains of somatic and visceral aetiologies make up the bulk of the cases of pain in AIDS. Recent work suggests that of the pains experienced by ambulatory patients with AIDS, approximately 33 per cent are somatic, 35 per cent are visceral, and 33 per cent are neuropathic. In addition, somatic, visceral, and neuropathic pains often occur concurrently, and neuropathic pain is not often the predominant pain.[21]

Multidimensional concept of pain in terminal illness

Pain, and especially pain in advanced cancer and AIDS, is not a purely nociceptive or physical experience, but involves complex aspects of human functioning including: personality, affect, cognition, behaviour, and social relations.[22] A more enlightened description of the pain resulting from a terminal illness coined by Cecily Saunders[23] is 'total pain', a label that attempts to describe the all-encompassing nature of this type of pain. It is important to note that the use of analgesic drugs alone does not always lead to pain relief.[24] In a recent study,[25] it has been demonstrated that psychological factors play a modest but important role in pain intensity. The interaction of cognitive, emotional, socio-environmental, and nociceptive aspects of pain shown in Fig. 1 illustrates the multidimensional nature of pain in terminal illness and suggests a model for multimodal intervention.[3] The challenge of untangling and addressing both the physical and psychological issues involved in pain is essential to developing rational and

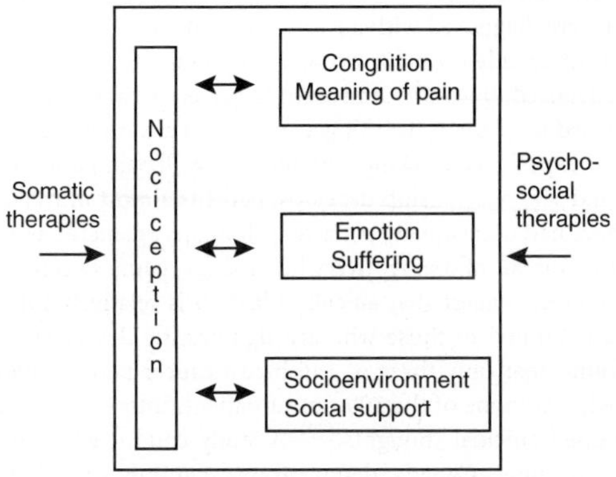

Fig. 1 The multidimensional nature of pain in terminal illness.

effective management strategies. Psychosocial therapies directed primarily at psychological variables have profound impact on nociception, while somatic therapies directed at nociception have beneficial effects on the psychological aspects of pain. Ideally, such somatic and psychosocial therapies are used simultaneously in the multidisciplinary approach to pain management in the terminally ill.[4]

Psychological factors in pain experience

The patient with cancer or AIDS faces many stressors during the course of illness including dependency, disability, and fear of painful death. Such fears are universal; however, the level of psychological distress is variable and depends on medical factors, social supports, coping capacities, and personality. Pain has profound effects on psychological distress in cancer patients, and psychological factors such as anxiety, depression, and the meaning of pain can intensify cancer pain experience. Daut and Cleeland[26] showed that cancer patients who attribute a new pain to an unrelated benign cause report less interference with their activity and pleasure than cancer patients who believe their pain represents progression of disease. Spiegel and Bloom[27] found that women with metastatic breast cancer experience more intense pain if they believe their pain represents spread of their cancer, and if they are depressed. Beliefs about the meaning of pain and the presence of a mood disturbance are better predictors of level of pain than is the site of metastasis.

In an attempt to define the potential relationships between pain and psychosocial variables, Padilla et al.[28] found that there were pain-related quality of life variables in three domains: (i) physical well-being; (ii) psychological well-being consisting of affective factors, cognitive factors, spiritual factors, communication, coping, and meaning of pain or cancer; and (iii) interpersonal well-being focusing on social support or role functioning. Patients who feel that their pain is related to their cancer report pain of greater intensity coupled with greater affective distress.[29] The perception of marked impairment in activities of daily living has been shown to be associated with increased pain intensity.[30,31] Measures of emotional disturbance have been reported to be predictors of pain in late stages of cancer, and cancer patients with less anxiety and depression are less likely to report pain.[32,33] Patients reported poorly controlled pain or higher overall levels of pain expressed significantly more existential concerns including fears about the future.[34] Patients who report negative thoughts about their personal or social competence report increased pain intensity and emotional distress in both cancer and AIDS patients.[31,32] In a prospective study of cancer patients, it was found that maladaptive coping strategies, lower levels of self-efficacy, and distress specific to the treatment or disease progression were modest but significant predictors of reports of pain intensity.[25] Patients who report that their episodes of pain is unpredictable, report greater psychological distress.[35] Rather than a homogeneous presentation, patients with cancer-related pain differ in their responses to pain. The classifications of 'dysfunctional', 'interpersonally distressed', and 'adaptive coping', categories used in chronic non-malignant pain also apply to patients with cancer pain. The recognition of different styles with which patients cope with pain suggests the importance of psychosocial evaluation of patients.[36] A strong association exists between numbers of concerns that patients endorsed and their psychological distress. Concerns about pain and treatment were particularly associated with depression.[37]

Psychological variables—such as the amount of control people believe they have over pain, emotional associations and memories of pain, fear of death, depression, anxiety, and hopelessness—also contribute to the experience of pain in people with AIDS and can increase suffering.[38] The negative thoughts related to pain are associated with greater pain intensity, psychological distress, and disability in ambulatory patients with AIDS.[30] Pain appears to have a profound impact on levels of emotional distress and disability. In a pilot study of the impact of pain on ambulatory HIV-infected patients,[39] depression was significantly correlated with the presence of pain. In addition to being significantly more distressed and depressed, those with pain were twice as likely to have suicidal ideation (40 per cent) as those without pain (20 per cent). HIV-infected patients with pain were more functionally impaired. Such functional interference was highly correlated to levels of pain intensity and depression. Those who felt that pain represented a threat to their health reported more intense pain than those who did not see pain as a threat. Patients with pain were more likely to be unemployed or disabled, and they reported less social support. Singer and colleagues[40] also reported an association among the frequency of multiple pains, increased disability, and higher levels of depression.

All too frequently, however, psychological variables are proposed to explain continued pain or lack of response to therapy when in fact medical factors have not been adequately appreciated. Often, the psychiatrist is the last physician to consult on a cancer or AIDS patient with pain. In that role one must be vigilant that an accurate pain diagnosis is made and be able to assess the adequacy of the medical analgesic management provided. Psychological distress in terminally ill patients with pain must initially be assumed to be the consequence of uncontrolled pain. Personality factors may be quite distorted by the presence of pain, and relief of pain often results in the disappearance of a perceived psychiatric disorder.[9,41]

Psychiatric disorders and pain in the terminally ill

There is an increased frequency of psychiatric disorders found in cancer patients with pain. In the Psychosocial Collaborative Oncology Group Study[42] on the prevalence of psychiatric disorders in cancer patients, of the patients who received a psychiatric diagnosis (see Table 1), 39 per cent reported significant pain, while only 19 per cent of patients without a psychiatric diagnosis had significant pain. The psychiatric disorders seen in cancer patients with pain include primarily adjustment disorder with depressed or anxious mood (69 per cent) and major depression (15 per cent). This finding of increased frequency of psychiatric disturbance in cancer pain patients has been reported.[43,44]

Epidural spinal cord compression (ESCC) is a common neurological complication of systemic cancer that occurs in 5–10 per cent of patients with cancer and can often present with severe pain. These patients are routinely treated with a combination of high-dose dexamethasone and radiotherapy. Patients who receive this high-dose regimen are exposed to as much as 96 mg a day of dexamethasone for up to a week, and continue on a tapering course for up to 3 or 4 weeks. Stiefel et al.[45] described the psychiatric complications seen in cancer patients undergoing such treatment for epidural spinal cord compression. Twenty-two per cent of patients with ESCC had a major depressive syndrome diagnosed as compared to 4 per cent in the comparison group. Also, delirium was much more common in the dexamethasone-treated patients with ESCC, with 24 per cent diagnosed with delirium during the course of treatment as compared to only 10 per cent in the comparison group.

Table 1 Rates of DSM-III psychiatric disorders and prevalence of pain observed in 215 cancer patients from three cancer centres

Diagnostic category	Number in diagnostic class	Percentage of psychiatric diagnoses	Number with significant pain[a]
Adjustment disorders	69	32	68
Major affective disorders	13	6	13
Organic mental disorders	8	4	8
Personality disorders	7	3	7
Anxiety disorders	4	2	4
Total with psychiatric diagnosis	101	47	39 (39%)
Total with no psychiatric diagnosis	114	53	21 (19%)
Total patient population	215	100	60 (28%)

[a] Score greater than 50 mm on a 100 mm VAS pain severity.

Cancer patients with advanced disease are a particularly vulnerable group. The incidence of pain, depression, and delirium increases with greater debilitation and advanced stages of illness.[46] Approximately 25 per cent of all cancer patients experience severe depressive symptoms, with the prevalence increasing to 77 per cent in those with advanced illness. The prevalence of organic mental disorders (delirium) among cancer patients requiring psychiatric consultation has been found to range from 25 to 40 per cent, and to be as high as 85 per cent during the terminal stages of illness.[47] Narcotic analgesics, such as meperidine, levorphanol, and morphine sulphate, can cause confusional states, particularly in the elderly and terminally ill.[48]

Breitbart and Passik[20] described the psychological impact of pain in an ambulatory AIDS population. AIDS patients with pain reported significantly greater depression and functional impairment than those without pain. Psychiatric disorders, in particular, the organic mental disorders such as AIDS dementia complex, can occasionally interfere with adequate pain management in the AIDS patients. Opioid analgesics, the mainstay of treatment for moderate to severe pain, may worsen dementia or cause treatment-limiting sedation, confusion, or hallucinations in patients with neurological complications of AIDS. The judicious use of psychostimulants to diminish sedation, and neuroleptics to clear confusional states can be quite helpful. Other psychiatric disorders that have an impact on pain management in the AIDS population include substance abuse and personality disorders.

Pain and suicide

Uncontrolled pain is a major factor in suicide and suicidal ideation in cancer and AIDS patients.[49–51] Cancer is perceived by the public as an extremely painful disease compared with other medical conditions. In Wisconsin, a study revealed that 69 per cent of the public agreed that cancer pain could cause a person to consider suicide.[52] The majority of suicides observed among patients with cancer had severe pain, which was often inadequately controlled or tolerated poorly.[53] Although relatively few cancer patients commit suicide, they are at increased risk.[52,54] Patients with advanced illness are at highest risk and are the most likely to have the complications of pain, depression, delirium, and deficit symptoms. Psychiatric disorders are frequently present in hospitalized cancer patients who attempt suicide. A review of the psychiatric consultation data at Memorial Sloan-Kettering Cancer Center showed that one-third of cancer patients who were seen for evaluation of suicide risk received a diagnosis of major depression; approximately 20 per cent met criteria for delirium and more than 50 per cent were diagnosed with an adjustment disorder.[49]

Thoughts of suicide probably occur quite frequently, particularly in the setting of advanced illness,[55] and seem to act as a steam valve for feelings often expressed by patients as 'If it gets too bad, I always have a way out'. It has been our experience working with terminally ill pain patients that once a trusting and safe relationship develops, patients almost universally reveal that they have had occasionally persistent thoughts of suicide as a means of escaping the threat of being overwhelmed by pain. Recent published reports, however, suggest that suicidal ideation is relatively infrequent in cancer and is limited to those who are significantly depressed. Silberfarb et al.[56] found that only three of 146 breast cancer patients had suicidal thoughts, whereas none of the 100 cancer patients interviewed in a Finnish study expressed suicidal thoughts.[57] A study conducted at St Boniface Hospice in Winnipeg, Canada, demonstrated that only 10 of 44 terminally ill cancer patients were suicidal or desired an early death, and all 10 were suffering from clinical depression.[58] At Memorial Sloan-Kettering Cancer

Center (MSKCC), suicide risk evaluation accounted for 8.6 per cent of psychiatric consultations, usually requested by staff in response to patients verbalizing suicidal wishes.[49] In the 71 cancer patients who had suicidal ideation with serious intent, significant pain was a factor in only 30 per cent of cases. In striking contrast, virtually all 71 suicidal cancer patients had a psychiatric disorder (mood disturbance or organic mental disorder) at the time of evaluation.[49]

We examined the role of cancer pain in desire for hastened death. Severity of clinical depression, hopelessness were significantly associated with suicidal ideation. In multivariate analyses, depression and hopelessness provided independent and unique contributions to the prediction of the desire for hastened death while social support and physical functioning added significant but smaller contributions.[59] In looking at 185 cancer pain patients involved in ongoing research protocols of the MSKCC Pain and Psychiatry Services,[60] suicidal ideation occurred in 17 per cent of the study population with the majority reporting suicidal ideation without intent to act. Interestingly, in this population of cancer patients who all had significant pain, suicidal ideation was not directly related to pain intensity but was strongly related to degree of depression and mood disturbance. Pain was related to suicidal ideation indirectly in that patients' perception of poor pain relief was associated with suicidal ideation. Perceptions of pain relief may have more to do with aspects of hopelessness than pain itself. Pain plays an important role in vulnerability to suicide; however, associated psychological distress and mood disturbance seem to be essential cofactors in raising the risk of suicide in cancer patients. Pain has adverse effects on patients' quality of life and sense of control and impairs the family's ability to provide support. Factors, other than pain, such as mood disturbance, delirium, loss of control, and hopelessness contribute to cancer suicide risk.[53] Frequency of suicidal ideation in one study was associated with poor well-being, depression, anxiety, and shortness of breath but not with other somatic symptoms such as pain, nausea, and loss of appetite.[61]

A study of men with AIDS in New York City[62] demonstrated a relative risk of suicide 36 times greater than that of males in the general population. Many of these patients had advanced AIDS with Kaposi's sarcoma and other potentially painful conditions. However, the role of pain in contributing to increased risk of suicide was not specifically examined. Our group at MSKCC has also examined the prevalence of suicidal ideation in an ambulatory AIDS population, and examined the relationship between suicidal ideation, depression, and pain.[63] Suicidal ideation in ambulatory AIDS patients was found to be highly correlated with the presence of pain, depressed mood (as measured by the Beck Depression Inventory), and low T4 lymphocyte counts. While 20 per cent of ambulatory AIDS patients without pain reported suicidal thoughts, over 40 per cent of those with pain reported suicidal ideation. Only two subjects in the sample ($n = 110$) reported suicidal intent. One of these two men was in the pain group; however, both scored quite highly on measures of depression. No correlations were observed between suicidal ideation and pain intensity or pain relief. The mean visual analogue scale measure of pain intensity for the group overall was 49 mm (range 5–100 mm), thus falling predominantly in the moderate range. As with cancer pain patients, suicidal ideation in AIDS patients with pain is more likely to be related to a concomitant mood disturbance than to the intensity of pain experienced. Although AIDS patients are frequently found to have suicidal ideation, these thoughts are more often context-specific, occurring almost exclusively during exacerbations of the illness often accompanied by severe pain or at times of bereavement.[63]

Inadequate pain management: assessment issues in the treatment of pain

While recent studies suggest that pain in cancer is still being undertreated,[64] pain in AIDS is dramatically undertreated. While still preliminary in nature, reports of dramatic undertreatment of pain in AIDS are appealing in the literature.[65,66] These studies suggest that opioid analgesics are underused in the treatment of pain in AIDS. Our group has reported[67] that, in our cohort of AIDS patients, only 6 per cent of individuals reporting pain in the severe range (8–10 on a numerical rating scale) received a strong opioid, such as morphine, as recommended in the WHO Analgesic Ladder. This degree of undermedication far exceeds published reports of undermedication of pain in cancer populations.[64] As with cancer, we have found that factors that influence undertreatment of pain in AIDS include gender (women are more undertreated), education, substance abuse history, and a variety of patient-related barriers.[67] While opioid analgesics are underused, it is also clear from our work and the work of others that adjuvant agents such as the antidepressants are also dramatically underused.[65,66,68] Only 6 per cent of subjects in a sample of AIDS patients reporting pain received an adjuvant analgesic drug (i.e. an antidepressant). This class of analgesic agents is a critical part of the WHO Analgesic Ladder and is vastly underused.

Inadequate management of pain is often due the inability to properly assess pain in all its dimensions.[2,4,8] All too frequently, psychological variables are proposed to explain continued pain or lack of response to therapy, when in fact medical factors have not been adequately appreciated. Other causes of inadequate pain management include: lack of knowledge of current pharmacy or psycho-therapeutic approaches; focus on prolonging life rather than alleviating suffering; lack of communication between doctor and patient; limited expectations of patients to achieve pain relief; limited capacity of patients impaired by organic mental disorders to communicate; unavailability of narcotics, doctors' fear of causing respiratory depression, and, most importantly, doctors' fear of amplifying addiction and substance abuse. In advanced cancer, several factors have been noted to predict the undermanagement of pain including: a discrepancy between physician and patient in judging the severity of pain; the presence of pain that physicians did not attribute to cancer; better performance status, age of 70 or over; and female sex.[64]

Fear of addiction affects both patient compliance and physician management of narcotic analgesics leading to undermedication of pain in cancer and AIDS patients.[3,8,69,70] Studies of the patterns of chronic narcotic analgesic used in patients with cancer have demonstrated that, although tolerance and physical dependence commonly occur, addiction (psychological dependence) is rare and almost never occurs in an individual without a history of drug abuse prior to cancer illness.[71] Escalation of narcotic analgesic use by cancer patients is usually due to progression of cancer or the development of tolerance. Tolerance means that a larger dose of narcotic analgesic is required to maintain an original analgesic effect. Physical dependence is characterized by the onset of signs and symptoms of withdrawal if the narcotic is suddenly stopped or a narcotic antagonist is administered. Tolerance usually occurs in association with physical dependence but does not imply psychological dependence; psychological dependence or addiction is not equivalent to physical dependence or tolerance and is a behavioural pattern of compulsive drug abuse characterized by a craving for the drug and overwhelming involvement in obtaining and using it for effects other than pain relief. The cancer pain patient with a history of intravenous opioid abuse presents an often unnecessarily difficult management problem. Macaluso et al.[70] reported on their experience in managing cancer pain in such a population. Of 468 inpatient cancer pain consultations, only eight (1.7 per cent) had a history of intravenous drug abuse, but none had been actively abusing drugs in the previous year. All eight of these patients had inadequate pain control and more than half were intentionally undermedicated because of concern by staff that drug abuse was active or would recur. Adequate pain control was ultimately achieved in these patients by using appropriate analgesic dosages and intensive staff education.

More problematic, however, is the management of pain in the growing segment of the AIDS population that is actively abusing intravenous drugs.[72] Such active drug use, in particular, intravenous opiate abuse, poses several pain treatment difficulties including: (i) high tolerance to narcotic analgesics; (ii) drug-seeking and manipulative behaviour; (iii) lack of compliance or reliability of patient history; and (iv) the risk of spreading HIV while high and disinhibited. Unfortunately, the patient's subjective report is often the best or only indication of the presence and intensity of pain as well as the degree of pain relief achieved by an intervention. Physicians who believe drug-seeking individuals are manipulating them are hesitant to use narcotic analgesics in appropriate dosages for adequate control of pain, often leading to undermedication. Most clinicians experienced in working with this population of AIDS patients recommend clear and direct limit setting. While this is an important aspect of the care of IV drug using AIDS patients, it is by no means the whole answer. As much as possible, clinicians should attempt to eliminate the issue of drug abuse as an obstacle to pain management by dealing directly with the problems of opiate withdrawal and drug abuse treatment. Often, specialized substance abuse consultation services are available to help manage such patients and initiate drug rehabilitation. One should avoid making the analgesic drugs the focus of a battle for control between the patient and physician, especially in terminal stages of illness. Err on the side of believing a patient when they complain of pain, and utilize your knowledge of the specific pain syndrome seen in AIDS patients to corroborate the patient's report if you feel it is unreliable.

The risk of inducing respiratory depression is too often overestimated and can limit appropriate use of narcotic analgesics for pain and symptom control. Bruera et al.[73] demonstrated that, in a population of terminally ill cancer patients with respiratory failure and dyspnea, administration of subcutaneous morphine actually improved dyspnoea without causing a significant deterioration in respiratory function. The adequacy of cancer pain management can be influenced by the lack of concordance between patient ratings or complaints of their pain and those made by caregivers. Persistent cancer pain is often ascribed to a psychological cause when it does not respond to treatment attempts. In our clinical experience, we have noted that patients who report their pain as 'severe' are quite likely to be viewed as having a psychological contribution to their complaints. Staff members' ability to empathize with a patient's pain complaint may be limited by the intensity of the pain complaint. Grossman et al.[74] found that while there is a high degree of concordance between patient and caregiver ratings of patient pain intensity at the low and moderate levels, this concordance breaks down at high levels. Thus, a clinician's ability to assess a patient's level of pain becomes unreliable once a patient's report of pain intensity rises above 7 on a visual analogue rating scale of 0 to 10. Physicians must be educated as to the limitations of their ability to objectively assess the severity of a subjective pain experience. Additionally, patient education is often a useful intervention in such cases. Patients are more likely to be believed and adequately treated if they are taught to request pain relief in a non-hysterical, business-like fashion.

Psychiatric management of pain in advanced disease

Optimal treatment of pain associated with advanced disease is multimodal and includes pharmacological, psychotherapeutic, cognitive–behavioural, anaesthetic, neuro-stimulatory, and rehabilitative approaches. Psychiatric participation in pain management involves the use of psychotherapeutic, cognitive–behavioural, and psychopharmacologic interventions, usually in combination, which are described below.

Psychotherapy and pain

The goals of psychotherapy with medically ill patients with pain are to provide support, knowledge, and skills (Table 2). Utilizing short-term supportive psychotherapy focused on the crisis created by the medical illness, the therapist provides emotional support, continuity, information, and assists in adaptation. The therapist has a role in emphasizing past strengths, supporting previously successful coping strategies, and teaching new coping skills such as: relaxation, cognitive coping, use of analgesics, self-observation, documentation, assertiveness, and communication skills. Communication skills are of paramount importance for both patient and family, particularly around pain and analgesic issues. The patient and family are the unit of concern, and need a more general, long-term, supportive relationship within the health-care system in addition to specific psychological approaches dealing with pain and dying, which a psychiatrist, psychologist, social worker, chaplain, or nurse can provide.

Table 2 Goals and forms of psychotherapy for pain in patients with advanced disease

Goals	Form
Support—provide continuity	Individuals—supportive/crisis intervention
Knowledge—provide information	Family—patient and family are the unit of concern
Skills—relaxation cognitive coping use of analgesics communication	Group—share experiences identify successful coping strategies

Psychotherapy with the dying patient in pain consists of active listening with supportive verbal interventions and the occasional interpretation.[75] Despite the seriousness of the patient's plight, it is not necessary for the psychiatrist or psychologist to appear overly solemn or emotionally restrained. Often, it is only the psychotherapist, of all the patient's caregivers, who is comfortable enough to converse lightheartedly and allow the patient to talk about his life and experiences, rather than focus solely on impending death. The dying patient who wishes to talk or ask questions about death and pain and suffering should be allowed to do so freely, with the therapist maintaining an interested, interactive stance. It is not uncommon for the dying patient to benefit from pastoral counselling. If a chaplaincy service is available, it should be offered to the patient and family. As the dying process progresses, psychotherapy with the individual patient may become limited by cognitive and speech deficits. It is at this point that the focus of supportive psychotherapeutic interventions shifts primarily to the family. In our experience, a very common issue for family members at this point is the level of alertness of the patient. Attempts to control pain are often accompanied by sedation that can limit communication between patient and family. This can sometimes become a source of conflict, with some family members disagreeing amongst themselves or with the patient about what constitutes an appropriate balance between comfort and alertness. It can be helpful for the physician to clarify the patient's preferences as they relate to these issues early so that conflict can be avoided and work related to bereavement can begin.

Group interventions with individual patients (even in advanced stages of disease), spouses, couples, and families are a powerful means of sharing experiences and identifying successful coping strategies. The limitations of using group interventions for patients with advanced disease are primarily pragmatic. The patient must be physically comfortable enough to participate and have the cognitive capacity to be aware of group discussion. It is often helpful for family members to attend support groups during the terminal phases of the patient's illness. Passik et al.[76] have worked with spouses of brain tumour patients in a psychoeducational group that has included spouses at all phases of the patient's illness. They have demonstrated how bereavement issues are often a focus of such interventions from the time of diagnosis on. The group members have benefit from one another's support into widowhood. The leaders have been impressed by the increased quality of patient care that can be given at home by the spouse (including pain management and all forms of nursing care) when the spouses engage in such support.

Psychotherapeutic interventions that have multiple foci may be most useful. Based upon a prospective study of cancer pain, cognitive behavioural and psychoeducational techniques based upon increasing support, self-efficacy, and providing education may prove to be helpful in assisting patients in dealing with increased pain.(77) Results of an evaluation of patients with cancer pain indicate psychological and social variables are significant predictors of pain. More specifically, distress specific to the illness, self-efficacy, and coping styles were predictors of increased pain.

Utilizing psychotherapy to diminish symptoms of anxiety and depression, factors that can intensify pain, empirically has beneficial effects on cancer pain experience. Spiegel and Bloom(78) demonstrated, in a controlled randomized prospective study, the effect of both supportive group therapy for metastatic breast cancer patients in general and, in particular, the effect of hypnotic pain control exercises. Their support group focused not on interpersonal processes or self-exploration, but rather on a series of themes related to the practical and existential problems of living with cancer. Patients were divided into two treatment groups and a control group. The treatment patients experienced significantly less pain than the control patients. Those in the group that combined a self-hypnosis exercise group showed a slight increase, and the control group showed a large increase in pain.

While psychotherapy in the cancer pain setting is primarily non-analytical and focuses on current issues, exploration of reactions to cancer often involve insights into earlier more pervasive life issues. Some patients choose to continue a more exploratory psychotherapy during extended illness-free periods or survivorship.

Cognitive–behavioural techniques

Cognitive–behavioural techniques can be useful as adjuncts to the management of pain in cancer and AIDS patients (Table 3). These techniques fall into two major categories: cognitive techniques and behavioural techniques. Such techniques include passive relaxation with mental imagery, cognitive distraction or focusing, progressive muscle relaxation, biofeedback, hypnosis, and music therapy.(41,79–81) The goal of treatment is to guide the patient towards a sense of control over pain. Some techniques are primarily cognitive in nature, focusing on perceptual and thought processes, and others are directed at modifying patterns of behaviour that help cancer patients cope with pain. Behavioural techniques for pain control seek to modify physiologic pain reactions, respondent pain behaviours, and operant pain behaviours (see Table 4 for definitions).

Primarily, cognitive techniques for coping with pain are aimed at reducing the intensity and distress that are part of the pain experience. This may be accomplished by the utilization of a number of techniques including the modification of thoughts the patient has about their pain or psychological distress, introduction of more adaptive coping strategies, and instruction in relaxation techniques. Cognitive modification (cognitive restructuring) is an approach derived from cognitive therapy for depression or anxiety and is based on how one interprets events and bodily sensation. It is assumed that patients have dysfunctional automatic thoughts that are consistent with underlying assumptions and beliefs. In both cancer and AIDS pain populations, negative thoughts about pain have been shown to be significantly

Table 3 Cognitive–behavioural techniques used by pain patients with advanced disease

Psychoeducation
Preparatory information
Self-monitoring
Relaxation
Passive breathing
Progressive muscle relaxation
Distraction
Focusing
Controlled by mental imagery
Cognitive distraction
Behavioural distraction
Combined techniques (relaxation and distraction)
Passive/progressive relaxation with mental imagery
Systematic desensitization
Meditation
Hypnosis
Biofeedback
Music therapy
Cognitive therapies
Cognitive distortion
Cognitive restructuring
Behavioural therapies
Modelling
Graded task management
Contingency management
Behavioural rehearsal

Table 4 Cognitive–behavioural techniques: definitions and descriptions

Behavioural therapy	The clinical use of techniques derived from the experimental analysis of behaviour, i.e. learning and conditioning for the evaluation, prevention, and treatment of physical disease or physiological dysfunction
Cognitive therapy	A focused intervention targeted at changing maladaptive beliefs and dysfunctional attitudes. The therapist engages the client in a process of collaborative empiricism, where these underlying beliefs are challenged and corrected
Operant pain	Pain behaviours resulting from operant learning or conditioning. Pain behaviour is reinforced and continues because of secondary gain, i.e. increased attention and caring
Respondent pain	Pain behaviours resulting from respondent learning or conditioning. Stimuli associated with prior painful experiences can elicit increased pain and avoidance behaviour
Cognitive restructuring	Redefinition of some or all aspects of the patient's interpretation of the noxious or threatening experience, resulting in decreased distress, anxiety, and hopelessness
Self-monitoring (pain diary)	Written or audiotaped chronicle that the patient maintains to describe specific agreed-upon characteristics associated with pain
Contingency management	Focusing of patient and family member responses that either reinforce or inhibit specific behaviours exhibited by the patient. Method involves reinforcing desired 'well' behaviours
Grade task assignments	A hierarchy of tasks, i.e. physical, cognitive, and behavioural, are compartmentalized and performed sequentially in manageable steps ultimately achieving an identified goal
Systematic desensitization	Relaxation and distraction exercises paired with a hierarchy of anxiety-arousing stimuli presented through mental imagery, or presented *in vivo*, resulting in control of fear

related to pain intensity, degree of psychological distress, and level of interference in functional activities.[30,31] By identifying and challenging dysfunctional automatic thoughts and underlying beliefs by restructuring or modifying thought processes, a more rational response to pain can occur.[79] Examples of such automatic thoughts that have been shown to worsen pain experience are: 'The intensity of my pain will never diminish' or 'Because my pain limits my activities, I am completely helpless'. Patients can be taught to recognize and interrupt such thoughts and proceed to develop a view of the pain experience as time-limited and themselves as functional despite periods in which they are limited.

Although cognitive restructuring may be a useful technique in the earlier stages of cancer and AIDS, the goals change in the palliative care context. In this setting the goal is not necessarily to change the patient's maladaptive thoughts but to utilize techniques designed to diminish the patient's frustration, anxiety, and anger. Helping patients to employ more adaptive coping strategies, that is, the avoidance of catastrophizing and encouraging an increase in problem-solving skills may be helpful at this stage.[82–84]

Aside from modifying dysfunctional thoughts and attitudes, the most fundamental behavioural technique is self-monitoring. The development of the ability to monitor one's behaviours allows a person to notice their dysfunctional reactions to the pain experience and learn to control them. Systematic desensitization (see Table 4) is useful in extinguishing anticipatory anxiety that leads to avoidant behaviours and in remobilizing inactive patients. Graded task assignment is essentially systematic desensitization as it is applied to patients who are encouraged to take small steps gradually so as to perform activities more readily. Contingency management is a method of reinforcing 'well' behaviours only; thus, modifying dysfunctional operant pain behaviours associated with secondary gain.[80,81]

Cognitive–behavioural interventions that are useful in the setting of advanced illness include a variety of techniques that range from preparatory information and self-monitoring to systematic desensitization and methods of distraction and relaxation.[85] Most often, techniques such as hypnosis, biofeedback, or systematic desensitization utilize both cognitive and behavioural elements such as muscular relaxation and cognitive distraction. A review of non-pharmacological strategies suggests that although behavioural interventions can be helpful in managing a variety of distressing physical and psychological symptoms, there is increasing evidence that these methods are not equally effective. Hypnotic-like methods, including relaxation, suggestion, and distracting imagery hold the greatest promise although research on the usage of these techniques to control pain is scant.[86–87] The combined use of non-pharmacological and pharmacological pain management techniques with pediatric populations is especially recommended.[88]

Patient selection for cognitive–behavioural interventions for pain

Many cancer and AIDS patients fear that focus on their pain will distract their physicians from treating the underlying causes of their disease and consequently are highly motivated to learn and practice cognitive–behavioural techniques. These techniques are often effective not only in pain control, but in restoring a sense of self-control, personal efficacy, and active participation in their care. It is important to note that these techniques must not be used as a substitute for appropriate analgesic management of pain, but rather as part of a comprehensive multimodal approach. The lack of side-effects of these techniques makes them attractive in the palliative care setting as a supplement to already complicated medication regimens. The successful use of these techniques should never lead to the erroneous conclusion that the pain was of psychogenic origin and as such not 'real'. The mechanisms by which these cognitive and behavioural techniques relieve pain are not known; however, they all seem to share the elements of relaxation and distraction. Distraction or redirection of attention helps reduce awareness of pain, and relaxation reduces muscle tension and sympathetic arousal.[80]

Most patients with advanced illness and pain are appropriate candidates for useful application of these techniques; the clinician, however, should take into account the intensity of pain and the mental clarity of the patient. Ideal candidates have mild to moderate pain and can expect benefit, whereas patients with severe pain can expect limited benefit from psychological interventions unless somatic therapies can lower the level of pain to some degree. Confusional states interfere dramatically with a patient's ability to focus attention and thus limit the usefulness of these techniques.[81] Occasionally, these techniques can be modified so as to include even mildly cognitive impaired patients. These often involve the therapist taking a more active role by orienting the patient, creating a safe and secure environment, and evoking a conditioned response to the therapist's voice or presence.

Barriers to engaging patients in cognitive–behavioural therapies can be divided into physician/nurse-based barriers and patient-based barriers. The health-care provider who works with patients with advanced illness may have particular difficulty in becoming comfortable with the use of behavioural therapies. Pharmacotherapy is highly effective in the management of pain and seems simpler and easier to use by physicians than labour-intensive and time-consuming non-pharmacological interventions. Physicians and nurses have typical concerns about the practice of behavioural interventions such as: 'What if the patient laughs, doesn't buy it?' or 'It seems too theatrical, unscientific, non-medical; too New Age!' Overcoming such obstacles will be greatly rewarded. It is imperative that physicians working with patients with advanced illness be aware of the effective non-pharmacological interventions for pain available, and be able to make appropriate referrals to practitioners who can provide such interventions.

Patients themselves may be uncertain about the utility of behavioural therapies. Some may ask, 'How can breathing take away my pain?' They may be frightened by the word 'hypnosis' and its connotations. Hypnosis, as patients conceptualize it, is often associated with powerful and magical properties; however, some patients become frightened at the prospect of losing control or being under the influence of someone else. We generally attempt to introduce behavioural interventions only after we have been able to establish some rapport with a patient and engage them in an alliance with us. Occasionally, some patients may benefit from a discussion of the theoretical basis of these interventions; however, we stress that it is not important to understand why a technique works, but rather to use the technique that works. Apprehensions must be affirmed and dealt with. Patients must also feel in control of the process at all times and be reassured that they can stop at any time.

General instructions

A general approach to using cognitive–behavioural interventions with patients with advanced illness and pain involves the following: (i) assessment of the symptom; (ii) choosing a cognitive–behavioural strategy; and (iii) preparing the patient and the setting.

The main purpose of conducting a cognitive–behavioural assessment of pain is to determine what, if any, behavioural interventions are indicated.[71] One must initially engage the patient and establish a therapeutic alliance. A history of the pain symptom must be taken. One should review previous efforts to treat the patient's pain, and collect data regarding the nature of the pain and its impact on the patient and their family.

The assessment process will lead to a variety of potential behavioural interventions. Choosing the appropriate behavioural strategy involves taking into consideration the patient's medical condition, physical and cognitive limitations, as well as such issues as time constraints and practical matters. For instance, patients with cognitive impairment or delirium will probably be unable to keep a pain diary or employ techniques that involve cognitive manipulation.

Relaxation techniques

Several techniques can be used to achieve a mental and physical state of relaxation. Muscular tension, autonomic arousal, and mental distress exacerbate pain.[80,81] Some specific relaxation techniques include (a) passive relaxation focusing attention on sensations of warmth and decreased tension in various parts of the body, (b) progressive muscle relaxation involving active tensing and relaxing of muscles, and (c) meditation.

Other techniques that employ both relaxation and cognitive techniques include hypnosis, biofeedback, and music therapy and are discussed later in this chapter. A review of relaxation studies suggests that even though relaxation can lead to significantly lower pain sensations scores, there is insufficient evidence to confirm that relaxation can reduce chronic pain. Relaxation with imagery does, however, appear to have a positive effect on anxiety.[89–91]

Passive relaxation, focused breathing, and passive muscle relaxation exercises involve the focusing of attention systematically on one's breathing, on sensations of warmth and relaxation, or on release of muscular tension in various body parts. Verbal suggestions and imagery are used to help promote relaxation. Muscle relaxation is an important component of the relaxation response and can augment the benefits of simple focused breathing exercises, leading to a deeper experience of relaxation and self-control.

Progressive or active muscle relaxation involves the active tensing and relaxing of various muscle groups in the body, focusing attention on the sensations of tension and relaxation. Clinically, in the hospital setting, relaxation is most commonly achieved through the use of a combination of focused breathing and progressive muscle relaxation exercises. Once patients are in a relaxed state, imagery techniques can then be used to induce deeper relaxation and facilitate distraction from or manipulation of a variety of cancer-related symptoms.

The following script is a generic relaxation exercise, utilizing passive relaxation or focused breathing, that is based on and integrates the work of Erickson,[92] Benson,[93] and others.[81]

Script for passive relaxation (focused breathing)

Why don't you begin by finding a comfortable position. It could be in a bed or in a chair. Slowly allow your body to unwind and just let it go. That's it... I wonder if you can allow your body to become as calm as possible... just let it go, just let your body sink into that bed (or chair)... feel free to move or shift around in any way that your body needs to, to find that comfortable position. You need not try very hard, simply and easily allow yourself to follow the sound of my voice as you allow your body to find itself a safe, comfortable position to relax in.

If you like, (patient's name here), you can gently allow your eyes to close, just let the lids cover your eyes... allow your eyes to sink back deeply into their sockets... that's it, just let them go, falling back gently and deeply into their sockets as your lids begin to feel heavier and heavier. As you allow your head to fall back deeply into the pillow, feeling the weight of your head sinking into the pillow as you breath out, just breath out, one big breath. Slowly, if you can begin to turn your attention to your breathing. Notice your breath for a few moments, how much air you take in, how much air you let out, and just breath evenly and naturally, and with the sound of my voice I wonder if you can begin to take in more air, breathing in and out, in and out, that's it, gradually breathing in and out... in and out... breathing in calmness and quietness, breathing out tiredness and frustration, that's it... let it go, it's not important to you now... breathing in quietness and control, breathing out fear and tension... breathing in and out... in and out... you can enjoy breathing in this relaxed way for as long as you need to. You are peaceful now as you continue to observe your even and steady breathing that is allowing you to feel gentle and calm, breathing that is allowing you to feel a gentle calm, that's it, breathing relaxation in and tension out... in and out... breathing in quietness and control, breathing out tiredness and tension... that's it (patient's name here) as you continue to notice the quietness and stillness of your body, Why don't you take a few quiet moments to experience this process more fully.

It may be helpful for the clinician to mark the end of an exercise by increasing the pace, raising the volume of voice, and shifting position. Additionally, it is helpful for the clinician to both pace and model for the patient. This includes positioning yourself as similarly to the patient as possible (e.g. closing eyes, assuming a position of relaxation, and breathing at the same rate). If the patient exhibits any visible anxiety or agitation, this can be briefly explored verbally, and then, if appropriate, the exercise can be continued.

Script for active or progressive muscle relaxation

This exercise involves the patient actively tensing and then relaxing specific body parts. Once again, it may be helpful if the clinician paces and models for the patient.

Now, I wonder if you can tense up every muscle in your body... that's it, squeeze in the muscles... hold it, and then just let it go... once more, tense up your muscles... make them very tight and tense, hold it, hold it... and then breath out, and let your muscles relax, just let them go... Now, as your body begins to feel more and more relaxed, clench your jaw, squeeze it tight, clench it and then let it go... now open your mouth wide, as wide as it will go, stick out your tongue, stick it way out, hold it and then let it go. Feel your head becoming more and more relaxed, as it sinks down into the pillow, allowing all the tension and tightness to drift out of it ... Now, I wonder if you can lift up your shoulders, lift them up, up to your ears, hold them there, squeezing them tightly, squeeze, and then let them drop down, just let them go... and then once more lift them up... hold it... then let them go... as you feel all the tightness and tension in your shoulders begin to drain away... Now, I wonder if you can clench your hands into a fist, make a tight fist as your whole arm tightens, tense your arms as you squeeze in your fingers tighter and tighter... and now just let them go, once more now make a fist, a tight fist, hold it, and then let it go.

As with passive muscle relaxation, the clinician guides the patient through the exercise, requesting the patient to tense and release specific muscles in a progressive order.

Imagery/distraction techniques

Clinically, relaxation techniques are most helpful in managing pain when combined with some distracting or pleasant imagery. The use of distraction or focusing involves control over the focus of attention and can be used to make the patient less aware of the noxious stimuli.[94] One can employ imaginative inattention by picturing oneself on a beach. Mental distraction can be used and is similar to the practice of counting sheep to aid sleep. Keeping oneself busy is a form of behavioural distraction. Imagery, that is, using one's imagination while in a relaxed state, can be used to transform pain into a warm or cold sensation. One can also imaginatively transform the context of pain, that is, imagining oneself in battle on the football field instead of the hospital bed. Dissociated somatization can be employed by some patients whereby they imagine that a painful body part is no longer part of their body.[3,4,79,81] It is important to note that not every patient finds these techniques acceptable, and the therapist must try out a number of approaches to determine which are consistent with the patient's style.

Imagery (often referred to as guided imagery) is most effective when the specific image is obtained from the patient. The clinician may ask the patient to close his or her eyes and think of a place, an activity, or an experience where the patient felt most safe and secure. The clinician may provide suggestions for the patient such as a favourite beach scene, or a room in a house, or riding a bicycle in a state park. Once the patient identifies the scene, the clinician may ask the patient to elaborate upon the scene, asking for specific details such as the temperature, season, time of day, type of ocean (calm, or with big waves), etc. The clinician then utilizes this information and describes an image for the patient in detail. The skill is for the clinician to be as flexible and as creative as possible, and to elaborate upon the scene, utilizing all aspects of the senses and bodily sensations such as 'feel the suns rays touch your skin, allow your skin to feel warm and tingly all over...' or, 'breath in the fresh, clear air, allow it to fill your lungs with its freshness...' or, 'feel the fresh dew of the grass under your feet'. The clinician can focus on 'aromas in the garden' or the 'sounds of birds singing' always reminding the patient to breath evenly and steadily as he or she feels more and more relaxed and more and more in control. If possible, the clinician should avoid volunteering an image or scene for the patient because the clinician is unaware of the association or meaning the image may have for the patient. For example, a patient may have a fear of the water, and therefore a beach scene may invoke feelings of fear and loss of control.

Script for pleasant distracting imagery

Once you are in a comfortable position, I wonder if you can continue lying there with your eyes closed, continuing to breath in out... in and out to the sound of my voice. Let your mind wander... just let it go... and if any unwanted thoughts come into your mind, you can allow then to pass out as easily as they came in... You don't need them now... they are not important to you now. You have the ability to control your thoughts. You have the ability to be in control.

The clinician now begins to describe a specific image in detail as originally suggested by the patient.

Slowly, I wonder if you can allow your mind to travel . . . to travel far away to your favorite beach. The beach that you have many fond memories of. I wonder if you can imagine that it's almost the end of the day and the beach is deserted . . . and the sun, while setting, is still warm, as it beats down . . . and makes your skin feel tingly and warm all over. As you begin to walk on the sand, you can feel the granules underneath your feet. Step evenly and steadily along the sand. As you look around, you can see the different colors in the sky. You can see for miles off into the distance and you feel exhilarated and free because no one is around you. You are alone and in control. As you walk closer to the edge of the ocean the sand is becoming a little damp and you can feel the dampness underneath your feet—it feels refreshing. As you continue walking, you may notice a few odds and ends on the sand maybe something that the ocean brought in . . . some shells perhaps. They may be broken from being knocked against the rocks . . . or there may be a few bits of seaweed or some jellyfish. You stop to notice them as you walk past . . . marveling at the wonders of nature. As you get to the edge of the ocean, you can feel the tiny little ripples of water washing over your feet . . . bouncing over your feet making you feel light and fresh. The water is warm—it soothes your feet. Washing back and forth . . . back and forth. As you keep walking you see your rubber raft. This is your old dependable rubber raft. You get to the raft and you secure it in your hands and lie down on it letting your whole body sink into the raft—just let it go . . . that's it. Slowly you kick off as the raft begins to take you away. The ocean is very calm and very gentle. Your whole body begins to unwind and sink deeper and deeper into the raft as you feel more and more relaxed. This raft allows you to drift off . . . and underneath you can feel the ripples of the ocean . . . rocking back and forth . . . back and forth as you continue to float away evenly and gently. You can become aware of the sun beating down in your skin. You are aware of the sounds around you—you can hear the ocean washing against the rocks as the waves rock back and forth . . . back and forth. You can hear the gulls crying in the distance. There is a very tiny protected bay that you are floating away in. It is a very calm and peaceful day, and you are feeling more and more relaxed. You are in control now . . . and as you continue to sail away, all your troubles and problems wash right out of you. They're not important to you now. You don't need them now. What's important is that your whole body, from the tip of your toes all the way up to the top of your head, is relaxed and calm in this very safe and private place that is your own. You can continue to lie here as you rock back and forth . . . back and forth for as long as you need to.

When you are ready, you can slowly readjust yourself to the sound of my voice and I am going to count slowly backwards from 10 and with each count backwards, you can become more and more familiar with where you are. Perhaps when I get to number 5 you may want to open your eyes or you can keep then closed for as long as you need to. Ten, nine . . . —become aware of the sounds around you . . . eight, seven . . . become aware of the temperature of the room—how does it feel?, how does your body feel? . . . six, five . . . —you can open your eyes now if you want to or you can keep them closed . . . four, three, two, one. You can stay in this relaxed position for as long as you need to. When you feel ready you may slowly prepare to sit up.

Hypnosis

Hypnosis can be a useful adjunct in the management of cancer pain.[78,95–98] Hypnotherapy can be used effectively in the management of pain associated with invasive procedures.[86] In a controlled trial comparing hypnosis with cognitive–behavioural therapy in relieving mucositis following a bone marrow transplant, patients utilizing hypnosis reported a significant reduction in pain compared to patients who used cognitive–behavioural techniques.[77] The hypnotic trance is essentially a state of heightened and focused concentration, and thus it can be used to manipulate the perception of pain. The depth of hypnotizability may determine the effectiveness as well as the strategies employed during hypnosis. One-third of cancer patients are not hypnotizable, and it is recommended that other techniques be employed for them. Of the two-thirds of patients who are identified as being less, moderately, and highly hypnotizable, three principles underlie the use of hypnosis in controlling pain:[94] (a) use self-hypnosis; (b) relax, do not fight the pain; and (c) use a mental filter to ease the hurt in pain. Patients who are moderately and highly hypnotizable can often alter sensations in a painful area by changing temperature sensation or experiencing tingling. Less hypnotizable patients can often utilize an alternative focus by concentrating on a sensation in a non-affected body part or on a mental image of a pleasant scene. The main disadvantage of hypnosis for cancer patients is that the technique frequently requires more attentional capacity than these patients generally have. For paediatric patients, hypnosis and cognitive–behavioural skills are effective in managing the pain associated with procedure related pain.[99]

Biofeedback

Fotopoulos et al.[100] noted significant pain relief in a group of cancer patients who were taught electromyographic (EMG) and electroencephalographic (EEG) biofeedback-assisted relaxation. Only two of 17 were able to maintain analgesia after the treatment ended. A lack of generalization of effect can be a problem with biofeedback techniques. Although physical condition may make a prolonged training period impossible, especially for the terminally ill, most cancer patients can often utilize EMG and temperature biofeedback techniques for learning relaxation-assisted pain control.[88]

Music, aroma, and art therapies

Munro and Mount[101] have written extensively on the use of music therapy with cancer patients, documenting clinical examples and suggesting mechanisms of action. Music can often capture the focus of attention like no other stimulus, offers patients a new form of expression, and helps patients distract themselves from their perception of pain, while expressing themselves in meaningful ways.[102,103] Music therapy can be helpful in managing the discomfort associated with procedures.[104]

Aromas have been shown to have innate relaxing and stimulating qualities. Our colleagues at Memorial Hospital have recently begun to explore the use of aroma therapy for the treatment of procedure-related anxiety (i.e. anxiety related to MRI scans). Utilizing the scent, heliotropin, Manne et al.[105] reported that two-thirds of the patients found the scent especially pleasant and reported much less anxiety than those who were not exposed to the scent during MRI. As a general relaxation technique, aroma therapy may have an application for pain management, but this is as yet unstudied.

Art therapy allows the less verbally skilled adult or children to express the fears and concerns that they have in a more comfortable fashion. The creative experience can be used as both a important means of providing support and also as an avenue for providing patients with psychological insights into their experience.[106]

Psychotropic adjuvant analgesics for pain in the patient with advanced illness

The patient with advanced disease and pain has much to gain from the appropriate and maximal utilization of psychotropic drugs. Psychotropic drugs, particularly the tricyclic antidepressants, are useful as adjuvant analgesics in the pharmacological management of cancer pain and neuropathic pain. Table 5 lists the various psychotropic medications with analgesic properties, their routes of administration, and their approximate daily doses. These medications are not only effective in managing symptoms of anxiety, depression, insomnia, or delirium that commonly complicate the course of advanced disease in patients with cancer or AIDS who are in pain, but also potentiate the analgesic effects of the opioid drugs and have innate analgesic properties of their own.[107] A common use of adjuvant analgesics is to manage neuropathic pain. In this population, non-opioid adjuvant drugs that are neuroactive or neuromodulatory may be needed to complement opioid therapy. The primary adjuvant analgesics are anticonvulsant and antidepressant medications but a variety of other drugs are used.[108]

Table 5 Psychotropic adjuvant analgesic drugs for pain in patients with advanced disease

Generic name	Approximate daily dosage range (mg)	Route
Tricyclic antidepressants		
Amitriptyline	10–150	PO, IM, PR
Nortriptyline	10–50	PO
Imipramine	12.5–150	PO, IM
Desipramine	12.5–150	PO
Clomipramine	10–150	PO
Doxepin	12.5–150	PO, IM
Non-cyclic antidepressants		
Trazodone	25–300	PO
Fluoxetine	20–60	PO
Paroxetine	20–60	PO
Monoamide oxidase inhibitors		
Phenelzine	45–75	PO
Amine precursors		
L-Tryptophan	500–3000	PO
Psychostimulants		
Methylphenidate	2.5–20 b.i.d.	PO
Dextroamphetamine	2.5–20 b.i.d.	PO
Pemoline	18.75–75 b.i.d.	PO
Phenothiazines		
Fluphenazine	1–3	PO, IM
Methotrimeprazine	10–20 q6h	PO, IM, IV, SC
Butyrophenones		
Haloperidol	1–3	PO, IM, IV, SC
Pimozide	2–6 b.i.d.	PO
Atypical neuroloptics		
Olanzapine	2.5–20	PO
Antihistamines		
Hydroxyzine	50 q4–6h	PO, IM, IV
Benzodiazepines		
Alprazolam	0.25–2.0 t.i.d.	PO
Clonazepam	0.5–4 b.i.d.	PO

PO, per oral; IM, intramuscular; PR, parenteral; IV, intravenous; q6h, every 6 h; q4–6 h, every 4 to 6 h; t.i.d., three times a day; b.i.d., two times a day.

Antidepressants

The current literature supports the use of antidepressants as adjuvant analgesic agents in the management of a wide variety of chronic pain syndromes, including cancer pain.[109–116] While clinically useful as adjuvant analgesics in managing AIDS-related pain (e.g. HIV neuropathies), there are no published controlled clinical trials of antidepressants as analgesics.[72,117] Amitriptyline is the tricyclic antidepressant most studied, and proven effective as an analgesic, in a large number of clinical trials, addressing a wide variety of chronic pains.[118–122] Other tricyclic antidepressants that have been shown to have efficacy as analgesics include imipramine,[123–125] desipramine,[126,127] nortriptyline,[128] clomipramine,[129,130] and doxepin.[131] In a placebo controlled double-blind study of imipramine in chronic cancer pain, Walsh[132] demonstrated that imipramine had analgesic effects independent of its mood effects, and was a potent co-analgesic when used along with morphine. In general, the tricyclic antidepressants are utilized in cancer pain as adjuvant analgesics, potentiating the effects of opioid analgesics, and are rarely used as the primary analgesic.[114,132,134] Ventafridda et al.[114] reviewed a multicentre clinical experience with antidepressant agents (trazodone and amitriptyline) in the treatment of chronic cancer pain that included a deafferentation of neuropathic component. Almost all of these patients were already receiving weak or strong opioids and experienced improved pain control. A subsequent randomized double-blind study showed both amitriptyline and trazodone to have similar therapeutic analgesic efficacy.[114] Magni et al.[115] reviewed the use of antidepressants in Italian cancer centres and found that a wide range of antidepressants were used for a variety of cancer pain syndromes, with amitriptyline being the most commonly prescribed, for a variety of cancer pains. In nearly all cases, antidepressants were used in association with opioids. There is some evidence that there may be a subgroup of patients who respond differentially to tricyclics and therefore if amitriptyline fails to alleviate pain, another tricyclic should be tried.[134] The tricyclic antidepressants are effective as adjuvants in cancer pain through a number of mechanisms that include: (i) antidepressant activity;[109] (ii) potentiation or enhancement of opioid analgesia;[133,135,136] (iii) direct analgesic effects.[137]

The heterocyclic and non-cyclic antidepressant drugs such as trazodone, mianserin, maprotiline, and the newer serotinin-specific reuptake inhibitors fluoxetine and paroxetine may also be useful as adjuvant analgesics for cancer patients with pain; however, clinical trials of their efficacy as analgesics have been equivocal.[138–142] There are several case reports that suggest that fluoxetine may be a useful adjuvant analgesic in the management of headache,[143] fibrositis,[144] and diabetic neuropathy.[145] In a recent clinical trial, fluoxetine was shown to be no better than placebo as an analgesic in painful diabetic neuropathy.[146] Paroxetine is the first serotonin-specific re-uptake inhibitor shown to be a highly effective analgesic in the treatment of neuropathic pain,[147] and may be a useful addition to our armamentarium of adjuvant analgesics for cancer pain. Newer antidepressants such as sertraline, velafaxine, and nefazodone may also eventually prove to be clinically useful as adjuvant analgesics. Nefazodone, for instance, has been demonstrated to potentiate opioid analgesics in an animal model.[148] Recent randomized controlled trials suggest that fluoxetine and desipramine were effective and well-tolerated in improving depression and the quality of life in women with advanced cancer. Fluoxetine and other SSRIs may offer greater benefit to these patients as evidenced by greater improvements in quality of life measures.[149] At this point, it is clear that many antidepressants have analgesic properties. There is no definite indication that any one drug is more effective than the others, although the most experience has been accrued with amitriptyline, which remains the drug of first choice. In terms of appropriate dosage, there is evidence that the therapeutic analgesic effects of amitriptyline are correlated with serum levels just as the antidepressant effects are, and analgesic treatment failure is due to low serum levels.[118,119,150] A high-dose regimen of up to 150 mg of amitriptyline or higher is suggested.[121,151] As to the time course of onset of analgesia or with antidepressants, there appears to be a biphasic process that occurs with immediate or early analgesic effects that occur within hours or days[130,133,137] and later, longer analgesic effects that peak over a 4–6 week period.[118–120]

Treatment should be initiated with a small dose of amitriptyline for instance, that is, 10–25 mg at bedtime especially in debilitated patients, and increased slowly by 10–25 mg every 2–4 days towards 150 mg with frequent assessment of pain and side-effects until a beneficial effect is achieved. Maximal effect as an adjuvant analgesic may require continuation of drug for 2–6 weeks. Serum levels of antidepressant drug, when available, may also help in management to assure that therapeutic serum level's of drug are being achieved. Both pain and depression in cancer patients often respond to lower doses (25–100 mg) of antidepressant than are usually required in the physically healthy (100–300 mg), most likely because of impaired metabolism of these drugs. The choice of drug often depends on the side-effect profile, existing medical problems, the nature of depressive symptoms if present, and past response to specific antidepressants. Sedating drugs like amitriptyline are helpful when insomnia complicates the presence of pain and depression on a cancer patient. Anticholinergic properties of some of these drugs should also be kept in mind. Occasionally, in patients who have limited analgesic response to a tricyclic, potentiation of analgesia can be accomplished with the addition of lithium augmentation.[152] Tricyclic antidepressants have been shown to be effective as analgesics for mucositis when compared to opioids and for patients for whom opioids are contraindicated tricyclic antidepressants may be used.[153]

Monoamine oxidase inhibitors (MAOIs) are also less useful in the cancer setting because of dietary restriction and potentially dangerous interactions between MAOIs and narcotics such as meperidine. Amongst the MAOI drugs available, Phenelzine has been shown to have adjuvant analgesic properties in patients with atypical facial pain and migraine.[154,155]

Psychostimulants

The psychostimulants dextroamphetamine and methylphenidate are useful antidepressant agents prescribed selectively for medically ill cancer patients with depression.[156,157] Psychostimulants are also useful in diminishing excessive sedation secondary to narcotic analgesics, and are potent adjuvant analgesics. Bruera et al.[158–160] demonstrated that a regimen of 10 mg methylphenidate with breakfast and 5 mg with lunch significantly decreased sedation and potentiated the analgesic effect of narcotics in patients with cancer pain. Dextroamphetamine has also been reported to have additive analgesic effects when used with morphine in postoperative pain.[161] In a relatively low dose, psychostimulants stimulate appetite, promote a sense of well-being, and improve feelings of weakness and fatigue in cancer patients. Treatment with dextroamphetamine or methylphenidate usually begins with a dose of 2.5 mg at 8:00 a.m. and at noon. The dosage is slowly increased over several days until a desired effect is achieved or side-effects (overstimulation, anxiety, insomnia, paranoia, confusion) intervene. Typically, a dose greater than 30 mg per day is not necessary although occasionally patients require up to 60 mg per day. Patients usually are maintained on methylphenidate for 1–2 months, and approximately two-thirds will be able to be withdrawn from methylphenidate without a recurrence of depressive symptoms. Those who do recur can be maintained on a psychostimulant for up to 1 year without significant abuse problems. Tolerance will develop and adjustment of dose may be necessary. A strategy we have found useful in treating cancer pain associated with depression is to start a psychostimulant (starting dose of 2.5 mg of methylphenidate at 8 a.m. and noon) and then to add a tricyclic antidepressant after several days to help prolong and potentiate the short effect of the stimulant. Pemoline is a unique alternative psychostimulant that is chemically unrelated to amphetamine, but may have similar usefulness as an antidepressant and adjuvant analgesic in cancer patients.[162] Advantages of pemoline as a psychostimulant in cancer pain patients include the lack of abuse potential, the lack of federal regulation through special triplicate prescriptions, the mild sympathomimetic effects, and the fact that it comes in a chewable tablet form that can be absorbed through the buccal mucosa and thus used by cancer patients who have difficulty swallowing or have intestinal obstruction. In our clinical experience, pemoline is as effective as methylphenidate or dextroamphetamine in the treatment of depressive symptoms, and in countering the sedating effects of opioid analgesics. There are no studies of pemoline's capacity to potentiate the analgesic properties of opioids. Pemoline can be started at a dose of 18.75 mg in the fore-noon and at noon, and increased gradually over days. Typically, patients require 75 mg a day or less. Pemoline should be used with caution in patients with liver impairment, and liver function tests should be monitored periodically with longer-term treatment.[163]

Neuroleptics

Methotrimeprazine is a phenothiazine that is equianalgesic to morphine, has none of the opioid effects on gut motility, and probably produces analgesia through alpha-adrenergic blockade.[164] In patients who are opioid tolerant, it provides an alternative approach in providing analgesia by a non-opioid mechanism. It is a dopamine blocker and so has antiemetic as well an anxiolytic effects. Methotrimeprazine can produce sedation and hypotension and should be given cautiously by slow intravenous infusion. Other phenothiazines such as chlorpromazine and prochlorperazine (compazine) are useful as antiemetics in cancer patients, but probably have limited use as analgesics.[165] Fluphenazine in combination with TCAs has been shown to be helpful in neuropathic pains.[129] Haloperidol is the drug of choice in the management of delirium or psychoses in cancer patients, and has clinical usefulness as a co-analgesic for cancer pain.[165] Pimozide (Orap), a butyrophenone, has been shown to be effective as an analgesic in the management of trigeminal neuralgia, at doses of 4–12 mg per day.[166] Olanzapine has been used to treat unmanaged pain in the context of anxiety and mild cognitive impairment. Patients received 2.5–7.5 mg of olanzapine daily. Daily pain scores decreased; anxiety and cognitive impairment resolved.[167]

Anxiolytics

Hydroxizine is a mild anxiolytic with sedating and analgesic properties that are useful in the anxious cancer patient with pain.[168,169] This antihistamine has antiemetic activity as well. One hundred milligrams of parenteral hydroxizine has analgesic activity approaching 8 mg of morphine, and has additive analgesic effects when combined with morphine. Benzodiazepines have not been felt to have direct analgesic properties, although they are potent anxiolytics and anticonvulsants.[170] Some authors have suggested that their anticonvulsant properties make certain benzodiazepine drugs useful in the management of neuropathic pain. Recently, Fernandez et al.[171] showed that alprazolam, a unique benzodiazepine with mild antidepressant properties, was a helpful adjuvant analgesic in cancer patients with phantom limb pain or deafferentation (neuropathic) pain. Clonazepam (klonopin) may also be useful in the management of lancinating neuropathic pains in the cancer setting, and has been reported to be an effective analgesic for patients with trigeminal neuralgia, headache, and post-traumatic neuralgia.[172,173] With the use of midazolam by IV in a patient-controlled dosage, there was no reduction in the use of post-operative morphine requirements or in the patient's perception of pain.[174] Intrathecal midazolam in animal models, however, has been shown to potentiate morphine analgesia.[175]

Placebo

A mention of the placebo response is important in order to highlight the misunderstandings and relative harm of this phenomenon. The placebo response is common, and analgesia is mediated through endogenous opioids. The deceptive use of placebo response to distinguish psychogenic pain from 'real' pain should be avoided. Placebos are effective in a small percentage of patients for a short period of time only and are not indicated in the management of cancer pain.[2]

References

1. **Foley, K.M.** (1975). Pain syndromes in patients with cancer. In *Advances in Pain Research and Therapy* Vol. 2 (ed. J.J. Bonica, V. Ventafriddi, R.B. Fink, L.E. Jones, and J.D. Loeser), pp. 59–75. New York: Raven Press.
2. **Foley, K.M.** (1985). The treatment of cancer pain. *New England Journal of Medicine* **313**, 845.
3. **Breitbart, W. and Holland, J.** (1990). Psychiatric aspects of cancer pain. In *Advances in Pain Research and Therapy* Vol. 16 (ed. K.M. Foley et al.), pp. 73–87. New York: Raven Press.
4. **Breitbart, W.** (1989). Psychiatric management of cancer pain. *Cancer* **63**, 2336–42.
5. **Breitbart, W.** (1990). Psychiatric aspects of pain and HIV disease. *Focus: A Guide to AIDS Research and Counseling* **5**, 1–2.
6. **Massie, M.J. and Holland, J.C.** (1987). The cancer patient with pain: psychiatric complications and their mangement. *Medical Clinics of North America* **71**, 243–58.
7. **Fitzgibbon, D.R.** (2001). Cancer pain: management. In *Bonica's Management of Pain* 3rd edn. (ed. J.D. Loeser et al.), pp. 659–703. Philadelphia: Lippincott Williams & Wilkins.
8. **Twycross, R.G. and Lack, S.A.** *Symptom Control in Far Advanced Cancer: Pain Relief.* London: Pitman Brooks, 1983.
9. **Marks, R.M. and Sachar, E.J.** (1973). Undertreatment of medical inpatients with narcotic analgesics. *Annals of Internal Medicine* **78**, 173–81.

10. **Grond, S., Zech, D., Diefenbach, C., and Bischoff, A.** (1994). Prevalence and pattern of symptoms in patients with cancer pain: a prospective evaluation of 1635 cancer patients referred to a pain clinic. *Journal of Pain and Symptom Management* **9**, 372–82.

11. **Walsh, D., Donnelly, S., and Rybicki, L.** (2000). The symptoms of advanced cancer: relationship to age, gender, and performance status in 1000 patients. *Support Care Cancer* **8** (3), 175–9.

12. **Breitbart, W., McDonald, M.V., Rosenfeld, B., Passik, S.D., Hewitt, D., Thaler, H., and Portenoy, R.K.** (1996). Pain in ambulatory AIDS patients. I: Pain characteristics and medical correlates. *Pain* **68** (2–3), 315–21.

13. **Frich, L.M. and Borgbjerg, F.M.** (2000). Pain and pain treatment in AIDS patients: a longitudinal study. *Journal of Pain and Symptom Management* **19** (5), 339–47.

14. **Lebovits, A.H., Lefkowitz, M., McCarthy, D., Simon, R., Wilpon, H., Jung, R., and Fried, E.** (1989). The prevalence and management of pain in patients with AIDS. A review of 134 cases. *The Clinical Journal of Pain* **5**, 245–8.

15. **Newshan, G., Wainapel, S., and Schmitz, D.** Pain related syndromes and their treatment in persons with AIDS (Abstract). Eighth Annual Scientific Meeting of the American Pain Society, Phoenix, AZ, 1989.

16. **Levy, R.M., Bredesen, D.E., and Rosenblum, M.L.** (1985). Neurological manifestations of the AIDS experience at UCSF and review of the literature. *Journal of Neurosurgery* **62**, 475–95.

17. **Snider, W.D. et al.** (1983). Neurological complications of AIDS; analysis of 50 patients. *Annals of Neurology* **14**, 403–18.

18. **Cornblath, D.R. and McArthur, I.C.** (1988). Predominantly sensory neuropathy in patients with AIDS and AIDS-related complex. *Neurology* **38**, 794–6.

19. **Schofferman, J. and Brody, R.** (1990). Pain in far advanced AIDS. In *Advances in Pain Research and Therapy* Vol. 16 (ed. K.M. Foley et al.), pp. 379–86. New York: Raven Press.

20. **Breitbart, W. and Passik, S.** Pain in AIDS: prevalence and psychosocial impact (Abstract). Biopsychosocial Aspects of HIV Infection: 1st International Conference, Amsterdam, The Netherlands, September 22–25, 1991.

21. **Hewitt, D., Breitbart, W., Rosenfeld, B., McDonald, M., and Portenoy, R.** Pain syndromes in the ambulatory AIDS patient (Abstract). American Pain Society, 1994.

22. **Stiefel, F.** (1993). Psychosocial aspects of cancer pain. *Supportive Care in Cancer* **1**, 130–4.

23. **Saunders, C.M.** *The Management of Terminal Illness.* London: Hospital Medicine Publications, 1967.

24. **Hanks, G.W.** (1991). Opioid responsive and opioid non-responsive pain in cancer. *British Medical Bulletin* **47**, 718–31.

25. **Syrjala, K. and Chapko, M.** (1995). Evidence for a biopsychosocial model of cancer treatment-related pain. *Pain* **61**, 69–79.

26. **Daut, R.L. and Cleeland, C.S.** (1982). The prevalence and severity of pain in cancer. *Cancer* **50**, 1913–18.

27. **Spiegel, D. and Bloom, J.R.** (1983). Pain in metastatic breast cancer. *Cancer* **52**, 341–5.

28. **Padilla, G., Ferrell, B., Grant, M., and Rhiner, M.** (1990). Defining the content domain of quality of life for cancer patients with pain. *Cancer Nursing* **13**, 108–15.

29. **Smith, W.B., Gracely, R.H., and Safer, M.A.** (1998). The meaning of pain: cancer patients' rating and recall of pain intensity and affect. *Pain* **78** (2), 123–9.

30. **Payne, D., Jacobsen, P., Breitbart, W., Passik, S., Rosenfeld, B., and McDonald, M.** Negative thoughts related to pain are associated with greater pain, distress, and disability in AIDS pain. Presentation at the American Pain Society, Miami, Florida, 1994.

31. **Payne, D.** *Cognition in Cancer Pain.* Unpublished dissertation, 1995.

32. **McKegney, F.P., Bailey, C.R., and Yates, J.W.** (1981). Prediction and management of pain in patients with advanced cancer. *General Hospital Psychiatry* **3**, 95–101.

33. **Bond, M.R. and Pearson, I.B.** (1969). Psychological aspects of pain in women with advanced cancer of the cervix. *Journal of Psychosomatic Research* **13**, 13–19.

34. **Strang, P.** (1997). Existential consequences of unrelieved cancer pain. *Palliative Medicine* **11** (4), 299–305.

35. **Portenoy, R.K., Payne, D., and Jacobsen, P.** (1999). Breakthrough pain: characteristics and impact in patients with cancer pain. *Pain* **81** (1–2), 129–34.

36. **Turk, D.C., Sist, T.C., Okifuji, A., Miner, M.F., Florio, G., Harrison, P., Massey, J., Lema, M.L., and Zevon, M.A.** (1998). Adaptation to metastatic cancer pain, regional/local cancer pain and non-cancer pain: role of psychological and behavioral factors. *Pain* **74** (2–3), 247–56.

37. **Heaven, C.M. and Maguire, P.** (1998). The relationship between patients' concerns and psychological distress in a hospice setting. *Psycho-oncology* **7** (6), 502–7.

38. **Breitbart, W., Passik S., Rosenfeld, B., Portenoy R.K., McDonald, M., and Thaler, H.** Pain intensity and its relationship to functional interference in patients with AIDS (Poster). American Pain Society, 1994.

39. **Breitbart, W., Passik S., Bronaugh, T., Zale, C., Bluestine, S., and Gomez, M.** Pain in the ambulatory AIDS patient: prevalence and psychosocial correlates (Abstract). 38th Annual Meeting, Academy of Psychosomatic Medicine, 1991.

40. **Singer, E.J., Zorilla, C., Fahy-Chandon, B., Chi, S., Syndulko, K., and Teunteliotte, W.** (1993). Painful symptoms reported for ambulatory HIV-infected men in a longitudinal study. *Pain* **54**, 15–19.

41. **Cleeland, C.S. and Tearnan, B.H.** (1986). Behavioral control of cancer pain. In *Pain Mangement* (ed. D. Holzman and D. Turk), pp. 193–212. New York: Pergamon Press.

42. **Derogatis, L.R. et al.** (1983). The prevalence of psychiatric disorders among cancer patients. *Journal of the American Medical Association* **249**, 751–7.

43. **Ahles, T.A., Blanchard, E.B., and Ruckdeschel, J.C.** (1983). The multidimensional nature of cancer related pain. *Pain* **17**, 277–88.

44. **Woodforde, J.M. and Fielding, J.R.** (1970). Pain and cancer. *Journal of Psychosomatic Research* **14**, 365–70.

45. **Stiefel, F.C., Breitbart, W., and Holland, J.C.** (1989). Corticosteroids in cancer: neuropsychiatric complications. *Cancer Investigation* **7**, 479–91.

46. **Bukberg, J., Penman, D., and Holland, J.** (1984). Depression in hospitalized cancer patients. *Psychosomatic Medicine* **43**, 199–212.

47. **Massie, J.M., Holland, J.C., and Glass, E.** (1983). Delirium in terminally ill cancer patients. *American Journal of Psychiatry* **140**, 1048–50.

48. **Bruera, E. et al.** (1989). The cognitive effects of the administration of narcotics. *Pain* **39**, 13–16.

49. **Breitbart, W.** (1987). Suicide in cancer patients. *Oncology* **1**, 49–53.

50. **Breitbart, W.** (1990). Cancer pain and suicide. In *Advances in Pain Research and Therapy* Vol. 16 (ed. K.M. Foley et al.), pp. 399–412. New York: Raven Press.

51. **Sison, A., Eller, K., Segal, J., Passik, S., Breitbart, W.** Suicidal ideation in ambulatory HIV-infected patients: the roles of pain, mood, and disease status (Abstract). *Current Concepts in Psycho-oncology IV*, New York, October 10–12, 1991.

52. **Levin, D.N., Cleeland, C.S., and Dan, R.** (1985). Public attitudes toward cancer pain. *Cancer* **56**, 2337–9.

53. **Bolund, C.** (1985). Suicide and cancer: II. Medical and care factors in suicide by cancer patients in Sweden, 1973–1976. *Journal of Psychosocial Oncology* **3**, 17–30.

54. **Farberow, N.L., Schneidman, E.S., and Leonard, C.V.** Suicide among general medical and surgical hospital patients with malignant neoplasms. Medical Bulletin 9, Washington DC, US Veterans Administration, 1963.

55. **Massie, M., Gagnon, P., and Holland, J.** (1994). Depression and suicide in patients with cancer. *Joural of Pain and Symptom Management* **9** (5), 325–31.

56. **Silberfarb, P.M., Manrer, L.H., and Cronthamel, C.S.** (1980). Psychological aspects of neoplastic disease, I: Functional status of breast cancer patients during different treatment regimens. *American Journal of Psychiatry* **137**, 450–5.

57. **Achte, K.A. and Vanhkonen, M.L.** (1971). Cancer and the psych. *Omega* **2**, 46–56.

58. **Brown, J.H., Henteleff, P., Barakat, S., and Rowe, J.R.** (1986). Is it normal for terminally ill patients to desire death. *American Journal of Psychiatry* **143**, 208–11.

59. **Breitbart, W., Rosenfeld, B., Pessin, H., Kaim, M., Funesti-Esch, J., Galietta, M., Nelson, C.J., and Brescia, R.** (2000). Depression, hopelessness, and

desire for hastened death in terminally ill patients with cancer. *Journal of the American Medical Association* **284** (22), 2907–11.

60. **Saltzburg, D.** et al. The relationship of pain and depression to suicidal ideation in cancer patients (Abstract). ASCO Annual Meeting, San Francisco, May 21–23, 1989.
61. **Suarez-Almazor, M.E., Newman, C., Hanson, J., and Bruera, E.** (2002). Attitudes of terminally ill cancer patients about euthanasia and assisted suicide: predominance of psychosocial determinants and beliefs over symptom distress and subsequent survival. *Journal of Clinical Oncology* **20** (8), 2134–41.
62. **Marzuk, P., Tierney, H., Tardiff, K., Gross, G., Morgan, E., Hsu, M., and Mann, J.** (1988). Increased risk of suicide in persons with AIDS. *Journal of the American Medical Association* **259**, 1333–7.
63. **Rabkin, J., Remien, R., Katoff, L., and Williams, J.** (1993). Suicidality in AIDS long-term survivors: what is the evidence? *AIDS-Care* **5** (4), 401–11.
64. **Cleeland, C., Gonin, R., Hatfield, A., Edmonson, J., Blum, R., Stewart, J., and Pandya, K.** (1994). Pain and its treatment in outpatients with metastatic cancer. *New England Journal of Medicine* **330**, 592–6.
65. **Lebovits, A.K., Lefkowitz, M., and McCarthy, D.** (1989). The prevalence and management of pain in patients with AIDS. A review of 134 cases. *The Clinical Journal of Pain* **5**, 245–8.
66. **McCormack, J.P., Li, R., Zarowny, D., and Singer, J.** (1993). Inadequate treatment of pain in ambulatory HIV patients. *The Clinical Journal of Pain* **9**, 279–83.
67. **Breitbart, W., Passik, R., Rosenfeld, B., Portenoy, R., McDonald, M., and Thaler, H.** AIDS specific patient-related barriers to pain management (Poster). American Pain Society, 1994.
68. **Breitbart, W., Passik S., Rosenfeld, B., Portenoy, R., McDonald, M., and Thaler, H.** Undertreatment of pain in AIDS (Poster). American Pain Society, 1994.
69. **Charap, A.D.** (1978). The knowledge, attitudes, and experience of medical personnel treating pain in the terminally ill. *Mt Sinai Journal of Medicine* **45**, 561–80.
70. **Macaluso, C., Weinberg, D., and Foley, K.M.** Opiod abuse and misuse in a cancer pain population (Abstract). Second International Congress on Cancer Pain, Rye, New York, July 14–17, 1988.
71. **Kanner, R.M. and Foley, K.M.** (1981). Patterns of narcotic use in a cancer pain clinic. *Annals of the New York Academy of Science* **362**, 161–72.
72. **Breitbart, W. and Patt, R.** (1994). Pain management in the patient with AIDS. *Hematology/Oncology Annals* **2**, 391–9.
73. **Bruera, E., MacMillan, K., Pither, J., and MacDonald, R.N.** (1990). Effects of morphine on the dyspnea of terminal cancer patients. *Journal of Pain and Symptom Management* **5**, 341–4.
74. **Grossman, S.A., Sheidler, V.R., Sweden, K., Mucenski, J., and Piantadosi, S.** (1991). Correlations of patient and caregiver ratings of cancer pain. *Journal of Pain and Symptom Management* **6**, 53–7.
75. **Cassem, N.H.** (1987). They dying patient. In *Massachusetts General Hospital Handbook of General Hospital Psychiatry* 2nd edn (ed. T.P. Hackett and N.H. Cassem), pp. 332–52. Littleton MA: PSG Publishing Co. Inc.
76. **Passik, S., Horowitz, S., Malkin, M., and Gargan, R.** A psychoeducational support program for spouses of brain tumor patients (Abstract). Symposium on New Trends in the Psychological Support of the Cancer Patient, American Psychiatric Association Annual Meeting, New Orleans, LA, May 7–12, 1991.
77. **Syrajala, K., Cummings, C., and Donaldson, G.** (1992). Hypnosis or cognitive behavioral training for the reduction of pai and nausea during cancer treatment: a controlled trial. *Pain* **48**, 137–46.
78. **Spiegel, D. and Bloom, J.R.** (1983). Group therapy and hypnosis reduce metastatic breast carcinoma pain. *Psychosomatic Medicine* **4**, 333–9.
79. **Fishman, B. and Loscalzo, M.** (1987). Cognitive–behavioral interventions in the management of cancer pain: principles and applications. *Medical Clinics of North America* **71**, 271–87.
80. **Cleeland, C.S.** (1987). Nonpharmacologic management of cancer pain. *Journal of Pain and Symptom Control* **2**, 523–8.
81. **Loscalzo, M. and Jacobsen, P.B.** (1990). Practical behavioral approaches to the effective management of pain and distress. *Journal of Psychosocial Oncology* **8**, 139–69.
82. **Turk, D. and Fernendez, E.** (1990). On the Putative Uniqueness of cancer pain: do psychological principles apply? *Behaviour Research and Therapy* **28** (1), 1–13.
83. **Fishman, B.** (1990). The treatment of suffering in patients with cancer pain. In *Advances in Pain Research and Therapy* Vol. 16 (ed. K. Foley, J. Bonica and V. Ventafridda), pp. 301–16. New York: Raven Press.
84. **Jensen, M., Turner, J., Romano, J., and Karoly.** (1991). Coping with chronic pain: a critical review of the literature. *Pain* **47**, 249–83.
85. **Breitbart, W. and Holland, J.C.** (1988). Psychiatric complications of cancer. In *Current Therapy in Hematology Oncology-3* (ed. M.C. Brain and P.P. Carbone), pp. 268–74. Toronto and Philadelphia: B.C. Decker, Inc.
86. **Montgomery, G.H., Weltz, C.R., Seltz, M., and Bovbjerg, D.H.** (2002). Brief presurgery hypnosis reduces distress and pain in excisional breast biopsy patients. *International Journal of Clinical and Experimental Hypnosis* **50** (1), 17–32.
87. **Sellick, S.M. and Zaza, C.** (1998). Critical review of 5 nonpharmacologic strategies for managing cancer pain. *Cancer Prevention and Control* **2** (1), 7–14.
88. **Kazak, A.E., Penati, B., Brophy, P., and Himelstein, B.** (1998). Pharmacologic and psychologic interventions for procedural pain. *Pediatrics* **102** (1 Pt 1), 59–66.
89. **Carroll, D. and Seers, K.** (1998). Relaxation for the relief of chronic pain: a systematic review. *Journal of Advanced Nursing* **27** (3), 476–87.
90. **Wallace, K.G.** (1997). Analysis of recent literature concerning relaxation and imagery interventions for cancer pain. *Cancer Nursing* **20** (2), 79–87.
91. **Luebbert, K., Dahme, B., and Hasenbring, M.** (2001). The effectiveness of relaxation training in reducing treatment-related symptoms and improving emotional adjustment in acute non-surgical cancer treatment: a meta-analytical review. *Psycho-oncology* **10** (6), 490–502.
92. **Erickson, M.H.** (1959). Hypnosis in painful terminal illness. *American Journal of Clinical Hypnosis* **1**, 1117–21.
93. **Benson, H.** *The Relaxation Response.* New York: William Morrow, 1975.
94. **Broome, M., Lillis, P., McGahhe, T., and Bates, T.** (1992). The use of distraction and imagery with children during painful procedures. *Oncology Nursing Forum* **19**, 499–502.
95. **Spiegel, D.** (1985). The use of hypnosis in controlling cancer pain. *CA—A Cancer Journal for Clinicians* **4**, 221–31.
96. **Levitan, A.** (1992). The use of hypnosis with cancer patients. *Psychiatry and Medicine* **10**, 119–31.
97. **Tan, S.Y. and Leucht, C.A.** (1997). Cognitive–behavioral therapy for clinical pain control: a 15-year update and its relationship to hypnosis. *International Journal of Clinical and Experimental Hypnosis* **45** (4), 396–416.
98. **Douglas, D.B.** (1999). Hypnosis: useful, neglected, available. *American Journal of Hospice and Palliative Care* **16** (5), 665–70.
99. **Liossi, C. and Hatira, P.** (1999). Clinical hypnosis versus cognitive behavioral training for pain management with pediatric cancer patients undergoing bone marrow aspirations. *International Journal of Clinical and Experimental Hypnosis* **47** (2), 104–16.
100. **Fotopoulos, S.S., Graham, C., and Cook, M.R.** (1979). Psychophysiologic control of cancer pain. In *Advances in Pain Research and Therapy* Vol. 2 (ed. J.J. Bonica and V. Ventafridda), pp. 231–44. New York: Raven Press.
101. **Munro, S.M. and Mount, B.** (1978). Music therapy in palliative care. *Canadian Medical Association Journal* **119**, 1029–34.
102. **Schroeder-Sheker, T.** (1993). Music for the dying: a personal account of the new field of music thanatology—history, theories, and clinical narratives. *Advances* **9**, 36–48.
103. **Magill, L.** (2001). The use of music therapy to address the suffering in advanced cancer pain. *Journal of Palliative Care* **17** (3), 167–72.
104. **Chlan, L., Evans, D., Greenleaf, M., and Walker, J.** (2000). Effects of a single music therapy intervention on anxiety, discomfort, satisfaction, and compliance with screening guidelines in outpatients undergoing flexible sigmoidoscopy. *Gastroenterology Nursing* **23** (4), 148.
105. **Manne, S., Redd, W., Jacobsen, P., and Georgiades, I.** Aroma for treatment of anxiety during, MRI scans (Abstract). Symposium on New Trends in the Psychological Support of the Cancer Patient, American Psychiatric Association Annual Meeting, New Orleans, LA, May 7–12, 1991.

106. **Connell, C.** (1992). Art therapy as part of a palliative cancer program. *Palliative Medicine.* **6**, 18–25.

107. **Breitbart, W.** (1992). Psychotropic adjuvant analgesics for cancer pain. *Psycho-Oncology* **V**, 133–45.

108. **Farrar, J.T. and Portenoy, R.K.** (2001). Neuropathic cancer pain: the role of adjuvant analgesics. *Oncology* **15** (11), 1435–42, 1445, 1450–3.

109. **France, R.D.** (1987). The future for antidepressants: treatment of pain. *Psychopathology* **20**, 99–113.

110. **Getto, C.J., Sorkness, C.A., and Howell, T.** (1987). Antidepressants and chronic nonmalignant pain: a review. *Journal of Pain and Symptom Control* **2**, 9–18.

111. **Walsh, T.D.** (1983). Antidepressants and chronic pain. *Clinical Neuropharmacology* **6**, 271–95.

112. **Walsh, T.D.** (1990). Adjuvant analgesic therapy in cnacer pain. In *Advances in Pain Research and Therapy* Vol. 16 (ed. K.M. Foley et al.), pp. 155–65. Second International Congress on Cancer Pain. New York: Raven Press.

113. **Butler, S.** (1986). Present status of tricyclic antidepressants in chronic pain therapy. In *Advances in Pain Research and Therapy* Vol. 7 (ed. C. Benedetti et al.), pp. 173–96. New York: Raven Press.

114. **Ventafridda, V., Bonezzi, C., Caraceni, A., DeConno, F., Guarise, G., Ramella, G., Saita, L., Silvani, V., Tamburini, M., and Toscani, F.** (1987). Antidepressants for cancer pain and other painful syndromes with deafferentation component: comparison of Amitriptyline and Trazodone. *Italian Journal of Neurological Sciences* **8**, 579–87.

115. **Magni, G., Arsie, D., and DeLeo, D.** (1987). Antidepressants in the treatment of cancer pain. A survey in Italy. *Pain* **29**, 347–53.

116. **Onghena, P. and Van Houdenhove, B.** (1992). Antidepressant-induced analgesia in chronic non-malignant pain: a meta-analysis of 39 placebo-controlled studies. *Pain* **49**, 205–19.

117. **Lefkowitz, M. and Breitbart, W.** (1992). Chronic pain and AIDS. *Innovations in Pain Medicine* **36**, 2–3, 18.

118. **Max, M.B., Culnane, M., Schafer, S.C., Gracely, R.H., Walther, D.J., Smoller, B., and Dubner R.** (1987). Amitriptyline relieves diabetic-neuropathy pain in patients with normal and depressed mood. *Neurology* **37**, 589–96.

119. **Max, M.B., Schafer, S.C., Culnane, M., Smollen, B., Dubner, R., and Gracel, R.H.** (1982). Amitriptyline, but not lorazepam, relieves postherpetic neuralgia. *Neurology* **38**, 427–32.

120. **Pilowsky, I., Hallett, E.C., Bassett, D.L., Thomas, P.G., and Penhall, R.K.** (1982). A controlled study of amitriptyline in the treatment of chronic pain. *Pain* **14**, 169–79.

121. **Sharav, Y., Singer, E., Schmidt, E., Dione, R.A., and Dubner, R.** (1987). The analgesic effect of amitriptyline on chronic facial pain. *Pain* **31**, 199–209.

122. **Watson, C.P., Evans, R.J., Reed, K., Merskey, H., Goldsmith, L., and Warsh, J.** (1982). Amitriptyline versus placebo in post herpetic neuralgia. *Neurology* **32**, 671–3.

123. **Kvindesal, B., Molin, J., Froland, A., and Gram, L.F.** (1984). Imipramine treatment of painful diabetic neuropathy. *Journal of the American Medical Association* **251**, 1727–30.

124. **Young, R.J. and Clarke, B.F.** (1985). Pain relief in diabetic neuropathy: the effectiveness of imipramine and related drugs. *Diabetic Medicine* **2**, 363–6.

125. **Sindrup, S.H.** et al. (1989). Imipramine treatment in diabetic neuropathy: relief of subjective symptoms without changes in peripheral and autonomic nerve function. *European Journal of Clinical Pharmacology* **37**, 151–3.

126. **Max, M.B.** et al. (1991). Efficacy of desipramine in painful diabetic neuropathy: a placebo-controlled trial. *Pain* **45**, 3–10.

127. **Gordon, N., Heller, P., Gear, R., and Levine, J.** (1993). Temporal factors in the enhancement of morphine analgesic by desipramine. *Pain* **53**, 273–6.

128. **Gomez-Perez, F.J.** et al. (1985). Nortriptyline and fluphenazine in the symptomatic treatment of diabetic neuropathy. A double-blind cross-over study. *Pain* **23**, 395–400.

129. **Langohr, H.D., Stohr, M., and Petruch, F.** (1982). An open and double-blind crosover study on the efficacy of clomipramine (anafranil) in patients with painful mono- and polyneuropathies. *European Neurology* **21**, 309–15.

130. **Tiegno, M., Pagnoni, B., Calmi, A., Rigoli, M., Braga, P.C., and Panerai, A.E.** (1987). Chlorimipramine compared to pentazocine as a unique treatment in post-operative pain. *International Journal of Clinical and Pharmacological Research* **7**, 141–3.

131. **Hammeroff, S.R.** et al. (1982). Doxepin effects on chronic pain, depression and plasma opioids. *Journal of Clinical Psychiatry* **2**, 22–6.

132. **Walsh, T.D.** Controlled study of imipramine and morphine in chronic pain due to advanced cancer (Abstract). ASCO, Los Angeles, May 4–6, 1986.

133. **Botney, M. and Fields, H.C.** (1983). Amitriptyline potentiates morphine analgesia by direct action on the central nervous system. *Annals of Neurology* **13**, 160–4.

134. **Watson, C., Chipan, M., Reed, K., Evans, R., and Birket, N.** (1992). Amitriptyline versus maprotiline in postherpetic neuralgia: a randomized double-blind crossover trial. *Pain* **48**, 29–36.

135. **Malseed, R.T. and Goldstein, F.J.** (1979). Enhancement of morphine analgesics by tricyclic antidepressnts. *Neuropharmacology* **18**, 827–9.

136. **Ventafridda, V.** et al. (1990). Studies on the effects of antidepressant drugs on the antinociceptive action of morphine and on plasma morphine in rat and man. *Pain* **43**, 155–62.

137. **Spiegel, K., Kalb, R., and Pasternak, G.W.** (1983). Analgesic activity of tricyclic antidepressants. *Annals of Neurology* **13**, 462–5.

138. **Davidoff, G.** et al. (1987). Trazodone hydrochloride in the treatment of dysesthetic pain in traumatic myelopathy: a randomized, double-blind, placebo-controlled study. *Pain* **29**, 151–61.

139. **Costa, D., Mogos, I., and Toma, T.** (1985). Efficacy and safety of mianserin in the treatment of depression of woman with cancer. *Acta Psychiatrica Scandinavica* **72**, 85–92.

140. **Eberhard, G.** et al. (1988). A double-blind randomized study of clomipramine versus maprotiline in patients with idiopathic pain syndromes. *Neuropsychobiology* **19**, 25–32.

141. **Feighner, J.P.** (1985). A comparative trial of fluoxetine and amitriptyline in patients with major depressive disorder. *Journal of Clinical Psychiatry* **46**, 369–72.

142. **Hynes, M.D.** et al. (1985). Fluxoetine, a selective inhibitor of serotonin uptake, potentiates morphine analgesia without altering its descriminative stimulus properties or affinity for opioid receptors. *Life Sciences* **36**, 2317–23.

143. **Diamond, S. and Frietag, F.G.** (1989). The use of fluoxetine in the treatment of headache. *Clinical Journal of Pain* **5**, 200–1.

144. **Geller, S.A.** (1989). Treatment of fibrositis with fluoxetine hydrochloride (Prozac). *American Journal of Medicine* **87**, 594–5.

145. **Theesen, K.A. and Marsh, W.R.** (1989). Relief of diabetic neuropathy with fluoxetine. *DICP, The Annals of Pharmacotherapy* **23**, 572–4.

146. **Max, M.B., Lynch, S.A., Muir, J., Shoaf, S.E., Smoller, B., and Dubner, R.** (1992). Effects of desipramine, amitriptyline, and fluoxetine on pain in diabetic neuropathy. *New England Journal of Medicine* **326**, 1250–6.

147. **Sindrup, S.H., Gram, L.F., Brosen, K., Eshoj, O., and Mogenson, E.F.** (1990). The selective serotonin reuptake inhibitor paroxetine is effective in the treatment of diabetic neuropathy symptoms. *Pain* **42**, 135–44.

148. **Pick, C.G., Paul, D., Eison, M.S., and Pasternak, G.** (1992). Potentiation of opioid analgesia by the antidepressant nefazodone. *European Journal of Pharmacology* **211**, 375–81.

149. **Holland, J.C., Romano, S.J., Heiligenstein, J.H., Tepner, R.G., and Wilson, M.G.** (1998). A controlled trial of fluoxetine and desipramine in depressed women with advanced cancer. *Psychooncology* **7** (4), 291–300.

150. **McQuay, H., Carroll, D., and Glynn, C.** (1993). Dose–response for analgesic effect of amitriptyline in chronic pain. *Anesthesia* **48**, 281–5.

151. **Watson, C.P. and Evans, R.J.** (1985). A comparative trial of amitriptyline and zimelidine in post-herpetic neuralgia. *Pain* **23**, 387–94.

152. **Tyler, M.A.** (1974). Treatment of the painful shoulder syndrome with amitriptyline and lithium carbonate. *Canadian Medical Association Journal* **111**, 137–40.

153. **Ehrnrooth, E., Grau, C., Zachariae, R., and Andersen, J.** (2001). Randomized trial of opioids versus tricyclic antidepressants for radiation-induced mucositis pain in head and neck cancer. *Acta Oncologica* **40** (6), 745–50.

154. **Lascelles, R.G.** (1966). Atypical facial pain and depression. *British Journal of Psychology* **122**, 651.

155. **Anthony, M. and Lance, J.W.** (1969). MAO inhibition in the treatment of migraine. *Archives in Neurology* **21**, 263.

156. Fernandez, F. et al. (1987). Methylphenidate for depressive disorders in cancer patients. *Psychosomatics* **28**, 455–61.

157. Kaufmann, M.W., Murray, G.B., and Cassem, N.H. (1982). Use of psychostimulants in medically ill depressive patients. *Psychosomatics* **23**, 817–19.

158. Bruera, E., Chadwick, S., Brennels, C., Hanson, J., and MacDonald, R.N. (1987). Methylphenidate associated with narcotics for the treatment of cancer pain. *Cancer Treatment Reports* **71**, 67–70.

159. Bruera, E., Brenneis, C., Paterson, A.H., and MacDonald, R.N. (1989). Use of methylphenidate as an adjuvant to narcotic analgesics in patients with advanced cancer. *Journal of Pain and Symptom Management* **4**, 3–6.

160. Bruera, E., Fainsinger, R., MacEachern, T., and Hanson, J. (1992). The use of methylphenidate in patients with incident cancer pain receiving regular opiates: a preliminary report. *Pain* **50**, 75–7.

161. Forrest, W.H. et al. (1977). Dextroamphetamine with morphine for the treatment of post-operative pain. *New England Journal of Medicine* **296**, 712–15.

162. Breitbart, W. and Mermelstein, H. (1992). Pemoline: an alternative psychostimulant in the management of depressive disorders in cancer patients. *Psychosomatics* **33**, 352–6.

163. Nehra, A. et al. (1990). Pemoline associated hepatic injury. *Gastroenterology* **99**, 1517–19.

164. Beaver, W.T. et al. (1966). A comparison of the analgesic effect of methotrimeprazine and morphine in patients with cancer. *Clinical Pharmacology and Therapeutics* **7**, 436–46.

165. Maltbie, A.A. et al. (1979). Analgesia and haloperidol: a hypothesis. *Journal of Clinical Psychiatry* **40**, 323–6.

166. Lechin, F. et al. (1989). Pimozide therapy for trigeminal neuralgia. *Archives in Neurology* **9**, 960–4.

167. Khojainova, N., Santiago-Palma, J., Kornick, C., Breitbart, W., and Gonzales, G.R. (2002). Olanzapine in the management of cancer pain. *Journal of Pain and Symptom Management* **23** (4), 346–50.

168. Beaver, W.T. and Feise, G. (1976). Comparison of the analgesic effects of morphine, hydroxyzine and their combination in patients with post-operative pain. In *Advances in Pain Research and Therapy* (ed. J.J. Bonica and Albe-Fessard), pp. 533–57. New York: Raven Press.

169. Rumore, M. and Schlichting, D. (1986). Clinical efficacy of antihistamines as analgesics. *Pain* **25**, 7–22.

170. Coda, B., Mackie, A., and Hill, H. (1992). Influence of alprazolam on opioid analgesia and side effects during steady-stage morphine infusions. *Pain* **50**, 309–16.

171. Fernandez, F., Adams, F., and Holmes, V.F. (1987). Analgesic effect of alprazolam in patients with chronic, organic pain of malignant origin. *Journal of Clinical Psychopharmacology* **3**, 167–9.

172. Caccia, M.R. (1975). Clonazepam in facial neuralgia and cluster headache: clinical and electrophysiological study. *European Neurology* **13**, 560–3.

173. Swerdlow, M. and Cundill, J.G. (1981). Anticonvulsant drugs used in the treatment of lancinating pains: a comparison. *Anesthesia* **36**, 1129–34.

174. Egan, K., Ready, L., Nessly, M., and Greer, B. (1992). Self administration of midazolam for post-operative anxiety: a double blinded study. *Pain* **49**, 3–8.

175. Liao, J. and Takemori, A. (1990). Quantitative assessmentof antinociceptive effects of midazolam, amitriptyline, and carbamazepine alone and in combination with morphine in mice. *Anesthesiology* **73**, A753.

8.2.11 Difficult pain problems: an integrated approach

Russell K. Portenoy, Karen Forbes, David Lussier, and Geoffrey Hanks

Introduction

Roughly 80–90 per cent of pain due to cancer can be relieved relatively simply with oral analgesics and adjuvant drugs in accordance with the World Health Organization's (WHO) guidelines. The remaining 10–20 per cent are difficult to treat and a small proportion present formidable problems of management. These figures have not changed in the last 10 years since the first edition of this textbook, though there has been some progress in refining our approach to the most difficult problems. What has changed is that the general level of management of pain in cancer has improved and is improving as the knowledge and skills required to relieve uncomplicated pain is much more widely taught and learnt, particularly at an undergraduate or pre-registration level. In terms of potential gains in the relief of suffering due to cancer this remains a priority: to ensure that all those who need to know have the knowledge (and also the means to put that knowledge into practice) to allow them to effectively relieve uncomplicated cancer pain.

This chapter is about pain that is not easily relieved using a simple pharmacological approach: the 10–20 per cent of cancer patients who have difficult problems. Not surprisingly, just as the figures have not changed, the nature of the problems too have not. There have been important developments in the intervening years, with some new pharmacological agents and also new methods of delivering old drugs that have contributed to improved outcomes for patients.

Opioid-responsive and opioid poorly responsive pain

The most important drugs used in the pharmacological management of pain are the opioids, and when pharmacological treatment proves inadequate the focus has been on this group. However, the terminology used to describe pains that are not easily controlled with opioid analgesics is confusing. It is rarely the case that pain can be described as 'non-responsive' or 'resistant to opioids' because this implies on all or nothing phenomenon. Usually, pain in cancer responds at least partially to opioids and a preferable term is 'opioid poorly responsive pain'. A pragmatic clinical definition is that this is pain which is inadequately relieved by opioid analgesics given in a dose that causes intolerable adverse effects despite optimal measures to control them. The most common example is neuropathic pain. Some authorities have suggested that it is oxymoronic to classify pain according to drugs to which it does not respond. However, this terminology is now part of day-to-day clinical parlance and whilst being necessarily imprecise it communicates clearly the nature of the problem.

Morphine and alternative step 3 opioids appear to have no clinically relevant ceiling effect to analgesia. As the dose is raised analgesic effects increase as a log linear function. A point may be reached at which higher doses could theoretically produce greater analgesia but dose escalation is not possible because adverse effects supervene, thus effectively defining the responsiveness of the pain syndrome in that particular patient. It follows, therefore, that opioid responsiveness is a continuum that might be influenced by any of a large number of patient and drug related, as well as pain related, factors.

It is important to stress that a presumptive or tentative diagnosis of pain that is likely to be poorly responsive to opioids is not an indication to avoid the use of these drugs. Whatever the underlying cause of the pain the usual approach using the framework of the WHO method should be followed.

Paradoxical pain and morphine-3-glucuronide

In the last edition of the textbook we discussed the concept of paradoxical pain: a recently introduced term that had caused some confusion.[1] Paradoxical pain was first described as 'pain which ceases to be relieved or is worsened by further administration' of morphine or diamorphine.[2] The idea that pain in some patients could be made worse by continued administration of morphine conflicts with the substantial clinical experience that there is no arbitrary ceiling to the dose of morphine that may be required by an individual patient and that it is safe to titrate up the dose until pain relief is achieved or side-effects supervene. The suggestion, thus, raised anxiety about the potential harm that may be done if the morphine dose is titrated too far. The concept of paradoxical pain was based on a theory that in some patients the major metabolite of morphine, morphine-3-glucuronide (M3G) was produced in excessive amounts.[3] In the past, M3G has been assumed to be inert as is the case with most glucuronide metabolites.[4] Recent behavioural studies in rodents, however, suggested that M3G produces a functional antagonism of the analgesic effects of morphine and its active metabolite M6G.[5,6] There is also some evidence in animal models that M3G may be responsible for the central nervous system excitatory adverse effects seen with morphine, such as myoclonus.[7,8] The data suggesting an antagonistic effect of M3G were puzzling and difficult to interpret in the light of previous assumptions about the inactivity of this metabolite and evidence that it does not bind to opioid receptors.[9] This had been disputed by the authors of the concept of paradoxical pain but it does now seem clear that M3G does not bind to opioid receptors.[10] Data from electrophysiological animal models show no evidence of an antagonistic effect of M3G[11] and recent studies in human volunteers indicate that M3G appears to be devoid of significant activity.[12,13] In particular, there is no evidence of functional antagonism of morphine or M6G in humans and overall it seems that M3G plays no significant role in the pharmacodynamics of morphine.

In our previous discussion of paradoxical pain we concluded that 'it seems likely that both the concept of paradoxical pain as a distinct entity and the purported explanation are spurious'.[1] The most recent evidence supports this conclusion. What was described as paradoxical pain is 'opioid poorly responsive pain'. In some patients this uncontrolled pain may be complicated by delirium and hyperexcitability, characterized by multifocal myoclonus and other signs of central nervous system excitation (tremulousness and occasionally seizures), which may be associated not just with morphine but with other opioids too.

Opioid-irrelevant pain

In some patients, the complaint of pain is more a reflection of social, psychological, or spiritual turmoil than a result of physical injury or damage. Such pain is not best treated with morphine and has been characterized as 'opioid-irrelevant pain' by Hinton (quoted by Kearney).[14] Such pain may appear to be 'opioid poorly responsive pain'. It may dominate a particular individual or, more commonly, may form a component of many patients' complaints of pain. This emphasizes the need to keep in mind the concept of 'total pain', which encompasses physical, social, psychological, and spiritual factors, when managing cancer patients in pain. Patients whose pain remains a problem despite careful dose titration with an opioid analgesic, or who appear unduly sensitive to opioid adverse effects, need careful reassessment of the mechanisms underlying their pain with particular attention to possible psychological factors.

Difficult pain problems

In this chapter, we have selected examples of cancer pain that usually present the most difficult management problems. Each is illustrated by a case history that is based on a real patient. The reader will note some differences in clinical practice because these case histories come from Europe and North America. For example, hydromorphone is widely prescribed in the United States and Canada but has only recently become available in the United Kingdom, and is still relatively little used. These differences in detail should not obscure the overall approach to each problem and the principles of management.

Neuropathic pain

Patients with chronic neuropathic pain are over-represented amongst those who are refractory to routine analgesic measures, including opioid therapy.[15–17] The clinical challenge presented by such patients may be daunting, as illustrated by the following case.

Case history A 66-year-old man presented with progressive scapula pain. A computerized tomographic (CT) scan demonstrated a mass that arose from the lung apex and abutted the chest wall; enlarged lymph nodes were identified in the mediastinum. A needle biopsy revealed squamous cell carcinoma. Radiotherapy was scheduled and pain was effectively treated with an oxycodone/aspirin combination product. The pain was completely relieved by the radiotherapy.

Two months later, an intermittent stabbing pain began in the medial forearm. Within weeks severe aching in the elbow and burning sensations in the hand began. CT revealed that the apical mass had extended superiorly into the region of the brachial plexus. The mediastinal tumour had increased and there were new metastatic deposits in both lungs. Further antitumour therapy was offered but the patient declined.

Little pain relief was provided by the oxycodone/aspirin regimen, and the patient was switched to oral morphine in a dose of 30 mg 4-hourly. Pain continued to be severe and the morphine dose was gradually increased to 150 mg 4-hourly. The pain improved but sedation and confusion became intolerable. Morphine was discontinued and a trial of oral hydromorphone was begun in a dose equianalgesic to two-thirds of the dose of morphine. Pain relief was much improved although still inadequate and daytime sedation lessened. Higher doses, however, produced hallucinations without improving analgesia.

Oral hydromorphone was continued at the initial dose and amitriptyline was added in a dose of 10 mg nightly. There was no effect on pain but sedation and confusion worsened. The amitriptyline was discontinued and gabapentin was substituted, at an initial daily dose of 300 mg daily. This drug was better tolerated and the dose was gradually increased to 2700 mg daily in three divided doses. Improvement was noted with each dose increase and no side-effects occurred. At the highest dose, pain was still constant but its usual intensity was mild and severe episodes were both less intense and less frequent. The patient perceived these residual symptoms to be tolerable and therapy was continued.

Six weeks later, pain in the shoulder, elbow, and hand escalated rapidly. Nutritional status had been poor and the patient was troubled by progressive asthenia, dyspnoea on exertion, and cough. A small increase in the hydromorphone dose produced confusion and the patient was admitted to hospital. Dexamethasone was added at an initial dose of 10 mg followed by 2 mg twice daily. This decreased pain intensity and also improved appetite and the dyspnoea. After a few days, however, he became delirious and the dexamethasone was discontinued. Consecutive trials of mexiletine, carbamazepine, sodium valproate, and clonidine were then administered but each was limited to a relatively low dose due to the onset of worsening cognitive impairment. None of these trials improved pain control.

A stellate ganglion block was performed ipsilateral to the painful limb but produced no change in the pain. A percutaneous epidural catheter was then placed with the tip of the catheter situated just caudal to the cervical enlargement. A trial of morphine and then a morphine/local anaesthetic mixture was initiated. The dose of morphine was increased until confusion worsened without impact on the pain. The addition of the local anaesthetic initially yielded substantial improvement but this persisted for only 3 days. The patient developed a fever and the catheter was removed.

The risks and potential benefits of neurolytic procedures, including rhizotomy, cordotomy, and cingulotomy, were discussed with the patient, who refused invasive approaches. Following discussion with the patient and family, it was decided that the opioid dose would be increased and that neuroleptic or sedative drugs would be used to manage the delirium that would ensue. This was done and the patient was transferred to a hospice 2 weeks later, where he remained deeply sedated until his death a few days later.

The problem

The term 'neuropathic pain' is applied to a diverse group of syndromes in which the sustaining mechanisms for the pain are presumed to be related to aberrant somatosensory processes in the peripheral nervous system, central nervous system, or both. These pains are usually precipitated by overt injury to neural structures but, once established, are often far in excess of any overt peripheral pathology.

This category of pain syndromes is part of a broader taxonomy based on inferred pain mechanisms,[18] which also includes the so-called nociceptive pains and psychogenic pains. Nociceptive pain refers to pain that is perceived to be due to ongoing activation of primary afferent nerves that respond to noxious stimuli (nociceptors). These nerves innervate both somatic and visceral structures; somatic pain and visceral pain are considered subtypes. Psychogenic pain, subtypes of which may be described using an alternative psychiatric classification,[19] refers to pain that is at least partially sustained by primary psychological processes.

Although this approach to classification by inferred pain mechanism is undoubtedly a gross simplification of the complex pathophysiologies that result in chronic pain, it is clinically relevant and widely accepted by practitioners. As discussed below, such inferences can help guide patient assessment and therapeutic decision-making.

The patient in the case report described aching shoulder pain and dysaesthesiae ('unpleasant abnormal sensation'[20]) in the arm. The nature of these pains and the position and extent of the tumour mass suggest that the pain syndrome resulted from both nociceptive processes (activation of somatic nociceptors by direct infiltration of the chest wall) and neuropathic processes (caused by brachial plexus injury). The experience of multiple types of pain in the same patient is very common in the palliative care setting.[21] A psychological contribution also is probably quite common in such settings but was not prominent in this case. As time passed, the predominating and most challenging aspect of the pain was its neuropathic component.

The clinical challenge associated with the management of neuropathic pain derives from the observation that these pains may respond less well to opioid drugs than nociceptive pains. The patient described in the case report, for example, failed to respond satisfactorily to two opioids (morphine and hydromorphone) and the same opioid (morphine) by two routes of administration.

The observation that at least some types of neuropathic pain are relatively less responsive to opioid drugs has strong empirical support from both clinical studies[15–18,21–23] and experimental data.[24] Although there is no evidence to support the conclusion that neuropathic pains are generically 'opioid-resistant', it is likely that a neuropathic mechanism (or some types of neuropathic mechanisms) increases the likelihood of an unfavourable opioid response.[16,17]

Given the discouragement that many clinicians experience when encountering patients with neuropathic pain, it is important to emphasize that favourable responses to opioid drugs do occur in such cases. Indeed, clinical experience suggests that properly administered opioid therapy often yields a satisfactory outcome. This potential for a favourable opioid response has been demonstrated in surveys of patients with malignant and non-malignant pain,[15,25–27] pharmacokinetic–pharmacodynamic studies of opioid infusions in patients with diverse neuropathic pain syndromes,[23] and randomized controlled studies. The latter studies have shown that patients with different types of neuropathic pain can respond favourably to intravenous morphine[28] or fentanyl.[29] An intravenous infusion of morphine is more effective than intravenous lidocaine in patients with postherpetic neuralgia[30] and a recent double-blind randomized trial demonstrated that oral morphine is more effective than nortriptyline in the same condition.[31] Similar trials also have confirmed the efficacy of oxycodone and tramadol in postherpetic neuralgia and painful diabetic neuropathy.[32–34] Together, these observations strongly support the value of a trial of opioid therapy as a primary strategy in the treatment of neuropathic pain.

Clinical spectrum and pathophysiology

Neuropathic pains comprise numerous distinctive clinical entities that vary in presentation, specific pathophysiological factors, and, to a lesser extent, treatment.[35,36] Although taxonomies based on syndrome identification or lesion localization are often used, classification by putative mechanism[18] (Fig. 1) may be particularly useful in fashioning treatment strategies (see below). Such a classification begins with the division of neuropathic pains into those predominantly sustained by mechanisms in the peripheral nervous system and those sustained by mechanisms in the central nervous system. The evidence for this conceptualization, like that for the broader construct of neuropathic pain itself, is largely conjectural (Table 1) but clinically relevant. A syndrome-based classification of neuropathic cancer pain syndromes also may be useful[36] (Table 2).

Neuropathic pains sustained by a peripheral mechanism

A diverse group of neuropathic pains results from pathological processes that develop at the site of peripheral nerve injury. These pains may be divided into painful mononeuropathies and painful polyneuropathies. Syndromes characterized by intermittent stabbing pains, which can be

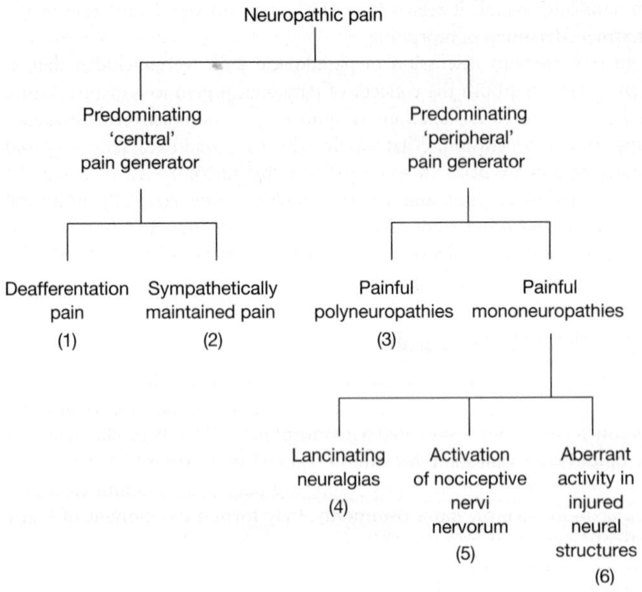

Fig. 1 Classification of neuropathic pains by inferred pathophysiology. (1) Can be precipitated by either peripheral or central nervous system injury. (2) Is most strongly associated with reflex sympathetic dystrophy/causalgia and may be considered a subclass of these syndromes; the possibility of this pathophysiology is suggested by the development of focal autonomic dysregulation (e.g. oedema, vasomotor disturbances), motor impairment, and trophic changes in the region of the pain, but is confirmed by improvement with sympathetic nerve block. (3) Multiple mechanisms probably involved. (4) The patterns of peripheral activity, or peripheral and central interaction, that yield the lancinating quality of these pains are unknown. (5) Nociceptive nervi nervorum (small afferents that innervate larger nerves) may account for neuropathic pain accompanying nerve compression or inflammation. (6) Injury to axons may be followed by neuroma formation, a source of aberrant activity likely to be involved in pain. (Adapted from Portenoy.[18])

Table 1 Types of evidence supporting the division of neuropathic pains into those with sustaining mechanisms for the pain located in the central nervous system and those with sustaining mechanisms for the pain located in the peripheral nervous system

Evidence	Caveat
Surveys of patients undergoing neurolysis suggest that some pains have a central mechanism that causes pain even after the painful part is denervated	Data are limited and published cases have selection bias; evidence that peripheral pains do reliably respond to neurolysis is meagre
Correlations in specific syndromes, e.g. abnormal activity in central nervous system structures of patients with deafferentation pain and similar activity on microneuronography of nerves proximal to neuroma	Correlations between findings and pain do not prove causality; there have been no simultaneous recordings from peripheral and central structures in man
Animal models suggest that there are changes following nerve injury that may be either central or peripheral, e.g. the neuroma model demonstrates characteristics, such as mechanosensitivity, that correspond to findings in humans with similar pathology	Relationship between animal models and chronic neuropathic pain in man is highly inferential; studies show that peripheral injury produces substantial changes in the central nervous system and that central nervous system injury may cause changes in the periphery

This division is inferred and its tentative nature is emphasized by noting the weaknesses in the supporting data. This model remains hypothetical.

Table 2 Classification of neuropathic cancer pain syndromes (Martin and Hagen[36])

Syndromes	Examples
Related to cancer	
Cranial nerves neuralgias	Base of skull or leptomeningeal metastases, head and neck cancers
Postherpetic neuralgia	
Mononeuropathy	Rib metastases with intercostal nerve injury
Other neuralgias	Along the distribution of any sensory nerve
Radiculopathy	Epidural mass, leptomeningeal metastases
Cervical plexopathy	Head and neck cancer with local extension, cervical lymph node metastases
Brachial plexopathy	Lymph node metastases from breast cancer or lymphoma, direct extension of Pancoast tumour
Lumbosacral plexopathy	Direct extension of colorectal cancer, cervical cancer, sarcoma, or lymphoma; breast cancer metastases
Paraneoplastic peripheral neuropathy	Small cell lung cancer
Central pain	Spinal cord compression
Related to therapeutic interventions	
Analgesic interventions	High-dose intrathecal and epidural injections of opioids
Epidural injection	
Post-surgical	Post-mastectomy, neck dissection, post-thoracotomy
Phantom pain	Post-amputation, post-mastectomy
Radiation therapy	Myelopathy, plexopathy, neuropathy
Chemotherapy	Peripheral neuropathy associated with vinca alkaloids, paclitaxel, cytarabine
Parenteral corticosteroids	Perineal burning sensation
Intrathecal methotrexate	Acute meningitic syndrome

termed 'lancinating neuralgias', may also be distinguished, since the unique clinical characteristics shared by these pains probably relates to a unique pathophysiology. Both painful polyneuropathies (such as that caused by neurotoxic chemotherapy) and painful mononeuropathies (such as the brachial plexopathy described in the case report) are common in the palliative care setting.

A variety of pathophysiological processes presumably underlie different peripheral neuropathic pain syndromes. The best studied are those associated with painful mononeuropathies. These may include activation of nociceptive nervi nervorum (small primary afferent nerves that invest the trunks of larger nerves) by compression or inflammation of the nerve, sensitization of the primary afferent neurone, and neuroma formation following axonal transection.[37–39] Studies of neuromas have demonstrated spontaneous electrical activity associated with pain reports in humans, as well as exaggerated responses to both mechanical deformation and some chemical stimuli, such as noradrenaline.[37]

Injury to peripheral nerve can cause persistent changes in the central nervous system, which may contribute further to the pain and produce hyperalgesia and allodynia. Indeed, a process of 'central sensitization' is likely to be pivotal in many cases of refractory neuropathic pain.[37,38,40,41] It can occur in any situation of prolonged or repeated activation of nociceptive C fibres. It appears to be a complex process that results from interactions between multiple receptors and both neurotransmitters and neuromodulators. Activation of *N*-methyl-D-aspartate receptors by excitatory amino acids released by primary afferent neurones is likely to be a pivotal process.[40,42]

The identification of a predominately peripheral pathogenesis for a neuropathic pain may have important therapeutic implications. Some of these pains may be relieved by a peripheral intervention, such as decompression of a nerve, resection of a neuroma, or proximal denervation via a neurolytic procedure.[38]

Neuropathic pains sustained by a central mechanism

Neuropathic pains primarily sustained by central nervous system mechanisms can be divided into two broad categories: the so-called deafferentation pains and the complex regional pain syndromes (also known as the reflex sympathetic dystrophy/causalgia syndromes).[35] The latter syndromes include an important subgroup–the sympathetically maintained pains (Fig. 1)—which appear to be sustained by efferent activity in the sympathetic nervous system. Clinical recognition of these types of neuropathic pain may suggest useful adjunctive strategies to conventional analgesic therapy.

Deafferentation pains

The deafferentation pains include a number of alternatively named syndromes, such as phantom pain, postherpetic neuralgia, root avulsion pain, anaesthesia dolorosa, and central pain.[35] Although these pains vary in the site of nerve injury, presentation, and response to some specific therapies, all are presumably sustained by abnormal processes in the spinal cord or brain. The specific pathophysiological processes are likely to be diverse and may include denervation hypersensitivity of central neurones, ectopic electrogenesis at sites of injured central neurones, changes in the receptive fields of central somatosensory neurones, and loss of central inhibitions.[43]

The remarkable observation that injury to a peripheral nerve can produce either a peripheral painful mononeuropathy (e.g. from neuroma formation) or a deafferentation syndrome (e.g. anaesthesia dolorosa or phantom pain) has important implications for the use of neurolytic procedures in the treatment of refractory pains. It is possible that neurolytic procedures that denervate the painful part could have markedly different results depending upon the underlying mechanisms sustaining the pain. A peripheral neuropathic pain may be more likely to be relieved by such a procedure and a deafferentation pain might be worsened. In the clinical setting, temporary local anaesthetic nerve blocks are often used to guide treatment when this consideration exists. Patients with neuropathic pain associated with a peripheral nerve lesion who fail to obtain a favourable response following blockade of the nerves between the painful site and the central nervous system are suspected of having pain sustained by central mechanisms and are not subjected to neurolysis. Unfortunately, given the reality of a placebo effect and the possibility that afferent input may be contributing to a centrally maintained pain to some extent, a favourable response to a local anaesthetic nerve block neither proves a peripheral mechanism nor predicts successful neurolysis.

Complex regional pain syndromes

The pain syndromes that have traditionally been labelled reflex sympathetic dystrophy or causalgia have been renamed complex regional pain syndrome (CRPS) type I and type II, respectively, by the International Association for the Study of Pain.(43) Although the term sympathetically maintained pain has also been used, this appellation is now preferred only when pain can be reliably relieved with sympathetic nerve block. Only some patients with complex regional pain syndrome have sympathetically maintained pain.

The diagnosis of CRPS type I (or reflex sympathetic dystrophy) may be offered when focal pain accompanied by autonomic dysregulation, motor impairment, and trophic signs occur after injury to bone, joint, or soft tissue.(44) The diagnosis of CRPS type II (or causalgia) is appropriate for the identical syndrome when it is precipitated by injury to a nerve trunk. In both cases the inciting injury may be minor and, in rare cases, the pain and associated features appear without recollection of a prior event.

The pain of CRPS is typically, but now always, dysaesthetic. It often includes a constant burning with intermittent paroxysms. The pain can be spontaneous or evoked by touch or movement. Allodynia, pain caused by light touch, may accompany a constant pain or be the most prominent complaint. The focal autonomic dysregulation may include swelling, vasomotor changes (pallor, erythema or cyanosis, livedo reticularis, or a focal increase or decrease in skin temperature), or sweating abnormalities. Motor phenomena, including stiffness, weakness, and abnormal involuntary movements (tremor, chorea, or dystonias), are common when the lesion involves an extremity. The so-called trophic changes, such as thinning of the skin, change in hair or nail growth, atrophy of subcutaneous tissues or muscle, or focal osteoporosis, may also occur.

In some cases, CRPS is suspected but the routine evaluation does not reveal the autonomic or trophic changes needed to establish the diagnosis. Autonomic dysfunction may be demonstrated using more sophisticated measures, such as thermography or quantitative sweat testing, and trophic changes may be assessed with bone scintigraphy, radiography, or magnetic resonance imaging.

Although a major analgesic response to sympathetic nerve block suggests that the pain is sympathetically maintained, the interpretation of a test that is performed in varying ways, often without confirmation of physiological change and almost never with a placebo control, is problematic.(45) There have been no studies that clarify the degree or duration of response necessary to attribute the pain to activity in the sympathetic nervous system. The use of a pharmacological approach to sympathetic block, specifically intravenous phentolamine infusion,(45,46) has recently been introduced as a more specific way of assessing sympathetic efferent function. This may be also difficult to interpret,(47,48) and may provide an alternative method for testing the response to sympathetic interruption, but does not increase the reliability of the clinical interpretation.

The varying response to sympathetic interruption among those with clinical findings consistent with CRPS underscores the complexity of the pathophysiology. These syndromes may actually reflect the end result of multiple mechanisms, only some of which involve the sympathetic nervous system. One recent analysis of the available literature(49) hypothesized that changes in the primary afferent neurones (mostly type C fibres) induced by inflammation or persistent stimulation results in central sensitization, which might be the basis of the development of CRPS type I. The trauma associated with a nerve lesion, and the consequent morphological, biochemical, and neurophysiological changes (including ectopic afferent activity), might induce central hyperexcitability and the development of CRPS type II. The focal autonomic changes may be epiphenomena of these more fundamental central processes. Another analysis suggested a fundamental role for visceral afferent neurones, which travel with the sympathetic nerves, in the pathogenesis of reflex sympathetic dystrophy.(50) Another hypothesis is that the sensitization of central neurones in the dorsal horn of the spinal cord is maintained by sympathetically driven activation of non-nociceptive primary afferent neurones, which themselves might be sensitized by peripheral trauma.(51)

Regardless of the underlying pathophysiology, the clinical recognition of CRPS has important implications by suggesting the potential therapeutic value of sympathetic interruption. The appearance of local autonomic dysregulation in a region of neuropathic pain is usually sufficient to suggest the diagnosis and justify diagnostic sympathetic blockade. Interruption of sympathetic efferent function is usually performed by sympathetic nerve block. In some cases the response is favourable enough to consider repeated sympathetic nerve blocks as a primary treatment approach. If nerve blocks cannot be performed, phentolamine infusion can be considered as a diagnostic approach, or other sympatholytic agents might be considered for therapeutic trials (see Chapter 8.2.6).

Management of neuropathic pain

Management of neuropathic pain, like other chronic pains encountered in the palliative care setting, begins with a comprehensive assessment.(52–54) This assessment characterizes the phenomenology of the pain, attempts to elucidate the underlying aetiology and likely pathophysiologies, and determines relevant medical and psychosocial disturbances that either help explain the nature of the pain or demand independent therapy. This assessment usually yields a complex understanding of a range of problems that together undermine quality of life.

The variable constellation of symptoms, medical problems, functional impairments, and psychosocial concerns often encountered in practice suggests the need for a multimodality strategy that targets a group of specific therapies for discrete problems identified by the comprehensive assessment. The use of one or more specific analgesic treatments is typically part of this strategy.

Similar to the management of other types of chronic pain, opioid therapy is considered to be the first-line approach for the treatment of moderate or severe neuropathic pain in the palliative care setting. Guidelines for optimal opioid therapy (discussed in Chapter 8.2.3) stress the need for individualization of the opioid dose through gradual titration to an endpoint defined by a favourable balance between analgesia and side-effects. This is particularly salient in the treatment of neuropathic pains, which may be less opioid responsive than other pains and thereby demonstrate a narrower therapeutic window. Hence, all patients with moderate or severe neuropathic pain should undergo a trial with an opioid drug, during which doses should be gradually escalated until either favourable effects occur or intolerable and unmanageable side-effects develop.

Failure with one opioid does not necessarily predict an inadequate response to another and trials of other opioids should be considered in the management of refractory cases.(27,55–57) The process of 'opioid rotation' is as relevant to the treatment of neuropathic pain as it is to the treatment of other types of pain.

Patients who do not obtain adequate analgesia with an opioid alone may be candidates for any of a large number of adjunctive approaches. These range from alternative drug therapies to a variety of invasive approaches.

Adjuvant analgesics

The use of the so-called adjuvant analgesics to treat neuropathic pain is now widely accepted. Numerous drugs in diverse drug classes have been recommended for this indication (Table 3). The pharmacology, indications, and dosing guidelines for these drugs are described in Chapter 8.2.5. Although the potential for favourable effects justifies sequential trials, the clinician must recognize the possibility of adverse effects in a population predisposed

Table 3 Adjuvant analgesics used in the management of neuropathic pain (see Chapter 8.2.5)

Drug class	Examples
Tricyclic antidepressants	Amitriptyline, nortriptyline, desipramine, doxepin, imipramine, clomipramine
Selective serotonin reuptake inhibitors	Paroxetine, citalopram, fluoxetine, sertraline, fluvoxamine
Noradrenaline serotonin reuptake inhibitors	Venlafaxine
Other antidepressants	Maprotiline, bupropion, trazodone
Anticonvulsants	Gabapentin, topiramate, carbamazepine, phenytoin, valproate, oxcarbazepine, lamotrigine, levetiracetam, pregabalin
Oral local anaesthetics	Mexiletine, tocainide, flecainide
Alpha-2 adrenergic agonists	Clonidine, tizanidine
N-Methyl-D-aspartate receptor antagonists	Dextromethorphan, ketamine
Gamma-aminobutyric acid (GABA) agonist	Baclofen
Corticosteroids	Dexamethasone, prednisone, prednisolone
Topical agents	Capsaicin, lidocaine patch, EMLA
Neuroleptics	Methotrimeprazine, pimozide
Miscellaneous	Calcitonin
Drugs for sympathetically maintained pain	Prazosin, propranolol, nifedipine

to complications by advanced age, concurrent organ dysfunction, and coadministration of drugs with additive side-effects. Trials must be implemented cautiously and monitoring should be intensified.

Anaesthetic approaches (see Chapter 8.2.6)

As discussed above, a trial of sympathetic blockade should be considered whenever the clinical findings suggest a CRPS in a patient with refractory pain. The patient with intractable pain due to malignant brachial plexopathy who develops swelling and erythema of the hand should not be assumed simply to have venous outflow or lymphatic obstruction but, rather, should be considered a potential case of CRPS that may respond to sympathetic nerve block. An experienced anaesthetist on the palliative care team can help optimize decisions about these invasive procedures.

Other anaesthetic techniques are also useful in patients with neuropathic pain. The simplest of these, trigger point injections, may ameliorate the myofascial pains that can be associated with the primary pain complaint. Trigger point injections are within the purview of all clinicians and are probably underused in the palliative care setting.

Occasionally patients with neuropathic pain obtain relatively long-lasting benefit from transient somatic nerve blocks using local anaesthetic. In these cases, blocks can be repeated at intervals. More often, however, local anaesthetic blocks produce short-lived relief. This type of response may suggest the potential value of subsequent neurolysis, particularly in patients with severe refractory pain and short life expectancies. Neurolysis may be reas-onable in these situations despite the concern, described previously, that worsening denervation could exacerbate the pain of an underlying deafferentation syndrome.

Patients with suspected neuroma (e.g. in a surgical scar) may benefit from direct injection of local anaesthetic into the site of the neuroma. Some of these patients gain long-term relief from neurolytic blockade at these sites.[58]

Intraspinal infusion techniques (or the so-called neuraxial analgesia) may be very useful in some patients with neuropathic pain. A recent randomized comparison of subarachnoid drug infusion via an implanted pump and systemic drug treatment in a population with cancer pain demonstrated better outcomes among those with the pump[59] and suggests an expanding role for this technology in the future. The usual indication for a trial of epidural or intrathecal opioid infusion is the development of intolerable central nervous system side-effects (somnolence or confusion) during escalation of a systemic opioid (see Chapter 8.2.6). Although the same type of relatively poorer opioid responsiveness that is observed during systemic drug administration may occur during neuraxial administration,[60] the intraspinal route offers options for combined therapy that may enhance effectiveness. The combination of an opioid and a local anaesthetic can benefit some patients with refractory neuropathic pain[61] and a placebo-controlled trial confirmed the value of epidural clonidine in the treatment of cancer-related neuropathic pain.[62] The use of intraspinal drug combinations in the treatment of refractory neuropathic pain, especially in patients with advanced illness, should be considered only by experienced practitioners who are able to implement and monitor these interventions.[63]

Neurostimulatory approaches

Non-invasive stimulatory approaches comprise counter-irritation (systematic rubbing of the painful part) and transcutaneous electrical nerve stimulation. Invasive approaches include acupuncture, percutaneous electrical nerve stimulation, dorsal column stimulation, and deep brain stimulation. All of these approaches have been used in the palliative care setting for patients with refractory neuropathic pain but only the non-invasive approaches are used commonly. Like the invasive anaesthetic approaches, invasive stimulatory approaches should be considered only by experienced practitioners, or a team of practitioners, who can evaluate the patient comprehensively, optimize non-invasive therapies, and integrate invasive procedures with other treatments.

Transcutaneous electrical nerve stimulation will initially benefit many patients but only a small minority continue to obtain relief from this approach beyond a period of weeks. Nonetheless, the morbidity is extremely low and the existence of an occasional patient who achieves remarkable benefit for prolonged periods impels consideration of a trial in all patients with refractory neuropathic pain (see Chapter 8.2.8). A trial of transcutaneous electrical nerve stimulation that recognizes individual differences in the response to this approach usually requires a period of weeks. The patient should attempt stimulation using various electrode placements, timing of treatment (minutes, hours, or continuously throughout the day), and stimulation parameters (frequency and amplitude of the waveform and stimulus intensity). In this way, the most effective stimulation regimen can be identified.

Rehabilitation therapies

Although the functional benefits possible through rehabilitative techniques are well recognized, the potential analgesic consequences from these treatments are not often appreciated. Physiotherapy may be able to forestall or reduce the myofascial complications that commonly exacerbate neuropathic pain. Occupational therapy may be able to identify methods that allow a patient to regain function without provoking painful episodes. Patients who experience relief only when a limb or torso is partially immobilized may achieve some measure of analgesia through the skilful use of an orthosis.

Surgical approaches

Surgical procedures that are sometimes considered for neuropathic pains include those designed to address nerve injury directly, such as resection of a neuroma or decompression of a peripheral nerve, and those designed to denervate the painful part, such as rhizotomy or cordotomy.[64,65] Clinical observations suggest that the latter procedures, the most useful of which is cordotomy, may be generally less efficacious for neuropathic pains than for nociceptive pains.[66] Nonetheless, some patients with short life expectancies and severe refractory neuropathic pains clearly benefit from surgical neurolysis of nerve pathways proximal to the painful site. Experienced clinicians weigh the risks and benefits in each case and use these approaches for carefully selected patients.

In some cases, the decision to try denervation opens the possibility of either an anaesthetic approach (neurolytic nerve block) or a surgical approach. For example, rhizotomy can be performed by epidural or subarachnoid instillation of a neurolytic solution or by surgical sectioning of the nerve root. There have been no comparative trials of any of these techniques and the selection of one or another is usually based on the medical status of the patient, technical considerations, or the availability of resources.

Psychological approaches

Specific cognitive approaches, such as hypnosis and distraction techniques, have been used to manage pain in the palliative care setting.[67] There have been no studies of these approaches in patients with neuropathic pains. Given the potential benefits and lack of risk, however, they should certainly be considered in cognitively intact patients, if the expertise exists to apply them.

Conclusion

The management of neuropathic pain syndromes is a compelling clinical challenge, the outcome of which is too often unsatisfactory. Given the variability of the medically ill patients who experience these syndromes, the lack of data about mechanisms and natural history, and the empirical methods used in management, it is remarkable that the outcome achieved with many patients is as favourable as it is. Further improvements depend on basic and clinical investigations that clarify the mechanisms and phenomenology of these syndromes, and provide data that allow a targeting of treatment according to underlying pathophysiology.

Breakthrough pain

Breakthrough pain refers to a transitory exacerbation of pain experienced by the patient who has relatively stable and adequately controlled baseline pain. In the palliative care population, the baseline pain is typically managed with opioid drugs, and breakthrough pain denotes brief periods during which the usual opioid regimen fails to provide adequate analgesia.

Case history A 72-year-old man with metastatic prostate cancer was receiving hormonal agents when he noted the insidious onset of progressive sacral pain. Metastases to the sacrum and pelvis had been previously documented and a pelvic CT scan revealed some progression of these lesions. Radiotherapy was administered to the painful site, which abolished the pain. He continued hormonal therapy and was asymptomatic for 6 months, at which time he again experienced the onset of pain in the sacrum and left ileum. CT revealed progression of the bony disease and extension of a tumour mass into the presacral soft tissues. The pain was initially controlled with a combination product containing paracetamol and codeine 30 mg. As the pain worsened, he was switched to controlled-release oxycodone 20 mg twice a day. This regimen yielded minimal residual pain except during periods of physical exertion.

Two months later, continuous aching pain increased and episodes of severe pain on sitting and walking began again. Intermittent perineal stabbing pains started soon after. The latter pains, which were paroxysmal and very brief, increased in frequency and intensity and soon became highly distressing. At first, an increase in the dose of the controlled-release oxycodone to 40 mg twice a day yielded a fairly good response, and the patient once again became pain-free except during periods of exertion. Within a week, however, stabbing perineal pains began again. During the ensuing 2 weeks, the oxycodone dose was gradually increased to 100 mg twice a day. As the dose of the oxycodone was raised the intermittent pains with activity became mild and the perineal stabbing pains became less frequent and severe. However, function was compromised during pain-free periods by sedation. Reduction in the oxycodone dose allowed the patient to think more clearly, but immediately resulted in an exacerbation of the stabbing pain.

Gabapentin and dexamethasone were added to the oxycodone regimen and eliminated the stabbing perineal pain. Within a month, however, the patient reported that the aching sacral pain began to flare intolerably upon sitting or standing for more than a few minutes. Pelvic CT revealed further bony destruction and a large presacral soft tissue mass. Chemotherapy was offered but refused and a surgical consultant could offer no solution.

Higher doses of oxycodone produced confusion and had no effect on the pain. Use of a supplemental oxycodone dose, which was to be taken only during exacerbations of pain, failed because pain onset was too abrupt and the patient would promptly recline when the pain occurred severely, thereby eliminating the need for the supplemental dose. The controlled-release oxycodone was discontinued and a trial of an alternative opioid, transdermal fentanyl, was initiated. There was no clinical improvement despite adjustment of the dose.

An epidural catheter was inserted. The transdermal fentanyl and gabapentin were continued at doses below those associated with cognitive impairment. Epidural administration of first morphine and then fentanyl failed to identify a dose that eliminated the breakthrough pain without producing an exacerbation of side-effects. A low concentration of a local anaesthetic, bupivicaine, was added to the epidural opioid but provided no additional relief. Higher concentrations of local anaesthetic ultimately provided enough relief for the patient to sit, but this treatment impaired the patient's ability to walk and produced an unacceptable numbness in the legs and perineum. The catheter was removed.

The options available to manage the refractory breakthrough pain were discussed with the patient. The use of epidural or subarachnoid neurolysis was rejected because of the likelihood of morbidity, specifically the loss of normal micturition and the possibility that the sensory changes and weakness that had been experienced during local anaesthetic instillation might be reproduced. The potential risks and benefits of other neurolytic procedures, including bilateral cordotomy and myelotomy, were discussed, and these options were compared with an alternative outcome in which the patient would accept a bed-bound existence.

The patient requested bilateral cordotomy and this was performed percutaneously in two steps during the following week. The response was initially excellent. The patient could sit and stand comfortably and walk short distances without pain. The opioid dose was reduced by half and cognition cleared fully.

The patient was discharged home and required no additional interventions until 2 months later, at which time the pain flared again. The patient was readmitted to hospital where re-evaluation showed a pathological fracture of the sacrum and newly apparent metastatic deposits in the liver. The dose of transdermal fentanyl was adjusted until the patient was comfortable at rest. The patient accepted the recommendation that he be confined to bed and he was discharged home, where he died 2 weeks later.

The problem

Although there is widespread clinical recognition that episodic or breakthrough pain can be a major impediment to function[15,68–70] and can be associated with significant psychological distress, there is no generally accepted nomenclature to describe the phenomenon, and its optimal management has not been well defined. Several definitions attempt to narrow the context for these pains. For example, the term 'breakthrough pain' may be used only when transient pains occur superimposed on a baseline pain controlled by an opioid regimen.[68,71,72] Alternatively, the term may be equated with 'incident pain', which is typically understood to be induced by some voluntary action of the patient. Researchers and clinicians from different countries may define breakthrough pain differently, as suggested by an international survey that reported significant variations in its prevalence across countries.[(73)] To facilitate the recognition and proper assessment and management of breakthrough pain, a broad definition is most useful: breakthrough pain is any acute transient pain that is severe and has an intensity that flares over baseline.[(74)] A consensus conference recently advocated the use of a broader term, such as episodic or transient pain.[(74)]

The patient described in the case report experienced two distinct types of breakthrough pain. The first, aching sacral pain on sitting or standing, could also be labelled as incident pain. It was attributable to the destructive lesion of the sacrum and its pathophysiology could be inferred to be nociceptive. The second pain, intermittent perineal stabbing, was most likely a neuropathic pain caused by tumour extension into the sacral plexus. It was not precipitated by a voluntary action and, therefore, would not be termed an incident pain. These two types of breakthrough pains were similar in their partial responsiveness to an opioid (both the increased baseline dose and the use of a supplemental dose) and could be distinguished by their differential response to an anticonvulsant, gabapentin.

This patient highlights the great variability in the presentation and aetiology of breakthrough pain. This variability, combined with a poor response to many of the routine pharmacological interventions used to manage more continuous baseline pain, complicates the treatment of breakthrough pains.

Clinical spectrum and pathophysiology

The epidemiology of breakthrough pain has been explored in numerous surveys during the past decade.[(68,70–76)] The prevalence of the phenomenon in these surveys varies with the definition used to identify it and the population investigated. In patients admitted to oncology units, the prevalence varies between 41 and 63 per cent. Similar figures have been reported for patients followed in an outpatient cancer pain clinic and a higher prevalence 89 per cent was noted among those enrolled in home care or inpatient hospice programmes. In a survey of hospice patients with diagnoses other than cancer, 63 per cent experienced breakthrough pain.[(77)] Overall, these surveys suggest that breakthrough pain is more likely to be a problem when disease is advanced and when baseline pain is relatively severe.[(70)] Interestingly, the recognition of breakthrough pain varies among countries, and is diagnosed most often in United States, Canada, Australia, New Zealand, and several European countries.[(73)]

Breakthrough pains are highly variable. The average daily frequency of pains ranges between 1.5 and 7. Occasional patients experience very frequent pains.[(68,75)] Most painful episodes are brief, lasting an average of 30 min; rare breakthrough pains persist for more than 1 h.[(72)] The onset of breakthrough pain is usually gradual, but very rapid onsets may occur. Among the rapid onset breakthrough pains are the lancinating neuralgias that characterize some neuropathic pain syndromes. Breakthrough pains are identified as somatic (33–45 per cent) more often than visceral (20–29 per cent), neuropathic (9–33 per cent), or mixed (16–20 per cent) pains.[(68,75,77)] Among those with cancer, approximately three-quarters of the pains are specifically related to a known neoplastic lesion, whereas up to 20 per cent are an effect of antineoplastic therapy and 4–19 per cent appear to be unrelated to the cancer or its treatment. As illustrated in the case report, many patients experience more than one type of breakthrough pain concurrently.

Most breakthrough pains represent a flare of a baseline pain, and share the characteristics and location of the baseline pain. Although the episodes of breakthrough pain are often unpredictable, precipitating events are sometimes identified. Approximately half of the episodes occur with a voluntary action and can thus be labelled as incident pain. These actions include moving in bed, walking, sitting, standing, touching the painful site, coughing, or swallowing. Some pains are also precipitated by non-volitional events, including bowel distension, ureteral distension, and regurgitation of analgesic medication.[(68)] Up to one-third of breakthrough pain episodes occur at the end of the dosing interval for an analgesic drug.[(68,72)]

Management of breakthrough pain

The management of breakthrough pain is accomplished through a combination of prescribed approaches and strategies fortuitously discovered by the patients themselves. The most frequent approach is the use of a supplemental dose of an opioid ('rescue' dose). In various surveys, 39–75 per cent of patients describe rescue dosing as an effective strategy.[(68,70,75,76)] Thus, the use of a rescue medication is extremely valuable but does not obviate the need for alternative approaches. One survey of hospice patients revealed that only 25 per cent of patients experiencing breakthrough pain were satisfied with the overall pain control, compared to 78 per cent of patients without breakthrough pain.[(77)]

A recent consensus conference highlighted the need for a more comprehensive management approach for breakthrough pain.[(74)] Due to the paucity of published data, the following management principles are mostly derived from clinical experience and expert recommendations.[(74,78)] Controlled clinical trials of therapeutic interventions for breakthrough pain are needed.

Comprehensive assessment

Similar to the evaluation of cancer pain in general,[(52–54)] the evaluation of breakthrough pains should characterize the pain itself and the clinical status of the patient. An understanding of the extent of disease and the physical, psychological, and social condition of the patient clarifies the overall approach to treatment.

Pain should be assessed in terms of intensity, location, frequency, quality, and duration. Precipitating and alleviating factors should be noted, among which is the relationship to the dosing of the baseline analgesic regimen. The breakthrough pain should be characterized as an acute worsening of the baseline pain or a distinct syndrome, and the mechanisms inferred to be sustaining the pain should be categorized as nociceptive, neuropathic, or mixed.[(74,78)]

Treatment of the underlying cause

Primary therapy directed at the cause of the breakthrough pain can eliminate the need for analgesic therapies but may be associated with considerable burden or risks for the patient. If such primary therapy is available, its appropriate use depends on many factors, including the extent of the disease, the general medical status of the patient, previous treatments, and the overriding goals of care. Treatment for the specific lesion associated with the breakthrough pain should be provided if it is feasible, does not subject the patient to excessive risk, and has a reasonable likelihood of reducing the frequency or intensity of the pain.

Local radiotherapy to a bone metastasis is the most common primary antineoplastic therapy used to address breakthrough pain.[(74,78)] If the radiated area is limited to one painful lesion, it is generally well tolerated, even in advanced cancer patients.

Although chemotherapy usually is not administered with the sole objective of pain control, the advent of newer agents may lead to an expanded role. Gemcitabine has been shown to improve quality of life and decrease pain in patients with inoperable, locally advanced, or metastatic adenocarcinoma of pancreas[(79,80)] and non-small cell lung cancer.[(81)] Similar results have been reported with mitoxantrone treatment of prostate cancer.[(82)] These chemotherapeutic agents are usually well tolerated in those with advanced cancer and the data suggest that they may be appropriate to address the problem of refractory pain in selected patients.

Palliative surgical interventions, such as stabilization of the spine or a long bone after pathological fracture, or decompression of an obstructed hollow viscus, also are considered in carefully selected cases. The risks and benefits of a procedure must be carefully assessed in the context of the goals of care.

Optimizing the analgesic regimen

The observation that some breakthrough pains only occur, or flare dramatically, at the end of the dosing interval suggests that these pains are related to the plasma concentration of the analgesic drug. For such pains, the maintenance of a higher plasma concentration throughout the dosing interval may resolve the problem.

It is likely that some breakthrough pains without a demonstrable relationship to the end of the dosing interval, such as those occurring in patients receiving opioid infusions, would also be responsive to an increase in dose. This speculation suggests that an adjustment in the regularly scheduled analgesic regimen is a reasonable intervention in all patients with breakthrough pain. If the regularly scheduled analgesic is an opioid, the dose should be increased until either favourable effects occur or intolerable and unmanageable side-effects supervene, which usually occurs during the intervals between the severe pains.(69) Breakthrough pains are often improved, but seldom eradicated, by this approach.

Primary analgesic approaches

Although many patients appear to benefit from the administration of primary treatments and adjustment of the scheduled analgesic regimen, most will require specific analgesic interventions directed at the breakthrough pain itself. At the present time, the selection and use of these approaches is also empirical.

'Rescue' dose

The use of a pharmacological 'rescue' dose is widely accepted in the management of breakthrough pain.(83,84) In this technique, a supplemental 'as required' dose of an analgesic drug is offered concurrently with the regularly scheduled analgesic drug. Due to the characteristics of breakthrough pains, the ideal supplemental medication should be absorbed quickly, have a rapid onset of analgesia, and a short duration of action, so that the effects of the medication resolve as the pain abates.(85) This drug can be a nonsteroidal anti-inflammatory drug (NSAID), but is more often an opioid. If the regularly scheduled opioid has a short half-life, the same drug should be selected for the rescue; if the regularly scheduled opioid has a long half-life or duration of effect (e.g. modified release oral morphine or methadone), an alternative short half-life drug should be used as the rescue.

If possible, the same route of administration should be used for both the rescue and the fixed scheduled dose. However, occasional patients find that the onset of action of an oral rescue dose is too slow to treat the breakthrough pain effectively. Parenteral administration of an opioid can be considered in this situation. The development of patient-controlled analgesia systems in ambulatory infusion devices capable of delivering continuous subcutaneous or intravenous infusion can, if available, expedite the administration of supplemental doses in those receiving opioid infusions. Patients can be provided with an ambulatory infusion device solely to have access to rescue doses that could be administered quickly and parenterally.

The advent of transmucosal formulations may be another method for the quick administration of a supplemental opioid dose. Any highly lipophilic drug may cross nasal or oral mucosal surfaces rapidly enough to meet the needs of patients who require a 'rescue' dose with a prompt onset of action.

An oral transmucosal fentanyl citrate (OTFC) formulation is now available in several countries and may be a useful alternative treatment for breakthrough pain. By avoiding first-pass metabolism through absorption across the oral mucosa, it allows a high bioavailability and rapid onset of action. The median time to the onset of pain relief is 5 min(86) and the peak plasma concentration is reached at about 22 min.(87) Despite a terminal elimination half-life of 7 h, drug redistribution into tissues makes its duration of action much shorter in most patients.(87) Studies have shown that individual titration of the OTFC dose (available in 200–1600 μg units) allows safe and effective pain control for most episodes of breakthrough pain in cancer patients.(88–91) Unexpectedly, in these studies there was no linear relationship between the effective dose of OTFC and the dose of the baseline opioid regimen, further justifying individualization of the dose in all cases.(88,91)

When appropriately titrated, OTFC usually is well tolerated. To reduce the risk of rapidly absorbed fentanyl, it is best to consider only when patients already are receiving an opioid regimen equivalent in dose to at least 60 mg of oral morphine (in 24 h) or 50 μg/h of transdermal fentanyl.(92) With the exception of tooth caries, which can occur with frequent use, side-effects are like other opioids. There is no drug accumulation with repeated doses(93) and it is safe to be used on a long-term basis at home by cancer patients.(94)

Other transmucosal formulations have been reported in case series. These have described the use of intranasal fentanyl(95) or sufentanil(96) as well as sublingual fentanyl.(97) The use of an intranasal formulation of butorphanol, available in the United States, is limited by the agonist–antagonist properties of this opioid. Similarly, buprenorphine is available in many countries as a sublingual formulation, but it is a partial agonist with a limited effective dose range. In the United Kingdom, sublingual dextromoramide is often employed as a rescue medication because it is potent and short-acting.

The studies of OTFC, which demonstrated no relationship between the effective size of the rescue dose and the baseline opioid dose, contradicted common clinical experience with other formulations, which generally supported the conclusion that the dose of an opioid rescue drug must be proportionate to the baseline opioid dose to optimize efficacy. Some clinicians begin with a dose roughly equivalent to 5–10 per cent of the total daily opioid intake, which is offered at short intervals, usually between 1 and 3 h, as needed. Another approach in patients receiving 4-hourly oral morphine is to use the same 4-hourly dose for breakthrough pain, administered as frequently as required (or in patients receiving twice daily controlled release morphine, the equivalent 4-hourly dose).

Regardless of the starting dose selected for the rescue medication, dose titration may be needed to optimize the effects. Titration of the rescue dose should be viewed as a key principle in the management of breakthrough pain. In practice, patients with breakthrough pain often are given inadequate doses of rescue medication because the prescribed rescue dose does not keep pace as the regular opioid dose is increased.

Guidelines for the timing of the supplemental dose are similarly empirical. Patients with predictable pain appear to benefit most from a rescue dose taken 30–60 min before the precipitating event. Treatment of unpredictable pains with a supplemental dose is most likely to be effective if the medication is administered as soon after the onset of the pain as possible.

Other pharmacological approaches

Strategies other than dose titration that are used to optimize the baseline opioid regimen also should be considered when prescribing rescue medication. Opioid rotation to identify the most effective rescue drug is a reasonable approach and the coadministration of an opioid and non-opioid might be valuable in selected patients. If escalation of the baseline regimen substantially reduces breakthrough pain but causes somnolence between episodes, coadministration of a psychostimulant also might be considered.(98,99) If somnolence or other side-effects preclude administration of an effective opioid regimen, neuraxial infusion might be tried, just as it might were the target problem baseline pain rather than breakthrough pain.(63)

The importance of the opioid rescue dose in the management of breakthrough pain should not obscure the potential benefits of other pharmacological approaches. For example, there is substantial evidence that patients with lancinating neuropathic breakthrough pains may respond well to the administration of an anticonvulsant drug or other specific agent (see Chapter 8.2.5). Similarly, some patients whose breakthrough pain is related to neoplastic invasion of bone or nerve trunk appear to benefit, at least temporarily, from the coadministration of a corticosteroid. Finally, the use of specific drugs to reduce the frequency of precipitating events, such as antitussives, laxatives, antiperistaltic drugs, or agents that reduce muscle spasm, should be considered.

Interventional approaches

Like neuraxial infusion, other interventional approaches may play a role in the management of refractory breakthrough pain. Although temporary neural blockade with local anaesthetic seldom provides long-lasting relief, successful blocks may suggest benefit from other approaches, including chemical neurolysis or continuous neural blockade via long-term regional local anaesthetic infusion (e.g. epidural, interscalene, or interpleural local anaesthetic infusion). Studies are needed to evaluate the safety and efficacy of these invasive approaches in the management of this problem.

Like chemical neurolysis, surgical denervation of the painful part can also be considered in selected patients with refractory breakthrough pain. As illustrated in the case report, risks and benefits must be carefully considered and discussed with the patient.

Several minimally invasive approaches have become available and may increase the utility of interventional strategies in selected patients. For example, percutaneous vertebroplasty consists of the percutaneous puncture of a vertebral body containing a bone metastasis, followed by injection of an acrylic polymer to provide bone augmentation and prevent further collapse. It may be effective in addressing refractory back pain with weight bearing.[100]

Non-pharmacological approaches

Non-pharmacological approaches also may be useful in patients with breakthrough pain. Physiotherapy, for example, may lessen the musculoskeletal complications that predispose to breakthrough pains, including foreshortening of immobilized muscles, joint ankyloses, and myofascial trigger points. Those patients with severe movement-related pain may be able to benefit from an orthosis that limits the movements that precipitate the pain. Psychological approaches may be used by some patients to reduce the impact of breakthrough pain. Patients with predictable pains may be particularly good candidates for cognitive approaches that assist in preparation for the pain.

Conclusion

Given the frequency of breakthrough pain in the palliative care setting, the clinician must be prepared to address the problem with specific interventions. Assessment is a critical first step in this process. Although the use of a rescue dose of analgesic is sufficient in many patients, some will not respond to this intervention and the use of other approaches must be considered. Surveys are needed to clarify the characteristics, causes, and impact of these pains and clinical trials are required to identify the most useful management approaches.

Pain in patients with impaired ability for self-report

Good pain management requires comprehensive pain assessment, implementation of a management plan in discussion with the patient and reassessment and evaluation. Clearly, such a model requires good communication between patients and their professional carers.

Pain is a very personal experience and some argue that patient self-report is the only way of assessing an individual's subjective experience.[101] There are clearly advantages to using self-report in a patient-centred model of care, however the patient's ability to self-report may be compromised. Many palliative care patients are elderly and frail. They may have impaired cognitive function due to age, co-existing dementia, previous stroke or their underlying malignant or non-malignant diagnosis. Their ability to communicate may be compromised by difficulties with vision, hearing, or speech, or by a decreased level of consciousness, particularly in the terminal phase. Clinicians, therefore, cannot rely solely on palliative care patients' self-report in assessing pain, since to do so might disadvantage a significant proportion of patients in their care.

Case history A 76-year-old woman with dementia presented with back pain. Investigations revealed bony metastases from an occult breast primary. She responded initially to tamoxifen, but then her general condition deteriorated and she developed increased pain on movement. She was adamant that she did not want to go to hospital and, therefore, no further investigations were done. She lived in a remote area of the country with her daughter; two other daughters lived in the same village.

Her general practitioner managed her pain with telephone advice from a hospice. It appeared that she responded to each increase in her opioid dose, but for progressively shorter periods of time, such that her opioid dose was escalating rapidly. Tablet burden became a problem and so her oral morphine was converted to diamorphine given subcutaneously via a syringe driver. Over a weekend her diamorphine dose was increased to 1500 mg over 24 h. She was reportedly still in pain, although drowsy, and her daughters decided to override their mother's previous objections and asked that she be admitted to the hospice for pain control.

She arrived at the hospice after a long and uncomfortable ambulance journey, accompanied by her daughters. As the ambulance attendants lifted her off the stretcher onto the bed she had a marked myoclonic jerk. Her daughters became distressed on seeing this, demanding that she was given something for her severe pain as soon as possible.

On examination she was very drowsy with almost continuous myoclonic jerks and was clinically opioid toxic. After much explanation her daughters allowed her syringe driver to be discontinued, and she was managed initially with as required parenteral analgesia for breakthrough pain. Two days later she was comfortable at rest on diamorphine 30 mg over 24 h and an NSAID, although she still had pain on movement. She was alert, disorientated in time and place, but knew she was not at home. Her daughters felt she would not have wanted to be referred for radiotherapy or further treatment. They understood that signs of opioid toxicity had been misinterpreted as pain and were very willing to continue to care for her at home, where she stayed until her death 3 weeks later.

The problem

Pain assessment instruments are usually divided into self-report and observational measures. Both verbal and non-verbal self-report instruments are in use; however, even self-report instruments that do not require the patient to use expressive language, for example, visual analogue and faces scales, still require language comprehension and the ability to transform the experience of pain into a language-based output.

The development of self-report of pain

Neonates and infants have yet to develop the language necessary to report pain, so observational pain assessment instruments are used in these children. Sophisticated measures of various aspects of behaviour such as the character of cry, facial expression, breathing, torso, arm and leg position, and arousal have been validated with respect to infant distress, differentiation between painful stimuli and analgesic efficacy, usually in the context of procedural pain such as heel prick, venesection, and lumbar puncture or bone marrow aspiration.[102]

In older children, pain assessment instruments appropriate to their cognitive development can be used. Those assessing them must also recognize that children's pain behaviour changes from being involuntary observable responses, to responses that are shaped by their family, social, and cultural context, but also by their experience of pain and the fear and anxiety it provokes in them. Children with prolonged pain experience, as in the palliative care setting, may adapt and complain less in response to a noxious stimulus or a procedure than a child with little pain experience.

As children become older and their language develops, self-report becomes more valid. Children's cognitive development at a given age is variable, so tools appropriate to the particular child's understanding are used. Most children have developed pain language and abstract thinking sufficient to use pain assessment tools validated in adults by the age of 9. Before this age, self-report is possible, usually using non-verbal instruments such as the Poker Chip Tool, representing up to four pieces of 'hurt' in acute pain[103] and the variety of faces scales. There has been much debate in the literature about whether faces scales measure pain or children's affective response to it, and whether their psychometric properties are valid. For instance, the anchor at the lower end of many faces scales represents a happy face, which many children are reluctant to use, since not being in pain does not necessarily mean that they are happy. An Expert Working Group of the European Association for Palliative Care (EAPC) recommends the Bieri Faces Scale, suggesting it is more sensitive to pain intensity than to the child's affective response as compared with other faces scales.[104,105] The EAPC Working Group also recommends that pain assessment in children should be multidimensional, incorporating self-report, behavioural and physiological measures, whilst acknowledging that physiological parameters may alter as a function of stress due to pain, as well as in response to pain itself.

Whilst it might be tempting to use behavioural pain scales developed for neonates or infants in adult palliative care patients unable to communicate in the terminal phase, it may not be appropriate to assume that an infant's pain behaviour is similar to a semi-conscious adult's, with a lifetime of learned, and thus modified, pain behaviour behind them.

Pain assessment in the elderly

Most of the studies on pain assessment in the elderly do not differentiate between malignant and non-malignant pain and are not specific to the palliative care setting. Pain is an under-diagnosed and under-managed problem in the elderly, reported in up to 50 per cent of those living in the community and up to 80 per cent of nursing home residents in the United States.[106] Approaches to improving the assessment and care of the elderly in long-term care include the development of Minimum Data Sets applicable to the nursing home setting. These have been applied in both North American and European settings. In the United States, the Minimum Data Set includes pain assessment instruments validated in younger adults and both established and research assessment instruments in cognitively impaired residents, with the aim of raising the profile and thus the management of pain in the elderly.[107] There is no published evidence thus far that they have improved the care of the many elderly residents in long-term care. Interestingly, there is no mention of the systematic assessment or recording of pain in a review published in 1999 of 50 assessment documents used for the 'comprehensive' assessment of older people receiving social care in the United Kingdom.[108]

Barriers to pain assessment and management in the elderly

Even in the cognitively intact elderly barriers to pain assessment include under-reporting by patients, co-morbidities complicating the clinical picture and caregivers' beliefs and attitudes about the reliability of patients' pain reporting, the prevalence of pain in the elderly, and the dangers of opioids in this patient group.

There may be a lack of congruence between patients' and carers' perceptions of pain; for example, in a study of 45 pairs of elderly residents and their usual nursing assistants in the United States, 49 per cent of residents reported pain in the last week. The nurses under-reported pain for 38 per cent of residents and over-reported for 24 per cent.[109]

Caregivers may also misinterpret pain behaviour. In a study of 42 American nursing home residents, both professional and family caregivers were confident about their ability to identify pain-related behaviours and the intensity of the elderly person's pain. However, their judgements correlated poorly with the resident's self-report.[110]

Even when pain is recognized, it may be under-managed, particularly in certain groups of patients. In a cross-sectional study of 49 971 nursing home residents in the United States over 3 years to 1995 using the SAGE database (Systematic Assessment of Geriatric drug use via Epidemiology), Minimum Data Set items were linked to nursing home drug use. Twenty-six per cent of residents reported daily pain. Of these patients, 25 per cent received no analgesics and residents over 85 years of age, men, the cognitively impaired, and racial minorities were over-represented in this group.[111]

Pain assessment in the cognitively impaired

Pain assessment and management is more complex in those with cognitive impairment where the ability to self-report may be decreased or absent. There is some evidence that individuals with cognitive impairment may perceive less pain; for instance, patients with Alzheimer's disease report less pain intensity and less pain affect than controls matched for age and the presence of painful conditions.[112] However, grimacing, moaning, restlessness, and changes in behaviour may be seen as part of an underlying psychiatric state, rather than pain behaviour, so that pain may be underestimated and inappropriately managed.

Many studies suggest that patients with cognitive impairment receive fewer analgesics than the cognitively intact elderly, even for surgical procedures such as repair of hip fracture.[113] Thus, there is evidence that pain is both underestimated and under-managed. The Expert Working Group of the EAPC concludes that there is currently no valid instrument for pain assessment in the cognitively impaired; however, some studies suggest that the assessment of pain in these patients can be improved using combinations of standard pain assessment instruments. For example, in a cross-sectional survey of 305 elderly nursing home residents, a combination of a visual analogue scale, a behaviour (faces) scale, and a pain descriptive scale improved the frequency of diagnosing pain in those over 85 years and the cognitively impaired as compared to the question 'do you have pain' used in the control group.[106] A further study included 90 patients over 55 years of age admitted to a subacute care facility in the United States. Patients were asked to rate their pain three times daily for 7 days using a five-point verbal rating scale, the Bieri faces scale, a 21-point box scale (a row of 21 boxes labelled from 0 to 100 in increments of five), and two vertical 21-point box scales (0–20) measuring pain intensity and pain unpleasantness. The authors conclude that older patients can accurately report their pain and that a 21-point box scale is most useful in this patient group, including those with mild to moderate cognitive impairment. For those with more severe cognitive impairment (Folstein Mini Mental State Examination scores mean 12 to 13) comprehension of a 0–10 scale may be impossible, although these patients fared no better with the shorter assessment instruments. Pain assessment in these individuals requires further research.[114]

Pain assessment in patients unable to self-report

The literature in patients with little or no ability to self-report, such as patients with severe learning disabilities, genetic or acquired brain damage, or severe cognitive impairment is sparse. Observation of physiological indices and pain behaviour is suggested, but these indicators may not be the same in those with and without severe cognitive impairment. What literature there is suggests that caregivers, including the parents of severely impaired children 'make use of many and varied non-verbal expressions for pain in the cognitively impaired'.[115] Knowledge of the person's non-pain state, interpretation of behaviour, clinical judgement, and intuition all play a part.[116]

Relevance in the palliative care setting

Patients with ability to self-report

Palliative care promotes the practice of holistic, patient-centred care, in which the assessment and management of pain and other symptoms is seen as core. Pain assessment instruments are commonly seen as research tools rather than being relevant to everyday practice. Where they are incorporated into routine assessment instruments such as the Memorial Symptom Assessment Score or the Edmonton Symptom Assessment System (ESAS) reports vary as to how many palliative care patients are able to complete them. In one study, in a palliative care unit in the United Kingdom, nearly half of the patients with advanced disease were unable to complete the

ESAS.[117] Radbruch and colleagues developed a Minimal Documentation System for patients within a palliative care unit with the aim of combining 'minimal burden for patients and staff with sufficient information content for outcome control and quality assurance'.[118] In this study of over 100 patients, 35 per cent of patients were cognitively impaired using a MMSE cut-off point of 21. Patients with low MMSE scores had many missing values using the Brief Pain Inventory and the SF-12, about 60 per cent could rate average and worst pain on a numerical rating scale, and 17 per cent of patients had to have their pain and other symptoms assessed by the physician. The authors conclude that for routine practice some patients will require numerical rating scales to be replaced by verbal categorical scales completed by the patient or at interview.

It is salutary to consider that the diagnosis of pain in certain groups of elderly patients was improved by completing assessment instruments rather than asking the question 'do you have pain?'. The literature from the care of the elderly setting suggests that the routine use of assessment instruments could increase the diagnosis of pain in both cognitively intact and mild-to-moderately cognitively impaired palliative care patients but that the assessment of those with moderate-to-severe cognitive impairment remains a challenge.

Patients with little or no ability for self-report

Further research is required into pain assessment in those patients with little or no ability for self-report, including patients in the terminal phase. Models for assessing pain in unconscious patients exist, such as those used in anaesthetized patients or for critically ill patients in intensive care units; however, since the mechanism of patients' decreased level of consciousness is very different it is questionable whether such models are appropriate. The literature suggests that patients' 'usual carers' knowledge of the patient is important; however, it is known that relatives' reports of patients' pain are influenced by their perception of their loved-one's distress and by their own distress.[119]

Hadjistavropoulos and Craig propose a communications model for understanding self-report and observational measures of pain.[120] They propose that pain is firstly an internal experience for an individual, which is then encoded in expressive behaviour, either behaviourally, or by reporting the experience in some way. This behaviour or report is then decoded by the observer. This decoding may be altered by the clarity of the message or by observer bias. In the terminal phase, this observer bias may be due to relatives' distress at the situation or professionals' expectations and beliefs about how much pain the patient is expected to have and what constitutes a 'good' or 'peaceful' death.

Strategies to coordinate and standardize practice, with the aim of improving the care of patients in the terminal phase, include the development of integrated care pathways for the dying patient.[121] The aim of care is for the patient to be pain free. In the care pathway being widely introduced in the United Kingdom, pain is recorded as (a) vocalized by the patient if they are conscious, (b) patient is pain-free on movement, or (c) the patient appears peaceful.[122] The simplicity of such a scoring system should mean it is easy to use. It is possible, however, that observer bias about expectations of the dying process will colour the assessment and recording of pain. Further research will be required to assess whether such pathways do improve the standard of pain assessment and management in the dying, or whether further formalization of the observation, clinical judgement, and intuition of those caring for dying patients is needed to standardize and improve patient care at the end of life.

Conclusion

There has been little research into the assessment and measurement of pain in adult patients with impaired ability to self-report. Research findings and experience with children in pain provide some analogies but cannot be easily translated to the management of such patients. In a palliative care context, knowledge of the person's non-pain state, interpretation of behaviour, and clinical judgement within the context of integrated care pathways for the dying should contribute to improved outcomes for these patients.

Rectal and bladder pain

Rectal and bladder pain are considered together here. Though there may be obvious differences in presentation and pathophysiology, there are a number of similarities. Tenesmus is 'ineffectual and painful straining at stool or in urinating' and may be difficult to treat, whether it arises from rectum or bladder. Occasionally patients experience excruciating spasms of pain in the rectum, or spasms of pain in the bladder or urethra. Less dramatic but more common is the poorly localized perineal pain, which may be associated with any intrapelvic malignancy.

Case history A 63-year-old retired chef presented with a 2-month history of lower abdominal pain and a change in bowel habit. Investigations demonstrated a mass in the rectum and he subsequently had an anterior resection of a 5-cm long rectal tumour. There was no macroscopic evidence of spread at laparotomy, but histological examination showed it to be an adenocarcinoma with local lymph node involvement (Duke's C). His postoperative course was uncomplicated. Adjuvant chemotherapy was advised but he declined.

He remained well for the next 15 months but then developed pain in the perineum extending across the left buttock and down the left posterior thigh. He was unable to sit in comfort for more than 10–15 min. The pain in the perineum, buttock, and posterior thigh was described as burning in character. He was constipated and said that he was fearful of opening his bowels as this caused a severe searing perineal and anal pain but at the same time he had a constant feeling of needing to open his bowels.

The distribution of his pain was thought to indicate involvement of S2 to S5 nerve roots, and a CT scan showed a local recurrence of the rectal carcinoma with associated bony erosion of the sacrum. A defunctioning colostomy was considered because of the severe pain on defaecation but the patient declined any further surgery.

Coproxamol (paracetamol 325 mg and dextropropoxyphene 32.5 mg) tablets, two 6-hourly, had not controlled his pain. He was started on morphine 10 mg 4-hourly together with dexamethasone 4 mg twice a day, with codanthramer (a combination of danthron and poloxamer) for his constipation. His morphine was titrated to 40 mg 4-hourly. This improved his pain and was well tolerated, apart from some temporary drowsiness, but he was still unable to sit for long periods. A course of radiotherapy, 30 Gy in 10 fractions over 14 days, was recommended and his morphine was gradually increased.

Following radiotherapy, he was sleeping well and able to sit for up to 1 h with comfort on a dose of morphine of 100 mg 4-hourly. His steroids were reduced over the next 3 weeks. With the reduction in dexamethasone, an NSAID, naproxen, was added as he began to complain of pain when walking, consistent with the bony erosion of his sacrum. His pain responded well to the naproxen.

Throughout this period, the patient and his wife needed considerable psychological support. This required frequent exploration, explanation, and reassurance provided mainly by his general practitioner and the community palliative care nurses who visited him at home. His general practitioner, who had known him for many years provided valuable insight into the psychodynamics of his family life. The patient had been very dependent throughout his adult life. Both he and his wife had consulted their general practitioner frequently over many years for a large variety of somatic symptoms. They had one daughter, who was now married and living away from home, whom they telephoned on average five or six times each day. This dependent behaviour was never challenged by their daughter. They had emigrated from Spain 30 years previously and despite this lapse of time their command of English was very poor, further increasing their dependence on their daughter.

Three months later, the patient's pain returned, as did the constant feeling that he needed to open his bowels. A further course of dexamethasone and escalating doses of morphine failed to produce acceptable relief. He was changed from morphine to oxycodone in increasing doses and his general level of pain was improved. The tenesmoid discomfort remained a problem and he also experienced intermittent severe spasmodic pain in his perineum. The possibility of a nerve block was discussed but he preferred to pursue alternative drug treatments. He was able to use oral transmucosal fentanyl citrate (OTFC) for the intermittent pain with good effect, but this was short-lived as his general condition deteriorated over the next few weeks (by now he was known to have extensive liver metastases) and he died 2 years after his original presentation.

The problem

In a series of 350 patients admitted to a hospice in the United Kingdom, 11 per cent had intrapelvic pain and in about half of these the pain was associated with cancer of the large bowel.[123] The incidence of colorectal cancer is generally increasing, mostly in the developed world and in the urban areas of the developing world,[124] and it remains the second most common cause of cancer death in Western societies. Surgical resection remains the main mode of treatment but, despite improvements in surgical and anaesthetic techniques, 5-year survival rates have changed little over the past 40 years. However, in recent years it has become clear that adjuvant chemotherapy and radiotherapy either alone or in combination may confer significant survival advantage for a proportion of patients. The use of chemotherapy and radiotherapy may also improve both quality of life and survival in patients with recurrent or metastatic disease. In recent years, there has been a huge growth in our understanding of the molecular biology of cancer and colorectal cancer has been a specific focus for much of this work. This holds great promise for the future.

Pain is a frequent problem in patients with recurrent disease and the most common site of pain is in the rectum (even after surgical resection—so-called 'phantom' rectal pain). The descriptions of the pain in the series described above tended to fall into two categories: either a constant feeling of fullness (a 'tenesmoid' pain) or a severe spasmodic or searing pain.[123]

The incidence of bladder tenesmoid pain and painful bladder spasm in a palliative care population has not been accurately documented. These pains may be associated with bladder or other pelvic tumours, stones or blood clots, infection or retention, or with an indwelling urinary catheter (see Chapter 8.10).

Pathophysiology

Rectal pain rarely occurs in isolation but is usually a component of a complex clinical picture as illustrated by the case history. The patient described here had symptomatic problems that were similar in a number of respects to those of the patient described in the first section of this chapter, but the underlying pathology was quite different. This emphasizes the need for careful assessment of each patient in order to devise an appropriate and individualized treatment strategy. This man's pain also had both nociceptive and neuropathic components and, in addition, was complicated by the searing anorectal and perineal pain associated with defaecation and his anxious mental state.

Intermittent anorectal pain of this nature or anorectal spasmodic pain resembles proctalgia fugax and, as in that condition, the precise mechanism underlying the pain is unclear. Spasm of the levator ani and coccygeal musculature or of the anal sphincter itself are probable contributors and may result from direct tumour invasion of the muscles or may be due to involvement of the sacral plexus. The spasms of pain may occur spontaneously or may be precipitated by a full rectum or defaecation.

Rectal tenesmoid pain is usually less severe but is still sufficient to cause considerable distress, and is more likely to be continuous in nature rather than intermittent. It is usually associated with progressively enlarging pelvic tumour and tends to be made worse by anything that increases pressure within the pelvis, such as constipation or sitting.

Since the precise cause of anorectal spasmodic pain or tenesmoid pain is not understood, it is only possible to speculate on their anatomical and physiological basis. Both somatic and autonomic neuronal pathways are implicated. Excessive contraction of smooth muscle or distension of a hollow viscus will give rise to pain transmission in afferent fibres accompanying autonomic nerves, whereas surrounding inflammation may result in pain impulses transmitted in somatic afferents. The anal sphincter has both smooth muscle and skeletal muscle components, and both may be subject to spasm.

Perineal pain, which follows abdominoperineal resection of the rectum for the treatment of carcinoma (other than that arising immediately after surgery), is an early sign of recurrence. In a prospective study of 177 patients, Boas and colleagues describe two underlying causes for perineal pain after rectal amputation.[125] These were either local recurrence of tumour or neuronal deafferentation following surgical excision of the pudendal nerve supply to the lower rectum and anus. Their data indicate that late development of perineal pain is a highly significant indicator of tumour recurrence. It is more likely to respond to analgesic drugs than early onset pain, which is more often neuropathic in nature.

Bladder tenesmoid pain is similar to rectal tenesmus and may also be caused by enlarging pelvic tumour arising from within the bladder or from some other pelvic organ. Urinary retention and urinary tract infection may cause similar discomfort but are generally dealt with more easily.

Management: rectal pain

Careful assessment is the basis of effective management. Because rectal tenesmus or the constant feeling of needing to defaecate is often difficult to treat pharmacologically, it is particularly important that the temporal characteristics of the pain and aggravating and relieving factors are clearly identified. Sometimes perineal discomfort may be relieved or ameliorated by simple manoeuvres or changes in behaviour or lifestyle and ergonomic advice and aids from an occupational therapist may be more helpful than frequent changes in the drug regimen.

The patient described was fearful of opening his bowels because this precipitated excruciating pain. In this situation, it is particularly important to pay close attention to keeping the stool soft and maintaining a regular bowel motion.

This patient had considerable psychological problems complicating his pain symptoms. It would be misleading to make generalizations about psychological components of anorectal pain, but this association of symptoms is not unusual and needs always to be kept in mind and dealt with appropriately.

Antitumour therapy

Pelvic radiotherapy should be considered in patients with symptomatic recurrent colorectal cancer who have not already had pelvic irradiation, and in other patients with intrapelvic malignancies where tumour mass or infiltration is causing pain or other symptoms. Chemotherapy is also occasionally helpful in this situation.

Analgesics

Conventional analgesics used in the usual manner are the basis of analgesic management of rectal pain. This patient illustrates a recurring theme of this chapter, which is that patients with difficult pain invariably present complicated clinical problems involving both nociceptive and non-nociceptive pain. In this case, the nociceptive (bone and tumour) pain and the neuropathic pain in the perineum, buttock, and thigh were initially well controlled with opioid analgesics. Other strategies were subsequently required for the movement-related bone pain, the dysaesthetic perineal pain, and the spasmodic anorectal pain.

Adjuvant drugs

The burning dysaesthetic pain involving the perineum, left buttock, and left posterior thigh in this patient was presumed to result from compression of the sacral nerve roots by tumour or from malignant infiltration of the nerves and nerve roots of the sacral plexus. The management of such neuropathic pain is outlined in the early part of this chapter. In this patient corticosteroids were used to good effect.

The mode of action of corticosteroids when used in this way is presumed to be essentially mechanical—nerve compression is relieved by a reduction in inflammatory oedema and hyperaemia surrounding a tumour or within an infiltrated nerve bundle (though other systemic effects of corticosteroids may contribute).[126] This means that if a trial of steroids is successful, treatment with pelvic radiotherapy should be considered as a next step.

In the patient described, the combination of opioid analgesics, corticosteroids, and then radiotherapy controlled his pain. After some 3 months, his pain returned and then his complaints were dominated by a continuous midline perineal pain (no longer burning in nature) and severe anorectal spasms. Two approaches to management were considered: further pharmacological manipulation or invasive anaesthetic techniques.

The history and clinical characteristics of these pains suggested that the perineal pain was partly nociceptive (caused by enlarging tumour within the tight tissue planes of the pelvis) and partly neuropathic (resulting from damage to the sacral plexus or nerve roots). The pain due to muscle spasm was presumed to be mainly smooth muscle generated, but with a possible skeletal muscle cramp-like component. This constellation of different pains with different underlying mechanisms made the choice of the next treatment strategy particularly difficult. It was felt that time was short and that a good response to 'conventional' adjuvants was unlikely (particularly as far as the spasmodic pain was concerned). Other possible drug treatments were considered.

The belladonna alkaloids atropine and hyoscine and related synthetic and semisynthetic antimuscarinic drugs, such as dicyclomine and flavoxate, have a direct smooth muscle relaxant effect. The problem with this group of drugs is that when used in doses that have a significant spasmolytic effect, they invariably produce troublesome anticholinergic effects, and this limits their usefulness. There is little documented information about the use of these drugs to treat rectal tenesmus or spasm but they are invariably tried as treatment options become progressively limited. In the United Kingdom, hyoscine butylbromide is widely used to treat visceral pain, colic and tenesmoid pains.[127]

Calcium channel blocking agents have also been used as antispasmodic agents[128] and diltiazem has specifically been reported to relieve the pain of proctalgia fugax.[129] As yet no controlled studies have been published, but these reports open up another potential therapeutic option for a symptom that may be unresponsive to any currently available remedy.

Anaesthetic procedures

The sympathetic nervous system may be specifically involved in mediating rectal pain. In one series of patients with rectal tenesmoid pain, bilateral chemical lumbar sympathetic block produced complete relief in 10 out of 12 patients.[130] This procedure is discussed in more detail in Chapter 8.2.6, but it is a safe technique associated with low morbidity and should be considered at an early stage in the management of rectal tenesmus or any other pelvic visceral distension pain. A similar but more selective technique of superior hypogastric plexus block may be also effective in the management of pelvic pain.[131]

Midline perineal pain resulting from pelvic malignancy may be effectively relieved by a neurolytic saddle block. Traditionally, this has been carried out with a hyperbaric agent such as phenol and it is claimed that in experienced hands this can be accomplished without affecting the bladder. However, a small series of nine patients treated with intrathecal phenol for perianal and perineal pain highlights the limitations of this technique.[132] The duration of pain relief was short (17.8 days) and there was a significant incidence of serious adverse effects, including permanent urinary retention in two patients. This procedure is now infrequently used. An alternative technique for intractable perineal pain is blockade of the ganglion impar (the ganglion of Walther or sacrococcygeal ganglion)[133] but there are few published data on efficacy and adverse effects with this technique. Cryoanalgesia also may be effective in the relief of perineal pain.[134] A needle cryoprobe is inserted through the sacrococcygeal ligament and into the sacral canal. Repeated freeze cycles produce anaesthesia of the lower sacral nerve roots.

None of these techniques were felt appropriate for this patient. In recent years, there has been an accelerating move away from neurodestructive techniques. This reflects greater sophistication of pharmacological management and a wider choice both of opioids and adjuvant analgesics. One inevitable consequence of this trend is that it is sometimes difficult to find practitioners with the necessary skills and experience to carry out these procedures in the now relatively few instances where they might be considered.

Management: bladder pain

The emphasis of this section is on the management of bladder tenesmoid pain and bladder spasm.

The first step is to identify potentially remediable causes of bladder pain. Infection or direct irritation by catheter, tumour, debris, or blood clot should all be dealt with appropriately. Where the underlying cause cannot be treated, or where symptoms persist despite appropriate action, symptomatic remedies are applied.

Analgesics

Once again a conventional approach should be adopted as the baseline, progressing from non-opioid analgesics to opioids.

Adjuvants

Corticosteroids may have a place where symptoms are related to tumour mass, but generally have a limited application in bladder pain management.

NSAIDs may be effective in the management of detrusor instability caused by increased bladder activity.[135] This use was prompted by the observation that the prostaglandins PGE2 and F2α stimulate strips of human bladder muscle *in vitro*.[136] Thus, there is a theoretical basis for using NSAIDs in the management of bladder pain, particularly spasm, because of their prostaglandin-synthetase-inhibitory action. NSAIDs also have intrinsic analgesic actions. A trial of an NSAID (in conjunction with opioid analgesics) should be the first option in the management of bladder tenesmus or spasm.

Other pharmacological treatments are generally unsatisfactory. The smooth-muscle relaxant drugs dicyclomine and flavoxate have been mentioned above and are frequently employed, usually with little success, as are the postganglionic anticholinergic agents propantheline and emepronium bromide (now withdrawn in the United Kingdom). The last two are more likely to cause anticholinergic adverse effects such as dry mouth, blurred vision, and urinary retention. The theoretical basis for the use of all these atropine-like drugs is that they block the parasympathetic control of the bladder. Thus, they can lower intravesicular pressure, increase capacity, and reduce the frequency of urinary bladder contractions.[137]

Oxybutynin hydrochloride is a tertiary amine similar to dicyclomine and flavoxate that has been shown to be effective in a variety of unstable bladder conditions.[138] Topical administration by instillation into the bladder may enhance its beneficial effects whilst reducing systemic anticholinergic effects[139] (and this route may also be preferable for administration of other drugs with similar actions such as atropine and phentolamine[140]). A more recent quaternary ammonium compound, trospium, is also claimed to have a more favourable therapeutic ratio after systemic administration with less anticholinergic effects because it does not easily cross the blood–brain barrier.[141] Unfortunately, with all of these drugs it is easier to demonstrate significant effects on objective urodynamic parameters than symptomatic relief in patients with painful bladder spasm.

Pyridium (phenazopyridine) and methylene blue are azo dyes that are said to have analgesic effects on bladder and urinary tract mucosa. These drugs have been used in a non-specific way to treat dysuria and bladder and urethral pain, but there is little information about their efficacy. Neither is now available in the United Kingdom.

In recent years, there have been reports of the analgesic effects of intravesical local anaesthetics[142] and capsaicin[143] in various painful bladder conditions, and the former is certainly worth trying in patients with painful bladder or urethral spasm associated with an indwelling catheter.

Bupivacaine, 20 ml of 0.25 per cent solution instilled for 20 min, is recommended[144] but has not been subjected to investigation in controlled trials.

A recent report of a 57-year-old man with carcinoma of the bladder and prostate, experiencing 'excruciating bladder spasms radiating from his suprapubic area into both groins and pelvis' describes dramatic relief following the use of intravesical diamorphine (10 mg in 20 ml of saline instilled intravesically 4-hourly).[145] The pain was relieved within hours of the first instillation and he remained pain free. The patient had previously been taking sustained release oral morphine (which was continued) and had had trials of oxybutynin, amitriptyline, gabapentin, corticosteroids, clonazepam, and intravesical bupivacaine for the bladder spasm without success. The explanation for the profound local analgesic effect of diamorphine in a patient receiving systemic opioids is unclear. The authors of this report were able to identify only one study describing the use of intravesical morphine[146] and one other reference to such use.[147] The patient described was taught to perform intermittent self-catheterization and instil the diamorphine himself. His suprapubic catheter was removed and he was discharged home.

Anaesthetic procedures

No anaesthetic procedure has proved itself to be particularly useful in the management of bladder tenesmus or bladder spasm, though spinal administration of opioids may be preferable to systemic analgesics.[148]

Conclusion

Rectal and bladder tenesmus and spasm remain difficult, and sometimes intractable, problems. As with most pain problems in palliative care an integrated approach using drug and non-drug measures will usually produce some amelioration of these symptoms but not infrequently patients are left with troublesome residual pain and discomfort. Whilst these types of pain represent a small proportion of those encountered in cancer patients, for those involved they may be a continuing source of misery. There is still much scope for improvements in management.

Abdominal pain

Abdominal pain is common in advanced cancer patients. In one series of patients with advanced cancer being followed at home, 45 per cent had abdominal pain.[149] Pancreatic pain is considered here as an example of visceral abdominal pain, which may be difficult to manage with conventional analgesics.

Case history A 49-year-old businessman had been an insulin-dependent diabetic since the age of 18. He presented with malaise, loss of appetite, weight loss of 10 lb (4.5 kg) over 3 months, and vague abdominal discomfort, which was worse after eating and was later associated with a gnawing ache in the lower thoracic region in the midline. The patient tried resting after meals but he noted that the pain was sometimes intensified when he was recumbent, with relief on sitting up. He became jaundiced and a CT scan revealed a mass in the head of the pancreas. Laparotomy confirmed the diagnosis of pancreatic cancer and multiple small hepatic metastases were noted. A choledochojejunostomy was carried out.

Postoperative abdominal pain was controlled with parenteral morphine. Coeliac plexus block was performed on the sixth day with total relief of back pain but he continued to experience epigastric pain. The patient was converted to oral morphine plus ibuprofen and was subsequently discharged home.

Over the next 3 weeks his morphine requirements increased. He was treated with palliative radiotherapy together with 5-fluorouracil. Ibuprofen was discontinued and prednisolone, megestrol, and methylphenidate were added to the regimen. The patient enjoyed satisfactory pain control for 6 weeks and felt sufficiently well to take a sea voyage. However, during the last week of his holiday, his pain increased. On his return he was readmitted to hospital with severe epigastric pain. He alternated between periods of confusion and agitation and excessive sedation secondary to increments in morphine therapy. He was converted to a continuous subcutaneous infusion of hydromorphone. Methylphenidate was discontinued and the steroid dose was reduced. He was still confused 2 days later but did not appear to be in pain. He gradually recovered his mental faculties and was switched back to oral morphine but his general condition deteriorated and he died 5 weeks later.

The problem

Adenocarcinoma of the exocrine pancreas is a disease of industrialized countries and its incidence has increased in the last 45 years. For unknown reasons, this upward trend has stabilized in the last decade but the outlook for patients remains very poor. About 80–90 per cent of patients with pancreatic cancer will die within a year of diagnosis, and less than 5 per cent will be alive 5 years after diagnosis.[150]

Pain is common but not inevitable, occurring in 75–90 per cent of patients at some stage, often at presentation.[151] Pain from carcinoma of the pancreas usually responds to conventional analgesic drugs. Control may be achieved but the scenario often rapidly changes, requiring consideration of other modalities of therapy in addition to analgesics.

Pathophysiology: abdominal pain

Abdominal pain often puzzles the clinician because the pathophysiology of visceral nociception is poorly defined. Thus, perplexing presentations and responses to therapy are common. Abdominal pain is by nature more difficult to assess than cutaneous pain. The patient readily identifies cutaneous sensation, localizes it with precision, and describes it in terms that separate pain from other cutaneous sensations. We do tend not to confuse itch or cutaneous pressure with pain.

In contrast, abdominal pain, particularly in its early chronic stages, is often vaguely located and difficult to describe. This is not surprising since, except for satiety and rectal sensations, visceral neurones normally mediate digestive events that do not require conscious perception.[152] Visceral pain is often associated with other unpleasant sensations, which, while not painful, cause great distress. The patient may say, 'I think I have pain, but what bothers me is the feeling of fullness in my stomach and nausea. It makes me feel very weak'. The patient's confusion and uncertainty is mirrored by that of neurophysiologists. Arguments continue about whether specific bowel nociceptors exist and the mechanisms of referred pain.

Stimuli that elicit pain in other parts of the body may not be nociceptive when applied to the viscera. For example, intestinal cutting, burning, or point pressures will not produce acute pain. Electrical stimulation (an unnatural process that is probably not clinically relevant), bowel or duct distension (a very relevant stimulus), and application of various chemicals will cause pain in normal subjects. However, if a viscus is inflamed, stimuli that are normally non-painful, such as pressure, will cause pain that is accentuated if the stimulus is applied for a period of time over a large tissue area.

Thus, we have a model where summation occurs and pain sensations that are poorly appreciated at the onset become agonizing if pain remains unrelieved. As visceral pain intensifies, it tends to localize.

Localization often occurs because of disease extension to a somatically innervated tissue such as the parietal peritoneum. However, distension studies in normal subjects show that localization will occur even in the absence of somatic nerve involvement. The classic sites of localization are well identified for many organs and disorders. Gallbladder pain localizing in the right upper quadrant is one example. Bladder pain presenting in both the hypogastric (suprapubic) area and sacrum, ulcer pain in the epigastrium, renal colic, and testicular torsion provide other commonly recognized patterns.

Involvement of somatic nerves (defined as those serving the parietal peritoneum, muscles surrounding the abdomen, associated bone and connective tissue, and skin) will help localize the site of disease. A classic example is the localization of pain in the right lower quadrant following inflammation of the parietal peritoneum in association with an inflamed appendix.

Pain will also be referred to somatic structures without direct involvement of somatic nerves. Perhaps the best recognized example of this mechanism is the occurrence of ipsilateral shoulder and scapula pain due to phrenic nerve stimulation by diaphragmatic irritation. Other common patterns include right flank pain following renal colic and pain in the T10–L2 back area with pancreatic disease.

The nature of referred pain is not clearly established. Pertinent factors include the possible presence of 'dichotomizing' sensory nerves with endings in both visceral and somatic tissues and, at the spinal cord level, wide ramifications of visceral nerves whose axons also interact with neurones receiving somatic nerve input. As a result, the higher brain centres assign pain to the region from which sensory inputs are normally received.

Recent reviews have highlighted the complex neurophysiology of visceral pain and the subtleties of its clinical presentation:(153,154)

1. Visceral pain is very commonly associated with activation of autonomic reflexes, which, in turn, can evoke intense and highly unpleasant associated symptoms (such as nausea and weakness), which may present a confusing picture.
2. The quality or intensity of pain does not differentiate visceral pain arising from different anatomical sites.
3. Resonant 'vicious circles' probably exist whereby pain arising from a distended, inflamed viscus promotes abnormal gut function, which, in turn, accentuates pain. For example, a partially obstructed bowel may induce smooth muscle contractions, which, in turn, increase distension and pain. Clinically, dull, abdominal pain interspersed with crampy, severe, episodic pain may be described.
4. The onset of visceral pain may lag behind the stimulus as sensitization of sensory nerves plus persistence of the disease process must be present before pain is recognized.
5. Hyperalgesia may be present over body surfaces to which visceral pain is referred.
6. Visceral pain cannot be evoked from all viscera and is not always linked to visceral injury.

So, abdominal pain may present in varied and surprising ways.

Cancer-induced abdominal pain

An intra-abdominal neoplasm can cause pain through a variety of mechanisms. Growth within a closed space (such as the liver) can stretch a capsule. A tumour partially obstructing the bowel can distend an adjacent loop of bowel with consequent local inflammation, release of cytokines and other inflammatory mediators, and secondary occurrence of smooth muscle spasm or incoordinate action, which may add a crampy pain component. Parietal pain may be caused by direct tumour invasion. If tumours invade ducts such as the common bile duct or the large pancreatic duct, inflammation, distension, and consequent pain will occur. Within the pancreas the problem is sometimes compounded by the release outside the ducts of pancreatic enzymes, further inflammation, and increased pain.

Regardless of the anatomical site, a combination of distortion, inflammation, smooth muscle abnormality, and ultimately neuronal hypersensitivity is commonly associated with cancer.

Abdominal pain—AIDS

Abdominal pain, which is often non-specific in nature and not clearly related to intra-abdominal pathology, is also encountered in patients with AIDS.(155) Here, the aetiology of pain is even less clear than pain associated with cancer. Abdominal cramps are seen in association with enteritis and ileitis.(156) On occasion retroperitoneal adenopathy or tumour involvement of the bowel wall, in particular Kaposi's sarcoma, may be found. However, Kaposi tumours are usually asymptomatic.(157) Sclerosing cholangitis may cause upper abdominal pain, while pancreatitis may occur in patients receiving pentamidine, didanosine, or dideocytidine.(156) Often a specific cause cannot be determined. Neuropathies are common in patients with AIDS, but a syndrome of painful visceral neuropathy has not been clearly delineated.

Management

Continuing with the example of pancreatic cancer, dull aching pain will occur in most patients, with a higher incidence in those with involvement of the pancreatic body or tail. The pain is usually in the epigastrium but diffuse non-localizing abdominal pain or radiation to the back is common. Our patient showed a feature sometimes indicative of pancreatic pain—an increase of pain on recumbency with improvement on changing positions.

Anorexia, general malaise, and 'indigestion' are common accompanying symptoms. Depression is frequently associated with pancreatic cancer with a disproportionate incidence compared with other abdominal tumours with similar presentation, for example, stomach cancer.(158) While the patient's awareness of the presence of an undiagnosed serious illness no doubt contributes to the inordinate rate of depression in pancreatic cancer, it also probably represents a true paraneoplastic syndrome of unknown aetiology. All these factors need to be taken into account alongside specific attention to the pain.

Antitumour therapy

Surgery is the only curative treatment for carcinoma of the pancreas but only a small proportion of patients (less than 20 per cent) are suitable. There is no evidence that the lives of patients with pancreatic cancer are prolonged by chemotherapy or radiotherapy. As noted at the beginning of this section, the prognosis is poor and cancer of the pancreas has the lowest 5-year survival of all cancers.(150)

Does therapy influence pain? Choledochojejunostomy is commonly performed to relieve bile duct pressure and obstruction, while gastrojejunostomy is sometimes carried out to prevent or alleviate duodenal obstruction. Both palliative procedures can obviously improve patient comfort and delay or obviate catastrophe. Their specific effect on pain is not defined, although many surgeons feel that relief of duct obstruction will also improve pancreatic pain.

Chemotherapy by itself is not analgesic in this condition, but 5-fluorouracil, which was the most commonly employed agent for gastrointestinal cancers, has radiosensitizing actions in the laboratory. It is often used in combination with radiation therapy. The evidence at hand suggests that 5-fluorouracil combined with radiotherapy is superior to radiotherapy alone, relieving pain in 30–40 per cent of patients for an uncertain period.(159) The patient may, however, pay a price for pain relief with increased nausea and anorexia. In a single controlled trial, gemcitabine proved superior to 5-fluorouracil (which was ineffective as a single agent) in relieving pain in a subset of patients.(160)

In the case of the patient described, therapy was reasonably well tolerated and he enjoyed good pain control following radiation treatment. However, during this time he was also treated with steroids and followed closely in the clinic and at home with frequent titration of analgesics.

Analgesics

Oral opioids are the long-term anchor of pain management in cancer of the pancreas. They can be used at the same time as interventional techniques such as coeliac plexus block or radiotherapy. If these last procedures are effective, opioids can readily be tapered.

The patient received conventional oral opioid therapy with good effect throughout his illness. Morphine contributed to his sedation and confusion but it is likely that this episode was exacerbated by adjuvant drugs. When the patient presented in a confusional state, he was switched from oral morphine to subcutaneous hydromorphone and it was anticipated that good pain control would be achieved at lower equivalent doses of hydromorphone with a consequent reduction in opioid side-effects.

It is uncertain whether this manoeuvre actually helped the patient. His pain did improve, his mind cleared, and he was able to take oral morphine

Table 4 Guidelines for the management of upper abdominal cancer pain

Consider a coeliac plexus block
At laparotomy
Percutaneous
Use concomitant analgesic therapy
Opioids
NSAIDs
Corticosteroids
Consider trial of chemoradiotherapy (careful framing of objectives and assessments)
Adjuvant drugs
Methylphenidate
If oversedation
Antidepressants
Use not proven
Help both pain and depression?
Adjuvant non-pharmacological techniques
Behavioural therapy
Imagery
Hypnosis
Distraction
Epidural opioids in centres with established programmes

once again. Probably the simplification of his adjuvant medication plus, possibly, resolution of a superimposed acute pain event were primarily responsible for the improvement.

The ideal sequence for using opioids, coeliac plexus block or antitumour therapy has not been determined in clinical trials. Our practice follows the sequence outlined in Table 4. We prefer to carry out a coeliac plexus block at the onset of severe pancreatic cancer pain as the results of the blocks are reasonable, we believe that associated opioid therapy may be more easily maintained at low doses, and the length of pain relief spans the trajectory of illness in this disorder with a very short survival time after diagnosis. We are more selective in patients with other types of upper abdominal cancer where results are less consistent and where life expectancy may be longer.

This patient's confusion in the latter weeks of his life raises the question of treatment with spinal opioids. Theoretically, the use of epidural opioids would reduce the risk of opioid-associated adverse effects. Whether their use is associated with reduced end-stage delirium is not known, although the hypothesis is eminently reasonable. Randomized trials comparing spinal and subcutaneous opioids in the management of abdominal pain are needed.

Adjuvant drugs

NSAIDs have a proven benefit in pancreatic cancer pain.(161) Patients should receive a trial of an NSAID, if not contra-indicated. Alternatively, corticosteroids may be used for short-term pain control (but the possibility of steroid-induced diabetes should be kept in mind).

The dose of morphine required for pain control in this patient caused distressing sedation, which responded to methylphenidate. The methylphenidate, along with the corticosteroids, may have contributed to subsequent dysphoria and confusion.

Pancreatic cancer patients have an increased incidence of depression, and one might think that antidepressants might relieve both the depression and associated pain. This is an intriguing concept that has not been tested. In view of the high incidence of often-missed depression,(158) the concomitant use of antidepressants with analgesic properties should be considered in patients with pancreatic pain.

The patient also received a progestational agent, megestrol, for anorexia. He benefited from this drug with an increase in appetite and stabilization of weight for a 6- to 8-week period.

Anaesthetic procedures: coeliac plexus block

The pain fibres from the pancreas travel primarily with the sympathetic afferents. Therefore, they will gather in the coeliac plexus before dispersing as part of the superior and middle thoracic splanchnic nerves entering the spinal cord. A neurolytic block of the coeliac plexus is a standard technique in the management of pancreatic pain and other upper abdominal pain associated with malignancy.(162–164) In expert hands, destruction of the coeliac plexus causes few major acute or long-term harmful sequelae. Postural hypotension may occur transiently because of sympathetic nerve damage; a postblock deafferentation syndrome has occasionally been recognized, probably due to the spread of the injected alcohol to somatic nerves. Rarely, serious neurological sequelae (paraplegia, leg weakness) occur, again due to inadvertent diffusion of alcohol or phenol beyond the plexus. Sympathetic pancreatic nerve stimulation increases enzyme release. Theoretically, patients may actually benefit from reduced stimulus to pancreatic enzyme production and associated pancreatitis.

Randomized controlled trials studying percutaneous coeliac plexus block are uncommon. A recent attempt at meta-analysis(165) summarized 24 studies but only one randomized controlled trial (with an enrolment of only 20 patients) that compared coeliac plexus block with analgesic drugs.(166) The meta-analysis of all 24 studies reported 'good to excellent pain relief' in 89 per cent of patients immediately post-procedure, with partial to complete maintenance of pain control for 90 per cent of patients at 3 months after the procedure. While transient hypotension or diarrhoea were common, major adverse effects occurred in only 2 per cent of patients. A recent study assessed the effectiveness of coeliac plexus block in relation to the location of the primary tumour, the head or tail, and body of the pancreas as the predictor variable.(167) The data show that patients with cancer of the head of the pancreas had much more pronounced and longer lasting pain relief after coeliac plexus block compared with patients with cancer of the body and tail of the pancreas (mean 119 versus 65 days, and a response rate of 92 versus 29 per cent).

If percutaneous blocks are usually successful, should the surgeon block the coeliac plexus at laparotomy? Lillemoe describes a randomized trial comparing operative block using 50 per cent alcohol and placebo.(168) This study reports not only on the effects of a block on established pain but also on the role of coeliac plexus block in preventing pain. The patients who had an alcohol block had a significant reduction in pain scores and a delay in the subsequent return of pain. If free of pain at the time of the alcohol block patients remained free of pain for a significant period compared with the saline (placebo) group. They required lower doses of opioids if pain eventually developed. Lillemoe estimated that the necessary operative exposure added 5 min to the time of surgery; an increase in postoperative morbidity did not occur.

Our patient had only partial relief of pain following coeliac plexus block; the posterior component disappeared but an anterior abdominal pain remained untouched. His cancer was in the head of the pancreas so a good response was more likely according to the study reported above.(167) Incomplete relief may relate to an incomplete block. Alternatively, as some vagal afferents also transmit pain impulses,(169) perhaps vagal transmission was responsible for our patient's residual pain.

As is the case with all surgical interventions, results are 'operator dependent'. The excellent results for coeliac plexus block reported in the literature arise presumably from experienced groups. In the authors' opinion, patients requiring laparotomy for pancreatic cancer will benefit from contact with surgeons skilled and interested in carrying out intra-operative palliative procedures. For the increasing numbers of patients who have a diagnosis of inoperable cancer established without laparotomy, early consideration of a percutaneous block is desirable if they have moderate to severe pain. Recent studies of thoracoscopic splanchnicectomy suggest that it is effective in relieving pancreatic pain.(170,171) It is a minimally invasive technique with low morbidity but so far there has been limited experience.

New approaches

A trial of oral pancreatic enzymes relieved pain in 50 per cent of patients in an open non-randomized trial.(172) Giving trypsin may reduce hyperstimulation of the pancreas by cholecystokinin, thus reducing local inflammation. These results need confirmation.

The results of cytotoxic chemotherapy are disappointing and have stimulated an interest in hormonal therapy for pancreatic cancer. Treatment with octreotide (a synthetic somatostatin analogue) may confer a survival advantage without producing objective tumour shrinkage, to patients with a variety of advanced gastrointestinal cancers.[173] Somatostatin may inhibit sensory neurones. A trial of epidural somatostatin in postoperative pain demonstrated analgesic effects,[174] although another study of subcutaneous octreotide failed to demonstrate a general analgesic effect.[175] In this series one patient with post-prandial pancreatic pain did respond.

Conclusion

Pancreatic pain represents one of the few situations in cancer pain management where an invasive procedure, coeliac plexus block, should be considered at an early stage. Upper abdominal pain of other aetiology may also benefit from this block and other minimally invasive techniques such as thoracoscopic splanchnicectomy show some promise for the future. However, as always, this procedure represents only one part of a comprehensive strategy including anticancer therapy, analgesics, adjuvant drugs, and non-drug treatments.

References

1. **Hanks, G., Portenoy, R.K., MacDonald, N., and Forbes, K.** (1998). Difficult pain problems. In *Oxford Textbook of Palliative Medicine* 2nd edn (ed. D. Doyle, G.W.C. Hanks, and N. MacDonald), pp. 454–77. Oxford: Oxford University Press.
2. **Morley, J.S., Miles, J.B., Wells, J.C., and Bowsher, D.** (1992). Paradoxical pain. *Lancet* **340**, 1045.
3. **Bowsher, D.** (1993). Paradoxical pain. *British Medical Journal* **306**, 473.
4. **Hanks, G.W.** (1991). Morphine pharmacokinetics and analgesia after oral administration. *Postgraduate Medical Journal* **67** (Suppl. 2), S60–3.
5. **Smith, M.T., Watt, J.A., and Cramond, T.** (1990). Morphine-3-glucuronide—a potent antagonist of morphine analgesia. *Life Sciences* **47**, 579–85.
6. **Gong, Q.-L., Hedner, J., Bjorkman, R., and Hedner, T.** (1992). Morphine-3-glucuronide may functionally antagonise morphine-6-glucuronide induced antinociception and ventilatory depression in the rat. *Pain* **48**, 249–55.
7. **Yaksh, T.L. and Harty, G.J.** (1987). Pharmacology of the allodynia in rats evoked by high dose intrathecal morphine. *Journal of Pharmacology and Experimental Therapeutics* **244**, 501–7.
8. **Labella, F.S., Pinsky, C., and Havlicek, V.** (1979). Morphine derivatives with diminished opiate receptor potency show enhanced central excitatory activity. *Brain Research* **174**, 263–71.
9. **Shimomura, K. et al.** (1971). Analgesic effect of morphine glucuronides. *Tohuku Journal of Experimental Medicine* **105**, 45–52.
10. **Bartlett, S.E. and Smith, M.T.** (1995). The apparent affinity of morphine-3-glucuronide for mu_1-opioid receptors results from morphine contamination: demonstration using HPLC and radioligand binding. *Life Sciences* **57**, 609–15.
11. **Hewett, K., Dickenson, A.H., and McQuay, H.J.** (1993). Lack of effect of morphine-3-glucuronide on the spinal antinociceptive action of morphine in the rat: an electrophysicological study. *Pain* **53**, 59–63.
12. **Penson, R.T., Joel, S.P., Bakhshi, K., Clark, S.J., Langford, R.M., and Slevin, M.L.** (2000). Randomised placebo-controlled trial of the activity of the morphine glucuronides. *Clinical Pharmacology and Therapeutics* **68**, 667–76.
13. **Penson, R.T., Joel, S.P., Clark, S., Gloyne, A., and Slevin, M.L.** (2001). Limited phase I study of morphine-3-glucuronide. *Journal of Pharmaceutical Sciences* **90**, 1810–16.
14. **Kearney, M.K.** (1990). Experience in a hospice with patients suffering cancer pain. In *Opioids in the Treatment of Cancer Pain* (ed. D. Doyle), pp. 69–74. Royal Society of Medicine Services International Congress and Symposium Series. No 146. London: RSM Services Ltd.
15. **Moulin, D.E. and Foley, K.M.** (1990). A review of a hospital-based pain service. In *Advances in Pain Research and Therapy* Vol. 16 (ed. K.M. Foley, J.J. Bonica, and V. Ventafridda), pp. 413–28. Second International Congress on Cancer Pain. New York: Raven Press.
16. **Bruera, E., MacMillan, D., Hanson, J., and MacDonald, R.N.** (1989). The Edmonton staging system for cancer pain: preliminary report. *Pain* **37**, 203–10.
17. **Mercadante, S., Maddaloni, S., Roccella, S., and Salvaggio, L.** (1992). Predictive factors in advanced cancer pain treated only by analgesics. *Pain* **50**, 151–5.
18. **Portenoy, R.K.** (1991). Issues in the management of neuropathic pain. In *Towards a New Pharmacotherapy of Pain* (ed. A. Basbaum and J.-M. Besson), pp. 393–416. New York: John Wiley and Sons.
19. **American Psychiatric Association.** *Diagnostic and Statistical Manual of Mental Disorder* 4th edn. Washington DC: American Psychiatric Association, 1994.
20. **Merskey, H. and Bogduk, N.**, ed. *Classification of Chronic Pain* 2nd edn. Seattle: IASP Press, 1994.
21. **Cherny, N.I. et al.** (1994). Opioid responsiveness of cancer pain syndromes caused by neuropathic or nociceptive mechanisms: a combined analysis of controlled single dose studies. *Neurology* **44**, 857–61.
22. **Arner, S. and Meyerson, B.A.** (1988). Lack of analgesic effect of opioids on neuropathic and idiopathic forms of pain. *Pain* **33**, 11–23.
23. **Portenoy, R.K., Foley, K.M., and Inturrisi, C.E.** (1990). The nature of opioid responsiveness and its implications for neuropathic pain: new hypotheses derived from studies of opioid infusions. *Pain* **43**, 273–86.
24. **Mao, J.J., Price, D.D., and Mayer, D.J.** (1995). Experimental mononeuropathy reduces the antinociceptive effects of morphine: implications for common intracellular mechanisms involved in morphine tolerance and neuropathic pain. *Pain* **61**, 353–64.
25. **Urban, B.J., France, R.D., Steinberger, D.L., Scott, D.L., and Maltbie, A.A.** (1986). Long-term use of narcotic/antidepressant medication in the management of phantom limb pain. *Pain* **24**, 191–7.
26. **Zenz, M., Strumpf, M., and Tryba, M.** (1992). Long-term opioid therapy in patients with chronic nonmalignant pain. *Journal of Pain and Symptom Management* **7**, 66–77.
27. **Galer, B.S., Coyle, N., Pasternak, G.W., and Portenoy, R.K.** (1992). Individual variability in the response to different opioids: report of five cases. *Pain* **49**, 87–91.
28. **McQuay, H.J. et al.** (1992). Opioid sensitivity of chronic pain: a patient-controlled analgesia method. *Anaesthesia* **47**, 757–67.
29. **Dellemijn, P.L. and Vanneste, J.A.** (1997). Randomized double-blind active-placebo-controlled crossover trial of intravenous fentanyl in neuropathic pains. *Lancet* **349**, 753–8.
30. **Rowbotham, M.C., Reisner, L., and Fields, H.L.** (1991). Both intravenous lidocaine and morphine reduce the pain of postherpetic neuralgia. *Neurology* **41**, 1024–8.
31. **Raja, S.N. et al.** (2002). Opioids versus antidepressants in postherpetic neuralgia: a randomized, placebo-controlled trial. *Neurology* **59**, 1015–21.
32. **Harati, Y. et al.** (1998). Double-blind randomized trial of tramadol for the treatment of the pain of diabetic neuropathy. *Neurology* **50**,1842–6.
33. **Watson, C.P.N. and Babul, N.** (1998). Efficacy of oxycodone in neuropathic pain: a randomized trial in postherpetic neuralgia. *Neurology* **50**, 1837–41.
34. **Sindrup, S.H. et al.** (1999). Tramadol relieves pain and allodynia in poly-neuropathy: a randomized, double-blind, controlled trial. *Pain* **83**, 85–90.
35. **Portenoy, R.K.** (1996). Neuropathic pain. In *Pain: Theory and Practice* (ed. R.K. Portenoy and R.M. Kanner) pp. 83–125. Philadelphia: FA Davis.
36. **Martin, L.A. and Hagen, N.A.** (1997). Neuropathic pain in cancer patients: mechanisms, syndromes, and clinical controversies. *Journal of Pain and Symptom Management* **14**, 99–117.
37. **Devor, M. and Seltzer, Z.** (1999). Pathophysiology of damaged nerves in relation to chronic pain. In *Textbook of Pain* 4th edn. (ed. P.D. Wall and R. Melzack), pp. 129–64. London: Churchill Livingstone.

38. **Fields, H.F., Baron, R., and Rowbotham, M.C.** (1999). Peripheral neuropathic pain: an approach to management. In *Textbook of Pain* 4th edn. (ed. P.D. Wall and R. Melzack), pp. 1523–48. London: Churchill Livingstone.

39. **Scadding, J.W.** (1999). Peripheral neuropathies. In *Textbook of Pain* 4th edn. (ed. P.D. Wall and R. Melzack), pp. 815–34. London: Churchill Livingstone.

40. **Dickenson, A.H., Matthews, E.A., and Suzuki, R.** (2001). Central nervous system mechanisms of pain in peripheral neuropathy. In *Progress in Pain Research and Management Series. Neuropathic Pain: Pathophysiology and Treatment* Vol. 21 (ed. P.T. Hansson, H.L. Fields, R.G. Hill, and P. Marchettini), pp. 85–106. Seattle: IASP Press.

41. **Woolf, C. and Mannion, R.** (1999). Neuropathic pain: aetiology, symptoms, mechanisms and management. *Lancet* **353**, 1959–64.

42. **Fisher, K., Coderre, T.J., and Hagen, N.A.** (2000). Targeting the *N*-Methyl-D-asparate receptor for chronic pain management: preclinical animal studies, recent clinical experience and future research directions. *Journal of Pain and Symptom Management* **20**, 358–73.

43. **Fields, H.L. and Hill, R.G.** (2001). Neuropathic pain: the near and far horizon. In *Progress in Pain Research and Management Series. Neuropathic Pain: The Near and Far Horizon* Vol. 21 (ed. P.T. Hansson, H.L. Fields, R.G. Hill, and P. Marchettini), pp. 251–64. Seattle: IASP Press.

44. **Schwartzman, R.J. and McLellan, T.L.** (1987). Reflex sympathetic dystrophy: a review. *Archives of Neurology* **44**, 555–61.

45. **Dellemijn, P.L.I., Fields, H.L., Allen, R.R., McKay, W.R., and Rowbotham, M.C.** (1994). The interpretation of pain relief and sensory changes following sympathetic blockade. *Brain* **117**, 1475–87.

46. **Raja, S.N., Treede, R.D., Davis, K.D., and Campbell, J.N.** (1991). Systemic alpha-adrenergic blockade with phentolamine: a diagnostic test for sympathetically-maintained pain. *Anesthesiology* **74**, 691–8.

47. **Verdugo, R.J. and Ochoa, J.L.** (1994). Sympathetically-maintained pain. I. Phentolamine block questions the concept. *Neurology* **44**, 1003–10.

48. **Fine, P.G., Roberts, W.J., Gillette, R.G., and Child, T.R.** (1994). Slowly developing placebo responses confound tests of intravenous phentolamine to determine mechanisms underlying idiopathic chronic low back pain. *Pain* **56**, 235–42.

49. **Janig, W.** (2001). CRPS-I and CRPS-II: a strategic view. In *Progress in Pain Research and Management Series. Complex Regional Pain Syndrome* Vol. 22 (ed. R.N. Harden, R. Baron, and W. Janig), pp. 3–15. Seattle: IASP Press.

50. **Schott, G.D.** (1994). Visceral afferents: their contribution to 'sympathetic dependent' pain. *Brain* **117**, 397–413.

51. **Roberts, W.J.** (1986). A hypothesis on the physiological basis for causalgia and related pains. *Pain* **24**, 297–311.

52. **Cleeland, C.S.** (1990). Assessment of pain in cancer: measurement issues. In *Advances in Pain Research and Therapy* Vol. 16 (ed. K.M. Foley, J.J. Bonica, and V. Ventafridda), pp. 47–55. Second International Congress on Cancer Pain. New York: Raven Press.

53. **Gonzales, G.R., Elliot, K.J., Portenoy, R.K., and Foley, K.M.** (1991). The impact of a comprehensive evaluation in the management of cancer pain. *Pain* **47**, 141–4.

54. **Cherny, N.I. and Portenoy, R.K.** (1999). Cancer pain: principles of assessment and syndromes. In *Textbook of Pain* 4th edn. (ed. P.D. Wall and R. Melzack), pp. 1017–64. London: Churchill Livingstone.

55. **MacDonald, N., Der, L., Allan, S., and Champion, P.** (1993). Opioid hyper-excitability: the application of alternate opioid therapy. *Pain* **53**, 353–5.

56. **Cherny, N.I.** (1996). Opioid analgesics: comparative features and prescribing guidelines. *Drugs* **51**, 713–37.

57. **Cherny, N.I.** (2001). The pharmacological management of cancer pain. *European Journal of Cancer* **37** (Suppl. 7), S265–78.

58. **Kirvela, O. and Nieminen, S.** (1990). Treatment of painful neuromas with neurolytic blockade. *Pain* **41**, 161–5.

59. **Smith, T.J.** et al. (2002). Randomized clinical trial of an implantable drug delivery system compared with comprehensive medical management for refractory cancer pain: impact on pain, drug-related toxicity, and survival. *Journal of Clinical Oncology* **20**, 4040–9.

60. **Arner, S. and Arner, B.** (1983). Differential effects of epidural morphine in the treatment of cancer-related pain. *Acta Anesthesiologica Scandinavica* **29**, 32–6.

61. **Sjoberg, M.** et al. (1991). Long-term intrathecal morphine and bupivacaine in 'refractory' cancer pain. *Acta Anesthesiologica Scandinavica* **35**, 30–43.

62. **Eisenach, J.C., DuPen, S., Dubois, M., Miguel, R., and Allin, D., and The Epidural Clonidine Study Group (USA)** (1995). Epidural clonidine analgesia for intractable cancer pain. *Pain* **61**, 391–400.

63. **Mercadante, S.** (1999). Problems of long-term spinal opioid treatment in advanced cancer patients. *Pain* **79**, 1–13.

64. **Gybels, J.M. and Sweet, W.H.** *Neurosurgical Treatment of Persistent Pain.* Basel: Karger, 1989.

65. **Arbit, E.** *Management of Cancer-Related Pain.* Mount Kisco NY: Futura, 1993.

66. **Willis, W.D.** (1994). Central plastic responses to pain. In *Proceedings of the 7th World Congress on Pain* (ed. G.F. Gebhart, D.L. Hammond, and T.S. Jensen), pp. 301–24. Seattle: IASP Press.

67. **Fishman, B. and Loscalzo, M.** (1987). Cognitive-behavioral interventions in the management of cancer pain: principles and applications. *Medical Clinics of North America* **71**, 271–88.

68. **Portenoy, R.K. and Hagen, N.A.** (1990). Breakthrough pain: definition, prevalence and characteristics. *Pain* **41**, 273–82.

69. **Hanks, G.W.** (1988). The pharmacological treatment of bone pain. *Cancer Surveys* **7**, 87–101.

70. **Portenoy, R.K., Payne, D., and Jacobsen, P.** (1999). Breakthrough pain: characteristics and impact in patients with cancer pain. *Pain* **81**, 129–34.

71. **Fine, P.G. and Busch, M.A.** (1998). Characterization of breakthrough pain by hospice patients and their caregivers. *Journal of Pain and Symptom Management* **16**, 179–83.

72. **Gomez-Batiste, X.** et al. (2002). Breakthrough cancer pain: prevalence and characteristics in patients in Catalonia, Spain. *Journal of Pain and Symptom Management* **24**, 45–52.

73. **Caraceni, A. and Portenoy, R.K.** (1999). An international survey of cancer pain characteristics and syndromes. *Pain* **82**, 263–74.

74. **Mercadante, S.** et al. (2002). Episodic (breakthrough) pain: consensus conference of an expert working group of the European Association for Palliative Care. *Cancer* **94**, 832–9.

75. **Petzke, F.** et al. (1999). Temporal presentation of chronic cancer pain: transitory pains on admission to a multidisciplinary pain clinic. *Journal of Pain and Symptom Management* **17**, 391–401.

76. **Zeppetella, G.** (2000). An assessment of the safety, efficacy, and acceptability of intranasal fentanyl citrate in the management of cancer-related breakthrough pain: a pilot study. *Journal of Pain and Symptom Management* **20**, 253–8.

77. **Zeppetella, G.** (2001). Prevalence and characteristics of breakthrough pain in patients with non-malignant terminal disease admitted to a hospice. *Palliative Medicine* **15**, 243–6.

78. **Portenoy, R.K.** (1997). Treatment of temporal variations in chronic cancer pain. *Seminars in Oncology* **24** (Suppl. 16), S7–12.

79. **Burris, H.A., III** et al. (1997). Improvements in survival and clinical benefit with gemcitabine as first-line therapy for patients with advanced pancreas cancer: a randomized trial. *Journal of Clinical Oncology* **15**, 2403–13.

80. **Storniolo, A.M.** et al. (1999). An investigational new drug treatment program for patients with gemcitabine: results for over 3000 patients with pancreatic carcinoma. *Cancer* **85**, 1261–8.

81. **Jassem, J.** et al. (2002). A phase II study of gemcitabine plus cisplatin in patients with advanced non-small cell lung cancer: clinical outcomes and quality of life. *Lung Cancer* **35**, 73–9.

82. **Tannock, I.F.** et al. (1996). Chemotherapy with mitoxantrone plus prednisone or prednisone alone for symptomatic hormone-resistant prostate cancer: a Canadian randomized trial with palliative endpoints. *Journal of Clinical Oncology* **14**, 1756–64.

83. **Jacox, A.** et al. *Management of Cancer Pain. Clinical Practice Guideline No. 9.* ANCPR Publication No. 94-0592. Rockville MD: Agency for Health Care Policy and Research, US Department of Health and Human Services, Public Health Service, 1994.

84. **American Pain Society.** *Principles of Analgesic Use in the Treatment of Acute Pain and Cancer Pain* 3rd edn. Skokie Ill.: American Pain Society, 1992.

85. **Cleary, J.F.** (1997). Pharmacokinetic and pharmacodynamic issues in the treatment of breakthrough pain. *Seminars in Oncology* **24** (Suppl. 16), S13–19.

86. **Lichtor, J.L.** et al. (1999). The relative potency of oral transmucosal fentanyl citrate compared with intravenous morphine in the treatment of moderate to severe postoperative pain. *Anesthesia and Analgesia* **89**, 732–8.

87. **Streisand, J.** et al. (1991). Absorption and bioavailability of oral transmucosal fentanyl citrate. *Anesthesiology* **75**, 223–31.

88. **Christie, J.M.** et al. (1998). Dose-titration, multicenter study of oral transmucosal fentanyl citrate for the treatment of breakthrough pain in cancer patients using transdermal fentanyl for persistent pain. *Journal of Clinical Oncology* **16**, 3238–45.

89. **Coluzzi, P.H.** et al. (2001). Breakthrough cancer pain: a randomized trial comparing oral transmucosal fentanyl citrate (OTFC®) and morphine sulfate immediate release (MSIR®). *Pain* **91**, 123–30.

90. **Farrar, J.T.** et al. (1998). Oral transmucosal fentanyl citrate: randomized, double-blinded, placebo-controlled trial for treatment of breakthrough pain in cancer patients. *Journal of the National Cancer Institute* **90**, 611–16.

91. **Portenoy, R.K.** et al. (1999). Oral transmucosal fentanyl citrate (OTFC) for the treatment of breakthrough pain in cancer patients: a controlled dose titration study. *Pain* **79**, 303–12.

92. **Rospond, R.M.** (1999). A new transmucosal fentanyl for breakthrough cancer pain. *Cancer Practice* **7**, 317–20.

93. **Egan, T.D.** et al. (2000). Multiple dose pharmacokinetics of oral transmucosal fentanyl citrate in healthy volunteers. *Anesthesiology* **92**, 665–73.

94. **Payne, R.** et al. (2001). Long-term safety of oral transmucosal fentanyl citrate for breakthrough cancer pain. *Journal of Pain and Symptom Management* **22**, 575–83.

95. **Zeppetella, G.** (2000). Nebulized and intranasal fentanyl in the management of cancer-related breakthrough pain. *Palliative Medicine* **14**, 57–8.

96. **Jackson, K., Ashby, M., and Keech, J.** (2002). Pilot dose finding study of intranasal sufentanil for breakthrough and incident cancer-associated pain. *Journal of Pain and Symptom Management* **23**, 450–2.

97. **Zeppetella, G.** (2001). Sublingual fentanyl citrate for cancer-related breakthrough pain: a pilot study. *Palliative Medicine* **15**, 323–8.

98. **Cox, J.M. and Pappagallo, M.** (2001). Modafinil: a gift to portmanteau. *American Journal of Hospice and Palliative Care* **18**, 408–10.

99. **Wilwerding, M.B., Loprinzi, C.L., Mailliard, J.A., O'Fallon, J.R., Miser, A.W., van Haelst, C., Barton, D.L., Foley, J.F., and Athmann, L.M.** (1995). A randomized, crossover evaluation of methylphenidate in cancer patients receiving strong narcotics. *Supportive Care in Cancer* **3**, 135–8.

100. **Jensen, M.E. and Kallmes, D.E.** (2002). Percutaneous vertebroplasty in the treatment of malignant spine disease. *Cancer Journal* **8**, 194–206.

101. **Craig, K.D.** (1998). The facial display of pain. *Measurement of Pain in Infants and Children* (ed. G.A. Finlay and P.J. McGrath), In *Progress in Pain Research and Management*, vol. 10, pp. 103–22. Seattle: IASP Press.

102. **McGrath, P.J.** (1998). Behavioural measures of pain. *Measurement of Pain in Infants and Children* (ed. G.A. Finlay and P.J. McGrath), In *Progress in Pain Research and Management*, vol. 10, pp. 83–102. Seattle: IASP Press.

103. **Hester, N.K.** (1979). The preoperational child's reaction to immunization. *Nursing Research* **28**, 250–5.

104. **Caraceni, A.** et al. (2002). Pain measurement tools and methods in clinical research in palliative care: recommendations of an Expert Working Group of the European Association of Palliative Care. *Journal of Pain and Symptom Management* **23**, 239–55.

105. **Bieri, D., Reeve, R.A., Champion, G.D., Addicoat, L., and Ziegler, J.B.** (1990). The faces pain scale for the self assessment of pain experienced by children. *Pain* **41**, 139–50.

106. **Kamel, H.K., Phlavan, M., Malekgoudarzi, B., Gogel, P., and Morley, J.E.** (2001). Utilizing pain assessment scales increases the frequency of diagnosing pain among elderly nursing home residents. *Journal of Pain and Symptom Management* **21**, 450–5.

107. **Stein, W.M.** (2001). Pain in the nursing home. *Clinics in Geriatric Medicine* **17**, 575–94.

108. **Stewart, K., Challis, D., Carpenter, I., and Dickinson, E.** (1999). Assessment approaches for older people receiving social care: content and coverage. *International Journal of Geriatric Psychiatry* **14**, 147–56.

109. **Horgas, A.L. and Dunn, K.** (2001). Pain in nursing home residents. Comparison of residents' self-report and nursing assistants' perceptions. *Journal of Gerontological Nursing* **27**, 44–53.

110. **Weiner, D., Peterson, B., and Keefe, F.** (1999). Chronic pain associated behaviours in the nursing home: resident versus caregiver perceptions. *Pain* **80**, 577–88.

111. **Won, A., Lapone, K., Gambass, G., Bernabei, R., Mor, V., and Lipsitz, L.A.** (1999). Correlates and management of non-malignant pain in the nursing home. SAGE study group. Systematic Assessment of Drug Use via Epidemiology. *Journal of the American Geriatrics Society* **47**, 936–42.

112. **Scherder, E., Bouma, A., Barkent, M., and Rahman, O.** (1999). Alzhemier patients report less pain intensity and pain affect than non-demented elderly. *Psychiatry* **62**, 265–72.

113. **Morrison, R.S. and Siu, A.L.** (2000). A comparison of pain and its treatment in advanced dementia and cognitively intact patients with hip fracture. *Journal of Pain and Symptom Management* **19**, 240–8.

114. **Chibnall, J.T. and Tait, R.C.** (2001). Pain assessment in cognitively impaired older adults: a comparison of four scales. *Pain* **92**, 173–86.

115. **Abu-Saad, H.H.** (2001). Challenge of pain in the cognitively impaired. *Lancet* **356**, 1867–8.

116. **Davies, D. and Evans, L.** (2001). Assessing pain in people with profound learning disabilities. *British Journal of Nursing* **10**, 513–16.

117. **Rees, E., Hardy, J., Ling, J., Broadley, K., and A'Hern, R.** (1998). The use of the Edmonton Symptom Assessment Scale (ESAS) within a palliative care unit in the UK. *Palliative Medicine* **12**, 75–82.

118. **Radbruch, L., Sabatowski, R., Loick, G., Jonen-Thielemann, Kasper, M., Gondek, B., and Lehmann, K.A.** (2000). Cognitive impairment and its influence on pain and symptom assessment in a palliative care unit: development of a Minimal Documentation System. *Palliative Medicine* **14**, 266–76.

119. **Redinbaugh, E.M., Baum, A., DeMoss, C., Fello, M., and Arnold, R.** (2002). Factors associated with the accuracy of family caregiver estimates of patient pain. *Journal of Pain and Symptom Management* **23**, 31–8.

120. **Hadjistavropoulos, T. and Craig, K.D.** (2002). A theroretical framework for understanding self-report and observational features of pain: a communications model. *Behaviour Research and Therapy* **40**, 551–70.

121. **Ellershaw, J., Smith, C., Overill, S., Walker, S.E., and Aldridge, J.** (2001). Care of the dying: setting standards for symptom control in the last 48 hours of life. *Journal of Pain and Symptom Management* **21**, 12–17.

122. **Ellershaw, J., Foster, A., Murphy, D., Shea, T., and Overill, S.** (1997). Developing an integrated care pathway for the dying patient. *European Journal of Palliative Care* **4**, 203–7.

123. **Baines, M. and Kirkham, S.R.** (1989). Cancer pain. In *Textbook of Pain* 2nd edn. (ed. P.D. Wall and R. Melzack), pp. 590–7. Edinburgh: Churchill Livingstone.

124. **Potter, J.D.** *Food, Nutrition and the Prevention of Cancer: A Global Perspective.* Washington: World Cancer Research Fund/American Institute for Cancer Research, 1997.

125. **Boas, R.A., Schug, S.A., and Acland, R.H.** (1993). Perineal pain after rectal amputation: a 5-year follow-up. *Pain* **52**, 67–70.

126. **McQuay, H.** (1988). Pharmacological treatment of neuralgic and neuropathic pain. *Cancer Surveys* **7**, 141–59.

127. **Twycross, R. and Wilcock, A.**, ed. *Symptom Management in Advanced Cancer.* Abingdon: Radcliffe Medical Press Ltd, 2001.

128. **Castell, D.O.** (1985). Calcium channel blocking agents for gastrointestinal disorders. *American Journal of Cardiology* **55**, 210B–13B.

129. **Boquet, J., Moore, N., Lhuintre, J.P., and Boismare, F.** (1986). Diltiazem for proctalgia fugax. *Lancet* **i**, 1493.

130. **Bristow, A. and Foster, J.M.G.** (1988). Lumbar sympathectomy in the management of rectal tenesmoid pain. *Annals of the Royal College of Surgeons of England* **70**, 38–9.

131. **Plancarte, R., Amescua, C., Patt, R.B., and Aldrete, J.A.** (1990). Superior hypogastric plexus block for pelvic cancer pain. *Anesthesiology* **73**, 236–9.
132. **Lynch, J., Zech, D., and Grond, S.** (1992) The role of intrathecal neurolysis in the treatment of cancer-related perianal and perineal pain. *Palliative Medicine* **6**, 140–5.
133. **de Leon-Casasola, O.A.** (1997). Regional anesthetic techniques for the management of cancer pain. In *Techniques in Regional Anesthesia and Pain Management* Vol. 1 (ed. W. Urmey), pp. 27–31. Philadelphia PA: WB Saunders.
134. **Evans, P.J.D., Lloyd, J.W., and Jack, T.M.** (1981). Cryoanalgesia for intractable perineal pain. *Journal of the Royal Society of Medicine* **74**, 804–9.
135. **Cardozo, L.D. and Stanton, S.L.** (1980). A comparison between bromocriptine and indomethacin in the treatment of detrusor instability. *Journal of Urology* **123**, 399–401.
136. **Abrams, P. and Feneley, R.** (1976). The action of prostaglandins on the smooth muscle of the human urinary tract *in vitro*. *British Journal of Urology* **47**, 909–15.
137. **Brown, J.H.** (1990). Atropine, scopolamine and related antimuscarinic drugs. In *The Pharmacological Basis of Therapeutics* 8th edn. (ed. A.G. Gilman, T.W. Rall, A.S. Nies, and P. Taylor), pp. 150–65. New York: Pergamon.
138. **Kirkali, Z. and Whitaker, R.H.** (1987). The use of oxybutynin in urological practice. *International Urology and Nephrology* **19**, 385–91.
139. **Brendler, C.B., Radebaugh, L.C., and Mohler, J.L.** (1989). Topical oxybutynin chloride for relaxation of dysfunctional bladders. *Journal of Urology* **141**, 1350–2.
140. **Ekstrom, B., Andersson, K.-E., and Mattiasson, A.** (1993). Urodynamic effects of intravesical instillation of atropine and phentolamine in patients with detrusor hyperactivity. *Journal of Urology* **149**, 135–8.
141. **Madersbacher, H., Stohrer, M., Richter, R., Burgdorfer, H., Hachen, H.J., and Murtz, G.** (1995). Trospium chloride versus oxybutynin: a randomised double-blind, multicentre trial in the treatment of detrusor hyperreflexia. *British Journal of Urology* **75**, 452–6.
142. **Holmang, S., Aldenborg, F., and Hedelin, H.** (1994). Extirpation and fulguration of multiple superficial bladder tumour recurrences under intravesical lignocaine anaesthesia. *British Journal of Urology* **73**, 177–80.
143. **Barbanti, G., Maggi, C.A., Beneforti, P., Baroldi, P., and Turini, D.** (1993). Relief of pain following intravesical capsaicin in patients with hypersensitive disorders of the lower urinary tract. *British Journal of Urology* **71**, 686–91.
144. **Kaye, P.** *A to Z of Hospice and Palliative Medicine.* Northampton: EPL Publications, 1992, p. 184.
145. **McCoubrie, R. and Jeffery, M.A.** (2003). Intravesical diamorphine for bladder spasm. *Journal of Pain & Symptom Management* **25**, 1–2.
146. **Duckett, J.W.** et al. (1997). Intravesical morphine analgesia after bladder surgery. *Journal of Urology* **1574**, 1407–9.
147. **Twycross, R.** (2001). Urinary symptoms. In *Symptom Management in Advanced Cancer* 3rd edn. (ed. R. Twycross), pp. 91–301. Oxford: Radcliffe Medical Press.
148. **Olshwang, D., Shapiro, A., Perlberg, S., and Magora, F.** (1984). The effect of epidural morphine on ureteral colic and spasm of the bladder. *Pain* **18**, 97–101.
149. **Mercadante, S.** (1994). Prevalence, causes, and mechanisms of pain in home-care patients with advanced cancer. *Pain Clinic* **7**, 131–6.
150. **Russell, R.C.G., Ross, P.J., and Cunningham, D.C.** (2002). Cancer of the pancreas. In *Oxford Textbook of Oncology* 2nd edn. (ed. R.L. Souhami, F. Tannock, P. Hohenberger, and J.-C. Horiot), pp. 1603–26. Oxford: Oxford University Press.
151. **Kelsen, D.P.** et al. (1995). Pain and depression in patients with newly diagnosed pancreas cancer. *Journal of Clinical Oncology* **13**, 748–55.
152. **Mayer, E.A.** (1995). Gut feelings: what turns them on? *Gastroenterology* **108**, 927–40.
153. **Ness, T.J. and Gebhart, C.F.** (1990). Visceral pain: a review of experimental studies. *Pain* **41**, 167–234.
154. **Cervero, F. and Laird, J.M.A.** (1999). Visceral pain. *Lancet* **353**, 2145–8.
155. **Schofferman, J.** (1988). Pain: diagnosis and management in the palliative care of AIDS. *Journal of Palliative Care* **4**, 46–50.
156. **O'Neill, W.M. and Sherrard, J.S.** (1993). Pain in human immunodeficiency virus disease: a review. *Pain* **54**, 3–14.
157. **Friedman, S.L., Wright, T.L., and Altman, D.F.** (1985). Gastrointestinal Kaposi's sarcoma in patients with acquired immunodeficiency syndrome. Endoscopic and autopsy findings. *Gastroenterology* **89**, 102–8.
158. **McDaniel, J.S.** et al. (1995). Depression in patients with cancer. Diagnosis, biology and treatment. *Archives of General Psychiatry* **52**, 89–99.
159. **Moertel, C.E.** et al. (1981). Therapy of unresectable pancreatic carcinoma: a randomised comparison of high dose radiation alone, moderate dose radiation and high dose radiation plus 5-FU. *Cancer* **48**, 1705–10.
160. **Burris, H.A., III** et al. (1997). Improvements in survival and clinical benefit with gemcitabine as first line therapy for patients with advanced pancreas cancer: a randomised trial. *Journal of Clinical Oncology* **15**, 2403–13.
161. **Moertel, C.G.** et al. (1971). Aspirin and pancreatic cancer pain. *Gastroenterology* **60**, 552–3.
162. **Hanna, M., Peat, S.J., Woodham, M.J., Latham, J., Gouliaris, A., and Di Vadi, P.** (1989). The use of coeliac plexus blockade in patients with chronic pain. *Palliative Medicine* **4**, 11–16.
163. **Lema, M.J.** (1998). Invasive procedures for cancer pain. *Pain Clinical Update* **vi**, 1–8.
164. **Nicosia, F. and Mercadante, S.** (1998). Current indications of neurolytic blocks in cancer pain. *Current Pain and Headache Reports* **2**, 175–80.
165. **Eisenberg, E., Carr, D.B., and Chalmers, T.C.** (1995). Neurolytic coeliac plexus block for treatment of cancer pain: a meta-analysis. *Anesthesia and Analgesia* **80**, 290–5.
166. **Mercadante, S.** (1993). Celiac plexus block versus analgesics in pancreatic cancer pain. *Pain* **52**, 187–92.
167. **Rykowski, J.J. and Hilgier, M.** (2000). Efficacy of neurolytic celiac plexus block in varying locations of pancreatic cancer: influence on pain relief. *Anesthesiology* **92**, 347–54.
168. **Lillemoe, M.D.** et al. (1993). Chemical splanchnicectomy in patients with unresectable pancreatic cancer. A prospective randomized trial. *Annals of Surgery* **217**, 447–57.
169. **Mayer, E.A. and Gebhart, G.F.** (1994). Basic clinical aspects of visceral hyperalgesia. *Gastroenterology* **107**, 271–93.
170. **Le Pinpec Barthes, F.** et al. (1998). Thoracoscopic splanchnicectomy for control of intractable pain in pancreatic cancer. *Annals of Thoracic Surgery* **65**, 810–13.
171. **Olak, J. and Gore, D.** (1996). Thoracoscopic splanchnicectomy: technique and case report. *Surgical Laparoscopy and Endoscopy* **6**, 228–30.
172. **Ihse, I. and Permerth, J.** (1990). Enzyme therapy and pancreatic pain. *Acta Chirurgica Scandinavica* **156**, 281–3.
173. **Cascinu, S., Del Ferro, E., and Catalano, G.** (1995). A randomized trial of octreotide vs best supportive care only in advanced gastrointestinal cancer patients refractory to chemotherapy. *British Journal of Cancer* **71**, 97–101.
174. **Taura, P.** et al. (1994). Epidural somatostatin as an analgesic in upper abdominal surgery: a double-blind study. *Pain* **59**, 135–40.
175. **De Conno, F.** et al. (1994). Subcutaneous octreotide in the treatment of pain in advanced cancer patients. *Journal of Pain and Symptom Management* **9**, 34–8.

8.3 Gastrointestinal symptoms

8.3.1 Palliation of nausea and vomiting

Kathryn A. Mannix

Introduction

Nausea and vomiting are unpleasant symptoms that are reported as highly distressing by sufferers.[1,2] The symptoms are separate, but related, and arise in many conditions including cancer, AIDS, and hepatic or renal failure.[3,4] Nausea and vomiting commonly cause misery for people with advanced cancer (40–70 per cent patients) and despite major advances in antiemetic drug development in the last two decades, the incidence and severity of these symptoms is largely unchanged.[1,2,5,6]

The neurophysiology of the vomiting reflex is well established in experimental animals,[7,8] and is being better understood in man.[9,10] Intervention aimed at reducing nausea and vomiting must take into account the cause of the symptoms and the central emetogenic pathways involved. Thus, treatment requires knowledge of these pathways, careful assessment of the patient, and prescribing tailored to the cause of the symptoms and to the patient's individual needs.

The distress caused by the experience of nausea and, to a lesser extent, vomiting, is less well understood. The physiological processes can be partly extrapolated from animal models but the management of a nauseated patient also demands empathy, supportive care, and attention to the patient's concerns, in addition to any pharmacological intervention deemed appropriate.

Pathways involved in emesis

Central pathways involved in emesis

Emesis is mediated centrally by two separate 'centres'. Whilst these are anatomically distinct in experimental animals, in man the pathways are more diffuse.

The chemoreceptor trigger zone (CTZ) is located in the area postrema, in the floor of the fourth ventricle, where there is effectively no blood–brain barrier. Chemosensitive nerve cell projections are bathed by cerebrospinal fluid (CSF), which is in chemical equilibrium with blood in the fenestrated local capillaries. The nature of the chemoreceptors in the CTZ remains obscure. Neural pathways project from the CTZ to the nucleus of the tractus solitarius and the reticular formation in the medulla oblongata: these structures are the location of the 'vomiting centre'.[7,8,11]

There may be a central anti-emetic tone sustained by medullary neurones, inhibition of which potentiates the CTZ.[12] An enkephalinergic pathway has been hypothesized: displacement of enkephalins from their receptors by naloxone[10] or opioids[13] may reduce antiemetic tone, as may inhibition of enkephalin synthesis by chemotherapy.[14] This interesting hypothesis would help to explain, for example, the different emetogenic potentials of chemotherapeutic agents according to the point at which they interrupt cellular protein synthesis. The presence of medullary antiemetic tone and its influence on the CTZ remains speculative.

The vomiting centre (VC) is a diffuse, interconnecting neural network that integrates emetogenic stimuli with parasympathetic and motor efferent activity to produce the vomiting reflex. This is a complex reflex with respiratory, salivary, vasomotor, and somatic motor components: the VC acts as a central pattern generator. It has been proposed that sequential activation of various components of the VC, with amplification at each step, is required to trigger vomiting.[11] Nausea in the absence of vomiting may arise from stimuli that excite the VC without sufficient amplification to trigger the vomiting cascade.[7,15] Thus, nausea usually accompanies the prodromal autonomic effects that precede vomiting. However, the degree of nausea cannot be predicted by the accompanying autonomic changes, for example, the relative reduction in gastric contraction.[7] Also, nausea is not always relieved by vomiting: this usually indicates continuing excitation of the central emetogenic pathway.

A preliminary report of involvement of the inferior frontal gyrus of the human cerebral cortex in the sensation of nausea is intriguing.[16] This area is association cortex, and such cortical involvement would help to explain the highly aversive nature of nausea.

The VC receives afferents from the cerebral cortex and higher brainstem, thalamus and hypothalamus, the vestibular system, and via the vagus and splanchnic nerves, the pharynx, gastrointestinal tract, and serosae. There is also input from the CTZ, which can only initiate vomiting via the VC (Fig. 1).[7,17,18]

At least 17 potential neurotransmitters or receptors have been identified in the CTZ and nucleus of the tractus solitarius. These include dopamine, serotonin, histamine, opioid, cannabinoid, and neurokinin receptors. The principal receptors at the CTZ are dopamine type 2 (D_2); at the VC the principal receptors are muscarinic cholinergic (Ach_m) and histamine type 1 (H_1). Both sites exhibit serotonin type 3 ($5HT_3$) receptors, and serotonin type 2 ($5HT_2$) receptors appear to be important in the VC.[12] Neurokinin type 1 (NK_1) receptors are widely distributed in the central nervous system, and particularly in those areas of the brainstem involved in emesis.[15]

Afferent pathways involved in emesis

The interrelationship between CTZ, VC, and their various afferent inputs is summarized in Fig. 1. The major afferent neural pathway from the body to the central structures is the vagus, with additional input via the splanchnic nerves, sympathetic ganglia, and the glossopharyngeal nerve. The vagus itself is stimulated via mechanoreceptors and chemoreceptors in the gastrointestinal tract, serosae, and viscera.[12,18–20]

The VC receives descending fibres from higher centres, which may stimulate or inhibit activation of the emetic cascade. Most vagal afferents terminate at the VC, but there is some vagal input to the CTZ.

Projections from the vestibular nuclei, which mediate emesis, are incompletely understood; the CTZ may be involved, although D_2 antagonists are not potent in motion sickness.[21] H_1 and Ach_m antagonists are more potent: they are thought to act on first-order vestibular neurones. Opioids can potentiate sensitivity of the labyrinth.[22]

Choosing an antiemetic

Before prescribing drugs, care should be taken to reduce the stimulus to nausea from the patient's environment. This includes avoidance of cooking smells, attention to unpleasant odours (e.g. from an infected, necrotic tumour), and presentation of small, attractive meals. Cool, fizzy drinks are more palatable than still or hot drinks. Many patients experience a taste change so that previously innocuous foods taste nauseating.

Selection of an appropriate antiemetic strategy involves seven steps, namely:

1. identify the likely cause(s) of nausea and/or vomiting;
2. identify the pathway by which each cause triggers the vomiting reflex (Fig. 1);
3. identify the neurotransmitter receptor involved in the identified pathway;
4. choose the most potent antagonist to the receptor identified—the binding affinity of a particular antagonist predicts its antiemetic efficacy[23,24] (Table 1);
5. choose a route of administration that ensures that the drug reaches its site of action—this often excludes the oral route;
6. titrate the dose carefully, review the patient frequently, give the antiemetic regularly;

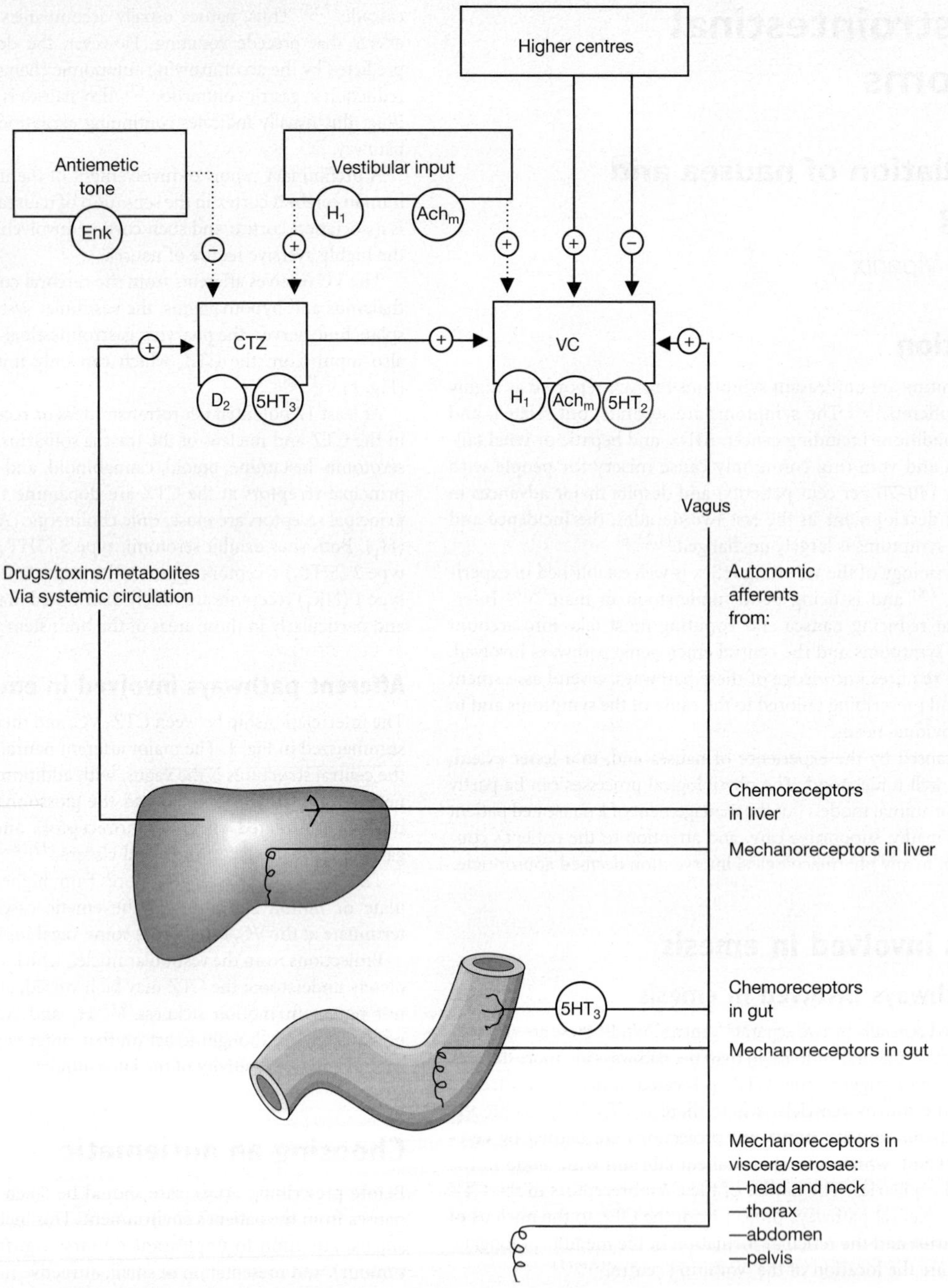

Fig. 1 The interrelationship between CTZ, VC, and their afferent inputs. —, established connections; ---, postulated connections; CTZ, chemoreceptor trigger zone; VC, vomiting centre; Enk, enkephalinergic pathways. *Receptors*: D_2, dopamine type 2; $5HT_{2,3}$, serotonin types 2,3; Ach_m, muscarinic cholinergic; H_1, histamine type 1.

7. if symptoms persist, review the likely cause(s): additional treatment may be required for an overlooked cause, or alternative treatment may be suggested by a different cause becoming apparent.

If several different receptors are involved, use of a potent antagonist for each receptor is preferable to use of one drug that weakly antagonizes several receptors. NK_1 receptor antagonists would act at several sites, but their commercial development is still awaited.

Antiemetic drugs available

A wide variety of antiemetic drugs is available. Those that have potent, receptor-specific action are summarized in Table 1. The antiemetic efficacy and side-effects of a drug can be predicted by its binding affinity for particular receptors.[23,24]

Drugs with receptor-specific action

Dopamine (D_2) antagonists

Of the dopamine (D_2) antagonists, haloperidol is the most potent at the CTZ.[23] Metoclopramide and domperidone, whilst having some CTZ antidopaminergic activity, act potently in the gut to antagonize D_2 and stimulate $5HT_4$ receptors. Local acetylcholine release, mediated by the $5HT_4$ receptor, appears to play an important role in reversing gastroparesis and bringing about normal peristalsis in the upper gastrointestinal tract.

Table 1 Receptor-specified antiemetics of use in palliative care

Drug	Receptor and site (see text)	Indications	Dosage and routes	Side-effects	Notes
Butyrephenones Haloperidol	D_2 -CTZ	Opioid induced N; chemical/ metabolic N	1.5–5.0 mg/day; po, sc (occ up to 20 mg/day)	Dystonias Dyskinesia Akathisia	Side-effects unusual at low doses
Prokinetic agents Metoclopramide	D_2 -CTZ D_2 -GIT $5\text{-}HT_4$ -GIT	Gastric stasis; ileus	10–30 mg 2–4 hourly po, sc, iv	Dystonias Akathisia Oesophageal spasm; colic in GI obstruction	Prolonged half-life in renal failure
	$5\text{-}HT_3$ -CTZ $5\text{-}HT_3$ -GIT (at high doses)	Chemotherapy	N/A	Frequent at high doses	Superseded by $5HT_3$ antagonists
Domperidone	D_2 -CTZ D_2 -GIT	Gastric stasis; ileus	10–30 mg po 4–8 hourly 30–90 mg pr 4–8 hourly	Colic if GIT obstructed; oesophageal pain	Extrapyramidal side-effects are rare
Cisapride	$5\text{-}HT_4$ (potentiation) -GIT Ach -GIT	Gastric stasis; ileus	10 mg po 6–8 hourly 30 mg pr 6–8 hourly	Abdominal cramps; diarrhoea; cardiac arrhythmias particularly with systemic azole antifungals	Prokinetic throughout GIT
Phenothiazines (including prochlorperazine chlopromazine, thiethylperazine)	D_2 -CTZ D_2 -GIT H_1, Ach, α_1 Ad: -VC, -CNS, -GIT, -CVS		Prochlorperazine: 5–20 mg po, 12.5–25 mg im, 25 mg pr 6–8 hourly Chlorpromazine: 25–50 mg im 4–6 hourly	Vary according to spectrum of receptor blockade: see text	Not recommended for routine use, but see text
Levomepromazine	$5HT_2$ -VC H_1 -VC D_2, α_1 Ad: -CTZ, -GIT, -CVS, -CNS	Intestinal obstruction, peritoneal irritation; nausea of unknown aetiology; vestibular causes; raised ICP	5–12.5 mg/24 hourly po, sc	Drowsiness at higher doses	Long half-life: once-daily injection may suffice
Antihistamines Cyclizine Cinnarizine Diphenylhydramine Promethazine	H_1 -VC -vestibular afferents -brain substance		Cyclizine: 25–50 mg 8 hourly po/sc/pr Only cyclizine is tolerated by sc injection	Dry mouth; blurred vision (rare); sedation Cyclizine: skin irritation at sc injection sites in some patients	Cyclizine is least sedative therefore the drug of choice
Diphenylhydramine Promethazine	Ach_m -VC				
Anticholinergics Hyoscine (scopolamine) hydrobromide	Ach_m -VC -GIT	Intestinal obstruction; peritoneal irritation; raised ICP; excess secretions	200–400 μg 4–8 hourly subling/sc 500–1500 μg/72 h transdermal patches	Dry mouth; ileus; urinary retention; blurred vision; occasionally agitation	Useful if N and V coexist with colic
$5\text{-}HT_3$ antagonists Granisetron Ondansetron Tropisetron	$5\text{-}HT_3$ -GIT -CTZ -(VC)	Chemotherapy; abdominal radiotherapy; postoperative nausea and vomiting	Granisetron: 3 mg slowly iv up to 8 hourly; odansetron: 8 mg po or slowly iv 8 hourly; tropisetron: 5 mg po or slowly iv daily	Headache in 30%; constipation; diarrhoea	Effectiveness increased by combination with dexamethasone

CTZ = chemoreceptor trigger zone; VC = vomiting centre; GIT = gastrointestinal tract; ICP = intracranial pressure; N = nausea; V = vomiting; po = by mouth; pr = by rectum; sc = by subcutaneous injection; iv = by intravenous injection; im = by intramuscular injection; occ = occasionally.

At high doses, metoclopramide blocks $5HT_3$ receptors in the CTZ and gut; extrapyramidal side-effects are common and this mode of use has been superseded by development of specific $5HT_3$ antagonists for cancer chemotherapy-induced emesis.[25]

Any agent that is prokinetic may induce colic in an obstructed intestine.

Phenothiazines

The phenothiazines are less potent D_2 antagonists. They have varying antagonist activity at other receptors which predicts their side-effects (e.g. chlorpromazine—α_1 adrenergic receptor—may cause hypotension and sedation; diphenhydramine, a phenothiazine antihistamine—Ach_m receptor—may cause sedation and dry mouth). Extrapyramidal reactions occur with all of the D_2 antagonists, although the incidence with domperidone is extremely low.[24] Levomepromazine blocks a wide spectrum of receptors at higher doses; it is highly sedative and causes hypotension but it is a useful antiemetic at lower doses (5–12.5 mg/24 h by mouth or subcutaneous infusion). Circumstantial evidence suggests that $5HT_2$ blockade may mediate levomepromazine antiemetic activity.[26] The binding affinity of low-dose levomepromazine for its $5HT_2$ receptor suggests that it is likely to be a potent antiemetic at the VC; its lower affinity for D_2 receptors may nevertheless make it a broad-spectrum antiemetic. Comparative clinical trials are awaited.

Antihistamines and anticholinergics

The antihistamines act on H_1 receptors in the VC and on vestibular afferents.[21,22] Only cyclizine is suitable for subcutaneous injection. Cyclizine is less sedative than the anticholinergic hyoscine (scopolamine) hydrobromide, which blocks Ach_m receptors in the VC and peripherally.[19,22] Hyoscine hydrobromide can be given sublingually, subcutaneously, and transdermally. Its side-effects are those of parasympathetic blockade, which may be beneficial (drying of secretions, reduction of colic) or troublesome (dry mouth, ileus, urinary retention, blurred vision). Drowsiness is not uncommon.

Hyoscine butylbromide does not have central antiemetic action. In the gut, however, its anticholinergic properties reduce peristalsis and inhibit exocrine secretions, thus contributing to the palliation of colic and nausea in intestinal obstruction.[27] Glyopyrrolate, a powerful peripheral anticholinergic drug with similar potency to atropine but little penetration into the central nervous system, may be used as an alternative to hyoscine butylbromide.

$5HT_3$ receptor antagonists

The discovery of selective $5HT_3$ receptor antagonists caused a revolution in antiemetic prescribing in oncology and a massive drive for the perfect antidote to chemotherapy-induced emesis. The initial early promise of this class of drugs in the 1980s has proved successful for acute-onset emesis in chemotherapy, although later-onset nausea remains a problem.[13,19,25,28–33]

Although extremely effective for cancer chemotherapy-induced emesis and becoming established for radiotherapy-induced emesis, no place has been demonstrated for $5HT_3$ antagonists in the management of nausea and vomiting from other causes. They do not reverse nausea mediated by dopamine pathways (e.g. opioid induced) and they remain largely untested in the nausea and vomiting syndromes associated with advanced cancer and AIDS. Some role in postoperative emesis is claimed for them and ondansetron is licensed in the United Kingdom for this indication. Benefit is probably only to be expected in 25 per cent of patients, and is no greater than with droperidol or metoclopramide.[35]

$5HT_3$ receptors have been demonstrated in the CTZ and VC centrally, and on terminals of vagal afferents in the gut peripherally. The bulk of human serotonin is located within entrochromaffin cells in the gut wall; this serotonin is released and metabolized locally in response to various insults including direct abdominal irradiation and highly emetogenic chemotherapy.[9,18,23,24,36,73] Release appears to be by active secretion, although it is not blocked by octreotide.[9] The emetogenic action of serotonin derived from enterochromaffin cells appears to be by direct stimulation of local vagal $5HT_3$ receptors: high abdominal vagotomy abolishes emesis induced by abdominal irradiation, and blood serotonin levels are rarely raised during emesis, although raised urinary levels of the serotonin metabolite 5-hydroxindole acetic acid reflect the timing and severity of emesis after chemothe-rapy.[19,36] $5HT_3$ antagonists block vagal afferent activity. A reflex increase in vagal efferent activity may be caused, and this has been shown to give rise to temporary (and inconsequential) bradyarrhythmias in patients receiving repeated doses of these drugs, although not in healthy volunteers.[37,38]

Several $5HT_3$ antagonists are currently available (see Table 1). Of these, dolasetron and its major metabolite, and granisetron are the most specific $5HT_3$ receptor antagonists, ondansetron and tropisetron both showing some affinity for other receptors including α-adrenergic, other 5HT and opioid μ receptors. In clinical trials that have compared granisetron, ondansetron, and tropisetron, there appears to be little to choose between them, although patients who expressed a preference consistently preferred granisetron. All are licensed for use in children, and adverse effects are few. Evidence-based antiemetics guidelines issued by the American Society of Clinical Oncology make no distinction between the different agents available, suggesting that cost should dictate local practice. They also recommend the use of cheaper oral preparations rather than intravenous treatment as first line.[25]

Other antiemetic drugs

Corticosteroids

Corticosteroids are known to possess intrinsic antiemetic properties and to enhance the effect of other antiemetics.[25,39] Their mechanism of action is unclear and may be multiple. Corticosteroids may enhance antiemetic tone in the medulla by:

1. reducing the permeability of the blood–brain barrier to chemicals that antagonize medullary antiemetic tone, such as chemotherapy agents;
2. depleting the inhibitory amine γ-aminobutyric acid (GABA) in medullary antiemetic neurones;
3. reducing leu-enkephalin release in the brainstem.[13]

In addition, the anti-inflammatory effects of corticosteroids can reduce tumour mass, thereby reducing the stimulus to emesis from peripheral autonomic stretch receptors or from intracranial tumours.

Cannabinoids

Anecdotal reports of a lower incidence of chemotherapy-induced emesis amongst marijuana smokers led to clinical trials of cannabinoids. Synthetic cannabinoids with and without psychotropic effects are antiemetic, although cannabis may be more effective than its synthetic analogues.[40]

The recent identification of a brain-stem cannabinoid receptor suggests a site of action of these compounds;[41] ligands for this receptor are arachidonic congeners, dubbed anandamides.[42] However, some antiemetic effects of synthetic cannabinoids are reversed by naloxone, raising the possibility that some of their mechanism of action is via opioid μ receptors.[13]

The use of the currently licensed cannabinoids is limited by psychotomometic side-effects, particularly dysphoria in the elderly. This effect can be reduced by low-dose phenothiazines but the resulting drowsiness may undermine any therapeutic advantage of the cannabinoids.[43] Euphoria is more common than dysphoria in younger patients, and there are reports of the successful use of nabilone for intractable nausea in AIDS patients, who tend to be younger than adults with cancer, and in children receiving chemotherapy.[44–46] Larger studies are needed to assess the value of cannabinoids for emesis in advanced disease.

Benzodiazepines

Benzodiazepines have been used in chemotherapy antiemetic combinations. Although they have little antiemetic potency *per se*, in drug combinations they reduce anxiety and akathisia, and reduce the likelihood of anticipatory nausea. These drugs are sedative and sometimes amnesic when used in effective doses, which limits their usefulness for patients with chronic nausea.[28,47,48]

Octreotide

Octreotide is a long-acting somatostatin analogue that exerts wide-ranging potent inhibition of endocrine and exocrine secretions and promotes reabsorption of electrolytes in the gut; there is clinical evidence of both inhibition and restoration of normal gastrointestinal transit.(49,50) Its combination of effects can be useful in palliating emesis caused by intestinal obstruction: inhibition of exocrine secretion in the gut reduces distension, thus diminishing the stimulus to nausea and to colic.(51–53) Subcutaneous infusion is useful during titration to establish the effective dose; for patients with a longer prognosis, a long-acting depot injection may be an alternative.

Propofol

Propofol, an intravenous anaesthetic agent, has been noted to protect against postoperative emesis.(54,55) Recent work shows that subhypnotic doses of propofol have antiemetic action in post-anaesthetic and chemotherapy-induced emesis.(56–58) The duration of antiemetic action of an intravenous low-dose bolus outlasts the very short duration of hypnosis that would be introduced by a far larger dose, suggesting that hypnosis or anxiolysis are not the mechanisms of antiemetic action. Propofol has a widespread central nervous system depressant effect and it is possible that its antiemetic action is at a subcortical level, in either the CTZ or within the VC complex. The observation that propofol is less successful as an antiemetic following vagal-stimulating abdominal surgery suggests that its site of action may be the CTZ.

Opioids

Opioids can induce or block emesis in experimental models; both actions can be antagonized by naloxone. It has been proposed that δ and/or κ opioid receptors are emetogenic, whilst μ receptors are antiemetic. Experimentally, intravenous fentanyl in subanaesthetic doses abolishes emesis due to morphine, cisplatin, and copper sulphate, an effect which is reversed by naloxone.(59) In clinical practice, the nauseating properties of the opioids are well known: it remains to be seen whether more μ-specific drugs can be developed, and whether these may have any role as antiemetics.

Substance P

Substance P is found in high concentrations in the CTZ and VC. It binds to a specific receptor, neurokinin 1 (NK_1). After initial exciting reports about the beneficial effects of NK_1 receptor antagonists in the 1990s, there has been little evidence of further development of this class of agents. NK_1 receptor antagonists showed efficacy in reducing both acute-onset and the more problematic delayed-onset emesis in patients receiving chemotherapy, when added to currently available agents.(32–34) There is also a suggestion of benefit for postoperative nausea and vomiting.(60) NK_1 receptor antagonists appear to have a broad spectrum of action for diverse causes of emesis in animals, but similar studies have not been undertaken in man.

Non-drug measures of palliation of nausea and vomiting

Psychological techniques

Most of the authoritative research on psychological techniques for palliation of emesis has been conducted amongst chemotherapy patients, which is not analogous to the situation of nauseated patients with disease which is not amenable to chemotherapy. However, these studies have shown that patients can learn techniques such as progressive muscle relaxation and guided mental imagery, and use these during the stress of chemotherapy with good effect.(61–63) Cognitive therapy has been used to help relieve the psychological morbidity arising from physical symptoms in advanced cancer.(64) The possibility of adapting such techniques for the needs of nauseated patients with advanced diseases warrants further exploration (see Chapter 8.2.8) (see also Chapter 8.17).

Transcutaneous electrical nerve stimulation (See chapter 8.2.8)

Transcutaneous electrical nerve stimulation (TENS) has been shown to enhance the effect of antiemetic drugs: the TENS effect is blocked by naloxone, suggesting that it is mediated by endogenous opioid peptides.(65) (see Chapter 8.2.9).

Acupuncture and acupressure (See chapter 8.2.9)

Acupuncture and acupressure have been shown to augment the effect of antiemetics during chemotherapy, and to reduce postoperative nausea and vomiting. The benefit of acupuncture is lost if administered under general anaesthetic.(66) Acupressure prolongs the effect of acupuncture, and the use of TENS in place of traditional acupuncture needles at the P6 acupuncture point is a practical technique for self-use by patients, being only slightly less effective than the use of traditional needles.(67,68) The P6 (Neiguan) acupuncture point is located in the midline of the palmar aspect of each wrist, approximately 3 cm from the palmar crease.

Clinical syndromes associated with nausea and vomiting

Table 2 summarizes some common or important causes of nausea and vomiting in palliative care patients. They are grouped according to the pathway that mediates emesis, and are similarly grouped in the following discussion.

It must be emphasized, however, that in advanced disease nausea and vomiting may have more than one cause, stimulating symptoms via more than one pathway. Sometimes, apparently appropriate treatment fails to relieve symptoms, necessitating a search for additional and less obvious causes. Sometimes, a cause cannot be identified: into this category are likely to fall those with cancer-associated autonomic failure. Growth factors and other tumour products may be emetogenic; their actions are still only partly understood, but it is likely that such factors would act via the CTZ. Tumours arising outside the areas described in the table may generate emesis via the same pathways, for example, head and neck tumours cause pressure effects which trigger autonomic relays to the VC. The key to good management of nausea and vomiting is a high index of suspicion, an understanding of the pathways involved, and the setting of realistic goals.

Chemical causes of emesis

Drug-induced nausea may arise by chemical action at the CTZ, by serotonin release in the gut, through gastrointestinal irritation or gastric stasis, or a combination of these (Table 3).

Transient nausea mediated by the CTZ accompanies the introduction or increase of morphine in about one-third of patients;(69) these patients will benefit from haloperidol, a central D_2 antagonist, during this period. In the United Kingdom and New Zealand, haloperidol is used with good effect; in Northern America metoclopramide is often used as an alternative although it has weaker central anti-D_2 activity. The appearance of nausea with other opioid toxicity manifestations (small pupils, drowsiness, myoclonic jerks) in a patient taking morphine who was previously tolerant of the same dose of morphine may herald the onset of renal insufficiency: the opioid should be reduced in dose and/or frequency. An alternative opioid may be prescribed, at equinalgesic dose, provided it does not rely on renal excretion of active metabolites (see Chapter 8.2.3). A proportion of patients experience opioid-induced gastric stasis. Tolerance to this does not develop; a prokinetic agent is required, sometimes in high doses, if change to a different opioid is ineffective or not possible.

Cytotoxic-induced nausea is mediated by the CTZ and by $5HT_3$ receptors on vagal gut afferents. Selective blockade of $5HT_3$ receptors in the gut is highly effective for immediate-onset emesis;(25) these drugs may also act as the CTZ. Adding antiemetics that work at other sites enhances the

Table 2 Common syndromes involving nausea and vomiting in patients requiring palliative care (supplementary information in text)

Syndrome	Causes	Key features	Pathway and receptors	Treatment possibilities
Chemically induced nausea	◆ Drugs: opioids, digoxin, anticonvulsants, antibiotics, cytotoxics ◆ Toxins: food poisoning, ischaemic bowel, e.g. gut obstruction, ? tumour products ◆ Metabolic: organ failure, hypercalcaemia, ketoacidosis	Of drug toxicity or of underlying disease, plus constant nausea, variable vomiting	Chemical action stimulates D_2 ($\pm 5HT_3$) in CTZ Chemotherapy → serotonin release in GI tract → 5-HT_3 receptors on vagus	◆ Stop or reduce the offending drug ◆ Treat the underlying cause ◆ Haloperidol ◆ $5HT_3$ antagonists for chemotherapy or direct abdominal irradiation
Gastric stasis	◆ Anticholinergic drugs, opioids ◆ Ascites ◆ Hepatomegaly ◆ Peptic ulcer ◆ Gastritis ▪ Stress ▪ Drugs ▪ Radiotherapy ◆ Autonomic failure	Epigastric pain, fullness, nausea, early satiety, flatulence, acid reflux, hiccup, large volume vomits, (possibly projectile) gastric regurgitation, other features of autonomic failure	Gastric mecho-receptors ↓ vagal afferents ↓ VC H_1; Ach_m	◆ Treat the underlying causes ◆ Prokinetic agents ◆ Reduce gastric secretions: ▪ H_2 blocker, ▪ Omeprazole, ▪ Octreotide ◆ Aid eructation: dimethicone
Stretch/distortion of GI tract	◆ Constipation ◆ Intestinal obstruction ◆ Mesenteric metastases	Altered bowel habit, nausea, vomiting, may be faeculent, colic	Gut/serosal mechanoreceptors ↓ vagal afferents ↓ VC	◆ Treat underlying cause ◆ Active bowel management ◆ Corticosteroids may reduce the size of tumour mass
Serosal stretch/irritation	◆ Liver metastases ◆ Ureteric obstruction ◆ Retroperitoneal cancer	Of underlying condition, nausea, occasional vomiting	H_1; Ach_m	◆ Cyclizine ◆ Hyoscine hydrobromide if bowel paralysis is acceptable
Irritation of GI tract	◆ e.g. cryptospordiosis	Profuse diarrhoea, nausea, occasional vomiting		
Raised intracranial pressure/meningism	◆ Cerebral oedema ◆ Intracranial tumour ◆ Intracranial bleeding ◆ Meningeal infiltration by tumour ◆ Skull metastases ◆ Cerebral infection (AIDS)	Headache, (diurnal); papilloedema, photophobia may be absent. Nausea may be diurnal; neurological signs may be absent	May be direct stimulation of cerebral H_1 Meningeal mechanoreceptors ↓ VC H_1; Ach_m	◆ Treat underlying cause ◆ High-dose corticosteroids may reduce cerebral oedema/mass size ◆ Cyclizine ◆ Levomepromazine
Movement-associated emesis	◆ Opioids (more common in ambulant patients) ◆ Gut distortion ◆ Gastroparesis → passive regurgitation	Nausea and/or sudden vomits on movement/turning in bed	Opioid-induced sensitivity of vestibular afferents H_1; Ach_m Gut mechanoreceptors ↓ vagal afferents ↓ VC H_1; Ach_m	◆ Treat the underlying cause ◆ Nasogastric aspiration in terminal gastroparesis ◆ Cyclizine ◆ Cinnarizine ◆ Hyoscine hydrobromide

Table 2 Continued

Syndrome	Causes	Key features	Pathway and receptors	Treatment possibilities
Anxiety-induced emesis	◆ Anxiety ▪ about self ▪ about others ▪ about disease ▪ about symptoms ◆ Anticipatory emesis with cytotoxics	'Waves' of nausea, ± vomiting, reminders trigger nausea; may be relieved by distraction	Cortex ↓ VC H_1; Ach_m	◆ Address the anxiety ◆ Psychological techniques ◆ Relaxation ◆ Benzodiazepines may be useful

D_2 = dopamine type 2 receptor; 5-HT_3 = serotonin type 3 receptor; H_1 = histamine type 1 receptor; Ach_m = muscarinic cholinergic receptor; CTZ = chemoreceptor trigger zone; VC = vomiting centre; GI = gastrointestinal.

Table 3 Causes of drug-induced nausea

Mechanism	Drugs	
Activation of chemo-receptor trigger zone	Opioids Digoxin Anticoagulants	Cytotoxics Imidazoles Antibiotics
Gastrointestinal irritation	Non-steroidal anti-inflammatory drugs Iron supplements	Antibiotics Cytotoxics
Gastric stasis	Tricyclics Phenothiazines	Opioids Anticholinergics

effectiveness of treatment, particularly for delayed-onset emesis. Combinations of $5HT_3$ antagonist with a corticosteroid and/or benzodiazepine have been particularly effective, with 65–89 per cent complete control of symptoms in patients receiving cisplatin.[25,28,30]

Metabolic causes of nausea include organ failure and hypercalcaemia, which may progress insidiously. Nausea can be controlled using a central D_2 blocker: higher doses of haloperidol may be required (5–20 mg daily) with a consequently higher incidence of extrapyramidal side-effects. These respond to antimuscarinic drugs such as procyclidine and benztropine, which may be given by slow intravenous injection for relief of acute dystonias.

Gastrointestinal causes of emesis

Pharyngeal irritation may cause retching, nausea, or cough-induced vomiting. The oropharynx is richly innervated by the glossopahryngeal nerve and vagus, and is highly sensitive to touch. Tenacious sputum or candida overlying the pharyngeal mucosa can stimulate the VC via these afferents; AIDS patients may also have mucosal lesions of cytomegalovirus or herpes simplex. Appropriate antimicrobial therapy is indicated for infections of mouth, pharynx, oesophagus, or respiratory tract. Sticky sputum may be loosened by inhalations, and irritating nocturnal cough causing retching and disturbed sleep may be palliated by application of local anaesthetic spray to the pharynx (with appropriate caution about eating and drinking for the next few hours).

Delayed gastric emptying may arise from physiological abnormalities or mechanical resistance to emptying. Mechanical resistance includes ascites, hepatomegaly, prepyloric inflammation, duodenal ulceration or tumour, and pancreatic cancer. Resistance may be partial or there may be complete obstruction. Physiological abnormalities include anticholinergic effects of drugs (Table 3), including opioids, and autonomic failure. The symptoms are listed in Table 2; they may not all occur and the diagnosis can easily be missed.

Complete gastric outlet obstruction is managed as high intestinal obstruction (see Chapter 8.3.4). Other causes of delayed emptying are managed by attention to:

1. *Anxiety:* listening to concerns, explanation of cause of vomiting and plan of treatment.
2. *Optimizing gastric emptying:* the prokinetic agents metoclopramide and domperidone normalize the rate of gastric and upper intestinal peristalsis, increase lower oesophageal tone (thus reducing reflux), and relax the pylorus; gastric and upper intestinal transit time is shortened. The prokinetic agent cisapride increases the rate of peristalsis throughout the gastrointestinal tract. It was withdrawn in the United Kingdom because of concerns about cardiotoxicity, but remains available on a named-patient basis.
3. *Reducing stimulus to gastric stretch:* reduction in volume of meals and drinks and inhibition of gastric secretion using H_2 blockers, proton-pump inhibitors, or octreotide will reduce gastric stretch, thus reducing both the phrenic nerve irritation which gives rise to hiccup and the vagal stimulation which gives rise to nausea and pain.

Two adverse effects of the prokinetic agents are noteworthy. In a partially obstructed intestine, prokinetic agents may induce colic. Gastric colic may have a long periodicity mimicking ulcer or tumour-related pain. Action of prokinetic agents in the lower oesophagus may provoke oesophageal spasm; typically, this is retrosternal and may mimic angina pectoris. Oesophageal spasm may be relieved by sublingual glyceral trinitrate.

Stretch and distortion of the gastrointestinal tract activates mechanoreceptors in the bowel wall; similar receptors are present in visceral capsules and in parietal serosal surfaces. Their afferent input is to the VC via the vagus and splanchnic nerves. Mechanoreceptors may be triggered by tumour distorting an organ, stretching or directly invading serosa or mesentry, or by increased transmural pressure in a hollow viscus proximal to a site of obstruction, for example, ureter or colon. This is, therefore, a common complication of advanced intra-abdominal, retroperitoneal, or pelvic malignancy. Local inflammation may potentiate afferent nerve receptors in the gastrointestinal tract, mediating emesis in bowel infections such as cryptosporidiosis in AIDS patients.

If reversal of the cause of emesis is not possible, nausea may be palliated by using antiemetics active at the VC. Control of vomiting may be more difficult to achieve with obstruction in the gastrointestinal tract: this is discussed in more detail in Chapter 8.3.4.

Constipation with resultant colonic stretch is assumed to be a common cause of nausea and anorexia in advanced disease, although there are no studies to prove this. Management is of the constipation, although antiemetics acting at the VC may help to reduce the nausea. Anticholinergic agents should be avoided as they will exacerbate the constipation.

Cranial causes of emesis

Raised intracranial pressure may present with nausea and vomiting before headache is apparent. Meningeal irritation can also trigger emesis. Clinical associations are with intracerebral tumours (primary and secondary), bone metastases to skull (base of skull metastases may give rise to cranial nerve symptoms and signs), intracranial bleeding, and cerebral oedema. High-dose corticosteroids are the treatment of choice; an antiemetic acting at the VC may be necessary in addition. Palliative radiotherapy should be considered.

Other causes of emesis

Movement-associated emesis may be triggered by distorted or distended viscera exerting increased traction upon their mesentery during movement. Movement-associated nausea may also occur as a side-effect of opioids, related to increased vestibular sensitivity. This centrally-mediated emesis must be distinguished from passive regurgitation of gastric contents during movements of a terminally ill patient, which is usually related to gastroparesis; temporary passage of a nasogastric tube to aspirate the stomach dry of fluid and gas may be necessary to relieve this symptom.

Anxiety-induced emesis is a common experience in health. The patient with advanced disease may be able to identify anxiety as the trigger to nausea, or carers may notice an association between symptoms and stressful situations or conversations. Other causes of emesis must be excluded as far as possible before attributing nausea and vomiting to anxiety. Treatment is by identifying anxiety as a trigger and then working collaboratively with the patient to increase relaxation, identify and challenge anxiety-provoking thoughts, and establishing workable coping strategies.(62,64) Benzodiazepines may be useful as short-term adjuvants: it is preferable to select a benzodiazepine with a longer half-life given as a single, evening dose (e.g. diazepam) to prevent as required use of anxiolytics, which is unlikely to be helpful. Some patients benefit from tricyclic antidepressants with secondary anxiolytic properties, for example, amitriptyline. All these drugs reduce a patient's ability to concentrate and can therefore reduce a patient's ability to learn or practise psychotherapeutic techniques.(61)

Anticipatory emesis is a conditioned response in some patients who have suffered nausea and/or vomiting provoked by cytotoxic drugs. Any reminder of their previous experience may trigger emesis, including television pictures of hospitals, hospital smells, or visits by hospital personnel. It can be refractory to treatment and is best avoided by control of emesis from the first cycle of chemotherapy. Management is as for anxiety-induced emesis. Systematic desensitization has also been used successfully in these patients.(61,62)

Intractable nausea

As with pain, the pathways of emesis are probably incompletely documented. Identification of triggers and administration of receptor-specific antiemetics was successful in 93 per cent of patients in a well-conducted study,(19) but a minority remain for whom nausea continues unabated. There are few published data about these patients. Amongst cachexic patients with chronic nausea, Bruera's group have identified a high incidence of autonomic failure.(70)

Appropriate goal-setting is important. It is unwise to expect or to promise total relief of nausea and vomiting. Most patients will be content with major relief of nausea, even if intermittent vomiting continues, provided they have been led to expect this as a possible outcome. It may be helpful to grade emesis or to use a tool to measure change, in order to assess response to treatment. Patients' perceptions are different from those of nurses observing them, and there is a need for an agreed tool for measurement of nausea and vomiting.(71,72)

When apparently appropriate measures have failed to relieve symptoms, and combinations of antiemetics directed at different receptors have proved ineffective, empirical use of levomepromazine may offer relief to some patients. Good clinical trials of therapy for such patients are necessary.

Future developments

Progress has been made in the recognition of nausea as an important symptom that must be evaluated separately from vomiting. This has improved the quality of the data emerging from chemotherapy-related emesis and postoperative nausea and vomiting studies.

The development of tools for self-evaluation of symptoms by patients, and the identification of biological markers for emesis, would enhance the evaluation of antiemetic strategies. Good, controlled trials of therapy are still awaited, including further outcome studies of receptor-based prescribing to expand earlier work.

The potential for the development of broad spectrum antiemetics is intriguing, particularly levomepromazine and the NK_1 receptor antagonists. Multicentre studies will be necessary to produce sufficient numbers of patients for robust studies of clinical outcomes in a palliative care population.

References

1. **Dunlop, G.M.** (1989). A study of the relative frequency and importance of gastrointestinal symptoms, and weakness in patients with far advanced cancer. *Palliative Medicine* **4**, 37–43.
2. **Meuser, T.** et al. (2001). Symptoms during cancer pain treatment following WHO guidelines: a longitudinal follow-up study of symptom prevalence, severity and etiology. *Pain* **93**, 247–57.
3. **Bliss, J.M., Robertson, B., and Selby, P.J.** (1992). The impact of nausea and vomiting upon quality of life measures. *British Journal of Cancer* **66**, S14–23.
4. **Coates, A.** et al. (1983). On the receiving end—patient perception of the side-effects of cancer chemotherapy. *European Journal of Cancer* **19**, 203–8.
5. **Grond, S., Zech, D., Diefenbach, C., and Bischoff, A.** (1994). Prevalence and pattern of symptoms in patients with cancer pain: a prospective evaluation of 1635 cancer patients referred to a pain clinic. *Journal of Pain and Symptom Management* **9**, 372–82.
6. **Fainsinger, R., Miller, M., Bruera, E., Hanson, J., and Maceachern, T.** (1991). Symptom control during the last week of life on a palliative care unit. *Journal of Palliative Care* **7**, 5–11.
7. **Borison, H.L. and Wang, S.C.** (1953). Physiology and pharmacology of vomiting. *Pharmacological Reviews* **5**, 192–230.
8. **Wang, S.C.** (1965). Emetic and antiemetic drugs. In *Physiological Pharmacology: a Comprehensive Treatise* (ed. W.S. Root and F.G. Hofman), Vol. II, pp. 255–328. New York: Academic Press.
9. **Cubeddu, L.X., Hoffman, I.S., Fuenmayor, N.T., and Malave, J.J.** (1992). Changes in serotonin metabolism in cancer patients: its relationship to nausea and vomiting induced by chemotherapeutic drugs. *British Journal of Cancer* **66**, 198–203.
10. **Costello, D.J. and Borison, H.L.** (1972). Naloxone antagonises narcotic self-blockade of emesis in the cat. *Journal of Pharmacology and Experimental Therapeutics* **203**, 222–30.
11. **Davis, C.J., Harding, R.K., Leslie, R.A., and Andrews, P.L.R.** (1986). The organisation of vomiting as a protective reflex. In *Nausea and Vomiting: Mechanisms and Treatment* (ed. C.J. Davis, G.V. Lake-Bakaar, and D.G. Grahame-Smith), pp. 65–75. Berlin: Springer-Verlag.
12. **Lang, I.M.** (1999). Noxious stimulation of emesis. *Digestive Diseases and Sciences* **44** (Suppl.), 58S–63S.
13. **Harris, A.L. and Cantwell, B.M.J.** (1986). Mechanisms and treatment of cytotoxic-induced nausea and vomiting. In *Nausea and Vomiting: Mechanisms and Treatment* (ed. C.J. Davis, G.V. Lake-Bakaar, and D.G. Grahame-Smith), pp. 78–93. Berlin: Springer-Verlag.
14. **Harris, A.L.** (1982). Cytotoxic therapy-induced vomiting is mediated via enkephalin pathways. *Lancet* **i**, 714–16.
15. **Edwards, C.M.** (1988). Chemotherapy induced emesis—mechanisms and treatment. A review. *Journal of the Royal Society of Medicine* **81**, 658–62.
16. **Miller, A.D., Rowley, H.A., Roberts, T.P.L., and Kucharczyk, J.** (1996). Human cortical activity during vestibular and drug-induced nausea detected using, M.S.I. In *New Directions in Vestibular Research* (ed. S.M. Highstein, B. Cohen, and J.A. Büttner-Ennever), pp. 670–2. Ann NY Acad Ser 781.
17. **Lichter, I.** (1993). Which antiemetic? *Journal of Palliative Care* **9**, 42–50.
18. **Willems, J.L. and Lefebvre, R.A.** (1986). Peripheral nervous pathways involved in nausea and vomiting. In *Nausea and Vomiting: Mechanisms and Treatment* (ed. C.J. Davis, G.V. Lake-Bakaar, and D.G. Grahame-Smith), pp. 56–64. Berlin: Springer-Verlag.
19. **Lichter, I.** (1993). Results of antiemetic management in terminal illness. *Journal of Palliative Care*, **9**, 19–21.
20. **Andrews, P.L.R., Davis, C.J., Bingham, S., Davidson, H.I.M., Hawthorn, J., and Maskell, L.** (1990). The abdominal visceral innervation and the emetic reflex: pathways, pharmacology and plasticity. *Canadian Journal of Physiology and Pharmacology* **68**, 325.

21. **Stott, J.R.R.** (1986). Mechanisms and treatment of motion illness. In *Nausea and Vomiting: Mechanisms and Treatment* (ed. C.J. Davis, G.V. Lake-Bakaar, and D.G. Grahame-Smith), Berlin: Springer-Verlag.
22. **Gutner, L.B., Gould, W.J., and Batterman, R.C.** (1952). The effects of potent analgesics upon vestibular function. *Journal of Clinical Investigation* **31**, 259–66.
23. **Peroutka, S.J. and Snyder, S.H.** (1982). Antiemetics: neurotransmitter binding predicts therapeutic actions. *Lancet* **ii**, 658–9.
24. **Ison, P.J. and Peroutka, S.J.** (1986). Neurotransmitter receptor binding studies predict antiemetic efficacy and side effects. *Cancer Treatment Reports* **70**, 637–41.
25. **Gralla, R.J.** et al. (1999). for the American Society of Clinical Oncology Recommendations for the use of antiemetics: evidence-based, clinical practice guidelines. *Journal of Clinical Oncology* **17**, 2971–94.
26. **Twycross, R., Barkley, G.D., and Hallwood, P.M.** (1997). The use of low dose levomepromazine (methotrimeprazine) in the management of nausea and vomiting. *Progress in Palliative Care* **5**, 49–53.
27. **DeConno, F., Caraceni, A., Zecca, E., Spondi, E., and Ventafridda, V.** (1992). Continuous subcutaneous infusion of hyoscine butylbromide reduces secretions in patients with gastrointestinal obstruction. *Journal of Pain and Symptom Management* **6**, 484–6.
28. **Kris, M.G.** (1992). Rationale for combination antiemetic therapy and strategies for the use of ondansetron in combinations. *Seminars in Oncology* **19**, 61–6.
29. **Roberts, J.J. and Priestman, T.H.** (1993). A review of ondansetron in the management of radiotherapy-induced emesis. *Oncology* **50**, 173–9.
30. **Yarker, Y.E. and McTavish, D.** (1994). Granisetron: an update of its therapeutic use in nausea and vomiting induced by antineoplastic therapy. *Drugs* **48**, 761–93.
31. **Gardner, C.J.** et al. (1995). The broad-spectrum anti-emetic activity of the novel non-peptide tachykinin NK_1 receptor antagonist GR 203040. *British Journal of Pharmacology* **116**, 3158–63.
32. **Navari, R.M.** et al. (1999). Reduction of cisplatin-induced emesis by a selective neurokinin 1 receptor antagonist. L-754,030 Antiemetic Trials Group. *New England Journal of Medicine* **340**, 190–5.
33. **Rizk, A.N. and Hesketh, P.J.** (1999). Antiemetics for cancer chemotherapy-induced nausea and vomiting. A review of agents in development. *Drugs in Research and Development* **2**, 229–35.
34. **Hesketh, P.J.** et al. (1999). Randomised phase II study of the Neurokinin 1 receptor antagonist CJ-11, 974 in the control of cisplatin induced emesis. *Journal of Clinical Oncology* **17**, 338–43.
35. **Tramer, M.R., Moore, R.S., Reynolds, D.J.M., and McQuay, H.J.** (1997). A quantitative systematic review of ondansetron in established post-operative nausea and vomiting. *British Medical Journal* **314**, 1088–92.
36. **Cubeddu, L.X., O'Connor, D.T., and Parmer, R.J.** (1995). Plasma chromogranin A: a marker of serotonin release and of emesis associated with cisplatin chemotherapy. *Journal of Clinical Oncology* **13**, 681–7.
37. **Watanabe, H., Hasegawa, A., Shinozaki, T., Arita, S., and Chigira, M.** (1995). Possible cardiac side effects of granisetron, an antiemetic agent, in patients with bone and soft-tissue sarcomas receiving cytotoxic chemotherapy. *Cancer Chemotherapy Pharmacology* **35**, 278–82.
38. **Upward, J.W., Archbold, B.D.C., Link, C., Pierce, D.M., Allan, A., and Tasker, T.C.G.** (1990). The clinical pharmacology of granisetron (BRL 43694), a novel specific $5HT_3$ antagonist. *European Journal of Cancer* **26**, S12–15.
39. **Aapro, M.S.** (1991). Present role of corticosteroids as antiemetics. In *Recent Results in Cancer Research.* Vol. 121, pp. 91–100. Berlin: Springer-Verlag.
40. **Doblin, R.E. and Kleiman, M.A.R.** (1991). Marijuana as antiemetic medicine: a survey of oncologists' experiences and attitudes. *Journal of Clinical Oncology* **9**, 1314–19.
41. **Devane, W.A.** et al. (1992). Isolation and structure of a brain constituent that binds to the cannabinoid receptor. *Science* **258**, 1946–9.
42. **Feldman, R.S., Meyer, J.S., and Quenzer, L.F.** *Principles of Neuropsychopharmacology.* Sunderland MA: Sinauer, 1997.
43. **Cunningham, D.** et al. (1985). Nabilone and prochloperazine: a useful combination for emesis induced by cytotoxic drugs. *British Medical Journal* **291**, 864–5.
44. **Flynn, J. and Hanif, N.** (1992). Nabilone for the management of intractable nausea and vomiting in terminally staged AIDS. *Journal of Palliative Care* **8**, 46–7.
45. **Green, S.T., Nathwani, D., Goldbery, D.J., and Kennedy, D.H.** (1989). Nabilone as effective therapy for intractable nausea and vomiting in AIDS. *British Journal of Clinical Pharmacology* **28**, 494–5.
46. **Dalzell, A.M., Bartle, H.M., and Lylleyman, J.S.** (1986). Nabilone: an alternative antiemetic for cancer chemotherapy. *Archives of Disease in Childhood* **61**, 502–5.
47. **Potanovich, L.M.** et al. (1993). Midazolam in patients receiving anticancer chemotherapy and antiemetics. *Journal of Pain and Symptom Management* **8**, 519–24.
48. **Gordon, C.J.** et al. (1989). Metoclopramide vs metoclopramide and lorazepam: superiority of combined therapy in the control of cisplatin-induced mesis. *Cancer* **63**, 578–82.
49. **Fallon, M.T.** (1994). The physiology of somatostatin and its synthetic analogue, octreotide. *European Journal of Palliative Care* **1**, 20–2.
50. **Soudah, H.C., Hasler, W.L., and Chung, O.** (1991). Effect of octreotide on intestinal motility and bacterial overgrowth in scleroderma. *New England Journal of Medicine* **325**, 1461–7.
51. **Riley, J. and Fallon, M.** (1994). Octreotide in terminal malignant obstruction of the gastrointestinal tract. *European Journal of Palliative Care* **1**, 23–5.
52. **Mercadante, S.** et al. (1993). Octreotide in relieving gastrointestinal symptoms due to bowel obstruction. *Palliative Medicine* **7**, 295–9.
53. **Khoo, D., Riley, J., and Waxman, J.** (1992). Control of emesis in bowel obstruction in terminally ill patients. *Lancet* **339**, 375–6.
54. **Raftery, S. and Sherry, E.** (1992). Total intravenous anaesthesia with propofol and alfentanyl protects against postoperative nausea and vomiting. *Canadian Anaesthetists' Society Journal* **39**, 37–40.
55. **Barst, S.** et al. (1990). Anesthesia for pediatric cancer patients: ketamine, etomidate, or propofol? *Anaesthesiology* **73**, A1114.
56. **Borgeat, A., Wilder-Smith, O., Forni, M., and Suter, P.M.** (1994). Adjuvant propofol enables better control of nausea and emesis secondary to chemotherapy for breast cancer. *Canadian Journal of Anaesthetists* **41**, 117–19.
57. **Scher, C.S. and McDowall, R.H.** (1992). Use of propofol for the prevention of chemotherapy-induced nausea and emesis in oncology patients. *Canadian Anaesthetists' Society Journal* **39**, 170–2.
58. **Borgeat, A., Wilder-Smith, O.H.G., Saiah, M., and Rifat, K.** (1992). Subhypnotic doses of propofol possess direct antiemetic properties. *Anaesthesia and Analgesia* **74**, 539–41.
59. **Baines, N.M., Bunce, K.T., Naylor, R.J., and Rudd, J.A.** (1991). The actions of fentanyl to inhibit drug-induced emesis. *Neuropharmacology* **30**, 1073–83.
60. **Diemmunsch, P.** (1999). Antiemetic activity of the NK_1 receptor antagonist GR 205171 in the treatment of established postoperative nausea and vomiting after major gynaecological surgery. *British Journal of Anaesthesia* **82**, 274–6.
61. **Burish, T.G. and Tope, D.M.** (1992). Psychological techniques for controlling the adverse side effects of cancer chemotherapy: findings from a decade of research. *Journal of Pain and Symptom Management* **7**, 287–301.
62. **Fallowfield, L.J.** (1992). Behavioural interventions and psychological aspects of care during chemotherapy. *European Journal of Cancer* 28A, S39–41.
63. **Contach, P.H.** (1991). Use of nonpharmacological techniques to prevent chemotherapy-related nausea and vomiting. *Recent Results in Cancer Research* **121**, 101–7.
64. Adjuvant psychological therapy in advanced cancer. In *Psychological Therapy for Patients with Cancer: a New Approach,* S. Moorey and S. Greer. Oxford: Heinemann, 1989.
65. **Saller, R., Hellenbrecht, D., Bühring, M., and Hess, H.** (1986). Enhancement of the antiemetic action of metoclopramide against cisplatin-induced emesis by transdermal electrical nerve stimulation. *Journal of Clinical Pharmacology* **26**, 115–19.
66. **Vickers, A.J.** (1996). Can acupuncture have specific effects on health? A systematic review of acupuncture antiemesis trials. *Journal of the Royal Society of Medicine* **89**, 308–11.
67. **Dundee, J.W. and Yang, J.** (1991). Prolongation of the antiemetic action of P6 acupuncture by acupressure in patients having cancer chemotherapy. *Journal of the Royal Society of Medicine* **83**, 360–2.

68. **Dundee, J.W., Yang, J., and McMillan, C.** (1991). Noninvasive stimulation of the P6 (Neiguan) antiemetic acupunture point in cancer chemotherapy. *Journal of the Royal Society of Medicine* **84**, 210–12.
69. **Compora, E.** et al. (1991). The incidence of narcotic-induced emesis. *Journal of Pain and Symptom Management* **6**, 428–30.
70. **Bruera, E.** et al. (1987). Chronic nausea and anorexia in advanced cancer patients: a possible role for autonomic dysfunction. *Journal of Pain and Symptom Management* 2, 19–21.
71. **Olver, I.N., Matthews, J.P., Bishop, J.F., and Smith, R.A.** (1994). The roles of patient and observer assessments in antiemetic trials. *European Journal of Cancer* **30A**, 1223–7.
72. **Herrstedt, J.** (1994). We still need common criteria for the assessment of nausea and vomiting. *European Journal of Cancer* **30A**, 1217.
73. **Scarantino, C.W., Ornitz, R.D., Hoffman, L.G., and Anderson, R.F.** (1994). On the mechanisms of radiation-induced emesis: the role of serotonin. *International Journal of Radiation Oncology, Biology and Physics* **30**, 825–30.

8.3.2 Dysphagia, dyspepsia, and hiccup

Claud Regnard

Dysphagia

Definition

Dysphagia is difficulty in transferring liquids or solids from the mouth to the stomach.

Incidence

The incidence of dysphagia varies considerably depending on the cause and stage of disease. In a large series of nearly 7000 patients at St Christopher's Hospice, London, the overall incidence was 23 per cent,[1] although in a later series of 800 patients the incidence was only 12 per cent.[2] The incidence of dysphagia in patients with head and neck cancer depends on the site of the problem, being as low as 4 per cent in anterior oral lesions, rising to 100 per cent with postcricoid lesions.[3,4] Laryngeal and hypopharyngeal tumours produce the most severe problems.[5] In the motor neurone disease of amyotrophic lateral sclerosis the incidence of dysphagia is about 60 per cent,[6] but, despite its progressive nature, it is a fallacy that aspiration is a common cause of death in this condition.[7] Sixty-three per cent of patients with Parkinson's disease and 47 per cent of patients with multiple sclerosis have objective evidence of swallowing difficulty.[8,9] Swallowing becomes slower with age.[10] Older people may therefore be more vulnerable to disturbances of swallowing, which may explain why 55 per cent of a group of nursing home patients had swallowing problems.[11]

Anatomy and physiology

Although the path taken by fluids and food to the stomach is direct, the mechanism to achieve a smooth and easy passage is complex. It requires intact anatomy, normal mucosa, normal functioning of five cranial nerves and the brainstem, the co-ordination of the cortex, limbic system, basal ganglia, cerebellum, and brain stem centres involved in respiration, salivation, and motor function. Thirty-four skeletal muscles are involved. This complexity reflects the biological necessity for respiration and nutrition, with respiration taking priority. Swallowing comprises four distinct phases.[12] The first two are voluntary; the latter two reflexive:

1. *Oral preparatory phase:* food is mixed with saliva and chewed to break down larger particles.
2. *Oral swallowing phase:* the lips are closed to prevent leakage and the anterior tongue retracts and elevates in a wave that pushes the bolus into the oropharynx.
3. *Pharyngeal phase:* this is triggered by the bolus reaching the posterior tongue. The larynx closes, breathing stops, and the larynx elevates to seal with the epiglottis and vocal cords to protect the airway and prevent aspiration. A peristaltic wave moves the bolus into the oesophagus in under 1 s. These complex actions are necessary to protect the airway because the pharynx is a shared passage for air and food.
4. *Oesophageal phase:* reflex peristalsis carries the bolus down the oesophagus, the lower oesophageal sphincter relaxes, and the bolus enters the stomach.

Mechanisms and causes

Any disruption of normal anatomy and physiology may result in dysphagia and consequently there are many causes, sometimes with several concurrent (Table 1).[15] Mechanical obstruction is generally caused by cancer. Tumours of the mouth and upper pharynx cause early symptoms, while those of the lower pharynx and oesophagus are often silent at first. Food will collect proximally and may spill over into an unprotected airway (Fig. 1). Stricture formation may occur following surgery,[13] radiotherapy, or because of gastro-oesophageal reflux disease.

In the absence of mechanical obstruction, severe dysphagia due to functional disturbance can occur. For example, inability to raise the posterior tongue because of tumour infiltration may allow food to trickle into the pharynx and into an unprotected airway. Fibrosis following surgery or radiotherapy can also seriously disrupt the swallowing phases, but radiation dosage and volume is not related to the incidence, onset, or severity of dysphagia.[14] Nerve damage is another factor and perineural spread of and neck cancers can be demonstrated at autopsy in nearly 90 per cent of patients at post-mortem.[16] In life, this is often associated with dysaesthesia and pain, particularly in the territories of cranial nerves 5 and 9. Damage to cranial nerves 7, 9, 10, and 12 disturbs the pharyngeal phase of swallowing, often accompanied by aspiration.[17] Perineural vagal and sympathetic invasion combined with local fibrosis and tumour infiltration can cause severe functional dysphagia, which is indistinguishable from gross mechanical obstruction.[16] Pharyngeal and laryngeal sensory loss caused by cancer-related damage of the superior laryngeal nerve will cause silent aspiration. Other neurological and neuromuscular disorders listed in Table 1 can cause severe dysphagia, including the motor neurone diseases (e.g. amyotrophic lateral sclerosis),[6,7] Parkinson's disease,[8,18] multiple sclerosis,[9] and Huntingdon's disease. The mechanisms causing dysphagia in such conditions are complex. Mechanisms suggested in Parkinson's disease, for example, include a defect in a non-dopaminergic pathway from the medulla causing laryngeal dysmotility,[19,20] and disturbance of the oral phase due to bradykinesia.[21]

Loss of structures through surgery has varying effects. For example, hemilaryngectomy will rarely cause swallowing problems if the epiglottis is preserved, and yet a unilateral supraglottic laryngectomy is likely to result in a chronic swallowing disability.[22] Oesophageal spasm causes functional obstruction and, if intense, can cause severe central chest pain indistinguishable from ischaemic cardiac pain.[23] Spasm of the lower oesophageal sphincter or the cricopharyngeal muscle can be caused by anxiety,[24] but there is no evidence that dysphagic patients without obvious physical cause have psychological profiles that are different from patients with physical causes of dysphagia.[25] Drugs are another cause of dysphagia,[26,27] while severe functional dysphagia can occur as a rare complication of hypercalcaemia.[28]

Mucosal inflammation due to infection, radiotherapy, or chemotherapy may cause painful dysphagia (odynophagia). Candida may affect the mouth,

Table 1 Causes of dysphagia related to advanced disease

Caused by disease process	*Associated with advanced disease*
Obstruction by mass lesion in mouth, pharynx, or oesophagus	Dry mouth
Infiltration or fibrosis of walls of mouth, pharynx, or oesophagus causing reduced motility ± damage to nerve plexus	Mucosal infection of mouth, pharynx, or oesophagus (candidiasis, apthous ulceration, herpes simplex, herpes zoster, cytomegalovirus)
External compression (e.g. mediastinal tumour)	Dental caries
Perineural tumour spread	Extreme weakness (patient moribund)
Upper motor neurone damage (cerebral tumour or infarction)	Hypercalcaemia (rare)
Lower motor neurone damage (motor neurone disease, multiple sclerosis, cranial nerve palsy)	*Concurrent disease*
Motor or sensory cranial nerve palsy (tumour at base of skull, leptomeningeal infiltration, brainstem metastases or infarction)	Benign stricture
Cerebellar damage (infarction, surgery, tumour, paraneoplastic)	Reflux oesophagitis (hiatus hernia, gastric stasis)
Neuropathy (paraneoplastic)	Functional (non-ulcer) dysmotility dyspepsia
Neuromuscular dysfunction (myasthenic-myopathic syndrome, polymyositis, dermatomyositis, Parkinsonism, Huntingdon's disease)	Pain (mucosal, soft tissue, dental, bone)
Cerebral cortex damage (stroke, tumour, dementia)	Brain injury (trauma, infection, hypoxia)
Caused by treatment	*Factors that may worsen swallowing*
Surgery (loss of structure, motor loss, sensory loss, fibrosis, fistula)	Old age
Radiotherapy (fibrosis, reduced saliva, mucosal inflammation)	Lack of time to eat
Chemotherapy (mucosal inflammation)	Missing teeth
Drugs, by causing abnormal motility or dry mouth (e.g. neuroleptics, metoclopramide, anticholinergic drugs)	Poor environment
	Uninteresting, tepid food
	Insufficient staff to help
	Drowsiness
	Withdrawal (depression, fear)
	Dry mouth (anxiety)

Updated from ref. 15, with permission.

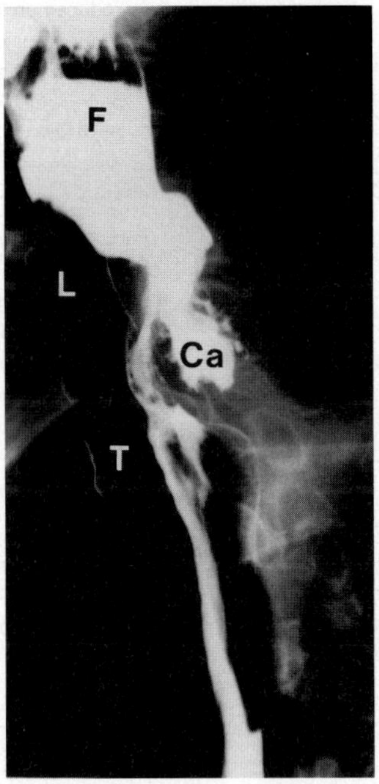

Fig. 1 Lateral view of barium swallow showing an ulcerating squamous cell carcinoma of the upper oesophagus (Ca) with poor pharyngeal emptying demonstrated by the presence of a fluid level in the pharynx (F). Laryngeal (L) and tracheal (T) aspiration of barium can be seen.

pharynx, and oesophagus and may present as a reddened mucosa, angular stomatitis, pale patches of chronically infected epithelium, or the classical white patches that leave an erythematous area when rubbed away. Oral candida is found in only 50 per cent of patients with oesophageal candidiasis.(29) The 'moth-eaten' appearances of oesophageal ulceration on barium swallow are characteristic of candida, herpes simplex, or cytomegalovirus infection. Infection in advanced cancer is usually mild, but can be severe and extensive in patients with AIDS. Painful swallowing for any reason can disrupt one or more swallowing phases sufficiently to reduce oral intake.

A number of factors can worsen or precipitate swallowing difficulties. Concurrent disease causing pain or dry mouth will cause difficulties. Brain injury can cause dysphagia and this is well recognized in stroke where anterior or periventricular white matter damage is more likely to result in aspiration.(30) Excessive drowsiness, disinterest, and weakness will result in a poor oral preparatory phase with leakage of food from the mouth, drooling, and possibly aspiration because of delayed or absent triggering of the swallowing reflex. Ageing has a number of effects that affect swallowing. Missing teeth make the oral preparation phase more difficult,(31) swallowing is slower,(10) and there is reduced sensitivity in the mouth and pharynx.(32,33) Inadequate staffing can increase the risk of dehydration in dysphagic patients,(34) while the urge to swallow can be greatly diminished by a poor environment, tepid food temperatures, or uninteresting food.

Evaluation

History

The patient's description can provide useful information (Table 2).(15) Difficulty with certain food consistencies provides some information but is far less specific than is commonly believed.(35) For example, although obstructing lesions generally produce dysphagia for solids initially with progression to liquids later, neuromuscular disorders may well cause dysphagia for both solids and liquids more or less simultaneously. In contrast to information about food consistency, localization by the patient of an obstruction is very accurate and in one series of 1000 patients, 99 per cent of patients accurately localized the anatomical site of the problem.(12) It is also important to know which head positions a patient prefers (Table 2). A detailed treatment history is essential, especially for current drugs, previous surgery, and past radiotherapy. A number of assessment tools, scales, and questionnaires have been developed to assess dysphagia.(36–43)

Examination

A basic evaluation can be carried out by the doctor and nurse but if abnormalities are found, a full assessment and further investigation should be organized by a speech and language therapist with a special interest in

Table 2 Evaluation of dysphagia: history

Information provided	Possible interpretation
Patient tilts head down during swallowing	Delayed swallowing reflex or poor laryngeal closure
Patient throws head back during swallowing	Problem with oral swallowing phase, usually due to problems with tongue movement
Difficulty with solids in triggering swallowing	Poor tongue control
Difficulty with liquids	Poor tongue control, reduced/absent swallowing reflex, severe obstruction, muscular incoordination, soft palate paralysis, or fixation
Food sticks—will indicate site	Obstruction: patient accurately localizes level of obstruction
Frequent nasal regurgitation	Palatal dysfunction
Lack of awareness where food is during swallowing	Sensory loss

Updated from ref. 15, with permission.

Table 3 Evaluation of dysphagia: examination

Observation	Possible interpretation
Stridor—'rough' wheeze from upper airway	Airway narrowing—needs urgent treatment
Abnormal mucosa (dry, ulcerated, or infected) or teeth (missing or damaged)	Mucosal dryness/pain or dental problems causing dysphagia
Leakage from mouth, drooling	Poor lip closure, reduced lip sensation, abnormal tongue movement, or reduced/absent swallowing reflex
Bites cheeks or tongue	Reduced lip or tongue sensation
Food collecting in mouth	Poor lip, buccal, or tongue control
Prolonged chewing or food collecting in vallecula or pyriform fossae	Reduced/absent swallowing reflex
Patient washes food down with a drink or pushes food in with finger	Reduced tongue control
Coughing, choking before swallowing	Laryngeal penetration due to poor tongue control or delayed or absent swallowing reflex
Coughing, choking during swallowing	Laryngeal penetration due to reduced airway protection
Poor or absent laryngeal elevation on swallowing	Poorly protected airway
Coughing, choking after swallowing	Laryngeal penetration due to reduced pharyngeal emptying, reduced laryngeal elevation, cricopharyngeus dysfunction, pharyngeal or oesophageal obstruction, or tracheo-oesophageal fistula
Voice changes	
Inability to say 'pa'	Poor lip closure
Inability to say 'ta'	Poor movement of anterior tongue
Inability to say 'ka'	Poor movement of posterior tongue
'Hot potato' voice	Vallecular tumours
'Breathy' voice or hoarseness	Recurrent laryngeal nerve palsy
Nasal escape speech	Lower motor neurone lesion
'Donald Duck' speech	Upper motor neurone lesion
Flaccid, fasciculating tongue	Lower motor neurone lesion
Small, spastic tongue	Upper motor neurone lesion
Bedside swallowing test	
Oropharyngeal transit time >1 s	Dysphagia present
'Gargle' type voice or 'bubbling' heard through stethoscope on neck	Penetration or aspiration of food/fluid into larynx
Drop in SaO_2 on pulse oximetry	Aspiration below vocal cords into airway
Unable to feel cold mirror	Sensory loss in area tested
Gag reflex	No relationship with dysphagia—not used in assessment

Updated from ref. 15, with permission.

swallowing disorders. A non-specialist examination can be done at the bedside (see Table 3). Examination includes evaluation of the relevant cranial nerves, looking for evidence of muscle weakness (e.g. drooling or leakage of food, food collecting on palate, or lateral sulci), checking for stridor, observing any jaw misalignment during chewing, assessing lip closure by rapidly repeating a syllable such as 'pa', and checking the condition of the teeth and mucosa. Anterior tongue movement is observed easily and posterior tongue movement can be checked by rapidly repeating the syllable 'ka'. Tongue strength and tone can be assessed by asking the patient to push against the examiner's gloved finger and it is generally possible to differentiate between lower motor neurone (bulbar) lesions and upper motor neurone (pseudobulbar) lesions. A laryngeal mirror can be used when checking for mucosal sensation and then used to look for food debris or a pathological condition. A further useful examination is a test swallow using consistencies that the patient finds easiest to swallow. This also allows the examiner to feel if the larynx is rising. The oropharyngeal transit time is measured from the first tongue movement to the last laryngeal movement. Times of more than 1 s are abnormal and in two studies this screening test gave a sensitivity of 80 per cent and a specificity of 54 per cent in stroke patients, and a specificity of 86 per cent in general medical patients.(44,45) It is sensitive enough to identify patients with a simple, viral sore throat.(46) Coughing or choking indicates that fluid or food has penetrated the larynx, although the absence of coughing does not exclude penetration, while its presence does not imply that laryngeal contents have been aspirated into the airway.(47) Similarly, a 'gargle' quality to the voice after swallowing suggests penetration but not aspiration, while its absence does not exclude either penetration or aspiration.(48) In contrast, if oxygen saturation (SaO_2) is monitored during swallowing using pulse oximetry, a reduction in SaO_2 after a swallow is a good indicator that fluid or food has been aspirated.(49,50) Contrary to popular belief, the presence or absence of the gag reflex does not reflect on the patient's ability to swallow.(12,51,52) In the motor neurone disorders the pharyngeal response is brisk rather than depressed.(53)

Investigation

Although examination may uncover the cause of dysphagia in the oral preparatory phase, accurate evaluation of the remaining phases is best done radiologically. For example, aspiration will be missed on clinical evaluation in 40 per cent of patients.(12) Videofluoroscopy under the direction of a swallowing therapist has become the gold standard of assessing dysphagia, but weakness, immobility, and cognitive impairment can prevent its use,(51,54) while differing protocols can limit its value.(55) Nasal endoscopy is a new alternative that can be used at the bedside and is particularly good at identifying laryngeal penetration, anatomical abnormalities, and cranial neuropathies.(54,56)

Management

Clinical decisions for dysphagia

- Is hydration and/or feeding appropriate?
- Is a complete obstruction present?
- Is nutritional support required for surgery or chemotherapy?
- Is mucosal infection or a dry mouth present?
- Could drugs be a cause?
- Is pain affecting swallowing?

- Is anti-cancer treatment indicated?
- Is peritumour oedema present?
- Is aspiration causing troublesome symptoms?
- Is dysphagia persisting?
- Is non-oral feeding needed for more than 1 month?

Is hydration and/or feeding appropriate?

Those patients with a very short prognosis (day to day deterioration or faster) are unlikely to need or want feeding and hydration by any route (see Chapter 18). With slower deterioration, non-oral hydration is appropriate in many patients with severe dysphagia. In amyotrophic lateral sclerosis nasogastric tube feeding does not improve survival or distressing symptoms, and sometimes causes new problems.(57)

The appropriateness of medically assisted feeding and hydration depends on:

1. speed of deterioration;
2. patient's opinion;
3. opinion of family/partner;
4. opinion of caring staff;
5. potential advantages of feeding and/or hydration;
6. feasibility of an alternative route;
7. potential disadvantages of the route chosen.

In cases of doubt it is often possible to delay for several days or even weeks. It is easier not to start a treatment than to stop it a short time later.

Is a complete obstruction present?

If hydration is appropriate but there is complete obstruction, non-oral hydration will be required. Parenteral nutrition is rarely appropriate in the last weeks or days of a person's life. Endoscopic dilatation of the obstruction relieves dysphagia in over half of patients but, in malignant obstructions, improvement generally lasts less than 2 weeks.(58) Endoscopic dilatation is therefore used mostly as a short-term measure before radiation, intubation, laser resection, or local injection of alcohol or cisplatin. Single-dose intraluminal radiation (brachytherapy) of oesophageal cancer has a similar initial response rate to endoscopic dilatation, but improvement is maintained for a median of about 4 months.(59) Endoscopic stenting provides another option and self-expanding metal stents are now preferred to plastic stents as they are easier to insert, stay patent for longer, and have fewer complications.(60–63) Such stents can provide effective palliation with median survival times of 4 months (range 1–24 months) when combined with laser therapy to remove any recurrent, over-growing tumour.(64) Covered expandable prostheses are better if palliating a fistula or perforation.(65)

Endoscopic laser therapy produces better relief of dysphagia than intubation,(66,67) but the median survival of 4 months is the same as with brachytherapy and metal stents.(68) Photodynamic therapy (using a laser directed at tumour previously sensitized by a systemic injection of photosensitizer) in one series of 65 patients resulted in relief of dysphagia in all patients and a similar median survival of 6 months.(69) If laser is not available, then an alternative method is to cause tumour necrosis by local injection of ethanol,(70,71) or cisplatin.(72)

Is nutritional support required for surgery or chemotherapy? (see Chapter 8.4.3)

Parenteral nutrition may be indicated before surgery or chemotherapy and PEGs are often used in oral cancer patients prior to surgery or radiotherapy or to support them over the operative period.

Is mucosal infection or a dry mouth present? (see Chapter 8.12)

The commonest mucosal infection is candidiasis. Effective treatments are ketoconazole 200 mg once daily for 5 days, or a single dose of 150 mg fluconazole, the latter being useful when compliance is difficult.(73) Persistent or recurrent candidiasis will require longer courses, that is, 14 days, and immunosuppressed patients may require long-term prophylaxis with fluconazole 50–100 mg daily.(74) Extensive herpes simplex or zoster infections should be treated promptly with systemic acyclovir 200 mg every 4 h for 5 days. Extensive apthous ulceration can be helped by tetracycline 250 mg as a 2-min mouthwash three times a day. Chlorhexidine has been recommended to improve oral hygiene,(75) but chlorhexidine causes taste alteration, can damage oral mucosa, and some randomized trials have failed to show a bene-fit in mucositis caused by treatments such chemotherapy.(76) Together with the oral discomfort that occurs on application, chlorhexidine is not a panacea in the oral care of patients with advanced disease. Thalidomide may be an alternative for persistent apthous ulceration in AIDS patients.(77)

If the cause of a dry mouth cannot be reversed, local measures are helpful, for example, petroleum jelly to the lips, iced drinks, or semi-frozen fruit juices (e.g. pineapple or cranberry), and regular mouth care. Artificial salivas (methylcellulose or porcine mucin) can help if used several times every hour. Glycerin or lemon should be avoided as the former dehydrates the mucosa and the latter soon exhausts the salivary glands. Chewing gum has been suggested as a way of stimulating saliva.(75) Pilocarpine stimulates salivation but doses need to be kept low to minimize adverse effects.(78) When patients in the same study where given a choice, they felt pilocarpine was no better than a mucin-based saliva substitute. Previous work has shown that porcine mucin was felt by patients to be no better than water.(79) It seems that what patients find most helpful are sprays containing water or cool, pleasant drinks.

Could drugs be a cause?

Drugs can cause a dry mouth (anticholinergic drugs, opioids), and occasionally oesophageal spasm (neuroleptic drugs, metoclopramide). In these circumstances, the dose should be reduced if possible or an alternative drug prescribed.

Is pain affecting swallowing?

Mucosal pain in the mouth can be eased by topical analgesics such as choline salicylate gel or benzydamine mouthwash, which are topical non-steroidal anti-inflammatory drugs with a mild local anaesthetic action. Increased local anaesthesia can be obtained with local anaesthetic lozenges or spray 15 min before eating or drinking. This is also helpful if there is oesophageal pain on swallowing. Pain caused by widespread ulceration secondary to infection, chemotherapy, or radiotherapy is eased with a mucosal protective agent such as sucralfate suspension.(80) Having excluded or treated mucosal infection, the soft tissues need to be considered, particularly in patients with head and neck cancer. The rapid onset of pain over a few hours in such patients may well be caused by infection, but with little or no outward signs. Treatment with oral flucloxacillin and metronidazole resolve the infection and the pain within 24 h. Other causes of pain affecting bone, soft tissues, or nerve are treated as described elsewhere (see Chapter 8.2).

Is anti-cancer treatment indicated?

This is most commonly intraluminal radiation.(59) Chemotherapy is sometimes helpful in patients with advanced head and neck cancers.

Is peritumour oedema present?

In the absence of infection, corticosteroids may offer the possibility of easing dysphagia by reducing luminal obstruction, extramural compression, or nerve compression. Patients with dysphagia related to head and neck tumours may respond in the short term to dexamethasone.(66) This will occur only if oedema is present, but since there is no simple way of assessing this, treatment is often empirical. Dexamethasone 8 mg daily orally or 4 mg parenterally is a typical starting dose and can be given as a single oral or subcutaneous dose. Any beneficial effect may be present only for a few days or weeks but this is helpful, for example, in a patient awaiting radiotherapy.

Is aspiration causing troublesome symptoms?

Penetration of small amounts of food or fluid into the larynx commonly occurs in dysphagia and is also seen in some people who are not dysphagic.(81) In contrast, aspiration of food or fluid past the vocal cords into the airway is not seen in healthy people, but is seen in dysphagic patients, occurring in 33 per cent of stroke patients with dysphagia.(81) Even in patients who aspirate, however, 40 per cent do so silently without clinical signs or symptoms, their aspiration only being visible with videofluoroscopy or nasal endoscopy.[12] This challenges the commonly held view that aspiration is always dangerous and life-threatening, and suggests that the airways can cope with small amounts of aspirated material. This view is supported by the observation that dysphagia is only a modest risk factor for aspiration pneumonia, and that other factors such as smoking, tube feeding, and immobility are more important.[82,83] Consequently, in advanced disease aspiration need only be of concern if it is causing symptoms such as coughing, respiratory embarrassment, or repeated chest infections.

Is dysphagia persisting?

Simple changes to feeding can be helpful (see Fig. 2). If the problem persists, and if less than 10 per cent of swallowed material is aspirated, then a swallowing therapist can advise on a wide range of treatments.[84] Table 4 gives examples of the different types of therapy that can be offered. Direct, indirect, and facilitation techniques need to be managed by a swallowing therapist, but compensatory treatment is applicable to any setting and can be instituted by a wide range of professionals. Imaginative food preparation and presentation are vital if unappetizing homogeneous brown sludge is to be avoided during each mealtime. Even soft diets can be transformed with care and imagination (Table 5). Chilled foods are pleasant and patients with neurological dysfunction find them easier to swallow. Someone with poor muscular control of the head can be helped by stabilizing the head with pillows or a lightweight chin support.[85] Patients may need help with feeding, allowing them to concentrate on swallowing, while the helper concentrates on positioning and transferring the food from plate to mouth.[86] The patient needs to be helped into a comfortable position and allowed to pause for a few minutes

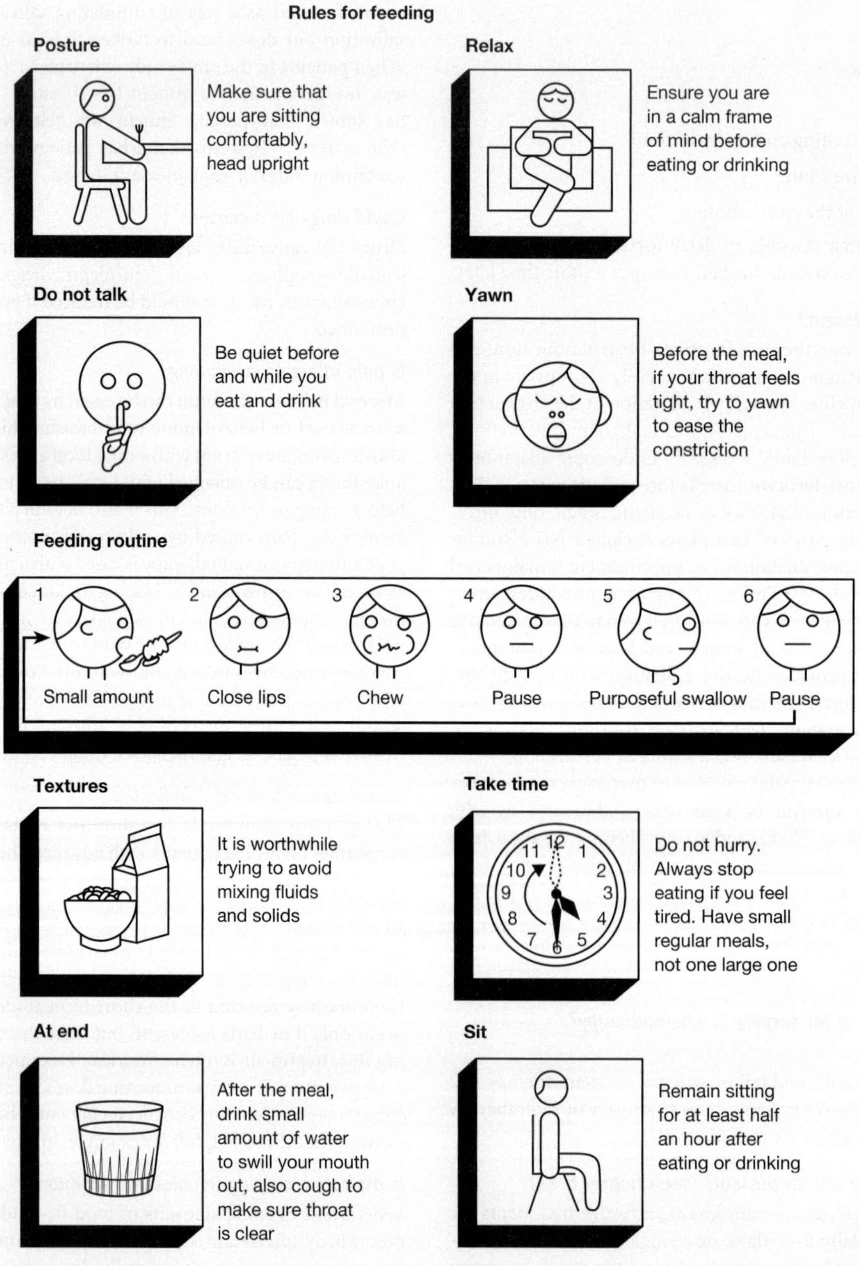

Fig. 2 Helpful hints to aid feeding in patients with dysphagia. (Reproduced with permission of Speech and Language Therapy, Frenchay Hospital, Bristol, United Kingdom.)

Table 4 Types and examples of swallowing therapy[84]

Type of therapy	Brief description	Example(s)
Facilitation techniques		
Postural changes	Alter angle of head to encourage gravity to alter the flow of food or fluid	Tilting head down to prevent premature spilling of bolus into pharynx Tilting head to the stronger side to direct bolus away from a unilateral pharyngeal paralysis
Swallowing manoeuvres	Altering the natural pattern of swallowing to facilitate a safer swallow	Multiple swallows to clear residue from laryngeal opening Supraglottic swallow (breath hold before and during swallow, followed by immediate cough or forceful exhalation of breath) to clear residue from laryngeal opening
Indirect techniques		
Strengthening and manipulation exercises	Range of motion and resistance exercises to improve muscle function	Prevention of muscle fibrosis after surgery or radiotherapy
Direct techniques		
Sensory stimulation	Used to enhance sensory input (temperature, taste, and pressure) prior to swallowing	Used in patients with reduced sensation or coordination
Compensatory treatment		
Food characteristics	Alteration of texture, taste, temperature, and amount of food and fluid	Adjusting textures and amounts to individuals, whilst maintaining taste, variation, and attractiveness of food and drink
Time and environment	Ensuring an environment appropriate for the individual	Providing time, whilst ensuring variety of temperatures in an environment that is dedicated to feeding
Positioning and help	Ensuring posture is suitable and sufficient help is available	Stabilizing the head with pillows if head control is poor Ensuring sufficient staff to help patients who cannot feed themselves

before eating (Fig. 2). Spectacles and hearing aids should be in place and in good working order. Dentures should also be in place, even if chewing is not required. The helper should face the patient so that they can see each other. Small amounts of food or drink should be given slowly. The technique advised by the swallowing therapist is then followed and its effect observed.

Is non-oral feeding needed for more than 1 month?

If the oropharyngeal transit time is longer than 10 s, or if more than 10 per cent of swallowed is aspirated, non-oral feeding is often the best option. The indications and contraindications for non-oral feeding are shown in Table 6.

Standard nasogastric tubes are uncomfortable for more than a few days, whereas fine bore tubes are well tolerated for a week or more but are more difficult to replace if displaced. Contrary to common belief, nasogastric tubes do not protect patients from aspiration.[87,88] Nasogastric tubes may even worsen aspiration by markedly increasing oropharyngeal secretions.[57] This may explain why survival was no better in patients receiving nasogastric tube feeding in a study of 1386 patients over 65 years with cognitive impairment.[87] In contrast, another large study suggested that tube feeding did modestly increase survival in nursing home residents, but patients were not all cognitively impaired and initially less disabled than in the previous study.[89] This suggests that early use of non-oral feeding can be helpful, but when patients suffer from multiple clinical problems nasogastric feeding offers few advantages.

Parenteral feeding has few indications and several contraindications that invariably preclude its use in end-stage disease. Because of these problems there has been a search for better alternatives. A pharyngostomy is probably the simplest to insert and maintain,[90] but has never been widely accepted, cannot be used in luminal obstructions of the pharynx or oesophagus, and is unsatisfactory for patients with motor neurone disease.[91] Consequently, a gastrostomy tube is now commonly used when non-oral feeding and hydration is needed for more than a few weeks. A tube can be inserted either endoscopically under sedation and local anaesthetic (percutaneous endoscopic gastrostomy—PEG)[92,93] or percutaneously under fluoroscopic control after distending the stomach with air or carbon dioxide through a temporary nasogastric tube (percutaneous fluoroscopic gastrostomy—PFG).[94,95] Gastrostomies are usually well tolerated and feeding and hydration through a gastrostomy improves nutrition more effectively than the nasogastric route.[96] Complications are usually limited to skin infection, tube blockage, or tube displacement, but more serious problems such as peritonitis can occur.[97] PEG insertion can be done as a day case.[98] However, it is common practice for patients to remain in hospital for 4–5 days until their bowels are coping with the increased nutrition and the patient and carers are confident of managing feeds and the support of a PEG team is invaluable in ensuring success and providing follow-up. Patients with a gastrostomy are easily managed at home.[99]

Table 5 Tomato bavrois with yellow pepper coulis

Contents	
Beef tomatoes	5
Caradom	1
Whipped cream	140 ml
Beaten egg whites	2
Chopped fresh basil leaves	5
Sheets of leaf gelatine	4
Maxijul powder	60 g
Yellow peppers	2
Butter	30 g
Pinch of salt and pepper	

Nutritional content: 169 kcal, 3 g protein, 11 g fat

Instructions

1. Remove the inside of the tomato
2. Puree the inside of the tomato with caradom, Maxijul, and chopped basil
3. Warm the pureed tomato and basil in a pan; then add gelatine
4. When the mixture is nearly set, add whipped cream and beaten egg whites
5. Gently mix without beating, and then pipe into the tomato skin
6. To make the yellow pepper coulis:
   - chop the yellow pepper
   - place in a pan with the butter
   - place the lid on the pan
   - cook gently for 1–2 min until tender
7. Place the tomato on the yellow pepper coulis, and then garnish with fresh basil leaves

David Taylor and Neil Bosomworth, St Oswald's Hospice, Newcastle-upon-Tyne, United Kingdom, 1994.

Table 6 Indications and contraindications for choosing a non-oral feeding route

All non-oral routes	Parenteral route (peripheral long line, central venous line)	Enteral route (nasogastric tube, pharyngostomy, gastrostomy, jejunostomy)
Indications		
Oral + pharyngeal transit time >10 s	Complete pharyngeal or oesophageal obstruction	Long-term use (>1 week)
Failure to modify swallowing technique during treatment to improve muscle control	Short term use (<1 week)	
	Anatomical or functional bowel loss	
Nutritional support for surgery or chemotherapy		
Contraindications		
Rapid deterioration	Presence of sepsis	Nasogastric tube: nasal, pharyngeal, or oesophageal obstruction; cosmetic appearance
Dysphagia due to exhaustion, debility or weakness caused by malignancy	Limited or no access to biochemical monitoring	Pharyngostomy: recently irradiated neck or local tumour
	Limited or no access to a parenteral nutrition team	
Psychological need of staff or family to provide 'active treatment'	Poor home circumstances	Gastrostomy: gastric tumour
	Long-term use (>1 week)	
	Superior vena caval obstruction	

Based on ref. 9, with permission.

Other considerations

The psychological impact of dysphagia can be profound. This is not surprising because from childhood we are taught that we must eat if we are to keep well and strong, making dysphagia a tangible threat. Anxiety, anger, fear, and depression may result or be exacerbated and will need support and management (Chapter 8.17). Non-oral hydration and feeding can cause additional problems for the patient and family—both resistance to starting or distress at stopping. The patient's choices come first, followed by sensitive communication with partner and relatives, and between staff. Problems with deciding on the right treatment are usually either due to uncertainty about prognosis or a failure of communication. The law is always a last resort for situations where there is honest uncertainty about the right way forward (Chapter 3.5).

If the patient cannot swallow saliva adequately, drooling is likely to be an embarrassing and troublesome problem. Anticholinergic drugs are helpful and transdermal hyoscine (scopolamine) hydrobromide is convenient, delivering 500 μg over 3 days. Radiation of the salivary glands also helps; 4–5 Gy are given initially, repeated if necessary 3 weeks later. In practice, however, this is rarely indicated.

It is inevitable that nutritional deficiencies are a risk in these patients. There is little information on the effect of nutritional deficiencies in patients with terminal illness. Consequently, we do not know which specific deficiencies need to be corrected. Until more data are available, it is necessary to rely on advice from a dietician/nutritionist (see Chapters 8.4.3 and 15.3). It is important, however, to avoid a rigid scientific approach which places major burdens on the patient in terms of nutritional demands and/or financial cost.

Key points for dysphagia

- Swallowing can be disrupted by changes in mucosal health, muscle control, sensory changes, and anatomical disturbances.
- Dysphagia is commonest in mucosal damage, cancers of the larynx, hypopharynx, and oesophagus, and in a range of neurological conditions.
- Patients accurately localize obstructions, but food consistency preferences is less useful.
- A simple bedside screening examination can be carried out by any professional, but the gag reflex does not reflect the ability to swallow.
- Further examination and investigations should be managed by a speech therapist specializing in swallowing problems.
- Clinical decisions can be used to guide management and help tailor treatment to the individual patient.

Dyspepsia

Definition

The Greek term dyspepsia means bad (dys) digestion (peptin) and is often linked with the Latin-derived term indigestion, an equally vague term. Over the past 25 years, new definitions of dyspepsia have emerged at the rate of almost one each year.(100) This reflects the difficulty of defining a term that describes a syndrome whose symptoms share very different pathologies. There is now agreement that dyspepsia is *not* air swallowing, biliary pain, chronic pancreatitis, or irritable bowel disease—all conditions that in the past have been given a 'dypepsia' label. Some believe that gastro-oesophageal reflux disease (GORD) should not be considered as dyspepsia,(100) but this view is not so clear in other classifications.(101)

The current view is that dyspepsia is a syndrome whose symptoms arise in the upper gastrointestinal tract and are unrelated to defaecation.(100) Dyspepsia encompasses a range of symptoms that vary in intensity and onset and are not present in every patient or in every episode, although upper abdominal pain is the commonest feature (see Table 7).(101) There is still disagreement about what should be included in a classification of dyspepsia, but from studies of patients' symptoms there are three distinct types of dyspepsia (Table 7) to which can be added gastro-oesophageal reflux:

1. Structural (organic) dyspepsia for which a structural change can be demonstrated, for example, a gastric ulcer. This type of dyspepsia is due to acid-related disease of the upper gastrointestinal tract.
2. Functional, non-ulcer dyspepsia, which is due to dysmotility of the upper gastrointestinal tract, of which there are two distinct types:
   - gastric/duodenal dysmotility;
   - oesophageal dysmotility.
3. GORD due to reflux of gastric contents into the oesophagus sufficient to cause mucosal damage and symptoms.(184)

Incidence

Dyspepsia is common,(102) but the incidence depends on the criteria used to define this syndrome. In one survey, 42 per cent of patients attending a community clinic were identified as having dyspepsia by their general practitioners, but a validated dyspepsia questionnaire agreed with the general practitioner's opinion in little more than half of cases.(103) When dyspeptic patients were selected using a questionnaire this gave a prevalence of 12 per cent.(104) In the general population, of those fully investigated, about one-third had a peptic ulcer, one-third had no obvious abnormality, and one-third had a variety of other diagnoses.(105) Chronic duodenal ulceration occurs in 10–15 per cent of the general population.(106) The risk of ulcer complications among all non-steroidal anti-inflammatory drug

Table 7 Symptoms of structural and functional dyspepsia (correlation of symptoms with three types of dyspepsia)

Structural (organic) dyspepsia	Functional (non-ulcer) dyspepsia	
Acid-related dyspepsia	**Gastric/duodenal dysmotility dyspepsia**	**Oesophageal dysmotility dyspepsia**
High positive correlations, i.e. symptom likely to be present (%)		
Symptoms listed in descending order of correlation score, i.e. from highest to lowest		
Epigastric pain (63)	Nausea (32)	Pain after meals (36)
Pain relieved by antacids (37)	Morning vomiting (5)	Dysphagia (3)
Acid regurgitation (42)	Pain relieved by vomiting (13)	
Heartburn (26)		
Pain in the night (41)		
High negative correlations, i.e. symptom likely to be absent (%)		
Other abdominal pain (25)	—	Pain relived by food (29)
Low correlations, i.e. symptom likely to be present for reasons other than dyspepsia (%)		
Symptoms listed in descending order of correlation score, i.e. from highest to lowest		
Pain relieved by food (29)	Pain in the morning (17)	Weight loss (4)
Upper abdominal pain (36)	Weight loss (4)	Heartburn (26)
Pain relieved by stool or flatus (25)	Loose stools (23)	Nausea (32)
Pain relived by vomiting (13)	Heartburn (26)	Pain relived by antacids (37)
Loose stools (23)	Pain relived by antacids (37)	Pain in the night (41)
Bloating (42)	Pain in the night (41)	Loose stools (23)

Prepared from data in ref. 101.

Percentages are from a survey of 7270 unselected patients presenting to general practitioners with dyspepsia.

(NSAID) users is between 25 and 35 per cent with 1200 deaths each year in the United Kingdom from non-aspirin NSAIDs.(107) Functional dyspepsia (i.e. dyspepsia without apparent organic cause) is seen in about 25 per cent of the normal population and is therefore common in patients with advanced disease. It may account for up to 70 per cent of patients presenting with symptoms of dyspepsia.(108)

Mechanisms and causes

There are many causes of dyspepsia in advanced disease (Table 8).

Structural (organic), acid-related dyspepsia

The end-result in this type of dyspepsia is mucosal damage, either because of direct damage (e.g. radiotherapy), compromised mucosal protection (e.g. NSAIDs), or delayed mucosal healing (e.g. corticosteroids).

Non-steroidal anti-inflammatory drugs

NSAIDs are the most widely reported drug cause of adverse effects and they have been described as representing a major health problem.(107) The mechanism of NSAID damage to the gastric and duodenal mucosa is by inhibiting the enzyme cyclo-oxygenase-1 (COX-1) that synthesizes prostaglandins E_2 and I_2 that are normally protective to the mucosa.(107,109) There is also some evidence that NSAIDs may slow the healing of existing ulcers,(110) and this may be mediated by inhibition of cyclo-oxygenase-2 (COX-2).(111) Most NSAIDs inhibit both enzymes, although some such as diclofenac preferentially inhibit COX-2, while newer NSAIDs are specific COX-2 inhibitors. These actions are a systemic, not a local effect, so that remote administration of a NSAID does not reduce the risk.(112) A paradoxical and potentially dangerous effect is that the anti-inflammatory action of NSAIDs can mask ulcer pain, delaying diagnosis and treatment. There is a linear increase in the risk of ulcer complications as the dose of NSAID increases,(113) and a difference in risk between NSAIDs with ibuprofen and diclofenac having approximately one-fourth of the risk of piroxicam and ketoprofen.(114) In contrast, age and *Helicobacter pylori* infection appear to be independent and less important risk factors. The newer, selective COX-2 NSAIDs produce fewer clinically significant ulcers,(115) but still share some of the adverse effects of non-selective NSAIDs such as salt and water retention and delayed ulcer healing.(110,116)

Table 8 Causes of dyspepsia in advanced disease

Caused by the disease process	Associated with advanced disease
Acid related	*Acid related*
Mucosal damage, e.g. gastric carcinoma	Mucosal damage, e.g. oesophageal candidiasis or CMV
Excessive acid production (→ ulceration), e.g. gastrinoma in Zollinger–Ellison syndrome	
Dysmotility	*Dysmotility*
Small stomach capacity, e.g. large stomach cancer or massive ascites	Minimal food and fluid intake
Gatroparesis (e.g. paraneoplastic autonomic neuropathy)	Depression/anxiety
Caused by treatment	**Concurrent disease**
Acid related	*Acid related*
Physical irritant (→ gastritis), e.g. iron, metronidazole, tranexamic acid	Chronic peptic ulcer disease
Loss of mucosal protection (→ gastropathy), e.g. NSAIDs	*H. pylori* infection
Delayed mucosal healing, e.g. corticosteroids, NSAIDs	Gastro-oesophageal reflux disease (GORD)
Radiotherapy to lumbar spine or epigastrium (→ mucosal damage)	*Dysmotility*
Dysmotility	Functional (non-ulcer) dyspepsia
Postsurgical, e.g. gastrectomy	Alcoholism
Delayed gastric emptying, e.g. anticholinergics, opioids, cisplatin	Uraemia
Reduced tone of lower oesophageal sphincter	Diabetes mellitus

Corticosteroids

Evidence suggests that the conventional view that corticosteroids cause ulceration can be attributed to the risks due to concurrent use of NSAIDs.(117,118) Although this is a view that is still considered uncertain and controversial,[119] the concurrent use of a corticosteroid in doses equivalent to 10 mg or more of prednisolone per day increases the risk of ulcer haemorrhage by a factor of nearly 15.[117]

Peptic ulcer disease

Although NSAIDs can cause acute ulceration, there is much less evidence of their role in chronic ulceration. The strongest causal link with peptic ulceration is *H. pylori* infection.[120]

Functional (non-ulcer) dysmotility dyspepsia

This type of dyspepsia has no relationship to *H. pylori* infection,[120,121] but there is evidence of oesophageal and gastric transit delay.[122] Most cases of squashed stomach syndrome[1] and cancer associated dyspepsia syndrome[123] are probably examples of dysmotility exacerbated by opioid-induced delayed gastric emptying and/or gross hepatomegaly and/or gross ascites. A few cancer patients complain of marked early satiety (a sensation that the stomach if full soon after eating) and/or other dyspeptic symptoms without any obvious predisposing cause.[124] In cancer, this probably relates to paraneoplastic visceral autonomic neuropathy,[125] but it may also be a mechanism in non-cancer patients.[126] There is often associated evidence of impaired autonomic control of the cardiovascular system mani-festing, for example, as postural hypotension.[126,127] Many drugs have an adverse effect on lower oesophageal sphincter tone and the use of morphine and other opioids may lead to reflux secondary to delayed gastric emptying. Lower oesophageal tone can be decreased by alcohol, nicotine, caminatives (mint, anise, dill), anticholinergics, meperidine, benzodiazepines, nitrates and calcium channel blockers; and can be increased by antacids, prokinetic drugs (metoclopramide, domperidone), and parasympathomimetics (e.g. bethanechol). Psychiatric disorders, mainly depression and anxiety, have been observed in over half of patients with functional oesophageal dysmotility dyspepsia, rising to nearly 80 per cent if pain was absent as a feature, suggesting the possibility that long-term distress, anxiety, and depression can influence functional dyspepsia symptoms.[128] Chronic alcoholism and uraemia are two further conditions that have been shown to reduced gastric activity,[129,130] and both are known to be associated with dyspepsia.

Gastro-oesophageal reflux disease

While some reflux is normal, repeated exposure of the lower oesophagus to gastric contents has been considered to be reflux disease once mucosal damage occurs that can be visualized on endoscopy.[131] Most reflux occurs after food during the day, but the change to severe oesophagitis is accelerated by nocturnal reflux of acidic gastric contents.[131] However, the symptoms of GORD do not equate with endoscopic evidence of oesophagitis is suggested,[184] and this may explain the disagreement over its inclusion as a cause of dyspepsia. GORD therefore seems to be a syndrome consisting of classic symptoms of heartburn (especially on bending and lying flat) and epigastric pain, with atypical symptoms of vomiting, dental enamel erosion, cardiac pain, respiratory symptoms (e.g. nocturnal postprandial asthma), and ear, nose and throat problems (e.g. hoarseness).[184]

Evaluation

A study in 7270 patients with abdominal symptoms showed three distinct symptom patterns relating to dyspepsia (Table 7).[101] Structural, acid-related dyspepsia was most likely to be accompanied by pain restricted to the epigastrium, pain relief with antacids, acid regurgitation, heartburn, and pain at night. Two functional (non-ulcer) types of dysmotility were identified. Gastric and/or duodenal dysmotility had nausea, together with vomiting that occurred in the morning and relieved any pain. Oesophageal dysmotility had pain after meals (but not relieved by food) and dysphagia as the main features. Other symptoms were present, but showed a low correlation with any one type of dyspepsia. GORD was not included in this study, but its main features of heartburn, regurgitation, and occasionally dysphagia (due to a stricture or mucosal oedema) overlap with the symptoms of structural dyspepsia and oesophageal dysmotility dyspepsia.[131]

It is important to differentiate between these conditions because the treatment differs. Careful history-taking and clinical examination generally indicate which type is predominant. Investigations are now reserved for patients who have not responded to initial treatment with antacids of antisecretory drugs.[185] The most important investigation is to test for *H. Pylori* infection by laboratory serum immunoabsorbant assay, stool antigen test, or ^{13}C-urea breath test. Endoscopy is needed if alarm symptoms are present (see below), symptoms persist, or the *H. pylori* test is positive. Barium studies are necessary only in a few patients.

Management

General

As always, treatment begins with explanation. There may be need for advice on diet, smoking, and alcohol. The causal role, if any, of medication should be discussed. Some patients keep over-the-counter proprietary 'indigestion' tablets or mixture in the home. The use of these for occasional dyspepsia can be supported provided the discomfort is relieved. One remedy in the United Kingdom, however, contains aspirin (Alka-Seltzer) and should be discouraged.

Clinical decisions for dyspepsia

- Are there any alarm symptoms?
- Do the symptoms suggest acid-related dyspepsia?
- Do the symptoms suggest a dysmotility dyspepsia?
- Is the dyspepsia persisting?

Are there any alarm symptoms?

A number of symptoms should prompt urgent admission to hospital for investigation:

- rapid clinical deterioration;
- persistent vomiting causing dehydration or electrolyte disturbance;
- vomiting fresh or altered blood (bleeding ulcer or severe gastritis);
- malaena (upper gastrointestinal haemorrhage);
- persistent and worsening pain (perforation or other intra-abdominal crisis);
- severe dysphagia (oesophageal obstruction).

Some patients will be too ill from their advanced disease to benefit from hospital admission, while others will choose not to be treated. These patients will require adequate analgesia, antiemetics, comfort, and company for their last days and hours (see Chapter 18).

Do the symptoms suggest acid-related dyspepsia?

If the features for acid-related dyspepsia in Table 7 are present then the following actions need to be taken.

Any existing ulceration or mucosal damage needs to be treated and a recent systematic review supports the use of antacid proton pump inhibitors in dyspepsia.[132] Omeprazole 20 mg or lansoprazole 30 mg once daily are both effective in treating chronic peptic ulceration and NSAID ulceration. Higher doses can be used for resistant ulceration. Sucralfate is a mucosal protective agent that is effective at both preventing and healing peptic ulceration,[133] including NSAID-induced dyspepsia and ulceration.[134] It is also an efficient haemostatic agent that will reduce or stop gastric bleeding.[135] Of the two commonly available antisecretory H_2-receptor antagonists, ranitidine is preferable to cimetidine because the likelihood of drug interactions is much less. An initial dose of 300 mg at bedtime for 2 weeks followed by 150 mg at bedtime is generally sufficient. Cimetidine (but not ranitidine) inhibits methadone metabolism and on occasion this has resulted in respiratory depression and coma.[136]

Drug medication needs to be reviewed to stop or change the formulation of physical irritants such as iron. If the patient is taking an NSAID then several options are available:

1. Start a preventative drug. Omeprazole 20 mg once daily has been shown to be more effective than misoprostol 400 μg 12-hourly in preventing NSAID ulceration.[137] However, the same study showed that for gastric erosions, misoprostol was more effective. Misoprostol sometimes causes diarrhoea, but this has the advantage that it can be used as a 'co-laxative' in constipated patients. H_2-receptor antagonists prevent NSAID-related duodenal ulceration, but they do not prevent NSAID-related gastric ulceration.[138]
2. Find an alternative NSAID that is less irritant—patients who experience dyspepsia with flurbiprofen, for example, may not with diflunisal or naproxen, or vice versa.
3. Reduce the NSAID dose.
4. Changing to a shorter-acting drug such as ibuprofen.
5. Prescribing a physical mucosal protective agent such as sucralfate.
6. Substitute regular paracetamol.

Do the symptoms suggest a dysmotility dyspepsia?

If the features for dysmotility dyspepsia in Table 7 are present then a prokinetic drug needs to be started.[139] Tumour-related gastroparesis also benefits from a prokinetic.[140,141] The choice lies between metoclopramide (dopamine antagonist and 5-HT_4 agonist) and domperidone (dopamine antagonist).[142] All trigger a cholinergic system in the myenteric plexus. Despite its dual mechanism of action, metoclopramide is not more potent than domperidone when used in standard doses, that is, 10 mg 6–8 hourly.[143,144]

A review of the drugs taken may reveal causes of reduced motility. It may be possible to stop replacement of anticholinergic drugs with alternatives (e.g. tricyclic antidepressant to a serotonin selective reuptake inhibitor antidepressant). Morphine and other opioids impede the release of neuronal acetylcholine, and slow gastric emptying. Metoclopramide 10 mg partly and cisapride completely corrects this,[145] but cisapride has now been withdrawn because of its effect of prolonging the QT interval. Data are not available for domperidone. The maximum plasma concentration of morphine after slow-release 20 mg is little affected by metoclopramide 10 mg.[146] Paradoxically, sedation was noted after metoclopramide[146] suggesting that metoclopramide may have its own central sedative effect.

If dyspepsia is associated with a small stomach capacity, patients should be advised to separate their main fluid from their main solid intake, and to eat 'small and often', that is, take five or six small meals/snacks during the day rather than two or three big meals. Patients with a small stomach capacity may benefit from an antiflatulant after meals to help clear space in a relatively overfull stomach. An example of a defoaming antiflatulent is silica activated dimethicone/simethicone as in the proprietary preparations Asilone and Maolox Plus.[147]

Is the dyspepsia persisting?

Other causes of mucosal damage need to be considered. Malignant ulceration will cause pain and may either need a mucosal protective agent such as sucralfate, or a local anaesthetic such as oxetacaine (in the antacid preparation Mucaine). Mucosal damage due to infection such as candida, CMV, or herpes can be extensive and will need specific antimicrobial treatment.

GORD also needs to be considered. An antacid containing simethicone is superior to a plain antacid in the management of reflux oesophagitis.[148] Proton pump inhibitors are effective for treatment and maintenance of acid reflux.[149] If bile salts are being refluxed then hydrotalcite (magnesium aluminium carbonate hydrate) is a naturally occurring antacid that reversibly binds bile acids but needs an acid medium, so would be much less effective in combination with proton pump inhibitors or after gastrectomy.[150] At higher bile acid concentrations, cholestyramine is more efficacious than hydrotalcite.[151] No dose regimen for this condition has been established but it is suggested that 2 g (half a sachet) four times a day (after meals and at bedtime) might be tried.[152] There is a likelihood of steatorrhoea and, if treatment is long continued, supplements of fat-soluble vitamins A, D, E, and K should be considered.

Key points on dyspepsia

- Dyspepsia is a vague term, but the current view is that it consists of two types: acid-related causes visible on endoscopy and abnormal motility of the upper gastrointestinal tract.
- Gastro-oesophageal reflux disease is now considered to be a separate condition, but its symptoms overlap those of dyspepsia.
- NSAIDs are a major cause of dyspepsia.
- Alarm symptoms (clinical deterioration, bleeding, severe dysphagia, or persistent pain) should prompt urgent admission, unless they are too ill from their advanced disease or they choose not to receive further treatment.
- Acid-related dyspepsia is best treated with a proton pump inhibitor.
- The risk of NSAID ulceration is reduced most by proton pump inhibitors—H_2 antagonists do not prevent gastric ulceration.
- Dysmotility dyspepsia is best treated by a prokinetic such as metoclopramide.
- If dyspepsia persists consider mucosal ulceration, mucosal infection, or gastro-oesophageal reflux.

Hiccup

Definition

Hiccup is a pathological respiratory reflex characterized by spasm of one or both sides of the diaphragm, resulting in sudden inspiration and closure of the glottis. Accessory muscles of respiration (anterior scalene, intercostal, abdominal) are occasionally involved.[153]

Incidence

Occasional hiccup is such a common human experience that it only warrants designation as a symptom when it is severe and intractable.[154] Over a 28-year period at the Mayo Clinic, 220 patients reported hiccup lasting for more than 2 days.[155] The incidence of troublesome hiccup in terminal disease is not known. Children are more prone to hiccups than adults and in one series of 200 children premedicated with midazolam prior to minor surgery, 22 per cent developed hiccups.[156] It shows a circadian rhythm, being more common in the evening.[157]

Mechanisms and causes

In the Mayo clinic series,[155] 82 per cent of those with hiccups were men. Of the 220 patients with hiccup, 66 per cent had medical problems, 22 per cent were diagnosed as having a psychological cause, and 18 per cent were postoperative. Specific diagnoses included cerebrovascular and coronary heart disease (20 per cent), hiatus hernia (15 per cent), duodenal ulcer (5 per cent), and metabolic disturbances (5 per cent), which were mainly diabetes mellitus and uraemia. Many had two concurrent disorders. In terminal disease, clinical experience suggests that gastric distension is the commonest cause. Other relatively common causes include diaphragmatic irritation, and toxicity (uraemia or infection). Less common causes include phrenic nerve irritation and CNS tumour. Hiccup is occasionally the presenting symptom of neoplasms of the brain stem and oesophagus.[158,159] Persistent hiccup occurs, therefore, in association with one or more of many diseases (Table 9). In addition, a wide variety of drugs have been reported as causing hiccup, with some of the same drugs being reported to cure hiccup (Table 10).

Hiccup is generally considered to be pathological because it appears to serve no useful function.[160] Because of an association with eating, it has been suggested that hiccup may serve to shift food lodged in the oesophagus.[161] The relationship of hiccup to gastric distension, however, probably explains this association. Hiccup appears to be a reflex that is not under direct cortical control and there is evidence that it penetrates all stages of sleep, although it is modified by different sleep stages.[157,162] The fact that the pharynx is the cross-over point for both air and food/fluid suggests powerful mechanisms exist to favour only one at a time. This 'singleness of action' was proposed over 75 years ago[163] and more recently it has been suggested that a failure of this control is the cause for hiccup.[157] This theory suggests that the brainstem complex which closes the glottis is never activated at the same time as the brainstem complex which stops respiration—one is inhibited while the other is activated and vice versa. In pathological situations the two are activated together. This hypothesis is supported by two observations: (a) the two complexes are next to each other in the dorsal part of the lower medulla;[157] and (b) damage to the part of the medulla containing these two complexes can result in severe and intractable hiccup.[164–167] The reported benefits of drugs that reduce CNS excitation such as benzodiazepines and anticonvulsants suggest that they are suppressing an abnormal reciprocating circuit between the two centres.[157] The reflex arc for hiccup is more extensive however:[157,168)]

1. *From periphery to centre (afferent pathway):* vagus nerve, phrenic nerve, or thoracic sympathetic fibres.
2. *The central connections:* the inspiratory and glottis control centres in the posterior lower medulla. In addition, there may be connections to the phrenic nerve nuclei, reticular formation, and hypothalamus.
3. *From centre to periphery (efferent pathway):* primarily the phrenic nerve to diaphragm. Occasional patients continue to hiccup despite surgical section of both phrenic nerves.[155] In these patients, the efferent pathway will involve the accessory muscles of respiration.

The receptors involved in this reflex arc are not known, but the nature of the drugs that both cause and treat hiccups (Table 10) suggest that dopamine, serotonin, opioid, calcium channel, and GABA pathways may be involved.[169]

Evaluation

There is no difficulty recognizing the presence of persistent hiccups, although only the patient can decide how troublesome it is to them. Rarely, hiccup is a major cause of distress,[170] interrupting talking, eating, and sleeping, and resulting in weight loss, exhaustion, anxiety, and depression. In such situations treatable causes need to be found. Knowing the past surgical history and the current extent of any tumour from examination or recent scans can help identify the possibility of local pressure or damage to the vagus nerve, phrenic nerve, or to the lower medulla. Symptoms of acid-related dyspepsia (Table 7) may identify a gastritis, or symptoms suggesting GORD. A history of dysphagia, or pain on swallowing (odynophagia), may suggest oesophageal mucosal damage (infection, tumour), oesophageal dysmotility dyspepsia, or physical obstruction. Feeling full after only a little food (early satiety), epigastric fullness, and heartburn suggest gastric distension, while vomiting with brief or little nausea (together with relief after vomiting) suggests reduced gastric emptying. Chest examination and a bedside urine test will check for chest or urine infections, while testing for faecal occult blood in the faeces will check for upper gastrointestinal bleeding. An electrocardiogram will help to identify cardiac ischaemia. Blood biochemistry will check for causes such as hyponatraemia, hypocalcaemia, uraemia, and myocardial infarction. In advanced disease, it is unusual to carry out more complex investigations for hiccup.

Management

Clinical decisions for hiccup

- Are the hiccups troublesome to the patient?
- Is infection present?
- Is a drug the cause?
- Is a biochemical cause present?
- Is peritumour oedema a likely cause?
- Are the hiccups persisting?

Are the hiccups troublesome to the patient?

Hiccups can be mild and intermittent and may respond to simple physical treatments. Stimulation of the pharynx with a plastic or rubber suction

Table 9 Selected causes of hiccups in advanced disease[154,155]

Caused by the disease process	Associated with advanced disease
Irritation of the vagus nerve	*Irritation of the vagus nerve*
Hepatomegaly	Pneumonia
Intra-abdominal tumour	Bowel obstruction
Oesophageal tumour	Oesophageal irritation (e.g. infection, stent)
Prostatic cancer	Gastrointestinal bleeding
Irritation of the phrenic nerve	Hydronephrosis
Mediastinal tumour or sarcoid	Urinary tract infection
Tumour involving diaphragm	*Irritation of the phrenic nerve*
Cervical tumour	Pleurisy or empyema
Central nervous system	*Central nervous system*
Intracranial tumours	Encephalitis
Brainstem lesions (tumour, infarct, multiple sclerosis)	Toxic (renal failure)
	Hyponatraemia
	Psychological
Caused by treatment	**Concurrent disease**
Irritation of the vagus nerve	*Irritation of the vagus nerve*
Surgery	Pancreatitis
Gastric distension	Oesophageal reflux
Gastritis	Oesophageal obstruction
Irritation of the phrenic nerve	Coronary occlusion
Surgery	*Irritation of the phrenic nerve*
	Subphrenic abscess
Central nervous system	*Central nervous system*
Drugs (e.g. corticosteroids)	Basilar arterial insufficiency
Hypocalcaemia (e.g. due to bisphosphonates)	Head Injury
Hypocapnia (e.g. due to opioids)	Meningitis
	Toxic (alcohol)
	Multiple sclerosis

Table 10 Drug causes and treatments of hiccup

Reported drug causes of hiccup	Reported drug treatments of hiccup
Corticosteroids (dexamethasone, prednisolone, methylprednisolone)	Anticonvulsants (carbamazepine, gabapentin, valproate)
Chemotherapeutic drugs (cisplatin, etoposide)	Calcium channel blockers (nifedipine, nimodipine)
Dopamine antagonists (perphenazine)	Corticosteroids (dexamethasone, prednisolone, methylprednisolone)
Megestrol acetate	Dopamine antagonists (chlorpromazine, haloperidol, droperidol)
Methyldopa	Ketamine
Nicotine	Marijuana
Opioids (diamorphine, hydrocodone)	SSRI antidepressants (sertraline)
Skeletal muscle relaxants (chlordiazepoxide, diazepam, midazolam)	Skeletal muscle relaxants (chlordiazepoxide, baclofen, midazolam)

catheter was successful in the treatment of hiccup in 84 out of 85 patients, 65 of whom were anaesthetized.[171] Stimulation of the pharynx by an oral catheter is equally effective. The nasal route is better tolerated in conscious patients.[172] Nebulized saline every 4 h has been used successfully in one patient whose hiccup failed to respond to various drugs.[173] Palatal massage is also successful in stopping hiccup.[174] A cotton-wool 'bob' is inserted into the mouth and used to massage the anterior soft palate in the midline for about 1 min. Other 'folk' remedies involve pharyngeal stimulation such as the rapid ingestion of two heaped teaspoons of granulated sugar, the rapid ingestion of two glasses of liqueur, swallowing dry bread, swallowing crushed ice, drinking from the wrong side of a cup, or a cold key dropped down the collar of one's shirt or blouse.[175] Other remedies such as breath holding and rebreathing into a bag are also physiological since the resultant hypercapnia has a central depressant effect and blocks the central component of the reflex.[176] Deep breathing and chest physiotherapy also may disrupt the repetitive diaphragmatic spasms.

If the patient is very distressed by the hiccups,[170] then some interim intervention is needed. Titrated parenteral midazolam is effective,[177] starting with 1 mg intravenously or 2.5 mg subcutaneously and repeated at 2-min intervals for the intravenous route and 15-min intervals for the subcutaneous route until the hiccups settle, but short of producing sedation. The midazolam can be continued as a continuous subcutaneous infusion using doses of 30–120 mg/24 h.[177] This then gives time to find a reversible cause or an alternative, oral treatment.

Is infection present?

Infections in the chest, urine, or affecting the oesophageal mucosa are treated conventionally with appropriate antimicrobials. For oesophageal mucosal damage, pain can be helped with local anaesthetic lozenges or spray, 15 min before eating or drinking.

Is a drug the cause?

The onset of hiccups after starting a new drug (taking into account the time for that drug to reach a steady blood level—usually 3 half-lives) suggests that drug as a cause and a therapeutic trial of stopping the drug is worthwhile. Some drugs have been reported to both cause and treat hiccups (corticosteroids, dopamine antagonists, and benzodiazepines) suggesting that if these drugs are suspected, rather than being stopped, their dose should be adjusted, initially down.

Is a biochemical cause present?

Renal failure may be irreversible unless stenting or haemodialysis is possible. Hypocalcaemia after treatment with bisphosphonates is unusual, but is easily treated with 10 ml (2.25 mmol) calcium gluconate 10 per cent solution followed by a continuous infusion of 40 ml (9 mmol) daily. Hyponatraemia severe enough to cause hiccups needs to be investigated. If it is due to inappropriate ADH secretion, democycline can be used. Fluid restriction is only a short-term solution and infusion of hypertonic saline should not be used as it can cause pontine haemorrhage.

Is peritumour oedema a likely cause?

If tumour is compressing surrounding structures, the use of dexamethasone may reduce peritumour oedema and so relieve pressure. Doses of 8 mg orally (or 4 mg subcutaneous) once in the morning is a reasonable starting dose. Higher doses are only needed if very urgent oedema reduction is needed or lower doses have failed.

Are the hiccups persisting?

Unusual causes such as brainstem lesions need to be considered, but treatment is needed to relieve the hiccups.

If gastric distension is suspected, a 2-d trial of a defoaming antiflatulent (e.g. silica activated dimethicone/simethicone in Asilone, Maalox-Plus) before or after meals and at bedtime should be considered. With more troublesome hiccup, a combination of simethicone and a prokinetic drug (metoclopramide, domperidone) should be used. At some centres, peppermint water is used as first-line treatment. Although this facilitates belching by relaxing the lower oesophageal sphincter, it does not have a defoaming action on the gastric contents. It is therefore probably less effective than a defoaming antiflatulent, although no controlled trials have been reported. The concurrent use of metoclopramide and peppermint should be discouraged; there is little sense in deliberately combining two drugs with opposing actions on the lower oesophageal sphincter. A defoaming antiflatulent and enhanced belching is preferable to a permanently relaxed oesophageal sphincter.

There is now increasing evidence of the effectiveness of baclofen, although the numbers of patients in studies is small.[178,179] It is effective in doses as small as 5–10 mg twice a day, although occasionally 20 mg three times a day have been necessary.[179] Alternatives that have been reported (usually as single case reports) are:

- gabapentin 300–600 mg orally 8-hourly;[180]
- nifedipine 10–20 mg orally or sublingually 8-hourly;[170,181]
- haloperidol 3 mg orally at bedtime, but other regimes have been suggested.[182]

Although widely used in the past, chlorpromazine can no longer be recommended because of its adverse effects. In the event of hiccups that continue to be troublesome, intravenous midazolam can be used as described in the first clinical decision above. Although destroying the efferent arc of the hiccup reflex by crushing one or both phrenic nerves might seem an attractive option for resistant cases, this has never been necessary in the author's experience. Phrenic nerve stimulation is another possible option.[183] Osteopaths sometimes treat hiccup with traction of a leg. This relaxes the ipsilateral psoas muscle and may also terminate spasm of the diaphragm. This may also explain why physical activity sometimes brings about a cessation of hiccups.

Key points for hiccup

- Hiccup may be due to an abnormal reciprocating circuit between inspiratory and swallowing centres in the lower medulla, caused by stimulation or damage to the vagus nerve, the phrenic nerve, or the brainstem.
- A wide variety of diseases and conditions can cause hiccup—reversible causes need to be considered.
- Simple physical treatments are often effective.
- In persistent hiccup, baclofen is the drug of choice, with parenteral midazolam being used for intractable cases of distressing hiccup.

Acknowledgements

The author would like to recognize and thank Dr Robert Twycross who authored previous editions of this chapter, and on which this updated chapter is based. The author is also grateful to the following who offered helpful comments on the text: Dr Ken Matthewson, Gastroenterologist, and Sue Clark, Head Speech and Language Therapist, Royal Victoria Hospital, Newcastle upon Tyne.

References

1. **Twycross, R.G. and Lack, S.A.** *Control of Alimentary Symptoms in Far Advanced Cancer.* Edinburgh: Churchill Livingstone, 1986.
2. **Sykes, N.P., Baines, M., and Carter, R.L.** (1988). Clinical and pathological study of dysphagia conservatively managed in patients with advanced malignant disease. *Lancet* **2**, 726–8.
3. **Robertson, M.S. and Hornibrook, J.** (1982). The presenting symptoms of head and neck cancer. *New Zealand Medical Journal* **95**, 337–41.
4. **Aird, D.W., Bihari, J., and Smith, C.** (1983). Clinical problems in the continuing care of head and neck cancer patients. *Ear Nose and Throat Journal* **62**, 10–30.
5. **Stenson, K.M., MacCracken, E., List, M., Haraf, D.J., Brockstein, B., Weichselbaum, R., and Vokes, E.E.** (2000). Swallowing function in patients with head and neck cancer prior to treatment. *Archives of Otolaryngology and Head and Neck Surgery* **126**, 371–7.

6. **Saunders, C., Walsh, T.D., and Smith, M.** *A Review of 100 Cases of Motor Neurone Disease in a Hospice.* London: Edward Arnold, 1981.
7. **O'Brian, T., Kelly, M., and Saunders, C.** (1992). Motor neurone disease: a hospice perspective. *British Medical Journal* **304**, 471–3.
8. **Fuh, J.L., Lee, R.C., Lin, C.H., Wang, S.J., Chiang, J.H., and Liu, H.C.** (1997). Swallowing difficulty in Parkinson's disease. *Clinical Neurology and Neurosurgery* **99**, 106–12.
9. **Thomas, F.J. and Wiles, C.M.** (1999). Dysphagia and nutritional status in multiple sclerosis. *Journal of Neurology* **246**, 677–82.
10. **Rademaker, A.W., Pauloski, B.R., Colangelo, L.A., and Logemann, J.A.** (1998). Age and volume effects on liquid swallowing function in normal women. *Journal of Speech, Language and Hearing Research* **41**, 275–84.
11. **Kayser-Jones, J. and Pengilly, K.** (1999). Dysphagia among nursing home residents. *Geriatric Nursing* **20**, 77–82.
12. **Logemann, J.A.** *Evaluation and Treatment of Swallowing Disorders.* San Diego: College Hill Press, 1983.
13. **Duranceau, A., Jamieson, G., and Hurwitz, A.L.** (1976). Alteration in esophageal motility after laryngectomy. *American Journal of Surgery* **131**, 30–5.
14. **Wu, C.H., Hsaio, T.Y., Ko, J.Y., and Hsu, M.M.** (2000). Dysphagia after radiotherapy: endoscopic examination of swallowing in patients with nasopharyngeal carcinoma. *Annals of Otology, Rhinology and Laryngology* **109**, 320–5.
15. **Regnard, C.F.B.** (1988). Dysphagia. In *Clinical Oncology: Contemporary Palliation of Difficult Symptoms* (ed. T. Bates), pp. 327–55. London: Balliere Tindall.
16. **Carter, R., Pittam, M., and Tanner, N.** (1982). Pain and dysphagia in patients with squamous carcinomas of the head and neck: the role of perineural spread. *Journal of the Royal Society of Medicine* **75**, 598–606.
17. **Perie, S., Coiffier, L., Laccourreye, L., Hazebroucq, V., Chaussade, S., and St Guily, J.L.** (1999). Swallowing disorders in paralysis of the lower cranial nerves: a functional analysis. *Annals of Otology, Rhinology and Laryngology* **108**, 606–11.
18. **Logemann, J., Blonsky, R.E., and Boshes, B.** (1975). Dysphagia in parkinsonism. *Journal of the American Medical Association* **231**, 69–70.
19. **Leopold, N.A. and Kagel, M.C.** (1997). Laryngeal deglutition movement in Parkinson's disease. *Neurology* **48**, 373–6.
20. **Hunter, P.C., Crameri, J., Austin, S., Woodward, M.C., and Hughes, A.J.** (1997). Response of parkinsonian swallowing dysfunction to dopaminergic stimulation. *Journal of Neurology, Neurosurgery and Psychiatry* **63**, 579–83.
21. **Nagaya, M., Kachi, T., Yamada, T., and Igata, A.** (1998). Videoflurographic study of swallowing in Parkinson's disease. *Dysphagia* **13**, 95–100.
22. **Weaver, A.W. and Fleming, S.M.** (1978). Partial laryngectomy: analysis of associated swallowing disorders. *American Journal of Surgery* **136**, 486–9.
23. **Vantrappen, G., Janssens, J., and Ghillebert, G.** (1987). The irritable oesophagus—a frequent cause of angina-like pain. *Lancet* **1**, 1232–4.
24. **Rogers, A.I., Abrams, K.S., and Presley, D.** (1980). Can emotional stress induce esophageal spasm in man? *Gastroenterology* **78**, 1246.
25. **Kim, C.H., Hsu, J.J., Williams, D.E., Weaver, A.L., and Zinsmeister, A.R.** (1996). A prospective psychological evaluation of patients with dysphagia of various etiologies. *Dysphagia* **11**, 34–40.
26. **Lobo, A.J. and Dickinson, R.J.** (1987). Oropharyngeal dyskinesia induced by prochlorperazine. *British Medical Journal* **295**, 333.
27. **Stones, M., Kennie, D.C., and Fulton, J.D.** (1990). Dystonic dysphagia associated with fluspirilene. *British Medical Journal* **301**, 668–9.
28. **Grieve, R. and Dixon, P.** (1983). Dysphagia: a further symptom of hypercalcaemia. *British Medical Journal* **286**, 1935–6.
29. **Trier, J.S. and Bjorkman, D.J.** (1984). Esophageal, gastric and intestinal candidiasis. *American Journal of Medicine* **77**, 39–43.
30. **Daniels, S.K. and Foundas, A.L.** (1999). Lesion localization in acute stroke patients with risk of aspiration. *Journal of Neuroimaging* **9** (2), 91–8.
31. **Hildebrandt, G.H., Dominguez, L., Schork, M.A., and Loesche, W.J.** (1997). Functional units, chewing, swallowing and food avoidance among the elderly. *Journal of Prosthetic Dentistry* **77**, 588–95.
32. **Caruso, A.J. and Max, L.** (1997). Effects of aging on neuromotor processes of swallowing. *Seminars in Speech and Language* **18**, 181–92.
33. **Aviv, J.E.** (1997). Effects of aging on sensitivity of the pharyngeal and supraglottic areas. *American Journal of Medicine* **103** (5A), 74S–76S.
34. **Kayser-Jones, J., Schell, E.S., Porter, C., Barbaccia, J.C., and Shaw, H.** (1999). Factors contributing to dehydration in nursing homes: inadequate staffing and lack of professional supervision. *Journal of the American Geriatrics Society* **47**, 1187–94.
35. **Logemann, J.A.** (1985). Aspiration in head and neck surgical patients. *Annals of Otology, Rhinology and Laryngology* **94**, 373–6.
36. **McHorney, C.A., Bricker, D.E., Kramer, A.E., Rosenbek, J.C., Robbins, J., Chignell, K.A., Logemann, J.A., and Clarke, C.** (2000). The SWAL-QOL outcomes tool for oropharyngeal dysphagia in adults: I. Conceptual foundation and item development. *Dysphagia* **15**, 115–21.
37. **McHorney, C.A., Bricker, D.E., Robbins, J., Kramer, A.E., Rosenbek, J.C., and Chignell, K.A.** (2000). The SWAL-QOL outcomes tool for oropharyngeal dysphagia in adults: II. Item reduction and preliminary scaling. *Dysphagia* **15**, 134–5.
38. **Salassa, J.R.** (1999). A functional outcome swallowing scale for staging oropharyngeal dysphagia. *Digestive Diseases* **17**, 230–4.
39. **Dray, T.G., Hilliel, A.D., and Miller, R.M.** (1998). Dysphagia caused by neurologic deficits. *Otolayngologic Clinics of North America* **31**(3), 507–24.
40. **O'Neil, K.H., Purdy, M., Falk, J., and Gallo, L.** (1999). The Dysphagia Outcome and Severity Scale. *Dysphagia* **14**, 139–45.
41. **Logemann, J.A., Veis, S., and Colangelo, L.** (1999). A screening procedure for oropharyngeal dysphagia. *Dysphagia* **14**, 44–51.
42. **Wallace, K.L., Middleton, S., and Cook, I.J.** (2000). Development and validation of a self-report symptom inventory to assess the severity of oral-pharyngeal dysphagia. *Gastroenterology* **118**, 678–87.
43. **O'Loughlin, G. and Shanley, C.** (1998). Swallowing problems in the nursing home: a novel training exercise. *Dysphagia* **13**, 172–83.
44. **DePippo, K.L., Holas, M.A., and Reding, M.J.** (1994). The Burke dysphagia screening test: validation of its use in patients with stroke. *Archives of Physical and Medical Rehabilitation* **75**, 1284–6.
45. **Smithard, D.G. and Crockford, C.** (1997). The swallow test. *RCSLT Bulletin* January, 7–8.
46. **Hughes, T.A. and Wiles, C.M.** (1996). Measurement of swallowing in patients with sore throats. *Clinical Otolaryngology and Allied Sciences* **21**, 305–7.
47. **Logemann, J.A.** (1999). Do we know what is normal and abnormal airway protection? *Dysphagia* **14**, 233–4.
48. **Warms, T. and Richards, J.** (2000). 'Wet voice' as a predictor of penetration and aspiration in oropharyngeal dysphagia. *Dysphagia* **15**, 84–8.
49. **Sherman, B., Nisenboum, J.M., Jesberger, B.L., Morrow, C.A., and Jesberger, J.A.** (1999). Assessment of dysphagia with the use of pulse oximetry. *Dysphagia* **14**, 152–6.
50. **Collins, M.J. and Bakheit, A.M.** (1997). Does pulse oximetry reliably detect aspiration in dysphagic stroke patients? *Stroke* **28**, 1773–5.
51. **Farell, Z. and O-Neill, D.** (1999). Towards better screening and assessment of oropharyngeal swallow disorders in the general hospital. *Lancet* **354**, 355–6.
52. **Hughes, T.A. and Wiles, C.M.** (1996). Palatal and pharyngeal reflexes in health and in motor neurone disease. *Journal of Neurology, Neurosurgery and Psychiatry* **61**, 96–8.
53. **Leder, S.B.** (1996). Gag reflex and dysphagia. *Head and Neck* **18**, 138–41.
54. **Bastian, R.W.** (1998). Contemporary diagnosis of the dysphagic patient. *Otolaryngologic Clinics of North America* **31**, 489–506.
55. **O'Donaghue, S. and Bagnall, A.** (1999). Videofluoroscopic evaluation in the assessment of swallowing disorders in paediatric and adult populations. *Folio Phoniatrica et Logopedica* **51**, 158–71.
56. **Broniatowski, M., Sonies, B.C., Rubin, J.S., Bradshaw, C.R., Speigel, J.R., Bastian, R.W., and Kelly, J.H.** (1999). Current evaluation and treatment of patients with swallowing disorders. *Otolaryngology—Head and Neck Surgery* **120**, 464–73.
57. **Scott, A.G. and Austin, H.E.** (1994). Nasogastric feeding in the management of severe dysphagia in motor neurone disease. *Palliative Medicine* **8**, 45–9.
58. **Aste, H., Munizzi, F., Martines, H., and Pugliese, V.** (1985). Esophageal dilation in malignant dysphagia. *Cancer* **11**, 2713–15.
59. **Brewster, A.E., Davidson, S.E., Makin, W.P., Stout, R., and Burt, P.A.** (1995). Intraluminal brachytherapy using the high dose rate microselectron in the palliation of carcinoma of the oesophagus. *Clinical Oncology* **7**, 102–5.

60. Sanyka, C., Corr, P., and Haffejee, A. (1999). Palliative treatment of oesophageal carcinoma—efficacy of plastic versus self-expandable stents. *South African Medical Journal* **89**, 640–3.

61. Birch, J.F., White, S.A., Berry, D.P., and Veitch, P.S. (1998). A cost–benefit comparison of self-expanding metal stents and Atkinson tubes for the palliation of obstructing esophageal tumours. *Diseases of the Esophagus* **11**, 172–6.

62. Ell, C., Hochberger, J., May, A., Fleig, W.E., and Hahn, E.G.H. (1994). Coated and uncoated self-expanding metal stents for malignant stenosis in the upper GI tract: preliminary clinical experiences with wallstents. *American Journal of Gastroenterology* **89**, 1496–500.

63. Tytgat, G.N.J. and Tytgat, S. (1994). Esophageal endoprosthesis in malignant stricture. *Journal of Gastroenterology* **29**, 80–4.

64. Singhvi, R., Abbasakoor, F., and Manson, J.M. (2000). Insertion of self-expanding metal stents for malignant dysphagia: assessment of a simple endoscopic method. *Annals of the Royal College of Surgeons of England* **82**, 243–8.

65. Bartelsman, J.F., Bruno, M.J., Jensema, A.J., Haringsma, J., Reeders, J.W., and Tytgat, G.N. (2000). Palliation of patients with esophagogastric neoplasms by insertion of a covered expandable, modified Gianturico-Z endoprosthesis: experiences in 153 patients. *Gastrointestinal Endoscopy* **51**, 134–8.

66. Carter, R., Smith, J.S., and Anderson, J.R. (1992). Laser recanalization versus endoscopic intubation in the palliation of malignant dysphagia: a randomized prospective study. *British Journal of Surgery* **79**, 1167–70.

67. Lewis-Jones, C.M., Sturgess, R., and Ellershaw, J.E. (1995). Laser therapy in the palliation of dysphagia in oesophageal malignancy. *Palliative Medicine* **9**, 327–30.

68. Savage, A.P., Baigrie, R.J., Cobb, R.A., Barr, H., and Kettlewell, M.G. (1997). Palliation of malignant dysphagia by laser therapy. *Diseases of the Esophagus* **10**, 243–6.

69. Moghissi, K., Dixon, K., Thorpe, J.A., Stringer, M., and Moore, P.J. (2000). The role of photodynamic therapy (PDT) in inoperable oesophageal cancer. *European Journal of Cardio-Thoracic Surgery* **17**, 95–100.

70. Nwokolo, C.U., Payne-James, J.J., and Silk, D.B.A. (1994). Palliation of malignant dysphagia by ethanol induced tumour necrosis. *Gut* **35**, 299–303.

71. Carazzone, A., Bonavina, L., Segalin, A., Ceriani, C., and Peracchia, A. (1999). Endoscopic palliation of oesophageal cancer: results of a prospective comparison of Nd:YAG laser and ethanol injection. *European Journal of Surgery* **165**, 351–6.

72. Monga, S.P., Wadleigh, R., Sharma, A., Adib, H., Strader, D., Singh, G., Harmon, J.W., Berlin, M., Monga, D.K., and Mishra, L. (2000). Intratumoral therapy of cisplatin/epinephrine injectable gel for palliation in patients with obstructive esophageal cancer. *Americal Journal of Clinical Oncology* **23**, 386–92.

73. Regnard, C. (1994). Single dose fluconazole versus five day ketoconazole in oral candidiasis. *Palliative Medicine* **8**, 72–3.

74. Rabeneck, L. and Laine, L. (1994). Esophageal candidiasis in patients infected with the human immunodeficiency virus. *Archives of Internal Medicine* **154**, 2705–10.

75. Lucas, V.S., Roberts, G.J., Dixon, J.M., Hockley, P.M., and Thornhill, D.A. (1998). Mouth care and skin care in palliative medicine. *British Medical Journal* **316**, 1246–7.

76. Dodd, M.J. et al. (1996). Randomized clinical trial of chlorhexidine versus placebo for prevention of oral mucositis in patients receiving chemotherapy. *Oncology Nurse Forum* **23**, 921–7.

77. Youle, M., Clarbour, J., and Farthing, C. (1989). Treatment of resistant apthous ulceration with thalidomide in patients positive for HIV antibody. *British Medical Journal* **298**, 432.

78. Davies, A.N., Daniels, C., Pugh, R., and Sharma, K. (1998). A comparison of artificial saliva and pilocarpine in the management of xerostomia in patients with advanced cancer *Palliative Medicine* **12**, 105–11.

79. Sweeny, M.P., Bagg, J., Baxter, W.P., and Aitchison, T.C. (1997). Clinical trial of a mucin-containing oral spray for treatment of xerostomia in hospice patients. *Palliative Medicine* **11**, 225–32.

80. Solomon, M.A. (1986). Oral sucralfate suspension for mucositis. *New England Journal of Medicine* **314**, 29–32.

81. Robbins, J.A., Coyle, J., Rosenbek, J., Roecker, E., and Wood, J. (1999). Differentiation of normal and abnormal airway protection during swallowing using the penetration-aspiration scale. *Dysphagia* **14**, 228–32.

82. Langmore, S.E., Terpenning, M.S., Schork, A., Chen, Y., Murray, J.T., Lopatin, D., and Loesche, W.J. (1998). Predictors of aspiration pneumonia: how important is dysphagia? *Dysphagia* **13**, 69–81.

83. Loeb, M., McGeer, A., McArthur, M., Walter, S., and Simor, A.E. (1999). Risk factors for pneumonia and other lower respiratory tract infections in elderly residents of long-term care facilities. *Archives of Internal Medicine* **159**, 2058–64.

84. Poertner, L.C. and Coleman, R.F. (1998). Swallowing therapy in adults. *Otolaryngologic Clinics of North America* **31**, 561–79.

85. Unsworth, J. *Coping with the Disability of Established Disease.* London: Chapman & Hall Medical, 1994.

86. Hargrove, R. (1980). Feeding the severely dysphagic patient. *Journal of Neurosurgical Nursing* **12**, 102–7.

87. Mitchell, S.L., Kiely, D.K., and Lipsitz, L.A. (1997). The risk factors and impact on survival of feeding tube placement in nursing home residents with severe cognitive impairment. *Archives of Internal Medicine* **157**, 327–32.

88. Finucane, T.E. and Bynum, J.P.W. (1996). Use of tube feeding to prevent aspiration pneumonia. *The Lancet* **348**, 1421–4.

89. Rudberg, M.A., Egleston, B.L., Grant, M.D., and Brody, J.A. (2000). Effectiveness of feeding tubes in nursing home residents with swallowing disorders. *Journal of Parenteral and Enteral Nutrition* **24**, 97–102.

90. Meehan, S.E., Wood, R.A.B., and Cuschieri, A. (1984). Percutaneous cervical pharyngostomy: a comfortable and convenient alternative to protracted nasogastric intubation. *American Journal of Surgery* **148**, 325–30.

91. Leighton, S.E.J., Burton, M.J., Lund, W.S., and Cochrane, G.M. (1994). Swallowing in motor neurone disease. *Journal of the Royal Society of Medicine* **87**, 801–5.

92. Ashby, M., Game, P., Devitt, P., Britten-Jones, R., Brooksbank, M., Davy, M., and Keam, E. (1991). Percutaneous gastrostomy as a venting procedure in palliative care. *Palliative Medicine* **5**, 147–50.

93. Boyd, K.J. and Beeken, L. (1994). Tube feeding in palliative care: benefits and problems. *Palliative Medicine* **8**, 156–8.

94. Laing, B., Smithers, M., and Harper, J. (1994). Percutaneous fluoroscopic gastrostomy: a safe option? *Medical Journal of Australia* **161**, 308–10.

95. Myssiorek, D., Siegel, D., and Vambutas, A. (1998). Fluoroscopically placed gastrostomies in the head and neck patient. *Laryngoscope* **108**, 1557–60.

96. Norton, B., Homer-Ward, M., Donelly, M.T., Long, R.G., and Holmes, G.K.T. (1996). A randomised prospective comparison of percutaneous endoscopic gastrostomy and nasogastric tube feeding after dysphagic stroke. *British Medical Journal* **312**, 13–16.

97. Kimber, C.P. and Beasley, S.W. (1999). Limitations of percutaneous endoscopic gastrostomy in facilitating eneteral nutrition in children: review of the shortcomings of a new technique. *Journal of Paediatric and Child Health* **35**, 427–31.

98. Mandal, A., Steel, A., Davidson, A.R., and Ashby, C. (2000). Day-case percutaneous endoscopic gastrostomy: a viable proposition? *Postgraduate Medical Journal* **76**, 157–9.

99. Campos, A.C.L., Butters, M., and Meguid, M.M. (1990). Home enteral nutrition via gastrostomy in advanced head and neck cancer patients. *Head and Neck* **12**, 137–42.

100. Chiba, N. (1998). Definitions of dyspepsia: time for a reappraisal. *European Journal of Surgery Supplement* **583**, 14–23.

101. Meinechie-Schmidt, V. and Christensen, E. (1998). Classification of dyspepsia. *Scandinavian Journal of Gastroenterology* **33**, 1262–72.

102. Grainger, S.L., Klass, H.J., Rake, M.O., and Williams, J.G. (1994). Prevalence of dyspepsia: the epidemiology of overlapping symptoms. *Postgraduate Medical Journal* **70**, 154–61.

103. Moayyedi, P., Duffett, S., Braunholtz, D., Mason, S., Richards, I.D., Dowell, I.D., and Axon, A.T. (1998). The Leeds Dyspepsia Questionnaire: a valid tool for measuring the presence and severity of dyspepsia. *Alimentary Pharmacology and Therapeutics* **12**, 1257–62.

104. Woodward, M., Morrison, C.E., and McColl, K.E. (1999). The prevalence of dyspepsia and use of antisecretory medication in North Glasgow: role of *Helicobacter pylori* vs. lifestyle. *Alimentary Pharmacology and Therapeutics* **13**, 1505–9.

105. **Editorial** (1986). Non-ulcer dyspepsia. *Lancet* **1**, 1306–7.

106. **Misiewicz, J.J. and Pounder, R.E.** (1996). Peptic ulceration. In *Oxford Textbook of Medicine* 3rd edn. on CD-ROM (ed. D.J. Weatherall, J.G.G. Ledingham, and D.A. Warrell), pp. 1877–91. Oxford: Oxford University Press and Electronic Publishing B.V.

107. **Hawkey, C.J.** (2000). Non-steroidal anti-inflammatory drug gastropathy. *Gastroenterology* **119**, 521–35.

108. **Lambert, R.** (1999). Digestive endoscopy: relevance of negative findings. *Italian Journal of Gastroenterology and Hepatology* **31**, 761–72.

109. **Hull, M.A., Brough, J.L., and Hawkey, C.J.** (1999). Expression of cyclooxygenase-1 and -2 by human gastric endothelial cells. *Gut* **45**, 529–36.

110. **Schmassmann, A., Peskar, B.M., Stettler, C., Netzer, P., Stroff, T., Flogerzi, B., and Halter, F.** (1998). Effects of prostaglandin endoperoxide synthetase-2 in chronic gastrointestinal ulcer models in rats. *British Journal of Pharmacology* **123**, 795–804.

111. **Horie-Sakata, K., Schimida, T., Hiraishi, H., and Terano, A.** (1998). Role of cyclooxygenase 2 in hepatocyte growth factor-mediated gastric epithelial restitution (Suppl. 1). *Journal of Clinical Gastroenterology* **27**, S40–6.

112. **Kelly, J.P., Kaufman, D.W., Jurgelon, J.M., Sheehan, J., Koff, R.S., and Shapiro, S.** (1996). Risk of aspirin-associated major upper-gastrointestinal bleeding with enteric-coated or buffered product. *Lancet* **348**, 1413–16.

113. **Wolfe, M.M., Lichtenstein, D.R., and Sing, G.** (1999). Gastrointestinal toxicity of non-steroidal anti-inflammatory drugs. *New England Journal of Medicine* **340**, 1888–99.

114. **Henry, D., Lim, L.L.-Y., Garcia Rodriquez, L.A., Gutthann, S.P., Carson, J.L., Griffen, N., Savage, R., Logan, R., Moride, Y., Hawkey, C., Hill, S., and Fries, J.T.** (1996). The ability in risk of gastrointestinal complications with individual non-steroidal anti-inflammatory drugs: results of a collaborative meta-analysis. *British Medical Journal* **312**, 1563–6.

115. **Langman, M.J., Jensen, D.M., Watson, D.J., Harper, S.E., Xhao, P.-L., and Quan, H.** (1999). Incidence of upper gastrointestinal perforations, symptomatic ulcers and bleeding (PUBS). Rofecoxib compared to NSAIDs. *Journal of the American Medical Association* **282**, 1929–33.

116. **McAdam, B.F., Catella-Lawson, F., Mardini, I.A., Kapoor, S., and Lawson, J.A.** (1999). Systemic biosynthesis of prostacyclin by cyclooxygenase (COX)-2: the human pharmacology of a selective inhibitor of COX-2. *Proceedings of the National Academy of Sciences of the USA* **11** (96), 5890.

117. **Piper, J.M., Ray, W.A., Daugherty, M.R., and Griffen, M.R.** (1991). Corticosteroid use and peptic ulcer disease: role of nonsteroidal anti-inflammatory drugs. *Annals of Internal Medicine* **114**, 735–40.

118. **Hochain, P., Berkelmans, I., Czernichow, P., Duhamel, C., Tranvouez, J.L., Lerebours, E., and Colin, R.** (1995). Which patients taking non-aspirin non-steroidal anti-inflammatory drugs bleed? A case–control study. *European Journal of Gastroenterology and Hepatology* **7**, 419–26.

119. **Weil, J., Langamn, M.J.S., Wainwright, P., Lawson, D.H., Rawlins, M., Logan, R.F.A., Brown, T.P., Vessey, M.P., Murphy, M., and Colin-Jones, D.G.** (2000). Peptic ulcer bleeding: accessory risk factors and interactions with non-steroidal anti-inflammatory drugs. *Gut* **46**, 27–31.

120. **Childs, S., Roberts, A., Meineche-Scmidt, V., de Wit, N., and Rubin, G.** (2000). The management of *Helicobacter pylori* infection in primary care: a systematic review of the literature. *Family Practice* **17** (Suppl. 2), S6–11.

121. **Talley, N.J., Janssens, J., Lauritson, K., Racz, I., and Bolling-Sternevald, E.** (2000). Eradication of *Helicobacter pylori* in functional dyspepsia: randomised double blind placebo controlled trial with 12 month's follow up. The Optimal Regimen Cures Helicobacter Dyspepsia (ORCHID) Study Group. *British Medical Journal* **318**, 833–7.

122. **Chaudhuri, S., Santra, A., Dobe, P.B., Das, A.S., Dasgupta, J., Roay, A., and Mazumder, D.N.** (2000). Esophageal and gastric dysmotility. *Indian Journal of Gastroenterology* **19**, 109–11.

123. **Nelson, K., Walsh, T., O'Donovan, P., Sheehan, F., and Falk, G.** (1993). Assessment of upper gastrointestinal motility in the cancer-associated dyspepsia syndrome (CADS). *Journal of Palliative Care* **9**, 27–31.

124. **Armes, P.J., Plant, H.J., Allbright, A., Silverstone, T., and Slevin, M.L.** (1992). A study to investigate the incidence of early satiety in patients with advanced cancer. *British Journal of Cancer* **65**, 481–4.

125. **Bruera, E., Catz, Z., Hooper, R., Lentle, B., and MacDonald, R.N.** (1987). Chronic nausea and anorexia in advanced cancer patients: a possible role for autonomic dysfunction. *Journal of Pain and Symptom Management* **2**, 19–21.

126. **Muth, E.R., Koch, K.L., and Stern, R.M.** (2000). Significance of autonomic nervous system activity in functional dysypepsia. *Digestive Diseases and Sciences* **45**, 854–63.

127. **Bruera, E., Chadwick, S., MacDonald, N., Fox, R., and Hanson, J.** (1986). Study of cardiovascular autonomic insufficiency in advanced cancer patients. *Cancer Treatment Reports* **70**, 1383–7.

128. **Handa, M., Mine, K., Yamamoto, H., Tsutsui, S., Hayashi, H., Kinkawa, N., and Kubo, C.** (1999). Esophageal motility and psychiatric factors in functional dyspepsia with or without pain. *Digestive Diseases and Sciences* **44**, 2094–8.

129. **Pfaffenbach, B., Adamek, R.J., Hagemann, D., Scaffstein, J., and Wegener, M.** (1998). Gastric emptying and antral myoelectrical activity in chronic alcoholics with dyspepsia. *Hepato-Gastroenterology* **45**, 1165–71.

130. **Ko, C.W., Chang, C.S., Lien, H.C., Wu, M.J., and Chen, G.H.** (1998). Gastric dysrhythmia in uremic patients on maintenance hemodialysis. *Scandinavian Journal of Gastroenterology* **33**, 1047–51.

131. **Dent, J.** (1996). Diseases of the oesophagus. In *Oxford Textbook of Medicine* 3rd edn. on CD-ROM (ed. D.J. Weatherall, J.G.G. Ledingham, and D.A. Warrell), pp. 1865–76. Oxford: Oxford University Press and Electronic Publishing BV.

132. **Delaney, B.C., Innes, M.A., Deeks, J., Wilson, S., Oakes, R., Moayyedi, P., Hobbs, F.D., and Forman, D.** (2002). Initial management strategies for dyspepsia. *Cochrane Database of Systematic Reviews (computer file)* **2**, CD001961.

133. **Lam, S.K.** (1990). Why do ulcers heal with sucralfate? *Scandinavian Journal of Gastroenterology* **25** (Suppl. 173), 6–16.

134. **Caldwell, J.R., Roth, S.H., Wu, W.G., Semble, E.L., Castell, D.D., Heller, M.D., and March, W.H.** (1987). Sucralfate treatment of nonsteroidal anti-inflammatory drug-induced gastrointestinal symptoms and mucosal damage. *American Journal of Medicine* **83** (Suppl. 3B), 74–82.

135. **Regnard, C.F.B. and Mannix, K.** (1990). Palliation of gastric carcinoma haemorrhage with sucralfate. *Palliative Medicine* **4**, 329–30.

136. **Sorkin, E. and Ogawa, C.** (1983). Cimetidine potentiation of narcotic action. *Drug Intelligence and Clinical Pharmacy* **17**, 60–1.

137. **Hawkey, C.J., Karrasch, J.A., Szcepanski, L., Walker, D.G., Barkun, A., Swanell, A.J., and Yeomans, N.D. for the Omeprazole vs Misoprostol for NSAID-Induced Ulcer Management (OMNIUM) Study Group** (1998). Omeprazole compared with misoprostol for ulcers associated with non steroidal anti inflammatory drugs. *New England Journal of Medicine* **338**, 727–34.

138. **Koch, M., Capurso, L., Dezi, A., Ferrario, F., and Scarpignato, C.** (1995). Prevention of NSAID-induced gastroduodenal mucosal injury: meta-analysis of clinical trials with misoprostol and H_2 antagonists. *Digestive Diseases* **1**, 62–74.

139. **Twycross, R.G.** (1995). The use of prokinetic drugs in palliative care. *European Journal of Palliative Care* **4**, 141–5.

140. **Shivshanker, K., Bennett, R.W., and Haynie, T.P.** (1983). Tumor-associated gastroparesis: correction with metoclopramide. *American Journal of Surgery* **145**, 221–5.

141. **Kris, M.G., Yeh, S.D.J., Gralla, R.J., and Young, C.W.** (1985). Symptomatic gastroparesis in cancer patients. A possible cause of cancer-associated anorexia that can be improved with oral metoclopramide. *Proceedings of the American Society of Clinical Oncology* **4**, 267.

142. **Sanger, G.J. and King, F.D.** (1988). From metoclopramide to selective gut motility stimulants and 5HT3 receptor antagonists. *Drug Design and Delivery* **3**, 273–95.

143. **Loose, F.D.** (1979). Domperidone in chronic dyspepsia: a pilot open study and a multicentre general practice crossover comparison with metoclopramide and placebo. *Pharmatheripeutica* **2** (3), 140–6.

144. **Moriga, M.** (1981). A multicentre double blind study of domperidone and metoclopramide in the symptomatic control of dyspepsia. In *Progress with Domperidone. A Gastrokinetic and Anti-emetic Agent* (ed. G. Touse), pp. 77–9. London: Royal Society of Medicine.

145. **Rowbotham, D., Bamber, P., and Nimmo, W.** (1988). Comparison of the effect of cisapride and metoclopramide on morphine-induced delay in gastric emptying. *British Journal of Clinical Pharmacology* **26**, 741–6.

146. **Manara, A.R., Shelly, M.P., Quinn, K., and Park, G.R.** (1988). The effect of metoclopramide on the absorption of oral controlled release morphine. *British Journal of Clinical Pharmacolology* **25**, 518–21.

147. **Bernstein, J. and Kasich, M.** (1974). A double-blind trial of simethicone in functional disease of the upper gastrointestinal tract. *Journal of Clinical Pharmacology* **14**, 614–23.

148. **Ogilvie, A.L. and Atkinson, M.** (1986). Does dimethicone increase the efficacy of antacids in the treatment of reflux oesophagitis? *Journal of the Royal Society of Medicine* **79** (10), 584–7.

149. **Jasperson, D., Diehl, K.L., Schoeppner, H., Geyer, P., and Martens, E.** (1998). A comparison of omeprazole, lansoprazole and pantoprazole in the maintenance treatment of severe reflux disease. *Alimentary Pharmacology and Therapeutics* **12**, 49–52.

150. **Watters, K.J., Murphy, G.M., Tomkin, G.H., and Ashford, J.J.** (1979). An evaluation of the bile acid binding and antacid properties of hydrotalcite in hiatus hernia and peptic ulceration. *Current Medical Research Opinion* **6**, 85–7.

151. **Llewellyn, A.F., Tomkin, G.H., and Murphy, G.M.** (1977). The binding of bile acids by hydrotalcite and other antacid preparations. *Pharmaceutica Acta Helvetiae* **52**, 1–5.

152. **Keeckner, F.S., Stahler, E.J., Hartzell, G., and Eicher, W.P.** (1972). Esophagitis and gastritis secondary to bile reflux. *Gastroenterology* **62**, 890.

153. **Nathan, M.D., Leshner, R.T., and Keller, A.P.** (1980). Intractable hiccups. *Laryngoscope* **90**, 1612–18.

154. **Launois, S., Bizec, J., Whitelaw, W., Cabane, J., and Derenne, J.** (1993). Hiccup in adults: an overview. *European Respiratory Journal* **6**, 563–75.

155. **Souadjian, J.V. and Cain, J.C.** (1968). Intractable hiccup: etiologic factors in 220 cases. *Postgraduate Medicine* **43**, 72–7.

156. **Marhofer, P., Glaser, C., Krenn, C.G., Grabner, C.M., and Semsroth, M.** (1999). Incidence and therapy of midazolam induced hiccups in paediatric anaesthesia. *Paediatric Anaesthesia* **9**, 295–8.

157. **Askenasy, J.J.M.** (1992). About the mechanism of hiccup. *European Neurology* **32**, 159–63.

158. **Stotka, V.L., Barclay, S.J., Bell, H.S., and Clare, F.B.** (1962). Intractable hiccough as the primary manifestation of brain stem tumor. *American Journal of Medicine* **32**, 313–15.

159. **Kaufman, H.J.** (1982). Hiccups: an occasional sign of esophageal obstruction. *Gastroenterology* **82**, 1443–5.

160. **Fodstad, H. and Nilsson, S.** (1993). Intractable singultus: a diagnostic and therapeutic challenge. *British Journal of Neurosurgery* **7**, 255–62.

161. **Wagner, H.S. and Stapczynski, J.S.** (1982). Persistent hiccups. *Annals of Emergency Medicine* **11**, 24–6.

162. **Askenasy, J.J.** (1988). Sleep hiccup. *Sleep* **11**, 187–94.

163. **Liddell, E.G.T. and Sherrington, C.** (1925). Further observations on myotatic reflexes. *Proceedings of the Royal Society of London (Biology)* **97**, 267–83.

164. **Moretti, R., Torre, P., Antonello, R.M., Nasuelli, D., and Cazzato, G.** (2000). Gabapentin as a drug therapy of intractable hiccup due to vascular lesion. *Nuova Rivista di Neurologica* **10**, 58–62.

165. **Ward, B.A. and Smith, R.R.** (1994). Hiccups and brainstem compression. *Journal of Neuroimaging* **4**, 164–5.

166. **Chang, Y.Y., Wu, H.S., Tsai, T.C., and Liu, J.S.** (1994). Intractable hiccup due multiple sclerosis: MR imaging of medullary plaque. *Canadian Journal of Neurological Sciences* **21**, 271–2.

167. **Musumeci, A., Cristofori, L., and Bricolo, A.** (2000). Persistent hiccup as presenting symptom in medulla oblongata cavernoma: a case report and review of the literature. *Clinical Neurology and Neurosurgery* **102**, 13–17.

168. **Rousseau, P.** (1994). Hiccups in terminal disease. *American Journal of Hospice and Palliative Care* **11** (6), 7–10.

169. **Lauterbach, E.C.** (1999). Hiccup and apparent myoclonus after hydrocodone: review of the opiate-related hiccup and myoclonus literature. *Clinical Neuropharmacology* **22**, 87–92.

170. **Mukhopadhyay, P., Osman, M.R., Wajima, T., and Wallace, T.I.** (1986). Nifedipine for intractable hiccups. *New England Journal of Medicine* **314**, 1256.

171. **Howard, R.S.** (1992). Persistent hiccups. *British Medical Journal* **305**, 1237–8.

172. **Salem, M.R., Baraka, A., Rattenborg, C.C. and Holaday, D.A.** (1967). Treatment of hiccups by pharyngeal stimulation in anesthetized and conscious subjects. *Journal of the American Medical Association* **202**, 126–30.

173. **De Ruysscher, D., Spaas, P., and Specenier, P.** (1996). Treatment of intractable hiccup in a terminal cancer patient with nebulized saline. *Palliative Medicine* **10**, 166–7.

174. **Goldsmith, A.** (1983). A treatment for hiccups. *Journal of the American Medical Association* **249**, 1566.

175. **Lamphier, T.A.** (1977). Methods of management of persistent hiccup (singultus). *Maryland State Medical Journal* November, 80–1.

176. **Saitto, C., Gristina, G., and Cosmi, E.V.** (1982). Treatment of hiccups by continuous positive airway pressure (CPAP) in anesthetized subjects. *Anesthesiology* **57**, 345.

177. **Wilcock, A. and Twycross, R.** (1997). Midazolam for intractable hiccup. *Journal of Pain and Symptom Management* **12**, 59–61.

178. **Guelaud, C., Similowski, T., Bizec, J.L., Cabane, J., Whitelaw, W.A., and Derenne, J.P.** (1995). Baclofen therapy for chronic hiccup. *European Respiratory Journal* **8**, 235–7.

179. **Ramirez, F.C. and Graham, D.Y.** (1992). Treatment of intractable hiccup with baclofen: results of a double-blind randomized, cross-over study. *American Journal of Gastroenterology* **87**, 1789–91.

180. **Petroianu, G., Hein, G., Syegmeier-Petroianu, A., Bergler, W., and Rufer, R.** (2000). Gabapentin 'add-on therapy' for idiopathic chronic hiccup (ICH). *Journal of Clinical Gastroenterology* **30**, 321–4.

181. **Lipps, D.C., Jabbari, B., Mitchell, M.H., and Daigh, J.D.** (1990). Nifedipine for intractable hiccups. *Neurology* **40**, 531–2.

182. **Ives, T.J., Fleming, M.F., Weart, C.W., and Block, D.** (1985). Treatment of intractable hiccups with intramuscular haloperidol. *American Journal of Psychiatry* **142**, 1368–9.

183. **Aravot, D.J., Wright, G., Rees, A., Maiwand, O.M., and Garland, M.H.** (1989). Non-invasive phrenic nerve stimulation for intractable hiccups. *Lancet* **2**, 1047.

184. **de Caestecker, J.** (2001). ABC of the upper gastrointestinal tract. Oesophagus: heartburn. *British Medical Journal* **323**, 736–9.

185. **Logan, R. and Delaney, B.** (2001). ABC of the upper gastrointestinal tract. Implications of dyspepsia for the NHS. *British Medical Journal* **323**, 675–7.

8.3.3 Constipation and diarrhoea

Nigel Sykes

Constipation

Definition

Constipation is the passage of small, hard faeces infrequently and with difficulty. Individuals vary in the weight they give to the different components of this definition when assessing their own constipation and may introduce other factors, such as flatulence, bloating, or a sensation of incomplete evacuation.

Less than 1 per cent of a healthy British population[1] or 5 per cent of a North American one[2] fail to defaecate at least three times a week. These findings have informed what are sometimes referred to as the 'Rome criteria',[3] which are often used to define constipation for research or drug regulatory purposes; the presence of two or more of the following symptoms for at least three months:

- straining at least 25 per cent of the time;
- hard stools at least 25 per cent of the time;
- incomplete evacuation at least 25 per cent of the time;
- two or fewer bowel movements per week.

In practice, the bowel frequency criterion is often given most importance, but the validity of this in a palliative care or general population is doubtful. There is evidence that many people feel constipated when still not meeting the Rome criteria.[4,5]

Prevalence of constipation

The first National Health and Nutrition Examination Survey in the United States found that 8 per cent of men and 21 per cent of women reported themselves to be constipated.(6) In a British survey 10 per cent overall said they were constipated,(1) but again the gender difference was consistent. Both self-reported constipation and laxative consumption increase with ageing.

Physical illness is a risk factor for constipation: 63 per cent of elderly people in hospital have been found to be constipated, compared with 22 per cent of the same age group living at home.(7) Constipation is more common in people terminally ill with cancer than in those dying of other causes,(8) and about 50 per cent of patients admitted to British hospices complain of it. This is an under-estimate of the problem, as some patients will already be receiving effective laxative therapy. It has been reported to rival or exceed pain as a cause of distress. Depression is a risk factor for constipation in population surveys,(6) but results of a depression rating scale used on British hospice patients do not correlate with indices of constipation.

Pathophysiology

Intestinal motility

Small and large intestines each have their own characteristic motility patterns, but throughout the gut most muscle movements do not propel the contents but mix them. This facilitates enzymatic and bacterial breakdown of food and absorption of the resulting nutrients and of water.

Bursts of propagated motor activity occur in the small gut every 90–120 min. This activity is associated with increased gastric, pancreatic, and biliary secretion and is suggested to represent a cleansing mechanism for the small intestine. Feeding abolishes the regularity of this pattern, resulting in an increased variability of the rate of transit of luminal contents. Motor activity in the fed state is apparently random and presumably performs the function of mixing the gut contents in order to allow digestion and absorption of nutrients. Resumption of regular propagated activity correlates closely with the end of gastric emptying; both are delayed by larger or more fatty meals,(9) again suggesting that adequate facilities for digestion are being provided.

The colon shows much less frequent episodes of forward peristalsis, which result in mass movements of gut contents. Manometry suggests this activity occurs about six times per day, but is grouped into two peaks, a larger one associated with wakening and breakfast and a smaller one associated with midday meal.(10) The frequency is reduced by inactivity.(11)

Food residues normally spend 1–2 h in the small intestine, but 2–3 days in the colon. In constipation, colonic transit may be greatly prolonged: nearly half of a hospice population had transit times of between 4 and 12 days.(12)

Gut muscle layers form a syncytium through which depolarization spreads from pacemaker areas. The myenteric nerve plexus co-ordinates motility, which is also under external neuronal influence, particularly via the parasympathetic system. High spinal cord transection mainly abolishes the motility response to food, but low cord or pelvic outflow lesions produce colonic dilation and slowing of transit in the descending and distal transverse colon.

Autonomic neuropathy has been implicated in some cases of chronic constipation and in constipation related to diabetes mellitus. The suggestion has been made that autonomic neuropathy occurring as a non-metastatic manifestation of malignancy might contribute to constipation in patients with advanced cancer,(13) but definite evidence has yet to appear.

Immunocytochemical work in animals has revealed multiple putative transmitter peptides and amines in myenteric neurones. The two principal neurotransmitters involved in the control of peristalsis appear to be acetylcholine (ACh) and vasoactive intestinal peptide (VIP). Peristalsis movements have two components, ascending contraction and descending relaxation; ACh mediates the first of these and VIP the second. Anticholinergic drugs tend to constipate because they control part of the peristaltic complex. Both ACh and VIP neurones are modulated by other agents of which endogenous opioids are one group.

Fluid and electrolyte handling

About 7 l of fluid enters the jejunum daily from gastric, salivary, pancreatic, and biliary secretions, to which is added a further 1.5 l of dietary fluid. Approximately 75 per cent of the total volume is absorbed in the small intestine and all but about 150 ml of the remainder in the colon. The difference between constipation and diarrhoea in terms of fluid excretion is around 100 ml/day, implying a remarkably precise control of water absorption in the colon. The maximal colonic absorptive capacity is 4.5–5 l/day, and hence there is wide tolerance of fluctuations in ileal output, but small variations in colonic absorption can produce diarrhoea. There is no evidence that constipation is accompanied by increased water absorption save by virtue of the extended time contents remain in the gut.

Gut fluid absorption is an active process, chiefly dependent on electrogenic Na^+ transport by the Na^+/K^+-ATPase system at the basolateral surface of the enterocytes. Fluid also follows neutral absorption of Cl^- in exchange for HCO_3, and of NaCl. Na^+ is also co-transported with glucose and amino acid molecules. At the mucosal surface, a cyclic AMP-dependent system mediates Cl^- and consequently fluid, secretion.

Non-absorbed solutes retain water in the lumen by osmosis, but luminal factors can also influence active transport. Short-chain fatty acids increase absorption and bile acids, prostaglandins, bacterial toxins, and some laxatives stimulate secretion. Accordingly, diarrhoea can sometimes be relieved by a bile acid-binding resin or a prostaglandin inhibitor.

Electrolyte, and hence, water, transport is under neuronal control. The basic secretory condition of intestinal epithelium is cholinergic, mediated through changes in intracellular calcium concentrations. Anticholinergic agents and hypercalcaemia tend to constipate and hypocalcaemia tends to cause diarrhoea.

Lipophilic agents, such as bile salts, could stimulate villous nerve endings directly, but it has been proposed that epithelial 'receptor' cells mediate a defence response of increased secretion and peristalsis to water-soluble toxins.(14) Endogenous opioids inhibit this defence response experimentally and although the physiological significance of such modulation is unclear, it may be a component of exogenous opioids' action in infective and perhaps other forms of diarrhoea (Table 1).

Defaecation

During defaecation, abdominal pressure is raised by contraction of the abdominal muscles against a closed glottis, a process facilitated by assuming a squatting position. This pressure is transmitted to the rectum and tends to expel a stool positioned in the rectal ampulla. However, once defaecation has been initiated, stools from the length of the descending colon can be expelled without abdominal contraction. Such effortless expulsion is probably due to an anocolonic reflex that produces distal colonic contraction in response to anal contact with passing stool. The effort required to pass a stool is inversely proportional to its size, accounting for the straining involved in passing a small, constipated stool.(15)

Normal defaecation depends on the ability of upper anal canal receptors to detect the presence of stool, and on the relaxation of the involuntary internal anal sphincter and of puborectalis, which also exerts a sphincter function. These actions are abolished by lower motor neurone lesions to

Table 1 Opioid effects on the gut

Increased tone in ileocaecal and anal sphincters
Reduced peristaltic component of motility in small intestine and colon
Increased electrolyte and water absorption in small intestine, and colon during induced diarrhoea
Restoration of colonic capacitance after intracaecal fat infusion
Impaired defaecation reflex
Reduced sensitivity to distention
Increased internal anal sphincter tone

produce loss of rectal sensation, decreased rectal tone, and inability to defaecate. Upper motor neurone lesions also destroy rectal sensation, but leave intact both reflex relaxation of the internal sphincter and the anocolonic reflex. Hence, many patients with high spinal lesions learn to initiate defaecation by digital stimulation of the anal canal.

Mechanisms of the contribution of opioids to constipation

Opioid analgesics, specifically morphine, are probably the largest single identifiable constipating influence in palliative care patients. Sixty-three per cent of such patients *not* taking morphine required laxatives, a figure similar to that found in the ill elderly,[7] but 87 per cent of those receiving morphine needed them and used a higher average dose.[16] There appeared to be the type of dose–response relationship between morphine and constipation that might be expected from a drug–receptor interaction, although with considerable scatter.

Exogenous opioids are well known to constipate, not by relaxing intestinal muscle but by suppressing forward peristalsis and raising sphincter tone (Table 1). These effects are apparent in both the small and the large intestines. If sufficiently severe, the clinical results on the gut of opioid analgesia produce functional colonic obstruction, a situation whose symptoms have been called the 'narcotic bowel syndrome',[17] but which appears simply to represent severe constipation.

Opioid receptors are present on gut smooth muscle and at all levels of nervous input to the intestine, mu- and delta-receptors apparently being the most important in motility, the former predominating in the myenteric plexus and the latter in the submucous plexus. In animals, gut opioid effects involve both central and peripheral receptors, but only peripheral opioid activity has been confirmed in man. This does not imply that parenterally administered opioids are not constipating: it has been shown in man that subcutaneous morphine slows transit and reduces stool frequency.[18] No doubt opioid receptors in the gut wall can be reached not just by opioids in the lumen but also in the circulation.

Endogenous opioids have been shown to be involved in the modulation of other neurotransmitters, notably ACh and VIP, which are involved in control of peristalsis. Human studies using naloxone suggest that endogenous opioids may exert a basal control of gut motility[18] and, clinically, oral naloxone has been reported to improve idiopathic constipation[19] and constipation in geriatric patients.[20] Although these results are in line with some animal data they require confirmation and further work with more specific antagonists to clarify the contribution of different opioid receptor populations.

Experimentally, mu_2-receptor-mediated opioid actions such as delaying of intestinal transit show less development of tolerance than mu_1-mediated analgesia does.[21] The development of clinical tolerance to morphine-induced constipation remains to be quantified: 28 palliative care patients followed up for over 2 months did not differ significantly from 470 shorter-lived patients in morphine or laxative consumption, but did have higher stool frequencies and somewhat lower use of enemas and suppositories. Their median laxative dose had risen over the review period but by much less than had their median morphine dose.[16] In a smaller study, 12 patients survived for 6 months. Among them were four who required no laxatives despite taking morphine, sometimes in substantial amounts. It is not clear whether these four patients had never needed laxatives or whether they had at some point been able to give them up, that is, whether they had become tolerant to the constipating effect of morphine or whether they lay at one extreme of a morphine dose–response curve for constipation.[22]

Opioids may vary in their constipating potency. There is now reasonable evidence that transdermal fentanyl is somewhat less constipating than morphine,[23] possibly because of the smaller doses that have to be given in order to achieve CNS penetration. Reduction in laxative use has also been reported after changing from morphine to methadone, but to date only on a case history basis.[24] Clearly, formal trials are needed.

A physiological role for endogenous opioids in defaecation has yet to emerge, but exogenous opioids inhibit anorectal sphincteric relaxation and diminish anorectal sensitivity (Table 1). Both actions exacerbate constipation. As anorectal sensitivity decreases with age, the constipating effects of opioid therapy are likely to be more pronounced in the elderly.

Table 2 Causes of constipation in palliative medicine

Malignancy
Directly due to tumour
Intestinal obstruction due to (i) tumour in the bowel wall; (ii) external compression by abdominal or pelvic tumour
Damage to lumbosacral spinal cord, cauda equina or pelvic plexus
Hypercalcaemia
Due to secondary effects of disease
Inadequate food intake
Low fibre diet
Dehydration
Weakness
Inactivity
Confusion
Depression
Unfamiliar toilet arrangements
Drugs
Opioids
Drugs with anticholinergic effects:
Hyoscine
Phenothiazines
Tricyclic antidepressants
Antiparkinsonian agents
Antacids (calcium and aluminium compounds)
Diuretics
Anticonvulsants
Iron
Antihypertensive agents
Vincristine
Concurrent disease
Diabetes
Hypothyroidism
Hypokalaemia
Hernia
Diverticular disease
Rectocoele
Anal fissure or stenosis
Anterior mucosal prolapse
Haemorrhoids
Colitis

Causes of constipation in palliative medicine

Constipation in patients with progressive disease is usually multifactorial; for instance, an ill person with poor food intake, impaired mobility, and a requirement for opioid analgesia has three reasons to be constipated. A list of the constipating factors most relevant to palliative medicine is given in Table 2. Of these, the most important are the secondary effects of disease and the use of opioids.

Clinical manifestations and diagnostic considerations in constipation

History

It is important to clarify a complaint of constipation by a careful history. The degree to which constipation pre-dated the present illness should be established, as this may justify wider investigations. Whether it was construed by the patient as constipation or not, the prior stool pattern should be elicited as a basis for comparison. Some necessary questions for taking a constipation history are suggested in Table 3.

Occasionally, the patient reports a trick that aids defaecation: a finger inserted in the vagina implies the presence of a rectocoele, a finger in the rectum to push away a flap suggests a solitary rectal ulcer, and pressure exerted behind the anus assists defaecation if the levator muscles are weak. All these are distinct from the digital rectal evacuation to which many constipated patients are forced to resort.

Such symptoms as abdominal pain, bloating, flatulence, nausea, malaise, headache, and halitosis are associated by some patients with constipation, but are non-specific and mostly can occur also with diarrhoea. It is the frequency and difficulty of defaecation that are the basis for the diagnosis of constipation.

Assessment tools for constipation

In palliative care constipation is important as a symptom, and hence it is the patient's perspective that is most valid. However, the widely accepted 'Rome criteria'[3] invite the measurement of objective outcomes that are taken to be indicators of the severity of constipation. Whether they also reflect the impact of disordered bowel function upon the patient is much less clear (Table 4). The correlation of the objective assessment of stool appearance with bowel transit time has been validated in a palliative care population,[12] and is a non-invasive, technology-free method of assessing this key indicator of intestinal function.

An objective indicator of the presence of constipation is a plain abdominal radiograph. A scoring system to describe the amount of stool present was described and tested by Bruera et al.[25] in a palliative care study. Similar systems of more or less complexity have been described by Barr[26] and others, and are claimed to show high inter-observer reliability and good correlation with stool frequency. Radiographs are of course a static measure of current faecal loading and give no information about the speed of transit or about performance of different colonic segments. In a large paediatric study, Barr scores showed poor correlation with transit time and too great a variability to be reliable in diagnosing chronically constipated subjects.[27] On the other hand, scoring of pre- and post-intervention radiographs could aid objectivity of assessment in the badly needed trials of the efficacy of suppositories and enemas in palliative care.

Subjective measures of constipation, which assess patients' reports of their bowel function without externally measurable criteria, take the form of visual analogue (VAS) or adjectival scales, or of questionnaires. A discrete response modification of the VAS and an adjectival scale have each been found to have validity and to be easy to use in a palliative care setting.[28] Since up to about 10 per cent of palliative care patients have diarrhoea, whose commonest cause in this setting is an excess of laxatives, it is appropriate that any subjective measure includes the ability to assess not only constipation but also diarrhoea as well. This is easily arranged with VAS and adjectival scales, but is lacking in the questionnaires that have been validated for the assessment of constipation.

Perhaps the best-established constipation questionnaire is the Constipation Assessment Scale (CAS) of McMillan and Williams.[29] This is an eight-item scale validated on cancer, although not specifically palliative care, patients. Completion time averages 2 min. The Constipation Scoring System also has eight items, and when tested on 50 constipated and 50 non-constipated patients it predicted the presence of constipation correctly in 96 per cent of cases.[30] Unlike the CAS, it has not been shown to distinguish between severities of constipation, although it seems likely that it would do so.

The PAC-SYM and PAC-QOL are related questionnaires directed at the patient's perspective on constipation.[31] The PAC-SYM has three subscales related to stool symptoms, rectal symptoms and abdominal symptoms, and has been validated on a large ($n = 216$) sample of chronically constipated subjects but not a cancer or palliative care population. The PAC-QOL is a constipation-specific quality of life measure. The PAC-SYM contains no assessment of diarrhoea, although the PAC-QOL has a bowel frequency rating. Several other bowel function rating scales exist but are either derived from one of those already mentioned or are not specific to constipation.

Examination

Abdominal examination and, unless there has been a recent full evacuation, rectal examination, are vital, and will help to avoid the major pitfalls in the diagnosis of constipation in palliative medicine. These are:

Impaction, presenting as diarrhoea, often with incontinence. This occurs characteristically in elderly patients in whom inattention to the need to defaecate, confusion, or rectal insensitivity leads to the formation of a large faecal mass that is impossible to pass spontaneously. Faecal material higher in the colon is broken down into semi-liquid form by bacterial

Table 3 History-taking in constipation

When were the bowels last opened?
What were the characteristics of the last stool, e.g. loose or formed; thin and ribbon-like or small, hard pellets?
Was straining necessary for defaecation?
Was defaecation painful?
How characteristic of recent bowel actions was the last stool?
What is the usual stool frequency now?
Does the patient feel a need to defaecate but is unable to do so (suggests hard stool or rectal obstruction)?
Is the urge to defaecate largely absent (suggests colonic inertia)?
Does the stool emerge part way through a bulging anal outlet after significant straining (suggests haemorrhoids)?
Is there blood or mucus in the stool (suggests tumour obstruction or haemorrhoids)?
Is there blood or mucus in the stool (suggests tumour obstruction or haemorrhoids or both)?

Table 4 Methods of objective assessment of constipation

Parameter	Test	Comments
Bowel frequency	Counting episodes of defaecation	Patient diary recording or clinical observation are more accurate than recall. Often only 'satisfactory' episodes of defaecation are counted, but who decides
	Stool-free interval	72-h periods without defaecation are counted.[57] May be more clinically relevant than simple bowel frequency
Whole intestinal transit time	Radio-opaque markers	Requires minimal specialized equipment, but cumbersome[28]
	Scintigraphy	Specialist facilities required
	Radio-telemetry	Can demonstrate regional contributions to transit time
	Stool consistency	Non-invasive, quick. Shape of stools can be graded, and can be estimated reliably either by patients or staff. Shown to correlate well with transit time in palliative care patients[12]
Small bowel transit time	Lactulose-hydrogen breath test	More rapid than any direct measure of whole intestinal transit
Extent of facal loading	Radiography	Rapid. Gives only a static measure of intestinal function. Scoring methods have been devised, but show poor correlation with other tests

action and seeps past the mass, appearing as diarrhoea and, if the closing pressure of the anal sphincters has been exceeded by the mass, faecal leakage, or incontinence. Ninety-eight per cent of faecal impactions are said to occur in the rectum and although it is probable that opioid analgesia alters this distribution, rectal examination will diagnose the great majority.

Intestinal obstruction by tumour or adhesions. Known intra-abdominal malignant deposits, previous intestinal surgery, alternating constipation and diarrhoea, gut colic, and nausea and vomiting combine to suggest the presence of intestinal obstruction. A similar picture can, however, occur in severe constipation of which the 'narcotic bowel syndrome' following use of opioid analgesia is probably one manifestation. The distinction is important, as attempts to clear 'constipation', which is actually obstruction by use of stimulant laxatives, can cause severe pain.

Nausea. Some patients rapidly experience nausea, with or without vomiting, in the presence of intestinal hold-up.[32] Unexplained nausea or vomiting should prompt enquiry and examination for constipation.

Abdominal pain. The effort of colonic muscle to propel hard faeces commonly leads to abdominal pain, frequently colicky in nature. History and examination usually suggest the cause of the pain, but constipation is still sometimes 'treated' with morphine. Such pain may be particularly marked—and difficult to diagnose—where abdominal or pelvic tumour exists, presumably as a result either of pressure on the tumour from distended gut or because of partial intestinal obstruction.

Palpation of the abdomen may reveal faecal masses in the line of the descending colon and even that of the more proximal colon and caecum. The distinction between tumour and faecal masses can be hard to make. Faeces will usually indent, if the patient will tolerate sufficiently firm pressure, and may give a crepitus-like sensation because of entrained gas. They also move, given time. Sometimes, an abdominal radiograph is needed to distinguish tumour from stool, but this is uncommon.

Digital examination of the rectum may reveal a hard mass of impacted faeces. The clinical picture, however, may be of faecal leakage. Alternatively, the complete absence of stool implies colonic inertia. Rectal examination may also uncover rectal tumour, a rectocoele, solitary rectal ulcer, or anal stenosis. A lax anal sphincter may indicate spinal cord damage associated with colonic hypotonia. If a rectocoele or compression from pelvic tumour masses is suspected, vaginal examination may be justifiable.

Examination of the stool can be useful. Small, hard pellets suggest slow colonic transit, ribbon-like stools suggest stenosis or haemorrhoids, and blood or mucus suggests tumour, haemorrhoids, or co-existing colitis.

Urinary incontinence. Faecal impaction is well-recognized as a precipitant of urinary incontinence in the elderly, and the recent onset of incontinence should indicate abdominal and rectal examination as the first investigative steps.

Investigations

Investigations are rarely needed in the assessment of constipation in palliative medicine. Abdominal radiography may distinguish between constipation and obstruction if there is persisting doubt, but is rarely necessary and should certainly not be a standard procedure.

Blood tests are confirmatory rather than a screening procedure, but if the clinical picture is suggestive, corrected calcium levels and thyroid function tests should be performed.

Management approaches

Prophylaxis

The aetiologies of constipation in patients with progressive disease (Table 1) suggest several prophylactic measures (Table 5). First of all, there should be good general symptom control, without which no other measures are possible. A key stimulus to colonic peristalsis and defaecation is activity[11] and hence patients should be encouraged and enabled to be as mobile as their physical limitations allow.

Constipated stools have relatively low water content, rendering them hard and difficult to pass. This tendency will be exacerbated if the individual is dehydrated and an adequate fluid intake is therefore helpful. The overall comfort of the person must be kept in view, however, and constipation does not justify the use of parenteral infusions. Rather, the policy must be to enhance oral intake by encouragement and the provision of drinks the patient likes—men frequently identify beer as a laxative in its own right.

Ill people have small appetites and what food they do eat tends to be low in fibre. Dietary fibre deficiency has been linked with constipation in Western society, but individuals with severe constipation are not fibre deficient and their gut function responds poorly to added fibre.[33] Work with radiotherapy patients in Oxford suggested that an increase in stool frequency of 50 per cent would require an approximately 450 per cent mean increase in dietary fibre, well beyond the tolerance of most subjects.[34] Hence, although opportunities should be taken to raise the fibre content of patients' diets, this alone will not correct severe constipation and the priority remains that food should be as attractive as possible to the person who is expected to eat it.

Doctors should know which drugs are likely to cause constipation (Table 2) and either avoid them or make a laxative available at the time of first prescription, without waiting until constipation is established.

Institutional lack of privacy for defaecation and the use of bed pans, which impose an inappropriate posture and greatly increase the pressure required to expel a stool, create an environment conducive to constipation. There is evidence that practised patients adapt to such indignities, but it should be a priority to allow patients privacy and the use of a lavatory, or at least a commode, for defaecation.

Use of oral laxative agents

Despite prophylaxis, the majority of patients with advanced disease require laxatives. Nearly 80 per cent of hospice cancer patients need laxatives; this applies to 63 per cent of our patients who do not receive strong opioid analgesia and 87 per cent of those who do, the former figure being similar to the reported prevalence of constipation in a hospitalized, elderly population with non-malignant disease.[7]

Laxative agents may be divided into those that predominantly soften the stool and those that predominantly stimulate gut peristalsis (Table 6). However, any drug that softens stool also increases its bulk and thus reflexly stimulates colonic peristalsis. Agents that directly stimulate gut muscle contraction are known also to enhance intestinal fluid secretion and so

Table 5 Prophylaxis of constipation

Maintain good general symptom control
Encourage activity
Maintain adequate oral fluid intake
Maximize the fibre content of the diet
Anticipate constipating effects of drugs, altering treatment or starting a laxative prophylactically
Create a favourable environment

Table 6 Oral laxative classification

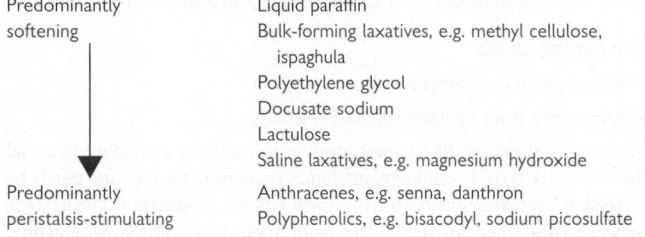

Predominantly softening	Liquid paraffin
	Bulk-forming laxatives, e.g. methyl cellulose, ispaghula
↓	Polyethylene glycol
	Docusate sodium
	Lactulose
	Saline laxatives, e.g. magnesium hydroxide
Predominantly peristalsis-stimulating	Anthracenes, e.g. senna, danthron
	Polyphenolics, e.g. bisacodyl, sodium picosulfate

improve stool consistency. Nevertheless, there is evidence that the combination of softener and stimulant is effective at a lower total dose than a predominantly softening agent alone and causes fewer adverse effects than a predominantly peristalsis-stimulating agent given singly.[35]

The acceptability of laxative therapy will be maximized if previously satisfactory drugs are not changed unnecessarily, even if they are not the unit's standard prescription, and if the patient's preference regarding the choice of a solid or liquid laxative, sweet or less sweet, is heeded. Clinical criteria guide the selection of the class of laxative, but within most classes there are options that can reflect the patients' wishes.

The aim of laxative therapy is comfortable defaecation, not any particular frequency of evacuation. No single laxative dose is adequate for everyone, and many patients are subjected to both rectal interventions and an inadequate oral dose of laxative. The dose needs to be titrated against the response and the advent of adverse effects, remembering the latent period of action of the drug concerned, and should be increased prophylactically if, say, opioids are introduced or their dose is being substantially increased.

As in chronic pain, so in chronic constipation, therapy should be regular, not intermittent. Low doses of laxative are best given at night, but higher doses will need to be divided, usually morning and evening, but sometimes more often. Diarrhoea usually settles promptly by suspending therapy for 24 h and resuming one dose level down.

Lubricant laxatives

Preparation: liquid paraffin.

Starting dose: 10 ml daily.

Mechanism: liquid paraffin lubricates the stool surface and softens the stool by penetration allowing easier passage.

Latency of action: 1–3 days.

Uses: liquid paraffin has been blamed for many adverse effects. Most relevant to palliative medicine are the lipoid pneumonia, which may follow paraffin inhalation, and the propensity to cause leakage of oily faecal material with consequent embarrassment and perianal irritation.

There seems no justification for reliance on liquid paraffin as the sole laxative. However, its emulsion with magnesium hydroxide, which contains only 25 per cent paraffin, has not been associated with the above adverse effects and has been recommended as an effective and cheap laxative preparation.[36]

Surfactant laxatives

Preparations: docusate sodium, poloxamer.

Starting dose: docusate sodium 300 mg daily.

Mechanism: these agents act as detergents to increase water penetration, and hence softening, of the stool. Docusate also promotes water, sodium, and chloride secretion in the jejunum and colon;[37] there is a clinical impression that at higher doses it may stimulate peristalsis.

Latency of action: 1–3 days.

Use: docusate is available alone or in combination with danthron (Codanthrusate) or bisacodyl. Poloxamer is marketed only in combination with danthron (Codanthramer). Docusate's ability as a laxative has been questioned, as it failed to increase colonic output of solids or water in healthy volunteers.[38] However, docusate has been found to be more effective than placebo in clinical trials in elderly or chronically ill patients.[39] Poloxamer has been claimed to be an effective laxative, but in clinical practice there is no opportunity to separate its benefits from those of the danthron with which it is combined. Docusate alone has failed to win popularity in British hospice practice.

Bulk-forming agents

Preparations: bran, methyl cellulose, ispaghula.

Starting doses: bran 8 g daily, others 3–4 g daily.

Mechanism: these agents increase stool bulk partly by providing material that resists bacterial breakdown and hence remains in the gut, and partly by providing a substrate for bacterial growth and gas production. The balance between these mechanisms varies from agent to agent. Non-digestible polythene particles will enhance stool bulk and shorten transit time, presumably by a reflex response to stretch or direct mechanical irritation. However, it appears that transit is speeded especially as a result of fermentation and is to some degree independent of stool bulking action.[40]

Latency of action: 2–4 days.

Use: bulking agents are 'normalizers' rather than true laxatives: they will soften a hard stool but make firmer a loose one. Effective in mild constipation, they are less helpful in palliative medicine for three main reasons. First, they need to be taken with ample water (at least 200–300 ml); this and their consistency are unacceptable to many ill patients. Second, if taken with inadequate water, a viscous mass may result, which can complete an incipient malignant obstruction. Third, their effectiveness in severe constipation is doubtful.

Osmotic laxatives

Preparations: lactulose, mannitol, and sorbitol.

Starting dose: 15 ml bd.

Mechanism: these agents are not broken down or absorbed in the small gut, where as a result they exert an osmotic influence to retain water in the lumen. Bacterial degradation in the colon produces short-chain organic acids, which lower the intestinal pH, possibly stimulating peristalsis, and increasing stool bulk by enlargement of the microbial mass. These acids are absorbed and so the osmotic effect does not extend throughout the colon.

Latency of action: 1–2 days.

Use: lactulose is the most popular single laxative in British hospices and probably in British general hospitals too, where its expense has caused concern. It significantly increases faecal weight, volume, water, and frequency but if used alone in opioid-induced constipation often requires to be given in doses that result in bloating and colic. Flatulence is a problem for about 20 per cent of patients. Its sweet taste is sickly to some. There are suggestions that tolerance to its laxative effects may occur, presumably through changes in bacterial flora. Mannitol and sorbitol are less used as oral preparations, but sorbitol has been reported to be as effective as lactulose, cheaper and less nauseating.[41]

Saline laxatives

Preparations: magnesium hydroxide or sulphate, sodium sulphate.

Starting doses: 2–4 g daily.

Mechanism: these agents are poorly absorbed and, unlike lactulose, exert an osmotic influence throughout the gut. They also increase intestinal water secretion and appear directly to stimulate peristalsis. Magnesium and sulfate ions are the most potent. It has been suggested that saline laxatives' actions are mediated by cholecystokinin (CCK)[42] but other releasers of CCK, such as calcium, lack a purgative effect.

Latency of action: 1–6 h (dose dependent).

Use: saline laxatives, especially magnesium sulphate, can produce an undesirably strong purgative action. Except as a last resort they are therefore not regularly used in ill patients. Magnesium hydroxide is less potent than the sulphate and, either alone or as an emulsion with liquid paraffin, deserves re-evaluation as a cheaper alternative to lactulose and other more popular preparations.[36]

Polyethylene glycol (PEG)

Starting doses: for constipation, two sachets daily, dissolved in 250 ml water. For faecal impaction, eight sachets per day in 1 l of water.

Latency of action: higher doses 1–3 days, longer for lower doses.

Mechanism: PEG is a non-absorbed, non-degraded polymer prepared in an iso-osmotic solution (with sodium bicarbonate and sodium and potassium chlorides) to avoid electrolyte disturbance. It, therefore, provides a source of non-absorbed fluid, which can then exert a softening effect on the bowel contents. Stool weight is increased in proportion to the total mass of PEG ingested.[43] It accelerates gut transit and can provide an oral treatment for faecal impaction[44] and chronic constipation.[45] However, large volumes may be needed. Culbert et al.[44] used 500 ml bd of 110 g/L PEG solution for up to 3 days in impacted elderly patients. The full dose was managed by

12 out of 16 patients on day 1, six out of eight on day 2, and one out of two on day 3. Fifteen of the 16 passed a good volume of stool with ease. The PEG solution was consumed in an average of 143 (75–300) min. Corazziari's 'small volume' approach used a total of 500 ml daily over 4 weeks.[45]

Use: for those patients who can tolerate the volumes involved, PEG can be either their routine laxative or, at higher doses, can relieve faecal impaction without recourse to suppositories or enemas. Trial evidence of the effectiveness and acceptability of PEG in palliative care is pending.

Anthracene and polyphenolic laxatives

Preparations: anthracenes: senna, danthron; polyphenolics: bisacodyl, sodium picosulphate.

Starting doses: senna 15 mg daily, danthron 50 mg daily, bisacodyl 10 mg daily, and sodium picosulphate 5 mg daily.

Mechanism: these drugs directly stimulate the myenteric plexus to induce peristalsis; their action can be abolished by local anaesthetic infiltration of the mucosa. Colonic electromyography in man following oral senna shows an increase in myoelectrical activity of the type seen in diarrhoea. Net absorption of water and electrolytes in the colon is reduced, partly through inhibition of Na^+, K^+-ATPase and probably also by stimulation of cAMP, prostaglandin E_2, and perhaps serotonin synthesis. The effects on water and electrolyte transport may be relatively more important for polyphenolic agents than for the anthraquinones.[46]

Senna contains anthraquinone glycosides, which are almost inactive as laxatives but are converted by colonic bacteria to the active aglycone forms. In consequence, activity is concentrated almost entirely in the colon. The aglycones are absorbed to a limited degree and secreted in the bile, but this circulation is more important for danthron and the polyphenolic agents, which undergo glucuronidation and can then be reconverted in the gut to active drug, prolonging the agents' action.

Latency of action: 6–12 h (bisacodyl suppository 15–60 min).

Uses: senna is the most popular laxative in British hospices after lactulose, and the two drugs are often used in combination. This is a logical practice, lactulose providing a relatively greater stool softening effect and senna a relatively greater peristalsis-stimulating effect. Danthron is available in combination with a surfactant agent, either docusate (Codanthrusate) or poloxamer (Codanthramer, which is available in two strengths with differing proportions of the constituents, the higher strength containing three times as much danthron as the lower but five times as much poloxamer). Both Codanthrusate and Codanthramer are available as a capsule or a suspension. It should be noted that in the standard strength of codanthramer one capsule is equal to 5 ml suspension, but in the higher strength one capsule is the equivalent of only 2.5 ml of the suspension. Equal proportions of senna liquid and lactulose are significantly more potent than standard codanthramer, but are probably less potent than higher strength codanthramer.[47] Sodium picosulphate is formulated as a single strength elixir.

Any of the anthraquinones or polyphenolics can cause severe purgation, with colicky abdominal pains. This can generally be avoided by dose titration and combined use of a more specific stool-softening agent. They are valuable where there is evidence of colonic inertia.

Morphine is known to antagonize the water and electrolyte effects of senna[48] and it has been suggested that there is a relatively fixed relationship between a dose of codeine and that of senna, which will counteract the resulting constipation.[49] This may be true for a given individual taking relatively low doses of opioid analgesia, but increase of opioid dosage does not proportionately increase constipation.[16] Also, effective doses of polyphenolic laxatives show four- to eightfold variation between individuals[50] and the same seems true of the anthraquinones.

Both classes of agent have been implicated in causing myenteric plexus damage,[51] but neither this nor danthron's unconvincing association with carcinogenicity in rats is sufficient to influence their use in palliative medicine. Patients should, however, be warned of the pink discoloration of the urine that danthron can cause and watch kept for the perianal rash it may precipitate, especially in incontinent patients.

Use of rectal laxatives

The use of rectal laxatives is undignified for the patient and may be unpleasant for staff, but their short latency of action is satisfying for both parties, who may in consequence come to rely heavily on them.

Rectal laxatives may be given either as suppositories or enemas, the latter usually being used as second-line therapy or for rectal impaction. Any rectal intervention may precipitate defaecation by stimulation of the ano-colonic reflex, but more specific mechanisms of action parallel those of oral agents.

Lubricant rectal laxatives

Enemas: arachis oil, olive oil.

Use: these agents are normally used as retention enemas overnight to allow evacuation or manual removal of hard faeces impacted in the rectum. Naturally, their efficacy depends on the patient's ability to retain the oil.

Osmotic rectal laxatives

Suppositories: glycerine.

Enema: sorbitol.

Use: glycerine softens stools by osmosis and is also lubricant. Any stimulation of colonic contraction is presumably mechanical. Sorbitol is a constituent of several proprietary micro-enemas.

Surfactant rectal laxatives

Enemas: sodium docusate, sodium lauryl sulphoacetate, sodium alkyl sulphacetate.

Uses: docusate elixir can be used as an enema, but all the above agents are included in different proprietary mini-enemas to aid stool softening by aiding water penetration of the faecal mass.

Saline rectal laxatives

Suppositories: sodium phosphate.

Enemas: sodium phosphate, sodium citrate.

Uses: in rectal use these agents are claimed to release bound water from faeces, but, as with oral saline laxatives, may stimulate rectal or distal colonic peristalsis, an action that is presumably aided when an extended enema tube is used to place the liquid as high as possible in the rectum. Repeated use of phosphate enemas can cause hypocalcaemia and hyperphosphataemia. Phosphate enemas can also produce rectal gangrene in ill patients with a history of haemorrhoids.[52] Hence care should be taken in their use.

Sodium phosphate is available in an effervescent base as a suppository (Carbalax). The resultant production of gas is intended to assist defecation, although as rectal distension by gas is readily distinguishable from that by stool the rationale is unclear.

Polyphenolic rectal laxative

Suppositories: bisacodyl suppositories, 5 mg (paediatric), 10 mg (adult).

Use: alone among rectal laxative preparations, bisacodyl suppositories act principally by promoting colonic peristalsis. Their latency of action is claimed to be 15–60 min, compared with 6–12 h orally. The difference is probably due to bisacodyl's immediate conversion to its active desacetyl form by colonic flora in the rectum. As activity depends on bisacodyl reaching the rectal mucosa, care should be taken so that stool does not separate the suppository from the rectal wall.

Bisacodyl suppositories are sometimes inserted in an empty rectum to 'bring the stool down'. A plausible rationale exists for this practice but its efficacy relative to use of oral laxatives, or even a high phosphate enema, is untested.

Selection of rectal laxatives

As with oral laxatives, there are few data on the comparative efficacy of rectal laxatives. One study showed the following percentages of patients achieving defaecation within an hour of the rectal intervention: phosphate enema 100 per cent, mini-enema (Micralax) 95 per cent, bisacodyl suppository 66 per cent, and glycerine suppository 38 per cent.[53] The approximately equal effectiveness of phosphate and mini-enemas,[54] the speed of action of mini-enemas,[55] and the superiority of bisacodyl suppositories over glycerine suppositories[56] have been confirmed elsewhere. The volume (about 130 ml) and potential adverse effects of phosphate enemas mean that, if an enema is required, the much smaller (5 ml), rather cheaper, and nearly as effective mini-enema, of which various proprietary products are available, is preferable. If a constipated patient simply requires assistance with an initial evacuation, suppositories may be adequate if only moderate softening is required. A combination of a bisacodyl and a glycerine suppository is often used, as is that of an enema followed by suppositories. Both practices are logical, but no data yet exist to show what advantages they may hold or which categories of patient may benefit.

If none of the rectal laxatives mentioned proves adequate to remove impacted faeces, rectal lavage with normal saline can be performed. This is cumbersome and messy, requiring about 8 l of (preferably) warmed saline. Tap water should not be used because of the risk of circulatory overload and neither should soap and water, which is irritant to the rectal mucosa and can cause hyperkalaemia if a potassium-based soap is employed. In practice, most units will prefer in these circumstances to follow the softening action of an oil retention enema with a manual removal of faeces, under cover of diazepam sedation if necessary.

Whenever rectal laxatives have been needed, the doses and types of oral laxatives being taken by the patient should be reappraised and if possible modified to obviate further rectal measures.

A guideline for laxative therapy

It would be desirable to produce an evidence-based guideline for the use of laxatives in palliative care. However, Medline and Embase literature searches (from the initiation of the databases to 2001) reveal only three randomized controlled trials of laxatives conducted in this patient group, together with another carried out in healthy volunteers using a model of opioid-induced constipation.[35] Of the clinical trials, one claimed to find a difference in effectiveness[47] and the others did not.[57,58] Because of differing designs and end-points, it is not possible to make a synthesis from these studies. The volunteer study found that all the preparations tested could relieve constipation, but the most favourable combination of medication burden and adverse effects arose from a combination of stimulant and softening types.

We are therefore still in the position of extrapolating evidence from other fields of medicine. Three possibly relevant systematic reviews of laxatives have been published: one looks at trials in chronic constipation[59] and the other, which is an extension of it, focuses on constipation in the elderly.[60] Seventeen out of 36 admissible trials in the first review and nine out of 20 in the second involved fibre-based preparations, which may be inappropriate for routine use in patients with advanced cancer. Both reviews conclude that laxatives and fibre improve bowel frequency by about 1.5 bowel movements per week compared with placebo. Neither was able to find evidence that any particular group of laxatives was more effective than another. The third review[61] addresses the effectiveness of laxatives in adults generally and reaches similar conclusions, although it draws attention to the cost implications of the lack of comparative data, that is, start with the cheapest laxative as there is no evidence that expensive ones are any better.

There is therefore no single correct way of selecting and employing laxatives, but one rational approach is summarized below. Naturally these situations may succeed one another.

1. *Exclude intestinal obstruction:* if in doubt use only laxatives with a predominantly softening action, for example, lactulose, sodium docusate, in order to avoid causing colic. Do not use bulking agents.
2. *If the rectum is impacted with hard faeces* spontaneous evacuation is unlikely to be possible without local measures to soften the faecal mass, for example, glycerine suppositories, olive, or arachis oil enema. It still may be necessary to perform a manual rectal evacuation, for which sedation or additional analgesia is often required. Alternatively, saline rectal lavage can be given.
3. *If the rectum is loaded with soft faeces* a predominantly peristalsis-stimulating laxative, for example, senna, may be effective alone. If there is rectal discomfort, a mini-enema may assist the initial defaecation. Frequent review is essential, as there is a likelihood that a stool-softening laxative will be required later as well, given either separately, for example, lactulose, or as in combination preparation, for example, codanthrusate, codanthramer.
4. *If there is little or no stool in the rectum,* a peristalsis-stimulating laxative is the drug of choice, for example, senna, but the stools are likely to be hard and it is a reasonable policy to use a stool-softening laxative in addition, for example, lactulose, or a combination preparation, for example, codanthrusate, codanthramer.

New developments and alternative approaches

There is much scope for further work on the comparative efficacy and palatability of conventional laxatives. However, several new developments or alternative approaches are worth mentioning.

There is interest in the use of prokinetic agents to accelerate intestinal transit. Cisapride, which acts by enhancing acetylcholine release from myenteric neurones through $5HT_4$ receptor agonism, is better than placebo in improving stool consistency and frequency in idiopathic constipation.[62] It has, however, been withdrawn from the market in the United Kingdom. Metoclopramide, which also increases gastrointestinal motility by interaction with gut $5HT_4$ receptors, has been shown to be effective in the so-called 'narcotic bowel syndrome' when given by continuous subcutaneous infusion.[63] Oral metoclopramide has not found a place in routine laxative treatment and is less potently prokinetic than cisapride.

As an antibiotic, oral erythromycin causes diarrhoea on about 50 per cent of occasions.[64] Apart from altering the balance of the gut flora, erythromycin acts as an agonist at motilin receptors, which are responsible for initiating the migrating motor complex in the small bowel. Motilin receptors are also present elsewhere in the gut and erythromycin reduces transit time in the right colon in healthy humans.[65] However, colonic activity was not stimulated in a group of chronically constipated individuals,[66] and so whether erythromycin and related macrolides that also possess a 14-carbon lactone ring will be effective laxatives or predominantly antireflux agents remains to be seen.

Morphine-induced constipation can be counteracted by an opioid antagonist given orally because a major part of the opioid effect on the human gut is mediated peripherally rather than centrally. Naloxone has shown success experimentally in patients receiving strong opioid analgesia.[67,68] Oral naloxone has a systemic availability of under 1 per cent, due to first pass hepatic metabolism, allowing a laxative effect without reversal of analgesia or generalized withdrawal. However, although non-controlled studies have shown response rates of 67–82 per cent, opioid withdrawal or return of pain has occurred in 13–30 per cent of people. A major multicentre randomized controlled trial of naloxone has recently been abandoned because of reported lack of efficacy. Quaternary derivatives of opioid antagonists, which do not cross the blood–brain barrier, may be an alternative to the use of naloxone itself and methylnatrexone has shown early promise.[69]

Further work is needed to clarify the role of opioid antagonists as laxatives.

The specific cholecystokinin (CCK) antagonist loxiglumide, given orally, significantly accelerated colonic transit in healthy volunteers.[70] This seems an unexpected finding as CCK itself increases colonic motor activity and can cause purgation. Clarification is needed.

Another possible therapeutic avenue for the management of opioid-induced constipation is suggested by the finding that in mice L-arginine reduces intestinal slowing produced by morphine. This perhaps occurs by the release of nitric oxide, which has been identified as a neuromodulator in the gut.[71]

Herbal medicine knows of many plants with laxative properties. Chrysanthemum stems and rhubarb have both been investigated recently as they contain anthraquinones, similar to the constituents of senna. Patients may prefer such treatments to pharmaceutical laxatives.

Diarrhoea

Definition

Diarrhoea is the passage of frequent loose stools with urgency. Objectively, it has been defined as the passage of more than three unformed stools within a 24-h period. Patients, however, may describe as 'diarrhoea' a single loose stool, frequent small stools of normal or even hard consistency, or faecal incontinence. As with constipation, therefore, a complaint of diarrhoea requires careful clarification.

Prevalence

Diarrhoea is a complaint of 7–10 per cent of cancer patients on admission to a hospice and 6 per cent of similar patients in hospital. It is, therefore, a far less common problem in palliative medicine than constipation when cancer patients are being considered, but 27 per cent of symptomatic HIV-infected patients have been reported to suffer diarrhoea.[72] (For management of HIV-related diarrhoea, see Chapters 10.2 and 10.3.)

Clinical manifestations and diagnostic considerations

Diarrhoea persisting for over 3 weeks is said to be chronic and is often linked to serious organic disease. Most diarrhoea is acute, lasting only a few days, and is generally the result of gastrointestinal infection (Table 7), possibly including overgrowth by *Candida.*

However, the commonest cause of diarrhoea in palliative medicine is an imbalance of laxative therapy.[73] This particularly occurs when laxative doses have been increased to clear a backlog of constipated stool. The diarrhoea normally settles within 24–48 h if laxatives are temporarily stopped, after which they should be reinstated at a lower dose. Meanwhile the diarrhoea may be distressing, especially if it leads to faecal incontinence.

Table 7 Causes of diarrhoea in palliative medicine

Drugs	
	Laxatives
	Antacids
	Antibiotics
	Chemotherapy agents, esp. 5-fluorouracil
	NSAID, esp. mefenamic acid, diclofenac, indomethacin
	Mitomycin
	Iron preparations
	Disaccharide-containing elixirs
Radiation	
Obstruction	
	Malignant
	Faecal impaction
	Narcotic bowel syndrome
Malabsorption	
	Pancreatic carcinoma
	Gastrectomy
	Ileal resection
	Colectomy
Tumour	
	Colonic or rectal carcinoma
	Pancreatic islet cell tumours
	Carcinoid tumours
Concurrent disease	
	Diabetes mellitus
	Hyperthyroidism
	Inflammatory bowel disease
	Irritable bowel syndrome
	Gastrointestinal infection
Diet	
	Bran
	Fruit
	Hot spices
	Alcohol

A variety of other common drugs can also precipitate diarrhoea, either commonly, as in the case of antacids and antibiotics, or idiosyncratically, as in the case of non-steroidal anti-inflammatory agents or iron preparations. Sorbitol, used as a sweetener in some 'sugar-free' elixirs, is easily overlooked as a cause of diarrhoea in sensitive patients. Those receiving enteral feeding appear particularly prone, sorbitol being more than twice as likely to be the cause of diarrhoea as the feed itself.[74]

Malignant intestinal obstruction and faecal impaction are the next most common causes of diarrhoea in this patient group. Complete intestinal obstruction produces intractable constipation, but partial obstruction may present with either diarrhoea or alternating diarrhoea and constipation. This clinical picture can also result from severe constipation caused by opioid analgesia, where it has been dubbed the 'narcotic bowel syndrome'.[17] Faecal impaction results in fluid stool leaking past the mass, often with anal leakage or incontinence. In elderly patients hospitalized for non-malignant disease, faecal impaction can account for 55 per cent of instances of diarrhoea,[75] emphasizing the need for careful attention to regular laxative therapy in any ill, relatively immobile population.

Radiotherapy involving the abdomen or pelvis is liable to cause diarrhoea, with a peak incidence in the second or third week of therapy and continuing for some time after cessation of the course. Damage to intestinal mucosa by radiation results in the release of prostaglandins and the malabsorption of bile salts, both of which increase peristaltic activity. Chronic radiation enteritis rarely presents as diarrhoea. Uncommonly, another iatrogenic cause of diarrhoea relevant to palliative care is coeliac plexus blockade, which can be associated with the onset of profuse, long-lasting watery diarrhoea. This possibly results from anatomical variations in the innervation of the gut so that in certain individuals interruption of the coeliac plexus has an excessive influence on bowel activity.[76]

Malabsorption sufficient to cause diarrhoea may occur in carcinoma of the head of the pancreas or after gastrectomy or ileal resection. Failure of pancreatic secretion leads to reduced fat absorption and consequent steatorrhoea. Gastrectomy can also produce steatorrhoea, presumably as a result of poor mixing of food with pancreatic and biliary secretions. However, the accompanying vagotomy causes increased faecal secretion of bile acids in some patients resulting in increased water and electrolyte secretion in the colon and hence a chologenic diarrhoea, compounding the problem.

Ileal resection reduces the gut's ability to reabsorb bile acids, of which up to 97 per cent are normally recirculated, again producing chologenic diarrhoea, which is characteristically watery and explosive. If less than 100 cm of terminal ileum is removed, fat malabsorption generally does not occur, as the liver can compensate for the increased biliary loss. A resection of over about 100 cm results in relative bile acid deficiency and hence fat malabsorption, exacerbating the diarrhoea. Ileal resection produces a disaccharidase deficiency proportional to the length of removed and thus an osmotic diarrhoea due to carbohydrate malabsorption.

Partial colectomy produces little, if any, persistent diarrhoea. However, total or almost total colectomy results in a high volume of liquid effluent that rapidly diminishes over 7–10 days but still remains at 400–800 ml/day owing to the small intestine's inability to compensate fully for the loss of the colon's water absorbing capacity. For this reason an ileostomy is normally fashioned. Such patients require an average of an extra litre of water per day and about 7 g of extra salt to compensate, with special care needed in hot weather. Iron and vitamin supplementation is also indicated. Similar symptoms can also result from an enterocolic fistula, caused either by cancer or as a result of operation.[77] Alteration of gut anatomy by surgery may also promote diarrhoea through bacterial overgrowth.

A colonic or rectal tumour can precipitate diarrhoea through causing partial intestinal obstruction, or loosen stools through increased mucus secretion. Rarely, endocrine tumours cause a secretory diarrhoea. The WDHA syndrome (watery diarrhoea hypokalaemia achlorhydria) is associated with tumours of the pancreatic islet cells and of the sympathetic nervous system, including the adrenal glands, and can occur with bronchogenic carcinomas. VIP is thought to be the causative hormone both here and in the diarrhoea of the Verner–Morrison syndrome encountered in childhood ganglioneuroblastoma. Diarrhoea occurs also in the

Zollinger– Ellison syndrome, seen with pancreatic islet cell tumours secreting gastrin, and in carcinoid tumours, where serotonin, prostaglandins, bradykinin, and VIP secretions have all been implicated.[78]

Apart from concurrent gastrointestinal disease (Table 6), the ability of dietary factors to cause diarrhoea should be remembered. Excessive dietary fibre may produce diarrhoea and fruits may do so both by this means and by their content of specific laxative factors.

Assessment

A complaint of diarrhoea demands a careful history, detailing first of all the frequency of defaecation, the nature of the stools, and the time course of the problem. Together, these often indicate the diagnosis. Defaecation described as 'diarrhoea', which occurs only once or twice a day, suggests anal incontinence. Profuse watery stools are characteristic of colonic diarrhoea, whereas the pale, fatty, offensive stools of steatorrhoea indicate malabsorption due to a pancreatic or small intestinal cause. The sudden advent of diarrhoea following a period of constipation, perhaps with little warning of impending defaecation, should raise the suspicion of faecal impaction.

Both current and recent medication should be sought. If laxatives are to blame, the error may be of insufficiently regular therapy, resulting in alternating constipation and diarrhoea, or an excessive dose. Too much of a predominantly peristalsis-stimulating laxative tends to produce colic and urgency, and too much of a predominantly stool-softening agent may cause faecal leakage, although at high doses lactulose and docusate have the ability to produce colic and watery diarrhoea in some patients.

Examination and investigations

Examination should exclude the possibilities of faecal impaction and intestinal obstruction, and should therefore include rectal examination and abdominal palpation for faecal masses. If there is doubt, an abdominal radiograph will make the distinction, but this is rarely necessary.

Steatorrhoea is generally clearly suggested in the history and readily confirmed on examination of the stool. Persistent watery diarrhoea, without systemic, upset which would suggest an infective cause, may be more difficult to diagnose. If in doubt, the stool osmolality and sodium and potassium concentrations should be measured. The anion gap, the difference between the stool osmolality and double the sum of the cation concentrations, is over 50 mmol/l in osmotic diarrhoea, because of the presence of an additional non-absorbed solute, for example, a disaccharide from a medicinal elixir. An anion gap of below 50 mmol/l shows secretory diarrhoea, resulting from active secretion of fluid and electrolytes, as in the WDHA syndrome. Ileal resection gives rise to a mixed picture, which will become purely secretory if the patient can be fasted.

In any persistent diarrhoea, haematology and blood chemistry should be checked. Diarrhoea occurring within 3 days of in-patient admission may be due to community-acquired bacterial enteric pathogens such as *Salmonella*, *Shigella*, or *Campylobacter*, or to viral infection. After this point the infection is likely to have originated in the in-patient unit and stool culture is usually unrewarding; repeating the culture does not improve the diagnostic yield.[79] *Clostridium difficile* is the most commonly detected cause of nosocomial diarrhoea and is identified by immunoassay of its toxins.

Management approaches

Supportive treatment

Other than in HIV infection, diarrhoea in palliative medicine is rarely of sufficient degree or duration to cause significant risk through dehydration. If rehydration *is* needed the oral route is superior to the intravenous. Proprietary rehydration solutions, containing appropriate electrolyte concentrations and a source of glucose to facilitate active electrolyte transport across the gut wall, are adequate for all but the most severe diarrhoea. Any diarrhoea will benefit from a diet of clear liquids, such as flat lemonade or ginger ale, and simple carbohydrates, as in toast or crackers. Some infective causes of diarrhoea cause transient lactase deficiency and so milk should be avoided in these circumstances. Protein and, later, fats are reintroduced gradually to the diet as the diarrhoea resolves.

Specific treatment

Specific treatments exist for several causes of diarrhoea (Table 8). Pancreatin is a combination of amylase, lipase, and protease, which is available in several forms for pancreatic enzyme replacement. The effective dose varies widely between individuals and it may be more effective if gastric acidity is reduced with an H_2-receptor antagonist, in which case enteric-coated preparations should not be used.

Cholestyramine is a bile acid-binding resin that is effective in controlling chologenic diarrhoea provided ileal resection has not been too extensive. It is often found unpalatable. Both cholestyramine[80] and aspirin[81] have been claimed to be effective in radiation-induced diarrhoea.

Carcinoid syndrome diarrhoea often responds to general antidiarrhoeals, but peripheral serotonin antagonists, such as methysergide or the less toxic cyproheptadine, have been claimed to be effective against more severe diarrhoea and, sometimes, the accompanying malabsorption.[78] $5HT_3$ antagonists may also have a role in this type of diarrhoea.[82]

Metronidazole is the recommended antibiotic for *C. difficile* diarrhoea, and can reasonably be tried also in situations where diarrhoea is suspected to be due to bacterial overgrowth, where it may produce a prompt resolution.

General treatment

Non-specific antidiarrhoeal agents are numerous, but are either absorbent, adsorbent, mucosal prostaglandin inhibitors, opioids, or somatostatin derivatives. These agents may make illness due to *Shigella* and *C. difficile* worse and so should be used with caution if these organisms are known to be present, or if there is blood in the stool or fever.

Absorbent agents

Preparations: bulk-forming agents, for example, methyl cellulose; pectin.

Mechanism: these agents absorb water to form a gelatinous or colloidal mass that gives a thicker consistency to loose stools. Water is held between the fibres in the case of bulk-forming agents, which are better regarded as 'stool normalizers than either laxative or antidiarrhoeal preparations'. Pectin produces a viscous colloidal solution with both absorbent and adsorbent properties.

Uses: bulk-forming agents may have a delay of up to 48 h in onset of antidiarrhoeal action and are poorly tolerated in ill patients. They have proved useful in the management of colostomies but exacerbate electrolyte loss from ileostomies.

The use of pectin against diarrhoea is time-honoured. It can be prepared simply from grated raw apple, but is sometimes combined with the adsorbent kaolin in proprietary antidiarrhoeal mixtures. There is some evidence of effectiveness in children.[83]

Adsorbent agents

Preparations and dose: kaolin, 2–6 g 4 hourly; chalk, 0.5–5 g 4 hourly; attapulgite, 1.2 g stat, 1.2 g after each loose stool up to 8.4 g/day.

Mechanism: adsorbents non-specifically take up dissolved or suspended substances, such as bacteria, toxins, and water, on to their surfaces. All are naturally occurring minerals, kaolin being hydrated aluminium silicate and attapulgite a hydrated magnesium aluminium silicate. The adsorptive capacity of a molecule depends on its surface area and attapulgite, having a three-layered crystalline structure, is claimed in consequence to have

Table 8 Specific treatments for diarrhoea in palliative medicine

Fat malabsorption: pancreatin (may be more effective if H_2 antagonist given before meals)
Chologenic diarrhoea: cholestyramine, 4–12 g tds
Radiation diarrhoea: cholestyramine 4–12 g tds, or aspirin
Zollinger–Ellison syndrome: H_2-antagonist, e.g. ranitidine, initially 150 mg tds
Carcinoid syndrome: cyproheptadine, initially 12 mg daily; methysergide, 12–20 mg/day
Pseudomembranous colitis: vancomycin 125 mg qds; metronidazole 400 mg tds
Ulcerative colitis: mesalazine 1.2–2.4 g/day steroids

33 times the adsorbent capacity of kaolin. How this translates into relative therapeutic efficacy is unknown.

Uses: attapulgite is used alone, but both kaolin and chalk are available in mixtures with morphine, the British Pharmacopoeia formulation of chalk with opium mixture containing considerably more morphine (5 mg/10 ml) than that of kaolin with morphine (0.7 mg/10 ml). Any difference in antidiarrhoeal effectiveness between the mixtures is surely due to this factor. Indeed, there is no evidence, despite their popularity, of any significant antidiarrhoeal effectiveness of either kaolin or chalk apart from that of the opiate with which they may be combined. Kaolin is also available in combination with pectin; there is the same dearth of evidence for efficacy.

Attapulgite has, however, been shown to be better than placebo in acute diarrhoea although significantly less effective than loperamide.(84)

Adsorbents may be appropriate for mild, non-specific acute diarrhoea in a healthy population. Their at best modest effectiveness, and the quite large volumes of a rather unattractive liquid that may have to be taken, make them unsuitable for general use in palliative medicine.

Mucosal prostaglandin inhibitors

Preparations and doses: aspirin, 300 mg 4 hourly, up to 4 g/day; mesalazine, 1.2–2.4 g/day; bismuth subsalicylate, 525 mg half-hourly up to 5 mg/day.

Mechanism: prostaglandins increase intestinal water and electrolyte secretion, and prostaglandin inhibitors (with exceptions such as mefenamic acid and indomethacin) reduce secretion. Bismuth subsalicylate is said to have a direct antimicrobial effect on enterotoxigenic *Escherichia coli.*(85) The active constituent of mesalazine is 5-amino-salicylic acid.

Uses: apart from bismuth subsalicylate, which is used for treatment of non-specific acute diarrhoea, these agents are used as specific anti-diarrhoeal treatments, aspirin for radiation-induced diarrhoea, and mesalazine in ulcerative colitis. All these agents are contraindicated in patients sensitive to salicylate, and the bismuth compound in its upper dose range can produce toxic blood salicylate levels.

Opioid agents

Preparations and doses: codeine, 10–60 mg 4 hourly, duration of action: 4–6 h. Diphenoxylate, 10 mg stat, then 5 mg 6 hourly, duration of action 6–8 h. Loperamide, 4 mg stat, then 2 mg after each loose stool up to 16 mg per day, duration of action 8–16 h.

Mechanism: the opioids act via specific gut opioid receptors to reduce peristalsis in the colon. They also preserve the fasting pattern of motility in the small intestine after food intake. Their effects on water and electrolyte secretion in man at therapeutic doses are unconvincing. Loperamide is capable of reducing ileal calcium fluxes by a mechanism that is not inhibited by naloxone, but the contribution of this effect to its clinical activity is undetermined. Opioids increase anal sphincter pressure and loperamide and codeine have been shown to improve continence in patients with diarrhoea suffering from faecal incontinence;(86) diphenoxylate is less effective, even at the same stool frequency.

Alone of the three, loperamide given orally does not reach or cross the blood–brain barrier significantly. In animal studies the relative specificity for antidiarrhoeal as opposed to analgesic effects for codeine, diphenoxylate, and loperamide was 5.24, 23.7, and greater than 552, respectively. The specificity for morphine was 6.45.(87) Although the recommended maximum daily dose of loperamide is 16 mg, volunteers have received 54 mg/day without ill-effects. Below its recommended maximum of 20 mg/day, diphenoxylate rarely gives significant systemic opioid effects, but does so at doses of 40 mg/day or more. As a result, it is available only in combination with atropine in order to limit its abuse potential.

In man, approximate equivalent antidiarrhoeal doses are 200 mg/day of codeine, 10 mg/day of diphenoxylate, and 4 mg/day of loperamide.(73)

Uses: the opioids are the mainstay of general antidiarrhoeal treatment in palliative medicine. A requirement for morphine analgesia may obviate the need for any additional antidiarrhoeal medication. Loperamide is the opioid antidiarrhoeal of choice, being significantly more effective than diphenoxylate or codeine and with few adverse effects in adults. In children, it has been reported to cause ileus-like conditions, irritability, drowsiness, and signs of opioid toxicity, and more caution is therefore required in its use. For persistent diarrhoea regular therapy can be given, the dose being titrated against the clinical response. The drug's duration of action means that administration can often be twice daily. Loperamide 8–12 mg/day significantly reduces ileostomy output,(88) but in some severe chronic diarrhoeas the required dose may need to be higher than usually recommended.

Codeine is prone to cause systemic opioid effects, but has the merit of cheapness, which encourages some units to use it for mild diarrhoea. In addition, despite the research evidence, clinical experience suggests that the individual response to opioids for diarrhoea can be as idiosyncratic as that for pain, and in some patients codeine has superior antidiarrhoeal properties to the other opioids without causing excessive nausea or drowsiness.

Diphenoxylate is at least as expensive as loperamide in equi-effective doses and appears to hold no advantages.

Somatostatin analogues

Preparations: octreotide: 300–600 mcg/24 h by subcutaneous infusion (British National Formulary recommendation—see notes below). Lanreotide: 30 mg intramuscularly every 14 days.

Mechanism: somatostatin is produced in intestinal D cells and acts on gut epithelial receptors to inhibit secretion and peristalsis. The native form has a short half-life but analogues have been created that are capable of extended activity.

Uses: octreotide has been shown to be effective in cryptosporidial diarrhoea and diarrhoea due to the carcinoid, Zollinger–Ellison, and Verner–Morrison syndromes as well as to ileostomy(89) or enterocolic fistula.(77) Subcutaneous injection of octreotide may be painful, but continuous subcutaneous infusion is generally well tolerated and the drug can be combined with morphine, diamorphine, haloperidol, midazolam, or hyoscine without apparent loss of efficacy.(89) Mixing with cyclizine may cause precipitation.

Although it is still not licensed in the United Kingdom for indication, octreotide is now established as an effective therapy for severe secretory diarrhoea, particularly that related to HIV infection, where doses up to 1500 mcg/24 h have been found necessary.(90) It also improves symptoms of malignant intestinal obstruction in up to 85 per cent of cases at doses that are usually within the range of 300–600 mcg/24 h. Although this principally relates to the incidence of vomiting, partial obstruction may produce diarrhoea and a trial of octreotide for this symptom is appropriate in these circumstances. However, expert consensus has recommended octreotide dose titration as high as 2400 mcg/24 h for chemotherapy-induced diarrhoea.(91)

Lanreotide has a far more prolonged duration of action which, while being a valuable quality for stable conditions such as the acromegaly which is its primary indication, makes it inflexible for use in the continually changing clinical situations of palliative care. However, it has the advantage of requiring neither frequent injections nor an infusion device.

New developments

Calcium carbonate 3.6 g/day reduced stool frequency by a mean of 49 per cent and faecal wet weight by 50 per cent over 12 weeks in 15 post-gut-resection patients. No change in plasma calcium concentrations was found.(92) Results in healthy subjects have been variable. Oral calcium supplements precipitate free bile acids and fatty acids in the colon. As bile acids and fatty acids inhibit colonic absorption and stimulate fluid and electrolyte secretion, this may be calcium's mode of action.

There is increasing interest in the use of probiotics, or beneficial microorganisms, for the management of diarrhoea, among other conditions. *Lactobacillus* spp. are the most commonly used. To date there is limited evidence that they can be effective in infective diarrhoea in adults.(93)

The pathogenesis of diarrhoea frequently involves neurohumoral mechanisms controlling water secretion, with a notable role for 5-hydroxytryptamine (5-HT), substance P, and VIP.(94) Antagonists to 5-HT and substance P may prove clinically useful in the future and peptide YY, which reduces intestinal fluid secretion, has been used experimentally in humans.(95)

References

1. Connell, A.M., Hilton, C., Irvine, G., Lennard-Jones, J.E., and Misiewicz, J.J. (1965). Variation in bowel habit in two population samples. *British Medical Journal* **ii**, 1095–9.
2. Drossman, D.A., Sandler, R.S., McKee, D.C., and Lovitz, A.J. (1982). Bowel patterns among subjects not seeking health care. *Gastroenterology* **83**, 529–34.
3. Thompson, W.G. et al. (1999). Functional bowel disorders and functional abdominal pain. *Gut* **45** (Suppl. 2): 1143–7.
4. Herz, M.J., Kahan, E., Zalevski, S., Aframian, R., Kuznitz, D., and Reichman, S. (1996). Constipation: a different entity for patients and doctors. *Family Practice* **13**, 156–9.
5. Ashraf, W., Park, F., Lof, J., and Quigley, E.M. (1996). An examination of the reliability of reported stool frequency in the diagnosis of idiopathic constipation. *American Journal of Gastroenterology* **91**, 26–32.
6. Everhart, J.E., Go, V.L., Johannes, R.S., Fitzsimmons, S.C., Roth, H.P., and White, L.R.A. (1989). A longitudinal survey of self-reported bowel habits in the United States. *Digestive Diseases and Sciences* **34**, 1153–62.
7. Wigzell, F.W. (1969). The health of nonagenarians. *Gerontologia Clinica* **11**, 137–44.
8. Cartwright, A., Hockey, L., and Anderson, J.L. *Life Before Death*. London: Routledge and Kegan Paul, 1973.
9. Madsen, J.L. and Dahl, K. (1990). Human migrating myoelectric complex in relation to gastrointestinal transit of a meal. *Gut* **31**, 1003–5.
10. Bassotti, G. and Gaburri, M. (1988). Manometric investigation of high-amplitude propagated contractile activity of the human colon. *American Journal of Physiology* **255**, G660–4.
11. Holdstock, D.J., Misiewicz, J.J., Smith, T., and Rowlands, E.N. (1970). Propulsion (mass movements) in the human colon and its relationship to meals and somatic activity. *Gut* **11**, 91–9.
12. Sykes, N.P. (1990). Methods of assessment of bowel function in patients with advanced cancer. *Palliative Medicine* **4**, 287–92.
13. Bruera, E. (1989). Autonomic failure in patients with advanced cancer. *Journal of Pain and Symptom Management* **4**, 163–6.
14. Lundgren, O. (1988). Nervous control of intestinal transport. *Baillieres Clinical Gastroenterology* **2**, 85–106.
15. Read, N.W. and Timms, J.M. (1986). Defaecation and the pathophysiology of constipation. *Clinics in Gastroenterology* **15**, 937–65.
16. Sykes, N.P. (1998). The relationship between opioid use and laxative use in terminally ill cancer patients. *Palliative Medicine* **12**, 375–82.
17. Sandgren, J.E., McPhee, M.S., and Greenberger, N.J. (1984). Narcotic bowel syndrome treated with clonidine. *Annals of Internal Medicine* **101**, 331–4.
18. Kaufman, P.N., Krevsky, B., Malmud, L.S., Maurer, A.H., Somers, M.B., Siegel, J.A., and Fisher, R.S. (1988). Role of opiate receptors in the regulation of colonic transit. *Gastroenterology* **94**, 1351–6.
19. Kreek, M.J., Schaefer, R.A., Hahn, E.F., and Fishman, J. (1983). Naloxone, a specific opioid antagonist, reverses chronic idiopathic constipation. *Lancet* **i**, 261–2.
20. Kreek, M.J., Paris, P., Bartol, M.A., and Mueller, D. (1984). Effects of short term oral administration of the specific opioid antagonist naloxone on fecal evacuation in geriatric patients. *Gastroenterology* **86**, 1144.
21. Ling, G.S., Paul, D., Simontov, R., and Pasternak, G.W. (1989). Differential development of acute tolerance. *Life Sciences* **45**, 1627–36.
22. Fallon, M. and Hanks, G. (1999). Morphine, constipation and performance status in advanced cancer patients. *Palliative Medicine* **13**, 159–60.
23. Radbruch, L., Sabatowski, R., Loick, G., Kulbe, C., Kasper, M., Grond, S., and Lehmann, K.A. (2000). Constipation and the use of laxatives: a comparison between transdermal fentanyl and oral morphine. *Palliative Medicine* **14**, 111–19.
24. Daeninck, P.J. and Bruera, E. (1999). Reduction in constipation and laxative requirements following opioid rotation to methadone. *Journal of Pain and Symptom Management* **18**, 303–9.
25. Bruera, E., Suarez-Almazor, M., Velasco, A., Bertolino. M., MacDonald, S.M., and Hanson, J. (1994). The assessment of constipation in terminal cancer patients admitted to a palliative care unit. *Journal of Pain and Symptom Management* **9**, 515–19.
26. Barr, R.G., Levine, M.D., Wilkinson, R.H., and Mulvihill, D. (1979). Occult stool retention: a clinical tool for its evaluation in school aged children. *Clinical Pediatrics* **18**, 674–9.
27. Benninga, M.A., Buller, H.A., Staalman, C.R., Gubler, F.M., Bossuyt, P.M., van der Plas, R.N., and Taminiau, J.A. (1995). Defaecation disorders in children, colonic transit time versus the Barr score. *European Journal of Paediatrics* **154**, 277–84.
28. Sykes, N.P. (2001). Methods for clinical research in constipation. In *Symptom Research: Methods and Opportunities. An Interactive Textbook* (ed. M. Max and J. Lynn). Bethesda: National Institutes of Dental and Craniofacial Research. Available at URL: www.symptomresearch.com/chapter_3/index.htm. Accessed 18 July 2003.
29. McMillan, S.C. and Williams, F.A. (1989). Validity and reliability of the Constipation Assessment Scale. *Cancer Nursing* **12**, 183–8.
30. Agachan, F., Chen, T., Pfeifer, J., Reissman, P., and Wexner, S.D. (1996). A constipation scoring system to simplify evaluation and management of constipated patients. *Diseases of the Colon and Rectum* **39**, 681–5.
31. Frank, L., Kleinman, L., Farup, C., Taylor, L., and Miner, P. (1999). Psychometric validation of a constipation assessment questionnaire. *Scandinavian Journal of Gastroenterology* **34**, 870–7.
32. Twycross, R.G. and Lack, S.A. (eds) (1986). Constipation. In *Control of Alimentary Symptoms in Far Advanced Cancer*, pp. 166–207. London: Churchill Livingstone.
33. Muller-Lissner, S.A. (1988). Effect of wheat bran on weight of stool and gastrointestinal transit time: a meta-analysis. *British Medical Journal* **296**, 615–17.
34. Mumford, S.P. (1986). Can high fibre diets improve the bowel function in patients on a radiotherapy ward? Cited in: Twycross, R.G. and Lack, S.A. *Control of Alimentary Symptoms in Far Advanced Cancer*, p. 183. Edinburgh: Churchill Livingstone.
35. Sykes, N.P. (1997). A volunteer model for the comparison of laxatives in opioid-induced constipation. *Journal of Pain and Symptom Management* **11**, 363–9.
36. Bateman, D.N. and Smith, J.M. (1988). A policy for laxatives. *British Medical Journal* **297**, 1420–1.
37. Moriarty, K.J., Fairclough, P.D., Clark, M.L., and Dawson, A.M. (1982). Inhibition of glucose and water absorption in the human jejunum by dioctyl sodium sulphosuccinate: a prostaglandin-mediated phenomenon? *Gut* **23**, A443.
38. Chapman, R.W., Sillery, J., and Saunders, D.R. (1984). Dioctyl sodium sulphosuccinate, 300 mg daily, does not increase human ileal or colonic output. *Gut* **25**, A1156.
39. Hyland, C.M. and Foran, J.D. (1968). Dioctyl sodium sulphosuccinate as a laxative in the elderly. *Practitioner* **200**, 698–9.
40. Read, N.W. (1990). Motility: functional diseases. *Current Opinion in Gastroenterology* **6**, 9–13.
41. Lederle, F.A., Busch, D.L., Mattox, K.M., West, M.J., and Aske, D.M. (1990). Cost-effective treatment of constipation in the elderly: a randomised double-blind comparison of sorbitol and lactulose. *American Journal of Medicine* **89**, 597–601.
42. Harvey, R.F. and Read, N.W. (1975). Mode of action of the saline purgatives. *American Heart Journal* **89**, 810–13.
43. Hammer, H.F., Santa Ana, C.A., Schiller, L.R., and Fordtran, J.S. (1989). Studies of osmotic diarrhea induced in normal subjects by ingestion of PEG and lactulose. *Journal of Clinical Investigation* **84**, 1056–62.
44. Culbert, P., Gillett, H., and Ferguson, A. (1998). Highly effective new oral therapy for faecal impaction. *British Journal of General Practice* **48**, 1599–600.
45. Corazziari, E., Badiali, D., Habib, F.I., Reboa, G., Pitto, G., Mazzacca, G., Sabbatini, F., Galeazzi, R., Cilluffo, T., Vantini, I., Bardelli, E., and Baldi, F. (1996). Small volume isosmotic polyethylene glycol electrolyte balanced solution (PMF-100) balanced solution in treatment of chronic non-organic constipation. *Digestive Diseases and Sciences* **41**, 1636–42.
46. Leng-Peschlow, E. (1989). Effects of sennosides A + B and bisacodyl on rat large intestine. *Pharmacology* **38**, 310–18.
47. Sykes, N.P. (1991). A clinical comparison of laxatives in a hospice. *Palliative Medicine* **5**, 307–14.

48. **Verhaeren, E.H., Geeraerts, V.C., and Lemli, J.** (1987). The antagonistic effect of morphine on rhein-stimulated fluid, electrolyte and glucose movements in guinea-pig perfused colon. *Journal of Pharmacy and Pharmacology* **39**, 39–44.

49. **Maguire, L.C., Yon, J.L., and Miller, E.** (1981). Prevention of narcotic-induced constipation. *New England Journal of Medicine* **305**, 1651.

50. **Brunton, L.L.** (1985). Laxatives. In *The Pharmacological Basis of Therapeutics* 7th edn. (ed. A.G. Gilman, L.S. Goodman, T.W. Rall, and F. Murad), pp. 994–1003. New York: Macmillan.

51. **Joo, J.S., Ehrenpreis, E.D., Gonzalez, L., Kaye, M., Breno, S., Wexner, S.D., Zaitman, D., and Secrest, K.** (1998). Alterations in colonic anatomy induced by chronic stimulant laxatives: the cathartic colon revisited. *Journal of Clinical Gastroenterology* **26**, 283–6.

52. **Sweeney, J.L., Hewett, P., Riddell, P., and Hoffmann, D.C.** (1986). Rectal gangrene: a complication of phosphate enema. *Medical Journal of Australia* **144**, 374–5.

53. **Sweeney, W.J.** The use of disposable microenema in obstetrical patients. *Proceedings of a Symposium on the Clinical Evaluation of a New Disposable Microenema*, New Brunswick, New Jersey, June 1963, pp. 7–8.

54. **Postlethwait, R.W.** (1965). Microenema as evacuant before proctoscopy. *Current Therapeutic Research* **7**, 7–9.

55. **Lieberman, W.** (1964). Rapid patient preparation for sigmoidoscopy by microenema. *American Journal of Proctology* **15**, 138–41.

56. **Mandel, L. and Silinsky, J.** (1960). Bisacodyl (Dulcolax): an evacuant suppository. A controlled therapeutic trial in chronically ill and geriatric patients. *Canadian Medical Association Journal* **83**, 384–7.

57. **Agra, Y., Sacristan, A., Gonzalez, M., Ferrari, M., Portuges, A., and Calvo, M.J.** (1998). Efficacy of senna versus lactulose in terminal cancer patients treated with opioids. *Journal of Pain and Symptom Management* **15**, 1–7.

58. **Ramesh, P.R., Suresh Kumar, K., Rajagopal, M.R., Balachandran, P., and Warrier, P.K.** (1998). Managing morphine-induced constipation: a controlled comparison of an Ayurvedic formulation and senna. *Journal of Pain and Symptom Management* **16**, 240–4.

59. **Tramonte, S.M., Brand, M.B., Mulrow, C.D., Amato, M.G., O'Keefe, M.E., and Ramirez, G.** (1997). The treatment of chronic constipation in adults: a systematic review. *Journal of General Internal Medicine* **12**, 15–24.

60. **Petticrew, M., Watt, I., and Sheldon, T.** (1997). Systematic review of the effectiveness of laxatives in the elderly. *Health Technology Assessment* **1**, 1–52.

61. **NHS Centre for Reviews and Dissemination** (2001). Effectiveness of laxatives in adults. *Effective Health Care* **7** (1), 1–12.

62. **Muller-Lissner, S.A.** (1987). Treatment of chronic constipation with cisapride and placebo. *Gut* **28**, 1033–8.

63. **Bruera, E., Brenneis, C., Michand, M., and MacDonald, N.** (1987). Continuous subcutaneous infusion of metoclopramide for treatment of narcotic bowel syndrome. *Cancer Treatment Reports* **71**, 1121–2.

64. **Shanson, D.C., Akash, S., Harris, M., and Tadayon, M.** (1985). Erythromycin stearate 1.5 g, for the oral prophylaxis of streptococcal bacteraemia in patients undergoing dental extraction: efficacy and tolerance. *Journal of Antimicrobial Chemotherapy* **15**, 83–90.

65. **Hasler, W., Heldsinger, A., Soudah, H., and Owyang, C.** (1990). Erythromycin promotes colonic transit in humans: mediation via motilin receptors. *Gastroenterology* **98**, A358.

66. **Bassotti, G., Chiaroni, G., Vantini, I., Morelli, A., and Whitehead, W.E.** (1998). Effect of different doses of erythromycin on colonic motility in patients with slow transit constipation. *Zeitschrift fur Gastroenterologie* **36**, 209–13.

67. **Culpepper-Morgan, J.A.** et al. (1992). Treatment of opioid-induced constipation with oral naloxone: a pilot study. *Clinical Pharmacology and Therapeutics* **52**, 90–5.

68. **Sykes, N.P.** (1996). An investigation of the ability of oral naloxone to correct opioid-related constipation in patients with advanced cancer. *Palliative Medicine* **10**, 135–44.

69. **Yuan, C.S., Foss, J.F., Osinski, J., Toledano, A., Roizen, M.F., and Moss, J.** (1997). The safety and efficacy of oral methylnaltrexone in preventing morphine-induced delay in oral-cecal transit time. *Clinical Pharmacology and Therapeutics* **61**, 467–75.

70. **Meyer, B.M.** et al. (1989). Role of cystokinin in regulation of gastrointestinal motor functions. *Lancet* **ii**, 12–15.

71. **Calignano, A., Moncada, S., and Di Rosa, M.** (1991). Endogenous nitric oxide modulates morphine-induced constipation. *Biochemical Biophysical Research Communications* **181**, 889–93.

72. **Rolston, K.V., Rodriguez, S., Hernandez, M., and Bodey, G.P.** (1989). Diarrhoea in patients infected with HIV. *American Journal of Medicine* **86**, 137–8.

73. **Twycross, R.G. and Lack, S.A.** (1986). Diarrhoea. In *Control of Alimentary Symptoms in Far Advanced Cancer* pp. 208–29. London: Churchill Livingstone.

74. **Edes, T.D., Walk, B.E., and Austin, J.L.** (1990). Diarrhoea in tube-fed patients: feeding formula not necessarily the cause. *American Journal of Medicine* **88**, 91–3.

75. **Kinnunen, O., Janhonen, P., Salokannel, J., and Kivela, S.L.** (1989). Diarrhoea and faecal impaction in elderly long-stay patients. *Zeitschrift Gerontologie* **22**, 321–3.

76. **Dean, A.P. and Reed, W.D.** (1991). Diarrhoea—an unrecognised hazard of coeliac plexus block. *Australian and New Zealand Journal of Medicine* **21**, 47–8.

77. **Mercadante, S.** (1992). Treatment of diarrhoea due to enterocolic fistula with octreotide in a terminal cancer patient. *Palliative Medicine* **6**, 257–9.

78. **Norton, J.A., Doppman, J.L., and Jensen, R.T.** (1989). Cancer of the endocrine system. In *Cancer: Principles and Practice of Oncology* 3rd edn. (ed. V.T. DeVita, S. Hellman, and S.A. Rosenberg), pp. 1269–344. Philadelphia: Lippincott.

79. **Chitkara, Y.K., McCasland, K.A., and Kenefic, L.** (1996). Development and implementation of cost-effective guidelines in the laboratory investigation of diarrhea in a community hospital. *Archives of Internal Medicine* **156**, 1445–8.

80. **Condon, J.R., South, M., Wolveson, R.L., and Brinkley, D.** (1996). Radiation diarrhoea and cholestyramine. *Postgraduate Medical Journal* **54**, 838–9.

81. **Mennie, A.T., Dalley, V.M., Dinneen, L.C., and Collier, H.O.** (1975). Treatment of radiation-induced gastrointestinal distress with acetylsalicylate. *Lancet* **ii**, 942–3.

82. **Saslow, S.B., Scolapio, J.S., Camilleri, M., Fortsrom, L.A., Thomforde, G.M., Burton, D.D., Rubin, J., Pitot, H.C., and Zinsmeister, A.R.** (1998). Medium-term effects of a new $5HT_3$ antagonist, alosetron, in patients with carcinoid diarrhoea. *Gut* **42**, 628–34.

83. **de la Motte, S., Bose-O'Reilly, S., Heinisch, M., and Harrison, F.** (1997). Double-blind comparison of an apple pectin-chamomile extract preparation with placebo in children with diarrhoea. *Arzneimittel-Forschung* **47**, 1247–9.

84. **DuPont, H.L., Ericsson, C.D., DuPont, M.W., Luna, A.C., and Mathewson, J.J.** (1990). A randomized, open-label comparison of nonprescription loperamide and attapulgite in the symptomatic treatment of acute diarrhoea. *American Journal of Medicine* **88** (Suppl. 6A), 205–35.

85. **Graham, D.Y., Evans, M.K., and Gentry, L.O.** (1983). Double-blind comparison of bismuth subsalicylate and placebo in prevention and treatment of ETEC-induced diarrhoea in volunteers. *Gastroenterology* **85**, 1017–22.

86. **Palmer, K.R., Corbett, C.L., and Holdsworth, C.D.** (1980). Double-blind cross-over study comparing loperamide, codeine and diphenoxylate in the treatment of chronic diarrhoea. *Gastroenterology* **79**, 1272–5.

87. **Awouters, F., Niemeegers, C.J.E., and Janssen, P.A.J.** (1983). Pharmacology of antidiarrhoeal drugs. *Annual Review of Toxicology and Pharmacology* **23**, 279–301.

88. **Ruppin, H.** (1987). Review: loperamide—a potent antidiarrhoeal drug with actions along the alimentary tract. *Alimentary Pharmacology and Therapeutics* **1**, 179–90.

89. **Riley, J. and Fallon, M.T.** (1994). Octreotide in terminal malignant obstruction of the gastrointestinal tract. *European Journal of Palliative Care* **1**, 23–5.

90. **Romeu, J., Miro, J.M., Sirera, G., Mallolas, J., Arnal, J., Valls, M.E., Tortosa, F., Clotet, B., and Foz, M.** (1991). Efficacy of octreotide in the management of chronic diarrhoea in AIDS. *AIDS* **5**, 1495–9.

91. **Harris, A.G., O'Dorisio, T.M., Woltering, E.A., Anthony, L.B., Burton, F.R., Geller, R.B., Grendell, J.H., Levin, B., and Redfern, J.S.** (1995). Consensus statement: octreotide dose titration in secretory diarrhea. Diarrhea Management Consensus Development Panel. *Digestive Diseases and Sciences* **40**, 1464–73.

92. Steinbach, G., Lupton, J., Reddy, B.S., Lee, J.J., Kral, J.G., and Holt, P.R. (1996). Calcium carbonate treatment of diarrhoea in intestinal bypass patients. *European Journal of Gastroenterology and Hepatology* **8**, 559–62.
93. De Roos, N.M. and Katan, M.B. (2000). Effects of probiotic bacteria on diarrhea, lipid metabolism and carcinogenesis: a review of papers published between 1988 and 1998. *American Journal of Clinical Nutrition* **71**, 405–11.
94. Farthing, M.J. (2000). Novel targets for the pharmacotherapy of diarrhoea: a view for the millenium. *Journal of Gastroenterology and Hepatology* **15** (Suppl.), G38–45.
95. Playford, R.J., Domin, J., Beacham, J., Parmar, K.B., Tatemoto, K., Bloom, S.R., and Calam, J. (1990). Preliminary report: role of peptide YY in defence against diarrhoea. *Lancet* **335**, 1555–7.

General references

Derby, S. and Portenoy, R.K. (1997). Assessment and management of opioid-induced constipation. In *Topics in Palliative Care* Vol. 1 (ed. R.K. Portenoy and E. Bruera), pp. 95–112. New York: Oxford University Press.
Twycross, R.G. and Lack, S.A. *Control of Alimentary Symptoms in Far Advanced Cancer.* Edinburgh: Churchill Livingstone, 1986.
Walsh, T.D. and O'Shaughnessy, C. (1989). Diarrhoea. In *Symptom Control* (ed. T.D. Walsh), pp. 99–116. Oxford: Blackwell.

8.3.4 Pathophysiology and management of malignant bowel obstruction

Carla Ripamonti and Sebastiano Mercadante

Introduction

Malignant bowel obstruction (MBO) is a well-recognized complication in advanced cancer patients with abdominal and pelvic malignancy. Although it may develop at any time in the disease, it occurs most frequently at the advanced stage, with the highest incidence ranging from 5.5 to 42 per cent in ovarian carcinoma. Bowel obstruction occurs in 4.4–24 per cent of patients with colorectal cancer.[1–7] It has been reported in patients with other advanced cancers, ranging from 3 to 15 per cent of cases. Clinical settings, admission criteria of the palliative care unit, diagnosis parameters, or clinical evaluation may explain these differences.[8–10]

Mechanisms of bowel obstruction

Bowel obstruction may be a presenting feature of intra-abdominal malignancy or a feature of recurrent disease or other pathology in patients with a history of malignancy. The aetiology may be benign in 10–48 per cent of cases at operation, caused by adhesions or radiation enteritis, or malignant with single site, multiple site or diffuse disease.

Primary cancer, relapse after surgery, chemotherapy or radiotherapy, associated pathologies, and diffuse carcinomatosis may cause bowel obstruction with different mechanisms.[11] Such phenomena are often concomitant.

The enlargement of the primary tumour or recurrence of abdominal masses, fibrosis, or adhesions may produce extrinsic occlusion of the lumen. Polypoidal lesions or annular narrowing due to dissemination may cause an intraluminal occlusion of the lumen. Infiltration of the intestinal muscles or superimposed inflammation may produce intramural occlusion of the lumen. Intestinal motility disorders due to a deranged extrinsic neural control of viscera may produce delay in intestinal transit, resulting in a clinical picture similar to bowel obstruction, namely pseudo-obstruction. Concomitant diseases, such as diabetes, para-neoplastic syndromes, or previous gastric surgery, may contribute to dysmotility of this kind.

Contributing factors are constipation, due to illness and/or to drugs such as anticholinergics and opioids. Pain due to opioid-induced constipation, wrongly treated with increased doses of opioids, may result in faecal impaction producing signs of bowel obstruction.[12]

Pathophysiology

An occlusion of the lumen prevents or delays the propulsion of the intestinal contents from passing distally. The accumulation of non-absorbed secretions produces abdominal distension and a colicky activity to surmount the obstacle in an early stage, corresponding to a sub-obstructive state, possibly still reversible. Although there is little or no through-movement of intestinal contents, the bowel continues to contract with increased uncoordinated peristaltic activity. As a consequence, the bowel becomes distended, stimulating intestinal fluid secretion, thus creating a vicious cycle of distension-secretion, further stretching the bowel wall. Moreover, in bowel obstruction the abnormally increased flora may also produce gases in the small intestine, contributing to the distension.[13]

This hypertensive state in the lumen will produce damage with a consequent inflammatory response. This inflammatory response involves activation of the cycloxygenase pathway and the release of prostaglandins, potent secretagogues either by a direct effect on enterocytes or enteric nervous reflex.[13] Vasoactive intestinal polypeptide (VIP) might be released into the portal and peripheral circulation and mediate local intestinal and systemic pathophysiological alterations as hyperaemia and oedema of the intestinal wall and an accumulation of fluid in the lumen thanks to its stimulating effects.[14,15] Hypoxia, caused by the reduction in venous drainage from the obstructed segment interfering with oxygen consumption, is the primary stimulus for VIP release as well as intraluminal bacterial overgrowth. High portal levels of VIP are known to cause hypersecretion and splanchnic vasodilatation.[16] Experimental studies have shown that higher VIP content is present in the duodenal tissue when compared to colonic tissue content. This may also explain the finding of redistribution of blood flow between the obstructed segment and the distal sites. Alterations of the auto-regulatory local and neuro-humoral control mechanisms of the splanchnic flow are the basis of the appearance of multiple organ failure syndrome caused or worsened by systemic hypotension commonly observed in the late stage of bowel occlusion.[17] Fluids and electrolytes are sequestered in the gut wall and in its lumen (third space) in the presence of vasodilatation contributing to hypotension and sepsis leading to multi-organ system failure, the cause of death in patients with bowel obstruction.

The hypovolaemic state may induce functional renal failure due to a decrease in the renal flow and, as a consequence, glomerular filtration. Oliguria, azotaemia, and haemoconcentration may accompany dehydration. Metabolic disorders in intestinal obstruction depend on the site and duration of the obstruction and are caused by dehydration, electrolyte losses, and disorders of acid–base balance.[18] The respiratory pattern will depend on the level of obstruction. Metabolic alkalosis, hypochloraemia, and hypokalaemia will be features of a high-level obstruction due to a prevalent loss of gastric secretions. In a low-level obstruction, there will be deficiencies of chloride, sodium, potassium, bicarbonates owing to intestinal stasis of biliary, pancreatic, intestinal, as well as gastric secretions.[11] There will be acidosis due to ischaemic lesions or septic complications.[19] The increased abdominal distension reduces the venous return and may impair pulmonary ventilation as a result of elevation of the diaphragm.

Sepsis will occur in the late stages of bowel obstruction, probably as a result of bacterial action. It consists of the passage of toxins from the intestinal contents passing through the intestinal wall into the lymphatic and systemic circulation. This phenomenon results from the increase in endoluminal pressure, stasis, and intestinal ischaemia, together with intestinal gangrene and perforation, commonly observed in the late stages of persisting bowel obstruction. The time course of these events is variable, occurring over several days in malignant mechanical bowel obstruction.

Diagnosis

The level of obstruction determines the different patterns of symptoms. The progression may be slow or fast, from partial obstruction to complete occlusion, each producing a different spectrum of symptoms, differing intensity of suffering, and ultimate outcome. Accumulation and increased production of secretion produce the principal symptoms, namely abdominal pain and distension, vomiting and constipation (Fig. 1). However, distension may be minimal in both jejunal involvement or fixed tumours extensively infiltrating the small bowel. In the presence of a high level of obstruction, such as in stomach, duodenum, pancreas, or jejunum, vomiting develops early and in larger volumes. Nausea is persistent or occasionally subsides temporarily after an episode of vomiting. Continuous pain is due to a visceral mass growth compressing the intestine, intestinal distension, or hepatomegaly, while severe superimposed colic above the obstruction, in the small or large intestine, may worsen the distress. This activity is variable in intensity and site due to distension proximal to the obstruction. In large bowel obstruction, the pain is less intense and occurs at longer intervals.

Dry mouth is invariably associated with the other symptoms, and is the consequence of severe dehydration and metabolic alterations, as well as pharmacological interventions such as anticholinergic drugs. No evacuation of faeces and no passing of flatus are typical features of complete obstruction. The eventual appearance of *paradoxical diarrhoea* results from leakage of faecal fluid from faecal impaction, generally in large bowel obstruction.

The diagnosis of intestinal obstruction is established or suspected on clinical grounds and usually confirmed with plain abdominal radiography demonstrating fluid levels. Contrast radiography may help in defining the site and the extent of obstruction. Barium is not absorbed and may interfere with subsequent diagnostic studies. Gastrografin is preferable, because it offers a similar radiological definition and in some circumstances is useful in restoring the intestinal transit in reversible obstruction. Abdominal CT scan is useful in evaluating the global extent of disease, which may be important in a subsequent therapeutic decision. It is often very difficult to differentiate between complete and partial bowel obstruction.[20]

Management of intestinal obstruction

Therapeutic strategies

The management of patients with MBO is one of the greatest challenges facing physicians who care for cancer patients. In the face of a clearly incurable situation, significant patient discomfort and suffering must be balanced by the need to simplify the care of those patients with a short time to live. While surgery must remain the primary treatment for MBO, it is now recognized that there is a group of patients with advanced disease or poor general condition who are unfit for surgery and who require alternative management to relieve distressing symptoms.

Self-expanding metallic stents are an option in the management of MBO at the level of the gastric outlet, proximal small bowel, and colon. Medical treatment by continuous subcutaneous or intravenous administration of analgesics, antisecretary drugs, and/or antiemetics has been shown to be an effective approach for controlling pain, nausea, and vomiting in patients with inoperable MBO. Nasogastric suction or percutaneous gastrostomy may be considered for the patients with refractory symptoms or upper MBO that does not respond satisfactorily to pharmacological measures.[20]

Surgery

Surgical treatment can palliate symptoms of MBO and may include bypass procedures such as entero–entero anastomosis, enterocolon anastomosis, or the creation of an external stoma. The surgical technique used depends on the type and site of obstruction.[21] Palliative surgical intervention

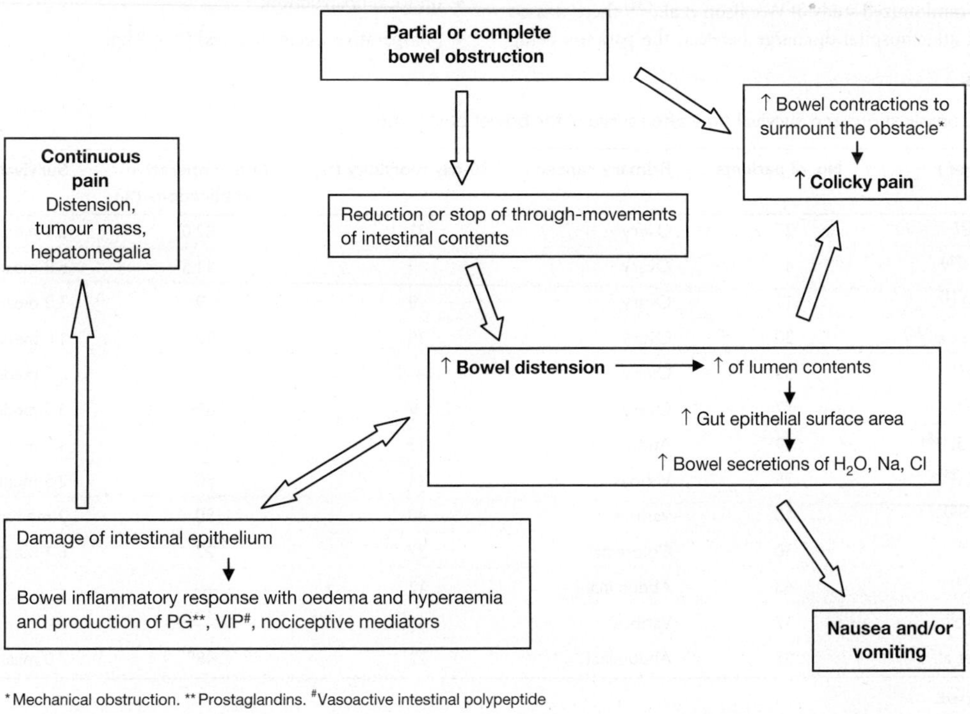

Fig. 1 Causes of symptoms in malignant bowel obstruction.

should be considered when relief of obstructive symptoms is not achieved with 48–72 h of conservative, medical management.[22,23]

The guidelines for conservative versus surgical treatment in patients with advanced cancer are still conflicting.[20,24] In much of the surgical literature, benefit from surgery is defined as at least 60 days of survival after operation. The literature lacks uniformity in outcome assessment, and quality of life, symptom control, and patient comfort are not described in most publications. In the study by Lund et al.,[2] for example, 56 per cent of patients survived 60 days after operation, but 43 per cent of this group manifested intermittent symptoms of incomplete and complete intestinal obstruction until death. In a large percentage of cases surgery can lead to further complications. It has to be asked if the short-term technical resolution of the obstruction is really the primary objective of management.

Table 1 reviews the operative mortality rate (defined as death from any cause within 30 days of the operation), the morbidity, and the length of survival after surgery for bowel obstruction according to publications from 1989 to 1997. Published data show that, in advanced cancer, the operative mortality is 9–40 per cent; with complication rates varying from 9 to 90 per cent.[1,2,18,24–34]

Complications of surgery

The most frequent complications are wound infections and/or wound dehiscence, sepsis, enterocutaneous fistula, further obstruction, peritoneal abscess, anastomosis dehiscence, gastrointestinal (GI) bleeding, pulmonary embolus, and deep venous thrombosis.

Benefits of surgery

The type of obstruction (partial versus complete) and the surgical procedure used (bypass versus resection and reanastomosis) have no significant effect on the outcome.[35,36] In the series of Piver et al.,[36] the survival was primarily related to the response to postoperative chemotherapy rather than the type of surgery performed.

As can be seen in the Table 1, recently published results are no better than those published in the past; improvements in surgical techniques and perioperative care appear not to influence the outcome. However, the lack of improved outcomes can be attributed to changes over time in the severity of the conditions of the patients coming in, as opposed to how they are managed. In the non-randomized study of Woolfson et al.,[34] there was no difference in survival after hospital discharge between the patients being operated on and those receiving conservative treatment. Long-term survival rates in both groups of patients were poor (median 1 month). The grade of the primary tumour and genitourinary cancers seemed to be associated with a more acceptable outcome whereas operative treatment was not correlated with a good outcome. The authors conclude that the value of operative intervention for MBO in patients with cancer is derived more from the possibility of a benign cause than alleviation of the consequences of carcinomatosis.

Patient selection for surgery

Since surgical palliation in advanced cancer patients is a complex issue, the decision to proceed with surgery must be carefully evaluated for each individual patient. The decision should be made by the doctors together with the patient and family members. In patients with known intra-abdominal recurrence of disease, however, operative intervention must be carefully weighed in the light of the limited survival, prolonged hospitalization necessary, the high morbidity and mortality, and the possibility that surgery may fail to resolve the obstruction.

In cancer patients, bowel obstruction is rarely an emergency and strangulation is uncommon; thus, there is time to monitor the clinical situation, undertake appropriate radiological investigations, to consider the poor prognostic criteria of surgical benefits before deciding for or against surgery. Table 2 shows the clinical parameters coming from retrospective studies and indicating low likelihood of clinical benefit from surgical management of MBO.[3–7,20,26,28,29,33,35,37,38,40–42]

According to Krebs and Goplerud,[4] the operative mortality rate was 44 per cent in the group of patients with ovarian carcinoma and two or more of factors numbered 3, 4, 5, 7; and it was significantly higher than the 13 per cent operative mortality among 32 patients who had no more than one risk factor. In the study of Jong et al.,[27] successful palliation (defined as patient survival >60 days after surgery, ability to return home, and relief of obstruction postoperatively >60 days) was significantly associated with four prognostic factors:

- absence of palpable abdominal or pelvic masses;
- volume of ascites less than 3 l;
- unifocal obstruction;
- preoperative weight loss less than 9 kg.

Table 1 Complications and survival time after surgery for bowel obstruction

Authors (ref.)	No. of patients	Primary cancer	30-day mortality (%)	Other operative complications (%)	Survival (months)
Lund et al.[2]	25	Ovary	32	32.0	2.0 median
Rubin et al.[25]	43	Ovary	9	11.5	6.8 mean
Beattie et al.[1]	11	Ovary	9	9	7.0 mean
van Oojen et al.[26]	20	Ovary	30	90	1.0 median
Jong et al.[27]	53	Ovary	—	42[a]	3.0 median
Sun et al.[32]	57	Ovary	9	39[b]	3.0 median
Turnbull et al.[28]	89	Abdominal	13	44	4.5 mean
Butler et al.[29]	25	Various	24	50	2.5 median
Chan et al.[18]	10	Various	40	80	2 median
Lau et al.[30]	30	Colorectal	37	27	6.1 median
Tang et al.[31]	43	Abdominal	12	—	—
Yazdi et al.[33]	17	Various	41	—	—
Woolfson et al.[34]	32	Abdominal	22	48[b]	7.0 mean

— not reported.

[a] Died with signs and symptoms of persistent or recurrent bowel obstruction.

[b] Continued to have some obstructive symptoms or recurrence of intestinal obstruction.

In the presence of favourable prognostic factors, the choice of the surgical approach should be based on certain conditions, what the aims of treatment are, and expected survival (Table 3).

Proximal bowel decompression

Proximal bowel decompression may be achieved either by nasogastric suction or drainage or by venting gastrostomy.

Short-term nasogastric tube (NGT) drainage is useful in achieving decompression of the stomach and/or intestine, before surgery or while a therapeutic decision is being made. This approach is generally not recommended for long-term drainage since NGT is uncomfortable for the patient (Table 4), the distress caused by the tube could increase the volume of air swallowed and it may provoke many complications.[43–45]

Prolonged nasogastric suction should only be considered for patients

- when pharmacological therapy for symptom control is ineffective;
- when gastrostomy cannot be carried out;
- as a temporary measure to reduce large volumes of secretions before starting pharmacological treatment;
- during the first days of such treatment.

Gastrostomy is a much more acceptable and well-tolerated method for the mid to long-term decompression of the obstructed GI tract.[46] Intermittent venting of the gastrostomy allows the patient to continue oral intake and maintain an active lifestyle without the inconvenience of a nasal tube. Gastrostomy provides patients the satisfaction of resuming oral intake of some foods, giving them significant psychological benefit.

Gastrostomy can be inserted operatively or percutaneously either by an endoscopic or ultrasound guided approach. Tube gastrostomy at the time of surgical exploration is the traditional method of long-term gastric decompression. It adds little time or morbidity to the surgical procedure, and should be done whenever the intraoperative impression is that complete bowel obstruction may be prolonged, permanent, or imminent.[47] Previous surgery or massive carcinomatosis may make placement of the gastrostomy difficult or dangerous, but every effort should be made to place a gastrostomy at the time of exploration if the clinical situation warrants one.

Percutaneous gastrostomy (PG) is the insertion of a tube into the stomach through the abdominal wall under fluoroscopic, ultrasound, or endoscopic guidance.[48,49] The addition of transcutaneous ultrasonography at the time of endoscopy permits accurate localization of the optimal site for PEG placement in patients with diffuse intra-abdominal disease and multiple

Table 2 Prognostic indicators of low likelihood of clinical benefit from surgery of MBO[a]

1.	Obstruction secondary to cancer[29]
2.[b]	Intestinal motility problems due to diffuse intraperitoneal carcinomatosis[5,7,26,28,37]
3.[c]	Widespread tumour[4]
4.[c]	Patients over 65[4] in association with cachexia[6,37]
5.[b]	Ascites requiring frequent paracentesis[4–7,26,33,38]
6.[c]	Low serum albumin level[6] and low serum pre-albumin level[39]
7.[c]	Previous radiotherapy of the abdomen or pelvis[3,4]
8.	Patients with nutritional deficits[40,41]
9.[b]	Diffuse palpable intra-abdominal masses[6,26] and liver involvement
10.[c]	Distant metastases, pleural effusion, or pulmonary metastases[4,35,38]
11.[b]	Multiple partial bowel obstruction with prolonged passage time on radiograph examination[6,38]
12.[c]	Elevated blood urea nitrogen levels, elevated alkaline phosphatase levels, advanced tumour stage, short diagnosis to obstruction interval[6,38]
13.[c]	Poor performance status[42]
14.[b]	A recent laparotomy which demonstrated that further corrective surgery was not possible[20]
15.[b]	Previous abdominal surgery which showed diffuse metastatic cancer[20]
16.[b]	Involvement of proximal stomach[20]
17.[c]	Extra-abdominal metastases producing symptoms which are difficult to control (e.g. dyspnoea)[20]

[a] Data from retrospective studies.

[b] Absolute contraindications = each is a 'stand-alone'.

[c] Relative contraindications (Ripamonti et al.[20]).

Table 4 Complications of prolonged nasoenteric intubation

Psychological distress
Pain
Epistaxis
Tube misplacement
Frequent spontaneous expulsions
Spontaneous migration of the tip of the tube
Nasal/pharyngeal irritation
Nasal cartilage erosion
Impairment of the function of the gastroesophageal sphincter causing or exacerbating oesophageal reflux
Oesophagitis
Oesophageal perforation, bleeding, strictures
Aspiration pneumonia
Pulmonary intubation
Interfere with coughing to clear pulmonary secretions
Otitis media
Tracheal-bronchial misplacement
Occlusions necessitating flushing or replacement

Source: refs 43–45.

Table 3 Patients with a previous good performance status: surgical evaluation, indications, and problems

	SNG	Gastrostomy	Stent	Surgery	Octreotide
Indications	Preparation for surgery (possibly avoided) Contraindication for gastrostomy	Long-term drainage in otherwise inoperable patients with prolonged expected survival	Postponing surgery	Benign cause Recent occurrence Survival expectancy: >2 months Good performance status Exclusion of contraindication criteria	Preparation to surgery
Problems	Uncomfortable for long-term use	Hospitalization TPN (Total parenteral nutrition)	Multiple levels of obstruction	Mortality–morbidity, hospitalization	

prior surgeries.[50,51] The procedure may be performed under intravenous sedation and local anesthesia.[52] Overall, this approach has been reported to control nausea and vomiting due to bowel obstruction in 83–93 per cent of cases.[53–58]

PG should be avoided in patients with portal hypertension, large volume ascites, in those predisposed to bleed, those taking anticoagulants, and those with active gastric ulceration.[46] Other relative contraindications are multiple previous abdominal surgeries, carcinomatosis, colostomy, or open/infected abdominal wounds.

In some patients with gastric outlet or proximal small bowel obstruction, some authors have described experience with the insertion of a draining gastrostomy with a concurrent feeding jejunostomy.[59]

Self-expanding metallic stents

In recent years, there has been growing experience in the use of expandable metallic stents in the management of obstruction in the gastric outlet, proximal small bowel, and colon.

These stents may be useful in the management of

- patients with advanced metastatic disease;
- patients who are at poor surgical risk;
- patients presenting with large bowel obstruction in which decompression by a stent allows treatment of coexisting medical complications to enable surgery to be carried out at a later date, after staging of the disease and thorough colonic preparation.[60]

Acute obstruction

The use of colorectal stents to alleviate acute MBO, followed by single-stage bowel resection and re-anastomosis is an application that is now well documented.[61] This technique can be palliative or can serve as an adjunct to curative resection. The goal is to convert an emergent procedure to a safer, elective operation and one that can be curative. In the report of Mainar et al.,[62] in 83 per cent of the patients, the clinical and radiological findings of bowel obstruction resolved within 24 h after stent placement. Six days after complete resolution of the colonic obstruction most patients underwent a single-stage surgical intervention. Preoperative stent placement is of additional value in patients with coexisting electrolyte imbalance, dehydration, or hyperglycaemia because the stent allows for optimal patient condition before surgery.

Post-placement evaluation includes a water-soluble contrast-enhanced enema examination and abdominal radiographs to evaluate stent placement and patency and to exclude perforation.

Gastroduodenal stenosis

Malignant duodenal obstruction is most commonly secondary to neoplastic invasion but more frequently due to extrinsic compression from carcinoma of the head of the pancreas or from compression by lymphadenopathy. Internal stenting of the lesion may be indicated in patients unfit for general anaesthesia and/or surgery or in patients unfit for a laparoscopic drainage procedure such as gastroenterostomy because of ascites and/or peritoneal metastases. Flexible, self-expanding metallic stents may be inserted using radiological or endoscopic techniques. The major limiting factor using the endoscopic technique is the inability to pass the endoscope through the stricture.

Several authors report relief of malignant gastric and/or duodenal obstruction in the majority of patients treated by per-oral endoscopic stent placement or via percutaneous insertion.[63–70] Most patients had immediate benefit and were able to eat small amounts of food without vomiting. No recurrence of gastric outlet obstruction was noted in the follow-up period of 1–5 months.[65,67,68]

As with any procedure, complications are possible. The major complications reported are gastric ulceration, bowel perforation after balloon dilatation of the stent, and stent migration.

According to some less recent reports, however, complications such as chest pain, blockage, gastro-oesophageal reflux, migration, perforation, and delayed massive bleeding occur in about 40–53 per cent of the patients.[71–73]

Contraindications to stenting Contraindications for the placement of a self-expanding stent are the presence of multiple stenoses and peritoneal carcinomatosis located distally in the small bowel that may not have been diagnosed at the preprocedural radiological examination because of the severity of the duodenal stenosis. Failure to relieve the obstruction may be secondary to an inability to cross the stricture, incomplete opening of the stent, or stent malposition that fails to traverse the entire stricture. In this case it is necessary to apply additional stents across the remaining obstruction.

Colon stenosis

The tumour site influences the decision regarding which patients are candidates for stent placement. Seventy per cent of colon and rectal cancers are left-sided and are considered accessible to stent placement.[62]

Various authors have reported good results after insertion of colonic stents in colorectal obstruction.[60,62,74–80]

Complications, which include perforation, bleeding, and stent migration, have been reported in fewer than 3 per cent of cases,[62,74–76] and only in a few patients treated with self-expanding mesh stents was there a recurrent obstruction due to tumour growth.[80] Temporary incontinence may be observed.[80] In the series of Canon et al.,[81] stent placement was successful in two out of four patients who needed a standard bowel cleansing before surgical resection with primary anastomosis and in five out of nine patients who had a stent as palliation of non-resectable tumours. Although colonic obstruction was relieved in 12 of 13 patients, seven (54 per cent) had some type of complication.

Mainar et al.[62] recommend self-expandable stents instead of balloon-expandable stents due to the risk of bowel perforation secondary to the excessive manipulation of balloon dilation on the friable tumour. According to Feretis et al.,[77] one of the possible disadvantages of the method may be the difficulty of treating tumour bleeding, since laser and thermal methods of haemostasis cannot be safely applied to a tumour that is covered by an endoprosthesis.

Normal bowel contractions could cause stent migration, especially if the stent diameter is too small, if the stent length is too short, or if the stent is placed too distal in the lesion. The migration into the rectal ampulla can result in obstruction and in painful spasm. According to Wholey et al.,[82] it is possible to retrieve stents from the rectum using fluoroscopic guidance.

According to Canon et al.,[81] before a patient is selected as a candidate for having an expandable metal stent placed in the colon, three factors are determined:

- the location of the lesion within the colon;
- the length of the tumour;
- the presence or absence of a synchronous carcinoma.

Thus, meticulous evaluation of the digestive tract downstream is mandatory to avoid pointless stent placement.

Further studies are necessary to identify those patients with advanced and terminal cancer and MBO who may have some benefit in terms of symptom control and quality of life after these procedures.

Pharmacological treatment in inoperable malignant bowel obstruction

The pharmacological management of MBO in inoperable patients focuses on the relief of nausea and vomiting, pain, and other possible distressing symptoms. It principally consists of an association of antiemetics, antisecretory drugs, and analgesics. This approach has been found successful in both in-patients and out-patients. The drugs of choice vary to a certain extent between countries and centres, depending on personal clinical experiences, drug availability, and costs, pending controlled studies which would give clear therapeutic guidelines.

Vomiting may be controlled either symptomatically, using antiemetic drugs with a specific central effects, or with anticholinergic drugs able to reduce gastrointestinal secretions. In the last years, steroids and somatostatin analogues have been successfully used as antisecretory–anti-inflammatory drugs, according to the most up-to-date views of the pathophysiology of bowel obstruction. Clinical practice recommendations for the management of MBO in patients with end-stage cancer have recently been published by the Working Group of the European Association for Palliative Care.[20]

Route of administration

As oral administration is unreliable in most patients with nausea and/or vomiting, in the presence of bowel obstruction, an alternative route, mainly the parenteral one, is mandatory. A continuous subcutaneous infusion allows a constant drug infusion with minimal discomfort to the patient. In the presence of a preexisting venous line, intravenous route will be the route of choice. Although a continuous infusion is preferable, a nylon needle can be inserted to deliver drugs subcutaneously as boluses at fixed intervals, according to the characteristics of the drug chosen. Morphine, haloperidol, cyclizine, and octreotide appear to be compatible in different combinations and can be mixed in the same syringe[20,83–87] (Table 5). Rectal and sublingual administration can occasionally be used. Finally, some drugs, such as fentanyl and scopolamine, may be also administered by the transdermal route.

Drugs

Figure 2 shows the drugs and their dosages used to control nausea and vomiting in bowel obstructed patients according to the data of ref. 20.

Antiemetics

Among the antiemetics, parenteral metoclopramide has been used successfully in patients with mainly functional or incomplete obstruction with no colicky pain rather than mechanical bowel obstruction. Metoclopramide (10 mg/4 h subcutaneously) used with dexamethasone has been the drug of choice for patients with incomplete bowel obstruction.[10] However, its use is not recommended in *complete* mechanical bowel obstruction as it may increase colic and vomiting.[8] Other antiemetics include haloperidol and the phenothiazines. Their use, while effective in most circumstances, has only been reported in anecdotal experiences in patients with inoperable bowel obstruction, and refer to clinical practice in different palliative care centres. Haloperidol, administered in varying doses, either intravenously or subcutaneously, titrated against the effect, is a specific antidopaminergic drug causing less sedation and having less anticholinergic effects compared with the phenothiazines. Among the phenothiazines, methotrimeprazine, chlorpromazine, and prochlorpromazine are commonly used. The two latter drugs may produce skin irritation when administered as a subcutaneous infusion.[20,88]

Antisecretory drugs

Anticholinergic drugs, such as hyoscine butylbromide and glycopyrrolate, may reduce vomiting by virtue of their antisecretory effects. Their anticholinergic activity decreases the tone and peristalsis in smooth muscle and the secretory activity of mucosal cells by a competitive inhibition of muscarinic receptors and by impairment of ganglionic neural transmission. Many open studies have demonstrated that this class of drugs may be effective in controlling GI symptoms in inoperable MBO, in combination with other drugs.[8,89–93] In comparison with scopolamine hydrobromide, these drugs have poor central nervous system penetration, so they are unlikely to produce central adverse effects. However, this class of drugs acts on the myenteric cholinergic

Table 5 Drug combinations in syringe drivers: compatibility and stability of opioids with antiemetics

	Concentration	Antiemetics	Concentration (mg/ml)	Notes
Opioids tested in 5% dextro				
Fentanyl citrate	25 mcg/ml	Atropine sulfate	0.4 undiluted	All the opioid solutions were compatible for at least 48 h with all the antiemetic tested[84]
Hydromorphone HCl	0.5 mg/ml	Diphenidramine HCl	2.0	
Methadone HCl	1.0 mg/ml	Haloperidol lactate	0.2	
Morphine sulfate	1.0 mg/ml	Hydroxyzine HCl	4.0	
		Methotrimeprazine	0.2	
		Metoclopramide HCl	5.0 undiluted	
		Scopolamine hydrobromide	0.05	
Opioids tested in distilled water				
Morphine sulfate	25 mg/ml	+Metoclopramide	25	Stable and compatible for 7 days
Hydromorphone HCl	10–20 mg/ml	+Metoclopramide	15	
Hydromorphone HCl	10 mg/ml	+Methotrimeprazine	10	
Morphine sulfate	20 mg/ml	+Haloperidol	2.0	Percipitable formulation[85]
Hydromorphone HCl	10–15 mg/ml	+Haloperidol	2.0	
Morphine sulfate	15 mg/ml	+Dexamethasone	0.02	No significant chemical degradation after 7 days at room temperature[83]
Morphine sulfate	15 mg/ml	+Metoclopramide	1.0	
Morphine sulfate	15 mg/ml	+Haloperidol	0.2	
Diamorphine	20–50–100 mg/ml	+Haloperidol	2.0	Stable and compatible after 7 days[86]
Diamorphine	20–50–100 mg/ml	+Haloperidol	3.0	
Diamorphine	20–50 mg/ml	+Haloperidol	4.0	
Diamorphine	50–100 mg/ml	+Cyclizine	4.0	Stable and compatible for 7 days[86]
Diamorphine	20 mg/ml	+Cyclizine	10.0	
Diamorphine	9 mg/ml	+Cyclizine	30.0	
Diamorphine	10 mg/ml	+Cyclizine	40.0	Stable and compatible for 48 h
Diamorphine	10 mg/ml	+Cyclizine	30.0	
Diamorphine	12 mg/ml	+Cyclizine	50.0	
Diamorphine	20 mg/ml	+Cyclizine	26.0	
Diamorphine	20 mg/ml	+Cyclizine	18.0	
Diamorphine	50 mg/ml	+Cyclizine	10.0	

Reproduced with permission from *Supportive Care in Cancer* (ref. 20).

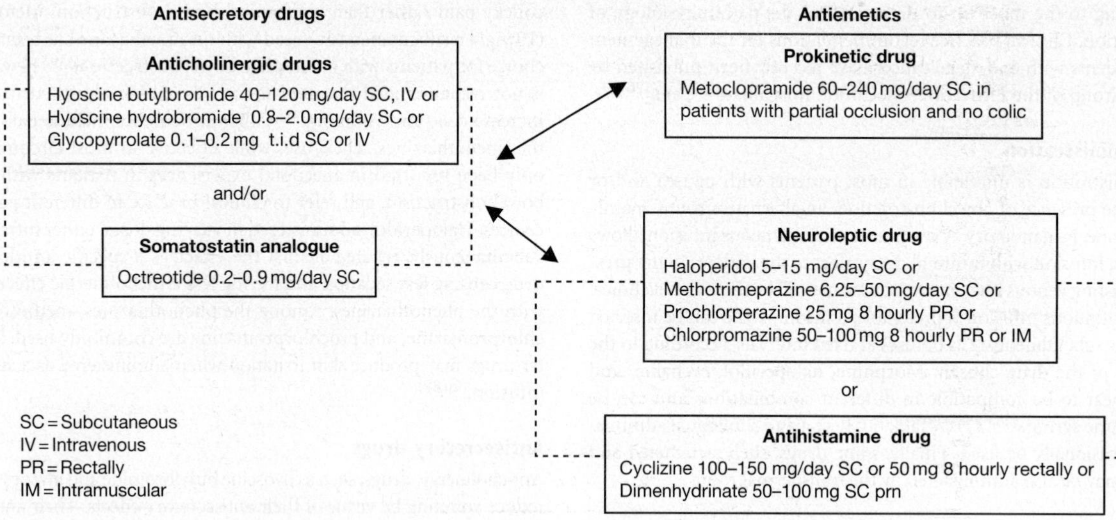

Fig. 2 Drugs to control nausea and vomiting in bowel obstruction. The dosages of the different drugs have been reported in ref. 20. (Reproduced with permission from Ripamonti et al. (2001). *Supportive Care in Cancer* **9**, 223–33.)

endings to reduce their activity, without influencing other intestinal processes which have been found to have a relevant influence on the absorption and secretion of water and salts at the level of the intestinal lumen. Moreover, these agents also possess important haemodynamic and thermoregulatory effects.

Octreotide

This is a synthetic analogue of somatostatin, with a duration of action of 8–12 h and has been used in the management of the symptoms of bowel obstruction. In relation to somatostatin, octreotide has been shown to have the same biological effects, but greater specificity and potency in the inhibition of release of certain hormones[94–98] and to be longer acting (half-life 90–120 min) with a peak of action at 2 h and a duration of 12 h.[99,100] Octreotide can be administered by continuous subcutaneous or intravenous infusion or by bolus parenteral injection. Octreotide inhibits the release of several GI hormones, thereby reducing gastric, pancreatic, biliary, and intestinal secretions, slowing down intestinal motility, and decreasing splanchnic blood flow, whilst at the same time increasing the absorption of water and electrolytes.[101] The rationale for using this drug can be explained by the mechanisms involved in the cascade of events presented in the section on Pathophysiology. Because the major morbidity of bowel obstruction relates to intestinal distension, electrolyte losses, and ischaemia, many experimental studies have been carried out to evaluate such features in animals treated with somatostatin or octreotide with respect to those treated with placebo.[102–106]

Table 6 shows the pre-clinical studies carried out to evaluate the role of somatostatin and octreotide in animal models of bowel obstruction.[103–105] Such experimental studies suggest that the principal mechanism of fluid secretion in bowel obstruction depends on VIP-induced inflammatory events.[75,16] VIP is released locally in the gut wall in the presence of ischaemia.[107] Octreotide has been shown to have a potent anti-VIP effect, resulting in the inhibition of intestinal secretion.[14] In an experimental preparation of rabbit ileum, the pro-absorptive effect of octreotide occurred without alterations in vascular resistance and was independent of systemic hormone interaction, thereby supporting a direct effect of octreotide on intestinal ionic transport.[94]

Clinical studies have proven the benefits of octreotide in different clinical conditions. The preoperative use of octreotide administered at the dose of 0.3 mg/day for 2–5 days in cancer patients undergoing surgery for bowel obstruction, caused by extrinsic occlusion of the lumen, prevented the typical anatomical changes, such as oedema, vessel congestion, or necrosis of the bowel above the obstruction due to the accumulation of fluids in the lumen, commonly observed during surgery. Moreover, the study of some samples of the intestine above and below the obstruction showed a normal anatomical and biochemical pattern.[108] The prophylactic use of octreotide in cancer patients with recurrent episodes of obstruction was successful in maintaining or restoring the intestinal transit even for prolonged periods of time.[109] These preliminary results were confirmed in a randomized, double-blind clinical trial carried out on 54 consecutive patients with mechanical bowel obstruction. Patients who received somatostatin preoperatively required surgery less often than patients who did not receive the drug. Moreover, severe dilatation and necrosis of the bowel proximal to the area of obstruction was significantly less frequent as compared with those patients who did not receive somatostatin preoperatively.[110]

On the basis of these experiences, octreotide could be considered in an early phase, in the presence of intermittent states of obstruction, or preoperatively to improve the surgical conditions and prevent postoperative complications.

Many uncontrolled studies report octreotide to be effective in relieving gastrointestinal symptoms in definitive MBO,[111–115] even in patients in whom hyoscine butylbromide had failed. The only two randomized studies published on the pharmacological treatment of GI symptoms due to inoperable bowel obstruction demonstrated that octreotide in doses of 0.3 mg daily was significantly more effective and had a shorter onset of action than hyoscine butylbromide in doses of 60 mg daily in reducing the intensity of nausea and the number of vomiting episodes,[93] and the amount of gastrointestinal secretion, allowing for removing the nasogastric tube previously inserted.[92] On the other hand, the association of the two drugs may reduce GI secretions and vomiting in patients whenever one drug alone proves ineffective.[116]

Octreotide is an expensive drug and its cost–benefit ratio should be carefully considered, especially for prolonged treatment. In many countries, the cost of 0.3 mg octreotide is the equivalent of US$ 37.73 whereas the cost of 60 mg hyoscine butyl bromide is US$ 1.35. The cost of a drug should be interpreted in the widest possible sense, however. The cost of a drug should be measured against the drug's ability to achieve rapid improvement of GI symptoms, which themselves affect admission to an in-patient unit and the length of hospitalization, in addition to the improved quality of life of the patient.

Steroids

The anti-inflammatory activity of steroids may reduce peri-tumoural oedema associated with a malignant lesion, thereby helping to resolve the obstruction and leading to consequent symptom relief. Steroids have been shown

Table 6 Pre-clinical studies on the role of somatostatin/octreotide in bowel obstruction

Author(s)	End-point	Type of study	Results
Mulvihill et al.[105]	To evaluate the effect of S on intestinal ions and water transport in reducing intestinal distension due to B ob	Anaesthetized rabbit model of closed-loop ileal Ob, the animal received S immediately after induced Ob or 6 h after, or received only hydration. After 24 h the animals were sacrificed and the intestine was examined	The animals that received S immediately or after 6 h presented, respectively, a sevenfold and fivefold reduction in fluid with respect to the control group In both groups treated with S, there was a significant reduction in luminal Na and K output compared to the control group in the closed-loop segments and in proximal bowel Tissue damage (mucosal necrosis, intramural haemorrhage, inflammation) was found in the closed-loop segment in the control group only
Yamaner et al.[106]	To compare the effects of OCT and saline and to observe anatomic and physiologic changes in the obstructed bowel	In 10 Wistar albino rats, two equal doses of OCT (7 μg/kg/day subacute) were administered with respect to the same volume of saline on the healing of bowel anastomosis	The diameter of the obstructed bowel increased significantly in the control group Na and K losses were significantly less in OCT group Ischaemic changes were more evident in the control group
Guiro' et al.[104]	To evaluate the water and ions absorption and secretion in animals treated with OCT (100 μg/kg) and the same volume of saline t.i.d.	120 Wistar rats were randomly assigned to six pathology groups: three B ob including complete, partial, complete with strangulation and three mesenteric vascular occlusions including partial permanent, total permanent, total temporary	OCT was shown: to reduce intestinal secretion and increase intestinal absorption in all the pathologies analysed except for total permanent intestinal ischaemia
Gittes et al.[103]	To verify the hypothesis that OCT reduces mortality	Mouse model of lethal small B ob	Improvement in survival of mice with proximal small B ob treated with OCT with respect to placebo

S, somatostatin; OCT, octreotide; B ob, bowel obstruction; Ob, obstruction; Na, sodium; K, potassium.

Table 7 Patients with a poor performance status with contraindications for surgical approach. Indications for the use of symptomatic drugs

	Antiemetics	Metoclopramide	Steroids	Hyoscine	Octreotide	SNG
Indications	Symptom control	Functional subobstruction	Subobstructive states Symptom control	Symptom control	Subobstructive states Symptom control	Pts unresponsive to pharmacological treatment Temporary measure
Problems		Stop in definitive or complete obstruction				Uncomfortable for long-term use

to increase water and salt absorption, thus reducing the net balance of water and electrolytes in the intestinal content. For this reason, this class of drugs can be considered as antisecretary agents.

Steroids have been found to be effective in MBO in a series of studies.[117,118] A recent meta-analysis of these studies showed a trend towards resolution of bowel obstruction using the corticosteroid dexamethasone in doses ranging from 6 to 16 mg/day intravenously with minimal morbidity, although this result did not achieve statistical significance.[119]

Analgesics

Most patients presenting symptoms from bowel obstruction are on strong opioids, usually morphine, at the time of diagnosis. The dose of opioids should be titrated against the effect, and most usually be administered parenterally, according to the WHO guidelines. In patients with subsequent episodes of subacute obstruction to which opioids may negatively contribute, it may be useful to choose the drug on the basis of presumed selectivity of distribution at the intestinal sites. Morphine tends to accumulate in intestinal tissues, interacting with local opioid receptors. It has been reported that more lipophilic drugs, like methadone and fentanyl, may limit their presence at the opioid intestinal receptors.[120,121] Experimental studies showed a more favourable constipation/analgesia ratio of fentanyl relative to morphine.[122] This is probably a reflection of the lipophilic properties of fentanyl. Some papers seem to indicate that transdermal fentanyl as well as methadone may have less constipating effects or may require lower laxative doses in comparison with morphine.[123–125] Moreover, switching from morphine to methadone improves GI tolerability[126] as well as switching the route of the opioid administration.[127]

On the other hand, the use of NSAIDs may allow for a reduction of constipation induced by opioids[128] and may result in improvement in the opioid bowel syndrome.[129]

The main recommendations for the use of symptomatic drugs or their combination, according to the aim of care and specific clinical conditions in patients with negative prognostic factors for surgery, are shown in Table 7.

Hydration and nutrition

The main goal of parenteral nutrition is to maintain or restore the patient's nutritional status and to correct or prevent malnutrition and its related symptoms.[130] The role of parenteral nutrition in the management of patients with inoperable bowel obstruction should be carefully considered on the basis of several factors. It rests on the ability to demonstrate genuine benefit for the patients.[131] The question is whether it improves quality of life and does not merely lengthen survival. Parenteral nutrition may prolong survival but can also lead to complications, add further suffering, and make prolonged hospitalization necessary.[132]

In some circumstances in which bowel obstruction is temporary and can spontaneously resolve, rehydration is of value in maintaining an appropriate nutrient intake until a therapeutic action has an effect. However, in most cases this practice is unnecessary and may worsen the patient's burden. It is often employed as a psychological measure at the insistence of relatives. In most cases, parenteral nutrition is interrupted after an appropriate explanation about the short prognosis and the evidence of no benefit.[133] Therefore, the routine use should be avoided when it is designed solely to prolong life. Parenteral nutrition should not be undertaken without a full discussion with the patient and family members. Only those patients who strongly support this decision after a clear explanation should be offered this approach. A home care programme for such patients requires active participation of the patient's caregiver and the involvement of skilled nurses, pharmacists, and physicians.

Most patients with bowel obstruction are dehydrated, due to a steel fluid syndrome of water and electrolytes at the intestinal level and poor oral intake of fluids. The correction of this status does not have any effect on dry mouth and thirst, as the intensity of these symptoms seem to be independent of the amounts of fluids administered either by oral or parenteral route.[20,134] A high level of hydration may result in more bowel secretions. On the other hand, the intensity of nausea was significantly lower in patients treated with moderate amounts of water (>500 ml/day), probably due to the prevention of metabolic derangement associated with severe dehydration and reduction of stimulation of the chemoreceptor trigger zone.[92,93] Administration of 1–1.5 l/day of solution containing electrolytes and glucose may be useful in preventing symptoms due to metabolic derangement.

Hypodermoclisis is a valid alternative to intravenous administration of fluids for patients with poor vein availability or without a central venous catheter.[135] Providing sips of oral fluids, frequent attention to mouth care, and sucking ice cubes are of paramount importance in relieving dry mouth, commonly associated with the use of anticholinergics drugs.[20]

Conclusions

Bowel obstruction should be carefully evaluated by experienced physicians, considering individual and prognostic factors, as well as life expectancy. Different options may be chosen depending on the goals of intervention, and the modalities of occurrence of bowel obstruction, as well as the patient's conditions. Involvement of patients and family members in this therapeutic decision-making is mandatory, based on clear information about the clinical status and the possible evolution of the clinical course. Further controlled studies on large numbers of patients are needed, looking at the problems from the epidemiological and prognostic point of view. Comparative trials performed at different stages of bowel obstruction could make an important contribution to defining the best treatments in potentially reversible conditions as well as established MBO. Specifically, in inoperable MBO the use of steroids or a combination of drugs, such as steroids with octreotide, or steroids with hyoscine butylbromide, should be investigated to improve gastrointestinal symptoms. The role and the level of hydration to administer to these patients should be assessed in studies with an appropriate design on a large number of patients.

References

1. **Beattie, G.J., Leonard, R., and Smyth, J.F.** (1989). Bowel obstruction in ovarian carcinoma: a retrospective study and review of the literature. *Palliative Medicine* **3**, 275–80.
2. **Lund, B.** et al. (1989). Intestinal obstruction in patients with advanced carcinoma of the ovaries treated with combination chemotherapy. *Surgery, Gynecology & Obsterics* **169**, 213–18.
3. **Castaldo, T.W.** et al. (1981). Intestinal operations in patients with ovarian carcinoma. *American Journal of Obstetrics and Gynecology* **139**, 80–4.
4. **Krebs, H.B. and Goplerud, D.R.** (1983). Surgical management of bowel obstruction in advanced ovarian carcinoma. *Obstetrics and Gynecology* **61**, 327–30.
5. **Larson, J.E.** et al. (1989). Bowel obstruction in patients with ovarian carcinoma: analysis of prognostic factors. *Gynecologic Oncology* **35**, 61–5.
6. **Fernandes, J.R., Seymour, R.J., and Suissa, S.** (1988). Bowel obstruction in patients with ovarian cancer: a search for prognostic factors. *American Journal of Obstetrics and Gynecology* **158**, 244–9.
7. **Gallick, H.L.** et al. (1986). Intestinal obstruction in cancer patients. An assessment of risk factors and outcome. *The American Surgeon* **52**, 434–7.
8. **Baines, M., Oliver, D.J., and Carter, R.L.** (1985). Mechanical management of intestinal obstruction in patients with advanced malignant disease: a clinical and pathological study. *Lancet* **II**, 990–3.
9. **Mercadante, S.** (1995). Bowel obstruction in home care cancer patients: four years of experience. *Supportive Care in Cancer* **3**, 190–3.
10. **Fainsinger, R.L.** et al. (1994). Symptom control in terminally ill patients with malignant bowel obstruction. *Journal of Pain and Symptom Management* **9**, 12–18.
11. **Mercadante, S.** (1997). Assessment and management of mechanical bowel obstruction. In *Topics in Palliative Care* Vol. 1 (ed. R.K. Portenoy and E. Bruera), pp. 113–30. New York NY: Oxford University Press.
12. **Glare, P. and Lickiss, J.N.** (1992). Unrecognized constipation in patients with advanced cancer. A review for therapeutic disaster. *Journal of Pain and Symptom Management* **7**, 369–71.
13. **Mercadante, S.** (1995). Pain in inoperable bowel obstruction. *Pain Digest* **5**, 9–13.
14. **Nellgard, P., Bojo, L., and Cassuto, J.** (1995). Importance of vasoactive intestinal peptide and somatostatin for fluid losses in small-bowel obstruction. *Scandinavian Journal of Gastroenterology* **30**, 464–9.
15. **Nellgard, P. and Cassuto, J.** (1993). Inflammation as a major cause of fluid losses in small-bowel obstruction. *Scandinavian Journal of Gastroenterology* **28**, 1035–41.
16. **Basson, M.D.** et al. (1989). Does vasoactive intestinal polypeptide mediate the pathophysiology of bowel obstruction? *American Journal of Surgery* **157**, 109–15.
17. **Neville, R.** et al. (1991). Vascular responsiveness in obstructed gut. *Diseases of the Colon and Rectum* **34**, 229–35.
18. **Chan, A. and Woodruff, R.K.** (1992). Intestinal obstruction in patients with widespread intra-abdominal malignancy. *Journal of Pain and Symptom Management* **7**, 339–42.
19. **Scott Jones, R. and Schirmer, B.D.** (1989). Intestinal obstruction, pseudo-obstruction and ileus. In *Gastrointestinal Disease* (ed. M.H. Sleisinger and J.S. Fordtran), pp. 369–81. Philadelphia: JB Lippincott Co.
20. **Ripamonti, C.** et al. (2001). Clinical-practice recommendations for the management of bowel obstruction in patients with end-stage cancer. *Supportive Care in Cancer* **9**, 223–33.
21. **Welch, J.P.** *Bowel Obstruction.* Philadelphia: WB Saunders, 1990.
22. **Krebs, H.B. and Goplerud, D.R.** (1984). The role of intestinal intubation in obstruction of the small intestine due to carcinoma of the ovary. *Surgery, Gynecology & Obstetrics* **158**, 467–9.
23. **Walsh, H.P.J. and Schofield, P.F.** (1984). Is laparotomy for small bowel obstruction justified in patients with previously treated malignancy? *British Journal of Surgery* **71**, 933–4.
24. **Feuer, D.J.** et al. (1999) Systematic review of surgery in malignant bowel obstruction in advanced gynaecological and gastrointestinal cancer. *Gynecologic Oncology* **75**, 313–22.
25. **Rubin, S.C.** et al. (1989). Palliative surgery for intestinal obstruction in advanced ovarian cancer. *Gynecologic Oncology*, **34**, 16–19.
26. **van Oojen, B.** et al. (1993). Surgical treatment or gastric drainage only for intestinal obstruction in patients with carcinoma of the ovary or peritoneal carcinomatosis of other origin. *Surgery, Gynecology & Obstetrics* **176**, 469–73.
27. **Jong, P., Sturgeon, J., and Jamieson, C.G.** (1995). Benefit of palliative surgery for bowel obstruction in advanced ovarian cancer. *Canadian Journal of Surgery* **38** (5), 454–7.

28. **Turnbull, A.D.M., Guerra, J., and Starners, H.F.** (1989). Results of surgery for obstructing carcinomatosis of gastrointestinal, pancreatic, or biliary origin. *Journal of Clinical Oncology* **7**, 381–6.
29. **Butler, J.A.** et al. (1991). Small bowel obstruction in patients with a prior history of cancer. *The American Journal of Surgery* **162**, 624–8.
30. **Lau, P.W. and Lorentz, T.G.** (1993). Results of surgery for malignant bowel obstruction in advanced, unresectable, recurrent colorectal cancer. *Diseases of the Colon and Rectum* **36** (1), 61–4.
31. **Tang, E., Davis, J., and Silberman, H.** (1995). Bowel obstruction in cancer patients. *Archives of Surgery* **130**, 832–7.
32. **Sun, X., Li, X., and Li, H.** (1995). Management of intestinal obstruction in advanced ovarian cancer: an analysis of 57 cases. *Chung Hua Chung Liu Tsa Chih* **17**, 39–42.
33. **Yazdi, G.P., Miedema, B.W., and Humphrey, L.J.** (1996). High mortality after abdominal operation in patients with large-volume malignant ascites. *Journal of Surgical Oncology* **62**, 93–6.
34. **Woolfson, R.G., Jennings, K., and Whalen, G.F.** (1997). Management of bowel obstruction in patients with abdominal cancer. *Archives of Surgery* **132**, 1093–7.
35. **Tunca, J.C., Buchler, D.A., Mack, E.A., Ruzicka, F.F., Crowley, J.J., and Carr, W.F.** (1981). The management of ovarian-cancer-caused bowel obstruction. *Gynecologic Oncology* **12**, 186–92.
36. **Piver, M.S.** et al. (1982). Survival after ovarian cancer induced intestinal obstruction. *Gynecologic Oncology* **13**, 44–9.
37. **Aabo, K.** et al. (1984) Surgical management of intestinal obstruction in the late course of malignant disease. *Acta Chirurgica Scandinavica* **150**, 173–6.
38. **Glass, R.L. and LeDuc, R.J.** (1973). Small intestinal obstruction from peritoneal carcinomatosis. *American Journal of Surgery* **125**, 316–17.
39. **Rapin, Ch.H.** et al. (1990). Pour une meilleure qualite' de vie en fin de vie: nutrition et hydratation. *Age et nutrition* **1**, 22–8.
40. **Clarke-Pearson, D.L.** et al. (1987). Surgical management of intestinal obstruction in ovarian cancer. I. Clinical features, postoperative complications, and survival. *Gynecologic Oncology* **26**, 11–18.
41. **Clarke-Pearson, D.L.** et al. (1988). Surgical management of intestinal obstruction in ovarian cancer II. Analysis of factors associated with complications and survival. *Archives of Surgery* **123**, 42–5.
42. **Weiss, S.M., Skibber, J.M., and Rosato, F.E.** (1984). Bowel obstruction in cancer patients: performance status as a predictor of survival. *Journal of Surgical Oncology* **25**, 15–17.
43. **Pictus, D., Marx, M.V., and Weyman, P.J.** (1988). Chronic intestinal obstruction: value of percutaneous gastrostomy tube placement. *American Journal of Radiology* **150**, 295–7.
44. **Rees, R.G.P.** et al. (1988). Spontaneous transpylorus passage and performance of fine bore polyurethane feeding under a controlled clinical trial. *Journal of Parenteral and Enteral Nutrition* **12**, 469–71.
45. **Ripamonti, C.** et al. (1996). Role of enteral nutrition in advanced cancer patients: indications and contraindications of the different techniques employed. *Tumori* **82**, 302–8.
46. **Forgas, I., Macpherson, A., and Tibbs, C.** (1992). Percutaneous endoscopic gastrostomy. The end of the line for nasogastric feeding? *British Medical Journal* **304**, 1395–6.
47. **Gleeson, N.C.** et al. (1994). Gastrostomy tubes after gynecologic oncologic surgery. *Gynecologic Oncology* **54**, 19–22.
48. **Malone, J.M.** et al. (1986). Palliation of small bowel obstructon by percutaneous gastrostomy in patients with progressive ovarian carcinoma. *Obstetrics and Gynecology* **68**, 431–3.
49. **George, J.** et al. (1990). Percutaneous endoscopic gastrostomy: a two year experience. *Medical Journal of Australia* **152**, 17–20.
50. **Vargo, J.J.** et al. (1993). Ultrasound-assisted percutaneous endoscopic gastrostomy in a patient with advanced ovarian carcinoma and recurrent intestinal obstruction. *American Journal of Gastroenterology* **88** (11), 1946–8.
51. **Cannizzaro, R.** et al. (1995). Percutaneous endoscopic gastrostomy as a decompressive technique in bowel obstruction due to abdominal carcinomatosis. *Endoscopy* **27**, 317–20.
52. **Adelson, M.D. and Kazowits, M.H.** (1993). Percutaneous endoscopic drainage gastrostomy in treatment of gastrointestinal obstruction from intraperitoneal malignancy. *Obstetrics and Gynecology* **81**, 467–9.
53. **Herman, L.L., Hoskins, W.J., and Shike, M.** (1992). Percutaneous endoscopic gastrostomy for decompression of the stomach and small bowel. *Gastrointestinal Endoscopy* **38**, 314–18.
54. **Schwab, K.S.** et al. (1993). Percutaneous endoscopic gastrostomy for decompression in patients with malignant carcinomatosis and radiation enteritis. *Gastrointestinal Endoscopy* **39**, 288A.
55. **Noyer, C.** et al. (1993). Percutaneous endoscopic gastrostomy (PEG): gastric decompression in patients with carcinomatosis. *Gastrointestinal Endoscopy* **39**, 282A.
56. **Marks, W.H., Perkal, M.F., and Schwartz, P.E.** (1993). Percutaneous endoscopic gastrostomy for gastric decompression in metastatic gynecologic malignancies. *Surgery, Gynecology & Obstetrics* **177**, 573–6.
57. **Cunningham, M.J.** et al. (1995). Percutaneous gastrostomy for decompression in patients with advanced gynecologic malignancies. *Gynecologic Oncology* **59**, 273–6.
58. **Campagnutta, E.** et al. (1996). Palliative treatment of upper intestinal obstruction by gynecological malignancy: the usefulness of percutaneous endoscopic gastrostomy. *Gynecologic Oncology* **62**, 103–5.
59. **Sriram, K., Sridhar, K., and Sridhar, R.** (1996). Gastroduodenal decompression and simultaneous nasoenteral nutrition: 'extracorporeal gastrojejunostomy' (clinical conference) [published erratum appears in *Nutrition* 1996, **12** (10), 747]. *Nutrition* **12**, 440–1.
60. **Wallis, F.** et al. (1998). Self-expanding metal stents in the management of colorectal carcinoma—a preliminary report (see comments). *Clinical Radiology* **53**, 251–4.
61. **Lamah, M.** et al. (1998). The use of rectosigmoid stents in the management of acute large bowel obstruction. *Journal of the Royal College of Surgeons, Edinburgh* **43**, 318–21.
62. **Mainar, A.** et al. (1996). Colorectal obstruction: treatment with metallic stents. *Radiology* **198**, 761–4.
63. **Scott-Mackie, P.** et al. (1997). The role of metallic stents in malignant duodenal obstruction. *British Journal of Radiology* **70**, 252–5.
64. **Pinto, I.T.** (1997). Malignant gastric and duodenal stenosis: palliation by peroral implantation of a self-expanding metallic stent. *Cardiovascular and Interventional Radiology* **20**, 431–4.
65. **Park, H.S.** et al. (1999). Upper gastrointestinal tract malignant obstruction: initial results of palliation with a flexible covered stent. *Radiology* **210**, 865–70.
66. **Keymling, M.** et al. (1993). Relief of malignant duodenal obstruction by percutaneous insertion of a metal stent. *Gastrointestinal Endoscopy* **39** (3), 439–41.
67. **Feretis, C.** et al. (1997). Duodenal obstruction caused by pancreatic head carcinoma: palliation with self-expandable endoprostheses. *Gastrointestinal Endoscopy* **46**, 161–5.
68. **de Baere, T.** et al. (1997). Self-expanding metallic stents as palliative treatment of malignant gastroduodenal stenosis. *American Journal of Roentgenology* **169**, 1079–83.
69. **Sebastian, J.J.** et al. (1997). Duodenal obstruction secondary to a metastasis from an adenocarcinoma of the cecum: a case report. *American Journal of Gastroenterology* **92**, 1051–2.
70. **Howden, C.W. and Woods, B.L.** (1995). Self-expanding metal stents for palliative treatment of malignant biliary and duodenal stenoses. *Gastrointestinal Endoscopy* **42**, 104–5.
71. **Song, H.Y.** et al. (1994). Covered, expandable esophageal metallic stent tubes: experiences in 119 patients. *Radiology* **193**, 689–95.
72. **Saxon, R.R.** et al. (1995). Treatment of malignant esophageal obstructions with covered metallic Z stents: long-term results in 52 patients. *Journal of Vascular and Interventional Radiology* **6**, 747–54.
73. **Feins, R.H.** et al. (1996). Palliation of inoperable esophageal carcinoma with the Wallstent endoprosthesis. *Annals of Thoracic Surgery* **62**, 1603–7.
74. **Arnell, T.** et al. (1998). Colonic stents in colorectal obstruction. *American Surgery* **64**, 986–8.
75. **Tejero, E.** et al. (1997). Initial results of a new procedure for treatment of malignant obstruction of the left colon. *Diseases of the Colon and Rectum* **40**, 432–6.

76. **Saida, Y.** et al. (1996). Stent endoprosthesis for obstructing colorectal cancers. *Diseases of the Colon and Rectum* **39**, 552–5.
77. **Feretis, C.** et al. (1996). Palliation of large-bowel obstruction due to recurrent rectosigmoid tumor using self-expandable endoprostheses. *Endoscopy* **28**, 319–22.
78. **Vandervoort, J.** et al. (1996). Self-expanding metal stent for obstructing adenocarcinoma of the sigmoid. *Gastrointestinal Endoscopy* **44**, 739–41.
79. **Rey, J.F., Romanczyk, T., and Greff, M.** (1995). Metal stents for palliation of rectal carcinoma: a preliminary report on 12 patients. *Endoscopy* **27**, 501–4.
80. **Dohomoto, M., Hunerbein, M., and Schlag, P.M.** (1997). Application of rectal stents for palliation of obstructing rectosigmoid cancer. *Surgical Endoscopy* **11**, 758–61.
81. **Canon, C.L.** et al. (1997). Treatment of colonic obstruction with expandable metal stents: radiologic features. *American Journal of Roentgenology* **168**, 199–205.
82. **Wholey, M.H.** et al. (1997). Retrieval of migrated colonic stents from the rectum. *Cardiovascular and Interventional Radiology* **20**, 477–80.
83. **Swanson, G.** et al. (1989). Patient-controlled analgesia for chronic cancer pain in the ambulatory setting. A report of 177 patients. *Journal of Clinical Oncology* **7**, 1903–8.
84. **Chandler, S.W., Trissel, L.A., and Weinstein, S.M.** (1996). Combined administration of opioids with selected drugs to manage pain and other cancer symptoms: initial safety screening for compatibility. *Journal of Pain and Symptom Management* **12**, 168–71.
85. **Storey, P.** et al. (1990). Subcutaneous infusions for control of cancer symptoms. *Journal of Pain and Symptom Management* **5**, 33–41.
86. **Grassby, P.F. and Hutchings, L.** (1997). Drugs combinations in syringe drivers: the compatibility and stability of diamorphine with cyclizine and haloperidol. *Palliative Medicine* **11**, 217–24.
87. **Mercadante, S.** (1995). Tolerability of continuous subcutaneous octreotide used in combination with other drugs. *Journal of Palliative Care* **4**, 14–16.
88. **Twycross, R.** et al. (1998). Nausea and vomiting in advanced cancer. *European Journal of Palliative Care* **5**, 39–45.
89. **Ventafridda, V.** et al. (1990). The management of inoperable gastrointestinal obstruction in terminal cancer patients. *Tumori* **76**, 389–93.
90. **De Conno, F.** et al. (1991). Continuous subcutaneous infusion of hyoscine butylbromide reduces secretions in patients with gastrointestinal obstruction. *Journal of Pain and Symptom Management* **6**, 484–6.
91. **Davis, M. and Furste, A.** (1999). Glycopyrrolate: a useful drug in the palliation of mechanical bowel obstruction. *Journal of Pain and Symptom Management* **18**, 153–4.
92. **Ripamonti, C.** et al. (2000). Role of octreotide, scopolamine butylbromide and hydration in symptom control of patients with inoperable bowel obstruction having a nasogastric tube. A prospective, randomized clinical trial. *Journal of Pain and Symptom Management* **19**, 23–34.
93. **Mercadante, S.** et al. (2000). Comparison of octreotide and hyoscine butylbromide in controlling gastrointestinal symptoms due to malignant inoperable bowel obstruction. *Supportive Care in Cancer* **8**, 188–91.
94. **Anthone, G.J.** et al. (1990). Direct proabsorptive effect of octreotide on ionic transport in the small intestine. *Surgery* **108** (6), 1136–42.
95. **Fallon, M.T.** (1994). The physiology of somatostatin and its synthetic analogue, octreotide. *European Journal of Palliative Care* **1**, 20–2.
96. **Penn, R.D.** et al. (1992). Octreotide, a potent new non-opiate analgesic for intrathecal infusion. *Pain* **49**, 13–14.
97. **Pless, J.** et al. (1986). Chemistry and pharmacology of SMS 201-995, a long acting octapeptide analogue of somatostatin. *Scandinavian Journal of Gastroenterology* **21**, 54–64.
98. **Roberts, W.G., Fedorak, R.N., and Chang, E.B.** (1988). *In vitro* effects of the long-acting somatostatin analogue SMS 201-995 on electrolyte transport by the rabbit ileum. *Gastroenterology* **94**, 1343–50.
99. **Reichlin, S.** (1983). Somatostatin. II. *New England Journal of Medicine* **309**, 1556–63.
100. **Reichlin, S.** (1983). Somatostatin. I. *New England Journal of Medicine* **309**, 1495–501.
101. **Mercadante, S.** (1994) The role of octreotide in palliative care. *Journal of Pain and Symptom Management* **9**, 406–11.
102. **Cullen, J.J., Eagon, J.C., and Kelly, K.A.** (1994). Gastrointestinal peptide hormones during postoperative ileus. Effect of octreotide. *Digestive Diseases and Sciences* **39** (6), 1179–84.
103. **Gittes, G.K.** et al. (1992). Improvement in survival of mice with proximal small bowel obstruction treated with octreotide. *American Journal of Surgery* **163** (2), 231–3.
104. **Guiro', F.F., Bertolini, G., and Salas, J.V.** (1999). Improvement in the intestinal processes of hydroelectrolytic absorption and secretion in abdominal pathologies of surgical interest treated with SMS 201-995: experimental protocol. *Surgery Today* **29** (5), 419–30.
105. **Mulvihill, S.J.** et al. (1988). The effect of somatostatin on experimental intestinal obstruction. *Annals of Surgery* **207** (2), 169–73.
106. **Yamaner, S., Bugra, D., Muslumanoglu, M., Bulut, T., Cubukcu, O., and Ademoglu, E.** (1995). Effects of octreotide on healing of intestinal anastomosis following small bowel obstruction in rats. *Diseases of the Colon and Rectum* **38** (3), 308–12.
107. **Modlin, I.M., Bloom, S.R., and Mitchell, S.C.** (1978). Plasma vasoactive intestinal polypeptide (VIP) levels and intestinal ischemia. *Experientia* **34**, 535–6.
108. **Mercadante, S.** et al. (1996). Octreotide prevents the pathological alterations of bowel obstruction in cancer patients. *Supportive Care in Cancer* **4**, 393–4.
109. **Mercadante, S., Kargar, J., and Nicolosi, G.** (1997). Octreotide may prevent definitive intestinal obstruction. *Journal of Pain and Symptom Management* **13**, 352–5.
110. **Bastounis, E.** et al. (1989). Somatostatin as adjuvant therapy in the management of obstructive ileus. *Hepato-Gastroenterology* **36** (6), 538–9.
111. **Mercadante, S. and Maddaloni, S.** (1992) Octreotide in the management of inoperable bowel obstruction in terminal cancer patients. *Journal of Pain and Symptom Management* **7**, 496–8.
112. **Mercadante, S.** et al. (1993). Octreotide in relieving gastrointestinal symptoms due to bowel obstruction. *Palliative Medicine* **7**, 295–9.
113. **Khoo, D., Riley J., and Waxman, J.** (1992). Control of emesis in bowel obstruction in terminally ill patients. *Lancet* **339**, 375–6.
114. **Riley, J. and Fallon, M.T.** (1994). Octreotide in terminal malignant obstruction of the gastrointestinal tract. *European Journal of Palliative Care* **1**, 23–8.
115. **Mangili, G.** et al. (1996). Octreotide in the management of bowel obstruction in terminal ovarian cancer. *Gynecologic Oncology* **61**, 345–8.
116. **Mercadante, S.** (1998). Scopolamine butylbromide plus octreotide in unresponsive bowel obstruction. *Journal of Pain and Symptom Management* **16** (5), 278–9.
117. **Hardy, J.** et al. (1988). Pifalls in placebo-controlled trials in palliative care: dexamethasone for the palliation of malignant bowel obstruction. *Palliative Medicine* **12**, 437–42.
118. **Laval, G.** et al. (2000). The use of steroids in the management of inoperable intestinal obstrution in terminal cancer patients: do they remove the obstruction? *Palliative Medicine* **14**, 3–10.
119. **Feuer, D.J.** et al. (1999). Systematic review and meta-analysis of corticosteroids for the resolution of malignant bowel obstruction in advanced gynaecological and gastrointestinal cancers. *Annals of Oncology* **10**, 1035–41.
120. **Mercadante, S.** (2001). What is the opioid of choice? *Progress in Palliative Care* **9**, 190–3.
121. **Mercadante, S., Sapio, M., and Serretta, R.** (1997). Treatment of pain in chronic bowel subobstruction with self-administration of methadone. *Support Care in Cancer* **5**, 327–9.
122. **Hazen, L.** et al. (1999) The constipation-inducing potential of morphine and transdermal fentanyl. *European Journal of Pain* **3** (Suppl. A), 9–15.
123. **Ahmedzai, S. and Brooks, D.** (1997). Transdermal fentanyl versus sustained-release oral morphine in cancer pain: preference, efficacy, and quality of life. *Journal of Pain and Symptom Management* **13**, 254–61.
124. **Radbruck, L.** et al. (2000). Constipation and the use of laxatives: a comparison between transdermal fentanyl and oral morphine. *Palliative Medicine* **14**, 111–19.
125. **Mancini, I.L.** et al. (2000). Opioid type and other clinical predictors of laxatives dose in advanced cancer patients: a retrospective study. *Journal of Palliative Medicine* **3**, 49–56.
126. **Mercadante, S.** et al. (2001). Switching from morphine to methadone to improve analgesia and tolerability in cancer patients: a prospective study. *Journal of Clinical Oncology* **19**, 2898–904.

127. Cherny, N. et al. (2001). Strategies to manage the adverse effects of oral morphine: an evidence-based report. *Journal of Clinical Oncology* **19**, 2542–54.
128. Mercadante, S. et al. (2002). A randomised controlled study on the use of anti-inflammatory drugs in patients with cancer pain on morphine therapy: effects on dose-escalation and pharmacoeconomical analysis. *European Journal of Cancer* **38**, 1358–63.
129. Joishy, S.K. and Walsh, D. (1998). The opioid-sparing effects of intravenous ketorolac as an adjuvant analgesic in cancer pain: application in bone metastases and the opioid bowel syndrome. *Journal of Pain and Symptom Management* **16**, 334–9.
130. Bozzetti, F. et al. (1996). Guidelines on artificial nutrition versus hydration in terminal cancer patients. *Nutrition* **12**, 163–7.
131. Cozzaglio, L. et al. (1997). Outcome of cancer patients receiving home parenteral nutrition. *Journal of Parenteral and Enteral Nutrition* **21**, 339–42.
132. Philip, J. and Depczynski, B. (1997). The role of total parenteral nutrition for patients with irreversible bowel obstruction secondary to gynecological malignancy. *Journal of Pain and Symptom Management* **13**, 104–11.
133. Mercadante, S. (1995). Parenteral nutrition at home. *Journal of Pain and Symptom Management* **10**, 476–80.
134. Burge, F.I. (1993). Dehydration symptoms of palliative care cancer patients. *Journal of Pain and Symptom Management* **8**, 454–64.
135. Fainsinger, R.L. et al. (1994). The use of hypodermoclysis for rehydration in terminally ill cancer patients. *Journal of Pain and Symptom Management* **9**, 298–302.

8.3.5 Jaundice, ascites, and hepatic encephalopathy

Krikor Kichian and Vincent G. Bain

Jaundice

The presence of jaundice in the terminally ill patient usually portends a rapid demise; nevertheless, it is important to understand the different underlying mechanisms and causes so that a rational approach can be planned. In some cases, symptomatic treatment of associated symptoms such as pruritus is the only therapeutic goal whereas in others, a more aggressive approach such as placement of a biliary stent through a malignant stricture may facilitate a markedly improved quality and perhaps even duration of life. The appearance of jaundice in a terminally ill patient serves as an obvious marker of a severe underlying illness; family, friends, and acquaintances may become alarmed and naturally suspect the gravity of the illness. The successful resolution of jaundice can therefore have positive psychological and palliative effects that cannot be overestimated. It is important to take a general approach to the patient with jaundice to avoid making the error of equating jaundice with end-stage, untreatable disease. We must endeavour to identify those patients whose jaundice can be reversed by relatively simple measures such as stopping a hepatotoxic medication and those who might benefit from relief of obstructive jaundice. Clearly, jaundice is not always a direct result of massive infiltration of the liver with malignancy.

Pathophysiology of jaundice

Jaundice can be classified as shown in Table 1 into pre-hepatic, hepatic, and post-hepatic disorders. Although not completely comprehensive, it includes conditions most likely to be encountered in cancer patients and thereby

Table 1 Classification of jaundice

Pre-hepatic	Hepatic	Post-hepatic
Gilbert's disease	Massive tumour infiltration	Malignant
Haemolysis	Viral hepatitis	Pancreas
Ineffective erythropoiesis	Hepatotoxic drugs (including alcohol)	Ampullary
Haematoma	Cholestasis	Cholangiocarcinoma
	Total parenteral nutrition	Metastatic lymph nodes
	Sepsis	Benign
	Drugs	Gallstones
	Ischaemia	Chronic pancreatitis
	Hepatic artery thrombosis	Biliary stricture
	Left ventricular failure	
	Venous outflow block	
	Severe right heart failure	
	Veno-occlusive disease	
	Budd–Chiari syndrome	

provides a useful framework for an orderly approach to the patient with jaundice. A pre-hepatic derangement is defined by an imbalance between the liver's capacity to take up unconjugated bilirubin and the amount being presented from the blood. As the term implies, it is not a hepatic problem at all; common examples include haemolysis, ineffective haematopoiesis, and Gilbert's disease, all of which are characterized by unconjugated hyperbilirubinaemia.

Hepatic causes of jaundice form the largest and most heterogeneous group (see Table 1). Any interference with the liver's capacity to excrete conjugated bilirubin into the biliary system will result in jaundice. In general, this may be secondary to widespread necrosis of hepatocytes (hepatocellular injury) or 'functional' (non-obstructive) impairment of biliary excretion (cholestasis). Extensive hepatic infiltration with malignant cells causes jaundice and is associated with a median survival of only 1 month.[1] In the western world, this is usually due to metastatic disease from primaries in the gastrointestinal tract (colon, pancreas, stomach), breast, lung, or haematologic malignancies.[1] In rare instances, metastatic liver disease may even present as fulminant hepatic failure.[2] Viral hepatitis must always be considered, particularly in patients receiving blood products who are at risk of infection with hepatitis C virus.[3] The risk of acquiring hepatitis C (previously non-A, non-B hepatitis) from unscreened blood products was previously 10 per cent; the routine screening of donors with the hepatitis C virus immunoassay has substantially reduced this risk. Chronic hepatitis B is widely prevalent especially in Asians; withdrawal of immunosuppressive chemotherapeutic agents may precipitate liver failure in chronic hepatitis B virus carriers.[4] Patients with widespread cancer, like other immunosuppressed individuals, are also at risk of viral hepatitis caused by cytomegalovirus and herpes simplex virus.

Numerous medications can lead to hepatic injury.[5] This usually leads to elevated serum liver enzymes in the absence of jaundice; however, several medications can cause severe hepatocellular injury or cholestasis with jaundice. Examples include commonly used agents such as halothane, erythromycin, amoxicillin/potassium clavulanate, alpha methyldopa, isoniazid, prochlorperazine, and chlorpromazine as well as numerous cancer chemotherapeutic agents such as the C-17 alkylated steroids, methotrexate, and rarely chlorambucil. Jaundice induced by any of the commonly used sedatives or analgesics (including acetaminophen at recommended dosage) would be extremely rare.

Intra-hepatic cholestasis may be defined as a reduction of bile excretion in the absence of extra-hepatic biliary obstruction. Many causes have been identified and cholestasis is often multifactorial; drugs, total parenteral nutrition, sepsis, and the post-operative state may all contribute. Cholestatic jaundice is generally less serious than jaundice secondary to extensive hepatocellular necrosis; however, if it persists, fat malabsorption and fat soluble vitamin deficiency may ensue.

The liver is a highly vascular organ receiving approximately 20–25 per cent of the cardiac output from its dual vascular supply of the portal vein

(70 per cent) and hepatic artery (30 per cent). Reduced cardiac output secondary to severe impairment of left ventricular function or prolonged hypotension from any cause may lead to hepatic injury;[6] however, in most instances, clinically significant hepatic injury is absent. Similarly, thrombosis of the hepatic artery secondary to catheterization, damage at surgery, or tumour invasion is usually a clinically silent event. In some instances, however, patients develop severe right upper quadrant pain, a marked rise of serum transaminases (often greater than 10 000 IU/l) and later, jaundice. Portal vein thrombosis may also occur secondary to tumour invasion or hyper-coagulable states but usually does not lead to jaundice providing hepatic function is not otherwise compromised.

Blood coming into the liver from the hepatic artery or portal vein percolates through the hepatic sinusoids then passes through the central hepatic veins and exits the liver through the hepatic veins into the inferior vena cava. Obliteration of the small intra-hepatic veins, termed veno-occlusive disease, has been associated with radiation, 6-thioguanine, azathioprine, herbal medication, and graft versus host disease following allogeneic bone marrow transplantation. Patients rapidly develop ascites, tender hepatomegaly, and with progression, jaundice. A similar clinical picture results from the Budd–Chiari syndrome, which follows thrombosis of the main hepatic veins as they enter the inferior vena cava. Budd–Chiari syndrome may complicate hypercoagulable states associated with malignancy or it may result from direct tumour invasion particularly by hepatocellular carcinoma or renal, adrenal, and atrial tumours. The clinical syndrome may develop insidiously or rapidly. Thrombosis may also involve the inferior vena cava, which is heralded by massive dependant oedema.

Post-hepatic jaundice results from high-grade obstruction to biliary flow at the level of the extra-hepatic bile ducts. Malignant causes include cancer of the pancreas, ampullary carcinoma, cholangiocarcinoma and enlarged lymph nodes at the porta hepatis, but benign causes must also be considered. Gallstones in the common bile duct, acute or chronic pancreatitis, and biliary strictures secondary to previous surgery or hepatic intra-arterial chemotherapy with 5-fluorouracil[7] may also cause obstructive jaundice.

Diagnostic approach

History and physical examination are of paramount importance in narrowing the lengthy differential diagnosis of jaundice and in directing its investigation. It is particularly important to inquire about prior liver disease, alcohol intake, medications, and risk factors for hepatitis. In most patients, jaundice will be painless; however, the presence of associated abdominal pain is compatible with rapid hepatic capsular distention (e.g. Budd–Chiari syndrome), biliary colic, or pancreatic carcinoma where posterior radiation and exacerbation by recumbency is typical. Dark or tea-coloured urine results from conjugated hyperbilirubinaemia and is therefore absent in pre-hepatic causes of jaundice. Acholic stools suggest a hepatic or post-hepatic problem; intermittently acholic stools may be caused by gallstones whereas acholic stools that persist suggests malignant obstruction or a primarily hepatic process such as viral hepatitis. Chills and fever suggest cholangitis but may occasionally accompany acute viral hepatitis. Pruritus is more common with extra-hepatic obstruction or cholestasis but like fatigue, it is not of great diagnostic value.

Deep jaundice is easily detected but more subtle degrees of jaundice will only be appreciated by careful inspection of the sclera and oral mucus membranes under natural light; this assumes even greater importance in dark-skinned individuals. Lymphadenopathy, stigmata of chronic liver disease (e.g. vascular spider naevi and palmar erythema), and oedema are important associated findings. Abdominal examination may reveal hepatomegaly, which, if massive, is highly suggestive of direct tumour involvement. Viral hepatitis is associated with a smooth surfaced, tender liver, whereas irregularity of the edge suggests neoplasia or cirrhosis. A palpable gallbladder is compatible with extra-hepatic obstruction. Other abdominal masses should be carefully sought. The presence of an arterial bruit over the liver points to hepatoma. Ascites is consistent with hepatic venous outflow obstruction, cirrhosis of any cause, or peritoneal carcinomatosis.

Blood tests

Liver function tests (LFTs), or more appropriately, liver injury tests, are frequently helpful in assessing the cause and severity of hepatic dysfunction. Although a mixed or intermediate pattern is often seen, derangement of LFTs can be broadly divided into two patterns suggesting either hepatocellular injury or cholestasis/obstruction. Hepatocellular injury is characterized by a markedly increased aspartate transaminase (AST) or alanine transaminase (ALT) and a variably increased bilirubin level; typical examples include viral hepatitis or injury induced by drugs such as halothane or isoniazid. Intra-hepatic cholestasis and biliary obstruction are both associated with normal or only minimally elevated AST and a raised bilirubin. An increased serum alkaline phosphatase is a rather constant finding in obstructive jaundice but varies greatly in different types of cholestasis. Many variations exist particularly before a given disease process is completely manifest; for example, with early incomplete biliary obstruction, the bilirubin will still be normal whereas the alkaline phosphatase will be elevated.

Numerous other blood tests add supplemental information to the above basic LFTs. Bilirubin fractionation is useful in patients with hyperbilirubinaemia but a normal AST and alkaline phosphatase. A predominant increase in the unconjugated bilirubin fraction is compatible with a pre-hepatic disorder such as Gilbert's disease or haemolysis, both of which are associated with only low-grade hyperbilirubinaemia (less than 120 mmol/l). Since both fractions are increased in hepatic and post-hepatic jaundice, bilirubin fractionation is of little diagnostic aid in most patients with jaundice. Although a rising serum lactic dehydrogenase (LDH) is often considered a particularly poor prognostic sign, a multivariate analysis of prognostic variables in 175 patients with hepatic metastasis secondary to colorectal carcinoma did not show independent predictive value; other LFTs including serum alkaline phosphatase, bilirubin, and albumin were highly significant predictors of survival.[8] Either a 5′ nucleotidase or a gamma glutamyl transpeptidase (GGT) determination are useful to confirm the hepatic source of an elevated serum alkaline phosphatase especially in patients with the potential for bony metastasis. Patients with evidence of hepatocellular injury should undergo serologic testing for viral hepatitis particularly types B and C.

Imaging

Non-invasive imaging techniques are of paramount importance in the assessment of jaundice.[9] Abdominal ultrasound, computed tomography (CT) scanning, magnetic resonance imaging (MR), endoscopic ultrasonography, and scintiscanning have been studied extensively, are widely available, and are inherently safe.

Ultrasound and CT scanning

Abdominal ultrasound is an exceedingly useful first investigation in cases of suspected biliary obstruction. Distal common bile duct obstruction, for example, secondary to ampullary carcinoma or pancreatic carcinoma, will result in dilatation of the extra-hepatic biliary tree including the gallbladder and usually the intra-hepatic ducts as well. More proximal lesions, for example, cholangiocarcinoma at the hilum, will result in intra-hepatic bile duct dilatation only. Although the site and nature of the obstruction are usually visualized, this technique may be limited in the following circumstances: obscured visualization of a distal obstructing lesion secondary to duodenal gas; sub-optimal examination in the obese; and detection of ductal gallstones where 50 per cent may be overlooked even by experienced radiologists. In addition to detecting obstruction, ultrasound is valuable for the identification of primary and secondary hepatic tumours, occlusion of the hepatic veins in Budd–Chiari syndrome, and in insuring patency of the hepatic artery and portal vein. This versatility makes the abdominal ultrasound the imaging procedure of first choice in the investigation of jaundice. Abdominal CT provides similar information to ultrasound; biliary obstruction and hepatic tumours are readily diagnosed and in particular CT scanning with intravenous contrast enhancement is of special value in the evaluation of hepatic masses. Considering the greater cost of a CT scan, it is best used as a supplement when ultrasound is inconclusive.

Magnetic resonance cholangiopancreatography (MRCP)

In recent years, MRCP has gained approval as a useful diagnostic tool in the evaluation of pancreaticobiliary ductal abnormalities. MRCP is non-invasive and does not require injection of contrast. It provides optimal contrast between the hyperdense signal of bile and the hypodense signal of solid organs and blood. The quality of images of biliary pathologic conditions obtained by using MRCP now approach those obtained by percutaneous transhepatic cholangiography and endoscopic retrograde cholangiopancreatography (ERCP).[10,11] Despite its advantage as a non-invasive diagnostic tool, MRCP has some inherent limitations in evaluating fine details of the bile duct wall and in differentiating benign from malignant obstruction.[12] The addition of conventional T1 and T2 weighed MR imaging has been demonstrated as a way to improve the diagnostic sensitivity of MRCP.[13] Given that an MR study of the upper abdomen would be indicated for the evaluation and staging of malignant lesions involving the hepatobiliary system, a combination study of MR with MRCP has been proposed as a convenient and complete diagnostic study.[14]

Endoscopic ultrasonography (EUS)

Endoscopic ultrasonography is the latest diagnostic tool that can be used to assess extra-hepatic cholestasis.[15] EUS involves endoscopic positioning of an ultrasound probe adjacent to the pancreas permitting the operator to visualize local anatomic details. EUS is capable of detecting small lesions that can be missed by conventional ultrasound and CT.[16] Moreover, recent advances, which have enabled EUS to be coupled with fine needle aspiration (FNA), have extended the usefulness of this modality to obtaining tissue diagnosis.[17] EUS, although more invasive, was demonstrated to be as accurate as MR imaging in the diagnosis of extra-hepatic biliary obstruction.[18] The advantage of EUS and EUS-guided FNA in pancreatic malignancies is that it provides TN staging information while procuring a tissue diagnosis and assessing local invasion without subjecting the patient to unnecessary surgery.[19] Currently, the lack of experience and unavailability of EUS in most centres limits the full potential of this tool.

Iminodiacetic acid scintograms

Scintiscans employing technetium-labelled iminodiacetic acid (IDA) derivatives (e.g. HIDA scan) can usually make a reliable distinction between hepatocellular dysfunction in which there is poor hepatic uptake of the isotope and extra-hepatic obstruction, which is characterized by hepatic isotope uptake but lack of secretion into small bowel.[20] IDA scintograms have not been utilized widely as initial imaging techniques, however, because of poor anatomical resolution compared to ultrasound and CT scanning and due to occasional failure of obstructed livers to concentrate the isotope leading to an erroneous impression of hepatocellular injury. Nevertheless, IDA scintograms are useful in special circumstances such as to demonstrate a bile leak or to prove biliary obstruction has been relieved (e.g. by stent placement) when the ducts are still dilated.[20]

Cholangiography

Despite the recent advances of MRCP and EUS technology in visualization of hepato-biliary lesions, in many centres where these tools are not readily available, patients with suspected or demonstrated obstruction undergo cholangiography for an assessment of the obstructive lesion. A percutaneous transhepatic cholangiogram (PTC) will successfully opacify the biliary system in over 95 per cent of obstructed patients; serious adverse effects including bleeding, biliary leakage, and sepsis occur in less than 5 per cent.[21] In patients with severe ascites or coagulopathy, endoscopic retrograde cholangiopancreatography (ERCP) is preferred. ERCP is particularly valuable in individuals with suspected pancreatic disease since a pancreatogram can also be obtained. Further, ERCP has the advantage of not only opacifying the biliary system but could also serve for endoscopic biliary drainage. In experienced hands, a satisfactory ERCP will be obtained in 80–90 per cent of cases; periampullary diverticulae, previous Bilroth II gastrectomy, papillary stenosis, or tumour make the procedure more technically difficult. Side-effects occur in 3 per cent of cases and include pancreatitis and cholangitis.[22] Local expertise is also a factor when choosing the most appropriate type of cholangiogram.

Liver biopsy

Liver biopsy is reserved for highly selected patients with unexplained jaundice or LFT abnormalities in whom obstruction has been excluded or is unlikely. In each individual case, the possible benefits of accurate diagnosis must be weighed against the risk of biopsy. The most important and potentially lethal complication of liver biopsy is haemorrhage. An experience with almost 10 000 liver biopsies described non-fatal haemorrhage in 0.24 per cent and fatal haemorrhage in 0.11 per cent.[23] Risk factors for haemorrhage included advancing age, number of passes with the biopsy needle, female sex, and notably, the presence of malignancy. Aspirin and other non-steroidal anti-inflammatory drugs induce platelet dysfunction, which may predispose to bleeding; aspirin should be stopped 10 days prior to biopsy. Where liver biopsy is being used as an aid in the diagnosis of infection with hepatic involvement, tissue must also be sent for special stains and cultures for fungal, viral, mycobacterial, and bacterial pathogens. In the diagnosis of metastatic liver disease, diagnostic yield is increased using ultrasound-guided or laparoscopic-directed biopsy.[24]

Management

In view of the vast array of causes of jaundice in the palliative care patient, it is important to first consider remediable yet potentially rapidly fatal conditions such as ascending cholangitis. This condition is usually amenable to antibiotic therapy following endoscopic or surgical relief of obstruction. The majority of patients under consideration, however, have jaundice secondary to massive hepatic infiltration with tumours. Nevertheless, the occasional patient has an enlarged lymph node at the porta hepatis, which may be responsive to radiotherapy or biliary stenting. Chemotherapy will be a consideration in some patients with potentially responsive tumours including breast cancer, small cell carcinoma of the lung, testicular and ovarian carcinomas and lymphomas; however, most patients have relatively resistant tumours including gastrointestinal adenocarcinomas, malignant melanoma, and non-small cell lung carcinomas. The combined use of radiation and chemotherapy has also been generally disappointing.[25]

The use of general measures can greatly add to patient comfort. Patients feel better with the correction of severe anaemia with blood transfusion. Management of pruritus is also an important consideration in patients with malignant biliary obstruction.

Pruritus (Fig. 1)

The mechanism of pruritus in cholestasis is unknown. Although bile acids have been widely implicated, other possible mediators include histamine, kallikreins, prostaglandins, substance p, and more recently, endogenous opioids[26] and serotonin.[27] Whatever the stimulus, peripheral neurofilaments are activated with transmission of an impulse via unmyelinated C fibres and the spinothalamic tract to the thalamus and cerebral cortex. Although pruritus is most frequently encountered in patients with malignant biliary obstruction, it is also seen in other neoplastic conditions including polycythemia rubra vera, Hodgkin's lymphoma, systemic mastocytosis, Waldenstrom's macroglobulinemia, multiple myeloma, mycosis fungoides, carcinoid syndrome, and various forms of carcinoma.

Pruritus is occasionally refractory to treatment but can usually be at least diminished by the use of general, local, and systemic therapies. As a general measure, an air-conditioned and humidified environment may be useful since cool temperatures, humidity, and reduced cutaneous perspiration lower the itch threshold. Local measures include the use of moisturising agents (e.g. oatmeal and oil bath), astringents such as Calamine, and the use of steroids creams. Topically applied tricyclic antidepressants such as doxepin have been used because of their histamine inhibiting action with some evidence of benefit in dermatitis but their effect in obstructive jaundice with pruritus is unknown.[28]

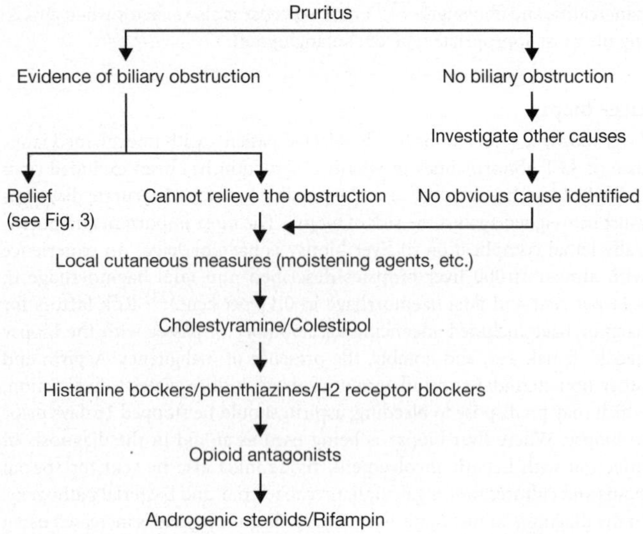

Fig. 1 An alogrithm for the management of pruritus. A trial of systemic agents is recommended starting with the drugs with the least side-effects.

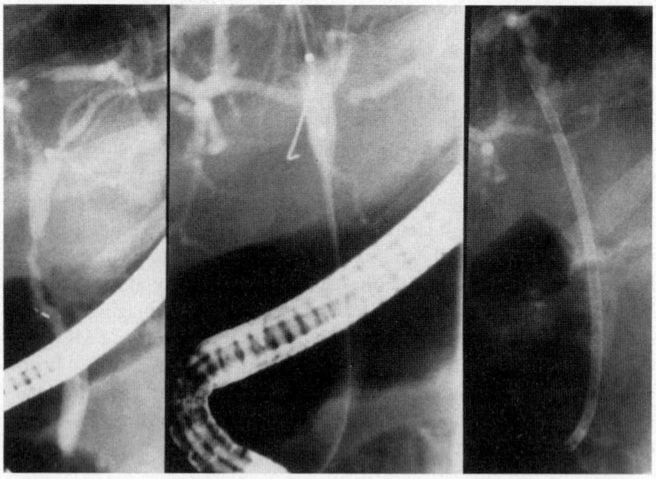

Fig. 2 These cholangiograms are from a 61-year-old male with obstructive jaundice and pruritus. A high-grade stricture is shown in the common hepatic duct in the left panel. In the middle panel, the stricture is being dilated with a balloon catheter passed over a guidewire. In the right panel, a large (11.5 French) stent has been placed across the stricture from the duodenum up to the proximal intrahepatic ducts to maintain biliary drainage. His pruritus resolved within 24 h and his jaundice cleared by 10 days.

Numerous systemic therapies have been tried, although few have been subjected to critical analysis. Most of the drugs used are suggested on the basis of uncontrolled clinical experience or extrapolation from other non-malignant conditions associated with pruritus. Antihistamines are not uniformly effective, but may be beneficial in some patients. Hydroxyzine and cyproheptadine are felt to be the most useful in this class. Similarly, phenothiazines such as trimeprazine and prochlorperazine have been widely recommended. Both the antihistamines and phenothiazines likely act by depressing the central nervous system rather than a specific peripheral effect. H2-receptor blockers (particularly cimetidine) have been recommended, but are likely ineffective as single-agent therapies. Bile acid resins such as cholestyramine and colestipol are effective agents in the management of cholestatic pruritus.(29) These basic polystyrenes decrease the absorption of many substances from the gut and in the process inhibit the reabsorption of bile acids. Cholestyramine at a dose of 4 g one to six times daily is particularly effective in providing relief from pruritus. However, at high doses, cholestyramine may impair absorption of a variety of medications as well as fat-soluble vitamins by reducing intestinal luminal concentrations of bile acids below a critical micellar level. Fat-soluble vitamin supplementation and adjustment of medication dosages are recommended with cholestyramine therapy. Compliance is a major problem with the use of bile acids as these drugs are relatively unpalatable and can induce constipation.

Opioid antagonists hold great promise for the relief of pruritus but beware of precipitating a withdrawal-like syndrome in patients receiving opioid analgesia.(26) Both parenteral naloxone and oral nalmefene and naltrexone appear to be effective.(30,31) Recently, both naloxone and naltrexone were shown to effectively decrease pruritus in small but controlled cross-over trials.(32,33)

There is considerable clinical experience with androgenic steroids, such as methyl testosterone, which will usually relieve pruritus within 1 week.(26) Norethandrolone and stanozolol may be helpful in some patients but are not widely available. Paradoxically, these sex steroids may themselves cause cholestasis and worsen jaundice and should be used only in extreme cases. Rifampin has been useful in alleviating pruritus in chronic cholestasis secondary to primary biliary cirrhosis(34) and other cholestatic disorders.(35) Its mechanism of action is unknown, but may relate to its ability to inhibit bile acid uptake into hepatocytes, thereby minimizing bile acid toxicity and preventing release of other putative 'pruritogens'. Rifampin use is limited by its potential for hepatitis and idiosyncratic reactions. When pruritus is severe, general and local measures should be combined with systemic drug treatment. Cholestyramine should be tried first since it is most likely to be effective. Histamine (H1-receptor) blockers and phenothiazines should generally be tried next because they are relatively free of serious side-effects. Opioid antagonists and/or an H2-receptor blocker such as cimetidine can be added if required. Androgenic steroids or rifampin can be tried if these first-line therapies fail. Since pruritus can be particularly bothersome at night, adequate sedation is a useful added measure. It should be emphasized, however, that pruritus is most effectively palliated by relief of biliary obstruction where possible.

Relief of biliary obstruction

Patients with biliary obstruction secondary to pancreatic carcinoma, cholangiocarcinoma, and less frequently metastatic disease develop jaundice and pruritus and are at risk of ascending cholangitis. Surgical bypass or non-operative stenting (percutaneous or endoscopic) of the malignant stricture provides effective palliation (Fig. 2). These procedures should be performed early for best results and may prolong life, but this is unproven. Surgical bypass is usually achieved by performing either a cholecystojejunostomy or a choledochojejunostomy; the latter may provide superior relief of obstruction.(36) Surgical treatment is associated with a low incidence of recurrent jaundice and furthermore, in patients with pancreatic carcinoma, it provides the opportunity to perform a gastroenterostomy for prophylaxis against future duodenal obstruction that will otherwise develop in 20–40 per cent of patients. However, biliary enteric anastomosis is associated with an operative mortality as high as 33 per cent(37) and a significant hospital stay. This invasive approach is not well suited to older and less-well patients who will suffer a particularly high operative morbidity and mortality. Percutaneous transhepatic stent placement is associated with a high risk of sepsis, biliary leakage, and haemorrhage and superior results have been reported using endoscopically placed stents.(38–40) Furthermore, external drainage for pre-operative decompression prior to surgical biliary bypass is associated with a higher mortality than immediate surgery.(41) Nevertheless, difficult strictures including those involving the hepatic hilum sometimes require transhepatic drainage or a combined approach with a guide wire passed by the percutaneous, transhepatic route through the obstruction into the duodenum followed by endoscopic stent placement over the wire.

Results using stents placed endoscopically continue to improve as experience accumulates.(42,43) Early reports mostly included patients considered non-operable with the most advanced disease and therefore shortest life expectancy. Randomized controlled trials have compared bypass surgery to endoscopic stent placement for the relief of unresectable malignancy involving the bile ducts (principally, pancreatic carcinoma and cholangiocarcinoma).[44–46] The results suggest that endoscopic stent placement is associated with less procedure-related mortality and lower short-term morbidity and mortality than surgery. Readmission rates, however, were higher secondary to stent clogging requiring replacement and duodenal obstruction requiring surgery. Both provided excellent palliation of obstruction but long-term survivals were similar in endoscopically and surgically treated patients. A retrospective cost analysis has compared endoscopic/radiologic stent placement to surgical bypass.[47] Total costs including all medical costs from diagnosis to death were 50 per cent higher in the surgical group despite similar survivals in the two groups.

Despite the widespread use of endoscopically placed plastic stents for relief of malignant obstructions, a major hurdle for patient care remains the relatively rapid occlusion rates of the stents (average patency duration 3 months). Clogging of plastic stents occurs as a result of the formation of bacterial biofilm, which adheres to the stent side holes and common bile duct wall. In addition, bacterial enzymatic activity leads to the formation and deposition of crystals promoting sludge in the stent lumen.[48,49] Attempts to prolong stent patency by the use of prophylactic antibiotics and cholerectic agents (ursodeoxycholic acid) have proven to be largely ineffective strategies.[50,51] Other approaches that have been tested to decrease the frequency of changing plastic stents include the use of larger diameter stents (endoscopic accessory channel limits the internal diameter diameter of a plastic stent to 12 French), better stent positioning, the use of different materials (Teflon or polyethylene), and the use of different shaped stents.[52–55] Despite these efforts, the duration of patency of plastic stents has not significantly improved. An important advance to reduce stent clogging utilizes expandable metal stents of several available types that can be inserted via the endoscopic or percutaneous transhepatic route.[56] These metallic stents have small diameters before placement, which permits them to be easily placed, but subsequently expand to 10 mm or 30 French, which reduces their incidence of occlusion by bacterial biofilm. These new types of stents are expensive, but this is blunted by a reduced need for reintervention due to stent clogging. Cost analysis studies determined that metallic stents were more cost-effective in patients who survived longer than 4–6 months.[57] The drawback of metallic stents is that they cannot be removed easily and may, therefore, compromise resectional surgery should that still be an option. The problem of tumour ingrowth between the struts of the stent is being addressed by new coatings such as silicone and metal stents without an open framework;[58,59] however, tumour extension beyond the end of the stents remains as a real problem.

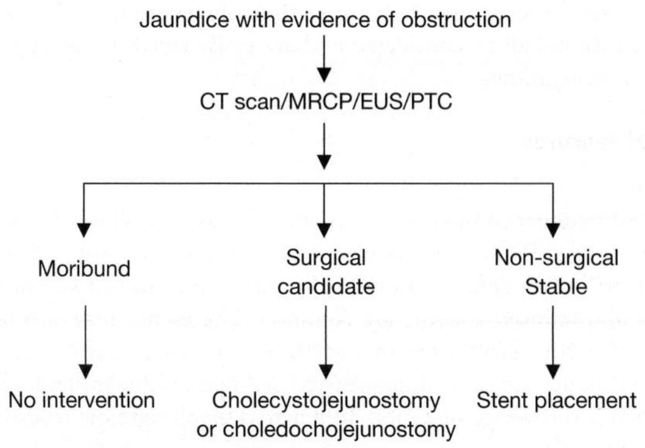

CT = computed tomography
MRCP = magnetic resonance cholangiopancreatograghy
EUS = endoscopic ultrasound
PTC = percutaneous transhepatic cholangiogram

Fig. 3 An algorithm for the palliation of obstructive lesions.

In summary (Fig. 3), the following general guidelines can be adopted for palliation of obstructive jaundice. Fit patients with small tumours as determined by CT or MRCP should undergo laparotomy to establish unresectability and for biliary enteric bypass; many with pancreatic carcinoma will also be candidates for gastroenteric anastomosis for prophylaxis against future duodenal obstruction.[60] ERCP with endoscopic stenting is now considered the first line of therapy for obstructive jaundice in patients who have larger lesions or who are not fit for surgery. Moribund patients and those with a very limited life-span should simply be kept comfortable with analgesia and sedation.

Hepatic abnormalities in AIDS (see also Chapter 10.2)

Despite a lack of hepatic trophism for HIV, hepatic abnormalities are very common in AIDS and have been the subject of several reviews.[61–63] Liver disease in AIDS seldom progresses to liver failure; however, clinicians caring for AIDS patients must be familiar with the associated spectrum of liver disease so that treatable conditions can be recognized.

The more frequently encountered afflictions of the liver in AIDS are summarized in Table 2. Due to shared risk factors, AIDS patients are at increased risk for chronic hepatitis secondary to hepatitis B virus and hepatitis C virus; however, because of marked impairment of cellular immune function, hepatic damage is usually limited for hepatitis B.[64] Hepatitis C may be more aggressive in this setting.[64] The liver may be involved secondarily by Kaposi's sarcoma or lymphoma, the two commonest malignancies seen in AIDS. Hepatic amyloidosis has been reported in intravenous drug users with AIDS possibly secondary to chronic suppurative skin infections resulting from dirty needles.[65] A wide variety of fungal and protozoal organisms may infect the liver; however, *Mycobacterium avium*-intracellular is the commonest opportunistic pathogen detected histologically.[63] As in any patient with hepatic abnormalities, the possibility of a hepatotoxic reaction to self-prescribed or prescription drugs must be considered; such reactions are more common in those with underlying liver disease such as viral hepatitis. AIDS patients are frequently on investigational drugs, which may have unknown hepatotoxic potential. Indeed, fulminant hepatic failure was reported with the use of 2′,3′ dideoxyinosine, indinavir, and didanosine, in a patient with AIDS.[66] Finally, a wide array of biliary changes have been described in AIDS patients often in association with cryptosporidial or CMV infection.[67,68] The clinical spectrum of disease in these patients includes papillary stenosis, sclerosing cholangitis (focal strictures and dilatation of intrahepatic and extrahepatic ducts), combined sclerosis of the duct and papillary stenosis, and long strictures of the extrahepatic ducts. The clinical manifestations of AIDS cholangiopathy vary from classic cholangitis and may be limited to isolated right upper quadrant pain.[69] There will be, although blunted, biochemical evidence of biliary stasis with a CD4 count well below 100 cells/mm^3.

Table 2 Classification of AIDS hepatopathy

Viral hepatitis
Hepatitis B virus, hepatitis C virus, hepatitis D virus, cytomegalovirus, Epstein–Barr virus, herpes simplex virus
Malignancy
Kaposi's sarcoma, lymphoma
Amyloidosis
Opportunistic infection
Mycobacteria, *Pneumocystis carina*, cryptococcus
Drug reactions
Trimethoprim/sulfamethoxazole, isoniazid, zidovudine (AZT), ketoconazole pentamidine, ddl
Biliary tract disease
Sclerosing cholangitis, biliary stricture, papillary stenosis, acalculous cholecystitis

The temptation to aggressively investigate hepatic abnormalities in AIDS must be tempered by the fact that no effective treatment exists for many of the conditions listed in Table 2. Viral hepatitis is best diagnosed serologically and can often be managed without resort to liver biopsy. The presence of hepatic malignancy can often be surmized from the existence of malignancy elsewhere. Abdominal ultrasound supplemented with CT scanning, if necessary, is useful for the detection of focal masses and to determine the presence of biliary dilatation secondary to obstruction. Biliary dilatation is best investigated by ERCP, where if required, a therapeutic procedure can be performed concomitantly such as endoscopic sphincterotomy for papillary stenosis.[70]

In selected patients, use of special stains and cultures on liver biopsy specimens in addition to histologic examination provides a unique opportunity for the diagnosis of a wide variety of infectious and other conditions. Liver biopsy will reveal diagnostic findings in about 50 per cent of AIDS patients with abnormal LFTs;[71] however, in some instances, this will only confirm infections involving more readily accessible extra-hepatic sites. Liver biopsy will have greatest diagnostic yield when reserved for those patients with unexplained fever, persistently elevated serum alkaline phosphatase, or hepatomegaly.[62] Risk of bleeding should be minimized by checking coagulation status, platelet count, and bleeding time where indicated. Specific and effective therapy is seldom available; however, establishing a diagnosis will prevent further potentially invasive investigation and allows the patient's symptoms to be specifically addressed.

Ascites

The appearance of ascites in a patient with malignancy has always been considered an unfortunate event both in terms of patient comfort and its prognostic implications; 1-year survival 40 per cent, 3-year survival less than 10 per cent. It has also been the source of considerable distress for the physician because it places him/her in the unenviable position of having to chose between a variety of therapeutic options that carry appreciable morbidity and mortality rates yet for the most part have not been documented to be efficacious on the basis of data derived from prospective, randomized, controlled trials. Fortunately, the long-standing reluctance of investigators to design and enrol patients with terminal malignancies in such trials has given way to the realization that these data an essential for providing the most appropriate and compassionate care for these unfortunate individuals. As a result, in recent years there have been significant advances in the understanding, diagnosis, and treatment of patients with malignant ascites. These advances have resulted in a more rationale approach to diagnostic interventions and an expanding list of safer, more effective therapeutic options.

Incidence of malignant ascites

Malignancy is the underlying cause of ascites in approximately 10 per cent of all cases of ascites and 15–50 per cent of patients with malignancy will develop ascites.[72,73] Certain tumours are especially likely to result in malignant ascites. For example, the association with ovarian cancer is particularly strong with 30 per cent of ovarian cancer patients having ascites at presentation and over 60 per cent at the time of death.[74] Other cancers that not uncommon result in malignant ascites including cancers of the endometrium, breast, large bowel, stomach, and pancreas, which account for approximately 80 per cent of all cases of malignant ascites.[74] Less common causes include mesothelioma, non-Hodgkin's lymphoma, prostatic carcinoma, multiple myeloma, and melanoma.[75]

Classification and pathogenesis of malignant ascites (Fig. 4)

For diagnostic and therapeutic reasons, malignant ascites can be classified into four relatively distinct subtypes. In the 'central' form of malignant ascites, which constitutes approximately 15 per cent of all cases, the tumour invades the hepatic parenchyma resulting in compression of the portal venous and/or lymphatic systems. The ascites that ensues resembles that formed as a result of primary liver disease, that is, elevated hydrostatic

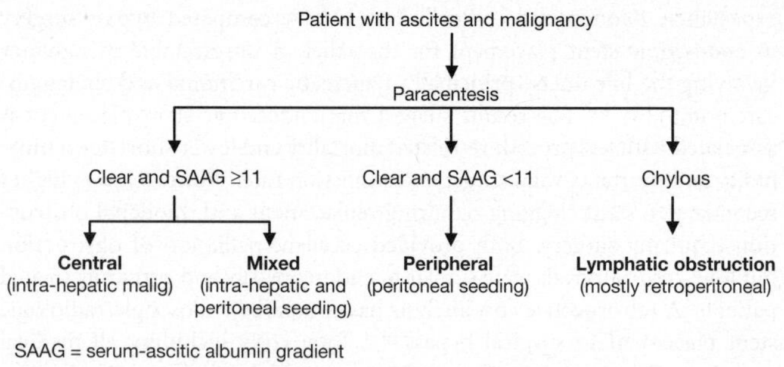

Fig. 4 An algorithm to classify malignant ascites.

pressure combined with decreased oncotic pressure. In central malignant ascites, however, the decreased oncotic pressure is more the result of limited protein intake and the catabolic state associated with cancer rather than defective hepatic protein synthesis.

In the 'peripheral' form of malignant ascites, which constitutes 50 per cent of cases, deposits of tumour cells are found on the surface of the parietal or visceral peritoneum. As with central ascites, the formation of ascites is largely the result of mechanical interference with venous and/or lymphatic drainage but in this instance the blockage is at the level of the peritoneal space rather than the liver parenchyma. Experimentally, reduced efflux of peritoneal fluid precedes increased fluid influx.[76] There are data to suggest that vasoactive substances released from peritoneal tumour implants and non-malignant monocytes or macrophages increase capillary permeability and thereby contribute to ascites formation.[75,77]

A third form of malignant ascites could be considered a 'mixed' form in which tumour is present both in the liver and on the peritoneal surface. In this form of ascites, which constitutes 15 per cent of all cases, fluid accumulation is the result of combined central and peripheral pathophysiologic processes.

The fourth type of malignant ascites is 'chylous malignant ascites' where tumour infiltration of the retroperitoneal space causes obstruction of lymphatic flow through the lymph nodes and/or pancreas. Leakage from the lymphatic channels as a result of direct tumour invasion may also be operative in this form of malignant ascites.

Differential diagnoses

Not all ascites that develop in patients with malignancy is the result of malignancy. Pre-existing advanced liver disease with portal hypertension, portal venous thrombosis, congestive heart failure, nephrotic syndrome, pancreatitis, tuberculosis, hepatic venous obstruction, and bowel perforations should all be considered and are easily ruled out by appropriate clinical investigations.

Clinical features

History

The most frequent complaints of patients with ascites, whether it be malignant or non-malignant in nature, is abdominal bloating and pain.[78] Patients will often describe an unexplained increase in belt size or weight. Nausea and reduced appetite are common. The ascites may also result in increased reflux symptoms of heartburn or 'waterbrash'. When pronounced, ascites can cause dyspnoea and orthopnoea due to elevation of the diaphragms or leakage of ascitic fluid across diaphragmatic fenestrae into the pleural space.

Physical findings

Two litres of ascitic fluid must be present for bulging of the flanks to be appreciated on physical examination.[78] When the ascites is more extensive, abdominal or inguinal hernia, scrotal oedema, and abdominal venous engorgement may appear.[79] A bruit in the abdomen of a patient with malignant ascites indicates a hypervascular tumour such as hepatocellular carcinoma, carcinoid islet cell, leiomyosarcoma, or metastases from a renal cell carcinoma.

Extra abdominal findings may include decreased sweating due to third space fluid losses, pleural effusions in approximately 5 per cent of individuals with the majority of these being right sided, peripheral oedema that develops as a result of low protein concentrations in the circulation and mechanical impairment of IVC flow, displacement of the cardiac apex in a superiolateral direction, and distension of the neck veins due to increased right atrial and thoracic pressure.[79]

Radiologic findings

Plain films of the abdomen characteristically demonstrate hazy or ground glass features, distended and separated loops of bowel, poor definition of the abdominal organs, and loss of the psoas muscle shadows.[78,80]

In general, ultrasound and CT scans of the liver are equally adept at identifying free peritoneal fluid.[81] A collection of fluid around the edge of the liver or in Morrison's pouch are the typical findings with both techniques. It has been reported that gallbladder wall thickness on ultrasound examination may be useful in distinguishing malignant (non-thickened wall) from non-malignant (thickened or double wall) ascites.[82] This is because the gallbladder wall becomes thickened in response to the hypoproteinemia associated with chronic liver disease or nephrotic syndrome.

Ultrasound may demonstrate a number of abnormalities that serve to heighten the suspicion of malignancy in a patient with ascites. These include visualization of peritoneal metastasis, matted bowel loops, echogenic ascitic fluid, omental matting, lymphadenopathy, or other masses including hepatic metastasis.[83] A negative ultrasound, CT scan, and fluid cytology does not exclude malignant ascites. Laparoscopy will document malignancy in up to 50 per cent of such cases.[84]

Advances in MR imaging technology, including faster pulse sequence, breath hold imaging, and the use of intravenous contrast agents, and surface coils, have made this tool available for screening and diagnosis of malignant ascites.[85] A recent prospective study comparing helical CT to MR imaging for surveillance of extra-hepatic malignancies with subsequent surgical correlation demonstrated that MR imaging depicted more sites of tumour and was particularly advantageous for the peritoneum, mesentery, and bowel.[85]

Paracentesis

A diagnostic paracentesis of 50–100 ml of fluid should be performed in every case of newly diagnosed ascites. Before proceeding with the procedure, potential complications should be considered and explained to the patient or next of kin. The most common complication following paracentesis is continued leakage from the puncture site but more serious complications include perforated viscera with or without associated haemorrhage and peritonitis.[86] In the absence of midline scars, a site midway between the umbilicus and symphysis pubis should be chosen to minimize the risk of perforation and haemorrhage. The right or left flank (well down from the liver and spleen, respectively) in the mid-anterior axillary line can serve as alternate sites. Ultrasound is helpful to guide paracentesis in difficult cases.

The appearance of the ascitic fluid obtained at paracentesis may provide some indication of the underlying nature of the problem. For example, bile-stained fluid suggests malignancy or a recent traumatic tap or biopsy.[87] A milky appearance that stains sudan black positive indicates chylous ascites.[88] Turbid or purulent ascites is consistent with pyogenic or malignant causes.[78,79] Mucinous ascites may be found in patients with pseudomyxoma peritonei, or peritoneal metastasis from colloid carcinoma of the stomach or colon.[78] Bloody ascites is frequent with malignancy, but also occurs with tuberculosis.

A number of laboratory tests have been advocated to establish the cause(s) of ascites. Of these, cytology, cell count, gram stain with culture, and protein (albumin) concentrations have emerged as the most useful.

Cytology It is stated that cytologic examination of ascitic fluid is positive in only 50 per cent of cases where malignancy is the cause.[87] However, this disappointing figure almost certainly reflects the contribution of patients with non-peripheral forms of malignant ascites to most study populations. Indeed, by excluding patients with central or chylous ascites and submitting larger volumes (1 l) for analysis, the results of ascitic fluid cytologic examinations in patients with peripheral or mixed malignant ascites is between 80 and 100 per cent.[89] False positive results are uncommon in experienced laboratories but when they do occur are often due to exfoliated mesothelial cells resembling malignant cells.[90]

Peritoneal biopsy is less sensitive for diagnosing malignancy (50 per cent) than tuberculosis (100 per cent), which once again may reflect the heterogeneity of malignant ascites study populations.[91]

Cell counts Cell counts are employed to rule out bacterial peritonitis. A leucocyte count greater than 500–750 cells/mm^3 and a neutrophil count greater than 250–500 cells/mm^3 are consistent with infection.[92] Monocytosis in the ascitic fluid is often seen in patients with tuberculosis infection of the peritoneal space. Quantitatively, subjecting cells to flow cytometry can be useful to measure their DNA content, which allows identification of cell populations with abnormal quantities of DNA and provide information on cellular proliferative activity. The DNA index could be used to diagnose malignancy in samples where conventional cytopathological exams are negative.[93]

Gram stain and culture A combination of gram stain and direct inoculation of 10 ml of ascitic fluid into aerobic and anaerobic blood culture tubes at the patient's bedside result in positive identification of the causative organism in approximately 90 per cent of cases compared to only 40 per cent when conventional ascitic fluid culture methods are employed.[94]

Protein and albumin concentrations In a patient with malignancy and no underlying hepatic, cardiac, or renal disease, an ascitic fluid protein concentration of less than 2.5 g/dl or 50 per cent that of serum protein ('transudative ascites') is suggestive of central or mixed malignant ascites. If on the other hand, the ascitic fluid protein concentration is greater than 2.5 g/dl or 50 per cent that of serum protein ('exudative ascites') peripheral malignant ascites is more likely.[72] One must keep in mind, however, that ascitic fluid protein concentrations should not be interpreted in isolation. For example, the use of diuretics or albumin infusions prior to paracentesis will increase ascitic fluid protein concentrations and thereby transform transudative ascites to an exudative pattern.[95,96] Similarly, large intravenous infusions of crystalloid will decrease ascitic fluid protein concentrations and in the process transform an exudative ascites to a transudative pattern.[97] A more useful test for determining the type of malignant ascites is the difference between serum and ascitic albumin concentrations where a difference of less than 11 g/l is consistent with peripheral malignant ascites whereas values greater than 11 g/l suggest either central or mixed malignant ascites.[98] In essence, an ascitic-serum difference greater than 11 denotes portal hypertension secondary to hepatic metastasis.

Tests that have been reported to be useful in distinguishing malignant from non-malignant ascites include raised levels of ascitic fluid fibronectin,[99] isoamylase,[100] lactic dehydrogenase,[101] alpha fetoprotein,[72] carcinoembryonic antigen,[102] beta-human chorionic gonadotrophin,[102] ovarian cancer-associated antigen 125,[103] ferritin,[104] cholesterol and triglyceride concentrations.[105,106] Unfortunately, in each case the overlap between malignant and non-malignant groups as well as between the different types of malignant ascites particularly those with central and mixed forms is such that these tests are often unhelpful individually. A recent study investigated telomerase activity (an enzyme thought to be responsible for preventing cellular senescence in malignancy) as an assay to differentiate between malignancy-related and non-malignant ascites.[107] Telemerase activity was reported to have a sensitivity of 76 per cent and specificity of 95.7 per cent in detecting malignant ascites. In the non-malignant group telemerase activity was found in only 4.3 per cent of cases. It remains to be seen whether this test will be have a practical application for routine diagnosis of ascites.

Treatment

Treatment for malignant ascites consists of instituting palliative measures without the expectation that survival might be altered. Exceptions include patients with ovarian cancer in whom survival can be prolonged with surgical intervention and adjuvant therapy,[78] and patients with malignant ascites secondary to lymphoma who respond to radiation and/or chemotherapy.[78] Hormonally sensitive malignancies such as some breast cancers also deserve separate consideration.

Medical therapy

As for ascitic patients with advanced liver disease, patients with the central form (hepatic metastasis with portal hypertension) of malignant ascites often have increased renal sodium and water retention. Therefore, restriction of their sodium intake to 100 mmol/day or less is indicated.[105] Fluid restriction is reserved for patients with moderate to severe hyponatraemia, for example, less than 125 mmol/l. Spironolactone (100–400 mg/day) is the diuretic of choice but frusemide (40–80 mg/day) may be required to initiate a diuresis. Care must be taken to avoid over-diuresis, which can precipitate electrolyte imbalances, hepatic encephalopathy, and pre-renal failure. There is no theoretical reason to expect sodium and fluid restriction or diuretics to be of use in patients with peripheral (peritoneal tumour spread) or chylous forms of malignant ascites and a recent clinical series has borne this out. Furthermore, diuretic complications were frequent in this patient subgroup.[108] However, a trial of sodium restriction and diuretics may prove worthwhile in patients with the mixed form of malignant ascites. A low fat diet and an increase in medium-chain triglyceride intake may be useful in patients with chylous ascites.[88,109]

Therapeutic paracentesis

Large-volume paracentesis significantly shortens the hospital stay for patients with tense ascites (from a mean of 30 to 10 days) without increasing morbidity or mortality when compared to medical therapy.[110] The removal of 5 l/day until the abdomen is 'dry' is generally well tolerated by patients, particularly those with peripheral oedema who call upon their peripheral reserve of fluid for rapid restoration of effective circulating volume.[111] If it is available and affordable, intravenous albumin (6 g/l of ascitic fluid removed) should be provided[112,113] and will effectively reduce the complications of hypovolaemia, pre-renal failure, and hyponatraemia. Total paracentesis, which consists of complete drainage of all ascitic fluid at one session, affords the ascitic patient the most prompt relief from their discomfort and the earliest possible discharge from hospital,[114,115] but it is important to stress that the data generated to date on large or total volume paracentesis have been derived from patients with non-malignant ascites. Whether the same promising results can be extrapolated to patients with malignant ascites remains to be determined. A reasonable approach is to remove 5–10 l of ascitic fluid to provide symptomatic relief. This can usually be accomplished on an outpatient basis. It is, however, recognized that in many places albumin is either not available or, if available, not affordable for many palliative care patients.

Peritoneovenous shunts

Peritoneovenous shunts drain ascitic fluid from the peritoneal space into the internal jugular vein. A properly functioning shunt limits the need for dietary/fluid restrictions, diuretics and hospitalizations for paracentesis. The shunt can be inserted during a 30–60 min procedure under local anaesthesia. The original studies in cirrhotics with the Denver or LeVeen shunts (the former having a pressure sensitive valve-chamber that can be manipulated manually by the patient) resulted in palliation for 75–85 per cent of patients who survived the shunt procedure.[116,117] Unfortunately, the results in patients with malignant ascites have been less impressive, presumably due to the high protein concentrations and decreased flow obtained with the peripheral form of malignant ascites.[118,119] Shunt-related operative mortality figures in patients with advanced liver disease are significantly higher (30 per cent) than for patients with malignant ascites (15 per cent), suggesting that operative mortality is primarily due to advanced liver disease rather than the shunt per se.[117] Morbidity rates are high (40–60 per cent) in all patients who require this form of therapy.[117,119] Some of the more serious complications include disseminated intravascular coagulation (DIC) (50 per cent), upper gastrointestinal bleeds (45 per cent), sepsis (20 per cent), pulmonary oedema (14 per cent), thrombo-embolism (10 per cent), as well as superior vena caval thrombosis, pneumonia, hepatic coma, and neoplastic seeding of subcutaneous tissue but not systemic spread.[116,117] In patients with malignant ascites, DIC may be less frequent.[120] Less serious (but common complications) include shunt malfunction and ascitic fluid leakage around the insertion site. Removal of at least 50–70 per cent of ascitic fluid and/or replacement with normal saline at the time of shunt insertion will significantly decrease shunt related morbidity and mortality.[118] Prophylactic antibiotic should be used perioperatively in all patients. Specific contraindications to shunt therapy include haemorrhagic or proteinaceous (>45 g/l) ascitic fluid, patients with recent or recurrent bacterial peritonitis or encephalopathy, bilirubin values above 100 μmol/l, advanced coagulopathy, large oesophageal varices, and kidney failure. In brief, severely ill patients are poor candidates for this procedure.

Surgical intervention

Surgical intervention for malignant ascites has met with only limited success. Novel therapies have focused on intent to treat protocols with a multimodal approach where extensive cytoreductive surgery (peritonectomy) is followed by post-operative intraperitoneal antiblastic agents combined with intraperitoneal heathing, so-called hyperthermic intra-peritoneal intra-operative chemotherapy.[121] The rationale for this approach is that debulking surgery by itself was demonstrated to be ineffective in prolonging survival from peritoneal carcinomatosis even when combined with adjuvant intravenous chemotherapy.[122] On the other hand, the delivery of intraperitoneal chemotherapy allowed the direct application of high concentrations of drugs while incurring minimal systemic exposure, but was again not found to improve disease-free survival compared to conventional therapy.[123] The application of intraperitoneal hyperthermic therapy in combination with intraperitoneal chemotherapy stemmed from animal research which demonstrated that 41–43°C heat applied post-operatively does not only have antiblastic properties but also sensitizes neoplastic cells to the action of antimitotic agents.[124] The application of this approach is at its infancy, but so far the initial experience has demonstrated improved survival in patients with limited carcinomatosis of the peritoneum.[125] Standardization of techniques, cost analysis, and randomized control studies on patients with histologically identical tumours represent some of the challenges that remain before the more widespread application of this treatment.

Pharmacologic therapy

Radioactive isotopes were the first agents to be employed in an attempt to decrease ascitic fluid formation.[126] Although favourable responses were reported (30–70 per cent of cases) with ^{63}Zn, ^{198}Au, and ^{32}P, the high incidence of side-effects (50 per cent) including nausea, pain, fever and in the case of ^{198}Au, bone marrow suppression, as well as the risk of radiation exposure to hospital staff eventually limited their use.[126–129] Moreover, these agents are expensive, have a short half-life, and due to radiation safety requirements are confined to use by large treatment centres. As a result, radioisotopes eventually gave way to trials of sclerosing agents (nitrogen mustard, quinacrine, doxorubicin), mild irritants (bleomycin, tetracycline, cisplatin), and non-sclerosant agents (methotrexate, thiotepa, 5-fluorouracil). Recently, there was an evaluation of the feasibility and pharmakokinetics of suramin, an agent originally designed as an antiparasitic that has been characterized to have properties that inhibit lipid growth factors. The continous intraperitoneal infusion of this agent will target lipid containing as well as peptide growth factors involved in the proliferation of intraperitoneal malignancy.[130] The results achieved with the variety of agents described above are difficult to interpret due to the differences in the parameters of response, small number of patients involved, retrospective nature of the studies, and lack of comparative data.[131–136] Due to the potential toxicity of these agents when given intraperitoneally, it seems prudent to avoid their use until the results of prospective controlled clinical trials are available.

Biological agents such as intraperitoneal alpha or beta interferon have been used for malignant ascites in uncontrolled trials. Response rates approximating 40 per cent at 1 month have been reported with recurrence in the majority by 3 months.[129] Side-effects include flu-like symptoms, local pain, and fever, but generally these agents were well tolerated. A preliminary positive experience with intraperitoneal recombinant tumour necrosis factor alpha in malignant ascites has been reported as well.[137] A review of intracavitary treatments for malignant effusions has been published.[129]

A logical approach to the management of malignant ascites therefore starts with sodium restriction and diuretics particularly in those with the central form of ascites (liver metastasis) or a serum-ascitic albumin concentration difference greater than 11 g/l. Non-responding patients will benefit from either repeated paracentesis or possibly insertion of a peritoneovenous shunt; however, there are significant risks with the latter. Most intraperitoneal agents remain unproven, but some of the biologic agents (alpha or beta interferon, tumour necrosis factor alpha) hold promise and controlled trials are awaited.

Hepatic encephalopathy

Hepatic encephalopathy is a complex neuropsychiatric syndrome characterized by disturbance of consciousness, personality, and intellect together with altered neuromuscular activity and EEG abnormalities. It arises most frequently in patients with end-stage cirrhosis from any cause but may also occur in patients with extensive hepatic metastasis. Many cirrhotics are not liver transplant candidates and will benefit from the measures described below for cancer patients. In fact, most of the research underlying our current treatments for hepatic encephalopathy was conducted in cirrhotic patients.

Unlike malignant ascites, hepatic encephalopathy is often considered an almost welcome event in the course of the terminally ill patient. Its onset often marks the beginning of a process wherein anxiety and discomfort are attenuated and give way to a peaceful state of repose. The major task facing the physician caring for terminally ill patients with hepatic encephalopathy is to determine whether treatment of the encephalopathy will result in a meaningful survival period or a lightening of the mental state that only serves to allow the patient to become more aware of their suffering.

Pathogenesis

The pathogenesis of hepatic encephalopathy remains unclear. Hypotheses regarding ammonia, false neurotransmitters, and GABAergic neurotransmission abnormalities all leave a number of important questions and observations unanswered.[138] The most recent hypothesis implicates endogenous benzodiazepine-like compounds that have been found in increased concentrations in the central nervous system of patients with liver failure.[139] These compounds may increase GABAergic neurotransmission that is inhibitory to the brain. Perhaps there is no one encephalopathogenic factor but rather a combination of many if not all the hitherto proposed compounds. A review of this subject cites mounting evidence for 'neurotransmission failure' possibly as a result of chronic central nervous system exposure to ammonia.[140]

Diagnosis

Clinical features

The most common presenting features of hepatic encephalopathy are drowsiness, reversal of day/night sleep patterns, and difficulty with concentration. As the encephalopathy becomes more advanced, confusion may develop. By this time, abnormalities in spatial appreciation, as reflected by inability of the patient to draw concentric circles or five pointed stars become evident. Other physical signs may include *fetor hepaticus* (an odd, sweetish smell of breath secondary to increased mercaptan concentrations), hyperactive tendon reflexes, and, ultimately, decerebrate posturing. The speech of the encephalopathic patient is slow, slurred, and monotonous. Asterixis, an often sought and important clinical feature of hepatic encephalopathy, is tested by fixed extension of the forearms, dorsiflexion of the wrists, and fanning of the digits with eyes opened and then closed. A rapid, forward flexion of the hands at the metacarpophalangeal joints reflects decreased afferent (proprioceptive) input to the reticular activating system. Once the encephalopathy has advanced to the stage of coma, asterixis, like many of the other motor abnormalities, is no longer present. Prior to overt hepatic encephalopathy more sensitive tests such as psychometric testing, standard electroencephalograms, or visual evoked potential responses may detect subclinical abnormalities.

Laboratory tests

Biochemical tests

Hepatic encephalopathy is associated with a series of biochemical abnormalities that include elevated plasma ammonia, aromatic amino acids, short-chain fatty acids, mercaptan levels, and decreased plasma branched-chain amino acid concentrations.[141] Of these, the plasma ammonia levels (venous or arterial) are most useful since they are markedly elevated in 90 per cent of encephalopathic patients while only rarely elevated beyond two to three times normal in other conditions that alter cerebral function. Despite helping to distinguish hepatic encephalopathy from other causes of confusion, ammonia levels do not correlate well with the course or the severity of the illness.

Non-biochemical tests

Psychometric tests have been used in diagnosing early (preclinical) hepatic encephalopathy.[142,143] These tests have also been found to be helpful in following the course of the disease, a feature that is becoming increasingly important as new therapeutic modalities are being considered. Of the many psychometric tests that can be applied, the Reitan trail-making or number connection test has achieved the most popularity.[144] This test involves having the patient connect a series of scattered numbers from 1 to 50 while being timed with a stop watch. Their time is compared to standards established for normal, mild, moderate, and severe encephalopathy. It is more sensitive than most other psychometric tests including the five-pointed-star construction test, signature test, or subtraction-of-serial-sevens test and is easier to quantitate. Proton magnetic resonance spectroscopy is very sensitive in the diagnosis of both subclinical and overt hepatic encephalopathy using clinical and neuropsychiatric testing as the gold standard.[145] The specificity of this technique using encephalopathic patients due to a variety of other disturbances has not been established.

The EEG abnormalities observed in patients with hepatic encephalopathy are non-specific. Similar if not identical changes are seen in patients with encephalopathy secondary to advanced renal disease or other severe metabolic disturbances that are common with advanced malignancy. Nonetheless, the presence of low-frequency, high-amplitude waveforms in a patient with advanced liver disease, a decreased level of consciousness, and no alternative explanation for the latter finding is strong supportive evidence for the diagnosis of hepatic encephalopathy.[146] Moreover, the extent of the abnormality on EEG correlates well with the patient's clinical status. Although problems with specificity are common, the sensitivity of EEGs are excellent. Indeed, abnormalities compatible with hepatic encephalopathy may be present well prior to the appearance of clinical features and may remain abnormal once clinical features have resolved. In clinical practice, however, the diagnosis is usually made without an EEG on the basis of typical clinical findings in a patient with liver disease or extensive hepatic metastasis.

Differential diagnosis

Table 3 lists disorders that may be difficult to distinguish from hepatic encephalopathy. Fortunately, clinical examination and simple laboratory and/or radiological investigations will often identify their presence. A high index of suspicion is required to consider and exclude these possibilities.

Table 3 Differential diagnosis of hepatic encephalopathy

Metabolic	Organ failure	Toxic	Intracerebral
Hypoglycaemia	Cardiac	Drugs	Haemorrhage/infarct
Hyponatraemia	Respiratory	Sedatives	Metastasis
Hypoxia	Renal	Tranquillizers	Meningitis
Hyperosmolar coma		Hypnotics	Abscess
		Alcohol withdrawal	
		Wernicke–Korsakoff's syndrome	

Treatment

Consideration should first be given to precipitants of encephalopathy. The three most common precipitating factors are prerenal azotemia secondary to aggressive use of diuretics and/or persistent vomiting/diarrhoea; over use of tranquillizers, sedatives, or analgesics; and overt or covert gastrointestinal haemorrhage from varices, peptic ulceration, or gastritis.[147] Other precipitating factors include an increased dietary protein intake, hypokalaemic alkalosis (often secondary to diuretics), bacterial infection, and constipation. While searching for and treating these precipitating factors a number of non-specific therapeutic interventions can be employed. A stepwise approach to hepatic encephalopathy is provided in Table 4.

The removal of protein breakdown products from the gut is helpful since gut-derived toxins (e.g. ammonia) play an important role in the pathogenesis. This can be achieved by reducing protein in the diet to approximately 40 g/day, by administering non-absorbable antibiotics active against gram negative and anaerobic intestinal bacteria and by the use of purgatives. Following protein restriction, the usual approach is to add a non-absorbable disaccharide such as lactulose or lactitol in a dose sufficient to induce one to two loose stools per day. A meta-analysis examining the published randomized controlled trials comparing these two cathartics concluded that they are equally efficacious in the treatment of hepatic encephalopathy and that they have similar side-effect profiles.[148] Nevertheless, patients generally prefer lactitol over lactulose because of better palatability and less flatulence.

In patients not responding to the above measures, a non-absorbable antibiotic can be added, such as neomycin,[149] metronidazole, or rifaximine.[150] This will reduce intraluminal generation of ammonia and possibly other neurotoxins.

Enteral or parenteral administration of branched-chain amino acids have been studied as both treatment of hepatic encephalopathy (replacement of missing neurotransmitters) and a way to supplementation of essential amino acids with protein restricted diets.[151] A meta-analysis of the various studies could not justify the use of parenteral branched-chain amino acids as the treatment had marginal benefit on mental status and dubious benefit on mortality. On the other hand, the supplementation of branched-chain amino acids to a protein-restricted diet enabled the delivery of protein requirements and the maintenance of a positive nitrogen balance without exacerbating the ongoing encephalopathy.[152] Randomized controlled studies with long follow-up are required to further assess the benefit of these therapies.

Table 4 Stepwise approach to hepatic encephalopathy

Stop all sedatives, tranquillizers, hypnotics
Correct any precipitating factors: Azotaemia GI bleeding Hypokalaemia/alkalosis Excessive dietary protein Infection Constipation
Exclude other causes of encephalopathy (Table 3)
Reduce dietary protein to 40 g/day (0.5 g/kg)
Add lactulose or lactitol (oral, nasogastric, or by enema)
If response inadequate, add a non-absorbable antibiotic, e.g. neomycin, metronidazole, rifaximine
Other measures Flumazenil Sodium benzoate Branched-chain amino acids

A randomized controlled trial has shown sodium benzoate, a food preservative and ammonia-lowering agent, to be as effective as lactulose in hepatic encephalopathy at a lower cost;[153] however, clinical experience with sodium benzoate is still limited.

Benzodiazepine antagonists, such as flumazenil, have been used therapeutically by their ability to interfere with the binding of endogenous, benzo-diazepine-like ligands to their receptor sites on the GABA receptor complex. These agents have been shown to reverse hepatic encephalopathy in animal models, and to induce marked and rapid, but transient, improvements in humans with chronic liver disease and encephalopathy. Randomized trials of flumazenil in cirrhotics were conducted in patients with low-grade as well as high-grade encephalopathy. One milligram of flumazenil delivered intravenously improved symptoms of encephalopathy in only a select population of patients with high-grade encephalopathy with minimal effects in patients with low-grade disease.[154,155] The current use of this agent remains experimental particularly in patients with malignancy. Possible applications include patients in whom the cause of encephalopathy is unclear, patients having received benzodiazepine, and possibly to provide prognostic information.

Finally, there have been a flurry of reports recently describing subclinical encephalopathy (SHE) and the benefit of treating this population. The diagnosis SHE is made when a patient performs poorly on psychometric tests in the absence of clinical symptoms of encephalopathy.[156] The diagnosis of SHE has also been demonstrated by prolonged latency of auditory evoked potential.[157] SHE predisposes patients to clinical encephalopathy and has been linked to poor functional capacity.[157,158] Further, recent reports demonstrate that treatment of SHE with lactulose can prevent the transformation to clinical encephalopathy.[159] While the data support screening cirrhotic patients for SHE, there are no studies to support the surveillance and treatment of SHE in patients with malignant liver disease.

References

1. **Jaffe, B.M., Donegan, W.L., Watson, F., and Spratt, J.S.** (1968). Factors influencing survival in patients with untreated liver metastases. *Surgery, Gynaecology and Obstetrics* **127**, 1–11.
2. **Myszor, M.F. and Record, C.D.** (1990). Primary and secondary malignant disease of the liver and fulminant hepatic failure. *Journal of Clinical Gastroenterology* **12**, 441–6.
3. **Choo, Q.L., Kuo, G., Weiner, A.J., Overby, L.R., Bradley, D.W., and Houghton, M.** (1989). Isolation of a cDNA clone derived from a blood-borne non-A, non-B viral hepatitis genome. *Science* **244**, 359–62.
4. **Pinto, P.C., Hu, E., Bernstein-Singer, M., Pinter-Brown, L., and Govindarajan, S.** (1990). Acute hepatic injury after the withdrawal of immunosuppressive chemotherapy in patients with hepatitis B. *Cancer* **65**, 878–84.
5. **Bass, N.M. and Ockner, R.K.** (1990). Drug induced liver disease. In *Hepatology. A Textbook of Liver Disease* (ed. D. Zakim and T.D. Boyer), pp. 754–91. Philadelphia: WB Saunders Co.
6. **Cohen, J.A. and Kaplan, M.M.** (1978). Left sided heart failure presenting as hepatitis. *Gastroenterology* **74**, 583–7.
7. **Shea, W.J., Demas, B.E., Goldberg, H.I., Hohn, D.C., Ferrell, L.D., and Kerlan, R.K.** (1986). Sclerosing cholangitis associated with hepatic arterial FUDR: radiographic–histologic correlation. *American Journal of Roentgenology* **146**, 717–21.
8. **Lahr, C.J. et al.** (1983). A multifactorial analysis of prognostic factors in patients with liver metastases from colorectal carcinoma. *Journal of Clinical Oncology* **1**, 720–6.
9. **Dick, R. and Dooley, J.** (1987). Jaundice in adults. In *Imaging in Hepatobiliary Disease* (ed. J. Dooley, R. Dick, M. Viamonte Jr, and S. Sherlock), pp. 3–36. Oxford: Blackwell.
10. **Chan, Y.L. et al.** (1996). Choledocholithiasis: comparison of MR cholangiography and endoscopic retrograde cholangiography. *Radiology* **200**, 85–9.

11. **Regan, F., Fradin, J., Khazan, R., Bohlman, M., and Magnuson, T.** (1996). Choledocholithiasis: evaluation with MR cholangiography. *American Journal of Roentgenology* **167**, 1441–5.
12. **Adamek, H.E.** et al. (1998). A prospective evaluation of magnetic resonance cholangiography in patients with suspected bile duct obstruction. *Gut* **43**, 680–3.
13. **Kim, M.-J., Mitchell, D.G., Ito, K., and Outwater, E.K.** (2000). Biliary dilatation: differentiation of benign from malignant causes—value of adding conventional MR imaging to MR cholangiopancreatography. *Radiology* **214**, 173–81.
14. **Pavone, P., Laghi, A., and Passariello, R.** (1999). MR cholangiopancreatography in malignant biliary obstruction. *Seminars in Ultrasound, CT, and MRI* **20**, 317–23.
15. **Brugge, W.R.** (1988). Endoscopic ultrasonography: the current status. *Gastroenterology* **115**, 1315–22.
16. **Palazzo, L.** et al. (1993). Endoscopic ultrasonography in the diagnosis and staging of pancreatic adenocarcinoma: results of a prospective study with comparison to ultrasonography and CT scan. *Endoscopy* **25**, 143–50.
17. **Chang, K.J.** et al. (1994). Endoscopic ultrasound-guided fine needle aspiration. *Gastrointestinal Endoscopy* **40**, 694–700.
18. **Materne, R.** et al. (2000). Extrahepatic biliary obstruction: magnetic resonance imaging compared with endoscopic ultrasound. *Endoscopy* **32**, 3–9.
19. **Chang, K.** et al. (1997). The clinical utility of endoscopic ultrasound (EUS) guided fine needle aspiration (FNA) in the diagnosis and staging of pancreatic carcinoma. *Gastrointestinal Endoscopy* **45**, 387–93.
20. **Drane, W.E.** (1991). Nuclear medicine techniques for the liver and biliary system. Update for the 1990s. In *The Radiologic Clinics of North America: Imaging of the Liver and Biliary Tree* Vol. 29, pp. 1129–50. Philadelphia: WB Saunders Co.
21. **Mueller, P.R., VanSonnenberg, E., and Simeone, J.F.** (1982). Fine needle transhepatic cholangiography. Indication and usefulness. *Annals of Internal Medicine* **97**, 567–72.
22. **Bilbao, M.K., Dotter, C.T., Lee, T.G., and Katon, R.M.** (1976). Complications of ERCP. A study of 10 000 cases. *Gastroenterology* **70**, 314–20.
23. **McGill, D.B., Rakela, J., Zinsmeister, A.R., and Ott, B.J.** (1990). A 21 year experience with major hemorrhage after percutaneous liver biopsy. *Gastroenterology* **99**, 1396–400.
24. **Jori, G.P. and Peschle, C.** (1972). Combined peritoneoscopy and liver biopsy in the diagnosis of hepatic neoplasm. *Gastroenterology* **63**, 1016–19.
25. **Ajlouni, M.I., Merrick, H.W., Skeel, R.T., and Dobelbower R.R. Jr.** (1990). Concomitant radiation therapy and constant infusion FUDR for unresectable hepatic metastases. *American Journal of Clinical Oncology* **13**, 532–5.
26. **Khandelwal, M. and Malet, P.F.** (1994). Pruritus associated with cholestasis. A review of pathogenesis and management. *Digestive Diseases and Sciences* **39**, 1–8.
27. **Richardson, B.P.** (1990). Serotonin and nociception. *Annals of the New York Academy of Sciences* **600**, 511–20.
28. (1994). Doxepin cream for pruritus. *Medical Letter on Drugs and Therapeutics*, **36**, 99–100.
29. **Datta, D. and Sherlock, S.** (1963). Treatment of pruritus of obstructive jaundice with cholestyramine. *British Medical Journal* **1**, 216.
30. **Bergasa, N.V.** et al. (1992). A controlled trial of naloxone infusions for the pruritis of chronic cholestasis. *Gastroenterology* **102**, 544–9.
31. **Jones, E.A. and Bergasa, N.V.** (1992). The pruritus of cholestasis and the opiod system. *Journal of the American Medical Association* **268**, 3359–62.
32. **Wolfghagen, F.H.** et al. (1997). Oral naltrexone treatment for cholestatic pruritus: a double-blind, placebo-controlled study. *Gastroenterology* **113**, 1264.
33. **Bergasa, N.V.** et al. (1998). Open-label trial of oral nalmefene therapy for the pruritus of cholestasis. *Hepatology* **27**, 679.
34. **Ghent, C.N. and Carruthers, S.G.** (1988). Treatment of pruritus in primary biliary cirrhosis with rifampin. Results of a double-blind crossover randomized trial. *Gastroenterology* **94**, 488–93.
35. **Gregorio, G.V., Ball, C.S., Mowat, A.P., and Mieli-Vergani, G.** (1993). Effect of rifampicin in the treatment of pruritus in hepatic cholestasis. *Archives of Disease in Childhood* **69**, 141–3.
36. **Rosemurgy, A.S., Burnett, C.M., and Wasselle, J.A.** (1989). A comparison of choledochoenteric bypass and cholcystoenteric bypass in patients with biliary obstruction due to pancreatic cancer. *American Surgeon* **55**, 55–60.
37. **Schouten, J.T.** (1986). Operative therapy for pancreatic carcinoma. *American Journal of Surgery* **151**, 626–30.
38. **Joseph, P.K., Bizer, L.F., Sprayregen, S.S., and Gliedman, M.L.** (1986). Percutaneous transhepatic biliary drainage. Results and complications in 81 patients. *Journal of the American Medical Association* **255**, 2763–7.
39. **Speer, A.G.** et al. (1987). Randomized trial of endoscopic versus percutaneous stent insertion in malignant obstructive jaundice. *Lancet* **2**, 57–62.
40. **Smith, A.C.** et al. (1994). Randomised trial of endoscopic versus percutaneous stent insertion in malignant obstructive jaundice. *Lancet* **344**, 1655–60.
41. **McPherson, G.A.D., Benjamin, I.S., Hodgson, H.J.F., Bowley, N.B., Allison, D.J., and Blumgart, L.H.** (1984). Preoperative percutaneous transhepatic biliary drainage: the results of a controlled trial. *British Journal of Surgery* **71**, 371–5.
42. **England, R.E.** et al. (2000). A prospective randomised multicenter trial comparing 10F Teflon Tannenbaum stents with 10F polyethylene Cotton–Leung stents in patients with malignant common duct strictures. *Gut* **46**, 395–400.
43. **Pereira-Lima, J.C.** et al. (1996). Endoscopic biliary stenting for palliation of pancreatic cancer: results, survival predictive factors, and comparison of 10-French with 11.5 French gauge stents. *American Journal of Gastroenterology* **21**, 79–84.
44. **Andersen, J.R., Sorensen, S.M., Kruse, A., Rokkjaer, M., and Matzen, P.** (1989). Randomized trial of endoscopic endoprosthesis versus operative bypass in malignant obstructive jaundice. *Gut* **30**, 1132–5.
45. **Shepherd, H.A., Royle, G., Ross, A.P., Diba, A., Arthur, M., and Colin-Jones, D.** (1988). Endoscopic biliary endoprosthesis in the palliation of malignant obstruction of the distal common bile duct: a randomized trial. *British Journal of Surgery* **75**, 1166–8.
46. **Dowsett, J.F.** et al. (1989). Malignant obstructive jaundice: a prospective randomized trial of bypass surgery versus endoscopic stenting. *Gastroenterology* **96**, A128.
47. **Brandabur, J.J.** et al. (1988). Nonoperative versus operative treatment of obstructive jaundice in pancreatic cancer: cost and survival analysis. *American Journal of Gastroenterology* **83**, 1132–9.
48. **Sung, J.Y., Leung, J.W., Shaffer, E.A., Lam, K., and Costerton, J.W.** (1993). Bacterial biofiilm, brown pigmented stone and blockage of biliary stents. *Journal of Gastroenterology and Hepatology* **8**, 28–34.
49. **Yu, J.L., Andersson, R., and Ljungh, A.** (1996). Protein adsorption and bacterial adhesion to biliary stent material. *Journal of Surgical Research* **62**, 69–73.
50. **Barrioz, T., Ingrand, P., Besson, I., deLedinghen, V., Silvain, C., and Beauchant, M.** (1994). Randomised trial of prevention of biliary stent occlusion by ursodeoxycholic acid plus norflaxacin. *Lancet* **334**, 581–2.
51. **Ghosh, S. and Palmer K.** (1994). Prevention of biliary stent occlusion using cyclical antibiotics and ursodeoxycholic acid. *Gut* **35**, 1757–9.
52. **Kadakia, S.C. and Starnes, E.** (1992). Comparison of 10F French gauge stent with 11.5 French gauge stent in patients with biliary tract diseases. *Gastrointestinal Endoscopy* **38**, 454–9.
53. **Liu, Q., Khay, G., and Cotton, P.B.** (1998). Feasibility of stent placement above the sphincter of Oddi ('inside-stent') for patients with malignant biliary obstruction. *Endoscopy* **30**, 687–90.
54. **Hoffman, B.J., Cunningham, J.T., Marsh, W.H., O'Brien, J.J., and Watson, J.** (1994). An *in vitro* comparison of biofilm formation on various biliary stent material. *Gastrointestinal Endoscopy* **40**, 581–3.
55. **Rey, J.F., Maupetit, P., and Greff, M.** (1985). Experimental study of biliary endoprosthesis efficiency. *Endoscopy* **17**, 145–8.
56. **Lameris, J.S. and Stoker, J.** (1994). Metal stents for malignant biliary obstruction. *Digestive Diseases* **12**, 161–9.
57. **Yeoh, K.G., Zimmermman, M.J., Cunningham, J.T., and Cotton, P.B.** (1999). Comparative costs of metal versus plastic biliary stent strategies for malignant obstructive jaundice by decision analysis. *Gastrointestinal Endoscopy* **49**, 466–71.
58. **Shim, C.S.** et al. (1998). Preliminary results of a new covered biliary metal stent for malignant biliary obstruction. *Endoscopy* **30**, 345–50.

59. **Baron T.** (2001). Expandable metal stents for the treatment of cancerous obstruction of the gastrointestinal tract. *New England Journal of Medicine* **344** (22), 1681–7.
60. **Cotton, P.B.** (1989). Nonsurgical palliation of jaundice in pancreatic cancer. *Surgical Clinics of North America* **69**, 613–27.
61. **Lebovics, E., Thung, S.N., Schaffner, F., and Radensky, P.W.** (1985). The liver in the acquired immunodeficiency syndrome: a clinical and histologic study. *Hepatology* **5**, 293–8.
62. **Schneiderman, D.J., Arenson, D.M., Cello, J.P., Margaretten, W., and Weber, T.E.** (1987). Hepatic disease in patients with the acquired immune deficiency syndrome. *Hepatology* **7**, 925–30.
63. **Cappell, M.S.** (1991). Hepatobiliary manifestations of the acquired immune deficiency syndrome. *American Journal of Gastroenterology* **86**, 1–15.
64. **Herrero, M.E.** (2001). Hepatitis B and C co-infection in patients with HIV. *Reviews of Medical Virology* **11**, 253–70.
65. **Osick, L.A.** et al. (1993). Hepatic amyloidosis in intravenous drug abusers and AIDS patients. *Journal of Hepatology* **19** (1), 79–84.
66. **Brau, N., Leaf, H.L., Wiecsoref, R.L., and Margolis, D.M.** (1997). Severe hepatitis in three AIDS patients treated with indinavir. *Lancet* **349** (9056), 924–5.
67. **Bouche, H., Housset, C., and Dumont, J.L.** (1993). AIDS-related cholangitis: diagnostic features and course in 15 patients. *Journal of Hepatology* **17**, 34–9.
68. **Cello, J.P.** (1989). Acquired immunodeficiency syndrome cholangiopathy: spectrum of disease. *American Journal of Medicine* **86**, 539–46.
69. **Nash, J.A. and Cohen, S.A.** (1997). Gallbladder and biliary tract disease in AIDS. *Gastroenterology Clinics of North America* **26**, 323–35.
70. **Gordon, S.C.** et al. (1986). The spectrum of liver disease in the acquired immunodeficiency syndrome. *Journal of Hepatology* **2**, 475–84.
71. **Cappell, M.S., Schwartz, M.S., and Biempica, L.** (1990). Clinical utility of liver biopsy in patients with serum antibodies to the human immunodeficiency virus. *American Journal of Medicine* **88**, 123–30.
72. **Runyon, B.A., Hoefs, J.C., and Morgan, T.R.** (1988). Ascitic fluid analysis in malignancy-related ascites. *Hepatolology* **8**, 1104–9.
73. **Runyon, B.A.** (1982). Ascites. In *Diseases of the Liver* 7th edn. (ed. L. Schiff and E.R. Schiff), pp. 990–1015. Philadelphia PA: Lippincott.
74. **Lifshitz, S.** (1982). Ascites, pathophysiology and control measures. *International Journal of Radiation Oncology, Biology and Physiology* **8**, 1423–6.
75. **Garrison, R.N., Kaelin, L.D., Heuser, L.S., and Galloway, R.H.** (1986). Malignant ascites: clinical and experimental observations. *Annals of Surgery* **203**, 644–51.
76. **Nagy, J.A., Herzberg, K.T., Dvorak, J.M., and Dvorak, H.F.** (1993). Pathogenesis of malignant ascites formation: initiating events that lead to fluid accumulation. *Cancer Research* **53**, 2631–43.
77. **Yeo, K.T.** et al. (1993). Vascular permeability factor in guinea pig and human tumour and inflammatory effusions. *Cancer Research* **53**, 2912–18.
78. **Tabbarah, H.J. and Casciato, D.A.** (1990). Malignant effusions. In *Cancer Treatment* (ed. C.M. Haskell), pp. 815–25. Philadelphia PA: WB Saunders.
79. **Sherlock, S.** (1993). Ascites. In *Diseases of the Liver and Biliary System* 9th edn. (ed. S. Sherlock and J. Dooley), pp. 114–31. Oxford: Blackwell Scientific Publications.
80. **Keeffe, E.J., Gagliardi, R.A., and Pfister, R.C.** (1967). The roentgenographic evaluation of ascites. *American Journal of Roentgenology* **101**, 388–96.
81. **Callen, P.W., Marks, W.M., and Filly, R.A.** (1979). Computed tomography and ultrasonography in the evaluation of the retroperitoneum in patients with malignant ascites. *Journal of Computer Assisted Tomography* **3**, 581–4.
82. **Huan, Y.S., Lee, S.D., Wu, J.C., Wang, S.S., Lin, H.C., and Tsai, Y.T.** (1989). Utility of sonographic gallbladder wall patterns in differentiating malignant from cirrhotic ascites. *Journal of Clinical Ultrasound* **17**, 187–92.
83. **Goerg, C. and Schwerk, W.B.** (1991). Malignant ascites: sonographic signs of peritoneal carcinomatosis. *European Journal of Cancer* **27**, 720–3.
84. **Inadomi, J.M., Kapur, S., Kinkhabwala, M., and Call, J.P.** (2001). The laparoscopic evaluation of ascites. *Gastrointestinal Endoscopy Clinics of North America* **1**, 79–91.
85. **Low, R.N. and Francis, I.R.** (1997). MR imaging of the gastrointestinal tract with IV gadolinium and diluted barium oral contrast media compared with unenhanced MR imaging and CT. *American Journal of Roentgenology* **169**, 1051–9.
86. **Low, R.N., Semelka, R.C., Worawattanakul, S., Alzate, G.D., and Sigeti, J.S.** (1999). Extrahepatic abdominal imaging in patients with malignancy: comparison of MR imaging and helical, CT, with subsequent surgical correlation. *Amecican journal of Roentgenology* **210**, 625–32.
87. **Runyon, B.A.** (1986). Paracentesis of ascitic fluid: a safe procedure. *Archives of Internal Medicine* **146**, 2259–61.
88. **Malden, L.T. and Tattersall, M.H.N.** (1986). Malignant effusions. *Quarterly Journal of Medicine* **227**, 221–39.
89. **Press, O.W., Press, N.O., and Kaufman, S.D.** (1982). Evaluation and management of chylous ascites. *Annals of Internal Medicine* **96**, 358–64.
90. **Anonymous** (1981). Diagnosis of ascites. *British Medical Journal* **282**, 1499.
91. **Levine, H.** (1967). Needle biopsy of peritoneum in exudative ascites. *Archives of Internal Medicine* **120**, 542–5.
92. **Yang, C.Y.** et al. (1985). White count, pH and lactate in ascites in the diagnosis of spontaneous bacterial peritonitis. *Hepatology* **5**, 85–90.
93. **Both, C.T., de Mattos, A.A., Neumann, J., and Reis, M.D.** (2001). Flow cytometry in the diagnosis of peritoneal carcinomatosis. *American Journal of Gastroenterology* **96**, 1605–9.
94. **Runyon, B.A.** (1988). Spontaneous bacterial peritonitis: an explosion of information. *Hepatology* **8**, 171–5.
95. **Hoefs, J.C.** (1981). Increase in ascites white blood cell and protein concentrations during diuresis in patients with chronic liver disease. *Hepatology* **1**, 249–54.
96. **Dykes, P.W.** (1961). A study of the effects of albumin infusions in patients with cirrhosis of the liver. *Quarterly Journal of Medicine* **30**, 297.
97. **Mankin, H. and Lowell, A.** (1948). Osmotic factors influencing the formation of ascites in patients with cirrhosis of the liver. *Journal of Clinical Investigation* **27**, 145.
98. **Mauer, K. and Manzione, N.C.** (1988). Usefulness of serum-ascites albumin difference in separating transudative from exudative ascites. Another look. *Digestive Diseases and Sciences* **33**, 1208–12.
99. **Adamsen, S., Jonsson, P., Brodin, B., Lindberg, B., and Jorpes, P.** (1991). Measurement of fibronectin concentration in benign and malignant ascites. *European Journal of Surgery* **157**, 325–8.
100. **Kosches, D.S., Sosnowik, D., Lendvai, S., and Bank, S.** (1989). Unusual anodic migrating isoamylase differentiates selected malignant from nonmalignant ascites. *Journal of Clinical Gastroenterology* **11**, 43–6.
101. **Boyer, T.D., Kahn, A.N., and Reynolds, T.B.** (1978). Diagnostic value of ascitic fluid lactic dehydrogenase, protein and WBC levels. *Archives of Internal Medicine* **138**, 1103–5.
102. **Couch, W.D.** (1981). Combined effusion fluid tumour marker assay, carcinoembroyonic antigen (CEA) and human chorionic gonadotropin (hCG), in the detection of malignant tumours. *Cancer* **48**, 2475–9.
103. **Bergmann, J.F., Bidart, J.M., George, M., Beaugrand, M., Levy, V.G., and Bohuon, C.** (1987). Elevation of CA 125 in patients with benign and malignant ascites. *Cancer* **59**, 213–37.
104. **Kourouras, J., Boura, P., Tsapas, G., Charsis, K., Magoula, I., and Tsakiri, I.** (1993). Value of ascitic fluid ferritin in the differential diagnosis of malignant ascites. *Anticancer Research* **13**, 2441–5.
105. **Jungst, D., Gerbes, A.L., Martin, R., and Paumgartner, G.** (1986). Value of ascitic lipids in the differentiation between cirrhotic and malignant ascites. *Hepatology* **6**, 239–43.
106. **Colloredo-Mels, G.** et al. (1991). Fibronectin, cholesterol and triglyceride ascitic fluid concentrations in the prediction of malignancy. *Italian Journal of Gastroenterology* **23**, 179–86.
107. **Tangkijvanich, P., Tresukosol, D., Sampatanukul, P., Sakdikul, S., Voravud, N., Mahachai, V., and Mutirangura, A.** (1999). Telomerase assay for differentiating between malignancy-related and nonmalignant ascites. *Clinical Cancer Research* **5**, 2470–5.
108. **Pockros, P.J., Esrason, K.T., Nguyen, C., Dugue, J., and Woods, S.** (1992). Mobilization of malignant ascites with diuretics is dependent on ascitic fluid characteristics. *Gastroenterology* **103**, 1302–6.
109. **Lewis J.W. Jr. and Storer, E.H.** (1979). The management of iatrogenic chylous ascites. *Henry Ford Hospital Medical Journal* **27**, 140–2.
110. **Gines, P.** et al. (1987). Comparison of paracentesis and diuretics in the treatment of cirrhotics with tense ascites: results of a randomized study. *Gastroenterology* **93**, 234–41.

111. **Kao, H.W., Rakov, N.E., Savage, E., and Reynolds, T.B.** (1985). The effect of large volume paracentesis on plasma volume—a cause of hypovolemia? *Hepatology* **5**, 403–7.

112. **Liebowitz, H.R.** (1962). Hazards of abdominal paracentesis in the cirrhotic patient (Part III). *New York State Journal of Medicine* **62**, 2223–9.

113. **Pinto, P.C., Amerian, J., and Reynolds, T.B.** (1988). Large-volume paracentesis in nonedematous patients with tense ascites: its effect on intravascular volume. *Hepatology* **8**, 207–10.

114. **Panos, M.Z.** et al. (1990). Single, total paracentesis for tense ascites: sequential hemodynamic changes and right atrial size. *Hepatology* **11**, 662–7.

115. **Tito, L.** et al. (1990). Total paracentesis associated with intravenous albumin management of patients with cirrhosis and ascites. *Gastroenterology* **98**, 146–51.

116. **Gines, P., Arroyo, V., and Rodes, J.** (1989). Treatment of ascites and renal failure in cirrhosis. *Bailliere's Clinical Gastroenterology* **3**, 165–86.

117. **Epstein, M.** (1980). The LeVeen shunt for ascites and hepatorenal syndrome. *New England Journal of Medicine* **302**, 628–30.

118. **Holm, A., Halpern, N.B., and Aldrete, J.S.** (1989). Peritoneovenous shunt for intractable ascites of hepatic, nephrogenic, and malignant causes. *American Journal of Surgery* **158**, 162–6.

119. **Soderlund, C.** (1986). Denver peritoneovenous shunting for malignant or cirrhotic ascites. A prospective consecutive series. *Scandinavian Journal of Gastroenterology* **21**, 1167–72.

120. **Gough, I.R. and Balderson, G.A.** (1993). Malignant ascites. A comparison of peritoneovenous shunting and non-operative management. *Cancer* **71**, 2377–82.

121. **Pilati, P., Rossi, C.R., Mocellin, S., Foletto, M., Scagnet, B., Pasetto, L., and Lise, M.** (2001). Multimodal treatment of peritoneal carcinomatosis and sarcomatosis. *European Journal of Surgical Oncology* **27**, 125–34.

122. **Brennan, M., Casper, E., and Harrison, L.** (1997). Soft? tissue carcinoma. In *Cancer Principles and Practice of Oncology* (ed. V.T. De Vita, S. Hellman, and S.A. Rosemberg), p. 1738. New York: Lippincott-Raven Press.

123. **Sugarbaker, P., Gianola, F.J., Speyer, J.C., Wesley, R., Barofski, I., and Meyers, C.E.** (1985). Prospective, randomized trial of intravenous versus intraperitoneal-fluorouracil in patients with advanced primary colon or rectal cancer. *Surgery* **98**, 414–21.

124. **Meyn, R.E., Corry, P.M., Fletcher, S.E., and Demetriades.** (1980). Thermal enhancement of DNA damage in mamalian cells treated with cis-diaminodichloroplatinum. *Cancer Research* **40**, 1136–9.

125. **Fujimoto, S., Takahashi, M., Mutou, T., Kobayashi, K., Toyosawa, T., Isawa, E., Sumida, M., and Ohkubo, H.** (1997). Improved mortality rate of gastric carcinoma patients with peritoneal carcinomatosis treated with intraperitoneal hyperthermic chemoperfusion combined with surgery. *Cancer* **79**, 884–90.

126. **Myers, C.E. and Collins, J.M.** (1983). Pharmacology of intraperitoneal chemotherapy. *Cancer Investigation* **1**, 395–407.

127. **Dybicki, J., Balchum, O.J., and Meneelly, GR.** (1959). Treatment of pleural and peritoneal effusion with intracavitary colloidal radiogold (^{198}Au). *Archives of Internal Medicine* **104**, 802–15.

128. **Jacobs, M.L. and Duarte, M.D.** (1958). Radioactive colloidal chromic phosphate to control pleural effusion and ascites. *Journal of the American Medical Association* **166**, 597–9.

129. **Gebbia, N.** et al. (1994). Intracavity treatment of malignant pleural and peritoneal effusions in cancer patients. *Anticancer Research* **14**, 739–46.

130 **Westermann, A.M., Dubbelman, R., Baars, J.P., Moolenaar, W.H., Beijnen, J.H., and Rodenhuis, S.** (2000). Feasibility and pharmacokinetics of intraperitoneal suramin in advanced malignancy. *Cancer Chemotherapy and Pharmacology* **46**, 57–62.

131. **Andersen, A.P. and Brincker, H.** (1968). Intracavitary thiotepa in malignant pleural and peritoneal effusions. *Acta Radiological Therapy Physics Biology* **7**, 369–77.

132. **Bayly, T.C.** et al. (1978). Tetracycline and quinacrine in the control of malignant pleural effusions. *Cancer* **41**, 1188.

133. **Fracchia, A.A., Knapper, W.H., Carey, J.T., and Farrow, J.H.** (1970). Intrapleural chemotherapy for effusion from metastatic breast cancer. *Cancer* **26**, 626.

134. **Tattersall, M.H.N., Fox, R.M., Newlands, E.S., and Woods, R.L.** (1979). Intracavitary doxorubicin in malignant effusions. *Lancet* **1**, 390.

135. **Keffort, R.F., Woods, R.L., Fox, R.M., and Tattersall, M.H.N.** (1980). Intracavitary adriamycin, nitrogen mustard and tetracycline in the control of malignant effusions. A randomized study. *Medical Journal of Australia* **2**, 447–8.

136. **Suhrland, L.G. and Weisberger, A.S.** (1965). Intracavitary 5-fluorouracil in malignant effusions. *Archives of Internal Medicine* **116**, 431–3.

137. **Rath, U.** et al. (1991). Effect of intraperitoneal recombinant human tumour necrosis factor alpha on malignant ascites. *European Journal of Cancer* **27**, 121–5.

138. **Weissenborn, K.** (1992). Recent developments in the pathophysiology and treatment of hepatic encephalopathy. *Bailliere's Clinical Gastroenterology* **6**, 609–30.

139. **Jones, E.A., Basile, A.S., Yurdaydin, C., and Skolnich, P.** (1993). Do benzodiazepine ligands contribute to hepatic encephalopathy? *Advances in Experimental Biology and Medicine* **341**, 57–69.

140. **Mousseau, D.D. and Butterworth, R.F.** (1994). Current theories on the pathogenesis of hepatic encephalopathy. *Proceedings of the Society for Experimental Biology and Medicine* **206**, 329–44.

141. **Hoyumpa, A.M. Jr. and Schenker, S.** (1982). Perspectives in hepatic encephalopathy. *Journal of Laboratory and Clinical Medicine* **100**, 477–87.

142. **Elsass, P., Lund, Y., and Ranek, L.** (1978). Encephalopathy in patients with cirrhosis of the liver: a neuropsychological study. *Scandinavian Journal of Gastroenterology* **13**, 241–7.

143. **Rikkers, L., Jenko, P., Rudman, D., and Freides, D.** (1978). Subclinical hepatic encephalopathy: detection, prevalence and relationship to nitrogen metabolism. *Gastroenterology* **75**, 462–9.

144. **Conn, H.O.** (1977). Trailmaking and number-connection test in the assessment of mental state in portal systemic encephalopathy. *Digestive Diseases and Sciences* **22**, 541–50.

145. **Ross, B.D.** et al. (1994). Subclinical hepatic encephalopathy: proton MR spectroscopic abnormalities. *Radiology* **193**, 457–63.

146. **Parsons-Smith, B.G., Summerskill, W.H.J., Dawson, A.M., and Sherlock, S.** (1957). The electroencephalograph in liver disease. *Lancet* **2**, 867–71.

147. **Conn, H.O.** (1993). Hepatic encephalopathy. In *Diseases of the Liver* 7th edn. (ed. L. Schiff and E.R. Schiff), pp. 1036–60. Philadelphia: J.B. Lippincott.

148. **Camma, C., Fiorello, F., Tine, F., Marchesini, G., Fabbri, A., and Pagliaro, L.** (1993). Lactitol in treatment of chronic hepatic encephalopathy. A meta-analysis. *Digestive Diseases and Sciences* **38**, 916–22.

149. **Dawson, A.M., McLaren, J., and Sherlock, S.** (1957). Neomycin in the treatment of hepatic coma. *Lancet* **2**, 1263–8.

150. **Bucci, L. and Palmieri, G.C.** (1993). Double-blind, double-dummy comparison between treatment with rifaximin and lactulose in patients with medium to severe degree hepatic encephalopathy. *Current Medical Research & Opinion* **13**, 109–18.

151. **Naylor, C.D., O'rourke, K., Detski, A.S., and Baker, J.P.** (1989). Parenteral nutrition with branched–chain amino acids in hepatic encephalopathy. *Gastroenterology* **97**, 1033–42.

152. **Bianchi, G.P.** et al. (1993). Vegetable vs animal protein diet in cirrhotic patients with chronic encephalopathy. A randomized cross-over comparison. *Journal of Internal Medicine* **233**, 385–92.

153. **Sushma, S., Dasarathy, S., Tandon, R.K., Jain, S., Gupta, S., and Bhist, M.S.** (1992). Sodium benzoate in the treatment of acute hepatic encephalopathy: a double blind randomized trial. *Hepatology* **16**, 138–44.

154. **Gyr, K.** et al. (1996). Evaluation of the efficacy and safety of flumazenil in the treatment of portal systemic encephalopathy: a double blind, randomised, placebo controlled multicentre study. *Gut* **39**, 319–24.

155. **Barbero, G.** et al. (1998). Flumezenil for hepatic encephalopathy Grade III and IVa in patients with cirrhosis: an Italian multicentre double-blind, placebo-controlled, cross over study. *Hepatology* **28**, 374–8.

156. **Das, A., Dhiman, R.K., Saraswat, V.A., Verma, M., and Naik, S.R.** (2001). Prevalence and natural history of subclinical hepatic encephalopathy in cirrhosis. *Journal of Gastroenterology and Hepatology* **16**, 531–5.

157. **Sexena, N., Bhatia, M., Joshi, Y.K., Garg, P.K., and Tandon, R.K.** (2001). Auditory P300 event related potentials and number connection test for the

evaluation of subclinical hepatic encephalopathy in patients with cirrhosis of the liver: a follow-up study. *Journal of Gastroenterology and Hepatology* **16**, 322–7.

158. **Groeneweg, M.** et al. (1998). Subclinical hepatic encephalopathy impairs daily function. *Hepatology* **28**, 45–9.
159. **Dhiman, R.K.** et al. (2000). Efficacy of lactulose in cirrhotic patients with subclinical hepatic encephalopathy. *Digestive Diseases and Sciences* **45**, 1549–52.
160. **Cowling, M.G. and Adam, A.N.** (2001). Internal stenting in malignant biliary obstruction. *World Journal of Surgery* **25**, 355–61.
161. **Knyrim, K., Wagner, H.J., Pausch, J., and Vakil, N.** (1993). A prospective randomised controlled trial of metal stents for malignant obstruction of the common bile duct. *Endoscopy* **25**, 207.
162. **Sutton, R., Phil, D., Slavin, J.P., and Neoptolemos, J.P.** (2001). Invited commentary. *World Journal of Surgery* **25**, 355–61.

8.4 Nutrition in palliative medicine

8.4.1 Pathophysiology of the anorexia/cachexia syndrome

Florian Strasser

Introduction

Most of the patients seen by a palliative care service experience a loss of body weight, a decrease of appetite, a reduction in the level of energy, fatigue, and weakness. Other associated symptoms or stressors may occur, such as chronic nausea, early satiety, change in body image, or psychological distress of the patients or their loved ones.(1) These features can be manifest in a variety of diseases, including progressive cancer,(2) AIDS,(3) chronic heart,(4) liver,(5) or renal failure,(6) chronic obstructive pulmonary disease (COPD),(7) or cystic fibrosis.(8) Likewise, in patients with acute or chronic infections(9) some of these characteristics may be observed.

The term anorexia/cachexia syndrome (ACS) is used mostly for cancer patients, in contrast to the terms HIV-wasting disease or cardiac cachexia. Nevertheless, the pathogenesis and manifestations of these diseases overlap, even though variable metabolic, neuroendocrine, or anabolic modifications may occur, and variable characteristics of the inflammatory state may be observed. Therefore in this chapter the term ACS is used and refers to the different cachexia or wasting syndromes. The term failure to thrive refers mainly to children's malnutrition caused by dietary, organic, and social factors,(10) whereas the term sarcopenia is used to describe the loss of muscle mass and strength with age.(11)

Several factors besides ACS can lead to weight loss, anorexia, fatigue, or associated symptoms. An important factor, for example, is impaired oral intake due to altered integrity or function of the gastrointestinal tract, leading to starvation. These aggravating factors may be paraphrased as secondary anorexia/cachexia (Table 1), in contrast to the primary ACS, which is a 'metabolic' disorder (Table 2, Fig. 1). The primary ACS is 'directly' caused by the underlying disease and complex metabolic, neuroendocrine, and anabolic modifications that occur in the context of an ongoing altered inflammatory state (Table 3, Fig. 2).

Table 1 Aggravating factors/secondary anorexia/cachexia (mainly cancer-related)

(A) Starvation/malnutrition
Impaired oral intake
Stomatitis, taste alterations, zinc deficiency
Dry mouth (xerostomia), dehydration
Dysphagia, odynophagia
Severe constipation
Bowel obstruction
Autonomic failure
Vomiting
Severe pain, dyspnoea, depression
Cognitive impairment/delirium
Social and financial obstacles
Impaired gastrointestinal absorption
Malabsorption
Exocrine pancreatic insufficiency
Chronic severe diarrhoea
Significant loss of proteins
Frequent drainage of ascites or pleural fluid punctions
Nephrotic syndrome
(B) Loss of muscle mass
Prolonged inactivity (bed rest, microgravity), deconditioning
Growth hormone deficiency, hypogonadism, aging, sarcopenia
(C) Other catabolic states
Chronic and acute infections
Treatment with proinflammatory cytokines
Chronic heart failure (cardiac cachexia), lung disease, or renal failure
Poorly controlled diabetes mellitus, liver cirrhosis
Hyperthyroidism

Table 2 Alterations in primary anorexia/cachexia (mainly cancer-related) compared with starvation

	Primary anorexia/cachexia	Starvation
Energy expenditure/lean body mass	⇑	⇓
Protein synthesis		
overall	⇑	⇓
muscle proteins	⇓	⇓
acute-phase proteins	⇑	⇔
Proteolysis		
muscle proteins	⇑⇑	⇑
Lipogenesis	⇓	⇓
Lipolysis	⇑	⇑⇑
Glucose turnover	⇑	⇓
Ketone bodies	⇓	⇑
Leptin	⇔⇓	⇓
Neuropeptide Y	⇔⇑	⇑
Ghrelin	?	?
Testosterone	⇔⇓	⇓
Growth hormone/IGF-I	⇔⇓	⇓
Thyroxine (T4)	⇔	⇓
Cortisol	⇑	⇓

This chapter aims to provide an update on the evolving understanding of anorexia/cachexia in different diseases, with a focus on patients with advanced cancer. The chapter will review briefly the potential causes of secondary anorexia/cachexia, discuss the three mechanisms (metabolic, neuroendocrine, and anabolic) which are altered or involved in primary

ACS, the role of cytokines and the immune system as well as of tumour-derived cachectic factors, and finally potential implications of the pathogenesis of anorexia/cachexia on clinical assessment, treatment, and decision-making.

Causes for secondary anorexia/cachexia

In most patients suffering from primary ACS aggravating factors may contribute to weight loss, anorexia, fatigue, or other associated symptoms. The presence of these factors can be obvious, such as transient anorexia because of severe pain. On the other hand, it may be difficult to distinguish, for example, between a concurrent subacute infection and primary ACS. Many of the aggravating factors are reversible, and can be conceptualized under the term secondary anorexia/cachexia. Many patients present with one or more of these factors, in addition to primary ACS. For example, a patient with advanced cancer and primary ACS might suffer also from chronic heart failure (cardiac cachexia) or chronic renal failure (renal cachexia). Secondary anorexia/cachexia may be divided in three groups (Table 1).

Starvation

The first group of secondary anorexia/cachexia is a form of starvation or malnutrition, caused by impaired oral intake secondary to both altered function of the gastrointestinal tract and interfering symptoms or loss of proteins through body fluids. The energy expenditure is reduced, proteins are conserved, and ketone bodies are utilized as an energy source. The result is weight loss, mostly at the expense of body fat. These features contrast to the alterations seen in primary ACS. Table 2 refers to the metabolic alterations in cancer-related primary ACS, compared to starvation. Starvation itself might impact the immune function or neuroendocrine regulation. Healthy adults die from starvation after a nitrogen loss of 35 per cent of the

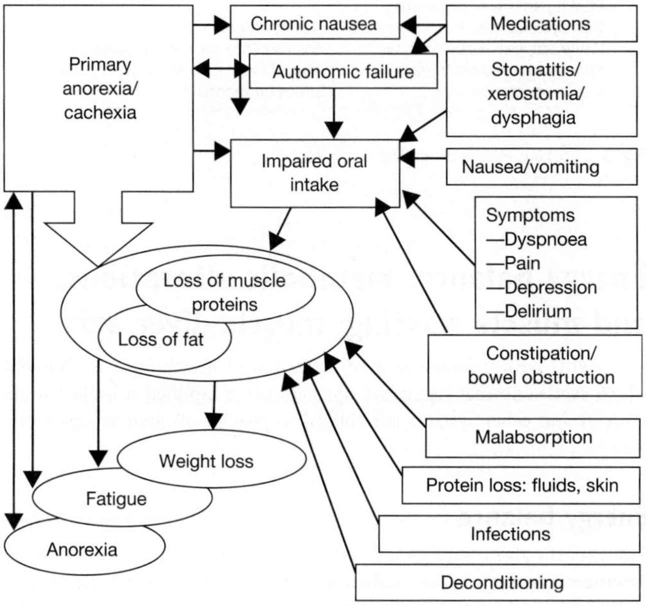

Fig. 1 Interplay of the primary anorexia/cachexia (mainly cancer-related anorexia/cachexia) syndrome and aggravating factors of anorexia/cachexia (secondary anorexia/cachexia).

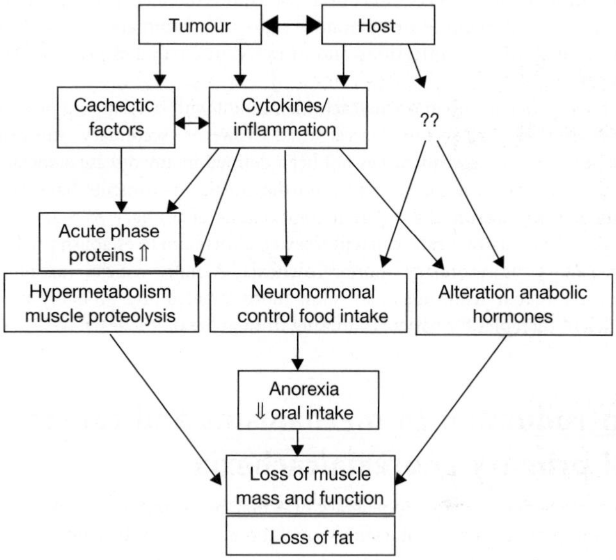

Fig. 2 Main elements of the pathogenesis of primary anorexia/cachexia in cancer patients.

Table 3 Comparison of different diseases associated with primary anorexia/cachexia syndrome

	Clinical manifestation		Mechanism mediating the anorexia/cachexia syndrome			Causative factors	
	Weight loss	Anorexia	Metabolism	Neurohormonal	Anabolic hormones	Cytokines	PIF/LMF
Cancer (Cancer ACS)	+++	++	+++	++	+	+++	+++
AIDS (HIV-wasting)	+++	+	++	++	+++	+++	?
Chronic heart failure (Cardiac cachexia)	++	+	+	++	++	++	?
Chronic renal failure (Renal cachexia)	++	+	+	+	++	++	?
Elderly patients (Sarcopenia)	++	(+)	−	+	++	(+)	?

ideal weight, that is, after 60–75 days, despite adequate adipose reserves, since the protein mass is the major determinant of starvation.[12] An estimate for dying from starvation equals about 15–30 days for patients with progressive, terminal cancer. If patients have in addition a systemically activated immune system caused by circulating cytokines, such as during infections (systemic inflammatory response syndrome), the time to death will decrease further.

Deconditioning

The second group describes the loss of muscle tissue in the absence of primary ACS, as a consequence of decreased muscle activity because of immobility (occurring, e.g., during prolonged bed rest) or microgravity. This phenomenon has been called deconditioning. The failure to increase muscle mass in children (subgroup of failure to thrive) or the involuntary loss of muscle in elderly people (sarcopenia) despite adequate nutrition might be related to the phenomenon of deconditioning.

Infections

The final group contains concomitant acute or chronic infections, causing a catabolic state.[9] In clinical reality, it is often difficult in patients presenting with clinical or laboratory signs of inflammation to sort out the contribution of infections and of cytokine-mediated primary ACS (see below).

Most patients with anorexia/cachexia present with overlapping primary ACS and secondary anorexia/cachexia. However, secondary anorexia/cachexia and its assessment has not been defined in any disease associated with anorexia/cachexia. Currently no diagnostic instruments have been validated to measure the different components of primary ACS and secondary anorexia/cachexia. Current research efforts aim to establish predictive factors for secondary anorexia/cachexia. A more concise taxonomy of the different syndromes may allow more targeted and probably more efficient therapies for patients suffering from anorexia/cachexia.

Introduction to mechanisms and causes of primary anorexia/cachexia

The mechanisms leading to primary ACS may be summarized under three overlapping groups of alterations (metabolic, neuroendocrine, or anabolic), whereas the most common cause for primary ACS are immune alterations including (proinflammatory) cytokines. Tumour-derived cachectic glycoproteins might also be an important causal factor, at least in patients with cancer.

In the different diseases leading to primary ACS these three mechanisms and causative factors might be observed. However, in the various diseases the relative contribution of each mechanism and causative factor (mainly the extent of inflammation or circulating cytokines) may be different (Table 3). In patients with advanced cancer, for example, active cancer cells and their interactions with the host cause several overlapping syndromes of anorexia/cachexia. Both hypermetabolism with metabolic alterations in the 'muscle–liver axis' (adapted term as proposed by Argiles et al.[13]) are present, as well as neuroendocrine alterations in the 'gut–brain axis' (term as proposed by Meguid et al.[14]). However, research from other wasting conditions, such as cardiac cachexia or AIDS-wasting, has highlighted the role of the family of growth hormones and anabolic hormones. This 'endocrine–muscle/somatotropic axis' is of growing interest for cancer ACS also, and will be given more weight here (Table 3). The immune alterations causing primary ACS are complex and involve not only systemic effects, which may be measurable in the blood, but also predominantly local effects, including the brain and muscles (Fig. 3). However, in the different diseases associated with primary ACS other, or associated, causal factors are currently explored, such as tumour-derived cachectic glycoproteins.

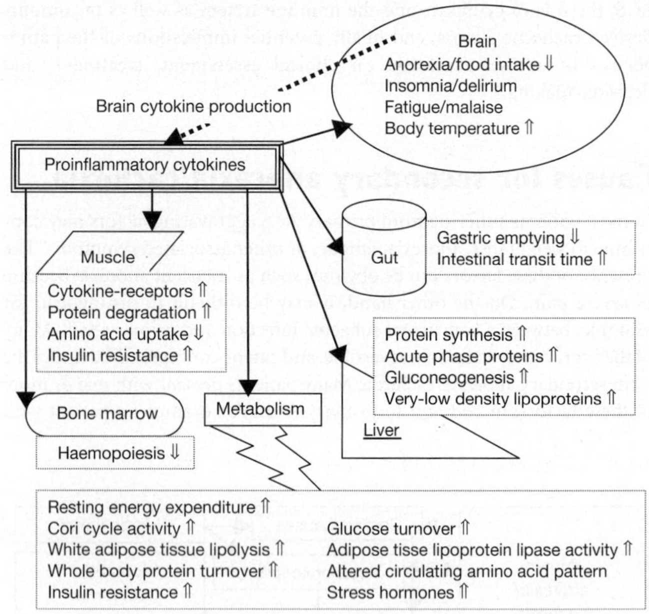

Fig. 3 Cytokine effects on different organs.

Energy balance, metabolic alterations, and muscle wasting: muscle–liver axis

In patients with primary ACS an activation of metabolism is observed, which evades normal regulatory mechanisms. Simplified it looks like the muscles and other systems are obliged to provide all their energy to the liver[13] (Table 4).

Energy balance

The reports about energy expenditure (EE) in patients with ACS are heterogenous. Reasons for conflicting results may include: (i) differences of resting EE and total EE, influenced by physical activity; (ii) variable methods of measuring EE (bicarbonate–urea, or whole-body indirect calorimetry); (iii) unclear data about energy costs of feeding; (iv) heterogeneous patient populations; and (v) calculating EE in relation to body weight rather than lean body mass. However, more precise approaches to measurement demonstrated that the energy expenditure[15] in relation to lean body mass is indeed increased in cancer anorexia/cachexia.[16] This hypermetabolic state is followed by a preterminal hypometabolism.

Carbohydrate metabolism

The glucose turnover is increased, including both the rates of hepatic gluconeogenesis[17] and the activity of futile cycles, such as recycling via lactate (Cori cycle).[18] The insulin secretory response is delayed in ACS without a major difference in overall magnitude. This results in a delayed clearance of glucose. A relative glucose intolerance and insulin resistance is present with a decreased muscle insulin-stimulated glucose uptake. This is most likely a result of impaired insulin responsiveness, rather than an abnormal insulin sensitivity, suggesting a post-receptor defect in insulin action.[19,20] The anabolic effects of insulin on skeletal muscle are abolished during inflammation[21] or infusion of TNF-alpha, indicating an insulin resistance regarding protein synthesis. In addition, increases in counter-regulatory hormones, such as glucagon or glucocorticoids, also seem to be involved.[17] The concentration of ketone bodies, which seem to inhibit muscle proteolysis in starvation, is decreased through impaired ketogenesis and increased peripheral uptake. However, in patients with chronic heart failure blood ketone bodies are elevated in proportion to the severity of cardiac dysfunction and neurohormonal activation (noradrenaline, growth hormone, interleukin-6).[22]

Lipid metabolism

In adipose tissue during primary ACS the glucose transport and *de novo* lipogenesis is inhibited and lipolysis activated.[23] In contrast in the liver lipogenesis is increased, and hypertriglyceridaemia is present. Carnitine is involved in transporting long-chain fatty acids into the mitochondrial matrix. However, at the present time its role in cancer cachexia remains to be elucidated. In tumour-bearing rats the hepatic mitochondrial outer-membrane carnitine palmitoyltransferase I (CPT I) was reported to be unaffected by the presence of the extra-hepatic tumour, whereas the mitochondrial inner-membrane carnitine palmitoyltransferase II (CPT II) activity was markedly decreased.[24]

During cachectic states an increase in brown adipose tissue thermogenesis is reported. The uncoupling protein-1 (UCP-1) or thermogenin uncouples oxidative phosphorylation in the mitochondrial compartment leading to energy released as heat rather than used for ATP-synthesis. The recently described UCP-2 and UCP-3 are elevated in skeletal muscle during tumour growth.[25]

Protein metabolism

Whole-body protein turnover is increased in cachexia in association with progressive disease.[26] Protein synthesis shifts from normal muscle protein and other tissue protein synthesis to increased hepatic protein synthesis. The muscle fibrillar synthesis and the overall muscle amino acid uptake is reduced. A downregulation of the MyoD mRNA[27] has been reported, and DNA fragmentation is increased, suggesting apoptosis.[28] The proteolysis of myofibrils is increased, provided mostly by the activated ATP–ubiquitin–proteasome system.[29] The two other proteolytic pathways (lysosomal cathepsins, calpains), are not upregulated, rather they are decreased.[30] The ATP–ubiquitin–proteasome system seems to be a common final pathway, with probable involvement of a lipoxygenase metabolite, both for muscle loss in starvation and cachexia.[31] The liver-protein synthesis is reprioritized with increased production of acute phase proteins (serum-amyloid A, C-reactive protein, haptoglobin, fibrinogen, among others), but decreased albumin synthesis.[32] The presence of acute phase protein reaction correlates with survival in cancer patients.[33] The circulating amino acid pattern changes in catabolic conditions.[13] The turnover of branched-chain amino acids (leucine, isoleucine, valine), which are normally poorly metabolized in the liver, but well in the muscle, is increased. The muscle increases the production of alanine and glutamine. Alanine is an alternative glycolytic endproduct to lactate for safe transport of 3C-ketoacids to the liver. The turnover of glutamine increases in order to provide a major source for energy as well as for nucleic acid synthesis, and also for storage of nitrogen as an alternative to ammonia.[34] Feeding, without modification of the complex metabolic alterations, was reported to increase only the synthesis of muscle protein without influencing proteolysis,[35] and to accelerate the acute phase protein synthesis while not influencing albumin synthesis.[36] Several of these metabolic abnormalities, such as increased energy expenditure[3,37] or insulin resistance,[38] are reported in patients with primary ACS other than cancer, such as AIDS-wasting or cardiac cachexia.

Table 4 Interrelationship between skeletal muscle and liver in ACS

Muscle	
Proteolysis	⇑
Glucagon-synthesis	⇑
Alanine-synthesis	⇑
BCAA[a]-uptake	⇑
Muscle-protein synthesis	⇓
Lactate-production	⇑
Ketone bodies utilization	⇓
Liver	
Acute phase protein synthesis	⇑
Alanine and glucagon uptake (liver unable to process BCAA)	⇑
Very-low density lipoproteins	⇑

[a] BCAA: branched-chain amino acids (leucine, isoleucine, valine).

Neurohumoral circuits and food intake: gut–brain axis

Food intake and consequently energy homeostasis is regulated by a highly complex process involving taste sensation, neural, and humoral signals from the gastrointestinal tract and neurotransmitters and peptides in the hypothalamus or other brain regions[39] (Fig. 4).

Psychosocial and spiritual distress

These can influence the sensation of hunger, appetite, or satiety, culminating in expression of total suffering.[40] This cause of anorexia may be unrecognized, even when a careful assessment for causes of secondary anorexia/cachexia is performed.

Satiety and adiposity signals from the periphery to the brain

Satiety signals

Such signals from the upper gastrointestinal tract, the liver, and from peptides such as cholecystokinin (CCK) are transmitted through the vagus nerve and sympathetic fibres to the autonomic centres of the hindbrain and possibly to the forebrain. The vagus transmits meal-related signals (mechanical, chemical, hormonal) elicited by nutrient contact with the gastrointestinal tract to sites in the central nervous system that mediate ingestive behaviour.[41] The vagus also seems to be important in mediating anorexic effects of some,[42] but not all,[43] proinflammatory cytokines produced in the peritoneum.

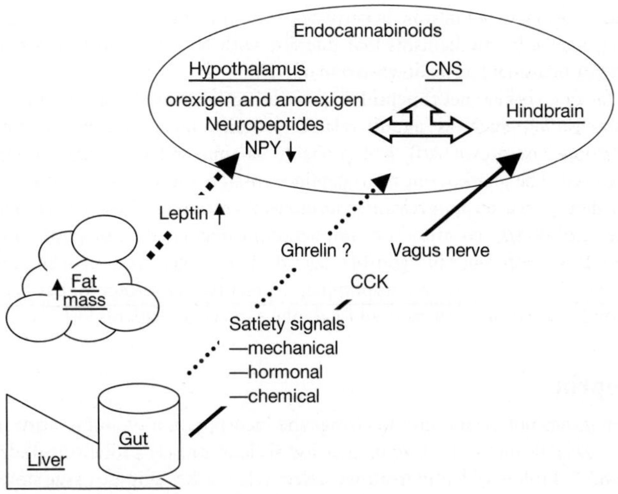

Fig. 4 Aspect of neurohumoral regulation of food intake. CNS, Central nervous system; NPY, Neuropeptide; CCK, Cholecystokinine.

Ghrelin

This is a recently discovered hormone produced predominantly by the stomach; smaller amounts are formed in the bowel, pituitary, and hypothalamus.[44] Ghrelin has adipogenic and orexigenic effects, which are independent of its ability to stimulate growth hormone secretion.[45] Chronic administration of ghrelin was reported to improve left ventricular dysfunction and attenuates development of cardiac cachexia in rats with heart failure.[46] Ghrelin was found to have gastroprokinetic activity, as well as orexigenic activity through action on the hypothalamic neuropeptide Y (NPY) receptor, which was lost after vagotomy.[47] Ghrelin expression in the stomach was found to be increased by fasting but decreased by administration of leptin, as well as by interleukin-1beta. In nine human volunteers intravenous ghrelin was found to promote appetite and food intake compared to placebo (saline), but did not influence gastric emptying.[48]

Adiposity signals

Peripheral adiposity signals are provided by leptin[49] (secreted by adipocytes) and insulin (secreted by the endocrine pancreas in proportion to adiposity). They are proposed to stimulate catabolic pathways (mediated by melanocortins) and inhibit anabolic pathways (NPY, agouti-related protein). They can act in the gastrointestinal tract[50] and centrally.

Hypothalamus and central nervous system control of food intake

Hypothalamus

In the hypothalamus several neuropeptide-containing pathways mediating leptin and insulin action are under investigation.[51]

Neuropeptide-Y

NPY is an anabolic signalling molecule. NPY expression is stimulated by falls in circulating concentrations of insulin and leptin, both of which inhibit the hypothalamic NPY neurons.[52] NPY is expressed in a subset of hypothalamic neurons, which also express leptin receptors (OB-Rb). Increased hypothalamic NPY expression is reported in underfed and insulin-deficient diabetic rats, suggesting a role in stimulating hunger and hyperphagia. However, mice lacking NPY have been found with intact feeding responses to leptin.[53] A recent study with cachectic (weight loss of 19 per cent compared to pair-fed controls) MAC16-tumour-bearing rats reported a normal regulation of leptin (decreased concentration in relation to loss of fat tissue, upregulation of hypothalamic OB-Rb mRNA), insulin (reduction in both groups), and NPY (increase of hypothalamic NPY mRNA).[54] These results suggest that in anorexia/cachexia related to cancer, a normal hypothalamic hyperphagic response to weight loss is overridden, maybe by mechanisms that interfere with NPY transport or release and/or neuronal targets downstream of NPY.

Several other neuropeptides promoting increased energy intake (*orexigenic*), such as agouti-related protein, melanin-concentrating hormone, or orexin A/B, and probably galanin and noradrenaline are involved. The *anorexigenic* neuropeptides entail α-melanocyte-stimulating hormone, corticotropin-releasing hormone, thyrotropin-releasing hormone, interleukin-1β, cocaine- or amphetamine-regulated transcript, and probably serotonin, glucagon-like peptide 1, neurotensin, urocortin, and others.[39,51] Levels of free tryptophan, a precursor of serotonin, has been found to correlate with reduced food intake in cancer patients.[55]

Leptin

Leptin has not been found to change the incorporation of amino acids in the skeletal muscle *in vitro* or increase skeletal muscle protein degradation.[56] Prolonged leptin treatment selectively reduces adipose tissue stores while the muscle mass remains unaffected.[57] It is possible that a deficiency in leptin could contribute to immune dysfunction.[58] TNF-α has been shown to directly regulate leptin secretion of adipocytes *in vitro*, providing cytokine-induced hyperleptinemia.[59] However, the opposite findings are also reported.[60] Leptin levels are increased in some models of inflammation.[61,62] In patients undergoing elective surgery a positive correlation was reported for acute phase response and plasma leptin.[63] However, in patients with cancer-related anorexia/cachexia the leptin concentrations seem to be decreased, rather than increased, when compared with healthy controls.[64,65] A recent study reported an inverse correlation of increased IL-6 with decreased leptin in 16 advanced cancer patients.[66] In 73 patients with 'incurable' cancer a greater than 50 per cent decline in appetite during the last 2 months and lower values of NPY were found than in historic controls, but no difference in leptin or cholecystokinin-8 levels[67] were detected.

Endocannabinoid system

Cannabinoid receptor type 1 (CB1) receptor knockout mice eat less than their wild-type littermates, and the CB1 antagonist SR141716A reduces food intake in wild-type but not in knockout mice. Defective leptin signaling is associated with elevated hypothalamic, but not cerebellar, levels of endocannabinoids (in obese db/db and ob/ob mice and Zucker rats) and acute leptin treatment of normal rats and ob/ob mice reduces anandamide and 2-arachidonoyl glycerol in the hypothalamus. These findings may indicate that endocannabinoids in the hypothalamus can tonically activate CB1 receptors to maintain food intake and form part of the neural circuitry regulated by leptin.[68] The endocannabinoid system was found to play a vital role in milk suckling, and hence in growth and development during the early stages of mouse life. The endocannabinoid 2-arachidonoyl glycerol is found in human milk. The administration of the CB1 antagonist SR141716A to newborn mice resulted in death within a week. This effect was reversed by feeding the mice Δ-9-THC, which binds to CB1 receptors, but not by cannabidinol, which binds to the CB2 receptor.[69]

Melanocortin signaling system

The central melanocortin signaling system was found to remain active in cachectic tumour-bearing rats, despite marked loss of body weight. This system would be expected to be downregulated to conserve energy stores. The intracerebroventricular injection of SHU9119, a melanocortin receptor antagonist, was found to increase food intake and promote weight gain in cachectic tumour-bearing rats, but not in their pair-fed controls. Interestingly, intracerebroventricular injection of both ghrelin and NPY did not improve oral intake or result in weight gain.[70]

Autonomic failure

Changes in autonomic nerve function (autonomic failure) may contribute to ACS. In 43 patients with advanced (locally recurrent or metastatic) breast cancer 52 per cent of cardiovascular autonomic insufficiency tests were abnormal, in contrast to healthy controls (20 patients) with 7 per cent abnormal tests. In cancer patient's abnormal tests were correlated with decreased performance status, malnutrition, and increased basal heart rate.[71] In five patients with advanced breast, thyroid, and prostate cancers, complaining of unexplained chronic nausea and anorexia, an increased mean gastric emptying time in association with abnormal cardiovascular autonomic tests were reported.[72] Several of the symptoms of autonomic disorders, which are briefly discussed below, are present in patients with advanced cancer: orthostatic abnormalities (postural hypotension), male sexual dysfunction, urinary incontinence, gastrointestinal symptoms (gastroparesis, pseudo-bowel obstruction, diarrhoea, constipation), and sleep dysfunction, suggesting a potential role of autonomic disorders in patients with advanced cancer.

The autonomic nervous system, through the sympathetic and parasympathetic pathways, supplies and influences every organ in the body. It closely integrates vital processes, such as blood pressure and body temperature.[73] Autonomic disorders are an increasingly recognized group of diseases, which may be localized (e.g. Horner's syndrome, Holmes–Adie pupil) or systemic. Three groups of systemic primary dysautonomia (pure autonomic failure, Parkinson's disease with autonomic failure, multiple-system atrophy, including Shy–Drager syndrome with pure orthostatic hypotension) have been defined.[74]

The symptoms of autonomic disorders have been proposed to be grouped into nine domains: orthostatic; secretomotor, including sudomotor; male sexual dysfunction; urinary; gastrointestinal, including gastroparesis; diarrhoea; constipation; pupillomotor, including visual symptoms; vasomotor; reflex syncope; and sleep function.[75]

Several gastrointestinal diseases may be linked to autonomic disorders. Primary enteric neuropathies may cause gastrointestinal motor dysfunction.[76] Idiopathic slow transit constipation has been hypothesized to be a consequence of pelvic autonomic dysfunction. Altered autonomic function also has been involved in patients with gastroesophageal reflux disease, as well as functional disorders, such as irritable bowel syndrome or functional dyspepsia.

Secondary autonomic disorders may include autonomic neuropathy secondary to neurotoxic treatments, or as a consequence of degenerative neuropathies associated with diabetes mellitus or amyloidosis.[77] Tumour invasion of the sympathetic ganglia can result in pseudo-obstruction. Spinal cord pathology may also cause autonomic neuropathy. Gastrointestinal forms of a paraneoplastic neurological syndrome (such as polymyositis and Eaton–Lambert syndrome) may represent secondary autonomic failure. Paraneoplastic gastrointestinal motor dysfunction can precede diagnosis of the cancer by many months.[78]

Growth hormone, IGFs, anabolic (androgenic) hormones: somatotropic axis

The complex system of growth hormone (GH), insulin-like growth factors (IGFs), and anabolic (androgenic) hormones has been observed to be altered in patients with catabolic illnesses, contributing to wasting of lean body mass.[79] Among the diseases associated with primary ACS, these changes and their treatment have been best studied in patients with AIDS-wasting, and to a far lesser extent in cancer patients. A possible reason might be that alterations of the somatotropic axis are a more prominent feature in AIDS primary ACS compared to cancer primary ACS, where metabolic and neuroendocrine alterations are more predominant. Alternatively it might be argued that due to (outdated[80]) concerns about tumour growth stimulation by GH, the investigation of this axis is underexplored in cancer patients.

Growth hormone/IGFs

Regulation

GH promotes nitrogen retention and improves the nitrogen balance. These anabolic effects on protein metabolism are mediated primarily through an increase in protein synthesis.[81] It is unclear, how GH acts directly on the skeletal muscle to stimulate its growth. The GH receptor mRNA is present on skeletal muscle, but specific binding of GH to skeletal muscle or to myoblasts in culture remains to be clearly demonstrated.

Circulating GH acts on the liver to stimulate expression of the IGF-I and IGFBP3 genes, resulting in increased levels of these proteins in the circulation, and it stimulates expression of IGF-I genes in skeletal muscle. However, skeletal muscle IGF-I expression can be elevated in the absence of GH.

IGFs are mitogens, which play a pivotal role in regulation of cell proliferation, differentiation, and apoptosis. These effects are mediated through the IGF-I receptor, at least six IGF-binding proteins (IGFBP), and IGFBP proteases.[82]

IGF-I and IGF-II stimulate many anabolic responses in myoblasts, as they do in other cell types, and are critical factors in skeletal muscle development, regeneration, and hypertrophy. Since the skeletal muscle fibres are incapable of DNA synthesis, muscle growth and regeneration relies on proliferation and subsequent differentiation of undifferentiated skeletal muscle precursor cells, the myoblasts. IGF-I and IGF-II have the unusual property of stimulating both proliferation and differentiation of myoblasts.[83]

The effects of IGFs are significantly modulated by IGFBPs secreted by myoblasts. Insulin-like growth factor-binding protein-1 (BP-1) is a multifunctional protein that binds IGF-I in solution and integrins on the cell surface. BP-1 was shown to inhibit IGF-I-mediated protein synthesis by binding to IGF-I, and, acting independently of IGF-I, inhibit protein degradation.[84]

Myoblasts also express sufficient amounts of autocrine IGF-II to stimulate myogenesis. Autocrine expression of IGFs is widely seen in cells responding to mitogenic stimuli, they may be seen as extracellular second messengers mediating many actions of agents that stimulate cell proliferation.

Interesting findings are reported from rats flying in space: in the microgravity environment their muscle weight decreased 19–24 per cent, paralleled by increased myostatin/beta-actin mRNA ratios, increased myostatin protein levels, decreased IGF-II mRNA, unchanged IGF-I mRNA, and unchanged proteolysis markers (3-methyl histidine, ubiquitin mRNA, proteasome 2C mRNA),[85] suggesting a downregulation of protein synthesis without activation of proteolysis.

Systemic inflammation (sepsis) and GH/IGFs

Catabolic illnesses induce a decrease in protein synthesis and an increase in proteolysis, as discussed above. These alterations in protein metabolism during catabolic diseases are found to be paralleled by an acquired resistance to GH and GH-mediated induction of IGF-I.[86] It is assumed that increased levels of inflammatory cytokines can inhibit the effects of GH on target tissues. Accordingly, GH has been found to have reduced effectiveness in retarding protein catabolism in septic patients and is associated with increased mortality in critically ill patients.[87]

Likewise, IGF-I was decreased in sepsis,[88] whereas its binding protein (IGFBP-1) is over-expressed and accumulates in skeletal muscle during catabolic illnesses. Muscle protein synthesis was reported decreased in association with endotoxins.[89] In muscle cells of burned rats IGF-I treatment both *in vitro* and *in vivo* was shown to block the catabolic response.[90] However, this effect was not seen in muscles from septic rats incubated *in vitro* with IGF-I, even at high hormone concentrations, suggesting development of IGF-I resistance.[91] In contrast to the inability of IGF-I to inhibit proteolysis, protein synthesis was found to be stimulated by intravenous IGF-I even during sepsis.[92] Likewise, the administration of a binary complex of IGF-I complexed with IGF binding protein-3 (IGFBP-3) attenuated the sepsis-induced inhibition of protein synthesis.[88] Accordingly *in vivo* experiments in septic rats revealed a reversal of the decreased muscle protein synthesis by IGF-I, but no effect on the increased myofibrillar muscle protein breakdown, even though a reduction of ubiquitin and $E2_{14k}$ mRNA levels was achieved.[93]

GH/IGFs in primary ACS

In primary ACS a decrease of IGF-I is consistently reported in patients with cancer, cardiac cachexia, and AIDS, whereas few studies focused on GH alterations.

In 21 cachectic patients with chronic heart failure, an increase in total GH and immunologically intact GH, and a decrease in GH-binding protein, IGF-BP3 and IGF-I, was found, compared to 51 non-cachectic patients with chronic heart failure and 26 healthy control subjects.[94]

In 20 patients with lung cancer and weight loss an association between loss of body cell mass and IGF-I was found, in addition to a correlation with inflammation.[95]

From advanced breast cancer patients decreased IGF-I levels are reported, which seem to increase during treatment with megestrol acetate. In those patients an increased IGFBP-3 protease activity was found and may account for the decreased IGF-I levels. The same group demonstrated, in 128 patients with newly diagnosed breast cancer, positive correlations of an increased IGFBP-3 proteolysis associated with invasive cancer compared with DCIS/benign conditions, with tumour mass, as well as with presence of metastases and stage, but a negative correlation with IGF-I and IGF-II.[96] In 16 patients with metastatic breast cancer treated with diethylstilboestrol (5 mg, three times daily) a significant decrease of IGF-I, IGF-II, free IGF-I, IGFBP-2, IGFBP-3, and IGFBP-3 protease activity was found, but there was a significant increase of IGFBP-1, and IGFBP-4.[97]

Administration of GH was observed to increase lean body mass in patients with cardiac cachexia,[98] aging,[99] chronic obstructive pulmonary disease,[100] or AIDS wasting.[101] Results from IGF-I substitution are available only from studies in rats, where a reduction of weight loss is reported during starvation, diabetes, or during dexamethasone treatment. Only preliminary data are available from patients with cancer-related ACS, allowing no conclusion as to whether GH supplementation may reduce skeletal muscle loss (see Chapter 8.4.4).

Anabolic (androgenic) steroids

The effects of testosterone and its (mostly) less androgenic derivatives (e.g. nandrolone, oxandrolone, fluoxymesterone, oxymetholone, stanazolol, danazol, methandrostenolone) are mediated by only one androgen receptor. Testosterone levels gradually decrease as a normal consequence of aging, and can lead to a decrease of bone mass, reduced bone marrow activity, causing anaemia, reduced muscle strength, and diminished sexual function in men and in women.[102] In addition behavioural and cognitive deficits have been found to be associated with hypogonadism.[103] In women normal values of testosterone are not well defined, that is, in postmenopausal states. In women a syndrome of relative androgen deficiency has been proposed. It has been suggested to be associated with alterations in mood, and energy, as well as sexual function.[104]

Testosterone used in supraphysiologic doses was found to enhance muscle size and strength in eugonadal men.[105] Testosterone replacement in hypogonadal men, such as elderly patients, was reported to increase lean body mass,[106] and in some, but not all studies, bone mineral density, haematocrit, prostate volume, self-reported sense of energy and sexual function, muscle size, and strength. The merits of hormone replacement in a normal ageing population are presently debated.

Serum testosterone levels are decreased in primary ACS associated with HIV-infection, probably mostly due to hypogonadotropic hypogonadism.[107] In HIV-infected men serum testosterone levels are lower in those with weight loss,[107] correlate with deficits in muscle mass, low Karnofsky scores, and disease progression.[108,109] Likewise low testosterone levels were found in female HIV patients.[110] Therapy with testosterone or its derivatives was found to be beneficial in HIV-infected patients, that is, resulting in an increase of lean body mass and other improvements in some studies (muscle size and strength, haemoglobin), in both hypogonadal and eugonadal patients. Likewise beneficial effects of testosterone therapy have been reported from HIV-infected women (see Chapter 8.4.4). Interestingly exercise was found in one study to increase body weight, muscle mass and strength in hypogonadal HIV-infected men to the same amount as testosterone replacement, and the combination of both did not increase the gain.[111]

The prevalence of hypogonadism in cancer-related primary ACS is not well known. These patients may have hypogonadism due to impaired hypothalamic-pituitary axis function, anorexia/cachexia, antineoplastic treatments, or opioid therapy.[112] Preliminary reports documented lower testosterone levels in more than half of the patients with advanced cancer.[113] In 44 adult male patients with disseminated cancer, 82 per cent were less than 90 per cent of their ideal body weight, 66 per cent had decreased serum testosterone.[114] In 36 patients with pancreatic adenocarcinoma or other malignancies serum testosterone was found to be lower than in 29 patients with non-malignant conditions.[115] In 20 male patients with lung cancer the patients with weight loss less than 10 per cent had higher serum testosterone values (21.5 ± 5.6 nmol/l) than those with weight loss greater than 10 per cent (13.2 ± 7.5 nmol/l), and a correlation between testosterone and loss of lean body mass was found.[95] In patients with advanced cancer only three clinical trials with anabolic (androgenic) hormones are reported. The treatments, two with nandrolone decanoate alone and in combination with chemotherapy and one with fluoxymesterone, had a minor effect on improving weight loss (see Chapter 8.4.4).

Chronic renal failure is associated with gonadal dysfunction, which is probably principally due to aberrant neuroendocrine regulation of GnRH secretion.[116] Therapy with anabolic androgenic steroids has been found to be beneficial in patients with chronic renal failure; for example, nandrolone was reported to improve lean body mass, function, and fatigue compared with placebo.[117]

Likewise in patients with COPD levels of free testosterone are reported decreased, both in patients without and with concurrent corticosteroid treatment.[118] Preliminary studies report that treatment with anabolic steroids increases fat-free mass in patients with ACS associated with COPD,[119] including male patients undergoing long-term glucocorticoid treatment.[120]

Alterations of the beta-2 adrenergic system have rarely been described in primary ACS, but animal and human data suggest a therapeutic role of beta-2-adrenergic agonists, which have anabolic effects. They were found to promote muscle growth/hypertrophy and muscle strength, paralleled by a reduction of the body fat component, without requiring an increased food intake or exercise. In tumour-bearing animals a normalization of protein breakdown rates was achieved by beta-2-agonists through a decrease in hyperactivation of the ATP–ubiquitin-dependent proteolytic pathway. However, in heart-failure-related primary ACS no effect of sustained-released salbutamol was found on muscle strength or fatigue in a small study (see Chapter 8.4.4).

In critically-ill patients thyroid function may be altered, manifest by the transient sick-euthyreot syndrome, where TSH, T3, as well as T4 are lowered. Administration of intraarterial TNF-alpha was reported to cause the euthyreot-sick syndrome.[121] However, in patients with cancer-related ACS, even though patients are often sick, preliminary data suggest a syndrome different from the euthyreot-sick syndrome. No decrease of T3 and T4, despite an ongoing catabolic state, was observed in cancer ACS, whereas TSH levels seem not to be altered.[122] Likewise in patients with HIV infection unusual prolonged maintenance of normal T3 levels was reported.[123]

Cytokines

Countless studies implicate cytokines in the pathogenesis of primary ACS in several diseases. For example, in patients with lung cancer a correlation of weight loss and height-adjusted lean body mass with sTNFR-p55 and sTNFR-p75 (soluble tumour necrosis factor receptors, respectively, of molecular masses 55 and 75 kDa), but not with IL-6, was found.[95] In patients with non-small-cell lung cancer a positive correlation between

Table 5 Proinflammatory and anti-inflammatory cytokines

Proinflammatory cytokines
Interleukin-1
Interleukin-6
Tumour necrosis factor-α
Interferon-γ
Anti-inflammatory cytokines
Interleukin-4
Interleukin-9
Interleukin-10
Interleukin-12
Interleukin-15
Soluble TNF receptor

sTNF-55 and resting energy expenditure was shown.[124] A correlation between increased serum IL-6 and weight loss was found in patients with non-small-cell lung cancer.[125] Other examples are patients with chronic heart failure, in whom increased TNF-alpha levels were associated with exercise intolerance and neurohormonal (catecholamine) activation,[126] as well as geriatric patients, for whom a correlation between the reduction of cytokine levels (TNFR-p55, TNFR-p75, sIL-2R, IL-6) after megestrol acetate treatment and fat-free mass was reported.[127] However, the relative role of proinflammatory cytokines in the pathogenesis of primary ACS may be different in the various diseases, with variable alterations of the three main mechanisms (axis) (Table 5).

Acute phase response as a physiological mechanism

Several of the clinical and metabolic features of the ACS may resemble a sustained or protracted acute phase response. The acute phase response is a physiological reaction of adult mammals towards tissue damage or infection. It involves a variety of rapid systemic changes, including a profound change in the synthesis of plasma proteins, hypermetabolism, fever, chills, somnolence, and anorexia. The acute phase response is mediated by proinflammatory cytokines, such as IL-6, IL-1, as well as TNF-alpha, IFN-gamma, or leukaemia inhibitory factor. The role of T-cell helper 1 and helper 2 subsets remains to be elucidated in primary ACS.

Proinflammatory cytokines mimic features of primary ACS

TNF-alpha administration can promote weight loss, increased energy expenditure, anorexia, acute phase protein response, increased thermogenesis, alterations in lipid metabolism and adipose tissue dissolution, insulin resistance, muscle wasting including activation of the ATP-dependent ubiquitin–proteasome pathway, inhibition of the myogenic differentiation, protein breakdown, and increased branched chain amino acid metabolism. In tumour-bearing mice, a soluble pegylated 55-kDA TNF-alpha receptor construct improved food intake and led to weight gain compared to a vehicle-treated control group.[128] In contrast in rats bearing the Yoshida AH-130 acites hepatoma, treatment with goat anti-mTNF-alpha IgG did not affect weight loss but decreased protein degradation rates in heart, liver, and gastrocnemius muscle.[129]

IL-6 is an inductor of the acute phase response,[124] but seems to have few effects on TNF-alpha.[130] Whether IL-6 directly causes muscle catabolism or an induction of weight loss is controversial. Some groups found an involvement of IL-6 in experimental cachexia,[131] whereas others found that IL6 did not cause weight loss in normal mice, but was associated with an increased acute phase protein production.[132] In mice bearing the colon-26 adenocarcinoma, serum IL-6 was associated with progression of cachexia, and administration of anti-IL6 immunoglobulin reduced the loss of gastrocnemius muscle.[133] The role of IL-6 may therefore be an epiphenomenon of the host cytokine cascade, mediating increased acute phase protein production, rather than being the key element in mediating muscle wasting and cachexia. However, blood levels of IL-6[134] or of acute phase proteins[33] in patients with anorexia/cachexia correlate with weight loss and survival.

IFN-gamma and IL-1 were found to have procachectic activity, including the activation of muscle proteolysis.[135] In 64 patients with pancreatic adenocarcinoma and in 101 healthy controls it was observed that the possession of a genotype resulting in increased IL-1b production was associated with shortened survival and increased serum CRP level.[136]

In vivo data from cytokine gene knockout mice showed that weight loss from implanted experimental tumours was not improved by knockout of the host cytokines TNF-alpha, IL12, or interferon-gamma, but that the host cytokine IL-6 could play a role in promoting an acute phase response. These data may suggest that these host cytokines could be less important in promoting primary ACS than tumour-derived factors.[137]

Limitations of blood levels to assess cytokine effects

Systemic blood levels of cytokines only partially reflect their local effects. Paracrine–autocrine interactions within organs can sustain cytokine production independently of cytokine concentrations in the circulation. Besides the systemic effects of proinflammatory cytokines during an acute phase response, their locally mediated effects are increasingly recognized, such as upregulation of cytokine receptors of muscle cells or central nervous system effects of cytokines, as discussed below.

This may explain why the association of increased TNF-alpha levels in the blood of cancer patients with primary ACS is not consistent: some studies report a correlation of TNF-alpha with weight loss,[138,139] while others do not.[140,141] Technical problems in measuring TNF-alpha and other cytokines may explain some of these inconsistent results. However, in patients with cachexia caused by parasitic infections increased TNF-alpha concentrations were technically detectable 15 years ago.[142] Since many cytokines are very short lived in the blood, increasingly, cytokine receptors, such as the soluble TNF-alpha receptors (sTNF-R55 and 75), are monitored[95,126] instead.

Local cytokine effects in the brain

The central nervous effects of peripherally administrated cytokines (IL-2, interferon-alpha, TNF-alpha) are well-known side effects of these treatments. Peripheral inflammatory responses, such as those caused by infections or cytokine administration, are associated with increased brain cytokine synthesis and release.[143] The phenomenon of anorexia, as observed during anorexia/cachexia, may be therefore directly related to peripheral cytokines acting in the brain. Besides systemic effects of cytokines on the brain, local cytokine effects have been shown in animal models. For example, athymic mice were injected intracerebrally with human A431 epidermoid carcinoma or OVCAR3 ovarian carcinoma and developed anorexia and weight loss within 7–10 days before a large tumour developed.[144] In contrast mice injected intraperitoneally or subcutaneously developed tumours without evidence of anorexia. Likewise intra-cerebral injected GBLF glioma cells, used as a control, did not induce cachexia until day 20, when the tumour was large. Measurement of cytokines in the brain revealed that the carcinoma cells produced (human) cytokines, such as IL-1, IL-6, TNF-alpha, and LIF. Of the brain cytokines originating from the host (murine), only IL-6 was increased in the A431-bearing mice. The described effects occurred exclusively locally in the brain, since serum levels of both murine (host) and human (tumour) cytokines were not predictive of cancer cachexia development. Administration of IL-6 receptor monoclonal antibody, concomitant with tumour cells, resulted in increased survival and in partial attenuation of the signs of wasting. However, this confirmation of the direct IL-6 effect on the brain was found only in the OVCAR3-bearing animals.

Cytokines and muscle

Diverse aspects of skeletal muscle function are regulated by proinflammatory cytokines. For example, it has been shown that TNF-alpha, which activates NF-κB, (i) prevented immature myoblasts from differentiating into major myotubes, (ii) suppressed differentiated myotubes from synthesizing myosin, and (iii) inhibited the synthesis of mRNA encoding the myogenic transcription factor, myo-D, in muscle.[27] The muscle cytokine receptors mediating these functions have recently been characterized. Skeletal muscle of rats was found to express low levels of mRNAs encoding receptors for IL-1, IL-6, interferon, and TNF-alpha. These cytokine receptors were induced by intraperitoneal administration of both endotoxin and TNF-alpha.[145] The capacity of the muscle for receptor induction provides therefore a mechanism for amplification of cytokine responses at the muscle level.

The recently discovered naturally occurring interleukin-15, which has 'IL-2-like' stimulatory activity on T cells, was reported to exert a preventative effect on muscle protein wasting in animal models,[146] illuminating further the complexity of the cytokine–muscle interactions.[137]

Corticosteroids

The role of cortisol in propagation of ACS is not well established. Elevated levels of cortisone and glucagon have been shown in patients with cancer.[122] However, in 20 patients with lung cancer no association between loss of lean body mass and cortisol was reported.[95] Patients with COPD experience increased weight loss during corticosteroid treatment.[7] Infusion of cortisol can cause protein loss, acute phase protein response, increased energy expenditure, and glucose intolerance. Cytokines can trigger circulating cortisol levels and induce proteolysis. *In vivo* data from a mice model failed to show an improvement in weight loss after treatment with mifepristone/RU486, an anticortisol medication.[147]

Tumour-derived catabolic factors

Effective antineoplastic treatments obviously not only shrink (or eliminate) the tumour but also improve tumour-related morbidity. Indeed, there is a growing body of literature documenting the symptomatic effect of antineoplastic treatments, besides the 'classical' oncological outcome measurements (such as response rate, survival, time to progression). For several paraneoplastic phenomena tumour-derived products have been identified and their specific effects have been demonstrated. Recently tumour-derived products mediating anorexia/cachexia have been characterized.

Proteolysis-inducing factor (PIF) is a sulfated glycoprotein detectable in the urine of cancer patients experiencing weight loss.[148] PIF was reported to be associated with an accelerated rate of weight loss in patients with tumours of the pancreatic head, when compared with patients, where PIF was not detectable in urine, who had less weight loss.[149]

Another research group has demonstrated the expression of PIF on tumour tissue from gastrointestinal cancers and has also found detectable PIF in urine associated with weight-loss.[150] Initially PIF, which is a 24-kDa protein, was believed to be a lipid-mobilizing factor,[151] but this is now not thought to be the case.[152]

PIF directly initiates muscle protein degradation, through activation of ATP–ubiquitin–dependent proteolysis,[153] and decreases protein synthesis.[154] These direct effects of PIF, inducing protein as well as muscle catabolism *in vitro* (rat model of cachexia), were found to follow a bell-shaped dose–response with a decrease of effect at higher doses of PIF and tumour burden, respectively. The rapid weight loss caused by PIF was found to be associated with a significant decrease in the weight of the spleen and soleus and gastrocnemius muscle, but with no effect on the weight of the heart or the kidney.[155] The above-described effects were found to be reversible by treatment with specific antibodies against PIF.[154,156]

The exact site of PIF-induced protein degradation is under investigation. PIF induces an accumulation of ubiquitin–protein conjugates in weight-loosing mice.[154] PIF also induces (*in vitro* data from C_2C_{12} myoblasts) an increased release of arachidonic acid with a dose–response curve parallel to that of protein degradation,[154] and arachidonic acid was shown to be rapidly metabolized to prostaglandins E_2, $F_2\alpha$, and 15-HETE (hydroxy-eicosatetraaenoic acid). The role of prostaglandin E_2 in mediating cachexia is under investigation. Increased protein degradation of extremity muscles by prostaglandins was suggested decades ago. In contrast, both in normal and in septic rats no inhibition of the proteolytic rate was achieved by PG_2.[153] Since 15-HETE produced *in vitro* a significant increase in protein degradation with the same bell-shaped dose curve as that produced by PIF, it has been suggested that the effect of PIF could be mediated by an increased synthesis of 15-HETE.[155]

Substantial binding of PIF is reported only for skeletal muscle and liver, as cited by Cabal-Manzano et al.[150] In hepatocyte cultures PIF was found to activate NF-κB resulting in increased IL-8 and IL-6 production, as well as the STAT3 pathway, which is involved in the acute phase protein response.[157] However, in clinical studies, PIF expression and the association with weight loss were found to be independent of the acute phase response.[148]

In summary, some of the above-discussed features of primary ACS, such as metabolic alterations, match observations made about the effects of PIF. At the present time the role of PIF in ACS other than cancer remains to be elucidated.

Lipid mobilizing factor (LMF) has been demonstrated in the serum and urine of cachetic cancer patients, which caused the immediate release of glycerol when intubated with epididymal adipodicytes. LMF was found to also correlate with the extent of weight loss as well as with the response to chemotherapy.[149,151] LMF, a 43-kDa protein, is believed to counteract the two major mechanisms proposed to account for the decrease in body lipids in cancer cachexia, mainly the inhibition of the clearing enzyme lipoprotein lipase, which prevents adipocytes from extracting fatty acids from plasma lipoproteins for storage, as well as the direct stimulation of triglyceride hydrolysis in adipocytes by activation of triglyceride lipase. LMF was reported to induce lipolysis in white adipose tissue by stimulation of cAMP production, mediated possibly through a beta-adrenergic receptor.[158]

The plasma levels of TNF-alpha, IL-5, IL-8, and IL-6 were higher in 24 patients with advanced cancer and elevated parathyroid hormone-related protein (*PTHrP*) than in 26 cancer patients with normal PTHrP. PTHrP was found to correlate with blood levels of IL-6 and TNF-alpha. Anti-PTHrP monoclonal antibodies (Mabs) improved hypercalcaemia, and the author suggests, that when compared with the effects of bisphosphonates and calcitonin, Mab had an effect also on symptoms (food intake, drinking, weight, behaviour) unrelated to hypercalcaemia.[159] PTHrP may therefore be seen as another tumour-derived procachectic factor.

Evolving pathogenesis of the ACS: clinical implications

An understanding of why patients with advanced incurable illnesses lose weight and appetite, and the implications for treatment are still evolving.

Recognition of primary ACS

Patients with advanced incurable illnesses, aware of their weight loss and decreased appetite, consequently express concerns about not eating enough. Fatigue and declining performance status is intuitively associated with insufficient nutritional intake. This belief about the cause of anorexia/cachexia triggers family members to insist on a sufficient amount of the right type of food for their loved one. Likewise, health care professionals did base the concept of providing parenteral or enteral nutrition on the observation, that cancer patients who lose weight really have decreased calorie intake and that they lose fat tissue. Anorexia/cachexia, at least in patients with cancer, was believed to be the result of a nutritional deficit caused by the combination of decreased energy intake due to tumour-related factors, which acted at the satiety centre in the central nervous system, as well as increased energy consumption by the tumour. However, attempts to increase (only) nutritional intake, including aggressive nutritional therapies, did not significantly improve clinical outcomes. The sometimes-achieved weight gain by nutritional therapy was barely associated with an increase in lean body mass, but more with an increase in body water and fat.[160] Nutritional therapy remained controversial in patients with cancer, and was usually found not to be beneficial in patients with far-advanced disease.[161,162]

Pharmacological treatment of the primary ACS

Consequently, the nature of a primary ACS was considered and attempts were made to manipulate the metabolic, neuroendocrine, and anabolic alterations. Disease-modifying treatments, such as antineoplastic therapies for cancer or antiretroviral therapy for AIDS often improve primary ACS. In addition, pharmacological treatments of primary ACS were established. For patients with cancer-related primary ACS three evidence-based therapies are now available (corticosteroids, progestins, and prokinetics) and several new promising drugs (thalidomide, omega-3-fatty acids, ATP, cannabinoids, melatonin) are in the stage of randomized-controlled trials. The options for patients with AIDS-related primary ACS include growth hormone and 9-D-THC. However, not all patients with primary ACS benefit from pharmacological treatments for several reasons. They may suffer from a relevant aggravating factor for anorexia/cachexia (Table 2, Fig. 1). Or they may belong to a subgroup of patients with a distinct primary ACS with variable importance of the pathogenetic mechanism (Fig. 2, Table 3). For example, a cancer patient suffering from a primary ACS involving mostly the somatotropic axis may not profit from appetite-stimulation alone, but may be from anabolic treatments. However, the existence of subgroups of primary ACS remains hypothetical at the present time; in reality it may be impossible to distinguish overlapping anorexia/cachexia conditions in patients with advanced incurable illnesses. A third reason, for a limited benefit from pharmacological treatment for primary ACS, is the individual vulnerability to side-effects, which requires a careful decision-making considering meaningful (symptomatic) outcomes (discussed in the next three chapters).

Identification of aggravating factors of anorexia/cachexia with a starvational component

There is an important subset of patients with anorexia/cachexia, who seem to benefit from nutritional interventions. These patients can be described as those having a relevant starvational component of anorexia/cachexia. Or, in other words, they have relevant aggravating factors contributing to weight loss and anorexia, for example, secondary anorexia/cachexia. Examples of patients with an important actual or predicted starvational component of anorexia/cachexia are patients with (i) bowel obstruction (and slow-growing tumours), (ii) undergoing radiotherapy for head and neck cancers (often presenting with severe dysphagia), (iii) with inadequate dietary intake because of interfering symptoms or psychosocial and financial factors, (iv) undergoing surgery (i.e. upper gastrointestinal tract cancer), and (v) treated in high-dose chemotherapy protocols.

Comprehensive nutritional approaches may therefore be beneficial for some patients with anorexia/cachexia. Clinicians may treat pharmacological the primary ACS ('fix the engine'), but provide inadequate nutritional intake ('give fuel to the engine'). Likewise, social, psychological, economical, and neurological conditions contributing to impaired nutritional intake may be underrecognized.

However, for the diagnosis and assessment of the relative importance of a starvational component of anorexia/cachexia no current assessment instruments are available. Such instruments, which are under development, would facilitate the identification of patients with anorexia/cachexia, which have a higher likelihood of response to nutritional support.

Multidimensional treatment approaches

Current research aims on the one hand to better characterize the primary ACS, maybe allowing the targeting of interventions at multiple, different sites of action, resulting in either individualized therapies of subgroups or the development of combined treatment strategies. On the other hand efforts are made to improve the recognition and characterization of aggravating factors of anorexia/cachexia.

Conclusion

The pathophysiology of anorexia/cachexia is complex and multidimensional. Further characterization of the mechanism and causes of the primary ACS, involving metabolic, neurohormonal, and anabolic alterations, as well as inflammatory responses and specific procachectic molecules, is required for the optimization of therapies. The active screening and assessment of aggravating and reversible factors of anorexia/cachexia, considering multiple (physical, psychosocial, economical, and existential) dimensions, including an estimation of the starvational component of anorexia/cachexia, is crucial for a balanced decision-making.

Further reading

Energy balance, metabolic alterations, and muscle wasting: muscle–liver axis

Argiles, J.M., Busquets, S., and Lopez-Soriano, F.J. (2001). Metabolic interrelationships between liver and skeletal muscle in pathological states. *Life Science* **69** (12), 1345–61.

Tisdale, M.J. (2000). Biomedicine. Protein loss in cancer cachexia. *Science* **289** (5488), 2293–4.

Baracos, V.E. (2001). A deadly combination of anorexia and hypermetabolism. *Current Opinion in Clinical Nutrition and Metabolic Care* **4** (3), 175–7.

Hasselgren, P.O. and Fischer, J.E. (2001). Muscle cachexia: current concepts of intracellular mechanisms and molecular regulation. *Annals of Surgery* **233** (1), 9–17.

Neurohormonal circuits and food intake: gut–brain axis

Schwartz, M.W., Woods, S.C., Porte, D. Jr., Seeley, R.J., and Baskin, D.G. (2000). Central nervous system control of food intake. *Nature* **404** (6778), 661–71.

Ahima, R.S. and Osei, S.Y. (2001). Molecular regulation of eating behavior: new insights and prospects for therapeutic strategies. *Trends in Molecular Medicine* **7** (5), 205–13.

Meguid, M.M., Yang, Z.J., and Gleason, J.R. (1996). The gut–brain brain–gut axis in anorexia: toward an understanding of food intake regulation. *Nutrition* **12** (Suppl. 1), S57–62.

Schwartz, G.J. (2000). The role of gastrointestinal vagal afferents in the control of food intake: current prospects. *Nutrition* **16** (10), 866–73.

Wren, A.M., Seal, L.J., Cohen, M.A., Brynes, A.E., Frost, G.S., Murphy, K.G., Dhillo, W.S., Ghatei, M.A., and Bloom, S.R. (2001). Ghrelin enhances appetite and increases food intake in humans. *Journal of Clinical Endocrinology and Metabolism* **86** (12), 5992.

Growth hormone, IGFs, anabolic (androgenic) hormones: somatotropic axis

Basaria, S., Wahlstrom, J.T., and Dobs, A.S. (2001). Anabolic-androgenic steroid therapy in the treatment of chronic diseases. *Journal of Clinical Endocrinology and Metabolism* **86** (11), 5108–17.

Frost, R.A. and Lang, C.H. (1998). Growth factors in critical illness: regulation and therapeutic aspects. *Current Opinion in Clinical Nutrition and Metabolic Care* **1** (2), 195–204.

Cytokines

Plata-Salaman, C.R. (2000). Central nervous system mechanisms contributing to the cachexia–anorexia syndrome. *Nutrition* **16** (10), 1009–12.

Argiles, J.M. and Lopez-Soriano, F.J. (2000). New mediators in cancer cachexia. *Nestle Nutrition Workshop Series & Clinical Performance Programme* **4**, 147–62 (see also discussion 163–5).

Tumour-derived cachectic factors

Tisdale, M.J. (2000). Catabolism of skeletal muscle proteins and its reversal in cancer cachexia. *Nestle Nutrition Workshop Series & Clinical Performance Programme* **4**, 135–43 (see also discussion 144–6).

References

1. **Holden, C.M.** (1991). Anorexia in the terminally ill cancer patient: the emotional impact on the patient and the family. *The Hospice Journal* **7**, 73–84.
2. **Walsh, D., Donnelly, S., and Rybicki, L.** (2000). The symptoms of advanced cancer: relationship to age, gender, and performance status in 1000 patients. *Supportive Care in Cancer* **8**, 175–9.

3. **Schwenk, A.** et al. (1996). Resting energy expenditure, weight loss, and altered body composition in HIV infection. *Nutrition* **12**, 595–601.
4. **Anker, S.D.** et al. (1997). Wasting as independent risk factor for mortality in chronic heart failure. *Lancet* **349**, 1050–3.
5. **Roongpisuthipong, C.** et al. (2001). Nutritional assessment in various stages of liver cirrhosis. *Nutrition* **17**, 761–5.
6. **Mitch, W.E.** (1998). Robert H Herman Memorial Award in Clinical Nutrition Lecture, 1997. Mechanisms causing loss of lean body mass in kidney disease. *The American Journal of Clinical Nutrition* **67**, 359–66.
7. **Creutzberg, E.C.** et al. (2000). Characterization of nonresponse to high caloric oral nutritional therapy in depleted patients with chronic obstructive pulmonary disease. *American Journal of Respiratory and Critical Care Medicine* **161**, 745–52.
8. **Marchand, V.** et al. (2000). Randomized, double-blind, placebo-controlled pilot trial of megestrol acetate in malnourished children with cystic fibrosis. *Journal of Pediatric Gastroenterology and Nutrition* **31**, 264–9.
9. **Macallan, D.C.** et al. (1998). Whole body protein metabolism in human pulmonary tuberculosis and undernutrition: evidence for anabolic block in tuberculosis. *Clinical Science (London)* **94**, 321–31.
10. **Altemeier, W.A. III.** (2000). What is happening to children with failure to thrive? *Pediatric Annals* **29**, 531 (see also p. 534).
11. **Gallagher, D.** et al. (2000). Weight stability masks sarcopenia in elderly men and women. *American Journal of Physiology, Endocrinology and Metabolism* **279**, E366–75.
12. **Cherel, Y.** et al. (1992). Relationships between lipid availability and protein utilization during prolonged fasting. *Journal of Comparative Physiology. B. Biochemical, Systemic, and Environmental Physiology* **162**, 305–13.
13. **Argiles, J.M., Busquets, S., and Lopez-Soriano, F.J.** (2001). Metabolic interrelationships between liver and skeletal muscle in pathological states. *Life Science* **69**, 1345–61.
14. **Meguid, M.M., Yang, Z.J., and Gleason, J.R.** (1996). The gut–brain brain–gut axis in anorexia: toward an understanding of food intake regulation. *Nutrition* **12**, S57–62.
15. **Gibney, E.** et al. (1997). Total energy expenditure in patients with small-cell lung cancer: results of a validated study using the bicarbonate–urea method. *Metabolism* **46**, 1412–17.
16. **Falconer, J.S.** et al. (1994). Cytokines, the acute-phase response, and resting energy expenditure in cachectic patients with pancreatic cancer. *Annals of Surgery* **219**, 325–31.
17. **Leij-Halfwerk, S.** et al. (2000). Altered hepatic gluconeogenesis during L-alanine infusion in weight-losing lung cancer patients as observed by phosphorus magnetic resonance spectroscopy and turnover measurements. *Cancer Research* **60**, 618–23.
18. **Tayek, J.A.** (1992). A review of cancer cachexia and abnormal glucose metabolism in humans with cancer. *Journal of the American College of Nutrition* **11**, 445–56.
19. **Barber, M.D.** et al. (2000). Metabolic response to feeding in weight-losing pancreatic cancer patients and its modulation by a fish-oil-enriched nutritional supplement. *Clinical Science (London)* **98**, 389–99.
20. **Yoshikawa, T.** et al. (2001). Insulin resistance in patients with cancer: relationships with tumor site, tumor stage, body-weight loss, acute-phase response, and energy expenditure. *Nutrition* **17**, 590–3.
21. **Jurasinski, C., Gray K., and Vary, T.C.** (1995). Modulation of skeletal muscle protein synthesis by amino acids and insulin during sepsis. *Metabolism* **44**, 1130–8.
22. **Lommi, J.** et al. (1996). Blood ketone bodies in congestive heart failure. *Journal of the American College of Cardiology* **28**, 665–72.
23. **Vlassara, H.** et al. (1986). Reduced plasma lipoprotein lipase activity in patients with malignancy-associated weight loss. *Hormone and Metabolic Research* **18**, 698–703.
24. **Seelaender, M.C.** et al. (1998). Carnitine palmitoyltransferase II activity is decreased in liver mitochondria of cachectic rats bearing the Walker 256 carcinosarcoma: effect of indomethacin treatment. *Biochemistry and Molecular Biology International* **44**, 185–93.
25. **Busquets, S.** et al. (2001). Hyperlipemia: a role in regulating UCP3 gene expression in skeletal muscle during cancer cachexia? *FEBS Letters* **505**, 255–8.
26. **Melville, S.** et al. (1990). Increased protein turnover despite normal energy metabolism and responses to feeding in patients with lung cancer. *Cancer Research* **50**, 1125–31.
27. **Guttridge, D.C.** et al. (2000). NF-kappaB-induced loss of MyoD messenger RNA: possible role in muscle decay and cachexia. *Science* **289**, 2363–6.
28. **van Royen, M.** et al. (2000). DNA fragmentation occurs in skeletal muscle during tumor growth: a link with cancer cachexia? *Biochemical and Biophysical Research Communications* **270**, 533–7.
29. **Attaix, D.** et al. (1999). Adaptation of the ubiquitin–proteasome proteolytic pathway in cancer cachexia. *Molecular Biology Reports* **26**, 77–82.
30. **Busquets, S.** et al. (2000). Calpain-3 gene expression is decreased during experimental cancer cachexia. *Biochimica et Biophysica Acta* **1475**, 5–9.
31. **Whitehouse, A.S. and Tisdale, M.J.** (2001). Downregulation of ubiquitin-dependent proteolysis by eicosapentaenoic acid in acute starvation. *Biochemical and Biophysical Research Communications* **285**, 598–602.
32. **Fearon, K.C.H.** et al. (1998). Albumin synthesis rates are not decreased in hypoalbuminemic cachectic cancer patients with an ongoing acute-phase protein response. *Annals of Surgery* **227**, 249–54.
33. **Wigmore, S.J.** et al. (2001). Acute-phase protein response, survival and tumour recurrence in patients with colorectal cancer. *British Journal of Surgery* **88**, 255–60.
34. **De Blaauw, I.** et al. (1997). Increased whole-body protein and glutamine turnover in advanced cancer is not matched by an increased muscle protein and glutamine turnover. *The Journal of Surgical Research* **68**, 44–55.
35. **Bozzetti, F.** et al. (2000). Effect of total parenteral nutrition on the protein kinetics of patients with cancer cachexia. *Tumori* **86**, 408–11.
36. **Barber, M.D.** et al. (2000). Liver export protein synthetic rates are increased by oral meal feeding in weight-losing cancer patients. *American Journal of Physiology, Endocrinology and Metabolism* **279**, E707–14.
37. **Toth, M.J.** et al. (1997). Daily energy requirements in heart failure patients. *Metabolism* **46**, 1294–8.
38. **Swan, J.W.** et al. (1997). Insulin resistance in chronic heart failure: relation to severity and etiology of heart failure. *Journal of the American College of Cardiology* **30**, 527–32
39. **Schwartz, M.W.** et al. (2000). Central nervous system control of food intake. *Nature* **404**, 661–71.
40. **Clark, D.** (1958–1967). 'Total pain', disciplinary power and the body in the work of Cicely Saunders. *Social Science & Medicine* **49**, 727–36.
41. **Schwartz, G.J.** (2000). The role of gastrointestinal vagal afferents in the control of food intake: current prospects. *Nutrition* **16**, 866–73.
42. **Konsman, J.P. and Dantzer, R.** (2001). How the immune and nervous systems interact during disease-associated anorexia. *Nutrition* **17**, 664–8.
43. **Porter, M.H.** et al. (1998). Vagal and splanchnic afferents are not necessary for the anorexia produced by peripheral IL-1beta, LPS, and MDP. *American Journal of Physiology* **275**, R384–9.
44. **Horvath, T.L.** et al. (2001). Minireview: ghrelin and the regulation of energy balance-a hypothalamic perspective. *Endocrinology* **142**, 4163–9.
45. **Nakazato, M.** et al. (2001). A role for ghrelin in the central regulation of feeding. *Nature* **409**, 194–8.
46. **Nagaya, N.** et al. (2001). Chronic administration of ghrelin improves left ventricular dysfunction and attenuates development of cardiac cachexia in rats with heart failure. *Circulation* **104**, 1430–5.
47. **Asakawa, A.** et al. (2001). Ghrelin is an appetite-stimulatory signal from stomach with structural resemblance to motilin. *Gastroenterology* **120**, 337–45.
48. **Wren, A.M.** et al. (2001). Ghrelin enhances appetite and increases food intake in humans. *Journal of Clinical Endocrinology and Metabolism* **86**, 5992.
49. **Friedman, J.M. and Halaas, J.L.** (1998). Leptin and the regulation of body weight in mammals. *Nature* **395**, 763–70.
50. **Matson, C.A. and Ritter, R.C.** (1999). Long-term CCK-leptin synergy suggests a role for CCK in the regulation of body weight. *American Journal of Physiology* **276**, R1038–45.
51. **Wisse, B.E. and Schwartz, M.W.** (2001). Role of melanocortins in control of obesity. *Lancet* **358**, 857–9.

52. **Baskin, D.G.** et al. (1999). Insulin and leptin: dual adiposity signals to the brain for the regulation of food intake and body weight. *Brain Research* **848**, 114–23.

53. **Erickson, J.C., Clegg, K.E., and Palmiter, R.D.** (1996). Sensitivity to leptin and susceptibility to seizures of mice lacking neuropeptide Y. *Nature* **381**, 415–21.

54. **Bing, C.** et al. (2001). Cachexia in MAC16 adenocarcinoma: suppression of hunger despite normal regulation of leptin, insulin and hypothalamic neuropeptide Y. *Journal of Neurochemistry* **79**, 1004–12.

55. **Cangiano, C.** et al. (1994). Cytokines, tryptophan and anorexia in cancer patients before and after surgical tumor ablation. *Anticancer Research* **14**, 1451–5.

56. **Carbo, N.** et al. (2000). Short-term effects of leptin on skeletal muscle protein metabolism in the rat. *The Journal of Nutritional Biochemistry* **11**, 431–5.

57. **Muzzin, P.** et al. (1996). Correction of obesity and diabetes in genetically obese mice by leptin gene therapy. *Proceedings of the National Academy of Sciences of the United States of America* **93**, 14804–8.

58. **Lord, G.M.** et al. (1998). Leptin modulates the T-cell immune response and reverses starvation-induced immunosuppression. *Nature* **394**, 897–901.

59. **Finck, B.N. and Johnson, R.W.** (2000). Tumor necrosis factor-alpha regulates secretion of the adipocyte-derived cytokine, leptin. *Microscopy Research and Technique* **50**, 209–15.

60. **Yamaguchi, M.** et al. (1998). Autocrine inhibition of leptin production by tumor necrosis factor-alpha (TNF-alpha) through TNF-alpha type-I receptor *in vitro*. *Biochemical and Biophysical Research Communications* **244**, 30–4.

61. **Mantzoros, C.S.** et al. (1997). Leptin concentrations in relation to body mass index and the tumor necrosis factor-alpha system in humans. *Journal of Clinical Endocrinology and Metabolism* **82**, 3408–13.

62. **Sarraf, P.** et al. (1997). Multiple cytokines and acute inflammation raise mouse leptin levels: potential role in inflammatory anorexia. *The Journal of Experimental Medicine* **185**, 171–5.

63. **Moses, A.G.** et al. (2001). Leptin and its relation to weight loss, ob gene expression and the acute-phase response in surgical patients. *British Journal of Surgery* **88**, 588–93.

64. **Wallace, A.M., Sattar, N., and McMillan, D.C.** (1998). Effect of weight loss and the inflammatory response on leptin concentrations in gastrointestinal cancer patients. *Clinical Cancer Research* **4**, 2977–9.

65. **Simons, J.P.** et al. (1997). Plasma concentration of total leptin and human lung-cancer-associated cachexia. *Clinical Science (London)* **93**, 273–7.

66. **Mantovani, G.** et al. (2001). Serum values of proinflammatory cytokines are inversely correlated with serum leptin levels in patients with advanced stage cancer at different sites. *Journal of Molecular Medicine* **79**, 406–14.

67. **Jatoi, A.** et al. (2001). Neuropeptide Y, leptin, and cholecystokinin 8 in patients with advanced cancer and anorexia: a North Central Cancer Treatment Group exploratory investigation. *Cancer* **92**, 629–33.

68. **Di Marzo, V.** et al. (2001). Leptin-regulated endocannabinoids are involved in maintaining food intake. *Nature* **410**, 822–5.

69. **Fride, E.** et al. (2001). Critical role of the endogenous cannabinoid system in mouse pup suckling and growth. *European Journal of Pharmacology* **419**, 207–14.

70. **Wisse, B.E.** et al. (2001). Reversal of cancer anorexia by blockade of central melanocortin receptors in rats. *Endocrinology* **142**, 3292–301.

71. **Bruera, E.** et al. (1986). Study of cardiovascular autonomic insufficiency in advanced cancer patients. *Cancer Treatment Reports* **70**, 1383–7.

72. **Bruera, E.** et al. (1987). Chronic nausea and anorexia in advanced cancer patients: a possible role for autonomic dysfunction. *Journal of Pain and Symptom Management* **2**, 19–21.

73. **Mathias, C.J.** (1997). Autonomic disorders and their recognition. *New England Journal of Medicine* **336**, 721–4.

74. **Consensus Committee of the American Autonomic Society and the American Academy of Neurology** (1996). Consensus statement on the definition of orthostatic hypotension, pure autonomic failure, and multiple system atrophy. *Neurology* **46**, 1470.

75. **Suarez, G.A.** et al. (1999). The Autonomic Symptom Profile: a new instrument to assess autonomic symptoms. *Neurology* **52**, 523–8.

76. **De Giorgio, R.** et al. (2000). Primary enteric neuropathies underlying gastrointestinal motor dysfunction. *Scandinavian Journal of Gastroenterology* **35**, 114–22.

77. **Corbo, M. and Balmaceda, C.** (2001). Peripheral neuropathy in cancer patients. *Cancer Investigation* **19**, 369–82.

78. **Lee, H.R.** et al. (2001). Paraneoplastic gastrointestinal motor dysfunction: clinical and laboratory characteristics. *American Journal of Gastroenterology* **96**, 373–9.

79. **Frost, R.A. and Lang, C.H.** (1998). Growth factors in critical illness: regulation and therapeutic aspects. *Current Opinion in Clinical Nutrition and Metabolic Care* **1**, 195–204.

80. **Fiebig, H.H., Dengler, W., and Hendriks, H.R.** (2000). No evidence of tumor growth stimulation in human tumors *in vitro* following treatment with recombinant human growth hormone. *Anticancer Drugs* **11**, 659–64.

81. **Jenkins, R.C. and Ross, R.J.** (1996). Growth hormone therapy for protein catabolism. *The Quarterly Journal of Medicine* **89**, 813–19.

82. **Yu, H. and Rohan, T.** (2000). Role of the insulin-like growth factor family in cancer development and progression. *Journal of the National Cancer Institute* **92**, 1472–89.

83. **Florini, J.R., Ewton, D.Z., and Coolican, S.A.** (1996). Growth hormone and the insulin-like growth factor system in myogenesis. *Endocrine Reviews* **17**, 481–517.

84. **Frost, R.A. and Lang, C.H.** (1999). Differential effects of insulin-like growth factor I (IGF-I) and IGF-binding protein-1 on protein metabolism in human skeletal muscle cells. *Endocrinology* **140**, 3962–70.

85. **Lalani, R.** et al. (2000). Myostatin and insulin-like growth factor-I and -II expression in the muscle of rats exposed to the microgravity environment of the NeuroLab space shuttle flight. *The Journal of Endocrinology* **167**, 417–28.

86. **Jenkins, R.C. and Ross, R.J.** (1996). Acquired growth hormone resistance in catabolic states. *Bailliere's Clinical Endocrinology and Metabolism* **10**, 411–19.

87. **Takala, J.** et al. (1999). Increased mortality associated with growth hormone treatment in critically ill adults. *New England Journal of Medicine* **341**, 785–92.

88. **Svanberg, E.** et al. (2000). IGF-I/IGFBP-3 binary complex modulates sepsis-induced inhibition of protein synthesis in skeletal muscle. *American Journal of Physiology, Endocrinology and Metabolism* **279**, E1145–58.

89. **Lang, C.H.** et al. (2000). Endotoxin-induced decrease in muscle protein synthesis is associated with changes in eIF2B, eIF4E, and IGF-I. *American Journal of Physiology, Endocrinology and Metabolism* **278**, E1133–43.

90. **Fang, C.H.** et al. (1998). Treatment of burned rats with insulin-like growth factor I inhibits the catabolic response in skeletal muscle. *American Journal of Physiology* **275**, R1091–8.

91. **Hobler, S.C.** et al. (1998). IGF-I stimulates protein synthesis but does not inhibit protein breakdown in muscle from septic rats. *American Journal of Physiology* **274**, R571–6.

92. **Jurasinski, C.V. and Vary, T.C.** (1995). Insulin-like growth factor I accelerates protein synthesis in skeletal muscle during sepsis. *American Journal of Physiology* **269**, E977–81.

93. **Fang, C.H.** et al. (2000). Insulin-like growth factor I reduces ubiquitin and ubiquitin-conjugating enzyme gene expression but does not inhibit muscle proteolysis in septic rats. *Endocrinology* **141**, 2743–51.

94. **Anker, S.D.** et al. (2001). Acquired growth hormone resistance in patients with chronic heart failure: implications for therapy with growth hormone. *Journal of the American College of Cardiology* **38**, 443–52.

95. **Simons, J.P.** et al. (1999). Weight loss and low body cell mass in males with lung cancer: relationship with systemic inflammation, acute-phase response, resting energy expenditure, and catabolic and anabolic hormones. *Clinical Science (London)* **97**, 215–23.

96. **Helle, S.I.** et al. (2001). Plasma insulin-like growth factor binding protein-3 proteolysis is increased in primary breast cancer. *British Journal of Cancer* **85**, 74–7.

97. **Helle, S.I.** et al. (2001). Alterations in the insulin-like growth factor system during treatment with diethylstilboestrol in patients with metastatic breast cancer. *British Journal of Cancer* **85**, 147–51.

98. **Osterziel, K.J.** et al. (1998). Randomised, double-blind, placebo-controlled trial of human recombinant growth hormone in patients with chronic heart failure due to dilated cardiomyopathy. *Lancet* **351**, 1233–7.
99. **Papadakis, M.A.** et al. (1996). Growth hormone replacement in healthy older men improves body composition but not functional ability. *Annals of Internal Medicine* **124**, 708–16.
100. **Burdet, L.** et al. (1997). Administration of growth hormone to underweight patients with chronic obstructive pulmonary disease. A prospective, randomized, controlled study. *American Journal of Respiratory and Critical Care Medicine* **156**, 1800–6.
101. **Schambelan, M.** et al. (1996). Recombinant human growth hormone in patients with HIV-associated wasting. A randomized, placebo-controlled trial. Serostim Study Group. *Annals of Internal Medicine* **125**, 873–82.
102. **Morley, J.E.** (2001). Anorexia, body composition, and ageing. *Current Opinion in Clinical Nutrition and Metabolic Care* **4**, 9–13.
103. **Wang, C.** et al. (1996). Testosterone replacement therapy improves mood in hypogonadal men—a clinical research center study. *The Journal of Clinical Endocrinology and Metabolism* **81**, 3578–83.
104. **Lobo, R.A.** (2001). Androgens in postmenopausal women: production, possible role, and replacement options. *Obstetrical & Gynecological Survey* **56**, 361–76.
105. **Bhasin, S.** et al. (1996). The effects of supraphysiologic doses of testosterone on muscle size and strength in normal men. *New England Journal of Medicine* **335**, 1–7.
106. **Snyder, P.J.** et al. (2000). Effects of testosterone replacement in hypogonadal men. *Journal of Clinical Endocrinology and Metabolism* **85**, 2670–7.
107. **Dobs, A.S.** et al. (1996). Serum hormones in men with human immunodeficiency virus-associated wasting. *Journal of Clinical Endocrinology and Metabolism* **81**, 4108–12.
108. **Grinspoon, S.** et al. (1996). Loss of lean body and muscle mass correlates with androgen levels in hypogonadal men with acquired immunodeficiency syndrome and wasting. *Journal of Clinical Endocrinology and Metabolism* **81**, 4051–8.
109. **Arver, S.** et al. (1999). Serum dihydrotestosterone and testosterone concentrations in human immunodeficiency virus-infected men with and without weight loss. *Journal of Andrology* **20**, 611–18.
110. **Grinspoon, S.** et al. (1997). Body composition and endocrine function in women with acquired immunodeficiency syndrome wasting. *Journal of Clinical Endocrinology and Metabolism* **82**, 1332–7.
111. **Bhasin, S.** et al. (2000). Testosterone replacement and resistance exercise in HIV-infected men with weight loss and low testosterone levels. *Journal of the American Medical Association* **283**, 763–70.
112. **Abs, R.** et al. (2000). Endocrine consequences of long-term intrathecal administration of opioids. *Journal of Clinical Endocrinology and Metabolism* **85**, 2215–22.
113. **Blackman, W.R.** et al. (1988). Comparison of the effects of lung cancer, benign lung disease, and normal aging on pituitary-gonadal function in men. *Journal of Clinical Endocrinology and Metabolism* **66**, 88–95.
114. **Chlebowski, R.T. and Heber, D.** (1982). Hypogonadism in male patients with metastatic cancer prior to chemotherapy. *Cancer Research* **42**, 2495–8.
115. **Todd, B.D.** (1988). Pancreatic carcinoma and low serum testosterone; a correlation secondary to cancer cachexia? *European Journal of Surgical Oncology* **14**, 199–202.
116. **Handelsman, D.J. and Dong, Q.** (1993). Hypothalamo-pituitary gonadal axis in chronic renal failure. *Endocrinology and Metabolism Clinics of North America* **22**, 145–61.
117. **Johansen, K.L., Mulligan, K., and Schambelan, M.** (1999). Anabolic effects of nandrolone decanoate in patients receiving dialysis: a randomized of the controlled trial. *Journal of the American Medical Association* **281**, 1275–81.
118. **Kamischke, A.** et al. (1998). Testosterone levels in men with chronic obstructive pulmonary disease with or without glucocorticoid therapy. *European Respiratory Journal* **11**, 41–5.
119. **Schols, A.M.** et al. (1995). Physiologic effects of nutritional support and anabolic steroids in patients with chronic obstructive pulmonary disease. A placebo-controlled randomized trial. *American Journal of Respiratory and Critical Care Medicine* **152**, 1268–74.
120. **Reid, I.R.** et al. (1996). Testosterone therapy in glucocorticoid-treated men. *Archives of Internal Medicine* **156**, 1173–7.
121. **Feelders, R.A.** et al. (1999). Characteristics of recovery from the euthyroid sick syndrome induced by tumor necrosis factor alpha in cancer patients. *Metabolism* **48**, 324–9.
122. **Knapp, M.L.** et al. (1991). Hormonal factors associated with weight loss in patients with advanced breast cancer. *Annals of Clinical Biochemistry* **28**, 480–6.
123. **Lambert, M.** (1994). Thyroid dysfunction in HIV infection. *Bailliere's Clinical Endocrinology and Metabolism* **8**, 825–35.
124. **Staal-van den Brekel, A.J.** et al. (1997). The effects of treatment with chemotherapy on energy metabolism and inflammatory mediators in small-cell lung carcinoma. *British Journal of Cancer* **76**, 1630–5.
125. **Scott, H.R.** et al. (1996). The relationship between weight loss and interleukin 6 in non-small-cell lung cancer. *British Journal of Cancer* **73**, 1560–2.
126. **Cicoira, M.** et al. (2001). High tumour necrosis factor-alpha levels are associated with exercise intolerance and neurohormonal activation in chronic heart failure patients. *Cytokine* **15**, 80–6.
127. **Yeh, S.S.** et al. (2001). The correlation of cytokine levels with body weight after megestrol acetate treatment in geriatric patients. *The Journals of Gerontology. Series A, Biological Sciences and Medical Sciences* **56**, M48–54.
128. **Torelli, G.F.** et al. (1999). Use of recombinant human soluble TNF receptor in anorectic tumor-bearing rats. *American Journal of Physiology* **277**, R850–5.
129. **Costelli, P.** et al. (1993). Tumor necrosis factor-alpha mediates changes in tissue protein turnover in a rat cancer cachexia model. *Journal of Clinical Investigation* **92**, 2783–9.
130. **Banks, R.E.** et al. (2000). Subcutaneous administration of recombinant glycosylated interleukin 6 in patients with cancer: pharmacokinetics, pharmacodynamics and immunomodulatory effects. *Cytokine* **12**, 388–96.
131. **Strassmann, G.** et al. (1992). Evidence for the involvement of interleukin 6 in experimental cancer cachexia. *The Journal of Clinical Investigation* **89**, 1681–4.
132. **Yasumoto, K.** et al. (1995). Molecular analysis of the cytokine network involved in cachexia in colon 26 adenocarcinoma-bearing mice. *Cancer Research* **55**, 921–7.
133. **Fujita, J.** et al. (1996). Anti-interleukin-6 receptor antibody prevents muscle atrophy in colon-26 adenocarcinoma-bearing mice with modulation of lysosomal and ATP-ubiquitin-dependent proteolytic pathways. *International Journal of Cancer* **68**, 637–43.
134. **Martin, F.** et al. (1999). Cytokine levels (IL-6 and IFN-gamma), acute phase response and nutritional status as prognostic factors in lung cancer. *Cytokine* **11**, 80–6.
135. **Llovera, M.** et al. (1998). Different cytokines modulate ubiquitin gene expression in rat skeletal muscle. *Cancer Letters* **133**, 83–7.
136. **Barber, M.D.** et al. (2000). A polymorphism of the interleukin-1 beta gene influences survival in pancreatic cancer. *British Journal of Cancer* **83**, 1443–7.
137. **Cahlin, C.** et al. (2000). Experimental cancer cachexia: the role of host-derived cytokines interleukin (IL)-6, IL-12, interferon-gamma, and tumor necrosis factor alpha evaluated in gene knockout, tumor-bearing mice on C57 Bl background and eicosanoid-dependent cachexia. *Cancer Research* **60**, 5488–93.
138. **Bossola, M.** et al. (2000). Serum tumour necrosis factor-alpha levels in cancer patients are discontinuous and correlate with weight loss. *European Journal of Clinical Investigation* **30**, 1107–12.
139. **Karayiannakis, A.J.** et al. (2001). Serum levels of tumor necrosis factor-alpha and nutritional status in pancreatic cancer patients. *Anticancer Research* **21**, 1355–8.
140. **Socher, S.H.** et al. (1988). Tumor necrosis factor not detectable in patients with clinical cancer cachexia. *Journal of the National Cancer Institute* **80**, 595–8.
141. **Maltoni, M.** et al. (1997). Serum levels of tumour necrosis factor alpha and other cytokines do not correlate with weight loss and anorexia in cancer patients. *Supportive Care in Cancer* **5**, 130–5.
142. **Scuderi, P.** et al. (1986). Raised serum levels of tumour necrosis factor in parasitic infections. *Lancet* **2**, 1364–5.
143. **Plata-Salaman, C.R.** (2000). Central nervous system mechanisms contributing to the cachexia-anorexia syndrome. *Nutrition* **16**, 1009–12.
144. **Negri, D.R.** et al. (2001). Role of cytokines in cancer cachexia in a murine model of intracerebral injection of human tumours. *Cytokine* **15**, 27–38.
145. **Zhang, Y.** et al. (2000). Cytokines and endotoxin induce cytokine receptors in skeletal muscle. *American Journal of Physiology, Endocrinology and Metabolism* **279**, E196–205.

146. **Carbo, N.** et al. (2001). Interleukin-15 mediates reciprocal regulation of adipose and muscle mass: a potential role in body weight control. *Biochimica et Biophysica Acta* **1526**, 17–24.
147. **Llovera, M.** et al. (1996). Muscle hypercatabolism during cancer cachexia is not reversed by the glucocorticoid receptor antagonist RU38486. *Cancer Letters* **99**, 7–14.
148. **Todorov, P.** et al. (1996). Characterization of a cancer cachectic factor. *Nature* **379**, 739–42.
149. **Wigmore, S.J.** et al. (2000). Characteristics of patients with pancreatic cancer expressing a novel cancer cachectic factor. *British Journal of Surgery* **87**, 53–8.
150. **Cabal-Manzano, R.** et al. (2001). Proteolysis-inducing factor is expressed in tumours of patients with gastrointestinal cancers and correlates with weight loss. *British Journal of Cancer* **84**, 1599–601.
151. **McDevitt, T.M.** et al. (1995). Purification and characterization of a lipid-mobilizing factor associated with cachexia-inducing tumors in mice and humans. *Cancer Research* **55**, 1458–63.
152. **Tisdale, M.J.** (2000). Catabolism of skeletal muscle proteins and its reversal in cancer cachexia. *Nestle Nutrition Workshop Series. Clinical & Performance Programme* **4**, 135–43.
153. **Lorite, M.J.** et al. (2001). Activation of ATP-ubiquitin-dependent proteolysis in skeletal muscle *in vivo* and murine myoblasts *in vitro* by a proteolysis-inducing factor (PIF). *British Journal of Cancer* **85**, 297–302.
154. **Smith, H.J., Lorite, M.J., and Tisdale, M.J.** (1999). Effect of a cancer cachectic factor on protein synthesis/degradation in murine C2C12 myoblasts: modulation by eicosapentaenoic acid. *Cancer Research* **59**, 5507–13.
155. **Lorite, M.J.** et al. (1998). Mechanism of muscle protein degradation induced by a cancer cachectic factor. *British Journal of Cancer* **78**, 850–6.
156. **Tisdale, M.J.** (2000). Biomedicine. Protein loss in cancer cachexia. *Science* **289**, 2293–4.
157. **Watchorn, T.M.** et al. (2001). Proteolysis-inducing factor regulates hepatic gene expression via the transcription factors NF-(kappa)B and STAT3. *FASEB Journal* **15**, 562–4.
158. **Islam-Ali, B.** et al. (2001). Modulation of adipocyte G-protein expression in cancer cachexia by a lipid-mobilizing factor (LMF). *British Journal of Cancer* **85**, 758–63.
159. **Ogata, E.** (2000). Parathyroid hormone-related protein as a potential target of therapy for cancer-associated morbidity. *Cancer* **88**, 2909–11.
160. **Klein, S.** et al. (1997). Nutrition support in clinical practice: review of published data and recommendations for future research directions. Summary of a conference sponsored by the National Institutes of Health, American Society for Parenteral and Enteral Nutrition, and American Society for Clinical Nutrition. *American Journal of Clinical Nutrition* **66**, 683–706.
161. **Bozzetti, F.** et al. (1996). Guidelines on artificial nutrition versus hydration in terminal cancer patients. European Association for Palliative Care. *Nutrition* **12**, 163–7.
162. **Winter, S.M.** (2000). Terminal nutrition: framing the debate for the withdrawal of nutritional support in terminally ill patients (Review). *American Journal of Medicine* **109**, 723–6.

8.4.2 Clinical assessment and decision-making in cachexia and anorexia

Robin L. Fainsinger and Jose Pereira

Introduction

At the most basic level, this chapter will outline an approach to assessment of appetite, caloric intake, and nutritional status. This will cover the spectrum from simple bedside assessments, to more complicated patient recordings, laboratory tests, and sophisticated technical procedures. Cachexia and anorexia do not exist in isolation in any individual patient, and the potential complex interplay of associated symptoms will be explored. Careful and accurate assessment is essential before applying therapeutic options that may be at our disposal. Decision-making in this regard requires a rational use of options given the background of supportive evidence for benefit and careful application to the circumstances of the specific individual patient and family.

However, as we consider these various aspects, there are some other underlying issues we need to keep in mind. Our current definitions of palliative care generally do not describe the certainties or acknowledge the ambiguities of the boundaries of palliative care.(1) Palliative care is clearly not limited to cancer populations alone; however, the problems of cachexia and anorexia are most commonly described in patients with advanced cancer and to a lesser extent AIDS.(2) Certainly most of the research and literature on palliative care in this area has focused on the cancer population. Some aspects of the approach that we have developed in this patient population may well be applicable to other palliative care populations, although we need to keep in mind that the underlying pathophysiology may well vary.(3)

We also need to avoid having our use of treatment approaches hampered by the often quoted statement that 'palliative care neither hastens nor postpones death'.(1) Indeed, some of the potential therapeutic options in this area may well prolong life in a meaningful and important manner that has clear benefits for patients and families.

A simple definition of anorexia implies a loss of appetite and reduced caloric intake,(2) while cachexia can be defined as an involuntary weight loss of more than 10 per cent of premorbid weight, associated with loss of muscle and visceral protein and lipolysis.(4) Although these definitions are reasonably clear, there may well be circumstances of clinical uncertainty. Patients and families may not always agree on the significance or severity of decreased appetite and caloric intake. Similarly, there are no firm criteria to define a diagnosis of cachexia where weight loss and alterations in laboratory values do not necessarily correlate.

We commonly refer to the 'cachexia/anorexia syndrome' as one of the most frequent and devastating problems affecting patients with advanced cancer.(5) However, just as cachexia does not necessarily correlate with tumour stage or burden, cachexia may not correlate with anorexia.(4) Indeed, cachexia may occur long before the patient or family notices any loss of appetite. The extent to which cachexia and anorexia derive from identical pathophysiologies is beyond the scope of this chapter, and while certainly in the latter stages of advanced diseases they are commonly associated, it would be unwise to assume that they necessarily always appear in tandem.

Assessment of appetite

Various scales, including visual, numerical, and verbal rating scales, have been used in clinical and research settings to assess patients' subjective sense of appetite.(6,7) Patients may be asked how they would describe their appetite from very poor to very good and to represent it on these scales. Anorexia and weight loss, as perceived by a patient, should be assessed within the context of other symptoms. The Edmonton System Assessment Scale (ESAS), a series of visual analogue or numerical rating scales to assess the severity of up to nine symptoms, is one method.(8) Dudgeon et al., assessing the application of the ESAS in patients in an inpatient palliative care unit,(9) found that anorexia as a symptom did not change much over time. This challenges the need to assess it as frequently as other symptoms such as pain and shortness of breath in patients with very advanced disease who have limited life expectancy.

In addition to assessing appetite, other subjective approaches may be used to assess the impact of treatments. These may include simply asking patients whether or not their appetite has increased since the treatment or trial was commenced.(10) The data can be transposed to a categorical scale to obtain more quantitative data. Perceived improvement in quality of life following management of appetite and nutrition has been evaluated in the research setting.[11,12] Subjects in these studies have been asked questions such as: 'Do you enjoy eating more or less since the start of the treatment?' 'Do you think this treatment has been of benefit to you?' 'To what extent has your appearance changed since starting the treatment?'

Assessment of caloric intake

Most methods that assess food and caloric intake rely mainly on retrospective reporting or prospective dietary record keeping. Retrospective determination relies on the accuracy of recall and self-reporting by the patients and/or their main caregivers.[13,14] Recall of up to 3 days has been shown to be relatively reliable. In prospective dietary keeping, all the foods and fluids can be weighed just before they are eaten and the caloric intake then calculated using previously published tables that correlate food weights with caloric values for each foodstuff. Apart from measuring energy-yielding foods, this method requires that several days of assessment be completed in order to obtain a dependable estimate of intake.[15] A less accurate method relies on patients comparing their food quantities relative to standardized portions or household measures without having to actually weigh their food.[16]

An alternative method that has been successfully used in research[17] calls for trained proxies such as nurses and volunteers to estimate, as a percentage, individual food portions consumed by patients.[18] In this method, Bruera and colleagues demonstrated a good correlation between this and actual caloric intake, and also found it to be more reliable than the 24-h recall method.

The assessment of dietary and caloric intake is discussed in more detail in a separate chapter in this book.

Assessment of nutritional status and body composition

A number of methods have been used to assess the nutritional status of patients with progressive diseases such as cancer and AIDS.[14] These are listed in Tables 1 and 2. Many of them have been used exclusively in the research setting. Some require sophisticated equipment and expertise that is not widely available, thereby limiting their widespread clinical use. Others are receiving increasing attention in the clinical setting.

Nutritional status is conventionally assessed by means of a combination of assessment method, in both the clinical and the research settings.[11]

Subjective global assessment of nutrition (SGA)

The subjective global assessment (SGA) questionnaire is a standardized instrument developed to assess nutritional status in an easy, non-invasive, and cost-effective manner.[19] Patients are rated into three groups: (a) a well-nourished group (SGA-A); (b) a group that is moderately malnourished or has borderline malnutrition (SGA-B); and (c) a group that is severely malnourished (SGA-C). SGA-A denotes stable weight or increasing weight due to improvement in symptoms; SGA-B signifies weight loss up to 10 per cent during the last 6 months and eating less than usual; and SGA-C denotes greater than 10 per cent weight loss in last 6 months and, in addition, obvious physical signs of malnutrition. The SGA has been validated in surgical patients and a modified form has been developed for use in cancer patients.[20] The SGA is divided into six sections. These are weight history, food intake (as perceived by patients over the month prior to the assessment), symptoms, functional capacity (as perceived by patients over month prior to assessment), problems that have kept the patient from eating (in the 2 weeks prior to the assessment, e.g. early satiety, poor appetite, vomiting), disease and its relation to nutritional requirements and physical examination. Thoresen and colleagues recently evaluated the SGA in a palliative setting and found it to be a useful and easy method for assessment of nutrition in the palliative setting and can be used as a screening tool.[21] The original SGA called for patients to recall their weight at 6 and 12 months prior to the assessment date. Thoresen and colleagues found that patients were not able to recall that far back and therefore substituted this with the items 'unintentional weight loss', 'pre-diagnosis weight', and 'time and magnitude of body weight loss'. The SGA correlated highly to the objective nutritional criteria and the mean values of triceps skinfold and mid-upper arm muscle circumference (MAMC). The investigators reported the SGA to be a valid and easily applied tool for the screening and assessment of nutritional status in patients with advanced disease. While they were not able to pronounce the study a formal validation of the SGA because of the lack of reliable 'gold standards', they did nevertheless find the tool a useful screening tool to detect malnutrition in patients with advanced cancer.

Table 1 Methods to assess nutritional status and body composition

Method	Currently being used in clinical setting	Currently being used in research	Has potential for more widespread clinical use
Anthropometric testing			
Body weight	+	+	+
Skinfold thickness		+	+
Mid-upper arm circumference		+	+
Dynamometry		+	
Infrared interactance		+	
Whole-body bio-impedance and electroconductivity		+	+
Imaging with computed tomography (CT), magnetic resonance (MRI), or ultrasound (US)		+	
Dual energy X-ray absorptiometry/dual photon absorptiometry		+	?
Neutron activation analysis (NAA)			
Whole-body potassium estimation		+	
Total-body water estimation		+	
Laboratory tests (see Table 2)			

?, Potential clinical role.

Table 2 Laboratory methods to assess nutritional status and body composition

Methods	Rationale	Limitations	Currently being used in clinical setting	Currently being used in research	Has potential for more widespread clinical use
Albumin	Provides index of advanced disease	Not specific to cachexia: other problems may cause hypoalbuminaemia	+	+	
Urinary creatinine and Creatinine/Height Index (CHI)	Indirect estimate of muscle mass			+	+
Cytokines levels (interleukin-1, interleukin-6, gamma interferon, protein cachexia factor)	Recognized protagonists in cachexia syndrome	Levels do not correlate with weight loss		+	?
C-reactive protein (CRP)	Marker of pro-inflammatory cytokine activity	Not specific to cachexia			?
Lymphocytic function (total T-cells, T-helper cells, natural killer cells, CD20 count, CD40 count, CD4/CD8 ratio)	Lean body weight mass leads to decreased performance of the immune system	Not specific to cachexia syndrome		+	
Haemoglobin		Non-specific			
Electrolyte abnormalities (potassium, magnesium, histadine)		Non specific			

?, Potential clinical role.

Anthropometric tests

Anthropometric tests rely mainly on three parameters: body weight, skinfold thickness, and mid-arm circumference. Accuracy is improved by combining more than one anthropometric measure.[22]

Body weight

Body weight, an index of body mass, is generally the easiest nutritional parameter to assess. Consequently, it is often used in clinical and research settings.[7,23] It is clinically more meaningful to determine the percentage of total body weight loss rather than measuring total weight. A reduction of at least 10 per cent of the body weight is often used as a criterion in cachexia studies.[24,25] Weight loss of greater than 5–10 per cent has been associated with reduced survival and higher rates of infections.[26] Serial measurements of individual patients may be useful in select patients.[27] These may be compared with their pre-morbid weight, if that information is available. Patients' weights may also be compared against population-based tables.[28] The presence of ascites, oedema, or increased tumour mass may affect body weight. When weighing patients, scales should be accurately calibrated and thin clothing worn. The body mass index (BMI) is not sensitive enough to detect malnutrition when its values exceed 20.[21]

Skinfold thickness

Skinfold thickness provides an estimation of body fat.[23,29,30] Measurements can be obtained from the triceps, biceps, subscapular, and suprailiac skinfolds. Skinfold thickness is measured by pinching the skin and subcutaneous fat between a pair of calipers. These are standardized to deliver consistent pressure over a standard area. The total body fat is then calculated by comparing the skinfold thickness with body density data determined from large population studies. A caveat is that these tables are derived largely from young healthy subjects. Reliability depends on accurate and consistent siting of the calipers.

Mid-upper arm circumference

The mid-upper arm circumference (MUAC), in combination with the triceps skinfold thickness (TSF), can be used to derive the mid-arm muscle circumference.[23] The mid-arm muscle circumference (MAMC) is an index of the body's muscle mass, an indicator of protein reserve. The MAMC is calculated by using the MUAC and the TSF.[31,32]

In a study of patients with recently diagnosed non-small-cell cancer of the lung, Ferrigno and Buccheri found that the anthropometric measures have a marginal prognostic value compared with other prognostic factors such as functional status, but may be significant predictors of survival, although not independently of other prognostic factors that included physical and biochemistry parameters.[33] Patients with higher values of arm circumference had significantly longer survival than patients with lower values.

Dynamometry

Dynamometry is the measurement of muscle strength. This is often done by measuring hand grip or shoulder muscle strength. Although it has been used peri-operatively[27,34,35] as an indirect index of nutritional status, its validity in this context may be challenged. A recent study by Knols and colleagues found the reproducibility of strength measurements with a hand-held pull-gauge dynamometer in patients with cancer was poor.[36]

Infrared interactance

Infrared light, when directed at different parts of the body and tissues, reflects and transmits to varying degrees, depending on the tissue.[37] Calculations based on calibrated standards are then used to estimate total body fat.

Whole-body bioimpedance and electroconductivity

This safe and quick method is based on the measurement of resistance of the body to the flow of an alternating electrical current.[38,39] Lean tissue, which is high in conducting water and electrolyte content, conducts electricity far better than adipose tissue. Electrodes are placed at the extremities on the non-dominant side of the body. Baumgartner et al. have demonstrated that only one limb can be used.[38] A small current is passed through the body and resistance is calculated from the voltage change acros the body. Total body water is then calculated and the fat-free mass computed on the basis that 73 per cent of it is water. However, since it measures resistance at the extremities, it is less accurate in assessing changes in body composition in central body regions such as the viscera or abdomen. Increasingly, this method is being used in studies involving patients with cancer and AIDS.[11,23,40] Conslick et al. have showed that bioimpedance is as accurate as anthropometric tests.[39] Equipment, primarily scales, that measure bioimpedance rapidly are becoming more easily available and may be increasingly used in both the clinical and research settings in the future.

In contrast, measuring electroconductivity requires that patients be placed in an electromagentic field and the change in impedance measured. Prediction equations have been made to estimate the lean body mass.[41]

Computed tomography (CT), magnetic resonance (MRI), and ultrasound imaging

These techniques are used to visualize both adipose tissue and non-fat tissue in those parts of the body that are scanned. Equations have been derived to calculate the total and visceral adipose tissue.[42] Seidel and colleagues have demonstrated that CT imaging is as accurate as anthropometric tests.[43] High costs, the need for specialized equipment, and the exposure of patients to small doses of ionizing radiation relegates this test to the research context. Unlike CT scanning, there is no radiation with MRI scanning. Seidel et al. compared this form of imaging with CT scanning and found that the two methods are comparable in accuracy.[44] As with CT scanning, this is a costly method and many patients dislike it or experience claustrophobia. Ultrasound scanning has also been used to estimate total adipose tissue.[16]

Dual energy X-ray absorptiometry/dual photon absorptiometry

This method, widely used for measuring bone density, may also be used to estimate the percentage of body fat in non-bone tissues and the lean body mass,[45] and determine total-body water content.[46] Although this method is gaining popularity as a simple, relatively non-invasive method of assessing body content,[11,27] some caution has been advised about its accuracy and predictability.[47]

Neutron activation analysis (NAA)

This technique allows for the accurate and direct measurement of a variety of the elements of body composition, including nitrogen, calcium, and sodium.[16] The individual is irradiated by a beam of neutrons. These are caught by the target elements within the body and decay over time. As they decay they emit gamma energy that can be counted by spectrograph analysis. Total body nitrogen, one of several parameters that can be calculated, provides an index of the lean body mass (mainly muscle mass). It is an expensive test that requires special training and equipment.

Whole-body potassium estimation

Total-body potassium is a sensitive index of lean body mass. Potassium is an intracellular cation that is not found in adipose tissue. The body naturally contains the potassium isotope ^{40}K. The gamma irradiation it emits can be measured using a whole-body counter. Lean body mass can be derived from total-body potassium (68.1 mEq of potassium per kilogram of lean body mass[11,48,49]). Newer counters, unlike their older predecessors, do not require shielding and are therefore less costly.

Total-body water estimation

The individual ingests or is injected with an isotope (^{18}O, hydrogen, deuterium, and tritium) and the concentration excreted or eliminated through breath, urine, or plasma water is then determined.[50]

Laboratory tests

Hypoalbuminaemia is often used at the bedside as an indicator of advanced disease,[51] particularly in patients with cancer. Serum albumin provides an index of visceral protein status.[52] Hypoalbuminaemia occurs as acute phase reactants such as fibrinogen and C-reactive protein serum levels increase, resulting in the loss of somatic proteins.[46,53] The level of serum albumin may be affected by a variety of conditions, including inflammatory reactions of any cause, severe liver disease, and dehydration. It has been suggested that serum albumin should be considered more as an indicator of illness or as a prognostic factor than a major indicator of nutritional status.[54] Serum proteins are probably not as sensitive markers of nutritional status as the anthropometric measures.[21]

The role of other rapid turnover proteins such as thyroxin-binding prealbumin as indicators of nutritional status is unclear. It has been suggested that these are sensitive to changes in nutritional status.

Creatinine phosphate is largely located in skeletal muscles. Therefore, urinary creatinine and creatinine/height index (CHI) may be used to estimate muscle mass.[11,55] Urinary creatinine excretion, averaged over a few days, is multiplied by a constant of 18 kg of muscle per gram of urinary creatinine and indexed for height to determine the percentage of predicted muscle mass.[56,57] During the test period patients receive meat-free diets.

Several cytokines are implicated as mediators of the cachexia process, among which are tumour necrosis factor alpha (TNF-α), interleukin-1, interleukin-6, and gamma interferon, as well as other factors such as leukaemia inhibitory factor and tumour-derived factors such as lipid-mobilizing factor and protein-mobilizing factor.[53,58–60] While there has been some interest in the clinical setting in using serum levels of tumour necrosis factor alpha and other cytokines as markers for the presence of cachexia syndrome, their serum levels do not correlate with weight loss or anorexia in cancer patients. However, most studies have failed to measure increased circulating TNF-α levels in cachectic cancer patients.[60–63] In addition, other factors such as a very short plasma half-life may make detection of TNF-α activity very difficult.[64]

There is increased interest in measuring C-reactive protein (CRP) as a marker for pro-inflammatory cytokine activity *in vivo*.[23] It has been noted that in patients with advanced pancreatic cancer receiving no specific intervention, CRP tends to rise with disease progression.[65] Some $n-3$ polyunsaturated fatty acids such as eicosapentaenoic acid (EPA) are immunomodulatory and have been shown to suppress the production of pro-inflammatory cytokines such IL-1 and TNF by peripheral blood mononuclear cells from healthy volunteers.[66,67] In a pilot study, there was a significant decrease in C-reactive protein and increase in body weight in patients with gastrointestinal cancer treated with a combination of megestrol acetate and ibuprofen for 6 weeks.[68] Laboratory studies of weight-losing pancreatic cancer patients receiving EPA have demonstrated suppression of peripheral blood mononuclear cells (PBMC) IL-6 production and an associated reduction in the ability of the patients' PBMC supernatants to stimulate CRP production by the human liver.[23,67] However, it must be noted that CRP is a non-specific pro-inflammatory substance and many other factors may result in increased production. Moreover, the level at which CRP becomes abnormal with respect to cachexia has not been established. The bedside clinical applications of this test are therefore as of yet unclear, but do show promise.

Lean body weight loss leads to decreased performance of the immune system.[4] There has therefore been interest in assessing lymphocytic function (including total T-cells, T-helper cells, T-suppressor cells, natural killer cells, CD20 and CD40 counts, and CD4/CD8 ratios), particularly in the context of assessing treatments such as 3-omega fatty acids and thalidomide.[23] However, tumour–host interactions are complex and it is unclear whether these parameters have clinical value with respect to assessing nutritional status.[62]

Several other laboratory tests have been used to assess nutritional status. Abnormalities such as anaemia, hypokalaemia, hypomagnesaemia, and lactic acidosis are sometimes used as indirect indices of nutritional function. As nutritional indices they are not by themselves specific. 3-Methyl histadine excretion as a marker of muscle protein breakdown has been evaluated but not used much in the clinical setting[11,27,69] and warrants evaluation. Total urinary nitrogen excretion is sometimes used.[70,71] Grinspoon and colleagues, in their study assessing androgen therapy in patients with

AIDS-related wasting, measured total urinary nitrogen excretion from consecutive 24-h collections averaged over 3 days.[11] Calorie and protein intake were monitored on a daily basis and nitrogen intake was derived from total protein intake divided by a constant of 6.25 mg of protein per gram of nitrogen. This group of investigators also evaluated resting energy expenditure by indirect calorimetry.

Assessing impact of treatments on quality of life

Most of the assessments discussed thus far are used to evaluate nutritional status and the effect of treatments, largely in the context of research but occasionally also in the clinical setting. While increased appetite, food intake, and weight gain might be considered sufficient benefits of therapy, these benefits are of substantially greater value if they are associated with parallel improvement in patient-rated well-being and quality of life. Some additional benefits that may be of relevance include enhanced mood, improved sense of well-being, improved body image, ability to derive pleasure from eating, and social benefits derived from increased ability to enjoy a meal with family or friends.[72] Unfortunately, there exists a dearth of well-established and psychometrically validated instruments to evaluate subjective benefits associated with improvement in target symptoms such as appetite, food intake, and weight gain. With this in mind, Cella and colleagues developed and validated the Bristol–Myers Anorexia/Cachexia Recovery Instrument (BACRI), a tool to quantify patient perception of benefit in areas such as decreased concern over weight and appearance, increased pleasure in eating, and increased global perception of quality of life.[72] The instrument was validated in an HIV population with wasting treated with megesterol acetate.

One of the most important aspects of evaluation in the clinical setting is to assess the patient and family's understanding of what the symptom or problem means to them.[73] For many, loss of weight or appetite may signify progressive disease, thereby eliciting or exacerbating their psychological distress. There is often the fear of starving to death. These fears need to be addressed. Explaining, in non-technical terms, the difference between the starving model and disease-related cachexia syndrome, may be helpful to reduce or avert the feelings of guilt that may arise when patients do not eat or families find themselves unable to feed the patient. The hallmark of cancer- or AIDS-related cachexia is the disproportionate and excessive loss of lean tissue along with fat loss, brought about by profound alterations in metabolism. Mediators such as cytokines and proteolysis-inducing factor induce these alterations. In contrast, starvation is characterized by a preferential loss of adipose tissue and a relative preservation of lean tissue. Weight loss is primarily due to inadequate caloric intake and specific mediators are not generally implicated.[74]

Symptoms associated with cachexia

As the multi-dimensional aspects of the total pain experience have been well recognized for many years, the multi-dimensional and associated problems of cachexia in advanced disease need to be recognized.[75] In addition to the well-recognized association with anorexia, other associations commonly recognized include asthenia, chronic nausea, and psychological symptoms. Less commonly acknowledged problems may be the inter-play with oral complications, pain syndromes, and dyspnoea. Family studies demonstrated that the cachexia/anorexia/asthenia complex ranks high in the physical causes of suffering and contribution to psychosocial distress.[76] Although it may be apparent that symptom associations are common, the pattern of these relationships and specific symptom inter-play has not been systematically investigated.[77] Nevertheless, given the diagnostic and therapeutic implications of these interactions, appropriate assessment and application of treatment options will require an attempt to clarify possible associations in individual clinical circumstances. An approach to the assessment of potential associations has been outlined:[77]

1. symptoms are concurrent but unrelated in aetiology;
2. symptoms are concurrent and related to the same pathological process;
3. symptoms are concurrent and the second symptom is directly or indirectly a consequence of a pathological process initiated by the first symptom;
4. symptoms are concurrent and the second symptom is a consequence or side-effect of therapy directed against the first symptom.

Anorexia

Anorexia has been associated with disorders of all systems. It represents a consistent clinical manifestation during infections, chronic pain, and cancer. It has been reported that anorexia was the second most common symptom in 78 per cent of cancer patients during their last year of life. Nevertheless, it only ranked 10th in 'distressing' symptoms, suggesting that other problems may often be seen as more important to patients and families.[78]

Anorexia may be associated with endocrine, gastrointestinal, hepatic, pancreatic, biliary, renal, pulmonary, cardiovascular, connective tissue, immune, haematological, neurological, and psychiatric disorders. Thus, anorexia is often a non-specific but prominent clinical manifestation of an extensive variety of clinical problems.[79] All of the above diseases are commonly associated not only with long-term anorexia, but simultaneously or subsequently with cachexia. It is postulated that various mechanisms are involved in the anorexia observed during disease, including cytokine action. However, it is interesting to note that a study with the main objective of demonstrating an association between serum levels of four cytokines and clinical features of cachexia did not reveal a statistically significant correlation between circulating levels of these substances and weight loss or anorexia.[62] Nevertheless, clinical experience does suggest that the presence of gastrointestinal symptomatology is related to anorexia, and that anorexia is related to cachexia.[77,79]

It is worth noting that anorexia generally does not cause physical discomfort unless accompanied by nausea. Nevertheless, the impact of resulting physical and psychological effects can certainly be significant. Anorexia may be associated or result in cachexia or malnutrition, contribute to fatigue, and cause psychological symptoms. Quality of life often suffers with cultural and family expectations relating to food intake.[77]

Asthenia

Fatigue or generalized weakness is now recognized as one of the most frequent symptoms in cancer and many other chronic illnesses. The lack of focus on asthenia may be partially explained by the lack of recognized standards of assessment and a nihilistic attitude to treatment options. The prevalence of asthenia in cancer patients has been estimated at more than 80 per cent in those receiving chemotherapy, and over 70 per cent in patients with advanced cancer.[80–82] It has been recognized that in the majority of patients asthenia is likely the result of cachexia rather than an independent problem.[24] Nevertheless, there may be clinical situations where this relationship is not as interdependent. This possible hypothesis is underlined by the association of asthenia with non-malignant conditions where cachexia is less evident such as the chronic fatigue syndrome or major depressive disorders. In addition, asthenia may be a significant problem in some malignancies with a low prevalence of cachexia such as breast cancer or lymphomas.

Rehabilitation groups have noted the association of multiple symptoms and decreased physical function.[32] Patients living with advanced cancer may benefit from enhanced mobility and self-care, although it is certainly uncertain to what degree rehabilitation interventions can stem the tide of functional decline that accompanies advancing malignancy.[83] Nevertheless, given the successful results in other advanced and end-stage diseases such as AIDS and chronic obstructive lung disease, it seems reasonable to assume that some advanced cancer patients may benefit.

Certainly there have been some promising results in both cancer patients receiving acute management[84] and terminal cancer patients admitted to an in-patient hospice.[85] The latter study appeared to demonstrate that while rehabilitation cannot eliminate the inevitable progressive decline, it can certainly attenuate and decelerate the decline in some patients. Nevertheless, the degree to which rehabilitation interventions may improve function and symptom management such as anorexia and cachexia in terminally patients remains unclear.[86]

The impact of treatments such as aerobic conditioning, strengthening, increasing flexibility, and mechanical efficiency on immune status and cytokine regulation in the cancer population may be important.[87] The possibility that exercise may down-regulate interleukin-1 or other myotoxic cytokines was suggested.[87]

Nausea

Chronic nausea is recognized as a highly prevalent and distressing symptom in terminal cancer.[88] There are multiple potential aetiologies including autonomic failure, medications such as opioids, metabolic abnormalities, and constipation. The relationship between specific gastrointestinal symptoms such as nausea and weight loss has seldom been studied.[77] However, there are some data to support the clinical impression that symptom complexes related to gastrointestinal function may contribute to the development of cachexia. There is recognition that these interactions should be considered in clinical practice, have likely received minimal attention despite a high prevalence, and that future studies should attempt to clarify the overlapping association.[77,88]

Oral complications

Oral cavity disorders can have a tremendous impact on the quality of life of patients with advanced cancer and other non-malignant chronic end-stage disease. These lesions can result in great interference with both physical and psychological function. In addition to causing a loss of appetite and decreased oral intake, there certainly is the possibility in chronically untreated situations to develop associated malnutrition and aggravate cachexia.

Oral complications can include fungal, viral, and bacterial infections. Other problems include neutropenic ulcers, medication and radiotherapy-induced stomatitis, xerostomia, and taste alterations. Although there may be no controlled clinical data supporting a direct association between oral cavity complications of advanced illness and cachexia, it has been considered self-evident that such a relationship exists.[89]

Psychosocial issues

There have been reports to demonstrate that there is a clear association with cachexia, anorexia, and asthenia and a significant psychological impact.[73] These problems are often seen as a sign of impending death by patient and family, and may be a source of conflict between the patient and family in a patient unable to eat. Weight loss can certainly have considerable impact on a patient's body image.

Appetite is recognized as being extremely sensitive to mood changes, which are common at the time of diagnosis or disease recurrence. The differential diagnosis between a major depression and a physical origin of anorexia can be difficult. While anorexia and cachexia may result from a physical pathology, depression may be the prime cause of anorexia and subsequent weight loss, or anorexia and cachexia may produce a resulting depression given the perceived poor prognosis of an advanced illness.

Pain

The association of cachexia and asthenia in causing a progressive physical decline is well recognized.[87] The attendant effects caused by immobility, soft tissue and joint stiffness, decubitus ulceration, and resulting complaints of physical discomfort are common. Cachexia has also been noted as an aggravating mechanism in the development of ascites and lower limb oedema, with resulting complaints of pain.[90]

Dyspnoea

A study by Dudgeon and Lertzman[91] attempted to better understand the responsible pathophysiological mechanisms underlying dyspnoea in terminal cancer patients. In this group of 100 terminally ill cancer patients, a significant finding was the very low maximum inspiratory pressure suggesting severe respiratory muscle weakness may contribute significantly to dyspnoea in this patient population. A subsequent study by the same group[92] attempted to characterize the factors that may contribute to respiratory muscle weakness demonstrated in the earlier study. Although nutritional status as determined by the percentage of weight loss and serum albumin were not significantly correlated with respiratory muscle weakness, further study was felt warranted to clarify the degree to which dyspnoea may be a clinical expression of overwhelming cachexia and asthenia causing muscle weakness.

Rational use of therapeutic options

The high prevalence of cachexia and anorexia in advanced cancer patients has long been recognized,[93,94] and has resulted in increasing interest in this area of patient management.[5] Management suggestions have included clarifying goals of treatment, dietary counselling, enteral and parenteral nutrition, and a variety of pharmacological alternatives. Anecdotal and research reports on these different modalities have been reviewed by many authors.[74,76,95–106] Recommendations from these reviews, as well as reports on the practical application of these guidelines reveal a composite picture of how the management of the cachexia/anorexia syndrome is approached. Nevertheless, the average practitioner looking after advanced cancer patients may often find these reports difficult to translate into a practical rational approach. Conflicting conclusions, uncertain or unproven value of different treatment options, cost of treatment, likelihood of benefit to individual patients, and varying cultural and economic circumstances around the world all need to be taken into consideration. As has been pointed out:[76] 'At present, a "heap of facts" garnered by research workers working in disparate areas is available to the clinical investigator concerned with cancer cachexia. The web connecting these observations in a coherent mosaic, however, remains to be fully woven.'

Goals of treatment

Tchekmedyian[95] states that intervention goals need to be defined prior to instituting therapy. The major features requiring evaluation in advanced cancer patients are symptom control and comfort. Loprinzi[97] comments that it is unlikely that any of the therapeutic options will have a significant impact on patient survival. Nevertheless, effective treatment could improve quality of life in a similar fashion to effective management of pain or nausea. Bruera[94,98] has been hopeful that successful treatment may result in improvements in both life expectancy and quality of life. However, as cure of the underlying cancer is not possible in a majority of advanced cancer patients, other objectives become important. Rather than focusing on traditional outcomes such as survival, tumour response, and treatment toxicity, improvements should be monitored in measures such as anorexia and asthenia, patient and/or family satisfaction, and functional and nutritional status.[2,107]

MacDonald et al.[76] noted that as family studies have demonstrated that cachexia and related problems rank near the top of physical causes of suffering and psychosocial distress, cancer research outcome measures should emphasize improvement in function and satisfaction with therapy. Nelson et al.[100] state that as cure is not a realistic goal in the majority of advanced cancer patients, treatment should emphasize improving quality of life. The main target symptoms would be improving appetite and food intake. Ottery[101,102] emphasizes that the goals of treatment are to support nutritional status, body composition, functional status, and quality of life. Early intervention is considered crucial as attempts to reverse severe nutritional depletion are seldom successful. Rimmer[78] notes that the importance of anorexia and cachexia to the patient and family must be assessed separately and potential for a source of conflict identified and addressed. Support of the patient and family may be all that is required.

The common theme of treatment goals is clearly 'quality of life'. This translates into the goal of relieving nausea, improving appetite and maintaining or gaining weight, and psychosocial support and education to assist the patient and family in understanding and accepting the benefits and limits of treatment intervention.

Dietary support

Dieticians can play a useful role in assessing nutritional status, dietary needs, and providing advice to patients and their families.[103,108] This provides support in patient management by increasing comfort and food safety, and consideration of economic circumstances while attempting to maximize nutrition. The value of a dietician and dietary counselling is endorsed in most management recommendations as a reasonable approach.[78,94–96,98,99] Obviously, there will be limitations to dietary counselling,[96] with the increasing caloric count following nutritional counselling having been noted to fall to baseline levels after 3 weeks.[94]

A more optimistic view has been expressed[101,102] with the proposal for a specialized nutritional clinic and a multidisciplinary approach including a dietician, physician, and oncology clinical nurse specialist. Using this approach, it was claimed that 70 per cent of patients were able to maintain or gain weight, while maintaining or improving visceral protein status.

In a review of designer diets in cancer,[109] it was noted that in palliative care patients there were no clinical data to document beneficial effects of long-term nutritional support with designer diets. The basis for improvement in nutritional support would be a better understanding of the metabolism of advanced cancer patients. Bosaeus et al.[110] studied a group of 297 cancer patients to analyse dietary intake in relation to resting energy expenditure and reported weight loss. The results demonstrated that weight loss could not be accounted for by diminished dietary intake and that the expected up-regulation of dietary intake in response to elevated energy expenditure is frequently lost in cancer patients. As a result, cachexia could be explained by the uncoupling of food intake to energy expenditure rather than by primary alterations in appetite. Nevertheless, there has been renewed enthusiasm for the potential interventions of dietitians based on reports suggesting the attenuation of weight loss after dietary supplementation with fatty acids fed orally to patients with advanced pancreatic cancer either as fish oil capsules or fish oil supplemented enteral formula. Reported beneficial effects included slowing or reversal of weight loss, increased appetite, and improved quality of life.[23,67,111–114]

The importance of a dietician in the interdisciplinary palliative care approach is widely accepted and described by many palliative care programmes.[115–117] Nevertheless, this is not universal as there are other examples of interdisciplinary palliative care teams that have not included a dietitian.[118–120]

However, it is important to recognize that there is a lack of formal evaluation by dietary groups of the benefit obtained by specific structured dietary counselling in managing the cachexia/anorexia found in palliative care populations. This noted deficit resulted in the organization of a Society for Nutritional Oncology Adjuvant Therapy to design prospective nutritional trials.[101,102]

Enteral/parenteral nutrition

Much of the comment on supplemental nutrition in palliative care populations has tended to focus on advanced cancer patients, and report enteral and parenteral nutrition as similar management options. This oversimplification is further complicated by the involvement of palliative care groups in a variety of non-malignant patient populations.

A critical review of the evidence for enteral nutrition in critically ill patients reported that there was evidence that enteral nutrition may have a favourable impact on gastrointestinal immunological function and infectious morbidity.[121] A prospective multi-centre trial,[122] to evaluate the tolerance of critically ill patients to early intragastric enteral feedings, reported this as a safe and feasible approach in the majority of patients. The incidence of pneumonia was 10 per cent.

Noting that nutritional support has become a standard of care for hospitalized patients, a meta-analysis attempted to clarify whether total parenteral nutrition affected morbidity and mortality in critically ill patients.[123] While total parenteral nutrition may have a positive effect on nutritional endpoints and minor complications, the overall conclusion was that there was no benefit on mortality or major complication rates. A similar meta-analysis explored the relationship between total parenteral nutrition and complication and death rates in surgical patients. The conclusion was that given the potential of increased costs and complications associated with use of TPN and no apparent reduction in mortality or length of stay, further studies were needed to confirm any benefit to this treatment approach.[124]

MacDonald et al.[76] comment that most cancer patients lose weight due to complex metabolic changes that do not respond to calorie replacement via the enteral or parenteral route. Nevertheless, all weight changes in cancer patients do not necessarily result from the cachexia/anorexia syndrome. Some patients may lose weight due to starvation that may respond to calorie supplementation. Very few reports state categorically that there is never a place for enteral and parenteral nutrition in managing cachexia/anorexia. Bozzetti[125] stated that enteral nutrition may help cancer patients with weight loss aggravated by fistulas, short bowel obstruction, and vomiting or malabsorption due to the tumour or treatment. Bruera [94,98,99,104] noted that enteral nutrition is less expensive than parenteral nutrition, and that the former may be useful in patients with head and neck or oesophageal cancer, who are unable to swallow but continue to complain of appetite and hunger. In addition, although no significant benefit from parenteral nutrition given to advanced cancer patients has been demonstrated, issues such as quality of life, strength, performance status, and psychological benefits have not been adequately assessed. Mercadante[126] notes that the failure of conventional parenteral nutrition to improve clinical outcomes in patients with cancer may be related to the fact that standard formulations do not address or reverse abnormalities of metabolism that result in cancer cachexia. The difficulty is to identify those patients who are at risk for malnutrition and at the same time identify the subset of patients who will benefit clinically from parenteral nutrition. The choice of nutritional support depends on the aetiology of the malnutrition, planned therapy, patient preferences, and survival expectations. The indications for parenteral nutrition are limited and routine use should be discouraged.

A review of 70 prospective randomized clinical trials, evaluating the clinical efficacy of enteral and parenteral nutrition in cancer patients, concluded that if this method of nutritional support has therapeutic benefit, it is very small or limited to a subset of patients.[127] An editorial comment[128] on this review[127] noted that it is disappointing that we are still unable to provide successful nutritional support to malnourished cancer patients, but nevertheless 'Although we have been unable to solve the fundamental problem of how best to nutritionally support these cancer patients who have become wasted, we should continue to seek answers to these elusive questions.' Other reports have suggested that caution on the consensus of lack of benefit from parenteral nutrition is warranted, due to defects in the reported trials.[100,129] Problems include small patient numbers, varying degrees of nutritional deficit and duration of parenteral nutrition, and differences in the cancer diagnosis.

Although health care professionals working with advanced cancer patients generally agree on the limitations of enteral and parenteral nutrition, there are some reports advocating a less pessimistic position.[130–133]

A committee of experts under the auspices of the European Association for Palliative Care[106] developed guidelines to assist clinicians to make reasonable decisions on nutritional support for terminally ill cancer patients. It was acknowledged that part of the controversy relates to the definition of terminal patients, and difficulty in predicting life expectancy and potential response to vigorous nutritional support. A three-step process was proposed. The first step involved assessment of (a) oncological/clinical condition, (b) symptoms, (c) expected survival, (d) hydration and nutritional status, (e) oral nutrient intake, (f) psychological profile, (g) gastrointestinal function and potential route of administration, and (h) special services available for nutritional support. The second step involves an overall assessment of the pros and cons for an individual patient. The third step involves periodic reevaluation of the treatment approach.

Although recommendations and guidelines on enteral and parenteral nutrition are plentiful, accurate reporting of how these recommendations have been put into practice by palliative care groups are less frequent. Bruera and MacDonald(94) reported experience with 106 consecutive cancer patients with a variety of tumours undergoing aggressive chemotherapy for symptomatic or curative intent. Continued weight loss was seen in 25 patients despite dietary counselling and enteral nutrition via gastric tube. Outcome and success of treatment were not reported. Mercadante(134) reported the experience of a palliative care programme in Palermo, Italy, with the use of parenteral nutrition. Thirteen of the 1150 patients (1.1 per cent) followed at home during a 5-year period received parenteral nutrition. All patients had advanced cancer with survival time after initiation of treatment ranging from 3 to 121 days. Eleven of the 13 patients survived for 33 days or less. It was noted that while parenteral nutrition is not the usual practice of this group, special circumstances do arise where use is considered appropriate. Decision-making can be complicated by patient or family inability to accept an absence of an alternative when oral feeding is not possible, difficulty in stopping parenteral nutrition previously started in hospital, and adverse psychological impact of treatment withdrawal for some patients and families.

A report of 278 inpatients seen for palliative care consultation in an acute care hospital setting over a 1-year period noted only two of these patients received parenteral nutrition (0.7 per cent).(135) As described in the report, one of these patients was deemed to benefit from nutritional supplementation due to the indolent nature of the patient's disease. In the second patient no nutritional benefit was expected, and the main indication was the psychological difficulty the patient and family experienced in agreeing to discontinue the parenteral nutrition. The ethical implications of instituting this treatment raises difficult questions regarding patient autonomy, beneficence, non-maleficence, and justice.(136)

Howard(137) has documented a more common use of enteral and parenteral nutrition in the United States in a report on the clinical outcome of 2168 active cancer patients receiving home nutritional support. Of them, 1672 received home parenteral nutrition, with 1296 receiving home enteral nutrition. Survival figures document 28 per cent of the cancer patients on parenteral nutrition and 32 per cent of the patients on enteral nutrition alive at 1 year. Ninety per cent of deaths were due to the cancer diagnosis, 9 per cent other medical conditions, and less than 1 per cent from complications related to the nutritional support. In Europe, parenteral nutrition is reportedly used in about two persons per million, as compared to the United States where it is 80 persons per million. Howard concluded that:

1. patients 'cured' of cancer clearly benefit from parenteral nutrition;
2. those patients surviving more than 1 year with 'active' cancer probably have slow growing or potentially curable diseases in whom parenteral nutrition is clearly justified;
3. the majority of 'active' cancer patients receiving nutritional support died in 6–9 months, making the appropriateness of treatment in this patient group less clear;
4. increased use of home nutritional support in the United States may result from increased public awareness of treatment availability resulting in increased patient and family demands, increased training of health care professionals providing this treatment, and willingness of health insurers to pay particularly if more expensive hospital admissions may be shortened.

The differing viewpoints on the benefits and management of nutritional support for palliative care patients highlight the ethical dilemmas in the decision-making process.(138,139) Does a patient have the right to demand a medically futile treatment (autonomy)? Will nutritional support do good or harm (beneficence and non-malificence)? What are the society limitations in determining access to health care and treatment costs (justice)?

Pharmacological management

Corticosteroids,(140–143) progestational agents,(10,17,144–149) cyproheptadine,(150–152) hydrazine sulfate,(153–156) cannabinoids,(157–161) pentoxifylline,(162–164) thalidomide,(165) and fatty acids,(23,67,112–114) have all been studied to demonstrate their potential usefulness in the pharmacological management of cachexia and anorexia. These studies have been predominantly in patients with advanced cancer or AIDS, and have been extensively reviewed. The conclusions highlight similarities and differences.

Loprinzi(74,96,97,144) concludes that progestational agents and corticosteroids have a place in the management of advanced cancer patients with cachexia and anorexia. He argues that it would be reasonable to choose an inexpensive corticosteroid in patients with a poor prognosis expected to survive a short period of days to a few weeks. For planned long-term use of weeks to months, an agent such as megestrol acetate would be more appropriate in a dose range of 160–800 mg/day. The dose would vary depending on risk of thrombo-embolic complications and medication costs.

Nelson et al.(100) considered metoclopramide as the first-line agent for appetite stimulation due to the association of delayed gastric emptying and gastroparesis in advanced cancer patients. Dexamethasone was suggested if a more rapid effect is required with doses of 4–8 mg/day. Megestrol acetate may be useful for less-advanced cancer patients not requiring rapid results, with a recommended starting dose of 160 mg/day titrated upwards as necessary. Cannabinoids may be better tolerated by patients with experience with the drug who may be more comfortable with possible side-effects.

Davis and Dickerson(4) suggested a four-step pharmacological approach based on existing data including evidenced base trials for megesterol acetate and dexamethasone, and single-arm trials with dronabinol, fatty acids, thalidomide, and melatonin. The first step should include treatment of potentially reversible causes of anorexia, anxiety, constipation, depression, dysphagia, nausea and vomiting, oral complications, and pain. Step two is consideration of reduced appetite associated with early satiety or evidence of gastroparesis, resulting in a trial of metoclopramide in the range of 60–120 mg/day. Step three would be a trial of megesterol acetate starting at 160 mg/day and titrating up to 800 mg/day in a patient with a relatively good prognosis. An alternative would be dexamethasone 8–10 mg twice a day in patients with a poor prognosis. Step four would be consideration of a trial of other promising agents such as dronabinol 2.5 mg two to three times per day, melatonin 20–40 mg/day, thalidomide 100 mg at bedtime, and eicosapentaenoic acid 2 gm/day.

Reports by other authors have suggested an approach very similar to that outlined above.(2,77,79,107) Although the published results of pharmacological management with megesterol acetate and corticosteroids are encouraging, a note of caution(166) is suggested as patients with advanced disease with poor performance status and limited prognosis are unlikely to have been recruited to the clinical trials published to date. As a result, conclusions in these reports might reflect an unrealistic and over-optimistic view of the benefits of pharmacological management.

There have been reports from palliative care groups, documenting their prescribing patterns.(167–172) However, these reports provide little information on how commonly pharmacological management is instituted for cachexia and anorexia in palliative care populations. The evidence available suggests that gastric motility agents such as metoclopramide, or appetite enhancing medications such as dexamethasone may be the preferred initial step. The use of these agents and the infrequent use of megestrol acetate or cannabinoids may reflect the affordability and multi-purpose benefit of the former options compared to the latter.(105)

Clinical considerations

A growing body of evidence and opinion suggests that early recognition of nutritional compromise (before patients become significantly wasted), followed by early nutritional and pharmacological interventions, may delay or decelerate weight loss.(21) Combining treatments such as the 3-omega fatty acids and megestrol acetate, along with attention to minimizing muscle deconditioning through exercise, may slow the cachexia process in some individuals early in their disease process.(76) Thoresen et al., in their evaluation of the Subjective Gobal Assessment of Nutrition Tool, observed that severe loss of body weight occurred in both patients with normal body weight and in overweight patients.(21) This emphasizes the need for regular assessments of nutritional status and for developing strategies for nutritional intervention before weight loss becomes serious. The purpose of screening is to identify those patients with mild or moderate malnutrition, before the patient has become overtly wasted and thus be able to attempt to prevent or slow down further deterioration.

Multidimensional assessments are required.(173) Key clinical questions need to be addressed, including an evaluation of the extent and aggression of disease. A combination of subjective and objective measurements and tests are optimal. These should be practical at the bedside and not add to patient burden. An assessment of food intake is essential and serial body weight measurements, despite their limitations, should be encouraged in the early stages of disease. The SGA shows promise as a simple, bedside screening tool. It includes an assessment of body weight, changes in weight, and problems that may contribute to compromised nutrition. Additional anthropometric measurements such as skinfold thickness and upper-arm circumference should be considered. Basic laboratory parameters such as albumin level, interpreted in the context of the other parameters, should be added to the assessment. A creatinine/height index may also be useful. Future studies should look at the feasibility of adding additional tests such as whole-body bio-impedance and electroconductivity to the evaluation,

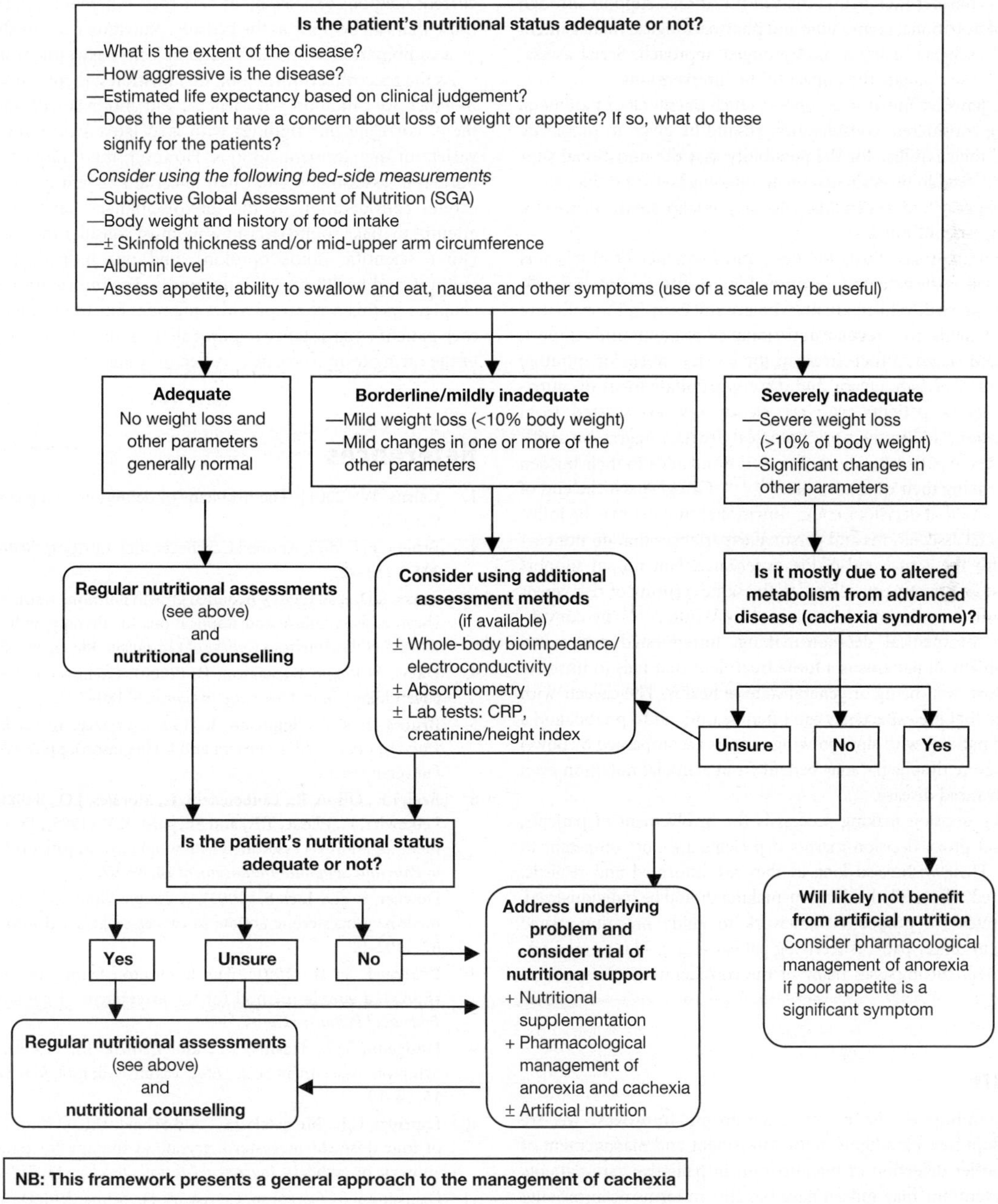

Fig. 1 Cachexia in palliative oncology patients: a proposed approach to clinical decision-making.

especially as advances in technology bring these tests closer to the bedside. The clinical utility of a parameter such as CRP as a rough indicator of the presence of altered metabolic states should be evaluated further.

Weight loss is not invariably attributable to the cachexia syndrome. Thoresen and colleagues have categorized the causes of malnutrition as primary or secondary.[21] Primary factors are largely related to the metabolic changes associated with the cachexia syndrome, while secondary causes include difficulties with swallowing (e.g. as a result of a localized cancer of the head and neck) and obstruction of the gastrointestinal tract by locally advanced disease or the side-effects of treatment. Nutritional intervention in patients suffering from weight loss due to secondary factors may differ from that implemented in patients with weight loss primarily due to the loss of appetite and patients whose weight loss is primarily due to advanced cachexia syndrome. The assessment should therefore also attempt to identify secondary causes of weight loss.

When it is unclear as to whether or not there is nutritional compromise, clinicians should consider therapeutic trials of nutritional support through a combination of nutritional counselling and pharmacological management of anorexia and cachexia, using a multipronged approach. Serial assessments are essential to evaluate the impact of the interventions.

Where more aggressive nutritional support (such as enteral or parenteral feeding) is being considered, consideration should be given to preparing the patients and their families for the possibility that the nutritional supplementation will need to be evaluated on an ongoing basis and that, some time in the future, may lose its benefits. This may ameliorate the distress of a treatment being discontinued.

A flexible approach that adjusts the need and frequency of nutritional assessments, as well as the extent of nutritional interventions, across the illness trajectory, is needed. While patients who are still early in the palliative continuum may benefit from regular nutritional assessments and support, patients in the end stages of their lives (in the last few weeks or months) require a different approach. Overly and disproportionate focus on nutritional assessments in patients who are clearly severely wasted from advanced disease may add to their psychological distress. Aggressive artificial nutrition in these patients is most often futile and adds to their burden rather than improving their quality of life.[127,174] Caregivers at the end of life need to be aware that decisions about nutritional support may be influenced by emotional associations and personal experiences that do not correspond well with the actual end-of-life experience. Nutritional support should be viewed as a treatment, subject to the same scrutiny of risk versus benefits as any other treatment. As expressed by Winter,[174] 'by conventional standards of medical decision-making, unrequested nutritional support of terminally ill patients is a futile treatment that fails to improve prognosis, comfort, well-being or general state of health'. The caveats with this approach are that life expectancy can often be difficult to predict and a small number of patients with slow growing cancers accompanied by bowel obstruction or severe dysphagia, may benefit from artificial nutrition even in the face of advanced disease.

Inherent in the decision-making process is the involvement of patients, their families, and proxy decision-makers if patients are not competent to make decisions. Their wishes, so long as they are informed and realistic, should be respected. Above all, the decision-making should be individualized.

Figure 1 represents a proposed framework to guide nutrition-related decision-making in cancer patients receiving palliative care. This framework, although not tested, encompasses many of the considerations discussed in this chapter.

Conclusion

As our understanding of the cachexia syndrome improves, we are challenged to adopt new paradigms in the assessment and management of this problem. Earlier detection of malnutrition in palliative care patients and earlier interventions may indeed have benefits in terms of improving quality of life and even prolonging life. Regular screening and assessments of nutritional status, before patients start experiencing severe weight loss, is required. Increasingly, palliative care teams are being called upon to see patients who are much earlier in the illness trajectory. Much of our experience has been gained in the context of terminal or end-of-life care. Consequently, we need to be aware that our decision-making framework may be biased towards caring for patients in the last few months of their lives where aggressive treatments and artificial nutrition have been shown, with a few exceptions, to be largely futile and burdensome. Our thinking needs to be broadened to more adequately address the needs of those patients who are earlier in their disease trajectory.

However, continuing these assessments in the presence of very advanced disease and profound wasting, will likely add to our patients' burden and distress. A flexible approach that adjusts the need and frequency of nutritional assessments, as well as the extent of nutritional interventions across the illness trajectory is therefore needed.

Assessment is complicated by the complexity of the problem at hand and current methods of assessment have their inherent limitations, particularly those that can be done at the bedside. Nutritional status should be assessed by a combination of subjective and objective assessment methods.

As the preceding information demonstrates, there is no shortage of ways in which we can approach cachexia and anorexia with methods of assessment, correlate our findings with associated symptoms, and consider a variety of management options. However, the frailty of our patients, the burden of assessment, and often uncertain benefit of treatment, demands careful consideration by the interdisciplinary health care team. As we attempt to make sound decisions we must consider the knowledge available (some scientific, some opinion), and our individual socio-economic, cultural, and health care circumstances. The information contained in the chapters in this section provides a guide, but the unique individuality of each patient circumstance requires all the skill, experience, and compassion of the caring team to create a 'coherent mosaic'.[76]

References

1. **Cairns, W.** (2001). The problems of definitions. *Progress in Palliative Care* **9** (5), 187–9.

2. **Bruera, E.** (1997). Anorexia, cachexia, and nutrition. *British Medical Journal* **315**, 1219–22.

3. **Anker, S.D.** et al. (2001). Acquired growth hormone resistance in patients with chronic heart failure and implications for therapy with growth hormone. *Journal of the American College of Cardiology* **38** (2), 443–52.

4. **Davis, M.P. and Dickerson, D.** (2000). Cachexia and anorexia: cancer's covert killer. *Supportive Care in Cancer* **8**, 180–7.

5. **Bruera, E. and Higginson, I.** (1996). Preface. In *Cachexia–Anorexia in Cancer Patients* (ed. E. Bruera and I. Higginson), pp. V–VI. Oxford: Oxford University Press.

6. **Beal, J.E., Olson, R., Laubenstein, L., Morales, J.O., Bellman, P., Yangco, B., Lefkowitz, L., Plasse, T.F., and Shepard, K.V.** (1995). Dronabinol as a treatment for anorexia associated with weight loss in patients with AIDS. *Journal of Pain and Symptom Management* **10**, 89–97.

7. **Downer, S. and Joel, S.** (1993). A double-blind placebo controlled trial of medroxyprogesterone acetate in cancer cachexia. *British Journal of Cancer* **67**, 1102–5.

8. **Bruera, E.** et al. (1991). The Edmonton Symptom Assessment System (ESAS): a simple method for the assessment of palliative care patients. *Journal of Palliative Care* **7**, 6–9.

9. **Dudgeon, D.J., Harlos, M., and Clinch, J.J.** (1999). The Edmonton Symptom Assessment Scale (ESAS) as an audit tool. *Journal of Palliative Care* **15**, 14–19.

10. **Loprinzi, C.L., Michalak, J.C., and Schaid, D.L.** (1993). Phase 3 evaluation of four doses of megesterol acetate as therapy for patients with cancer anorexia or cachexia. *Journal of Clinical Oncology* **11**, 762–7.

11. **Grinspoon, S., Corcoran, C., Askari, H., Schoenfeld, D., Wolf, L., Burrows, B., Walsh, M., Hayden, D., Parlman, K., Anderson, E., Basgoz, N., and**

Klibanski, A. (1998). Effects of androgen administration in men with the AIDS wasting syndrome. A randomized, double-blind, placebo-controlled trial. *Annals of Internal Medicine* **129**, 18–26.

12. **Oster, M.H.** et al. (1994). Megesterol acetate in patients with AIDS and cachexia. *Annals of Internal Medicine* **121**, 400–8.
13. **Willcox, J.** et al. (1984). Prednisolone as an appetite stimulant in patients with cancer *British Medical Journal* **288**, 27.
14. **Bruera, E.** et al. (1984). Association between malnutrition and caloric intake, emesis, psychological depression, glucose taste and tumor mass. *Cancer Treatment Reports* **6**, 873–5.
15. **Bingham, J.** (1987). The dietary assessment of individuals; methods accuracy, new techniques and recommendations. *Nutrition Abstracts Review* **57**, 705–42.
16. **Burman, R. and Chamberlain, J.** (1996). The assessment of the nutritional status, caloric intake, and appetite of patients with advanced cancer. In *Cachexia–Anorexia in Cancer Patients* (ed. E. Bruera and I. Higginson), pp. 83–93. New York: Oxford University Press.
17. **Bruera, E., MacMillan, K., Hanson, J., Juehn, N., and MacDonald, R.N.** (1990). A controlled trial of megestrol acetate on appetite, caloric intake, nutritional status, and other symptoms in patients with advanced cancer. *Cancer* **66**, 1279–82.
18. **Bruera, E.** et al. (1986). Caloric intake assessment in advanced cancer patients: a comparison of three methods. *Cancer Treatment Reports* **79**, 981–3.
19. **Detsky, A.S.** et al. (1987). What is subjective global assessment of nutritional status? *Journal of Parenteral and Enteral Nutrition* **11**, 8–13.
20. **Ottery, F.D.** (1996). Definitions of standardised nutritional assessment and interventional pathways in oncology. *Nutrition Supplement* **12**, S15–19.
21. **Thoresen, L.** et al. (2002). Nutritional status of patients with advanced cancer: the value of using the subjective global assessment of nutritional status as a screening tool. *Palliative Medicine* **16**, 33–42.
22. **Symreng, T. and Anderberg, B.** (1983). Nutritional assessment and clinical course in 112 elective surgical patients. *Acta Chirurgica Scandinavica* **149**, 657–62.
23. **Wigmore, S.J., Barber, M.D., Ross, J.A., Tisdale, M., and Fearon, K.C.H.** (2000). Effect of oral eicosapentoic acid on weight loss in patients with pancreatic cancer. *Nutrition and Cancer* **3**, 177–84.
24. **Neuenschwander, H. and Bruera, E.** (1996). Asthenia–cachexia. In *Cachexia–Anorexia in Cancer Patients* (ed. E. Bruera and I. Higginson), pp. 57–75. New York: Oxford University Press.
25. **Donnelly, S. and Walsh, T.D.** (1995). The symptoms of advanced cancer. *Seminars in Oncology* **22**, 67–72.
26. **Wheeler, D.A., Muurhainen, N., Launer, C., Gilbert, C., and Bartsch, G.** Change in body weight (wt) as a predictor of death and opportunistic infections (OC) in HIV. International Conference on AIDS; 7–12 July 1996, Vancouver, British Columbia. Abtract Tu.B 2383: 332.
27. **Strawford, A., Barbieri, T., Van Loan, M., Parks, E., Catlin, D., Barton, N., Neese, R., Christiansen, M., King, J., and Hellerstein, M.K.** (1999). Resistance exercise and supraphysiologic androgen therapy in eugonadal med with HIV-related weight loss. A randomized controlled trial. *Journal of the American Medical Association* **281**, 1282–90.
28. (1983). Metropolitan height and weight tables. *Statistical Bulletin of the Metropolitan Life Foundation* **64**, 3–11.
29. **Durnin, J.V.G.A. and Womersley, J.** (1973). Body fat assessed from total body density and its estimation from skinfold thickness: measurements on 481 men and women from 16 to 72 yrs. *British Journal of Nutrition* **32**, 77–97.
30. **Lohman, T.G.** (1981). Skinfolds and body density and their relation to body fatness: a review. *Human Biology* **53**, 181–225.
31. **Jelliffe, D.B.** *The Assessment of the Nutritional Status of the Community.* Geneva, Switzerland: World Health Organization, 1996 (WHO Monograph 53).
32. **Heymsfield, S.B.** (1982). Anthropometric measurement of muscle mass: revised equations for calculating bone free arm muscle area. *American Journal of Clinical Nutrition* **36**, 680–90.
33. **Ferrigno, D. and Buccheri, G.** (2001). Anthropometric measurements in non-small-cell lung cancer. *Supportive Care in Cancer* **9**, 522–7.
34. **Griffin, C.D.M. and Clark, R.G.** (1984). A comparison of the Sheffield prognostic index with forearm muscle dynamometry in patients from Sheffield undergoing major abdominal and urological surgery. *Clinical Nutrition* **3**, 147–51.
35. **Hunt, D.R., Rowlands, B.J., and Johnston, D.** (1985). Handgrip strength: a simple prognostic indicator in surgical patients. *Journal of Parenteral and Enteral Nutrition* **9**, 701–4.
36. **Knols, R.H.** et al. (2002). Isometric strength measurement for muscle weakness in cancer patients: reproducibility of isometric muscle strength measurements with a hand-held pull-gauge dynamometer in cancer patients. *Supportive Care in Cancer* **10**, 430–8.
37. **Lakuski, H.C.** (1987). Methods of assessment of human body composition traditional and new. *American Journal of Clinical Nutrition* **46**, 537–56.
38. **Baumgartner, R.N., Chumlea, W.C., and Roche, A.F.** (1989). Estimation of body composition from bioelectric impedance of body segments. *American Journal of Clinical Nutrition* **50**, 221–6.
39. **Conslick, E.A.** et al. (1992). Predicting body composition from anthropometry and bioimpedance. *American Journal of Clinical Nutrition* **55**, 1051–9.
40. **Hannan, W.J., Cowen, S.J., Plester, C.E., Fearon, K.C.H., and de Beaux, S.C.** (1995). Comparison of bioimpedance spectroscopy and multi-frequency bioimpedance analysis for the assessment of extracellular and total body water in surgical patients. *Clinical Science* **89**, 651–8.
41. **Presta, E.** et al. (1983). Measurement of total body electrical conductivity: a new method for estimating body composition. *American Journal of Clinical Nutrition* **37**, 735–9.
42. **Kvist, H.** et al. (1988). Predictive equations of total and visceral adipose tissue columes derived from measurements with C-T scanning in adult men and women. *American Journal of Clinical Nutrition* **48**, 1351–61.
43. **Seidell, J.C.** et al. (1987). Assessment of intra-abdominal fat: relation between anthropometry and C-T scanning. *American Journal of Clinical Nutrition* **45**, 7–13.
44. **Seidell, J.C. Bakker, C.J.G., van der Kooy, K.** (1990). Imaging techniques for measuring adipose-tissue distribution: a comparison between computerised tomography and 1.5-T magnetic resonance. *American Society of Clinical Nutrition* **52**, 953–5.
45. **Mazess, R.B.** et al. (1990). Dual energy X-ray absorptiometry for total body and regional bone mineral and soft-tissue composition. *American Journal of Clinical Nutrition* **51**, 1106–12.
46. **Kushner, R.F. and Schoeller, D.A.** (1986). Estimation of total body water by bioelectrical impedance analysis. *American Journal of Clinical Nutrition* **44**, 417–24.
47. **Roubenoff, R.** et al. (1993). Use of dual energy X ray absorptiometry in composition studies; not yet a gold standard. *American Journal of Clinical Nutrition* **58**, 589–91.
48. **Forbes, G.B. and Lewis, A.M.** (1956). Total sodium, potassium and chloride in adult man. *Journal of Clinical Investigation* **35**, 596–600.
49. **Pierson, N.J.J.R., Wang, J., and Thorton, J.C.** (1984). Body potassium by four pi-K counting; an anthropometric correction. *American Journal of Physiology* **246**, 234–9.
50. **Schoeller, D.A.** et al. (1980). Total body water measurement in humans with 18-O and 2H water. *American Journal of Clinical Nutrition* **33**, 2686–93.
51. **Vigano, A., Dorgan, M., Buckingham, J., Bruera, E., and Suarez-Almazor, M.E.** (2000). Survival prediction in terminal cancer patients: a systematic review of the medical literature. *Palliative Medicine* **14**, 363–74.
52. **Starker, P.M., Gump, F.E., and Askanazi, J.** (1982). Serum albumin levels as an index of nutritional support. *Surgery* **91**, 194–9.
53. **Tisdale, M.** (1997). Biology of cachexia. *Journal of the National Cancer Institute* **89**, 1763–73.
54. **Shenkin, A.** et al. (1996). Laboratory assessment of protein-energy status. *Clinica Chimica Acta* **253**, S5–9.
55. **Forbes, G.B. and Bruning, G.J.** (1976). Urinary creatinine excretion and lean body mass. *American Journal of Clinical Nutrition* **29**, 1359–66.
56. **Heymsfield, S.B., Arteaga, C., McManus, C., Smith, J., and Moffitt, S.** (1983). Measurement of muscle mass in humans: validity of the 24-hour urinary creatinine method. *American Journal of Clinical Nutrition* **37**, 478–94.
57. **Mendez, J. and Buskirk, E.R.** (1971). Creatinine-height index. *American Journal of Clinical Nutrition* **24**, 385–6.

58. **Cariuk, P., Lorite, M.J., Field, W.N., Wigmore, S.J., and Tisdale, M.J.** (1997). Induction of cachexia in mice by a product isloated from the urine of cachectic cancer patients. *British Journal of Cancer* **76**, 606–13.
59. **Tisdale, M.** (1999). Wasting in cancer. *Journal of Nutrition* **129**, 2435–65.
60. **Tisdale, M.** (1998). New cachexia factors. *Current Opinion in Clinical Nutrition and Metabolic Care* **1**, 253–6.
61. **Socher, S.H., Martinez, D., Craig, J.B., Kuhn, J.G., and Oliff, A.** (1988). Tumor necrosis factor not detectable in patients with clinical cancer cachexia. *Journal of the National Cancer Institute* **80**, 595–8.
62. **Maltoni, M., Fabbri, L., Nanni, O., Scarpi, E., Pezzi, L., Flammi, E., Riccoban, A., Derni, S., Pallotti, G., and Amadori, D.** (1997). Serum levels of tumour necrosis factor alpha and other cytokines do not correlate with weight loss and anorexia in cancer patients. *Supportive Care in Cancer* **5**, 130–5.
63. **Fearson, K., Barber, M., Falconer, J., McMillan, D., Ross, J., and Preston, J.** (1999). Pancreatic cancer as a model: inflammatory mediators, acute-phase response and cancer cachexia. *World Journal of Surgery* **23**, 584–8.
64. **Socher, S.H., Martinez, D., Craig, J.B., Kuhn, J.G., and Oliff, A.** (1988). Tumor necrosis factor not detectable in patients with clinical cancer cachexia. *Journal of National Cancer Institute* **80**, 595–8.
65. **Falconer, J.S.** et al. (1995). The acute-phase protein response and survival duration of patients with advanced pancreatic cancer. *Cancer* **75**, 2077–82.
66. **Endres, S.** et al. (1989). The effect of dietary supplementation with $n-3$ polyunsaturated fatty acids on the synthesis of interleukin-1 and tumor necrosis factor by mononuclear cells. *New England Journal of Medicine* **320**, 265–71.
67. **Wigmore, S.J., Fearon, K.C.H., Maingay, J.P., and Ross, J.A.** (1997). Down-regulation of the acute phase response in patients with pancreatic cancer cachexia receiving oral eicosapentaenoic acid is mediated via suppression of interleukin-6. *Clinical Science* **92**, 215–21.
68. **McMillan, D.C., O'Gorman, P., Fearon K.C.H., and McArdie, C.S.** (1997). A pilot study to megesterol acetate and ibuprofen in the treatment of cachexia in gastrointestinal cancer patients. *British Journal of Cancer* **78**, 788–90.
69. **Long, C.L., Haverburg, L., and Young, V.R.** (1975). Metabolism of 3-methylhistidine in man. *Metabolism* **24**, 929–35.
70. **Spiekerman, A.M.** (1993). Proteins used in nutritional assessment. *Clinics in Laboratory Medicine* **13**, 353–69.
71. **Shils, M.E., Olson, J.A., and Shike, M.**, ed. *Modern Nutrition in Health and Disease.* Philadelphia: Lea & Febiger, 1994, pp. 829–34.
72. **Cella, D.F., Von Roenn, J., Lloyd, S., and Browder, H.P.** (1995). The Bristol–Myers Anorexia/Cachexia Recovery Instrument (BACRI): a brief assessment of patients' subjective response to treatment for anorexia/cachexia. *Quality of Life Research* **4**, 221–31.
73. **Higginson, I. and Winget, C.** (1996). Psychological impact of cancer cachexia on the patient and family. In *Cachexia–Anorexia in Cancer Patients* (ed. E. Bruera and I. Higginson), pp. 172–83. Oxford: Oxford University Press.
74. **Loprinzi, C.L.** (2001). Current management of cancer-associated anorexia and weight loss. *Oncology* **15**, 497–510.
75. **Bruera, E. and Higginson, I.** (1996). Practical concepts for clinicians. In *Cachexia–Anorexia in Cancer Patients* (ed. E. Bruera and I. Higginson), pp. 184–9. Oxford: Oxford University Press.
76. **MacDonald, N., Alexander, R., and Bruera, E.** (1995). Cachexia–anorexia–asthenia. *Journal of Pain and Symptom Management* **10**, 151–5.
77. **Ingham, J. and Portenoy, R.** (1996). Cachexia in context: the interactions among anorexia, pain, and other symptoms. In *Cachexia–Anorexia in Cancer Patients* (ed. E. Bruera and I. Higginson), pp. 158–71. Oxford: Oxford University Press.
78. **Rimmer, T.** (1998). Treating the anorexia of cancer. *European Journal of Palliative Care* **5** (6), 179–81.
79. **Plata-Salaman, C.R.** (1996). Anorexia during acute and chronic disease. *Nutrition* **12**, 69–78.
80. **Irvine, D.M.** et al. (1991). A critical appraisal of the research literature investigating fatigue in the individual with cancer. *Cancer Nursing* **14** (4), 188–99.
81. **Bruera, E. and MacDonald, N.** (1988). Asthenia in patients with advanced cancer. *Journal of Pain and Symptom Management* **3** (1), 9–14.
82. **Bruera, E.** et al. (1987). Association between involuntary muscle function and asthenia, nutritional status, lean body mass, psychometric assessment and tumor mass in patients with advanced breast cancer. *Proceedings of the American Society of Clinical Oncology* **6**, 261.
83. **Cheville, A.** (2001). Rehabilitation of patients with advanced cancer. *Cancer* **92**, 1039–48.
84. **Dimeo, F.C.** et al. (1997). Aerobic exercise in the rehabilitation of cancer patients after high dose chemotherapy autologous peripheral stem cell transplantation. *Cancer* **79**, 1717–22.
85. **Yoshioka, H.** (1994). Rehabilitation for the terminal cancer patient. *American Journal of Physical Medicine and Rehabilitation* **73**, 199–206.
86. **Santiago-Palma, J. and Payne, R.** (2001). Palliative care and rehabilitation. *Cancer* **92**, 1049–52.
87. **Gerber, L.H.** (2001). Cancer rehabilitation into the future. *Cancer* **92**, 975–9.
88. **Pereira, J. and Bruera, E.** (1996). Chronic nausea. In *Cachexia–Anorexia in Cancer Patients* (ed. E. Bruera and I. Higginson), pp. 23–37. Oxford: Oxford University Press.
89. **Ripamonti, C., Shanotto, A., and DeConno, F.** (1996). Oral complications of advanced cancer. In *Cachexia–Anorexia in Cancer Patients* (ed. E. Bruera and I. Higginson), pp. 38–56. Oxford: Oxford University Press.
90. **Campbell, C.** (2001). Controlling malignant ascites. *European Journal of Palliative Care* **8** (5), 187–90.
91. **Dudgeon, D.J. and Lertzman, M.** (1998). Dyspnea in the advanced cancer patient. *Journal of Pain Symptom Management* **16**, 212–19.
92. **Dudgeon, D.J., Lertzman, M., and Askew, G.R.** (2001). Physiological changes and clinical correlation of dyspnea in cancer out-patients. *Journal of Pain and Symptom Management* **21**, 373–9.
93. **Curtis, E.B., Krech, R., and Walsh, T.D.** (1991). Common symptoms in patients with advanced cancer. *Journal of Palliative Care* **7**, 25–9.
94. **Bruera, E. and MacDonald, R.N.** (1988). Nutrition in cancer patients: an update and review of our experience. *Journal of Pain and Symptom Management* **3**, 133–40.
95. **Tchekmedyian, N.S.** (1993). Clinical approaches to nutritional support in cancer. *Current Opinion in Oncology* **5**, 633–8.
96. **Loprinzi, C.L., Goldberg, R.M., and Burnham, N.L.** (1992). Cancer-associated anorexia and cachexia. *Drugs* **43**, 499–506.
97. **Loprinzi, C.L.** (1995). Management of cancer anorexia/cachexia. *Supportive Care in Cancer* **3**, 120–2.
98. **Bruera, E.** (1993). Is the pharmacological treatment of cancer cachexia possible? *Supportive Care in Cancer* **1**, 298–304.
99. **Bruera, E. and Fainsinger, R.L.** (1993). Clinical management of cachexia and anorexia. In *Oxford Textbook of Palliative Medicine* (ed. D. Doyle, G. Hanks, and N. MacDonald), Chapter 4.3.6, pp. 330–7. Oxford: Oxford University Press.
100. **Nelson, K., Walsh, D., and Sheehan, F.A.** (1994). The cancer anorexia-cachexia syndrome. *Journal of Clinical Oncology* **12**, 213–25.
101. **Ottery, F.D.** (1994). Cancer cachexia. *Cancer Practice* **2**, 123–31.
102. **Ottery, F.D.** (1995). Supportive nutrition to prevent cachexia and improve quality of life. *Seminars in Oncology* **22**, 98–111.
103. **Shaw, C.** (1992). Nutritional aspects of advanced cancer. *Palliative Medicine* **6**, 105–10.
104. **Vigano, A. and Bruera, E.** (1996). Enteral and parenteral nutrition in cancer patients. In *Cachexia–Anorexia in Cancer Patients* (ed. E. Bruera and I. Higginson), pp. 110–27. Oxford: Oxford University Press.
105. **Fainsinger, R.L.** (1996). Pharmacological approach to cancer anorexia/cachexia. In *Cachexia–Anorexia in Cancer Patients* (ed. E. Bruera and I. Higginson), pp. 128–40. Oxford: Oxford University Press.
106. **Amadori, D.** et al. (1996). Guidelines on artificial nutrition versus hydration in terminal cancer patients. *Nutrition* **12**, 163–7.
107. **Bruera, E.** (1998). Pharmacological treatment of cachexia: any progress? *Supportive Care in Cancer* **6**, 109–13.
108. **Maillet, J.O. and King, D.** (1993). Nutritional care of the terminally ill adult. In *Nutrition and Hydration in Hospice Care* (ed. C. Gallagher-Allred and M.O. Amenta), pp. 37–54. New York: Haworth Press.
109. **Imoberdorf, R.** (1997). Immuno-nutrition: designer diets in cancer. *Supportive Care in Cancer* **5**, 381–6.

110. **Bosaeus, I.** et al. (2001). Dietary intake and resting energy expenditure in relation to weight loss in unselected cancer patients. *International Journal of Cancer* **93** (3), 380–3.
111. **Barber, M.D.** et al. (2000). Metabolic response to feeding in weight-losing pancreatic cancer patients and its modulation by a fish-oil-enriched nutritional supplement. *Clinical Science* **98** (4), 389–99.
112. **Barber, M.D.** et al. (1999). Fish-oil enriched nutritional supplement attenuates progression of the acute-phase response in weight-losing patients with advanced pancreatic cancer. *Journal of Nutrition* **129**, 1120–5.
113. **Wigmore, S.J.** et al. (1997). Changes in nutritional status associated with unresectable pancreatic cancer. *British Journal of Cancer* **75**, 106–9.
114. **Wigmore, S.J.** et al. (1996). The effect of polyunsaturated fatty acids on the progress of cachexia in patients with pancreatic cancer. *Nutrition* **12**, S27–30.
115. **Fainsinger, R., Bruera, E., Miller, M.J., Hanson, J., and MacEachern, T.** (1991). Symptom control during the last week of life on a palliative care unit. *Journal of Palliative Care* **7** (1), 5–11.
116. **Ajemian, I.** (1993). The interdisciplinary team. In *Textbook of Palliative Medicine* (ed. D. Doyle, G. Hanks, and N. MacDonald), Chapter 2.2, pp. 17–28. Oxford: Oxford University Press.
117. **Coyle, N.** (1995). Supportive care program, pain service, Memorial Sloan-Kettering Cancer Centre. *Supportive Care in Cancer* **3**, 161–3.
118. **Meier, M.L. and Neuenschwander, H.** (1995). Hospice—a home care service for terminally ill cancer patients in southern Switzerland. *Supportive Care in Cancer* **3**, 389–92.
119. **de Stoutz, N. and Glaus, A.** (1995). Supportive and palliative care of cancer patients at Kantonsspital St Gallen, Switzerland. *Supportive Care in Cancer* **3**, 221–6.
120. **Stuart-Harris, R.** (1995). Sacred Heart Hospice: An Australian centre for palliative medicine. *Supportive Care in Cancer* **3**, 280–4.
121. **Heyland, D.K., Cook, D.J., and Guiatt, G.H.** (1993). Enteral nutrition in the critically ill patient: a critical review of the evidence. *Intensive Care Medicine* **19**, 435–42.
122. **Heyland, D.K.** et al. (1999). How well do critical ill patients tolerate early, intragastric enteral feeding? Results of a prospective, multi-centre trial. *Nutrition in Clinical Practice* **14**, 23–8.
123. **Heyland, D.K., MacDonald, S., and Keefe, L.** (1998). Total parenteral nutrition in the critical ill patient. A meta-analysis. *Journal of American Medical Association* **280**, 2013–19.
124. **Heyland, D.K.** et al. (2001). Total parenteral nutrition in the surgical patient: a meta-analysis. *Canadian Journal of Surgery* **44** (2), 102–10.
125. **Bozzetti, F.** (1994). Is enteral nutrition a primary therapy in cancer patients? *Gut* **1**, S65–8.
126. **Mercadante, S.** (1998). Parenteral versus enteral nutrition in cancer patients: indications and practice. *Supportive Care in Cancer* **6**, 85–93.
127. **Klein, S. and Koretz, R.L.** (1994). Nutrition support in patients with cancer: What do to the data really show? *Nutrition in Clinical Practice* **9**, 91–100.
128. **Bloch, A.S.** (1994). Feeding the cancer patient: Where have we come from. where are we going? *Nutrition in Clinical Practice* **9**, 87–9.
129. **Mattox, T.W.** (1993). Drug use evaluation approach to monitoring use of total parenteral nutrition: a review of criteria for use in cancer patients. *Nutrition in Clinical Practice* **8**, 233–7.
130. **Grant, J.P.** (1995). On enteral nutrition during multimodality therapy in upper gastrointestinal cancer patients. *Annals of Surgery* **221**, 325–6.
131. **Daly, J.M., Weintraub, F.N., and Shou, J.** (1995). Enteral nutrition during multimodality therapy in upper gastrointestinal cancer patients. *Annals of Surgery* **221**, 327–38.
132. **King, L.A.** et al. (1993). Outcome assessment of home parenteral nutrition in patients with gynecologic malignancies: what have we learned in a decade of experience? *Gynecologic Oncology* **51**, 377–82.
133. **Echenique, N.M.** (1999). Home nutrition support of advanced cancer patients with gastrointestinal obstruction or dysfunction. *Nutrition and Clinical Practice* **14**, 36–7.
134. **Mercadante, S.** (1995). Parenteral nutrition at home in advanced cancer patients. *Journal of Pain and Symptom Management* **10**, 476–80.
135. **Fainsinger, R.L. and Gramlich, L.M.** (1997). Case report: how often can we justify parenteral nutrition in terminally ill cancer patients. *Journal of Palliative Care* **13**, 48–51.
136. **Latimer, E.** (1991). Caring for seriously ill and dying patients: philosophy and ethics. *Canadian Medical Association Journal* **144**, 859–64.
137. **Howard, N.** (1993). Home parenteral and enteral nutrition in cancer patients. *Cancer* **72**, 3531–41.
138. **Fainsinger, R., Chan, K., and Bruera, E.** (1992). Total parenteral nutrition for a terminally ill patient? *Journal of Palliative Care* **8** (2), 30–2.
139. **Sharp, J.W. and Roncagli, T.** (1993). Home parenteral nutrition in advanced cancer. Ethical and psychosocial aspects. *Cancer Practice* **1**, 119–24.
140. **Willcox, J.** et al. (1984). Prednisolone as an appetite stimulant in patients with cancer. *British Medical Journal* **200**, 37.
141. **Bruera, E., Roca, E., Cedaro, L., Carroro, S., and Chacon, R.** (1985). Action of oral methylprednisolone in terminal cancer patients: a prospective randomized double-blind study. *Cancer Treatment Reports* **69**, 751–4.
142. **Robustelli Della Cuna, G., Pellegrini, A., and Piazzi, M.** (1989). Effect of methylprednisolone sodium succinate on quality of life in pre-terminal cancer patients: a placebo controlled multi-center study. *European Journal of Cancer and Clinical Oncology* **25**, 1817–21.
143. **Popiela, T., Lucchi, R., and Giongo, F.** (1989). Methylprednisolone as palliative therapy for female terminal cancer patients. *European Journal of Cancer and Clinical Oncology* **25**, 1823–9.
144. **Loprinzi, C.L.** et al. (1999). Randomized comparison of megesterol acetate versus dexamathasone versus fluoxymesterone for the treatment of cancer anorexia/cachexia. *Journal of Clinical Oncology* **17** (10), 3299–306.
145. **Loprinzi, C.L.** et al. (1990). Controlled trial of megestrol acetate for the treatment of cancer, anorexia and cachexia. *Journal of the National Cancer Institute* **82**, 1127–32.
146. **Tchekmedyian, S.** et al. (1992). Megestrol acetate in cancer anorexia and weight loss. *Cancer* **69**, 1268–74.
147. **Loprinzi, C.L.** et al. (1993). Body-composition changes in patients who gain weight while receiving megestrol acetate. *Journal of Clinical Oncology* **11**, 152–4.
148. **Maltoni, M.** et al. (2001). High dose progestins for the treatment of cancer anorexia-cachexia syndrome: a systematic review of randomized clinical trials. *Annals of Oncology* **12** (3), 289–300.
149. **Bruera, E.** et al. (1998). Affectiveness of megestrol acetate in patients with advanced cancer: a randomized, double-blind, cross-over study. *Cancer Prevention and Control* **2** (2), 74–8.
150. **Kardinal, C.** et al. (1990). A controlled trial of cyproheptadine in cancer patients with anorexia and/or cachexia. *Cancer* **65**, 2657–62.
151. **Lexchin, J.** (1994). Appetite stimulant claim deleted from label. *Canadian Family Physician* **40**, 20–2.
152. **Durbin, R.L.** (1994). Response. *Canadian Family Physician* **40**, 22.
153. **Loprinzi, C.L.** et al. (1994). Randomized placebo-controlled evaluation on hydrazine sulfate in patients with advanced colorectal cancer. *Journal of Clinical Oncology* **12**, 1121–5.
154. **Loprinzi, C.L., Goldberg, R.M., and Su, J.Q.** (1994). Placebo-controlled trial of hydrazine sulfate in patients with newly diagnosed non-small-cell lung cancer. *Journal of Clinical Oncology* **12**, 1126–9.
155. **Kosty, M.P.** et al. (1994). Cisplatin, vinblastine, and hydrazine sulfate in advanced non-small-cell lung cancer; a randomized placebo-controlled, double-blind phase III study of the cancer and leukemia group B. *Journal of Clinical Oncology* **12**, 1113–20.
156. **Herbert, V.** (1994). Three stakes in hydrazine sulfate's heart, but questionable cancer remedies, like vampires, always rise again. *Journal of Clinical Oncology* **12**, 1107–8.
157. **Lane, M.** et al. (1991). Dronabinol and prochlorperazine in combination for treatment of cancer chemotherapy-induced nausea and vomiting. *Journal of Pain and Symptom Management* **6**, 352–9.
158. **Wadleigh, R.** et al. (1990). Dronabinol enhancement of appetite and cancer patients. *Proceedings of the American Society of Oncology* **9**, 331.
159. **Gorter, R.** (1991). Management of anorexia–cachexia associated with cancer and HIV infection. *Oncology* **5** (Suppl. 9), 13–17.
160. **Nelson, K.** et al. (1994). A phase II study of delta-nine-tetrahydrocannabinol for appetite stimulation in cancer-associated anorexia. *Journal of Palliative Care* **10**, 14–18.
161. **Beal, J.E.** et al. (1997). Long term efficacy and safety of dronabinol for acquired immunodeficiency syndrome-associated anorexia. *Journal of Pain and Symptom Management* **14**, 7–14.

162. **Dezube, B.J.** et al. (1990). Pentoxifylline and well-being in patients with cancer. *Lancet* **335**, 662.
163. **Dezube, B.J., Sherman, M.L., and Friadovich-Keil, J.L.** (1993). Down-regulation of tumor necrosis factor expression by pentoxifylline in cancer patients: a pilot study. *Cancer Immunotherapy* **36**, 57–60.
164. **Goldberg, R.M.** et al. (1995). Pentoxifylline for treatment of cancer anorexia and cachexia? A randomized, double-blind placebo-controlled trial. *Journal of Clinical Oncology* **13**, 2856–9.
165. **Bruera, E.** et al. (1999). Thalidomide in patients with cachexia due to terminal cancer: preliminary report. *Annals of Oncology* **10** (7), 857–9.
166. **Davis, C.L. and Hardy, J.R.** (1994). Palliative care. *British Medical Journal* **308**, 1359–62.
167. **Curtis, E.B. and Walsh, T.D.** (1993). Prescribing practices of a palliative care service. *Journal of Pain and Symptom Management* **8**, 312–16.
168. **Twycross, R.G., Bergi, S., John, S., and Lewis, K.** (1994). Monitoring drug use in palliative care. *Palliative Medicine* **8**, 137–43.
169. **Drummond, S.H.** et al. (1996). National survey of drug use in palliative care. *Palliative Medicine* **10**, 119–24.
170. **Dickerson, D.** (1999). The 20 essential drugs in palliative care. *European Journal of Palliative Care* **6** (4), 130–5.
171. **Mercadante, S., Fulfaro, F., and Casuccio, A.** (2001). Pattern of drug use by advanced cancer patients followed at home. *Journal of Palliative Care* **7** (1), 37–40.
172. **Watanabe, S., Fainsinger, R.L., and Bruera, E.** (1995). Commonly prescribed medications in advanced cancer patients. *Journal of Palliative Care* **11** (3), 70.
173. **Baker, J.P., Detsky, A.S., and Mendelson, R.A., Wolman, S.L., Wesson, D.E. and Jeejcebhoy, K.N.** (1984). Evaluating the accuracy of nutritional assessment techniques applied to hospitalized patients. *Journal of Parenteral and Enteral Nutrition* **8**, 153–9.
174. **Winter, S.M.** (2000). Terminal nutrition: framing the debate for the withdrawal of nutritional support in terminally ill patients. *American Journal of Medicine* **109**, 723–6.

8.4.3 Dietary and nutritional aspects of palliative medicine

Isobel Davidson and Rosemary Richardson

> Mealtimes are no longer a pleasure. It is sometimes difficult to decide what to have for a meal. My husband gets anxious my bones are sticking out.
>
> (Cancer patient)

Introduction

To any health care professional or lay person the provision of nourishment is probably thought of as a fundamental component of care. Yet, despite often Herculean efforts on the part of the professional, the patient, and his/her carers, the majority of patients with incurable conditions fail to achieve an energy intake that is sufficient to sustain or arrest aggressive weight loss. This failure to achieve anabolism (maintain body weight) underlines the necessity to understand the complex interplay of immune, metabolic, and endocrine events that contribute to the pathophysiology of cachexia and anorexia (see Chapter 8.4.1). It is only through an appreciation of the sequelae of events in cachexia and anorexia that appropriate and effective nutritional intervention strategies may begin to be identified.

The anorexia that accompanies incurable non-malignant disease (i.e. advanced respiratory, cardiac and neurological diseases, and AIDS) has, to date, received little attention and is accepted as an inevitable consequence of end-stage disease. As a result reliance is often placed on translating what has been learned about the aetiology and management of cachexia and anorexia in neoplastic disease to other groups.

In palliative care, patients frequently report a significant loss of the body's endogenous energy reserves (adipose and lean tissue) which may be paralleled by the progression of their disease (i.e. pancreatic insufficiency, gastrointestinal obstruction, bowel dysfunction, severe dysphagia, and/or tumour growth). Consideration of the nutritional aspects of advanced progressive disease may be viewed by some clinicians as being of little importance and/or ineffective in improving nutritional status. For example, the initiation of aggressive nutritional support (enteral or parenteral) for cancer patients has failed to reverse loss of lean tissue[1] and distressingly the use of parenteral nutrition has been shown to have a deleterious effect on survival and infection rate.[2]

For the patient and their carer anorexia and the ravages of weight loss have been cited as one of the most troubling symptoms of their disease.[3,4] In a study that used 38 specific questions to determine the prevalence of symptoms in 100 patients, pain was the symptom reported with greatest frequency (89 per cent), followed by weight loss (58 per cent), anorexia (55 per cent), constipation (40 per cent), and early satiety (40 per cent). Severity of symptoms was also rated in this study and all patients had lost more than 10 per cent of their preillness weight; anorexia, early satiety, and constipation were rated as severe or moderate in 82, 75, and 60 per cent, respectively, of this cohort.

In palliative care it is from the patient's perspective and that of their carer that the nutritional manifestations of their disease appear to have a powerful impact on wellbeing. Nutrition is a central part of everyone's daily life; it is the focus of social interaction where food is associated with times of celebration or commiseration, bringing those we are close to together. This is perhaps brought into perspective by the experience of patients and carers themselves.[5,6]

> It was so frightening for me to see her lose weight. I knew something was drastically wrong. I blame myself for not feeding her the right things[6]
>
> (Carer whose wife had advanced cancer)

> at first cooking was difficult; since I've had cancer we have radically changed what we eat[5]
>
> (Cancer patient)

These quotes powerfully describe the impact that the deterioration in nutritional status has on patients with advanced cancer and are likely to be echoed by patients with other pathologies.

The incidence of undernutrition in patients with terminal disease is estimated to be half to three-quarters of this population. It has been shown to detrimentally impact on survival and quality of life[7] and thus it is disappointing that the provision of adequate nutrients has proved an ineffective treatment modality. Nevertheless, it has directed those interested in the nutritional wellbeing of patients to examine more subtle approaches to nutritional management. These should serve to take advantage of our understanding of the metabolic events accompanying cachexia and anorexia and the impact these have on the normal physiological determinants of nutrient intake.

Sensory determinants of energy intake

The clinical presentation of sensory aberration in palliative medicine is frequently reported by patients but is rarely a primary focus of investigation. Although it is overt changes in the special senses such as taste and smell which are usually reported it is the gastrointestinal autonomic sensory nerves which inhibit the tonic drive to eat and thus mediate the sensation of satiety.

Sensation in the gastrointestinal tract triggered by the stimulus of food plays a major role in determining energy intake. The stimulus of food may induce either inhibition of food intake, commonly known as satiety, or stimulate further ingestion of food increasing energy intake. The positive influences on energy intake are primarily determined by the palatability of food presented and mediated by the cranial nerves innervating the oro-nasal areas, which includes the olfactory, glossopharyngeal, and facial nerves. Whereas, the negative or satiety-inducing effects of food are dictated by the autonomic sensory nerves innervating the proximal gastrointestinal tract and liver and are contained within the afferent arm of the vagus nerve. These autonomic afferents induce satiation (stopping eating) and maintain satiety (inhibition of eating) by influencing the hypothalamic feeding areas.

Gastrointestinal sensory vagal afferents are activated by the volume of food ingested as well as its composition and subsequently its utilization as macronutrients, primarily carbohydrate and fat, from which energy as adenosine triphosphate (ATP) is ultimately derived (see Table 1). It is the complex relationship between these mechanisms and the cognitive influences orchestrated by central feeding centres, which dictate energy intake and associated ingestive behaviour, such as meal frequency and duration (see Fig. 1). The dynamics of the system are such that alterations in the flow of nutrients, metabolites, immunomodulators, or endogenous mediators will have a significant impact on energy intake. In advanced cancer and other wasting disorders such as acquired immune deficiency syndrome (AIDS) the suppression of energy intake is a significant factor in perceived changes of quality of life in these groups.

It is evident that a low energy intake, when combined with hypermetabolism, will accelerate loss of energy stores. Despite attempts to reverse this phenomenon there have been relatively few reports of energy balance being successfully achieved. This may be partly due to not only the heterogeneity of the patients under study, in terms of primary diagnosis and stage of disease, but also the poor understanding of the neural and humoral influences determining energy intake and the modulation of these events which occurs with the presence of advanced disease.

Table 1 Physiological and pathophysical roles of the vagus

Sensory functions	*Motor functions*
Fullness	Gastric secretion
CCK-mediated satiety	Pancreatic secretion
Hepatic ATP sensor	Gastrointestinal motility
Physiological function	*Pathophysical manifestation*
Post-absorptive nutrient monitor	Gastric stasis/nausea
Hepatic energy sensor	Chemotherapy/radiotherapy-induced vomiting
Satiety (fullness and incretin mediated)	Appetite-suppressing effects (via IL1β)

Smell and taste

The alterations in taste and smell, which accompany advanced disease, have been extensively reported, primarily in patients with cancer.[8,9] However, more recently alterations in taste have been reported in patients with other advanced wasting diseases (e.g. AIDS)[10] and appear to have both a peripheral and central component. The influence of chemotherapy or radiotherapy regimens in cancer may provide an explanation for the loss of taste perception or perhaps the reported distortion of taste perception, such as the 'metallic' or even 'cotton wool' taste of food,[11] where there is loss of renewable taste receptor cells.[12,13] It does not explain the reported reduction in taste (bitter) thresholds,[14,15] which suggests an increased sense of gustation is paralleled by active weight loss. A similar phenomenon appears to exist with respect to olfaction,[16] where a heterogeneous group of advanced cancer patients in palliative care correctly identified more odours than their age-matched counterparts (see Fig. 2).

Physiological stimulation of gustation and olfaction by food in healthy individuals appears primarily to be a positive influence on intake, so long as the food itself is palatable. This is commonly a focus of attempts to improve energy intake (see Chapter 13.3). However, during the time course of a normal eating episode this positive influence wains[17] and subjects undergo sensory-specific satiety whereby the pleasure and desire for specific foods decreases.[18]

In patients with enhanced sensory perception this may induce early sensory satiety and consequently reduce energy intake. It may be the case that this is further exacerbated by attempts of well-meaning carers to improve energy intake in cachectic patients by providing highly palatable favourite meal options, thus further contributing to reduced meal duration and reduced intake. This highlights the practical problems of feeding patients with an on-going metabolic disorder.

Since this sensitization of taste and smell occurs only in weight-losing patients it has been suggested that mediators of the inflammatory response in cachexia (primarily IL6, TNFα, and IL1β) may be neuromodulators of olfactory and gustatory stimuli. There have been attempts to correlate subjective or perceived changes in taste with plasma levels of cytokines, and whilst more recently identified mediators of muscle degradation (e.g. proteolysis inducing factor) may increase the likelihood of significant findings such a simple correlation does not imply a cause–effect relationship.

Experimental evidence in animals reveals the upregulation of neural activation in the chorda tympani following injection of lipopolysaccharide.[19] This model acts to induce an inflammatory response and if paralleled in humans would magnify the effects of signalling from the glossopharyngeal

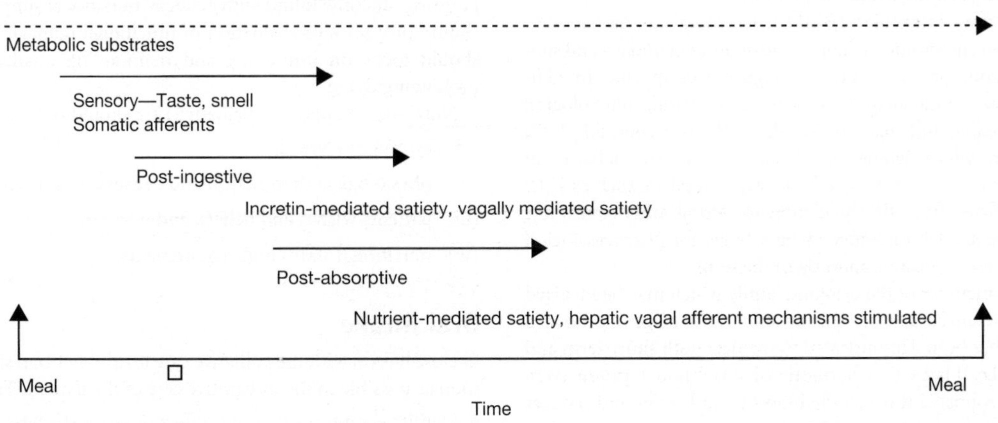

Fig. 1 Pre- and post-prandial influences on satiety.

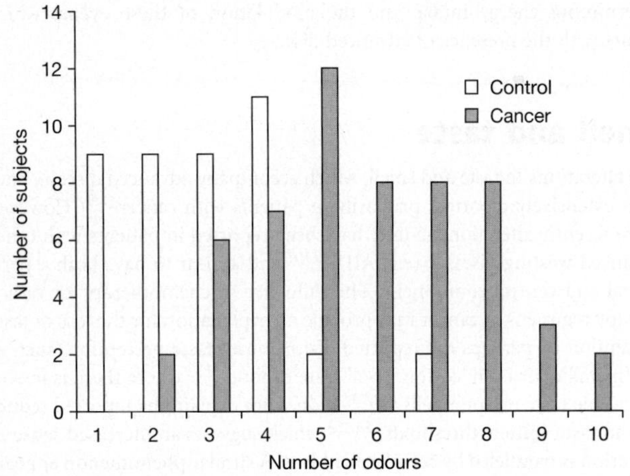

Fig. 2 A study of heterogeneous group of advanced cancer patients in palliative care.

and facial nerves. For normal and enhanced perception of orosensation normal mucosal architecture of the taste receptor cells and supportive structures is required. This will not always be the case in patients who have undergone recent chemotherapy or radiotherapy.

Perceived changes in taste and smell reported by palliative care patients are not uniform. This may be partly influenced by prescribed medications which may affect sensory stimulation or perception of taste and smell.(20) Whether the degree and direction (inhibited or stimulated) of taste and smell aberrations predict energy intake, or what is probably more important, predict the degree to which energy intake may be increased remains unclear. In addition the degree to which these aberrations in olfaction and gustation affect the hedonics of eating is likely to be a significant factor, impacting directly on quality of life.

Appetite

While objective measures may be used to assess aberrations in taste and smell, this is not the case for changes in subjective feelings such as appetite. Loss of appetite (anorexia) is commonly reported in patients and may be evident at diagnosis. The progression of anorexia may be rapid and parallel disease progression thereby contributing to a patient's decreased energy intake and weight loss. The mechanisms of anorexia during active disease or infection may be a consequence of the production of cytokines which elicit communication between the neural pathways responsible for appetite regulation and the immune system. These are also mediators of the altered metabolism in wasting disorders (see Chapter 8.4.1).

One of these cytokines, interleukin 1β (ILβ), acts rapidly on the vagus(21) which communicates sensory information to the brain stem initially and subsequently to the hypothalamus, the ultimate regulator of appetite. In addition, the vagus nerve is intimately involved in co-ordinating physiological responses during feeding and may provide the pathway responsible for a number of symptoms which manifest in advanced disease (see Table 1). In addition to effecting changes in the gut–brain axis, cytokines such as IL1β may also be transported from the circulation to central areas controlling appetite.(22) This avenue will undoubtedly be a target for pharmacological manipulation of disease-associated anorexia in the future.(23)

Leptin is another member of the cytokine family which may be involved in the anorexia of advanced disease. This protein of the *ob* gene produced from the adipocyte has been demonstrated to regulate both short-term and long-term food intake. It is a satiety hormone which, although produced in the periphery, is transported through the blood brain barrier and reduces food intake and increases energy expenditure.

Elevated production of leptin has been reported in inflammatory diseases. However, in cachexia associated with pancreatic cancer circulating leptin levels are reported to be lower than in health.(24) This alone does not preclude a role for leptin in the anorexia of other wasting disorders(25) where a central hypothalamic involvement may be contributory. However, the afferent limb of the leptin pathway appears intact in advanced disease of the prostrate.(26) Despite these results, further elucidation of leptin physiology provides the potential for modulation of both sides of the energy balance equation.

Suppression of appetite may be influenced by biochemical correlates of tumour and host metabolism as described above. In addition this reduction in appetite may have a psychological basis and some drugs used in symptom control may also affect food intake.(27)

The benefit gained from drug administration in alleviation of poor appetite may arise from direct central orexigenic effects or from relief of symptoms contributing indirectly to development of anorexia. The pharmacological management is reviewed in Chapter 8.4.4.

The management of poor appetite in palliative care, however, should not solely focus on the use of pharmacological agents. Alcohol has long been used as an aperitif and appetite stimulant. Providing there are no contraindications alcohol consumption (e.g. two glasses of wine) may serve to not only promote energy intake but may also serve as a palatable and sociable approach to improve food intake.

As with so many aspects of nutritional care in palliative medicine resolution of decreased appetite requires consideration of the following:

- symptom control,
- attention to the presentation and timing of meals, and
- involvement of patient and relatives to identify food preference and food aversions.

Nutritional management strategies

If food intake is to be optimized the sensory and metabolic sequelae must be assessed and anticipated. This includes consideration of delivery of nutrients, effects on body weight (stabilization or improvement), and attenuating loss of lean body mass.

A reduction in spontaneous dietary intake is ubiquitous in patients receiving palliative care. Symptoms of disease (i.e. cachexia syndrome, taste changes, dysphagia, dementia, nausea, vomiting, diarrhoea) and in some cases therapeutic modalities (i.e. palliative radiotherapy, opioids) may affect the quantity and quality of nutrients consumed. Disease progression and symptom-induced weight loss pose formidable problems. Though the use of parenteral or enteral tube feeding can increase energy intake and attenuate weight loss, it is evident that improvements in nutritional status are merely reflected in fat mass but no demonstrable benefits in outcome.(28) In other words, an approach that simply increases energy intake is unlikely to achieve any significant clinical benefits.

However, in the current health care climate the focus is on clinical governance, clinical effectiveness, and patient-centred care. The disappointing outcome found with artificial nutritional support in palliative care should prompt a re-evaluation of nutritional management. The approach should focus on improving and maintaining quality of life and avoid prolonging dying.

Nutritional support in palliative care should reflect:

(i) symptom control,

(ii) physiological dysfunction and delivery of nutrients,

(iii) patients wishes and beliefs, and

(iv) nutritional status and requirements.

Oral intake

In close liaison with the palliative care team a dietitian should be involved as soon as possible in the integrative care of the patient. Their role is to:

- identify symptoms that may affect intake and advise on ways of improving intake,
- determine current nutritional intake (quantity) and taste changes,

Table 2 Energy and nutrient intakes of cancer patients compared with recommended values[a]

	Mean	RDA[b]
Energy (kcal)	1178	2150
Protein (g)	42	54
Fat (g)	46	—
Carbohydrate (g)	155	—

[a] Adapted from ref. 30.

[b] RDA = recommended daily allowance.

- advise the care team on appropriate nutritional regimens, and
- inform the care team on patient's progress.

The determination of patients' dietary intake relies on the accuracy of self reporting by the patient and/or their informal or formal carers. Although underreporting is reported among overweight individuals this is generally not the case in undernourished patients.(29)

The dietitian is skilled in elucidating an accurate dietary history and subsequently compares patient intakes to recommended daily intakes of macro and micronutrients. For many patients there is a deficit in energy intake which cumulatively results in deterioration in nutritional status. In one of the few studies that used the 3-day weighed technique to determine nutritional intake in cancer patients(30) it was found that energy and protein intakes were 55 and 78 per cent of recommended values, respectively (Table 2).

Factors that may affect oral intake

Taste

The physiological mechanisms involved in the manifestation of aberrant taste found in patients with metabolically actively disease (i.e. cancer, AIDS) has already been reviewed in this chapter. Altered taste and smell can reduce intake, contribute to poor nutritional status, and alter the cephalic responses that normally act positively to optimize nutrient intake and meet host requirements.

Whilst, taste changes have been extensively reported in neoplastic disease,(8) it is evident that altered taste and smell are also found in HIV patients.(31) Interestingly, in this study of 40 HIV patients, significantly higher taste and smell detection thresholds were found when compared with matched controls. Additionally, it appeared that this blunting of taste and smell worsened with disease progression. Factors implicated in the deterioration of taste and smell include the disease process, opportunistic infections, and medications. This appears to be at odds with the profile of olfactory change in cancer.(16)

Indeed the profile of taste changes found in cancer patients appears to be complex, with a third of patients having a reduction in their perception of sweet taste. The detection of bitter taste in some patients is heightened and may account for aversion to foods such as meat and coffee.(32) Work from our own group (Table 3) shows that the energy and macronutrient intake of a group of cancer patients with changes in bitter taste sensitivity is higher when compared with a group of age-matched controls without taste changes.

Altered taste is likely to have a differential effect on patients and underlines the importance of individual patient management. For example, this may involve the exclusion of foods patients have only recently found to be unpleasant and unappetizing.

Xerostomia

Xerostomia or oral dryness is a common and distressing symptom. Not surprisingly, a lack of saliva makes swallowing difficult and patients may complain of burning and soreness. Xerostomia also predisposes to oral infections. The principal causes of xerostomia are drugs (anticholingeric drugs, some antidepressants, opioids, sedatives, and diuretics) and dehydration.(33) The presence of dry mouth is likely to reduce dietary intake with patients tolerating only fluids.

Table 3 Nutrient intake of cancer patients with or without heightened taste for bitter [mean ± (SEM)]

	Heightened taste for bitter ($n = 25$)	No change in taste ($n = 70$)
Energy	4.6 (0.4)	3.2 (0.7)
Fat (g)	49 (9.0)	40 (6.0)
Fat energy (%)	44 (1.0)	44 (2.0)
Protein (g)	43 (7.0)	30 (4.0)
Protein energy (%)*	18 (1.0)	15 (1.0)
Carbohydrate (g)	105 (18.0)	83 (11.0)
Carbohydrate energy (%)	39 (1.0)	40 (2.0)

* $P < 0.05$ between cancer patients and control subjects.

Table 4 Management of xerostomia

Review patient's history and medications
If possible consider changes to drug regimens
Mouth care
Review diet if patient's mouth is sore and encourage energy dense protein rich fluids. Avoid fruit juices
Encourage gustatory and masticatory stimulation by making hard sweets or sugar-fee gum available
In severe cases the use of parasympathomimetic drugs to increase flow of saliva may be considered
Use of saliva substitutes

The treatment and resolution of xerostomia aims to alleviate distressing symptoms in order to improve the enjoyment of food and improve dietary intake (Table 4). The management of patients with xerostomia, as with almost all areas of care, requires an integrated approach (see Chapter 8.12).

Dysphagia

Patients who may develop dysphagia include those with motor neurone disease, Parkinson's disease, Alzheimer's disease, Huntingdon's chorea, progressive multiple sclerosis, and head and neck cancer. Dysphagia is often one of the first symptoms of motor neurone disease, and a great fear for those patients is that they will choke to death while eating. As Parkinson's disease advances patients are more likely to have swallowing problems and interestingly it appears that in patients without dementia a more aggressive approach to dietary management is used.(34) (See Chapter 10.6.)

The severity of dysphagia varies considerably, some patients may have mild swallowing problems requiring minor food modifications (altered texture) whereas others with severe dysphagia are unable to tolerate even thickened liquids. For those patients unable to swallow enough to maintain hydration or nutrition, endoscopic placement of a percutaneous gastrostomy (PEG) may be considered. While artificial nutrition support has a place in dysphagia management the clinical team and patient may wish to re-evaluate long-term treatment goals.

The assessment of swallowing is normally undertaken by a speech and language therapist (see Chapter 15.5); their evaluation will determine the dietary prescription. The most widely used approach to dysphagia diets is through a series of graded dietary consistencies (Table 5).

Care must be taken in the presentation of these meals but availability of thickening agents has allowed food moulding to significantly improving aesthetic appeal. It should be remembered that the liquid content of these modified diets tends to be higher and acts to dilute nutritional content, nutrient fortification may, therefore, be required.

Table 5 Diets used in nutritional management of dysphagia

Dysphagia	Food modification
Stage IV	Soft diet
Stage III	Soft diet + liquids
Stage II	Puree base, thickening agent, some liquids
Stage I	Puree diet, thickening agent, no liquids

Artificial nutrition support

Despite efforts to improve patients' oral intake many are unable to consume sufficient energy (protein, fat, carbohydrate) to arrest progressive weight loss. This anorexia may be due to the presence of cachexia and can be accompanied by increasing functional disability, (i.e. dysphagia, dementia, gastrointestinal dysfunction, obstruction). In such cases artificial nutrition support, either enteral using a nasogastric tube or PEG, or total parenteral nutrition (TPN) may be considered. Prior to embarking on aggressive nutritional therapy the potential benefit in terms of symptom relief and quality of life must be weighed against the added burden this therapy will have on the patient and their family.

As the majority of patients receive artificial nutrition support at home, it should not be initiated without careful deliberation and there should be some tangible benefit. Determination of measurable and appropriate benefits of artificial nutrition support in palliative care requires robust investigation. An assumption if often made that improvement in nutritional status will increase functional ability and in turn quality of life but there is little evidence to substantiate this hypothesis. This failure to unequivocally show benefit may, in part, be due to the difficulties of isolating the effect of nutritional support per se from other confounding variables such as disease progression, survival time, psychological state, and cognitive impairment.

In fact it may be that the initiation of artificial nutrition support is associated with increased discomfort and risk of treatment-related complications (gastric distension, reflux, infections, aspiration, fluid overload). There is a need to improve determinants of outcome for patients receiving artificial nutrition support.

A 5-year survey of patients in the United Kingdom[(35)] receiving home artificial nutritional support reports that the majority of patients receiving this therapy have neurological disease. In 1996, 2957 patients were included in the survey. Seven per cent had motor neurone disease, 5–6 per cent multiple sclerosis, and 2.2 per cent Parkinson's disease. This profile has changed little and by the year 2000, of the 6629 patients registered on home enteral feeding 4–5 per cent had motor neurone disease, 3.6 per cent multiple sclerosis, and 3.2 per cent Parkinson's disease. Whilst there has been an increase in the number of patients with cancer registered for home enteral feeding rising from 12 per cent in 1996 to 17.5 per cent in 2000, less than 5 per cent of home parenteral nutrition (HPN) patients in 2000 had neoplastic disease. A proportion of the cancer patients receiving HPN may have had curable disease but this is not clear from the data. This is important as the use of HPN in terminal cancer is particularly controversial.

Interestingly, when the HPN registers from different countries are considered there is significant geographical variation in the use of HPN in cancer. A European survey of 5000 HPN patients conducted under the auspices of the European Society of Parenteral and Enteral Nutrition[(36)] found that cancer patients receiving HPN accounted for 60 per cent of patients in the Netherlands, 27 per cent in Spain, and 8 per cent in Belgium. The reasons for this variation may be clinical preference, cultural or religious factors, and also the setting where HPN was commenced. For example, patients may start HPN in the acute sector but subsequent cessation of this treatment in the palliative care setting may be complicated.

Survey information on patients receiving home enteral and HPN is of interest but it does not exclusively focus on issues relevant to palliative care. In particular, more information on the direct impact artificial nutrition support has on the patient and their carers is required. This approach would permit identification of areas of care where greater education and support was required. For example, in a 5-year prospective review of 417 patients receiving home enteral nutrition[(37)] it was found that over half had dysphagia related to neurological impairment or cancer. The majority of these patients were fed via a PEG, a route that was a major cause of distress for the patient. This highlights the importance of a full understanding of what is involved in home artificial nutritional support. Furthermore, only 42 per cent were alive at 1 year with 35 per cent dying after 1 month of enteral feeding. This emphasizes the need for careful selection of patients who will benefit from artificial nutrition as an active treatment.

Enteral nutrition

Enteral nutrition is a method of delivering nutrients (macro and micronutrients) to the gastrointestinal tract through a nasogastric, gastrostomy, or jejunostomy tube. The route of feeding will depend on the clinical features of disease (e.g. head and neck obstruction) and, wherever possible, patient choice. Today, a PEG is frequently used in the nutritional support of palliative care patients. It is particularly useful in those patients with a risk of aspiration, for example, motor neurone disease. For many patients, the presence of a nasogastric tube is aesthetically unacceptable whereas the endoscopic placement of a relatively discreet 'button' gastrostomy carries a low complication rate and allows patients to carry on daily activities albeit limited.

Education of the patient and his/her informal carer is central to maintaining the patency of the tube (nasogastric or gastrostomy), to keeping the gastrostomy site clean and dry and in the delivery of the feed. The feed prescription should be sufficient to meet requirements and may be calculated from predictive equations[(38)] and dietary reference values.[(39)]

There is an extensive range of commercial feeding regimens available and the majority of patients can tolerate whole protein regimens. The energy content of enteral feeds is usually 1.0–1.5 kcal ml and are nutritionally complete in volumes of 1500–2000 ml/day; although, this should be checked with the dietitian. For those patients with deterioration of their gastrointestinal absorptive capacity, a peptide or elemental regimen may be deemed more appropriate. Unlike the monitoring of patients oral intake determination of actual intake from enteral feeding is more objective, and provided the prescription is met the patient should be driven into positive energy balance.

Despite enteral nutrition improving nutritional intake it does not appear to bring about repletion of the functional component of body composition (body cell mass). This appears to be the case not only with cancer and AIDS but also in chronic neurological disorders where dysphagia rather than cachexia is the indication for starting enteral feeding.[(41)] The influence of enteral nutrition on clinical outcome and quality of life in chronic neurological disease remains to be investigated.

Parenteral nutrition

Parenteral nutrition delivers nutrients directly into the circulation, avoiding problems for patients with gastrointestinal dysfunction, major resection, and obstruction. Catheters for parenteral feeding may be inserted centrally or peripherally, and complete nutrient solutions containing lipid, dextrose, amino-acids, vitamins, minerals, and trace elements are delivered either continuously or cyclically (8–12 h/day). The procedure for catheter insertion, catheter care, prescription of feeds, and monitoring is beyond the scope of this chapter. Parenteral nutrition is up to 10 times more expensive and not as physiologically normal when compared with enteral feeding. In addition it carries a significantly greater complication risk (i.e. metabolic, infective).

There is little evidence to justify the use of parenteral nutrition in palliative care and reports have focused on patients receiving curative anticancer treatment and patients with AIDS. One study[(42)] examined the use of parenteral nutrition in terminally ill cancer patients where 156 patients received TPN as an adjunctive therapy and 11 patients received TPN as a supportive therapy (nutrition and hydration). In both groups the quality of life (pain, activities of daily living, ability to take oral diet) continued to deteriorate and had no influence on outcome (discharge, death). In end-stage AIDS TPN improved weight gain when compared with AIDS patients with a central catheter not used for feeding. TPN did not, however, have any positive effects on length of hospital stay and quality of life indicators.[43]

Parenteral nutrition has proved disappointing in terms of increasing patients' lean body mass and improving quality of life. Nutritional support of palliative care patients predominantly centres on the provision of enteral nutrition. Whilst the use of feeding regimens, to date, has not clearly demonstrated benefit the inclusion of novel substrates or nutraceuticals may attenuate muscle loss in cachexia, but more data are required.

Loss of lean body mass and body weight in palliative care patients is driven not only by a reduced energy intake because of anorexia but also because of enhanced breakdown of body energy stores. Agents which alleviate muscle wasting or promote anabolism have been extensively studied in recent years (see Chapter 8.4.4).

Ethical issues

Administration of nutrients and fluid constitutes medical treatment and as with any other therapeutic agent may be refused by competent patients (see Chapter 3.3). Maintaining only fluid intake may potentially prolong the dying process. Since fluid ingestion is such an habitual action patients have been reported to have forgotten to cease intake[44] even when a clear desire to stop oral intake has been demonstrated.

The question of determining competency of the patient to make a decision, understand the choices available, and communicate a decision, in addition to appreciating the consequences of the choice made, are relevant to nutritional and dietary intervention. The patients' ability in relation to the entire decision-making process and underlying rational basis are key to whether nutritional therapy should be instigated or continued.

There may be difficulty in affirming the option for refusal of oral intake or the fact that it is actively voluntary. However, the withdrawal of oral nutrition may be a distressing decision for carers and family to accept.

Decisions to continue nutritional support may be made more difficult depending on the progression of the disease per se. This is a problem evident in progressive neurological illnesses such as motor neurone disease, Alzheimers disease, and Creutzfeld–Jacob disease. In the terminal stages of such disorders the likelihood of recumbency and inability to communicate increases. This compounds the problem of withdrawal of nutritional support where there is considerable uncertainty as to whether it is possible to inform the patient of choices affecting their treatment and may be impossible to hear the voice of patients in end of life care. Where tube feeding results in the development of clinical problems for which they may have been instigated (e.g. aspiration pneumonia), it has been proposed[45] that this may be considered a clear clinical decision to withdraw artificial nutritional support.

Current available techniques (see Chapter 15.3) have the potential to prolong life but not necessarily the quality of that life. The decision to instigate artificial nutritional support may initially be made with identifiable and achievable goals, including the potential to improve nutritional status and achieve a return to oral intake. However, in patients such as those institutionalized with severe Alzheimer's disease these goals are clearly unachievable and the evidence for any benefit of enteral feeding in these cases is not proven.[46]

References

1. **Evans, W.K.** et al. (1987). A randomised trial of oral nutritional support versus ad lib nutritional intake during chemotherapy for advanced colorectal and non-small cell lung cancer. *Journal of Clinical Oncology* **5**, 113–24.
2. **Klein, S.** (1993). Clinical efficacy of nutritional support in patients with cancer. *Oncology* **7**, 87–92.
3. **Curtis, E., Krech, R., and Walsh, T.D.** (1991). Common symptoms in patients with advanced cancer. *Journal of Palliative Care* **7**, 25–9.
4. **Holden, C.M.** (1991). Anorexia in the terminally ill cancer patient: the emotional impact on the patient and the family. *Hospital Journal* **7**, 73–84.
5. **Van der Molen, B.** (2000). Relating information needs in the cancer experience. *European Journal of Cancer Care* **9**, 41–7.
6. **Jatoi, A. and Loprinzi, C.L.** (2001). An update: cancer associated anorexia as a treatment target. *Clinical Nutrition and Metabolic Care* **4**, 179–82.
7. **Ovesen, L.** (1994). Anorexia in patients with cancer with special references on it's association with early changes in food intake behaviour: chemotherapeutic treatment and adjuvant enteral nutrition. *International Journal of Oncology* **5**, 889–99.
8. **DeWys, W.D. and Walters, K.** (1975). Abnormalities of taste sensation in cancer patients. *Cancer* **36**, 1888–96.
9. **Williams, L.R. and Cohen, M.H.** (1978). Altered taste threshold in lung cancer. *American Journal of Clinical Nutrition* **31**, 122–5.
10. **Graham, C.S.** (1995). Taste and smell losses in HIV infected patients. *Physiology and Behaviour* **58**, 287–93.
11. **Wickham, R.** et al. (1999). Taste changes experienced by patients receiving chemotherapy. *Oncology Nursing Forum* **26**, 697–706.
12. **Ovesen, L., Hanibal, J., and Sorensen, M.** (1991). Taste thresholds in patients with small-cell lung cancer. *Journal of Cancer Research and Clinical Oncology* **117**, 70–2.
13. **Ripamonti, C.** et al. (1998). A randomised controlled clinical trial to evaluate the effects of zinc sulphate on cancer patients with taste alterations caused by head and neck irradiation. *Cancer* **82**, 1938–45.
14. **Ovesen, L.** et al. (1991). Electrical taste detection thresholds and chemical smell detection thresholds in patients with cancer. *Cancer* **68**, 2260–5.
15. **Pattison, R.M.** et al. (1997). Impact of altered taste sensitivity on dietary intake of patients with advanced cancer. *Proceedings of the Nutrition Society* **56**, 314A.
16. **Davidson, H.I.M., Pattison, R.M., and Richardson, R.A.** (1998). Clinical undernutrition states and their effects on taste. *Proceedings of the Nutrition Society* **57**, 633–8.
17. **Rogers, P. and Mela, D.** (1998). Sensory responses food preferences and macronutrient selection. In *Food and Obesity the Psychobiological Basis of Appetite and Weight Control.* London: Chapman and Hall.
18. **Rolls, E.T. and Rolls, J.H. (1996)**. Olfactory sensory specific satiety in humans. *Physiology and Behaviour* **61**, 461–73.
19. **Phillips, L.M. and Hill, D.L.** (1997). Novel regulation of peripheral gustatory function by the immune system. *American Journal of Physiology* **271**, R857–62.
20. **Schiffman, S.** (1998). Effect of psychotropic drugs on taste responses in young and elderly persons. *Annals of the New York Academy of Sciences* **855**, 732–7.
21. **Konsman, J.P. and Dantzer, T.** (2001). How the immune and nervous systems interact during disease-associated anorexia. *Nutrition* **17**, 664–8.
22. **Konsman, J.P.** et al. (2000). The vagus nerve mediates behavioural depression, but not fever, in response to peripheral immune signals; a functional anatomical analysis. *European Journal of Neuroscience* **12** (12), 4434–46.
23. **Marks, D., Ling, N., and Cone, R.D.** (2001). Role of the central melanocortin system in cachexia. *Cancer Research* **61**, 1432–8.
24. **Brown, D.R., Berkowitz, D.E., and Breslow, M.** (2001). Weight loss is not associated with hyperleptinaemia in humans with pancreatic cancer. *The Journal of Clinical Endocrinology and Metabolism* **86**, 162–6.
25. **Simons, J.P.** et al. (1997). Plasma concentration of total leptin and human lung-cancer associated cachexia. *Clinical Science* **93**, 273–7.
26. **Nowicki M., Bryc, W., and Kokot, F.** (2001). Hormonal regulation of appetite and body mass index in patients with advanced prostate cancer treated with combined androgen blockade. *Journal of Endocrinology Investigation* **24**, 31–6.
27. **Feuz, A. and Rapin, C.H.** (1994). An observational study of the role of pain control and food adaptation of elderly patients with terminal cancer. *Journal of the American Dietetic Association* **94**, 767–70.
28. **Shike, M.** et al. (1984). Changes in body composition in patients with small cell lung cancer. The effect of total parenteral nutrition as an adjunct to chemotherapy. *Annals of International Medicine* **101**, 303–9.

29. **McDiarmid, J. and Blundell, J.E.** (1997). Dietary under-reporting: what people say about recording their food intake. *European Journal of Clinical Nutrition* **51**, 199–200.
30. **Holmes, S. and Dickerson, W.T.** (1991). Food intake and quality of life in cancer patients. *Journal of Nutritional Medicine* **2**, 359–68.
31. **Heald, A.E., Pieper, C.F., and Schiffman, S.S.** (1998). Taste and smell complaints in HIV infected patients. *AIDS* **12**, 1667–77.
32. **Vickers, Z.M., Nielsen, S.S., and Theologides, A.** (1981). Food preferences of patients with cancer. *Journal of the American Dietetic Association* **79**, 441–5.
33. **Sweeney, M.P. and Bragg, J.** (2000). The mouth and palliative care. *American Journal of Hopsice and Palliative Care* **2**, 118–24.
34. **Bine, J.E., Frank, E.M., and McDade, H.L.** (1995). Dysphagia and dementia in subjects with Parkinson's disease. *Dysphagia* **10**, 160–4.
35. **British Artificial Nutrition Survey (BANS)**. *Trends in Artificial Nutrition Support in the UK During 1996–2000.* British Association of Parenteral and Enteral Nutrition. Maidenhead UK: Ed Eliah Pubs., 2001.
36. **Van Gossum, A. et al.** (1999). Home parenteral nutrition in adults: a European multicentre survey in 1997, ESPEN home artificial nutrition working group. *Clinical Nutrition* **18**, 135–40.
37. **Schneider, S.M. et al.** (2001). Outcome of patients treated with home enteral nutrition. *Journal of Parenteral and Enteral Nutrition* **25**, 203–9.
38. **Schofield, W.N.** (1985). Predicting basal metabolic rate: new standards and review of previous work. *Human Nutrition* **39c**, 5–41.
39. **Department of Health**. *Dietary Reference Values for Food Energy and Nutrients for the United Kingdom.* London: HMSO, 1991.
40. **Kohler, D.P.** (2000). Nutritional alterations with HIV infection. *Journal of Acquired Immune Deficiency Syndrome* **25**, S81–7.
41. **Palmo, A. et al.** (2001). Home artificial nutrition in chronic neurological disorders. *Clinical Nutrition* **20**, 29–33.
42. **Torelli, G., Campos, A., and Meguid, M.** (1999). Use of TPN in terminally ill cancer patients. *Nutrition* **15**, 665–7.
43. **Edwards, W. et al.** (1997). Efficacy of total parenteral nutrition in a series of end-stage AIDS patients: a case control study. *AIDS Patient Care* **11**, 323–9.
44. **Terman, S.A.** (2001). Determining the decision-making capacity of a patient who refused food and water. *Palliative Medicine* **15**, 55–60.
45. **Campbell-Taylor, I. and Fisher, R.H.** (1987). The clinical case against tube feeding in palliative care of the elderly. *Journal of the American Geriatrics Society* **34**, 1100–4.
46. **Chouinard, J.** (2000). Dysphagia in Alzheimer disease: a review. *Journal of Nutrition Health and Aging* **4**, 214–17.

8.4.4 Pharmacological interventions in cachexia and anorexia

Eduardo Bruera and Catherine Sweeney

Introduction

Cachexia occurs with a number of chronic illnesses, including cancer, AIDS, congestive heart failure (CHF) and chronic obstructive pulmonary disease (COPD). Cancer cachexia is now known to be the result of a complex interaction between tumour and host factors. Clinical assessment in a given patient should be multidimensional, looking at potential underlying causes and the effects and interactions of cachexia with a variety of physical and psychological symptoms. Cachexia occurs in approximately 80 per cent of patients with cancer.[1,2] Cancer cachexia is associated with reduced survival and decreased tolerance to both radiation and chemotherapy in cancer patients.[3]

The pathophysiology and assessment of cachexia has been discussed elsewhere in this book, some aspects of nutritional intervention have also been discussed. Since cachexia has devastating consequences at multiple symptom levels and nutritional approaches are of limited value in most patients, pharmacological interventions are routinely considered.

This chapter will mainly focus on pharmacological management of cachexia in cancer patients. In the chapter we will discuss established and emerging agents of potential benefit in the management of cachexia; in addition we will discuss agents sometimes used that have limited or no proven efficacy. This will be followed by some clinical information on decision-making regarding pharmacological interventions in cachexia management.

General principles

One of the main challenges in the management of cachexia is to properly define reasonable outcomes for nutritional and pharmacological interventions. Generally pharmacological interventions are aimed at improving symptom complexes. Table 1 outlines the symptom complexes associated with cachexia. Of these symptoms anorexia, chronic nausea and asthenia, and fatigue can be improved without changes in actual body mass, while improvement of altered body image requires increase in body fat and or body mass. The main purpose of pharmacological treatment at the present time is to improve the symptoms of anorexia and chronic nausea. The management of gastrointestinal symptoms such as nausea, vomiting, and constipation are discussed in detail elsewhere in this book. Some of the agents used in the management of anorexia and chronic nausea are also capable of significantly decreasing the level of asthenia. Management of fatigue and asthenia is discussed in Chapter 8.5. Unfortunately, with current available therapies, only a minority of patients experience a significant body weight gain and therefore psychological distress associated with a negative body image is usually not reduced by pharmacological interventions.

In a minority of patients such as those with slow-growing tumours accompanied by bowel obstruction or severe dysphagia, nutritional deprivation or starvation can be the main mechanism of weight loss and cachexia. In these patients the use of enteral or parenteral nutrition may improve survival.[4]

Established agents

A number of pharmacological agents have established roles in the management of cachexia. Table 2 summarizes agents that have been found in randomized controlled trials to improve symptom complexes associated with cachexia.

Metoclopramide

Metoclopramide is an antidopaminergic drug with a central antiemetic effect. It also has a prokinetic effect that promotes gastric emptying. It is

Table 1 Symptom complexes associated with cachexia

Anorexia
Chronic nausea
Early satiety
Asthenia/fatigue
Changes in body Image

Table 2 Established pharmacological agents for the management of symptom complexes associated with cachexia

Metoclopramide
Progestational agents (megestrol acetate, medroxyprogesterone acetate)
Corticosteroids (short-term)

particularly effective for patients who complain of chronic nausea.[5] Metoclopramide has been demonstrated to be effective in reversing tumour-associated gastroparesis and nausea associated with advanced cancer.[6–10] Patients with nausea due to autonomic failure or opioid therapy often respond well to regular use of oral or subcutaneous metoclopramide with significant improvement in appetite and food intake.[7,10]

One problem with the administration of metoclopramide is its short elimination half-life, which necessitates frequent administration to provide optimal relief of nausea. Clinical trials support the view that sustained metoclopramide concentrations are required to suppress nausea and vomiting and possibly other gastrointestinal symptoms associated with advanced cancer.[8–10] As a result some patients require frequent administration or continuous infusions for optimal results.[11] In a recent study, 26 cancer patients with a greater than 1 month history of dyspepsia were randomized to receive either controlled-release metoclopramide 40 mg 12 hourly or placebo for 4 days.[8] Patients were then crossed over to the alternative treatment for another 4 days. On the last day of each treatment phase nausea was significantly lower in the controlled-release metoclopramide group compared with placebo. Controlled-release metoclopramide was well tolerated and adverse events did not differ between treatments and placebo groups. In another study immediate-release metoclopramide 20 mg 6 hourly was compared with controlled-release metoclopramide 40 mg 12 hourly in patients with advanced cancer and chronic nausea. Nausea scores by day 3 of treatment were significantly lower for patients who received controlled release as compared to immediate-release metoclopramide.[10] Metoclopramide occasionally causes acute dystonic reactions; these are more common in younger patients, especially in young men.

Progestational drugs

Significant weight gain was reported in patients in trials using progestational drugs as therapy for hormone-responsive tumours.[12,13] This weight gain occurred with or without tumour response and prompted investigators to look at these drugs for the treatment of cachexia. Megestrol acetate has been the most commonly studied progestational agent in the management of cachexia. Several controlled trials have found that megestrol acetate is capable of reducing nausea, improving appetite, or increasing caloric intake in patients with advanced cancer.[14–26] Similar findings have been reported for patients with AIDS-related cachexia.[20] In addition, a number of these studies found improvement in nutritional variables, such as body weight, calf circumference, or increased serum thyroid binding pre-albumen levels, in cachectic cancer patients treated with megestrol acetate.[14–22] Megestrol acetate was administered in various doses ranging from 160 to 1600 mg over study periods of between 1 week and 4 months. Loprinzi et al.[19] in a randomized controlled trial involving 342 patients looked at the effect of various doses of megestrol acetate ranging from 160 to 1280 mg daily. A dose-related benefit on appetite, caloric intake, body weight gain (mostly fat), and sensation of well being was found with an optimal dose of approximately 800 mg/day. Recent studies involving terminally ill patients have demonstrated rapid (within 10 days) symptomatic improvement (appetite, fatigue, and general well being) from lower doses of megestrol (160–480 mg/day) when compared with placebo without any significant change in nutritional status.[25,26] These studies suggest that megestrol has beneficial symptomatic effects by mechanisms other than weight gain.

Adverse effects are likely to be dose related[27] and high doses of megestrol may be expensive. It is therefore justifiable to start the patient on a lower dosage (300–480 mg/day) and to titrate the dose upwards according to clinical response. Other progestational agents such as medroxyprogesterone acetate have also shown symptomatic and nutritional advantages, though these have been less frequently studied.[28–30]

The mechanism of action of progestational agents is currently unclear and may be related to glucocorticoid or anabolic activity as well as effects on cytokine release. Recent research suggests that megestrol acetate is capable of inducing appetite via stimulation of neuropeptide-y in the hypothalamus.[31] Modulation of calcium channels in the ventromedial hypothalamus may also be involved.[32] There is some evidence that medroxyprogesterone acetate may inhibit the activity of some cytokines such as interleukin-1, interleukin-6, and tumour necrosis factor (TNF).[33]

Both megestrol and medroxyprogesterone can induce thromboembolic phenomena, breakthrough bleeding, peripheral oedema, hyperglycaemia, hypertension, Cushing's syndrome, alopecia, adrenal suppression, and adrenal insufficiency, particularly if the drug is abruptly discontinued.[34,35] In clinical trials patients rarely need to discontinue these drugs for treatment-related side effects. However, one study with patients receiving antineoplastic therapy for non-small-cell lung cancer (NSCLC) showed that giving megestrol might decrease survival and increase the rate of thromboembolic disease (9 per cent with megestrol acetate versus 2 per cent with placebo).[36]

Corticosteroids

Several double blind randomized controlled trials have demonstrated the symptomatic effect of different types and dosages of corticosteroids for cancer cachexia.[37–41] Most research has shown a beneficial effect on symptoms such as appetite, food intake, sensation of well being, and performance status. These beneficial effects appear to be limited in duration to 2–4 weeks. The majority of studies have failed to demonstrate significant gain in body weight. The best type and dose of corticosteroids have not been established, but most authors have used doses ranging from 20 to 40 mg of prednisone or equivalent.

The mechanism of effect on appetite, energy, and well being is unclear; it may be related to central euphoriant activity in addition to effects on prostaglandin metabolism or the inhibition of cytokine release.[42,43] Corticosteroids also have non-specific antiemetic effects that again are not well understood. Corticosteroids have been found to be useful in combination with metoclopramide in the management of chronic nausea in cancer patients.[9,44] Corticosteroids are also useful in the management of other symptoms that may co-exist with nausea in advanced cancer patients, such as pain and asthenia.[37,40,45] Despite the wide range of potential side effects of corticosteroids their use in advanced cancer patients is becoming widely accepted. Due to their short lasting but significant symptomatic benefits, these drugs can be useful in patients whose expected survival is short. Alternatively they can be used for a short period of time and weaned off.

Emerging drugs

As the understanding of the pathophysiology of cancer cachexia evolves it appears that it is associated with a number of tumour- and host-related circulating by-products, altered inflammatory response, abnormalities in muscle and fat metabolism, and abnormalities in the regulation of appetite. In recent years a number of drugs have been found to have effects on various aspects of these different mechanisms of cachexia. Table 3 summarizes drugs with a potentially beneficial effect in the management of cancer cachexia. Further clinical studies are required to assess the potential benefits of these agents in the treatment of cachexia.

Table 3 Emerging pharmacological agents for the management of symptom complexes associated with cachexia

Thalidomide
Omega-3-fatty acids
Growth hormone/IGFs
Androgenic anabolic steroids
Cannabinoids
Melatonin
Beta 2-adrenergic blockers
NSAIDS
ATP

Cannabinoids

Appetite stimulation and increased body weight are well-recognized effects of the chronic use of marijuana and its derivatives.[46] Several different cannabinoids have been identified. Delta-9-tetra-hydro-cannabinol (dronabiol, THC) and nabilone have been used as mild to moderately effective antiemetic agents in cancer patients for some years.[47,48] A randomized controlled trial of 139 patients with AIDS cachexia comparing oral dronabinol 2.5 mg twice a day with placebo showed a significant improvement in appetite, mood, and decreased nausea; but no body weight gain was observed in patients taking the active drug.[49]

There is some evidence supporting a beneficial effect on cachexia in cancer patients. In a double blind crossover study of THC in advanced cancer patients 16 of 34 patients were evaluable for weight gain. Significant weight gain was observed during a 1-week treatment period with oral THC (0.1 mg/kg three times daily) when compared with the placebo treatment period. Six of 20 patients who did not complete the trial did so because of side effects while on THC.[50] In an open pilot study of 42 cancer patients treated with doses of THC 2.5 mg daily, 5 mg daily, 2.5 mg twice daily, or 5 mg twice daily there was a significant reduction in weight loss in both groups receiving treatment twice daily.[51] Significant improvement in appetite (measured on a visual analogue scale) was observed in the group receiving 2.5 mg twice daily. Ten patients discontinued the study early due to side effects; eight of these came from the 5 mg daily and twice daily groups. An open label study of THC (2.5 mg three times daily) in 19 patients with cancer-associated anorexia found that 8 of 13 evaluable patients reported improved appetite.[52] The effects of THC in cachectic cancer patients appear to be limited. In a recent study comparing megestrol acetate with THC in cancer patients with weight loss megestrol acetate had more of an effect on anorexia than THC did. A combination of megestrol acetate and THC was not better than megestrol acetate alone.[53] A randomized, double blind, placebo-controlled multicentre study is currently underway to compare the effects of cannabis extract with THC 2.5 mg and cannabidiol 1 mg twice daily with isolated THC 2.5 mg twice daily or placebo.

Some of the main limitations of these agents, as potential appetite stimulants in cancer patients, are their central adverse effects of somnolence, confusion, and perceptual disturbances.[49] These adverse effects may be even more severe in cachectic cancer patients with borderline cognitive function who are frequently receiving opioids and other psychotropic drugs. More research is needed to look at the longer-term effects of cannabinoids on anorexia and cachexia in cancer patients and to compare the effects of various cannabinoids.

Thalidomide

Thalidomide was used during the 1950s as a mild anxiolytic, hypnotic, and antiemetic agent. It was removed from the market after it was found to cause severe teratogenesis when administered to pregnant women. In recent years it has been found to have complex immunomodulatory effects, including inhibition of TNFα.[54–56] Its mechanism of action in cachexia is unclear but may be related to this effect on TNFα.

Thalidomide has been found to be effective in halting and reversing weight loss in AIDS-associated cachexia.[57–60] In a randomized double blind, placebo-controlled study of 64 evaluable male patients with AIDS-associated wasting significant weight gain was observed in patients treated for 8 weeks with thalidomide 100 and 200 mg/day.[59] Approximately half the weight gain was fat-free mass, as measured by bioimpedance analysis. Thalidomide treatment was associated with mild to moderate fevers and rashes. No significant change occurred in CD4+ cell counts, neutrophil counts, or TNFα levels in the active treatment groups. In a randomized, double blind, placebo-controlled study of 28 patients with advanced HIV disease, treatment with thalidomide 100 mg four times daily was associated with reversal of wasting and preservation of performance status.[60]

A pilot study of thalidomide 100 mg/day in 37 evaluable cancer patients resulted in an improvement in appetite, sensation of well being, nausea, and insomnia after 10 days of treatment.[61] This improvement was greater than that observed in a historical control group treated with megestrol 480 mg/day. These findings suggest that thalidomide may exert multiple symptomatic effects in this very ill population and provides justification for randomized controlled trials of low dose thalidomide on appetite, calorie intake, and nutritional status for patients with cancer cachexia. The effects of thalidomide on other variables such as wellbeing, fatigue, insomnia, and chronic nausea should also be assessed.

Melatonin

Melatonin has been found to reduce the circulating levels of TNF in patients with advanced cancer.[62–64] A study in 100 patients with untreatable metastatic solid tumours comparing melatonin with best supportive care found a reduction in the number of patients with more than 10 per cent body weight loss.[64] In addition to the potential beneficial effect on cancer cachexia, melatonin may have beneficial effects on fatigue in patients receiving chemotherapy.[65] Since this drug is well tolerated when administered orally, placebo-controlled trials in advanced cancer patients are justified.

Non-steroidal anti-inflammatory drugs

Non-steroidal anti-inflammatory drugs (NSAIDS) can reduce mediators of the inflammatory response such as interleukin-6.[66] Ibuprofen has been found to reduce resting energy expenditure and acute phase protein production in cancer patients.[67] Animal studies have found that inhibition of prostaglandin synthesis by the use of NSAIDS may attenuate tumour progression and reduce cancer cachexia.[68,69] In a recent study the cyclooxygenase-2 inhibitor meloxicam was found to inhibit tumour growth and attenuate cachexia in tumour-bearing mice.[70] In addition, the proteolytic effect of proteolysis-inducing factor (PIF) on mouse myoblasts was attenuated by meloxicam.

Some preliminary studies in humans have suggested that ibuprofen can produce body weight gain, reduce the production of C-reactive protein, and even prolong survival in undernourished patients with metastatic solid tumours.[71,72] McMillan et al.[73] compared megestrol acetate (160 mg three times daily) plus placebo three times daily with megestrol acetate (160 mg three times daily) plus ibuprofen (400 mg three times daily) in 73 patients with gastrointestinal malignancies in a randomized controlled trial. The megestrol acetate/ibuprofen group had significant weight gain (median 2.3 kg) compared with weight loss (median 2.8 kg) in the megestrol acetate/placebo group. The megestrol acetate/ibuprofen group had significant improvement in quality of life scores. Appetite improved in both groups. Further randomized, placebo-controlled trials are needed in order to better clarify the potential role of NSAIDS in patients with cancer cachexia.

Omega-3 fatty acids

Unsaturated fatty acids can be categorized as omega-3 fatty acids, omega-6 fatty acids, and omega 9-fatty acids. The omega-3 fatty acids include eicosapentanoic acid (EPA), docosahexanoic acid (DHA), docosapentanoic acid, and alpha-linoleic acid. EPA is one of the major omega-3 fatty acid constituents of fish oil.

Polyunsaturated fatty acids modulate immune function and the inflammatory response by mechanisms that are not fully understood.[74,75] In patients with colorectal cancer, supplementation with omega-3 and omega-6 fatty acids 4.8 g/day significantly decreased circulating levels of TNF, interleukin-1, interleukin-2, interleukin-4, interleukin-6, and interferon-gamma after 2 months of treatment.[76] A randomized, placebo-controlled trial of fish oil (18 g omega-3 polyunsaturated fatty acids) plus vitamin E in 60 severely ill cancer patients with solid tumours found that fish oil treatment prolonged survival. Both treatment arms consisted of 15 well-nourished and 15 malnourished patients. In malnourished patients fish oil had significant immunomodulatory effects.[77] There have been reports of improvement in a number of inflammatory conditions with fish oil supplementation, including rheumatoid arthritis, inflammatory bowel disease, and asthma.[74] In addition, omega-3 fatty acids have been found to inhibit lipolysis and proteolysis in a cancer cachexia model.[78,79] EPA may attenuate the effects of PIF.[78] EPA has also been found to have an antitumour effect in an animal model.[79]

Omega-3 fatty acid preparations containing EPA appear to have a beneficial effect on weight gain in weight-losing cancer patients.[80–82] Significant weight changes were observed by Wigmore et al. in 18 patients with unresectable pancreatic cancer treated with fish oil supplementation (capsules containing 18 per cent EPA and 12 per cent DHA) at a median fish oil dose of 12 g/day.[80] Prior to treatment patients had a median weight loss of 2.9 kg/month; at a mean of 3 months after fish oil was started there was a median weight gain of 0.3 kg/month accompanied by a significant but temporary reduction in acute phase proteins. Wigmore et al.[81] also studied the effect of EPA on weight loss in 26 weight-losing patients (median pretreatment weight loss of 2.0 kg/month) with advanced pancreatic cancer. High-purity EPA (95 per cent pure) was used with a starting dose of 1 g/day and increased over 4 weeks to a maintenance dose of 6 g/day. After 4 weeks of supplementation a significant median weight gain of 0.5 kg was observed and stabilization of weight persisted over the 12-week study period. EPA was well tolerated with five patients experiencing side effects that were possibly due to EPA. In a study looking at the effect of an oral nutritional supplement enriched with EPA in weight-losing patients (median pretreatment rate of weight loss 2.9 kg/month) dietary intake increased by almost 400 kcal/day and significant weight gain was observed at 3 (median 1 kg) and 7 (median 2 kg) weeks.[82] Performance status and appetite were significantly increased at 3 weeks.

In a dose-finding study of fish oil (capsules containing EPA 378 mg/g, DHA 249 mg/g, and smaller amounts of omega 6 fatty acids) in patients with cancer cachexia the maximum tolerated dose of this preparation was 0.3 g/kg/day.[83] The dose-limiting side effects were gastrointestinal in origin, mainly diarrhoea. Other side effects included abnormal taste, abnormal body smell, belching, and flatulence.

Randomized controlled trials are required in order to better characterize the role of various preparations containing omega-3 fatty acids in the management of cachexia.

Beta 2-adrenergic agonists

Beta 2-adrenergic agonists have anabolic effects. In cachexia research clenbuterol has been the most commonly studied beta 2-adrenergic agonist. Recent studies suggest a positive effect from beta 2-adrenergic agonists on muscle mass in tumour-bearing rats.[84–86] An advantage of this drug is that in animal studies the effects on muscle preservation seem to occur without the need for either exercise or increased food intake.[85]

One randomized controlled trial in patients undergoing knee surgery found that clenbuterol was able to significantly improve relative muscle strength when compared with placebo.[87] However, the effects of beta 2-adrenergic agonists on muscle are not well defined in patients with muscle abnormalities. In patients with CHF muscle abnormalities including atrophy are common.[88] In a randomized placebo-controlled trial of 12 men with CHF slow-release salbutamol 8 mg twice daily for 3 weeks was not found to increase skeletal muscle bulk, strength or fatigue.[89]

The effects of beta 2-agonists on cachexia in humans have not been studied and should be addressed in future research. The adverse effects (nervousness, tachycardia, muscle tremors, and headaches) may be limiting factors in conducting clinical trials in cancer patients.

Androgenic anabolic steroids

For many years athletes wanting to enhance muscle growth and strength have used androgenic anabolic steroids (AAS) such as testosterone and its derivatives (e.g. nandrolone, oxandrolone). Supraphysiological doses of testosterone have been found to increase fat-free mass and muscle size and strength in normal men.[90]

Administration of AAS to hypogonadal men has been found to increase lean body mass.[91–93] Hypogonadism is common in HIV/AIDS patients.[94] Several studies have looked at the effects of AAS in patients with HIV-associated wasting.[95–101,102–104] A beneficial effect has been observed on lean body mass or weight gain in many studies.[95–101] Grinspoon et al.[97] found that testosterone administration resulted in sustained increases in lean body mass during 1 year of therapy in hypogonadal men with AIDS wasting. The beneficial effects of AAS is not restricted to hypogonadal men with HIV wasting; beneficial effects on weight and lean body mass have been observed in eugonadal patients with HIV wasting.[100,101] A pilot study in 59 women with HIV-associated wasting found that transdermal testosterone (at a dose of 150 μg/day for 12 weeks) was associated with significant weight gain when compared with placebo.[104] However, a dose of 300 μg/day was not associated with weight gain. In addition to benefits on body composition, AAS may have beneficial effects on haemoglobin concentrations.[93,96]

AASs have been found to have a beneficial effect on weight gain and lean body mass in patients with wasting associated with a variety of other chronic diseases such as renal failure and COPD.[105–107]

AASs have not been comprehensively studied in the management of cancer cachexia. In a randomized study patients with unresectable NSCLC received chemotherapy alone or chemotherapy plus nandrolone 200 mg weekly for 4 weeks.[108] There was a trend for less severe weight loss in the group treated with nandrolone. In a double blind, placebo-controlled trial of 40 patients who had surgery for oesophageal cancer no therapeutic benefit on weight was observed after low dose nandrolone treatment (five injections of nandrolone 50 mg were given over a 3-month period).[109] A recent randomized controlled trial in cachetic cancer patients found that fluoxymesterone was significantly less effective than both dexamethasone and megestrol acetate in symptomatic measures such as appetite and nutritional variables.[110] Randomized controlled trials should be conducted in advanced cancer patients suffering from cachexia and hypogonadism.

Growth hormone and insulin-like growth factors

Growth hormone (GH) has an anabolic effect that is thought to be primarily the result of promotion of protein synthesis.[111] GH stimulates the induction of the insulin-like growth factor-1 (IGF-1) gene[112] and IGF stimulates myoblast proliferation and differentiation.[113] Acquired GH resistance occurs in catabolic patients.[114,115] IGF-1 levels may be decreased in cancer cachexia and may respond to treatment with megestrol acetate.[116]

Animal studies have shown that GH supplementation results in increased carcass weight, muscle weight, and muscle protein content in protein-fed, tumour-bearing animals.[117] Possible tumour growth stimulation by GH is a concern. Evidence from animal models and *in vitro* studies does not indicate that this is a problem.[117,118] A number of studies have shown anabolic benefit and increases in lean body mass from GH treatment in AIDS-related wasting[119,120] and it is approved in the United States for this indication.

Similar long-term studies have not been conducted in patients with cancer cachexia. In a metabolic study of 28 cancer patients GH and a short-term infusion of insulin reduced skeletal muscle protein loss.[121] A short-term (3 days) study of GH treatment in 10 cancer patients did not find an anabolic response in those patients who were malnourished.[122] One randomized controlled trial looked at the effects of total parenteral nutrition alone, in combination with GH, and in combination with GH and insulin in patients with upper gastrointestinal malignancies undergoing surgery.[123] In both groups receiving GH there was an improvement in the whole body net protein balance. The potential effects of GH on cancer cachexia and tumour growth need to be evaluated by future research.

There are case reports of increased muscle mass, strength, and exercise tolerance following GH treatment in cachectic patients with CHF and of increased weight gain and fat-free mass in a malnourished patient with chronic respiratory disease treated with GH.[124–126] In an animal study ghrelin (a novel GH-releasing peptide) was found to attenuate the development of cardiac cachexia in rats with CHF.[127] Further studies should look at the effects of GH treatment in patients with cachexia-related chronic cardiac and respiratory illness.

In an animal model IGF-1 has been found to reduce weight loss due to starvation.[128] In the future, treatment with IGF-1 may offer possibilities in the management of cachexia.

Adenosine triphosphate

Adenosine triphosphate (ATP) has been investigated as an antineoplastic agent in recent years. In a phase II study of 15 patients with NSCLC it was noted that a mean weight gain of 1.3 kg occurred during treatment with ATP.[129] Prior to treatment mean recent weight loss was 1.6 kg. Patients were treated with at least three 96-hour infusions of ATP 50 µg/kg/min or higher. Side effects of chest pain and dyspnoea led to discontinuation of treatment in five patients. Tumour response to ATP was very poor. In a trial of 58 patients with advanced NSCLC randomized to receive either 10–30-hour ATP infusions or no treatment, a beneficial effect on weight (no weight loss when compared with a mean weight loss of 1 kg in the control group per 4 week interval) and muscle strength was observed in the group treated with ATP.[130] A study looking at the effects of ATP infusion on gluconeogenesis and glucose turnover in patients with NSCLC found that glucose turnover was similar in those receiving high dose ATP infusions, low dose ATP infusions, and those in the control group.[131] In between ATP infusions glucose turnover was significantly lower in patients receiving high dose ATP infusions than in those receiving low dose ATP and control NSCLC patients and was similar to that in healthy subjects.

In animal studies ATP levels have been found to be lower in those with tumours.[132,133] Intraperitoneal injection of ATP or adenosine 5′ monophosphate has been found to inhibit tumour growth and host weight loss in tumour-bearing animals.[134]

The mechanism of action of ATP is not fully understood and its breakdown product adenosine may play a role in its metabolic effects.[135] The potential effects of ATP and possibly adenosine on weight loss in cancer cachexia should be further investigated in future research. In addition, side effects should be better characterized in this patient population.

Drugs of limited proven efficiency

Hydrazine sulphate

This drug was initially developed to attempt to inhibit gluconeogenesis. Improved appetite and nutritional status were reported in initial studies.[136–138] This prompted three large randomized placebo-controlled trials.[139–141] None of the three trials found evidence of symptomatic improvement or body weight gain; however, they did find significant toxicities and reduced quality of life measures in patients who were randomized to receive hydrazine sulphate when compared with placebo. At the present time there is no justification for further research on this agent. However, it continues to be widely used as an alternative therapy, both in North America and in Europe.

Cyproheptadine

Cyproheptadine is an antiserotonergic drug with appetite-stimulating effects. It is still used in some Latin American and European countries as an appetite stimulant. A randomized controlled trial in patients with cancer cachexia found a mild positive effect on appetite and food intake without any body weight gain.[142] It is likely to be of limited usefulness in patients with cancer cachexia due to side effects that include sedation.

Decision-making on pharmacological interventions

The current complex view of the pathophysiology of cachexia has led to the possibility of intervention at several levels. In most cancer patients, cachexia results from a number of major metabolic, neuroendocrine, and anabolic abnormalities associated with altered immune function and increased inflammation. In patients with HIV infection similar complex mechanisms are involved. Table 4 summarizes potential mechanisms of action of established and emerging drugs in the management of anorexia and cachexia. Further research into the clinical effects and better understanding of mechanisms of action of both established and emerging agents should facilitate decision-making in the pharmacological management of cachexia. The complex pathophysiology of cachexia indicates that a combination of drugs that interfere with the pathophysiology of anorexia and cachexia at different levels (such as an anabolic agent combined with an anti-inflammatory agent) may allow management of anorexia and cachexia to be optimized. Future research should address the possibility of combination therapy for the symptom complexes of anorexia and cachexia.

Table 4 Possible mechanisms of action of established and emerging pharmacological agents in the management of cachexia

Possible mechanism	Agent
Central nervous system effects	Metoclopramide Corticosteroids Progestational agents Cannabinoids Thalidomide
Modulate immune response/reduce inflammation	Corticosteroids Progestational agents Polyunsaturated fatty acids Thalidomide Melatonin NSAIDS ATP
Anabolic effect	Growth hormone/insulin growth factor-1 Androgenic anabolic agents Beta 2-adrenergic agents ATP
Stimulate gastrointestinal motility/increase gastric emptying	Metoclopramide

Pharmacological management of cachexia should be part of a more general approach to symptom management. The intensity of symptom complexes associated with cachexia varies from one patient to another, mostly due to the co-existence of other more severe symptoms. Not all patients consider anorexia a major problem nor do they require the same level of symptomatic intervention. In addition, some symptoms such as psychological distress associated with body image can only be reversed if weight gain is induced. Therefore, pharmacological interventions aimed exclusively at anorexia or chronic nausea may not be considered adequate for these patients. Decision-making regarding pharmacological interventions should be based on careful patient assessment.

A pharmacological approach in isolation will not allow optimum management of this devastating symptom. Progressive cachexia causes great psychological and social distress for many patients and their families. Patients and relatives often believe that cachexia is due to lack of calorie intake. Adequate counselling of patients and families will help to reduce the anxiety of family members that their relative is 'starving to death'. An explanation that neither enteral nor parenteral nutrition nor increased oral intake is likely to achieve the goals of improved survival, appetite, or weight gain in patients with advanced cancer-related cachexia is often needed. However, nutritional counselling alone may be capable of improving the daily calorie intake in a majority of patients. The addition of currently available pharmacological interventions may increase the effectiveness of nutritional counselling to improve calorie intake.

In recent years progress has been made in the pharmacological management of anorexia and cachexia. Several emerging agents offer the potential to further improve pharmacological management of the symptom complexes associated with cachexia. In the future optimum management may include the use of a number of complementary pharmacological agents.

References

1. **Ma, G. and Alexandar, H.R.** (1998). Prevalence and pathophysiology of cancer cachexia. In *Topics in Palliative Care* (ed. E. Bruera and R.K. Portenoy), pp. 91–129. New York: Oxford University Press.
2. **Dunlop, R.** (1996). Clinical epidemiology of cancer cachexia. In *Cachexia–Anorexia in Cancer Patients* (ed. E. Bruera and I. Higginson), pp. 76–82. Oxford: Oxford University Press.
3. **Dewys, W.D.** et al. (1980). Prognostic effect of weight loss prior to chemotherapy in cancer patients. Eastern Cooperative Oncology Group. *American Journal of Medicine* **69**, 491–7.
4. **Bozzetti, F.** et al. (1996). Guidelines on artificial nutrition versus hydration in terminal cancer patients. European Association for Palliative Care. *Nutrition* **12**, 163–7.
5. **Pereira, J. and Bruera, E.** (1996). Chronic nausea. In *Cachexia-Anorexia in Cancer Patients* (ed. E. Bruera and I. Higginson), pp. 23–37. Oxford: Oxford University Press.
6. **Kris, M.G.** et al. (1985). Symptomatic gastroparesis in cancer patients: a possible cause of cancer associated anorexia (abstract). *Proceedings of the American Society of Clinical Oncology* **4**, 267.
7. **Shivshanker, K., Bennett, R.W., Jr., and Haynie, T.P.** (1983). Tumor-associated gastroparesis: correction with metoclopramide. *American Journal of Surgery* **145**, 221–5.
8. **Bruera, E.** et al. (2000). A double-blind, crossover study of controlled-release metoclopramide and placebo for the chronic nausea and dyspepsia of advanced cancer. *Journal of Pain and Symptom Management* **19**, 427–35.
9. **Bruera, E.** et al. (1996). Chronic nausea in advanced cancer patients: a retrospective assessment of a metoclopramide-based antiemetic regimen. *Journal of Pain and Symptom Management* **11**, 147–53.
10. **Bruera, E.** et al. (1994). Comparison of the efficacy, safety, and pharmacokinetics of controlled release and immediate release metoclopramide for the management of chronic nausea in patients with advanced cancer. *Cancer* **74**, 3204–11.
11. **Bruera, E.** et al. (1987). Continuous Sc infusion of metoclopramide for treatment of narcotic bowel syndrome (letter). *Cancer Treatment Reports* **71**, 1121–2.
12. **Cruz, J.M.** et al. (1990). Weight changes in women with metastatic breast cancer treated with megestrol acetate: a comparison of standard versus high-dose therapy. *Seminars in Oncology* **17**, 63–7.
13. **Tchekmedyian, N.S.** et al. (1986). Appetite stimulation with megestrol acetate in cachectic cancer patients. *Seminars in Oncology* **13**, 37–43.
14. **Erkurt, E., Erkisi, M., and Tunali, C.** (2000). Supportive treatment in weight-losing cancer patients due to the additive adverse effects of radiation treatment and/or chemotherapy. *Journal of Experimental and Clinical Cancer Research* **19**, 431–9.
15. **Bruera, E.** et al. (1990). A controlled trial of megestrol acetate on appetite, caloric intake, nutritional status, and other symptoms in patients with advanced cancer. *Cancer* **66**, 1279–82.
16. **Loprinzi, C.L.** et al. (1990). Controlled trial of megestrol acetate for the treatment of cancer anorexia and cachexia. *Journal of the National Cancer Institute* **82**, 1127–32.
17. **Tchekmedyian, N.S.** et al. (1992). Megestrol acetate in cancer anorexia and weight loss. *Cancer* **69**, 1268–74.
18. **Heckmayr, M. and Gatzemeier, U.** (1992). Treatment of cancer weight loss in patients with advanced lung cancer. *Oncology* **49** (Suppl. 2), 32–4.
19. **Loprinzi, C.L.** et al. (1993). Phase III evaluation of four doses of megestrol acetate as therapy for patients with cancer anorexia and/or cachexia. *Journal of Clinical Oncology* **11**, 762–7.
20. **Schmoll, E.** et al. (1991). Megestrol acetate in cancer cachexia. *Seminars in Oncology* **18**, 32–4.
21. **Feliu, J.** et al. (1992). Usefulness of megestrol acetate in cancer cachexia and anorexia. A placebo-controlled study. *American Journal of Clinical Oncology* **15**, 436–40.
22. **Azcona, C.** et al. (1996). Megestrol acetate therapy for anorexia and weight loss in children with malignant solid tumours. *Alimentary Pharmacology and Therapeutics* **10**, 577–86.
23. **Beller, E.** et al. (1997). Improved quality of life with megestrol acetate in patients with endocrine-insensitive advanced cancer: a randomised placebo-controlled trial. Australasian Megestrol Acetate Cooperative Study Group. *Annals of Oncology* **8**, 277–83.
24. **Gebbia, V., Testa, A., and Gebbia, N.** (1996). Prospective randomised trial of two dose levels of megestrol acetate in the management of anorexia-cachexia syndrome in patients with metastatic cancer. *British Journal of Cancer* **73**, 1576–80.
25. **Bruera, E.** et al. (1998). Effectiveness of megestrol acetate in patients with advanced cancer: a randomized, double-blind, crossover study. *Cancer Prevention and Control* **2**, 74–8.
26. **De Conno, F.** et al. (1998). Megestrol acetate for anorexia in patients with far-advanced cancer: a double-blind controlled clinical trial. *European Journal of Cancer* **34**, 1705–9.
27. **Kornblith, A.B.** (1993). Effect of megestrol acetate on quality of life in a dose-response trial in women with advanced breast cancer. The Cancer and Leukemia Group B. *Journal of Clinical Oncology* **11**, 2081–9.
28. **Simons, J.P.** et al. (1996). Effects of medroxyprogesterone acetate on appetite, weight, and quality of life in advanced-stage non-hormone-sensitive cancer: a placebo-controlled multicenter study. *Journal of Clinical Oncology* **14**, 1077–84.
29. **Lelli, G.** et al. (1983). The anabolic effect of high dose medroxyprogesterone acetate in oncology. *Pharmacological Research Communications* **15**, 561–8.
30. **Downer, S.** et al. (1993). A double blind placebo controlled trial of medroxyprogesterone acetate (MPA) in cancer cachexia. *British Journal of Cancer* **67**, 1102–5.
31. **McCarthy, H.D.** et al. (1994). Megestrol acetate stimulates food and water intake in the rat: effects on regional hypothalamic neuropeptide Y concentrations. *European Journal of Pharmacology* **265**, 99–102.
32. **Costa, A.M.** et al. (1995). Residual Ca^{2+} channel current modulation by megestrol acetate via a G-protein alpha s-subunit in rat hypothalamic neurones. *Journal of Physiology* **487**, 291–303.
33. **Mantovani, G.** et al. (1997). Medroxyprogesterone acetate reduces the *in vitro* production of cytokines and serotonin involved in anorexia/cachexia and emesis by peripheral blood mononuclear cells of cancer patients. *European Journal of Cancer* **33**, 602–7.
34. **Steer, K.A., Kurtz, A.B., and Honour, J.W.** (1995). Megestrol-induced Cushing's syndrome. *Clinical Endocrinology (Oxford)* **42**, 91–3.
35. **Subramanian, S.** et al. (1997). Clinical adrenal insufficiency in patients receiving megestrol therapy. *Archives of Internal Medicine* **157**, 1008–11.
36. **Rowland, K.M.** et al. (1996). Randomized double-blind placebo-controlled trial of cisplatin and etoposide plus megestrol acetate/placebo in extensive-stage small-cell lung cancer: a North Central Cancer Treatment Group study. *Journal of Clinical Oncology* **14**, 135–41.
37. **Moertel, C.G.** et al. (1974). Corticosteroid therapy of preterminal gastrointestinal cancer. *Cancer* **33**, 1607–9.
38. **Willox, J.C.** et al. (1984). Prednisolone as an appetite stimulant in patients with cancer. *British Medical Journal (Clinical Research Edition)* **288**, 27.
39. **Della Cuna, G.R., Pellegrini, A., and Piazzi, M.** (1989). Effect of methylprednisolone sodium succinate on quality of life in preterminal cancer patients: a placebo-controlled, multicenter study. The Methylprednisolone Preterminal Cancer Study Group. *European Journal of Cancer and Clinical Oncology* **25**, 1817–21.
40. **Bruera, E.** et al. (1985). Action of oral methylprednisolone in terminal cancer patients: a prospective randomized double-blind study. *Cancer Treatment Reports* **69**, 751–4.
41. **Popiela, T., Lucchi, R., and Giongo, F.** (1989). Methylprednisolone as palliative therapy for female terminal cancer patients. The Methylprednisolone

Female Preterminal Cancer Study Group. *European Journal of Cancer and Clinical Oncology* **25**, 1823–9.

42. **Fainsinger, R.** (1996). Pharmacological approach to cancer anorexia and cachexia. In *Cachexia–Anorexia in Cancer Patients* (ed. E. Bruera and I. Higginson), pp. 128–40. Oxford: Oxford University Press.
43. **Plata-Salaman, C.R.** (1991). Dexamethasone inhibits food intake suppression induced by low doses of interleukin-1 beta administered intracerebroventricularly. *Brain Research Bulletin* **27**, 737–8.
44. **Bruera, E.D.** et al. (1983). Improved control of chemotherapy-induced emesis by the addition of dexamethasone to metoclopramide in patients resistant to metoclopramide. *Cancer Treatment Reports* **67**, 381–3.
45. **Watanabe, S. and Bruera, E.** (1994). Corticosteroids as adjuvant analgesics. *Journal of Pain and Symptom Management* **9**, 442–5.
46. **Foltin, R.W., Fischman, M.W., and Byrne, M.F.** (1988). Effects of smoked marijuana on food intake and body weight of humans living in a residential laboratory. *Appetite* **11**, 1–14.
47. **Frytak, S.** et al. (1979). Delta-9-tetrahydrocannabinol as an antiemetic for patients receiving cancer chemotherapy. A comparison with prochlorperazine and a placebo. *Annals of Internal Medicine* **91**, 825–30.
48. **Lucas, V.S. and Laszlo, J.** (1980). Delta 9-tetrahydrocannabinol for refractory vomiting induced by cancer chemotherapy. *Journal of the American Medical Association* **243**, 1241–3.
49. **Beal, J.E.** et al. (1995). Dronabinol as a treatment for anorexia associated with weight loss in patients with AIDS. *Journal of Pain and Symptom Management* **10**, 89–97.
50. **Regelson, W.** et al. (1976). Tetrahydrocannbinol as an efective antidepressant and appetite-stimulating agent in advanced cancer patients. In *The Pharmacology of Marijuana: A Monograph of the National Institute of Drug Abuse* (ed. M.C. Braude and S. Szara), pp. 763–76. New York: Raven.
51. **Plasse, T.F.** et al. (1991). Recent clinical experience with dronabinol. *Pharmacology Biochemistry and Behavior* **40**, 695–700.
52. **Nelson, K.A., Walsh, D., and Sheehan, F.A.** (1994). The cancer anorexia–cachexia syndrome. *Journal of Clinical Oncology* **12**, 213–25.
53. **Jatoi, A.** et al. (2002). Dronabiol versus megestrol acetate versus combination therapy for cancer-associated anorexia: A North Central Cancer Treatment Group Study. *Journal of Clinical Oncology* **20** (2), 567–73.
54. **Kaplan, G.** (1994). Cytokine regulation of disease progression in leprosy and tuberculosis. *Immunobiology* **191**, 564–8.
55. **Schuler, U. and Ehninger, G.** (1995). Thalidomide: rationale for renewed use in immunological disorders. *Drug Safety* **12**, 364–9.
56. **Tramontana, J.M.** et al. (1995). Thalidomide treatment reduces tumor necrosis factor alpha production and enhances weight gain in patients with pulmonary tuberculosis. *Molecular Medicine* **1**, 384–97.
57. **Haslett, P.** et al. (1977). The metabolic and immunologic effects of short-term thalidomide treatment of patients infected with the human immunodeficiency virus. *AIDS Research and Human Retroviruses* **13**, 1047–54.
58. **Klausner, J.D.** et al. (1996). The effect of thalidomide on the pathogenesis of human immunodeficiency virus type 1 and *M. tuberculosis* infection. *Journal of Acquired Immune Deficiency Syndrome and Human Retrovirology* **11**, 247–57.
59. **Kaplan, G.** et al. (2000). Thalidomide for the treatment of AIDS-associated wasting. *AIDS Research and Human Retroviruses* **16**, 1345–55.
60. **Reyes-Teran, G.** et al. (1996). Effects of thalidomide on HIV-associated wasting syndrome: a randomized, double-blind, placebo-controlled clinical trial. *AIDS* **10**, 1501–7.
61. **Bruera, E.** et al. (1999). Thalidomide in patients with cachexia due to terminal cancer: preliminary report. *Annals of Oncology* **10**, 857–9.
62. **Lissoni, P.** et al. (1994). Role of the pineal gland in the control of macrophage functions and its possible implication in cancer: a study of interactions between tumor necrosis factor-alpha and the pineal hormone melatonin. *Journal of Biological Regulators and Homeostatic Agents* **8**, 126–9.
63. **Braczkowski, R.** et al. (1995). Modulation of tumor necrosis factor-alpha (TNF-alpha) toxicity by the pineal hormone melatonin (MLT) in metastatic solid tumor patients. *Annals of the New York Academy of Sciences* **768**, 334–6.
64. **Lissoni, P.** et al. (1996). Is there a role for melatonin in the treatment of neoplastic cachexia? *European Journal of Cancer* **32A**, 1340–3.
65. **Lissoni, P.** et al. (1999). Decreased toxicity and increased efficacy of cancer chemotherapy using the pineal hormone melatonin in metastatic solid tumour patients with poor clinical status. *European Journal of Cancer* **35**, 1688–92.
66. **McMillan, D.C.** et al. (1995). Effect of extended ibuprofen administration on the acute phase protein response in colorectal cancer patients. *European Journal of Surgical Oncology* **21**, 531–4.
67. **Wigmore, S.J.** et al. (1995). Ibuprofen reduces energy expenditure and acute-phase protein production compared with placebo in pancreatic cancer patients. *British Journal of Cancer* **72**, 185–8.
68. **Gelin, J., Andersson, C., and Lundholm, K.** (1991). Effects of indomethacin, cytokines, and cyclosporin A on tumor growth and the subsequent development of cancer cachexia. *Cancer Research* **51**, 880–5.
69. **Tessitore, L., Costelli, P., and Baccino, F.M.** (1994). Pharmacological interference with tissue hypercatabolism in tumour-bearing rats. *Biochemical Journal* **299**, 71–8.
70. **Hussey, H.J. and Tisdale, M.J.** (2000). Effect of the specific cyclooxygenase-2 inhibitor meloxicam on tumour growth and cachexia in a murine model. *International Journal of Cancer* **87**, 95–100.
71. **Lundholm, K.** et al. (1994). Anti-inflammatory treatment may prolong survival in undernourished patients with metastatic solid tumors. *Cancer Research* **54**, 5602–6.
72. **McMillan, D.C.** et al. (1997). A pilot study of megestrol acetate and ibuprofen in the treatment of cachexia in gastrointestinal cancer patients. *British Journal of Cancer* **76**, 788–90.
73. **McMillan, D.C.** et al. (1999). A prospective randomized study of megestrol acetate and ibuprofen in gastrointestinal cancer patients with weight loss. *British Journal of Cancer* **79**, 495–500.
74. **Calder, P.C.** (2001). Polyunsaturated fatty acids, inflammation, and immunity. *Lipids* **36**, 1007–24.
75. **Kelley, D.S.** (2001). Modulation of human immune and inflammatory responses by dietary fatty acids. *Nutrition* **17**, 669–73.
76. **Purasiri, P.** et al. (1994). Modulation of cytokine production *in vivo* by dietary essential fatty acids in patients with colorectal cancer. *Clinical Science (Colch.)* **87**, 711–17.
77. **Gogos, C.A.** et al. (1998). Dietary omega-3 polyunsaturated fatty acids plus vitamin E restore immunodeficiency and prolong survival for severely ill patients with generalized malignancy: a randomized control trial. *Cancer* **82**, 395–402.
78. **Tisdale, M.J.** (1996). Inhibition of lipolysis and muscle protein degradation by, E.P.A in cancer cachexia. *Nutrition* **12**, S31–3.
79. **Beck, S.A., Smith, K.L., and Tisdale, M.J.** (1991). Anticachectic and antitumor effect of eicosapentaenoic acid and its effect on protein turnover. *Cancer Research* **51**, 6089–93.
80. **Wigmore, S.J.** et al. (1996). The effect of polyunsaturated fatty acids on the progress of cachexia in patients with pancreatic cancer. *Nutrition* **12**, S27–30.
81. **Wigmore, S.J.** et al. (2000). Effect of oral eicosapentaenoic acid on weight loss in patients with pancreatic cancer. *Nutrition and Cancer* **36**, 177–84.
82. **Barber, M.D.** et al. (1999). The effect of an oral nutritional supplement enriched with fish oil on weight-loss in patients with pancreatic cancer. *British Journal of Cancer* **81**, 80–6.
83. **Burns, C.P.** et al. (1999). Phase I clinical study of fish oil fatty acid capsules for patients with cancer cachexia: cancer and leukemia group B study 9473. *Clinical Cancer Research* **5**, 3942–7.
84. **Carbo, N.** et al. (1997). Comparative effects of beta 2-adrenergic agonists on muscle waste associated with tumour growth. *Cancer Letters* **115**, 113–18.
85. **Choo, J.J.** et al. (1990). Effects of the beta 2-adrenoceptor agonist, clenbuterol, on muscle atrophy due to food deprivation in the rat. *Metabolism* **39**, 647–50.
86. **Costelli, P.** et al. (1995). Muscle protein waste in tumor-bearing rats is effectively antagonized by a beta 2-adrenergic agonist (clenbuterol). Role of the ATP–ubiquitin-dependent proteolytic pathway. *Journal of Clinical Investigation* **95**, 2367–72.
87. **Maltin, C.A.** et al. (1993). Clenbuterol, a beta-adrenoceptor agonist, increases relative muscle strength in orthopaedic patients. *Clinical Science (Colch.)* **84**, 651–4.

88. **Minotti, J.R.** et al. (1993). Skeletal muscle size: relationship to muscle function in heart failure. *Journal of Applied Physiology* **75**, 373–81.
89. **Harrington, D., Chua, T.P., and Coats, A.J.** (2000). The effect of salbutamol on skeletal muscle in chronic heart failure. *International Journal of Cardiology* **73**, 257–65.
90. **Bhasin, S.** et al. (1996). The effects of supraphysiologic doses of testosterone on muscle size and strength in normal men. *New England Journal of Medicine* **335**, 1–7.
91. **Katznelson, L.** et al. (1996). Increase in bone density and lean body mass during testosterone administration in men with acquired hypogonadism. *Journal of Clinical Endocrinology and Metabolism* **81**, 4358–65.
92. **Tenover, J.S.** (1992). Effects of testosterone supplementation in the aging male. *Journal of Clinical Endocrinology and Metabolism* **75**, 1092–8.
93. **Wang, C.** et al. (2000). Transdermal testosterone gel improves sexual function, mood, muscle strength, and body composition parameters in hypogonadal men. Testosterone Gel Study Group. *Journal of Clinical Endocrinology and Metabolism* **85**, 2839–53.
94. **Dobs, A.S.** et al. (1988). Endocrine disorders in men infected with human immunodeficiency virus. *American Journal of Medicine* **84**, 611–16.
95. **Bhasin, S.** et al. (2000). Testosterone replacement and resistance exercise in HIV-infected men with weight loss and low testosterone levels. *Journal of the American Medical Association* **283**, 763–70.
96. **Bhasin, S.** et al. (1998). Effects of testosterone replacement with a nongenital, transdermal system, Androderm, in human immunodeficiency virus-infected men with low testosterone levels. *Journal of Clinical Endocrinology and Metabolism* **83**, 3155–62.
97. **Grinspoon, S.** et al. (1999). Sustained anabolic effects of long-term androgen administration in men with AIDS wasting. *Clinical Infectious Dieases* **28**, 634–6.
98. **Grinspoon, S.** et al. (1998). Effects of androgen administration in men with the AIDS wasting syndrome. A randomized, double-blind, placebo-controlled trial. *Annals of Internal Medicine* **129**, 18–26.
99. **Hengge, U.R.** et al. (1996). Oxymetholone promotes weight gain in patients with advanced human immunodeficiency virus (HIV-1) infection. *British Journal of Nutrition* **75**, 129–38.
100. **Strawford, A.** et al. (1999). Resistance exercise and supraphysiologic androgen therapy in eugonadal men with HIV-related weight loss: a randomized controlled trial. *Journal of the American Medical Association* **281**, 1282–90.
101. **Wagner, G.J. and Rabkin, J.G.** (1998). Testosterone therapy for clinical symptoms of hypogonadism in eugonadal men with AIDS. *International Journal of STD and AIDS* **9**, 41–4.
102. **Coodley, G.O. and Coodley, M.K.** (1997). A trial of testosterone therapy for HIV-associated weight loss. *AIDS* **11**, 1347–52.
103. **Dobs, A.S.** et al. (1999). The use of a transscrotal testosterone delivery system in the treatment of patients with weight loss related to human immunodeficiency virus infection. *American Journal of Medicine* **107**, 126–32.
104. **Miller, K.** et al. (1998). Transdermal testosterone administration in women with acquired immunodeficiency syndrome wasting: a pilot study. *Journal of Clinical Endocrinology and Metabolism* **83**, 2717–25.
105. **Johansen, K.L., Mulligan, K., and Schambelan, M.** (1999). Anabolic effects of nandrolone decanoate in patients receiving dialysis: a randomized controlled trial. *Journal of the American Medical Association* **281**, 1275–81.
106. **Ferreira, I.M.** et al. (1998). The influence of 6 months of oral anabolic steroids on body mass and respiratory muscles in undernourished COPD patients. *Chest* **114**, 19–28.
107. **Schols, A.M.** et al. (1995). Physiologic effects of nutritional support and anabolic steroids in patients with chronic obstructive pulmonary disease. A placebo-controlled randomized trial. *American Journal of Respiratory and Critical Care Medicine* **152**, 1268–74.
108. **Chlebowski, R.T.** et al. (1986). Influence of nandrolone decanoate on weight loss in advanced non-small cell lung cancer. *Cancer* **58**, 183–6.
109. **Darnton, S.J.** et al. (1999). The use of an anabolic steroid (nandrolone decanoate) to improve nutritional status after esophageal resection for carcinoma. *Diseases of the Esophagus* **12**, 283–8.
110. **Loprinzi, C.L.** et al. (1999). Randomized comparison of megestrol acetate versus dexamethasone versus fluoxymesterone for the treatment of cancer anorexia/cachexia. *Journal of Clinical Oncology* **17**, 3299–306.
111. **Jenkins, R.C. and Ross, R.J.** (1996). Growth hormone therapy for protein catabolism. *Quarterly Journal of Medicine* **89**, 813–19.
112. **Mathews, L.S., Norstedt, G., and Palmiter, R.D.** (1986). Regulation of insulin-like growth factor I gene expression by growth hormone. *Proceedings of the National Academy of Science* **83**, 9343–7.
113. **Florini, J.R., Ewton, D.Z., and Coolican, S.A.** (1996). Growth hormone and the insulin-like growth factor system in myogenesis. *Endocrine Reviews* **17**, 481–517.
114. **Jenkins, R.C. and Ross, R.J.** (1996). Acquired growth hormone resistance in catabolic states. *Baillieres Clinical Endocrinology and Metabolism* **10**, 411–19.
115. **Bentham, J., Rodriguez-Arnao, J., and Ross, R.J.** (1993). Acquired growth hormone resistance in patients with hypercatabolism. *Hormone Research* **40**, 87–91.
116. **Frost, V.J.** et al. (1996). Effects of treatment with megestrol acetate, aminoglutethimide, or formestane on insulin-like growth factor (IGF) I and II, IGF-binding proteins (IGFBPs), and IGFBP-3 protease status in patients with advanced breast cancer. *Journal of Clinical Endocrinology and Metabolism* **81**, 2216–21.
117. **Bartlett, D.L., Stein, T.P., and Torosian, M.H.** (1995). Effect of growth hormone and protein intake on tumor growth and host cachexia. *Surgery* **117**, 260–7.
118. **Fiebig, H.H., Dengler, W., and Hendriks, H.R.** (2000). No evidence of tumor growth stimulation in human tumors *in vitro* following treatment with recombinant human growth hormone. *Anticancer Drugs* **11**, 659–64.
119. **Krentz, A.J.** et al. (1993). Anthropometric, metabolic, and immunological effects of recombinant human growth hormone in AIDS and AIDS-related complex. *Journal of Acquired Immune Deficiency Syndromes* **6**, 245–51.
120. **Schambelan, M.** et al. (1996). Recombinant human growth hormone in patients with HIV-associated wasting. A randomized, placebo-controlled trial. Serostim Study Group. *Annals of Internal Medicine* **125**, 873–82.
121. **Wolf, R.F.** et al. (1992). Growth hormone and insulin reverse net whole body and skeletal muscle protein catabolism in cancer patients. *Annals of Surgery* **216**, 280–8.
122. **Tayek, J.A. and Brasel, J.A.** (1995). Failure of anabolism in malnourished cancer patients receiving growth hormone: a clinical research center study. *Journal of Clinical Endocrinology and Metabolism* **80**, 2082–7.
123. **Berman, R.S.** et al. (1999). Growth hormone, alone and in combination with insulin, increases whole body and skeletal muscle protein kinetics in cancer patients after surgery. *Annals of Surgery* **229**, 1–10.
124. **O'Driscoll, J.G.** et al. (1977). Treatment of end-stage cardiac failure with growth hormone. *Lancet* **349**, 1068.
125. **Cuneo, R.C.** et al. (1989). Cardiac failure responding to growth hormone. *Lancet* **1**, 838–9.
126. **Pichard, C.** et al. (1999). Treatment of cachexia with recombinant growth hormone in a patient before lung transplantation: a case report. *Critical Care Medicine* **27**, 1639–42.
127. **Nagaya, N.** et al. (2001). Chronic administration of ghrelin improves left ventricular dysfunction and attenuates development of cardiac cachexia in rats with heart failure. *Circulation* **104**, 1430–5.
128. **O'Sullivan, U.** et al. (1989). Insulin-like growth factor-1 (IGF-1) in mice reduces weight loss during starvation. *Endocrinology* **125**, 2793–4.
129. **Haskell, C.M.** et al. (1998). Phase II study of intravenous adenosine 5′ triphosphate in patients with previously untreated stage IIIB and stage IV non-small cell lung cancer. *Investigational New Drugs* **16**, 81–5.
130. **Agteresch, H.J.** et al. (2000). Randomized clinical trial of adenosine 5′ triphosphate in patients with advanced non-small-cell lung cancer. *Journal of the National Cancer Institute* **92**, 321–8.
131. **Agteresch, H.J.** et al. (2000). Effects of ATP infusion on glucose turnover and gluconeogenesis in patients with advanced non-small-cell lung cancer. *Clinical Science (Colch.)* **98**, 689–95.
132. **Tsuburaya, A.** (1995). Energy depletion in the liver and in isolated hepatocytes of tumor-bearing animals. *Journal of Surgical Research* **59**, 421–7.
133. **Hochwald, S.N.** et al. (1996). Depletion of high energy phosphate compouds in the tumor-bearing state and reversal after tumor resection. *Surgery* **120**, 534–41.
134. **Rapaport, E. and Fontaine, J.** (1989). Generation of extracellular ATP in blood and its mediated inhibition of host weight loss in tumor-bearing mice. *Biochemical Pharmacology* **38**, 4261–6.

135. **Agteresch, H.J.** et al. (1999). Adenosine triphosphate: established and potential clinical applications. *Drugs* **58**, 211–32.
136. **Tayek, J.A., Heber, D., and Chlebowski, R.T.** (1987). Effect of hydrazine sulphate on whole-body protein breakdown measured by 14C-lysine metabolism in lung cancer patients. *Lancet* **2**, 241–4.
137. **Chlebowski, R.T.** et al. (1987). Hydrazine sulfate in cancer patients with weight loss. A placebo-controlled clinical experience. *Cancer* **59**, 406–10.
138. **Chlebowski, R.T.** et al. (1990). Hydrazine sulfate influence on nutritional status and survival in non-small-cell lung cancer. *Journal of Clinical Oncology* **8**, 9–15.
139. **Loprinzi, C.L.** et al. (1994). Randomized placebo-controlled evaluation of hydrazine sulfate in patients with advanced colorectal cancer. *Journal of Clinical Oncology* **12**, 1121–5.
140. **Loprinzi, C.L.** et al. (1994). Placebo-controlled trial of hydrazine sulfate in patients with newly diagnosed non-small-cell lung cancer. *Journal of Clinical Oncology* **12**, 1126–9.
141. **Kosty, M.P.** et al. (1994). Cisplatin, vinblastine, and hydrazine sulfate in advanced, non-small-cell lung cancer: a randomized placebo-controlled, double-blind phase III study of the Cancer and Leukemia Group B. *Journal of Clinical Oncology* **12**, 1113–20.
142. **Kardinal, C.G.** et al. (1990). A controlled trial of cyproheptadine in cancer patients with anorexia and/or cachexia. *Cancer* **65**, 2657–62.

8.5 Fatigue and asthenia

Catherine Sweeney, Hans Neuenschwander, and Eduardo Bruera

Introduction

Fatigue is the most frequent symptom in patients with advanced cancer. Various studies have reported its prevalence to be between 60 and 90 per cent in cancer patients.[1–5] Prevalence of fatigue varies depending on diagnostic criteria used and patient populations studied.

In the past asthenia was used to describe a subjective sensation and fatigue used to describe a symptom precipitated by effort. However, the terms are currently often used in the same context. The terms asthenia and fatigue are assumed to be synonymous for the purpose of this chapter and fatigue will generally be used.

Fatigue includes three different major symptoms:

1. easy tiring and reduced capacity to maintain performance;
2. generalized weakness, defined as the anticipatory sensation of difficulty in initiating a certain activity; and
3. mental fatigue, defined as the presence of impaired mental concentration, loss of memory, and emotional lability.[6,7]

Fatigue occurs both as a result of cancer and its treatment. The onset of fatigue may precede the diagnosis of cancer or it may occur at any stage in the course of the illness. It may first occur or be exacerbated following treatment of cancer with chemotherapy, radiotherapy, or surgery and may be present for prolonged periods of time following these treatments.[8] In patients with advanced cancer it usually co-exists with a number of other symptoms that may include pain, anorexia, nausea, vomiting, dyspnoea, difficulty sleeping, anxiety, or depression.

Fatigue can interfere with a patient's ability to perform physical and social activities. It may influence patients' decision-making regarding future treatment and lead to refusal of potentially curative treatment.

Over recent years as the management of other symptoms such as pain, dyspnoea, and nausea in palliative care patients has improved there has been an increased awareness of the importance of fatigue as symptom deserving of attention.

The purpose of this chapter is to highlight the importance of fatigue and asthenia in palliative care, to discuss pathophysiology, assessment, and management in the context of palliative care patients, and to stimulate an interest in research into this prevalent and troublesome symptom. Most of the evidence presented in this chapter relates to studies in cancer patients. However, similar principles can be applied to fatigue in patients with HIV infection and cardiac conditions resulting in fatigue with advanced cancer.

Pathophysiology

In the majority of patients with advanced cancer the aetiology of fatigue is unclear. The basic mechanisms by which fatigue is caused are not well understood and in addition, several possible underlying causes of fatigue exist in most patients. Occasionally one predominant abnormality is present and appears to be the main contributor to the symptom; however, in most cases several abnormalities and other symptoms are present that may contribute to the genesis of fatigue.

In patients with cancer a complex interaction occurs between tumour and host. This interaction which is not well understood can result in fatigue in several ways. Table 1 outlines mechanisms by which tumours have the potential to directly or indirectly produce fatigue in patients with advanced cancer. Figure 1 summarizes contributors to fatigue in cancer patients.

Tumour- and host-derived factors

Tumours can produce lipolytic and proteolytic factors capable of interfering with host metabolism. These factors are believed to play a role in the development of cancer cachexia.[9] The relationship between cachexia and fatigue is discussed below. The presence of a tumour can induce the production of a number of inflammatory cytokines such as tumour necrosis factor alpha, interleukin-1, interleukin-6, and interleukin-2 by host macrophages and lymphocytes. These cytokines are involved in the production of anorexia–cachexia syndrome and are discussed in detail elsewhere in this book. Similarly, there may be release and/or induction of substances by the tumour that lead to fatigue.[10,11] For example, if blood from a fatigued subject is injected into a rested subject, manifestations of fatigue are produced.

Abnormalities of muscle

Impaired muscle function may be one of the main underlying mechanisms in fatigue. The cause of these muscular abnormalities may relate, in part, to

Table 1 Mechanisms by which tumours may directly or indirectly cause fatigue

Direct effects	Induced host factors	Accompanying factors
Lipolytic factors	Tumour necrosis factor	Cachexia
Proteolytic factors	Interleukin-1	Infection
Tumour degradation products	Interleukin-6	Anaemia
Invasion of brain or pituitary gland by tumour or metastases		Hypoxia Metabolic dehydration Neurological disorders Endocrine disorders Paraneoplastic Psychological issues

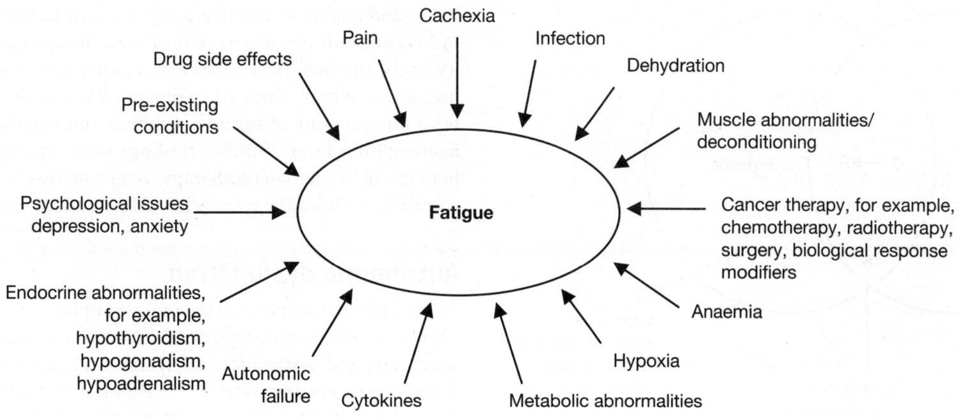

Fig. 1 Contributors to fatigue.

known abnormalities in cytokine production, but the production of other fatigue-inducing substances by the tumour or the host has been postulated. Muscle alterations in tumour-bearing patients are well known. Cachexia leads to a loss of muscle and fat. This at least may partially explain the relationship between cachexia and fatigue. However, tumour-bearing patients can have muscle abnormalities even in the presence of normal caloric intake and a constant body weight and lean body mass. Tumour-free muscle tissue of cancer patients has been found to contain excessive amounts of lactate.[(12)] It is unclear whether lactate is part of the pathogenic mechanism of weakness or a consequence of it. Atrophy of type-II muscle fibres has been suggested to be a systemic effect of cancer even in early or non-metastatic stages.[(13)] Tumour-free muscle from tumour-bearing animals show alterations in the activity of various enzymes, distribution of isoenzymes, and synthesis and breakdown of myofibrillar and sarcoplasmic proteins.[(10)] Our group found impaired maximal strength, decreased relaxation velocity, and increased fatigue after electrical stimulation of the abductor pollicis muscle via the ulnar nerve in patients with breast cancer when compared with normal controls.[(14)]

Myopathies can also be caused by medications used in cancer patients. Corticosteroids can cause loss of muscle mass and cyclosporine has been implicated as a cause of mitochondrial myopathy.[(15)]

Deconditioning

Prolonged bed rest and immobility leads to loss of muscle mass and reduced cardiac output. This deconditioning result in reduced endurance for exercise and activities of daily living and may be compounded by other muscle abnormalities in patients with cancer.[(16,17)] Recent studies have found that endurance exercise training can reduce fatigue and improve physical performance in cancer patients undergoing chemotherapy[(18)] and in patients who have undergone bone marrow or autologous stem cell transplantation.[(19,20)] Exercise may have a beneficial effect on muscle mass and cardiovascular fitness. In a randomized controlled trial of patients who underwent high dose chemotherapy and peripheral blood stem cell transplantation, significantly higher haemoglobin concentrations were found in the exercise group than in the control group. Improved physical performance can also result in improved mood, self-esteem and less anxiety.[(21)]

Over-exertion

Over-exertion is a frequent cause of fatigue in non-cancer patients.[(22)] It should also be considered in young cancer patients who are receiving aggressive antineoplastic treatment, such as radiotherapy and chemotherapy, and who are trying to maintain their social and professional activities. Research in sports medicine has shown that for prolonged endurance it is important to provide muscles with adequate substrate (carbohydrate loading). Unfortunately, cancer patients frequently present with abnormalities in muscle metabolism that may not allow an adequate utilization of this substrate.[(23)] In addition, sports medicine researchers have recently been addressing the role of neurotransmitters such as serotonin or choline as mediators of fatigue and depression in athletes suffering from over-exertion.[(23)] Anecdotal evidence suggests that in some of these patients' fatigue may disappear after 48 h of treatment with antidepressants of the serotonin-specific reuptake inhibitor group.[(23)] These findings could provide a key to future therapeutic approaches for fatigue.

Central nervous system abnormalities

The mechanisms by which fatigue is perceived or induced at the central nervous system (CNS) level are poorly understood. It has been suggested that the reticular activating system is responsible for the control of the experience of fatigue. The reticular activating system receives descending stimuli from the cortex on a feedback system based on ascending information from a number of sensory organs.[(24)] Chronic stimuli such as pain may generate fatigue through unremitting reticular stimulation. It has also been suggested that physiological fatigue might have an important protective function against over-exertion. Cancer fatigue could be due to a breakdown of this particular mediated mechanism and by environmental and cortical stimuli, and/or humeral factors.

Primary or secondary tumours involving the CNS and leading to invasion of brain tissue, and in particular of the pituitary gland, with resulting endocrine abnormalities appear to be possible mechanisms by which tumours may induce fatigue in cancer patients. Disturbance of cognitive function may be caused by fatigue but may also contribute to fatigue. Brain tumours can cause cognitive dysfunction, and other tumours such as small-cell lung cancer can affect brain function by the production of hormones or neurotransmitters.[(25)] Antineoplastic treatments such as chemotherapy and radiotherapy and other drugs such as opioids and corticosteroids used to treat complications of cancer can have effects on the CNS.[(26–28)] It has been observed that more than 70 per cent of patients receiving cranial radiotherapy for acute lymphoblastic leukaemia experience fatigue, depression, and some somnolence.[(26)] Research is needed to improve the understanding of the mechanisms causing fatigue at CNS level.

Relationship between fatigue and cachexia

Fatigue and cachexia coexist in the great majority of patients with advanced cancer. It is likely that malnutrition is a major contributor to fatigue. The loss of muscle mass resulting from progressive cachexia provides a reason for profound weakness and fatigue. As previously discussed, even in the presence of normal protein and caloric intake and normal body weight, structural and biochemical muscle abnormalities are found in cancer patients.[(12,29,30)] Similar abnormalities would explain fatigue associated

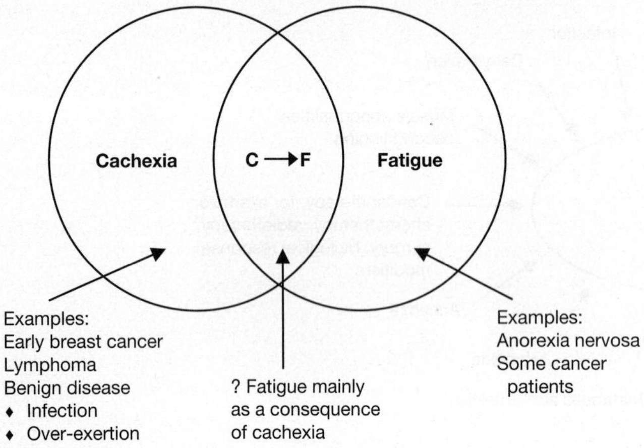

Fig. 2 Possible relationship between fatigue and cachexia.

with chronic cardiac and respiratory disease. Some metabolic abnormalities related to cachexia are specifically responsible for muscle breakdown. These include an increased concentration of cathepsin-D (a lysosomal enzyme involved in the intracellular degradation of macromolecules).[31]

However, profound fatigue can exist in the absence of significant weight loss. Fatigue is common in patients with breast cancer and lymphomas in which prevalence of cachexia is low. In non-malignant conditions such as chronic fatigue syndrome or depression profound fatigue is generally not associated with malnutrition. Our group found no correlation between fatigue and nutritional status or weight in a population of breast cancer patients.[32] On the other hand, severe malnutrition without fatigue can be observed in patients with anorexia nervosa and in some patient populations with solid tumours. Figure 2 illustrates the potential relationship between cachexia and fatigue.

It has been proposed that anorexia and fatigue may be part of an expression of the major metabolic abnormalities that occur in cancer patients, rather than simply an expression of malnutrition per se.[33] This situation would be similar to that experienced when a catabolic state occurs, such as a viral infection or in the early postoperative period. In these conditions, patients experience anorexia and fatigue that is secondary to the metabolic abnormalities and not a cause of those abnormalities. Some interventions used for the treatment of cancer cachexia, such as corticosteroids and progestational agents, have been found to be effective in the management of fatigue. The mechanisms by which these agents ameliorate cachexia and fatigue are not well understood. Current pharmacological interventions for cachexia are discussed elsewhere in this book. (See Chapters 8.4.3 and 8.4.4.)

Infection

Fatigue is frequently associated with infections, particularly when infections are recurrent or protracted. It may occur as a prodromal symptom, and it may outlast the infection by weeks or even months.[34,35] In patients with cancer the presence of immunosuppresion as a result of the cancer itself or cancer treatment increases the risk of infection and its complications. Chronic infection and cancer induce the same mediators for cachexia, including tumour necrosis factor alpha.[11] It can be hypothesized that they might share similar mediators for fatigue as well.

Anaemia

Anaemia is prevalent in cancer patients. Common causes of anaemia in cancer patients include myelosupression by chemotherapeutic agents, iron deficiency, bleeding, haemolysis, nutritional deficiencies, and anaemia of chronic disease. Severe anaemia (haemoglobin < 8 g/dl) is known to be a cause of profound fatigue. In patients receiving chemotherapy there is evidence that treating less severe anaemia improves energy levels, activity levels, and quality of life. In a prospective, open label study of epoetin-alfa in 2342 anaemic patients receiving chemotherapy mean energy levels, activity levels, and quality of life were found to improve with increases in mean haemoglobin levels from approximately 9 to 11 g/dl.[36] The improvements were independent of tumour response and correlated with increases in haemoglobin levels. Similar findings were reported in a study of 2289 patients receiving chemotherapy. Again increases in haemoglobin were correlated with improvements in energy, activity, and quality of life.[37]

Autonomic dysfunction

Autonomic dysfunction is a common complication of advanced cancer.[38] This syndrome includes postural hypotension, occasional syncope, fixed heart rate, and gastrointestinal symptoms such as nausea, anorexia, and diarrhoea or constipation.[38,39] Postural hypotension has been documented in patients with a subset of severe chronic fatigue syndrome.[40] The association between fatigue and autonomic dysfunction has not been established in cancer patients and should be investigated in future research.

Psychological issues

Anxiety, depression, and stress can all contribute to fatigue. In non-cancer patients who present with fatigue, the final diagnosis is psychological in almost 75 per cent of cases (depression, anxiety, and other psychological disorders).[41] While some depressive symptoms are frequent in cancer patients, only a minority or patients develop adjustment disorders and a small percentage present with major depressive or anxiety disorders.[42,43] The diagnosis of a major depressed episode in patients with advanced cancer is difficult because of the frequent presentation with neuro-vegetative and somatic symptoms that are part of the disease itself. The diagnosis should rely more on the presence of psychological and cognitive signs and symptoms.[44] These are discussed elsewhere in this book. Patients presenting with an adjustment disorder or a major depressive disorder can have fatigue as one of the prevalent symptoms. Some authors have found an association between fatigue and mood changes in patients with breast cancer that they have attributed to a combination of the disease and its therapy.[45]

Metabolic and endocrine disorders

Endocrine disorders such as diabetes mellitus, Addison's disease, and hypothyroidism, and electrolyte disorders such as hyponatremia, hypokalaemia, and hypercalcaemia are possible causes of fatigue and in many instances have relatively simple and effective treatments.

Interest in hypogonadism as a cause of fatigue and loss of muscle mass has increased in recent years as a result of the prevalence of these symptoms in HIV-positive men. Testosterone deficiency results in loss of muscle mass, fatigue, reduced libido, and reduced haemoglobin.[46] Androgen insufficiency in cancer patients can result from the anorexia-cachexia syndrome.[47] In addition, cancer therapies such as chemotherapy and radiotherapy can result in hypogonadism. Hormonal ablative therapy has been found to double the incidence of fatigue in patients with prostate cancer.[48] In patients with testosterone insufficiency due to HIV disease and other causes, treatment with androgenic anabolic steroids including testosterone and its derivatives has been found to increase muscle mass,[49–52] improve energy and libido,[49] and increase haemoglobin levels.[49,53] Androgenic anabolic steroids are regularly used for the treatment of hypogonadism in HIV-positive men. The effects of treating hypogonadism in cancer patients have not been well studied.

Abnormalities of the hypothalamic–pituitary–adrenal (HPA) axis involving corticotrophin-releasing factor have been postulated as another possible endocrine-related cause of fatigue. Corticotrophin-releasing factor is increased in situations of stress and may cause fatigue.[54] The HPA axis is activated by stress and hyperactivity can lead to depression.[55] However, reduced HPA activity has been postulated as a possible cause of chronic fatigue syndrome.[56] Further research is needed to clarify the role of abnormalities of the HPA in the genesis of fatigue.

Paraneoplastic neurological syndromes

Paraneoplastic neurological syndromes are rare, but are important to recognize since many of these syndromes may precede the clinical presentation of a malignancy. They may be partially reversible with primary treatment of the tumour. Table 2 summarizes some of the paraneoplastic neurological syndromes associated with fatigue.[57]

Other symptoms

Pain and other symptoms such as dyspnoea and nausea when poorly controlled may exacerbate fatigue. Poorly controlled symptoms may lead to insomnia, depression, and anxiety which in turn can contribute to fatigue.

Side effects of cancer treatment

Both antineoplastic therapies and treatment of symptoms and conditions caused by cancer can cause or aggravate fatigue. Worsening of fatigue is common during chemotherapy and radiotherapy.[58–61] The mechanisms by which these treatment modalities cause fatigue are not fully understood. Radiotherapy can result in anaemia, diarrhoea, anorexia, and weight loss, all of which may contribute to fatigue. In addition, radiotherapy can result in chronic pain, which may also contribute to fatigue. Chemotherapy commonly causes anorexia, nausea, vomiting, and anaemia. Immunosupression secondary to chemotherapy predisposes patients to infection. Breast cancer patients who undergo adjuvant chemotherapy or autologous bone marrow transplantation appear to experience fatigue for months to years after completion of treatment.[62] Patients who have local treatment only do not appear to suffer the same degree of long-term fatigue.

Biological response-modifying agents such as interferon alpha causes fatigue in 70 per cent of patients who receive this treatment.[63] Fatigue is the most important dose-limiting side effects in patients receiving biological response-modifying treatments.

Opioids such as morphine have significant effects on the reticular system and are capable of inducing sedation, cognitive changes, and fatigue in some patients. In addition, anxiolytics, hypnotics, and other drugs may cause sedation and fatigue. Table 3 outlines cancer therapies and drugs that frequently contribute to fatigue in patients with cancer.

In summary, fatigue is a complex syndrome with multiple contributing causes in addition to the well-known metabolic and muscle abnormalities it shares with cancer cachexia.

Table 2 Paraneoplastic neurological syndromes associated with fatigue

Syndrome	Comment
Progressive multifocal leucoencephalopathy	Leukaemia, lymphoma
Paraneoplastic encephalomyelitis	70% lung, 30% others
Amyotrophic lateral sclerosis	
Subacute motor neuropathy	Proximal or distal, often asymmetric (e.g. following irradiated lymphoma)
Subacute necrotic myelopathy	Mainly lung cancer
Peripheral paraneoplastic neurological syndrome	Often preceeds the primary, similar to Guillain–Barre
Ascending acute polyneuropathy (Guillain–Barre)	Lymphoma
Neuromuscular paraneoplastic syndromes:	
Dermatomyositis, polymyositis	Associated with malignangy in about 50% (onset within 1 year)
Eaton–Lambert syndrome	Strongly associated with small-cell lung cancer Can preceed tumour by months Improves with successful treatment
Myasthenia gravis	Thymoma (30%), lymphoma

Table 3 Cancer therapies and medications that commonly contribute to fatigue

Chemotherapeutic agents
Radiotherapy
Biological response (modifiers, e.g. interferon)
Opioids
Hypnotics
Anxiolytics
Antihistamines
Antiemetics
Antihypertensives

Assessment

Assessment of fatigue should involve evaluation of severity of fatigue, onset, duration, level of interference with everyday life, associated psychological or social problems, and possible underlying causes.

Fatigue is essentially a subjective sensation, and at present no 'gold standard' tool exists for its assessment. Its multidimensional nature adds to the complexity of assessment. Table 4 outlines some assessment tools for fatigue; several others exist. Functional capacity tests attempt to determine the objective function that the patient is capable of performing when subjected to a standard task such as treadmill, bicycle, or prolonged driving in a simulator. These test have been used in the assessment of drugs used for cardiovascular and respiratory diseases and in the assessment of drug effects on professions that involve a sustained task such as drivers or pilots. These types of assessments tend to be highly reproducible. However, they are of very limited value in cancer care and research as they are very difficult for the advanced cancer patient to perform. Task-related fatigue tests attempt to assess the fatigue induced by standard tasks. Assessment using performance status is the most commonly used in oncology. Two popular tools: the European Cooperative Oncology Group[66] and the Karnofsky Performance Status[65] consist of a physician's rating of the patient's functional capabilities after a regular medical consult. The Edmonton Functional Assessment Test (EFAT)[67] is performed by a physiotherapist and attempts to determine functional status of the patient, in addition to the various obstacles to clinical performance. Subjective measures of fatigue are generally considered to be the most relevant in clinical practice and in clinical trials. Visual analogue scales, numerical scales, the Functional

Table 4 Assessment approaches for fatigue

Functional capacity	**Task-related fatigue**
Treadmill performance (speed, duration)	Visual analogue/numerical rating scale Pearson and Byars Fatigue Feeling
Number of errors (pilot, driver)	Checklist[64]
Performance status	**Subjective assessment tools**
Karnofsky Performance Status[65]	Visual analogue/numerical rating scale
European Cooperative Oncology Group[66]	Functional Assessment of Cancer Therapy-Anaemia[68]
Edmonton Functional Assessment Tool[67]	Piper Fatigue Scale[69] Brief Fatigue Inventory[70]

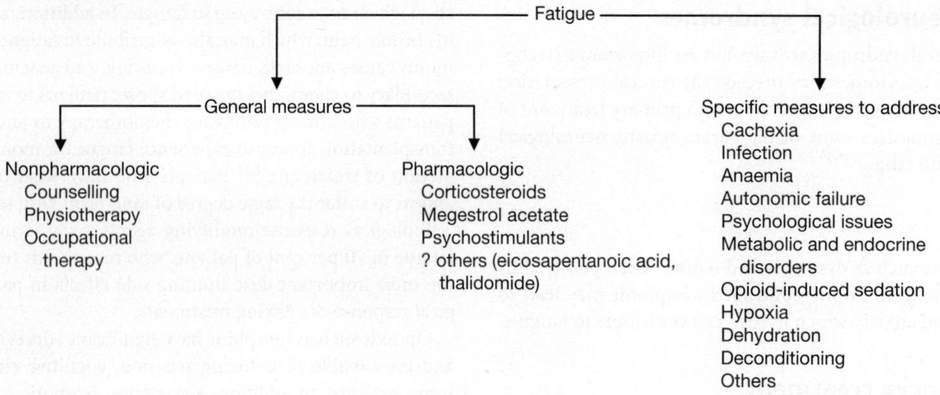

Fig. 3 Therapeutic approach to managing fatigue.

Assessment of Cancer Therapy-Anaemia (FACT-An),[68] the Piper Fatigue Scale (PFS),[69] and the Brief Fatigue Inventory (BFI)[70] have been validated and can be used in both pharmacological and non-pharmacological studies. In addition to these tools there are validated functional assessments in many quality of life questionnaires.

Tools that are multidimensional are generally preferred as they give a broader picture of the problem and can highlight general and specific management approaches that may benefit a specific patient. Examples of multidimensional assessments of fatigue include EFAT, PFS, and FACT-An.

Assessment of fatigue also involves assessment of possible underlying causes including those factors included in Fig. 1. This involves careful systems review and psychological assessment, detailed physical examination, and blood tests to look for anaemia, electrolyte or endocrine abnormalities. Multiple causes should be suspected in all patients and the possible impact of various factors should be assessed.

Screening for fatigue

Patients may not report fatigue spontaneously as they may believe it has to be put up with or that it may delay or prevent cancer treatment and physicians may fail to screen for fatigue as they may be unsure that they can treat it effectively.[4,71] The recently published guidelines of the National Comprehensive Cancer Network Fatigue Practice Guidelines Panel recommends that patients are screened for presence and severity of fatigue at initial doctor contact and that ongoing assessments be made.[72] They suggest that screening designates fatigue as mild, moderate, or severe (on a 0–10 numerical rating scale 1–3 is considered mild, 4–6 moderate, and 7–10 severe). Mild fatigue would be reevaluated on an ongoing basis, moderate or severe fatigue would undergo more focused assessment and intervention.

Management

Since fatigue is a complex multidimensional symptom it is crucial for an adequate therapeutic approach to identify and prioritize the different underlying factors. Alterations in fatigue over time may demonstrate a relationship with a particular factor (e.g. an increase following growth in tumour size, a change of medication, or a reduction in haemoglobin concentration). This temporal pattern underlines the importance of continuous assessment and monitoring of symptoms and signs in palliative medicine. In planning the therapeutic approach it is also important to answer the following questions:

1. is fatigue a symptom of primary importance for this patient?
2. what are the major, probable causes?
3. are there therapeutic measures available with reasonable cost/benefit ratio?

The intervention may have a purpose of either decreasing the intensity of fatigue or allowing the patient to express the maximal possible level of function with a stable level of fatigue, or both. In palliative care the satisfactory treatment of a symptom such as fatigue does not mean that it is mandatory to eliminate it completely. Even minor improvements can be enough to shift fatigue into a less relevant level in the patient's priority symptom list.

In a given patient it is impossible to determine with certainty whether or not an identified problem is a major contributor to fatigue or is simply a coexisting problem. Therefore, it is of great importance to measure the intensity of fatigue and the patient's performance before and after treating any contributing factor. For example, fatigue should be measured before and after correcting hypercalcemia or treating anaemia. This can be done in a number of ways, including using a simple numerical scale (0 = best, 10 = worst) or a visual analogue scale (0 = best, 100 = worst imaginable). If the level of fatigue does not improve after correction of an underlying abnormality is clear that further treatment of that abnormality will not result in improvement of fatigue in the future.

Figure 3 outlines some general and specific measures that may be useful in the management of fatigue in cancer patients. In many patients there will be no identified reversible causes. A number of effective pharmacological and non-pharmacological approaches are available for these patients. General measures include pharmacological and non-pharmacological approaches that may reduce energy expenditure or reduce levels of fatigue. Specific measures attempt to address underlying abnormalities that are thought to be contributing to fatigue in an individual patient.

General measures

Non-pharmacological approaches

Counselling can be very useful for both patients and families. Patients frequently underestimate the side effect burden at the beginning of chemotherapy. In one study 8 per cent of patients expected tiredness though 86 per cent experienced it.[73] This suggests a significant information gap that may reduce the ability to develop realistic expectations. Counselling and informing the patient of the possible causes of fatigue and the type of therapeutic options available may provide the patient the opportunity to develop realistic expectations. As disease progresses the patient will be required to adapt to progressive limitations in physical function and activity. The family will need to have realistic goals for the patient.

If patients are empowered by correct information and counselling they may combat fatigue by:

1. adapting activities of daily living by reducing housework, enlisting to help with physical duties;
2. spending more time in bed or alternatively taking some exercise if deconditioning is considered to be a contributor to the fatigue;

3. rearranging schedules within the day depending on fatigue patterns;
4. requesting changes in medications perceived to be causing loss of energy; and
5. avoiding expending energy on unnecessary activities.

Deconditioning due to inactivity has been discussed earlier. A physiotherapist can suggest suitable exercises and encourage increased activity. This may have beneficial effects both from physical and psychosocial perspectives. In addition a physiotherapist can provide passive movements to maintain flexibility and decrease painful tendon retraction in immobile patients. Occupational therapies can allow patients to remain safe and more active at home by providing extremely useful resources such as ramps, wheelchairs and walkers, elevated toilets, safe bathrooms, and hospital beds. In addition, patients and families can be provided with useful tips for mobilization and for the prevention of further muscle atrophy, tendon retraction, and pressure ulcers.

Pharmacological treatments

In patients with fatigue of unknown origin and those in who specific treatment is not available a number of non-specific pharmacological interventions have been proposed.

Corticosteroids

A number of studies have suggested that corticosteroids decrease fatigue in cancer patients. In a randomized, controlled, double blind crossover trial both patients and investigators identified methylprednisolone 32 mg/day as more effective than placebo in reducing levels of fatigue.(74) Two multicenter European trials have confirmed the effect of corticosteroid therapy in fatigue.(75,76) In addition to beneficial effects on fatigue, corticosteroids can have beneficial effects on several other symptoms such as nausea, appetite, and pain that are common in patients with advanced cancer.

The mechanism of action of corticosteroids on fatigue is unknown. The inhibition of tumour or tumour-induced substances, as well as central euphoriant effects are potential mechanisms.(74) The effects of these drugs are probably not due to their demonstrated appetite simulation since corticosteroids do not result in significant improvements of nutritional status.

Unfortunately the duration of effect is generally limited to between 2 and 4 weeks. In addition, corticosteroids cause metabolic abnormalities and serious long-term toxicity, including osteoporosis, myopathies, and increased risk of infections. Therefore, long-term treatment should generally be avoided. The best type and dose of corticosteroids have not been established. Most studies have used doses equivalent to approximately 40 mg/day of prednisone.

Megestrol acetate

Recent studies involving terminally ill patients have demonstrated rapid (within 10 days) improvement in fatigue and general well being in patients treated with megestrol acetate(160–480 mg/day) as compared to placebo without any significant change in nutritional status.(77,78) The mechanism of action of progestational agents is currently unclear and may be related to glucocorticoid or anabolic activity as well as effects on cytokine release.

Other agents of potential benefit in the management of cachexia

Other pharmacological agents such as thalidomide and omega-3 fatty acids that are of potential benefit in the management of cachexia may have a beneficial effect on fatigue. Thalidomide was found to preserve performance status in a randomized, double blind, placebo-controlled study of 28 patients with advanced HIV disease and cachexia.(79) A pilot study of thalidomide 100 mg/day in 37 evaluable cancer patients with cachexia resulted in an improvement in sensation of well being and after 10 days of treatment.(80) In a study looking at the effect of an oral nutritional supplement enriched with eicosapentanoic acid (EPA) (an omega-3 fatty acid found in fish oil) in weight-losing cancer patients, performance status was significantly improved after 3 weeks of treatment.(81) Further research is needed to study potential beneficial effects of these agents on fatigue in cancer patients.

The treatment of malnutrition as a cause of fatigue in the specific situation of cancer patients remains controversial. Malnourished patients are known to have significant levels of fatigue. However, it has not been clearly demonstrated that attempts to reverse the level of malnutrition result in significant improvement in the level of fatigue.(82,83)

Specific measures

As previously discussed fatigue is often multicausal and may appear as a consequence of other conditions such as cachexia, infection, or anaemia. Any intervention capable of reversing an underlying contributor should result in an improvement in fatigue. It is useful in any given patient to consider all possible contributing factors with the aim of identifying reversible causes. Reversible causes such as dehydration, metabolic disorders, or severe anaemia may coexist with non-reversible causes.

Infections should be treated appropriately. Factors leading to recurrent infections should be addressed where possible.

In patients with anaemia assessment of the underlying cause is important, as it may influence the choice of treatment. Treatment may also be influenced by the acuity with which anaemia develops. Severe anaemia (haemoglobin < 8 g/dl) is usually treated with blood transfusion. There is evidence as discussed earlier that patients with less severe anaemia also benefit from increased haemoglobin levels.(36,37) Epoetin-alfa at a dose of 10 000 units three times weekly increasing to 20 000 units three times weekly depending on response has been found to be effective in patients receiving chemotherapy.(37) Gabrilove et al.(84) found that weekly dosing with 40 000 units of epoetin-alfa (increased to 60 000 units depending on response after 4 weeks) produced clinical benefits similar to treatment with a three times weekly regimen. A recent systematic review of controlled clinical trials of epoetin treatment of anaemia associated with cancer therapy found that only studies with mean baseline haemoglobin concentrations of 10 g/dl or less reported significant benefits of treatment on quality of life.(85) The main disadvantages of epoetin-alfa include the cost and the delay of 4–8 weeks until an increase of 1–2 g/dl is observed in haemoglobin concentration, with resulting symptomatic improvement. This is particularly relevant in palliative care patients who have short life expectancy. In addition to transfusion or treatment with epoetin-alfa, treatment of underlying contributors to anaemia, such as iron deficiency, is important to help prevent the recurrence of anaemia. Further studies are needed to confirm the benefits of treating mild to moderate anaemia in cancer patients who are not receiving chemotherapy, particularly in those with advanced disease.

Autonomic failure in patients with diabetes and neurological disorders has been effectively managed by midodrine, a specific alpha 1 sympathomimetic agent.(86,87) This drug might be of interest in patients with severe cancer-related fatigue in whom autonomic failure is found to be present. Randomized controlled trials of this drug have not been conducted in cancer patients.

Counselling should be considered for patients with adjustment disorders, depression, anxiety, and coping difficulties. Patients with major depression should be treated with antidepressant medication. The choice of antidepressant depends on other patient factors. Selective serotonin reuptake inhibitors are commonly used and have fewer side effects than tricyclic antidepressants. In patients with problematic insomnia as part of the depression, an agent such as a tricyclic antidepressant that causes sedation may be preferred. An alternative is to consider using a psychostimulant such as methylphenidate, pemoline, or dextroamphetamine to treat depression. Psychostimulants have been found to be effective antidepressants and are also useful in the treatment of opioid-induced sedation.(88,89). An advantage of psychostimulants is their rapid onset of antidepressant effect, usually apparent within a few days. Disadvantages include neurotoxic side effects, possible development of tolerance, and potential for addiction.

Psychostimulants have also been found to be effective in treating fatigue related to opioid-induced sedation. Randomized controlled trials have shown that methylphenidate and dextroamphetamine are capable of antagonizing the sedating effect of opioids when compared with placebo.[90–92] However, a randomized controlled trial of mazindol for the treatment of fatigue in advanced cancer patients found no significant improvement in either fatigue or activity, and significant neurotoxicity occurred. At the present time there is not enough evidence to consider the use of psychostimulants for the general management of fatigue in patients who do not have evidence of opioid-related sedation.

Modafinil is a novel psychostimulant that appears to have a mode of action different from that of the amphetamine derivatives.[93] It is licensed for the treatment of narcolepsy. It appears to have less abuse potential than amphetamines.[94] It has been found to reduce fatigue in healthy individuals during sustained mental work and may have fewer side effects than D-amphetamine.[95] A retrospective case series of seven patients who had partial or no response to an antidepressant suggests that modafinil may augment antidepressant treatment and reduce fatigue in these patients.[96] Research is needed to explore whether or not modafinil is an effective alternative to amphetamine derivatives in the treatment of opioid-induced sedation.

Metabolic disorders such as hypercalcaemia, hyponatremia, and hypokalaemia should be corrected where possible. Endocrine deficiencies such as hypothyroidism and Addison's disease require treatment with hormone replacement. Testosterone replacement therapy can be considered for patients with hypogonadism. Future studies are needed to look at the effects of testosterone replacement in cancer patients with fatigue and to determine which patients are most likely to benefit from treatment.

Other possible contributors should be considered and treated. The list of prescribed drugs should be monitored regularly to prevent fatigue as an iatrogenic effect. Dehydration and hypoxia should be managed as appropriate and treatment of underlying cardiac or respiratory conditions should be optimized.

Fatigue in cancer patients is now accepted as a symptom that should be studied in its own right. In the past it was accepted as a symptom that was an inevitable consequence of cancer and its treatment. In order to improve treatment, a better understanding of many aspects of fatigue is needed. Identification of tumour or tumour-induced factors that cause fatigue is important. Assessment and staging tools that are valid and reliable are needed to assist in clinical practice and research. The role of nutritional interventions along with those of a number of commonly used agents such as megestrol acetate and corticosteroids needs to be more thoroughly investigated. The potential of agents such as EPA, thalidomide, and an abolic steroids needs to be explored in studies where fatigue is a primary endpoint. The role of psychostimulants, including modafinil, should be further researched and the importance of rest and exercise should be clarified.

References

1. **Bruera, E.** (1998). Research into symptoms other than pain. In *Oxford Textbook of Palliaitve Medicine* (ed. D. Doyle, G. Hanks, and N. MacDonald), pp. 179–85. Oxford: Oxford University Press.
2. **Coyle, N.** et al. (1990). Character of terminal illness in the advanced cancer patient: pain and other symptoms during the last four weeks of life. *Journal of Pain and Symptom Management* **5**, 83–93.
3. **Cella, D.F.** et al. (1993). The functional assessment of cancer therapy scale: development and validation of the general measure. *Journal of Clinical Oncology* **11**, 570–9.
4. **Vogelzang, N.J.** et al. (1997). Patient, caregiver, and oncologist perceptions of cancer-related fatigue: results of a tripart assessment survey. The Fatigue Coalition. *Seminars in Hematology* **34**, 4–12.
5. **Portenoy, R.K.** et al. (1994). Symptom prevalence, characteristics and distress in a cancer population. *Quality of Life Research* **3**, 183–9.
6. **Theologides, A.** (1982). Asthenia in cancer. *American Journal of Medicine* **73**, 1–3.
7. **Bruera, E. and MacDonald, R.N.** (1988). Asthenia in patients with advanced cancer. Issues in symptom control. Part 1. *Journal of Pain and Symptom Management* **3**, 9–14.
8. **Berglund, G.** et al. (1991) Late effects of adjuvant chemotherapy and postoperative radiotherapy on quality of life among breast cancer patients. *European Journal of Cancer* **27**, 1075–81.
9. **Tisdale, M.J.** (1998). New cachexic factors. *Current Opinion in Clinical Nutrition and Metabolic Care* **1**, 253–6.
10. **Theologides, A.** (1986). Anorexins, asthenins, and cachectins in cancer. *American Journal of Medicine* **81**, 696–8.
11. **Beutler, B. and Cerami, A.** (1987). Cachectin: more than a tumor necrosis factor. *New England Journal of Medicine* **316**, 379–85.
12. **Holroyde, C.P.** et al. (1979). Lactate metabolism in patients with metastatic colorectal cancer. *Cancer Research* **39**, 4900–4.
13. **Warmolts, J.R.** et al. (1975). Type II muscle fibre atrophy (II-atrophy): an early systemic effect of cancer. *Neurology* **2**, 374.
14. **Bruera, E.** et al. (1988). Muscle electrophysiology in patients with advanced breast cancer. *Journal of the National Cancer Institute* **80**, 282–5.
15. **Tirdel, G.B.** et al. (1998). Metabolic myopathy as a cause of the exercise limitation in lung transplant recipients. *Journal of Heart and Lung Transplantation* **17**, 1231–7.
16. **Germain, P., Guell, A., and Marini, J.F.** (1995). Muscle strength during bedrest with and without muscle exercise as a countermeasure. *European Journal of Applied Physiology and Occupational Physiology* **71**, 342–8.
17. **Levine, B.D., Zuckerman, J.H., and Pawelczyk, J.A.** (1997). Cardiac atrophy after bed-rest deconditioning: a nonneural mechanism for orthostatic intolerance. *Circulation* **96**, 517–25.
18. **Dimeo, F.C.** et al. (1999). Effects of physical activity on the fatigue and psychologic status of cancer patients during chemotherapy. *Cancer* **85**, 2273–7.
19. **Dimeo, F.** et al. (1997). Effects of aerobic exercise on the physical performance and incidence of treatment-related complications after high-dose chemotherapy. *Blood* **90**, 3390–4.
20. **Dimeo, F.** et al. (1996). An aerobic exercise program for patients with haematological malignancies after bone marrow transplantation. *Bone Marrow Transplant* **18**, 1157–60.
21. **Dimeo, F.C.** (2001). Effects of exercise on cancer-related fatigue. *Cancer* **92**, 1689–93.
22. **Plum, F.** (1988). Asthenia, weakness and fatigue. In *Cecil Textbook of Medicine* (ed. J. Wyngaarden and L. Smith), p. 2044. Philadelphia PA: WB Saunders.
23. **Burnfoot, A.** (1994). The brain connection. *Runners World* **29**, 70–5.
24. **Grandjean, E.P.** (1970). Fatigue. *American Industrial Hygeine Association Journal* **31**, 401–11.
25. **Valentine, A.D. and Meyers, C.A.** (2001). Cognitive and mood disturbance as causes and symptoms of fatigue in cancer patients. *Cancer* **92**, 1694–8.
26. **Proctor, S.J., Kernaham, J., and Taylor, P.** (1981). Depression as component of post-cranial irradiation somnolence syndrome. *Lancet* **1**, 1215–16.
27. **Schagen, S.B.** et al. (1999). Cognitive deficits after postoperative adjuvant chemotherapy for breast carcinoma. *Cancer* **85**, 640–50.
28. **Schagen, S.B.** et al. (2001). Neurophysiological evaluation of late effects of adjuvant high-dose chemotherapy on cognitive function. *Journal of Neurooncology* **51**, 159–65.
29. **Beck, S.A., Mulligan, H.D., and Tisdale, M.J.** (1990). Lipolytic factors associated with murine and human cancer cachexia. *Journal of the National Cancer Institute* **82**, 1922–6.
30. **Smith, K.L. and Tisdale, M.J.** (1993). Mechanism of muscle protein degradation in cancer cachexia. *British Journal of Cancer* **68**, 314–18.
31. **Beck, S.A. and Tisdale, M.J.** (1987). Production of lipolytic and proteolytic factors by a murine tumor-producing cachexia in the host. *Cancer Research* **47**, 5919–23.
32. **Bruera, E.** et al. (1989). Association between asthenia and nutritional status, lean body mass, anemia, psychological status, and tumor mass in patients with advanced breast cancer. *Journal of Pain and Symptom Management* **4**, 59–63.
33. **Bruera, E.** (1992). Current pharmacological management of anorexia in cancer patients. *Oncology (Huntington)* **6**, 125–30.

34. **Jones, J.F.** et al. (1985). Evidence for active Epstein–Barr virus infection in patients with persistent, unexplained illnesses: elevated anti-early antigen antibodies. *Annals of Internal Medicine* **102**, 1–7.
35. **Straus, S.E.** et al. (1985). Persisting illness and fatigue in adults with evidence of Epstein–Barr virus infection. *Annals of Internal Medicine* **102**, 7–16.
36. **Glaspy, J.** et al. (1997). Impact of therapy with epoetin alfa on clinical outcomes in patients with nonmyeloid malignancies during cancer chemotherapy in community oncology practice. Procrit Study Group. *Journal of Clinical Oncology* **15**, 1218–34.
37. **Demetri, G.D.** et al. (1998). Quality-of-life benefit in chemotherapy patients treated with epoetin alfa is independent of disease response or tumor type: results from a prospective community oncology study. Procrit Study Group. *Journal of Clinical Oncology* **16**, 3412–25.
38. **Bruera, E.** et al. (1986). Study of cardiovascular autonomic insufficiency in advanced cancer patients. *Cancer Treatment Reports* **70**, 1383–7.
39. **Henrich, W.L.** (1982). Autonomic insufficiency. *Archives of Internal Medicine* **142**, 339–44.
40. **Calkins, H. and Rowe, P.C.** (1998). Relationship between chronic fatigue syndrome and neurally mediated hypotension. *Cardiology Reviews* **6**, 125–34.
41. **Adams, R.** (1993). Anxiety, depression, asthenia and personality disorders. In *Harrison's Principles of Internal Medicine* (ed. R. Petersdorf, R. Adams, and E. Brawnnald), pp. 68–75. New York: McGraw-Hill.
42. **Derogatis, L.R.** et al. (1993). The prevalence of psychiatric disorders among cancer patients. *Journal of the American Medical Association* **249**, 751–7.
43. **Hayes, J.R.** (1991). Depression and chronic fatigue in cancer patients. *Primary Care* **18**, 327–39.
44. **Breitbart, W., Chochinov, H., and Passik, S.** (1998). Psychiatric aspects of palliative care. In *Oxford Textbook of Palliative Medicine* (ed. D. Doyle and G.W. Hanks), pp. 933–54. Oxford: Oxford University Press.
45. **Piper, B.F.** (1993). Fatigue. In *Pathophysiological Phenomena in Nursing: Human Responses to Illness* (ed. V. Carrieri, A. Lindsey, and C. West), pp. 279–302. Philadelphia PA: WB Saunders.
46. **Basaria, S., Wahlstrom, J.T., and Dobs, A.S.** (2001). Clinical review 138: Anabolic-androgenic steroid therapy in the treatment of chronic diseases. *Journal of Clinical Endocrinology and Metabolism* **86**, 5108–17.
47. **Todd, B.D.** (1988). Pancreatic carcinoma and low serum testosterone; a correlation secondary to cancer cachexia? *European Journal of Surgical Oncology* **14**, 199–202.
48. **Stone, P.** et al. (2000). Fatigue in patients with prostate cancer receiving hormone therapy. *European Journal of Cancer* **36**, 1134–41.
49. **Snyder, P.J.** et al. (2000). Effects of testosterone replacement in hypogonadal men. *Journal of Clinical Endocrinology and Metabolism* **85**, 2670–7.
50. **Bhasin, S.** et al. (1997). Testosterone replacement increases fat-free mass and muscle size in hypogonadal men. *Journal of Clinical Endocrinology and Metabolism* **82**, 407–13.
51. **Bhasin, S.** et al. (1998). Effects of testosterone replacement with a nongenital, transdermal system, Androderm, in human immunodeficiency virus-infected men with low testosterone levels. *Journal of Clinical Endocrinology and Metabolism* **83**, 3155–62.
52. **Grinspoon, S.** et al. (1998). Effects of androgen administration in men with the AIDS wasting syndrome. A randomized, double-blind, placebo-controlled trial. *Annals of Internal Medicine* **129**, 18–26.
53. **Wang, C.** et al. (2000) Transdermal testosterone gel improves sexual function, mood, muscle strength, and body composition parameters in hypogonadal men. Testosterone Gel Study Group. *Journal of Clinical Endocrinology and Metabolism* **85**, 2839–53.
54. **Gutstein, H.B.** (2001). The biologic basis of fatigue. *Cancer* **92**, 1678–83.
55. **Checkley, S.** (1996). The neuroendocrinology of depression and chronic stress. *British Medical Bulletin* **52**, 597–617.
56. **Scott, L.V. and Dinan, T.G.** (1999). The neuroendocrinology of chronic fatigue syndrome: focus on the hypothalamic-pituitary-adrenal axis. *Functional Neurology* **14**, 3–11.
57. **Warenius, H.M.** (1989). Paraneoplastic neurological syndromes. In *The Clinical Neurology of Old Age* (ed. R. Tallis), pp. 323–34. New York: John Wiley and Sons Ltd.
58. **Greene, D.** et al. (1994). A comparison of patient-reported side effects among three chemotherapy regimens for breast cancer. *Cancer Practice* **2**, 57–62.
59. **Stone, P.** et al. (2001). Fatigue in patients with cancers of the breast or prostate undergoing radical radiotherapy. *Journal of Pain and Symptom Management* **22**, 1007–15.
60. **Irvine, D.** et al. (1994). The prevalence and correlates of fatigue in patients receiving treatment with chemotherapy and radiotherapy. A comparison with the fatigue experienced by healthy individuals. *Cancer Nursing* **17**, 367–78.
61. **Blesch, K.S.** et al. (1991). Correlates of fatigue in people with breast or lung cancer. *Oncology Nursing Forum* **18**, 81–7.
62. **Jacobsen, P.B. and Stein, K.** (1999). Is fatigue a long-term side effect of breast cancer treatment? *Cancer Control* **6**, 256–63.
63. **Jones, T.H., Wadler, S., and Hupart, K.H.** (1998). Endocrine-mediated mechanisms of fatigue during treatment with interferon-alpha. *Seminars in Oncology* **25**, 54–63.
64. **Pearson, P.G. and Byars, G.E.** *The Development and Validation of a Checklist Measuring Subjective Fatigue. H556115.* School of Aviation, USAF, Randolf AFB, TX, 1956.
65. **Karnofsky, D.A. and Burchenal, J.H.** (1949). The clinical evaluation of chemotherapeutic agents in cancer. In *Evaluation of Chemotherapeutic Agents* (ed. C.M. Macleod), pp. 191–205. New York: Columbia University Press.
66. **Zubrod, C.G.** et al. (1960). Appraisal of methods for the study of chemotherapy of cancer in man: comparative therapeutic trial of nitrogen mustard and triethylene thiophosphoramide. *Journal of Chronic Disease* **11**, 7–33.
67. **Kaasa, T.** et al. (1997). The Edmonton Functional Assessment Tool: preliminary development and evaluation for use in palliative care. *Journal of Pain and Symptom Management* **13**, 10–19.
68. **Cella, D.** (1997). The Functional Assessment of Cancer Therapy-Anemia (FACT-An) Scale: a new tool for the assessment of outcomes in cancer anemia and fatigue. *Seminars in Hematology* **34**, 13–19.
69. **Piper, B.F.** et al. (1998). The revised Piper Fatigue Scale: psychometric evaluation in women with breast cancer. *Oncology Nursing Forum* **25**, 677–84.
70. **Mendoza, T.R.** et al. (1999). The rapid assessment of fatigue severity in cancer patients: use of the Brief Fatigue Inventory. *Cancer* **85**, 1186–96.
71. **Kirsh, K.L.** et al. (2001). I get tired for no reason: a single item screening for cancer-related fatigue. *Journal of Pain and Symptom Management* **22**, 931–7.
72. **Mock, V.** (2001). Fatigue management: evidence and guidelines for practice. *Cancer* **92**, 1699–707.
73. **Love, R.R.** et al. (1989). Side effects and emotional distress during cancer chemotherapy. *Cancer* **63**, 604–12.
74. **Bruera, E.** et al. (1985). Action of oral methylprednisolone in terminal cancer patients: a prospective randomized double-blind study. *Cancer Treatment Reports* **69**, 751–4.
75. **Della Cuna, G.R., Pellegrini, A., and Piazzi, M.** (1989). Effect of methylprednisolone sodium succinate on quality of life in preterminal cancer patients: a placebo-controlled, multicenter study. The Methylprednisolone Preterminal Cancer Study Group. *European Journal of Cancer and Clinical Oncology* **25**, 1817–21.
76. **Popiela, T., Lucchi, R., and Giongo, F.** (1989). Methylprednisolone as palliative therapy for female terminal cancer patients. The Methylprednisolone Female Preterminal Cancer Study Group. *European Journal of Cancer and Clinical Oncology* **25**, 1823–9.
77. **Bruera, E.** et al. (1998). Effectiveness of megestrol acetate in patients with advanced cancer: a randomized, double-blind, crossover study. *Cancer Prevention and Control* **2**, 74–8.
78. **De Conno, F.** et al. (1998). Megestrol acetate for anorexia in patients with far-advanced cancer: a double-blind controlled clinical trial. *European Journal of Cancer* **34**, 1705–9.
79. **Reyes-Teran, G.** et al. (1996). Effects of thalidomide on HIV-associated wasting syndrome: a randomized, double-blind, placebo-controlled clinical trial. *AIDS* **10**, 1501–7.
80. **Bruera, E.** et al. (1999). Thalidomide in patients with cachexia due to terminal cancer: preliminary report. *Annals of Oncology* **10**, 857–9.

81. **Barber, M.D.** et al. (1999). The effect of an oral nutritional supplement enriched with fish oil on weight-loss in patients with pancreatic cancer. *British Journal of Cancer* **81**, 80–6.
82. **Koretz, R.L.** (1984). Parental nutrition: is it oncologically logical? *Journal of Clinical Oncology* **2**, 534–8.
83. **Evans, W., Macmillan, K., and Daly, J.** (1986). A randomized study of standard or augmented oral nutritional support versus ad lib nutrition intake in patients with advanced cancer (Abstract). *Clinical and Investigative Medicine* **9**, 127.
84. **Gabrilove, J.L.** et al. (2001). Clinical evaluation of once-weekly dosing of epoetin alfa in chemotherapy patients: improvements in hemoglobin and quality of life are similar to three-times-weekly dosing. *Journal of Clinical Oncology* **19**, 2875–82.
85. **Seidenfeld, J.** et al. (2001). Epoetin treatment of anemia associated with cancer therapy: a systematic review and meta-analysis of controlled clinical trials. *Journal of the National Cancer Institute* **93**, 1204–14.
86. **Fouad-Tarazi, F.M., Okabe, M., and Goren, H.** (1995). Alpha sympathomimetic treatment of autonomic insufficiency with orthostatic hypotension. *American Journal of Medicine* **99**, 604–10.
87. **Wright, R.A.** et al. (1998). A double-blind, dose-response study of midodrine in neurogenic orthostatic hypotension. *Neurology* **51**, 120–4.
88. **Olin, J. and Masand, P.** (1996). Psychostimulants for depression in hospitalized cancer patients. *Psychosomatics* **37**, 57–62.
89. **Masand, P.S. and Tesar, G.E.** (1996). Use of stimulants in the medically ill. *Psychiatric Clinics of North America* **19**, 515–47.
90. **Bruera, E.** et al. (1987). Methylphenidate associated with narcotics for the treatment of cancer pain. *Cancer Treatment Reports* **71**, 67–70.
91. **Bruera, E.** et al. (1989). Influence of the pain and symptom control team (PSCT) on the patterns of treatment of pain and other symptoms in a cancer center. *Journal of Pain and Symptom Management* **4**, 112–16.
92. **Bruera, E.** et al. (1992). The use of methylphenidate in patients with incident cancer pain receiving regular opiates. A preliminary report. *Pain* **50**, 75–7.
93. **Broughton, R.J.** et al. (1997). Randomized, double-blind, placebo-controlled crossover trial of modafinil in the treatment of excessive daytime sleepiness in narcolepsy. *Neurology* **49**, 444–51.
94. **Anonymous** (2000). Randomized trial of modafinil as a treatment for the excessive daytime somnolence of narcolepsy: US Modafinil in Narcolepsy Multicenter Study Group. *Neurology* **54**, 1166–75.
95. **Pigeau, R.** et al. (1995). Modafinil, d-amphetamine and placebo during 64 hours of sustained mental work. I. Effects on mood, fatigue, cognitive performance and body temperature. *Journal of Sleep Research* **4**, 212–28.
96. **Menza, M.A., Kaufman, K.R., and Castellanos, A.** (2001). Modafinil augmentation of antidepressant treatment in depression. *Journal of Clinical Psychiatry* **61**, 378–81.

8.6 Clinical management of anaemia, cytopenias, and thrombosis in palliative medicine

A. Robert Turner

Introduction

Many palliative care patients have haematological problems. Supportive therapy often includes management of anaemias or other cytopenias. Transfusion support can provide gratifying relief of symptoms and improvement in overall quality of life permitting resumption of pleasurable activities. Thrombosis problems are also frequent in palliative care patients. Acute and chronic venous thrombosis, coagulopathy, and venous insufficiency can all be managed to the benefit of the patient. As with transfusion therapy for cytopenias, anticoagulation can provide effective palliation. This chapter emphasizes a practical approach intended to maximize quality of life.

Marrow failure

Many patients in palliative care have had extensive prior treatment with myelotoxic chemotherapy and/or radiation treatments. Some patients will have bone marrow failure related to infiltration of the marrow by their cancer. Marrow failure can present as an isolated cytopenia, such as a reduced platelet count, a reduced total white cell count, or an anaemia, but the key feature of the clinical presentation of such a patient is their inability to respond to haemorrhage, by increasing their production of young red blood cells (reticulocytosis); to sepsis, by increasing production of white cells; or to thrombocytopenia by increasing production of platelets. Transfusion of red cells or platelets may be needed on a regular basis to counteract symptoms of anaemia or purpuric bleeding. Patients may have become reliant on transfusion during the acute phase of their treatment leading to difficult ethical dilemmas.[1]

Anaemia

Anaemia is the most prevalent manifestation of marrow failure and is a common problem in patients receiving palliative care producing significant symptoms which include:

- easy fatigability, reduced mental acuity, anorexia;
- dyspnoea, exacerbation of angina, headache; and
- postural hypotension, oedema.

To the extent that these symptoms are caused by anaemia, correction to a more normal haemoglobin will result in dramatic relief. Fortunately, several therapeutic options exist but, first, the cause of the anaemia must be determined. This may be challenging since the aetiology of anaemia is often multifactorial.

The differential diagnosis of anaemia in a patient seen in a palliative care setting is different from the differential diagnosis of patients with anaemia in a general medical context. The major entities which should be considered are: (several of these causes of anaemia may be occurring in an individual patient)

- anaemia of chronic disorders,
- acute and chronic haemorrhage,
- marrow suppression,
- malnutrition,
- haemolysis, and
- underlying chronic or congenital anaemia.

Anaemia of chronic disorders[2–4]

This is a hypoproliferative anaemia which is unresponsive to haematinic therapy. Severe anaemia is unusual but transfusions are sometimes required to maintain the patient's activity levels. The anaemia of chronic disorders (ACD) is caused by an immunological reaction to the presence of a malignancy or an inflammation. Several cytokines are released in this reaction. Interleukin 1 (IL-1β), is one of a large family of glycoprotein hormones which carries signals from various types of leucocytes to other types of white cells. IL-1β, previously known as endogenous pyrogen, is released by macrophages. It interacts with other cytokines, such as tumor necrosis factor (TNFα) and gamma interferon (IFγ), to mediate an immune response. IL-1β affects the haematological system in many ways. One of these is to impede the transfer of iron molecules from storage sites in the reticuloendothelial system to red cell precursors. This results in the paradoxical situation of iron deficient erythropoiesis occurring in a marrow replete with iron. IL-1β also causes stimulation of splenic macrophages which leads to hypersplenism and a shortened red cell survival. TNFα and IFγ both impair red cell precursor proliferation. Interleukin 6 (IL-6), another proinflammatory cytokine, is upregulated in malignant disorders causing a low-grade anaemia as well as decreased serum albumin.

The diagnosis of ACD is often based on the exclusion of other forms of anaemia. However, ACD should always be considered in the palliative care setting. The anaemia will be slightly microcytic or near the lower limits of the mean corpuscular volume. The reticulocyte count will be low reflecting a reduced marrow output. The serum ferritin is normal as the patient's iron stores are not reduced. Serum iron studies should be interpreted carefully. The serum iron may be low but the total iron binding capacity (transferrin) is also low and the iron saturation is greater than 15 per cent. (In iron deficiency, the total iron binding capacity would be elevated resulting in a very low iron saturation index.) Modest elevations of indirect bilirubin and lactate dehydrogenase (LDH) and slight reduction of serum haptoglobin are the result of mild haemolysis and ineffective erythropoiesis. Red cell survival is shortened but this test should not be part of routine investigations.

Acute and chronic haemorrhage[5–8]

Haemorrhage can occur due to bleeding from neoplastic lesions within the gastrointestinal tract, the upper and lower respiratory tract, or the genitourinary system. Less commonly, haemorrhage can occur within tumour masses or around a pathological fracture. This bleeding can be acute and massive, resulting in a rapid depletion of intravascular volume and consequent shock. More commonly, the bleeding is of a chronic nature with a loss of a few millilitres of blood daily. Chronic loss of blood can lead to iron deficiency. In most cases, the chronic blood loss is obvious from the presence of blood in bodily fluids but occasionally tests for occult blood or endoscopic examinations are necessary to determine the presence and site of the bleeding.

The first priority is to control the bleeding if practical. This may be accomplished surgically, endoscopically, or by radiation of the bleeding lesion. Medical therapy (H_2 antagonists such as ranitidine, or a proton pump inhibitor, omeprazole, or misoprostol or sucralfate) may be helpful for some patients with chronic haemorrhage who are bleeding from non-neoplastic lesions within the gastrointestinal tract such as chronic peptic ulcer. Patients whose chronic bleeding has led to iron deficiency can be treated with an orally administered simple iron salt such as ferrous sulphate or ferrous gluconate (300 mg two to three times daily). Intravenous administration of 1–2 g of iron is a very useful way to provide a reserve of iron when oral iron preparations cannot be tolerated or are poorly absorbed. Transfusion therapy will be discussed in a separate section below.

Chronic haemorrhage can also be seen in patients with thrombocytopenia secondary to marrow failure or coagulation factor deficiencies due to liver failure or disseminated intravascular coagulation (DIC) (see below). Extensive ecchymoses are often evident in patients whose platelet count is less than 50×10^9/l or whose prothrombin time or activated partial thromboplastin time is prolonged. These patients tend to have a gradual drop in their haemoglobin levels without gross evidence of blood in the stool or other body fluids.

An important cause of anaemia in patients in any type of institutional setting is chronic bloodletting for laboratory testing purposes. Each vial of blood that is drawn represents 7–10 ml of whole blood. Routine, repetitive laboratory testing should be limited.

Marrow suppression[9]

Patients who have had extensive treatments with myelotoxic chemotherapy or radiation, or whose marrow has been infiltrated with metastatic cancer, myelodysplasia, or fibrosis will not be able to produce red blood cells on demand. Thrombocytopenia may lead to purpura and haemorrhage. If the neutrophil count is less than 0.5×10^9/l, neutropenic sepsis is a risk.

The presence of a leucoerythroblastic blood reaction (the presence of immature red blood cells and immature white blood cells in the peripheral blood) as well as the presence of tear drop-shaped red cells points to the presence of metastasis or fibrosis within the bone marrow. A bone marrow aspirate and biopsy can document the metastasis or fibrosis but a bone marrow examination is rarely done in a palliative care setting since the test is uncomfortable and there are few therapies which would benefit the patient beyond transfusion support.

Malnutrition[10]

Most patients in a palliative care setting have protein and/or calorie malnutrition. Along with protein/calorie malnutrition, there will be deficiencies in the dietary intake of haematologically important nutrients such as iron or folic acid. Iron deficiency usually results from chronic or acute haemorrhage and not from malnutrition alone, but patients can readily become deficient in folic acid if they have not had it in their diet for 4–6 weeks. Patients with chronic anaemias, rapidly growing tumours, and prior treatment with folic antagonists such as methotrexate are at especially high risk for this easily correctable deficiency. Folic acid, 5 mg daily, can be administered orally or subcutaneously.

Deficiencies of iron should be suspected when the mean cell size is reduced. A serum ferritin test should be done to establish the diagnosis as ACD often causes a very similar microcytic picture. Folic acid deficiency should be suspected in a patient who has a macrocytic anaemia. It can be confirmed by doing a red cell folate assay. Other important causes of a macrocytic anaemia in a patient in palliative care include liver disease and B_{12} deficiency.

Chronic protein malnutrition can lead to a generalized hypoproteinemia that is often accompanied by a normocytic anaemia and marrow failure. The anaemia in these patients may respond to improvement in overall nutrition if the cachexia–anorexia syndrome is not present.

Chronic haemolysis[11,12]

Haemolysis is rarely a major contributor to anaemia in the palliative care setting. Some neoplasms are associated with haemolysis such as chronic lymphocytic leukaemia, non-Hodgkin's lymphomas, thymomas, and adenocarcinomas of diverse origins. Haemolysis should be suspected in the patient who has a progressive anaemia and in whom chronic haemorrhage cannot be documented. The laboratory evaluation of these patients may show an elevated LDH, indirect bilirubin, and a reduction in serum haptoglobin. Because of the effects of concomitant ACD and/or marrow failure, a reticulocytosis may not be seen despite active haemolysis.

Three general types of haemolysis can be seen in these patients. They are:

- immune haemolysis (Coomb's positive or cold agglutinin),
- microangiopathic haemolytic anaemia, and
- hypersplenism.

Immune haemolysis is due to the presence of an immunoglobulin or complement on the surface of red cells causing red cell lipsis or macrophage engulfment in the reticulo-endothelial system. The Coomb's test (direct antiglobulin test or the cold agglutinin screen) detects the immunoglobulin or complement. If active haemolysis is occurring, there will be evidence of red cell breakdown (including elevation of red cell-derived LDH) and evidence of increased haemoglobin release (i.e. increased indirect bilirubin and decreased haptoglobin). An examination of peripheral blood may show spherocytes or agglutinated red cells.

Immune haemolysis not due to cold agglutinin may be treated with corticosteroids (prednisolone, 0.5–1.0 mg/kg). Other forms of treatment include splenectomy or the use of immunosuppressive drugs such as cyclophosphamide or azathioprine but they are not often utilized in the palliative care setting. Cold agglutinin haemolysis does not respond to corticosteroids or splenectomy. Transfusions are the mainstay of therapy.

Microangiopathic haemolytic anaemia may be seen when there is destruction of the red cell membrane as it passes through abnormal vasculature within a tumour or in a disorder sometimes associated with vascular neoplasms or chemotherapy agents such as mitomycin C. There are striking changes noted in the peripheral blood of these patients, and prominent red cell fragmentation is seen. The therapy of these disorders has been unrewarding.

Hypersplenism is a disorder in which an enlarged or overactive spleen causes an increased rate of destruction of red blood cells and other blood elements. This disorder can be treated with splenectomy or by radiation to the spleen. The latter approach may be attractive in palliative care when the general condition of the patient would make surgery difficult. Surgical advances have made laparoscopic splenectomy much less traumatic than removing a spleen through a laparotomy incision.

Chronic or congenital haematological disorders[13,14]

Patients receiving palliative care bring with them a variety of medical disorders. Some of these can be associated with anaemia and should not be disregarded in the differential diagnosis of anaemia in the palliative care patient. Examples of chronic disorders include rheumatological diseases, inflammatory bowel disorders, or chronic infections. Perhaps the most common cause of chronic anaemia in the world is the presence of α- or β-thalassemia trait. Thalassemia trait will cause a chronic anaemia marked by the presence of severe microcytosis and target cells in the peripheral blood. It can be confused with iron deficiency or ACD. Many patients with thalassemia trait will have a positive family history. β-Thalassemia trait can be diagnosed by demonstrating an elevation in the proportion of haemoglobin A_2 on haemoglobin electrophoresis.

General approach to the diagnosis of anaemia

In the palliative care setting, anaemia is very common and is almost always multifactorial in aetiology (Table 1). Any patient who has a neoplasm or chronic infection will have some degree of anaemia of chronic disorders. Many of these patients will also have chronic haemorrhage and marrow failure. Haemolysis and malnutrition occur in a minority of patients but need to be recognized since the therapeutic options will be influenced. Laboratory investigation needs to be individualized to each patient depending upon their prognosis and the likelihood of remediable causes of the anaemia. The peripheral blood smear often gives very valuable clues as to the diagnosis and the cause of anaemia. Estimates of iron stores using a serum ferritin and the demonstration of immune haemolysis with the direct antiglobulin test (Coomb's) are commonly used. A bone marrow examination is done infrequently.

Table 1 Approach to the diagnosis of anaemia in a palliative care setting

Anaemias	Diagnosis	Therapy
ACD	Exclude other causes	Transfuse Erythropoietin
Haemorrhage	Determine site	Control haemorrhage Block H_2 receptor (if from peptic ulcer)
Marrow failure	Marrow examination	Transfuse
Malnutrition	Iron, folate levels	Increase calories Iron or folate
Haemolysis	Coomb's test, cold agglutinin haptoglobin, LDH, indirect bilirubin, blood smear	Prednisolone Splenectomy Transfuse

Transfusions in the palliative care setting

In the past, for many patients, transfusion therapy represented the extent of palliation. Transfusion of packed red cells remains a very important part of the comprehensive care of palliative care patients. In addition to red cells, platelets and plasma components can also be administered. Advances in the delivery of transfusions in the home setting have expanded greatly the number of patients whose quality of life is improved. Guidelines for transfusion are given in Table 2.

Indications for transfusion of red blood cells[15–19]

Red blood cells provide two important factors to patients: oxygen transport to tissues from the lung is augmented and intravascular volume expansion is provided. Other blood products provide superior means to produce plasma volume expansion and will be discussed later. Red cell concentrates can only provide oxygen carrying capacity.

This discussion will deal exclusively with the provision of red cell concentrates in the chronically anaemic patient. The management of acute haemorrhage will not be dealt with here.

The most important factor in determining the need for red cell transfusion in the patient with chronic anaemia is the presence or absence of symptoms attributable to the anaemia. Patients who have developed their anaemia chronically will tolerate levels of haemoglobin much lower than that tolerated by patients suffering an acute haemorrhage. Therefore, no specific guidelines can be given as to the degree of anaemia which necessitates transfusion. If the patient is symptomatic from dyspnoea, angina, postural hypotension, headache, or peripheral oedema and there are no other medical explanations for these symptoms, the patient should be transfused.

One can anticipate the progression of anaemia in many patients in the palliative care setting. Patients who have marrow failure develop anaemia at the rate of approximately 1 g/dl/week. It is common to transfuse these patients at a rate of three to four units of red cells every 3–4 weeks.

In estimating the number of units required it is convenient to aim for a post-transfusion haemoglobin of 11–12 g/dl. Each unit of packed red cells administered to an adult will result in a rise in haemoglobin concentration of 1 g/dl. In a patient with a haemoglobin of 8 g, a transfusion of three to four units will raise the haemoglobin concentration to 11–12 g/dl.

Three types of complications can be seen with red blood cell transfusion in the palliative care setting; they are: volume overloading, febrile/urticarial reactions, and iron overloading.

Many patients in a palliative care setting have a compromised cardiovascular system which will not tolerate the rapid addition of several hundred

Table 2 Transfusion guidelines

Product	Transfusion trigger	Comments
Red blood cells	Symptoms Hb < 8 g/dl	Watch for fluid overload
Platelet concentrate	Symptoms (no critical no.)	Tranexamic acid may help
Albumin	If diuresis needed	
Frozen plasma	Prothrombin time (PT) International normalized ration (INR) > 5	Vitamin K helpful
Cryoprecipitate	Fibrinogen < 1.0 g/l	L-Deamino-8-D-arginine vasopressin (DDAVP) if von Willebrand's

millilitres of fluid. Each red cell unit provides the equivalent of approximately 450 ml of fluid. Three units therefore have in excess of 1200 ml. Volume overload problems can be avoided by administering a small amount of frusemide (furosemide) (20 mg) with alternate units and by administering the blood slowly. Each unit can be administered over a period of 3–4 h. It is advisable to administer no more than two units per day.

Febrile and urticarial reactions used to occur frequently in patients receiving blood products because of the presence of white blood cells in the transfused product carrying HLA antigens to which the patient has become immunized. Most transfusion services are now providing red cell (and platelet) concentrates that have been subjected to leucodepletion. These leucodepleted products are a significant improvement in transfusion therapy. Most patients do not require premedication with antihistamines or paracetamol (acetaminophen). Occasional patients continue to have febrile reactions to blood products. These patients are likely sensitized to proteins in the plasma. These reactions can be attenuated with an antihistamine such as diphenhydramine (50 mg) or by the use of washed red cells or platelets.

Iron overload is not often a concern in the palliative care setting since it does not become evident until between 50 and 75 units of red cells have been transfused to the patient. Each unit of blood adds 250 mg of iron to the patient's iron stores. Patients with more than 20 g of iron in their stores are at risk for haemosiderosis. Haemosiderosis can cause heart and liver dysfunction or failure of pancreatic endocrine function. The best way to avoid the problem of haemosiderosis is to transfuse red blood cells only when the patient's symptoms demand it. Iron chelation therapy (desferrioxamine) can remove iron from patient stores but is very rarely indicated in the palliative care setting.

Infectious complications of blood transfusion have been minimized by recent improvements in the screening of blood donations. AIDS, hepatitis B, hepatitis C, HTLV-1/2, and syphilis can be screened for and the risk of these infections arising from a blood transfusion prepared in a blood bank with these procedures in place are minimal. In most situations, the benefit of improved quality of life with the transfusion of red blood cells would outweigh the potential risk from infectious complications. Although there is some experimental evidence that transfusion might induce immunosuppression and enhance the growth of neoplasms, this complication of transfusion is not of practical importance in this setting and patients should not be denied the benefit of red cell transfusion because of this theoretical disadvantage. The removal of white cells in the leucodepletion process would also reduce the risk of immunosuppression.

Erythropoietin and other pharmacological agents[13,20–22]

Erythropoietin (Epo), a hormone made in the kidney, stimulates red cell production in the marrow. Its use during chemotherapy treatments has been shown to reduce the need for red cell transfusions and to improve patients' quality of life, in particular in counteracting fatigue. Epo also appears to potentiate radiation effects on the uterine cervix and head and neck cancers. There have been intriguing suggestions in the data from quality of life studies that Epo can counteract deleterious effects of cytokines causing ACD and cachexia–anorexia syndrome and prolong survival.

If Epo were not so expensive, there would be little disagreement over its use during active cancer chemotherapy or radiotherapy but it is only 'cost-effective' compared to transfusions when large litigation costs relating to transfusion liability are factored in.

In the palliative care setting, reduction of fatigue and anaemia symptoms, and the avoidance of transfusions is unlikely to shift the cost equation in favour of routine use of Epo.

Other pharmacological agents sometimes used to control these symptoms include androgens such as danazol or halotestin and modest doses of prednisolone. Little or no scientific data supports their use and hormone-related exacerbation of thrombosis or tumour growth must always be considered.

Transfusion of other blood products

Platelets[23]

Thrombocytopenia may be due to extensive marrow involvement by the neoplasm, immune reactions, DIC, an enlarged spleen, or extensive myelotoxic therapy. Platelet counts of less than 50×10^9/l can be associated with bleeding problems. If the patient has a platelet count of less than 50×10^9/l and is bleeding, transfusion of five units of platelet concentrate may be helpful in curtailing the bleeding for a short period of time. In most patients in the palliative care setting, thrombocytopenia is a chronic problem. Some patients with chronic purpura will have less bleeding with the use of an antifibrinolytic medication such as tranexamic acid (1000 mg, three times daily).

Albumin[24]

Many patients in a palliative care setting are hypoalbuminemic. This is not an indication for the transfusion of albumin. Albumin should be administered only when there is a need for an acute expansion of plasma volume, such as when acute diuresis is necessary. There is no use in transfusing albumin to the patient with chronic hypoalbuminemia for 'nutritional' purposes. In most cases, hypoalbuminemia is a feature of the cachexia–anorexia syndrome (see Chapters 8.4.1 and 8.4.2).

Other plasma components[25]

Fresh plasma and cryoprecipitate should be used only when a specific and documented bleeding diathesis remediable by plasma or cryoprecipitate is present. Examples of this would be the correction of a prolonged prothrombin time due to liver failure or warfarin anticoagulation by frozen plasma or the correction of an abnormal bleeding time due to a deficiency of von Willebrand's factor (vWf) by cryoprecipitate. DDAVP (desmopressin), 20 μg intravenously, is a useful way to raise vWf activity, if required. DDAVP is helpful in reducing the bleeding diathesis, due to diminished vWf, seen in chronic renal failure.

Thrombosis[26–32]

There is a well-known association between cancer and hypercoagulability. Thrombophlebitis is quite common is cancer patients. Hypercoagulability may have preceded the diagnosis of cancer and patients who have cancer-related hypercoagulability have a worse prognosis than those patients whose cancer is not associated with hypercoagulability. There are some types of cancers which appear to have a particular predilection to induce hypercoagulability: prostate, pancreas, breast, and ovary. It is thought that cancer-related thrombosis results from inactivation of the coagulation cascade as well as an inhibition of anticoagulant protein and fibrinolysis.

Another issue related to cancer-related hypercoagulability is whether anticoagulation would prolong survival by 'treating' the underlying malignant disease. Warfarin, heparin, fibrinolytics, and antiplatelet agents disrupt the growth of cancer cells *in vitro* and also impair the metastatic process. Patients treated with chemotherapy and warfarin or low molecular weight heparin (LMWH) seem to have a survival benefit. A practical question for palliative medicine research to resolve is whether anticoagulation extends the lives of patients not receiving chemotherapy or radiation therapy.

Acute deep venous thrombosis

Acute deep venous thrombosis can produce painful swelling of a lower limb, or less commonly, an upper limb. Extension and embolization of these clots can occur if the clotting is present above the popliteal fossae. An important complication is pulmonary embolization. This may contribute to the cause of death in the majority of patients with end-stage cancer. Other patients will have a very painful swelling of the entire limb (phlegmasia cerulea dolens).

The diagnostic and therapeutic approaches have to be individualized to each patient's circumstances. If the decision to treat has been made, the deep venous thrombosis should be documented by venography, plethmysography, or Doppler studies. The presence or absence of pulmonary embolism can be difficult to establish with certainty and routine diagnostic imaging tests available for this condition (such as ventilation perfusion scans) are not very specific. A high-resolution CT scan of the chest is the most specific.

The therapy of acute deep venous thrombosis usually involves the administration of a bolus of 5000 units of heparin followed by a continuous i.v. infusion of 18 units/kg of heparin hourly. Sufficient heparin should be infused to raise the activated partial thromboplastin time (aPTT) to between 60 and 90 s. Oral warfarin should be started at a dose of 5–10 mg and continued daily until the prothrombin time International normalized ratio, (PT INR) is between 2 and 3. Once a therapeutic PT INR is achieved, the heparin can be discontinued and the warfarin continued indefinitely.

The decision to use heparin is often a complex one. Many of these patients have major or minor contraindications to the use of heparin. Major contraindications include active gastrointestinal haemorrhage, active bleeding from some other site, an intracranial neoplasm, and uncontrolled hypertension. Minor contraindications include a past history of gastrointestinal haemorrhage, retinopathy, and the presence of bleeding disorders. It is the author's approach to recommend full anticoagulation in most patients without major contraindications whose prognosis exceeds a few days and who are having significant symptoms from the deep venous thrombosis.

LMWHs, such as dalteparin or enoxaparin, have the dual advantage of requiring much less monitoring than warfarin or whole heparin and being administered by once daily subcutaneous injections. These expensive agents may be useful in the palliative care setting where blood letting should be minimized for patient comfort.

Venocaval filters may prevent pulmonary embolization in patients with recurrent deep venous thrombosis receiving anticoagulant therapy or in patients with major contraindications to anticoagulation but are associated with painful engorgement of both lower limbs.

Chronic venous thrombosis

Patients with neoplastic lesions obstructing veins or with a hypercoagulability related to disseminated malignancy can have chronic venous thrombosis. Two therapeutic approaches are suggested for these patients: chronic warfarin and subcutaneous whole heparin or LMWH.

Chronic warfarin therapy can be administered quite safely if the prothrombin time is monitored closely. The PT INR should be checked every 1–2 weeks after establishment of the initial therapeutic dose. The INR should be kept within 2 to 3. Some patients will have continued thrombosis despite maintenance therapy with coumarins and an INR between 2 and 3. In some of those patients, increasing the warfarin dose so that the INR is between 3 and 4 will be successful in controlling the thrombotic tendency but many of those patients will have bleeding complications. If warfarin therapy has to be reversed rapidly, the administration of three to four units of fresh plasma and 10 mg of vitamin K will bring the PT INR back to baseline rapidly.

In those patients who continue to have thrombotic problems despite warfarin therapy, subcutaneous whole heparin or LMWH should be considered. This approach involves subcutaneous injection of whole heparin twice daily or LMWH once daily. Many patients can self-administer heparin and it does not necessarily involve increased use of medical personnel. An adjusted dose of whole heparin or a standard dose of LMWH should be utilized. For whole heparin, a starting dose of 10 000–15 000 units is given every 12 h and adjusted such that the aPTT is prolonged to approximately 50 s, 6 h after the subcutaneous injection is given. If the patient has been receiving intravenous heparin therapy, the total dose administered over a 24-h period can be used as a guide to selecting the initial subcutaneous dose. Half of the total 24-h dose is administered each 12 h. Standard prophylactic and therapeutic doses for each LMWH are listed in prescribing information sheets.

Trousseau's syndrome is a migratory polyphlebitis affecting superficial veins primarily but also causing venous and arterial clotting. It is seen in patients with disseminated bronchogenic tumours or adenocarcinomas. It can be very bothersome and may not be adequately treated with either warfarin or subcutaneous heparin. Indomethacin at a dose of 25 mg, three to four times daily, is a useful adjunct in these patients, but gastrointestinal side effects must be monitored.

Table 3 Anticoagulation guidelines

Thrombosis issue	Strategy
Acute DVT/PE	Full dose i.v. heparin Warfarin → PT INR 2–3
Chronic DVT	Warfarin → PT INR 2–3 LMWH once daily s.c.
Contraindication to anticoagulation	IVC filter
Cancer hypercoagulability	Warfarin → PT INR 2–3 LMWH (prophylactic dose)
Superficial thrombophlebitis	Aspirin, indomethacin

Guidelines for anticoagulation are given in Table 3. Chronic DIC may be seen in patients with metastatic prostatic carcinoma as well as some other solid tumors and haematological neoplasms.[7,33] Chronic DIC is produced by an activation of the clotting process but the result is the consumption of the components of the clotting system. Thrombocytopenia, hypofibrinogenaemia, and prolongation of the PT INR and aPTT are commonly present. Chronic DIC can lead to troublesome bleeding. Effective therapy is difficult when the underlying neoplasm cannot be eradicated or suppressed in the case of hormone sensitive prostate cancer. If therapeutic measures are to be utilized, emphasis should be placed upon augmenting the fibrinogen levels with cryoprecipitate and transfusing platelets when there is thrombocytopenic bleeding. Heparin is rarely used now.

References

1. **Chiu, T.Y.** et al. (2000). Ethical dilemmas in palliative care: a study in Taiwan. *Journal of Medical Ethics* **26**, 353–7.
2. **Bron, D., Meuleman, N., and Mascaux, C.** (2001). Biologic basis of anemia. *Seminars in Oncology* **28** (2 Suppl. 8), 1–6.
3. **Fuchs, D.** et al. (1994). Inhibitory cytokines in patients with anaemia of chronic disorders. *Annals of the New York Academy of Sciences* **718**, 344–6.
4. **Ershler, W.B. and Keller, E.T.** (2000). Age-associated increased interleuken-6 gene expression late-life diseases and frailty. *Annual Review of Medicine* **51**, 245–70.
5. **Hillman, R.S. and Hershko, C.** (2001). Acute blood loss anemia. In *Williams Hematology* 6th edn. (ed. E. Beutler, M.A. Lichtman, B.S. Coller, and T.J. Kipps), pp. 677–82. New York: McGraw-Hill.
6. **Fairbanks, V.F. and Beutler, E.** (2001). Iron deficiency. In *Williams Hematology* 6th edn. (ed. E. Beutler, M.A. Lichtman, B.S. Coller, and T.J. Kipps), pp. 447–70. New York: McGraw-Hill.
7. **Schwartzberg, L.S. and Holbert, J.M.** (1988). Hemorrhagic and thrombotic abnormalities of cancer. *Critical Care Clinics* **4** (1), 107–28.
8. **Smoller, B.R. and Kruskall, M.S.** (1986). Phlebotomy for diagnostic laboratory tests in adults. Pattern of use and effect on transfusion requirements. *New England Journal of Medicine* **314**, 1233–5.
9. **Erslev, A.J.** (2001). Anaemia associated with marrow failure. In *Williams Hematology* 6th edn. (ed. E. Beutler, M.A. Lichtman, B.S. Coller, and T.J. Kipps), pp. 477–9. New York: McGraw-Hill.
10. **Smith, J.S. and Souba, W.W.** (2001). Nutritional support. In *Cancer, Principles and Practice of Oncology* 6th edn. (ed. V.T. DeVita, Jr., S. Hellman, and S.A. Rosenberg), pp. 3012–31. Philadelphia PA: Lippincott Williams & Wilkins.
11. **Rytting, M., Worth, L., and Joffe, N.** (1996). Hemolytic disorders associated with cancer. *Hematology and Oncology Clinics of North America* **10**, 365–76.

12. **Ruggenenti, P. and Remuzzi, G.** (1991). Thrombotic microangiopathies. *Critical Reviews in Oncology Hematology* **11**, 243–65.
13. **Ludwig, H.** et al. (1994). Prediction of response to erythropoietin treatment in chronic anaemia of cancer. *Blood* **84**, 1056–63.
14. **Weatherall, D.J.** (2001). The thalassemias. In *Williams Hematology* 6th edn. (ed. E. Beutler, M.A. Lichtman, B.S. Coller, and T.J. Kipps), pp. 547–80. New York: McGraw-Hill.
15. **Menitove, J.E.** (1999). Red cell transfusion therapy in chronic anemia. In *Transfusion Therapy: Clinical Principles and Practice* 6th edn. (ed. P.D. Muntz), pp. 1–12. Bethesda MD: AABB Press.
16. **Office of Medical Applications of Research** (1988). National Institute of Health Consensus Development Conference on Red Blood Cell Transfusion. Perioperative red blood cell transfusion. *Journal of the American Medical Association* **260**, 2700–3.
17. **Vanvakas, E.C. and Blajchman, M.A.** (2001). Universal WBC reduction: the case for and against. *Transfusion* **41**, 691–712.
18. **Gabutti, V. and Borgna-Pignatti, C.** (1994). Clinical manifestations and therapy of transfusional haemosiderosis. *Bailliere's Clinical Haematology* **7**, 919–40.
19. **Jinger, Y. and Shvartzman, P.** (1998). The feasibility and advisability of administering home blood transfusions to the terminally ill patient. *Journal of Palliative Care* **14**, 46–8.
20. **Cella, D.** (1998). Factors influencing quality of life in cancer patients: anemia and fatigue. *Seminars in Oncology* **25**, 43–6.
21. **Turner, R.** et al. (2001). Erythropoietin alfa in cancer patients: Evidence-based guidelines. *Journal of Pain and Symptom Management* **22**, 954–65.
22. **Littlewood, T.J.** et al. (2000). Possible relationship of hemoglobin levels with survival in anemic patients receiving chemotherapy. *Proceedings of ASCO* **19**, 605a.
23. **Strauss, R.G.** (1995) Clinical perspectives of platelet transfusion: defining the optimal dose. *Journal of Clinical Apheresis* **10**, 124–7.
24. **Sub-committee of the Victorian Drug Usage Advisory Committee** (1992). Human albumin solutions: consensus statements for use in selected clinical situations. *Medical Journal of Australia* **157**, 340–3.
25. **Maltz, G.S., Siegel, J.E., and Carson, J.L.** (2000). Hematologic management of gastrointestinal bleeding. *Gastroenterology Clinics of North America* **29**, 169–87.
26. **Letai, A. and Kuter, D.J.** (1999). Cancer, coagulation and anticoagulation. *Oncologist* **4**, 443–9.
27. **Falonga, A. and Donati, M.B.** (2001). Pathogenesis of thrombosis in patients with malignancy. *International Journal of Hematology* **73**, 137–44.
28. **Raskob, G.E., Hull, R.D., and Pineo, G.F.** (2001). Venous thrombosis. In *Williams Hematology* 6th edn. (ed. E. Beutler, M.A. Lichtman, B.S. Coller, and T.J. Kipps), pp. 1735–42. New York: McGraw-Hill.
29. **Kakkar, A.K. and Williamson, R.C.** (1999). Prevention of venous thromboembolism in cancer patients. *Seminars in Thrombosis and Hemostasis* **25**, 239–43.
30. **Sorensen, H.T.** et al. (2000). Prognosis of cancer associated with venous thromboembolism. *New England Journal of Medicine* **343**, 1846–50.
31. **Bona, R.D., Hickey, A.D., and Wallace, D.M.** (1997). Efficacy and safety of oral anticoagulation in patients with cancer. *Thrombosis and Haemostasis* **78**, 137–46.
32. **Breddin, H.R.** et al. (2001) for the CORTES Investigators. Effects of a low-molecular weight heparin on thrombus regression and recurrent thromboembolism in patients with deep-vein thrombosis. *New England Journal of Medicine* **344**, 626–31.
33. **Colman, R.W. and Rubin, R.N.** (1990). Disseminated intravascular coagulation due to malignancy. *Seminars in Oncology* **17**, 172–86.

8.7 Pruritus and sweating in palliative medicine

Mark R. Pittelkow and Charles L. Loprinzi

Introduction

Itching (pruritus) and sweating (perspiration, diaphoresis) are physiological functions of the skin that normally serve human existence well. Itching is the sensory input arising from the skin and mucous membranes that alerts man to potentially harmful insults from physical, chemical, and biological sources. The reflex of scratching is closely linked to the perception of itch, and in most situations functions effectively as an aversive motor response to relieve the sensation and protect the skin. Similarly, sweating is a well-developed and finely coordinated sudomotor response designed to regulate body temperature and prevent hyperthermia.

However, both pruritus and sweating have the potential to function aberrantly and develop into pathological conditions that create significant suffering and morbidity. Since these skin responses encompass both normal and abnormal functions, effective treatments to alleviate or eliminate the pathological component are challenging. In this chapter we provide a practical overview of the normal function and pathophysiology of pruritus and sweating, and offer a variety of therapeutic options and general comforting measures for patients experiencing these maladies.

Pruritus

Terminology

Itch and pruritus are terms used to described both physiological and pathological sensory perception. Itch is a distinctive and common cutaneous sensation that arises from the superficial layers of the skin and mucous membranes. It is often fleeting, and the sensation may pass relatively unnoticed since the reflex action of scratching is largely involuntary and typically relieves the temporary discomfort.

Itch (itching, itchy, or itchiness) and pruritus (from the Latin *prurire*, to itch) are generally considered to have equivalent meanings. Itch and related descriptions such as 'terrible itching' are terms commonly used by the patient to convey this distinctive symptom. However, subtle differences in the terminology of itch and pruritus have evolved in the medical literature. In this respect, the terms itch and pruritus have been used to characterize the spectrum of unique cutaneous sensations ranging from the physiological response to severe pathological symptoms.[1–5] Physiological itch is the short-lived cutaneous response to the usual events of living, while pruritus is more closely associated with pathological itch.[1,2] Use of the term pruritus represents the symptomatic level or quality of itch that is defined as an intense cutaneous discomfort occurring with pathological change in the skin or body and eliciting vigorous scratching.

The definition of pruritus or itch is subjective and not entirely precise. Although the general sensation is well known and implicitly understood, many patients with more severe symptoms assimilate itch with various other discomforting or unpleasant sensation. The term itch frequently encompasses a range of descriptive or qualifying terms such as tickle, prickle, pins and needles, burning, stinging, chafed, raw, aching, and even 'painful' sensations.[2]

To avoid confusion and to focus on the palliative medicine perspective, the terms itch and pruritus are used interchangeably to describe this pathological symptom. Patients experiencing pruritus may develop this symptom only mildly and transiently, or itching may be so severe and unrelenting that it preoccupies and completely disrupts their daily existence. It must be recognized that itch or pruritus is variable in its perceived quality and intensity. As with pain, the perception and tolerance of pruritus and the response to this sensation depends significantly on the individual's physical and emotional states, the functional level of activity, adaptive coping mechanisms, and the overall outlook. Attempts to develop questionnaires that assess severity of pruritus have been developed based on modified pain questionnaires.[6] These quantitative measuring tools will be useful to better standardize symptoms and treatment responses.

Anatomy and physiology

Pruritus is a discrete sensation and a primary sensory modality arising from the activation and integration of cutaneous sensory neural receptors, afferent pathways, and central nervous system processing centres[7] (Fig. 1). In the past itch was considered to be a low-threshold form or submodality of pain based on various clinical and experimental observations. Both pain and itch are induced by noxious stimuli and therefore are designated 'nociceptive'.

A prevailing theory was that itch and pain were related sensations that differed only in the strength of the stimulus, with itch being a response to a weak stimulus and pain being elicited by a stronger stimulus. Further investigation of pain and pruritus not only revealed similarities but also clearly demonstrated the distinctive differences between these two sensations. Recent research has conclusively demonstrated that itch and pain are represented by distinct nerve fibres. Itch neurons are specific type C fibres in skin, each having a wide innervation territory, thin axon, and very low conduction velocity.[8] The central neural pathway for itch has also been recently localized to spinothalamic lamina I neurons that are selectively sensitive to histamine.[9]

Many definitions of pruritus specifically include the reflex action of scratching. Scratching illustrates the distinctive sensation of pruritus, and the scratching reflex is routinely elicited and intimately coupled to itch. Scratching is regarded as a protective reflex, much as withdrawal (flexion) and guarding are comparable reflexes in response to painful stimuli.

Pruritogenic stimuli

Pruritus is induced in skin by various stimuli. Both exogenous and endogenous factors have the capacity to elicit itch.[10,11] Most experimental and spontaneous triggering factors are mediated via the exogenous or external route. Cutaneous sensory nerves which convey the pruritic signal become activated through the application of either physical or chemical stimuli to the skin (Fig. 2). Many physical stimuli induce pruritus, including pressure, thermal stimulation, low-intensity electrical stimulation, formation of suction blisters, and epicutaneous application of caustic substances.

Chemical stimuli include histamine, proteases, prostaglandins, and neuropeptides.[7] Delivery of histamine to the upper layers of skin by injection or iontophoresis has been a quantitative and reproducible method of examining pruritus experimentally. Histamine is also secreted in skin by mast cells. It acts directly on free nerve endings in skin.

Proteases such as trypsin, chymotrypsin, papain, and kallikrein have the ability to induce pruritus when injected into skin. For example, the spicules of the plant cowage (*Mucuna pruriens*) contain an endopeptidase. These fine spicules are an active ingredient of itching powder and induce an itching sensation when they penetrate into the epidermal layers or dermoepidermal junction of skin. Other natural proteases produced in cells and tissues of the body or by microorganisms such as bacterial or fungal microflora of the skin also have the potential to induce pruritus.

Mediators of pruritus

The nerve fibres that conduct signals representing itch are located predominantly at the epidermal–dermal junction and have free endings extending into the epidermis.[10] Many of these nerve fibres contain neuropeptides such as substance P, neurokinin A, and calcitonin gene-related peptide (CGRP) (Fig. 2). Other neuropeptides contained in nerves deeper in the dermis and located around blood vessels include vasoactive intestinal peptide (VIP) and neuropeptide Y. Substance P, which is the best-characterized pruritogenic neuropeptide, is a sensory transmitter of nociception. It is localized to sensory nerve endings in the skin and is abundant in the prevertebral ganglia, the dorsal roots of the spinal cord, and the brain. Administration of substance P intrathecally causes intense scratching that can be blocked by an antagonist. Nerve fibres containing substance P appear to transmit direct synaptic sensory impulses for the itch sensation.

Capsaicin, an alkaloid derived from the common pepper plant, is a well-known stimulant of erythema and pain when applied to mucous membrane or skin. It depletes substance P from the sensory nerves and excites the type C polymodal nerve fibres conveying pain. However, after initial stimulation, capsaicin blocks C fibre conduction and mediates neuronal toxicity which eventually decreases fibre density. These activities of capsaicin have stimulated the use of this agent for the treatment of pruritus.[12]

Neuromediators directly influence vascular permeability and erythema (Fig. 2). They also activate release of other mediators such as interleukins, prostaglandins, bradykinin, serotonin, and histamine from infiltrating

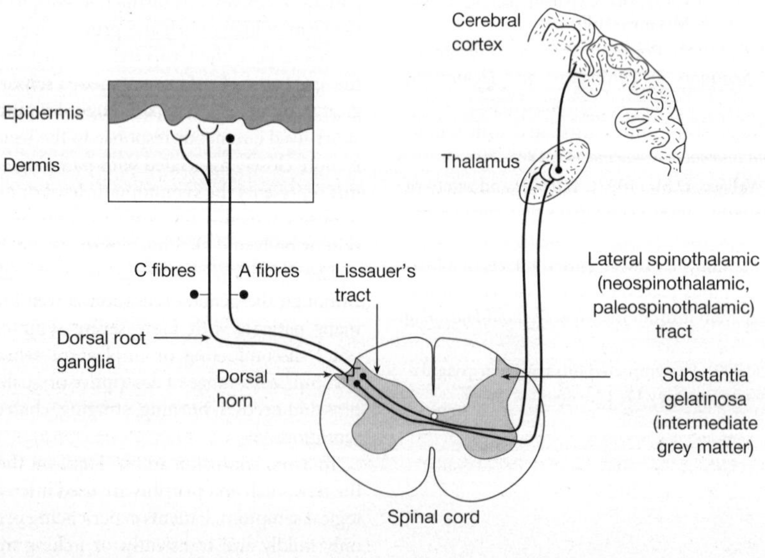

Fig. 1 Pathway for transmission of itch sensation. The C fibres terminate in substantia gelatinosa. Spinothalamic relay axons cross and ascend contralaterally at the spinal level of entering sensory neurones. Larger-diameter A fibres and other interneuronal and central pathways may modulate signalling information. (Modified with permission from refs 2 and 10.)

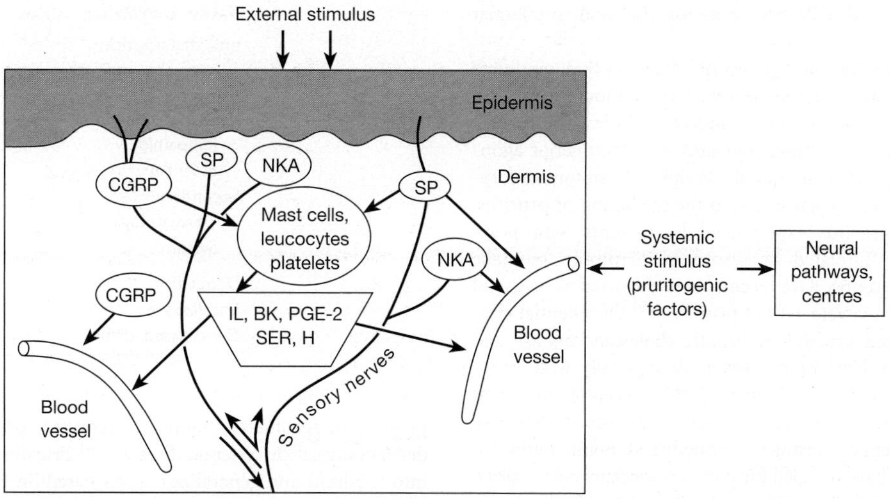

Fig. 2 Stimuli of itch in skin or at peripheral and central neural sites. External or endogenous (systemic) routes of activation trigger nerve fibre stimulation in the skin and the release of neuropeptides including substance P (SP), neurokinin A (NKA), and calcitonin gene-related peptide (CGRP). These mediators trigger inflammatory cells in the skin to release histamine (H), bradykinins (BK), serotonin (S), interleukins (IL), and prostaglandin E_2 (PGE-2). Vascular permeability, inflammatory cell infiltration, and nerve stimulation are evoked by stimuli. (Modified with permission from ref. 10.)

leucocytes and tissue-localized mast cells. Together, these neural and cellular mediators induce the sensation of itch, augment local activation of inflammatory responses that often accompany itch, and create areas of hyper-responsiveness around the primary stimulus zone for itch. For example, the phenomenon of 'itchy skin' (alloknesis) may be due to regional hyper-responsiveness as well as a lowering of the threshold to itch stimuli at the level of the spinal cord. Additionally, neuromediator release is probably augmented through antidromic nerve stimulation.

Cutaneous neural input

Human skin is supplied principally by nerve fibre networks composed of A and D myelinated fibres and thin type C unmyelinated fibres. Afferent type C fibres include C mechanoreceptors, cold thermoreceptors, C polymodal, and C itch nociceptors. Itch is primarily conveyed by the C itch fibres which represent approximately 15–20 per cent of unmyelinated nerve fibres in skin. The remaining polymodal C fibres constitute about 80 per cent of all afferent C fibres (Fig. 1). The exact location and unique identity of the itch receptor is unknown, but it is likely resides in free nerve endings.

Itch, therefore, is separate from the slow, aching, dull, or burning pain that is conducted by type C polymodal fibres.[(13,14)] Myelinated A delta nociceptors conveying sharp pain also have been identified. Physiological and pharmacological studies have shown that separate independent sensory channels conduct itch and pain stimuli. The latency between stimulation and onset of the sensation of pain coincides with the relatively low rates of conduction (2 m/s) by the neurones that serve these sensory functions. Itch fibres have very slow velocities of 0.5–0.7 m/s.[(8,9)] Some investigators have suggested separating 'itch' into the 'pricking' sensation carried by myelinated fibres and the 'burning' sensation conveyed by unmyelinated fibres. This classification of sensations correlates with the two different systems of sensation described by Head[(15)] in 1905 as the epicritic or specific well-defined sensation that mediates spontaneous itch and the protopathic or diffuse poorly localized sensation that conveys the perception of itchy skin. On the basis of current scientific knowledge pain and itch are largely separable cutaneous sensations. However, there is evidence of secondary neuron interactions with 'itch-specific' fibres being suppressed by coactivation of pain nociceptors using agents such as capsaicin.

In addition to the external or exogenous pathway for initiation of the itch sensation, there is considerable clinical evidence for the endogenous activation of pruritus.[(1–5)] (Fig. 2). The endogenous route for stimulation of pruritus represents a major and clinically relevant pathway; however, it is poorly understood. The potential sites of stimulation (the peripheral nervous system, the spinal cord, and/or the central nervous system), the inciting agents and mediators, and the relative overlap of exogenous versus endogenous activation pathways remain to be clearly delineated and applied effectively in the clinical setting. The systemic or endogenous stimuli for itch have been only partially characterized, and the biochemical causes for pruritus associated with a spectrum of systemic illnesses, including metabolic disease, organ failure, and various malignancies, continue to be ill-defined and vexing problems.

Several substances have been shown to mediate different or opposing effects on itch when tested experimentally. Their activities depend on the route of administration and their specific responses at the peripheral, spinal cord, and/or central nervous system levels. These observations support the concept of itch as a neural message that is interpreted in the context of signal reception, transmission, and modulation at each level of the nervous system.

Opioid and serotonergic mediators

Opioids are one example of substances that exert separate and potentially disparate responses in modulating the transmission and perception of itch and pain at different levels of the nervous system.[(2,16)] Uncovering the existence of central opioid receptors led to the discovery of encephalins, endogenous pentapeptides that bind to these receptors. Opioids are powerful analgesics that mimic the effects of encephalins. However, opioids mediate both excitatory and modulatory effects on pruritus at several levels. At the spinal level, encephalins released from short spinal interneurones and opioids stimulate an inhibitory presynaptic signal transmitted to primary afferents that modulates secondary transmission of itch. However, within some regions of the central nervous system, opioids directly trigger itch. Clinically, intrathecal or epideral morphine has been known to induce localized or generalized itching. At the peripheral level within skin, opioids stimulate mast cell degranulation and release of histamine which produces itch. Furthermore, based on the recent identification and characterization of itch-specific primary nerve fibres, opioids may induce itching by blocking the painful stimuli that suppress activity of central itch neurons.

Central activation of itch by opioids appears to play a dominant role in some diseases, since opioid antagonists have been shown to exert significant antipruritic effects.[(16,17)] The parenterally administered opioid antagonist naloxone inhibits induction of itch following histamine injection of skin. Pruritus of cholestatic liver disease (primary or secondary biliary cirrhosis) can be dramatically reduced with naloxone or the oral antagonist nalmephene.[7,18]

Serotonergic compounds are another group of agents that modulate effects on pruritus primarily at the peripheral level, although receptors for serotonin are present in the peripheral and central nervous systems. Cutaneous injection but not intravenous infusion of a serotonergic agonist increases the scratching reflex in animals. Peripheral serotonin receptors in humans are presumed to play a role in the mediation of pruritus. Temperature-dependent pruritus experienced by patients with polycythaemia vera may be stimulated by serotonin. Serotonin reuptake inhibitors, specifically paroxetine, have recently been reported to be useful for treatment of polycythemia vera-related pruritus.[19] Of potential clinical significance, generalized pruritus of hepatic cholestatic disease and chronic renal insufficiency have been relieved dramatically with intravenous administration of the type 3 serotonin ($5\text{-}HT_3$) receptor antagonist ondansetron.[20,21] However, other recent placebo-controlled studies have refuted this finding in uraemic pruritus.[22] Nonetheless, opioid and serotonin receptor antagonists have revealed the complex mechanisms involved in transmitting signals for pruritus at the peripheral and central nervous system levels.

Pathogenic correlates in management of pruritus

The similarity of the symptoms of exogenous and endogenous forms of pruritus has prompted empirical use of similar treatment measures for both types of conditions. Frequently, however, effective therapy for pruritus caused by one condition is not particularly beneficial for pruritis of another cause. Also, treatments that ameliorate or relieve pruritus induced by exogenous agents have limited or minimal effects on alleviating pruritus of endogenous cause. This is probably related to the site and mode of activity of these treatments and their limitations in targeting the receptors, mediators, or central neural pathways that control expression of endogenous versus exogenous pruritus.

The nuclei of the afferent C itch and polymodal nerves reside in the dorsal root ganglia and axon extensions that synapse in the dorsal horn of the substantia gelatinosa (Fig. 1). Secondary neurones cross the spinal cord to the contralateral spinothalamic tract of the venterolateral quadrant before ascending to the thalamus. Lamina I of the spinothalamic tract contains type C itch fibres.[9] There is also evidence in animals that pathways in addition to the anterolateral system can transmit pruritogenic stimuli. Both the ventral posterior inferior nucleus and the ventral periphery of the ventral posterior lateral nucleus of the thalamus contain itch fibres projecting from lamina I.[9] The synaptic neurones within the thalamus project to the somatosensory cortex of the postcentral gyrus. Scratching is the spinal reflex in response to itching but also has input from higher neural centres.

Perception of itch has the potential to be modulated at the level of the spinal cord and, probably at other levels, by additional neural input as described for pain by Melzak and Wall.[23] The description of 'a gate control system that modulates sensory input from the skin before it evokes pain perception' can also be applied to the perception of itch.

A fibre impulse conduction is self-regulated by a negative feedback pathway that tends to dampen continued firing. It also interrupts summation of sensations of itch and pain conveyed by the C itch and polymodal fibres. The 'gate' has the ability to control neural transmission. Gate closure is envisaged to produce inhibition at the spinal cord level such that stimulation of A fibres by scratching would induce or enhance inhibition of conduction. Although the gate-control theory has been intensively evaluated and revised over the past three decades and its operational functionality has been challenged, practical application based on this theory appears to have been made in the control of pain and itch using transcutaneous electrical nerve stimulation.[24,25]

Clinical evaluation and treatment of pruritus

The clinical approach to pruritus can present a considerable diagnostic as well as therapeutic challenge. To formulate a simple clinical strategy for diagnosis and treatment of pruritus, pathological itch can be classified as primary or secondary (Table 1). Secondary pruritus is caused by either dermatological or systemic disease.[1–4] Pruritus can be further separated into localized and generalized forms based on the location and extent of body surface involvement. In most cases, localized pruritus is due to cutaneous infections or other regionalized expressions of dermatological disease.

Table 1 Pruritus: causes and distribution

Aetiology
Primary
Idiopathic
Essential
Secondary
Dermatological
Systemic
Distribution
Localized
Generalized, diffuse

Generalized or diffuse pruritus typically presents more troublesome symptoms for the patient and a greater challenge for the physician. Diffuse pruritus is usually related to a dermatological or systemic disorder affecting the entire skin surface. However, even pruritus which is generalized or diffuse exhibits symptoms that may be accentuated and localized to certain regions of the body, and these symptoms may fluctuate, migrate, or extend over time.

Primary pruritus

Primary or idiopathic pruritus is identified in the majority (more than 70 per cent) of patients where dermatological disease (secondary pruritus) has been excluded as a cause for itching.[26] Idiopathic pruritus may be fairly limited in extent and intensity. Symptoms can be reasonably controlled by conscientious skin care and topical soothing measures. However, other cases of primary pruritus prove to be quite extensive, severe, and chronic. The diagnosis of primary pruritus is established following a thorough medical and dermatological evaluation to exclude secondary causes of itching.

Evaluation and management of idiopathic pruritus is frequently a frustrating experience for the patient and physician as possible causes and beneficial treatments are sought. When no clear aetiology is delineated, both the patient and physician may experience disappointment. With severe idiopathic pruritus, there is also lingering uncertainty whether an occult disease, particularly malignancy, may eventually be uncovered. However, several clinical studies have shown that only a small percentage of patients referred to dermatologists for generalized pruritus will develop a malignancy during follow-up evaluation.[26,27] The majority manifest haematological malignancies, particularly lymphomas, and therefore periodic clinical surveillance is warranted. However, the duration and severity of chronic primary pruritus may be sufficiently debilitating for palliative intervention and the identification of effective therapies to become the principal goals.

Secondary pruritus—dermatological

Secondary pruritus is associated with a variety of disorders including both dermatological and systemic diseases (Tables 2 and 3). For example, contact dermatitis is a common characteristic skin disease that has itching and scratching as its hallmarks. Table 2 lists the major dermatological entities that are accompanied by pruritus. Some disorders, such as scabies, insect bites, folliculitis, and allergic contact dermatitis, are caused by exogenous agents that elicit pruritus. Other conditions, including atopic dermatitis, bullous pemphigoid, lichen planus, psoriasis, and urticaria, are endogenously mediated inflammatory skin conditions that exhibit variably intense symptoms of pruritus.

The mechanisms that induce itching have been partially characterized for some of these disorders. Specific inflammatory cell types, such as mast cells, lymphocytes, and eosinophils, play important roles in the pathogenesis of specific diseases and the development of pruritus. Neuropeptides, cytokines, and proteases, among other mediators, are the main cellular products initiating pruritus (Fig. 3). These mediators probably act in addition to specific neurotransmitters which directly convey a pruritogenic signal to the itch receptor. Treatment of the specific skin condition and elimination of any offending exogenous agent(s) typically alleviate the symptoms of pruritus. When dealing with pruritus which may be skin related, it is crucial to identify and classify any primary skin lesions and obtain appropriate skin sample specimens or skin biopsies. This information

Table 2 Skin diseases associated with pruritus

Aquagenic pruritus
Atopic dermatitis (eczema)
Bullous pemphigoid
Contact dermatitis
Cutaneous T-cell lymphoma (mycosis fungoides, Sézary's syndrome)
Dermatitis herpetiformis
Drugs (dermatitis medicamentosa)
Folliculitis
Graver's disease
Insect bites
Lichen planus
Lichen simplex chronicus
Mastocytosis
Miliaria
Pediculosis
Pityriasis rosea
Prurigo
Prurigo nodularis
Pruritus ani and vulvae
Psoriasis
Scabies
Sunburn
Systemic parasitic infection (onchocerciasis, trichinosis, echinococcosis)
Urticaria, dermographism
Xerosis

Table 3 Systemic disorders associated with pruritus

Biliary and hepatic disease Biliary atresia Primary biliary cirrhosis Sclerosing cholangitis Extrahepatic biliary obstruction Cholestasis of pregnancy Drug-induced cholestasis
Chronic renal failure—uraemia
Drugs Opioids Amphetamines Cocaine Acetylsalicylic acid Quinidine Niacinamide Etretinate Other medications Subclinical drug sensitivity
Endocrine diseases Diabetes insipidus Diabetes mellitus Parathyroid disease Thyroid disease (hypothyroidism, thyrotoxicosis)
Haematopoietic diseases Hodgkin's and non-Hodgkin's lymphoma Cutaneous T-cell lymphoma (mycosis fungoides, Sézary's syndrome) Systemic mastocytosis Multiple myeloma Polycythaemia vera Iron-deficiency anaemia
Infectious diseases Syphilis Parasitic HIV Fungal
Malignancy Breast, stomach, lung, etc. Carcinoid syndrome
Neurological disorders Distal small-fibre neuropathy Stroke Multiple sclerosis Tabes dorsalis Brain abscess/tumours Psychosis, psychogenic causes Delusions of parasitosis

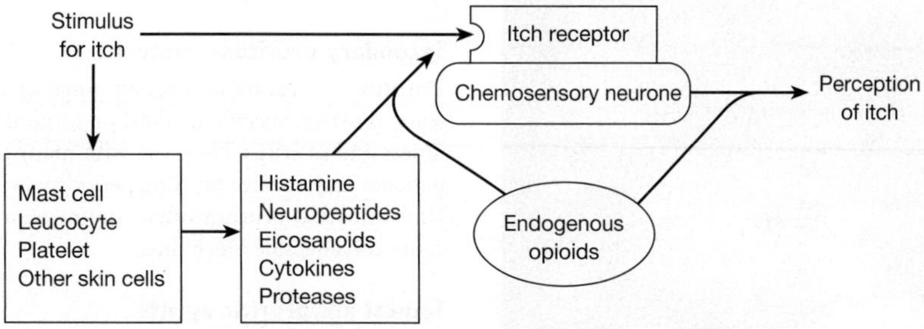

Fig. 3 Factors mediating itch: direct or indirect activation of itch receptor by specific pruritogens. The itch signal is transmitted to a chemosensory neurone which is activated and conveys perception centrally in the nervous sytem. Endogenous opioids, among other factors, modulate pruritogenic signals. (Modified with permission from ref. 2.)

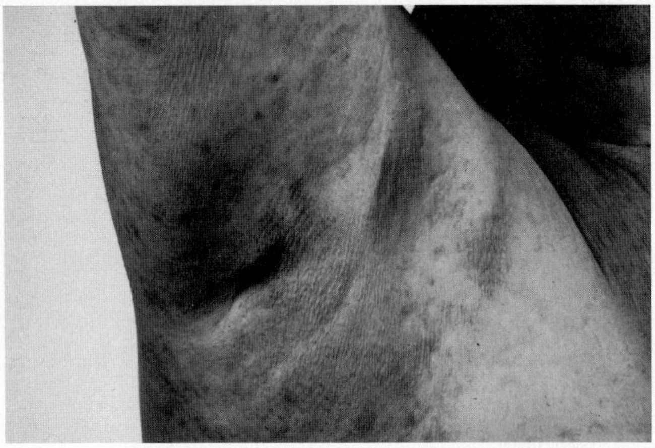

Fig. 4 Scabies: erythematous papules, crusts, and excoriations. Mite burrows can be identified under magnification.

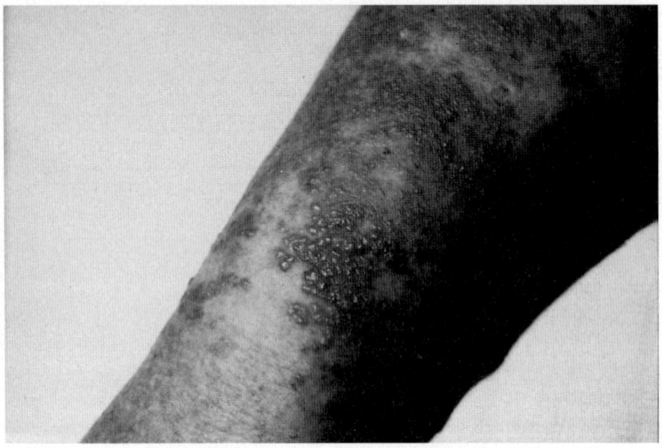

Fig. 5 Acute dermatitis: erythema, scaling, and blister formation due to allergy after application of triple antibiotic ointment containing neomycin.

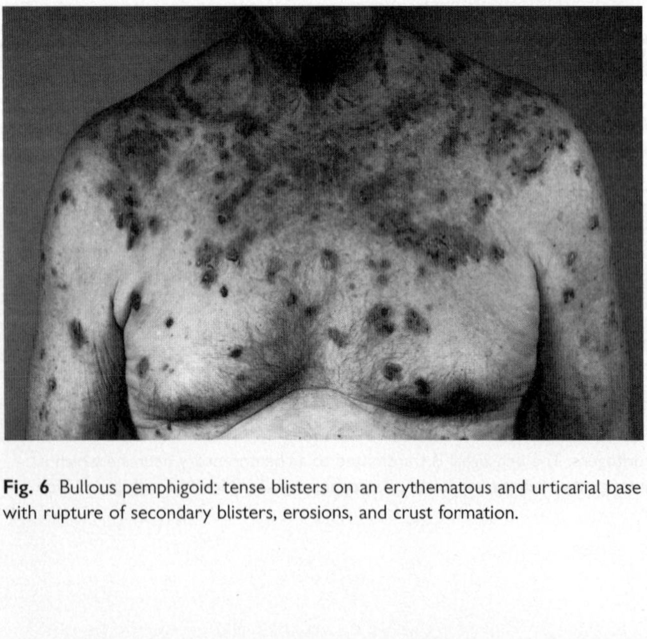

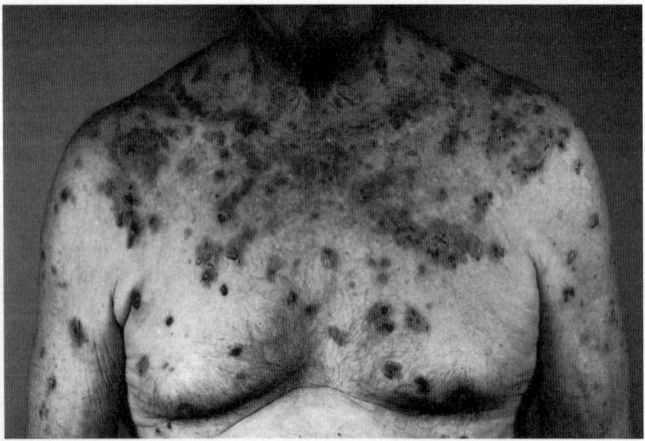

Fig. 6 Bullous pemphigoid: tense blisters on an erythematous and urticarial base with rupture of secondary blisters, erosions, and crust formation.

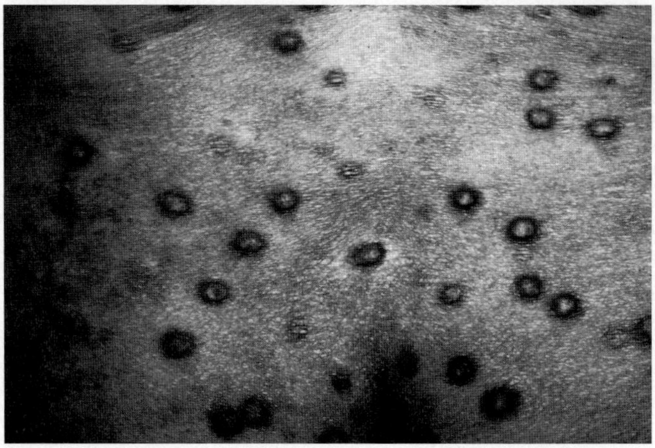

Fig. 7 Prurigo nodularis: discrete firm pruritic globular nodules over the sacral area which often have a verrucous crust and an excoriated surface.

is often very helpful in establishing a diagnosis. The correct diagnosis and appropriate therapy for dermatological disorders should be sought through specialist consultation and is well described in standard dermatology textbooks.

Cutaneous diseases which cause pruritus should not be overlooked. For example, unrelenting pruritus caused by scabies infestation, sometimes lasting for months to years, has been mistakenly attributed to concurrent malignancy (Fig. 4). Other cutaneous infections, irritant or allergic contact dermatitis (Fig. 5), or autoimmune blistering diseases such as bullous pemphigoid (Fig. 6) have been repeatedly observed to develop during the course of malignancies or other systemic illnesses. By recognizing that pruritus is due to a supervening dermatological condition, prompt and appropriate treatment can be instituted and the skin disease and pruritus both resolve. Therefore the periodic evaluation and re-evaluation of the causes of idiopathic or poorly controlled pruritus may uncover new information that will significantly benefit total patient care and improve overall comfort.

Some dermatological conditions provide instructive lessons on the aetiology and limitations of managing pruritus. For example, prurigo nodularis is a distinctive pruritic dermatosis that can be chronic and is often recalcitrant to therapy.[28] The symptom of pruritus appears to play a more central role in the pathogenesis and propagation of this disease. The pruritus of prurigo nodularis largely localizes to the nodular lesions that appear to develop and become more prominent as a result of scratching (Fig. 7). Cutaneous nerve elements are accentuated within the lesions and are often difficult to block effectively or eliminate. These factors probably account for the refractory nature of the condition to various treatments. Clinical and therapeutic observations on prurigo nodularis potentially have aetiological and practical relevance to non-dermatological disorders that are associated with pruritus since some of these conditions may also be quite refractory to many therapeutic measures directed at alleviating the itch.

Secondary pruritus—systemic

Pruritus is a feature of a broad range of systemic diseases (Table 3). For some diseases, specific medical or surgical treatment provides cure of the illness and pruritus. However, with many of the chronic systemic diseases, patients may survive for long periods with adequate control of the illness. Unfortunately, pruritus often continues to be a major symptom and may cause considerable morbidity.

Topical antipruritic agents

A variety of topical medications have been developed through the years to provide symptomatic relief of itching.[29,30] Many of the active ingredients have long been known to ease the symptoms of itch. A list of the common therapeutic antipruritic lotions, creams, and gels, together with their active

Table 4 Topical antipruritic agents

Preparation	Active ingredient
Dodd's lotion	Phenol, glycerine, zinc oxide
Lerner's lotion	Ethyl alcohol, glycerine, zinc oxide
Pamscol	Phenol, acetylsalicylic acid
Sarna	Menthol, camphor, phenol
Schamberg's lotion	Menthol, phenol, zinc oxide
Topic gel	Benzl alcohol, ethyl alcohol, methol, phenol
Wibi lotion	Menthol
Crude coal tar 3%–10% solution	Crude coal tar
Caladryl	Diphenhydramine, calamine, camphor
Pramosone, Prax	Pramoxine
Quotane	Dimethisoquin
EMLA	Lignocaine, prilocaine
Lignocaine patch	Lignocaine
Zonalon	Doxepin
Zostrix	Capsaicin

Modified from ref. 30.

Table 5 Pruritus therapies

Anti-inflammatory agents
- Corticosteroids
- H_1, H_2, H_3 blocking agents
- Salicylates
- Cromolyn
- Thalidomide

Vasoactive drugs
- α-Blockers
- β-Blockers (e.g. propranolol)

Central and peripheral nervous system agents
- Anaesthetic agents
  - Lignocaine etc.
  - Propofol
- Antidepressant agents (tricyclic, SSRI[34])
  - Neuroleptic agents
  - Tranquillizing agents
  - Sedatives
  - Opioid antagonists (naloxone, naltrexone, nalmephene)
  - Serotonin antagonists (ondestranon)

Sequestrants
- Cholestyramine
- Charcoal
- Heparin (IV)

Miscellaneous
- Disease-specific drugs and therapies
  - Cholestatic disease[35]: rifampicin, methyltestosterone ursodeoxycholic acid, partial external biliary diversion[30,36–38]
  - Uraemia: erythropoietin, parathyroidectomy, ultraviolet B phototherapy[39–41]
  - Polycythaemia vera: α-interferon,[42] paroxetine[19]
  - Neurofibromatosis (neurofibroma): ketotifen[43]
- Phototherapy: ultraviolet A, ultraviolet B, photochemotherapy (PUVA)[30,41]

Transcutaneous nerve stimulation[24,25]

Plasma exchange, apheresis[30]

Acupuncture[30]

Psychotherapy, biofeedback, relaxation techniques[30]

ingredients, is given in Table 4. Topical medications are not convenient to apply to the entire body surface on a routine basis, but even patients with more generalized pruritus often have localized areas of accentuated itching that are more troublesome to control. Therefore topical agents have a role in treating both regionalized accentuation of generalized pruritus and localized itching.

Phenol in dilute solution (0.5–2 per cent) alleviates pruritus by anaesthetizing cutaneous nerve endings. Phenol is potentially neurotoxic and hepatotoxic, and should be avoided in pregnancy and in infants under 1 year of age. Menthol and camphor relieve itching by counter-irritant and anaesthetic properties. Menthol (typically 0.25–2 per cent, but can be as high as 16 per cent) produces a cool sensation, and camphor (typically 1–3 per cent, but can be as high as 9 per cent) exerts similar effects. Zinc oxide, coal tars, calamine, glycerine, and salicylates also have been used in many preparations with reported benefit, although their specific modes of action have not been elucidated.

Pramoxine hydrochloride is a topical anaesthetic similar to dyclonine that has been used as the sole ingredient or has been compounded with hydrocortisone or menthol and is available as an aerosol, foam, cream, gel, or lotion. Newer anaesthetic prescription medications include EMLA cream, a combination of the caine drugs lignocaine (lidocaine) and prilocaine which are absorbed transcutaneously and produce anaesthesia as well as abolish itch. Lignocaine patches (Lidoderm) are also available that can be applied to problematic pruritic areas.[31] Doxepin has been demonstrated to be effective in relieving the itch of skin disease and may be useful for pruritus of various aetiologies. Capsaicin has been reported to be effective in localized neurogenic pruritus of various causes and has demonstrated benefit in other conditions accompanied by itch. Initial applications of the medication produce burning sensations and other discomfort. The patient must be alerted to these sensations and coaxed to continue if sustained use is planned and benefit is to be obtained.

Systemic therapies and other treatments

A plethora of systemic medications and various other modalities have been used in the treatment of pruritus.[1,4,5,30,32,33] These agents are organized and listed in Table 5 according to their standard pharmacological activities. On examining this list, it becomes apparent that no drug has ever been successfully developed, tested, and produced exclusively or even primarily for pruritus. This fact alone reveals the potential difficulties that are encountered in the pharmacological treatment of chronic and severe cases of pruritus. All too frequently, patients requiring palliative relief from intractable itching are subjected to trials of various medicines in an attempt to discover which one 'works best' for them. With persistence and luck, a particular drug or modality can be identified that offers benefit and has tolerable side-effects. Combinations of systemic and topical agents often seem to provide the best relief. Clinical experience has also shown that certain medications or treatment modalities seem to provide more consistent benefit for specific types of secondary pruritus, as is the case for ultraviolet B (UVB) phototherapy and the pruritus of chronic renal failure. Unfortunately, few controlled clinical studies have ever been conducted on the palliative management of pruritus, and a well-developed and simple clinical management strategy does not exist. Therefore, as outlined above, the practical aspects of establishing the probable cause(s), selecting a treatment, and assessing its benefit, side-effects, and potential risks must all be addressed routinely as part of the process of providing palliative care for the patient with pruritus. In addition, several simple measures can be adopted to give patients and their skin some relief from the anguish of itching and the injury of scratching.

Pruritus of malignancy

Itching associated with malignancy presents special challenges and dilemmas. It can be among the most severe and recalcitrant forms of secondary pruritus. Patients with malignancy-associated pruritus represent a significant percentage of those requiring palliation, and many may manifest this symptom at some time during their illness. However, the frequency, chronicity, and severity of pruritus associated with malignancy and its response to treatment are difficult parameters to determine, and they have not been examined systematically and reported in the literature. For example, the percentage of patients for whom the symptoms of itching have been relieved by primary treatment of the malignancy versus those who have benefited from symptomatic therapies has not been defined in this population of patients. As a result, a single, specific, and effective treatment plan for pruritus of malignancy is not available.

Symptomatic skin care

Patients with itching of malignancy may manifest different types of pruritic skin lesions that warrant individualized therapies. Many patients will demonstrate excoriations due to scratching and injury of the skin from fingernails or other implements (brushes etc.) (Fig. 8). Other patients show discrete papular, crusted, or excoriated lesions more characteristic of prurigo (Fig. 9). As a routine, close trimming and filing of sharp edges of fingernails as well as wearing cotton gloves, if necessary, are initial steps to minimize further skin injury. Tepid (not too warm or too hot) baths are usually soothing and temporarily relieve the itch. Patients often relate that a hot bath or shower feels more relaxing and offers symptom relief, but the itch is worse afterwards due in part to vasodilation and the accentuated neural response of cutaneous heating. Immediately following the bath and a light towelling, the patient or caregiver should lubricate the skin with a fragrance-free cream-base emollient containing phenol or menthol if this is found to be beneficial. Applying a cream results in better maintenance of skin hydration and lessens the chance of further aggravation of pruritus from xerosis. Wearing clothing that is loose fitting, less irritating (e.g. avoid wools), and minimizes heat retention and sweating (e.g. avoid synthetics) can also be helpful in lessening the frequency and intensity of itch. Cotton fabric clothing usually meets these requirements.

For patients with numerous excoriations and crusting due to scratching, application of tap water wet dressings (or cotton long underwear soaked in water) to the affected areas several times daily for 1 to 2 h provides temporary relief and hastens healing of injured skin. A low- to medium-potency corticosteroid cream containing 1–2.5 per cent hydrocortisone can be applied to the skin prior to the wet dressings for topical anti-inflammatory action. A more potent corticosteroid such as triamcinolone 0.05–0.1 per cent in a cream base can be used for 7–10 days as needed on an intermittent basis, but prolonged use should be avoided to prevent atrophy and bruising of the skin, secondary skin infections, or hypothalamic–pituitary–adrenal suppression.

Oral corticosteroids

Various systemic anti-inflammatory agents are useful in the management of pruritus. Oral corticosteroids often improve the symptoms of itching for patients with primary or secondary pruritus. In many patients, the specific activity is unknown. The corticosteroid may inhibit release of pruritogens, inflammatory factors, or neuromediators, or it may block pruritogen activity or alter its metabolism. As with topical steroids, prolonged use has significant adverse side-effects. However, in cases where the duration of treatment is limited, an oral corticosteroid can provide much sought relief of itching.

Antihistamines

Antihistamines are another class of agent that offers benefit in treatment of itching. More than 30 different antihistaminic compounds of at least six different classes are available over the counter or by prescription. Although antihistamines provide minimal benefit for some patients with problematic itching such as that associated with Hodgkin's disease, obstructive jaundice, or uraemic pruritus, they have a good safety profile and should be used at full dose to attempt amelioration of pruritus. For example, pruritis is an early manifestation of HIV infection, and antihistamines, sometimes at high dosages, are used to control symptoms. Studies have shown superior efficacy of sedating over low-sedating antihistamines for relieving itch. Low-sedating antihistamines (e.g. fexofenadine, cetirizine, loratadine) should be reserved for the histamine-mediated whealing disorders that are accompanied by pruritus. Longer-acting antihistamines with central nervous system sedation are preferred for control of itch. These include chlorpheniramine, diphenhydramine, clemastine, hydroxyzine, and cyproheptadine. Agents of different classes should be tried if an antihistamine of one class is not effective. Sometimes, combination of agents from different classes is efficacious when a single agent is ineffective.

Other drug therapies

Cromones and thalidomide are anti-inflammatory agents that have been reported to be useful in pruritus associated with several different types of

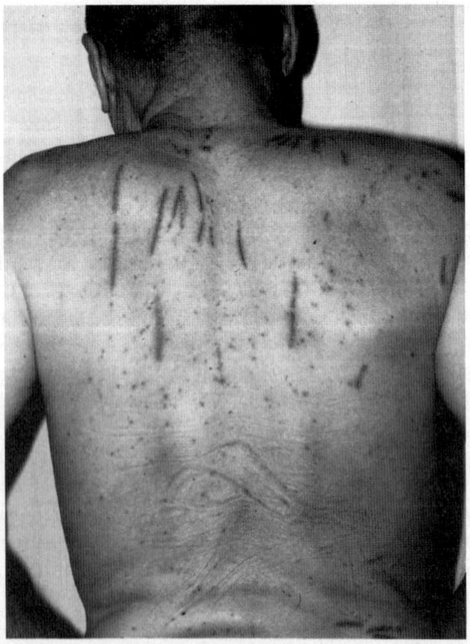

Fig. 8 Linear excoriations, erosions, and crusts resulting from unrelenting pruritus and scratching by a patient with small cell carcinoma of the lung.

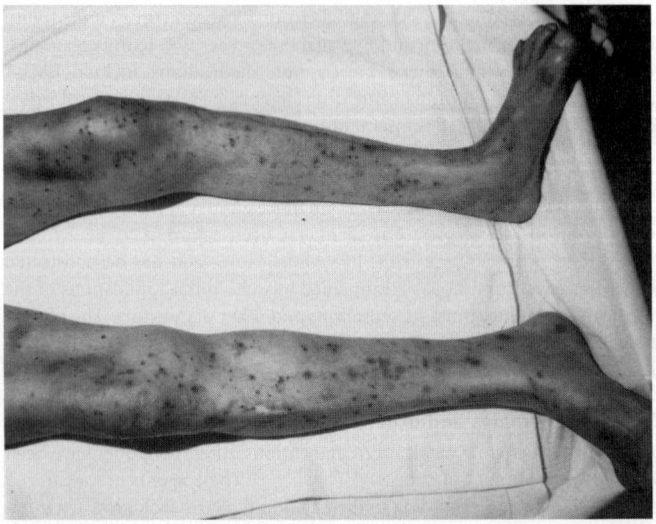

Fig. 9 Discrete, crusted, and haemorrhagic prurigo-like lesions accompanying generalized pruritus of chronic renal failure and diabetes mellitus.

chronic or malignant disease. Disodium chromoglycate improves the flushing and pruritus of systemic mast cell disease.[44] It also has been reported to improve the pruritus of Hodgkin's disease when other therapies have failed.[45] Thalidomide has been found to relieve the intractable pruritus and development of skin lesions in prurigo nodularis.[46] More recently, thalidomide (100 mg/day) was found to produce significant relief of uraemic pruritus.[47] This drug is used primarily in the treatment of leprosy reactions and graft-versus-host disease. Because of its neuropathic and teratogenic side-effects, thalidomide is not routinely available for prescription. However, selected patients who require only a limited course of therapy and can be monitored regularly may be candidates for thalidomide when an alternative medication is sought.

Many drugs have effects on the peripheral or central nervous system, and some of these agents have been found to be very useful in the treatment of itching from many causes. Anaesthetic agents administered by the intradermal, intravenous, or intra-arterial routes have effects similar to topical anaesthetics in blocking sensory input and transmission, including the sensation of pruritus. Parenteral lignocaine (200 mg in 100 ml saline by an intra-arterial line) alleviates refractory pruritus in hepatic cholestasis and chronic renal failure.[48,49] Hypotension, cardiovascular effects, seizures and psychosis are possible side-effects. Recently, the anaesthetic sedative propofol, used at subhypnotic doses (15 mg) daily when itch was most severe or by continuous infusion at 1–1.5 mg/kg/h, produced significant reduction in pruritus due to cholestatic disease of pancreatic neoplasia, hepatic and bile duct metastasis, cholangitis, and primary biliary cirrhosis.[50,51] A rapid onset of action within 5–10 min was observed. Propofol also relieves pruritus from spinal morphine administration, and it is postulated that propofol blocks effects of opioid-like pruritogens at the spinal level.[52] Parenterally administered agents such as lignocaine, propofol, and naloxone are of relatively limited use in chronic pruritus. However, if acute severe episodes of pruritus become incapacitating, these agents can often provide much sought relief and re-establish some measure of symptom control.

Antidepressant drugs, including doxepin, amitriptyline, nortriptyline, and imipramine, have antihistaminic effects as well as psychoactive and analgesic properties that make them useful in the management of various pain and itch states. Serotonin reuptake inhibitors such as paroxetine have demonstrated significant actitvity in controlling recalcitrant types of pruritus, especially secondary to polycythemia vera,[19] as well as various other advanced cancers.[34] Neuropathic pain with protopathic features of diffuse burning itch as well as the sensation of pain is improved by chronic antidepressant treatment.[53] These medications may also benefit patients with pruritus where depression appears to be playing a role in the prominence or severity of symptoms.[54] Neuroleptic medications, including pimozide and haloperidol as well as risperidone, drugs useful in the management of delusions of parasitosis, may play a therapeutic role in some clinical situations. Although not indicated for the primary treatment of organic pruritus, these agents may be useful when patients exhibit delusional ideation in conjunction with their disease process. Treatment improves the symptoms of psychosis and diminishes the mental fixation on pruritus.[54]

Sedative medications such as diazepam have been shown to be ineffective in reducing experimental itch, although mechanically induced pruritus was eliminated with this agent.[33,55] Sedatives in conjunction with other antipruritic agents appear to offer greater relief if the patient is experiencing anxiety as part of the chronic pruritic reaction. In addition to the sedative effects of antihistamines such as hydroxyzine, doxepin, and diphenhydramine, specific anxiolytic agents, including buspirone, clomipramine, and benzodiazepines such as alprazolam, can be used when anxiety appears to be playing a role in magnifying the symptoms of pruritus. Long-term treatment with benzodiazapines should be avoided as there is a risk of habituation.[54]

The opioid and serotonin antagonists, as reviewed earlier, have been found to be very effective in selected types of chronic pruritus. The opioid antagonists have been evaluated most extensively in the clinical setting of pruritus of cholestasis where they show significant benefit in symptom relief.[17,56] Naloxone must be administered parenterally. Naltrexone and nalmephene are orally active agents which may be useful as longer-term therapeutic agents for chronic pruritus. Some studies have clearly demonstrated benefit for cholestatic pruritus,[35] though randomized, blinded and placebo-controlled studies in uraemic pruritus seem to indicate no significant improvement in symptoms.[57] Serotonin (5-HT) antagonists are few in number and less well evaluated in pruritus. However, the 5-HT_3 receptor antagonist ondestranon shows promise as the first in a new class of agents to alleviate the symptoms of generalized pruritus in patients with cholestasis and chronic renal failure,[20,21] although recent studies have refuted its efficacy in uraemic pruritus.[22]

Sequestrants such as cholestyramine or charcoal administered orally or heparin administered by intravenous infusion have been reported to be helpful in the treatment of obstructive biliary pruritus.[30] Cholestyramine was also observed to improve itching in polycythaemia vera and uraemia. These treatments may be useful as adjuvant or alternative therapies during the management of chronic pruritus due to these diseases.

A variety of miscellaneous therapies are listed in Table 5, which also includes additional disease-specific medications reported to benefit chronic pruritus and other treatment modalities such as phototherapy, transcutaneous nerve stimulation, plasma exchange, and acupuncture. Pertinent references reporting the benefit of specific therapies are cited for each modality. For example, several medications and physical modalities have been found to relieve the pruritus of chronic renal failure. Despite our lack of knowledge regarding specific pruritogenic factors and their expression and activity in chronic renal failure, UVB phototherapy often provides symptomatic relief. UVB phototherapy is well tolerated, has few side-effects, and can be administered at many dermatological practices or regional clinical phototherapy centres. A combination of narrow band UVB and crotamiton has been reported to alleviate pruritus of metastatic breast carcinoma to the skin.[58] Erythropoetin and thalidomide have been reported to improve uraemic pruritus. Interferon-α and rifampicin have been found to be effective for polycythemia vera and malignant cholestatic pruritus, respectively.[59,60] Parenteral lignocaine is typically reserved for severe recalcitrant episodes of pruritus in uraemic patients unresponsive to other measures.

The multitude and variety of medications and sundry other therapeutic modalities reviewed in this chapter attest to the magnitude, severity, and chronicity of pruritus. All these drugs and therapies have been successful, to some extent, in ameliorating or abolishing this troublesome symptom. In managing the symptom of pruritus as well as the disease, it behoves the physician to make the best possible assessment of the specific physical and emotional factors that may be contributing to the intensity and character of a patient's problem of itch. With reassurance, flexibility, creativity, persistence, and a demonstrated concern by the physician, most patients will find relief and comfort.

Sweating

Anatomy and physiology

Sweating is a physiological sudomotor response of skin that has pathological counterparts. Abnormalities of sweating can be classified in terms of quantitative or qualitative dysfunction. From the perspective of palliative care, the most troublesome sudomotor symptoms relate to inappropriate or excessive sweating which occurs as part of malignant disease or its treatment. To understand the aetiological factors contributing to abnormal sweating and its palliative management, the anatomy and physiology of the peripheral and central thermoregulatory systems of the human are presented and reviewed.

Sweating or perspiration is a unique function of the skin of humans and apes that allows evaporative heat loss and regulation of body temperature in a hot environment or during physical exertion. Other mammals must pant, seek a cooler location, rest, or splash the skin with water to lower body temperature thermally. The crucial function and efficiency of sweat production is witnessed in individuals with the inherited disorder anhidrotic ectodermal hypoplasia who are unable to rely on evaporative heat loss through

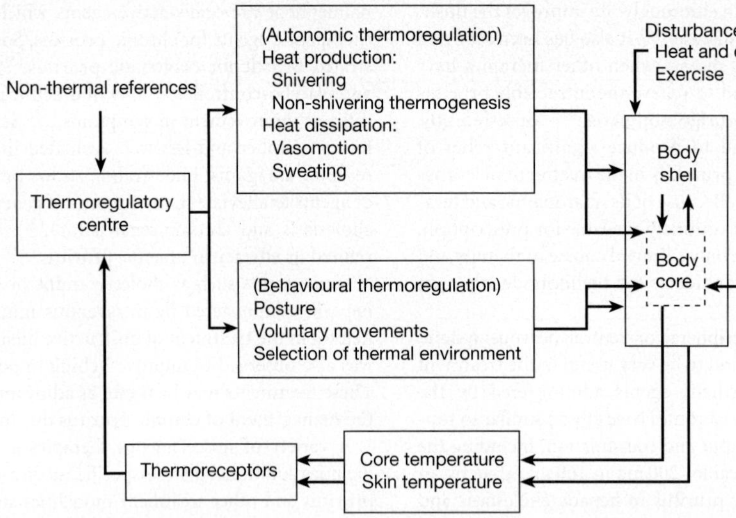

Fig. 10 The human thermoregulatory system. (Reproduced with permission from ref. 61.)

sweating. Physical inactivity, a cool ambient environment, or wetting the clothing or skin with water substitutes for sweating in order to achieve thermoregulation. Another group of persons particularly susceptible to the adverse consequences of thermal stress are young infants and the sedentary elderly who fail to sweat sufficiently and are also more likely to develop and succumb to hyperthermia.

Temperature regulation

Sweating is an important component of the elaborate thermoregulatory system of humans that is shown diagrammatically in Fig. 10.[(61)] The hypothalamus integrates inputs from central and peripheral thermoreceptors with the efferent response mechanisms, particularly sweating. The two types of thermosensitive neurones, warm-sensitive and cold-sensitive, are located in the preoptic and anterior hypothalamus (POAH). Warm-sensitive neurones respond to a rise in peripheral body temperature and are more abundant than cold-sensitive neurones which are activated by a decrease in peripheral temperature.

Body temperature is sensed at several crucial sites within the body, including specific thermoreceptors in the skin, spinal cord, and brainstem as well as thermal responses from the abdominal viscera. The POAH integrates thermal information from these sites and others in the body. Body temperature appears to be regulated to match a set-point. An abnormal upward shift of the set-point is believed to be the mechanism for production of fever. Additional control of the central thermoregulatory centre is mediated at several other sites in the brain with projections to the POAH, including the midbrain reticular formation, the raphe nucleus, the amygdala, the hippocampal formation, the sulcal prefrontal cortex, and the medial forebrain bundle. Thermoregulatory control of the hypothalamus can be modified by higher brain activity such as sleep, mental stress, and emotional excitement.

Hypercapnia, plasma osmolality, intravascular volume changes, and dehydration also alter the body temperature and set-point. Chemical mediators, including neurotransmitters such as catecholamines and acetylcholine and the eicosanoid prostaglandin E, play central roles in the control of normal thermoregulation as well as in the expression of fever. Hypothalamic peptides, including thyrotropin-releasing hormone, bombesin, neurotensin, ACTH, and vasopressin, are also important in the modulation of central thermoregulation.

Autonomic control

The afferent input and efferent responses of thermoregulation are complex but are intimately coupled and controlled by both peripheral and central

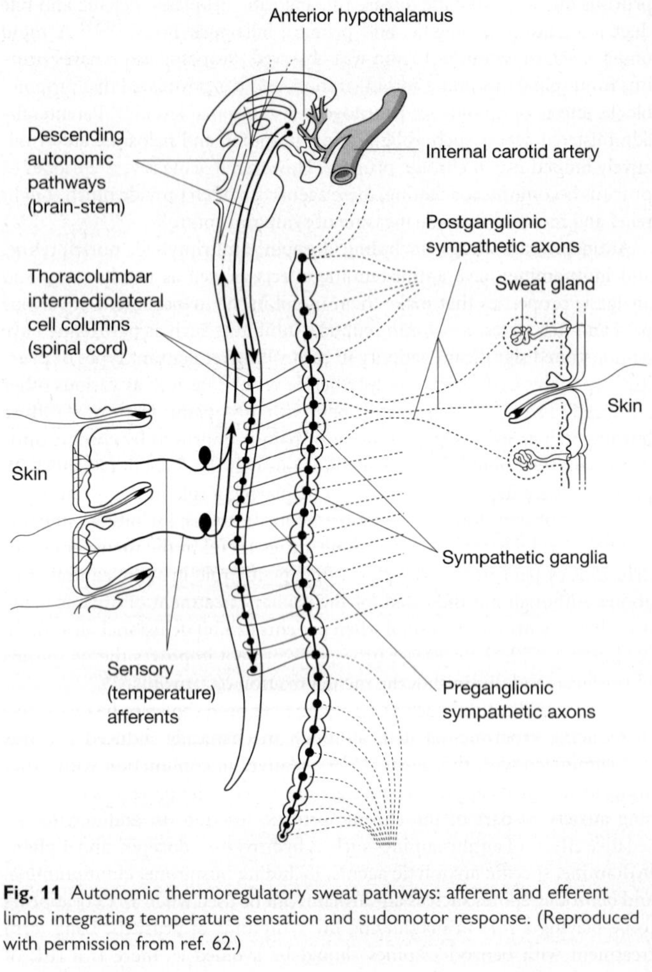

Fig. 11 Autonomic thermoregulatory sweat pathways: afferent and efferent limbs integrating temperature sensation and sudomotor response. (Reproduced with permission from ref. 62.)

mechanisms (Fig. 11). The main thermoregulatory response affecting vasomotion and sweating is mediated through the autonomic system. The cutaneous vasculature is innervated mainly by adrenergic vasoconstrictor nerve fibres. Vasodilation and constriction are coordinated with sweating responses and interact to control blood flow and dissipate or preserve body heat. Sympathetic efferent pathways descend from the hypothalamus through the brainstem to the spinal cord and the preganglionic neurones. From here the fibres exit the cord and enter the sympathetic chain. Postganglionic sympathetic axons innervate sweat glands, blood vessels, and pilomotor muscles in skin. Eccrine glands are innervated by cholinergic fibres. Sweating is produced by both thermal and mental stimulation of eccrine glands, but the distribution and inciting factors causing the sudomotor response are different. Thermal sweating results from excess temperature that is perceived by the body. A local thermal stimulus will generate a uniform sweat response over the body surface while sparing the palms and soles.

The palms and soles show a baseline sweat pattern in the waking state, and mental excitement and stress will increase the rate. This response is called mental sweating. Mental sweating is controlled by the cerebral neocortex limbic system as well as by the hypothalamus. Thermal and mental sweating have some overlap in their central control but are also coordinated independently. General body surface sweating can be affected by various mental stresses. Mental sweating may augment or depress the thermal response of sweating over the body surface, but always increases sweating of the palms and soles. Axillary and, in some individuals, forehead sweating have a lower threshold to stimulation and are often active when there is no thermal sweating elsewhere.

Thermal sweating normally occurs uniformly over the body. Various factors, including body position, exercise, dehydration, sweat gland blood flow, ambient humidity, gender, and age, have also been shown to exert significant effects on the distribution, rate of production, activation thresholds, and other functional aspects of sweating. These factors must be taken into consideration in determining whether sweating responses are physiological or pathological.

Hyperhidrosis

In considering the palliative aspects of sweat dysfunction, most patients are typically bothered by hyperhidrosis (excessive sweating) or the distinctive symptom of nocturnal diaphoresis (night sweats).[63] A variety of underlying disorders contribute to localized or generalized hyperhidrosis (Table 6). Hyperhidrosis can be further classified as primary or secondary. It also should be appreciated that it may be a compensatory response to anhidrosis at other body sites (Fig. 12). Therefore the cause of hyperhidrosis should be determined if possible, and attempts should be made to alleviate underlying abnormalities that may induce pathological states of excessive or insufficient sweat production.

Clinical evaluation

Determination of sweating abnormalities can be based on the clinical history and examination, or on more comprehensive evaluations such as thermoregulatory sweat testing or specific measurements such as quantitative sudomotor axon reflex tests (QSART).[62] QSART measures the pattern of sweat response and discriminates whether abnormalities in sweat production are pre- or postganglionic. Postganglionic abnormalities demonstrate alterations in the QSART while disturbances at the preganglionic level typically spare QSART function.

Thermoregulatory sweat testing assesses the integrity of the peripheral and central sympathetic sudomotor pathways.[62] Thermal stimulation is achieved by raising the skin temperature and the central or core body temperature. An environmentally controlled cabinet that warms the ambient air temperature to 45–50°C and also heats the skin with infrared lamps is used to raise central (oral or tympanic membrane) temperature and skin temperature to levels that stimulate sweating. Sweating on the skin surface is visualized with a special indicator powder containing iodinated corn starch, iodine solution, or alizarin-red-containing corn starch and sodium carbonate. Reduced or absent sweating can be delineated clearly (Fig. 12), and the distribution and extent of sweat loss is useful in further characterizing potential pathological abnormalities of the pre- or postganglionic pathways (Fig. 13) or the end organ, that is, the sweat glands (Fig. 14).

Disruption of the sympathetic chain or white rami produces localized loss of sweating as can be seen with a Pancoast tumor involving the apical lung (Fig. 13). In contrast, irritation of the sympathetic chain by encroachment of a neoplasm such as bronchial carcinoma, mesothelioma, or osteoma may also produce ipsilateral hyperhidrosis.[64] Stroke rarely causes contralateral hyperhidrosis if large infarcts affect both the superficial and deep cerebral structures. Basilar artery strokes have been known to produce focal symmetrical sweating.

Table 6 Hyperhidrosis

Localized hyperhidrosis	Generalized hyperhidrosis
Essential (primary)	Systemic illness
Neurogenic	Phaeochromocytoma
Spinal cord disease	Thyrotoxicosis
Peripheral neuropathy	Hypopituitarism
Cerebrovascular disease (stroke)	Diabetes insipidus
Intrathoracic neoplasms or masses	Diabetes mellitus
Unilateral circumscribed	Acromegaly
Cold-induced	Hypoglycaemia
Associated with cutaneous lesions	Carcinoid syndrome
Gustatory	Menopause
	Tuberculosis
	Lymphoma
	Endocarditis
	Angina
	Malignancy
	Nocturnal
	Episodic
	Medication-induced

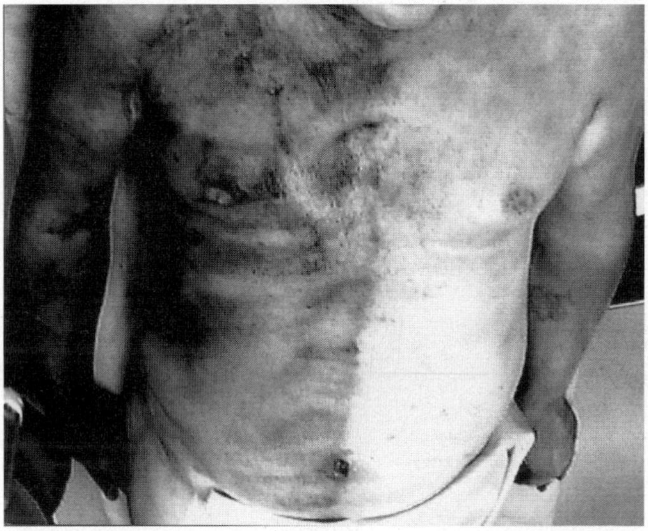

Fig. 12 Compensatory hyperhidrosis resulting from hemitruncal anhidrosis measured by thermoregulatory sweat testing (sweat indicated by dark areas). (Courtesy of Dr R. Fealey, Mayo Clinic.)

Generalized or regionalized hyperhidrosis

Generalized hyperhidrosis occurs with various systemic diseases, including endocrine disorders, menopause, infections, lymphomas and other cancers, carcinoid syndrome, and drug withdrawal.[65] Endocrine disturbances observed to cause excessive sweating include acromegaly, diabetes mellitus, diabetes insipidus, hypopituitarism, hypoglycaemia thyrotoxicosis, and phaeochromocytoma. Drugs reported to cause hyperhidrosis include opioid analgesics such as morphine, diamorphine, methadone, butorphanol,

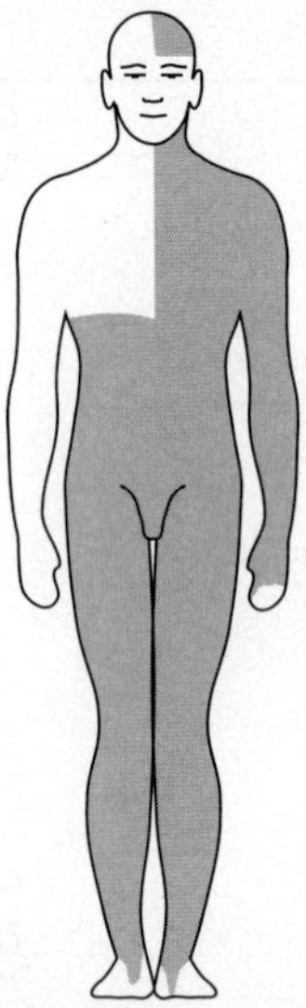

Fig. 13 Anhidrosis (light-coloured areas) of the right head, upper trunk, and upper extremity due to a right-sided Pancoast tumour. Distal sweat loss is due to peripheral neuropathy. (Reproduced with permission from ref. 62.)

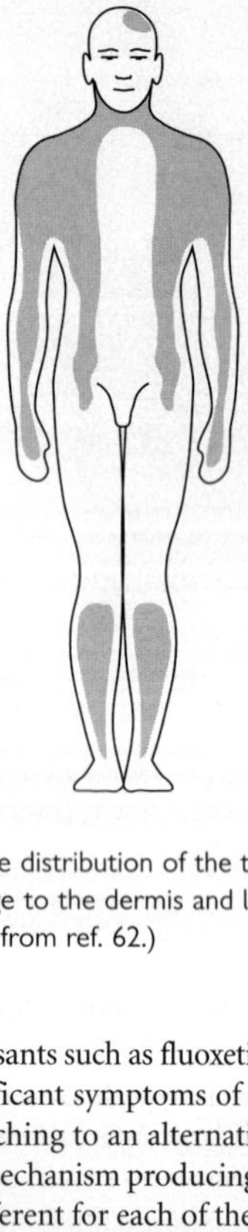

Fig. 14 Loss of sweating in the distribution of the truncal radiation port. Anhidrosis is caused by damage to the dermis and loss of sweat gland function. (Reproduced with permission from ref. 62.)

and pentazocine, antidepressants such as fluoxetine, acyclovir, and naproxen. If patients experience significant symptoms of sweat excess as a result of a particular medication, switching to an alternative drug may provide significant relief. Although the mechanism producing hyperhidrosis is not clearly understood and may be different for each of these causes, a downward shift of the set-point of the POAH could stimulate inappropriate sweating.

The patient may confuse excessive regionalized sweating with generalized hyperhidrosis. Compensatory hyperhidrosis may occur within normal sweat-producing areas of the skin in response to anhidrosis that involves other areas of the skin. The patient may not notice the loss of sweating, but, rather, experiences discomfort from the exaggerated sweating response. In this case, detection of the underlying cause of the loss of sweating would guide further treatment and appropriate management for symptomatic hyperhidrosis.

Treatment of sweating

The management of hyperhidrosis is based on identifying the primary cause underlying the abnormal sweat response as well as eliminating any potential aggravating factors that may further augment sweating. Primary hyperhidrosis will not be considered in the discussion of the palliative management of sweating. A variety of therapies offer benefit in treatment of primary hyperhidrosis but are not usually applicable to management of secondary hyperhidrosis.(66) For primary localized hyperhidrosis, endoscopic thoracic sympathectomy or botulinum toxin injections into the affected skin regions are the most popular therapies.(67,68)

Hot flushes

Hot flushes are a prominent cause of excessive sweating in patients with cancer. A detailed discussion of the proposed pathophysiological mechanisms for this problem is outside the scope of this chapter but can be found elsewhere.(69–71) Hot flushes classically occur in menopausal women and are associated with oestrogen depletion. Breast cancer survivors are not exempt from this clinical problem; in fact, they are more at risk for several reasons. First, adjuvant chemotherapy given to premenopausal women can frequently result in premature ovarian failure with all the sequelae of oestrogen-depletion problems; second the commonly used anti-oestrogen, tamoxifen, causes hot flushes as its most common toxicity; third, general clinical practice has been to deny hormone replacement therapy to these women because of theoretical concerns that oestrogen replacement might harm them.

Given that breast cancer is a commonly diagnosed cancer whose incidence is rising, particularly among younger women, and that hot flushes are a very common clinical problem, what therapeutic options are available? Potential options can be grouped into two classes: hormonal and non-hormonal. We will consider non-hormonal options first.

To date, the most effective studied non-hormonal antidote for hot flushes is venlafaxine. A four-arm placebo-controlled double-blinded clinical trial demonstrated that a venlafaxine dose of 75 mg/day decreased hot flushes by approximately 60 per cent, compared to a hot flush reduction of approximately 25 per cent in a placebo group.(72) From this investigation, it is recommended that venlafaxine be started at a dose of 37.5 mg/day for a week and consider increasing this up to 75 mg/day. Higher doses of venlafaxine did not appear to be more beneficial for reducing hot flushes in the randomized dose-seeking trial.(72) There are other antidepressants which also appear to have efficacy against hot flushes. These include paroxetine(73) and fluoxetine.(74) Several other similar newer antidepressants are being evaluated for their potential efficacy against hot flushes.

A number of other non-hormonal compounds have been studied as a means for alleviating hot flushes in patients. These include the antihypertensive medication clonidine,(75,76) Bellergal (a combination product of belladonna alkaloids and phenobarbital),(77) black cohosh,(78) and vitamin E.(79) None of these medications appear to work as well as the newer antidepressants do. In addition, some of them (e.g. clonidine) have bothersome toxicities which limit their utility.

There is one non-hormonal agent which appears to be quite promising but is awaiting definitive study. This is gabapentin. There is one published case series which suggests that it is quite beneficial for alleviating hot flushes.(80) Information should be available over the next couple of years regarding its true efficacy and toxicity status in this regard.

What about hormonal agents? First, let us discuss soy. Soy products contain phytoestrogens. Based on preliminary reports suggesting that soy *might* be beneficial for reducing hot flushes, placebo-controlled trials have been conducted. To date, the placebo-controlled trials suggest that soy products do not have any more efficacy against hot flushes than does a placebo.(81) A group of hormonal agents which does have efficacy against hot flushes are progestational drugs. Progestational agents appear to have as much efficacy against hot flushes as does estrogen therapy.(82) Although arguments can be made that there are no data which clearly demonstrate that progestational agents are any safer to use in breast cancer survivors than is estrogen, there are also no data to clearly indicate that progestational agents cause harm in these patients. Nonetheless, because of concerns about hormonal agents, it is reasonable to try non-hormonal agents prior to utilizing progestational agents such as megestrol acetate. When megestrol acetate is utilized, a low dose is recommended. Forty milligrams per day is a usual starting dose for the first month. Following this, the dose can frequently be decreased down to 20 mg/day.(82)

The use of oestrogen can sometimes be considered for treatment of hot flushes, or other clinical problems associated with oestrogen depletion, in breast cancer survivors. Although this may sound heretical to many, there is much uncertainty about the theoretical risks of oestrogen replacement therapy on breast cancer, and many potential benefits are ascribed to oestrogen replacement therapy in women. Instead of denying oestrogen therapy to all breast cancer survivors and thus being governed by the 'knee-jerk' response that 'oestrogen should never be used in a patient with a history of breast cancer', the pros and cons of the use of this therapy should be individualized in breast cancer survivors in the same manner as should be done in women in general.(83) This topic is the focus of substantial research efforts at present, and it is hoped that new insights into this matter should become apparent in the near future.

Another group of cancer patients who suffer from hot flushes are men who have had androgen ablation therapy for prostate cancer. Hot flushes affect approximately 75 per cent of such men and can be a very substantial problem.(70,71) A placebo-controlled trial demonstrated that clonidine does not appear to decrease hot flushes in men.(84) However, low-dose megestrol acetate alleviates hot flushes in men as well as it does in women.(82) It should be noted that megestrol acetate has occasionally been associated with rising PSA concentrations, however.(85) Lastly, venlafaxine appears to help hot flushes in men as well as it does in women,(86) so it is reasonable to try this agent first, saving progestational agents for patients who do not get relief from venlafaxine.

Treatment of other causes of sweating

Another cause of sweating is related to fever. Sweating is a physiological response to fever, and documented fevers that elicit diaphoresis either during or following the episodes need to be investigated and treated appropriately. Sweating can be a prominent clinical problem in patients with advanced cancer who have tumour fever. Antipyretic agents such as aspirin and paracetamol (acetaminophen) appear to reduce fever by resetting the POAH set-point, and these agents improve symptoms, including sweating, that are associated with fever. At times, however, patients with tumour fever are relatively asymptomatic while they are febrile, but they may perspire and chill during defervescence. A simple solution to this problem is to discontinue antipyretic medications. Asymptomatic fever may continue but symptomatic periods of defervescence decrease. Another method of treating tumour fever is to use non-aspirin-containing non-steroidal anti-inflammatory drugs (NSAIDs) such as naproxen. These drugs can be remarkably successful in alleviating tumour fevers and associated sweating.(87–89) While the efficacy may cease after a period of weeks or months, switching to another NSAID may again induce defervescence.(87)

Sweating may be a chronic and prominent concern for many patients who do not have any malignancy or infectious aetiology. Even in patients with malignancy, where antipyretic therapies have either been instituted or discontinued to attempt symptom relief, diaphoresis may continue to be a major symptom. Various medications, including H_2-antagonists, have been tried empirically in attempts to provide relief. Although a specific mechanism of action is not well defined and documented clinical trials are lacking, clinical experience has indicated marked benefit from cimetidine (400–800 mg twice daily) in both idiopathic and malignancy-associated sweating. Whether other newer H_2-blockers exhibit a better or worse clinical response is not known.

Thalidomide is another medication that may exert significant benefit in reducing sweating as well as improving other symptoms and syndromes of advanced cancer, such as cachexia, nausea, and insomnia.(90) Both low-dose (100 mg orally every night) and high-dose (300 mg twice daily) thalidomide have been reported to improve sweating in the majority of affected patients.(91,92) Thalidomide has been shown to reduce tumor necrosis factor-α production as well as modulate other interleukins and cytokines. Besides peripheral neuropathy, severe constipation, headache, cutaneous eruptions-skin sloughing, and oedema have been reported. However, the relative safety of the drug in advanced cancer favours judicious use. It is hoped that improved therapies will follow as the peripheral and central neural controls of sweating become better understood.

References

1. **Winkelmann, R.K. and Muller, S.A.** (1964). Pruritus. *Annual Reviews of Medicine* **15**, 53–64.
2. **Bernhard, J.D.** *Itch: Mechanisms and Management of Pruritus.* New York: McGraw-Hill, 1994.
3. **Winkelmann, R.K.** (1961). Dermatological clinics. 1. Comments on pruritus related to systemic disease. *Mayo Clinic Proceedings* **36**, 187–96.
4. **Gilchrest, B.A.** (1982). Pruritus: pathogenesis, therapy, and significance in systemic disease states. *Archives of Internal Medicine* **142**, 101–5.
5. **Denman, S.T.** (1986). A review of pruritus. *Journal of the American Academy of Dermatology* **14**, 375–92.
6. **Yosipovitch, G.** et al. (2001). A questionnaire for the assessment of pruritus: validation in uremic patients. *Acta Dermatologica Venereologia* **81**, 108–11.
7. **Greaves, M.W., and Wall, P.D.** (1996). Pathophysiology of itching. *Lancet* **348**, 938–40.
8. **Schmelz, M.** et al. (1997). Specific C-receptors for itch in human skin. *Journal of Neuroscience* **17**, 8003–8.
9. **Andrew, D. and Craig, A.D.** (2001). Spinothalamic lamina I neurons selectively sensitive to histamine: A central neural pathway for itch. *Nature Neuroscience* **4**, 72–7.
10. **Wallengren, J.** (1993). The pathophysiology of itch. *European Journal of Dermatology* **3**, 643–7.
11. **Hägermark, O.** (1992). Peripheral and central mediators of itch. *Skin Pharmacology* **5**, 1–8.
12. **Bernstein, J.E.** (1992). Capsaicin and substance P. *Clinics in Dermatology* **9**, 497–503.
13. **Winkelmann, R.K.** (1988). Cutaneous sensory nerves. *Seminars in Dermatology* **7**, 236–68.
14. **Handwerker, H.O., Forster, C., and Kirchhoff, C.** (1991). Discharge patterns of human C-fibres induced by itching and burning stimuli. *Journal of Neurophysiology* **66**, 307–15.
15. **Head, H.** (1905). The afferent nervous system from a new aspect. *Brain* **28**, 99–115.
16. **Lowitt, M.H. and Bernhard, J.D.** (1992). Pruritus. *Seminars in Neurology* **12**, 374–84.
17. **Bergasa, N.V.** et al. (1995). Effects of naloxone infusions in patients with the pruritus of cholestasis. *Annals of Internal Medicine* **123**, 161–7.
18. **Khandelwal, M. and Malet, P.F.** (1994). Pruritus associated with cholestasis: a review of pathogenesis and management. *Digestive Diseases Sciences* **39**, 1–7.
19. **Diehn, F. and Tefferi, A.** (2001). Pruritus in polycythaemia vera: prevalence, laboratory correlates and management. *British Journal of Haematology* **115**, 619–21.
20. **Schworer, H. and Ramadori, G.** (1993). Treatment of pruritus: a new indication for serotonin type 3 receptor antagonists. *Clinical Investigation* **71**, 659–62.
21. **Raderer, M., Muller, C., and Scheithauer, W.** (1994). Ondansetron for pruritus due to cholestasis. *New England Journal of Medicine* **330**, 1540.
22. **Ashmore, S.D.** et al. (2000). Ondansetron therapy for uremic pruritus in hemodialysis patients. *American Journal of Kidney Disease* **35**, 827–31.
23. **Melzack, R. and Wall, P.D.** (1965). Pain mechanisms: a new theory. *Science* **150**, 971–9.
24. **Carlsson, C.-A.** et al. (1975). Electrical transcutaneous nerve stimulation for relief of itch. *Experientia* **31**, 191.

25. **Monk, B.E.** (1993). Transcutaneous electronic nerve stimulation in the treatment of generalized pruritus. *Clinical and Experimental Dermatology* **18**, 67–8.
26. **Paul, R., Paul, R., and Jansen, C.T.** (1987). Itch and malignancy prognosis in generalized pruritus: a 6-year-follow-up of 125 patients. *Journal of the American Academy of Dermatology* **16**, 1179–82.
27. **Kantor, G.R. and Lookingbill, D.P.** (1983). Generalized pruritus and systemic disease. *Journal of the American Academy of Dermatology* **9**, 375–8.
28. **Doyle, J.A.** et al. (1979). Prurigo nodularis: a reappraisal of the clinical and histological features. *Journal of Cutaneous Pathology* **6**, 392–403.
29. **Arndt, K.A., Bowers, K.E., and Chuttani, A.R.** *Manual of Dermatological Therapeutics: With Essentials of Diagnosis* 5th edn. New York: Little Brown, 1995, pp. 145–8, 317–22.
30. **Fransway, A.F. and Winkelmann, R.K.** (1988). Treatment of pruritus. *Seminars in Dermatology* **7**, 310–25.
31. **Devers, A. and Galer, B.S.** (2000). Topical lidocaine patch relieves a variety of neuropathic pain conditions: An open-label study. *Clinical Journal of Pain* **16**, 205–8.
32. **Winkelmann, R.K.** (1982). Pharmacologic control of pruritus. *Medical Clinics of North America* **66**, 1119–33.
33. **Lorette, G. and Vaillant, L.** (1990). Pruritus: current concepts in pathogenesis and treatment. *Drugs* **39**, 218–23.
34. **Zylicz, Z., Smits, C., and Krajnik, M.** (1998). Paroxetine for pruritus in advanced cancer. *Journal of Pain and Symptom Management* **16**, 121–4.
35. **Jones, E.A. and Bergasa, N.V.** (2000). Evolving concepts of the pathogenesis and treatment of the pruritus of cholestasis. *Cancer Journal of Gastroenterology* **14**, 33–40.
36. **Ghent, C.N. and Carruthers, S.G.** (1988). Treatment of pruritus in primary biliary cirrhosis with rifampin. *Gastroenterology* **94**, 488–93.
37. **Gregorio, G.V.** et al. (1993). Effect of rifampicin in the treatment of pruritus in hepatic cholestasis. *Archives of Disease in Childhood* **69**, 141–3.
38. **Whitington, P.F. and Whitington, G.L.** (1988). Partial external diversion of bile for the treatment of intractable pruritus associated with intrahepatic cholestasis. *Gastroenterology* **95**, 130–6.
39. **Marchi, S.** et al. (1992). Relief of pruritus and decreases in plasma histamine concentrations during erythropoietin therapy in patients with uremia. *New England Journal of Medicine* **326**, 969–74.
40. **Hampers, C.** et al. (1986). Disappearance of uraemic itching after subtotal parathyroidectomy. *New England Journal of Medicine* **279**, 695–700.
41. **Gilchrist, B.** et al. (1977). Relief of uraemic pruritus with ultraviolet phototherapy. *New England Journal of Medicine* **297**, 136–8.
42. **Finelli, C.** et al. (1993). Relief of intractable pruritus in polycythemia vera with recombinant interferon alfa. *American Journal of Hematology* **43**, 316–18.
43. **Riccardi, V.M.** (1993). A controlled multiphase trial of ketotifen to minimize neurofibroma-associated pain and itching. *Archives of Dermatology* **129**, 577–81.
44. **Soter, N.A., Austin, K.F., and Wasserman, S.I.** (1979). Oral disodium cromoglycate in the treatment of systemic mastocytosis. *New England Journal of Medicine* **301**, 465–9.
45. **Leven, A.** et al. (1979). Sodium cromoglycate and Hodgkin's pruritus. *British Medical Journal* **2**, 896.
46. **Winkelmann, R.K.** et al. (1984). Thalidomide treatment of prurigo nodularis. *Acta Dermatologica Venereologica* **64**, 412–17.
47. **Silva, S.R.B.** et al. (1994). Thalidomide for the treatment of uraemic pruritus: a crossover randomized double-blind trial. *Nephrology* **67**, 270–3.
48. **Levy, M. and Catalano, R.** (1985). Control of common physical symptoms other than pain in patients with terminal disease. *Seminars in Oncology* **12**, 411–30.
49. **Tapia, L.** et al. (1977). Pruritus in dialysis patients treated with parenteral lidocaine. *New England Journal of Medicine* **296**, 261–2.
50. **Borgeat, A., Wilder-Smith, O.H.G., and Mentha, G.** (1993). Subhypnotic doses of propofol relieve pruritus associated with liver disease. *Gastroenterology* **104**, 244–7.
51. **Borgeat, A.** et al. (1994). Intractable cholestatic pruritus after liver transplantation–management with propofol. *Transplantation* **58**, 727–30.
52. **Borgeat, A.** et al. (1992). Subhypnotic doses of propofol relieve pruritus induced by epidural and intrathecal morphine. *Anesthiology* **76**, 510–12.
53. **Willner, C. and Low, P.A.** (1993). Pharmacologic approaches to neuropathic pain. In *Peripheral Neuropathy* 3rd edn. (ed. P. Dyck et al.), pp. 1700–20. Philadelphia PA: Saunders.
54. **Fried, R.G.** (1994). Evaluation and treatment of 'psychogenic' pruritus and self-excoriation. *Journal of the American Academy of Dermatology* **30**, 993–9.
55. **Hagermark, K.O.** (1973). Influence of antihistamines, sedatives and aspirin on experimental itch. *Acta Dermatologica Venereologia* **53**, 363–8.
56. **Jones, E.A. and Bergasa, N.V.** (1990). The pruritus of cholestasis: from bile acids to opiate agonists. *Hepatology* **11**, 884–7.
57. **Pauli-Magnus, C.** et al. (2000). Naltrexone does not relieve uremic pruritus: Results of a randomized, double-blind, placebo-controlled crossover study. *Journal of the American Society of Nephrology* **11**, 514–19.
58. **Holme, S.A. and Mills, C.M.** (2001). Crotamiton and narrow-band UVB phototherapy: Novel approaches to alleviate pruritus of breast carcinoma skin infiltration. *Journal of Pain and Symptom Management* **22**, 803–5.
59. **Lengfelder, E., Berger, U., and Hehlmann, R.** (2000). Interferon alpha in the treatment of polycythemia vera. *Annals of Hematology* **79**, 103–9.
60. **Price, T.J., Patterson, W.K., and Olver, I.N.** (1998). Rifampicin as treatment for pruritus in malignant cholestasis. *Support Care Cancer* **6**, 533–5.
61. **Ogawa, T. and Low, P.** (1992). Autonomic regulation of temperature and sweating. In *Clinical Autonomic Disorders: Evaluation and Management* (ed. P.A. Low), pp. 79–91. Boston MA: Little Brown.
62. **Fealey, R.D.** (1992). The thermoregulatory sweat test. In *Clinical Autonomic Disorders: Evaluation and Management* (ed. P.A. Low), pp. 217–29. Boston MA: Little Brown.
63. **Lea, M.J. and Aber, R.C.** (1985). Descriptive epidemiology of night sweats upon admission to a university hospital. *Southern Medical Journal* **78**, 1065–7.
64. **Walsh, J.C., Low, P.A., and Allsop, J.L.** (1976). Localized sympathetic overactivity: an uncommon complication of lung cancer. *Journal of Neurology, Neurosurgery and Psychiatry* **39**, 93–5.
65. **Freeman, R., Waldorf, H.A., and Dover, J.S.** (1992). Autonomic neurodermatology (Part II): disorders of sweating and flushing. *Seminars in Neurology* **12**, 394–407.
66. **White, J.W.** (1986). Treatment of primary hyperhidrosis. *Mayo Clinic Proceedings* **61**, 951–6.
67. **Vallieres, E.** (2001). Endoscopic upper thoracic sympathectomy. *Neurosurgery Clinics of North America* **12**, 321–7.
68. **Heckmann, M., Ceballos-Baumann, A.O., and Plewig, G.** (2001). Botulinum toxin A for axillary hyperhidrosis (excessive sweating). *New England Journal of Medicine* **344**, 488–93.
69. **Casper, R.F. and Yen, S.S.C.** (1985). Neuroendocrinology of menopausal flushes: An hypothesis of flush mechanism. *Clinical Endocrinology* **22**, 293–312.
70. **Charig, C.R. and Rundle, J.S.** (1989). Flushing: Long-term side effect of orchiectomy in treatment of prostatic carcinoma. *Urology* **33**, 175–8.
71. **Quella, S., Loprinzi, C.L., and Dose, A.M.** (1994). A qualitative approach to defining 'hot flashes' in men. *Urological Nursing* **14**, 155–8.
72. **Loprinzi, C.L.** et al. (2000). Venlafaxine in management of hot flashes in survivors of breast cancer: A randomised controlled trial. *Lancet* **356**, 2059–63.
73. **Stearns, V.** et al. (2000). A pilot trial assessing the efficacy of paroxetine hydrochloride (Paxil) in controlling hot flashes in breast cancer survivors. *Annals of Oncology* **11**, 17–22.
74. **Loprinzi, C.L., Quella, S.K., and Sloan, J.A.** (1999). Preliminary data from a randomized evaluation of fluoxetine (Prozac) for treating hot flashes in breast cancer survivors. *Breast Cancer Research and Treatment* **57**, 34 (abstract).
75. **Goldberg, R.M.** et al. (1994). Transdermal clonidine for ameliorating tamoxifen-induced hot flashes. *American Society of Clinical Oncology* **12**, 155–8.
76. **Pandya, K.J.** et al. (2000). Oral clonidine in postmenopausal patients with breast cancer experiencing tamoxifen-induced hot flashes: a University of Rochester Cancer Center Community Clinical Oncology Program study. *American College of Physicians* **132**, 788–93.
77. **Bergmans, M.G.M.** et al. (1987). Effect of Bellergal Retard on climacteric complaints: A double-blind, placebo-controlled study. *Maturitas* **9**, 227–34.

78. **Jacobson, J.** et al. (2001). Randomized trial of black cohosh for the treatment of hot flashes among women with a history of breast cancer. *Journal of Clinical Oncology* **19**, 2739–45.
79. **Barton, D.L.** et al. (1998). Prospective evaluation of vitamine for hot flashes in breast cancer survivors. *Journal of Clinical Oncology* **16**, 495–500.
80. **Guttuso, T.** (2000). Gabapentin's effects on hot flashes and hypothermia. *Neurology* **54**, 2161–3.
81. **Quella, S.K.** et al. (2000). Evaluations of soy phytoestrogens for the treatment of hot flashes in breast cancer survivors: a North Central Cancer Treatment Group trial. *Journal of Clinical Oncology* **18**, 1068–74.
82. **Loprinzi, C.L.** et al. (1994). Megestrol acetate for the prevention of hot flashes. *New England Journal of Medicine* **331**, 347–52.
83. **Col, N.F.** et al. (2001). Hormone replacement therapy after breast cancer: a systematic review and quantitative assessment of risk. *Journal of Clinical Oncology* **19**, 2357–63.
84. **Loprinzi, C.L.** et al. (1994). Transdermal clonidine for ameliorating post-orchiectomy hot flushes. *Journal of Urology* **151**, 634–6.
85. **Burch, P.A. and Loprinzi, C.L.** (1999). Prostate specific antigen (PSA) decline after withdrawal of low-dose megestrol acetate. Letter to the Editor. *Journal of Clinical Oncology* **17**, 1987–8.
86. **Quella, S.K.** et al. (1999). Pilot evaluation of venlafaxine for the treatment of hot flashes in men undergoing androgen ablation therapy for prostate cancer. *Journal of Urology* **162**, 98–102.
87. **Tsavaris, N.** et al. (1990). A randomized trial of the effect of three non-steroid anti-inflammatory agents in ameliorating cancer-induced fever. *Journal of Internal Medicine* **228**, 451–5.
88. **Chang, J.C. and Gross, H.M.** (1984). Utility of naproxen in the differential diagnosis of fever of undetermined origin in patients with cancer. *American Journal of Medicine* **76**, 597–603.
89. **Chang, J.C. and Hawley, H.B.** (1995). Neutropenic fever of undetermined origin (N-FUO): why not use the naproxen test? *Cancer Investigation* **13**, 448–50.
90. **Peuckmann, V., Fisch, M., and Bruera, E.** (2000). Potential novel uses of thalidomide: Focus on palliative care. *Drugs* **60**, 273–92.
91. **Deaner, P.B.** (2000). The use of thalidomide in the management of severe sweating in patients with advanced malignancy: Trial report. *Palliative Medicine* **14**, 429–31.
92. **Eisen, T.G.** (2000). Thalidomide in solid tumors: the London experience. *Oncology* **14**, 17–20.

8.8 Palliative medicine in malignant respiratory diseases

Kin-Sang Chan, Michael M.K. Sham, Doris M.W. Tse, and Anne Berit Thorsen

Introduction

> The Lord God formed man from the dust of the ground and breathed into his nostrils the breath of life, and man became a living creature
>
> Genesis

A breath is a vital sign of a living creature. When one dies, one expires. A breath, however, serves more than physiological purposes. A sigh often carries unspeakable messages from the inner being. Hence the essence of a breath is filled with physiological, psychological, and spiritual signals.

Everyday, millions of people throughout the world are distressed by breathlessness and other respiratory symptoms, resulting from the highly prevalent lung cancer and pulmonary metastasis. Besides, millions are sighing from their suffering.

Breathing, an automatic activity which one undergoes hundreds of millions of cycles throughout one's life, is mostly effortless. However, when the respiratory system is compromised by diseases, every breath becomes laborious. Dyspnoea, cough, sputum, and haemoptysis are the key symptoms that our patients with malignancies face. Current clinical experiences reveal that dyspnoea is a prevalent symptom, especially when approaching death, yet sub-optimally controlled.

Care for patients at the end of life aims at maximizing quality of remaining lives, sustaining the will to live and finally achieving good death. For patients with respiratory malignancy, these goals can only be achieved when distresses related to respiratory symptoms are addressed. The sub-optimal outcome of dyspnoea control calls for a deeper understanding of its pathophysiological basis. A systematic approach to evaluate dyspnoea, a deep understanding of the multidimensionality of the symptoms, and the exploration of new treatment modalities will hopefully open new horizon to improve the quality of remaining lives.

Factors that relate to the 'will to live' are often complex and deep-seated in an individual. A recent study has shed new insight on factors that predict the will to live.[(1)] The four predictors are depression, anxiety, shortness of breath, and sense of well being. Dyspnoea becomes a critical factor affecting the will to live while approaching death.

Good dying is not a natural gift for patients with terminal illnesses. The capability of the palliative care team to relieve the respiratory distress, the ability to empower patients and their families to exercise their decisions and self-control, while balancing the benefit and risk of treatment, is the science and art of caring.

Dyspnoea

Definition of dyspnoea

Dyspnoea is the term generally applied to unpleasant or uncomfortable respiratory sensations experienced by individuals. The American Thoracic Society defines dyspnoea as 'a subjective experience of breathing discomfort that consists of qualitatively distinct sensations that vary in intensity'.[(2)] The experience is derived from interaction among physiological, psychological, social, and environmental factors, and may induce secondary physiological and behavioral responses.[(2)]

No matter how one defines dyspnoea, it is still a very personal experience of the patient. Dyspnoea encompasses multiple sensations, as illustrated by dyspnoea descriptor studies on patients with various chronic cardiopulmonary diseases. They described the sensation with different clusters of descriptors. For example, chronic obstructive pulmonary disease (COPD) was characterized by 'heavy, gasping, hunger, and effort', whereas asthma was characterized by 'effort, tight, exhalation, deep, and concentration'.[(3)] The descriptors were also unique for the underlying disease, though different conditions shared some of the descriptors, indicating sharing pathophysiology.[(3)]

Dyspnoea is a term we use for a symptom that patients often describe as breathlessness. In the following text, the two are used interchangeably. When dyspnoeic patients were asked to describe this symptom, various phrases had been used, reflecting the unpleasant and fearful sensation of dyspnoea. Notable examples include 'short of breath', 'hard to move air', 'not getting enough air', 'tired or fatigue', 'chest tightness', 'sense of filling up' or 'drowning', 'somebody taking the breath away', 'choking', 'panting', and 'gasping', and 'sense of suffocation'.[(4–6)]

Pathophysiology of dyspnoea

Control of breathing

The respiratory rhythm is under the automatic control of the respiratory centre in the medulla, that integrates afferent inputs from the chemoreceptors and other receptors from the airway, lung, and chest wall. The motor outputs of the brainstem can also be influenced by voluntary control from the cerebral cortex, which modifies the breathing pattern of the individual.

Mechanisms of dyspnoea

The possible mechanisms of dyspnoea include: (i) increase afferent input from chemoreceptors and lung receptors, (ii) increase sense of respiratory effort, and (iii) afferent mismatch.

Chemoreceptors

The central chemoreceptors, situated within the medulla, are sensitive to small changes in pH of cerebral spinal fluid resulting from diffusion of carbon dioxide (CO_2) from the blood. The peripheral chemoreceptors are situated on the carotid body and aortic body that respond primarily to changes in PO_2 in the blood, and PCO_2, but to a lesser degree.

Hypoxia and hypercapnia are postulated to be associated with sensations of dyspnoea via central or peripheral chemoreceptors. When patients with COPD were given supplemental oxygen, dyspnoea improved out of proportion to the reduction in ventilation. Thus, the alleviation of dyspnoea could only be partially accounted for by the decrease in ventilation. Hypoxia might be a stimulus for dyspnoea on its own.[7] However, some patients with hypoxia do not have dyspnoea, many patients with dyspnoea are not hypoxic. The role of hypoxia awaits clarification.

For the role of PCO_2, earlier studies showed that hypercapnia did not produce dyspnoea in the absence of respiratory muscle activity. However, in more recent studies on quadriplegic subjects[8] or in volunteers paralyzed by neuromuscular blocker,[9] hypercapnia induced the sensation of dyspnoea. This suggests that dyspnoea induced by hypercapnia occurs independently of any associated increase in respiratory activity. Patients with chronic hypercapnia and metabolic compensation may have little dyspnoea at rest.

The relative potency of hypercapnia and hypoxia as dyspnogenic stimuli remains uncertain.[10]

Upper airway and pulmonary receptors

Mechanoreceptors that reside in the airway, lung, and chest wall may contribute to the control of breathing. There are three groups of lung receptors: (i) the slowly adapting stretch receptors in the airways respond to lung inflation and participate in the termination of inspiration, (ii) the rapidly adapting or irritant receptors in airway epithelium respond to a variety of mechanical and chemical stimuli and mediate bronchoconstriction, and (iii) the C fibres (juxta-pulmonary or J) receptors located in the alveolar wall and blood vessels respond to interstitial congestion. Stimulation of different receptors may occur in different diseases. For example, stimulation of irritant receptors occurs in asthma, stimulation of J receptors occurs in pulmonary oedema, lymphangitis carcinomatosis, pneumonia, and pulmonary embolism. However, the exact role of lung receptors in the pathogenesis of dyspnoea remains uncertain.

Clinical observation suggests that upper airway and facial receptors modify the sensation of dyspnoea. Patients sometimes notice a decrease in dyspnoea when sitting by a fan or open window.[11] There are also mechanoreceptors in the joints, tendons, and muscle of the chest wall that may influence the sensation of dyspnoea.

Sense of respiratory effort

Respiratory muscles play an important role in the mechanism of dyspnoea. When the outgoing motor command is sent to the respiratory muscles, a corollary discharge is sent from the motor cortex or possibly brainstem respiratory centre to the sensory cortex, producing a sense of effort. The sense of effort is related to the ratio of the pressure generated by respiratory muscles to the maximum pressure-generating capacity of the muscles.[10] The sense of respiratory effort increases whenever the central motor command to the respiratory muscles is increased. This occurs when the muscle load is increased, or the muscles are weakened by fatigue, paralysis, or an increase in lung volume. Dyspnoea that can possibly be explained by increased sense of effort include that experienced by patients with obstructive airway diseases (e.g. COPD and asthma) and restrictive lung diseases (e.g. interstitial lung disease and respiratory muscle weakness).

Afferent mismatch

According to the theory of length–tension inappropriateness, there should be an appropriate relationship between the tension in the muscle and the resulting displacement. The sensation of dyspnoea may reflect the detection of displacement that is less than that expected.[12] A study has found that at a given PCO_2, constraining tidal volume and breathing frequency increased dyspnoea. This is in line with the theory of length–tension inappropriateness. Dyspnoea is related to voluntary inhibition of muscle shortening resulting in a displacement less than that expected.[13] The concept of length–tension inappropriateness has been refined to incorporate the general concept of afferent mismatch. It is believed that instead of being directly related to muscular activities, dyspnoea is experienced when there is a mismatch between the outgoing motor command to the respiratory muscles and the incoming afferent information.[10]

Dyspnoea in cancer patients—magnitude of the problem

Dyspnoea occurs commonly in cancer. It is also frequently of enough significant intensity, even towards the end of life, to cause great distress to our patients.

Frequency and intensity of dyspnoea

The prevalence of dyspnoea varies with the site of primary cancers, the stage of the disease, and other factors. The reported prevalence ranges from 19 to 64 per cent in patients with heterogeneous cancers.[14–21] Symptoms that exceed dyspnoea in frequency are pain, anorexia or eating problems, tiredness, and weakness. Dyspnoea of moderate to severe intensity occurs in 19–55 per cent in these patients.

For patients with primary lung cancer, dyspnoea is more common and more severe, when compared with those having heterogeneous cancers.[22–24] The prevalence of dyspnoea is as high as 85 per cent and above for both small-cell lung carcinoma (SCLC) and non-small-cell lung carcinoma (NSCLC) at presentation.[24] Up to 50 per cent of patients with SCLC and 60 per cent with NSCLC suffer from dyspnoea of at least moderate intensity. Though the number and severity of symptoms increase with decreased performance status, dyspnoea remains one of the four commonest symptoms. In another series of lung cancer patients, dyspnoea and cough were the most common and most severe symptoms on presentation, affecting three quarters of all patients, and half of which were of at least moderate intensity.[23] Longitudinal follow up revealed that dyspnoea became more common towards death despite the effort of palliation. In general, dyspnoea and cough were less well palliated than haemoptysis and chest pain. In another study on symptoms of 100 lung cancer patients,[22] dyspnoea of all intensities was found in 70 per cent, that of moderate and severe intensity in 47 per cent, and ranked second among all symptoms.

Multiple factors are found to be related to prevalence and intensity of dyspnoea[14–16,19] (Table 1).

Dyspnoea in the terminal weeks

In the National Hospice Study,[14] the prevalence of dyspnoea increased from 49 to 64 per cent during the last 6 weeks of life. Higginson and McCarthy[25] reported that 15.1 per cent of advanced cancer patients had dyspnoea as the main symptom on referral, and 21 per cent of all patients developed dyspnoea as the main and most severe symptom towards death. Similarly, Conill et al.[26] found that dyspnoea occurred in 39.8 per cent of

Table 1 Factors related to prevalence and intensity of dyspnoea

Prevalence
Site of primary—lung, breast, colorectal(14,15,19)
Metastases to lung or pleura(14,15,19)
Lung irradiation(19)
Past history of cardiac or pulmonary diseases(14,19)
Low performance status(14,19)
Smoking(14,19)
Exposure to asbestos, coal dust, cotton dust, grain dust(19)
Intensity
Lung involvement—primary or secondary(19)
Metastases to mediastinum, hila, ribs(19)
Anxiety(16,37)
Fatigue or tiredness(16)
Vital capacity(16)
Maximum inspiratory pressure (MIP)(16)

advanced cancer patients on presentation, but increased to 46.6 per cent in the last week of life. For the very terminally ill who died within a day after admission into a palliative care unit, Heyse-Moore et al.(15) had noted dyspnoea in over three-quarters of them.

Towards the end of life, or as the functional status of the patient decreases, there is a tendency for dyspnoea to become more problematic in terms of frequency and intensity.(14,15,23,25–27) Mercandante et al.(27) reported that the incidence as well as the intensity of dyspnoea increased progressively as Karnofsky Performance Scale (KPS) fell below 60 and peaked at KPS 30 and 20.

Distress of patients with dyspnoea

Dyspnoea appears to be a symptom of great distress as reported by breathless cancer patients in qualitative studies.(4–6) This is not surprising as two of these studies are performed on lung cancer patients, who often have more severe dyspnoea.(4,6) Breathlessness was often reported as the most troublesome or awful symptom, and perceived as life threatening. Hence, one can appreciate why breathlessness can substantially affect patients' quality of life.

Impact on physical well being

Many other physical symptoms occur together with dyspnoea. When patients suffer from breathlessness, nearly all of them have fatigue as well. Poor concentration, loss of appetite, pain, and loss of memory are present in the majority. Other symptoms include sweating, constipation, nausea, insomnia, voice problem, and difficulty in weight bearing.

Impact on emotional well being

The course of dyspnoea is often chronic and interspersed with severe attacks, which are associated with great emotional impact. As the symptom is perceived as life threatening, anxiety, nervousness, fear, or even panic is commonly reported. Quantitative studies have demonstrated the association of anxiety with the intensity of dyspnoea.(16,37) Other emotions reported include depression, anger, helplessness, and loneliness. Many patients think that they are not supported by staff and have to develop their own strategies to combat this distressing symptom all by themselves.(4,5)

Impact on functional and social well being

Breathlessness is a major barrier to all activities, including that of daily living, inside and outside the house. Simple activities such as eating, bathing, or even answering a phone may be affected. Patients have to slow down, move less, or transfer the activities to others. Majority are socially isolated and unable to enjoy going out or even reading. Sexual life and the usual role in the family cannot be fulfilled. Many patients feel that their future is hopeless, with a strong sense of isolation and dependence.(4–6)

Impact of dyspnoea on survival

Knowing the prognosis in relation to the occurrence of dyspnoea will facilitate the formulation of care plans and help the patient to make an informed choice of management strategies. Many workers had reported positive correlation of dyspnoea with poor survival.(14,15,28–31)

Dyspnoea has been included as one of the factors in prognostic prediction models designed by Pirovano et al.(31) and Morita et al.(30) The palliative prognostic score derived by Pirovano et al.(31) consists of six variables: clinical prediction of survival, KPS, anorexia, dyspnoea, total white blood count, and lymphocyte percentage. The total score can predict the probability of survival at 30 days. Morita et al.(30) reported a prognostic model with a combination of factors of performance status, oedema, dyspnoea at rest, and delirium, which could predict survival for 3 and 6 weeks with a sensitivity of 85 and 79 per cent, and specificity of 84 and 72 per cent, respectively.

The prognosis of acute dyspnoeic cancer patients presenting as a medical emergency is often our concern. In a study of 122 cancer patients who attended an emergency department with dyspnoea, lung cancer patients survived significantly shorter as compared with patients with other cancers.(32) Dyspnoea appeared to be an ominous clinical sign among lung cancer patients and a clinical marker for the terminal phase of their disease. In another report, four risk factors were identified for imminent death in cancer patients presented with acute dyspnoea, and predicted a survival of less than 2 weeks. Rapid respiratory rate above 28/min is one of them.(33)

Classification of dyspnoea in advanced cancer

The causes of dyspnoea in advanced cancer are listed in the flow chart, and they can be classified by the following approaches.

Local cardiopulmonary causes versus systemic causes

Cardiopulmonary causes are the main causes of dyspnoea, and among them parenchymal infiltration and malignant pleural effusion are common. In the National Hospice study(14) on 1754 advanced cancer patients, among those who were dyspnoeic, 39 per cent had lung or pleural involvement; 34 and 24.3 per cent had cardiac and non-malignant respiratory diseases, respectively. In another series of 100 cancer patients presenting with dyspnoea, radiological findings included parenchymal abnormality in 54 per cent, hilar/mediastinal adenopathy in 30 per cent, pleural effusion in 36 per cent, lymphangitis carcinomatosis in 8 per cent, and normal in 9 per cent.(34) Occasionally, paucity in physical and chest radiograph abnormalities may not account for the degree of dyspnoea. This can occur in patients who have major airway obstruction, superior vena cava syndrome, pericardial effusion, lymphangitis carcinomatosis, and pulmonary hypertension.

Systemic causes such as anaemia, ascites, hepatomegaly, and respiratory muscle weakness may occur concomitantly. They should be looked for when there is no apparent cardiopulmonary cause for the dyspnoea, or the degree of dyspnoea is disproportionate to the extent of cardiopulmonary embarrassment. In the National Hospice Study,(14) 23.9 per cent of dyspnoeic patients had neither cardiac nor lung causes identified, and debilitation of cancer had been postulated as the underlying cause.

Malignant versus paramalignant, non-malignant

The local cardiopulmonary causes and the systemic causes can be further classified into cancer-related or non-related causes, which affect the prognosis. Malignant causes are related to the direct effect of cancer, whereas paramalignant causes are due to the indirect effect of tumour (e.g. predisposition to infection and thromboembolism) or related to cancer treatment. In many cancer patients, concomitant medical illnesses such as COPD and heart problems are common.

Classification according to physiological impairment

Dyspnoea can also be classified according to physiological impairment, which may affect dyspnoea management. The physiological parameters concerned include spirometry, maximum inspiratory pressure (MIP), and oxygen saturation.

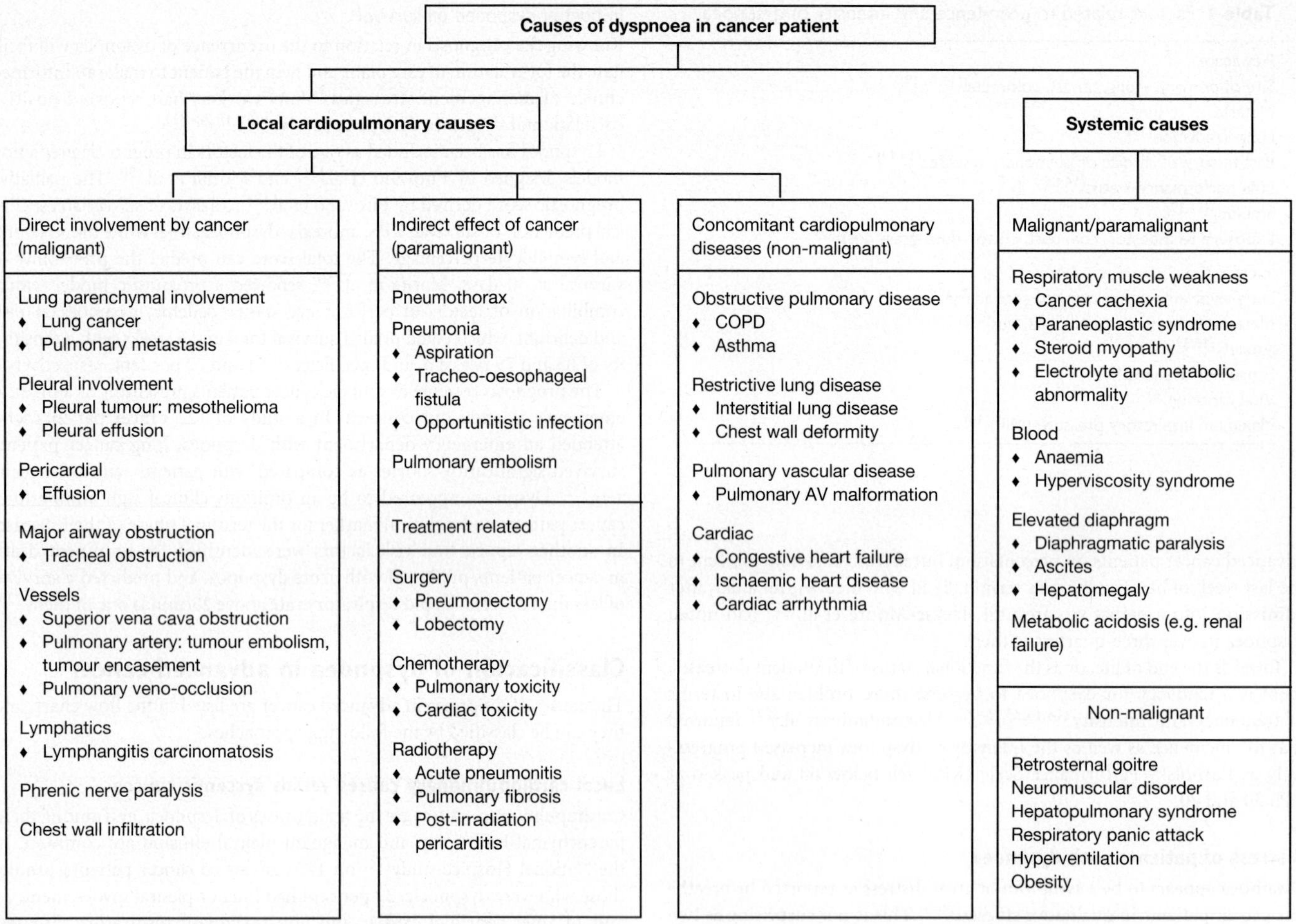

Abnormal lung function pattern is common in cancer patients, and treatable airflow obstruction can be easily missed. In one study, 49 per cent of lung cancer patients were found to have airflow obstruction, which had a strong association with the breathlessness rating. However, only 14.4 per cent of patients received bronchodilator therapy.(35) However, no correlation between dyspnoea and lung function impairment was observed in other studies and the presence of multiple underlying causes may account for the poor correlation.(34,36,37) In these studies, abnormal lung function pattern was reported in a majority of patients, ranging from 75 to 98 per cent, though the relative percentages of different patterns vary quite a lot.

In advanced cancer patients, respiratory muscle weakness may contribute to dyspnoea. The MIP, a measure of the respiratory muscle strength, was lower than normal (mean = -16 cm H_2O) in a group of cancer patients with dyspnoea.(34) In another group of patients with at least moderate dyspnoea, MIP was found to be an independent correlate of intensity of dyspnoea.(16)

Identification of the presence of hypoxia may have an implication on the management of dyspnoea though results from existing studies are conflicting.(38,39) In one study, up to 40 per cent of dyspnoeic patients with cancer were found to be hypoxic.(34) The contribution of correcting hypoxia to the palliation of dyspnoea awaits further studies.

Table 2 Classification of dyspnoea in a cancer patient

Classification	
Local or systemic	Cardiopulmonary Systemic
Casual relationship with tumour	Malignant Paramalignant Non-malignant
Lung function pattern	Obstructive Restrictive Mixed
Oxygen saturation	Hypoxic Non-hypoxic

Example:
A cancer patient with history of COPD and with malignant pleural effusion: the causes of dyspnoea can be classified to be (i) cardiopulmonary (pleural effusion), (ii) malignant in origin, (iii) obstructive impairment from COPD, and restrictive impairment from pleural effusion, and (iv) hypoxic or non-hypoxic, depending on the oximetry or blood gases

Clinical approach to advanced cancer patient with dyspnoea

Before one formulates the care plan for an advanced cancer patient with dyspnoea, the clinical approach comprises (i) identification of all the underlying causes of dyspnoea, including the specific causes or the dyspnoea syndromes, by detailed history taking, physical examination, and selected investigations; and (ii) assessment of the symptom of dyspnoea qualitatively and quantitatively.

Identification of underlying causes of dyspnoea

Elucidation of all the underlying causes of dyspnoea guides its treatment, but this is often limited by the compromised performance status and limited prognosis. A summary of the above approach in classification and its illustration by a clinical example is shown in Table 2.

Multiple causes are commonly present to account for dyspnoea in advanced cancer patients. In one study, patients had a median of five factors contributing to dyspnoea. In that study, 40 per cent were identified as hypoxic, 52 per cent found to have bronchospasm, and 20 per cent anaemia.[34] To optimize results of palliation, one should try to address all underlying causes.

Identifying specific dyspnoea syndromes

It is useful to identify specific causes of dyspnoea. We define these specific causes of dyspnoea as dyspnoea syndromes, as each has its own distinct clinical features, and can be caused by more than one underlying diseases. For each syndrome, there is a specific treatment approach. Major dyspnoea syndromes in cancer, as illustrated in the latter part of the text, include: (i) pleural effusion, (ii) pleural tumour, (iii) pericardial effusion, (iv) major airway obstruction, (v) superior vena cava syndrome, (vi) lymphangitis carcinomatosis, (vii) pulmonary embolism, (viii) respiratory muscle weakness, (ix) chest infection, and other miscellaneous causes.

History, physical examination, and investigation

Elucidation of all the underlying causes relies on good history (Table 3), detailed physical examination (Table 4), and carefully selected investigations.

Investigations

Investigations should be carefully selected to guide specific treatment. First line investigations include haemoglobin level, oxygen saturation by oximetry, and chest radiograph. Oximetry is non-invasive and enables us to

Table 3 History findings in cancer patients with dyspnoea

Smoking	
Occupational exposure	Asbestos, cotton wool
Drug history	Beta blocker, non-steroidal anti-inflammatory drugs (NSAIDs) precipitating heart failure Long-term steroid use causing respiratory muscle weakness
Past anticancer treatment	Chemotherapy agents with cardiopulmonary toxicity Radiation to lung and mediastinum
Concomitant medical illness	COPD, asthma, heart disease, anxiety
Associated respiratory symptoms	Cough, sputum, haemoptysis, wheeze, stridor Pleuritic chest pain (e.g. pleural effusion, pneumothorax, pulmonary embolism) Severe chest wall pain (e.g. tumour invasion, mesothelioma)
Special patterns of dyspnoea	Nocturnal or early morning dyspnoea (e.g. asthma) Orthopnoea, for example congestive heart failure, superior vena cava syndrome, gross ascites, diaphragmatic paralysis and respiratory muscle weakness Platyspnoea, that is, worsening of dyspnoea on sitting up, for example, pulmonary arteriovenous malformation, hepatopulmonary syndrome

Table 4 Physical examination findings in cancer patients with dyspnoea

General examination	Pallor, plethora, cyanosis, engorged neck and upper chest wall veins, leg oedema, cachexia, muscle wasting Retrosternal goitre, tense ascites, hepatomegaly
Respiratory system	
Abnormal chest wall expansion	Localized decreased expansion Wasted accessory respiratory muscle and insucking intercostal muscle (e.g. respiratory muscle weakness)
Abnormal breathing pattern	Prolonged expiration (e.g. COPD) Rapid shallow breathing (e.g. restrictive lung disease) Paradoxical breathing (e.g. upper airway obstruction, respiratory muscle weakness) Hyperventilation (e.g. panic attack) Kussmaul breathing in acidosis
Breath sounds	Stridor or inspiratory noise in major airway obstruction Expiratory wheeze in COPD Silent chest in the presence of severe dyspnoea (e.g. in critical airway stenosis, severe asthma, respiratory muscle weakness)
Cardiac system	
Pulse	Paradoxical pulse (defined by an inspiratory fall of systolic pressure of 10 mmHg or more) in pericardial effusion
Jugular venous pressure	Raised in heart failure, cardiac tamponade, pulmonary embolism, and cor pulmonale
Heart sounds	Gallop rhythm in heart failure Muffled in massive pericardial effusion

Table 5 Chest radiograph interpretation in dyspnoeic cancer patients

Anatomical site	X-ray findings	Possible causes of dyspnoea
Parenchymal	Lung masses	Primary or secondary lung tumours
	Infiltration	Pneumonia
	Collapse consolidation	Major airway obstruction
		Pulmonary embolism
	Reticular shadow	Lymphangitis carcinomatosis
		Radiation-related lung injury
		Chemotherapy-related lung injury
Pleural	Blurring of costophrenic angle	Pleural effusion
	Subpulmonary effusion mimic raised diaphragm	
	Pseudotumour	
	Opacification of whole lung field	
	Pleural base opacity	Pleural tumour
	Pleural calcification	
Trachea and major airway	Deviation	Massive pleural effusion
		Lung collapse
	Narrowing	Endobronchial tumour
		Mediastinal mass, including retrosternal goitre
Mediastinum	Mediastinal shift	Massive pleural effusion
		Lung collapse
	Mediastinal widening	Mediastinal mass, including mediastinal lymphadenopathy
		SVCO
Diaphragm	Elevation	Diaphragmatic paralysis
		Diaphragmatic muscle weakness
		Phrenic nerve paralysis
		Gross hepatomegaly
		Tense ascites
		Subpulmonary effusion
Cardiac shadow	Cardiomegaly	Pericardial effusion
		Congestive heart failure
		Cor pulmonale
Pulmonary vessels	Enlarged pulmonary conus	Pulmonary hypertension
Normal chest radiograph	Pulmonary causes	Major airway obstruction
		SVCO
		Pulmonary embolism
		Lymphangitis carcinomatosis
	General causes	Respiratory muscle weakness
		Anaemia
		Ascites
		Metabolic acidosis
		Hyperventilation
		Obesity

differentiate whether the patient is hypoxic or not. Chest radiograph may be informative in defining specific dyspnoea syndromes (Table 5).

Second line investigations are non-invasive but are more expensive, and may not be available in every palliative care setting. Echocardiogram and Doppler ultrasound will be helpful or even diagnostic in examining the pleura, pericardium, heart, and veins. Though most cases of obstructive airway diseases can be diagnosed by clinical examination, bedside spirometry is often helpful when diagnosis is subtle. A flow volume loop is a simple, fast, and non-invasive investigation to look for upper airway obstruction.

The third line investigations should be considered in highly selected cases, and subject to availability of resource and benefit versus burden analysis. Computerized tomography of thorax or ventilation perfusion scan is indicated if the outcome will be modified by the results. The computerized tomography may be valuable in diagnosing conditions that cannot be confirmed on the chest radiograph, for example, pulmonary embolism, major airway obstruction, superior vena cava obstruction, and lymphangitis carcinomatosis. Bedside MIP can be performed for detection of inspiratory muscle weakness in patients who can cooperate. It should be made more readily available.

Assessment of dyspnoea

Good measurement of dyspnoea remains a challenge to palliative care workers, and will not be possible without an understanding of the nature of the symptom.

Dyspnoea as a multidimensional symptom

Dyspnoea is a subjective and complex sensation that does not correlate consistently with lung function tests.(36) Like other cancer symptoms, dyspnoea is multidimensional. It has long been recognized that measuring a symptom only by its frequency and intensity is far from adequate.(40) Distress is another distinct dimension that has to be addressed, and is one that is most reliable when reported by the patient. The clinical framework for assessing the symptom of dyspnoea, as described in the following section, has also taken into consideration the dimensions that will affect the interpretation of the symptom of dyspnoea by the patient.

Framework for clinical assessment of dyspnoea

Results from various studies including semi-structured interviews of dyspnoeic cancer patients have provided valuable information, and hence insights, on how dyspnoea can be assessed in qualitative terms.[4–6] Inconsistency in knowledge of the staff on dyspnoea, and patients' unwillingness to report their breathlessness because they think professionals will not understand, are barriers to good assessment of dyspnoea. Often dyspnoea is unnoticed by the staff as patients try to limit their activity or stay quiet to cope with dyspnoea.[5]

In order to formulate effective interventional strategy that is individualized for the dyspnoeic patient concerned, listening to the patient's own unique experience and understanding its impact on the patient is an important prerequisite.[6] Any standardized scale for grading dyspnoea cannot be a substitute for this, but may play a role in the quantitative assessment. The recently developed Breathlessness Assessment Guide for assessing dyspnoea and formulating interventional strategies illustrates an example of such guided approach. It has incorporated open-ended questions on various dimensions of the symptom and a modified Medical Research Council dyspnoea scale to measure the functional impairment.[41] The following table (Table 6) suggests the clinical framework for assessing dyspnoea, including the qualitative dimensions and the quantitative assessment of intensity by a measuring scale, for example, visual analogue scale (VAS).

Dyspnoea measuring scales

For purposes of research or measurement of outcome of intervention of dyspnoea, various dyspnoea measuring scales have been employed. In deciding on the scale to be used, one has to define the objective of measurement (e.g. for research, formulation of an intervention strategy, assessment of effectiveness of intervention), and therefore the dimensions that have to be measured. The burden of the test on both the patient and the staff is always an important consideration especially when a battery of scales is employed. Moreover, concomitant symptoms, poor performance status, and emotional distress of facing a demanding test can affect the patient's acceptance of the assessment.[42]

Scales measuring multiple symptoms including dyspnoea

In these global measuring scales, dyspnoea is being measured together with other common cancer symptoms in various dimensions. For example, in the Edmonton Symptom Assessment System (ESAS), nine cancer-related symptoms are reported by patient or by staff.[43] Support Team Assessment Schedule (STAS), is a five-point or seven-point scale that can measure

Table 6 Framework for clinical assessment of dyspnoea in cancer

Past dyspnoea experience	Past history of chronic pulmonary or cardiac diseases History of emergency admissions due to dyspnoea Experience of dyspnoea after the diagnosis of cancer History of frightening experience of dyspnoea
Description of dyspnoea or breathlessness	The sensation is most accurate when self-described by the patient (e.g. 'short of breath', 'difficulty in breathing', 'hard to move air', 'fatigue', 'suffocation', 'not enough air going through', 'tightness', 'filling up or drowning', 'choking', 'taking the breath away from me', 'could be my last breath')
Severity of dyspnoea	Rating scale, e.g., VAS to give the most severe score, least severe score, and average score for most of the time
Precipitating factors for dyspnoea	Physical activities or posture Mechanical factors (e.g. crying and laughing) Environmental factors (e.g. bad weather, pollens, and smoke) Emotional factors (e.g. anxiety, frustration, excitement, and fear)
Trajectory of dyspnoea	Chronic or intermittent Characteristics of each dyspnoeic episode (e.g. initial phase of increasing dyspnoea, plateau phase, declining phase) Duration and frequency of attack, interval between attacks
Concurrent symptoms	Respiratory symptoms (e.g. cough, haemoptysis) General symptoms (e.g. fatigue, loss of concentration, loss of appetite, pain, insomnia, sweating)
Impact on emotional well being	Unpleasant emotions (e.g. anxiety, depression, anger, helplessness, nervousness, fear, loneliness, sense of isolation)
Impact on functional well being	Note the indoor and outdoor activities and ADL that have to be stopped, slow down, modified, or transferred to others
Impact on social well being	Impact on sexual life, performing usual roles, recreational activities, and the degree of isolation
Behavioural coping strategies	Immediate coping strategies to relieve dyspnoea (e.g. positioning, moving more slowly, posture, use of medications, pursed-lip breathing) Long-term adaptive strategies (e.g. decrease, slow down, modification, or advanced planning of activities), home modification, breathing strategy, avoidance of precipitants, improving ventilation, relaxation techniques, diversional activities
Emotional coping strategies	Acceptance, stay calm, avoid being alone, avoid thinking about it, seek support from family

dyspnoea in terms of intensity, frequency, and its interference with activity.[25] Some other scales, such as the Symptom Distress Scale (SDS) and the Rotterdam Symptom Checklist (RSCL), focus on the symptom distress. In SDS, 11 cancer symptoms are being assessed by 13 items.[44] RSCL is a patient-reported instrument that measures physical symptom distress, psychological distress, activity level, and overall quality of life.[45] To address the multidimensionality of cancer symptoms, a multidimensional scale, Memorial Symptom Assessment Scale (MSAS) has been developed. It is a 32-item, patient-reported scale that measures three factors of symptoms, including frequency, severity, and distress of symptoms.[46]

Scales for measuring single symptom of dyspnoea

Some relatively simpler tools can be used for assessing intensity of dyspnoea in isolation, though they can also be applied to other cancer symptoms. For example, VAS has been commonly used for measuring the intensity of dyspnoea. Another scale often used for measuring intensity is the verbal rating scale (e.g. none, mild, moderate, severe) or the Likert-type scale. Application is relatively easy, even in cancer patients who have lost their mobility.

Recently, the Cancer Dyspnoea Scale (CDS) has been validated in lung cancer patients for measuring dyspnoea. It is a 12-item, brief, self-reported scale. Three factors are being measured, including the sense of effort, anxiety, and discomfort. The total dyspnoeic score has good correlation with VAS and Borg Scale. The sensitivity of the scale to changes after intervention was not validated in this study.[47]

There is another group of scales for assessing dyspnoea related to function or activity (Table 7). Most of the instruments are developed for and validated in patients with chronic respiratory diseases, but the shuttle walking test[42] and the reading numbers aloud test have been studied in cancer patients.[48] In these scales, dyspnoea is rated against a specific task or graded exercise, or the functional impairment is being measured. For patients with poor performance status or who are dyspnoeic at rest, these tests may not be applicable, nor sensitive enough to detect the effect of intervention. The effect of coexisting symptoms that also have a limiting effect on the functional activity, for example, pain, cannot be separated out.

Management of dyspnoea syndromes

Malignant pleural effusion

Malignant pleural effusion is often a sign of advanced malignancy. In one autopsy study, malignant effusions were found in 15 per cent of cancer patients.[53] Currently, lung and breast carcinoma account for two-thirds of the primaries in malignant pleural effusion.[57,65] Other common primaries are gastrointestinal tumour, ovarian tumour, and lymphoma. In 5–10 per cent of cases, the primary site of tumour cannot be located.[54] Mesothelioma is however found on the rising trend.[55] Malignant effusion results predominantly from obstruction and disruption of lymphatic channels by malignant cells. Vascular endothelial growth factor, a potent angiogenic mediator and promoter of endothelial permeability, is postulated to play a part in the formation of malignant effusion and local tumour growth.[56]

Pleural effusion in a patient with known malignancy is mostly due to pleural metastases. It can also be due to paramalignant causes, which include the local effect of tumour (e.g. bronchial obstruction with pneumonia or atelectasis, lymphatic obstruction, and venous obstruction as in superior vena cava syndrome) or systemic complications such as pulmonary embolism and hypoalbuminaemia.[57] Non-malignant causes of pleural effusion like congestive heart failure, liver cirrhosis, nephrotic syndrome, and infection such as tuberculosis, can occur concomitantly.

Pleural effusion is not equal to malignant pleural spread. A diagnostic thoracocentesis should be contemplated. In the absence of evidence otherwise, exudative effusion can be assumed to be malignant in patients with disseminated disease. In 5–15 per cent of malignant pleural effusion, it has features of transudation that can be caused by concomitant heart failure, hypoalbuminaemia, lymphatic obstruction, or atelectasis of lung. The majority of paramalignant effusions are transudative except in parapneumonic effusion and post-irradiation pneumonitis.[57]

The chest radiograph can provide useful information. In massive pleural effusion, contralateral mediastinal shift is expected. An ipsilateral mediastinal shift may indicate bronchial obstruction with atelectasis or

Table 7 Dyspnoea measuring scales referring to activities or functional impairment

Instrument	Description
Modified Borg Scale[49]	Self-reported scale, quick and easy to use Assess dyspnoea perception by 12 grades produced at a specific time point after performing a specific task
Baseline Dyspnoea Index (BDI)[50]	Measure dyspnoea in three categories 1. Functional impairment (grade 0–4) 2. Magnitude of task to evoke dyspnoea (grade 0–4) 3. Magnitude of effort to evoke dyspnoea (grade 0–4)
Transitional Dyspnoea Index (TDI)[50]	Measures the change in each of the three categories measured from −3 (major deterioration) to +3 (major improvement) in seven grades
Modified Dyspnoea Index[51]	Modification of BDI and TDI, with enhanced precision of rating and separated scores for home and work settings
Medical Research Council (MRC) dyspnoea scale	Measures the degree to which various activities will stimulate dyspnoea, which is graded in five points
Shuttle Walking Test[42]	The patient walks at a speed provided by an external pacemaker Rated by the measurement of the total distance walked[a]
Oxygen-Cost diagram (OCD)[52]	Measures the level of daily activity at which the dyspnoea is not tolerable using a 100 mm vertical VAS line with descriptive phrases of everyday activities placed at various points, which correspond with the oxygen requirements
Reading Numbers Aloud Test[48]	The patient instructed to read numbers aloud as quickly and as clearly as they can for 60 s, five times Dyspnoea rated by the maximum number of numbers read and the numbers read per breath after five readings[a]

[a] Study on advanced cancer patients.

a trapped lung from pleural encasement. In cases of apparent massive effusion with no mediastinal shift, it may signify mediastinal tumour infiltration or an extensive lung consolidation which mimics pleural effusion.[58] In cases of cardiomegaly, coexisting pericardial effusion has to be ruled out.

Clinical approach to malignant pleural effusion

Malignant pleural effusions can be managed by systemic chemotherapy if the tumour is chemosensitive. Neoplasms that tend to be chemotherapy responsive include breast cancer, SCLC, and lymphoma. Effusions associated with prostate, ovary, thyroid, and germ-cell neoplasm may also be chemotherapy responsive.[57] Otherwise, symptomatic drainage of the fluid becomes the mainstay of treatment. Consider other coexisting conditions that contribute to dyspnoea and treat accordingly, if the dyspnoea cannot be relieved by drainage of pleural fluid.

Prognosis of malignant pleural effusion

The overall prognosis of malignant pleural effusion is generally poor. Most will have a median survival of 3–6 months.[59] Positive correlation factors for survival include type of primary tumour, extent of metastasis, pleural pH,[62] and performance status.[61] Lowering of pleural fluid pH to less than 7.3 and glucose level to less than 3.3 mmol/l may indicate an increased tumour mass and has been suggested as a negative predictor of survival.[62] However, this has not been substantiated by other studies. In a recent meta-analysis of 417 cases by Heffner et al.[59] pleural fluid pH threshold of 7.28 or lesser was found to have the highest independent prediction of survival duration. However, only 24.8, 38.9, and 54.4 per cent of patients who died at 1, 2, and 3 months were classified correctly using pH as predictor. In another study, only KPS was predictive of survival, but not pleural fluid pH, pleural fluid glucose, and extent of pleural carcinomatosis.[61]

Failure of lung expansion—trapped lung syndrome

Failure of full lung expansion may result from bronchial obstruction or trapped lung. Trapped lung is caused by tumour encasement on pleura, creating a vacuum space so that pleural effusion ensues. The properties of the effusion in trapped lung are borderline between a transudate and exudate.[57] Chest radiographs may show an absence of contralateral mediastinal shift with a large effusion. Trapped lung should be suspected when the pleural pressure falls more than 20 cm H_2O per litre of effusion removed.[63] Clinical suspicion arises when a pleural effusion recurs rapidly and requires repeated aspiration. When a lung fails to expand after chest drain insertion in the presence of trapped lung, failure of pleurodesis is an expected outcome.

Symptomatic management of malignant pleural effusion

Factors to be considered in the symptomatic treatment of pleural effusion include: (i) whether or not pleural effusion accounts for the dyspnoea, (ii) whether the pleural effusion is recurrent, (iii) whether the lung is re-expansible, and (iv) whether the patient has a reasonable prognosis. The treatment options include: (i) repeated thoracocentesis, (ii) chemical pleurodesis, (iii) chronic indwelling pleural catheter, and (iv) pleuroperitoneal shunt.

Thoracocentesis

Thoracocentesis should be considered when the patient with pleural effusion has symptoms such as dyspnoea, cough, or chest discomfort. Needle thoracocentesis is usually performed in the hospital setting where supportive facilities are readily available for managing complications such as pneumothorax. The advisable site of thoracocentesis is anterior to the mid-axillary line to avoid pain on lying flat in case local deposits occur. The recommended amount of fluid aspirated will be less than 1–1.5 l so as to prevent re-expansion pulmonary oedema.[57] The finding of contralateral mediastinal shift on chest radiograph may imply significant pressure effect from the effusion. An early aspiration may be helpful in preventing sudden deterioration. In the case of ipsilateral mediastinal shift towards the side of the pleural effusion, which may suggest atelectasis or trapped lung, a therapeutic tapping of less than 300 ml can be tried. Aspiration should be abandoned if there is increasing dyspnoea, chest discomfort, and persistent cough during the procedure. Alternatively, monitoring and keeping the pleural pressure at not less than −20 m H_2O will minimize the risk of re-expansion pulmonary oedema.[57] In case of failure in aspiration, ultrasound can help in localizing a loculated effusion or in identifying organized effusion. Routine chest radiograghs for detecting pneumothorax after needle thoracocentesis may not be required if the procedure is smooth and the patient has no deterioration of symptoms during or after the procedure.[269] The risk of pneumothorax will be minimized if aspiration is performed with a small needle, guided by ultrasound,[270] and with caution if the patient is likely to have trapped lung. If pleurodesis is not contemplated after aspiration, tube thoracostomy should be avoided. If effusion recurs shortly with symptoms, pleurodesis can be considered with tube thoracostomy. In patients with a poor performance or limited prognosis of several weeks, repeated needle aspiration is the preferred option.

Chemical pleurodesis

Chemical pleurodesis should be considered in recurrent malignant pleural effusion if the following conditions are satisfied:

- relief of dyspnoea after thoracocentesis,
- full lung expansion after tube thoracostomy, and
- satisfactory performance status and prognosis of the patient.[63]

Many workers would only consider pleurodesis if the estimated survival is longer than a month.

Low pleural fluid pH of less than 7.2 had been used as a guide to predict the failure of pleurodesis. However, a recent meta-analysis of 417 cases revealed that pleural fluid pH was a weak predictor of successful pleurodesis.[60] In this series, 65 per cent of patients in the lowest quartile of pH (6.7–7.26) had successful pleurodesis compared to 88 per cent of patient who had a pH of 7.27 or more.

Many sclerosing agents have been used for chemical pleurodesis, including antibiotics, antineoplastics, biological response modifiers (e.g. interferon, *Corynebacterium parvum*), and others. The choice of agent depends on its efficacy, accessibility, safety, ease of administration, and cost.[64] Currently, the most common agents used are the tetracycline group, bleomycin, and talc.[65] Walker-Renard et al. reviewed chemical pleurodesis from 1966 to 1992, in 1168 patients treated with these agents.[66] The overall success rate, as defined by non-recurrence of effusion on clinical examination or chest radiograph, was 93 per cent in talc (153 in 165), 67 in tetracycline (240 in 359), 72 in doxycyline (43 in 60), and 54 in bleomycin (108 in 199). The success rate with non-antineoplastic fibrotic agents was higher than that with an antineoplastic agent (75 versus 44 per cent).[66] Other studies have also reported the high success rate of talc, from 80 to more than 90 per cent.[57,65] However, prospective controlled studies comparing the efficacy of different agents have shown inconsistent results (Table 8).

The most common side effects reported were chest pain and fever. Chest pain was reported in 7, 40, 14, and 28 per cent, and fever in 16, 31, 19, and 24 per cent of talc, doxycycline, tetracycline, and bleomycin pleurodesis, respectively.[66] Tetracycline is not commercially available now, and is substituted by doxycycline and minocycline. The commonly prescribed dosage was 500 mg for doxycyline, 60 units for bleomycin, and not more than 5 g for talc.[57] The main concerns for bleomycin are cost and side effects from systemic absorption. Talc has the advantage of low cost and high efficacy. Talc slurry by tube thoracostomy, which has a similar efficacy as thoracoscopic talc poudrage,[67] is a favourable choice in advanced cancer patients. However, adult respiratory distress syndrome (ARDS) has been reported in a small number of patients with the use of talc, an uncommon but potentially fatal side effect.[68] Most cases of ARDS have been associated with the doses in excess of 5 g of talc.[65] Preparation of talc should fulfill the requirement of sterilization, particle size, and being asbestos free.[70] More ideal agents

Table 8 Randomized controlled studies of chemical pleurodesis in malignant pleural effusion

Author	Agents	No. of patients studied	Success rate At 30 days	At 90 days
Ruckdeshel et al., 1991[71,72]	Ble/Tet	74	Ble: 64% Tet: 33% P = 0.023	Ble: 70% Tet: 47% P = 0.047
Hartman et al., 1993[73]	Talc powder Ble/Tet	106	Tal: 97% Ble: 64% Tet: 33% All P < 0.05	Tal: 95% Ble: 70% Tet: 47% All P < 0.05
Emad and Rezaicen, 1996[74]	Tet vs Ble vs Ble + Tet	57	Tet: 90% Ble: 60% Tet + Ble: 95% P = 0.06	Tet: 68% Ble: 47% Tet + Ble: 95% P = 0.006
Diacron et al., 2000[75]	Ble/Talc powder	31	Ble: 59% Tal P: 87% P = 0.12	Ble: 41% Tal: 87% P = 0.01
Studies with no significant difference detected between agents investigated				
Yim et al., 1996[67]	Talc slurry/Talc powder	57	Tal S: 89% Tal P: 96% (NS)	
Zimmer et al., 1997[76]	Ble/Talc slurry	29	B: 79% Tal S: 90% (NS)	
Noppen et al., 1997[77]	Ble/Talc slurry	26	B: 75% Tal S: 78.6% (NS)	
Martinez-Moragon et al., 1997[78]	Ble/Tet	62	Ble: 45% Tet: 52%(NS)	
Patz et al., 1998[79]	Ble/Dox (small-bore catheter)	29	Ble: 72% Dox: 79% (NS)	
Ong, 2000[80]	Ble/Talc slurry	38	B: 70% Tal S: 89% (NS)	

Ble, bleomycin; Tet, tetracycline; Tal S, talc slurry; Tal P, talc powder; Dox, doxycyline.

such as silver nitrate are being explored for future use.[69] The current recommended agent for pleurodesis is therefore either talc slurry, a drug of the tetracycline group, or talc poudrage, depending on local availability of agents, thoracoscopy service,[65] and the patient's general condition.

Smaller bore size intercostal tubes were shown to be equally effective as conventional large-bore tubes in several non-controlled studies[57] and a randomized study.[81] Radiological confirmation of complete re-expansion is a prerequisite for pleurodesis. The sclerosing agent of choice is added to 50–100 ml of sterile normal saline. The chest drain is clamped for 1 h, and then subsequently reconnected to 20 cm H_2O suction. Suction is applied until the 24-h output is less than 150 ml.[57] Rotation of the patient following intrapleural administration of sclerosing agent is no longer considered necessary, as the agent is dispersed throughout the pleural space within seconds as demonstrated by radiolabelled tetracycline. Adequate analgesics should be given parentally or intrapleurally to minimize the pleuritic chest pain that occurs during pleurodesis.

When chemical pleurodesis fails

Chemical pleurodesis may fail resulting in recurrent pleural effusion. If trapped lung is excluded, a second pleurodesis performed by either talc slurry or thoracoscopic talc poudrage is an option. A chronic indwelling pleural catheter has been demonstrated in a randomized study to be equally effective as doxycyline pleurodesis.[82] The catheter can be managed in the out-patient setting with shortened hospitalization. It is also a convenient and effective means for providing symptomatic relief for trapped lung.[83] Pleuroperitoneal shunt had been performed in a large series of 160 patients with trapped lung and recurrent effusion.[84] No intraoperative mortality was reported and median survival was 7.7 months. Repeat thoracocentesis would be the choice for a patient with short expected survival.

Pleural tumour—mesothelioma

Managing patients with malignant mesothelioma presents multiple challenges for the health care team. Until the emergence of a new breakthrough in treatment, it is uniformly a fatal disease with poor response to treatment. More patients are expected to die from malignant mesothelioma in the coming years, as a delayed effect occurs decades after exposure to asbestos. Moreover, the clinical course tends to be accompanied by physical symptoms that are difficult to manage, and there are complex psychosocial factors that are related to the occupational nature of the disease.

Malignant mesothelioma is inexorably progressive except in the few patients who have undergone curative surgery. The median survival reported ranged from 8 to 14 months.[85] Its propensity to infiltrate the neighbouring structures, especially the lung, diaphragm, chest wall, and mediastinum renders complete resection impossible. Malignant mesothelioma is relatively resistant to radiotherapy. Until now, there has been no randomized trial comparing survival or symptom control in patients treated with chemotherapy or best supportive care. Palliative care remains the most important component of care.

A history of exposure to asbestos can be obtained in about 87 per cent of cases in United Kingdom.[86] In subjects heavily exposed to asbestos early in their working life, more than one in 10 may die of mesothelioma.[85] Projections suggests that the number of men dying from mesothelioma in

Western Europe each year will increase in the next 20 years, from 5000 in 1998 to about 9000 in 2018, and then decline. Over the next 35 years, there will be a total of a quarter of a million people dying from the disease in Europe.(55) Men born around 1945–1950 in European countries and in the late 1920s in America will have the highest risk. In the United States, approximately 3000 patients die of mesothelioma each year, as many as from Hodgkin's disease.(87)

Management of dyspnoea in malignant mesothelioma

Most patients with malignant mesothelioma require symptom palliation from the time of diagnosis onwards. The most common symptoms are dyspnoea, chest pain, and cough. Dyspnoea is often due to multiple causes that include:

1. pleural effusion which occurs in 95 per cent of patients and at an earlier stage of disease,
2. pleural encasement which causes restrictive lung or trapped lung in severe cases,
3. cardiac tamponade caused by pericardial involvement,
4. mediastinal structure invasion, for example, superior vena cava, pulmonary vessels encroachment,
5. pulmonary fibrosis from asbestos exposure, and
6. cardiopulmonary diseases among patients who are chronic smokers.

Pleural effusion becomes a key management issue for the majority of patients. Early pleurodesis, either by a medical or surgical approach, is preferable to repeated thoracocentesis for inoperable patients.(85) Various chemical agents had been used for pleurodesis. When using talc poudrage by thoracoscopy, the response rate of 78.8 per cent at 1 month was reported in 88 patients.(88) Another study of 117 patients showed a response rate of 81 per cent for oxytetracycline and 86.2 per cent for *Corynebacterium parvum*.(89)

Thoracoscopic pleurectomy could be performed within a short operating time for control of pleural effusion provided trapped lung and heavily diseased visceral pleura were absent.(90) Pleuroperitoneal shunt had been performed for cases with trapped lung.(91) In the largest series, 36 cases of mesothelioma with trapped lung had undergone this procedure with a median survival of 10.1 months.(84) Common complications reported were shunt occlusion and infection. A chronic indwelling catheter had been used in mesothelioma with recurrent pleural effusion.(82,83) Stenting is preferable to radiotherapy for superior vena cava obstruction as the response to radiotherapy is poor.(85) Radiotherapy is seldom useful in the control of dyspnoea.(85) Prophylactic radiotherapy has a role in prevention of local chest wall deposits after needle aspiration or biopsy.

Malignant pericardial effusion and cardiac tamponade

The clinical diagnosis of malignant pericardial effusion is now facilitated with an echocardiogram. Most result from malignant spread in the advanced stage. Lung cancer is the most common primary, accounting for one-third or more of the cases at autopsy and in clinical studies.(92–95) Breast cancer is the second commonest, other common primaries are leukaemia and lymphoma. Melanoma also has a high propensity for metastases to the heart. Adenocarcinoma is the most common cell type, followed by squamous cell carcinoma.(93)

Other causes are related to cancer treatment, including irradiation to mediastinum or to the thyroid, chemotherapy with anthracycline drugs, and immunosuppression predisposing to infective pericarditis. In idiopathic cases, the underlying cause cannot be found.(96) However, as the gross appearance and biochemistry of the pericardial fluid are not diagnostic, malignancy cannot be excluded by a negative biopsy and cytology.

Diagnosing cardiac tamponade

Heightening the index of suspicion is crucial to early diagnosis. Helpful points are

1. awareness of the common primary tumours involved,
2. getting a good history of previous cancer therapy,
3. looking specifically for signs of cardiac tamponade that may be subtle, and
4. watching for cardiomegaly in chest radiograph which may be obscured by concomitant pleural effusion which is present in about two-thirds of the cases with pericardial effusion.(94,97)

To confirm the diagnosis, echocardiogram is the investigation of choice.

Management of pericardial effusion and cardiac tamponade

There is no consensus on the best modality of treatment for malignant pericardial effusion as there is a lack of randomized controlled trials comparing different approaches. Despite this limitation, the following can serve as guidelines:

1. If possible, pericardial fluid should be drained promptly to relief the symptoms.
2. Prevention of recurrence is indicated unless the patient has a very short lifespan.
3. Availability of resources and local preferences affect the choice of treatment.

A medical approach, that is, pericardiocenteses and sclerosis, is favoured as a safer procedure in the ill patients by some who only use surgical procedure for rescue purpose; and the surgical approach is favoured by others because of better results in long-term control.

Pericardiocentesis and sclerosis

Pericardiocentesis gives prompt relief of symptoms, but recurrence is common if sclerosis is not performed.(98) Tetracycline prevented recurrence in three-quarters of the cases.(94) Now other agents such as doxycycline and minocycline have been used as substitutes as tetracycline is no longer commercially available. Pain during the procedure is a problem, other complications being arrhythmia, fever, pericardial rub, and catheter blockade.(94,97) Bleomycin, when compared with doxycycline in a controlled trial, gave equally good results, and pain was not a problem.(97) Many other chemotherapeutic agents have been reported to be effective in small studies or as case reports.

Surgical procedures under local anaesthesia

These include subxiphoid pericardiotomy and percutaneous balloon pericardiotomy. Subxiphoid pericardiotomy gives good immediate relief, and provides long-term control in over 90 per cent of cases. It provides a chance for pericardial biopsy and examination, with low operative morbidity and mortality.(95,96) In percutaneous balloon pericardiotomy, the balloon is introduced with a guide wire and inflated to tear the pericardium, so that fluid can drain into pleural cavity.(99)

Surgical procedures under general anaesthesia

These procedures require the patient to be haemodynamically stable, and therefore not suitable for rapid relief. Rigid pericardioscopy has been performed via the subxyphoid route for drainage, cleansing, exploration, and obtaining an adequate biopsy.(100) Video-assisted thoracoscopy has been employed for patients with coexisting pleural or lung pathology.(101) Other procedures such as pleuropericardiotomy and pericardectomy are major operations.

Superior vena cava obstruction

Superior vena cava obstruction (SVCO) is a condition in which venous return of blood from the head, upper limb, and thorax to the right atrium is interrupted by obstruction of the SVC, which is situated in a confined space in the superior mediastinum. About 90 per cent of cases are due to tumours. Bronchogenic carcinoma is the commonest primary responsible, with small cell being the leading histology, accounting for 40 per cent of cases caused by lung cancer.(102) Non-Hodgkin's lymphoma is the second most common primary. Metastates are most commonly from breast cancer. SVCO can also be due to paramalignant causes such as prolonged central venous line insertion for chemotherapy and radiotherapy to the thorax. Other non-malignant causes include fibrosing mediastinitis associated with histoplasmosis and cardiac pacemaker.

SVCO can result from direct luminal occlusion by tumour, external compression, fibrosis, or thrombosis (e.g. due to partial obstruction by tumour, presence of nidus such as venous catheter, pacemaker wire).(103)

Several collateral systems are interconnected, with the azygos–hemiazygos system being the main collateral pathway. Greater degrees of collateral development occur with greater extent of obstruction and concomitant occlusion of the azygos system.(104) The severity of clinical features also depends on the speed of obstruction. The clinical signs and symptoms are the net effect of the venous hypertension, the impairment of venous circulation, the development of venous collaterals, and the underlying pathology.(104) The patient may complain of dyspnoea, cough, orthopnoea, facial oedema, headache, and dizziness. A florid picture may include facial and arm swelling, neck vein distention, upper body plethora, glossal oedema, and cerebral oedema. The features may be alarming and distressing to the patient, but the syndrome itself is seldom life-threatening. However, when the pathology causing SVCO is also compressing the trachea, there is a potential threat of major airway obstruction.(102,104,105)

Investigations

Chest radiography may show widening of the superior mediastinum and associated pulmonary lesions, and pleural effusion.(106) Pleural effusion is present in about one-quarter of patients due to thoracic lymphatic obstruction and venous hypertension.(106) Contrast-enhanced computed tomography provide detailed information on the location and extent of occlusion of SVCO, the mechanism of obstruction, the collateral development, and guidance for planning of radiotherapy.(104) Venography is useful in revealing intraluminal thrombus and collateral formation, and for decision-making on interventions like bypass surgery, angioplasty, stent insertion, and/or thrombolysis.(104,107) Other investigations that could be performed depend on local availability of resources, for example, MRI and nuclear venography.

Obtaining the diagnosis or histology before treatment is important if this is not yet available, as this affects the choice of treatment. SVCO is seldom an emergency or life-threatening condition,(102,103,105,108) and investigations can be carried out without serious complications or increased mortality.(102,103,108)

Treatment

The objective of treatment of SVCO is to relieve the symptoms by reducing the obstruction, which may be mediated or accompanied by reduction in tumour mass. Radiotherapy or chemotherapy is most commonly used, depending on histology. Stent insertion has also emerged as an effective intervention for rapid relief of symptoms. Surgical bypass is uncommonly used for cancer patients. For patients with documented thrombus, it can be lysed or removed by thrombolytic therapy, using streptokinase or urokinase, or by thrombectomy.(109) In some patients, eventual collateral development may bring about symptom relief in those without regaining patency of SVC.(102)

General measures can be initiated before specific treatment. These include propping up the patient, diuretic, and steroid therapy. Dexamethasone at a daily dose of 16 mg can be given, and then gradually tapered. It is advisable to avoid the SVC drainage field in giving subcutaneous injections or infusions.

Radiotherapy is often the treatment of choice when the tumour is not chemosensitive. In one study,(106) radiotherapy as primary treatment for SVCO provided excellent and good relief in 70 per cent of patients with bronchogenic carcinoma and in 95 per cent of patients with lymphoma. In one retrospective review of 125 patients,(110) most patients showed good symptomatic response to radiotherapy alone. Good symptomatic response was reported in 50 per cent, with an excellent or complete response in 15–23 per cent of bronchogenic carcinoma. For lymphoma, good to excellent symptomatic response was reported in more than 90 per cent of patients.(110) Radiotherapy is generally well tolerated, with dysphagia from oesophagitis as the main side effect.(106,110)

Chemotherapy is particularly effective for chemosensitive tumours like small cell tumour of the lung and lymphoma. In SCLC, chemotherapy with or without radiotherapy has produced excellent palliation. In one retrospective study on 724 SCLC patients, of which 87 had SVCO, intensive chemotherapy had given complete or partial symptomatic response in 81 per cent of patients.(108) Non-Hodgkin's lymphoma causing SVCO may respond to both chemotherapy and radiotherapy.

Stent insertion has emerged as an effective method for relief of SVCO. Stenting has a role when SVCO is unresolved or recurs after radiotherapy and chemotherapy. Its role as the first line treatment for SVCO has not been established as there has been no prospective controlled trial to compare this with other conventional modalities. Arguments favouring the use of stents include rapid relief of symptoms and no interference with subsequent chemotherapy or radiotherapy.(111,112) Recurrence of symptoms can occur with tumour invasion or thrombosis, and can be dealt with by repeated stenting, thrombolysis, clot aspiration through venous catheter, or balloon dilatation.(113) The use of anticoagulation with and after the procedure is not standard. Other assistive procedures have been performed before stenting, for example, lysis of thrombus and balloon dilatation for tight stenosis.(107)

Studies have demonstrated that SCLC patients with SVCO did not have a shorter survival compared with those without SVCO. Urban et al.(108) reported the median survival to be 42 and 40 weeks for those with and without SVCO, respectively. The survival is, in fact, closely related to that of the underlying cancer. Patients with lymphoma and breast cancer survive longer than those with lung cancer.(102)

Major airway obstruction

Major airway obstruction is defined here as airway obstruction from the level of the larynx to the level of the lobar bronchi. It can be a life-threatening cause of dyspnoea, but is potentially reversible. It can present as acute respiratory distress or even asphyxiation, or insidiously masquerade as asthma or COPD.

Causes of major airway obstruction

In advanced cancer patients, major airway obstruction often results from occlusion by endoluminal tumours (e.g. bronchogenic carcinoma and carcinoid tumour) or due to extrinsic compression by tumours or mediastinal masses. Narrowing of the airway can also result from bilateral vocal cord paralysis or a stricture as a complication of endobronchial intubation, brachytherapy, or tracheostomy. Non-malignant causes of airway obstruction include displacement of tracheostomy tube or stent, retention of sputum, foreign body, Ludwig's angina, retrosternal goitre, and angioneurotic oedema.

Clinical features

The most common presentations of major airway obstruction include dyspnoea, cough, obstructive pneumonia, and haemoptysis. The following features may suggest the presence of upper airway obstruction:

1. inspiratory noise or stridor,
2. worsening of dyspnoea in the recumbent position,
3. dyspnoea with paradoxical breathing pattern,
4. wheeze not responding to bronchodilators,
5. lung collapse, and
6. persistent cough or haemoptysis with normal chest radiograph.

A high kV chest radiograph can show up tracheal narrowing, while a lung function test may reveal a truncated inspiratory or expiratory flow volume loop. Computerized tomography of the thorax can confirm the diagnosis and determine the nature of obstruction. In cases of life-threatening dyspnoea, an emergency bronchoscopic examination can provide a rapid diagnosis.

Management

The management of major airway obstruction in advanced cancer patients depends on the underlying mechanism of obstruction and the patient's performance status. Simple causes such as sputum retention in airway stent or kinking of a tracheostomy tube should be ruled out. In acute situations, endobronchial lesions can be treated by rigid bronchoscopic debulking, laser therapy, and electrocautery, and extrinsic compression by stenting. In sub-acute cases, other endoluminal therapies like cryotherapy, brachytherapy, and photodynamic therapy, which require longer time to take effect, can be considered; and for extrinsic compression, external irradiation or brachytherapy are alternatives to stenting.[114] The median survival of patients receiving different endobronchial modalities is similar, and in the range of 4–6 months.[247] If the patient's condition precludes therapeutic bronchoscopy, external irradiation can be a choice. Steroids may temporarily decrease the dyspnoea.

Interventional bronchoscopic procedures

Laser is commonly performed to relieve obstruction due to endoluminal lesion. It provides rapid relief, and can be repeated if indicated. The neodynium-yttrium aluminium garnet (Nd-YAG) laser is most commonly used for tracheobronchial lesions. Contraindications include extrinsic obstruction, coagulation disorders, tumour invading or close to a major vessel. The success rate reported in several large series is approximately 80 per cent. In a large series of 1838 patients with bronchogenic carcinoma, immediate patency of the airway was achieved in 93 per cent.[115] For long-standing bronchial obstruction of more than 4–6 weeks, re-expansion of the involved lung is unlikely. It is a safe procedure in expert hands, with low morbidity and mortality.[115] Complications include bleeding and tissue perforation. Electrocautery was reported as a cheaper alternative to laser in some cases and may gain popularity in future.[116]

The main indication for cryotherapy in advanced cancer is relief of obstruction due to endoluminal tumours, and is reported to be effective in 60 per cent.[117,118] When compared with laser, it may be safer for distal lesions because of the lower risk of perforation, and is usually well tolerated. However, its effect is not immediate. Two or more treatments are often needed.[119]

Endobronchial stents are used mainly for extrinsic compression involving trachea, carina, and main bronchus.[115] The rate of symptom relief rate is high, ranging between 78 and 98 per cent.[114] It can be used with the combination of other bronchoscopic procedures such as laser or brachytherapy. There are two main types of endobronchial stents in use today: the tube silicone stent and the expandable metallic stent. Potential complications of silicone stents include stent migration, formation of granulation tissue, and inspissation of secretion. Metallic stents are fairly expensive and formation of granulation tissue is common at both ends of the stent.[114]

Radiotherapy

Radiotherapy is commonly employed for symptom palliation for dyspnoea, cough, haemoptysis, and obstructive pneumonia as caused by major airway tumours.

In two studies by the Medical Research Council in the United Kingdom,[120,121] patients with untreated, symptomatic, inoperable NSCLC were randomized to receive radiation at different fractionations and dosages. The recommended regimen for palliation was two fractions of 8.5 Gy delivered 1 week apart; and for those with poor performance status, a single fraction of 10 Gy.[121] Success of palliation was reported to be 48–65 per cent for cough, 72–86 per cent for haemoptysis, and 59–80 per cent for chest pain.[120,121]

Brachytherapy, as given via a fibreoptic bronchoscope, has the advantage of limiting the radiation to the tumour tissue, and may be repeated in case of tumour recurrence or initiated after failure of conventional therapy. Good palliation is achieved in 88–99 per cent of haemoptysis and 60–87 per cent for dyspnoea. Cough is less well controlled, with improvement in only 30–85 per cent.[122–124]

Brachytherapy can be given alone or in combination with external irradiation, laser therapy, or cryotherapy. Brachytherapy given after laser or cryotherapy may prolong survival compared with laser or cryotherapy alone.[125] A randomized controlled study was performed comparing external irradiation (30 or 60 Gy) with external irradiation plus endobronchial brachytherapy (two fractions of 7.5 Gy) in inoperable NSCLC.[126] The combined treatment group had a higher rate of re-expansion of collapsed lung from main bronchus obstruction, but there was no statistical difference in the response rate for dyspnoea, cough, haemoptysis, and chest pain.

Recently, the first United Kingdom randomized trial comparing endobronchial brachytherapy (15 Gy) and external irradiation (30 Gy over 10–12 days) in the palliative treatment of inoperable NSCLC was published.[127] There was no significant difference between the brachytherapy and external irradiation in the palliation of major symptoms as assessed at 8 weeks; dyspnoea was relieved in 38 and 49 per cent, cough was relieved in 45 and 65 per cent, and haemoptysis was relieved in 71 and 90 per cent, respectively. However, external beam irradiation provided better overall and more sustained palliation with fewer retreatments and a modest gain in survival time.

The most common complications of endobronchial brachytherapy are radiation bronchitis and bronchial stenosis.[122] Fatal haemoptysis was reported after brachytherapy in up to 50 per cent in a small series.[128] However, a recent review of 2842 patients revealed that the mean rate of fatal haemoptysis was 10.3 per cent[122] which is similar to the rate of fatal haemoptysis from central lung cancer, regardless of treatment. The two randomized controlled studies by Stout et al.[127] and Langendijk et al.[126] also showed no statistically significant difference in fatal haemorrhage rate after external irradiation compared with that after brachytherapy.

Pulmonary lymphangitis carcinomatosis

Pulmonary lymphangitis carcinomatosis is characterized by diffuse involvement of pulmonary lymphatics with tumour thrombi,[129] which may be due to tumour microembolization or retrograde spread from involved lymph nodes. Lymphangitis carcinomatosis may also be a late manifestation of pulmonary arterial tumour embolism, with secondary invasion of the lymphatics. The clinical and radiological features of pulmonary arterial tumour embolism and lymphangitis carcinomatosis are similar. Pulmonary hypertension has also been reported, and is thought to be due to obliteration and compression of the pulmonary vasculature by adjacent lymphatics.[130]

Approximately 6–8 per cent of patients with pulmonary metastases develop lymphangitis carcinomatosis. The commonest histological type is adenocarcinoma. The site of primary can be in the lung, breast, and others. Patients with lymphangitis carcinomatosis usually have a poor prognosis, and less than half of the patients survived 3 months in a review.[131]

Clinical features

Symptoms and signs can be non-specific. Patients can present with exertional dyspnoea, cough, fever, chills, night sweats, chest pain, and haemoptysis.

On examination, patients may be tachypnoeic, tachycardiac, and cyanotic with non-specific chest signs.

Chest radiographic changes are variable, though typically described as widespread linear, micronodular (less than 3 mm), or reticulonodular interstitial infiltrates. Larger nodules (up to 1 cm) may also be present.(132) Many other features are reported, and they are either non-specific or may mimic other cardiopulmonary conditions. These findings include Kerley A and B lines, hilar lymphadenopathy, thickening of fissures, perihilar haze, consolidation, reduced lung volume, or a miliary pattern.(129)

High-resolution computerized tomography is helpful in differentiating lymphangitis carcinomatosis from other interstitial lung diseases. The typical feature is a polygonal pattern with beading or nodular interstitial thickening and uneven thickening of the bronchovascular bundle. Among patients with lymphangitis carcinomatosis, computerized tomography scan diagnosis has been reported to be correct in 85 per cent. Whether this may obviate the need for confirmation with a biopsy is still controversial.(129)

Treatment

For most patients, dyspnoea is a predominant symptom and symptomatic treatment is required. Corticosteroids have been shown to produce transient subjective improvement in anecdotal reports.(130,131) A reported starting dosage of dexamethasone is 8–12 mg/day.(133)

Specific oncological treatment with chemotherapy has been tried with success in patients with tumours sensitive to these treatments, such as carcinoma of breast and ovary.(132) Hormonal therapy with bilateral orchidectomy, oestrogen, or aminoglutethimide has induced remission and improved symptoms, radiographic appearance, and lung functions of patients with carcinoma of prostate with lymphangitis carcinomatosis.(131)

Pulmonary embolism in cancer patients (see Chapter 8.6)

Cancer patients are prone to develop venous thromboembolism for various reasons.(134) Firstly, venous stasis can result from immoblization or compression by tumours. Secondly, tumour cells are known to express procoagulants, and host tissues also express procoagulant activities in response to tumour.(134) Liver dysfunction as in massive involvement by tumour can result in decreased clearance of activated coagulation factors. Thirdly, cancer treatment can increase thrombotic tendency. These include administration of antineoplastic agents or hormonal agents (tamoxifen, steroid), radiotherapy, surgery, bone marrow transplantation, and placement of central catheter.(134,135)

Reported clinical incidence of deep vein thrombosis (DVT) and pulmonary embolism (PE) in cancer ranges from 1 to 15 per cent, and even higher in autopsies.(134,135) Thrombotic events are most common in mucin-producing tumours of gastrointestinal tract. Others are lung, breast, ovary, and primary brain tumours. Because of the high prevalence of lung cancer, it is the tumour most commonly associated with clinical thromboembolic events.(134)

Diagnosing PE

PE is often underdiagnosed in clinical settings. Investigations performed in cancer patients will be the same as those in the non-cancer group,(135) though in palliative care setting, the extent of investigations is often limited by the consideration of the burden of the tests and the life expectancy of the patient.

Basic tests that should be performed include blood gases, electrocardiography, and chest radiography. They are poor at specific diagnosis of PE, but can help to exclude other diagnoses.(136) The PIOPED investigators found that in 383 patients with PE, 12 per cent had normal CXR. Findings were non-specific, with atelectasis being the commonest. Others were prominent central markings, pleural effusion, oligaemia, enlarged hilum, and raised hemidiaphragm.(137)

Specific investigations aimed at supporting or refuting a diagnosis of PE include ventilation/perfusion (V/Q) scan, echocardiogram, pulmonary angiogram, spiral computed tomography, and magnetic resonance imaging. Tests for confirming DVT may help by inferring presence of PE in suspected patients—compression or colour flow Doppler ultrasonography, ascending contrast venography, and radioisotope studies.(136) However, compression ultrasonogram may be misleading in patients with inguinal masses.(135)

As for the V/Q scan, a normal scan is helpful in excluding PE, whereas a high probability scan is indicative of PE.(138) However, when the scan is indeterminate or low probability but the clinical condition is highly suspicious, other investigations such as spiral computed tomography or pulmonary angiogram are indicated.(136) In cancer patients, lung tumour compressing on pulmonary vessels may mimic PE on V/Q scan.(135)

Spiral computed tomography emerges as a sensitive, specific, and non-invasive test for diagnosing PE,(139) and for confirming diagnosis in those with indeterminate V/Q scan.(136) Its accuracy is lower for peripheral emboli. Whether spiral computed tomography can replace V/Q scan remains to be determined.(139) Pulmonary angiogram is the reference standard but is invasive.(136)

Management of pulmonary embolism in cancer

In patients with incurable cancer, the decision whether to treat with anticoagulation is a difficult one. A survey among United Kingdom palliative physicians showed that 98 per cent of them would consider anticoagulation if considered approriate.(140) Careful weighing of risks and benefits is important in individual cases. Though anticoagulation may improve symptoms and prolong life, it may bring discomfort and sufferings like the burden of injections, blood taking, and bleeding. When PE occurs near the end of life, symptomatic treatment of dyspnoea, pain, and cough may be the most appropriate.

Anticoagulation treatment

This includes initial heparinization with unfractionated heparin (UFH) or low molecular weight heparin (LMWH) in the acute stage, followed by maintenance anticoagulation. This is the standard treatment for patients who are not severely haemodynamically compromised or after thrombolysis.(141) Before anticoagulation, a baseline platelet count, partial thromboplastin time (aPTT) and prothrombin time (PT) should be checked. UFH can be given by intravenous infusion at a body weight-based dosage or subcutaneously. The dose of UFH is adjusted to prolong the aPTT to a range that corresponds to a plasma concentration of 0.2–0.4 U/ml by protamine titration, or at 1.5–2.5 times the pretreatment value.(141)

UFH is being progressively replaced by LMWH nowadays, which is as effective and safe as UFH in the treatment of acute pulmonary embolism.(142) LMWH has better bioavailability, more predictable anticoagulant response, and less complications like bleeding, osteoporosis, and thrombocytopaenia.(143) It has a longer duration of action and some can be given subcutaneously once a day. Moreover, it is given at a dose adjusted to body weight and monitoring is normally not needed, except for patients with renal failure or with morbid obesity.(143) These advantages reduce the burden of treatment in our cancer patients.

For maintenance therapy, anticoagulation is switched to warfarin after at least 5 days of UFH or LMWH, even when the target International normalized ratio (INR) is reached earlier, as time is required for clearance of coagulation factors already present in plasma.(141) The goal is to keep the INR at 2.0–3.0. However, the use of warfarin may be inconvenient and problematic in advanced cancer patients as the INR can fluctuate despite frequent monitoring. Laboratory errors, dietary factors, altered warfarin metabolism by liver disorder, and co-administration of other drugs may contribute to this.(140,144) A quarter of workers have shifted to LMWH because of the risk of bleeding associated with warfarin.(140) Continuation with LMWH as maintenance, which is safe, effective, and well tolerated, may be a better option in advanced cancer patients. There are no standardized trials on prolonged anticoagulation in cancer patients. However, as it is reasonable to consider cancer patients as having continuing risks, anticoagulation may have to be given indefinitely.[135]

Thrombolytic therapy and caval filters

Thrombolytic therapy is mainly reserved for patients with severely compromised circulation, or in those who fail to respond to a conventional anticoagulation regimen.[141] Major bleeding is a concern, and contraindications to thrombolytics include recent history of major operation and stroke, bleeding tendency, active internal bleeding, and intracerebral and intraspinal diseases.[141] The recombinant tissue plasminogen activators (rt-PA), urokinase and streptokinase, are similar in their efficacy or bleeding complication rates. Thrombolytic therapy may still be effective when administered 10–14 days after the onset of PE.[141]

For cancer patients, bleeding at tumour sites, in particular intracranial lesions, can be dangerous.[135] Randomized trials on assessment of risk of bleeding from intracranial tumours are lacking. Some will recommend venous interruption by vena caval filter to prevent PE in such cases, as in other cases where anticoagulation is contraindicated. Complications include oedema of lower limbs and perforation of vena cava.[135] Lastly, catheter or surgical embolectomy are major procedures which need careful consideration before being embarked upon.

Respiratory muscle weakness

While respiratory muscle weakness is a well-established cause of dyspnoea among non-malignant conditions, its role in advanced cancer has only been reported recently. Among advanced cancer patients with dyspnoea, a significant proportion have no identifiable underlying parenchymal, pleural, or other cardiopulmonary diseases, and this was reported in one study in 24 per cent of the 1754 terminal cancer patients who had dyspnoea.[14] It was postulated that dyspnoea in this group might be due to 'debility of terminal cancer' which included general muscle weakness and associated medical complications. Studies showing the positive correlation between dyspnoea and poor performance status also suggested that general causes other than local lung or cardiac, might contribute to dyspnoea.[27,29]

The role of respiratory muscle weakness in causing dyspnoea among the terminally ill patients, as indicated by a low MIP, was reported recently by Dudgeon and Bruera. In a prospective study of 100 dyspnoeic cancer patients, VAS of shortness of breath and anxiety, bedside spirometry, MIP, chest radiography, and arterial blood gases were assessed. The median MIP of -16 cm H_2O was grossly lower than the quoted normal value of -50 cm H_2O. It was suggested that grossly abnormal maximum inspiratory pressure might contribute significantly to the restrictive pattern of the respiratory impairment.[34]

In another prospective study on 144 ambulatory terminally ill cancer patients, 40 per cent of patients who reported moderate dyspnoea (defined by VAS $\geq$ 30/100) had normal chest radiography. Multivariate analysis in patients with moderate to severe dyspnoea demonstrated that anxiety and MIP were independent correlates of the intensity of dyspnoea.[16] The finding suggested the possible contributory role of respiratory muscle weakness in causing dyspnoea.

However, Dudgeon reported another prospective study on 76 oncology out-patients who have moderate to severe dyspnoea, the median MIP was higher than the previous study, (median: -55 cm H_2O); and MIP was not correlated with dyspnoea VAS.[37] This may reflect the fact that patients in this study did not have as severe respiratory muscle weakness.

Causes of respiratory muscle weakness

In advanced cancer, multiple factors may contribute to respiratory muscle weakness. Possible causes include:

- metabolic causes and electrolyte disturbances;
- drugs-related causes like steroid myopathy, aminoglycosides, and clofibrate;
- anorexia–cachexia syndrome;
- paraneoplastic manifestations of malignancy; and
- concurrent medical illnesses such as COPD and sepsis.

In the study by Dudgeon, et al.[37] of patients who have low MIP, diaphragmatic excursion, haemoglobin, serum phosphate, oxygen saturation, total lung capacity, forced vital capacity, and the vital capacity percentage predicted were found to explain 58 per cent of variance in MIP in the multivariate model. In COPD patients, it was shown that respiratory muscle strength was closely associated with body weight and lean body mass.[145] Nutritional factors also contributed to the pathogenesis of respiratory insufficiency.[146] Anorexia–cachexia syndrome is present in a high proportion of advanced cancer patients with body weight loss arising from loss of muscle and fat (see Chapters 8.4.2–8.4.4). Proinflammatory cytokines like interleukin 1, interleukin 6, tumour necrosis factor α, interferon α, and interferon γ are postulated to be responsible for the increased catabolism and decreased synthesis of skeletal muscle. Recently, a transcription factor, nuclear factor kappa β (NF-KB), a mediator of skeletal muscle wasting in cachexia was reported as the pathogenic factor. It is activated by tumour necrosis factor, which in turn suppress MyoD, a transcription factor that is needed in increasing myofibril formation.[147]

Respiratory steroid myopathy has been well reported.[148] Acute steroid myopathy can occur after a high dose of steroid. Chronic steroid myopathy occurred after prolonged treatment with moderate dosage.[149] In a prospective study of steroid myopathy in cancer patients, nine out of 15 patients developed peripheral muscle weakness. Of these nine patients, eight experienced a significant decline in respiratory function, with symptomatic dyspnoea developing in four. The muscle weakness developed within 15 days and was significantly related to the cumulative dose of steroid. Respiratory muscle weakness could occur when proximal limb muscle remained strong and it could be reversed with the reduction or discontinuation of steroid.[150]

Lambert–Eaton myasthenic syndrome (LEMS), an autoimmune channelopathy associated with cancer, often presents with proximal weakness. Pathogenesis involves antibodies targeted at voltage-gated calcium channel.[151] One report suggested that mild to moderate diaphragmatic weakness could be discovered by measurement of trans-diaphragmatic pressures.[152] In some instances, LEMS could present with respiratory failure.[153]

Clinical approach

Respiratory muscle weakness is easily missed especially in the presence of other causes of dyspnoea.[154] Clinical breathlessness occurs after the respiratory muscle strength is lowered to a quarter of the normal. The following clinical features may suggest the presence of respiratory muscle weakness:

1. paradoxical abdominal breathing pattern,
2. hypoventilation,
3. dyspnoea in supine position or when sitting in water, and
4. dyspnoea with no underlying lung or cardiac causes.[155]

Investigations

The choice of investigations for respiratory muscle weakness should be individualized. The following tests can be considered.[155] Chest radiography may show bilateral elevated diaphragm. Fluoroscopy examination with short submaximal sniff test may reveal paradoxical movement in case of diaphragmatic weakness or paralysis. The characteristic lung function test is that of reveal restrictive pattern with a normal or raised carbon monoxide transfer. A fall in supine vital capacity exceeding 25 per cent may suggest diaphragmatic weakness. These tests may be difficult to perform especially when patient is too weak. The accuracy of the test is subjected to variation in effort and skill. Other tests like nasal pressure, sniff trans-diaphragmatic pressure, phrenic nerve stimulation, and magnetic stimulation may not be appropriate in advanced cancer patients.

Treatment

The treatment approach to respiratory muscle weakness include:

- withdrawal of toxic medications like steroids;
- correction of metabolic and electrolytes disturbances such as hypokalaemia, hypophosphataemia, hypomagnesaemia, hypoxia, and anaemia;
- prescribing drugs that improve respiratory function such as inotrophic agents;
- prescribing drugs that stimulate muscle growth;[(272)]
- respiratory muscle support; and
- the treatment of underlying medical disorders.[(272)]

Many agents have been reported to have inotrophic action, such as phosphodiesterase inhibitors and antioxidant drugs.[(272)] Theophylline has been demonstrated to improve respiratory muscle function in patients with COPD[(273)] but its effect in cancer is unknown. Anabolic steroids and insulin-like factor-1 (IGF-1) have been used in non-cancer patients,[(272)] but may not be applicable or even be detrimental for cancer patients. Respiratory support in the form of non-invasive positive pressure ventilation (NIPPV) is an established treatment in neuromuscular conditions.[(156)] Its role in symptom control in the palliative setting remains to be explored. Treatment for underlying medical disorders, especially cancer cachexia syndrome, remains a challenge. Possible research directions in the future may include the exploration of treatment that inhibit NF-KB, targeting the pathogenesis of cancer cachexia syndrome.[(157)]

Infection of the chest

Infection of the respiratory tract is common in advanced cancer patients. In one study, it accounted for 22.9 per cent of infections in a palliative care unit.[(158)] Predisposing factors to infection include airway obstruction, increased risk for aspiration, impaired immunity, and underlying chest diseases.

Clinical approach

The patient's prognosis, the reversibility of the underlying causes of the chest infection, the predicted efficacy of the antibiotics, the goals of treatment, and patient's preference will contribute to the management decision of chest infections. Management ranges from symptomatic control to intensive treatment with antibiotics, hospitalization, and specific treatment of reversible factors, for example, radiotherapy for bronchial obstruction. When the patient has very limited prognosis, symptomatic management such as control of fever and management of sputum may be appropriate. Antibiotics alter little the course of the terminal events. However, antibiotics are often indicated if the patient has a favourable prognosis.

The choice of antibiotics is usually guided by the predicted organisms and the local antibiotics sensitivity pattern. Routine sputum culture may not be required unless drug resistance or organisms not covered by empiric antibiotics is suspected.[(159)] For community acquired pneumonia, the likely organisms include *Streptococcus pneumoniae*, *Haemophilus influenzae*, *Staphylococcus aureus*, *Mycoplasma pneumoniae*, and *Chlamydia pneumoniae*. Penicillin-resistant or drug-resistant *Pneumococcus* (DRSP) infections are becoming an increasing problem in many countries. Patients who live in nursing home have a higher chance of Methicillin-resistant *Staphylococcus aureus*. For patients who are frail, nursing home residents, and with history of repeated hospitalization, the likely infective organisms are aerobic Gram-negative organisms. These include Enterbacteriaceae such as *Escherichia coli*, *Klebsiella* spp., or even *Pseudomonas aeruginosa*.[(159)] Fungal infection may occur in patients who are neutropaenic or with history of steroid usage. Likelihood of infection with *Influenza*, *Legionella*, or *Mycobacterium tuberculosis*, depends on the prevalence rate.

Before the initiation of antibiotic therapy, its aim, whether to prolong survival or for symptomatic relief for cough, fever, and sputum should be clarified. The option of antibiotics to cover community acquired organisms include β-lactam antibiotics such as high dose amoxicillin, amoxicillin/calvulanate plus macrolide or doxycycline; or antipneumococcal fluroquinolone which can cover DRSP.[(159)] Second or third generation cephalosporin can be used for Gram-negative infection other than *Pseudomonas*. In case of *Pseudomonas* infection, choice of antibiotics include anti-pseudomonal penicillin or third generation cephalosporins like ceftazidime plus aminoglyside or fluroquinolone.[(271)]

Antipyretic treatment is often provided to patients with fever to promote comfort. The management of sputum will be described in the section of sputum and airway secretion and under Physiotherapy (see Chapter 15.4). When parapneumonic pleural effusion develops with worsening of dyspnoea, thoracocentesis can be done.

Aspiration

Aspiration is the inhalation of oropharyngeal or gastric contents into the larynx and lower respiratory tract. Our natural defence against aspiration depends on intact swallowing or the protection of the airway during swallowing by nearby structures, and an effective cough reflex. Many factors predispose advanced cancer patients to aspiration. These include general factors like old age, impaired conscious level, impaired cough or gag reflex, near-supine position during feeding, and local factors like cranial nerve palsy, structural diseases of larynx and pharynx, for example, head and neck tumour, vocal cord palsy, problems of major airways such as tracheostomy tube, tracheo-oesophageal fistula, and oesophageal or gastric obstruction. Aspiration can give rise to chemical pneumonitis when gastric content is aspirated, pneumonia when colonized oropharyngeal secretion is aspirated, or asphyxiation if the airway is obstructed.[(160)]

Assessment of risk of aspiration

Bedside assessment including testing of cough and gag reflex is unreliable. A comprehensive swallowing assessment by a speech therapist will provide more information. Videofluoroscopy is the gold standard test, and it helps to identify the best food consistency. If this is not available, it can be presumed that swallowing fluid is most difficult.[(161)]

Choking after feeding is a clue, but cough may be absent in those with silent aspiration. Noisy breathing, cough, or dyspnoea at night may be due to accumulation of oropharyngeal secretions due to suppressed cough reflex by sedatives, hypnotics, or opioids. In the chest radiograph, infiltrations involving posterior segment of the upper lobes, apical basal (superior), or the basal segments of the lower lobes may suggest aspiration as the cause of pneumonia.

Management of aspiration

The importance of good oral care cannot be over-emphasized in the prevention of aspiration pneumonia. The following precautions should be taken during oral feeding: adopt an upright position, divide food into small boluses, feed slowly, ask patient to tuck the chin to the chest and swallow repeatedly. The food can be prepared in the best consistency as defined by videofluoroscopy, or by thickening the fluid taken. It is of utmost importance that the family members should be educated on the correct method of feeding.[(161)]

If oral feeding becomes impossible due to recurrent aspiration or irreversible predisposing factors, one may have to consider feeding through nasogastric or gastrostomy tube. However, both are not absolute protection for aspiration, and the gastrostomy tube is not superior to the nasogastric tube in this regard. Aspiration from colonized oral secretions may still occur, so vigorous oral care should be continued.

When saliva accumulates in the oropharynx due to a swallowing problem, medications may be given to reduce the secretion. Antimuscarinic agents, most commonly hyoscine (scopolamine) hydrobromide, can be given subcutaneously, or, in some countries, transdermally. Glycopyrrolate, compared with scopolamine, is more potent in decreasing salivary secretion, causes less sedation or paradoxical agitation, and has a longer duration of action.[162]

Preferred antibiotics for aspiration pneumonia involving anaerobic organisms include β-lactam/β-lactamase inhibitor or clindamycin. For patients who are frail or with a history of repeated hospitalization, coverage for Gram-negative organisms by anti-*Pseudomonas* penicillins and second or third generation cephalosporins is recommended.

Pulmonary tuberculosis

Tuberculosis is not uncommon in patients with advanced cancer, especially in high prevalence countries. The presentation may be atypical, especially in older patients. The single most useful test is sputum smear examination for acid-fast bacilli, and hospices/palliative care units should have access to this test. In places where multiresistant tuberculosis is prevalent, drug sensitivity testing should be performed.

If treatment is considered, it should consist of at least three standard antituberculosis drugs, namely isoniazid, rifampicin, and pyrazinamide.[163] In areas where multiresistant tuberculosis is common, medications should be modified according to the resistance pattern. Early treatment is important for prevention of cross infection.

Miscellaneous syndromes

Anaemia (see Chapter 8.6)

Anaemia is common among cancer patients and one study reported an incidence of 20 per cent in dyspnoeic cancer patients.[34] Multiple causes may contribute to anaemia, but potentially reversible ones should be looked for, for example, iron deficiency and haemolytic anaemia that may be steroid responsive.

Blood transfusion is often given to relieve weakness and dyspnoea caused by anaemia in cancer patients.[164] In a study where blood transfusion was given for haemoglobin of 8 g/l or lesser, with or without severe fatigue or dyspnoea, 51.4 per cent of patients reported subjective improvement with transfusion.[165] The relief of symptoms did not have any significant relationship with pretransfusion haemoglobin level or performance status. Survival was shorter for the group with no improvement (18.2 days versus 77.3 days). Transfusion of patients who had a survival of only a few weeks might not provide significant symptom relief. Another report showed a highly significant improvement in the VAS of breathing at 2 days after transfusion was given to anaemic patients with dyspnoea, and the benefit persisted at 14 days.[164] Recombinant human erythropoietin has been used in cancer patients undergoing chemotherapy, but its cost, availability in some countries, and the limited prognosis of the patient limit its role in terminally ill cancer patients.

Pulmonary hypertension

If the apparent cause of dyspnoea in advanced cancer is not found, the clinical signs of right heart disease, an enlarged pulmonary conus, and cardiomegaly on chest radiograph may suggest pulmonary hypertension to be the possible cause of dyspnoea. Doppler echocardiogram confirms the diagnosis. Common causes include Cor pulmonale secondary to chronic lung disease, and PE. Rarer causes of pulmonary hypertension that may occur in cancer patients include pulmonary tumour microembolism, lymphangitis carcinomatosis, and extrinsic compression of pulmonary arteries.

In pulmonary tumour microembolism, reported cases had marked pulmonary hypertension that could be rapidly fatal. The tumour embolism causes vascular occlusion not by a direct effect, but by local activation of coagulation and fibrocellular intimal thickening.[166] In a few reports of bronchogenic carcinoma, which compressed on pulmonary arteries, percutaneous intravascular stent restored the perfusion.

Hyperventilation

Hyperventilation is physiologically defined as breathing in excess of the metabolic needs of the body.[167] It is characterized by tachypnoea with low blood CO_2 level. Causes of hyperventilation include central neurogenic hyperventilation, hyperventilation syndrome, and organic causes of hyperventilation. Central neurogenic hyperventilation has been described in cerebral tumour, especially cerebral lymphoma.[168] Panic disorder is well described in patients with COPD.[169] Its prevalence in dyspnoea cancer patients is not reported. Respiratory symptoms of hyperventilation include dyspnoea, tightness of chest, suffocation, and inability to sigh.[167] In a study, the hyperventilation provocation test was positive in 20.9 per cent of cancer patients, indicating the contributory role of hyperventilation in cancer patients with dyspnoea.[170] As for organic causes of hyperventilation, acidosis is a common cause, and patients can present with air hunger. Acidosis can result from renal failure of various causes, including obstructive uropathy due to tumours in the urinary tract, pelvis, or retroperitoneal space.

Symptomatic management of dyspnoea

Non-pharmacological approach

A non-pharmacological approach to the management of dyspnoea emerges from the paradigm shift from understanding of dyspnoea as a symptom of mainly physical dimension to one that is multidimensional. Its application in day-to-day practice, however, requires a change in the model of care from a pharmacotherapy-centred approach to a biopsychosocial and 'patient-empowerment' approach.

The core concept of non-pharmacological intervention consists of an integrative model in which the psychological experience of breathlessness is considered inseparable from the physical aspects of the symptom.[171] The key intervention strategies consist of detail assessment, psychosocial support, breathing control, and problem-focused and emotional-focused coping. The success of this model depends on the patent's ability to learn, to cope, and ultimately feel self-empowered to deal with the dyspnoeic episodes. A multidisciplinary approach is pivotal.

There have been two recent randomized controlled studies looking into the effectiveness of non-pharmacological intervention. One was performed in 20 NSCLC patients.[171] Interventions included weekly sessions of counselling, breathing retraining, relaxation, and coping and adaptation strategies provided by a nurse research practitioner over 3–6 weeks. Improvement was confirmed in the intervention group compared with the control group. Distress from breathlessness was improved by a median of 53 per cent, breathlessness at worst by 35 per cent and functional capacity by 21 per cent, while the distress of the control group was worsened by a median of 10 per cent.

A larger scale multicentered randomized controlled trial was conducted in 119 patients diagnosed with lung cancer or mesothelioma, who had completed the first line treatment for their diseases and reported breathlessness.[172] Patients in the intervention group attended a weekly nursing clinic for up to 8 weeks. Interventions included (i) detailed assessment, (ii) advice and support provided to patients and families on management of dyspnoea, (iii) exploration of the meaning of breathlessness, (iv) training in breathing control techniques, (v) goal setting to complement breathing and relaxation techniques and management of functional and social activities, and (vi) early recognition of problems warranting pharmacological and medical intervention. Results showed that the intervention group improved significantly at 8 weeks in 5 of the 11 items assessed: breathlessness at best, WHO performance status, level of depression, and two Rotterdam Symptom checklist measures (physical symptom distress and breathlessness). Significant improvement was also seen in the three items of activities: climbing stairs, walking outdoor, and shopping. The findings confirmed that patients who received interventions had improvements in breathlessness and depression, and could maintain the performance status throughout the 8 weeks of intervention.

Strategy of non-pharmacological intervention

A detailed assessment of dyspnoea is important for the planning of non-pharmacological intervention. The clinical framework for assessment of dyspnoea as illustrated earlier in this chapter highlights the necessary information to be gathered. It is important to document the triggers for breathlessness, including the physical activities, environmental, or emotional factors. The overall strategy of non-pharmacological approach is outlined in Table 9.

Psychosocial support and empowerment

Breathlessness often is an emotion-loaded experience associated with fear, anxiety, helplessness, panic, or depression. Patients may have feelings of impending death during the acute dyspnoeic attack. A sense of loss, emotional loneliness secondary to impaired daily activity, or loss of social roles is frequently encountered. Therefore, empathetic listening to the details of the history and evaluating their significance to the person is of paramount importance. Understanding the distress and suffering caused by the breathlessness is pivotal for assessment, as well as provision of psychological support to the patients and their families. Giving relevant and optimal information related to the disease and underlying causes of breathlessness may alleviate many unknown anxieties. This is especially important when dyspnoea is due to non-malignant causes. Advice and support should be given to the patients and the carers who often face tremendous stress in handling daily dyspnoeic episodes. Education on medications and respiratory equipment will empower the patients and families for self-management. The availability of a home care team or a 'hot line' service will support the patient when the symptom is at its worst.

Control breathlessness techniques

Controlled breathing techniques include positioning, pursed-lip breathing (PLB), breathing exercises, and coordinated breathing training. Positioning is the simplest and most common adopted strategy to relieve dyspnoea. Classically, the patient is instructed to lean forward with arms bracing a chair or knees with the upper body supported. This positioning has been demonstrated to improve ventilatory capacity.[173]

PLB has frequently been practised by patients with COPD. Patients inhale through their nose for several seconds with their mouths closed; they then exhale slowly for 4–6 s through pursed lips held in a whistling or kissing position. PLB should be performed during exercise and whenever dyspnoea is triggered. Studies showed the PLB could relieve perception of dyspnoea, increase tidal volume, decrease respiratory rate, and improve gas parameters in patients with chronic chest ailments.

Activities or emotions can often bring about dyspnoeic episodes. This dyspnoeic attack if severe can bring fear and precipitate a respiratory panic attack, as uncoordinated breathing can further worsen ventilation. Training in coordinated breathing during dyspnoeic attacks may be effective in aborting the respiratory panic attack.

Simple measures like cold facial stimulation by a flow of cold air onto the face has been shown to reduce the sense of breathlessness.[11] The use of cold air with a fan can be a simple measure to relieve dyspnoea. Further, airflow over the face and nasal mucosa during oxygen administration may improve dyspnoea.

Emotional and problem-focused coping

Various strategies can be employed to enhance emotional coping during the dyspnoeic episode, for example, relaxation technique,

Table 9 Non-pharmacological intervention for dyspnoea in advanced cancer patients

Intervention goals	Intervention strategy and modalities
Detailed assessment of breathlessness	Dyspnoea assessment chart (Table 6)
Support for patients and their families on ways of managing breathlessness	Patient education Psychological support Support for respiratory equipment Patient group Day care centre
Exploring perception of patient and family on breathlessness and their disease	Explore anxiety, fear, and panic attack associated with breathlessness attack Explain causes of breathlessness and its meaning Discuss prognosis of disease Explore effects of breathlessness on daily living and social role Work on losses related to disease deterioration
Control of breathlessness training	Posture and positioning Breathing retraining: pursed-lip breathing, coordinated breathing Use of cool air or electric fan
Emotional coping during dyspnoea episode	Relaxation technique Desensitization Distraction, visual imagery
Problem focused coping: maximizing functional activities	Guided mastery technique Exercise training Training in activities of daily living Energy conservation techniques Home environment modification Arrangement for home respiratory equipment and adaptive device (e.g. oxygen concentrator, portable oxygen, wheelchair) Advance planning of daily activities
Early recognition of attacks requiring drug or medical intervention	Support from home care team Education and drug supervision

distraction, and visual imagery. Problem-focused coping strategies can include strategies to maximize functional activities, densensitization, and guided mastery.[175] Dyspnoeic patients often adopt a dyspnoea–fear–avoidance pattern, which leads to a vicious cycle of progressive inactivity. With guided mastery, patients' activities can be gradually increased under the supervision of a therapist with fear and anxiety being addressed. This technique may be helpful in relieving dyspnoea in advanced cancer patients.

When the symptom of dyspnoea is getting more severe, planning of daily activities in advance is often desirable. Pacing of breathing with activity, energy conservation techniques, and home modification can maintain the patient's basic activities of daily living. Sometimes home respiratory equipment or mobility aids, for example, oxygen concentrator and wheelchair, may be required for symptom relief and to maximize the functional capabilities, and this can be very important in alleviating the social isolation due to dyspnoea.

Oxygen therapy

Oxygen therapy has been widely used in acute hypoxaemic conditions. Long-term oxygen therapy has been documented and adopted as a standard therapy in patients with COPD with hypoxia.[176,177] The physiological benefits of long-term oxygen include improvement in survival, pulmonary haemodynamics,[176,178] exercise capacity, and neuropsychological function, and decrease in the sensation of dyspnoea.[176]

The goal of oxygen therapy in palliative care setting is mainly the relief of dyspnoea. The other physiological benefits of oxygen are uncertain in advanced cancer patients. In a study of 100 dyspnoeic cancer patients,[34] 40 per cent had hypoxia. It has been shown that dyspnoea in the terminally ill does not correlate with the degree of hypoxaemia.[16] However, the pathophysiology of dyspnoea in cancer patient, as we have seen, is often complex. Other than hypoxia, many cancer patients suffer from restrictive lung impairment that leads to increase in respiratory effort. Probably this can account for the poor correlation between dyspnoea and hypoxia.

There are several randomized controlled studies on the effect of oxygen on dyspnoea and exercise tolerance in patients with COPD and interstitial lung disease. Five out of six controlled studies in COPD patients showed a positive symptomatic benefit with oxygen.

In advanced cancer patients, two randomized controlled crossover studies have been performed to compare the effect of oxygen and air on dyspnoea. Bruera et al. reported a double-blind study on 12 hypoxemic cancer patients comparing air and oxygen at 5 l/min.[179] Oxygen is significantly better than air in terms of oxygen saturation, respiratory effort, respiratory rate, and the dyspnoea VAS score. All the patients and the investigators consistently preferred oxygen to air.

However, in another single-blind study on 38 patients, Booth et al. reported that air was just as effective as oxygen at 4 l/min in relieving dyspnoea.[39] Baseline dyspnoea VAS score was significantly reduced after administration of either air ($P < 0.001$) or oxygen ($P < 0.001$). There was no significant difference in the mean VAS scores between the two groups, though the improvement with oxygen was quantitatively greater and its effect appeared to carry over into the air phase. The improvement in dyspnoea with oxygen could not be predicted from the baseline hypoxic level. However, in Booth's study, only six patients had a SaO_2 below 90 per cent. The conclusions from these two studies are conflicting, but the patients recruited are different in terms of oxygen saturation. The effect of oxygen on dyspnoeic cancer patient requires further evaluation, especially separating the hypoxic from the non-hypoxic patients.

As an interim practical guideline, it is reasonable to prescribe supplemental oxygen in dyspnoeic cancer patients with saturation less than 90 per cent. Its effect on relieving dyspnoea can then be monitored. For any advanced cancer individual who is non-hypoxic, a trial of oxygen or air by the method of *N* of 1 trial may help to guide oxygen therapy.[179] Patient can put on either air or oxygen sequentially to evaluate its effect in relieving dyspnoea.

Oxygen delivery

Overprescription of supplemental oxygen can suppress ventilation resulting in hypercapnia and CO_2 narcosis. This can occur when the patient is only monitored by pulse oximetry and not by blood gas parameters. The patient can become progressively somnolent despite good oxygen saturation. When this occurs, oxygen flow should be lowered to maintain the SaO_2 at around 90 per cent, with the mental status or the blood gases of the patient being monitored.

Nasal oxygen cannulae are more comfortable and convenient than the oxygen mask as the former does not impede speech, communication, or eating. In the case of refractory hypoxia despite high oxygen flow, the effectiveness of oxygen delivery can be enhanced by a reservoir nasal cannula (oximizer or oximizer pendant). This reservoir device has a pouch that stores 20 ml of oxygen during expiration, which will be delivered as a bolus at the onset of inspiration in the subsequent breath.[174]

The oxygen concentrator is a convenient way of delivering oxygen in the home setting. The flow is usually limited to a maximum of 5 l/min for most models. An oxygen cylinder is an alternative when the oxygen concentrator is not readily available. A portable cylinder enables patient to continue with some outdoor activities. Extra oxygen flow of 1 l/min can be added during activity or sleep. The patient's abstinence from smoking is a prerequisite for oxygen therapy because of the fire hazard.

Opioids for symptomatic management of dyspnoea

The presence of opioid terminals and neuronal bodies in the respiratory nuclei strongly suggests that endogenous opioid has a modulatory role in the function of the nuclei. Opioid receptors are found in high densities in the brain stem. The Mu receptor clearly has an inhibitory influence on respiration, the delta receptor has a modest effect, the kappa has little, and the sigma receptor may stimulate respiration.[180] Opioid receptors, the conventional (μ, κ, δ) and the non-conventional ones, are also found widely distributed in the lung.

Exogenous opioids have been used for reducing dyspnoea, but the site of possible action is unknown.[181] A central site of action is possible. Administration of exogenous opioid leads to a dose-dependent reduction in minute ventilation leading to increase in PCO_2, and a depression of the ventilatory response to CO_2 demonstrated by displacement of the CO_2 response curve to the right, or reduction in slope, or both.[180] However, in clinical studies, it has been shown that relief of dyspnoea is possible *without* an increase in CO_2. This suggests that other sites or mechanisms are involved.[182] Another mechanism proposed is through modulation of perception or anxiety by the opioid. Lastly, opioids may act peripherally on lung receptors. This is suggested by the fact that studies have shown a beneficial effect of nebulized morphine on dyspnoea, and this has occurred with low systemic bioavailability. Activation of these local lung receptors inhibits release of acetylcholine which induces bronchial constriction and mucus secretion, or may activate a J receptor-mediated reflex with beneficial pulmonary consequence.[181]

Use of morphine for relieving dyspnoea in non-cancer groups (see Chapter 10.4)

Opioids, both strong and weak, have been studied in non-cancer groups, including patients with COPD,[183–191] interstitial lung diseases,[192] patients with advanced diseases,[193] and normal subjects.[194] Results are controversial.

The following studies have demonstrated effectiveness of dihydrocodeine and morphine in relieving dyspnoea in COPD patients. Oral dihydrocodeine

Table 10 Studies on using opioids for relieving dyspnoea in cancer patients

Author	Sample	Study design	Regime	Findings
Bruera et al., 1993[182]	10 Cancer patients on regular morphine subcutaneously	Crossover, placebo-controlled trial	Intermittent SC morphine as needed at 50% higher than regular dose	Good response in 90% None had respiratory suppression
Allard et al., 1999[206]	33 Terminally ill cancer patients already on PO or SC morphine	Randomized, double-blind, continuous sequential trial	Single additional dose of regular morphine by 25 or 50% of regular dose	VAS for dyspnoea improved significantly, same for both doses
Davis et al., 1996[202]	79 Advanced cancer patients	Randomized, double-blind, controlled trial	Single predetermined dose of 5–50 mg nebulized morphine compared with normal saline	Improvement in dyspnoea VAS, no significant difference between morphine and control No drop in PFR or drowsiness reported
Mazzocato et al., 1999[205]	Nine cancer patients	Randomized, crossover, double-blind controlled trial	Single dose SC morphine	Effective with minimal side effects
Peterson et al., 1996[200]	Eight terminally ill	Controlled trial	Regular doses of 2.5–5 mg of nebulized morphine compared with normal saline	No added value in adding nebulized morphine to those who are already on PO or SC morphine
Zeppetella, 1997[201]	17 Cancer patients four opioid naïve	Uncontrolled study	Regular doses of nebulized morphine at 10–40 mg Q4H for 48 h	16 (94%) Improved after 24 h, but no further improvement at 48 h Well tolerated
Tanaka et al., 1999[199]	15 Cancer patients	Uncontrolled open study	Single dose of 20–40 mg nebulized morphine	Effective in 8 patients Increase to 40 mg had no effect on the result No major side effects
Farncombe et al., 1994[204]	54 Advanced cancer patients on regular oral opioid form	Retrospective chart review	Regular doses of nebulized morphine given at 5–30 mg Q4H Also nebulized hydromorphone, codeine, and anilerdine	Subjective improvement in dyspnoea, exercise tolerance, well-being in 34 (63%)
Boyd and Kelly, 1997[196]	15 Advanced cancer patients, four had COPD	Open, uncontrolled study	Given MST 10 mg BD or increase original dose by 30%	Nine completed study Three improved Two deteriorated Four progressive dyspnoea
Breura et al., 1990[211]	20 Terminal cancer patients	Open, uncontrolled study	Five opioid naïve patients on 5 mg SC 15 Opioid constant patient given 2.5 times their regular dose SC	19 (95%) Improved in dyspnoea VAS No respiratory suppression
Cohen et al., 1991[197]	Eight terminal lung cancer	Open, uncontrolled study	IVI bolus of 1–2 mg morphine every 5–10 min till effective, then followed by IV infusion of a mean dose of 5.6 mg/h	Six good relief Five had somnolence Seven died Two received naloxone
Quelch et al., 1997[203]	Four advanced cancer patients	Case reports	20–50 mg nebulized morphine Q4H	Subjective improvement in dyspnoea, exercise tolerance, and well being
Ventafridda et al., 1990[198]	Five cancer patients	Case reports	10 mg morphine IMI + chlorpromazine 25 mg IMI	Improvement subjectively

has been reported to be useful in reducing breathlessness in COPD patients in several double-blind, randomized crossover trials.[183,184,186] Nebulized morphine was reported to increase exercise endurance,[188] and oral morphine at a dose of 0.8 mg/kg was shown to improve exercise tolerance,[187] but with somnolence as the major side effect.

However, in more recent studies, use of nebulized morphine has not been found to be useful in reducing dyspnoea in patients with COPD,[185,189–191] interstitial lung disease,[192] advanced diseases,[193] and normal subjects.[194] In another study, oral diamorphine was reported as not useful in reducing dyspnoea in COPD patients.[195]

Opioids for dyspnoea in advanced cancer patients

While enhancing exercise endurance may be beneficial to patients with chronic respiratory diseases, the primary goal of treatment of dyspnoeic cancer patients must be alleviation of the symptom. It is debatable whether the results in COPD patients can be extrapolated to cancer patients. There are relatively few controlled trials in cancer patients, and most of these studies involved a small number of patients (Table 10). Unlike the use of opioid for cancer pain, there is no general consensus on the optimum starting dose, the best regimen (e.g. intermittent or continuous), and the best route of administration of opioid in alleviation of dyspnoea. In these studies, morphine was the most commonly used, and had been administered through various routes, including oral,(196) subcutaneous,(182) intravenous,(197) intramuscular,(198) and nebulized form.(199–204) Intermittent or continuous administration of morphine had been employed.

Use of systemic morphine in cancer

Systemic morphine has been shown to be effective in controlling dyspnoea in a few controlled studies. One used oral morphine as a supplementary dose of 25–50 per cent of the stable, analgesic dose.(206) Three studies had reported usefulness of subcutaneous morphine in controlling dyspnoea, one given as a single supplementary dose of 25–50 per cent of the stable dose,(206) one given as intermittent doses at 50 per cent higher than regular dose,(182) the other at a single dose of 5 mg or 50 per cent higher than the stable dose.(205) In these studies, major adverse effects including respiratory suppression were not reported.

In other uncontrolled studies, systemic morphine had been used in an oral sustained-release form(196) and as an intravenous infusion.(197) In the former study, three out of nine patients did show some improvement, but somnolence was a problem.(196) In the latter study using continuous infusion of morphine, six out of eight had relief, but somnolence and respiratory suppression was significant.(197)

Use of nebulized morphine in cancer

Giving morphine via a nebulizer has the potential advantage of reducing adverse effects because of low systemic bioavailability. The systemic bioavailability of nebulized morphine varied from 9 to 35 per cent when given with mechanical ventilation,(207) but was only 5 per cent with compressed air nebulizer.(208) Peak plasma concentration of morphine is reached at a fast rate, much more rapidly than when given orally.(208)

In cancer patients, there are no controlled trials to support the use of nebulized morphine. In two controlled studies, nebulized morphine, when given at a single dose of 5–50 mg(202) or 2.5–5 mg,(200) did not produce any significant results when compared with the control group. Nebulized morphine was, however, reported to be useful in a few uncontrolled studies. In these studies, nebulized morphine was given at a dose of 10–40 mg(201) and 5–30 mg 4 hourly,(204) or at a single dose of 20 or 40 mg.(199)

Nebulized morphine is generally well tolerated, though some may complain of claustrophobia with the mask and a bitter taste.(201) None of the studies reported major side effects with nebulized morphine, such as excessive somnolence, respiratory suppression, and bronchospasm. (The worry about the side effect of bronchospasm is based on the fact that morphine is known to induce histamine release.)

Use of other opioids via nebulized route in cancer

Nebulized fentanyl, hydromorphone, codeine, and anileridine have been used for relief of dyspnoea in cancer patients, but not in controlled studies. Their value in clinical use awaits further confirmation.(204,209)

Recommendation

Despite morphine being widely used in controlling dyspnoea, there are no controlled trials to compare the efficacy of various routes of administration, the starting dose, and the optimal dosage. Based on the above evidences, it is reasonable to increase the dose of regular (analgesic) morphine, orally or subcutaneously, by 25–50 per cent to control dyspnoea. For those who are opioid naïve, a starting dose of 5 mg is a reasonable choice. The choice of regimen (i.e. intermittent or continuous) may depend on the profile of the dyspnoeic episodes of individual patients. Needless to say, it is important to monitor the side effects of somnolence and respiratory suppression, especially for those who are on regular morphine.

Nebulized morphine has been tried in various studies as mentioned above.(199–202) Major side effects were not associated with the use of nebulized morphine in these studies, but clinical benefits are reported in a few uncontrolled trials only. A recent systematic review of the literature does not support the use of nebulized opioid in control of dyspnoea in terminally illness(264) as good evidence for its therapeutic effect from well designed trials are lacking. In this review, majority of the studies were not performed in cancer patients. Further studies with standardized opioid regimens and standardized outcome measures are required to determine the efficacy of nebulized morphine in controlling dyspnoea in terminal cancer patients. Until the role of opioid receptors in the lung and the mechanism whereby opioid receptors reduces dyspnoea are clearly elucidated, the relative role of peripheral and central action of opioid remains uncertain.

Other drugs for symptomatic management of dyspnoea

Psychotropic agents

Anxiety and especially panic disorder appear to be more common in patients with respiratory diseases.(169,212) Hyperventilation syndrome is reported to be common in advanced cancer patients.(170)

Benzodiazepines are commonly given for symptomatic control of dyspnoea in advanced cancer. Anxiolytics have the potential to relieve dyspnoea by depressing hypoxia or hypercapnia ventilatory responses and alter the emotional response to dyspnoea. However, several small-scale controlled studies performed in COPD and in healthy volunteers gave inconsistent results and anxiolytics tends to be poorly tolerated.(2) Benzodiazepines like alprazolam and lorazepam may have a potential role for dyspnoeic patients with a high component of anxiety or panic.(212) Lorazepam, diazepam, and midazolam are frequently prescribed empirically to relieve dyspnoea.(213) Tricyclic antidepressant and selective serotonin reuptake inhibitors are also reported as effective antipanic and anxiolyic agents.(212)

Several randomized controlled studies of phenothiazines for the control of dyspnoea were conducted in patients with COPD. Studies involving promethazine and chlorpromazine gave conflicting results.(214–216) Intravenous or *per rectum* chlorpromazine was reported to be effective in controlling dyspnoea and restlessness in the advanced cancer patients.(217)

Buspirone, a nonbenzodiazepine anxiolytic drug that produced conflicting results in COPD, has not been studied in cancer patients.

Bronchodilators

Airflow obstruction in cancer patients is under-diagnosed and undertreated.(35) An obstructive lung function pattern is commonly found in dyspnoeic cancer patients.(34) Inhaled beta$_2$-agonist, either in short acting or the rapid onset long acting form, can produce a fast onset bronchodilator effect in asthma patients. An anticholinergic drug is the first choice for COPD patients. They have a slower onset of action and can be given with beta$_2$-agonist.(218) Theophylline can be used as a third line drug, with a potential role of enhancing diaphragmatic strength and endurance. As the therapeutic margin is narrow, reduction of dosage is advised in patients with impaired liver function.

Corticosteroids

Steroids are widely used for symptomatic treatment of dyspnoea in cancer patients, but the efficacy has not been evaluated in controlled studies. Steroids have a definite role in the treatment of asthma and in the subgroup of steroid-responsive COPD patients.[218] Steroids are also used empirically for relieving dyspnoea in conditions such as major airway obstruction, SVCO, and lymphangitis carcinomatosis.

Steroids may cause weakness in proximal and respiratory muscles, which aggravates the immobility and dyspnoea.[133,150] The dose should be tailed down to the lowest effective dose or stopped if ineffective.

Others

Nebulized lignocaine has been tried for relieving dyspnoea as a means to anaesthetize the airway receptors. Studies involving interstitial lung disease and cancer patients both gave negative results.[219,220] Hence, it is not recommended for dyspnoea relief.

Cough in cancer patients

Prevalence of cough

Cough has a prevalence of 47–86 per cent in lung cancer and 23–37 per cent in general cancer patients. Cough of moderate to severe intensity occurred in 13 per cent of general cancer patients[20,46] and in 17–48 per cent of lung cancer patients.[22–24] In lung cancer, cough is one of the most common symptoms.

Cough reflex—receptors and pathway

Impulses in the afferent pathway are transmitted mainly via the vagus. Input from the higher cortex is likely as cough can be voluntarily suppressed or initiated.

Receptors for cough belong mainly to the group of rapidly adapting pulmonary stretch receptors (RAR). Pulmonary and bronchial C fibre receptors may also have a role. The RAR is polymodal and heterogeneous, responding to a variety of mechanical (inflation and deflation, dust, mucus, foreign body) and chemical (noxious gas, smoke, capsaicin) stimuli; and to inflammatory and immunological mediators (acetylcholine, histamine, serotonin, prostaglandin, bradykinin, substance P). RAR are widely distributed in the airways except beyond the respiratory bronchioles. When stimulated, they can cause cough, bronchoconstriction, mucus secretion, and a spectrum of respiratory reflexes depending on the site and characteristics of the receptors.[221–223]

Afferent pathways relay signals to the cough centres diffusely located in the medulla.[221] The motor efferent then goes to the inspiratory and expiratory muscles through the phrenic and other spinal motor nerves, and to the larynx and bronchial tree through the recurrent laryngeal branches of the vagi.

Physiology of cough

Cough efficiency relies on the high expiratory pressure and airflow velocity generated to expel mucus and droplets, which in turn depends on the optimal function of the respiratory muscles, closure of the glottis, dynamic compression of the major airways, the mucus properties, and mucociliary clearance. However, in cancer patients, cough can be ineffective for various reasons (Table 11).

Causes of cough in cancer patients

Chronic cough in the general population is due to multiple causes in up to 93 per cent. In cancer, it is likely that multiple causes and hence multiple mechanisms are responsible[221,224] (Table 12).

Impact of cough on cancer patients

Cough may serve to expel mucus, sputum, fluid, foreign body from the airway, or indicate a pathological process. More often, cough is a nuisance or distress to the patient by causing exhaustion, excessive sweating, and insomnia. However, in the presence of other concomitant symptoms of cancer, and due to the fact that cough is often intermittent, its impact may not be readily recognized.

In normal subjects, due to the high intrathoracic pressure and high energy generated during cough, many physical complications like syncope, hernia, incontinence, rib fractures, and pneumothorax have been reported.[221] In a study of the impact of chronic cough on the quality of life in the general population, exhaustion and life-style changes have been shown to have significant correlation with the Sickness Impact Profile Score.[225] Few studies, however, quantitatively examined the distress caused by cough in cancer patients. In one series of 240 cancer patients, of which 21.3 per cent has lung cancer, cough was present in 33 per cent. Among all patients, 13 per cent had moderate to severe cough and 18 per cent of all patients suffered from severe distress from cough.[20]

Management of cough in cancer

In the general population, treating cough is highly successful if the underlying cause is identified. In cancer, the principle of being caused-directed in symptom treatment still holds true, although the search for a specific cause may be limited by the burden of investigations. The management of cough can therefore be categorized into (i) specific treatment of the underlying causes (Table 13), (ii) enhancing effectiveness of cough when indicated, and (iii) suppression of cough.

Table 12 Causes of cough in cancer

Non-malignant	Cancer-related
Post-nasal drip syndrome (PNDS)	Major airway or endobronchial lesions
Asthma	Pleural disease—effusion, mesothelioma
Gastroesophageal reflux (GERD)	Lung parenchymal infiltration
Chronic bronchitis	Aspiration (e.g. head and neck tumour, tracheoesophageal fistula, vocal cord paralysis)
Post-infectious	
Angiotensin-converting enzyme inhibitor (ACEI)	Lymphangitis carcinomatosis
Eosinophilic bronchitis	Pericardial effusion
Bronchiectasis	Radiation-induced fibrosis
Heart failure	Chemotherapy-induced fibrosis
	Pneumonia
	Microembolism

Table 11 Factors leading to ineffective cough in cancer patients

Muscle factor	General debility	Anaemia, weakness, impaired conscious level
	Weakness of respiratory muscles	Cachexia syndrome, steroid myopathy
	Neurological problem	Spinal cord compression
	Ineffective use of respiratory muscles	Weakness of abdominal muscles, gross ascites, hepatomegaly
Airway factor	Vocal cord problem	Paralysis
	Non-compressible airway	Tumour, stent insertion
Mucus factor	Reduction of water content of mucus	Reduced fluid intake, effect of drugs
Mucociliary factor	Impaired mucociliary function	Smoking

Table 13 Specific treatment of cough

Cause	Treatment
Endobronchial tumours	Steroid, laser, cryotherapy
Tracheo-oesophageal fistula	Stent insertion
Lymphangitis carcinomatosis	Steroid
Post-irradiation lung damage	Steroid
Pleural and pericardial effusion	Fluid aspiration
Aspiration pneumonia	Antibiotics, prevention of aspiration
Congestive heart failure	Diuretics
Asthma	Bronchodilators, steroid
Post-nasal drip syndrome (PNDS)	Antihistamine
Gastrooesophageal reflux (GERD)	H_2 blocker, proton pump inhibitor, diet modification
Eosinophilic bronchitis	Steroid

When the aim is to improve the cough mechanism, for example, in the case of copious sputum in chest infections, chest physiotherapy, assisted cough manoeuvre, and improving hydration can be helpful, but evidence on clinical outcome measures is lacking.(221) Pharmacological treatment by protussive agents is discussed in next section. When the underlying cause is not reversible or treatable, cough can be suppressed using various agents.

Agents used for suppressing cough in cancer

Opioid

All opioids have antitussive effect, and codeine is the prototype drug used for suppressing cough. The central cough centre is the likely site of action, and 5HT is also postulated to be involved. The action of the opioid is not through sedation, as equally sedative drugs are not antitussive, and blocking the 5HT reduced the antitussive effect but not the sedative effect of morphine.(221)

Codeine can be given 15–30 mg every 4 h.(224) Hydrocodone is a metabolite of codeine, but causes less neuropsychological problems and constipation. It is preferred to codeine by some and is given at a dose of 5–10 mg 4 hourly.(226)

Dextromethorphan

Dextromethorphan is the dextro isomer of the codeine congener of levorphanol. It is a centrally acting non-opioid antitussive that has been shown to be effective in randomized controlled trials, but tends to cause fewer side effects on the gastrointestinal tract and the central nervous system.(228) The dose recommended is 15–30 mg orally four times a day.(224)

Benzonatate

This is a peripheral acting drug related to the local anaesthetic group of procaine, which dampens the activity of the stretch receptors. Benzonatate acts in 15–20 min and its effect can last for 3–8 h. Doses of 100–200 mg tid have been used as a second choice for treatment of cough when hydrocodone failed.(226,227) The patient should be instructed not to chew the capsule to avoid local anaesthetic effect in the oropharynx.(229)

Levodropropizine

Levodropropizine, like benzonatate, acts on the periphery by modulation of C fibre activity. In one multicentre, parallel group, randomized, double-blind controlled study comparing levodropropizine (75 mg tid) and dihydrocodeine (10 mg tid) for treatment of cough in lung cancer, both were equally effective in controlling cough, but somnolence was significantly less in the levodropropizine group (8 versus 22 per cent).(230)

Sodium cromoglycate

Sodium cromoglycate is believed to have an inhibitory action on C fibres. In a double-blind randomized controlled trial, sodium cromoglycate given at 2 puffs bid (total 40 mg/day) significantly reduced cough in lung cancer patients without significant side effects.(231)

Lignocaine

Lignocaine has been reported to be useful in preventing cough during bronchoscopy and other surgical procedures, probably by acting on the afferent C fibres. In cancer patients, evidence from RCT is lacking, but nebulized lignocaine has been suggested for cough control.(224) The duration of action was reported to vary from 6 h to 5 days when used in a lung cancer patient.(232) Some workers suggest giving 5 ml of 0.25 per cent (12.5 mg) bupivacaine Q4H.(233) In giving nebulized lignocaine, it is recommended to stop oral intake, preferably 4 h before, and for a minimum of 2 h afterwards, or till the local anaesthetic effect wears off.

Sputum and mucus secretion in cancer patients

Airway secretion refers to mucus secreted by the submucosal glands and goblet cells, and which will become purulent in the presence of inflammation or infection. The airway secretion can accumulate due to increased production, decreased mucociliary clearance, and ineffective cough reflex.(234) These occur in patients who are chronic smokers, who have underlying pulmonary diseases like chronic bronchitis and bronchiectasis, who have tumours causing partial airway obstruction, or who have tracheo-oesophageal fistulae. Factors contributing to ineffective cough in cancer patients are listed in Table 11.

Excessive airway secretion distresses the cancer patients by interfering with normal sleep, inducing cough, predisposing to infection, and increasing dyspnoea by further compromising the airway. The embarrassment on the airway depends on the physical properties of the secretion, including volume and tenacity. These vary from the tenacious or inspissated sputum in the dehydrated and debilitated terminally ill, to the very watery voluminous secretion in bronchorrhoea.

On physical examination, noisy breathing and crepitations may be heard, indicating a moist lung. However, moist lung from various causes, for example, airway secretion with or without infection, aspiration of saliva, accumulation of blood from haemoptysis, pulmonary oedema not being easily differentiated, especially when the 'secretion' is not expectorated out for examination.

Improve clearance of sputum

Clearance of sputum can be improved by alteration of rheology to render mucus more fluid or by other measures to enhance expectoration. They include general measures like hydration, improving nutrition, bronchopulmonary hygiene physical therapy, improving the cough mechanism, suctioning, and pharmacological protussive therapy. However, clinical evidences of those non-pharmacological measures are generally lacking, and their use should be determined by balancing the burden and clinical benefit individually. Protussive agents are used for liquefying sputum, and again, not all of them are shown to improve sputum clearance. As sputum volume increases with these agents, an intact cough reflex is needed to clear them up.

With loss of water content, mucus become more tenacious. Fluid intake should be encouraged, and steam inhalation can be given to moisten the inhaled air. Fluid given parenterally may be more burdensome to patients and carers. Bronchopulmonary hygiene and physical therapy makes use of physical forces to remove lung secretions manually. Postural drainage may be effective, but chest percussion and vibration give no additional benefit.[235] Other active measures include forced exhalation, delivery of positive expiratory pressure, a flutter device to create vibrations in the airway, and assisted cough manoeuvre by applying compression on the upper abdomen.[221] Sometimes gentle suction may be required to clear up the secretions.

Pharmacological protussive therapy refers to the use of agents that improve cough clearance of sputum. Examples include drugs like beta-agonists, hypertonic saline, cysteine derivatives, for example, carbocysteine, *N*-acetylcysteine, bromhexine, amiloride, erdosteine, and the newer drug recombinant human DNase (rhDNase). Beta-agonists can be delivered by inhalers or by nebulizers which require minimal coordination. Cysteine derivatives serve to liquefy the lung secretions by altering physical properties. Hypertonic saline inhalation induces liquid influx from epithelium into the mucus. Guaifenesin enhances the output of secretions in the respiratory tract by reducing the surface tension and adhesiveness of the mucus. rhDNase breaks down the DNA which is secreted by neutrophils during infection and makes the sputum viscous.[221,236–238]

Bronchorrhoea

By definition, patients with bronchorrhoea produce more than 100 ml of watery sputum per day.[241] However, a daily production of up to 9 l has been reported in the literature.[239] Bronchorrhoea can be due to non-malignant causes like endobronchial tuberculosis, asthma, and relapsing polychondritis; but in advanced cancer patients, it is mostly likely due to the malignancy, especially lung cancer. Bronchioloalveolar carcinoma is frequently reported,[240] but the condition may also arise from pulmonary metastases from other tumours.

The impact on the patient is mainly due to the large volume of secretion involved. It has been reported that the patient had to bend forward constantly to expectorate the sputum.[239] It can cause cough, disturbance to sleep, airway obstruction, dehydration, and electrolyte disturbance.[241]

Management

Management of bronchorrhoea includes general supportive measures to maintain fluid balance and to promote comfort, and measures to decrease the sputum production. It is advisable to monitor the fluid status, electrolyte imbalance, and renal function to guide fluid replacement.

Specific oncological treatment with radiotherapy and chemotherapy has been used to alleviate bronchorrhoea, but the effect is variable.

Different agents have been used for decreasing the secretion with variable success. Anticholinergic drugs given in various routes often fail to improve bronchorrhoea.[239,241] Corticosteroids have been shown to improve bronchorrhoea in asthma but not in cancer.[239] Erythromycin inhibits the synthesis and secretion of a mucus secretagogue from pulmonary macrophages, and has been used to treat bronchorrhoea with variable outcome.[242] Cyclooxygenase-2 has been implicated in the pathogenesis of bronchorrhoea, and blockade with inhaled indomethacin has been reported to improve bronchorrhoea, dyspnoea, and hypoxaemia.[240] Octreotide has also been shown to cause temporary reduction in bronchorrhoea sputum.[241]

Haemoptysis

Haemoptysis, or coughing up blood, is often an alarming symptom to patients and their families. It can occur at any time during the illness, and occasionally, is a terminal event.

Causes of haemoptysis in cancer

The causes of haemoptysis in cancer patient are multiple, and are categorized into malignant, paramalignant, and non-malignant causes. Malignant causes include lung cancer, tumour involving major airway, like tracheal tumour, pulmonary carcinoid, endobronchial metastasis, haemic malignancy, and fistula formation between tumour and vessels. Paramalignant causes include cancer-related coagulopathy, thrombocytopenia, disseminated intravascular coagulopathy, and pulmonary embolism. Non-malignant causes include infection, for example, tuberculosis, bronchiectasis, and drug-related causes, for example, anticoagulation.

Among all cancers, bronchogenic carcinoma is the most common cause of haemoptysis. In a large retrospective autopsy analysis of 877 cases of lung cancer,[243] the overall incidence of haemoptysis was 19.3 per cent. Twenty-nine patients (3.3 per cent) had massive terminal haemoptysis, which was strongly associated with squamous cell carcinoma (82.8 per cent), cavitation (48.3 per cent), and major airway involvement (51.7 per cent major bronchus, 41.4 per cent lobar or segmental bronchus, 6.9 per cent peripheral). However, non-lethal haemoptysis was not associated with any one histological type. Of NSCLC patients referred for palliative radiotherapy, 47 per cent were referred for haemoptysis.[120] Most of them had mild to moderate haemoptysis, and massive haemoptysis as a terminal event occurred in 3.3 per cent.

Haemoptysis from malignant tracheal tumour is less common when compared with bronchogenic carcinoma. The most common endobronchial metastases reported are from breast, colon, and renal cell carcinoma. Bronchial carcinoid is well known to be located in central airways and haemoptysis is reported in one-quarter of the patients.[244]

In haematological malignancies, fungal pneumonia was strongly associated with fatal haemoptysis,[245] with fungal invasion of blood vessels, vascular thrombosis, and extensive haemorrhagic infarction as the underlying pathology.

Among non-malignant causes, inflammatory causes like bronchiectasis and tuberculosis are the most common causes.

Clinical approach to cancer patients with haemoptysis

Before deciding on the modality of treatment, one has to assess the severity of bleeding, the risk of recurrent haemoptysis, and the cause and the site of bleeding. Available treatment modalities include:

1. general management and pharmacological therapy,
2. specific oncological treatment (e.g. radiotherapy),
3. invasive interventions—bronchoscopic procedure, endobronchial therapies, and bronchial artery embolization in the case of massive bleeding, and
4. palliative treatment of fatal haemoptysis.

The severity of haemoptysis will guide the prognosis and further therapy. Massive haemoptysis carries a grave prognosis with risks of respiratory failure, haemodynamic disturbance, and even death. The outcome is affected by the rate of bleeding, baseline ventilatory reserve, and haemodynamic disturbance. A milder degree of haemoptysis may sometimes precipitate acute respiratory failure in a respiratory cripple.

Localization of the sites and source of bleeding may define the best modality of treatment for stopping the bleeding. Bleeding can come from an endobronchial site or alveolar level; at either site, it could come from the bronchial or pulmonary circulation. For major haemoptysis, the bleeding often comes from bronchial arteries and collaterals from systemic circulation.

Baseline investigations include complete blood count, electrolytes, renal and liver function tests, prothrombin time, and activated partial thromboplastin time. Chest radiography may identify the sites of tumours, cavitatory lesions, and lung atelectasis in the case of endobronchial obstruction. Computed tomography may show central airway tumour, cavitatory lesions, or identify bronchiectasis in patients with a normal chest radiograph. In the case of significant haemoptysis, localization of the site of bleeding is often necessary to guide specific therapy. The option of bronchoscopic examination of the airway needs careful weighing of benefit, burden, and prognosis.

General management

Haemoptysis is, understandably, often alarming to the patient and the family. The symptom is so visible and is associated with fears. It is always worthwhile to find out what the bleeding means to the patient and the family. Communication with the patient about the causes of the haemoptysis, the prognosis, and the treatment plan will alleviate much anxiety.

Specific treatment is required for concomitant medical conditions. A course of antibiotics is appropriate if there is increased purulent sputum. A cough suppressant may decrease the distress and lessen the haemoptysis.

In the case of major haemoptysis, general management includes positioning of patients with their bleeding site down to prevent drowning of the other lung segments, correction of hypoxaemia, coagulopathy, and hypovolaemia. Haemostatic agents, for example, tranexamic acid or aminocaproic acid, are frequently used empirically but beneficial effect has not been documented by well-conducted study. In a report on the management of tumour-associated bleeding,(246) the bleeding was controlled in 14 out of 16 patients by using a haemostatic agent.

Oncological treatment: radiotherapy

Haemoptysis is an indication for radiotherapy. In prospective trials of palliative external beam irradiation, successful palliation of haemoptysis was reported in 74–97 per cent of patients.(247) In the Medical Research Council randomized trial of palliative radiotherapy for inoperable NSCLC, haemoptysis was palliated in 81–86 per cent. The recommended regimen is two fractions of 8.5 Gy given 1 week apart or one fraction of 10 Gy if the patient has a poor performance status.(120,121)

Brachytherapy has the advantage of delivering high dose radiotherapy exactly to the bleeding site and less to the rest of the lung. It can be given repeatedly and after failure with conventional radiotherapy. However, bronchoscopy is needed for every radiotherapy session. Success rate in palliation of haemoptysis was reported to be 88 per cent and higher.(122–124)

Invasive intervention for massive haemoptysis

The prognosis of massive haemoptysis is poor without specific treatment, which requires a careful weighing of the risks versus benefits for each patient. If the episode happens as the very end-stage of the disease, comfort with minimal intervention will be appropriate. If invasive intervention *is* considered, bronchoscopy is usually needed to locate the source of bleeding. Bronchoscopic procedures include insertion of balloon catheter(248) and installation of iced saline.(249) Fibrinogen-thrombin(250) has also been used with success. For visible lesions in the trachea and proximal bronchi, laser, cryotherapy, or electrocautery treatment is useful (see under 'Major airway obstruction').

Massive bleeding is more likely to come from the high-pressure bronchial arteries, which may be stopped by embolization with the aid of bronchoscopy and angiography. The immediate and long-term success rate is high in non-cancer patients.(251) This procedure has been performed in cancer-related haemoptysis.(252)

Management of fatal haemoptysis

Massive haemoptysis in cancer patients is uncommon, but when it happens, it impacts on patients, relatives, and staff. If a patient is at risk of massive haemoptysis, it is essential to establish a plan of action.(253) The family needs to be informed, psychologically prepared, with possible treatment options discussed. If a massive life-threatening haemoptysis occurs, sedation to relieve the distress should be given as soon as possible. Midazolam can be given intravenously or via the subcutaneous route. Diazepam given *per rectal* is an alternative. Morphine can also lessen the dyspnoea and distress. The patient should be accompanied by staff all the time, and a dark green or red towel used to cover the patient and, hopefully, reduce the visual impact. Keeping an 'emergency box' with the necessary drugs and towels in the ward facilitates timely intervention of such crisis.

The psychological impact of a patient dying from massive haemoptysis is enormous. Family members, other patients, and the staff who witness the event, will all be affected. Immediate support and attention should be given to the family and other patients. It is important that support will also be given to the staff after the incident.

Chest pain

Chest pain is a common symptom of malignancies involving the respiratory system. Different types of chest pain are described that include: (i) pleural pain, (ii) chest wall pain, (iii) deep visceral pain, (iv) neuropathic chest pain, and (v) costopleural syndrome.

Pleural pain is chest pain associated with breathing without local tenderness. It can be caused by cancer invading pleura, malignant pleural effusion, chest infection, pneumothorax, PE, or as a side effect from pleurodesis. Chest wall pain is characterized by local tenderness. The causes include local chest wall invasion by tumour, vertebral metastasis, rib erosions, or metastasis. Deep visceral pain is often a dull ache in character and poorly localized. It can be caused by intrathoracic spread involving trachea, oesophagus, pericardium, and SVC. Neuropathic pain is characterized by allodynia, burning sensation, shooting pain, dysaesthesia, and sensory loss, often over the sensory distribution of the affected nerve. Neuropathic chest pain can be caused by intercostal nerve infiltration in vertebral erosion, brachial plexus infiltration in Pancoast's tumour, radiculopathy or spinal cord compression in epidural deposits, thoracic Herpes Zoster or post-thoracotomy syndrome. As neuropathic pain can be a sign of epidural deposits, a full neurological examination is warranted to look for spinal cord compression.

Costopleural syndrome

The costopleural syndrome results from tumour invasion of the pleura, soft tissue, or ribs, often with entrapment of the thoracic intercostal, autonomic nerves, and brachial plexus. The most common underlying tumours are lung cancer and mesothelioma. A study reported that 58 per cent of mesothelioma presented with pain.(254) Costopleural irritation causes a sharp aching or burning sensation usually overlying the pathological lesion, and is aggravated by deep breathing, coughing, and movement. Central lesions of the diaphragmatic pleura cause localized sharp or aching pain in the shoulder or ridge of the trapezius. Involvement over the muscular portion of the diaphragm causes a referred dull ache to the upper lumbar region of the back and the upper two-thirds of the abdomen. Tumour infiltration of the cupola of the lung produces pain in the upper interscapular or vertebral area and in the medial aspect of the arm. Mediastinal pleural invasion produces pain deep in the central portion of the chest and also in the shoulder and trapezius regions.(255)

Costopleural pain may not be adequately controlled by opioid alone. Co-analgesics like NSAIDs, anticonvulsants, and tricyclic antidepressants can be added to control the bony and neuropathic components of pain. Radiotherapy is effective for pain control in 50 per cent cases of mesothelioma.(85) Interventional pain treatment is an option when drugs fail. For a larger area of involvement, intrapleural, epidural, or intrathecal analgesic may be attempted.(85) Percutaneous cervical cordotomy at C1/C2 level has been performed for patients with refractory pain and reported to cause reduction in pain in 83 per cent of patients.(256)

Palliative sedation for refractory respiratory symptoms

Palliative sedation is often considered a last option for relieving suffering that arises from refractory symptoms. With the possible risk of respiratory depression with sedation, its role in the management of refractory dyspnoea remains to be carefully defined. Towards death, unlike pain, a significant proportion of patients are still facing uncontrolled dyspnoea. This may reflect our limited ability to control dyspnoea until better treatment strategies evolve from a more thorough understanding of the symptom. 'Refractoriness', being not an absolute phenomenon, should be defined and its underlying causes carefully assessed. The management of patients with refractory dyspnoea is a situation that every palliative care physician has to struggle with, balancing the medical and ethical imperatives. The adoption of palliative sedation as a last resort may reflect the great desire of the physician to address uncontrolled suffering by every effort. Respiratory side effects may not be present, and therefore sedation should not be withheld due to disproportionate fear of respiratory depression. However, when the risk of respiratory depression becomes genuine, the benefits, risks, and the ethical principle of 'double effects' must be carefully considered. Without the indication and the intention of sedation being clearly defined, there is always a concern that liberal use of palliative sedation may fall into the slippery slope of 'slow euthanasia'.

Use of palliative sedation in hospices

The frequency of use of sedation for refractory symptoms is highly variable in hospices/palliative care units, as well as the indications (Table 14). Dyspnoea is often reported as one of the most common symptoms requiring sedation.[265] However, in a recent multicentre study, it was found that the need to sedate dyspnoeic patients varied widely among the different hospice units.[258] This may be due to the difference in the condition of patients, prescription habit, culture, social values, and hospice policies. Even the definition of sedation, be it terminal or palliative, seems to be different among different authors.

Sedation has been prescribed intermittently or continuously, maintained as mild or deep, depending on the need. Mild sedation, however, may aggravate weakness and dyspnoea. When sedation is given near the end of life, it may be reasonable to continue the sedation till death to avoid recurrence of distressing symptoms. When time and the situation allows, reversal of sedation for reviewing the symptoms is an option.

Midazolam is one of the most commonly used drugs for sedation for refractory symptoms. It is short and fast acting, and plasma concentrations of midazolam correlate well with the subcutaneous infusion rates, facilitating titration against clinical response. Other drugs used include opioids, other benzodiazepines, and major tranquillizers. The route of administration may be subcutaneous, intravenous, intramuscular, rectal, or oral (Table 14).

Considerations for palliative sedation

Sedation for refractory symptoms has been considered by some to be a form of 'slow euthanasia'. This is especially so in patients with respiratory problems, who are considered to be more predisposed to the respiratory depressant effect of sedatives and opioids. Nevertheless, recent evidence shows that use of opioids and sedatives in the last days of life for various indications are not associated with a shortened survival.[210,259,261,266,267]

Careful considerations should be taken before deciding on palliative sedation which may have undesirable side effects. This is especially important for this controversial means of relieving suffering, which has a risk of being given too liberally. The decision should be based on the conditions that the symptom is refractory, the patients and families are fully involved in the decision making, the benefits of sedation should outweigh the risks and burden, and that sedation is a means of relieving distressing symptom, and not the ultimate goal of treatment.

Cherny and Portenoy defined a symptom as refractory when it is perceived that further interventions (i) will not bring adequate relief, (ii) will be associated with intolerable morbidity, and (iii) are unlikely to bring relief within a reasonable time frame. Expert consultation and team involvement is advisable before considering a symptom refractory.[268] They also underscored the importance of distinguishing a 'refractory' symptom from a 'difficult' symptom.

Not all patients and their family members seek sedation for the relief of symptoms, even when death draws near. The therapeutic goal in symptom control is usually relief of distress with preserved function. Sedation results in a loss of interactional function which may not be acceptable to some patients and families. The patients and their families have to be involved in the discussion, and the patient's consent must be obtained. They have to be reassured that as sedation is only a means of treatment, it will be under constant review, and both continuation and reversal of sedation can be considered if deemed appropriate.

Dyspnoea is refractory to treatment in some patients despite all efforts. While breathlessness may escalate as death is approaching, patients often fear that their physicians will abandon them and will not be present to relieve their sufferings when they are dying. As a last resort of alleviating suffering, the practice of palliative sedation respects sanctity of life with the sacrifice of consciousness. A good death always contains an intrinsic personal perspective. For patients who choose relieving dyspnoea while

Table 14 Studies on palliative sedation for refractory symptoms including respiratory distress

Author	Type of study and findings
Ventafridda et al., 1990[210]	Prospective, 120 patients, 63 need sedation for uncontrollable symptoms, 33 of 63 had dyspnoea[a]
McIver et al., 1994[217]	Prospective, 82 deaths, 20 (24.4%) received palliative sedation till death, 10 (50%) for dyspnoea
Morita et al., 1999[257]	Prospective, 71 sedated patients Sedated patients accounted for 45% of all deaths. Dyspnoea as main symptom for sedation (41%)
Fainsinger et al., 2000[258]	Prospective, multicentred Need to sedate: 15% in Israel ($n = 100$, 0 for dyspnoea), 29% in Durban ($n = 94$, 13% for dyspnoea), 36% in Cape Town ($n = 93$, 12% for dyspnoea), 22% in Madrid ($n = 100$, 2% for dyspnoea)
Chiu et al., 2001[259]	Prospective, 276 patients, 251 died, 70 (27.9%) required sedation, dyspnoea in 16 (22.8%)[a]
Morita et al., 1996[260]	Retrospective, 143 patients, 69 (48.3%) sedated, dyspnoea accounted for 49%, intermittent sedation until death in 44%
Stone et al., 1997[261]	Retrospective, 115 patients 31% in hospice, 21% in general hospital required sedation. Dyspnoea was an indication for sedation in six patients (20%)[a]
Fainsinger et al., 1998[262]	Retrospective, 76 patients 23 (30%) sedated, three for dyspnoea (13%)
Chater et al., 1998[263]	Survey of experts, 100 sedated patients Respiratory distress accounted for 19% Only 50% of patients and 60% of relatives involved in decision-making of sedation

[a] No difference in survival between sedated and non-sedated patients.

trading off conciousness, palliative sedation remains an option. For those patients who decline sedation despite overwhelming discomforts, it remains for the palliative care workers to hold, to accompany, and to walk with the patients in their last journey.

The extent and depth of suffering of our patients living and dying with respiratory symptoms is enormous. This suffering calls for a greater attention to be given to these patients. To achieve a better quality of life and quality of death, a concerted effort of good clinical care, education, and research remains our challenge in the coming days.

References

1. **Chochinov, H.M.** et al. (1999). Will to live in the terminally ill. *Lancet* **354**, 816–19.
2. **American Thoracic Society** (1999). Dyspnea. Mechanisms, assessment, and management: a consensus statement. *American Journal of Respiratory and Critical Care Medicine* **159**, 321–40.
3. **Simon, P.M.** et al. (1990). Distinguishable types of dyspnoea in patients with shortness of breath. *American Review of Respiratory Disease* **142**, 1009–14.
4. **Brown, M.L.** et al. (1986). Lung cancer and dyspnoea: the patient's perception. *Oncology Nursing Forum* **13**, 19–24.
5. **Roberts, D.K., Thorne, S.E., and Pearson, C.** (1993). The experience of dyspnoea in late-stage cancer. *Cancer Nursing* **16**, 310–20.
6. **O'Driscoll, M., Corner, J., and Bailey, C.** (1999). The experience of breathlessness in lung cancer. *European Journal of Cancer Care* **8**, 37–43.
7. **Lane, R.** et al. (1987). Arterial oxygen saturation and breathlessness in patients with chronic obstructive airways disease. *Clinical Science* **72**, 693–8.
8. **Banzett, R.B.** et al. (1989). 'Air hunger' arising from increased PCO_2 in mechanically ventilated quadriplegics. *Respiratory Physiology* **76**, 53–67.
9. **Banzett, R.B.** et al. (1990). 'Air hunger' from increased PCO persists after complete neuromuscular block in humans. *Respiratory Physiology* **81**, 1–17.
10. **Manning, H.L. and Schwartzstein, R.M.** (1999). Dyspnea and the control of breathing. In *Control of Breathing in Health and Disease* (ed. M.D. Altose and T. Kamakami). New York: Marcel Dekker.
11. **Schwartzstein, R.M.** et al. (1987). Cold facial stimulation reduces breathlessness induced in normal subjects. *American Review of Respiratory Disease* **136**, 58–61.
12. **Campbell, E.J.M. and Howell, J.B.L.** (1963). The sensation of breathlessness. *British Medical Bulletin* **19**, 36–40.
13. **Chonan, T.** et al. (1987). Effects of voluntary constraining of thoracic displacement during hypercapnia. *Journal of Applied Physiology* **63**, 1822–8.
14. **Reuben, D.B. and Mor, V.** (1986). Dyspnoea in terminally ill cancer patients. *Chest* **89**, 234–6.
15. **Heyse-Moore, L.H., Ross, V., and Mullee, M.A.** (1991). How much of a problem is dyspnoea in advanced cancer? *Palliative Medicine* **5**, 20–6.
16. **Bruera, E.** et al. (2000). The frequency and correlates of dyspnoea in patients with advanced cancer. *Journal of Pain and Symptom Management* **19**, 357–62.
17. **Curtis, E.B., Krech, R., and Walsh, D.** (1991). Common symptoms in patients with advanced cancer. *Journal of Palliative Care* **7**, 25–9.
18. **Donnelly, S. and Walsh, D.** (1995). The symptoms of advanced cancer: identification of clinical and research priorities by assessment of prevalence and severity. *Journal of Palliative Care* **11**, 27–32.
19. **Dudgeon, D.J.** et al. (2001). Dyspnoea in cancer patients: prevalence and associated factors. *Journal of Pain and Symptom Management* **21**, 95–102.
20. **Chang, V.T.** et al. (2000). Symptom and quality of life survey of medical oncology patients at a veterans affairs medical center. *Cancer* **88**, 1175–83.
21. **Lo, R.S.** et al. (1999). Prospective study of symptom control in 133 cases of palliative care inpatients in Shatin Hospital. *Palliative Medicine* **13**, 335–40.
22. **Krech, R.L.** et al. (1992). Symptoms of lung cancer. *Palliative Medicine* **6**, 309–15.
23. **Muers, M.F. and Round, C.E.** (1993). Palliation of symptoms in non-small cell lung cancer: a study by the Yorkshire Regional Cancer Organisation Thoracic Group. *Thorax* **48**, 339–43.
24. **Hopwood, P. and Stephens, R.J.** (1995). Symptoms at presentation for treatment in patients with lung cancer: implications for the evaluation of palliative treatment. The Medical Research Council (MRC) Lung Cancer Working Party. *British Journal of Cancer* **71**, 633–6.
25. **Higginson, I. and McCarthy, M.** (1989). Measuring symptoms in terminal cancer: are pain and dyspnoea controlled? *Journal of the Royal Society of Medicine* **82**, 264–7.
26. **Conill, C.** et al. (1997). Symptom prevalence in the last week of life. *Journal of Pain and Symptom Management* **14**, 328–31.
27. **Mercadante, S., Casiccio, A., and Fulfaro, F.** (2000). The course of symptom frequency and intensity in advanced cancer patients followed at home. *Journal of Pain and Symptom Management* **20**, 104–12.
28. **Hardy, J.R.** et al. (1994). Prediction of survival in a hospital-based continuing care unit. *European Journal of Cancer* **30A**, 284–8.
29. **Maltoni, M.** et al. (1995). Prediction of survival of patients terminally ill with cancer. *Cancer* **75**, 2613–22.
30. **Morita, T.** et al. (1999). Do hospice clinicians sedate patients intending to hasten death? *Journal of Palliative Care* **15**, 20–3.
31. **Pirovano, M.** et al. (1999). A new palliative prognostic score: a first step for the staging of terminally ill cancer patients. *Journal of Pain and Symptom Management* **17**, 231–49.
32. **Escalante, C.P.** et al. (1996). Dyspnoea in cancer patients. Etiology, resource utilisation, and survival-implications in a managed care world. *Cancer* **78**, 1314–19.
33. **Escalante, C.P.** et al. (2000). Identifying risk factors for imminent death in cancer patients with acute dyspnoea. *Journal of Pain and Symptom Management* **20**, 318–25.
34. **Dudgeon, D.J. and Lertzman, M.** (1998). Dyspnoea in the advanced cancer patient. *Journal of Pain and Symptom Management* **16**, 212–19.
35. **Congleton, J. and Muers, M.F.** (1995). The incidence of airflow obstruction in bronchial carcinoma, its relation to breathlessness, and response to bronchodilator therapy. *Respiratory Medicine* **89**, 291–6.
36. **Heyse-Moore, L.H., Beynon, T., and Ross, V.** (2000). Does spirometry predict dyspnoea in advanced cancer? *Palliative Medicine* **14**, 189–95.
37. **Dudgeon, D.J., Lertzman, M., and Askew, G.R.** (2001). Physiological changes in clinical correlations of dyspnoea in cancer outpatients. *Journal of Pain and Symptom Management* **21**, 373–9.
38. **Bruera, E.** et al. (1993). Effects of oxygen on dyspnoea in hypoxaemic terminal-cancer patients. *Lancet* **342**, 13–14.
39. **Booth, S.** et al. (1996). Does oxygen help dyspnoea in patients with cancer? *American Journal of Respiratory and Critical Care Medicine* **153**, 1515–18.
40. **McDaniel, R.W. and Rhodes, V.A.** (1995). Symptom experience. *Seminars in Oncology Nursing* **11**, 232–4.
41. **Corner, J. and O'Driscoll, M.** (1999). Development of a breathlessness assessment guide for use in palliative care. *Palliative Medicine* **13**, 375–84.
42. **Booth, S. and Adams, L.** (2001). The shuttle walking test: a reproducible method for evaluating the impact of shortness of breath on functional capacity in patients with advanced cancer. *Thorax* **56**, 146–50.
43. **Bruera, E.** et al. (1991). The Edmonton Symptom Assessment System (ESAS): a simple method for the assessment of palliative care patients. *Journal of Palliative care* **7**, 6–9.
44. **McCockle, R. and Young, K.** (1978). Development of a symptom distress scale. *Cancer Nursing* **1**, 373–8.
45. **de Haes, J.C., van Kippenberg, F.C.E., and Neijt, J.P.** (1990). Measuring psychological and physical distress in cancer patients: Structure and application of the Rotterdam Symptom Checklist. *British Journal of Cancer* **62**, 1034–8.
46. **Portenoy, R.K.** et al. (1994). The memorial Symptom Assessment Scale: an Instrument for the Evaluation of symptom prevalence, characteristics and distress. *European Journal of Cancer* **30A**, 1326–36.
47. **Tanaka, K.** et al. (2000). Development and validation of the Cancer Dyspnoea Scale: a multidimensional, brief, self-rating scale. *British Journal of Cancer* **82**, 800–5.
48. **Wilcock, A.** et al. (1999). Reading numbers aloud: a measure of the limiting effect of breathlessness in patients with cancer. *Thorax* **54**, 1099–103.
49. **Burdon, J.** et al. (1982). The perception of dyspnoea in asthma. *American Review of Respiratory Disease* **126**, 825.

50. **Mahler, D.A.** et al. (1984). The measurement of dyspnoea. Contents, interobserver agreement, and physiologic correlates of two new clinical indexes. *Chest* **85**, 751–8.
51. **Stoller, J.K., Ferranti, R., and Feinstein, A.R.** (1986). Further specification and evaluation of a new clinical index for dyspnea. *American Review of Respiratory Disease* **134**, 1129–34.
52. **McGavin, C.R.** et al. (1978). Dyspnoea, disability, and distance walked: Comparison of estimates of exercise performance in respiratory disease. *British Medical Journal* **2**, 241.
53. **Rodriguez-Panadero, F., Borderas, N.F., and Lopez, M.J.** (1989). Pleural metastatic tumours and effusions. Frequency and pathogenic mechanisms in a post-mortem series. *European Respiratory Journal* **2**, 366–9.
54. **Chernow, B. and Sahn, S.A.** (1977). Carcinomatous involvement of the pleura: an analysis of 96 patients. *American Journal of Medicine* **63**, 695–702.
55. **Peto, J.** et al. (1999). The European mesothelioma epidemic. *British Journal of Cancer* **79**, 666–72.
56. **Cheng, D.** et al. (1999). Vascular endothelial growth factor in pleural fluid. *Chest* **116**, 760–5.
57. **American Thoracic Society** (2000). Management of malignant pleural effusions. *American Journal of Respiratory and Critical Care Medicine* **162**, 1987–2001.
58. **Sahn, S.A.** (1998). Malignancy metastasis to the pleura. *Clinics in Chest Medicine* **19**, 351–61.
59. **Heffner, J.E., Nietert, P.J., and Barbieri, C.** (2000). Pleural fluid pH as a predictor of survival for patients with malignant pleural effusions.*Chest* **117**, 79–86.
60. **Heffner, J.E., Nietert, P.J., and Barbieri, C.** (2000). Pleural fluid pH as a predictor of pleurodesis failure. *Chest* **117**, 87–95.
61. **Burrows, C.M., Mathews, W.C., and Colt, H.G.** (2000). Predicting survival in patients with recurrent symptomatic malignant pleural effusions: and assessment of the prognostic values of physiologic, morphologic, and quality of life measures of extent of disease. *Chest* **117**, 73–8.
62. **Sahn, S.A. and Good, J.T., Jr.** (1988). Pleural fluid pH in malignant effusions, diagnostic, prognostic, and therapeutic implications, *Annals of Internal medicine* **108**, 345–9.
63. **Rodriguez-Panadero, F.** (1997). Current trends in pleurodesis. *Current Opinion in Pulmonary Medicine* **3**, 319–25.
64. **Grossi, F.** et al. (1998). Management of malignant pleural effusions. *Drugs* **55**, 47–58 (Review).
65. **Antunes, G. and Neville, E.** (2000). Management of malignant pleural effusions. *Thorax* **55**, 981–3 (Review).
66. **Walker-Renard, P.B., Vaughan, L.M., and Sahn, S.A.** (1994). Chemical pleurodesis for malignant pleural effusions. *Annals of Internal Medicine* **120**, 56–64.
67. **Yim, A.P.** et al. (1996). Thoracoscopic talc insufflation versus talc slurry for symptomatic malignant pleural effusion. *Annals of Thoracic Surgery* **62**, 1655–8.
68. **Light, R.W.** (2000). Talc should not be used for pleurodesis. *American Journal of Respiratory and Critical Care Medicine* **162**, 2024–6 (Review).
69. **Vargas, F.S., Carmo, A.O., and Teixeira, L.R.** (2000). A new look at old agents for pleurodesis: nitrogen mustard, sodium hydroxide, and silver nitrate. *Current Opinion in Pulmonary Medicine* **6**, 281–6.
70. **Kennedy, L.** et al. (1995). Sterilization of talc for pleurodesis. Available techniques, efficacy, and cost analysis. *Chest* **107**, 1032–4.
71. **Ruckdeschel, J.C.** et al. (1991). Intrapleural therapy for malignant pleural effusion: a randomised comparison of bleomycin and tetracycline. *Chest* **100**, 1528–35.
72. **Moffett, M.J. and Ruckdeschel, J.C.** (1992). Bleomycin and tetracycline in malignant pleural effusions: a review. *Seminars in Oncology* **19**, 59–62 (Review).
73. **Hartman, D.L.** et al. (1993). Comparison of insufflated talc under thoracoscopic guidance with standard tetracycline and bleomycin pleurodesis for control of malignant pleural effusions. *Journal of Thoracic Cardiovascular Surgery* **105**, 743–7.
74. **Emad, A. and Rezaian, G.R.** (1996). Treatment of malignant pleural effusions with a combination of bleomycin and tetracycline. A comparison of bleomycin or tetracycline alone versus a combination of bleomycin and tetracycline. *Cancer* **78**, 2498–501.
75. **Diacon, A.H.** et al. (2000). Prospective randomized comparison of thoracoscopic talc poudrage under local anesthesia versus bleomycin instillation for pleurodesis in malignant pleural effusions. *American Journal of Respiratory and Critical Care Medicine* **162**, 1445–9.
76. **Zimmer, P.W.** et al. (1997). Prospective randomized trial of talc slurry versus bleomycin in pleurodesis for symptomatic malignant pleural effusions. *Chest* **112**, 430–4.
77. **Noppen, M.** et al. (1997). A prospective, randomized study comparing the efficacy of talc slurry and bleomycin in the treatment of malignant pleural effusions. *Acta Clinical Belgium* **52**, 258–62.
78. **Martinez-Moragon, E.** et al. (1997). Pleurodesis in malignant pleural effusions: a randomized study of tetracycline versus bleomycin. *European Respiratory Journal* **10**, 2380–3.
79. **Patz, E.F., Jr.** et al. (1998). Sclerotherapy for malignant pleural effusions: a prospective randomized trial of bleomycin versus doxycycline with small-bore catheter drainage. *Chest* **113**, 1305–11.
80. **Ong, K.C.** (2000). A comparative study of pleurodesis using talc slurry and bleomycin in the management of malignant pleural effusions. *Respirology* **5**, 99–103.
81. **Parulekar, W.** et al. (2001). Use of small-bore versus large-bore chest tubes for treatment of malignant pleural effusions. *Chest* **120**, 19–25.
82. **Putnam, J.B.** et al. (1999). A randomised comparison of indwelling pleural catheter and doxycline pleurodesis in the management of malignant pleural effusion. *Cancer* **86**, 1992–9.
83. **Pien, G.W.** et al. (2001). Use of an implantable pleural catheter for trapped lung syndrome in patients with malignant pleural effusion. *Chest* **119**, 1641–6.
84. **Genc, O.** et al. (2000). The long-term morbidity of pleuroperitoneal shunts in the management of recurrent malignant effusions. *European Journal of Cardiothoracic Surgery* **18**, 143–6.
85. **British Thoracic Society Standard of Care Committee** (2001). Statement on malignant mesothelioma in the United Kingdom. *Thorax* **56**, 250–65.
86. **Yates, D.H.** et al. (1997). Malignant mesothelioma in south east England: clinicopathological experience of 272 cases. *Thorax* **52**, 507–12.
87. **Lee, Y.C.** et al. (2000). Management of malignant pleural mesothelioma: a critical review. *Current Opinion in Pulmonary Medicine* **6**, 267–74.
88. **Viallat, J.R.** et al. (1996). Thoracoscopic talc poudrage pleurodesis for malignant effusions. A review of 360 cases. *Chest* **110**, 1387–93.
89. **Senyigit, A.** et al. (2000). Comparison of the effectiveness of some pleural sclerosing agents used for control of effusions in malignant pleural mesothelioma, a review of 117 cases. *Respiration* **67**, 623–9.
90. **Waller, D.A., Morritt, G.N., and Forty, J.** (1995). Video-assisted thoracoscopic pleurectomy in the management of malignant pleural effusion. *Chest* **107**, 1454–6.
91. **Petrou, M., Kaplan, D., and Goldstraw, P.** (1995). Management of recurrent malignant pleural effusions. The complementary role talc pleurodesis and pleuroperitoneal shunting. *Cancer* **75**, 801–5.
92. **Thurber, D.L.** et al. (1962). Secondary malignant tumours of the pericardium. *Circulation* **XXVI**, 228–41.
93. **Klatt, E.C. and Heitz, D.R.** (1990). Cardiac metastases. *Cancer* **65**, 1456–9.
94. **Maher, E.A., Shepherd, F.A., and Todd, T.J.R.** (1996). Pericardial sclerosis as the primary management of malignant pericardial effusion and cardiac tamponade. *Journal of Thoracic and Cardiovascular Surgery* **112**, 637–43.
95. **Wilkes, J.D.** et al. (1995). Malignancy-related pericardial effusion. *Cancer* **76**, 1377–87.
96. **Campbell, P.T.** et al. (1992). Subxiphoid pericardiotomy in the diagnosis and management of large pericardial effusions associated with malignancy. *Chest* **101**, 938–43.
97. **Liu, G.** et al. (1996). Prospective comparison of the sclerosing agents doxycycline and bleomycin for the primary management of malignant pericardial effusion and cardiac tamponade. *Journal of Clinical Oncology* **14**, 3141–7.
98. **Celermajer, D.S.** et al. (1991). Pericardiocentesis for symptomatic malignant pericardial effusion: a study of 36 patients. *Medical Journal of Australia* **154**, 19–22.

99. **Ziskind, A.A.** et al. (1993). Percutaneous balloon pericardiotomy for the treatment of cardiac tamponade and large pericardial effusions: description of technique and report of the first 50 cases. *Journal of American College of Cardiology* **21**, 1–5.
100. **Porte, H.L.** et al. (1999). Pericardoscopy for primary management of pericardial effusion in cancer patients. *European Journal of Cardiothoracic Surgery* **16**, 287–91.
101. **Geissbuhler, K.** et al. (1998). Video-assisted thoracoscopic pericardial fenestration for loculated or recurrent effusions. *European Journal of Cardiothoracic Surgery* **14**, 403–8.
102. **Ahmann, F.** (1984). A reassessment of the clinical implications of the superior vena caval syndrome. *Journal of Clinical Oncology* **2**, 961–9.
103. **Schraufnagel, D.E.** et al. (1981). Superior vena caval obstruction, is it a medical emergency? *American Journal of Medicine* **70**, 1169–74.
104. **Baker, G.L. and Barnes, H.J.** (1992). Superior vena cava syndrome: etiology, diagnosis, and treatment. *American Journal of Critical Care* **1**, 54–64.
105. **Yellin, A.** et al. (1990). Superior vena cava syndrome. *American Review of Respiratory Disease* **141**, 1114–18.
106. **Perez, C.A., Presant, C.A., and Van Amburg, A.L., 3rd** (1978). Management of superior vena cava syndrome. *Seminars in Oncology* **5**, 123–34.
107. **Jackson, J.E. and Brooks, D.M.** (1995). Stenting of superior vena caval obstruction. *Thorax* **50** (1S), S31–6.
108. **Urban, T.** et al. (1993). Superior vena cava syndrome in small-cell lung cancer. *Archives of Internal Medicine* **153**, 384–7.
109. **Gray, B.H.** et al. (1991). Safety and efficacy of thrombolytic therapy for superior vena cava syndrome. *Chest* **99**, 54–9.
110. **Armstrong, B.A.** et al. (1987). Role of irradiation in the management of superior vena cava syndrome. *International Journal of Radiation Oncology, Biology, and Physics* **13**, 531–9.
111. **Nicholson, A.A.** et al. (1997). Treatment of malignant superior vena cava obstruction: metal Stents or radiation therapy. *Journal of Vascular and Interventional Radiology* **8**, 781–8.
112. **Tanigawa, N.** et al. (1998). Clinical outcome of stenting in superior vena cava syndrome associated with malignant tumours. *Acta Radiologica* **39**, 669–74.
113. **Hochrein, J.** et al. (1998). Percutaneous stenting of superior vena cava syndrome: a case report and review of the literature. *American Journal of Medicine* **104**, 78–84.
114. **Seijo, L.M. and Sterman, D.H.** (2001). Interventional pulmonology. *New England Journal of Medicine* **344**, 740–9.
115. **Cavaliere, S.** et al. (1996). Endoscopic treatment of malignant airway obstructions in 2,008 patients. *Chest* **110**, 1536–42.
116. **Coulter, T.D. and Mehta, A.C.** (2000). The heat is on: impact of endobronchial electrosurgery on the need for Nd-YAG laser photoresection. *Chest* **118**, 516–21.
117. **Walsh, D.A.** et al. (1990). Bronchoscopic cryotherapy for advanced bronchial carcinoma. *Thorax* **45**, 509–13.
118. **Maiwand, M.O.** (1999). The role of cryosurgery in palliation of tracheobronchial carcinoma. *European Journal of Cardiothoracic Surgery* **15**, 764–8.
119. **Mathur, P.N.** et al. (1996). Fiberoptic bronchoscopic cryotherapy in the management of tracheobronchial obstruction. *Chest* **110**, 718–23.
120. **Lung Cancer Working Party** (1991). Inoperable non-small-cell lung cancer (NSCLC) a medical research council randomized trial of palliative radiotherapy with two fractions or ten fractions. *British Journal of Cancer* **63**, 265–70.
121. **Lung Cancer Working Party** (1992). A Medical Research Council (MRC) randomized trial of palliative radiotherapy with two fractions or a single fraction in patients with inoperable non-small-cell lung cancer (NSCLC) and poor performance status. *British Journal of Cancer* **65**, 934–41.
122. **Speiser, B.L.** (1999). Brachytherapy in the treatment of thoracic tumors. Lung and esophageal. *Hematological Oncology Clinics of North Americia* **13**, 609–34.
123. **Chang, L.F.** et al. (1994). High dose rate afterloading intraluminal brachytherapy in malignant airway obstruction of lung cancer. *International Journal of Radiation Oncology, Biology, and Physics* **28**, 589–96.
124. **Gollins, S.W.** et al. (1994). High dose rate intraluminal radiotherapy for carcinoma of the bronchus: outcome of treatment of 406 patients. *Radiotherapy & Oncology* **33**, 31–40.
125. **Shea, J.M.** et al. (1993). Survival of patients undergoing Nd:YAG laser therapy compared with Nd:YAG laser therapy and brachytherapy for malignant airway disease. *Chest* **103**, 1028–31.
126. **Langendijk, H.** et al. (2001). External irradiation versus external irradiation plus endobronchial brachytherapy in inoperable non-small cell lung cancer: a prospective randomized study. *Radiotherapy in Oncology* **58**, 257–68.
127. **Stout, R.** et al. (2000). Clinical and quality of life outcomes in the first United Kingdom randomized trail of endobronchial brachytherapy (intraluminal radiotherapy) versus external beam radiotherapy in the palliative treatment of inoperable non-small cell lung cancer. *Radiotherapy in Oncology* **56**: 323–7.
128. **Khanavkar, B.** et al. (1991). Complications associated with brachytherapy alone or with laser in lung cancer. *Chest* **99**, 1062–5.
129. **Munk, P.L.** et al. (1988). Pulmonary lymphangitic carcinomatosis: CT and pathologic findings. *Radiology* **166**, 705–9.
130. **Sawin, S.W.** et al. (1995). Recurrent squamous cell carcinoma of the cervix with pulmonary lymphangitic metastasis. *International Journal of Gynaecology and Obstetrics* **48**, 85–90.
131. **Bruce, D.M., Heys, S.D., and Eremin, O.** (1996). Lymphangitis carcinomatosa: a literature review. *Journal of Royal College of Surgeons Edinburgh* **41**, 7–13.
132. **Ikezoe, J.** et al. (1995). Pulmonary lymphangitic carcinomatosis: chronicity of radiographic findings in long-term survivors. *American Journal of Roentgenology* **165**, 49–52.
133. **Hardy, J.R.** et al. (2001). A prospective survey of the use of dexamethasone on a palliative care unit. *Palliative Medicine* **15**, 3–8.
134. **Green, K.B. and Silverstein, R.L.** (1996). Hypercoagulability in cancer. *Haematology and Oncology Clinics of North America* **10**, 499–530.
135. **Durica, S.S.** (1997). Venous thromboembolism in the cancer patient. *Current Opinion in Haematology* **4**, 306–11.
136. **Tai, N.R.M., Atwai, A.S., and Hamilton, G.** (1999). Modern management of pulmonary embolism. *British Journal of Surgery* **86**, 853–68.
137. **Worsley, D.F.** et al. (1993). Chest radiographic findings in patients with acute pulmonary embolism: observations from the PIOPED study. *Radiology* **189**, 133–6.
138. **The PIOPED investigators** (1990). Value of the ventilation/perfusion scan in acute pulmonary embolism, results of the prospective investigation of pulmonary embolism diagnosis (PIOPED). *Journal of the American Medical Association* **263**, 2753–9.
139. **De Monye, W. and Pattynama, P.M.T.** (2001). Contrast-enhanced spiral computed tomography of the pulmonary arteries: an overview. *Seminars in Thrombosis and Hemostasis* **27**, 33–9.
140. **Johnson, M.J. and Sherry, K.** (1997). How do palliative physicians manage venous thromboembolism? *Palliative Medicine* **11**, 462–8.
141. **Riedel, R.** (2001). Acute pulmonary embolism. 2. Treatment. *Heart* **85**, 351–60.
142. **Simonneau, G.** et al. (1997). A comparison of low-molecular weight heparin with unfractionated heparin for acute pulmonary embolism. *New England Journal of Medicine* **337**, 663–9.
143. **Hirsh, J.** et al. (1998). Heparin and low-molecular-weight heparin: mechanisms of action, pharmacokinetics, dosing considerations, monitoring, efficacy and safety. *Chest* **114**, 489S–510S.
144. **Ansell, J.** et al. (2001). Managing oral anticoagulant therapy. *Chest* **119**, 22S–38S.
145. **Nishimura, Y.** et al. (1995). Relationship between respiratory muscle strength and lean body mass in men with COPD. *Chest* **107**, 1232–6.
146. **Aldrich, T.K.** (1993). Nutritional factors in the pathogenesis and therapy of respiratory insufficiency in neuromuscular diseases. *Monaldi Archives of Chest Disease* **48**, 327–30 (Review).
147. **Guttridge, D.C.** et al. (2000). NF-kappaB-induced loss of MyoD messenger RNA: possible role in muscle decay and cachexia. *Science* **289**, 2363–6.
148. **Gallagher, C.G.** (1994). Respiratory steroid myopathy. *American Journal of Respiratory and Critical Care Medicine* **150**, 4–6.
149. **Dekhuijzen, P.N. and Decramer, M.** (1992). Steroid-induced myopathy and its significance to respiratory disease: a known disease rediscovered. *European Respiratory Journal* **5**, 997–1003.

150. **Batchelor, T.T.** et al. (1997). Steroid myopathy in cancer patients. *Neurology* **48**, 1234–8.
151. **Takamori, M.** (1999). An autoimmune channelopathy associated with cancer: Lambert–Eaton myasthenic syndrome. *Internal Medicine* **38**, 86–96 (Review).
152. **Laroche, C.M.** et al. (1989). Respiratory muscle weakness in the Lambert–Eaton myasthenic syndrome. *Thorax* **44**, 913–18.
153. **Yamada, A.** et al. (1990). Eaton–Lambert syndrome manifested by respiratory failure associated with small cell carcinoma of the lung. *Rinsho Shinkeigaku* **30**, 780–3 (in Japanese).
154. **Moxham, J.** (1997). Bilateral diaphragmatic weakness: a late complication of radiotherapy. *Thorax* **52**, 828–9 (Commentary).
155. **Polkey, M.I., Green, M., and Moxham, J.** (1995). Measurement of respiratory muscle strength. *Thorax* **50**, 1131–5 (Review).
156. **Leger, P.** et al. (1994). Nasal intermittent positive pressure ventilation. Long-term follow-up in patients with severe chronic respiratory insufficiency. *Chest* **105**, 100–5.
157. **Mitch, W.E. and Price, S.R.** (2001). Transcription factors and muscle cachexia: is there a therapeutic target? *Lancet* **357**, 734–5.
158. **Vitetta, L., Kenner, D., and Sali, A.** (2000). Bacterial infections in terminally ill hospice patients. *Journal of Pain and Symptom Management* **20**, 326–34.
159. **American Thoracic Society** (2001). Guideline on the management of adults with community-acquired pneumonia. *American Journal of Respiratory and Critical Care Medicine* **163**, 1730–54.
160. **Marik, P.E.** (2001). Primary care: aspiration pneumonitis and aspiration pneumonia. *New England Journal of Medicine* **344**, 665–71.
161. **Pannunzio, T.G.** (1996). Aspiration of oral feedings in patients with tracheostomies. *AACN Clinical Issues* **7**, 560–9.
162. **Bennett, M.I.** (1996). Death rattle: an audit of hyoscine (scopolamine) use and review of management. *Journal of Pain and Symptom Management* **12**, 229–33.
163. **American Thoracic Society** (1994). Treatment of tuberculosis and tuberculosis infection in adults and children. *American Journal of Respiratory and Critical Care Medicine* **149**, 1359–74.
164. **Gleeson, C. and Spencer, D.** (1995). Blood transfusion and its benefits in palliative care. *Palliative Medicine* **9**, 307–13.
165. **Monti, M.** et al. (1996). Use of red blood cell transfusions in terminally ill cancer patients admitted to a palliative care unit. *Journal of Pain and Symptom Management* **12**, 18–22.
166. **Von Herbay, A.** et al. (1990). Pulmonary tumor thrombotic microangiopathy with pulmonary hypertension. *Cancer* **66**, 587–92.
167. **Folgering, H.** (1999). The hyperventilation syndrome. In *Control of Breathing in Health and Disease* (ed. M.D. Altose and T. Kamakami), pp. 633–60. New York: Marcel Dekker.
168. **Pauzner, R.** et al. (1989). High incidence of primary cerebral lymphoma in tumor-induced central neurogenic hyperventilation. *Archives in Neurology* **46**, 510–12.
169. **Karajgi, B.** et al. (1990). The prevalence of anxiety disorders in patients with chronic obstructive pulmonary disease. *American Journal of Psychiatry* **147**, 200–1.
170. **Heyse-Moore, L.H.** (1993). *On dyspnoea in advanced cancer.* MD Thesis, University of Southampton.
171. **Corner, J.** et al. (1996). Non-pharmacological intervention for breathlessness in lung cancer. *Palliative Medicine* **10**, 299–305.
172. **Bredin, M.** et al. (1999). Multicentre randomized controlled trial of nursing intervention for breathlessness in patients with lung cancer. *British Medical Journal* **318**, 901–4.
173. **Banzett, R.B.** (1988). Bracing arms increase the capacity for sustained hyperpnea. *American Review of Respiratory Disease* **138**, 106–9.
174. **Tiep, B.L., Burns, M., and Hererra, J.** (1989). A new pendant oxygen-conserving cannula which allows pursed lips breathing. *Chest* **95**, 857–60.
175. **Carrieri-Kohlman, V.** et al. (1993). Desensitization and guided mastery: treatment approaches for the management of dyspnoea. *Heart and Lung* **22**, 226–34.
176. **Nocturnal Oxygen Therapy Trial Group** (1980). Continuous or nocturnal oxygen therapy in hypoxemic chronic obstructive lung diseases. *Annals of Internal Medicine* **93**, 391–8.
177. **Weitzenblum, E., Apprill, M., and Oswald, M.** (1992). Benefit from long-term O_2 therapy in chronic obstructive pulmonary disease patients. *Respiration* **59** (Suppl. 2), 14–17.
178. **Medical Research Council Working Party** (1981). Long term domiciliary oxygen therapy in chronic hypoxic cor pulmonale complicating chronic bronchitis and emphysema. *Lancet* **I**, 681–6.
179. **Bruera, E., Schoeller, T., and MacEachern, T.** (1992). Symptomatic benefit of supplemental oxygen in hypoxemic patients with terminal cancer: the use of the N of 1 randomized controlled trail. *Journal of Pain and Symptom Management* **7**, 365–8.
180. **Florez, J.** (1993). Opioid, respiration and vomiting. In *Opioids* (ed. A. Hertz). Berlin: Springer.
181. **Zebraski, S.E., Kochenash, S.M., and Raffa, R.B.** (2000). Lung opioid receptors: pharmacology and possible target for nebulized morphine in dyspnea. *Life Sciences* **66**, 2221–31.
182. **Bruera, E.** et al. (1993). Subcutaneous morphine for dyspnea in cancer patients. *Annals of Internal Medicine* **119**, 906–7.
183. **Woodcock, A.A.** et al. (1981). Effects of dihydrocodeine, alcohol and caffeine on obstructive lung disease and normal blood gases. *New England Journal of Medicine* **305**, 1611–16.
184. **Woodcock, A.A., Johnson, M.A., and Geddes, D.M.** (1982). Breathlessness, alcohol, and opiates. *New England Journal of Medicine* **306**, 1364–4.
185. **Masood, A.R., Reed, J.W., and Thomas, S.H.L.** (1995). Lack of effect of inhaled morphine on exercise-induced breathlessness in chronic obstructive pulmonary disease. *Thorax* **50**, 629–34.
186. **Johnson, M.A., Woodcock, A.A., and Geddes, D.M.** (1983). Dihydrocodeine for breathlessness in 'pink puffers'. *British Medical Journal* **286**, 675–7.
187. **Light, R.W.** et al. (1989). Effects of oral morphine on breathlessness and exercise tolerance in patients with chronic obstructive pulmonary disease. *American Review of Respiratory Disease* **139**, 126–33.
188. **Young, I.H., Daviskas, E., and Keena, V.A.** (1989). Effect of low dose nebulised morphine on exercise endurance in patients with chronic lung disease. *Thorax* **44**, 387–90.
189. **Jankelson, D.** et al. (1997). Lack of effect of high doses of inhaled morphine on exercise endurance in chronic obstructive pulmonary disease. *European Respiratory Journal* **10**, 2270–4.
190. **Beauford, W.** et al. (1993). Effects of nebulized morphine sulfate on the exercise tolerance of the ventilatory limited COPD patient. *Chest* **104**, 175–8.
191. **Leung, R., Hill, P., and Burdon, J.** (1996). Effect of inhaled morphine on the development of breathlessness during exercise in patients with chronic lung disease. *Thorax* **51**, 596–600.
192. **Harris-Eze, A.O.** et al. (1995). Low-dose nebulized morphine does not improve exercise in interstitial lung disease. *American Journal of Respiratory and Critical Care Medicine* **152**, 1940–5.
193. **Noseda, A.** et al. (1997). Disabling dyspnoea in patients with advanced disease: lack of effect of nebulised morphine. *European Respiratory Journal* **10**, 1079–83.
194. **Masood, A.R.** et al. (1995). Effects of inhaled nebulized morphine on ventilation and breathlessless during exercise in healthy man. *Clinical Science (London)* **88**, 447–52.
195. **Eiser, N.** et al. (1991). Oral diamorphine: lack of effect on dyspnoea and exercise tolerance in the 'pink puffer' syndrome. *European Respiratory Journal* **4**, 926–31.
196. **Boyd, K.J. and Kelly, M.** (1997). Oral morphine as symptomatic treatment of dyspnoea in patients with advanced cancer. *Palliative Medicine* **11**, 277–81.
197. **Cohen, M.H.** et al. (1991). Continuous intravenous infusion of morphine for severe dyspnea. *Southern Medical Journal* **84**, 229–34.
198. **Ventafridda, V., Spoldi, E., and De Conno, F.** (1990). Control of dyspnea in advanced cancer patients. *Chest* **98**, 1544.
199. **Tanaka, K.** et al. (1999). Effect of nebulized morphine in cancer patients with dyspnea: a pilot study. *Japanese Journal of Clinical Oncology* **29**, 600–3.
200. **Peterson, G.M.** et al. (1996). Pilot study of nebulised morphine for dyspnoea in palliative care patients. *Australian Journal of Hospital Pharmacy* **26**, 545–7.
201. **Zeppetella, G.** (1997). Nebulized morphine in the palliation of dyspnoea. *Palliative Medicine* **11**, 267–75.

202. **Davis, C.L.** et al. (1996). Single dose randomised controlled trial of nebulised morphine in patients with cancer related breathlessness. *Palliative Medicine* **10**, 64–5.
203. **Quelch, P.C., Faulkner, D.E., and Yun, J.W.S.** (1997). Nebulized opioids in the treatment of dyspnea. *Journal of Palliative Care* **13**, 48–52.
204. **Farncombe, M., Chater, S., and Gillin, A.** (1994). The use of nebulized opioids for breathlessness: a chart review. *Palliative Medicine* **8**, 306–12.
205. **Mazzocato, C., Buclin, T., and Rapin, C.H.** (1999). The effects of morphine on dyspnea and ventilatory function in elderly patients with advanced cancer: a randomized double-blind controlled trial. *Annals of Oncology* **10**, 1511–14.
206. **Allard, P.** et al. (1999). How effective are supplementary doses of opioids for dyspnea in terminally ill cancer patients? A randomized continuous sequential clinical trial. *Journal of Pain and Symptom Management* **17**, 256–65.
207. **Chrubasik, J.** et al. (1988). Absorption and bioavailability of nebulized morphine. *British Journal of Anaesthesia* **61**, 228–30.
208. **Masood, A.R. and Thomas, S.H.L.** (1996). Systemic absorption of nebulized morphine compared with oral morphine in healthy subjects. *British Journal of Clinical Pharmacology* **41**, 250–2.
209. **Sham, M.K.** (1996). Inhaled fentanyl in the control of dyspnoea in advanced cancer. *Abstracts of 3rd Hong Kong International Cancer Congress*, 13–16 November, Hong Kong, H50.3.
210. **Ventafridda, V.** et al. (1990). Symptom prevalence and control during cancer patients' last days of life. *Journal of Palliative Care* **6**, 7–11.
211. **Bruera, E.** et al. (1990). Effects of morphine on the dyspnoea of terminal cancer patients. *Journal of Pain and Symptom Management* **5**, 341–4.
212. **Smoller, J.W.** (1996). Panic anxiety, dyspnoea, and respiratory disease. Theoretical and clinical considerations. *American Journal Respiratory Critical Care Medicine* **154**, 6–17.
213. **Davis, C.L.** (1997). ABC of palliative care: breathlessness, cough, and other respiratory symptom. *British Medical Journal* **315**, 931–4.
214. **Stark, R.D., Gambles, S.A., and Lewis, J.A.** (1981). Methods to assess breathlessness in healthy subjects: a critical evaluation and application to analyse the acute effects of diazepam and promethazine on breathlessness induced by exercise or by exposure to raised levels of carbon dioxide. *Clinical Science (London)* **61**, 429–39.
215. **O'Neill, P.A., Morton, P.B., and Stark, R.D.** (1985). Chlorpromazine—a specific effect on breathlessness. *British Journal of Clinical Pharmacology* **19**, 793–7.
216. **Woodcock, A.A., Gross, E.R., and Geddes, D.M.** (1981). Drug treatment of breathlessness: contrasting effects of diazepam and promethazine in pink puffers. *British Medical Journal* **283**, 343–6.
217. **McIver, B., Walsh, D., and Nelson, K.** (1994). The use of chlorpromazine for symptom control in dying cancer patients. *Journal of Pain and Symptom Management* **9**, 341–5.
218. *Global Initiative for Chronic Obstructive Lung Disease.* National Institutes of Health, Publication no. 2701A. Washington DC: National Institute of Health, 2001.
219. **Winning, A.J., Hamilton, R.D., and Guz, A.** (1988). Ventilation and breathlessness on maximal exercise in patients with interstitial lung disease after local anaesthesia aerosal inhalation. *Clinical Science* **74**, 275–81.
220. **Wilcock, A., Corcoran, R., and Tattersfield, A.E.** (1994). Safety and efficacy of nebulised lignocaine in patients with cancer and breathlessness. *Palliative Medicine* **8**, 35–8.
221. **Irwin, R.S.** et al. (1998). Managing cough as a defense mechanism and as a symptom. *Chest* **114**, 133S–81S.
222. **Sant'Ambrogio, G. and Widdicombe, J.** (2001). Reflexes from airway rapidly adapting receptors. *Respiration Physiology* **125**, 33–45.
223. **Widdicombe, J.G.** (1996). Sensory neurophysiology of cough reflex. *Journal of Allergy and Clinical Immunology* **98**, S84–90.
224. **Cowcher, K. and Hanks, G.W.** (1990). Long-term management of respiratory symptoms in advanced cancer. *Journal of Pain and Symptom Management* **5**, 320–30
225. **French, C.L.** et al. (1998). Impact of chronic cough on quality of life. *Archives of Internal Medicine* **158**, 1657–61.
226. **Homsi, J.** et al. (2000). Hydrocodone for cough in advanced cancer. *American Journal of Hospice & Palliative Care* **17**, 342–6.
227. **Doona, M. and Walsh, D.** (1997). Benzonatate for opioid-resistant cough in advanced cancer. *Palliative Medicine* **12**, 55–8.
228. **Hagen, N.A.** (1991). An approach to cough in cancer patients. *Journal of Pain and Symptom Management* **6**, 257–62.
229. **Walsh, D.** et al. (2000). Symptom control in advanced cancer: important drugs and routes of administration. *Seminars in Oncology* **27**, 69–83.
230. **Luporini, G.** et al. (1998). Efficacy and safety of levodropropizine and dihydrocodeine on nonproductive cough in primary and metastatic lung cancer. *European Respiratory Journal* **12**, 97–101.
231. **Moroni, M.** et al. (1996). Inhaled sodium cromoglycate to treat cough in advanced lung cancer patients. *British Journal of Cancer* **74**, 309–11.
232. **Louie, K., Bertolino, M., and Fainsinger, R.** (1992). Management of intractable cough. *Journal of Palliative Care* **8**, 46–8.
233. **Twycross, R., Wilcock, A., and Thorp, S.** *Palliative Care Formulary.* Oxford: Radcliffe Medical Press, 1998.
234. **Sorenson, H.M.** (2000). Managing secretions in dying patients. *Respiratory Care* **45**, 1355–64.
235. **Jones, A.P. and Rowe, B.H.** (2002). Bronchopulmonary hygiene physical therapy for chronic obstructive pulmonary disease and bronchiectasis. *The Cochrane Database Systematic Review* **2**, CD000045.
236. **Wills, P. and Greenstone, M.** (2002). Inhaled hyperosmolar agents for bronchiectasis. *The Cochrane Database Systematic Review* **1**, CD002996.
237. **Clarke, S.W.** (1987). Management of mucus hypersecretion. *European Journal of Respiratory Disease* **71**, S136–44.
238. **Crockett, A.J.** et al. (2001). Mucolytics for bronchiectasis. *The Cochrane Database Systematic Review* **1**, CD001289.
239. **Hidaka, N. and Nagao, K.** (1996). Bronchioloalveolar carcinoma accompanied by severe bronchorrhea. *Chest* **110**, 281–2.
240. **Tamaoki, J.** et al. (2000). Inhaled indomethacin in bronchorrhea in bronchioloalveolar carcinoma: role of cyclooxygenase. *Chest* **117**, 1213–14.
241. **Lembo, T. and Donnelly, T.J.** (1995). A case of pancreatic carcinoma causing massive bronchial fluid production and electrolyte abnormalities. *Chest* **108**, 1161–3.
242. **Marom, Z.M. and Goswami, S.K.** (1991). Respiratory mucus hypersecretion (bronchorrhea): a case discussion—possible mechanism(s) and treatment. *Journal of Allergy Clinical Immunology* **87**, 1050–5.
243. **Miller, R.R. and McGregor, D.H.** (1980). Hemorrhage from carcinoma of the lung. *Cancer* **46**, 200–5.
244. **Fink, G.** et al. (2001). Pulmonary carcinoid, presentation, diagnosis and outcome in 142 cases in Isreal and review of 640 cases from the literature. *Chest* **119**, 1647–51.
245. **Panos, R.J.** et al. (1988). Factors associated with fatal hemoptysis in cancer patients. *Chest* **94**, 1008–13.
246. **Dean, A. and Tuffin, P.** (1997). Fibrinolytic inhibitors for cancer associated bleeding problems. *Journal of Pain and Symptom Management* **13**, 20–4.
247. **Detterbeck, F.C., Jones, D.R., and Morris, D.E.** (2001). Palliative treatment of lung cancer. In *Diagnosis and Treatment of Lung Cancer. An Evidence-Based Guide for the Practicing Clinician* (ed. F.C. Detterbeck et al.), pp. 419–36. Philadelphia PA: WB Saunders.
248. **Freitag, L.** et al. (1994). Three years experience with a new balloon catheter for the management of haemoptysis. *European Respiratory Journal* **7**, 2003–7.
249. **Conlan, A.A.** et al. (1983). Massive hemoptysis. Review of 123 cases. *Journal of Thoracic Cardiovascular Surgery* **85**, 120–4.
250. **Tsukamoto, T., Sasaki, H., and Nakamura, H.** (1989). Treatment of haemoptysis patients by thrombin and fibrinogen-thrombin infusion therapy using a fiberoptic bronchoscope. *Chest* **96**, 473–6.
251. **Jean-Baptiste, E.** (2000). Clinical assessment and management of massive hemoptysis. *Critical Care Medicine* **28**, 1642–7.
252. **Fernando, H.C.** et al. (1998). Role of bronchial artery embolization in the management of hemoptysis. *Archives of Surgery* **133**, 862–6.
253. **Gagnon, B.** et al. (1998). Palliative management of bleeding events in advanced cancer patients. *Journal of Palliative Care* **14**, 50–4.
254. **Matthews, A.W.** (1992). A survey of malignant mesothelioma in Portmouth 1982–1991. *Thorax* **47**, 851–2.

255. **Gavrin, J.R.** (2001). Chest pain from other disorder including cancer. In *Bonica's Management of Pain* (ed. J.D. Loeser), pp. 1210–14. Lippincott: Williams & Wilkins.

256. **Jackson, M.B.** et al. (1999). Percutaneous cervical cordotomy for the control of pain in patients with pleural mesothelioma. *Thorax* **54**, 238–41.

257. **Morita, T.** et al. (1999). Do hospice clinicians sedate patients intending to hasten death? *Journal of Palliative Care* **15**, 20–3.

258. **Fainsinger, R.L.** et al. (2000). A multicentre international study of sedation for uncontrolled symptoms in terminally ill patients. *Palliative Medicine* **14**, 257–65.

259. **Chiu, T.Y.** et al. (2001). Sedation for refractory symptoms of terminal cancer patients in Taiwan. *Journal of Pain and Symptom Management* **21**, 467–72.

260. **Morita, T., Inoue, S., and Chihara, S.** (1996). Sedation for symptom control in Japan: the importance of intermittent use and communication with family members. *Journal of Pain and Symptom Management* **12**, 32–8.

261. **Stone, P.** et al. (1997). A comparison of the use of sedatives in a hospital support team and in a hospice. *Palliative Medicine* **11**, 140–4.

262. **Fainsinger, R.L.** et al. (1998). Sedation for uncontrolled symptoms in a South African hospice. *Journal of Pain and Symptom Management* **16**, 145–52.

263. **Chater, S.** et al. (1998). Sedation for intractable distress in the dying—a survey of experts. *Palliative Medicine* **12**, 255–69.

264. **Jennings, A.L.** et al. (2001). Opioids for the palliation of breathlessness in terminal illness. *The Cochrane Database Systematic Review* **4**, CD002066.

265. **Sales, J.P.** (2001). Sedation and terminal care. *European Journal of Palliative Care* **8**, 97–100.

266. **Thorns, A. and Sykes, N.** (2000). Opioid use in the last week of life and the implications for end-of-life decision making. *Lancet* **356**, 398–9.

267. **Morita, T.** et al. (2001). Effects of high dose opioids and sedatives on survival in terminally ill cancer patients. *Journal of Pain and Symptom Management* **21**, 282–9.

268. **Cherny, N.I. and Portenoy, R.K.** (1994). Sedation in the management of refractory symptoms: guidelines for evaluation and treatment. *Journal of Palliative Care* **10**, 31–8.

269. **Aleman, C.** et al. (1999). The value of chest roentgenography in the diagnosis of pneumothorax after thoracentesis. *American Journal of Medicine* **107**, 340–3.

270. **Raptopoulos, V.** et al. (1991). Factors affecting the development of pneumothorax associated with thoracentesis. *American Journal of Roentgenology* **156**, 917–20.

271. **American Thoracic Society** (1995). Hospital-acquired pneumonia in adults. *American Journal of Respiratory and Critical Care Medicine* **153**, 1711–25.

272. **Decramer, M.** (1996). Respiratory muscle pharmacology. *Monaldi Archives of Chest Disease* **6**, 499–503.

273. **Vaz Fragoso, C.A. and Miller, M.A.** (1993). Review of the clinical efficacy of theophylline in the treatment of chronic obstructive pulmonary disease. *American Review of Respiratory Disease* **147**, S40–7.

8.9 Skin problems in palliative medicine

8.9.1 Medical aspects

Ian C. Pearson and Peter S. Mortimer

Introduction

As the largest and most exposed organ it is not surprising that the skin rarely escapes problems in any chronically sick patient. These problems are generally minor, but can be debilitating and uncomfortable, and distressing due to their visibility. The general condition, and particularly nutritional status of the patient, will be reflected in the skin. Limited healing powers mean minor and usually reversible skin conditions become major problems in the chronically sick patient.

No branch of medicine is more reliant on clinical acumen and less dependent on the laboratory than dermatology. As a window on general health all professional carers need to recognize the skin signs of internal disease, such as purpura of thrombocytopaenia or scurvy, excoriation due to itching in renal and liver diseases, or pigmentation due to Addison's disease.

The skin performs a number of vital functions and it is when these fail that problems arise.

1. The skin is a barrier between the body and its environment—'to keep in what should be in', particularly water, electrolytes, and other body constituents, 'and to keep out what is out', namely noxious materials and biological hazards such as infection. The skin also has to be physically resilient and prevent the effects of mechanical injury, such as pressure, stretching, or scratching. The success of this barrier depends on the integrity of the epidermis through the close cohesion of the stratum corneum cells sealed by surface lipids. The dermis provides support to the epidermis, both nutritionally and physically. A change in the blood supply or in the quality of collagen or elastic fibres impairs this support function and limits the ability of the skin to resist injury from pressure or stretch and to repair wounds.

2. Control of body temperature is effected by the skin. The skin blood supply is far in excess of metabolic requirements because of this thermoregulatory role. Extensive cutaneous disease can lead to the shunting of most of the cardiac output through the skin to the detriment of critical organs such as the kidney; simultaneously the excessive demands on the heart can precipitate high output cardiac failure. These events are more likely in the elderly or chronically sick patient.

3. The skin is a major sensory organ. Cutaneous sensation allows orientation in relation to the environment. This is particularly important in the cancer patient where nerve damage from cancer (e.g. paraplegia) or its therapy (e.g. drug-induced neuropathy) exposes the skin to undetected damage and allows development of a chronic wound. Sedating opioid drugs may compound this situation. Anaesthetized skin is more prone to ulceration akin to the situation in diabetes and leprosy.

4. The skin normally has excellent powers of regeneration in the form of wound and tissue repair. This process is usually quick and efficient due mainly to the blood supply. Ill health and catabolic states such as cancer cachexia particularly impair this process.

5. Vitamin D production occurs in the skin. Calcium homeostasis may be compromised by prolonged periods indoors which should therefore be avoided in chronically sick patients.

Internal homeostasis relies on all these skin functions. A weakened skin barrier is almost inevitable in the sick, debilitated patient predisposing to dehydration, dermatitis, infection, and ulceration. The effects of neoplasia and chronic infection mimic those of dehydration and malnutrition. The skin is dry and ichthyotic leading to a lack of suppleness in the stratum corneum which readily cracks (asteatosis). Dermatitis, which can be itchy and sore, supervenes. Anaemia, oedema, and sore tongue reflect the catabolic state. Pressure points are particularly vulnerable and dermatitis may well lead to ulceration. Poor wound healing properties mean these areas are slow to recover. Management of skin disorders in palliative care must therefore first and foremost address aspects of general welfare such as hydration, nutrition, and hygiene. The likelihood of serious skin problems will then be greatly reduced.

Primary tumours

Primary skin cancer is rarely a problem in the patient with advanced malignant disease.

Primary malignant melanoma is optimally treated with wide local excision, often even in the presence of metastatic disease, to avoid cutaneous complications. Local spread can produce unsightly nodules which may ulcerate or fungate. Treatment by simple excision is usually appropriate but radiotherapy or laser treatment can be effective palliation.[1,2]

Basal cell carcinoma is common and may co-exist by chance or occur in a previously irradiated field. Treatment only becomes necessary when complications of ulceration, bleeding, or even smell supervene. In these cases excision under local anaesthetic or radiotherapy should be considered.

Cutaneous squamous cell carcinoma can be the source of metastatic spread, particularly in immunosuppressed individuals, such as renal transplant recipients. Usually the primary tumour has been satisfactorily treated but occasionally recurrent local tumour may develop ulceration, bleeding, or infection. Radiotherapy will usually control symptoms.

Kaposi's sarcoma is a predominantly cutaneous malignancy. The classic form usually presents as slow-growing purple nodules on the ankles of elderly men of Eastern European or Mediterranean origin. Local spread occurs slowly up the limb and prognosis is good. The endemic form occurs in African children and adults who develop multiple vascular lesions with gross oedema. Prognosis is less favourable. Epidemic or AIDS-associated Kaposi's sarcoma is associated with a profound defect of cell-mediated immunity and extra-cutaneous involvement. This form may respond to highly active antiretroviral therapy (HAART) which increase CD4 counts.[3] Similarly Kaposi's sarcoma in patients with non-HIV-associated immunosuppression, such as renal transplant recipients, is often aggressive with extra-cutaneous involvement. Regression is seen if immunosuppression is relieved. The epidemiology of Kaposi's sarcoma reflects an infective cause. The isolation of human herpes virus 8 from all clinical subtypes of Kaposi's sarcoma suggests this as the aetiologic agent. The lymphangiogenic ligand vascular endothelial growth factor-C potently stimulates the proliferation of Kaposi's sarcoma cells thus suggesting a lymphatic origin and/or differentiation of the tumour cells.[4]

Treatment reflects the clinical subtype. Simple excision may be appropriate in classical cases and tumours are radiosensitive. More extensive disease may warrant systemic chemotherapy, such as oral etoposide.[5] Similar treatments can be employed in the other variants of Kaposi's sarcoma but response is less durable. In AIDS-related Kaposi's sarcoma HAART may be effective and can be combined with treatments such as interferon alpha.[6]

Cutaneous T-cell lymphoma (mycosis fungoides) characteristically persists for years in the skin alone and only in the terminal phase will systemic involvement occur. Problems arise from tumour ulceration with secondary infection and bleeding. Death may occur from septicaemia, particularly as host immunity becomes compromised. There is a general trend in Europe towards a palliative approach to treatment from an early stage in the disease. A large proportion of patients with mycosis fungoides are frail, elderly, and likely to succumb either to general medical problems or to over-enthusiastic therapy. Photochemotherapy (PUVA) may keep the disease in check but radiotherapy, either electron-beam or conventional X-rays, is most effective in eradicating tumours. The indolent nature of many cases means no survival benefit is conferred by more aggressive treatment regimens at an early stage. Chemotherapy is reserved for those with recalcitrant disease or extracutaneous involvement.[7] Pruritus may be troublesome but symptomatic relief can be provided by topical steroids and antihistamines.

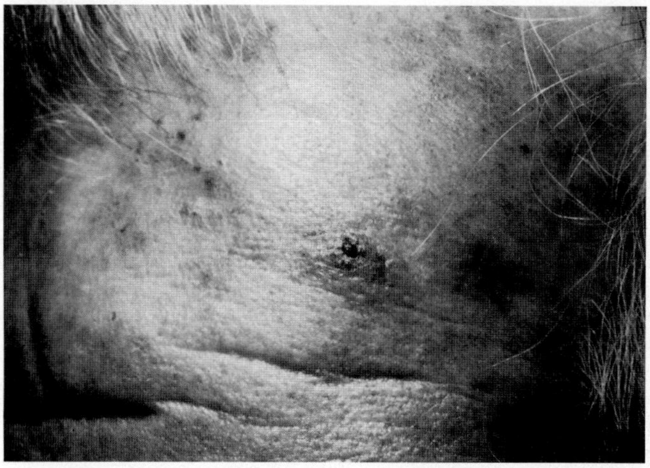

Fig. 1 Angiosarcoma: the bruised appearance with ill-defined borders is typical of this tumour.

Angiosarcoma (Fig. 1) is rare and occurs most commonly on the head and neck in elderly patients as a slowly spreading bruise. Prognosis is poor due to rapid invasion of local structures beyond clinical tumour margins. Some success has been reported with biopsy-guided excision followed by radiotherapy.[8]

Skin metastases and fungating wounds

Skin infiltration with the development of ulceration or a fungating wound can be a distressing problem for the cancer patient. At one extreme is the patient with melanoma in whom a metastatic nodule may be a constant visual reminder of disease progression. At the other is the patient with extensive fungating breast carcinoma. Good palliative management should aim to relieve both the associated physical and psychological burden.

Metastatic malignant tumours

Most malignant tumours can produce cutaneous metastases. Commonest sites for these are abdomen (including umbilicus), chest wall, and head and neck. The commonest primary tumours are gastrointestinal and pulmonary in males and breast in females.[9] The skin is involved by metastases in 4 per cent of malignant tumours and generally this is a poor prognostic sign. Occasionally, however, histological or immunohistochemical analysis of a cutaneous metastasis may reveal a previously unknown tumour.

Direct invasion of the skin usually presents with ulceration or inflammation. The most frequent cause is carcinoma of the breast which may present in a number of ways. Paget's disease of the nipple represents the most reliable sign of underlying malignancy and is caused by carcinoma of the breast. Direct extension of cancer cells into the nipple and areola presents as inflammation and anatomical distortion. Extramammary Paget's disease usually presents as an exudative plaque in the anogenital region, and is more common in elderly women. Histology is of a cutaneous adenocarcinoma and underlying adnexal, gastrointestinal, and genital malignancies are often found.[10]

Inflammatory carcinoma of the breast may mimic cellulitis—carcinoma erysipeloides—with spreading sheets of erythema and oedema (Fig. 2). A lack of systemic upset and failure to respond to antibiotics should arouse suspicion and a biopsy should reveal carcinoma cells in the dermis or lymphatics with associated inflammation. This type of cancer is difficult to eradicate and exhibits a slowly progressive natural history during which time the patient is remarkably well. Contiguous spread leads to the whole upper trunk being enveloped. Induration ensues and the skin and subcutaneous tissues become hard (cancer *en cuirasse*). Dermal lymph stasis results in elephantiasic skin changes with hyperkeratosis and papillomatosis. Occasionally a scirrhous dermal reaction similar to localized scleroderma (morphoea) occurs or the skin becomes crusted and itchy due to dermatitis. Very potent topical steroid preparations are required for symptom control. As such cases are often refractory or unsuitable for conventional treatment newer topical agents such as miltefosine are being evaluated.[11]

Specific cutaneous infiltrations may be seen with haematological malignancies. This occurs commonly with lymphoma and also with leukaemia, particularly the prolymphocytic type.

The scalp is a site where metastases may present (e.g. renal cell carcinoma) and may go unnoticed until hair loss occurs. Alopecia neoplastica (Fig. 3) produces scarring and therefore permanent hair loss even with tumour regression. Early discussion with an appliance officer skilled in the provision of wigs may be vital to maintain patient self-esteem.

Although skin deposits often indicate wide dissemination of cancer, removal of lesions whenever possible is indicated. Excision of solitary deposits together with treatment of the primary tumour may give worthwhile remission. Similarly, early removal of skin deposits when small may avoid later problems.

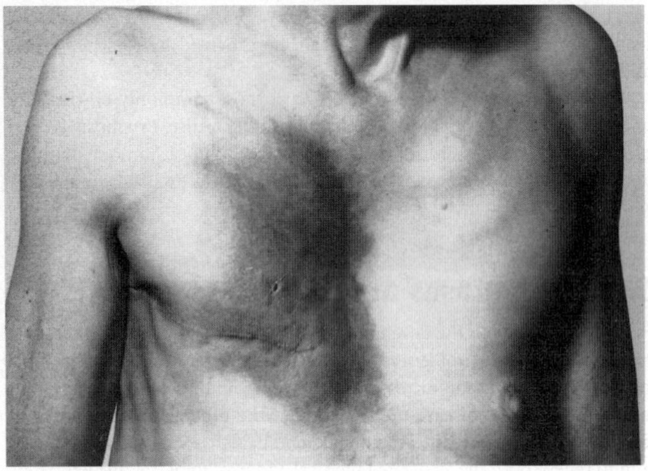

Fig. 2 Carcinoma erysipeloides: the fixed erythema resembling cellulitis/erysipelas is due to dermal infiltration with breast cancer.

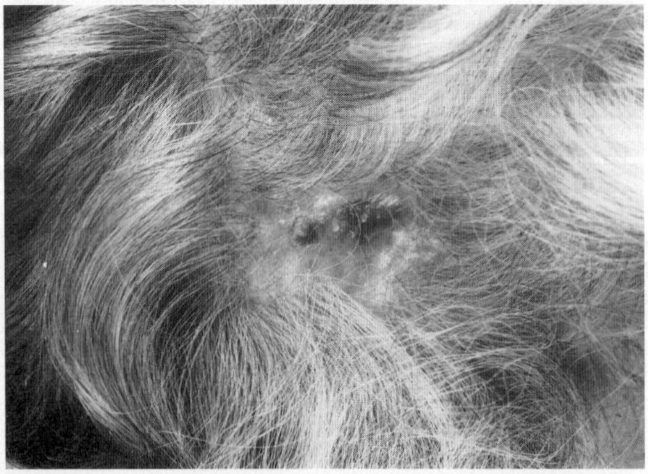

Fig. 3 Alopecia neoplastica: tumour infiltration of the scalp, in this case with breast cancer, gives rise to a scarring alopecia.

Malignant wounds

Little information exists in the medical literature on malignant wounds. Breast cancer is the most common neoplasm to fungate (ulceration with proliferation) but can occur with most other tumours, including lung, stomach, head and neck, colon, bladder, melanoma, and lymphoma. Local extension of malignancy or embolization by vascular or lymphatic spread results in a tumour mass which compromises tissue viability. Local blood flow together with oxygen and nutrient supply to the extracellular fluids is impaired. Tumour angiogenesis forms an inefficient and vulnerable microcirculation within the invading tumour. All these factors lead to tumour infarction and necrosis. Anaerobic organisms flourish in the inaccessible necrotic tissues and release volatile fatty acids as a metabolic end product. These give rise to the characteristic offensive smell.

Ulcerated skin lesions quickly become colonized by aerobic pathogens. Purulent discharge, spreading erythema, or pain indicate the need for microbiological culture of skin swabs. Appropriate systemic antibiotic treatment is required if clinical deterioration occurs. *Staphylococcus aureus* is a common cause of secondary infection which can be overcome with topical treatment (e.g. mupirocin cream). Gram-negative organisms are often found colonizing wounds in anogenital sites and require specific antibiotic treatment. A greenish-hue to wounds may suggest *Pseudomonas* spp. superinfection which may respond to locally applied silver sulphadiazine. Potassium permanganate baths or wet-dressings may help prevent re-infection.

The presence of ulcerating malignant wounds is usually associated with advanced disease and poor prognosis. However, cutaneous T-cell lymphoma may present with ulcerating tumours but prognosis is excellent following treatment. Similarly primary tumours of breast or melanoma may be amenable to curative procedures. Histopathological assessment is therefore indicated for all fungating tumours and essential for correct treatment planning. Even with advanced disease conventional treatment (surgical resection and reconstruction, radiotherapy, chemotherapy, or biological therapy) may reduce symptoms by decreasing tumour bulk and can sometimes lead to healing. Tumours resistant to therapeutic measures require local palliation. Radiotherapy, if suitable, can reduce bleeding and discharge. The nursing management of fungating wounds is discussed in the following chapter.

Non-metastatic cutaneous manifestations of malignancy

There are many examples of skin changes associated with internal malignancy but not due to direct infiltration (Table 1); only a few are reliable markers of underlying disease. Their importance depends on their specificity in guiding the physician along the correct path of investigation. With paraneoplastic syndromes removal of the offending tumour usually results in clearance of skin signs, whereas recurrence of skin manifestations indicates tumour relapse. Often, however, the cancer is metastatic by the time skin signs appear. Equally, cutaneous problems are likely to persist as the cancer progresses.

Cutaneous manifestations may present in three ways:

1. A genetically determined syndrome with a cutaneous component in which there is also an inherent predisposition to neoplasia.
2. A cutaneous marker of exposure to a carcinogen.
3. A group of cutaneous syndromes which appear to represent a response from the neoplasm itself—the paraneoplastic dermatoses.

Genetic syndromes

Progress in molecular biology is allowing the identification of familial cancer syndromes and their causative genes. Identifying these syndromes,

Table 1 Non-metastatic cutaneous manifestations of malignancy

Non-specific cutaneous markers	Paraneoplastic dermatoses	Genetic syndromes with a predisposition to cancer
Pallor	Acanthosis nigricans	Familial melanoma
Pigmentation	Erythema gyratum repens	Naevoid basal cell carcinoma syndrome
Pruritus	Dermatomyositis	Xeroderma pigmentosum
Acquired ichthyosis	Acquired hypertrichosis lanuginosa	Cowden's disease
Exfoliative dermatitis	Migratory thrombophlebitis	Gardner's syndrome
Erythroderma	Pyoderma gangrenosum	Muir-Torre syndrome
Erythema annulare centrifugum	Acute febrile neutrophilic dermatosis	MEN type 1
Erythema multiforme	Subcorneal pustular dermatosis	MEN type 2A + 2B
Erythema nodosum	Cutaneous amyloid	Neurofibromatosis 1
Urticaria	Pemphigus	Neurofibromatosis 2
Panniculitis	Endocrine malignancies	Tuberous sclerosis
Vasculitis	Carcinoid flushing	Familial tylosis
Dermatitis herpetiformis	Glucagonoma (necrolytic migratory erythema)	
Acquired epidermolysis bullosa		
Porphyria cutanea tarda	Unilateral lymphoedema	
Deep venous thrombosis	Leser-Trelat sign	
Erythromelalgia	Paraneoplastic acrokeratosis	
Clubbing of nails		
Arsenical keratoses		
Bowen's disease of covered skin		

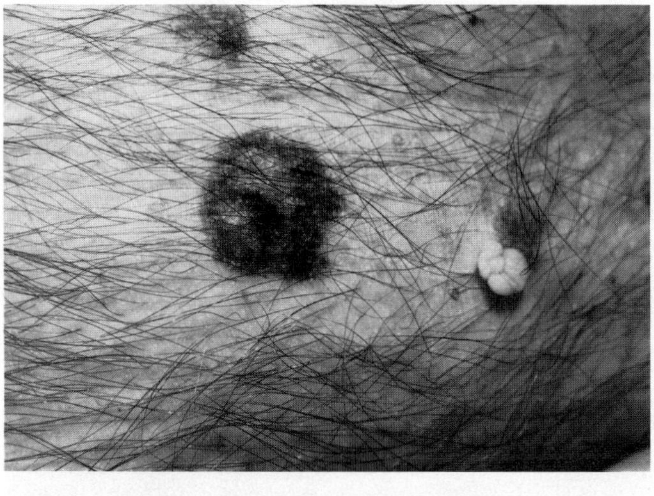

Fig. 4 Dysplastic naevus: a large atypical-looking naevus which characteristically occurs on the trunk and is usually multiple.

even in dying patients, allows screening and counselling of relatives, often at a time of high anxiety. Familial melanoma (familial atypical mole melanoma syndrome) is characterized by numerous atypical moles (Fig. 4) and multiple cutaneous melanomas. A subset of these cases show mutations in the CDKN2A gene on chromosome 9p21 which increases susceptibility to internal malignancies such as pancreatic cancer.[(12)]

Naevoid basal cell carcinoma (NBCCS) syndrome is an autosomal dominant condition in which multiple basal cell carcinomas develop from a young age. Associated findings are palmar pits, mandibular keratocysts, and an increased frequency of internal malignancy, particularly medulloblastoma.[(13)] Mutations have been found in the PATCHED gene, a highly conserved tumour suppressor, in families with NBCCS and in somatic DNA from basal cell carcinomas and internal malignancies.[(14)]

Xeroderma pigmentosum is characterized by photosensitivity, early onset of cutaneous malignancies, and increased risk of internal malignancy. Inheritance is autosomal recessive due to a group of genes integral to DNA repair after UV radiation damage.

The above-mentioned three are all familial cancer syndromes in which cutaneous malignancy is a main feature. Table 2 illustrates genetic conditions with skin signs indicative of a predisposition to internal malignancy.

Exposure to carcinogens

Heavy nicotine staining is a simple example of a skin sign of the most important chemical carcinogen in man. Other signs include X-ray damage to the skin, particularly if it occurred many years previously, because it suggests increased risk of cancer in the skin and underlying tissues such as thyroid or bone marrow. Arsenic-induced keratoses (Fig. 5) on the sides and palmar apects of the fingers associated with truncal Bowen's disease (cutaneous squamous cell cancer in situ) and superficial basal cell carcinomas convey an increased risk of internal neoplasia, particularly bronchial. Vinyl chloride-induced scleroderma-like skin changes are associated with angiosarcoma of the liver and peripheries. Increased occupational safety means such exposure is becoming increasingly rare in the developed world although this may continue where environmental safety is poor.

Paraneoplastic syndromes

Acanthosis nigricans developing in adult life in the absence of obesity or endocrinopathy is invariably associated with an internal neoplasm. Epidermal papillomatous thickening with hyperkeratosis leads to a velvety pigmented rash with a predilection for flexures of the neck, axillae, and groins. More extensive involvement occurs in the paraneoplastic form including mucous membranes and mucocutaneous junctions (Fig. 6). Irritation may be severe and hair may be shed. About 80–90 per cent of cases are associated with an intra-abdominal adenocarcinoma, gastric carcinoma being the most common. In most cases acanthosis nigricans and cancer are diagnosed at the same time and prognosis is poor. However, skin changes may precede the malignant diagnosis. Treatment is generally ineffective and cutaneous changes rarely regress with treatment of the internal malignancy.

Benign acanthosis nigricans is associated with insulin resistance. High insulin levels are thought to non-specifically activate insulin-like growth

Table 2 Genetic conditions with skin signs indicative of a predisposition to internal malignancy[15]

Genetic syndrome	Cutaneous findings	Inheritance and *candidate genes*	Related malignancy
Cowden's disease	Multiple hamartomas	AD *PTEN*	Breast, thyroid, colon
Gardner's syndrome	Epidermal cysts, lipomas, neurofibromas	AD *APC*	Intestinal polyps
Muir-Torre syndrome	Sebaceous tumours	AD *hMSH2*	Colorectal, genitourinary, breast, haematologic, head + neck
MEN type 1	Angiofibromas, collagenomas, CALM, lipomas, necrolytic migratory erythema	AD *MEN1*	Parathyroid adenomas, pituitary adenomas, gastrointestinal endocrine, carcinoids
MEN type 2A + 2B	2A-pruritic foci 2B-mucosal neuromas	AD *RET*	Medullary thyroid carcinoma, phaeochromocytoma
Neurofibromatosis 1	>6 CALM, flexural freckling, neurofibromas, iris hamartomas	AD *NF1*	Neurofibrosarcoma, optic gliomas, astrocytoma, CML, ALL
Neurofibromatosis 2	Neurofibromas, schwannomas	AD *F2*	Acoustic neuromas
Tuberous sclerosis	Hypopigmented macules, facial angiofibromas, periungal fibromas, collagenomas	AD *TSC1* *TSC2*	CNS tubers
Familial tylosis	Palmo-plantar keratoderma	AD *TOC*	Oesophageal carcinoma

AD, autosomal dominant; CALM, café au lait macules; MEN, multiple endocrine neoplasia.

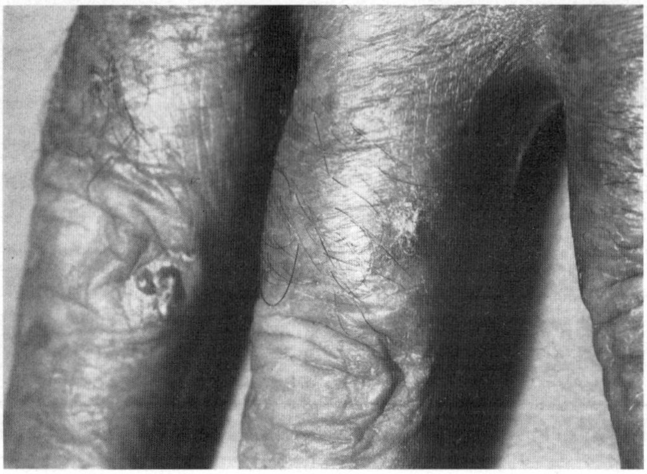

Fig. 5 Arsenical keratoses characteristically occur on the sides of the digits.

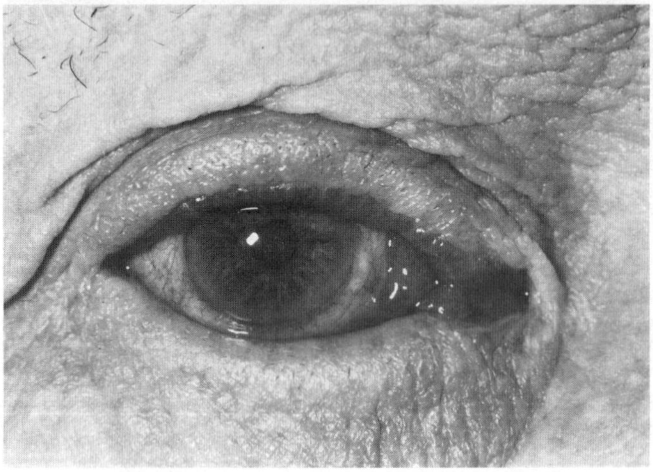

Fig. 6 Acanthosis nigricans of the conjunctiva is a rare but pathognomonic sign of underlying malignancy.

factor receptors which promote cellular growth. In the malignant form these receptors may also be activated non-specifically by tumour-derived factors, for example, transforming growth factor-α.[16]

Tripe palms, a thickened velvety appearance to the palms and occasionally soles, is accompanied by acanthosis nigricans in three out of four cases.[17] Importantly, however, almost half of cases of tripe palms precede a malignant diagnosis, meaning all cases need a thorough work up, particularly for pulmonary and gastric neoplasms.

A sudden increase in the size and number of seborrhoeic keratoses in association with internal malignancy, usually gastric adenocarcinoma or lymphoma is known as the sign of Leser-Trelat. The skin changes do not require treatment unless cosmetically unacceptable, and may recede with cancer-directed therapy.

Erythema gyratum repens has a characteristic, striking appearance. Migrating whorls of annular erythema and scaling give a pattern resembling woodgrain. Association with underlying malignancy, particularly breast and lung, is frequent but not invariable. Resolution of the rash follows treatment of the underlying malignancy.

Necrolytic migratory erythema occurs in the glucagonoma syndrome, with glucose intolerance, high serum glucagon level, and weight loss and is caused by a tumour of the pancreatic islet α-cells. The rash is highly specific and presents as migrating annular erythema coalescing to a serpiginous pattern. Bullae, crusts, and erosions may be seen as the necrotic epidermis migrates. The rash follows a relapsing, remitting course but resolves with treatment of the underlying neoplasm. Cases associated with metastatic disease may be treated with octreotide.[18]

Dermatomyositis often predates cancer diagnosis and is associated with a three fold increase of all malignancies.[19] The classical clinical findings are erythema (deep red or 'heliotrope' colour) and swelling of periorbital skin, cheeks, and forehead with linear violaceous plaques on the dorsal aspects of fingers and hands (Gottron's pads). The rash is photosensitive (Fig. 7) but can occur at any time of year on light-exposed sites. Periungal erythema, nailfold telangiectasia, and ragged cuticles are also typical (Fig. 8). Symmetrical proximal muscle weakness and a raised creatine kinase (CK) is typical but not invariable. Polymyositis similarly affects proximal muscles without the rash. It is associated, although less strongly, with underlying malignancy. Dermatomyositis is associated most commonly with ovarian, lung, gastric, colorectal and pancreatic cancers, and non-Hodgkin's lymphoma. Geographic incidence of associated malignancies may vary, nasopharyngeal cancer being most common in Chinese patients.[20] Underlying malignancies may be curable and therefore thorough screening is vital, even in younger adults. This vigilance should be maintained throughout follow-up as dermatomyositis may precede cancer diagnosis by years.

The aetiology may be tumour antigens sharing common antigenic determinants with skin and muscle, such that the immune response directed at tumour inadvertently attacks host tissues. Serum from affected patients can be shown to contain complement fixing antibodies to their own tumour. Alternatively immunologically competent neoplastic cells, such as lymphocytes, may synthesize damaging autoantibodies. Interestingly patients with cancer-associated dermatomyositis are less likely to have myositis-specific antibodies and raised CK than those without cancer.[21]

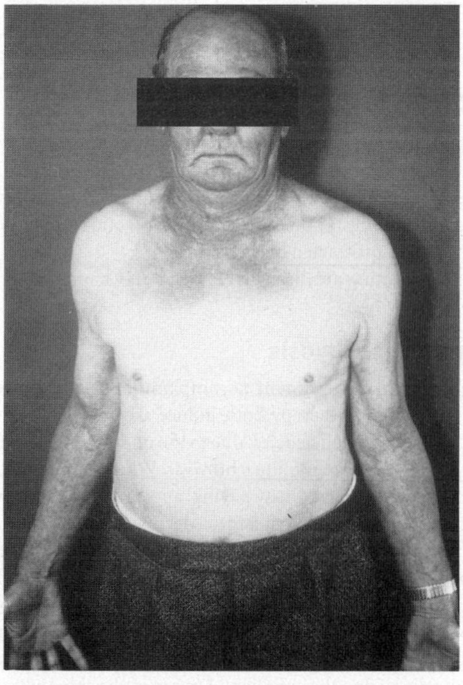

Fig. 7 The photosensitivity rash of dermatomyositis in a patient with carcinoma of the stomach.

Treatment rests initially with removal of the cause. The course is variable but relapse may signal recurrence of underlying disease. Poor prognostic factors include increasing age, pulmonary, and oesophageal involvement. Rest is essential in the acute phase. Corticosteroid treatment is required in almost all cases, often at high doses (prednisolone 60–120 mg). Dose reduction should parallel clinical response. A maintenance dose of 5–15 mg may be required for many months. Immunosuppression with antimetabolites such as azathioprine may be inadvisable in cancer-associated cases.

Acquired ichthyosis (Fig. 9) is associated with internal malignancy, most commmonly with Hodgkin's disease.[22] Widespread dry, flaky skin resembling fish-scales (*ichthos* = fish) should not be confused with asteatosis (no lipid; dry, cracked skin) which is common particularly on the lower legs. No differentiation can be made from ichthyosis due to underlying lymphoma and that seen with other systemic disorders, including malnutrition,

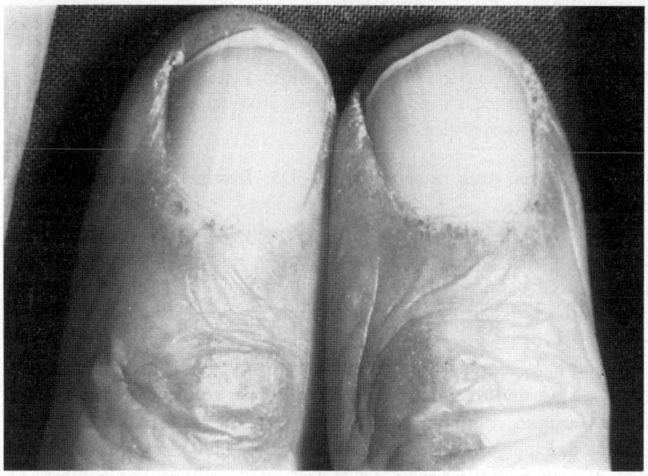

Fig. 8 Nail-fold telangiectasiae and ragged nail folds of dermatomyositis.

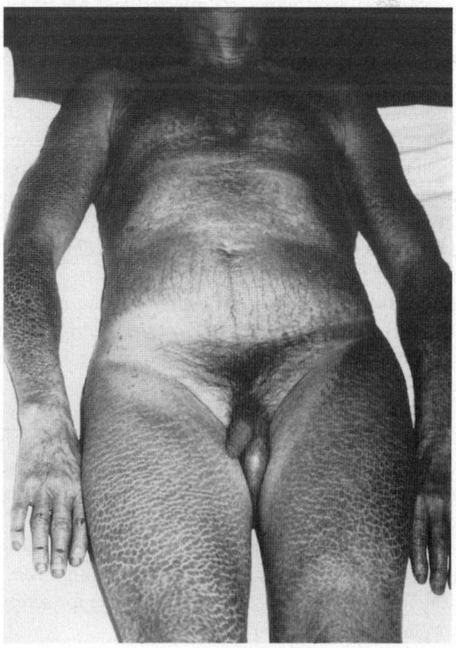

Fig. 9 Acquired ichthyosis associated with lymphoma.

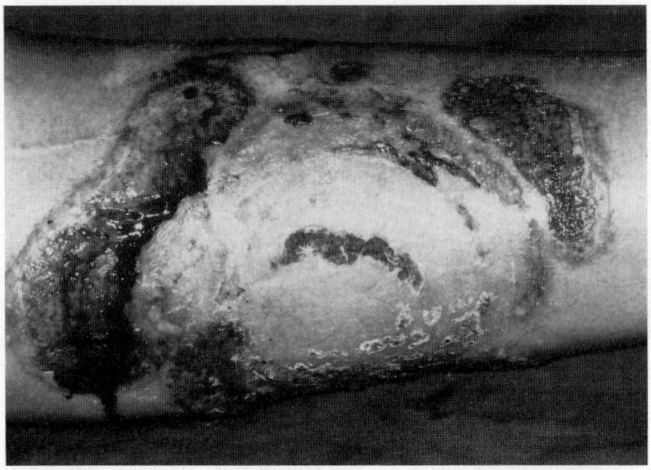

Fig. 10 Pyoderma gangrenosum is an inflammatory ulcer which usually develops on the lower limb and is associated with myeloproliferative disorders. The blue-black necrotic spreading edge is typical.

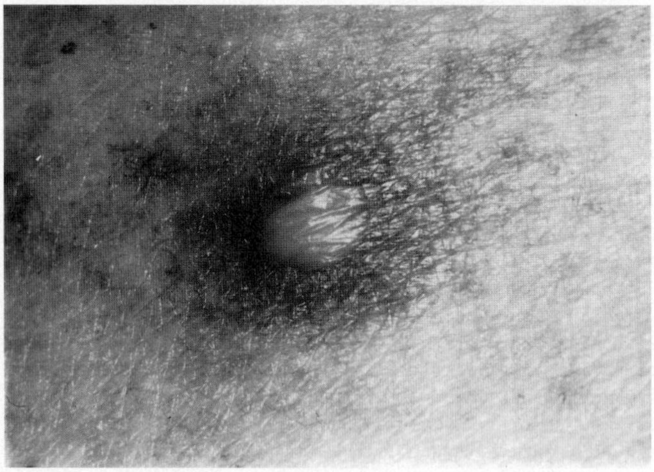

Fig. 11 The sterile pustules of subcorneal pustular dermatosis (Sneddon Wilkinson disease) are often flaccid and contain a fluid level (of pus).

cancer cachexia, drug reactions, and AIDS. Treatment is directed at the underlying cause.

Acquired hypertrichosis lanuginosa ('malignant down') presents with excessive growth of fine, silky lanugo-like hair, at first over the face, but can progress to the entire body. It is seen with malignancy, particularly carcinoma of the bronchus, but also with drug ingestion, thyrotoxicosis, and shock.[23]

Pyoderma gangrenosum (Fig. 10) is mostly seen with inflammatory bowel disease and rheumatoid arthritis but 7 per cent of cases have or will develop cancer, commonly acute myelogenous leukaemia.[24] A painful pustule develops with a centrifugally spreading blue-black rim of inflammation with central necrosis. These are usually solitary and painful and respond to high dose steroids but exclusion of other diagnoses, particularly infection, is necessary first.

Paraneoplastic pemphigus occurs most commonly with B-cell lymphoproliferative disorders. Intra-epithelial blistering occurs due to antibodies directed against desmogleins 1 and 3 in desmosomal junctions between keratinocytes. Mucous membranes are affected and life-threatening pulmonary involvement may be seen. Prognosis is poor and clinical course is independent of that of the underlying malignancy. Relief may be achieved with corticosteroids and cyclosporin or cyclophosphamide.[25]

Sweet's syndrome (acute febrile neutrophilic dermatosis) is characterized by fever, neutrophilia, and tender erythematous plaques or nodules, usually on the proximal limbs and upper body. The characteristic histopathology is infiltration of the dermis by polymorphonuclear leukocytes. Although usually idiopathic, 20 per cent of cases are cancer associated, usually with myeloproliferative disorders. Symptoms and rash resolve promptly with systemic corticosteroids.

Subcorneal pustular dermatosis (Fig. 11) is a rare disease frequently associated with myeloma, particularly of IgA type. Multiple sterile pustules occur in waves around axillae and flanks and there is a characteristic response to dapsone.

Vascular dermatoses. Migratory thrombophlebitis (Trousseau's syndrome) was first described with gastrointestinal malignancies and is a reflection of the hypercoagulant state of neoplasia. Although described with most malignancies, it is seen most commonly with solid tumours, and these are often occult.

An episode of deep venous thrombosis is associated with a significantly higher frequency of malignancy in the first 6 months from diagnosis. Simple clinical and diagnostic methods are adequate for screening; more extensive investigation is not cost-efficient.[26]

Vasculitis, presenting as palpable purpura, is secondary to underlying malignancy in 5 per cent of cases, particularly haematological disease.

Erythromelalgia is characterized by erythema, heat, and intense burning pain of extremities and in adult-onset is associated with myeloproliferative disease in 20 per cent of cases.

Other paraneoplastic dermatoses exist but are less specific than the above mentioned. Digital clubbing may denote malignancy, particularly if seen in association with hypertrophic osteoarthropathy. Bazex's syndrome (acrokeratosis neoplastica) refers to an acral distribution of psoriasiform lesions (most commonly nose, ears, hands and feet) which are refractory to treatment and all reported cases were associated with malignancy, mostly squamous cell carcinomas of upper aerodigestive tract.

Primary amyloidosis is associated with multiple myeloma and disorders of immunoglobulin metabolism. The mucocutaneous features are periorbital purpura, waxy papules on eyelids, lips, tongue, buccal mucosa and flexures, and macroglossia. Episodic cutaneous flushing, particularly in association with systemic symptoms such as diarrhoea, should prompt screening for a carcinoid tumour.

Skin conditions

Pallor, pigmentation, pruritus, and purpura are common in advanced malignant disease. Immunoparesis and general debilitation predispose cancer patients to infections, particularly candidiasis, herpes simplex, and zoster. Atypical manifestations of common infections may deceive, for example, severe and protracted herpes simplex.

Pruritus and sweating are discussed in detail in Chapter 8.7.

Dry skin and ichthyosis

Xerosis or dry skin is a frequent accompaniment of advanced cancer. Chemotherapy and radiotherapy both induce skin dryness which may be permanent. Nutritional deficiencies, due to the underlying malignancy, give rise to a dry, fine scaling resembling ichthyosis. When the superficial layer of the epidermis cracks giving a 'crazy paving' appearance itching and inflammation supervene (so-called asteatotic dermatitis) (Fig. 12). If this is allowed to progress profound dermatitis with weeping and oedema can ensue, particularly on the shins. The regular application of emollients and use of soap substitutes limits this process. Recommended applications include 50 per cent liquid paraffin in 50 per cent white soft paraffin or emulsifying ointment. Severe scaling can be treated by the addition of 2 per cent salicylic acid to the emollient. Drying of the skin may also exacerbate pre-existing skin conditions such as atopic dermatitis or allow it to re-emerge in patients predisposed.

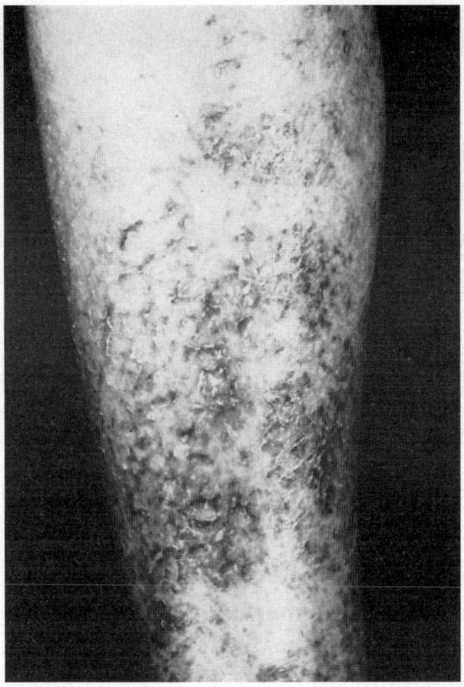

Fig. 12 Asteototic dermatitis: drying of the epidermis results in a loss of flexibility within the stratum corneum; splits develop and dermatitis is established.

Research into the components and maintenance of the epidermal barrier are likely to provide new therapies to prevent skin drying which is a feature of both ageing and advanced cancer.

Erythroderma and exfoliative dermatitis

Erythroderma (red skin all over) reflects widespread skin inflammation and may result directly from underlying disease, for example, Sezary syndrome (T-cell lymphoma/leukaemia), a drug eruption, or exacerbation of a pre-existing skin disease, such as atopic dermatitis or psoriasis. The patient is often systemically unwell and may need high-dependency care. There is increased insensible fluid loss and electrolyte disturbance with loss of temperature control. Accurate fluid resuscitation is vital especially in elderly or frail patients. Secondary infection is common and prophylactic antibiotics may be warranted, even without neutropaenia. If the skin is markedly exudative or secondarily infected potassium permanganate baths are safe and often helpful. Apart from addressing the underlying cause, therapy should include emollients, topical or systemic corticosteroids if appropriate, and oral antihistamines for itch.

Exacerbation of skin diseases

New cancer treatments such as immunomodulation and biologic therapies are likely to result in the emergence of new skin conditions or reactivation of known diseases. Psoriasis, for example, is related to cytokine release and γ-interferon use can provoke an outbreak.

Equally, all the psychological and physical effects of cancer and its treatment can unearth latent skin disease such as psoriasis or atopic dermatitis. The relapsing and remitting nature of these skin diseases often makes association with a stressful life event difficult to prove.

Seborrheic dermatitis is characterized by red, flaky skin over central face, eyebrows, ears, scalp, and central chest. Stress contributes but immunosuppression, such as seen in AIDS, can cause florid symptoms. An underlying fungal aetiology means treatment with oral fluconazole or itraconazole may be successful. Topical treatments then maintain remission, for example, 2 per cent sulphur 2 per cent salicylic acid in 1 per cent hydrocortisone cream. A number of other skin diseases, for example, psoriasis can worsen in association with HIV infection and AIDS, and AIDS patients may be more likely to develop drug eruptions.

Hair and nail changes

Nail changes can occur with malignant disease but are mostly related to therapy. Clubbing (see above), although not specific, is associated with underlying malignancy—metastatic or primary bronchopulmonary cancer, pleural and mediastinal tumours, including lymphoma, and oesophageal, gastric, and colonic cancer.

Cancer patients are prone to hair loss as 'telogen effluvium' (acute moult) the mechanism of which is unclear. A single insult such as fever, surgery, haemorrhage, sudden starvation, emotional stress, or drugs leads to an acute moult of the hair some 3–9 months later, which is self-limiting. Nutritional deficiencies such as iron or protein may also lead to hair loss which is ongoing unless the deficiency is corrected.

Alopecia mucinosa is associated with cutaneous T-cell lymphoma. The late stage of Sezary syndrome may give rise to diffuse alopecia due to infiltration. In widespread pruritus, for example, in Hodgkin's disease, alopecia may result from repeated rubbing and scratching.

Cutaneous aspects of cancer treatment

Cancer treatment frequently involves the skin, whether it be for intravenous access for chemotherapy or as a tissue through which radiotherapy is delivered. Extravasation of chemotherapeutic agents and radiation can both result in major skin problems, including necrosis. In general these complications can be avoided with care.

Reactions to chemotherapy

Patients receiving systemic chemotherapy also receive a host of supportive treatments which make attributing skin changes to specific agents difficult. However, there are a number of skin and mucous membrane reactions which occur repeatedly with particular regimens. Most commonly seen are alopecia and mucositis. Oral inflammation occurs as a direct toxic effect of chemotherapy, particularly antimetabolites, due to the high mitotic index of oral epithelium. This is noted most commonly 4–7 days post-chemotherapy. Indirectly, bone marrow suppression by chemotherapy leads to infection or haemorrhage of the oral mucosa at 10–14 days. In both cases prevention with meticulous oral hygiene is vital. Prophylactic use of antifungal or antibacterial oral rinses is often recommended. Treatment is essentially supportive. Topical local anaesthetic preparations may be effective, but systemic analgesia is often required. Fever and pain suggest infection and should be treated systemically with antifungals, antibiotics, or antiviral therapy.

Acral erythema (palmoplantar dysaesthesia syndrome), particularly noted with cytarabine, starts as numbness and tingling of the palms and/or soles. Erythema develops which progresses to blistering and finally desquamation[27] (Fig. 13). The reaction occurs days after chemotherapy and resolves in a fortnight. The mechanism is poorly understood and differentiation from acute graft versus host disease (GVHD) can be difficult clinically and histologically. A similar desquamating reaction can occur in the flexures of patients receiving systemic chemotherapy, and may be due to direct toxicity. Accumulation of toxic metabolites in the sweat ducts may explain localization to the palms, soles, and flexures.

Localized or generalized hyperpigmentation of skin and nails can be seen after chemotherapy with, for example, busulphan, cyclophosphamide, or cisplatin.[28] Patients who have previously been given radiotherapy can develop dermatitis at previously irradiated sites when given cytotoxics, so-called radiation recall. Phototoxicity and UV recall including inflammation of solar keratoses, have been documented with agents such as fluorouracil

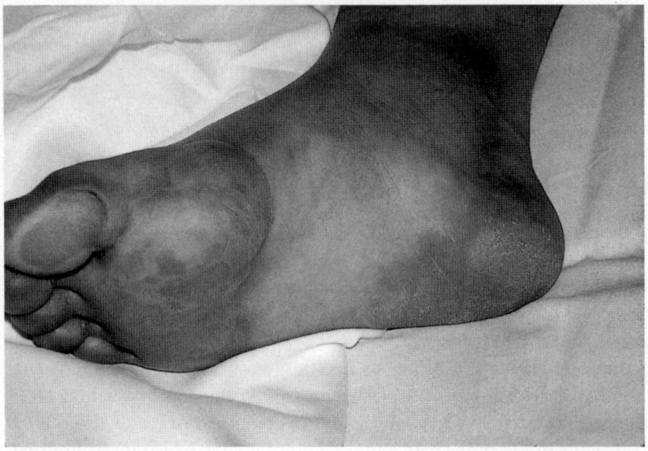

Fig. 13 Acral erythema—palm and sole erythema with desquamation due to direct chemotherapy toxicity.

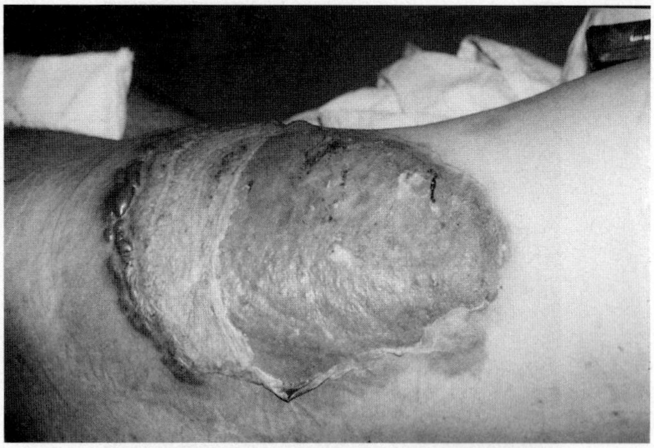

Fig. 14 Chronic recalcitrant herpes simplex in a patient with malignancy.

and methotrexate.[29] Cytotoxic agents, particularly bleomycin, may also enhance the cutaneous toxicity of radiation when given concomitantly.

Drug eruptions are an extremely common event in patients being treated for malignancy. This is partly due to polypharmacy but also because immunosuppressed individuals are more easily sensitized. A similar paradox is seen in HIV infection. Cytotoxic agents themselves can produce hypersensitivity reactions, including urticaria, erythema multiforme, and toxic epidermal necrolysis. More common is the maculopapular exanthem in patients immmunosuppressed and on a number of antibiotic agents. Rarely is the rash specific but it usually takes 7–10 days to appear (or 24–48 h if previously sensitized) allowing an intelligent guess of the culprit to be made. Rechallenge would identify the true cause but is rarely ethical in advanced cancer. Sometimes the interaction of two drugs or between drug and disease prompt the rash, as is the case with the morbilliform eruption seen from ampicillin if given to patients with infectious mononucleosis or lymphatic leukaemia. Not all drug reactions are allergic in origin. Certain drugs, such as opioids and radiocontrast media, may release mast cell mediators and lead to urticaria. High dose corticosteroids, particularly dexamethasone, cause acneiform and pustular eruptions. Resolution without treatment is slow and a 6-week course of tetracycline or erythromycin may be required. Two entities described with chemotherapeutic agents and diagnosed on clinical and histological grounds are neutrophil eccrine hidradenitis and syringosquamous metaplasia. Both are rare and self-limiting. The cutaneous eruption of lymphocyte recovery is described following marrow ablative chemotherapy, and is thought to be due to the return of immunocompetent lymphocytes to the peripheral circulation. A widespread maculopapular rash becoming confluent, with associated fever, is seen and clears over 4–5 days.

Hair and nail changes

Alopecia is the commonest cutaneous side-effect of chemotherapy treatment. Cytotoxic agents arrest mitosis in the hair papilla leading to weakness and fracturing of the hair shaft. This is a form of anagen alopecia, and continued therapy can lead to total hair loss. Combination therapies are more likely to produce this than larger doses of a single agent. Regrowth of hair is expected after treatment but can be of different colour or hair type. The use of scalp cooling to avoid hair loss has met with mixed results but is contraindicated in conditions associated with scalp metastasis and haematologic malignancy.

The commonest nail change with chemotherapy is Beau's lines. These are transverse white (or pigmented) grooves or lines across the nail plate occurring after each chemotherapy course. Arrested nail growth with chemotherapy may result in a horizontal break (onychomadesis) and subsequent shedding. More specific changes may be seen with particular agents, for example, mitoxantrone-induced onycholysis.[30]

Cutaneous manifestations of immunosuppressive therapy

Immunosuppressive and immunomodulation therapies are increasingly used in neoplastic disease. Cutaneous effects can be predictable but may be unusual in presentation and refractory to standard therapy. Advanced cancer patients are also immunosuppressed and similar problems arise.

The cutaneous complications of systemic corticosteroids are Cushing's syndrome, skin atrophy, striae, telangiectasia, hirsutism, and acne. Cyclosporin causes hypertrichosis and gingival hypertrophy. In general there is an increased susceptibility to infection and increased incidence of malignancy, particularly skin malignancy.

Common infections such as herpes simplex may present atypically (Fig. 14) and require high dose antiviral therapy. Viral infections, such as herpes simplex, varicella zoster, and cytomegalovirus may reactivate with immunosuppression necessitating prophylactic antiviral therapy. Furunculosis, impetigo, and cellulitis of bacterial aetiology occur more frequently and appropriate microbiological investigations are vital to monitor for antibiotic resistance. Tuberculosis and atypical mycobacterial infections may reactivate in the skin and biopsies may need to be sent for extended culture.

Mucocutaneous candidiasis is common, particularly with broad spectrum antibiotic use, and occurs in the intertriginous areas and mucous membranes. More widespread cutaneous candidiasis results in numerous small pustules with a superficial scaling margin. Treatment with oral fluconazole or itraconazole is recommended.

Dermatophyte (ringworm) fungal infection may present as subcutaneous nodules or extensive conventional infection, with or without nail involvement. Treatment if indicated is with once daily oral terbinafine.

Infestations such as scabies may present without itch. The crusted (Norwegian) variety with heavy mite infestation is more common in the immunosuppressed. Treatment is with 5 per cent permethrin cream and needs to be applied all over (and repeated in 7 days). The crusted form is highly contagious and close relations and nursing staff may also need treatment.

Skin and internal neoplasms may arise due to immunosuppressive therapy, particularly if prolonged after bone marrow transplantation. Kaposi's sarcoma and skin cancers, particularly squamous cell carcinoma, are increased in incidence. More aggressive behaviour of these malignancies is seen, necessitating a high level of awareness and swift treatment.

Radiation reactions[31]

In most cases radiotherapy must traverse the skin to gain access to the target tissue. In some cases, for example, breast cancer, it may be pertinent to treat the skin to avoid recurrence. X-rays produce acute and late radiation reactions and as with UV there is great individual variation in tissue response. Previously the acute reaction of erythema and oedema occurring 2–3 weeks into a fractionated course was used as a guide to dosage. Once set in motion moist desquamation usually supervenes and treatment is symptomatic, with moisturisers and good nursing care.

Increased understanding of radiobiology now minimizes side effects to bystander tissues. Modern megavoltage radiotherapy delivers maximal dose at a greater depth avoiding the acute skin reaction. However, late reactions may still occur. Clinically this manifests as telangiectatic, atrophic skin with underlying fibrosis. These areas show less compliance and resilience, allowing ulceration in sites of trauma and moisture. Increasing age and UV exposure may be additive and accelerate atrophy, necrosis, and secondary malignant change.

There may be difficulty distinguishing recurrent tumour, an X-ray induced neoplasm or radionecrotic ulceration. The latter is associated with severe pain. Breast cancer recurring within a previously irradiated field may ulcerate, fungate or enhance sclerosis (carcinoma *en cuirasse*), or produce papillomata which readily weep and bleed. The most common radiotherapy-induced tumour is the basal cell carcinoma and this can be multiple. Excision is technically difficult in sclerotic skin and as progression is slow a 'wait and watch' policy can usually be adopted. Sarcomas and atypical fibroxanthomas may also occur in previously irradiated fields.

Rarely *de novo* skin disease may localize to an area of radiotherapy treatment. Bullous pemphigoid and localized scleroderma(32) have been reported in this context.

GVHD

This is a multisystem disorder where the skin is often involved. It is an immunological assault by immunocompetent cells engrafted into a host unable to reject them. Most commonly it occurs in allogeneic bone marrow transplant recipients. Two forms of the disease exist—an acute and a chronic form. The acute form is closely linked to histocompatibilty of donor and recipient, occurring more frequently with increased major histocompatibility complex (MHC) mismatch;(33) 10–20 days post-transplantation fever and a non-specific maculopapular rash occur. The rash can progress to a widespread bullous form and associated mucous membrane changes, resembling toxic epidermal necrolysis. Diarrhoea and liver dysfunction often co-exist and need monitoring. Strategies to avoid acute GVHD include careful MHC matching of donor and recipient, donor T-cell depletion, and pretreatment with immunosuppressives such as cyclosporin. A lower incidence of acute and chronic GVHD may be seen with transplants of cord blood or peripheral stem cells.

Chronic GVHD is more likely to be seen in the palliative care setting. The skin is the main organ involved and can vary from a change resembling lichen planus to features of systemic sclerosis. Chronic GVHD occurs at least 3 months post-transplantation but is more common after acute GVHD. A particularly disabling form (Fig. 15) results in cutaneous sclerosis, contractures, malabsorption, wasting, alopecia, skin ulceration, and death. There is marked resemblance to connective tissue disease, dry eyes and dry mouth may be seen, so can liver dysfunction, immunosuppression, and lung fibrosis. Mortality approaches 50 per cent at 10 years and is higher in patients with progressive disease (acute GVHD evolving into chronic GVHD), and lung involvement.(34) Treatment with agents, such as prednisolone and azathioprine, used in connective tissue disease, have been associated with clinical improvement, particularly in combination. Newer agents such as tacrolimus, mycophenolate mofetil, and antitumour necrosis factor are under investigation. UV irradiation and psoralen can lead to resolution of skin disease, which has led to the effective use of extra-corporeal photochemotherapy as an adjunct in refractory acute and chronic GVHD.(35)

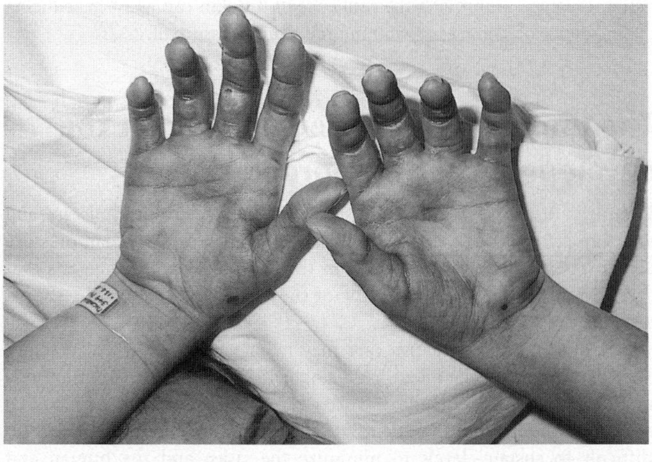

Fig. 15 Chronic GVHD: progressive widespread sclerotic changes in the skin lead to joint contractures, alopecia, sores, and eventually death.

References

1. **Kirova, Y.M.** et al. (1999). Radiotherapy as palliative treatment for metastatic melanoma. *Melanoma Research* **9** (6), 611–13.
2. **Strobbe, L.J., Niewig, O.E., and Kroon, B.B.** (1997). Carbon dioxide laser for cutaneous melanoma metastases: indications and limitations. *European Journal of Surgical Oncology* **23** (5), 435–8.
3. **Wit, F.W.** et al. (1998). Regression of AIDS-related Kaposi's sarcoma associated with clearance of human-herpes virus 8 from peripheral blood mononuclear cells following initiation of antiretroviral therapy. *AIDS* **12**, 218–19.
4. **Skobe, M.** et al. (1999). Vascular endothelial growth factor-C (VEGF-C) and its receptors KDR and flt-4 are expressed in AIDS-associated Kaposi's sarcoma. *Journal of Investigative Dermatology* **113** (6), 1047–53.
5. **Brambilla, L.** et al.(1994). Mediterranean Kaposi's sarcoma in the elderly: a randomized study of oral etoposide versus vinblastine. *Cancer* **74**, 2873–8.
6. **Dezube, B.J.** (2000). New therapies for the treatment of AIDS-related Kaposi's sarcoma. *Current Opinion in Oncology* **12** (5), 445–9.
7. **Kim, Y.H. and Hoppe, R.T.** (1999). Mycosis fungoides and the Sezary syndrome. *Seminars in Oncology* **26**, 276–89.
8. **Bullen, R.** et al. (1998). Angiosarcoma of the head and neck managed by a combination of multiple biopsies to determine tumour margin and radiation therapy. *Dermatologic Surgery* **24** (10), 1105–10.
9. **Kanitakis, J.** (1993). Cutaneous metastases of internal carcinomas. *Presse medicale* **22** (13), 631–6.
10. **Chanda, J.J.** (1985). Extramammary Paget's disease: prognosis and relationship to internal malignancy. *Journal of the American Academy of Dermatology* **13** (6), 1009–14.
11. **Terwogt, J.M.** et al. (1999). Phase II trial of topically applied miltefosine solution in patients with skin-metastasized breast cancer. *British Journal of Cancer* **79** (7–8), 1158–61.
12. **Goldstein, A.M.** et al. (1995). Increased risk of pancreatic cancer in melanoma-prone kindreds with $p16^{INK4}$ mutations. *New England Journal of Medicine* **333**, 970–4.
13. **Gorlin, R.J.** (1987). Naevoid basal cell carcinoma syndrome. *Medicine* **66**, 98–110.
14. **Johnson, R.L.** et al. (1996). Human homolog of patched, a candidate gene for the basal cell naevus syndrome. *Science* **272**, 1668–71.
15. **Tsao, H.** (2000). Update on familial cancer syndromes and the skin. *Journal of the American Academy of Dermatology* **42**, 939–69.
16. **Ellis, D.L.** et al. (1987). Melanoma, growth factors, acanthosis nigricans, the sign of Leser-Trelat, and multiple achrocordons. *New England Journal of Medicine* **317**, 1582–7.
17. **Cohen, P.R.** et al. (1989). Tripe palms and malignancy. *Journal of Clinical Oncology* **7**, 669–78.
18. **Boden, G.** et al. (1986). Treatment of inoperable glucagonoma with the long-acting somatostatin analogue SMS 201-995. *New England Journal of Medicine* **314** (26), 1686–9.
19. **Hill, C.L.** et al. (2001). Frequency of specific cancer types in dermatomyositis and polymyositis: a population based study. *Lancet* **357**, 96–100.

20. **Peng, J.C., Sheen, T.S., and Hsu, M.M.** (1995). Nasopharyngeal carcinoma with dermatomyositis: an analysis of 12 cases. *Archives of Otolaryngology, Head and Neck Surgery* **121** (11), 1298–301.
21. **Fudman, E.J. and Schnitzer, T.J.** (1986). Dermatomyositis without creatine kinase elevation: poor prognostic sign. *American Journal of Medicine* **80**, 329–32.
22. **Kurzrock, R. and Cohen, P.R.** (1995). Mucocutaneous paraneoplastic manifestations of haematologic malignancies. *American Journal of Medicine* **99** (2), 207–16.
23. **Kurzrock, R. and Cohen, P.R.** (1995). Cutaneous paraneoplastic syndromes in solid tumours. *American Journal of Medicine* **99** (6), 662–71.
24. **Powell, F.C. et al.** (1985). Pyoderma gangrenosum: a review of 86 patients. *Quarterly Journal of Medicine* **55**, 173–86.
25. **Nousari, H.C. and Anhalt, G.J.** (1999). Pemphigus and bullous pemphigoid. *Lancet* **354**, 667–72.
26. **Naschitz, J.E. et al.** (1996). Diagnosis of cancer associated vascular disorders. *Cancer* **77** (9), 1759–67.
27. **Baack, B.R. and Burgdorf, W.H.C.** (1991). Chemotherapy induced acral erythema. *Journal of the American Academy of Dermatology* **24**, 457–61.
28. **Susser, W.S. et al.** (1999). Mucocutaneous reactions to chemotherapy. *Journal of the American Academy of Dermatology* **40**, 367–98.
29. **Bataille, V. et al.** (1996). Inflammation of solar keratoses following systemic 5-fluorouracil. *British Journal of Dermatology* **135**, 478–80.
30. **Creamer, J.D., Mortimer, P.S., and Powles, T.J.** (1995). Mitozantrone induced onycholysis. *Clinical and Experimental Dermatology* **20**, 459–61.
31. **Spittle, M.F.** (1986). Ionizing radiation. In *Textbook of Dermatology* (ed. A. Rook et al.), pp. 625–6. Oxford: Blackwell Scientific.
32. **Colver, G.B. et al.** (1989). Post irradiation morphoea. *British Journal of Dermatology* **120**, 831–5.
33. **Klingebiel, T. and Schlegel, P.G.** (1998). GVHD: Overview on pathophysiology, incidence, clinical and biological features. *Bone Marrow Transplantation* **21** (Suppl. 2), S45–9.
34. **Ratanatharathorn, V. et al.** (2001). Chronic graft versus host disease: clinical manifestations and therapy. *Bone Marrow Transplantation* **28** (2), 121–9.
35. **Greinix, H.T. et al.** (1998). Successful use of extracorporeal photochemotherapy in the treatment of severe acute and chronic graft-versus host disease. *Blood* **92** (9), 3098–104.

8.9.2 Nursing aspects

Patricia Grocott and Carol Dealey

Introduction

Skin problems are almost inevitable in patients receiving palliative care for multiple, progressive pathologies. The focus of this chapter is the nursing care of patients with a weakened skin barrier and the management of wounds caused by particular diseases and conditions that are prevalent in palliative care. The general principles of nursing care proposed are based substantially on those adopted for the care of the elderly. The rationale for this approach is three fold. First, ageing is associated with a number of skin problems that are derived from a weakened skin barrier. Second, problems in advanced disease are largely attributable to skin that is weakened by general effects of chronic disease, such as malnutrition, dehydration, and immobility.[1] Third, a systematic review of the literature on the level of need for palliative care indicates that the incidence of cancer, respiratory, circulatory, and nervous diseases, all of which may be responsible for skin damage, is high in the older age group.[2] The management of wounds in palliative care can be complicated because of the advanced nature of the underlying disease or condition. As yet the subject is under-researched and therefore not fully formalized into rational standards of care supported by appropriate protocols and products. The general principles of nursing care described may therefore have to be adapted to meet individual patient needs.

The nursing care of patients with a weakened skin barrier

There are many factors that predispose palliative care patients to skin problems; if they are taken into account when taking a history and assessing the patient it may be possible to mitigate their effects. Nursing care is clearly not able to prevent and resolve all the problems of advanced disease, for example, immobility and anorexia. However, dedicated interventions to prevent morbidity resulting from these problems, for example, pressure ulcers and dry skin conditions, may be possible.

Skin care

Ensuring that patients are able to meet their hygiene needs is a fundamental aspect of nursing care. However, this is more than ensuring that patients are clean. A key focus of skin care is the prevention or treatment of dry skin, as patients receiving palliative care will have dry skin for a variety of reasons. For example, the skin in older people is thinner and less elastic, partly because there is less collagen in the dermis and it is of poorer quality.[1,3] Repeated washing following incontinence may result in dry skin over the perineum and buttocks. Particular problems of dry skin in palliative care may be a consequence of radiotherapy or may be associated with anorexia.[4] Dry skin also predisposes patients to pruritis due to loose skin scales.

There are a number of simple measures to prevent or treat dry skin.[3] They include general measures such as ensuring that patients avoid too much heat, as it has a drying effect on the skin, and that they drink ample amounts of water. Simple moisturizers should be applied liberally and frequently to the skin. They may be in the form of bland emollients, which form a barrier on the skin, preventing evaporation and sealing in moisture, or humectants that are able to attract and hold water on the skin surface. Alternatives to cleansing with soap and water should be considered if the skin dryness is due to repeated washing following incontinence.[5] An emollient that includes an additional barrier such as zinc will help to prevent excoriation from urine and faeces. Vigorous movements should be avoided, especially with fragile skin, as it may tear. Overall the reasons for using moisturisers are to improve patient comfort and to increase tissue resilience. Improving the resilience of the skin can assist in reducing the incidence of skin tears[6] and in preventing pressure ulcers.[7]

The impact of advanced disease on the development of skin problems

The focus of this section includes the problems of advanced disease and their impact on the development of skin problems, in particular, pressure ulcers. The Department of Health in the United Kingdom suggests that pressure ulcers are a key indicator of the quality of care provided by a hospital.[8]

Patients receiving palliative care may be at particular risk of pressure ulcer development. The dilemmas facing palliative care in relation to pressure ulcer prevention include: the extent to which pressure damage can be avoided without eroding patient autonomy; raising the costs of care to 'difficult to sustain' levels to minimize the risks; and the human and financial costs of not preventing pressure damage.

Aetiology of pressure ulcers

Pressure ulcers are caused by a combination of extrinsic factors, and factors that are intrinsic to the patient.[1] The intrinsic factors associated with pressure ulcer development have been identified using multivariate analysis in a number of cohort studies, which have been reviewed and analysed.[9] Five factors were consistently implicated in the studies: age, mobility, nutrition, perfusion, and skin status.

Extrinsic factors

Pressure

Pressure is considered to be the key causal factor in pressure ulcer development.[1] However, it is the length of time and the intensity of the pressure that ultimately results in tissue damage.[10] Localized external pressure over a bony prominence results in compression of the soft tissue. If the pressure is greater than capillary closing pressure then this is followed by localized ischaemia and, subsequently, tissue destruction if the pressure is prolonged. Bony prominences such as the sacrum, ischial tuberosities, heels, and elbows are particularly vulnerable to pressure damage.

Friction

Friction forces occur when two surfaces rub against each other, such as when a patient is dragged rather than lifted. The result is superficial damage with stripping of the epidermis. Friction forces are increased in the presence of moisture.

Shear

Shearing causes tissue distortion and tearing of blood vessels. Gebhardt[11] has argued that shearing is a factor in pressure damage because pressure is not applied uniformly and results in tissue distortion and ultimately tearing. Patients who constantly slide down in their bed or chair are particularly vulnerable to shearing damage.

Intrinsic factors

Mobility

In their review, Nixon and McGough[9] found that 10 of the 11 cohort studies identified impaired mobility to be both a significant and an independent predictor of pressure ulcer development. Patients who are bed or chair fast are particularly vulnerable to pressure damage. Equally, patients who do not move because of inadequate pain control or who are sedated by hypnotics, anxiolytics, antidepressants, and opioid analgesics will also be at risk. Neurological deficit may be associated with impaired mobility, for example, patients with spinal injury or degeneration. Loss of sensation impacts on the normal desire to move to relieve pressure.

Age

A number of studies have found older age to be associated with an increased incidence and prevalence of pressure ulcers.[12] Allman[13] suggests that the reasons for this may be multifactorial and linked to both age-related skin changes, which reduce tissue tolerance, and also increased morbidity and disease, which can affect mobility.

Nutrition-related factors

There is controversy as to whether poor nutritional status is a causal factor in pressure ulcer development. In one study,[14] patients with a good appetite were 3–4 times less likely to develop pressure ulcers than those with a poor appetite. However, there was a stronger association with older age where the risk was 10-fold higher than for younger patients. In a recent review, nutrition-related factors were identified as an independent risk factor in 8 of 11 studies. However, there was considerable variation between the studies as to how this was measured, which partly explains the continuing lack of clarity in this area. Logic might suggest that the skin of a patient with poor appetite who has lost weight and is dehydrated will have less resilience than someone with a normal appetite, and will thus be more vulnerable to pressure damage. As yet there is insufficient evidence to determine the precise role of nutrition in pressure ulcer aetiology.

Perfusion

Poor perfusion results in a lowering of capillary closing pressure and increases vulnerability to pressure, but again there is no clearly defined cause–effect relationship between pressure ulcers and perfusion.[9]

Skin status

Healthy individuals are able to tolerate considerable insult to the skin without developing tissue damage. This is because healthy skin is resilient. A number of factors can reduce skin tolerance and increase the risk of pressure damage. Age, poor nutrition, and weight loss have already been mentioned. Another factor to consider is incontinence[15] which can cause skin maceration and increase friction. Repeated cleansing of the skin causes excessive drying, which can also adversely affect skin tolerance.

Prevention of pressure ulcers

The most effective strategy for pressure ulcer prevention is to identify those at risk and to implement appropriate prevention strategies. There are several published clinical guidelines,[16,17] the most recent from the National Institute for Clinical Excellence (NICE),[18] and they will be used as the framework for discussing this topic. Details of the guidelines can be found in Tables 1–5. In addition education for health care professionals, patients, and carers is essential to ensure effective planning and implementation of prevention strategies. The advent of Clinical Nurse Specialists in Tissue Viability has had a major impact on the education and advice available at a local level.[1] Health care professionals can also access a wide range of study days, conferences, and courses to cover the topics listed in Table 5.

Obviously prevention is as important for patients receiving palliative care as for other patient groups and should continue until patients are in the last days of life. The human and financial costs are too great not to do so. However, prevention strategies may have to be adapted to meet individual

Table 1 Guidance for identifying patients at risk of developing pressure ulcers[a]

Risk assessment should be carried out by personnel who have undergone appropriate training to recognize risk factors
Risk assessment should be carried out within 6 h of admission to care episode or if there is a change in condition
Risk assessment should be documented and be accessible to all members of the inter-disciplinary team
Risk calculators should be used as an aide-memoire—not replace clinical judgement
Risk assessment includes recognizing the specific intrinsic and extrinsic factors within an individual that can potentially result in pressure ulcer development

[a] Guideline on pressure ulcer risk assessment and prevention. NICE Inherited Clinical Guideline B, April 2001, www.nice.org.uk.

Table 2 Skin inspection guidance[a]

Skin inspection should occur regularly and the frequency should be determined by individual patient need
Skin inspection should include assessment of the most vulnerable to pressure damage. Typically this would include bony prominences such as heels, sacrum, and ischial tuberosities. Other areas should be inspected as necessitated by the patient's condition
Where possible, individuals who are willing and able should be given education and encouraged to inspect their own skin
Individuals who are wheelchair users should use a mirror to inspect the areas that they cannot see easily or get others to inspect them
Health care professionals should be aware of the clinical signs of incipient skin damage, including those found in darkly pigmented skin Skin changes should be documented immediately

[a] Guideline on pressure ulcer risk assessment and prevention. NICE Inherited Clinical Guideline B, April 2001, www.nice.org.uk.

Table 3 Positioning guidance[a]

At risk patients should be repositioned regularly, the frequency should be determined by individual patient need and skin status, not ritual
Repositioning should take overall patient condition into consideration
Patients at acute risk of developing pressure ulcers should not sit out in chairs for more than 2 h
Repositioning schedules should be agreed with the individual and recorded
Individuals and/or their carers who are both willing and able should be taught how to reposition themselves
Care should be taken to reduce friction and shear when using manual handling devices and no manual handling apparatus should be left under the individual after use

[a] Guideline on pressure ulcer risk assessment and prevention. NICE Inherited Clinical Guideline B, April 2001, www.nice.org.uk.

Table 4 Guidance for pressure-redistributing equipment[a]

There is inadequate information on the cost-effectiveness of pressure-redistributing equipment to provide guidance for health care professionals at this time
Water-filled gloves, synthetic sheepskins, genuine sheepskins, and doughnut-type devices should not be used as pressure-relieving aids
Seating assessments should be carried out by trained assessors
Advice from trained assessors with acquired specific knowledge and expertise should be sought about correct seating positions
Positioning of individuals who spend substantial periods of time in a chair or wheelchair should take into account distribution of weight, postural alignment, and support of feet
No seat cushion has been shown to perform better than another

[a] Guideline on pressure ulcer risk assessment and prevention. NICE Inherited Clinical Guideline B, April 2001, www.nice.org.uk.

need. For example, it is of little use to plan a regimen of repositioning a patient from side to side if that patient has severe dyspnoea and gross oedema associated with end-stage heart failure. Such a patient would be better nursed on a low-air-loss bed, which would allow the patient to sit upright whilst providing pressure redistribution.

In the final stages of life when signs of peripheral circulatory failure are becoming evident, and the patient is distressed when moved, patient

Table 5 Guidance for education and training[a]

All health care professionals should have relevant education and training
Health care professionals with recognized training in pressure ulcer management should cascade their knowledge and skill to their local colleagues
An interdisciplinary approach should be used
Training and education programmes should include: risk factors for pressure ulcer development, pathophysiology of pressure ulcer development, the limitations and potential applications of risk assessment tools, skin assessment, skin care, selection of pressure-redistributing equipment, use of pressure-redistribution equipment, maintenance of pressure-redistributing equipment, methods of documenting risk assessments and prevention activities, positioning to minimize pressure, shear, and friction damage, including the correct use of manual handling devices, roles and responsibilities of inter-disciplinary team members in pressure ulcer management, policies and procedures regarding transferring individuals between care settings, and patient education and information giving
Patients and carers who are able and willing should be informed and educated about risk assessment and resulting prevention strategies
Patient/carer education should include providing information on the following: the risk factors associated with them developing pressure ulcers, the sites that are of the greatest risk to them of pressure damage, how to inspect skin and recognize skin changes, how to care for skin, methods for pressure relief/reduction, where they can seek further advice and assistance should they need it, emphasize the need for immediate visits to a health care professional should signs of damage be noticed

[a] Guideline on pressure ulcer risk assessment and prevention. NICE Inherited Clinical Guideline B, April 2001, www.nice.org.uk.

comfort should take precedence over pressure-relieving interventions that may cause additional distress to a dying patient.

The principles of pressure ulcer prevention are: risk assessment, skin assessment and care, positioning, and the use of pressure-relieving equipment.

Identifying patients at risk of developing pressure ulcers

Accurate assessment of pressure ulcer risk requires both skill and good clinical judgement. One reason why the use of risk assessment tools is so popular is that they are a useful aid to clinical judgement, especially for less-experienced staff. However, there are many different tools available which possibly reflects the fact that none is applicable to all patient groups. For example, Chaplain[19] set out to ensure effective use of an established tool but subsequently concluded that it did not adequately reflect the risks of patients requiring palliative care. She and her colleagues ultimately developed a tool specifically for this patient group.

There are major issues that face palliative care practitioners in relation to respecting patient autonomy, care planning, and resource management when the risks of pressure ulcer development can be assessed.[19] These issues are explored further in the following strategy for pressure ulcer prevention in palliative care.

Skin assessment and care

The skin should be assessed for signs of dryness, fragility, and decreased turgour as well as incipient signs of pressure damage. Assessment of the skin is, however, often inadequate and poorly documented. It is important that skin status is recorded whether or not there is any pressure damage. Strategies for the care of the skin are described in the section on 'Skin care'.

The appropriate use of repositioning and equipment strategies for pressure ulcer prevention in palliative care requires significant skill, expertise, and judgement. The NICE guidelines[18] reflect the lack of hard evidence to underpin this area of patient care. For example, on the subject of positioning, the guidance is that patients should be repositioned regularly, and that the frequency should be determined by individual need, not ritual (see Table 3). With regard to equipment, there is currently a lack of adequate information on the cost-effectiveness of pressure-redistributing equipment (see Table 4).

Positioning

Repositioning is a key nursing strategy for pressure ulcer prevention. Reduced numbers of staff, manual handling regulations, and the increased use of pressure redistributing equipment have all impacted on the use of this strategy. There is also greater awareness, as evident in the NICE guidelines (Table 3), of the need to move away from the ritualistic regimens of the past to an approach where individual need is addressed. It must also be acknowledged that patients need to be moved for reasons other than pressure relief. When planning a repositioning schedule those factors must also be taken into consideration. A key requirement is to achieve a balance between respecting individual preferences and meeting needs in relation to pressure relief. Failure to do so can have disastrous consequences as the following case history illustrates.

Case study The patient had advanced prostate cancer and developed spinal cord compression with hemiplegia including complete loss of motor function, sensation, bowel and bladder functions. He was initially nursed in the community. His family and community nurses tried to introduce a pressure-relieving strategy but the patient insisted on sitting out in a chair for long periods. He developed grade 4 pressure ulcers on both buttocks (extensive destruction involving muscle and tendon with exposed bone) and was admitted to a hospice (Fig. 1). He was nursed on a low-air-loss bed to prevent further pressure damage. The ulcers were surgically debrided of necrotic tissue, leaving residual ischaemic tissue at the base of both wounds. The wound management goals at this point were to further debride the wounds, to eliminate the heavy colonization by methicillin-resistant *Staphylococcus aureus* and *Pseudomonas aeruginosa*, and promote healing. Wound management was, however, complicated by faecal incontinence. Steps to manage his bowel function with a regular regimen of enemas failed when he developed diarrhoea as a side-effect of antibiotic treatment, which was needed for repeated chest infections. An anal plug (Coloplast Ltd) may have helped to control the faecal flow. However, this appliance was not available in the United Kingdom at that time. The incontinence forced lengthy dressing changes that were repeated several times a day. This disturbance of the wounds, together with progressive deterioration in the patient's condition, meant that little progress was made in healing the ulcers. He became progressively depressed and withdrawn. He died 4 months after the onset of pressure ulceration. The nurses who cared for him were so distressed by this patient's circumstances they required counselling for some time after his death.

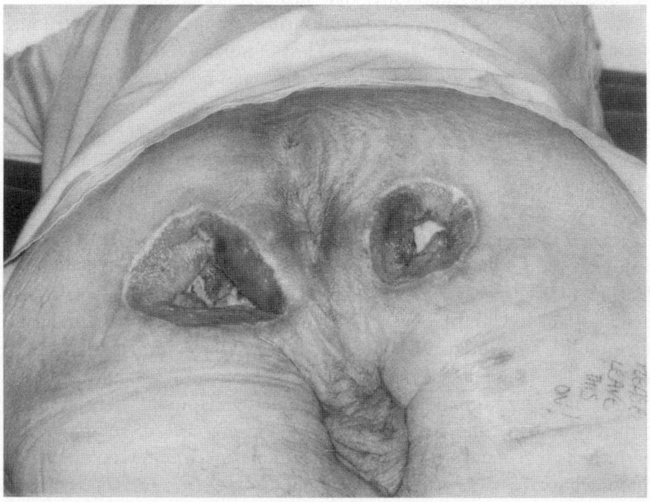

Fig. 1 Grade 4 pressure ulcers.

The above case history illustrates that risk assessment needs to take account of any medical conditions that the patient may be predisposed to, in order to take prompt action to manage the condition. In the case of advanced prostate cancer, spinal cord compression with consequent paraparesis is a recognized complication and one that may be reversed if emergency treatment is commenced in good time. Rapid onset of paraplegia and loss of sphincter function may not, however, be recoverable.[20] The patient and family need to be alerted to key signs of altered sensation and function to speed diagnosis and prevent paralysis. If paralysis cannot be prevented the patient and family need to receive clear information about the consequences of paralysis, pressure ulcer development in particular, as described in the NICE guidelines (Table 5). Interpersonal and communication skills are essential to put such information across in a way that does not inappropriately alarm the individuals concerned but gives enough information so that appropriate choices about management and care can be made.

The case history describes the circumstances when patient autonomy prevailed with disastrous consequences for the individual and his family. There were significant resource and cost implications for the hospice concerned. In addition, the burden of care to the nurses had a physical and psychological impact that took time to resolve.

Use of equipment

There is a wide range of pressure-redistributing equipment available. When selecting equipment for individual use a number of factors have to be considered, the most important of which is to provide adequate pressure relief. At the same time, the selected equipment should allow the patient to remain as mobile and independent as possible. The care setting may also impact on selection, particularly if there are limitations in the types of equipment available. Consideration also needs to be given to seating as well as equipment for use on the bed, especially for patients who may sit in a chair for long periods or are more comfortable in a reclining chair than a bed.

Overall, pressure ulcer prevention in palliative care is a complex issue and one that requires skilled assessment and resources, together with interpersonal and communication skills so that individual autonomy is respected and patients make informed decisions about their care. As described above, pressure ulcers have been used as a key indicator of quality of nursing care. However, pressure damage may not be altogether preventable in the final days of life, and some level of pressure damage may be accepted to avoid repositioning a patient who is distressed by this intervention.

Pressure ulcer management

When a patient develops pressure ulcers it is helpful to identify the critical event that resulted in tissue damage. Many patients receiving palliative care can be at considerable risk of pressure damage for long periods of time without injury. It is easy to assume that the ulcer is due to further deterioration of the patient's condition and this may indeed be true for some. But there may also be a cause that can be easily eliminated. For example, the cushion the patient sits on for long periods of time may be worn out and needs replacing; or an outing in a car lasting several hours without the use of a pressure-redistributing cushion may result in avoidable skin damage.

Even a heavy cold can increase patient vulnerability to pressure damage, rendering normal prevention strategies ineffective. Good education of health care professionals, patients, and carers can prevent some of these problems in the first instance, or at least ensure early detection of pressure damage to prevent an ulcer deteriorating. If an ulcer is detected whilst the skin is still intact, the damage may be reversible.

Grading of pressure ulcers

The use of a grading tool is very helpful for describing the severity of pressure ulcers. There are number of different tools described in the literature with grades ranging from 0 to 6. They all have a common feature in that the higher the grade the deeper the sore.(1) Table 6 provides an example of a widely used grading tool. Recognition of a grade 1 ulcer can be problematic, especially in those with dark skin. It may also be difficult to determine the level of damage in patients with unbroken skin who have signs of 'bruising' beneath the surface of the skin. The National Pressure Ulcers Advisory Panel (NPUAP) in the United States has recently produced a new definition for a grade 1 pressure ulcer which takes account of these difficulties:

A stage 1 pressure ulcer is an observable pressure related alteration of intact skin whose indicators, as compared to the adjacent or opposite area on the body, may include changes in one or more of the following:

- skin temperature (warmth or coolness)
- tissue consistency (firm or boggy feeling) and/or
- sensation (pain, itching).

The ulcer appears as a defined area of persistent redness in lightly pigmented skin, whereas in darker skin tones, the ulcer may appear with persistent red, blue, or purple hues.(21)

Wound management

The reader is directed to other texts cited at the end of this chapter, which cover this topic in greater detail than is possible here. The principles of wound management involve adequate assessment of the patient and wound, the setting of appropriate goals, and evaluating progress. Determining appropriate goals for patients at the end of their lives is especially important. If healing is not the goal of treatment then it may be more appropriate to address specific patient issues, such as prevention and management of excessive exudate or odour. An example might be a dying patient with necrotic pressure ulcers on his heels. If there is no exudate, then it would be best to leave the ulcers exposed and dry as this causes less distress to the patient than frequent dressing changes.

Table 6 An example of a pressure ulcer grading tool[a]

Grade	Description
Grade 1	Non-blanchable erythema of intact skin. Discoloration of the skin, warmth, oedema, induration, or hardness may also be used as indicators, especially on individuals with darker skin
Grade 2	Partial thickness skin loss involving epidermis, dermis, or both. The ulcer is superficial and presents clinically as an abrasion or blister or both
Grade 3	Full thickness skin loss involving damage to or necrosis of subcutaneous tissue that may extend to, but not through underlying fascia
Grade 4	Extensive destruction, tissue necrosis, or damage to muscle, bone, or supporting structures with or without full thickness skin loss

[a] Taken from: European Pressure Ulcer Advisory Panel, *Pressure Ulcer Treatment Guidelines*, EPUAP, Oxford, 1998. (The European Pressure Ulcer Advisory Panel has left the above Guidelines in the public domain so all or part of them are freely available for use.)

Prevention strategies

If the patient already has a prevention plan it must be reviewed. Further measures are likely to be necessary, particularly up-grading the level of pressure-redistributing equipment. For example, if the patient has been on an alternating air overlay and develops a pressure ulcer, more sophisticated equipment such as an alternating air mattress may be more appropriate. Low-air-loss beds and air-fluidized beds have all been shown to be effective in healing pressure ulcers. However, they are costly items that require considerable space, so are not practical for use in all health care settings.(1)

The management of pressure ulcers requires skills in assessment as well as treatment. Clear documentation is also required to detail the assessment, describe the goals of care with the supporting rationale and the plan of care. This will enable reliable evaluation of progress towards meeting goals.

Fungating wound management

Aetiology

Fungating malignant wounds are caused by infiltration of the skin and its supporting blood and lymph vessels by tumour cells. They may arise from locally advanced tumours, metastatic, or recurrent growths. Unless amenable to anticancer treatments the infiltration extends and the wounds advance. There is the potential for massive damage to the skin through a combination of proliferative growth, loss of vascularity, and ulceration. The loss of vascularity is a major source of the problems associated with these wounds because of the loss of tissue viability and consequent necrosis.(22) Anaerobic and aerobic bacteria proliferate in these conditions and are probably the sources of the malodour and exudate that are commonly associated with these wounds.(23)

Uncontrolled tumour fungation

Any tumour can cause fungation, and tumour progression through the skin is diverse. Fungating breast cancer can present as extensive cutaneous infiltration of the chest wall, proud nodules or deep necrotic ulceration with proliferative growth of the ulcer margins (Figs 2–4).

Carcinomas of the ovary, caecum, and rectum, which infiltrate the anterior wall of the abdomen, may present initially as small raised nodules which develop into necrotic 'cauliflower-like' structures (Fig. 5).

Carcinomas of the rectum and genitourinary tract can cause protruding perineal growths, gross deformity, and loss of normal function, which may include fistulae involving the bladder, vagina, and bowel (Fig. 6).

Head and neck tumours can advance aggressively and result in significant disfigurement (Fig. 7).

In addition, extensive areas of the skin may be eroded in conditions such as advanced cutaneous T-cell lymphoma and malignant melanoma.

The location of the fungating tumour is critical and, arguably, more important than the type of cancer in determining the approaches to symptom control and local wound management. There are related symptoms that may also increase morbidity and management problems. These include: pain and loss of function attributable to pressure of the tumour on surrounding structures, cutaneous pain and irritation, recurrent infection, swelling as a consequence of impaired capillary and lymphatic drainage, fistula, and sinus formation. Patients with perineal tumours may also have difficulty walking and sitting because of the presence of solid tumour, perineal oedema, and lymphoedema. Head and neck tumours may erode into the buccal cavity necessitating enteral feeding.

Uncontrolled fungating wounds can take over the patient's life with leakage of exudate, and excessive soiling, dressing changes, and laundry. After the patient's death, family bereavement can be protracted if life has

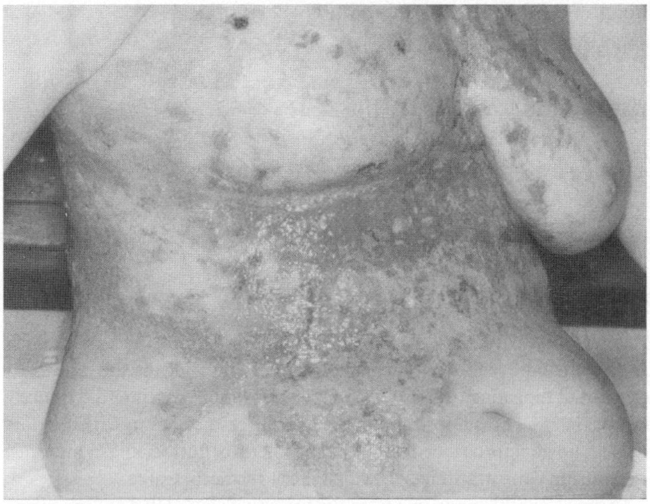

Fig. 2 Extensive cutaneous infiltration of the chest wall from a carcinoma of the breast.

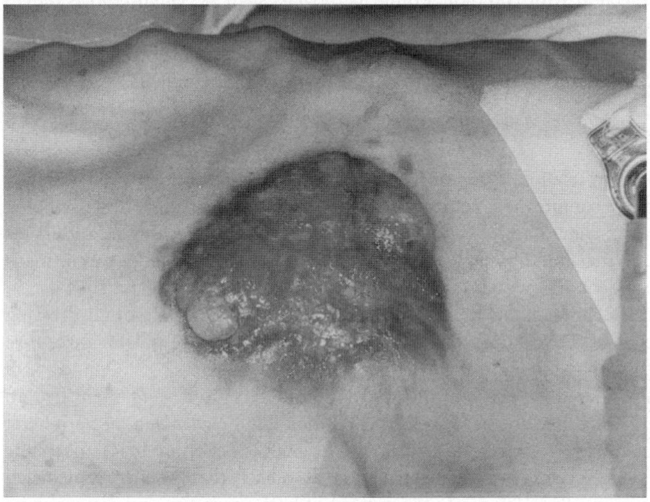

Fig. 3 Fungating nodule from a carcinoma of the breast.

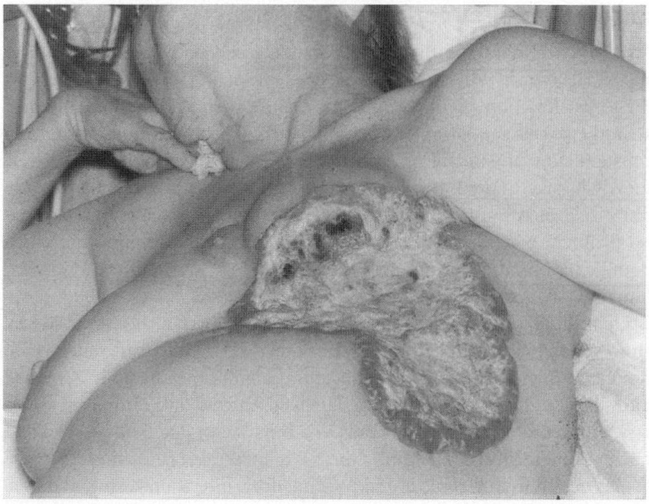

Fig. 4 Deep necrotic ulceration and fungating ulcer margins from a carcinoma of the breast.

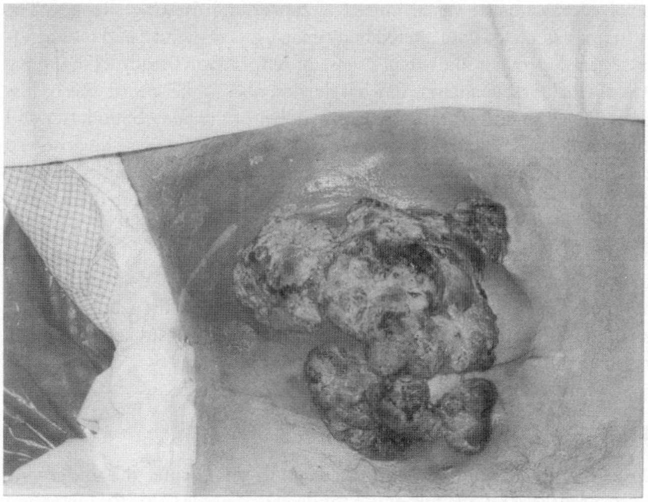

Fig. 5 Infiltration of the anterior wall of the abdomen from a carcinoma of the rectum.

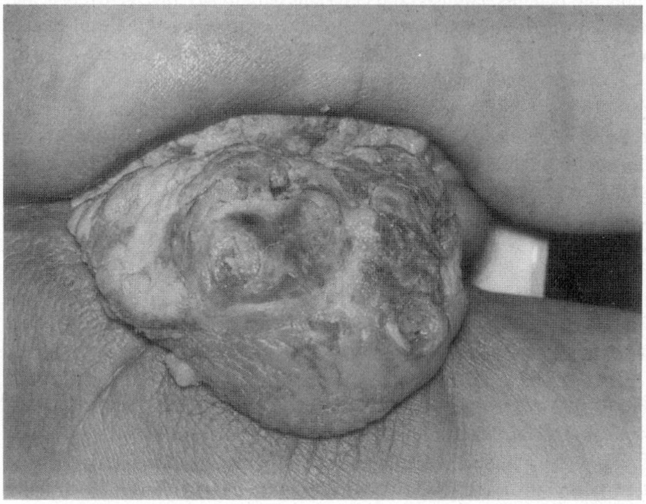

Fig. 6 Protruding fungating growth in the perineum from a carcinoma of the rectum.

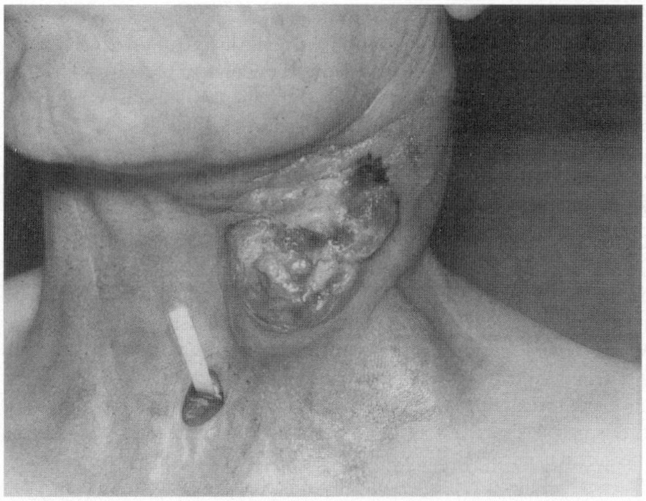

Fig. 7 Fungating and ulcerating nodule on the neck from a carcinoma of the larynx.

revolved around the visual impact of cancer and dressing changes. The suffering associated with altered body image, loss of dignity, and independence can destroy an individual's sense of self. Lawton's study of the dying process includes an analysis of what she describes as the special case of loss of bodily autonomy, through the breakdown of the body boundaries and associated smell, and the loss of self. In these circumstances she observed patients and families withdraw from each other, with the patients withdrawing further into a form of 'social death' some time before their 'physical death'. When symptom control measures and the application of wound dressings restored body boundaries she also observed that patients regained their autonomy.[24] In order to promote and sustain patient and family autonomy the management of fungating wounds therefore requires dedicated, skilled commitment by the interdisciplinary team and adequate resource provision, with a key role for wound dressings.

Management

As for the other skin problems discussed in this chapter the underlying cause of the wound, the tumour in this instance, needs to be diagnosed and treated. If the tumour is sensitive to treatment (radiotherapy or chemotherapy), significant reduction in tumour size and healing of the skin can be achieved. Unfortunately tumour recurrence with fungation is not uncommon and patients, families, and clinicians have to face this recurrence, and all the problems of living with and managing the fungating tumour, over again.

The prevalence of fungating tumours is unknown, as these data are not recorded in population-based cancer registries. When they occur they present an enormous challenge to clinicians. The patients may absorb a disproportionate share of available resources, including clinical time, dressings, and medications, over a lengthy period. Clinical oncologists are particularly challenged by patients who are reluctant to abandon contact with them in the hope that a treatment may be found. They absorb clinical time that, arguably, should be devoted to new patients and those who are in treatment. This suggests that palliative care teams need to take a lead in developing care pathways for patients with fungating tumours, and accessing appropriate resources for them.

The mainstays of the palliative management of fungating wounds, identified by Dunlop,[25] include symptom control measures, both local and systemic, together with wound dressings. In addition patient care may include stoma and lymphoedema management and enteral feeding. Palliative care teams therefore need to acquire a broad range of skills to manage the complex problems that arise when local tumour growth is uncontrolled. With a combination of specialist skills, symptom control measures, and wound dressings it is possible to reduce, measurably, the physical and psychosocial problems, and therefore the overall impact of the fungating wound on patients and families.

There are, however, limitations in the performance of dressing systems that are currently available. These need to be addressed urgently so that the patients' needs are accommodated. The limitations will be discussed in the section on 'Local wound management' later in this chapter.

Assessment and evaluation

Using the TELER® system of treatment evaluation (Treatment Evaluation by Le Roux's method) a tool has been developed to aid clinical assessment, documentation, and evaluation of fungating wounds.[26,27] A paper describing the validation of the system is published (Grocott, 2001) on the World Wide Wounds website, www.worldwidewounds.com. TELER is a system of clinical note taking. It includes indicators of dressing performance, optimal wound management, and symptom control. The indicators define patient-centred goals of care in relation to a fungating wound and measure the outcomes. An example of a TELER indicator is given in Box 1. The system reflects principles of palliative care whereby patients play a key role in identifying, understanding, and assessing their own problems and goals of care.

Box 1 TELER indicator for odour

0 = Odour is obvious in the house/clinic/ward
1 = Odour is obvious at arm's length from the patient
2 = Odour is obvious at less than arm's length from the patient
3 = Odour is detected at arm's length
4 = Odour is detected by the patient only
5 = No odour

Symptom control measures

This textbook covers a wide range of symptom control measures which could contribute to the overall management of fungating disease. The management of fungating tumours is complex and requires an interdisciplinary approach.[28] The symptom control measures that are outlined below include novel approaches to the management of intractable symptoms, used during Grocott's study,[29] which merit further research.

The major problems arising from the fungating wound that require symptom management include: pain, soreness and irritation from excoriated skin conditions, pruritis, odour, and spontaneous bleeding and haemorrhage.

These problems may be interrelated, for example, heavy colonization and infection with common wound pathogens such as *Staphylococcus aureus* and *Pseudomonas* can cause pain, odour, bleeding, and rapid extension of the wound. It is therefore important to reach an accurate diagnosis of concurrent problems in order to initiate appropriate treatments.

Pain

Pain in relation to fungating wounds may be multifactorial. For example, nerve compression from a bulky solid tumour may result in acute stabbing nerve pain. Macerated skin conditions may give rise to stinging and irritation that is additional to the nerve compression. Interventions for the management of nerve pain are described elsewhere in this textbook. The focus in this chapter is on topical measures administered at a wound dressing change. Topical opioids are increasingly being used to palliate nociceptive pain and stinging from damaged and ulcerated skin.[30–32] Opioids were considered to act centrally until opioid receptors were identified in inflamed peripheral tissues, and the possible mechanisms of peripheral opioid analgesia were described.[33] The analgesic effect of topical morphine is sustained at low doses, which makes it unlikely that the effect is mediated systemically.[31] Topical preparations of both morphine and diamorphine are used. Diamorphine may be preferred in the United Kingdom because of its much greater solubility.

Excoriated skin conditions

As already described in this chapter exudate and body fluids that are in sustained contact with the skin cause predictable and inevitable damage to the skin with consequent inflammation and pruritis. Topical creams and anaesthetic gels must form a barrier for the skin that can withstand the constant flow of exudate or effluent from fungating wounds. Otherwise they will have limited effect in preventing or treating these particularly distressing and persistent problems. Excoriated skin conditions are a particular problem with perineal fungating tumours. The problems are compounded if oil-based creams are used as these interfere with the absorbent function of continence pads.

Lignocaine preparations are used for their local anaesthetic effects. However, they are short acting and the preparations contain alcohol, which can cause intense stinging on application. Lignocaine is readily absorbed into the systemic circulation from damaged mucosa and caution is necessary with repeated application to avoid adverse central nervous system and cardiovascular effects. In addition the use of lignocaine is restricted because of the possibility of clinically important drug interactions, for example, with antiarrthymics, beta-blockers, diuretics, and ulcer-healing drugs such as cimetidine.[34]

Two new options have been shown to overcome some of the above limitations and assist healing of macerated skin, principally because fluids do not readily displace them. The first is an unlicensed novel local anaesthetic gel (Lutrol with lignocaine), identified by McGregor et al.(35) and evaluated further by Naylor et al.(36) As this preparation forms a sustained barrier to the skin the applications, and therefore the lignocaine dosage, can be monitored carefully. A study is needed to evaluate the Lutrol with and without lignocaine to determine whether the therapeutic effect of the preparation lies in its barrier properties rather than being related to the local anaesthetic.

The second includes alcohol and lignocaine-free barrier products (e.g. 3M Cavilon®; Cavilon; 3M Durable Barrier Cream®; SuperSkin®—Vernacare). The latter preparations are licensed and readily available in the United Kingdom. To maintain skin integrity it is crucial that the barrier product is commenced immediately a problem of uncontrolled body fluids is identified and that the barrier is applied with scrupulous attention to cover the area of skin that is vulnerable to breakdown. The barrier needs to be re-applied with sufficient frequency so that it is sustained. The manufacturers of the commercial products give guidance on the frequency of re-applications. Clinical and patient judgements also need to be included in the management plan. The type of effluent that is uncontrolled is a further key factor in determining the frequency of applications. For example, saliva, upper intestinal material, or faecal material may require more frequent re-applications than wound exudate because the respective alkalinity and acidity and the presence of digestive enzymes in these fluids renders them particularly toxic to the skin.(36,37)

Cutaneous irritation

This is an intense noxious sensation attributed to the activity of the tumour, particularly in inflammatory breast disease and cutaneous infiltration. Zylicz et al.(38) have reported that it is generally not responsive to antihistamines, and tricyclic antidepressants may be too toxic. A series of case studies by Zylicz et al.(39) indicates that paroxetine, a serotonin reuptake inhibitor, is effective in the control of pruritis of different aetiologies, with doses titrated to individual patient need. In addition, Grocott(40) found that the use of transcutaneous electrical nerve stimulation (TENS) was a useful nonpharmacological intervention (see Chapter 8.2.8).

Odour

The sources of odour related to fungating wounds include devitalized necrotic tissue that is heavily colonized with aerobic and anaerobic bacteria. Deep-seated tissue necrosis with a sinus exit in the skin presents particularly difficult odour management problems because of the limitations in delivering a therapeutic agent to the necrotic site. In addition effluent from fistulae can be malodorous, a faecal fistula is an obvious example. Management of fistulae with stoma devices is outlined elsewhere in this chapter. However the location and size of fungating wounds can present intractable problems. In these circumstances clinicians need to devise imaginative, in some situations unorthodox, approaches to managing distressing odour.

Patients and families do not always acknowledge odour, and their ability to conduct normal social relationships is not affected. The clinical and research experiences of the authors are that it is not helpful if professionals conclude that such patients and families are 'in denial' and attempt to impose odour management strategies on the individuals concerned. Immense damage can be done to individual coping strategies and patients can rapidly lose their sense of self. Clearly the perception of odour is highly individual and clinicians need to have the means to prevent and control odour caused by advanced disease.

When the usual approaches to odour management, discussed below, are not successful there is a case to be made for novel approaches. In advanced disease, such as fungating cervical and perineal cancer, when the management of effluent as well as offensive exudate are problems, patients have been nursed on air-fluidized beds with incontinence sheets to catch effluent and gel sheet dressings placed over the fungating lesions (Novogel, Ford Medical in the United Kingdom; Elastogel, SouthWest Technologies in the United States and Continental Europe). The gel sheets assist in blocking the odour, as well as in absorbing exudate and preventing adherence of bedclothes. The air-fluidized bed maintains the patient on a full pressure-relieving surface that, additionally, removes leaked body fluids through a filter system where they are converted into powder form and any micro-organisms are killed. The use of such a bed can greatly facilitate the nursing management of advanced fungating disease.

The use of a decontamination suit may also be helpful to prevent malodorous volatile substances from reaching the environment. In one instance a patient was nursed in an adapted decontamination suit in the final days of life to contain the odour from progressively necrotic lower limbs, which was a major problem to the patient. In addition Moyle(41) has described in detail the use of activated fan-assisted air suction devices, which draw malodorous air through a large volume of activated charcoal, and can contribute to managing the difficult problem of unpleasant odours.

As to conventional approaches there are four main options for the management of odour:

- systemic antibiotics,
- topical metronidazole,
- charcoal dressings, and
- debridement of devitalized tissue, colonized by aerobic and anaerobic bacteria, to remove the source of the odour-forming bacteria.

There are, however, limitations to the above approaches largely attributable to the size and eccentric shape of the wounds, the liquefaction of dead tissue, and the management of consequent exudate. These limitations are discussed below.

Systemic antibiotics

The logic behind the use of systemic antibiotics is that they will reduce bacterial colonization and thereby control the offensive odour from volatile metabolic end products. One of the limitations of systemic antibiotics is the increasing incidence of antibiotic resistance, though resistance to metronidazole amongst anaerobes is uncommon.(42) A further limitation is their acceptability to patients, which may be challenged by gastric side-effects, for example. Some authorities suggest that side-effects may be avoided at low doses (metronidazole 200 mg twice daily as opposed to 400 mg three times a day), without losing the odour-reducing effect.(34)

Topical metronidazole

Topical metronidazole may be an effective alternative to systemic administration.(23,43) However, in extensive necrotic wounds a sufficient inhibitory concentration of metronidazole to deodorize may not be reached because of a mismatch between the amount of gel applied and the size of the wounds. The proprietary gels are expensive. In the United Kingdom for example, a 15 g tube can cost 7–8 £. A further limitation of the topical route is a lack of tissue penetration to bacteria located below the surface of large wounds. The site of the wound, for example, the perineum, may also affect the efficacy of the topical gel, which is lost to the absorbent dressings and pads.

Activated charcoal

Laboratory studies demonstrate that activated charcoal dressings act as filters to adsorb the volatile malodorous chemicals from the wound.(44) One of the commercially available charcoal dressings is impregnated with silver and may have bacteriostatic properties in addition to adsorbing odour-forming molecules (Actisorb Silver 220, Johnson & Johnson Advanced Wound Care). Grocott(45) and Thomas(46) explored the lack of correlation between *in vitro* and *in vivo* dressing performance unless these dressings can be fitted as a sealed unit. If they cannot, the volatile malodorous chemicals simply escape into the air and the dressing has a limited, if any, effect on odour. The study by Suarez et al.(47) suggests that airtight charcoal garments may overcome this limitation when the wounds are extensive or sited in body curves that are difficult to dress.

Debridement of necrotic tissue

Surgical debridement of dead tissue is generally not an option for fungating wounds because of the bleeding potential. The use of a vacuum-assisted closure system to clear necrotic tissue and slough and drain exudate is also contraindicated because the system promotes neovascularization and cell mitosis, and may therefore stimulate tumour growth.[41]

Autolytic debridement with topical hydrating materials may be appropriate, but the clinical gains need to be assessed critically. As with pressure ulcer management, patients with extensive wounds covered with intact eschar may not benefit from debridement if life expectancy is short and the consequent exudate profuse.

Honey and enzymatic debriding agents are novel forms of autolytic debridement. In Grocott's (1999) study preparations of a krill enzyme and Manuka honey debrided the lesions and reduced odour significantly. The krill enzyme was derived from an arctic shrimp (Phairson Medical Ltd).

Honey is an ancient remedy in wound care that is undergoing laboratory and clinical evaluation to compare its performance with modern dressing materials. The studies by Cooper and Molam[48] and Dunford et al.[49] demonstrate that, *in vitro* and *in vivo*, honey has potent antibacterial activity and may be effective in clearing heavy colonization and infection. It also has a debriding action, an anti-inflammatory action, and stimulates angiogenesis, granulation, and epithelialization in healing wounds. The antibacterial activity in honey is attributed to hydrogen peroxide, which is continuously produced by enzyme action when honey is diluted, but remains below the level that causes an inflammatory effect. Some honeys additionally contain plant-derived antibacterial agents: honey from some *Leptospermum* species, for example Manuka honey, has a very high concentration of such agents.

Manuka honey was used for a patient with wet necrotic fungating tumours on the abdomen. Odour was reduced from TELER codes 0 (odour was obvious in the house/clinic/ward) to 3 (odour is detected at arm's length) in 10 days of daily applications (see Box 1). The wet necrosis was also beginning to separate. The data collection ceased at this point as the patient was dying. However, the significance of this outcome to the patient and her family was that odour was no longer obvious in the house, but contained in the bedroom where the dressings were changed.[29]

A potential limitation of any approach to promote autolysis is an inevitable increase in exudate as the devitalized tissue is liquefied and separated from the wound bed. This exudate has to be contained with wound dressings, otherwise the patients experience a further unpleasant problem or the aggravation of an existing problem. The management of exudate is discussed further in relation to local wound management.

Overall effective management of odour centres on removing the underlying cause, together with methods of preventing the odour-forming substances from reaching or invading the environment. Further research is clearly indicated for all four approaches to the management of odour to narrow the gap between what is theoretically possible and what is usually achieved.

Bleeding

Fungating tumours are friable and thus abnormal, fragile blood vessels are prone to rupture. However, it is important not to assume that a recurrent bleeding problem is attributable to the tumour alone. Critical assessment of the bleeding problem will assist in distinguishing between spontaneous bleeding from damaged blood vessels and bleeding from dressing adherence or inappropriately vigorous cleaning techniques.

Spontaneous bleeding

Radiotherapy and embolization are used to control recurrent spontaneous bleeding. It is therefore important to maintain open lines of communication with an oncology centre so that a rapid referral for emergency control of bleeding can be made. In addition a low blood platelet count may predispose the patient to bleeding. Platelet transfusions may be legitimate palliative measures to limit the bleeding potential.

Topical measures, such as adrenaline 1 : 1000 and silver nitrate sticks are also recommended as emergency measures.[25,34,50] These topical applications need to be used with caution as they can cause unwanted side-effects. For example, liberal use of adrenaline, which is vasoconstrictive, could cause tissue necrosis: the application of a silver nitrate stick to control bleeding from a fungating nodule on the neck cauterized the bleeding point but the sero-sanguinous exudate that trickled down the patient's chest as the silver nitrate was applied also cauterized the healthy skin. Surgical haemostatic sponges (e.g. Spongostan, Johnson & Johnson Advanced Wound Care) are alternative, emergency measures for controlling fast capillary bleeding that are easily administered by patients and families. The sponges may appear expensive on a unit cost basis, but cost effective when compared with the expense of an emergency admission to hospital. The topical application of sucralfate suspension has also been identified as a cost effective and simple method of controlling bleeding.[51]

Overall these approaches can reduce the fear of bleeding and give patients and families a degree of control over both spontaneous bleeds and those that arise during dressing changes. Clearly a catastrophic arterial bleed will be fatal and profoundly disturbing for all who witness it. However, this event is remarkably rare and the authors' experience to date is that patients are relieved when bleeding from the tumour is discussed and local measures, as described in this chapter, are explained and provided.

Bleeding at dressing changes

Attention to the following can reduce the likelihood of bleeding at the dressing changes:

- dressing application and removal techniques,
- maintenance of humidity at the wound/dressing interface, and
- cleaning techniques that do not include swabbing (e.g. gentle irrigation).

In addition to the above, the use of fibrous dressings, for example, alginates and carboxymethylcellulose, should be avoided. An anomaly in the performance of fibrous alginates, promoted as haemostatic dressings, was observed for friable fungating wounds. When capillaries are visible to the naked eye on the surface of these wounds mechanical damage and bleeding was repeatedly observed with the use of fibrous materials.[29] Alternative non-fibrous systems are described below.

Local wound management

The focus in this section on local wound management is exudate. The management of exudate is illustrated in Fig. 8[29] and this section is based on the study by Grocott.[29]

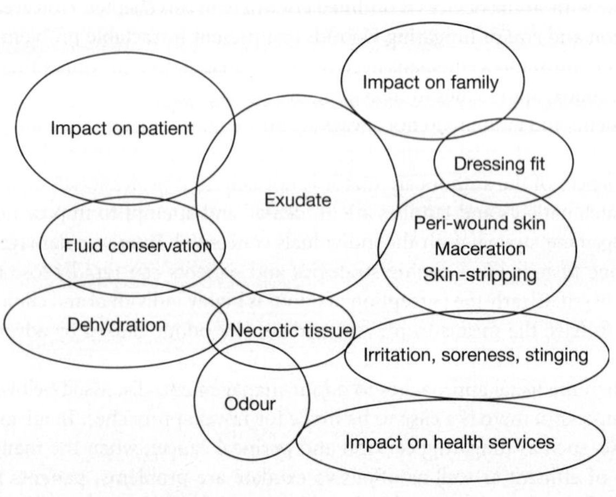

Fig. 8 Pivotal position of exudate.

In response to a question concerning the day to day experiences of living with a fungating wound patients described themselves as 'living in a laundry' and unable to meet social goals because of the embarrassment of soiled clothes. The impact on the family was evident in the number of visits made by them to community doctors and pharmacists to maintain supplies of dressings. Their personal lives were further eroded by the need to wait in for community nurses to change dressings, or they took on this responsibility themselves. When the problems continued over an extended period, for example, over 2 years, the relatives once bereaved were not always able to pick up their lives again. The impact on the health services was seen in the disproportionate amount of resources expended, as mentioned earlier in this chapter. In addition the frustration for the nurses of trying to manage intractable wound-related problems with inadequate resources was immense and caused significant distress. Dressing fit was crucial. Unless the dressings fitted well, exudate inevitably leaked. In once instance, the overlap of 14–15 dressings, 10 × 20 cm in size, to cover the chest wall was not only impractical and inefficient, but could take up to 2 h of experimentation on the patient. This exercise was repeated on a daily basis and became an increasingly unacceptable, but unavoidable, intrusion on the patient concerned.

Exudate also damaged the peri-wound skin through maceration effects, and macerated skin was further damaged by friction and trauma from dressing products, those with adhesive in particular.

Stinging, irritation, and soreness accompanied the maceration effects and, additionally, aggravated the tumour-related symptoms of cutaneous pain and irritation. When exudate was not controlled, or it was predicted to be a problem to control, it was difficult to embark on treatments to debride the necrotic tissue autolytically because, as indicated above, exudate is an endpoint of autolysis. Without debridement, odour management was in turn inefficient.

Retention of exudate under semi-occlusive and occlusive wound dressings resulted in accumulation and leakage. Conversely, uncontrolled venting of moisture with gauze products resulted in a lack of moisture at the dressing/wound interface, with consequent dressing adherence, trauma, and bleeding on removal.

With the focus on exudate management, eight dressing systems were evaluated in the study in terms of their expected fluid handling capabilities (see Table 7). Systems one to seven comprise materials that are fully permeable, occlusive, semi-occlusive, and semi-permeable. System eight comprises the continence products for patients with perineal wounds.

System eight comprises continence products that are a different form of medical device from sterile dressings. Exudate and effluent need to be removed from the skin to prevent maceration, soreness, and stinging which arise when a wet pad is held against the skin. To achieve this the pads need to have a fluid 'lock-in' system across the whole of the pad, not just in a central strip. The pads should be used in conjunction with the barrier products mentioned in the section on 'Excoriated skin conditions', avoiding oily skin creams and emollients that interfere with the absorption of exudate or effluent into the pad.

Table 7 Dressing systems

Dressing system	Description
System one	Two dressing layers: a non-adherent primary contact layer, a permeable gauze pad, and fixation tape/garment
System two	Two dressing layers: a fibrous alginate layer, a permeable gauze pad, and fixation tape
System three	A single composite dressing in the form of a vapour permeable foam dressing
System four	A single composite dressing in the form of an occlusive hydrocolloid or glycerine gel sheet
System five	Two dressing layers: a flat sheet or amorphous hydrogel in conjunction with a secondary fixation layer of HMVTR film
System six	Three dressing layers: a non-adherent primary contact layer, a permeable gauze pad in conjunction with a fixation layer of HMVTR film
System seven	Two dressing layers: a fibrous (soft) or a non-fibrous (hard) alginate/hydrofibre material in conjunction with a fixation layer of HMVTR film
System eight	Continence products with fluid 'lock-in' systems

The evaluation of systems one to seven reveals that current practice in wound care, including the manufacturing focus for wound dressings, is based on Winter's[52] theory of moist wound healing (MWHT). However, MWHT explains the profound influence on epithelialization of restricting the evaporation of water from the wound surface. It does not explain exudate management in chronic wounds, such as fungating wounds.[29]

There is currently a reliance on the absorptive capacity of a dressing, which also conserves humidity and moisture, to manage exudate and prevent adherence. This is not, however, an efficient method of managing excess exudate, particularly when there are inevitable problems fitting dressings to the extensive, eccentrically shaped wounds and curved body surfaces illustrated in this chapter.

There is therefore a gap in the provision of wound dressings for exudate management that needs to be filled if the needs of patients with exuding fungating wounds are to be met. Systems are required with the following key components:

- non-adherence (to prevent traumatic removal),
- wet strength (to facilitate complete dressing removal),
- absorptive capacity (for rapid uptake of exudate),
- fluid dispersion and retention properties (for optimal fluid handling, prevention of maceration), and
- venting capacity for excess fluid (for optimal fluid handling and dressing use).

There may also be a case to be made for hydrophobic systems that oppose the attraction of fluid to the wound surface, for example, when hydrophilic materials are applied.

Crucially the dressings need to fit the size and site of the wound. The current convention of pre-sized dressings (10 × 10 cm, 15 × 20 cm) is difficult to work with when wounds do not fit the sizes and shapes that are available. The availability of dressings in metre rolls, for example, would substantially advance the management of wounds on the chest wall, abdomen, and limbs. The use of adhesives and the configuration of the adhesive on films and tapes are also critical to prevent skin stripping.

Three options were identified in Grocott's[29] study to control exudate based on the above five components. The first is made up of dressings that are commercially available. The second and third require dressings that were evaluated in the author's study but are not commercially available at the time of writing.

Two-layer permeable system (System one)

- Non-adherent layer (e.g. Mepitel by Mölnlycke Healthcare Ltd)
- Absorbent layer (e.g. Mesorb by Mölnlycke Healthcare Ltd, or a simple dressing pad)
- Secured by non-adhesive retention products (e.g. Tapeless products by MediPlus Ltd).

The principles underpinning the system are that a perforated non-adherent layer protects the wound surface and permits passage of exudate to an absorbent and permeable layer. Clinical judgement is needed to determine if the exudate needs to be managed with a superabsorbent or a simple pad. With both of these types of dressing pads excess moisture is vented through the back surface of the dressing. The retention garment holds the dressings in place without the need for adhesive products.

Two-layer system with controlled permeability (System seven)

- Fibrous (soft) or a non-fibrous (hard) alginate/hydrofibre material
- High moisture transfer (HMVTR) fixation film

The principles underpinning the second option is that the primary wound contact layer is in precise contact with the exuding wound surfaces, rapidly absorbs exudate, and transfers the excess to the secondary fixation layer which has a high moisture vapour transfer rate to vent the excess fluid (HMVTR > 10 000 g/m^2/24 h). This system is not appropriate for effluent or sinus fluid. The latter require a system such as system six described below, or fluid collection devices such as stoma pouches. System seven is appropriate for extensive areas of skin loss and deep necrotic ulcers with heavy exudate. The primary wound contact layer for the deep ulcers needs to be one of the ranges of fibrous cavity fillers. If leakage occurs it is usually slight and in sites such as the groin, the pubic region, and the axilla. This system is non-bulky and may be more cosmetically acceptable to the patients than dressing pads. It can be fitted to some head and neck wounds. Overall specific design work is needed to develop applications for head and neck wounds, the groin, pubic region, and axilla to minimize fiddling and experimenting on the patients, which is difficult to avoid, when fitting dressings to these sites.

Three-layer system with controlled permeability (System six)

- Non-adherent layer (e.g. Mepitel by Mölnlycke Healthcare Ltd)
- Absorbent layer (e.g. a simple dressing pad)
- HMVTR fixation film.

This system comprises a primary wound contact layer, or barrier product, a simple gauze pad with a fixation layer that has a HMVTR < 10 000 g/m^2/24 h to support the venting of excess fluid from the back surface of the pad. This system can manage effluent and sinus fluid in circumstances when a stoma pouch or wound management system cannot be fitted. The frequency of the changes will depend on the amount of fluid loss. For a patient with an abdominal sinus, for example, the system could be left in situ for more than 24 h, though 24 h was probably optimal to renew the barrier protection to the skin. Materials with levels of moisture vapour transfer above 12 000 g/m^2/24 h are not readily available in the United Kingdom currently. However, there is a logical place for high venting capacity materials in the portfolio of wound dressings.

In summary, the mainstays of the palliative management of fungating wounds are symptom control measures and wound dressings. Both are crucial to the physical and psychological care of patients and families and, if effective, can preserve patient dignity, autonomy, and an individual's sense of self. As indicated in this chapter there are currently significant limitations in the management of necrosis, odour, and the application of dressings to fungating lesions, particularly in relation to exudate management.

Fistula management

A fistula is an abnormal track that communicates between two hollow organs. An enterocutaneous fistula is a connection between a hollow organ and the skin. There are multiple causes of fistulae, for example, they may develop as a complication of surgery, infection, radiotherapy, and progressive malignant disease.

The nursing care of patients with fistulae follows substantially the principles of stoma care. These principles are listed below and the reader is referred to the relevant chapter on stoma management (Chapter 15.7) and the following references (1, 36, 53). The focus of this section on fistula management includes circumstances when it is not possible to fit stoma appliances.

Summary of the principles of fistula management

- Prevention of skin excoriation with barrier products;
- collection of effluent in closed stoma devices or wound manager devices (e.g. Convatec® Wound Manager);
- management of odour in a closed device; the use of odour-neutralizing sprays when bags are emptied and changed;
- nutrition and fluids to maintain a balance between intake and loss, which may require enteral or parenteral feeding; and
- supportive care to protect the patient's sense of self, autonomy, and ability to socialize.

The location of the fistula may preclude the application of a stoma device. Clinicians are challenged in these circumstances to find novel approaches to manage the lesions, as the following case study illustrates. The focus was to contain the secretions and exudate in order to maximize the patient's independence.

Case study The patient had a carcinoma of the floor of the mouth and local fungation on two sites (Figs 9 and 10). The lesion on the chin communicated with the buccal cavity. It therefore discharged saliva and secretions as well as exudate. The patient required feeding via a gastrostomy tube. Fitting dressings to both lesions was extremely difficult, and compounded by facial swelling that developed overnight and drained spontaneously during the day. Fixation materials aggravated the swelling problem. An unorthodox approach was adopted to fit dressings to the lesions to contain the secretions, and maximize this patient's autonomy and ability to spend time with his young family. A make up artist was involved and a latex prosthesis was developed to hold absorbent dressings, for example, alginates and foams. A barrier product (3M Cavilon) was applied to extensive areas of the neck and upper chest wall to prevent excoriation. The prosthesis was applied with medical adhesives and removed with hypoallergenic solvents (Hollister Ltd). This approach was a partial success. However, significant design work is needed to develop dressing systems for general applications of dressings to the head and neck.

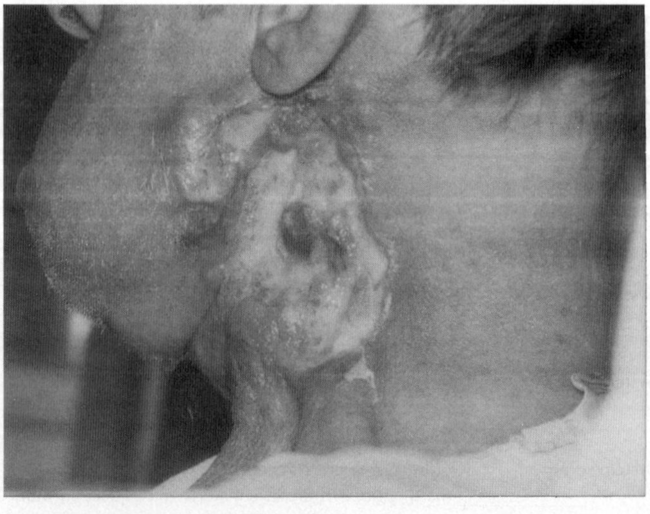

Fig. 9 Ulcerating and fungating lesion on the neck from a squamous cell carcinoma of the floor of the mouth.

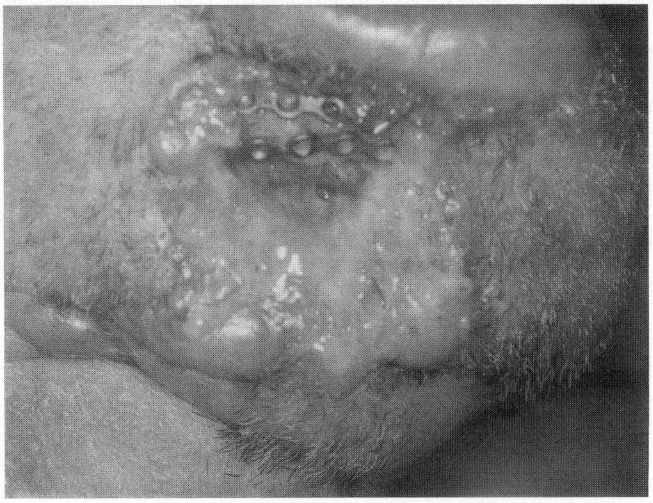

Fig. 10 Ulcerating lesion on the chin, communicating with the buccal cavity.

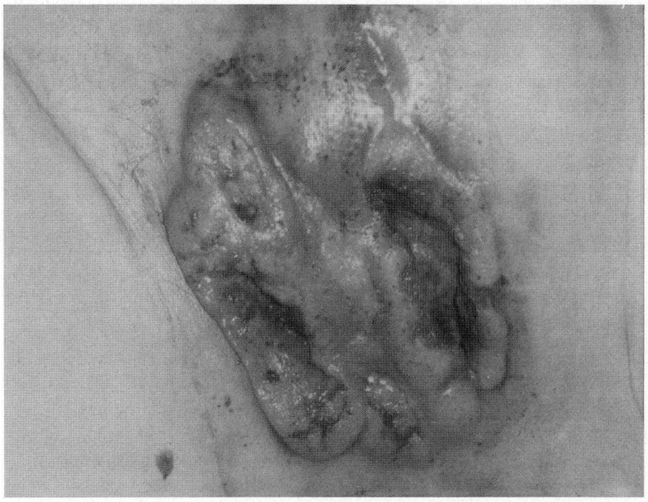

Fig. 11 Multiple faecal fistulae from a squamous cell carcinoma of the anterior abdominal wall.

As the underlying cause of the fistula advances, for example, malignant growth, or the patient's general condition deteriorates with progressive destruction of an already weakened skin it may become increasingly difficult to apply stoma devices as the following case study illustrates.

Case study This patient had multiple enterocutaneous fistulae between the colon and the skin, which discharged faecal fluid (Fig. 11). The fistulae arose from a fungating squamous cell carcinoma of the skin, which was attributed to a long-standing irritant discharge from a mucous stoma from previous bowel surgery.[(29)] Initially the individual fistulae were isolated using paediatric stoma appliances. However, as the fungation extended it became increasingly difficult to keep the appliances in situ, not least because the lesions were sited on the lower abdomen close to the groin and therefore affected by leg movements. The patient lost confidence in the appliances arguing that if the appliance lifted there was nothing to stem the flow of the faecal effluent. A non-adherent silicone mesh dressing (Mepitel, Mölnlycke Healthcare Ltd) was applied over the lesions and overlapped to the healthy skin surrounding the lesions to keep the dressing in place and prevent dependent leakage of effluent. A simple dressing pad was fitted over the silicone layer and fixed with waterproof tape. The patient changed the dressing pads when they were heavily soiled. The silicone dressing was only changed when the apertures were clogged with debris, every 4–7 days. The silicone dressing protected the skin, minimized the need for cleaning, and assisted in preventing further breakdown from the excoriating faecal fluid. It also assisted in containing the effluent within the pad by preventing lateral and dependent dispersion.

The patient found that it was crucial to avoid constipation. Otherwise normally patent sections of the bowel were filled with hard stool and faecal flow increased significantly through the fistulae, with inevitable aggravation of the management problems. Being a long-standing ostomist he and his wife had worked out a routine for dietary and fluid intake with the occasional softening aperient. When he required opioids for pain control he increased his intake of softening aperients.

Overall conclusions

This chapter has focused on the nursing care of patients with advanced disease who have a weakened skin barrier and on the management of specific wound types. The management of wounds in palliative care is under-researched and therefore not fully formalized into rational standards of care supported by appropriate products and protocols. The general literature on care of the elderly was substantially drawn on to support principles of nursing care of patients with skin problems, because ageing and advanced disease are both associated with problems derived from a weakened skin barrier and reduced mobility.

References

1. **Dealey, C.** *The Care of Wounds. A Guide for Nurses* 2nd edn. Oxford: Blackwell Science, 1999.
2. **Franks, P.J.** et al. (2000). The level of need for palliative care: a systematic review of the literature. *Palliative Medicine* **14**, 93–104.
3. **Palmissano, C. and Norman, R.A.** (2000). Geriatric dermatology in chronic care and rehabilitation. *Dermatology Nursing* **12**, 116–23.
4. **Fincham Gee, C.** (1994). A healthy skin. *Nursing Standard* **8** (Suppl.), 3–8.
5. **Dealey, C. and Keogh, A.** (1998). A randomised study comparing the triple care cleanser. In *Proceedings of the 7th European Conference on Advances in Wound Management* (ed. D. Leaper, C. Dealey, P.J. Franks et al.) **7**, London: EMAP Healthcare Ltd. pp. 59–60.
6. **Mason, S.R.** (1997). Type of soap and the incidence of skin tears among residents of a long-term care facility. *Ostomy and Wound Management* **43**, 26–30.
7. **EPUAP.** *Pressure Ulcer Treatment Guidelines.* Oxford: European Pressure Ulcer Advisory Panel, 1998.
8. **DoH.** *Pressure Sores: A Key Quality Indicator.* London: Department of Health, 1993.
9. **Nixon, J. and McGough, A.** (2001). Principles of patient assessment: screening for pressure ulcers and potential risk. In *The Prevention and Treatment of Pressure Ulcers* (ed. M. Morison), Edinburgh: Harcourt Publishers Ltd.
10. **Reswick, J.B. and Rogers, J.** (1976). Experience at Ranchos Los Amigos Hospital with devices and techniques to prevent pressure sores. In *Bedsore Biomechanics* (ed. R.M. Kenedi, J.M. Cowden, and J.T. Scales), pp. 301–3. London: Macmillan Press.
11. **Gebhardt, K.** (1995). What causes pressure sores? *Nursing Standard* **9** (Suppl. 31), 48–51.
12. **Bergstrom, N. and Braden, B.** (1992). A prospective study of pressure sore risk among institutionalised elderly. *Journal of the American Geriatrics Society* **40**, 747–8.
13. **Allman, R.M.** (1997). Pressure ulcer prevalence, incidence, risk factors, and impact. *Clinics in Geriatric Medicine* **13**, 421–36.
14. **Perneger, T.V.** et al. (1998). Hospital-acquired pressure ulcers: risk factors and use of preventive devices. *Archives of Internal Medicine* **158**, 1940–5.
15. **Schnelle, J.F.** et al. (1997). Skin disorders and moisture in incontinent nursing home residents: intervention implications. *Journal of the American Geriatrics Society* **45**, 1182–8.

16. **AHCPR.** *Pressure Ulcers in Adults: Prediction and Prevention.* Rockville USA: Agency for Healthcare Policy and Research, London, 1992.
17. **EPUAP.** (1998). A policy statement on the prevention of pressure ulcers from the European Pressure Ulcer Advisory Panel. *British Journal of Nursing* **7**, 888–90.
18. **NICE.** *Pressure Ulcer Risk Assessment and Prevention.* London: National Institute of Clinical Excellence, 2001.
19. **Chaplain, J.** (2000). Pressure sore risk assessment in palliative care. *Journal of Tissue Viability* **10**, 27–31.
20. **Twycross, R.** *Symptom Management in Advanced Cancer* 2nd edn. Oxford: Radcliffe Medical Press, 1997.
21. **NPUAP.** *Stage 1 Assessment in Darkley Pigmented Skin.* Reston: National Pressure Ulcer Advisory Panel, 1998.
22. **Mortimer, P.** (1998). Skin problems in palliative care: medical aspects. In *Oxford Textbook of Palliative Medicine* (ed. D. Doyle, G.W.C. Hanks, and N. MacDonald), pp. 617–27. Oxford: Oxford Medical Publications.
23. **Thomas, S. and Hay, N.P.** The anti-microbial properties of two metronidazole medicated dressings to treat malodorous wounds. *The Pharmaceutical Journal* **246**, 261–6.
24. **Lawton, J.** *The Dying Process. Patients' experiences of palliative care.* London: Routledge, 2000.
25. **Dunlop, R.** *Cancer: Palliative Care.* London: Springer, 1998.
26. **Le Roux, A.A.** (1995). TELER: The Concept. *Physiotherapy* **79**, 755–8.
27. **Grocott, P.** (1997). Evaluation of a tool used to assess the management of fungating wounds. *Journal of Wound Care* **6**, 421–4.
28. **Miller, C.** (1998). Skin problems in palliative care: nursing aspects. In *Oxford Textbook of Palliative Medicine* (ed. D. Doyle, G.W.C. Hanks, and N. MacDonald), pp. 642–56. Oxford: Oxford Medical Publications.
29. **Grocott, P.** *An Evaluation of the Palliative Management of Fungating Malignant Wounds in a Multiple-Case Study Design.* Unpublished PhD Thesis, King's College. London: University of London, 2000.
30. **Back, I.N. and Finlay, I.** (1995). Analgesic effect of topical opioids on painful skin ulcers. *Journal of Pain and Symptom Control* **10**, 493.
31. **Krajnik, M. and Zylicz, Z.** (1997). Topical morphine for cutaneous cancer pain. *Palliative Medicine* **11**, 326.
32. **Krajnik, M.** et al. (1999). Potential uses of topical opioids in palliative care–report of 6 cases. *Pain* **80**, 121–5.
33. **Stein, C.** (1994). Interaction of Immune-Competent Cells and Nociceptors. In *7th World Congress on Pain* (ed. G. Gebhardt, D.L. Hammond, and T.S. Jensen), pp. 285–97. Seattle USA: IASP Press.
34. **Twycross, R.A., Wilcock, A., and Thorp, S.** *PCFI Palliative Care Formulary.* Oxford: Radcliffe Medical Press, 1998.
35. **Macgregor, K.J.** et al. (1994). Symptomatic relief of excoriating skin conditions using a topical thermoreversible gel. *Palliative Medicine* **8**, 76–7.
36. **Naylor, W.D., Laverty, D., and Mallet, J.**, ed. *The Royal Marsden Hospital Handbook of Wound Management in Cancer Care.* Oxford: Blackwell Science, 2001.
37. **Breckman, B.** (1998). Stoma Management. In *Oxford Textbook of Palliative Medicine* (ed. D. Doyle, G.W.C. Hanks, and N. MacDonald), pp. 839–45. Oxford: Oxford Medical Publications.
38. **Zylicz, Z. and Krajnik, M.** (1999). [Pruritus in cancer: uncommon, but sometimes worse than the pain]. *Nederlands Tijdschrift voor Geneeskunde* **143**, 1937–40.
39. **Zylicz, Z.** et al. (1998). Paroxetine for pruritus in advanced cancer. *Journal of Pain and Symptom Management* **16**, 121–4.
40. **Grocott, P.** (2000). Palliative management of fungating malignant wounds. *Journal of Community Nursing* **14**, 31–40.
41. **Moyle, J.** (1998). The management of malodour. *European Journal of Palliative Care* **5**, 148–51.
42. **Hampson, J.P.** (1996). The use of metronidazole in the treatment of malodorous wounds. *Journal of Wound Care* **5**, 421–6.
43. **Newman, V., Allwood, M., and Oakes, R.A.** (1989). The use of metronidazole to control the smell of malodorous lesions. *Palliative Medicine* **3**, 303–5.
44. **Thomas, S.** et al. (1998). Odour-absorbing dressings. *Journal of Wound Care* **7**, 246–50.
45. **Grocott, P.** (1998). Odour absorbing dressings: 1. *Journal of Wound Care* **7**, 340.
46. **Thomas, S.** (1998). Odour-absorbing dressings: 1. *Journal of Wound Care* **7**, 340.
47. **Suarez, F.L., Springfield, J., and Levitt, M.D.** (1998). Identification of gases responsible for the odour of human flatus and evaluation of a device purported to reduce this odour. *Gut* **43**, 100–4.
48. **Cooper, R. and Molan, P.** (1999). The use of honey as an antiseptic in managing Pseudomonas infection. *Journal of Wound Care* **8**, 161–9.
49. **Dunford, C.** et al. (2000). The use of honey in wound management. *Nursing Standard* **15**, 63–8.
50. **Hoy, A.** (1993). Other symptom challenges. In *The Management of Terminal Malignant Disease* (ed. C. Saunders and N. Sykes). London: Edward Arnold.
51. **Regnard, C. and Tempest, S.** *A Guide to Symptom Relief in Advanced Disease* 4th edn. London: Hochland & Hale, 1998.
52. **Winter, G.D.** (1962). Formation of the scab and rate of epithelialisation of superficial wounds in the skin of the young domestic pig. *Nature* **193**(4182), 293–4.
53. **Pringle, W.** (1995). The management of patients with enterocutaneous fistulas. *Journal of Wound Care* **4**, 211–13.

Further reading

Dealey, C. *The Care of Wounds. A Guide for Nurses* 2nd edn. Oxford: Blackwell Science, 1999.

Grocott, P. (1997). Evaluation of a tool used to assess the management of fungating wounds. *Journal of Wound Care* **6**, 421–4.

Grocott, P. and Cowley, S. (2001). The palliative management of fungating malignant wounds–generalising from multiple-case study data using a system of reasoning. *International Journal of Nursing Studies* **3**, 533–46.

Morison, M. *The Prevention and Treatment of Pressure Ulcers.* Edinburgh: Harcourt publishers, Ltd., 2001.

8.9.3 Lymphoedema

Peter S. Mortimer and Caroline Badger

The scope of the problem

Lymphoedema is best defined as tissue swelling due to a failure of lymph drainage.[1,2] It may be primary in type due to an inherent or congenitally determined problem of lymph drainage, or secondary to obliteration or obstruction of lymph channels from extrinsic factors such as infection, surgery, or radiation. Lymphoedema remains an enigma because its basic pathophysiology is poorly understood. It is difficult to induce experimentally, and the reason for the long latent period from lymphatic damage during cancer therapy to onset of swelling is unknown.

Lymphoedema is considered rare, but chronic swelling due to oedema, particularly of the lower extremities, is a common disorder. The chief function of the lymphatic system is the control of extracellular fluid volume and content. Therefore, it is a safety valve for the prevention of oedema—any oedema—and it follows that all forms of oedema concern the lymphatic system.

Clinical teaching categorizes oedema into that associated with heart failure, with renal failure, or with venous obstruction, rather than considering it from a physiological standpoint, namely the balance between capillary filtration and lymph drainage. This latter approach not only simplifies understanding but indicates the pivotal role of lymph drainage in all forms of oedema. Oedema frequently develops from either an excess of capillary filtrate with normal but overloaded regional lymphatics, as occurs in heart failure, renal failure, hypoproteinaemia, and chronic venous disease, or from a defective lymphatic system with an unaltered lymph load (lymphoedema). Chronic oedema rarely arises solely from a failure of one system; usually several factors combine to disturb the fine balance of forces controlling extracellular fluid volume. For example, in advanced pelvic cancer, lymphatic obstruction may coexist with inferior vena caval obstruction to generate gross lower limb swelling, but additional hypoproteinaemia and obstructive uropathy may further fuel the oedematous state.

There is little information on the prevalence of chronic oedema in general or of lymphoedema (oedema caused primarily and predominantly from lymphatic obstruction) in cancer patients. There are two main explanations for this: first the diagnosis of lymphoedema is not as straightforward as would at first appear, and second the problem has been relatively neglected. During the era of the Halstead radical mastectomy, the incidence of lymphoedema was variously reported at between 6.7 and 62.5 per cent.[(3,4)] Since the extensive review by Hughes and Patel in 1966,[(5)] there has been one paper[(6)] that examined the risk of arm swelling in 200 breast cancer patients attending for regular review. Objective lymphoedema (a difference in limb volume of more than 200 ml) was present in 25.5 per cent overall, but the incidence after axillary clearance plus radiotherapy was significantly greater (38.3 per cent). A questionnaire survey revealed a 28 per cent lifetime prevalence of arm swelling in 1077 patients treated for unilateral breast cancer in one health district.[(7)] When extrapolated to 20 000 new cases of breast cancer per year for a condition that is incurable, this indicates a sizeable clinical problem. No equivalent data exist for lower-limb swelling following cancer therapy.

Pathophysiology

Comparative physiology

Research on experimental animals has not provided an adequate explanation for the chronic postoperative lymphoedema that may follow either mastectomy or radical block dissection of the groin in humans. The latter procedure is a useful example because its effects are not usually complicated by later radiotherapy. Some lymphoedema of the leg occurs in about 10 per cent of patients, yet a similar procedure carried out in animals (usually dogs, rabbits, or sheep) does not cause such effects. In order to produce lymphoedema in the hind limbs of animals one must do much more than perform a simple lymphadenectomy; all tissues except the major artery, vein, and long bone must be divided and fibrogenic silica dust should be distributed throughout the wound for good measure.[(8)] Even then, despite these gross mutilations and later fibrosis, genuine lymphoedema will not occur in every case. A better method involves the total blockage of both the superficial and deep lymphatic networks by the direct instillation of Neoprene latex,[(9)] but this, too, is hardly relevant to the clinical situation.

What can account for this difference between animals and humans? There are several partial and unconvincing explanations. Perhaps the fact that man walks upright on two legs puts an additional burden on fluid return from these limbs, which is not shared by quadrupeds. Also, surgeons carrying out a block dissection of the groin will deliberately strive to excise the lymph nodes with as wide a margin of normal subcuticulum as possible. Inevitably, this will lead to a gap of several inches between the cut ends of the afferent and efferent lymphatic vessels of the nodes. An equivalent operation in experimental animals (which are nearly all smaller than humans) leaves a gap of at most a few centimetres, which can be made good rapidly by the vigorous regeneration that proceeds from the cut ends of the lymphatic vessels.[(10)] *De facto*, the lymphatic vessels of humans seem to have less regenerative capacity than those of animals, but it is not known whether this is genuine intrinsic deficiency or merely reflects the greater absolute distances that may be involved. When such uncertainties exist about such a relatively simple situation, a real understanding of what happens after mastectomy, for example, must be even more elusive.

The surgical procedures used in the treatment of cancer of the breast are various and are often followed by radiotherapy. Sometimes radiotherapy is the main treatment. Obviously, patients with confirmed cancer of the breast who are treated by surgery alone usually undergo a procedure that includes the excision of many lymph nodes and lymphatic vessels. Any lymphoedema that occurs later is assumed to have an aetiology similar to that described above in relation to inguinal–iliac lymphadenectomy. However, the incidence of lymphoedema is greatest when the insult of radiotherapy is added to the injury of less radical surgery in the axilla. Although large doses of radiotherapy cause no immediate change in the structure or function of peripheral lymphatic vessels, the irradiated lymph nodes of sheep soon begin to show unequivocal fibrosis[(11)] and later defects in the function of cutaneous lymphatic vessels have been detected in irradiated pigs.[(12)] These facts, together with the observation that radiotherapy for cancer of the breast can alone cause lymphoedema, leave no doubt that irradiation can damage the lymphatic system severely. Several factors probably operate: the postirradiation fibrosis of nodes may obstruct lymph flow directly, the irradiation may damage the mechanisms that control the intrinsic rhythmic contractility of lymphatic vessels, and, where lymphatic vessels have been cut or removed, the irradiation may inhibit the cell division necessary for their regeneration. In addition, irradiation may increase the general fibrosis in the mastectomy wound and thus create a mechanical barrier to those lymphatic vessels still capable of regeneration. In other words, the irradiation substitutes for the fibrogenic silica dust used to cause lymphoedema in experimental animals. Unfortunately, it is impossible to describe these effects in quantitative terms, and so there is no means of ranking them in order of importance.

A central difficulty is the very great variation in the amount of postirradiation fibrosis that occurs in different species of experimental animals or even between different inbred strains of the same species. In addition, it is often practically impossible to expose experimental animals to the accurate regional fractionated irradiation that is given to human patients in clinical radiotherapy protocols. It is also true that the anatomy of the regional lymphatic systems differs a great deal. Whereas the lymphatic vessels from the breast of the human female may drain into between 20 and 30 individual lymph nodes the (much larger) mammary glands of sheep and cattle often drain into only one. These difficulties and differences are not the only ones that preclude any accessible animal model from relating directly to the human situation.

Clinical lymphoedema may not appear in the affected limb for months or even years after the primary treatment. This may be explained partly by the so-called 'die-back' of lymphatic vessels. The basis of this phenomenon is the progressive centrifugal atrophy of those lymphatic vessels that remained intact after the original therapeutic onslaught. As usual, the cause of this is unknown. In some cases, no doubt, progressive fibrosis and contraction of irradiated tissues may be an important factor, but this cannot apply when the condition occurs in non-irradiated patients. It is a matter of common observation that frank lymphoedema may occur only after one or more episodes of inflammatory 'cellulitis' and lymphangitis in the affected limb, which seem to erode further the already parlous structure and function of the remaining lymphatic vessels.

Capillary dynamics

The flux of fluid from blood vessel (capillary) to interstitial space is determined by the balance of osmotic and hydrostatic forces across the capillary wall. In a steady state (where there is no swelling) there should be no net movement of fluid (plus protein and solutes), but in reality there is, and this net flow is counterbalanced by the lymph drainage. As lymph contains macromolecules, in particular protein, obstruction to lymph drainage will result in a gradual build-up of protein within the tissues. By attracting water, osmotic forces will lead to swelling. This represents traditional thinking with regard to the pathophysiology of clinical lymphoedema.

In reality, the situation is probably far more complicated. Recent work in breast-cancer-related arm swelling has shown that lymphoedematous fluid does not possess the high concentration of protein previously supposed, although the total mass of protein trapped within the swollen limb is considerable.(13) The relative increase in interstitial water is not explained by lymphatic obstruction alone and suggests other haemodynamic disturbances. One unexpected finding which needs further confirmation is a lower plasma osmotic pressure in the lymphoedema patients compared with matched breast cancer patients without swelling. This would result in a reduced absorptive capacity of the vascular compartment for water, and oedema would be encouraged.

Other abnormalities discovered so far, which would tend to enhance capillary filtration and thus place extra demands on an already vulnerable lymph drainage, are increased limb blood flow and venous outflow obstruction. Over 50 patients with post-surgery/radiotherapy swollen arm were examined using pulsed and colour duplex ultrasound.(14,15) All had had total or partial mastectomy and 85 per cent had received radiotherapy. Arterial blood flow was increased by over 50 per cent in more than half the patients studied.(14) Fifty per cent had obstructed or narrowed subclavian or axillary veins, and colour duplex ultrasound clearly demonstrated collaterals that were not visualized on conventional grey-scale images. A further 25 per cent of patients had normal venous anatomy but abnormal venous flow patterns. Subclavian vein thrombosis, which was clinically unsuspected, was demonstrated in two cases.(15) Thus, serious macrovascular abnormalities, which would further contribute to oedema formation, seem to exist in the majority of these patients.

Inflammation

If lymphatic obstruction is the sole cause of lymphoedema, then why does swelling not occur immediately following lymphadenectomy or radiotherapy in all patients undergoing cancer therapy? Following venous obstruction, venous collaterals develop readily to permit satisfactory venous drainage, and so there is no reason to believe that lymphatic vessels behave any differently provided that a sufficient incentive to lymph drainage, for example, muscle pump activity, is maintained (see below). Mention has already been made of the difficulties in creating experimental lymphoedema, and so lymphatic vessel regeneration must be considered efficient on the whole. Extensive scar formation and tissue fibrosis following radiotherapy or wound infection are all known to discourage lymph vessel reanastomosis. Collateral lymph drainage routes may be damaged by X-rays even if they lie outside the field of irradiation.(12) Inflammatory processes may easily cause intraluminal obliteration of lymphatic vessels due to lymphangitis or lymphangiothrombosis. Infections such as bacterial lymphangitis and cellulitis are the major culprits and may herald the onset of lymphoedema.

Movement

Lymphatics rely almost entirely on local tissue movement for lymph propulsion. Lymph capillaries and precollectors possess no smooth muscle in the vessel wall. Lymph movement into and along these smallest peripheral vessels is largely a passive process dependent on changes in local hydrostatic and osmotic pressures; it is only the larger contractile lymphatic collectors and trunks which actively pump lymph. A common but poorly documented form of peripheral oedema results from a combination of immobility and dependency. Immobility leads to chronic lymph stasis,(2) which is compounded by enhanced lymph formation from venous hypertension in a dependent lower limb. This clinical syndrome is most vividly seen in infirm patients who are confined to a chair, day and night, by heart and respiratory failure. The phrase 'armchair legs' has been coined to describe this syndrome, for which the clinical appearances are indistinguishable from lymphoedema.(1) An alternative term is 'dependency syndrome'. Chronic oedema arises under similar circumstances in paralysed limbs and with severe arthritis where the combination of immobility and dependency prevail.

Tumour

Tumour rarely presents as lymphoedema except in circumstances of advanced cancer, for example, cancer of the prostate. For this to occur, infiltration with carcinoma or lymphoma has to be extensive as lymph flow is maintained surprisingly well through malignant nodes. More commonly, lymphoedema is a manifestation of recurrent cancer when lymph transport capacity has already been compromised through previous cancer therapy. Skin infiltration with tumour, particularly carcinoma of the breast, frequently targets in and around dermal lymphatic vessels. Expansion of the lymphatic vessel permits bidirectional growth of tumour throughout the lymph network. Extensive infiltration of skin and subcutaneous lymphatic vessels produces profound obstruction and tense oedema, leading to a firm to hard consistency of the tissues, the so-called carcinoma en cuirasse. Fibrosis and elephantiasis soon ensue.

Clinical manifestations

Lymphoedema most commonly affects an anatomical region drained by regional lymph glands. Less commonly, a more localized area may be affected owing to damage to smaller, more peripheral lymphatic collectors. Swelling tends to occur in those non-compartmentalized tissues where expansion is possible, such as the subcutis. The overlying skin tends to suffer secondarily as a result of back pressure from obstructed proximal lymphatic vessels 'downstream'—the so-called 'dermal backflow'. Limbs are affected most by lymphoedema simply because of the limited exit route. Lymph drainage of the adjoining quadrant of the trunk is equally affected, but the possibilities for collateral drainage are that much greater. Nevertheless, close inspection of the upper trunk in any case of arm lymphoedema secondary to axillary intervention will reveal some truncal lymphoedema, usually in the anterior and posterior axillary folds.

Lymphoedema differs from all other forms of oedema in the changes that it generates in the skin and subcutaneous tissues. Enhanced skin creases, increased tissue turgor, hyperkeratosis, and papillomatosis are most obvious in circumstances where peripheral lymphatics are overloaded and severely obstructed (Fig. 1). This occurs most commonly in lower-limb lymphoedema and malignant infiltration of skin lymphatic vessels, and the clinical diagnosis of lymphoedema depends almost entirely on these changes in skin and subcutaneous tissue. Stemmer(16) described the useful sign of thickened skin folds of the toes which prevent pinching of the skin, particularly at the base of the second toe (Fig. 2).

Traditionally, lymphoedema is described as brawny oedema that does not readily pit. Whilst this may be generally true, pitting is a most unreliable sign as many cases of lymphoedema will exhibit easy displacement of tissue fluid on pressure. Most forms of oedema respond to elevation and diuretics, but lymphoedema does not, except in the very early stages or

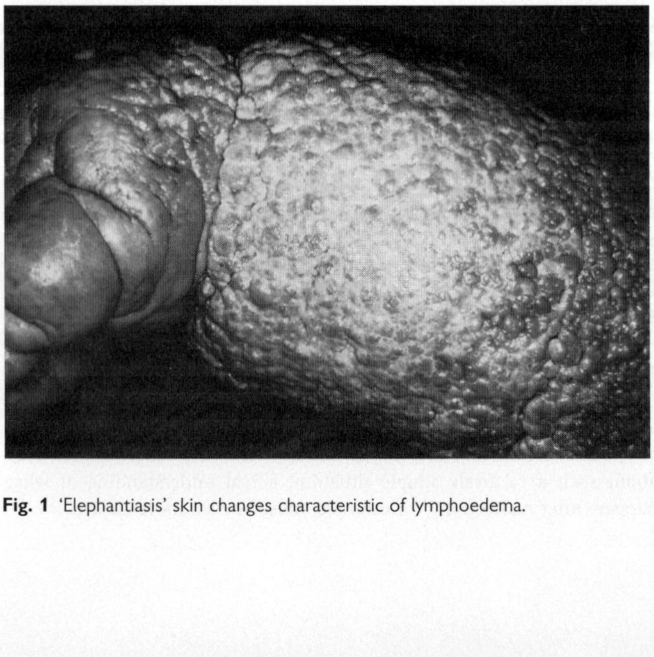

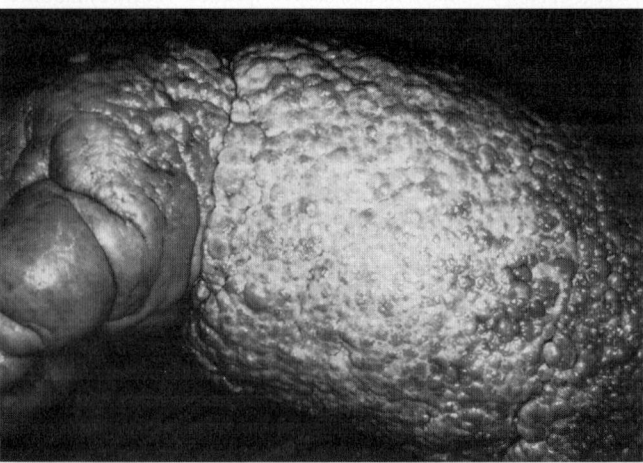

Fig. 1 'Elephantiasis' skin changes characteristic of lymphoedema.

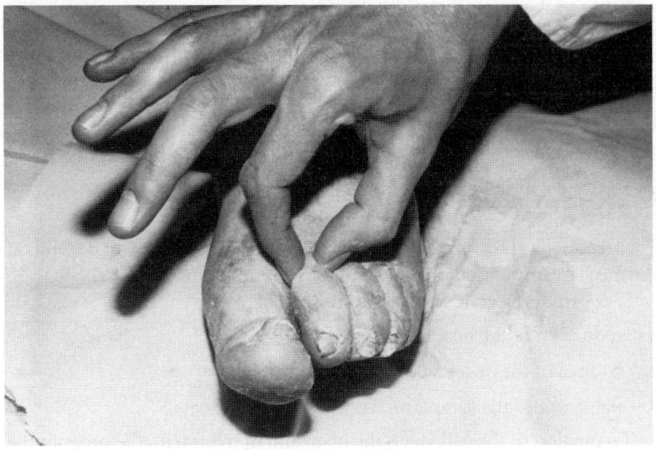

Fig. 2 Stemmer's sign: the thickened skin and subcutaneous tissues prevent pinching of a fold of skin at the base of the second toe.

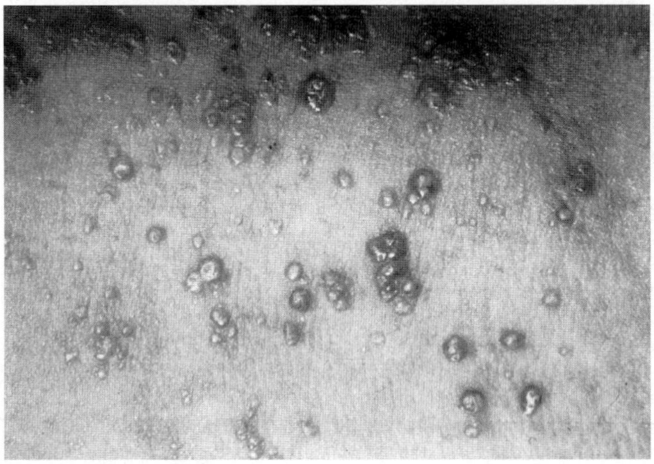

Fig. 3 Acquired lymphangiomas: lymph 'blisters' due to dilated superficial dermal lymphatic vessels.

when compounded by increased capillary filtration. Indeed, chronic swelling that does not reduce significantly after overnight elevation is likely to be lymphatic in origin.

Dilatation of upper dermal lymphatic vessels to the extent whereby they visibly bulge on the skin surface as lymph 'blisters' is referred to as lymphangiectasia. Such lesions can appear anywhere on a lymphoedematous limb, but occur more commonly in areas of subcutaneous fibrosis, perhaps within or close to radiation damage (Fig. 3). From time to time the lymph blisters release lymph on to the skin surface and serve as a portal of entry for infection. With time, organization of lymphangiectatic or dilated surface lymphatic vessels results in papillomatosis.

There is one specific and characteristic complication of lymphoedema, and that is recurrent erysipelas or cellulitis. The patient feels constitutionally unwell, as if influenza is starting, and within 8–24 h redness and tenderness appear in the lymphoedematous area. Swelling invariably increases, and may remain even after the resolution of the attack. Because of the failure to isolate an organism in the majority of cases, the bacterial aetiology of all such cases has been brought into question. Under normal circumstances, the lymphatic system contains and handles any infection regionally between the portal of entry and the lymph node. Presumably, an impaired lymph drainage route permits more rapid dissemination of microorganisms within the tissues and into the blood, leading to constitutional upset before any

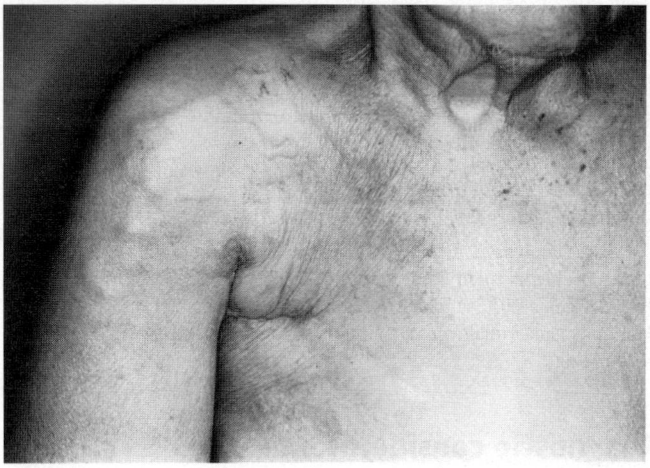

Fig. 4 Visibly dilated collateral veins around the shoulder indicative of venous outflow obstruction.

signs of inflammation are evident. All infections—viral, fungal, and bacterial—seem more common in lymphoedema, but data on true incidence are lacking. Indeed, fungal infection (*Tinea pedis*) is almost invariable at some time in lower-limb lymphoedema.

There is a small but significant risk of the development of a secondary malignancy within chronic lymphoedema. The most infamous is lymphangiosarcoma (Stewart–Treves syndrome), but other tumours including squamous cell carcinoma, lymphoma, melanoma, and malignant fibrous histiocytoma have been described. The favoured theory for the association of chronic lymphoedema and subsequent malignancy is altered immune surveillance in the affected region.[17] Kaposi's sarcoma is frequently associated with lymphoedema, but the tumour usually antedates the onset of the swelling. Lymphoedema may facilitate the local spread of the primary tumour, for example, in melanoma. This is presumably because the obstructed and dilated lymphatics allow free bidirectional spread of tumour cells within the vessel lumen.

When the clinician is presented with chronic asymmetrical oedema, for example, arm swelling in a breast cancer patient, there is a tendency to diagnose lymphoedema automatically. As discussed in the section on pathophysiology, there may be several underlying factors contributing to oedema. All breast cancer patients who have had axillary intervention, whether it be simple node sampling or full axillary clearance plus radiotherapy, will have lymph drainage impairment, albeit in different degrees of severity. Therefore, the addition of hypoalbuminaemia, venous outflow obstruction, neurological deficit, or restricted joint movements may, in the face of compromised lymph drainage, tip the balance in favour of tissue oedema. Thus, the development of lymphoedema depends upon the dynamic interplay of all these factors.

A full clinical assessment should bear all these possibilities in mind. Venous outflow obstruction may manifest with dilated collateral veins around the shoulder and on the chest wall (Fig. 4). In addition, the brachial vein may be distended permanently or perhaps only in certain arm positions. Sometimes the skin may appear rather cyanosed or mottled, further signs of compromised venous drainage.

Poor shoulder movements will not only lead to a limb that is held in a dependent position, but the lack of use will limit the activation of the muscle pump, which is so important for both lymph and venous drainage.

Neurological deficit usually results from brachial plexus neuropathy either from radiation damage or tumour compression/infiltration. The reduced mobility and dependency of the arm will encourage swelling, as seen so often in patients who are paralysed following a stroke. Therefore, a careful neurological examination is important. Progressive neurological signs may be the first clue to axillary recurrence of tumour.

Similar problems occur in lower-limb lymphoedema, but venous hypertension with consequent increased capillary filtration coexists more frequently. Apart from the recurring theme of a dependent and immobile limb, the risk of silent deep vein thrombosis is much greater in the leg. In addition, pelvic tumours may compress or infiltrate the main collecting veins including the inferior vena cava. Thrombosis may then ensue. Venous outflow obstruction will manifest with dilated skin venules and a cyanotic congested look to the skin. Haemorrhage into the skin may occur and collateral veins may be evident on the abdomen or flanks.

Severe pain is never the result of lymphoedema alone, and usually indicates other problems such as bone metastases or nerve infiltration. Profound venous obstruction or deep vein thrombosis can also be painful. Lymphoedema usually causes symptoms of discomfort, heaviness, tightness, or bursting.

Diagnostic considerations

The diagnosis of lymphoedema is not always straightforward. *In vivo* visualization of lymphatic vessels (lymphangiography) and nodes (lymphography) using a radiographic contrast medium remains the gold standard for demonstrating lymphatic vessel abnormalities. However, the technique is invasive and difficult to perform in the presence of oedema. Only subcutaneous lymphatics as large as, or larger than, the collectors can be opacified, except in pathological circumstances when dermal backflow occurs and smaller skin lymphatics become visible. Lymphangiography is rarely if ever justified for the investigation of oedema in the cancer patient.

The need for more functional information rather than simply anatomical detail, as contrast lymphography provides, has seen the emergence of quantitative lymphoscintigraphy (isotope lymphography). The dynamics of lymph flow as depicted by radiocolloid uptake and transit via lymphatic vessels can be studied using a gamma camera with a large field of view. The tracer is administered by interstitial injection, which obviates the need for direct cannulation of peripheral lymphatic vessels. Transit times and time–activity curves calculated from regions of interest (e.g. over nodes) permit quantitative analysis. Quantitative lymphoscintigraphy (isotope lymphography) has proved useful in the differential diagnosis of chronic limb swelling by detecting lymphatic insufficiency.[18] The main lymph drainage routes can be identified. Lymphatic obstruction results in retrograde lymph flow to cutaneous lymphatics (dermal backflow). Thus, various subgroups of lymphoedema can be identified without recourse to conventional lymphography, and in this way it is possible to identify subtle or incipient lymphoedema and lymphatic insufficiency in cases of chronic oedema of compound origin. Obviously, if total or partial lymphadenectomy has taken place, nodal radioactivity cannot be used as an index of lymph drainage function! In such cases, the fractional removal rate of tracer from the injection site has to be used for functional assessment of lymph drainage.

The overriding consideration in the investigation of lymphoedema must be the quest for underlying malignancy, if not already known. Its exclusion is not always straightforward or guaranteed by negative results. Therefore, the possibility must always be borne in mind.

Sometimes tumour may be present within the lymphoedema. This is not infrequently the case with inflammatory breast carcinoma, and a simple skin biopsy may put the clinical problem into context.

A major advance in the investigation of the venous system has been the development of colour duplex ultrasound.[15] The colour facility permits imaging of vessels not previously visible and indicates direction of flow. Consequently, flow disturbances indicative of venous obstruction and thrombi can be readily identified by non-invasive means. If access to colour duplex facilities is limited then conventional venography has to be performed if venous abnormalities are suspected. This procedure is not only invasive but is difficult to perform in the presence of oedema.

Magnetic resonance imaging (MRI) produces the best soft tissue images and is theoretically useful for distinguishing between fat and water, a common clinical conundrum in the differential diagnosis of lymphoedema. MRI can demonstrate a number of characteristic features in lymphoedema including a thickened skin and a honeycomb pattern in the subcutaneous tissues.[19] MRI is also useful for distinguishing pure lymphoedema from swelling caused by expansion of the sub-fascial compartment following a deep vein thrombosis. MRI and CT are of course helpful in excluding infiltrative tumour as a cause of swelling.

Management

The treatment of lymphoedema in the palliative care setting will depend on the mechanisms underlying the development of oedema.[20]

There are three main approaches to treatment:

1. reduction of the oedema;
2. control of the oedema;
3. palliation of the symptoms associated with oedema.

If reduction of the oedema is the main aim of treatment, the programme of care will usually consist of a combination of bandaging, movement, and manual lymph drainage. Reduction must then be followed by a maintenance programme if the benefits are to be long-lasting.

Control of the oedema means maintaining the status quo, whether that be a smaller limb with drained tissues, as is the case following reduction treatment, or preserving the current state of the limb with the aim of preventing the situation from worsening. The treatments that form a standard part of this approach are compression hosiery and exercise. These treatments are not expected to make a significant impact on the size of any but the mildest, pitting oedemas such as venous or gravitational oedema but should be sufficient to hold the situation.

Palliation is undertaken when reduction and/or control of the swelling is either no longer possible or no longer appropriate and is aimed at reducing common symptoms of a feeling of heaviness in the limb, tension and pressure in the oedematous tissues, a deep aching in the limb, as well as aching and discomfort in supporting muscles and joints. In situations such as these, individual treatment components may be selected and used to ease specific symptoms.

Oedema that occurs in a palliative care setting will not necessarily require a palliative approach to treatment, it may be just as appropriate to consider reduction or control of swelling particularly if the oedema is not the result of local malignancy. The four steps outlined in Fig. 5 are suggested as a guide to making decisions about the best approach to treatment.

Establish the cause and type of oedema

Patients with advanced cancer will often have a number of different causes for their oedema. A distinction should be made between oedema of central origin, such as that due to heart failure, and oedema due to peripheral causes such as local damage from surgery or radiotherapy. The former need medical interventions while the latter can largely be managed using nursing interventions.

Consider the patient's circumstances

Factors that need to be taken into account are such things as the patient's life expectancy and the presence of other problems that co-exist with the oedema. A limited life expectancy of a few weeks will usually call for less intensive measures to be used. Problems such as paralysis, nausea, fungating tumour,

Guide to the selection of treatment

1. Establish the cause and type of oedema
2. Consider the patient's circumstances
3. Consider the patient's wishes
4. Establish the likely outcome of treatment

Fig. 5 Steps to take before deciding on the approach to treating oedema in advanced disease.

or pain may be more pressing, making a focus on the oedema inappropriate.

Establish the key outcomes

If the specific mechanism underlying the oedema can be manipulated by treatment, then there is a reasonable chance of gaining control of the oedema. If the cause cannot be influenced, then it is unlikely that any lasting impact will be made on the oedema. Thus, a patient with spinal cord compression and oedema in the lower limbs may well respond to elevation and compression of the limbs. A patient with oedema resulting from cutaneous recurrence of melanoma, on the other hand, is unlikely to see much of a reduction in his oedema if the tumour obstructing the skin lymphatics is not amenable to treatment, although some degree of control may be possible. Should the tumour respond to treatment, then a corresponding improvement in oedema is likely, until the tumour advances again.

The patient's wishes

Careful questioning will elicit to what extent the oedema is a problem for the patient. Areas that need to be explored are: the degree to which oedema impedes mobility or function and whether this causes distress; the degree to which oedema contributes to any discomfort; the extent of any psychological distress associated with the oedema. Having elicited what the patient considers the main problems to be, the various options for treatment and the patient's expectations of any treatment should be explored and these matched against the likely outcomes of treatment.

Drug therapy

Drug therapy for lymphoedema is extremely disappointing. Diuretics achieve little more than relief of symptoms of tightness in a congested limb and do not improve swelling. Nevertheless, their use may be justified in cases of very tense oedema particularly if the oedema has been exacerbated by the administration of fluid-retaining drugs. Care must be taken as fluid may be mobilized from everywhere but the offending limb, leaving a chronically ill patient with a reduced plasma volume, hypotension, and altered electrolyte status.

In advanced cancer, it is not unusual for both venous and lymphatic obstruction to occur, for example, with extensive abdominal and pelvic tumour. In this situation potent diuretics may be necessary to achieve some symptom relief. High-dose steroids are also justified if, by reducing tumour bulk, venous and lymphatic channels can be re-opened, albeit temporarily.

Claims(21) that benzopyrones such as oxerutins are effective in the treatment of lymphoedema are not supported by any good-quality evidence. While experimental work has shown that these drugs have vasoactive properties, suggesting that their action is through influencing capillary protein flux and filtration rather than lymph flow,(22) but there is insufficient clinical trial data to enable useful conclusions to be reached about their clinical use.

Physical therapy treatment: principles and rationale

The four main principles of treatment are care of the skin, external support or compression, movement, and massage.(23)

Care of the skin

One of the characteristic features of lymphoedema is an increased risk of local infections due to the locally compromised immune system. Since the skin in oedematous areas is particularly vulnerable to trauma, its care is an essential component of treatment. The focus is on keeping the skin supple, intact, and well-hydrated. Oil-based creams rather than water-based lotions are preferred. Oedematous limbs should be washed daily and care should be taken when drying, particularly between the toes. The use of soap should be discouraged and non-soap cream cleansers used instead. It is best to stick to unscented products so as to avoid irritation of the skin. A regular check should be made for tinea pedis and any signs of this treated promptly. Salicylic acid ointment is useful for removing the rough, hyperkeratotic areas of skin common in long-standing lymphoedema.

External support and compression

Support may be defined as 'the retention and control of tissue without the application of compression'.(24) When using external support, pressure is achieved by the tissue pushing against the material that has been applied, much as the tissues of the foot press against the leather of a shoe. Compression, on the other hand, results from forces in the applied material pulling in against the tissues: in other words, the tension in the material causes pressure to be exerted beneath it. The key difference between these two methods of generating pressure lies in the resulting pattern of pressure rather than the degree of pressure: support results in relatively high working pressure against low resting pressure—for this reason it is well-tolerated overnight, for example, while the pressure under compressive materials varies very little between active and resting states.

Broadly speaking, elastic hosiery will generate compression while short-stretch bandages generate support. Hosiery is generally used to maintain the size of a limb but can have a reducing effect on mild or soft oedema, while bandages are more effective than hosiery at reducing swelling even in cases of solid or gross oedema but can also be applied with less tension to produce control or maintenance of oedema.

Bandages

The technique used in the treatment of oedema is that of a system of layers.(25) Tubular stockinette is first applied to the limb to protect the skin from any chafing effects. Next, a layer of padding is applied to protect the joint flexures and to even out any distortion in the shape of the limb, thus providing a smooth profile on which to bandage. Finally, bandages are applied to give an evenly graduated pressure, high distally reducing to low proximally up the length of the limb. When the objective is reduction of the oedema, the bandages are left in place around the clock and reapplied every 24 h to ensure the maintenance of adequate pressure. Treatment is carried out daily until the limb size has reached a satisfactory level when compression hosiery can be fitted to maintain the improvement. In situations where the maintenance of high levels of pressure is not critical and where the principal aim is to support and alleviate discomfort arising from distension of the tissues the bandages may be left in place for longer periods than this. However, bandaging should never result in trauma to the skin and it is wise to check the condition of the skin regularly, particularly when bandaging patients with reduced sensation in the affected limb.

The indications for using bandages in place of hosiery include gross swelling, fragile or damaged skin, lymphorrhoea, and significant distortion in limb shape. In all other cases hosiery is to be preferred since it is less time-consuming to apply, less bulky, and involves less disturbance to the patient.

Hosiery

The availability of off-the-shelf hosiery in a wide range of sizes, designs, and compression classes mean that most patients can be fitted. Shaped tubigrip has a useful role to play in containing soft pitting oedema and layers can be added to increased pressure when this is desirable. It is best used on arms or lower legs rather than full-length on the leg since it has a tendency to roll over at the top causing constriction in the area of the groin. Antiembolism stockings have no part to play in either reducing or controlling swelling since their purpose in simply to improve venous return.

Movement

The presence of oedema in a limb reduces mobility in the affected joints and often hampers free movement of the limb owing to the increased weight. There is an understandable tendency for the patient to be reluctant to move the affected limb and to support a swollen arm, for instance, in a sling. This can result in the joints becoming fixed and encourages pooling of fluid and increased discomfort. Emphasis on improving or simply preserving any residual movement in the swollen limb by regular gentle mobilization and exercise will help to promote the drainage of fluid(26) and to minimize joint stiffness. The use of slings should be discouraged and a collar and cuff substituted. This system is preferable because the weight of the arm is distributed across the patient's back not around the neck; it supports the arm at the wrist to a level just sufficient to relieve the weight from the affected shoulder and avoids immobilizing the arm with the elbow flexed. When the patient is sitting or resting the cuff should be removed and the arm supported outstretched on pillows high enough to relieve the pressure on the shoulder. There is no need to elevate the limb beyond the horizontal nor is there any advantage to be gained from doing so.

Massage

A very gentle form of massage is used to encourage the movement of lymph from congested oedematous areas to areas of the body where it can drain normally.[25,26] The amount of pressure used when massaging should only be enough to move the skin and tissues beneath the hand. It should not cause the skin to redden. The skin should be free of oils, creams, or talcum powder when massaging.

Specific problems

Infection

Some patients are prone to recurrent acute inflammatory episodes (cellulitis) in the swollen limb. Antibiotics started at the peak of the attack are probably of little use and the emphasis is on prevention. Daily low dose penicillin-V is recommended as a prophylactic for patients experiencing recurrent attacks. Treatment with hosiery or bandages should be postponed until an attack has resolved and the patient should be advised to elevate and rest the affected limb.

Lymphorrhoea

Lymphorrhoea is the term used to describe the leakage of lymph through a break in the skin. It can occur as a result of accidental trauma to the skin, or because of an acute onset or exacerbation of oedema when the skin is not able to stretch quickly enough to accommodate swelling, or if acquired lymphangiomata are present. Lymphorrhoea requires prompt action since it increases the risk of infection. Pressure applied to the affected limb and maintained over 24–48 h will usually resolve the leakage. Bandages are the most convenient and effective method of treatment. Ensure that the limb is clean and apply a thick sterile pad to the leaking area with a layer of paraffin gauze beneath it to prevent the pad from adhering. Then, bandage the limb in the usual way. Change the wet bandages as often as necessary and maintain the pressure around the clock. Once the leakage has resolved compression hosiery will need to be applied to control the swelling and prevent further leakage.

Fragile skin

Acute onset or exacerbation of swelling, particularly in the legs of elderly or debilitated patients, often results in disruption of the capillaries leading to bruising or small tears in the skin that appear as fine red streaks or cracks. The skin looks taut and shiny and is extremely fragile. In these cases bandages are the most suitable approach to treatment until the condition of the skin improves, since the application and removal of close-fitting hosiery carries the risk of further trauma.

Cutaneous tumour infiltration

Tumour involving the skin of the oedematous limb further impairs lymph drainage by obstructing collateral lymph drainage routes through the skin. Pressure in the limb is increased and the tissues become tense and hard. The skin is often discoloured and inflamed in appearance. Breakdown of the skin is common and is often accompanied by weeping from areas of tumour or from lymph blisters that have formed. Most patients find relief from the intense feeling of pressure in the tissues when a counter-pressure is applied to the limb. Bandaging is the simplest way of achieving the necessary support and has the added advantage of being easy to apply over any necessary dressings. Be guided by what the patient finds comfortable with when choosing the amount of pressure to use since the aim here is to alleviate discomfort and not necessarily to force fluid out of the limb.

Venous obstruction

Venous blood flow may be compromised by tumour, or by thrombosis or by a combination of the two. Swelling of a limb due to vein thrombosis generally eases as the clot resolves and is not usually an indication for the application of compression or support. However, if a blood clot develops in a lymphoedematous limb an extra burden is placed on the already impaired lymph drainage routes and the subsequent increase in swelling may not resolve as easily. Compression can safely be applied in the case of thrombus developing in the upper limb usually with considerable effect on the reduction of limb size. In the case of deep vein thrombosis in the lower limb or obstruction to blood flow by tumour, support to the limb will help the associated discomfort and is more appropriate than the use of compression. Once again either bandages or one of the lower classes of compression hosiery (i.e. Class 1 stockings) can be used.

Tumour in the abdomen or pelvis

Tumour in the abdomen or pelvis may result in the compression or occlusion of venous blood flow and a resulting backlog of fluid in the lower limbs, the genitals, and the tissues of the lower trunk. Depending on the level and degree of obstruction oedema can extend as far up the body as the axillae. Obviously, any treatment that results in a reduction in the size of the tumour will lead to a corresponding improvement in the degree of oedema. If this is not possible a trial of high-dose steroids and diuretics may bring some relief: in theory reducing peri-tumour swelling and thereby to some degree relieving the compression of the blood vessels should allow some improvement in the drainage of fluid.

Although the oedema in the legs may be soft, pitting, and easily displaced, there is little to be gained from reducing their size: fluid will be forced into the already congested tissues of the trunk adding to the patient's discomfort. Hosiery in the weakest class of compression (Class 1) will give a feeling of support to the tissues. Stockings that come in the form of tights may give support to the genital area but these can be difficult to apply; thigh length stockings with long-line supportive underwear over the top works just as well and is easier to cope with. Maternity panty-hose can be a particularly useful alternative if the patient has ascites or finds pressures on the abdomen uncomfortable.

Gentle massage can be used to encourage whatever drainage is possible. Massage should start above the level of the swelling, concentrating on areas such as the axillae and the supra-clavicular fossae and move gradually down the trunk. This can have the effect, albeit short-term, of easing tightness in the oedematous tissues and many patients find it soothing and comforting. Massage can be performed as often as the patient likes and it is something that can be taught to visiting relatives and friends, who benefit from the feeling of involvement in the patient's care.

Midline oedema

Midline oedema refers to swelling affecting the head and the neck or the genitals. Swelling of the head and neck is rarely seen and its presence suggests local tumour. Genital oedema is commonly seen in patients with abdominal or pelvic tumour. It can be precipitated if either bandages or more commonly pneumatic compression are used to treat leg swelling in patients with obstructive lower limb oedema. Treatment of both these sites is difficult. In the case of head and neck swelling regular, gentle massage performed several times a day is the only feasible option; supportive underwear and even bandages can be added to massage to treat genital swelling.

Dependency/immobility oedema

Oedema secondary to dependency or immobility is common in elderly or very debilitated patients who often spend long periods sitting in a chair or wheelchair with their legs down. In the absence of movement there is no propulsion to the flow of lymph and if the limb is positioned in a dependent position gravitational forces encourage pooling of fluid. Brachial plexus damage leading to weakness and disuse of the limb can also result in the formation of oedema in the dependent arm. This kind of oedema is often ignored until inevitably problems develop.

The typical picture is of grossly puffy feet and ankles with dry and flaking skin. There are often bruises and small injuries to the legs from knocks on surrounding furniture; the weight of the swollen legs adds to the patient's immobility and they are often more clumsy and unstable on their feet as a result. There is frequently copious weeping from these injuries as well as from the lymph blisters that can form. This constant wetting of the skin together with the fact that swelling makes it difficult to fit slippers or shoes means that the legs and feet are often icy cold to the touch.

Treatment should begin by resolving any weeping with bandages. Compression hosiery will usually reduce this pitting oedema and should be combined with elevation of the limbs when the patient is seated. Regular movement of the limbs, either passive or active, will promote the drainage of fluid and the limitation of fluid formation by employing the muscle pump.

Neurological deficit

If a neurological deficit is present in the limb, there is an additional problem besides that of dependency oedema. The reduction or absence of sensation greatly increases the risk of injury. Great care must be taken when applying any pressure to avoid accidental trauma or constriction of blood flow; the joints and fingers are particularly vulnerable. Since the patient will be unable to report feelings of constriction or pain, regular checks should be made to see that any hosiery or bandage is not rolling over at the top or gathering in joint flexures. The temperature and colour of the tips of the toes or fingers must also be checked and the skin inspected for signs of friction or breakdown.

References

1. **Mortimer, P.S.** (1990). Investigation and management of lymphoedema. *Vascular Medicine Review* **1**, 1–20.
2. **Mortimer, P.S. and Regnard, C.F.** (1986). Lymphostatic disorders. *British Medical Journal* **293**, 347–8.
3. **Handley, W.S.** (1908). Lymphangioplasty: new method for relief of brawny arm of breast-cancer and for similar conditions of lymphatic origin. *Lancet* **i**, 783–5.
4. **Lobb, A.W. and Harkins, H.N.** (1949). Postmastectomy swelling of the arm with note on the effect of segmental resection of axillary vein at time of radical mastectomy. *Western Journal of Surgery* **57**, 550–7.
5. **Hughes, J.H. and Patel, A.R.** (1966). Swelling of the arm following mastectomy. *British Journal of Surgery* **53**, 4–15.
6. **Kissin, M.W., Querci della Rovere, G., Easton, D., and Westbury, G.** (1986). Risk of lymphoedema following the treatment of breast cancer. *British Journal of Surgery* **73**, 580–4.
7. **Mortimer, P.S.** et al. (1996). The prevalence of arm oedema following treatment for breast cancer. *Quarterly Journal of Medicine* **89**, 377–80.
8. **Drinker, C.K., Field, M.E., and Homans, J.** (1934). The experimental production of oedema and elephantiasis as a result of lymphatic destruction. *American Journal of Physiology* **108**, 509–20.
9. **Calnan, J.S.** (1971). Lymphatics in the swollen leg. In *The Scientific Basis of Medicine* (ed. I. Gilliland and J. Francis), pp. 349–64. London: Athlone Press.
10. **Gray, J.H.** (1939–40). Studies of the regeneration of the lymphatic vessels. *Journal of Anatomy* **74**, 309–35.
11. **Hall, J.G.** The function of the lymphatic system in immunity. PhD Thesis, Australian National University, 1964.
12. **Mortimer, P.S., Simmonds, R., Rezvani, M., Robbins, M., Ryan, T.J., and Hopewell, J.W.** (1991). Time-related changes in lymphatic clearance in pig skin after a single dose of 18 Gy of X-rays. *British Journal of Radiology* **64**, 1140–6.
13. **Bates, D.O., Levick, J.R., and Mortimer, P.S.** (1994). Starling pressures in the human arm and their alteration in postmastectomy oedema. *Journal of Physiology* **477** (2), 355–63.
14. **Svensson, W.E., Mortimer, P.S., Tohno, E., and Cosgrove, D.O.** (1994). Increased arterial inflow demonstrated by Doppler ultrasound in arm swelling following breast cancer treatment. *European Journal of Cancer* **30**, 661–4.
15. **Svensson, W.E., Mortimer, P.S., Tohno, E., and Cosgrove, D.** (1994). Colour Doppler demonstrates venous flow abnormalities in breast cancer patients with chronic arm swelling. *European Journal of Cancer* **30**, 657–60.
16. **Stemmer, R.** (1976). Ein klinisches Zeichen zur fruhund differential Diagnose des Lymphodems. *VASA* **5** (3), 261–2.
17. **Schreiber, H.** et al. (1979). Stewart–Treves syndrome: a lethal complication of post mastectomy lymphoedema and regional immune deficiency. *Archives of Surgery* **114**, 82–5.
18. **Proby, C.M., Gane, J.N., Joseph, A.E., and Mortimer, P.S.** (1990). Investigation of the swollen limb with isotope lymphography. *British Journal of Dermatology* **123**, 29–37.
19. **Liu, N-F. and Warg, C.G.** (1998). The role of magnetic resonance imaging in the diagnosis of peripheral disorders. *Lymphology* **31**, 1119–27.
20. **Badger, C.** (1987). Lymphoedema: management of patients with advanced cancer. *Professional Nurse* **2** (4), 100–2.
21. **Casley-Smith, J.R., Gwn Morgan, R., and Piller, N.B.** (1993). Treatment of lymphoedema of the arms and legs with 5,6-benzo-[X]-pyrone. *New England Journal of Medicine* **329**, 1158–63.
22. **Michel, C.C., Blumberg, S., and Clough, G.** (1988). Hydroxyethyl rutosides reduced the increased permeability which follows perfusion of frog capillaries with protein free solutions. *International Journal of Microcirculation: Clinical and Experimental* Special Issue, 544.
23. **Foldi, E., Foldi, M., and Weissleder, H.** (1985). Conservative treatment of lymphoedema of the limbs. *Angiology* **36**, 171–80.
24. **Thomas, S.** (1990). Bandages and bandaging: the science behind the art. *Care Science and Practice* **8** (2), 56–60.
25. **Badger, C. and Twycross, R.G.** *Management of Lymphoedema—Guidelines.* Oxford: Sobell Study Centre, 1988.
26. **Leduc, O., Peeters, A., and Bourgeois, P.** (1990). Bandages: scintigraphic demonstration of its efficacy on colloidal protein reabsorbtion during muscle activity. In *Progress in Lymphology* Vol. 12 (ed. M. Nishi, S. Uchino, and S. Yabuki), pp. 421–3. Amsterdam: Excerpta Medica.

8.10 Genito-urinary problems in palliative medicine

Richard W. Norman and Greg Bailly

Introduction

The genitourinary system may produce a variety of disturbing symptoms or life-threatening conditions in patients receiving palliative care. Unilateral or bilateral ureteral obstructions occur commonly in association with primary or secondary malignancies involving the retroperitoneum and pelvis. This can lead to pain and/or impaired renal function. Lower-tract obstruction may be associated with benign or malignant conditions involving the bladder neck, prostate, or urethra. Anticholinergic drugs, frequently prescribed for patients receiving palliative care, may be responsible for voiding dysfunction and may need modification of type or dosage. Interaction between the bladder and other pelvic organs may be significant and can lead to fistula formation. Haematuria requires investigation to determine whether it is of upper- or lower-tract origin and, if severe, will need intervention.

This chapter is concerned with the practical aspects of symptom control in patients receiving palliative care and suffering from urinary tract dysfunction; arguably the most difficult management decision is choosing the right option in the context of the patient's total situation. Factors to consider include the patient's pre-morbid health and preference status, adequacy of symptom control, disease progression, and the burden versus the benefit balance of investigation and intervention. Emphasis is placed on less aggressive, non-invasive therapies, in keeping with the general condition of these patients. Decisions to recommend more complex, invasive procedures may be appropriate but should always be based on the quality of life anticipated, stage of the disease, and reasonable likelihood of symptomatic improvement.

Pathophysiology and factors governing voiding

The bladder wall is composed of a mesh of smooth muscle fibres which become organized in layers at the bladder neck (detrusor muscle). The outer layer extends throughout the length of the female urethra (Fig. 1)[1] and to the distal aspect of the prostate in the male, where its arrangement (circular/spiral) is responsible for the major involuntary sphincter (Fig. 2).[2] The middle circular layer ends at the bladder neck and contributes to sphincteric function. Internal fibres remain longitudinal and extend to the distal end of the urethra in the female and the prostate in the male. Converging, they form the muscle of the vesical neck, which contributes to urinary continence.

The bladder receives its principal nerve supply from one paired somatic and two paired autonomic nerves. The hypogastric nerves, arising from lumbar spinal segments, mediate sympathetic activity, while the pelvic nerves, derived from S2–S4, contain parasympathetic fibres. The pudendal nerves (S2–S4) primarily serve as a conduit for non-autonomic fibres. With distension of the bladder wall, stretch receptors trigger pelvic nerve fibres which, unless inhibited by higher centres, will lead to a parasympathetic motor response and bladder contraction (Fig. 3).

The voluntary external sphincter is made up of striated muscle, which is located between the layers of the urogenital diaphragm. In the male, these fibres are concentrated at the distal aspect of the prostate; in the female, they are found mainly in relation to the middle third of the urethra. Smooth muscle investing the vesical neck and posterior urethra is under sympathetic control, mediated through the hypogastric nerve with thoracolumbar origin (T11–L2). Norepinephrine is the neurotransmitter in this sympathetic release. The external sphincter is under pudendal nerve control (S2–S4) and influenced by autonomic as well as somatic innervation from the pelvic floor. All are coordinated by higher centres to initiate or inhibit bladder emptying.

Satisfactory voiding requires an unobstructed passage from the bladder to the urethral meatus, in addition to a functioning detrusor muscle, an intact bladder wall, and integrity of the nerves initiating and coordinating detrusor and sphincteric activities. Stimulation of the parasympathetic bladder nerves causes contraction of the detrusor muscle and relaxation of the bladder neck sphincter. Stimulation of the sympathetic system (T10–T12, L1) has the reverse effect.

Neurological damage associated with metastases to the spine and epidural space causing spinal cord compression or nerve root injury secondary to tumour infiltration may interfere with voiding. Drugs required for control of pain and other symptoms in patients with advanced cancer also have an important impact on bladder function. Anticholinergic drugs can interfere by causing contraction of the bladder neck sphincter and relaxation of the detrusor muscle. Drugs with such effects which are frequently used in patients with advanced cancer include phenothiazines, haloperidol, antihistamines, and tricyclic antidepressants. Opioid drugs have little impact on bladder function unless combined with other problems, for example, faecal impaction, which, when significant, adds an obstructive component by pressure on the urethra. Particular caution is indicated in the use of these drugs in the elderly and in patients who have pre-existing early bladder outlet obstruction and coexisting immobility.

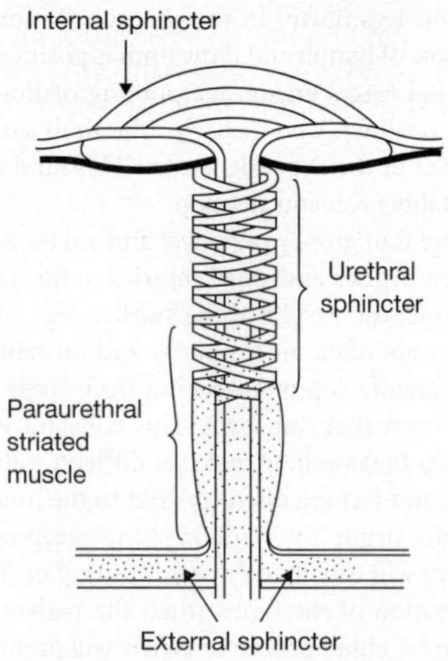

Fig. 1 Sphincter arrangement in the female.

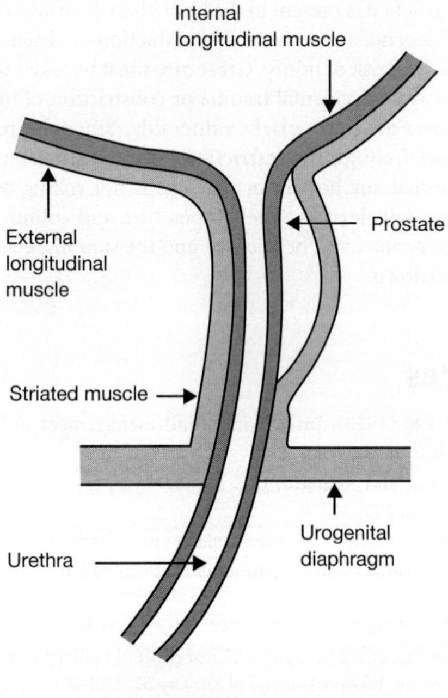

Fig. 2 Sagittal section of the male urethra.

Bladder outlet obstruction with distension produces great physical distress which may be masked in the elderly and in patients taking opioid drugs and neuroleptic agents. Confusion is a common presentation, particularly in the elderly. This may result from the physical discomfort or as a result of metabolic disturbances from impaired renal function. In the evaluation of dysfunction, the anatomical and functional integrities of the bladder and urethra should be considered. Spinal cord or nerve root damage should be ruled out. The patient's drug profile must be reviewed. If possible, drugs with anticholinergic effects should be eliminated or their dosages reduced. Constipation should be considered. Biochemical abnormalities which may increase urinary flow must be remembered—hypercalcaemia, hyperglycaemia, and diabetes insipidus should be excluded.

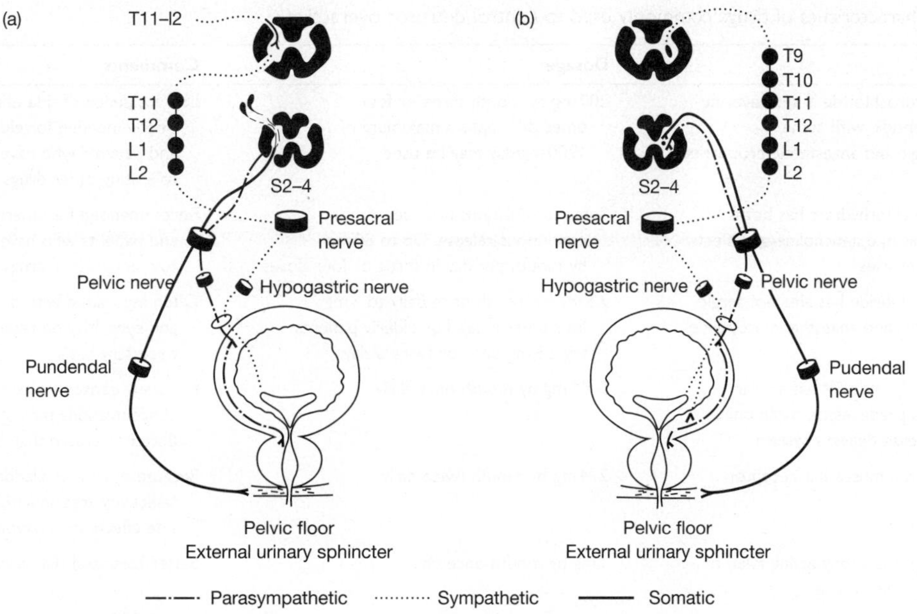

Fig. 3 Innervation of bladder and sites of drug activity.

Urinary incontinence

Involuntary loss of urine or urinary incontinence is described as total, overflow, urgency, or stress. In patients with advanced malignant disease, total urethral incontinence or extraurethral loss from urinary fistulae are the most common and significant. Proper management is very important as incontinence predisposes to perineal rashes, pressure ulcers, urinary tract infections, urosepsis, falls, and fractures.

Total urethral incontinence

This is associated with sphincteric incompetence. Direct tumour invasion, surgical intervention, or loss of innervation from spinal cord or nerve root damage represents the usual responsible factors in patients in palliative care. Direct visualization confirms the urethral nature of the loss. Endoscopic examination and/or urodynamic evaluation may be necessary to establish a diagnosis. The presence of other motor or sensory abnormalities suggesting spinal cord or nerve root damage may provide the necessary evidence to implicate a neurological deficit. Management usually entails use of an indwelling Foley catheter in women and condom drainage or a penile clamp in men. If the condom or penile clamp is not well tolerated, a Foley catheter would be the next choice. Although artificial sphincters are being used with increasing frequency, their use in patients with active and advanced malignant disease is ordinarily inappropriate.

Overflow incontinence

This type of urinary incontinence is associated with bladder outlet or urethral obstruction. Initially associated with the acute distress of acute retention, voiding occurs in small amounts and without control. The bladder is distended and usually palpable except in the very obese or in patients with pelvic masses or extensive lymphoedema involving the lower abdominal wall.

Catheterization is indicated. Definitive treatment must be individualized and may include surgical or other interventional techniques to correct the obstruction, long-term dependence on an indwelling catheter, intermittent catheterization, or an intraurethral stent.

Urgency incontinence

Detrusor overactivity is associated with increased spontaneous activity of detrusor smooth muscle, leading to excessive detrusor force in relation to urethral sphincter tone. The urge is sudden and urinary loss may be severe. The impaired mobility of patients in a palliative care setting may be an aggravating factor in preventing them from reaching the toilet in time. Causes include intrinsic and extrinsic tumours which produce irritation of the bladder wall, particularly in the region of the trigone and vesical neck. It may also be associated with inflammatory changes from physical agents (e.g. previous radiation), drugs (e.g. cyclophosphamide), or bacteria. An irritable bladder producing urgency incontinence may be of non-specific type or related to lack of inhibition from neural deficiency, as seen in association with cerebrovascular insufficiency. It usually responds to anticholinergic therapy, such as oxybutynin 2.5 mg orally two to three times per day. In the elderly, a single low dose daily is recommended and 'as necessary' dosing considered. If this is not tolerated other drugs can be considered to reduce detrusor overactivity (Fig. 3, Table 1).

Stress incontinence

Stress incontinence consists of involuntary urethral loss of urine associated with increased intraabdominal pressure from coughing, sneezing, jumping, laughing, or, in severe cases, even walking. It is associated with faulty urethral support, wherein the increased intravesical pressure cannot be resisted. This does not usually represent a major problem in patients in palliative care. Surgery is the usual treatment but it is unlikely to be appropriate in patients with advanced cancer. If not contraindicated by other conditions, treatment with an alpha agonist such as phenylpropandamine (50–100 mg/day in divided doses),[3] or a tricyclic antidepressant, such as imipramine, may be appropriate (Fig. 3, Table 1). Long-term catheterization may be necessary in severe cases.

Extraurethral incontinence

Urinary fistulae are covered elsewhere in the chapter.

Table 1 Characteristics of drugs commonly used to control detrusor overactivity

Action	Dosage	Comments
Flavoxate hydrochloride is a papaverine-like antispasmodic with some anticholinergic and anaesthetic properties	200 mg by mouth three or four times daily upto a maximum of 1200 mg/day may be used	Low incidence of side effects. Recommended for elderly patients and patients who have trouble tolerating other drugs
Dicyclomine chlorhydrate has both musculotropic and anticholinergic effects on smooth muscles	Some formulations provide continuous-release. Up to 80 mg by mouth per day in three or four doses	Recommended for elderly patients and patients who have trouble tolerating other drugs
Oxybutynin chloride has anticholinergic, antispasmodic, and anaesthetic properties	2.5 mg by mouth once daily to 5 mg four times a day. For elderly patients try 2.5 mg once or twice a day	Often associated with dry mouth and eyes. May be taken on a necessary basis
Oxybutynin chloride ER has similar actions as its predecessor, oxybutinin, but slow release delivery system	5–15 mg by mouth once daily	Relatively constant plasma concentrations throughout 24 h. Better tolerated than oxybutynin
Tolterodine is a muscarinic receptor antagonist	2–4 mg by mouth twice daily	Because of greater bladder selectivity, less anticholinergic side effects than oxybutynin
Tolterodine LA is a long-acting form of its precessor, tolterodine	4 mg by mouth once daily	Better tolerated than tolterodine
Propantheline bromide is a cholinergic receptor competitor	From 7.5 mg by mouth once daily to 15 mg by mouth four times a day. Where absorption in the digestive tract is incomplete up to 30 mg by mouth four times a day may be necessary	Frequent dosing usually required
Imipramine chlorhydrate is a tricyclic antidepressant with anxiolytic, anticholinergic, direct musculotropic, and adrenergic properties. It also has mild anaesthetic and antihistamine effects. Inhibits the noredrenaline reuptake at presynaptic nerve terminals lesions	Increase gradually to about 25 mg twice daily, but up to a maximum of 200 mg/day can be used if necessary	Imipramine should not be given along with MAO inhibitors
Belladonna/opium suppositories have analgesic, anticholinergic, and antispasmodic properties. Because of their potential addictiveness, they should only be used over the short term, e.g., to control pain and bladder spasm after bladder or prostate surgery	One suppository every 3–4 h as required	Useful in management of bladder spasms in those who can not tolerate medication orally

Investigation and management of sudden urinary stoppage

Sudden and marked decrease in urinary output can be both a distressing and potentially lethal problem for patients if it persists and is associated with the metabolic abnormalities characteristic of acute renal failure. Complete cessation of urinary output usually implies obstruction of either the lower urinary tract at the level of the bladder neck, prostate, or urethra or upper-tract obstruction of both ureters or obstruction of a single functioning kidney.

Lower-tract obstruction as a cause of sudden urinary stoppage

Most patients who develop urinary retention will have had some milder, usually progressive, symptoms of obstruction, including hesitancy, decreased urinary stream, and inability to empty the bladder satisfactorily. Symptoms of urinary frequency, nocturia, incontinence, and urinary tract infection may also be apparent. Past history of urethral instrumentation, injury, or infection may point towards the development of a urethral stricture. A history of anticholinergic or α-adrenergic drug use may be a contributing factor. On physical examination, these patients are usually restless and uncomfortable due to a painfully overfilled bladder—usually one is able to see, palpate, and percuss the distended organ. Attention should be paid to the urethral meatus, to rule out significant meatal stenosis, and to the entire length of the urethra, to identify areas of scarring or induration which could imply stricture or tumour formation. Rectal examination is imperative in order to assess the size and consistency of the prostate gland. Firm irregularities may be indicative of cancer of the prostate.

The most appropriate treatment at this time is passage of a urethral catheter to drain the bladder. If this is impossible, insertion of a suprapubic catheter will permit satisfactory bladder drainage and allow relief of symptoms until further definitive endoscopic assessment of the lower urinary tract can be arranged. It is important that the subsequent urinary output of these patients be measured on an hourly basis for several hours to ensure that they do not develop a significant post-obstructive diuresis. Although most of these patients with prostatic enlargement will benefit from a limited transurethral prostatectomy, sometimes referred to as a 'channel TURP', careful case selection is advised because this population of patients often have increased risk of bleeding, clot retention, infection, and persistent failure to void. Alternatives to prostatectomy include intraurethral stent,[4] transurethral microwave therapy, transurethral needle ablation, and holmium laser enucleation. Medical therapy, such as the use of α-blockers and 5α-reductase inhibitors, has gained in popularity for the management of men with symptomatic benign prostatic hyperplasia but is not indicated in men with refractory urinary retention.

Case study A 79-year-old man presented with mild obstructive voiding symptoms and lower back discomfort. He underwent a digital rectal examination and cystoscopy which confirmed the presence of a large necrotic nodular prostatic tumour mass with invasion into the right side of the trigone. Biopsies confirmed poorly differentiated adenocarcinoma of the prostate. Renal ultrasound was consistent with right-sided hydronephrosis and a bone scan showed diffuse metastases. Serum prostate specific antigen measured 987 ng/ml. He was treated with total androgen blockade with some improvement in his voiding symptoms and back discomfort. Three months later, he suffered a myocardial infarction. Two weeks following discharge he went into urinary retention and, despite attempts at catheter removal, was unable to void spontaneously. He found the catheter very uncomfortable, but because of his recent cardiovascular problem, he was not felt to be a suitable candidate for a transurethral resection of the prostate. He was treated by placement of an intraurethral stent (Fig. 4) under local anaesthesia and subsequently voided normally.

Comment

There are an increasing number of alternatives for the management of bladder outlet obstruction and it is important to individualize therapy for a specific patient. In this particular case, it was possible to treat this man's problem in a palliative fashion and improve his quality of life without the catheter, despite his serious underlying malignant and cardiovascular diseases.

Bilateral ureteric obstruction as a cause of sudden urinary stoppage

Acute renal failure secondary to bilateral ureteric obstruction is a common problem in palliative care. Obstruction in the cancer patient may be secondary to tumour invasion, compression of the ureter by retroperitoneal tumour, encasement of the ureter by retroperitoneal or pelvic lymph nodes involved with metastatic disease, or, rarely, by direct metastases to the ureter. In 75 per cent of patients within this group, an underlying malignant disorder will be diagnosed.[5] In almost one-half, the development of bilateral ureteric obstruction is the initial manifestation of the underlying cancer. About three-quarters of the tumours are pelvic in origin; the most common in women is carcinoma of the cervix, and in men, carcinoma of the prostate. The most frequent benign diagnosis is retroperitoneal fibrosis.[6]

Common symptoms are a lack of urinary output and abdominal pain. Acute ureteral obstruction usually causes flank pain and colic typical of urolithiasis. Chronic renal obstruction is usually a silent event that is often detected as hydronephrosis with atrophy of the renal cortex on upper abdominal imaging. Physical examination may reveal evidence of flank masses or tenderness. The bladder will not be distended and the urethra should be unremarkable. The importance of an adequate rectal and pelvic examination is emphasized in view of the anticipated causes of obstruction.

Because the obstruction may have been progressing over several days prior to causing complete urinary stoppage, most of these patients will reveal laboratory evidence of acute renal failure with elevated levels of serum creatinine and potassium, metabolic acidosis, and fluid overload, and as a result, investigation and treatment become urgent. Intravenous pyelography is contraindicated in acute renal failure, but renal ultrasonography can be extremely useful in identifying both kidneys and the degree of obstruction. Occasionally, it may show obstructing stones in the upper ureter or renal pelvis. More recently, unenhanced spiral computed tomography has become an effective and safe initial imaging tool in the evaluation of renal obstruction, providing more useful information than ultrasonography.[7]

Regardless of the method used to acutely relieve bilateral renal obstruction, these patients must be observed closely for changes in their potassium and creatinine levels, as well as the volume of urinary output, following relief of obstruction which often is followed by a diuresis. If fluid and electrolyte abnormalities are severe, it may be necessary to arrange early temporary haemodialysis to correct life-threatening problems.

In the presence of bilateral ureteric obstruction, cystoscopy and bilateral retrograde pyelograms are usually done next. These studies can reveal abnormalities within the urinary bladder, such as a primary or secondary tumour involving the trigone, and will outline the ureters to define the level, and often the cause, of the ureteric obstruction. Once this has been accomplished, an indwelling ureteric stent can be passed, under cystoscopic control, up the ureter such that one end lies within the renal pelvis and the other within the bladder.[8] This would usually be attempted on both sides if feasible and both kidneys appear to have reasonable potential for regaining function (Fig. 5). When single stents have failed, placement of two parallel stents simultaneously in extrinsically obstructed ureters may

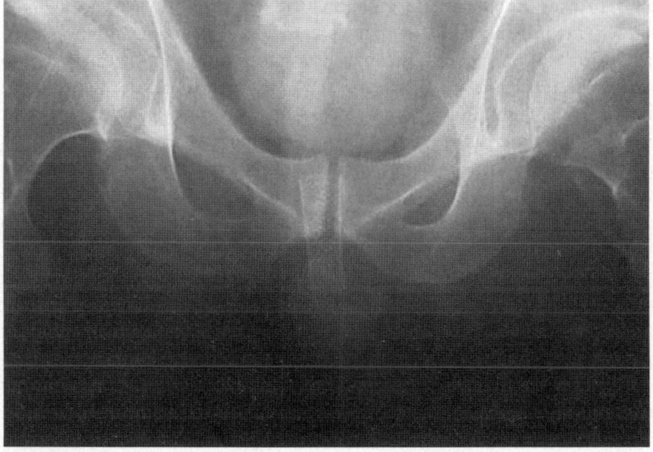

Fig. 4 Urethral stent bridging prostatic urethra.

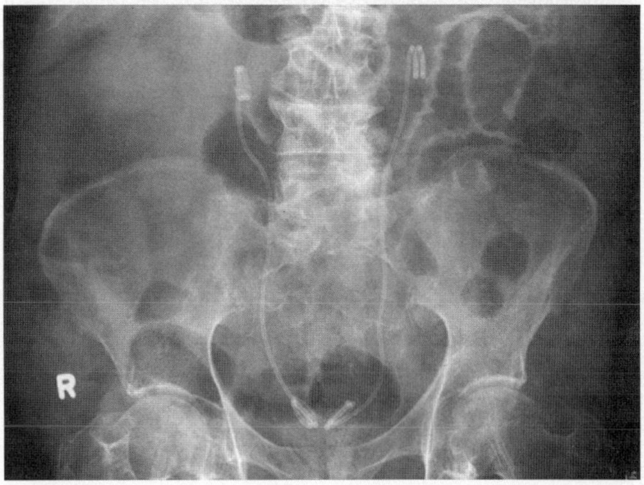

Fig. 5 Bilateral ureteric stents draining obstructed ureters secondary to bladder cancer.

improve drainage of the kidney.[9] Others have described the placement of self-expandable metallic mesh stents as an alternative to traditional ureteric stents, although experience is limited.[10–12]

In circumstances in which it is impossible to endoscopically position ureteric stents, one would proceed to percutaneous placement of a nephrostomy tube under ultrasound guidance. Antegrade nephrostograms can then be performed to localize the site and extent of obstruction (Fig. 6). Nephrostomy tubes can sometimes be replaced by antegrade insertion of ureteric stents and eliminate the need for an external drainage device. If indwelling stents are not successful, long-term management of obstruction can be provided by several means. Percutaneous nephrostomy tubes are often difficult to manage for many patients because the posterior exit site increases the risk of displacement, infection, and blockage. Subcutaneous tunnelling of nephrostomy tubes obviates these problems.[13] The procedure may be done with local anaesthesia and conscious sedation, as conventional 8F tubes are replaced by larger 12F tubes under fluoroscopic guidance. Each tube is tunnelled subcutaneously anteriorly where it exits through a common opening in the skin in the right lower quadrant (Fig. 7(a)–(d)). The patient can manage the urinary drainage with an external ostomy appliance and drainage bag. Tube exchange is performed every 3 months on an outpatient basis.

Once a ureteral stent or nephrostomy tube is placed, subsequent management requires close follow-up, including periodic monitoring of renal function and periodic stent or tube placement (every 4–6 months). If a specific treatment, for example, radiation or chemotherapy, eliminates the lesion responsible for the obstruction, then removal of the nephrostomy tubes or stents can be done, provided imaging studies confirm that the kidneys are draining freely. In advanced prostate cancer patients, androgen blockade is an important palliative treatment which may reduce tumour volume and induce ureteric patency, eliminating the need for long-term stents or tubes.

In situations where this scenario is the result of long-term progression of an underlying malignancy, active intervention at this stage may not be warranted. Posed with a difficult ethical question, the physician and patient must consider the benefits of facilitating treatment and palliation of symptoms versus merely prolonging the patient's suffering. This option should be discussed with the patient and family. In cases where this is the initial manifestation of underlying cancer, therapy is usually tailored towards the underlying malignancy in the hope of relieving the obstruction. Ordinarily, definitive surgical intervention would be entertained only in this situation.

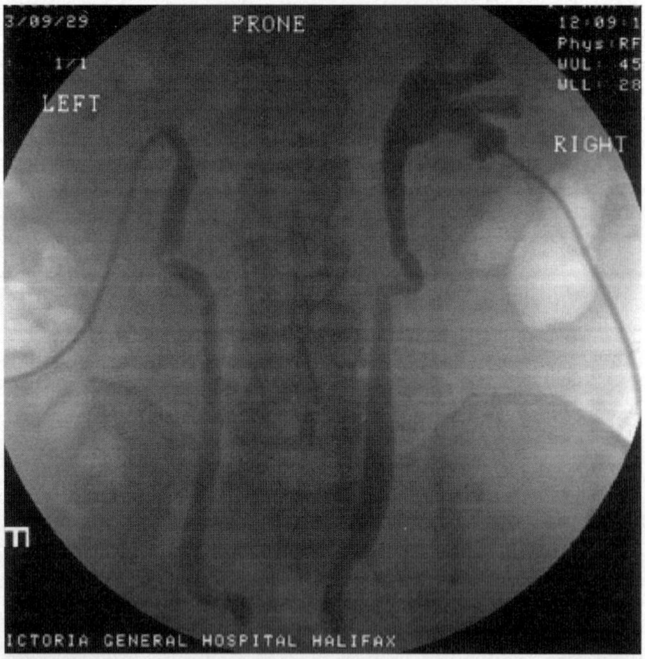

Fig. 6 Bilateral nephrostograms demonstrate complete obstruction of both ureters by prostate cancer.

Case study A 79-year-old man with advanced metastatic prostate cancer treated with total androgen blockade, presented to hospital with a 1-month history of increasing fatigue, anorexia, nausea, vomiting, and decreased urine output. On examination he was tachypneic, and had an elevated JVP, bilateral pulmonary rales, and significant paedal oedema. Digital rectal exam revealed a large, hard, nodular prostate. Investigations showed a creatinine of 988 mmol/l, potassium of 7.2 meq/l, and bicarbonate of 9 meq/l. Renal ultrasound revealed severe bilateral hydronephrosis and normal parenchymal thickness. Electrolyte disturbances were treated medically and the patient had urgent insertion of percutaneous nephrostomy tubes bilaterally (Fig. 6). Over the next 5 days, electrolytes and creatinine returned to normal. Cystoscopy was performed and showed infiltration of the trigone by tumour with obliteration of the ureteric orifices making it impossible to insert ureteric stents in a retrograde fashion. Attempted antegrade placement was also unsuccessful. After discussion with the patient, the nephrostomy tubes were tunnelled subcutaneously and urine drainage was managed with an ostomy appliance (Fig. 7(d)). The patient managed well for 16 months before succumbing to his disease from diffuse metastatic disease.

Comment

Most patients who have advanced inoperable pelvic mailignancy with significant bilateral ureteric obstruction should be managed initially with ureteric stents. With recurrent obstruction or failure of stent insertion, appropriate management may include subcutaneously tunnelled nephrostomy tubes if the obstruction is anticipated to be indefinite.

Unilateral ureteric involvement by underlying malignancy

Because of their long length through either side of the retroperitoneum, the ureters are susceptible to involvement by a wide variety of primary and secondary malignancies. In many cases this can be insidious and asymptomatic; in other instances the effect can be sudden and associated with significant discomfort. In either case, the presence of ureteric obstruction is usually established by intravenous pyelography, renal ultrasonography, or computerized tomography of the abdomen. These studies may also give further clues to the possible underlying cause of obstruction.

Physical examination of the abdomen, pelvis, and rectum is critical and may provide important information that will assist in determining the underlying problem. Because of the presence of obstruction and the associated decrease in renal function, intravenous pyelography may fail to demonstrate the site of blockage. Many patients, therefore, will require cystourethroscopy and a retrograde study. This will provide important information in terms of the site, degree, and cause of obstruction.

If the involved side is symptomatic, or if the contralateral side is absent or non-functioning, cystoscopic placement of an indwelling ureteric stent is useful in providing temporary relief of the obstruction while further investigation and treatment can be established. When this is impossible, percutaneous placement of an indwelling nephrostomy tube can be a useful means of drainage and can permit injection of dye into the upper tract further to define the site and degree of obstruction. Antegrade stenting or subcutaneous tunnelling may be considered for patient comfort. In general, the ultimate outcome in these circumstances will be dictated by the underlying disease. Open surgical therapy to divert the urine or to lyse the ureters is not usually indicated in the face of advanced underlying malignancy. Assuming the contralateral kidney to be functioning reasonably

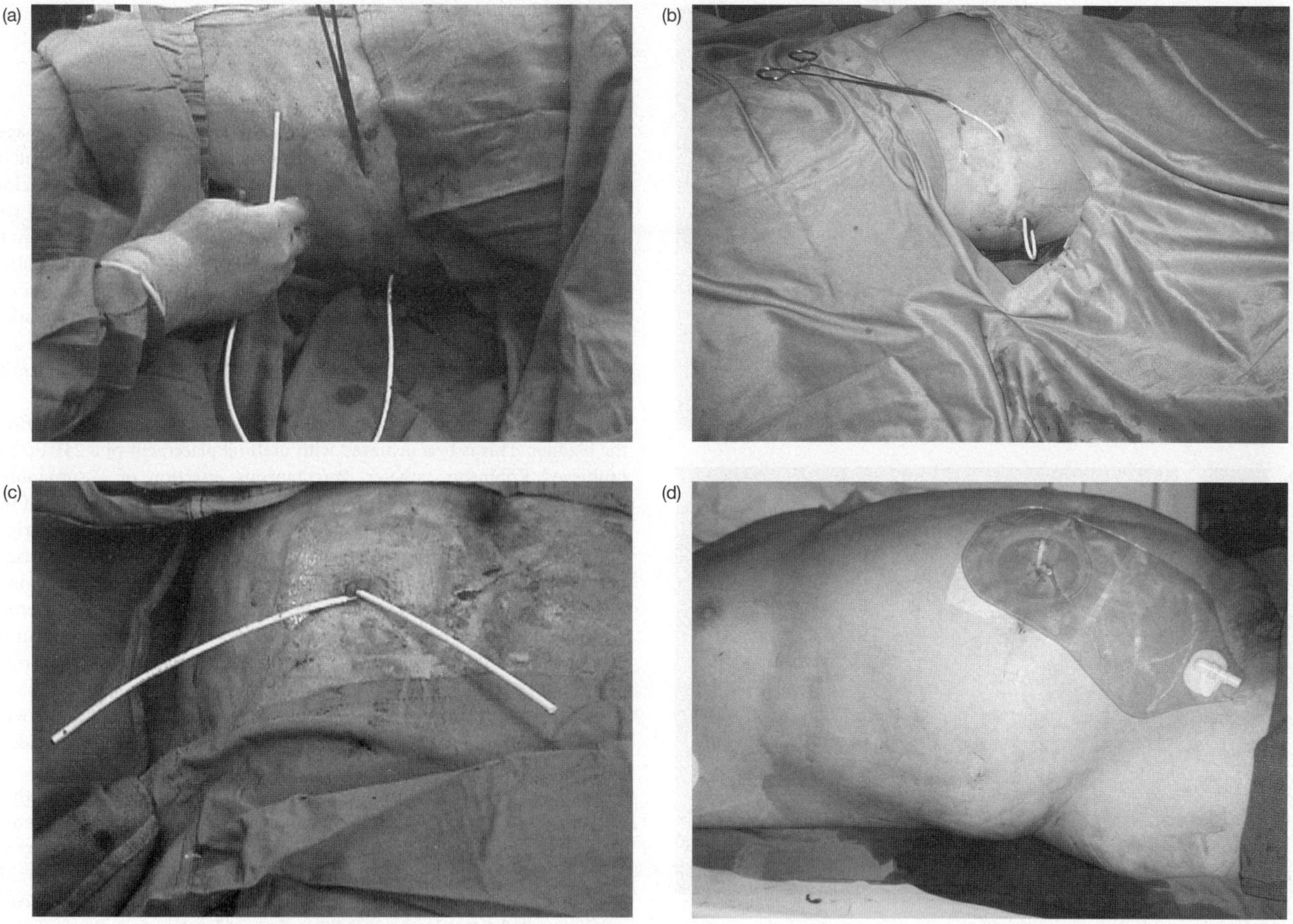

Fig. 7 Operative steps in placement of subcutaneously tunnelled nephrostomy tubes. (a) Instrument is passed subcutaneously into a 1-cm stab wound in the left anterior flank and will be brought out through another stab wound posteriorly beside the nephrostomy tube. (b) Left nephrostomy tube is being pulled out through the anterior incision. This will be repeated until the left and right tubes are brought out through a single site in the right lower quadrant. (c) Both nephrostomy tubes have been tunnelled subcutaneously and are exiting through a single stab wound in the right lower quadrant. (d) The nephrostomy tubes have been cut so that 2 cm protrude from the skin and they can easily be inserted into and covered by an appliance.

well, it is sometimes necessary to remove the involved, obstructed kidney if it continues to be symptomatic, despite satisfactory internal or external drainage. This is often better tolerated than a heroic attempt at reconstruction. In circumstances where the obstructed kidney is completely asymptomatic and the contralateral kidney is functioning well, intervention is usually not required.

Case study A 57-year-old man complained of some mild fullness and discomfort in the right flank for 6 weeks. Past history revealed that he had undergone an abdominoperineal resection for carcinoma of the rectum 2 years previously. At that time, the surgical margins were clear and the lymph nodes were negative. Current investigations included a renal ultrasound which showed high-grade ureteric obstruction on the right side with a normal left kidney. Cystoscopy and a right retrograde pyelogram confirmed the presence of marked obstruction of the lower end of the right ureter, secondary to an extrinsic mass. An abdominal and pelvic computerized tomography scan were consistent with liver metastases, right hydroureteronephrosis, and a large right pelvic mass encasing the lower end of the ureter (Fig. 8(a) and (b)). Attempts at insertion of a ureteric stent were unsuccessful and in view of the fact that the patient was coping well, it was decided to perform no further interventions to the right kidney or ureter.

Comment

There are a number of endoscopic and percutaneous approaches to the obstructed ureter, but when a patient has a variety of other underlying problems it is not always appropriate to intervene unless there are significant symptoms. In this situation, the patient was reasonably comfortable and it was decided not to get involved in any more complicated interventional procedures.

Haematuria

Haematuria is a frequent symptom and sign of underlying urological disease but the degree of bleeding does not always correlate with the seriousness of the underlying condition.[14] Although a specific cause for asymptomatic microscopic haematuria can often not be determined, it may signal the presence of an underlying malignancy. It is important, therefore,

(a)
(b)

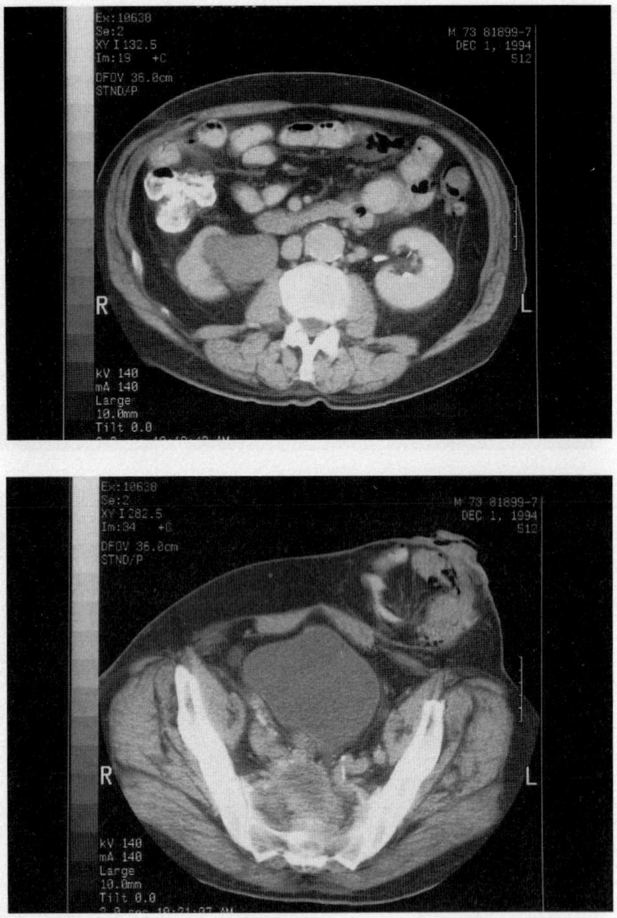

Fig. 8 CT scan showing (a) obstructed and dilated right renal pelvis and (b) large tumour mass behind the bladder and obstructing the right ureter.

that all degrees of newly diagnosed haematuria be assessed. A key feature in the history relates to whether the urine has been previously examined and whether the presence of blood is a new and persistent finding. Other associated symptoms, such as dysuria and urinary frequency and urgency, may point towards a urinary tract infection which can be diagnosed with an adequate urinalysis and urine culture, or less commonly malignant invasion of the bladder diagnosed endoscopically. Use of non-steroidal anti-inflammatory drugs and aspirin has been associated with microhaematuria. Danthron, a common component of laxatives used in palliative care, may tint alkaline urine a harmless pink or orange and cause confusion. Lower abdominal or flank discomfort may point towards abnormalities in the bladder, ureter, or kidney as the cause. Unfortunately, physical examination often fails to provide satisfactory clues. In these patients, an intravenous pyelogram will allow assessment of the upper tracts in terms of presence, function, and drainage. Although the bladder is also seen, small lesions within it can be missed radiographically and complete cystourethroscopy is indicated when upper-tract radiological procedures do not establish a diagnosis. Specific therapy will be directed towards individual abnormalities.

One of the most frightening symptoms is the sudden onset of gross haematuria. This may simply mean the passage of brown- or red-coloured urine, or it could involve the passage of large clots or the development of clot retention or colic. Either will require prompt urological consultation. In the palliative care setting, knowledge of the site an underlying malignancy, possibility of a major coagulation disorder, history of cyclophosphamide use, or prior pelvic irradiation may be significant. In less urgent cases, investigations as described above would be necessary.

Lower tract

Patients with clot retention require immediate intervention and management prior to the initiation of specific studies. Most of these patients will be frightened and uncomfortable due to bladder distension from blood clots and urine. Usually they are extremely restless and unable to remain still because of discomfort, but in rare cases bleeding may have been sufficient to cause hypotension and shock. On physical examination the distended bladder can be seen, palpated, and percussed. Tenderness or a mass in either flank may hint at an upper-tract cause for the bleeding. Rectal examination is important in men to assess the size and consistency of the prostate and pelvic and rectal examinations are important in women to try to identify a pelvic abnormality.

Adequate initial management requires complete evacuation of clots from the bladder. This is best achieved with urethral placement of a 24F or 26F multieyed Robinson catheter. Percutaneous insertion of a suprapubic catheter is contraindicated in the presence of clot retention because of the inability to place a catheter of satisfactory size to provide adequate irrigation and the potential for seeding of the percutaneous tract by an unsuspected bladder carcinoma. Once the urethral catheter has been passed into the bladder, vigorous irrigation with water or saline, using a Toomey syringe, will usually permit removal of all clots. Bladder irrigation can be very uncomfortable and may require additional analgaesia. Manual irrigation should be continued until no further clots are obtained and the backflow is clear. At this stage the Robinson catheter should be replaced with a 22F or 24F three-way indwelling catheter and continuous bladder irrigation should be established using cold water or saline.

Unsuccessful attempts at initial placement of a satisfactory urethral catheter, or continued bleeding and recurrent obstruction of the irrigating catheter, are specific indications for early endoscopic evaluation. Recurrent obstruction of the urethral catheter is usually related either to the persistence of clots or to significant continuous bleeding. Cystourethroscopy permits complete evaluation of the entire penile and prostatic urethra as well as the bladder. In these circumstances it is important to rule out causes of obstruction and to identify sites of bleeding. The larger and more rigid cystoscope or resectoscope sheath (compared with the urethral catheter) allows improved evacuation of bladder clots. In the majority of instances this type of bleeding will be caused by local disease involving either the bladder or the prostate. Depending upon the specific circumstances, small and isolated bleeding sites can be cauterized or fulgurated at this time, but usually there is a requirement for transurethral resection of specific lesions to stop the bleeding and to obtain tissue for histological diagnosis. When these procedures have been completed, continuous bladder irrigation is established using an indwelling three-way Foley catheter.

Significant or recurrent haematuria may be the result of a condition known as haemorrhagic cystitis, defined as an acute or insidious diffuse bladder inflammation with haemorrhage. In cancer patients, metabolites of chemotherapeutic agents (e.g. cyclophosphamide), bladder injury secondary to radiation therapy, and viral infections account for the vast majority of cases. If the bleeding is refractory to these conservative measures, bladder instillations with formalin under general anaesthesia and direction of a urologist,[15,16] silver nitrate (100 cc of 0.5–1.0 per cent in sterile water instilled for 10–20 min followed by saline irrigation and repeated as necessary),[16] alum (1 per cent solution of the ammonium salt of aluminium in sterile water administered by continuous bladder irrigation over 12–24 h),[16] or epsilon aminocaproic acid[17] may be tried. Haemorrhagic cystitis secondary to cyclophosphamide responds to intravesical instillation of carboprost tromethane, an F2-α prostaglandin in more than 50 per cent of cases.[18] Bleeding from established radiation cystitis may respond to hyperbaric oxygen and chronic or recurrent episodes may benefit from oral pentosan polysulphate.[19,20] On the other hand, local irradiation of the bladder can be palliative in the presence of unresectable cancer and oral tranexamic acid may be helpful, but can cause clot formation and retention. Rarely, it is necessary to resort to surgical intervention, such as hypogastric artery ligation or embolization, or proximal urinary diversion with or without cystectomy.

Upper tract

Occasionally gross haematuria is not due to local bladder pathology but due to upper-tract bleeding. Cystoscopy under these circumstances is again useful in confirming the side from which the blood is coming, and in permitting removal of bladder clots. Retrograde pyelography is occasionally useful under these circumstances, but it should be remembered that many apparent filling defects within the ureter or renal pelvis at these times often represent blood clots.

The next investigation would be an intravenous pyelogram, if renal function is satisfactory, or a renal ultrasound if not. The most likely causes of upper-tract bleeding, under these circumstances, would be the presence of renal tumour, such as a renal cell carcinoma or transitional cell carcinoma of the renal pelvis or ureter, or a stone. Rarely, a specific cause will not be identified with these studies and it may be necessary to progress to renal arteriography. Selective injections permit optimal visualization of the intrarenal vasculature and can identify small arteriovenous malformations, small neoplasms, or renal vein varices. Occasionally, even the renal arteriogram will be normal, despite continued gross haematuria, and in these circumstances ureteroscopy can be helpful to identify the specific site of haemorrhage, which can be biopsied and/or cauterized.

In the event that a renal tumour is identified, appropriate management requires metastatic work-up and, if this is negative, a radical nephrectomy is performed. Radical nephroureterectomy with removal of a bladder cuff is usually indicated if it is a transitional cell lesion of the upper tract.

Occasionally the chest radiograph, abdominal computerized tomography scan, or bone scan will confirm the presence of metastases which would obviate the need for radical surgery. In these circumstances, therapeutic arteriography with the injection of pharmacodynamic agents and/or clot or gelfoam can be used to control bleeding. If bleeding persists, palliative nephrectomy may be required despite the presence of metastases.(21)

Urinary fistulae

A fistula (from the Latin word *pipe*) is a non-anatomic connection between two epithelial lined organs and is commonly related to inflammation, both benign and malignant in nature. In patients with underlying malignancy, the symptoms associated with urinary tract fistulae can be devastating. The psychological distress and physical afflictions associated with these problems can make patients, their families, and their care givers distraught and give them a sense of hopelessness. The four most common urinary fistulae are vesicoenteric, vesicovaginal, urethrocutaneous, and rectourethral.

Vesicoenteric fistulae

Fistulization between the bladder and the alimentary tract can involve any segment of bowel. Usually the problem is secondary to colonic malignancy or diverticulitis or small bowel inflammatory disease. Rarely, the primary problem originates from the bladder. The most common complaint associated with vesicoenteric fistulae is dysuria (73 per cent), which almost always precedes the development pneumaturia, that is, the passage of gas or froth in the urine (65 per cent).(22) Because of a connection between the bowel and urinary tract, many patients will suffer from persistent urinary tract infections, particularly when the colon is involved. The urine usually has a foul odour. In circumstances where the connection is large, patients may be aware of passing particulate faecal matter in the urine. Physical examination may reveal the presence of an associated bowel-related mass from underlying disease, but it is often non-contributory. Diagnostic confirmation of a fistula may be difficult. Cystoscopy confirms the diagnosis in 30–67 per cent of cases.(23) One usually observes a localized area of erythema and bullous inflammation at the fistulous site, which is frequently high on the posterior wall. Small amounts of stool may be seen extruding from the involved area. The remainder of the bladder may or may not appear inflamed. Occasionally the fistulous site may be so small that it cannot be appreciated at the time of endoscopy, and in these circumstances a variety of other tests, including cystography (sensitivity 32–56 per cent), intestinal barium studies from above or below, visible contrast media, oral ^{51}Cr-labelled sodium chromate,(24) and/or oral or rectal charcoal(23) or indocyanine green solution(25) may be required to identify the abnormal communication. CT scan and MRI are the most sensitive methods used to detect enterovesical fistulae. Overall, CT scanning with oral and rectal contrast, together with cystoscopy, should be adequate to demonstrate an enterovesical fistula in most cases.(26)

Management of enterovesical fistulae is usually dictated by the underlying bowel disease, and patient comorbidity. Ideally, the segment of bowel and bladder are removed together and remaining healthy bowel and bladder integrity are re-established. If this is not technically feasible, intestinal diversion may redirect enough of the faecal stream to reduce the urinary symptoms to a tolerable level. In rare circumstances when massive bladder involvement is present, a total cystectomy, with or without complete pelvic exenteration, and ileal conduit urinary diversion may be necessary. Placement of bilateral percutaneous nephrostomy tubes, with subsequent tunnelling, is sometimes performed to divert the urine.

Case study An 83-year-old woman with severe, chronic obstructive lung disease was admitted to hospital with pneumonia. She deteriorated rapidly and required endotracheal intubation and ventilation. She was treated with antibiotics, bronchodilators, and steroids and eventually required a tracheostomy. Although she remained alert and was able to communicate with sign language, mouthing of words, and writing, it was impossible to wean her from the respirator. As a result she had difficulty mobilizing. Three weeks later, her urine developed a foul smell and was noted to contain large particles of faeces. Cystoscopic evaluation revealed a large fistula arising from the posterior aspect of the bladder in the midline, above the trigone. Barium enema confirmed a large colovesical fistula (Fig. 9). She was not felt to be a candidate for a major surgical procedure because of her underlying respiratory difficulties and she was therefore treated with a defunctioning colostomy.

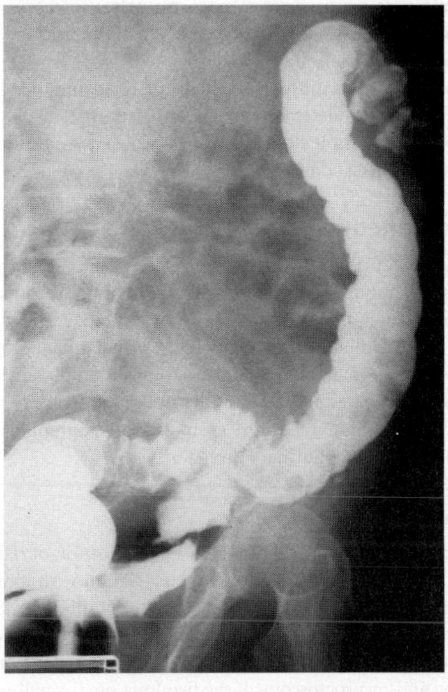

Fig. 9 Barium enema showing large vesicoenteric fistula originating in sigmoid colon.

Comment

In a healthy patient, an enterovesical fistula would be treated with bowel resection and closure of the bladder. In the palliative care setting, the optimal therapy is often not possible because of underlying restrictions on choices because of the idiosyncrasies of the patients. In this case, it was felt that the patient would not tolerate any further insult to her tenuous respiratory status and the minimal procedure of faecal diversion was carried out to eliminate the faecaluria and associated symptomatology.

Vesicovaginal urinary fistulae

Most vesicovaginal fistulae are the result of gynaecological surgery or local trauma.[27] The characteristic symptom is leakage of urine from the bladder into the vagina. Routine physical examination is usually unrewarding, although occasionally one may be able to identify a large fistulous site on pelvic examination. Intravenous pyelography is necessary to exclude the presence of ureteric involvement in the fistula. The latter is usually heralded by associated evidence of associated obstruction or significant displacement of the ureter. Cystoscopy will allow characterization of the vesicovaginal fistula in terms of size, site, and multiplicity. It is usually present low on the posterior wall, but the demonstration of proximity to a ureteric orifice is crucial to planning corrective surgery. Escape of irrigating fluid from the vagina while filling the bladder confirms the diagnosis. Vaginoscopy may be confirmatory. When the fistula is small it is occasionally helpful to place a vaginal pack and then fill the bladder with methylene blue to demonstrate the connection. In circumstances where the cause of the fistula is not obvious, a biopsy of the involved area at the time of cystoscopy is imperative to establish a specific diagnosis.

In the absence of underlying malignancy or other significant pathology, small fistulae occasionally close spontaneously following 4–6 weeks of urethral or suprapubic catheter drainage. Usually it will be necessary to proceed with a surgical repair and this can be accomplished vaginally or transabdominally, with interposition of an omental pedicle graft. Success of surgical management is dependent upon gentle and selective tissue handling, layered closure, lack of tension along suture lines, use of absorbable sutures, use of suprapubic catheter drainage of the bladder post-operatively, and administration of appropriate antibiotics peri-operatively.[28]

In circumstances where there is extensive pelvic disease, which is not manageable by surgical reconstruction or requiring anterior or pelvic exenteration, urinary diversion may be required.

When the patient has diffuse metastases or is unable to tolerate major surgery, placement of bilateral percutaneous nephrostomy tubes, with or without subcutaneous tunnelling, may be indicated as a means of diverting the urine and restoring continence.

Urethrocutaneous fistulae

Urethrocutaneous urinary fistulae are most frequently a complication of hypospadias repair, but may be the result of primary or secondary urethral or penile malignancies. Patients complain of a localized penile mass and drainage of urine through the fistulous site. Ultimate management usually requires a proximal, total, or partial penectomy with subsequent adjuvant surgical or pharmacological therapy as necessary. In those patients who are not candidates for definitive therapy, a percutaneous suprapubic cystostomy would be the ideal form of urinary diversion.

Rectourethral fistulae

Rectourethral fistulae occur most often as a complication of radical prostatectomy, but they are seen occasionally in association with locally invasive prostatic or rectal cancer. Most patients will complain of the passage of urine *per rectum* and/or pneumaturia and the passage of faecal material *per urethram*. The diagnosis is usually confirmed at the time of cystourethroscopy and/or proctoscopy. If the fistulous site is small, it may occasionally close spontaneously following a temporary diverting colostomy and bladder catheterization. If this is unsuccessful and there is no obvious persisting local malignancy, surgical repair is indicated. If persistent malignancy is present, the optimal treatment for the underlying malignancy should be determined and urinary and/or faecal diversion may be necesssary.

Urethral catheters

The indwelling urethral catheter remains one of the most useful and commonly used urological instruments. Its primary uses are to provide continuous drainage of urine from the bladder in patients who are unable to void spontaneously or who suffer from marked urinary incontinence not amenable to condom drainage. Occasionally, urethral catheters are used as a means of assessing the degree of bladder emptying, irrigating blood clots from the bladder, and measuring hourly urine output.

The most frequently used urethral catheters are made from latex rubber and are blunt-tipped. These have one channel for draining the urine and another smaller channel for inflating the balloon which prevents displacement of the catheter. Because of a tendency towards encrustation, irritation, and infection, a variety of new hydrophilic polymers have been developed to improve catheter biocompatibility. These lubricious coatings provide protection against irritation of urethral mucosa, help to minimize encrustation, and enhance patient comfort. Their effectiveness has reduced the need for more expensive silicone catheters. Silver-impregnated catheters, antibiotic-coated catheters, and electrified catheters may diminish bacteriuria for a few days, but are costly and have no role in long-term catheterization.[29]

A critical factor to be considered when choosing the catheter is the size. Most are labelled with respect to the measurement of the outer circumference of the catheter. The most frequently used system is the F-scale and conversion to the diameter of the catheter is possible by remembering that each number of the F-scale equals 0.33 mm. In the usual situation of using an indwelling urethral catheter, one would use a 16F or a 18F. Catheters smaller than this are less useful because of their tendency to coil up in the urethra during passage and to obstruct with bladder debris. It is best to minimize bladder irritation by using 5 or 10 ml balloons.

In patients for whom urethral catheterization is difficult, it is useful to fill the urethra with 10 ml of 2 per cent lignocaine (lidocaine) jelly; one should allow 5 min for this to take effect. This lubricates the urethra, allows the external sphincter to relax, and decreases some of the discomfort. Occasionally, a curved or Coudé catheter can be used to simplify passage through the external sphincter and prostatic urethra or bladder neck.

When it is impossible to pass a urethral catheter to drain a distended bladder, a suprapubic drainage system can be used. There are many kits to permit placement of a suprapubic catheter, but the principles of the technique involve placing the patient in a slight Trendelenburg position, treating the suprapubic area with an appropriate antiseptic, infiltrating a small area of skin 5 cm above the pubis in the midline with a local anaesthetic, and using a syringe and needle to aspirate urine through this area to confirm the position of the distended bladder. Once this had been accomplished, a plastic trocar and sheath can be passed through the same tract into the bladder. The trocar is then removed and the indwelling catheter passed through the sheath, which is then withdrawn or peeled away. The catheter is sutured in place and left indwelling. This can be an extremely important technique in patients with extensive urethral stricture disease.

The incidence of urinary tract infections in patients with indwelling urinary catheters is related to the duration of catheterization.[30] This acquired bacteriuria occurs at a rate of about 5–10 per cent per day of catheterization, with 50 per cent of patients bacteriuric within 10–14 days, and virtually all by 6 weeks.[31] Since it is impossible to eliminate catheter-associated infections, and the bacterial flora changes rapidly in patients with chronic indwelling urethral catheters, treatment of asymptomatic bladder bacteriuria or funguria is not recommended.[32] Antibiotic prophylaxis simply promotes the emergence of antibiotic-resistant microbes. Because of the risk of blockage and encrustation and formation of stones on the catheter, it is recommended that it be changed every 4–6 weeks, although the ideal frequency is not known. Patients whose catheter's block are metabolically different from patients without blocked catheters and should receive fresh catheters at 7–10 days to avoid obstruction.[33] It would be appropriate to use a short course of antibiotics around the time of manipulation; the authors use an oral fluoroquinolone for 24 h when changing a catheter has been difficult or traumatic. In some instances, if patients are physically able to or if they have assistance, it can be beneficial to initiate a programme of regular intermittent clean catheterization to maintain low urinary residuals. This technique is useful in both males and females.[34] The frequency may be individualized, depending on bladder capacity. This type of protocol is associated with fewer urinary tract infections and obviates the problems of a long-term indwelling catheter.

Having an intravesical balloon inflated with 5 cc of water as the mechanism of preventing displacement, these urethral catheters may produce considerable bladder irritation and discomfort in some patients, and occasionally, loss of urine around the catheter. Bladder spasms are described as intermittent episodes of excruciating suprapubic discomfort, often associated with leakage of small amounts of urine through the urethra alongside the catheter when the bladder contracts. These can often be reduced by using a catheter with a smaller balloon or evacuating some of the fluid within the balloon. This tip is especially useful if a 30 cc balloon was used initially. In patients in whom this does not provide symptomatic improvement, the use of belladonna and opium (B and O) suppositories *per rectum* every 4 h or low-dose oxybutynin 2.5 mg orally two times per day can be helpful. There is a tendency to treat urine leakage secondary to bladder spasms by increasing the size of the catheter and balloon; this is counterproductive and tends to aggravate the underlying problem.

Failure of the catheter balloon to deflate after aspiration of its contents has been attempted, is not uncommon and can make removal of the catheter difficult or impossible. Gentle passage of a ureteric wire stylet along the inflation channel will puncture the balloon and correct the problem.[35]

Pain

Renal colic

Pain associated with urinary dysfunction represents one of the most distressing types of acute pain. In the absence of personal experience as sufferer or observer, it is unlikely that the distress of severe ureteric colic can be appreciated fully. Induced by acute ureteric obstruction, usually a stone or blood clot, pain in renal distribution is thought to be due to capsular distension. The severe colicky-type pain, which is probably due to ureteric muscle spasm, extends from the costovertebral angle, along the course of the ureter, and radiates to the ipsilateral testis or labium. The associated autonomic outpouring is reflected in a characteristic response associated with severe restlessness, pallor, and diaphoresis. An intravenous opioid, such as morphine, or an intramuscular injection of a non-steroidal anti-inflammatory drug such as ketorolac or diclofenac are effective in relieving this discomfort.[36] Under-dosing is a common error and should be avoided, but, keep in mind that non-steroidal anti-inflammatory drugs may be associated with numerous side effects, including renal failure, gastrointestinal bleeding, and platelet dysfunction, and they must be used with care in the palliative population, especially those with underlying urinary tract obstruction.

Bladder pain

This may be identified as obstructive or irritative.

Obstructive

Chronic distension of the bladder, developing over a period of weeks or months, is usually associated with little more than a sense of fullness in addition to the symptoms of chronic urinary retention. Overflow incontinence may occur. On the other hand, acute retention of sudden onset will produce agonizing lower abdominal pain, severe restlessness, and a constant and compelling urge to void. If the obstruction is not relieved spontaneously or by passage of a catheter, the acute urge will gradually subside but bladder distension will persist. Symptoms, particularly in the elderly and those on opioid drugs, may be masked. Confusion may be the major presenting symptom.

Irritative symptoms

Inflammation of the bladder is most often due to infection and symptoms consist of excessive urinary frequency, dysuria, and urgency incontinence. Dysuria at the end of voiding suggests prostatic origin in the male and trigone in the female.

Irritative bladder symptoms are frequently associated with external radiation and with certain chemotherapeutic agents, such as cyclophosphamide. Idiopathic detrusor instability and central neurological disease may also be responsible. Metabolic abnormalities producing polyuria should be excluded. Intravesical or extravesical tumours may produce irritative bladder symptoms and, along with other agents, may be responsible for the development of bladder spasms, which comprise an exquisitely painful sensation felt mainly in the bladder region. These spasms are due to severe contraction of the detrusor muscle responding to some irritation, usually on the trigone. In addition to tumour, infection, radiation, and calculi may be responsible—irritation is often associated with an indwelling catheter, particularly with encrustation. Treatment of this condition is covered under the section on 'Catheters'.

References

1. **Hutch, J.A.** (1967). A new theory of the anatomy of the internal urinary sphincter and the physiology of micturition. IV. The urinary sphincteric mechanism. *Journal of Urology* **97**, 705–12.
2. **Hutch, J.A. and Rambo, O.A.** (1967). A new theory of the anatomy of the internal urinary sphincter and the physiology of micturition. III. Anatomy of the urethra. *Journal of Urology* **97**, 696–704.
3. **Urinary Incontinence Guideline Panel.** *Urinary Incontinence in Adults: Clinical Practice Guidelines, AHCPR Pub. No. 92-0038.* Rockville MD: Agency for Health Care Policy and Research, Public Health Service, US Department of Health and Human Services, March, 1992.
4. **Chiou, R.K.** et al. (1996). Long-term outcome of prostatic stent treatment for benign prostatic hyperplasia. *Urology* **48**, 589–93.
5. **Feng, M.I., Bellman, G.C., and Shapiro, C.E.** (1999). Management of ureteral obstruction secondary to pelvic malignancies. *Journal of Endourology* **13**, 521–4.
6. **Norman, R.W.** et al. (1982). Acute renal failure secondary to bilateral ureteric obstruction: review of 50 cases. *Canadian Medical Association Journal* **127**, 601–4.
7. **Koelliker, S.L. and Cronan, J.J.** (1997). Acute urinary tract obstruction: imaging update. *Urology Clinics of North America* **24**, 571–82.
8. **Andriole, G.L.** et al. (1984). Indwelling double-J ureteral stents for temporary and permanent urinary drainage: experience with 87 patients. *Journal of Urology* **131**, 239–41.
9. **Lui, J.S. and Hrebinko, R.L.** (1998). The use of two ipsilateral ureteric stents for relief of ureteral obstruction from extrinsic compression. *Journal of Urology* **159**, 179–81.
10. **Ahmed, M.** et al. (1999). Metal mesh stents for ureteral obstruction caused by hormone resistant carcinoma of prostate. *Journal of Endourology* **13**, 221–4.
11. **VanSonnenberg, E.** et al. (1994). Malignant ureteral obstruction: treatment with metal stents—technique, results, and observations with percutaneous untraluminal US. *Radiology* **191**, 765–8.
12. **Pauer, W. and Lugmayr, H.** (1992). Metallic wallstents: a new therapy for extrinsic ureteral obstruction. *Journal of Urology* **148**, 281–4.
13. **Wilcox, D.T., De Bruyn, R., and Mouriquand, P.D.** (1999). The tunnelled nephrosotmy tube. *BJU International* **83**, 506–7.

14. **Mariani, A.J.** et al. (1989). The significance of adult hematuria: 1000 hematuria evaluations including a risk-benefit and cost-effectiveness analysis. *Journal of Urology* **141**, 350–5.

15. **Donahue, L.A. and Frank, I.N.** (1989). Intravesical formalin for hemorrhagic cystitis: analysis of therapy. *Journal of Urology* **141**, 809–12.

16. **DeVries, C.R. and Freiha, F.S.** (1990). Hemorrhagic cystitis: a review. *Journal of Urology* **143**, 1–9.

17. **Singh, I. and Laungani, G.B.** (1992). Intravesical epsilon aminocaproic acid in management of intractable bladder hemorrhage. *Urology* **40**, 227–9.

18. **Levine, L.A. and Jarrard, D.F.** (1993). Treatment of cyclophosphamide-induced hemorrhagic cystitis with intravesical carboprost tromehamine. *Journal of Urology* **149**, 719–23.

19. **Norkool, D.M.** et al. (1993). Hyperbaric oxygen therapy for radiation-induced hemorrhagic cystitis. *Journal of Urology* **150**, 332–4.

20. **Mathews, R.** et al. (1999). Hyperbaric oxygen for radiation induced hemorrhagic cystitis. *Journal of Urology* **161**, 435–7.

21. **Flanigan, R.C.** (1987). The failure of infarction and/or nephrectomy in stage IV renal cell cancer to influence survival or metastatic regression. *Urology Clinics of North America* **14**, 757–62.

22. **McNamara, M.J.** et al. (1990). Surgical treament of enterovesical fistulas in Crohn's disease. *Diseases of the Colon and Rectum* **33**, 271–6.

23. **Pontari, M.A.** et al. (1992). Diagnosis and treatment of enterovesical fistulae. *American Surgery* **58**, 258–63.

24. **Lippert, M.C., Teates, C.D., and Howards, S.S.** (1984). Detection of enteric-urinary fistulas with a non-invasive quantitative method. *Journal of Urology* **132**, 1134–6.

25. **Sou, S.** et al. (1999). Preoperative detection of occult enterovesical fistulas in patients with Crohn's disease: efficacy of oral or rectal administration of indocyanine green solution. *Diseases of the Colon and Rectum* **42**, 266–70.

26. **Manganiotis, A.N., Banner, M.P., and Malkowicz, S.B.** (2001). Urologic complications of Crohn's Disease. *Surgery Clinics of North America* **81**, 197–215.

27. **Leach, G.E. and Trockman, B.A.** (1998). Surgery for vesicovaginal and urethrovaginal fistula and urethral diverticulum. In *Campbell's Urology*. 7th edn. (ed. P.C. Walsh et al.), pp. 1135–53. Philadelphia PA: WB Saunders.

28. **Turner-Warwick, R.** (1986). Urinary fistulae in the female. In *Campbell's Urology* 5th edn. (ed. P.C. Walsh et al.), pp. 2718–38. Philadelphia PA: WB Saunders.

29. **Cravens, D.D. and Zweig, S.** (2000). Urinary catheter management. *American Family Physician* **61**, 369–76.

30. **Platt, R.** et al. (1986). Risk factors for nosocomial urinary tract infection. *American Journal of Epidemiology* **124**, 977–85.

31. **Sedor, J. and Mulholland, S.G.** (1999). Hospital-acquired urinary tract infection associated with the indwelling catheter. *Urology Clinics of North America* **26**, 821–8.

32. **Yoshikawa, T.T., Nicolle, L.E., and Norman, D.C.** (1996). Management of complicated urinary tract infection in older patients. *Journal of the American Geriatric Society* **44**, 1235–41.

33. **Kunin, C.M., Chin, Q.F., and Chambers, S.** (1987). Indwelling urinary catheters in the elderly: relation of 'catheter life' to formation of encrustations in patients with and without blocked catheters. *American Journal of Medicine* **82**, 405–11.

34. **Wyndaele, J.J. and Maes, D.** (1990). Clean intermittent self catheterization: a 12 year follow-up. *Journal of Urology* **143**, 906–8.

35. **Browning, G.G., Barr, L., and Horsburgh, A.G.** (1984). Management of obstructed balloon catheters. *British Medical Journal* **289**, 89–91.

36. **Oosterlinck, W.** et al. (1990). A double-blind single dose comparison of intramuscular ketorolac tromethamine and pethidine in the treatment of renal colic. *Journal of Clinical Pharmacology* **30**, 336–41.

8.11 Head and neck cancer

Barbara A. Murphy, Anthony Cmelak, Steven Bayles, Ellie Dowling, and Cheryl R. Billante

Introduction

By convention, head and neck cancer refers to tumours arising from the epithelial lining of the upper aerodigestive track. This includes patients with tumours of the oral cavity, larynx, pharynx, paranasal sinuses, and salivary glands. There are approximately 50 000 cases of head and neck cancer diagnosed annually within the United States.(1) The vast majority of tumours (>90 per cent) are squamous cell carcinomas. Due to the higher rate of smoking and heavy drinking in males, this type of cancer affects men disproportionately. Nasopharyngeal carcinoma (NPC), while less frequent in the United States and in Europe, is the second most common malignancy in Southeast Asia.(2) NPC, which is associated with Epstein–Barr virus,(3) has a distinct natural history and specific treatment issues. Nonetheless, both squamous and non-squamous cancers of the head and neck share many of the same symptom control issues.

Patients with head and neck cancer experience a wide array of palliative problems. Symptoms may be related to the tumour, acute toxicities of treatment or the long-term sequella of therapy. Although some symptoms are common to all cancers, head and neck cancer patients experience a host of unique problems which require special consideration. In addition, palliation is a major issue throughout the disease trajectory. Symptoms are usually present at the time of diagnosis and remain problematic through the terminal phase. For those patients who are cured, long-term biopsychosocial sequella may persist for years. Thus, assessment and treatment of palliative issues is an intrinsic and vital component of care for the head and neck cancer patient. This chapter will address the palliative issues unique to head and neck cancer patients. It has been divided into four sections: (1) a review of presenting symptoms, initial evaluation, and contemporary treatment; (2) quality of life and psychosocial issues; (3) functional deficits (speech and voice); and (4) symptom control issues specific to head and neck cancer. The reader is referred to other chapters in this text to address general symptom control problems.

Presenting symptoms, initial evaluation, and treatment

Presenting symptoms

As with all patients being evaluated for malignancy, patients with carcinoma arising in the head and neck region demand a comprehensive history and physical examination. A complete history should be obtained with particular attention to type and duration of symptoms. Presenting symptoms are often the result of encroachment of normal structures within the upper aerodigestive system and may be predictive of the primary tumour's location. Symptoms of hoarseness, for example, would implicate laryngeal involvement, whereas dysphagia may be more indicative of hypopharyngeal or oropharyngeal involvement. Many patients' complaints early in the disease process may mimic routine complaints seen in a primary care physician's office, such as sore throat, nasal congestion, hoarseness, swollen glands, and earache. Symptoms not spontaneously resolving or improving within 3 weeks with conservative measures warrant additional attention and specialty evaluation, particularly in patients with clear risk factors of smoking and alcohol use. Attention should be given to more subtle symptoms such as otalgia with no evidence of ear disease, for this may represent referred pain from a lesion of the upper aerodigestive tract. Conductive hearing loss with a unilateral serous otitis media is highly suggestive of a nasopharyngeal mass obstructing the eustachian tube. More ominous symptoms of airway obstruction, oral bleeding and hemoptysis deserve emergent assessment.

Physical examination

A thorough examination involves inspection and palpation of each region of the head and neck. Initial assessment of the skin and scalp area may identify cutaneous malignancies. A complete cranial nerve exam is necessary since patients with advanced carcinomas may display signs of perineural spread or extension into the skull base. Otoscopy is performed to assess for the possibility of serous effusion, which may herald a mass in the nasopharynx obstructing the eustachian tube. Unilateral serous otitis media in an adult demands direct visualization of the nasopharynx. Nasal exam begins with anterior rhinoscopy to assess the vestibule, turbinates, and septum. The oral cavity is then inspected for mucosal abnormalities. Ulceration and leukoplakia are suspicious for malignancy. Bimanual palpation of the oral cavity and the oropharynx is essential to identify submucosal masses that are not visualized by surface change to the mucosa and to assess for contiguous extension of visible primaries. Tumours of the base of tongue and tonsil are often missed because they are not immediately evident on simple oral visualization but can oftentimes be identified by palpation of a firm mass within the region. Fixation of tumour to the mandible and loose dentition are indicative of bony involvement. Trismus may be the result of extension of tumour into the deep pterygomaxillary space. Visualization of the larynx is either accomplished with a mirror examination or more commonly with a fibreoptic scope. The use of a fibreoptic scope through a transnasal route also allows for additional inspection of the nasopharynx and posterior soft palate as well as the larynx and hypopharyngeal inlet. Attention should be given to subsites of laryngeal involvement and the impact that any tumour has on vocal cord mobility, for this ultimately will impact overall tumour stage. The neck is then palpated with attention to nodal basins. The parotids, suboccipital, submental, jugulodigastric and paratracheal nodes are bimanually palpated and any mass is characterized by its size, location, consistency, and mobility. Fixation of nodal metastasis often suggests extracapsular extension with potential involvement of the carotid artery or deep neck musculature, which may be unresectable.

Radiographic and laboratory assessment

CT scans and MRIs are routinely used in the assessment of head and neck carcinoma. MRI imaging can be valuable in assessing skull base involvement and perineural spread of tumour, while CT scans are more useful for bone evaluation and nodal assessment. Work-up must include an evaluation for potential distant metastatic disease. Chest radiographs are used as a routine screening tool; however, additional CT scan of the chest may be warranted in advanced stage disease with large and multiple nodal metastasis. A complete metabolic profile with attention to liver function tests is valuable. Elevations in liver enzymes may prompt CT evaluation of the abdomen for potential hepatic metastasis. Elevations of alkaline phosphatase may herald bony metastasis and warrant bone scanning. PET scans have had a growing role in assessing head and neck carcinomas, most particularly in the assessment of the unknown primary and as a surveillance tool for patients treated with organ preserving chemoradiation protocols, but their routine use is still not defined.

Endoscopy

Operative endoscopy in the form of laryngoscopy, bronchoscopy, and esophagoscopy is commonly performed to completely assess extension of tumour not easily viewed in the office. Patients with a known head and neck primary carcinoma additionally carry a 5–15 per cent risk of a synchronous primary elsewhere in the aerodigestive tract necessitating inspection of these sites. Additionally, due to the complexity and overlap of mucosal folds within the oral cavity, oropharynx, pharynx, and hypopharynx, standard images often fail to delineate the exact location of a tumour. For example, a tumour arising on the postcricoid aspect of the larynx on CT scan cannot be differentiated from a tumour arising on the posterior pharyngeal wall behind the larynx because these two surfaces are in contact with one another. Operative endoscopy offers the opportunity to manipulate the region, lift the larynx off the posterior pharyngeal wall, and define the site of origin and extent of the tumour. Mapping of the tumour becomes critical in assessing the ability to resect the tumour and defining the potential defect that would be created so a reconstructive effort may be planned.

Treatment and outcome

Upon completion of the initial evaluation, the tumour is characterized based on stage and the site of origin. The staging process must be carried out in a thorough and deliberate fashion since both treatment and outcome are heavily dependent on the extent of disease and the site of primary. Patients with early stage tumours ($T_{1-2}N_0M_0$) have a cure rate of between 70 and 90 per cent with either radiation or surgery.[4] Unfortunately, the majority of patients present with locally advanced disease (T_{3-4} or N+). Historically, patients with *locally advanced*, disease were divided into surgically resectable and unresectable groups. Patients with resectable disease were treated with surgery followed by radiation therapy to eliminate microscopic residual disease. Depending on the stage and the site of primary, 3-year survival for patients with resectable locally advanced disease was 30–70 per cent. In select patients, surgical based treatment was found to lead to severe functional compromise. Patients at particular risk for poor functional outcome with a surgical approach included those patients with laryngeal, hypopharyngeal, and base-of-tongue primaries. For patients with *unresectable disease*, radiation therapy was utilized as a single modality. Results of treatment with radiation alone was poor (2-year survival 5–20 per cent). Clinical research over the past two decades has focused on the use of altered fractionation radiation therapy, induction chemotherapy followed by radiation (ICR), and concomitant chemoradiation (CCR) as: (1) a means to avoid morbid surgical procedures; and (2) to improve survival in patients with advanced, unresectable disease.[5]

Recent studies have confirmed the efficacy of chemoradiation as a tissue sparing treatment option for patients with locally advanced resectable carcinomas (stage III or stage IV disease). Two seminal randomized phase III studies have been reported which directly compared surgery followed by radiation versus tissue sparing therapy with ICR: the Veterans Affairs Laryngeal Cancer Study Group[6] and the EORTC hypopharynx trial.[7] Results demonstrated equivalent survival between the chemoradiation and surgical treatment arms. Forty-two to 64 per cent of patients were able to avoid laryngectomy with ICR. More recently, the ECOG reported the results of a randomized phase III comparison of radiation alone, ICR, and CCR in patients with laryngeal carcinomas. The results demonstrated equivalent overall survival for all three treatment arms; however, larynx preservation was achieved in 55, 65, and 85 per cent of patients respectively. The difference in larynx preservation between radiation alone and CCR was statistically significant. Thus, CCR has become the standard method for treatment of HNC patients who wish to undergo function sparing therapy. The added role of induction chemotherapy or hyperfractionated radiation has yet to be determined.

CCR has also been extensively investigated in patients with unresectable disease. A number of phase III trials have been reported a clinically meaningful and statistically significant survival advantage with CCR compared to radiation alone.[8–23] In addition, three meta-analyses (two literature-based and one patient-based) evaluating the role of chemotherapy in the primary treatment of squamous carcinoma of the head and neck, have now been reported.[24–26] All three identified a survival advantage for patients receiving CCR. Data from Bourhis reported a 19 per cent relative risk reduction and an absolute survival benefit of 8 per cent at 5 years ($p = 0.0001$).[26] Thus, both randomized phase III trials and three meta-analyses demonstrate superior survival and local control rates for patients treated with concomitant chemoradiation.

Of note, CCR is associated with increase in both acute and long-term toxicities. The clinician is, therefore, challenged to provide sufficient symptom control to ensure completion of this aggressive therapy. In addition, attempts to minimize long-term sequella of treatment through rehabilitation, nutritional counselling and general support services is mandatory.

Quality of life and psychosocial issues

Quality of life

There are four core domains included in health-related quality of life (QOL): function, emotional, social, and physical well being. The treatment of head and neck cancer can have a tremendous impact on all four parameters. Historically, QOL research in HNC patients has been limited by: (1) lack of adequate tool; (2) lack of prospective data collection with appropriate baseline and long term follow-up; (3) inadequate power due to small sample size; and (4) heterogeneous patient selection and lack of treatment uniformity. Over the past decade, numerous tools have been developed to assess QOL in patients with cancer. The two most commonly used are the Functional Assessment of Cancer Therapy (FACT/FACIT)[27] and the European Organization for Research into the Treatment of Cancer Quality of Life Questionnaire for Head and Neck Cancer (EORTC QLQ-30). Both of these instruments have head and neck subscales which address disease specific symptoms. The sensitivity, reliability, validity, and responsiveness to change of these tools have been well summarized in a recent review of QOL instruments for HNC.[28] Prospective QOL assessments using these and other validated tools are now being reported. These studies have provided intriguing results. Of particular interest are studies that: (1) evaluate the long-term effects of surgery, radiation, or chemoradiation; (2) compare surgical to radiation based approaches; and (3) evaluate the outcome of function preservation therapies. To date, little QOL data is available in patients with metastatic, refractory or terminal disease.

Long-term QOL outcome with HNC therapy

Regardless of the treatment approach used, patients with HNC experience an initial drop in QOL post-treatment. The QOL then rises slowly towards baseline levels as acute symptoms abate, function improves, and as patients adapt to new physical limitations. Using the University of Washington QOL tool (UW-QOL), Rogers et al.[29] assessed pretreatment QOL in 48 patients undergoing surgical resection for oral cavity tumours. QOL was reassessed at 3 and 12 months. Twenty-five of 29 surviving patients completed the 1-year post-treatment assessment. The results demonstrate a drop in overall QOL 3 months after primary surgery with a return to pre-treatment levels at 12 months. Investigators were able to identify prognostic indicators for poor outcome which included: more advanced stage, the need for adjuvant radiation and anterior oral cavity lesions.[29] Similarly, Murry et al.[30] reported the QOL outcome of 58 patients treated with intra-arterial chemoradiation for organ preservation. Overall QOL and physical/functional parameters worsened with therapy. At 6 months, overall QOL had improved above baseline. The degree of QOL improvement was site specific with laryngeal and hypopharyngeal cancer patients showing improved QOL, while QOL was unchanged for patients with oral cavity tumours. This study was limited by the relatively low number of patients who completed the 6 month assessment ($n = 27$).[30]

QOL with function preservation therapy

The role of function preservation therapy has been hotly debated over the past two decades. Current data would indicate that surgical and radiation-based approaches provide similar survival. Thus, the impact of function preservation on QOL and functional outcome is crucial for making treatment decisions. In an analysis of 46 of 65 surviving patients treated on the VA laryngeal preservation protocol, patients treated with function preservation had improved in mental health and emotional domains.[31] Similarly, Larto et al.[32] compared the QOL of patients with laryngeal tumors treated with radiation versus radiation plus concomitant chemotherapy. Acute toxicities were worse for patients receiving combined modality therapy but long-term QOL outcome parameters were improved. The investigators hypothesized that patients treated with combined modality therapy had a higher rate of larynx preservation which resulted in an improvement in QOL. Weymuller evaluated QOL in 210 consecutive patients treated with either primary surgery or radiation. Composite QOL scores were *not* affected by treatment method (surgery versus chemoradiation) with the exception of 12 patients with advanced laryngeal cancer.[33] In this cohort, QOL was better for patients treated with chemoradiation (achieved statistical significance at 2 years). Karnell et al.[34] assessed QOL in patients 2–12 months post-treatment using the Head and Neck Health Status Assessment Inventory. Results demonstrated voice and swallowing to be the two most predictive factors for overall QOL with correlation coefficient of 0.61 for voice and 0.48 for eating ($R^2 = 0.4647$). Unfortunately, the sample size was small ($n = 62$) and treatment was mixed (surgery, RT or both). Thus, the bulk of currently available data would support the hypotheses that function preservation therapy results in better long-term QOL.

QOL as a means of evaluation of physical function and symptom control

Although it has long been recognized that the patients with HNC are profoundly affected by both their tumour and their treatment, it is only of late that the extent of disability, function loss, and social dysfunction have begun to be appreciated. This is largely due to the growing quality of life data that highlights previously unrecognized problems. In a recent report by de Graff et al.[35] 153 patients with HNC were assessed at baseline, 6 and 12 months post-treatment using the EORTC QLQ-30/HN-35 and the Center for Epidemiologic Studies Depression scale. They identified two pre-treatment factors, depression and poor physical function, that were associated with poor post-treatment physical and psychological function. This study was well conducted and methodologically sound; however, the patient population was heterogeneous (patients with all stages of disease and all treatment modalities were included). In a cross-sectional assessment of 65 HNC patients more than 6 months post-therapy, Epstein reported pain in 58 per cent, mood disorders in more than 50 per cent, interference in social activities in 60 per cent, adverse effects on financial status 57 per cent, and limitations of work/housework for 41.5 per cent. Although quality of life studies do not provide solutions to the many symptom control problems faced by HNC patients, they do provide insight which will allow the design and testing of interventions.

Comorbid disease

Primary risk factors for HNC include smoking and drinking, both of which may lead to the development of comorbid disease. Using the Modified Medical Comorbidity Index, a modification of the Kaplan–Feinstein Index, Piccirillo[36] reported that 21 per cent of head and neck cancer patients have moderate to severe comorbid disease. Table 1 summarizes the results of four studies comparing the 5-year survival of HNC patients with and without significant comorbid disease. Patients with significant comorbid disease are less likely to tolerate therapy and appear to have a worse treatment outcome. Furthermore, alcoholism is an independent risk factor for survival in HNC.[37] Thus, an extensive medical evaluation is mandatory for all patients prior to initiating therapy.

Socioeconomic status

In addition to complex medical problems, patients with HNC have significant psychosocial issues. After treatment, patients often experience prolonged treatment side effects and increasing social isolation. Using QOL questionnaires, Epstein et al.[42] reported on the psychosocial effect of HNC on a cohort of patients who had completed therapy. Moderate or severe adverse effects were reported on social interactions (44.6 per cent), family interactions (44.6 per cent) and finances (56.9 per cent). In addition, the prevalence of 'significant' psychological symptoms was high, with irritability (13.4 per cent), tension (15.2 per cent), depression (12.3 per cent), and worry (16.9 per cent) predominating. In a separate study reported by D'antonio,[43] 20 per cent of HNC patients who had completed therapy had either moderate or severe depression. For patients who undergo disfiguring

Table 1 Survival based on comorbid status using the Kaplan–Feinstein Grading System

Study	Site	Patient number	5-year overall survival (%)	
			Comorbidities	No comorbidities
Feinstein et al.[38]	Larynx	192	15	54
Piccirillo et al.[39]	Larynx	193	15	74
Pugliano et al.[40]	Oropharynx	281	18	40
Pugliano et al.[41]	Oral cavity	277	10	49

Table 2 Survival and economic status in HNC patients

Income group	Survival (%)
Quintile 1	65.4
Quintile 2	60.1
Quintile 3	60.6
Quintile 4	60.3
Quintile 5	51.7

surgery, diminished self image can result in further increase in social isolation and diminished QOL.[44,45]

Unfortunately, HNC patients frequently have few resources to cope with complex array of medical and psychological problems. In a study of the long term psychosocial implications of surgery for head and neck cancer patients, over half of patients were unable to return to work after treatment.[46] The financial implications for the patient and the patient's family may be significant. Inadequate resources may impact on both QOL and survival. In a recent report from Canada, patients with a lower socioeconomic status had worse treatment outcomes than patients with a higher socioeconomic status. The cause-specific 5-year survival was from 65.4 per cent in the highest quintile compared to 51.7 per cent in the lowest quintile (CL 11.1–16.3) (Table 2).[47] Providing adequate medical and psychosocial support for HNC patients can challenge the treatment team. Aggressive social work involvement is needed from the time of diagnosis and throughout treatment to aid the patient and the treatment team and optimize therapeutic outcome.

Functional deficits: swallowing and voice (see Chapter 15.5)

Head and neck cancer may profoundly affect two vital life functions: swallowing and vocalization. Abnormalities in swallowing and voice may be the result of either progressive tumour or treatment-related sequella.[48,49] Functional damage due to tumour may be irreparable; however, investigators have attempted to identify therapies which optimize outcome. 'Function preservation' or 'tissue sparing' treatment is directed at providing patients with a curative treatment that limits function loss. Techniques which have been investigated as potential function sparing approaches include: function sparing surgery, altered fractionation radiation therapy, and CCR.[5]

For early stage diseases, both surgery and radiation-based function preservation approaches have become standard treatment options.[50] Radiation therapy as a single modality has long been utilized as a treatment for patient with stage I, stage II, and good risk stage III squamous carcinomas of the larynx. Over the past two decades, surgical function sparing therapies have been also become popular. Such techniques include: microflap resection of carcinoma *in situ*, partial cordotomy, total cordotomy, supraglottic laryngectomies, and hemilaryngectomies. As with single modality radiation therapy, the majority of function-sparing surgical approaches have demonstrated feasibility in patients with early stage disease. While surgery and radiation have long been accepted as function sparing approaches for early stage disease (stage I and stage II), it is only within the past decade that function-preserving approaches using ICR or CCR have been utilized in locally advanced head and neck carcinomas (stage III and stage IV). As data has accumulated, concern has been expressed that tissue-preserving therapy may not result in good functional outcome, particularly in patients treated with aggressive regimens.[42] Thus, there is tremendous interest in the evaluation and comparison of functional outcome for patients treated with either a surgical or radiation-based approach. The outcome parameters of the most vital interest are swallowing and voice.

When addressing functional issues in patients with HNC one must frame the discussion in a meaningful manner. It is often helpful to distinguish functional impairment from disability and handicap. Most HNC patients have an amazing ability to adapt to functional deficits. However, functional deficits may lead to disability (effect of dysfunction on self) or handicap (effect of dysfunction in relationship to others). More often than not, physicians are unaware of the extent and severity of functional deficits, disabilities, and handicaps experienced by their patients.[51] Rehabilitation services can more effectively identify the type and extent of functional deficits. In selected patients, therapy can be undertaken to improve function and minimize the disability and handicap resulting from function loss.

Swallowing

Swallow function and dysfunction

Swallowing is a complex series of mechanical processes that allows for nutritional intake. It can be broken down into several phases: oral, pharyngeal, and oesophageal. The oral phase can be described as having two separate components: the oral preparation phase and the oral transport phase.[52] During the oral phase, the lips and tongue play a vital role in oral bolus preparation and bolus propulsion to the oropharynx. During the subsequent pharyngeal phase, the tongue acts as the driving force for the food bolus while a complex sequence of physiologic processes propels the bolus towards the oesophagus. These physiologic processes include: (1) closure of the velopharyngeal port; (2) elevation and anterior movement of the larynx and hyoid; (3) closure of the larynx at the level of the true and false vocal cords and epiglottis; and (4) opening of the upper oesophageal sphincter allowing for bolus passage into the oesophagus.[53] The pharyngeal phase takes about 800 ms from entry of the pharynx to exit into the oesophagus.[54] The oesophageal phase, which typically lasts 8–20 s, begins at the cricopharyngeal juncture or upper oesophageal sphincter and ends at the gastroesophageal juncture or lower oesophageal sphincter. Oesophageal peristalsis carries the bolus to the stomach.

Deficits in any one of these phases can result in significant levels of disability. Swallowing dysfunction may require patients to substantially alter the consistencies and type of foods they ingest. These dietary changes may lead to nutritional deficits and the numerous complications of malnutrition. Furthermore, functional deficits may lead to handicaps such as inability to eat in public or at social gatherings. The most severe complication of swallowing dysfunction is aspiration. Patients who aspirate are at risk for pneumonia. In the stroke population, aspiration results in 40 000 deaths per year.[55] The number of deaths due to aspiration in the HNC population is unknown. Lundy et al.[56] reported on 166 consecutive patients referred for swallowing evaluation with various underlying medical problems. Eighty patients had neurologic problems, 38 medical problems and 33 HNC. HNC patients had the highest rate of aspiration with a total of 76 versus 49 per cent for patients with a neurologic diagnosis and 43 per cent of patients who had a medical diagnosis. Thus, it is likely that aspiration is a significant and frequently unrecognized problem in the HNC population. It is imperative that physicians are aware of the possibility of aspiration in this patient population and that appropriate evaluation and therapy be undertaken when indicated.

Assessment of swallowing dysfunction

Various instrumental techniques have been used to study swallowing, including electromyography, manometry, scintigraphy, ultrasound, endoscopy, and videofluoroscopy. The most commonly used technique in the clinical setting and what is considered 'the gold standard' for swallowing assessment is the videofluoroscopy, also referred to as the modified barium swallow study (MBSS). The MBSS provides information on oral and pharyngeal transit deficits as well as the presence, and most importantly etiology of aspiration. The MBSS also provides information to the clinician regarding the effectiveness of diet modification and compensatory strategies that may be utilized to improve swallowing safety and function.

Pre-treatment swallowing abnormalities

To clearly understand the effect of therapy on swallowing abnormalities in HNC patients, prospective longitudinal studies are needed. Unfortunately, few studies have been conducted in this manner. The majority of studies are cross-sectional evaluations of swallowing function after therapy has been completed. Thus, baseline data is missing. Stenson et al.[57] undertook an analysis of HNC patients prior to treatment in order to provide insight into the baseline swallowing abnormalities. The tools selected for assessment were the MBSS and the Swallowing Performance Status Scale (SPSS). The SPSS is a global assessment tool for reporting the results of a MBSS. It is rated on a scale of 1 (normal) to 7 (severe impairment—requires PEG tube). As expected, the type of impairment was site specific with oral cavity and oropharynx tumours manifesting oral impairment, larynx and hypopharynx tumours manifesting pharyngeal impairment, and hypopharyngeal tumours manifesting oesophageal impairment. The degree of impairment was site specific with hypopharyngeal and laryngeal patients experiencing the most impaired swallowing with a SPSS score of 4.1 and 3.7, respectively. Similarly, patients with hypopharyngeal and laryngeal carcinomas were the most likely to experience aspiration (80 and 67 per cent respectively). Interestingly, there was no association between T-stage or overall stage and swallowing dysfunction. The high rate of baseline swallowing dysfunction underscores the need for prospective trials in order to clearly ascertain the long-term effects of treatment.

Post-treatment swallowing abnormalities

Patients who undergo surgery of an organ involved in swallowing may expect some alteration in function. The degree of functional deficit is largely dependent on the extent of surgery. McConnel et al.[58] evaluated 30 patients who underwent resection of oral cavity cancers. The percentage of oral and tongue base resected were the only parameters prognostic for swallowing outcome. This has been confirmed by other investigators.[59] In addition to extent of resection, Logemann and Bytell[60] demonstrated that the degree of swallowing dysfunction was also related to the site of resection. Patients undergoing floor of mouth or tongue base resections had more swallowing difficulty than those undergoing supraglottic laryngectomies.[60] Adjuvant radiation may worsen postoperative swallowing by increasing edema, fibrosis and xerostomia.[61] Finally, the method of reconstruction may also effect functional outcome.

Swallowing abnormalities have also been noted in patients who undergo primary radiation therapy. These deficits can be divided into abnormalities related to acute toxicities and those associated with long-term effects. Acutely during therapy, patients develop severe mucosal ulcers and soft tissue edema. These result in painful swallowing and dysphagia. Acute toxicities resolve slowly within 4–12 weeks of completing therapy. Late effects may begin to appear simultaneous with the resolution of acute toxicities. Persistent oedema and the development of fibrosis result in mechanical alterations in swallow function. Swallowing abnormalities can be seen in the oral preparation, oral, pharyngeal, and oesophageal phases. The most commonly identified swallowing abnormalities include: decreased tongue base retraction, decreased laryngeal elevation, decreased epiglottic inversion, decreased pharyngeal wall motion and aspiration. Fortunately, in many cases, patients are able to tolerate oral diets with various modifications to prevent aspiration and improve swallow efficiency.[62]

Recently, considerable effort has been directed at attempts to identify patients who are at risk for poor swallowing function after radiation-based therapy. Kendall et al.[63] conducted a study of swallowing function in patients 12 months after primary radiation therapy. Although flawed by the lack of baseline measurements, they demonstrated abnormal swallowing in all patients. Of significance, the tongue base tumours were found to have a high incidence of aspiration. This has been confirmed by other investigators. Using the Head and Neck Radiotherapy Questionnaire and a swallowing questionnaire, Murry et al.[30] identified disease site as a predictor for swallowing outcome after aggressive treatment with intra-arterial chemoradiation for organ preservation. In addition to site specificity as potential predictors for swallowing outcome, retrospective studies of primary radiation therapy demonstrate a worse functional outcome for patients with a higher T-stage. Risk factors for poor functional outcome may also include a patient's characteristics which reflect general health and psychosocial support.

Of interest, patients often attribute difficulty swallowing to xerostomia. Logemann et al.[64] evaluated the effect of xerostomia on bolus transport in patients treated with chemoradiation. Although patients with xerostomia perceived swallowing deficits, bolus transport was unaffected.[64] Xerostomia does affect mastication and oral manipulation of dry food.[65]

Various techniques are available for swallowing therapy and rehabilitation; however, the role of swallowing therapy in head and neck cancer patients remains to be clarified. Issues that require further study include: (1) the optimal techniques for specific deficits; (2) timing of therapy (does pre-treatment versus post-treatment intervention improve outcome?); (3) duration of therapy; and (4) identification of those most likely to benefit. Dejonckere reported the results of a retrospective analysis of swallowing function in 88 patients who have completed therapy: 87 per cent were treated with surgery with or without post-operative radiation and 13 per cent were treated with radiation. Post-treatment, all patients underwent evaluation of swallowing function followed by rehabilitation. Rehabilitation lasted less than 12 weeks for 45 per cent of patients and less than 24 weeks for 78 per cent of patients. Patients underwent reassessment post-treatment. There was a marked improvement in swallowing function ($p = 0.0001$) post-treatment. Nine of 82 patients had significant swallowing abnormalities post rehabilitation. While this study does not have a control arm and some degree of improvement over time should be expected, it appears that swallowing therapy does improve outcome.

Voice

The ability to communicate is a critical human function and vocalization is our most important communication method. Without an intact voice, patients often become isolated and experience a marked decrease in their social interactions. Furthermore, conducting activities of daily living may be difficult without vocal ability. Treatment of HNC often necessitates resection of structures critical to the production of normal speech, resonance, and voice. Further, resection of a malignancy may require sacrifice of the nerve supply which innervates these structures, leaving the patient with paralysis of the tongue, pharynx, palate, or larynx. In general, the greater the extent of resection, the more severe the resultant communication disorder. Primary or adjuvant radiation may also affect vocalization. The speech–language pathologist is an integral member of the multidisciplinary team which carries out the comprehensive care and complex rehabilitation of these patients. Listed below are brief descriptions of the voice abnormalities noted in HNC patients. For further information on evaluation and treatment, please see Chapter 15.5 on Speech and Language Therapy.

Disordered speech

Lip

Most early lip lesions can be effectively treated with resection or radiation therapy. Small local wedge shaped defects can be closed primarily. More serious tissue deficits can be reconstructed with pedicle flaps.[66] This may results in altered articulation of bilabial sounds /b, p, m/, and labiodental sounds /f,/v/. Injury to the second and third branches of the trigeminal nerve disrupts sensation to the lips, while motor function is supplied by a branch of CN VII (upper lip) or marginal mandibular nerve (lower lip). Labial paralysis prevents normal articulation of related sounds.

Tongue

Reconstruction of lingual tissue defects are usually achieved with primary closure or local, regional, or distant flaps. In the case of minor deficits, speech and swallowing can be largely preserved. However, in the case of advanced disease, total glossectomy severely alters articulation. In such cases, the focus of speech therapy is to maximize remaining function through range of motion and flexibility drills, and to devise alternative articulatory placements for affected speech sounds. In cases where disability is extreme, an augmentative system of communication, such as computerized speech is indicated. A prosthesis may be helpful in rehabilitating the communication of the glossectomy patient. Involvement or sacrifice of the hypoglossal nerve creates a unilateral lingual paralysis. Dysarthria, weak and imprecise articulation, is the resulting speech disability.

Teeth

Loss of or extraction of teeth associated with tumour involvement or radiation therapy, or mandibular osteoradionecrosis, can negatively impact articulation and overall intelligibility. Lingual and labiodental placements may be modified and speech therapy may provide compensatory articulatory postures.

Hard palate

Hard palate defects resulting from maxillary involvement of tumor potentially affect the production of lingua-alveolar sounds [t, d, n, l] and lingual-palatal sounds [sh, zh, ch, j]. Often a flap is used to close the defect. Alternatively, the team prosthodontist can design an obturator to cover and seal the defect to generally normalize articulation of these sounds.[66]

Disordered resonance

During speech production, the soft palate makes contact with the posterior pharyngeal wall to separate the nasal and oral cavities, and allow for normal articulation of 'plosive' consonants such as /p, b, k, g, t, d, ch, sh/. In the patient with unilateral palatal paralysis, the inability of the soft palate to contact the posterior pharyngeal wall creates a constant air leak in the vocal tract. The abnormal leak of air through the nose during speech production results in a hypernasal quality to the voice. When severe, the patient's speech may be distorted to the point of being unintelligible.[67] Vocal volume is abnormally soft, because as much as 10 dB of sound is lost through the nose.[68] When a malignancy requires surgical resection of the soft palate, the resulting tissue deficit creates velopharyngeal insufficiency. Similarly, when tumour involvement or its removal necessitates disruption of cranial nerves IX or X, the resulting unilateral palatal paralysis creates a velopharyngeal gap.

There are several options to restore velopharyngeal closure if the neurologic input to these structures is intact. When the velopharyngeal gap is minimal, behavioural therapy may facilitate over articulation of speech sounds sufficient to reduce nasality and optimize intelligibility.[69] However, in the case of a moderately sized or large gap, a surgical solution for velopharyngeal incompetence is indicated. Gaps of small to moderate size have been managed with a pharyngeal wall implant, which moves the posterior pharyngeal wall into range of contact with soft palate elevation. Silicone, Teflon, and collagen have been used, but migration of these substances has been a concern.[70,71] The most popular surgical solution has traditionally been a pharyngeal flap. In this procedure, a superiorly based flap from the posterior pharyngeal wall is sutured to the velum to bridge the space and obturate the gap.

In the case of palatal paralysis following involvement or sacrifice of the vagus nerve for skull base tumors, a palatal adhesion effectively eliminates hypernasality and nasal regurgitation. In this procedure, the paralysed side of the soft palate is sutured to the posterior pharyngeal wall to close the gap between the oral and nasal cavities.[72] Alternatively, a palatal lift prosthesis can be fashioned to place the soft palate in a position favourable to assist velopharyngeal contact. In the most severe cases of velopharyngeal incompetence, where a lack of tissue prevents a flap procedure, a speech bulb/obturator can be fitted by the prosthodontist. The appliance fills the velopharyngeal space as the lateral pharyngeal walls move to snugly surround the bulb.[73]

Disordered voice

Neurologic abnormalities

The voice disorder resulting from laryngeal paralysis is extremely debilitating. Most patients present with a very soft, breathy voice quality or even a whisper.[74] Attempts to force enough vocal volume to be heard results in rapid fatigue of laryngeal and respiratory muscles, and patients may avoid communication because of the effort required. The lack of volume is very problematic or potentially dangerous for patients who work in a noisy environment or who must communicate with hard-of-hearing family members. Professional voice users, such as teachers or salespeople may be unable to fulfil the vocal demands of their work, and may find their career in jeopardy.

In patients with unilateral vocal fold paralysis, medialization laryngoplasty is performed to reposition the immobile vocal fold into a more favourable midline position to allow contact with its contra lateral, mobile partner.[75] A small silastic implant is placed lateral to the paralysed vocal fold, which pushes the muscle toward the laryngeal midline. Improved vocal fold contact restores voice and prevents aspiration. Studies have documented that voice quality is normal or better following phonosurgery.[76,77] Injection of collagen has been recommended for vocal fold immobility.[78] Numerous other materials have been evaluated for vocal fold immobility. New concern over potential bioreaction has prompted testing of autologous materials. Injection of fat tissue has been found to improve glottal closure in case of laryngeal paresis;[79,80] however, its abbreviated life span of less than 12 months has been corroborated histologically.

Surgical organ preservation procedures

Operative procedures which spare some glottic structures and mobility yield varying voice results. Vocal cordectomy or cordotomy remove a portion of the sound source of phonation, and create a breathy dysphonia. When a malignancy involves one vocal fold and surrounding structures, a vertical hemilaryngectomy may provide a mechanism for voicing; the uninvolved vocal fold vibrates against the tissue of the neolarynx, preserving a functional voice. In the case of supraglottic tumour, the entire laryngeal vestibule may be excised, with the membranous vocal folds left intact to provide for phonation.[81] When laryngeal cancer requires a supracricoid laryngectomy, all laryngeal structures above the level of the glottis are removed as well as the membranous vocal folds. In general, one or both mobile arytenoid cartilages are spared.[82] The arytenoids approximate on adduction and make contact with the base of tongue to produce a vibratory source and generate 'voice'. In general, the voice quality is very breathy and low-pitched. Finally, the near total-laryngectomy requires removal of an entire hemilarynx and the anterior two-thirds of the contra lateral hemilarynx. The laryngeal remnant is not sufficient to allow normal air exchange, so a permanent tracheostoma is constructed.[83] A tracheopharyngeal tract is created to form a vibratory source for sound production. Voice quality is very similar to that achieved with a tracheoesophageal voice prosthesis.

Total laryngectomy

There are several options for rehabilitation of communication in the patient who undergoes total laryngectomy. An artificial larynx (electrolarynx) is a device which provides an external sound source. The most common type of electrolarynx is a small, handheld machine which is placed against the neck or into the mouth with a tubular adapter. The patient's articulation of speech sounds is superimposed over the robotic sound source to produce a mechanical-sounding voice. The greatest advantage of the electrolarynx is that it provides immediacy of communication. With minimal training on placement and overarticulation, the patient can begin to 'speak' in the perioperative period.[84] A second type of speech method is the use of oesophageal speech. This requires a long commitment to therapy but allows for greatest communicative independence. In this method, air is pumped via swallow or inhaled into the cervical oesophagus and immediately exhaled. The pharyngoesophageal segment is vibrated by the expelled air and sound is produced, similar to a controlled belch.[85] Generally, the patient can produce a few syllables per air change. Some patients become quite proficient at this, and not have to rely on a mechanical or prosthetic device to communicate. Creation of a tracheoesophageal tract allows insertion of a one-way valve. With the stoma occluded, air from the lungs is shunted through the prosthesis and into the oesophagus. The air vibrates tissue in the superior aspect of the oesophagus to produce sound.[86] The patient uses the sound to articulate audible voice. The advantage of prosthetic speech over esophageal speech is that the patient removes the device periodically for cleaning. More recently, the development of indwelling prostheses allows a patient to wear the device for several months without removal.

Specific symptom control issues

Airway control

The impact that advanced head and neck carcinoma has on the aerodigestive system often leads to progressive airway compromise. The inability to swallow and handle secretions or breath as a direct result of extension of tumour into the airway presents one of the most distressing symptoms of progressive disease. The airway must be divided into multiple levels—the nasal cavity, nasopharynx, oral cavity, oropharynx, larynx, extrathoracic and intrathoracic trachea, and lungs. Obstruction can occur in any area along the airway and the symptoms and treatment differ depending on the level of obstruction. Initial assessment of the airway begins with an observation of breathing pattern to determine grossly the level of airway obstruction. Mouth breathing with normal inspiratory and expiratory duration and without noise may be indicative of purely nasal obstruction; whereas, sonorous mouth breathing without stridor would suggest obstruction at the level of base of tongue or oral cavity that could be immediately palliated with a nasal trumpet and upright positioning until more definitive procedure could be performed. Inspiratory or biphasic stridor is more indicative of a fixed laryngotracheal obstruction, which will likely require bypass, most often in the form of a tracheostomy. Anxiety, agitation, confusion, and claustrophobia are all signs of progressive hypercarbia and air hunger resulting from obstruction and immediate intervention is warranted. Flexible fibre-optic laryngoscopy can be performed to further assess the mass effect of the tumour and its overall degree of obstruction. Laryngoscopy also permits a determination as to whether a patient may be amenable to intubation in the event of complete airway loss. Additional factors such trismus, and neck immobility from prior radiation or direct tumour involvement may however complicate intubation, and a tracheostomy under local anaesthetic may be simpler than an attempted intubation which may result in loss of the airway due to inability to expose the larynx. If the tumour is extremely friable, then a tracheostomy under local anaesthetic may be more prudent to avoid manipulation of the tumour. Ultimately for patients with known incurable disease, an honest discussion with the patient about the potential future need for tracheostomy and early placement may avoid emergent intervention under duress.

The most common and definitive procedure that can be offered is a tracheostomy. This can be performed under local or general anaesthesia. An incision is made approximately 1–2 cm below the cricoid cartilage, either vertically or horizontally. The strap muscles of the neck are reflected laterally to provide access to the trachea. If the thyroid isthmus is encountered, it may be ligated or reflected superiorly or inferiorly for exposure of the trachea. The trachea is generally entered between tracheal rings 2 and 3, however, may be entered lower if necessary to bypass any subglottic extension of tumour. Tracheostomy tubes come in a variety of sizes and shapes depending on the individual vendor, however, most generally have three components—an outer cannula, an inner cannula, and an obturator. The obturator is placed through the outer cannula to provide a smooth tip to allow for easy insertion. Once the tracheostomy has been inserted, the obturator is removed and an inner cannula is inserted into the outer cannula. The inner cannula can be removed frequently to facilitate cleaning and prevent plugging of the tracheostomy. The initial tracheostomy change should be performed by the surgeon, but after a mature tract has formed, usually within 1–2 weeks, the tracheostomy can be changed with ease by the patient or care provider. The tracheostomy is maintained patent by encouraging patients to cough. Additional saline lavage and deep suctioning can also clear secretions and should be done routinely initially every 4 h and as needed. Patients often need supplemental humidification to thin secretions when they have a tracheostomy, for the natural humidification provided by airflow through the mouth and nose is lost when the upper airway is bypassed. A bedside humidifier, humidified trach collar, and frequent instillation of saline drops through the tracheostomy can provide the necessary humidification. The addition of mucolytics such as guaifenesin or nebulized Mucomyst may be of added benefit to patients with thick secretions, which are difficult to clear. Added modifications to tracheostomy tubes include high volume low-pressure cuffs. A cuffed tube is initially placed at the time of surgery to prevent any blood from passing distally into the airway, Cuffed tracheostomy tubes, however, are usually only necessary for patients requiring positive pressure ventilation, which requires a seal of the trachea to achieve the necessary pressure. A common misconception is that patients need a cuffed tube to prevent aspiration of secretions around the tracheostomy tube from above. Inflation of a cuff places pressure on the posterior common party wall between the trachea and oesophagus, and this added obstruction to the oesophagus can actually induce greater secretion pooling and potentiate aspiration to a degree. In general after a mature tract has formed, a cuffless tracheostomy tube can be used in the cancer patient, which will permit enough collateral flow around the tube, if appropriately sized, to allow a patient to occlude the lumen with a finger or a passy-muir valve and still speak. Another modification to the tracheostomy tube is the addition of a fenestrated opening in the canula to permit added airflow past the trach with occlusion of the lumen. This design is meant to enhance glottal airflow with occlusion and improve speech. However, fenestrations in the trach tube often create a rough surface, which incite granulation tissue formation in the airway that can be problematic. The added benefit of a fenestrated tube is often minimal and should be used only with reservation.

Nutrition (see also Sub-section 8.4)

Nutritional deficits are present in a high per cent of patients with newly diagnosed or recurrent HNC. Malnutrition is often multi-factorial in nature. Careful assessment and treatment of weight loss and the institution of preventive measures during therapy are mandatory to optimize therapeutic outcome. Clinical trials have demonstrated that weight loss at the time of diagnosis is prognostic for survival and ability to tolerate treatment.[87–89] Further studies have demonstrated that aggressive nutritional intervention can minimize weight loss and decrease treatment related toxicity.[90] Thus, aggressive nutritional intervention is an important component of care for HNC patients. In addition, the presence of cytokines known to be associated with cancer cachexia (tumour necrosis factor and Interleukin-6) may carry prognostic value.[91]

Prior to instituting therapy, the causes of weight loss should be identified and treatable causes must be attended to quickly. Decreased oral intake may be caused by a wide array of functional problems including oral pain, difficulty swallowing, or mechanical obstruction caused by the tumour.[92] Patients with oral pain due to cancer should be given adequate pain medications. If functional abnormalities are present, a swallowing evaluation and swallowing therapy may prove beneficial. In patients with mild to moderate swallowing deficits, soft, puréed foods and liquid supplements can stabilize weight loss. Patients with severe swallowing difficulty require more aggressive therapy such as placement of a PEG feeding tube.

Weight loss secondary to treatment is almost universal with the exception of patients with small lesions amenable to surgical resection or lesions requiring a small radiation port. Patients who have extensive surgical procedures and are expected to have difficulty swallowing usually have a PEG tube placed. In this setting, PEG tubes have demonstrated a decrease in length of hospital stay and diminished complication rate when compared to nasogastric (NG) tubes.[93] Patients undergoing primary radiation therapy or combined chemoradiation may develop severe mucositis which results in a profoundly diminished oral intake. In a report by Newman et al.[94] patients undergoing aggressive chemoradiotherapy lost an average of 10 per cent body weight during therapy. The aggressive use of PEG feeding tubes can minimize weight loss during therapy and improve QOL. In a study reported by Tyldesley et al.,[95] patients who received an elective PEG tube prior to radiation therapy had a 3 per cent weight loss at week 6 of therapy versus 9 per cent in the control group. The difference was maintained at 3 months (3 versus 12 per cent).[95] The use of a nasogastric tube should be avoided since patients with HNC usually require prolonged nutritional support and NG tubes may exacerbate radiation induced mucositis.

Post-treatment, nutrition remains a major issue of concern for many patients. There are numerous factors that contribute to the dietary alterations noted in post-treatment HNC patients: (1) swallowing abnormalities due to tumour or treatment; (2) xerostomia from salivary gland radiation inhibits food bolus formation; (3) dental extractions alter the ability to chew solid foods; (4) alterations in taste cause food aversions; (5) mucosal sensitivity causes pain. These factors lead to decreased food intake with or without restriction in the consistencies and type of foods ingested.[96] Adaptations may result in micronutrient deficits that have heretofore been unrecognized. The early identification of patients with swallowing abnormalities and nutritional deficits may enable physicians to make appropriate referrals to ancillary services (i.e. Speech Pathology and Nutritional Services). Ideally, physicians would be able to use a self-report measure (questionnaire) to screen patients who have completed therapy to identify those at risk for swallowing and nutritional problems. Currently available head and neck quality of life tools have not been demonstrated to provide this type of information. Other factors which must be considered in the nutritional assessment include comorbid diseases which impact on nutritional status, the adequacy of socioeconomic support, and the presence of alcohol abuse. It is important to identify all factors contributing to malnutrition in order establish an effective treatment plan.

In addition to the functional and treatment related causes of weight loss, patients with locally advanced, metastatic, or recurrent disease may also have cancer cachexia. Through yet unclear pathways, cancers are able to profoundly affect the normal metabolic pathways resulting in a loss of lean muscle and adipose tissue. The resultant state of weight loss is termed 'cancer cachexia'. It is beyond the scope of this chapter to discuss the characteristics and possible etiologies for cancer cachexia. However, several excellent reviews have been published recently and the reader is referred to these briefs and to the chapter on Cachexia and Asthenia for further review.[97–99]

Pain

Pain in the patient with HNC is a multi-dimensional symptom complex with physical, emotional, and cultural factors contributing to the overall pain experience. All of these factors must be addressed in order to provide adequate palliation. It is beyond the scope of this chapter to review the basics of cancer pain management. The reader is referred to the chapter on Pain elsewhere in this text. There are, however, specific problems that confront HNC patients that merit special attention.

Grond[100] reported on the type of pain experienced by HNC patients prior to, during, and after treatment. Of 167 patients studied, 138 (83 per cent) patients had pain due to tumour. Of 138 patients with tumour-related pain, 80 per cent had soft tissue pain, 20 per cent had bone pain and 35 per cent had neuropathic pain. Head and neck tumours are often deeply ulcerative causing severe somatic pain. Irritation of an ulcerative tumour by movement from speech or swallowing can diminish function and make pain control a challenge. Tumour invasion into nerves either peripherally or at the level of the base of skull can lead to refractory pain syndromes as well as debilitating neurologic deficits. Tumors such as adenoid cystic carcinoma may track along peripheral nerves (perineural invasion) and into nerve roots resulting in painful peripheral neuropathies.[101] Finally, maxillofacial pain thought to be due to benign processes such as sinusitis, temporomandibular joint dysfunction, or maxillofacial neuralgias can be the first manifestation of carcinomas.[102–108] Determining the etiology of pain in the head and neck patient requires familiarity with anatomy and often calls for consultation with the treating otolaryngologist and neuroradiologist.

Patients undergoing surgical resection will experience post-operative pain which should be treated per recommendations in the AHCCPR Clinical Practice Guidelines for Acute Pain Management.[109] Adequate treatment of post-operative pain in HNC patients can present specific challenges. Tracheostomy tube placement, loss of speech function, or severe oral pain may make it difficult to for patients to effectively communicate with caregivers, thus interfering with pain assessment. As patients recuperate, post-operative pain subsides. However, it is import to emphasize that chronic postoperative pain is common in the head and neck population. In a report by Chaplin and Morton,[110] 26 per cent of patients had pain 2 years after completing therapy. Pain was described as moderate or severe in 14 per cent of patients. Predictors for chronic pain included: pain at 3 months post-treatment and neck dissection. Peripheral nerves may be damaged during resection resulting in the development of neuropathic pain. Less commonly, patients may have associated syncopal episodes.[111] Patients may also develop contractures and tissue scaring in the neck and shoulders. This can lead to severe and debilitating musculoskeletal dysfunction with resultant pain. The degree of musculoskeletal pain may be determined by the extent of surgery or amount of adjuvant radiation therapy used for treatment. For example, Short et al.[112] demonstrated that sparing of the spinal accessory nerve during neck dissection resulted in diminished postoperative shoulder pain. The utilization of non-pharmacologic interventions to prevent and treat this sequella is extremely important. Physical therapy consultation can help guide patients in exercises which can decrease contractures and preserve function and range of motion.[113] Heat, massage, and relaxation techniques can help alleviate muscle spasm.

Radiation therapy may be used as primary treatment or as adjuvant therapy in the post-operative setting. In general, the dose of radiation therapy used for the treatment of HNC is high (70 Gy for primary treatment and 50–60 Gy for adjuvant therapy). These doses are expected to result in significant damage to the mucous membranes, soft tissue, and skin. The severity of symptoms is usually related to the size of the radiation field and the area involved. Patients with large fields, and those receiving radiation to the oral cavity experience severe debilitating mucositis and radiation dermatitis. The treatment of mucositis-induced pain requires close and frequent monitoring. It is imperative that pain treatment be aggressive. A small study reported from the Medical College of Wisconsin demonstrated that daily nursing assessment with aggressive treatment of mucositis resulted in decreased pain, improved sleep and eating, and a better energy level when compared to historical controls.[114] During the first 2–3 weeks of radiation therapy, oral discomfort is usually mild. The use of topical lidocaine solution and mixed opioid/non-opioid tablets such as Lortab or Percocet is usually adequate. By week 4–5, oral and dermal pain begins to increase substantially. At the same time, patients' ability to swallow decreases substantially.[115] Fentanyl patches are a very convenient method for administering long-acting narcotics in this patient population. Short-acting liquid narcotics should be used for breakthrough pain. If patients are unable to tolerate oral nutrition or medications, a PEG tube should be placed as quickly as possible to ensure adequate nutrition as well as palliation. Patients with large tumours requiring extensive radiation ports should have a PEG placed prior to starting therapy. Pain due to radiation mucositis takes weeks to months to resolve. Although detailed epidemiologic data regarding chronic post-radiation pain is lacking, there are a significant cohort of patients with persistent pain months to years after completion of therapy.[110]

Pain due to local recurrence is a major palliative issue in terminal HNC patients. More importantly, it may be the first symptom indicating recurrent disease. In a recent report by Smit et al.[116] pain was the first symptom indicative of recurrence in 70 per cent of patients, with a median lag time of 4 months between the onset of pain and the diagnosis of recurrent disease. Thus, new onset pain in a previously treated HNC patient should be carefully investigated.

Mucositis (see also Chapter 8.12)

Oral and pharyngeal mucositis is the most devastating acute complication of radiotherapy for HNC. Oral mucosa undergoes constant regeneration through a process, whereby the cells at the basal layer mature, migrate to the surface layer and exfoliate. This process requires approximately 14 days. Radiation-induced mucositis is a result of mitotic death in the basal layer resulting in an inability to replace the naturally exfoliated apical layer of cells at the mucosal surface. Mucositis usually begins after 10–14 days which corresponds with the loss of regenerative capabilities in the basal mucosa. Clinically, the initial observation is a transient patchy white discoloration of the mucosa followed by a confluent deep erythema and pseudomembrane formation.(117) The most severe manifestation is frank ulceration of the mucosa. Mucositis may be exacerbated by accelerated radiation fractionation,(118) concurrent chemotherapy(16) superinfection with *Candida albicans* or abnormal bacteria flora.(119) In addition to causing pain, mucositis impairs eating, swallowing, and speech. When severe, mucositis may lead to hospitalization for malnutrition or dehydration, and may result in interruptions in treatment. Overwhelming data indicate that breaks in treatment decrease local control and overall survival, thus treatment breaks due to mucositis must be avoided.(120) A plethora of traditional treatments for oropharyngeal mucositis have been reported, but rarely have these been substantiated or corroborated by rigorous well-controlled studies. For further information on treatment of mucositis and other oral cavity lesions, please see the chapter on Oral care.

Xerostomia (see also Chapter 8.12)

Xerostomia can be a severe and permanent complication of external beam radiation therapy. It results from damage to the acinar cells and stromal matrix of the major and minor salivary glands. The degree of xerostomia is related to the amount of salivary gland tissues within the radiation port and the radiation dose delivered. The sparing of at least one salivary gland can significantly reduce sequella of radiation therapy to the oral cavity. Damage to the acinar cells is evident at low doses of radiation therapy. Salivary gland function, both stimulated and unstimulated, drops rapidly to 5–30 per cent of normal within the first 2–3 weeks of therapy and remains low (<10 per cent of normal) following completion of radiation for a prolonged period of time.(121–124) In general, recovery of function is slow and partial. With the use of combined chemo- and radiation therapy, the severity of xerostomia may be worsened.

Saliva is vital for normal oral function.(125) Symptoms due to hyposalivation are numerous and can profoundly decrease quality of life. Saliva plays an important role in moistening food to allow bolus formation. Even mild xerostomia can result in a significant decrease in the variety and types of food that patients can eat. Difficulty forming a food bolus makes deglutition difficult. Patients, therefore, avoid eating and may loose a substantive amount of weight. Saliva maintains oral flora, thus preventing the development of dental caries. It lubricates mucosal membranes allowing normal speech and swallowing. Finally, xerostomia results in mucosal irritation and pain. The irritation can be extremely severe at night and in dry conditions. A number of therapeutic interventions can be attempted to improve symptoms of xerostomia and its associated complications. Unfortunately, currently available drugs are only modestly effective. Identification of new, active agents for the prevention and treatment of xerostomia are urgently needed.

Patients with severe xerostomia usually carry water with them to swish and swallow on a frequent basis. The soothing effect is short lived. Patients with severe xerostomia may drink litres of fluid daily merely for comfort purposes. The use of a sodium bicarbonate rinse can help maintain dental hygiene as well as sooth the mucosal surface. A number of commercial salivary gland substitutes are available. Although some patients find these products useful, the majority of patients fail to find significant benefit.

With increasing use of primary radiation therapy +/− chemotherapy for treatment of squamous carcinomas of the head and neck, attention has turned to methods for ameliorating treatment-related toxicity. Prevention of xerostomia has been an area of active clinical research. Several agents merit mention because they are now approved for and commonly used in the treatment of xerostomia.

Pilocarpine is a parasympathomimetic that acts as a muscarinic agonist. It has a time to peak effect of 1 h (unstimulated salivation) and a duration of effect of between 3 and 5 h. Pilot trials demonstrated promising results with pilocarpine for the treatment of xerostomia.(126,127) Subsequently, two double-blind controlled trials were undertaken to confirm the efficacy of pilocarpine in the treatment of radiation-induced xerostomia. Johnson et al.(128) reported on 207 patients who received ~4000 cGy with at least one parotid gland within the radiation port. Patients were randomly assigned to placebo or pilocarpine at one of two doses (5 and 10 mg tabs t.i.d.).(128) Results demonstrated an improvement in xerostomia related symptoms for both the 5 and 10 mg tablet. The results of the objective saliva production were less clear. In a study conducted by LeVeque et al.(129) in 162 patients with radiation-induced xerostomia, similar results were reported. In both trials, the most common side effects include sweating, nausea, rhinitis, chills, flushing, urinary frequency, dizziness, and asthenia. Thus, pilocarpine at a dose of 5 mg PO t.i.d.–q.i.d. may produce a modest but significant subjective improvement in oral symptoms related to xerostomia with generally mild side effects. Symptom relief was maximal at 4 months and a prolonged drug trial may be required to determine efficacy in a given patient. Pilocarpine is also being investigated as a prophylactic treatment during radiation therapy. Small phase II trials have demonstrated a reduction in radiation-induced xerostomia when patients received pilocarpine during radiation therapy.(130) Confirmatory phase III trials are currently underway.

Amifostine (WR-2721) is a free radical scavenger that has been investigated for its potential to protect cells from chemotherapy and radiation-induced DNA damage. Amifostine has been FDA approved for reduction in xerostomia in patients undergoing postoperative radiation treatment for HNC when the radiation port includes a large segment of salivary gland tissue (>75 per cent of both salivary glands included in the radiation port). In a randomized trial of 315 patients receiving post-op radiation therapy, patients receiving amifostine 200 mg/m^2 15–30 min prior to each fractionation of radiation had a significantly decreased rate of grade 2 or greater xerostomia. The rate of acute xerostomia dropped from 78 to 51 per cent ($p < 0.0001$) and late xerostomia dropped from 57 to 35 per cent ($p = 0.0016$). Side effects to amifostine are significant with hypotension reported in 15 per cent of patients. Therefore, work is ongoing to evaluate the relative effectiveness and toxicity of subcutaneous administration. Furthermore, the ability of amifostine to protect against xerostomia in patients being treated with concomitant chemo radiation has yet to be determined.

Auditory function

HNC patients may experience a decrease in hearing as a result of therapy. Sensorineural hearing loss may result from therapy with either radiation or systemic chemotherapy agents such as cisplatin. In a longitudinal study of hearing loss in patients treated with radiation or radiochemotherapy for nasopharyngeal carcinoma,(131) 31 per cent of patients had a measurable sensorineural hearing deficit 3 months after completing therapy. Hearing deficits improved over time in only 40 per cent of patients. Older patients (>50 years of age) and patients with pre-treatment hearing deficits were more likely to develop measurable sensorineural hearing loss. Concomitant chemotherapy did not worsen hearing outcome. Rarely, destruction of the inner ear apparatus by infiltrative tumours results in sensorineural hearing loss. Patients with a clinically significant sensorineural hearing loss should be referred for hearing aids. Middle ear effusions are a common cause of non-sensorineural hearing loss and should be identified and treated appropriately.

Taste alteration

The majority of tastes buds are located on the tongue. They may also be found scattered throughout the upper aerodigestive system. Taste buds are composed of 50 to 100 receptor cells with associated support cells. Receptor cells transmit signals to the intrageminal nerve fibers which carry information to the brain. Loss of taste may be caused by a wide variety of medical illnesses and pharmaceutical agents including many chemotherapy drugs.[132] Radiation therapy, which is an integral part of treatment for all patients with locally advanced disease, may result in severe and permanent alteration in taste sensation. The exact mechanism of radiation induced taste alteration remains to be elucidated. Taste alteration may begin 2–3 days after initiating therapy and taste bud degeneration may be seen 6–7 days after starting radiation therapy. Accumulated doses over 6000 cGy may be associated with permanent damage.

Extensive clinical studies evaluating the long-term effects of radiation on taste sensation are lacking; however, it is clear that loss of taste may have a profound effect on nutritional status and quality of life. Patients may describe an inability to take nutrition orally due to severe loss of taste or altered taste sensation. The taste of food may become noxious resulting in nausea and vomiting. Taste slowly returns for the majority of patients weeks to months after the completion of therapy. However, some patients have a permanent alteration in taste sensation.

Wound care, fistulas, and carotid rupture

With the advancement in reconstructive techniques in the past two decades, our ability to handle larger and more complex wounds in the head and neck has improved. Regional and distant tissue transfer techniques have expanded the ability to cover vital organs such as the carotid artery and bring well vascularized tissue into a contaminated operative field that can resist infection and post-operative radiation therapy. In general, if distant tissue is used to reconstruct a wound created by resection of a tumour, the blood supply to that tissue is preserved by isolating the tissue on a pedicle artery and vein. If the tissue is simply rotated on its pedicle to reach the defect, it is called a pedicled flap, such as a pectoralis muscle or the latissimus muscle flap. If the vascular pedicle has to be divided to allow movement of the flap from a remote site, such as the fibula, then the arterial and venous blood supply must be re-established through a microvascular anastamosis in the neck and this is referred to as a free flap. In all cases, the reconstruction, particularly in the immediate postoperative period, is solely dependent on its blood supply and careful attention must be given to placing any dressings around the neck, which may compress the pedicle vessels. Tracheostomies are typically sewn in place to avoid a circumferential dressing around the neck until the wound appears to be sealed.

Despite newer reconstructive techniques, patients who have undergone prior radiation therapy or combined chemo-radiation therapy are at greater risk for wound breakdown as a result of the small vessel arteritis that reduces oxygen tissue exchange in the area. Additionally, patients' preoperative nutritional status and smoking history complicate their wound healing capacity. Pharyngocutaneous fistulas may result from wound breakdown if a watertight seal of the pharynx cannot be maintained. Patients who have had a breech of the pharynx during their resection are often maintained with nasogastric feedings to limit the contamination of the suture lines for 1–2 weeks. Fistula formation is usually heralded by erythema of the neck, tenderness, and low-grade fevers. The saliva in the neck must be drained and the path of drainage directed away from the carotid artery. Saliva, with its digestive enzymes, has the ability to necrose the great vessels resulting in life threatening hemorrhage. Additionally, exposure of the vessels to the external environment leads to desiccation and potential carotid rupture. Exposure of the neck vessels as a result of loss of overlying skin or fistula formation represents a surgical emergency. The vessels should be covered with saline soaked gauze until vascularized tissue can be placed over the vessels. Any continuous bleeding from an exposed area must be taken seriously for it may herald an early leak from the carotid artery and surgical exploration to repair the vessel may be necessary.

If a fistula does form, and the great vessels are not exposed, the wound can often be managed conservatively until secondary healing occurs. The patient should continue to be fed through a non-oral route to minimize contamination. The wound should be packed with wet to dry gauze dressings twice a day or more frequently if contamination is excessive.

In patients who have unresectable disease in the neck, ulceration of the tumour with necrotic debris may become problematic. Tumour hygiene can be achieved through gentle debridement with hydrogen peroxide. Desiccating powders may be applied if wound remains moist. Intermittent use of antibiotics to cover anaerobic floral contaminants will often assist with sterilizing the field and assist with odour control. Oral hygiene can be maintained with use of a water pik at low settings to debride tissue. Use of frequent mouth rinses with saline and soda or formal preparations such as Peridex can assist in cleansing as well.

A carotid rupture is an uncommon but catastrophic complication of HNC and its therapy. Carotid rupture may occur in patients undergoing extensive resection, external beam radiation therapy, brachytherapy, or those with recurrent/advanced cancers of the neck. Although initial retrospective reviews in the 1950s and 1960s demonstrated rates of carotid rupture as high as 14 per cent,[133] the numbers are much lower with contemporary treatment methods.[134] The investigators at MSKCC reviewed the data of 2346 patients undergoing head and neck surgical procedures between 1994 and 1995. Only one case of carotid rupture was identified.[135] When possible, patients with carotid rupture should undergo evaluation with angiography. In patients with controlled tumour (i.e. the post-operative setting), aggressive intervention with surgery or invasive radiologic procedures are indicated. Unfortunately data on the success of radiologic procedures (i.e. balloon occlusion and embolization) are scant.[136] In one series reported by Citardi et al.[137] 12 patients with carotid rupture were treated with endovascular occlusion. All 12 patients survived without nuerologic sequelae. In patients will terminal disease, palliative measures are usually undertaken.

Osteoradionecrosis

Mandibular osteoradionecrosis (ORN) is one of the most serious complications from head and neck irradiation. The incidence varies depending upon total radiation dose,[138] fractionation, volume irradiated,[139] follow-up time, the status of dentition, and reporting institution.[140–144] It is more common in edentulous patients, however, ORN is often reported as occurring after dental extractions following irradiation.[145,146] The pathogenesis of ORN include a decrease in cellularity, suppressed osteoblastic activity, disorganization of the bone remodelling apparatus, avascularity, and fibrosis that leads to poor wound healing after dental trauma and an increased risk of secondary infection from bacterial flora.[147] ORN can ultimately result in exposure of bone, fistula formation, or pathologic fracture. Radiographic signs include crestal bone irregularity, density changes, osteolysis, obvious sequestration, and frank pathologic fracture. Since tissue changes induced by radiation are long-term and the risk of dental trauma is lifelong, careful attention must be paid to the dentition and gingiva before, during, and after radiation treatment. Current standards for dental care were developed at a Consensus Development Conference on Oral Complications of Cancer Therapies[148] and were reported as a monograph by the National Cancer Institute.[149]

Prevention

Before initiation of treatment, all patients scheduled to receive high dose ($\geq$50 Gy) radiation to one or both jaws should be evaluated by a skilled dentist familiar with radiation side effects. Panoramic radiographs are essential for the evaluation. All grossly diseased maxillary and mandibular teeth should be extracted immediately, and alveolar tori trimmed and carefully smoothed so that primary closure of the mucosa can be performed under little no tension. Antibiotic prophylaxis should be used, and a minimum of 14 days (preferably 21 days) should be allowed for healing prior to onset of radiation.[133]

Following treatment, prevention of ORN has naturally evolved around minimizing trauma or local irritants that have been shown to precipitate the process. Periodontal disease has been shown to be a major predisposing factor, particularly when dental extractions are performed in a portion of the previously irradiated jaw.[150] Although a certain number of cases will arise spontaneously in spite of conscientious care, the patient can be instructed on ways to decrease overall risk. A correlation between higher ORN and continued tobacco and alcohol use has been reported.[151] Improvement of salivary function with sialogogues such as pilocarpine hydrochloride[152] and bromhexine[153] can decrease bacterial decay. Daily use of fluoride via trays or liquids before bedtime are effective in minimizing dental carries. Diseased teeth should be maintained, if possible, through meticulous endodontic therapy with or without coronal recontouring (crown amputation). It has been shown that endodontic management of teeth in previously irradiated cancer patients does not increase the risk of ORN.[154] For periodontally involved or cariously unrestorable teeth, the retention of roots (with or without endodontic therapy) and the use of overdentures are preferable to extractions.[155]

Treatment of established ORN

Treatment of ORN via the *nonsurgical* route prior to the use of hyperbaric oxygen (HBO) therapy consists of improving oral hygiene and removing local irritants like alcohol and tobacco. Irrigation, packing, and systemic antibiotics may also be useful. Pentoxifylline, a methylxanthine derivative introduced in 1984 for the treatment of intermittent claudication and venous stasis ulcers, has been shown to improve erythrocyte flexibility and increase tissue oxygen levels. It has been helpful in promoting healing of radiation soft tissue necrosis, fibrosis, and atrophy due to head and neck irradiation.[156,157] Unfortunately, a randomized trial in the United States comparing pentoxifylline (400 mg every 8 h) to best supportive care for patients with ORN closed before completion due to poor accrual. HBO therapy was shown to be an effective treatment for ORN in 1975.[158] Early ORN (stage I) without fractures of fistulae may be cured by HBO alone. A suggested regimen is 30 dives of 90 min at 2.5 atm.[159]

If conservative measures fail or in advanced cases (stage II or III), then HBO in combination with surgical management is necessary. In stage III ORN, Marx reported good results using 30 dives HBO followed by transoral alveolar sequestrectomy with a primary mucosal closure.[145] Adjunctive HBO is recommended, varying from 10 to 30 dives. Others have reported good results using 5–10 pre-operative dives of 2.5–2.8 atm for 90–120 min, followed by 5–7 dives post-operatively.[160] In severe cases (stage III), 30 dives have been recommended followed by resection, using tetracycline fluorescence under ultraviolet light or the presence of bleeding bone to determine margins. Stabilization of the mandible with either an extraskeletal pin or maxillofacial fixation is usually necessary. HBO is then performed until a healthy mucosal closure is seen (usually 20–30 dives). It has been advocated that reconstruction can be accomplished 10 weeks later, using HBO pre-operatively for 20 dives, then operating strictly from a transcutaneous approach to avoid oral contamination. Ten additional dives are recommended post-operatively.

Dermatitis and soft tissue damage

Similar to oral mucositis, patients receiving treatment will external beam radiation can develop severe dermal and soft tissue reactions. Acute radiation dermatitis usually begins 2–3 weeks after therapy is initiated. The first manifestation of radiation dermatitis is erythema with mild oedema. As treatment progresses, the skin may begin to blister, ulcerate, and slough. As with mucositis, radiation dermatitis can be graded according to a variety of toxicity scales. The severity of radiation induced dermal damage may increase if chemotherapy is given concomitantly. In addition, patients with tracheostomy tubes in place may have increased irritation and ulceration. Acute radiation induced dermal damage begins to heal within 2–4 weeks after radiation is completed.

Long-term sequella of radiation develop 2–4 months after completion of therapy. Patients often develop a fibrous soft tissue mass in the submental region or anterior neck. The fibrous mass usually begins to involute over 3–6 months. However, its development is often frightening to patients who interpret the development of such an abnormality as a recurrence of cancer. Patients may also develop contracted fibrotic skin within the radiation port. Many years after treatment, atrophy of the soft tissues of the neck may result in a 'pencil neck' appearance. Radiation or surgical induced damage to lymphatic and vascular drainage in the neck can result in bothersome facial oedema and swelling. Use of steroids, diuretics, or massage may diminish symptoms; however, they are often refractory to treatment.

Laboratory abnormalities

Hypothyroidism

After primary surgery, neck dissection or radiation therapy, patients frequently develop hypothyroidism. Routine follow-up should include a careful history and physical exam directed towards signs or symptoms of hypothyroidism. Periodic monitoring with a serum TSH is appropriate for any patient who has received aggressive therapy for locally advanced disease. For recommendations regarding treatment of hypothyroidism, please reference the American Thyroid Association Standards of Care Committee guidelines.[161]

Hypercalcemia

Hypercalcemia is common in patients with squamous carcinoma of the head and neck. The majority of patients' tumours express parathyroid-hormone-related protein (PTHrP) which causes release of calcium from the skeleton.[162] Although an occasional patient with curable locally advanced squamous carcinoma of the head and neck will present with hypercalcemia, the majority of patients have metastatic disease. Treatment of the underlying disease should be attempted where possible. Intravenous hydration, diuretics, bisphosphonates, and other pharmacologic agents should be used as indicated by the clinical setting.

Anaemia

Anaemia is a common presenting haematologic abnormality in patients with HNC and may worsen throughout the course of radiation or chemoradiation. Compelling data in a number of tumour sites, including HNC, demonstrate that anemia is a strong predictor for outcome with radiation-based treatment regimens.[163–166] It is hypothesized that low numbers of circulating red blood cells may increase the fraction of cancer cells that are hypoxic. Hypoxic tumour cells are resistant to radiation therapy. Thus, anaemia may lead to increased radiation resistance. In a recent analysis of RTOG 8527, patients were randomly assigned to radiation alone or radiation plus Etanidazole (a radiation sensitizing agent).[167] Primary analysis demonstrated no survival advantage to concomitant therapy with Etanidazole.[154,168] A secondary analysis was conducted to evaluate the association between pre-treatment anaemia and overall survival local regional control and radiation therapy complications. Results of this study indicated that patients with a normal haemoglobin (>14.5 g/ml in men and >13 g/ml in women) had a statistically significant improvement in overall survival and local regional control. The survival advantage for normal haemoglobin level persisted at 5 years. In addition to the survival and local regional control advantage, late toxicity was diminished in patients with a normal haemoglobin level at initiation of therapy. Additional studies confirm the predictive value of haemoglobin level on treatment outcome. Fein et al.[169] reported on pre-treatment haemoglobin level with patients undergoing radiation therapy for $T_{1/2}$ squamous carcinoma of the glottic larynx. The 2-year local control in patients with a haemoglobin of less than 13 g/dl was 66 per cent ($p = 0.018$). For patients with a haemoglobin of more than 13/g/dl, the 2-year local control was 95 per cent. For normal and abnormal haemoglobin levels, similarly 2-year survival was 46 and 88 per cent respectively ($p < 0.001$). Overgaard et al.[170] reported on predictive factors for outcome of radiation therapy for laryngeal and pharyngeal carcinoma. Nine hundred and fifty patients received primary irradiation in doses ranging from 60 to 68 Gy in 6–7 weeks. Pre-treatment haemoglobin was associated with tumour control and survival in patients with pharyngeal and supraglottic tumours. The RTOG is undertaking a randomized trial of radiation therapy (with or without concomitant chemotherapy) +/− erythropoietin to evaluate its ability ameliorating radiation induced hematologic toxicity and enhance treatment efficacy.

Routine symptom screening for HNC patients

The symptom control issues in HNC can be overwhelming. In the busy Oncology clinic, the physician does not always have time to do an extensive review of systems to uncover all of the symptom control issues for each patient. In order to effectively identify and palliate symptoms, a tumour-specific symptom questionnaire is necessary. Using a two-stage card sort method, investigators at Vanderbilt developed a screening tool which is now routinely used in the Head and Neck clinic for all patients undergoing treatment or who are in the immediate post-treatment phase. This tool includes questions that address nutrition, swallowing, aspiration, mucositis, mucus production, and pain. Initial studies demonstrate content validity when compared to the FACT-HN, PSS-HN, and the EORTC HN35. More importantly, it is an effective clinical aid for the treating physician.

Conclusions

Patients with HNC suffer from a variety of cancer and treatment related symptom control problems. Some of the palliative issues are unique to the head and neck population. Optimal palliation requires a multimodality team of physicians, nurses, social workers, dentists, physical therapists, and speech/swallowing therapists in order to address the multitude of needs. Since many of these patients have poor social support systems, the treatment team may need to spend substantially more time with the patient to ensure adequate symptom palliation. The added effort and attention can result in improved cure rates, diminished long-term side effects and decreased existential distress for the patient and family. For those patients who are destined to die of their disease, adequate medical support can mean the difference between an agonizing death and one that is both physically and emotionally comfortable.

Appendix

Head and neck staging

Stage grouping*			
Stage 0	Tis	N0	M0
Stage I	T1	N0	M0
Stage II	T2	N0	M0
Stage III	T3	N0	M0
	T1	N1	M0
	T2	N1	M0
	T3	N1	M0
Stage IVA	T4	N0	M0
	T4	N1	M0
	Any T	N2	M0
Stage IVB	Any T	N3	M0
Stage IVC	Any T	Any N	M1

* T stage is dependent on the primary site.

Regional lymph nodes (N)

NX Regional lymph nodes cannot be assessed

N0 No regional lymph node metastasis

N1 Metastasis in a single ipsilateral lymph node, 3 cm or less in greatest dimension

N2 Metastasis in a single ipsilateral lymph node, more than 3 cm but not more than 6 cm in greatest dimension; or in multiple ipsilateral lymph nodes, none more than 6 cm in greatest dimension; or in bilateral or contralateral lymph nodes, none more than 6 cm in greatest dimension

- N2a Metastasis in single ipsilateral lymph node more than 3 cm but not more than 6 cm in greatest dimension
- N2b Metastasis in multiple ipsilateral lymph nodes, none more than 6 cm in greatest dimension
- N2c Metastasis in bilateral or contralateral lymph nodes, none more than 6 cm in greatest dimension

N3 Metastasis in a lymph node more than 6 cm in greatest dimension

Distant metastasis (M)

MX Distant metastasis cannot be assessed

M0 No distant metastasis

M1 Distant metastasis

References

1. *Cancer Facts and Figures 2000.* Atlanta GA: American Cancer Society, 2000.
2. **Fandi, A.** et al. (1994). Nasopharyngeal cancer: epidemiology, staging, and treatment. *Seminars in Oncology* **21** (3), 382–97.
3. **Pathmanathan, R.** et al. (1995). Clonal proliderations of cells infected with Epstein–Barr virus in preinvasive lesions related to nasopharyngeal carcinoma. *New England Journal of Medicine* **333**, 693–8.
4. **Shah, J.P. and Lydiatt, W.** (1995). Treatment of cancer of the head and neck. *CA: A Cancer Journal for Clinicians* **45** (6), 352–68.
5. **Cmelak, A., Murphy, B.A., and Day, T.** (1999). Combined-modality therapy for locoregionally advanced head and neck cancer. *Oncology* **5**, 1–9.
6. **Department of Veterans Affairs Laryngeal Cancer Study Group** (1991). Induction chemotherapy plus radiation compared with surgery plus radiation in patients with advanced laryngeal cancer. *New England Journal of Medicine* **324**, 1685–90.
7. **Lefebvre, J., Chavalier, D., and Luboinski, B.** (1996). Larynx preservation in pyriform sinus cancer: preliminary results of a European organization for research and treatment of cancer phase II trail. *Journal of the National Cancer Institute* **88**, 890–9.
8. **Shanta, V. and Krishnamurthi, S.** (1980). Combined bleomycin and radiotherapy in oral cancer. *Clinical Radiology* **31**, 617–20.
9. **SECOG** (1986). A randomized trail of combined multidrug chemotherapy and radiotherapy in advanced squamous cell carcinoma of the head and neck. *European Journal of Surgical Oncology* **12**, 289–95.
10. **Fu, K., Philips, T., and Silverberg, I.** (1987). Combined RT and CT with bleomycin in advanced inoperable head and neck cancer: update of the Northern California Oncology Group randomized trial. *Journal of Clinical Oncology* **5** (9), 1410–18.
11. **Weissberg, J., Son, Y., and Papac, R.** (1989). Randomized clinical trial of mitomycin C as an adjunct to radiotherapy in head and neck cancer. *International Journal of Radiation Oncology, Biology, Physics* **17**, 3–9.
12. **Adelstein, D., Sharan, V., and Earle, A.** (1990). Simultaneous versus sequential combined technique for head and neck cancer. *Cancer* **65**, 1685–91.
13. **Sanichiz, R., Milla, A., and Torner, J.** (1990). Single fraction per day versus two fractions per day versus radiochemotherapy in the treatment of head and neck cancer. *International Journal of Radiation Oncology, Biology, Physics* **19**, 1347–50.

14. **Merlan, M., Couro, R., and Maigino, G.** (1990). Combined chemotherapy and radiation therapy in advanced inoperable squamous cancer of the head and neck. The final report of a randomized trial. *Cancer* **19**, 915–21.

15. **Merlano, M., Vitale, V., and Rosso, R.** (1992). Treatment of advanced squamous-cell carcinoma of the head and neck. *New England Journal of Medicine* **327**, 1115–21.

16. **Wendt, T., Granbenbauer, G., and Rodel, C.** (1998). Simultaneous radiochemotherapy versus radiotherapy alone in advanced head and neck cancer: a randomized multicenter study. *Journal of Clinical Oncology* **16** (4), 1318–24.

17. **Adelstein, D.** et al. (2000). A phase III comparison of standard radiation therapy (RT) versus RT plus concurrent cisplatin (DDP) versus split-course RT plus CCP and 5-flurouracil (5FU) in patients with unresectable squamous cell head and neck cancer (SCHNC): an intergroup study. *Proceedings of the American Society of Clinical Oncology* **19**, 411A (Abstract # 1624).

18. **Brizel, D., Sauer, R., and Wnnenmacher, W.** (1998). Randomized trial of radiation +/− amifostine in patients with head and neck cancer. *Proceedings of the American Society of Clinical Oncology* **17**, 386a.

19. **Al-Sarraf, M., Lebland, M., and Gig, P.** (1998). Chemo-radiotherapy (CT-RT) versus radiotherapy (RT) in patients (PTS) with advanced nasopharyngeal cancer (NPC). Intergroup (0099) (SWOG 8892, RTOG 8817, ECOG 2388) phase III study: progress report. *Proceedings of the American Society of Clinical Oncology* **17** (Abstract # 1483).

20. **Zakotnik, B., Smid, L., and Budhina, M.** (1998). Concomitant radiotherapy with mitomycin C and bleomycin compared with radiotherapy alone in inoperable had and neck cancer: final report. *International Journal of Radiation Oncology, Biology, Physics* **41**, 1121–7.

21. **Dobrowsky, W.** et al. (1998). Continuous hyperfractionated accelerated radiotherapy with/without mitomycin C in head and neck cancer *International Journal of Radiation Oncology, Biology, Physics* **42**, 803–6.

22. **Jeremic, B.** et al. (2000). Hyperfractionated radiation therapy with or without concurrent low-dose cisplatin in locally advanced squamous cell carcinoma of the head and neck: a prospective randomized trial. *Journal of Clinical Oncology* **18**, 1458–64.

23. **Lo, T., Wiley, A., and Ansfield, F.** (1976). Combined radiation therapy and 5-flurouracil for advanced squamous cell carcinoma of the oral cavity and oropharynx: a randomized study. *American Journal of Roentgenology* **126**, 229–35.

24. **El-Sayed, S. and Nelson, N.** (1996). Adjuvant and adjunctive chemotherapy in the management of squamous cell carcinoma of the head and neck region. A meta-analysis of prospective and randomized trials. *Clinical Oncology* **14**, 838–47.

25. **Munro, A.** (1995). Meta-analysis of chemotherapy in head and neck cancer. *British Journal of Cancer* **71**, 83–91.

26. **Bourhis, J., Pignon, J., and Designe, L.** (1998). Meta-analysis of chemotherapy in head and neck cancer (MHACH-NC): loco-regional treatment versus same treatment + chemotherapy (CT). *Proceedings of the American Society of Clinical Oncology* **17** (Abstract # 1486).

27. **Cella, D.** et al. (1993). The functional assessment of cancer therapy (FACT) scale: development and validation of a general measure. *Journal of Clinical Oncology* **11**, 570–9.

28. **Ringash, J. and Bezjak, A.** (2001). A stuctured review of quality of life instruments for head and neck cancer patients. *Head & Neck* **23**, 201–13.

29. **Rogers, S.** et al. (1999). The University of Washington Head and Neck Cancer Measure as a predictor of outcome following primary surgery for oral cancer. *Head & Neck* **21**, 394–401.

30. **Murry, T.** et al. (1998). Acute and chronic changes in swallowing and quality of life following intraarterial chemoradiation for organ preservation in patients with advanced head and neck cancer. *Head & Neck* **20**, 31–7.

31. **Terrell, J., Fisher, S., and Wolf, G.** (1998). Long-term quality of life after treatment of laryngeal cancer. *Archives of Otolaryngology—Head & Neck Surgery* **124**, 964–71.

32. **Larto, M.** et al. (1998). A randomized trial comparing radiation therapy alone with chemoradiotherapy for squamous cell cancer of the head and neck (SCHNC): Quality of life (QOL) assessment. *Proceedings of the American Society of Clinical Oncology* **17**, 382a (Abstract # 1460).

33. **Weymuller, E.** et al. (2000). Quality of life in patients with head and neck cancer. *Archives of Otolaryngology—Head & Neck Surgery* **126**, 329–35.

34. **Karnell, L., Funk, G., and Hoffman, H.** (2000). Assessing head and neck cancer patient outcome domains. *Head & Neck* **22**, 6–11.

35. **de Graeff, A.** et al. (2000). Pretreatment factors predicting quality of life after treatment for head and neck cancer. *Head & Neck* **22**, 398–407.

36. **Piccirillo, J.** (2000). Importance of comorbidity in head and neck cancer. *Laryngoscope* **110**, 593–602.

37. **Deleyiannis, F.** et al. (1996). Alcoholism: independent predictor of survival in patients with head and neck cancer. *Journal of the National Cancer Institute* **88**, 542–9.

38. **Feinstein, A.** et al. (1977). Cancer of the larynx: a new staging system and a re-appraisal of prognosis and treatment. *Journal of Chronic Diseases* **30**, 277–305.

39. **Piccirillo, A.** et al. (1994). New clinical severity staging system for cancer of the larynx five year survival rates. *The Annals of Otology, Rhinology, and Laryngology* **103**, 83–92.

40. **Pugliano, F.** et al. (1997). Clinical-severity staging system for oropharyngeal cancer five year survival rates. *Archives of Otolaryngology—Head & Neck Surgery* **123**, 1118–24.

41. **Pugliano, F., Piccirillo, J., and Zequeira, M.** (1999). Clinical-severity staging system for oral cavity cancer. *Archives of Otolaryngology—Head & Neck Surgery* **120**, 38–45.

42. **Epstein, J.B.** et al. (1999). Quality of life and oral function following radiotherapy for head and neck cancer. *Head & Neck* **21**, 1–11.

43. **D'Antonio, L.L.** et al. (1998). Relationship between quality of life and depression in patients with head and neck cancer. *Laryngoscope* **108**, 806–11.

44. **Shapiro, P.A. and Kornfeld, D.S.** (1987). Psychiatric aspects of head and neck cancer surgery. *The Psychiatric Clinics of North America* **10** (1), 87–100.

45. **DeBoer, M.F.** et al. (1999). Physical and psychosocial correlates of head and neck cancer: a review of the literature. *Otolaryngology—Head and Neck Surgery* **120**, 427–36.

46. **David, D.J. and Barritt, J.A.** (1982). Psychosocial implications of surgery for head and neck cancer. *Symposium on Social and Psychological Considerations in Plastic Surgery* **9** (3), 327–36.

47. **Boyd, C.** et al. (1999). Associations between community income and cancer survival in Ontario, Canada and the United States. *Journal of Clinical Oncology* **17**, 2244–55.

48. **Simpson, C.B.** et al. (1997). Speech outcomes after laryngeal cancer management. *Otolaryngologic Clinics of North America* **30** (2), 189–206.

49. **Blaylock, D.** (1997). Speech rehabilitation after treatment of laryngeal carcinoma. *Otolaryngologic Clinics of North America* **30** (2), 179–88.

50. **NCCN Practice Guidelines for Head and Neck Cancer** (1998). *Oncology* **3**, 39–147.

51. **Perry, A. and Shaw, M.** (2000). Evaluation of functional outcomes (speech, swallowing and voice) in patients attending speech pathology after head and neck cancer treatment(s): development of a multi-centre database. *J. Larygol. Otol.* **114**, 605–15.

52. **Perlman, A.** (1994). Disordered swallowing. In *Diagnosis in Speech-Language Pathology* (ed. H. Morris and D. Spriestersback), pp. 361–82. San Diego: Singular Publishing Group.

53. **Logemann, J.** Evaluation and Treatment of Swallowing Disorders. Austin TX: Pro-ed, 1998.

54. **McConnel, F.** et al. (1988). Timing of major events of pharyngeal swallowing. *Archives of Otolaryngology—Head & Neck Surgery* **114**, 1413–18.

55. **Aviv, J.** et al. (1996). Supraglottic and pharyngeal sensory abnormalitites in stroke patients with dysphagia. *The Annals of Otology, Rhinology, and Laryngology* **105**, 92–7.

56. **Lundy, D.** et al. (1999). Aspiration: cause and implications. *Otolaryngology—Head and Neck Surgery* **120**, 474–8.

57. **Stenson, K.** et al. (2000). Swallowing function in patients with head and neck cancer prior to treatment. *Archives of Otolaryngology—Head & Neck Surgery* **126**, 371–7.

58. **McConnel, F., Logemann, J., and Rademaker, A.** (1994). Surgical variables affecting postoperative swallowing efficiency in oral cancer patients: a pilot study. *Laryngoscope* **104**, 87–90.

59. **Hirano, M.** et al. (1992). Dysphagia following various degrees of surgical resection for oral cancer. *The Annals of Otology, Rhinology, and Laryngology* **101**, 1992.

60. **Logemann, J. and Bytell, D.** (1979). Swallowing disorders in three types of head and neck surgical patients. *Cancer* **44**, 1095–105.

61. **Pauloski, B.** et al. (1998). Speech and swallowing in irradiated and nonirradiated postsurgical oral cancer patients. *Otolaryngology—Head and Neck Surgery* **118**, 616–24.

62. **Dowling, E.R., Murphy, B., and Cmelak, A.** (2001). Swallowing deficits in patients treated with combined chemoradiation for locally advanced head and neck cancer. *Proceedings of the American Society of Clinical Oncology* **20**, 227a.

63. **Kendall, K.A.** et al. (1998). Structural mobility in deglutition after single modality treatment of head and neck carcinomas with radiotherapy. *Head & Neck* **20**, 720–5.

64. **Logemann, J.** et al. (2001). Effects of xerostomia on perception and performance of swallow function. *Head & Neck* **23**, 317–21.

65. **Hamlet, S.** et al. (1997). Mastication and swallowing in patients with post-irradiation xerostomia. *International Journal of Radiation Biology* **37**, 789–96.

66. **Baker, S.** (1990). Current management of cancer of the lip. *Oncology* **4** 107–20.

67. **Hardin, M., VanDemark, D., and Morris, H.** (1990). Long-term speech results of cleft palate speakers with marginal velopharyngeal competence. *Journal of Communication Disorders* **23**, 401–16.

68. **McWilliams, B., Morris, H., and Shelton, R.** *Cleft Palate Speech.* St Louia: C.V. Mosby Company, 1994.

69. **Nylen, B.** (1961). Cleft palate speech. *Acta Radiologica. Supplementum* 203.

70. **Blocksma, R.** (1963). Correction of velopharyngeal insufficiency by silastic pharyngeal implant. *Plastic and Reconstructive Surgery* **31**, 268.

71. **Lewy, R., Cole, R., and Wepman, J.** (1965). Teflon injection in the correction of velopharyngeal insufficiency. *The Annals of Otology, Rhinology, and Laryngology* **74**, 874.

72. **Netterville, J. and Vrabed, J.** Unilateral palatal adhesions for paralysis after high vagal injury. *Archives of Otolaryngology—Head & Neck Surgery* **120**, 218–21.

73. **Johnson, J., Aramany, M., and Myers, E.** (1983). Palatal neoplasms: reconstruction considerations. *Otolaryngologic Clinics of North America* **16**, 441.

74. **Colton, R. and Casper, J.** *Understanding Voice Problems.* Baltimore MD: Williams & Williams, 1996.

75. **Issihiki, N.** et al. (1974). Thyroplasty as a new phonosurgical technique. *Acta Otolaryngologica* **78**, 451–7.

76. **Netterville, J.** et al. (1993). Silastic medializaton and arytenoid adduction: the Vanderbilt experience. A review of 116 phonosurgical procedures. *The Annals of Otology, Rhinology, and Laryngology* **102** (6), 413–24.

77. **Wanamaker, J., Netterville, J., and Ossoff, R.** (1993). Phonosurgery: silastic medialization for unilateral vocal fold paralysis. *Operation Techniques in Otolaryngology Head & Neck Surgery* **4** (3), 207–17.

78. **Ford, C., Bless, D., and Loftus, J.** (1992). Role of injectable collagen in the treatment of glottic insufficiency: a study of 119 patients. *The Annals of Otology, Rhinology, and Laryngology* **101** (3), 237–47.

79. **Shindo, M., Saretsky, L., and Rice, D.** (1996). Autologous fat injection for unilateral vocal fold paralysis. *The Annals of Otology, Rhinology, and Laryngology* **105** (8), 602–6.

80. **Mikaelian, D., Lowry, L., and Sataloff, R.** (1991). Lipoinjection for unilateral vocal cord paralysis. *Laryngoscope* **101**, 465–8.

81. **Bocca, E., Pignataro, O., and Oldini, C.** (1983). Supraglottic laryngectomy: 30 years of experience. *The Annals of Otology, Rhinology, and Laryngology* **92**, 14–19.

82. **Levine, P.** et al. (1997). Management of advanced-stage cancer. *Otolaryngologic Clinics of North America* **30** (1), 101–12.

83. **DeSanto, L., Pearson, B., and Olsen, K.** (1989). Utility of near-total laryngectomy for supraglottic, pharyngeal, base-of-tongue, and other cancers. *The Annals of Otology, Rhinology, and Laryngology* **98** (1), 2–7.

84. **Keith, R. and Thomas, J.** *A Handbook for the Laryngectomy* 4th edn. Austin TX: Pro-ed, 1996.

85. **Case, J.** *Clinical Management of Voice Disorders.* Rockville MD: Aspen Publishers Inc., 1984, pp. 237–84.

86. **Singer, M. and Blom, E.** (1980). Tracheostoma valve for postlaryngectomy voice rehabilitation. *The Annals of Otology, Rhinology, and Laryngology* **91**, 576–8.

87. **Dewys, W.** et al. (1980). Prognostic effect of weight loss prior to chemotherapy in cancer patients. *American Journal of Medicine* **69**, 491–7.

88. **Hammerlid, E.** et al. (1998). Malnutrition and food intake in relation to quality of life in head and neck cancer patients. *Head & Neck* **20**, 540–8.

89. **Brookes, G.B.** (1985). Nutritional status—a prognostic indicator in head and neck cancer. *Otolaryngology—Head and Neck Surgery* **93**, 69–74.

90. **Lopez, M.J.** et al. (1994). Nutritional support and prognosis in patients with head and neck cancer. *Journal of Surgical Oncology* **55**, 33–6.

91. **Scheur, V.B.-d.v.d.** et al. (2000). Survival of malnourished head and neck cancer patients can be predicted by human leukocyte antigen-DR expression and interleukin-6/tumor necrosis factor-alpha response of the monocyte. *Journal of Parenteral and Enteral Nutrition* **24**, 329–36.

92. **Minasian, A. and Dwyer, J.T.** (1998). Nutritional implications of dental and swallowing issues in head and neck cancer. *Oncology* **12**, 1155–62.

93. **Gibson, S. and Wenig, B.** (1992). Percutaneous endoscopic gastrostomy in the management of head and neck carcinoma. *Laryngoscope* **102**, 977–81.

94. **Newman, L. A.** et al. (1998). Eating and weight changes following chemoradiation therapy for advanced head and neck cancer. *Archives of Otolaryngology—Head & Neck Surgery* **124**, 589–92.

95. **Tyldesley, S.** et al. (1996). The use of radiologically placed gastrostomy tubes in head and neck cancer patients receiving radiotherapy. *International Journal of Radiation Oncology, Biology, Physics* **36** (5), 1205–9.

96. **Murphy, B.** et al. (2002). Dietary intake and adaptations in head and neck cancer patients treated with chemo radiation. *Proceedings of the American Society of Clinical Oncology* **21**, 234a (Abstract # 932).

97. **Bunn, P.** (1998). Cancer and acquired immunodeficiency syndrome wasting syndromes: current and future therapies. *Seminars in Oncology* **25**, 1–3.

98. **Heber, D. and Tchekmedyian, N.** (1999). Cancer cachexia and anorexia. In *Nutritional Oncology* (ed. D. Heber, G.L. Blackburn, and V.L.W. Go), pp. 537–46. San Diego: Academic Press.

99. **Tisdale, M.J.** (1997). Biology of cachexia. *Journal of the National Cancer Institute* **89**, 1763–73.

100. **Grond, S.** (1993). Validation of World Health Organization guidelines for pain relief in head and neck cancer. *The Annals of Otology, Rhinology, and Laryngology* **102**, 342–8.

101. **Boerman, R.** et al. (1999). Trigeminal neuropathy secondary to perineural invasion of head and neck carcinomas. *Neurology* **53**, 213–16.

102. **Trumpy, I.G. and Lyberg, T.** (1993). Temporomandibular joint dysfunction and facial pain caused by neoplasms. *Oral Surgery, Oral Medicine, and Oral Pathology* **76**, 149–52.

103. **Cohen, S.G. and Quinn, P.D.** (1988). Facila trismus and myofacial pain associated with infections and malignant disease. *Oral Surgery, Oral Medicine, and Oral Pathology* **65**, 538–44.

104. **Bullitt, E., Tew, J., and Boyd, J.** (1986). Intracranial tumors in patients with facial pain. *Journal of Neurosurgery* **64**, 865–71.

105. **Huntley, T. and Wiesenfeld, D.** (1994). Delayed diagnosis of the cause of facial pain in patients with neoplastic disease: a report of eight cases. *Journal of Oral and Maxillofacial Surgery* **52**, 81–5.

106. **Gouda, J.J. and Brown, J.A.** (1997). Atypical facial pain and other pain syndromes. *Neurosurgical Clinics of North America* **8** (1), 87–100.

107. **Donlon, W.C. and Jacobson, A.L.** (1984). Maxillofacial pain **30**, 151–63.

108. **Thaller, S. and Thaller, J.** (1990). Head and neck symptoms. Is the problem in the ears, face, neck, or oral cavity? *Postgraduate Medicine* **87**, 75–86.

109. **Carr, D., Jacox, A., and Chapman, C.** Acute Pain Management: Operative or Medical Procedures and Trauma. Clinical Practice Guideline No. 1. AHCPR Pub. No. 92-0032. Rockville MD: Agency for Health Care Policy and Research, Public Health Service, US Department of Health and Human Services, 1992.

110. **Chaplin, J.M. and Morton, R.P.** (1999). A prospective, longitudinal study of pain in head and neck cancer patients. *Head & Neck* **21**, 531–7.

111. **Butler, J.D. and Miles, J.** (1998). Dysaesthetic neck pain with syncope. *Pain* **75**, 395–7.

112. **Short, S.O.** et al. (1984). Shoulder pain and function after neck dissection with or without preservation of the spinal accessory nerve. *American Journal of Surgery* **148**, 478–82.

113. **Barrett, N.V.J.** et al. (1988). Physical therapy techniques in the treatment of the head and neck patient. *Journal of Prosthetic Dentistry* **59**, 343–6.

114. **Jannjan, N., Weissman, D., and Pahule, A.** (1992). Improved pain management with daily nursing intervention during radiation therapy for head and neck carcinoma. *International Journal of Radiation Oncology, Biology, Physics* **23**, 647–52.

115. **Epstein, J.B. and Stewart, K.H.** (1993). Radiation therapy and pain in patients with head and neck cancer. *Oral Oncology, European Journal of Cancer* **29**, 191–3.

116. **Smit, M.** et al. (2001). Pain as sign of recurrent disease in head and neck squamous cell carcinoma. *Head & Neck* **23**, 372–5.

117. **Reynolds, R.** (1998). Treatment-induced mucositis: an old problem with new remedies. *British Journal of Cancer* **77** (10), 1689–95.

118. **Saunders, M., Dische, S., and Barrett, A.** (1996). Randomized multicentre trials of CHART versus conventional radiotherapy in head and neck and non small cell lung caner: an interim report. *British Journal of Cancer* **73**, 1455–62.

119. **Eschwege, F., Sncho-Garnier, H., and Gerard, G.** (1988). Ten-year results of randomized trial comparing radiotherapy and concomitant bleomycin to radiotherapy alone in epidermoid carcinomas of the oropharynx: experience of the European Organization for Research and Treatment of Cancer. *National Cancer Institute Monographs* **6**, 275–8.

120. **Wong, W.W.** et al. (1994). Time-dose relationship for local tumor control following alternate week concomitant radiation and chemotherapy of advanced head and neck cancer. *International Journal of Radiation Oncology, Biology, Physics* **29**, 153–62.

121. **Liu, R.P.** et al. (1990). Salivary flow rates in patients with head and neck cancer—5 to 25 years after radiotherapy. *Oral Surgery, Oral Medicine, and Oral Pathology* **70**, 724–9.

122. **Marunick, M.** et al. (1991). The effect of head and neck cancer treatment on whole salivary flow. *Journal of Surgical Oncology* **48**, 81–6.

123. **Frazen, L.** et al. (1992). Parotid gland function during and following radiotherapy of malignancies in the head and neck. *British Journal of Cancer* **28**, 457–62.

124. **Cheng, V.S.** et al. (1981). The function of the parotid gland following radiation therapy for head and neck cancer. *International Journal of Radiation Oncology, Biology, Physics* **7**, 253–8.

125. **Mandel, D.D.** (1989). The role of saliva in maintaining oral homeostasis. *The Journal of the American Dental Association* **119**, 298–304.

126. **Wolff, A.** et al. (1990). Pretherapy interventions to modify salivary dysfunction. *National Cancer Institute Monographs* **9**, 87–90.

127. **Vladez, I.H.** et al. (1993). Use of pilocarpine during head and neck radiation therapy to reduce xèrostomia and salivary dysunction. *Cancer* **1993**, 848–51.

128. **Johnson, J.T.** et al. (1993). Oral pilocarpine for post-irradiation xerostomia in patients with head and neck cancer. *New England Journal of Medicine* **329**, 390–5.

129. **LeVeque, F.G.** et al. (1993). A multicenter, randomized, double-blind placebo-controlled-titration study of oral pilocarpine for treatment of radiation-induced xerostomia in head and neck cancer patients. *Journal of Clinical Oncology* **11**, 1124–31.

130. **LeVeque, F.** et al. (1996). Salivary gland sheltering using concurrent pilocarpine (PC) in irradiated head and neck cancer patients. *Proceedings of the American Society of Clinical Oncology* **15**, 1665.

131. **Ho, W.-K.** et al. (1999). Long-term sensorineural hearing deficit folowing radiotherapy in patients suffering from nasopharyngeal carcioma: a prospective study. *Head & Neck* **21**, 547–53.

132. **Nelson, G.M.** (1998). Biology of taste buds and the clinical problem of taste loss. *The Anatomical Record (New Anatomy)* **253**, 70–8.

133. **Marks, J.** et al. (1978). Pharyngeal wall cancer: an analysis of treatment results, complications, and patterns of failure. *International Journal of Radiation Oncology, Biology, Physics* **4**, 587–93.

134. **Gall, A.** et al. (1977). Complications following surgery for cancer of the larynx and hypopharynx **39**, 626.

135. **Downey, R.** et al. (1999). Critical care for the severely ill head and neck patient. *Critical Care Medicine* **27** (1), 95–7.

136. **Lam, H.** et al. (2001). Internal carotid artery hemorrhage after irradiation and osteoradionecrosis of the skull base. *Otolaryngology—Head & Neck Surgery* **125** (5), 522–7.

137. **Citardi, M., Chaloupka, J., and Son, Y.** (1995). Management of carotid artery rupture by monitored endovascular therapeutic occlusion (1988–1994). *Laryngoscope* **105**, 1086–92.

138. **Fujita, M.** et al. (1996). An analysis of mandibular bone complications in radiotherapy for T1 and T2 carcinoma of the oral tongue. *International Journal of Radiation Oncology, Biology, Physics* **34** (2), 333–9.

139. **Beumer, J., Curtis, T., and Morrish, R.** (1976). Radiation complications in edentulous patients. *Journal of Prosthetic Dentistry* **36**, 193–302.

140. **Wang, C.** (1972). Management and prognosis of squamous cell carcinoma of the tonsillar region. *Radiology* **104**, 667–71.

141. **Murray, C., Herson, J., and Daly, T.** (1980). Radiation necrosis of the mandible: a 10-year study, part 1. Factors influencing the onset of necrosis. *International Journal of Radiation Oncology, Biology, Physics* **6**, 543–8.

142. **Larson, D., Lindberg, R., and Lane, E.** Major complications of radiotherapy in cancer of the oral cavity and oropharynx. *American Journal of Surgery* **146**, 531–6.

143. **Coffin, F.** (1983). The incidence and management of ostesoradionecrosis of the jaws following head and neck radiotherapy. *Journal of Radiological Protection* **56**, 851–7.

144. **Emami, B.** et al. (1987). Reirradiation of recurrent head and neck cancers. *Laryngoscope* **97**, 85–8.

145. **Withers, H., Peters, L., and Taylor, J.** (1995). Late normal tissue sequela from radiation therapy for carcinoma of the tonsil: patterns of fractionation study of radiobiology. *International Journal of Radiation Oncology, Biology, Physics* **33**, 563–8.

146. **Silverman, S.J.** (1999). Current concepts in the management of oral/dental adverse sequelae of head and neck radiotherapy. In *Radiation Injury—Advances in Mangement and Prevention* Vol. 32 (ed. J. Meyers and J. Vaeth). Karger.

147. **Savostin-Ashling, I. and Silverman, S.** (1996). Effects of therapeutic radiation on microvasculature of the human mandible. *Oral Surgery, Oral Medicine, Oral Pathology, Oral Radiology, and Endodontics* **81**, 506–7.

148. **Freidman, R.** (1990). Osteoradionecrosis: causes and prevention. *National Cancer Institute Monographs* **9**, 145–9.

149. Consensus statement: oral complications of cancer therapies. (1990). *National Cancer Institute Monographs* **9**, 3–8.

150. **Rosenberg, S.** (1990). Chronic dental complications. *National Cancer Institute Monographs* **9**, 173–7.

151. **Kluth, E., Jain P., and Stutchell, R.** (1987). A study of factors contributing to the development of osteonecrosis of the jaws. *Journal of Prosthetic Dentistry* **58**, 78–82.

152. **Greenspan, D. and Daniels, T.** (1987). Effectiveness of pilocarine in postradiation xerstomia. *Cancer* **59**, 1123–5.

153. **Manthorpe, R., Frost-Larsen, K., and Isager, H.** (1980). Sjögren's syndrome treated with bromhexine: a reassessment. *British Journal of Medicine* **280**, 1356.

154. **Seto, B., Buemer, J., and Kagawa, T.** (1985). Analysis of endodontic therapy in patients irradiated for head and neck cancer. *Journal of Prosthetic Dentistry* **51**, 314–17.

155. **McDermott, I. and Rosenberg, S.** (1984). Overdentures for the irradiated patient. *Journal of Prosthetic Dentistry* **51** (3), 314–17.

156. **Hussey, D. and Feidland, J.** (1991). Second report of a pilot study of pentoxifyllline in the treatment of late radiation necrosis. In *Workshop on Pentoxifylline Leukocyte Cytokines L Potential Therapeutic Uses*, Scottsdale, A7.

157. **Futran, N., Trotti, A., and Gwende, C.** (1997). Pentoxifylline in the treatment of radiation-related soft tissue injury: preliminary observations. *Laryngoscope* **107**, 391–5.

158. **Mainous, E. and Har, G.** (1975). Osteoradionecrosis of the mandible. *Archives of Otolaryngology—Head & Neck Surgery* **101**, 173–7.

159. **Marx, R.** (1983). A new concept in the treatment of osteoradionecrosis. *Journal of Oral and Maxillofacial Surgery* **41**, 351–7.

160. **Aitasalo, K.** et al. (1983). A modifed protocol for early treatment of osteomyelitis and osteoradionecrosis of the mandible. *Head & Neck* **20**, 411–17.

161. **Singer, P.** et al. (1995). Treatment guidelines for patients with hyperthyroidism and hypothyroidism. Standards of Care Committee. American Thyroid Association. *Journal of the American Medical Association* **173**, 80–1.

162. **Wysolmerski, J. and Broadus, A.** (1994). Hypercalcemia of malignancy: the central role of parathyroid hormone-related proteins. *Annual Review of Medicine* **45**, 189–200.

163. **Dische, S., Suanders, M.I., and Warburton, M.** (1986). Hemoglobin, radiation, morbidity and survival. *International Journal of Radiation Oncology, Biology, Physics* **12**, 1335–7.

164. **Vijakumar, S.** et al. (1993). Effect of subcutaneous recombinant human erythropoietin in cancer patients receiving radiotherapy: preliminary results of a randomized, open-labeled, phase II trial. *International Journal of Radiation Oncology, Biology, Physics* **26**, 721–9.

165. **Fazekas, J.** et al. (1987). Failure of misonidazole-sensitized radiotherapy to impact upon outcome among stage III-IV squamous cancers of the head and neck. *International Journal of Radiation Oncology, Biology, Physics* **13**, 1155–60.

166. **Overgaard, J.** et al. (1989). Misonidazole combined with split-course radiotherapy in the treatment of invasive carcinoma of larynx and pharynx: report from DAHANCA 2 study. *International Journal of Radiation Oncology, Biology, Physics* **16**, 1065–8.

167. **Lee, D.-J.** et al. (1995). Results of an RTOG phase III trial (RTOG-85-27) comparing radiotherapy plus etanidazole with radiotherapy alone for locally advanced head and neck carcinomas. *International Journal of Radiation Oncology, Biology, Physics* **32** (3), 567–76.

168. **Lee, W.R.** et al. (1991). Anemia is associated with decreased survival and increased locoregional failure in patients with locally advanced head and neck carcioma: a secondary analysis of RTOG 85-27. *International Journal of Radiation Oncology, Biology, Physics* **42**, 1069–75.

169. **Fein, D.A.** et al. (1995). Pretreatment hemoglobin level influences local control and survival of T1-T2 squamous cell carcinomas of the glottic larynx. *Journal of Clinical Oncology* **13**, 2077–83.

170. **Overgaard, J.** et al. (1986). Primary radiotherapy of larynx and pharynx carcinoma—an analysis of some factors influencing local control and survival. *International Journal of Radiation Oncology, Biology, Physics* **12**, 515–21.

8.12 Mouth care

Franco De Conno, Alberto Sbanotto, Carla Ripamonti, and Vittorio Ventafridda

Introduction

Lesions of the oral cavity have a great impact on the quality of life of patients with advanced cancer. Such lesions cause considerable morbidity and interfere a great deal with both physical and psychological functions. Perhaps most importantly, these complications impair oral nutrition with a variety of consequences, including malnutrition, anorexia, and cachexia. In addition, psychological disturbances relate to the role that the oral cavity plays in communication, social life, and pleasures associated with eating.

Oral hygiene

Good oral hygiene is fundamental to the well being of cancer patients. Its purpose is to:

1. keep lips and oral mucosa clean, soft, and intact, as far as possible;
2. remove plaque and debris;
3. prevent oral infection, decay, periodontal disease, and halitosis;
4. relieve oral pain and discomfort and increase or maintain oral intake;
5. prevent further damage to the oral mucosa in patients undergoing antineoplastic and pharmacological treatments;
6. minimize psychological distress and social isolation and increase family involvement; and
7. maintain the patient's dignity even as death is approaching.

Oral cavity examination (Table 1), should be carried out routinely during the patient's stay in hospital or hospice or at home and should follow a fixed schedule of at least twice a week (Table 2). Daily brushing with a soft-bristle toothbrush, use of unwaxed dental floss, and rinsing with a mild solution of sodium bicarbonate (one teaspoonful per large cup of water), form the basis of good oral hygiene. A thick paste of sodium bicarbonate and a few drops of warm water can be applied by the patient with a soft toothbrush in a 'pat and push' manner into the gingival sulcus and around the teeth. This technique is an effective complementary regimen to mechanical plaque debridement for reducing sulcus/pocket

Table 1 Factors to be considered before oral cavity examination

Local
Oral hygiene (methods, products used)
Previous/actual dental diseases (periodontopathy, decay)
Dentures (type, cleaning methods)
Local pain
Haemorrhages
Ulceration (infections, trauma, tumour)
Xerostomia
Taste alterations
Dysphagia
Local tumour
Previous/current chemotherapy/local radiotherapy and/or surgery
Oxygen therapy, breathing by mouth
Previous/current infections (viral, bacterial, mycotic)
Systemic
Drugs (steroids, antibiotics, anticholinergic, chemotherapy)
Dehydration
Cachexia syndrome
Diabetes, hypothyroidism
Immunological diseases
Nutritional status

Table 2 Oral cavity: routine examination

Equipment: examination gloves, light, tongue depressor, hand mirror

1. External examination of the lips, degree of mouth opening
2. Remove dentures (if present)
3. Observe the state of the following structures:
   —the hard and soft palate
   —the pillars of the fauces and pharynx
   —the internal side of the cheeks
   —the oral vestibule and outer part of the gums
   —the upper side of the tongue
   —the lower part of the tongue, the floor of the mouth, and of inner part of the gums
   —the state of the teeth
   —the state of any denture

Table 3 Care of dentures

Reline dentures if they are loose
Brush and clean well after meals
Remove dentures overnight and leave them (non-metal) in an antiseptic solution (1% sodium hypochlorite)
Brush metal dentures with povidone–iodine solution
If dentures are stained, soak in warm water with a commercial denture cleaner[a] (brushing and rinsing before reinserting)
If oropharyngeal candidiasis is present, leave dentures in nystatin suspension

[a] Many disinfectant solutions can also promote certain microbial growth if left to stagnate for more than 24 h.

organisms and improving periodontal health.[1,2] Commercial mouthwashes may be helpful, but patients with stomatitis may have to avoid products containing alcohol, lemon, and glycerine as well as dentifrices with an abrasive action.

Many patients wear partial or complete dentures. Cachectic patients may find that their dentures are loose and ill-fitting, with consequent abrasions and ulcerations of soft tissue, and pain. Some principles for the care of dentures are presented in Table 3. A careful oral examination is important to maintain good hygiene.

Importance of saliva for oral health

Saliva is a major protector of the tissues and organs of the mouth. In its absence both the hard and soft tissues of the oral cavity may be severely damaged, with an increase in ulcerations, infections such as candidiasis,[3] and dental decay.[4,5]

About 1000–1500 ml of saliva are produced daily by the parotid, submaxillary, and sublingual glands and by small, minor salivary glands of the oral cavity. Salivary pH is about 6–7, favouring the digestive action of a salivary enzyme, α-amylase. Saliva is composed of a serous part (α-amylase), devoted to starch digestion, and a mucous component which acts as a lubricant. It is saturated with calcium and phosphate and is necessary for maintaining healthy teeth. The bicarbonate content of saliva enables it to buffer and produces the conditions necessary for the digestion of plaque which holds acids in contact with teeth.[6] Moreover, saliva helps with bolus formation and lubricates the throat for the easy passage of food. The organic and inorganic components of the salivary secretions have a protective potential. They act as a barrier to irritants and a means of removing cellular and bacterial debris. Saliva contains various components involved in defence against bacterial and viral invasion, including mucins, lipids, secretory immunoglobulin, lysozymes, lactoferrin, salivary peroxidase, and myeloperoxidase.

Amylase originates from the salivary glands; its production is reduced by gland damage, as occurs following radiotherapy.[7] Lysozyme, lactoferrin, and myeloperoxidase are all present in polymorphonuclear leucocytes, which may release these molecules into the saliva. Lysozyme and lactoferrin are also synthesized in acinar cells. The activity of these molecules is increased following oral inflammation.[8,9] Although the minor glands only produce approximately 10 per cent of the total salivary output, they account for 70 per cent of the total mucin in saliva.[10] This substance protects the oral tissues from chemical and mechanical trauma and infections, and lubricates the oral membranes.[11] Raised serum and salivary immunoglobulin concentrations have been found in patients with oral cancer.[12,13] These may result from the production of soluble immunostimulatory tumour-associated antigens by such patients.

Numerous other factors are also important in the preservation of the oral mucosa.[14] In frogs, the presence of magainins, intrinsic protective components of the skin, has been described recently. Similar substances may have a protective role for mammalian mucosa.[15]

Table 4 Causes of xerostomia

1. Reduced salivary secretion caused by —radiotherapy of the head and neck regions —surgery in the buccal and submandibular regions —drugs —obstruction, infection, aplasia, malignant destruction of salivary glands —encephalitis, brain tumours, neurosurgical operations, autonomic pathways destruction —hypothyroidism —autoimmune diseases —sarcoidosis
2. Widespread erosion of buccal mucosa caused by —cancer —chemotherapy, radiotherapy, immunodeficiency —stomatitis —viral, bacterial, and fungal oral infections
3. Dehydration caused by —anorexia —diarrhoea —fever —O_2 therapy —breathing by mouth —large bedsores and/or ulcers —vomiting —polyuria —haemorrhage —diabetes insipidus —difficulty in swallowing
4. Depression, anxiety

Xerostomia

Xerostomia is the subjective feeling of dryness of the mouth, not always accompanied by a detectable decrease in saliva flow.[16,17] In general, unstimulated whole salivary flow rates of less than 0.1 ml/min are considered low and indicative of xerostomia.[18] It is a symptom that receives little attention and so its prevalence may be underestimated. In one series of patients with advanced cancer receiving care in the community or in hospice setting 88 per cent reported dry mouth of a mean intensity of $6.2 \pm$ SD 2.21 (mean $\pm$ SD) on a 1–10 scale.[19]

In a study of 529 adults in a primary care setting, the prevalence of xerostomia was 29 per cent.[17] Women were more frequently affected and there was a positive correlation with age. Few data are available on the frequency of xerostomia in patients with advanced cancer, although 30 per cent of patients beginning a palliative care programme described it as 'a lot' and 'awful'.[20] It was a specific complaint in 40 per cent of a sample of patients at the time of admission to a hospice, but probably all patients suffer from a dry mouth at some point during the terminal stage of cancer.[21] Causes of xerostomia are listed in Table 4.

A variety of symptoms may be associated with the feeling of oral dryness. In the study of Sreebny et al.[17] the symptoms most frequently present (in 48 per cent or more of the xerostomic subjects) were: the need to do something to keep the mouth moist, the need to get up at night to drink water, and difficulty with speech. Other problems included:

1. having to keep fluids at the bedside,
2. a reduction in taste acuity,
3. difficulty with chewing dry foods,
4. burning and tingling sensations on the tongue,
5. the presence of cracks or fissures at the corners of the lips, and
6. difficulty in swallowing.

These symptoms contribute to anorexia, loss of weight, and cachexia. Dental prostheses will frequently traumatize the vulnerable mucosa, leading to further difficulty in mastication and reduced intake of food.(22)

Xerostomia due to radiotherapy

Patients treated with radiotherapy for oral or head and neck cancer often suffer from xerostomia from the beginning of treatment. Radiation can affect one or both parotid glands and the submandibular salivary glands, resulting in a marked diminution in the normal salivary flow(23–29) as a consequence of inflammation and degeneration of the acini and ducts,(24–30) connective tissue,(31) and vascular components of the salivary glands. The most important factor affecting salivary flow after a curative dose of radiotherapy seems to be the volume of the major salivary glands irradiated,(23) particularly the parotid as it is more radiosensitive than the other major salivary glands.(32–34) The flow rate of an irradiated parotid gland is almost negligible after only two treatments of 2.25 Gy each.(35) When 100 per cent of the parotid gland is irradiated, no saliva can be produced; however, exclusion of 10–20 per cent of the gland from the radiation field allows the continued production of saliva.(32) A sharp decrease in salivary flow usually occurs after the first week of radiotherapy with a dose of about 10 Gy.(29,33,36) The decrease in the flow rate continues throughout the treatment, which may lead to persistent xerostomia.(29,33) While one study noted a partial return of salivary flow 8 months after the end of radiotherapy,(28) others found minimal, if any, improvement some years after radiotherapy.(37,38)

Irradiation of the salivary glands causes saliva to become more viscous,(7,25,30,39) and more acidic, with a loss of organic and inorganic components.(40,41) Production of the aqueous component of whole saliva is much more sharply depressed than that of the protein component during xerostomia. Therefore, the capacity of saliva to act as a barrier against irritating substances or to remove bacterial and cellular debris is reduced. The bicarbonate content also diminishes,(7,25,30) further impairing the cleansing action of saliva and there is an increase in the salivary content of Na^+, Cl^-, Mg^{++}, and protein.(25,30,34) The reduction in salivary flow, together with these qualitative changes, can alter the oral microbial flora and result in increased growth of *Streptococcus, Lactobacillus,* and *Candida.* These often irreversible changes can rapidly damage dental structures and increase tooth decay.(26,40)

In patients undergoing radiotherapy, tooth decay can be rapid and lesions can be manifest within 3–6 months.(25) The process of decay may cause pain in the oral cavity, adding to the suffering of the patient. Loss of already decaying teeth causes further difficulty in mastication, which, when added to xerostomia, may cause difficulty in swallowing and digestion. Saving the minor oral glands may play an important role in protection against new colonization by micro-organisms(7,34,43,44) or against tooth decay.(42,45,46)

Apart from flow rate measurements, the level of α-amylase seems to be the best indicator of salivary gland function during radiotherapy, whereas albumin and lactoferrin are good indicators of the inflammatory reactions often related to irradiation.(7) To assess long-term xerostomia in patients receiving parotid-sparing radiation therapy for head and neck cancer a self-reported xerostomia-specific questionnaire was recently elaborated.(47)

Drug-induced xerostomia

A large number of drugs cause dryness of the mouth, including tricyclic antidepressants, antihistamines, anticholinergic drugs, anticonvulsants, antipsychotics, hypnotics, β-blockers, and diuretics.(7,48,49,52) They may reduce the flow of saliva directly or indirectly and some have a parasympatholytic effect. In the study of Sreebny et al.(51) almost 60 per cent of those patients with a dry mouth were taking drugs known to cause this symptom.

The intake of xerostomia-inducing medications is positively correlated with age and with the total number of drugs taken daily(50,51) and it is highest among institutionalized patients.(50) Reduced salivation in the elderly may be related to drug use rather than to age.

Xerostomia was not generally recognized as a side-effect of morphine(53) but clinical experience suggested that it was a common problem in cancer patients treated with morphine. Ventafridda et al.(54) observed a significantly higher incidence of dry mouth following treatment with oral aqueous morphine than with methadone or controlled-release morphine tablets.(55) Another study, carried out for a 2-month period after initial treatment, noted that dry mouth was present 35 per cent of the time during treatment with an anti-inflammatory and/or adjuvant drugs, 36 per cent of the time during treatment with weak opioids and/or adjuvants, and 51 per cent of the time during treatment with strong opioids and/or adjuvants.(56) White et al.(53) also describe a highly significant association between the use of morphine and xerostomia, and it seems clear now that dryness of the mouth is a common side effect of oral morphine.

Other factors which may contribute to xerostomia

Dehydration

Advanced cancer patients are often dehydrated (Table 4), with consequent thirst and dry mouth.(57) There have been no controlled clinical trials which have demonstrated any relief of xerostomia following hydration, and the use of parenteral hydration in the palliative care setting remains controversial. A recent study(58) did not show any association between the severity of thirst and fluid intake in palliative care patients. When present, symptoms related to dehydration seem to be manageable with simple measures, such as oral fluids or ice chips and lubrication of the lips.(59) The therapy of dehydration-induced xerostomia can be specific (Table 5) or exclusively palliative (Table 6).

Decreased mastication

Mastication plays an important role in the regulation of salivary secretion, its effects being mediated through somatic afferent nerves of the oral mucosa and in the periodontal tissues. Patients taking a liquid diet or with immobilized jaws following oral surgery show a significant decrease in salivary flow.(18) No data are available concerning decreased salivation in enterally fed patients or those with a gastrostomy or affected by trismus.

Psychological factors

Psychological factors, including anxiety, are known to reduce salivary flow. Hyposalivation and xerostomia may be observed in patients suffering from depression.(60)

Table 5 Specific therapies for oral complications

Xerostomia
2% citric acid solution(16)
75–100 mg nicotinic acid more than once per day(21)
Dihydroergotamine(203)
Pilocarpine(68–71)
Antholetrithione ANTT(72)
ANTT + pilocarpine(31)
Xerostomia caused by drugs
Reduce the dosage and/or change the drug if possible
Application of fluoride gel to avoid dental damage
Xerostomia caused by systemic dehydration
Correct the cause
Increase the liquid intake by mouth
Hypodermoclysis (not endstage patients)
Make use of intravenous hydration in selected patients
Decay
Good dental hygiene
Gargle with saline, peroxide, or solutions of baking soda(42, 204, 205)
Daily application of fluoride gel(42, 204, 205)
Dental treatment

Table 6 Palliative therapy for xerostomia

Oral hygiene every 2 h
Humidified air
Suck: ice cubes, vitamin C tablets, frozen tonic water[21]
Chew: sugarless chewing gum, lemon sugar candy, acid substances, pieces of pineapple[21]
Artifical saliva: ◆ glycerin, cologel, normal saline (1 : 1 : 8) ◆ carboxymethylcellulose, sorbitol, water, sodium fluoride, menthol, minerals, and chlorhexidine ◆ methylcellulose + lemon essence + water[21] ◆ hydrophilic chewing gum which releases artifical saliva with a remineralizing effect[206] ◆ mucin-containing artificial saliva based on bovine salivary gland extract[207]
Dentures which include a reservoir for the release of artificial saliva[208]

Prevention and treatment of xerostomia

The regimen currently used by the authors involves good oral hygiene, the prevention and treatment of infections such as candidiasis by administration of clotrimazole or fluconazole (especially in high-risk patients such as those undergoing high-dose corticosteroid therapy or radiotherapy for head and neck cancer), and a review of the drug regimen to avoid the use of drugs that may induce xerostomia.

Xerostomia after radiation therapy may be the most difficult to treat since irreversible damage to the salivary glands may occur. Seikaly and colleagues in a prospective non-randomized study of patients with head and neck cancer, transferred one submandibular gland from the side of the neck with the least risk of metastases to the submental area during neck dissection. This technique successfully prevented radiation-induced xerostomia.[61]

Current therapy for chronic xerostomia includes the use of saliva substitutes or salivary stimulants. Water, glycerine preparations, and artificial saliva are used as substitutes for saliva, while sialogogues, sugarless sweets, and chewing gum stimulate the production of saliva.[62] Many commercial products are available for use primarily as a gargle to relieve the symptoms of xerostomia. Rarely do they improve the problem but only a small number of controlled clinical studies have been performed. Artificial preparations of saliva that contain mucin provide substantially more symptomatic relief to patients with xerostomia than do conventional, non-mucin substitutes.[63–67]

Currently available therapies for xerostomia are listed in Table 5. Pilocarpine, an alkaloid, functions primarily as a muscarinic–cholinergic agonist, and has potent effects on both smooth muscle and exocrine tissues. It has been shown to stimulate salivary flow and increase salivation in patients treated by radiotherapy and in those with Sjögren's syndrome.[68–72] The peak secretory effects of pilocarpine are assumed to occur within 1 h after its intake.[69] Controlled studies have been carried out on the use of oral pilocarpine for radiation-induced xerostomia.[69–71,73–75] All these studies show that pilocarpine produces clinically significant benefits with acceptable side-effects. Best results are obtained with continuous treatment for more than 8 weeks with doses greater than 2.5 mg three times a day. A 5.0-mg three times a day regimen produces the best clinical results when both efficacy and side-effects are considered. Higher doses (10 mg three times a day) can increase clinical benefits; however, an increase in side-effects (mainly moderate sweating) may occur. Pilocarpine-treated patients require lesser amounts of artificial saliva; furthermore, patients treated with pilocarpine report that improvements in xerostomia, comfort, and speaking occur immediately. Pilocarpine is contraindicated in patients subject to bronchospasm or who have pre-existing bradycardia. A recent French trial evaluated the action of pilocarpine hydrochloride against xerostomia and the relationship of the response to dose/volume radiotherapy parameters.[76] The response to pilocarpine was independent of the dose of radiotherapy suggesting that pilocarpine acts primarily by stimulating minor salivary glands and may be of benefit to patients with severe xerostomia regardless of the radiotherapy dose.

Anethole-trithione (Sialor, Sulfarlem) seems to act directly on the secretory cells of the salivary glands. Some studies have found it to improve salivary flow, while others have not.[77] Epstein and Schubert reported a phase I–II trial of the combined use of pilocarpine and anethole-trithione in patients who had not responded with increased saliva production to either agent alone.[31] A statistically significant increase in salivary volume and improved symptoms were reported. Seemingly the anethole-trithione prepared the salivary glands cells for the stimulation provided by pilocarpine. Acupuncture has been shown recently to be effective in patient with pilocarpine-resistant xerostomia after radiotherapy.[78]

Dietary advice includes the ingestion of foods with a high moisture content and the drinking of plenty of liquids with meals to facilitate mastication.

Infections

In comparison to normal subjects, the oral flora of patients with advanced cancer more often includes yeasts (83 per cent), coliforms (49 per cent), and coagulase-positive staphylococci (28 per cent).[79] Such data indicate a loss of resistance to colonization of the oral mucosa in terminal cancer patients. Many predisposing factors for candidiasis may be present, including antibiotics and immunosuppressive agents,[80] nutritional factors,[81] and low salivary rates.[82,83] Increased oral coliforms have been reported in several groups of compromised patients, including those on cytotoxic therapy for malignant disease,[84] patients who have received radiotherapy for oral and laryngeal cancer,[85] and those with acute leukaemia.[86] Perhaps the release of endotoxin by Gram-negative bacilli may be responsible for oral soreness and clinical inflammation of the oral mucosa.[87] Microbial factors, such as adhesion and interbacterial interference, exogenous factors, including antimicrobial chemotherapy, and miscellaneous host factors, such as xerostomia,[79] seem to play an important part in the loss of resistance to bacterial colonization.

Fungal infections

Candidiasis is the most common fungal infection seen in cancer patients.[88] *Candida* species are reported to be present in the normal oral flora of 40–60 per cent of the population.[89] In healthy asymptomatic subjects *Candida* is usually present in the vegetative form (blastospore); when pathogenic it can also exist in a hyphal form. Positive cultures are obtained from about 75 per cent of asymptomatic hospital patients; this proportion can reach 89 per cent if repeated cultures are obtained over a period of time.[57,83]

Clinically evident candidiasis developed in up to 27 per cent of patients admitted to an oncology ward.[90] Oropharyngeal candidiasis can be the source of regional and systemic dissemination, particularly in granulocytopenic and immunosuppressed patients.[91]

The primary pathogen is *Candida albicans*, but other *Candida* species and other fungi, including *Aspergillus*, may be involved. The development of clinically evident oral candidiasis depends on local and/or systemic factors commonly involved in other oral infections and symptoms (Table 7). The role of xerostomia and drugs (such as steroids) should be emphasized; about 40 per cent of patients receiving adrenal corticosteroid therapy and about 30 per cent of those receiving antibiotics, develop oropharyngeal candidiasis.[92] Oral *Candida* infection usually presents as acute pseudomembranous candidiasis (thrush), acute atrophic candidiasis (or acute erythematous candidiasis), chronic atrophic (or chronic erythematous) candidiasis, chronic hyperplastic candidiasis, or candidal cheilosis (Table 8).

Other clinical presentations are seen more rarely.[93,94] Thrush appears as a white–yellowish plaque, which is easily wiped off, leaving a bleeding, painful surface. The acute atrophic form is often related to broad-spectrum antibiotics; white plaques are minimal and painful lesions of the oral mucosa and depapillation of the dorsum of the tongue are present. Chronic

Table 7 Main factors involved in fungal infections of oral cavity

1. *Local factors*
   - Wearing dentures
   - Xerostomia
   - Saliva composition alterations[a]
   - Oral mucosa disruption[b]
   - Microbial alterations
   - Reduced mechanical debridement[c]
   - Previous infections
   - Poor oral hygiene
2. *Systemic factors*
   - Diabetes
   - Immunosuppression
   - Medical therapies (e.g. steroids)
   - Nutritional status alterations

[a] Mainly proteins and electrolytes.
[b] Radiotherapy, chemotherapy, surgery, cancer.
[c] Comatose patients, enterally/parenterally fed patients, trismus, etc.

Table 8 Common clinical pictures of oral candidiasis

Type	Signs/symptoms (see text for more details)
Thrush (acute pseudomembranous form)	Typical white–yellowish plaques. Usually accompanied by tenderness, burning, dysphagia, dysgeusia
Acute atrophic	More generalized red lesions, tongue depapillation. Dysgeusia usually present
Chronic atrophic	Bright red surface (denture print); often accompanied by angular cheilitis, which can be moderately painful and bleeding. Dysgeusia usually present
Chronic hyperplastic	Usually resembles leukoplakia. Symptoms are usually absent

atrophic candidiasis is characterized by erythema and oedema, usually localized to the part of the palatal mucosa in contact with dentures. This particular form of candidiasis occurs in up to 65 per cent of elderly individuals who wear complete maxillary dentures and is more common in women. Individuals with denture-related chronic atrophic candidiasis often also have angular cheilitis characterized by soreness, redness, and cracks at the corners of the mouth. It can be either erosive or granular in type; habitual licking of the corners of the mouth and a reduction in the vertical dimensions of the lower third of the face, due to edentia, play a major role in this clinical form. Chronic candidal infections are also capable of producing a hyperplastic clinical picture which can resemble leucoplakia, especially when occurring in the retrocommissural area; its role as a precancerous lesion remains open to debate.[(95)]

In patients with advanced cancer a cytological diagnosis is not generally necessary; when indicated, a wet-mounted potassium hydroxide preparation or Gram stain may be performed. Immunofluorescent techniques are less useful.[(96)]

Both topical and systemic treatments are available, and they can be used together in more severe cases. Nystatin suspension (100 000 U/ml, 4–6 ml every 6 h) is the classic, topical treatment of oral candidiasis but results can sometimes be disappointing.[(97,98)] (Its action is limited to the time of contact with the mucosal surface; consequently ice lollies made of nystatin diluted with water are a soothing and effective alternative). Any combination with chlorhexidine reduces its activity.[(99)] Clotrimazole lozenges (10 mg five times a day) have good antimycotic activity, even in nystatin-resistant patients.[(100,101)] Clotrimazole is well tolerated and inexpensive[(102)] and seems to be an effective drug for the prevention of oropharyngeal candidiasis.[(103)] Miconazole, an imidazole derivative, is another suggested topical treatment, and is very effective in the form of lozenges (250 mg four times daily) or gel (two to four times daily),[(104,105)] although the taste of lozenges may be found unpleasant. Amphotericin B lozenges can also be used for oral candidiasis, but are not as effective as clotrimazole and miconazole.[(106)] Intravenous amphotericin is not indicated in the treatment of oral candidal infection, due to the low concentrations that are achieved in saliva.[(107)]

Table 9 Weekly costs of some antifungal drugs

Drug	Daily dosage	Cost ($)
Nystatin suspension (100 000 U/ml)	24 00 000 U	8.00
Miconazole (oral gel 2%)	12 ml	19.00
Ketoconazole (capsules 200 mg)	200 mg	9.00
Fluconazole (capsules 50 mg)	50 mg	40.00

Among systemic treatments, ketoconazole (200 mg once daily)[(108,109)] has largely been replaced by the new triazole derivatives, such as fluconazole (50–150 mg once daily) and itraconazole (100–200 mg once daily), which have fewer side-effects. These are well absorbed by the gastrointestinal tract, and have a long half-life, allowing once daily administration. Their spectrum of action is wide; they are active against many different fungi, and hence are useful in the treatment of oropharyngeal candidiasis and systemic and deep fungal infections.[(110–115)] Side-effects are minimal. Fluconazole treatment of oropharyngeal candidiasis (50 g once daily for 7–14 days) is possibly more effective than traditional treatments such as nystatin and ketoconazole,[(114)] and its once-a-day schedule makes it an attractive alternative for patients with advanced cancer. A recent controlled trial, comparing fluconazole versus clotrimazole troche (lozenge), showed a superior capacity of fluconazole in preventing oesophageal and oropharyngeal candidiasis in patients with advanced HIV infection;[(116)] the presence of breakthrough episodes of infections in 10.6 per cent of patients taking fluconazole, raises the possibility of the development of a resistance to this antifungal agent.[(117)] Table 9 shows the relative costs for a 1-week course of the different antifungal drugs. Specific treatment must be accompanied by good oral hygiene.

Bacterial infections

Few data are available concerning bacterial infections in advanced or terminal cancer patients.[(118)] Periodontal disease is very common in the healthy population: about 70–80 per cent of adults are affected by minor periodontitis. About 15 per cent of those between the ages of 60 and 64 are affected by more severe levels of periodontal destruction.[(119)] Studies in patients with acute leukaemia suggest that periodontal disease may be an important cause of death during myelosuppression.[(120–122)] While the common oral flora is characterized by a prevalence of Gram-positive bacteria, xerostomia, chemotherapy, radiotherapy, and immunosuppression cause a shift of oral flora towards Gram-negative colonization.[(123)] The presence of heterogeneous flora, including *Candida* and other species, makes bacterial cultures difficult to interpret, and interactions between bacteria and fungi contribute to the adherence and colonization of host tissues by microorganisms.[(124)] Small haemorrhages, pain localized to the peridontium, and fever can be present, especially during chemotherapy. Secondary infection can be present in nearby[(121,122)] structures and radiographic signs of periapical abscess may exist.

Table 10 Causes of poor oral hygiene and treatment

Pain
If possible, treat the basic cause
Good titration of systemic analgesic drugs
Analgesic gargles with:
◆ benzydamine hydrochloride 0.15%, 15 ml every 2 h
◆ Xylocaine viscous 2%, 5–15 ml every 4 h
◆ Xylocaine spray 10%, every 4 hr
◆ diphenhydramine hydrochloride elixir 12.5 mg/5 ml and aluminum hydroxide in equal parts up to 30 ml every 2 hr
◆ choline salicylate dental paste 8.7%, every 3–4 h on the oral and perioral lesions
◆ aluminum hydroxide and lignocaine 2% in equal parts
◆ dyclonine hydrochloride
◆ cetacaine (benzocaine) 20% solution
◆ systemic analgesics
◆ avoid alcohol and lemon containing mouthwashes
Haemorrhage
Treat the basic cause (e.g. thrombocytopaenia)
Avoid using toothbrush and dental floss
Use a low-pressure dental jet and/or a gauze pad wrapped around a finger or a disposable sponge (toothette) moistened in a mild solution of baking soda and water
Gargles with:
◆ saline solution
◆ hexetidine 0.1%
◆ sodium perborate
◆ chlorhexidine 0.2%
◆ povidone–iodine 1%
◆ bicarbonate of soda
◆ cetylpyridinium
◆ H_2O_2 3–6% in water 1 : 4
Gargles or soaked gauzes with antihaemorrhagic drugs:
◆ thrombin 1–2 g/day
◆ tranexamic acid 2–4 g/day
Debility or unconsciousness
Assisted oral hygiene by using a brush, gargles, spray, dental jet, cotton swabs moistened with mouthwash, gauze
Lips cracking prevention (petroleum jelly)
Room humidifier

The treatment of bacterial infections depends first on adequate hygiene[125–127] (Table 10, Fig. 1). Periodontal probing and scaling could possibly reduce postchemotherapy oral complications:[128–130] the exact role of these treatments in advanced cancer patients has to be evaluated. In acute periodontal infection, broad-spectrum antibiotic therapy is usually initiated, followed by more specific therapy based on the bacterial cultures, if possible and if indicated. Teeth debridement with 2 per cent hydrogen peroxide and frequent rinsing are helpful. Povidone iodine and chlorhexidine 0.2 per cent mouthwashes can be added to the oral hygiene schedule, especially in the presence of fungating cancer lesions. In a palliative care setting pain treatment, usually with non-steroidal anti-inflammatory drugs and topical treatments may play an important role.

Viral infections

Herpes simplex, cytomegalovirus, varicella zoster, and Epstein–Barr virus are the main causes of viral infections of the oral cavity.[131] Herpes simplex virus type 1 is the most common in patients receiving cancer chemotherapy; the reported incidence ranges from about 11 to about 65 per cent[132,133] and different studies suggest a strong correlation of oral mucositis with isolation of herpes simplex virus.[134–136] Oral lesions due to herpes simplex appear to represent recurrent rather than primary infection. There are no data on the incidence of this infection in patients with advanced disease.

Herpetic infections appear as yellowish lesions, which are easily removed from the mucosa and are extremely painful; vesicles can also appear on the lips (cold sores) and fever, anorexia, and malaise may coexist. In severe infections, pain can be so intense as to produce complete dysphagia. The diagnosis of herpes simplex virus infection is mainly clinical: some difficulties can arise from the presence of other oral infections. When needed, exfoliative cytology permits an accurate diagnosis (95 per cent) in a short time.[137] The infection should be differentiated from aphthous ulcers: a history of vesicles preceding ulcers, a location on hard gingiva and hard palate, and crops of lesions are indicative of herpetic infection rather than aphthous ulcers.

Specific treatment of the herpes infection is provided by acyclovir, which can be administered intravenously, with few side-effects, although patients must be hydrated and creatinine clearance monitored.[138–141] Venous extravasation must be avoided. Lymphocyte counts greater than 600 mm^3 and monocyte counts greater than 250 mm^3 have been shown to be necessary for infection to resolve in patients with haematological malignancy.[142] Acyclovir can be employed also for prophylaxis in patients undergoing antineoplastic chemotherapy: screening for anti-HSV antibodies might be useful in order to identify patients at high risk for herpes simplex virus infection.[143] In patients with advanced cancer, the oral and topical route (5 per cent acyclovir ointment) are better employed (Table 10, Fig. 1). Control of associated infections and oral hygiene are necessary. Chlorhexidine (0. 2 per cent twice daily rinsing) may be beneficial with herpes simplex virus type 1 infection.[144] Extraoral lesions may become secondarily infected: topical antibiotics are then indicated.

Neutropenic ulcers

Severe neutropenia (neutrophil count less than 100 mm^3) is very often complicated by mouth ulcers:[145] up to 50 per cent of admissions to hospital with acute leukaemia suffer from this complication.[146] The epidemiology of neutropenic ulcers in patients with advanced solid tumours is unknown. In about one-third of cases neutropenic ulcers can be traced to some local factors—drug toxicity, herpes simplex virus infection, leukaemia infiltration, trauma, or haemorrhage—but the remainder have no identifiable cause.[145,146] Ulcers appear as one or more lesions, characterized by few signs of inflammation, regular margins, and a yellowish appearance; they are not easily removed.[135,146]

Recovery of the neutrophil count is essential for healing.[120] Topical symptomatic measures, such as hydrocortisone pellets or other corticosteroid preparations, and oral hygiene are necessary. Concurrent oral infections have to be specifically treated and prevented. The role of granulocyte macrophage colony-stimulating factor (GM-CSF) is still a matter of study: the high cost is an important limiting factor for a palliative care setting. Thalidomide, a sedative drug withdrawn from the market 30 years ago because of its teratogenic and neurotoxic effects, has been recently used for the treatment of a variety of ulcerative and immunological conditions, especially for recurrent aphthous stomatitis in HIV patients.[147,148] Its role in the treatment of neutropenic ulcers in cancer patients is not known.

Drug- and radiotherapy-induced stomatitis

The epidemiology of these conditions is complicated by the scarcity of data and the fact that other pathogenetic factors may coexist, complicating the exact diagnosis.

Drug-induced stomatitis

Mucositis induced by chemotherapy is a common side-effect of cancer treatment: approximately 40 per cent of patients receiving chemotherapy develop an oral problem related to treatment and patients with haematological malignancies develop oral problems at two or three times the rate of

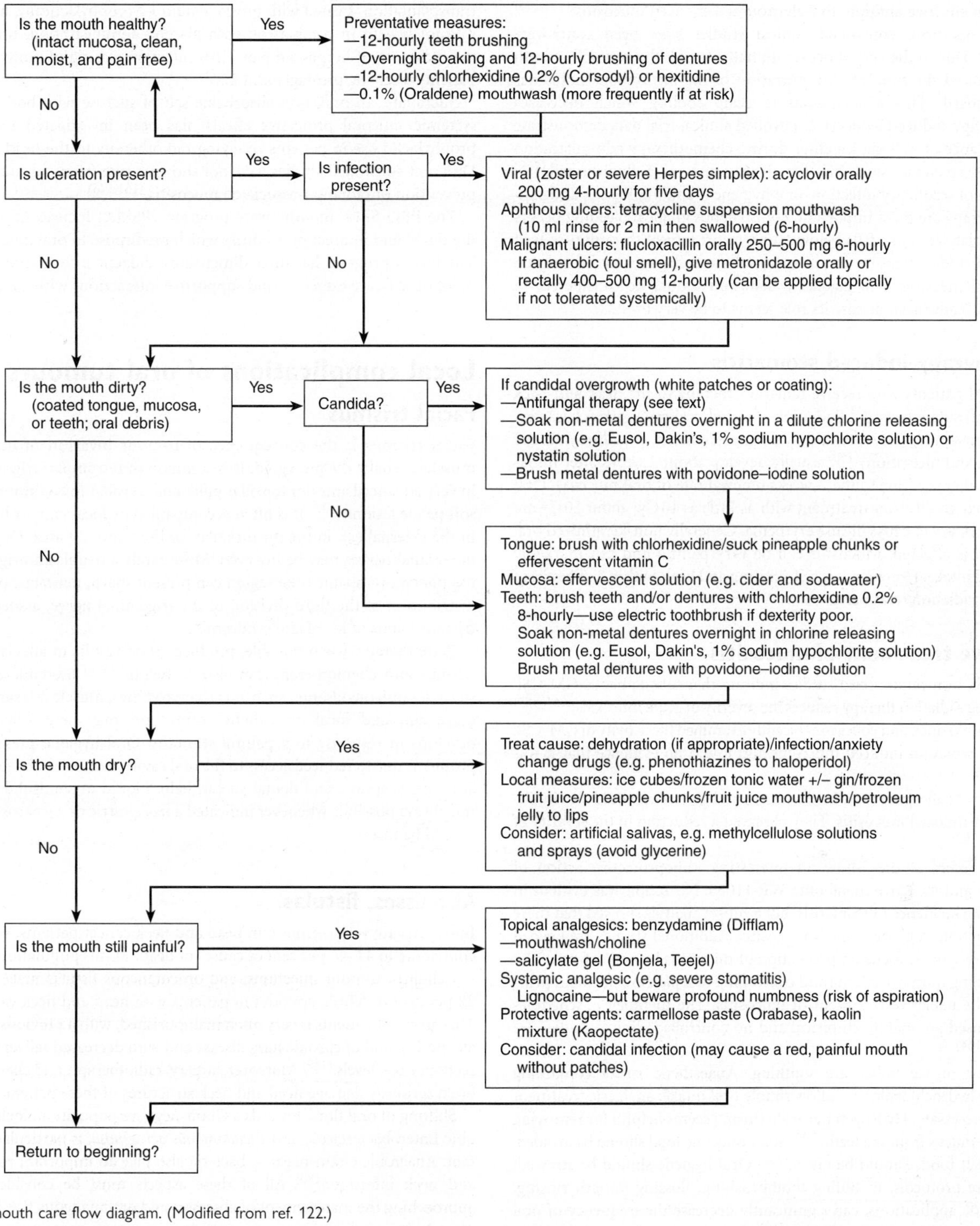

Fig. 1 A mouth care flow diagram. (Modified from ref. 122.)

patients with solid tumours. In patients undergoing bone marrow transplants, more than 75 per cent may experience troublesome mucositis.[149–152] Patients with poor oral health have a higher risk of oral infections following chemotherapy.[153,154]

Stomatotoxicity generally results from the non-specific inhibitory effect of the chemotherapeutic agents on mitosis of the rapidly dividing cells of the oral epithelium (direct toxicity). The reduction of the renewal rate of the mucosa results in atrophic changes and ulceration.[154] Mucositis most often affects the non-keratinized oral mucosa, including the cheek, soft palate, lips, ventral surface of the tongue, and the floor of the mouth. It occurs about 5–7 days after drug administration, often a few days before the patient's haematological nadir. Thus, the mucosal disruption provides a portal of entry for micro-organisms at the time of maximum myelosuppression, and may be accompanied by haemorrhages.

A wide variety of agents may product direct toxicity: notable examples include 5-fluorouracil, methotrexate, and doxorubicin.[150] In general, mucositis is dose-related: drug administration in divided doses, rather than as a bolus, can reduce this problem.

Specific treatment of the oral lesions induced by chemotherapy is almost non-existent:[117] early pilot studies suggested that allopurinol mouthwash could be an effective antidote to 5-fluorouracil-induced mucositis;[155,156] recent results from controlled clinical studies have been controversial.[157,158] Due to the very short serum half-life of 5-fluorouracil, mouth cooling around the time of administration of the intravenous bolus has been proposed. This is analogous to scalp cooling which decreases chemotherapy-induced alopecia. Controlled clinical trial data demonstrate the importance of sucking ice chips during chemotherapy administration in patients receiving short-half-life drugs, such as 5-fluorouracil.[159] Prevention of secondary infection, oral hygiene (Table 10, Fig. 1), and supportive therapy are most important. Spontaneous gingival bleeding occurs when the platelet count falls below 10 000 mm^3: topical thrombin-soaked gauze held under pressure or microcrystalline collagen may be helpful. When local measures fail, platelet transfusion should be considered: in patients with advanced disease its role seems to be very limited.

Radiotherapy-induced stomatitis

Virtually all patients who receive radiation therapy to the head and neck develop oral side-effects.[41] Radiation-induced oral mucositis (characterized by xerostomia, taste alterations, diffuse erythema, pseudomembrane formation, and ulceration)[160] usually develop about 2 weeks after initiation of the therapy (due to the 2-weeks renewal rate of oral mucosa). Oral soreness may result from treatment with as little as 10 Gy; about 20 Gy are usually necessary to cause diffuse erythema. Generally non-keratinized oral epithelium is affected. Mucositis can be very painful and can markedly reduce oral intake. However, it is self-limiting and heals within 2–3 weeks of the end of radiation treatment.

Palliative treatment of mucositis

Some small, non-randomized studies indicate that subcutaneous GM-CSF given during radiation therapy reduces the severity of acute mucositis.[161–163] However, Makkonen and colleagues recently examined the activity of GM-CSF to prevent radiation induced mucositis and found no evidence that it was effective.[161]

Huang and colleagues examined whether oral glutamine could also inhibit radiation-induced mucositis. They observed a reduction in the severity of mucositis.[162]

Several recent studies show an interesting radioprotective action of amifostine and its active metabolite WR-11065. No action was evident in reducing the incidence of stomatitis, but a subset analysis showed that there was a reduction in grade 3 and 4 mucositis. Additional studies are needed with a more specific focus on prevention of mucositis by amifosfine.[163]

Minimizing mucosal trauma and controlling oral pain are the main principles of the palliative treatment of mucositis. The therapeutic schedules currently used are mainly empirical and no controlled clinical studies are available.[164]

Ice chips or ice lollies are soothing. Anaesthetic rinses containing lignocaine hydrochloride may allow simple oral intake; analgesic treatment is usually necessary. Hydrogen peroxide rinsing seems helpful for removing debris and mucus from the teeth.[140] Spicy or acidic food should be avoided; soft, low salt foods should be given.[165] Oral hygiene should be stressed: mouth care protocols, including toothbrushing, flossing, mouth rinsing, and fluoride applications, can significantly decrease the frequency of oral complications (Table 10, Fig. 1).[166–168] Concurrent oral infections, especially candidiasis, should be energetically treated.

Severe oral pain may require systemically administered medications. Morphine or methadone can be administered orally or parenterally.[169] In bone-marrow transplant recipients, where severe mucositis is often present, continuous intravenous unfusion of morphine is used routinely with good results.[170] Patient-controlled analgesia seems to obtain the same results as continuous infusion, with less morphine consumption and less sedation and difficulty in concentrating.[171] Results of prostaglandin E2 administration for treatment of mucositis in patients undergoing chemotherapy and/or radiotherapy or bone marrow transplantation are controversial.[172,173] In a randomized double-blind clinical trial, patients undergoing bone marrow transplantation, treated with prostaglandin E2 prophylactically, had no significant benefit in comparison with placebo administration. Importantly, the incidence of herpes simplex virus infection was significantly higher in patients receiving prostaglandin E2.[174]

Sucralfate, an oral, non-absorbable salt of sucrose with both local and systemic mucosal protective effects, has been investigated for possible prophylactic use in patients receiving radiotherapy to the head and neck. Different controlled studies have not shown a significant advantage in the prevention of radiation-associated mucositis.[161,176]

The PRO-SELF mouth aware program (PSMA) focuses on decreasing the direct and indirect morbidities which predispose to oral mucositis.[175] The PSMA program has three dimensions: didactic information, development of self-care exercises, and supportive interactions with a nurse.

Local complications of oral tumours

Facial trismus

Facial trismus is the consequence of tumour invasion of masticatory muscles, usually the pterygoid. It is common in retromolar trigone lesions, in very advanced anterior tonsillar pillar and tonsillar fossa tumours, and in soft palate lesions.[177] It is often accompanied by local pain or by pain felt in the external ear, in the preauricular, or the temporal area. Occasionally, the cranial nerves may be involved. More rarely a neoplasm originating in the pharygotympanic tube region can present sharp, neuralgic pain in the distribution of the third division of the trigeminal nerve, associated with trismus (sinus of Morgagni syndrome).

Radiotherapy, when possible, produces good results in alleviating facial trismus and chemotherapy can also be helpful.[178] Systemic analgesics, steroids, anticonvulsants (such as carbamazepine), muscle relaxants such as diazepam, and local anaesthetic infiltration may help when trismus develops in response to a painful stimulus. Oral hygiene presents many problems due to reduced access to the oral cavity. Cotton swabs soaked with antiseptics, sprays, and dental jet can help. Liquid or semisolid feeding is not always possible: whenever indicated a nasogastric or a gastrostomy tube should be inserted.

Abscesses, fistulas

Infections are very common in head and neck cancer patients, reported to contribute to 44–46 per cent of causes of death in this population.[179]

Cellulitis, tumour infections, and orocutaneous fistulas make up about 22 per cent of febrile episodes in patients with head and neck cancers.[179] This group of patients is very often malnourished, with a previous history of alcoholism and of chronic lung disease and with decreased salivary flow and secretory IgA levels.[149] Moreover surgery, radiotherapy, and chemotherapy often seriously damage head and neck structures of these patients.

Shifting of oral flora, towards a Gram-negative population, including aerobic Enterobacteriaceae and *Pseudomonas aeruginosa*, is particularly important. Anaerobic Gram-negative bacteria also play an important role in head and neck infection.[180] All of these aspects must be considered when approaching the management of abscesses and orocutaneous fistulas. A simple povidone-iodine solution is a sufficient preventive measure in patients at risk for developing secondary bacterial infections. The same antiseptics can be used as oral medication when an abscess is already present. In the presence of signs of sepsis or of local pain or discharge, broad-spectrum antibiotics, including metronidazole, should be administered.[180] Patient's relatives should be carefully instructed about medication and possible emergencies, such as massive haemorrhages (Table 10).

Tumour discharge

Many oral cavity tumours discharge, causing problems in swallowing and dysphagia and creating a chronic bad taste in the mouth. Radiotherapy may help this symptom, reducing the tumour mass and its secretions, but if this is not possible, local measures must be applied. Frequent rinsing with hydrogen peroxide can help by removing tumour debris. Benzydamine hydrochloride rinse can reduce the colonization of the oral cavity and help patients to cleanse the mouth.[181] Prevention and treatment of other oral problems such as candidiasis is very important (Table 10, Fig. 1).

Taste alteration

Taste alteration occurs as a reduction in taste sensitivity (hypogeusia), an absence of taste sensation (ageusia), or a distortion of normal taste (dysgeusia). The incidence of these symptoms is unknown, but according to Twycross between 25 and 50 per cent of cancer patients have a diminished taste sensation.[182] Our clinical experience suggests that taste alterations are hardly ever reported spontaneously by the patients, but many will report it as a reason for loss of appetite if specifically questioned. Patients typically report that 'the food is tasteless' or 'the food is bitter'.

Taste is mediated through the taste buds, each of which contain about 50 cells and are continuously renewed. The number of taste buds decreases with age. They are found on the tongue, soft palate, pharynx, larynx, epiglottis and uvula, lips and cheeks, and in the upper third of the oesophagus. The tongue is most sensitive to sweetness on the anterior surface and tip, to salt and sour tastes on the two lateral sides, and to bitter tastes on the circumvillate papillae on the posterior surface. Sour and bitter taste are perceived most acutely on the palate; salt and sweet are most sensitive on the tongue. The pharynx has decreased sensitivity to all four tastes.

The cells of the taste buds are provided with microvilli in direct communication with the oral cavity through an apical pore. A protein (the gate-keeper) regulates the quantity of stimuli that pass through the pore per unit of time. Changes in these protein molecules are controlled by the equilibrium of metals, and zinc in particular is associated with hypogeusia and anorexia.[183–185]

Taste information is sent by way of the fifth, seventh, ninth, and tenth cranial nerves to the medulla (nucleus of the tractus solitarius), and from there through pons and thalamus to the cortical area subserving taste. Information in this pathway is also projected to the lateral hypothalamus. A lesion in any one of these areas can alter taste perception.[186]

The effect of cancer on taste is unknown. Potential causes of taste alteration are listed in Table 11. Taste abnormalities in cancer patients may be correlated with the site or extent of the tumour, independent of the histological type. A positive correlation exists between weight loss and the presence of abnormal taste sensation.[187] Disturbances in taste can also alter digestion because stimulation of taste organs can increase salivary and pancreatic flow, gastric contractions, and bowel motility.[186] There is also an association between advanced disease and an abnormality in the recognition of sugar and urea. A higher concentration of sweetness is needed for the solution to be recognized.[187]

Williams and Cohen[187] demonstrated elevated thresholds for recognition of sour (HCl), but not bitter (urea), sweet (sucrose), or salt (NaCl) in a group of patients with lung cancer who were tested before receiving chemotherapy or radiotherapy. An elevated threshold of detection for all four basic tastes was reported in a group of patients with laryngeal cancer who were examined before laryngectomy.[188,189]

Taste alterations have been reported as a consequence of radiotherapy for tumours in the head and neck regions. This effect may be due to damage to the microvilli of the taste cells or to reduced salivation. Taste loss is not observed until radiation doses of 20 Gy have been administered.[190,191] At doses of 20–40 Gy taste loss increases rapidly and a dose of 60 Gy causes a relative taste loss of over 90 per cent.[190] Mossman et al.[38] demonstrated that curative courses of radiotherapy for tumours of the head and neck resulted in long-term changes in taste and salivary function; the maximum tolerance doses resulting in a 50 per cent complication rate 5 years after treatment were estimated to be 40–65 Gy for xerostomia and 50–65 Gy for taste loss.

In most instances, taste acuity is partially restored between 20 and 60 days after radiotherapy and is fully restored within 2–4 months. Three weeks after initiation of radiotherapy, detection of bitter and salty tastes show the earliest and greatest impairment, with sensitivity to sweet tastes being least affected. Drugs[192] administered to cancer patients may also alter taste. Although about 80 different drugs have been associated with taste alterations,[193] many of these have been reported as a cause only once.

Zinc deficiency has been noted as a potential cause of anorexia, dysgeusia, or hypogeusia. Plasma zinc levels have been found to be reduced in patients with bronchial carcinoma compared to the healthy population, and the zinc level in leukaemic cells appears to be lower than that in normal white blood cells.[194] The administration of zinc has been reported to correct abnormalities of taste in some patients,[195,196] and copper and nickel have also been used with good result in clinical trials. Patients treated prophylactically with 25 mg of oral zinc four times a day prior to radiotherapy developed less severe hypogeusia than those given radiotherapy without zinc treatment. Zinc must be administered in the middle of a meal to reduce potential gastrointestinal symptoms.[196] Controlled clinical trials need to be carried out to document the potential for zinc administration in cancer patients.

Patients suffering from taste alterations need good oral hygiene, treatment to increase salivation, and the withdrawal of drugs that can induce or increase the symptoms. Patients can sometimes take hot food with a strong smell, the addition of lemon, pineapple, or vinegar being useful if stomatitis or mouth ulcers are not present.

Table 11 Causes to taste alteration

Local disease of the mouth and tongue caused by cancer
Partial glossectomy
Tobacco usage
Elimination of the olfactory component of taste after laryngectomy
Surgical removal of the palate
Damage to the nervous system following surgery or cerebral lesions
Alteration of the cell renewing, or cell regenerating cycle ◆ malnutrition ◆ radiotherapy ◆ drugs ◆ metabolic disturbances ◆ xerostomia ◆ stomatitis and oral infections ◆ endocrine factors (thyroidectomy, hypophysectomy, adrenalectomy)
Modification in the receptor cells due to alteration of saliva by metabolic agents, drugs, radiation
Dental pathology
Bad dental hygiene

Sialorrhea

Sialorrhea (excessive salivation) is uncommon in advanced cancer patients but can cause discomfort, inconvenience, and social embarrassment as well as irritation of lips, commissure, and chin. The most frequent causes are:

1. oral pain (apthous ulcers),
2. local irritants (ill-fitting dentures),
3. drugs (lithium, cholinesterase inhibitors, cholinergic agonists),
4. psychosis,
5. epilepsy,
6. radical mandibular resection procedures, and
7. recurrent oral cancer which suspends the mouth in an open position.[197–200]

In a controlled clinical trial, a single dose of 0.02 mg/kg of hyoscine (scopolamine) hydrobromide solution, rinsed in the mouth for 5 min before swallowing, reduced non-stimulated and paraffin-stimulated salivation at 60 min by 81 and 80 per cent, respectively. The heart rate of these patients increased significantly when compared with those given placebo and subjective sedation and relaxation were experienced by most of the volunteers.[198] Clinically useful sedative and antisialogogue effects can be produced by oral and transdermal administration of hyoscine (scopolamine) hydrobromide solution.[201] No data are available about the long-term use of this drug in patients suffering from sialorrhea. Mier et al. in a placebo-controlled double-blind cross-over dose-ranging study demonstrated that glycopyrrolate is effective in the control of excessive sialorrhea in children with developmental disabilities.[202]

Halitosis

Halitosis (unpleasant or bad breath), occurs when exhaled air is combined with foul-smelling substances coming from various sections of the respiratory tract or from the upper digestive tract.[203] No epidemiological data are available about the incidence and prevalence of this symptom in cancer patients. Table 12 shows the most important causes of halitosis.

Between 56 and 85 per cent of the cases of halitosis are a consequence of diseases of the oral cavity.[204,205] A careful history and examination of the oral cavity, sinuses, and the upper respiratory tract must be carried out to exclude inflammatory, infective, or neoplastic conditions.[206,207]

When the sensation of halitosis is subjective, without objective evidence, it is necessary to investigate neurological or psychiatric illness. Sometime, dysgeusia or dysosmia can cause these disturbances. Hygiene measures, mainly use of a toothbrush and dental floss, are extremely important.[205]

Table 12 Causes of halitosis

Diseases of the oral cavity
Poor oral hygiene, xerostomia, periodontal disease
Dental plaque, decay, cancer, bleeding gums
Tongue coating
Acute necrotizing ulcerative gingivitis
Gingivostomatitis (herpes virus, candidosis)
Inflammatory-suppurative phenomena
Diseases of the respiratory tract
Infection of the nose, tongue, nasal sinuses, pharynx, lungs
Tonsillar abscess, necrotic ulcers
Chronic rhinitis and rhinopharyngitis
Pharyngeal-laryngeal cancer with superinfection
Bronchiectasis, lung abscess
Abscess-forming lung cancer
Diseases of the digestive tract
Oesophageal diverticula, hiatal hernia, gastric stasis
Gastric stagnation due to pyloric stenosis and/or cancer with/without regurgitation, dyspepsia
Altered secretion or bile-composition, colon stasis
Metabolic failure
Diabetic ketoacidosis (sweet acetone breath)
Uraemia (ammoniacal smell)
Severe hepatic insufficiency (foetor hepaticus)
Drugs
Causing xerostomia and/or taste alteration
Anticancer drugs causing oral complications
Dimethylsulfoxide, antibiotics
Amyl nitrite, chloral hydrate, or iodine-based drugs
Foods
Garlic, onions, leeks, radishes
Meat, fish

The diet plays an important role in the genesis of halitosis. Some substances, such as garlic, leeks, onions, and alcohol contain volatile products which are absorbed by the intestinal wall and then excreted through the lungs. Alcohol also causes a decrease in salivary flow. The sulphur-containing amino acids in meat and fish can cause halitosis. A decreased intake of food can deplete body fat stores, with acidosis and ketosis giving an acetone odour. The role of smoking is controversial, but may modify the oral environment, exerting a local effect upon the oral mucosa. Oral rinses, such as 0.2 per cent aqueous chlorhexidine gluconate, are helpful.[208]

The treatment of halitosis is summarized in Table 13. It is necessary to give individual drug treatment according to the causes and the general condition of the patient.

Educational and prevention programmes

Health professionals involved in cancer management should be trained in the prevention, assessment, and treatment of oral problems.

An oral disease prevention programme for patients receiving radiation and chemotherapy should be available at every institution involved in cancer care: oral hygiene should not be a matter for only advanced or terminally ill patients. A dental team involved in early dental referral (before treatment) and long-term maintenance, as well as family-oriented education and motivation programmes, are necessary to enhance patient understanding and compliance.

In 1985, the National Institute of Dental Research (National Institutes of Health, Bethesda, MD) developed a programme for enhancing the oral health care of cancer patients undergoing therapy.[169] The programme focussed on: the potential deleterious effects of medical treatment, the benefits of oral preparation by the dental team and patient oral health regimens.

In a retrospective study conducted on 440 patients with malignancies other than those of the head and neck, Sonis and Kunz[166] showed that the frequency of oral problems was reduced from 38.7 to 10.5 per cent after the introduction of a dental team referral system.

Table 13 Treatment of halitosis

General measures
Oral hygiene:
Toothbrushing, tongue scraping, and dental flossing
Dietary advice
Reduce alcohol intake and smoking
Denture care
Specific measures
Oral and upper airway
—systemic and/or topical antibiotics and local antiseptics (e.g povidone–iodine mouthwash, chlohexidine 0.2%, hydrogen peroxide 1%)
Xerostomia
—see Tables 5, 6
Oral bleeding
—see Table 10
Gastric stasis
—prokinetic drugs (metoclopramide, domperidone)
Dyspepsia
—reduce fat intake and administer enzymatic products specific for lipid digestion (e.g. ursodeoxycholic acid 50–150 mg before meals)
Pulmonary infection
—cultured sputum examination
—start broad-spectrum antibiotic and/or antifungal drugs while waiting for culture results (metronidazole)
Drugs
—discontinue use of drugs causing the symptom, if possible

Table 14 Family education programme

The importance of oral hygiene in advanced and terminal cancer
Family-oriented oral cavity examination
The correct use of toothbrushes, dental floss, gauzes, toothette, gloves
Different mouthwashes: preparation, indication, and uses
The main oral complications of advanced cancer patients General Specific to their relative
Personalized oral care programme (centred on the patient and his family)
Dietary and behavioral advice (e.g if mucositis, dysgeusia, xerostomia)
Oral care in the unconscious patient

Table 15 Future research

Perform epidemiological studies, evaluating the incidence and prevalence of oral cavity problem in patients with advanced cancer, including the role of pre-existing infections (e.g. HSV)
Define the impact of oral complications on the quality of life of patients with advanced and terminal cancer
Develop quantifiable and reproducible criteria for assessing and classifying oral cavity pathologies in patients with advanced and terminal cancer
Define the importance of long-term oral side-effects of anticancer therapies and their optimal planning, according to these aspects (e.g. radio therapy-fractionation schedules, different kinds of destructive and/or reconstructive surgery)
Study the interactions between oral cavity problems and different systemic conditions present in advanced cancer (e.g. cachexia, anorexia, malnutrition)
Develop controlled studies in patients with advanced cancer, completely integrated with antineoplastic therapies
Develop appropriate evaluation methods for xerostomia and its treatment
Define and develop appropriate diagnostic tools for oral care in patients with advanced cancer
Develop and determine the role of oral care protocols in the palliative care setting
Develop adequate education tools to get the family involved in their relative's oral care
Determine the preventive and therapeutic role of the different antifungal drugs according to their administration schedules, to their compliance, their side-effects, and costs
Perform clinical studies evaluting the oral complications of drugs currently used in palliative care (e.g. steroids, morphine, anticholinergic drugs)
Evaluate the role of biological response modifiers in preventing oral complications due to antineoplastic treatment performed in patients with advanced cancer
Evaluate the topical and systemic treatments for the prevention and cure of taste alterations
Evaluate the role of systemic hydration in the management of xerostomia
Conduct controlled studies to define and select topical and systemic analgesics for mucositis
Evaluate the different treatments for the management of fistulas, abscesses, and fungating tumours, in head and neck cancers
Develop prevention and treatment strategies for oral problems feasible within developing countries
Develop new specific treatments for oral cavity problems

The family must be involved in the patient's oral care, especially in a palliative care setting, when patients are often unable to take care of themselves. The palliative care team should have a teaching programme for oral care: this can be applied during hospice and/or hospital admissions and continued during home care (Table 14). It is essential to involve relatives actively in this programme, training them in the main oral hygiene measures, in the presence of the team. A range of different teaching aids is preferable: videos, booklets, group sessions, and slides (see Section 6).

Conclusions

Many aspects of oral care need to be better defined. A greater effort has to be made in both the oncological and the palliative care settings. The main areas of research should include the epidemiology of oral complications, their impact on quality of life, evaluation tools, and controlled clinical studies. Table 15 indicates the main directions for future research.

References

1. **Daeffler, R.** (1981). Oral hygiene measures for patients with cancer III. *Cancer Nursing* **2**, 29–35.
2. **Rosling, B.G.** et al. (1983). Microbiological and clinical effects of topical subgingival antimicrobial treatment on human periodontal disease. *Journal of Clinical Periodontology* **10**, 487–514.
3. **Tapper-Jones, L., Aldred, M., and Walker, D.M.** (1980). Prevalence and intraoral distribution of *Candida albicans* in Sjögren's syndrome. *Journal of Clinical Pathology* **33**, 282–7.
4. **Markitziu, A.** et al. (1982). Prevention of caries progress in xerostomic patients by topical fluoride applications: a study *in vivo* and *in vitro*. *Journal of Dentistry* **10**, 248–53.
5. **Grad, H., Grushka, M., and Yanover, L.** (1985). Drug-induced xerostomia—the effect and treatment. *Canadian Dentistry Association Journal* **4**, 296–301.
6. **Bahn, S.L.** (1972). Drug-related dental destruction. *Oral Surgery* **33**, 49–54.
7. **Makkonen, T.A.** et al. (1986). Changes in the protein composition of whole saliva during radiotherapy in patients with oral or pharyngeal cancer. *Oral Surgery* **62**, 270–5.
8. **Mandel, I.D.** (1980). Sialochemistry in diseases and clinical situations affecting salivary glands. *CRC Critical Reviews in Clinical and Laboratory Science* **11**, 321–66.
9. **Tenovuo, J.** et al. (1986). Antimicrobial factors in whole saliva of human infants. *Infection and Immunity* **51**, 49–53.
10. **Milne, R.W. and Dawes, C.** (1973). The relative contributions of different salivary glands to the blood group activity of whole saliva in humans. *Vox Sanguinis* **25**, 298–307.
11. **Tabak, L.A.** et al. (1982). Role of salivary mucins in the protection of the oral cavity. *Journal of Oral Pathology* **11**, 1–17.
12. **Mandel, M.A., Dvorak, K., and DeCosse, J.J.** (1973). Salivary Immunoglobulins in patients with oropharyngeal and bronchopulmonary carcinoma. *Cancer* **31**, 1408–13.
13. **Brown, A.M.** et al. (1975). The association of the IgA levels of serum and whole saliva with the progression of oral cancer. *Cancer* **35**, 1154–62.
14. **Wolff, A.** et al. (1990). Oral mucosal status and major salivary gland function. *Oral Surgery, Oral Medicine, Oral Pathology* **70**, 49–54.
15. **Zasloff, M.** (1987). Magainins, a class of antimicrobial peptides from *Xenopus* skin: isolation, characterization of two active forms, and partial cDNA sequence of a precursor. *Proceedings of the National Academy of Sciences of the United States of America* **84**, 5449–53.
16. **Spielman, A.** et al. (1981). Xerostomia—diagnosis and treatment. *Oral Medicine* **51**, 144–7.
17. **Sreebny, L.M. and Valdini, A.** (1988). Xerostomia. Part I: Relationship to other oral symptoms and salivary gland hypofunction. *Oral Surgery, Oral Medicine, Oral Pathology* **66**, 451–8.
18. **Sreebny, L.M. and Valdini, A.** (1987). Xerostomia. A neglected symptom. *Archives of Internal Medicine*, **147** 1333–7.

19. **Oneschuk, D., Hanson, J., and Bruera, E.** (2000). A survey of mouth pain and dryness in patients with advanced cancer. *Support Care Cancer* **8**, 372–6.

20. **Ventafridda, V.** et al. (1990). Quality-of-life assessment during a palliative care programme. *Annals of Oncology* **1**, 415–20.

21. **Twycross, R.G. and Lack, S.A.**, ed. *Control of Alimentary Symptoms in far Advanced Cancer. The mouth* Vol. 2, pp. 12–39. Edinburgh: Churchill Livingstone, 1986.

22. **Chen, M.S. and Daly, T.E.** (1980). Xerostomia and complete denture retention. *Oral Health* **70**, 27–9.

23. **Makkonen, T.A. and Nordman, E.** (1987). Estimation of long-term salivary gland damage induced by radiotherapy. *Acta Oncologica* **26**, 307–12.

24. **Anderson, M.W., Izutsu, K.T., and Rice, J.C.** (1981). Parotid gland pathophysiology after mixed gamma and neutron irradiation of cancer patients. *Oral Surgery* **52**, 495–500.

25. **Brown, L.R., Dreizen, S., and Rider, I.** (1976). The effect of radiation-induced xerostomia on saliva and serum lysozyme and immunoglobulin levels. *Oral Surgery* **41**, 83–92.

26. **Carl, W., Schaff, N.G., and Chen, T.Y.** (1972). Oral care of patients irradiated for cancer of the head and neck. *Cancer* **30**, 448–53.

27. **Dreizen, S.** et al. (1977). Prevention of xerostomia-related dental caries in irradiated cancer patients. *Journal of Dental Research* **56**, 99–104.

28. **Eneroth, C.M., Henrikson, C.O., and Jakobsson, P.A.** (1972). Effect of fractionated radiotherapy on salivary gland function. *Cancer* **30**, 1147–53.

29. **Wescott, W.B.** et al. (1978). Alterations in whole saliva flow rate induced by fractionated radiotherapy. *American Journal of Roentgenology* **130**, 145–9.

30. **Dreizen, S.** et al. (1976). Radiation-induced xerostomia in cancer patients. Effect on salivary and serum electrolytes. *Cancer* **38**, 273–8.

31. **Epstein, J.B. and Schubert, M.M.** (1987). Synergistic effect of sialagogoues in management of xerostomia after radiation therapy. *Oral Surgery, Oral Medicine, Oral Pathology* **64**, 179–82.

32. **Cheng, V.S.T.** et al. (1981). The function of the parotid gland following radiation therapy for head and neck cancer. *International Journal of Radiation Oncology, Biology, Physics* **7**, 253–8.

33. **Wescott, W.B., Starcke, E.N., and Shannon, I.L.** (1981). Some factors influencing salivary function when treating with radiotherapy. *International Journal of Radiation Oncology, Biology, Physics* **7**, 535–41.

34. **Kuten, A.** et al. (1986). Oral side effects of head and neck irradiation: correlation between clinical manifestations and laboratory data. *International Journal of Radiation Oncology, Biology, Physics* **12**, 401–5.

35. **Shannon, I.L., Trodhal, J.N., and Starcke, E.N.** (1978). Radiosensitivity of the human parotid gland. *Proceedings of the Society of Experimental Biology and Medicine* **157**, 50–3.

36. **Shannon, I.L.** (1981). Management of head and neck irradiated patients. In *Saliva and Salivation* (ed. T. Zelles), pp. 313–20. Oxford: Pergamon Press.

37. **Liu, R.P.** et al. (1990). Salivary flow rates in patients with head and neck cancer 0.5 to 25 years after radiotherapy. *Oral Surgery, Oral Medicine, Oral Pathology* **70**, 724–9.

38. **Mossman, K., Shatzman, A., and Checharick, J.** (1982). Long-term effects of radiotherapy on taste and salivary function in man. *International Journal of Radiation Oncology, Biology, Physics* **8**, 991–7.

39. **Dudiak, L.A.** (1987). Mouth care for mucositis due to radiation therapy. *Cancer Nursing* **10**, 131–40.

40. **Carl, W.** (1980). Dental management of head and neck cancer patients. *Journal of Surgical Oncology* **15**, 265–81.

41. **Beumer, J., Curtis, T., and Harrison, R.E.** (1979). Radiation therapy of the oral cavity: sequelae and management. *Head and Neck Surgery* **1**, 301–2.

42. **Wescott, W.B., Starcke, E.N., and Shannon, I.L.** (1975). Chemical protection against postirradiation dental caries. *Oral Surgery* **40**, 709–19.

43. **Heimdahl, A. and Nord, C.E.** (1985). Colonization of oropharynx with pathogenic micro-organisms—a potential risk factor for infection in compromized patients. *Chemotherapia* **4**, 186–91.

44. **Marks, J.E.** et al. (1981). The effects of radiation on parotid salivary function. *International Journal of Radiation Oncology, Biology, Physics* **7**, 1013–19.

45. **Crawford, J.M., Taubman, M.A., and Smith, D.J.** (1975). Minor salivary glands as a major source of secretory immunoglobulin A in the human oral cavity. *Science* **190**, 1206–9.

46. **Hensten-Petersen, A.** (1975). Biological activities in human labial and palatine secretions. *Archives of Oral Biology* **20**, 107–9.

47. **Eisbruch, A.** et al. (2001). Xerostomia and its predictors following parotid-sparing irradiation of head-and-neck cancer. *Internation Journal of Radiation Oncology, Biology, Physics* **50** 695–704.

48. **Bennett, D.R., McVeigh, S., and Rodgers, B.**, ed. *AMA Drug Evaluations* 5th edn. Chicago IL: American Medical Association, 1983.

49. **Goodman, G.A.** et al., ed. *The Pharmacological Basis of Therapeutics* 8th edn. New York: Pergamon Press, 1990.

50. **Handelman, S.L.** et al. (1986). Prevalence of drugs causing hyposalivation in an institutionalized geriatric population. *Oral Surgery, Oral Medicine, Oral Pathology* **62**, 26–31.

51. **Sreebny, L.M., Valdini, A., and Yu, A.** (1989). Xerostomia. Part II. Relationship to nonoral symptoms, drugs, and diseases. *Oral Surgery, Oral Medicine, Oral Pathology* **68**, 419–27.

52. **Sreebny, L.M. and Schwartz, S.S.** (1986). Reference guide to drugs and dry mouth. *Gerodontology* **5**, 75–99.

53. **White, I.D.** et al. (1989). Morphine and dryness of the mouth. *British Medical Journal* **298**,1222–3.

54. **Ventafridda, V.** et al. (1986). A randomized study on oral morphine and methadone in the treatment of cancer pain. *Journal of Pain and Symptom Management* **1**, 203–7.

55. **Ventafridda, V.** et al. (1989). Clinical observations on controlled-release morphine in cancer pain. *Journal of Pain and Symptom Management* **4**, 124–9.

56. **Ventafridda, V.** et al. (1987). A validation study of the WHO method for cancer pain relief. *Cancer* **59**, 850–6.

57. **Baines, M.J.** (1984). Control of other symptoms. In *The Management of Terminal Disease* 2nd edn. (ed. C. Saunders), London: Edward Arnold.

58. **Burge, F.I.** (1993). Dehydration symptoms of palliative care cancer patients. *Journal of Pain and Symptom Management* **8**, 454–64.

59. **McCann, R.M., Hall, W.J., and Groth-Juncker, A.** (1994). Comfort care for terminally ill patients. The appropriate use of nutrition and hydration. *Journal of the American Medical Association* **272**, 1263–6.

60. **Mathew, R.J., Weinman, M., and Claghorn, J.L.** (1979). Xerostomia and sialorrhea in depression. *American Journal of Psychiatry* **136**, 1476–7.

61. **Seikaly, H.** et al. (2001). Submandibular gland transfer: a new method of preventing radiation-induced xerostomia. *Laryngoscope* **111** (2), 347–52.

62. **Levine, M.J.** et al. (1987). Artificial salivas: present and future. *Journal of Dental Research* **66**, 693–8.

63. **'S-Gravenmade, E.J., Roukema, P.A., and Panders, A.K.** (1974). The effect of mucin-containing artificial saliva on severe xerostomia. *International Journal of Oral Surgery* **3**, 435–9.

64. **Duxbury, A.J., Thakker, N.S., and Wastell, D.G.** (1989). A double-blind cross-over trial of a mucin-containing artificial saliva. *British Dental Journal* **166**, 115–20.

65. **Vissink, A.** et al. (1986). Wetting properties of human saliva and saliva substitutes. *Journal of Dental Research* **65**, 1121–4.

66. **Vissink, A.** et al. (1987). The efficacy of mucin-containing artificial saliva in alleviating symptoms of xerostomia. *Gerodontology* **6**, 95–101.

67. **Visch, L.L.** et al. (1986). A double-blind crossover trial of CMC- and mucin-containing saliva substitutes. *International Journal of Oral and Maxillofacial Surgery* **15**, 395–400.

68. **Greenspan, D.** (1979). The use of pilocarpine in irradiation-induced xerostomia. *Journal of Dental Research* **58**, 420–3.

69. **Fox, P.C.** et al. (1986). Pilocarpine for the treatment of xerostomia associated with salivary gland dysfunction. *Oral Surgery* **61**, 243–8.

70. **Schuller, D.E.** et al. (1989). Treatment of radiation side effects with oral pilocarpine. *Journal of Surgical Oncology* **42**, 272–6.

71. **Greenspan, D. and Daniels, T.E.** (1987). Effectiveness of pilocarpine in postradiation xerostomia. *Cancer* **59**, 1123–5.

72. **Epstein, J.B., Decoteau, W.E., and Wilkinson, A.** (1983). Effect of sialor in treatment of xerostomia in Sjögren's syndrome. *Oral Surgery* **56**, 495–9.

73. **LeVeque, F.G.** et al. (1993). A multicenter, randomized, double-blind, placebo-controlled, dose-titration study of oral pilocarpine for treatment of

radiation-induced xerostomia in head and neck cancer patients. *Journal of Clinical Oncology* **11**, 1124–31.

74. **Johnson, J.T.** et al. (1993). Oral pilocarpine for post-irradiation xerostomia in patients with head and neck cancer. *New England Journal of Medicine* **329**, 390–5.
75. **Rieke, J.W.** et al. (1995). Oral pilocarpine for radiation-induced xerostomia: integrated efficacy and safety results from two prospective randomized clinical trials. *International Journal of Radiation Oncology, Biology, Physics* **31**, 661–9.
76. **Horiot, J.C.** et al. (2000). Post-radiation severe xerostomia relieved by pilocarpine: a prospective French cooperative study. *Radiotherapy in Oncology* **55** (3), 233–9.
77. **Greenspan, D.** (1990). Management of salivary dysfunction. *National Cancer Institute Monographs* **9**, 159–61.
78. **Johnstone, P.A.S.** et al. (2001). Acupuncture for pilocarpine-resistant xerostomia following radiotherapy for head and neck malignancies. *International Journal of Radiation Oncology, Biology, Physics* **50**, 353–7.
79. **Jobbins, J., Bagg, J., Parsons, K., Finlay, I., Addy, M., and Newcombe, R.G.** (1992). Oral carriage of yeasts, coliforms and staphylococci in patients with advanced malignant disease. *Journal of Oral Pathology and Medicine* **21**, 305–8.
80. **Macfarlane, T.W. and Samaranayake, L.P.** (1986). Systemic infections. In *Oral Manifestations of Systemic Disease* 2nd edn. (ed. J.H. Jones and D.K. Mason), pp. 339–86. London: Ballière Tindall.
81. **Samaranayake, L.P.** (1986). Nutritional factors and oral candidosis. *Journal of Oral Pathology* **15**, 61–5.
82. **Aldred, M.J.** et al. (1991). Oral health in the terminally ill: a cross sectional pilot survey. *Specialist Care in Dentistry* **11**, 59–62.
83. **Finlay, I.G.** (1986). Oral symptoms and candida in the terminally ill. *British Medical Journal* **292**, 592–3.
84. **Samaranayake, L.P.** et al. (1984). The oral carriage of yeasts and coliforms in patients on cytotoxic therapy. *Journal of Oral Pathology* **13**, 390–3.
85. **Martin, M.V., Al-Tikriti, U., and Bramley, P.** (1981). Yeasts flora of the mouth and skin during and after irradiation for oral and laryngeal cancer. *Journal of Medical Microbiology* **14**, 457–61.
86. **Wahlin, Y.B. and Holm, A.K.** (1988). Changes in the oral microflora in patients with acute leukaemia and related disorders during the period of induction therapy. *Oral Surgery, Oral Medcine, Oral Pathology* **65**, 411–17.
87. **Spijkervet, F.K.L.** et al. (1990). Mucositis prevention by selective elimination of oral flora in irradiated head and neck cancer patients. *Journal of Oral Pathology and Medicine* **19**, 486–9.
88. **Bodey, G.P.** (1984). Candidiasis in cancer patients. *American Journal of Medicine* **77D**, 13–19.
89. **Epstein, J.B., Truelove, E.L., and Izutzu, K.T.** (1984). Oral candidiasis: pathogenesis and host defense. *Reviews of the Infectious Diseases* **6**, 96–106.
90. **Yeo, E.** et al. (1985). Prophylaxis of oropharingeal candidiasis with clotrimazole. *Journal of Clinical Oncology* **3**, 1668–71.
91. **De Gregorio, M.W.** et al. (1984). Fungal infections in patients with acute leukemia. *American Journal of Medicine* **73**, 543–8.
92. **Bodey, G.P., Samonis, G., and Rolston, K.** (1990). Prophylaxis of candidiasis in cancer patients. *Seminars in Oncology* **17**, 24–8.
93. **Dreizen, S.** (1984). Oral candidiasis. *American Journal of Medicine* **77D**, 28–33.
94. **Samaranayake, L.P. and Yacob, H.B.** (1990). The classificaion of oral candidosis. In *Oral Candidosis* (ed. L.P. Samaranayake and T.W. MacFarlane), pp. 124–31. London: Wright.
95. **Regezi, J.A. and Sciubba, J.J.**, ed. (1989). White lesions. In *Oral pathology: Clinical-Pathologic Correlations.* Philadelphia PA: WB Saunders **3**, 84–124.
96. **Lynch, D.P. and Gibson, D.K.** (1987). The use of Calcofluor white in the histopathologic diagnosis of oral candidiasis. *Oral Surgery, Oral Medicine, Oral Pathology* **63**, 698–703.
97. **Barret, A.P.** (1984). Evaluation of nystatin in prevention and elimination of oropharyngeal candida in immunosuppressed patients. *Oral Surgery* **58**, 148–51.
98. **DeGregorio, M.W., Lee, M.W., and Ries, C.A.** (1982). Candida infections in patients with acute leukemia: ineffectiveness of nystatin prophylaxis and relationship between oropharyngeal and systemic candidiasis. *Cancer* **50**, 2780–4.
99. **Barkvoll, P. and Attramadal, A.** (1989). Effect of nystatin and chlorexidine digluconate on Candida Albicans. *Oral Surgery, Oral Medicine, Oral Pathology* **67**, 279–81.
100. **Kirkpatrick, C.H. and Alling, D.W.** (1978). Treatment of chronic oral candidiasis with clotrimazole troches: a controlled clinical trial. *New England Journal of Medicine* **299**, 1201–3.
101. **Yeo, B.S. and Bodey, G.P.** (1979). Oropharyngeal candidiasis treated with a troche form of clotrimazole. *Archives of Internal Medicine* **139**, 656–7.
102. **Quintiliani, R.** et al. (1984). Treatment and prevention of oropharyngeal candidiasis. *American Journal of Medicine* **10**, 44–8.
103. **Meunier, F., Paesmans, M., and Autier, P.** (1994). Value of antifungal prophylaxis with antifungal drugs against oropharyngeal candidiasis in cancer patients. *Oral Oncology, European Journal of Cancer* **30B**, 196–9.
104. **Roed-Petersen, B.** (1978). Miconazole in the treatment of oral candidiasis. *International Journal of Oral Surgery* **7**, 558–63.
105. **Brincker, H.** (1976). Treatment of oral candidiasis in debilitated patients with miconazole—a new potent antifungal drug. *Scandinavian Journal of Infectious Diseases* **8**, 117–20.
106. **de Vries-Hospers, G.H. and van der Waaij, D.** (1980). Salivary concentrations of amphotericin B following its use as an oral lozenges. *Infection* **8**, 63–5.
107. **Holbrook, W.P.** (1979). Sensitivity of *Candida albicans* from patients with chronic oral candidiasis. *Postgraduate Medical Journal* **55**, 692–4.
108. **Symoens, J.** et al. (1980). An evaluation of two years of clinical experience with ketoconazole. *Reviews of the Infectious Diseases* **2**, 674–82.
109. **Hughes, W.T.** et al. (1983). Ketoconazole and candidiasis: a controlled study. *Journal of Infectious Diseases* **147**, 1060–3.
110. **Saag, M.S. and Dismukes, W.E.** (1988). Azole antifungal agents: emphasis on new triazoles. *Antimicrobial Agents and Chemotherapy* **32**, 1–8.
111. **Heykants, J.** et al. (1987). The pharmacokinetics of itraconazole in animals and man: an overview. In *Recent Trends in the Discovery, Development and Evaluation of Antifungal Agents* (ed. R.A. Fromtling), pp. 223–4. Barcelona: J.R. Prou Science Publ.
112. **Cauwenbergh, G.** et al. (1987). Itraconazole in the treatment of human mycoses: Review of three years of clinical experience. *Reviews of the Infectious Diseases* **9**, S146–52.
113. **Humphrey, M.J., Jevenson, S., and Tarbit, M.H.** (1985). Pharmacokinetic evaluation of UK-49858, a metabolically stable triazole antifungal drug, in animals and humans. *Antimicrobial Agents and Chemotherapy* **28**, 648–53.
114. **DeWit, S.** et al. (1989). Comparison of fluconazole and ketoconazole for oropharyngeal candidiasis in AIDS. *Lancet* **1**, 746–8.
115. **Dupont, B. and Drouhet, E.** (1988). Fluconazole for the treatment of fungal diseases in immunosuppressed patients. *Annals of the New York Academy of Sciences* **544**, 564–70.
116. **Powderly, W.G.** et al. (1995). A randomized trial comparing fluconazole with clotrimazole troches for the prevention of fungal infections in patients with advanced human immunodeficency virus infection. *New England Journal of Medicine* **332**, 700–5.
117. **Cameron, M.L.** et al. (1993). Correlation of *in vitro* fluconazole resistance of Candida isolates in relation to therapy and symptoms of individual seropositive for human immunodeficency virus type 1. *Antimicrobial Agents and Chemotherapy* **37**, 2449–53.
118. **Poland, J.M.** (1987). Stomatitis and specific oral infections of the oncologic patients. *American Journal of Hospice Care*, **Sep/Oct**, 30–2.
119. **Epidemiology and Oral Disease Prevention Program, National Institute of Dental Research.** *Oral Health of United States Adults: the National Survey of Oral Health in US Employed Adults and Seniors, 1985–86: National Findings.* Bethesda, MD: Department of Health and Human Services, Public Health Service, National Institutes of Health, 1987 (NIH publication no. 87–2868).
120. **Lockart, P.B. and Sonis, S.T.** (1979). Relationship of oral complications to peripheral blood leukocyte and platelets count in patients receiving cancer chemotherapy. *Oral Surgery, Oral Medicine, Oral Pathology* **48**, 21–8.
121. **Overholsen, C.D.** et al. (1982). Periodontal infections in patients with acute non lymphocytic leukemia: prevalence of acute exacerbations. *Archives of Internal Medicine* **142**, 551–4.

122. **Peterson, D.E. and Overholsen, C.D.** (1981). Increased morbidity associated with oral infections in patients with non acute lymphocytic leukemia. *Oral Surgery, Oral Medicine, Oral Pathology* **51**, 390–3.

123. **Minah, G.E.** et al. (1986). Oral succession of gram-negative bacilli in myelosuppressed cancer patients. *Journal of Clinical Microbiology* **24**, 210–13.

124. **Peterson, D.E.** et al. (1990). Effect of granulocytopenia on oral microbial relationships in patients with acute leukemia. *Oral Surgery, Oral Medicine, Oral Pathology* **70**, 720–3.

125. **Daeffler, R.** (1980). Oral hygiene measures for patients with cancer I. *Cancer Nursing* Oct, 347–56.

126. **Daeffler, R.** (1980). Oral hygiene measures for patients with cancer II. *Cancer Nursing* Dec, 427–32.

127. **Regnard, C. and Fitton, S.** (1989). Mouth care: a flow diagram. *Palliative Medicine* **3**, 67–9.

128. **Slots, J.** et al. (1979). Periodontal therapy in humans. *Journal of Periodontology* **50**, 495–509.

129. **Weikel, D.S.** et al. (1989). Incidence of fever following invasive oral interventions in the myelosuppressed cancer patient. *Cancer Nursing* **12**, 265–70.

130. **Peterson, D.E.** (1983). Dental Care. In *Supportive Care of the Cancer Patient* (ed. P.H. Wiernik), pp. 145–71. New York: Futura Pub.

131. **Barret, A.P.** (1986). A long term prospective clinical study of orofacial herpes simplex virus infection in acute leukemia. *Oral Surgery, Oral Medicine, Oral Pathology* **61**, 149–52.

132. **Rand, H.R., Kramer, B., and Johnson, A.C.** Cancer chemotherapy and associated symptomatic stomatitis and the role of herpes simplex virus. *Cancer* **50**, 1262.

133. **Barret, A.P.** (1987). A long term prospective clinical study of oral complications during conventional chemotherapy for acute leukemia. *Oral Surgery, Oral Medicine, Oral Pathology* **63**, 313–16.

134. **Montgomery, R.T., Redding, S.W., and Le Maistre, C.F.** (1986). The incidence of oral herpes simplex virus infection in patients undergoing cancer chemotherapy. *Oral Surgery, Oral Medicine, Oral Pathology* **61**, 238–42.

135. **Beattie, G.** et al. (1989). Herpes simplex virus, Candida Albicans and mouth ulcers in neutropenic patients with non-haematological malignancy. *Cancer Chemotherapy and Pharmacology* **25**, 75–6.

136. **Bergmann, O.J., Mogensen, S.C., and Ellegard, J.** (1990). Herpes simplex virus and intraoral ulcers in immunocompromised patients with haematological malignancies. *European Journal of Clinical Microbiology and Infectious Disease* **9**, 184–90.

137. **Barret, A.P.** et al. (1986). The value of exfoliative cytology in diagnosing of oral herpes infection in immunosuppressed patients. *Oral Surgery, Oral Medicine, Oral Pathology* **62**, 175–8.

138. **Dreizen, S.** et al. (1982). Oral infections associated with chemotherapy in adults with acute leukemia. *Postgraduate Medical Journal* **71**, 133–46.

139. **Hann, J.M.** et al. (1983). Acyclovir prophylaxis against herpes virus infections in severely immunocompromised patients: a randomised double blind study. *British Medical Journal* **287**, 384–8.

140. **Sheperd, I.P.** (1978). The management of the oral complications of leukemia. *Oral Surgery, Oral Medicine, Oral Pathology* **45**, 543–8.

141. **Leflore, S., Anderson, P.L., and Fletcher, C.V.** (2000). A risk-benefit evaluation of acyclovir for the treatment and prophylaxis of herpes simplex virus infections. *Drug Safety* **23** (2), 131–42.

142. **Epstein, J.B.** et al. (1990). Clinical study of herpes simplex virus infection in leukemia. *Oral Surgery, Oral Medicine, Oral Pathology* **70**, 38–43.

143. **Carrega, G.** et al. (1994). Herpes simplex virus and oral mucositis in children with cancer. *Support Care-Cancer* **2**, 266–9.

144. **Park, J.B. and Park, N.H.** (1989). Effect of chlorexidine on the *in vitro* and *in vivo* herpes simplex virus infection. *Oral Surgery, Oral Medicine, Oral Pathology* **67**, 149–53.

145. **Barret, A.P.** (1987). Neutropenic ulceration—a distinctive clinical entity. *Journal of Periodontology* **58**, 51–5.

146. **Barret, A.P.** (1987). Long term prospective clinical study of neutropenic ulceration in acute leukemia. *Journal of Oral Medicine* **42**, 102–5.

147. **Revuz, J.** et al. (1990). Crossover study of thalidomide vs placebo in severe recurrent aphthous stomatitis. *Archives of Dermatology* **126**, 923–7.

148. **Paterson, D.L.** et al. (1995). Thalidomide as treatment of refractory aphthous ulceration related to human immunodeficiency virus infection. *Clinical Infectious Diseases* **20**, 250–4.

149. **Johnson, F.M.G.** (2001). Alteration in taste sensation. *Cancer Nursing* **24**, 149–55.

150. **Sonis, S.T.** (1989). Oral complications of cancer therapy. In *Cancer—Principles and Practice of Oncology* 3rd edn.(ed. V.T. De Vita, Jr, S. Hellman, and S.A. Rosenberg), pp. 2144–52. Philadelphia. PA: J.B. Lippincott Co.

151. **Beck, S.** (1979). Impact of a systematic oral care protocol on stomatitis after chemotherapy. *Cancer News* **2**, 185–99.

152. **Raber-Durlacher, J.E.** et al. (2000). Oral mucositis in patients treated with chemotherapy for solid tumors: a retrospective analysis of 150 cases. *Support Care Cancer* **8** (5), 366–71.

153. **Greenberg, M.S.** et al. (1982). The orak flora as a source of septicemia in patients with acute leukemia. *Oral Surgery, Oral Medicine, Oral Pathology* **53**, 32–6.

154. **Guggenheimer, J.** et al. (1977). Clinico-pathologic effects of cancer chemotherapeutic agents on human buccal mucosa. *Oral Surgery, Oral Medicine, Oral Pathology* **44**, 58–63.

155. **Lynch, M.A. and Ship, I.I.** (1977). Initial oral manifestations of leukemia. *Journal of the American Dental Association* **75**, 932–40.

156. **Clark, P.I. and Slevin, M.L.** (1985). Allopurinol mouthwash and 5-fluoruracil-induced oral toxicity. *European Journal of Surgical Oncology* **11**, 267–8.

157. **Dose, A.M.** et al. (1989). A controlled evaluation of an allopurinol mouthwash as prophylaxis against 5-fluoruracil (5-FU)-induced stomatitis: a North Central Treatment Group and Mayo Clinic Study. *Proceedings of the American Society of Clinical Oncology* **8**, 341.

158. **Porta, C., Moroni, M., and Nastasi, G.** (1994). Allopurinol mouthwashes in the treatment of 5-Fluorouracil-induced stomatitis. *American Journal of Clinical Oncology* **17**, 246–7.

159. **Mahood, D.J.** et al. (1991). Inhibition of fluorouracil-induced stomatitis by oral cryotherapy. *Journal of Clinical Oncology* **9**, 449–52.

160. **Reynolds, W.R., Hickey, A.J., and Feldman, M.I.** (1980). Dental management of the cancer patient receiving radiation therapy. *Clinical and Preventive Dentistry* **2**, 5–9.

161. **Makkonen, T.A.** et al. (2000). Granulocyte macrophage-colony stimulating factor (GM-CSF) and sucralfate in prevention of radiation-induced mucositis: a prospective randomized study. *International Journal of Radiation Oncology, Biology, Physics* **46**, 525–34.

162. **Huang, E.Y.** et al. (2000). Oral glutamine to alleviate radiation-induced oral mucositis: a pilot randomized trial. *International Journal of Radiation Oncology, Biology, Physics* **46** (3), 535–9.

163. **Bennett, C.L.** et al. (2001). Economic analysis of amifostine as adjunctive support for patients with advanced head and neck cancer: preliminary results from a randomized phase II clinical trial from Germany. *Cancer Investigations* **19** (2), 107–13.

164. **De Conno, F.** et al. (1989). Oral complications in patients with advanced cancer. *Journal of Palliative Care* **5**, 7–15.

165. **Bruya, M.A. and Maderia, N.P.** (1975). Stomatitis after chemotherapy. *American Journal of Nursing* **75**, 1349–52.

166. **Sonis, S.T. and Kunz, A.** (1988). Impact of improved dental services on the frequency of oral complications of cancer therapy for patients with non-head-and-neck malignancies. *Oral Surgery, Oral Medicine, Oral Pathology* **65**, 19–22.

167. **Dudjak, L.A.** (1987). Mouth care for mucositis due to radiation therapy. *Cancer Nursing* **10**, 131–40.

168. **Borowsky, B.** et al. (1994). Prevention of oral mucositis in patients treated with high-dose chemotherapy and bone marrow transplantation: a randomised controlled trial comparing two protocols of dental care. *Oral Oncology, European Journal of Cancer* **30B**, 93–107.

169. **Wright, W.E.** et al. (1985). An oral disease prevention program for patients receiving radiation and chemotherapy. *Journal of the American Dental Association* **110**, 43–7.

170. **Hill, H.F.** et al. (1990). Self-administration of morphine in bone-marrow transplant patients reduces drug requirements. *Pain* **40**, 121–9.

171. **Mackie, A.M., Coda, B.C., and Hill, H.F.** (1991). Adolescents use patient-controlled analgesia effectively for relief from prolonged oropharyngeal mucositis pain. *Pain* **46**, 265–9.

172. **Kuhrer, I.** et al. (1986). Topical PGE2 enhances healing of chemotherapy-associated mucosal lesions. *Lancet* **1**, 623.

173. **Porteder, H.** et al. (1988). Local prostaglandin E2 in patients with oral malignancies undergoing chemo-and radiotherapy. *Journal of Cranio-Maxillo-Facial Surgery* **16**, 371–4.

174. **Labar, B.** et al. (1993). Prostaglandin E2 for prophylaxis of oral mucositis following BMT. *Bone Marrow Transplant* **11**, 379–82.

175. **Larson, P.J.** et al. (1998). The PRO-SELF Mouth Aware program: an effective approach for reducing chemotherapy-induced mucositis. *Cancer Nursing* **21**, 263–8.

176. **Etiz, D.** et al. (2000). Clinical and histopathological evaluation of sucralfate in prevention of oral mucositis induced by radiation therapy in patients with head and neck malignancies. *Oral Oncology* **36**, 116–20.

177. **Million, R.R., Cassini, N.J., and Clark, J.R.** (1989). Cancer of the head and neck. In *Cancer—Principles and Practice of Oncology* 3rd edn. (ed. V.T. De Vita, Jr, S. Hellman, and S.A. Rosenberg), pp. 488–590. Philadelphia PA: J.B. Lippincott.

178. **Hussain, M.** et al. (1991). The role of infection in the morbidity and mortality of patients with head and neck cancer undergoing multimodality therapy. *Cancer* **67**, 716–21.

179. **Barret, A.P.** (1988). Metronidazole in the management of anaerobic neck infection on acute leukemia. *Oral Surgery, Oral Medicine, Oral Pathology* **66**, 287–9.

180. **Epstein, J.B. and Stevenson-Moore, P.** (1988). Benzydamine hydrochloride in prevention and management of pain in oral mucositis associated with radiation therapy. *Oral Surgery, Oral Medicine, Oral Pathology* **62**, 145–8.

181. **Twycross, R.G. and Lack, S.A.**, comps. (1986). Taste change. *Control of Alimentary Symptoms in Far Advanced Cancer*, vol. 4, pp. 57–65. Edinburgh: Churchill Livingstone.

182. **Gray, H.** *Anatomy, Descriptive and Surgical*, 15th edn. New York: Bounty Books, 1977.

183. **Guyton, A.C.** *Textbook of Medical Physiology*, 5th edn. Philadelphia PA: WB Saunders, 1976.

184. **Murray, R.G.** (1971). Ultrastructure of taste receptors. In *Handbook of Sensory Physiology* (ed. L.M. Beidler), pp. 31–5. New York: Springer.

185. **Schiffman, S.S.** (1983). Taste and smell in disease. *New England Journal of Medicine* **308**, 1275–9.

186. **DeWys, W.D. and Walters, K.** (1975). Abnormalities of taste sensation in cancer patients. *Cancer* **36**, 1888–96.

187. **Williams, L.R. and Cohen, M.H.** (1978). Altered taste thresholds in lung cancer. *American Journal of Clinical Nutrition* **31**, 122–5.

188. **Kashima, H.K. and Kalinowski, B.** (1979). Taste impairment following laryngectomy. *Ear, Nose, and Throat Journal* **58**, 88–92.

189. **Mossman, K.L.** (1986). Gustatory tissue injury in man: radiation dose response relationship and mechanisms of taste loss. *British Journal of Cancer* **53**, 9–11.

190. **Herrmann, Th., Adamski, K., and Stefan, M.** (1984). Storungen von Speichelproduktion und Geschmacksempfindung nach Bestrahlung intramuscular oropharyngeal Bereich. *Radiobiology Radiotherapy* **25**, 621–9.

191. **Mossman, K.L. and Henkin, R.I.** (1978). Radiation-induced changes in taste acuity in cancer patients. *International Journal of Radiation Oncology, Biology, Physics* **4**, 663–70.

192. **Willonghby, J.M.** (1983). Drug-induced abnormalities of taste sensation. *Adverse Drug Reaction Bulletin* **100**, 368–71.

193. **Davies, K.J.T., Musa, M., and Dormandy, T.L.** (1986). Measurements of plasma zinc in malignant disease. *Journal of Clinical Pathology* **21**, 359–65.

194. **Henkin, R.I. and Brandley, D.F.** (1970). Hypogeusia corrected by Ni++ and Zn++. *Life Science* **9**, 701–9.

195. **Henkin, R.I.** et al. (1971). Idiopathic hypogeusia with dysgeusia, hyposmia and dysosmia: a new syndrome. *Journal of the American Medical Association* **217**, 434–40.

196. **Henkin, R.I.** (1972). Prevention and treatment of hypogeusia due to head and neck irradiation. *Journal of the American Medical Association* **220**, 870–1.

197. **Mullins, W.M., Gross, C.W., and Moore, J.M.** (1979). Long-term follow-up of tympanic neurectomy for sialorrhea. *Laryngoscope* **89**, 1219–23.

198. **Lieblich, S.** (1989). Episodic supersalivation (idiopathic paroxysmal sialorrhea): description of a new clinical syndrome. *Oral Surgery, Oral Medicine, Oral Pathology* **68**, 159–61.

199. **Donaldson, S.R.** (1982). Sialorrhea as a side effect of lithium: a case report. *American Journal of Psychiatry* **139**, 1350–1.

200. **Markkanen, Y.J. and Pihlajamaki, K.** (1987). Oral scopolamine Hydrobromide solution as an antisialagogic agent in dentistry. *Oral Surgery, Oral Medicine, Oral Pathology* **63**, 417–20.

201. **Markkanen, Y.J., Lauren, L., and Peltomaki, T.** (1987). Serum antimuscarinic activity after a single dose of oral scopolamine hydrobromide solution measured by radioreceptor assay. *Oral Surgery, Oral Medicine, Oral Pathology* **63**, 534–8.

202. **Mier, R.J., Bachrach, S.J., and Lakin R.C.** et al. (2000). Treatment of sialorrhea with glycopyrrolate. *Archives of Pediatric Adolescent Medicine* **154**, 1214–18.

203. **Molinari, F.** (1987). Notes on gastroenterology from symptom to therapy. In *Halitosis* (ed. R. Cheli), pp. 25–8. Florence: Boehringer Ingelheim.

204. **Attia, E.L. and Marshall, G.L.** (1982). Halitosis. *Canadian Medical Assocation Journal* **126**, 1281.

205. **Scully, C., Porter, S., and Greenman, J.** (1994). What to do about halitosis. *British Medical Journal* **308**, 217–18.

206. **Richardson, H.C. and Prichard, A.J.N.** (1994). Managing halitosis (letter). *British Medical Journal* **308**, 652.

207. **Parmar, S.C. and Naik, P.C.** (1994). Remember the tongue (letter). *British Medical Journal* **308**, 652.

208. **Rosenberg, M.** (1992). Halitosis—the need for further research and education. *Journal of Dental Research* **71**, 424.

Further reading

National Cancer Institute. *Consensus Development Conference on Oral Complications of Cancer Therapies: Diagnosis, Prevention, and Treatment.* Bethesda MD: US Department of Health and Human Services, 1990 (Monographs 9).

Twycross, R.G. and Lack, S.A., ed. *Control of Alimentary Symptoms in Far Advanced Cancer.* Edinburgh: Churchill Livingstone, 1986.

8.13 Endocrine and metabolic complications of advanced cancer

Mark Bower and Sarah Cox

Introduction

Advanced malignancy produces endocrine and metabolic complications in two ways. Firstly, the primary tumour or its metastases may interfere with the function of endocrine glands, kidneys, or liver by invasion or obstruction. Secondly, tumours may give rise to remote effects without local spread. Many of these paraneoplastic syndromes arise due to secretion of hormones, cytokines, and growth factors by tumours. Paraneoplastic syndromes also arise when normal cells secrete products in response to the presence of tumour cells. For example, antibodies produced in this fashion are responsible for many paraneoplastic neurological syndromes, including cerebellar degeneration, Lambert–Eaton myasthenic syndrome, and paraneoplastic retinopathy.

This chapter reviews the pathogenesis, epidemiology, and management of the commonest paraneoplastic endocrinopathies and concludes with a brief discussion of the management of diabetes mellitus, renal failure, and liver failure in the context of advanced malignancy.

Paraneoplastic syndromes

Hypercalcaemia

Hypercalcaemia is the commonest life-threatening metabolic disorder associated with cancer. It usually occurs in patients with advanced disseminated malignancy and produces a number of distressing symptoms. The treatment of hypercalcaemia of malignancy frequently ameliorates these symptoms, and for this reason the diagnosis should always be sought.

Pathogenesis

Three related mechanisms contribute to hypercalcaemia:

1. increased osteoclastic bone resorption,
2. decreased renal clearance of calcium, and
3. enhanced absorption from the gut.

All three processes occur in malignancy and in different circumstances; each contributing to a greater or lesser extent. Bone resorption in malignant hypercalcaemia is universal and may be related to both local cytokine and prostaglandin production in response to metastases and humoral factors produced by tumours. It is mediated by osteoclasts which are multinucleated giant cells derived from the fusion of macrophages and reside in Howship's lacunae of bone. Osteoclasts resorb bone at their ruffled border where cellular proton pumps secrete hydrogen and chloride ions that dissolve hydroxyapatite and liberate bicarbonate and calcium phosphate into the blood stream. In addition, osteoclasts produce lytic proteases, including lysosomal proteases, metalloproteinases, and cystine proteases that dissolve bone matrix.

Decreased renal calcium excretion occurs with low glomerular filtration rates and/or increased tubular reabsorption of calcium in response to parathyroid hormone or its relatives. Increased gastrointestinal absorption of calcium in response to elevated levels of 1,25-dihydroxycholecalciferol (1,25$(OH)_2D_3$, calcitriol) resulting from ectopic production of this vitamin by haematological neoplasms occurs rarely.

Cytokines

Hypercalcaemia in the context of bone metastases occurs due to osteoclastic bone resorption mediated by locally produced osteoclast-activating factors and osteoclast-recruiting factors that promote proliferation and maturation of osteoclast progenitors. These factors lead to the uncoupling of the usual homeostatic balance between osteoclastic bone resorption and osteoblastic bone formation. Several cytokines with osteoclast-activating actions have been identified, including transforming growth factor (TGF), interleukin-1 (IL-1), interleukin-6 (IL-6), interleukin-11 (IL-11), tumour necrosis factor (TNF), stem cell factor (SCF), granulocyte macrophage colony stimulating factor (GM-CSF), and macrophage colony stimulating factor (M-CSF or CSF-1). All these cytokines cause bone resorption *in vitro* in organ cultures of foetal rat long bones or neonatal mouse calvariae.

Prostaglandins

Prostaglandin E_2 causes osteoclastic bone resorption *in vitro* and directly stimulates osteoclasts. Although occasional tumours produce large quantities of prostaglandins, levels do not correlate with hypercalcaemia, and inhibitors of prostaglandin synthesis rarely lower serum calcium in malignant hypercalcaemia.[1] Prostaglandins may play a part in local osteolysis but appear to have only a limited role in hypercalcaemia of malignancy.

Parathyroid hormone

In most cases of malignancy-associated hypercalcaemia cytokine-mediated osteoclastic bone resorption appears to be the dominant factor; however, in up to 20 per cent of cases no bone metastases are present: so-called humoral hypercalcaemia of malignancy. In these patients ectopic secretion of factors by the tumour accounts for the disturbance of calcium homeostasis. Humoral hypercalcaemia of malignancy resembles primary hyperparathyroidism, biochemically, with hypercalcaemia, hypophosphataemia, renal phosphate wasting, increased tubular resorption of calcium, and enhanced osteoclastic bone resorption. However, the ratio of deoxypyridinoline to osteocalcin which is normal in primary hyperparathyroidism is markedly raised in malignancy-associated hypercalcaemia.[2] Early suggestions of ectopic parathyroid hormone (PTH) secretion by tumours have not been supported by radioimmunoassay and gene expression studies; although very occasional cases of true ectopic secretion of PTH have been described in nonparathyroid tumours.

Parathyroid hormone-related protein

Parathyroid hormone related protein (PTHrP) is a 16-kDa peptide that resembles PTH in bioactivity but has a different immunoreactivity. PTHrP (1–141) has four times the bioactivity of PTH and competitive binding assays show that it acts via the same receptor: the PTH receptor 1, a large heptahelical G-protein coupled membrane spanning receptor that binds PTH and PTHrP with equal affinity. In addition to the actions on calcium metabolism, PTHrP acts as a mitogen in rat carcinoma models[3] and the expression of PTHrP is upregulated by *H-ras* and *v-src* oncogenes.[4] Whilst PTH is only expressed in parathyroid glands, PTHrP gene expression is found in several tissues, including keratinocytes, placenta, breast tissue, parathyroid glands, foetal liver, and brain. The physiological roles of PTHrP have been elucidated chiefly from knock-out mice experiments. PTHrP appears to play a central role in endochondrial bone formation promoting chondrocyte proliferation. The PTHrP driven chondrocyte proliferation is in equilibrium with cartilage differentiation which is stimulated by the Indian hedgehog Protein, the human homologue of a secreted patterning protein of Drosophila fruit flies.[5,6] In addition, PTHrP has been implicated in breast morphogenesis and transplacental calcium flux.[7]

Early studies demonstrated that PTHrP immunoperoxidase staining is strongly positive in human squamous cell carcinomas from various sites.[8] Moreover PTHrP mRNA expression was detected in all tumours obtained from patients with humoral hypercalcaemia of malignancy but not in any of those from normocalcaemic control patients with cancer.[9] Serum levels of PTHrP measured by immunoassay have revealed elevated levels (>2.5 pg/ml) in cancer patients with hypercalcaemia.[10] Thus PTHrP assays may facilitate the diagnosis of the cause of hypercalcaemia.[11] PTHrP may also have a limited role as a prognostic tumour marker, predicting the development of bone metastases in women with breast cancer.[12]

At least 80 per cent of patients with solid tumours and hypercalcaemia have elevated serum levels of PTHrP,[13] including over 60 per cent of patients with bone metastases.[14] Antibodies to PTHrP alleviate hypercalcaemia in animal models of humoral hypercalcaemia of malignancy,[15,16] and it has been reported that serum levels of PTHrP fell in parallel with serum calcium in three patients with humoral hypercalcaemia of malignancy who had successful curative surgery.[17] Nevertheless, PTHrP cannot explain all the biochemical findings in humoral hypercalcaemia of malignancy. In contrast to primary hyperparathyroidism, there is impaired intestinal calcium absorption, low 1,25 $(OH)_2D_3$ levels, and osteoclastic bone resorption is far more prominent. These features suggest that other factors (probably cytokines) have an important role in humoral hypercalcaemia of malignancy even in the absence of bone metastases.

Vitamin D

The majority of cases of humoral hypercalcaemia of malignancy are associated with impaired gut absorption of calcium and low levels of vitamin D. However, a number of cases of Hodgkin's disease have been reported in which ectopic production of 1,25 $(OH)_2D_3$ resulted in hypercalcaemia.[18] Elevated levels of 1,25 $(OH)_2D_3$ have been reported with other lymphoproliferative disorders and the mechanism is thought to involve extra-renal hydroxylation of 25$(OH)D_3$ by 1 alpha-hydroxylase.[19] Tumour-related vitamin D excess causing increased gut absorption of calcium has implications for therapy. Hypercalcaemia of malignancy is usually associated with low absorption and dietary calcium restriction is unnecessary; however, with elevated 1,25 $(OH)_2D_3$ levels, a low calcium diet is needed to control hypercalcaemia.

Epidemiology

Ten per cent of cancer patients develop hypercalcaemia and malignancy accounts for about half the cases of hypercalcaemia amongst hospital inpatients. Hypercalcaemia occurs most frequently with myeloma (up to 50 per cent of patients), breast, lung, and renal cancers, and up to 20 per cent of cases occur in the absence of bone metastases. Most patients with hypercalcaemia of malignancy have disseminated disease and 80 per cent die within 1 year. The prognosis is grave with a median survival of 3–4 months. Thus hypercalcaemia is usually a complication of advanced disease and its treatment should be directed at symptom palliation. Occasionally patients with myeloma or metastatic breast cancer present with hypercalcaemia.

Clinical features

The clinical manifestations of hypercalcaemia are myriad and many symptom which may have been attributed to the underlying malignancy may resolve on correction of the hypercalcaemia. Although the severity of symptoms is not correlated with degree of elevation of serum calcium, most patients initially develop malaise and lethargy, followed by thirst nausea, and constipation before neurological (drowsiness and confusion) and cardiological features appear (Table 1). A diagnosis of hypercalcaemia can only be made by biochemical investigation and so all symptomatic patients with malignancy should have their serum calcium measured if treatment is likely to be appropriate.

Treatment

In parallel with the advances in the understanding of the pathogenesis of hypercalcaemia in the late 1980s and early 1990s came improvements in therapy. These new therapies are more effective, less toxic, and easier to administer and represent a major improvement in palliative therapy for cancer patients. The treatment of hypercalcaemia should be determined on the basis of attributable symptoms and the corrected serum calcium calculated from the formula:

$$\text{Corrected calcium} = \text{measured calcium} + [(40 - \text{serum albumin (g/l)}) \times 0.02]$$

Rehydration followed by the administration of calcium-lowering agents is the mainstay of therapy. Low calcium diets are unpalatable, impractical, and exacerbate malnutrition, and have no place in palliative therapy. Drugs promoting hypercalcaemia (thiazides diuretics, vitamins A and D) should be withdrawn.

Table 1 Clinical features of hypercalcaemia of malignancy

General	Gastrointestinal	Neurological	Cardiological
Dehydration	Anorexia	Fatigue	Bradycardia
Polydipsia	Weight loss	Lethargy	Atrial arrhythmias
Polyuria	Nausea	Confusion	Ventricular arrhythmias
Pruritis	Vomiting Constipation Ileus	Myopathy Hyporeflexia Seizures Psychosis Coma	Prolonged P–R interval Reduced Q–T interval Wide T waves

Intravenous fluids

Dehydration due to polyuria and vomiting is a prominent feature of hypercalcaemia and intravenous rehydration is the mainstay of acute therapy for severe or symptomatic hypercalcaemia. Although large volumes of fluid will lower serum calcium, patients rarely achieve normocalcaemia, and careful monitoring to avoid fluid overload is necessary. In view of this, 2–3 l/day of fluid is now the accepted practice with daily serum electrolyte measurement to prevent hypokalaemia and hyponatraemia. Loop diuretics are often prescribed as an adjunct to intravenous fluids and cause calciuresis. However, there is little evidence of any benefit and they may exacerbate hypovolaemia, hypokalaemia, and hypomagnesaemia and are best avoided.

Corticosteroids

Glucocorticoids have been widely used in cancer-related hypercalcaemia and rapidly inhibit osteoclastic bone resorption *in vitro* in addition to reducing calcium absorption from the gut. However, their limited benefit to patients is chiefly due to tumour responsiveness to the cytostatic effects of steroids. They are most effective in myeloma, lymphoma, leukaemia, and occasionally in breast cancer when hypercalcaemia occurs as a flare effect caused by endocrine therapy. The role of steroids in severe hypercalcaemia is limited to haematological malignancies and oral prednisolone 40–100 mg/day is usually effective in these circumstances.

Bisphosphonates

Bisphosphonates are synthetic pyrophosphate analogues characterized by a phosphorus–carbon–phosphorus bond, making them resistant to enzymatic hydrolysis. They reduce bone resorption by directly inhibiting osteoclast function, leading to the disappearance of the ruffled border, decreased acid production, and altered enzyme activity.[20,21] Bisphosphonates bind hydroxyapatite crystals with a high affinity and affect osteoclast recruitment and activation. They are highly effective in controlling hypercalcaemia of malignancy causing a gradual fall in serum calcium over a few days. Etidronate is a first generation bisphosphonate that has weak activity and requires repeated infusions over 3 days.[22] Clodronate has been shown to be more effective than placebo (in the only randomized controlled study) and may be administered as a single 1.5 g infusion over 4 h.[23] However, the most commonly prescribed bisphosphonate is pamidronate which may be administered as a single infusion of 30–90 mg according to the corrected serum calcium at 1 mg/min (Table 2). Lower doses (30 mg) have been shown to be equally effective but higher doses (60–90 mg) have a longer duration of control lasting up to 4 weeks. A randomized trial has shown that pamidronate is superior to clodronate in terms of the duration of normocalcaemia achieved.[24,25] Maintenance therapy with oral bisphosphonates has been reported for both etidronate and clodronate: however, their low bioavailability and considerable gastrointestinal toxicity limit their value in this context. Bisphosphonates do not alter PTHrP levels or renal calcium reabsorption and so they may fail to control humoral hypercalcaemia of malignancy without bone metastases.[26] Indeed, there is a correlation between the responsiveness to pamidronate in humoral hypercalcaemia and the plasma PTHrP level. Non-responders have levels above 75 pg/ml and so PTHrP measurement may allow the identification of patients requiring higher doses of bisphosphonates and increased dose frequency.[27]

Table 2 Pamidronate dosage for the management of hypercalcaemia of malignancy

Corrected serum calcium (mmol/l)	Dosage of pamidronate
<3.0	30 mg in 250 ml N/S[a] over 30 min
3.0–3.5	60 mg in 250 ml N/S over 60 min
>3.5	90 mg in 500 ml N/S over 90 min

[a] N/S, normal (0.9%) saline.

A number of third generation bisphosphonates have been developed in an attempt to enhance oral bioavailability and reduce gastrointestinal toxicity. Of the numerous new bisphosphonates, only ibandronate (4 mg intravenous infusion over 2 h)[28] and zoledronate[29] have been shown to be effective in studies in humoral hypercalcaemia of malignancy. Recently zoledronate has been found to achieve a normal corrected serum calcium in more patients, faster and for longer than pamidronate, in addition to requiring only a 15-min infusion.[30] In addition to these actions, intravenous bisphosphonates have valuable analgesic activity in patients with metastatic bone pain, and reduce skeletal morbidity in patients with breast cancer and myeloma.[31]

Calcitonin

Calcitonin is secreted by the parafollicular cells of the thyroid gland although its physiological role in calcium homeostasis remains undefined. In much larger doses calcitonin reduces osteoclastic bone resorption and increases calciuresis, thereby reducing serum calcium. It is effective in around a third of patients and usually causes a fall in calcium within 4 h (compared to 48 h for bisphosphonates) but normocalcaemia is rare. Doses of up to 8 IU/kg salmon calcitonin may be injected subcutaneously or intramuscularly every 6 h and this therapy has minimal toxicity (nausea is the most frequent problem; occasional hypersensitivity reactions are seen).

Calcitonin and calcitonin gene-related peptide (CGRP) are produced by alternate exon splicing from the same gene on chromosome 11p15.5 close to the PTH gene. Calcitonin expression is regulated by serum calcium via the same calcium sensing receptor that controls PTH secretion. Calcitonin acts via a heptahelical G protein-coupled receptor expressed by osteoclasts and osteoblasts, whilst CGRP also acts through a separate receptor as a neurotransmitter and vasodilator. Both may be produced by tumours but no clinical syndrome has been attributed to their production and conversely athymic patients who produce no calcitonin have no disturbance of calcium metabolism. Although production of calcitonin and CGRP is common in many tumours, its main value to the oncologist is as a tumour marker for medullary cell carcinoma of the thyroid and multiple endocrine neoplasia type II.

Plicamycin

Plicamycin (formerly mithramycin), a cytotoxic antibiotic, is toxic to osteoclasts by blocking RNA synthesis and hence reduces bone resorption, producing prompt and effective lowering of serum calcium. It is administered as an intravenous bolus or 2 h infusion at a dosage of 25 mg/kg. It produces normocalcaemia within 3 days in 80 per cent of patients and is usually repeated weekly. The disadvantage of this highly effective treatment is its toxicity; cumulative nephrotoxicity and hepatotoxicity occur and thrombocytopenia is common; nausea is frequent and may be reduced when plicamycin is given as an infusion. It is rarely employed.

Phosphates

Oral phosphates may be effective in mild hypercalcaemia by a combination of effects on calcium metabolism. The usual recommended dose is 0.5–3 g/day phosphate (as sodium cellulose phosphate powder) and this frequently causes nausea and diarrhoea. Intravenous phosphate is a highly effective therapy for acute life-threatening hypercalcaemia and the onset of its hypocalcaemic action is more rapid than any other agent. However, the severe toxicity of parenteral phosphate includes extensive extraskeletal calcification and has lead to the abandoning of this therapy in all but exceptional cases. Recommended dosing is 1.5 g (50 mmol) elemental phosphate diluted in 1 l of saline over 6–8 h and should preferably be given in intensive care where the patient's cardiac and renal function can be monitored closely.

Gallium nitrate

Gallium nitrate is incorporated into bone, rendering hydroxyapatite less soluble.[32] It directly inhibits bone resorption without killing osteoclasts and is not associated with the nausea or myelosuppression caused by plicamycin. Gallium is highly effective, producing normocalcaemia in 80 per cent of patients with hypercalcaemia of malignancy. Two randomized double-blind trials have demonstrated the superiority of gallium over calcitonin[33] and etidronate.[34] The main drawback of gallium is that it requires continuous intravenous infusion (100–200 mg/m^2 per day) for 5 days and it causes nephrotoxicity. Gallium nitrate is not licensed in the United Kingdom.

Future approaches

Passive immunization with monoclonal antibodies against PTHrP reduces serum calcium in nude mice bearing human tumour xenografts secreting PTHrP.[35] Osteoprotegerin is a physiological inhibitor of osteoclast differentiation that is produced by osteoblasts. It acts by blocking osteoclast differentiation factor or RANKL (receptor activator of NF-kappaB ligand).[36,37] In murine models of malignancy-associated hypercalcaemia osteoprotegerin reduces serum calcium faster and further than pamidronate.[38] Herbimycin A, an antibiotic which inhibits *src* tyrosine kinase, reduces osteoclastic bone resorption *in vitro* and hypercalcaemia in mouse model systems.[39,40] Osteoclasts bind proteins *in vitro* via integrins that recognize the arginine-glycine-arspartate tripeptide sequence. Kistrin is a snake venom protein containing arginine-glycine-arspartate which inhibits bone resorption *in vitro* and osteoclast activity *in vivo*. Kistrin infusion restored normocalcaemia in hypercalcaemic mice.[41] The vitamin D analogue EB1089 does not enhance calcium absorption but downregulates PTHrP expression and inhibits hypercalcaemia in animal models[42] Calcium sensor mimetics or calcimimetics are small organic molecules that potentiate the effect of calcium on the calcium receptor and suppress PTH secretion. Calcimimetics have been used successfully in primary and secondary hyperparathyroidism.[43] All these and other approaches may yield clinical advances in the management of hypercalcaemia.

Treatment summary

Symptomatic or severe hypercalcaemia requires intravenous rehydration with 2–3 l/day followed by a single infusion of pamidronate at 1 mg/min according to the corrected serum calcium. This combination will control hypercalcaemia in most patients simply, promptly, and with minimal toxicity. The majority of patients will remain normocalcaemic for 2–4 weeks with encouragement of oral hydration. In the absence of effective treatment of the malignancy, however, hypercalcaemia will recur and the serum calcium should be rechecked every 3–4 weeks. Maintenance pamidronate infusions over 2 h can be managed on an outpatient basis. Zoledronate may well replace pamidronate in routine clinical practice because of its advantages. Second line therapy for humoral hypercalcaemia of malignancy resistant to bisphosphonates should probably be with gallium nitrate where this is available.

Cushing's syndrome

Clinically overt Cushing's syndrome caused by ectopic secretion of adrenocorticotrophic hormone (ACTH) by non-endocrine-derived tumours is rare. However, the production of pro-opiomelanocortin (POMC)-derived peptides by tumours is not uncommon and the rarity of clinical signs and symptoms reflects the subtle and complex control of hormone production from this gene. Usually, symptoms arise as a consequence of excessive ACTH production by tumours through uncontrolled gene expression following promoter switches or transcription activation. The mRNA transcripts may be of altered lengths and give rise to different POMC peptides by variations in protein cleavage and glycosylation.

Pathogenesis

The POMC gene is located at p23 on the short arm of chromosome 2 and includes three exons and three putative promoter sites which are active to varying degrees in different tissues (Fig. 1). The expression of the POMC gene is influenced by glucocorticoids which suppress transcription and corticotrophin which stimulates transcription via cAMP. Glucocorticoids act by binding to a steroid hormone receptor which in turn binds a

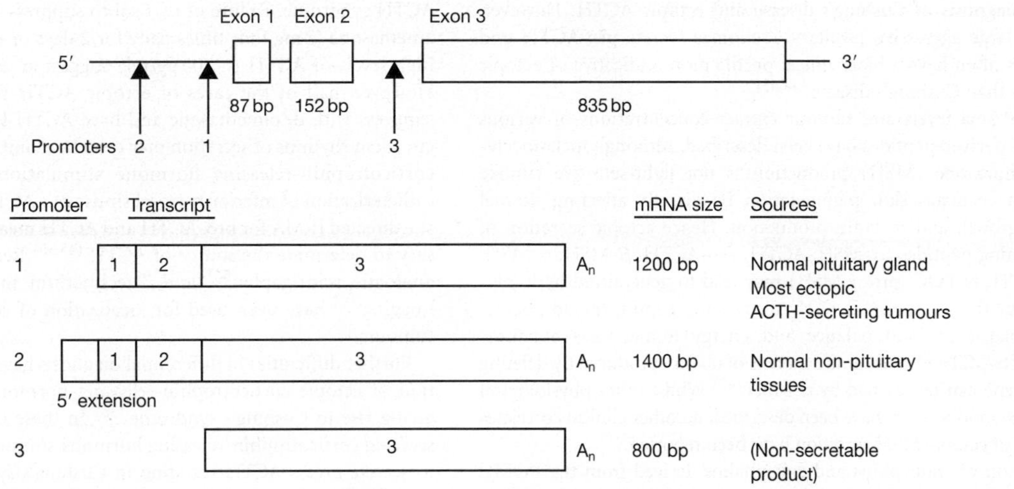

Fig. 1 The molecular biology of pro-opiomelanocortin gene expression.

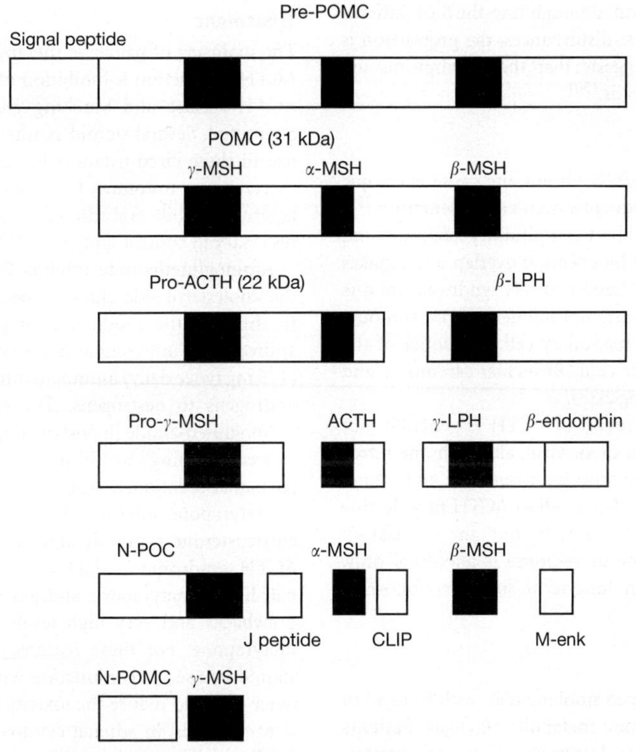

Fig. 2 Pro-opiomelanocortin (POMC)-derived peptides. Abbreviations: POMC, pro-opiomelanocortin; MSH, melanocyte stimulating hormone; LPH, lipotropin; POC, pro-opiocortin; CLIP, corticotropin-like intermediate lobe peptide; enk, enkephalin.

glucocorticoid inhibitory element sequence of POMC gene. In this way steroids downregulate POMC transcription only when it is driven by promoter 1, yielding the 1200-base transcript, and this may account for the failure of steroids to suppress ectopic ACTH production by some tumours where alternative promoters are active.

Post-translational processing of POMC peptide gives rise to a large number of different peptides, many of which have been detected in tumour extracts and cell lines. Some of these peptides have also been identified in patients' plasma and are biologically active (Fig. 2). Following the development of monoclonal antibodies to these peptides, high specificity two-site immunoradiometric assays (IRMA) have been introduced. IRMA is able to discriminate between ACTH and its larger precursors (pro-ACTH and POMC). This methodology has been used to demonstrate that most patients with ectopic ACTH secrete pro-ACTH, which has only 5 per cent of the steroidogenic activity of ACTH 1–39, whilst patients with pituitary adenomas produce normal 1200 base POMC transcripts and the peptide product undergoes normal proteolysis and glycosylation culminating in the secretion of ACTH 1–39. Thus, two-site directed IRMA may help in the differential diagnosis of Cushing's disease and ectopic ACTH. However, occasionally large aggressive pituitary adenomas secrete pro-ACTH and these patients often have a biochemical profile more indicative of ectopic ACTH rather than Cushing's disease.(44,45)

Elevated plasma levels and tumour extract concentrations of various other POMC-derived peptides have been described. Although melanocyte-stimulating hormone (MSH) production is not light-sensitive (unlike melatonin) it regulates skin pigmentation by directly affecting dermal melanocyte growth and melanin production. Hence ectopic secretion of MSH-containing peptides (α-MSH, ACTH, pro-ACTH, β-MSH, γ-MSH, β-LPH, γ-LPH, N-POC, pro-γ-MSH) may lead to generalized hyperpigmentation but this symptom is rarely distressing. Leptin, the adipocyte-derived regulator of food balance and energy homeostasis enhances expression of α-MSH(46) and mouse models of obesity produced by deleting the POMC gene can be rescued by α-MSH.(47) Whilst other physiological roles for α-, β-, and γ-MSH have been described, no other clinical correlates in the setting of ectopic MSH secretion have been reported.

The secretion of endorphins and enkephalins derived from the POMC gene occurs frequently in conjunction with ectopic ACTH secretion.(48,49) Numerous clinical effects within the central nervous system have been postulated for these endogenous opioids that bind G-protein-coupled receptors, inhibiting net cAMP synthesis by antagonizing adenyl cyclase and activating phosphodiesterase. However, these opioid molecules cross the blood-brain barrier with difficulty and although one-third of patients with Cushing's syndrome have psychiatric disturbances, the proportion is lower in Nelson's syndrome which suggests that these symptoms are related to excess steroids rather than opioids.(50)

Epidemiology

In up to 20 per cent of cases of Cushing's syndrome the cause is ectopic ACTH secretion by a tumour which is frequently occult at presentation.(51) For this reason the differential diagnosis between pituitary adenoma and ectopic ACTH is important clinically but biochemical overlap often makes this difficult. More than half the cases of ectopic ACTH syndrome are due to small-cell lung cancer, with carcinoid tumours and neural crest tumours (phaeochromocytoma, neuroblastoma, medullary cell carcinoma of the thyroid) accounting for a further 15 per cent. Bronchial carcinoids and thymomas make up most of the remaining cases.

In small-cell lung cancer, ectopic secretion of ACTH is generally not thought to be correlated with either stage or survival, although one retrospective analysis suggested an association with poor outcome and a high incidence of infectious complications.(52) The levels of ACTH may decline in response to chemotherapy or radiotherapy,(53) but any correlation between declining ACTH levels and tumour response is anecdotal only, and elevation of ACTH may persist in long-term survivors following chemotherapy.(54)

Clinical features

The typical presentation is of a middle-aged smoking man with features of severe hypercortisolism and hypokalaemic metabolic alkalosis. Patients have muscle weakness or atrophy, oedema, hypertension, mental changes, glucose intolerance, and weight loss. When ectopic ACTH production arises from a more benign tumour (e.g. bronchial carcinoid or thymoma) the other classical features of Cushing's syndrome may be present, including truncal obesity, moon facies, and cutaneous striae often making the clinical distinction from pituitary-dependant Cushing's disease impossible. Furthermore, biochemical tests do not always reliably differentiate a pituitary from an ectopic tumour as the source of ACTH.

Diagnosis

In addition to the clinical features, the diagnosis of Cushing's syndrome may be confirmed by elevated urinary free cortisol, loss of diurnal variation of plasma cortisol, and failure of cortisol suppression in the low dose dexamethasone (2 mg) test. After establishing the diagnosis, an elevated plasma ACTH supports the diagnosis of pituitary adenoma or ectopic ACTH syndrome. Failure of cortisol to suppress following high dose dexamethasone (2 mg four times daily for 2 days or 8 mg overnight) and very high levels of ACTH (>200 pg/ml) suggest an ectopic source of ACTH. However, half of the cases of ectopic ACTH from carcinoid tumours suppress with dexamethasone and have ACTH levels in the lower range; circadian rhythms of secretion may even be maintained. In difficult cases, a corticotrophin-releasing hormone stimulation test, selective venous catheterization of inferior petrosal sinus with ACTH estimations, and two-site directed IRMA for pro-ACTH and ACTH measurements may be necessary to determine the source of ACTH.(45,55) Recently both somatostatin analogue scintigaphy(56) and ^{99}technetium methoxyisobutylisonitrile imaging(57) have been used for localization of ectopic ACTH-producing tumours.

Further difficulties in differential diagnosis have arisen with the description of ectopic corticotrophin-releasing hormone secretion by tumours giving rise to Cushing's syndrome.(58) In these circumstances ectopically secreted corticotrophin-releasing hormone stimulates the normal pituitary to secrete excess ACTH resulting in Cushing's syndrome. A patient with medullary carcinoma of the thyroid developed Cushing's syndrome due to ectopic production of a bombesin-like peptide that is thought to stimulate ACTH secretion by pituitary corticotrophs; providing a further diagnostic complication.

Treatment

The mainstay of palliative therapy for Cushing's syndrome due to ectopic ACTH production is inhibition of steroid synthesis although inhibition of ACTH release and blocking glucocorticoid receptors have also been attempted. Several steroid synthesis inhibitors are available and successful use in these circumstances has been reported with aminoglutethamide, metyrapone, mitotane, ketoconazole, and octreotide. On rare occasions laparoscopic bilateral adrenalectomy or adrenal artery embolization may be necessary to control symptoms.(55)

Aminoglutethamide inhibits 20,22-desmolase enzyme which catalyses the cholesterol side chain cleavage which gives rise to δ5-pregnenolone. In this way the production of glucocorticoids, mineralocorticoids, and androgens is inhibited at higher doses (1.5–3 g/day) whilst at lower doses (125 mg twice daily) aminoglutethamide inhibits aromatase which converts androgens to oestrogens. The latter is responsible for the efficacy of aminoglutethamide in post-menopausal breast cancer. The high doses used to treat Cushing's syndrome are associated with considerable toxicity, in particular sedation, ataxia, and rashes.

Metyrapone inhibits 11-β-hydroxylase, the final step in cortisol and corticosterone synthesis and has been shown to be effective in ectopic ACTH syndrome at doses of 250–750 mg four times a day. The short half-life of metyrapone and gastrointestinal toxicity (chiefly nausea) are drawbacks and very high levels of ACTH may over-ride the effects of metyrapone. For these reasons it has been suggested that metyrapone should be used in conjunction with low dose aminoglutethamide (250 mg twice daily) to reduce the toxicities of both compounds.(59)

Mitotane is an adrenal cytotoxic, structurally related to the insecticide DDT, which irreversibly inhibits 11-β-hydroxylase and 18-hydroxylase, thus reducing glucocorticoid, mineralocorticoid, and androgen production. It produces focal atrophy and necrosis of the zona fasiculata and zona reticularis. Doses of 1–12 g/day in four divided doses have been used and it is also active against primary adrenal tumours. Mitotane is a toxic drug with gastrointestinal side-effects (anorexia, nausea, vomiting, diarrhoea) reported in 80 per cent of patients and lethargy and somnolence in 40 per cent.(60)

The imidazole antifungal ketoconazole inhibits cytochrome P450-dependent steroid hydroxylases and case reports document its successful use in Cushing's syndrome due to ectopic ACTH secretion.(61,62) The potential side effects include nausea, headaches, pruritic rashes, and liver failure. Bromocriptine has also been advocated for use in these circumstances. Bromocriptine acts on dopamine-2 receptors, inhibiting cAMP production and decreasing POMC expression *in vitro* but it is rarely successful *in vivo*.(63)

The suppression of ectopic ACTH secretion by the administration of octreotide, a long-acting somatostatin analogue has been documented. The mechanism of this action is unknown but may reflect the wide distribution of somatostatin receptors on tumours and the diverse endocrine effects of somatostatin.(64) However, somatostatin analogues occasionally cause a paradoxical rise in plasma ACTH and cortisol levels in patients with ectopic ACTH production and so a preliminary evaluation of their therapeutic efficacy is suggested.(65)

Mifepristone (RU-486) is a progesterone partial agonist that inhibits the separation of heat shock protein (hsp90) from the progesterone receptor. Case reports describe symptomatic improvement in Cushing's syndrome patients although it has yet to be used in ectopic ACTH secretion.(45) Antisense oligonucleotide complimentary to a region of β-endorphin reduced the synthesis of POMC-derived peptides *in vitro* and this approach may prove fruitful in the future.(66)

Treatment summary

The first line therapy in these patients should be aminoglutethamide 250 mg twice daily and metyrapone 2507 mg four times daily used together. The efficacy of treatment should be monitored and this is most easily achieved by measuring 24 h urinary cortisol excretion. As levels return to normal in these patients hormone replacement therapy is frequently necessary. Regimens similar to those used in Addison's disease should be used (e.g. hydrocortisone 20 mg at 0800 hours and 10 mg at 1800 hours, fludrocortisone 0.05–0.15 mg daily). Mitotane is second line therapy although it should be used as first line therapy in patients with primary adrenal tumours. Mitotane is currently not licensed in Europe but may be obtained from the United States.

Syndrome of inappropriate antidiuresis

Hyponatraemia is a common finding in association with advanced malignancy and many factors may contribute, including cardiac and hepatic failure, hyperglycaemia, diuretics, and the sick cell syndrome. However, the detection of concentrated urine in conjunction with hypo-osmolar plasma suggests abnormal renal free water excretion and the presence of the syndrome of inappropriate antidiuresis (SIAD). This acronym is more suitable than 'SIADH' since there is no vasopressin secretion in approximately 15 per cent of cases.(67)

Pathogenesis

The vasopressin gene lies on human chromosome 20 and comprises three exons encoding a transcript of 700 base pairs. The peptide product includes the nine amino acid arginine vasopressin (AVP) and a 90-amino acid peptide, vasopressin-specific neurophysin II (NP II). This peptide complex is flanked by an N-terminal signal peptide and a C-terminal glycoprotein (absent in the oxytocin–NP I peptide). The AVP–NP II polypeptide is transported by axonal streaming from its site of synthesis in the supraoptic and paraventricular nuclei of the hypothalamus to the posterior pituitary gland. The peptide is cleaved and secreted by the posterior pituitary to produce a nonapeptide (arginine vasopressin) and the 10-kDa transport peptide (NP II). This molecular mechanism is mimicked by oxytocin–NP I whose gene is adjacent on chromosome 20p13 but in mirror image orientation. Mutations in NP II are linked to autosomal dominant neurohypophyseal diabetes insipidus.

Epidemiology

In most cases of SIAD there is either stimulation of hypothalamic-pituitary secretion of AVP or a direct effect on distal nephrons. However, in malignancy-related SIAD, tumours secrete ectopic AVP or vasopressin-like peptides.(68) This has been demonstrated *in vitro* in cell lines and tumour extracts and *in vivo* in plasma. SIAD is most frequently associated with small-cell lung cancer or carcinoid tumours but has also been described in pancreatic, oesophageal, prostatic, and haematological malignancies. In one series of 523 patients with small-cell lung cancer 9 per cent had clinically evident SIAD, 32–44 per cent had elevated AVP detectable by radioimmunoassay, and 53–68 per cent had abnormal renal handling of water loads.(69,70) In another study 58 per cent of small-cell lung cancer patients had raised plasma neurophysins (NP I, 14 per cent; NP II, 44 per cent),(71) although the high incidence of vasopressin/oxytocin gene expression in lung cancer is confined to neuroendocrine tumours(72) and both normal and abnormal gene products are found.(73) Prognosis, stage at diagnosis, and response to chemotherapy are similar in small-cell lung cancer patients with and without SIAD.(74) Furthermore, although correction of hyponatraemia may correlate with tumour response to chemotherapy(75,76) complete restoration of normal renal water handling is rare even when complete remissions are achieved.(77)

Clinical features

Significant symptoms of hyponatraemia appear at plasma sodium levels below 125 mmol/l with confusion progressing to stupor, coma, and seizures as levels fall. Nausea, vomiting, and focal neurological deficits may also occur. The clinical features depend on both the levels of plasma sodium and the rate of decline; with gradual falls in sodium the brain cells are able to compensate against cerebral oedema by secreting potassium and other intracellular solutes. Asymptomatic hyponatraemia therefore suggests chronic SIAD rather than acute SIAD. The division into chronic and acute SIAD is of therapeutic importance as their management differs.(78)

Diagnosis

The diagnosis of SIAD requires the demonstration of plasma hyponatraemia and hypo-osmolality in the presence of concentrated urine and normal extracellular fluid volume (Table 3).

There are a number of causes of SIAD, including ectopic AVP production by tumours, and several may play a role in hyponatraemia in patients with advanced malignancy. Pulmonary, meningeal, and cerebral infections are common causes and drug-induced SIAD may also present in patients with cancer. Most drugs cause SIAD by stimulating hypophyseal secretion of AVP, although prostaglandin synthesis inhibitors directly inhibit renal tubular excretion of free water. The list of drugs implicated is long and includes morphine, phenothiazines, tricyclic antidepressants, and non-steroidal anti-inflammatory drugs, all frequently used in palliative care, as well as the cytotoxic drugs vincristine and cyclophosphamide, and nicotine. The possibility of drug-related SIAD should always be considered before invoking ectopic AVP secretion by tumours and in most cases the hyponatraemia resolves when the drug is stopped. When SIAD presents with no identifiable cause, a thorough search for occult malignancy (especially small-cell lung cancer) should be undertaken, as SIAD may be the presenting symptom and may precede radiological evidence by up to 1 year.(79)

Table 3 Diagnosis of syndrome of inappropriate diuresis (SIAD)

Essential criteria to establish this diagnosis are

- Plasma hypo-osmolality (plasma osmolality <275 mosm/kg H_2O and plasma sodium <135 mmol/l)
- Concentrated urine (plasma osmolality >100 mosm/kg H_2O)
- Normal plasma/extracellular fluid volume
- High urinary sodium (urine sodium >20 mEq/l) on a normal salt and water intake
- Exclude (i) hypothyroidism, (ii) hypoadrenalism, and (iii) diuretics

Supportive criteria for this diagnosis are

- Abnormal water load test (unable to excrete >90% of a 20-ml/kg water load in 4 h, and/or failure to dilute urine to osmolality <100 mosmol/kg H_2O)
- Elevated plasma AVP

Treatment

The management of SIAD depends upon the rate of onset of hyponatraemia and the presence of neurological complications. Acute SIAD with an onset over 2–3 days and falls in serum sodium in excess of 0.5 mmol/l/day are associated with neurological sequelae and require prompt correction by intravenous hypertonic saline. In contrast, the mainstay of therapy for chronic asymptomatic SIAD is fluid restriction and inhibition of tubular reabsorption of water with drugs such as demeclocycline.

Acute hyponatraemia with neurological symptoms has a mortality of 5–8 per cent, partly reflecting the underlying pathology. Rapid correction of hyponatraemia by intravenous hypertonic saline causes central pontine myelinosis often with additional extrapontine myelinosis. Central pontine myelinosis usually presents 1–2 days after correcting hyponatraemia with quadriparesis and bulbar palsy and is related to the rapidity of correction of sodium. A safe balance between overzealous correction causing irreversible myelinosis and the considerable mortality of uncorrected SIAD is required.(80,81) Hypertonic saline infusions should correct serum sodium at a rate of 0.5 mmol/l/h(82) although a correction rate of up to 2 mmol/l/h is said to be safe.(83) The total rise in serum sodium should not exceed 25 mmol/l and correction should stop once the serum sodium exceeds 120 mmol/l and symptoms have resolved. To achieve a correction rate of 0.5 mmol/l/h requires 0.3 × body weight in kg (mmol Na^+ /h). Hypertonic (twice normal) saline solution of 1.8 per cent contains 0.3 mmol/l Na^+. So the correct rate of infusion is 1 ml/kg body weight per hour of 1.8 per cent sodium chloride.(84)

The mainstay of treatment of chronic asymptomatic SIAD is fluid restriction. It is suggested that intake is restricted to 500 ml/day or the daily urine output should be less 500 ml/day. This should include all fluids and takes several days to influence the hyponatraemia. In the context of palliative care, fluid restriction is frequently undesirable as it is unpleasant for patients and onerous for their carers. Alternative strategies for chronic SIAD include the use of distal nephron inhibitors preventing water reabsorption and osmotic diuretics.

The tetracycline analogue demeclocycline (desmethylchlortetracycline) causes nephrogenic diabetes insipidus by inhibiting vasopressin-induced cAMP formation in distal tubules and is used in the treatment of chronic SIAD. Demeclocycline administered orally in two divided doses equivalent to 900–1200 mg/day will reverse chronic SIAD gradually over 3–4 days and should be followed by a maintenance dosage of 600–900 mg/day. The main side-effects of demeclocycline are gastrointestinal disturbances and hypersensitivity reactions, although reversible nephrotoxicity may occur with prolonged use, especially when hepatic function is impaired. Lithium carbonate, which has a similar effect on tubular water reabsorption, has also been used in the treatment of SIAD but is not recommended as its efficacy is less consistent and its toxicity is greater.

Urea acts as an osmotic diuretic increasing free water excretion and in addition reduces natriuresis by increasing intramedullary urea levels. It is effective in controlling SIAD when given both intravenously and orally. Oral urea should be given once daily in a dose of 30 g dissolved in orange juice to mask the taste. There is no need to fluid restrict patients treated with oral urea because of its diuretic properties.(85)

The development of vasopressin analogues which may act as specific antagonists is underway and these may hold the key to the control of SIAD in the future. A series of oral non-peptide antagonists of vasopressin receptor subtypes have been synthesized, including selective V2 receptor antagonists that lead to dose-dependent diabetes insipidus in animals.(86) This class of drugs has been christened aquaretics in recognition of their different mechanism of diuresis compared to the saliuretic actions of more familiar diuretics such as frusemide.(87)

Atrial natriuretic peptide

Atrial natriuretic peptide (ANP) is secreted by atrial monocytes and acts to regulate natriuresis and diuresis via the kidney and adrenals. A role for ectopic or inappropriate ANP secretion had been proposed to account for cases of SIAD when vasopressin is undetectable.(88) Elevated serum levels of ANP in small-cell lung cancer patients with SIAD have been demonstrated in conjunction with raised AVP, where ANP may be contributing to the hyponatraemia. A patient with small-cell lung cancer and hyponatraemia with elevated ANP and undetectable AVP has been reported and it was proposed that inappropriate ANP was the cause of the SIAD: however, the source of ANP was not demonstrated.(89) More recently ectopic production of ANP has been identified by radioimmunoassay in various neuroendocrine tumours.(90) The natriuretic peptide family is now known to include three peptides; atrial natriuretic peptide, brain natriuretic peptide, and C-type natriuretic peptide, which act via two gyuanylyl cyclase receptors and a third peptide clearance receptor.(91) The exact role of natriuretic peptides in SIAD remains to be established and ANP inhibitors may in the future have a place in treating SIAD.(92)

Non-islet cell tumour hypoglycaemia

Tumour-related hypoglycaemia is a frequent complication of beta islet cell tumours of the pancreas which secrete insulin, but occurs uncommonly with non-islet cell tumours. Although ectopic insulin secretion has been documented in a woman with cervical cancer,(93) most non-islet cell tumours produce hypoglycaemia by increased glucose use by tumours, secretion of insulin-like factors, and failure of the normal compensatory mechanisms.(94)

Pathogenesis

Increased glucose utilization by tumours has been documented in association with anaerobic metabolism by measuring arteriovenous differences in glucose concentrations. Daily glucose consumption by tumours may reach 200 g/kg per day. In addition, hepatic glucose production falls despite normal glycogen stores, producing an acquired glycogen storage disease which may contribute to hypoglycaemia. Furthermore, suppression of other compensatory mechanism, including growth hormone and glucagon secretion is believed to play a role.

Insulin-like growth factors (IGFs) (formerly named somatomedins) are a family of peptides involved in cellular growth, differentiation, and metabolism, that cross-react with insulin in both bioassay and radioreceptor assay but may be differentiated from insulin by radioimmunoassay. Two IGFs have been characterized and both have sequence homology with insulin but act via different receptors. High levels of expression of IGF-2 transcripts have been detected in non-islet cell tumours associated with hypoglycaemia, indeed elevated plasma IGF-2 levels are found in 40 per cent of these tumours. Moreover, it is an aberrant precursor form of IGF-2 that is usually found in plasma in these patients that includes the E domain that is normally cleaved from pro-IGF-2 during intracellular peptide processing in a manner analogous to the conversion of pro-insulin to insulin and it is worth recalling that pro-insulin rather than insulin dominates in the plasma of patients with insulinomas. IGF-2 (formerly somatomedin A) binds at least two receptors: an insulin-receptor-like tyrosine kinase for which IGF-1 is also a ligand, and the mannose-6-phosphate receptor. IGF-2 expression is induced by human placental lactogen, especially during foetal life where the expression of IGF-2 and its type 2 receptor are reciprocally modulated by genomic imprinting. Unlike insulin, the IGFs are bound to at least six plasma IGF-binding proteins. At high levels of IGF-2 there is a specificity spill-over so that lower affinity binding to the insulin receptor occurs and this may mediate hypoglycaemia. In addition suppression of counter-regulatory hormones, including growth hormone and glucagon, is a feature of non-islet cell hypoglycaemia. IGF-2 suppresses growth hormone secretion and thus reduces the production of IGF binding proteins by the liver.(95) Decreased IGF binding protein levels permit free IGF-2 levels to rise, leading to the inhibition of hepatic glucose release and stimulation of peripheral glucose uptake. The role of IGFs, their binding proteins and their receptors in the pathogenesis of cell transformation is under close scrutiny.(96) Rarely other mechanisms contribute to non-islet cell hypoglycaemia including the development of autoantibodies to the insulin receptor in Hodgkin's disease,(97,98) as well as overwhelming hepatic destruction.

Epidemiology

Non-islet cell tumours associated with hypoglycaemia are usually large (average 2.4 kg), retroperitoneal, or intrathoracic, often with liver invasion and following a protracted time-course over several years. Histologically these tumours are 45–65 per cent mesenchymal (mesothelioma, neurofibroma, fibrosarcoma, leiomyosarcoma, rhabdomyosarcoma, neurofibrosarcoma, haemangiopericytoma, and spindle cell carcinoma), 20 per cent hepatoma, 5–10 per cent adrenal carcinoma (chiefly androgen-secreting), and 5–10 per cent gastrointestinal tumours. Unlike other endocrine complications of malignancy, hypoglycaemia is very rarely associated with lung cancer.

Clinical features

Hypoglycaemia may be a presenting symptom but more commonly occurs in the terminal stages of the disease. The clinical manifestations are associated with cerebral hypoglycaemia and secondary secretion of catecholamines. Neurological findings include agitation, stupor, coma, and seizures which usually follow exercise or fasting and occur most often in the early morning and late afternoon. Focal neurological deficits may be present especially when cerebral circulation is poor.

Tumour-related hypoglycaemia should be differentiated from other causes of hypoglycaemia, including drugs (e.g. sulphonylureas), hypoadrenalism, hypopituitarism, and liver failure. In advanced malignancy the most common cause of hypoglycaemia is continued oral hypoglycaemic medication in long-standing diabetics.

Treatment

The reversal of life-threatening or symptomatic hypoglycaemia initially requires intravenous glucose infusion. Hyperosmolar glucose solutions in excess of 10 per cent should be administered via central lines; serum glucose levels require frequent monitoring to ensure optimal correction of hypoglycaemia. Up to 2000 g/day may be required to control tumour-related hypoglycaemia. Debulking surgery and effective chemotherapy frequently improve paraneoplastic hypoglycaemia and should therefore be considered even in a palliative context. Dietary supplementation with frequent feeding, including during the night, may control symptoms of mild paraneoplastic hypoglycaemia. Corticosteroids in high doses, parenteral glucagon, and human growth hormone have all been of benefit in some patients, whilst diazoxide, which inhibits insulin secretion, and somatostatin have been ineffective. Arterial embolization of tumours may also be used to palliate paraneoplastic hypoglycaemia.

Future approaches

The discovery of the role of IGFs in the pathogenesis of non-islet cell tumour hypoglycaemia suggests that antagonists of these peptides may become useful as therapy and may reduce the dependence on continuous glucose infusions to control hypoglycaemia in these circumstances.

Enteropancreatic hormone syndromes

Enteropancreatic hormone production is relatively uncommon in malignant disease. A variety of clinical syndromes occur associated with hormone secretion by endocrine tumours of the pancreas and less frequently by tumours arising in other organs. The majority of pancreatic islet cell tumours are malignant (with the exception of most insulinomas) and metastases are frequently present at diagnosis. Surgical excision of small localized tumours is optimal treatment and unresectable malignant secretory tumours may respond to chemotherapy. However, in many patients the distressing clinical manifestations arising from excessive secretion of gastrointestinal peptides require palliation and this may be difficult to achieve. These tumours often secrete more than one polypeptide hormone and may switch their hormone production during follow-up. Furthermore, many molecular species of the hormones, including precursor peptides with varying bioactivity, may be found in the circulation.

Treatment

The clinical manifestations listed according to the major hormone product of secretory endocrine tumours are shown in Table 4 along with the palliative endocrine manoeuvres that may control them. The control of insulinoma-related hypoglycaemia is similar to the management of paraneoplastic hypoglycaemia (see above), except that diazoxide may be a valuable additional agent in insulinoma. Diazoxide inhibits insulin release from beta islet cells but may cause salt and water retention and so is usually prescribed with chlorothiazide. Palliation of acid hypersecretion in Zollinger–Ellison syndrome is most effectively achieved by proton pump inhibitors, although other drugs including high dose histamine H_2 receptor antagonists may be useful. The symptomatic control of other secretory tumors has been revolutionized by the introduction of long-acting somatostatin analogues.

Somatostatin is a widely distributed 14 amino acid cyclic neuroendocrine peptide which plays an inhibitory role in homeostatic mechanisms of the nervous system, gastrointestinal tract, and both endocrine and exocrine pancreas. A single gene on chromosome 3 encodes somatostatin which is translated as the 116-amino acid pre-pro-somatostatin that includes a signal peptide. Extensive post-translational processing yields SOM-14, the biologically active form. SOM-14 acts via at least five somatostatin receptors that activate G proteins, which in turn reduce adenyl cyclase activity, decrease conductance of voltage-sensitive calcium channels, activate potassium channels, and stimulate tyrosine kinase activity.[(99)] Somatostatin has a short duration of action, requires intravenous administration, and following infusion, rebound hypersecretion of hormones may occur. These shortcomings have been overcome by the use of the synthetic analogue octreotide, an eight amino acid analogue that is given by sub-cutaneous injection. Octreotide acts on three of the somatostatin receptor subtypes and appears to exert its clinical effect via binding to receptor subtype 2.[(99)]

The control of clinical symptoms associated with enteropancreatic hormone hypersecretion, including profuse diarrhoea, hypokalaemia, hypoglycaemia, peptic ulceration, necrolytic skin lesions, and even Cushing's syndrome, can be achieved by 100–450 mg octreotide subcutaneously daily in many patients with endocrine pancreatic tumors. The response to octreotide seems to depend upon the presence of somatostatin receptors on the tumours and this has been exploited for tumour localization using *in vivo* scintigraphy with labeled octreotide.[(100)] Somatostatin analogues provide valuable symptom palliation in insulinomas, glucagonomas, gastrinomas, VIPomas, and GRFomas but there is little evidence to suggest that they control tumour growth. Resistance may develop with chronic use of octreotide and this is thought to occur due to the emergence of tumour cells lacking somatostatin receptors. Octreotide therapy is well tolerated; although initially abdominal cramps and diarrhoea may occur, significant steatorrhoea and malabsorption have not been observed.

Carcinoid syndrome

Carcinoid tumours arise from enterochromaffin cells principally in the gastrointestinal tract, pancreas, and lungs but occasionally in the thymus and gonads. The incidence of these uncommon neoplasms is 1.5 per 100 000. The carcinoid syndrome develops in 6–18 per cent of patients with these tumours and these patients almost invariably have hepatic metastases.[(99,101,102)] The features of carcinoid tumours vary by their sites of origin and are shown in Table 5.

The cardinal feature of the carcinoid syndrome is the combination of diarrhoea and flushing, which occurs in at least 75 per cent of patient, and may be associated with asthma, endomyocardial fibrosis, and pellagra. One-third of patients develop cardiac manifestations which are late complications, typically involve the right side of the heart, and lead to pulmonary valve stenosis and tricuspid valve regurgitation. Asthma and pellagra are less common. The pellagroid rash is thought to arise secondary to the diversion of tryptophan for 5-hydroxytryptamine (5HT) synthesis rather than nicotinamide production.[(103)] The clinical features are mediated by several potentially active substances secreted by the tumours, including 5HT, 5-hydroxytryptophan, kallikrein, tachykinins (substance P, neuropeptide K), prostaglandins,

Table 4 Clinical manifestations of secretory endocrine tumours

Tumour	Major feature	Minor feature	Common sites	Malignant	MEN associated	Palliative therapies
Insulinoma	Neuroglycopenia (confusion, fits)	Permanent neurological deficits	Pancreas (β cells)	10%	10%	Frequent feeding Glucose Glucagon Diazoxide and chlorothiazide Octreotide
Gastrinoma (Zollinger–Elison syndrome)	Peptic ulceration	Diarrhoea, Weight loss Malabsorption Dumping	Pancreas (D cells) Duodenum	40–60%	25%	Gastrectomy Proton pump inhibitor H2 receptor antagonists Octreotide
VIPoma (WDHA or Werner-Morrison syndrome)	Watery diarrhoea Hypokalaemia Achlorhydria	Hypercalcaemia Hyperglycaemia Hypomagnesaemia	Pancreas (A–D cells) Neuroblastoma SCLC Phaeochromocytoma	40%	<5%	Octreotide Glucocorticoids
Glucagonoma	Migratory necrolytic erythema Mild diabetes mellitus Muscle wasting Anaemia	Diarrhoea Thromboembolism Stomatitis Hypoaminoacidaemia Encephalitis	Pancreas (α cells)	60%	<5%	Octreotide Oral hypoglycaemics
Somatostatinoma	Diabetes mellitus Cholelithiasis Steatorrhoea Malabsorption	Anaemia Diarrhoea Weight loss Hypoglycaemia	Pancreas (β cells)	66%	Case reports only	—
GRFoma	Acromegaly	—	Pancreas	?	Case reports only	Octreotide
PPoma	None	Diarrhoea Hypokalaemia Achlorhydria Weight loss	Pancreas (interacinar F cells)	40%	25%	—

Abbreviations: MEN, multiple endocrine neoplasia; SCLC, small-cell lung cancer; VIP, vasoactive intestinal polypeptide; GRF, growth hormone releasing factor; PP, pancreatic polypeptide; H2, histamine type 2; WDHA, watery diarrhoea, hypokalaemic achlorhydria.

Table 5 Comparison of carcinoid tumours by site of origin

	Foregut	Midgut	Hindgut
Site	Respiratory tract, pancreas, stomach, proximal duodenum	Jejunum, ileum, appendix, Meckle's diverticulum, ascending colon	Transverse and descending colon, rectum
Tumour products	Low 5HTP, multihormones[a]	High 5HTP, multihormones[a]	Rarely 5HTP, multihormones[a]
Blood	5HTP, histamine, multihormones[a], occasionally ACTH	5HT, multihormones[a], rarely ACTH	Rarely 5HT or ACTH
Urine	5HTP, 5HT, 5HIAA, histamine	5HT, 5HIAA	Negative
Carcinoid syndrome	Occurs but is atypical	Occurs frequently with metastases	Rarely occurs
Metastasises to bone	Common	Rare	Common

Abbreviations: 5HT, 5-hydroxytryptamine (serotonin); 5HTP, 5-hydroxytryptophan; 5HIAA, 5-hydroxyindole acetic acid.

[a] Multihormones include tachykinins (substance P, substance K, neuropeptide K), neurotensin, PYY, enkephalin, insulin, glucagon, glicentin, VIP, somatostatin, pancreatic polypeptide, ACTH, α-subunit of human chorionic gonadotrophin.

catecholamines, and histamine. The diagnosis is usually established by measuring the urinary excretion of 5-hydroxyindoloacetic formed by the action of monoamine oxidase on 5HT. However, platelet 5HT levels are a more sensitive diagnostic test (and are unaffected by diet[104]). Tumour localization may be achieved using somatostatin receptor scintigraphy or by positron emission tomography scanning after injecting ^{11}C-labeled 5-hydroxytryptophan.[105]

The pharmacological control of carcinoid syndrome is primarily directed at inhibiting the synthesis, release, and peripheral action of circulating tumour products, principally 5HT. The choice of drugs remains empirical in view of the varied profiles of active substances released by different tumours. Parachlorophenylalanine and methyldopa block 5HT synthesis but are poorly tolerated and, therefore, now rarely used. At least 16 5HT receptors have been cloned and most have been found to be G-protein coupled, although the $5HT_3$ receptor is a ligand-gated ion channel. The development of selective 5HT receptor ligands and antagonists will allow the investigation of the physiological roles of each receptor. However, the relevance of the different receptors in the clinical manifestations of carcinoid syndrome remains uncertain and is obscured by the secretion of multiple products by these tumours. Of the drugs which block $5HT_2$ receptors, cyproheptadine (4–7 mg thrice daily) improves diarrhoea in 60 per cent of patients and flushing in 47 per cent. The mean duration of response to cyproheptadine is 8 months. In contrast, ketanserin (40–160 mg once daily) ameliorates flushing in 50 per cent but only 20 per cent find relief from diarrhoea. Selective $5HT_3$ receptor inhibitors have been shown to reduce diarrhoea in carcinoid syndrome. Metoclopramide and cisapride are believed to stimulate gastric motility via the $5HT_4$ receptor and antagonists of this receptor, which are in development, may prove useful in the palliation of carcinoid syndrome.

Somatostatin analogues are considered by most physicians to be the first line treatment of choice for patients with carcinoid syndrome. Octreotide in doses of 50–150 μg two or three times daily, subcutaneously reduces 5HT secretion and its peripheral action and is valuable in controlling both flushing and diarrhoea in the carcinoid syndrome. It produces initial relief of symptoms in 80 per cent of patient.[106] Sandostatin LAR and lanreotide, a related peptide, are long-acting analogues that have been found to be efficacious.[107–109] A reduction in tumour rarely occurs, however, and the effects of treatment diminish with time.

Palliative debulking surgery may be offered to selected patients with metastatic disease as it can delay the development of the carcinoid syndrome. Hepatic artery embolization similarly can be employed and may produce good symptom palliation.[110] Chemotherapy and alpha interferon have also been used successfully to palliate symptoms in carcinoid syndrome.[99,105] Finally, ^{131}I-met-iodobenzylguanidine (^{131}I-MIBG) has been used in patients with disabling symptoms in whom other therapeutic options have failed.[111]

Palliation of the clinical manifestations of carcinoid syndrome includes symptomatic therapy of diarrhoea (codeine phosphate, loperamide, or diphenoxylate), β_2 adrenergic agonists for wheezing, and avoiding precipitating factors to reduce flushing (including alcohol and some foods).

Phaeochromocytoma

Phaeochromocytomas arise from the chromaffin cells of the sympathetic nervous system most frequently in the adrenal medulla but occasionally from sympathetic ganglia. Phaeochromocytomas commonly secrete norepinephrine and epinephrine but in some cases significant quantities of dopamine are also produced. The catecholamines cause intermittent, episodic, or sustained hypertension and other clinical manifestations including anxiety, tremor, palpitations, sweating, flushing, headaches, gastrointestinal disturbances, and polyuria. These symptoms are all attributable to excessive adrenergic stimulation, and when surgery and chemotherapy are unable to control the disease, palliative treatment is usually achieved by α and β adrenergic receptor blockade. However, these tumours may elaborate and secrete other peptide hormones which may cause symptoms refractory to adrenergic inhibition, but this is rare. Initial treatment should be α blockade to control hypertension (e.g. phenoxybenzamine 10 mg twice daily and gradually increasing the dosage until symptoms are palliated) followed by β blockade to control tachycardia (e.g. propranolol 20–80 mg three times daily). This combination will control symptoms in most patients with malignant phaeochromocytoma. If palliation is not achieved despite full adrenergic receptor blockade, α-methylparatyrosine (250 mg twice daily increasing up to 4 g/day) may be used. α-Methylparatyrosine is a competitive inhibitor of tyrosine hydroxylase, the rate limiting enzyme in catecholamine synthesis, and reduces catecholamine production by up to 75 per cent but it is poorly tolerated due to sedation, extrapyramidal effects, and diarrhoea. The noradrenaline analogue MIBG is taken up by catecholamine synthesising tissues and ^{131}I-MIBG is useful for imaging phaeochromocytomas. At higher doses ^{131}I-MIBG may be used as therapy for phaeochromocytoma and neuroblastoma and it reduces catecholamine synthesis in patients with malignant phaeochromocytoma.[112]

Gonadotrophin secretion

Follicle stimulating hormone, luteinizing hormone, and human chorionic gonadotrophin (hCG) may be secreted by pituitary, trophoblastic, or germ cell tumours and ectopically by tumours arising in other organs. All three gonadotrophins are dimeric glycoproteins sharing the same β subunit with thyroid stimulating hormone but each has a unique α subunit that confers biological activity. The overproduction by tumours of gonadotrophins may result in precocious puberty in children, secondary amenorrhoea in women, gynaecomastia in men, and rarely, hyperthyroidism. hCG is a valuable tumour marker for detecting and monitoring therapy in trophoblastic and germ cell tumours.

Precocious puberty

Central precocious puberty occurs with central nervous system tumours secreting gonadotrophins which activate the hypothalamic-pituitary axis. Incomplete or peripheral precocious puberty may result from hCG secretion by germinomas, teratomas, chorioepitheliomas, and hepatomas and oestrogen or testosterone production by adrenal, testicular (Leydig cell), and ovarian (granulosa thecal cell) tumours. The treatment of precocious puberty includes psychological counselling for boys with increased aggression and excessive masturbation. Medical therapy is required to control both the psychosocial aspects and sustained effects on skeletal maturation. Central precocious puberty is amenable to gonadotrophin-releasing-hormone analogues which, following an initial phase of stimulation, lead to pituitary gonadotrophin receptor desensitization resulting in suppressed luteinizing hormone and follicle-stimulating-hormone secretion. The management of incomplete precocious puberty is more difficult and requires the use of antiandrogens (e.g. cyproterone acetate and spironolactone) and inhibitors of androgen synthesis (e.g. ketoconazole and finasteride).

Amenorrhoea

Secondary amenorrhoea in women with cancer may occasionally be a consequence of gonadotrophin, prolactin, oestrogen, or androgen-secreting tumours although iatrogenic causes are far commoner. The vasomotor symptoms associated with menopause may be palliated by hormone replacement therapy and dyspareunia caused by vaginal atrophy may be alleviated by topical oestrogen preparations.

Gynaecomastia

Gynaecomastia results from elevation in the oestrogen:androgen ratio which may be either a consequence of decreased androgen production or activity or increased oestrogen formation (usually by peripheral aromatization of circulating androgens to oestrogens). In men with advanced cancer, gynaecomastia is most often a consequence of drug therapy: chemotherapy (alkylating agents, vinca alkaloids, nitrosoureas), antiemetics (metoclopramide and phenothiazines), antiandrogens (cyproterone acetate, flutamide, bicalutamide), or gonadotrophin-releasing-hormone analogues (goserelin, leuprorelin). Occasionally other drugs are implicated or tumour secretion of oestrogens or gonadotrophins may be responsible.

Testicular Leydig-cell tumours and feminizing adrenocortical tumours may secrete oestrogens whilst peripheral aromatization is a feature of Sertoli cell tumours, trophoblastic germ cell tumours, and sex cord tumours of the testes and hepatocellular cancers. The elevated, circulating oestrogen levels induce ductal, lobular, and alveolar growth of the breast leading to gynaecomastia. hCG-secreting tumours (including testicular tumours, trophoblastic tumours, non-small-cell lung cancers, hepatoma, and islet cell tumours of the pancreas) stimulate oestradiol production by interstitial and Sertoli cells of the testes resulting in gynaecomastia. Symptomatic therapy for gynaecomastia should include discontinuation of any incriminated drugs and treatment of the primary tumour. Tamoxifen, clomiphene, topical dihydrotestosterone, and danazol have all been used with some success, as have liposuction, subcutaneous mastectomy, and low dosage radiotherapy for palliation of painful gynaecomastia.[113,114]

Hyperthyroidism

On account of the structural similarities to thyroid stimulating hormone, hCG has intrinsic thyrotropic action via a thyroid-stimulating-hormone-receptor spill-over effect.[115] Clinically overt hyperthyroidism caused in thus way only occurs with tumours secreting very large quantities of hCG, usually trophoblastic tumours.[116] The hyperthyroidism resolves after surgical removal of the tumour, and so palliation of the hyperthyroidism should be with drugs (e.g. carbimazole) rather than with radioactive iodine or thyroidectomy.

Prolactin

Ectopic prolactin secretion from non-pituitary tumours is very rare and uncommonly causes galactorrhoea. Small-cell lung cancer and renal cell cancer have been associated with elevated prolactin levels although the mechanism remains uncertain. Elevated serum prolactin is a poor prognostic indicator in women with breast cancer[117] and prolactin promotes the growth *in vitro* of human breast cancer cells. Galactorrhoea due to ectopic prolactin production may be treated by the dopaminergic agonist bromocriptine.

Oxytocin

The molecular biology of oxytocin resembles that of AVP with similar genes, precursor proteins, and transport by axonal streaming. Furthermore, ectopic secretion of both oxytocin and its carrier protein NP I have been demonstrated in small-cell lung cancer, usually in conjunction with ectopic AVP production. Although water intoxication and hyponatraemia may follow oxytocin infusions in women with obstetric problems, ectopic oxytocin secretion is not thought to contribute to SIAD or any other clinical symptoms.

Pyrexia

Pyrexia is a common feature of terminal cancer and is usually attributable to infection or drugs. In only 5 per cent of cases is the fever directly related to the cancer.[118] Malignancy accounted for only 7 per cent of cases in a series of 199 patients with pyrexias of unknown origin.[119] Paraneoplastic pyrexia is a diagnosis of exclusion established after other causes of fever have been ruled out. Hodgkin's disease, renal cell adenocarcinoma, lymphoma, leukaemia, hepatoma, myxoma, and osteogenic sarcoma account for most cases of paraneoplastic fever.

Pathogenesis

Pyrexia is a consequence of endogenous pyrogenic cytokines (including TNF, IL-1, IL-6, and interferons) stimulating the organum vasculosum of the lamina terminalis which lacks a blood-brain barrier. This results in the synthesis and release of prostaglandin E_2 from the preoptic anterior hypothalamus which mediates thermal homeostasis. Resetting the thermostatic set point by 1–4°C enhances macrophage killing of bacteria and also impairs replication of micro-organisms.[120–122] Tumour-related pyrexia is thought to be a consequence of cytokine production by neoplastic cells or by normal cells in response to tumour presence. Evidence for the former includes TNF-α production in Hodgkin's disease, which may be localized by *in vitro* hybridization to the Reed Sternberg cell.[123] Furthermore, the abnormal lymphocytes in Castleman's disease (an angiofollicular lymph node hyperplasia related to lymphoma and associated with fever) produce IL-6. After complete surgical excision of these tumours circulating plasma IL-6 is no longer detectable and symptoms resolve. In addition, anti-IL-6 receptor antibody therapy has been shown to be a useful therapy for multicentric Castleman's disease.[124] A similar mechanism has been elucidated in phaeochromotyoma where tumour cells produce IL-6 resulting in paraneoplastic pyrexia which resolves with tumour resection.[125] In addition, raised serum levels of TNF-α, IL-1, and IL-6 are found in patients with renal cell carcinoma and serum IL-6 may be used as a tumour marker in these patients.[126]

Therapy

Definitive therapy of the tumour will resolve paraneoplastic pyrexias in most cases of Hodgkin's disease and many lymphomas. Sponging, ice-packs, and fans may often relieve discomfort. Pharmacological agents such as paracetamol, aspirin, non-steroidal anti-inflammatory drugs, and steroids are effective antipyretics.[127] Advances in the understanding of the pathogenesis of paraneoplastic pyrexia propose a role for cytokine antagonists in therapy. The development of IL-1 false receptors is an attractive approach to cytokine-induced pyrexia that has already been usurped in nature by vaccinia virus: vaccinia secretes virally encoded IL-1 receptors that compete with endogenous IL-1 receptors on T-lymphocytes thus attenuating the host response to infection including pyrexia.[128] Similarly strategies based upon IL-1 receptor antagonists including IL-1ra, which is structurally related to IL-1 have been explored in paraneoplastic pyrexia along with strategies aimed at blocking IL-6 signalling.[129,130]

Non-paraneoplastic complications

Hyperglycaemia

The prevalence of hyperglycaemia in cancer patients is higher than in the general population. It has repeatedly been claimed that diabetes mellitus is a risk factor for the development of pancreatic cancer. However, a multicentre study involving 720 patients failed to confirm this.[131] Several mechanisms may contribute to hyperglycaemia in advanced cancers including increased gluconeogenesis and Cori cycle activity (conversion of muscle-derived lactate to glucose), diminished glucose tolerance and turnover, and insulin resistance.[132] These changes may arise as a consequence of hepatic dysfunction, altered glucose metabolism by tumour cells, and the secretion of insulin antagonists. Furthermore, the frequent use of corticosteroids in palliative medicine may contribute since one in five patients on high dose steroids will develop steroid-induced diabetes mellitus.

The conventional treatment of diabetes advocates tight control of blood sugar to delay the onset of diabetic complications, including neuropathy, retinopathy, and nephropathy. In contrast the aims of therapy in palliative care are to minimize symptoms associated with hypoglycaemia or marked hyperglycaemia. For this reason a wider range of blood sugar is acceptable and close blood glucose monitoring is unnecessary.

Weight loss and anorexia reduce the need for hypoglycaemic agents as cancer progresses, and strict dietary restrictions are unnecessary and burdenserve. Oral hypoglycaemic drugs can usually be reduced or stopped in non-insulin-dependent diabetics without symptomatic hyperglycaemia ensuing. Similarly, the insulin requirements of insulin-dependent diabetics with advanced malignancy reduce and insulin regimens can usually be simplified to once daily, long-acting insulin such as human mixed insulin zinc suspensions (e.g. Human monotard, Humulin lente) or human crystalline insulin zinc suspensions (e.g. human Ultratard, Humulin Zn). Blood sugars may be allowed to stay on the high side to prevent the distressing symptoms of hypoglycaemia. Where possible, monitoring should be performed by urinalysis rather than by blood sampling. Steroid-induced diabetes, which occurs frequently in advanced cancer, is usually asymptomatic and requires no therapy; however, if polyuria and polydipsia develop a short-acting sulfonylurea may be useful (e.g. gliclazide 40–80 mg once daily.)

Renal failure

Renal failure is a common feature of advanced malignancy and many aetiological factors play a role in its pathogenesis (see Table 6). In the context of incurable malignant disease reversible causes may be addressed but aggressive treatment such as renal replacement therapy is usually not appropriate.

Potentially reversible metabolic causes of renal failure include urate nephropathy, hypercalcaemia, and tumour lysis syndrome. Prerenal and obstructive renal failure may be reversible although treatment may not be appropriate if the patient is very frail and antitumour options have been exhausted.[133] Tumour infiltration can sometimes be unproved if effective anticancer therapy is available as in newly diagnosed lymphoma.

Symptomatic management is important. Patients may experience nausea, vomiting, drowsiness, and confusion as the kidneys fail. Dry mouth and anorexia are often present anyway as a consequence of advanced cancer but may be exacerbated by renal impairment. Appropriate and sensitive explanation to the patient and family should be accompanied by medication to relieve any unpleasant symptoms. In the context of renal failure doses of some medications may need to be reduced or stopped to avoid drug accumulation or deterioration of renal function. Patients already receiving renal dialysis for pre-existing chronic renal failure usually chose to continue this until it becomes impractical.

Obstructive nephropathy may cause colicky pain in addition to the non-specific symptoms of renal failure. Although analgesics and antispasmodics may ameliorate the pain, longer lasting relief of symptoms can be achieved with percutaneous nephrostomy. This procedure, performed under sedation, can be followed by antegrade catheterization of the ureters. Nephrostomy tube insertion is an invasive procedure and is appropriate in selected cases where prognosis may be longer or antitumour treatment is planned.

Liver failure

Liver failure in cancer patients is usually a consequence of biliary obstruction, very extensive hepatic metastases, or drug therapy, although a paraneoplastic hepatopathy has been described in patients with renal cell adenocarcinoma.[134] After excluding drug causes, it is important to differentiate obstructive and parenchymal causes as the approach to palliation differs.

Obstructive jaundice may be differentiated from other causes by the detection of urinary bilirubin in the absence of urinary urobilinogen using dipstick testing. Biliary obstruction may be confirmed by ultrasonography and drainage may be undertaken to relieve jaundice and associated symptoms (anorexia, nausea, pruritus) (see Chapter 8.7). Biliary drainage may be obtained by percutaneous transhepatic biliary drainage or endoscopic retrograde biliary drainage, and both techniques provide good palliation.

Hepatic failure due to massive metastases may produce jaundice, pruritis, anorexia, liver capsule pain, ascites, disturbances of haemostasis, malabsorption, and electrolyte disturbances, culminating in hepatic encephalopathy. The palliative treatment of liver failure needs to be tailored to the particular symptoms of each patient. Liver capsule pain may be helped by non-steroidal anti-inflammatory drugs and corticosteroids together with conventional analgesics. Symptoms of functional gastric outlet obstruction may be helped by metoclopromide before meals. Nausea secondary to liver failure may require centrally acting antiemetics such as haloperidol. Pruritus may be reduced by using emollients and night sedation. Naltrexone and stanozolol have also been found to be effective in pruritus from intrahepatic cholestasis and obstructive jaundice, respectively. If the cause is obstructive then stenting provides the most effective palliation.

Hepatic encephalopathy is thought to be due to an excess of γ-aminobutyric acid activity, ammonia, and other toxins in the central nervous system. Conventional therapies for hepatic encephalopathy include restriction of dietary protein and sodium, bowel clearance with magnesium sulphate enemas and lactulose, as well as bowel sterilization with neomycin in an attempt to reduce ammonia production by gut microflora. Since hepatic encephalopathy is a terminal event in the context of advanced malignancy, these unpleasant treatments are rarely appropriate. The main symptom of encephalopathy is confusion, and after establishing the cause of confusion, familiar company, a light and quiet environment, and a regular routine should be provided together with explanation, reassurance, and reorientation. Sedation may be necessary if the patient is agitated. Under these circumstances, haloperidol (1.5–5 mg) or levomepromazine (6.25–150 mg) may be given orally or subcutaneously, and will also have an antiemetic action (see also Chapter). The combination of portal hypertension and abnormal coagulation in liver failure predisposes to gastrointestinal haemorrhage. Major haemorrhage should usually be managed symptomatically (Chapter).

Table 6 Causes of renal failure in malignancy

1. Infiltration by tumour
2. Fluid depletion
3. Electrolyte imbalance
   - —Uric acid (tumour lysis syndrome)
   - —Hypercalcaemia
   - —Paraprotein (e.g. myeloma)
   - —Amyloid (e.g. myeloma)
   - —Lysozyme (e.g. acute myelomonocytic leukaemia)
   - —Mucoprotein (e.g. pancreatic adenocarcinoma)
   - —Nephrogenic diabetes insipidus (e.g. leiomyosarcoma)
4. Urinary tract obstruction
5. Iatrogenic
   - —Chemotherapy
   - —Radiotherapy
6. Paraneoplastic
   - —Membranous glomerulonephritis (e.g. carcinomas)
   - —Minimal change glomerulonephritis (e.g. Hodgkin's disease)
   - —Membranoproliferative glomerulonephritis (e.g. non-Hodgkin's lymphoma)
7. Pre-existing chronic renal failure

Lactic acidosis

Type B lactic acidosis is a rare complication of malignancy which presents clinically with hyperventilation and hypotension. In most cases the underlying malignancy is haematological. Increased lactate production by tumour cells owing to uncoupled oxidative phosphorylation and glycolysis, and reduced lactate clearance due to liver dysfunction have both been implicated in the pathogenesis of malignancy-associated lactic acidosis. The diagnosis is established biochemically by the combination of wide anion gap acidosis and raised plasma lactate (>2 mEq/l). Intravenous isotonic (26 per cent) sodium bicarbonate may be used to correct the metabolic acidosis but should only be used if effective anticancer therapy is available and appropriate to be attempted.[135]

References

1. **Laforga, J., Vierna, J., and Aranda, F.** (1994). Hypercalcaemia in Hodgkin's disease related to prostaglandin synthesis. *Journal of Clinical Pathology* **47**, 567–8.
2. **Nakayama, K.** et al. (1996). Differences in bone and vitamin D metabolism between primary hyperparathyroidism and malignancy-associated hypercalcemia. *Journal of Clinical Endocrinology and Metabolism* **81**, 607–11.
3. **Benitez-Verguizas, J. and Esbrit, P.** (1994). Proliferative effect of parathyroid hormone related protein on the hypercalcaemic Walker 256 carcinoma cell line. *Biochemical and Biophysical Research Communication* **198**, 1281–9.

4. **Li, X. and Drucker, D.** (1994). Parathyroid hormone related peptide is a downstream target for *ras* and *src* activation. *Journal of Biological Chemistry* **269**, 6263–6.
5. **Vortkamp, A.** et al. (1996). Regulation of rate of cartilage differentiation by Indian hedgehog and PTH-related peptide. *Science* **273**, 613–22.
6. **Lanske, B.** et al. (1996). PTH/PTHrP receptor in early development and Indian hedgehog-regulated bone growth. *Science* **273**, 663–6.
7. **Epstein, F.** (2000). The physiology of parathyroid hormone related protein. *New England Journal of Medicine* **342**, 177–85.
8. **Danks, J.** et al. (1989). Parathyroid hormone-related protein of cancer: immunohistochemical localisation in cancers and in normal skin. *Journal of Bone and Mineral Research* **4**, 273–8.
9. **Honda, S.** et al. (1988). Expression of parathyroid hormone-related protein mRNA in tumours obtained from patients with humoral hypercalcaemia of malignancy. *Japanese Journal of Cancer Research* **79**, 677–83.
10. **Budayr, A.** et al. (1989). Increased serum levels of a parathyroid hormone-like protein in malignancy-associated hypercalcaemia. *Annals of Internal Medicine* **111**, 807–12.
11. **Hutchesson, A.** et al. (1993). Parathyroid hormone-related protein as a tumour marker in humoral hypercalcaemia associated with occult malignancy. *Postgraduate Medical Journal* **69**, 640–2.
12. **Bouizar, Z.** et al. (1993). Polymerase chain reaction analysis of parathyroid hormone-related protein gene expression in breast cancer patients and occurrence of bone metastases. *Cancer Research* **53**, 5076–8.
13. **Wysolmerski, J. and Broadus, A.** (1994). Hypercalcaemia of malignancy: the central role of parathyroid hormone-related protein. *Annual Review of Medicine* **45**, 189–200.
14. **Grill, V.** et al. (1991). Parathyroid hormone-related protein: elevated levels in both humoral hypercalcemia of malignancy and hypercalcemia complicating metastatic breast cancer. *Journal of Clinical Endocrinology and Metabolism* **73**, 1309–15.
15. **Kukreja, S.** et al. (1988). Antibodies to parathyroid hormone-related protein lower serum calcium in athymic mouse models of malignancy associated hypercalcaemia of cancer. *Journal of Clinical Investigation* **82**, 1798–802.
16. **Henderson, J.** et al. (1990). Effects of passive immunization against parathyroid hormone (PTH)-like peptide and PTH in hypercalcaemic tumour-bearing rats and normocalcaemic controls. *Endocrinology* **127**, 1310–18.
17. **Burtis, W.** et al. (1990). Immunocytochemical characterisation of circulating parathyroid hormone-related protein in patients with humoral hypercalcaemia of malignancy. *New England Journal of Medicine* **322**, 1106–12.
18. **Jacobsen, J.** et al. (1989). Humoral hypercalcaemia in Hodgkin's disease. Clinical and laboratory evaluation. *Cancer* **63**, 917–23.
19. **Davies, M.** et al. (1994). Abnormal synthesis of 1,25-dihydroxyvitamin D in patients with malignant lymphoma. *Journal of Clinical Endocrinology and Metabolism* **78**, 1202–7.
20. **Sato, M.** et al. (1991). Bisphosphonate action. Aldendronate localization in rat bone and effects on osteoclast ultrastructure. *Journal of Clinical Investigation* **88**, 2095–105.
21. **Zimolo, Z., Wesolowski, G., and Rodan, G.** (1995). Acid extrusion is induced by osteoclast attachment to bone Inhibition by aledronate and calcitonin. *Journal of Clinical Investigation* **96**, 2324–33.
22. **Gucalp, R.** et al. (1992). Comparative study of pamidronate disodium and etidronate disodium in the treatment of cancer-related hypercalcaemia. *Journal of Clinical Oncology* **10**, 134–42.
23. **O'Rourke, N.** et al. (1993). Effective treatment of malignant hypercalcaemia with a single intravenous infusion of clodronate. *British Journal of Cancer* **67**, 560–3.
24. **Purohit, O.** et al. (1995). A randomised double-blind comparison of intravenous pamidronate and clodronate in the hypercalcaemia of malignancy. *British Journal of Cancer* **72**, 1289–93.
25. **Vinholes, J.** et al. (1997). Evaluation of new bone resorption markers in a randomized comparison of pamidronate or clodronate for hypercalcemia of malignany. *Journal of Clinical Oncology* **15**, 131–8.
26. **Walls, J.** et al. (1994). Response to intravenous bisphosphonate therapy in hypercalcaemic patietns with and without bone metastases: the role of parathyroid hormone-related protein. *British Journal of Cancer* **58**, 556–7.
27. **Wimalwansa, S.** (1994). Significance of plasma PTH-rp in patients with hypercalcaemia of malignancy treated with bisphosphonate. *Cancer* **73**, 2223–30.
28. **Ralston, S.** et al. (1997). Dose-response study of ibandronate in treatment of cancer-associated hypercalcaemia. *British Journal of Cancer* **75**, 295–300.
29. **Body, J.** et al. (1999). A dose-finding study of zoledronate in hypercalcemic cancer patients. *Journal of Bone and Mineral Research* **14**, 11557–61.
30. **Major, P.** et al. (2001). Zoledronic acid is superior to pamidronate in the treatment of hypercalcemia of malignancy: a pooled analysis of two randomised controlled clinical trial. *Journal of Clinical Oncology* **19**, 558–67.
31. **Body, J.** et al. (1998). Current use of bisphosphonates in oncology. *Journal of Clinical Oncology* **16**, 3890–9.
32. **Bockman, R.** et al. (1990). Distribution of trace levels of therapeutic gallium in bone as mapped by synchrotron X-ray microscopy. *Proceedings of the National Academy of Sciences of the United States of America* **87**, 4149–53.
33. **Warrell, R.** et al. (1988). A randomised double-blind study of gallium nitrate versus calcitonin for acute treatment of cancer-related hypercalcaemia. *Annals of Internal Medicine* **108**, 669–74.
34. **Warrell, R.** et al. (1991). A randomised double-blind study of gallium nitrate compared to etidronate for acute control of cancer related hypercalcemia. *Journal of Clinical Oncology* **9**, 1467–75.
35. **Sato, K.** et al. (1993). Passive immunisation with anti-parathyroid hormone-related protein monoclonal antibody markedly prolongs survival time of hypercalcemic nude mice bearing transplanted human PTHrP-producing tumours. *Journal of Bone and Mineral Research* **8**, 849–60.
36. **Lacey, D.** et al. (1998). Osteoprotegerin ligand is a cytokine that upregulates osteoclast differentiation and activation. *Cell* **93**, 165–76.
37. **Kong, Y.** et al. (1999). OPGL is a key regualtor of osteoclastogenesis, lymphocyte development and lymph node organogenesis. *Nature* **397**, 315–23.
38. **Capparelli, C.** et al. (1999). Comparison of osteoprotegerin and pamidronate in a murine model of humoral hypercalcemia of malignancy. *Journal of Bone and Mineral Research* **14** (Suppl. 1), S163.
39. **Yoneda, T.** et al. (1993). Herbimycin A, a pp60c-src tyrosine kinase inhibitor, inhibits osteoclastic bone resorption *in vitro* and hypercalcemia *in vivo*. *Journal of Clinical Investigation* **91**, 2791–5.
40. **Moriyama, K.** et al. (1996). Herbimycin A, a tyrosine kinase inhibitor, impairs hypercalcemia associated with a human squamous cancer producing interleukin-6 in nude mice. *Journal of Bone and Mineral Research* **11**, 905–11.
41. **King, K.** et al. (1994). Effects of kistrin on bone resorption *in vitro* and serum calcium *in vivo*. *Journal of Bone and Mineral Research* **9**, 381–7.
42. **El Abdaimi, K.** et al. (1999). Reversal of hypercalcemia with the vitamin D analogue EB1089 in a human model of squamous cancer. *Cancer Research* **59**, 3325–8.
43. **Goodman, W.** et al. (2000). A calcimimetic agent lowers plasma parathyroid hormone levels in patients with secondary hyperparathyroidism. *Kidney* **58**, 436–45.
44. **Hale, A.** et al. (1985). A case of pituitary-dependent Cushing's disease with clinical and biochemical features of ectopic ACTH syndrome. *Clinical Endocrinology* **22**, 479–88.
45. **Orth, D.** (1995). Cushing's syndrome. *New England Journal of Medicine* **332**, 791–803.
46. **Friedman, J. and Halaas, J.** (1998). Leptin and the regulation of body weight in mammals. *Nature* **395**, 763–70.
47. **Yaswen, L.** et al. (1999). Obesity in the mouse model of pro-opiomelanocortin deficiency responds to peripheral melanocortin. *Nature Medicine* **5**, 1066–70.
48. **Pullan, P.** et al. (1980). Ectopic production of methionine enkephalin and beta endorphin. *British Medical Journal* **280**, 758–9.
49. **Chatikhine, V.** et al. (1994). Expression of opiod peptides in cells and stroma of human breast cancer and adenofibromas. *Cancer Letter* **77**, 51–6.
50. **Jeffcoate, W.** et al. (1979). Psychiatric manifestations of Cushing's syndrome: response to lowering plasma cortisol. *Quarterly Journal of Medicine* **48**, 465–72.
51. **Howlett, T.** et al. (1986). Diagnosis and management of ACTH-dependent Cushing's syndrome: a comparison of the features in ectopic and pituitary ACTH production. *Clinical Endocrinology (Oxford)* **24**, 699–713.

52. **Delisle, L.** et al. (1993). Ectopic corticotropin syndrome and small-cell carcinoma of the lung. Clinical features, outcome, and complications. *Archives of Internal Medicine* **153**, 746–52.
53. **Abeloff, M., Trump, D., and Baylin, S.** (1981). Ectopic adrenocortiotrophin (ACTH) syndrome and small cell carcinoma of the lung: assessment of clinical implications in patients on combination chemotherapy. *Cancer* **48**, 1082–7.
54. **Hansen, M., Hammer, M., and Hammer, L.** (1980). ACTH, ADH and calcitonin concentrations as markers of response and relapse in small cell carcinoma of the lung. *Cancer* **46**, 2062–7.
55. **Boscaro, M.** et al. (2001). Cushing's syndrome. *Lancet* **357**, 783–91.
56. **de Herder, W.** et al. (1994). Somatostatin receptor scintigraphy: its value in tumor localization in patients with Cushing's syndrome caused by ectopic corticotropin or corticotropin-releasing hormone secretion. *American Journal of Medicine* **96**, 305–12.
57. **Jacobsson, H.** et al. (1994). Techetium-99 methoxyisobutylisonitrile localizes an ectopic ACTH-producing tumour: case report and review of the literature. *European Journal of Nuclear Medicine* **21**, 582–6.
58. **Carey, R.** et al. (1984). Ectopic secretion of corticotrophin-releasing factor as a cause of Cushing's syndrome: a clinical, morphologic and biochemical study. *New England Journal of Medicine* **311**, 13–20.
59. **Child, D.** et al. (1976). Drug control of Cushing's syndrome. Combined aminoglutethamide metyrapone therapy. *Acta Endocrinology* **82**, 330–41.
60. **Wajchenberg, B.** et al. (2000). Adrenocortical carcinoma. Clinical and laboratory observations. *Cancer* **88**, 711–36.
61. **Hoffman, D. and Boigham, B.** (1991). The use of ketoconazole in ectopic adrenocorticotropic hormone syndrome. *Cancer* **67**, 1447–9.
62. **Winquist, EW.** et al. (1995). Ketoconazole in the management of paraneoplastic Cushing's syndrome secondary to ectopic adrenal corticotropin production. *Journal of Clinical Oncology* **13**, 157–64.
63. **Farrell, W.** et al. (1992). Bromocriptine inhibits pro-opiomelanocortin mRNA and ACTH precursor secretion in small cell lung cancer cell lines. *Journal of Clinical Investigation* **90**, 705–10.
64. **Woodhouse, N.J.** et al. (1993). Acute and long-term effects of octreotide in patients with ACTH-dependent Cushing's syndrome. *American Journal of Medicine* **95**, 305–8.
65. **Rieu, M.** et al. (19931). Paradoxical effect of somatostatin analogues on the ectopic secretion of corticotropin in two cases of small cell lung carcinoma. *Hormone Research* **39**, 207–12.
66. **Spampinato, S.** et al. (1994). Inhibition of proopiomelanocortin expression by an oligonucleotide complementary to beta-endorphin mRNA. *Proceedings of the National Academy of Sciences of the United States of America* **91**, 8072–6.
67. **Verbalis, J.** (1989). Hyponatraemia. *Balliere's Clinical Endocrinology and Metabolism* **3**, 499–530.
68. **Smitz, S.** et al. (1988). Identification of vasopressin-like peptides in the plasma of a patient with the syndrome of inappropriate secretion of antidiuretic hormone and an oat cell carcinoma. *Acta Endocinology (Copenhagen)* **119**, 567–74.
69. **Hansen, M., Hammer, M., and Hummer, L.** (1980). Diagnostic and therapeutic implications of ectopic hormone production in small cell lung cancer. *Thorax* **35**, 101–6.
70. **Comis, R., Miller, M., and Ginsberg, S.** (1980). Abnormalities in water homeostasis in small cell anaplastic lung cancer. *Cancer* **45**, 2414–21.
71. **North, W.** et al. (1988). Neurophysins as tumour markers for small cell carcinoma of the lung. A cancer and leukemia group B evaluation. *Cancer* **62**, 1343–7.
72. **Friedmann, A., Memoli, V., and North, W.** (1993). Vasopressin and oxytocin production by non-neuroendocrine lung carcinomas: an apparent low incidence of gene expression. *Cancer Letter* **75**, 79–85.
73. **Friedmann, A.** et al. (1994). Products of vasopressin gene expression in small cell carcinoma of the lung. *British Journal of Cancer* **69**, 260–3.
74. **List, A.** et al. (1986). The syndrome of inappropriate secretion of antidiuretic hormone in small cell lung cancer. *Journal of Clinical Oncology* **4**, 1191–8.
75. **Cohen, M.** et al. (1978). Chemotherapy rather than demeclocycline for inappropriate secretion of antidiuretic hormone. *New England Journal of Medicine* **298**, 1423.
76. **Vanhees, S., Paridaens, R., and Vansteenkiste, J.** (2000). Syndrome of inappropriate antidiuretic hormone associated with chemotherapy-induced tumour lysis in small cell lung cancer: case report and review of the literature. *Annals of Oncology* **11**, 1061–5.
77. **Srensen, J.** et al. (1987). Syndrome of inappropriate antidiuresis in small cell lung cancer. Classification and effect of tumour regression. *Acta Medica Scandanavica* **222**, 155–61.
78. **Hojer, J.** (1994). Management of symptomatic hyponataemia: dependence on the duration of development. *Journal of Internal Medicine* **235**, 497–501.
79. **Cohen, I., Warren, S., and Skowsky, W.** (1984). Occult pulmonary malignancy in syndrome of inappropriate ADH secretion with normal ADH levels. *Chest* **86**, 929–31.
80. **Chitmans, F. and Meinders, A.** (1990). Management of severe hyponatremia: rapid or slow correction. *American Journal of Medicine* **88**, 161–6.
81. **Sterns, R.** (1990). The treatment of hyponatremia: first do no harm. *American Journal of Medicine* **88**, 557–60.
82. **Sterns, R.** (1987). Severe symptomatic hyponatremia: treatment and outcome. *Annals of Internal Medicine* **107**, 656–64.
83. **Ayus, J., Olivero, J., and Frommer, J.** (1982). Rapid correction of severe hyponatremia with intravenous hypertonic saline solution. *American Journal of Medicine* **72**, 43–8.
84. **Adrogue, H. and Madias, N.** (2000). Hyponatremia. *New England Journal of Medicine* **342**, 1581–9.
85. **Decaux, G.** et al. (1993). 5-year treatment of the chronic syndrome of inappropriate secretion of ADH with oral urea. *Nephron* **63**, 468–70.
86. **Fujisawa, G.** et al. (1993). Therapeutic efficacy of non-peptide ADH antagonist OPC-31260 in SIADH rats. *Kidney International* **44**, 19–23.
87. **Mayinger, B. and Hensen, J.** (1999). Nonpeptide vasopressin antagonists: a new group of hormone blockers entering the scene. *Experimental and Clinical Endocrinology and Diabetes* **107**, 157–65.
88. **Cogan, E.** et al. (1986). High levels of atrial natriuretic factor in SIADH. *Lancet* **ii**, 1258–9.
89. **Kamoi, K.** et al. (1987). Hyponatremia in small cell lung cancer. Mechanisms not involving inappropriate ADH secretion. *Cancer* **60**, 1089–93.
90. **Yoshinaga, K.** et al. (1994). Production of immunoreactive atrial natriuretic polypeptide in neuroendocrine tumors. *Cancer* **73**, 1292–6.
91. **Levin, E., Gardner, D., and Samson, W.** (1998). Natriuretic peptides. *New England Journal of Medicine* **339**, 321–8.
92. **Morishita, Y.** et al. (1992). HS-142-1, a novel nonpeptide atrial natriuretic peptide (ANP) antagonist, blocks ANP-induced renal responses through a specific interaction with guanylyl cyclase-linked receptors. *European Journal of Pharmacology* **225**, 203–7.
93. **Kiang, D., Baner, G., and Kennedy, B.** (1973). Immunoassayable insulin in carcinoma of the cervix. *Cancer* **31**, 801–5.
94. **Gorden, P.** et al. (1981). Hypoglycaemia associated with non-islet cell tumor and insulin-like growth factors. *New England Journal of Medicine* **305**, 1452–5.
95. **Marks, V. and Teale, J.** (1998). Tumours producing hypoglycaemia. *Endocrine-Related Cancer* **5**, 111–29.
96. **Yu, H. and Rohan, T.** (2000). Role of the insulin-like growth factor family in cancer development and progression. *Journal of the National Cancer Institute* **92**, 1472–89.
97. **Braund, W.** et al. (1987). Autoimmunity to insulin receptor and hypoglycaemia in patients with Hodgkin's disease. *Lancet* **i**, 237–40.
98. **Walters, E.** et al. (1987). Hypoglycaemia due to an insulin-receptor antibody in Hodgkin's disease. *Lancet* **i**, 241–3.
99. **Kulke, M. and Mayer, R.** (1999). Carcionid tumours. *New England Journal of Medicine* **340**, 858–68.
100. **Lamberts, S.** et al. (1990). Parallel in vivo and in vitro detection of functional somatostatin receptors in human endocrine pancreatic tumours: consequences with regard to diagnosis, localization and therapy. *Journal of Clinical Investigation* **71**, 566–74.
101. **Feldman, J.** (1987). Carcinoid tumours and syndrome. *Seminars in Oncology* **14**, 237–46.
102. **Modlin, I. and Sandor, A.** (1997). An analysis of 8305 cases of carcinoid tumors. *Cancer* **79**, 813–29.

103. **Vinik, A.** et al. (1989). Clinical features, diagnosis and localization of carcinoid tumours and their management. *Gastroenterology Clinics of North America* **18**, 865–96.

104. **Kema, I.** et al. (1992). Influence of a serotonin and dopamine rich diet on platelet serotonin content and urinary excretion of biogenic amines and their metabolites. *Clinical Chemistry* **38**, 1730–6.

105. **Jensen, R.** (2000). Carcinoid and pancreatic endocrine tumors: recent advances in molecular pathogenesis, localization and treatment. *Current Opinion in Oncology* **12**, 368–77.

106. **Kvols, L. and Reub, J.** (1993). Metastatic carcinoid tumours and the malignant carcinoid syndrome. *Acta Oncologica* **32**, 197–201.

107. **Di Bartolomeo, M.** et al. (1996). Clinical efficacy of octreotide in the treatment of metastatic neuroendocrine tumors: a study by the Italian Trials in Medical Oncology Group. *Cancer* **77**, 402–8.

108. **Ruszniewski, P.** et al. (1996). Treatment of the carcinoid syndrome with the long-acting somatostatin analogue lanreotide: a prospective study in 39 patients. *Gut* **39**, 279–83.

109. **Rubin, J.** et al. (1999). Octreotide acetate long-acting formulation versus open label subcutaneous octreotide acetate in malignant carcinoid syndrome. *Journal of Clinical Oncology* **17**, 600–6.

110. **Moertel, C.** et al. (1993). Hepatic arterial occlusion alone and sequenced with chemotherapy in the management of patients with advanced carcinoid tumors and islet cell carcinomas. *Annals of Internal Medicine* **120**, 302–9.

111. **Taal, B.** et al. (1996). Palliative effect of metaiodobenzylguanidine in metastatic carcinoid tumors. *Journal of Clinical Oncology* **14**, 1829–38.

112. **Shapiro, B.** (1993). Uses of MIBG in catecholamine-secreting tumours. *Balliere's Clinical Endocrinology and Metabolism* **7**, 500–7.

113. **Wilson, J.** (1991). Gynaecomastia-a continuing dilemma. *New England Journal of Medicine* **324**, 334–5.

114. **Braunstein, G.** (1993). Current concepts: gynaecomastia. *New England Journal of Medicine* **328**, 490–5.

115. **Fradkin, J.** et al. (1989). Specificity spillover at the hormone receptor — exploring its role in human disease. *New England Journal of Medicine* **320**, 640–5.

116. **Giralt, S.** et al. (1992). Hyperthyroidism in men with germ cell tumors and high levels of beta-human chorionic gonadotrophin. *Cancer* **69**, 1286–90.

117. **Dowsett, M.** et al. (1983). Prognostic significance of serum prolactin levels in advanced breast cancer. *British Journal of Cancer* **47**, 763–9.

118. **Petersdorf, R.** (1965). Fever and cancer. *Hospital Medicine* **1**, 2–10.

119. **Knockaert, D.** et al. (1992). Fever of unknown origin in the 1980s. *Archives of Internal Medicine* **152**, 51–5.

120. **Saper, C. and Breder, C.D.** (1994). Seminars in Medicine of the Beth Israel Hospital, Boston: the neurologic basis of fever. *New England Journal of Medicine* **330**, 1880–6.

121. **Netea, M., Kullberg, B., and Van der Meer, J.** (2000). Circulating cytokines as mediators of fever. *Clinical Infectious Diseases* **31**, S178–84.

122. **Blatteis, C., Sehic, E., and Li, S.** (2000). Pyrogens sensing and signaling: old views and new concepts. *Clinical Infectious Diseases* **31**, S168–77.

123. **Kretschmer, C.** et al. (1990). Tumor necrosis factor alpha and lympho-toxin production in Hodgkin's disease. *American Journal of Pathology* **137**, 341–51.

124. **Nishimoto, N.** et al. (2000). Improvement in Castleman's disease by humanized anti-interleukin-6 receptor antibody therapy. *Blood* **95**, 56–61.

125. **Fukumoto, S.** et al. (1991). Phaeochromocytoma with pyrexia and marked inflammatory signs: a paraneoplastic syndrome with possible relation to interleukin 6 production. *Journal of Clinical Endocrinology and Metabolism* **73**, 871–81.

126. **Dosquet, C.** et al. (1994). Tumour necrosis factor α, interleukin 1b and interleukin 6 in patients with renal cell carcinoma. *European Journal of Cancer* **30**, 1589–97.

127. **Styrt, B. and Sugarman, B.** (1990). Antipyresis and fever. *Archives of Internal Medicine* **150**, 1589–97.

128. **Alcami, A. and Smith, G.** (1992). A soluble receptor for interleukin-1β encoded by vaccinia virus: a novel mechanism of virus modulation of the host response to infection. *Cell* **71**, 153–67.

129. **Eisenberg, S.** et al. (1991). Interleukin 1 receptor antagonist is a member of the interleukin 1 gene family: evolution of a cytokine control mechanism. *Proceedings of the National Academy of Sciences of the United States of America* **88**, 5232–6.

130. **Coceani, F.** et al. (1992). Interleukin-1 receptor antagonist: effectiveness against interleukin-1 fever. *Canadian Journal of Physiology and Pharmacology* **70**, 1590–6.

131. **Gullo, L.** et al. (1994). Diabetes and the risk of pancreatic cancer. *New England Journal of Medicine* **331**, 81–4.

132. **Nelson, K., Walsh, D., and Sheehan, F.** (1994). The cancer anorexia-cachexia syndrome. *Journal of Clinical Oncology* **12**, 213–25.

133. **Garrick, M. and Mayer, R.** (1978). Acute renal failure associated with neoplastic disease and its treatment. *Seminars in Oncology* **5**, 155–65.

134. **Cronin, R.** et al. (1976). Renal cell carcinoma: unusual systemic manifestations. *Medicine* **55**, 291–311.

135. **Doolittle, G.** et al. (1988). Malignancy-associated lactic acidosis. *Southern Medical Journal* **81**, 533–6.

8.14 Neurological problems in advanced cancer

Augusto Caraceni, Cinzia Martini, and Fabio Simonetti

Introduction

Neurological complications in advanced cancer are frequent, therefore an adequate neurological assessment must always be part of patient evaluation in palliative medicine.

Pain, a frequent occurrence in AIDS and cancer, is a traditional focus of palliative medicine. It always requires neurological evaluation to clarify the pathophysiology and cause. Correct diagnosis of the pain syndrome is necessary in order to achieve successful treatment and anticipate complications.

Among the major general neurological syndromes and symptoms, intracranial hypertension, seizures, and delirium are described first in some detail because of their impact in terms of symptomatic management and because they occur frequently in advanced cancer. Special complications of advanced malignancies are also reviewed in the following section of the chapter to guide neurological assessment of these patients.

Intracranial hypertension

General aspects

Intracranial pressure (ICP) is not constant but depends on systemic blood pressure, venous pressure, and intrathoracic pressure. In adults, the values of ICP range from 5 to 15 mmHg, from 2.4 to 4.2 mmHg in neonates, and from 10 to 15 mmHg in children. Patients with intracranial space-occupying lesions tolerate pressure values around 15–22 mmHg. When ICP reaches 30 mmHg, electrical brain activity decreases and signs of hypoperfusion occur. An ICP of 60 mmHg usually causes death. Exceptions to these general rules are benign intracranial hypertension and communicating hydrocephalus. In both cases, high pressure values are not associated with displacement of brain structures and are therefore relatively better tolerated.

Intracranial content is made of: brain 80 per cent (= in adults 1400 g), blood 10 per cent (32–58 ml), and cerebrospinal fluid (CSF) 10 per cent. Total CSF quantity amounts to 140 ml (23 ml in the cerebral ventricles, 37 ml in the sub-arachnoidal intracranial space, and 80 ml in the spine). In children, CSF quantity varies from 65 to 140 ml. CSF is actively reabsorbed and produced at a rate of about 0.35 ml/min, which accounts for a 4-times-a-day turn over.

Intracranial masses increase the intracranial content. If this occurs by a slow progressive process brain distortion and herniation can occur at least temporarily without an increase in ICP due to compensation mechanisms, such as enhanced CSF reabsorption and increased drainage through the lymphatic and circulatory system. When these mechanisms are insufficient or if the process is particularly acute, ICP rises rapidly and may cause death without causing brain distortion or herniation.

Clinical findings

The clinical picture of ICP is characterized by an altered state of consciousness, headache, nausea and vomiting, papilloedema and, at times, focal signs. An altered state of consciousness is the most frequent sign, starting with psychomotor retardation, slowing of verbal and motor responses, and progressing to stupor and coma. Headache is severe, diffuse, more intense in the supine position, and in the morning immediately after awakening. It can also wake the patient from sleep, is worsened by head movements, cough, and the Valsalva manoeuvre.

Nausea and vomiting are frequent. Vomiting may be projectile especially in children with posterior fossa lesions. Papilloedema is a specific sign of ICP but it can often be absent especially in the elderly. Among focal signs the most frequent are due to paralysis of the abducent nerve (which, due to its long intracranial course, is particularly sensitive to traction) sensory-motor signs in general and seizures. The 'sunset' sign (Collier's sign) may be seen in children: eyelid retraction and eyes rotated downward due to compression of the pretectal region. Also in children, it is important to emphasize that non-specific findings are not uncommon. ICP may manifest as irritability, labile mood, negativism, or aggressive or hostile behaviours. Two specific situations can be found in ICP that have particular clinical implications, acute pressure symptoms that can precede severe deterioration and cerebral herniation that is an already decompensating process.

Acute pressure symptoms

Acute pressure symptoms (Table 1) are due to the spontaneous sudden increase of ICP occurring for seconds to minutes caused by three types of ICP waves described in 1960 by Lundberg[1,2] (Table 2). Clinical changes occur only with the A waves, but these wave forms are relevant to explain the transition from a compensating to an unstable condition. A and B waves are both responsible of this process.

Table 1 Signs and symptoms of ICP waves

Altered state of consciousness, agitation, delirium
Headache, neck-pain
Focal or generalized seizures
Cerebellar fits (opistotonus)
Decerebration (hypertonus, extension, and intrarotation of four limbs)
Amaurosis, midriasis
II, IV, VI nerve paralysis, conjugated eye deviation
Nystagmus, tinnitus
Myoclonus of face and limb muscles
Dysarthria, dysphagia
Pyramidal signs, paresthesias
Cardiovascular or respiratory disturbances, yawning
Hyperthermia, face cyanosis, flushing, pallor, sweating
Nausea, vomiting, hiccup, sialorrhoea, diarrhoea, incontinence

Herniation

Cerebral herniation is the displacing of the brain or part of it within the cranial box structures. This phenomenon is usually described by topographic and anatomical criteria as central, sub-falcial, uncal, and cerebellar tonsil herniation. We describe the most frequent occurrences.[3]

Central herniation syndrome

Clinical findings are characterized by a progressive compression of the cerebral structure of the diencephalon and brainstem due to the pressure cone originating in the upper brain structure forcing in an up-down direction the intracranial content. In the diencephalic stage of compression, the conscious level starts to deteriorate, Cheyne–Stokes respiration is apparent, pupils are miotic and react to light, eye-doll phenomenon is present. Pyramidal signs are present, paratonic rigidity (opposition to forced extension of limbs, also called gegenhalten), painful stimuli induce decorticate rigidity (upper arm flexion and lower limb extension) initially contralaterally to the lesion then bilaterally. When mesencephalic and pontine damage occur, coma is complete, respiratory rhythm is deranged, pupils are fixed in intermediate position, oculovestibular manoeuvres are abnormal and decerebral rigidity occurs. The terminal stage is characterized by signs of pons and medullary compromise with a profound state of coma, ataxic breathing, fixed pupils, and absence of eye-doll phenomenon. Flaccidity and response to pain stimuli may be present with upper limb flexion but inconsistent and there is flaccidity of the lower limbs.

Uncal herniation

Uncal herniation is the displacement of the temporal lobe or part of it underneath the cerebellar tentorium. Neurological signs are first due to compression of the structures homo-lateral to the lesion against the free edge of the tentorium cerebelli. Initially, the homo-lateral pupil is affected due to compression or traction of the homo-lateral III cranial nerve, the pupil is midriatic not reacting or slowly reacting to light but, more rarely, the compression may occur on the opposite side, and the contra-lateral III nerve may be affected. At times an oval pupil homo- or, more rarely, contra-lateral to the lesion can be a sign of impending herniation. Visual field defects can be caused by compression of the homo-lateral posterior cerebral artery. Subsequently consciousness deteriorates, hyperventilation is followed by Cheyne–Stokes breathing, complete paralysis of the homolateral III cranial nerve, eye-doll response is abnormal, painful stimulation evokes decortical response homo-laterally to the lesion and decerebral response contra-laterally.

Cerebellar herniation

This is due to the descent of cerebellar structures through the occipital foramen. The syndrome can be preceded by occipital or frontal headache, vomiting, hiccup, followed by an altered state of consciousness, abnormality of breathing, and sometimes 'cerebellar fits' characterized by opistotonus and episodes of decerebration.

Table 2 Three types of ICP waves

A waves—recurrent plateau waves, reaching 50–100 mmHg, duration 5–20 s, associated with deterioration in clinical signs. Onset of new signs and symptoms are indicative of a reduced compensating capacity of ICP
B waves—of shorter duration, rhythmical, 0.5–2 per min, of variable amplitude, lower than 50 mmHg. They are related to respiratory movements and are also indicative of reduced compliance
C waves—small oscillations, rhythmical at about 6 per min, with amplitude of only 20 mmHg, and related to intracranial transmission of the arterial pulse

Brain oedema and treatment of increased ICP

Brain oedema

In both primary and secondary brain tumours, oedema is the cause of increased ICP. The underlying pathogenic mechanism is the loss of osmotically active substances such as albumin from the circulatory system into the brain interstitial tissue caused by dysfunction of the blood–brain barrier within the tumour and in the surrounding tissue.

The classic classification of Klatzo[4] recognizes:

Vasogenic oedema: an increase of the extra-cellular space caused by increased capillary permeability. Any lesion affecting the blood–brain barrier can cause this type of oedema.

Cytotoxic oedema: an increase of intracellular volume, caused by ischaemic or hypoxic cellular damage. Cellular dysfunction of the ion pump system produces intracellular accumulation of sodium followed by extracellular fluid entrance. It is now referred to as cellular swelling.

Interstitial oedema: an increase of the extracellular space due to blockade of CSF re-absorption at any level.

Osmotic oedema: an increase of the water content of the brain parenchyma caused by plasma hypo-osmolarity, occurring in water intoxication or in SIADH.

The last two conditions are rare and do not apply to tumour-induced brain oedema which is mainly sustained, at least initially, by vasogenic mechanisms.

Treatment of increased ICP

Conservative management of cerebral oedema has two main goals: maintenance of cerebral perfusion and reduction of vasogenic oedema.[5,6]

Cerebral perfusion pressure (CPP) CPP depends on arterial pressure and ICP. CPP = (mean arterial pressure) − (mean ICP). Mean ICP is about equal to the mean venous cerebral pressure. If CPP decreases, the increase of ICP can rapidly cause cerebral damage. The risk of maintaining a high CPP is to worsen vasogenic oedema. Present guidelines suggest therefore maintaining CPP at about 50 mmHg in adults and 40 mmHg in children. While it is unlikely that monitoring CPP is feasible or desirable in most palliative care situations, the theoretical implications and clinical consequences of the underlying pathophysiological mechanisms, are relevant.

Reduction of vasogenic oedema

Positioning: A neutral head position should be adopted with the head at least 30° above the heart to facilitate venous drainage.

Hyperventilation: By reducing P_{CO_2} and causing vasoconstriction, intracranial blood flow is reduced.[7] Often patients hyperventilate spontaneously, but in emergencies if the patient can cooperate, he or she can be asked to hyperventilate for a few minutes. Assisted ventilation is employed in intensive care and P_{CO_2} should be kept at 20–25 mmHg. These interventions will be seldom necessary or feasible in palliative care.

Infusion of hypertonic solutions: Rapid reduction of ICP and cerebral oedema with hypertonic solutions has been utilized since 1925[8] despite the fact that the mechanism of action is not yet completely understood. Hyperosmolar solutions include magnesium sulphate (obsolete), urea (obsolete), glycerol,[9] sorbitol, hypertonic NaCl solutions, and mannitol.

Mannitol: Mannitol is the most commonly used agent.[10,11] Its activity is based on creating an osmolar gradient between blood and brain extracting water from the cerebral compartment. There are a number of other actions associated with the therapeutic effect of mannitol which include a diuretic effect, an increase in red cell deformability and a rapid reduction of the diameter of arterioles and small veins of the brain surface.

Routes and schedules of mannitol administration: After oral administration only a small fraction of mannitol is absorbed. After IV infusion the aim is to achieve concentrations higher than 5 mmol/l, which is osmotically active and persists for 4–6 h.

Mannitol is not metabolized and is excreted by the kidneys. With moderate reduction of glomerular filtration it accumulates in the central compartment. Usually more water than sodium is eliminated with mannitol, resulting in hypovolemia and hyponatremia. There is no interaction between mannitol and glucose metabolism.

Mannitol 18 or 20 per cent solutions are used and the suggested dose regimens are 0.25–1 g/kg in 15–30 min every 6 (0.25 g/kg) or 12 (1 g/kg) h (both in adults and children). The regimen can vary according to the severity of symptoms. If symptoms are severe and for a rapid onset of action 1 g/kg can be given in 30 min For a less urgent intervention and to have a more long-lasting effect, 0.5–1 g/kg can be given in 60 min.

Daily doses vary from 1 to 4 g/kg and should never be higher than 150–200 g/day. Renal disease, and congestive heart failure contraindicate the use of mannitol. Intracerebral haemorrhage is also a contraindication. However, if there is severe associated intracranial hypertension, with cerebral herniation and brain stem compression the patient should be considered for surgical decompression. Mannitol therapy should never extend for more than 3–4 days. Salt and water balance should be carefully monitored to avoid dehydration and hypotension. Hyper-osmolality should also be prevented by cessation of therapy at values of 320 mosmol/kg.

Mannitol rebound effect: Longer-term therapies are at risk of a rebound effect that is in part a consequence of the osmotic agents entering the intracranial compartment with inversion of the osmotic gradient between blood, extracellular fluid, and brain. It may also result in increased intracranial pressure.[10]

Conclusions: Mannitol is an important drug in the treatment of intracranial hypertension but needs careful handling to achieve maximum benefit and least inconvenience. The decision to treat the patient with hypertonic solutions has to be based on an accurate diagnosis of intra-cranial hypertension. The radiological finding of 'oedema' in patients without specific symptoms is not a sufficient basis for osmotic therapy.

Corticosteroids

After the early observation by Galicich and French of the anti-peritumoral oedema effect of dexamethasone,[12] corticosteroids have gained wide application in neuro-oncology.[13] Dexamethasone does not reduce the water content of the swelling brain tissue (as mannitol does). Indeed a reduction of ICP does not occur before 48–72 h, while it is common to observe a clinical improvement within the first 24 h. The mechanism of action is fundamentally based on the ability of this drug to block the outflow of haematic components from the capillary bed into the brain tissue at the site of blood–brain barrier damage.

Doses and administration schedules of corticosteroids have never been established by specific guidelines. It is therefore worthwhile considering the relative potency of the different drugs and their pharmacokinetics and pharmacodynamics[14] (Table 3). Biological half-life and not plasma half-life should guide dosing schedules.

Dexamethasone is found in higher concentrations within the CSF compared with prednisolone because it is less bound to plasma proteins. This should be taken into account when switching from one to another steroid in addition to the potency data shown in Table 3. The dose of dexamethasone used in metastatic or primary brain tumours varies according to the

Table 3 Relative potency of different drugs

	Equipotency based on anti-inflammatory activity	Biological half-life (h)	Plasma half-life (h)
Hydrocortisone	1	8–12	
Prednisone	4	12–36	3–4
Methylprednisolone	5	12–36	1.5–3
Dexamethasone	25	36–54	2–5
Bethamethasone	30	36–54	5–7

Sodium retention activity is 1 for hydrocortisone, 0.5 for prednisone and methylprednisolone, and 0 for bethamethasone and dexamethasone.

Table 4 Side-effects of corticosteroids

Infections (especially relevant if associated with chemotherapy): reactivation of TB, candida, pneumocystis pneumonia
Metabolic disturbances: hyperglycaemia, electrolyte imbalances, fluid retention, hyperlipidaemia
Dystrophic reaction: delay in wound healing, purpura, dermal atrophy, acne
Myopathy:[20] weakness affects mainly the pelvic girdle muscles, but also head flexor and shoulder muscles are affected. Muscle enzymes and EMG are normal. On the contrary, cretinuria is elevated. Myopathy occurs as early as 2 weeks of starting dexamethasone, manifesting with difficulties in climbing stairs and standing from a sitting position. Some authors suggest that substitution with non-fluorinated steroids (methylprednisolone or prednisone) is effective in reducing myopathic effects
Bone: Osteoporosis probably due to the reduced intestinal absorption of calcium and reduced tubular reuptake with increased calciuria. These mechanisms cause hypocalcaemia which reflects on parathyroid activation and subsequent increased bone re-absorption. Phenobarbital causes osteopathy so it is preferable to use different anticonvulsants in combined therapies Aseptic bone necrosis (usually of the femoral head). Two hypotheses have been proposed to explain this complication. Fat embolism due to altered lipid metabolism and osteomedullary ischaemia. Bone necrosis has been seen after relatively short-term treatment with dexamethasone (cumulative doses of 220 mg)[21]
GI side-effects: Peptic ulcer disease: the use of steroids alone in patients in good general condition is not associated with damage to the GI tract. There are, however, specific risk factors that are associated with peptic ulceration and bleeding, such as, very high doses, systemic neoplasm, previous peptic ulcer, and combined use of NSAIDs.[22] It is also well known that patients with intracranial lesions are at risk of GI bleeding.[23] Prophylaxis with proton pump inhibitors is therefore suggested in patients at increased risk Hiccup: chronic hiccup has been observed in association with the use of dexamethasone or high-dose methylprednisolone. The physiopathology of this effect is unknown[24,25]
Psychiatric effects:[26] Euphoria with mild insomnia Hyperalert reaction: anxiety can be associated with confusion Steroid psychosis: can have hypomanic, depressive, and psychotic features with high inter- and intraindividual variability. This reaction is usually seen within 2 weeks of therapy at doses above 40 mg of prednisone per day. The steroid dose should be tapered and symptoms usually subside spontaneously in about 3 weeks
Anaphylaxis: has been observed after IV methylprednisolone[27]
Ocular toxicity: glaucoma,[28] cataract[29]
Perineal burning sensation[30]
Endocrine effects: adrenal suppression is seen after ten days of therapy with doses in excess of 7.5 mg prednisone per day. It is therefore useful to follow some practical suggestions to minimize this effect:[31] Morning administration matches the physiological zenith of ACTH secretion while evening administration favours the inhibition of ACTH secretion Single administration should be preferred and when possible on alternate days Before withholding therapy it would be important to check adrenal function (assessment of morning cortisol levels and response to ACTH stimulation)
Steroid withdrawal syndrome: this syndrome can occur with sudden discontinuation of therapy and includes, pseudo-rheumatism, headache, lethargy, nausea, vomiting, post-ural hypotension, papilloedema[32]
Epidural lipomatosis: this complication can cause slowly developing spinal cord compression[33]
Pseudo-tumour cerebri: papilloedema and headache can occur without focal neurological signs and normal CSF. It has been described in patients with Addison's disease and after steroid withdrawal and it has also been reported after chronic steroid use[34,35]

clinical findings and degree of oedema from 4 mg every 6 h to 96 mg/day in patients with more severe symptoms. Once or twice daily administration is consistent with the drug's pharmacokinetic profile. At least one study shows that also once daily administration is enough to control neurological symptoms due to brain metastases.[15]

In children, the suggested initial dose of dexamethasone is 1 mg/kg followed by doses of 0.4–1 mg/kg 6-hourly. Clinical experience suggests that in case of need higher doses can be administered safely.

In some centres, immuno-competent patients with brain tumours being treated with long-term steroids receive prophylactic therapy for *Pneumocystis carinii* pneumonia (one double strength tablet of trimethoprim–sulphamethoxazole on three consecutive days each week).[16–18]

It is common for steroids to be continued indefinitely for no good reason.[19] Continuation of steroid therapy of any type must always be under constant review and should be tapered and discontinued when clinical benefit is exceeded by side-effects. Steroid side-effects are significant and some of them may add to the disability of patients in palliative care (e.g. weakness due to myopathy). Table 4 lists the side effects of corticosteroids, not all of which are relevant to short term management of symptoms in palliative care. But many can seriously impact on the quality of life of patients and require careful balancing with therapeutic effects.

Epilepsy in patients with brain tumours

Seizures are not infrequently encountered in palliative medicine. They may be caused by metastatic cerebral lesions in advanced cancer, by AIDS, or as a consequence of metabolic derangement or of drug toxicity. While non-structural causes of seizures are quite common,[36,37] they occur in 25 per cent of patients with brain metastases.[38]

Seizure definition and classification

Epileptic seizures are classified according to their electroencephalographic (EEt) features as partial seizures when an initiating focus can be identified in a specific brain area and generalized seizures when the seizure seems to have bilateral onset. Focal seizures can evolve into generalized tonic–clonic seizures, and in this case the term secondary generalized seizures is used.[35] Depending on the level of consciousness during attacks, seizures can be classified as follows:

- *Simple partial seizures,* which are associated with a normal level of consciousness. Only a selective area of the cortex participates in the seizure activity causing symptoms that depend on the function of that part of the cortex. Therefore, partial motor, sensory, autonomic, and affective seizures are possible. At times when symptoms of this kind precede the onset of a generalized seizure they are called an 'aura'.

- *Complex seizures* are associated with impaired consciousness. The main clinical presentations of complex seizures include, absence seizures, partial complex seizures, and generalized tonic–clonic seizures.
  - *Absence (petit mal) seizures* are typical of infancy, can last for 5–10 s and can occur ten to hundreds of times a day. The patient stops whatever they are doing, with fixed unresponsive eyes. If the seizure lasts for more than 10 s he or she can blink or smack lips repetitively. Atypical absences can be of longer duration and can be associated with flaccidity or muscle rigidity. They usually begin after age of five.
  - *Partial complex seizures* combine focal symptoms with an altered state of consciousness. These are the most common type of seizures seen in adults and probably the most common also in palliative care. The patient seems awake but no contact with the environment is possible. He/she does not answer questions appropriately, eyes can be fixed, or rolling purposelessly around, the patient is immobile or engaged in repetitive behaviours (motor automatisms), repeats words or sentences, grimacing, snapping fingers, chewing, running, or undressing. If physically restrained, he/she can become hostile or aggressive. These attacks can be preceded by auras that are equivalent to simple partial seizures. The seizure lasts on average 3 min and is followed by a post-ictal phase. Post-ictal symptoms include somnolence, delirium, and headache and can last for several hours. After complete recovery, the patient has no recall of the event, but sometimes may remember the aura.
  - *Generalized tonic–clonic (grand mal) seizures* start with a sudden loss of consciousness, at times accompanied by shouting (due to forced air expiration by sudden contraction of the diaphragm). Diffuse muscle rigidity follows and cyanosis, after 1-min myoclonus and muscle fasciculations occur for 1–2 min In this phase, the patient can bite his or her tongue. At the end, the post-ictal phase presents with deep sleep, slow deep breathing, and the patient gradually awakens often complaining of headache.

Absence and tonic–clonic seizures are the most typical clinical presentation of generalized seizures which include also *clonic seizures*; with rhythmic contractions of upper limb, neck, and face muscles; *myoclonic seizures* with brief segmental contractions of the limbs, occurring alone or in clusters without loss of consciousness; *tonic seizures* with sudden generalized muscle rigidity associated with loss of consciousness and falls; and *atonic seizures* with sudden loss of muscle tone.

Treatment[35,39]

Prophylactic anticonvulsant treatment in patients with brain tumours or metastases is controversial and in fact very few studies have addressed the efficacy of prophylactic anticonvulsant therapy in patients with brain tumours. In non-controlled clinical series prophylactic treatment has not been shown to give any advantage.[40,41] One randomized clinical trial confirmed that in patients with brain metastases who had never had seizures prophylactic treatment did not prevent seizure development.[42] In patients with primary brain tumours without seizures, it is suggested that anticonvulsant therapy be withdrawn 1 week after surgery.[43] Metastases from melanoma,[44] choriocarcinoma, and cancer of the testis are more often associated with seizures, possibly because these lesions are often haemorrhagic and, in the case of melanoma, tend to invade the grey matter. All anticonvulsants have potentially serious side-effects and many interact with chemotherapeutic drugs and steroids. They are also sedative and produce cognitive impairment.[38,45–47] Prophylaxis is therefore only recommended in patients who have already had a seizure or in patients with melanomas.[38] Seizures worsen brain oedema;[48] therefore, in patients who develop new seizures in spite of anticonvulsant therapy it is advisable to optimize antioedema therapies before modifying anticonvulsant regimen.

Pharmacological therapy

The general characteristics of anticonvulsants are summarized in Table 5 together with the recommended range of plasma concentrations if available. Blood levels of some anticonvulsants must be monitored because of the unpredictability of metabolic changes and drug interactions, although it must be remembered that clinical response and not blood levels should guide dosage.

Phenytoin is the first line drug in simple and complex partial seizures and in generalized tonic–clonic seizures. It is widely used in neuro-oncology. Dosing can vary from 4 to 8 mg/kg/day in two to three daily administrations preferably after eating.

Phenytoin has some drawbacks. Blood levels of phenytoin are quite variable as a consequence of the administration of many other drugs interfering with liver metabolism, absorption, or protein binding. Interactions have been demonstrated with cyclosporin, cisplatinum, and paclitaxel. Significant pharmacokinetic interaction is found with concurrent dexamethasone which can reduce phenytoin plasma levels by 50 per cent. Advantages of phenytoin are the lack of sedative effects, and good tolerability at higher than recommended doses.

Side-effects due to chronic use are ataxia, GI disturbances, gingival hypertrophy, hirsutism, osteoporosis, and megaloblastic anaemia. Severe allergic reactions involving rash, hypersensitivity reactions, liver toxicity, and myelo-suppression have been reported, but are rare.

Phenobarbitone is available in oral and parenteral formulations. It is effective in both partial and generalized tonic–clonic seizures. It is metabolized by liver cytochrome P450, and has very slow plasma clearance (4–5 days), that can be affected by liver disease. It is a safe drug with a wide therapeutic index but it can cause drowsiness, ataxia, and severe rash (Stevens–Johnson syndrome and toxic epidermal necrolysis (Lyell syndrome)). It interferes with the metabolism of several chemotherapy agents and in chronic use is associated with pseudo-rheumatism which can worsen the symptoms of a concurrent steroid-induced osteoporosis.

Sodium valproate is active in most types of generalized seizure (tonic, myoclonic, absence, tonic–clonic) including secondary generalized partial seizures. Doses start at 250–500 mg/day and are increased by 250 mg/week up to 1000–3000 mg/day. In children, the initial dose is 10–15 mg/kg/day, increased by the same incremental doses. Common side-effects are tremors, sedation, ataxia, GI symptoms, and thrombocytopenia. Liver enzymes and blood ammonia can be increased. Severe liver toxicity can occur (usually in the first 6 months of therapy) most cases occurring in children and in association with other anticonvulsants.

Carbamazepine is only available in oral formulations. It is effective in the treatment of simple and complex partial seizures, and in tonic–clonic

Table 5 Main therapeutic dosing schedules of anticonvulsants

Drug	Therapeutic daily dose	Schedule	Plasma levels
Phenytoin	4–8 mg/kg	q8h–q12h	10–20 µg/ml
Phenobarbital	1–5 mg/kg	qhs	15–40 mg/ml
Sodium valproate	1000–3000 mg; 30–60 mg/kg[a]	q12h	50–100 mg/ml
Carbamazepine	400–1200 mg; 20 mg/kg[a]	q8h–q12h	4–12 mg/ml
Oxcarbazepine	400–1800 mg	q8h–q12h	—
Clonazepam	1–3 mg	q8h	—
Gabapentin	1200–1800 mg	q8h	—
Topiramate	200–400 mg; 5–9 mg/kg[a]	q12h	—
Lamotrigine	200–500 mg	q12h	—

[a] Paediatric dose.

generalized seizures. Doses should start low at 200 mg/day, increasing by 200 mg per week (Table 5). Acute intoxication can cause stupor and coma, convulsions, and respiratory depression. After chronic administration, sedation, vertigo, ataxia, diplopia, and myelo-suppression can occur. Severe myelotoxicity is found (one case of aplastic anaemia per 200 000 patients).

Oxcarbazepine is chemically related to carbamazepine, but with less pharmacological interaction liability because of lower liver enzyme inducing potential. Its mechanism of action seems also linked to sodium channel modulation. It is approved for partial seizures in adults both as mono- and add-on therapy. Side-effects are similar to carbamazepine but it is usually better tolerated. Initial dose ranges from 300–600 mg in two to three daily administration and is usually titrated up to 600–1800 mg/day.

Clonazepam is approved by the FDA for the prophylaxis of absence, atypical absence and myoclonic epilepsy. It can also be used as a temporary treatment to control and prevent seizures not controlled by ongoing therapy. In children initial doses start with 0.01–0.03 mg/kg/day and are increased by 0.25–0.5 mg every 3 days. The most relevant side-effect is sedation. Paradoxical excitation is rare.

Gabapentin is approved for supplemental therapy of partial seizures with or without secondary generalization.[49] Its use is facilitated by the lack of binding to plasma protein and of pharmacological metabolic interferences. Elimination is renal and influenced only by renal function. Usual daily doses are given in Table 5 but doses 2–3 times higher than recommended in children and as high as 3600–6000 mg/day in adults have been used without severe side-effects. Gabapentin is also considered effective as a single agent in epilepsy but its use in neuro-oncology has never been studied. Side-effects include ataxia, weight gain, and dizziness.

Topiramate is indicated in partial and generalized seizures in children and adults. Initial dose should be low (25 mg) and increased by 25–50 mg/week. Minimal full daily doses range from 200 to 400 mg. In children the initial dose is 0.5–1 mg/kg/day, increased weekly by the same amount up to 5–9 mg/kg. Main side-effects are of the central type, sedation, unsteadiness, memory, and concentration problems.

Lamotrigine is available as an oral preparation. Its use has been approved for partial seizures in adults in association with other drugs. It is effective also as monotherapy and also for the treatment of absence seizures. It is metabolized by the liver and has significant interactions with all the classic anticonvulsants (phenobarbitone, phenytoin, carbamazepine). Cases of severe rashes including Stevens–Johnson syndrome have been observed and are related to a rapid titration of the drug dose. With slow initiation of therapy, the risk of skin rash is comparable with that seen with phenytoin. The risk is increased in patients younger than 16 years of age, with rapid dose escalation and in association with sodium valproate. It is therefore important to titrate the dose slowly with weekly increments of 25 or 50 mg up to 300–500 mg/day. In patients who are already taking liver enzyme-inducing antiepileptic drugs (with the exception of sodium valproate) the starting dose should be 50 mg/day for 2 weeks, then increased by 100 mg/day (in two divided doses) to a maintenance dose of 300–500 mg/day. If added to a sodium valproate containing regimen, lamotrigine should be started at 25 mg every other day for 2 weeks and titrated even more carefully.

Conclusions

Prophylactic therapy of seizures in patients with brain metastases should not be undertaken if the patient has never had seizures, except in patients with melanoma. The ideal drug for palliative care is not easy to establish as the classic anticonvulsants cause a variety of metabolic interactions and significant side-effects. Among the newer drugs there is little experience in this indication. The need for slow titration schedules limits the usefulness of topiramate and lamotrigine, and lamotrigine is also a strong inducer of liver enzymes.

Status epilepticus

In adults and in children over the age of five, a seizure lasting more than 5 min or two or more seizures occurring without complete recovery of consciousness in between are defined as status epilepticus (SE).[50]

Clinical characteristics

Depending on the type of seizures SE can be defined as

1. Tonic–clonic SE;
2. Tonic SE;
3. Clonic SE (only in children);
4. Myoclonic SE;
5. Simple partial SE or SE epilepsia partialis continua (without impairment of consciousness).

Non-convulsive status epilepticus (NCSE). This particular condition is characterized by EEG seizure activity without convulsive activity. It is a significant cause of impaired consciousness in patients with complex toxic–metabolic encephalopathies, occurring in 8 per cent of comatose patients according to recent data.[51] According to some authors most patients with altered state of consciousness and mild motor signs have EEG findings compatible with SE. NCSE can manifest as absence type NCSE and as partial complex NCSE.

Partial complex NCSE is a particularly challenging situation. Seizure activity fluctuates and recurs often originating from temporal cortical areas and causes a confusional state with variable clinical findings. This condition can be continuous, with long-lasting delirium, with or without psychotic behaviours and automatisms, and, in this case, is sustained by continuous focal seizures, or discontinuous with recurrent partial complex seizures, but with recovery of consciousness between the single seizure episodes. Clinical aspects may be baffling with minimal abnormalities in answering questions but affective manifestations of fear or paranoid ideation. Duration can vary from 30 min to 2 weeks. In 40 per cent of cases, the episode is shorter than 24 h; in another 40 per cent, the episode lasts from 1 to 10 days. One case reported a partial complex status lasting for 7.5 months.[52]

Treatment[50,53]

The first priority is that cardio-circulatory and respiratory function are supported. Intravenous infusion of benzodiazepines and phenytoin are the first line pharmacological approaches. Treatment has a high rate of success (80 per cent) if initiated within 30 min. If delayed for more than 2 h these drugs fail in 60 per cent of cases (Table 6).

Characteristics of drugs used in SE

The drugs used for the acute control of epileptic seizures also have other indications in palliative care when they are used primarily for their sedative effects.

Lorazepam[54,55] is considered the drug of choice. Mean time to clinical effect is 3 min, half-life is 10–15 h but effective brain levels are maintained for 8–24 h. It has no active metabolites. It should be infused IV not faster than 2 mg/min. It is rapidly absorbed after rectal administration. Intramuscular (IM) administration is not recommended. In acute administration the main risk is respiratory depression.

Diazepam enters the brain in a few seconds but because of its high lipid solubility, redistribution to all body tissues is rapid with a consequent fall of brain concentrations. Its anticonvulsant effect is therefore very brief and a second dose may be necessary after only 20–30 min. Rectal formulations are available. Recommended doses are 10 mg in adults and 5 mg (0.5 mg/kg) in children. Rectal administration at these doses does not cause respiratory depression. After IM administration, absorption is very variable and unpredictable and this route should generally be avoided.

Midazolam[56,57] is water soluble, has a very short half-life, and has no active metabolites. Its onset of action is 3 min after IV administration, 5 and 15 min, respectively, after IM and oral administration. The good IM and SC absorption are an important advantage in cases of difficult venous access. In refractory SE, the initial dose is 0.2 mg/kg, followed by 0.05–0.5 mg/kg/h IV infusion. In older patients, it is better to start off with lower doses of 1–2 mg.

Phenytoin.[58,59] Its onset of action is short (10–20 min), it has no sedative effects, does not cause respiratory depression, and has a long

Table 6 Algorithm for the management of SE

Minutes	Intervention
0–5	Diagnosis, airway–breathing–circulation, venous access, blood glucose, and oximetry
6–9	If hypoglycaemia or if the blood glucose is not available, thiamine 100 mg IV followed by 50 ml glucose 50%, in children 2 ml/kg glucose 25%
10–20	*Lorazepam* 0.1 mg/kg. Infusion rate 2 mg/min to total dose of 8 mg for adults; children 0.05–0.5 mg/kg, infusion rate to total of 4 mg or *Diazepam* 0.15–0.25 mg/kg, infusion rate 5 mg/min to 20 mg total dose in adults *Diazepam can be repeated after 5 min and phenytoin should always be given afterwards. Phenytoin is now considered a second choice line
20+	*If not effective* *Phenytoin* 20 mg/kg, maximum infusion rate 50 mg/min, in adults, or 1 mg/kg/min in children. Dilute in saline as recommended in text (monitoring of cardiac frequency and blood pressure); phosphophenytoin can be administered with an infusion rate up to 150 mg/min
>60	*If SE persists* Give an additional phenytoin dose of 5 mg/kg and repeat if needed until reaching a total maximum dose of 30 mg/kg *If not effective* *Phenobarbitone* 20 mg/kg at 60 mg/min IV infusion. Apnoea can occur especially if the patient has already been treated with benzodiazepines *If status persists* *Phenobarbitone additional dose 5–10 mg/kg* *If status persists it is defined as* *Refractory status epilepticus* to be managed by intensive care units with the following alternative drugs a) *Pentobarbitone* 3–12 mg/kg loading dose, followed by 1–10 mg/kg/h infusion; b) *Idazolam* 0.2 mg/kg, 0.1–0.6 mg/kg/h; c) *Propofol* 1–2 mg/kg IV in 5–10 min, 2–10 mg/kg/h; d) *Sodium valproate* 60–70 mg/kg IV; e) *Diazepam* 50 mg diluted in 250 cm^3 of saline* 1 ml/kg/h (2 mg/kg/h); *Solution should be freshly prepared every 6 h

Modified from refs 16 and 63.

duration of action. It should be used in benzodiazepine-refractory SE by IV infusion, not more than 50 mg/min. In elderly patients, the dose should be reduced to 15 mg/kg. After a loading dose has been infused (Table 6), the duration of the therapeutic effect is about 24 h. Blood levels can be checked 120 min after the end of the infusion. A loading dose of 15–20 mg/kg can be also administered orally but poor gastric tolerability limits the use of this route in some patients.

After diluting phenytoin in saline, the solution should be infused within 1 h. A concentration of 6.7 mg/ml (1000 mg/130 ml) is suggested although the drug is stable in solutions of up to 10 mg/ml. Side-effects may be related to excessively fast infusion rates, as may be required in emergency situations and include cardiac arrhythmias, arterial hypotension and CNS depression. The 'purple glove syndrome' is due to the high pH of the drug (−13) causing local toxicity at the site of infusion which manifests with blue discolouration, and distal oedema, 2 h after administration.

Propofol[57,60] has an effect on GABA receptors similar to that of benzodiazepines and barbiturates. Its use requires intensive care support and is reserved for cases of SE which are refractory to standard treatment. Hypotensive effects should be carefully managed.

Phenobarbitone is an option if benzodiazepines and phenytoin fail. The peak clinical effect is delayed for 20–60 min after administration.

Thiopentone is highly lipid soluble and for this reason undergoes rapid redistribution, resulting in a state of coma that is less prolonged than with phenobarbitone. It is partially metabolized to pentobarbital. Thiopentone lowers ICP but is associated with severe hypotension, oedema, ileus, sepsis, immune suppression, and an increase in P_{CO_2}. Awakening is complicated by long-lasting side-effects and recovery of function has a very long and variable profile: recovery of motor function occurs within 1–72 h after the end of treatment, eye-opening after 1–3 days, cognitive function 2–18 days.

Pentobarbitone is an alternative to thiopentone.

Sodium valproate. The availability of a parenteral formulation of valproate provides an alternative to phenytoin. At least one report confirms the efficacy and safety of valproate infusion in high doses (20 mg/kg, IV infusion rate from 30 to 555 mg/min), in patients with repetitive seizures.[61]

Table 7 Conditions associated with motor and behavioural abnormalities

Psychiatric disturbances: somatoform reactions, anxiety panic attacks, psychotic dissociative episodes, Munchausen syndrome
Cardiovascular disorders: syncope, arrhythmia, transient ischaemic attacks (TIA)
Headache: emicrania complicata, emicrania basilare
Movement disorders: tremor, diskinesia, tic, myoclonus
Parasomnias and sleep disturbances: nightmares, somnambulism, narcolepsy, cataplexy, nocturnal paroxysmal dystonia
Gastrointestinal symptom: nausea or colic
Delirium

Differential diagnosis

It is important to keep in mind that acute conditions with an altered state of consciousness, at times associated with motor or behavioural abnormalities are often erroneously considered seizures. The most frequent of these conditions are listed in Table 7.[62]

Delirium

Definition

Delirium has been defined as a transient organic brain syndrome characterized by the acute onset of disordered attention and cognition, accompanied

Table 8 DSM IV criteria for diagnosing delirium due to a general medical condition

A.	Disturbance of consciousness with reduced ability to focus, sustain, and shift attention
B.	Change in cognition (such as memory deficit, disorientation, language disturbances, or perception disturbances not better explained by a pre-existing stabilized or evolving dementia)
C.	The disturbance develops over a short period of time and tends to fluctuate during the course of the day
D.	There is evidence from the history, physical examination or laboratory findings that the disturbance is caused by the direct physiological consequences of a general medical condition

by disturbances of cognition, psychomotor behaviour, and perception.(64,65) Delirium is considered to be a single taxonomic entity,(64) and the DSM-IV proposes specific diagnostic criteria for its diagnosis (Table 8).(65)

The terms 'encephalopathy' and 'acute confusional state' have been used by neurologists to describe acute changes in mental status.(3,66) As a consequence, a dichotomous tendency exists between the psychiatric and neurology literature. This dualism is usually only semantic.

Delirium has been described also by Engels and Romano as a syndrome of cerebral insufficiency.(67) It is considered to be a stereotyped response of the brain to a spectrum of differing insults and has been viewed as a state on the continuum between normal wakefulness and stupor and coma.

The EEG of patients with delirium, regardless of the aetiology of the delirium, demonstrates a generalized symmetric slowing of the EEG with reduction of the alpha rhythm and an increase in delta and theta frequencies.(67) These changes are not dissimilar to those found in stages of the sleep pattern. In general, the degree of EEG slowing correlates with a decrease in arousal. In some conditions, EEG fast wave activity, beta activity, is also present.(68) This activity is more prevalent in delirium characterized by hyperactive phenomena, such as delirium tremens.

Clinical applications of diagnostic criteria

The diagnosis of delirium requires that consciousness and attention are assessed together with cognitive function and performance. This is best done by systematically using instruments that are sensitive to the derangement of these areas of brain function. The Mini Mental State Examination (MMSE) is the most widely used and known method. It is also a simple instrument to facilitate bedside patient assessment. It can be used for assessing cognitive function keeping in mind that it is not a diagnostic tool. In fact, the MMSE is not specific for delirium but generally for cognitive failure, as can be found in dementia and in delirium to mention only the two most important differential diagnoses.(69,70)

The Confusion Assessment Method in contrast is a diagnostic system that can be used to apply the DSM criteria for the diagnosis of delirium and is very sensitive and specific when applied by trained personnel.(71,72)

The Delirium Rating Scale (DRS)(73,74) and the Memorial Delirium Assessment Scale (MDAS)(75) are instruments specifically designed to assess delirium and its severity that can be used to evaluate the full range of symptoms occurring in patients with delirium and to grade their severity.(70)

Symptoms and signs fluctuate and the diagnosis may be overlooked if careful attention is not paid to the changes in mental status examination over time. Additionally, subtle changes frequently precede the onset of delirium. These minor symptoms and behavioural changes may go unnoticed, only to be recalled later in family or staff interviews. A patient may be restless, anxious, depressed, irritable, angry, or emotionally labile. These symptoms are not specific for a diagnosis. Each of them may be a manifestation of an adjustment disorder, may represent a symptom of delirium, or may be a consequence of any of a large number of conditions, including dementia.

In the early stages of, or while recovering from delirium, isolated disturbances may be found that alone may not fulfil the criteria for a diagnosis of delirium. Findings frequently include daytime somnolence with night-time insomnia, and subtle mood and personality changes and hallucinations.

The first of the DSM diagnostic criteria for delirium relates to disturbance of consciousness and impaired attention. This disturbance can be highly variable, characterized by increased or decreased arousal, or merely by distractibility and reduced responsiveness. Three clinical variants of delirium have been described based on the type of arousal disturbance: hypoalert–hypoactive, hyperalert–hyperactive, and mixed type (with fluctuations from hypoalert to hyperalert).(76,77)

Attention disturbances are manifest not only by the level of arousal but also by changes in the patient's ability to concentrate, which can be subtle. Attention disturbances may be evidenced by an inability to maintain a conversation or to attend to its flow, language abnormalities and difficulties in writing.(78)

The second DSM criterion for delirium relates to the presence of changed cognition, for example, disorientation, memory deficits, and disturbances of language, reasoning, and perception. It is important to recognize that a diagnosis of delirium may be established in the presence of any one of these cognitive abnormalities. The best way to assess globally this area is by using a comprehensive method such as the MMSE as already suggested.

Language abnormalities are frequently present in delirium and are often compounded by the presence of incoherent reasoning. Language may lack fluency and spontaneity, and conversation may be prolonged and interrupted by long pauses or repetitions. The language may reflect an inability to find the correct word or to name objects (anomia) and may be characterized by 'passepartout' words (non-specific phrases that substitute for specific language, for example, 'you know what I mean'), perseveration, stereotypes, and cliches. Writing abilities are affected early and more severely than other language-related skills.(79–82) Delirium affects reasoning and patients frequently demonstrate irrelevant or rambling thinking, abnormal conceptualization, and altered insight with anosognosia.

Perceptual abnormalities and delusions are not considered by the MMSE and may be typical of delirium especially in some sub-types, in particular delirium tremens and hyperactive deliria in general. They can be systematically assessed by using the DRS and the MDAS. Delusions may be associated with hallucinations. These delusions are frequently poorly organized and characterized by paranoid features, which may incorporate themes that relate, for example, to homicide, imprisonment, or jealousy. Occupational delusions are among the most common with the patient locating himself or herself in a familiar time and space and attending to usual activities. Lipowski describes 'the law of the unfamiliar mistaken for the familiar'(64) and suggests that perceptions are influenced by the emotional colour of the situation and the patient's personality characteristics.(83)

Delirium can significantly interfere with family and staff understanding of patient's suffering. A recent small study of 14 patients with cancer pain and severe cognitive failure found that during episodes of agitated cognitive failure, pain intensity as assessed by a nurse was significantly higher than the patient's assessment had been before and after the episode.(84) Upon complete recovery, none of these patients recalled having had any discomfort during the episode.

The third and fourth criteria for diagnosis of delirium relates to the time course and organic aetiology of the disturbance. For diagnosis, there must be evidence confirming that the disturbance has developed over a short period of time and tends to fluctuate during the course of the day. Fluctuation in the clinical manifestations of delirium is usually apparent in disturbance of the sleep–wake cycle. Patients usually experience insomnia and may be agitated at night and somnolent during the day. As noted previously, this change in sleep pattern is often found to be among the prodromal symptoms of the syndrome. The phenomenon known as 'sundowning' refers to the worsening of symptoms toward evening and probably has more to do with sleep–wake abnormalities than with environmental factors.

In addition to mental status changes, described above, neurological examination may identify findings associated with diffuse brain dysfunction, such as multifocal myoclonus and asterixis. Some findings may be relatively specific for one or more aetiologies. For example, tremulousness is typical of alcohol withdrawal states; miosis and mydriasis suggest opioid toxicity and anticholinergic toxicity, respectively; and tachypnoea may be a manifestation of a central process, or of sepsis or hypoxaemia.

Frequency

According to very old data, in hospitalized cancer patients, the prevalence of organic brain syndromes is 4 per cent.[85] No prevalence data are available for the general cancer population by using a more specific definition of delirium. More recently, delirium prevalence has been studied in the elderly, patients in the post-operative period, and patients presenting to the emergency room.[86,87] Altered mental state is the second most common reason for neurological consultation at a tertiary cancer centre.[88] In patients admitted to inpatient hospice or to home palliative care programmes, prevalence of delirium is about 30 per cent.[89,90]

In a study by Gagnon et al. 18 (20 per cent) of 89 cancer patients consecutively hospitalized for terminal care were delirious on screening at admission and, among the 71 who were free of delirium at admission, the incidence of confirmed delirium was 32 per cent.[91] In a similar population, 104 patients in an acute palliative care unit in a university-affiliated teaching hospital, Lawlor et al. diagnosed delirium in 44 patients (42 per cent), and of the remaining 60, delirium developed in 27 (45 per cent).[92] Reversal of delirium occurred in 46 (49 per cent) of 94 episodes in 71 patients and terminal delirium occurred in 46 (88 per cent) of the 52 deaths.[92]

Underdiagnosing is often a problem.[93] In the emergency room setting, for example, one study demonstrated that only 6 per cent of delirium diagnoses were detected by the emergency room physician.[94] In a series of elderly medical patients, the physicians' diagnoses correctly identified only eight of 47 patients as being delirious or acutely confused.[95]

Aetiologic factors in delirium and multifactorial risk model

Risk factors

The socio-demographic and disease-related factors that may predispose to delirium or predict its occurrence have not been documented in cancer patients. The studies that have investigated delirium in the oncology setting have generally sought to address the spectrum and prevalence of a range of psychiatric diagnoses rather than to address factors involved in specific diagnoses, such as delirium. As a consequence, the number of delirious cancer patients that has been studied has not been large enough to allow investigators to draw conclusions that relate to predictive factors. In one recent study dyspnoea, anorexia, presence of brain metastases, performance status, and physician estimate prediction of survival were associated with the diagnosis of delirium but only univariate statistics were applied.[90]

Inouye and Charpentier have proposed a multifactorial model for delirium in the hospitalized elderly that may be relevant in the cancer population.[96–98] The model involves the interaction between 'baseline

Table 9 Aetiological factors implicated in the onset of delirium in patients with cancer

Primary CNS tumour
Secondary CNS tumour
Brain metastases
Meningeal metastases
Non-metastatic complications of cancer
Metabolic encephalopathy due to hepatic, renal, or pulmonary failure
Electrolyte abnormalities
Glucose abnormalities
Infections
Haematological abnormalities
Nutritional deficiency (thiamine, folic acid, vitamin B12 deficiency)
Vasculitis
Paraneoplastic neurological syndromes
Toxicity of antineoplastic therapies
Chemotherapy: methotrexate, cisplatin, vincristine, procarbazine, asparaginase, citosina arabinoside, 5-fluorouracil, ifosfamide, tamoxifene (rare), etoposide (high doses), nitrosurea (high doses or arterial route)
Radiation to brain
Acute and delayed encephalopathy
Toxicity of other drugs
Anticholinergics: belladonna alkaloids, scopolamine, atropine, hyoscine
Drugs with established anticholinergic activity: tricyclic antidepressants, diphenhydramine, promethazine, triesifenidile, chlorpromazine, and other neuroleptics: hyoscine butylbromide
Anxiolytics, hypnotics
Steroids, opioids, digitalis, cyprofloxacine, acyclovir, gancyclovir, NSAIDs, anticonvulsants, H2 blockers (cimetidine, ranitidine, famotidine), omeprazole, interferons, interleukins, cyclosporin, levodopa, lithium
Other diseases not related to neoplasms
CNS diseases or trauma
Cardiac disease
Lung disease
Endocrinopathy
Alcohol or drug abuse or withdrawal

vulnerability' and 'precipitating factors or insults'.[97] In this model, baseline vulnerability is defined by the predisposing factors present at the time of admission to hospital, and the precipitating factors are the noxious insults that occurred during hospitalization. Patients who have high baseline vulnerability may develop delirium with any precipitating factor, whereas those with low baseline vulnerability will be more resistant to the development of delirium, even with noxious insults. The factors that Inouye et al. specifically demonstrated to be contributory to baseline vulnerability in the elderly include visual impairment, severe illness, cognitive impairment, and an elevated serum urea nitrogen/creatinine ratio of 18 or greater (dehydration).[96] Other studies have implicated risk factors including: each of the aforementioned factors, age, dementia, depression, alcohol abuse, the pre-operative use of anticholinergic drugs, poor functional status, and markedly abnormal preoperative serum sodium, potassium, or glucose levels.[86,99–101] Certain medications have also been implicated as risk factors for delirium, including neuroleptics, opioids, and anticholinergic drugs[86,99] especially drugs with potential anticholinergic effects.[102]

Aetiology

In cancer patients, the potential aetiologies of delirium, as distinct from 'risk factors', may be divided into direct effects related to tumour involvement and indirect effects. The latter category includes drugs, electrolyte imbalance, cranial irradiation, organ failure, nutritional deficiencies, vascular complications, paraneoplastic syndromes, and many other factors (Table 9).

A survey of 140 confused cancer patients referred initially for a neurology consultation demonstrated multiple potential aetiology in most cases.[103] A single cause of the altered mental status was found in 31 per cent of patients, whereas 69 per cent had multiple causes; the median number of probable contributing factors in each patient was 3. Drugs, especially opioids, were associated with altered mental status in 64 per cent of patients, metabolic abnormalities in 53 per cent, infection in 46 per cent, and recent surgery in 32 per cent. A structural brain lesion was the sole cause of encephalopathy in 15 per cent of patients. Lateralizing neurological signs were found in 41 per cent of patients, and of those 42 per cent had cerebral metastases. Importantly, however, it was noted that 25 per cent of patients without lateralizing signs who had neuro-imaging had a focal cerebral lesion defined as a cause or a contributory factor to the delirium. Two-thirds of the patients in this survey recovered cognitive function when the cause of the delirium was treated.

In a second study, Lawlor et al. studied a population of 104 patients with advanced cancer admitted to a palliative care unit.[92] In this population, as in the previous study,[103] population, the median number of precipitating factors was 3, and 49 per cent of patients had delirium that was reversible. Psychoactive medications, predominantly opioids were precipitating factors that were independently associated with reversibility of the delirium but the authors concluded that often times more than one factor (e.g. opioid medication *and* dehydration) requires attention if the delirium is to be reversed.[92] Other studies have demonstrated that drug interactions and metabolic failure (especially renal impairment) can produce unexpected toxicities especially in the patient with advanced disease.[104–106]

Cognitive compromise is likely the most common symptom and sign at the presentation of brain[107] and leptomeningeal metastases.[108,109] Paraneoplastic encephalitis, that can be associated with Anti-Hu and other antineuronal antibodies, should also be considered, albeit rare, as a cause, of delirium.[110]

Non-convulsive epileptic status, that can occur in association with complex metabolic problems and also with ifosfamide encephalopathy, is a condition that can also result in altered consciousness manifesting with delirium.[111] EEG can be used to confirm this diagnosis which is likely to be more frequent than suspected.[51]

Finally, it is important to recognize that many factors contributing to delirium are potentially reversible, and these are often underestimated in this population. These factors include, among others, dehydration,[112] borderline renal function, infections, metabolic causes, drug withdrawal, psychoactive medications, and the accumulation of opioid metabolites.[92,113,114]

General assessment recommendations

Clinical assessment should include careful physical and neurological examination. Specific mental status assessment can follow the above-mentioned recommendations and can be helped by the systematic use of the MMSE, DRS, or MDAS and also by screening with the CAM. Aetiological screening should follow the rational stepwise implementation of a number of procedures that may be appropriate or totally inappropriate depending on the patient's condition, wishes, prognosis, and therefore, on goals of care (Table 10). The completeness of the list is not inconsistent with a policy of avoiding in practice any further evaluation in the individual case.

EEG techniques may be useful in the study of delirium, clarifying the differential diagnosis and severity, and providing a better method for serial monitoring.[115] EEG findings, specifically decreased alpha and increased delta and theta frequencies, have been demonstrated to correlate with low MMSE scores in delirious patients.[116] The utility of EEG in the differential diagnosis of delirium has also been demonstrated in the differentiation of non-convulsive status epilepticus from delirium and several specific diagnostic entities. For example, the EEG associated with delirium produced by high-dose ifosfamide shows rhythmic complexes typical of seizure-like activity, in contrast to generalized symmetric slowing of the EEG considered to be typical of other types of delirium.[111]

Treatment

Aetiological interventions are aimed at correcting, infectious and toxic-metabolic causes or risk factors as reviewed in Table 10. Symptomatic management is often required both in reversible and irreversible cases and is based on non-pharmacological and pharmacological therapies.

Environmental intervention

A calm, quiet environment is important to allow for potential recovery and to help the patient to reorient to time and space (a visible clock, calendar,

Table 10 Screening process for delirium aetiology in advanced cancer

Toxic factors	Bedside screen of medication profile Urine or blood drug screening
Sepsis	Temperature Blood/urine and other cultures for infection screen Leukocyte count Urinalysis Red cell count
Glucose-oxidative brain deficiency	Pulse oximetry Blood gases and acid-base balance Blood glucose
Electrolyte imbalances	Serum electrolytes (Na, K, Cl, Mg, Ca)
Renal failure	Urea, creatinine, creatinine clearance
Liver failure	Liver function tests Ammonia
CNS vascular, infectious or structural lesion	DIC screening and coagulation profile CSF examination: blood, glucose, proteins, lymphocytes, leucocytes, malignant cells, culture Brain CT or MRI
Paraneoplastic disease	Autoantibodies Anti-Hu, Yo, Ma, etc.
Cofactor deficiency malnutrition	B12 levels—administer B1 1 g/day[a]
Endocrine dysfunction	Thyroid hormone and TSH Adrenal function

[a] The determination of B1 levels is problematic. Our practice is to supplement B1 to every patient with poor nutritional status.

Table 11 Pharmacological therapy of delirium (Doses and schedules are intended for general guidance. Each case will need specific dose adjustment.)

Haloperidol; oral	0.5–5 mg every 8–12 h; a dose of 2 mg/day can be efficacious in mild cases
Haloperidol; SC, IM, or IV	0.5–2 mg per dose titrating dose to clinical effect hourly IV infusion 0.2–1 mg/h with careful titration to clinical effect can be used in difficult cases. ECG monitoring is recommended
Chlorpromazine; oral, IM, or IV	12.5–50 mg every 8–12 h. More sedating, anticholinergic, and hypotensive effects
Clozapine; oral	12.5–50 mg at night (monitoring of blood cell count is needed) very sedative, has less extrapyramidal effects than other neuroleptics
Risperidone; oral	From 0.5–1 mg/day up to 2–4 mg/day. In the elderly, has less extrapyramidal effects
Olanzapine; OS	5 mg qhs to be titrated up to clinical effect
Lorazepam; oral, SL, or IV	0.5–2 mg every 4–8 h if sedating anxiolytic effects required
Midazolam; SC or IV	20–100 mg 24 h IV or SC continuous infusion for sedation in refractory cases. 3–5 mg IV priming dose if rapid sedation is required. Start IV infusion with 1 mg/h, dose should be frequently titrated to effect
Promazin; IM or IV	50 mg every 8–12 h; antihistamine very sedative; useful if sedation desired

well-known object from the patient's house), good light. A recent study demonstrated that systematic reorientation and risk-modifying protocol can reduce the incidence of delirium among elderly hospitalized patients.(98) Presence in the room of family members can be very important.

Communication with patient and family

A close collaboration between staff and family is fundamental. Special attention needs to be focused on communication with the patient and the family. Family members are particularly stressed by observing the change of the patient's usual behaviour and by the communication barrier. The family has to be informed about the role of therapies, characteristics of delirium, its relationship with the disease conditions, potential for reversibility, short-term prognosis, and fluctuation of cognitive function.

In the hospice care of terminally ill patients, both at home or in an institution, goals of care need to be discussed and the level of patient suffering assessed and explained to family members. Family members who are overwhelmed by caring needs may require disproportionate interventions for relieving what they interpret as the patient suffering, or pain. Often this behaviour can swing from requests to withdraw medication to advocating sedation and is often compounded by personal problems in facing suffering, and death.

It is very important to clarify the role of symptomatic therapies. It is customary to blame opioid medications for mental changes that are indeed caused by the complex interaction of several factors. This idea is often reinforced by previous experiences, and by current erroneous medical beliefs and can result in the relatives feeling guilty for administering therapies that they believe related to the change of mental status. There are cases, such as the one presented, where aetiology cannot be established and decisions about using drugs that may contribute to the delirium is based on the priority of providing symptom control and comfort care.

In front of the patient it is important to show empathy and to ask simple questions ('Do you feel confused?'). While consciousness level fluctuates the patient needs to be reassured. Logic and rational communication skills should be substituted by more direct nonverbal communication skills. Communication with a well-known family member should be favoured and should focus more on affective aspects than on cognition and try to distract from delusional experiences and interpretations.

Pharmacological therapy

Agitated delirium often requires pharmacological treatment to control behaviours that could result in harm for the patient and others, and to treat hallucinations or delusions that may be contributing to patient suffering. The treatment of hypoactive deliria is more debatable and will depend on individual clinical judgement.

The first choice drug is haloperidol(117,118) since it has lower sedating potency and less anticholinergic and cardiovascular effects than other neuroleptics. Table 11 gives guidelines for the use of haloperidol and alternative drugs.

These guidelines are general and should be adapted to the clinical situation case by case. Haloperidol has been used via IV infusion although it is not licensed for that route of administration.(118) Very high IV doses up to 1200 mg per day have been safely administered. In our experience, therapeutic effects are seen at usual doses of 2–5 mg/day; difficult cases may require higher doses or sedation with other drugs. Careful titration of the dose at the bedside is the most important recommendation to improve outcome. ECG monitoring should be performed during haloperidol therapy to monitor possible prolongation of the Q-T interval that can occasionally intervene with most neuroleptics. Cases of torsade de pointe have been described with haloperidol administration via IV and oral routes.(119,120) Droperidol and chlorpromazine can be used for more sedative effects. Recently, risperidone, clozapine, and olanzapine have been used in cases of delirium.

Benzodiazepine can worsen delirium especially in the elderly(117) and are not to be used in hepatic encephalopathy. Their use should be limited to the treatment of delirium due to alcohol withdrawal where they are considered first choice drugs. Benzodiazepines can also be added in cases of delirium when anxiolytic and sedative effects are considered particularly desirable or in cases unresponsive to neuroleptic medications.

Often, delirium in cancer patient with terminal disease requires more than a single drug treatment. In one case series of 39 patients, only 20 per cent of cases could be managed by haloperidol alone.(121) When sedation is the goal of therapy and especially in patients with severe symptoms such as pain, haemorrhage, or dyspnoea complicated by delirium the combination of an opioid with a neuroleptic and an antihistamine such as promethazine can be particularly effective.

Neurological complications of cancer

Neurological complications are estimated to occur in up to 20 per cent of patients with cancer.(122) In a large consultation survey conducted at a comprehensive cancer centre, the most frequent complaints were pain and altered mental status (Table 12).(88)

Brain metastases

Pathology

Intracranial metastases are found at autopsy in about 25 per cent of patients who died of cancer.(123) Other common intracranial lesions involve the

Table 12 Cancer and cancer treatment related neurological diagnoses in 851 patients with cancer[a]

Diagnosis	Percentage
Brain metastasis	15.9
Metabolic or drug related encephalopathy	10.2
Pain associated with bone metastasis	9.9
Epidural tumour	8.5
Tumour plexopathy	5.8
Leptomeningeal metastasis	5.1
Chemotherapy peripheral neuropathy	3.2
Radiculopathy	2.7
Base-of-skull metastasis	2.7
Seizures due to metastasis	2.7
Seizures not due to metastasis	1.8
Paraneoplastic syndromes	1.2
Intracranial haemorrhage related to thrombocytopenia	1.3
Radiation myelopathy	1.2
Radiation plexopathy	1.1
Intracranial haemorrhage from tumour	0.6

[a] Modified from Clouston et al., 1992.[88] A total of 1042 diagnoses were given with up to three per patient. Among the non-cancer-related diagnoses, cerebrovascular disease, headache, and degenerative spine disease were the most common diagnoses.

skull and meninges. The choroid plexus and the pituitary are less commonly affected. There is evidence that the incidence of brain metastases and leptomeningeal metastases is increasing, because of better control of systemic disease and longer survival allowing 'sanctuary' cells in the central nervous system to grow and cause symptoms.[38] Lung cancer, melanoma, and breast cancer are the primary tumours most frequently associated with metastatic spread to the brain parenchyma. Tumours such as melanoma usually cause multiple lesions, while breast cancer more often causes single lesions (some 50 per cent of breast cancer patients have a single lesion and 20 per cent two lesions). It is important to bear this in mind when planning surgery or focal radiation treatment.

Brain metastases usually originate from tumours via neoplastic emboli. Tumour emboli lodge in the white matter at the grey/white matter junction where they grow as spherical masses displacing, rather than infiltrating, the brain and causing symptoms by various mechanisms. They usually involve the watershed territories at the end of the arterial supply. In general, their distribution in the brain relates to the cerebral vasculature and thus the supratentorial regions are more often affected (85 per cent of all central nervous system metastases). However, vasculature is not the only factor to influence the metastatic process. For example, some pelvic tumours tend to metastasize to the posterior fossa and the cerebellum (53 per cent of central nervous system metastases from pelvic tumours, excluding gastrointestinal tumours).

Brain metastases can cause symptoms by compression, local destruction, irritation of brain tissue, brain oedema, and bleeding. The most common effect of a metastatic lesion is brain oedema and increased ICP. Focal symptoms can be due to oedema or bleeding, other typical presentations include cognitive failure, seizures, and the syndrome of intracranial hypertension, that are discussed in specific sections of this chapter.

Clinical course

Median survival is about 2 months from diagnosis if no treatment is given, depending on tumour type.[124,125] Brain metastases are often the direct cause of death (a common situation in breast cancer patients)[125] but

Table 13 Symptoms and signs due to cerebral metastases in 162 patients

Symptoms	Percentage	Signs	Percentage
Headache	53	Hemiparesis	66
Focal weakness	40	Impaired cognition	77
Mental change	31	Unilateral sensory loss	27
Seizures	15	Papilloedema	26
Ataxia	20	Ataxia	24
Aphasia	10	Aphasia	19

From Posner (1980).[107]

patients responding to brain radiotherapy usually die of their systemic disease.

Signs and symptoms at presentation are listed in Table 13. Symptoms can present progressively and deceptively, or alternatively, can be sudden and 'stroke-like'. It should be remembered that in many patients formal neurological tests of strength and mental function will reveal signs of changes in the central nervous system that are not otherwise apparent.[7]

Headache is an important symptom—usually of a full aching quality and moderate intensity. It is caused by compression or traction of intracranial pain-sensitive structures. With supratentorial lesions it is often bifrontal, although it can occur on one side—always that of the tumour. Headache occurs more frequently and is more severe with infratentorial lesions and in this case is referred to the nuchal region and the neck.[8]

ICP is not always elevated but when it is clinical features are distinctive as explained in Chapter 8.15.

Treatment general

Options should include the provision of supportive treatment only.[126] Decisions should be taken after considering:

1. the type of cancer and its sensitivity to radiation and chemotherapy;
2. the neurological status of the patient;
3. the extent of systemic disease and its associated symptoms and the expected quality of life.

Surgery is indicated only for single metastases with limited or no systemic disease, especially with radioresistant tumours.[125–128] Whole brain irradiation produces neurological improvement in the majority of patients but survival after treatment is only 4–6 months (see Chapter 8.1.2).[129] Metastases from breast and lung cancers usually have a better response to radiotherapy, showing both clinical and radiological improvement. Metastases from melanoma and colonic and renal carcinomas often do not show radiological changes even where clinical improvement occurs. Treatment should never be withheld solely on the basis of histology, however, because, on occasion, lesions from radioresistant tumours do respond.

Newer techniques for focal radiation may benefit selected cases.[130] Focal brain irradiation or 'radiosurgery' can have a role in treating single, or occasionally two, brain metastases in combination with whole brain irradiation; the aim being eradication of disease from the brain. Radiosurgery is suggested as a substitute for surgery in this strategy.[131] Radioresistant histology was not found to affect outcome.[131] In advanced cases where a shorter course of treatment and a shorter expected latency for improvement of symptoms are greatly preferred, radiosurgery can be used for palliation of single or double lesions in the brain. It can also be used in cases where there is recurrence in the brain after whole brain irradiation. The indications for and role of focal brain irradiation remain to be clearly defined.[16]

Corticosteroids

Treatment with steroids is recommended for all symptomatic patients with brain metastases or tumour. Their main therapeutic effect is probably related to partial restoration of the blood–brain barrier which is disrupted by the tumour, thus reducing oedema. Steroids are also recommended for all patients undergoing brain irradiation. Treatment should start 48 h before radiation. A traditional regimen is dexamethasone 16 mg/day in four divided doses, although a recent study demonstrated that a regiment of 4 mg daily throughout the duration of radiation therapy (28 days) with subsequent discontinuation works as well and has fewer side-effects.(15) We recommend starting with a 16 mg daily dose in stable patients undergoing radiation and to commence tapering the steroid dose during the second week of radiation. Tapering should be gradual (2–4 mg every fifth day).

Higher doses can be given acutely if symptoms recur (16 mg/day) or if there are signs of increased intracranial pressure or cerebral herniation (10–100 mg IV). The dose should always be tapered to the minimum required for symptom control. Dexamethasone taper and discontinuation should always be attempted after completion of radiation treatment since in most patients steroids are not necessary to preserve neurological function.(19)

Spinal cord compression

Pathology

This complication is usually due to extrinsic compression of the cord from the epidural space secondary to extension of adjacent bony or soft tissue lesions. Less commonly, spinal cord compression can be due to intradural and intramedullary metastases. Intradural spinal cord compression arises from meningeal metastases presenting as a single mass compressing the cord(132) instead of the more frequent diffuse pattern of leptomeningeal disease (see below). Intramedullary metastases are rare and are due to direct haematogenous dissemination to the cord or to invasion from meningeal disease.

Other causes of epidural compression include epidural abscess or haemorrhage, herniated disc, and other rare epidural masses (such as epidural lipomatosis), and extramedullary haematopoiesis. Cauda equina and conus medullaris lesions have similar pathophysiology and clinical implications and are therefore considered here.

Most cases of epidural spinal cord compression in cancer are caused by a vertebral body metastasis invading the epidural space posteriorly and compressing the spinal cord or cauda equina structures. Another common cause is the invasion of the epidural space, through the intervertebral foramina, by a paraspinal lesion. This mechanism occurs typically in lymphoma and neuroblastoma, and in these cases the absence of a bony lesion on radiography can be misleading. Very rarely, spinal cord syndromes are due to epidural or cord metastases. Metastases from breast, lung, and prostate cancers more often affect the thoracic spine whereas the lumbar spine is more often affected by metastases from colorectal and other pelvic tumours.

Clinical course

Spinal cord compression occurs in 5–10 per cent of cases of cancer.(133,134) It is a neurological emergency as functional outcome is dependent on the degree of neurological impairment at diagnosis and initial response to therapy. Other factors important in prognosis are tumour histology and rate of progression of the neurological symptoms. The importance of early diagnosis cannot be over-emphasized; symptoms are usually present for some weeks before neurological emergency occurs. Pain precedes other neurological symptoms in almost every case but diagnosis is often delayed until the onset of symptoms and signs of myelopathy. In one series, there was an interval of more than 1 week between the onset of neurological symptoms and surgery in 52 per cent of patients.(135,136)

Pain of long duration which suddenly changes its characteristics should prompt re-evaluation and spine imaging. Pain in a crescendo pattern is particularly worrying, as is Lhermitte's sign (a tingling shock-like sensation passing down the arms or trunk when the neck is flexed),(137) pain aggravated by lying down and the Valsalva manoeuvre, and radiculopathy.

Lhermitte's sign, also described as 'barber's chair sign' in the British literature, can also be precipitated by sudden limb movements, coughing, sneezing, or may occur spontaneously. It is due to demyelination or compression of the posterior column of the spinal cord in the cervical or upper thoracic regions. Lhermitte's sign is frequent in multiple sclerosis but it is not uncommon in cancer and its differential diagnosis should include benign or relatively benign conditions such as transient radiation myelopathy, cisplatin polyneuropathy, or severe complications such as cord compression and progressive radiation myelopathy.(138)

Diagnosis

Signs of myelopathy usually begin in the lower extremities with weakness, paraesthesiae, and sensory loss starting in the feet and moving proximally. They are helpful in defining the level of the compression (Table 14). Emergency imaging of the spinal cord and canal should be carried out in patients with cancer and back pain who have symptoms of myelopathy. Ideally, this should be done when the characteristic back pain is noted.(139–142)

Other clinical and radiological characteristics are often associated with epidural invasion. In patients with back pain and bone changes on spine radiograph, epidural invasion has occurred in 60–70 per cent of cases,(139,140,142) and in 80 per cent of cases where there is vertebral collapse of more than 50 per cent.(143) In patients with radiculopathy, there is epidural invasion in 60 per cent of cases. Ninety per cent of patients with radiculopathy and bone changes on radiograph have epidural invasion.(139,140,142) However, in cases of lymphoma, radiographs which show no bony changes may be seriously misleading and false-negative results can be as high as 70 per cent.(144)

Table 14 Localizing signs with spinal cord lesions

Sign	Clinical level		
	Cord	**Conus and epiconus medullaris**	**Cauda equina**
Motor	Paraparesis usually flaccid Pyramidal signs can be present	If epiconus involved L5-S3 weakness If conus S2–S3 weakness	Never pyramidal signs Often asymmetrical weakness
Reflex	Absent or hyperactive	Patellar hyperactive Ankle hypoactive	Hypoactive Asymmetrical
Babinski	Usually present	Present only if lesion of epiconus	Never present
Sensory	Symmetrical level of dermatomal level sensory loss (locates compression within two dermatomes above the sensory level)	If conus S2–S5 'saddle' sensory loss If epiconus L4–S5	Asymmetrical findings in the lower extremities and perineum
Sphincter control	Can be initially preserved	Early involved sometimes selectively	Can be preserved

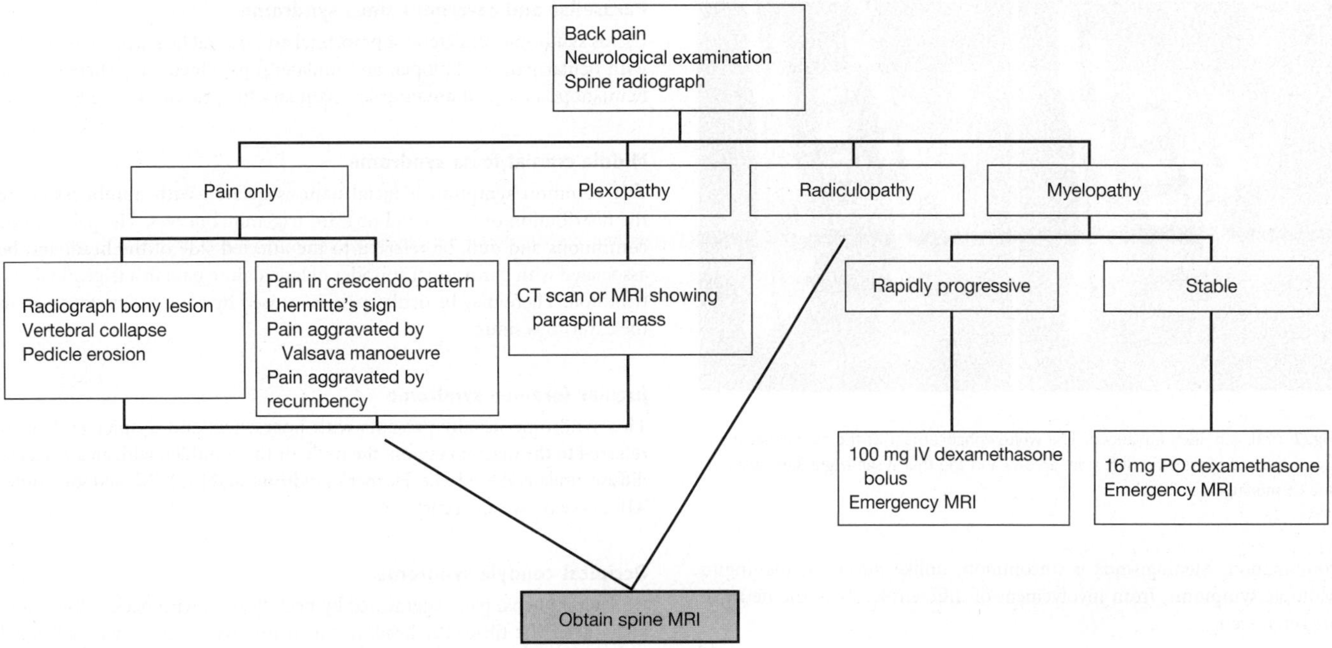

Fig. 1 Algorithm for the evaluation of back pain in the patient with cancer.

A positive bone scan without clinical changes is associated with epidural invasion in only 17 per cent of patients.[142]

Figure 1 summarizes the clinical and radiological findings which should prompt either immediate treatment or spinal cord imaging with magnetic resonance imaging (MRI), the results of which will dictate the treatment modality.[16,139,140,142,145] Although MRI is the best imaging procedure in these patients myelography or computerized tomography (CT) myelography still has a place when MRI is unavailable.[146–148] There may be multiple lesions and the whole spine should be evaluated.

Treatment (see also Chapter 8.1.2)

High-dose steroids and radiation should be offered to all patients where feasible.[149,150] Steroids can reduce pain, preserve neurological function, and improve functional outcome after definitive treatment.[151] Dexamethasone in high doses is recommended for high-degree lesions as shown by MRI or myelographic block (80 per cent or more) or with rapidly progressing myelopathy. A low-dose regimen should be used for low-degree lesions as shown by MRI or myelography or with stable or slowly progressing myelopathy. The high-dose regimen includes an initial intravenous bolus of 100 mg followed by a tapering schedule of 96 mg orally for 3 days and subsequent halving of the dose every third day until the end of radiation treatment.[152] The use of high doses for epidural spinal cord compression has been questioned[153] but experimental data favour this method.[16]

In the past, posterior laminectomy and radiation were the most used treatment modalities. Review of the literature and one randomized trial shows no advantage for posterior laminectomy plus radiation over the use of radiation alone.[16,154,155] and indeed posterior laminectomy can aggravate spine instability and neurological compromise.[156] A more rational surgical approach for anteriorly compressing lesions is vertebral body resection,[157,158] but the procedure requires intact vertebral elements above and below the affected level to stabilize the spine after surgery. Surgery is the first choice where the site of the primary tumour is unknown, where there is relapse after radiation treatment, and in cases of spinalinstability or vertebral displacement. It should also be considered when neurological symptoms progress during radiotherapy, in plegia of rapid onset, or where tumours are not radiosensitive.[16]

An evaluation of overall results of radiation and posterior laminectomy showed that ambulatory patients retained ambulation, and about half of paraparetic patients regained ambulation, while paraplegic patients rarely recovered.[16] Some series showed impressive results with vertebral resection. In one series, 13 of 36 paraplegic patients regained ambulation.[159] However, the numbers of patients are still too small to assess the benefits of this type of surgery. Prognosis and expected quality of life should influence the decision; it seems certainly worthwhile in some cases.

Leptomeningeal metastases

Pathology

Leptomeningeal metastases (also known as carcinomatous meningitis or meningeal carcinomatosis) are caused by the dissemination of cancerous cells throughout the sub-arachnoid space. Such cells can reach the meninges through the general circulation or the perineural spaces along nerve roots, by direct invasion from epidural lesions, or by direct seeding from existing brain tumours.[160] Meningeal involvement can be multifocal or diffuse and visible nodes or microscopic infiltration may result.

Clinical course

Leptomeningeal metastases were once considered an unusual complication of systemic cancer (1–8 per cent of cases at autopsy)[123,161] but these are increasingly seen nowadays, usually as a result of breast or lung cancer, lymphoma, leukaemia, or melanoma. Life expectancy is usually short, ranging from 3 to 6 months in patients who have received intensive treatment. Many patients are not offered treatment and their survival is shorter.[162,163]

The central and peripheral nervous systems are usually both involved and exhibit variable clinical syndromes. The pathophysiology includes abnormality in the flow and absorption of cerebrospinal fluid which can result in hydrocephalus,[164] direct involvement of the cranial and peripheral nerve meningeal sheets, competition with brain metabolism, invasion of the brain parenchyma, and ischaemia.

The most common symptoms are headache, change in mental status, and radicular-type pain[165,166] but cranial nerve involvement, seizures, polyradiculopathy, and cauda equina syndrome also occur in varying

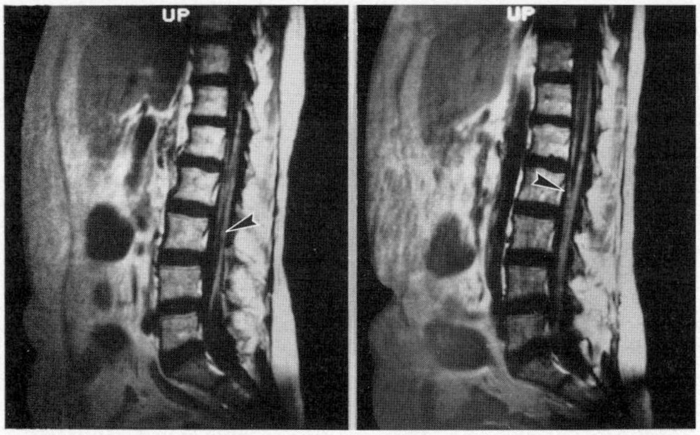

Fig. 2 MRI, gadolium enhanced. The white enhancement of the meningeal sheath around the cauda equina (left side, arrow) and the thecal sac (right side, arrow) due to meningeal infiltration.

combination. Meningismus is uncommon, unlike infectious meningitis. Multiple symptoms, from involvement of different levels of the neuraxis, are often seen.

Diagnosis

Diagnosis is usually made from examination of the CSF;[165,167] contrast-enhanced MRI can also be useful (Fig. 2), as the only sign of leptomeningeal metastases may be slight enhancement of the meninges with paramagnetic contrast due to blood–brain barrier disruption. In these circumstances, repeated spinal taps are required to identify malignant cells.

While malignant cells may not be apparent in the first sample of cerebrospinal fluid, other abnormalities are usually found such as high opening pressure, high protein content, increased white cell count, or low glucose content. In one series, only 3 per cent of the first samples were completely normal.[165] Other markers and immunocytochemical techniques have not been found to have clinical value.[16]

Therapy

Traditionally, treatment modalities have been based on a combination of corticosteroids, radiotherapy, and intrathecal chemotherapy. Systemic chemotherapy may also be helpful in some cases with appropriate tumour histology. In one series, only 23 per cent of treated patients could be regarded as long-term survivors. Intrathecal chemotherapy did not achieve better results than systemic chemotherapy (median survival 23 months),[163] and caused a treatment-related leucoencephalopathy in 58 per cent of cases. The role of intrathecal chemotherapy therefore requires prospective study.

Base of the skull and cranial nerve syndromes

Lesions at the base of the skull are commonly caused by metastasis of breast, prostate, and other tumours[168] and also result from local invasion by advanced head and neck tumours.[169] Symptoms secondary to bone lesions are commonly associated with alterations of cranial nerve function. Headache at the site of the lesion or referred to the vertex or to the entire affected side of the head is also frequent.[168,170,171] The best imaging procedure for all these syndromes is CT scan with bone window studies. Treatment with radiation is indicated, to control pain and neurological dysfunction.

Orbital syndrome

Progressive retro-orbital and supraorbital pain characterizes this syndrome, which may also be associated with blurred vision and diplopia. Chemosis, proptosis, external ophthalmoplegia, ipsilateral papilloedema, and sensory loss (in a trigeminal distribution) are common.

Parasellar and cavernous sinus syndrome

In this syndrome, unilateral supraorbital and frontal headache is associated with ocular palsies, diplopia, and unilateral papilloedema. There may be hemianopsia or quadrantanopsia, secondary to optic chiasm compression.

Middle cranial fossa syndrome

The common symptom is facial pain associated with numbness along the distribution of the second or third trigeminal nerves. The pain can be continuous and dull, be referred to the affected side of the head, and be associated with paroxysmal episodes of lancinating pain in a trigeminal distribution. There may be ocular palsies, caused by contiguous extension to the cavernous sinus.

Jugular foramen syndrome

This syndrome usually presents with hoarseness and dysphagia. Pain is referred to the mastoid region, the neck, or the shoulder, with an associated diffuse, unilateral headache. Horner's syndrome and IX, X, XI, and sometimes XII, nerve palsy can occur.

Occipital condyle syndrome

Unilateral nuchal pain, aggravated by neck flexion, with neck stiffness and a characteristic tilt of the head, occur in this syndrome. There is limited movement of the head and tenderness over the occipitocervical junction. The XI and XII nerves are often affected.

Clivus syndrome

While vertex headache may occur the pain can often be referred behind the eye, radiating posteriorly to the occiput. XI and XII nerve dysfunction is the most common finding but other lower cranial nerves (VI–IX) can be affected. Symptoms can occur on one or both sides.

Sphenoid and ethmoid sinus syndromes

These usually present with bilateral frontal headaches, nasal congestion and discharge, and diplopia secondary to VI nerve involvement.

Other cranial neuropathy syndromes

Glossopharyngeal nerve

The typical patient has throat and neck pain which radiates to the ear and is aggravated by swallowing. Pharyngeal and other carcinomas of the neck can present with odynophagia with reflex otalgia. Severe pain may be associated with syncope.[172] Although it has been described with leptomeningeal disease,[173] it commonly results from local nerve infiltration in the neck or base of the skull.

Trigeminal nerve

The most common presentation is a constant dull, well-localized pain related to the underlying disease of bone and other somatic structures, and associated with paroxysmal episodes of lancinating or throbbing pain. Lesions of the middle and posterior fossa can present with classical trigeminal neuralgia.[174] However, metastases at the base of the skull or leptomeningeal metastases can both produce atypical facial pain.[175] Atypical trigeminal pain and sensory abnormalities in the peripheral distribution of the V nerve, occasionally associated with incomplete lesions of the VII nerve, have been reported with different facial neoplasms.[176–178]

Involvement of the mental nerve does not usually produce pain but can cause the 'numb chin syndrome'. This is a sign of bony disease of jaw or foramen ovale, but can also be found with tumours of the base of the skull or leptomeninges and local perineural spread of lip carcinoma. The symptom can occur months before the discovery of a bony lesion.[179]

Radiculopathy

Radiculopathy is usually caused by leptomeningeal metastases, or by the compression of nerve roots by vertebral or paraspinal lesions. The pain of a root lesion is usually focal and radiates in the distribution of the affected root. It is sometimes difficult to distinguish a polyradiculopathy from a plexus lesion and in these cases the neurological assessment can be expanded to include electrical studies of the paraspinal muscles, thus identifying the level of the lesion. CT and MRI are useful for imaging non-bony paraspinal lesions. MRI is necessary for imaging the epidural space.

Herpes zoster and post-herpetic neuralgia are common in patients with cancer(180) and should always be considered in the differential diagnosis of painful radiculopathies.

Cervical plexopathy

Infiltration of the cervical plexus by tumour can be a result of compression by head and neck neoplasms or can occur from metastasis to cervical nodes. Symptoms usually include local lancinating or dysaesthetic pain referred to the retro-auricular and nuchal areas, the shoulder, and the jaw. Sensory abnormalities define the affected (greater auricular and greater occipital) nerves.(169) The differential diagnosis should include post-radical neck dissection syndrome. The diagnosis may be difficult because of the major postoperative and postradiation changes often found in these patients.

CT or MRI scans are appropriate, and imaging of the cervical spine and paraspinal structures is very important in distinguishing between bony lesions, cervical radiculopathy, and epidural spinal cord compression.

Brachial plexopathy

Five per cent of the neurological consultations at a comprehensive cancer centre were found to be initiated by brachial plexopathy.(88) It occurs most often with breast and lung carcinoma and with lymphoma. The plexus can be compressed or infiltrated by tumour lying in contiguous structures, such as axillary or supraclavicular nodes or apex of the lung. Pain is the first symptom in 85 per cent of patients,(181) preceding other neurological symptoms or signs by weeks or months.

Breast and lung malignancies typically affect the lower plexus (C7–T1) (Fig. 3) and cause pain in the shoulder, elbow, hand, and the fourth and fifth finger. Lung tumours can affect the intercostobrachial nerve, giving rise to a pain syndrome and associated sensory disturbances in the axilla (C8–T1–T2).(182) The upper brachial plexus (C5–C6) can also be affected, especially by breast cancer, when pain is usually referred to the paraspinal region, shoulder, biceps region, elbow, and hand; burning dysaesthesia in the index finger or thumb is common. The hallmark of the syndrome is the neuropathic nature of the pain with numbness, paraesthesia, allodynia, and hyperaesthesia.

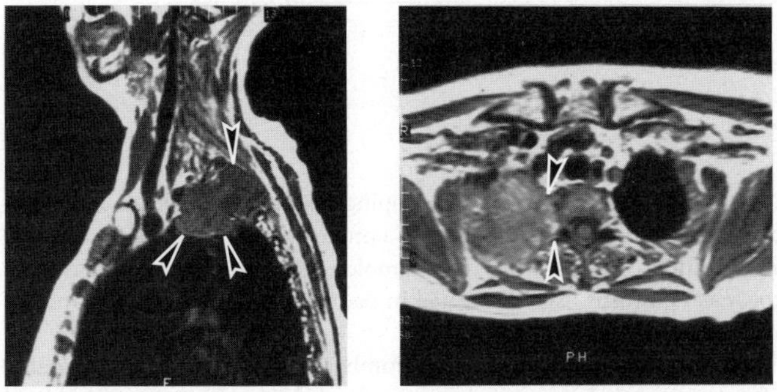

Fig. 3 MRI image. Lung tumour in the upper lobe compressing the lower trunk of the brachial plexus. Pain was reported in the inner aspect of the arm and paraesthesiae in the 5th and 4th finger. Left side: the arrows show the tumour mass invading the tissue planes in the area of the brachial plexus. Right side: the tumour is invading the left upper lobe, the arrows show the tumour invading one thoracic vertebral body. Reproduced with permission from Caraceni, A. (1996). Clinicopathologic correlates of common cancer pain syndromes. *Hematology and Oncology Clinics of North America* **10,** 57–78.

CT scan with narrow sections and contrast enhancement is effective in imaging soft tissue and bony structures in the plexus area. All patients with symptoms of brachial plexopathy should have a scan of the contiguous paravertebral region before radiation therapy, since extension of disease in this region is common (13/41 cases in one series). MRI is particularly useful in imaging the contiguous epidural space. While use of both techniques can give helpful complementary information in doubtful cases, sometimes neither is helpful even in cases of proven metastatic plexopathy.(183,184) Comparative data on specificity and sensitivity of the two techniques is lacking.

Epidural invasion will eventually occur in some patients with brachial plexopathy—six out of 41 in one series (Fig. 4).(185) Imaging of the epidural space is essential when patients develop Horner's syndrome, panplexopathy, vertebral body erosion, or a paraspinal mass detected on CT scan. These are often hallmark symptoms of tumour progression into the epidural space.(185)

Radiation fibrosis is important in the differential diagnosis of brachial plexopathy in cancer (Table 15), particularly in patients who have had radiotherapy and who present with upper plexus signs. Pain is often less prominent in patients with radiation-induced plexopathy.

Electrodiagnostic studies are helpful in distinguishing radiation-induced plexopathies from malignant invasion.(186) Sometimes, this differential diagnosis is difficult. MRI and CT scans may fail to distinguish fibrosis from tumour—in this case, surgical exploration of the plexus is necessary to rule out fibrosis, a new primary tumour, a radiation-induced tumour, or recurrent cancer.(181)

Lumbosacral plexopathy

Lumbosacral plexopathy is one of the most disabling complications of cancer. Although it is commonly associated with colorectal, cervical, and other pelvic malignancies (bladder, uterus, prostate, sarcoma, lymphoma) it can also be caused by breast or lung cancer or melanoma. Retroperitoneal

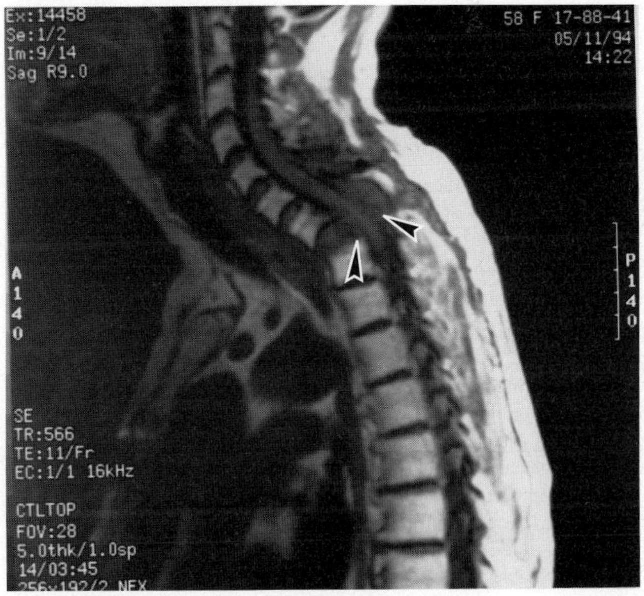

Fig. 4 MRI image in the same case as shown in Fig. 3. The tumour is invading the epidural canal and compressing the spinal cord. Reproduced with permission from Caraceni, A. (1996). Clinicopathologic correlates of common cancer pain syndromes. *Hematology and Oncology Clinics of North America* **10,** 57–78.

Table 15 Differential diagnosis of brachial plexopathy

	Tumour infiltration	Radiation fibrosis
Incidence of pain	89%	18%
Severity of pain	Severe in 98%	Mild to moderate
Dose of radiotherapy	—	>6000 cGy large fractions (>1900 cGy/day)
Latency	Not indicative	>6 months <5 years
Course	Progressive neurological dysfunction Pain progression with dysaesthetic quality C7–T1 distribution[a]	Progressive weakness Pain stabilizing with onset of weakness C5–C6 distribution
Horner	Can be present	Absent
CT scan findings[b]	Mass with tissue infiltration	Diffuse infiltration of tissue planes
MRI scan findings[b]	High signal intensity mass on T2-weighted images	Low signal intensity lesion on T_2-weighted images
Electromyography findings	Denervation no myochimia	Myochimia

[a] The distribution of the neurological findings can be helpful in some cases but it is not always indicative (see text for more details).

[b] The use of both techniques may provide complementary information. No method is totally credible in differentiating fibrosis from tumour.(184)

Table 16 Clinical findings in lumbosacral plexopathy due to cancer

	Upper plexopathy	Lower plexopathy	Panplexopathy
Local pain	Lower abdomen	Buttock, perineum	Lumbosacral
Referred pain	Flank, iliac crest	Hip and ankle	Variable
Radicular pain	Anterolateral thigh	Posterolateral thigh, leg	Variable
Paraesthesiae	Anterior thigh	Perineum, thigh, sole	Anterior thigh, leg, foot
Motor and reflex changes	L2–L4 Proximal leg weakness Patella reflex	L5–S1 Distal leg weakness Ankle reflex	L2–S2 Weakness can affect different muscle groups and reflexes
Sensory loss	Anterolateral thigh	Posterior thigh, sole	Anterior thigh, leg
Tenderness	Lumbar	Sciatic notch, sacrum	Lumbosacral
Positive SLRT			
Direct	50%	50%	83%
Reverse	15%	50%	83%
Leg oedema	41%	37%	83%
Rectal mass	25%	43%	15%
Anal sphincter weakness	0	50%	0

SLRT = straight leg raising test or Lasegue manoeuvre.

Modified from Jaeckle et al. (1985),(188) with permission.

tumours (e.g. sarcoma, metastatic nodal tumours) may affect the lumbosacral plexus or its roots more proximally.

The presenting symptom in almost all cases (93 per cent)(187) is pain in the buttocks or the legs; it often precedes other symptoms by weeks or months. It is usually followed by numbness, paraesthesia, weakness, and, later, leg oedema. The pain is usually aching or pressure-like in quality, and is rarely burning or dysaesthetic. In Jaeckle's series,(188) an upper plexopathy (L1–L4) was found in about one-third of cases, a lower plexopathy (L4–S1) in one-half of cases, and panplexopathy (L1–S3) in about 20 per cent (Table 16).

Other structures can be involved. These include roots of the plexus or contiguous structures, the sympathetic chain,(189) and psoas muscle.(190) Selective involvement of the L1, iliohypogastric, ilioinguinal, or genitofemoral nerves can produce pain and paraesthesia in the inguinal and scrotal region.

A sacral plexopathy, often overlapping a sacral polyradiculopathy, can be produced from direct extension of a presacral mass invading the sacrum, as sometimes occurs with rectosigmoid and bladder carcinomas. The coccygeal plexus is usually affected in patients with sphincter dysfunction and perineal 'saddle' sensory loss.

Tumour is often found in the lumbar vertebrae, sacrum, or pelvis of patients with lumbosacral plexopathy (45/76 patients) and epidural extension is also common, especially with retroperitoneal tumours. Hydroureter or hydronephrosis is extremely common at diagnosis.(187,188)

Lumbosacral plexopathy can occur after pelvic irradiation. Thomas et al.(187) reported that radiation-induced lumbosacral plexopathy very rarely presents with pain and has a median latency of 5 years from radiotherapy. Motor involvement is bilateral in 80 per cent of cases and electromyography can be a useful diagnostic tool. Other differential diagnoses include leptomeningeal carcinomatosis, cauda equina compression, and non-cancer-related causes of lumbar plexopathy—for example iliopsoas muscle haemorrhage or abscess, aortic aneurysm, idiopathic acute lumbosacral neuritis, and post-surgical compressive lesions, which often present as mononeuropathies.

MRI and CT scanning both image the lumbosacral plexus effectively. CT gives more information on the bony structures, while MRI is more accurate for soft tissues. The assessment should extend from L1 through the true pelvis,(184) and should include the spine and adjacent pelvic soft tissues.

Mononeuropathy

Mononeuropathy is less common than plexopathy or radicular lesions. It is caused by compression or infiltration of a nerve by bony lesions or by soft tissue masses in the limbs. Obturator,(191) femoral, and sciatic neuropathies are seen when tumour involves the soft tissue along the nerve distribution in the pelvis and thigh. Peroneal mononeuropathy can occur with bony lesions of the head of the fibula and sarcoma of the popliteal fossa. Ulnar and radial neuropathies result from bony lesions in the elbow or humerus.(192) These mononeuropathies must be distinguished from traumatic or compressive lesions, or from nutritional–metabolic lesions of nerves. Intercostal nerve neuropathy from invasion of the chest wall is the most common of the mononeuropathies caused by cancer.

Treatment of peripheral nerve compression

Radiation is indicated for all cases of plexopathy, neuropathy, and radiculopathy caused by tumour compression. Lesions caused by radioresistant tumours, such as sarcomas, are unlikely to respond. However, the results of radiotherapy in brachial plexopathy have been disappointing with only 46 per cent of patients reporting relief from pain in a retrospective series.(181)

Management of pain is often difficult in these syndromes; opioids are indicated and adjuvants for neuropathic pain should be used for specific indications. Clinical experience suggests that dexamethasone can be particularly effective for pain due to compression and oedema of peripheral nerves.

Peripheral neurolytic blocks, with alcohol or phenol, can be considered for severe arm and leg pain in patients with advanced plexus lesions. These blocks are sometimes associated with significant side-effects such as paresis and incontinence.(193) Sacral root blockade with phenol for perineal pain caused by root invasion is more acceptable when patients already have established urinary and rectal sphincter dysfunction. Late onset dysaesthesia may occur in long-term survivors (see Chapter 8.2.6).

Percutaneous cordotomy is feasible for the pain of lumbosacral plexopathy. Brachial plexopathy is more difficult to treat with cordotomy because the cervical dermatomes up to C4 must be included. This is technically difficult and increases the risk of respiratory depression and neurological sequelae. A short prognosis (6 months to 1 year) is required to avoid long-term post-cordotomy dysaesthetic pain (see Chapter 8.2.7).(194–196)

Peripheral polyneuropathy

Polyneuropathy in cancer patients can be caused by neurotoxicity of chemotherapy, metabolic nutritional deficiency, or paraneoplastic syndromes; the aetiology of the condition is summarized in Table 17.(197,198) Sub-clinical dysfunction of small and large sensory fibres can be demonstrated with quantitative sensory testing in 30–40 per cent of cancer patients.(199)

Peripheral neuropathy is characterized by a stocking–glove distribution of negative sensory (hypoaesthesia) and positive sensory symptoms, including painless paraesthesia or distressing burning dysaesthesia, allodynia, and hyperalgesia. Early sensory loss and later motor signs (weakness) are characteristic of some drug-induced sensorimotor neuropathies (vincristine, paclitaxel). Sensory involvement can be selective in neuropathies associated with cisplatin or paraneoplastic syndromes. Often the only early sign of polyneuropathy is reduction or loss of the ankle reflex. Muscle cramps may be associated with neuropathy and can sometimes be

Table 17 Polyneuropathies and peripheral neuropathies

Related to cancer
Myeloma associated neuropathies
Paraneoplastic sensory neuronopathy (Denny–Brown)
Sensory–motor peripheral neuropathy
Nutritional factors (cachexia-associated neuromyopathy[a])
Cancer related metabolic dysfunction: hepatic, renal
Infiltration of peripheral nerves (lymphomas, leukaemias)[b]
Vascular (haemorrhagic or ischaemic) peripheral nerve lesion[b]
Related to chemotherapy and radiation
Vincristine
Vinblastine
Vinorelbine
Cisplatin
Oxelipletin
Paclitaxel
Suramin
Radiation to limbs with worsening of vincristine neuropathy
Non-cancer related
Metabolic dysfunction: diabetes

[a] Very frequent.

[b] Mononeuritis multiplex.

Table 18 Muscle cramps in cancer

Aetiology	Number of patients
Peripheral neuropathy	22
Root and plexus pathology	17
Polymyositis	2
Hypomagnesaemia	1
Unknown	9

Modified from Steiner, I. and Siegal, T. (1989). Muscle cramps in cancer patients. *Cancer* **63**, 574–7, with permission.

prominent symptoms in vincristine neuropathy.(200) Muscle cramps are relatively frequent in cancer (see Table 18 for different aetiologies).

Paraneoplastic sensory neuropathy and sensory neuropathy caused by vincristine or paclitaxel is often more painful than that caused by cisplatin. Cisplatin induces a sensory neuronopathy mainly affecting the cells of the dorsal root ganglia with predominant involvement of the large fibre functions (proprioception) which causes sensory ataxia rather than pain. Vinca alkaloids and paclitaxel produce a mostly sensory axonopathy with some motor component.

Clinical examination is usually sufficient for diagnosis although nerve conduction studies and electromyography can be used.(201) Treatment is palliative, with analgesics and adjuvants (see Chapter 8.2.5).

Cerebrovascular disorders in patients with cancer

Cerebrovascular disease in patients with cancer is not uncommon. It is often tumour related, either as a direct effect of the tumour or its treatment or as an indirect effect of coagulation changes. Coronary and cerebral arteriosclerosis is less common in patients dying of cancer than in the general population.(16) In one study, cerebrovascular lesions were found at autopsy in 15 per cent of cases(202) and half of these patients had clinical symptoms related to the pathological findings. There were 500 vascular lesions, of which 244 were haemorrhagic and 256 ischaemic. Only 72 of the ischaemic lesions were related to atherosclerosis and nine haemorrhages were hypertensive, the remaining lesions being related to tumour-associated conditions. Haemorrhagic diatheses (thrombocytopenia, disseminated intravascular coagulation) or hypercoagulability states are common causes.

Cerebral haematoma is more common than subarachnoid haemorrhage and is the complication most frequently seen in leukaemia. Ischaemic complications caused by thrombotic emboli due to non-bacterial thrombotic endocarditis are a frequent finding at autopsy in patients with advanced cancer but are difficult to demonstrate *in vivo* since transoesophageal echocardiography is required.[203,204] Treatment with heparin is recommended.[16]

Multiple microinfarcts can produce a global encephalopathy associated with mild disseminated intravascular coagulation, but with no laboratory abnormalities, in patients with leukaemia, lymphoma, or breast cancer.[205] Other syndromes are listed in Table 19.[206–211]

Paraneoplastic syndromes

The pathogenesis of remote effects of systemic cancer on the nervous system is unknown, although autoimmune processes are seen in many syndromes and autoantibody determinations are sometimes helpful in diagnosis.[161,212,213] Paraneoplastic syndromes are rare, probably affecting less than 1 per cent of patients with cancer (see also Table 1), even if the most commonly associated neoplasms, such as small-cell lung cancer and ovarian cancer are considered.[198] Some classic paraneoplastic syndromes can be recognized and diagnosed with confidence (Table 20). Cerebellar degeneration associated with ovarian and lung cancer, or peripheral neuronopathy and limbic encephalitis associated with small-cell tumours of the lung are relatively stereotyped clinico-pathological entities associated with the presence of specific autoantibodies (anti-Yo for cerebellar degeneration and anti-Hu for neuronopathy with encephalomyelitis).[16] Opsoclonus–myoclonus and Lambert–Eaton myasthenic syndrome occurring in children with neuroblastomas and in small-cell lung cancer, respectively, are also classic in their presentation. However, many syndromes present with varying symptoms, affecting the brain and cranial nerves, spinal cord and dorsal root ganglia, and peripheral nerves and muscles, and pose a difficult diagnostic problem.[16] There is little in the literature on these syndromes, although the term encephalomyelitis is reserved by some authors for those patients with evidence of widespread neurological dysfunction without findings predominantly in one particular area.[212,213]

In general, neurological symptoms develop acutely and are severe. Subtle, long-lasting symptoms are not usually caused by paraneoplastic syndrome. Examination of CSF and immunofluorescence techniques for testing circulating autoantibodies can aid diagnosis. MRI scans are usually normal.[214]

The clinical course is independent of that of the original tumour, which in 50 per cent of cases is found after the onset of neurological symptoms, and is often small and slow growing with a relatively benign course.[16] Remission of the neurological symptoms only occasionally follows treatment of the tumour. Spontaneous remissions have been seen but the syndrome is usually irreversible.[16] The results of treatment are poor; steroids and plasmapheresis are not effective except in the Lambert–Eaton syndrome, where plasmapheresis is indicated.

Lambert–Eaton myasthenic syndrome presents with muscle weakness and fatiguability. Proximal muscles are affected and bulbar musculature usually spared. Strength initially improves with exercise and examination can therefore be ambiguous since power can improve during testing, although weakness recurs after continuous effort. Fifty per cent of patients have dry mouth and impotence. The diagnosis is made by electromyography, with a classic finding of small compound action potentials which increase with exercise. Repetitive stimulation at a low and high rate produces a decrease and increase in the compound action potential, respectively.

The syndrome is caused by a reduced release of acetylcholine from presynaptic membranes. Most patients have autoantibodies which react with the calcium channels at the cholinergic synapse level. The Lambert–Eaton syndrome is the only paraneoplastic syndrome for which an autoimmune pathogenesis has been proved with animal models. It often responds to immunosuppression and plasmapheresis.

Table 19 Cerebrovascular complications of cancer

Central nervous system complication	Mechanism
Cerebral haemorrhage	Intratumoural bleeding[a] Disseminated intravascular coagulation[b] Coagulopathy[b] Leukostasis[c]
Subdural haematoma	Dural metastases[d] Coagulopathy[d]
Embolic infarct	Non-bacterial thrombotic endocarditis[d] Tumour embolism[d] Fungal embolism[b]
Sinus thrombosis	Dural, bony tumour[d] Coagulopathy[d] L-asparaginase[b]
Thrombotic microinfarcts	Disseminated intravascular coagulation[b,d]

[a] Associated with cerebral and leptomeningeal tumour.

[b] Associated with leukaemia/lymphoma.

[c] Only found with leucocytes ≥ 100 000.

[d] Associated with solid tumours.

Table 20 Paraneoplastic neurological syndromes

Lambert–Eaton myasthenic syndrome
Sub-acute cerebellar degeneration
Sub-acute sensory neuronopathy
Opsoclonus–myoclonus
Motor neuronopathy (with lymphoma)
Limbic encephalitis

Adverse neurological effects of anticancer therapy

Surgery, chemotherapy, or radiation can cause neurological syndromes.[16,215] They are discussed in greater detail elsewhere in this textbook (see Chapter 8.1.1). In particular, irradiation of the brain can produce multiple acute and chronic adverse effects;[216] acute effects include worsening of neurological symptoms, somnolence, and Lhermitte's sign, and the main chronic effect is dementia caused by radiation necrosis and leucoencephalopathy.

Neuropathic pain syndromes

Neuropathic pain syndromes include those in which the pain process is thought to be sustained by a lesion in the peripheral or central nervous system. Abnormal processing of the somatosensory signal at peripheral and/or central level is thought to play a major role in the pathogenesis of the pain.[217] The pathophysiology of neuropathic pain conditions has been widely studied and various experimental mechanisms have clinical relevance. All suggest an abnormal function in the periphery (mainly the nociceptor) and in the central component of the pain pathways (the spinothalamic neurones in the dorsal horn and the spinothalamic tract).[218–220] These mechanisms may not be totally specific for the known neuropathic syndromes; they may also be involved in non-neuropathic chronic pain conditions (see Chapters 8.2.1 and 8.2.2).[217–221]

Table 21 lists the most clearly defined neuropathic pain syndromes. In cancer patients, many treatment-related syndromes can produce neuropathic pain and many cases of compression or infiltration by tumour have the same neuropathic mechanism and clinical features. Some authors report that pain caused by compression is more often aching and severe (nociceptive nerve pain), but with less neurological dysfunction, while invasive lesions cause more dysaesthetic sensation, burning pain, paraesthesia, or neuralgic pain (neuropathic pain).[222]

All neuropathic syndromes have some factors in common, albeit variably so (Table 22). Symptoms caused by the neurological lesion will depend on its location and will affect function accordingly, but the lesion will always involve the sensory system (sometimes selectively) when there is neuropathic pain. The sensory systems most affected are pain and temperature; less commonly vibration and two-point discrimination are affected. This is consistent with the observation that in painful peripheral neuropathies small fibres, which subserve pain and temperature sensation, are more often involved, whereas in central lesions associated with pain the spinothalamic system is more often affected.[223–227]

Manifestations vary with the underlying cause. Allodynia, for example, is typical of post-herpetic neuralgia (87 per cent of cases in one study)[225] but is not always present in central pain after stroke (57 per cent)[224,228] and is rarely present in central pain caused by multiple sclerosis.[227]

Table 21 Neuropathic pain syndromes

Painful peripheral neuropathies
Painful mononeuropathies
Plexopathies
Phantom limb pain
Post-herpetic neuralgia
Avulsion of the brachial plexus
Injury to the spinal cord
Cerebrovascular lesion to the thalamus, subcortical, or cortical structures
Syringomyelia
Sympathetically maintained pain syndromes, reflex sympathetic dystrophy

Table 22 Common sensory neurological findings in neuropathic pain

Spontaneous pain
Burning, shooting, lancinating
Negative findings
Hypoaesthesia to touch and vibratory stimulation
Hypoalgesia to pinprick
Hypoaesthesia to thermal (warm and cold) stimuli
Enhanced thermal pain threshold to quantitative sensory testing
Positive findings
Paraesthesiae
Abnormal non-painful sensations
Dysaesthesias
Abnormal uncomfortable sensations
Allodynia
Painful sensation evoked by a non-noxious stimulus
Hyperalgesia
Exaggerated response to a noxious stimulus
Hyperpathia
Exaggerated painful response to a noxious or non-noxious stimulus e.g., when the burning pain evoked by light touching (= allodynia) outlasts for seconds or minutes the duration of the stimulus

Painful polyneuropathies

A number of polyneuropathies can be painful. Many are characterized by axonal damage of the sensory fibres, particularly small diameter fibres important for temperature and pain sensation. They include diabetic neuropathy, AIDS-related neuropathy, alcohol–nutritional neuropathy, toxic neuropathies caused by thallium and arsenic, and some rare hereditary neuropathies.[229] Paraneoplastic sensory neuronopathy, in which all sensory modalities are affected, is also painful. Other peripheral nerve lesions which produce pain are more heterogeneous. This group includes leprous neuritis, Guillain–Barré syndrome, compression of spinal roots, and brachial neuritis.

Post-herpetic neuralgia

Post-herpetic neuralgia is a common cause of neuropathic pain, occurring in the dermatomal distribution of previous herpes zoster infection; the condition is usually defined as pain persisting 1 month after herpes zoster. It is more common in the elderly patient and in patients with cancer, particularly those with disease of the midthoracic dermatomes and of the ophthalmic branch of the trigeminal nerve. Pain is referred to the affected dermatomes; common symptoms are constant burning or aching pain, intermittent paroxysmal spontaneous episodes of lancinating pain, and pain induced by otherwise innocuous tactile and thermal stimulation (allodynia). Pathological examination shows pronounced lesions in the dorsal root ganglia sometimes extending into the spinal cord.[230] Clinical and quantitative sensory testing shows hypalgesia and hypaesthesia to touch, vibration, pinprick, and thermal stimulation in the affected dermatomes in all cases. Often pain is most severe where hyperaesthesia is most marked. Allodynia and hyperaesthesia are also commonly present.[225,231] After 12 months or more, spontaneous resolution of the pain will occur in many patients.[232] A comprehensive review of available treatment can be found in the literature.[233]

The treatment of neuropathic pain is also reviewed elsewhere in this textbook (Chapter 8.2.10). Tricyclic antidepressants have an established role in the treatment of this difficult pain syndrome but recent researches suggest that opioids are also effective analgesics in post-herpetic neuralgia;[234] topical capsaicin can be helpful in some cases, but is often poorly tolerated,[235] and topical lignocaine (lidocaine) proved effective in a recent double-blind controlled trial.[236] Local anaesthetic blockade is temporarily effective while sympathetic block proved totally ineffective.[237] *N*-methyl-D-aspartate receptor antagonists are the subject of ongoing experimental trials.[238]

Sympathetically maintained pain

Reflex sympathetic dystrophy (RDS or complex regional pain syndrome type 1 according to the new taxonomy)[239] and causalgia (or complex regional pain syndrome type 2)[239] are terms defining pain with associated dysautonomic and trophic changes following a soft tissue injury (RDS) or injury to a major mixed or sensory nerve (causalgia). It has been observed that patients with these syndromes benefit, sometimes, from sympathetic blockade, thus supporting the hypothesis that the sympathetic nervous system adversely mediates them.[240] However, the pathogenesis of sympathetically-mediated neuropathic pain syndromes remains unclear.[239–243] In controlled clinical experience, the efficacy of sympathetic blockade in neuropathic pain is unpredictable and disappointing,[237,244,245] as is regional sympathetic blockade with guanethidine.[246] It is difficult, therefore, to identify patients who might benefit from a sympathetic block, and it has been suggested that a test block be used in those patients showing signs of vasomotor and/or trophic changes in the affected area (see Chapters 8.2.6 and 8.2.7).[219]

References

1. **Lundberg, N.** (1960). Continuous recording and control of ventricular fluid pressure in neurosurgical practice. *Acta Psychiatrica et Neurologica Scandinavica* **36** (Suppl. 149).

2. **Ingwar, D. and Lundberg, N.** (1961). Paroxismal symptoms in intracranial hypertension, studies with ventricular fluid pressure recording and electroencefalography. *Brain* **84**, 446–59.
3. **Plum, F. and Posner, J.B.** *The Diagnosis of Stupor and Coma*, Vol. 19. Philadelphia: F.A. Davis, 1980.
4. **Klatzo, I.** (1967). Neuropathological aspects of brain edema. *Journal of Neuropathology and Experimental Neurology* **26**, 1–14.
5. **Rosner, M., Rosner, S., and Johnson, A.** (1995). Cerebral perfusion pressure: management protocol and clinical results. *Journal of Neurosurgery* **83**, 949–62.
6. **Robertson, C.** (2001). Management of cerebral perfusion pressure after traumatic brain injury. *Anesthesiology* **95**, 1513–17.
7. **Lundberg, N., Kjallquist, A., and Bien, C.** (1959). Reduction of increased intracranial pressure by hyperventilation. *Acta Psychiatrica et Neurologica Scandinavica* **34** (Suppl. 139).
8. **Howe, H.** (1925). Reduction of normal cerebrospinal fluid pressure by intravenous administration of hypertonic solutions. *Archives of Neurology and Psychiatry* **14**, 315–26.
9. **Rottenberg, D., Hurwitz, B., and Posner, J.** (1977). The effect of oral glycerol on intraventricular pressure in man. *Neurology* **27**, 600–8.
10. **Nau, R.** (2000). Osmotherapy for elevated intracranial pressure. A critical reappraisal. *Clinical Pharmacokinetics* **38**, 23–40.
11. **Lyons, M. and Meyer, F.** (1990). Cerebrospinal fluid physiology and the management of increased intracranial pressure. *Mayo Clinic Proceedings* **65**, 684–707.
12. **Galicich, J.H. and French, L.A.** (1961). Use of dexamethasone in the treatment of cerebral edema resulting from brain tumors and surgery. *American Practitioner and Digest of Treatment* **12**, 169–74.
13. **Koehler, P.** (1995). Use of corticosteroids in neuro-oncology. *Anticancer Drugs* **6**, 19–33.
14. **Schimmer, B. and Parker, K.** (2001). Adrenocorticotropic hormone: adrenocortical steroids and their synthetic analogs; inhibitors of the synthesis and actions of adrenocortical hormones. In *Goodman & Gilman's The Pharmacological Basis of Therapeutics* (ed. J.G. Hardman and L.E. Limbird), pp. 1649–77. New York: McGraw-Hill.
15. **Vecht, C.J., Hovestadt, A., Verbiest, H.B.C., van Vliet, J.J., and van Putten, W.L.J.** (1994). Dose–effect relationship of dexamethasone on Karnofsky performance in metastatic brain tumor: a randomized study of doses of 4, 8, 16 mg per day. *Neurology* **44**, 675–80.
16. **Posner, J.B.** Neurologic complications of cancer. *Contemporary Neurology Series*, Vol. 45. Philadelphia: F.A. Davis, 1995.
17. **Sepkowitz, K.A., Brown, A.E., Telzak, E.E., Gottlieb, S., and Armstrong, D.** (1992). Pneumocystis carinii pneumonia among patients without AIDS at a cancer hospital. *Journal of the American Medical Association* **267**, 832.
18. **Slivka, A.** et al. (1993). Pneumocystis carinii pneumonia during steroid taper in patients with primary brain tumors. *American Journal of Medicine* **94**, 216–19.
19. **Twycross, R.** (1992). Corticosteroids in advanced cancer. *British Medical Journal* **305**, 969–70 (editorial; comment).
20. **Batchelor, T., Taylor, L., Thaler, H., Posner, J., and DeAngelis, L.** (1997). Steroid myopathy in cancer patients. *Neurology* **48**, 1234–8.
21. **McCluskey, J. and Gutteridge, D.** (1982). Avascular necrosis of bone after high doses of dexamethasone during neurosurgery. *British Medical Journal* **284**, 333–4.
22. **Ellershaw, J.** (1994). Corticosteroids and peptic ulceration. *Palliative Medicine* **8**, 313–19.
23. **Cushing, H.** (1932). Peptic ulcers and the interbrain. *Surgery, Gynecology and Obstetrics* **55**, 1–35.
24. **LeWitt, P., Barton, N., and Posner, J.** (1982). Hiccup with dexamethasone therapy. *Annals of Neurology* **12**, 405–6.
25. **Baethge, B.A. and Lidsky, M.D.** (1986). Intractable hiccups associated with high-dose intravenous methylprednisolone therapy. *Annals of Internal Medicine* **104**, 58–9.
26. **Vanelle, J.-M., Aubin, F., and Michel, F.** (1990). Les complications psychiatriques de la corticotherapie. *La Revue du Praticien* **40**, 556–8.
27. **Freedmann, M., Schocket, A., Chapel, N., and Gerber, J.** (1981). Anaphylaxis after intravenous methylprednisolone administration. *Journal of the American Medical Association* **245**, 607–8.
28. **Garbe, E., LeLorier, J., Boivin, J.-F., and Suissa, S.** (1997). Risk of ocular hypertension or open-angle glaucoma in elderly patients on oral glucocorticoids. *Lancet* **350**, 979–82.
29. **Cumming, R., Mitchell, P., and Leeder, S.** (1997). Use of inhaled corticosteroids and the risk of cataracts. *New England Journal of Medicine* **337**, 8–14.
30. **Baharav, E., Harpaz, D., Mittelman, M., and Lewinski, U.** (1986). Dexamethasone-induced perineal irritation. *New England Journal of Medicine* **314**, 315–16.
31. **Helfer, E. and Rose, L.** (1989). Corticosteroids and adrenal suppression. Characterising and avoiding the problem. *Drugs* **38**, 838–45.
32. **Dixon, R.A. and Christy, N.P.** (1980). On the various forms of corticosteroid withdrawal syndrome. *American Journal of Medicine* **68**, 224–30.
33. **Jalladeau, E., Carpentier, A., Napolitano, M., and Delattre, J.-Y.** (2000). Lipomatosi epidurale cortico-induite. *Revue Neurologique* **156**, 517–19.
34. **Walker, A. and Adamkiewicz, J.** (1964). Pseudotumor cerebri associated with prolonged corticosteroid therapy. *Journal of the American Medical Association* **188**, 779–84.
35. **Victor, M. and Ropper, A.** *Adams and Victor's Principles of Neurology.* New York: McGraw-Hill, 2001.
36. **Delanty, N., Vaughan, C., and French, J.** (1998). Medical causes of seizures. *Lancet* **352**, 383–90.
37. **Martinez-Rodriguez, J.** et al. (2001). Nonconvulsive status epilepticus associated with cephalosporins in patients with renal failure. *American Journal of Medicine* **111**, 115–19.
38. **Posner, J.B.** (1992). Management of brain metastases. *Revue Neurologique* **148**, 477–87.
39. **McNamara, J.** (2001). Drugs effective in the therapy of the epilepsies. In *Goodman & Gilman's The Pharmacological Basis of Therapeutics* (ed. J.G. Hardman and L.E. Limbird), pp. 521–47. New York: McGraw-Hill.
40. **Cohen, N., Strauss, G., Lew, R., Silver, D., and Recht, L.** (1988). Should prophylactic anticonvulsants be administered to patients with newly-diagnosed cerebral metastases? A retrospective analysis. *Journal of Clinical Oncology* **6**, 1621–4.
41. **Franceschetti, S.** et al. (1990). Influence of surgery and antiepileptic drugs on seizures symptomatic of cerebral tumours. *Acta Neurochirurgica* **103**, 47–51.
42. **Glantz, M.** et al. (1994). Double blind randomized, placebo-controlled trial of anticonvulsants prophylaxis in adults with newly diagnosed brain metastases. *Proceedings of the American Society of Clinical Oncologists* **13**, 176.
43. **Glantz, M.** et al. (2000). Practice parameter: anticonvulsivant prophylaxis in patients with newly diagnosed brain tumors. *Neurology* **54**, 1886–93.
44. **Hagen, N.A. Cirrincione, C., Thaler, H.T., and DeAngelis, L.** (1990). The role of radiation therapy following resection of single brain metastasis from melanoma. *Neurology* **40**, 158–60.
45. **Delattre, J., Safai, B., and Posner, J.B.** (1988). Erythema multiforme and Stevens–Johnson syndrome in patients receiving cranial irradiation and phenythoin. *Neurology* **38**, 194–8.
46. **Taylor, L.P. and Posner, J.B.** (1989). Phenobarbital rheumatism in patients with brain tumor. *Annals of Neurology* **25**, 92–4.
47. **Posner, J.B.** (1992). Supportive care in the neuro-oncology patient. In *Management in Neuro-oncology* (ed. J. Hildebrand), pp. 89–103. Berlin: Springer-Verlag.
48. **Gabor, A., Brooks, A., Scobey, R., and Parsons, G.** (1984). Intracranial pressure during epileptic seizures. *Electroencephalography and Clinical Neurophysiology* **57**, 497–506.
49. **Perry, J. and Sawka, C.** (1996). Add-on gabapentin for refractory seizures in patients with brain tumours. *Canadian Journal of Neurological Sciences* **23**, 128–31.
50. **Shorvon, S.** *Status Epilepticus. Its Clinical Features and Treatment in Children and Adults.* Cambridge: Cambridge University Press, 1994.
51. **Towne, A.** et al. (2000). Prevelence of nonconvulsive status epilepticus in comatose patients. *Neurology* **54**, 340–5.
52. **Roberts, M. and Humphrey, P.** (1988). Prolonged complex partial status epilepticus: a case report. *Journal of Neurology, Neurosurgery, and Psychiatry* **51**, 586–92.
53. **Chapman, M., Smith, M., and Hirsch, N.** (2001). Status epilepticus. *Anesthesia* **56**, 648–59.

54. **Treiman, D.** et al. (1998). A comparison of four treatments for generalized convulsive status epilepticus. *New England Journal of Medicine* **339**, 792–8.

55. **Alldredge, B.** et al. (2001). A comparison of lorazepam, diazepam, and placebo for the treatment of out-of-hospital status epilepticus. *New England Journal of Medicine* **345**, 631–7.

56. **Yoshikawa, H., Yamazaki, S., Abe, T., and Oda, Y.** (2000). Midazolam as a first-line agent for status epilepticus in children. *Brain & Development* **22**, 239–42.

57. **Prasad, A., Worral, B., Bertram, E., and Bleck, T.** (2001). Propofol and midazolam in the treatment of refractory status epilepticus. *Epilepsia* **42**, 380–6.

58. **Wheless, J.** (1998). Pediatric use of intravenous and intramuscular phenytoin: lesson learned. *Journal of Child Neurology* **13**, s11–14.

59. **Meek, P.** et al. (1999). Guidelines for nonemergency use of parenteral phenytoin products: proceedings of an expert panel consensus process. Panel on Nonemergency Use of Parenteral Phenytoin Products. *Archives of Internal Medicine* **159**, 2639–44.

60. **Begemann, M., Rowan, A., and Tuhrim, S.** (2000). Treatment of refractory complex-partial status epilepticus with propofol: case report. *Epilepsia* **41**, 105–9.

61. **Limdi, N. and Faught, E.** (2000). The safety of rapid valproic acid infusion. *Epilepsia* **41**, 1342–5.

62. **Krumholz, A.** (1999). Nonepileptic seizures: diagnosis and management. *Neurology* **52**, s76–83.

63. **Pellock, J.** (1999). Status epilepticus. In *Pediatric Neurology. Principles & Practice* (ed. K. Swaiman and S. Ashwal), pp. 683–91. St Louis Baltimora: Mosby, 1999.

64. **Lipowski, Z.J.** *Delirium: Acute Confusional States.* New York: Oxford University Press, 1990, p. 490.

65. **American Psychiatric Association.** *Diagnostic and Statistical Manual of Mental Disorders*, 4th edn. Text revision. DSM IV-TR. Washington DC: American Psychiatric Press, 2000.

66. **Adams, R.D. and Victor, M.** *Principles of Neurology.* New York: McGraw-Hill, 1997.

67. **Engel, G.L. and Romano, J.** (1959). Delirium: a syndrome of cerebral insufficiency. *Journal of Chronic Diseases* **9**, 260–77.

68. **Itil, T. and Fink, M.** (1968). EEG and behavioral aspects of the interaction of anticholinergic hallucinogens with centrally active compounds. *Progress in Brain Research* **28**, 149–68.

69. **Crum, R.M., Anthony, J.C., Basset, S.S., and Folstein, M.F.** (1993). Population-based norms for the Mini-Mental State Examination by age and educational level. *Journal of the American Medical Association* **269**, 2386–91.

70. **Grassi, L.** et al. (2001). Assessing delirium in cancer patients: the Italian versions of the Delirium Rating Scale and the Memorial Delirium Assessment Scale. *Journal of Pain and Symptom Management* **21**, 59–68.

71. **Inouye, S.K., van Dyck, C.H., Alessi, C.A., Balkin, S., Siegal, A.P., and Horwitz, R.I.** (1990). Clarifying confusion: the confusion assessment method. A new method for detection of delirium. *Annals of Internal Medicine* **113**, 941–8.

72. **Inouye, S.K., Foreman, M.D., Mion, L.C., Katz, K.H., and Cooney, L.M.J.** (2001). Nurses' recognition of delirium and its symptoms: comparison of nurse and researcher ratings. *Archives of Internal Medicine* **161**, 2467–73.

73. **Trzepacz, P.T., Baker, R.W., and Greenhouse, J.** (1988). A symptom rating scale for delirium. *Psychiatry Research* **23**, 89–97.

74. **Trzepacz, P.T., Mittal, D., Torres, R., Kanary, K., Norton, J., and Jimerson, N.** (2001). Validation of the delirium rating scale-revised-98: comparison with the delirium rating scale and the cognitive test for delirium. *Journal of Neuropsychiatry and Clinical Neurosciences* **13**, 229–42.

75. **Breitbart, W., Rosenfeld, B., Roth, A., Smith, M.J., Cohen, K., and Passik, S.** (1997). The Memorial Delirium Assessment Scale. *Journal of Pain and Symptom Management* **13**, 128–37.

76. **Liptzin, B. and Levkoff, S.E.** (1992). An empirical study of delirium subtypes. *British Journal of Psychiatry* **161**, 843–5.

77. **Meagher, D., O'Hanlon, D., O'Mahony, E., Casey, P., and Trzepacz, P.** (1998). Relationship between etiology and phenomenologic profile in delirium. *Journal of Geriatric Psychiatry and Neurology* **11**, 146–9; discussion 157–8.

78. **Wallesch, C.W. and Hundsaltz, A.** (1994). Language function in delirium: a comparison of single word processing in acute confusional state and probable Alzheimer's disease. *Brain & Language* **46**, 592–606.

79. **Chedru, F. and Geschwind, N.** (1972). Writing disturbances in acute confusional state. *Neuropsychologia* **10**, 343–53.

80. **Baranowski, S.L. and Patten, S.B.** (2000). The predictive value of dysgraphia and constructional apraxia for delirium in psychiatric patients. *Canadian Journal of Psychiatry* **45**, 75–8.

81. **Macleod, A.D. and Whitehead, L.E.** (1997). Dysgraphia in terminal delirium. *Palliative Medicine* **11**, 127–32.

82. **Chedru, F. and Geschwind, N.** (1972). Disorders of higher cortical functions in acute confusional states. *Cortex* **8**, 395–411.

83. **Wolf, H.G. and Curran, D.** (1935). Nature of delirium and allied states. The disergastic reaction. *Archives of Neurology and Psychiatry* **33**, 1175–215.

84. **Bruera, E., Fainsinger, R.L., Miller, M.J., and Kuehn, N.** (1992). The assessment of pain intensity in patients with cognitive failure: a preliminary report. *Journal of Pain and Symptom Management* **7**, 267–70.

85. **Derogatis, L.R., Morrow, G.R., Fetting, J., Penman, D., Piasetsky, S., and Schmale, A.M.** (1983). The prevalence of psychiatric disorders among cancer patients. *Journal of the American Medical Association* **249**, 751–7.

86. **Francis, J., Martin, D., and Kapoor, W.N.** (1990). A prospective study of delirium in hospitalized elderly. *Journal of the American Medical Association* **263**, 1097–101.

87. **Levkoff, S.E.** et al. (1992). Delirium. The occurence and persistence of symptoms among elderly hospitalized patients. *Archives of Internal Medicine* **152**, 334–40.

88. **Clouston, P.D., De Angelis, L., and Posner, J.B.** (1992). The spectrum of neurological disease in patients with systemic cancer. *Annals of Neurology* **31**, 268–73.

89. **Minagawa, H., Yosuke, U., Yamawaki, S., and Ishitani, K.** (1996). Psychiatric morbidity in terminally ill cancer patients. *Cancer* **78**, 1131–7.

90. **Caraceni, A.** et al. (2000). The impact of delirium on the short-term prognosis of advanced cancer patients. *Cancer* **89**, 1145–8.

91. **Gagnon, P., Allard, P., Masse, B., and DeSerres, M.** (2000). Delirium in terminal cancer: a prospective study using daily screening, early diagnosis and continuous monitoring. *Journal of Pain and Symptom Management* **19**, 412–26.

92. **Lawlor, P.G.** et al. (2000). Occurrence, causes and outcome of delirium in patients with advanced cancer. *Archives of Internal Medicine* **160**, 786–94.

93. **Farrell, K.R. and Ganzini, L.** (1995). Misdiagnosing delirium as depression in medically ill elderly patients. *Archives of Internal Medicine* **155**, 2459–64.

94. **Lewis, L.M., Miller, D.K., Morley, J.E., Nork, M.J., and Lasater, L.C.** (1995). Unrecognized delirium in ED geriatric patients. *American Journal of Emergency Medicine* **13**, 142–5.

95. **Johnson, J.C., Kerse, N.M., Gottlieb, G., Wanich, C., Sullivan, E., and Chen, K.** (1992). Prospective versus retrospective methods of identifying patients with delirium. *Journal of the American Geriatrics Society* **40**, 316–19.

96. **Inouye, S.K., Viscoli, C.M., Horwitz, R.I., Hurst, L.D., and Tinetti, M.E.** (1993). A predictive model for delirium in hospitalized elderly medical patients based on admission characteristics. *Annals of Internal Medicine* **119**, 474–81.

97. **Inouye, S.K. and Charpentier, P.A.** (1996). Precipitating factors for delirium in hospitalized elderly persons. Predictive model and interrelationship with baseline vulnerability. *Journal of the American Medical Association* **275**, 852–7.

98. **Inouye, S.K.** et al. (1999). A multicomponent intervention to prevent delirium in hospitalized older patients. *New England Journal of Medicine* **340**, 669–76.

99. **Schor, J.D.** et al. (1992). Risk factors for delirium in hospitalized elderly. *Journal of the American Medical Association* **267**, 827–31.

100. **Williams-Russo, P., Urquhart, B.L., Sharrock, N.E., and Charlson, M.E.** (1992). Postoperative delirium: predictors and prognosis in elderly orthopedics patients. *Journal of the American Geriatrics Society* **40**, 759–67.

101. **Marcantonio, E.R.** et al. (1994). A clinical prediction rule for delirium after elective noncardiac surgery. *Journal of the American Medical Association* **271**, 134–9.

102. **Tune, L., Carr, S., Cooper, T., Klug, B., and Golinger, R.C.** (1993). Association of anticholinergic activity of prescribed medications with

postoperative delirium. *Journal of Neuropsychiatry Clinical Neurosciences* 5, 208–10.

103. **Tuma, R. and DeAngelis, L.M.** (2000). Altered mental status in patients with cancer. *Archives of Neurology* **57**, 1727–31.
104. **Stiefel, F. and Morant, R.** (1991). Morphine intoxication during acute reversible renal insufficiency. *Journal of Palliative Care* **7**, 45–7.
105. **Fainsinger, R., Schoeller, T., Boiskin, M., and Bruera, E.** (1993). Palliative care round: cognitive failure (CF) and coma after renal failure in a patient receiving captopril and hydromorphone. *Journal of Palliative Care* **9**, 53–5.
106. **Bortolussi, R.** et al. (1994). Acute morphine intoxication during high-dose recombinant Interleukin-2 treatment for metastatic renal cell cancer. *European Journal of Cancer* **30A**, 1905–7.
107. **Posner, J.B.** (1980). Clinical manifestations of brain metastasis. In *Brain Metastasis* (ed. L. Weiss, H. Gilbert, and J. Posner), pp. 189–207. The Hague: Martinus Nijhoff.
108. **Weitzener, M.A., Olofson, S.M., and Forman, A.D.** (1995). Patients with malignant meningitis presenting with neuropsychiatric manifestations. *Cancer* **76**, 1804–8.
109. **Formaglio, F. and Caraceni, A.** (1998). Meningeal metastases clinical aspects and diagnosis. *Italian Journal of Neurological Sciences* **19**, 133–49.
110. **Voltz, R.** et al. (1999). A serologic marker of paraneoplastic limbic and brain-stem encephalitis in patients with testicular cancer. *New England Journal of Medicine* **340**, 1788–95.
111. **Wengs, W.J., Talwar, D., and Bernard, J.** (1993). Ifosfamide-induced nonconvulsive status epilepticus. *Archives of Neurology* **50**, 1104–5.
112. **Seymour, D.G., Henschke, P.J., Cape, R.D.T., and Campbel, A.J.** (1980). Acute confusional states and dementia in the elderly: the role of dehydration volume depletion, physical illness and age. *Age and Ageing* **9**, 137–46.
113. **Bruera, E.** (1991). Severe organic brain syndrome. *Journal of Palliative Care* **7**, 36–8.
114. **de Stoutz, N.D., Tapper, M., and Faisinger, R.L.** (1995). Reversible delirium in terminally ill patients. *Journal of Pain and Symptom Management* **10**, 249–53.
115. **Jacobson, S. and Jerrier, H.** (2000). EEG in delirium. *Seminars in Clinical Neuropsychiatry* **5**, 86–92.
116. **Koponen, H., Partanen, J., Paakkonen, A., Mattila, E., and Rikkinen, P.J.** (1989). EEG spectral analysis in delirium. *Journal of Neurology, Neurosurgery, and Psychiatry* **52**, 980–5.
117. **Breitbart, W., Marotta, R., Platt, M.M., Weisman, H., Derevenco, M., and Grau, C.** (1996). A double-blind trial of haloperidol, chlorpromazine and lorazepam in the treatment of delirium in hospitalized AIDS patients. *American Journal of Psychiatry* **153**, 231–7.
118. **American Psychiatric Association.** (1999). Practice guideline for the treatment of patients with delirium. *American Journal of Psychiatry* **156**, 1–20.
119. **Wilt, J.L., Minnema, A.M., Johnson, R.F., and Rosenblum, A.M.** (1993). Torsade de pointes associated with the use of intravenous haloperidol. *Annals of Internal Medicine* **119**, 391–4.
120. **Jackson, T., Ditmanson, L., and Phibbs, B.** (1997). Torsade de pointes and low-dose oral haloperidol. *Archives of Internal Medicine* **157**, 2013–15.
121. **Stiefel, F., Fainsinger, R., and Bruera, E.** (1992). Acute confusional states in patients with advanced cancer. *Journal of Pain and Symptom Management* **7**, 94–8.
122. **Gilbert, M.R. and Grossman, S.A.** (1986). Incidence and nature of neurologic problems in patients with solid tumor. *American Journal of Medicine* **81**, 951–4.
123. **Posner, J.B. and Chernik, N.L.** (1978). Intracranial metastases from systemic cancer. *Advances in Neurology* **19**, 575–87.
124. **Chang, D.B., Yang, P.C., Luh, K.T., Kuo, S.H., and Lee, L.N.** (1992). Late survival of non-small cell lung cancer patients with brain metastases. *Chest* **101**, 1293–7.
125. **Boogerd, W., Vos, V.W., Hart, A.A.M., and Baris, G.** (1993). Brain metastases in breast cancer; natural history, prognostic factors and outcome. *Journal of Neuro-oncology* **15**, 165–74.
126. **Hoang-Xuan, K. and Delattre, J.** (1992). Treatment of brain metastases. In *Management in Neuro-oncology* (ed. J. Hildebrand), pp. 23–39. Berlin: Springer-Verlag.
127. **Patchel, R.A.** et al. (1990). A randomized trial of surgery in the treatment of single metastases to the brain. *New England Journal of Medicine* **322**, 494–500.
128. **Haaxma-Reiche, H.** et al. (1992). The outcome of single brain metastasis after treatment with irradiation alone or combined with neurosurgery. *Annals of Neurology* **32**, 286–7.
129. **DeAngelis, L.** (1994). Management of brain metastases. *Cancer Investigation* **12**, 156–65.
130. **Phillips, M.H., Stelzer, K.J., Griffin, T.W., Mayberg, M.R., and Winn, H.R.** (1994). Stereotactic radiosurgery: a review and comparison of methods. *Journal of Clinical Oncology* **12**, 1085–99.
131. **Alexander, E.I.** et al. (1995). Stereotactic radiosurgery for the definitive, treatment of brain metastases. *Journal of the National Cancer Institute* **87**, 34–40.
132. **Perrin, R.G., Livingston, K.E., and Aarabi, B.** (1982). Intradural extramedullary spinal metastasis. A report of 10 cases. *Journal of Neurosurgery* **56**, 835–7.
133. **Lewis, D.W., Packer, R.J., and Raney, B.** (1986). Incidence, presentation and outcome of spinal cord disease in children with systemic cancer. *Pediatrics* **78**, 438.
134. **Barron, K.D.** et al. (1959). Experience with metastatic neoplasms involving the spinal cord. *Neurology* **9**, 91–100.
135. **Shaw, M.D.M., Rose, J.E., and Paterson, A.** (1980). Metastatic extradural malignancy of the spine. *Acta Neurochirurgica* **52**, 113–20.
136. **Gilbert, R.W., Kim, J.H., and Posner, J.B.** (1978). Epidural spinal cord compression from metastatic tumor: diagnosis and treatment. *Annals of Neurology* **3**, 40–51.
137. **Kanchandani, R. and Howe, J.G.** (1982). Lhermitte's sign in multiple sclerosis: a clinical survey and review of the literature. *Journal of Neurology, Neurosurgery and Psychiatry* **45**, 308–12.
138. **Ventafridda, V., Caraceni, A., Martini, C., Sbanotto, A., and De, C.F.** (1991). On the significance of Lhermitte's sign in oncology. *Journal of Neuro-oncology* **10**, 133–7.
139. **Rodichok, L.D.** et al. (1981). Early diagnosis of spinal epidural metastases. *American Journal of Medicine* **70**, 1181–8.
140. **Rodichok, L.D.** et al. (1986). Early detection and treatment of spinal epidural metastases: the role of myelography. *Annals of Neurology* **20**, 696.
141. **Portenoy, R.K., Lipton, R.B., and Foley, K.M.** (1987). Back pain in the cancer patient: an algorithm for evaluation and management. *Neurology* **37**, 134–8.
142. **Portenoy, R.K.** et al. (1989). Identification of epidural neoplasm. Radiography and bone scintigraphy in the symptomatic and asymptomatic spine. *Cancer* **64**, 2207–13.
143. **Graus, F., Krol, G., and Foley, K.M.** (1986). Early diagnosis of spinal epidural metastasis: correlation with clinical and radiological findings. *Proceedings of the American Society of Clinical Oncology* **5**, abstract 1047.
144. **Haddad, P., Thaell, J.F., Kiely, J.M., Harrison, E.G., and Miller, R.H.** (1976). Lymphoma of the spinal epidural space. *Cancer* **38**, 1862–6.
145. **Caraceni, A.** (1988). Compressioni midollari metastatiche: diagnosi e terapia. *Argomenti di Oncologia* **9**, 45–52.
146. **Carmody, R.F., Yang, P.J., Seeley, G.W., Seeger, J.F., Unger, E.C., and Johnson, J.E.** (1989). Spinal cord compression due to metastatic disease: diagnosis with MR imaging versus myelography. *Radiology* **173**, 225–9.
147. **Hagen, N., Stulman, J., Krol, G., Foley, K.M., and Portenoy, R.K.** (1989). The role of myelography and magnetic resonance imaging in cancer patients with symptomatic and asymptomatic epidural disease. *Neurology* **39**, 309.
148. **Hagenau, C.** et al. (1987). Comparison of spinal magnetic resonance imaging and myelography in cancer patients. *Journal of Clinical Oncology* **5**, 1663–9.
149. **Ingham, J., Beveridge, A., and Cooney, N.J.** (1993). The management of spinal cord compression in patients with advanced malignancy. *Journal of Pain and Symptom Management* **8**, 1–6.
150. **Boogerd, W. and van der Sande, J.J.** (1993). Diagnosis and treatment of spinal cord compression in malignant disease. *Cancer Treatment Reports* **19**, 129–50.
151. **Sorensen, P.S.** et al. (1994). Effect of high-dose dexamethasone in carcinomatous metastatic spinal cord compression treated with radiotherapy. A randomized trial. *European Journal of Cancer* **30A**, 22–7.

152. **Greenberg, H.S., Kim, J., and Posner, J.B.** (1980). Epidural spinal cord compression from metastatic tumor: results with a new treatment protocol. *Annals of Neurology* **8**, 361–6.

153. **Vecht, C.J., Haaxma-Reiche, H., van Putten, W.L.J., de Visser, M., Vries, E.P., and Twijnstra, A.** (1989). Initial bolus of conventional versus high-dose dexamethasone in metastatic spinal cord compression. *Neurology* **39**, 1255–7.

154. **Young, R.F., Post, E.M., and King, G.A.** (1980). Treatment of spinal epidural metastases. Randomized prospective comparison of laminectomy and radiotherapy. *Journal of Neurosurgery* **53**, 741–8.

155. **Findlay, G.F.** (1984). Adverse effects of the management of malignant spinal cord compression. *Journal of Neurology, Neurosurgery, and Psychiatry* **47**, 761–8.

156. **Findlay, G.F.** (1987). The role of vertebral body collapse in the management of malignant spinal cord compression. *Journal of Neurology, Neurosurgery, and Psychiatry* **50**, 151–4.

157. **Harrington, K.D.** (1984). Anterior cord decompression and spinal stabilization for patients with metastatic lesions of the spine. *Journal of Neurosurgery* **61**, 107–17.

158. **Cooper, P.R., Errico, T.J., Martin, R., Crawford, B., and Di, B.T.** (1993). A systematic approach to spinal reconstruction after anterior decompression for neoplastic disease of the thoracic and lumbar spine. *Neurosurgery* **32**, 1–8.

159. **Harrington, K.D.** (1988). Anterior decompression and stabilization of the spine as treatment for vertebral collapse and spinal cord compression from metastatic cancer. *Clinical Orthopaedics* **233**, 177–97.

160. **Kokkoris, C.P.** (1983). Leptomeningeal carcinomatosis. How does cancer reach the pia-arachnoid? *Cancer* **51**, 154–60.

161. **Henson, R.A. and Urich, H.** *Cancer and the Nervous System*. Boston MA: Blackwell Scientific Publications, 1982, pp. 100–19, 368–405.

162. **Sause, W.T.** et al. (1988). Whole brain radiation and intrathecal methotrexate in the treatment of solid tumor leptomeningeal metastases—a southwest oncology group study. *Journal of Neuro-oncology* **6**, 107–12.

163. **Siegal, T., Lossos, A., and Pfeffer, M.R.** (1994). Leptomeningeal metastases. Analysis of 31 patients with sustained off-therapy response following combined-modality therapy. *Neurology* **44**, 1463–9.

164. **Chamberlain, M.C.** (1995). Comparative spine imaging in leptomeningeal metastases. *Journal of Neuro-oncology* **23**, 233–8.

165. **Wasserstrom, W.R., Glass, J.P., and Posner, J.B.** (1982). Diagnosis and treatment of leptomeningeal metastasis from solid tumors: experience with 90 patients. *Cancer* **49**, 759–72.

166. **Kaplan, J.G., Portenoy, R.K., Pack, D.R., and DeSouza, T.** (1990). Polyradiculopathy in leptomeningeal metastasis: the role of EMG and late response studies. *Journal of Neuro-oncology* **9**, 219–24.

167. **Fleisher, M., Wasserstrom, W.R., Schold, S.C., Schwartz, M.K., Melamed, M.R., and Posner, J.B.** (1981). Lactic dehydrogenase isoenzymes in cerebrospinal fluid in patients with systemic cancer. *Cancer* **47**, 2654–9.

168. **Greenberg, H.S.** et al. (1981). Metastasis to the base of the skull: clinical findings in 43 patients. *Neurology* **31**, 530–7.

169. **Vecht, C.J., Hoff, A.M., Kansen, P.J., de Boer, M., and Bosch, D.A.** (1992). Types and causes of pain in cancer of the head and neck. *Cancer* **70**, 178–84.

170. **Foley, K.M.** (1979). Pain syndromes in patients with cancer. In *Advances in Pain Research and Therapy* Vol. 2 (ed. J.J. Bonica and V. Ventafridda), pp. 59–75. New York: Raven Press.

171. **Foley, K.M.** (1979). The management of pain of malignant origin. In *Current Neurology* Vol. 2 (ed. H.D. Tyler, P.M. Dawson), pp. 279–302. New York: Raven Press.

172. **Weinstein, R.E., Herec, D., and Friedman, J.H.** (1986). Hypotension due to glossopharyngeal neuralgia. *Archives of Neurology* **40**, 90–2.

173. **Sozzi, C., Marotta, P., and Piatti, L.** (1987). Vagoglossopharyngeal neuralgia with syncope in the course of carcinomatous meningitis. *Italian Journal of Neurological Science* **8**, 271–6.

174. **Cheng, T.M., Cascino, T.L., and Onofrio, B.M.** (1993). Comprehensive study of diagnosis and treatment of trigeminal neuralgia secondary to tumors. *Neurology* **43**, 2298–302.

175. **DeAngelis, L.M. and Payne, R.** (1987). Lymphomatous meningitis presenting as atypical cluster headache. *Pain* **30**, 211–16.

176. **Carter, R.L., Pittam, M.R., and Tanner, N.S.B.** (1982). Pain and dysphagia in patients with squamous carcinomas of the head and neck: the role of perineural spread. *Journal of the Royal Society of Medicine* **75**, 598–606.

177. **Clouston, P.D., Sharpe, D.M., Corbett, A.J., Kos, S., and Kennedy, P.J.** (1990). Perineural spread of cutaneous head and neck cancer. Its orbital and central neurologic complications. *Archives of Neurology* **47**, 73–7.

178. **Brazis, P.W., Vogler, J.B., and Shaw, K.E.** (1991). The 'numb cheek-limb lower lid' syndrome. *Neurology* **41**, 327–8.

179. **Burt, R.K., Sharfam, W.H., Karp, B.I., and Wilson, W.H.** (1992). Mental neuropathy (Numb chin syndrome). A harbinger of tumor progression or relapse. *Cancer* **70**, 877–81.

180. **Rusthoven, J.J.** et al. (1988). Risk factors for varicella zoster disseminated infection among adult cancer patients with localized zoster. *Cancer* **62**, 1641–6.

181. **Kori, S.H.** et al. (1981). Brachial plexus lesions in patients with cancer 100 cases. *Neurology* **31**, 45–50.

182. **Marangoni, C., Lacerenza, M., Formaglio, F., Smirne, S., and Marchettini, P.** (1993). Sensory disorder of the chest as presenting symptom of lung cancer. *Journal of Neurology, Neurosurgery, and Psychiatry* **56**, 1033–4.

183. **Castagno, A.A. and Shuman, W.P.** (1987). MR imaging in clinically suspected brachial plexus tumor. *American Journal of Roentgenology* **149**, 1219–22.

184. **Krol, G.** (1993). Evaluation of neoplastic involvement of brachial and lumbar plexus: imaging aspects. *Journal of Back and Musculoskeletal Rehabilitation* **3**, 35–43.

185. **Cascino, T.L., Kori, S., Krol, G., and Foley, K.M.** (1983). CT scan of brachial plexus in patients with cancer. *Neurology* **33**, 1553–7.

186. **Harper, C.M., Thomas, J.E., Cascino, T.L., and Litchy, W.J.** (1989). Distinction between neoplastic and radiation-induced brachial plexopathy, with emphasis on EMG. *Neurology* **39**, 502–6.

187. **Thomas, J.E., Cascino, T.L., and Earl, J.D.** (1985). Differential diagnosis between radiation and tumor plexopathy of the pelvis. *Neurology* **35**, 1–7.

188. **Jaeckle, K.A., Young, D.F., and Foley, K.M.** (1985). The natural history of lumbosacral plexopathy in cancer. *Neurology* **35**, 8–15.

189. **Dalmau, J., Graus, F., and Marco, M.** (1989). 'Hot and dry foot' as initial manifestation of neoplastic lumbosacral plexopathy. *Neurology* **39**, 871–2.

190. **Stevens, M.J. and Gonet, Y.M.** (1990). Malignant psoas syndrome: recognition of an oncologic entity. *Australasian Radiology* **34**, 150–4.

191. **Rogers, L.R., Borkowski, G.P., Albers, J.W., Levin, K.H., Barohn, R.J., and Mitsumoto, H.** (1993). Obturator mononeuropathy caused by pelvic cancer: six cases. *Neurology* **43**, 1489–92.

192. **Martini, C.** Sindromi dolorose da Cancro. Univerita' degli Studi di Milano, Facolta' di Medicina a Chirurgia, Scuola di Specializzazione in Oncologia, 1991.

193. **Ventafridda, V. and Martino, G.** (1976). Clinical evaluation of subarachnoid neurolytic blocks in intractable cancer pain. In *Advances in Pain Research and Therapy* (ed. J.J. Bonica et al.), pp. 699–703. New York: Raven Press.

194. **Ischia, S., Ischia, A., Luzzani, A., Toscano, D., and Steele, A.** (1985). Results up to death in the treatment of persistent cervico-thoracic (Pancoast) and thoracic malignant pain by unilateral percutaneous cervical cordotomy. *Pain* **21**, 339–55.

195. **Sanders, M. and Zuurmond, W.** (1995). Safety of unilateral and bilateral percutaneous cervical cordotomy in 80 terminally ill cancer patients. *Journal of Clinical Oncology* **13**, 1509–12.

196. **Ventafridda, V. and Caraceni, A.** (1994). Cancer pain. In *Current Review of Pain* (ed. P. Prithvi Raj), pp. 156–78. Philadelphia: Current Medicine.

197. **Posner, J.B.** (1991). Paraneoplastic syndromes. *Neurologic Clinics* **9**, 919–36.

198. **Delattre, J.Y. and Posner, J.B.** (1989). Neurological complications of chemotherapy and radiation therapy. In *Neurology and General Medicine* (ed. M.J. Aminoff), pp. 365–87. New York: Churchill Livingstone.

199. **Lipton, R.B.** et al. (1991). Large and small fibre type sensory dysfunction in patients with cancer. *Journal of Neurology, Neurosurgery, and Psychiatry* **54**, 706–9.

200. **Siegal, T.** (1991). Muscle cramps in the cancer patient: causes and treatment. *Journal of Pain and Symptom Management* **6**, 84–91.

201. **Chaudhry, V., Rowinsky, E.K., Sartorius, S.E., Donehower, R.C., and Cornblath, D.R.** (1994). Peripheral neuropathy from taxol and cisplatin

combination chemotherapy. Clinical and electrophysiological studies. *Annals of Neurology* **35**, 304–11.

202. **Graus, F., Rogers, L., and Posner, J.B.** (1985). Cerebrovascular complications in patients with cancer. *Medicine* **64**, 16.
203. **Barrow, K.D., Sigueira, E., and Hirano, A.** (1960). Cerebral embolism caused by nonbacterial thrombotic endocarditis. *Neurology* **10**, 391.
204. **Rogers, L.H., Cho, E.S., Kempin, S., and Posner, J.B.** (1987). Cerebral infarction from non-bacterial thrombotic endocarditis. A clinical and pathological study including the effects of anticoagulation. *American Journal of Medicine* **83**, 746.
205. **Collins, R.C., Al-Mondhiry, H., Chernik, N.L., and Posner, J.B.** (1975). Neurologic manifestations of intravascular coagulation in patients with cancer. A clinicopathological analysis of 12 cases. *Neurology* **25**, 795.
206. **Frits, R.D., Forkner, C.E., Freirich, E.J., Frei, E., and Thomas, L.B.** (1959). The association of fatal intracranial hemorrhage and 'blastic crisis' in patients with acute leukemia. *New England Journal of Medicine* **261**, 59.
207. **Lossos, A. and Siegal, T.** (1992). Spinal subarachnoid hemorrage associated with leptomeningeal metastases. *Journal of Neuro-oncology* **12**, 167–71.
208. **Sigsbee, B., Deck, M.D.F., and Posner, J.B.** (1979). Non-metastatic superior sagittal sinus thrombosis complicating systemic cancer. *Neurology* **29**, 139.
209. **Mandybur, T.I.** (1977). Intracranial hemorrhage caused by metastatic tumors. *Neurology* **27**, 650.
210. **Shimamura, K., Oka, K., Nakazawa, M., and Kojima, M.** (1983). Distribution patterns of microthrombi in disseminated intravascular coagulation. *Archives of Pathology & Laboratory Medicine* **107**, 543–7.
211. **Posner, J.B.** Cerebrovascular disorders in patients with cancer. Neuro-oncology V: Recent advances in diagnosis and treatment. Syllabus of the postgraduate course Memorial Sloan Kettering Cancer Center. New York: Memorial Sloan Kettering Cancer Center, 1992.
212. **Graus, F. and Rene, R.** (1992). Clinical and pathological advances on central nervous system paraneoplastic syndromes. *Revue Neurologique* **148**, 496–501.
213. **Posner, J.B.** (1992). Pathogenesis of central nervous system paraneoplastic syndromes. *Revue Neurologique* **148**, 502–12.
214. **Glantz, M.J., Biran, H., Myers, M.E., Gockerman, J.P., and Friedberg, M.H.** (1994). The radiographic diagnosis and treatment of paraneoplastic central nervous system disease. *Cancer* **73**, 168–75.
215. **Tuxen, M.K. and Werner Hansen, S.** (1994). Neurotoxicity secondary to antineoplastic drugs. *Cancer Treatment Reviews* **20**, 191–214.
216. **Crossen, J.R., Garwood, D., Glatsein, E., and Neuwelt, E.A.** (1994). Neurobehavioral sequelae of cranial irradiation in adults: a review of radiation-induced encephalopathy. *Journal of Clinical Oncology* **12**, 627–42.
217. **Elliot, K.J.** (1994). Taxonomy and mechanisms of neuropathic pain. *Seminars in Neurology* **14**, 195–205.
218. **Devor, M. and Rappaport, H.** (1990). Pain and pathophysiology of damaged nerve. In *Pain Syndromes in Neurology* (ed. H. Fields), pp. 47–83. London: Butterworths.
219. **Fields, H.L. and Rowbotham, M.C.** (1994). Multiple mechanisms of neuropathic pain: a clinical perspective. In *Proceedings of the 7th World Congress on Pain, Progress in Pain Research and Management* Vol. 2 (ed. G.F. Gebhart, D.L. Hammond, and T.S. Jensen), pp. 437–54. Seattle: IASP Press.
220. **Gonzales, G.R.** (1994). Central pain. *Seminars in Neurology* **14**, 255–62.
221. **Devor, M. et al.** (1991). Group Report: Mechanisms of neuropathic pain following peripheral injury. In *Towards a New Pharmacotherapy of Pain* (ed. A. Basbaum, and J.-M. Besson), pp. 417–40. New York: John Wiley & Sons.
222. **Asbury, A.K. and Fields, H.L.** (1984). Pain due to peripheral nerve damage: an hypothesis. *Neurology* **34**, 1587–90.
223. **Boivie, J., Leijon, G., and Johanson, I.** (1989). Central post-stroke pain—a study of the mechanisms through analyses of the sensory abnormalities. *Pain* **37**, 173–85.
224. **Leijon, G., Boivie, J., and Johanson, I.** (1989). Central post-stroke pain—neurological symptoms and pain characteristics. *Pain* **36**, 13–25.
225. **Nurmikko, T. and Bowsher, D.** (1990). Somatosensory findings in postherpetic neuralgia. *Journal of Neurology, Neurosurgery, and Psychiatry* **53**, 135–41.
226. **Asbury, A.K.** (1990). Pain in generalized neuropathies. In *Pain Syndromes in Neurology* (ed. H. Fields), pp. 131–41. London: Butterworth.
227. **Osterberg, A., Boivie, J., Holmgren, H., Thuomas, K., and Johanson, I.** (1994). The clinical characteristics and sensory abnormalities of patients with central pain caused by multiple sclerosis. In *Proceedings of the 7th World Congress on Pain, Progress in Pain Research and Management* Vol. 2 (ed. G.F. Gebhart, D.L. Hammond, and T.S. Jensen), pp. 789–96. Seattle: IASP Press.
228. **Boivie, J.** (1992). Hyperalgesia and allodynia in patients with CNS lesions. In *Hyperalgesia and Allodynia* (ed. W. Willis), pp. 363–73. New York: Raven Press.
229. **Dyck, P.J., Low, P.A., and Stevens, J.C.** (1983). 'Burning feet' as the only manifestation of dominantly inherited sensory neuropathy. *Mayo Clinic Proceedings* **58**, 426–9.
230. **Watson, C.P. and Deck, J.P.** (1993). The neuropathology of herpes zoster with particular reference to postherpetic neuralgia and its pathogenesis. Herpes zoster and postherpetic neuralgia. In *Pain Reseach and Clinical Management* Vol. 8 (ed. C.P.N. Watson), pp. 139–57. Amsterdam: Elsevier.
231. **Watson, C.P.N., Evans, R.J., Watt, V.R., and Birkett, N.** (1988). Postherpetic neuralgia: 208 cases. *Pain* **35**, 289–97.
232. **Watson, C.P.D.** (1990). Postherpetic neuralgia clinical features. In *Pain Syndromes in Neurology* (ed. H.L. Fields), pp. 223–38. London: Butterworths.
233. **Rowbotham, M.C.** (1994). Postherpetic neuralgia. *Seminars in Neurology* **14**, 247–54.
234. **Rowbotham, M.C., Reisner, L., and Fields, H.L.** (1991). Both intravenous lidocaine and morphine reduce the pain of postherpetic neuralgia. *Neurology* **41**, 1024–8.
235. **Watson, C.P.N., Evans, R.J., and Watt, V.R.** (1988). Postherpetic neuralgia and topical capsaicin. *Pain* **33**, 333–40.
236. **Rowbotham, M.C., Davies, P.M., and Fields, H.L.** (1995). Topical lidocaine gel relieves postherpetic neuralgia. *Annals of Neurology* **37**, 246–53.
237. **Nurmikko, T., Wells, C., and Bowsher, D.** (1991). Pain and allodynia in postherpetic neuralgia: role of somatic and sympathetic nervous systems. *Acta Neurologica Scandinavica* **84**, 146–52.
238. **Eide, P.K., Jorum, E., Stubhaug, A., Bremnes, J., and Breivik, H.** (1994). Relief of post-herpetic neuralgia with the n-methyl-d-aspartic acid antagonist ketamine: a double-blind cross-over comparison with morphine and placebo. *Pain* **58**, 347–54.
239. **Stanton-Hicks, M., Janig, W., Hassenbusch, S., Haddox, J.D., Boas, R., and Wilson, P.** (1995). Reflex sympathetic dystrophy: changing concepts and taxonomy. *Pain* **63**, 127–33.
240. **Backonia, M.** (1994). Reflex sympathetic dystrophy/sympathetically mantained pain/causalgia: the syndrome of neuropathic pain with dysautonomia. *Seminars in Neurology* **14**, 563–71.
241. **Perl, E.R.** (1994). Causalgia and reflex sympathetic dystrophy revisited. Touch, temperature and pain in health and disease: mechanisms and assessment. In *Progress in Pain Research and Management* Vol. 3 (ed. J. Boivie, P. Hansson, and U. Lindblom), pp. 231–48. Seattle: IASP Press.
242. **Campbel, J.N., Meyer, R.A., Davis, K.D., and Raja, S.N.** (1991). Sympathetically mantained pain: a unifying hypothesis. In *Hyperalgesia and Allodynia* (ed. W. Willis), pp. 141–9. New York: Raven Press.
243. **Schott, G.D.** (1994). Visceral afferents: their contribution to 'sympathetic dependent' pain. *Brain* **117**, 397–413.
244. **Verdugo, R.J. and Ochoa, J.L.** (1994). 'Sympathetically maintained pain.' I. Phentolamine block questions the concept. *Neurology* **44**, 1003–10.
245. **Verdugo, R.J., Campero, M., and Ochoa, J.L.** (1994). Phentolamine sympathetic block in painful neuropathies. II. Further questioning of the concept of 'sympathetically maintained pain'. *Neurology* **44**, 1010–14.
246. **Jadad, A.R., Carroll, D., Glynn, C.J., and McQuay, H.J.** (1995). Intravenous regional sympathetic blockade for pain relief in reflex sympathetic dystrophy: a systematic review of the literature and a randomized double-blind crossover study. *Journal of Pain and Symptom Management* **10**, 13–20.

8.15 Brain tumours

Claudia Bausewein, Gian Domenico Borasio, and Raymond Voltz

Introduction

Patients with primary brain tumours comprise about 2 per cent of all new cases of cancer.[1] However, their incidence is rising—due to unknown factors—with an incidence of 5–15/100 000 per year currently.[2] Primary brain tumours comprise several histological entities, from more benign forms such as ependymomas to very malignant tumours such as glioblastoma multiforme (GBM) with a poor prognosis[3] (Table 1). Some tumours, for example, astrocytomas, may over time develop in to more malignant forms.[2]

Depending on the histology, different disease modifying therapeutic options exist. Most patients undergo surgery, radiotherapy, chemotherapy, or a combination of treatments, but the chances of cure are very low.[4] The average life expectancy of a patient with GBM is between several weeks and several months after post-operative radiotherapy.[4] Few patients survive 2 years.[3] Most so-called long-term survivors of GBM are likely to have had a mistaken histological diagnosis.[5]

In most countries, patients with brain tumours are usually seen by neurologists and neurosurgeons who are not familiar with basic medical, legal, and ethical issues in palliative care.[6] Given the lack of curative treatments and the short life expectancy of most patients, good palliative care is essential, beginning with the time of diagnosis.

Communication

Patients and families should be informed early in the course of the disease that the tumour—depending on its localization—is likely to cause cognitive impairment with consequent limitations in decision-making and legal capacity. In most patients, communication becomes progressively more difficult during the course of the disease because of dysphasia, confusion, somnolence, or all of these. Therefore, end-of-life issues like tube feeding, life-sustaining treatments, resuscitation, or discontinuation of steroids must be discussed early, and the patients should be encouraged to formulate an advance directive and name a health care proxy.[7,8]

Caring for patients and relatives

Psycho-social issues play a major role in the care of brain tumour patients. Patients not only have to face their life-threatening disease but also possible change of their personality, as well as cognitive and functional deficits. Patients commonly experience feelings of shock, anxiety, despair, anger, fear, and sadness at the time of diagnosis.[9] Most patients with malignant glioma seem unaware or are only partly aware of their poor prognosis, while their relatives appear more aware and more distressed.[10] Brain tumour patients seldom seem to reach a state of acceptance of the disease, possibly due to progressive cognitive dysfunction.[9]

The psychological burden for relatives becomes higher during the course of the disease. The relatives feel progressively estranged from the patient and often experience the social death of the patient long before the actual death. Therefore, the family needs special attention, counselling, and care from the multidisciplinary team, and they should be involved in medical decisions and care from the beginning.

Organization of care

Patients with primary brain tumours are diagnosed in most cases by a neurologist, and then receive treatment from a neurosurgeon and radiotherapist for tumour-specific treatment. As the disease progresses, however, these specialists tend to withdraw from care. Sometimes patients are then returned to the neurologist for chemotherapy. In areas where palliative care is available, there is a frequent misconception that brain tumour patients have no treatable symptoms and that their life expectancy is too long for a hospice or palliative care unit.[11] However, patients with brain tumours and their families have multidimensional problems requiring early involvement of a multiprofessional and interdisciplinary team, including physiotherapy, occupational therapy, and speech therapy. This effort is usually coordinated by the GP, with the support of the neurologist or the palliative care specialist.

Symptom control

Symptoms in patients with primary brain tumours are either related to raised intracranial pressure or to the direct impingement of the tumour on brain structures.[12] Concurrent and inter-related causes of raised intracranial pressure include the expanding tumour mass, cerebral oedema, and impaired absorption of cerebrospinal fluid.

Headache

About 60 per cent of brain tumour patients suffer from headaches during the course of their disease, 20 per cent in the initial stages. Relatively few patients experience the 'classic' brain tumour headache with nausea and vomiting on awakening, easing off after rising.[13] Most patients complain of a dull generalized headache similar to tension headache, while a few describe a migraine-type headache.[14] Headaches are caused by traction on

Table 1 Histological types and prognosis of primary brain tumours

		Incidence	Median survival (months)		
			Age ≤20 years	Age 21–64 years	Age ≥65 years
Astrocytic tumours	Pilocytic astrocytoma WHO I	10% of astrocytic tumours most common in children			
	Diffuse astrocytomas WHO II	10–15% of astrocytic tumours		22.6	4.0
	Anaplastic astrocytomas WHO III				
	Glioblastoma multiforme WHO IV	50–60% of astrocytic tumours 12–15% of all intracranial neoplasms	9.9	10.8	3.5
Oligodendroglial tumours	Oligodendroglioma WHO II			97.3	13.9
Ependymal tumours	Ependymoma		96.5		
	Medulloblastoma			74	

(*Modified from:* Davis, F.G., Freels, S., Grutsch, J., Barlas, S., and Brem, S. (1998). *Journal of Neurosurgery* **88** (1), 1–10; and Kleihues, P. and Lavence, W.K. *Pathology and Genetics: Tumours of the Nervous System*. Lyon: IARC Press, 2000.)

pain-sensitive structures such as meninges, cranial nerves, and venous sinuses due to raised intracranial pressure. They often correlate with the degree of raised intracranial pressure, cerebral oedema, or shift of midline structures, but not with the size of the tumour mass itself.(13) Severe pain of acute onset may signify a rapid rise in intracranial pressure, for example, haemorrhage into the tumour. Corticosteroids play an important role in the treatment of headaches caused by brain tumours.(15) The steroid dose needs to be titrated against the severity of the headaches.(7) If steroids alone are not sufficient, analgesic therapy is necessary. There is no reason to with old opioids in patients with brain tumours. Cognitive impairment in more advanced stages makes pain assessment difficult. Physical signs such as rubbing of the head or moaning may be taken as indication of underlying headache.(7)

Steroids are important in symptom management of patients with brain tumours. They reduce the raised intracranial pressure by reducing vasogenic peritumoural oedema.(15) The effect of steroids on headache, impaired consciousness, nausea and vomiting, and neurological deficits is often dramatic and usually within days but is often not long-lasting. This needs to be explained in advance to patients and relatives, together with the fact that steroids have no influence on tumour progression.

There are no clear guidelines regarding dose, type of steroid, or duration of treatment.(15) In a randomized controlled trial in patients with brain tumours, doses of 4 mg dexamethasone per day were as effective as 16 mg/day but caused less side-effects.(16) Prescription and dosage of steroids should be reviewed regularly.(15,17) Many patients seem to be maintained on too high a dose of steroids for too long, which may lead to severe side-effects including Cushing's syndrome, psychosis, and myopathy. In the case of acutely raised intracranial pressure, we recommend starting treatment with high doses (16–24 mg/day, given in the morning and at midday, not in the evening to prevent sleep disturbances), and quickly reducing them after symptom control has been achieved to the lowest tolerated dose, which is often as low as 2 mg/day. Extract from *Boswellia serrata* (H15, 1200–3600 mg/day) may be tried alternatively or in combination with steroids.(18) In our experience, about half of the patients report a positive effect. The main side-effects observed are nausea and vomiting.

Dysphagia

Patients with primary brain tumours may develop dysphagia as a consequence of cranial nerve or bulbar palsy. In contrast to dysphagia due to obstruction, it is easier for patients with neurogenic dysphagia to swallow solids than fluids. Aspiration and malnutrition are the main complications of dysphagia and a percutaneous endoscopic gastrostomy should be considered.

Cognitive and behavioural dysfunction

Patients with brain tumours develop cognitive dysfunction at a much earlier stage than other patients with terminal illness. Patients present with a variety of symptoms ranging from attention deficit to personality changes and psychiatric problems. In particular, relatives need to be warned that paranoid features may be strong and deeply distressing. A specific problem which may be a cause for admission is the reversal of sleep patterns. The patient sleeps by day and is awake all night.

In all cases of sudden onset or worsening of behavioural or cognitive dysfunction, a non-convulsive status epilepticus needs to be ruled out (see Chapter 8.14). If agitation or delirium ensue, neuroleptic treatment is warranted (see Chapter 8.14 for details), but it must be kept in mind that neuroleptics lower the seizure threshold. Due to its sedating properties, levomepromazine may be an alternative to haloperidol as a first-line treatment.

The most common types of cognitive dysfunction are summarized in Table 2. Brain imaging and laboratory tests may be necessary to identify the

Table 2 Types and causes of cognitive and behavioural dysfunction in brain tumour patients

Type	Description	Anatomical localization	Treatment
Anosognosia	Inability to accept the reality of one's illness	Posterior parietal non-dominant hemisphere	Acceptance and explanation to the relatives
Aphasia	Difficulty in speaking and/or understanding (see Table 3)	Dominant (usually left) parietotemporal hemisphere	Speech therapy (if slow course)
Apraxia	Inability to plan and perform complex movements	Parietal lobes	Occupational therapy to improve activities of daily living
Neglect	Loss of interest in one side of the body	Non-dominant (usually right) parietal hemisphere	Occupational therapy, neuropsychological training (of limited value if rapid progression)
Memory loss	Short-term memory is usually affected first	Hippocampus, temporal lobes	As above
Attention deficit	Insidious onset, fluctuations	Frontoparietal lobes	As above
Apathy	May be so severe as to simulate unconsciousness	Frontal lobes	As above
Affective disinhibition	Loss of distance, inadequate emotional expression	Frontal lobes	Psycho-social adjustment, explanation to the family
Personality change	May range from apathy to aggression; very troublesome for relatives; often presenting symptom	Variable	Psycho-social adjustment, explanation to the family
Psychosis	May present with hallucinations and/or paranoid ideas	Variable; consider steroid-induced psychosis	Neuroleptics; beware of lowered seizure threshold!
Depression	May mimic cognitive dysfunction (pseudodementia)	N/A	Psychotherapy (consider family therapy), antidepressants
Delirium	May be hypo- or hyperactive	Generalized, often metabolic or drug induced	Treat the cause if possible (see Chapter 8.14)

cause and assess its potential for reversibility with treatment. Fluctuation of these symptoms is common.

Speech and language problems

Disturbed speech and language are important symptoms in patients with brain tumours. About one third of patients with high-grade gliomas have speech deficits at first presentation, requiring early access to speech therapy.[19] One must distinguish between dysphasia (Table 3), a loss of production or comprehension of spoken and/or written language (cortical dysfunction), and dysarthria (Table 4), a disturbance in articulation (dysfunction of brainstem, cranial nerves, or muscles). Comprehension of dysphasic patients is normally worse than anticipated. Questions should be asked slowly and clearly. It is important to develop a yes/no code or to find alternative strategies like pointing, writing, or painting. Patients with fluent dysphasia should be slowed down, those with hesitant speaking should be encouraged. Patience, time, and empathy are necessary. In patients with severe dysarthria, communication boards or electronic aids might be necessary to support communication. Patients should have early access to a speech therapist (see Chapter 15.5).

Seizures

Seizures are a frequent problem in patients with brain tumours. In about one-third, a seizure is the presenting symptom leading to the diagnosis, and about half of the patients will experience seizures during the course of their illness.[12] They must be differentiated from other forms of involuntary movements, such as myoclonus (e.g. with opioid therapy), drug-induced hyperkinesias (e.g. with haloperidol), or movement patterns related to terminal elevation of intracranial pressure (see Chapter 8.14).

Seizures should be described in detail according to what happens to the patient, as this approach localizes the epileptogenic regions of the cortex best.[20] In an acute seizure, care must be taken that the patient does not hurt him/herself. A single generalized tonic–clonic seizure, which usually lasts around 3–5 min, requires no acute anticonvulsant therapy. However, a status epilepticus warrants aggressive therapy because of its high mortality (see Chapter 8.14).

The use of prophylactic anticonvulsant therapy in brain tumour patients is controversial.[12] A recent practice parameter from the American Academy of Neurology advises against routine anticonvulsant prophylaxis in newly diagnosed brain tumour patients.[21] Short-term anticonvulsant therapy should be prescribed after brain surgery (for 1 week) or before administering iodinated contrast medium for CT scans. This is not necessary before administering gadolinium prior to MRI scanning.[22] Long-term prophylaxis seems reasonable after a first seizure has occurred, but not before.

The choice of anticonvulsant is influenced by several factors:

1. *Time factor:* If a rapid onset of effect is needed, for example, for status epilepticus, IV lorazepam, clonazepam, midazolam, or diazepam may be used (for a detailed discussion of the treatment of status epilepticus, see Chapter 8.14). Diazepam is also available for rectal administration. Sodium valproate and phenytoin are both available as IV preparations and can be used in benzodiazepine-refractory status epilepticus or when oral anticonvulsant administration is not possible. With all other drugs which are available only orally it may take several days before therapeutic levels are reached.
2. *Drug interactions:* Anticonvulsants such as phenytoin and carbamazepine may lower serum levels of other medications such as corticosteroids or chemotherapy, and vice versa. Increasing the doses of the medication may compensate for this effect but increases the danger of reaching toxic levels, especially with phenytoin as this drug has non-linear pharmacokinetics. Drug toxicity from anticonvulsants may mimic tumour symptoms such as ataxia, double vision, or gait disturbance. Sodium valproate or newer anticonvulsants such as levetiracetam do not interact with other medication to that extent.[23]
3. *Efficacy and side-effects:* Anticonvulsant drug doses should be increased until no more seizures occur, or side-effects appear. Here, the upper limit of drug levels is of less clinical value than generally acknowledged. Sometimes, patients have side-effects long before this 'upper limit' is reached, others have no side-effects even above it. Patients, not serum levels, should be treated. Carbamazepine may be switched abruptly to the newer agent oxcarbazepine at a 1 : 1 basis, once side-effects occur,

Table 3 Dysphasia

	Comprehension	Speaking	Reading/writing
Global dysphasia	Disturbed	Repetition of syllables instead of words	Totally disturbed
Wernicke's dysphasia	Disturbed	Nonsensical but fluent disfigurement of words	Similar to comprehension and speaking
Broca's dysphasia	Good	Hesitant, telegraphic style, grammar disturbed	Similar to comprehension and speaking
Amnestic dysphasia	Hardly disturbed	Difficulty in wording, correct construction of sentences	Hardly disturbed

Table 4 Dysarthria

Type of dysarthria	Localization	Clinical feature
Cortical	Motor cortex, descending motor pathway	Reduced articulation, often combined with dysphasia
Suprabulbar corticobulbar	Descending motor pathways	'Staccato' speech
Extrapyramidal system	Basal ganglia	Low voice, stuttering
Cerebellar	Cerebellum	Scanning speech (abnormal separation of syllables)
Bulbar	Brainstem	Hollow, unarticulated

and then oxcarbazepine may be increased as this generally is less toxic.[23] Carbamazepine may have an adverse effect on late radiation toxicity.[24] Another severe side-effect, especially relevant for brain tumour patients, is the so-called Stevens–Johnson syndrome (potentially lethal multiform exsudating erythema) in patients receiving phenytoin, and sometimes carbamazepine, who have received cranial irradiation and are on decreasing doses of steroids.[25]

Mobility problems

In patients with brain tumours, mobility may be impaired due to hemiplegia, increasing weakness or obesity after long-term treatment with steroids. Problems with coordination may evolve from ataxia. Steroid myopathy affecting proximal muscles of legs and arms occurs often even after short-term treatment. Patients then find it difficult to get up from a chair or climb steps.

Any small gain in mobility decreases the need for care and increases the independence of the patient. In consequence, he/she might be able to stay longer at home and the burden for the relatives might be less. Physiotherapy and occupational therapy should be organized early on and adapted to the patient's actual situation, abilities, and skills (see Chapter 15.4).

Specific issues in the terminal phase

Little is known about the terminal phase of patients with brain tumours. In a retrospective study, the main symptoms in the last 72 h were somnolence (84 per cent), pain (33 per cent), death rattle (18 per cent), seizures (9 per cent), and restlessness (9 per cent).[26] In this series, a peaceful death was observed in 85 per cent of the patients. Reasons for a non-peaceful death were uncontrolled symptoms such as pain, epileptic seizures, and dyspnoea.

With increasing weakness and unconsciousness, the patients are not able to take medication orally. Therefore, alternative routes such as transdermal, rectal, or subcutaneous administration of drugs necessary for symptom control (such as analgesics and antiemetics) have to be planned in advance of the terminal phase.

Most brain tumour patients are on long-term steroids. When their condition deteriorates it has to be decided whether to increase the dose or to discontinue the treatment. An increase in the dose of steroids should be limited to 5–7 days. If no effect is seen within that time, the dose should be reduced again.[17] In dying patients who cannot take oral medication, continuation of steroids might prolong the dying phase, while discontinuation might lead to exacerbation of cerebral oedema (unlikely if the fluid intake is reduced) and to adrenal insufficiency (unlikely to result in significant suffering). Thus, parenteral continuation of steroids in the dying phase is rarely appropriate or necessary.[7] If steroids are discontinued, intensified symptom monitoring is required. Increasing the analgesic, antiemetic, and anticonvulsant medication may be necessary.

References

1. **Prados, M.D. and Levin, V.** (2000). Biology and treatment of malignant glioma. *Seminars in Oncology* **27** (3 Suppl. 6), 1–10.
2. **Kleihues, P. and Cavenee, W.K.** *Pathology and Genetics: Tumours of the Nervous System*. Lyon: IARC Press, 2000.
3. **Davis, F.G., Freels, S., Grutsch, J., Barlas, S., and Brem, S.** (1998). Survival rates in patients with primary malignant brain tumours stratified by patients age and tumour histological type: an analysis based on Surveillance, Epidemiology and End Results (SEER) data, 1973–1991. *Journal of Neurosurgery* **88** (1), 1–10.
4. **Blomgren, H.** (1996). Brain tumours. *Acta Oncologica* **35** (Suppl. 7), 16–21.
5. **Morita, M., Rosenblum, M.K., Bilsky, M.H., Fraser, R.A., and Rosenfeld, M.R.** (1996). Long-term survivors of glioblastoma multiforme: clinical and molecular characteristics. *Journal of Neurooncology* **27** (3), 259–66.
6. **Carver, A.C., Vickrey, B.G., and Bernat, J.L.** (1999). End-of-life-care: a survey of US neurologists, attitudes, behaviour and knowledge. Neurology **53**, 284–93.
7. **Peterson, K.** (2001). Brain tumours. In *Neurologic Clinics: Palliative Care* Vol. 19, No. 4 (ed. A. Carver and K.M. Foley), pp. 887–90. Philadelphia PA: WB Saunders Company.
8. **Voltz, R., Akabayashi, A., Reese, C., Ohi, G., and Sass, H.-M.** (1998). End-of-life decisions and advance directives in palliative care: a crosscultural survey of patients and health care professionals. *Journal of Pain and Symptom Management* **16**, 153–62.
9. **Adelbratt, S. and Strang, P.** (2000). Death anxiety in brain tumour patients and their spouses. *Palliative Medicine* **14**, 499–507.
10. **Davies, E., Clarke, C., and Hopkins, A.** (1996). Malignant cerebral glioma II: perspectives of patients and relatives on the value of radiotherapy. *British Medical Journal* **313**, 1512–16.
11. **Behar, R. and Abu Rkih, R.** (2001). Does the patient with a primary brain tumour need hospice? *European Journal of Palliative Care* (abstracts of the 7th Congress of EAPC: 120).
12. **Posner, J.B.** (1995). Neurologic complications of cancer. *Contemporary Neurology Series*. Philadelphia PA: F.A. Davis Company.
13. **Forsyth, P.A. and Posner, J.B.** (1993). Headaches in patients with brain tumours. *Neurology* **43**, 1678–83.
14. **Glantz, M.J., Burger, P.C., and Friedman, A.H.** (2001). Treatment of radiation-induced nervous system injury with heparin and warfarin. *Neurology* **44**, 2020–7.
15. **Kirkham, S.** (1988). The palliation of cerebral tumours with high-dose dexamethasone: a review. *Palliative Medicine* **2**, 27–33.
16. **Vecht, C.J., Hovestadt, A., Verbiest, H.B., van Vliet, J., and van Putten, W.** (1994). Dose–effect relationship of dexamethasone on Karnofsky performance in metastatic brain tumours: a randomized study of doses of 4, 8 and 16 mg per day. *Neurology* **44** (4), 675–80.
17. **Twycross, R.** (1994). The risks and benefits of corticosteroids in advanced cancer. *Drug Safety* **11**, 163–78.
18. **Streffer, J.R., Bitzer, M., Schabet, M., Dichgans, J., and Weller, M.** (2001). Response of radiochemotherapy-associated cerebral edema to a phytotherapeutic agent, H15. *Neurology* **56**, 1219–21.
19. **Thomas, R., O'Connor, A.M., and Ashley, S.** (1995). Speech and language disorders in patients with high grade glioma and its influence on prognosis. *Journal of Neurooncology* **23** (3), 265–70.
20. **Luders, H., Acharya, J., Baumgartner, C., Benbadis, S., Bleasel, A., Burgess, R., Dinner, D.S., Ebner, A., Foldvary, N., Geller, E., Hamer, H., Holthausen, H., Kotagal, P., Morris, H., Meencke, H.J., Noachtar, S., Rosenow, F., Sakamoto, A., Steinhoff, B.J., Tuxhorn, I., and Wyllie, E.** (1999). A new epileptic seizure classification based exclusively on ictal semiology. *Acta Neurologica Scandinavica* **99** (3), 137–41.
21. **Glantz, M.J., Cole, B.F., Forsyth, P.A., Recht, L.D., Wen, P.Y., Chamberlain, M.C., Grossman, S.A., and Cairncross, J.G.** (2000). Practice parameter: anticonvulsant prophylaxis in patients with newly diagnosed brain tumours. Report of the Quality Standards Subcommittee of the American Academy of Neurology. *Neurology* **54** (10), 1886–93.
22. **Telfeian, A.E., Philips, M.F., Crino, P.B., and Judy, K.D.** (2001). Postoperative epilepsy in patients undergoing craniotomy for glioblastoma multiforme. *Journal of Experimental and Clinical Cancer Research* **20** (1), 5–10.
23. **McAuley, J.W., Biederman, T.S., Smith, J.C., and Moore, J.L.** (2002). Newer therapies in the drug treatment of epilepsy. *Annals of Pharmacotherapy* **36** (1), 119–29.
24. **Nieder, C., Leicht, A., Motaref, B., Nestle, U., Niewald, M., and Schnabel, K.** (1999). Late radiation toxicity after whole brain radiotherapy: the influence of antiepileptic drugs. *American Journal of Clinical Oncology* **22** (6), 573–9.
25. **Eralp, Y., Aydiner, A., Tas, F., Saip, P., and Topuz, E.** (2001). Stevens–Johnson syndrome in a patient receiving anticonvulsant therapy during cranial irradiation. *American Journal of Clinical Oncology* **24** (4), 347–50.
26. **Bausewein, C., Hau, P., Borasio, G.D., and Voltz, R.** How do patients with brain tumours die? Submitted for publication.

8.16 Sleep in palliative care

Michael J. Sateia and Robert B. Santulli

Introduction

Sleep disorders have been recognized for centuries as a frequent complication of medical illness. The last several decades have produced an explosive growth in our knowledge and understanding of sleep physiology and pathophysiology. Unfortunately, the practical application of this knowledge has been slow in reaching the majority of health care providers, including those in palliative medicine. However, examination of the literature on this subject does suggest a growing recognition on the part of clinicians that attention to patients' sleep is a necessary and an important aspect of care in this population. A good night's sleep may provide the palliative care patient an invaluable respite from the worries and pain of the day, and may allow him to meet the next day with renewed energy and motivation. In this chapter, we review basic aspects of sleep and sleep disorders, particularly as they apply to palliative care, and discuss strategies for the evaluation and treatment of these conditions.

Sleep physiology

Human sleep is a complex and dynamic physiologic function, the nature of which we have only begun to unravel. Contrary to the historical view of sleep as a passive state of little medical interest or relevance, it has become increasingly clear that sleep is an active condition that is affected by waking physiological and psychological states and which, in turn, has significant effects on those waking conditions. This is particularly true in the case of major medical illnesses in which marked perturbations in somatic and psychological functions may result in severe disruption of sleep and concomitant waking complications.

Normal sleep consists of two distinct states. Non-rapid eye movement (NREM) sleep (stages 1–4) accounts for approximately 75 per cent of the night; the remainder consists of rapid eye movement (REM) or 'dreaming' sleep. In the NREM sleep of the healthy young adult, stage 1 (light sleep) normally represents only 5–10 per cent of total sleep, stage 2 (medium sleep) represents approximately 50 per cent, and stages 3/4 (deep sleep) represent about 20 per cent. These stages, along with the REM stage of sleep, repeat themselves in cyclical fashion through the night. The deepest stages of sleep occur predominantly during the first half of sleep, while REM periods are significantly longer and more intense during the second half of the night. NREM sleep is a period of relative physiological and cognitive quiescence, quite distinct from REM sleep, which is characterized by muscle atonia, dreaming, and autonomic variability. The last-mentioned characteristic includes periodic increases in pulse, blood pressure, and respiration, as well as increased cerebral blood flow, decreased temperature regulation, and erection activity in males. The sleep–wake cycle is a component of the body's overall circadian rhythm. As such, its timing is synchronized with other biological rhythms including temperature oscillation and cortisol and growth hormone secretion. Onset and maintenance of normal sleep patterns are dependent on the satisfaction of a number of conditions. These include appropriate timing of sleep within the 24-h circadian rhythm, an adequate level of physical comfort, an acceptable sleeping environment, an intact central nervous system function, and relative absence of psychological distress and psychophysiologic arousal.

The restorative functions of sleep are dependent on a well-organized and reasonably uninterrupted structure or 'sleep architecture'. In many medical conditions, as well as with advancing age, there is a tendency towards lighter sleep, with an increase in stage 1 and decrease in stages 3/4. The percentage of REM sleep remains relatively constant in a healthy elderly population but is typically decreased when cognitive impairment or certain other medical conditions are present. Sleep often becomes more fragmented, with increased awakenings through the night. Disturbances of this nature result in complaints from affected patients of poor sleep and associated daytime consequences.

Classification of sleep disorders

Sleep disorders are classified according to the International Classification of Sleep Disorders of the American Sleep Disorders Association.[1] This system categorizes sleep disorders into three primary groups: (i) dyssomnias, (ii) parasomnias, and (iii) sleep disorders secondary to medical or psychiatric conditions. Dyssomnias include primary disorders that result in disturbance of the quantity, quality, or timing of nocturnal sleep as well as those conditions that are associated with excessive daytime sleepiness. Dyssomnias may be related to intrinsic factors (e.g. obstructive sleep apnoea, narcolepsy, or 'primary' insomnias) or to extrinsic factors (drugs, medications, or environmental conditions). Parasomnias are events or conditions that are caused or exacerbated by sleep, such as nightmares, sleep terrors, or enuresis. For the purposes of this chapter, we shall focus on primary patient complaints—most often insomnia or excessive sleepiness.

Insomnia

In clinical practice, insomnia can be defined as a subjective complaint by the patient of poor sleep. This definition encompasses complaints of insufficient sleep, difficulty initiating or maintaining sleep, interrupted sleep, poor quality or 'non-restorative' sleep, or sleep which occurs at the wrong time in the day–night cycle. Insomnia is a symptom, not a diagnosis. It is incumbent upon the clinician to clarify the nature of the complaint and to consider potential aetiologies. In the case of insomnia associated with medical conditions there are often a number of contributing factors which give rise to a patient's sleep disturbance. These include physiological, psychological, and environmental factors. Among the most common physiological determinants are pain, toxic and metabolic disturbance, medications, sleep-related breathing disorder (e.g. obstructive and central sleep apnoea, nocturnal asthma), movement disorders, and diseases of the central nervous system. Depression and anxiety are leading psychological causes of insomnia. Environmental circumstances such as unfamiliar surroundings, frequent interruptions, or noise are particularly important factors for patients in hospital. The most frequent causes of insomnia among terminally ill patients are outlined in Table 1.

Sleep deprivation may result in a broad spectrum of physiological and psychological changes, which vary according to the degree and type of deprivation. The changes most frequently described include progressive fatigue, sleepiness, impairment of concentration, and irritability.[2,3] Individuals who are chronically sleepy as a result of physiological disruption of night-time sleep frequently become depressed.[4] Sleep, particularly the deepest stages of NREM, may play a critical role in tissue restoration.[5] This observation is supported by the finding that a musculoskeletal pain syndrome may be experimentally induced by repetitive sleep interruption.[6] Of particular interest in cancer or AIDS patients is the observation that sleep deprivation results in alterations of immune system function.[7] Morley et al.[8] noted that immune activation has a stimulating effect on slow-wave sleep (presumably mediated, at least in part, by cytokine production) and, conversely, that slow-wave sleep enhances immune function. They speculated that sleep may be a factor in recuperative processes, including recovery from infection. More recent studies have demonstrated alterations in natural killer cell activity associated with sleep deprivation[9,10] Savard et al., assessing women at risk for cervical cancer, demonstrated that satisfaction with sleep quality was positively associated with levels of helper T cells and cytotoxic/suppressor T cells.[11] Others have reported declines in interleukin levels (IL-6) with sleep loss.[12]

Excessive daytime sleepiness

Excessive sleepiness is a common and frequently overlooked symptom, particularly among patients with serious medical illness. Because sleepiness

Table 1 Common causes of insomnia in the terminally ill

Depression	Major depressive illness related to loss, chronic pain, effects of tumour on central nervous system, metabolic/endocrine disturbance
Anxiety	Adjustment disorder or generalized anxiety related to fears of illness, procedures, pain or death; medication; direct effects on central nervous system
Cognitive impairment disorder	Delirium secondary to medication, metabolic derangement, direct involvement of central nervous system, or non-specific delirium-inducing factors
Pain	Related to direct tumour effects, diagnostic or treatment interventions, non-specific causes
Nausea and vomiting	Associated with chemotherapy, medications or primary gastrointestinal disturbance
Respiratory distress	Dyspnoea due to hypoxia and/or anxiety, obstructive sleep apnoea
Medications	Stimulants, bronchodilators, steroids, some antihypertensives, activating antidepressants; withdrawal or rebound from sedative hypnotics or analgesics
Psychophysiological insomnia	Caused by conditional arousal response, negative expectations and poor sleep hygiene
Sleep–wake schedule disorder	Associated with disruption of normal schedule, excessive time in bed or napping, disturbed nocturnal sleep
Periodic limb movement/ restless legs syndrome	Secondary to sedative hypnotic withdrawal, antidepressant medication, anaemia, uraemia, leukaemia, diabetes mellitus, peripheral neuropathy, iron deficiency

renders many individuals more quiet and 'compliant', medical staff and other care providers are often not motivated to identify sleepiness as a problem. As Kubler-Ross[13] points out, health professionals may actually encourage daytime sedation as a means of dealing with their own discomfort with the dying patient. While some degree of daytime sedation can be desirable in certain cases, this is by no means uniformly the case. Excessive somnolence is potentially quite a disabling symptom that may further compromise already tenuous function in the terminally ill. The sleepy patient is inactive, poorly motivated, and less capable of participating in treatment. The ability to attend to and thereby retain information is compromised. Social interactions, which may be of great importance in the final weeks or months of life, become seriously impaired. Depression, irritability, and withdrawal are also potential complications of pathological sleepiness.

Sleepiness must be distinguished from more general and vague complaints of 'tiredness' and 'fatigue', which are very common among patients receiving palliative care. Specifically, it must be determined to what extent an individual experiences drowsiness or episodes of irresistible sleepiness, especially under circumstances of physical inactivity, or takes naps during normal waking hours. The most widely employed scale for assessment of subjective sleepiness is the Epworth Sleepiness Scale, an eight-item measure of sleep tendency in various settings.[14] When appropriate, an objective measure of pathological sleepiness, the Multiple Sleep Latency Test,[15] can be utilized. Diagnostic difficulty may arise in the final stages of disease when the distinction between excessive somnolence and alteration of consciousness associated with delirium becomes blurred.

There are many potential causes of excessive sleepiness in this population. They include insufficient or disturbed nighttime sleep, medication (analgesic, sedative-hypnotic, antidepressant, and chemotherapeutic), metabolic disorders, and disruption of the sleep–wake schedule. In some cases, subjective sleepiness may occur as a form of psychological with-drawal or as an atypical symptom of depressive illness. For many patients, the aetiology is multifactorial. A careful review of potential causes must be conducted in order to identify the source(s) of the complaint. Most importantly, it is essential that the clinician does not dismiss excessive sleepiness as an inevitable part of terminal illness but rather approaches it as a treatable symptom.

Disorders of the sleep–wake schedule

Maintenance of a normal sleep pattern is dependent on adherence to a well-established schedule of sleep and wakefulness. Because of frequent disruptions of nighttime sleep, an absence of usual daytime schedule demands, and relative inactivity during normal waking hours, terminally ill individuals are particularly prone to disturbances of the sleep–wake schedule. When night sleep has been poor, there is an inclination to delay the hour of rising and/or to engage in lengthy daytime naps. While these practices are understandable, they pose a problem in that the onset of sleep may be significantly delayed on the subsequent night. This, in turn, results in further delays in morning rising times and increased daytime napping. Ultimately, there is a pronounced difficulty in falling asleep until early morning hours, with subsequent sleep often stretching into the early afternoon. This disturbance is referred to as delayed sleep phase syndrome. In other cases, the fatigue and sedation so often associated with major medical illness may give rise to advancement of the normal sleep–wake schedule, resulting in early morning awakening (advanced sleep phase syndrome), coupled with evening sleepiness and/or earlier bedtimes. For some, a normal sleep–wake rhythm disappears altogether and is replaced by a pattern of multiple shorter sleep periods that are interspersed with wakefulness throughout the 24-h cycle.

These disorders may result in complaints of insomnia or excessive sleepiness, depending on the nature of the schedule disturbance and the particular focus of the patient. In addition to the dysfunction and frustration that these disorders engender for the patient, the burden imposed on care givers can be substantial in that they are required to respond to the needs of a patient who is awake at all hours.

Circadian rhythm disorders of the type described may respond to straightforward efforts at regularization of the sleep–wake schedule and adherence to proper sleep hygiene, as described later in this chapter. Short-term treatment with hypnotic medications may be helpful in regularizing the circadian rhythm in certain patients. Bright light therapy and melatonin, administered at the appropriate time, may advance or delay sleep phase.[16–18] For some patients, the more formal behavioural approach of 'chronotherapy' (e.g. progressive delay of sleep phase) is required to correct the rhythm disturbance.[19]

Sleep in cancer

Patients with malignant disease consider sleep disturbance an important and troubling symptom. Women with metastatic breast cancer rated sleep in the highest quartile of quality of life items[20] while patients undergoing radiation therapy ranked sleep disturbance as one of the 10 most troubling difficulties associated with their illness.[21] Current data suggests that sleep is disturbed in 50 per cent or more of those with advanced cancer, particularly when pain is a complicating factor.[22–26] The prevalence of sleep disturbance in cancer patients has been reviewed by Savard and Morin.[27] They note that comparisons of insomnia/sleep disturbance data across these studies are difficult in light of the variability in definitions and measurement devices. They add that, in their own analysis of 300 women with breast cancer (non-metastatic), 51 per cent reported insomnia symptoms but only 19 per cent met specific criteria for the full 'insomnia syndrome'. Of these, about one in three described the onset of sleep problems as occurring after the cancer diagnosis.

Despite the fact that insomnia occurs on an almost nightly basis for many patients, they often do not report the problem to their physicians, assuming that there is little that can be done to help. Engstrom et al.

found that 85 per cent of cancer patients with sleep disturbance did not discuss the problem with a health care provider.[28] The same population reported that physicians and other health care providers generally did not ask about sleep-related problems.

Patients with cancer sleep less at night and are more likely to sit, lie down, and sleep during the day than normals.[29] Beszterczey and Lipowski found that 45 per cent of a mixed group of cancer patients referred for radiotherapy had a total sleep time of less than 50 h week, while 23 per cent slept for less than 40 h per week.[30] A comparison of sleep in their patients with that in an independent group of mixed medical and surgical patients revealed less sleep in the patients with neoplastic disease. Other comparisons between cancer patients and those with non-malignant disease or normal controls have yielded mixed results. Lamb found no difference between the sleep of newly diagnosed cancer patients and a group with non-malignant medical illness.[31] Another survey which compared patients with cancer with cardiac patients and normal controls indicated that the cancer group had no less difficulty falling asleep than cardiac patients, but they reported significantly more problems in maintaining sleep than either of the two comparison groups.[32] Approximately 30 per cent of the cancer patients with sleep maintenance complaints described pain as a cause of awakening. Interpretation of this study is complicated by the use of hypnotics or analgesics in a higher percentage (33 per cent) of the cancer group. Engstrom et al. found that about half of the patients with sleep problems experienced the disturbance on an almost nightly basis.[28] Midcycle awakening was the most common symptom, followed by insufficient sleep and difficulty getting back to sleep. Reports of sleep problems correlated with a pre-morbid history of sleep disturbance. These nocturnal disturbances may be associated with any of the factors listed in Table 1 although pain is of particular importance in cancer patients.

The only laboratory-based study of sleep in cancer patients to date is that of Silberfarb et al.[33] who provided a preliminary report on a group of 14 patients with unresectable lung cancer. Nine patients were self-described 'good sleepers' and five were 'poor sleepers'. All patients were studied for three consecutive nights in a sleep laboratory. The groups did not differ with respect to sleep efficiency, sleep latency, or distribution of sleep stages, with the exception that good sleepers spent a significantly greater amount of time in stages 3/4 (delta) sleep. The authors suggest that, for cancer patients, the subjective appraisal of quality of sleep may relate to the amount of time spent in delta sleep, although both groups spent so little time in deep sleep that this explanation should be considered preliminary.

In a continuation of the aforementioned study, the sleep of 17 patients with unresectable lung cancer and 15 with breast cancer (in various stages of their disease) was compared to that of 32 insomniacs without medical illness and an equal number of normal controls.[34] All cancer patients were ambulatory and, for the most part, only mildly impaired by their illness, with mean Karnofsky ratings of 85.4 and 92.8 for the lung and breast cancer groups, respectively. Overall, cancer patients slept as long as the controls and significantly longer than the insomniacs. Patients with breast cancer were not distinguishable from controls on polysomnographic variables. Lung cancer patients achieved total sleep times that were comparable with those of the controls by spending significantly more time in bed. However, their sleep was clearly more disturbed, with prolonged latency to stage 2 sleep, lower sleep efficiency, increased stage 1, and increased awakenings through the night. Curiously, and in contradistinction to the usual reports of insomniacs, the lung cancer group under-reported the sleep disturbance, denying the presence of sleep problems despite polysomnographic evidence to the contrary. Psychological questionnaires and interviews suggested that the differences observed were not a function of psychological disturbance which was, in fact, not evident in this group of cancer patients.

Sleepiness and fatigue

Daytime fatigue and sleepiness may occur as a result of tumour effects (e.g. mediated by cytokines), treatment, or disturbance of quantity, quality, or timing of nocturnal sleep. There is very little documentation of sleepiness as a symptom in patients with terminal malignancies or other end-stage disease. One survey found that about 40 per cent of cancer patients described sleeping at unusual times (mid-morning/afternoon). Munro et al.[21] noted 'sleeping more than usual' as one of the most troublesome symptoms of patients undergoing radiation therapy, although others found no increase in subjective sleepiness, as measured by the Epworth Sleepiness Scale, during radiation therapy for prostate cancer.[35] Excessive sedation is described in association with opioid analgesics[36–38] and some forms of chemotherapy.[39,40] Other aetiologies of sleepiness in cancer patients, including breathing disturbance, movement disorder, and sleep–wake schedule disturbances are discussed elsewhere.

Fatigue in cancer patients accounts for a significant degree of functional disability. It is important to note that fatigue is not synonymous with sleepiness, the latter being associated with a somewhat more circumscribed set of aetiologies. Nevertheless, sleep–wake disturbances do account for a portion of the fatigue experienced by cancer patients. The United States National Comprehensive Cancer Network Guidelines include sleep disturbance as a primary factor associated with fatigue, along with pain, anaemia, emotional distress, and hypothyroidism.[41] Significant associations between sleep disturbance and severe fatigue have been noted in two samples of breast cancer survivors.[42,43] Berger and Farr also reported a strong association between nighttime awakenings and cancer-related fatigue.[44] Investigation of patients undergoing radiation treatments revealed substantial increases in fatigue during therapy, apparently unre-lated to depression or sleepiness.[35] Clearly, fatigue in this population is a multifactorial problem that requires careful assessment and a multifaceted therapeutic approach. Causes, correlates, and management of fatigue in cancer patients have been reviewed by Groopman.[45] (see also Chapter 8.5)

Sleep in HIV/AIDS (see also Chapter 10.2)

Sleep disorders are common in HIV-infected patients. Fatigue, daytime sleepiness, and difficulties initiating and maintaining sleep have been described.[46,47] Sixty per cent of HIV-infected patients reported dissatisfaction with the quality of sleep, while about one in four described sleep as 'poor' or 'very poor'.[48] In another investigation, nearly three-quarter of outpatients with HIV/AIDS met criteria for insomnia.[49] Occurrence of insomnia correlated with depression, anxiety, cognitive impairment, night sweats, chills, and headaches. Likewise, Nokes and Kendrew described sleep impairment in HIV patients, as measured by Pittsburgh Sleep Quality Index scores.[50] As with cancer patients, these problems appear to go largely unrecognized by health care providers. The severity of sleep disturbance and associated daytime dysfunction is correlated with progression of the disease. Darko et al.[46] postulate that the debilitating fatigue of these patients may be related to elevated levels of somnogenic humoral factors such as interferon, tumour necrosis factor, and interleukin-1.

Sleep has been studied in a number of HIV-infected patients, including some with clinical manifestations of AIDS. In a series of reports, Norman et al.[51–53] reported alterations in the sleep of asymptomatic HIV-infected males. These patients demonstrated an increase in total slow-wave sleep, particularly as a result of increased slow-wave sleep in the second half of the night, when compared with normal controls. Seven of 10 patients in one study complained of excessive sleepiness, although daytime nap studies yielded objective evidence of pathological sleepiness in only one. These investigators speculated that sleep changes might represent early changes in the central nervous system associated with the infection or an adaptation to bolster immune response. Similar findings were reported by White et al. who noted correlation between CD4 T cell counts and increase in delta sleep during the last half of the night.[54] They found no evidence of pathological daytime sleepiness.

Cytokine production has been identified as a potential source of enhanced nocturnal slow-wave activity as well as daytime sleepiness in HIV patients. This theory is supported by the findings of Darko et al. who noted that, in 6/10 HIV patients, fluctuations in the levels of tumour necrosis factor-alpha (TNF-alpha) were coupled to peak periods of slow-wave activity in sleep.[55] The likelihood of this association was proportional to the

CD4 cell count, suggesting that, as patients became more ill and cell counts dropped, this physiological coupling declines and, with it, slow-wave sleep.

The sleep of patients whose disease has progressed beyond earlier stages of HIV infection is more likely to be disturbed. St Kubicki et al.[56] described disturbance of sleep including decreased percentages of slow-wave sleep in patients with diagnosed cerebral disease. Others have reported lighter sleep, with increased stage 1, increased awakening, and lower sleep efficiencies in HIV/AIDS patients.[57] Numerous immuno-logical, endocrinological, and metabolic factors have been identified as potential causes of this sleep disturbance.

Sleep disturbance has also been described in association with treatment for HIV/AIDS. Insomnia has been reported as a side effect of AZT,[58,59] although others have questioned this association.[47,57] Severe sleepiness when receiving a combination of AZT and acyclovir[60] has also been observed. One polysomnographic investigation of sleep in HIV patients taking zidovudine found no significant alterations in sleep physiology compared to that of unmedicated HIV patients.[61]

As noted, the sleep changes in HIV-infected individuals may vary widely according to the stage of disease and its complications. The sleep of asymptomatic infected persons as described by Norman et al. is probably quite different from that in late-stage AIDS with attendant neoplastic or infectious manifestations. Likewise, the presence of depression, anxiety, and cerebral involvement, particularly AIDS dementia complex, is likely to have major impact on the sleep of these patients, although this issue has not been fully clarified. Hintz et al., noting estimates of a 10–20 per cent incidence of depression in HIV-positive patients, reported on the response to antidepressant treatment in 90 such patients.[62] Their investigation revealed that decreased sleep was a particularly prominent finding that distinguished this population from a depressed HIV-negative group.

Factors contributing to sleep disorder

Depression (see also Chapter 8.17)

Sleep disturbance is a hallmark of major depression. It is generally held that 90 per cent or more of depressed patients exhibit abnormalities of their sleep patterns. Although early morning awakening is most commonly associated with depression, difficulty initiating sleep and repeated awakenings are not uncommon, particularly in a population in which the depression is associated with medical illness and its attendant complications. Current evidence indicates that specific abnormalities can be identified in the sleep EEG of primary depressive patients. These include disturbances in the continuity of sleep, decreased latency to the first REM sleep period, and diminished slow-wave sleep (stages 3/4).[63] The extent to which these findings are valid in depression associated with or secondary to medical disorders, particularly those of palliative care patients, is not clear. What is certain is that the sleep disturbance experienced by depressed terminally ill patients is a major source of concern, frustration, and added disability.

Studies to date indicate that depression is common among cancer patients. The manner in which 'depression' has been assessed varies widely from one investigator to another, making comparisons of prevalence difficult. Depressive illness accounts for approximately 50 per cent of psychiatric consultations in cancer patients.[64] Investigation of psychiatric disorders in Japanese cancer patients found that sleep disorders were the second most common reason for initiation of a psychiatric consultation, and that these patients showed high rates of depression, anxiety, and cognitive disturbance.[65] Studies of self-reported depressive symptoms indicate 'moderate' to 'severe' symptoms in 25–50 per cent of cancer patients.[66,67] Derogatis et al.[68] reported a prevalence of approximately 6 per cent for major depressive disorder assessed by DSM III criteria, with an additional 25 per cent diagnosed as having adjustment disorder with depressed or mixed features. Bukberg et al.[69] found a prevalence rate of 42 per cent for moderate to severe depression in cancer patients in hospital. A review of mood disorders in cancer patients identified prevalence rates of 4.5–58 per cent.[70] In those with advanced disease, the rates were 23–58 per cent. The variation in these numbers is clearly a reflection of differences in diagnostic criteria used to identify depression as well as the difficulties inherent in diagnosing mood disorder in patients with medical illnesses (see below).

These prevalence statistics suggest that depression is a very significant cause of sleep pathology in the terminally ill. In light of this, it is surprising to find that antidepressant medication is administered to a relatively small percentage of cancer patients. A 1970s multicentre study of psychotropic drug utilization by the Psychosocial Collaborative Oncology Group (PSYCOG) found that antidepressant medications accounted for only 1 per cent of all psychotropic prescriptions.[71] In the study of Bukberg et al., in which 42 per cent of patients met criteria for depression, only 6 per cent were receiving an antidepressant.[69] Jaeger et al.[72] found that 10 per cent of patients with advanced cancer (life expectancy less than 3 months) received antidepressants. This higher rate of administration may reflect a greater degree of overt psychological distress among the terminally ill. More recent data suggests that this situation has not improved greatly. Review of antidepressant prescriptions in over 1000 patients receiving palliative care for cancer demonstrated that only 10 per cent received antidepressant medications from the palliative care team and that the majority of these were administered this medication only in the last two weeks of life, when it was unlikely to have much effect.[73]

The under-usage of antidepressant medication may, to some extent, be a function of the complications of establishing a diagnosis of depression in palliative care patients. There is ample room for debate regarding the distinction between appropriate grief and clinical depression. In addition, uncertainty exists regarding the use of somatic symptoms (including sleep) in establishing the diagnosis of depression, inasmuch as such symptoms may be a function of the medical disorder. Some evidence suggests that sleep-related symptoms may be of particular importance in identifying depressive illness in cancer patients. Analysis of the association between insomnia and depression, anxiety, and pain revealed that insomnia was closely correlated with depression and anxiety.[30] In an effort to address the issue of specificity of somatic symptoms in the diagnosis of depression in cancer patients, one group of investigators found that, with the exception of insomnia, somatic symptoms did not distinguish the patients with depression from the non-depressed cancer population.[69] Although no statistical analysis is offered, the data strongly suggest that early, middle, and late insomnia were significantly more diagnostic of depression. In contrast to the above findings, Plumb and Holland reported that depressed patients with malignant disease did not manifest significantly greater insomnia than their next of kin, and reported less insomnia than a psychiatric group with depression and suicide attempt.[67] Unfortunately, these results do not make clear whether these findings are indicative of little insomnia among the cancer patients or a relatively high degree of insomnia in the next-of-kin.

There is no specific evidence regarding the efficacy of antidepressant medications in the treatment of insomnia associated with depression in the terminally ill. First generation antidepressant medications, particularly the more sedating compounds such as amitriptyline, doxepin, and trazodone, have been effective in the treatment of chronic pain syndromes which are frequently accompanied by depression and insomnia.[74–76] Patients with combined pain, depression, and insomnia may benefit not only from sedative and antidepressant effects of tricyclic medication, but also from the analgesic activity of these compounds.[77] More recent generation antidepressants may offer some advantages in terms of fewer side effects and higher compliance rates. For those patients with insomnia complaints, more sedating compounds such as mirtazapine (which can also stimulate appetite) or nefazodone may be appropriate. In patients who are already sedated from opioid or other sources, less sedating/more stimulating medications such as fluoxetine or buproprion may be better choices. There is no clear consensus with regard to greater efficacy for a particular antidepressant or group of antidepressants in cancer patients. Various studies have suggested efficacy of tricyclics,[78] possible superiority of fluoxetine versus tricyclics in advanced cancer,[79] and lack of significant improvement with fluoxetine.[80] A review of antidepressant efficacy for depression in medical illnesses, including cancer, suggested efficacy for both tricyclics and SSRIs, with a trend towards greater effectiveness but also higher dropout rates with tricyclics.(81)

The available literature makes it clear that depression is a common cause of insomnia among patients with advanced malignancies and that this aspect of their condition frequently goes unrecognized or untreated. Insomnia is an important diagnostic marker for depressive illness that must not be overlooked, particularly in light of the fact that effective treatment is available.

Anxiety

Although there has been little specific investigation of the relationship between terminal illness, specifically cancer, and anxiety symptoms, the available literature supports the common-sense conclusion that anxiety is a frequent complication among these patients.(31,66,68) Anxiety symptoms may be directly related to aspects of the patient's medical condition or treatment. Pain is frequently associated with increased anxiety. Early delirium, withdrawal from analgesics or sedative-hypnotics, and shortness of breath can frequently result in anxiety symptoms. Among patients with significant anxiety, sleep disturbance is common. Battelli et al.(82) reported that 63 per cent of cancer patients with anxiety had insomnia.

Fears that are masked by distractions during the daylight hours may come rapidly to the fore once the patient is left with nothing but the stillness of night. Anxieties regarding the illness itself, concerns about forthcoming procedures, worries regarding family or financial matters are but a few of the tensions which can disrupt the onset or maintenance of sleep. Pain may be exacerbated during the night (owing to inadequate medication and lack of distraction), giving rise to further anxiety about the meaning of the pain as a possible sign of advancing disease. For patients in the final stages of their illness, the prospect of sleep may provoke anxieties about the possibility that they will never awaken.

As sleeplessness ensues, additional anxiety often arises over the inability to fall asleep. A vicious cycle is set in motion in which the patient with an initially transient insomnia disturbance develops a negative expectation regarding sleep and begins to dread the prospect of another tension- and frustration-laden night in bed. The bed thus becomes a powerful conditioned stimulus for escalating anxiety and arousal that prevents the onset of sleep. For patients who are not ambulatory and are unable to 'escape', this dilemma may be particularly difficult. The combination of heightened internal arousal and conditioned anxiety gives rise to a chronic condition of self-propagating sleep disturbance that is referred to as psychophysiological insomnia. The disturbance may be accompanied by an increase in muscle tension, sympathetic arousal, and unrelenting cognitive activity. As sleep steadily worsens, daytime anxiety and rumination regarding the inability to obtain a restful night may intervene.

The sleep of patients with diagnosed anxiety disorders has not been studied in great detail. Laboratory studies have revealed prolonged sleep latency, decreased sleep efficiency (the percentage of time in bed which is spent asleep), increased awake time during the night, decreased deep sleep, and higher percentages of light sleep.(83,84) In addition to the alteration of sleep architecture, specific anxiety-related disturbances such as nocturnal anxiety attacks or nightmares may occur.(85) Nightmares are dream anxiety episodes which ordinarily arise from REM sleep. They are accompanied by awakening from sleep with a sense of dread or terror and a moderate level of autonomic arousal. The frightening dream content is recalled in detail upon awakening. Nightmares may occur as a complication of severe anxiety or other psychiatric illness, administration of drugs, or use of certain medications such as some antidepressants, β-blockers, L-dopa, or reserpine.

Non-pharmacological therapeutic measures including support, reassurance, proper sleep hygiene and behavioural techniques such as relaxation training, may help to ameliorate the sleep disturbance associated with anxiety. Benzodiazepines have been effective in treating anxiety-related insomnia. Battelli et al. found that 80 per cent of patients with insomnia were sleeping normally after 2 weeks of treatment with lorazepam.(82) Diazepam has also been used with similar beneficial effects, although many patients experienced daytime sedation. Psychotherapy, benzodiazepines, and tricyclic medication have all been employed with some success in the treatment of recurrent nightmares.

Cognitive impairment disorders

Numerous investigations have revealed that cognitive dysfunction, particularly delirium, is common among cancer patients.(64,86) The incidence of delirium is particularly high among those in the terminal stages of illness.(87) Disturbance of the sleep–wake schedule is an intrinsic component of delirium. As described by Lipowski,(88) wakefulness during the daytime hours is typically reduced, while nighttime often brings increased alertness and agitation. As a result, the normal circadian rhythm may be reversed or severely disrupted in this population. The multiple aetiologies of delirium in patients with terminal malignancies have been reviewed elsewhere.(89,90) Sleep deprivation itself may predispose to the development of delirium.(91) Polysomnographic studies of delirium have been limited to withdrawal states,(92) and the applicability of these findings to the sleep of patients with delirium due to other causes is uncertain.

Dementia, while less commonly a direct result of cancer, may be encountered in terminally ill patients,(68) particularly in the geriatric population. This disorder is often associated with nocturnal delirium (sundowning). Sleep studies of dementia patients reveal increased sleep latencies, lighter sleep, reduced REM sleep, and increased awakening after sleep onset.(93,94)

The sleep disturbance associated with cognitive impairment disorders can be exceedingly difficult to manage. Accurate diagnosis is the first step. Delirium often goes unrecognized, particularly in its early stages, and may be mistaken for depression or anxiety in some patients. Attempts to treat or control the specific causes of delirium, particularly medication, constitute the primary approach. Efforts to prevent excessive sleep during the daytime are advisable. Patients with cognitive dysfunction may sleep better in a lit room, where disorientation and agitation are minimized. Conventional hypnotic medications have typically been avoided, because they may aggravate delirium. The usual pharmacological treatment for patients with non-drug-related delirium and disruptive behaviour is low dose neuroleptic medication such as haloperidol 0.5–2.0 mg or risperidone 0.5–1.0 mg. In patients whose agitation is largely limited to the nighttime, it is often helpful to begin administration of the medication in the late afternoon before agitation begins to escalate. Benzodiazepine and related medication (discussed later in this chapter) should be used with caution in light of the potential for aggravation of cognitive disturbance, but may be therapeutic. Subcutaneous midazolam has been used effectively in terminal patients with delirium or agitation when other agents were not helpful.(95,96)

Pain

A number of issues must be taken into consideration in assessing the relationship between pain and sleep in terminally ill patients. What are the effects of pain on sleep? How does sleep deprivation affect pain threshold and perception? What intervening variables, such as psychiatric disorders, influence the relationship between pain and sleep?

Numerous studies of cancer patients indicate that up to 50 per cent experience significant pain. In individuals with advanced cancer, estimates rise to 60–90 per cent.(97–99) These data, along with observations regarding the effects of pain on sleep in other conditions and indications that pain is often inadequately treated, suggest that pain plays an important role in sleep disturbance among cancer patients. Of 200 patients referred for treatment to a cancer pain clinic, 124 (61 per cent) reported that pain interrupted sleep.(100) Dorrepaal and colleagues evaluated pain experience and management in a group of 240 cancer patients in hospital.(101) They found that upon admission, 37 per cent of patients with pain reported that it interfered with sleep onset, while 65 per cent complained of difficulty in maintaining sleep through the night because of pain. Similarly, 56 per cent of 91 lung and colon cancer patients stated that pain interfered 'moderately' or 'greatly' with sleep.[102] An investigation of the influence of cancer-related pain on various quality of life indicators revealed that 58 per cent of cancer patients woke during the night because of pain.[103] Pain intensity has also been demonstrated to correlate inversely with total hours of sleep in patients with advanced cancer.[104]

Donovan et al. examined the issue of pain in hospitalized patients and the effects of inadequate analgesia.[105] In this mixed group, which consisted of predominantly non-cancer patients with acute or chronic pain, 61 per cent reported that they were awakened by pain. The patients were receiving an average of less than 25 per cent of the total analgesic dosage ordered. It should be noted that the cancer patients in this population did not differ from the non-cancer patients with respect to incidence or severity of pain.

Pain models and related variables

Understanding the effects of pain on sleep provides further insight into this problem. In assessing peak pain-related symptoms, Kinsman et al.[106] reported that 60 per cent of the group complained of frequent sleep disturbance. In a population of patients attending a pain clinic, sleep was characterized as 'poor' by 70 per cent of the group.[107] The poor sleepers reported greater pain intensity, less total sleep time, and a tendency towards greater disability. Pain intensity and depression were the only significant predictors of sleep disturbance, leading the investigators to speculate that degree of insomnia may serve as a useful marker for pain intensity. Closs found that pain was the most common factor resulting in sleep disturbance in post-operative patients. Pain relief was the most effective intervention for improving sleep maintenance.[108]

Animal models of chronic pain demonstrate an increase in wakefulness, a shift to lighter stages of NREM sleep, reduction in paradoxical (REM) sleep, and fragmentation of sleep.[109,110] A loss of the normal diurnal variation of the sleep–wake cycle was also noted. Similar polysomnographic findings have also been described in humans with rheumatic and other pain conditions.[111,112]

The observation of increased sleep disturbance in patients with pain does not, in itself, establish a direct cause and effect relationship between these variables. It is quite possible that intervening factors, particularly psychological distress, may play an important role. For example, it has been reported that the incidence of pain among cancer patients with psychiatric disorder is twice that of those without such disorder.[113] This may reflect the fact that patients with pain are also likely to have more advanced illness and therefore to be more susceptible to depression or cognitive impairment disorders. Nevertheless, it is apparent that comorbidity of this nature (i.e. psychiatric illness) may have as much responsibility for the sleep disturbance as the pain per se. Beszterczey and Lipowski[30] described decreased total sleep time in a group of cancer patients referred for radiation therapy. Analysis revealed that the insomnia correlated far better with the degree of depression and anxiety than with pain. A more recent study of sleep in chronic pain patients indicated that presleep cognitive arousal was more predictive of poor sleep than pain severity itself. Thus, while pain may be an important determinant of sleep disturbance, other factors, some of which co-vary with pain, may be of equal importance.

Sleep deprivation and pain

In order to understand fully the relationship between sleep and pain, it is necessary to address the question of how sleep deprivation affects pain perception and, in turn, to what extent improvement in sleep might produce a beneficial response with respect to pain. Hicks et al.[114] reported that pain threshold in rats is decreased in response to deprivation of REM sleep, and that the effect persisted for up to 96 h following the deprivation. This may be related to the fact that opioid receptor binding decreases after sleep deprivation.[115] It has been shown that sleep deprivation lowers pain threshold in human controls.[3,116] Likewise, reversal of sleep deprivation produces significant increases in threshold.[116] Burn patients reported higher levels of background pain during the nighttime and this correlated strongly with poor sleep quality.[117] In addition, poor sleep quality predicted higher levels of pain on the following day. Repeated interruptions of sleep induced experimentally result in a pain syndrome which is akin to fibromyalgia.[6] The work of Moldofsky and others related to fibromyalgia syndrome suggests that sleep may play an important role in pain modulation and that disturbance of sleep might predispose to the development of rheumatic pain disorder by interference with the tissue-restorative functions of NREM sleep in particular. The relationship of these findings to pain of other origins is uncertain.

Clinical experience suggests that patients whose coping skills are enhanced by improved sleep are in a far better position to maintain optimal function despite their pain and, perhaps, to perceive the pain as less severe. This notion is supported by reports from hospital patients with acute and chronic pain that sleep helped to reduce their pain.[105] Moreover, administration of delta-sleep-inducing peptide to chronic pain patients resulted in reduction of pain and associated symptoms of depression.[118]

Effects of pain treatment

It is clear that improved control of pain results in better sleep. One notable advance in this area has been the use of controlled-release opioid for pain control. Hanks et al. describe improved sleep in a group of advanced cancer patients in response to crossover from aqueous morphine sulfate administered 4 hourly to controlled-release morphine.[37] Ventafridda et al. reported that mean total sleep time was doubled in patients with cancer pain treated according to the WHO guidelines.[119] Similar observations have been described by other investigators.[36,120] Comparisons of controlled-release morphine and transdermal fentanyl have demonstrated improved sleep with both medications.[121–123] One study suggested that the transdermal fentanyl may be associated with somewhat less daytime sedation and poorer sleep quality than controlled-release morphine.[123]

Significant improvements in sleep have also been reported with the use of non-steroidal anti-inflammatory drugs (NSAIDs) in advanced cancer pain.[124] Carrol et al.[125] demonstrated that a combined regimen of methadone, NSAID, tricyclics, and hydroxyzine produced marked improvement in pain and sleep in patients not responsive to single drug therapy. For patients refractory to all other routes of opioid administration, combined, long-term intrathecal morphine and bupivacaine have produced prolonged improvement in sleep and pain.[126] A multidisciplinary approach which included various combinations of oral and epidural opioids, non-opioid analgesics, antidepressants, benzodiazepines, anticonvulsants, and nerve blocks produced an almost 80 per cent reduction in the number of cancer patients whose sleep was interrupted by pain.[100] In appropriate circumstances, continuous infusion and/or patient-controlled analgesia will be superior to immediate release oral opioids in fostering sustained sleep. A comparison of the effects of a mild sedative with those of a mild analgesic on sleep in non-cancer patients demonstrated that the analgesic was most important in improving sleep for those with pain.[127] The pharmacological effects of opioids on sleep physiology and wakefulness are discussed below.

In summary, pain is a frequent and often inadequately treated symptom of cancer and other terminal illnesses that is an important factor contributing to the development and maintenance of sleep disturbance. Sleep deprivation, in turn, may exacerbate pain problems and compromise the already tenuous function of patients receiving palliative care. Intervening variables such as depression and anxiety play a contributory role. Improved control of pain can result in marked improvement in sleep disturbance and thereby greatly improve the quality of life.

Medication

Discussion of the effects of medication on sleep in palliative care must include attention to those medications that interfere with normal sleep, as well as those that result in excessive or undesirable sedation. The effects of specific hypnotic medication are discussed later in this chapter.

Relatively little attention has been given to the effects of chemotherapy agents on sleep. Some studies demonstrate an association between chemotherapy, poor sleep, and increased fatigue in cancer patients.[128,129]

Shapiro has pointed out that certain chemotherapeutic agents may produce insomnia as a result of their potential for inducing nausea or cognitive dysfunction.[130] Clinical experience suggests that corticosteroids produce sleep disturbance, although this has not been well documented. Steroids do appear to decrease REM sleep,[131] but the clinical implications of this are uncertain. Methylxanthine derivatives (bronchodilators) are well known for their stimulant properties and may disturb sleep severely. Certain antihypertensives, such as methyldopa and propranolol, have been reported to cause insomnia; the latter also associated with nightmare activity in some patients. Central nervous system stimulants, sometimes advocated for their ability to counteract opioid-induced sedation, have clear potential for disrupting sleep when given too close to bedtime, as do certain types of antidepressants (e.g. monoamine oxidase inhibitors, fluoxetine, protriptyline, or bupropion). Withdrawal from sedative-hypnotic medication is also a potentially important cause of insomnia.

Psychotropic agents

Excessive sleepiness and associated daytime impairment may severely compromise the function of patients already impaired by other aspects of their disease. The most common offending agents are psychotropic medications prescribed for anxiety, sleep, depression, or control of nausea. Older patients with medical illness are particularly vulnerable to excess sedation due to drug accumulation as a result of delayed metabolism and excretion. Sedating antidepressants such as amitriptyline, doxepin, or trazodone may result in daytime sleepiness, even when given at bedtime. Phenothiazines and other dopamine antagonists used in the treatment of nausea due to chemotherapy may be very sedating. This is especially true for aliphatic and piperidine compounds, but less so for piperazine derivatives and butyrophenones. H_1 antagonists are common sources of daytime sleepiness, although this appears to be less true for H_2 antagonists that have less effect on the central nervous system.

Opioids

The effects of opioids on sleep and wakefulness are complex and appear to include both stimulant and sedative properties.[132] Initial doses of morphine administered to non-dependent addicts decrease total sleep but increase drowsiness. With chronic usage, sleep latency is decreased but the total time awake after sleep onset is somewhat increased. Although drowsiness is a feature of acute morphine administration, this appears to abate with chronic usage. The effects of opioids on sleep structure vary with duration of usage. The most prominent initial effect is suppression of REM activity. However, this is less evident with longer-term administration. The effects on NREM sleep vary according to type of drug, length of usage, and specific sleep stage. There is some evidence to suggest that daytime psychomotor performance is slowed as a result of opioid administration[133] but other data showing minimal or no effects of opioids.

Although these data are of some use in understanding the effects of opioid analgesics on sleep, it should be noted that they are based largely on studies of subjects who were not medically ill or in pain. As already discussed, effective analgesia clearly results in improved sleep for pain patients, and any alterations of 'normal' sleep which may be induced by medication are surely outweighed by the benefits attributable to relief of pain. Likewise, while opioids can produce some degree of daytime drowsiness, particularly in the earlier phases of administration, this is not always the case and, in some, may be considered a potentially unavoidable sequela of adequate pain relief. While the clinician should attempt to strike an appropriate balance in this regard, sufficient analgesia must take precedence. Effective strategies for control of daytime sedation with stimulant medications have been described.[134,135]

Respiratory disorder

Respiratory disturbance in sleep is a common cause of sleep disorder. Obstructive sleep apnoea is associated primarily with heavy snoring and excessive daytime sleepiness, although some patients report frequent nocturnal awakening. The syndrome is observed more commonly in older patients and those who are obese. There is no clear connection between obstructive sleep apnoea and malignancy, although it should be noted that patients whose upper airway structure or function is compromised directly as a result of tumour mass or indirectly through treatment might be predisposed to the development of obstruction during sleep. This has been described in patients with parapharyngeal tumour mass,[136,137] medulloblastoma,[138] and in those who have undergone mandibulectomy without reconstruction.[139] In patients with AIDS, daytime sleepiness has been described in association with sleep apnoea due to tonsillar hypertrophy.[140] Perhaps of greater importance for the majority of cancer patients is the fact that respiratory depressant medications, particularly opioid analgesics, can exacerbate this condition. Etches described severe respiratory depression associated with patient-controlled opioid analgesia.[141] Pre-existing sleep apnoea and concomitant use of sedatives-hypnotics were associated with the development of respiratory compromise. Central sleep apnoea has also been noted to occur with malignancy.[142] Sleep apnoea frequently goes unrecognized and may be a source of major compromise of function (due to sleepiness and attendant neuropsychological factors) in terminally ill patients.

Dyspnoea is a disturbing symptom for some palliative care patients, particularly those with primary lung cancer or pulmonary metastases. Pulmonary involvement may give rise to complaints of insomnia through two primary mechanisms. Patients describe the sensation of breathlessness as psychologically disturbing and have difficulty initiating or maintaining sleep as a result of heightened arousal associated with this anxiety. Studies of patients with chronic obstructive pulmonary disease also suggest that severe hypoxia and/or hypercapnoea, as well as chronic cough, may play a role in determining sleep disturbance. Decreased total sleep time, increased light sleep, multiple arousals, and decreased REM sleep have been reported in such patients.[143] Non-pharmacological treatment (e.g. relaxation training) for heightened arousal associated with breathlessness may aid sleep. Nocturnal oxygen supplementation is indicated for hypoxic patients. Pharmacological treatment with benzodiazepines may be used cautiously in patients without major blood gas alterations, but is contraindicated in more severely hypoxic or hypercapnoeic patients.

Gastrointestinal disorders

Nausea and vomiting following certain forms of chemotherapy can disrupt sleep and impair quality of life.[144] Some terminally ill patients report nocturnal diarrhoea or discomfort associated with chronic constipation as a cause of repeated sleep disruption. These complications may occur as a result of autonomic dysfunction, medication, or other forms of treatment. Gastro-oesophageal reflux is commonly aggravated during sleep, giving rise to epigastric pain, heartburn, and cough, with repeated disruption of sleep.

Hospital admission

It is well known that admission to hospital can be associated with marked disruption of sleep.[145–147] Although in most studies this issue has been examined in patients in surgical and intensive care units, it stands to reason that other seriously ill patients also experience frequent interruptions of sleep as a direct result of the hospital environment. Potential interruptions include intrusions by staff to monitor vital signs, check lines and equipment, or administer medications, excessive noise or light, or difficulties experienced by other patients occupying the same room. Under these circumstances sleep may become highly fragmented and total sleep time markedly reduced, giving rise to increased napping and disturbance of the sleep–wake cycle. Efforts by staff to minimize such disrupting factors are likely to result in improved sleep.[148]

Other conditions affecting sleep and wakefulness

Numerous other disorders may contribute to poor sleep in the terminally ill. Nutritional deficiency has not been well studied, although investigations of patients with anorexia nervosa suggest that a strong link exists between starvation and sleep disturbance.[149] Thus, nutritional deficiency may contribute to sleep disturbance in terminal cancer patients. Nocturia is a common source of repetitive awakening in patients receiving diuretics. Similarly, patients may suffer from frequent nocturnal headaches that disrupt sleep.

Endocrine disturbance can give rise to sleep disorder.[150] A specific endocrine issue that has been identified as a significant cause of sleep disturbance is that of hot flushes. Carpenter et al. reported that 65 per cent of post-menopausal breast cancer patients experienced hot flushes.[151] Among those with hot flushes, 86 per cent had some form of nocturnal hot flushes. Studies of post-menopausal women have demonstrated that hot flushes are associated with sleep disruption and that treatment with hormone replacement therapy (HRT) improves sleep.[152] Unfortunately, HRT may be contraindicated in the population of breast cancer patients, who are most susceptible to this problem.

There is limited, and largely anecdotal, information relating specific cancers to sleep disorders. Symptoms of narcolepsy/cataplexy have been described in association with midbrain or brainstem tumours, including those in the region of the third ventricle.[153,154] Centrally mediated respiratory disorders which disrupt sleep have been described in patients with brainstem tumours.[155] It seems certain that other primary malignancies or metastases of the central nervous system may affect sleep indirectly, through cerebral oedema, or directly through structures subserving sleep. An understanding of such effects awaits further investigation.

Other primary sleep disorders may occur in terminally ill patients. The most notable of those not mentioned elsewhere in this chapter are restless legs syndrome (RLS) and periodic limb movement in sleep (PLMS). RLS is a waking dysaesthesia, most often localized to the calves, which occurs primarily in evening hours. The major manifestation of this dysaesthesia is an irresistible urge to move the legs. RLS may interfere with sleep onset or maintenance, as well as cause the sufferer great torment while waking. PLMS, often observed in patients with RLS, consists of repetitive, stereotyped leg and/or arm movements that occur at intervals of 20–40 s during sleep, typically in clusters throughout the night. The repetitive movements may result in frequent arousals during sleep, leading to complaints of light or non-restorative sleep, sleep maintenance disturbance, and/or daytime sleepiness. Potential aetiologies of the disorders are noted in Table 1, although they are frequently idiopathic. These conditions will respond to correction of the underlying causative factor, when one can be identified. In idiopathic cases, dopamine agonists/L-dopa or clonazepam may be efficacious. Opioid and gabapentin have also been successful in the treatment of refractory cases.

Evaluation

The most serious and fundamental problem in the identification of sleep disorders is that patients are frequently never asked about their sleep. When complaints are offered by the patient, they are too often dismissed by clinicians out of ignorance or therapeutic nihilism. It is essential that health care practitioners recognize the importance of adequate sleep and alertness to the psychological, social, and physical well being of their patients. Two basic questions should be asked of all patients as a component of the general systems review: How are you sleeping at night? Are you excessively sleepy during the day? When sleep-related complaints are elicited, a more detailed history is required. As previously emphasized, insomnia and hypersomnolence are not diagnoses—they are symptoms. The aetiology of these complaints must be established before any reasonable treatment approach can be constructed. The basic principles of evaluation are outlined in Table 2.

A complaint of 'insomnia' may arise as a result of several different types of sleep-related disturbance. Although reports of difficulty in initiating or maintaining sleep are most often associated with insomnia, other factors such as the perceived quality of sleep, timing of the sleep–wake cycle, or total duration of sleep may also give rise to a complaint of poor sleep. Since these varied presentations may suggest different causative factors, an effort must be made to clarify these components of the disorder. It is helpful to identify the context in which the sleep disturbance began, with consideration of possible precipitating factors. Elaboration of the influence of intervening variables, including treatment efforts, may also yield useful information regarding aetiology. The patient's 24-h schedule must be determined. Sleep disorders clinicians frequently employ sleep logs for this purpose. Such logs typically include information regarding bedtime, sleep latency (time to onset of sleep), number of awakenings, length of awakenings, time of final awakening, estimated total sleep time, and perceived quality of sleep. Entries concerning daytime naps, unusual daytime activities, medications, drugs, and alcohol are included as well. Some patients report that the mere process of completing such a log helps them to identify conditions unfavourable to sleep.

Table 2 Evaluation of sleep disorders

Identify the primary complaint: insomnia, excessive sleepiness, parasomnia, (abnormal event), sleep–wake schedule disturbance
Characterize the complaint: difficulty initiating sleep, recurrent nocturnal awakening, insufficient total sleep, non-restorative sleep, advanced or delayed sleep onset, excessively long sleep, chronic drowsiness, sleep attacks
Document the sleep–wake cycle: sleep logs including nighttime sleep schedule, naps, activities, medications
Identify possible precipitants of disturbance: information from patient and spouse or family members (see Table 1)
Consider the particular sleep requirements of the patients: short/average/long sleepers, variation in sleep habits with age and situation
Medical and neuropsychiatric history
Substance use: medication, alcohol, drugs, caffeine, nicotine
Physical examination and laboratory data
Polysomnography, particularly in elderly medically ill patients with excessive sleepiness or those with histories suggesting underlying physiological disturbance
Multiple Sleep Latency Test; evaluation of excessive daytime sleepiness

Difficulty falling asleep is often associated with negative expectations regarding sleep, specific anxieties, ruminations, and, in some cases, heightened physiologic arousal (increased heart rate, respiratory rate, or muscle tension). In a medically ill population, physical factors, most notably pain, may interfere with the onset of sleep. In order to gain an understanding of associated patterns of cognition, affect, and behaviour that may further contribute to delayed sleep onset, it is necessary to determine what the patient thinks, feels, and does during the time in bed prior to sleep initiation. Identification of anxieties regarding the course of their illness, upcoming procedures, family matters, and death is of particular importance in terminally ill patients.

When patients have difficulty maintaining sleep, an effort must be made to identify possible precipitants for the awakenings. Although psychological factors, particularly depression, may contribute to awakening and difficulty in returning to sleep, midcycle awakening should increase the clinician's suspicion of an underlying physiological cause. Failure to provide analgesia of sufficient dosage and duration often results in awakening due to pain. Other readily identifiable causes such as nocturia, respiratory disturbance (sleep apnoea, congestive heart failure, primary or metastatic pulmonary disease), headache, or non-specific musculoskeletal discomfort must be sought. Repeated awakenings may be associated with specific sleep-related conditions such as periodic movements in sleep, sleep apnoea, nightmares, or sleep terrors. Disease of the central nervous system can result in severe disruption of the normal sleep–wake architecture and inability to maintain sound sleep for any length of time.

Some patients report that they do not feel rested despite what seems to be a normal amount of sleep. This 'non-restorative' pattern of sleep has been associated with repeated intrusion of alpha (7–12 Hz) activity in the sleep EEG, particularly during NREM sleep. Steady-state disturbance (such as pain) or frequent episodic abnormalities (such as movement disorder) may give rise to such sleep disturbance and concomitant daytime complaints of fatigue, poor concentration, and sleepiness in the absence of overt difficulty initiating or maintaining sleep.

In evaluating complaints of insomnia, the clinician must keep in mind that the duration of normal sleep varies significantly from person to person. The 'normal' amount of sleep for a given individual is best defined as that amount which is required to achieve adequate daytime alertness, concentration, and energy. This may be difficult to assess in terminally ill patients and, for this reason, it is necessary to rely on the patient's premorbid sleep history to determine how many hours of sleep that individual can reasonably expect. A complaint of insomnia should include evidence of impairment of daytime function that is attributable to insufficient or poor quality sleep. Lacking such evidence, it may be that the patient is a 'short-sleeper', that is, someone who requires less than the average amount of sleep for a person of that age. Likewise, there are some individuals who may complain of fatigue and sleepiness in spite of obtaining what the clinician assumes to be a normal amount of sleep. These patients may be 'long-sleepers' whose sleep need is greater than average. Although no systematic investigation has been conducted, it seems plausible that a need for extra sleep may arise in conditions of systemic illness.

For some patients, the complaint of insomnia may be more related to the timing of sleep in the 24-h cycle. Specifically, patients may complain of difficulty in falling asleep although, once asleep, they are capable of achieving an appropriate amount of sleep. This and other sleep–wake rhythm disorders have been discussed earlier in this chapter.

A careful review of medication, drugs, and alcohol usage is a crucial component in assessing complaints of insomnia and excessive sleepiness. The role of medication has been discussed. Patients who are experiencing difficulty sleeping may resort to alcohol in an effort to alleviate their symptoms. Although sufficient amounts of alcohol will ultimately induce sleep onset, sleep during later stages of the night is often light and marked by frequent awakenings and increased autonomic arousal. Alcohol may also aggravate sleep-related breathing disorders. Caffeine is an obvious, but surprisingly overlooked, cause of sleep disturbance. In assessing its role, one must be aware of the fact that some individuals experience marked and prolonged arousal in response to even small quantities of caffeine. Nicotine has also been demonstrated to have similar disruptive effects on sleep.

The physical examination and laboratory data must also be considered an essential part of the evaluation of patients with sleep disorder. Particular attention must be paid to the evaluation of pain and to the neurological, endocrine, and cardiopulmonary examinations. General laboratory screening should include a full blood count and biochemistry as well as screening for nutritional deficiency, endocrine disturbance, and medication levels.

Electrophysiologic evaluation (polysomnography) is an important element in the assessment of sleep disorders. However, such studies should clearly be used in a judicious manner for patients receiving palliative care. Nevertheless, when proper indications exist, the information gained from such studies may allow dramatic improvements in the quality of life. Standard polysomnography typically includes monitoring of sleep EEG, submental EMG, eye movement, airflow, respiratory effort, oxygen saturation, ECG, and leg movements, with additional parameters as indicated. An adequate diagnostic study can usually be accomplished in one night, with minimum discomfort or inconvenience for the patient. Such studies are most useful when an underlying physiological disturbance, such as periodic limb movement or sleep-disordered breathing, is suspected. Further characterization of abnormal events (parasomnias) or medical conditions in sleep may also be productive. Polysomnography is not indicated in the routine assessment of primary insomnia or insomnia due to mental disorders such as depression or anxiety. When complaints of daytime fatigue or sleepiness are present, daytime nap studies (Multiple Sleep Latency Test) can provide an objective determination of the degree of true sleepiness, as well as shedding light on certain specific diagnoses, such as narcolepsy.

Treatment

The treatment of sleep disorders must be carefully tailored according to the aetiology of the condition and the particular needs and situation of the patient. Just as there are usually a number of contributing factors in the genesis and maintenance of a sleep disorder, treatment must also be multifactorial. When insomnia or excessive sleepiness is secondary to another medical or psychiatric condition, the primary condition must be accurately identified and treated before there can be any reasonable expectation of improvement in sleep. However, it must also be recognized that secondary psychophysiologic complications may forestall amelioration of the disorder even when the primary condition has been adequately addressed. These conditioned factors must also be treated. By definition, it is not possible to abolish the primary disease process for palliative care patients, but it is usually feasible to control aspects of the process in a manner that will have a positive impact on sleep.

Sleep hygiene

Most people are aware of the common-sense rules and behaviours for promoting good sleep. Nevertheless, failure to adhere to these guidelines is an almost ubiquitous component of many sleep disorders. The problems in this area are so common that the International Classification of Sleep Disorders nosology now includes a separate diagnosis for 'Inadequate Sleep Hygiene', although it should be understood that disturbances in this area more often exist as a complication of some other sleep disorder. Adequate sleep is dependent on the proper internal (psychophysiologic) and external (environmental) circumstances. In effect, the rules of sleep hygiene attempt to operationalize these conditions. Suggestions for sleep hygiene in palliative care patients are summarized in Table 3.

Excessive arousal in bed is a frequent cause and effect of insomnia. For the terminally ill patient who carries multiple concerns to bed, the level of

Table 3 Sleep hygiene for palliative care patients

Maintain as regular a sleep–wake schedule as possible, particularly with respect to the hour of morning awakening
Avoid unnecessary time in bed during the day; for bedridden patients, provide as much cognitive and physical stimulation during daytime hours as conditions permit
Nap only as necessary and avoid napping in the late afternoon and evening, whenever possible
Keep as active a daytime schedule as possible: this should include social contacts and, when able, light exercise
Minimize nighttime sleep interruptions due to medication, noise, or other environmental conditions
Avoid lying in bed for prolonged periods at night in an alert and frustrated or tense state; read or engage in other relaxing activity (out of bed, when appropriate) until drowsiness ensues
Remove unpleasant conditioned stimuli, such as clocks, from sight and sound
Identify problems and concerns of the day before trying to sleep, and address these issues with an active problem-solving approach
Avoid stimulating medication and other substances (e.g. caffeine, nicotine), particularly in the hours before bedtime
Maintain adequate pain relief through the night, preferably with long-acting analgesics
Use sleep medication as indicated after proper evaluation of the sleep problem and avoid overusage

arousal may be quite pronounced. Lying in bed, mind racing, agitated and tense, there is little possibility that the patient will fall asleep soon. Remaining in bed at this point becomes distinctly frustrating and most certainly counterproductive. However, this is often what patients with insomnia do, either by choice or, in the case of non-ambulatory patients, because they have no option. Under the mistaken impression that they are 'resting' (which is seldom the case), or because getting out of bed is a sign of defeat, they remain in bed, sometimes for hours, fully awake. When this occurs on a regular basis for weeks or months, the bed becomes associated not with relaxation and sleep but, rather, with frustration and tension. In time, the mere sight of the bed evokes increased arousal. At this point, the patient's worst fear has become a self-fulfilling prophecy.

When an individual is unable to fall asleep within a reasonable period (best defined by the sleeper, but typically within 30 min), he should get out of bed and engage in some relaxing activity until he feels ready to sleep. For patients who require assistance to get out of bed, this presents a problem. In such cases, some provision should be made to allow for some relaxing activity (e.g. reading, music, television, or hand-work) in bed. It is most important that the focus be turned away from a pressure to fall asleep. Other stimuli may also come to evoke a response of wakefulness. One of the most common is the clock. When unable to fall asleep, or following an awakening, patients often stare at the clock. In time, the clock becomes a very powerful reminder of their inability to fall asleep. This and other such conditioned stimuli must be identified and removed from sight or sound.

Palliative care patients are especially susceptible to alterations of their normal schedules. Because of fatigue, immobility, discomfort, or lack of motivation, the daytime level of activity is often severely curtailed. When this occurs, the division between day and night becomes blurred. This is particularly true if napping and time in bed are a significant part of the daily routine. Lacking many of the usual environmental cues (*zeitgebers*) that serve to strengthen basic circadian rhythms, the affected individual is no longer well entrained to an organized sleep–wake rhythm. As a result, the sleep pattern may become chaotic and unpredictable. The solution to this problem is to take steps to reinforce the basic rest/activity–sleep/wake cycle. A regular hour of bedtime and arising is the most essential part of this. Complete avoidance of daytime napping and recumbent rest are not realistic for very sick patients, but such time should be as limited as possible and scheduled such that there is a prolonged 'up time' prior to bedtime. A programme of physical activity and cognitive and social stimulation will underscore day–night differences and strengthen biological rhythms. Although vigorous physical exercise is not usually possible in this population, mild exercise, even in a sitting or recumbent position, may be helpful. However, physical stimulation should be avoided in the pre-bedtime hours as this may interfere with sleep onset.

It is frequently the case that patients manage to avoid anxieties during the day by means of distraction, only to be inundated by them in bed. Therefore, it is important to address anxieties, concerns, and disappointments in a direct fashion during waking hours, thus allowing the person to put these feelings to rest prior to bedtime. Identifying these issues, considering what they themselves can do about problems, seeking information, assistance, and support from others, and, finally, accepting those aspects of a situation that cannot be changed must all be a part of this process.

The sleeping environment cannot be overlooked as a potential source of sleep disturbance. Medically ill patients who are receiving some type of institutional care often experience frequent interruptions of sleep as a result of staff activities, background noise, lighting, or other factors. It is necessary to identify environmental circumstances of this nature and seek solutions in conjunction with the patient. For example, some patients prefer a darker sleeping environment while others, particularly those with some degree of cognitive disturbance, find a partially lit room to be orienting and reassuring. Hospital beds may assist some patients in attaining comfortable positions not possible in standard beds. For individuals who are not ambulatory and require special assistance in meeting minimal needs, it will be reassuring to have access to necessary articles at the bedside as well as a reliable means of calling for assistance.

Substances such as caffeine, nicotine, and alcohol, which may interfere with sleep, have been discussed. The relationship between sleep and food intake is not clear. Some patients find a snack at bedtime comforting, while others insist that food before bedtime promotes wakefulness. L-Tryptophan, found in higher concentrations in certain foodstuffs, has been promoted as a potential sleep aid, although laboratory studies indicate only modest results.[156]

Non-pharmacological treatment of insomnia

Cognitive-behavioural treatment has emerged as a mainstay in the treatment of insomnia that is due wholly or in part to heightened cognitive or physiological arousal and poor sleep hygiene. Reviews and meta-analyses of this subject are available.[157–160] There is no single most effective behavioural approach. Successful application depends most on appropriate matching of treatment modality and patient characteristics.

Successful applications of behavioural techniques for control of sleep disturbance in cancer patients have been reported. Cannici et al.[161] described the use of muscle relaxation training in 15 patients with insomnia 'secondary to cancer'. They reported a significant reduction in sleep latency and increase in total sleep time for the treatment group following 3 days of relaxation training. Anecdotal reports indicate that other behavioural approaches, including hypnosis[162] and somatic focus/imagery training,[163] have been effective for insomnia in cancer patients. In a related vein, behavioural interventions are frequently employed for patients with cancer pain and chronic pain syndromes.[164,165] Currie and others demonstrated effectiveness of a multicomponent cognitive-behavioural approach to insomnia in chronic pain patients, with maintenance of gains after 3 months.[166] This aspect of treatment, which is highly relevant to sleep disturbance, is reviewed in Chapter 8.2.10.

Numerous specific techniques are included in the cognitive-behavioural approach. Some have proven more effective than others in the management of insomnia. Progressive muscle relaxation therapy has been used widely in the treatment of insomnia, although meta-analysis does not suggest a high degree of effectiveness when used alone. This approach is based largely on the assumption that excessive muscle tension is an important component of sleep disturbance. This assumption appears to be true for some, but not all, insomniacs. Relaxation exercises may accomplish more than simple alleviation of muscle tension. The process of focusing on relaxation may, in effect, block the cognitive factors such as worry, apprehension, and rumination that serve to maintain wakefulness. Relaxation training can be accomplished by means of a bedside tape-recorded training session, although patients with more severe chronic insomnia may require the intervention of a skilled behavioural therapist.

Biofeedback is a potentially useful technique in the treatment of insomnia. The specific focus of the feedback may be muscle tension, skin conductance, or vasomotor tone, the ultimate goal being to teach the patient how to recognize and achieve a state of relaxation. Psychophysiologic assessment prior to biofeedback may help to direct the training at the most appropriate function. Other behavioural approaches such as hypnosis, autogenic training, systematic desensitization, or meditation may be helpful for some patients.

The previously noted observation that many patients with insomnia spend excessive time in bed in a waking and aroused state, thus establishing an undesirable association between bed and inability to sleep, has given rise to two behavioural interventions with the greatest demonstrated effectiveness. Sleep restriction, described by Spielman et al.[167] is designed to limit the amount of time that a person spends in bed in a waking state. The patient is instructed to determine the average total sleep time per night at baseline by means of sleep logs. That amount of time then becomes the maximum allowable time in bed. Once subjects are able to sleep for 90 per cent or more of the time in bed on five consecutive nights, sleep time is increased by 15 min and the same trial is repeated. In stimulus control therapy[168] the patient is, in effect, instructed to use the bed only for sleeping. If unable to sleep, the patients must remove themselves from the bed and do something else until sleepy, at which time a return to the bed is permitted. This same procedure is repeated as often as necessary through the night. Both of these approaches can be quite stressful on patients in their early phases and may result in some initial sleep deprivation, rendering them of limited practicality in very sick patients.

Finally, supportive brief psychotherapy contacts that allow the patient to ventilate hopes and fears can be most helpful. Although some of the therapeutic time may be spent in discussion of the sleep problem per se, it is unwise to allow this to become the sole focus. It is advisable for the therapist to turn the patient's attention towards anxieties, conflicts, or disappointments that inevitably arise during the terminal period of illness. A practical, problem-solving approach to these matters is particularly appropriate at this stage of the disease.

Pharmacological treatment

The conventional wisdom regarding the use of hypnotic medications for the treatment of insomnia is that they should be largely limited to short-term use. This approach is predicated on concern regarding tolerance, dosage escalation, psychological addiction, and physical dependency. While such concerns are valid under any circumstance, they are of less importance in the population of palliative care patients for whom life expectancy is limited and symptom relief is the primary goal. It is clear from data previously cited that hypnotic medications are used very frequently in cancer patients. Unfortunately, these data do not provide information about the specific medications used, their effectiveness, appropriateness, or their side effects. Depending on which medications are prescribed, their dosage, and their indications, hypnotics may greatly enhance the quality of remaining life in the terminally ill, or may further complicate an already difficult period.

Benzodiazepines

Benzodiazepine, imidazopyridine (zolpidem), pyrazolopyrimidine (zaleplon), and cyclopyrrolone (zopiclone) hypnotics are the standard medications of choice in the treatment of transient or short-term insomnia. Before such drugs are prescribed, however, the clinician must carefully consider the differential diagnosis in an effort to rule out other treatable aetiologies for the sleep disturbance. Having done so, it is then reasonable to consider use of a hypnotic as a component of a comprehensive treatment approach to insomnia. Such an approach should also incorporate non-pharmacological elements, as previously described.

Several factors must be considered in employing hypnotic medication. These include: the short- and long-term effectiveness of the drug, its rate of absorption and metabolism, and the potential risks or side effects. Characteristics of selected hypnotics, and other benzodiazepines often employed as hypnotics, are summarized in Table 4. These medications, as a group, have a reasonably well-established record of effectiveness in the short-term treatment of insomnia. Studies report reductions in sleep latency and wake time after sleep onset.(169,170) There has been substantial controversy over the issue of long-term effectiveness of these medications. At present, they are recommended primarily for short-term usage.

Table 4 Characteristics of benzodiazepines and other hypnotic drugs

Medication	Dosage[a]	Elimination half-life[b]	T_{max}[b]	Active metabolities	Comments[c]
Rapid elimination					
Triazolam[d]	0.125	2–4	1.0	No	Promote rapid sleep onset with minimal accumulation of drug over time; may be less effective for sleep maintenance problems; rebound insomnia, anterograde amnesia, untoward drug reactions described with triazolam
Zolpidem	5	1.5–4	1.0–1.5	No	
Zaleplon	5	1.0	0.5–1.0	No	
Zopiclone	3.75	5–6	0.5–2.0	±	Manufacturer suggests zaleplon may be taken for middle of the night insomnia but not less than four hours before morning awakening N-oxide metabolite of zopiclone has low pharmacological activity
Intermediate elimination					
Temazepam[e]	10–15	8–13	1.5	No	Promote sleep onset/maintenance; slower absorption may be a factor in treating sleep onset difficulty; minimal accumulation
Lorazepam	0.5 mg	12–15	2.0	No	
Slow elimination					
Flurazepam	15 mg	47–100 (*n*-desalkyl-flurazepam)	1.0	Yes	Effective for sleep onset and maintenance; may be effective over 2 nights or more after single dosage; daytime sedation; performance decrements; drug accumulation; especially in elderly or those with delayed metabolism
Quazepam	7.5[f]	29–73 (*n*-desalky-flurazepam)	2.0	Yes	

[a] Recommended starting dosage in elderly and medically ill patients.

[b] Elimination half-life and T_{max} represent estimated averages for healthy adults.

[c] All benzodiazepines carry potential for dosage escalation and for psychological and physical dependence.

[d] Not available in Norway and the United Kingdom.

[e] Elimination rate partially dependant on capsule form.

[f] Manufacturer recommends initial dosage of 15 mg with reduction to 7.5 mg after 1–2 nights.

Most benzodiazepines, as well as the non-benzodiazepine hypnotics, are absorbed rather quickly, reaching peak concentrations within approximately 1 h or less. Triazolam, temazepam, and flurazepam have been the most widely used, the latter much less so in recent years due to its long half-life and potential for accumulation. Lorazepam and oxazepam have not been extensively studied as hypnotic medications, but are frequently used as such. The rate of absorption of lorazepam, oxazepam, and temazepam may be slightly slower than the most rapidly absorbed benzodiazepines, such as diazepam. The half-life of flurazepam's major active metabolite (*n*-desalkyl flurazepam) is in excess of 50 h, resulting in significant accumulation when the compound is used on a nightly basis. For this reason, the use of flurazepam has declined markedly since the introduction of shorter-acting agents. The non-benzodiazepine hypnotics zolpidem and zaleplon as well as the benzodiazepine triazolam (triazolam has been removed from the market in certain countries) are rapidly metabolized to inactive compounds. Zaleplon's ultra-short elimination half-life of about 1 h makes it potentially suitable for middle of the night usage, provided that there are at least 4 h before time of arising. Zopiclone, not currently marketed in the United States, is also rapidly absorbed and has an active metabolite with low levels of pharmacological activity. Temazepam, lorazepam, and oxazepam have intermediate half-lives ranging from about 8 to 15 h. These figures have been established for healthy adults. It is essential to recognize that rate of metabolism may be substantially slower in medically ill and elderly patients, predisposing to greater accumulation of the drug and daytime carry-over effects.

The benefits that may be achieved through the use of hypnotic medication in palliative care patients must be weighed against the potential for complications and side effects associated with their use. Perhaps the most common undesirable effect is that of daytime sedation and performance decrement. In populations of otherwise healthy insomnia patients, there is clear evidence that longer-acting benzodiazepines, such as flurazepam, are associated with significant deficits in daytime performance. However, some question exists as to the relevance of the psychomotor tasks on which these findings are based to the population of palliative care patients. Long-acting hypnotics may have daytime carry-over antianxiety effects that may be beneficial for some patients. Performance decrement and daytime sedation are not prominent characteristics of shorter-acting hypnotics. Benzodiazepines and similar drugs may also predispose to nocturnal confusion, particularly in individuals with baseline cognitive dysfunction. Likewise, respiratory disturbance in sleep, most prominent in geriatric patients, may be exacerbated by hypnotic medication.

In prescribing hypnotic medication, the clinician must consider the complication of rebound insomnia. Extensive data suggests that the shortest-acting benzodiazepines (e.g. triazolam) predispose to transient insomnia following abrupt withdrawal of the medication, even after short-term use.[171] It has also been suggested that these medications may result in increased daytime anxiety and morning insomnia. These phenomena do not appear to be present with long-acting benzodiazepines and have not been clearly demonstrated with the non-benzodiazepine hypnotics. The clinical safety of these agents has been well established. Their lethality in the absence of other central nervous system depressants is very low. When any of these medications are discontinued after regular usage, clinicians must be mindful of the possibility of withdrawal symptoms and taper medications appropriately.

Other sleep medications

A number of medications other than standard hypnotics have been employed in the treatment of insomnia. Barbiturates, although effective in short-term treatment, result in rapid development of tolerance and are more lethal in overdose situations. These medications, and similar barbiturate-like compounds, are no longer recommended in the treatment of sleep disturbance. Chloral hydrate appears to have moderate short-term efficacy but is more toxic than benzodiazepines. Sedating antidepressant drugs have assumed a more important role in the treatment of various forms of insomnia and non-restorative sleep in the past decade. These medications have the advantage that they can be administered over long periods of time without concern regarding physiological addiction. Sedating tricyclics such as amitriptyline or doxepin, administered in lower dosages (10–50 mg) than are typically required for treatment of major depression, may be helpful adjuncts. Anticholinergic side-effects and daytime sedation can be problematic, especially in the medically ill. Delirium, due to central anticholinergic activity, is a potential complicating factor, as is lethality in overdose situations. Secondary amine tricyclics such as desipramine or nortriptyline, although somewhat less sedating, may be beneficial and produce fewer anticholinergic complications. Trazodone is a sedating heterocyclic antidepressant that has milder anticholinergic effects and a somewhat shorter half-life than most tricyclics. This medication, administered typically in dosages of 25–75 mg, has become widely used as a sleep aid. Newer generation sedating antidepressants such as nefazodone and mirtazapine may be effective sleep aids but are used primarily in treatment of depressed persons with insomnia. Low dose antidepressant medications have also been employed for the treatment of non-restorative sleep.

Melatonin has received widespread attention as a treatment for insomnia and other sleep disorders. The popularity of melatonin in recent years has far exceeded the scientific basis for its use as a treatment for all types of insomnia. Melatonin has been effectively used in the treatment of sleep–wake schedule disorders and has clear phase-shifting capability.[172–174] There is also evidence that indicates potential benefit from melatonin treatment of insomnia in the elderly, who may exhibit decreased melatonin secretion as a result of aging.[175,176] No large scale controlled trials have yet demonstrated effectiveness of melatonin for the symptomatic treatment of insomnia. It should also be recognized that 'off the shelf' preparations for insomnia are not regulated as a drug in many countries and, as a result, the contents and source of the material may not be identifiable by the consumer. Finally, users should be aware that melatonin is a potent hormone with a variety of physiological effects, including reproductive and cardiovascular. While the ultimate clinical effects of exogenous melatonin are not known, some degree of caution seems advisable.

The choice of a particular pharmacological treatment for insomnia must be based on the particular situation in which it will be used. Considerations include the nature of the insomnia, the expected duration of treatment, potential side effects, including daytime sedation and performance decrement, and patient tolerance. Once initiated, it is most important to determine efficacy and complications and adjust dosage or type of medication accordingly.

Choice of hypnotics in the elderly and infirm

The choice of a hypnotic medication in the elderly or the infirm must be predicated on achieving a careful balance between therapeutic efficacy and adverse consequences, for which this population is particularly at risk. A number of studies suggest that the use of sedative-hypnotics in the elderly is associated with increased risk of falls, hip fracture, and cognitive impairment.[177–179]

Alterations in drug sensitivity and pharmacokinetics among the elderly and sick must be taken into account in prescribing. Older patients may have heightened sensitivity to hypnotic medications compared to younger persons, even at comparable plasma levels. In addition, drug clearance of at least some benzodiazepines is decreased in the elderly.

Benzodiazepines and their active metabolites which undergo oxidative metabolism in the liver (e.g. diazepam, quazepam-flurazepam/desalkylflurazepam, alprazolam, and triazolam) are cleared more slowly in the elderly, whereas those drugs which are directly metabolized to inactive substances (e.g. zolpidem, zaleplon, temazepam, oxazepam, lorazepam) show little change in rate of clearance in the elderly compared with younger age groups.[180] Furthermore, epidemiological evidence suggests a relationship between longer-acting benzodiazepine hypnotics and risk of injury.[181] These data would seem to suggest that the optimal choice of hypnotic in the elderly and debilitated would be a shorter-acting drug which undergoes direct inactivation.

Concerns about sensitivity and drug accumulation have prompted manufacturers and clinicians to recommend lower dosages of these medications in elderly patients and those with severe medical illness. Recommended starting dosages for these populations are included in Table 4. Although nightly use of benzodiazepine or other hypnotics may be appropriate for patients in the terminal phase of illness, short-term, intermittent use may suffice and will minimize the possibility of drug accumulation. Aggravation of existing cognitive impairment, risk of fall and injury, worsening of nocturnal respiratory disturbance, and unwanted daytime sedation with its attendant impact on mood and behaviour are particular concerns in the elderly and infirm.

The metabolism of heterocyclic antidepressants may be substantially slowed in medically ill and older patients. Low starting dosages should be utilized and the potential for accumulation must be recognized. Development of excessive sedation, orthostatic hypotension, cardiotoxicity, and anticholinergic side effects are the major risks associated with elevated plasma levels of several of these agents.

Sleep in family and care providers (see Chapter 12.2)

Palliative care includes attention to the needs and difficulties of the patient's family and other care providers. This is certainly true with respect to sleep disturbances, which are common in this group. Focus on these problems for family care givers is especially important because sleep disruption and fatigue may contribute to loss of hope.[182] Grief, anxiety, and depression are frequently cited psychological disturbances which may cause insomnia among relatives.[183] Carter and Chang noted that 95 per cent of cancer care givers reported severe sleep problems, as measured by the Pittsburgh Sleep Quality Index.[184] These problems affected all aspects of sleep and were associated with evidence of clinical depression in over half of the group. For those providing direct care, frequent nighttime interruptions to attend to the patient fragment sleep and, in time, can result in psychophysiological insomnia. Care providers may feel compelled to 'keep one eye open' through the night so as not to miss a call for assistance.

Inquiries about the sleep patterns of family should be a component in assessing how well the palliative care system is succeeding. Discussion of sleep hygiene issues, practical problem solving approaches to reducing nighttime interruptions, and consideration of short-term use of a benzodiazepine hypnotic may be appropriate. For some, antidepressant medication is indicated. While it is clearly not advisable to employ sedating medication or antidepressants as a means of inhibiting normal grief, it must also be recognized that sleep deprivation and its sequelae may significantly interfere with the quality of relationships in the palliative care period and complicate bereavement following the patient's death.

References

1. **American Sleep Disorders Association.** *International Classification of Sleep Disorders, Revised: Diagnostic and Coding Manual.* Rochester MN: American Sleep Disorders Association, 1997.
2. **Roth, T.** et al. (1974). The effects of sleep deprivation on mood. *Sleep Research* **3**, 154.
3. **Johnson, Lc.** (1969). Psychological and physiological changes following total sleep deprivation. In *Sleep: Physiology and Pathology* (ed. A. Kales), pp. 206–20. Philadelphia PA: Lippincott.
4. **Millman, R.P.** et al. (1989). Depression as a manifestation of obstructive sleep apnea: reversal with nasal continuous positive airway pressure. *Journal of Clinical Psychiatry* **50** (9), 348–51.
5. **Oswald, I.** (1980). Sleep as a restorative process. *Progress in Brain Research* **53**, 279–88.
6. **Moldofsky, H. and Scarisbrick, P.** (1976). Induction of neurasthenic musculoskeletal pain syndrome by selective sleep stage deprivation. *Psychosomatic Medicine* **38**, 35–44.
7. **Moldofsky, H.** et al. (1989). Effects of sleep deprivation on immune function. *Federation of American Societies for Experimental Biology Journal* **3**, 1972–7.
8. **Morley, J.E.** et al. (1987). Neuropeptides: conductors of the immune orchestra. *Life Sciences* **41** (5), 527–44.
9. **Heiser, P.** et al. (2000). White blood cells and cortisol after sleep deprivation and recovery sleep in humans. *European Archives of Psychiatry and Clinical Neuroscience* **250** (1), 16–23.
10. **Irwin, M.** et al. (1994). Partial sleep deprivation reduces natural killer cell activity in humans. *Psychosomatic Medicine* **56** (6), 493–8.
11. **Savard, J.** et al. (1999). Association between subjective sleep quality and depression on immunocompetence in low-income women at risk for cervical cancer. *Psychosomatic Medicine* **61** (4), 496–507.
12. **Redwine, L.** et al. (2000) Effects of sleep and sleep deprivation on interleukin-6, growth hormone, cortisol, and melatonin levels in humans. *Journal of Clinical Endocrinology and Metabolism* **85** (10), 3597–603.
13. **Kubler-Ross, E.** (1973). On the use of psychopharmacologic agents for the dying patient and the bereaved. In *Psycho-pharmacological Agents for the Terminally Ill and Bereaved* (ed. I.K. Goldberg, S. Malitz, and A. H. Kutscher), pp. 3–6. New York: Columbia University Press.
14. **Johns, M.W.** (1991). A new method for measuring daytime sleepiness: the Epworth sleepiness scale. *Sleep* **14** (6), 540–5.
15. **Carskadon, M.A.** et al. (1986). Guidelines for the Multiple Sleep Latency Test (MSLT): a standard measure of sleepiness. *Sleep* **9**, 519–24.
16. **Chesson, A.L.** et al. (1999). Practice parameters for the use of light therapy in the treatment of sleep disorders. Standards of Practice Committee, American Academy of Sleep Medicine. *Sleep* **22** (5), 641–60.
17. **Kamei, Y.** et al. (2000). Melatonin treatment for circadian rhythm sleep disorders. *Psychiatry and Clinical Neuroscience* **54** (3), 381–2
18. **Okawa, M.** et al (1998) Melatonin treatment for circadian rhythm sleep disorders. *Psychiatry and Clinical Neuroscience* **52** (2), 259–60.
19. **Czeisler, C.A.** et al. (1981) Chronotherapy: resetting the circadian clocks of patients with delayed sleep phase insomnia. *Sleep* **4**, 1–21.
20. **Sutherland, H.J., Lockwood, G.A., and Boyd, N.F.** (1990). Ratings of the importance of quality of life variables: therapeutic implications for patients with metastatic breast cancer. *Journal of Clinical Epidemiology* **43** (7), 661–6.
21. **Munro, A.J.** et al. (1989). Distress associated with radiotherapy for malignant disease: a quantitative analysis based on patient's perceptions. *British Journal of Cancer* **60** (3), 370–4.
22. **Krech, R.L. and Walsh, D.** (1991). Symptoms of pancreatic cancer. *Journal of Pain and Symptom Management* **6** (6), 360–7.
23. **Portenoy, R.K.** et al. (1994). Symptoms prevalence, characteristics and distress in a cancer population. *Quality of Life Research* **3** (3), 183–9.
24. **Grond, S.** et al. (1994). Prevalence and pattern of symptoms in patients with cancer pain: a prospective evaluation of 1635 cancer patients referred to a pain clinic. *Journal of Pain and Symptom Management* **9** (6), 372–82.
25. **Ginsburg, M.L.** et al. (1995). Psychiatric illness and psychosocial concerns of patients with newly diagnosed lung cancer. *Canadian Medial Association Journal* **152** (5), 701–8.
26. **Walsh. D., Donnelly. S., and Rybicki, L.** (2000). The symptoms of advanced cancer: relationship to age, gender, and performance status in 1000 patients. *Supportive Care in Cancer* **8** (3), 175–9.
27. **Savard, J. and Morin, C.M.** (2001). Insomnia in the context of cancer: a review of a neglected problem. *Journal of Clinical Oncology* **19** (3), 895–908.
28. **Engstrom, C.A.** et al. (1999). Sleep alterations in cancer patients. *Cancer Nursing* **22** (2), 143–8.
29. **Malone, M., Harris, A.L., and Luscombe, D.K.** (1994). Assessment of the impact of cancer on work, recreation, home management and sleep using a general health status measure. *Journal of the Royal Society of Medicine* **87**, 386–9.
30. **Beszterczey, A. and Lipowski, Z.J.** (1997). Insomnia in cancer patients. *Canadian Medical Association Journal* **116**, 355.
31. **Lamb, M.A.** (1982). The sleeping patterns of patients with malignant and nonmalignant diseases. *Cancer Nursing* **5**, 389–96.
32. **Kaye, J., Kaye, K., and Madow, L.** (1983) Sleep patterns in patients with cancer and patients with cardiac disease. *Journal of Psychology* **114**, 107–13.
33. **Silberfarb, P.M.** et al. (1985). Insomnia in cancer patients. *Social Science and Medicine* **20** (8), 849–50.

34. **Silberfarb, P.M.** et al. (1993). Assessment of sleep in patients with lung cancer and breast cancer. *Journal of Clinical Oncology* **11** (5), 997–1004.

35. **Monga, U.** et al. (1999). Prospective study of fatigue in localized prostate cancer patients undergoing radiotherapy. *Radiation Oncology Investigations* **7** (3), 178–85.

36. **Lapin, J.** et al. (1989). Guidelines for use of controlled-release oral morphine in cancer pain management. *Cancer Nursing* **12** (4), 202–8.

37. **Hanks, G.W.** et al. (1987). Controlled release morphine tablets: a double-blind trial in patients with advanced cancer. *Anaesthesia* **42** (8), 840–4.

38. **Wilwerding, M.B.** et al. (1995). A randomized, crossover evaluation of methylphenidate in cancer patients receiving strong narcotics. *Supportive Care in Cancer* **3** (2), 135–8.

39. **Smedley, H.** et al. (1983). Neurological effects of recombinant human interferon. *British Medical Journal* **286** (6361), 262–4.

40. **Harris, A.L., Powles, T.J., and Smith, I.E.** (1982). Aminoglutethimide in the treatment of advanced post-menopausal breast cancer. *Cancer Research* **42** (8 Suppl.), 3405S–8S.

41. **Mock, V.** et al. (2000). NCCN practice guidelines for cancer-related fatigue. *National Comprehensive Cancer Network Proceedings* **14** (11A), 151–61.

42. **Bower, J.E.** et al. (2000). Fatigue in breast cancer survivors: occurrence, correlates, and impact on quality of life. *Journal of Clinical Oncology* **18** (4), 743–53.

43. **Okuyama, T.** et al. (2000). Factors correlated with fatigue in disease-free breast cancer patients: application of the Cancer Fatigue Scale. *Supportive Care in Cancer* **8** (3), 215–22.

44. **Berger, A.M. and Farr, L.** (1999) The influence of daytime inactivity and nighttime restlessness on cancer-related fatigue. *Oncology Nursing Forum* **26** (10), 1663–71.

45. **Groopman, J.E.** (1998). Fatigue in cancer and HIV/AIDS. *Oncology* **12** (3), 335–44.

46. **Darko, D.F.** et al. (1992). Fatigue, sleep disturbance, disability, indices of progression of HIV infection. *American Journal of Psychiatry* **149** (4), 514–20.

47. **Moeller, A.A.** et al. (1991). Self-reported sleep quality in HIV infection: correlation of the stage of infection and zidovudine therapy. *Journal of Acquired Immunodeficiency Syndrome* **4** (10), 1000–3.

48. **Cohen, F.L.** et al. (1996). Sleep in men and women infected with human immunodeficiency virus. *Holistic Nursing Practice* **10** (4), 33–43.

49. **Rubinstein, M.L. and Selwyn, P.A.** (1998). High prevalence of insomnia in an outpatient population with HIV infection. *Journal of Acquired Immunodeficiency Syndrome* **19** (3), 260–5.

50. **Nokes, K.M. and Kendrew, J.** (2001). Correlates of sleep quality in persons with HIV disease. *Journal of the Association of Nurses in AIDS Care* **12** (1), 17–22.

51. **Norman, S.E.** et al. (1992). Sleep disturbances in men with asymptomatic human immunodeficiency (HIV) infection. *Sleep* **15** (2), 150–5.

52. **Norman, S.E.** et al. (1990). Sleep disturbances in HIV-infected homosexual men. *AIDS* **4** (8), 775–81.

53. **Norman, S.E.** et al. (1988). Sleep disturbances in HIV-seropositive patients. *Journal of the American Medical Association* **260** (7), 922.

54. **White, J.L.** et al. (1995). Early central nervous system response to HIV infection: sleep distortion and cognitive-motor decrements. *AIDS* **9** (9), 1043–50.

55. **Darko, D.F.** et al. (1995). Sleep electroencephalogram delta-frequency amplitude, night plasma levels of tumour necrosis factor alpha, and human immunodeficiency virus infection. *Proceedings of the National Academy of Science* **92** (26), 12080–4.

56. **St Kubicki, H.** et al. (1988). AIDS-related sleep disturbances—a preliminary report. In *HIV and Nervous System* (ed. St. H. Kubicki, H. Henkes, H. Bienzle, and H.D. Pokle), pp. 97–105. Stuttgart: Gustar Fischer.

57. **Wiegand, M.** et al. (1991). Alterations of nocturnal sleep in patients with HIV infection. *Acta Neurologica Scandinavica* **83** (2), 141–2

58. **Harris, P.F. and Careres, C.A.** (1988). Azidothymidine in the treatment of AIDS. *New England Journal of Medicine* **318**, 250.

59. **Richman, D.D.** et al. (1987). The toxicity of azidothymidine (AZT) in the treatment of patients with AIDS and AIDS-related complex. A double-blind, placebo-controlled trial. *New England Journal of Medicine* **317**, 192–7.

60. **Bach, M.C.** (1987). Possible drug interaction during therapy with azidothymidine and acyclovir for AIDS. *New England Journal of Medicine* **316**, 547.

61. **Moeller, A.A.** et al. (1992). Effects of zidovudine on EEG sleep in HIV-infected men. *Journal of Acquired Immunodeficiency Syndrome* **5** (6), 636–7.

62. **Hintz, S.** et al. (1990). Depression in the context of human immunodeficiency virus infection: implications for treatment. *Journal of Clinical Psychiatry* **51** (12), 497–501.

63. **Benca, R.M.** (2000). Mood disorders. In *Principles and Practice of Sleep Medicine* 3d edn. (ed. M.H. Kryger, T. Roth, and W.C. Dement), pp. 1140–57. Philadelphia. PA: WB Saunders.

64. **Levine, P., Silberfarb, P.M., and Lipowski, Z.J.** (1978). Mental disorders in cancer patients. *Cancer* **42**, 1385–91.

65. **Akechi, T.** et al. (2001). Psychiatric disorders in cancer patients: descriptive analysis of 1721 psychiatric referrals at two Japanese cancer center hospitals. *Japanese Journal of Clinical Oncology* **31** (5), 188–94.

66. **Craig, T.J. and Abeloff, M.D.** (1974). Psychiatric symptomatology among hospitalized cancer patients. *American Journal of Psychiatry* **131** (12), 1323–27.

67. **Plumb, M.M. and Holland, J.** (1977). Comparative studies of psychological function in patients with advanced cancer-I. Self-reported depressive symptoms. *Psychosomatic Medicine* **39** (4), 264–76.

68. **Derogatiss, L.R.** et al. (1983). The prevalence of psychiatric disorders among cancer patients. *Journal of the American Medical Association* **249** (6), 751–7.

69. **Bukberg, J., Penman, D., and Holland, J.C.** (1984). Depression in hospitalized cancer patients. *Psychosomatic Medicine* **46** (3), 199–212.

70. **Breitbart, W.** et al. (1995). Neuropsychiatric syndromes and psychological symptoms in patients with advanced cancer. *Journal of Pain and Symptom Management* **10** (2), 131–41

71. **Derogatis, L.R.** et al. (1979). A survey of psychotropic drug prescriptions in an oncology population. *Cancer* **44** (5), 1919–29.

72. **Jaeger, H.** et al. (1985). A survey of psychotropic drug utilization by patients with advanced neoplastic disease. *General Hospital Psychiatry* **7**, 353–60.

73. **Lloyd-Williams, M., Friedman, T., and Rudd, N.** (1999). A survey of antidepressant prescribing in the terminally ill. *Palliative Medicine* **13** (3), 243–8

74. **Walsh, T.D.** (1983). Antidepressants in chronic pain. *Clinical Neuropharmacology* **6**, 271–95.

75. **Hameroff, S.R.** et al. (1984). Doxepin's effects on chronic pain and depression: a controlled study. *Journal of Clinical Psychiatry* **45** (3 Pt. 2), 47–53.

76. **Hameroff, S.R.** et al. (1982). Doxepin effects on chronic pain, depression and plasma opioids. *Journal of Clinical Psychiatry* **43** (8 Pt. 2), 22–7.

77. **Spiegel, K., Kalb, R., and Pasternak, G.W.** (1983). Analgesic activity of tricyclic antidepressants. *Annals of Neurology* **13**, 462–5.

78. **Kugaya, A.** et al. (1999). Successful antidepressant treatment for five terminally ill cancer patients with major depression, suicidal ideation and a desire for death. *Supportive Care in Cancer* **7** (6), 432–6.

79. **Holland, J.C.** et al. (1998). A controlled trial of fluoxetine and desipramine in depressed women with advanced cancer. *Psycho-Oncology* **7** (4), 291–300.

80. **Cheer, S.M. and Goa, K.L.** (2001) Fluoxetine: a review of its therapeutic potential in the treatment of depression associated with physical illness. *Drugs* **61** (1), 81–110.

81. **Gill, D. and Hatcher, S.** (2000). Antidepressants for depression in medical illness. *Cochrane Database of Systematic Reviews* (4), CD001312.

82. **Battelli, T.** et al. (1976). Anxiety therapy in the neoplastic patient. *Current Medical Research and Opinion* **4** (3), 185–8.

83. **Reynolds, C.F.** et al. (1983). EEG sleep in outpatients with generalized anxiety: a preliminary comparison with depressed outpatients. *Psychiatry Research* **8**, 81–9.

84. **Rosa, R.R., Bonnet, M.H., and Kramer, M.** (1983). The relationship of sleep and anxiety in anxious subjects. *Biological Psychology* **16**, 119–26.

85. **Neuhas, W.** et al. (1994). Psychological disease adjustment in breast cancer patients. *Geburtshilfe und Frauenheilkunde* **54** (10), 564–8.

86. **Massie, M.J., Holland, J., and Glass, E.** (1983). Delirium in terminally ill cancer patients. *American Journal of Psychiatry* **140** (8), 1048–50.

87. **Fasinsinger, R.** et al. (1991). Symptom control during the last week of life on a pallative care unit. *Journal of Pallative Care* **7** (1), 5–11.

88. **Lipowski, Z.J.** (1987). Delirium (acute confusional state). *Journal of the American Medical Association* **258** (13), 1789–92.
89. **Posner, J.B.** (1979). Neurological complications of systemic cancer. *Medical Clinics of North America* **63**, 783–800.
90. **Silberfarb, P.M.** (1988). Psychiatric treatment of the patient during cancer therapy. *CA: A Cancer Journal for Clinicans* **38** (3), 133–7.
91. **Sofer, D.J.** (1970). The concomitant effects of mild sleep loss and an anticholinergic drug. *Psychopharmacologia (Berin.)* **17**, 425–33.
92. **Evans, J.I. and Lewis, S.A.** (1968). Sleep studies in early delirium and during drug withdrawal in normal subjects and the effect of phenothiazines on such states. *Electro-encephalography and Clinical Neurophysiology* **25**, 508–9.
93. **Prinz, P.N.** et al. (1983). Sleep EEG and mental function changes in senile dementia of the Alzheimer's type. *Neurobiology of Aging* **3**, 361–70.
94. **Reynolds, C.F.** et al. (1985). EEG sleep in elderly depressed, demented and healthy subjects. *Biological Psychiatry* **20**, 431–42.
95. **Stiefel, F., Fainsinger, R., and Breura, E.** (1992). Acute confusional states in patients with advanced cancer. *Journal of Pain and Symptom Management* **7** (2), 94–8.
96. **Burke, A.L.** et al. (1991). Terminal restlessness—its management and the role of midazolam. *Medical Journal of Australia* **155** (7), 485–7.
97. **Panutti, F.** et al. (1979). The role of endocrine therapy for the relief of pain due to cancer. In *Advances in Pain Research and Therapy* Vol. 2 (ed. J.J. Bonica and V. Ventafridda), pp. 59–77. New York: Raven Press.
98. **Twycross, R.G. and Fairfields, S.** (1982) Pain in far advanced cancer. *Pain* **14**, 303–10.
99. **Bonica, J.J.** (1979). Importance of the problem. In *Advances in Pain Research and Therapy* Vol. 2 (ed. J.J. Bonica and V. Ventafridda), pp. 1–12. New York: Raven Press.
100. **Banning, A., Sjogren, P., and Henriksen, H.** (1991). Treatment outcome in a multi-disciplinary cancer pain clinic. *Pain* **47**, 129–34.
101. **Dorrepaal, K.L., Aaronson, N.K., and van Dam, F.S.** (1989). Pain experience and pain management among hospitalized cancer patients. *Cancer* **63**, 593–8.
102. **Portenoy, R.K.** et al. (1992). Pain in ambulatory patients with lung or colon cancer. Prevalence, characteristics, and effect. *Cancer* **70** (6), 1616–24.
103. **Strang, P. and Quarner, H.** (1990). Cancer-related pain and its influence on quality of life. *Anticancer Research* **10**, 109–12.
104. **Tamburini, M.** et al. (1987). Semantic descriptors of pain. *Pain* **29** (2), 187–93.
105. **Donovan, M., Dillon, P., and McGuire, L.** (1987). Incidence and characteristics of pain in a sample of medical-surgical inpatients. *Pain* **30** (1), 69–78.
106. **Kinsman, R.** et al. (1989). Multidimensional analysis of peak pain symptoms and experiences. *Psychotherapy and Psychosomatics* **51** (2), 101–12.
107. **Pilowsky, I., Crettenden, I., and Townley, M.** (1985). Sleep disturbance in pain clinic patients. *Pain* **23** (1), 27–33.
108. **Closs, S.J.** (1992). Patients' night-time pain, analgesic provision and sleep after surgery. *International Journal of Nursing Studies* **29** (4), 381–92.
109. **Landis, C.A., Levine, J.D., and Robinson, C.R.** (1989). Decreased slow-wave and paradoxical sleep in a rat chronic pain model. *Sleep* **12** (2), 167–77.
110. **Carli, G.** et al. (1987). Differential effects of persistent nociceptive stimulation on sleep stages. *Behavioural Brain Research* **26**, 89–98.
111. **Wittig, R.M.** et al. (1982). Disturbed sleep in patients complaining of chronic pain. *Journal of Nervous and Mental Disease* **170** (7), 429–31.
112. **Moldofsky, H., Lue, F.A., and Smythe, H.A.** (1983). Alpha EEG and morning symptoms in rheumatoid arthritis. *Journal of Rheumatology* **10**, 373–9.
113. **Breitbart, W.** (1989). Psychiatric management of cancer pain. *Cancer* **63**, 2336–42.
114. **Hicks, R.A.** et al. (1979). Pain thresholds in rats during recovery from REM sleep deprivation. *Perceptual and Motor Skills* **48**, 687–90.
115. **Fadda, P., Tortorella, A., and Fratha, W.** (1991) Sleep deprivation decreases μ and delta opioid receptor binding in the rat limbic system. *Neuroscience Letters* **129**, 315–17.
116. **Onen, S.H.** et al. (2001). The effects of total sleep deprivation, selective sleep interruption and sleep recovery on pain tolerance thresholds in healthy subjects. *Journal of Sleep Research* **10** (1), 35–42.
117. **Raymond, I.** et al. (2001). Quality of sleep and its daily relationship to pain intensity in hospitalized adult burn patients. *Pain* **92** (3), 381–8.
118. **Larbig, W.** et al. (1984). Therapeutic effects of delta-sleep-inducing peptide (DSIP) in patients with chronic, pronounced pain episodes. A clinical pilot study. *European Neurology* **23** (5), 372–85.
119. **Ventafridda, V.** et al. (1987). A validation study of the WHO method for cancer pain relief. *Cancer* **59** (4), 850–6.
120. **Goughnour, B.R., Arkinstall, W.W., and Steward, J.H.** (1989). Analgesic response to single and multiple doses of controlled-release morphine tablets and morphine oral solution in cancer patients. *Cancer* **63** (11 Suppl.), 2294–7.
121. **Wong, J.O.** et al. (1997). Comparison of oral controlled-release morphine with transdermal fentanyl in terminal cancer pain. *Acta Anaesthesiologica Sinica* **35** (1), 25–32.
122. **Payne, R.** et al. (1998). Quality of life and cancer pain: satisfaction and side effects with transdermal fentanyl versus oral morphine. *Journal of Clinical Oncology* **16** (4), 1588–93.
123. **Ahmedzai, S. and Brooks, D.** (1997). Transdermal fentanyl versus sustained-release oral morphine in cancer pain: preference, efficacy, and quality of life. *Journal of Pain and Symptom Management* **13** (5), 254–61
124. **Corli, O., Cozzolino, A., and Scaricabarozzi, I.** (1993). Nimesulide and diclofenac in the control of cancer-related pain. Comparison between oral and rectal administration. *Drugs* **46** (Suppl. 1), 152–5.
125. **Carrol, E.N.** et al. (1994) A four-drug regimen for head and neck cancers. *Laryngoscope* **104**, 694–700.
126. **Sjoberg, M.** et al. (1994). Long-term intrathecal morphine and bupivacaine in patients with refractory cancer pain. *Anesthesiology* **80** (2), 284–97.
127. **Smith, G.M. and Smith, R.H.** (1985). Effects of doxylamine and acetaminophen on post-operative sleep. *Clinical Pharmacology and Therapeutics* **37** (5), 549–57.
128. **Berger, A.M. and Higginbotham, P.** (2000). Correlates of fatigue during and following adjuvant breast cancer chemotherapy: a pilot study. *Oncology Nursing Forum* **27** (9), 1443–8.
129. **Broeckel, J.A.** et al. (1998). Characteristics and correlates of fatigue after adjuvant chemotherapy for breast cancer. *Journal of Clinical Oncology* **16** (5), 1689–96.
130. **Shapiro, W.** (1980). Sleep behaviour among narcoleptics and cancer patients. *Behavioral Medicine* **7**, 14–21.
131. **Gillin, J.C.** et al. (1972). Acute effect of a glucocorticoid on normal human sleep. *Nature (London)* **237**, 398–9.
132. **Kay, D.C. and Samiuddin, Z.** (1988). Sleep disorders associated with drug abuse and drugs of abuse. In *Sleep Disorders: Diagnosis and Treatment* (ed. R.L. Williams, I. Karacan, and C.A. Moore), pp. 315–71. New York: Wiley.
133. **Nicholson, A.N., Bradley, C.M., and Pascoe, P.A.** (1989). Medications: effect on sleep and wakefulness. In *Principles and Practice of Sleep Medicine* (ed. M.H. Kryger, T. Roth, and W.C. Dement), pp. 228–36. Philadelphia PA: WB Saunders.
134. **Bruera, E.** et al. (1992). The use of methylphenidate in patients with incident cancer pain receiving regular opiates. A preliminary report. *Pain* **50** (1), 75–7.
135. **Wilwerding, M.B.** et al. (1995) A randomized, crossover evaluation of methylphenidate in cancer patients receiving strong narcotics. *Supportive Care in Cancer* **3** (2), 135–8
136. **Veitch, D., Rogers, M., and Blanshard, J.** (1989). Pharyngeal mass presenting with sleep apnea. *Journal of Laryngology and Otology* **103** (10), 961–3.
137. **Zorick, F.** et al. (1980) Exacerbation of upper airway sleep apnea by lymphocytic lymphoma. *Chest* **77**, 689–90.
138. **Greenough, G., Sateia, M., and Fadul, C.E.** (1999) Obstructive sleep apnea syndrome in a patient with medulloblastoma. *Neuro-Oncology* **1**, 2889–91.
139. **Panje, W.R. and Holmes, D.K.** (1984) Mandibulectomy without reconstruction can cause sleep apnea. *Laryngoscope* **94** (12 Pt. 1), 1591–4.
140. **Epstein, L.J.** et al. (1995). Obstructive sleep apnea in patients with human immunodeficiency virus (HIV) disease. *Sleep* **18** (5), 368–76.
141. **Etches, R.C.** (1994) Respiratory depression associated with patient-controlled analgesia: a review of eight cases. *Canadian Journal of Anaesthesia* **4** (2), 125–32.
142. **Thomas, M., von Eiff, M., and van de Loo, J.** (1993). Central sleep apnea syndrome as a cause of impaired wakefulness in multiple myeloma. *Deutshe Medizinische Wochenschrift* **118** (51–52), 1884–8.

143. **Flenley, D.C.** (1989). Chronic obstructive pulmonary disease. In *Principles and Practice of Sleep Medicine* (ed. M.H. Kryger, T. Roth, and W.C. Dement), pp. 601–10. Philadelphia PA: WB Saunders.

144. **Osoba, D.** et al. (1997). Effect of postchemotherapy nausea and vomiting on health-related quality of life. *Supportive Care in Cancer* **5** (4), 307–13.

145. **Dlin, B.M.** et al. (1971). The problems of sleep and rest in the intensive care unit. *Psychosomatics* **12**, 155–63.

146. **Broughton, R. and Baron, R.** (1973). Sleep of acute coronary patients in an open ward type intensive care unit. *Sleep Research* **2**, 144.

147. **Topf, M. and Thompson, S.** (2001). Interactive relationships between hospital patients' noise-induced stress and other stress with sleep. *Heart and Lung* **30** (4), 237–43.

148. **Fabizan, L. and Gosselin, M.D.** (1982). How to recognize sleep deprivation in your ICU patient and what to do about it. *Canadian Nurse* **78** (4), 20–3.

149. **Crisp, A.H.** (1980). Sleep, activity, nutrition and mood. *British Journal of Psychiatry* **137**, 1–7.

150. **Regestein, Q.R.** (1987) Sleep disorders in the medically ill. In *Principles of Medical Psychiatry* (ed. A. Stoudemire and B.S. Fogel), pp. 271–305. New York: Grune and Stratton.

151. **Carpenter, J.S.** et al. (2001). Circadian rhythm of objectively recorded hot flashes in postmenopausal breast cancer survivors. *Menopause.* **8** (3), 181–8.

152. **Polo-Kantola, P.** et al. (1998). When does estrogen replacement therapy improve sleep quality? *American Journal of Obstetrics and Gynecology* **178** (5), 1002–9.

153. **Anderson, M. and Salmon, M.V.** (1977) Symptomatic cataplexy. *Journal of Neurology, Neurosurgery and Psychiatry* **40**, 186–91.

154. **Stashl, S.M.** et al. (1980). Continuous cataplexy in a patient with a midbrain tumour: the limp man syndrome. *Neurology* **30**, 1115–18.

155. **Jaeckle, K.A.** et al. (1990) Central neurogenic hyperventilation: pharmacological intervention with morphine sulfate and correlative analysis of respiratory, sleep, and ocular motor dysfunction. *Neurology* **40**, 715–20.

156. **Hartmann, E.** (1977). L-Tryptophan: a rational hypnotic with clinical potential. *American Journal of Psychiatry* **134**, 366–70.

157. **Hauri, P.J. and Sateia, M.J.** (1985). Nonpharmacological treatment of sleep disorders. In *American Psychiatric Association Annual Review* Vol. 4 (ed. R.E. Hales and A.J. Frances), pp. 361–78. Washington DC: American Psychiatric Press.

158. **Morin, C.M. and Kwentus, J.A.** (1988). Behavioral and pharmacological treatments for insomnia. *Annals of Behavioral Medicine* **10** (3), 91–100.

159. **Morin, C.M., Culbert, J.P., and Schwartz, S.M.** (1994). Nonpharmacological interventions for insomnia: a meta-analysis of treatment efficacy. *American Journal of Psychiatry* **151** (8), 1172–80.

160. **Murtagh, D.R. and Greenwood, K.M.** (1995). Identifying effective psychological treatments for insomnia: a meta-analysis. *Journal of Consulting and Clinical Psychology* **63** (1), 79–89.

161. **Cannici, J., Malcolm, R., and Peck, L.A.** (1983). Treatment of insomnia in cancer patients using muscle relaxation training. *Journal of Behavior Therapy and Experimental Psychiatry* **14** (3), 251–6.

162. **LaClave, L.J. and Blix, S.** (1989). Hypnosis in the management of symptoms in a young girl with malignant astrocytoma: a challenge to the therapist. *International Journal of Clinical and Experimental Hypnosis* **37** (1), 6–14.

163. **Stam, H.J. and Bultz, B.D.** (1986). The treatment of severe insomnia in a cancer patient. *Journal of Behavior Therapy and Experimental Psychiatry* **17** (1), 33–7.

164. **Fishman, B. and Loscalzo, M.** (1987). Cognitive-behavioral interventions in management of cancer pain: principles and applications. *Cancer Pain* **71** (2), 271–87.

165. **Morin, C.M., Kowatch, R.A., and Wade, J.B.** (1989). Behavioral management of sleep disturbances secondary to chronic pain. *Journal of Behavior Therapy and Experimental Psychiatry* **2** (4), 295–302.

166. **Currie, S.R.** et al. (2000) Cognitive-behavioral treatment of insomnia secondary to chronic pain. *Journal of Consulting and Clinical Psychology* **68** (3), 407–16.

167. **Spielman, A.J., Saskin, P., and Thorpy, M.J.** (1983) Sleep restriction: a new treatment of insomnia. *Sleep Research* **12**, 286.

168. **Bootzin, R.R. and Nicassio, P.N.** (1978). Behavioral treatments of insomnia. In *Progress in Behavior Modification* Vol. 6 (ed. M. Hersen, R. Eisler, and P. Miller), pp. 1–45. New York: Academic Press.

169. **Dement, W.C.** et al. (1978) Prolonged use of flurazepam: a sleep laboratory study. *Behavioral Medicine* **5**, 25–31.

170. **Spinweber, C.L. and Johnson, L.C.** (1982). Effects of triazolam (0.5 mg) on sleep, performance, memory and arousal threshold. *Psychopharmacology* **76**, 5–12.

171. **Vogel, G.** et al. (1975). The effect of triazolam on the sleep of insomniacs. *Psychopharmacology* **41** (1), 65–9.

172. **Dawson, D., Encel, N., and Lushington, K.** (1995). Improving adaptation to simulated night shift: timed exposure to bright light versus daytime melatonin administration. *Sleep* **18** (1), 11–21.

173. **Attenburrow, M.E.** et al. (1995). Melatonin phase advances circadian rhythm. *Psychopharmacology* **121** (4), 503–5.

174. **Lewy, A.J.** et al. (1995). Melatonin marks circadian phase position and resets the endogenous circadian pacemaker in humans. *Ciba Foundation Symposium* **183**, 303–17.

175. **Garfinkel, D.** et al. (1995). Improvement of sleep quality in elderly people by controlled-release melatonin. *Lancet* **346**, 541–4.

176. **Haimov, I.** et al. (1995). Melatonin replacement therapy of elderly insomniacs. *Sleep* **18** (7), 598–603.

177. **Robbins, A.S.** et al. (1989). Predictors of falls among elderly people. *Archives of Internal Medicine* **149**, 1628–33.

178. **Ray, W.A.** et al. (1987). Psychotropic drug use and the risk of hip fracture. *New England Journal of Medicine* **316**, 363–9.

179. **Larson, E.B.** et al. (1987) Adverse drug reactions associated with global cognitive impairment in elderly persons. *Annals of Internal Medicine* **107**, 169–73.

180. **Greenblatt, D.J., Harmatz, J.S., and Shader, R.I.** (1991) Clinical pharmacokinetics of anxiety and hypnotics in the elderly. *Clinicial Pharmacokinetics* **21**, 165–77.

181. **Ray, W.A., Griffin, M.R., and Downey, W.** (1989). Benzodiazepines of long and short elimination half-life and the risk of hip fracture. *Journal of the American Medical Association* **262**, 3303–7.

182. **Herth, K.** (1993). Hope in the family caregiver of terminally ill people. *Journal of Advanced Nursing* **18**, 538–48.

183. **Sawyer, M.G.** et al. (1993). A prospective study of the psychological adjustment of parents and families of children with cancer. *Journal of Paediatrices and Child Health* **23** (5), 352–6.

184. **Carter, P.A. and Chang, B.L.** (2000). Sleep and depression in cancer caregivers. *Cancer Nursing* **23** (6), 410–15.

8.17 Psychiatric symptoms in palliative medicine

William Breitbart, Harvey Max Chochinov, and Steven D. Passik

Introduction

Often, it is not death that is feared, but rather the process that leads to death. Images of suffering, or dying in isolation, can be foremost on the minds of those with terminal illness. Unaddressed physical and psychiatric symptoms often interact and impact negatively on quality of life. Therefore, the prompt recognition and effective treatment of both psychiatric and physical symptoms becomes critically important to the well being of the patient with advanced disease. In general, palliative care specialists are quite expert at managing a broad spectrum of difficult and complex physical symptoms. Managing psychiatric complications (such as anxiety, delirium, depression, suicide, and desire for hastened death) and difficult psychosocial issues (such as bereavement, loss, family dysfunction) facing patients with terminal illness and their families, however, can test the limits of even the most skilled and experienced palliative medicine practitioner. It is for this reason that a multidisciplinary approach to the management of the patient with advanced disease has gained broad acceptance. A psychiatrist or psychologist can play a vital role as a member of such a treatment team. This role includes the assessment and treatment of the psychiatric complications of terminal illness and the application of psychological and psychiatric techniques to the management of physical symptoms. This chapter is designed to both provide psychiatric consultants with a knowledge base specific to terminal illness, and to give the palliative medicine practitioner a framework for approaching psychiatric issues in palliative care. The interested reader is referred to another Oxford University Press textbook, edited by two of the authors of this chapter, entitled the Handbook of Psychiatry in Palliative Medicine[1] for a more extensive review.

Prevalence of psychiatric disorders in the terminally ill

The patient with advanced disease faces many stressors during the course of illness, including fears of a painful death, disability, disfigurement, and dependency. While such concerns are universal, the level of psychological distress is quite variable depending on personality, coping ability, social support, and medical factors. The Psychosocial Collaborative Oncology Group determined the prevalence of psychiatric disorders seen in 215 cancer patients (ambulatory or hospitalized, with a wide range of cancer diagnoses and stages of disease) in three cancer centres utilizing the criteria from the Diagnostic and Statistical Manual III classification of disorders.[2] About half (53 per cent) of the patients evaluated were adjusting normally to the stresses of cancer with no diagnosable psychiatric disorder; however, 47 per cent had clinically apparent psychiatric disorders. Of the 47 per cent who had psychiatric disorders, 68 per cent had reactive anxiety and depression (adjustment disorders with depressed or anxious mood), 13 per cent had major depression, 8 per cent had an organic mental disorder (delirium).

Cancer patients with advanced disease are a particularly vulnerable group in terms of the development of psychiatric complications.[1–4] The incidence of pain, depression, and delirium all increase with higher levels of physical debilitation and advanced illness.[5–10] Approximately 25 per cent of all cancer patients experience severe depressive symptoms, with the prevalence increasing to 77 per cent in those with advanced illness.[7] The prevalence of organic mental disorders (delirium) among cancer patients requiring psychiatric consultation has been found to range from 25 to 40 per cent and as high as 85–88 per cent during the terminal stages of illness.[3,9,10] Opioid analgesics such as meperidine, levorphanol, and morphine sulfate, commonly cause acute confusional states, particularly in the elderly and terminally ill.[9,10] Cancer patients with pain are twice as likely to develop a psychiatric disorder than patients without pain. Of the patients who received a psychiatric diagnosis, 39 per cent reported significant pain. In contrast, only 19 per cent of patients without a psychiatric diagnosis had significant pain.[2] The psychiatric diagnoses of these patients with pain were predominantly adjustment disorder with depressed or mixed mood (69 per cent) and major depression in 15 per cent. This finding of increased frequency of psychiatric disturbance in cancer patients with pain has been reported by others, including Ahles et al.[11] and Woodforde et al.[12]

In a recent study, Minagawa et al.[4] using the Structured Clinical Interview for DSM-III-R (SCID) to evaluate the incidence of psychiatric disorders in a sample of 109 terminally ill cancer patients admitted to a palliative care unit, found that 53.7 per cent of patients met criteria for a specific psychiatric disorder (this finding is similar to the rate of 47 per cent found in earlier studies of general cancer patient populations). The most common psychiatric disorders among the terminally ill cancer patients were: delirium (28 per cent), dementia (10.7 per cent), adjustment disorders (7.5 per cent), amnestic disorder (3.2 per cent), major depression (3.2 per cent), and generalized anxiety disorder (1.1 per cent). This study dramatically under-represents the prevalence of depression in patients with advanced disease. The sample studied consisted of patients in the last week or two of life. Delirium and organic mental disorders were thus developing rapidly in this sample, masking pre-existing depression and other disorders that were likely present up to the stage of disease where delirium overwhelmed the clinical picture. While the palliative care literature has data on the prevalence of psychiatric disorders in cancer and AIDS patients (see below), data regarding the prevalence of psychiatric disorders in patients with end-stage heart, lung, liver, or neurodegenerative disorders is almost completely lacking.

Early descriptions of the prevalence of psychiatric disorders in patients with human immunodeficiency virus (HIV) disease and/or AIDS suggested rather significant rates of anxiety, depression, cognitive impairment disorders, and risk for suicide.[13–16] Tross and Hirsh,[13] in 1988, reported the prevalence of psychiatric disorders in an ambulatory sample of 279 patients with AIDS spectrum disorders. The study included asymptomatic gay men, gay men with AIDS-related complex (ARC), and gay men with AIDS. All patients with organic mental disorders or obvious neurologic impairment were excluded. Men with ARC showed the greatest distress and frequency of psychiatric disorder. Three-quarters of the men with ARC, one-half of the AIDS patients, and two-fifths of the asymptomatic gay men were diagnosed as having a psychiatric disorder. The most common psychiatric diagnosis was adjustment disorder, seen in two-thirds of AIDS patients and more than half of patients with ARC. Depression was present in one-quarter of the entire study population. Patients with AIDS thus have quite comparable, if not higher, levels of psychiatric distress than cancer patients. There is a higher prevalence of psychiatric disorders seen in homosexual men (with or without HIV infection) as compared to the heterosexual men or the general population.[14] Atkinson et al.[14] found that homosexual men had higher lifetime rates of substance abuse, affective disorders, and anxiety disorders than the general population that may have predated their HIV infection.

There have been several reports of psychiatric diagnoses seen in AIDS patients who were hospitalized and more seriously ill. Karina et al. reported that of 357 patients hospitalized with AIDS, 49 (14 per cent) had at least one psychiatric diagnosis.[15] These patients were hospitalized an average 60 days longer than AIDS patients without such psychiatric illnesses. Differences in medical morbidity could not account for longer length of stay. Barbuto et al.[16] reviewed the psychiatric consultation data collected on 65 hospitalized patients with AIDS. Psychiatric consultations were most frequently requested to evaluate depressive symptoms, suicidal risk, and behaviour related to CNS impairment by delirium or dementia. In this study organic mental disorders, adjustment disorders, anxiety disorders, and affective disorders ranked in order of decreasing prevalence. Eighty per cent of AIDS patients, given a functional psychiatric diagnosis, had the diagnosis changed to an organic mental disorder as illness progressed and cognitive impairment became more obvious. Perry and Tross[17] reported on the prevalence of psychiatric disorders seen in medically hospitalized AIDS patients at New York Hospital. Sixty five per cent of patients were diagnosed with an organic mental disorder, and 17 per cent were diagnosed with major depression. The organic mental disorders seen were predominantly AIDS dementia complex (ADC) and delirium, often in combination. Perry[18] later reported in 1999 that between 65 and 80 per cent of AIDS patients develop some type of organic mental disorder during the course of illness.

Over the last decade, the epidemiology of the AIDS epidemic, particularly in developed countries has changed from a disease of homosexual men to a disease of injection drug users and their sexual partners. In addition the introduction of protease inhibitors in the late mid-1990s began to change the medical course of HIV disease. With the widespread introduction of highly active antiretroviral therapies, mortality rates among patients with advanced HIV disease have declined dramatically, and this has had an impact on the prevalence of psychiatric disorders, primarily cognitive impairment disorders such as AIDS-related dementia. Despite these advances in AIDS therapies, substantially elevated rates of major depression and substance abuse were consistently observed. Rabkin et al.[19] reported rates of major depression of about 10 per cent, rates of anxiety disorders in the 8–13 per cent range, and current drug use disorders in the 14–17 per cent range. In addition, recent surveys of psychological and physical symptom burden in ambulatory AIDS patients[20] are rather significant. Vogl et al.[20] report that ambulatory AIDS patients have an average of 17 symptoms on the Memorial Symptom Assessment Scale, with the most prevalent symptoms including: worrying (86 per cent), fatigue (85 per cent), sadness (82 per cent), and pain (76 per cent). Like cancer patients, patients with AIDS were more likely to have symptoms of psychological distress as disease advanced and when pain was a co-morbid symptom.

Controlling psychiatric symptoms

Anxiety in the patient with advanced illness

The terminally ill patient presents with a complex mixture of physical and psychological symptoms in a context of a frightening reality. Thus the recognition of anxious symptoms requiring treatment can be challenging. Patients with anxiety complain of tension or restlessness, or they exhibit jitteriness, autonomic hyperactivity, vigilance, insomnia, distractibility, shortness of breath, numbness, apprehension, worry, or rumination. Often the physical or somatic manifestations of anxiety overshadow the psychological or cognitive ones, and are the symptoms that the patient most often presents.[21] The consultant must use these symptoms as a cue to inquire about the patient's psychological state, which is commonly one of fear, worry, or apprehension. The assumption that a high level of anxiety is inevitably encountered during the terminal phase of illness is neither helpful nor accurate for diagnostic and treatment purposes. In deciding whether to treat anxiety during the terminal phase of illness, the patient's subjective level of distress is the primary impetus for the initiation of treatment. Other considerations include problematic patient behaviour such as non-compliance due to anxiety, family and staff reactions to the patient's distress, and the balancing of the risks and benefits of treatment.[22]

Prevalence studies of anxiety, primarily in cancer populations, report a higher prevalence of mixed anxiety and depressive symptoms rather than anxiety alone.[22] Prevalence of anxiety increases with advancing disease and decline in the patient's physical status.[19] Brandenberg et al.[23] reported that 28 per cent of advanced melanoma patients were anxious compared to 15 per cent of controls. Anxiety, like fever, is a symptom in this population that can have many etiologies. Anxiety may be encountered as a component of an adjustment disorder, panic disorder, generalized anxiety disorder, phobia, or agitated depression. Additionally, in the terminally ill cancer patient, symptoms of anxiety are most likely to arise from some medical complication of the illness or treatment such as organic anxiety disorder, delirium, or other organic mental disorders.[3,7,21,22] Hypoxia, sepsis, poorly controlled pain, and adverse drug reactions such as akathisia or withdrawal states are specific entities which often present as anxiety. Patients who had been managed for long periods of time with relatively high doses of benzodiazepines or opioid analgesics for the control of anxiety or pain, often become tolerant or physically dependent upon these drugs. During the terminal phase of illness, when patients become less alert, there is a tendency to minimize the use of sedating medications. It is important to consider the need to slowly taper benzodiazepines and opioid analgesics in order to prevent acute withdrawal states. Withdrawal states in terminally ill patients often present first as agitation or anxiety and become clinically evident days later than might be expected in younger, healthier patients due to impaired metabolism. Benzodiazepine withdrawal, for example, can present first as agitation or anxiety, though the diagnosis is often missed in terminally ill patients, and especially the elderly, where physiologic dependence on these medications is often unrecognized.[24] In the dying patient, anxiety can represent impending cardiac or respiratory arrest, pulmonary embolism, electrolyte imbalance, or dehydration.[25]

Despite the fact that anxiety in terminal illness commonly results from medical complications, it is important not to forget that psychological factors related to death and dying or existential issues, play a role in anxiety, particularly in patients who are alert and not confused.[21,22] Patients frequently fear the isolation and separation of death. Claustrophobic patients may be afraid of the idea of being confined and buried in a coffin. These issues can be disconcerting to consultants who may find themselves at a loss for words that are consoling to the patient. Nonetheless, one should not avoid eliciting these concerns, listening empathically to them, and enlisting pastoral involvement where appropriate.

The specific treatment of anxiety in the terminally ill often depends on aetiology, presentation, and setting. An example of how the specific aetiology of the anxious symptom is important is the case of hypoxia. Anxiety associated with hypoxia and dyspnoea in a patient with diffuse lung metastases is most responsive to treatment with oxygen and opioid analgesics. If the same patient's presentation included hallucinations and agitation, a neuroleptic would be added to the regimen. In the hospital setting, an arterial blood gas (ABG) can confirm the diagnosis of hypoxia. However, the good clinician caring for the terminally ill patient at home may conclude on clinical grounds that hypoxia is present and therefore would treat anxiety associated with it in an identical fashion to that in the hospital. An ABG provides confirmatory information but is not essential to considering and treating hypoxia and so may be unnecessary when attempting to maximize the patient's comfort.

Pharmacologic treatment of anxiety in the terminally ill

The pharmacotherapy of anxiety in terminal illness (see Table 1) involves the judicious use of the following classes of medications: benzodiazepines, neuroleptics (typical and atypical), antihistamines, antidepressants, and opioid analgesics.[3,7,21,22,26]

Benzodiazepines

Benzodiazepines are the mainstay of the pharmacologic treatment of anxiety in the terminally ill patient. The shorter-acting benzodiazepines, such as lorazepam, alprazolam, and oxazepam, are safest in this population. The selection of these drugs avoids toxic accumulation due to impaired metabolism in debilitated individuals.[27] Lorazepam, oxazepam, and temazepam are metabolized by conjugation in the liver and are therefore safest in patients with hepatic disease. This is in contrast to alprazolam and other benzodiazepines which are metabolized through oxidative pathways in the liver that are more vulnerable to interference with hepatic damage. The disadvantage of using short-acting benzodiazepines is that patients often experience breakthrough anxiety or end of dose failure. Such patients benefit from switching to longer-acting benzodiazepines such as diazepam or clonazepam. Dying patients often benefit from parenteral administration of these drugs. Common dosage regimens include: lorazepam 0.5–2.0 mg, PO, IV, or IM, 3–6 h; alprazolam 0.25–1.0 mg, PO, TID–QID; diazepam 2.5–10 mg, PO, PR, IM, or IV Q 3–6 h; clonazepam 1–2 mg, PO, BID–TID. Dying patients can be administered diazepam rectally when no other route is available, with dosages equivalent to oral regimens. Rectal diazepam[28] has been used widely in the palliative care field to control anxiety, restlessness, and agitation associated with the final days of life.

Midazolam, a very short-acting, water-soluble benzodiazepine, is usually administered as an intravenous infusion in critical care settings where sedation is the goal in an agitated or anxious patient on a respirator. Midazolam may also prove useful in controlling anxiety and agitation in terminal phases of illness.[28–30] Unlike diazepam, midazolam has a short duration of action and seems to be less irritating to subcutaneous tissues when given by subcutaneous infusion. Since it is several times as potent as diazepam, starting doses should be low and careful monitoring of effects should be initiated. Doses ranging from 2 to 10 mg/day have been found to be safe and effective for most patients. However, doses as high as 30–60 mg/day have been reported.[31] Clonazepam, a longer-acting benzodiazepine, has been found

Table 1 Anxiolytic medications used in patients with advanced disease

Generic name	Approximate daily dosage range (mg)	Route[a]
Benzodiazepines		
Very short acting		
Midazolam	10–60 per 24 h	IV, SC
Short acting		
Alprazolam	0.25–2.0 TID–QID	PO,SL
Oxazepam	10–15 TID–QID	PO
Lorazepam	0.5–2.0 TID–QID	PO, SL IV, IM
Intermediate acting		
Chlordiazepoxide	10–50 TID–QID	PO, IM
Long acting		
Diazepam	5–10 BID-QID	PO, IM, IV, PR
Clorazepate	7.5–15 BID-QID	PO
Clonazepam	0.5–2.0 BID-QID	PO
Non-Benzodiazepines		
Buspirone	5.0–20 TID	PO
Neuroleptics		
Haloperidol	0.5–5.0 Q 2–12 h	PO, IV, SC, IM
Methotrimeprazine	10–20 Q 4–8 h	IV, SC, PO
Thioridazine	10–75 TID–QID	PO
Chlorpromazine	12.5–50 Q 4–12 h	PO, IM, IV
Atypical neuroleptics		
Olanzapine	2.5–20 Q 12–24 h	PO
Risperidone	1.0–3.0 Q 12–24 h	PO
Quetiapine fumarate	25–200 Q 12–24 h	PO
Antihistamine		
Hydroxyzine	25–50 Q 4–6 h	PO, IV, SC
Tricyclic antidepressants		
Imipramine	12.5–150 h	PO, IM
Clomipramine	10–150 h	PO

[a] PO, *peroral*; IM, intramuscular; PR, *per rectum*; IV, intravenous; SC, sub-cutaneous; SL, sub-lingual; BID, two times a day; TID, three times a day; QID, four times a day. Parenteral doses are generally twice as potent as oral doses, intravenous bolus injections, or infusions should be administered slowly.

to be extremely useful in the palliative care setting for the treatment of anxiety, depersonalization, or derealization in patients with seizure disorders, brain tumours, and mild organic mental disorders. Patients who experience end of dose failure with recurrence of anxiety on shorter-acting drugs also find clonazepam helpful. It is not uncommon to switch patients from alprazolam to clonazepam when attempting to taper off alprazolam. Clonazepam is also useful in patients with organic mood disorders who have symptoms of mania, and as an adjuvant analgesic in patients with neuropathic pain.(32–34)

Fears of causing respiratory depression should not prevent the clinician from using adequate dosages of benzodiazepines to control anxiety. The likelihood of respiratory depression is minimized when one utilizes shorter-acting drugs, increases the dosages in small increments in a carefully monitored setting, and ultimately switches to longer acting drugs.

Non-benzodiazepine anxiolytics

Typical neuroleptics, such as thioridazine and haloperidol, and some of the newer atypical neuroleptics, such as olanzapine, are useful in the treatment of anxiety when benzodiazepines are not sufficient for symptom control.(19) They are also indicated when an organic aetiology is suspected or when psychotic symptoms such as delusions or hallucinations accompany the anxiety. Neuroleptics are perhaps the safest class of anxiolytics in patients where there is legitimate concern regarding respiratory depression or compromise. Typically haloperidol 0.5–5 mg, PO, IV, or SC, Q 2–12 h, is sufficient to control anxious symptoms and avoid excessive sedation. Lower potency neuroleptics such as thioridazine (10–25 mg, PO, TID) are effective anxiolytics and can help with insomnia and agitation. Methotrimeprazine (10–20 mg, every 4–8 h, IM, IV, or SC) is a phenothiazine with unique analgesic and anxiolytic properties that is often used for the treatment of pain and anxiety in the dying patient.(35,36) Its side effects include sedation, anticholinergic symptoms and hypotension. Intravenous administration by slow infusion is preferable to avoid problems with hypotension. Chlorpromazine (12.5–50 mg, PO, IM, or IV, Q 4–12 h) has similar side effects that limit its application in this setting. However, it can be useful in patients where sedation is desirable. With typical neuroleptic drugs, such as those listed above, one must be aware of the potential for extrapyramidal side effects (particularly when patients are taking additional neuroleptics for antiemetic purposes) and the remote possibility of neuroleptic malignant syndrome. Tardive dyskinesia is rarely a concern given the generally short-term usage and low dosages of these medications in this population.(37) Typical neuroleptics all share the same properties of non-specific and potent CNS dopamine blocking activity. Atypical neuroleptics such as risperidone, olanzapine, and quetiapine may have the same anxiolytic properties as typical neuroleptics, but with significantly lower frequency of extrapyramidal side effects or tardive dyskinesia.

Hydroxyzine is an antihistamine with mild anxiolytic, sedative, and analgesic properties. It is particularly useful when treating anxious, terminally ill cancer patients with pain. One hundred milligrams of hydroxyzine given parenterally has analgesic potency equivalent to 8 mg of morphine and potentiates the analgesic effects of morphine.(38) As an anxiolytic, 25–50 mg of hydroxyzine Q 4–6 h PO, IV, or SC is effective.

Tricyclic, heterocyclic, and second generation antidepressants are the most effective treatment for anxiety accompanying depression and are helpful in treating panic disorder.(39–41) Guidelines for their use are discussed in the section on 'Depression'. Their usefulness is often limited in the dying patient due to anticholinergic and sedative side effects. Very often the consultant is faced with the task of relieving symptoms in a short period of time and so drugs that require a period of weeks to achieve therapeutic effect are unsatisfactory.

Opioid drugs such as the narcotic analgesics are primarily indicated for the control of pain. However, these drugs are also effective in the relief of dyspnoea due to cardiopulmonary processes and the anxiety associated with them.(42) Opioid drugs are particularly useful in the treatment of dying patients who are in respiratory distress. Continuous intravenous infusions of morphine or other narcotic analgesics allow for careful titration and control of respiratory distress, anxiety, pain, and agitation.(43) Occasionally one must maintain the patient in a state of unresponsiveness in order to maximize comfort. When respiratory distress is not a major problem, it is preferable to use the opioid drugs solely for analgesic purposes and to add more specific anxiolytics (such as the benzodiazepines) to control concomitant anxiety.

Buspirone, is a non-benzodiazepine anxiolytic that is useful along with psychotherapy in patients with chronic anxiety or anxiety related to adjustment disorders. The onset of anxiolytic action is delayed in comparison to the benzodiazepines, taking 5–10 days for relief of anxiety to begin. Since buspirone is not a benzodiazepine, it will not block benzodiazepine withdrawal, and so one must be cautious when switching from a benzodiazepine to buspirone. The effective dose of buspirone is 10 mg orally three times a day.(44) Because of its delayed onset of action and indication for use in chronic anxiety states, buspirone may be of limited usefulness to the clinician treating anxiety and agitation in the terminally ill.

Non-pharmacologic treatment of anxiety in terminally ill patients

Non-pharmacologic interventions for anxiety and distress include supportive psychotherapy and behavioral interventions that are used alone or in combination. Brief supportive psychotherapy is often useful in dealing with both crisis-related issues as well as existential issues confronted by the terminally ill.[45] Psychotherapeutic interventions should include both the patient and family, particularly as the patient with advanced illness becomes increasingly debilitated and less able to interact. Mental health professionals can assist in seeing that the emotional needs of patients and families are met during the terminal phase of illness. Such needs include continuous, updated information regarding the disease status and treatment options available. This information must be delivered repeatedly and with sensitivity as to what they are currently prepared and able to hear and absorb. Families, especially, require a great deal of reassurance that they and the medical staff have done everything possible for the patient. The goals of psychotherapy with the patient are to establish a bond that decreases the sense of isolation experienced with terminal illness, to help the patient face death with a sense of self worth, to correct misconceptions about the past and present, to integrate the present illness into a continuum of life experiences, and to explore issues of separation, loss, and the unknown that lies ahead. The therapist should emphasize past strengths and support previously successful ways of coping. This helps the patient mobilize inner resources, modify plans for the future, and perhaps even accept the inevitability of death.

It is during the terminal phase of illness that we have the greatest opportunity to affect the process of adaptation to loss. Mental health professionals must extend their supportive stance to include both the patient and family. Anticipatory bereavement is a common experience which allows patients, loved ones, and health care providers the opportunity to mentally prepare for the impending death. Patients and family members should be encouraged to use this period to reconcile differences, extend important final communications, and re-affirm feelings and wishes. It is a time is of vital importance that can often set the tone for the subsequent bereavement course.[46]

Relaxation, guided imagery, and hypnosis may help reduce anxiety and thereby increase the patient's sense of control. Most patients with advanced illness are still appropriate candidates for useful application of behavioural techniques despite physical debilitation. In assessing the utility of such interventions for a terminally ill patient, the clinician should, however, take into account the mental clarity of the patient. Confusional states interfere dramatically with a patient's ability to focus attention and thus limit the usefulness of these techniques.[3] Occasionally these techniques can be modified so as to include even mildly cognitive impaired patients. This often involves the therapist taking a more active role by orienting the patient, creating a safe and secure environment, and evoking a conditioned response to the therapist's voice or presence. A typical behavioural intervention for anxiety in a terminally ill patient would include a relaxation exercise combined with some distraction or imagery technique. Typically the patient is first taught to relax with passive breathing accompanied by either passive or active muscle relaxation. Once in such a relaxed state, the patient is taught a pleasant, distracting imagery exercise. In a randomized study comparing a relaxation technique with alprazolam in the treatment of anxiety and distress in non-terminally ill cancer patients, both treatments were demonstrated to be quite effective for mild to moderate degrees of anxiety or distress. The drug intervention (alprazolam) was more effective for greater levels of distress or anxiety and had more rapid onset of beneficial effect.[47] Relaxation techniques can be prescribed concurrently with anxiolytic medications in highly anxious cancer patients.

Depression in patients with advanced illness

The prevalence of depression in cancer patients ranges from 10 to 25 per cent and increases with higher levels of disability, advanced illness, and pain.[3,8,48,49] Two recent studies of the prevalence of major depression in terminally ill cancer patients receiving care in palliative care units suggest that the prevalence of depression in patients during the last weeks to months of life ranges from 9 to 18 per cent.[48,50] Risk factors associated with depression have been identified for the general population and patients with advanced disease. Certain types of cancer are associated with an increased incidence of depression. Patients with pancreatic cancer, for example, are more likely to develop depression than patients with other types of intra-abdominal malignancies.[51] Family history of depression and history of previous depressive episodes further increase the risk of developing a depressive episode in the context of advanced cancer. Many studies have also found a correlation between depression, pain, and functional status.[52] Tumours by their origin or metastases to the CNS can cause depressive symptoms.[53] In addition, any evaluation of depression must also include an examination of medications and physical conditions that may be the cause of depression. Corticosteroids,[54] chemotherapeutic agents,[55–58] (vincristine, vinblastine, asparaginase, intrathecal methotrexate, interferon, interleukin) amphotericin,[59] whole brain radiation,[60] CNS metabolic-endocrine complications,[61] and paraneoplastic syndromes,[62,63] can present as depression, and addressing these factors must precede initiation of treatment. Recent reports suggest that loss of meaning and low scores on measures of spiritual well being are associated with higher levels of depressive symptoms, suggesting that the relationship between existential distress and depression in terminal illness warrants further investigation.[64]

Assessment of depression in the terminally ill

Depressed mood and sadness can be appropriate responses as the terminally ill patient faces death. These emotions can be manifestations of anticipatory grief over the impending loss of one's life, health, loved ones, and autonomy. Despite this, major depressive syndrome is a common mental health problem arising in the palliative care setting. Depression is under-diagnosed and under-treated. Depression significantly diminishes quality of life and complicates symptom control, resulting in more frequent admission to inpatient care setting. The under-diagnosis of depression in the palliative care setting relates to the minimization of these symptoms by clinicians, the concern that severely medically ill patients will not be able to tolerate the side effects or drug interactions associated with the initiation of antidepressant therapy, and the difficulties of accurately diagnosing depression in the terminally ill.[65]

The DSM-IV criteria for major depressive disorder, the most severe and well-documented diagnosis within the depression spectrum, are shown in Table 2. They include two core criterion symptoms, depressed mood and anhedonia, a marked loss of interest or pleasure in activities. In order to qualify for the diagnosis, a patient must exhibit one of these core symptoms, along with at least four other symptoms from the criterion list. A critical problem associated with diagnosing depression in medically ill patients' lies with the issue of how best to interpret the physical/somatic symptoms of depression.

Table 2 DSM-IV symptoms of major depression and substitute symptoms suggested by Endicott

DSM-IV criteria	Substitute symptoms
Depressed mood most of the day	
Markedly diminished interest or pleasure in all or almost all activities most of the day	
Weight loss or gain, or decreased or increased appetite	Depressed appearance, tearfulness
Insomnia or hypersomnia decreased	Social withdrawal, talkativeness
Psychomotor agitation or retardation	
Fatigue or loss of energy	Brooding, self-pity, or pessimism
Feeling of worthlessness or excessive or inappropriate guilt	
Diminished ability to think or concentrate, or indecisiveness	Lack of reactivity, cannot be cheered up
Recurrent thoughts of death, or suicidal ideation or planning or a suicide attempt	

Five different approaches to the diagnosis of major depression have been proposed: an inclusive approach—includes all symptoms whether or not they may be secondary to advanced illness or treatment; an exclusive approach—deletes and disregards all physical symptoms from consideration, not allowing them to contribute to the diagnosis; an aetiologic approach—the clinician attempts to determine if the physical symptom is due to illness or treatment or due to a depressive disorder; a substitutive approach—where physical symptoms of uncertain aetiology are replaced by other non-somatic symptoms.(66) This approach is best exemplified by the Endicott Substitution Criteria also listed in Table 2. Finally, a fifth approach involves requiring a higher threshold number of diagnostic criteria symptoms to make a diagnosis (seven rather than five). This approach is best exemplified by Chochinov et al.(49) who studied the prevalence of depression in a cohort of 130 terminally ill patients in a palliative care facility. They reported that 9.2 per cent met Research Diagnostic Criteria (RDC) for major depression when using high-severity thresholds for RDC criteria A symptoms (equivalent to the symptom threshold judgments specified in DSM-IV). This approach yielded the identical prevalence of major depression whether or not one included somatic symptoms in the diagnostic criteria or used Endicott revised criteria.(66) (involving replacement of somatic symptoms with non-somatic alternatives). While concern has been raised about the non-specificity of somatic symptoms in the medically ill, these results—along with those of other recent investigations(67,68)—indicate that their inclusion may not overly influence the diagnostic classification of major depression.

The diagnostic interview remains the most commonly used clinical tool and should directly assess commonly accepted criteria in addition to relying more on the psychological or cognitive symptoms of major depression (H). The diagnosis of a major depressive syndrome in a terminally ill patient often relies more on the psychological or cognitive symptoms of major depression (worthlessness, hopelessness, excessive guilt, and suicidal ideation), rather than the neuro-vegetative or somatic signs and symptoms of major depression. The strategy of relying on the psychological or cognitive signs and symptoms of depression for diagnostic specificity is itself not without problems. How is the clinician to interpret feelings of hopelessness in the dying patient when there is no hope for cure or recovery? Feelings of hopelessness, worthlessness, or suicidal ideation must be explored in detail. While many dying patients lose hope of a cure, they are able to maintain hope for better symptom control. For many patients hope is contingent on the ability to find continued meaning in their day to day existence. Hopelessness that is pervasive and accompanied by a sense of despair or despondency is more likely to represent a symptom of a depressive disorder. Similarly patients often state that they feel they are burdening their families unfairly, causing them great pain and inconvenience. Those beliefs are less likely to represent a symptom of depression than if the patient feels that their life has never had any worth, or that they are being punished for evil things they have done. Suicidal ideation, even rather mild and passive forms, is very likely associated with significant degrees of depression in terminally ill cancer patients.(69,70)

Numerous assessment methods for depression including diagnostic classification systems, structured interview, and screening instruments have been used in research, as enumerated in Table 3. Unfortunately, few studies of depression in terminally ill or advanced cancer patients have used such research assessment methods to date. Recently, Chochinov et al.(71) studied brief screening instruments to measure depression in the terminally ill. His group compared the performance of four brief screening measures for depression in a group of terminally ill patients. The methods compared included (i) a single-item interview assessing depressed mood—'Have you been depressed most of the time for the past two weeks?', (ii) a two-item interview assessing depressed mood and loss of interest in activities, (iii) a visual analogue scale for depressed mood, and (iv) the 13-item Beck depression inventory. Semi-structured diagnostic interviews were administered to 197 patients receiving palliative care for advanced cancer. The interview diagnoses served as the standard against which the screening performance of the four brief screening methods was assessed. As reported in other depression screening studies, the self-report instruments (i.e. the Beck and the mood visual analogue scale) demonstrated a low positive predictive value (0.27 and 0.17, respectively) and a high negative predictive value (0.96 and 0.92, respectively). Most noteworthy, the single-item interview question, 'Have you been depressed most of the time for the past two weeks?', correctly identified the diagnosis of every patient, while not misidentifying any patient, substantially outperforming the questionnaire and visual analogue measures. Brief screening measures for depression are thus important clinical tools for terminally ill patients. The performance of the single-item interview, which essentially asks patients if they are depressed, speaks to the importance of mood inquiry in this particularly vulnerable patient population.

Table 3 Assessment methods for depression in patients with advanced disease

Diagnostic classification systems
Diagnostic and Statistical Manual DSM-III, III-R, IV
Endicott Substitution Criteria
Research Diagnostic Criteria (RDC)
Structures diagnostic interviews
Schedule for Affective and Schizophrenia (SADS)
Diagnostic Interview Schedule (DIS)
Structured Clinical interview for DSM-IIIR (SCID)
Screening instruments—self-report
General Health Questionnaire-30 (GHQ)
Hospital Anxiety and Depression Scale (HADS)
Beck Depression Inventory—13 items (BDI)
Visual Analogue Scale for Depressed Mood

Passik and colleagues recently demonstrated that clinical depression is under-recognized in cancer patients, but that the Zung Depression Rating Scale could be utilized effectively by oncologists and nurses as a rapid screening tool for depression in advanced cancer patients, and that oncologists could be easily trained to diagnose and initiate further evaluation and treatment of clinical depression in advanced cancer patients.(72–76)

Management of depression in the terminally ill

Depression in cancer patients with advanced disease is optimally managed utilizing a combination of supportive psychotherapy, cognitive-behavioural techniques, and antidepressant medications.(48) Psychotherapy and cognitive-behavioural techniques are useful in the management of psychological distress in cancer patients, and have been applied to the treatment of depressive and anxious symptoms related to cancer and cancer pain. Psychotherapeutic interventions, either in the form of individual or group counselling, have been shown to effectively reduce psychological distress and depressive symptoms in cancer patients.(45,77,78) Cognitive-behavioural interventions, such as relaxation and distraction with pleasant imagery, have also been shown to decrease depressive symptoms in patients with mild to moderate levels of depression.(47) Psychopharmacological interventions (i.e. antidepressant medications) (see Table 4), however, are the mainstay of management in the treatment of cancer patients with severe depressive symptoms who meet criteria for a major depressive episode.(48) The efficacy of antidepressants in the treatment of depression in cancer patients has been well established.(40,48,79–81)

Pharmacologic treatment of depression in the terminally ill

Any treatment for major depression in the terminally ill will be less effective if given in a context devoid of psychotherapeutic support. Although both psychotherapy and cognitive-behavioural therapy have proven effective in reducing psychological distress and mild to moderate depressive symptomatology in the cancer setting, pharmacotherapy is the mainstay for treating terminally ill patients meeting diagnostic criteria for major depression.(44,65) Factors such as prognosis and the timeframe for treatment may play an

Table 4 Antidepressant medications used in patients with advanced disease

Generic name	**Approximate daily dosage range** (mg)	**Route**[a]
Tricyclic antidepressants		
Amitriptyline	10–150	PO, IM, PR
Doxepin	12.5–150	PO, IM
Imipramine	12.5–150	PO, IM
Desipramine	12.5–150	PO, IM
Nortriptyline	10–125	PO
Clomipramine	10–150	PO
Serotonin-specific reuptake inhibitors		
Fluoxetine	20–160	PO
Sertraline	50–200	PO
Paroxetine	10–60	PO
Citalopram	10–60	PO
Fluvoxamine	50–300	PO
Serotonin–norepinephrine reuptake inhibitor		
Venlafaxine	75–225	PO
Serotonin 2 antagonists/serotonin reuptake inhibitors		
Trazodone	25–300	PO
Nefazodone	100–600	PO
Norepinephrine and dopamine reuptake blockers		
Buproprion	200–450	PO
Buproprion—SR[b]	150–300	PO
Heterocyclic antidepressants		
Maprotiline	50–75	PO
Amoxapine	100–150	PO
Psychostimulants		
Dextroamphetamine	2.5–20 BID	PO
Methylphenidate	2.5–20 BID	PO
Pemoline	37.5–75 BID	PO, SL[c]
Modafinil	50–400	PO
Monoamine oxidase inhibitors		
Isocarboxazid	20–40	PO
Phenelzine	30–60	PO
Tranylcypromine	20–40	PO
Moclobemide	100–600	PO
Benzodiazepines		
Alprazolam	0.25–2.0 TID	PO
Lithium carbonate	600–1200	PO

[a] PO, *peroral*; IM, intramuscular; PR, *per rectum*; BID, two times a day; TID, three times a day; intravenous infusions of a number of tricyclic antidepressants are utilized outside of the United States. This route is, however, not FDA approved.

[b] SR, sustained release.

[c] Comes in chewable tablet form that can be absorbed without swallowing.

important role in determining the type of pharmacotherapy for depression. A depressed patient with several months of life expectancy can afford to wait the 2–4 weeks it may take to respond to a serotonin reuptake inhibitor or a tricyclic antidepressant. The depressed dying patient with less than 3 weeks to live may do best with a rapid-acting psychostimulant.[65,82,83] Patients who are within hours to days of death and in distress are likely to benefit most from the use of sedatives or narcotic analgesic infusions.

Tricyclic antidepressants

Tricyclic antidepressants (TCAs) have been the cornerstone for treating depression in the general cancer setting since the early 1960s. Their application specifically to the terminally ill, however, requires a careful risk–benefit ratio analysis. Although nearly 70 per cent of patients treated with a tricyclic for non-psychotic depression can anticipate a positive response, these medications are associated with a side effect profile which can be particularly troublesome for terminally ill patients.[65,84] They have multiple pharmacodynamic actions accounting for these side effects, including blockade of muscarinic cholinergic receptors, alpha-adrenoceptor blockade, and H_1 histamine receptor blockade. The tertiary amines (amitriptyline, doxepin, imipramine) have a greater propensity to cause side effects than do secondary amines (nortriptyline, desipramine).[85] The secondary amines are thus often a preferable choice for the terminally ill.

The anticholinergic side effects can include constipation, dry mouth, and urinary retention. To avoid exacerbating symptoms associated with genitourinary outlet obstruction, decreased gastric motility, or stomatitis, a relatively non-anticholinergic tricyclic, such as desipramine or nortriptyline, is a reasonable choice. Those patients who are receiving medication with anticholinergic properties (such as pethidine, atropine, diphenhydramine, phenothiazines) are at risk for developing an anticholinergic delirium, and thus antidepressants which are potently anticholinergic should be avoided.[86] The anticholinergic actions of TCAs can also cause serious tachycardia which can be problematic for terminally ill patients with cardiac insufficiency. The quinidine-like effects of TCAs can also lead to arrhythmias by virtue of their ability to delay conduction via the His-Purkinje system[87] (associated with nonspecific ST–T changes and T waves on the electrocardiograph). These effects are particularly concerning for those terminally ill patients with pre-existing conduction defects, especially second or third degree heart block.

Alpha1-blockade is associated with postural hypotension and dizziness. This can be of particular concern for the frail volume depleted patient who, because of these side effects, is at risk for falls and possible fractures. Nortriptyline and protriptyline are the TCAs least associated with alpha1-blockade. H_1 histamine receptor blockage is associated with sedation and drowsiness. For dying patients already exposed to a variety of sedating agents (e.g. narcotic analgesics, antiemetics, anxiolytics, neuroleptics) TCAs such as amitriptyline and doxepin are the most likely to accentuate the overall cumulative sedating effects of these medications.

TCAs should be started at low doses (10–25 mg qhs) and increased in 10–25 mg increments every 2–4 days, until a therapeutic dose is attained or side effects become a dose limiting factor. Depressed cancer patients often achieve a therapeutic response at significantly lower doses of TCAs (25–125 mg) than are necessary in the physically well (150–300 g).[44] There is also evidence to suggest that patients with advanced cancer achieve higher serum tricyclic levels at modest doses.[88] In order to minimize drug toxicity and more carefully guide the process of drug titration, prescribing tricyclics (desipramine, nortriptyline, amitriptyline, imipramine) with well-established therapeutic plasma levels may be advantageous.[89] Desipramine and nortriptyline are generally better tolerated in this population than is amitriptyline or imipramine.

The choice of which specific TCA to use depends on a variety of factors, including the nature of the underlying terminal medical condition, the characteristics of the depressive episode, past responses to antidepressant therapy, and the specific drug side effect profile. Those patients who present with agitation and insomnia may respond favourably to more sedating tricyclics (amitriptyline, doxepin). For the terminally ill depressed patient, the choice of TCA is made on the basis of a side effect profile which will be least incompatible with the patient's overall medical condition. Most tricyclics are available as rectal suppositories for patients who are no longer able to take medication orally. Outside of the United States, certain tricyclics are given as intravenous infusion.[90] Although not very practical, amitriptyline, imipramine, and doxepin can also be given intramuscularly.[48,65]

It must be borne in mind that a therapeutic response to TCAs (as with all antidepressants) has a latency time of 3–6 weeks. For the terminally ill depressed patient whose life expectancy is anticipated to be less than this, psychostimulants may offer a more viable, rapid response alternative.

Serotonin-specific reuptake inhibitors

The selective serotonin reuptake inhibitors (SSRIs) now have an important role in the pharmacotherapy of depression in the medically ill and those with advanced cancer and AIDS.[48,65,82,91] They have been found to be as effective in the treatment of depression as the tricyclics[92,93] and have a number of features which may be particularly advantageous for the terminally ill. The SSRIs have a very low affinity for adrenergic, cholinergic, and histamine receptors, thus accounting for negligible orthostatic hypotension, urinary retention, memory impairment, sedation, or reduced awareness.(94) They have not been found to cause clinically significant alterations in cardiac conduction and are generally favourably tolerated along with a wider margin of safety than the TCAs in the event of an overdose. They do not therefore require therapeutic drug level monitoring.

Most of the side effects of SSRIs result from their selective central and peripheral serotonin reuptake inhibition. These include increased intestinal motility (loose stools, nausea, vomiting, insomnia, headaches, and sexual dysfunction). Some patients may experience anxiety, tremor, restlessness, and akathisia (the latter is relatively rare but it can be problematic for the terminally ill patient with Parkinson's disease).(95) These side effects tend to be dose related and may be problematic for patients with advanced disease.

There are five SSRIs currently being marketed, including fluoxetine, sertraline, paroxetine, citalopram, and fluvoxamine. With the exception of fluoxetine, whose elimination half-life is 2–4 days, the SSRIs have an elimination half-life of about 24 h. Fluoxetine is the only SSRI with a potent active metabolite, norfluoxetine, whose elimination half-life 7–14 days. Fluoxetine can cause mild nausea and a brief period of increased anxiety as well as appetite suppression that usually lasts for a period of several weeks. Some patients can experience transient weight loss, but weight usually returns to baseline level. The anorectic properties of fluoxetine have not been a limiting factor in the use of this drug in cancer patients. Fluoxetine and norfluoxetine do not reach a steady state for 5–6 weeks, compared with 4–14 days for paroxetine, citalopram, fluvoxamine, and sertraline. These difference are important, especially for the terminally patient in whom a switch from an SSRI to another antidepressant is being considered. If a switch to a monamine oxidase inhibitor is required, the washout period for fluoxetine will be at least 5 weeks, given the potential drug interactions between these two agents. Since fluoxetine has entered the market, there have been several reports of significant drug–drug interactions.(96,97) Until it has been studied further in the medically ill, it should be used cautiously in the debilitated dying patient. Paroxetine, citalopram, fluvoxamine, and sertraline on the other hand require considerably shorter washout periods (10–14 days) under similar circumstances.

All the SSRIs have the ability to inhibit the hepatic isoenzyme P450 11D6, with sertraline and citalopram being least potent in this regard. Citalopram appears to be the SSRI with the least potential for serious drug–drug interactions. This is important with respect to dose/plasma level ratios and drug interactions, since the SSRIs are dependent upon hepatic metabolism. For the elderly patient with advanced disease, the dose response curve for sertraline appears to be relatively linear. On the other hand, particularly for paroxetine (which appears to most potently inhibit cytochrome P450 11D6), small dosage increases can result in dramatic elevations in plasma levels. Paroxetine, and to a somewhat lesser extent fluoxetine, appear to inhibit the hepatic enzymes responsible for their own clearance.(98) The co-administration of these medications with other drugs that are dependent on this enzyme system for their catabolism (e.g. tricyclics, phenothiazines, type IC antiarrhythmics, and quinidine) should be done cautiously. Fluvoxamine has been shown in some instances to elevate the blood levels of propranolol and warfarin by as much as twofold, and should thus not be prescribed together with these agents.

SSRIs can generally be started at their minimally effective doses. For the terminally ill, this usually means initiating therapy at approximately half the usual starting dose used in an otherwise healthy patient. For fluoxetine, patients can begin on 5 mg (available in liquid form) given once daily (preferably in the morning) with a range of 10–40 mg/day; given its long half-life, some patients may only require this drug every second day. Paroxetine can be started at 10 mg once daily (either morning or evening) for the patient with advanced disease, and has a therapeutic range of 10–40/day. Fluvoxamine, which tends to be somewhat more sedating, can be started at 25 mg (in the evenings) and has a therapeutic range of 50–300 mg. Sertraline can be initiated at 50 mg, morning or evening, and titrated within a range of 50–200 mg/day. Citalopram can be initiated at 10 mg per day and titrated up to a dose of 40–60 mg/day. If patients experience activating effects on SSRIs, they should not be given at bedtime but rather moved earlier into the day. Gastrointestinal upset can be reduced by ensuring the patient does not take medication on an empty stomach.(48,65)

Serotonin–norepinephrine reuptake inhibitor

Venlaflaxine (Effexor), is the only antidepressant in this class. It is a potent inhibitor of neuronal serotonin and norepinephrine reuptake and appears to have no significant affinity for muscarinic, histamine, or alpha1-adrenergic receptors. Some patients may experience a modest sustained increase in blood pressure, especially at doses above the recommended initiating dose. Compared with the SSRIs, its protein binding (<35 per cent) is very low. Few protein binding induced drug interactions are thus expected. Like other antidepressants, Venlaflaxine should not be used in patients receiving monamine oxidase inhibitors. Its side effect profile tends to generally be well tolerated with few discontinuations. While there is currently no data addressing at its use in the terminally ill depressed patient, its pharmacokinetic properties and side effect profile suggest it may have a role to play.(48,65,82)

Serotonin 2 antagonists/serotonin reuptake inhibitors

Nefazodone and trazodone are chemically related antidepressants that block post-synaptic 5-HT_2 receptors. Nefazodone is much less sedating than trazodone, but more likely to cause gastrointestinal activation. Nefazodone can be started at a dose of 50 mg at bedtime and titrated up to a range of 100–500 mg/day. Nefazodone does not have significant sexual side effects. If given in sufficient doses (100–300 mg/day), Trazodone can be an effective antidepressant. Although its anticholinergic profile is almost negligible it has considerable affinity for alpha1-adrenoceptors and may thus predispose patients to orthostatic hypotension and its problematic sequelae (i.e. falls, fractures, head injuries). Trazedone is very sedating and in low doses (100 mg qhs) is helpful in the treatment of the depressed cancer patient with insomnia. It is highly serotonergic and its use should be considered when the patient requires adjunct analgesics effect in addition to antidepressant effects. Trazodone has little effect on cardiac conduction but can cause arrhythmias in patients with premorbid cardiac disease.(99) Trazodone has also been associated with priapism and should thus be used with caution in male patients.(100) It is highly sedating with drowsiness being its most common adverse side effect. In smaller doses it can thus be used as an effective sedative hypnotic.

Norepinephrine and dopamine reuptake blockers

Buproprion has not been studied extensively in patients with advanced disease. However, one might consider prescribing buproprion if patients have a poor response to a reasonable trial of other antidepressants. Buproprion may have a role in the treatment of the psychomotor retarded depressed terminally ill patient as it has energizing effects similar to the stimulant drugs.(101,102) However, because of the increased incidence of seizures, in patients with CNS disorders, bupropion has a limited role in the oncology population. Buproprion and its sustained release form buproprion SR have also been used recently as an adjunct to smoking cessation interventions, but this experience has generally limited to patients with earlier stages of cancer or in healthy populations.(48,65,82)

Mirtazapine is the 6-aza analogue of the tetracyclic antidepressant mianserin. Mirtazapine enhances central noradrenergic and serotonergic activities with blockade of central presynaptic alpha2 inhibitory receptors and post-synaptic serotonin 5-HT_2 and 5-HT_3 receptors. It compares favourably with amitriptyline and trazodone, with further studies needed to compare the clinical efficacy of mirtazapine to serotonin reuptake inhibitors. Mirtazapine improves appetite resulting in weight gain, which is desirable in cancer patients. In addition, the marked sedative effect of this medication proves quite useful in patients with sleeping difficulties.(48,65,82)

Heterocyclic antidepressants

The heterocyclic antidepressants have side effect profiles that are similar to the TCAs. Maprotiline should be avoided in patients with brain tumours and in those who are at risk for seizures since the incidence of seizures is increased with this medication.[103] Amoxapine has mild dopamine blocking activity. Hence, patients who are taking other dopamine blockers (e.g. antiemetics) have an increased risk of developing extrapyramidal symptoms and dyskinesias.[104] Mianserin (not available in the United States) is a serotonergic antidepressant with adjuvant analgesic properties that is used widely in Europe and Latin America. Costa et al.[81] showed mianserin to be a safe and effective drug for the treatment of depression in cancer.

Psychostimulants

The psychostimulants (dextroamphetamine, methylphenidate, pemoline, and modafinil) offer an alternative and effective pharmacologic approach to the treatment of depression in the terminally ill.[83,105–117] These drugs have a more rapid onset of action than the SSRIs and are often energizing. They are most helpful in the treatment of depression in cancer patients with advanced disease and those where dysphoric mood is associated with severe psychomotor slowing and even mild cognitive impairment. Ocassionally treatment with an SSRI and a psychostimulant may be initiated concurrently so that patients with depression may receive the immediate benefits of the psychostimulant drug until the 1–2 weeks necessary for an SSRI to begin to work pass. At that point the psychostimulant may be withdrawn as symptoms of depression are monitored. A decision at that point can be made to either continue without the psychostimulant (if the SSRI has begun to take effect) or the psychostimulant drug can be restarted and continued. Psychostimulants have been shown to improve attention, concentration, and overall performance on neuropsychological testing in the medically ill.[118] In relatively low dose, psychostimulants stimulate appetite, promote a sense of well being, and improve feelings of weakness and fatigue in cancer patients. Treatment with dextroamphetamine or methylphenidate usually begins with a dose of 2.5 mg at 8 : 00 AM and at noon. The dosage is slowly increased over several days until a desired effect is achieved or side effects (overstimulation, anxiety, insomnia, paranoia, confusion) intervene. Typically a dose greater than 30 mg/day is not necessary although occasionally patients require up to 60 mg/day. Patients usually are maintained on methylphenidate for 1–2 months, and approximately two-thirds will be able to be withdrawn from methylphenidate without a recurrence of depressive symptoms. Those who do recur can be maintained on a psychostimulant for up to 1 year without significant abuse problems. Tolerance will develop and adjustment of dose may be necessary. An additional benefit of such stimulants as methylphenidate and dextroamphetamine are that they have been shown to reduce sedation secondary to opioid analgesics and provide adjuvant analgesics in cancer patients.[119] Common side effects of stimulants include nervousness, overstimulation, mild increase in blood pressure and pulse rate, and tremor. More rare side effects include dyskinesias or motor tics as well as a paranoid psychosis or exacerbation of an underlying and unrecognized confusional state.

Pemoline is a unique psychostimulant chemically unrelated to amphetamine. It is a less potent stimulant with little abuse potential.[109] Advantages of pemoline as a psychostimulant in cancer patients include the lack of abuse potential, the lack of federal regulation through special triplicate prescriptions, the mild sympathomimetic effects, and the fact that it comes in a chewable tablet form that can be absorbed through the buccal mucosa and be used by cancer patients who have difficulty swallowing or have intestinal obstruction. Pemoline appears to be as effective as methylphenidate or dextroamphetamine in the treatment of depressive symptoms in terminally ill cancer patients.[120] Pemoline can be started at a dose of 18.75 mg in the morning and at noon, and increased gradually over days. Typically patients require 75 mg a day or less. Pemoline should be used with caution in patients with liver impairment, and liver function tests should be monitored periodically with longer-term treatment.[121]

Recently modafinil, a new and novel psychostimulant, was approved for use in the United States for the treatment of excessive daytime sleepiness due to narcolepsy and other medical conditions. Although more controlled studies need to be completed, early case series reports suggest its efficacy as an antidepressant.[114–117] Modafinil is a novel psychostimulant, whose mechanism of action is unclear, that does not have a similar pharmacological profile to the other sympathomimetic amines. Although modafinil may produce euphoric effects and has been shown to be reinforcing at high doses in monkeys during clinical trials, the subjective effects of modafinil are markedly different from those of amphetamine and methylphenidate. This suggests that modafinil may not have the same abuse liability as those drugs. Because of this lower abuse potential, modafinil is a Schedule IV prescription.[114–117] A recent case series by Menza et al.[114] showed modafinil to be a useful augmenting agent in treatment resistant depression, particularly when patients complain of fatigue as one of their symptoms. In this series, modafinil was used in combination with a number of different antidepressants and anticonvulsants, including SSRIs, buproprion, venlafaxine, and divalproex. The addition of modafinil was well tolerated and led to a marked reduction in depressive symptoms in all seven patients. Modafinil should be given in the morning and can be started at a dose of 100 mg for most patients. Starting at 50 mg is advisable for elderly or frail patients. The dose can then be titrated upwards. In his case series, Menza's modal dose was 200 mg. However, modafinil can be used in doses up to 400 mg/day. Modafinil may be a useful alternative to other psychostimulants for patients who are unable to tolerate or for whom the usual psychostimulants are contraindicated (e.g. in that modafinil is less sympathomimetic, has less potential for adverse cardiovascular effects, for example, tachycardia, lowers seizure threshold very minimally if at all, and has very low abuse potential).

Monamine oxidase inhibitors

In general monoamine oxidase inhibitors (MAOIs) MAOIs have been considered a less desirable alternative for treating depression in the terminally ill. Patients who receive MAOIs must avoid foods rich in tyramine, sympathomimetic drugs (amphetamines, methylphenidate), and medications containing phenylpropranolamine and pseudoephedrine.[95] The combination of these agents with MAOIs may cause hypertensive crisis, leading to strokes and fatalities. MAOIs in combination with opioid analgesics have also been reported to be associated with myoclonus and delirium, and must therefore be used together cautiously.[65] The use of meperidine while on MAOIs is absolutely contraindicated and can lead to hyperpyrexia, cardiovascular collapses, and death. MAOIs can also cause considerable orthostatic hypotension. Avoiding this minefield of adverse interactions can be particularly problematic for the terminally ill. It is not surprising that MAOIs tend to be reserved in this patient population for those who have shown past preferential responses to them for treatment of their depression.

The new reversible inhibitors of monoamine oxidase-A (RIMAs) may reduce some of the problems associated with the older MAOIs (tranylcypromine, isocarboxazide). There are no studies on the role of RIMAs in the depressed terminally ill but there are interesting theoretical reasons to suggest they may eventually have a larger role to play than the non-selective MAOIs. RIMAs selectively inhibit MAO-A enzyme, therefore leaving MAO-B enzyme available to deal with any tyramine challenge. Moclobemide, a RIMA recently introduced onto the Canadian market, appears to be loosely bound to the MAO-A receptor and is thus relatively easily displaced by tyramine from its binding sight. It has a very short half-life which further reduces the possibility of any prolonged adverse effects, for example, hypertensive crisis. Dietary restrictions avoidant of tyramine-containing foods are thus not required. The side effect profile of moclobemide is far more favourable than non-selective MAOIs and tends to be well tolerated. Although the risk of hypertensive crisis is significantly reduced, it is not, however, entirely eliminated. Agents such as meperidine, procarbazine, dextromethorphan, or other ephedrine-containing agents are still best avoided. Its short half-life requires that moclobemide be administered two times daily, with a total dosage range of 150–600 mg daily. Co-administration with cimetidine will increase its plasma concentration thus requiring appropriate dosage adjustments. While RIMAs may offer some advantages in the terminally ill depressed patient over tranylcypromine and isocarboxazid, they will likely remain a second line choice to other available non-MAOI antidepressants.

Lithium carbonate

Patients who have been receiving lithium carbonate, prior to a cancer illness, should be maintained on it throughout their cancer treatment, although close monitoring is necessary in the preoperative and post-operative periods when fluids and salt may be restricted.[100] Maintenance doses of lithium may need reduction in seriously ill patients. Lithium should be prescribed with caution for patients receiving *cis*-platinum because of the potential nephrotoxicity of both drugs. Several authors have reported possible beneficial effects from the use of lithium in neutropenic cancer patients. However, the functional capabilities of these leukocytes have not been determined. The stimulation effect appears to be transient; no mood changes have been noted in these patients.[122,123]

Benzodiazepines

The triazolobenzodiazepine alprazolam has been shown to be a mildly effective antidepressant as well as an anxiolytic. Alprazolam is particularly useful in cancer patients who have mixed symptoms of anxiety and depression. Starting dose is 0.25 mg three times a day, effective doses are usually in the range of 4–6 mg daily.[47]

Electroconvulsive therapy

Occasionally, it is necessary to consider electroconvulsive therapy (ECT) for depressed cancer patients who have depression with psychotic features or in whom treatment with antidepressants pose unacceptable side effects. The safe effective use of ECT in the medically ill has been reviewed by others.[44]

Non-pharmacologic treatment of depression in terminally Ill patients

Supportive psychotherapy is a useful treatment approach to depression in the terminally ill patient. Psychotherapy with the dying patient consists of active listening with supportive verbal interventions and the occasional interpretation.[102] Despite the seriousness of the patient's plight, it is not necessary for the psychiatrist or psychologist to appear overly solemn or emotionally restrained. Often it is only the psychotherapist, of all the patient's care givers, who is comfortable enough to converse lightheartedly and allow the patient to talk about their life and experiences, rather than focus solely on impending death. The dying patient who wishes to talk or ask questions about death should be allowed to do so freely, with the therapist maintaining an interested, interactive stance. It is not uncommon for the dying patient to benefit from pastoral counselling. If a chaplaincy service is available, it should be offered to the patient and family.

A number of psychotherapies, other than supportive psychotherapy, have been described as potentially useful in the treatment of depressive symptoms and distress in a palliative care population. A review of the applications of interpersonal, existential, life narrative, and group psychotherapy intervention in the palliative care population is available to the reader.[1,124] Recently, several novel psychotherapies have been developed and are being tested in the treatment of depression, hopelessness, loss of meaning, and demoralization. Two examples of such developing psychotherapies include: Meaning-Centered psychotherapy[125] and Dignity-Conserving care.[126]

Suicide, assisted suicide, and desire for hastened death in the terminally ill

Suicide, suicidal ideation, and desire for hastened death are all important and serious consequences of unrecognized and inadequately treated clinical depression. While clinical depression has been demonstrated to be a critically important factor in desire for hastened death (through suicide or other means), understanding more fully why some patients with a terminal illness wish or seek to hasten their death remains an important element in the practice of palliative care. Despite the continued legal prohibitions against assisted suicide, a substantial number of patients think about and discuss those alternatives with their physicians, family, and friends.[127]

Suicide

Cancer patients are at increased risk of suicide relative to the general population, particularly in the terminal stage of illness. Factors associated with increased risk of suicide in patients with advanced disease[69,70] are listed in Table 5. Patients with advanced illness are at highest risk, perhaps because they are most likely to have such cancer complications as pain, depression, delirium, and deficit symptoms. Psychiatric disorders are frequently present in hospitalized cancer patients who are suicidal. A recent review of the psychiatric consultation data from Memorial Sloan-Kettering Cancer Center showed that one-third of suicidal cancer patients had a major depression, about 20 per cent suffered from a delirium, and 50 per cent were diagnosed with an adjustment disorder with both anxious and depressed features at the time of evaluation.[69,70]

Table 5 Suicide vulnerability factors in patients with advanced disease

Pain, suffering aspects
Advanced illness, poor prognosis
Depression, hopelessness
Delirium, disinhibition
Control, helplessness
Pre-existing psychopathology
Substance/alcohol abuse
Suicide history, family history
Fatigue, exhaustion
Lack of social support, social isolation

Cancer patients commit suicide most frequently in the advanced stages of disease.[128–131] Eighty-six per cent of suicides studied by Farberow et al.[132] occurred in the preterminal or terminal stages of illness, despite greatly reduced physical capacity. Poor prognosis and advanced illness usually go hand-in-hand. It is thus not surprising that in Sweden, those who were expected to die within a matter of months were the most likely to commit suicide. Of 88 cancer suicides, 14 had an uncertain prognosis, and 45 had a poor prognosis.[103] With advancing disease, the incidence of significant cancer pain increases. Uncontrolled pain in cancer patients is a dramatically important risk factor for suicide. The vast majority of cancer suicides in several studies showed that these patients had severe pain which was often inadequately controlled and poorly tolerated.[128,132]

Depression is a factor in 50 per cent of all suicides. Those suffering from depression are at 25 times greater risk of suicide than the general population.[133,134] The role depression plays in cancer suicide is equally significant. Approximately 25 per cent of all cancer patients experience severe depressive symptoms, with about 6 per cent fulfilling DSM-III criteria for the diagnosis of major depression.[45,49] Among those with advanced illness and progressively impaired physical function, symptoms of severe depression rise to 77 per cent.[7] Depression also appears to be important in terms of patient preferences for life-sustaining medical therapy. Ganzini et al. reported that among elderly depressed patients, an increase in desire for life-sustaining medical therapies followed treatment of depression in those subjects who had been initially more severely depressed, more hopeless, and more likely to overestimate the risks and to underestimate the benefits of treatment.[135] They concluded that while patients with mild to moderate depression are unlikely to alter their decisions regarding life-sustaining medical treatment in spite of treatment for their depression, severely depressed patients—particularly those who are hopeless—should be encouraged to defer advance treatment directives. In these patients, decisions about life-sustaining therapy should be discouraged until after treatment of their depression.

Hopelessness is the key variable that links depression and suicide in the general population. Further, hopelessness is a significantly better predictor of completed suicide than is depression alone.[136] In a recent study[137] Chochinov et al. demonstrated that hopelessness was correlated more highly with suicidal ideation in terminally ill cancer patients than was the level of depression. With the typical cancer suicide being characterized by advanced illness and poor prognosis, hopelessness is commonly experienced.

In Scandinavia, the highest incidence of suicide was found in cancer patients who were offered no further treatment, and no further contact with the health care system.[128,131] Being left to face illness alone creates a sense of isolation and abandonment that is critical to the development of hopelessness. The prevalence of organic mental disorders among cancer patients requiring psychiatric consultation has been found to range from 25 to 40 per cent,[2,138] reaching as high as 85 per cent during the terminal stages of illness.[9] While earlier work suggested that delirium was a protective factor in regard to cancer suicide,[129] clinical experience has found these confusional states to be a major contributing factor in impulsive suicide attempts, especially in the hospital setting.

Loss of control and a sense of helplessness in the face of cancer are important factors in suicide vulnerability. Control refers to both the helplessness induced by symptoms or deficits due to cancer or its treatments, as well as the excessive need on the part of some patients to be in control of all aspects of living or dying. Farberow et al. noted that patients who were accepting and adaptable were much less likely to commit suicide than cancer patients who exhibited a need to be in control of even the most minute details of their care.[132] This need to control may be prominent in some patients and cause distress with little provocation. However, it is not uncommon for cancer-related events to induce a great sense of helplessness even in those who are not typically controlling individuals. Impairments or deficits induced by cancer or cancer treatments include loss of mobility, paraplegia, loss of bowel and bladder functions, amputation, aphonia, sensory loss, and inability to eat or swallow. Most distressing to patients is the sense that they are losing control of their minds, especially when they are confused or sedated by medications. The risk of suicide is increased in cancer patients with such physical impairments, especially when accompanied by psychological distress and disturbed interpersonal relationships due to these deficit factors.[132]

Fatigue, in the form of emotional, spiritual, financial, familial, communal and other resource exhaustion increases risk of suicide in the cancer patient.[70] Cancer is now often a chronic illness. Increased survival is accompanied by increased numbers of hospitalizations, complications, and expenses. Symptom control thus becomes a prolonged process with frequent advances and setbacks. The dying process also can become extremely long and arduous for all concerned. It is not uncommon for both family members and health care providers to withdraw prematurely from the cancer patient under these circumstances. A suicidal patient can thus feel even more isolated and abandoned. The presence of a strong support system for the patient that may act as an external control of suicidal behaviour reduces risk of cancer suicide significantly.

Holland[139] advises that it is extremely rare for a cancer patient to commit suicide without some degree of premorbid psychopathology that places them at increased risk. Farberow et al.[129] described a large group of cancer suicides as the 'Dependent Dissatisfied'. These patients were immature, demanding, complaining, irritable, hostile, and difficult ward management problems. Staff often felt manipulated by these patients and became irritable due to what they saw as excessive demands for attention. Suicide attempts or threats were often seen as 'hysterical' or manipulative. Consultation data from Memorial Sloan-Kettering on suicidal cancer patients showed that half had a diagnosable personality disorder.[170]

The frequency of suicide attempts in cancer patients has not been well studied. While the frequency of suicidal thinking in the cancer setting may be in question, its relationship to suicide attempts or completions is clearer. Bolund[128] reports that half of all Swedish cancer suicides had previously conveyed suicidal thoughts or plans to their relatives. In addition, many of the completed cancer suicides had been preceded by an attempted suicide. This is consistent with the statistics of suicide in general, which show that a previous suicide attempt greatly increases the risk of completed suicide.[140–142] A family history of suicide is of increasing relevance in assessing suicide risk.

Suicidal ideation

Thoughts of suicide probably occur quite frequently, particularly in the setting of advanced cancer, and seem to act as a steam valve for feelings often expressed by patients as 'if it gets too bad, I always have a way out'. Once they develop a trusting and safe relationship, patients almost universally reveal occasional persistent thoughts of suicide as a means of escaping the threat of being overwhelmed by cancer. Recent published reports, however, suggest that suicidal ideation is relatively infrequent in cancer and is limited to those who are significantly depressed. Silberfarb et al.[143] found that only three of 146 breast cancer patients had suicidal thoughts, while none of the 100 cancer patients interviewed in a Finnish study expressed suicidal thoughts.[144] A study conducted at St Boniface Hospice in Winnipeg, Canada, demonstrated that only 10 of 44 terminally ill cancer patients were suicidal or desired an early death, and all 10 were suffering from clinical depression.[145]

At Memorial Hospital, suicide risk evaluation accounted for 8.6 per cent of psychiatric consultations, usually requested by staff in response to a patient verbalizing suicidal wishes.[70] Among 185 cancer patients with pain studied at Memorial Hospital, suicidal ideation was found in 17 per cent of the study population.[70] The actual prevalence of suicidal ideation may be considerably higher in that patients often disclose these thoughts only after a stable, ongoing physician–patient relationship has been established.

Assessment and management of the suicidal terminally ill patient

Assessment of suicide risk and appropriate intervention are critical. Early and comprehensive psychiatric involvement with high-risk individuals can often avert suicide in the cancer setting.[116] A careful evaluation includes a search for the meaning of suicidal thoughts as well as an exploration of the seriousness of the risk. The clinician's ability to establish rapport and elicit a patient's thoughts are essential as he or she assesses history, degree of intent, and quality of internal and external controls. One must listen sympathetically, not appearing critical or stating that such thoughts are inappropriate. Allowing the patient to discuss suicidal thoughts often decreases the risk of suicide. The myth that asking about suicidal thoughts 'puts the idea in their head', is one that should be dispelled, especially in cancer.[127] Patients often reconsider and reject the idea of suicide when the physician acknowledges the legitimacy of their option and the need to retain a sense of control over aspects of their death.

The suicide vulnerability factors (Table 5) should be utilized as a guide to evaluation and management. Once the setting has been made secure, assessment of the relevant mental status and adequacy of pain control can begin. Analgesics, neuroleptics, or antidepressant drugs should be utilized when appropriate to treat agitation, psychosis, major depression, or pain. Underlying causes of delirium or pain should be addressed specifically when possible. Initiation of a crisis-intervention-oriented psychotherapeutic approach, mobilizing as much of the patient's support system as possible is important. A close family member or friend should be involved in order to support the patient, provide information, and assist in treatment planning. Psychiatric hospitalization can sometimes be helpful but is usually not desirable in the terminally ill patient. Thus, the medical hospital or home is the setting in which management most often takes place. While it is appropriate to intervene when medical or psychiatric factors are clearly the driving force in a cancer suicide, there are circumstances when usurping control from the patient and family with overly aggressive intervention may be less helpful. This is most evident in those with advanced illness where comfort and symptom control are the primary concerns.

Ultimately the palliative care clinician may not be able to prevent all suicides in all terminally ill patients that he or she cares for. The emphasis of intervention should be to aggressively attempt to prevent suicide that is driven by the desperation of uncontrolled physical and psychological symptoms such as uncontrolled pain, unrecognized delirium, and unrecognized and untreated depression. Prolonged suffering caused by poorly controlled symptoms can lead to such desperation, and it is the appropriate role of the palliative care team to provide effective management of physical and psychological symptoms as an alternative to desire for death, suicide, or request for assisted suicide by patients.

Requests for assisted suicide

A growing body of literature has emerged on the type of physical and psychological concerns that may give rise to a desire for hastened death and request for assisted suicide. Even if relatively little empirical research has addressed this issue, especially with medically ill patients, some authors found rates of support for legalization of assisted-suicide that were roughly comparable to those published in studies on the general population. In a survey study done by Breitbart et al., 64 per cent of AIDS patients supported assisted-suicide legalization.[(146)] In another study 55 per cent of terminally ill AIDS patients indicated a possible interest in assisted suicide. In a 1996 study of oncology patients, 25 per cent of cancer patients reported that they had thought seriously about euthanasia and 12 per cent had discussed this option with their physicians.[(147)] A number of social variables, such as fear of becoming a burden to family and friends and experience with the death of a friend or family, have been significant predictors of interest in assisted suicide among ambulatory patients with AIDS.[(146)] This joins a growing evidence of research demonstrating an important relationship between social support and desire for death, when no relationship was found with pain, physical symptoms, or stage of disease.[(127)]

Desire for hastened death

Desire for hastened death may be thought of as a unifying construct underlying requests for assisted suicide or euthanasia, as well as suicidal thoughts in general. Literature has emerged on the type of physical and psychological concerns that may give rise to a desire for hastened death. Several studies have demonstrated that depression plays a significant role in the terminally ill patient's desire for hastened death. The precise intensity of this association between depression and desire for hastened death is still being investigated. Chochinov et al. found that of 200 terminally ill patients in a palliative care facility, 44.5 per cent acknowledged at least a fleeting desire to die—these episodes were brief and did not reflect a sustained or committed desire to die.[(148)] However, 17 patients (8.5 per cent) reported an unequivocal desire for death to come soon and indicated that they held this desire consistently over time. Among this group, 10 (58.8 per cent) received a diagnosis of depression, compared to a prevalence of 7.7 per cent in patients who did not endorse a genuine, consistent desire for death. Patients with depression were approximately six to seven times more likely to have a desire for hastened death than patients without depression. Patients with a desire for death were also found to have significantly more pain and less social support than those patients without a desire for death. Breitbart et al.[(50)] recently studied the relationships between depression, hopelessness, and desire for death in a sample of 92 terminally ill cancer patients. Sixteen patients (17 per cent) were classified as having a high desire for death, based on their scores on a validated self report measure of desire for hastened death called the Schedule of Attitudes Toward Hastened Death,[(149,150)] and 16 per cent met criteria for a current major depressive episode. Of the patients who met criteria for major depressive episode, seven (47 per cent) were classified as having a high desire for hastened death while only 12 per cent without a desire for death met criteria for depression. Thus, patients with a major depression were four times more likely to have a high desire for hastened death. In addition, Breitbart and his colleagues found that both depression and hopelessness, characterized as a pessimistic cognitive style rather than an assessment of one's poor prognosis, appear to be unique and synergistic determinants of desire for hastened death.[(46)] No significant association with the presence or the intensity of pain was found. Desire for hastened death also appears to be primarily a function of psychological distress and social factors such as social support, spiritual well being, quality of life and perception of oneself as a burden to others. Recent data suggest that among dying patients 'will to live', as measured with a visual analogue scale, tends to fluctuate rapidly over time and is correlated with anxiety, depression, and shortness of breath as death approaches.[(151)]

Interventions for desire for hastened death and despair at the end of life

The response of a clinician to despair at the end of life as manifest by a patient's expression of desire for death or request for assisted suicide has important and obvious implications on all aspects of care which impact on patients, family, and staff.[(152)] These issues must be addressed both rapidly and thoughtfully, offering the patient a non-judgmental willingness to engage in a discussion of the factors that contribute to the suffering and despondency that leads patients to express such a desire for death. Some investigators speak of this suffering in using such terms as 'spiritual' suffering, 'demoralization', loss of 'dignity', 'loss of meaning'[(125,153–156)] and have developed interventions based on these concepts/themes.

Palliative care practitioners have begun to deal with the issue of spirituality in the dying and interventions for spiritual suffering. Rousseau[(153)] outlines an approach for the treatment of spiritual suffering which is composed of the following steps: (i) controlling physical symptoms, (ii) providing a supportive presence, (iii) encouraging life review to assist in recognizing purpose value and meaning, (iv) exploring guilt, remorse, forgiveness, reconciliation, (v) facilitating religious expression, (vi) reframing goals, and (vii) encourage meditative practices, focus on healing rather than cure. Rousseau has presented an approach to spiritual suffering that is an interesting blend of basic psychotherapeutic principles.

Psychotherapeutic techniques that are particularly adaptive to psychotherapy with the dying, such as life narrative and life review, are also included. There is an emphasis on facilitating religious expression and confession that in fact may be extremely useful to many patients, but is not applicable to all patients and not necessarily an intervention that many clinicians feel comfortable providing. What Rousseau's work suggests is that novel psychotherapeutic interventions aimed at improving spiritual well being, sense of meaning, and diminishing hopelessness, demoralization, and distress are critically necessary to develop at this stage in the development of palliative medicine.

Kissane et al.[(154)] have described a syndrome of 'demoralization' in the terminally ill which they propose is distinct from depression, and consists of a triad of hopelessness, loss of meaning, and existential distress expressed as a desire for death. It is associated with life-threatening medical illness, disability, bodily disfigurement, fear, loss of dignity, social isolation, and feelings of being a burden. Because of the sense of impotence and hopelessness, those with the syndrome predictably progress to a desire to die or commit suicide. Kissane et al. describe a treatment approach for demoralization syndrome.[(154)] This approach emphasizes a multidisciplinary, multimodal approach consisting of: (i) ensuring continuity of care and active symptom management; (ii) ensuring dignity in the dying process; (iii) utilizing various types of psychotherapy to help sustain a sense of meaning, limit cognitive distortions, and maintain family relationships (i.e. meaning-based, cognitive-behavioral, interpersonal, and family psychotherapy interventions); (iv) use of life review and narrative, and attention to spiritual issues; and (v) pharmacotherapy for co-morbid anxiety, depression, and delirium.

Ensuring 'dignity' in the dying process is a critical goal of palliative care. Despite use of the term 'dignity' in arguments for and against a patient's self-governance in matters pertaining to death, there is little empirical research on how this term has been used by patients who are nearing death. Chochinov et al.[(155)] examined how dying patients understand and define the term 'dignity', in order to develop a model of dignity in the terminally ill (see Fig. 1). A semi-structured interview was designed to explore how patients cope with their advanced cancer and to detail their perceptions of dignity. Three major categories emerged from a detailed qualitative analysis, including illness-related concerns (concerns that derive from or are related to the illness itself, and threaten to or actually do impinge on the patient's sense of dignity); dignity conserving repertoire (internally held qualities or personal approaches or techniques that patients use to bolster or maintain their sense of dignity); and social dignity inventory (social concerns or relationship dynamics that enhance or detract from a patient's sense of dignity). These broad categories and their carefully defined themes and sub-themes form the foundation for an emerging model of dignity amongst the dying. The concept of dignity and the notion of dignity-conserving care offer a way of understanding how patients face advancing terminal illness, and presents an approach that clinicians can use to explicitly

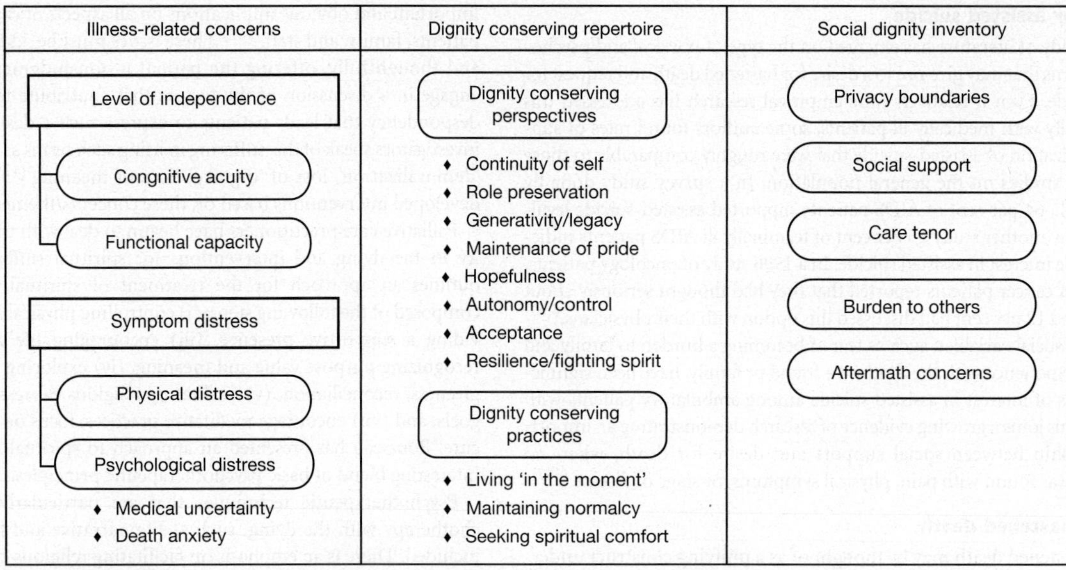

Fig. 1 Major dignity categories, themes, and sub-themes.

target the maintenance of dignity as a therapeutic objective, and principle of bedside care for patients nearing death. Chochinov, in fact, describes his technique of 'dignity conserving care' in a recent review[126] which interested readers can read for further details.

Interventions for hopelessness, loss of meaning and purpose in the terminally ill are of particular importance when addressing the issues of desire for death and despair at the end of life. Breitbart and colleagues[125,156] have developed an intervention they term 'meaning-centred' group psychotherapy for advanced cancer patients; an intervention based on the concepts and principles of Viktor Frankl's writings and logotherapy. The intervention is designed to help patients with advanced cancer sustain or enhance a sense of meaning, peace, and purpose in their lives even as they approach the end of life. Meaning-centred group psychotherapy is a manualized, 8-week (1.5 h weekly sessions) intervention which utilizes a mixture of didactics, discussion, and experiential exercises that focus around particular themes related to meaning and advanced cancer. The session themes include: Session 1—Concepts of Meaning and Sources of Meaning; Session 2—Cancer and Meaning; Session 3—Meaning and Historical Context of Life; Session 4—Storytelling, Life Project; Session 5—Limitations and Finiteness of Life; Session 6—Responsibility, Creativity, Deeds; Session 7—Experience, Nature, Art, Humor; Session 8—Termination, Goodbyes, Hopes for the Future. Patients are assigned readings and homework that are specific to each session's theme and which are utilized in each session. While the focus of each session is on issues of meaning/peace and purpose in life in the face of advanced cancer and a limited prognosis, elements of support and expression of emotion are inevitable in the context of each group session (but limited by the focus on experiential exercises, didactics and discussions related to themes focusing on meaning). Currently this intervention is undergoing a randomized controlled trial for efficacy.

Most palliative care clinicians believe that aggressive management of physical and psychological symptoms and syndromes that have been demonstrated to contribute to desire for death will naturally prevent such expressions of distress or requests for assisted suicide. For instance, there is a general consensus that individuals with a major depression can be effectively treated in the context of terminal illness. No research has yet addressed if such treatment for depression directly influences desire for hastened death. There are currently two large trials in cancer and AIDS populations examining this specific question.[50] Because depression and hopelessness are not identical constructs (although highly correlated) clinical interventions, such as those described above, developed to more specifically address hopelessness and related constructs such as dignity, loss of meaning, demoralization, and spiritual suffering or distress will be important to empirically test and utilize in general palliative care practice if they prove effective.

Cognitive disorders in the terminally ill

Cognitive failure is unfortunately all too common in patients with advanced illness. The Diagnostic and Statistical Manual of Mental Disorders, Fourth Edition (DSM-IV)[157] divides cognitive disorders into the sub-categories of: (i) delirium, dementia, amnesic, and other cognitive disorders; (ii) mental disorders due to a general medical condition (including mood disorder, anxiety disorder, and personality change due to a general medical condition); and (iii) substance-related disorders. While virtually all of these mental syndromes can be seen in the patient with advanced cancer, the most common include delirium, dementia, and mood and anxiety disorders due to a general medical condition. Lipowski[158] categorized organic mental disorders into those that were characterized by general cognitive impairment (i.e. delirium and dementia) and those where cognitive impairment was rather selective or limited (i.e. amnesic disorder, organic hallucinosis, and organic mood disorder). With organic mental disorders where cognitive impairment is selective, limited, or relatively intact, the more prominent symptoms tend to consist of either anxiety, mood disturbance, delusions, hallucinations, or personality change. For instance, the patient with mood disturbance meeting criteria for major depression, who is severely hypothyroid or on high-dose corticosteroids is most accurately diagnosed as having a mood disorder due to a general medical condition or substance-induced mood disorder, respectively (particularly if organic factors are judged to be the primary aetiology related to the mood disturbance). Similarly, the patient with hyponatremia, or the patient on acyclovir for CNS herpes who is experiencing visual hallucinations but has an intact sensorium with minimal cognitive deficits, is more accurately diagnosed as having a psychotic disorder due to a general medical condition or a substance-induced psychotic disorder, respectively.

In spite of very little being known about the neuropathogenesis of delirium, its symptoms suggest that it is a dysfunction of multiple regions of the brain.[159] Delirium has been characterized as an aetiologically

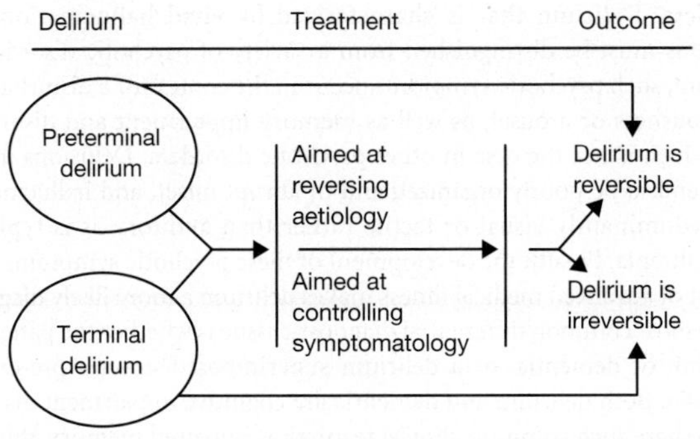

Fig. 2 Overview of delirium management.

non-specific, global, cerebral dysfunction characterized by concurrent disturbances of level of consciousness, attention, thinking, perception, memory, psychomotor behaviour, emotion, and the sleep–wake cycle. Disorientation, fluctuation, or waxing and waning of these symptoms, as well as acute or abrupt onset of such disturbances are other critical features of delirium. Delirium, in contrast with dementia, is conceptualized as a reversible process. Reversibility of the process of delirium (Fig. 2) is often possible even in the patient with advanced illness; however, it may not be reversible in the last 24–48 h of life. This is most likely due to the fact that irreversible processes such as multiple organ failure are occurring in the final hours of life. Delirium occurring in these last days of life is often referred to as terminal restlessness or terminal agitation in the palliative care literature.

At times it is difficult to differentiate delirium from dementia since they frequently share such common clinical features as impaired memory, thinking, judgment, and disorientation. Dementia appears in relatively alert individuals with little or no clouding of consciousness. The temporal onset of symptoms in dementia is more sub-acute or chronically progressive, and one's sleep–wake cycle seems less impaired. Most prominent in dementia are difficulties in short- and long-term memory, impaired judgment, and abstract thinking as well as disturbed higher cortical functions (such as aphasia and apraxia). Occasionally one will encounter delirium superimposed on an underlying dementia, such as in the case of an elderly patient, an AIDS patient, or a patient with a paraneoplastic syndrome. Clinically, we often utilize a number of scales or instruments that aid us in the diagnosis of delirium, dementia, or cognitive failure.

Delirium in the terminally ill: prevalence, diagnosis, assessment, and management

Prevalence of delirium

Delirium is the most common and serious neuropsychiatric complication in the patient with advanced illness. Cognitive disorders, and delirium in particular, have enormous relevance to symptom control and palliative care. Delirium is highly prevalent in cancer and in AIDS patients with advanced disease, particularly in the last weeks of life, with prevalence rates ranging from 25 to 85 per cent.[(9,160–166)] Delirium is one of the most common mental disorders encountered in general hospital practice. Knight and Folstein[(167)] estimated that 33 per cent of hospitalized medically ill patients have serious cognitive impairments. Massie et al. found delirium in 25 per cent of 334 hospitalized cancer patients seen in psychiatric consultation and in 85 per cent (11 of 13) of terminal cancer patients.[(9)] Pereira et al. found the prevalence of cognitive impairment in cancer inpatients to be 44 per cent, and just prior to death, the prevalence rose to 62.1 per cent.[(168)] Delirium also occurs in up to 51 per cent of post-operative patients.[(158,169)] The incidence of delirium is currently increasing, which reflects the growing numbers of elderly, who are particularly susceptible.[(158)] Studies of elderly patients admitted to medical wards estimate that between 30 and 50 per cent of patients 70 years or older showed symptoms of delirium at some point during hospitalization.[(170–174)] Elderly patients who develop delirium during a hospitalization have been estimated to have a 22–76 per cent chance of dying during that hospitalization.[(175)]

Delirium is associated with increased morbidity in the terminally ill, causing distress in patients, family members, and staff.[(161,176,177)] In a recent study of the 'delirium experience' of terminally ill cancer patients, Breitbart et al.[(176)] found that 54 per cent of patients recalled their delirium experience after recovery from delirium. Factors predicting delirium recall included the degree of short-term memory impairment, delirium severity, and the presence of perceptual disturbances (the more severe the less likely recall). Distress related to the episode of delirium was rated by patients, spouses/care givers, and nurses on a 0–4 numerical rating scale (with 4 being most severe). Patients averaged a rating of 3.2, spouses 3.75, and nurses a 3.2. The most significant factor predicting distress for patients was the presence of delusions. Patients with hypoactive delirium were just as distressed as patients with hyperactive delirium. Predictors of spouse distress included the patients' Karnofsky Performance Status (the lower the Karnofsky, the worse the spouse distress), and nurse distress included delirium severity and perceptual disturbances. Delirium can interfere dramatically with the recognition and control of other physical and psychological symptoms such as pain[(178–180)] in later stages of illness. Often a preterminal event, delirium is a sign of significant physiologic disturbance, usually involving multiple medical aetiologies, including infection, organ failure, medication side effects (including opioids), as well as extremely rare paraneoplastic syndromes.[(54,166,181–183)] Lawlor et al.[(184)] recently reported on their experience in the management of delirium in advanced cancer patients in a palliative care unit. While 42 per cent of patients had delirium upon admission to their palliative care unit, terminal delirium occurred in 88 per cent of the deaths. Unfortunately delirium is often under-recognized or misdiagnosed, and inappropriately treated or untreated in terminally ill patients. Impediments to progress in the recognition and treatment delirium have included confusion regarding terminology and lack of consistency in utilizing diagnostic classification systems. In addition, the signs and symptoms of delirium can be diverse and are sometimes mistaken for other psychiatric disorders such as mood or anxiety disorders. Practitioners caring for patients with life-threatening illnesses must be able to diagnose delirium accurately, undertake appropriate assessment of aetiologies, and be knowledgeable about the benefits and risks of the pharmacologic and non-pharmacologic interventions currently available in managing delirium among the terminally ill.

Diagnosing delirium

The clinical features of delirium are quite numerous and include a variety of neuropsychiatric symptoms that are also common to other psychiatric disorders such as depression, dementia, and psychosis.[(185)] Clinical features of delirium include prodromal symptoms (restlessness, anxiety, sleep disturbance, and irritability), rapidly fluctuating course, reduced attention (easily distractible), altered arousal, increased or decreased psychomotor activity, disturbance of sleep–wake cycle, affective symptoms (emotional lability, sadness, anger, and euphoria), altered perceptions (misperceptions, illusions, delusions—poorly formed—and hallucinations), disorganized thinking and incoherent speech, disorientation to time, place, or person, and memory impairment (cannot register new material). Neurologic abnormalities can also be present during delirium, including cortical abnormalities (dysgraphia, constructional apraxia, dysnomic aphasia), motor abnormalities (tremor, asterixis, myoclonus, and reflex and tone changes), and electroencephalogram abnormalities (usually global slowing). It is this protean nature of delirious symptoms, the variability and fluctuation of clinical findings, and the unclear and often contradictory definitions of the syndrome that have made delirium so difficult to diagnose and treat.

Table 6 lists the DSM-IV[(157)] criteria for delirium. The essential defining features of delirium, based on DSM-IV criteria, have shifted, from the extensive list of typical symptoms and abnormalities described above, to a focus on the two essential concepts of disordered attention (arousal) and cognition (while continuing to recognize the importance of acute onset and organic aetiology). Associated phenomena such as psychomotor behavioral changes, perceptual disturbances, hallucinations, or delusions are no longer viewed as essential to the diagnosis of delirium. Delirium is now conceptualized primarily as 'a disorder of arousal and cognition'[186] in contrast to dementia, which is a disorder of cognition (with no arousal disturbance). It is this disorder of the arousal system, with consequent disturbances in level of consciousness and attention, that is pathognomonic of delirium and is, in part, the basis for classifying delirium into several subtypes.

Sub-types of delirium

Three clinical sub-types of delirium, based on arousal disturbance and psychomotor behaviour, have been described. These sub-types included the 'hyperactive' (hyperarousal, hyperalert, or agitated) sub-type, the 'hypoactive' (hypoarousal, hypoalert, or lethargic) sub-type, and a 'mixed' sub-type with alternating features of hyperactive and hypoactive delirium.[186,187] Researchers[188] suggest that the hyperactive form is most often characterized by hallucinations, delusions, agitation, and disorientation, while the hypoactive form is characterized by confusion and sedation, but is rarely accompanied by hallucinations, delusions, or illusions. In addition, there is evidence suggesting that specific delirium sub-types may be related to specific aetiologies of delirium, may have unique pathophysiologies, and may have differential responses to treatment.[34,35] It is estimated that approximately two-thirds of deliria are either of the hypoactive or mixed sub-type, hence, the prototypically agitated delirious patient most familiar to clinicians is actually a minority of the deliria which occur.[187–189]

Differential diagnosis

Many of the clinical features and symptoms of delirium can be also be associated with other psychiatric disorders such as depression, mania, psychosis, and dementia. For instance, delirious patients, not uncommonly, may exhibit emotional (mood) disturbances such as anxiety, fear, depression, irritability, anger, euphoria, apathy, and mood lability. Delirium, particularly the 'hypoactive' sub-type, is often initially misdiagnosed as depression. Symptoms of major depression, including altered level of activity (hypoactivity), insomnia, reduced ability to concentrate, depressed mood, and even suicidal ideation, can overlap with symptoms of delirium making accurate diagnosis more difficult. In distinguishing delirium from depression, particularly in the context of advanced disease, an evaluation of the onset and temporal sequencing of depressive and cognitive symptoms is particularly helpful. Importantly, the degree of cognitive impairment in delirium is much more severe and pervasive than in depression, with a more abrupt temporal onset. Also, in delirium the characteristic disturbance in arousal or consciousness is present, while it is usually not a feature of depression. Similarly, a manic episode may share some features of delirium, particularly a 'hyperactive' or 'mixed' sub-type of delirium. Again, the temporal onset and course of symptoms, the presence of a disturbance of consciousness (arousal) as well as of cognition, and the identification of a presumed medical aetiology for delirium are helpful in differentiating these disorders. Delirium that is characterized by vivid hallucinations and delusions must be distinguished from a variety of psychotic disorders. In delirium, such psychotic symptoms occur in the context of a disturbance in consciousness or arousal, as well as memory impairment and disorientation, which is not the case in other psychotic disorders. Delusions in delirium tend to be poorly organized and of abrupt onset, and hallucinations are predominantly visual or tactile rather than auditory as is typical of schizophrenia. Finally, the development of these psychotic symptoms in the context of advanced medical illness makes delirium a more likely diagnosis.

The most common differential diagnostic issue is whether the patient has delirium, or dementia, or a delirium superimposed upon a pre-existing dementia. Both delirium and dementia are cognitive impairment disorders and so share such common clinical features as impaired memory, thinking, judgment, and disorientation. The patient with dementia is alert and does not have the disturbance of consciousness or arousal that is characteristic of delirium. The temporal onset of symptoms in dementia is more sub-acute and chronically progressive, and one's sleep–wake cycle seems less impaired. Most prominent in dementia are difficulties in short- and long-term memory, impaired judgment, and abstract thinking as well as disturbed higher cortical functions (such as aphasia and apraxia). Occasionally one will encounter delirium superimposed on an underlying dementia such as in the case of an elderly patient, an AIDS patient, or a patient with a paraneoplastic syndrome. Delirium, in contrast with dementia, is conceptualized as a reversible process. Reversibility of the process of delirium is often possible even in the patient with advanced illness; how-ever, it may not be reversible in the last 24–48 h of life. This is most likely due to the fact that irreversible processes such as multiple organ failure are occurring in the final hours of life. Delirium occurring in these last days of life is sometimes referred to as 'terminal delirium' in the palliative care literature.

Table 6 DSM-IV criteria for delirium

Delirium due to a general medical condition
1. Disturbance of consciousness (i.e. reduced clarity of awareness of the environment) with reduced ability to focus, sustain, or shift attention
2. Change in cognition (such as memory deficit, disorientation, language disturbance, or perceptual disturbance) that is not better accounted for by a pre-existing, established, or evolving dementia
3. The disturbance develops over a short period of time (usually hours to days) and tends to fluctuate during the course of the day
4. There is evidence from the history, physical examination, or laboratory findings of a general medical condition judged to be aetiologically related to the disturbance

Delirium screening/diagnostic scales

A number of scales or instruments have been developed which can aid the clinician in rapidly screening for cognitive impairment disorders (dementia or delirium) or in establishing a diagnosis of delirium[190–198] (see Table 7). Such scales have been described and their relative strengths and weaknesses reviewed elsewhere.[195,199] Perhaps most helpful to clinicians are the Mini-Mental State Examination (a cognitive impairment screening tool) and several delirium diagnostic/rating scales, including the Delirium Rating Scale, the Delirium Rating Scale—Revised 98, the Confusion Assessment Method, the Abbreviated Cognitive Test for Delirium, and the Memorial Delirium Assessment Scale. These tools are described briefly below.

Table 7 Assessment methods for delirium in cancer patients

Diagnostic classification systems
DSM-IV
ICD-9, ICD-10
Diagnostic interviews/instruments
Delirium Symptom Interview[190] (DSI)
Confusion Assessment Method[201] (CAM)
Delirium rating scales
Delirium Rating Scale[196] (DRS)
Delirium Rating Scale—Revised 98[200] (DRS-R-98)
Confusion Rating Scale[197] (CRS)
Saskatoon Delirium Checklist[195] (SDC)
Memorial Delirium Assessment Scale[191] (MDAS)
Abbreviated Cognitive Test for Delirium[202] (CTD)
Cognitive impairment screening instruments
Mini-Mental State Exam[192] (MMSE)
Short Portable Mental Status Questionnaire[198] (SPMSQ)
Cognitive Capacity Screening Examination[202] (CCSE)
Blessed Orientation Memory Concentration Test[194] (BOMC)

Mini-Mental State Examination

The Mini-Mental State Examination (MMSE)[197] is useful in screening for cognitive failure, but does not distinguish between delirium or dementia. The MMSE provides a quantitative assessment of the cognitive performance and capacity of a patient, and is a measure of severity of cognitive impairment. It is also most sensitive to cortical dementias such as Alzheimer's disease, and less sensitive in detecting sub-cortical deficits such as those found in AIDS dementia. The MMSE assesses five general cognitive areas, including orientation, registration, attention and calculation, recall and language. Although a score of 23 or less has generally been considered the cutoff score for cognitive impairment, a three-tiered system is now often utilized suggesting that a score of 24–30 indicates no impairment, 18–23: mild impairment, and 0–17: severe impairment.

Delirium Rating Scale

The Delirium Rating Scale (DRS), developed by Trzepacz et al.[196] is a 10-item clinician-rated symptom rating scale for diagnosing delirium. The scale is based on DSM-III-R diagnostic criteria for delirium and is designed to be used by the clinician to identify delirium, and distinguish it reliably from dementia, or other neuropsychiatric disorders. Each item is scored by choosing one best rating and carries a numerical weight chosen to distinguish the phenomenological characteristic of delirium. A score of 12 or greater is diagnostic of delirium.

Delirium Rating Scale—Revised 98

The Delirium Rating Scale—Revised 98 (DRS-R-98) is a revision of the DRS. The DRS-R-98 has 13 severity and three diagnostic items with descriptive anchors for each rating level. It includes more items than the DRS and was designed for phenomenological and treatment research, though it can be used clinically. The DRS-R-98 is a valid, sensitive, and reliable instrument for rating delirium severity. It has advantages over the original DRS for repeated measures and phenomenological studies due to its enhanced breadth of symptoms and separation into severity and diagnostic sub-scales.[200]

Confusion Assessment Method

The Confusion Assessment Method (CAM)[201] is a nine-item delirium diagnostic scale utilizing the DSM-III-R criteria for delirium, which can be administered rather quickly by a trained clinician. A unique and helpful feature of the CAM is that the CAM also can be given using a simplified diagnostic algorithm that includes only four items of the CAM, that is designed for rapid identification of delirium by non-psychiatrists. The four-item algorithm requires the presence of: acute onset and fluctuating course, inattention, and either disorganized thinking or altered level of consciousness.

Abbreviated Cognitive Test for Delirium

The Abbreviated Cognitive Test for Delirium[202] was recently developed as a tool to help identify delirium in patients in the intensive care unit setting who have limited ability to communicate verbally. This brief tool utilizes visualization span and recognition memory for pictures as two of nine content scores that produces a total score that reliably identifies delirium and can discriminate delirium from dementia, depression, and schizophrenia.

Memorial Delirium Assessment Scale

The Memorial Delirium Assessment Scale (MDAS) is a 10-item delirium assessment tool (see Table 8) validated among hospitalized inpatients with advanced cancer and AIDS.[191] The MDAS is both a good delirium diagnostic screening tool as well as a reliable tool for assessing delirium severity among patients with advanced disease. A cutoff score of 13 is diagnostic of delirium. The MDAS has advantages over other delirium tools in that it is both a diagnostic as well as a severity measure that is ideal for repeated assessments and for use in treatment intervention trials. Recently, Lawlor et al.[203] further examined the clinical utility and validation of the MDAS in a population of advanced cancer patients in a palliative care unit. These investigators found the MDAS to be useful in this population, and found that a cutoff score of 7 out of 30 yielded the highest sensitivity (98 per cent) and specificity (76 per cent) for a delirium diagnosis in this palliative care population.

Table 8 Items from the Memorial Delirium Assessment Scale (MDAS)

1.	Reduced level of consciousness (awareness)
2.	Disorientation
3.	Short-term memory impairment
4.	Impaired digit span
5.	Reduced ability to maintain and shift attention
6.	Disorganized thinking
7.	Perceptual disturbance
8.	Delusions
9.	Decreased or increased psychomotor
10.	Sleep-wake cycle disturbance (disorder of arousal)

Management of delirium in the terminally ill

The standard approach to the managing delirium in the medically ill, and even in those with advanced disease, includes a search for underlying causes, correction of those factors, and management of the symptoms of delirium.[37,50,51] The desired and often achievable outcome is a patient who is awake, alert, calm, cognitively intact, not psychotic, and communicating coherently with family and staff. In the terminally ill patient who develops delirium in the last days of life ('terminal' delirium), the management of delirium is in fact unique, presenting a number of dilemmas, and the desired clinical outcome may be significantly altered by the dying process.

Assessment of aetiologies of delirium

When confronted with a delirium in the terminally ill or dying patient, a differential diagnosis should always be formulated as to the likely aetiology(ies). There is an ongoing debate as to the appropriate extent of diagnostic evaluation that should be pursued in a dying patient with a terminal delirium.[204,207] Most palliative care clinicians would undertake diagnostic studies only when a clinically suspected aetiology can be identified easily, with minimal use of invasive procedures, and treated effectively with simple, interventions that carry minimal burden or risk of causing further distress. Diagnostic work-up in pursuit of an aetiology for delirium may be limited by either practical constraints such as the setting (home, hospice) or the focus on patient comfort, so that unpleasant or painful diagnostics may be avoided. Most often, however, the aetiology of terminal delirium is multifactorial or may not be determined. Bruera et al.[161] report that an aetiology is discovered in less than 50 per cent of terminally ill patients with delirium. When a distinct cause is found for delirium in the terminally ill, it is often irreversible or difficult to treat. Studies, however, in patients with earlier stages of advanced cancer have demonstrated the potential utility of a thorough diagnostic assessment.[161,179] When such diagnostic information is available, specific therapy may be able to reverse delirium. One study found that 68 per cent of delirious cancer patients could be improved, despite a 30-day mortality of 31 per cent.[162] Another found that one-third of the episodes of cognitive failure improved following evaluation that yielded a cause for these episodes in 43 per cent.[161]

In a recent prospective study of delirium in patients on a palliative care unit,[184] investigators reported that the aetiology of delirium was multifactorial in the great majority of cases. Even though delirium occurred in 88 per cent of dying patients in the last week of life, delirium was reversible in approximately 50 per cent of episodes. Causes of delirium that were most associated with reversibility included dehydration and psychoactive/opioid medications. Hypoxic and metabolic encephalopathy were less likely to be reversed in terminal delirium. The diagnostic work-up should include an assessment of potentially reversible causes of delirium. A full physical examination should assess for evidence of sepsis, dehydration, or major organic failure. Medications that could contribute to delirium should be reviewed. A screen of laboratory parameters will allow assessment of the possible role of metabolic abnormalities, such as hypercalcemia, and other problems, such as hypoxia or disseminated intravascular coagulation. Imaging studies of the brain and assessment of the cerebrospinal fluid may be appropriate in some instances.

Delirium can have multiple potential aetiologies (see Table 9). In patients with advanced cancer, for instance, delirium can be due either to the direct effects of cancer on the central nervous system (CNS), or to indirect CNS effects of the disease or treatments (medications, electrolyte imbalance, failure of a vital organ or system, infection, vascular complications, and pre-existing cognitive impairment or dementia).[161,184] Given the large numbers of drugs cancer patients require, and the fragile state of their physiologic functioning, even routinely ordered hypnotics are enough to tip patients over into a delirium. Narcotic analgesics such as levorphanol, morphine sulfate, and meperidine, are common causes of confusional states, particularly in the elderly and terminally ill. Chemotherapeutic agents known to cause delirium include methotrexate, fluorouracil, vincristine, vinblastine, bleomycin, BCNU, *cis*-platinum, asparaginase, procarbazine, and the glucocorticosteroids.[54–60,180] Except for steroids, most patients receiving these agents will not develop prominent CNS effects. The spectrum of mental disturbances related to steroids includes minor mood lability, affective disorders (mania or depression), cognitive impairment (reversible dementia), and delirium (steroid psychosis). The incidence of these disorders range from 3 to 57 per cent in non-cancer populations, and they occur most commonly on higher doses. Symptoms usually develop within the first 2 weeks on steroids, but in fact can occur at any time, on any dose, even during the tapering phase.[179] These disorders are often rapidly reversible upon dose reduction or discontinuation.[179]

Non-pharmacologic interventions

In addition to seeking out and potentially correcting underlying causes for delirium, symptomatic and supportive therapies are important.[162,163,177,206] In fact, in the dying patient they may be the only steps taken. Fluid and electrolyte balance, nutrition, vitamins, measures to help reduce anxiety and disorientation, interactions with and education of family members may be useful. Measures to help reduce anxiety and dis-orientation (i.e. structure and familiarity) may include a quiet, well-lit room with familiar objects, a visible clock or calendar, and the presence of family. Judicious use of physical restraints, along with one-to-one nursing observation may also be necessary and useful.

Recently, Inouye et al.[208] reported on a successful multicomponent intervention program to prevent delirium in hospitalized older patients. They focused on a set of risk factors that were highly predictive of delirium in the elderly which included: pre-existing cognitive impairment, visual impairment, hearing impairment, sleep deprivation, immobility, dehydration, and severe illness. Interventions directed at constant reorientation, correction of hearing and visual impairment, reversal of dehydration, and early mobilization appeared to significantly reduce the number and duration of episodes of delirium in hospitalized older patients. The applicability of these interventions and the likelihood that they would prevent delirium in the terminally ill, particularly in the last days of life, is likely minimal.

Table 9 Causes of delirium in patients with advanced disease

Direct central nervous system (CNS) causes
Primary brain tumour
Metastatic spread to CNS
Seizures
Indirect causes
Metabolic encephalopathy due to organ failure
Electrolyte imbalance
Treatment side effects from
chemotherapeutic agents
steroids
radiation
narcotics
anticholinergics
antiemetics
antivirals
Infection
Haematologic abnormalities
Nutritional deficiencies
Paraneoplastic syndromes

Pharmacologic interventions in delirium

Supportive techniques alone are often not effective in controlling the symptoms of delirium, and symptomatic treatment with neuroleptics or sedative medications are necessary (Table 10). Neuroleptic drugs (dopamine blocking drugs) such as haloperidol, are utilized frequently as antiemetics in the medical setting; however, only 0.5–2 per cent of hospitalized cancer patients, for instance, receive haloperidol for the management of the symptoms of delirium.[209,210] In terminally ill populations, as many as 17 per cent receive an antipsychotic for agitation or psychological distress, despite an estimated prevalence of delirium ranging from 25 per cent in the hospitalized cancer patient to 85 per cent in the terminally ill.[211,212]

Neuroleptics

Haloperidol, a neuroleptic drug that is a potent dopamine blocker, is often the drug of choice in the treatment of delirium in patients with advanced disease.[1,212–219] Haloperidol in low doses, 1–3 mg/day, is usually effective in targeting agitation, paranoia, and fear. Typically 0.5–1.0 mg haloperidol (PO, IV, IM, SC) is administered, with repeat doses every 45–60 min titrated against target symptoms.[204,220,221] An intravenous route can facilitate rapid onset of medication effects. If intravenous access is unavailable, one can start with intramuscular or sub-cutaneous administration and switch to the oral route when possible. The majority of delirious patients can be managed with oral haloperidol. Parenteral doses are approximately twice as potent as oral doses. Delivery of haloperidol by the sub-cutaneous route is utilized by many palliative care practitioners.[161,222] Low doses of neuroleptic medication is usually sufficient in treating delirium in elderly terminally ill patients. In general, doses need not exceed 20 mg of haloperidol in

Table 10 Medications in managing delirium in patients with advanced disease

Generic name	Approximate daily dosage range[a]	Route
Neuroleptics		
Haloperidol	0.5–5 mg every 2–12 h	PO, IV, SC, IM
Thioridazine	10–75 mg every 4–8 h	PO
Chlorpromazine	12.5–50 mg every 4–12 h	PO, IV, IM
Methotrimeprazine	12.5–50 mg every 4–8 h	IV, SC, PO
Molindone	10–50 mg every 8–12 h	PO
Droperidol	0.625 mg–2.5 mg every 4–8 h	IV, IM
Atypical neuroleptics		
Olanzapine	2.5–20 mg every 12–24 h	PO
Risperidone	1–3 mg every 12–24 h	PO
Quetiapine	25–200 mg every 12–24 h	PO
Benzodiazepines		
Lorazepam	0.5–2.0 mg every 1–4 h	PO, IV, IM
Midazolam	30–100 mg every 24 h	IV, SC
Anesthetics		
Propofol	10–70 mg every hour Upto 200–400 mg/h	IV

[a] Parenteral doses are generally twice as potent as oral doses; IV, intravenous infusions or bolus injections should be administered slowly; IM, intramuscular injections should be avoided if repeated use becomes necessary; PO, oral forms of medication are preferred; or SC, subcutaneous infusions are generally accepted modes of drug administration in the terminally ill.

a 24-h period; however, there are those that advocate high doses (upto 250 mg/24 h of haloperidol usually intravenously) in selected cases.(215)

A common strategy in the management of symptoms related to delirium is to add parenteral lorazepam to a regimen of haloperidol.(223,224) Lorazepam (0.5–1.0 mg Q 1–2 h PO or IV), along with haloperidol may be more effective in rapidly sedating the agitated delirious patient, and may help minimize extrapyramidal side effects associated with haloperidol.(224) An alternative strategy is to switch from haloperidol to a more sedating neuroleptic such as chlorpromazine (see Fig. 3). In a double-blind, randomized comparison trial of haloperidol, chlorpromazine, and lorazepam, Breitbart et al. demonstrated that lorazepam alone, in doses up to 8 mg in a 12-h period, was ineffective in the treatment of delirium and in fact contributed to worsening delirium and cognitive impairment.(160) Both neuroleptic drugs, however, in low doses (approximately 2 mg of haloperidol equivalent/24 h), were highly effective in controlling the symptoms of delirium (dramatic improvement in DRS scores) and improving cognitive function (dramatic improvement in MMSE scores). In addition, both haloperidol and chlorpromazine were demonstrated to significantly improve the symptoms of delirium in both the 'hypoactive' as well as the 'hyperactive' subtypes of delirium.(160) Methotrimeprazine, a phenothiazine neuroleptic with properties similar to chlorpromazine, is often utilized parenterally (intravenously or by subcutaneous infusion) to control confusion and agitation in terminal delirium.(225) Dosages range from 12.5 to 50 mg every 4–8 h up to 300 mg/24 h for most patients, including the elderly where doses at the lower end of the range are preferable. Hypotension and excessive sedation are potential limitations of this drug; however, methotrimeprazine has the advantage of also being an analgesic, equipment to morphine, through non-opioid mechanisms.(225)

Atypical neuroleptics

Several new, atypical, antipsychotic agents with less or more specific dopamine blocking effects (less risk of extrapyramidal side effects or tardive dyskinesia) are now available and include such agents as clozaril, risperidone, and olanzapine.(226–230) Risperidone has been useful in the treatment of dementia and psychosis in AIDS patients at doses of 1–6 mg/day, suggesting safe use in patients with delirium.(229) There are a limited number of published studies of the use of these agents in the treatment of delirium.(227–230) Breitbart et al.(230) recently published a large ($n = 82$) open trial of olanzapine for the treatment of delirium in hospitalized patients with advanced cancer. Olanzapine was highly effective in the treatment of delirium, resolving delirium in 76 per cent of patients, with no incidence of extrapyramidal side effects. Several factors were found to be significantly associated with poorer response to olanzapine treatment for delirium, including age over 70, history of dementia, and hypoactive delirium. The average starting dose was in the 2.5–5 mg range and patients were given up to 20 mg/day of olanzapine. Sedation was the most common side effect. Many palliative care clinicians are using risperidone in low doses (e.g. 0.5–1.0 mg twice a day, orally) as well as olanzapine (2.5–20 mg/day in divided doses) in the management of delirium in terminally ill patients, particularly in those who have a demonstrated intolerance to the extrapyramidal side effects of the classic neuroleptics.(231) Currently, a limitation on the use of these new agents is the lack of availability of these agents in parenteral formulations. Figure 3 illustrates an algorithm that has been developed for use by the Memorial Sloan-Kettering Cancer Center Psychiatry Service, for the management of delirium in hospitalized cancer patients.

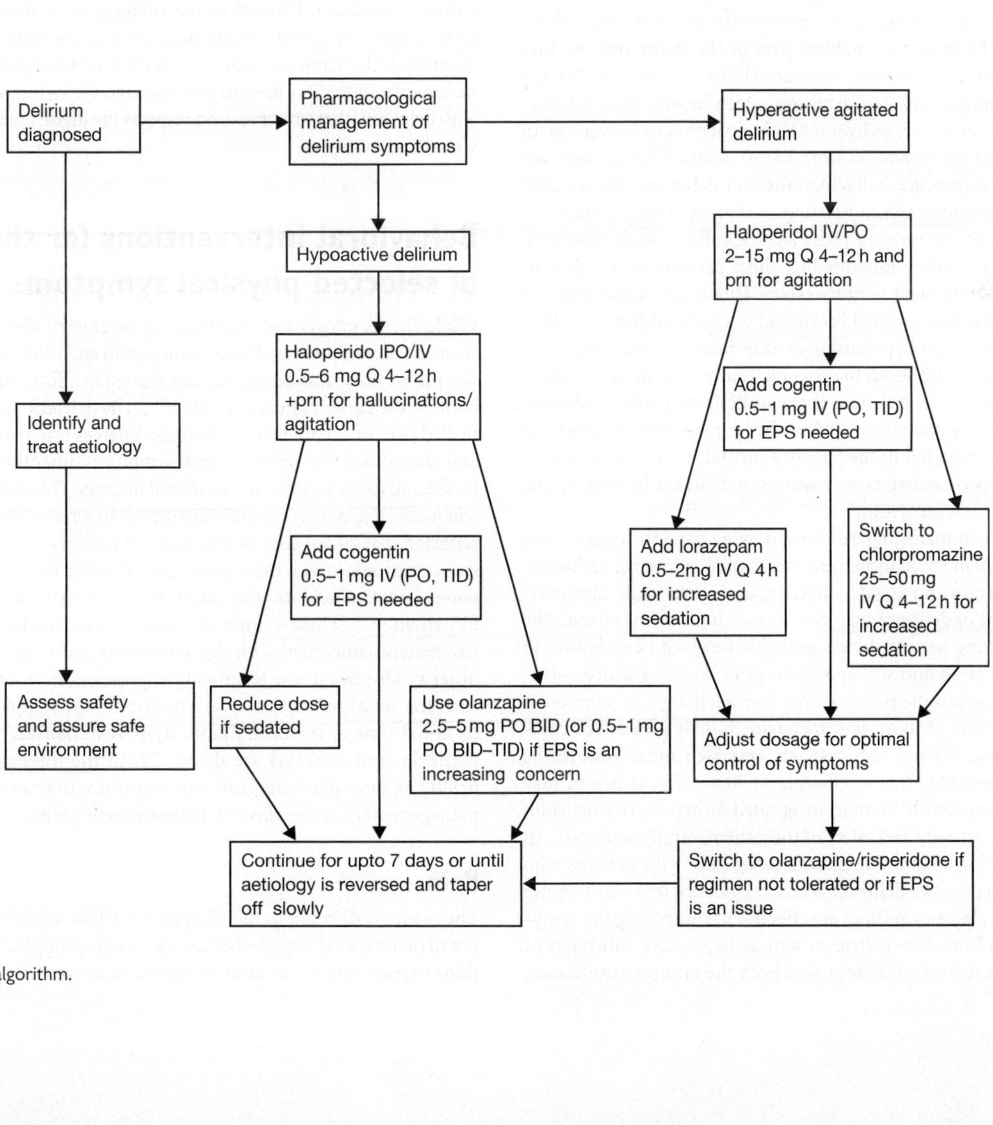

Fig. 3 The delirium algorithm.

While neuroleptic drugs such as haloperidol are most effective in diminishing agitation, clearing the sensorium, and improving cognition in the delirious patient, this is not always possible in delirium which complicates the last days of life. Processes causing delirium may be ongoing and irreversible during the active dying phase. Ventafridda et al.[232] and Fainsinger et al.[180] have reported that a significant group (10–20 per cent) of terminally ill patients experience delirium that can only be controlled by sedation to the point of a significantly decreased level of consciousness. Lawlor et al.[184] report that at least 50 per cent of terminal delirium is reversible. The goal of treatment with such agents as midazolam, propofol, and to some extent methotrimeprazine, is quiet sedation only. Midazolam, given by subcutaneous or intravenous infusion in doses ranging from 30 to 100 mg/24 h can be used to control agitation related to delirium in the terminal stages.[29,30] Propofol, a short-acting anaesthetic agent, has also begun to be utilized primarily as a sedating agent for the control of agitated patients with 'terminal' delirium. In several case reports of propofol's use in terminal care, an intravenous loading dose of 20 mg of propofol was followed by a continuous infusion of propofol with initial doses ranging from 10 to 70 mg/h, and with titration of doses up to as high as 400 mg/h over a period of hours to days in severely agitated patients.[233,234] Propofol has an advantage over midazolam in that the level of sedation is more easily controlled and recovery is rapid upon decreasing the rate of infusion.[233]

Controversies in the management of terminal delirium

Several aspects of the use of neuroleptics and other pharmacologic agents in the management of delirium in the dying patient remain controversial in some circles. Some have argued that pharmacologic interventions with neuroleptics or benzodiazepines are inappropriate in the dying patient. Delirium is viewed by some as a natural part of the dying process that should not be altered. In particular, there are clinicians who care for the dying who view hallucinations and delusions which involve dead relatives communicating with or in fact welcoming dying patients to heaven, as an important element in the transition from life to death. Clearly, there are many patients who experience hallucinations and delusions during delirium that are pleasant and in fact comforting, and many clinicians question the appropriateness of intervening pharmacologically in such instances. Another concern that is often raised is that these patients are so close to death that aggressive treatment is unnecessary. Parenteral neuroleptics or sedatives may be mistakenly avoided because of exaggerated fears that they might hasten death through hypotension or respiratory depression. Many are unnecessarily pessimistic about the possible results of neuroleptic treatment for delirium. They argue that since the underlying pathophysiologic process often continues unabated (such as hepatic or renal failure), no improvement can be expected in the patient's mental status. There is concern that neuroleptics or sedatives may worsen a delirium by making the patient more confused or sedated.

Clinical experience in managing delirium in dying patients suggests that the use of neuroleptics in the management of agitation, paranoia, hallucinations, and altered sensorium is safe, effective, and often quite appropriate.[223] Management of delirium on a case by case basis seems wisest. The agitated, delirious dying patient should probably be given neuroleptics to help restore calm. A 'wait and see' approach, prior to using neuroleptics, may be appropriate with some patients who have a lethargic or somnolent presentation of delirium, or those who are having frankly pleasant or comforting hallucinations. Such a 'wait and see' approach must however be tempered by the knowledge that a lethargic or hypoactive delirium may very quickly and unexpectedly become an agitated or hyperactive delirium that can threaten the serenity and safety of the patient, family, and staff. An additional rationale for intervening pharmacologically with patients who have a lethargic or hypoactive delirium is recent evidence that neuroleptics (i.e. haloperidol and chlorpromazine) are effective in controlling the symptoms of delirium in both hyperactive as well as hypoactive sub-types of delirium.[160] In fact neuroleptics improved both the arousal disturbance, as well as cognitive functioning in patients with hypoactive delirium. Also, some clinicians suggest that hypoactive delirium may respond to psychostimulants or combinations of neuroleptics and stimulants.[235,236] Similarly, hallucinations and delusions during a delirium that are pleasant and comforting can quickly become menacing and terrifying. It is important to remember that by nature, the symptoms of delirium are unstable, and fluctuate over time.

Finally, perhaps the most challenging of clinical problems is management of the dying patient with a 'terminal' delirium that is unresponsive to standard neuroleptic interventions, whose symptoms can only be controlled by sedation to the point of a significantly decreased level of consciousness. Before undertaking interventions such as midazolam or propofol infusions, where the best achievable goal is a calm, comfortable, but sedated and unresponsive patient, the clinician must first take several steps. The clinician must have a discussion with the family (and the patient if there are lucid moments when the patient appears to have capacity) eliciting their concerns and wishes for the type of care that can best honour their desire to provide comfort and symptom control during the dying process. The clinician should describe the optimal achievable goals of therapy as they currently exist. Family members should be informed that the goal of sedation is to provide comfort and symptom control, and not to hasten death. They should also be told to anticipate that sedation may result in a premature sense of loss, and that they may feel their loved one is in some sort of limbo state, not yet dead, but yet no longer alive in the vital sense. The distress and confusion that family members can experience during such a period can be ameliorated by including the family in the decision-making and emphasizing the shared goals of care. Sedation in such patients is not always complete or irreversible; some patients have periods of wakefulness despite sedation, and many clinicians will periodically lighten sedation to reassess the patient's condition. Ultimately, the clinician must always keep in mind the goals of care and communicate these goals to the staff, patients, and family members. The clinician must weigh each of the issues outlined above in making decisions, on how to best manage the dying patient who presents with delirium, that preserves and respects the dignity and values of that individual and family.

Behavioral interventions for the control of selected physical symptoms

While the diagnosis and treatment of psychiatric disorders in the patient with advanced illness is of importance, pain and other troublesome physical symptoms must also be aggressively treated in efforts aimed at the enhancement of the patient's quality of life.[237] The deleterious influence of uncontrolled pain on a patient's psychological state is often intuitively understood and recognized. However, physical symptoms other than pain can go undetected and cause significant emotional distress. This distress often dissipates when effective management is instituted. In a recent study, Coyle et al.[238] reported that 70 per cent of terminally ill patients have three or more physical symptoms other than pain. This finding replicates those of earlier papers that elucidate the multiple problems facing the terminally ill patient.[239] These symptoms must be assessed by the psychologist or psychiatrist concerned with the assessment and treatment of affective and other syndromes in the terminally ill population. In other chapters of this text, the management of a variety of physical symptoms experienced in terminal illness, including pain, dyspnoea, nausea, vomiting, asthenia, cachexia, and anorexia are discussed. In the following section, we will briefly review psychological interventions that may be useful in the management of some selected distressing symptoms.

Pain

The reader is directed to the Chapter 8.2.10 for a detailed discussion of the use of behavioural, psychotherapeutic, and psychopharmacologic interventions in pain control. In brief, behavioural interventions are effective in the management of acute procedures-related cancer pain, and as an adjunct in the management of chronic cancer pain.[240,241] Hypnosis, biofeedback, and multicomponent cognitive behavioural interventions have been used to provide comfort and minimize pain in adults, children, and adolescents undergoing bone marrow aspirations, spinal taps, and other painful procedures.[242–244] Typically, behavioural interventions utilized in the management of acute procedure-related pain employ the basic elements of relaxation and distraction or diversion of attention. In chronic cancer pain, cognitive-behavioural techniques are most effective when they are employed as part of a multimodal, multidisciplinary approach.[221] Adequate medical assessment and management of cancer pain is essential. Mild to moderate levels of residual pain can be effectively managed with behavioural techniques that are quite similar to those used for anxiety, phobias, and anticipatory nausea and vomiting. Relaxation techniques are utilized to help the patient achieve a relaxed state. Once in a relaxed state, the cancer patient with pain can use a variety of imagery techniques, including pleasant distracting imagery, transformational imagery, and dissociative imagery.[221] Transformational imagery involves the imaginative transformation of either the painful sensation itself, or the context of pain, or both. Patients can imaginatively transform a sensation of pain in their arm, for instance, into a sensation of warmth or cold. They can use such imagery as 'dipping their arm into a bucket of cold spring water', or 'into a vat of warm honey'. Such techniques can also be used to alter the context of the pain. Dissociative imagery or dissociated somatization refers to the use of one's imagination to disconnect or dissociate from the pain experience. Specifically, patients can sometimes imagine that they leave their pain racked body in bed and walk about for 5–10 min pain free. Patients can also imagine that a particularly painful part of their body becomes disconnected or dissociated from the rest of them, resulting in a period of freedom from pain. These techniques can provide much needed respite from pain. Even short periods of relief from pain can break the vicious pain cycle that entraps many cancer patients.

Anorexia and weight loss (see Sub-section 8.4)

Cancer patients and their families find weight loss demoralizing, perplexing, and distressing. Weight loss and anorexia in the terminally ill patient are complex problems that can arise from a number of sources. While most often a variety of medical factors account for the anorexia and cachexia associated with terminal illness, psychological and psychiatric factors may also play a role in the aetiology of anorexia and weight loss. Among the most frequent of such causes are anxiety, depression, and conditioned food aversions.[245]

The treatment of anorexia and weight loss begins with the identification and correction of its reversible causes. For example, when uncontrolled opioid-induced nausea is identified as a key factor in a patient's inability to eat, adding an antiemetic may completely control the subsequent anorexia. Once specific causes have been ruled out or corrected, subsequent treatment relies upon environmental manipulations.[239] Frequent administration of favourite foods, nutritional supplements, and fluids can reverse weight loss.

When poor appetite is a symptom of underlying major depression or significant anxiety, psychopharmacologic interventions with antidepressants and anxiolytics are indicated. Conditioned nausea and vomiting is often quite responsive to relaxation training and other behavioural techniques.[246] These interventions can be employed even by patients with advanced disease if their sensorium is clear and they are capable of concentrating.

Behavioural interventions are commonly used to treat a variety of eating disorders in cancer patients, including conditioned anorexia, swallowing difficulties, and nausea and vomiting. Dixon[247] reported on a study of 55 nutritionally at-risk cancer patients who were randomized to four intervention groups. One group received nutritional support alone, the other received relaxation training only, a third group received both supplementation and relaxation, and the fourth group was a no intervention control. Weight gain was greatest for the relaxation groups who were taught deep abdominal breathing, autosuggestion, progressive relaxation, and imagery. Campbell et al.[248] showed that a relaxation and imagery exercise program was associated with weight gain and improvement in performance status. Conditioned difficulties with eating, swallowing, and nausea have been managed successfully with systematic desensitization.[249,250] Hypnosis has been utilized in children with cancer[251] resulting in improved appetite and weight gain.

Asthenia/fatigue

Asthenia or fatigue is defined as generalized weakness, and physical or mental fatigue. Studies suggest that as many as two-thirds of advanced cancer patients complain of fatigue. Unfortunately, a treatable cause of asthenia will be identified and corrected in only a minority of cases. The role of psychiatric factors in the presentation of asthenia in the dying cancer patient is small in comparison to that of physical factors. However, psychiatric factors are probably enlisted too often by frustrated house staff who have seen a number of treatments fail, and then view the patient's continuing malaise as a sign of depression. More likely the cause of asthenia arises from some of the following aetiologies: malnutrition, infection, profound anaemia, metabolic abnormalities, and reactions to medication. Chemotherapeutic agents and radiotherapy are frequently employed as palliative therapies in patients with advanced cancer. Both can cause significant weakness that may resolve after treatment is completed.

The psychological and psychiatric treatment of patients with fatigue includes patient and family education (especially to address the non-psychological nature of the problem in many cases). An ongoing supportive relationship which permits the patient to express fears and concerns about the meaning of continued weakness and to address distorted ideas that they may have about its prognostic significance is critically important.[252] Some patients who suffer with temporary fatigue from chemotherapy or radiotherapy feel that their weakness is a sign of imminent death. The literature in support of the pharmacotherapy of fatigue in cancer patients is largely anecdotal. Some patients respond to steroids (methylprednisone, 15–30 mg daily) with improvement in mood, appetite, and physical well being. Unfortunately, this response tends to be fleeting. Also problematic is the fact that prolonged use of steroids can exacerbate weakness by causing proximal myopathy. Steroids have several other potentially distressing adverse effects including severe psychiatric syndromes such as organic mood syndromes and delirium. Psychostimulants have been used in the treatment of asthenia with good results.[253] In a randomized, double-blind, placebo-controlled trial, Breitbart et al.[235] demonstrated that the psychostimulants methylphenidate and pemoline were superior to placebo and provided clinically significant improvement in fatigue amongst a sample of ambulatory AIDS patients. The average dose of methylphenidate was approximately 50 mg/day and 100 mg/day for pemoline; minimal side effects and weight gain was noted with the stimulant drugs. Selected patients do respond well to amphetamine, methylphenidate, or pemoline, and it is thus appropriate to use stimulants not only for depressive syndromes but also for the asthenia/weakness syndrome. Despite the appetite suppressing effects of amphetamine-like drugs, stimulants often improve energy and appetite in fatigued terminally ill patients.

Nausea and vomiting

Approximately 50 per cent of patients with advanced cancer experience nausea and vomiting during the course of their illness.[239,254] Common causes of nausea and vomiting in cancer patients include radiation, medications, toxins, metabolic derangements, obstruction of the gastrointestinal tract, and chemotherapy. During the course of chemotherapy, many patients become sensitized to the treatment, develop phobic-like reactions, and even develop conditioned responses to stimuli in the hospital setting. As a result of being conditioned by the experience of profound nausea and vomiting secondary to highly emetic chemotherapy agents, patients report being nauseated in anticipation of treatment. A conservative estimate of the prevalence of anticipatory nausea and vomiting (ANV) is at least 33 per cent.[255] The factors that increase the likelihood of developing ANV are as follows: (i) severity of post-treatment nausea and vomiting (high density, duration, and frequency); (ii) a pattern of increasing nausea and vomiting; and (iii) receiving highly emetic drugs (*cis*-platinum) or combinations of chemotherapies.[256]

Given the relationship between intensity of post-chemotherapy nausea and vomiting and the development of ANV, the efficacy of antiemetic regimens in the management of these symptoms becomes increasingly important. Antiemetic drugs are the mainstay of managing chemotherapy-induced nausea and vomiting in patients with advanced disease. Several antiemetic drugs have dopamine blocking properties and so can cause a variety of extrapyramidal side effects. Akathisia is a common extrapyramidal symptom experienced by the patient as an intense inner sense of restlessness, often accompanied by outward manifestations of agitation. This is often confused with anxiety related to illness by physicians and nurses. Patients can often differentiate feelings of anxiety and nervousness from a sense of motor restlessness. Additionally, akathisia is often accompanied by other extrapyramidal symptoms such as mild tremor or cogwheel rigidity. Treatment of akathisia secondary to antiemetics may involve lowering the dose of the antiemetic, switching to a non-dopamine blocking agent such as ondansetron, or the addition of a benzodiazepine or an anticholinergic agent.

Rapid onset, short-acting benzodiazepines are helpful in controlling ANV once it has developed. Alprazolam has been shown to be clinically effective in reducing ANV in doses of 0.25–0.5 mg TID to QID, given for 1–2 days prior to chemotherapy.[257] Behavioural control of anticipatory nausea and vomiting has proven to be highly effective.[254] The techniques that have been studied include relaxation training with guided imagery, video game distraction (in children), and systematic desensitization. It is unclear whether muscular relaxation or cognitive-attentional distraction is the key element in the efficacy of some of these techniques. Chemotherapy nurses trained in these techniques can remarkably improve the quality of life in chemotherapy patients.

Insomnia (see Chapter 8.16)

Behavioral interventions have been successfully applied to the treatment of insomnia in cancer patients. Cannici et al.[258] studied 15 patients suffering from secondary insomnia due to cancer, and showed a marked reduction in mean sleep onset latency after progressive muscle relaxation training. Stam and Bultz[259] showed an increase in duration of sleep utilizing relaxation and imagery techniques. Such techniques are useful non-pharmacologic interventions that help keep medication use to a minimum. Occasionally sleep disturbance in cancer patients may be due to a concomitant psychiatric disorder such as depression or delirium. Obviously in these cases specific treatment for the underlying disorder is a preferred approach. Pharmacotherapy utilizing benzodiazepines, neuroleptics, or antidepressants may also be indicated when sleep disturbance is due to medication side effects or some other organic aetiology.

Conclusion

As the possibility of cure or prolongation of life becomes remote in the care of the patient with advanced cancer or AIDS, the focus of treatment shifts to symptom control and enhancement of quality of life. Such patients are uniquely vulnerable to both physical and psychiatric complications. The high prevalence of distressing physical symptoms, such as pain, make the assessment of psychiatric symptoms difficult. It is critical that physicians and nurses working in the palliative care setting recognize the unique knowledge and skills of psychiatrists and psychologists and the contributions they can make to the care of the terminally ill patient. The role of the psychiatrist, or other mental health professional, in the care of the terminally ill or dying patient is critical to both adequate symptom control and integration of the physical, psychological, and spiritual dimensions of human experience in the last weeks of life. To be most effective in this role, the psychiatrist must not only have specialized knowledge of the psychiatric complications of terminal illness and the existential issues confronted those at the end of life, but also must be familiar with the common physical symptoms that plague the patient with advanced disease and contribute so dramatically to suffering.

References

1. **Chochinov, H.M.C. and Breitbart, W.**, ed. *Handbook of Psychiatry in Palliative Medicine*. New York: Oxford University Press, 2000.
2. **Derogatis, L.R. et al.** (1983). The prevalence of psychiatric disorders among cancer patients. *Journal of the American Medical Association* **249**, 751–7.
3. **Breitbart, W. et al.** (1995). Neuropsychiatric syndromes and psychological symptoms in patients with advanced cancer. *Journal of Pain and Symptom Management* **10**, 131–41.
4. **Minagawa, H. et al.** (1996). Psychiatric morbidity in terminally ill cancer patients. *Cancer* **78**, 1131–7.
5. **Foley, K.M.** (1985). The treatment of cancer pain. *New England Journal of Medicine* **313**, 84–95.
6. **Chochinov, H.M.C.** (2000). Psychiatry and the terminally ill. *Canadian Journal of Psychiatry* **45**, 143–50.
7. **Breitbart, W., Jaramillo, J.R., and Chochinov, H.M.C.** (1998). Palliative and terminal care. In *Psycho-Oncology* (ed. J.C. Holland et al.), pp. 437–49. New York: Oxford University Press.
8. **Bukberg, J., Penman, D., and Holland, J.** (1984). Depression in hospitalized cancer patients. *Psychosomatic Medicine* **43**, 199–212.
9. **Massie, M.J., Holland, J.C., and Glass, E.** (1983). Delirium in terminally ill cancer patients. *American Journal of Psychiatry* **140**, 1048–50.
10. **Lawlor, P.G. et al.** (2000). Occurrence, causes and outcomes of delirium in patients with advanced cancer. *Archives of Internal Medicine* **160**, 786–94.
11. **Ahles, T.A., Blanchard, E.B., and Ruckdeschel, J.C.** (1983). The multi-dimensional nature of cancer related pain. *Pain* **17**, 277–88.
12. **Woodforde, J.M. and Fielding, J.R.** (1970). Pain and cancer. *Journal of Psychosomatic Research* **14**, 365–70.
13. **Tross, S. and Hirsch, D.A.** (1988). Psychological distress and neuropsychological complications of HIV infection and AIDS. *American Psychologist* **43**, 929–34.
14. **Atkinson, J.H., Grant, I., and Kennedy, C.J.** (1988). Prevalence of psychiatric disorders among men infected with human immunodeficiency virus. *Archives of General Psychiatry* **45**, 859–64.
15. **Karina, K. et al.** (1994). Psychiatric comorbidity and length of stay in hospitalized AIDS patients. *American Journal of Psychiatry* **151**, 1475–8.
16. **Barbuto, J., Fleishman, S., and Holland, J.** (1987). *Prevalence of Psychiatric Disorders in AIDS Patients. Current Concepts in Psycho-Oncology and AIDS.* Memorial Sloan-Kettering Cancer Center, 17–19 September.
17. **Perry, J.S.W. and Tross, S.** (1984). Psychiatric problems of AIDS inpatients at the New York Hospital: a preliminary report. *Public Health Reports* **99**, 200–5.
18. **Perry, S.W.** (1990). Organic mental disorders caused by HIV: update on early diagnosis and treatment. *American Journal of Psychiatry* **147**, 696–710.
19. **Rabkin, J. et al.** (1997). Prevalence of axis I disorders in an AIDS cohort: a cross-sectional, controlled study. *Comprehensive Psychiatry* **38**, 146–54.
20. **Vogl, D. et al.** (1999). Symptom prevalence, characteristics, and distress in AIDS outpatients. *Journal of Pain and Symptom Management* **18**, 253–62.
21. **Holland, J.C.** (1989). Anxiety and cancer: the patient and family. *Journal of Clinical Psychiatry* **50**, 20–5.
22. **Massie, M.J. and Payne, D.K.** (2000). Anxiety in palliative care. In *Handbook of Psychiatry in Palliative Medicine* (ed. H.M.C. Chochinov and W. Breitbart), pp. 63–74. New York: Oxford University Press.
23. **Brandenberg, Y., Bolund, C., and Sigurdardotti, V.** (1992). Anxiety and depressive symptoms at different stages of malignant melanoma. *Psycho-oncology* **1**, 71–8.
24. **Whitcup, S.M. and Miller, F.** (1987). Unrecognized drug dependence in psychiatrically hospitalized elderly patients. *Journal of American Geriatric Society* **35**, 297–301.
25. **Strain, J.J., Liebowitz, M.R., and Klein, D.F.** (1981). Anxiety and panic attacks in the medically ill. *Psychiatry Clinics of North America* **4**, 333–48.

26. **Wald, T.** et al. *Rapid Relief of Anxiety in Cancer Patients with Both Alprazolam and Placebo* Vol. 34.4. Washington DC: American Psychiatric Press, 1994–1995.
27. **Hollister, L.E.** (1986). Pharmacotherapeutic considerations in anxiety disorders. *Journal of Clinical Psychiatry* **47**, 33–6.
28. **Twycross, R.G. and Lack, S.A.** (1984). *Therapeutics in Terminal Disease.* London: Pitman, pp. 99–103.
29. **Bottomley, D.M. and Hanks, G.W.** (1990). Subcutaneous midazolam infusion in palliative care. *Journal of Pain and Symptom Management* **5**, 259–61.
30. **Mendoza, R.** et al. (1987). Midazolam in acute psychotic patients with hyperarousal. *Journal of Clinical Psychiatry* **48**, 291–3.
31. **De Sousa, E. and Jepson, A.** (1988). Midazolam in terminal care. *Lancet* **1**, 67–8.
32. **Chouinard, G., Young, S.N., and Annable, L.** (1983). Antimanic effect of clonazepam. *Biological Psychiatry* **18**, 451–66.
33. **Keck, P., McElroy, S., and Nemeroff, C.** (1992). Anticonvulsants in the treatment of bipolar disorder. *The Journal of Neuropsychiatry and Clinical Neurosciences* **4**, 395–405.
34. **Walsh, T.D.** (1990). Adjuvant analgesic therapy in cancer pain. In *Advances in Pain Research and Therapy* Vol. 16 (ed. K.M. Foley, J.J. Bonica, and V. Ventafridda), pp. 155–66. Second International Congress on Cancer Pain. New York: Raven Press.
35. **Beaver, W.T.** et al. (1966). A comparison of the analgesic effect of methotrimeprazine and morphine in patients with cancer. *Clinical and Pharmacological Therapy* **7**, 436–46.
36. **Oliver, D.J.** (1985). The use of methotrimeprazine in terminal care. *British Journal of Clinical Practice* **39**, 339–40.
37. **Breitbart, W.** (1986). Tardive dyskinesia associated with high dose intravenous metaclopramide. *New England Journal of Medicine* **315**, 518.
38. **Beaver, W.T. and Feise, G.** (1976). Comparison of the analgesic effects of morphine, hydroxyzine and their combination in patients with postoperative pain. In *Advances in Pain Research and Therapy* (ed. J.J. Bonica and Albe-Fessard), pp. 553–7. New York: Raven Press.
39. **Liebowitz, M.R.** (1985). Imipramine in the treatment of panic disorder and its complications. *Psychiatry Clinics of North America* **8**, 37–47.
40. **Massie, M.J. and Popkin, M.K.** (1998). Depression. In *Psycho-oncology* (ed. J.C. Holland et al.), pp. 518–41. New York: Oxford University Press.
41. **Mavissakalian, M.** (1993). Combined behavioral and pharmacological treatment of anxiety disorders. In *American Psychiatric Press Review of Psychiatry* Vol. 12. Washington DC: American Psychiatric Press.
42. **Bruera, E.** et al. (1990). Effects of morphine on the dyspnoea of terminal cancer patients. *Journal of Pain and Symptom Management* **5**, 341–4.
43. **Portenoy, R.K.** et al. (1986). Intravenous infusions of opioids in cancer pain: clinical review and guidelines for use. *Cancer Treatment Reports* **70**, 575–81.
44. **Robinson, D., Napoliello, M.J., and Schenk, J.** (1988). The safety and usefulness of buspirone as an anxiolytic drug in elderly versus young patients. *Clinical Therapy* **10**, 740–6.
45. **Massie, M.J., Holland, J.C., and Straker, N.** (1989). Psychotherapeutic interventions. In *Handbook of Psycho-oncology: Psychological care of the Patient with Cancer* (ed. J.C. Holland and J.H. Rowland), pp. 455–69. New York: Oxford University Press.
46. **Chochinov, H.M.C. and Holland, J.C.** (1989). Bereavement. In *Handbook of Psycho-oncology: Psychological Care of the Patient with Cancer* (ed. J.C. Holland and J.H. Rowland), pp. 612–27. New York: Oxford University Press.
47. **Holland, J.C.** et al. (1991). A randomized clinical trial of alprazolam versus progressive muscle relaxation in cancer patients with anxiety and depressive symptoms. *Journal of Clinical Oncology* **9**, 1004–11.
48. **Wilson, K.G.** et al. (2000). Diagnosis and Management of Depression in Palliative Care. In *Handbook of Psychiatry in Palliative Medicine* (ed. H.M.C. Chochinov and W. Breitbart), pp. 25–44. New York: Oxford University Press.
49. **Chochinov, H.M.C.** et al. (1994). Prevalence of depression in the terminally ill: effects of diagnostic criteria and symptom threshold judgments. *American Journal of Psychiatry* **151** (April), 4.
50. **Breitbart, W.** et al. (2000). Depression, hopelessness, and desire for hastened death in terminally ill patients with cancer. *Journal of the American Medical Association* **284**, 2907–11.
51. **Holland, J.C.** et al. (1986). Comparative psychological disturbance in pancreatic and gastric cancer. *American Journal of Psychiatry* **143**, 982–6.
52. **E. Spiegel, D., Sands, S., and Koopman, C.** (1994). Pain and depression in patients with cancer. *Cancer* **74**, 2570–8.
53. **F. Lynch, M.E.** (1995). The assessment and prevalence of affective disorders in advanced cancer. *Journal of Palliative Care* **11**, 10–18.
54. **Stiefel, F.C., Breitbart, W., and Holland, J.C.** (1989). Corticosteroids in cancer: neuropsychiatric complications. *Cancer Investigation* **7**, 479–91.
55. **Young, D.F.** (1982). Neurological complications of cancer chemotherapy. In *Neurological Complications of Therapy: Selected topics* (ed. A. Silverstein), pp. 57–113. New York: Futura Publishing.
56. **Holland, J.C., Fassanellos, and Ohnuma, T.** (1974). Psychiatric symptoms associated with L-asparaginase administration. *Journal of Psychiatric Research* **10**, 165.
57. **Adams, F., Quesada, J.R., and Gutterman, J.U.** (1984). Neuropsychiatric manifestations of human leukocyte interferon therapy in patients with cancer. *Journal of the American Medical Association* **252**, 938–41.
58. **Denicoff, K.D.** et al. (1987). The neuropsychiatric effects of treatment with interleukin-w and lymphokine-activated killer cells. *Annals of Internal Medicine* **107** (3), 293–300.
59. **Weddington, W.W.** (1982). Delirium and depression associated with amphotericin B. *Psychosomatics* **23**, 1076–8.
60. **DeAngelis, L.M., Delattre, J., and Posner, J.B.** (1989). Radiation-induced dementia in patients cured of brain metastases. *Neurology* **39**, 789–96.
61. **Breitbart, W.B.** (1989). Endocrine-related psychiatric disorders. In *The Handbook of Psycho-oncology: The Psychological Care of the Cancer Patient* (ed. J. Holland and J. Rowland), pp. 356–66. New York: Oxford University Press.
62. **Posner, J.B.** (1988). Nonmetastatic effects of cancer on the nervous system. In *Cecil's Textbook of Medicine* (ed. J.B. Wyngaarden and L.H. Smith), pp. 1104–7. Philadelphia PA: WB Saunders.
63. **Patchell, R.A. and Posner, J.B.** (1989). Cancer and the nervous system. In *The Handbook of Psycho-oncology: The Psychological Care of the Cancer Patient* (ed. J. Holland and J. Rowland), pp. 327–41. New York: Oxford University Press.
64. **G. Nelson, C.J.** et al. (2002). Spirituality, religion, and depression in the terminally ill. *Psychosomatics* **43**, 213–20.
65. **H. Block S.** (2000). Assessing and managing depression in the terminally ill patient. *Annals of Internal Medicine* **132**, 209–18.
66. **Endicott, J.** (1983). Measurement of depression patients with cancer. *Cancer* **53**, 2243–8.
67. **Kathol, R.G.** et al. (1990). Diagnosis of major depression in cancer patients according to four sets of criteria. *American Journal of Psychiatry* **147**, 1021–4.
68. **Zimmerman, M., Coryell, W.H., and Black, D.W.** (1990). Variability in the application of contemporary diagnstic criteria: endogenous depression as an example. *American Journal of Psychiatry* **147**, 1173–9.
69. **Breitbart, W.** (1990). Cancer pain and suicide. In *Advances in Pain Research and Therapy* Vol. 16 (ed. K. Foley et al.), pp. 399–412. New York: Raven Press.
70. **Breitbart, W.** (1987). Sucide in cancer patients. *Oncology* **1**, 49–53.
71. **Chochinov, H.M.C.** et al. (1997). Are you depressed? Screening for depression in the terminally ill. *American Journal of Psychiatry* **154**, 674–6.
72. **Passik, S.** et al. (1998). Oncologists' recognition of depression in their patients with cancer. *Journal of Clinical Oncology* **16**, 1594–600.
73. **McDonald, M.** et al. (1999). Nurses' recognition of depression in patients with cancer. *Oncology Nursing Forum* **10**, 185–93.
74. **Dugan, W.** et al. (1998). Use of the Zung self rating depression scale in cancer patients: feasibility as a screening tool. *Psycho-oncology* **7**, 483–93.
75. **Passik, S.** et al. (2000). Oncology staff recognition of depressive symptoms on videotaped interviews of depressed cancer patients: implications for designing a training program. *Journal of Pain and Symptom Management* **19**, 329–38.
76. **Passik, S.** et al. (2001). An attempt to employ the zung self-rating depression scale as a lab test to trigger follow-up in ambulatory oncology clinics: criterion validation and detection. *Journal of Pain and Symptom Management* **21**, 273–81.
77. **Spiegel, D., Bloom, J.R., and Yalom, I.D.** (1981). Group support for patients with metastatic cancer: a randomized prospective outcome study. *Archives of General Psychiatry* **38**, 527–33.

78. **Spiegel, D. and Bloom, J.R.** (1983). Group therapy and hypnosis reduce metastatic breast carcinoma pain. *Psychosomatic Medicine* **4**, 333–9.
79. **Rifkin, A.** et al. (1985). Trimipramine in physical illness with depression. *Journal of Clinical Psychiatry* **46**, 4–8.
80. **Purohit, D.R.** et al. (1978). The role of antidepressants in hospitalized cancer patients. *Journal of the Association of Physicians in India* **26**, 245–8.
81. **Costa, D., Mogos, I., and Toma, T.** (1985). Efficacy and safety of mianserin in the treatment of depression of women with cancer. *Acta Psychiatric Scand* **72**, 85–92.
82. **Tremblay, A. and Breitbart, W.** (2001). Psychiatric dimensions of palliative care. *Neurology Clinics* **19**, 949–67.
83. **Homsi, J.** et al. (2001). A phase II study of methylphenidate for depression in advanced cancer. *American Journal of Hospice and Palliative Care* **18**, 403–7.
84. **Davis, J.M. and Glassman, A.H.** (1989). Antidepressant drugs. In *Comprehensive Textbook of Psychiatry*, 5th edn. (ed. H.I. Kaplan and B.J. Sadock), Baltimore MD: Williams and Wilkins.
85. **Preskorn, S.H.** (1993). Recent pharmacologic advances in antidepressant therapy for the elderly. *American Journal of Medicine* **94** (Suppl. 5A).
86. **Breitbart, W. and Passik, S.D.** (1993). Psychiatric aspects of palliative care. In *Oxford Texbook of Palliative Medicine* (ed. D. Doyle, G.W. Hanks, and MacDonald), Oxford: Oxford University Press.
87. **Le Melledo, J.M. and Bradwejn, J.** (1993). Psychopharmacology of depression. In *Pharmacotherapy of Depression; Pharmanual* Vol. 20 (ed. Yvon D. Lapiere), pp. 25–46. Montreal: Chicago; Pharmalibri.
88. **Stoudemire, A. and Fogel, B.S.** (1987). Psychopharmacology in the medically ill. In *Principles of Medical Psychiatry* (ed. A. Stoudemire, B.S. Fogel, and F.L. Orlando), pp. 79–112. Grune and Stratton, Inc.
89. **Preskorn, S.H. and Jerkovich, G.S.** (1990). Central nervous system toxicity of tricyclic antidepressants: phenomenology, course, risk factors, and role of therapeutic drug monitoring. *Journal of Clinical Psychopharmacology* **10**, 88–95.
90. **Massie, M.J. and Holland, J.C.** (1984). Diagnosis and treatment of depression in the cancer patient. *Journal of Clinical Psychiatry* **42**, 25–8.
91. **Fisch, M.J.** et al. (2002). Fluoxetine versus placebo in advanced cancer outpatients: a placebo controlled, double-masked trial of the Hoosier Oncology Group. In *Proceedings of the 37th Annual Meeting of ASCO*, May 12–15, San Francisco, CA, abstract # 383A.
92. **Glassman, A.H.** (1984). The newer antidepressant drugs and their cardiovascular effects. *Psychopharmacological Bulletin* **20**, 272–9.
93. **Mendels, J.** (1987). Clinical experience with serotonin reuptake inhibiting antidepressants. *Journal of Clinical Psychiatry* **48** (Suppl.), 26–30.
94. **Cooper, G.L.** (1988). The safety of fluoxetine—an update. *British Journal of Psychiatry* **153**, 77–86.
95. **Preskorn, S. and Burke, M.** (1992). Somatic therapy for major depressive disorder: selection of an antidepressant. *Journal of Clinical Psychiatry* **53** (Suppl.), 1–14.
96. **Ciraulo, D.A. and Shader, R.I.** (1990). Fluoxetine drug–drug interactions. I. Antidepressants and antipsychotics. *Journal of Clinical Psychopharmacology* **10**, 48–50.
97. **Pearson, H.J.** (1990). Interaction of fluoxetine with carbamazepine. *Journal of Clinical Psychiatry* **51**, 126.
98. **Armstrong, S.C. and Cozza, K.L.** (2001). Consultation-liaison psychiatry drug–drug intractions update. *Psychosomatics* **42**, 269–72
99. **Rudorfer, M.V. and Potter, W.Z.** (1989). Anti-depressants. A comparative review of the clinical pharmacology and therapeutic use of the 'newer' versus the 'older' drugs. *Drugs* **37**, 713–38.
100. **Sher, M., Krieger, J.N., and Juergen, S.** (1983). Trazodone and priapism. *American Journal of Psychiatry* **140**, 1362–4.
101. **Shopsin, B.** (1983). Buproprion: a new clinical profile in the psychobiology of depression. *Journal of Clinical Psychiatry* **44**, 140–2.
102. **Peck, A.W., Stern, W.C., and Watkinson, C.** (1983). Incidence of seizures during treatment with tricyclic antidepressant drugs and buproprion. *Journal of Clinical Psychiatry* **44**, 197–201.
103. **Lloyd, A.H.** (1977). Practical consideration in the use of maprotiline (ludiomil) in general practice. *Journal of Internal Medical Research* **5**, 122–5.
104. **Ayd, F.** (1979). Amoxapine: a new tricyclic antidepressant. *International Drug Therapy Newsletter* **14**, 33–40.
105. **Fernandez, F.** et al. (1987). Methylphenidate for depressive disorders in cancer patients. *Psychosomatics* **28**, 455–61.
106. **Katon, W. and Raskind, M.** (1980). Treatment of depression in the medically ill elderly with methylphenidate. *American Journal of Psychiatry* **137**, 963–5.
107. **Kaufmann, M.W., Muarray, G.B., and Cassem, N.H.** (1982). Use of psychostimulants in medically ill depressed patients. *Psychosomatics* **23**, 817–19.
108. **Fisch, R.** (1985–1986). Metylphenidate for medical inpatients. *International Journal of Psychiatry in Medicine* **15**, 75–9.
109. **Chiarillo, R.J. and Cole, J.O.** (1987). The use of psychostimulants in general psychiatry. A reconsideration. *Archives of General Psychiatry* **44**, 286–95.
110. **Satel, S.L. and Nelson, C.J.** (1989). Stimulants in the treatment of depression: a critical overview. *Journal of Clinical Psychiatry* **50**, 241–9.
111. **Woods, S.W.** et al. (1986). Psychostimulant treatment of depressive disorders secondary to medical illness. *Journal of Clinical Psychiatry* **47**, 12–15.
112. **Burns, M.M. and Eisendrath, S.J.** (1994). Dextroamphetamine treatment for depression in terminally ill patients. *Psychosomatics* **35** (11), 80–2.
113. **Olin, J. and Masand, P.** (1996). Psychostimulants for depression in hospitalized cancer patients. *Psychosomatics* **37** (1), 57–61.
114. **Menza, M.A., Kaufman, K.R., and Castellanos, A.M.** (2000). Modafinil augmentation of antidepressant treatment in depression. *Journal of Clinical Psychiatry* **61**, 378–81.
115. **Gold, L.H. and Balster, R.L.** (1996). Evaluation of the cocaine-like discriminative stimulus effects and reinforcing effects of modafinil. *Psychopharmacology (Berlin)* **126**, 286–92.
116. **Warot, D.** et al. (1993). Subjective effects of modafinil, a new central adrenergic stimulant in healthy volunteers: a comparison with amphetamine, caffeine, and placebo. *European Psychiatry* **8**, 201–8.
117. **Cox, J.M. and Pappagallo, M.** (2001). Modafinil: a gift to portmanteau. *American Journal of Hospice and Palliative Medicine* **18**, 408–10.
118. **Fernandez, F.** et al. (1988). Cognitive impairment due to AIDS related complex and its response to psychostimulants. *Psychosomatics* **29**, 38–46.
119. **Bruera, E.** et al. (1987). Methylphenidate associated with narcotics for the treatment of cancer pain. *Cancer Treatment Reports* **71**, 67–70.
120. **Breitbart, W. and Mermelstein, H.** (1992). Pemoline: an alternative psychostimulant for the management of depressive disorders in cancer patients. *Psychosomatics* **33**, 352–6.
121. **Nehra, A.** et al. (1990). Pemoline associated hepatic injury. *Gastroenterology* **99**, 1517–19.
122. **Greenberg, D.B., Younger, J., and Kaufman, S.D.** (1993). Management of lithium in patients with cancer. *Psychosomatics* **34**, 388–94.
123. **Stein, R.S., Flexner, J.H., and Graber, S.E.** (1980). Lithium and granulocytopenia during induction therapy of acute myelogenous leukemia: update of an ongoing trial. *Advances in Experimental Medical Biology* **127**, 187–98.
124. **Cassem, N.H.** (1987). The dying patient. In *Massachusetts General Hospital Handbook of General Hospital Psychiatry*, 2nd edn. (ed. T.P. Hackett and N.H. Cassem), pp. 332–52. Littleton MA: PSG Publishing Co. Inc.
125. **W. Breitbart, W.** (2002). Spirituality and meaning in supportive care: spirituality and meaning-centered group psychotherapy interventions in advanced cancer. *Supportive Care in Cancer* **10**, 272–80.
126. **Chochinov, H.M.C.** (2002). Dignity-conserving care—a new model for palliative care. *Journal of the American Medical Association* **287**, 2253–60.
127. **Rosenfeld, B.** et al. (2002). Suicide, assisted suicide, and euthanasia in the terminally ill. In *Handbook of Psychiatry in Palliative Medicine* (ed. H.M.C. Chochinov and W. Breitbart), pp. 51–62. New York: Oxford University Press.
128. **Bolund, C.** (1973–1976). Suicide and cancer: II. Medical and care factors in suicide by cancer patients in Sweden. *Journal of Psychosocial Oncology* **3**, 17–30.
129. **Farberow, N.L., Schneidman, E.S., and Leonard, C.V.** Suicide among general medical and surgical hospital patients with malignant neoplasms. *Medical Bulletin 9*, Washington DC: US Veterans Administration, 1963.
130. **Fox, B.H.** et al. (1982). Suicide rates among cancer patients in Connecticut. *Journal of Chronic Diseases* **35**, 85–100.
131. **Louhivuori, K.A. and Hakama, J.** (1979). Risk of suicide among cancer patients. *American Journal of Epidemiology* **109**, 59–65.
132. **Farberow, N.L.** et al. (1971). An eight year survey of hospital suicides. *Suicide and Life-Threatening Behavior* **1**, 20.

133. **Robins, E.** et al. (1950). Some clinical considerations in the prevention of suicide based on 134 successful suicides. *American Journal of Public Health* **49**, 888–9.
134. **Guze, S. and Robins, E.** (1970). Suicide and primary affective disorders. *British Journal of Psychiatry* **117**, 437–8.
135. **Ganzini, L.** et al. (1994). The effect of depression treatment on elderly patients' preferences for life-sustaining medical therapy. *American Journal of Psychiatry* **151**, 1613–16.
136. **Beck, A.T., Kovacs, M., and Weissman, A.** (1975). Hopelessness and suicidal behavior: an overview. *Journal of the American Medical Association* **234**, 1146–9.
137. **Chochinov, H.M.C.** et al. (1998). Depression, hopelessness, and suicidal ideation in the terminally ill. *Psychosomatics* **39**, 366–70.
138. **Levine, P.M., Silberfarb, P.M., and Lipowski, Z.J.** (1978). Mental disorders in cancer patients. *Cancer* **42**, 1385–90.
139. **Holland, J.C.** (2003). Psychological aspects of cancer. In *Cancer Medicine,* 6th edn. (ed. J.F. Holland and E. Frei), pp. 1039–54. Philadelphia PA: Lea and Febiger.
140. **Zweig, R. and Hinrichsen, G.** (1993). Factors associated with suicide attempts by depressed older adults: a prospective study. *American Journal of Psychiatry* **150**, 1687–92.
141. **Dubovsky, S.L.** (1978). Averting suicide in terminally ill patients. *Psychosomatics* **19**, 113–15.
142. **Murphy, G.E.** (1977). Suicide and attempted suicide. *Hospital Practice* **12**, 78–81.
143. **Silberfarb, P.M., Maurer, L.H., and Cronthamel, C.S.** (1980). Psychosocial aspects of breast cancer patients during different treatment regimens. *American Journal of Psychiatry* **137**, 450–5.
144. **Achte, K.A. and Vanhkouen, M.L.** (1971). Cancer and the psyche. *Omega* **2**, 46–56.
145. **Brown, J.H.** et al. (1986). Is it normal for terminally ill patients to desire death? *American Journal of Psychiatry* **143**, 208–11.
146. **Breitbart, W., Rosenfeld, B., and Passik, S.D.** (1996). Interest in physician-assisted suicide among ambulatory HIV-infected patients. *American Journal of Psychiatry* **153**, 238–42.
147. **Emmanuel, E.J.** et al. (1996). Euthanasia and physician-assisted suicide: Attitudes and experiences of oncology patients, oncologists and the public. *Lancet* **347**, 1805–10.
148. **Chochinov, H.M.C.** et al. (1995). Desire for death in the terminally ill. *American Journal of Psychiatry* **152**, 1185–91.
149. **Rosenfeld, B.** et al. (1999). Measuring desire for death among patients with HIV/AIDS: the schedule of attitudes toward hastened death. *American Journal of Psychiatry* **156**, 94–100.
150. **Rosenfeld, B.** et al. (2000). The schedule of attitudes toward hastened death: measuring desire for hastened death in terminally ill cancer patients. *Cancer* **88**, 2868–75.
151. **Chochinov, H.M.C.** et al. (1999). Will to live in the terminally ill. *Lancet* **354**, 816–19.
152. **Breitbart, W., Chochinov, H.M.C., and Passik, S.** (1998). Psychiatric aspects of palliative care. In *Oxford Textbook of Palliative Medicine* (ed. D. Doyle, G.E.C Hanks, and N. McDonald), pp. 933–54. Oxford: Oxford University Press.
153. **Rousseau, P.** (2000). Spirituality and the dying patient. *Journal of Clinical Oncology* **18**, 2000–2.
154. **Kissane, D., Clarke, D.M., and Street, A.F.** (2001). Demoralization syndrome—a relevant psychiatric diagnosis for palliative care. *Journal of Palliative Care* **17**, 12–21.
155. **Chochinov, H.M.C.** et al. (2002). Dignity in the terminally ill: an empirical model. *Social Science and Medicine* **54**, 433–43.
156. **Greenstein, M. and Breitbart, W.** (2000). Cancer and the experience of meaning: a group psychotherapy program for people with cancer. *American Journal of Psychotherapy* **54**, 486–500.
157. **American Psychiatric Association.** *Diagnostic and Statistical Manual of Mental Disorders* 4th edn. Washington DC: American Psychiatric Association, 1994.
158. **Lipowski, Z.J.** (1990). *Delirium: Acute Confusional States.* New York: Oxford University Press.
159. **Lipowski, Z.J.** (1983). Transient cognitive disorders (delirium, acute confusional states) in the elderly. *American Journal of Psychiatry* **140**, 1426–36.
160. **Breitbart, W.** et al. (1996). A double-blind trial of haloperidol, chlorpromazine, and lorazepam in the treatment of delirium in hospitalized AIDS patients. *American Journal of Psychiatry* **153**, 231–7.
161. **Bruera, E.** et al. (1992). Cognitive failure in patients with terminal cancer: a prospective study. *Journal of Pain and Symptom Management* **7**, 192–5.
162. **Fainsinger, R. and Young, C.** (1991). Cognitive failure in a terminally ill patient. *Journal of Pain and Symptom Management* **6**, 492–4.
163. **Leipzig, R.** et al. (1987). Reversible narcotic associated mental status impairment in patients with metastatic cancer. *Pharmacology* **35**, 47–54.
164. **Levine, P.M., Silberfarb, P., and Lipowski, Z.J.** (1978). Mental disorders in cancer patients. *Cancer* **42**, 1385–91.
165. **Murray, G.B.** (1987). Confusion, delirium, and dementia. In *Massachusetts General Hospital Handbook of General Hospital Psychiatry* 2nd edn. (ed. T.P. Hackett and N.H. Cassem), pp. 84–115. Littleton MA: PSG Publishing.
166. **Posner, J.B.** (1979). Delirium and exogenous metabolic brain disease. In *Cecil Textbook of Medicine* (ed. P.B. Beeson, W. McDermott, and J.B. Wyngaarden), pp. 644–51. Philadelphia PA: WB Saunders.
167. **Knight, E.B. and Folstein, M.F.** (1977). Unsuspected emotional and cognitive disturbance in medical patients. *Annals of Internal Medicine* **87**, 723–4.
168. **Pereira, J., Hanson, J., and Bruera, E.** (1997). The frequency and clinical course of cognitive impairment in patients with terminal cancer. *Cancer* **79**, 835–41.
169. **Tune, L.E.** (1991). Post-operative delirium. *International Psychogeriatrics* **3**, 325–32.
170. **Gillick, M.R., Serrel, N.A., and Gillick, L.S.** (1982). Adverse consequences of hospitalization in the elderly. *Social Science in Medicine* **16**, 1033–8.
171. **Warsaw, G.A.** et al. (1982). Functional disability in the hospitalized elderly. *Journal of the American Medical Association* **248**, 847–50.
172. **Berman, K. and Eastham, E.J.** (1974). Psychogeriatric ascertainment and assessment for treatment in an acute medical ward setting. *Aging* **3**, 174–88.
173. **Seymour, D.J.** et al. (1980). Acute confusional states and dementia in the elderly: the role of dehydration/volume depletion, physical illness and age. *Aging* **9**, 137–46.
174. **Hodkinson, H.M.** (1973). Mental impairment in the elderly. *Journal of the Royal College of Physicians London* **7**, 305–17.
175. **Varsamis, J., Zuchowski, T., and Maini, K.K.** (1972). Survival rates and causes of death in geriatric psychiatric patients: a six year follow-up study. *Canadian Psychiatry Association Journal* **17**, 17–22.
176. **Breitbart, W., Gibson, C., and Tremblay, A.** (2002). The delirium experience: Delirium recall and delirium related distress in hospitalized patients with cancer, their spouses/caregivers, and their nurses. *Psychosomatics* **43**, 183–9.
177. **Trzepacz, P.T., Teague, G.B., and Lipowski, Z.J.** (1985). Delirium and other organic mental disorders in a general hospital. *General Hospital Psychiatry* **7**, 101–6.
178. **Bruera, E.** et al. (1992) The assessment of pain intensity in patients with cognitive failure: a preliminary report. *Journal of Pain and Symptom Management* **7** (5), 267–70.
179. **Coyle, N.** et al. (1994). Delirium as a contributing factor to 'Crescendo' pain: three case reports. *Journal of Pain and Symptom Management* **9**, 44–7.
180. **Fainsinger, R.** et al. (1991). Symptom control during the last week of life in a palliative care unit. *Journal of Palliative Care* **7**, 5–11.
181. **Bruera, E.** et al. (1989). The cognitive effects of the administration of narcotic analgesics in patients with cancer pain. *Pain* **39**, 13–16.
182. **Silberfarb, P.M.** (1983). Chemotherapy and cognitive defects in cancer patients. *Annual Review of Medicine* **34**, 35–46.
183. **Stiefel, F., Fainsinger, R., and Bruera, E.** (1992). Acute confusional states in patients with advanced cancer. *Journal of Pain and Symptom Management* **7**, 94–8.
184. **Lawlor, P.G.** et al. (2002). The occurrence, causes and outcomes of delirium in advanced cancer patients: a prospective study. *Archives of Internal Medicine* **160**, 786–94.

185. **Wise, M.G. and Brandt, G.T.** (1992). Delirium. In *Textbook of Neuropsychiatry* 2nd edn (ed. S.C. Yudofsky and R.E. Hales), pp. 89–107. Washington DC: American Psychiatric Press.
186. **Ross, C.A.** (1991). CNS arousal systems: possible role in delirium. *International Psychogeriatrics* **3**, 353–71.
187. **Lipowski, Z.J.** (1980). Delirium: acute brain failure in man. Springfield IL: Charles C Thomas, 1980.
188. **Breitbart, W.** et al. (1995). Neuropsychiatric syndromes and psychological symptoms in patients with advanced cancer. *Journal of Pain and Symptom Management* **10**, 131–41.
189. **Ross, C.A.** et al. (1991). Delirium: phenomenologic and etiologic subtypes. *International Psychogeriatrics* **3**, 135–47.
190. **Albert, M.S.** et al. (1991). The delirium symptom interview: an interview for the detection of delirium symptoms in hospitalized patients. *Journal of Geriatric Psychiatry and Neurology* **5**, 14–21.
191. **Breitbart, W.** et al. (1997). The Memorial Delirium Assessment Scale. *Journal of Pain and Symptom Management* **13**, 128–37.
192. **Folstein, M.F., Folstein, S.E., and McHugh, P.R.** (1975). 'Mini-mental status': a practical method for grading the cognitive state of patients for clinicians. *Journal of Psychiatric Research* **12**, 189–98.
193. **Jacobs, J.C.** et al. (1977). Screening for organic mental syndromes in the medically ill. *Annals of Internal Medicine* **86**, 40–6.
194. **Katzman, R.** et al. (1983). Validation of a short orientation-memory-concentration test of cognitive impairment. *American Journal of Psychiatry* **140**, 734–9.
195. **Levkoff, S.** et al. (1992). Review of research instruments and techniques used to detect delirium. *International Psychogeriatrics* **3**, 253–72.
196. **Trzepacz, P.T., Baker, R.W., and Greenhouse, J.** (1988). A symptom rating scale for delirium. *Psychiatric Research* **1**, 89–97.
197. **Williams, M.A.** (1991). Delirium/acute confusional states: evaluation devices in nursing. *International Psychogeriatrics* **3**, 301–8.
198. **Wolber, G.** et al. (1984). Validity of the short Portable Mental Status Questionnaire with elderly psychiatric patients. *Journal of Consultational and Clinical Psychology* **52**, 712–13.
199. **Smith, M.J., Breitbart, W.S., and Platt, M.M.** (1995). A critique of instruments and methods to detect, diagnose, and rate delirium. *Journal of Pain and Symptom Management* **10**, 35–77.
200. **Trzepacz, P.T.** et al. (1999). Validity of the Delirium Rating Scale—Revised-98 (DRS-R-98). Abstract #41. In *Proceedings of the 46th Annual Meeting of the Academy of Psychosomatic Medicine*, 18–21 November, New Orleans, LA.
201. **Inouye, B.K.** et al. (1990). Clarifying confusion: the confusion assessment method, a new method for detection of delirium. *Annals of Internal Medicine* **113**, 941–8.
202. **Hart, R.P.** et al. (1997). Abbreviated cognitive test for delirium. *Journal of Psychosomatic Research* **43**, 417–23.
203. **Lawlor, P.G.** et al. (2000). Clinical utility, factor analysis and further validation of the Memorial Delirium Assessment Scale (MDAS). *Cancer* **88**, 2859–67.
204. **American Psychiatric Association** (1999). Practice Guidelines for the Treatment of Patients with Delirium. *American Journal of Psychiatry* **156**, S1–20.
205. **Bruera, E.** (1991). Case report. Severe organic brain syndrome. *Journal of Palliative Care* **7**, 36–8.
206. **Lichter, I. and Hunt, E.** (1990). The last 48 hours of life. *Journal of Palliative Care* **6** (4), 7–15.
207. **Tuma, R. and DeAngelis, L.** (1992). Acute encephalopathy in patients with systemic cancer. *Annals of Neurology* **32**, 288–9.
208. **Inouye, B.K.** et al. (1999). A multicomponent intervention to prevent delirium in hospitalized older patients. *New England Journal of Medicine* **340**, 669–76.
209. **Derogatis, L.R.** et al. (1979). A survey of psychotropic drug prescriptions in an oncology population. *Cancer* **44**, 1919–29.
210. **Steifel, F., Kornblith, A., and Holland, J.** (1990). Changes in prescription patterns of psychotropic drugs for cancer patients during a 10-year period. *Cancer* **65**, 1048–53.
211. **Goldberg, G. and Mor, V.** (1985). A survey of psychotropic use in terminal cancer patients. *Psychosomatics* **26**, 745–51.
212. **Jaeger, H., Morrow, G., and Brescia, F.** (1985). A survey of psychotropic drug utilization by patients with advanced neoplastic disease. *General Hospice Psychiatry* **7**, 353–60.
213. **Akechi, T.** et al. (1996). Usage of haloperidol for delirium in cancer patients. *Support Care in Cancer* **4**, 390–2.
214. **Fernandez, F.** et al. (1988). Treatment of severe, refractory agitation with a haloperidol drip. *Journal of Clinical Psychiatry* **49**, 239–41.
215. **Fernandez, F, Levy, J.F., and Mansell, P.W.A.** (1989). Management of delirium in terminally ill AIDS patients. *International Journal of Psychiatry in Medicine* **19**, 165–72.
216. **Rosen, J.H.** (1979). Double-blind comparison of haloperidol and thioridazine in geriatric outpatients. *Journal of Clinical Psychiatry* **40**, 17–20.
217. **Smith, G.R., Taylor, C.W., and Linkons, P.** (1974). Haloperidol versus thioridazine for the treatment of psychogeriatric patients: a double-blind clinical trial. *Psychosomatics* **15**, 134–8.
218. **Thomas, H., Schwartz, E., and Petrilli, R.** (1992). Droperidol versus haloperidol for chemical restraint of agitated and combative patients. *Annals of Emergency Medicine* **21**, 407–13.
219. **Tsuang, M.M.** et al. (1971). Haloperidol versus thioridazine for hospitalized psychogeriatrics patients: double-blind study. *Journal of the American Geriatrics Society* **19**, 593–600.
220. **Breitbart, W.** (1988). Psychiatric complications of cancer. In *Current Therapy in Hematology Oncology-3* (ed. M.C. Brain and P.P. Carbone), pp. 268–74. Toronto: BC Decker.
221. **Breitbart, W.** (1989). Psychiatric management of cancer pain. *Cancer* **63**, 2336–42.
222. **Twycross, R.G. and Lack, S.A.** *Symptom Control in Far Advanced Cancer: Pain Relief.* London: Pitman Books, 1983.
223. **Breitbart, W.** (2001), Diagnoisis and management of delirium in the terminally ill. In *Topics in Palliative Care* Vol. 5 (ed. R. Portenoy and E. Bruera), pp. 303–21. New York: Oxford University Press
224. **Menza, M., Murray, G., and Holmes, V.** (1988). Controlled study of extrapyramidal reactions in the management of delirious medically ill patients: intravenous haloperidol versus intravenous haloperidol plus benzodiazepines. *Heart and Lung* **17**, 238–241.
225. **Oliver, D.J.** (1985). The use of methotrimeprazine in terminal care. *British Journal of Clinical Practice* **39**, 339–40.
226. **Baldessarini, R. and Frankenburg, F.** (1991). Clozapine: a novel antipsychotic agent. *New England Journal of Medicine* **324**, 746–52.
227. **Passik, S.D. and Cooper, M.** (1999). Complicated delirium in a cancer patient successfully treated with olanzipine. *Journal of Pain and Symptom Management* **17**, 219–23.
228. **Sipahimalani, A. and Massand, P.S.** (1998). Olanzipine in the treatment of delirium. *Psychosomatics* **39**, 422–30.
229. **Sipahimalani, A., Sime, R.M., and Masand, P.S.** (1997). Treatment of delirium with risperidone. *International Journal of Geriatric Psychopharmacology* **1**, 24–6.
230. **Breitbart, W., Tremblay, A., and Gibson, C.** (2002). An open trial of olanzapine for the treatment of delirium in hospitalized cancer patients. *Psychosomatics* **43**, 175–6.
231. **Breitbart, W., Chochinov, H.M.C., and Passik, S.** (1998). Psychiatric aspects of palliative care. In *Oxford Textbook of Palliative Medicine* 2nd edn. (ed. D. Doyle, G.E.C. Hanks, and N. MacDonald), pp. 933–54. Oxford: Oxford University Press.
232. **Ventafridda, V.** et al. (1990). Symptom prevalence and control during cancer patients' last days of life. *Journal of Palliative Care* **6**, 7–11.
233. **Mercadante, S., De Conno, F., and Ripamonti, C.** (1995). Propofol in terminal care. *Journal of Pain and Symptom Management* **10**, 639–42.
234. **Moyle, J.** (1995). The use of propofol in palliative medicine. *Journal of Pain and Symptom Management* **10**, 643–6.
235. **Fainsinger, R. and Bruera, E.** (1992). Treatment of delirium in a terminally ill patient. *Journal of Pain and Symptom Management* **7**, 54–6.
236. **Stiefel, F. and Bruera, E.** (1991). Psychostimulants for hypoactive-hypoalert delirium? *Journal of Palliative Care* **3**, 25–6.
237. **Bruera, E.** (1990). Symptom control in patients with cancer. *Journal of Psychosocial Oncology* **8**, 47–73.

238. **Coyle, N.** et al. (1990). Character of terminal illness in the advanced cancer patient: pain and other symptoms during the last four weeks of life. *Journal of Pain and Symptom Management* **5**, 83–93.

239. **Levy, M. and Catalano, R.** (1985). Control of common physical symptoms other than pain in patients with terminal disease. *Seminars in Oncology* **12**, 411–30.

240. **Fotopoulos, S.S., Graham, C., and Cook, M.R.** (1979). Psychophysiologic control of cancer pain. In *Advances in Pain Research and Therapy* Vol. 2. (ed. J.J. Bonica and V. Ventafridda), pp. 231–44. New York: Raven Press.

241. **Turk, D. and Rennert, K.** (1981). Pain and the terminally ill cancer patient: a cognitive-social learning perspective. In *Behavior Therapy in Terminal Care* (ed. H.J. Sobel), pp. 137–54. Cambridge: Ballinger.

242. **Hilgard, E. and LeBaron, S.** (1982). Relief of anxiety and pain in children and adolescents with cancer: quantitative measures and clinical observations. *International Journal of Clinical Experimental Hypnosis* **30**, 417–42.

243. **Jay, S., Elliott, C., and Varni, J.** (1986). Acute and chronic pain in adults and children with cancer: *Journal of Consulting and Clinical Psychology* **54**, 601–7.

244. **Kellerman, J.** et al. (1983). Adolescents with cancer: hypnosis for the reduction of acute pain and anxiety associated with medical procedures. *Journal of Adolescent Health Care* **4**, 85–90.

245. **Lesko, L.** (1989). Anorexia. In *Handbook of Psycho-oncology: Psychological Care of the Patient with Cancer* (ed. J.C. Holland and J. Rowland), pp. 434–43. New York: Oxford University Press.

246. **Redd, W.H., Andresen, G.V., and Minagawa, R.Y.** (1982). Hypnotic control of anticipatory emesis in patients receiving cancer chemotherapy. *Journal of Consulting and Clinical Psychology* **50**, 14–19.

247. **Dixon, J.** (1984). Effect of nursing interventions on nutritional and performance status in cancer patients. *Nursing Research* **33**, 330–5.

248. **Campbell, D.** et al. (1984). Relaxation: its effect on the nutritional status and performance status of clients with cancer. *Journal of the American Dietary Association* **84**, 201–4.

249. **Redd, W.H.** (1980). *In vivo* desensitization in the treatment of chronic emesis following gastrorintestinal surgery. *Behavior Therapy* **11**, 421–7.

250. **West, B. and Piccionne, C.** (1982). Cognitive-behavioral techniques in treating anorexia and depression in a cancer patient. *The Behavioral Therapist* **5**, 115–17.

251. **LeBaw, W.** et al. (1975). The use of self hypnosis by children with cancer. *American Journal of Clinical Hypnosis* **17**, 233–8.

252. **Bruera, E. and MacDonald, N.** (1988). Asthenia in patients with advanced cancer. *Journal of Pain and Symptom Management* **3**, 9–14.

253. **Breitbart, W.** et al. (2001). A randomized, double-blind, placebo-controlled trial of psychostimulants for the treatment of fatigue in ambulatory patients with human immunodeficiency virus disease. *Archives of Internal Medicine* **161**, 411–20.

254. **Barnes, M.** (1988). Nausea and vomiting in the patient with advanced cancer. *Journal of Pain and Symptom Management* **3**, 81–5.

255. **Morrow, G.R. and Morrell, B.S.** (1982). Behavioral treatment for the anticipatory nausea and vomiting induced by cancer chemotherapy. *New England Journal of Medicine* **307**, 1476–80.

256. **Jacobsen, P.B.** et al. (1988). Non pharmacologic factors in the development of post treatment nausea with adjuvant chemotherapy for breast cancer. *Cancer* **61**, 379–85.

257. **Greenberg, D.B.** et al. (1987). Alprazolam for phobic nausea and vomiting related to cancer chemotherapy. *Cancer Treatment Reports* **71**, 549–50.

258. **Cannici, J., Malcolm, R., and Peck, L.A.** (1983). Treatment of insomnia in cancer patients using muscle relaxant training. *Journal of Behavior Therapy and Experimental Psychiatry* **14**, 251–6.

259. **Stamm, H., Bultz, B., and Pittman, C.** (1986). Psychosocial problems and interventions in a referred sample of cancer patients. *Psychosomatic Medicine* **48**, 539–48.

9

Paediatric palliative medicine

9 Paediatric palliative medicine

9.1 Pain control

Patricia A. McGrath and Stephen C. Brown

Introduction

Pain control is an integral component of paediatric palliative care. Children may experience many different types of pain from invasive procedures, the cumulative effects of toxic therapies, progressive disease, or psychological factors. The pain is often complex with multiple sources, comprised of nociceptive and neuropathic components. In addition, several situational factors usually contribute to children's pain, distress, and disability. Thus, to adequately treat pain in children receiving palliative care, we must evaluate the primary pain sources and ascertain which situational factors are relevant for which children and families. Treatment emphasis should shift accordingly from an exclusive disease-centred framework to a more child-centred focus.

In this chapter, we describe a child-centred framework for understanding and controlling pain for children receiving palliative care. Pain control should include regular pain assessments, appropriate analgesics administered at regular dosing intervals, adjunctive drug therapy for symptom and side-effects control, and non-drug interventions to modify the situational factors that can exacerbate pain and suffering. Since much specific information on pain control (presented in Chapter 9.2) is also relevant for children, basic information on pathophysiology, pharmacology, and physical interventions is not repeated in this chapter. Instead, this chapter provides a complementary focus to the other contributions in this textbook by describing the unique nature of children's pain including the primary factors that affect their pain and quality of life, presenting guidelines for selecting and administering drug therapy in accordance with the nociceptive and neuropathic components, and recommending practical non-drug therapies for integration within a hospital, home, or hospice setting.

The nature of children's pain

Throughout the last decade, we have gained an increasing appreciation for the plasticity and complexity of children's pain. As with adults, children's pain is often initiated by tissue damage caused by noxious stimulation, but the consequent pain is neither simply nor directly related to the amount of tissue damage. Perhaps even more than in adults, differing pain responses to the same tissue damage are noted. The eventual pain evoked by a relatively constant noxious stimulus can be different depending on children's expectations, perceived control, or the significance that they attach to the pain.[1] Children do not sustain tissue damage in an isolated manner, devoid of a particular context, but actively interpret the strength and quality of any pain sensations, determine the relevance of any hurting, and learn how to interpret the pain by observing the general environment, especially the behaviour of other people. Children's perceptions of pain is defined by their age and cognitive level; their previous pain experiences, against which they evaluate each new pain; the relevance of the pain or disease causing pain; their expectations for obtaining eventual recovery and pain relief; and their ability to control the pain themselves. While plasticity and complexity are critical features for all pain perception, plasticity seems an even more important feature for controlling children's pain.

Much research has been conducted to identify the critical factors responsible for the plasticity of pain perception (for review see ref. 2). Animal behaviour studies, in which the physiological responses activated by a noxious stimulus are directly recorded, have demonstrated that certain factors, such as the primate's attention, the predictability of a painful stimulus, and the relevance of the stimulus can directly modify the intensity of the physiological responses evoked by a constant noxious stimulus. Parallel psychophysical studies, in which adults rate the painfulness of constant noxious stimuli in different contexts, have demonstrated that these same factors can modify the perceived intensity and unpleasantness of the consequent pain sensations. Psychologically mediated modulation of pain can occur at the earliest levels of pain processing, but also at the highest levels. Recent PET and functional MRI studies have demonstrated that painful stimulation activates different cortical regions—depending on an individual's expectations and attention.[3] Human studies evaluating the impact of environmental and psychological factors on the perception of experimentally induced pain have been conducted primarily in adults. However, results from the few laboratory studies conducted with children are consistent with those from adult studies.[4,5] In addition, much compelling evidence about the powerful mediating role of psychological factors in children's pain derives from clinical studies of acute, recurrent, and chronic pain. These studies highlight the need to recognize and evaluate the mediating impact of these factors in order to optimally control children's pain.

The model illustrated in Fig. 1 provides a framework for assessing these factors, based on our knowledge of the plasticity and complexity of children's pain. Some factors are relatively stable for a child, such as gender, temperament, and cultural background while other factors change progressively, such as age, cognitive level, previous pain experience, and family learning (listed in the open box in the figure). These child characteristics shape how children generally interpret and experience the various sensations caused by tissue damage. In contrast, the cognitive, behavioural, and emotional factors (listed in the shaded boxes) are not stable. They represent a unique interaction between the child and the situation in which the pain is experienced.[1,6] These situational factors can vary dynamically throughout the course of a child's illness, depending on the specific circumstances in which children experience pain. For example, a child receiving treatment for cancer will have repeated injections, portacatheter access, and lumbar punctures—all of which may cause some pain (depending on the analgesics, anaesthetics, or sedatives used). Even though the tissue damage from these procedures is the same each time, the particular set of situational factors for each treatment is unique for a child—depending on a child's (and parent's expectations), a child's (and parent's *and* staff's behaviours), and on a child's (and family's) emotional state. Although the causal relationship between an injury and a consequent pain seems direct

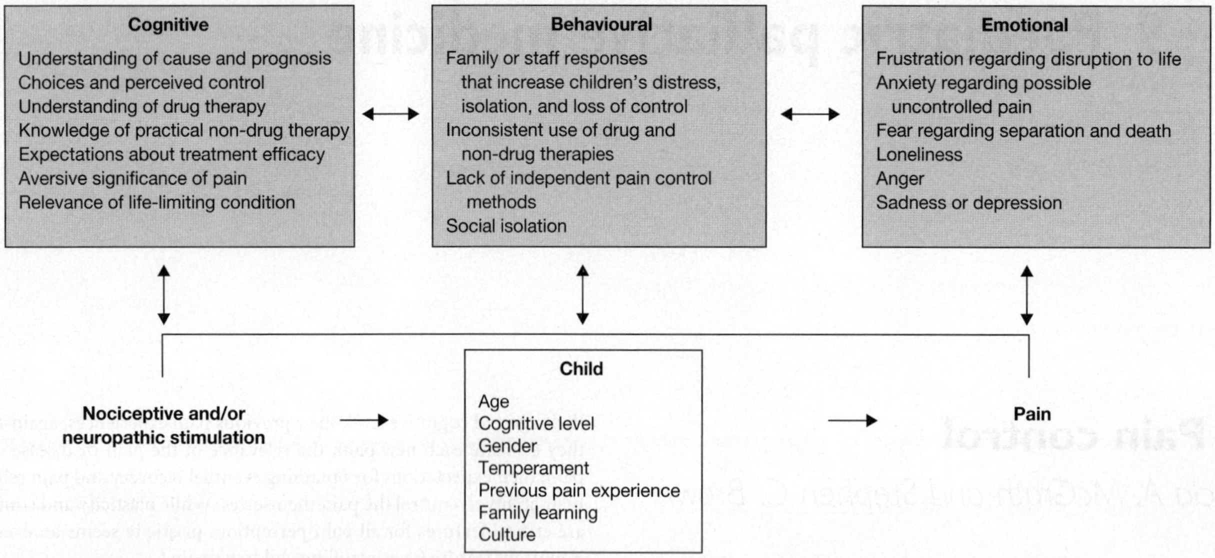

Fig. 1 A model depicting the situational factors that modify children's pain perception.

and obvious, what children understand, what they do, and how they feel all affect their pain. Certain factors can intensify pain, exacerbate suffering, or affect adversely a child's quality of life.[4] While parents and health care providers may be unable to change the more stable child characteristics, they can modify situational factors and dramatically improve children's pain and lives.

The impact of situational factors on children's pain

Cognitive factors include children's understanding about the pain source, their ability to control what will happen, their expectations regarding the quality and strength of pain sensations that they will experience, their primary focus of attention (that is distracted away from or focused primarily on the pain), and their knowledge of pain control strategies. In general, children's pain can be lessened by providing accurate age-appropriate information about pain, for example emphasizing the specific sensations that children will experience (such as the stinging quality of an injection, rather than the general hurting aspects), by increasing their control and choices, by explaining the rationale for what can be done to reduce pain, and by teaching them some independent pain reducing strategies.[1,7] For children receiving palliative care, key cognitive factors also include the relevance or meaning of their illness—particularly its life-threatening potential, their beliefs about death and their understanding of the significance of their lives.

Behavioural factors refer to the specific behaviours of children, parents, and staff when children experience pain and also encompass parents' and children's wider behaviours in response to a chronic pain problem or progressive illness. Common behavioural factors include children's distress or coping reactions (e.g. crying, using a pain control strategy, withdrawing from life) and parent's and health staff's subsequent reactions to them (e.g. displaying frustration, calmly providing encouragement for children to use pain control strategies, engaging them in conversation and activities).[4] They also include the extent to which children are physically restrained during invasive or aversive treatments and the broader physical and social restrictions on children's and family's lives as children become sicker. Distress behaviours and some altered behavioural patterns may initiate, exacerbate, or maintain children's pain. In general, as children's mental or physical activity increases, as children use coping and pain control methods, as their distress and disability behaviours decrease, and as staff and parental responses become more consistent in encouraging them to use pain control methods, their pain should lessen. Children receiving palliative care seem to report less pain, feel less distressed by pain, and have a higher quality of life when families and staff encourage them to remain engaged in life and live as fully as possible.

Emotional factors include parents' and children's feelings in response to pain, to the daily effects of the underlying illness or condition, and to the subsequent impact of the children's deaths on the family. Children's emotions affect their ability to understand what is happening, their ability to cope positively, their behaviours, and ultimately their pain. Children's immediate emotional reactions to pain may vary from a relatively neutral acceptance to annoyance, anxiety, fear, frustration, anger, or sadness. The specific emotions depend on the nature of the pain—type, cause, intensity, and duration—and its impact on their lives. In general, the more emotionally distressed children are the stronger or more unpleasant their pain. When children do not understand what is happening, when they lack control and do not know independent pain control strategies, their emotional distress increases and their pain intensifies. Similarly, when children's behaviours are restricted, when they are physically restrained during medical procedures, or when their usual daily activities and social interactions are disrupted, their emotional distress and pain can intensify. Children with life-threatening conditions may not understand what they are feeling or may be unable to verbalize their fears and anxieties. Yet, almost all children will become aware of differences in how their parents and families respond to them as they progress from receiving active curative treatments to receiving only palliative therapies. Even very subtle behavioural cues can still evoke fear, uncertainty, apprehension, or depression depending on children's ages and what they understand about death and separation. Thus, an essential component of pain control should be evaluating whether these emotions are exacerbating children's pain and distress and impairing the quality of their lives.

Situational factors in paediatric palliative care

Cognitive and emotional factors are the most salient situational factors that affect pain for children receiving palliative care. Children probably have already endured a prolonged period of intermittent pain, physical disability, and multiple aversive treatments. Children who were receiving curative therapies become more focused on the future consequences of their disease. Their thoughts, behaviours, and feelings change as they begin to understand that they are dying. Naturally, the type of support, information, and guidance children require also changes. While the impact is profound for all children and families, each child and family is unique with respect to their specific psychological, medical, social, and spiritual needs. All families experience anguish and grief, but they may also experience denial, anxiety, anger, guilt, frustration, and depression. It is essential that health professionals listen attentively and observe carefully not only to ensure that all the needs of both the child and family are met but also to resolve the myriad factors that can exacerbate children's pain and suffering. The primary situational factors in paediatric palliative care are listed in Table 1. This summary has evolved from our treatment of children referred to the pain clinic. Child and family factors are listed in italics; the factors that are relevant for health staff, as well as families, are listed in roman print.

The shift in care from curative to palliative therapies may signify to some children and families that health professionals are giving up on the child. Children and families must understand that stopping ineffective therapies is not giving up, but represents a rational decision based on children's best interests. Pain control is an essential component of palliative care.[8–14] Children and parents should not fear that health professionals have given up on controlling pain and aversive symptoms. Pain and all symptoms must be treated aggressively from the dual perspective of targeting the primary source of tissue damage and modifying the secondary contributing factors. Although most families receive accurate information about their disease and required treatments, few children or their parents receive concrete information about their pain, the factors that can attenuate or exacerbate it, a rationale for the interventions they receive, and training in effective non-drug pain control methods. The latter may be particularly important for children in palliative care, who have diminishing control in their lives. Children and their parents often do not understand that pain control therapies may vary in efficacy due to changing disease, the effects of other drugs, and situational factors. Thus, their confidence in certain pain control therapies can decrease, even though these therapies would effectively alleviate pain at another time. The fear of inadequate pain control places an enormous emotional burden on an already distressed child and family and can create a situation in which children's pain and disability intensifies.

Table 1 Situational factors in paediatric palliative care

Cognitive factors
Meaning of death
Inaccurate understanding
Impact of situational factors on pain and quality of life
Course of disease
Palliative versus curative therapy
Little independent control over pain
Limited choices
Expectation for continuing pain and suffering
Misunderstanding of drug therapy
Opioids
Dosing and administration
Criteria for evaluating effectiveness
Behavioural factors
Social withdrawal
Physical inactivity
Passive approach to pain control
Secondary gains
Stress reduction
Emotional denial
Parent or staff attention
Inappropriate drug management
Choice or mode of drug administration
Failure to aggressively treat opioid-related side-effects
Failure to evaluate pain sources and document pain level
Failure to use effective non-drug therapies
Emotional
Anxiety about
Dying and death
Suffering
Meaning of life
Fear of
Separation
Inadequate pain control
Increasing adverse symptoms
Impact on family
Anger
Sadness or depression
Distancing by staff and friends

Generally, children's physical activity has been progressively restricted due to the disability caused by their condition. Parents who encourage children to adopt passive patient roles, to behave differently than other children, and to depend primarily on others for pain control will undoubtedly create a situation wherein children's pain is maximized. Even when children are somnolent, it is possible to create some 'normal environment' in which children can participate and actively involve themselves during their alert periods. Children should live as fully as possible, even though they are also dying.

Children who experienced adverse physical effects from medication, such as hair loss and weight gain, may have become acutely self-conscious about their appearance. As a result, these children may have progressively withdrawn from social interactions with their peers because they anticipated negative reactions. Children become more distant from the people and activities that they had enjoyed. Moreover, many children may lose the opportunity to be regarded as unique individuals by the friends and classmates they value; instead, they are regarded increasingly as sick, different, or even dying. Their peers and their daily accomplishments (whether social, academic, or athletic) had provided special meaning about children's unique value in the world. While families emphasize children's value to them and to the world, children often lose the objective feedback they routinely received. The increased withdrawal and social isolation can exacerbate their pain and emotional distress. Their withdrawal may increase when treatment emphasis shifts from cure and palliation to palliation alone. Parents may 'close-in', spending even more exclusive time with the dying child as a closed family unit. While important for children and families, the exclusive focus on the family increases a child's social isolation and may cause more anxiety for some children—particularly when the family does not openly address children's concerns about death and dying. Inadvertently, the family may prevent children from interacting both with peers who can lessen their anxiety through play and conversation and also with health professionals who can help them to resolve their anxiety and fears about dying.

Children seem to know intuitively, even when dying has not been discussed directly with them. They fear separation and abandonment; some children may fear that their illness is a punishment. Dying children may feel frightened, isolated, and guilty unless they are able to openly express and resolve their concerns. Many observers have noted that children who are dying have a level of maturity 'far beyond their years'. It is essential to acknowledge and resolve their fears. Children should receive accurate information, consistent with their spiritual beliefs, presented in a calm reassuring manner. They may need concrete reassurance that they will not suffer when they die, that they will not be alone, and that their families will remember them. Unresolved emotions add anguish and may intensify their pain. (For the comprehensive care of the dying child, please see refs 11, 15–19.)

Optimal pain control for children

Pain control is an intrinsic component of paediatric palliative care. Since children may experience complex pains due to myriad physical and psychological

Table 2 Primary components of pain assessment

Sensory characteristics	*Cognitive factors*
Onset	Understanding of pain source
Location	Understanding of diagnosis, treatment, and prognosis
Intensity	Expectations
Quality	Perceived control
Duration	Relevance of disease or painful treatments
Spread to other sites (consistent with neurological pattern)	Knowledge of pain control
Radiation	*Behavioural factors*
Temporal pattern	General coping style
Accompanying symptoms	Learned pain behaviours
Medical/surgical	Overt distress level
Investigations conducted	Parent's behaviours
Radiological and laboratory results	Physical activities and limitations
Consult results	Social activities and limitations
Analgesic and adjuvant medications (type, dose, frequency, route, length of medication trial)	*Emotional factors*
Clinical factors	Frustration
Environmental features	Anxiety
Roles of medical and associated health professionals	Fear
Nature of interventions	Denial
Complementary and alternative therapy	Sadness
Documentation of pain	Anger
Criteria for determining analgesic effectiveness	Depression

factors, pain control must be child-centred rather than disease-centred. Health care providers must carefully evaluate the varied causes and contributing factors to select the most effective therapies for each child's pain.

Onset, location, intensity, quality, duration (or frequency, if recurring), spatial extent, temporal pattern, and accompanying physical symptoms are the key pain characteristics for assessment, as listed in Table 2. All these characteristics should be evaluated as part of the initial clinical examination, with pain intensity and any other characteristics that are clinically relevant for children monitored regularly. Children's descriptions about the nature of their pain (when self-report is available) complete the information obtained through radiological and laboratory investigations. Since several situational factors usually contribute to children's pain, distress, and disability, health care providers should evaluate the extent to which these may be relevant for a child—building on their knowledge of the child and family's previous experiences throughout the child's illness and their observations of the current situation.

In palliative care, the differential diagnosis of a child's pain is a dynamic process that guides our clinical management. We should select specific therapies to target the responsible central and peripheral mechanisms and to mitigate the pain-exacerbating impact of situational factors, recognizing that the multiple causes and contributing factors will vary over time. Drug therapies—analgesics, analgesic-adjuvants, and anaesthetics, are essential for pain control, but non-drug therapies—cognitive, physical, and behavioural, are also essential. As we monitor the child's improvement in response to the therapies initiated, we refine our pain diagnosis and treatment plan accordingly. Pain control is achieved practically by adjusting both drug and non-drug therapies in a rational child-centred manner based on the assessment process, as outlined by the treatment algorithm in Fig. 2. (The different therapies are described later in the chapter.) Controlling children's pain requires an integrated approach because many factors are responsible, no matter how seemingly clear cut the aetiology. Adequate analgesic prescriptions, administered at regular dosing intervals, must be complemented by a practical cognitive–behavioural approach to ensure optimal pain relief.

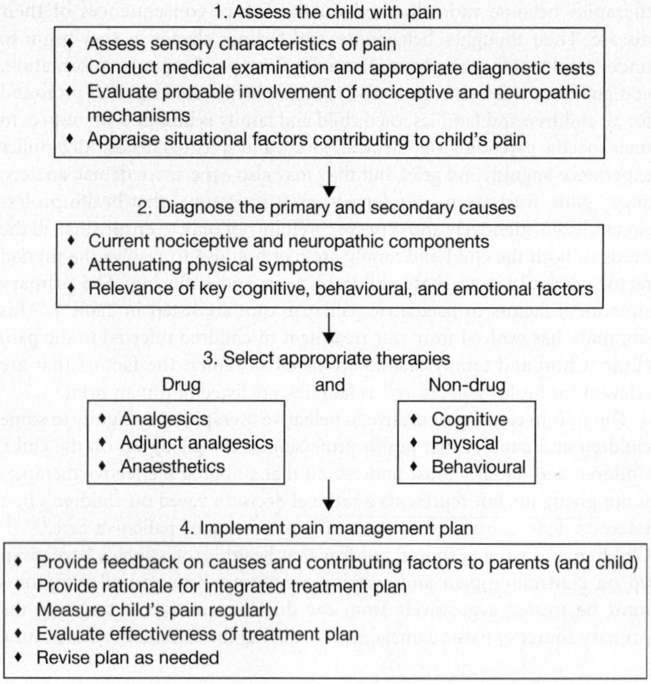

Fig. 2 A treatment algorithm for controlling children's pain.

Misconceptions regarding pain control in children

Several misconceptions have led to inadequate pain control in children as described in the following (revised from ref. 1).

Misconceptions about children's pain systems

Many health care providers continue to treat children's pain from an erroneous disease model perspective wherein pain is always proportional to the extent and severity of tissue damage. As a result of misconceptions about the plasticity and complexity of children's nociceptive systems, they focus on the primary source of noxious stimulation but not on all the causative and contributing factors that affect nociceptive processing. As a result of misconceptions about nociceptive and neuropathic components of pain, they fail to use the wide range of analgesic and analgesic-adjuvants available to control pain.

Misconceptions about the pharmacodynamics and pharmacokinetics of opioid analgesics

As a result of misconceptions about the pharmacodynamics and pharmacokinetics of opioid analgesics, health professionals do not always select the most appropriate drugs, doses, dosing intervals, or administration routes.

Misconceptions about the risk of addiction

Some health care providers and parents believe that opioid analgesics should be administered only as a last resort, to avoid drug addiction. They have not understood that Tolerance + Physical Dependence $\neq$ Addiction. As a result, children have not always received the potent analgesics required to relieve severe pain. Moreover, they may not understand that opioid related side effects should be treated aggressively so that the potential efficacy of these drugs for controlling pain is not compromised by adverse side-effects.

Misconceptions about the efficacy of non-drug therapies

Many health professionals do not realize that relatively simple non-drug strategies can lessen children's pain. As a result, they have not taught children or their parents how to use practical cognitive, physical, and behavioural strategies that are effective for reducing pain, distress, and pain-related disability. Similarly, they have not taught parents the importance of evaluating and modifying situational and familial factors to lessen children's pain.

Misconceptions about comprehensive pain control

Many health care providers believe that drug therapies are both necessary and sufficient to control children's pain. They have not prescribed non-drug therapies to supplement or complement analgesics, even when situational factors are impeding analgesic efficacy.

Misconceptions about pain assessment

Many health care providers do not know how to routinely assess children's pain levels or the factors that intensify their pain and distress. As a result, it may be difficult to evaluate the effectiveness of changes in drug therapy, complementary therapies, and situational factors.

Misconceptions about who is in charge of pain control

One individual should assume primary responsibility for ensuring that a child's pain is controlled adequately. Diffusion of responsibility among various health care providers leads to gaps in recognizing a child's pain and treating pain appropriately.

Misconceptions about the importance of consistent pain control

The medical specialties, which provide care to children throughout their illness, do not always adopt a consistent approach to pain assessment and pain control, similar to their consistent approach to disease diagnosis and medical treatment. The failure to regard pain control as important throughout a child's treatment can lead to difficulties for children in palliative care, whose previous experiences with inadequate pain management creates undue stress and anxiety for them and their parents.

Guidelines for assessment, analgesic selection and administration, and non-pharmacological interventions

The principles of analgesic therapy, the guidelines for drug administration, and the guidelines for a supportive cognitive–behavioural approach are those that should be followed in all paediatric palliative care, including the care of children with cancer, neurodegenerative diseases, and acquired human immunodeficiency virus (HIV) infection.

Evaluating children's pain

Pain assessment is an integral component of diagnosis and treatment for children. A thorough medical history, physical examination, and assessment of pain characteristics and contributing factors are necessary to establish a correct clinical diagnosis. Subsequent assessments of pain intensity enable us to determine when treatments are effective and to identify those children for whom they are most effective. Health care providers need pain measures that are convenient to administer and whose resulting pain scores provide meaningful information about children's pain experiences. An extensive array of pain measures have been developed and validated for use with infants, children, and adolescents.[20–22]

Like adult pain measures, children's pain measures are classified as physiological, behavioural, and psychological, depending on what is monitored—physical parameters (e.g. heart rate, sweat index, blood pressure, cortisol level), distress behaviours (e.g. grimaces, cries, protective guarding gestures), or children's own descriptions of what they are experiencing (e.g. words, drawings, numerical ratings). Physiological and behavioural measures provide indirect estimates of pain because health care providers must infer the location and strength of a child's pain solely from his or her responses. In contrast, psychological measures can provide direct information about the location, strength, quality, affect, and duration.

The criteria for an accurate pain measure are similar to those required for any measuring instrument. A pain measure must be valid, in that it measures a specific aspect of pain so that changes in pain ratings reflect meaningful differences in a child's pain experience. The measure must be reliable, in that it provides consistent and trustworthy pain ratings regardless of the time of testing, the clinical setting, or who is administering the measure. The measure must be relatively free from bias, in that children should be able to use it similarly, regardless of differences in how they may wish to please adults. The pain measure should be practical and versatile for assessing different types of pain (e.g. disease-related, procedural pain) in many different children (according to age, cognitive level, cultural background) and for use in diverse clinical and home settings.

Physiological and behavioural pain scales

Although physiological parameters can provide valuable information about a child's distress state, more research is required to develop a sensitive system for interpreting how these parameters reflect pain strength. At present, there are no valid physiological pain scales for children.

Most behavioural pain scales are checklists of the different distress behaviours that children exhibit when they experience a certain type of pain.[20,23,24] To develop these scales, trained health care providers carefully observe children when they are in pain (e.g. after surgery) and document any behaviours that seem caused by the pain. They then list these 'presumed pain' behaviours (e.g. crying, facial expression, limb rigidity) on an itemized checklist. Parents complete the pain scale by checking which of the listed behaviours they see when children are ill. On many scales, parents also rate the intensity of the behaviours. The intensity scores for each of the observed behaviours are summed to produce a composite pain score. Although most behavioural scales measure acute pain, recent attention is focused on the need to develop sensitive measures for children who are cognitively or physically impaired.[25]

The current behavioural scales may not be adequate for children receiving palliative care. The complexity of a child's disease or health condition, concomitant drug therapy, and the other distress sources in the health care environment, may limit children's ability to behave so that the pain score is not meaningful. Their pain behaviours may be very different from those of the children studied to develop the original scales. Moreover, the most salient pain behaviour might be very child-dependent and vary widely among different children or change throughout the course of their illness. At present, health care providers must use their content expertise and consult with parents to carefully consider which behaviour or behaviours are the most relevant indices of pain for a particular child. They can chart the presence and intensity of these behaviours (it is likely that these will be more subtle indices than on current standardized scales) and interpret them as an indirect measure of pain.

Psychological pain scales

Psychological or self-report pain scales directly capture an individual's subjective experience of pain. Interviews, questionnaires, adjective checklists, and numerous pain intensity scales are available for children, each with some evidence of validity and reliability.[20,26] Clinical interviews are ideally suited for learning about the sensory characteristics of pain, the aversive component, and contributing cognitive, behavioural, and emotional factors. Interviews should also include a simple rating scale to document pain strength. Children choose a level on the scale that best matches the strength of their own pain (i.e. a level on a number or thermometer scale, a number of objects, a mark on a visual analogue scale, a face from a series of faces varying in emotional expression, or a particular word from adjective lists). Pain intensity scales are easy to administer, requiring only a few seconds once children understand how to use them. Many of these scales yield pain scores on a 0–10 scale. Visual and coloured analogue scales are versatile for use with acute, recurrent, and chronic pain and provide a convenient and flexible pain measure for use in hospital and at home.

Health care providers must consider the age and cognitive ability of a child when selecting a pain scale. Most toddlers (approximately 2 years of age) can communicate the presence of pain, using words learned from their parents to describe the sensations they feel when they hurt themselves. They use concrete analogies to describe their perceptions. Gradually children learn to differentiate and describe three levels of pain intensity—'a little', 'some or medium', and 'a lot'. By the age of 5, most children can differentiate a wider range of pain intensities and many can use simple pain intensity scales.

Children's understanding and descriptions of pain naturally depend on their age, cognitive level, and previous pain experience. Children begin to understand pain through their own hurting experiences; they learn to describe the different characteristics of their pains (intensity, quality, duration, and location) in the same way that they learn specific words to describe different sounds, tastes, smells, and colours. Most children can communicate meaningful information about their pain. Gradually they develop an increasing ability to describe specific pain features—the quality (aching, burning, pounding, sharp), intensity (mild to severe), duration and frequency (a few seconds to years), location (from a diffuse location on their skin to more precise internal localization), and unpleasantness (mild annoyance to an intolerable discomfort). Children's understanding of pain and the language that they use to describe pain comes from the words and expressions used by their families and peers and from characters depicted in books, videos, and movies. (For a more extensive review of developmental factors in children's pain, see refs 1, 6, 27–31.)

Physicians should always ask children directly about their pain. Pain onset, location, frequency (if recurring), quality, intensity, accompanying physical symptoms, and pain related disability should be assessed as part of children's clinical examination. Health care providers should also assess relevant situational factors in order to modify their pain-exacerbating impact, especially the factors listed in Table 1.

Analgesic selection and administration

Pain control should include regular pain assessments, appropriate analgesics, and adjuvant analgesics administered at regular dosing intervals, adjunctive drug therapy for symptom and side-effects control, and non-drug therapies to modify the situational factors that can exacerbate pain and suffering. Analgesics include acetaminophen, non-steroidal anti-inflammatory drugs (NSAIDs), and opioids. Adjuvant analgesics include a variety of drugs with analgesic properties that were initially developed to treat other health problems, such as anticonvulsants and antidepressants. The use of adjuvant analgesics has become a cornerstone of pain control in paediatric palliative care. They are especially crucial when pain has a neuropathic component.

The guiding principles of analgesic administration are 'by the ladder', 'by the clock', 'by the child', and 'by the mouth'. 'By the ladder' refers to a three-step approach for selecting drugs according to their analgesic potency based on the child's pain level—acetaminophen to control mild pain, codeine to control moderate pain, and morphine for strong pain.[32] The ladder approach was based on our scientific understanding of how analgesics affect pain of nociceptive origins. If pain persists despite starting with the appropriate drug, recommended doses, and dosing schedule, move up the ladder and administer the next more potent analgesic. Even when children require opioid analgesics, they should continue to receive acetaminophen (and NSAIDs, if appropriate) as supplemental analgesics. The analgesic ladder approach is based on the premise that acetaminophen, codeine, and morphine should be available in all countries and that doctors and health care providers can relieve pain in the majority of children with a few drugs.

However, increasing attention is focusing on 'thinking beyond the ladder' in accordance with our improved understanding of pain of neuropathic origins.[33,34] Children should receive adjuvant analgesics to more specifically target neuropathic mechanisms. Regrettably, two of the main classes of adjuvant analgesics, antidepressants and anticonvulsants, have unfortunate names. Proper education of health care providers, parents, and children should lead to a wider acceptance and use of these medications for pain management. For example, amitriptyline may require 4–6 weeks to affect depression, but often requires only 1–2 weeks to affect pain. The newer classes of antidepressants, the selective serotonin reuptake inhibitors (SSRIs), may be beneficial to treat depression for a child with pain but have not been shown to be beneficial for pain management. The other main class of adjuvant analgesics are the anticonvulsants. The two principal medications used for this purpose in paediatrics are carbamazepine and gabapentin. With gabapentin, the main dose-limiting side-effect is sedation so that a slow titration to maximal dose is required. Because of its greater number of significant side-effects, the use of carbamazepine has decreased recently and the use of gabapentin has increased. We still await published studies to support the wide use of gabapentin.

NSAIDs are similar in potency to aspirin. NSAIDs are used primarily to treat inflammatory disorders and to lessen mild to moderate acute pain. They should be used with caution in patients with hepatic or renal impairment, compromised cardiac function, hypertension (since they may cause fluid retention, oedema), and a history of GI bleeding or ulcers. NSAIDs may also inhibit platelet aggregation and thus must be monitored closely in patients with prolonged bleeding times. Indications for NSAIDs are much narrower for children with cancer (due to the concern for bleeding problems) than for children with other painful conditions. Although acetaminophen should be considered the routine non-opioid analgesic for children with cancer, NSAIDs are effective for patients with bony metastases, who have adequate platelets.

Although the specific drugs and doses are determined by the needs of each child, general guidelines for drug therapies to control pain for children in palliative care have been developed through a Consensus Conference on the Management of Pain in Childhood Cancer, published as a supplement to *Pediatrics*,[35] in a monograph, *Cancer Pain Relief and Palliative Care for Children*,[14] and in clinical practice guidelines.[36–38] The drugs listed in this chapter are based on these sources and guidelines from our institution.[39] Recommended starting doses for analgesic medications to control children's disease-related pain are listed in Tables 3 and 4; starting doses for adjuvant analgesic medications to control pain, drug related side-effects, and other symptoms are listed in Table 5. (For further review of analgesics and adjuvant analgesics in children, see refs 34, 40–44.)

Children should receive analgesics at regular times, 'by the clock', to provide consistent pain relief and prevent breakthrough pain. The specific drug schedule (e.g. every 4 or 6 h) is based on the drug's duration of action and the child's pain severity. Although breakthrough pain episodes have been recognized as a problem in adult pain control, they may represent an even more serious problem for children. Unlike adults, who generally realize that they can demand more potent analgesic medications or demand more frequent dosing intervals, children have little control, little awareness of alternatives, and fear that their pain cannot be controlled. They may become progressively frightened, upset, and preoccupied with their symptoms. Thus, it is essential to establish and maintain a therapeutic window of pain relief for children.

Analgesic doses should be adjusted 'by the child'. There is no one dose that will be appropriate for all children with pain. The goal is to select a dose that prevents children from experiencing pain before they receive the next dose. It is essential to monitor the child's pain regularly and adjust analgesic doses as necessary to control the pain. The effective opioid dose to relieve pain varies widely among different children or in the same child at different times. Some children require massive opioid doses at frequent intervals to control their pain. If such large doses are necessary for effective pain control, and the side-effects can be managed by adjunctive medication so that children are comfortable, then the doses are appropriate. Children receiving opioids may develop altered sleep patterns so that they are awake at night, fearful and complaining about pain, and they sleep intermittently throughout the day. They should receive adequate analgesics at night with antidepressants or hypnotics as necessary to enable them to sleep throughout the night. To relieve severe ongoing pain, opioid doses should be increased steadily until comfort is achieved, unless the child experiences unacceptable side-effects such as somnolence or respiratory depression (Table 6).

'By the mouth' refers to the oral route of drug administration. Medication should be administered to children by the simplest and most effective route, usually by mouth. Since children are afraid of painful

Table 3 Non-opioid drugs for relieving cancer pain in children

Drug	Dosage	Comments
Acetaminophen	10–15 mg/kg PO, every 4–6 h	Lacks gastrointestinal and haematological side-effects; lacks anti-inflammatory effects (may mask infection-associated fever) Dose limit of 65 mg/kg/day or 4 g/day, whichever is less
Ibuprofen	5–10 mg/kg PO, every 6–8 h	Anti-inflammatory activity Use with caution in patients with hepatic or renal impairment, compromised cardiac function or hypertension (may cause flu retention, oedema), history of GI bleeding or ulcers, may inhibit platelet aggregation Dose limit of 40 mg/kg/day; max. dose of 2400 mg/day
Naproxen	10–20 mg/kg/day PO, divided every 12 h	Anti-inflammatory activity. Use with caution and monitor closely in patients with impaired renal function. Avoid in patients with severe renal impairment Dose limit of 1 g/day
Diclofenac	1 mg/kg PO, every 8–12 h	Anti-inflammatory activity. Similar GI, renal, and hepatic precautions as noted above for ibuprofen and naproxen Dose limit of 50 mg/dose

Note: Increasing the dose of non-opioids beyond the recommended therapeutic level produces a 'ceiling effect', in that there is no additional analgesia but there are major increases in toxicity and side-effects.

PO, by mouth; GI, gastrointestinal.

Table 4 Opioid analgesics: usual starting doses

Drug	Equianalgesic dose (parenteral)	Starting dose IV	IV : PO ratio	Starting dose PO/transdermal	Duration of action
Morphine	10 mg	Bolus dose = 0.05–0.1 mg/kg every 2–4 h Continuous infusion = 0.01–0.04 mg/kg/h	1 : 3	0.15–0.3 mg/kg/dose every 4 h	3–4 h
Hydromorphone	1.5 mg	0.015–0.02 mg/kg every 4 h	1 : 5	0.06 mg/kg every 3–4 h	2–4 h
Codeine	120 mg	Not recommended		1.0 mg/kg every 4 h (dose limit 1.5 mg/kg/dose)	3–4 h
Oxycodone	5–10 mg	Not recommended		0.1–0.2 mg/kg every 3–4 h	3–4 h
Meperidine[a]	75 mg	0.5–1.0 mg/kg every 3–4 h	1 : 4	1.0–2.0 mg/kg every 3–4 h (dose limit 150 mg)	1–3 h
Fentanyl[b]	100 μg	1–2 μg/kg/h as continuous infusion		25 μg patch	72 h (patch)
Controlled-release morphine[c,d]				0.6 mg/kg every 8 h or 0.9 mg/kg every 12 h	
Controlled-release hydromorphone[d]				0.18 mg/kg every 12 h	
Controlled-release codeine[d]				3 mg/kg every 12 h	
Controlled-release oxycodone[d]				0.3–0.6 mg/kg every 12 h	
Methadone	10 mg	0.1 mg/kg every 4–8 h	1 : 2	0.2 mg/kg every 4–8 h	12–50 h

Doses are for opioid naïve patients. For infants under 6 months, start at one-quarter to one-third the suggested dose and titrate to effect.

PO, by mouth; IV, intravenous.

Principles of opioid administration:

1. If inadequate pain relief and no toxicity at peak onset of opioid action, increase dose in 50% increments.
2. Avoid IM administration.
3. Whenever using continuous infusion, plan for hourly rescue doses with short onset opioids if needed. Rescue dose is usually 50–200% of continuous hourly dose. If greater than six rescues are necessary in 24-h period, increase daily infusion total by the total amount of rescues for previous 24 h ÷ 24. An alternative is to increase infusion by 50%.
4. To change opioids—because of incomplete cross-tolerance: if changing between opioids with short duration of action, start new opioid at 50% of equianalgesic dose. Titrate to effect. If changing between opioids from short to long duration of action (i.e. morphine to methadone), start at 25% of equianalgesic dose and titrate to effect.
5. To taper opioids—anyone on opioids over 1 week must be tapered to avoid withdrawal: taper by 50% for 2 days, and then decrease by 25% every 2 days. When dose is equianalgesic to an oral morphine dose of 0.6 mg/kg/day may be stopped. Some patients on opioids for prolonged periods, may require much slower weaning.

[a] Avoid use in renal impairment. Metabolite may cause seizures.

[b] Potentially highly toxic. Not for use in acute pain control.

[c] Use may be hampered by child's difficulty in swallowing large tablets.

[d] The widely equianalgesic doses in adults are used as guidelines in paediatric practice but have not been substantiated in children.

Table 5 Adjuvant analgesic drugs

Drug category	Drug, dosage	Indications	Comments
Antidepressants	Amitryptyline, 0.2–0.5 mg/kg PO. Titrate upward by 0.25 mg/kg every 2–3 days. Maintenance: 0.2–3.0 mg/kg Alternatives: nortriptyline, doxepin, imipramine, venlafaxine	Neuropathic pain (i.e. vincristine-induced, radiation plexopathy, tumour invasion, CRPS-1) Insomnia	Usually improved sleep and pain relief within 3–5 days Anticholinergic side-effects are dose-limiting. Use with caution for children with increased risk for cardiac dysfunction
Anticonvulsants	Carbamazepine, initial dosing: 10 mg/kg/day PO divided OD or BID. Maintenance: up to 20–30 mg/kg/day PO divided every 8 h. Increase dose gradually over 2–4 weeks Alternatives: phenytoin, clonazepam Gabapentin, 5 mg/kg/day PO. Titrate upward over 3–7 days. Maintenance: 15–50 mg/kg/day PO divided TID	Neuropathic pain, especially shooting, stabbing pain	Monitor for haematological, hepatic, and allergic reactions Side-effects: gastrointestinal upset, ataxia, dizziness, disorientation, somnolence
Sedatives, hypnotics, anxiolytics	Diazepam, 0.025–0.2 mg/kg PO every 6 h Lorazepam, 0.05 mg/kg/dose SL Midazolam, 0.5 mg/kg/dose PO administered 15–30 min prior to procedure; 0.05 mg/kg/dose IV for sedation	Acute anxiety, muscle spasm Premedication for painful procedures	Sedative effect may limit opioid use. Other side-effects include: depression and dependence with prolonged use
Antihistamines	Hydroxyzine, 0.5 mg/kg PO every 6 h Diphenhydramine, 0.5–1.0 mg/kg PO/IV every 6 h	Opioid-induced pruritus, anxiety, nausea	Sedative side-effects may be helpful
Psychostimulants	Dextroamphetamine, Methylphenidate, 0.1–0.2 mg/kg BID Escalate to 0.3–0.5 mg/kg as needed	Opioid-induced somnolence Potentiation of opioid analgesia	Side-effects include agitation, sleep disturbance, and anorexia Administer second dose in afternoon to avoid sleep disturbances
Corticosteroids	Prednisone, prednisolone, and dexamethasone dosage depends on clinical situation (i.e. dexamethasone initial dosing: 0.2 mg/kg IV. Dose limit 10 mg. Subsequent dose 0.3 mg/kg/day IV divided every 6 h)	Headache from increased intracranial pressure, spinal, or nerve compression; widespread metastases	Side-effects include oedema, dyspeptic symptoms, and occasional gastrointestinal bleeding

CRPS-1, complex regional pain syndrome, Type 1; PO, by mouth; IV, intravenous; SL, sublingual.

injections they may deny that they have pain or they may not request medication. When possible, children should receive medications through routes that do not cause additional pain. Although optimal analgesic administration for children requires flexibility in selecting routes according to children's needs, parenteral administration is often the most efficient route for providing direct and rapid pain relief. Since intravenous, intramuscular, and subcutaneous routes cause additional pain for children, serious efforts have been expended on developing more pain-free modes of administration that still provide relatively direct and rapid analgesia. Attention has focused on improving the effectiveness of oral routes. As an example, oral transmucosal fentanyl citrate (OTFC) provides rapid onset analgesia via a pleasant route for children with cancer receiving painful medical procedures. OTFC produces significant serum concentrations after 15–20 min.[45] Children aged 2–14 years have shown good cooperation and sedation when given OTFC as a premedication.[46,47] OTFC produced safe and effective analgesia for outpatient wound care in children and the taste was preferred to oral oxycodone.[48]

Many hospitals have restricted the use of intramuscular injections because they are painful and drug absorption is not reliable; they advocate the use of intravenous lines into which drugs can be administered directly without causing further pain. Topical anaesthetic creams should also be applied prior to the insertion of intravenous lines in children. The use of portacatheters has become the gold standard in paediatrics, particularly for children with cancer who require administration of multiple drugs at weekly intervals.

Continuous infusion has several advantages over intermittent subcutaneous, intramuscular, or intravenous routes. This method circumvents repetitive injections, prevents delays in analgesic drug administration, and provides continuous levels of pain control without children experiencing increased side-effects at peak level and pain breakthroughs at trough level. Continuous infusion should be considered when children have pain for which oral and intermittent parenteral opioids do not provide satisfactory pain control, when intractable vomiting prevents oral medications, when intravenous lines are not desirable, and when children would like to remain at home despite severe pain. Children receiving a continuous infusion should continue to receive 'rescue doses' to control breakthrough pain, as necessary. As outlined in Table 4, the rescue doses should be 50–200 per cent of the continuous infusion hourly dose. If children experience repeated breakthrough pain, the basal rate can be increased by 50 per cent or by the total amount of morphine administered through the rescue doses over a 24-h period (divided by 24 h).

Patient-controlled analgesia (PCA) enables children to administer analgesic doses according to their pain level. PCA provides children with a continuum of analgesia that is prompt, economical, not nurse dependent and a lower overall narcotic use.[49–54] It has a high degree of safety, allows for wide variability between patients and there is no delay in analgesic administration (for review, see ref. 49). It can now be regarded as a standard for the delivery of analgesia in children aged more than 5 years.[55] However, there are opposing views about the use of background infusions with PCA. Although they may improve efficacy, they may increase the occurrence of

Table 6 Opioid side-effects

Side-effect	Management
Respiratory depression	Reduction in opioid dose by 50%, titrate to maintain pain relief without respiratory depression
Respiratory arrest	Naloxone, titrate to effect with 0.01 mg/kg/dose IV/ETT increments or 0.1 mg/kg/dose IV/ETT, repeat PRN. Small frequent doses of diluted naloxone or naloxone drip preferable for patients on chronic opioid therapy to avoid severe, painful withdrawal syndrome. Repeated doses often required until opioid side-effect subsides
Drowsiness/sedation	Frequently subsides after a few days without dosage reduction; methylphenidate or dextroamphetamine (0.1 mg/kg administered twice daily, in the morning and mid-day so as not to interfere with night-time sleep). The dose can be escalated in increments of 0.05–0.1 mg/kg to a maximum of 10 mg/dose for dextroamphetamine and 20 mg/dose for methylphenidate
Constipation	Increased fluids and bulk, prophylactic laxatives as indicated
Nausea/vomiting	Administer an antiemetic (e.g. ondansetron, 0.1 mg/kg IV/PO every 8 h) Antihistamines (e.g. dimenhydrinate 0.5 mg/kg/dose every 4–6 h IV/PO) may be used. Pre-chemotherapy, Nabilone 0.5–1.0 mg PO and then every 12 h may also be used
Confusion, nightmares, hallucinations	Reassurance only, if symptoms mild. A reduced dosage of opioid or a change to a different opioid or add neuroleptic (e.g. haloperidol 0.1 mg/kg PO/IV every 8 h to a maximum of 30 mg/day)
Multifocal myoclonus; seizures	Generally occur only during extremely high dose therapy; reduction in opioid dose indicated if possible. Add a benzodiazepine (e.g. clonazepam 0.05 mg/kg/day divided BID or TID increasing by 0.05 mg/kg/day every 3 days PRN up to 0.2 mg/kg/day. Dose limit of 20 mg/day)
Urinary retention	Rule out bladder outlet obstruction, neurogenic bladder, and other precipitating drug (e.g. tricyclic antidepressant). Particularly common with epidural opioids. Change of opioid, route of administration, and dose may relieve symptom. Bethanechol or catheter may be required

IV, intravenous; PO, by mouth; ETT, endotracheal tube; PRN, as needed.

adverse effects such as nausea and respiratory depression. In a comparison of PCA with and without a background infusion for children having lower extremity surgery, the total morphine requirements were reduced in the PCA only group and the background infusion offered no advantage.[56] In another study comparing background infusion and PCA, children between 9 and 15 achieved better pain relief with PCA while children between 5 and 8 showed no difference.[57] Although data on the use of background infusions in combination with PCA for the paediatric palliative care patient is limited, our current standard is to add a background infusion to the PCA if the pain is not controlled adequately with PCA alone. The selection of opioid used in PCA is perhaps less critical than the appropriate selection of parameters such as bolus dose, lockout, and background infusion rate. The opioid choice may be based on adverse effect profile rather than efficacy. Clearly, patient controlled analgesia offers special advantages to children who have little control and who are extremely frightened about uncontrolled pain. PCA is as it states, patient controlled analgesia. When special circumstances require that alternate people administer the medication, we do allow both nurse and parent controlled analgesia. Under these circumstances, parents require our nurse educators to fully educate them on the use of PCA.

Fentanyl is a potent synthetic opioid, which like morphine binds to mu receptors. However, fentanyl is 75–100 times more potent than morphine. The intravenous preparation of fentanyl has been used extensively in children. A transdermal preparation of fentanyl was introduced in 1991 for use with chronic pain. This route provides a noninvasive but continuously controlled delivery system. Although limited data is available on transdermal fentanyl (TF) in children, its use is increasing for children with stable and chronic cancer pain. In a recent study, TF was well tolerated with effective pain relief in 11 of 13 children and provided an ideal approach for children where compliance with oral analgesics was problematic.[58] Children in palliative care were converted from oral morphine doses to TF; the investigators noted diminished side-effects and improved convenience with TF.[59] The majority of parents and investigators considered TF to be better than previous treatment. No serious adverse events were attributed to fentanyl, suggesting that TF was both effective and acceptable for children and their families. Similarly, no adverse effects were noted in a study of TF for children with pain due to sickle cell crisis.[60] This study showed a significant relationship between TF dose and fentanyl concentration; pain control with the use of TF was improved in seven of 10 patients in comparison to PCA alone. In a multicentre crossover study in adults, TF caused significantly less constipation and less daytime drowsiness in comparison to morphine, but greater sleep disturbance and shorter sleep duration.[61] Of those patients able to express a preference, significantly more preferred fentanyl patches. As with all opioids, fatal adult complications have been noted with the use of multiple transdermal patches.[62]

The use of regional techniques (epidural and spinal) for the administration of local anaesthetics and analgesics for children continues to be an integral part of pain control in children.[63] Experience from many centres suggests that these techniques can be extremely useful for children with advanced cancer with resulting pain that may be difficult to control by more conventional means. It is also feasible for children to receive epidural and spinal infusions at home on an extended basis.

When one undertakes the administration of potent analgesics and anaesthetics, whether by intravenous or a regional anaesthetic technique such as an epidural or spinal approach, appropriate monitoring must be paramount for the safety of our patients. This involves the education and training of staff; immediate availability of resuscitative drugs and equipment; and an accurate and timely pain record consisting of vitals signs, pain and sedation scores. A complete set of intravenous and epidural monitoring guidelines have been included in Table 7.

Dosing considerations for neonates and infants

Recent research on controlling pain in neonates has led to improved rational therapeutic regimens to provide safe and effective analgesia with a minimum of side-effects.[64–71] Neonates and infants require the same three categories of analgesic drugs as older children. However, the differences in pharmacokinetics and pharmacodynamics among neonates, pre-term infants, and full-term infants, warrant special dosing considerations for infants and close monitoring when they receive opioids. Acetaminophen can be safely administered to neonates and infants without concern for hepatotoxicity, when given for short courses at the recommended dose (10–15 mg/kg PO). The rate of absorption is slower in neonates and its plasma half-life prolonged, so peak serum concentrations are reached at approximately 60 min after an oral dose, and subsequent doses may be required after 6 h rather than 4 h. Acetaminophen does not cause respiratory depression and does not produce tolerance.

Table 7 Analgesia monitoring guidelines

Baseline assessment	
Obtain RR, HR, BP, O_2 saturation, sedation score, and pain score before administering a single or intermittent dose or initiating continuous infusion	
Intermittent intravenous administration	
RR, HR, BP, and sedation score every 5 min × 4, then every 30 min × 2, and then as per child's condition/pre-existing orders	
Pain score every 20–30 min	
Continuously monitor O_2 saturation only for children whose underlying condition predisposes them to respiratory depression	
Intravenous additive (to run over 15–20 min)	
RR, HR, BP, and sedation score every 10 min × 2, then every 30 min × 2, and then as per child's condition	
Pain score at completion of the flush, then every 30 min × 2, and then as per child's condition/pre-existing orders	
Continuously monitor O_2 saturation only for children whose underlying condition predisposes them to respiratory depression	
Continuous IV infusion/PCA	
RR, HR, BP, pain score, and sedation score every 1 h × 4, then RR and sedation score every 1 h, and then HR, BP, and pain score every 4 h	
Continuously monitor O_2 saturation and document reading every 1 h	
Intermittent epidural administration	
RR, HR, and BP every 5 min for the first 20 min following a bolus dose, and then RR and sedation score every 1 h	
HR, BP, pain score, and motor block score every 4 h	
Continuously monitor only for children whose underlying condition predisposes them to respiratory depression	
Continuous epidural infusion[a,b]	
RR, HR, BP, sedation score, pain score, and motor block score every 1 h × 4 h, then RR and sedation score every 1 h, and HR, BP, pain score, and motor block score every 4 h	
Continuously monitor O_2 saturation and document reading every 1 h	

[a] Opioids used with bupivacaine.

[b] After any change in drug dose, infusion rate or if transferred between patient care areas, return to assessments every 1 h for 4 h.

Continuous respiratory rate/apnoea monitoring may provide additional benefits for certain children who are receiving continuous opioid infusions by alerting the nurse to a decreasing respiratory rate. Respiratory rate monitoring is not, however, a substitute for frequent patient observation and vital sign monitoring

ECG monitoring is not routinely required, but may be ordered if the child's underlying condition predisposes them to ECG abnormalities.

Source: Adapted from 2001–2002 Drug Formulary, The Hospital for Sick Children, Toronto, Ontario.

Opioid analgesics are the mainstay of treatment for controlling severe pain in neonates. When compared to Table 4, the starting doses for opioid analgesics in infants under 6 months of age are one-quarter to one-third the suggested doses. As for children, the dosage and mode of administration of opioids needs to be titrated between the degree of analgesia required and a reasonable level of sedation. (Note: theoretically postulated long-term effects of opioid administration include the alteration of endogenous opioid receptor development but these effects are irrelevant in neonatal palliative care.) The drug clearance and the analgesic effects of morphine, fentanyl, sufentanil, and methadone for infants above the age of 6 months and children resemble those for young adults. Thus, the general clinical impression is that morphine and other opioids have a reasonable margin of safety and excellent efficacy for most children over 6 months of age with cancer pain. However, premature and term newborns show reduced clearance of most opioids. The widely observed sensitivity of new-borns to morphine is probably due to kinetic factors, including smaller volume of distribution, diminished clearance, immaturity of the blood–brain barrier, and increased sensitivity on a pharmacodynamic basis associated with the immaturity of ventilatory responses to hypoxaemia and hypercarbia. Therefore, opioids must be used more cautiously with infants under the age of 6 months and appropriate monitoring must be instituted. Proper dosing and careful monitoring will help minimize side-effects. Tolerance has significance only as a signal of receptor function or a potential indicator of withdrawal when therapy is discontinued.

Neonates who have pain severe enough to require opioids usually have an intravenous line in place. If a limited number of doses is needed and if intravenous access is not available, intramuscular or subcutaneous routes may be used occasionally in full term neonates. However, these routes are painful and not suitable for preterm neonates because of their sparse muscle mass and delicate skin. They are also not suitable for long-term pain management in term neonates because plasma levels and clinical effects are less controlled and difficult to titrate from intramuscular administrations. Similarly, intravenous doses may produce peak levels resulting in coma and respiratory depression with rapid decline in plasma levels, causing alternate periods of pain and analgesia. Thus, continuous intravenous infusion of opioids, producing constant blood levels and minimal fluctuations in analgesia, is the most effective route. The use of peripherally inserted central catheters (PICCs) has become standard practice for the neonate with difficult venous access or for the patient that may require access for a prolonged period. Anand et al. recommend a loading dose of 50 μg/kg followed by a continuous infusion of morphine at 10–20 μg/kg/h.[(64)] Further increases in the infusion rate may be required to titrate to clinical effect or with the development of tolerance. However, infants must be monitored carefully because most opioids have prolonged duration of action in neonates, so that continuous infusions can result in slow accumulation of the drug over time with high blood levels that may not be detected immediately.

The principal and potentially life-threatening side-effect of all opioid drugs is the dose-dependent respiratory depression leading to apnoea, which may be observed in infants and neonates at relatively low doses. This is advantageous in ventilated patients, but poses considerable challenges when using opioids for spontaneously breathing newborns. Opioid-induced respiratory depression can be reversed with naloxone, but the effect of the drug diminishes within 30 min so that repeated naloxone dosing may be required. If apnoea does occur, stimulation of the baby will usually elicit some respiratory effort temporarily while emergency arrangements are made to inject naloxone and provide respiratory support. Naloxone should be titrated to effect in increments of 10 μg/kg until a desired effect is obtained, or up to a total dose of 100 μg/kg. High doses of naloxone may produce a massive stress response from sudden nociception and withdrawal, or may result in undesirable fluid shifts. Following an effective dose of naloxone, the neonate should be monitored closely for at least 24 h. In fact, because plasma concentrations of morphine can increase in some neonates, even after an opioid infusion is discontinued, neonates require close monitoring for at least 24 h after morphine administration is discontinued.

Young infants, especially premature babies or those who have neurological abnormalities or pulmonary disease, are more susceptible to apnoea and respiratory depression when systemic opioids are used. The infants' metabolism is altered so that the elimination half-life is longer and there may be possible increased entry into the brain, due to immaturity of the blood–brain barrier. Both factors result in young infants having higher concentrations of opioids in the brain for a given dose than mature infants or adults. Thus, non-ventilated infants who are less than 1 year of age should be monitored closely when they receive opioids because extreme sedation and decreased respiratory effort may be difficult to assess. Institutions where neonates and infants are treated for cancer should train personnel in the safe and effective administration of analgesia and provide appropriate technologies for monitoring. Monitoring should include respiratory rate, heart rate, blood pressure, sedation score and pain score, as shown in Table 7.

Epidural analgesia is now widely used for infants with postoperative pain. The haemodynamic effects of major regional analgesia in infants with postoperative pain appear minimal. For paediatric epidural infusions, the standard local anaesthetic we use is bupivacaine in an infusion rate of 0.2–0.4 mg/kg/h. Epidural infusions that exceed the recommended rate may lead to convulsions. Epidural opioids such as morphine and fentanyl have been used successfully, even for very young infants with cancer. The proper use of infusions or intermittent doses of epidural opioids or local anaesthetics requires expertise and appropriate monitoring, as shown in Table 7.

Physical dependence, tolerance, and addiction

Physical dependence is defined as a state of adaptation that often includes tolerance and is manifested by a drug class specific withdrawal syndrome that can be produced by abrupt cessation, rapid dose reduction, decrease in the blood level of drug, and/or administration of an antagonist. Tolerance is a state of adaptation in which exposure to a drug induces changes that result in a diminution of one or more of the drug's effects over time. Addiction is a primary, chronic, neurobiological disease, with genetic, psychosocial, and environmental factors influencing its development and manifestations. It is characterized by behaviours that include one or more of the following four Cs: impaired Control over drug use, Compulsive use, continued use despite harm (Consequences), and Craving.[72]

The fear of opioid addiction in children has been greatly exaggerated. While physical dependence is common, gradual tapering protocols can control the withdrawal syndromes caused by an abrupt cessation of the medication. Physical dependence may develop in as short a period as 7–10 days. Tolerance is also an expected change to be seen and anticipated in children. There is no empirical evidence that children receiving opioid analgesics for pain control are at risk for addiction. In contrast, children who do not receive appropriate analgesic medications are probably more at risk for 'pseudoaddiction' by becoming excessively concerned about receiving their next medication dose in the hope that they might eventually relieve their suffering.

Parents, and occasionally staff, may have misconceptions about the use of potent opioids. Although the sensory characteristics of children's pain should be consistent with the known pattern from the presumed source of tissue injury, the source is not easily identified for all children. This is particularly true for children who have cancer, since there may be multiple sources of noxious stimulation due to disease and the effects of curative therapies. Yet, children's pain must be controlled, even when the specific aetiology is not yet determined. Otherwise, children become increasingly anxious, fearful, and distressed—beginning a cycle of increasing pain that will be more difficult to alleviate.

Parents are often anxious about opioids for their children, particularly when children require increased dose increments. Staff must educate parents that physical dependence and tolerance are very different from addiction. Parents will then understand that physical dependence and tolerance are normal drug effects; they do not mean that their children with pain have become addicted. Physical drug dependence is well recognized. When opioids are suddenly withdrawn, children may suffer from irritability, anxiety, insomnia, diaphoresis, rhinorrhoea, nausea, vomiting, abdominal cramps, and diarrhoea. These withdrawal symptoms can be prevented by the gradual tapering of an opioid. Even though children with severe pain require progressively higher and more frequent opioid doses due to drug tolerance, they should receive the doses they need to relieve their pain. However, children who require increased opioids to relieve previously controlled pain should be assessed carefully to determine whether the disease has progressed, since pain may be the first sign of advancing disease.

Therapists can use familiar analogies to explain dependence, tolerance, and addiction. For example parents are often accustomed to drinking coffee in the morning. They know that they will experience some noticeable effects without their usual caffeine intake, but they also know that they can withdraw from coffee by gradually lowering their daily consumption. The fact that their body is used to a certain amount of caffeine at certain times of the day means that they are dependent. Similarly, many people become accustomed to a certain level of salt for a food to taste 'salty'. After a while they may need to increase their salt intake if they want foods to taste the same, because their bodies have adjusted to or now tolerate the previous amount of salt so that it no longer has the same effect. In the same way, their children can become tolerant to a morphine dose so that they require a slightly higher dose to achieve the same pain reduction. These benign examples of a body's normal responses to substances often help parents understand that when opioids are prescribed for their children the effects of those drugs are well known, well understood, and will not lead to adverse effects, including addiction.

Opioid-related side-effects

The safe, rational use of opioid analgesics requires an understanding of their clinical pharmacology. The potent opioids that we use to treat children for palliative pain control have no fixed upper dosage limit. The dose can be increased as necessary to maximize pain control, as long as children do not experience dose-limiting side-effects (i.e. vomiting, respiratory depression). The goal should be titrating medication either up or down for maximum clinical effect. Side-effects must be anticipated and treated aggressively. Since opioids produce physical dependence and tolerance, doses must be increased over time to control pain. Doses must be adjusted according to the child's need depending on pain severity, prior analgesic medication use, and the bioavailability and drug distribution of the medication.

All opioids have a similar spectrum of side-effects. These well-known problems should be anticipated and treated whenever opioids are administered, so that children can receive pain control without suffering untoward effects. Children may not report all side-effects (i.e. constipation, dysphoria) voluntarily, so they should be asked specifically about these problems. Some side-effects may resolve within the first 1 or 2 weeks of initiating therapy as the child develops tolerance to them (e.g. nausea, vomiting, and drowsiness). The clinician must educate the patient about these problems and encourage them to give the medication an adequate trial. Slow titration may minimize this problem. Other side-effects may require aggressive treatment. If they persist despite appropriate interventions, conversion to an alternate opioid may be indicated. There is generally incomplete cross-tolerance between opioids, so that the guidelines for converting from one opioid to another is to begin at the lower dosing range, considering the presence or absence of central nervous system side-effects, and titrate upward. When used in therapeutic doses, opioids have not been demonstrated to cause long-term permanent organ toxicity. This makes them a safe choice for use in children. There is evidence that untreated severe chronic pain may cause cognitive impairment, which is improved with opioid therapy. The treatment of opioid side-effects is summarized in Table 6.

Non-drug therapies

Cognitive and behavioural approaches

An extensive array of non-drug therapies are available to treat children's pain, including counselling, guided imagery, hypnosis, biofeedback, behavioural management, acupuncture, massage, homeopathic remedies, naturopathic approaches, and herbal medicines. Non-drug therapies are generally regarded as safe, with few contra-indications for their use in otherwise healthy children. However, little is known about the safety and effectiveness of certain therapies for children in palliative care. In particular, almost no paediatric research has been conducted on many of the therapies regarded as complementary to traditional medical approaches. Thus, the efficacy of complementary therapies for treating children's pain is unknown, even though children are increasingly using complementary therapies.(73) In contrast, the evidence base supporting the efficacy of cognitive and behavioural approaches is strong.(4,5,14,74–85) These methods can mitigate some of the factors that intensify pain, distress, and disability for children in palliative care.

The primary cognitive and behavioural therapies are listed in Table 8. Cognitive therapies are directed at a child's beliefs, expectations, and coping abilities. They encompass a wide range of approaches from basic patient education to formal psychotherapy. Most children and families benefit from supportive counselling. Accurate information about what will happen and what children may feel should improve children's understanding, increase their control, lessen their distress, and reduce their pain.

In addition, health care providers can teach children how to use a few pain control methods to lessen pain and guide families to recognize the particular circumstances that exacerbate pain and distress. These methods provide children with some independent strategies—either to relieve mild pain or to complement the medication needed to relieve strong pain. Children should begin by learning a few basic methods. As they acquire confidence in using these methods, they seem to naturally adapt them to fit their personality or invent new equally effective methods. A therapist guides them throughout this process. Children should be interested and motivated in learning some independent pain control methods. They seem more adept than adults at using non-drug therapies, presumably because they are usually less biased than adults about their potential efficacy.

Distraction is a simple and effective pain control method. When children intently attend to something other than their pain, they can lessen its intensity and unpleasantness. Distraction is often incorrectly perceived as a simple diversionary tactic; the implication is that the pain is still there but the child is momentarily focused elsewhere. However, when children's attention is fully absorbed in some engaging topic or activity, distraction is a very active process that can reduce the neuronal responses to a noxious stimulus. Children do not simply ignore their pain, but are actually reducing it. The essential feature for achieving pain relief is a child's ability to attend fully to and concentrate on something else besides the pain. Therefore, the choice of a distraction is crucial and varies according to children's ages and interests. Young children usually need to be actively involved with their parents or peers, while older children and adolescents can distract themselves more independently. Children should work with their parents or a therapist to choose distracting activities that children can practically incorporate into their lives. Guided imagery is a specific method of distraction and attention. A health care provider guides children to concentrate fully on the image of an experience or situation. Children recall and vividly describe what they experienced—the colours, sounds, tastes, and feel of the situation. Children are guided to become as immersed in their image as if it were occurring in the present situation.

Table 8 Cognitive and behavioural therapies

Cognitive
Information
Choices and control
Supportive counselling
Counselling
Stress management
Attention and distraction
Guided imagery
Hypnosis
Behavioural
Simple exercise
Participation in activities
Desensitization training
Relaxation training
Biofeedback
Behavioural modification

There is considerable overlap among the interventions of attention/distraction, guided imagery, and hypnosis. Hypnosis usually begins with an induction procedure in which a child's full attention is focused gradually on the therapist and his/her suggestions. The therapist guides the child into a very relaxed physical and mental state, an altered level of consciousness—distinct from an alert or sleep state. The induction procedure typically includes guided imagery for children and progressive muscle relaxation for adolescents. The induction can be very simple for young children. They can be guided into a hypnotic state as they vividly imagine their favourite television shows, movies, books, or cartoon characters.(86–88) As they imagine an activity, scene or character, they gradually receive suggestions for relaxation, reduced anxiety, increased control, and pain reduction. The therapist provides consistent positive suggestions, rather than authoritative commands. The emphasis is on the child's own natural abilities, as in 'Notice that your back, legs (painful body areas) feels lighter, the heaviness and pain are starting to lessen. It seems as if your back doesn't hurt as much as before. You are doing well at turning down the pain switch'.

During a hypnotic state, individuals become extremely susceptible to suggestions, including suggestions for pain relief. Children become so involved in thoughts or ideas that they dissociate from a 'reality orientation'.(87) Hypnosis enables children to re-direct attention from the painful sensation or to reinterpret the sensation as something more pleasant/less aversive and/or less bothersome.(88) Like adults, children differ in their ability to be hypnotized. Children's ability to use their imagination is the key component in determining their hypnotic susceptibility.

Behaviour therapy is often used in combination with cognitive therapy. The goals are to lessen the specific behaviours (i.e. child, family, and staff) that may increase pain, distress, or disability, while concomitantly increasing healthy behaviours that engage children in living as fully as possible. Relaxation training is a common method used for children with chronic pain. Therapists train children how to achieve a state of mental and physical relaxation so that children can eventually relax independently when they experience pain or feel stressed and fearful about their condition. Therapists may use guided imagery, hypnosis, deep breathing, or progressive relaxation exercises to train children. Biofeedback is a useful tool for teaching children to recognize when their bodies are relaxed. Surface electrodes, attached to the skin or specific muscle groups, transform the electrical activity of the body into easily observable signals.

Pain control methods

Health professionals and parents can relieve children's pain, not only by administering analgesic drugs, but also by increasing their understanding and control, decreasing their emotional distress, and teaching them some simple methods to reduce their pain and anxiety. In addition to providing support and reassurance, parents can help children to understand what will happen, make choices, gain whatever control is possible within the setting, and independently use pain reducing methods. Thus, the family, as well as health professionals, share a fundamental role in managing their children's cancer pain. The key concept underlying the use of all analgesic and non-analgesic therapies for children is 'by the child', as described above.

Specific pain control methods that require the child to concentrate and focus attention should always be used for children with cancer pain. Beales noted critical differences between adults and children in their perceptions of pain, especially cancer pain.(89) Children's cancer pain seemed even less positively correlated with pathology than adults' cancer pain. Beales suggested that some of the psychological mechanisms involved in pain perception may be manipulated more easily in children than in adults, consistent with our clinical observations that children's cancer pain is more plastic than that of adults.[1,82] Children seem to possess an enhanced ability to absorb themselves completely in a task, game, or imagined event and thus, might be more able than adults to trigger endogenous pain-inhibitory mechanisms. Even very young children can easily learn to use a variety of practical pain control methods. The goals of therapy are to enable children to understand what is happening and to have something that they can actively do to lessen their anxiety, distress, and pain.

The specific methods selected depend on the age of the child, the type of pain experienced, and the resources available. Simple methods such as deep breathing, blowing bubbles, alternately tightening and relaxing their fists, squeezing their mother's hand, listening to stories or music, and imagining that they are in a pleasant setting can be very effective for reducing procedural-related pain, when used with appropriate analgesics. When possible, children should learn a few basic methods to reduce their pain and distress. They should not be encouraged to develop a false reliance on the magical benefits of any one method. Instead, they should understand that these practical methods relieve pain because they change the factors that usually increase pain and they help to restore normal sensory input.

All children should learn that pain from some procedures is generally less when they are able to choose the site and rub the area before and after the injection or finger prick. They should learn that pain is less when they are very relaxed. Progressive muscle relaxation with simple exercises in which they tense and relax their body limbs, and biofeedback can help to show them that any type of pain can be intensified if the muscles are always tightened. Children should learn that fear and anxiety can make them tense and increase pain. Then, they need practical tools to alleviate their fear about the cancer or their anxiety towards necessary treatments. Children and families must learn that what they think, how they behave, and how they feel affects their children's pain. Then they can begin to work independently and with staff to create additional non-drug pain control methods based on the child's interest, the cultural setting, and the availability of resources. Specific interventions should be selected and administered to children as part of a comprehensive pain programme, in the same manner as the most appropriate analgesics are selected and administered in adequate doses, at regular dosing intervals, through the most efficient routes.

Summary

Optimal pain control for children in palliative care requires an integrated treatment plan with both drug and non-drug therapies. However, the specific interventions must be selected after determination of the primary and secondary sources of noxious stimulation and after a thorough assessment of the unique situational, behavioural, emotional, and familial factors which affect a child's pain. It is impossible to adequately relieve children's pain from a unidimensional perspective, in which pain is considered as synonymous with the nature and extent of tissue damage. Childhood pain must be viewed from a multidimensional perspective because multiple sensory, environmental, and emotional factors are responsible for the pain—no matter how seemingly clear cut an aetiology. Treatment begins with a thorough assessment of these multiple factors, using structured interviews and standardized measures. Pharmacological, physical, and psychological strategies must be incorporated into a flexible intervention programme for children, in which parents and siblings form an essential component of treatment.

All analgesics should be selected 'by the ladder' and administered 'by the clock', 'by the child', and in an effective and painless route. Dosing intervals should be frequent enough to adequately control pain, so that children do not experience an alternating cycle of pain, drowsy analgesia, pain, etc. Children should also learn some simple pain control strategies so that they can reduce acute pain caused by invasive treatments and disease or therapy related pain. Adjuvant medications should be administered to control aversive symptoms and side-effects. Non-drug therapies should also be used to control pain.

Special problems in pain control may arise when children die at home, unless parents and medical and nursing teams communicate openly about the availability of potent analgesics and the flexibility of dosing routes and regimens. Parents may be unduly anxious because even small children, like adults with cancer, may require larger opioid doses at more frequent intervals. Parents' fears can lead them to deny the extent to which their children are in pain or children may fail to report pain because they do not want to further distress parents or because they fear injections.

Multiple sources of noxious stimulation are usually responsible for pain in dying children, as the disease progressively affects many systems. Increased disability, toxic side-effects of medication, physical impairment, and the emotional adjustment of children and their families can intensify pain and suffering. Like adults, children's pain affects the entire family and must be viewed within a broader context. Effective pain control is possible when the goals are to reduce or block nociceptive activity by attenuating responses in peripheral afferents and central pathways, activate endogenous pain inhibitory systems, and modify situational factors that exacerbate pain. Thus, the choice for pain control is not merely 'drug versus non-drug therapy', but rather a therapy that mitigates both the causative and contributing factors for pain. Pain management is a continuous dynamic process, since the disease state and factors that influence pain are not static. Different combinations of drug and non-drug therapies will be required at different times. Thus, health professionals must continually assume as much responsibility for monitoring and relieving children's pain as for medically managing their diseases. Children should not suffer. We have the knowledge to ensure that children receive adequate pain control, from the time they are diagnosed to their death. Parents' memories of their children should not be marred by memories that they experienced unrelieved pain.

Acknowledgement

We would like to acknowledge Shue Lin Loo for her excellent assistance in the preparation of this chapter.

References

1. **McGrath, P.A.** *Pain in Children: Nature, Assessment and Treatment.* New York: Guilford Publications, 1990.
2. **Price, D.D.** *Psychological Mechanisms of Pain and Analgesia.* Seattle WA: IASP Press, 1999.
3. **Casey, K.L. and Bushnell, M.C.**, ed. *Pain Imaging.* Seattle WA: IASP Press, 2000.
4. **McGrath, P.A. and Hillier, L.M.** (2003). Modifying the psychologic factors that intensify children's pain and prolong disability. In *Pain in Infants, Children and Adolescents* 2nd edn. (ed. N.L. Schechter, C.B. Berde, and M. Yaster), pp. 85–104. Baltimore MD: Lippincott Williams and Wilkins.
5. **Schechter, N.L., Berde, C.B., and Yaster, M.**, ed. *Pain in Infants, Children and Adolescents* 2nd edn. Baltimore MD: Lippincott Williams and Wilkins, 2002.
6. **Ross, D.M. and Ross, S.A.** *Childhood Pain: Current Issues, Research, and Management.* Baltimore MD: Urban and Schwarzenberg, 1988.
7. **McGrath, P.A. and deVeber, L.L.** (1986). The management of acute pain evoked by medical procedures in children with cancer. *Journal of Pain and Symptom Management* **1**, 145–50.
8. **Chafee, S.** (2001). Pediatric palliative care. *Primary Care* **28**, 365–90.
9. **American Academy of Pediatrics, Committee on Bioethics and Committee on Hospice Care** (2000). Palliative care for children. *Pediatrics* **106**, 351–7.
10. **Goldman, A.** (1998). ABC of palliative care: special problems of children. *British Medical Journal* **316**, 49–52.
11. **Goldman, A.**, ed. *Care of the Dying Child.* Oxford: Oxford University Press, 1994.
12. **Goldman, A., Frager, G., and Pomietto, M.** (2003). Pain and palliative care. In *Pain in Infants, Children and Adolescents* 2nd edn. (ed. N.L. Schechter,

C.B. Berde, and M. Yaster), pp. 539–63. Baltimore MD: Lippincott Williams and Wilkins.

13. **Frager, G.** (1997). Palliative care and terminal care of children. *Child and Adolescent Psychiatric Clinics of North America* **6**, 889–90.

14. **World Health Organization.** *Cancer Pain Relief and Palliative Care in Children.* Geneva: World Health Organization, 1998.

15. **Howell, D.A. and Martinson, I.M.** (1993). Management of the dying child. In *Principles and Practice of Pediatric Oncology* 2nd edn. (ed. P.A. Pizzo and D.G. Poplack), pp. 1115–24. Philadelphia PA: JB Lippincott.

16. **Davies, B. and Howell, D.** (1998). Special services for children. In *Oxford Textbook of Palliative Medicine* 2nd edn. (ed. D. Doyle, G.W.C. Hanks, and N. MacDonald), pp. 1078–84. Oxford: Oxford University Press.

17. **Sourkes, B.M.** (1996). The broken heart: anticipatory grief in the child facing death. *Journal of Palliative Care* **12**, 56–9.

18. **Stevens, M.M.** (1998). Care of the dying child and adolescent: family adjustment and support. In *Oxford Textbook of Palliative Medicine* 2nd edn. (ed. D. Doyle, G.W.C. Hanks, and N. MacDonald), pp. 1057–75. Oxford: Oxford University Press.

19. **Stevens, M.M.** (1998). Psychological adaptation of the dying child. In *Oxford Textbook of Palliative Medicine* 2nd edn. (ed. D. Doyle, G.W.C. Hanks, and N. MacDonald), pp. 1045–56. Oxford: Oxford University Press.

20. **McGrath, P.A. and Gillespie, J.** (2001). Pain assessment in children and adolescents. In *Handbook of Pain Assessment* 2nd edn. (ed. D.C. Turk and R. Melzack), pp. 97–118. New York: Guilford Press.

21. **Finley, G.A. and McGrath, P.J.**, ed. *Measurement of Pain in Infants and Children.* Seattle WA: IASP Press, 1998.

22. **Royal College of Nursing Institute.** *Clinical Guideline for the Recognition and Assessment of Acute Pain in Children: Recommendations.* London: Royal College of Nursing Institute, 1999.

23. **McGrath, P.J.** (1998). Behavioral measures of pain. In *Measurement of Pain in Infants and Children* (ed. G.A. Finley and P.J. McGrath), pp. 83–102. Seattle WA: IASP Press.

24. **Sweet, S.D. and McGrath, P.J.** (1998). Physiological measures of pain. In *Measurement of Pain in Infants and Children* (ed. G.A. Finley and P.J. McGrath), pp. 59–81. Seattle WA: IASP Press.

25. **Hunt, A.M., Goldman, A., Mastroyannopoulou, K., and Seers, K.** Identification of pain cues of children with severe neurological impairment. *Proceedings of the 9th World Congress on Pain.* Seattle WA: IASP Press, 1999, Abstract 84.

26. **Champion, G.D., Goodenough, B., von Baeyer, C.L., and Thomas, W.** (1998). Measurement of pain by self-report. In *Measurement of Pain in Infants and Children* (ed. G.A. Finley and P.J. McGrath), pp. 123–60. Seattle WA: IASP Press.

27. **Bush, J.P. and Harkins, S.W.**, ed. *Children in Pain: Clinical and Research Issues from a Developmental Perspective.* New York: Springer-Verlag, 1991.

28. **Gaffney, A., McGrath, P.J., and Dick, B.** (2003). Measuring pain in children: developmental and instrumental issues. In *Pain in Infants, Children and Adolescents* 2nd edn. (ed. N.L. Schechter, C.B. Berde, and M. Yaster), pp. 128–42. Baltimore MD: Lippincott Williams and Wilkins.

29. **McGrath, P.J. and Unruh, A.** *Pain in Children and Adolescents.* Amsterdam: Elsevier, 1987.

30. **Peterson, L., Harbeck, C., Farmer, J., and Zink, M.** (1991). Developmental contributions to the assessment of children's pain: conceptual and methodological implications. In *Children in Pain: Clinical and Research Issues from a Developmental Perspective* (ed. J.P. Bush and S.W. Harkins), pp. 33–58. New York: Springer-Verlag.

31. **Pichard-Leandri, E. and Gauvain-Piquard, A.**, ed. *La Douleur Chez l'Enfant.* Paris: Medsi/McGraw-Hill, 1989.

32. **World Health Organization.** *Cancer Pain Relief and Palliative Care.* Geneva: World Health Organization, 1990.

33. **Staats, P.S.** (1998). Cancer pain: beyond the ladder. *Journal of Back and Musculoskeletal Rehabilitation* **10**, 67–80.

34. **Galloway, K.S. and Yaster, M.** (2000). Pain and symptom control in terminally ill children. *Pediatric Clinics of North America* **47**, 711–46.

35. **Schechter, N.L., Altman, A., and Weisman, S.** (1990). Report of the Consensus Conference on the Management of Pain in Childhood Cancer. *Pediatrics* **86** (5 Pt 2), 826–31.

36. **Acute Pain Management Guideline Panel.** *Clinical Practice Guideline: Acute Pain Management in Infants, Children and Adolescents: Operative and Medical Procedures.* Rockville MD: Agency for Health Care Policy and Research, 1992.

37. **Consensus Panel.** *Pediatric Pain and Symptom Algorithms for Palliative Care.* Seattle WA: Children's Hospital, 1999.

38. **Jacox, A.** et al. *Management of Cancer Pain. Clinical Practice Guideline.* Rockville MD: Agency for Health Care Policy and Research, US Department of Health and Human Services, Public Health Service, 1994.

39. **The Hospital for Sick Children.** *Drug Formulary 2001–2002.* Toronto: The Hospital for Sick Children, 2002.

40. **Collins, J.J. and Weisman, S.J.** (2003). Management of pain in childhood cancer. In *Pain in Infants, Children, and Adolescents* 2nd edn. (ed. N.L. Schechter, C.B. Berde, and M. Yaster), pp. 517–39. Baltimore MD: Lippincott Williams and Wilkins.

41. **Krane, E.J., Leong, M.S., Golianu, B., and Leong, Y.Y.** (2003). Treatment of pediatric pain with nonconventional analgesics. In *Pain in Infants, Children, and Adolescents* 2nd edn. (ed. N.L. Schechter, C.B. Berde, and M. Yaster), pp. 225–41. Baltimore MD: Lippincott Williams and Wilkins.

42. **Maunuksela, E.L. and Olkkola, K.T.** (2003). Nonsteroidal anti-inflammatory drugs in pediatric pain management. In *Pain in Infants, Children, and Adolescents* 2nd edn. (ed. N.L. Schechter, C.B. Berde, and M. Yaster), pp. 171–81. Baltimore MD: Lippincott Williams and Wilkins.

43. **Yaster, M., Kost-Byerly, S., and Maxwell, L.G.** (2003). Opioid agonists and antagonists. In *Pain in Infants, Children, and Adolescents* 2nd edn. (ed. N.L. Schechter, C.B. Berde, and M. Yaster), pp. 181–225. Baltimore MD: Lippincott Williams and Wilkins.

44. **Yaster, M., Tobin, J.R., and Kost-Byerly, S.** (2003). Local anesthetics. In *Pain in Infants, Children, and Adolescents* 2nd edn. (ed. N.L. Schechter, C.B. Berde, and M. Yaster), pp. 241–65. Baltimore MD: Lippincott Williams and Wilkins.

45. **Schutzman, S.A., Liebelt, E., Wisk, M., and Burg, J.** (1996). Comparison of oral transmucosal fentanyl citrate and intramuscular meperidine, promethazine and chlorpromazine for conscious sedation of children undergoing laceration repair. *Annals of Emergency Medicine* **28**, 385–90.

46. **Dsida, R.M., Avram, M.J., Enders-Klein, C., Maddalozzo, J., and Cote, C.J.** (1998). Premedication of pediatric tonsillectomy patients with oral transmucosal fentanyl citrate. *Anesthesia and Analgesia* **86**, 66–70.

47. **Malviya, S., Voepel-Lewis, T., Huntington, J., Siewert, M., and Green, W.** (1997). Effects of anesthetic technique on side effects associated with fentanyl Oralet premedication. *Journal of Clinical Anesthesia* **9**, 374–8.

48. **Sharar, S.R., Carrougher, G.J., Selzer, K., O'Donnell, F., Vavilala, M.S., and Lee, L.A.** (2002). A comparison of oral transmucosal fentanyl citrate and oral oxycodone for pediatric outpatient wound care. *Journal of Burn Care Rehabilitation* **23**, 27–31.

49. **Gaukroger, P.B.** (1993). Patient-controlled analgesia in children. In *Pain in Infants, Children, and Adolescents* (ed. N.L. Schechter, C.B. Berde, and M. Yaster), pp. 203–12. Baltimore MD: Williams and Wilkins.

50. **Hill, H.F., Chapman, C.R., Kornell, J.A., Sullivan, K.M., Saeger, L.C., and Bendetti, C.** (1990). Self-administration of morphine in bone marrow transplant patients reduces drug requirement. *Pain* **40**, 121–9.

51. **Rodgers, B.M., Webb, C.J., Stergios, D., and Newman, B.M.** (1988). Patient-controlled analgesia in pediatric surgery. *Journal of Pediatric Surgery* **23**, 259–62.

52. **Shapiro, B., Cohen, D., and Howe, C.** (1991). Use of patient-controlled analgesia for patients with sickle cell disease. *Journal of Pain and Symptom Management* **6**, 176.

53. **Tahmooressi, J., Schmalzle, S., and Tobin, J.** (1991). Patient-controlled analgesia in the adolescent undergoing Cotrel-Dubosset Rod. *Journal of Pain and Symptom Management* **6**, 160.

54. **Webb, C.J., Paarlberg, J.M., and Sussman, M.** (1991). The use of a PCA device by parents or nurses for postoperative pain in children with cerebral palsy. *Journal of Pain and Symptom Management* **6**, 160.

55. **McDonald, A.J. and Cooper, M.G.** (2001). Patient-controlled analgesia: an appropriate method of pain control in children. *Paediatric Drugs* **3**, 273–84.

56. **McNeely, J.K. and Trentadue, N.C.** (1997). Comparison of patient-controlled analgesia with and without nighttime morphine infusion following

lower extremity surgery in children. *Journal of Pain and Symptom Management* **13**, 268–73.

57. **Bray, R.J., Woodhams, A.M., Vallis, C.J., Kelly, P.J., and Ward-Platt, M.P.** (1996). A double-blind comparison of morphine infusion and patient controlled analgesia in children. *Paediatric Anesthesia* **6**, 121–7.
58. **Noyes, M. and Irving, H.** (2001). The use of transdermal fentanyl in pediatric palliative care. *American Journal of Hospice and Palliative Care* **18**, 411–16.
59. **Hunt, A., Goldman, A., Devine, T., and Phillips, M.** (2001). Transdermal fentanyl for pain relief in a paediatric palliative care population. *Palliative Medicine* **15**, 405–12.
60. **Christensen, M.L., Wang, W.C., Harris, S., Eades, S.K., and Wilimas, J.A.** (1996). Transdermal fentanyl administration in children and adolescents with sickle cell pain crisis. *Journal of Pediatric Haematology and Oncology* **18**, 372–6.
61. **Ahmedzai, S. and Brooks, D.** (1997). Transdermal fentanyl versus sustained-release oral morphine in cancer pain: preference, efficacy, and quality of life. The TTS-Fentanyl Comparative Trial. *Journal of Pain and Symptom Management* **13**, 254–61.
62. **Edinboro, L.E., Poklis, A., Trautman, D., Lowry, S., Backer, R., and Harvey, C.M.** (1997). Fatal fentanyl intoxication following excessive transdermal application. *Journal of Forensic Science* **42**, 741–3.
63. **Wilder, R.T.** (2003). Regional anesthetic techniques for chronic pain management in children. In *Pain in Infants, Children and Adolescents* 2nd edn. (ed. N.L. Schechter, C.B. Berde, and M. Yaster), pp. 396–417. Baltimore MD: Lippincott Williams and Wilkins.
64. **Anand, K.J.S., Shapiro, B.S., and Berde, C.B.** (1993). Pharmacotherapy with systemic analgesics. In *Pain in Neonates* (ed. K.J.S. Anand and P.J. McGrath), pp. 155–98. New York: Elsevier.
65. **Anand, K.J.S. and McGrath, P.J.**, ed. *Pain in Neonates.* New York: Elsevier, 1993.
66. **Fitzgerald, M. and Howard, R.** (2003). The neurological basis of pediatric pain. In *Pain in Infants, Children, and Adolescents* 2nd edn. (ed. N.L. Schechter, C.B. Berde, and M. Yaster), pp. 19–43. Baltimore MD: Lippincott Williams and Wilkins.
67. **Franck, L.S. and Gregory, G.A.** (1993). Clinical evaluation and treatment of infant pain in the neonatal intensive care unit. In *Pain in Infants, Children, and Adolescents* (ed. N.L. Schechter, C.B. Berde, and M. Yaster), pp. 519–36. Baltimore MD: Williams and Wilkins.
68. **Greeley, W.J., Boyd, J.L.I., and Kern, F.H.** (1993). Pharmacokinetics of analgesic drugs. In *Pain in Neonates* (ed. K.J.S. Anand and P.J. McGrath), pp. 107–54. Amsterdam: Elsevier.
69. **Koren, G., Butt, W., Chinyanga, H., Soldin, S., Tan, Y.K., and Pape, K.** (1985). Postoperative morphine infusion in newborn infants: assessment of disposition characteristics and safety. *Journal of Pediatrics* **107**, 963–7.
70. **Collins, C., Koren, G., Crean, P., Klein, J., Roy, W.L., and MacLeod, S.M.** (1985). Fentanyl pharmacokinetics and hemodynamic effects in preterm infants during ligation of patent ductus arteriosus. *Anesthesia and Analgesia* **64**, 1078–80.
71. **Lynn, S.M. and Slattery, J.T.** (1987). Morphine pharmacokinetics in early infancy. *Anesthesiology* **66**, 136–9.
72. **Joney, R.D.** *Managing Pain: The Canadian Health Care Professional's Reference.* Healthcare and Financial Publishing, Rogers Media, 2002, pp. 64–6.
73. **Spigelblatt, L., Laine-Ammara, G., Pless, I.B., and Guyver, A.** (1994). The use of alternative medicine by children. *Pediatrics* **94**, 811–14.
74. **Dahlquist, L.M., Gil, K.M., Armstrong, F.D., Ginsberg, A., and Jones, B.** (1985). Behavioural management of children's distress during chemotherapy. *Journal of Behavioural Therapy and Experimental Psychiatry* **16**, 325–9.
75. **Dash, J.** (1980). Hypnosis for symptom amelioration. In *Psychological Aspects of Childhood Cancer* (ed. J. Kellerman), pp. 215–30. Springfield IL: Charles C. Thomas.
76. **Hartman, G.A.** (1981). Hypnosis as an adjuvant in the treatment of childhood cancer. In *Living with Childhood Cancer* (ed. J.J. Spinetta and P. Deasy-Spinetta), pp. 143–52. Toronto: CV Mosby Co.
77. **Hilgard, J.R. and LeBaron, S.** (1982). Relief of anxiety and pain in children and adolescents with cancer: quantitative measures and clinical observations. *International Journal of Clinical Experimental Hypnosis* **30**, 417–42.
78. **Hilgard, J.R. and LeBaron, S.** *Hypnotherapy of Pain in Children with Cancer.* Los Altos CA: William Kaufman, 1984.
79. **Jay, S.M., Elliott, C.H., Ozolins, M., Olson, R.A., and Pruitt, S.D.** (1985). Behavioural management of children's distress during painful medical procedures. *Behaviour Research and Therapy* **23**, 513–52.
80. **Katz, E.R., Kellerman, J., and Ellenberg, L.** (1987). Hypnosis in the reduction of acute pain and distress in children with cancer. *Journal of Pediatric Psychology* **12**, 379–94.
81. **LaBaw, W.L., Holton, C., Tewell, K., and Eccles, D.** (1975). The use of self-hypnosis by children with cancer. *American Journal of Clinical Hypnosis* **17**, 233–8.
82. **McGrath, P.A. and Hillier, L.M.** (2002). A practical cognitive–behavioral approach for controlling children's pain. In *Psychological Approaches to Pain Management* 2nd edn. (ed. D.C. Turk and R. Gatchel), pp. 534–52. New York: Guilford Press.
83. **Olness, K.** (1981). Imagery (self-hypnosis) as adjunct therapy in childhood cancer: clinical experience with 25 patients. *American Journal of Pediatric Hematology/Oncology* **3**, 313–21.
84. **Olness, K.** (1981). Hypnosis in pediatric practice. *Current Problems in Pediatrics* **12**, 1–47.
85. **Zeltzer, L. and LeBaron, S.** (1982). Hypnosis and nonhypnotic techniques for reduction of pain and anxiety during painful procedures in children and adolescents with cancer. *Journal of Pediatrics* **101**, 1032–5.
86. **Hall, H.** (1999). Hypnosis and pediatrics. In *Medical Hypnosis: An Introduction and Clinical Guide* (ed. R. Tennes), pp. 79–93. New York: Churchill Livingstone.
87. **LeBaron, S. and Zeltzer, L.K.** (1996). Children in pain. In *Hypnosis and Suggestion in the Treatment of Pain* (ed. J. Barber), pp. 305–40. New York: Norton.
88. **Olness, K. and Kohen, D.P.** *Hypnosis and Hypnotherapy with Children.* New York: Guilford Press, 1996.
89. **Beales, J.G.** (1979). Pain in children with cancer. In *Advances in Pain Research and Therapy* (ed. J.J. Bonica and V. Ventafridda), pp. 89–98. New York: Raven Press.

9.2 Symptom control in life-threatening illness

John J. Collins

Introduction

Dying children are often highly symptomatic and their symptom burden may increase with time, especially when the terminal phase is reached. This symptom burden consists of a matrix composed of physical, psychological, spiritual, and other factors. Although the entire matrix needs to be considered in the symptom assessment of the dying child, the reader is referred to the other sections that cover the psychological and cognitive, social, spiritual, and existential domains of caring for a dying child.

Physical symptoms may be caused by either the underlying illness, side-effects related to medical interventions and treatment, or to causes unrelated to either the primary disease or its treatment. The assessment and diagnosis of symptoms is fundamental to the clinical care of dying children. Palliative therapeutics should generally only be implemented once the underlying causative mechanisms have been established, since therapies directed at the primary cause may ultimately have a more effective outcome for symptom management.

Clinical assessment of symptoms is complemented by symptom measurement. Measurement refers to the application of some metric to a specific element of a symptom. The measurement of symptoms in children often utilizes formal scales that assess symptom intensity or frequency. Intensity is the most frequently measured dimension of pain, for example, and is often the dimension measured clinically to monitor success or otherwise of analgesic prescription.

Current status of symptom measurement in children with life-threatening illness

The progress in symptom control in adults receiving palliative care does not have a parallel experience in children. This is due, in part, to the paucity of symptom measures in children and explains the reliance of best practice in paediatric palliative care on the best evidence in adult palliative care. Most of the validated symptom assessment tools in paediatrics have focused on two common symptoms, pain and nausea. In contrast to instruments measuring nausea and vomiting, instruments measuring pain in children have largely been validated in predominantly the non-cancer setting. Few multidimensional symptom assessment scales exist for children. Systematic symptom assessment may be useful in assessing symptom burden as part of decision making towards palliative care and in future epidemiological studies of symptoms in dying children.

Instruments for the assessment of pain

Unidimensional self-report measures

Self-report measures of pain in children have largely focused on the assessment of pain severity. Generally, the data support the use of visual analogue scales or numerical rating scales for children over the age of 5. Visual analogue scales have been used in the assessment of paediatric cancer pain.[1,2] To use such scales, children must understand the concept of proportionality, be able to conceptualize their pain experience along a continuum, and be able to translate that understanding to the visual representations of the line and the anchors.

Similar strategies, such as Likert scales with anchor points of 1 ('no pain') and 5 ('extreme pain'), have been used to assess pain in children with cancer.[3] However, research on the use of verbal rating scales with children (9 years and older) has not clearly established the utility of this approach over visual analogue scales.[4] In the context of childhood cancer, other investigators have used visual cues, such as different pictures of a child's face which are graded from neutral or happy expressions (no pain) to sad/distressed expressions (extreme pain).[5,6]

Behavioural observation measures

The subjective distress of acute pain, particularly after traumatic medical procedures, often manifests itself in certain facial expressions, verbal, and motor responses. Behavioural methods for assessing pain in children require independent observers recording the physical behaviours of children in pain, as well as the frequency of their occurrence.[3,7,8] Observation methods have generally been used to obtain data on specific, treatment-related pain-distress reactions in children with cancer (e.g. bone marrow aspiration [BMA], lumbar puncture [LP], post-operative pain, etc.).

Gauvain–Piquard rating scale

The Gauvain–Piquard rating scale[9] is an observation scale designed for the assessment of chronic pain in paediatric oncology patients aged 2–6 years. The scale consists of 17 items, seven of which are related to pain assessment (antalgic rest position, spontaneous protection of painful areas, somatic complaints, the child points out painful areas, antalgic behaviour during movement, control exerted by child when moved, emotional reactions to medical examination of painful regions), six are related to depression (child retires 'into his shell', lack of expressiveness, lack of interest in surroundings, slowness and rarity of movements, signs of regression, social withdrawal), and four assess anxiety (nervousness/anxiety, ability to protest, moodiness/irritability, tendency to cry). Kappa statistics analysing the correlation between observers were low, ranging from 0.24 to 0.60.

Instruments for the assessment of nausea in children

A comparison of child and parental ratings of children's nausea and emesis symptoms was assessed among 33 children (aged 1.7–17.5 years, median 4.7 years) with acute lymphoblastic leukaemia receiving identical chemotherapy.[10] The measures utilized nausea and vomiting vignettes designed to assess the frequency and severity of nausea and emesis symptoms as reported by children and their parents based on the previous chemotherapy experience of the child.

The vignettes, based on the work of Zeltzer et al.,[11] consisted of 12 questions separately assessing nausea and emesis at three time intervals: prior to, during, and after chemotherapy. A five-point Likert-type rating scale ranging from 'not at all' to 'all the time' for the frequency items and from 'not bad' to 'real bad' on the severity items were employed. A composite nausea/vomiting score was determined by calculating the mean of the 12 frequency and severity items. This study demonstrated a significant correlation between child and parent ratings of nausea. Significant inter-rater correlations for nausea frequency and severity but not for emesis frequency or severity were found. Lastly, a rating scale for nausea and vomiting utilizing verbal descriptors was used in a series of assessment studies in children with cancer aged 5–18.[12–15] There was 80 per cent agreement between parent and child rating when they were assessed independently.

Multidimensional symptom assessment tools for children

The Memorial Symptom Assessment Scale (MSAS) 10–18 is a 30-item patient-rated instrument adapted from a previously validated adult version to provide multidimensional information about the symptoms experienced by children with cancer aged 10–18.[16] The analyses supported the reliability and validity of the MSAS 10–18 sub-scale scores as measures of physical, psychological, and global symptom distress, respectively. The majority of patients could easily complete the scale in a mean of 11 min.

A revised MSAS was created as an instrument for the assessment of symptoms children with cancer aged 7–12 years.[17] Validity was evaluated by comparison with the medical record, parental report, and concurrent assessment on visual analogue scales for selected symptoms. The data provide evidence of the reliability and validity of MSAS 7–12 and demonstrated that children with cancer as young as 7 years could report clinically relevant and consistent information about their symptom experience. The completion rate for MSAS 7–12 was high and the majority of children completed the instrument in a short period of time and with little difficulty. The instrument appeared to be age appropriate and may be helpful to older children unable to independently complete MSAS 10–18.

Symptom epidemiology in children with life-limiting illness

The child dying in hospital

Following the publication of recent data from the United States,[18] there has been an increasing awareness of the need for better symptom management of dying children. Wolfe et al.[18] found that 89 per cent of 103 parents whose children died of cancer in a hospital setting retrospectively reported that their children experienced 'a lot' or 'a great deal' from at least one symptom in their last month of life. In the children who were treated for specific symptoms, treatment was thought to be successful in only 27 per cent of those with pain and in only 16 per cent of those with dyspnoea.

A retrospective survey to describe the course of terminal care provided to 77 dying hospitalized children in terms of symptom assessment and management, and communication and decision-making, at the end of life was performed in Edmonton, Canada.[19] Eighty-three per cent of children died in intensive care settings (64/77), and 78 per cent (60/77) were intubated prior to their death. Opioid analgesia was provided in 84 per cent of all cases (65/77), six (8 per cent) patients had 'do not resuscitate' (DNR) orders preceding final hospital admission, and 56/71 (79 per cent) patients had documented discussion resulting in DNR decision during final hospital admission. Median time from DNR to death was less than 1 day. Decision-making regarding end-of-life issues in this paediatric population were deferred very close to the time of death, and only after no remaining curative therapy were available. Acuity of care was very high prior to death for most children. Children in this survey were rarely told that they were dying.

Another retrospective study examined symptom prevalence, characteristics, and distress of 30 children dying at the Children's Hospital, Westmead, Australia.[20] Symptoms and their characteristics during the last day of life were determined from an interview of a nurse who cared for that child during the last day of life using a symptom assessment instrument. The dominant disease process was cancer, while the most likely location of death was intensive care. The mean duration of the 'active phase of dying' was 25.2 h and the major physiological disturbances at this time were respiratory failure and encephalopathy. The mean ($\pm$SD) number of symptoms per patient was 11.1 $\pm$ 5.6 with significantly more ($p < 0.02$) symptoms for children dying on the ward (14.3 $\pm$ 6.1) compared to children dying in intensive care (9.5 $\pm$ 4.7). Six symptoms (lack of energy, drowsiness, skin changes, irritability, pain, and oedema of the extremities) occurred with a high prevalence (affecting 50 per cent or more of the children) in the last week of life. Symptoms in the last day of life even if they occurred with a high prevalence, frequency ('a lot' to 'almost always') or severity ('moderate' to 'very severe') were, in general, not associated with a high level of distress ('quite a lot' to 'almost always'). Lack of energy was the only symptom where over 30 per cent of children with the symptom had a high level of distress ('quite a bit' to 'very much'). The level of patient comfort as perceived from the medical notes indicated that the majority of children were 'always comfortable' to 'usually comfortable' in the last week (64 per cent), day (76.6 per cent), and hour (93.4 per cent) of life.[20]

In summary, the symptom burden of children dying in hospital is high. Ironically, in Drake et al.'s survey,[20] the symptom burden was significantly reduced in the intensive care unit where the most aggressive interventions were undertaken.

The child dying in an inpatient hospice

There are few epidemiological data on the symptoms experienced by children with life-limiting and life-threatening illness dying in a children's inpatient hospice unit. A retrospective survey of 30 children at a children's hospice indicated pain, secretions, dyspnoea, oral symptoms, and cough to be common problems for children in the last week of life.[21] This survey was dependent upon the report of carers, since many of the children were cognitively impaired. As such, this survey may be under reporting the frequency with which these symptoms occurred.

The symptoms of children with cancer

Children with cancer aged 10–18 were surveyed at Memorial Sloan Kettering, New York, for symptom prevalence and distress.[16] Symptom prevalence ranged from 49.7 per cent for lack of energy to 6.3 per cent for problems with urination (Table 1). The mean ($\pm$SD) number of symptoms per inpatient was 12.7 $\pm$ 4.9 (range, 4–26), significantly more than the mean 6.5 $\pm$ 5.7 (range, 0–28) symptoms per outpatient. Patients who had recently received chemotherapy had significantly more symptoms than patients who had not received chemotherapy for more than 4 months (11.6 $\pm$ 6.0 versus 5.2 $\pm$ 5.1), and those patients with solid tumours had significantly more symptoms than patients with either leukaemia, lymphoma, or central nervous system malignancies (9.9 $\pm$ 7.0 versus 6.8 $\pm$ 5.5 versus 6.8 $\pm$ 5.0 versus 8.0 $\pm$ 6.1) (Table 2). The most common symptoms (prevalence >35 per cent) were lack of energy, pain, drowsiness, nausea, cough, lack of appetite, and psychological symptoms (feeling sad, feeling nervous, worrying, feeling irritable). Of the symptoms with prevalence rates more than 35 per cent, those that caused high distress in more than one third of patients were feeling sad, pain, nausea, lack of appetite, and feeling irritable. These data confirm a high prevalence of symptoms overall and the existence of subgroups with high distress associated with one or multiple symptoms. Systematic symptom assessment may be useful in future epidemiological studies of symptoms and in clinical chemotherapeutic trials. Symptom epidemiology may also provide a focus for future clinical trials related to symptom management in children with cancer.

A survey of symptom prevalence and distress was performed in younger children aged 7–12.[17] Of the eight symptoms surveyed, the mean number of symptoms experienced by younger children was 1.9 ($\pm$ 1.6). Symptom prevalence during the 48 h prior to the completion of the questionnaire included: tiredness (35.6 per cent), pain (32.4 per cent), insomnia (31.1 per cent), itch (25.0 per cent), lack of appetite (22.3 per cent), worry (20.1 per cent), nausea (13.4 per cent), and sadness (10.1 per cent) (Table 3). More than half the children who endorsed pain as a symptom rated their pain as a 'medium amount' to 'a lot'. Although sadness was the least prevalent symptom, more than half of the patients who experienced it rated it as severe, frequent, and distressing. Tiredness and lack of appetite were less likely to be causes of high distress than pain, insomnia, itch, nausea, or worry.[17]

The epidemiology of intractable pain in children

Pain that cannot be relieved using conventional treatment is intractable. Intractable pain that does not respond to therapies beyond conventional practice is refractory. The relief of refractory pain may require a therapy that compromises consciousness. Intractable pain in childhood is rare and is usually seen in the setting of cancer pain. Intractable childhood cancer pain is usually associated with disease-related syndromes. It is rare, however, for a paediatric patient to have persistent tumour-related pain from diagnosis.[22] Disease-related pain often recurs at the time of tumour recurrence and when the cancer becomes unresponsive to treatment.

The opioid requirements of 199 children with terminal malignancy were examined in a retrospective study.[23] Twelve (6 per cent) of the patients in this study required therapies beyond conventional opioid pharmacotherapy. The majority of the patients had neuropathic pain as the basis of their intractability. Eleven of the patients had spinal cord compression, solid tumour metastatic to the spinal nerve roots, nerve plexus, or large peripheral nerve. Half of the patients had adequate analgesia with either regional anaesthesia or with opioid infusion alone. The remaining patients required the addition of sedation to control refractory pain.

Symptom management in children with life-threatening illness

The adequate, proficient, and timely management of symptoms in the dying child is of critical importance. Not only is it important from a humanitarian viewpoint, but also it is apparent that the memory of unrelieved symptoms in dying children may be retained in the memory of parents many years after their child has died.[18] It will be impossible for children and their families to negotiate the domains of psychological and spiritual care if physical symptomatology has not been adequately treated. The following outlines the management of the major symptoms experienced by children receiving palliative care. As few controlled studies of symptom management have been performed in childhood, many of the therapies used in children have been devised utilizing best practice for adults. The reader is referred to the adult section of this volume for the principles of management of unusual symptoms. An emphasis has been given in this

Table 1 Prevalence and characteristics of symptoms determined by the MSAS in 159 children with cancer[16]

Symptom	Overall prevalence (%)	Degree when symptom was present		
		Intensity Mod–VSev (%)[a]	Frequency A lot–AA (%)[b]	Distress QB–VM (%)[c]
Lack of energy	49.7	61.6	40.9	21.4
Pain	49.1	80.8	35.9	39.1
Feeling drowsy	48.4	64.0	34.6	18.6
Nausea	44.7	65.9	23.0	36.6
Cough	40.9	47.7	23.0	16.3
Lack of appetite	39.6	66.3	39.7	35.8
Feeling sad	35.8	59.6	17.5	39.5
Feeling nervous	35.8	56.1	28.1	23.7
Worrying	35.4	66.1	28.6	27.2
Feeling irritable	34.6	63.6	30.9	34.7
Itching	32.7	63.4	26.9	30.0
Insomnia	30.8	66.7	38.8	58.7
Dry mouth	30.8	50.2	28.6	23.5
Hair loss	28.3	66.6	NE	48.0
Vomiting	27.7	67.5	32.3	45.2
Weight loss	26.6	51.2	NE	25.0
Dizziness	24.5	55.2	15.4	21.9
Numbness/tingling in hands/feet	22.0	36.0	28.6	22.7
Sweating	20.3	54.7	25.0	10.8
Lack of concentration	20.1	54.5	21.9	30.3
Diarrhoea	20.1	61.6	28.1	33.4
Skin changes	20.1	68.8	NE	46.1
Dyspnoea	16.5	69.1	22.9	29.1
Change in the way food tastes	16.5	77.0	NE	30.4
'I don't look like myself'	15.8	76.0	NE	49.5
Mouth sores	13.9	59.2	NE	56.9
Difficulty swallowing	12.6	83.8	56.3	76.1
Constipation	13.8	81.8	NE	25.9
Swelling of arms/legs	12.0	52.8	NE	8.0
Problems with urination	6.3	90.0	70	45.0

[a] Percentage moderate to very severe.

[b] Percentage a lot to almost always.

[c] Percentage quite a bit to very much.

NE, not evaluated.

Reprinted by permission of Elsevier Science from 'The Memorial Symptom Assessment Scale (MSAS): validation study in children aged 10–18', by Collins, J.J., Byrnes, M.E., Dunkel, I., Foley, K.M., Lapin, J., Rapkin, B., Thaler, H.T., and Portenoy, R.K. *Journal of Pain and Symptom Management* **19** (5), 363–77, 2000, by the US Cancer Pain Relief Committee.

chapter to the palliative care emergencies of childhood. Less urgent symptoms have been discussed in alphabetical order.

The palliative care emergencies of childhood

Intractable pain

Pain that cannot be relieved using conventional treatment is intractable. Intractable pain that does not respond to therapies beyond conventional practice is refractory. The relief of refractory pain may require a therapy that compromises consciousness. The modalities of pain control for the management of intractable cancer pain in paediatric patients include opioid dose titration, adjuvant analgesics (covered in a previous section), regional anaesthesia, and sedation. Non-pharmacologic methods of pain control have a secondary role in the setting of intractable pain.

The paediatric pain crisis

The pain crisis in a child is an emergency and requires treatment beyond conventional means. A specific diagnosis must be made, as therapies directed at the primary cause may be more effective in the longer term. The management of intractable pain requires the clinician to be at the patient's bedside to titrate incremental intravenous doses every 10–15 min until

Table 2 Symptom prevalence (%) in four tumour types (n = 131)[16]

Symptom	Prevalence (%)			
	Leukaemia (n = 33)	Lymphoma (n = 26)	Solid tumour (n = 54)	CNS tumour (n = 18)
Lack of energy	43.8	50.0	53.7	66.7
Pain	43.8	26.9	63.0	50.0
Feeling drowsy	50.0	38.5	57.4	33.3
Nausea	43.8	34.6	53.7	50.0
Cough	34.4	38.5	48.1	22.2
Lack of appetite	28.1	30.8	51.9	33.3
Feeling sad	34.4	26.9	37.0	38.9
Feeling nervous	28.1	23.1	42.6	22.2
Worrying	31.3	36.0	37.0	22.2
Feeling irritable	34.4	34.6	38.9	27.8
Itching	40.6	15.4	35.2	38.9
Insomnia	28.1	30.8	29.6	27.8
Dry mouth	21.9	11.5	40.7	55.6
Hair loss	9.4	50.0	38.9	22.2
Vomiting	12.5	15.4	38.9	33.3
Weight loss	15.6	19.2	29.6	47.1
Dizziness	21.9	15.4	31.5	22.2
Numbness/tingling in hands/feet	25.0	34.6	16.7	22.2
Sweating	12.9	26.9	24.1	16.7
Lack of concentration	21.9	15.4	20.4	27.8
Diarrhoea	21.9	11.5	24.1	16.7
Skin changes	15.6	15.4	20.4	22.2
Dyspnoea	21.9	11.5	18.5	5.6
Change in the way food tastes	9.4	7.7	27.8	11.8
'I don't look like myself'	—	23.1	24.1	11.1
Mouth sores	9.4	15.4	20.4	5.9
Difficulty swallowing	3.1	3.8	18.5	11.1
Constipation	6.3	—	24.1	16.7
Swelling of arms/legs	6.3	15.4	14.8	11.8
Problems with urination	—	3.8	9.3	11.1

Reprinted by permission of Elsevier Science from 'The Memorial Symptom Assessment Scale (MSAS): validation study in children aged 10–18', by Collins, J.J., Byrnes, M.E., Dunkel, I., Foley, K.M., Lapin, J., Rapkin, B., Thaler, H.T., and Portenoy, R.K. *Journal of Pain and Symptom Management* **19** (5), 363–77, 2000, by the US Cancer Pain Relief Committee.

Table 3 Prevalence and characteristics of symptoms determined by the MSAS 7–12 in children with cancer aged 7–12[17]

Symptom	Overall prevalence (%)	Degree when symptom was present		
		Intensity Medium amt–a lot (%)	Frequency Medium amt–almost all the time (%)	Distress Medium amt–very much (%)
Lethargy	53 (35.6)	51	64	5
Pain	48 (32.4)	56	54	37
Insomnia	46 (31.1)	—	—	39
Itch	37 (25.0)	56	54	38
Lack of appetite	33 (22.3)	—	52	12
Worry	30 (20.1)	43	43	30
Nausea	20 (13.4)	—	45	65
Sadness	15 (10.1)	60	53	50

Reprinted by permission of Elsevier Science from 'The measurement of symptoms in young children with cancer: the validation of the Memorial Symptom Assessment Scale in children aged 7–12', by Collins, J.J., Devine, T.B., Dick, G., Johnson, E.A., and Kilham, H.K. *Journal of Pain and Symptom Management* **23** (1), 10–16, 2002, by the US Cancer Pain Relief Committee.

effective analgesia has been achieved. The analgesic effects of opioids increase in a log-linear function, with incremental opioid dosing required until either analgesia is achieved or somnolence occurs.[24] The total amount of opioid administered to achieve this reduction in pain intensity is considered the opioid loading dose. A continuous infusion of opioid may need to be commenced to maintain this level of analgesia, and the infusion rate is often based on the opioid administered as a loading dose.[24] An alternative to a continuous infusion of opioid is intermittent parenteral opioid, especially in the setting of an unpredictable pain syndrome.

'Rescues'

Rescues (or breakthrough doses) are additional doses of opioid incorporated into the analgesic regime to allow for additional analgesia if required by the patient. Rescue doses of opioid may be calculated as approximately 5–10 per cent of the total daily opioid requirement and may be administered orally every hour.[24] Given the frequency with which additional analgesia may be required for severe pain, it is often convenient for patients to self-administer opioids using a patient-controlled analgesia (PCA) device. The PCA device must be programmed to deliver an opioid dose at a pre-determined frequency, with a maximum total dose over a set time period. Post-operative data suggest that 7-year-old children of normal intelligence can use PCA effectively to provide analgesia.[25]

Opioid dose escalation

If pain can be controlled by the opioid-loading technique (above), then the subsequent opioid dose escalation may be calculated as follows:

1. If greater than approximately six rescue doses of opioid are required in a 24-h period, then the hourly average of this total daily rescue opioid should be added to the baseline opioid infusion. An alternative would be to increase the baseline infusion by 50 per cent.[24]
2. Rescue doses are kept as a proportion of the baseline opioid infusion rate and a re-calculated as between 50 and 200 per cent of the hourly basal infusion rate.[24]

Opioid switching (rotation or substitution)

The usual indication for switching to an alternative opioid is dose-limiting opioid toxicity. In the setting of the general paediatric oncology population, opioid rotation is required in approximately 10 per cent of patients (Ross Drake, unpublished data). In the setting of intractability, opioid dose escalation may be limited by opioid-related side-effects. An observation is that a switch from one opioid to another is often accompanied by change in the balance between analgesia and side-effects.[26] A favourable change in opioid analgesia to side-effect profile will be experienced if there is less cross-tolerance at the opioid receptors mediating analgesia than at those mediating adverse effects.[27]

Following a prolonged period of regular dosing with one opioid, equivalent analgesia may be attained with a dose of a second opioid that is smaller than that calculated from an equianalgesic table (see previous sections). An opioid switch is usually accompanied by a reduction in the equianalgesic dose (approximately 50 per cent for short half-life opioids).

In contrast to short half-life opioids, the doses of methadone required for equivalent analgesia after switching may be of the order of 10–20 per cent of the equianalgesic dose of the previously used short half-life opioid. A protocol for methadone dose conversion and titration has been documented for adults.[28]

Invasive approaches to intractable paediatric cancer pain

Anaesthetic approaches

In contrast to the adult population, the experience of using regional anaesthesia for children with intractable pain is limited. A retrospective study of children with terminal cancer[29] showed that regional anaesthesia is appropriate in a highly select subset of children. The indications for regional anaesthesia in this group were largely related to either dose-limiting side-effects of opioids or opioid unresponsiveness in patients where pain was confined to one region of the body. Rapid intravenous opioid dose reduction was required in some cases. Technique modifications appropriate to children have been recommended.[30] The recommendations included the use of sedation and the routine use of imaging for epidural insertion.

Neuro-surgical approaches

Experience with neuro-destructive procedures in children is limited. Matson described his experience with cordotomy in children[31] with intractable pain. It is unclear whether these cases may have been effectively managed by current pharmacologic techniques. In selected cases neurosurgical approaches to pain management may be appropriate.

Sedation as a therapeutic modality for intractable pain

The use of sedation in the setting of refractory pain generally assumes that therapies beyond the conventional have been utilized and that there is no acceptable means of providing analgesia without compromising consciousness. This trade-off between sedation and inadequate pain relief requires the consideration of the wishes of the child and his or her family. The ethical issues surrounding prolonged sedation in paediatrics, including the principle of double effect have been previously discussed.[32–34] The continuation of high-dose opioid infusions in these circumstances is recommended to avoid situations in which a patient may have unrelieved pain but inadequate clarity to express pain perception. A variety of drugs have been used in this setting, including barbiturates, benzodiazepines, and phenothiazines.[33]

Seizure control

Seizures in palliative care patients may be either recent in onset or part of a long-standing underlying seizure disorder. In the former situation, the onset will usually be frightening to patients and families and may be due to many possible causes (e.g. cerebral metastases, infection, metabolic disorder, hypoxia, etc.) which must be excluded as treatment directed at the primary causes may be appropriate whilst anticonvulsant therapy is implemented. In the latter situation, worsening seizure control in a patient with an underlying seizure disorder may indicate either disease progression or factors related to anticonvulsant dose, class, or administration which should be reviewed.

Refractory seizure control has been the subject of two recent reviews.[35,36] Initial treatment of status epilepticus in children typically consists of either diazepam or lorazepam, immediately followed by phenytoin or phenobarbitone.[35] Recently, buccal midazolam has been shown to be at least as effective as rectal diazepam in the acute treatment of seizures.[36] Administration via the mouth is more socially acceptable and convenient and may become the preferred treatment for long seizures that occur outside hospital.[36] The buccal dose is the same as the oral dose of midazolam used for sedation (0.3 mg/kg per dose, maximum dose 15 mg) and should be used as a single dose only.

Traditionally, refractory status epilepticus is treated with barbiturate coma or general anaesthetics, both of which require invasive cardiorespiratory and haemodynamic monitoring and are associated with significant complications. Midazolam has been effective in terminating seizures refractory to diazepam, lorazepam, phenytoin, and phenobarbitone in paediatric patients.[35]

Spinal cord compression

Spinal cord compression is an unusual complication of childhood cancer and occurs most likely late in a child's illness. Back pain, more often than abnormal neurologic signs or symptoms, is the usual initial presenting sign of spinal cord compression in children.[37] Spinal cord compression is an emergency, since adult data show that if treated whilst a patient is ambulatory, the probability of retaining ambulant status is 89–94 per cent.[38] The mainstays of management are firstly radiological diagnosis and treatment with radiotherapy for radio-sensitive tumour and corticosteroids.[39] Decompressive surgery, generally with resection of the vertebral body, may be indicated for patients with radio-resistant tumours and those whose disease progresses despite an initial trial of radiotherapy.

Bleeding

Although the fear of external bleeding is paramount in the minds of families and caregivers of children dying of either haematological malignancy or children dying of liver failure, massive external bleeding as a mode of death in childhood is uncommon. While some children with malignancy receive blood products indefinitely, this is not always feasible or appropriate. If the fear of external bleeding is overwhelming for families, this may influence their choice of location of the child's death and attitude towards blood product transfusion.

Terminal dyspnoea

Dyspnoea has been defined as uncomfortable awareness of breathing.[40] In the terminal phase, it is often highly distressing to patients and for families to watch. Terminal dyspnoea may be due to a variety, and perhaps combination, of causes. These include pulmonary metastases, intrinsic lung disease or infection, cardiac failure, acidosis, muscle weakness, etc. Again, diagnosis is important as this may influence choice of therapies. Non-invasive ventilation may be a viable choice for symptom management of dyspnoea related to muscle weakness, for example, and bronchospasm could be easily reversed with bronchodilators.

Most of the data on the management of terminal dyspnoea is from studies of adults with terminal malignancy. There are no data on the appropriate management of dyspnoea related to muscle weakness or complications of cystic fibrosis, for example. The goal of palliative therapies for terminal dyspnoea is to improve the patient's subjective sensation. A double-blind, cross-over trial studied the effects of supplemental oxygen on dyspnoea in adult patients with terminal cancer.[41] The subjective sensation of dyspnoea was improved in patients receiving supplemental oxygen. In addition, systemic opioid therapy[40,42] and cognitive–behavioural strategies[43] have been shown to be of benefit to patients with dyspnoea related to terminal malignancy. As anxiety is often a component of terminal dyspnoea, judicious prescription of a benzodiazepine may be warranted.

Secretions

The management of noisy secretions in an unconscious patient is aimed at reducing the distress of family, other patients, and staff. The sound of noisy secretions can be haunting to all concerned and should be given some priority by the attending clinician. While there is no standard of care for the management of noisy secretions, accepted management includes explanation to relatives, positioning, suction, and anticholinergics (e.g. hyoscine hydrobromide or glycopyrrolate).[44]

Terminal delirium

Delirium during the final phase of dying is one of the most distressing symptoms for caregivers to watch, especially if the delirium is agitated. The interpretation of the latter may be that the delirium is a manifestation of an internal existential angst. This latter interpretation is unlikely, since the aetiology of delirium in the setting of an actively dying patient is usually multifactorial with a physical rather psychological basis (e.g. hypoxia, metabolic derangement, central nervous system disease, infection, fever, etc.). Simple causes that can be corrected, hypoxia for example, should be excluded. As terminal delirium cannot be predicted, a therapeutic plan for its management should be considered in every dying child. The usually therapies consist of haloperidol for delirium per se with consideration of adding a benzodiazepine if there is agitation as well.

The palliation of other symptoms in childhood

Constipation

Although constipation is a relatively common symptom in children, it is more likely to be distressing to the child's caregivers than to the child.

Table 4 Guidelines for the management of opioid-induced constipation in children

Non-drug measures
Dietary change
Increase fluids
Increase physical activity
Principles of laxative prescription
By a pleasant route of administration (i.e. avoid per rectum administration)
Individualize to avoid side-effects
Around the clock dosing
Simple dosing regime
Laxative prescription[51]
1. Try a stimulant laxative first (e.g. senna 7.5 mg once or twice daily)
2. If this is ineffective, increase the dose
3. If this is ineffective, add lactulose (1 ml/kg/dose once or twice daily). This dose frequency may need to be increased
4. Bisacodyl suppository ± an enema may be required if the above fails to produce a response

Table 5 Nausea and vomiting: paediatric palliative care

Cause	Putative mechanism(s)[51]	Treatment
Gastrointestinal causes		
Poor mouth care	Cerebral cortex, vagus	Regular mouth care
Gastric irritation	Vagus	Exclude drug-related causes, consider prescription of H1 antagonists
Intestinal obstruction	Vagus	May require surgical opinion
Constipation	Vagus	Laxatives (see below)
Hepatic distension	Vagus	Depends on aetiology (e.g. frusemide for cardiac failure, dexamethasone for tumour-related causes)
Metabolic causes		
Renal failure	Chemoreceptor trigger zone (CTZ)	Consider antiemetics if more invasive therapies not appropriate
Hypercalcaemia	CTZ	If appropriate, consider hydration, diuretic (osteoclast inhibitors may also be appropriate)
CNS causes		
Raised intracranial pressure	Vomiting centre	Dexamethasone
Vestibulitis	Vestibular apparatus	Antihistamine
Treatment-related causes		
Medications (chemotherapy, opioids, etc.)	CTZ Vagus	Consider an opioid switch for dose-limiting side-effects
Psychological trigger		
Anxiety	Cerebral cortex	Consider cognitive–behavioural therapy
Emotional distress	Cerebral cortex	
Other causes		
Pain	Vagus	Treat the primary cause
Infection	CTZ, Vomiting centre	Treat the primary cause
Migraine headache	Vagus	Antimigraine therapies
Situational triggers (unpalatable food, etc.)	Cerebral cortex	Alter situation

The aetiology of constipation is often multifactorial and may include reduced physical activity, mechanical obstruction, metabolic derangement, poor diet and low fluid intake, bowel atony due to opioids, etc. Although unusual, bowel obstruction and faecal impaction must be excluded and treated urgently in any child presenting with constipation.

Generally, dietary changes are recommended in the first instance (increased vegetables and fruity, bulk, prune juice, etc.). In addition, attention should be given to hydration, mobility, and other activities of daily living. Chronic opioid therapy necessitates the prescription of a regular laxative. There is little evidence to guide the prescription of laxatives in children. Whilst there are emerging adult data to suggest oral naloxone may be appropriate for the management of opioid-induced constipation,[45] a senna and lactulose combination is often prescribed in the adult population.[46] It is not clear if a senna/lactulose combination is appropriate for children. Table 4 gives some guidelines for the management of opioid-induced constipation in children.

Fatigue

Fatigue is a common symptom of children with cancer[16–18,47] and one that is often highly distressing. The aetiology of fatigue in children dying of cancer may be due to a combination of factors including: anaemia, poor nutrition, insomnia, metabolic derangement, the increased work of breathing in patients with dyspnoea, side-effects of medication, and psychological factors.

In the assessment of fatigue in a child, and the matrix of its potential causes, it is important to establish if this symptom is distressing to the child and/or his/her family. If so, the potential remediable causes should be considered. Therapies directed at the primary cause should be instituted only if these therapies are not of substantial burden to the patient and/or his/her family. There are adult and limited paediatric data on the use of stimulant medication for the treatment of opioid-induced somnolence.[48–50] In children, it has become more common practice to switch opioids (see above) for somnolence as a dose-limiting side-effect of opioid therapy.

Insomnia

Sleep disturbance is common in children with life-threatening illness. In the context of cancer, insomnia is both prevalent and distressing to children and, by inference, distressing to caregivers (Table 1). The aetiology of insomnia is multifactorial and is often a combination of physical, psychological, and perhaps environmental factors. When depression is a factor, consideration should be given to psychotherapy and pharmacologic treatment. Fatigue often coexists with sleep disturbance. Lifestyle changes, including improved sleep hygiene and exercise may be helpful to improved sleep. Low-dose amitriptyline, if not contraindicated, is often a helpful pharmacologic agent for the management of insomnia in terminally ill children, particularly if pain is a symptom management issue.

Mouth care and hydration

Routine mouth care promotes patient comfort and ability to eat and drink, prevents halitosis, and helps identify problems such as dry mouth, candidiasis, and ulceration.[51] Lip emollients and mouthwashes are important therapies for mouth care. The sensation of a dry mouth may be due to local (e.g. mouth breathing, candidiasis, radiotherapy to salivary glands, etc.) and systemic causes (e.g. dehydration, anticholinergic drugs uraemia, etc.) and is often distressing. The issue of hydration in dying patients is a contentious issue. Small but frequent volumes of fluid to maintain insensible losses may be appropriate via the oral route. However, this may be impossible in some instances unless other routes of administration are considered.

Table 6 Anti-emetic drug therapy in paediatric palliative care

Drug category	Putative mechanism of action[51]	Drugs	Dosing regime	Route of administration	Side-effects/caution
Prokinetic drugs	Promote gastric emptying via a cholinergic mechanism. All act on the CTZ	Metoclopramide	0.15 mg/kg/dose 6–8 hourly prn	O/IV/IM/SC	Extrapyramidal side-effects more common in children
$5HT_3$ antagonists	Central action on CTZ and vomiting centre. Block serotonin receptors on vagal efferents in the bowel	Ondansetron	0.15 mg/kg/dose 8–12 hourly prn or 5 mg/m2/dose 8–12 hourly prn	O/IV	Dose limit 8 mg/dose
Corticosteroids	Probably act via peripheral mechanisms. Useful for chemotherapy related emesis	Dexamethasone	0.1–1.0 mg/kg/day 6–8 hourly prn	O/IV/SC[a]	Cushingoid effects with long-term use Gastric irritation Mood instability Poor contol of blood sugar levels
Antihistamines	Act on the vomiting centre	Cyclizine	0.8 mg/kg/dose 6 hourly prn	O/IV/SC	Anti-cholinergic side-effects, drowsiness Max. dose 50 mg
Neuroleptic drugs	Act on the CTZ	Haloperidol	10–50 μg/kg/day 8–12 hourly prn	O/SC	Extrapyramidal side-effects Drowsiness
Anticholinergic drugs	Act on the vomiting centre	Hyoscine hydrobromide (Scopolamine)	6–10 μg/kg/dose 6 hourly prn	O/IV/IM/SC	Maximum dose = 400 μg/dose
Benzodiazepines	Act on the cerebral cortex	Lorazepam	25–50 μg/kg/dose 6–8 hourly prn	O/IV	Drowsiness Max. dose 1 mg

[a] Incompatible in combination with many other drugs via SC route.

O, oral; SC, subcutaneous; IM, intramuscular; IV, intravenous; Prn, when required.

As with all therapies, the benefits and deficits of any intervention must be discussed with the patient and family before any therapeutic intervention is implemented.

Nausea and vomiting

Nausea and vomiting are not uncommon in children receiving palliative care. Nausea and vomiting occur when the vomiting centre in the brain is activated by any of the following: cerebral cortex (e.g. anxiety), vestibular apparatus, chemoreceptor trigger zone (CTZ), vagus nerve, or by direct action on the vomiting centre. A clear diagnosis must be sought as to aetiology as the list of potential causes is great and therapies different, depending on the putative mechanism (see Table 5).

Anti-emetic drug trials in children

Apart from pain, the only other symptom control therapies for which clinical trials have been undertaken in children are the antiemetics. Antiemetic drug trials have been conducted with an increasing degree of sophistication in this population, ranging from open label studies[52] to randomized double-blind cross-over studies.[53] Unfortunately, these studies are few in number, have a small number of recruited subjects, and may be flawed by virtue of the measures used. In addition, the context for most of these nausea and emesis drugs trials is related to cancer chemotherapy. Table 6 outlines one approach to anti-emetic prescription in children receiving palliative care. There are no data on the use of 5HT3 for non-chemotherapy/non-post-operative induced nausea and vomiting in children.

Summary

Symptom management is one of many domains of care of the dying child. A recent report[18] indicates that the memory of a dying child's symptomatology lingers for a long time in the memory of parents and caregivers. This same report, and others, indicates that the dying child is often highly symptomatic and these symptoms need to be prioritized and treated meticulously.

References

1. **Jay, S.M., Elliott, C., Katz, E., and Siegal, S.** (1987). Cognitive, behavioral, and pharmacologic interventions for children's distress during painful medical procedures. *Journal of Consulting and Clinical Psychology* **55**, 860–5.
2. **Elliott, C., Jay, S.M., and Woody, P.** (1987). An observational scale for measuring children's distress during medical procedures. *Journal of Pediatric Psychology* **12**, 543–51.
3. **LeBaron, S. and Zeltzer, L.** (1984). Assessment of acute pain and anxiety in children and adolescents by self-reports, observer reports and a behavior checklist. *Journal of Consulting and Clinical Psychology* **52**, 729–38.
4. **Savedra, M.** et al. (1982). How do children describe pain? A tentative assessment. *Pain* **14**, 95–104.
5. **Kuttner, L., Bowman, M., and Teasdale, M.** (1988). Psychological treatment of distress, pain and anxiety for children with cancer. *Developmental and Behavioral Pediatrics* **9**, 374–81.
6. **Manne, S.L.** et al. (1992). Adult and child interaction during invasive medical procedures: sequential analysis. *Health Psychology* **11**, 241–9.
7. **Jay, S.M., Elliott, C., Ozolins, M., Caldwell, S., and Pruitt, S.** (1985). Behavioral management of children's distress during painful medical procedures. *Behaviour Research and Therapy* **5**, 513–20.
8. **Jay, S.M., Ozolins, M., Elliott, C., and Caldwell, S.** (1983). Assessment of children's distress during painful medical procedures. *Health Psychology* **2**, 133–47.
9. **Gauvain-Piquard, A., Rodary, C., Rezvani, A., and Lemerle, J.** (1987). Pain in children aged 2–6 years: a new observational rating scale elaborated in a pediatric oncology unit: a preliminary report. *Pain* **31**, 177–88.
10. **Tyc, V.L.** et al. (1993). Chemotherapy induced nausea and emesis in pediatric cancer patients: external validity of child and parent ratings. *Developmental and Behavioral Pediatrics* **14** (4), 236–41.
11. **Zeltzer, L., LeBaron, S., Richie, D.M., and Reed, D.** (1988). Can children understand and use a rating scale to quantify somatic symptoms? Assessment of nausea and vomiting as a model. *Journal of Consulting Clinical Psychology* **56** (4), 567–72.
12. **Zeltzer, L., Kellerman, J., Ellenberg, L., and Dash, J.** (1983). Hypnosis for reduction of vomiting associated with chemotherapy and disease in adolescents with cancer. *Journal of Adolescent Health Care* **4** (77), 84.
13. **Zeltzer, L., LeBaron, S., and Zeltzer, P.M.** (1984). The effectiveness of behavioral intervention for reducing nausea and vomiting in children and adolescents receiving chemotherapy. *Journal of Clinical Oncology* **2**, 683–90.
14. **Zeltzer, L., LeBaron, S., and Zeltzer, P.M.** (1984). A prospective assessment of chemotherapy related nausea and vomiting in children with cancer. *American Journal of Pediatric Hematology/Oncology* **6**, 5–16.
15. **LeBaron, S. and Zeltzer, L.** (1984). Behavioral intervention for reducing chemotherapy-related nausea and vomiting in adolescents with cancer. *Journal of Adolescent Health Care* **5** (178), 182.
16. **Collins, J.J., Byrnes, M.E., Dunkel, I., Foley, K.M., Lapin, J., Rapkin, B., Thaler, H.T., and Portenoy, R.K.** (2000). The Memorial Symptom Assessment Scale (MSAS): validation study in children aged 10–18. *Journal of Pain and Symptom Management* **19** (5), 363–77.
17. **Collins, J.J., Devine, T.B., Dick, G., Johnson, E.A., and Kilham, H.K.** (2002). The measurement of symptoms in young children with cancer: the validation of the Memorial Symptom Assessment Scale in children aged 7–12. *Journal of Pain and Symptom Management* **23** (1), 10–16.
18. **Wolfe, J.** et al. (2000). Symptoms and suffering at the end of life in children with cancer. *New England Journal of Medicine* **342** (5), 326–33.
19. **McCallum, D.E., Byrne, P., and Bruera, E.** (2000). How children die in hospital. *Journal of Pain and Symptom Management* **20** (6), 417–23.
20. **Drake, R., Frost, J., and Collins, J.J.** (2003) The symptoms of dying children *Journal of Pain and Symptom Management* **25**, 1–10.
21. **Hunt, A.M.** (1990). A survey of signs, symptoms and symptom control in 30 terminally ill children. *Developmental Medicine and Child Neurology* **32**, 347–55.
22. **Miser, A.W.** et al. (1987). The prevalence of pain in a pediatric and young adult population. *Pain* **29**, 265–6.
23. **Collins, J.J., Grier, H.E., Kinney, H.C., and Berde, C.B.** (1995). Control of severe pain in terminal pediatric malignancy. *Journal of Pediatrics* **126** (4), 653–7.
24. **Cherny, N.I. and Foley, K.M.** (1996). Nonopioid and opioid analgesic pharmacotherapy of cancer pain. *Hematology/Oncology Clinics of North America* **10**, 79–102.
25. **Berde, C.B.** et al. (1991). Patient controlled analgesia in children and adolescents: a randomized, prospective comparison with intramuscular morphine for postoperative analgesia. *Journal of Pediatrics* **118**, 460–6.
26. **Galer, B.S.** et al. (1992). Individual variability in the response to different opioids: report of five cases. *Pain* **49**, 87–91.
27. **Portenoy, R.H., Gebhart, G.F., Hammond, D.I., and Jensen, T.S.**, ed. (1994). Opioid tolerance and responsiveness: research findings and clinical observations. In *Progress in Pain Research and Management* (ed. Gebhart et al.), pp. 615–19. Seattle: IASP Press.
28. **Inturrisi, C.E., Portenoy, R.K., Max, M., Colburn, W.A., and Foley, K.M.** (1990). Pharmacokinetic–pharmacodynamic relationships of methadone infusions in patients with cancer pain. *Clinical Pharmacology and Therapeutics* **47**, 565–77.
29. **Collins, J.J., Grier, H.E., Sethna, N.F., and Berde, C.B.** (1996). Regional anesthesia for pain associated with terminal malignancy. *Pain* **65**, 63–9.
30. **Berde, C.B.** (1989). Regional analgesia in the management of chronic pain in childhood. *Journal of Pain and Symptom Management* **4** (4), 232–7.
31. **Matson, D.D.** *Neurosurgery of Infancy and Childhood.* Springfield: Charles C. Thomas, 1969, p. 847.
32. **Truog, R.D., Berde, C.B., Mitchell, C., and Grier, H.E.** (1992). Barbiturates in the care of the terminally ill. *New England Journal of Medicine* **327**, 1678–82.
33. **Kenny, N.P. and Frager, G.** (1996). Refractory symptoms and terminal sedation in children: ethical issues and practical management. *Journal of Palliative Care* **12**, 40–5.

34. **Truog, R.D.** et al. (2002). Ethical considerations in pediatric oncology. In *Principles and Practice of Pediatric Oncology* 4th edn. (ed. P.A. Pizzo and D.G. Poplack), pp. 1411–30. Philadelphia: Lippincott Williams & Wilkins.
35. **Pellock, J.M.** (1998). Use of midazolam for refractory status epilepticus in pediatric patients. *Journal of Child Neurology* **13** (12), 581–7.
36. **Scott, R.C., Besag, F.M., and Neville, B.G.** (2002). Buccal midazolam and rectal diazepam for treatment of prolonged seizures in childhood and adolescence: a randomised trial. *Lancet* **353**, 623–6.
37. **Lewis, D., Packer, R., and Raney, B.** (1986). Incidence, presentation, and outcome of spinal cord disease in children with systemic cancer. *Pediatrics* **78**, 438–43.
38. **Loblaw, D.A. and Laperriere, N.J.** (1998). Emergency treatment of malignant extradural spinal cord compression: an evidence-based guideline. *Journal of Clinical Oncology* **16** (4), 1613–24.
39. **Abrahm, J.L.** (1999). Managment of pain and spinal cord compression in patients with advanced cancer. *Annals of Internal Medicine* **131** (1), 37–46.
40. **Bruera, E. MacEachern, T., Ripamonti, C., and Hanson, J.** (1993). Subcutaneous morphine for dyspnea in cancer patients. *Annals of Internal Medicine* **119** (9), 906–7.
41. **Bruera, E.** et al. (1993). Effects of oxygen on dyspnea in hypoxemic terminal cancer patients. *Lancet* **342** (8862), 13–14.
42. **Boyd, K.J. and Kelly, M.** (1997). Oral morphine as symptomatic treatment of dyspnoea in patients with advanced cancer. *Palliative Medicine* **11**, 277–81.
43. **Corner, J., Planth, H., Hern, R., and Bailey, C.** (1996). Non-pharmacological interventions for breathlessness in lung cancer. *Palliative Medicine* **10** (4), 299–305.
44. **Hughes, A.C., Wilcock, A., and Corcoran, R.** (1996). Management of 'Death Rattle'. *Lancet* **12** (6), 271–2.
45. **Culpepper-Morgan, J.A., Adelhardt, J., Foley, K.M., and Portenoy, R.K.** (1992). Treatment of opioid-induced constipation with oral naloxone: a pilot study. *Clinical Pharmacology and Therapeutics* **52**, 90–5.
46. **Abu-Saad, H.H. and Courtens, A.** (2001). *Journal of Pain and Symptom Management* **7**, 63–87.
47. **Hockenberry-Eaton, M.** et al. (1998). Fatigue in children and adolescents with cancer. *Journal of Pediatric Oncology Nursing* **15**, 172–82.
48. **Bruera, E., Faisinger, R., MacEachern, T., and Hanson, J.** (1992). The use of methylphenidate in patients with incident pain receiving regular opiates: a preliminary report. *Pain* **50**, 75–7.
49. **Bruera, E., Miller, M.J., Macmillan, K., and Kuehn, N.** (1992). Neuropsychological effects of methylphenidate in patients receiving a continuous infusion of narcotics for cancer pain. *Pain* **48**, 163–6.
50. **Yee, J.D. and Berde, C.B.** (1994). Dextroamphetamine or methylphenidate as adjuvants to opioid analgesia for adolescents with cancer. *Journal of Pain and Symptom Managment* **9**, 122–5.
51. **World Health Organization.** *Symptom Relief in Terminal Illness.* Geneva: World Health Organization, 1998.
52. **Pinkerton, C.R., Williams, D., Wooton, C., Meller, S.T., and McElwain, T.J.** (1990). 5-HT3 antagonist ondansetron—an effective outpatient antiemetic in cancer treatment. *Archives of Disease in Childhood* **65**, 822–5.
53. **Alvarez, O., Freeman, A., and Bedros, A.** (1995). Randomized double-blind cross-over ondansetron–dexamethasone versus ondansetron–placebo study for treatment of chemotherapy induced nausea and vomiting in pediatric patients with malignancies. *Journal of Pediatric Hematology and Oncology* **17** (2), 145–50.

9.3 Psychological adaptation of the dying child

Michael M. Stevens

What do children think and fear about death—particularly their own death? Do children who are dying develop insight to adjust and cope? These questions, currently amongst the most topical in psychosocial paediatrics, are clearly relevant to paediatric palliative medicine and are discussed in this chapter.

Psychological development of the normal child

An understanding of what sick children think and fear about death and how they adjust requires a brief discussion of how healthy children begin to think and form concepts including a concept of death.

Jean Piaget (1896–1980) is regarded as one of the most significant psychologists of the twentieth century. His stage theory of child development[1,2] describes the development of the child's intellect (thoughts, perceptions, judgement, reasoning) as an orderly hierarchical sequence of three major periods, each integrating and extending the previous one. This theory is widely used as a model in experimental child psychology (Table 1).

In the first period (sensorimotor intelligence, birth to 2 years), intellectual development begins with motor and sensory actions, which, by being repeated, become behavioural sequences. These form the basis for later intellectual structure. Piaget believed infants in this period are still unable to think or form concepts.

The second period (preparation and organization of concrete operations, early childhood to adolescence) consists of two stages, referred to as pre-operational thought and concrete operations. During the stage of pre-operational thought (age 2–7 years) the child is still unable to differentiate between the internal and external worlds (egocentricity), and has thoughts that do not follow logical rules. The child will attribute life and consciousness to inanimate objects (animistic thinking) and believes that inanimate objects can be commanded to obey actions or thoughts (magical thinking). This assists the child in making order out of the world and ascribing causes to events. The child will ascribe magical pre-logical explanations in discovering what differentiates life from death. The child will also believe that all objects and events in the world are manufactured to serve people (artificialism).

During the stage of concrete operations (age 7–12 years), the child gradually becomes less egocentrically orientated. Animistic, magical, and artificialistic thinking decrease and gradually disappear and the child comes to realize the personal nature of his or her views. Language and communication skills increase dramatically and the child acquires the concepts of conservation, space, time, and rate. The child's thinking becomes logical and influenced by the rules of disciplines such as arithmetic and mechanics. The child is concerned with the actual, rather than the hypothetical, and his or her reasoning will be connected as much as possible to beliefs based on direct observation. The child confronted by death will now know that animals and people do not die because a magic spell was put upon them that can be lifted, and will seek to discover what differentiates life from death.

During formal operations (adolescence to adulthood), previous cognitive structures and functions are integrated to achieve full intellectual capacities, including the ability to deal effectively with the world of abstract ideas.

The sequence of these periods will be orderly in all children, but children may differ widely in the ages at which they move through the sequence. Occasional reversions to a less-developed mode of thought will occur.

Table 1 The child's cognitive development and development of death concepts: recommendations for caregivers

Period/stage of cognitive development (Piaget)[a]	Life period[b]	Some major characteristics	Predominant death concepts	Recommendations for caregivers[c]
I. Period of sensorimotor intelligence	Infancy (0–2)	'Intelligence' consists of sensory and motor actions. No conscious thinking. Limited language[d], no concept of reality	No concept of death	Provide maximum physical relief and comfort
II. Period of preparation and organization of concrete operations				
1. Stage of pre-operational thought	Early childhood (2–7)	Egocentric orientation. Magical, animistic, and artificialistic thinking. Thinking is irreversible. Reality is subjective	Death is reversible: a temporary restriction, departure, or sleep	Minimize child's separation from parents. If parents unavailable, provide reliable and consistent substitute. Correct misperception of illness as punishment for bad thoughts or actions. Evaluate for feelings of guilt, rejection, anger, resentment of self or others
2. Stage of concrete operations	Middle childhood/ pre-adolescence (7–11/12)	Orientation ego-decentred. Thinking is limited to actual (although possibly absent) features of a situation rather than exploring abstract relationships and hypotheses. More adaptive thinking but confined to objects. No abstract reasoning. Understands conservation, reversibility. Multiple classification ability	Death is irreversible but capricious: external–internal physiological explanations	Evaluate for fears of abandonment, destruction, or body mutilation. Be truthful and open. Provide details about treatments. Reassure treatments are not punishments. Maintain access to peers. Foster child's sense of control, mastery
III. Period of formal operations	Adolescence and adulthood (12+)	Propositional and hypodeductive thinking. Generality of thinking. Reality is objective	Death is irreversible, universal, personal, but distant: natural, physiological, and theological explanations	Reinforce comfortable body image, self-esteem. Allow ventilation of anger. Provide privacy. Support reasonable measures for independence. Be clear, honest, and direct. Maintain access to peers. Consider mutual support groups

[a] Each stage includes an initial period of preparation and a final period of attainment; thus, whatever characterizes a stage is in the process of formation.

[b] There are individual differences in chronological ages.

[c] Adapted from ref. 3, Rando, T.A. *Grief, Dying and Death: Clinical Interventions for Caregivers*. Champaign IL: Research Press, 1984, pp. 385–91.

[d] By the end of their second year children, on the average, have attained a vocabulary of approximately 250–300 words. Adapted with permission from ref. 4.

The well child's concept of death and its development

The development of an understanding of death in the well child parallels Piaget's sequence of periods of cognitive development.

Specific cognitive achievements suggested as essential for understanding the various components of a concept of death include classification abilities (ability to categorize in hierarchies and to attend to multiple classifications simultaneously, e.g. a banana is yellow and long and belongs to the fruit family), the ability to focus on transformations as well as states, a linear notion of time, the ability to perform reversible operations (ability to follow a process from beginning to end and retrace steps back to the starting point), reciprocity skills (recognition that others may feel and/or think differently to oneself) that enable children to learn from the experience of others, increased objectivity, decreased egocentrism, and the universal application of rules. A child's concept of death will vary according to his or her level of cognitive development.

Maria Nagy conducted 484 assessments on 378 Hungarian children aged between 3 and 10 years in Budapest and its environs, using compositions written by those aged 7–10 years on the subject of death, drawings by those aged 6–10 years, and discussions with those aged 3–10 years. Her results were published in English in 1948,(5) although much of the work was done as early as 1936. Nagy found three stages of development of a concept of death:

1. Age 3–5 years: death seen as temporary and reversible, and not distinguished completely from life.
2. Age 5–9 years: death is personified and imagined as a separate person.
3. Age 9 years and upwards: death is seen as the cessation of corporal activities, and is universal and inevitable.

Sylvia Anthony studied definitions of the word 'dead' by 128 children.(6) Their responses fell into five categories:

1. apparent ignorance of the meaning of the word 'dead';
2. limited or erroneous concept;

3. no evidence of non-comprehension of the meaning of 'dead' but definition by reference to (a) associated phenomena that were not biologically or logically essential or (b) humans specifically but not other living things;
4. correct, essential, but limited reference;
5. general, logical, or biological definition or description.

As the child grew older, his or her concept of 'dead' changed in the order of the classification from (1) to (5). Anthony noted that immature death concepts take the form of oral fantasy. She also observed that fairy tales are full of such oral fantasy about death of a kind which is not death: Red Riding Hood's grandmother is eaten by the wolf and is later recovered from the beast's belly; Hansel and Gretel eat part of the witch's house, and she welcomes them inside but plans to cook and eat them.

Components of the child's concept of death: the current view

Although earlier studies have been valuable, it now appears that the child's concept of death is virtually complete by the age of 8 years. Studies have confirmed that different components of the child's concept of death are acquired at differing ages. In one study, 3-year-olds were found often to have some realization of death, but only at the age of 12 years would a child be likely to have an accurate idea of what a dead body would look like.(7)

In a review of three key components of a death concept,(8) it was concluded that, under at least some circumstances, young children think that death is reversible, attribute various life-defining functions to dead things, and think that certain individuals (often including themselves) will not die. Irreversibility, non-functionality, and universality are understood at roughly the same time (for most children between 5 and 7 years). In a second study(9) of the age of acquisition of seven of Kane's(7) components of the concept (separation, universality, causality, irrevocability, appearance of the body, insensitivity, and cessation of body function) in well children, about 60 per cent of the 5-year-olds, 70 per cent of the 6-year-olds, and 66 per cent of the 7-year-olds had complete or almost complete concepts. By the age of 8 and 9 years the figures were almost 100 per cent.

Some caution is required in comparing various studies of age of acquisition.

1. Differing statistical criteria are used by various investigators (e.g. a varying percentage of positive responses are defined to consider a concept acquired).
2. There are variations in the socioeconomic and educational standards of the children tested.
3. There are other influences related to the date of the particular study (e.g. the opportunity for the child to encounter death more commonly in the modern media).

The currently accepted components of the concept of death as summarized by Schonfeld(10) are presented in Table 2, with examples of incomplete understanding, and implications of incomplete understanding for adjustment to loss.

Development in well children of fears and anxieties concerning death

There are at least three views on how children acquire fears and anxieties about death.(12)

1. The psychoanalytic view suggests that death anxieties and fears in children and adults are derivatives of other anxieties and fears that develop in early life, principally separation anxiety, fear of object loss, fear of castration, fear of abandonment, and fears of physical immobility and the dark. Anthony(13) suggests that risk-taking behaviour such as 'dares' is one type of defence against such anxieties.
2. The cognitive view relates children's fears and anxieties about death to the stage of development of their concept of death. The young child may fear waking up after death and being trapped in the grave. After the child develops the concept of irreversibility of death, there will be a fear of its permanence.
3. The social learning view puts forward the idea that children's ideas and feelings are influenced by their experiences and by the observations of others. Thus, death fears and anxieties in children will be influenced by

Table 2 Concepts of death and implications of incomplete understanding for adjustment to loss

Component of death concept	Definition	Example of incomplete understanding	Implication of incomplete understanding
Irreversibility	The understanding that once a living thing dies, its physical body cannot be made alive again. Death as final, as irrevocable, as permanent	The child expects the deceased to return, as if from a trip	Failure to comprehend this concept prevents the child from detaching personal ties to the deceased, a necessary first step in mourning
Finality (non-functionality, dysfunctionality, cessation)	The understanding that all life-defining functions cease completely at death	The child worries about a buried relative being cold or in pain; the child wishes to bury food with the deceased	May lead to preoccupation with the physical suffering of the deceased and impair adjustment
Universality (inevitability)	The understanding that all living things die. Death as a natural phenomenon that no living being can escape indefinitely	The child views significant individuals (i.e. self, parents) as immortal	If the child does not view death as inevitable, he or she is likely to view death as punishment (either for actions or thoughts of the deceased, or the child) leading to excessive guilt and shame
Causality	A realistic understanding of the causes of death	Child who relies on magical thinking is apt to assume responsibility for death of a loved one by assuming that bad thoughts or unrelated actions were causative	Tends to lead to excessive guilt that is difficult for the child to resolve

Reproduced from ref. 10 with permission; additional data taken from refs 8 and 11.

their parents, as well as by siblings, peers, teachers, and relatives. Siblings and peers can provide 'information' about death that can be truly frightening. The media (particularly television), children's books, and fairy tales have also been noted to be significant influences.

Death education

Educating children about death has recently been advocated on the basis that it is desirable to promote conceptual development related to death and that death should be introduced as a general concept prior to the child's exposure to personal loss in order to lessen anxiety about death and assist more successful adjustment to loss.[11,14]

The sick child's perception of death

Although the survival rates for a variety of chronic illnesses have dramatically improved over the last 30 years, many children still do not survive. Thus, the issue of their concept of death is still pertinent. Anxiety about death is an issue for all chronically ill children, particularly those with leukaemia and other malignancies, whether or not they eventually survive.

Prior to 1970, most caregivers believed that unless a child was aged over 10 years, he or she was incapable of understanding death and therefore did not experience anxiety about it. It was felt that children did not need information about their disease and that they would be incapable of coping with the distress and anxiety of knowing that they were dying. A closed protective approach was advocated.[15–18]

Revised concepts of illness and death in children with leukaemia

In the late 1960s and early 1970s, pioneering work by Vernick and Karon,[19,20] Waechter,[21] and Bluebond-Langner[22] prompted a complete revision of this perspective.

The views of those advocating a closed protective approach were challenged bluntly for the first time in 1971 by the late Eugenia Waechter. In a key article[21] published in mid-1971, which was prepared from research on anxiety about death in terminally ill children conducted for her doctoral dissertation, Waechter reported on 64 children between the ages of 6 and 10 divided into four groups of equal size: those with a fatal disorder, those with a chronic non-fatal disease, those with a brief illness, and a group of well elementary school children who were not in hospital. A General Anxiety Scale for Children,[23] measuring concerns in many areas of living, was administered to each child. A set of eight pictures was also shown individually to each child and stories were requested in order to elicit fantasy expression of the child's concern regarding present and future body integrity and functioning. Four pictures were selected from the Thermatic Apperception Test.[24] Four others that were designed specifically for the study are reproduced in Fig. 1.

Parents of children in the first three groups were interviewed to assess how the quality and quantity of the fatally ill children's concerns about death were influenced by their previous experience with death, the religious devoutness within the family, the quality of maternal warmth towards them, and the opportunities that they had had to discuss their concerns or the

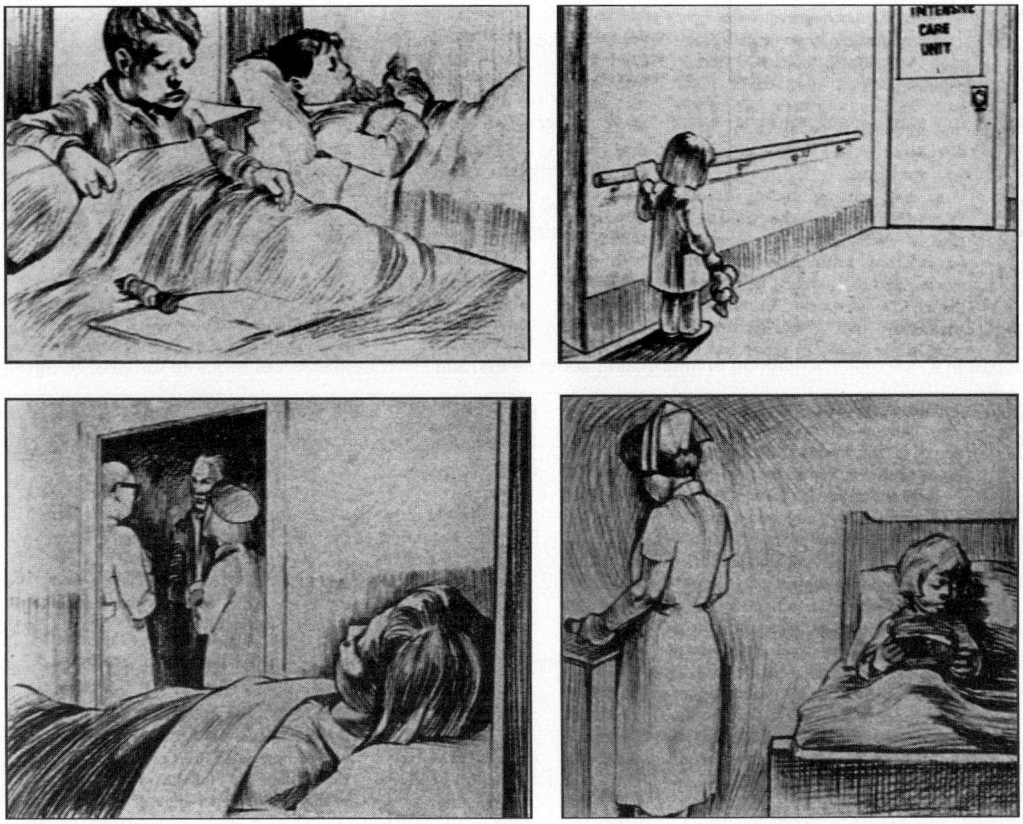

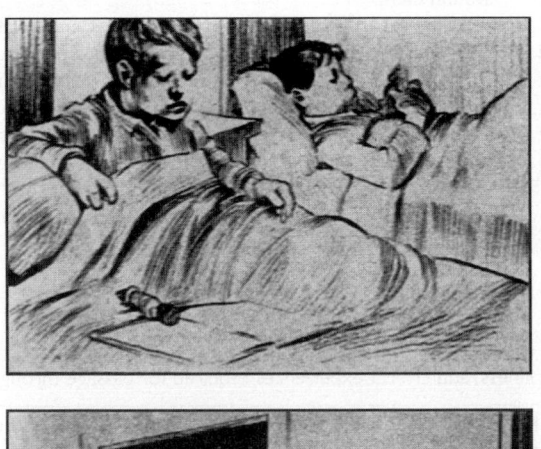

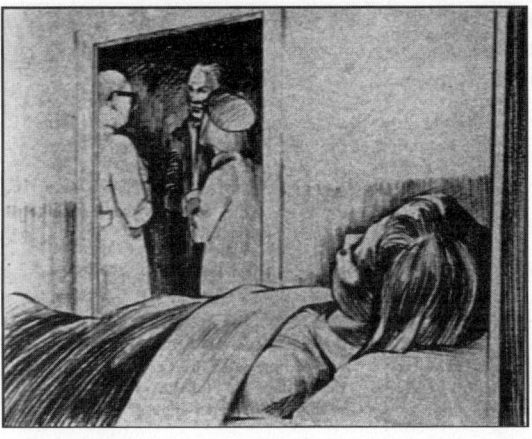

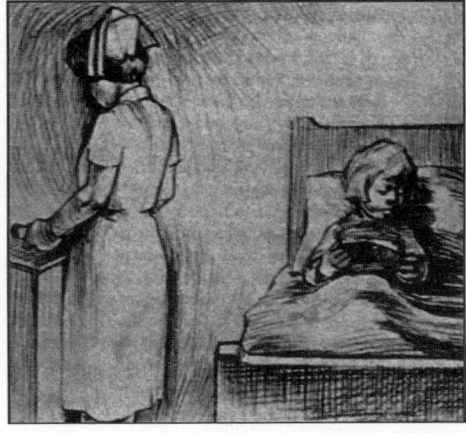

Fig. 1 Four specifically designed pictures used by Waechter to elicit fantasy expressions of concerns related to present and future body integrity from dying children aged 6–10 years. The children were asked to tell stories about the pictures. They often gave the characters their own diagnosis and symptoms and 63 per cent related their stories to death. (Reproduced with permission of the American Journal of Nursing Company.)

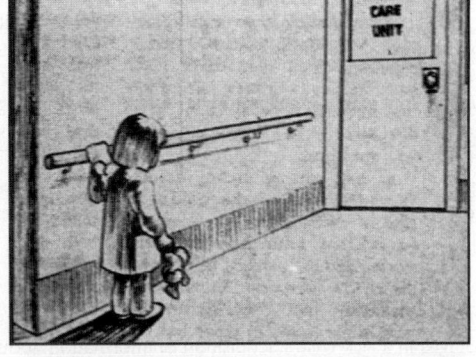

nature of their illness with their parents, professional personnel, or other meaningful adults.

Although only two of the 16 fatally ill children had been told their prognoses, the generalized anxiety was extremely high in all 16 cases, almost double that of the two comparison groups of children in hospital and three times that of healthy children. The children threatened with death discussed loneliness, separation, and death much more frequently in their fantasy stories. Waechter's most striking finding was the dichotomy between the children's degree of awareness of their prognosis, as inferred from their imaginative stories, and the parents' beliefs about their child's awareness. Only two of the 16 fatally ill children had discussed their concerns about death with their parents, yet 63 per cent of stories told by these children related to death. The children often gave the characters in the stories their own diagnoses and symptoms; they frequently depicted death in their drawings and occasionally they would express awareness of their prognoses to persons outside their immediate family. Waechter concluded that denial and protectiveness by adults may not be entirely effective in preventing these children from experiencing anxiety or in keeping their diagnosis and probable prognosis from them. She recommended that the child's questions and concerns should be dealt with in a way that did not further alienate and isolate the child from the parents and other meaningful adults.

In the early 1970s, Myra Bluebond-Langner, an anthropologist, confirmed and extended Waechter's research by conducting detailed, long-term observations of leukaemic children, their parents, and the various health professionals caring for them in the haematology/oncology clinic and ward of an American hospital. Her observations and conclusions, published in 1978,[22] together with those of Waechter, have been pivotal in changing the establishment's views on how to work most effectively with dying children.

Stages of acquisition of factual information about the disease (Bluebond-Langner)

Although parents and staff provided little or no information to the child about any aspect of the illness in the hope of lessening his or her anxiety, it was found that over time such children acquired information about their disease in five stages and that particular experiences were critical to passage through these stages. As the children passed through these stages, they also passed through five different definitions of themselves (Table 3).

The children's personal experiences were a much more significant determinant than age or intellectual ability in determining concepts of their sickness. Thus a 3- or 4-year-old child might know more about his or her prognosis than a very intelligent 9-year-old child.

Mutual pretence

Bluebond-Langner's research confirmed that not only did terminally ill children know they were dying before death became imminent, but they also kept such knowledge a secret, mainly to avoid upsetting their parents and to lessen the probability of being abandoned by loved ones or caregivers because of the anxieties that such disclosures might cause in the latter. Instead, the children, together with their parents and the caregivers, practised an elaborate ritual of mutual pretence, in which all parties defined the patient as dying but acted as if the patient was going to live (Table 4).

Interestingly, in the children studied by Bluebond-Langner, breaches in these rules did not lead to open awareness. Mutual pretence remained the dominant mode of interaction in all children studied, who practised it to the end.

Many patients practise mutual pretence because they find it the most comfortable way to relate to many staff members in the treatment team. The important thing is to be aware that it exists and that it is not a suitable medium for honest communication.

Other research on sick children's concepts of death, illness, and isolation

An evaluation of anxiety and withdrawal in children aged between 6 and 10 years who were terminally ill with leukaemia was conducted in 1974.[26,27] It was found that they appeared to be aware of the seriousness of their illness (even though they might not be yet capable of talking about this awareness in adult terms), expressed more anxiety than controls, and, of greater concern, perceived a growing psychological distance from those around them.

A later study[28] of concepts of death, illness, and isolation in 21 children with leukaemia aged between 4 and 9 years, conducted in 1988 in the United Kingdom, found no indications that the sick children interviewed had radically different concepts of death than have been shown by healthy children. Some of the perceptions of the sick children about themselves in hospital were worrying. The children's feelings of being alone, even with ample company, suggested deprivation of another sort. There was a large variation in the concept of death between individual children, particularly in those younger than 8 years.

Table 3 Stages in a sick child's acquisition of information about illness, and critical experiences required for passage through stages

Stage of acquisition of information	Child's information	Experience required for passage to this stage	Child's self-concept at this stage
First stage	'It' is a serious illness (not all know the name of the disease)	Parents being informed of diagnosis	I was previously well but am now seriously ill
Second stage	The names of the drugs used in treatment, how they are given, and their side-effects	Parents being informed that child is in remission, child speaking to other children at clinic	I am seriously ill and will get better
Third stage	Purposes of special procedures and additional treatments consequent to the side-effects of therapy, and the relationship between particular symptoms and procedures	The first relapse	I am always ill and will get better
Fourth stage	A larger perspective of the disease as an endless series of relapses and remissions	Several further relapses and remissions	I am always ill and will never get better
Fifth stage	The disease as a series of relapses and remissions, ending in death	Child learns of the death of an ill peer	I am dying

Adapted from ref. 22.

Table 4 Rules for practice of mutual pretence[a]

1.	All parties to the interaction should avoid dangerous topics
2.	Talk about dangerous topics is permissible as long as neither party breaks down
3.	All parties to the interaction should focus on safe topics and activities
4.	Props should be used to sustain the 'crucial illusion'
5.	When something happens, or is said which tends to expose the fiction that both parties are attempting to sustain, then each must pretend that nothing has gone awry
6.	All parties to the interaction must strive to keep the interaction normal
7.	All parties must strive to keep the interaction brief
8.	When the rules become impossible to follow and the breakdown of mutual pretence appears imminent, avoid or terminate the interaction

[a] Dying children, their parents, and caregivers are observed to adhere to these rules when practising mutual pretence. Data from refs 22 and 25.

The family's culture and environment and the child's concept of death

Little information is yet available to indicate how a child's concept of death will be affected by the family's culture and environment. However, there is a recurrent theme in the death literature that the way in which parents and others discuss death within the family will have a significant effect on the child's developing concept. Virtually all the literature encourages openness and honesty, and opportunity for the child to talk about the subject. Some predictions that could be tested by research can be attempted based on knowledge already available about how various cultures handle serious illness, dying, death, and mourning [see Table 4 in *Care of the dying child and adolescent: family adjustment and support* (Chapter 9.4)]. For instance, the Buddhist regards illness and death as a natural part of life, whereas the Aboriginal regards death as punishment or the result of evil magic. It is likely that the Buddhist child would have a different concept of death from that of the Aboriginal child, and would be less afraid of it and accept it more as a part of life. Some cultures, for example that of the Lebanese, are rich in mourning rituals but have a closed attitude to discussion of death. It is not yet known how Lebanese children who attend a relative's funeral or who are seriously ill themselves deal with the sudden massive displays of emotion that they witness without the benefit of discussion with other members of the family.

Guidelines for working with the dying child

Clearly, seriously ill and dying children are much more aware of their illness and prognosis than it is comfortable to acknowledge. They are known to harbour anxiety about their situation and are helped by the provision of age-appropriate information. Equipped with this knowledge, the caregiver can certainly be more attentive to the child's verbal and non-verbal communications and seek, where possible, to lessen the child's anxiety.

The emotional needs of the dying child are as follows:

- those of all children regardless of health;
- those arising from the child's reaction to illness and admission to hospital;
- those arising from the child's concept of death.

The following guidelines[29] can be used to help seriously ill children communicate the inner experiences related to their illness:

1. Before proceeding with communication, ascertain the child's own perception of the situation, taking into account his or her developmental level and experience.
2. Understand the child's symbolic language. Children often experience emotions without being able to put them into concepts or words, and young children can use symbolic language to communicate their worries.
3. Clarify reality and dispel fantasy. Children often have difficulty distinguishing between reality and fantasy and between actions and thoughts. A common fantasy of sick children is that of being responsible for the illness. Thus, admission to hospital and medical procedures are interpreted as punishment.
4. Encourage the expression of feelings. When children are allowed to express their anger, sadness, and anxiety, they are able to examine these feelings, place them in perspective, and gain control over them.
5. Promote self-esteem through mastery. The self-esteem of the child with cancer is threatened by pain, frustration, deprivation, changes in body image, and the possibility of death. As a result, his or her school attendance and peer relationships may both suffer. School is the ideal setting in which to encourage the child to communicate about his or her illness in a way that will promote self-esteem through mastery.
6. When approaching the child with cancer, make no assumptions about what the situation will entail. Be open to what each encounter can teach. Do not underestimate the child's ability to master life's challenges creatively and with humour and dignity.

A child who asks 'Am I going to die?' has already picked the person to ask. The wisest and best response is to be honest and confirm that such is the case. How one replies and the words one uses will vary greatly because the details of each child's situation and management, and the relationship with the caregiver asked the question, make every case unique. The important thing is to be honest, confirm that the answer to the question is 'yes', and stay with the child to deal with whatever specific concerns he or she may mention next. Like adults, children are concerned that they will be comfortable, safe, and not alone.

Recommendations for caregivers working with a terminally ill child are referred to in Table 1 and are also discussed in *Care of the dying child and adolescent: family adjustment and support* (Chapter 9.4).

Methods of assessing children's psychological adaptation

Art therapy and music therapy are both forms of expressive therapy that can be used for effective communication by the child. Both can also be used as effective measures of the child's psychological adaptation.

Art therapy

Children are natural artists and can express themselves with few inhibitions. The child's art may communicate what words cannot. While the therapist needs to understand the images produced by children, interpretations of their work are most reliable when provided by the children themselves.

Art therapy can be used to rechannel acting-out behaviour and aggression, provide periods of normality in the midst of frequent examinations, tests, and treatments, and provide opportunity for the children's expressions of creativity. Group art therapy provides opportunities for socializing and communication with peers and for countering feelings of withdrawal or isolation.

The art work of terminally ill children has been found to share common features and to follow particular trends. Objects and forms tend to move towards the upper left quadrant of a page as death approaches. An unusual treatment of a body area has corresponded to new areas of disease unsuspected by the medical staff. Pictures depicting extreme weather conditions have been noted frequently in the art work of terminally ill children: clouds, heavy rain, or snow (often with a brightly shining sun nearby) are said to indicate feelings of anxiety or of being overwhelmed. There may also be a decreased selection of bright colours as the disease progresses, reflecting decreased physical stamina and emotional energy. The interested reader is referred to a report[30] for a more detailed account of this useful medium for communication and assessment. (See also Chapter 15.6.)

Music therapy

Music therapy is also effective in uncovering and working through fears and anxieties related to death and mourning, and it offers the opportunity for creative acts. As illustrated by the case histories of one therapist working with children terminally ill with cancer,[31] music therapy may energize or relax, promote thought or distract, and provide an opportunity for expression. A variety of music therapy techniques, including song writing and selection, lyric substitution, improvization, and guided imagery, can all be used to encourage the child to release his or her fears through a creative act. Music may facilitate a therapeutic relationship, which in turn may supply the security and trust that enables the child to let go of his or her fears. Concerns that are too threatening to be talked about openly can be indirectly expressed during music-therapy activities.

The use of music therapy in paediatric settings is currently confined largely to the United States but, with the continuing encouragement of a small but growing number of advocates in other countries,[32] its application and acceptance in this field will extend elsewhere. (See also Chapter 15.2.)

Books about death for adults and children

There are a wide variety of books dealing with death in both fiction and non-fiction for children and parents, including such well-known works as *Little Women* by L.M. Alcott and *Charlotte's Web* by E.B. White. There is some difference of opinion about the usefulness of such material for working with children.[33–36] Such books are useful when they assist parents or health professionals in explaining aspects of death to a questioning child, particularly when they allow a dialogue on the subject to develop between parent and child. Lists of recommended titles for adults and children appear in Tables 5 and 6.

Table 5 Books for adults about death

Adams, D.W. *Childhood Malignancy: The Psychosocial Care of the Child and his Family.* Springfield IL: Charles C. Thomas, 1979
Adams, D.W. and Deveau, E.J. *Coping with Childhood Cancer—Where Do We Go From Here?* 3rd edn. Hamilton, Ontario: Kinbridge Publications, 1993
Deitrick, R. and Armstrong-Dailey, A. *Approaching Grief* (pamphlet). Children's Hospice International, 1850 M Street, NW, Suite 900, Washington DC 20036, USA
Grollman, E.A. *Talking About Death: A Dialogue Between Parent and Child.* Boston MA: Beacon Press, 1976
Martinson, I.M. *Home Care for the Dying Child: Professional and Family Perspectives.* New York: Appleton-Century-Crofts, 1976
McKissock, M. *Coping with Grief.* Australian Broadcasting Corporation, Box 8888, Crows Nest, NSW, 2065, Australia
Miles, M.S. *'The Grief of Parents'.* Privately printed, 1978. Available from Compassionate Friends Inc., PO Box 1347, Oak Brook, IL 60521, USA
Schiff, H.S. *The Bereaved Parent.* New York: Crown Publishers, 1977
Schulman, J.L. *Coping with Tragedy: Successfully Facing the Problem of a Seriously Ill Child.* Chicago: Follett Publishing, 1976
Sherman, M. *The Leukemic Child.* Washington DC: US Department of Health, Education & Welfare, Publication No. (NIH) 76–863, 1976
Stephens, S. *Death Comes Home.* New York: Morehouse-Barlow, 1973
Wass, H. and Corr, C.A., ed. *Helping Children Cope with Death: Guidelines and Resources* 2nd edn. Washington DC: Hemisphere, 1984
Wells, R. *Helping Children Cope with Grief—Facing a Death in the Family.* London: Sheldon Press, 1988
Zagdanski, D. *Something I've Never Felt Before—How Teenagers Cope with Grief.* Melbourne: Hill of Content Press, 1990

Table 6 Books for children about death

Alcott, L.M. *Little Women.* Boston: Little, Brown, 1968
Alex, M. and Alex, B. *Grandpa and Me.* Hertford UK: Lion Publishing, 1981
Bernstein, J.E. and Gullo, S.V. *When People Die.* New York: EP Dutton, 1977
Fassler, J. *My Grandpa Died Today.* New York: Human Sciences Press, 1971
Grollman, E.A. *Talking About Death—A Dialogue Between Parent and Child.* Boston MA: Beacon Press, 1976
White, E.B. *Charlotte's Web.* New York: Harper & Row, 1952
Zim, H. and Bleeker, S. *Life and Death.* New York: William Morrow, 1970

The terminally ill child at school

As a result of their illness, children with cancer will have acquired concepts and experiences of pain, loss, and grief, which will have changed them and distinguish them from their peers. Children who receive treatment for cancer encounter a loss of self-esteem. Their unusual situation requires them to deal with new and significant issues, occasionally with some anxiety, so that they may have less attention and energy for the day-to-day matters of school. They will be less assertive. They will be more reluctant than their healthy peers to attempt new concepts in which failure is possible because of the risk of losing more self-esteem through failure. Schooling for these children should always start out from areas and levels of competence in which they feel absolutely comfortable.[37]

Children who are terminally ill with cancer may continue to receive treatment, and in many cases will remain well enough to attend school for many months. Even though they may be in an advanced stage of their disease, it is very important for their self-esteem and sense of mastery over a deteriorating situation to continue to attend school when they wish to, if only for a few hours a day.

An explanation to the class about the child's illness will have been given by a member of the treatment team earlier in the course of the illness, usually soon after the diagnosis. At the outset, classmates are most frequently concerned about whether or not they can catch the disease from the patient.

In the event of the child becoming terminally ill, the child's teacher will have to confront and deal with the impending death of the child and the resulting effects on the classmates, other teachers, and students at the school. Under these circumstances, it is wise to have made some preparation beforehand. Discussion at a staff meeting might take place involving other teachers and the principal to examine their attitudes to death and dying. This would assist staff to formulate an appropriate plan which the child's teacher could then implement with the class. The teacher should also confer with the child's parents, who need to be involved in these plans.

The child's treatment team, particularly the hospital school teacher, will liaise with the school and the child's school teachers to maximize his or her educational opportunities. Terminally ill children may wish to be included and need to be treated as normally as possible. A bean chair or similar comfortable support in the corner of the classroom close to the focus of interest may enable such children to enjoy many hours of satisfaction, even though they may not be able to participate actively in all lessons. Deterioration is usually gradual and death is not expected to occur suddenly or unexpectedly, for example, during class. If the terminally ill student deteriorated rapidly or unexpectedly collapsed, there still would be sufficient time to take him or her home or to hospital with the parents and family.

Saying goodbye: the child's preparation for death

Children who are seriously or terminally ill will usually take steps to put their affairs in order. During her preparation for a mismatched bone marrow transplant, one of the author's patients completed tapestries bearing personal notes of thanks for the author and another doctor. These were presented after her death by her parents, who reported that she had discussed her funeral with her friends, requesting that her two closest girlfriends sing a favoured hymn.

Another patient, a teenage boy dying of progressive non-Hodgkin's lymphoma, summoned all the ward staff to his room to say goodbye to each. Later, with many of his friends present, he bequeathed one of his possessions to each, including his most cherished possession, a CB radio.

The following example from the author's department provides even more striking evidence of preparation for and acceptance of imminent death.

Case history

Patient A had acute non-lymphoblastic leukaemia diagnosed at age 13. Following relapse 18 months later, she proceeded to a mismatched bone marrow transplant 3 months after relapse, with her mother as the donor. Patient A died 5 weeks after the transplant.

A's mother reported that during her last few months, A spoke more about the possibility of death and of the need to plan for the disposal of her material possessions. After her relapse she frequently spoke of not wanting to die, mainly confiding her thoughts to her mother. She attended three healing masses and was noted to have fewer periods of depression afterwards. One of the pages from her notebook on which she recorded her observations of what she thought death would be like, is reproduced with the family's permission in Fig. 2.

A's mother reported A's great self-control as she planned for the possibility of not surviving the transplant. She asked that the family have a holiday together before the transplant, she asked if she owned her bedroom furniture and her piano, and about her right to make a will. Those attending her funeral were to wear bright colours. The service was to be held in her school chapel and the madrigal group of which she was a member was to sing a favourite hymn. A nominated a white coffin, named the clothing for her burial ('not a nightie, under any circumstances'), and asked that a family photograph, a Bible, and her rosary beads be placed in her coffin. She purchased a remembrance gift for her parents and wrote them a personal letter. She recorded herself playing a special piece of music on the piano. She asked her parents not to remain sad, to be kind and loving to each other, and always to stay together.

These examples show that dying children may respond in a manner well beyond their years.

The dying child's premonition of imminent death

Terminally ill children often know when they are about to die and may even share this information with their parents.

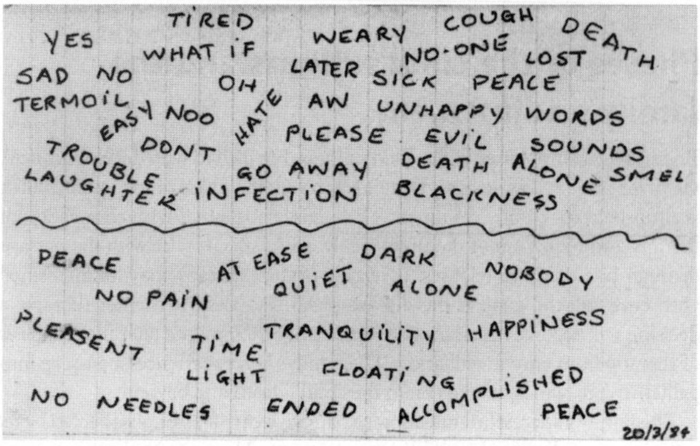

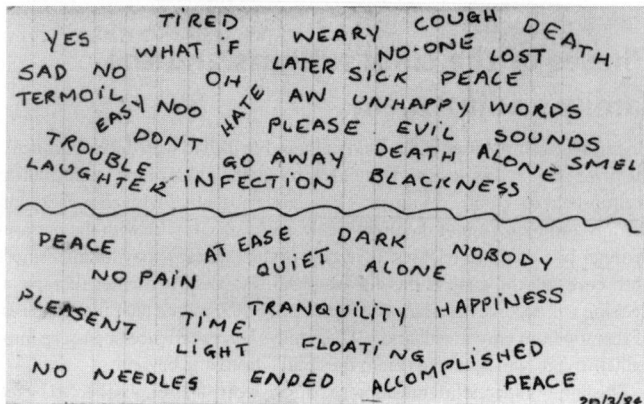

Fig. 2 A page from A's notebook recording her own observations of what she thought death would be like (reproduced with her parents' permission).

One of the author's patients, a 9-year-old boy, died suddenly shortly after the abrupt onset of severe interstitial pneumonitis 8 months after bone marrow transplant. His family owned one of a number of shops clustered in a marina, and their son was well known to the other tenants. After he had died, the parents learnt that he had spent time chatting with each and every tenant in the marina, on the day before his death.

Another of the author's patients, a 5-year-old boy with terminal acute lymphoblastic leukaemia, died at home. On the night he died, he came into his parents' bedroom. He explained that he did not quite know what to say to them and, instead, sang a familiar children's song, *Sing a Rainbow*.[38]

Needing permission to die

Young people who are dying may linger close to death for prolonged periods. They may simply need permission from their loved ones to die and will often die promptly when such permission is given. One of the author's patients, an 11-year-old boy with osteogenic sarcoma, was dying at home after a 5-year illness. Throughout his illness, he had demonstrated a notable tenacity to survive and willingness to endure continuing and painful treatment as long as it entailed some hope for further quality survival. After his death, his father reported that as the boy's death drew close, he lingered on in a coma for more than 7 days. An Aboriginal community nurse who was caring for the patient spoke with his father, informing him that the boy needed his parents' permission to die. The father and mother ushered the boy's grandmother and other relatives out of his room, sat down alone by the boy's bed, spoke to him of their love for him, and gave him their permission to die. The boy died peacefully a few hours later.

Future prospects in paediatric palliative care

One can anticipate ongoing studies on psychological aspects of death and dying in both well and sick children. The challenge for the caregiver will be to keep abreast of current thought and to respond to new principles of care as they become validated.

Conclusion: implications for staff

Staff caring for terminally ill children face similar stresses to those confronted by the family. Because the family's outlook is greatly influenced by the personality and reactions of the staff, a special degree of maturity and caring is required. Staff should remember to recognize their own limitations and the importance of the support an inter-disciplinary team approach can offer. Staff should be realistic in the goals they set and use supports available to them. Regular periods of leave, and interests and commitments outside the work-place, will all help to ensure a continuing effective level of care to those in need.

It is often asked how one could work in such an emotionally charged field, and the response (as most who work in this field will know) is that one enjoys the work and finds working with children such as these and their families rewarding, fascinating, frequently unpredictable, never boring, and always a privilege.

References

1. **Piaget, J. and Inhelder, B.** *The Psychology of the Child.* Translated from the French by Helen Weaver. New York: Basic Books, 1969.
2. **Singer, D. and Revenson, T.** *A Piaget Primer: How a Child Thinks.* New York: Universities Press, 1978.
3. **Rando, T.A.** *Grief, Dying and Death: Clinical Interventions for Caregivers.* Champaign IL: Research Press, 1984, pp. 385–91.
4. **Wass, H.** (1984). Concepts of death: a developmental perspective. In *Childhood and Death* (ed. H. Wass and C.A. Corr), pp. 4, 18. Washington DC: Hemisphere.

5. Nagy, M. (1948). The child's theories concerning death. *Journal of Genetic Psychology* **73**, 3–27.
6. Anthony, S. *The Discovery of Death in Childhood and After.* New York: Basic Books, 1972.
7. Kane, B. (1979). Children's concepts of death. *Journal of Genetic Psychology* **134**, 41–53.
8. Speece, M.W. and Brent, S.B. (1984). Children's understanding of death: a review of three components of a death concept. *Child Development* **55**, 1671–86.
9. Lansdown, R. and Benjamin, G. (1985). The development of the concept of death in children aged 5–9 years. *Child: Care, Health and Development* **11**, 13–20.
10. Schonfeld, D. (1989). Crisis intervention for bereavement support: a model of intervention in the children's school. *Clinical Pediatrics* **28**, 29.
11. Schonfeld, D.J. and Kappelman, M. (1990). The impact of school-based education on the young child's understanding of death. *Developmental and Behavioural Pediatrics* **11**, 247–52.
12. Wass, H. and Cason, L. (1984). Fears and anxieties about death. In *Childhood and Death* (ed. H. Wass and C.A. Corr), pp. 25–45. Washington DC: Hemisphere.
13. Anthony, S. *The Discovery of Death in Childhood and After.* New York: Basic Books, 1972, pp. 163–5.
14. McNeil, J. (1983). Young mothers' communication about death with their children. *Death Education* **6**, 323–39.
15. Knudson, A.G. and Natterson, J.M. (1960). Participation of parents in the hospital care of their fatally ill children. *Pediatrics* **26**, 482–90.
16. Morrissey, J.R. (1965). Death anxiety in children with a fatal illness. In *Crisis Intervention* (ed. H.J. Parad), pp. 324–38. New York: Family Service Association of America.
17. Natterson, J.M. and Knudson, A.G. (1960). Observations concerning fear of death in fatally ill children and their mothers. *Psychosomatic Medicine* **22**, 456–65.
18. Richmond, J.B. and Waisman, H.A. (1955). Psychologic aspects of management of children with malignant diseases. *American Journal of Diseases in Childhood* **89**, 42–7.
19. Vernick, J. and Karon, M. (1965). Who's afraid of death on a leukemia ward? *American Journal of Diseases of Children* **109**, 393–7.
20. Karon, M. and Vernick, J. (1968). An approach to the emotional support of fatally ill children. *Clinical Pediatrics* **7**, 274–80.
21. Waechter, E.H. (1971). Children's awareness of fatal illness. *American Journal of Nursing* **71**, 1168–72.
22. Bluebond-Langner, M. *The Private Worlds of Dying Children.* Princeton NJ: Princeton University Press, 1978.
23. Sarason, S.B. et al. *Anxiety in Elementary School Children.* New York: Wiley, 1960.
24. Murray, H.A. *Thermatic Apperception Test.* Cambridge MA: Harvard University Press, 1943.
25. Glaser, B. and Strauss, A. *Awareness of Dying: A Study of Social Interaction.* Chicago: Aldine, 1965.
26. Spinetta, J.J., Rigler, D., and Karon, M. (1974). Personal space as a measure of a dying child's sense of isolation. *Journal of Consulting and Clinical Psychology* **42**, 751–6.
27. Spinetta, J.J., Rigler, D., and Karon, M. (1973). Anxiety in the dying child. *Pediatrics* **52**, 841–5.
28. Clunies-Ross, C. and Lansdown, R. (1988). Concepts of death, illness and isolation found in children with leukaemia. *Child: Care, Health and Development* **14**, 373–86.
29. Adams-Greenly, M. (1984). Helping children communicate about serious illness and death. *Journal of Psychosocial Oncology* **2** (2), 61–72.
30. Schmitt, B.B. and Guzzino, M.H. (1985). Expressive therapy with children in crisis: a new avenue of communication. In *Hospice Approaches to Pediatric Care* (ed. C.A. Corr and D.M. Corr), pp. 155–77. New York: Springer.
31. Fagen, T.S. (1982). Music therapy in the treatment of anxiety and fear in terminal pediatric patients. *Music Therapy: Journal of the American Association for Music Therapy* **2**, 13–23.
32. Bright, R. *Grieving: A Handbook for Those who Care.* St Louis MO: MMB Music, 1986.
33. Corr, C.A. (1984). Books for adults. In *Childhood and Death* (ed. H. Wass and C.A. Corr), pp. 367–71. Washington DC: Hemisphere Publishing Corporation.
34. Wass, H. (1984). Books for children. In *Childhood and Death* (ed. H. Wass and C.A. Corr), pp. 373–6. Washington DC: Hemisphere Publishing Corporation.
35. Lamers, E. (1986). Books for adolescents. In *Adolescence and Death* (ed. C.A. Corr and J.N. McNeil), pp. 233–42. New York: Springer.
36. Aradire, C. (1976). Books for children about death. *Pediatrics* **57**, 372.
37. Stevens, M.M. (1996). Cancer in childhood. In *Physical as Anything: Collaborative Support for Students with Physical Disabilities and Medical Conditions* (ed. M.M. Stevens, J. Rayner, R. Turnell, B. Graham, D. Piper, and T. Smith). Sydney, NSW: NSW Dept of School Education.
38. Stevens, M. (1989). Palliative care in paediatrics. *Cancer Forum* **13**, 21–5.

Further reading

Corr, C.A. and Corr, D.M., ed. *Hospice Approaches to Pediatric Care.* New York: Springer, 1985. Influential treatise on application of principles of palliative care to children.

Foley, G.V. and Whittam, E.H. (1990). Care of the child dying of cancer: Part I. *CA—A Cancer Journal for Clinicians* **40**, 327–54. Concise and valuable overview of paediatric palliative care.

Pettle, M.S.A. and Lansdown, R.G. (1986). Adjustment to the death of a sibling. *Archives of Disease in Childhood* **61**, 278–83. Useful report of the experiences of siblings of a deceased child.

9.4 Care of the dying child and adolescent: family adjustment and support

Michael M. Stevens

This chapter discusses the family's adjustment during the experience of coping with the child's illness and impending death, and provides some suggestions for support by caregivers.

Phases of the child's illness and the family's adjustment

There are various phases in the child's illness. For a child who develops cancer, the first begins at diagnosis and extends through the phase of treatment, which is almost always curative in intent. This phase ends either with completion of therapy and follow-up of the presumably cured survivor, or with the passage through one or more relapses. If relapse occurs, therapy may be intensified with cure still the goal. If the disease progresses despite further therapy, a decision will become necessary to cease curative therapy and alter the emphasis of therapy from cure to palliation. The family then experiences a passage into palliative care, which extends on to the child's death and beyond.

The family's successful transition to palliative care is strongly affected by its experiences earlier in the child's management. The caregiver's attention to earlier aspects of the family's management does much to help the family cope with the child's palliative care and death. Hence, an evaluation of the family's experience will be given, along with suggestions for support in each phase.

The family can be regarded as a system of parts or components. Like any system, the family attempts to maintain a degree of balance and equilibrium, and each will have distinct patterns of communication, behaviour, roles, rules, and expectations. A family may be seen as an open system if family members have full freedom to communicate, boundaries between family members are flexible, and family rules are up to date and promote growth. In contrast, a family may be seen as a closed system if communication is restricted or indirect, boundaries are enmeshed, members are overly involved with and dependent on one another, and rules are too inflexible to allow change or permit growth.[1] Clearly, the experiences that each family encounters and the challenges generated will vary considerably.

Foundations for effective palliative care: the family's early experience

The quality of the family's experience in the earliest phase of the child's illness, in the first few weeks after diagnosis, is particularly important in determining later adjustment to palliative care, should that become necessary.

The initial treatment goals set for a child with cancer are almost always curative in intent. Considerable advances in surgery, radiotherapy, and particularly chemotherapy have occurred over the last 40 years. The advent of multi-institutional randomized trials of therapy for paediatric cancer in the United Kingdom, the United States, and elsewhere has led to encouraging improvements in the cure rate for many types of childhood cancer. About 75 per cent of children who develop the most common type of childhood cancer, acute lymphoblastic leukaemia, will be cured with current conventional therapy. Over 80 per cent of children who develop some of the most common paediatric solid tumours, including localized Wilms' tumour, localized non-Hodgkin's lymphoma, and Hodgkin's disease, will also be cured with current therapy. The outlook for others with less common types of leukaemia, certain cerebral tumours, disseminated neuroblastoma, and other solid tumours where detectable spread has occurred prior to diagnosis remains less favourable. Overall, about 75 per cent of today's young patients with malignant disease will be cured. The remainder will ultimately die of their disease and need palliative care.

At diagnosis the child should be referred to a paediatric institution offering skilled multimodal cancer therapy. Occasionally children may be very ill at the time of diagnosis and may almost immediately enter the terminal phase. However, for most children the emphasis of initial therapy will be strongly directed towards cure.

Communicating with the child's parents at diagnosis: foundation for successful palliative care

On receiving the diagnosis the child's parents always assume the worst, that their child is certainly going to die and soon. One of the goals of the initial consultations with the child's paediatrician and other significant caregivers is to readjust the parents' expectations to a more hopeful level in keeping with the child's actual prognosis.

However, there are other equally important goals in these initial consultations. Effective communication with the child's parents in the days after diagnosis is vital in laying the foundation for effective palliative care later, should that become necessary. If information, friendly encouragement, practical support, and hope have been made freely available to the family by the treatment team from the time of diagnosis, parents will be much more likely to cope successfully with palliative care than if they feel uninformed, misunderstood, and unsupported.

In interviews of 20 families of children who died of leukaemia in the mid-1960s, many of the parents described the events at diagnosis as the hardest blow they had to bear throughout the course of the child's illness. All families expressed appreciation for the frankness and honesty of the initial discussions with the treatment team, and eight specifically singled them out as one of the major sources of help.[2] Disagreements and misunderstandings arising from poor communication between paediatric patients with leukaemia, their parents, and physicians may be responsible for seemingly unusual or maladaptive coping by patients or families.[3]

The diagnosis of cancer in a child is a crisis for the child and the family. The parents will usually be stunned and disbelieving at the outset, and there will be an initial period of shock, confusion, and numbness. The parents will describe a feeling of being overwhelmed by the situation, or of feeling unable to function. There may be denial of the diagnosis, or intellectual acceptance of the diagnosis without any emotional release.

As the initial shock declines, a progressive testing of reality occurs. This is usually accompanied by feelings of anger, guilt, sadness, and depression. With no explanation of the cause of the child's cancer forthcoming, the parents may blame themselves or each other for a failure of some sort. They may hold themselves responsible by having 'passed the disease on' to the child. This will not be so except in cases of hereditary retinoblastoma or other rare family cancer syndromes. There is often guilt over a perceived delay in diagnosis and a sentiment that the illness would not have occurred had they sought attention earlier. They may also fear for the child's siblings or even themselves, lest they develop the same illness. There is a definite similarity between these early reactions at diagnosis and those experienced in the early phases of bereavement.

Effective communication with parents under these circumstances is always difficult and may fail even in skilled hands. Pointers to good communication early in therapy are provided in Table 1. As the child's therapy progresses and the parents meet more caregivers and other families who corroborate what the family has been told, parents develop trust in the treatment team and willingly cooperate. Longer-term pointers for good communication with parents are also provided in Table 1. Pointers for good communication with adolescents with cancer are provided later in this chapter.

Rarely, an assessment of the child's initial outlook (e.g. the presence of irreversible paralysis due to spinal metastases from disseminated rhabdomyosarcoma involving additional distant sites) may indicate that therapy is best not undertaken and a programme of palliative care adopted immediately. This requires that the treatment team not only develop an effective relationship with the child's family immediately but also move directly to the transition phase to palliative care.

Occasionally, a child may have a favourable prognosis, but the family will steadfastly refuse consent for potentially curative therapy. One has the option of adopting legal means to displace the parents' right to withhold consent. A decision about such action cannot be taken until the motives for the parents' actions have been discussed fully with them and an objective appraisal made of the child's prognosis and anticipated quality of life during therapy. One may decide that the treatment is in the child's best interests, although the consequences of such action on the family's relationship with the treatment team may be adverse (see Chapter 3.5).

Grandparents, siblings, and the child's school at diagnosis

The child's grandparents, brothers and sisters, family friends, and school will all be deeply disturbed by the diagnosis.

In one study of families' adaptation to a child's final illness, half the families studied considered that one or both sets of grandparents had become a burden or hindrance, but in many other families the grandparents offered considerable support. Negative interactions reflected to a considerable extent past relations between parents and grandparents.[2]

Grandparents benefit considerably from an early consultation with the child's physician, undertaken with the parents' consent soon after diagnosis. This allows any misconceptions or irrational guilt to be dealt with. The grandparents may subsequently become closely involved in the day-to-day care of their grandchild and thus provide support and practical assistance to the parents. Those grandparents who have coped well during the child's illness will also cope more successfully with bereavement after the child's death.

The caregiving team must pay special attention to the welfare of the sick child's siblings. A number of studies have documented that brothers and sisters of a seriously ill child undergo significant anxieties and stresses

Table 1 Pointers to good communication with parents of children with cancer[4]

Ensure that both parents are present for the initial consultation. This recognizes the importance of both parents and makes it less likely that one partner will misinterpret information
Interview parents in a quiet, comfortable room, with everyone seated
During important discussions, allow the parents to include a close friend or relative, who may recall information that parents forget
Have another member of the caregiving team, for example, the nurse, present to help identify areas for discussion
Give parents a clear description of their child's illness; identify the illness as cancer; use plain English
Emphasize that the parents did not cause the disease and could not have prevented it; that the disease is not hereditary (if that is so); that the diagnosis has been made without undue delay; and that effective therapy is available that has cured other children
Provide enough time so that parents can ask questions and not feel rushed. Encourage them to write down any points of concern as they occur for discussion at the next consultation. Seek feedback about what parents have understood from each consultation
On receiving the diagnosis, parents always assume that their child is going to die, and soon. Aim to readjust their expectations to a hopeful level, in keeping with the child's actual outlook
A written summary or tape-recording of the discussion may be helpful
With parental approval, involve the child in some of the early discussions to lessen his or her anxiety
Parents will be shocked initially and even disbelieving, then angry, guilty, and depressed. This limits their ability to absorb and retain information. Repeat information patiently over several consultations. In the beginning, do not provide detailed technical information that the family may misunderstand or forget
At an early stage, spend time with the patient's siblings and grandparents and liaise with the child's school to help allay anxiety and reduce family members' stress
Have the family meet a child with a similar diagnosis who has done well
Longer-term pointers Be easy to contact by parents
A patient-held medical record[5] provides the family with readily accessible information about their child's progress
Regular seminars, support meetings, and newsletters for parents of surviving and deceased patients improve parents' knowledge and help them feel supported
Have parents attending the treatment centre elect a liaison committee to assist in optimal patient management. The liaison committee is a group of elected members of the parent body who act as conductors of information between the oncology staff and the patients' families. This is achieved through a quarterly magazine, an annual parent seminar day, regular evening forums for parents, casual wine and cheese nights in different parts of the city, and meetings with the oncology staff during which the committee can act as parent advocates
Always allow parents hope, no matter how poor the outlook. Support the family in their current hope and help them maintain a realistic focus on what their child can still do

during the child's illness. Not only do they face the potential loss of their sibling, but also the loss of their family as they have known it and the loss of their parents' attention. This may engender feelings of being rejected by the parents and also resentment towards the dying child.

A study[6] of school-aged patients from 71 families attending a paediatric oncology clinic and their healthy siblings aged 6–16 years revealed that siblings of children with cancer have the same significant anxieties, fears for their own health, social isolation, and other stresses once thought to be peculiar to the patients themselves. The siblings' anxiety about their own health frequently found expression in physical symptoms. The siblings felt very isolated from their parents, from other family members, and from friends. Divisions in the family were caused by the patients' hospital admissions accompanied by the mother, while the fathers attempted to cope at home and with job responsibilities. The siblings were frequently found to be left at home, alone, worried, and cut off from reassurance and support. Despite the siblings' isolation and relative neglect, they were reluctant to express anger or negative feelings towards other family members.

Healthy adaptation for siblings would be encouraged by allowing them to participate in conferences with the physician, by directing parents' attention to their needs, and by encouraging them to visit the ward whenever the patient is in hospital.

The welfare of siblings of the dying child is discussed again later in this chapter.

Liaison with the child's school soon after diagnosis assists the family in re-establishing some degree of equilibrium during therapy. Ideally, with the parents' permission, a member of the treatment team should visit the school and provide the school's staff with relevant information about the child's illness and treatment. Precautions helpful to the child's therapy can be emphasized, such as the importance of minimizing exposure to varicella or morbilli, which may be lethal to the immunocompromised patient on chemotherapy. The child's classmates can be reassured, and arrangements can be made with the hospital's school for work to be sent to the hospital or home and for selected classmates to visit the child in hospital. Educational resources providing information about the child's illness and its treatment should be available to the parents[7] and the school.[8]

These measures will help to alleviate the anxiety of the child and family, and assist their attempts to regain control and some degree of normality in their day-to-day life.

Recognizing the family at risk

Families will be encountered that, for one reason or another, experience significant difficulties during the child's illness, for example, families already coping with physically or intellectually handicapped children, single-parent families, families where parents are separating at the time of the child's diagnosis, and families struggling because of financial difficulties, unemployment, or cultural or language difficulties.

Such families require extra help at diagnosis and during therapy to lessen the likelihood of additional crises other than those unavoidably linked to the child's diagnosis and treatment. Excessive criticism of health professionals already encountered earlier in the child's management indicates poor adjustment and the need for additional support. The family that places unreasonable demands on the treatment team needs to be recognized since compliance with all the family's requests may lead to conflict later. Some early agreement about level of service should be tactfully negotiated with such families in order to avoid problems.

Parent support groups in the early phases of the child's illness

Convincing documentation that parents of other leukaemic children are a source of support to parents was provided at least 30 years ago[2] and has been confirmed by others.[9,10] The author's team strongly believes in the value of parent support and has fostered the development of parent support groups both for families of children attending for treatment, and bereaved families. Families with newly diagnosed children are encouraged to contact these groups and to meet members of other families at periodic conferences or luncheons held at the hospital specifically for this purpose. Most families find the groups a valuable source of support, information, and practical assistance.

Transition to palliative care

The recognition that a child's leukaemia or cancer is entering a terminal phase after one or more unsuccessfully treated relapses heralds the onset of renewed stress for all concerned. Prior to this, the child will have been receiving chemotherapy and supportive treatment in a planned and methodical attempt at cure. During this time the child's cancer will have been under control and the child will have been reasonably or completely well. The family's shock, grief, and depression present at the time of diagnosis will have eased, although anxiety about the implications of relapse is constantly present in both parents and patients, even in those very long-term survivors already declared cured. Relapse and the eventual advent of palliative care plunges the family into renewed crisis.

All the reactions present at the original diagnosis resurface with heightened intensity, now overshadowed by the loss of hope implicit in relapse. The parents experience feelings of hopelessness and helplessness, coupled with grief, fear, depression, anger, and denial. Parents who constantly dread relapse and terminal care may express some sentiments of relief that the worst has at last occurred.

There is no easy way to convey bad news. All aids to communication employed at diagnosis and discussed previously become more important now. The paediatrician responsible for the child's cancer therapy should accept the responsibility of these painful consultations. One must be honest, frank, gentle, and sympathetic. The last requires a certain degree of empathy and therefore pain for the caregiving team.

Investigational or palliative therapy?

As described by Snyder,[11] there are several paths to follow for the child who is fatally ill at diagnosis or who has failed curative therapy and is entering a terminal phase.

One basic treatment plan is to give no medical or nursing treatment at all other than to enhance the physical, personal, and social comfort of the dying child. This plan may be very difficult for the treatment team to accept because it implies that the caregivers as well as their treatments have failed. Comfort measures, such as a manageable diet, pain control, and prevention or treatment of skin breakdown, are the only form of medical or nursing treatment provided.

A second plan is for palliative care, which places the highest priority on the control of pain in its broadest sense. Certain medications, chemotherapy protocols, irradiation, and even surgery may eventually result in a higher quality of remaining life for the child even though extension of life is not the goal of palliative care. The treatment team must consider carefully the enhanced quality of life after such palliative procedures when measured against their inherent discomfort. Recovery time must not use up long portions of the child's remaining life.

The third and most controversial plan is to administer investigational treatments that offer only a slight chance of cure and very frequently cause a significant increase in the pain and morbidity suffered by the child. This option is the only one that offers any chance at all of cure.

In explaining the implications of the terminal nature of the child's illness, the paediatrician will already have made a judgment that further therapy directed against the underlying cancer is not appropriate. This places a responsibility on the doctor to be fully informed of all recent advances in treatment, particularly those involving investigational agents or techniques of unproven activity against the disease involved. A decision by the child's paediatrician to change to palliative care should only be taken after full discussion of possible treatment options with the other team members. Occasional conflict will arise within the team over whether to proceed with investigational therapy or change to palliative care. While the need for trials of investigational therapy is not disputed, foremost consideration must be given to the anticipated benefits and disadvantages of the proposed therapy for the particular child. The need for a sensible advocate for the child within the treatment team is vital.

Making the transition to palliative care

Surprisingly, most families make the transition from curative to palliative therapy smoothly and effectively, even though it is an extremely demanding time for them. The time taken in earlier phases of the child's management to establish a trusting relationship between the child and family and the staff will be invaluable in helping them through this crisis. The caregiving team can help ensure this transition is made more successfully by providing the necessary information and support to assist the family's decisions. Most families are able to retain sufficient equilibrium to deal with the situation effectively. Information is most commonly relayed from the treatment team to the parents, who then convey it to the other members of the family. Maintenance of confidentiality at this stage is even more important than at diagnosis in order to allow the family to retain some control over how widely information is disseminated.

Parents need a careful and sympathetic explanation of the situation including available options for further therapy, so they can participate in the decisions being made. It is necessary that parents, and ultimately the patient and family, adjust to a shift in emphasis from cure to relief of symptoms. In acknowledging that the underlying disease will not be successfully eradicated, the goal of further treatment becomes that of ensuring optimal comfort and quality for each remaining day of the child's life.

The parents must be reassured that treatment failure is not their fault as there will be considerable guilt about previous minor and insignificant non-compliance with medication schedules. An estimate of how long the child is expected to live will be sought and should be provided. This may be only a matter of days when there is rapidly progressing infection or metabolic disturbance, or several months in a well child with a slowly growing tumour. A summary of the plan for the child's management during the terminal phase should be presented to the family and subsequently discussed with them by other members of the treatment team, all of whom play a role in the child's palliative care. Such a plan requires personal knowledge of the individual child.

It is best to inform the parents first without the child and give them time to adjust to the new situation before consulting directly with the child. The patient's brothers and sisters, grandparents, other relatives, and friends are also involved in the crisis. A brother or sister of the patient who has acted as a donor for a bone marrow transplant will face special difficulties, as will single parents and families hampered by cultural or language barriers. Allowance must be made for a wide range of reactions from families of different cultural backgrounds. Such reactions should not be allowed to prejudice the caregiving team's treatment of the child.

Occasionally, a family will refuse to accept the transition to palliative care. Such families will continue to insist that 'everything possible be done' and may seek alternate sources of therapy that may be of unproven benefit or even potentially harmful. The best approach is to continue discussing the issues objectively and patiently, emphasizing what is best for the child. The parents in such families may need to confront and acknowledge fears and other negative emotions relating to the potential loss of the child that may have been denied at diagnosis or in earlier phases of treatment.

Communicating with the child

Ill and dying children know a great deal more about their situation than might otherwise be thought. Furthermore, attempts to conceal the situation from them have been proven ineffective and damaging. Dying children invariably know the true situation from their past experiences in the treatment unit. Their own bodies provide strong additional clues that death may be imminent.

Consequently, it is essential to involve the child in at least some of the discussions about further management. With the consent of the parents one should consult directly with children over 5 or 6 years of age at this important phase of their management. A tactful but honest explanation as to why specific therapy is being discontinued should be given and ample opportunity for discussion of the implications provided. Children older than 6 or 7 years are often very matter-of-fact in their approach to their own situation.

The child's questions should be answered truthfully. The most difficult questions asked by the child may be directed to the parents or to a trusted member of the team other than the doctor and may be asked at a later time. Again, truthful answers are best. A child who asks a difficult question almost always knows the answer beforehand and is merely seeking confirmation to assess if it is permissible to discuss the subject with the person to whom the question has been directed. Failure to respond openly to such a question because of a fear of not coping deprives the child of a valuable opportunity for communication.

The child's perception and understanding of death will be influenced by chronological age, developmental level, individual personality, past experiences with death and loss, and the family's religious beliefs. It may be difficult for young children to express their fears. In particular, they fear separation from parents and loved ones, and sense and respond strongly to the level of anxiety surrounding them. Expressive play with art or music will assist them in working through and expressing their concerns, and they have a continuing need for reassurance and security. In not wishing to discuss painful matters and seemingly putting on a brave front, the child may in fact be seeking to protect the parents from further emotional turmoil for which he or she may feel responsible.

Communicating with the siblings

The young patient's brothers and sisters also face emotional difficulties during the terminal period. While grieving for the sick child, they may resent the lack of attention they receive because of the parents' preoccupation with him or her. This may lead to hostility towards the sick child and even a wish for his or her death. Later there may be guilt over these feelings. As with the parents, an opportunity for counselling by the child's doctor or other members of the treatment team to deal with some of these issues prior to the child's death will help to reduce disturbance afterwards.

The adolescent with a life-threatening illness

In times of crisis most adolescents require support to some extent from their parents, but also sufficient freedom to be able to experiment with coping with the challenge by themselves. Their response, typically, is that they want to be loved and supported, but not 'wrapped in cotton wool'.

Adolescents with a life-threatening illness may welcome the support from parents that may have developed during the crisis, yet will feel confused as to how best to be a 'normal adolescent' when an opportunity arises to spend time away from their parents. Rather than confide in their parents, they may prefer to confide in their peer group, particularly with peers who are in a similar situation, about their needs to experiment and for discussion of personal issues.

Much of the usual stress experienced by well adolescents is related to an inevitable struggle with developmental tasks, social changes, and relationships with family and peers. Adolescents with a life-threatening illness must deal not only with these challenges, but also with additional stresses associated with their illness, its treatment, and side-effects of therapy. How those around them react will have a significant effect on how successfully adolescents with a life-threatening illness cope and on their freedom to make their own choices.

Adolescents with a life-threatening illness react to crises occasioned by the normal process of growing up in a similar manner to their well peers. By remembering to consider the reactions and needs of adolescents with a life-threatening illness in the context of normal adolescence, a practical view may be gained of the problems they encounter and of potential solutions. Most terminally ill adolescents are more concerned about how their family and friends will be affected by their death, than about themselves. Further, they are not so much afraid of death, as of the process of dying. With patient and attentive listening, an accurate understanding is acquired of young persons' perceptions of death and of their own prognosis.

Phases of adolescence: implications of life-threatening illness

Adolescence is arbitrarily divided into early, middle, and late phases. Although in practice the boundaries between these phases may be blurred, some differences between phases are evident in key issues, behaviour, and relationships with peers and in the impact of a life-threatening illness.

The characteristics of adolescence and implications of a life-threatening illness in adolescence are summarized in Table 2.

Life-threatening illness and the early adolescent

Early adolescence generally occurs between the ages of 12 and 14 years in girls and 13 and 15 years in boys. This is a time of rapid physical growth and the onset of puberty. Early adolescents focus strongly on the development of their bodies. Membership of a peer group is very important.

Early adolescents with a life-threatening illness are most concerned about the effects of the illness on their physical appearance and mobility. Significant distress is common in adolescents with cancer if treatment results in weight gain, hair loss, scarring, or similar alterations to their physical appearance, which are perceived as drawing attention to their disability. Because privacy is all-important to early adolescents, large ward rounds are often excruciatingly embarrassing. Being less assertive than older adolescents, their concerns about such issues may go unrecognized.

Most early adolescents are still reliant on authority figures and are content to let parents act on their behalf. They do, however, wish to be involved in decisions and to have opportunities to talk with their doctor on their own.

Because many early adolescents are very disturbed by hospitals, the presence of familiar, friendly staff is all-important. Younger adolescents tend to rely on nursing or social work staff and parents to be their advocates, particularly with doctors.

The use of symbolic language is very common in this age group. Frequently, just giving voice to their thoughts reduces their anxiety. Encouraging them to do so will often be beneficial by helping them regain some control over their situation and to feel less overwhelmed. There is no need to force young people to confront their situation. If a carer listens to what is said, a gentle easing into the truth of the situation is possible.

Life-threatening illness and the middle adolescent

This period is defined as approximately 14–16 years of age for both females and males. Middle adolescents most commonly focus on attracting a boyfriend or girlfriend, emancipation from parents and authority figures, and increasing interaction with peers.

Middle adolescents with a life-threatening illness are most concerned about the effects the illness will have on their ability to attract a girlfriend or boyfriend, on their emancipation from parents and authority figures, and about being rejected by their peers. Time in hospital, and away from school, can severely interfere with social relationships and the acquisition of social skills. Social standing within a peer group can be threatened. The ability to attract a boyfriend or girlfriend can be reduced if illness or treatment affects the way a young person looks. Being different within a peer group can signal disaster for that adolescent. Fear of rejection by peers can lead to a number of adjustment problems, including a lowering of self-esteem, withdrawal, depression, and acting-out behaviours.

Non-compliance with medical treatments and lifestyle changes is highest in this age group. To young people in this age group, side-effects of treatment may be much more alarming than the threat of death. They understand the threat of death, but appear to make choices based on an unrealistic view of their invincibility.

With a life-threatening illness, middle adolescents often find themselves totally dependent on family again. This dependence and accompanying regression reduce self-esteem. A sense of personal autonomy is often compromised by admissions to hospital and frequent trips to clinics and specialists involved in routine treatment. As control issues are so important in middle adolescence, informed consent and open communication with authority figures involved in management is vital.

Life-threatening illness and the late adolescent

This period is defined as approximately 17–24 years for both females and males. Significant issues for the late adolescent include defining of careers, permanent relationships and life styles, increasing financial independence where this is possible, and separation from family.

Table 2 Characteristics of adolescence and implications of a life-threatening illness in adolescence[a]

Age	Early adolescence; 12–14 years (females), 13–15 years (males)	Middle adolescence; 14–16 years	Late adolescence; 17–24 years
Key issues and characteristics, focus	Focus on development of body Most pubertal changes occur Rapid physical growth Acceptance by peers Idealism Mood swings, contrariness, stubbornness, temper tantrums Day dreaming	Sexual awakening Emancipation from parents and authority figures Discovery of identity by testing limitations, boundaries Role of peer group increases	Defining and understanding functional roles in life in terms of: Careers Relationships Life styles
Social/relationships, behaviour	Skills in abstract thinking improve Foreseeing of consequences, planning for future Physical mobility prominent Energy levels high Appetite increased Social interaction mostly in groups Membership of a peer group very important	Relationships very narcissistic Risk-taking behaviour increases Intense peer interaction Most vulnerable to psychological problems	Increasing financial independence Planning for the future Establishment of permanent relationships Increasing time away from family
Relationships with adults	Parents and other authority figures still mostly respected As part of adjustment to new 'adult' bodies, may assert themselves as adults while still dependent on parents and caregivers Some testing out, e.g. with time away from home	Parental relationships strained Separation from family begins Some hero worship	Culmination of separation from family Increasing financial independence Sense of being equal to adults
Relationship with peers	Peers used as standards for measurement of developmental progress and assessment of 'normality' Comparisons of strength and prowess Friendships with same sex generally more important	Interaction with peers increases Questioning increases concerning who are one's friends and one's own identity and value Sexuality and sexual preference of more concern	Increasing experimentation with intimacy outside family
Impact of life-threatening illness	Concerns about physical appearance and mobility Privacy all-important Possible interference with normal cognitive development and learning (school absence, medication, pain, depression, fatigue) Comparison with peers hindered, making self-assessment of normality more difficult Possible lack of acceptance by peers Reliance on parents and other authorities in decision-making Hospitals perceived as very disturbing	Illness particularly threatening and least well tolerated at this stage Compromised sense of autonomy Emancipation from parents and authority figures impeded Interference with attraction of partner Fear of rejection by peers Limited interaction with peers may lead to social withdrawal Dependence on family for companionship and social support Hospitalization, school absences interfere with social relationships and acquisition of social skills Non-compliance with treatment	Absences from work, study Interference with plans for vocation and relationship Difficulties in securing employment and promotion at work Unemployment hinders achieving separation from family and financial independence Discrimination in employment, health cover, and life insurance Loss of financial independence and self-esteem Concerns about fertility and health of offspring

[a] Reprinted from Stevens, M.M. and Dunsmore, J.C. (1996). Adolescents who are living with a life-threatening illness. In *Helping Adolescents Cope with Death and Bereavement* (ed. C.A. Corr and D.E. Balk). New York: Springer, with permission from the publisher.

Late adolescents with a life-threatening illness are most concerned about the effects of the illness on their plans for career and relationships, and on their lifestyle. Time off work or away from study can interfere with work promotion and academic achievement. This in turn can have ramifications on economic independence and self-esteem. Job discrimination, and life insurance and health insurance rejection are also common. Illness and treatment can cause major social disruptions and increase dependence on parents, and thus interfere with the formation of intimate relationships. Some adolescents have to return home after having lived independently for a number of years.

Reproductive capabilities are reduced in some conditions, causing concern in this age group about intimate relationships and having children. Low energy or weakened physical capabilities can interfere with independence, economic security, and social flexibility. Questions from ill adolescents about fertility are common, even in the terminal stages of their illness. Sadness about possible loss of fertility, and loss, therefore, of the chance to live on through their children, can displace sadness over the prospect of death.

Significant losses mourned by adolescents with cancer

Being an adolescent and living with a life-threatening illness involves significant grieving, both at the onset of the illness, during its course and in its terminal phase. Not all of the losses are related to death or dying. Many are related to the process of having a chronic or debilitating illness.

For example, some significant losses mourned by adolescents with cancer are as follows.

Pre-diagnosis person

Adolescents with a serious illness often find themselves grieving for their former healthy selves. The onset of their illness prevents them from living in the style they enjoyed while well. The sick role makes them different because of feelings of weakness, lack of energy, and physical changes to their bodies. This can lower their standing within their peer group. One young person remarked, 'People don't treat me like the person I used to be'. Spontaneity is reduced and many young people, after diagnosis, question their place in the world, as in 'I wish it could just go back to the way it was'.

Body image

Amputation, hair loss, weight gain, weight loss, and other side-effects of treatment alter the young person's body image at a time when concerns about physical attractiveness and prowess are greatest. Compared with other age groups, the adolescent feels most the unpleasant and upsetting side-effects of radiotherapy and chemotherapy. Adolescents report how upset they felt when their hair fell out. This upset may not be evident to a casual observer at the time because many patients put on a brave front, but the pain of that experience is often expressed for many years. Loss of hair and related side-effects may have an isolating effect on the adolescent, because of the resultant self-imposed restriction on socializing and in some cases, rejection by peers. Use of cosmetic aids such as artificial limbs and wigs only superficially restores the adolescent's composure and confidence: the insult to their body image is internal and cannot be restored properly by an external prosthesis.

Health

Young people with a serious illness describe losing the perception by others that as a healthy person, one is independent, in control, and not unreasonably vulnerable to physical harm or emotional upset. This altered perception results instead in their being regarded as 'precious.' As one young person said, 'It's the "wrapped up in cotton wool" syndrome. My parents are paranoid about me catching infections and relapsing. "Don't be too late", they say, "You'll get sick".' Some continue to experience avoidance by others, including friends and parents of friends, long after treatment is completed because of fears of contagion.

School life

Young people are upset by missing out on developmentally important milestones associated with day-to-day life at school, such as sitting for exams, dating, poking fun at authority figures, and participation in group experimentation with risk behaviour (e.g. smoking, playing truant from school). Young men report the most disturbing losses as being associated with loss of prowess, loss of energy, not being able to take part in sports, and being seen as wimps. Girls experience losses resulting from school absence most strongly in a social context, for example, isolation from their 'group', missing out on the latest gossip, and activities with best friends.

Independence

Most adolescents test out and establish their independence between the ages of 12 and 18 years and attempt to identify their capabilities. The onset of a life-threatening illness during this stage makes it difficult for adolescents to become independent of parents and other authority figures. Ill adolescents are ambivalent about having to depend on parents for even their most basic care (e.g. changing of beds, toileting, washing, dressing, feeding). Considerable anger may be generated by the helplessness they experience over the loss of their independence. Matters are made worse if adolescents are treated unwittingly by staff of paediatric units in the same way as younger children. The dying adolescent's frustration may be taken out on a parent, usually the one that has been constantly at the bedside, by attempting to drive the parent away. If the attempt succeeds, or even seems likely to succeed, there is often an immediate plea for the parent to return. A young man aged 21 years who was dying said, 'I hate to see the sadness in my mother's eyes. She is also not well and yet she tries to do everything for me and fusses over everything like I'm five years old again. I want to scream at her but then I get scared she will leave me and no one will care for me then'.

Pre-diagnosis family

Following diagnosis of a life-threatening illness in a young person, family relationships may deteriorate or improve. Life in the family is no longer the same as it used to be. There is often a plea for life to return to the way it was.

Relationships with parents

The adolescent patient is often attempting to deal with feelings of anger and ambivalence about his or her parents. There is now doubt that eventual independence from the parents will be achieved. There are often concerns about the commitment of time and expense required by their parents, and about the demands placed on their own relationship. Roles within the family are often threatened.

Relationships with siblings

The patient's siblings may experience feelings of hostility and guilt. They may become angry because of all the attention given to their brother or sister and the various secondary gains that this can bring. They may be afraid of developing a similar illness. They may feel guilty, believing they have caused their brother's or sister's cancer because of some crisis that might have occurred at an earlier phase in their family life.

Relationships with girlfriends/boyfriends

Deterioration of the young person's appearance causes embarrassment. Ill adolescents frequently prefer to break off friendships, rather than risk causing their friends embarrassment or being abandoned by them. Their interest in sex appears to be similar to others their age, although those in relapse have commented on missing out on sexual experiences because of their physical appearance and low energy levels. Lack of opportunity for sexual intimacy is often not addressed by parents or caregivers of adolescents with a terminal illness.

Uncertainty about the future may adversely influence the development of a new relationship. The terminally ill young person may choose to break off a relationship with a partner to try and protect the partner from the pain of separation associated with death. Young people with a life-threatening illness do not want to be pitied. Their biggest fear is that someone may stay with them only because of pity.

Certainty about the future

The adolescent has a more mature concept of death and dying than does the younger child, being able to see the permanence of death and the finality of separation that it involves. The terminally ill adolescent mourns the loss of the future as well as of the past. It is in adolescence that life goals are becoming more strongly established in the mind. The adolescent senses this loss when confronting the possibility of death. It is difficult to predict with certainty which patients will be cured of their disease. The adolescent with cancer is left in a limbo of uncertainty about the results of treatment, often for many years after diagnosis and commencement of therapy. 'Living one day at a time' is a common dictum of adolescents with cancer.

Indicators of the future

A sense of worth in adolescence is linked to experiencing milestones along the journey to adulthood. If milestones such as examinations are missed due to illness, the young person's sense of worth may deteriorate. Adolescents who have been given a poor prognosis may experience difficulty in resuming studies after completion of treatment, if they perceive the likely duration of their survival to be limited. Other milestones include planning what one will do after leaving school, planning to have a family, planning for travel, and the attainment of increasing economic independence.

Hope

Young people living with a life-threatening illness have the same developmental needs as well adolescents. Young people facing death require opportunities to develop peer relationships, to experiment with different sides of their personalities, and to interact in the manner of their well peers. Frequently, young people who have been told that they may die soon report that people start to treat them as if they are already dead. As one 18-year-old said, 'They treat me like a non-person. It is as though I am in the coffin already and they are waiting to hammer in the final nails'. Hope becomes an essential ingredient for living successfully for these young people. Their hopes may not necessarily be for a cure or magical recovery, but more often for joy and for success with the challenges of living. One can be very clear about the implications of one's life-threatening illness and still maintain hope. One adolescent had on her bedroom wall, 'Be realistic. Plan for a miracle'.

Implications of life-threatening illnesses other than cancer in adolescence

Many of the implications for management of young people with cancer also apply to the management of young people with life-threatening illnesses other than cancer. However, the need for some modification is evident when specific diseases are discussed.

HIV/AIDS

Young people may acquire HIV/AIDS (see Chapter 10.3 on AIDS: aspects in children) because of sexual activity, or, in a relatively much smaller minority, drug misuse or medically acquired HIV/AIDS. Specific factors that further complicate the experience of young people with HIV/AIDS, as compared to other life-threatening illnesses, include the following.

Stigma—community fear and ignorance

The stigma associated with this diagnosis, which is related to community fear and ignorance, adversely colours many of the contacts that the young person has with others who are aware of the diagnosis.

Disclosure

Young gay men often need to disclose their homosexuality, as well as their antibody status, to their parents, siblings, peers, and health care workers when symptoms of HIV/AIDS develop and medical attention is required. There is also a legal requirement to disclose their status to intending sexual partners. This disclosure is frequently met with a very negative response, causes distress to all, and is described by young gay people as 'the double whammy'.(12) Similar distress is also experienced by young people with medically acquired HIV/AIDS.

Communication issues

Young people ill with HIV/AIDS express a fear that they will be treated differently or will be discriminated against by health care workers, because of the diagnosis. This concern commonly arises in the context of communication with the patient about the illness and plans for management.

Appearance and self-esteem

A healthy appearance ('healthiness, looking good, having a healthy body, going to gym') is considered crucial for self-esteem by young gay people, especially in organized gay communities in urban areas. The adverse effect on appearance both of HIV/AIDS-related illnesses such as Kaposi's sarcoma, and of treatment devices such as central venous catheters and subcutaneous injection portals, results in further social isolation, both from the gay community as well as family and friends.

Internalized guilt and blame

The young person with HIV/AIDS internalizes the homophobic thoughts and prejudices of others, manifested by convictions such as that if only one was not gay, the catastrophe of developing HIV/AIDS would not have happened. As one young gay person said, 'I always knew that because I was gay, something like this would happen'.

A poorer prognosis than with cancer

There is much less hope of survival for a young person with a diagnosis of HIV/AIDS than with cancer. One young gay person who was HIV-positive said, 'If only I had cancer then there'd be a chance. With HIV, there's no chance'.

Loss of friends within gay community

The young person with HIV/AIDS experiences repeated bereavements as friends within the gay community (not established through hospital-related contact) die from HIV/AIDS.

There is current concern by providers of health care for young people about the likelihood of an imminent and significant increase in the incidence of HIV/AIDS in young people. This concern is based on research such as that reported in North America(13) and Australia,(14) which indicates that the majority of university students have engaged in sexual intercourse by the end of their first year at university, that only a minority practice safe sex, and that a small but disturbing proportion are HIV-positive.

Cystic fibrosis

A diagnosis is commonly established early in childhood. Thus, young people with cystic fibrosis learn at an early age that their life-span is expected to be limited. Issues of dependency and of attaining goals in adolescence are experienced, as by young people with cancer. Denial is a common reaction in young patients with cystic fibrosis, evidenced, for example, by non-compliance with physiotherapy, diet, and other important components of long-term therapy.

Severe brain damage

Issues affecting the family may be more significant than those affecting the patient. Families of patients who are vegetative, apparently unresponsive, and totally dependent on them, may exhaust their reserves of energy in caring for such young people. These families will benefit from the patient receiving periodic respite care, to assist them in recharging their spiritual batteries. Families of such patients should be encouraged to remember that the patient may still be able to hear despite being unable to respond, and to continue talking to the patient at the bedside, even if about simple matters, such as what one is doing at that moment. These families may describe being in a dilemma of wanting the patient to die in order to be released, yet experiencing guilt over such feelings. Opportunities are required for these families to work through their anticipatory grieving. Just being able to discuss their feelings will assist them in the grieving process. Others will remain adamant that miracles do happen.

Catastrophic illness with short life-expectancy

When a catastrophic illness (e.g. motor vehicle accident, acute cardiomyopathy, viral meningitis, overwhelming sepsis) occurs in a previously well, young patient and death is imminent, issues of honesty with the young patient become important. Young people in this situation are very likely to suspect that they are about to die and deserve honesty from their caregivers to ensure, for example, that something they want to say or have done can be accomplished. Families in this situation are often required to make urgent and painful decisions about treatment or organ donation. Additional support may be required in such a death and also in removal of the deceased patient's body to the mortuary. The after-care of such families is as important as would have been the ongoing care of the young patient, had he or she survived.[15]

The family in palliative care: guidelines for support

As the child's palliative care commences, liaison must occur both within the treatment team and between it and the available support in the community. All members of the treatment team should be informed of the child's continuing condition and the plans for palliative care. Community resources must be mobilized to ensure that much of the child's care can be based at home. This is particularly important for families in isolated areas, where considerable distances exist between the family's home and local caregiving agencies and the palliative treatment team's hospital. As the programme of care commences, the parents will require further education about the ill child, particularly in practical matters such as maintenance of central lines and the nursing and biomedical equipment used in symptom control.

Home care versus hospital care—making the decision

As the emphasis of treatment shifts from cure to palliation and making the best of what time remains, care of the child at home becomes a priority for the family. Returning a terminally ill child to the home will support the family by keeping all its members together and allowing everyone to share in the child's care and provide mutual support. The home-care programme needs to be flexible to meet the needs of the individual family. Parents will need reassurance to help them cope with fears of having the child at home. Careful preparation and planning and securing lines of communication usually help allay these fears. The parents and older brothers and sisters will become primary caregivers in the home, and will need much support and encouragement from the treatment team.

With the change in emphasis from complex therapy to supportive care, the family's general practitioner may be pleased to become more closely involved in management and to provide much of the emotional support needed. Where possible, regular home visits by members of the treatment team (e.g. the community nurse consultant, the social worker, and the child's oncologist) will help to ensure that care is optimal. Regular telephone contact to discuss day-to-day difficulties also assists the parents in coping. Even with the best planning, care of the child at home may become too difficult because of parental exhaustion, stress, or development of symptoms requiring hospital admission (e.g. bleeding or recurrent seizures). The child may express a desire to return to the security of the hospital and the closer support of the medical team. Under these circumstances, a return to the treatment team's inpatient facility for respite care is preferable. A few days only may be required to allow the parents to rest. Longer periods may be necessary according to the wishes of the child and the family.

From a family's perspective, it is not easy to care for a terminally ill child. The strain and loneliness can be great. The advent of free-standing children's hospices, initially in the United Kingdom and more recently in Canada and Australia, provide a welcome alternative to hospitals for respite care for children and their families. A home-like atmosphere can be maintained more successfully in a children's hospice than in a hospital, while the burden of responsibility for the child's care can be temporarily transferred to hospice staff.

Benefits and disadvantages of home care

Care in the home offers the family the advantage of being together with the child in a secure, familiar, and comfortable environment. There is less disruption to family life. Nursing the child at home is perceived by parents as a positive experience. Siblings can participate in the child's care and their needs can be met more easily. The child's food preferences can be catered to more readily. There is greater privacy and freedom from the hospital environment, which holds unpleasant associations for the child. There is ready access to parents, brothers and sisters, friends, possessions, and pets. The parents will feel more in control since the whole family can participate in the child's care. By witnessing the child's gradual deterioration they will be able to face the approaching death more realistically. Family members are more likely to be present at the time of death and to grieve afterwards in an unhurried manner.

From the parents' perspective, the commonest difficulties of home care are watching the child's physical decline, coping with nights, handling fears of what will happen at the time of death, dealing with medical complications such as haemorrhage and seizures, and coping with domestic difficulties, including care of siblings.

Care in the hospital offers a greater degree of security for management of potentially frightening complications such as seizures or haemorrhage. However, the hospital may not be able to provide the same degree of privacy and informality that is available in the home.

An inquiry into the management of dying children and their families was conducted by the patient care review committee of a large Australian paediatric teaching hospital, and reported by Ashby and coworkers.[16] A 12-month sample of deaths of the hospital's patients was analysed, examining age at death, place of death, and cause of death. Fifteen hospital staff members and four parents were interviewed, and written submissions were received from 10 staff members and two parents. No anonymous contributions were received. During the 12-month period (July 1988–June 1989) there were 80 deaths, 66 in hospital and 14 at home. Of 22 cancer patients, 13 died in hospital and nine at home. Parents whose children had died and clinical staff were able to offer the committee many valuable and practical suggestions (Table 3).

Table 3 Suggestions from parents and staff on improving management of dying children and their families: results of an enquiry by a patient care review committee of a large Australian paediatric teaching hospital[16]

Provide better facilities including quiet rooms for communication, private grieving, rest, reflection, and privacy
Provide more sensitive body viewing, mortuary, autopsy, and funeral arrangements
Provide a more accessible chapel
Relocate telephones so that calls cannot be overheard
Provide better accommodation facilities for parents, better facilities for siblings, hot food available out of working hours, car parking
Provide facilities appropriate to the age of adolescent patients
Provide better in-service education for staff and information for families
Deal with issues well in advance to avoid crises
Ensure good communication and preparation over a period of time to allow smooth transition from curative to palliative to terminal management
Develop stronger links with palliative and hospice care teams, general practitioners, and community nurses

Evaluation of home-based care

Those working in paediatric palliative care commonly advocate the advantages of home care over hospital care for dying children. However, to date, there is little published information about how parents themselves actually perceive the care and support that they receive in this situation. An Australian study[17] provides information obtained from parents whose children died after receiving care at home. Recommendations for improved care of such children based on the parents' suggestions are as follows:

1. Families need to be able to opt for home-based, hospital-based, or hospice-based care for their child and receive adequate professional support to validate their choice. If circumstances change, the family needs to be able to change freely from one option to another. An integrated, coordinated programme of palliative care is required that offers these options.
2. Professional support needs to be available on a 24 hours a day, 7 days a week basis, so that medical and nursing needs of children receiving palliative care at home can be met at all times.
3. Parents providing care at home need to receive sufficient information about drug treatment and about what to expect. Adequate opportunities for communication with, and feed-back from, parents must be provided prospectively during home visits by members of the caregiving team.
4. Parents often benefit from speaking to another parent who has had a similar experience. Opportunities for such contact should be offered.
5. Parents require assistance with routine home duties to enable them to spend more time with their dying child. A coordinated volunteer service will fulfil this requirement.
6. Relief for parents at night is required to ensure adequate sleep. The presence of a non-professional volunteer may suffice but in some cases professional nursing skills will be required. Relief for parents by provision of respite care in hospital or hospice should also be available.
7. Readmission to hospital, when necessary, should be expedited. Parents, if they desire, should be permitted to remain the primary caregivers while their child is in hospital.
8. Local doctors and community nurses assisting families may need additional information about aspects of symptom control or nursing that are essential for successful management. This information can be provided via a case conference for all involved, by written instructions, and by ongoing contact between caregivers.

Each family needs to make its own decision about where care will be centred, without pressure one way or the other from the treatment team. The child's personal wishes should play a significant role in making this decision. Some parents and patients who initially feel that they will not be able to cope with death at home given good support will change their minds and subsequently manage successfully.

It is important to preserve hope at all stages during the terminal illness. To take away all hope will destroy a child's ability to live on from day to day and will foster feelings of hopelessness and helplessness. No matter how grim the situation, one should always strive to deal with matters with a positive attitude. The focus of hope changes over time, for example, from hope for cure to hope for a longer remission than last time, to hope that the child can be cared for at home, to hope that the child will die without pain. It is necessary to acknowledge the gradual accumulation of losses and the change in the focus of hope. The family should be supported in their current hope and helped to maintain a realistic focus on what the child can still do.

Guidelines for working with the dying child

The reader is encouraged to review the psychologic adaptation of the dying child as outlined in the chapter on Psychologic adaptation of the dying child.

For the infant too young to have a concept of death, one should aim to provide maximum physical relief and comfort. The child of 2–7 years of age will fear the separation from parents and other loved ones that death entails. Such separations should be minimized during the phase of palliative care. The child aged between 7 and 12 years will fear abandonment, destruction, and body mutilation. One should be open and honest and provide truthful explanations of symptoms and their management. Access to peers should be maintained, and the child's sense of control over his or her deteriorating body should be fostered.

Some members of the treatment team may feel less equipped to work directly with the dying child. Such members can direct their skills to working with the child's parents, helping them to cope more effectively with the situation. If one is uncomfortable working directly with the child, another caregiver that the child trusts should be involved.

Honesty and compassion must somehow be combined to alleviate the child's anxiety and preserve hope, as in the response of a colleague of the author during their haematology–oncology fellowship. One of his colleague's patients, a boy with non-Hodgkin's lymphoma who had experienced multiple relapses and was dying, arrived at the clinic with his mother. Despite receiving ample supportive care from the treatment team, in the middle of the reception area, he asked his mother tearfully whether he was going to die. The mother was unable to respond and looked to the author's colleague for assistance. She in turn promptly hugged him and said laughingly, 'Well, it looks like that might be the case, but you're certainly not going to die today'. In the midst of a busy clinic where no one was expecting such a question and no one else could respond, this doctor had the necessary presence of mind to respond quickly and honestly, establishing a beneficial conversation with the child.

To summarize, the emotional needs of the dying child include those of all children regardless of health, those arising from the child's reaction to illness and admission to hospital, and those arising from the child's concept of death.

Guidelines for working with the dying adolescent

The dying adolescent represents the greatest challenge to the caregiver.[18,19] It is necessary to reinforce the adolescent's self-esteem and body image, and allow adequate opportunity for ventilation of anger. The adolescent needs privacy and his or her sense of independence should be preserved as much as possible. Access to peers should be maintained and contact with mutual support groups may be helpful.

Pointers for improved communication with parents of children with cancer at diagnosis provided in Table 1 apply equally as well to adolescents with cancer. During interviews, young people may be intimidated by close eye to eye contact ('being eye-balled'); a side by side arrangement may be preferred. Interviews may be held effectively in settings other than a room, for example, a hospital coffee shop or garden. At an early stage, and with the patient's consent, spend time with the patient's partner as well as parents, siblings, and grandparents, and liaise with the patient's school or employer, to help allay anxiety. Encourage the young person to meet another young person who has or has had cancer and is doing well. In the longer term, another member of the caregiving team approved by the patient can be appointed as the patient's 'buddy', to be available for discussion, and to act as an advocate for the patient with the rest of the team. The patient and siblings should be encouraged to join a peer support organization.

How attentive listening and improved communication help

Much of the tension these adolescents experience can be released to assist them in successfully coping with their predicament, by simply permitting them to discuss their thoughts and feelings and share their dreams and frustrations. All too often, an issue of importance to the patient is ignored in the hope that it will go away. Denial is a coping strategy used by patients and carers alike. Health professionals and patients alike may not discuss important issues, fearing that doing so may 'open the flood-gates' and precipitate unacceptable levels of emotion. As one young person said, 'I thought if I started crying, I'd never stop!'.

In order to be able to listen to adolescents and discuss death and dying with them without putting up barriers, caregivers need to be aware of their own beliefs and fears about death. It is quite normal to have uncomfortable feelings surface when working with a young person who is facing death. But if one becomes overwhelmed by these feelings one will have little energy left to assist one's patients. Time out, and occasionally supervision, assist the caregiver to deal with a range of feelings, including sadness and anger, which emerge when dealing with the death of a young person and with past experiences of one's own that are brought to the surface at such times.

Negotiation and being offered choices

Adolescents value opportunities for negotiations concerning their treatment, whether early in the course of their illness, in follow-up, and for those who are dying, in palliative care. Being offered choices affords them a sense of control over their situation. In early phases of treatment, better compliance with therapy is likely. For those in palliative care, adverse emotions such as anger, frustration, depression, and anxiety will be lessened. Choices in even apparently mundane matters such as what to eat, wear, or watch on television, can boost morale effectively.

Recognition of small achievements

When one is required to redefine one's hopes from hope for cure to hope for prolonged survival with good quality, the positive value of small achievements becomes significant. Hope is better preserved if the ill adolescent's small achievements, from day to day, are acknowledged and respected.

Hospital and health care team issues

Adolescents prefer to be nursed in the company of their peers in an adolescent ward, rather than in a paediatric or adult ward. Hospital rules concerning visiting hours, rooming in, decoration of the patient's room, and related issues may need to be relaxed during hospital-based care of terminally ill patients, in order to foster a more home-like atmosphere.

Those caring for terminally ill adolescents must face the prospect of repeated losses and will frequently experience painful emotions including sadness, anger, frustration, and guilt. Caregivers must recognize their own limitations and use appropriate support within their institution or treatment team.

Jealousy and resentment may occur in staff who feel threatened by perceived intrusions into their area of responsibility by other health care professionals who are involved in the patient's care, or who feel displaced in the patient's affections. The patient's wishes and preferences should be respected and dialogue should occur between carers so that any conflict between carers may be lessened.

Occasional conflict will arise within the treatment team over whether to proceed with further attempts at curative therapy or change to palliative care. Foremost consideration must be given to the anticipated benefits and disadvantages of the proposed therapy for the patient. The need for a sensible advocate for the patient within the treatment team is vital.

Certain health professionals evoke striking affection, respect, and loyalty from their adolescent patients and develop close 'professional friendships'. These friendships are valued highly by patients. One adolescent said, 'It makes me feel that I'm alive that I affect someone else, it's not all one-sided'.

Leisure activities

Participation in activities such as camps affords chronically and terminally ill adolescents a valuable opportunity to escape from the tedium and concerns of their day-to-day routine. Recreational camps provide an ideal opportunity to mix socially with other teenagers and to have fun and take risks in a safe environment. Group discussions are easily arranged at camps. One to one discussions also are facilitated, because the teenagers are able to choose when, and with whom, they will talk. Camps afford a good opportunity for teenagers to talk informally amongst themselves and to become better acquainted with those who care for them, often seeing their health professionals in a different light for the first time. Self-esteem can be effectively built up by success with simple accomplishments.

Peer support and its value

Just as parents of other children with leukaemia or cancer are a source of support to parents, so too can young people with cancer or leukaemia offer helpful support and encouragement to each other. A young person with cancer should be encouraged to meet other young people who have or have had cancer and are doing well. Such contact helps to lessen feelings of social isolation and to maintain participation in social and leisure activities. Research is beginning to demonstrate the benefits for young people with cancer. However, further research is required into the value of peer support for young people with a life-threatening illness, and into the reasons why some young people prefer not to avail themselves of peer support.

Aids to the adolescent's communication with health professionals

Adolescents often benefit from having a focus other than the health professional, when discussing difficult issues. The use of photographs or photo albums, which enable the adolescent to talk about his or her family and friends, has been found to be very productive. Encouraging the writing of poems, letters (which may or may not be posted), or a journal, can all assist in the release of pent-up emotions, and help clarify issues and decisions that may need to be made.

Drawing as an aid to expression

Drawing is a creative activity that may be very therapeutic by facilitating non-verbal communication and enabling the release of emotions. Drawing assists adolescents in telling their stories.

Leaving behind a permanent record

When discussing their death and the effect their death may have on those that they love, many adolescents mention the importance of leaving behind some permanent record. Although painful for some, many adolescents who were dying have made a taperecording of messages for their friends and family, and some have made a video. Composing these messages in the company of a friend or counsellor may be less threatening, because a two-way conversation or interview is less artificial and often results in much more of the real personality of the young person being displayed. There may be much laughter, as well as more serious messages.

Because hope is so important to these adolescents, preparations such as these are often best completed while putting these tasks in the 'just in case' category. Discussion usually centres around all the energy that is required to suppress feelings of fear and anxiety associated with the possibility of dying. Nightmares are reported as common.

Often when adolescents have 'put their house in order', they find they can invest additional energy into living.

Guidelines for working with the parents

Sources of distress that parents face include the following:

The parental role

The parent must face not only the child's imminent death but also the perceived loss of part of himself or herself and must cope with the feeling of having failed as a parent. Feelings of loss of self-esteem are common.

The unnaturalness of a child predeceasing a parent

There may be strong feelings of guilt associated with surviving where one perceived as 'more worthy of life' is dying prematurely.

Societal reactions to the child's death

The approaching death is unnatural and threatening to the parents of other children. They fear the loss of their own child and withdraw, leaving the parents with little of the social support that is helpful in coping with the stresses of palliative care.

Loss of support of spouse

The threat of impending death strikes both parents simultaneously. Each is preoccupied with his or her own grief and is unavailable for support to the other. Each becomes vulnerable to feelings of anger or blame displaced by the other. One spouse may misinterpret the other's withdrawal and depression as rejection.

Parenting of remaining children

The parents are obliged to continue in the very role they are attempting to grieve for and relinquish. The surviving children serve as a painful reminder of the dying child. Feelings of hostility may be displaced onto the surviving children, leading to deepening guilt.

Identifying these issues and discussing them will help the parents focus on and talk about their feelings and deal more effectively with the issues confronting them.

The employment of one or both parents may be put at risk during the child's final illness. Simple liaison with the employer by the treatment team may be sufficient to obtain compassionate leave. The family may experience significant financial difficulties at this time because of loss of work and the increasing demands of the child's care. The assistance of supportive agencies and funds can often be obtained to help make ends meet and to have important bills paid on time. The practical difficulties involved in managing other children and the household may be significant. Grandparents or other members of the extended family may be available and willing to assist the parents with the care of other children and management of the household during this time.

The family will need adequate breaks from the stresses of caring for the child. Parents exhausted by care at home may benefit from the child receiving periods of respite care in hospital. The family may simply 'need permission' to take a break.

Occasionally, significant behavioural problems will occur in families attempting to deal with the stresses and threats of a terminal illness. The caregiving team must be alert to early signs of decompensation and make whatever interventions are required.

An example of extremely maladaptive behaviour has been described involving the childhood cancer patient and one parent, almost always the mother.[20] The child becomes so locked into an infantile tight-knit relationship with the mother that the two cannot be separated without panic. In some instances, the distress is more severe in the parent than the child. A rigid pattern of extreme mutual dependency develops, and together they withdraw socially. The parent and child may separate completely from the other parent and other children in the family. The patient sleeps with the mother and will usually exhibit classical school phobia. Typically, there is progressive social and physical isolation of the parent–child unit until the child dies, and then the parent makes a very poor later adjustment. Identification and intervention can do much to help with this significant problem.

Guidelines for working with the siblings

The following reactions have been noted[21] in the siblings of paediatric cancer patients:

1. the sibling may have his or her own private version of the causation of the patient's illness;
2. there may be misconceptions about the nature of the illness because of the lack of a visible focus of disease (e.g. in leukaemia compared to an amputation);
3. there may be misconceptions about the hospital clinic and the treatment programme;
4. there may be a fear of developing the same illness;
5. there may be guilt and shame relating to relief for not developing the illness, ambivalent feelings about the patient (envy, resentment over family's preoccupation with patient), and shame over the patient's disfigurement as marking the family as different;
6. there may be compromised academic and social functioning because of preoccupation with the stress of illness.

These emotions may lead the sibling to exhibit irritability, social withdrawal, academic underachievement, enuresis and acting-out behaviour.

The sibling bone marrow transplant donor

It has been recognized for some time that siblings who act as donors for bone marrow transplantation feel a responsibility for the outcome of the transplant and experience inappropriate feelings of guilt when graft-versus-host disease or other complications arise. At the outset they are required to undergo a bone marrow harvest, a painful procedure not primarily in the donor's interest. The sibling donor may also feel neglected and jealous when coping with the increased family disruption associated with the transplant. Less attention may be given to siblings by parents who are required to spend longer periods at hospital during the patient's admission.[22] If the transplant fails, the surviving donor will feel guilty for playing a seemingly easily identified role in the patient's death, if the death is due to severe graft-versus-host disease.

Donors' attitudes appear to differ in renal and bone marrow transplants. In renal transplants, the donor mourns the lost kidney, expresses concern about whether the patient will appreciate the sacrifice and take proper care of the donated organ, and focuses on anticipating personal gain such as military discharge or praise from the family.[23] The recipient of the kidney initially feels guilty about jeopardizing the life of the donor. In comparison, the bone marrow donor's reaction is of anxiety appropriate for any simple surgical procedure but with little concern for self. The direction of guilt is reversed, with the bone marrow donor usually experiencing significant guilt and the recipient showing either no guilt or expressing only mild concern that the donor had to be briefly admitted to hospital.

These family members require additional counselling and support to reverse and preferably prevent such misapprehensions.

Recommendations for parents

Suggestions that may help parents to assist the siblings of the ill child are given below:[24]

1. treat the children equally by taking into account each child's special needs;
2. keep in contact with the siblings during hospital stays with the ill child;
3. spend even limited time alone with the siblings;
4. permit the siblings to continue with their lives as normally as possible.

Counselling the sibling

Specific recommendations for the caregiver in counselling the sick child's sibling during the phase of palliative care include the following:

1. Give the sibling a clear and unambiguous concept of the child's illness and its cause.
2. Encourage the sibling to dispense with any erroneous concepts of the cause of the child's illness.
3. Allow the sibling to visit the clinic, meet staff caring for the child, and witness the child's treatment programme.
4. Assign the sibling helpful tasks in the child's home care.
5. Reassure the sibling that he or she will not develop the same illness (this is always slightly difficult, as the physician may have had personal experience of a sibling developing the same illness).
6. Provide the sibling with appropriate opportunities for ventilation (verbal and non-verbal) of feelings of resentment towards parents or the patient.
7. Liaise with the sibling's school.
8. Provide an opportunity for the sibling to 'say good-bye' as the child's death approaches.
9. Allow the sibling to attend the funeral along with the rest of the family if he or she wishes to do so. Children should not be forced to attend such events, and they need the freedom to participate to the degree they feel comfortable.

Support groups or discussion groups for siblings of children with cancer offer another source of support for working through such conflicts.

Many of the emotional reactions of the family of the terminally ill child are manifestations of anticipatory grief. It is well documented that the grieving process may commence prior to the patient's death. Anticipatory grieving is characterized by depression, a heightened concern for the terminally ill person, rehearsal of the death, and attempts to adjust to the consequences of the death. Anticipatory grief is discussed more fully in the section on Bereavement.

Roles of support groups in palliative phase

Parent support groups, which are of value in earlier phases of the child's illness, may assume special importance during the child's palliative care. Other parents who have already experienced the loss of a child may provide compassionate understanding and support, which can help the parents dealing with the approaching death of their own child. These groups may also provide practical assistance with cooking, housekeeping, shopping, child-minding, running errands, and other similar day to day tasks that otherwise may tax the ill child's family.

The child's impending death

Some time should be spent gently discussing with the parents the practical implications of the child's impending death. Members of the family will feel a need to make their final farewells to the child and should be encouraged to do so in whatever way each feels is appropriate. The child's condition usually deteriorates gradually and the parents are often considerably reassured to know that the death, when it occurs, will almost always be peaceful and free of fear and distress for the child. At this time the child will become more withdrawn and detached from those providing care. The family may need reassurance that this detachment is a normal part of the distancing and separation inherent in dying.

It is frequently difficult to predict when a terminally ill child who is approaching death will actually die. Children who are thought to be very near death can rally for a time. At the time the child was expected to die, the family may have worked through their anticipatory grief and will have considered themselves fully prepared for the child's death, only to find that the child's condition then improves for a further period of time. Family members may be unable at this stage to reinvest in emotional attachment to the child and may experience feelings of frustration or consternation that the much-expected death has not yet occurred.

Planning for the funeral

As the child's death draws near, the question of an autopsy should also be raised. There is considerable fear of and misconception about autopsies, and parents usually welcome some information to assist them in making a decision. Further, if there are significant and unanswered questions about the child's illness, an autopsy may provide information that will be of assistance to the parents during their bereavement. If an autopsy is planned after a death managed at home, provision must be made for the removal of the child's body from the home to the hospital. Parents should also be encouraged to give some thought to the child's funeral. They will be required to decide whether the child's body is to be buried or cremated, and will need to be in touch with a funeral director who will make the necessary preparations. Although seemingly difficult subjects, a small amount of planning in advance will later be regarded by the parents as valuable.

After the child dies, the family may benefit from a quiet time with the child's body. Hasty attempts to remove the body by well-meaning but uninformed staff or relatives are not to be encouraged. Brothers and sisters should be asked if they wish to see the child's body and allowed to do so. Family members who are excluded may harbour distressing fantasies of how the deceased looked after death and are deprived of the opportunity of 'saying good-bye'. Such issues may lead to considerable additional emotional disturbance during the period of bereavement. In effect, it is necessary to relearn practices that were considered perfectly familiar and desirable in earlier generations.

The family's culture: implications for palliative care

Culture is defined as the sum total of ways of living built up by a group of human beings, which is transmitted from one generation to another and includes language, ideas, beliefs, customs, taboos, and ceremonies.

It is important to note that in any culturally diverse society, customs and expectations surrounding the events of serious illness, dying, death, and mourning will vary. Members of a given culture will often maintain religious beliefs differing from those of the host country's predominant culture. There will usually be a strong overlap between religious and cultural practices, often with no distinction between the two made by the members of the culture themselves. Traditional practices within the culture will have been modified by the effects of mixing with other cultures, by the laws or practices of the host country's culture, and by the requirements of modern society.

The culture's customs and religious beliefs will have been learnt by experience and living rather than by learning per se. Thus, people of a given culture may find difficulty in explaining their particular beliefs, though they may still have deep significance to those practising them. Within any culture or religion, people will have their individual interpretations and beliefs. Understanding of the customs of other cultures assists those providing care to avoid causing needless offence or additional stress to patients and their families during palliative care and in the early days after the patient's death. Attitudes to serious illness, dying, death, and mourning in various cultures resident in Australia and New Zealand are summarized in Table 4.

Staff should ask the family in question about their particular beliefs and needs. Cultural requirements tend to be modified or relaxed by families in the case of an ill or deceased child in comparison with an adult.

Interestingly, there are striking parallels in the customs of quite disparate cultures with regard to attitudes to visitation of the dying, last rites, funeral and burial rites, and support of the bereaved during mourning. More research is required into the impact of culture on palliative care and bereavement, and into the influence of the family's culture and environment on the child's concept of death.

A coming of age for paediatric palliative care

It is encouraging to note that palliative care for children with life-limiting and terminal illnesses has 'come of age' since publication of the previous two editions of this textbook in 1993 and 1998. Growing recognition of the needs of gravely ill and dying children and their families, and of the significant differences in application of the principles of palliative care in paediatric and adult settings, has occurred progressively. Paediatric palliative medicine has emerged as a distinct paediatric sub-speciality, initially in the United Kingdom, and more recently in North America and Australia. Australia's first full-time position of staff paediatrician in pain and palliative care was established at The Children's Hospital at Westmead in Sydney in 1998.

The Association for Children with Life-Threatening or Terminal Conditions and their Families (ACT) serves as a national body in the United Kingdom representing children's palliative care in all settings. Children's hospices have continued to flourish in the United Kingdom where, in December 2001, there were 23 fully operational children's hospices, and 15 more at the building or planning stages. An Association of Children's Hospices was established in the United Kingdom in 1995. Revised guidelines for good practice in a children's hospice approved by all member organizations of the Association of Children's Hospices were published by the association in 2001.[25]

A guide to the development of children's palliative care services was published in 1997 by a joint working party of ACT and the Royal College of Paediatrics and Child Health.[26]

A joint briefing was published by the National Council for Hospice and Specialist Palliative Care Services, the Association for Children with Life-threatening or Terminal Conditions and their Families, and the Association of Children's Hospices, in 2001.[27] The principal recommendations of the joint briefing were:

- Children with different types of life-limiting illnesses should be considered and planned for as a discrete group.

Table 4 Serious illness, dying, death, and mourning in various cultures

Culture	Important perspectives	Cultural practices	Religious practices	Funeral practices
Australian Aboriginal[a]	Traditional view that death seen not as end of life but as last ceremony in present life. Urban Aboriginals may have a similar perspective on death and dying to non-Aboriginals. Importance of extended family. Relatives may be slow in coming to terms with reality of impending death. Senior members of extended family involved in decision-making. Deliberate slowness in making arrangements. Cultural/religious overlap and possible conflict between Aboriginal and non-Aboriginal beliefs and practices. Social rules for separation of male and female discourse and activity may require that patient is cared for by member of same sex. Also multiple avoidance rules determined by kin relationships, e.g. son-in-law/mother-in-law. Offence to use name of the deceased. Survivors with same name renamed. Photographs of deceased destroyed. Community involvement in dying process and funeral. Because of variations between communities, and even between families within a community, close and careful consultation is always required	Traditional belief that spirits of dead return to their places of origin as part of eternal stream of Dreamtime cycle. Disease and death may be seen as unnatural and resulting from evil magic by enemies identifiable by elders' inquests and interpretation of signs. However, contemporary Aboriginals (even remote tribes) known to relate to serious illness, dying, death, and mourning in similar ways to Western society. Relatives travel vast distances to visit sick or dying person or to attend funeral. Large undemanding gatherings at patient's home. Family may seek help of traditional healer. Personal space required. Discomfort in crowded and unfamiliar settings such as hospitals. Avoidance of eye contact by health professionals advisable as respect for personal space. In clinical encounter, Aboriginal people find it easier to talk about medical problems if the health professional first establishes a personal relationship with them	Spirits of the dead and burial grounds may be held in awe or fear by traditionally orientated Aboriginals. Many Aboriginals may use Christian rites, funeral, and burial services, sometimes in addition to traditional ceremonies. During terminal illness, family may ask healer to treat sufferer. Healer 'somebody spiritual'. Family relate to healer as person rather than to healer's status	Traditional practices included destroying possessions of the dead, burning of shelters, moving away of whole camp, names of dead not spoken. Essential that burial be in own territory and spirit sung properly to rest, with burial ceremonies lasting months or even years for an important person. Mummification by heat, body placed on platform or in hollow log, or cremation. Mourners painted with white clay, venting of grief in body laceration and wailing, widows observing prolonged food taboos and period of silence. Regional and tribal variations. Autopsy usually not permitted, offence to deceased person's spirit and integrity of body. If death at home, traditional practice of smoking out home after death to free spirit. All residents leave and do not re-enter after deceased's death until home smoked by selected person. May be deferred for months after death. Burial now almost universal. Little available literature or information on practices in urban or rural communities. Traditional ceremonies adapted widely in response to availability of technology, mortuaries, hospitals, Western medical care, and Christian beliefs
New Zealand Maori[b]	Events surrounding time of death are among the most sacred and important in Maori life. Traditional grieving and mourning practices affected significantly by influences of modern society. It is essential to acknowledge formally and make legitimate the contribution of traditional healers in the care of Maori patients. Bereaved family receive sustained support from relatives and friends	*He Kanohi kitea:* 'The seen face'. The Maoris believe it is much better to see a dying person whilst he or she is still alive. Friends, relatives, and family visit and gather at bedside prior to patient's death to pray. There is an obligation to visit especially for those closely related to patient. This may strain hospital resources	Reciting and chanting of special prayers at ill patient's bedside led by elders. Traditional belief that deceased person's spirit journeys to the Spirit World	There is a complex protocol governing commencement of formal mourning, preparation of the body for burial, and ceremonies held between death and interment. The body is not left unaccompanied during this time. Body lies in state on home *marae* (community gathering area). Paying of respects to deceased and bereaved with long speeches over 2–3 days after death. Church and graveside ceremony held on day of interment. Burial not cremation, preferably in family's traditional burial grounds. All who attend give gift of money (*koha*) to help with funeral expenses. Tramping of the deceased person's house by an elder after interment. Unveiling of memorial stone 1–5 years after burial
Chinese[c]	Death regarded as one of three great events in life, along with birth and marriage. Extended family valued. Many are superstitious, believing in evil spirits	Death and dying might not be discussed to avoid invoking bad luck on patient or speaker. Reluctance to visit dying for fear of consequences. Dying child's parents might avoid discussion of subject for fear of accelerating process. Wills not made. If death at home, deceased's remains must have direct and straight access to street, i.e. no corners (does not allow spirit free access to next life), may require temporary structural alterations to building. Acceptance of host country's and hospital's rules. Deceased's eyes not fully closed indicates final message left uncommunicated. Number 4 equated with death; similar phonetic sound	Multiple religions—Buddhism, Taoism, Confucianism, Christianity. Buddhist view of serious illness as result of past life (karma—fruits of action), emphasis on non-violence, brotherhood, meditation, and doctrine of rebirth. No special rites for dying but patient and family may wish to be visited by Buddhist monk. Important that prayers are said after death	Autopsy distasteful—usually refused. Buddhist regards souls as remaining in deceased's body for several days after death, thus crying avoided near body. After death, mantra recited to help spirit to be taken to better place. Washing of body with warm water. Food left for deceased 'food for journey'. Body dressed in layered longevity clothes. Usually burial. Funeral generally elaborate to speed spirit on its way. Wailing essential to denote proper mourning. Burning of paper cars, houses, and money to allow spirit a good time. Mourners dress humbly. Diviner often consulted for good aspect burial site. Monetary contributions to family for costs of funeral, burial. Money, food given to guests. Mourning for 49 days

Continued

Table 4 Continued

Culture	Important perspectives	Cultural practices	Religious practices	Funeral practices
Lebanese/Turkish[d]	Muslim practices and interpretation of beliefs vary from country to country. Turkish Muslims more open to Western practices than Lebanese. Muslim culture influences other religions in the country of origin (e.g. Catholicism). Equal proportion Muslim/Christian in Lebanon. Most Turks are Muslims. Strong expectations of gender roles. Strong identification with family mores. Preservation of family heart by women. Grief displayed openly and volubly	People's expectations of health care influenced by attitude that people with money receive best treatment. Tendency not to disclose diagnosis of serious illness to patient to prevent anxiety, e.g. one parent may request child's diagnosis withheld from spouse, both parents may request child not informed of deterioration. Cancer classified as male (benign) or female (malignant). Pork, alcohol, blood-based food, gelatin prohibited. Other meat permitted provided that it is killed according to Islamic law	Close mixing of genders restricted by religious regulations. Touching or observation of opposite sex disapproved. Ideally, female patient should be attended by female staff and male by male staff. Ritual washing and prayers required at five definite times each day even in debility. Fasting during holy month each year. Presence of religious elder (Iman) or Muslim over 18 years very important at death	Autopsy forbidden unless where suspicious circumstances, e.g. poisoning, murder. After death, eyes to be closed, lower jaw bound to head to avoid sagging, washing of body by Muslim with soap and warm water. After cleansing, body wrapped in white, placed in coffin, removed to mosque for burial prayer. Burial, not cremation, preferably in direct contact with ground. Body to be on right-hand side and facing Mecca. Crying during funeral and burial encouraged by most. Can be ritualized. Discouraged at graveside by some who say tears may drown the body. Mourning for 3 days (40 days by some Muslims). Family visited third, 40th day. House open 40 days. Widow indoors 130 days
Greek[e]	Strong identification with family unit. More pronounced in new country than in Greece because used as a method to 'survive'—people staying together for self-protection. Word 'cancer' not used. Often referred to as 'the disease' or 'the bad illness'. Belief that surgery (e.g. laparotomy) accelerates spread of cancer through the body	Strong overlap with religious practices. Wearing of black by bereaved: most women wear black, length of time varies (if husband has died, maybe for life), men do not wear black, may wear armband. Men may not shave for 40 days. Family does no cooking for 40 days, cooking done by extended family. Some cultural (and religious) beliefs based on superstition (e.g. belief in adverse consequences if 40-day observance broken)	Strong overlap with cultural practices. Strong belief in life after death, concepts of heaven and hell similar to other Christian religions. Important to maintain religious practices when ill. Access to sacraments important. In case of sudden death, last rites should be administered as soon as possible. If a child is sick, need for baptism may become important. Icons common near dying person—the saint after whom the patient is named or of the local church. Most Greeks are Greek Orthodox. A second church (Greek Community Church) has similar beliefs and practices	When a young girl dies, it is common that she be dressed as a bride for her burial. Services are advertized in the local Greek papers with a picture of the deceased. Poems are often written. Coffins are often open in church. Congregation files past, face of deceased may be kissed. Holy bread or special bread often taken by family to bless soul of deceased. Kolyva (boiled wheat) distributed to mourners leaving church. Burial not cremation. Meal after funeral (lunch or afternoon tea) including fish, dairy products rather than meat, which is regarded as a luxury. Mourners returning to home for meal wash hands at front door to 'wash death away'. Memorial services may be held after 9 and 40 days, 3, 6, 9, and 12 months, then annually

[a] Parbury, N. *Survival: a History of Aboriginal Life in New South Wales.* Sydney: Ministry of Aboriginal Affairs, 1986. Mobbs, R. In *Sickness and Health: The Sociocultural Context of Aboriginal Well-Being, Illness and Healing.* In *The Health of Aboriginal Australia* (ed. J. Reid and P. Trompf). Marrickville, NSW: Harcourt Brace Jovanovich Group (Australia) Pty Ltd, 1991, pp. 292–325. Ms R. Williams, Aboriginal Social Worker, The Royal Alexandra Hospital for Children, Camperdown, Sydney, September 1991. Dr G. Henderson, Visiting Research Fellow, Australian Institute for Aboriginal and Torres Strait Islander Studies, Canberra ACT, September 1991. Mr S. Houston, Administrator, Tharawal Aboriginal Health Service, Campbelltown NSW, September 1991. Professor J. Reid, Pro-Vice Chancellor (Academic), Queensland University of Technology, Brisbane Qld, October 1991.

[b] Na Paratene Ngata. *The Undiscovered Country: Customs of the Cultural and Ethnic Groups of New Zealand Concerning Death and Dying.* NZ Dept Health: 1986, Drs D. Mauger and J. Skeen, Auckland Hospital, Auckland NZ, 1991.

[c] Lee Sio Mong, *Spectrum of Chinese Culture.* Selangor Darul Ehsan, Malaysia: Pelanduk Publications, 1986. Drs M. Gett and A. Lam, Mr N. Lee, Camperdown. Ms B. Eng, British Columbia Children's Hospital, 1991.

[d] Circular, Islamic Funeral Services, 71 Wangee Road Lakemba, Sydney, April 1991. Mr I. Kurdi, Islamic Centre Lakemba, Sydney, September 1991. Dr M. Bashir, Camperdown, November 1991.

[e] Ms K. Karatasas, Oncology Social Worker, King George V Hospital, Camperdown, Sydney, April 1991.

Sources: Dr M. Stevens, Head, Oncology Unit and Ms P. Jones, previously Malcolm Sargent Social Worker, Oncology Unit, The Royal Alexandra Hospital for Children, Camperdown, Sydney, 1991.

- Children and families should receive a comprehensive package of care tailored to suit their individual needs.
- Every child with palliative care needs should have a multi-disciplinary children's palliative care team which should coordinate the many services involved in the care of the child and the family, and should include a 24-hour children's community nursing service.

As further significant evidence of the coming of age of palliative care for children, a comprehensive text book on paediatric palliative care is currently being planned by Oxford University Press.

Free-standing children's hospices have recently been established in two sites in Australia. Very Special Kids Inc., established in 1985, is a non-profit organization in Melbourne providing support by trained volunteers to families who have a child with a progressive life-limiting illness. Very Special Kids' House, opened in 1996, provides the amenities of a free-standing children's hospice to enhance the services provided by Very Special Kids Inc. The author's hospital, The Children's Hospital at Westmead, a tertiary level 350-bed paediatric referral hospital in Sydney, has established a 10-bed children's hospice, Bear Cottage, in Manly, Sydney. Bear Cottage opened in 2001. Bear Cottage offers free respite care and terminal care for children with life-limiting illnesses, and their families, from throughout New South Wales.

As these and other organizations adopt the principles of palliative care in the management of chronically and terminally ill children and adolescents, it will be important to plan and conduct as much relevant research as such programmes will reasonably permit.

Conclusion: implications for staff

Those providing care to dying children and their families face the prospect of repeated losses associated with the deaths of many of their patients. Caregivers must recognize their own limitations and use appropriate support within their institution or treatment team. A well-balanced and effective level of care can only be maintained by provision of adequate and regular periods of leave and by fulfilling interests outside the work-place.

There is a significant incidence of exhaustion and burnout in those caring for dying children and their families. It is gratifying to see a growing emphasis in the literature on the importance of spirituality and of nurturing and preserving right relationships for individuals, groups, and organizations, particularly those working in the field of health care, and in the restoration of wholeness and healing as valuable strategies for the long-term preservation of well-being in such carers. The interested reader is referred to an excellent discussion of this topic published in 2000.[28]

In an excerpt from her novel *George Beneath a Paper Moon*, appearing in an excellent article on the psychological care of children with malignant disease by Lansdown and Goldman,[29] Nina Bawden writes:

> The really unexpected happens so seldom that few of us know how to deal with it. We all move, for most of the time, in a small circle of known possibilities to which we have learned the responses. Outside this circle lies chaos; a dark land without guidelines.

Caring for children with malignant diseases, as Lansdown and Goldman add, involves helping them and their families to find some guidelines through the chaos.

References

1. **Rando, T.A.** *Grief, Dying and Death: Clinical Interventions for Caregivers.* Champaign IL: Research Press, 1984, pp. 327–8.
2. **Binger, C.M.** et al. (1969). Childhood leukemia: emotional impact on patient and family. *New England Journal of Medicine* **280**, 414–18.
3. **Mulhern, R.K., Crisco, J.J., and Camitta, B.M.** (1981). Patterns of communication among pediatric patients with leukemia, parents and physicians: prognostic disagreements and misunderstandings. *Journal of Pediatrics* **99**, 480–3.
4. **Stevens, M.M.** (1996). Palliative care for children dying of cancer: Psychosocial issues. In *Beyond the Innocence of Childhood (Volume 2): Helping Children and Adolescents Cope with Life-Threatening Illness and Dying* (ed. D.W. Adams and E.J. Deveau), pp 181–209. Amityville NY: Baywood Publishing Company.
5. **Stevens, M.M.** (1992). 'Shuttle Sheet': a patient-held medical record for pediatric oncology families. *Medical and Pediatric Oncology* **200**, 330–5.
6. **Cairns, N.U.** et al. (1979). Adaptation of siblings to childhood malignancy. *Journal of Pediatrics* **95**, 484–7.
7. **Adams, D.W. and Deveau, E.J.** *Coping with Childhood Cancer: Where Do We Go From Here?* Hamilton, Ontario: Kinbridge Publications, 1993.
8. **Stevens, M.M.** (1996). Cancer in childhood. In *Physical as Anything: Collaborative Support for Students with Physical Disabilities and Medical Conditions* (ed. M.M. Stevens, J. Rayner, R. Turnell, B. Graham, D. Piper, and T. Smith). Sydney NSW: NSW Dept. of School Education.
9. **Heffron, W.A., Bommelaere, K., and Masters, R.** (1973). Group discussions with the parents of leukemic children. *Pediatrics* **52**, 831–40.
10. **Klass, D.** (1985). Self-help groups: grieving parents and community resources. In *Hospice Approaches to Pediatric Care* (ed. C.A. Corr and D.M. Corr), pp. 241–60. New York: Springer.
11. **Snyder, C.C.** (1986). Nursing care of the child with cancer. In *Oncology Nursing* (ed. C.C. Snyder), pp. 247–97. Boston: Little, Brown.
12. **Schembri, A.M.** The Double Whammy: social work practice with HIV-positive young gay men. *Proceedings of Social Work and Adolescent Health Care Conference.* Prince of Wales Children's Hospital, Sydney, NSW, 1994.
13. **Fulton, R.** Children at risk because of AIDS. *Proceedings of the 10th International Conference on Death, Dying & Bereavement.* King's College, London, Ontario, 1992.
14. **Schembri, A.M.** 'Heads down and tails up': a report of the 1992 gay mens' welfare survey at the University of New South Wales. UNSW Student Guild, Sydney, NSW, 1992.
15. **Stevens, M.M. and Dunsmore, J.C.** (1996). Adolescents who are living with life-threatening illness. In *Handbook of Adolescent Death and Bereavement* (ed. C.A. Corr and D.E. Balk), pp. 107–35. New York: Springer.
16. **Ashby, M.A.** et al. (1991). An enquiry into death and dying at the Adelaide Children's Hospital: a useful model? *Medical Journal of Australia* **154**, 165–70.
17. **Collins, J.J., Stevens, M.M., and Cousens, P.** (1998). Home care for the child dying of progressive malignant disease: the parent's perception. *Australian Family Physician* **27**, 610–14.
18. **Stevens, M.M.** et al. (1983). Adolescent health—1: coping with cancer. *Australian Family Physician* **12**, 107–9.
19. **Stevens, M.M. and Dunsmore, J.C.** (1996). Helping adolescents who are coping with a life-threatening illness, along with their siblings, parents, and peers. In *Handbook of Adolescent Death and Bereavement* (ed. C.A. Corr and D.E. Balk), pp. 329–53. New York: Springer.
20. **Lansky, S. and Gendel, M.** (1978). Symbiotic regressive behavior patterns in childhood malignancy. *Clinical Pediatrics* **17**, 133–8.
21. **Sourkes, B.M.** (1980). Siblings of the pediatric cancer patient. In *Psychological Aspects of Childhood Cancer* (ed. J. Kellerman), pp. 47–69, Springfield IL: Charles C Thomas.
22. **Gardner, G.G., August, C.S., and Githens, J.** (1977). Psychological issues in bone marrow transplantation. *Pediatrics* **60**, 625–31.
23. **Fellner, C.H. and Marshall, J.R.** (1968). Twelve kidney donors. *Journal of the American Medical Association* **206**, 2703.
24. **Davies, B. and Martinson, I.M.** (1989). Care of the family: special emphasis on siblings during and after the death of a child. In *Pediatric Hospice Care: What Helps* (ed. B.B. Martin), pp. 189–90. Los Angeles CA: Children's Hospital of Los Angeles.
25. **Association of Children's Hospices** (2001). *Guidelines for Good Practice in a Children's Hospice.* Bristol, UK.
26. **Association for Children with Life-Threatening or Terminal Conditions and their Families/Royal College of Paediatrics and Child Health** (1997). *A Guide to the Development of Children's Palliative Care Services.*
27. **National Council for Hospice and Specialist Palliative Care Services/ Association for Children with Life-threatening or Terminal Conditions and**

their Families/Association of Children's Hospices. (2001). *Joint briefing.* NCHSPCS/ACT/ACH.

28. **Wright, S.G. and Sayre-Adams, J.** (2000). *Sacred Space—Right Relationship and Spirituality in Healthcare.* Edinburgh: Churchill Livingstone.
29. **Lansdown, R. and Goldman, A.** (1988). The psychological care of children with malignant disease. *Journal of Child Psychology and Psychiatry* **29**, 555–67.

Further reading

Adams, D.W. and Deveau, E.J., ed. *Beyond the Innocence of Childhood (Volume 1): Factors Influencing Children and Adolescents' Perceptions and Attitudes Toward Death.* Amityville NY: Baywood Publishing Company, 1996. A valuable contemporary collection of papers on the perceptions of death held by children and adolescents, and about societal and cultural influences on those perceptions.

Adams, D.W. and Deveau, E.J., ed. *Beyond the Innocence of Childhood (Volume 2): Helping Children and Adolescents Cope with Life-Threatening Illness and Dying.* Amityville NY: Baywood Publishing Company, 1996. A valuable contemporary collection of papers on helping children and adolescents cope with life-threatening illness and threat to their lives, and helping dying children and adolescents.

Adams, D.W. and Deveau, E.J., ed. *Beyond the Innocence of Childhood (Volume 3): Helping Children and Adolescents Cope with Death and Bereavement.* Amityville NY: Baywood Publishing Company, 1996. A valuable contemporary collection of papers on bereavement in children and adolescents.

Corr, C.A. and Balk, D.E., ed. *Handbook of Adolescent Death and Bereavement.* New York: Springer, 1996. A valuable contemporary collection of papers about death and bereavement in young people, and helpful interventions.

Corr, C.A. and Corr, D.M., ed. *Handbook of Childhood Death and Bereavement.* New York: Springer, 1996. A valuable contemporary collection of papers about death and bereavement in children, and helpful interventions.

Bluebond-Langner, M. *In the Shadow of Illness: Parents and Siblings of the Chronically Ill Child.* Princeton NJ: Princeton University Press, 1996. A comprehensive description of the reactions of family members when a child or young person has cystic fibrosis.

Goldman, A., ed. *Care of the Dying Child.* Oxford: Oxford University Press, 1994. A concise and contemporary textbook on paediatric palliative medicine by a leader in the field.

Buckman, R. and Kason, Y. *How to Break Bad News—A Guide for Health Care Professionals.* Baltimore MD: Johns Hopkins University Press, 1992. Useful information about how to break bad news.

Davies, B. *Shadows in the Sun: The Experiences of Sibling Bereavement in Childhood.* New York: Brunner & Mazel, 1998. Valuable descriptions of bereavement in siblings and helpful interventions.

9.5 Special consideration for children in palliative medicine

Betty Davies and Lizabeth-Sumner

Differences between palliative care for adult and children

The concept of *paediatric* palliative care is an extension of palliative care philosophy. Taken broadly, the phrase paediatric palliative care designates a programme or approach to care that seeks to maximize present quality of life by adapting principles of palliative care to children themselves, including newborn infants and adolescents, or their family members, and to other concerned persons who are coping with any of the following as they relate to a child: living with serious or life-threatening illness, the imminent likelihood of dying, or the aftermath of death.(1) Professional staff and volunteers in such programmes provide direct care and support and coordinate assistance from other sources to meet the total needs of this unique population.

Since the late 1960s, the adult palliative care movement has gradually increased in size and sophistication as a result of a growing awareness of the needs of terminally ill people and their families. Palliative care for adults has evolved to a stage where it is fairly well understood and is perceived as a reasonable option of care for individuals who may be suffering from an incurable illness. More recently, the ongoing development of palliative care for adults has been reflected in a surge of effort and initiatives in the areas of research, evaluation, and diversification of programme methodology. Palliative care for children, however, is in much earlier stages of societal acceptance, and is only beginning to receive its rightful place in the spectrum of health care services. The strongly held belief that 'children are not supposed to die' creates societal barriers to facing this reality. Children require specialized approaches and services to meet their unique needs, and they require a combination of specialized caregivers in addition to their family. Additionally, family members, especially siblings, have special unique needs and concerns. The needs and how they are met will vary greatly according to the characteristics and age of each child, the family, and caregivers involved.

The seriously ill child

Dependent status of child

As the child progresses from birth through adolescence to adulthood, the degree of his/her dependency is in constant flux, moving steadily towards the capability to be totally independent. This innate drive is impeded by serious illness, compounding stress and confusion for the child. Parents, overwhelmed by their fear of the impending loss of their child, cling more protectively and seek to be all things to him as a means of gaining some sense of control over their destiny. Younger children, dependent for all things, usually adjust accordingly, but adolescents may suffer greatly. At the stage they experience the greatest need for independence, privacy, and control, the authority of medicine, the over protectiveness of parents, and their own apprehension may add to the youth's burden and create conflict, both internally and with others. Additionally, this age group typically is given limited decision-making opportunities or authority. These circumstances can become opportunities for the palliative care team to facilitate alternate perspectives and approaches to children's experience of illness, treatment, and family responses.

Diagnosis

Children who could benefit from palliative care have different diagnoses than do most adults receiving palliative care. The common perception is that children's programmes are just for children dying of cancer, as is still the case for the majority of adult patients. With children however, only about 20 per cent of children admitted to palliative care programmes have cancer. The majority of children needing palliative care have a wide range of diagnoses including pulmonary disease, congenital anomalies, and progressive neurological, and metabolic disease, many with a range of associated mental and physical impairments. These diagnoses mean that a major focus of paediatric palliative care must be on the need for respite services due to the extended experience of illness. Most adult programmes admit patients who are within weeks to days of death. In contrast, children's programmes seek to admit children and their families as they progress through the various phases of the illness trajectory and into bereavement.(2) Accordingly, the length of stay may be considerably longer than is typical in adult programmes. In paediatrics, the emphasis is typically continuing life-prolonging interventions, 'buying time', and preserving hope. In the end, the quality of life for the child can be vastly improved even if the quantity of life cannot be dramatically changed, through the support and expertise of the palliative care team.

Legal and ethical status of children

In adult palliative care programmes, patient wishes are paramount and are given attention and protection. When caring for children, it is somewhat more difficult to determine whose wishes and goals are being followed or are directing the plan of care. Parents sometimes see the child's needs and options quite differently than the way the child sees them. Parents and various staff caregivers may also hold differing views. The age, cognitive level, and illness experience of the child must, of course, be taken into account. In addition, the child's legal status must be considered. As minors in the eyes of the law, children are subservient to the will of their parents under usual circumstances. This dictum has been challenged in the past decade, as the need for advocacy for the child has become more evident in the light of more sophisticated modalities of care and acknowledging children/adolescents do have decision-making capacity in some circumstances. Professionals are challenged to find ways seek the input, perspectives, and personal experience of the ill child as a guide for care giving decisions.[3] Traditionally, most professionals have had little training or experience in assuring their child's understanding of the disease process, treatment and therapies, identifying the child's personal goals, or exploring quality of life as defined by the patient/family's experience.

Ethical concerns, arising originally around the status of the foetus and, more recently, around organ donation and transplantation, recognize the child as an individual deserving of a voice in his/her own destiny.[4] Children themselves may voice a desire to refuse or discontinue life-sustaining treatments. If children are unable to speak for themselves, the ombudsman may intercede on their behalf to assure that the children's best interests are met. The hospice team can assist in ascertaining beliefs, values and concerns, related to their own goals of care and facilitate a discussion with parents and the health care team to unify perceptions. Despite the limits of legal rights and authority, children do need to be listened to. Their overt and covert communication must be noted to reveal their level of acceptance of the inevitability of their demise, their desire for more interventions or their ambivalence about the continuation of therapies, discouragement with how their life is impacted, and their quality of life as seen through their own eyes. In the situation of prenatal hospice, parents may decide on a palliative care approach during pregnancy, making incremental decisions about interventions, both medical and non-medical, at time of birth. Other challenging situations requiring legal or ethical considerations are children in foster care, withdrawal of ventilator support, hydration and/or nutrition. For further discussion of related ethical issues, see Chapter 3.5.

Family

Family size and experience

Families of young children tend to be more inclusive and extensive, and therefore, create a broader scope of impact than families of adult patients. Parents and grandparents are still living, siblings are often present, and school/neighbourhood friends are part of the affected family group, all requiring attention from the palliative team. Moreover, most family members will not have faced death of a child before so the task of meeting family needs requires special attention, skills, and considerable time. Siblings of the seriously ill child require focused attention and ongoing evaluation of support for their own needs, fears, concerns, and struggles both at home and at school. A child's illness changes the life of everyone in the family constellation.

Care provision

Most parents expect to care for their dependent children. Moreover, grief-filled parents seeking to assuage the anguish and pain of the possibility of death may compensate by trying to be all things at all times to their sick child and tend to resist help from outsiders. In addition, parents are coping with pre-existing psychosocial and emotional issues and conflicts within the family. The hospital environment, with its wide variety of caregivers, often puts parents in an ambiguous position where they appreciate the expert care but resent the control exerted over their child and themselves by authoritative professionals. Many parents, when inadvertently displaced from the bedside by well-meaning staff, have been electing to reclaim their autonomy by caring for their dying children at home, turning to home care support where available. More importantly, this choice may also indicate that parents identify home as the most appropriate setting to achieve any sense of normalcy as a family. It is essential that professional caregivers do not violate the relationship between parent and child; professionals must continuously reflect on their answer to the question, 'Whose need is this meeting? The parents'? Or my own?'. Professionals must create opportunities to strengthen parents' responsibility and authority in decisions and discussions related to their child's care and needs. Home-based palliative care programmes, as an adjunct to hospital care, are needed to provide skilled, accessible, and coordinated assistance in a sensitive and responsive manner in accordance with the parents' desires and child/family-directed goals.

Parents' need to 'be everything' and maintain control of their child's life helps dissipate their anguish and grief. Assisting the sick child, parents, and sibling alike gain control over the aspects of care and their own lives; experiencing choice contributes to a lessening of their intense feelings of powerlessness. There are many subtle yet significant decisions regarding care that can enhance or negatively impact the child's experience as a passive recipient or an active participant. Caregivers value and respect the child's experience by addressing such questions as: Does the child routinely get offered pre-medication for any painful procedure along with relaxation strategies to reduce fear and anxiety? Is care at home routinely offered or discussed as an option instead of deciding for the child/family that home care is not appropriate? Does the child want to master a particular aspect of care himself? Does the medical team 'talk over' the child as they discuss needs and changes? Has there been a discussion with the child regarding his/her desired place for the dying process and death to occur? Has there been discussion regarding the desired intensity of care related to specific symptoms and changes anticipated and their benefit/burden on the child? Are there friends who can be encouraged to visit? Are there simple changes in routines that might reduce anxiety or stress for the child? At all times, the care must fit the child, whether at home or in hospital, rather than fitting the child into the rigid structure of the setting.

Bereavement needs

As a rule, families suffer the death of a child more severely than the death of an adult. And, because of the composition of the family group and the differences in age of its members, there is potential for more disruption for a prolonged time following a child's death. Bereavement care must be a required programme component, with family-oriented support provided more frequently, to a more diverse group of bereaved family members, and for a longer time than in typical adult hospice programmes. Such care must be malleable enough to meet the needs of survivors of various cultures whose children had a range of conditions. The families of children who die outside of the typical palliative care model, such as in prenatal or infant death, do not consistently receive bereavement care, or do not have access to such care. The hospice model of care is uniquely the only one that automatically builds bereavement care into its scope of service. The support available may vary by programme but 'after care' is not routinely offered or available in many institutional settings or by traditional home care agencies. This is largely because of limited resources—human and financial, and the absence of reimbursement for such programmes. The practical limits of unit or field staff keeping up with the cumulative bereaved families, over time, along with current clients is finite. Institutions may have a protocol for use at the time of death and provide families with a packet of community and grief resources but the actual *mechanism* to ensure automatic and routine connections for follow-up does not usually exist. Parents who have a baby die receive keepsake items and often a memory box, but this same practice often does not exist in other paediatric settings, such as in emergency or intensive care units. Essential for optimal well-being and healing of family survivors is a seamless continuum of care (between settings and caregivers) that begins at diagnosis and continues through the illness experience where many losses are grieved and on into bereavement care after the child dies.

Caregivers

Knowledge base for adequate care

A natural result of the existing emphasis on adult palliative care is that there is little available research, experience, and knowledge pertaining to the principles and details of care for paediatric patients and their families. This is particularly apparent in the lack of accessible expertise and skills in strategies for pain and symptom management for the diverse ages and conditions of childhood, and for settings where children are cared for. Adapting existing knowledge to the care of children and seeking new approaches to the prevention and management of problems (physical, psychosocial, spiritual) and coordination of care should be major programme goals of any children's palliative care programme.

Caregivers also require extensive developmental and baseline knowledge of children and their perceptions of illness, death, and dying. Childhood development progresses through an orderly sequence of increasing comprehension, interpretation, and independence (see Chapter 9.3, Table 1). The ill child may be delayed in reaching his/her milestones, and with prolonged or serious illness, will likely regress. This does not mean, however, that strategies to facilitate the ill child's developmental progress can be ignored, since most children with serious illness seem to mature beyond their years in their perception of death and ability to cope.

Many adults assume that children are not affected to the same degree as are adults by serious illness, death, and grief because they are 'too young to understand', or because they 'will forget as time passes by'. Children may be less verbal and communicate their thoughts and feelings in different ways than adults, but it is not at all true that children are not affected by such events. Children are often not asked or approached appropriately to obtain their insights and perspectives; professional caregivers and parents often find greater comfort in talking with each other than with the children about sensitive topics, making assumptive decisions regarding care based on this exchange of information and sideline support.

Caregivers who are knowledgeable and experienced in childhood development are needed to assess and respond appropriately to the child's changing and evolving status and to design care plans appropriate to his/her goals and functional rather than chronological stage. Efforts need to be made to allow the child to assume control over optional aspects of care and decisions. Allowances need to be made to obtain a match between the child's desires and waning capabilities and his parents' expectations as well as the directives of the medical team. Communication with the ill child in accord with the level at which he/she is functioning will help the child express his/her feelings, needs, wishes, and fears more freely. A child's understanding of life and death, sickness and health, and self and non-self reflects his/her level of maturity along the developmental pathway (see Chapter 9.3, Table 3). Understanding the child's functional level permits the caregiver to provide the patient with as much control over his life and circumstances, as he is willing and able to handle. An approach that recognizes these patients are children *first* and seriously ill *second* helps to focus individualized priorities appropriately with the child and family. Sharing the developmental evaluation with the parents will enlighten them as they seek to cope with their child's behaviour and will reassure them that the regressive patterns are the expected norm.

The palliative care team assists the child and family to identify their goals and then works to help facilitate accomplishing them through ongoing communication among family and professionals and collaboration among all providers—both inpatient and home providers. The palliative care team, child/family, medical specialists, and primary care team all have contributions and perspectives to offer; a continuous feedback process must be organized for optimal communication to occur about such questions as: Do the parents (and child when appropriate) have the same understanding as the medical teams of the intent and purpose of the therapies/interventions? Have their mutual goals been evaluated for compatibility to achieve the desired outcome? Interventions and treatments may have a very different meaning or value placed on them by families than by professionals. Centralized coordination of care of all providers keep patient/family wishes uniformly centre stage, well understood, and actively pursued. Patient/family wishes should be driving the care planning process with input from the interdisciplinary health care team in order to create one voice for the family and relieve them of the burden of what seems to be 'running a business' of health care for their seriously ill child.

Teamwork

Special services for children require a highly skilled team that attends to the needs of each member of the family, and not only the patient.[5–7] Experienced caregivers must be closely attuned to the emotional, mental, spiritual, and physical stamina and resilience of the child's parents as well as siblings' responses to the illness and family changes. Paediatric personnel must acquire a thorough understanding of the family's lifestyle, personalities, spirituality and religion, cultural mores, and parent–child–sibling relationships. The ill child usually wants all care to be rendered by the parents, with whom he/she feel safest, but most children will respond to sensitive caregivers if the parents take the lead in accepting assistance from and demonstrating trust in the staff. As the legally responsible persons, all decisions regarding the dependent child rest with the parents. Their ability to function well and remain in charge will benefit from consistent support and guidance by an empathetic staff that incorporate the needs of all family members into the care plan and help the entire family to cope. Depending upon the duration and intensity of the child's illness, parents must either prepare for a sprint requiring courage and intense focus or a marathon of running the distance on an uphill and downhill course with unexpected turns that requires strength and endurance of body, spirit, and will. Parents tackle the situation without prior training or life experience to guide them. The team then must function as a coach—always guiding and supporting but never 'taking over' the course. Working parents require an approach from the palliative care team that fosters a sense of inclusiveness for both parents even when both are not available at the same time. Having the social worker/counsellor or chaplain meet regularly with the working parent later in the day, or at lunchtime, helps him/her feel connected to and perceived as part of the palliative care team. Such attention provides opportunity to clarify concerns and ask questions regarding the child's needs and their own. This can validate and reinforce their role as a parent when the burden of work, marriage, family, and a sick child become very heavy and isolating. Many families are additionally challenged with poverty, drug abuse, single parent households or grandparent caregivers—each of which has a different set of complexities.

Effective teamwork guides parents in reinvesting *some* of the energy singularly focused on a cure to a few short-term, realistic goals that can revitalize the spirit of the family. Hope has an intangible force that fuels the family through the unspeakable field of trials and sorrows and fears. As one parent said: 'It is hope that allows me to put one foot in front of the other each day, to keep me going at least for today, for this hour, this moment. Without hope, the weight of all this would paralyze me completely'. Hope allows families to raise their sights above the immediacy of their burdens and their fears of the present to the possibilities and opportunities that do exist, and to weave some small measure of 'normalcy' into their lives.

The pioneer efforts of Martinson in 1978, and later Lauer et al., demonstrated the value of the team concept in providing support to families.[8–12] This support permitted parents, even those living at a distance from the patient's hospital base, to be fully involved in the care of their child in the home, even choosing the place for death to occur. An important element of facilitating such involvement is careful planning ahead so that priorities are established and needless suffering is avoided. The resolution of a crisis or sudden change can serve as an opportunity for the team to help the family view it as a rehearsal of sorts for subsequent changes. Team members can encourage family members to discuss what they might do differently, what worked, and what can be prevented or anticipated for next time something similar happens. It might be as simple as improving communication between regular and after-hours staff, leaving more detailed, up to date information in the home or having a particular medication at hand. Using the 'teachable moments' as they arise gradually helps to mitigate the fears associated with parental anxiety of 'What will I do if something terrible happens?'

Successful palliation permits the child and family to share each day to the fullest degree possible, defining appropriate care plans with their caregivers. Bonds of trust, communication, and support with caregivers develop from the time of diagnosis and are essential to sustaining the child and family—for children, particularly when ill, do not adapt well to changes in caregivers, unless such changes are handled with great sensitivity and preparation.

Recruitment and retention of competent and sensitive caregivers is often difficult because of the personal pain and sadness associated with the impending death of a child (see Chapter 9.6). Staff needs to be protected from emotional exhaustion and depletion, as they must sustain the entire family in their supportive caregiving role as well as each other within the team. Adaptation to this specialty takes time, mentoring, and clinical supervision. In addition to the learning/coping needs of staff, managers have considerable responsibility to facilitate opportunities for thriving in this unique environment of care.

Location of care for children

In the provision of palliative care for children with life-limiting conditions, location of care is a major issue. At the onset, diagnosis and initial workup for a disease, the child may be hospitalized for lengthy periods of time as well as intermittently returning for exacerbations or additional treatments or procedures. Parents report this early phase as highly traumatic and stressful, requiring a depth of resources to be mobilized. Ideally, this is a relevant time for the palliative care team to be involved to ensure adequate attention to quality of life for the child and family, and to model an interdisciplinary holistic approach, in the early phase of treatment. Later, when options are limited or exhausted, the child facing the possibility of death and his/her parents reserve the right to select where his/her final days or weeks should be spent, and deserve the full endorsement and help of the caregiving staff to plan accordingly to accomplish this. Hospitals, the classic site over the past four decades, have become less essential since parents have become more knowledgeable and assertive in their active involvement in care, as pain control, and other symptom management strategies and support systems for the patient are now available in the home. However, admission should always be readily available for those families in need of the hospital/hospice for more acute clinical needs, episodes of exacerbation of illness or symptoms, fear of being a burden, for the sense of security and availability of sophisticated personnel,[13] or for individual cultural needs and wishes of the family. For home care to be successful, it is important to have an available means of immediate response in the home for sudden changes that may occur in order to prevent unnecessary suffering and/or unwanted hospitalization. For example, having an emergency kit of medications for anticipated/feared symptoms enables many parents to manage calm at home until the nurse arrives rather than waiting in panic, calling 911 or rushing to the ER.

It should be remembered that most paediatric deaths occur as a result of trauma; consequently, most children who die do so in hospitals. Applying the principles of palliative care to these children and their families is equally important.[14] Such family-focused care can contribute in meaningful ways to the experiences of children who die suddenly and unexpectedly and to their traumatized families. These children and families can benefit from brief yet intensive involvement of the palliative care team. Deliberate attention to the details of the child's and family's experience can shape the survivors' perceptions for years to come. Staff need to allow parents and even siblings the opportunity to be alone with the child, before death if possible, and then after the death in a private setting and for the time they feel is needed, before letting the child's body be taken away. Important rituals, memories, and keepsakes can be created at this very sorrowful time.

The child himself would rarely choose the hospital as his preference except when he senses his parents' inability to cope at home and to protect them, will subjugate his own wishes to theirs. Or, if the child perceives there is no alternative or recognizes the hospital is the desired site for higher acuity needs, or prefers care from trusted caregivers he may select the hospital for care. However, the child's dependent relationship within his family makes the isolation of the hospital, with separation from the familiar, undesirable for most children under any circumstance. In the final stages of a terminal illness, the emotional tensions of the despairing family and the potential subtle withdrawal of discomfited hospital staff including physicians can confuse and disturb the child, who may already be anxious. Ill children, and the families often perceive such changes as rejection and abandonment when the clinician's role is still essential even if cure is not attainable. This abandonment can trigger deeply hostile responses leading to intense conflicts, and even legal actions. Failure to maintain relationships with the family all the way through the experience can have dire consequences.

Whereas home would be the natural place for a child to want to spend his/her final days, this decision must be reached within the context of the family with awareness of the impact that the impending death will have on each member and with consideration given to the cultural mores of the family. The child's physical condition and possible emergency needs, available resources, and physical care-giving responsibilities must be anticipated, with plans in place, so that parents are prepared to cope with a sudden or unexpected change of status. Without the security of appropriate physical care in the home, the child's sense of safety and protection can be lost. Anxiety can easily escalate and exacerbate the physical symptoms. The decision for locus of care is weighty and should be made with serious attention to all aspects of family life and the ability of the chosen location to meet the quality of life expectations of the child and the parents.[15] Examination of the specific fears of the child and parents regarding care at home—or in the inpatient setting near death—can be discussed at a discharge planning conference. Typically, these are areas where parents will not want to feel out of control nor see their child suffer needlessly. For example, if parents' greatest and worst fear is sudden onset severe pain or acute shortness of breath, a plan can be made with the home care team to have a quick-acting medication available as a 'first responder' in the home. If severe bleeding is the fear and it is a distinct possibility, family members need to know what to look for and what to do in case of bleeding of a severe nature.

Home care is generally thought to be the best alternative for care of children with life-limiting illnesses.[16] Despite this emphasis, however, relatively few children in the industrialized world die at home. This may be due, in part, to certain conditions not being met; such conditions are requisite to paediatric home care.

Requirements for home care

Caregiver availability

Paediatric home care is feasible when a mother, father, or other responsible person is in the home and is able and willing to care for the child with some outside help and support. This is not surprising—caregiver availability and ability are major factors in determining feasibility for palliative home care for adult patients.[17] For families with children, it is not always possible for parents to be in the home consistently, especially since the once dominant scene, where the father went out to work and mother stayed home with the children, is now more and more a phenomenon of the past. In many households, both parents need to work. Various insurance programmes may relieve some of the burden and fears of job loss. But in all countries, including those with government insurance programmes, many smaller companies cannot afford to hold jobs open for extended periods of time. Employment requirements or benefits may force parents to be away from where they need to be to access needed care. The palliative care team may, at times, need to advocate for parents with employers, or keep employers informed as to the challenges the family faces.

Educated caregivers and professional staff

Caring for a seriously ill child at home places heavy responsibility on the parents, as well as the primary health care team who may rarely encounter dying children and often feel ill equipped to deal with the medical, emotional, or spiritual needs of the child and family. Moreover, since most health care professionals' education occurs in the hospital setting, most health care workers are neither comfortable with nor skilled at providing care in the home. Responding to changes in the home requires a very different approach. There is, therefore, a significant need for teaching both parents and health care professionals appropriate end of life care skills and resources. In addition to this, there is a scarcity of expertise and mentors in the evolving field of paediatric palliative care. Health care professionals often lack paediatric specific knowledge of pain and other complex symptom management strategies as the disease condition advances, knowledge about the actual disease trajectory for the wide range of paediatric diagnoses that are life-threatening, and how to meet needs across the paediatric spectrum: newborn through older adolescence and young adults.

Twenty-four-hour nurse availability

A third condition necessary for paediatric palliative homecare has been put forward by those who have implemented and evaluated such programmes.[16,18,19] These researchers concluded that the effectiveness of a programme depended upon a nurse being available 24 h a day, 7 days a week for professional consultation, support, and visits when necessary. For example, discharges from hospital to home may be precipitous and can occur at odd hours, requiring the availability of nursing staff to respond. Also important is nurses' being able to access medical consultation and pharmacy and ancillary team member support services as needed to provide optimal care to the child and family. This single component of consultation availability can become a most effective safety net in home care.

Respite visits

Providing home care to a seriously ill child often becomes impossible for families without the support of home care services and some form of respite care. With periodic respite from their caregiving burden and associated responsibilities, families gain a much-needed period of rest and revitalization and are better able to resume care, refreshed. Even a short period of respite helps maintain parents' endurance and resiliency. And, ill children themselves have reported that respite for their parents provides them with a welcome break from their parents. Respite care may be needed under other circumstances as well; for example, when a sibling or parent is ill, particularly if someone is ill with a contagious disease, which could spread to the already debilitated child. Few resources exist in most countries to meet this ongoing and significant demand. Insurers do not cover it and there are rarely the financial resources available for families to pay for this, so they go without, patching together some occasional relief through the kindness of friends or relatives. Through hospices, home visits of the home health aid can be of some relief for parents. In regions, such as the United Kingdom, where children's hospices provide respite care, families report the vital role of this service. Volunteers can also play a vital role in palliative care service, as companions for siblings, a listening ear for the child, or practical assistance for parents.

Coordination of services

It is critical that continuity of care be established and maintained so that families do not experience fragmented services or feelings of abandonment resulting from disruptive shifting of care between home and hospital and hospice. This same level of disruption can occur when communication is poor among the multiple specialists involved, various residents, and other staff who change over the length of illness. The goals of care, regardless of setting, diagnosis, or length of illness, are to normalize living to the degree possible, to optimize quality of life, and to create opportunities for living fully. To meet these goals, inpatient care must always be an option. Families may need assistance with symptom control or they may become increasingly anxious and need the reassurance of the familiar hospital and/or the quiet support of the hospice environment. Services offered between the various locations must be coordinated, with the child and family always supported to achieve their goals. The palliative care programme should ensure a seamless continuum of care—across settings, across caregivers, and over time.

Families are greatly reassured by the knowledge than an alternative exists if they find themselves unable to care for the child at home. They are further reassured when no guilt is attached to their choice for location of care. There is often an idealized notion that the 'best death' takes place at home, that everyone should die at home to have a 'good death'. Anyone who does not follow this path may be judged as failing in 'doing it right'. Nursing shortages now influence the landscape of home care for paediatrics. In the United States, the reimbursement for the comprehensive needs of children is woefully inadequate to cover the cost of care; multiple providers must compete for the allocation of coverage—often one agency at a time, causing families to choose between one needed service and another when they need both simultaneously. The unpredictability of the prognosis for widely ranging diagnoses makes it hard to identify when the child might benefit from palliative care—although it is proposed that it be from point of diagnosis through the illness and into bereavement. Coordination of services is also needed for children and families who do not change settings—the multitude of physicians and other professional caregivers who enter the child's life must be coordinated and organized so that families are not overwhelmed by sheer numbers of helpers and are clear as to who does what for the child. The suggestion of a 'cornerstone carer' or a care coordinator is a worthy one—where one key individual is identified as the family's primary contact person who ensures consistency of care while assisting them through the maze of other helpers.[20] Unfortunately, for children with non-traditional life-threatening illness—of which there are many—there are few, if any, centralized providers or organizations locally to advocate for the child's needs and to assist families to navigate the system.

Other supportive environments for children

School

Palliative care services for children need to take into consideration that school plays a vital role in the lives of children and conversely, children deeply impact their school communities. For many children, school is their second 'family' community that includes classmates, teachers, counsellors, school nurses, other parents, and teammates. Consequently, although palliative care currently only focuses primarily on children in the final stages of life, there may be many weeks to months of ups and downs and slow decline during which encouragement of the child to continue to attend school may give him/her satisfaction and even pleasure through participation in normal activities with his/her peers and through striving for personal goals. Schools are required to meet the needs of special needs children and yet they may not be equipped to meet the additional needs and issues surrounding a dying child in their midst. The child should be encouraged to participate although he/she should be the final judge of what he/she is able to do. For children who cannot attend school, home school assistance is another option that helps the child maintain connections with the classroom and fulfill a sense of accomplishment.

School conferences with representatives of the palliative care team can facilitate the ongoing desires of the child to attend school and, at the same time, integrate the health care team into the existing supports available at school. The nurse can speak to the child's classmates, be a resource to the teacher, and suggest ways to establish an emotionally and clinically safe environment for the child in the school. The school can also facilitate connection with the homebound child through the assistance of classmates and teachers with the palliative care team.

Day care

Day care programmes for daytime activities and companionship, increasingly utilized for adult patients with cancer and Alzheimer's disease, have not yet found widespread use in paediatrics, although such programmes are able to offer respite to parents and an opportunity for some freedom from surveillance and physical care for the significant number of children whose illness and terminal course is prolonged. For the pre-school child, day care provides the peer companionship, stimulation, and sense of belonging that school provides for the older child. St Mary's Hospital for Children in Bayside, New York, provides a stimulating day care programme for their handicapped children and has extended enrolment to some of the terminally ill children from the hospice unit no longer able to attend school.(21) Personal communication from several other hospital-based programmes indicates that a variety of day programmes for family respite are being explored but are still experimental.

Play therapy is a recognized modality of care for all children—play is the work of all children. When utilized in day care, as in the school system, activities need to be tailored to the child's level of function and endurance. Meaningful play is the ideal way to help the young patient express his feelings and reduce anxiety, anger, depression, and fears. Bibliotherapy, art, and music are also valuable techniques for helping children understand and express their reactions to the changes they experience physically, emotionally, socially, and spiritually. Child life specialists are often especially trained to assist with such techniques, but such professionals are currently not a standard component of hospice and palliative care. They may be accessed through paediatric clinical settings and, in some areas, are actually being integrated into adult hospital settings to better meet the emotional needs of children whose parents are ill.

Professional health care workers

People who have had previous experience with sick infants, children, and adolescents and their anxious parents best meet the many needs of the dying child. This is not to exclude those who wish to learn to relate to children who are seriously or terminally ill, but, since time is of the essence for these children, the dying child deserves access to skilled paediatric caregivers. The learning curve for becoming such a caregiver is slow for persons starting from no experience, as the process of integrating child development, child psychology, cultural, and religious influences, pathophysiology of the range of disease processes, therapeutic treatment modalities, pain control, and other symptom management is long and difficult. The care of a child receiving palliation demands the same commitment to excellence and the same level of monitoring and skilled intervention as does acute care. Currently, there are few resources and research-based clinical competencies for interdisciplinary team members in paediatric palliative care. The model required is one of mentoring over time based on best practice and current trends in clinical care. Most communities do not have this depth of local expertise and thereby rely on a scattered, fragmented approach. Unfortunately, many try to approach the care of these children as small adults and the results can be very negative from the family's point of view.

The nurse

In palliative care, the nurse emerges as the natural leader of the team in her role as coordinator of the plan of care. Time spent with the child and the ability to read his/her body language and incorporate pertinent pieces of scientific knowledge into an effective care plan equips the nurse with the ability to coordinate collaborative team efforts, which may significantly influence the emotional burden and stress and ease the coming events. The nurse must be mindful not to displace the parents in their need to care for their child and simultaneously not demand more of them than they can handle. In addition, the nurse serves as the 'control tower navigator', recognizing when to call in the strengths, services, and consultation of others. In times of limited resources or in areas less well endowed, the nurse may need to fill multiple roles as well as train volunteers to assist. Besides knowledge and skill in physical palliative care, the nurse must also weave the psychosocial and spiritual dimensions of the child's experience into her care as they are all closely intertwined and interconnected. The nurse has far more responsibility than simply 'body care'. It is equally important for the nurse to be keenly aware of her own limitations and to reflect on her own practice, and to take the time for self-care in order to provide ongoing optimal care.

The physician

Most seriously ill and dying children have been treated by multiple physician specialists. To optimize communication and facilitate supportive services, specialists need to work in close collaboration with the child's primary physician or paediatrician. With the transitioning of goals over time from curative to palliative care, parents need to know which one person will serve as their primary physician. Close collaboration between the physician and nurse is needed to achieve optimal symptom control and to provide continuity of care to the patient and reassurance to the family. Constancy of caregivers is essential, for as the child weakens he/she will relate well to fewer and fewer people, and be less open to strangers. As with adults in end-of-life care, the dying child's world shrinks as his/her disease progresses; the number of people interacting in his daily care and life declines also. The physician has a vital role in adapting treatment through the ongoing changes in condition and in anticipating what to expect as a result. Since the realm of palliative care extends from pre-natal diagnoses through adolescent medicine, a wide range of providers may participate in the direction of medical care. For example, the obstetrician or the genetic counsellor may be involved at various stages. In other situations, the paediatrician may be left out of the coordination of care during high acuity in hospital. The family paediatrician (or obstetrician) may be in a unique position to be the thread of continuity before and after the child's illness and death. The paediatrician may be caring for the siblings and the obstetrician may see the mother after the baby's death; each is in a unique position to evaluate the coping and need for support. Many parents find it very comforting to have a follow-up visit with the physician to review the cause of death, what happened and what implications there might be for future pregnancies or the other siblings.

The social workers

In the care of children with life-threatening diseases or conditions, the social worker plays many roles. As an experienced listener, the social worker prioritizes the problems and concerns of all involved parties and seeks to expedite solutions for them. Resources and pertinent information are provided, as is expert negotiation of management crises and bureaucratic obstacles. The social worker's contributions to and support of the family include facilitation of family conflict and communication. Social workers also can address sibling issues during the illness, assist and guide the family in memory-making activities and rituals, and facilitate expression of feelings and concerns. Social work services do not end with the death, but may, in some programmes, continue throughout the bereavement period. The social worker fulfills a valuable liaison role—parents, nurse, physician, psychologist, clergy, and others are well served by an experienced social worker. Social workers should also be available to families who are not receiving hospital-based care.

The clergy

The child tends to cling to and reflect the religious or spiritual beliefs, practices, and commitment of his/her family in accord with his/her age and level of comprehension. Whenever possible, a clergy person of the family's religious background should be recruited to collaborate with the team, in addition to the clergy usually associated with the palliative care team. Many clergy are well trained as counsellors, and the spiritual support and hope they provide, will be of comfort to the patient, siblings, parents, and the care team. Clergy provide formal rites, hear concerns, fears and confessions, offer counseling, serve as a non-judgemental companion on the journey, facilitate personalized rituals, and support the family in finding meaning in their experience, and most importantly, symbolize a link to an uncertain future.

The psychologist/psychiatrist

The mental health disciplines may more likely be involved early in the child's illness and are probably under-utilized later in the illness, but the family and the staff may well benefit from their continued support, or gain reassurance through clarification about the dying child's pattern of behaviour. Adolescents, often filled with anger, ambivalence, conflict, and resentment as well as fear, may benefit from the psychologist's role as a sounding board. Clinical consultation on escalating anger, behaviour problems and assessment for clinical depression, and substance abuse issues are also appropriate indicators for mental health clinicians' involvement in the child's care.

Other supportive resources

Parent/peer group support

When available, supportive family members are invaluable in rallying round the stricken family. However, not all parents have extended family members present; moreover, many parents find themselves socially and emotionally isolated as friends and family also struggle with their difficult situation. Parent/peer support groups become important to such parents, and become increasingly effective as parents adjust to their changed lives and identify with others who share similar challenges. Parent groups can be most beneficial if they provide parents with freedom to move in and out of the group until they find their own level of comfort and choose to participate with the group. Encouragement by caregivers, and sensitivity on their part to introduce parents likely to be compatible, smoothes the adjustment for parents and child and helps create a supportive ambience for all concerned. Consideration of confidentiality is important before the contact is made. Some families are fortunate to connect with other parents through a disease-specific organization but those whose children have rare or less familiar diseases, are more isolated. One alternative has been the explosion of Web-based supports where parents can often find others in a similar situation. However, caution is advisable since the information shared and the presented facts can sometimes be largely unsubstantiated and even harmful. Even still, the Internet has helped many families of children with progressive, life-limiting conditions.

Others

Flexibility and adaptability are key elements of palliative care staffing. To attain the goal of meeting the needs of the ill child and his family, the team needs to include, on an ad hoc basis, whoever is most capable of accomplishing each given task, or helping the child and family reach their goals. Classmates, teachers, coaches, scout leaders, or others may contribute to the ill child's sense of still belonging to a peer group and should be encouraged to participate in accord with the patient's wishes, emotional state, and physical reserves.

A fine line exists between responding to the child's wishes and exhausting him/her with excessive activities or ministrations. As the child's fatigue increases, and his/her attention span shortens, brevity and pacing become the order of the day. Memory-making and keepsake activities can be simple, requiring little energy and still help create and preserve special time and memories. As death approaches, physical comfort and freedom from pain and other symptoms will make a peaceful death more possible.

Volunteers have proven to be a valuable asset in staffing home, hospice, and inpatient care programmes. Volunteers should be well trained so that they augment the staff, benefit the family and in no way antagonize or inadvertently do harm to the patient and family. Volunteers can bring a fresh outlook to the scene, provide beneficial services to the child and family, and relieve parents and staff, providing them with respite from stress. In paediatric situations, volunteers are especially beneficial in providing attention and companionship to siblings.

Ombudsmen are invaluable in ascertaining that the child's point of view is heard and that decisions are made in his best interest. The parent–child relationship is of such magnitude that bringing in a third party is not common, but time has shown that utilizing an ombudsman as a 'neutral observer' may provide excellent service in prevention of miscommunication, particularly in acute care hospital settings where the environment predisposes to a focus on curative efforts.

The interdisciplinary team and spirituality

Care directed to the physical body without concern for the mind and spirit is incomplete and frequently ineffective. The child is inherently a spiritual being not yet fully burdened by the complexities of life. His/her religious orientation, imitative or parent-directed, may have limited meaning for him/her or may have powerful personal meaning for a particular child. The spiritual dimension or life force of the family imprints the child from birth and provides him/her with a model for developing his/her own person, values, and meanings. The strength of the family spirit becomes his strength, and his trust in the love and protection of his family sustains him, or vice versa. The pre-death awareness of children who are dying is a familiar experience for those who work with these children; they seem to demonstrate wisdom beyond their years and also have a sense of what is ahead. Children frequently achieve a sense of peace before their parents are nearing acceptance of the inevitability of the child's demise. Children are naturally very spiritual beings and can benefit greatly from the wise counsel and guidance of an experienced clinician. Spiritual care is not only appropriate but is an innate need of all persons, religious or not. In offering spiritual care, the caregiver goes the extra mile to seek out the inner person of the patient or family member, share their anguish, provide solace, and perhaps help them find meaning in their experience.[22]

Appreciation of the family's values, strengths, beliefs, and fears enhances the ability of the caregiver to encourage uninhibited communication on all matters and to offer constructive coping skills. The goal of spiritual care is to provide non-judgemental love and the promise of non-abandonment. Providing spiritual care transcends the empathetic communication used to meet the family's daily psychosocial needs and invokes a sharing of self through listening and presence when needed. Caregivers are challenged to reach beyond their personal religious belief system to help each family probe, access, and utilize its own religious ties and nurture them. For parents facing the loss of a child, the search for meaning is painful but inevitable as they struggle through guilt, defiance, anger, and potentially acceptance. The unconditional spiritual support of a caring person can be the glue that holds the family together through and beyond the death of their child.

Cost of paediatric palliative care

Palliative care must be quality care—efficient and yet cost-effective. In the field of paediatrics, particularly in life-threatening illnesses, no family would let cost deprive their child of life-saving care. Many exhaust all financial resources in the pursuit of additional treatments or possibility of a cure. Health professionals concerned with the dynamics of the whole family have long been aware of the devastating impact of serious and terminal illness on the needs of other members of the family. As technology has increased in sophistication, with its resultant escalation in costs, families are facing unbearable financial burdens, which impact on all the members. Families can become impoverished as a result.

The growth and success of the palliative care movement since the 1960s have been described as a social movement provoked by rising health care costs.[23,24] Certainly, the survival of the hospice philosophy of home care in a highly competitive hospital-dominated environment can be attributed in part to the need to control rising costs recognized by both provider and consumer. It would be inappropriate, however, if the intent of pioneer Dame Cicely Saunders and her associates—to relieve pain, alleviate symptoms, and provide comfort to those suffering in their final days of life—and the contributions of countless numbers of volunteers committed to palliative care were perceived to be driven primarily by money.

The outstanding advances in pain control made through research in pharmacology and neurology have been welcomed, but the price of these gains is to increase the cost of care which will need further evaluation to demonstrate if the benefits gained are truly cost-effective. Analysis of the elements of cost, the rightful assignment of charges, and the measurement of out-of-pocket costs must also include the savings in hospital costs, in-kind contributions of family and volunteers, and reduction in physical and mental health costs in survivors.(23,25)

Work by Birenbaum,(26) comparing hospital care and home care costs for children, indicates the importance of a breakdown of sub-categories of cost in order to identify the burden of cost to families using home care who must bear the higher out-of-pocket social costs and direct non-health costs. The literature reports a variety of conflicting observations, but in general seems to favour the position that home care in toto is less costly than hospital admission.(27) More definitive studies are needed to analyse actual costs in a prospective manner, since retrospective studies, even with diaries, are limited in their ability to capture many of the important details. In the United States, financial assistance for non-medical expenses is sorely needed as, increasingly, the financial burden can break an already emotionally strained marriage and/or leave the family with an insurmountable debt as well as an irreparable marital relationship. Definitive cost analyses will be essential to move the policy-makers to provide the additional financing needed for the current unacknowledged expenditures.

Children present a particularly poignant problem, especially in the United States where there is no national system of universal health insurance. Most young parents are poorly insured, if at all. Federal and state programmes for hospital therapeutic care may sustain the most impoverished, but little is available for comprehensive services. Both Bloom et al.(28) and Lansky et al.(29) have provided data suggesting that, although the family portions of the total costs may be only 5 per cent, on a per family basis this ill consume approximately 38 per cent of the gross annual family income.

Paediatric palliative care costs more than adult care, primarily because of the large number of specialized personnel needed to provide definitive paediatric care and support services to entire families and the need for care over an indeterminate length of time. Further studies on cost-effectiveness and cost–benefit of palliative care will be critical to its continued existence as an integral part of the health care system. Survival of palliative care hinges on cost wise management and hard evidence that the cost–benefit ratio is favourable.(30) Regular case review of a child's care, conducted by the palliative care team and medical specialists, can ensure the child is receiving treatments and interventions that are actually benefiting the patient, still in line with the expressed goals of the parent/child and are clinically indicated. Reviews serve as a check and balance so that care that is not working is not continued simply because the interdisciplinary team has not stopped to ask, 'Whose need is this meeting? Is this still appropriate treatment based on the child's condition? Does it enhance or at minimum maintain quality of life? Will it be continued at all cost until death?'.

Research and evaluation of palliative care

The opportunities for research in paediatric palliative care are unlimited, since well-controlled studies with significant data are minimal in most areas of the field. At the present time, there are very few paediatric centres or programmes able to conduct large-scale controlled evaluations on either the physical or behavioural aspects of palliative therapy or to provide validated outcome measures. Most hospice programmes are service oriented and lack the skill and resources for research. There is rarely a well-established relationship between the academic settings and the care provider systems for hospice or palliative care, which grossly limits the advancement of research in the care setting.

In palliative care, the quality of remaining life, regardless of its length, for the patient is primary and is a product of optimal relief of suffering and excellent symptom control.(31,32) Evaluation of quality of life is both complex and multifactorial. For children, most evaluation tools lack validation. One major difficulty has been separation of the child's statements and values from those of the parents. Paediatric patients present a demanding challenge to investigators in questions of design, measurement, analysis, and ethics.(33) The behaviour of a developing infant or child is in constant flux, with continuously changing norms. Children frequently present barriers to communication-limited comprehension, unpredictable behaviour, and capricious cooperation, which may frustrate efforts to evaluate even the most simple actions. In the adolescent age group, the natural rebelliousness and need for control are heightened by the teenager's anger at the injustice of a foreshortened life. The more tenuous the child's hold on life, the less inclined will the patient or family be to participate in any but the most necessary activities, and even the most cooperative will become resistant to measurements and evaluations which impinge on their remaining time. The researcher, in turn, feels guilty about adding to the burden of a family under such agonizing stress.

The problems of conducting randomized controlled studies of paediatric palliative care procedures seem overwhelming, given the wide diversity of the existing programmes, services, and personnel. Financial support from health agencies and foundations will continue only if there is hard evidence of the values to be realized by high-calibre palliative care. In the United States, there has been growing dissatisfaction with the peer review system of individual cases through chart audits as the major tool for monitoring outcomes and evaluating patient care. Satisfaction surveys as well are less than helpful to clearly define the benefit and effectiveness of care. Increasingly, funding sources are demanding more definitive monitoring, audit, and quality assurance. JCAHO's (Joint Commission on Accreditation of Health care Organizations) criteria for pain monitoring, etc. has set a standard that has been a catalyst for change in practice and hopefully, in care. Certification and licensing also require improved methods of documentation. Regulatory and reviewing bodies do not seem to take note of the lack of paediatric specific standards for hospice and home care. With children, clinical judgement, clouded by emotional overlay, may influence the evaluation and interfere with the orderly collection of comparative data needed for improved quantitative systems of review. The 1990 report of the Institute of Medicine, Medicare: *A Strategy for Quality Assurance* urged the use of data-driven studies to promote improved patient outcomes and mould clinical decision-making by meaningful feedback to both caregivers and consumers alike.(34)

Within the National Health Service of the United Kingdom, efforts to evaluate care have focused increasingly on cost. Audit tools, particularly performance indicators, used in the National Health Service compare one hospital with another rather than with established standards. For many hospitals, these indicators serve the same purpose as the diagnosis-related groups in the United States to encourage early discharge of patients who are incurable, with little concern for the patient's wishes or quality of care.

Such a dangerous trend threatens the care of children, for whom most terminal care continues to be hospital-based despite the growing trend for home as the site for the later stages of illness. For a variety of reasons, not all parents are capable of caring for their child in the later stages, especially without assistance, in the home, and in some cases the child's physical condition and needs are of such a magnitude that only hospital care will suffice. Comparisons of paediatric palliative care benefits in the United Kingdom and the United States have frequently shown different outcome conclusions, particularly when measured by patient satisfaction. These differences may reflect the variations in cultural backgrounds and social mores, despite a common language. Research questions should be addressed to infants, children, and youth across each age and developmental category, with the data analysed accordingly rather than amassed under the single euphemism of 'children'. Although there may be similar responses to research questions, regardless of age, the variations at each developmental milestone are of such a magnitude as to cloud the outcome if not carefully segregated before the fact. Additionally, cultural variations in child-rearing practices and subsequent child behaviour may be so different across countries that data will not be generalizable, but will have to be viewed and interpreted culturally.

Very few paediatric programmes have evaluated critical issues such as staff attitudes towards children dying in a 'do not resuscitate' status, patient-controlled opioid administration, acceptance of the parent as a co-caregiver, or, most basically, how, when, and by whom the decision should be made to move from curative to palliative care. In addition, many of the same questions need to be addressed to the child and his/her family in each of the different locations where a child might receive palliative care. Children, more than adults, react quite differently in various environments—a hospital, hospice home care, non-hospice home care, or a paediatric hospice facility.

Although Lauer et al. have demonstrated successful parental adaptation and psychological adjustment to the child dying at home, there are still many questions to be answered concerning when hospital admission is appropriate, and desired by all parties, and when an alternative is preferable to the patient and the family members.[10] Regardless of location, research is needed on the components and provisions of quality care during a child's final weeks.

If indeed, as earlier studies have shown, the child with terminal illness wants to be in his/her own home, further definitive research is needed to identify the ideal characteristics of successful home care. The coping mechanisms most useful to parents to handle the stress, the influence of various types of support services, the role reversal between parent and clinical caregivers, and the grief work necessary for each member of the family, as well as the patient, the benefit of extending hospice care principles into pregnancy with a potentially fatal pre-natal diagnosis are just a few of the issues requiring well-controlled studies.

The need for 'hospice' or specialist palliative care facilities for paediatric patients, an ongoing debate in the United Kingdom, deserves study in the light of criticisms regarding the use of limited resources for such highly specialized low-census centres.[35,36] Demographic research of regions or districts could better define the extent of the need for facilities offered in respite care to children with chronic disease and their parents. The marked difference in geography and population distribution in countries such as Canada, the United States, and Australia, compared with the United Kingdom, will require multisite studies of the similarities and disparities of styles, services, and staffing to render the findings applicable across countries. Now that alternative sites of care are available, it is incumbent upon the physician to justify using the precious numbered days of a child's life in hospital if other adequate alternatives, more preferable to the child, are available.

The future of paediatric palliative care

As medicine, with its increasingly sophisticated diagnostics and therapies has grown, the relentless pursuit of cure has riveted attention on disease and away from the patient. The ideal would be to have the patient at the centre point of the discussion. The medical graduate of the 1900s is poorly prepared to function competently in the presence of terminal illness, death, or bereavement.

The last half of the twentieth century saw a dramatic fall in morbidity and mortality in children, with improved survival rates for many diseases. Most families have never experienced the death of a child, and even the demise of elderly parents or relatives has occurred at a distance, in hospital or a nursing home. However, in contrast, many families over many generations have experienced a birth tragedy of one type or another and yet this type of death is still barely recognized as a valid reason for mourning in modern society. At a time when families have become less confident in their competence to care for their severely ill, the hospitals, beset with burgeoning costs to sustain the new technology, cannot assign expensive paediatric beds to patients needing non-reimbursable, symptom-directed palliation. The disincentive exists for pursuit of palliation when higher reimbursement ends when 'comfort care only' appears in the medical record. Patients in need of palliation are refused admission or are discharged prematurely to fend for themselves in an unprepared community environment or at the hands of their overwhelmed family members.

The community has tried to respond to the needs of such patients with significant improvement in broader services, increased availability of home care nursing, and the development of hospice programmes and facilities.[6,37] Collaborations between hospices and hospitals can extend the limited resources of both and extend the support further into the community. Community-based partnerships that seek to avoid duplication and identify unmet needs may actually reduce costs and the burden of responsibility. These previously mentioned limits may prevent those who are not curable from being discharged, but only if financing of their care can be procured and guaranteed. The equally difficult challenge of educating health professionals to recognize that medicine was designed to serve the patient, not the disease, and to perfect the skills necessary to provide compassionate care until death and into bereavement will be much harder to influence.

For children with chronic or prolonged illnesses, care during the final months and weeks of life should be provided, whenever possible, by the family in the home where the child is most secure. When the hospital must be used to provide special services and complex care, the parents should be incorporated into the care plan and remain with the young or very ill child. As quickly as possible the child whose life is limited needs to be returned to his/her home environment. During this terminal phase, the family will require physical, emotional, and spiritual support.

For parents, the decision to move their child from a course of further therapeutic care—the unfortunate interpretation from early hospice days that palliation replaces *all* treatment modalities—has been a serious drawback to timely and effective symptom control. It permeates the language of medicine through this 'all or none' mentality. Successful palliation often requires full utilization of chemotherapy, radiation, antibiotics, and even surgical intervention on occasion. The goal of palliation—to affect the best quality of life for the patient—will be best met by utilizing every means appropriate to alleviate the patient's symptoms. In fact, only the goals and the type of treatment changes, never a cessation of care. Asking parents to choose between continuing treatments or giving up is all too common in attempts to discuss transition to hospice care with parents. Even the most realistic parents cling to the hope that some event will transpire to prevent the death of their child.

Palliative care has served an even larger and more diverse group of patients as the public and professional acceptance of home care for irreversible and chronic illness has increased. The paediatric conditions previously excluded from most palliative care services by nature of the unpredictability of the date of death and the long terminal trajectory, namely cystic fibrosis, congenital anomalies and abnormalities, genetic disorders, neurodegenerative disorders, severe CNS impairment, metabolic disorders, cardiac disease, an array of rare and fatal disorders and most recently AIDS, are pressing for much needed support. With the removal of the original restrictive life expectancy limitation imposed by third party payers in the United States, they too can receive care throughout their lifespan that is forever changed by their diagnosis. The nature of each of these conditions will require special services and collaboration amongst the many disciplines and policy decision makers involved in their care to ensure for them the most optimal quality of life, throughout their lifetime. 'All living things have lifetimes. And lifetimes are really all the same, they have beginnings and endings . . . and there is living in between.' We must set our sights on the living and focus our collective energy to make the necessary improvements in service.

References

1. **Corr, C.A. and Corr, D.M.** (1988). In our opinion . . . What is pediatric hospice care? *Children's Health Care* **17**, 4–11.
2. **Frager, G.** (1996). Pediatric palliative care: building the model, bridging the gaps. *Journal of Palliative Care* **12** (3), 9–12.
3. **American Academy of Pediatrics, Committee on Bioethics** (1996). Ethics and the care of critically ill infants and children. *Pediatrics* **98**, 149–52.
4. **American Academy of Pediatrics, Committee on Bioethics** (1995). Informed consent, parental permission, and assent in pediatric practice. *Pediatrics* **95**, 314–17.
5. **Wilson, D.C.** (1985). Caring for dying children: general principles. In *Hospice Approaches to Pediatric Care* (ed. C.A. Corr and D.M. Corr), pp. 5–30. New York: Springer Publishing Company.
6. **Wallace, A.C. and Jackson, D.** (1995). Establishing a district palliative care team for children. *Child: Care, Health and Development* **21** (6), 383–5.
7. **Sumner, L.** (2001). Staff support in pediatric hospice care. In *Hospice Care for Children* 2nd edn. (ed. A. Armstrong-Dauky and S. Zarback), pp. 190–212. New York: Oxford University Press.
8. **Martinson, I.M., Armstrong, G.D., and Geis, D.P.** (1978). Home care for children dying of cancer. *Pediatrics* **62**, 106–13.
9. **Lauer, M.E.** et al. (1983). A comparison study of parental adaptation following a child's death at home or in the hospital. *Pediatrics* **71**, 107–11.
10. **Mulhern, R.K., Lauer, M.E., and Hoffman, R.G.** (1983). Death of a child at home or in the hospital: subsequent psychological adjustment of the family. *Pediatrics* **71**, 743–7.
11. **Lauer, M.E.** et al. (1986). Utilization of hospice/home care in pediatric oncology: a national survey. *Cancer Nursing* **9**, 102–7.
12. **Lauer, M.E.** et al. (1989). Long term follow-up of parental adjustment following a child's death at home or hospital. *Cancer* **63**, 988–94.
13. **Lauer, M.E. and Mulhern, R.K.** (1984). Home-care referral: parental self selection versus psychosocial predictors of capacity. *American Journal of Hospice Care* **1**, 35–8.
14. **Davies, B. and Steele, R.** (1998). Families in pediatric palliative care. In *Topics in Palliative Care* Vol. 3, (ed. R.K. Portenoy and E. Bruera), pp. 29–49. New York: Oxford.
15. **Singleton, R.** (1992). Palliative home care program for terminally ill children. *Leadership in Health Services* **1** (1), 21–7.
16. **Duffy, C.** et al. (1990). Home based palliative care for children. Part 2: The benefits of an established program. *Journal of Palliative Care* **6** (2), 8–14.
17. **Brown, P., Davies, B., and Martens, N.** (1990). Families in supportive care, Part II: Palliative care at home—a viable setting. *Journal of Palliative Care* **6**, 21–7.
18. **Martinson, I.M. and Enos, M.** (1985). The dying child: at home. In *Hospice Approaches to Pediatric Care* (ed. C.A. Corr and D.M. Corr), pp. 31–42. New York: Springer Publishing Company.
19. **Martin, B.B.** (1985). Home care for terminally ill children and their families. In *Hospice Approaches to Pediatric Care* (ed. C.A. Corr and D.M. Corr), pp. 65–86. New York: Springer Publishing Company.
20. **Stein, A.** et al. (1989). Life threatening illness and hospice care. *Archives of Disease in Childhood* **64**, 114–18.
21. **Grebin, B.** (2001). Palliative care in an inpatient hospital setting. In *Hospice Care for Children* 2nd edn. (ed. A. Armstrong Dauky and S. Zarback), pp. 313–22. New York: Oxford University Press.
22. **Davies, B.** et al. Addressing spirituality in pediatric hospice and palliative care. *Journal of Palliative Care* **1**, 59–67.
23. **Mor, V. and Kidder, D.** (1985). Cost savings in hospice: final results of the National Hospice Study. *Health Services Research* **20**, 407–22.
24. **Paradis, L.F.** (1988). An assessment of sociology's contributions to hospice: priorities for future research. *Hospice Journal* **4**, 57–71.
25. **Houts, P.** et al. (1984). Non-medical costs to patients and their families associated with outpatient chemotherapy. *Cancer* **53**, 2388–92.
26. **Birenbaum, L.K.** Cost of terminal care for families of children with cancer. *Phyllis F. Verhonick Nursing Research Conference, Delivering Nursing Care in the 90s: Growing Needs, Shrinking Resources.* Charlottesville VA, 6 April 1990.
27. **Bloom, B.S.** (1987). Is hospice care least expensive for the terminally ill? *Hospice Journal* **3**, 67–76.
28. **Bloom, B.S., Knorr, R., and Evans, A.** (1985). The epidemiology of disease expenses. *Journal of the American Medical Association* **253**, 2393–9.
29. **Lansky, S.B., Black, J.L., and Cairns, N.U.** (1983). Childhood cancer: medical costs. *Cancer* **52**, 762–6.
30. **Hill, F. and Oliver, C.** (1989). Hospice—an update on the cost of patient care. *Palliative Medicine* **3**, 119–24.
31. **Robbins, M.** *Evaluating Palliative Care: Establishing the Evidence Base.* Oxford: Oxford University Press.
32. **Scriven, M.** (1993). Hard-won lessons in program evaluation. *New Directions for Program Evaluation* **58**, 1–101.
33. **Moore, I.M. and Ruccione, K.** (1989). Challenges to conducting research with children with cancer. *Oncology Nursing Forum* **16**, 587–9.
34. **Institute of Medicine, Division of Health Care Services** (1990). In *Medicare: A Strategy for Quality Assurance* (ed. K.N. Lohr), pp. 5–48. Washington DC: National Academy Press.
35. **Chambers, T.L.** (1987). Hospices for children. *British Medical Journal* **295**, 1309–10.
36. **Wilkinson, J.M.** et al. (1987). Hospices for children? *British Medical Journal* **295**, 210–11 (Correspondence).
37. **Davies, B.** (1996). Assessment of need for a children's hospice program. *Death Studies* **20**, 247–68.

9.6 Bereavement issues and staff support

Betty Davies and Stacy Orloff

Bereavement: significance of the concept

Most children in developing countries die of infectious diseases; those in the more developed countries, because of advances in medical technology and delivery of health care, most often die of trauma. Despite such scientific progress, however, children continue to die of incurable disease such as cancer, congenital anomalies, and genetic defects. Though sometimes difficult to admit, the end result of the paediatric palliative care experience is the death of a child. A child's death is considered a greater loss because the child has not had the opportunity to live a full life as compared to the adult or aged individual; a child's death confounds our expectation that children will grow into adulthood and live a normal lifespan. A child's death confounds our hope that this child may be the one who recovers. All concerned—the parents, the child, the physician, and the other professionals involved in the care—face difficulties in acknowledging the death of a child. A child's death evokes in each one of us the 'inner bereaved child'; it reawakens those painful and repressed effects of separation and loss from our earliest development and makes for a rapid withdrawal from the pain involved. The purpose of this chapter is to bridge the gap between theory and practice and to offer some practical suggestions to assist parents and siblings following the death of a child from life-threatening illness, health care professionals with this emotion-filled experience, and the greater community that is affected by the death of the child.

Death of a child: impact on the family

The family provides for its members the necessary relationships, both in quality and intensity, out of which normal growth and development occur. Because of these relationships, the system behaves, not as a simple composition of independent elements, but coherently and inseparably as a whole. Following this perspective, illness or death in any family member is a potential assault on the family system. The death of a child, therefore, affects not only individual family members, but also the family unit as a whole.

Empty space

The death of a child creates an empty space for surviving family members, a sense in the family that there is always something missing.[1] Interviews with 49 families, 7–9 years after a death from childhood cancer, suggested that three patterns of grieving characterized family members' responses to this sense of emptiness: getting over it, filling the emptiness, and keeping the connection. Those families who placed emphasis on getting over the grief tended to have a somewhat concrete plan for putting the death of the child behind them. They accepted the death matter of factly as either God's will or as something we all have to face. The second group of families filled the empty space by keeping busy (e.g. building a new house) or by substituting other problems or situations to take their mind off their grief. They acknowledged the emptiness, but made an effort to fill up the space with activities. The largest number of families accepted the empty space though they tried never to forget or become very busy. They acknowledged the empty space, allowed it to exist, treasured their remaining children more, and valued life in general.

No pattern of grieving is suggested as superior to the others. The patterns only serve to emphasize that grief, for any family or family member, should not be expected to follow a specific path within specified time limits. Additional findings from this same study reported that the child's death requires individual reorganization and adjustments within the family system.[2] Changes in marital status and or the addition of other children required adjustments in the relationships of family members. Some changes were developmental in nature while others, according to the informants, were directly related to the death of the child. Regardless of the changes, however, a child's death is perceived as a significant event, a reference point to which all subsequent events can be related.

Levels of functioning

When a child dies, all aspects of family life are altered. How the family responds to and incorporates those changes are critical for all family members. Even before their child dies, families have characteristic ways of being in the world, responding to stress, sharing thoughts and feelings, and interacting with the external world. When a child is ill and dies, these characteristic ways of coping come into play. These coping strategies are more or less functional and help health care providers to understand the variability in family response.[3,4]

Communicating openly

Some families communicate freely in discussing the child's illness, death, and family members' responses following the death. Such discussion occurs in the presence of other family members, and all persons are allowed to express their own thoughts and feelings. Each member of the family offers a similar version of a story; there is an underlying sense of coherence among family members. Other families are more closed in that they do not have this freedom of expression. There may be considerable talk, but it is not focused on the questions being asked. Communication is limited or guarded; family members seem less connected to one another.

Dealing with feelings

Some families focus not only on events, but also on the thoughts and feelings associated with such events. As a result, they are more aware of the process; this awareness leads to action. The opposite is true for other families who are less able to focus on feelings and to anticipate potentially difficult occasions, such as special holidays, and consequently became stuck in their sadness.

Defining roles

Some families are more flexible in assuming new roles while acknowledging that no one could take the place of the child who died. Each family member is valued for himself and is perceived as an integral member of the group. In other families, roles are rigidly maintained; surviving siblings may be expected to fill the vacated role of 'older' child, or 'responsible' child, for example.

Utilizing resources

More functional families use a wide range of resources, accepting their vulnerabilities and their need for support. They seek out and request support from a variety of sources, and often express gratitude and satisfaction with the assistance they receive. Less functional families withdraw from sources of support, claiming that they are able to manage 'on their own' and sometimes denying the extent of their grief. They seem unable to communicate what their needs are, or what they want. Any assistance comes from formal sources rather than from informal networks of friends and family. They often feel angry and resentful due to their unfulfilled expectations.

Solving problems

Some families identify problems or difficulties as they occur, openly exchange information about the situation, and develop strategies for dealing with the problem. Input is sought from all family members and others, and creative solutions are developed. Other families approach problems by focusing on why the problem occurred, and on who was at fault, rather than on generating solutions. There is little sense that change is occurring.

Incorporating change

All families struggle with incorporating the past into the present; it takes considerable effort to incorporate the changes associated with the loss of a loved one. Some families are able to reflect on this process, and identify ways in which they are accommodating to the changes. Other families are resistant to reorganization; they seem static, lamenting that they will 'never be the same', and often feel stuck at being sad, depressed, angry, or resentful.

Assessing a family for ways of coping provides some direction for assisting grieving families. For example, in families where communication is closed, health care providers must make an effort to share information with all family members instead of relying on one member to convey the information to the others. Or, in families where anger and sadness prevail, health care providers must spend additional time listening to the distress and the perceived causes of the situation, while gently encouraging broader perspectives and insights. Most importantly, awareness of levels of family functioning helps care providers understand that different families cope in different ways. The goal is not to 'fix' families but to understand them and support them as much as possible.

Parental grief

The loss of a child through death is quite unlike any other loss known. In comparison with other individuals in different role relationships to the deceased (e.g. spouse, sibling, and child), the grief of parents is more intense, more complex, and longer lasting.[5,6] When a child dies, the parents feel each day as grey, hollow, empty; each day is a burden. Parents feel overwhelmed with feelings of anger, depression, uncontrollable tears, hopelessness, frustration, and fear for their remaining children. Parents can be reassured that the psychosomatic symptoms they experience are not congruent with mental illness. This reassurance is underscored by a study of parents 2 years after their child had died from cancer.[7] These parents presented a profile on a symptom checklist (Symptom Checklist 90—Revised) that was significantly different from the normal non-clinical and psychiatric outpatient group. This suggests that these bereaved mothers and fathers display a psychological pattern that is more symptomatic than normal, but less symptomatic than diagnosed outpatients. Despite the recognition of parental grief as an intensely difficult psychological experience, relatively few researchers have empirically addressed this issue. Study samples vary widely in composition and results have been contradictory. Four types of factors potentially related to bereavement outcome have been identified:

1. demographic factors;
2. factors related to parents' premorbid personalities or experiences;
3. factors related to the child's hospitalization or death;
4. post-death factors.[8]

It is also very important to note that most of this research has traditionally focused on mothers' grief. There are very few studies that have investigated the phenomenon of fathers' grief, though fathers are very much affected by their child's death. In one study,[9] mothers in five countries whose child had died from cancer indicated that fathers were having the most difficult time since the child's death. The mothers perceived that their husbands blamed themselves for the child's illness, could not easily express their feelings, and responded by working harder or through anger. In a pilot study focusing specifically on fathers' experiences,[10] these men described vulnerability and helplessness associated with their child's diagnosis of a life-threatening condition. All fathers in the study were actively involved in caregiving and many took time off work, or quit work, to care for their child. They each described how their own childhood lessons characterized their approach to life in general and to the illness and bereavement in particular. For example, one man remembered that when his father died, his grandmother told him that he would have to lead the family now. When his daughter became ill, he found himself not knowing how 'to lead' and felt very helpless. Fathers, like mothers in other studies, also had individual ways of coping with the situation; some found strength in faith, others benefited from 'lessons learned'.

Duration and intensity of grief

It has often been assumed that the pain of grief decreases with the passing of time. However, some studies[8,11] report that parents who had been grieving for longer than 2 years reported similar patterns to parents who had experienced a loss within the past 2 years and that parental grief appears to remain fairly intense for at least 4 years. These findings concur with more recent conceptualizations of grief as an active process that occurs over time[12] rather than as an event from which individuals 'recover'. Additional research also highlights an optimal time frame for a child's terminal illness as it relates to the parents' grief experience. Parents whose children died between 6 and 18 months after diagnosis seemed to be the most prepared for the death and had a better adjustment in the bereavement process[13] than those whose child lived for more than 18 months after diagnosis.

Survival guilt

The unique difficulties inherent in the loss of a child stem from the view that the death of a child is not only inappropriate in the context of living, but its tragic and untimely nature is also a basic threat to the function of parenthood. Parents feel victimized by the loss of their child, by the loss of their hopes and dreams, and by their own loss of self-esteem because they failed as parents in protecting their child. This victimization is sometimes referred to as survival guilt.[14] This phenomenon lends evidence as to why coming to terms with their loss may be a difficult task and why bereaved parents face so many more difficulties than other bereaved individuals. Thoughts of suicide, self-accusations, inconsolable grief, and withdrawal from family and friends are common parental reactions to the loss.

Complicated grief

The experience of parental grief is profound, affected by a myriad of factors that predispose parents to be exceptionally vulnerable to complicated or unresolved grief. Complicated bereavement is characterized by an inability to adapt to the loss and bring grieving to a satisfactory conclusion.[15] Research into the elements of complicated parental bereavement has been limited. It is inappropriate, therefore, to evaluate parental bereavement with traditional criteria. A new model of parental mourning must be developed. Until such a model is developed, the following behaviours remain the most useful for the clinician in assessing complicated bereavement. These behaviours, displayed years after the actual death, include, but are not limited to, maintaining the dead child's environment just as it was at the time of death, developing physical symptoms similar to those of the deceased, feeling unacceptable and intense sadness at various anniversary times, being unable to talk about the deceased child without intense reactivation of the feelings experienced at the time of the death.[16]

The marital dyad

Parents as individuals are affected by the death of their child; the marital dyad is also affected. Mothers and fathers may deal differently with expression of feelings, working and doing daily activities, relating to things that trigger memories of the deceased child, and searching for meaning in what has happened. One of the most difficult aspects of parental bereavement is that the death of a child strikes both partners in the marital dyad simultaneously and confronts them with the same overwhelming loss. Consequently, each partner's primary and most therapeutic source of support is taken away. The person to whom each would turn for support is confronting and working through his or her own grief.

Divorce

A common occurrence is that one spouse may misinterpret the behaviour of the other. The erroneous assumption that because partners suffer the same loss, they will experience the same grief, may set up unrealistic expectations that most likely will not be met. The expectation of going through the entire crisis together is often thwarted for bereaved parents. This in itself constitutes a loss for the couple as they may have been accustomed to pulling together through crises. When combined with other factors, this loss places additional burdens of grief, loss, and demands for adaptation on already over-burdened individuals. Such reactions have led to the assertion that there may be higher divorce rates in bereaved couples. However, the assumption that parental loss of a child invariably destroys the marital relationship is an erroneous interpretation of early research findings; these reports have failed to take into account normal divorce rates and longitudinal designs. Several studies[17–19] suggest that while stresses of childhood illness and subsequent death of the child are exceptionally high, and may exacerbate pre-existing marital discord, family relationships do not automatically have to be disrupted and end in divorce. In one study[2] of 56 families 7–9 years following a child's death from cancer, nine couples were divorced. Four of the nine divorced couples stated that the death of the child was a major factor contributing to their divorce. The other five couples did not attribute the divorce to the child's death but viewed it as a result of other problems that existed before the child was diagnosed with cancer.

Intimacy

The lack of synchronicity in grieving styles and grief experiences commonly results in dissimilar expectations and coping strategies. Husbands and wives may deal differently with expression of feelings, working, and doing daily activities, relating to things that trigger memories of the deceased, and searching for the meaning of what has happened. One problem frequently discussed is the inhibition of sexual response and intimacy in bereaved parents. This area of difficulty may be the result of fear related to having and losing other children and/or guilt over experiencing pleasure. It may also be a symptom of grief and/or depression experienced by one partner or both partners.[20] Fathers, uncomfortable in verbally communicating feelings, may use sexual intimacy as a means of seeking comfort from their partners. It is not uncommon for the couple to sustain some sexual difficulties for up to 2 years following a child's death because of disinterest or grief-related symptomatology in one partner or both partners. In fact, in one cross-sectional study of 54 bereaved parents,[21] the response pattern was characterized by a decrease in intensity of the grief experience in the second year following the child's death, followed by an increase in intensity in the third year. Mothers tended to exhibit more intense grief experiences and poorer subsequent adjustment than fathers. Parental bereavement may intensify rather than decline, over time.

Search for meaning

The death of a child is so profound that it ultimately sends bereaved parents into a deep and painful existential 'search for meaning' and this search may be a key factor in a positive 'growth' versus negative 'despair' resolution of the grief experience. Of the numerous comments made by 36 parents in one study,[22] 40 responses indicated a positive outlook, whereas only 13 responses were negative. Positive growth responses included: learning to live each day to the fullest; being more understanding of others; having a stronger faith; being aware of the precariousness of life; and being a better person in general. Focusing on the potential for growth when a child has died is meant in no way to minimize the deep and long-lasting pain of grief; rather, it is meant to point out the importance of channelling the pain and rage into meaningful endeavours that can contribute to recovery.

Sibling grief

Paediatric palliative care is focused on families; this implies that health care professionals must also pay attention to the needs of the siblings of children who die. The responses of children to the death of a sibling have not been extensively examined until recent years, yet to lose a brother or sister has potentially traumatic effects that last a lifetime. Davies[4] offers a comprehensive review of sibling bereavement research, with suggestions for interventions for children and the adults who care for them. She presents a model of sibling bereavement that emphasizes numerous variables must be taken into account when attempting to understand and assist grieving siblings. The model suggests that siblings exhibit four major responses to the death of a brother or sister: 'I hurt inside', 'I do not understand', 'I do not belong', and 'I am not enough'. The first two responses are similar to those most often described that focus on the behavioural/emotional reactions of children and the cognitive responses that result from children's developing understanding about death. Looking at the longer-term responses of siblings brought forth the additional two responses.

Sibling responses

'I hurt inside'

This response includes all the emotions typically associated with grief, and the behavioural manifestations of such emotions in children. Siblings may exhibit a wide range of behavioural problems after the death of a brother or sister. Many studies, however, define the behavioural changes seen in bereaved children as problematic, if not even pathological, although positive responses also have been identified. Problems have included a range of behaviours, attitudes, emotions, symptoms, cognitions, and diagnoses (Table 1). Often ignored in children are psycho-physiological responses such as headaches, general aches and pains, stomach cramps, and disruptions in eating and sleeping patterns. These are common in grieving adults, and so it is not surprising that grieving children experience them as well. Sleeping disturbances are common—children may not want to go to bed at night, especially if they shared a room with the deceased child; they may have bad dreams or nightmares, or walk in their sleep. Eating disturbances may include overeating or a loss of appetite. Anxiety may be evident, and school performance may deteriorate. Children will frequently complain of loneliness. Some bereaved children also feel guilty for the death of their sibling even when they held no responsibility for the death.

Bereaved children's hurt derives from the vulnerability of being human, of feeling love for, and attachment to their brothers or sisters, so that when they are gone, siblings miss them. The other three responses derive from the vulnerability that children experience from being dependent on the adults in their lives. How adults interact with children determines the degree to which siblings feel that they do not understand, do not belong, or are not enough.

'I do not understand'

This response is greatly influenced by a child's level of cognitive development. Younger children may not comprehend that their brother or sister is never coming back; they may not understand that death is forever. Children of all ages may be confused by the array of powerful feelings that surge within them; they may be mystified by the activity and reactions of others. They are confused and bewildered by all that is happening.

Table 1 Sibling responses to the death of a brother or sister from cancer[53]

Psychological
Fearful of own death and parents' death
Tearful
Anxiety (over people leaving, with new situations)
Loneliness
Angry outbursts or temper tantrums
Concerns about getting cancer
Attention-seeking from parents
Withdrawn (guarding feelings and thoughts)
Sadness
Daydreaming
Change in school performance (decreased concentration)
Physiological
Sleep disturbances (reluctant to go to bed, nightmares)
Eating disturbances (loss of appetite, lack of interest in food)
Bodily complaints (e.g. head aches, stomach aches, generalized aches)
Increased incidence of colds and influenza episodes
Frequent infections (urinary tract, respiratory tract)

'I do not belong'

When children feel left out of what is happening, they feel as if they 'do not belong'. In the aftermath of a child's death, siblings often want to help, but do not know how; or, if they try to help, their efforts are not acknowledged or are even criticized. When children verbalize their natural curiosity in the form of questions, and are ignored or told to be quiet, they get the message that they are inappropriate and they begin to feel as if they 'do not belong'. The reorganization of roles and responsibilities that accompany the death of any family member may leave the child feeling as if he has lost his place in the family. As well, bereaved children feel different from their non-bereaved peers, and this too contributes to feelings of not belonging.

'I am not enough'

Siblings' feelings of 'I am not enough' arise from perceptions that they should have been the one to die since, in their view, the deceased child was the parents' favourite, or was the smartest, the prettiest, or the 'best' in some way.[4,23] Moreover, siblings see their parents' distress, and creatively attempt to lift their parents' spirits by behaving very well or by overachieving in school, for example. It is difficult for parents to manage their own grief; their personal resources are stretched to the limit, but their other children want their parents to 'get back to normal'. When parents continue to grieve, siblings may feel as if their efforts are in vain. They can feel they are not enough to make their mom and dad happy ever again.

Influencing factors

The aforementioned responses do not occur in isolation but within a context of many interrelated variables. No one factor accounts for the total experience of any individual child. Three categories of factors come into play: individual, situational, and environmental. Individual factors include age, gender, temperament, and past experience with loss. For example, loss occurring at younger than 5 years of age or during early adolescence, and the presence of pre-existing psychological difficulties are warning signs for children at risk.

Situational factors, such as the circumstances of the illness and death, affect sibling responses. For example, siblings who witness considerable pain and suffering in the ill child may be more troubled than siblings of children who die peacefully.

Environmental factors include the pre-death relationship between siblings. Siblings who shared close relationships with their brother or sister tend to demonstrate more internalizing behaviour after the death of the child. Emotional closeness between siblings exerts a stronger influence on bereavement outcome than closeness in age, length of illness, or number of surviving children in the family. Health care professionals, therefore, need to be particularly sensitive to the needs of the children who shared a close relationship with their brother or sister. Environmental variables also include the social climate and functioning level of families, and the social context of the family. For example, the greater the degree of commitment, help, and support family members provide for one another, the fewer withdrawing and acting out behaviour reported for the bereaved children.[24] Furthermore, families with a greater emphasis on social, cultural, recreational, and religious involvement tended to have children with fewer behavioural problems following a sibling's death.[4,24]

Intervening conditions and consequences

Davies' model emphasizes that intervening conditions either facilitate or constrain how siblings deal with their grief. The most significant conditions seem to be the ways in which adults interact with the siblings. When adults comfort those siblings who are hurting, teach those who do not understand, include siblings so they feel as if they belong, and validate siblings' sense of worth, then those children are more likely to have increased self-esteem and maturity, to be more sensitive and empathetic, and better prepared to handle death. In contrast, when adults belittle children's expressions of hurt, disregard their questions and level of cognitive development, exclude them from day-to-day events and activities, and shame them for not understanding, or for not responding as the adults expect, then the siblings are more likely to feel invisible, insecure, and insignificant. The impact of the death casts a dark shadow far into siblings' future.[4]

Summary

The death of a child has a potentially traumatic impact on the family. The death induces profound parental grief, which affects parents as individuals and as marital partners; the death alters the behaviour of siblings. From the literature reviewed, it can be concluded that the death of a child is not something to 'get over'. Instead, it is an event that surviving parents, siblings, and other family members must learn to integrate into the ongoing fabric of their lives. Only by understanding this to be the case can health professionals offer the knowledgeable, sensitive, and long-term support that such families require.

Professional caregiver response

Helping a child die well, physically comfortable, and psychologically and spiritually at peace; helping parents cope with the experience of their child's death as well as they possibly can; helping siblings and other children close to the dying child master the experience to the full potential of their developmental level—each of these is a challenge to health care professionals personally and professionally. Caregivers absorb much of the same stress experienced by the family members of a dying child and experience similar conflict. This stress, and the associated disruption, pressure, and depletion require significant personal and professional effort at adaptation and balance. Furthermore, the death of a child characteristically leads to a core conflict in persons caring for the child—a tendency to overprotect and become over-involved with the child and an opposing tendency to move away from the child to protect oneself from painful involvement.

Showing compassion

In order for those in helping professions to function effectively—to 'enjoy' being a good doctor, nurse, social worker/counsellor, clergyman, lawyer, professionals must allow themselves to approach, and to a degree share, the distress of those they are attempting to help.[25,26] They must show compassion. Yet, when confronted with a dying child, professionals are sometimes compelled to respond with analysis, clinical judgement, and 'doing' behaviours in an effort to maintain some sense of control and composure.

However, compassion and control seem incompatible. Professionals vary widely in the extent to which they can retain their compassion. Two things are crucial: the magnitude of the distress and the individual's own confidence in his or her ability to cope with it. As long as professionals feel that their participation is worthwhile, they will find themselves able to tolerate high levels of disturbance in others without disengaging. Confidence in one's ability to cope with the distress of others can be, and normally is, obtained by a process of attunement. By repeated, reflective exposure, professionals gradually discover what they can do to alleviate distress and how much of it is inevitable and insurmountable. Interdisciplinary teams can serve as a wonderful support for the health care professional. Interdisciplinary teams provide health-care professionals a safe place in which to share their feelings and receive guidance—particularly when professional boundaries may be 'too close for comfort'.

Key attributes

Some health care professionals are more suitable than others for the demanding role of working with dying children and adolescents.[27,28] Those who are best suited to this role have specific personal attributes, including: a high tolerance for ambiguity, flexibility, and an appreciation for individual differences; good external support networks and a realistic awareness of personal limits; joie de vivre and sense of humour; an open communication style and tendency to value self-awareness as assets; empathy and a willingness to continually learn.[29,30] Perhaps the most basic characteristic is one's comfort with death. Becoming a clinical practitioner who can move towards instead of away from children who are dying does not come easily. Only by coming to terms with one's own thoughts and feelings about death and about children, is it possible to adapt philosophically to working with children who might die. Self-awareness is integral to effective care of the dying; caregivers need to be conscious of their own agendas as they interface with patient, family, team, and institution directions and goals.[31]

Health care provider–family relationships

The duration of relationships with patients who have long-term, chronic illness provides health care providers with both the opportunity and the obligation to establish relationships as persons as well as professionals. The nurse, counsellor, or physician may become a 'professional friend'. The relationship is a professional one—it is time limited, goal oriented, and patient centred with professional knowledge and skills employed on the patient's behalf.[32] However, the relationship may also assume some of the qualities usually described as part of a socially meaningful relationship. When the patient is a child, health care providers often become professional friends not only of the child but also of the family. As the child enters the terminal phase, the closeness of the relationship may enhance personal and professional distress. Professional boundaries are almost always tested. One study[33] described the 'struggle' nurses experience while caring for children with chronic, life-threatening illness who die. They struggle with grief but their expression of such distress was hampered by a code of conduct either self-imposed or imposed by their profession, their institution, or society in general. Nurses also struggled with moral distress when directives for painful, life-prolonging treatment for children in the dying process challenged their professional ethic to provide comfort for the patient.

Manifestations of stress: cost of caring

In a study of occupational stress in the care of the critically ill, the dying, and the bereaved, three major categories of stress—physical, psychological, and behavioural—were reported.[31] Of these, physical symptoms of stress were reported less often, and psychological symptoms were reported more often than behavioural ones. Furthermore, younger caregivers reported more symptoms of stress and fewer coping strategies than older caregivers. By being aware of the manifestation of stress, professionals can monitor their own responses, taking appropriate action when they begin to experience such symptoms. Appropriate actions include approaches at both institutional and personal levels. Much of the literature cites the paediatric ward as a potential source of ultimate frustration, anguish, and personal and professional stress for caregivers; however, only a limited number of studies describe the stress experienced by staff working with such children.(32,33) In one of these published studies that describes staff stress in a paediatric hospice setting,(32) a small but distinct subgroup of staff who manifested symptoms of psychological distress were characterized in two ways. First, they experienced relatively recent bereavement in their personal lives. Second, they failed to resolve their grief about a bereavement that had occurred some considerable time before. Deep distress can be rekindled when a trigger event echoes back to and resurrects a sense of personal loss. The very nature of the work serves as a constant reminder of their loss and may interfere with their own natural grieving.

Institutional actions

Within agencies, primary consideration must be given to staff selection. Individuals must want to work in paediatric palliative care, and must come with a repertoire of coping abilities developed through previous work and personal experiences. They must be trained in the care of dying children. On the whole, physicians, nurses, counsellors, and chaplains are inadequately prepared to care for the dying; education has emphasized life-saving activities, maintenance of personal control, and the avoidance of failure. The lack of accountability for psychosocial care has also contributed to this lack of education for all health professionals; for example, issues of 'patient safely' have only referred to physical aspects of the situation.

The need for systematic education for nurses was identified more than 20 years ago;(34) however, in the interim, few such programmes have been described and even fewer programmes have been evaluated.(35) There are similar findings in medical literature pertaining to the education of physicians.(36–38) Other allied health care professionals such as social workers/counsellors and chaplains are also not frequently provided quality end of life care education. The need for appropriate training in the care of the dying remains strong.(39,40)

Recent findings suggest that the milieu of the ward when a child died affects the nurse's grief.(33) When it was acknowledged how difficult it might be for the nurse when her patient died, the nurse felt supported and felt better able to resolve her grief. When nursing care goals were clearly established as palliative, nurses experienced less distress since they were able to focus on making the patient comfortable, and the family was satisfied with the care. The difficulty in an acute care setting, however, is that not all members of the team are able to acknowledge the child will not recover. As well, opportunities to brief, debrief, review, and analyse the situation in a safe, supportive environment with one another and with physician colleagues helped nurses cope with current and subsequent stresses in their practice settings.

Health care providers who provide home-based care (particularly hospice care) to dying children may also struggle when the child dies. The very nature of hospice work requires the health care professional to work in a very intimate environment with the ill child and family. Day in and day out, the home-care staff are providing care while sitting on the child's bed at home and seeing the family in their own environment. Families may be less guarded at home and home-care staff often witness feelings and behaviours that may not be as evident in the hospital. This experience may also allow the home-care staff to feel more at peace after the child's death as they have had the opportunity to see the child happy to be in his home.

The necessity of team building and support in interdisciplinary teamwork has been the focus of long-standing debate. There are three primary advantages to allowing staff as a group the time and means to understand and tackle the difficult issues that necessarily arise in any team.(41) First, understanding of interpersonal dynamics and pitfalls amongst the team will further the team's understanding of the families for whom they care. Second, while some may argue that teams are really too busy helping families to waste time on the unnecessary nicety of promoting understanding, the contrary is true in that time is saved. Prolonged and unresolved staff conflict saps and debilitates the individual and undermines his or her self-esteem, commitment, and efficiency. At its worst, it leads to high staff turnover with consequent fragmentation in care and delivery. Third, 'problems and difficulties encountered by those facing great distress have a way of echoing and reverberating in the service set up to help them, with the danger that a service inadvertently mirrors, and therefore remirrors, the very difficulties it aims to ease.'(41) Any group claiming to work as a team should show their battle scars. 'If they don't have them, they haven't worked as a team!'(42)

Personal actions

The person best equipped to deal with the care of the dying child is that person who has developed a wide repertoire or coping skills through exposure to previous life stressors, both personally and professionally. Conversely, professionals who deal with feelings of helplessness and passivity by excessive intellectualization, flight into activity, denial, projection, rationalization, or withdrawal is going to experience personal distress as well as finding themselves in the middle of considerable staff conflict.(26) Effective coping requires a high degree of self-awareness and personal responsibility. Personal approaches, therefore, must include developing outlets for physical and emotional expression, creating periods of solitude for reflection and integration, and finding meaning through one's personal philosophy.

Implications for practice

Helping the bereaved

According to the Committee for the Study of Health Consequences of the Stress of Bereavement,(43) health care providers and institutions are professionally and morally obligated to assist the bereaved by being sensitive to and knowledgeable about grief's impact. To carry out this role responsibly, they should be able to communicate about sensitive issues, to understand the nature of normal and abnormal bereavement reactions, and to be knowledgeable about community resources to which the bereaved can be referred for specialized help if needed. A recent review of models in the field of death, dying, and bereavement suggests the need to shift perspective from passive victimization to an opportunity for active processes whereby one can regain some measure of control and meaning in living with loss.(12,44) Limitations in the attention paid to the bereaved by health care professionals appear to derive from three factors:

1. their inadequate training about the nature of bereavement and their own personal feelings toward death;
2. the failure of health care institutions to acknowledge their responsibility for bereavement follow-up, the stress that caring for dying and bereaved persons puts on their staff, and the need for sufficient staff time for these activities;
3. the financial constraints imposed by the current structure of third-party reimbursement arrangements, particularly in the United States.

Despite these constraints, it is necessary for health professionals to formulate some approach to the bereaved because, whether they are trained or untrained, those who interact with a bereaved person will have an impact—negative or positive—on that individual. It is clearly more beneficial to families for the health care provider to be trained in bereavement. In recent years, there has been much more documentation in the literature addressing assessment and intervention strategies when working with bereaved individuals.(45–47) A limited number of studies examined the relationship between parental bereavement outcome and health care professionals' interventions prior to, at the time of, and after the child's death.(11,48) Results revealed that, in many cases, actions that were considered helpful or not helpful varied according to each individual's personal perceptions and situations. Due to the uniqueness of every parent's grieving response, health care professionals' interventions cannot simply be standardized but rather, must be individualized to meet the needs of each bereaved parent and each family. The most consistently helpful action was related to the attitude of the health care providers—showing a caring, concerned attitude and demonstrating an ability to be involved with parents.(48)

While one must always be weary of 'cookbook' approaches to grief counselling, consideration of some general principles for helping individuals may be beneficial. Any health care professional providing support to bereaved families must, at a minimum, have a basic understanding of the theoretical perspectives, particularly with regard to families who have had a child die. The goal for health care professionals is to help bereaved siblings (and parents) to integrate their losses in ways that are regenerative, rather than degenerative, in the continual unfolding of their lives.

Bereaved parents

Interventions by health care professionals begin by making contact with the parents and letting them know that the health care team is available to meet with them should they desire such contact. Parents often have many questions about the child's death, and the team members who are willing to discuss these sensitive issues provide a meaningful service to the family. Parents especially value contact with those care providers who cared directly for their child, and in particular with any health care provider who was with the child at the moment of death.

In working with bereaved parents, it is critical to maintain a family systems perspective, recognizing the impact of the death on family members and on their interactions with one another. Health care professionals are in a unique position to help families enhance their functioning following a death through offering insights that may provide them with different ways of being in the world. For example, the belongings of the deceased child have the potential of serving as memories, and the meaning associated with a particular belonging determines whether or not the belonging is kept.(49) Furthermore, memories may vary in meaning for individuals within the family. Memories may have a mutually held meaning for the family as a whole and private meanings for its individual members. Consequently, if asked, health care professionals must avoid telling families what to do with their child's belongings. Rather, they can encourage families to be aware of the subtle meanings associated with various belongings that serve as memories. For example, when visible mementos of their child (e.g. photographs) are displayed within a grouping of photos of all children in the family, a different message is conveyed than if the photo is the only one displayed. In the first instance, the surviving children perceive that the deceased child was 'one of the family'; in the second instance, they may perceive that the deceased child is the 'most important' child in the family. Siblings in the first instance are likely to feel more special than siblings in the second family. Also, the greater the discrepancy between the family's mutually held meaning of the memory and the individual's private meanings of the memory, the less the integration of the loss by the family and its individual members. It is important, therefore, to encourage family members to share openly their private meanings, and to help them realize that not having the same meanings and memories is acceptable.

The importance of effective communication has been recognized as an essential element in facilitating individual and family coping with childhood chronic, life-threatening illness. However, effective communication refers not just to the sharing of information but to the creation of a climate within the family that allows and encourages the expression of feelings. Several studies support the suggestion that parent–sibling communication differs before and after the death. Before the death, talking about the illness and death is related specifically to the events of day-to-day care. After the death, while open expression may pertain to many topics and areas of concern to family members, discussion about the feelings aroused by the death may be excluded. Similarly, the open expression of grief may not be supported, even in the most expressive families. This exclusion may not, and is usually not, conscious. Often, it is communicated implicitly by the lack of willingness to experience and openly express the painful emotions associated with grief. Therefore, it seems that parents, including those who communicated openly with their children before the death, need encouragement in communicating openly with their surviving children after the death so that the sadness and sorrow is shared and expressed. It is also important to assess the communication style of the extended family. For many families, grandparents, aunts and uncles, other family members, and close friends may live close by and have participated in the child's care. They are grieving also and how information is shared with this extended family is important for health care providers to know. All assessments must include a sensitivity and understanding of the family's cultural, religious, and spiritual background. It is not reasonable to use one standard as the measurement of effective communication with all families.

Almost all the evidence recommends professional intervention following the death of a child; the need for a trained professional in the area of bereavement seems evident. Follow-up by the care providers focuses on facilitating communication within the family, allowing parents to vent their anxieties and concerns, assessing the family's grief in order to promote the mental health of the family, and referring the parents to other useful resources. One major resource may be books written for bereaved parents. A most potent resource available, however, are specific support groups for bereaved parents, which provide ongoing social support. Options include groups such as The Compassionate Friends, an international self-help group for all types of bereaved parents; Candlelighters, a group for parents of children with cancer, or other local groups or organizations (such as hospices) devoted to helping bereaved parents; and, CRUSE, a grief counselling service offered throughout the United Kingdom. Through mutual sharing, learning, modelling, and support, these groups support parents in their grief.

Probably the most critical realization for health care providers who offer bereavement support to parents is that they cannot take away the parents' pain and suffering. Therefore, the follow-up offered must be supportive in nature, and provided over time. Professionals providing bereavement support may feel helpless in such situations, and want to do something more. Instead, they must value the 'gift of presence', of being there to share the pain. Table 2 provides a synthesis of principles and intervention strategies for working with bereaved parents.(50,51)

Bereaved siblings

Two critical assumptions provide the foundation for interventions with bereaved siblings.(4) First, health care providers must acknowledge the impact of a child's death on the surviving siblings. Until very recently, the focus of all attention has been the parents of the child who died; siblings have been relatively forgotten. Research into the long-term effects of sibling bereavement continues to validate the significance of this event for siblings.

Table 2 Principles and strategies for working with bereaved parents(15,51)

1. Make contact and assess the bereaved parents
2. Provide assurance that they can survive their loss, keeping in mind the parents' unique perspective
3. Provide times to grieve, remembering that grief has its own time
4. Facilitate the identification and expression of feelings, including anger, hostility, sadness, relief, and guilt
5. Encourage verbalization of thoughts and recollections of the deceased child; do not be afraid to mention the deceased child's name
6. Interpret 'normal' grieving behaviour and responses
7. Maintain a therapeutic and realistic perspective; do not rush to 'fix' the pain
8. Allow for individual differences relating to gender, age, personality, culture, ethnicity, religion, and characteristics of the death
9. Avoid analysing or interrupting parents' repeated stories and tears
10. Help to identify and resolve secondary losses, such as the hopes, dreams, and expectations the parents had for the deceased child
11. Examine defenses and coping strategies; carefully examine resistance to the grief process
12. Assist in finding sources of continuing support
13. Identify and refer 'pathology'
14. Interpret 'recovery' for them; correct unrealistic expectations of themselves and of the grief process

Health care professionals must be aware of the meaning of sibling responses. For example, children who demonstrate a pattern of behaviour which includes persistent sadness and withdrawal, decreased involvement in activities and hobbies, acting out, diminished self-esteem, and a loss of interest and achievement in school require individualized attention through referrals to the school counsellor or to a specialist in children's grief.

Many bereaved siblings have described their experience of participating in a specialized bereavement support group as an important part of their experience. Such bereavement groups may be helpful for any bereaved sibling not just those who show long-term psychological symptomatology. The number of grief groups for children has increased considerably during the past decade throughout North America, the United Kingdom, and Australia. Some groups are time-limited, offered for 6 or 8 weeks or over a weekend; others are open-ended and children may attend over many months. Most offer structured activities that form the basis for group discussion and individualized expression. The evaluation of one programme indicated that the children valued learning that they were 'not alone' in their thoughts and feelings; they were reassured by learning that they were as 'not different from other kids' as they had previously thought. The participants' parents perceived the group lessened their children's anxiety and acting-out behaviours.(52)

The second underlying assumption to helping siblings is that health care providers must understand that a child's parents are often the best ones to help their own children. However, parents grieving over the loss of a child seldom have the personal energy to provide their grieving children as much as support as the parents would like to give. Health care professionals must support parents in supporting their children. This is not to say, however, that direct contact with siblings is not helpful; indeed, direct interventions by caregivers can be particularly advantageous for older children who need a less emotionally involved adult with whom to discuss their concerns. Such children often avoid discussing their own grief with their parents because they are trying to protect their parents from further distress.

There is considerable similarity between the techniques used to help children cope with a dying sibling and those used to help children adjust to the death of a sibling. In both cases, in order to guide parents in supporting their other children, health care professionals must understand children's views of death, and must be aware of the normal responses of children to death. This information then serves as the foundation upon which parents' questions and concerns about their surviving children can be discussed. Communication with siblings needs to be open, and must take into account each child's individual needs and developmental level. For all children, however, parents and caregivers need to remember the CHILD when helping him or her to cope with grief (Table 3).

Table 3 Helping children cope with grief: remember the CHILD

C—Consider
Consider the unique situation of the child, his/her developmental capacity to understand, his/her thoughts, his/her feelings, his/her relationship to his sibling
A child is a child: do not expect a child to be 'the man around the house' or the 'little mother'; it is unfair to the child's future development and often limiting to the grieving process to assign inappropriate role responsibilities to the child.
H—Honesty
Use the 'd' word: death, die, dying
Realize that it is all right to not have all the answers
Avoid euphemisms—words which are confusing or have other meanings for the child
Avoid words such as gone away or went on a trip; expressions such as these can make everyday events—leaving on a vacation, going to work—very frightening for the child
Do not explain to a child that the dead person is sleeping; he/she will be afraid of sleeping
I—Involve
Let the child know what is happening; if possible, before the death occurs.
Give the child factual knowledge about the cause of death—especially the school-age child
Involve the child in saying good-bye to the dying and deceased—allow the child the choice to participate in the funeral to the level at which he/she is comfortable
L—Listen
Concentrate on discussing the stumbling block of the moment—too often when the subject is sensitive, adults want to rush ahead to explain and reassure in order to finish the conversation; rather, let the child talk through what is on his/her mind
Let the child know that it is all right to not want to talk to anyone anymore about the death for awhile
Give the child outlets for expressing his/her grief—art, drawing, play, writing letters, poetry, stories, hammering
Be aware of thoughts and fantasies children may have of being reunited with the person who has died; each child must be considered potentially at risk for suicide and any kind of communication that suggests this possibility should be promptly and fully evaluated; careful attention to any suggestion of suicidal risk, no matter what the age of the child, is essential.
Clarify that death is **not** the result of the child's action or thoughts; be attuned to magical thinking involved in the child's explanation of the death and correct it to avoid guilt and inappropriate grief reactions
D—Do it over and over again
Appropriately share your grief: realize that children cannot do grief work without permission and role models; children need to see an honest expression of emotions from adults accompanied by explanations and reassurances
Keep in mind the developmental capacities of the child and his/her age-related concerns and needs

Conclusion

Facing the impending death of a child is an experience like no other. The unnaturalness of a child's death compounds the pain, the sorrow, and the sadness. And yet, children too must face life-threatening illness. It is crucial that we pay attention to this experience. The loss of a child triggers profound grief in all those who knew and cared for the child—the parents, siblings, grandparents, teachers, nurses, doctors, social workers, and chaplains as well as other health providers who, on a daily basis, were witness to the plight of the child and his family. Health care professionals can do much to facilitate optimal bereavement outcomes in the child's family. Such individuals must realize the child's need to be cared for in a style that promotes comfort and dignity. In addition, such individuals must remember that the experiences of the family during the dying process will significantly affect their future lives as survivors. Professionals must be aware of the various reactions that comprise 'normal' grief in parents and siblings, recognizing that such reactions may be influenced by a variety of mediating factors, some of which have been identified. Further, health care professionals must be aware that the intensity of the immediate impact does seem to diminish over time but the long-term effects, though not easily identified or measured, lasts a lifetime.

health care professionals who choose to care for dying children and their families do not engage in this work without needing support themselves. This is a challenging field, one which demands that professionals struggle with the difficult task of maintaining balance and perspective. In addition, however, working with such children and their families provides meaning to life. Working with these children helps to give a clear perspective on what is really valuable. Working with these children helps us to grow, to develop as both persons and professionals. It has been said that all of us need to learn about our own mortality, limitations, and vulnerabilities. These children and their families teach these lessons well.

References

1. **McClowry, S.G.** et al. (1987). The empty space phenomenon: the process of grief in the bereaved family. *Death Studies* **11**, 361–74.
2. **Martinson, I.M.** et al. (1994). Changes over time: a study of family bereavement following childhood cancer. *Journal of Palliative Care* **10**, 19–25.
3. **Davies, B.** et al. (1986). Manifestations of levels of functioning in grieving families. *Journal of Family Issues* **7** (3) 297–313.
4. **Davies, B.** *Shadows in the Sun: Experiences of Sibling Bereavement in Childhood.* Philadelphia PA: Bruner/Mazell, 1999.
5. **Clayton, P., Desmarais, L., and Winokur, G.** (1968). A study of normal bereavement. *American Journal of Psychiatry* **125**, 168–78.
6. **Sanders, C.M.** (1979–80). A comparison of adult bereavement in the death of a spouse, child, and parent. *Omega* **10**, 303–22.
7. **Moore, I.M., Gilliss, C.L., and Martinson, I.M.** (1988). Psychosomatic symptoms in parents 2 years after the death of a child with cancer. *Nursing Research* **37**, 1046.
8. **Hazzard, A., Weston, L., and Gutteres, C.** (1992). After a child's death. Factors related to parental bereavement. *Developmental and Behavioral Pediatrics* **13**, 24–30.
9. **Davies, B.** et al. (1998). Experiences of mothers of children who died from cancer—a cross cultural perspective. *Cancer Nursing* **21** (5), 301–11.
10. **Davies, B.** (2001). *Fathers' Experiences in Pediatric Palliative Care.* Paper presented at International Conference on Death, Dying, and Bereavement, London, Ontario.
11. **Neidig, l.R. and Dalgas-Pelish, P.** (1991). Parental grieving and perceptions regarding health care professionals' interventions. *Issues in Comprehensive Nursing* **14**, 179–91.
12. **Attig, T.W.** (1991). The importance of conceiving of grieving as an active process. *Death Studies* **15**, 383–93.
13. **Rando, T.** *Readings in Pediatric Psychology.* New York: Plenum Press, 1993.
14. **Miles, M.S.** (1985). Helping adults mourn the death of a child. In *Issues in Comprehensive Pediatric Nursing* Vol. I (ed. H. Wass and C.A. Corr), pp. 219–41. Washington DC: Hemisphere Publishing.
15. **Worden, W.** *Grief Counseling and Grief Therapy: A Handbook for the Mental Health Practitioner.* New York: Springer, 1982.
16. **Foley, G.V. and Whittham, E.H.** (1991). Care of the child dying of cancer: Part II. *CA—A Cancer Journal for Clinicians* **41**, 52–64.
17. **Foster, D., O'Malley, E., and Koocher, G.P.** (1981). The parent interviews. In *The Damocles Syndrome: Psychosocial Consequences of Surviving Childhood Cancer* (ed. G.P. Koocher and E. O'Malley), pp. 86–100. New York: McGraw-Hill.
18. **Lansky, S.B.** et al. (1978). Childhood cancer: parental discord and divorce. *Pediatrics* **62**, 184–8.
19. **Spinetta, L., Swarner, L., and Sheoposh, L.** (1981). Effective parental coping following death of a child from cancer. *Journal of Pediatric Psychology* **6**, 251–63.
20. **Rando, T.A.** (1986). The unique issues and impact of the death of a child. In *Parental Loss of a Child* (ed. T.A. Rado), pp. 5–43. Champaign IL: Research Press.
21. **Rando, T.A.** (1983). An investigation of grief and adaptation in parents whose children have died from cancer. *Journal of Pediatric Psychology* **8**, 3–20.
22. **Miles, M.S. and Crandall, E.K.** (1983). The search for meaning and its potential for affecting growth in bereaved parents. *Health Values: Achieving High Level Wellness* **7**, 19–23.
23. **Martinson, I., Davies, B., and McClowry, S.** (1987). The long-term effects of sibling death on self-concept. *Journal of Pediatric Nursing* **2**, 227–35.
24. **Davies, B.** (1988). The family environment in bereaved families and its relationship to surviving sibling behaviour. *Children's Health Care* **17**, 22–30.
25. **Parkes, C.M.** *Bereavement: Studies of Grief in Adult Life* 2nd edn. New York: Tavistock Publications, 1986.
26. **Vachon, M.L.S. and Pakes, E.** (1985). Staff stress in the care of the critically ill and dying child. *Issues in Comprehensive Pediatric Nursing* **8**, 151–82.
27. **Davies, B. and Eng, B.** (1993). Factors influencing nursing care of children who are terminally ill: a selective review. *Pediatric Nursing* **19**, 9–14.
28. **Hilden, J.M.** et al. (2001). Attitudes and practices among pediatric oncologists regarding end-of-life care: results of the American Society of Clinical Oncology Survey. *Journal of Clinical Oncology* **19** (1), 205–12.
29. **Benoliel, J.Q.** (1986). The cancer patient's right to know and decide: an ethical perspective. In *Issues and Topics in Cancer Nursing* (ed. R. McCorkle and G. Hongladarom), pp. 5–17. Norwalk CN: Appleton-Century-Crofts.
30. **Zerwekh, J.Y.** (1984). Professional stress and distress. In *Hospice and Palliative Nursing Care* (ed. A.G. Blues and J.Y. Zerwekh), pp. 347–62. New York: Grune and Stratton.
31. **Vachon, M.L.S.** *Occupational Stress in the Care of the Critically Ill, the Dying and the Bereaved.* New York: Hemisphere Publishing, 1987.
32. **Woolley, H.** et al. (1989). Staff stress and job satisfaction at a children's hospice. *Archives of Disease in Childhood* **64**, 114–18.
33. **Davies, B.** et al. (1996). The experience of nursing care for chronically ill children who die. Final report. *Pediatric Nursing* **22**, 500–7.
34. **Quint, J.C.** *The Nurse and the Dying Patient.* New York: Macmillan, 1967.
35. **Degner, L.F. and Gow, C.M.** (1988). Evaluation of death education in nursing: a critical review. *Cancer Nursing* **11**, 151–9.
36. **Penney, J.C.** (1987). The evolution of a medical school curriculum in death and dying. *Journal of Palliative Care* **3**, 14–18.
37. **Irwin, W.G.** (1984). Teaching terminal care at Queen's University of Belfast. I-Course, sessional educational objectives and content. *British Medical Journal* **289**, 1509–11.
38. **Scofield, G.R.** (1989). Terminal care and the continuing need for professional education. *Journal of Palliative Care* **5**, 32–6.
39. **Hilden, J.H.** et al. (2001). Attitudes and practices among pediatric oncologists regarding end-of-life care: results of the 1998 American Society of Clinical Oncology Survey. *Journal of Clinical Oncology* **19** (10), 205–12.
40. **Papadatou, D.** (1997). Training health professionals in caring for dying children and grieving families. *Death Studies* **21** (6), 575–600.
41. **Stein, A. and Woolley, H.** (1994). Care for the carers. In *Care of the Dying Child* (ed. A. Goldman), pp. 164–81. Oxford: Oxford University Press.
42. **Mount, B.M. and Voyer, S.** (1980). Staff stress in palliative hospice care. In *The Royal Victoria Hospital Manual on Palliative Hospice Care* (ed. I. Ajemaian and B.M. Mount), p. 146. New York: Arno Press.
43. **Osterweiss, M., Solomon, F., and Green, M.**, ed. *Bereavement Reactions, Consequences, and Care. Report by the Committee for the Study of Health Consequences of the Stress of Bereavement, Institute of Medicine, National Academy of Sciences.* Washington DC: National Academy Press, 1984.
44. **Corr, C.A. and Doki, K.J.** (1994). Current models of death, dying and bereavement. *Critical Care Nursing Clinics of North America* **6**, 545–52.
45. **McCollum, A.** (1974). Counseling the grieving parent. In *Care of the Child Facing Death* (ed. L. Burton), pp. 177–88. London: Routledge & Kegan Paul.
46. **Pine, Y.R. and Brauer, C.** (1986). Parental grief: a synthesis of theory research, and intervention. In *Parental Loss of a Child* (ed. T.A. Rando), pp. 59–96. Champaign IL: Research Press.
47. **Rando, T.A.** *Grief; Dying, and Death: Interventions for Caregivers.* Champaign IL: Research Press, 1984.
48. **Hasse, K.E.** (1989). At the time of death: help for the child's parents. *Children's Health Care* **18**, 146–52.
49. **Davies, B.** (1987). Family responses to the death of a child: the meaning of memories. *Journal of Palliative Care* **3**, 9–15.
50. **Rando, T.A.** (1986). Individual and couples treatment following the death of a child. In *Parental Loss of a Child* (ed. T.A. Rando), pp. 341–414. Champaign IL: Research Press.
51. **Schmidt, L.** (1987). Working with bereaved parents. In *The Child and Family Facing Life-Threatening Illness* (ed. T. Krulik, B. Holaday, and I.M. Martinson), pp. 327–44. Philadelphia: JB Lippincott.
52. **Davies, B.** et al. (1999). *Family Voices: An Evaluation of the Impact of the Canuck Place Children's Hospice Program. Final Report to British Columbia Health Research Foundation.* Vancouver BC: Community Grants Program.
53. **Davies, B. and Martinson, I.M.** (1989). Care of the family: special emphasis on siblings during and after the death of a child. In *Pediatric Hospice Care: What Helps* (ed. B.B. Martin), pp. 186–99. Los Angeles: Children's Hospital of Los Angeles.

10

Palliative medicine in non-malignant disease

10 Palliative medicine in non-malignant disease

10.1 Introduction

Marie Fallon

The needs of patients with progressive, incurable, non-malignant disease and the needs of their families are similar to those of patients with advanced cancer. However, 30 years after the founding of the modern hospice movement, only a small minority of non-cancer patients access specialist palliative care services. There is, however, a significant difference in the degree of coverage between the United Kingdom and the United States. While the modern hospice movement was founded in 1967 by Dame Cecily Saunders, hospices for the care of the dying pre-dated the opening of St Christopher's Hospice. We know that the earliest examples of hospices in the mid-nineteenth century were associated with religious orders who had a mission to serve the dying poor. The early hospices made no distinction between the needs of patients dying from cancer and patients dying from non-malignant conditions. When St Christopher's Hospice was first opened, it was envisaged that the inpatient service would be available to patients with non-malignant diseases. This decision was informed, in part, by the evidence from Hinton's work published in 1963.(1) He found that patients dying from non-malignant diseases were just as likely to experience distressing symptoms as cancer patients, but were less likely to have these symptoms relieved. In practice, however, cancer remained the dominant diagnosis group with a small number of patients with motor neurone disease (amyotrophic lateral sclerosis, ALS).(2) Early experiences in hospices exposed the problems of indeterminate prognosis. Although some palliative care literature addresses specific needs of patients with non-malignant diseases, it was not until the emergence of AIDS in the mid-1980s that the hospice movement was widely confronted by the challenge of non-malignant conditions.(3) Several recent studies have maintained this challenge by emphasizing the unmet needs of patients with advanced disease with conditions other than cancer.(4–8)

Data collected by the UK National Council for Hospice and Specialist Palliative Care Services and St Christopher's Hospice show that more than 96 per cent of all patients receiving inpatient care, home care or day hospice care in the United Kingdom had a diagnosis of cancer in 1994–1995.(8) Christakis and Escarce reviewed the diagnosis of Medicare hospice beneficiaries who received specialist palliative care in five major states in 1990.(9) Of the 6451 patients involved in hospice programmes, 19.8 per cent had a non-cancer diagnosis. Congestive cardiac failure was the most common, followed by chronic obstructive pulmonary disease, stroke, dementia, and renal failure. There is evidence that in the United States the number of patients in a palliative care programme with a non-cancer diagnosis is rising, the figure for 1999 given as 36 per cent according to Librach (see Chapter 17.2). However, there is no evidence that such an increase is taking place in UK inpatient palliative care units or indeed in many other countries. There is, however, anecdotal evidence that increasing numbers of patients with non-malignant disease are now being referred to hospital palliative care teams in some parts of the United Kingdom.

The ingredients of specialist palliative care

The modern hospice movement was established, nurtured, and developed through a complex mixture of compassion, imagination, knowledge, conviction, creativity, and determination. The ability to listen, observe, learn, experiment, adapt, and listen again were essential qualities. Clearly, charismatic personalities were a fundamental part of this process. We can see that no readymade formula existed for specialist cancer palliative care, as indeed no formula exists for non-cancer palliative care and we know that the growth of cancer palliative care has been marked by its diversity. Palliative care provision for non-cancer patients will also take diverse forms, and already does so according to disease, patient, and family wishes, the health care system, and, importantly, those who provide continuing care for such patients at present. With the call for improved palliative care for all, including non-cancer patients, it is important to stand back and examine the following:

- the range of non-cancer diagnoses and problems that most commonly require palliative care;
- the professionals caring for the patients' with advanced non-malignant disease at present;
- voluntary groups;
- current practice and problems;
- research evidence for the management of specific problems and models of care;
- evolving natural history of non-cancer chronic illness (e.g. HIV disease with the advent of new life-prolonging treatments, and potentially multiple sclerosis and amyotrophic lateral sclerosis (ALS));
- research from palliative cancer care into physical symptom control, psychosocial care, and models of care to avoid the extension of management based purely on anecdotal experience into other areas of patient care;(10)
- problems in current cancer palliative care that may inform developments in palliative care of non-malignant disease;
- the background and characteristics of current practice of palliative care professionals, which clearly will influence the type of approach the profession will take to developing non-cancer palliative care.

Increasingly, more people in the developed world die from chronic rather than acute diseases. The percentage of the population over 65 has increased and will continue to increase. The main causes of mortality are: heart disease, cerebrovascular disorders, chronic respiratory disease, and cancer.

The above points will help to inform the fundamental question: should specialists provide palliative care for non-malignant disease, or should the principles of palliative care be promoted and adopted for all non-cancer patients with chronic, progressive disease? From this question flow other questions—if palliative care specialists, both doctors and nurses, should be the ones providing the palliative care, is the time coming when we shall have to have sub-specialties for the many non-malignant conditions, within palliative care? This would have important and far-reaching implications for recruitment and training, and raise the possiblity of de-skilling the specialists who usually care for such patients. Of course, as described elsewhere in this textbook, there are few countries where palliative medicine or palliative care nursing are recognized as specialties—most countries electing to promote and facilitate the teaching of the principles of pallative care throughout their caring professions. In this case, it must be questioned whether there are suffiient people with experience of providing palliative care for non-malignant conditions to be able to teach it, and if the answer is no, how is the necessary experience to be gained. Are fundamental changes needed in current palliative medicine training courses?

A number of key factors will influence the response to these questions. Not only will the education, skills, and attitudes of palliative care professionals play a large part. The knowledge and attitudes of the professionals currently looking after patients with non-cancer chronic progressive disease will need to be addressed if they too are to be better informed and trained in this care and know how to access and take full advantage of the skills of their specialist palliative medicine colleagues. The knowledge and attitudes of patients and family is important and, of course, last but not least, the issue that often drives the development of most services—financial support and the informed understanding of politicians and health-care planners, are all important. For some reason people have come to believe that cancer is the principal 'killer' in the world and the one associated with the worst pain and suffering. It will take considerable public education to change this perception. It is likely to take some time before many doctors, whether generalist or specialist, are as sensitive to the palliative care needs of their non-maligant patients as they currently are for their cancer patients.

It is the unequivocal view of the editors of this textbook that in terms of needs, care provision, and quality of care, there can be no distinction between the care of patients with malignant and non-malignant disease, hence the many chapters devoted to this in the book.

To further clarify the role of palliative care, let us look at some of the issues that arise in the chronic, progressive diseases.

Progressive neurological illness

In the United Kingdom, at least 75 per cent of inpatient palliative care units in a 1998 survey were involved in the care of ALS patients and while only 15 per cent of patients were referred for symptom control, many were found to have uncontrolled symptoms on assessment.[11] Research and experience has gone some way to inform the important role of specialist palliative care services in the provision of care to patients with neurodegenerative diseases and their families.[2] The causes of the neurodegenerative disorders including ALS are as yet unidentified and in general there are no known cures. Much research is concerned with gaining a greater understanding of the precise aetiologies and in developing disease-modifying drugs. Treatments such as Riluzol for ALS are being developed to slow the progression of the disease process and in the future it is not impossible that treatments may be developed to reverse or even cure such illnesses as ALS. However, while research for disease-modifying agents continues, patients must be offered an optimal level of palliation to ensure that they have the best possible quality of life. ALS has a prevalence of 4–6 per 100 000. While the peak incidence occurs between 60 and 70 years, it can affect patients aged from their late teens to the tenth decade. While part of the basic definition of palliative care is that it does not aim to either hasten death or prolong life, there is no doubt that the process of good palliation will not infrequently involve a prolongation of life and this also applies to chronic, progressive, non-cancer illness as well as cancer. Issues in ALS such as gastrostomy feeding or ventilatory support can clearly affect prognosis and survival of the patient as well as some aspects of quality of life. The range of issues affecting a patient with ALS and most other progressive neurological disorders very much mirror the issues affecting a patient with cancer. The issue of communicating the diagnosis in the broadest sense, along with symptom control, including pain, dysphagia, nutritional problems, salivary dribbling, breathlessness and upper respiratory problems, dysarthria, anarthria, communication difficulties, sometimes bladder dysfunction, and, of course, depression and/or anxiety, are all commonly encountered. The care of the family and the need for interdisciplinary team work remain vital. All these issues are addressed in Chapter 10.6.

Cardiac disease

Heart disease is a common cause of death and a major public health issue. Chronic heart failure and intractable angina are the most common chronic heart problems likely to benefit from palliative care. Heart failure is the only major cardiovascular disease with increasing prevalence, incidence, and mortality. It is mainly a disease of old age. In the United Kingdom, heart disease causes about 60 000 deaths per annum and the actual number of individuals with compromised cardiac function is expected to increase dramatically over the next few decades.[12] There are no data on the prevalence of refractory angina but it affects a minority of patients with coronary disease. It is expected that the number of patients will increase as the long-term prognosis of coronary artery disease improves. The care of patients with cardiac disease is complex from the point of view of managing the disease process, managing symptoms, physical and non-physical, and by the nature of the often uncertain prognosis, balanced with the risk of sudden death.

The only UK study to investigate symptoms in terminal heart disease was the 'Regional Study of Care for the Dying'.[13] This a population-based retrospective survey of a random sample of people dying in 20 English health districts in 1990. Sudden deaths were excluded. The study did not identify particular cardiac diagnostic groups. People who died from heart disease mainly did so in hospital and were reported to have experienced a wide range of symptoms, which were frequently distressing and often lasted for more than 6 months.[13,14] Poor quality of life was caused by distressing symptoms (in particular, low mood, anxiety, and incontinence) and the need for assistance with self-care. At least one in seven had symptom severity comparable to those of cancer patients managed in hospices or by specialist palliative care services.[14] Although half were thought to have known, or probably have known that they were dying, open communication with health professionals was rare.[15] The findings suggested that these patients might benefit from the expertise of palliative care and symptom control, psychological support, and open communication, with emphasis on maintaining quality of life. These issues are discussed further in Chapter 10.5.

Respiratory disease

In the United Kingdom, one-fourth of hospital admissions are due to respiratory disease and over half of these are due to COPD. Patients with COPD have two to four times the number of general practitioner consultations than patients with angina [British Thoracic Society (BTS) 1997]. In England and Wales, there are 250–300 deaths per 100 000 in the 64–84-year age group from COPD. The profile of palliation of COPD has been raised by guidelines from the BTS.[16] The BTS guidelines suggest a variety of practices that general practitioners need to consider, ranging from prevention, early detection to early management of severe COPD. In addition, they recommend that each District General Hospital should have a specified respiratory physician with responsibility for COPD with a specialized respiratory nurse attached to each District Hospital with responsibility for liaising with primary care over the care plan. It is also suggested that resources should be available to develop pulmonary rehabilitation and there should be provision for terminal and respite care for patients with the most severe COPD.

It should be remembered that the prognosis for patients with severe COPD can be worse than for patients with metastatic breast or prostate cancer. Further published work has pointed out that current service provision on COPD is focused on acute exacerbations and that there is a need to manage the health and social care interface more effectively, with a shift from reactive ad hoc provision.[17] These issues are addressed in Chapter 10.4.

Renal disease

Renal failure results from various diseases irreversibly damaging both kidneys resulting in uraemic symptoms. These are commonly nausea and vomiting, anorexia, tiredness, itching, weakness, decreased sexual function, and libido. Without dialysis or transplantation the patient would become comatose and die. In developed countries, there is nearly universal access to dialysis treatment. Consequently, the population of patients receiving dialysis support has steadily grown and aged over the last decade. The acceptance of sicker patients whose renal disease results from, or is associated with, more severe, co-morbid conditions, has also increased. These factors affect both the quality and length of patients lives. The annual mortality rate of patients on dialysis in the United States is approximately 25 per cent, which is clearly higher than that of AIDS or of most cancers.[18] Cardiovascular complications account for at least half of the deaths. It is easy to see that as well as all the physical symptom control issues to be managed there are, of course, significant psychosocial family and communication issues and, of course, the difficulties associated with end-of-life decision-making, particularly withdrawal of dialysis.

Liver disease

The profile of terminal chronic liver disease has been modified greatly in countries with active liver transplant programmes, and many patients do not develop the range of complications considered here. However, in the United Kingdom at least four people die from chronic liver disease for every one transplanted. In addition, those parts of the world with the highest incidence of liver disease have limited access to transplantation. Patients with end-stage liver disease have a number of symptoms and signs and a few patients may develop hepatocellular carcinoma. All patients will have ascites, jaundice, or encephalopathy as elements of their disease with the majority of patients having all three during the last days of life. In the terminal stages, good symptomatic management is essential. Bleeding from varices in the oesophagus or stomach is the final cause of death in about one third of those to die. There is a general consensus that optimal management plans for such patients and their families have not been adequately worked out by the staff looking after them but a willingness to discuss this with palliative care colleagues is growing (see Chapter 8.3.5).

Dementia

Dementia is among the commonest nursing home diagnosis where care is given by a mix of registered nurses and nursing care assistants. The focus of care is the resident and little provision is made for support of relatives or for bereavement care. The culture in which patients are looked after in the nursing home is one of encouraging 'normalization' and this is clearly not always appropriate for every patient and in particular for those who are actively dying. It would seem that a great deal of work is required to be done in nursing homes before adequate palliative care for the patients with dementia becomes the norm.

Stroke

Estimates of the number of people suffering from stroke and fatality rates vary significantly because of difficulties with recording the data. However, it is estimated that a typical health authority in England of 250 000 may expect 500 new strokes and 1000 recurrent strokes each year. In such an area, it would be expected that 1500 survivors of stroke would be living in the community, half of whom will have significant disability. Twelve per cent of stroke survivors will be admitted to institutional care within a year.[19] While it is difficult to get accurate figures of the numbers of people with strokes for whom palliative care may be appropriate (not least because of the lack of clarity about the role of palliative care in stroke), it can be concluded that approximately one-third of people having a stroke will have died within 2 years. Studies of prognostic indicators suggest people living with stroke but with poor prospects of functional recovery will have major medical, health related and social needs.[20] Patients with poor prognosis stroke will have a range of problems including communication difficulties, feeding, terminal care, and bereavement support. Stroke survivors living in the community, but functionally dependent on others, are likely to be concerned with coping with ongoing uncertainty and disability, incontinence, post-stroke pain, and depression. Their informal carers may need respite care. Clearly, patients with stroke raise difficult end-of-life dilemmas as well as other problems and there is no doubt that these are areas in which specialist palliative care has expertise. Research, however, into the needs of patients with stroke is surprisingly lacking.

HIV disease

Therapeutic advances have had enormous impact on the clinical course of HIV infection. When HIV/AIDS first emerged, it was a disease characterized by peaks and troughs. As immunity gradually faded, patients repeatedly faced life-threatening crises from successive, variably treatable opportunistic infections and malignancies, as part of a fairly rapid terminal phase. Initially, HIV was regarded as an infection and, therefore, curable, until with time it became obvious that all patients eventually died and palliation was, in fact, necessary. Control of symptoms and complications evolved and then with the introduction of anti-retroviral treatments, the possibility of disease control was seen. However, it was not until the latter part of the 1990s when combination therapies of reverse transcriptase and protase inhibitors and improved prophylactics were introduced that we saw the most dramatic change in HIV management. It was then that survival increased dramatically and inpatient bed use declined.[21] Clinicians and patients are now able to expect a longer term of survival with some centres now seeing HIV as a predominantly outpatient problem. Sadly, however, drug resistance will become more of a problem and as treatment fails, the need for greater palliative care input may change once again. In general, however, those who currently are in need of palliation are the late presenters who are usually those with the most complex social circumstances involving not just themselves but other family members. HIV/AIDS is a good example of how a disease process can fluctuate with time, how palliative care physicians need to work with HIV specialists, and how adaptability of the service must be in-built to cope with fluctuation.

Clearly, the situation in the developing world with HIV/AIDS—in particular Central and Southern Africa—is very different, with the only treatment being care, and palliation is obviously a pressing need. As in other chronic progressive diseases, maintaining quality of life with the minimum symptomatic load is essential for patients living with uncertainty and any symptom issues highlighted in studies are around pain.[22,23] Other symptoms include breathlessness, nausea, gastrointestinal disturbance, fatigue, and weight loss. However, there are some major differences between HIV/AIDS and other chronic progressive diseases, particularly the need for vigilance around reversible or treatable conditions.

Chronic non-malignant painful conditions such as sickle cell disease

It is estimated that the number of patients in the United Kingdom with sickle cell disease is more than 10 000.[24] The median life expectancy for men and women with homozygous sickle cell anaemia in the United States is 42 and 48 years, respectively.[25] The most common causes of death from sickle cell disease are pulmonary complications, cerebrovascular accidents, causes related to infection, acute splenic sequestration, and chronic organ damage and failure.[25,26] In patients over 20 years old, more frequent (more than three per year) episodes of painful crisis are associated with an increased mortality.[27] In the cooperative study of sickle cell disease, only 18 per cent of deaths were in patients with chronically obvious organ failure such as renal failure, congestive heart failure, or chronic stroke. Thirty-three per cent of patients died acutely during a sickle crisis, most commonly a pain crisis, acute chest syndrome, or acute stroke.[25] A cooperative study of sickle cell disease also reported that only 5.2 per cent of patients with sickle cell disease experienced 3–10 episodes of pain each year. From these data we could say that, while specialist palliative care based on symptom control would be required for a relatively small number of patients, many more patients would benefit from a palliative care approach to a varying extent at different points in their illness. The use of opioid analgesia in the management of pain due to sickle cell disease is worth a special mention. There is an incorrect perception that significant numbers of patients with sickle cell disease and pain are addicted to drugs such as pethidine and morphine. It has been reported that 9 per cent of American Haematologists and 22 per cent of Emergency Department Physicians thought that more than 50 per cent of adult sickle cell patients were addicted to strong opioids.[28] There are numerous other studies that confirm these findings. While the palliative care needs of sickle cell patients have not been clearly defined, there is undoubtedly a subgroup with a poor prognosis and frequent pain crises who would benefit from specialist palliative care involvement. Well-conducted research with this group of patients would be very beneficial (see Chapter 8.2.1).

Chronic non-malignant gastrointestinal pathologies

There is a group of patients who not uncommonly come to the attention of specialist palliative care services when it is felt that nothing else can be done. This includes patients with a history of inflammatory bowel disease, which is not necessarily currently active, motility disorders either inherited or acquired, patients with chronic complications of surgery, and rare diseases such as porphyria. They are not uncommonly labelled as difficult personalities with opioid dependence and often have a background of chronic pathology that has been perceived as being cured or quiescent. This group of patients suffer from great physical and non-physical morbidity, spend much time in hospital, or in their general practitioner's surgery/office, and are often incapacitated from the point of view of working and leading any sort of normal life. They are traditionally not well dealt with by any of the usual services available. They constitute a group of patients who may benefit from specialist palliative care involvement in parallel with their standard medical care for a limited period of time. Further exploration of this area is needed.

Other patient groups and care settings

It has long been recognized that care of the elderly and palliative care have many features in common. As demonstrated in Chapter 10.7, though relatively few patients in a care-of-the-elderly unit have malignant disease many need palliative care, which can usually be provided by the staff of the unit though occasionally a palliative medicine specialist may be needed.

Though few would normally speak of palliative care and intensive care in the same breath, there is a place for the principles of palliative care in an intensive care unit as Cohen and Prendergast explain in Chapter 10.8.

Conclusions

Some of the strong messages from the spectrum of non-cancer/chronic disease categories above are:

1. The spectrum of problems presented by chronic progressive, non-malignant disease is wide, with the intensity of physical, psychosocial, and spiritual suffering often as intense as in malignant disease.
2. Clinicians already involved in the care of these patients are all highly trained and skilled in the diagnosis and various aspects of the management of these diseases. They recognize the need for high-quality palliative care, many already working with Clinical Nurse Specialists and other professionals with specialist expertise in these areas.
3. No palliative care professional can have knowledge to a specialist level in even one of these areas, let alone several. They can, however, help to make more widely known, and encourage the adoption of, the principles of palliative care.
4. There appears to be a lack of evidence of systematic communication between palliative medicine as a specialty and the different specialties managing the diseases above. Palliative care needs assessments should be conducted jointly with various specialties.
5. Not surprisingly, there is a lack of research evidence into specific areas of symptom control in the various progressive non-malignant diseases and research into potential best models for looking after such patients in a compassionate and knowledgeable way.

It is evident that to avoid mistakes and to do our best for patients and families with a range of chronic, non-malignant disease, each with a very different disease trajectory, we need to go back to communication. We have useful glimpses of patient needs and more experience in some areas, for example, ALS. We need to set up a dialogue with the various specialties about how we can best explore a partnership to help with the optimization of patient care at every point during their illness and care for some patients as required at certain points in their illness. Clearly combined research is fundamental to taking this important area forward. For that, as for any research, funding will be needed and for that to be made available there will need to be a greater awareness of the need for the principles of palliative care to be applied to non-malignant disease.

References

1. **Hinton, J.** (1963). The physical and mental distress of the dying. *Quarterly Journal of Medicine* **32**, 1–21.
2. **O'Brien, T., Kelly, M., and Saunders, C.** (1992). Motor neurone disease: a hospice perspective. *British Medical Journal* **304**, 471–3.
3. **Wilkes, E.** *The Dying Patient: The Medical Management of Incurable and Terminal Illness.* Lancaster: MTP Press, 1982.
4. **Addington-Hall, J., Fakhoury, W., and McCarthy, M.** (1998). Specialist palliative care in nonmalignant disease. *Palliative Medicine* **12**, 417–27.
5. **Hockley, J.M., Dunlop, R.J., and Davies, R.J.** (1988). Survey of distressing symptoms in dying patients and their families in hospital and the response to a symptom control team. *British Medical Journal* **296**, 1715–17.
6. **Seale, C. and Cartwright, A.** *The Year before Death.* Aldershot: Avebury Press, 1994.
7. **Standing Medical Advisory Committee, Standing Nursing and Midwifery Advisory Committee**. *The Principles and Provision of Palliative Care.* London: SMAC, SNMAC, 1992.
8. **Addington-Hall, J.M.** *Reaching Out.* Report of the Joint NCHSPCS and Scottish Partnership Agency Working Party on Palliative Care for Patients with Non-Malignant Disease. London: National Council for Hospice and Specialist Palliative Care Services, 1997.
9. **Christakis, N.A. and Escarce, J.J.** (1996). Survival of Medicare patients after enrollment in hospice programs. *New England Journal of Medicine* **335**, 172–8.
10. **Bosanquet, N. and Salisbury, C.** *Providing a Palliative Care Service: Towards an Evidence-Base.* Oxford: Oxford University Press, 1999.
11. **Oliver, D. and Webb, S.** (2000). The involvement of specialist palliative care in the care of people with motor neurone disease. *Palliative Medicine* **14** (5), 427–8.
12. **Madsen, B.K.** et al. (1994). Chronic congestive heart failure. Description and survival of 190 consecutive patients with a diagnosis of chronic congestive heart failure based on clinical signs and symptoms. *European Heart Journal* **15**, 303–10.

13. **Addington-Hall, J.M. and McCarthy, M.** (1995). Regional study of care for the dying: methods and sample characteristics. *Palliative Medicine* **9**, 27–35.
14. **McCarthy, M., Lay, M., and Addington-Hall, J.** (1996). Dying from heart disease. *Journal of the Royal College of Physicians of London* **30**, 325–8.
15. **McCarthy, M., Addington-Hall, J.M., and Ley, M.** (1997). Communication and choice in dying from heart disease. *Journal of the Royal Society of Medicine* **90**, 128–31.
16. **BTS** (1997). Guidelines for the management of chronic obstructive pulmonary disease. *Thorax* **52** (Suppl. 5).
17. **Skilbeck, J.** et al. (1998). Palliative care in chronic obstructive airways disease: a needs assessment. *Palliative Medicine* **12**, 245–54.
18. **United States Renal Data System 1998 Annual Report** (1998). The Excerpts. *American Journal of Kidney Diseases* **32** (2), 51–213.
19. **Effective Health Care Bulletin**. *Stroke Rehabilitation*. Leeds: University of Leeds, 1992.
20. **Kwakkel, G.** et al. (1996). Predicting disability in stroke—a critical review of the literature. *Age and Ageing* **25**, 479–89.
21. **Aalen, O.** et al. (1999). New therapy explains the fall in AIDS incidence with a substantial rise in number of persons on treatment expected. *AIDS* **13**, 103–8.
22. **Breitbart, W.** (1996). Pain management and psychosocial issues in HIV and AIDS. *The American Journal of Hospice and Palliative Care* January/February, 21–9.
23. **Hewitt, D.** et al. (1997). Pain syndromes and aetiologies in ambulatory AIDS patients. *Pain* **70**, 117–23.
24. **Streetly, A., Maxwell, K., and Mejia, A.** Sickle Cell Disorders in Greater London: A Needs Assessment of Screening and Care Services. London: Bexley and Greenwich Health Authority, 1997.
25. **Platt, O.S.** et al. (1994). Mortality in sickle cell disease. Life expectancy and risk factors for early death. *New England Journal of Medicine* **330**, 1639–44.
26. **Gray, A.** et al. (1991). Patterns of mortality in sickle cell disease in the UK. *Journal of Clinical Pathology* **44**, 459–63.
27. **Platt, O.S.** et al. (1991). Pain in sickle cell disease: rates and risk factors. *New England Journal of Medicine* **325**, 11–16.
28. **Shapiro, B.S.** et al. (1997). Sickle cell related pain: perceptions of medical practitioners. *Journal of Pain and Symptom Management* **14** (3), 168–74.

10.2 AIDS in adults

Roger Woodruff and Paul Glare

The natural history of infection with the human immunodeficiency virus (HIV) is that it evolves over a period of years into the acquired immune deficiency syndrome (AIDS), which is uniformly fatal. The estimates made by the Joint United Nations Programme on HIV/AIDS (UNAIDS) demonstrate the enormity of the HIV/AIDS pandemic, reflecting mortality and morbidity of catastrophic proportions[1] (Table 1).

In developed countries, the introduction of effective antiretroviral therapy during the 1990s led to a reduction in both the incidence and mortality of AIDS.[1] But in less developed countries, where 95 per cent of the world's HIV-infected people live, the epidemic is having devastating effects. Few patients receive antibiotics for opportunistic infections, never mind effective antiretroviral therapy. Their life expectancy is less than patients in developed countries and there are already noticeable effects on national life expectancies and economic productivity.[1]

Table 1 UNAIDS estimates of the HIV/AIDS epidemic (December 2001)

People newly infected with AIDS in 2001	5 million
Total number of people living with HIV/AIDS	40 million
AIDS deaths in 2001	3 million
Total AIDS deaths since beginning of epidemic	22 million

Table 2 Probable source of HIV infection: United Kingdom data

	1986 (n = 2767), %	2000 (n = 3551), %
Male homosexual contact	72	39
Heterosexual contact	6	49
Injecting drug use	16	3
Mother to child	0	2
Blood/tissue or blood product treatment	3	1
Other/unknown	3	6

The first part of this chapter describes the clinical features of HIV infection and AIDS, and the opportunistic infections and malignancies with which they are associated, followed by a section outlining the treatment of pain and common symptoms. The final section deals with the role of palliative care in the management of HIV/AIDS, including the differences in delivering palliative care to patients with HIV/AIDS compared to diseases like cancer, the evolving interface between HIV medicine and palliative care, and the provision of appropriate palliative care for patients with advanced disease. The specifics of the treatments for HIV infection, the opportunistic infections, and the AIDS-related cancers are not detailed here as it is assumed a palliative care specialist would be working in collaboration with specialists in HIV medicine, infectious diseases, and oncology.

HIV infection and AIDS

Epidemiology

HIV infection is transmitted by sexual contact, by exposure to infected blood or blood products, body fluids or tissue, and by perinatal transmission from mother to child. HIV infection was first reported in 1981 in male homosexuals, but it soon became apparent that the disease was also occurring in injecting drug users (IDUs), in haemophiliacs, and other patients who had received infected blood or blood products, and in children born to women with the disease.

In developed countries, the majority of patients with HIV infection have been either male homosexuals or IDUs and these groups represent the majority of the people living with HIV infection. There has been a gradual increase in the incidence of HIV infection attributed to heterosexual activity and data from the United Kingdom (Table 2) show that heterosexual contact is now the most frequent probable route of infection, although it is noted that the majority of these infections were contracted outside the United Kingdom, mainly in Africa.[2] In Australia, about half of the cases attributed to heterosexual contact occurred in migrants from areas where HIV is endemic or their sexual partners.[3]

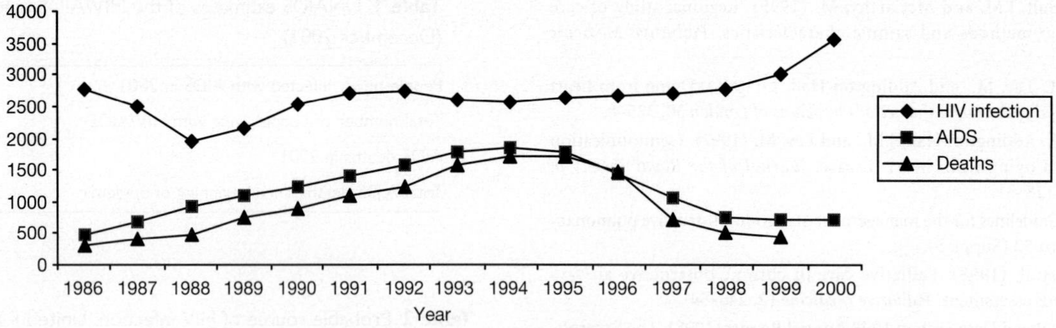

Fig. 1 Comparison over time of the numbers of patients with newly diagnosed HIV infection, newly diagnosed AIDS, and dying with HIV.[2]

The incidence of new cases of AIDS in developed countries began to fall in the early 1990s as a result of previously instituted public health policies and public education. The introduction of effective antiretroviral therapy in the mid-1990s led to a dramatic fall in both the incidence and mortality of AIDS[1,2] (Fig. 1). However, there has been no significant reduction in the frequency of new HIV infection over the last few years and the prevalence of HIV infection is continuing to increase. Data from the United Kingdom show an increasing incidence of new HIV infection over the last few years (Fig. 1), which has been attributed to an increase in unsafe sexual behaviours in the high-risk groups (male homosexuals and IDUs)[4] and to increasing spread to the heterosexual population.[5]

It is in less developed countries that the HIV/AIDS epidemic has reached alarming proportions. In sub-Saharan Africa, the Caribbean, and areas of South America, the disease is now transmitted primarily by heterosexual contact and there are increasing signs of similar changes in Asia. The situation is worst in some African countries where there are high rates of tuberculosis and HIV co-infection.[6] A dramatic recent increase in the numbers of HIV-infected IDUs has been reported in eastern Europe.[1]

Pathogenesis

HIV is a retrovirus, with a genome made up exclusively of RNA. Following introduction into the body, the virus binds to the CD4 surface receptors on CD4-positive T-lymphocytes and to a lesser extent on monocytes and macrophages. After gaining access to the cell, the enzyme reverse transcriptase produces a double-stranded DNA replica of the original RNA genome, which is then incorporated in the host cell genome. Activation of this material leads to production by the cell of large amounts of viral RNA, which is then processed to produce complete virus particles; HIV-derived protease is an important enzyme in this assembly process. Virions produced bud from the surface of the host cell and repeat the retroviral life cycle by infecting other CD4-positive cells.

CD4-positive T-lymphocytes serve as both essential regulators and effectors of the normal immune response. HIV infection leads to a progressive depletion of these cells, resulting in the progressive immunodeficiency that characterizes the disease.

Natural history

The natural history of HIV infection, without antiretroviral therapy, is that it progresses to AIDS and death over a period of about 10 years.[7] However, there is considerable individual variation with a few individuals dying of AIDS within months of the initial infection, whilst a few remain alive and well with only mild immunodeficiency more than 10 years after the initial infection.[8] There are no significant differences in the rate of disease progression or survival associated with sex, race, injection drug use, or other exposure category.[9–11] The differences in survival between developed and less developed countries relate to other factors including nutrition, the availability of antibiotics to treat and prevent opportunistic infections, co-infection with tuberculosis, and the availability of antiretroviral therapy.[1]

Phases of HIV infection

There is no universally accepted clinical staging system for HIV/AIDS. The different phases of the disease were originally shown to parallel the degree of immunodeficiency as measured by the numbers of CD4-positive T-lymphocytes (CD4) in the blood (Fig. 2). However, there are no sharp dividing lines and the different phases form part of a clinical continuum. The more recently introduced measurements of plasma HIV RNA or viral load have been shown to provide a more accurate assessment of disease progression and response to therapy. In general, plasma HIV RNA levels increase as the CD4 counts decrease, and the prognosis is most accurately defined using both the plasma HIV RNA and the CD4 count together.[12] High RNA titres predict rapid disease progression, whatever the CD4 count.[13] The plasma HIV RNA levels are reported to be lower in women[11] and perhaps in other groups,[14] but this is not associated with differences in the rate of progression to AIDS or survival.

Primary infection

Acute infection is characterized by a glandular fever-like illness, which typically occurs 2–4 weeks after infection.[15] Common manifestations include fever, fatigue, skin rash, myalgia, headache, pharyngitis, and lymphadenopathy. The illness usually lasts 10–14 days, following which there is return to normal clinical health.

Diagnosis is made by the detection of serum antibodies to HIV-specific proteins by an enzyme-linked immunosorbent assay (ELISA), which must be confirmed by immunoblotting (Western blot). Such antibodies are usually detectable within 4 weeks of inoculation and within the first few weeks of onset of clinical illness. The development of assays to detect HIV-specific RNA in plasma, which is often detectable before the appearance of antibodies, has greatly facilitated the diagnostic process.

Early immune deficiency

The second phase lasts an average of 4–5 years and is often asymptomatic. Some patients will develop autoimmune-type illnesses such as immune thrombocytopenic purpura (ITP), or Guillain-Barre syndrome and others develop persistent lymphadenopathy. Serial measurements during this phase show a gradual fall in CD4 lymphocyte count and a gradual rise in the HIV RNA titre.

Intermediate immune deficiency

The third or chronic symptomatic phase lasts an average of 4–5 years. During the first few years, the CD4 counts decline slowly and the HIV RNA titre continues to rise. The patients usually remain clinically well except for minor infections. Towards the end of this period, the CD4 lymphocyte counts decline more quickly and there is a parallel increase in the HIV RNA titres. More patients develop persistent lymphadenopathy and some develop AIDS-related malignancies. Antiretroviral therapy is usually started during this period.

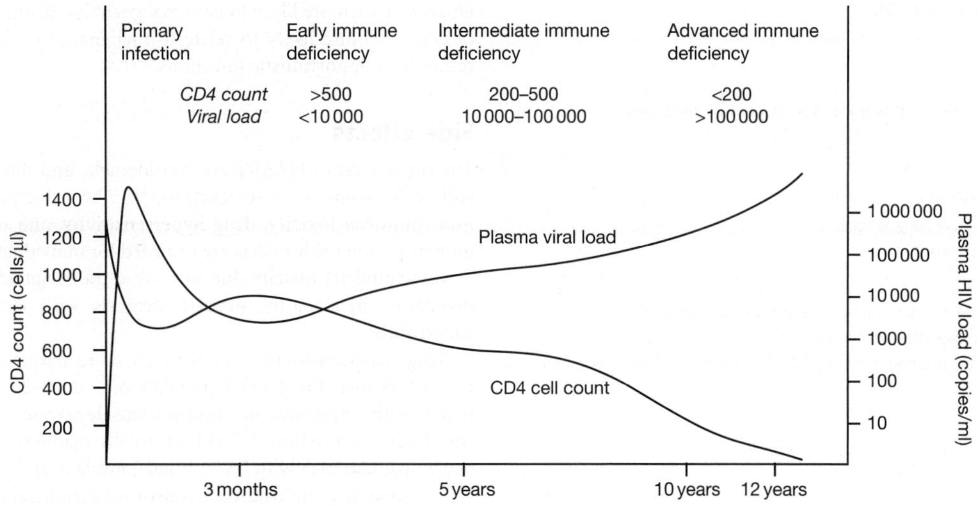

Fig. 2 Schematic representation of the natural history of HIV infection.

Table 3 AIDS-defining conditions

Candidiasis (oesophageal, tracheobronchial, or pulmonary)
Cervical cancer, invasive
Coccidioidomycosis (disseminated or extrapulmonary)
Cryptococcosis (extrapulmonary)
Cryptosporidiosis (>1 month)
Cytomegalovirus (retinitis, or other than liver, spleen, nodes)
Encephalopathy, HIV-related
Herpes simplex (ulceration >1 month, or oesophageal, pulmonary)
Histoplasmosis (disseminated or extrapulmonary)
Isosporiasis (>1 month)
Kaposi's sarcoma
Lymphoma (systemic or primary cerebral)
Mycobacterium tuberculosis, any site
Mycobacteria, other species (disseminated or extrapulmonary)
Pneumocystis carinii pneumonia
Salmonella septicaemia, recurrent
Toxoplasmosis, cerebral
Wasting syndrome due to AIDS

Advanced immune deficiency (AIDS)

The last phase or clinical AIDS may be defined by a CD4 lymphocyte count less that 200/µl or by the occurrence of AIDS-defining conditions as set out by the Centers for Disease Control and Prevention (CDC) in 1992[16] (Table 3). In a population of HIV-positive people, the CD4 count falls below 200/µl 1–2 years before AIDS-defining conditions develop, which has an obvious effect on the measurement of the survival of patients with AIDS. Prior to the use of antiretroviral therapy, survival from the time the CD4 lymphocyte count was less than 200/µl was 2–3 years, but only 1 year after the first AIDS-defining condition.[10,17]

The CDC definition of AIDS that is used in Western countries is not suitable for use in Africa or other parts of the developing world because the clinical manifestations may be different and because laboratory testing for HIV infection is often not available. Because of these difficulties, a WHO clinical case definition for AIDS was developed based on clinical conditions considered to have prognostic significance. It has relatively low sensitivity when compared to Western laboratory testing, but has the advantage of affordability and has been shown to have prognostic validity.[18,19]

Clinical course of AIDS

The clinical course of AIDS is characterized by the occurrence of opportunistic infections and AIDS-related constitutional symptoms (weight loss, fever, and diarrhoea). Some patients will develop AIDS-related malignancy or AIDS-related neurological disease. Antiretroviral therapy is continued and prophylaxis against other infections started. Patients suffer increasingly frequent infections that may become less responsive to therapy and from which they recover progressively less well. Serial measurements will show a continuing decline in the CD4 lymphocyte count and a corresponding rise in the HIV RNA titre.

The clinical course of AIDS follows a fluctuating course, punctuated by opportunistic infections requiring acute therapy, and there is considerable individual variation. The clinical course of AIDS has also been changed since the introduction of effective combination antiretroviral therapy. These factors complicate the timing and delivery of palliative care to these patients and underline the need for palliative care involvement long before the terminal phase, complementary to other medical care and not sequential to it. For patients who have failed antiretroviral therapy, or never had the opportunity to have it, the clinical course of AIDS can be broadly grouped into four phases that show the gradual shift in the goals of treatment with progression of the disease[20] (Table 4).

Antiretroviral therapy

Antiretroviral therapy has had a profound impact on the clinical course of HIV infection and AIDS. Following the introduction of zidovudine in the 1980s, a number of new drugs, of differing classes and mechanisms of action, have been developed (Table 5). The major changes occurred in the mid-1990s when the very potent protease inhibitors and a growing list of reverse transcriptase inhibitors enabled the development of combination therapy with three or four drugs aimed at durable suppression of viral replication. These combinations are collectively known as highly active antiretroviral therapy (HAART). The optimal use of these drugs—when they should be started and in what combination—remains the subject of on-going clinical research,[21] and regularly updated expert recommendations are available on the internet.[22] The search for more effective drugs is on-going.

Table 4 Clinical course of AIDS

Early stage
Recent diagnosis of AIDS
Good response to antiretroviral therapy and treatment of infections
Normal activities, work
Progressive stage
Increasing number and frequency of infections
Progressive weight loss, increasing fatigue
Capable of partial activity, work
Advanced stage
Increasing or constant infections, with poor response to treatment
Fatigue and debility seriously affect daily function
Active treatment should be stopped and the goal of treatment shifted to comfort
Terminal stage
Totally dependent
Death can be anticipated within days to a few months
Care is entirely comfort orientated

Table 5 Antiretroviral therapy

Reverse transcriptase inhibitors		Protease inhibitors
Nucleoside analogues	**Non-nucleoside analogues**	
Zidovudine	Nevirapine	Saquinavir
Didanosine	Delavirdine	Ritonavir
Zalcitabine	Efavirenz	Indinavir
Stavudine		Nelfinavir
Lamivudine		Amprenavir
Abacavir		Lopinavir/ritonavir

Effects

The introduction of HAART led to profound changes in the clinical features and outlook for patients with HIV/AIDS. Patients responding to HAART showed marked reduction in HIV RNA levels, often to undetectable levels, associated with increases in the CD4 count, often by several hundred cells/μl. This was associated with symptomatic improvement with increased appetite with weight gain as well as improved energy and well-being. This has translated into a prolongation of the time to the development of AIDS, and improved survival both after a diagnosis of AIDS and overall.(10,23,24) The magnitude of the effect parallels the intensity of the antiretroviral treatment, combination therapy being superior to monotherapy, and combination therapy that includes a protease inhibitor confers additional benefit.(25,26)

There is a dramatic reduction in the incidence of opportunistic infections in patients taking HAART(27–29) and patients with low or undetectable HIV RNA levels and significant and sustained increases in CD4 counts are able to safely stop prophylaxis for these infections.(30–32)

Treatment with HAART produces noticeable effects on the neurological disease of AIDS. Successful therapy leads to a reduction in the incidence of AIDS dementia(33) and there may be improvement in cognitive and neurological function,(34,35) AIDS dementia,(36) and progressive multifocal leukoencephalopathy.(37)

The pattern of AIDS-related malignancies has changed since the introduction of HAART. There has been a marked decrease in the incidence of Kaposi's sarcoma(38) and cerebral lymphoma,(33,39) but not in the incidence of systemic non-Hodgkin's lymphoma, Hodgkin's disease, or cervical cancer.(38–40)

The recovery of immune function following HAART may cause immune reconstitutions syndromes, caused by increased tissue inflammation directed against opportunistic infections or AIDS-related malignancies.(41,42)

HAART has changed the pattern of HIV disease. Patients responding to HAART are less likely to have an opportunistic infection as the AIDS-defining illness and are more likely to have malignant lymphoma. Similarly, the cause of death is more likely to relate to malignancy or chronic organ failure rather than opportunistic infections.(43)

Side effects

The side effects of HAART are considerable, and the majority of patients will suffer some adverse reaction.(44) The principal toxicities include mitochondrial toxicity, drug hypersensitivity, and lipodystrophy;(45,46) numerous other side effects are recorded for individual drugs.

Mitochondrial toxicity due to reverse transcriptase inhibitors includes myopathy, neuropathy, hepatic steatosis with lactic acidaemia, and pancreatitis.

Drug hypersensitivity occurs much more frequently in patients with HIV/AIDS than the general population, and 10–20 per cent of patients treated with amprenavir or a non-nucleoside reverse transcriptase inhibitor will develop a reaction.(45) This is usually manifest as a morbilliform or maculopapular rash with fever, fatigue, myalgia, and mucosal ulceration.

The lipodystrophy syndrome consists of peripheral lipoatrophy from the face and limbs with central fat accumulation in the abdomen and over the lower cervical spine (the so-called 'buffalo hump'), associated with hypertriglyceridaemia, hypercholesterolaemia, insulin resistance, and type II diabetes mellitus.

There are a large number of potential drug interactions both between different antiretroviral drugs and between antiretroviral drugs and other medications and recreational drugs.(45,47)

Small but significant numbers of patients fail to complete trials of HAART because of adverse events; others have difficulty with the complicated treatment regimens and adherence to HAART is often suboptimal.(48)

Limitations

HAART is not curative and is not effective for all patients. A proportion of patients will show no virological (reduced plasma HIV RNA levels) or immunological (increased CD4 counts) response and their disease will progress to AIDS and death. There is evidence of drug resistance in up to 27 per cent of people newly infected with HIV, who are unlikely to benefit from currently available HAART.(49,50) Other patients, particularly those with advanced disease at the time of starting drug therapy, may show a partial or transient response only,(51–53) following which their disease will progress. Even for patients who show an optimal response, viral rebound with increasing HIV RNA levels can occur within a year.(54,55) Reservoirs of HIV can be detected in peripheral blood mononuclear cells and in lymphoid tissue of patients with undetectable plasma HIV RNA levels(56–58) and discontinuation of HAART leads to rebound of the plasma HIV RNA levels within 3 weeks.(59)

The other limitations of HAART are that it is very expensive and that it is not available to the majority of people afflicted with HIV infection. It is to be hoped that continued research and development will result in therapy that is more effective and less toxic and, most importantly, affordable in developing countries where the great majority of people with HIV infection live.

HIV-associated infections

AIDS is characterized by the occurrence of multiple opportunist infections caused by a host of different pathogens. Regularly updated expert recommendations regarding diagnosis and treatment are available on the internet <http://www.aidsinfo.nih.gov>.(60)

Fungal infections

Pneumocystis carinii

Pneumocystis carinii pneumonia (PCP) occurred in about 85 per cent of patients with AIDS before PCP prophylaxis became standard. PCP usually presents with fever, dry cough, and progressive dyspnoea occurring over several weeks. Examination may be unremarkable or show tachypnoea and dry rales. Chest X-ray usually shows bilateral, symmetrical perihilar interstitial infiltrates. Diagnosis is by demonstration of the organism in an induced sputum specimen or bronchial washings.

Treatment

Treatment is with trimethoprim/sulphamethoxazole (TMP–SMX), given orally for mild and intravenously for moderate or severe infection. This is effective in the majority of patients although side effects are frequent. Some patients with severe infection will develop respiratory failure requiring mechanical ventilation and PCP still carries a significant mortality.[61] Patients who are allergic to TMP–SMX or have unresponsive disease can be treated with pentamidine or trimetrexate/folinic acid; alternatives for patients with less severe PCP include clindamycin/primaquine and trimethoprim/dapsone. Patients with PCP who are hypoxic should be treated with corticosteroids, started at the same time as antifungal therapy. This ameliorates or prevents the progressive hypoxia often seen 2–3 days after starting treatment and has been shown to significantly reduce both morbidity and mortality.[62]

Prophylaxis

Primary prophylaxis against PCP is recommended for any patient with a CD4 count less than 200/μl.[32,60] Standard therapy is with oral TMP–SMX. Patients unable to take this can be treated with dapsone, dapsone/pyrimethamine/folinic acid, or atovaquone. Aerosolized pentamidine is less effective than systemic therapy in preventing PCP and does not protect against extrapulmonary pneumocystis infections that may occur in patients with severe immunodeficiency. Indefinite secondary prophylaxis or maintenance therapy is required after infection with PCP, using the same medications as for primary prophylaxis. Patients treated with HAART with sustained CD4 counts more than 200/μl can safely discontinue primary or secondary PCP prophylaxis;[63,64] patients relapsing from HAART should restart prophylaxis when the CD4 count is 200/μl.

Candidiasis

Candida frequently causes oropharyngeal, oesophageal, and vaginal infection, but dissemination may occur with advanced immunodeficiency. Oropharyngeal candidiasis produces characteristic white plaques or may appear as smooth erythematous patches on the palate and tongue; it may also cause angular cheilosis with fissuring and cracking at the corners of the mouth. Diagnosis of oropharyngeal and vaginal candidiasis is made on clinical grounds and microbiological studies. Oesophageal candidiasis causes odynophagia, dysphagia, and substernal chest pain. The diagnosis is frequently made on clinical grounds, especially if there is oropharyngeal candidiasis; radiological studies and endoscopy are reserved for patients not responding to empiric therapy.

Treatment

Oropharyngeal infection is treated with topical therapy such as nystatin, amphotericin, or miconazole. Severe oral infection and oesophagitis are treated with fluconazole; itraconazole and ketoconazole are alternatives. Higher doses of fluconazole may be required for non-*albicans* infections. Occasionally, the development of multidrug resistance or disseminated infection necessitates therapy with intravenous amphotericin.

Prophylaxis

Prophylactic therapy for mucosal candidiasis is not usually recommended because of the effectiveness of treatment for acute disease. Daily or weekly fluconazole maintenance can be considered for patients with oesophageal candidiasis or recurrent mucosal infections not controlled with topical therapy.[60]

Cryptococcosis

Infection with *Cryptococcus neoformans* characteristically causes meningitis; pneumonia and skin infiltrates are the common extraneural lesions. Meningitis presents with fever and mild headache and meningeal signs are often absent; focal neurological signs and seizures are rare. The diagnosis is established by the demonstration of cryptococci or cryptococcal antigen in the CSF.

Treatment

Treatment is with amphotericin, with or without flucytosine, for 2 weeks, followed by fluconazole for 8–10 weeks.[65]

Prophylaxis

Life-long secondary prophylaxis or maintenance therapy with fluconazole is required.[32,60] It is uncertain whether this can be safely stopped in patients showing a sustained response to HAART.

Histoplasmosis

Infection with *Histoplasma capsulatum* occurs frequently in areas where the infection is endemic, particularly the central United States, Central and South America. The clinical features are non-specific and include fever, weight loss, and pneumonia. Diagnosis is made on bone marrow, liver or lymph node biopsy, or by culture of the organism from the blood, bone marrow, or sputum. Treatment is with itraconazole, which needs to be continued indefinitely.[60] Patients presenting with a septicaemic or meningitic illness should initially be treated with amphotericin.

Coccidioidomycosis

Infection with *Coccidioides immitis* occurs in the endemic areas of Latin America and the southwestern United States. In AIDS patients, coccidioidomycosis presents with malaise, fever, weight loss, and pneumonia. The diagnosis is established by demonstration of the organism in sputum or bronchial washings. Treatment is with amphotericin followed by indefinite maintenance therapy with either fluconazole or itraconazole.[60]

Penicilliosis

Infection with *Penicillium marneffei* is common in HIV-infected patients in Southeast Asia. It presents with fever, anaemia, and weight loss; skin lesions resembling molluscum contagiosum are common.[66] The diagnosis is made by isolation of the organism from blood, skin lesions, or bone marrow. Treatment is with amphotericin followed by itraconazole, which needs to be continued indefinitely.[67]

Aspergillosis

Infection with *aspergillus* species usually occurs in patients with advanced disease and severe immunodeficiency. Pulmonary infection causes focal or bilateral infiltrates and there may be cavitation. Treatment is with amphotericin but the mortality is high.[68]

Nocardiosis

Infection with *Nocardi* species may produce pneumonia, cerebral abscesses, or disseminated disease. It is treated with high doses of TMP–SMX similar to PCP, and continued TMP–SMX prophylaxis is required. *Nocardia* resistant to TMP–SMX are reported.[69] The widespread use of TMP–SMX prophylaxis for *Pneumocystis* may explain the relative infrequency of *Nocardia* infections in patients with AIDS.

Protozoal infections

Toxoplasmosis

Infection with *Toxoplasma gondii* is common and in normal individuals causes either no symptoms or a mild illness with fever and lymphadenopathy. Reactivation and dissemination of infection in patients with AIDS usually causes encephalitis. Cerebral toxoplasmosis presents with fever, headache, and focal neurological signs. Hemiparesis is the most common focal neurological sign and seizures are common. There may be an altered mental state with confusion and cognitive impairment, delusional behaviour or psychosis; some patients present in coma. The clinical diagnosis is made on the basis of positive serology for toxoplasma and the characteristic CT scan appearance of multiple, bilateral hypodense lesions that show ring enhancement with contrast. The definitive diagnosis can only be made on brain biopsy, which is usually reserved for patients not responding to appropriate therapy and those with a solitary lesion.

Treatment

Active treatment is with pyrimethamine/folinic acid and either sulphadiazine or clindamycin.

Prophylaxis

Primary prophylaxis is recommended for patients with CD4 lymphocytes less than 100/µl who are seropositive for toxoplasma. Treatment may be with TMP–SMX, or pyrimethamine/folinic/dapsone or atovaquone.[60] Seronegative patients are advised to avoid undercooked or raw meat, to ensure that all food is thoroughly washed, and to avoid any direct contact with animal or human faeces. Indefinite secondary prophylaxis or maintenance therapy is required and the combination of pyrimethamine/folinic acid/sulfadiazine is probably superior to other regimens and also provides adequate prophylaxis against *Pneumocystis* infection.[60] Patients having a sustained response to HAART with CD4 counts more than 100–150/µl can safely discontinue primary prophylaxis.[60]

Cryptosporidiosis

Infection with cryptosporidia causes a self-limited diarrhoeal illness in persons with normal immunity. In patients with AIDS, it causes severe enteritis with voluminous watery diarrhoea associated with colic, pain, anorexia, malaise, and weight loss. The infection may resolve spontaneously in patients with higher CD4 lymphocyte counts but patients with counts less than 100/µl can experience severe unremitting diarrhoea. The diagnosis is established by identification of the organism in the faeces.

Treatment

There is no consistently effective antimicrobial therapy. Azithromycin may reduce stool volume and lessen symptoms for some patients but does not eradicate the infection; paromomycin has been shown to be ineffective.[70] Successful treatment with HAART leads to resolution of the infection,[71] although it is likely to recur if the CD4 count falls.[72]

Prophylaxis

Patients with CD4 lymphocytes less than 200/µl should be advised to use only boiled water, as cryptosporidial infection is primarily water borne and infective oocysts are destroyed by boiling.[60] Rifabutin or clarithromycin taken for prophylaxis of *M. avium* infection may prevent cryptosporidiosis.[73]

Microsporidiosis

Infection with microsporidia causes a diarrhoeal illness similar to cryptosporidia. Diagnosis is made by identification of the organism in the stool or small bowel biopsy. Some patients respond to albendazole or fumagillin.[74]

Isosporiasis and cyclosporiasis

Infection with *Isospora belli* or *Cyclospora cayetanensis* causes a diarrhoeal illness similar to cryptosporidia. Diagnosis is made by identification of the organism in the stool or small bowel biopsy. Treatment is with TMP–SMX and continued maintenance therapy at a lower dose is recommended. Patients intolerant of TMP–SMX can be treated with ciprafloxacin or metronidazole.[75]

Giardiasis

Infection with *Giardia lamblia*, a frequent cause of the 'gay bowel syndrome' in homosexual men, may cause diarrhoea in patients with AIDS. Diagnosis is made by identification of the organism in the stool or small bowel biopsy. Treatment is with oral metronidazole.

Leishmaniasis

Infection with *Leishmania* species causes visceral leishmaniasis or kala-azar, probably as the result of recrudescence of previous asymptomatic infection. Coinfection with HIV and *Leishmania* has been reported in southern Europe and is likely to occur elsewhere as the HIV epidemic spreads. The clinical features include fever, hepatosplenomegaly, and anaemia. Diagnosis is made by identification of the parasite in the bone marrow or blood. Treatment is with pentavalent antimonials or amphotericin and continued suppressive therapy is necessary.[76,77]

Trypanosomiasis

American trypanosomiasis (*T. cruzi*; Chagas' disease) may be reactivated by coinfection with HIV, causing meningoencephalitis and cardiac disease.[78,79] Coinfection with HIV does not appear to exacerbate African trypanosomiasis (*T. brucei*; sleeping sickness).[79]

Bacterial infections

Mycobacterium tuberculosis

There is a markedly increased risk of tuberculosis (TB) in HIV-infected people.[80] Because of impaired cellular immunity, HIV-positive individuals are at increased risk of primary infection, reactivation of prior infection, or a second infection from exogenous sources. Whilst many cases of TB were thought to be reactivation of previous infections, it has now been demonstrated that new infection is responsible for up to half the cases in HIV-positive individuals.[80,81] TB has a detrimental affect on HIV infection and may accelerate the course of the disease.[80] In developing countries where TB is endemic, high rates of HIV co-infection are frustrating TB control programmes and the mortality from TB may be increasing.[6,82]

Clinical features

The clinical features are more likely to be atypical in patients with advanced immunodeficiency.[80] Patients with mild immunodeficiency (CD4 count >200/µl) usually present with typical features with upper lobe consolidation and cavitation and the tuberculin skin test is often positive. Since the introduction of HAART, more HIV-positive patients have presented with 'typical' features.[83] Patients with more severe immunodeficiency may present with non-specific symptoms of fever, weight loss, and fatigue, and are more likely to have atypical pulmonary disease with diffuse or lower zone infiltrates without cavitation; extra pulmonary disease occurs frequently and common sites of infection include lymph nodes, liver, bone marrow, and the central nervous system. The chest X-ray is usually abnormal, but 5 per cent of HIV-positive patients with positive sputum have a normal chest X-ray.[80] The diagnosis is made by identification of the organism in smears and cultures of sputum or other affected tissue.

Treatment

Specific recommendations regarding treatment of active infection vary in different countries. Some recommend quadruple therapy (isoniazid, rifampicin, pyrazinamide, and ethambutol) for at least 2 months followed by isoniazid and rifampicin for another 4 months, whilst others recommend that quadruple therapy be continued for longer periods. HIV-positive patients are likely to respond more slowly, and treatment should be continued until at least 4 months after cultures become negative.

There are complex interactions between antiretroviral drugs and the medications used for the treatment of TB.[60,80] Patients being treated for TB who are commenced on antiretroviral therapy may suffer a paradoxical worsening of their disease, due to intensification of the immune response to the infection; it is usually self-limited.

Highly drug-resistant strains of TB have been isolated from patients with AIDS. Outbreaks of nosocomial multidrug-resistant TB occurred in New York and Miami in the early 1990s with a mortality rate of up to 80 per cent in HIV-infected patients.[80] Stringent infection-control measures are required to control these outbreaks and prevent similar incidents. These organisms constitute a risk to others, including health-care workers and particularly other patients with HIV/AIDS.

Prophylaxis

Primary prophylaxis is recommended for HIV-positive patients if they have a positive tuberculin test, have had TB in the past, or have had recent contact with an infectious person.[84] Treatment with rifampicin/pyrazinamide for 2 months or isoniazid for 6–12 months is recommended.[85] The incidence of overt tuberculosis in HIV-positive patients given isoniazid prophylaxis is less after longer treatment.[86] Indefinite secondary prophylaxis or maintenance therapy with isoniazid should be given after the completion of acute therapy.[81,87]

Mycobacterium avium

Mycobacterium avium is an atypical mycobacterium that rarely causes disease in HIV-negative individuals, but between one-third and one-half of patients with AIDS and advanced immunodeficiency will develop disseminated *M. avium* complex (MAC) infection. Infection is usually manifest as a constitutional illness (with fever, malaise, anaemia, and weight loss) or gastrointestinal disease with chronic diarrhoea and abdominal pain sometimes associated with malabsorption and obstructive jaundice. The diagnosis is made by isolation of the organism from blood, bone marrow, or other tissue.

Treatment

Treatment is with ethambutol and either clarithromycin or azithromycin, which will lead to clinical and bacteriological improvement in half of the patients.[60,88] Patients commenced on HAART may present with high fevers and increased lymphadenopathy caused by an increased inflammatory response to previously asymptomatic MAC infection.[89]

Prophylaxis

Primary prophylaxis with either clarithromycin or azithromycin is recommended for patients with a CD4 count less than 50/μl.[60] Adding other drugs increases the risks of side effects and the potential for drug interactions without significantly improving efficacy. Patients treated for MAC require continuing therapy (secondary prophylaxis) with ethambutol and either clarithromycin or azithromycin. Patients showing a sustained response to HAART with CD4 counts more than 100/μl can have their prophylaxis withdrawn safely.[60]

Bacillary angiomatosis

Infection with the small gram negative bacilli, *Bartonella henselae* and *quintana*, occurs more frequently in patients with advanced immunodeficiency.[90] It presents as a few to many purple or red papules and nodules that may resemble Kaposi's sarcoma. The skin lesions may be the predominant manifestation of the infection or part of a systemic illness with fever, hepatitis, lymphadenopathy, and bone lesions. The diagnosis is made on biopsy. Treatment is with erythromycin or doxycycline. Treatment should be continued for 8 weeks for cutaneous disease, longer for visceral infection. Response may be dramatic but recurrence is common and maintenance therapy is often required.[60]

Pyomyositis

Muscle abscesses, usually caused by *Staphylococcus aureus*, cause local pain and tenderness. The creatine phosphokinase is normal. Diagnosis is made on microbiological studies and treatment is with appropriate antibiotics, initially given parentally, for a number of weeks.

Other bacterial infections

Bacterial infections are common in patients with AIDS because of HIV-related immunodeficiency, which may be compounded by neutropenia caused by antiretroviral therapy or chemotherapy. Infections are likely to be more severe than in immunocompetent individuals and there is a high incidence of bacteraemia. Recurrent infections are common because protective levels of antibodies fail to develop. Diagnosis is made on microbiological studies. Treatment is with appropriate antibiotics and, compared to patients without HIV infection, initial therapy may need to be given for a longer period. For some infections, notably salmonella, long-term suppressive therapy is required to prevent recurrence.

Viral infections

Cytomegalovirus (CMV)

Approximately half of the general population has serological evidence of previous infection with CMV. In patients with AIDS, the infection can reactivate and disseminate causing a variety of clinical problems including retinitis, colitis, encephalitis and myelitis, pneumonitis, and hepatitis. CMV retinitis occurs in about 20 per cent of patients with AIDS. It presents as diminished visual acuity that leads to blindness if untreated. The diagnosis is made on the characteristic fundal appearance of large yellowish-white granular areas with perivascular exudates and haemorrhages in a patient with HIV infection and antibodies to CMV. The diagnosis of CMV infection at other sites is made by demonstration of the characteristic viral inclusions on biopsy or the detection of CMV antigen or nucleic acid.

Treatment

Treatment of systemic infection is with parenteral ganciclovir, foscarnet, or cidofovir. Ganciclovir causes myelosuppression, foscarnet can be nephrotoxic, and cidofovir can cause uveitis and nephrotoxicity. Treatment of retinitis[60] is usually effective in preventing progression, but visual field defects present at the time of starting therapy do not improve. Ganciclovir can be given by intravitreal injection and ganciclovir implants have been developed for continuing intravitreal therapy. Systemic therapy is required in addition to the ganciclovir implant to provide protection for the other eye and other tissues. Treatment with ganciclovir implant and oral ganciclovir produces equivalent results to parenteral cidofovir, although the two treatments have different side-effect profiles.[91] Patients started on HAART may suffer severe intraocular inflammation or 'immune reconstitution uveitis' caused by increased immune response to CMV and which can lead to further loss of vision.[92]

Prophylaxis

Primary prophylaxis with oral ganciclovir can be considered for patients with CD4 counts less than 50/μl who have antibodies to CMV. Life-long secondary prophylaxis or chronic maintenance therapy is required.[60] Patients treated with HAART who achieve sustained elevation of the CD4 count to more than 100–150/μl can safely have prophylaxis withdrawn.[60]

Herpes simplex virus (HSV)

Herpes simplex viruses types 1 and 2 (HSV-1, HSV-2) cause recurrent herpetic lesions in the orolabial and anogenital regions. More than 95 per cent of patients with AIDS have serological evidence of previous infection with HSV and recurrent infections occur frequently. Recurrent HSV infections in patients with AIDS are likely to be more severe, with prolonged new lesion formation and delayed healing, associated with persistent local pain lasting several weeks. The frequency and the severity of the attacks increase with increasing immunodeficiency. Orofacial infection may commence with painful vesicles along the lips and spread to involve the oropharyngeal mucosa as well as adjacent areas of the face. Genital herpes causes proctitis (with pain, tenesmus, and mucosal ulceration), perianal infection (vesicle formation, pain, and ulceration), and may be associated with neurological symptoms in the distribution of the sacral plexus. HSV infection can also cause oesophagitis and encephalitis. The diagnosis is made on the basis of the clinical features and confirmed by direct microscopy and culture, or by the detection of viral antigen or nucleic acid in the affected tissue.

Treatment

Treatment is with aciclovir, which can usually be given orally. Therapy should be continued until all mucocutaneous lesions have crusted or re-epithelialised. Intravenous therapy is reserved for patients with severe infection or visceral involvement and those unable to take oral medication. Famciclovir and valaciclovir are also effective in the treatment of HSV infection; foscarnet or cidofovir are used for aciclovir-resistant HSV infection. Successful topical treatment has been reported with cidofovir,[93] imiquimod,[94] and foscarnet.[95] Patients suffering frequent attacks of HSV infection and those with severe immunodeficiency can be considered for continued maintenance therapy with oral aciclovir.

Varicella zoster virus (VZV)

Herpes zoster occurs in approximately 20 per cent of HIV infected patients and 20–30 per cent of these will have multiple attacks. Herpes zoster in patients with AIDS is more likely to involve multiple dermatomes and cutaneous lesions outside the affected dermatome(s) occur more frequently; healing times may be prolonged and bacterial superinfection is common. Herpes zoster is occasionally complicated by cutaneous dissemination (producing a disease indistinguishable from primary varicella or chicken pox), and less commonly by visceral dissemination that can cause pneumonitis, hepatitis, transverse myelitis, or encephalitis.[96] The diagnosis is made on the clinical features and confirmed by microscopy and culture or the detection of viral antigen.

Treatment

Treatment is with aciclovir, famciclovir, or valaciclovir. Therapy is continued for at least 7 days or until all external lesions are crusted. Intravenous therapy is used if there is evidence of dissemination. Foscarnet can be used for aciclovir-resistant VZV. Topical treatment of the rash is symptomatic and includes saline-soaked gauze pads or Burow's solution (aluminium acetate) for early, weeping lesions, and calamine lotion for pruritic, healing lesions. Secondary infection should be treated appropriately.

Molluscum contagiosum

This poxvirus infection causes multiple umbilicated papules with a predilection for the face (especially the eyelids) and the anogenital region. Diagnosis should be made by biopsy as a number of other benign and infective conditions may have a similar appearance. Treatment is with cryotherapy, electrocautery, curettage, or application of topical caustics. Repeated treatments are necessary as it is difficult or impossible to eradicate the infection. Successful topical treatment has been reported with cidofovir[97] and imiquimod.[98] The lesions may regress when antiretroviral therapy is given.[99]

Human papilloma virus (HPV)

HPV infection causes squamous papillomas or warts. Warts occur in greater numbers and in a wider distribution in patients with HIV infection, and this trend increases with progressive immunodeficiency. Treatment of warts is similar to molluscum with cryotherapy and the application of topical caustics. Successful topical treatment has been reported with cidofovir[100] and imiquimod.[98] In HIV-infected people, HPV infection in the anogenital region is associated with the increased incidence of anal cancer in men and cervical cancer in women.

JC virus

This papova virus infection causes progressive multifocal leukoencephalopathy (PML). It is discussed in the section on neurological disease.

HIV-related cancer

There is a greatly increased incidence of cancer in patients with HIV-AIDS. One-fourth of patients with AIDS develop cancer and it is a major contributory cause of death in about 15 per cent of patients. The cancers that occur with increased frequency can be broadly grouped by whether or not there is an increasing risk with increasing immunodeficiency.[101,102] Kaposi's sarcoma (KS), cerebral non-Hodgkin's lymphoma (NHL), and Hodgkin's disease (HD) occur with increasing frequency as the disease progresses, possibly related to the fact that they are believed to be caused by viral infection (human herpes virus type 8 (HHV8) in KS, Epstein–Barr virus (EBV) in lymphoma[103]). The human papilloma virus (HPV)-associated anal and cervical cancers occur with increased frequency in patients with HIV/AIDS but there is no increasing incidence with increasing immunodeficiency, suggesting the excess results from sexually acquired HPV infection and not because of immunodeficiency.[104] This grouping of AIDS-associated cancers is supported by observations following HAART therapy and from Africa. In developed countries, introduction of HAART has greatly reduced the incidence of KS and some lymphomas, but the incidence of cervical and anal cancers is unchanged;[39,105] in Africa, the incidence of KS and NHL are increasing rapidly but not cervical or anal cancer.[106,107]

Kaposi's sarcoma

Kaposi's sarcoma was a rarely reported malignancy before the AIDS epidemic but it is the most common cancer in HIV-infected persons.[108] In developed countries, the incidence of KS has fallen dramatically since the introduction of HAART. KS is caused by infection with the human herpes virus type 8.[109,110] It was originally thought that transmission was primarily via anal intercourse amongst homosexual men, but it is more likely that the transmission is via the salivary route to susceptible individuals.[110] In developed countries, KS is rare in HIV-infected women but in Africa it is seen in the two sexes almost equally and also in children and adolescents.[110,111]

AIDS-related KS is characterized by widespread lesions in the skin and mucous membranes and frequent visceral involvement. The skin lesions appear as red or purplish macules or nodules that usually increase in size and number with time. The lesions are usually multiple and may coalesce to form plaques of tumour. AIDS-related KS has a variable clinical course, depending primarily on the patient's immune status, ranging from a few indolent skin nodules to rapidly progressive systemic disease. Extracutaneous KS may involve any tissue but the common sites are the mucous membranes of the mouth and pharynx, the gastrointestinal tract, lymph nodes, and the lung. Gastrointestinal KS is usually asymptomatic but may cause obstruction and bleeding. Lymphatic involvement leads to local oedema. Pulmonary KS causes progressive dyspnoea and cough with a diffuse interstitial infiltrate on chest X-ray.[112] Pulmonary KS may respond less well to treatment than other visceral sites of involvement. The diagnosis is made by biopsy of the skin lesion or other involved tissue.

Treatment

Indications for treatment include cosmetic concerns for unsightly lesions, the palliation of symptoms for painful or bulky lesions and those causing oedema, and progressive systemic disease.

Local therapy

Local forms of therapy are of most use for non-bulky local disease. Local therapies employed include excision, cryotherapy, laser treatment, photodynamic therapy, intralesional injections of cytotoxic or sclerosing agents, and radiotherapy.[108] Radiotherapy, employing a variety of different treatment schedules, has a high response rate and local recurrence or progression is rare. However, radiotherapy is associated with more mucositis and soft tissue damage than would be expected in patients without AIDS. Topical treatment with alitretinoin[113] and docosanol[114] are reported.

Systemic therapy

Systemic therapy is indicated for widespread, bulky, or rapidly progressive disease. Chemotherapy with combinations such as doxorubicin, bleomycin, and vincristine produce only a modest response rate. Significantly better responses are seen with liposomal doxorubicin and paclitaxel.[108,115] Interferon has activity against KS, but its use is limited by toxicity; it is more effective given in high dose and in patients who do not have severe immunodeficiency.[108] Antiangiogenesis agents including thalidomide are reported to be effective.[116]

Non-Hodgkin's lymphoma

There is a greatly increased incidence of non-Hodgkin's lymphoma in patients with HIV infection that affects all risk groups. NHL may manifest as either systemic lymphoma or as a primary cerebral lymphoma. Epstein–Barr virus DNA has been isolated from most cerebral and some systemic NHL in patients with HIV infection.[103] Since the advent of HAART, there has been a significant fall in the incidence of primary cerebral lymphomas[33,105] and possibly systemic NHL of the immunoblastic type,[39] but there has been no significant change in the incidence of other types of systemic NHL.[40]

Primary cerebral lymphoma

Primary cerebral lymphomas are usually immunoblastic in type and occur in patients with advanced immunodeficiency (CD4 $<100/\mu l$, usually

<50/µl).[103] Patients present with headache in association with confusion, lethargy, and memory loss or there may be hemiparesis, cranial nerve abnormalities, and seizures. Meningeal and ocular involvement is common. Scanning demonstrates one or more mass lesions that may be difficult to distinguish from toxoplasmosis: toxoplasmosis presents as a solitary lesion in 20 per cent of cases and 50 per cent of cerebral lymphomas present with multiple lesions. Detection of EBV DNA in the cerebrospinal fluid is strongly indicative of cerebral lymphoma.[103] Definitive diagnosis is made on biopsy.

Treatment

Dexamethasone is given to reduce intracranial pressure. If there is significant neurological improvement and the patient is not too debilitated from other complications of AIDS, treatment with radiotherapy can be considered. However, despite apparently good clinical response rates with radiotherapy, the average life expectancy is only 1–4 months.[117,118] For patients who are comatose, those who do not improve with dexamethasone, and those severely debilitated from other effects of AIDS, radiotherapy is inappropriate. For the uncommon patient presenting with a good performance status and a CD4 count more than 200/µl, better results have been reported with combination chemotherapy and radiotherapy.[118]

Systemic NHL

Systemic NHL can occur at any time during HIV infection although the incidence rises as immunodeficiency increases. The majority of these tumours occur in patients with lower CD4 counts and are high-grade tumours associated with poor prognostic features.[119] The disease is usually widespread at the time of diagnosis with a high incidence of involvement of extranodal sites including the gastrointestinal tract, central nervous system, bone marrow, and liver. Severe constitutional symptoms including fevers, night sweats, and weight loss are common. Diagnosis is established on biopsy.

Treatment

Combination chemotherapy will alleviate pain and distressing systemic symptoms and stop weight loss in many patients, although less than half will achieve remission.[119,120] Few of the remissions are durable and the overall survival is inferior to non-AIDS patients, even after the introduction of HAART.[40,121] The use of G-CSF reduces the incidence of severe neutropenia and sepsis associated with treatment.[120,122] Patients presenting at an earlier stage with better performance status, higher CD4 counts, and less aggressive histology may do well with aggressive therapy.[120,122,123] Radiotherapy is used for localized disease and to treat areas of residual or bulky disease in patients responding to chemotherapy. The average survival is 6–9 months.

Hodgkin's disease

The incidence of Hodgkin's disease is increased two-to-five-fold in patients with HIV infection. Compared to patients without HIV infection, EBV DNA is detected more frequently in the tumour cells.[103] In patients with HIV infection, biopsy usually shows a more aggressive (mixed cellularity or lymphocyte depleted) histological type. The disease is usually disseminated (Stage III or IV) at diagnosis and extranodal involvement is frequent. Nearly all patients have constitutional 'B' symptoms.[124,125]

Treatment

Treatment is with combination chemotherapy, given with G-CSF to reduce myelotoxicity. However, whilst this may effectively palliate symptoms, response rates are poor and the median survival is usually less than a year.[124,125] Radiotherapy is used for local complications of the disease.

Cervical cancer

Women with HIV infection have an increased incidence of cervical intraepithelial neoplasia (CIN) and invasive carcinoma of the cervix (ICC), attributed to HPV infection. HIV-infected women are more likely to have persistent HPV infection that is more likely to include HPV subtypes known to be oncogenic, and the incidence increases with increasing immunodeficiency.[126,127] The incidence of CIN is increased compared to HIV-negative women, is more advanced at presentation, and the frequency increases with increasing immunodeficiency.[128,129] There is an increased incidence of ICC but the frequency is not related to progressive immunodeficiency[104] and has not decreased since the introduction of HAART.[130] Following standard treatment for ICC, the majority of HIV-infected women relapse and the median survival is less than a year.[131]

Anal cancer

Homosexual men have an increased incidence of anal HPV infection, anal intraepithelial neoplasia (AIN), and anal cancer. Patients who are HIV-positive are more likely to have heavy and persistent HPV infection and AIN, and the incidence of both increase with increasing immunodeficiency. AIN lesions do not regress after commencement of HAART[132] and the incidence of invasive anal cancer has not decreased.[104] AIN is more advanced at the time of presentation than in non-AIDS patients. AIN is treated by cryotherapy or electrocautery and regular follow-up. Invasive cancer is treated by combination chemoradiotherapy. However, invasive anal cancer in patients with HIV/AIDS presents in a more advanced state and has a higher recurrence rate and a poorer prognosis.[133]

Symptom control

Patients with AIDS experience many distressing physical and psychological symptoms and a high level of distress, which in turn have a significant effect on the quality of life.[134–136]

Patients with HIV/AIDS present a spectrum of symptoms and medical problems that involves every body system. The prevalence of symptoms in a series of patients with AIDS is shown in Table 6.[137] Some symptoms are

Table 6 Symptom prevalence in AIDS (Casey House Hospice, Toronto)

Symptom	Prevalence (%)
Anorexia/weight loss	91
Fatigue/weakness	77
Pain	63
Incontinence (urine/stool)	55
Shortness of breath	48
Confusion	43
Nausea/GI upset	35
Cough	34
Anxiety/depression	32
Visual loss	25
Skin breakdown	24
Constipation	24
Oedema	23
Psychological issues	18
Skin problems	17
Seizures	16
Fever	13
Potential for skin breakdown	4
Agitation	1

similar to those seen with cancer, some quite different. This section deals with the diagnosis and management of some of the common syndromes seen with AIDS, and the reader is referred to other sections of this book for more detailed discussion of symptoms that occur frequently in other diseases.

As with most medical problems in palliative care, symptoms are best managed by identifying and treating the underlying pathology, where this is possible and clinically appropriate.

All palliative treatment should be appropriate to the stage of the patient's disease and the prognosis. Over-enthusiastic therapy and patient neglect are equally deplorable. The prescription of appropriate therapy is particularly important in palliative care because of the additional unnecessary suffering that may be caused by inappropriately active therapy or by lack of treatment. The fluctuating course of AIDS, punctuated by episodes requiring acute interventions, can make decisions about appropriate therapy quite difficult.

Many symptoms in AIDS can be ameliorated by treatment with corticosteroids, but they have traditionally been withheld for fear of compromising immunity and predisposing to infection. For patients on HAART, a controlled study of prednisolone therapy (0.5 mg/kg/d for 8 weeks) showed the treatment was safe and had no deleterious effect on CD4 counts or HIV RNA levels.[138]

Pain

AIDS-related pain and cancer pain: similarities and differences

Pain is a common problem in patients with HIV infection, particularly when they progress to AIDS. AIDS-related pain has many similarities with cancer pain, particularly the increasing incidence with advancing disease and the impact on the quality of life (Table 7).

There are also significant differences that make AIDS-related pain more difficult to assess and treat[139] (Table 8). The pain syndromes that are common in HIV/AIDS are considered difficult pain problems when they occur in patients with cancer.[140] The assessment and treatment of pain may be complicated by psychosocial issues related to alternative lifestyles or intravenous drug use and the high incidence of psychiatric problems and dementia. There is less evidence for the efficacy of pharmacological therapies for AIDS-related pain than for cancer pain, and whilst there is substantial clinical experience in using strong opioids for AIDS-related pain, the level of evidence is only modest at the present time.

In developed countries, the advent of HAART has reduced the numbers of patients with AIDS and many patients with HIV infection can be maintained relatively well for a number of years. While pain is still a common symptom in these individuals, it is often of mild to moderate severity and not very distressing.

Table 7 Similarities between AIDS-related pain and cancer pain

Increasing incidence with disease progression
Moderate/severe in intensity
Profound effect on the quality of life
Usefully classified into pain due to (a) disease, (b) treatment, (c) debility, or (d) unrelated to disease or treatment
Multiple concurrent pains, the number increasing with disease progression
Under-treatment is problematic

Table 8 Differences between AIDS-related pain and cancer pain

Higher incidence of 'difficult to manage' pain syndromes e.g. neuropathic pain, abdominal pain, headache
Disease-specific therapy often appropriate even in advanced stages
More problems with polypharmacy, drug side effects, and interactions
Higher incidence of IDUs
Higher incidence of psychiatric disorders and dementia
Psychosocial problems associated with alternative lifestyles and other marginalized social groups
Lack of access to specialist pain clinics
Limited evidence for efficacy of analgesics

Incidence

Pain occurs frequently in patients with HIV/AIDS, the incidence increasing as the disease progresses. Pain is reported by about 25 per cent of patients in the 'asymptomatic' phase, 40–50 per cent of ambulatory patients with AIDS, and over 80 per cent of hospitalized patients with advanced disease.[134,139,141–144] The number of pains reported per patient also increases through the course of AIDS. Many patients with AIDS had pain rated to be moderate or severe, with significant impairment of activities of daily living.[141,143] A number of studies have documented the strong relationship between pain and psychological function, with pain being associated with increased levels of psychosocial distress, depression, hopelessness, and poorer quality of life.[142,144–146]

Pain in patients with AIDS may be acute or chronic. The types of pains were described in one series as 45 per cent somatic, 15 per cent visceral, 19 per cent neuropathic, and 4 per cent not defined.[147] In another report the anatomic site was recorded as extremities 32 per cent, head 24 per cent, upper gastrointestinal tract 23 per cent, and lower gastrointestinal tract 22 per cent.[143]

Cause

Pain may be caused by the HIV infection itself, the treatment, general debility, or an unrelated cause. Some examples are given in Table 9.

Assessment

The assessment of pain in HIV/AIDS is similar to the approach in patients with cancer (see Chapters 6.1 and 8.2.2). It requires a multidisciplinary approach to determine both the underlying cause of the pain and the psychosocial factors affecting the pain experience.

Patients with AIDS and pain have high levels of psychosocial and emotional distress and assessment for anxiety, depression, and other psychosocial problems is particularly important as these may greatly influence the severity or persistence of pain.

Table 9 Examples of causes of pain in AIDS

Pain due to HIV infection
HIV infection: neuropathy, arthropathy, aseptic meningitis
HIV-related infection: fungal, protozoal, viral, bacterial
HIV-related cancer: Kaposi's sarcoma, non-Hodgkin's lymphoma
Pain associated with treatment
Diagnostic procedures
Antiretrovirals: painful neuropathy, myopathy
Radiotherapy: mucositis
Pain related to debilitating disease
Pressure sores
Musculoskeletal pain secondary to inactivity, wasting
Constipation
Pain unrelated to HIV infection or treatment
Haemophiliac arthropathy

Treatment

Multi-modality therapy

As with cancer, the treatment of pain in patients with AIDS involves a number of different modalities, including analgesics and adjuvant analgesics, disease-specific therapy, invasive treatments, physical therapies, and psychosocial interventions (Table 10).

If an underlying cause can be defined, then it should be treated where possible and clinically appropriate. The best way to relieve pain caused by an opportunistic infection or malignancy is to treat the underlying pathology and such disease-specific therapy is often appropriate until the terminal stages.[139]

Treatment of pain in patients with AIDS includes management of any associated psychosocial problems. This may involve medications for anxiety or depression as well as non-pharmacological treatments directed at pain control such as relaxation exercises, supportive psychotherapy, and physical therapies.

Treatment with HAART lessens the number of patients progressing to AIDS but it does not reduce the incidence or severity of pain in patients with AIDS.[148]

Analgesics

The choice of analgesic depends on the type and severity of pain, and the WHO analgesic ladder, designed originally for the treatment of cancer pain, applies equally well to pain in AIDS. Patients with chronic pain should receive regular analgesics to both relieve the pain and prevent its recurrence.

The neuropathic pain that occurs frequently in AIDS, for which adjuvant analgesics should be used (see Chapter 8.2.5), has been the subject of a number of treatment trials. In a randomised trial, neither acupuncture nor amitriptyline was more effective than placebo.[149] A small randomized trial of mexiletine and placebo did not show mexiletine to be effective, but there was a remarkable placebo effect seen in this study.[150] A trial comparing amitriptyline, mexiletine, and placebo reported no benefit.[151] A randomized, double-blind, placebo-controlled trial of lamotrigine showed it to be effective for the treatment of painful peripheral neuropathy.[152] Gabapentin is also reported to be effective.[153] Other medications that have been trialled and found ineffective include peptide T,[154] vibratory counterstimulation,[155] and topical capsaicin.[156]

Patients requiring opioid analgesics should be treated by the oral route whenever possible, although patients with severe gastrointestinal disease may not absorb the medication. Oral slow-release morphine preparations are effective in AIDS patients.[157] Patients unable to take oral medication will require parenteral treatment or transdermal fentanyl.[158]

Table 10 Examples of different modalities for the treatment of AIDS-related pain

Disease-specific therapies
Treatment of opportunistic infections: antimicrobials
Anticancer therapy for HIV-related cancer: radiotherapy, chemotherapy
HAART
Analgesics
Non-opioids
Opioids
Adjuvant analgesics
Spinal analgesia
Invasive therapies, e.g. nerve blocks
Physical therapies, e.g. exercise, TENS
Psychosocial interventions
Management of anxiety, depression: medications, supportive psychotherapy
Supportive counselling
Group therapy
Non-pharmacological therapies, e.g. relaxation, meditation

Several important drug interactions may occur between opioid analgesics and other medications taken by patients with AIDS.[47] Opioid drugs inhibit the metabolism and increase the bioavailability and toxicity of zidovudine; this is managed by reducing the dose of zidovudine in patients on a stable opioid dose, but is more difficult to manage if opioids are being used intermittently. Rifampicin and rifabutin increase the metabolism of opioid drugs, particularly methadone, and can even precipitate physical withdrawal unless the dose of opioid is increased. Ritonavir causes a large reduction in the metabolism of methadone and fentanyl, and a moderate reduction in the case of codeine and tramadol, effects that will lead to opioid toxicity; the same drug may increase the metabolism of morphine and hydromorphone, necessitating an increased dose to maintain analgesia.

Barriers to treatment

Pain associated with AIDS is poorly treated. In a study from New York, 85 per cent of patients received inadequate analgesia as classified by the Pain Management Index (PMI) and only 8 per cent of patients with severe pain received a strong opioid analgesic. Women, IDUs, and less educated patients were most likely to be inadequately treated.[159] In another study, 57 per cent of patients who reported pain received no analgesia and only 22 per cent got an opioid drug.[142] The reason for this seems to lie with both patient and physician. A study of clinicians identified an admitted lack of knowledge about the treatment of pain and concerns about substance abuse as the most likely reasons for under treatment of pain in patients with AIDS.[160] In another study, the doctor underestimated the pain severity in 52 per cent of cases and this was more likely to occur when patients reported moderate or severe pain.[142] A study of patients showed they were apprehensive about taking analgesics because of fears about addiction and side effects. These barriers were most noticeable amongst the non-Caucasians, the less educated, and those with higher levels of psychosocial distress.[161]

Patients with a history of substance abuse

The principles of management of pain in IDUs and other patients with a history of substance abuse are no different from other patients although in practice treatment may be complicated by considerable tolerance to opioids and by the psychosocial problems that accompany substance abuse.

The incidence of pain in patients with a history of drug use is reported to be the same or a bit higher compared to those without such a history.[162,163] Reports of pain intensity and pain-related functional impairment were similar in the two groups.[162] However, the patients with a history of drug use were significantly more likely to receive inadequate analgesia, reported lower levels of pain relief, and suffered greater psychological distress.[162]

Pain in a patient with a history of substance abuse is carefully assessed as for any other patient. If opioid therapy is appropriate, the required dose is likely to be much higher than for other patients and needs to 'cover' what they were injecting or receiving on a maintenance program. Morphine is effective for the treatment of pain in patients with a history of drug use, but they require higher doses than patients without a history of drug use.[164] Oral medication such as methadone and slow-release morphine or transdermal fentanyl are preferred as they have a lower abuse potential. Patients on maintenance programmes receive methadone once a day to prevent withdrawal; this needs to be increased to 6- or 8-hourly for analgesia. Reports of increased pain and requests for increased doses need to be carefully assessed as some patients with a history of substance abuse are habitually manipulative. Some will require increased doses because of progressive physical disease and, as with patients without a history of substance abuse, some complaints of pain are really a manifestation of underlying psychosocial distress that requires skilled and sensitive management. For others, it may relate to psychological dependence and these patients are more likely to report 'loss' of prescribed drugs or prescriptions, make unsanctioned dose escalations, or be found to be obtaining opioids from multiple sources; boundaries may need to be set and specialists in the management of drug dependence should be involved.

Constitutional symptoms

Anorexia

There are many possible causes for anorexia, or a reduced desire to eat, in patients with AIDS (Table 11) and it may be a significant contributing factor to weight loss in some.

Treatment

The treatment of anorexia is that of the cause and many of those listed in Table 7 are amenable to some degree of palliation. The assistance of a dietitian may be invaluable.

Appetite stimulants

A number of appetite stimulants have been recommended. Corticosteroids will produce subjective improvement in appetite in the majority of patients, although the effect may last only a few weeks and the possibility that corticosteroids may further compromise immunity or predispose to infection has to be considered. Treatment with the progestogen, megestrol acetate, given in higher dosage (800 mg/d) has been shown in placebo-controlled studies to improve appetite and weight, although the weight gained is predominately fat;[165] lower doses may stimulate the appetite without leading to weight gain. Side effects are not insignificant and include fluid retention, oedema, and thrombosis.[166] The cannabis derivative, dronabinol, stimulates appetite but weight gain is minimal and troublesome side effects may occur, including dysphoria, dizziness, and sedation.[165]

Weight loss and wasting

Weight loss and wasting, defined as the involuntary loss of 10 per cent or more of the baseline body weight, occurs frequently in patients with AIDS. This may relate to reduced intake (related to anorexia, a functional blockage, or vomiting), malabsorption (caused by opportunistic infections, HIV enteropathy, or medications), increased energy expenditure, or hypogonadism.[167] There is evidence of increased energy expenditure in patients with HIV/AIDS during periods when the clinical condition is stable, exacerbated by the occurrence of opportunistic infections.[165] The documentation of increased energy expenditure during the asymptomatic, clinically quiescent, phase of HIV infection is in keeping with the knowledge that the HIV infection itself continues to progress during this period. Patients with AIDS and advanced cancer can develop a cachexia syndrome in which weight loss is primarily due to metabolic alterations induced by the tumour.

Significant weight loss in patients with AIDS is an ominous prognostic sign and has important psychological connotations. In the pre-HAART era, weight loss during the course of opportunistic infections was seldom completely regained. Progressive weight loss is associated with other clinical signs of progression of the HIV infection, and changes in the serum HIV RNA have now been shown to correlate with weight loss.[168] Weight loss has also been shown to correlate with depression and quality of life scores.[169]

The introduction of HAART has lessened the tendency to weight loss in patients with advanced HIV infection and has allowed some to regain lost weight. However, some patients continue to lose weight despite HAART therapy.[165]

Treatment

Treatment is directed at the underlying cause, where possible, and at the maintenance of weight. Patients with hypogonadism should receive physiological androgen replacement.[167] Optimal nutrition is crucial and the assistance of a dietitian is important.

Megestrol acetate, 800 mg/d, will increase body weight although the weight gained is primarily fat.[165] A randomized trial of megestrol, nandrolone, and dietary counselling reported that megestrol produced a significantly greater increase in weight, intake, and appetite than did the other two treatment arms, suggesting it may be the preferred agent in a palliative care setting.[170] Thalidomide leads to weight gain but has significant toxicity.[171] Testosterone has been shown to improve weight and muscle mass in both hypogonadal and eugonadal men and has few side effects;[165,172] continued therapy has been shown to result in sustained increases in lean body mass.[173] Treatment with the anabolic steroids, oxandrolone and nandrolone, produce similar weight gain to testosterone therapy, but may cause liver disease.[165] Treatment with recombinant human growth hormone leads to increased weight and lean body mass as well as improved performance; side effects include oedema, arthralgia, and myalgia.[165]

The use of total parenteral nutrition (TPN) has been shown to be effective in preventing weight loss and regaining weight lost in patients with continuing diarrhoea or evidence of malabsorption. The use of TPN in patients without malabsorption is ineffective.[165]

Many dietary and nutritional supplements have been advocated but few have shown significant benefit. A placebo-controlled study of the combination of β-hydroxy-β-methylbutyrate (a metabolite of leucine), L-glutamine and L-arginine was shown to significantly increase weight and lean body mass.[174]

Table 11 Causes of anorexia

Systemic infection	
Medications	Drugs for opportunistic infections Antiretrovirals Drugs for symptom palliation
Intracranial disease	Infection, malignancy, radiotherapy
Abnormal taste, smell	Stomatitis, xerostomia Radiotherapy, chemotherapy Medications
Gastrointestinal	Stomatitis, oesophagitis, enterocolitis Malignancy Opioid-related constipation, delayed gastric emptying Chemotherapy, abdominal radiotherapy Liver disease Medication-related nausea
Metabolic	Abnormalities of sodium, calcium, sugar Organ failure: liver, kidney, adrenal
Psychological	Anxiety, depression, confusion, dementia Fear of making diarrhoea worse
Organisational	Poor food preparation, presentation
Advanced cancer	
Pain	

Asthenia: weakness and fatigue

Asthenia is generalized weakness associated with fatigue and lassitude. There are many possible causes in patients with AIDS (Table 12).

Treatment is directed at the underlying cause, where possible. The management of the AIDS-related conditions that lead to asthenia are discussed elsewhere in this chapter. Patients responding to HAART may experience considerable improvement. Psychostimulants have also been shown to improve fatigue and quality of life in patients with AIDS.[175,176]

Neurological disease

Progressive neurological disease is one of the most debilitating features of AIDS. At least 40 per cent of patients have clinically significant CNS dysfunction and autopsies have shown CNS damage in up to 90 per cent of cases.[177] The common causes are listed in Table 13.[178]

Encephalopathy: disease involving the brain

Infection

The diagnosis and treatment of opportunistic infections involving the CNS are discussed in the section on infections. The clinical picture frequently includes altered mental state and diminished alertness. Diseases caused by HIV and JC virus infection are discussed below.

Primary cerebral lymphoma

The diagnosis and treatment of primary cerebral lymphoma, which may also cause alterations in mental state and consciousness, are discussed in the section on cancers.

Acute confusion or delirium

The investigation and management of acute confusion or delirium are discussed elsewhere (see Chapter 8.17). In patients with AIDS, there are a considerable number of potential causes and in many cases it is due to more than one cause. The most frequent causes relate to systemic infection and intracranial pathology. Metabolic encephalopathy also occurs frequently in patients with advanced disease due to hypoxia, electrolyte imbalance, and multi-organ failure. Drug toxicity, which includes illicit or recreational drugs as well as prescribed medications, is a frequent and reversible cause of confusion and is more likely in debilitated patients.

Neuroleptic drugs with antidopaminergic action should be used with care in patients with AIDS, who are particularly susceptible to the extra-pyramidal side effects.[179]

Table 12 Causes of generalized weakness and asthenia

Weight loss with muscle wasting	
Systemic infections	
Medications	Antiretrovirals Interferon Sedatives Other medications
Neuromuscular	Intracranial infection, malignancy Acute confusion or delirium Myelopathy, neuropathy, myopathy Overactivity, prolonged immobility
Metabolic	Hypogonadism Electrolyte imbalance, dehydration Renal, hepatic, adrenal failure Anaemia
Malnutrition	Inanition, malabsorption
Cancer	Chemotherapy, radiotherapy Cancer cachexia
Psychological	Anxiety, depression Dependency, boredom, insomnia

HIV encephalopathy (AIDS dementia complex)

HIV encephalopathy or AIDS dementia complex is a syndrome of subcortical dementia characterized by the triad of cognitive impairment, motor slowing, and behavioural dysfunction. An alternative name is the HIV-associated cognitive–motor complex. It is attributed to HIV infection of the CNS. The AIDS dementia complex is clinically evident in 25 per cent of patients with AIDS, although autopsy studies show changes in 80–90 per cent of patients. The incidence of AIDS dementia complex rises with increasing immunodeficiency. A clinical staging system for AIDS dementia complex is shown in Table 14.[178]

The clinical picture is one of progressive decline in cognitive ability and motor function. Initially, there may be difficulties with concentration or memory, reading, or performing complex tasks. It may cause the patient to be socially withdrawn and lead to an inappropriate diagnosis of depression.[180] Progression leads to complete intellectual disability. The initial signs of motor dysfunction include an unsteady gait or poor balance, tremor, and difficulty with rapid alternating movements. Progression leads to increasing weakness and an ataxic spastic paraparesis; urinary and faecal incontinence are common in the late stages. Some of these features are due to vacuolar degeneration in the spinal cord that is part of the AIDS dementia complex. Behavioural dysfunction manifests initially as apathy and lack of initiative;[181] occasionally, patients show agitation and mild mania. Progression leads to a vegetative state.

The diagnosis of HIV encephalopathy is made on clinical grounds and by exclusion of CNS infections and tumours and other potential causes (Table 15). The CT or MRI scan characteristically shows cerebral atrophy and the CSF findings are non-specific. The diagnosis requires mental state and neuropsychological examination; the HIV Dementia Scale (HDS) and the Executive Interview (EXIT) have been validated for the assessment of dementia in HIV/AIDS.[182]

Table 13 Neurological disease in AIDS

	Common	Uncommon
Brain: encephalopathy		
Focal brain disease	Toxoplasmosis Primary cerebral lymphoma JC virus (PML)	Tuberculosis Cryptococcosis VZV encephalitis Vascular disease
Diffuse brain disease	AIDS dementia complex (HIV) Metabolic encephalopathy CMV encephalopathy Toxoplasmosis	HSV encephalitis
Spinal cord: myelopathy	Vacuolar myelopathy (HIV)	VZV myelitis Lymphoma
Meninges	Cryptococcal meningitis Aseptic meningitis (HIV)	Lymphomatous meningitis Tuberculous meningitis Syphilitic meningitis
Peripheral nerve: neuropathy	Sensory polyneuropathy Herpes zoster (VZV) Demyelinating neuropathies Toxic neuropathy	Mononeuritis multiplex CMV polyradiculopathy
Muscle: myopathy	Polymyositis Toxic myopathy (zidovudine) Corticosteroid myopathy	

Table 14 Clinical staging of AIDS dementia complex

Stage	Characteristics
Stage 0 (normal)	Normal mental and motor function
State 0.5 (equivocal)	Minimal or equivocal symptoms of cognitive or motor function Normal capacity for work and activities of daily living (ADL) Normal gait and strength
Stage 1 (mild)	Unequivocal intellectual or motor impairment Able to do all but the more demanding work and ADL Can walk without assistance
Stage 2 (moderate)	Cannot work or perform demanding ADL Capable of basic self-care Ambulatory but may need a single support
Stage 3 (severe)	Major intellectual disability Cannot walk unassisted
Stage 4 (end-stage)	Nearly vegetative; mute or almost mute Rudimentary intellectual and social comprehension and response Paraparetic or paraplegic with urinary and faecal incontinence

Table 15 Causes of dementia

Related to HIV infection or treatment
AIDS dementia complex
CNS infection: JC virus, toxoplasmosis, tuberculosis, syphilis
Primary cerebral lymphoma
Obstructive hydrocephalus: infection, lymphoma
Radiotherapy
Unrelated to HIV infection or treatment
Alzheimer's disease
Alcoholic dementia
Cerebrovascular disease
Other: hydrocephalus, thyroid dysfunction, thiamine deficiency

Treatment with HAART leads to stabilization or improvement in neurological and cognitive function for a proportion of patients.[34,35,183,184] The introduction of HAART has reduced the incidence of HIV encephalopathy and dementia, although an increased proportion of new cases are being diagnosed when the CD4 count is still more than 200/μl.[33]

For patients who have failed to respond to HAART, or never had access to it, treatment is by symptomatic and supportive care (see Chapters 8.17 and 10.6). Patients with mild dementia may require no specific treatment unless a secondary acute confusional state develops. Patients with dementia will fare better in familiar surroundings, which should be simplified as much as possible to reduce demands on them. They are not kept in hospital unless necessary and their neuropsychiatric condition may improve after discharge home. In contrast to dementia occurring in patients without HIV infection, patients with AIDS dementia become progressively physically incapacitated as well as cognitively impaired and require increasing levels of support and assistance.

Progressive multifocal leukoencephalopathy (PML)

PML is an opportunistic infection caused by the JC virus, a ubiquitous human papova virus. It is reported to occur in 5 per cent of patients with AIDS and the untreated median survival is 6 months.[185]

Patients present with multiple and progressive focal neurological deficits without change in the level of consciousness. Focal neurological signs include hemiparesis, hemianopia, aphasia, and ataxia. The condition is progressive although spontaneous remissions are reported. Dementia, encephalopathy, and coma can occur in the later stages.

The MRI scan shows subcortical white matter lesions corresponding with the clinical abnormalities. Routine CSF examination usually shows non-specific changes, but the detection of JC virus DNA in the CSF is diagnostic in the appropriate clinical setting.

There has been no proven effective therapy for PML until recently. Treatment with cytosine arabinoside is ineffective[186] and topoisomerase is poorly tolerated. HAART is reported to reduce JC virus levels in the CSF, associated with neurological improvement or stabilization and improved survival.[37,187] HAART given in conjunction with cidofovir is more effective in reducing CSF JC virus levels, with improved neurological function and survival.[188]

Table 16 Headache

Aseptic meningitis (HIV)
Cerebral disease (including toxoplasmosis, lymphoma)
Meningeal disease (including cryptococcosis, tuberculosis, lymphoma)
Sinusitis
Migraine
Other causes of headache

Table 17 Causes of seizures

Infection	HIV, toxoplasmosis, cryptococcus, tuberculosis, JC virus (PML)
Tumour	Primary cerebral lymphoma
Metabolic	Hepatic encephalopathy, uraemia
Drug toxicity	Pethidine (meperidine)
Drug withdrawal	Opioids, barbiturates, alcohol, benzodiazepines

Aseptic meningitis (HIV meningoencephalitis)

Patients with AIDS may present with several weeks or months of generalized headache, with or without meningismus and photophobia, for which no cause other than HIV infection can be found. Aseptic meningitis may occur at the time of initial seroconversion but is more frequent as immunodeficiency progresses. Cerebral and meningeal diseases have to be excluded, as do other common causes of headache (Table 16). CSF examination is usually inconclusive. Treatment of aseptic meningitis or 'HIV headache' is symptomatic. Some patients are reported to respond to amitriptyline.

Seizures

Seizures are a relatively frequent complication of HIV infection and are reported to occur in up to 50 per cent of patients with AIDS dementia complex, 40 per cent of patients with cerebral toxoplasmosis, and 30 per cent of patients with primary cerebral lymphoma. Causes of seizures in AIDS patients are listed in Table 17, although no definite cause may be found in 20 per cent of patients.

The clinical features and investigation of seizures are discussed elsewhere (see Chapter 8.14). Seizures recur in up to 70 per cent of patients with AIDS, so anticonvulsant treatment should be instituted after the first episode. Patients with AIDS have an increased incidence of hypersensitivity reactions to phenytoin and carbamazepine may cause leucopenia; sodium valproate or clonazepam are better first-line drugs in this population. Careful observation is needed to ensure anticonvulsant therapy does not exacerbate liver disease. Protease inhibitors may markedly alter metabolism of some medications and anticonvulsant drug levels should be carefully monitored.

Spinal cord disease: myelopathy

Acute myelopathies

The causes of acute myelopathies include spinal cord compression by lymphoma, infection with VZV or other viruses, and bacterial or mycobacterial infections. If spinal cord compression is suspected, assessment and investigations must be carried out promptly, as the prognosis for recovery depends on the neurological function at the time of initiation of treatment. A MRI scan or CT myelogram are the investigations of choice. The CSF should be examined for evidence of infection or malignancy. The ability to detect viral and mycobacterial nucleic acids in CSF greatly facilitates the diagnostic process. Treatment of lymphoma and opportunistic infections are dealt with in the relevant sections (see above).

HIV myelopathy

About 20 per cent of patients with AIDS develop spinal cord disease. Vacuolar degeneration, thought to be due to HIV infection, may occur as part of the AIDS dementia complex. It presents initially as ataxia and progresses to cause spastic paraparesis with urinary and faecal incontinence. Other patients may develop a dorsal column syndrome with pure sensory ataxia or sensory myelopathy with paraesthesiae and dysaesthesiae in the lower limbs. Abnormalities are demonstrable on MRI scanning.[189] In contrast to the cerebral features of the AIDS dementia complex, spinal cord disease does not appear to respond to antiretroviral therapy. Treatment is supportive. Baclofen may attenuate spasticity, and painful dysaesthesias are treated with an adjuvant analgesic (see Chapter 8.2.5).

Peripheral neuropathy

Peripheral neuropathy occurs frequently in patients with HIV/AIDS.[190,191] The treatment of painful neuropathy with adjuvant analgesics is discussed in the section on pain in this chapter and elsewhere (see Chapter 8.2.5).

Distal sensory polyneuropathy

This produces a symmetrical tingling, numbness, and burning pain in the feet and may spread up the lower limbs with time. It is thought to be due to HIV infection. It is clinically manifest in one-third of AIDS patients and tests are abnormal in a further one-third. Antiretroviral therapy is not of benefit.

Toxic neuropathy

Didanosine, zalcitabine, and stavudine can produce painful peripheral neuropathy, usually when used in higher doses. The neuropathy will resolve a few weeks after discontinuation of the drugs. There are no tests available to determine whether a patient's neuropathy is drug related. Thalidomide also causes peripheral neuropathy.

Demyelinating polyneuropathy

This syndrome is characterized by progressive weakness, loss of reflexes, and mild sensory disturbances. It may be acute or chronic. The acute form resembles the Guillain–Barre syndrome and may occur at the time of seroconversion or during the phase of intermediate immune deficiency. Therapy, if required, is with plasmapheresis, intravenous immunoglobulin, or corticosteroids.

Mononeuritis multiplex

The acute onset of multiple nerve palsies that may be widespread and progressive is described in patients with AIDS. It is often due to CMV infection and may respond to therapy with ganciclovir or foscarnet.

CMV polyradiculopathy

This is a painful sensorimotor neuropathy that starts in the lumbosacral roots and progresses rostrally. Autonomic involvement with bowel and bladder dysfunction can occur. It is usually caused by CMV and may respond to therapy with ganciclovir or foscarnet.

Myopathy

HIV myopathy

Polymyositis with proximal muscle weakness and myalgia may occur in AIDS. It ranges in severity from a mild complaint to a severe illness with progressive weakness and pain. The creatine phosphokinase level is increased and the EMG abnormal. Muscle biopsy may show inflammatory changes. Treatment, if required, is with corticosteroids or intravenous immunoglobulin and physiotherapy.

Zidovudine myopathy

Patients treated with zidovudine for longer periods (usually more than a year) may develop proximal muscle weakness that is usually more marked in the lower limbs with wasting of the gluteal and thigh muscles. It may be difficult to distinguish from HIV polymyositis and inflammatory changes can be seen on biopsy. If zidovudine is suspected of causing myopathy, alternative antiretroviral therapy should be substituted. The myopathy usually resolves within 6–12 weeks of stopping zidovudine.

Corticosteroid myopathy

Patients treated with corticosteroids for more than a few weeks are at risk of developing proximal muscle weakness. The myopathy will improve within a few weeks of stopping the drug.

Eye disease

Conjunctivitis

Conjunctivitis is common in patients with AIDS and is usually due to infection (Table 18). Culture negative conjunctivitis occurs in about 10 per cent of patients with AIDS, which probably relate to allergy or systemic medications. Another 10 per cent of AIDS patients develop a dry eye syndrome, possibly related to autoimmunity or systemic medications. Conjunctivitis causes mild discomfort associated with watering, itching, and a gritty feeling in the eye. Vision is well preserved. Examination shows diffuse inflammation of the conjunctiva; a suppurative discharge suggests infection.

The treatment of conjunctivitis is with regular saline washes and appropriate antimicrobial therapy for specific infections. Aseptic conjunctivitis is treated with saline washes, cool compresses, and topical antibiotics to prevent bacterial infection. Dry eyes are treated with lubricant drops or artificial tears.

Keratitis

Keratitis or corneal inflammation is usually due to infection, the common causes being HSV, VZV, bacteria, fungi, and microsporidia. It is characterized by conjunctivitis, pain, photophobia, watering of the eye, and there is usually some blurring of vision. Infection with HSV is usually associated with signs of nasolabial infection and dendritic ulceration is seen on ophthalmological examination. Infection with VZV occurs in association with herpes zoster of the ophthalmic nerves and corneal ulceration is seen on examination. Herpetic infection is treated with topical aciclovir and corticosteroid. Other infections are treated appropriately.

Anterior uveitis

Anterior uveitis and iritis present as a painful red eye associated with photophobia. Formal ophthalmological assessment should be arranged. Causes include CMV, VZV, HSV, or other opportunistic infection, usually in conjunction with retinal involvement. Anterior uveitis occurs in a significant proportion of patients treated with rifabutin or cidofovir. If present,

Table 18 Conjunctival disease

Conjunctivitis	
Infective	HSV, VZV, bacterial
Non-infective	Allergy, medication side effects, radiotherapy (acute)
Dry eyes	Autoimmune, medication side effects, radiotherapy (late)
Tumour	Kaposi's sarcoma, squamous cell carcinoma

infection is treated appropriately. Drug-related uveitis is treated with topical corticosteroids and, if necessary, reducing the dose of the drug.

Retinal disease

Patients with AIDS who complain of visual disturbances should be assessed by an ophthalmologist, so that CMV retinitis can be diagnosed and treated before it causes blindness. CMV retinitis is seen most frequently in patients with a CD4 count less than 50/μl, and it is recommended that these patients have regular ophthalmological assessment.

Retinal abnormalities occur frequently in AIDS.[192] Cotton wool spots, seen in 50 per cent of patients, appear as hard white spots with irregular edges and are areas of retinal ischaemia caused by microvascular disease. CMV retinitis produces perivascular haemorrhage and exudates. *Pneumocystis carinii* causes raised yellow white plaques. Toxoplasma retinitis may look similar to CMV but usually occurs with cerebral toxoplasmosis. Herpetic infections cause multiple pale grey patches in the retina. CMV retinitis occurs in 25 per cent of patients with AIDS, the other infections less frequently.

Cotton wool spots do not compromise vision and do not require therapy. Appropriate antimicrobial therapy is given for the various infections as described in the section on infections.

Psychiatric disorders

Many patients with HIV/AIDS will experience psychiatric problems at some stage during the course of their illness. However, because of the high incidence of organic brain disease in patients with HIV/AIDS, all new psychiatric disorders should be considered to have an organic basis until proven otherwise.

Depression

A number of studies have reported that there is no increased risk of depression in HIV-positive people, although re-examination of these data by meta-analysis suggests the incidence of depression may be twice as high in HIV-infected people.[193] It has also been reported that more depressive symptoms and stress may lead to an acceleration of the course of HIV infection.[194]

The difficulties encountered in the diagnosis of depression in medically ill patients is discussed elsewhere (see Chapter 8.17). This is even more difficult in patients with HIV/AIDS because of the high incidence of organic brain disease. The symptoms upon which a diagnosis of depression is made in physically healthy individuals are shown in Table 19. These are not easily applicable to patients with HIV/AIDS, as both the cognitive and somatic symptoms may have an organic cause. For example, apathy has been ascribed as primarily related to neuropathology by some,[181] and to psychopathology by others.[195]

A number of different measures or scales have been validated for the diagnosis of depression in patients with HIV/AIDS,[196] although it has been suggested that deletion of the somatic symptoms increases the sensitivity of the ratings,[197] and that the use of self-report measures may significantly overestimate the true incidence of psychological illness.[198]

Table 19 Symptoms of depression

Psychological	Depressed mood Diminished interests or pleasure in activities Psychomotor agitation or retardation Diminished self-esteem, feelings of guilt Lack of concentration or indecision Thoughts of death or suicide
Somatic	Significant change in appetite and/or weight Insomnia or hypersomnia Fatigue and/or loss of energy

Most patients with HIV/AIDS will experience symptoms of depression at some time during their illness (Table 20). Depressive symptoms and anxiety occur as part of the normal psychological stress response at times of crisis such as treatment failure or disease progression. These reactions last 1–2 weeks and resolve spontaneously with time and appropriate support. Reactive depression or an adjustment disorder differs from the normal self-limited stress response in either degree or duration. Symptoms last longer than expected (more than 2 weeks) and may be more severe or intense, causing more disruption and interference with daily functioning, social activities, and relationships with others. Major or endogenous depression occurs in a small proportion of patients with HIV/AIDS. The symptoms are usually more severe than in reactive depression and the mood is incongruent with the disease outlook and does not respond to support, understanding, or distraction. Patients with acute confusional states (delirium) or dementia may exhibit features of depression. A number of drugs can also cause depressive symptoms, including corticosteroids, barbiturates, amphotericin, and interferon. In the case of delirium, dementia, and drug side effects, mental state examination will reveal evidence of organic brain dysfunction.

Treatment

If an organic brain syndrome is present, it is treated appropriately. Other problems causing or aggravating depression, particularly pain, should be treated. Patients with transient depressive symptoms occurring in response to acute crises usually require only good general supportive care. Psychotherapy is not usually required although relaxation training may be helpful if anxiety is pronounced.

A variety of different forms of psychotherapy have been reported for patients with HIV/AIDS. Cognitive-behavioural therapy has been reported to be of benefit.[199] In another study, either interpersonal psychotherapy or supportive psychotherapy together with imipramine were shown to be superior to supportive psychotherapy or cognitive-behavioural therapy alone.[200] Antidepressants are effective although side effects and drug interactions may be problematical. Tricyclic antidepressants may be effective but less well tolerated than newer SSRIs.[201,202] The difficulty interpreting the results of these trails is underlined by the observation that nearly half of the patients taking placebo in a trail of fluoxetine showed significant response.[203]

Three other forms of treatment have been used in patients with HIV/AIDS and depressive symptoms, the success of which suggests the possibility that a significant proportion of psychological symptomatology relates to neuropathology. First, treatment with psychostimulants (dextroamphetamine, methylphenidate, and pemoline) has been shown in placebo-controlled trials to significantly reduce levels of depression and psychological distress.[175,176] Second, a proportion of males with HIV/AIDS have hypogonadism and treatment with testosterone in blinded, placebo-controlled studies showed significant improvements in depression ratings.[204,205] Third, treatment with HAART, known to be of benefit to neuropsychological function, leads to significant improvement in depression scores.[206,207]

Demoralization syndrome

Demoralization is a prominent form of existential distress in which meaningless, hopelessness, and helplessness predominate and which may lead to a desire to die.[208,209] The diagnostic criteria are listed in Table 21 and it can be distinguished from depression in that demoralized patients

Table 20 Causes of depressive symptoms in patients with HIV/AIDS

Normal	Part of transient normal response to crises, stress
Adjustment disorder	Reactive depression ± reactive anxiety
Major depressive illness	
Organic brain syndromes	Acute confusion (delirium) Dementia Side effects of drugs

Table 21 Diagnosis of the demoralization syndrome

Symptoms of existential distress: meaninglessness, pointlessness, hopelessness
Sense of pessimism, helplessness, loss of motivation to cope differently, desire to die
Associated social isolation, alienation, or lack of support
Phenomena persist over more than 2 weeks

Table 22 Mania

Persistently elevated, expansive, or irritable mood
Unrealistically inflated self-esteem or grandiosity
Decreased need for sleep
Increased talkativeness
Flight of ideas or subjective experience that thoughts are racing
Easily distracted
Hyperactivity
Involvement in activities without regard to probable adverse consequences

can enjoy the present, their lack of hope being confined to the future. In the past, the features of this syndrome have probably been regarded as subclinical depression.

Demoralization can be actively treated with cognitive-behavioural therapy to counter the sense of pessimism and promote the setting of goals, meaning-based therapy that explores continued role and purpose, and supportive therapies to reduce feelings of isolation and dependence.

Anxiety

The assessment and management of anxiety is discussed in detail elsewhere (see Chapter 8.17). Anxiety occurs frequently in patients with HIV/AIDS.(210) Cognitive-behavioural stress management is reported to be effective.(211)

Psychosis

Mania and psychoses in patients with HIV/AIDS are usually attributable to organic brain disease or the effects of drugs (both medicinal and recreational). Presentation with psychosis occurs more frequently in patients with AIDS than in the earlier phases of HIV infection, and patients may show signs of cognitive impairment and have abnormalities on CT scanning of the brain.(212,213) Follow-up of these patients shows an increased incidence of cognitive impairment and AIDS dementia.(212,214)

Mania

The typical features of mania are listed in Table 22. In addition, there may be cognitive defects that may persist after resolution of the manic episode. In hypomania, the symptoms are not severe enough to cause serious impairment of social or occupational functioning and there are no psychotic features. In mania there is functional impairment and there may be psychotic features, including delusions, hallucinations, disorganized speech, and grossly disorganized or catatonic behaviour.

Initial therapy is with a potent neuroleptic. Any causative or precipitating factors related or organic brain disease or drugs are sought and treated appropriately. Continued therapy is with a lower potency neuroleptic or one of the mood altering drugs such carbamazepine or sodium valproate. Lithium therapy can be very difficult to manage in patients with advanced HIV infection and is not recommended.

Respiratory symptoms

The investigation and management of respiratory symptoms are dealt with elsewhere, including dyspnoea, cough, haemoptysis, pleural effusion, hoarseness, and terminal respiratory congestion (see Chapters 8.8 and 10.4).

Pneumonia

Treatment of pneumonia in patients with HIV infection and AIDS is with the appropriate specific antimicrobial therapy.(215) Treatment must be appropriate to the stage of the disease and the prognosis. Intensive therapy is only appropriate if it is felt that successful treatment of the infection will allow the patient to survive a significant period of time with reasonable quality of life. Treatment of *Pneumocystis carinii* and mycobacterial pneumonia is outlined in the section on opportunistic infections.

Table 23 Stomatitis: causative and predisposing factors

Causes	
Infection	
Fungal	Candida, other fungi
Bacterial	Gingivitis, periodontitis, other bacteria
Viral	HSV, CMV, HPV, hairy leukoplakia
Aphthous ulcers	
Radiotherapy	Direct mucosal damage, xerostomia
Chemotherapy	Direct mucosal damage, neutropenic sepsis
Predisposing factors	
Xerostomia	Diminished amount of less alkaline saliva
Poor oral hygiene	
Poor nutrition	Thin atrophic mucous membranes
Drugs	Steroids, antibiotics predispose to fungal infection
Cancer	Kaposi's sarcoma, non-Hodgkin's lymphoma

Gastrointestinal disease

Stomatitis

Stomatitis occurs frequently in AIDS, due to a variety of causes (Table 23).

The common symptoms are pain, altered taste, and halitosis. Severe stomatitis may prevent eating or drinking and cause difficulty taking medications. Infective stomatitis can be caused by a wide range or organisms, and as the clinical features are often atypical, appropriate microbiological studies and biopsies should be performed.

Candida usually presents in the pseudomembranous form (removable, creamy white plaques) but may manifest in an erythematous form (flat red patches) or cause angular cheilosis. HSV causes clusters of painful small vesicles that rupture and ulcerate, usually on keratinized mucosa (the hard palate or gingiva). VZV infection causes vesicles that coalesce to form large ulcers and always occurs in association with skin lesions involving the maxillary or mandibular branches of the trigeminal nerve. HPV infection can cause solitary or multiple nodules, which may be sessile or pedunculated and usually require biopsy for diagnosis. Oral CMV infection that occurs as part of systemic CMV disease causes ulcers that look necrotic with a white halo. Hairy leukoplakia is a white thickening of the oral mucosa that has a corrugated surface or 'hairy' appearance, typically occurring along the lateral margin of the tongue. It is an EBV-induced benign hyperplasia. Linear gingival erythema is a bacterial gingivitis that presents with a bright red band of erythema at the gingival margin, even in clean mouths. It may progress to a necrotizing ulcerative gingivitis and periodontitis in which there is rapid loss of gingival and periodontal tissues with destruction of supporting bone and loss of teeth; it is usually associated with severe pain. Bacillary angiomatosis causes vascular papular lesions in the mucosa that can mimic Kaposi's sarcoma. Aphthous ulcers are common and may be single or multiple, small or large, and are frequently recurrent. They occur on non-keratinized mucosa and have an erythematous margin. Kaposi's sarcoma presents as purplish lesions in the mucosa that may be raised or flat, single, or multiple. Non-Hodgkin's lymphoma may present as a painless swelling that may ulcerate.

Treatment

Preventive

All patients with advanced HIV infection and AIDS, particularly those receiving chemotherapy or radiotherapy, require a programme of preventive mouth care including regular mouth washing, attention to dental hygiene, and avoidance of very hot or very hard food. Prophylactic topical antifungal therapy should be considered for all patients with CD4 lymphocytes less than 200/μl. Addition of an antiseptic such as chlorhexidine reduces the incidence of bacterial stomatitis in myelosuppressed patients.

Treatment of pain

Mild to moderate pain can usually be managed using mouthwashes containing anaesthetic or analgesic agents, with or without oral analgesics. Severe pain is treated with opioid analgesics.

Specific therapy

Specific treatments for different causes of stomatitis are listed in Table 24. Candidal infection not responding to topical antifungal agents is treated with oral fluconazole. Aciclovir may improve the rate of healing of HSV lesions, and in higher dose VZV lesions. Hairy leukoplakia is not routinely treated and the response to oral aciclovir is usually short-lived. Linear gingival erythema is treated with regular mouth washing with either chlorhexidine or povidone-iodine. Necrotizing gingivitis requires plaque removal and local debridement, mouth washing with chlorhexidine or povidone-iodine, and oral antibiotic therapy with metronidazole or clindamycin. Aphthous ulcers are treated with topical steroid in orabase or a steroid mouthwash. Systemic steroids may be considered for severe aphthous ulcers or if there are also oesophageal lesions. Thalidomide (200 mg/d) is effective in the short-term treatment of aphthous ulcers but may cause somnolence, rash, and peripheral neuropathy.[216] Thalidomide taken intermittently at lower dose does not protect against recurrent aphthous ulcers.[217] Topical application of GM-CSF is reported to be effective for recalcitrant aphthous ulcers.[218]

Nausea and vomiting

The causes and management of nausea and vomiting are discussed elsewhere (see Chapter 8.3.1). In patients with AIDS, additional causes might include the side effects of medications (antiretrovirals, antimicrobials), opportunistic infections, malignancy, or infection affecting the central nervous system, and psychological factors. Management includes the identification and palliation of the cause, where possible, and antiemetics. There is an increased incidence of extrapyramidal side effects in patients with AIDS and the doses of antidopaminergic drugs should be kept as low as possible.[179] If a prokinetic drug is required, domperidone should be used in preference to metoclopramide as the former does not cross the blood–brain barrier.

Table 24 Treatment of stomatitis

Candida	Topical antifungal therapy, oral fluconazole
HSV, VZV	Oral aciclovir
CMV	Ganciclovir
HPV	Excision, cryotherapy, cautery, or laser therapy
Leukoplakia	High dose oral aciclovir
Other fungi	Antifungal therapy
Gingivitis	Chlorhexidine or povidone-iodine mouthwash
Periodontitis	Removal of necrotic tissue Chlorhexidine or povidone-iodine mouthwash Oral metronidazole or clindamycin
Other bacteria	Antibiotics selected on basis of culture results
Aphthous ulcers	Topical corticosteroid or corticosteroid mouthwash Thalidomide

Oesophagitis

The common causes of oesophagitis in AIDS are listed in Table 25. Oesophagitis causes pain on swallowing (odynophagia), some degree of difficulty with swallowing (dysphagia), and may produce anterior chest pain. Reflux oesophagitis causes characteristic burning retrosternal discomfort or 'heartburn'.

Barium examination will show mucosal irregularity or ulceration. Endoscopy to obtain biopsies and specimens for microbiological examination is frequently required. Candida infection produces white or yellow-white plaques, which may become confluent and cause oesophageal narrowing in severe cases; oropharyngeal infection is usually present. CMV infection produces either diffuse oesophagitis or multiple shallow ulcers; giant ulcers (>1 cm) are sometimes seen. Idiopathic ulcers, in which no pathogen can be identified, are typically large and shallow.

Treatment

Therapy includes treatment of infection, pain relief, measures to aid healing of ulceration, and avoidance of reflux (Table 26). In milder cases, thought to be due to candida because of the presence of oropharyngeal infection, radiological and endoscopic assessment may be delayed a few days to see if there is response to fluconazole. Idiopathic ulcers do not respond to the treatments used for infective oesophagitis but frequently respond to corticosteroids; thalidomide is also reported to be beneficial.[219]

Diarrhoea

Diarrhoea affects up to 90 per cent of patients with HIV infection and AIDS. The incidence increases with progressive immunodeficiency and

Table 25 Causes of oesophagitis

Infection	Candida, CMV, HSV
Idiopathic ulcers	
Radiation	Mucosal damage, predisposition to infection
Chemotherapy	Mucosal damage, predisposition to infection
Reflux oesophagitis	Raised intra-abdominal pressure (any cause) Prolonged recumbent posture Persistent vomiting Anticholinergic drugs, anticholinergic side effects of drugs

Table 26 Management of oesophagitis

Infection—specific antimicrobial therapy	
Candida	Fluconazole
CMV	Ganciclovir, foscarnet
HSV	Aciclovir
Idiopathic ulcers	
Corticosteroids, thalidomide	
Pain relief	
Topical local anaesthetics: oxethazaine, lignocaine, cocaine	
Oral analgesics (mild pain), parenteral opioids (severe pain)	
Antacids	
Dietary advice: liquid or semisolid diet, avoid very hot or cold foods	
Prevention and healing of ulceration	
Antacids combined with coating agent alginate	
Sucralfate	
Reduce gastric acid production: H_2-receptor antagonist, proton pump inhibitor	
Avoidance of reflux	
Reduce increased intra-abdominal pressure	
Dietary: avoid large meals, carbonated drinks, alcohol	
Posture: avoid stooping, lying flat	
Increase lower oesophageal sphincter tone: metoclopramide, cisapride	

there has been a marked reduction in the incidence in patients treated with HAART. In most cases it is due to an opportunistic infection (Table 27) and infection with more than one organism may occur at any given time. Non-infective causes (Table 28) also occur and both infection and infection-induced malabsorption may occur at the same time.[220]

Infective causes of diarrhoea can be broadly grouped by whether they cause enteritis or colitis (Table 27) although the distinction is not always clear and some organisms can affect all parts of the bowel. Small bowel disease is characterized by large volumes of watery diarrhoea associated with bloating and central abdominal pain. Colitis is associated with lower abdominal pain and cramping, urgency, and the frequent passage of small volumes of stool that often contains blood, mucous, and pus. The bacterial pathogens usually cause an acute diarrhoeal illness whilst infection with protozoa, viruses, and mycobacteria characteristically causes chronic diarrhoea.

Initial assessment includes microscopy and culture of three stool specimens. Tests for *Cl. difficile* toxin should be performed if there is a history of antibiotic use or pseudomembranous colitis is suspected. Blood cultures should be taken. If no pathogen is identified, endoscopy for biopsies and cultures should be considered: upper gastrointestinal endoscopy and small bowel biopsy are performed if the clinical features suggest enteritis, and sigmoidoscopy or colonoscopy is done for colitis-type diarrhoea. In a proportion of patients, no pathogen will be identified despite rigorous investigation. It has been suggested that some of these cases are due to HIV infection ('HIV enteropathy') but a causal association is unproven.

Treatment

Treatment of infection

After collection of stool specimens, patients should be given ciprofloxacin to which most enteric bacteria in HIV-positive patients are sensitive. Pseudomembranous colitis is treated with oral vancomycin. If a pathogen is identified, specific treatment is instituted, as described above in the section on infection. Maintenance therapy is necessary for some infections, particularly those more likely to occur when the CD4 count is less than 100/μl: CMV, MAC, cryptosporidia, microsporidia, and cyclospora.

Table 27 Infective causes of diarrhoea

Enteritis—predominantly small bowel	
Bacteria	*Mycobacterium avium, Salmonella* spp
Protozoa	Cryptosporidia, microsporidia, *Cyclospora* spp, *Isospora* spp, *Giardia lamblia*
Viruses	Enteroviruses, HIV
Colitis—predominantly colon	
Bacteria	*Campylobacter* spp, *Shigella* spp, *Yersinia* spp, *Aeromonas* spp, *Cl. difficile*
Protozoa	*Entamoeba histolytica*
Viruses	CMV, adenovirus, HSV

Table 28 Non-infective causes of diarrhoea

Dietary	Excess roughage, fibre; enteric supplements
Drugs	Laxatives, antibiotics, antiretrovirals, others
Haemorrhage	
Inflammation	Radiation, drugs
Cancer	Kaposi's sarcoma, non-Hodgkin's lymphoma
Lactose intolerance	
Steatorrhoea	Pancreatic insufficiency Biliary obstruction Bacterial overgrowth
Psychological	Anxiety

General measures

Maintenance of hydration is important except in the terminally ill. Commercially available soft drinks or oral rehydration solutions can be used. Intravenous rehydration may be necessary if diarrhoea is severe or if there is vomiting. Dietary modifications to both reduce diarrhoea and ensure adequate nutrition are important and the assistance of a dietician is useful. Patients with severe or prolonged diarrhoea may require consideration for enteral nutrition, either by nasogastric tube or percutaneous gastrostomy; patients with continuing diarrhoea and malabsorption benefit from TPN.[165] Drugs that may be causing or aggravating diarrhoea should be stopped, if possible.

Antidiarrhoeal agents

The opioid drugs such as loperamide, diphenoxylate, and codeine reduce diarrhoea by inhibiting peristalsis. Unless morphine or codeine is being given for analgesia, loperamide is the agent of choice. The hydrophilic bulking agents such as methylcellulose and ispaghula may reduce diarrhoea by absorbing excess fluid. Adsorbent agents such as the kaolin preparations are of questionable value and may interfere with absorption of other drugs. The somatostatin analogue, octreotide, reduces intestinal secretion and motility and is of benefit in a proportion of AIDS patients with diarrhoea.[221] It is more likely to help patients without a defined pathogen and recent studies suggest it may be more effective at higher doses. Acetorphan, an orally active encephalinase inhibitor, benefits some patients.[222] A compound isolated from a tropical plant, SP-303 (Provir), is reported to be effective in the treatment of diarrhoea in patients with AIDS.[223]

Anorectal disease

Anorectal disease is common in patients with AIDS, particularly male homosexuals (Table 29). Anorectal ulceration is most frequently caused by HSV, less often by CMV. Warts due to HPV infection are common. Proctitis is most frequently caused by chlamydia or gonorrhoea and less often by other bacterial infections, including syphilis. Kaposi's sarcoma, non-Hodgkin's lymphoma, and anal cancer can present as either mass lesions or ulceration. Idiopathic ulcers occur for which no pathogen can be identified, similar to idiopathic oesophageal ulcers. Fistulas, fissures, and haemorrhoids are common and may be caused or aggravated by local infections or severe diarrhoea. Assessment is by proctoscopy to view lesions and to obtain biopsies and specimens for microbiological studies. Examination should be thorough, including biopsy of any suspicious areas, given the high incidence of intraepithelial neoplasia in patients referred for benign conditions.[224]

Treatment is directed at the cause. Gonorrhoea is treated with amoxycillin, chlamydia with tetracycline, and HSV with oral aciclovir. Symptomatic measures including analgesia and stool softening (if appropriate) are instituted. Preparations for rectal use containing a local anaesthetic and corticosteroid can be of significant symptomatic benefit. Idiopathic ulcers respond to local or systemic corticosteroid and may respond to thalidomide.

Liver disease

Liver disease or abnormalities of liver function occur commonly and relate to pre-existing liver disease, infection, drug toxicity, or malignancy (Table 30). The infections that most commonly involve the liver are due to mycobacteria and CMV and occur as part of a systemic illness with fever and constitutional symptoms. Drug toxicity usually produces a diffuse hepatitic picture and ranges in severity from asymptomatic biochemical abnormalities to hepatic failure.

The history, other clinical features, and liver function tests may provide clues to the diagnosis. Imaging may show evidence of diffuse or focal liver

Table 29 Anorectal disease

Infection	Chlamydia, gonorrhoea, HSV, CMV, HPV, other bacteria
Cancer	Kaposi's sarcoma, non-Hodgkin's lymphoma, anal cancer
Other	Idiopathic ulcers, fissures, fistulas, haemorrhoids

disease or biliary pathology. Opportunistic infections can often be diagnosed by non-invasive means such as blood cultures. Liver biopsy may be necessary if the diagnosis cannot be made by other means.

Treatment

Treatment is directed at the underlying cause. Drugs causing toxicity are withdrawn or the dose modified. Infections are treated appropriately.

Co-infection with hepatitis viruses

In patients with AIDS, progressive immunodeficiency may lead to activation of hepatitis B (HBV) and hepatitis C (HCV) infections, and previously asymptomatic carriers may develop clinical hepatitis.(225) With HCV, this is associated with an increased incidence of progressive liver disease(226) and hepatocellular carcinoma is reported.(227) There are reports that HCV co-infection predisposes to more rapid progression to AIDS and death,(228,229) although others report no effect on survival.(230) Patients with HBV or HCV are less likely to tolerate treatment with protease inhibitors(231) and HCV patients respond less well to HAART.(232) Patients earlier in the course of their HIV infection and those who have responded to HAART should be considered for treatment of HBV and HCV, and control of HCV infection may facilitate the delivery of HAART.(233) However, in patients with AIDS who have either failed HAART or never had access to it, the HIV infection is regarded as the major determinate of their life expectancy and treatment of the hepatitis virus infection with interferon (with all its attendant toxicity) is not usually recommended.

Biliary disease

Sclerosing cholangitis and acalculous cholecystitis occur with increased frequency in patients with HIV/AIDS. They are related to an opportunistic infection in most cases; occasionally, strictures are due to malignant infiltration (Table 31).

Table 30 Causes of liver disease

Pre-existing liver disease	
Biliary disease	
Infection	*M. avium* CMV *M. tuberculosis* Cryptococcosis Histoplasmosis *P. carinii* *Rochalimaea henselae* Viral hepatitis B, C
Cancer	Kaposi's sarcoma Non-Hodgkin's lymphoma
Drugs	Antiretroviral, e.g. didanosine Antiviral, e.g. foscarnet Antifungal, e.g. ketoconazole Antimycobacterial, e.g. isoniazid Antiprotozoal, e.g. pentamidine
Complementary medications	
Recreational drugs	
Alcohol	

Table 31 Biliary disease

Sclerosing cholangitis ± papillary stenosis	CMV, cryptosporidia
Acalculous cholangitis	CMV, cryptosporidia, microsporidia
Biliary strictures	Infection, Kaposi's sarcoma, lymphoma, cholangiocarcinoma

Patients present with biliary-type abdominal pain that may be severe. Examination reveals fever and local tenderness. Liver function tests show progressive cholestasis. Imaging will usually show some dilatation of the biliary tree. In sclerosing cholangitis, endoscopic retrograde cholangiopancreatography (ERCP) may show multiple focal strictures and dilatations of both the intrahepatic and extrahepatic bile ducts, often associated with papillary stenosis at the ampulla. Large or solitary strictures suggest the possibility of malignancy.

Treatment

Sclerosing cholangitis is treated by endoscopic sphincterotomy and therapy directed at the underlying infection. This frequently provides good pain relief although the liver function tests may not improve significantly if there is continuing intrahepatic cholangitis. If severe or recurrent, acalculous cholecystitis is treated by cholecystectomy.

Haematological disorders

Anaemia

Up to 80 per cent of patients develop symptomatic anaemia during the course of HIV infection and AIDS, the incidence and severity increasing with progressive immunodeficiency.(234) Severe anaemia is associated with a poorer prognosis.(235)

The anaemia is frequently multifactorial (Table 32). For most patients with AIDS, anaemia is attributed to direct infection of the marrow by HIV. It is usually a diagnosis of exclusion, no other cause for anaemia being found. It has the features of an anaemia of chronic disease with normochromic, normocytic anaemia, a low reticulocyte count, and inappropriately low erythropoietin levels. Mycobacterial (*M. tuberculosis, M. avium*) and fungal (cryptococcosis, histoplasmosis, coccidioidomycosis) infections frequently involve the marrow. Infection with parvovirus B19, associated with transient aplasia in immunocompetent individuals, can cause severe and chronic anaemia in AIDS patients. Bone marrow infiltration occurs frequently with non-Hodgkin's lymphoma and Hodgkin's disease and the blood film may show a leucoerythroblastic picture. Cancer chemotherapy routinely causes a transient pancytopenia and a number of the drugs used in the treatment of HIV and opportunistic infections may also cause bone marrow suppression. Iron deficiency due to inadequate intake or bleeding produces a hypochromic, microcytic anaemia. Vitamin B12 or folate deficiency may occur secondary to intestinal malabsorption caused by infection and produce a macrocytic anaemia with megaloblastic changes in the marrow.

Iron deficiency anaemia will occur with significant bleeding at any site. The most frequent is bleeding from the gastrointestinal tract due to malignant infiltration or severe infection. Patients with haemophilia or severe thrombocytopenia are also at increased risk of haemorrhage.

Table 32 Causes of anaemia

Decreased red cell production
HIV infection
Opportunistic marrow infection
Marrow infiltration
Marrow suppression
Drugs: antiretrovirals, drugs for opportunistic infections
Chemotherapy
Radiation
Iron deficiency
Vitamin B12, folate deficiency
Red blood cell loss
Bleeding
Increased red cell destruction (haemolysis)
Infection
Drugs
Autoimmune

Table 33 Indications for blood transfusion for chronic anaemia

Hb < 80–90 g/l and symptomatic	
Hb 80–90 g/l and continued or likely haemorrhage	
	planned surgery
	planned radiotherapy
	planned chemotherapy
	serious infection
	doubt about symptomatic benefit
	unexplained weakness, fatigue, or dyspnoea
Hb > 90–100 g/l and symptomatic (cardiac or respiratory insufficiency)	

Table 34 Causes of thrombocytopenia

Diminished platelet production
HIV infection
Opportunistic infection of marrow
Malignant infiltration of marrow
Vitamin B12 or folate deficiency
Cancer treatment: chemotherapy, radiotherapy
Drugs
Increased platelet destruction
Immune thrombocytopenia (ITP)

Some degree of haemolysis (shortened red cell survival) occurs with many of the infections complicating AIDS. More severe haemolysis occurs when patients with G6PD deficiency are given sulfonamides or dapsone.

Treatment

Treatment of specific causes

Anaemia in patients with AIDS is frequently multifactorial and treatment is initially directed at specific causes, where possible. Bone marrow infection is treated with specific antimicrobial therapy; parvovirus B19 infection is treated with intravenous immunoglobulin.[236] Malignant lymphoma is treated with chemotherapy. Drug-induced bone marrow suppression requires consideration of dose reduction or use of different drugs. Iron, vitamin B12, and folate deficiencies are treated with replacement therapy. The underlying cause of bleeding is treated appropriately. The haemolysis associated with infections responds to treatment of the infection. Drug-induced haemolytic anaemia requires the offending drugs be withheld.

Transfusion

Decisions regarding blood transfusion depend on the speed of onset and the severity of the symptoms of anaemia. Acute anaemia due to blood loss or serious infection usually requires transfusion. Recommendations regarding transfusion for patients with chronic anaemia are summarized in Table 33. Patients without antibodies to CMV should receive CMV-negative blood. There is no benefit in using leucocyte-reduced red cell transfusions.[237]

Erythropoietin

Treatment of patients with AIDS and anaemia with recombinant human erythropoietin (EPO) leads to a significant rise in haemoglobin and improvement in the quality of life.[238] It is effective in patients with low endogenous erythropoietin levels (<500 IU/l) but may not produce improvement in patients with opportunistic infections or taking zidovudine. It is administered by subcutaneous injection (100 μg/kg) three times weekly and is well tolerated. EPO therapy is very expensive.

Lymphopenia

Progressive lymphopenia is the hallmark of HIV infection. Lymphopenia also occurs with chemotherapy, radiotherapy, and treatment with corticosteroids.

Neutropenia

HIV infection results in impaired neutrophil production, an effect that increases with progressive immunodeficiency. Neutropenia may also occur with marrow involvement by opportunistic infections or malignant infiltration. A considerable number of drugs used in the treatment of AIDS patients may cause neutropenia. Neutropenia predisposes to bacterial infection and also causes mucositis, particularly involving the gastrointestinal tract.

Treatment

Treatment of specific causes

Where possible, the specific cause is treated appropriately. Drug-related neutropenia requires consideration of dose reduction or the substitution of a different agent.

Growth factors

The neutrophil growth factors, G-CSF (granulocyte colony stimulating factor) and GM-CSF (granulocyte-macrophage colony stimulating factor), are effective in patients with persistent neutropenia and may allow other essential but myelotoxic medications to be continued. The CSFs are administered by daily subcutaneous injection; the usual starting dose is 5 μg/kg/d, although lower doses of the order of 1 μg/kg/d may be effective.[239] Side effects are few although the treatment is expensive. GM-CSF has been shown to augment HIV replication *in vitro* and, whilst there is no evidence that it has deleterious effect *in vivo*,[240,241] it is customary for patients receiving GM-CSF to be also on antiretroviral therapy.

Thrombocytopenia

Immune thrombocytopenia (ITP) may occur at any stage of HIV infection. Thrombocytopenia may also occur with various marrow disorders (Table 34). Thrombocytopenia related to HIV infection of the marrow increases in frequency and severity with progressive immunodeficiency.

Most patients with AIDS have mild thrombocytopenia and are asymptomatic. Bone marrow examination should be considered for patients with a platelet count less than 50×10^9/l for which the cause is not apparent. This will distinguish impaired production from increased peripheral destruction and will demonstrate any marrow pathology.

Treatment

Specific causes of diminished platelet production are treated, where possible. Antiretroviral therapy frequently produces improvement in the platelet count.

Treatment of more severe ITP in patients with HIV infection and AIDS is with corticosteroids, intravenous immunoglobulin, and splenectomy. Corticosteroids (e.g. prednisolone 0.5 mg/kg/d) produce improvement in 50–75 per cent of patients but thrombocytopenia frequently recurs when the dose is tapered. Intravenous immunoglobulin produces a response in 75–90 per cent of patients; the response is transient but is useful in patients who are bleeding or are scheduled for surgery. Splenectomy is reported to benefit 80 per cent of patients.[242]

Thrombotic thrombocytopenic purpura

Thrombotic thrombocytopenic purpura (TTP) is a rare condition characterized by severe thrombocytopenia, microangiopathic haemolytic anaemia, neurological signs, renal impairment, and fever. TTP occurs in patients with advanced HIV infection and AIDS, usually in association with opportunistic infections. Untreated, the condition is often rapidly fatal. Treatment is by plasma exchange with fresh frozen plasma.[243]

Skin disease

Skin disorders are extremely common in patients with HIV infection and AIDS. The frequency increases with progressive immunodeficiency and the lesions may be clinically more severe and respond less well to therapy. Atypical clinical presentations are common and skin biopsies are often necessary to establish the diagnosis.

Skin infections

Bacterial infections

Staphylococcal infection may present as folliculitis with pustules affecting the trunk, inguinal regions, and face, sometimes associated with severe pruritus. Other presentations include cellulitis, bullous impetigo, and ecthyma (punched-out ulcers, most frequently on the lower leg). Diagnosis is made on the clinical features and the results of cultures. Treatment is with appropriate antibiotics, and benzoyl peroxide washes or antibacterial soaps can be helpful. Patients with recurrent infections can be given a short course of rifampicin.

Bacillary angiomatosis presents as a few to many purple or red papules and nodules, which may resemble Kaposi's sarcoma or pyogenic infection. The diagnosis is made by biopsy. Treatment is with erythromycin or doxycycline.

Other bacterial infections, including syphilis and systemic mycobacterial infections, can produce unusual or atypical skin lesions. Biopsies and cultures are essential for diagnosis.

Viral infections

Infections with herpes simplex (HSV), varicella zoster (VZV), molluscum contagiosum, and human papilloma virus (HPV) are discussed in the section on infections.

Fungal infection

Infections with dermatophytes (fungi that infect the skin, hair, and nails) occur more frequently in patients with HIV infection and become more widespread and less responsive to treatment with progressive immunodeficiency. Tinea infections may be severe and widespread with prominent nail involvement. *Trichophyton rubrum* is a common cause of nail infection in patients with severe immunodeficiency and produces the characteristic proximal white subungual onychomycosis. Diagnosis is made by microscopy and culture.

Treatment is with topical antifungal agents including ketoconazole, clotrimazole, and terbinafine. More severe infections require systemic therapy using griseofulvin, an imidazole (ketoconazole, fluconazole, and itraconazole) or terbinafine. Oral therapy is more effective but more likely to cause side effects and drug interactions.

Candida usually affects the mouth and oesophagus but may also cause vulvovaginitis, balanitis, angular cheilosis, paronychia, and onychomycosis. Diagnosis is made on microscopy and culture

Skin lesions are common in patients with other systemic fungal infections. The lesions can resemble molluscum, making biopsy essential.

Parasitic infection

The mite that causes scabies, *Sarcoptes scabiei*, proliferates unchecked in patients with severe immunodeficiency, leading to heavy infestation that may involve much of the body surface. Diagnosis is by identification of mites or biopsy. Treatment is with topical benzyl benzoate, lindane, or permethrin, with or without oral ivermectin.[244,245] Close contacts of the patient must also be treated.

Skin disorders

Xerosis and ichthyosis

Xerosis or dry, fine scaling of the skin is common in AIDS. Treatment is symptomatic with topical moisturising applications. Ichthyosis, predominantly affecting the lower limbs, occurs in a quarter of patients with HIV infection. The skin is dry with a 'fish-scale' appearance. Treatment is with emollients to keep the skin as moist as possible; if scaling is severe, a keratolytic such as 2 per cent salicylic acid can be added to the emollient.

Seborrhoeic dermatitis

Seborrhoeic dermatitis is reported to occur in up to 90 per cent of patients with HIV infection, the incidence and severity increasing with progressive immunodeficiency. Erythematous patches covered with greasy scales characteristically occur on the face and scalp and may also involve the central chest, axillae, and groins. Treatment is with a topical corticosteroid preparation and antidandruff shampoos are useful for the scalp. The role of *Pitysporum orbiculare* in the causation of seborrhoeic dermatitis is controversial but the rash often responds well to ketoconazole cream in HIV-infected patients.

Psoriasis

Psoriasis typically presents as erythematous rounded plaques covered by silvery micaceous scale, predominantly affecting the elbows, knees, and scalp. In HIV-infected patients, the disease can be more severe and widespread and prove resistant to therapy; psoriatic arthritis is also more frequent. Treatment includes conventional topical tar products and topical corticosteroids, which may be ineffective in severe cases. Ultraviolet light therapy [either UV-A with psoralen (PUVA) or UV-B] is usually effective for patients with widespread disease. UV-B phototherapy is more widely used,[246] although it is reported the viral load may increase in patients who are not taking antiretroviral therapy who are treated with UV-B,[247] but not PUVA.[248] Other therapies include topical calcipotriol (a vitamin D analogue) and oral retinoid therapy with acitretin or etretinate. Methotrexate may compromise immune function and is not used.

Eosinophilic folliculitis

Eosinophilic folliculitis is a rare skin condition that occurs more frequently in patients with HIV infection. It presents with follicular and perifollicular urticarial papules and plaques scattered on the upper trunk, head and neck, and the upper arms, often associated with severe pruritus. Diagnosis is made on biopsy, which shows eosinophilic infiltration of the hair follicle. Treatment with antihistamines, topical corticosteroids, and ultraviolet light may be helpful. Some improve with itraconazole, suggesting an infective aetiology.

Hypersensitivity reactions

Photosensitivity

Patients with HIV infection are often very photosensitive and can suffer burns as a result of exposure to sunlight or radiation therapy. Treatment is with topical corticosteroids and discontinuance of any medications that may act as a photosensitiser. Advice should be given regarding the use of sunscreens and protective clothing.

Insect bite reactions

Mosquito and other insect bites can produce florid reactions in patients with HIV infection. Treatment is with antihistamines and topical corticosteroids and the avoidance of further bites by the use of insecticides, insect repellents, and protective clothing.

Drug reactions

Drug reactions are common in patients with AIDS and are usually due to sulfonamides or other antibiotics. The most common reaction is a widespread maculopapular rash; other patterns include urticaria, erythema multiforme and, less often, the Stevens–Johnson syndrome and toxic epidermal necrolysis. Mild reactions should be observed and may resolve. Symptomatic treatment is with antihistamines and topical corticosteroids. More severe reactions require withdrawal of the offending agent.

Other disorders

Arthropathy

Arthralgia occurs in about one-third of patients with HIV/AIDS for a variety of reasons.

HIV polyarthritis

A transient widespread mild polyarthralgia may occur at the time of seroconversion or during the 'asymptomatic' phase of HIV infection. Less frequently, a persistent symmetrical polyarthritis may develop in patients with advanced HIV infection or AIDS. If warranted, treatment is with NSAIDs.

HIV arthropathy

This is oligoarticular arthritis which involves large joints, predominantly the knees and ankles. It is non-erosive with few inflammatory changes in the synovial fluid. The onset is subacute, developing over 1–6 weeks, and it lasts 6 weeks to 6 months. Treatment with NSAIDs is often unhelpful but the condition usually responds to intra-articular corticosteroids.

Septic arthritis

Septic arthritis occurs relatively infrequently in patients with AIDS, given the high incidence of septicaemic illness. It can be caused by bacteria (e.g. *S. aureus*), mycobacteria, or fungi. Gonococcal infection may produce a widespread polyarthritis with mild joint swelling which is thought to be an immune reaction, or typical gonococcal arthritis with severe pain and swelling of a single joint and from which the organism can be cultured.

Reiter's syndrome

This is the triad of urethritis, arthritis, and conjunctivitis and may be triggered by sexually transmitted chlamydial infection. Persistent, painful, lower extremity oligoarthritis develops and may persist for months. Treatment is with NSAIDs and physiotherapy. Doxycycline is given if there is evidence of active chlamydial infection.

Psoriatic arthritis

Up to one-third of patients with HIV infection and psoriasis will develop psoriatic arthritis. It usually causes chronic, painful oligoarthritis involving the large joints in the lower limbs; sacroileitis, Achille's tendonitis, and plantar fasciitis may occur. Treatment is with NSAIDs and physiotherapy. Systemic steroids are avoided, if possible, because of the increased risk of infection. Methotrexate should be avoided because it may cause both myelosuppression and immunosuppression.

Renal failure

Renal impairment is most frequently caused by pre-renal factors and nephrotoxic drugs (Table 35). Drugs may cause renal damage by direct effects on renal cells, by precipitation in tubules, or as part of a hypersensitive reaction causing interstitial nephritis. Nephrotoxicity is more likely in dehydrated or debilitated patients, those with pre-existing renal impairment, or if two or more of the drugs are used at the same time.

Table 35 Causes of renal impairment in patients with HIV/AIDS

Pre-renal
Dehydration
Sepsis
NSAIDs
Renal
Glomerulonephritis
Immune complex proliferative glomerulonephritis
Focal and sclerosing glomerulosclerosis
Interstitial nephritis
Infections
Drug hypersensitivity
Nephrotoxic drugs
Antibiotics, antivirals, antiprotozoals, antifungals
Chemotherapy
Radiological contrast media
Radiation
Pyelonephritis
Post-renal
Ureteric obstruction by retroperitoneal lymphadenopathy

Two forms of glomerulonephritis are associated with HIV infection. A proliferative glomerulonephritis associated with immune complex deposition occurs and is thought to be due to HIV infection. It usually follows an indolent course with stable renal function over months or years. Focal and sclerosing glomerulosclerosis or HIV nephropathy is common in blacks and presents as a nephrotic syndrome progressing to renal failure in months.

The treatment of renal failure depends on the cause, the degree of impairment, and the stage of the patient's HIV illness. Pre-renal factors are corrected where possible. Care in prescribing potentially nephrotoxic drugs will reduce the incidence of reactions. If acute renal failure does occur, dialysis may be considered if this is appropriate to the stage of the patient's disease and general condition. Proliferative glomerulonephritis may require no therapy; dialysis may be considered if renal failure develops. Glomerulosclerosis responds to corticosteroid therapy.[249]

Gynaecological infections

Vaginal candidiasis

The incidence and severity of vaginal candidiasis increase with progressive immunodeficiency. Diagnosis is made on the clinical features and culture. Treatment is with topical nystatin or clotrimazole. Oral fluconazole is reserved for severe infections not responding to topical therapy. Maintenance therapy, either topical or systemic, can be considered for women with frequent infections.

Herpes simplex virus

The frequency and severity of ulcerative genital herpes increase with progressive immunodeficiency. Treatment is with aciclovir, followed by maintenance therapy for women with severe or frequent recurrences.

Aphthous ulceration

Giant idiopathic genital ulcers are uncommon but can be very painful. Diagnosis is by exclusion of all possible infective causes and malignancy. The pathogenesis may be similar to oesophageal aphthous ulcers, but the efficacy of steroids or thalidomide for genital ulceration is not documented.

Pelvic inflammatory disease

Pelvic inflammatory disease may be more severe in women with advanced immunodeficiency. Treatment is with standard antibiotic regimes incorporating anaerobic cover.

Human papilloma virus

Warts may become extensive and florid with advanced immunodeficiency. Treatment is with topical trichloroacetic acid or podophyllin or by cryotherapy, but the recurrence rate is high. Successful topical treatment has been reported with cidofovir[100] and imiquimod.[98]

Pregnancy

The majority of HIV-positive women are of childbearing age and much research has been conducted to reduce the risk of transmission from mother to child. The risk of infection *in utero* is probably dependent on the stage of the mother's infection, reflected by the CD4 count and plasma HIV RNA load. Risk factors during the perinatal period include the mother's CD4 count and a viral load, duration of ruptured membranes, maternal genital ulceration and HIV shedding, and the mode of delivery.[250,251] Breastfeeding is a well-documented mode of transmission.[252]

In developed countries, the risk of mother-to-child transmission can be reduced from about 30 per cent in untreated mother–child pairs to about 2 per cent with antiretroviral therapy given during the antenatal and neonatal periods, elective caesarean delivery, and avoidance of breastfeeding.[251,253] However, what constitutes optimal retroviral therapy in this situation, including minimizing adverse effects on the child, is uncertain.[253]

In developing countries, short courses of antenatal antiretroviral therapy have been shown to significantly reduce perinatal transmission.[253] In resource-poor situations in developing countries, avoidance of breastfeeding may jeopardize the health of the child; it has been shown that antiretroviral therapy during breastfeeding reduces the risk of transmission,[254] but continued therapy for the duration of breastfeeding may not be possible or feasible.

Palliative care and HIV/AIDS

HIV/AIDS has provided many challenges for palliative care and will continue to do so as the epidemic evolves. In developed countries, the role of palliative care in the management of patients with HIV/AIDS has at times been controversial and is again being questioned following the introduction of HAART.

During the early years of the epidemic, the concept of palliative care was resisted and equated with giving up hope. The patient population was young and there was a natural tendency for both patients and clinicians to pursue aggressive investigation and therapy right up until they died. Conventional palliative care, originally developed to cater for the diverse and multidisciplinary needs of the dying, with its emphasis on symptom control and psychological care, together with minimization of investigations and treatment, was not acceptable. Concerns were also expressed that palliative care services would discriminate against male homosexuals and IDUs.

By the early 1990s, before the advent of HAART, increasing numbers of patients and clinicians came to accept the value of palliative care, acknowledging that there comes a point when continuing to pursue active therapy is counterproductive to a patient concluding their life in a dignified, orderly, and meaningful way. Many patients with advanced AIDS were managed by palliative care services and a number of AIDS hospices were established. The major textbooks on HIV/AIDS even included a chapter dealing with palliative care and matters related to death and dying.

HAART has had a dramatic effect on HIV/AIDS in developed countries. Progression of HIV infection to AIDS has been slowed, as has the rate of progression of patients with AIDS, and the numbers dying of AIDS has fallen sharply (see Fig. 1). It has been argued that HIV/AIDS is now a chronic, stable problem—even possibly curable—with no need for palliative care and that talk of death and dying is unduly negative. Textbooks on HIV/AIDS no longer have chapters relating to palliative and terminal care. However, the long-term outlook for patients currently responding to HAART is unknown: there is increasing evidence of emerging drug resistance to HAART, and improved survival may be associated with an increased incidence of AIDS-related malignancies. In addition, not all patients will respond to HAART, others are unable to tolerate it, and some present late in the course of the disease and have a poorer prognosis even with HAART. It therefore seems likely that there will continue to be patients with advanced AIDS who will benefit from palliative care.

Palliative care has also evolved during the 20 years of the AIDS epidemic. In the past, palliative care has been regarded as primarily the care of the dying, to be employed when all avenues of treating the underlying disease are exhausted and further active medical treatment is considered inappropriate (Fig. 3).

More recently, the advantages of integrating palliative care with acute care have been explored in specialties such as oncology and HIV/AIDS. Even though HIV infection is incurable and ultimately fatal, its various manifestations are eminently treatable, and it is appropriate to provide pain relief, symptom control, and psychosocial support to patients with far-advanced disease while they continue to pursue disease-controlling therapies. Comprehensive symptomatic and supportive care, addressing all aspects of a patient's suffering and provided by an interdisciplinary team, should be made available for all patients with cancer or AIDS, long before the terminal phase of the illness. This treatment is complementary to (and not in competition with) all the active medical aspects of treatment, and should be integrated in a seamless manner with other aspects of the patient's care (Fig. 4); this has been termed the 'mixed management model' of end-of-life care.[255]

As well as expertise in pain and symptom control, palliative care brings to this partnership an interdisciplinary and holistic approach to care that is so important for the management of psychosocial problems but which is often lacking in modern disease-orientated medicine.

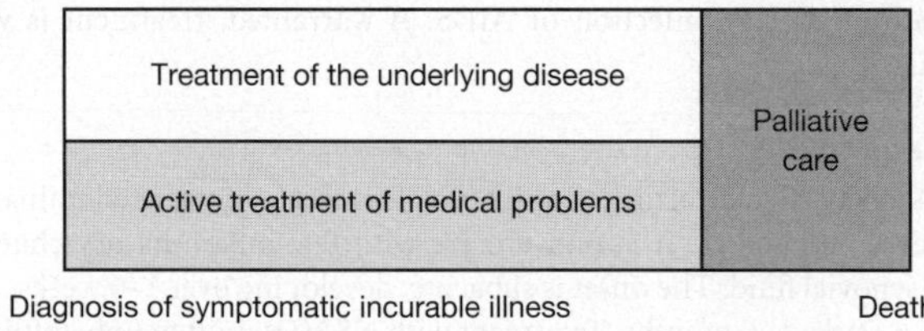

Fig. 3 A traditional view of palliative care. (Reproduced with permission from Woodruff, R. *Palliative Medicine—Symptomatic and Supportive Care for Patients with Advanced Cancer and AIDS* 3rd edn., Oxford University Press, 1999.)

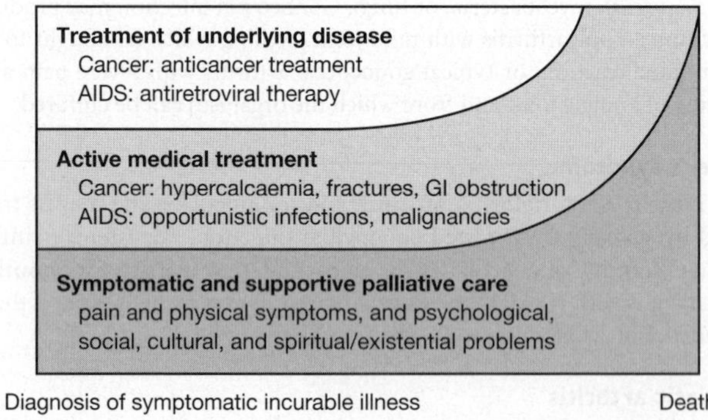

Fig. 4 Modern palliative care. Symptomatic and supportive palliative care is complementary to, and seamlessly integrated with, active treatment of the underlying disease. (Reproduced with permission from Woodruff, R. *Palliative Medicine—Symptomatic and Supportive Care for Patients with Advanced Cancer and AIDS* 3rd edn., Oxford University Press, 1999.)

The evolution of palliative care to provide services that are complementary to acute medical care earlier in the course of the disease, together with the observation that a proportion of patients with HIV infection will continue to progress to the advanced stages of AIDS, suggests that the need for palliative care in the management of patients with HIV/ AIDS will continue for the foreseeable future.[256,257]

The population of patients with HIV/AIDS in developed countries is also changing. Data from the United Kingdom (Table 2) shows that heterosexual contact is now the most frequent probable route of infection.[2] In developed countries, the incidence of HIV/AIDS is increasing in women, in minority and migrant populations, and in the socially disadvantaged. Palliative care stands to make a positive contribution to meeting the needs of this increasingly heterogeneous patient population.

Palliative care in resource-poor countries

The management of the HIV/AIDS epidemic in resource-poor countries of the developing world presents unparalleled challenges.[1,258]

In resource-poor countries, disease progression is more rapid and survival is shorter.[259,260] Poverty, malnutrition, and social inequalities are major co-factors in the epidemic in poorer countries. Gender inequality, in particular, has been singled out as the main reason that, globally, HIV infection is now more frequent in women than men.[1,261]

In resource-poor countries, basic health-care services may not be available, or cannot be accessed or afforded. Medications for opportunistic infections may be unavailable or unaffordable. The risk of transmission of HIV by blood transfusion remains high.[262] High rates of co-infection with TB complicate both epidemics in southern Africa.[6]

How resource-poor countries should address the problems of HIV/AIDS is much debated.[263,264] Prevention must remain a priority, requiring education of the population at large; voluntary testing and counselling is reported to be cost-effective.[265]

Treating HIV infection in resource-poor countries provides many challenges. It requires not only drugs but also the creation of a sustainable primary care system.[264,266,267] as well as programmes for identifying HIV-infected people before the terminal stage of the disease. Drug costs can be reduced and will lead to more widespread use.[267] To maximize the benefits and minimize the risks of drug-resistant disease, programmes will then be required to oversee optimal use and adherence, perhaps similar to the successful directly observed therapy (DOTS) programmes for tuberculosis.[266,267]

Even in the absence of antibiotic and antiretroviral therapy, there is much that palliative care can do to improve the quality of life of patients with AIDS.[268] Palliative care can promote basic medical care and symptom control, such as the use of opioids for pain control. Social supports can be strengthened and services accessed. Patients can be counselled and allowed to talk about how they feel, what to expect, and how they can help themselves. Families can be shown how to care for someone with AIDS, how to give emotional and spiritual support, and about safe waste disposal. Palliative care can help dispel fear and ignorance in carers and in the community, reducing the stigmatization that is often associated with AIDS.

Palliative care for advanced AIDS

Palliative care for patients with advanced or terminal AIDS is about quality of life and is directed at the alleviation of pain and physical symptoms as well as the assessment and management of psychological, social, and spiritual/existential problems. It also involves care and support of family members or partners, including bereavement follow-up. It requires a holistic approach to care and is best provided by a well-coordinated interdisciplinary team. It must be provided in a manner that shows respect for the individual patient—their dignity, their culture, their choices or wishes regarding treatment, and their goals and unfinished business. Continuity of care through the terminal illness is also very important.

Surveys of what patients believe constitutes quality end-of-life care report simpler, more specific concerns, focused on outcomes.[269] One study identified five domains: receiving adequate pain and symptom management, avoiding inappropriate prolongation of dying, achieving a sense of control, relieving burden, and strengthening relationships with loved ones.[270]

Palliative care for AIDS can be delivered in the patient's home or in a hospice or hospital—the principles and practices are the same. It is important that a palliative care consultation service be available in acute hospitals treating patients with AIDS.[271]

Palliative care for AIDS must accommodate the social and cultural background of the patients and provide service that is non-discriminatory and culturally sensitive.[272] In the United Kingdom, many new cases are occurring in immigrants who are socially disadvantaged, isolated, less aware of the health care to which they are entitled, and more likely to present only when symptomatic.[273] In the United States, the patients are disproportionately male, black, and poor.[274] There is lack of equitable access to palliative care services in both the United Kingdom and the United States.[275]

Medical care

The medical management of patients with AIDS is complicated by a number of factors related to the underlying disease. The population is younger, making the transition to palliative care and advance care planning more difficult. There may be uncertainties about the trajectory of the illness and the prognosis.[275] Patients may present with multiple and complex medical problems: as well as underlying AIDS, they may be suffering from one or more opportunistic infections, hepatitis B or C, side effects of HAART such as diabetes, and other unrelated medical conditions. There may also be a history of drug or alcohol abuse.

The palliative care of patients with AIDS also involves difficult decisions about such matters as aggressive investigation and treatment of complications, or the withdrawal of antiretroviral or infection prophylaxis therapies. These decisions have to be made with each individual patient and must be concordant with their goals, priorities, and expectations, albeit that these can change frequently.

Advance care planning

Advance care planning is the process of planning future medical care, particularly for the situation where patients may no longer be able to make their own decisions.[276] Such planning would be particularly appropriate to AIDS, given the high incidence of organic brain dysfunction in the later stages. However, only about 50 per cent of patients with HIV/AIDS have discussions about end-of-life care; the proportion is lower in non-whites, IDUs, and those with a lower educational level.[277] A study of barriers preventing such discussions suggests it may relate more to the clinicians than the patients.[278] Advance care planning in patients with advanced cancer has been said to foster feelings of personal resolution, but in patients with HIV/AIDS the response rate was low and it led to lessening of patients' overall satisfaction with care.[279]

Goals of care and appropriate treatment

Many difficult clinical and ethical problems can arise in the advanced and terminal stages of AIDS. These arise because on the one hand the underlying retroviral infection is incurable, progressive, and ultimately fatal, but on the other hand many of its manifestations, which are responsible for much of the morbidity and mortality of AIDS, are eminently treatable. However, as patients become increasingly weak and debilitated, whether some investigations and therapies are appropriate has to be questioned. Patients with advanced disease are less able to tolerate invasive procedures and are more likely to suffer side effects of medication. Whether or not there has been advance care planning, there needs to be an ongoing partnership of care between the patient and the treatment team, with honest and open communication, to define the goals of care. The physician must be able to convey prognosis, even with its uncertainties, and what it is reasonable for the patient to hope for. This allows patients to make informed decisions about their own care and treatment, and ensures that all decisions about therapy are individualized.

What constitutes medical futility is rarely unequivocal and can lead to disagreement. This may occur if there are misunderstandings about prognosis or if the physician or the patient is pursuing unrealistic goals, matters that can usually be resolved by discussion. One survey showed that the majority of patients accepted that the doctor was not obliged to talk about treatments considered futile.[280]

Decisions should be made according to what is in the patient's best interest and directed at the quality of life. Investigations and therapies should only be pursued if they will provide benefit to the patient in terms of quality of life or in the context of their goals and unfinished business.

Polypharmacy

Patients with AIDS are frequently taking multiple medications. These may include antiretroviral drugs, multiple medications for the treatment and prevention of opportunistic infections, medications for symptom control, as well as drugs for unrelated medical conditions. There is a high incidence of drug side effects and a significant risk of drug interactions.[45,47,281] Medications should be continually reviewed and those that are not essential or worthwhile discontinued.

Stopping antiretroviral therapy

Antiretroviral therapy given during the earlier phases of AIDS may be of great clinical benefit to the patient. However, in the advanced stages, it is possibly of no benefit and, as it is usually associated with significant clinical toxicity, a decision may have to be made about continuing treatment. This may constitute a major psychological and emotional step for the patient to take and requires careful and compassionate discussion. Many patients have a considerable psychological investment in continuing antiretroviral medication and a decision to discontinue it requires an acknowledgement of the state of their disease and prognosis.

Stopping infection prophylaxis

Patients with AIDS are frequently taking large numbers of tablets, many with significant side effects, as prophylaxis against various infections. As the disease progresses, the question arises as to when these treatments can be withdrawn. The decision is finally up to the patients and depends on their appreciation of the state of their disease, which in turn depends upon the adequacy of medical communication. A decision to discontinue prophylactic therapy should be based on the inconvenience and toxicity of the treatment, the likelihood that recurrent infection will occur within the patient's expected time of survival, and whether or not the symptoms of such infection can be adequately palliated.

Prophylactic therapy for candidiasis and HSV infection should be continued indefinitely or until the patient is unable to swallow. These medications are not associated with significant toxicity and painful or distressing infection may occur within days or a week or two of stopping the treatment. Prophylaxis for pneumocystis and toxoplasmosis with cotrimoxazole is relatively free of side effects and can be continued as long as the patient is taking oral medications. Prophylaxis for MAC infection usually involves multiple drugs with significant side effects; for patients with advanced or terminal AIDS the symptoms of *M. avium* infection may be better controlled with NSAIDs or corticosteroids than by the use of multiple antibiotics. Ganciclovir maintenance therapy for CMV retinitis is the most difficult for patients to discontinue, as half will develop significant deterioration of vision or blindness within a few weeks.

Treatment of infections

Whether or not to actively treat opportunistic infections can pose problems and, given uncertainty about the prognosis of the underlying disease, the decision is often made to proceed with treatment. However, the patient's wishes, their tolerance of the side effects of treatment, and their general condition (including signs of advanced disease or dementia) have all to be considered and the decisions individualized.

Parenteral nutrition

Whether or not patients with advanced disease and severe or chronic diarrhoea should receive parenteral hydration and nutrition can be problematic. Decisions need to be individualized and based both on the wishes of the patients and their general condition (excluding the effects of the diarrhoea). Parenteral nutrition is expensive and not without side effects and its use can lead to difficult decisions about discontinuation at a later stage.

Corticosteroids

The use of corticosteroids can be of major symptomatic benefit in patients with advanced AIDS. It may lead to significant improvement in neuropathic and musculoskeletal pain, headache, dyspnoea, nausea and anorexia, lethargy and weakness, fevers and sweats. Many patients experience a feeling of improved well-being. However, corticosteroids may further compromise immune function and predispose to infection. The decision to use corticosteroids usually requires that the patient has accepted a shift from disease control to symptom control and depends on whether the patient believes that the short-term benefits outweigh the possible risk of additional infection.

Terminal care

The final pathway of terminal AIDS is not very different to that of cancer. Although the duration of the terminal phase may be more variable, the last few days of life of AIDS involve debility and dependency, semi-consciousness, poor oral intake, and may feature generalized pain, restlessness, and rattling respiration. These symptoms respond to the usual measures, including subcutaneous analgesia, anxiolytics, and anticholinergics (see Chapter 18).

Infection control

In managing patients with AIDS, all blood and body substances should be regarded as infectious and standard precautions should be followed. This will protect caregivers from infection with HIV, hepatitis, and enteric pathogens. Gloves are worn if there is, or may be, exposure to blood, mucous membranes, non-intact skin, or any other body fluid or material. Cuts or abrasions on worker's hands should be covered with an occlusive waterproof dressing. Masks, including eye protection, are used if there is risk of splashing of blood or other body fluid; this includes the management of patients with chest infection who are coughing. Procedures should be established for the disposal of contaminated linen, equipment, and waste, and for the management of spillages of blood or body fluids. Care is required when implementing these procedures as excessive or unreasonable safety precautions can accentuate a patient's feelings of isolation and discrimination.

The estimated risk of contracting HIV infection from a percutaneous injury (such as a needle stick) is 0.3 per cent.[282] The risk of mucous membrane exposure (splashes) is much smaller and there are only two anecdotal reports of such infection and none were observed in prospective studies. There is no evidence for infection resulting from cutaneous exposure, such as spilling blood on intact skin. Workers who are immunosuppressed or have exfoliative dermatitis should seek advice before working with AIDS patients.

AIDS patients with pulmonary tuberculosis can pose a risk to healthcare workers, especially if the infection is drug-resistant.[283,284] The management of patients with TB should be in conjunction with respiratory and infectious disease specialists, and good-quality face masks that effectively filter the inspired air are required.

Infection control precautions must be continued after the patient's death. Tissue and fluid from the body remain infectious for days. There should be minimal handling of the body, which is placed in a special sealed plastic bag. Embalming is not performed. Further viewing of the body may not be possible and the bereaved should be made aware of this before the body is sealed away.

Psychosocial and spiritual/existential problems

Psychological problems

The psychological impact of AIDS on patients and their caregivers is enormous and the possible sources of psychological distress are legion (Table 36).

Psychological distress is often described simply in terms of anxiety and depression, but in practice a wide range of psychological reactions and physical symptoms may be manifest (Table 37).[285] Most importantly, it should be remembered that unresolved psychosocial and spiritual/existential problems may manifest clinically as pain and physical symptoms unresponsive to treatment. Depression, anxiety, and demoralization have been discussed in the section on psychiatric disorders.

Patients from the male homosexual community, IDUs, and immigrants from areas where HIV is heterosexually endemic may have experienced multiple previous bereavements as friends and family died of AIDS. This may serve to heighten their distress as their own health deteriorates.

Male homosexuals may be distressed by the visible deterioration in their physical appearance that occurs with AIDS. Their sexual orientation may not have been disclosed to their biological family and the boundaries established between their biological and social families are often breached in the face of a life-threatening illness. A life-threatening illness often exposes the conflicts and guilt relating to the homosexual lifestyle, but dealing with these conflicts is usually left until late in the disease and non-resolution may aggravate both physical symptoms and psychological distress. There is often great concern about the maintenance of confidentiality regarding the diagnosis, for fear of the repercussions it might have for them, their families or friends. Many homosexual communities have developed good support networks, but the fact that many have suffered multiple previous bereavements and that the carer may also be infected complicates their effectiveness. Male homosexual couples may need special legal advice to ensure the rights and financial security of the surviving partner.

Intravenous drug users often have poor social networks and have problems with poor nutrition and poor housing. Chaotic lifestyles and the continued use of mind-altering drugs, together with a negative perception of health institutions, often lead to problems with compliance.[286]

Table 36 Sources of psychological distress

Disease	Progressive disease, uncertain life expectancy Unrelieved pain and physical symptoms Disfigurement, disabilities Long illness leading to psychological exhaustion
Patient	Fear of pain, paralysis, dementia, death Loss (or fear of loss) of control, independence, dignity Loss (or fear of loss) of job, social position Helplessness, hopelessness Unfinished business: personal, interpersonal, financial Anxious personality: neuroticism, hypochondriasis
Treatment team	Poor communication, lack of information Lack of involvement in decisions regarding care Exclusion of caregivers, partners
Treatment	Side effects Multiple failed treatments Diagnostic delays Bureaucratic red-tape
Social	Stigmatization within family, communities, society Discrimination, alienation Need for confidentiality, secrecy Lack or failure of social supports, resources Multiple previous bereavements Financial hardship Disassociation of biological and social family Accessing appropriate care

Table 37 Some clinical features of psychological distress

Anxiety	Sadness, misery, remorse
Depression	Regression
Anger, frustration, irritability	Withdrawal
Hopelessness, despair	Passivity
Helplessness	Avoidance
Denial	Inappropriate compensation (joyful)
Guilt	Lack of co-operation with carers
Fear	Unresponsive pain or physical symptoms
Grief	

The increasing incidence of AIDS in minority and immigrant groups has highlighted problems related to accessing care and patients from these groups tend to take up services late in the course of their illness. These groups usually have low socioeconomic status, poor housing, and financial problems. Migrant groups may bring with them different perceptions of health and language barriers may complicate care.

Psychological distress may have a profound effect on quality of life and it is reported that high levels of stress and coping by denial are associated with disease progression.[(194)] HAART may have less effect on psychological distress than on physical health.[(148)]

Treatment includes support and counselling and the provision of appropriate services. A trial designed to enable patients to identify sources of stress and develop adapting coping responses led to improved emotional health.[(287)] Complementary therapies incorporating stress management may be useful.[(288)] Whether the patients are from the male homosexual or IDU communities, immigrants or other minority groups, support and counselling needs to be done in a culturally appropriate and sensitive manner.

Social problems

Social problems encountered in the management of patients with AIDS may relate to alternative life styles with disassociation of biological and social family or to the socioeconomic problems experienced by marginalized and minority groups. The high incidence of dementia in the terminal stage makes it important that matters of guardianship and wills are dealt with at a relatively early stage. Because of the discrimination that exists in society, the patient's privacy and confidentiality need to be protected. Patients with AIDS can have difficulty obtaining or keeping accommodation and some are homeless. Housing is a particular problem for otherwise well, younger patients with moderate to severe dementia; if alternative accommodation cannot be provided, long-term residential care for these individuals often falls on palliative care units. Social discrimination may lead to problems with employment.

The adequacy of, and satisfaction with, social supports can have significant effect on quality of life.[(289,290)] Interventions to improve social supports and services may be of great benefit.

Spiritual and existential problems

Questions pertaining to spiritual and existential issues, questions about meaning and purpose, may arise as the result of any life event, but occur most frequently in response to a life-threatening illness. Spiritual or existential distress may manifest clinically as a need to discuss issues or as pain and physical symptoms that respond poorly to appropriate therapy. The management of existential distress is discussed elsewhere (see Chapters 11 and 12.1). For patients with HIV/AIDS, therapy must be in a culturally appropriate manner.

Quality of life

A number of different tools have been developed to measure quality of life in patients with HIV/AIDS.[(289–292)]

Multiple bereavements

Multiple losses result in significant psychological, social, and spiritual problems, and facilitating grief work can reduce abnormal grieving reactions and promote effective coping skills.[(293)] A trial of a brief group intervention significantly reduced distress and assisted resolution of the grieving process.[(294)]

Euthanasia and physician assisted suicide

It is reported that more than half of patients with HIV/AIDS in developed countries consider physician-assisted suicide (PAS) or euthanasia.[(295,296)]

In the Netherlands, one-third of patients dying with AIDS receive euthanasia or PAS;[(297,298)] given the paucity of palliative care services in that country, it is unlikely these patients received any significant palliative care. In the San Francisco Bay area, a significant proportion of doctors looking after patients with HIV/AIDS admit to performing PAS;[(299)] these were mostly general practitioners who are likely to have had little or no training in palliative care. In Oregon, only one patient with HIV/AIDS is reported to have used the programme of legalized PAS.[(300)] Another study from the United States reported that 12 per cent of patients dying with AIDS were given increased doses of medications by their partner with the intention of hastening death.[(301)]

In contrast, a report from the Mildmay Mission Hospice, a specialist palliative care service caring for patients with AIDS in London, recorded only one request for euthanasia amongst 1800 admissions over a 3-year period.[(302)]

Requests for assisted death from patients with HIV/AIDS have been linked to psychological and psychosocial distress, and to poor control of pain and symptoms. It is documented that people with HIV/AIDS have a higher rate of psychiatric symptoms such as depression and a higher risk of suicide,[(303)] and pre-morbid and co-morbid psychiatric syndromes, as distinct from the physical and psychological consequences of the disease itself, have been advanced as a possible explanation of the high rate of suicide in men with HIV/AIDS.[(304)] Patients with HIV/AIDS may be susceptible to the demoralization syndrome[(208,209)] (see above).

The strongest predictors of interest in PAS are reported to be depression, hopelessness, experience with terminal illness in a family member or friend, and lack of social supports.[(295)] A study to validate the Schedule of Attitudes Toward Hastened Death in patients with HIV/AIDS showed good correlation with ratings of depression and psychological distress and also with pain intensity and physical symptom distress.[(305)]

A study of the origins of the desire for assisted death in people with HIV/AIDS suggests it is a way of limiting the loss of self due to personal disintegration. Such disintegration results from symptoms and loss of function, and from loss of community that is in turn due to the individual's inability to initiate and maintain personal relationships.[303]

These studies underline the importance of comprehensive palliative care in the treatment of patients with HIV/AIDS. All patients should have access to quality palliative care services, practised by interdisciplinary teams experienced in palliative care, and with attention to both the physical and psychosocial aspects of care. A request for euthanasia should be handled like any other distressing symptom occurring in the palliative care setting; it requires careful assessment, identification and treatment of the cause or causes where possible, and provision of comprehensive multidisciplinary symptomatic and supportive care.

References

1. **UNAIDS**, AIDS epidemic update, December 2001 www.unaids. org.
2. **Communicable Disease Surveillance Centre** (2000). *HIV and AIDS in the UK*. An Epidemiological Review, 2000.
3. **National Centre in HIV Epidemiology and Clinical Research** (2001). HIV/AIDS, Viral Hepatitis and Sexually Transmissible Infections in Australia, Annual Surveillance Report 2001. Sydney, NSW: National Centre in HIV Epidemiology and Clinical Research, The University of New South Wales.
4. **Scheer, S.** et al. (2001). Effect of highly active antiretroviral therapy on diagnoses of sexually transmitted diseases in people with AIDS. *Lancet* **357**, 432–5.
5. **Hader, S.L.** et al. (2001). HIV infection in women in the United States: status at the Millennium. *Journal of the American Medical Association* **285**, 1186–92.
6. **Harries, A.D.** et al. (2001). Deaths from tuberculosis in sub-Saharan African countries with a high prevalence of HIV-1. *Lancet* **357**, 1519–23.
7. **Collaborative Group on AIDS Incubation and HIV Survival** (2000). Time from HIV-1 seroconversion to AIDS and death before widespread use of highly-active antiretroviral therapy: a collaborative re-analysis. *Lancet* **355**, 1131–7.
8. **Learmont, J.C.** et al. (1999). Immunologic and virologic status after 14 to 18 years of infection with an attenuated strain of HIV-1. A report from the Sydney Blood Bank Cohort. *New England Journal of Medicine* **340**, 1715–22.
9. **Chaisson, R.E., Keruly, J.C., and Moore, R.D.** (1995). Race, sex, drug use, and progression of human immunodeficiency virus disease. *New England Journal of Medicine* **333**, 751–6.
10. **CASCADE Collaboration** (2000). Survival after introduction of HAART in people with known duration of HIV-1 infection. The CASCADE Collaboration. Concerted Action on SeroConversion to AIDS and Death in Europe. *Lancet* **355**, 1158–9.
11. **Sterling, T.R.** et al. (2001). Initial plasma HIV-1 RNA levels and progression to AIDS in women and men. *New England Journal of Medicine* **344**, 720–5.
12. **Mellors, J.W.** et al. (1997). Plasma viral load and CD4+ lymphocytes as prognostic markers of HIV-1 infection. *Annals of Internal Medicine* **126**, 946–54.
13. **Hennessey, K.A.** et al. (2000). AIDS onset at high CD4+ cell levels is associated with high HIV load. *AIDS Research and Human Retroviruses* **16**, 103–7.
14. **Saul, J.** et al. (2001). The relationships between ethnicity, sex, risk group, and virus load in human immunodeficiency virus type 1 antiretroviral-naive patients. *Journal of Infectious Diseases* **183**, 1518–21.
15. **Kahn, J.O. and Walker, B.D.** (1998). Acute human immunodeficiency virus type 1 infection. *New England Journal of Medicine* **339**, 33–9.
16. **Centers for Disease Control** (1992). 1993 revised classification system for HIV infection and expanded surveillance case definition for AIDS among adolescents and adults. *Morbidity and Mortality Weekly Report* **41**, 1–19.
17. **Mocroft, A.** et al. (1997). Survival after diagnosis of AIDS: a prospective observational study of 2625 patients. Royal Free/Chelsea and Westminster Hospitals Collaborative Group. *British Medical Journal* **314**, 409–13.
18. **Kassa, E.** et al. (1999). Evaluation of the World Health Organization staging system for HIV infection and disease in Ethiopia: association between clinical stages and laboratory markers. *AIDS* **13**, 381–9.
19. **Malamba, S.S.** et al. (1999). The prognostic value of the World Health Organization staging system for HIV infection and disease in rural Uganda. *AIDS* **13**, 2555–62.
20. **Expert Working Group on Integrated Palliative Care for Persons with AIDS** (1988). Summary of a report submitted to Health and Welfare, Canada. *Journal of Palliative Care* **4**, 76–86.
21. **Pomerantz, R.J.** (2001). Initiating antiretroviral therapy during HIV infection: confusion and clarity. *Journal of the American Medical Association* **286**, 2597–9.
22. **HIVATIS**, HIV/AIDS Treatment Information Service www.aidsinfo.nih.gov.
23. **Detels, R.** et al. (1998). Effectiveness of potent antiretroviral therapy on time to AIDS and death in men with known HIV infection duration. Multicenter AIDS Cohort Study Investigators. *Journal of the American Medical Association* **280**, 1497–503.
24. **Palella, F.J. Jr.** et al. (1998). Declining morbidity and mortality among patients with advanced human immunodeficiency virus infection. HIV Outpatient Study Investigators. *New England Journal of Medicine* **338**, 853–60.
25. **Hammer, S.M.** et al. (1997). A controlled trial of two nucleoside analogues plus indinavir in persons with human immunodeficiency virus infection and CD4 cell counts of 200 per cubic millimeter or less. AIDS Clinical Trials Group 320 Study Team. *New England Journal of Medicine* **337**, 725–33.
26. **Erb, P.** et al. (2000). Effect of antiretroviral therapy on viral load, CD4 cell count, and progression to acquired immunodeficiency syndrome in a community human immunodeficiency virus-infected cohort. Swiss HIV Cohort Study. *Archives of Internal Medicine* **160**, 1134–40.
27. **Sepkowitz, K.A.** (1998). Effect of HAART on natural history of AIDS-related opportunistic disorders. *Lancet* **351**, 228–30.
28. **Ledergerber, B.** et al. (1999). AIDS-related opportunistic illnesses occurring after initiation of potent antiretroviral therapy: the Swiss HIV Cohort Study. *Journal of the American Medical Association* **282**, 2220–6.
29. **Detels, R.** et al. (2001). Effectiveness of potent antiretroviral therapies on the incidence of opportunistic infections before and after AIDS diagnosis. *AIDS* **15**, 347–55.
30. **Currier, J.S.** (2000). Discontinuing prophylaxis for opportunistic infection: guiding principles. *Clinical Infectious Diseases* **30** (Suppl. 1), S66–71.
31. **Dworkin, M.S.** et al. (2000). Risk for preventable opportunistic infections in persons with AIDS after antiretroviral therapy increases CD4+ T lymphocyte counts above prophylaxis thresholds. *Journal of Infectious Diseases* **182**, 611–15.
32. **Kovacs, J.A. and Masur, H.** (2000). Prophylaxis against opportunistic infections in patients with human immunodeficiency virus infection. *New England Journal of Medicine* **342**, 1416–29.
33. **Sacktor, N.** et al. (2001). HIV-associated neurologic disease incidence changes: Multicenter AIDS Cohort Study, 1990–1998. *Neurology* **56**, 257–60.
34. **Price, R.W.** et al. (1999). Neurological outcomes in late HIV infection: adverse impact of neurological impairment on survival and protective effect of antiviral therapy. AIDS Clinical Trial Group and Neurological AIDS Research Consortium study team. *AIDS* **13**, 1677–85.
35. **Suarez, S.** et al. (2001). Outcome of patients with HIV-1-related cognitive impairment on highly active antiretroviral therapy. *AIDS* **15**, 195–200.
36. **Thurnher, M.M.** et al. (2000). Highly active antiretroviral therapy for patients with AIDS dementia complex: effect on MR imaging findings and clinical course. *American Journal of Neuroradiology* **21**, 670–8.
37. **Giudici, B.** et al. (2000). Highly active antiretroviral therapy and progressive multifocal leukoencephalopathy: effects on cerebrospinal fluid markers of JC virus replication and immune response. *Clinical Infectious Diseases* **30**, 95–9.
38. **Buchbinder, S.P.** et al. (1999). Combination antiretroviral therapy and incidence of AIDS-related malignancies. *Journal of Acquired Immune Deficiency Syndrome* **21** (Suppl. 1), S23–6.
39. **Appleby, P.** et al. (2000). Highly active antiretroviral therapy and incidence of cancer in human immunodeficiency virus-infected adults. *Journal of the National Cancer Institute* **92**, 1823–30.
40. **Matthews, G.V.** et al. (2000). Changes in acquired immunodeficiency syndrome-related lymphoma since the introduction of highly active anti-retro-viral therapy. *Blood* **96**, 2730–4.
41. **Behrens, G.M.** et al. (2000). Immune reconstitution syndromes in human immuno-deficiency virus infection following effective antiretroviral therapy. *Immunobiology* **202**, 186–93.

42. **DeSimone, J.A., Pomerantz, R.J., and Babinchak, T.J.** (2000). Inflammatory reactions in HIV-1-infected persons after initiation of highly active antiretroviral therapy. *Annals of Internal Medicine* **133**, 447–54.
43. **Sansone, G.R. and Frengley, J.D.** (2000). Impact of HAART on causes of death of persons with late-stage AIDS. *Journal of Urban Health* **77**, 166–75.
44. **Fellay, J.** et al. (2001). Prevalence of adverse events associated with potent antiretroviral treatment: Swiss HIV Cohort Study. *Lancet* **358**, 1322–7.
45. **Carr, A. and Cooper, D.A.** (2000). Adverse effects of antiretroviral therapy. *Lancet* **356**, 1423–30.
46. **Thiebaut, R.** et al. (2000). Lipodystrophy, metabolic disorders, and human immunodeficiency virus infection: Aquitaine Cohort, France, 1999. Groupe d'Epidemiologie Clinique du Syndrome d'Immunodeficience Acquise en Aquitaine. *Clinical Infectious Diseases* **31**, 1482–7.
47. **Piscitelli, S.C. and Gallicano, K.D.** (2001). Interactions among drugs for HIV and opportunistic infections. *New England Journal of Medicine* **344**, 984–96.
48. **Brook, M.G.** et al. (2001). Adherence to highly active antiretroviral therapy in the real world: experience of twelve English HIV units. *AIDS Patient Care STDS* **15**, 491–4.
49. **Little, S.J.** (2001). Is transmitted drug resistance in HIV on the rise? *British Medical Journal* **322**, 1074–5.
50. **UK Collaborative Group on Monitoring the Transmission of HIV Drug Resistance** (2001). Analysis of prevalence of HIV-1 drug resistance in primary infections in the United Kingdom. *British Medical Journal* **322**, 1087–8.
51. **Deeks, S.G.** et al. (1999). HIV RNA and CD4 cell count response to protease inhibitor therapy in an urban AIDS clinic: response to both initial and salvage therapy. *AIDS* **13**, F35–43.
52. **Piketty, C.** et al. (2001). Long-term clinical outcome of human immunodeficiency virus-infected patients with discordant immunologic and virologic responses to a protease inhibitor-containing regimen. *Journal of Infectious Diseases* **183**, 1328–35.
53. **Polis, M.A.** et al. (2001). Correlation between reduction in plasma HIV-1 RNA concentration 1 week after start of antiretroviral treatment and longer-term efficacy. *Lancet* **358**, 1760–5.
54. **Ledergerber, B.** et al. (1999). Clinical progression and virological failure on highly active antiretroviral therapy in HIV-1 patients: a prospective cohort study. Swiss HIV Cohort Study. *Lancet* **353**, 863–8.
55. **Mocroft, A.** et al. (2000). Immunological, virological and clinical response to highly active antiretroviral therapy treatment regimens in a complete clinic population. Royal Free Centre for HIV Medicine. *AIDS* **14**, 1545–52.
56. **Chun, T.W. and Fauci, A.S.** (1999). Latent reservoirs of HIV: obstacles to the eradication of virus. *Proceedings of the National Academy of Sciences of the USA* **96**, 10958–61.
57. **Orenstein, J.M.** et al. (1999). Lymph node architecture preceding and following 6 months of potent antiviral therapy: follicular hyperplasia persists in parallel with p24 antigen restoration after involution and CD4 cell depletion in an AIDS patient. *AIDS* **13**, 2219–29.
58. **Fischer, M.** et al. (2000). Residual HIV-RNA levels persist for up to 2.5 years in peripheral blood mononuclear cells of patients on potent antiretroviral therapy. *AIDS Research and Human Retroviruses* **16**, 1135–40.
59. **Harrigan, P.R., Whaley, M., and Montaner, J.S.** (1999). Rate of HIV-1 RNA rebound upon stopping antiretroviral therapy. *AIDS* **13**, F59–62.
60. **Centers for Disease Control and Prevention** (1999). 1999 USPHS/IDSA guidelines for the prevention of opportunistic infections in persons infected with human immunodeficiency virus: US Public Health Service (USPHS) and Infectious Diseases Society of America (IDSA). *Morbidity and Mortality Weekly Report* **48**, 1–66.
61. **Benfield, T.L.** et al. (2001). Prognostic markers of short-term mortality in AIDS-associated *Pneumocystis carinii* pneumonia. *Chest* **119**, 844–51.
62. **Bozzette, S.A.** et al. (1990). A controlled trial of early adjunctive treatment with corticosteroids for *Pneumocystis carinii* pneumonia in the acquired immunodeficiency syndrome. California Collaborative Treatment Group. *New England Journal of Medicine* **323**, 1451–7.
63. **Ledergerber, B.** et al. (2001). Discontinuation of secondary prophylaxis against *Pneumocystis carinii* pneumonia in patients with HIV infection who have a response to antiretroviral therapy. Eight European Study Groups. *New England Journal of Medicine* **344**, 168–74.
64. **Lopez Bernaldo de Quiros, J.C.** et al. (2001). A randomized trial of the discontinuation of primary and secondary prophylaxis against *Pneumocystis carinii* pneumonia after highly active antiretroviral therapy in patients with HIV infection. Grupo de Estudio del SIDA 04/98. *New England Journal of Medicine* **344**, 159–67.
65. **van der Horst, C.M.** et al. (1997). Treatment of cryptococcal meningitis associated with the acquired immunodeficiency syndrome. National Institute of Allergy and Infectious Diseases Mycoses Study Group and AIDS Clinical Trials Group. *New England Journal of Medicine* **337**, 15–21.
66. **Kurup, A.** et al. (1999). Disseminated *Penicillium marneffei* infection: a report of five cases in Singapore. *Annals of the Academy of Medicine, Singapore* **28**, 605–9.
67. **Supparatpinyo, K.** et al. (1998). A controlled trial of itraconazole to prevent relapse of Penicillium marneffei infection in patients infected with the human immunodeficiency virus. *New England Journal of Medicine* **339**, 1739–43.
68. **Holding, K.J.** et al. (2000). Aspergillosis among people infected with human immunodeficiency virus: incidence and survival. Adult and Adolescent Spectrum of HIV Disease Project. *Clinical Infectious Diseases* **31**, 1253–7.
69. **Jones, N.** et al. (2000). Nocardial infection as a complication of HIV in South Africa. *Journal of Infection* **41**, 232–9.
70. **Hewitt, R.G.** et al. (2000). Paromomycin: no more effective than placebo for treatment of cryptosporidiosis in patients with advanced human immunodeficiency virus infection. AIDS Clinical Trial Group. *Clinical Infectious Diseases* **31**, 1084–92.
71. **Maggi, P.** et al. (2000). Effect of antiretroviral therapy on cryptosporidiosis and microsporidiosis in patients infected with human immunodeficiency virus type 1. *European Journal of Clinical Microbiology and Infectious Diseases* **19**, 213–17.
72. **Carr, A.** et al. (1998). Treatment of HIV-1-associated microsporidiosis and cryptosporidiosis with combination antiretroviral therapy. *Lancet* **351**, 256–61.
73. **Holmberg, S.D.** et al. (1998). Possible effectiveness of clarithromycin and rifabutin for cryptosporidiosis chemoprophylaxis in HIV disease. HIV Outpatient Study (HOPS) Investigators. *Journal of the American Medical Association* **279**, 384–6.
74. **Molina, J.M.** et al. (2000). Trial of oral fumagillin for the treatment of intestinal microsporidiosis in patients with HIV infection. ANRS 054 Study Group. Agence Nationale de Recherche sur le SIDA. *AIDS* **14**, 1341–8.
75. **Verdier, R.I.** et al. (2000). Trimethoprim–sulfamethoxazole compared with ciprofloxacin for treatment and prophylaxis of *Isospora belli* and *Cyclospora cayetanensis* infection in HIV-infected patients. A randomized, controlled trial. *Annals of Internal Medicine* **132**, 885–8.
76. **Laguna, F.** et al. (1999). Treatment of visceral leishmaniasis in HIV-infected patients: a randomized trial comparing meglumine antimoniate with amphotericin B. Spanish HIV-Leishmania Study Group. *AIDS* **13**, 1063–9.
77. **Murray, H.W.** (1999). Kala-azar as an AIDS-related opportunistic infection. *AIDS Patient Care STDS* **13**, 459–65.
78. **Sartori, A.M.** et al. (1998). Follow-up of 18 patients with human immunodeficiency virus infection and chronic Chagas' disease, with reactivation of Chagas' disease causing cardiac disease in three patients. *Clinical Infectious Diseases* **26**, 177–9.
79. **Dedet, J.P. and Pratlong, F.** (2000). Leishmania, Trypanosoma and monoxenous trypanosomatids as emerging opportunistic agents. *Journal of Eukaryotic Microbiology* **47**, 37–9.
80. **Havlir, D.V. and Barnes, P.F.** (1999). Tuberculosis in patients with human immunodeficiency virus infection. *New England Journal of Medicine* **340**, 367–73.
81. **Sonnenberg, P.** et al. (2001). HIV-1 and recurrence, relapse, and reinfection of tuberculosis after cure: a cohort study in South African mineworkers. *Lancet* **358**, 1687–93.
82. **Dye, C.** et al. (1999). Consensus statement. Global burden of tuberculosis: estimated incidence, prevalence, and mortality by country. WHO Global Surveillance and Monitoring Project. *Journal of the American Medical Association* **282**, 677–86.
83. **Girardi, E.** et al. (2001). Changing clinical presentation and survival in HIV-associated tuberculosis after highly active antiretroviral therapy. *Journal of Acquired Immune Deficiency Syndrome* **26**, 326–31.

84. **Bucher, H.C.** et al. (1999). Isoniazid prophylaxis for tuberculosis in HIV infection: a meta-analysis of randomized controlled trials. *AIDS* **13**, 501–7.

85. **Gordin, F.** et al. (2000). Rifampin and pyrazinamide vs isoniazid for prevention of tuberculosis in HIV-infected persons: an international randomized trial. Terry Beirn Community Programs for Clinical Research on AIDS, the Adult AIDS Clinical Trials Group, the Pan American Health Organization, and the Centers for Disease Control and Prevention Study Group. *Journal of the American Medical Association* **283**, 1445–50.

86. **Fitzgerald, D.W.** et al. (2000). Active tuberculosis in individuals infected with human immunodeficiency virus after isoniazid prophylaxis. *Clinical Infectious Diseases* **31**, 1495–7.

87. **Fitzgerald, D.W.** et al. (2000). Effect of post-treatment isoniazid on prevention of recurrent tuberculosis in HIV-1-infected individuals: a randomised trial. *Lancet* **356**, 1470–4.

88. **Singer, J.** et al. (2000). Symptomatic and health status outcomes in the Canadian randomized MAC treatment trial (CTN010). Canadian HIV Trials Network Protocol 010 Study Group. *International Journal of STD and AIDS* **11**, 212–19.

89. **Race, E.M.** et al. (1998). Focal mycobacterial lymphadenitis following initiation of protease-inhibitor therapy in patients with advanced HIV-1 disease. *Lancet* **351**, 252–5.

90. **Mohle-Boetani, J.C.** et al. (1996). Bacillary angiomatosis and bacillary peliosis in patients infected with human immunodeficiency virus: clinical characteristics in a case–control study. *Clinical Infectious Diseases* **22**, 794–800.

91. **Jabs, D.A.** (2001). The ganciclovir implant plus oral ganciclovir versus parenteral cidofovir for the treatment of cytomegalovirus retinitis in patients with acquired immunodeficiency syndrome: The Ganciclovir Cidofovir Cytomegalovirus Retinitis Trial. *American Journal of Ophthalmology* **131**, 457–67.

92. **Deayton, J.R.** et al. (2000). Changes in the natural history of cytomegalovirus retinitis following the introduction of highly active antiretroviral therapy. *AIDS* **14**, 1163–70.

93. **Lalezari, J.** et al. (1997). A randomized, double-blind, placebo-controlled trial of cidofovir gel for the treatment of acyclovir-unresponsive mucocutaneous herpes simplex virus infection in patients with AIDS. *Journal of Infectious Diseases* **176**, 892–8.

94. **Gilson, R.J.** et al. (1999). A randomized, controlled, safety study using imiquimod for the topical treatment of anogenital warts in HIV-infected patients. Imiquimod Study Group. *AIDS* **13**, 2397–404.

95. **Javaly, K.** et al. (1999). Treatment of mucocutaneous herpes simplex virus infections unresponsive to acyclovir with topical foscarnet cream in AIDS patients: a phase I/II study. *Journal of Acquired Immune Deficiency Syndrome* **21**, 301–6.

96. **Gilden, D.H.** et al. (2000). Neurologic complications of the reactivation of varicella-zoster virus. *New England Journal of Medicine* **342**, 635–45.

97. **Meadows, K.P.** et al. (1997). Resolution of recalcitrant molluscum contagiosum virus lesions in human immunodeficiency virus-infected patients treated with cidofovir. *Archives of Dermatology* **133**, 987–90.

98. **Hengge, U.R.** et al. (2000). Self-administered topical 5% imiquimod for the treatment of common warts and molluscum contagiosum. *British Journal of Dermatology* **143**, 1026–31.

99. **Brown, C.W. Jr.** et al. (2000). Recalcitrant molluscum contagiosum in an HIV-afflicted male treated successfully with topical imiquimod. *Cutis* **65**, 363–6.

100. **Snoeck, R.** et al. (1995). Treatment of anogenital papillomavirus infections with an acyclic nucleoside phosphonate analogue. *New England Journal of Medicine* **333**, 943–4.

101. **Goedert, J.J.** et al. (1998). Spectrum of AIDS-associated malignant disorders. *Lancet* **351**, 1833–9.

102. **Frisch, M.** et al. (2001). Association of cancer with AIDS-related immunosuppression in adults. *Journal of the American Medical Association* **285**, 1736–45.

103. **Cohen, J.I.** (2000). Epstein–Barr virus infection. *New England Journal of Medicine* **343**, 481–92.

104. **Frisch, M., Biggar, R.J., and Goedert, J.J.** (2000). Human papillomavirus-associated cancers in patients with human immunodeficiency virus infection and acquired immunodeficiency syndrome. *Journal of the National Cancer Institute* **92**, 1500–10.

105. **Jones, J.L.** et al. (1999). Effect of antiretroviral therapy on recent trends in selected cancers among HIV-infected persons. Adult/Adolescent Spectrum of HIV Disease Project Group. *Journal of Acquired Immune Deficiency Syndrome* **21** (Suppl. 1), S11–17.

106. **Chokunonga, E.** et al. (1999). Aids and cancer in Africa: the evolving epidemic in Zimbabwe. *AIDS* **13**, 2583–8.

107. **Parkin, D.M.** et al. (1999). AIDS-related cancers in Africa: maturation of the epidemic in Uganda. *AIDS* **13**, 2563–70.

108. **Antman, K. and Chang, Y.** (2000). Kaposi's sarcoma. *New England Journal of Medicine* **342**, 1027–38.

109. **Campbell, T.B.** et al. (2000). Relationship of human herpesvirus 8 peripheral blood virus load and Kaposi's sarcoma clinical stage. *AIDS* **14**, 2109–16.

110. **Moore, P.S.** (2000). The emergence of Kaposi's sarcoma-associated herpesvirus (human herpesvirus 8). *New England Journal of Medicine* **343**, 1411–13.

111. **Thomas, J.O.** (2001). Acquired immunodeficiency syndrome-associated cancers in Sub-Saharan Africa. *Seminars in Oncology* **28**, 198–206.

112. **Aboulafia, D.M.** (2000). The epidemiologic, pathologic, and clinical features of AIDS-associated pulmonary Kaposi's sarcoma. *Chest* **117**, 1128–45.

113. **Bodsworth, N.J.** et al. (2001). Phase III vehicle-controlled, multi-centered study of topical alitretinoin gel 0.1% in cutaneous AIDS-related Kaposi's sarcoma. *American Journal of Clinical Dermatology* **2**, 77–87.

114. **Scolaro, M.J.** et al. (2001). The antiviral drug docosanol as a treatment for Kaposi's sarcoma lesions in HIV type 1-infected patients: a pilot clinical study. *AIDS Research and Human Retroviruses* **17**, 35–43.

115. **Nunez, M.** et al. (2001). Response to liposomal doxorubicin and clinical outcome of HIV-1-infected patients with Kaposi's sarcoma receiving highly active antiretroviral therapy. *HIV Clinical Trials* **2**, 429–37.

116. **Little, R.F.** et al. (2000). Activity of thalidomide in AIDS-related Kaposi's sarcoma. *Journal of Clinical Oncology* **18**, 2593–602.

117. **Bower, M.** et al. (1999). Treatment outcome in presumed and confirmed AIDS-related primary cerebral lymphoma. *European Journal of Cancer* **35**, 601–4.

118. **Chamberlain, M.C. and Kormanik, P.A.** (1999). AIDS-related central nervous system lymphomas. *Journal of Neurooncology* **43**, 269–76.

119. **Rossi, G.** et al. (1999). The International Prognostic Index can be used as a guide to treatment decisions regarding patients with human immunodeficiency virus-related systemic non-Hodgkin lymphoma. *Cancer* **86**, 2391–7.

120. **Ratner, L.** et al. (2001). Chemotherapy for human immunodeficiency virus-associated non-Hodgkin's lymphoma in combination with highly active antiretroviral therapy. *Journal of Clinical Oncology* **19**, 2171–8.

121. **Powles, T., Matthews, G., and Bower, M.** (2000). AIDS related systemic non-Hodgkin's lymphoma. *Sexually Transmitted Infections* **76**, 335–41.

122. **Remick, S.C.** et al. (2001). Oral combination chemotherapy in conjunction with filgrastim (G-CSF) in the treatment of AIDS-related non-Hodgkin's lymphoma: evaluation of the role of G-CSF; quality-of-life analysis and long-term follow-up. *American Journal of Hematology* **66**, 178–88.

123. **Gabarre, J.** et al. (2000). High-dose therapy and autologous haematopoietic stem-cell transplantation for HIV-1-associated lymphoma. *Lancet* **355**, 1071–2.

124. **Powles, T. and Bower, M.** (2000). HIV-associated Hodgkin's disease. *International Journal of STD and AIDS* **11**, 492–4.

125. **Levine, A.M.** et al. (2000). Chemotherapy consisting of doxorubicin, bleomycin, vinblastine, and dacarbazine with granulocyte-colony-stimulating factor in HIV-infected patients with newly diagnosed Hodgkin's disease: a prospective, multi-institutional AIDS clinical trials group study (ACTG 149). *Journal of Acquired Immune Deficiency Syndrome* **24**, 444–50.

126. **Sun, X.W.** et al. (1997). Human papillomavirus infection in women infected with the human immunodeficiency virus. *New England Journal of Medicine* **337**, 1343–9.

127. **Heard, I.** et al. (2000). Increased risk of cervical disease among human immunodeficiency virus-infected women with severe immunosuppression

and high human papillomavirus load(1). *Obstetrics and Gynecology* **96**, 403–9.

128. **Cardillo, M.** et al. (2001). CD4 T-cell count, viral load, and squamous intraepithelial lesions in women infected with the human immunodeficiency virus. *Cancer* **93**, 111–14.
129. **Davis, A.T.** et al. (2001). Cervical dysplasia in women infected with the human immunodeficiency virus (HIV): a correlation with HIV viral load and CD4+ count. *Gynecologic Oncology* **80**, 350–4.
130. **Dorrucci, M.** et al. (2001). Incidence of invasive cervical cancer in a cohort of HIV-seropositive women before and after the introduction of highly active antiretroviral therapy. *Journal of Acquired Immune Deficiency Syndrome* **26**, 377–80.
131. **Maiman, M.** et al. (1997). Cervical cancer as an AIDS-defining illness. *Obstetrics and Gynecology* **89**, 76–80.
132. **Palefsky, J.M.** (2000). Anal squamous intraepithelial lesions in human immunodeficiency virus-positive men and women. *Seminars in Oncology* **27**, 471–9.
133. **Cleator, S.** et al. (2000). Treatment of HIV-associated invasive anal cancer with combined chemoradiation. *European Journal of Cancer* **36**, 754–8.
134. **Vogl, D.** et al. (1999). Symptom prevalence, characteristics, and distress in AIDS outpatients. *Journal of Pain and Symptom Management* **18**, 253–62.
135. **Mathews, W.C.** et al. (2000). National estimates of HIV-related symptom prevalence from the HIV Cost and Services Utilization Study. *Medical Care* **38**, 750–62.
136. **Lorenz, K.A.** et al. (2001). Associations of symptoms and health-related quality of life: findings from a national study of persons with HIV infection. *Annals of Internal Medicine* **134**, 854–60.
137. **Foley, F.J. and Huggins, M.A.** (1994). AIDS palliative care. *Journal of Palliative Care* **10**, 133.
138. **McComsey, G.A.** et al. (2001). Placebo-controlled trial of prednisone in advanced HIV-1 infection. *AIDS* **15**, 321–7.
139. **Glare, P.A. and Cooney, N.J.** (1996). Managing HIV. Part 5: treating secondary outcomes. 5.19 HIV and palliative care. *Medical Journal of Australia* **164**, 612–15.
140. **Hanks, G.** et al. (1998). Difficult pain problems. In *Oxford Textbook of Palliative Medicine* 2nd edn. (ed. D. Doyle, G.W.C. Hanks, and N. MacDonald), Oxford: Oxford University Press.
141. **Breitbart, W.** et al. (1996). Pain in ambulatory AIDS patients. I: pain characteristics and medical correlates. *Pain* **68**, 315–21.
142. **Larue, F., Fontaine, A., and Colleau, S.M.** (1997). Underestimation and undertreatment of pain in HIV disease: multicentre study. *British Medical Journal* **314**, 23–8.
143. **Frich, L.M. and Borgbjerg, F.M.** (2000). Pain and pain treatment in AIDS patients: a longitudinal study. *Journal of Pain and Symptom Management* **19**, 339–47.
144. **Rotheram-Borus, M.J.** (2000). Variations in perceived pain associated with emotional distress and social identity in AIDS. *AIDS Patient Care in STDs* **14**, 659–65.
145. **Rosenfeld, B.** et al. (1996). Pain in ambulatory AIDS patients. II: impact of pain on psychological functioning and quality of life. *Pain* **68**, 323–8.
146. **Del Borgo, C.** et al. (2001). Multidimensional aspects of pain in HIV-infected individuals. *AIDS Patient Care in STDs* **15**, 95–102.
147. **Hewitt, D.J.** et al. (1997). Pain syndromes and etiologies in ambulatory AIDS patients. *Pain* **70**, 117–23.
148. **Brechtl, J.R.** et al. (2001). The use of highly active antiretroviral therapy (haart) in patients with advanced HIV infection. Impact on medical, palliative care, and quality of life outcomes. *Journal of Pain and Symptom Management* **21**, 41–51.
149. **Shlay, J.C.** et al. (1998). Acupuncture and amitriptyline for pain due to HIV-related peripheral neuropathy: a randomized controlled trial. Terry Beirn Community Programs for Clinical Research on AIDS. *Journal of the American Medical Association* **280**, 1590–5.
150. **Kemper, C.A.** et al. (1998). Mexiletine for HIV-infected patients with painful peripheral neuropathy: a double-blind, placebo-controlled, crossover treatment trial. *Journal of Acquired Immune Deficiency Syndromes and Human Retrovirology* **19**, 367–72.
151. **Kieburtz, K.** et al. (1998). A randomized trial of amitriptyline and mexiletine for painful neuropathy in HIV infection. AIDS Clinical Trial Group 242 Protocol Team. *Neurology* **51**, 1682–8.
152. **Simpson, D.M.** et al. (2000). A placebo-controlled trial of lamotrigine for painful HIV-associated neuropathy. *Neurology* **54**, 2115–19.
153. **La Spina, I.** et al. (2001). Gabapentin in painful HIV-related neuropathy: a report of 19 patients, preliminary observations. *European Journal of Neurology* **8**, 71–5.
154. **Simpson, D.M.** et al. (1996). Peptide T in the treatment of painful distal neuropathy associated with AIDS: results of a placebo-controlled trial. The Peptide T Neuropathy Study Group. *Neurology* **47**, 1254–9.
155. **Paice, J.A.** et al. (2000). Efficacy of a vibratory stimulus for the relief of HIV-associated neuropathic pain. *Pain* **84**, 291–6.
156. **Paice, J.A.** et al. (2000). Topical capsaicin in the management of HIV-associated peripheral neuropathy. *Journal of Pain and Symptom Management* **19**, 45–52.
157. **Kaplan, R.** et al. (1996). Sustained-release morphine sulfate in the management of pain associated with acquired immune deficiency syndrome. *Journal of Pain and Symptom Management* **12**, 150–60.
158. **Newshan, G. and Lefkowitz, M.** (2001). Transdermal fentanyl for chronic pain in AIDS: a pilot study. *Journal of Pain and Symptom Management* **21**, 69–77.
159. **Breitbart, W.** et al. (1996). The undertreatment of pain in ambulatory AIDS patients. *Pain* **65**, 243–9.
160. **Breitbart, W., Kaim, M., and Rosenfeld, B.** (1999). Clinicians' perceptions of barriers to pain management in AIDS. *Journal of Pain and Symptom Management* **18**, 203–12.
161. **Breitbart, W.** et al. (1998). Patient-related barriers to pain management in ambulatory AIDS patients. *Pain* **76**, 9–16.
162. **Breitbart, W.** et al. (1997). A comparison of pain report and adequacy of analgesic therapy in ambulatory AIDS patients with and without a history of substance abuse. *Pain* **72**, 235–43.
163. **Martin, C.** et al. (1999). Pain in ambulatory HIV-infected patients with and without intravenous drug use. *European Journal of Pain* **3**, 157–64.
164. **Kaplan, R.** et al. (2000). A titrated morphine analgesic regimen comparing substance users and non-users with AIDS-related pain. *Journal of Pain and Symptom Management* **19**, 265–73.
165. **Corcoran, C. and Grinspoon, S.** (1999). Treatments for wasting in patients with the acquired immunodeficiency syndrome. *New England Journal of Medicine* **340**, 1740–50.
166. **Sullivan, P.S.** et al. (2000). Epidemiology of thrombosis in HIV-infected individuals. The Adult/Adolescent Spectrum of HIV Disease Project. *AIDS* **14**, 321–4.
167. **Rietschel, P.** et al. (2000). Prevalence of hypogonadism among men with weight loss related to human immunodeficiency virus infection who were receiving highly active antiretroviral therapy. *Clinical Infectious Diseases* **31**, 1240–4.
168. **Lyles, R.H.** et al. (1999). Virologic, immunologic, and immune activation markers as predictors of HIV-associated weight loss prior to AIDS. Multicenter AIDS Cohort Study. *Journal of Acquired Immune Deficiency Syndrome* **22**, 386–94.
169. **Wagner, G.J. and Rabkin, J.G.** (1999). Development of the Impact of Weight Loss Scale (IWLS): a psychometric study in a sample of men with HIV/AIDS. *AIDS Care* **11**, 453–7.
170. **Batterham, M.J. and Garsia, R.** (2001). A comparison of megestrol acetate, nandrolone decanoate and dietary counselling for HIV associated weight loss. *International Journal of Andrology* **24**, 232–40.
171. **Kaplan, G.** et al. (2000). Thalidomide for the treatment of AIDS-associated wasting. *AIDS Research and Human Retroviruses* **16**, 1345–55.
172. **Grinspoon, S.** et al. (2000). Effects of testosterone and progressive resistance training in eugonadal men with AIDS wasting. A randomized, controlled trial. *Annals of Internal Medicine* **133**, 348–55.
173. **Grinspoon, S.** et al. (1999). Sustained anabolic effects of long-term androgen administration in men with AIDS wasting. *Clinical Infectious Diseases* **28**, 634–6.
174. **Clark, R.H.** et al. (2000). Nutritional treatment for acquired immunodeficiency virus-associated wasting using beta-hydroxy beta-methylbutyrate,

glutamine, and arginine: a randomized, double-blind, placebo-controlled study. *Journal of Parenteral and Enteral Nutrition* **24**, 133–9.

175. **Wagner, G.J. and Rabkin, R.** (2000). Effects of dextroamphetamine on depression and fatigue in men with HIV: a double-blind, placebo-controlled trial. *Journal of Clinical Psychiatry* **61**, 436–40.
176. **Breitbart, W.** et al. (2001). A randomized, double-blind, placebo-controlled trial of psychostimulants for the treatment of fatigue in ambulatory patients with human immunodeficiency virus disease. *Annals of Internal Medicine* **161**, 411–20.
177. **Jellinger, K.A.** et al. (2000). Neuropathology and general autopsy findings in AIDS during the last 15 years. *Acta Neuropathology (Berlin)* **100**, 213–20.
178. **Price, R.W.** (1999). Management of the neurological complications of HIV-1 infection and AIDS. In *Management of the Neurological Complications of HIV-1 Infection and AIDS* (ed. M.A. Sande and P. Volberding), Philadelphia: WB Saunders.
179. **Hriso, E.** et al. (1991). Extrapyramidal symptoms due to dopamine-blocking agents in patients with AIDS encephalopathy. *American Journal of Psychiatry* **148**, 1558–61.
180. **Stern, Y.** et al. (2001). Factors associated with incident human immunodeficiency virus-dementia. *Archives in Neurology* **58**, 473–9.
181. **Castellon, S.A., Hinkin, C.H., and Myers, H.F.** (2000). Neuropsychiatric disturbance is associated with executive dysfunction in HIV-1 infection. *Journal of the International Neuropsychology Society* **6**, 336–47.
182. **Berghuis, J.P., Uldall, K.K., and Lalonde, B.** (1999). Validity of two scales in identifying HIV-associated dementia. *Journal of Acquired Immune Deficiency Syndrome* **21**, 134–40.
183. **Cohen, R.A.** et al. (2001). Neurocognitive performance enhanced by highly active antiretroviral therapy in HIV-infected women. *AIDS* **15**, 341–5.
184. **Stankoff, B.** et al. (2001). Clinical and spectroscopic improvement in HIV-associated cognitive impairment. *Neurology* **56**, 112–15.
185. **Berger, J.R. and Major, E.O.** (1999). Progressive multifocal leukoencephalopathy. *Seminars in Neurology* **19**, 193–200.
186. **Hall, C.D.** et al. (1998). Failure of cytarabine in progressive multifocal leukoencephalopathy associated with human immunodeficiency virus infection. AIDS Clinical Trials Group 243 Team. *New England Journal of Medicine* **338**, 1345–51.
187. **Dworkin, M.S.** et al. (1999). Progressive multifocal leukoencephalopathy: improved survival of human immunodeficiency virus-infected patients in the protease inhibitor era. *Journal of Infectious Diseases* **180**, 621–5.
188. **De Luca, A.** et al. (2000). Cidofovir added to HAART improves virological and clinical outcome in AIDS-associated progressive multifocal leukoencephalopathy. *AIDS* **14**, F117–21.
189. **Chong, J.** et al. (1999). MR findings in AIDS-associated myelopathy. *American Journal of Neuroradiology* **20**, 1412–16.
190. **Wulff, E.A., Wang, A.K., and Simpson, D.M.** (2000). HIV-associated peripheral neuropathy: epidemiology, pathophysiology and treatment. *Drugs* **59**, 1251–60.
191. **Kolson, D.L. and Gonzalez-Scarano, F.** (2001). HIV-associated neuropathies: role of HIV-1, CMV, and other viruses. *Journal of the Peripheral Nervous System* **6**, 2–7.
192. **Cunningham, E.T. Jr. and Margolis, T.P.** (1998). Ocular manifestations of HIV infection. *New England Journal of Medicine* **339**, 236–44.
193. **Ciesla, J.A. and Roberts, J.E.** (2001). Meta-analysis of the relationship between HIV infection and risk for depressive disorders. *American Journal of Psychiatry* **158**, 725–30.
194. **Leserman, J.** et al. (2000). Impact of stressful life events, depression, social support, coping, and cortisol on progression to AIDS. *American Journal of Psychiatry* **157**, 1221–8.
195. **Rabkin, J.G.** et al. (2000). Relationships among apathy, depression, and cognitive impairment in HIV/AIDS. *Journal of Neuropsychiatry and Clinical Neurosciences* **12**, 451–7.
196. **Cockram, A.** et al. (1999). The evaluation of depression in inpatients with HIV disease. *Australian and New Zealand Journal of Psychiatry* **33**, 344–52.
197. **Kalichman, S.C., Rompa, D., and Cage, M.** (2000). Distinguishing between overlapping somatic symptoms of depression and HIV disease in people living with HIV-AIDS. *Journal of Nervous and Mental Disease* **188**, 662–70.
198. **Richardson, M.A.** et al. (1999). Effects of depressed mood versus clinical depression on neuropsychological test performance among African American men impacted by HIV/AIDS. *Journal of Clinical and Experimental Neuropsychology* **21**, 769–83.
199. **Lee, M.R.** et al. (1999). Cognitive-behavioral group therapy with medication for depressed gay men with AIDS or symptomatic HIV infection. *Psychiatric Services* **50**, 948–52.
200. **Markowitz, J.C.** et al. (1998). Treatment of depressive symptoms in human immunodeficiency virus-positive patients. *Archives of General Psychiatry* **55**, 452–7.
201. **Elliott, A.J. and Roy-Byrne, P.P.** (1998). Major depressive disorder and HIV-1 infection: a review of treatment trials. *Seminars in Clinical Neuropsychiatry* **3**, 137–50.
202. **Elliott, A.J.** et al. (1998). Randomized, placebo-controlled trial of paroxetine versus imipramine in depressed HIV-positive outpatients. *American Journal of Psychiatry* **155**, 367–72.
203. **Rabkin, J.G., Wagner, G.J., and Rabkin, R.** (1999). Fluoxetine treatment for depression in patients with HIV and AIDS: a randomized, placebo-controlled trial. *American Journal of Psychiatry* **156**, 101–7.
204. **Grinspoon, S.** et al. (2000). Effects of hypogonadism and testosterone administration on depression indices in HIV-infected men. *Journal of Clinical Endocrinology and Metabolism* **85**, 60–5.
205. **Rabkin, J.G., Wagner, G.J., and Rabkin, R.** (2000). A double-blind, placebo-controlled trial of testosterone therapy for HIV-positive men with hypogonadal symptoms. *Archives of General Psychiatry* **57**, 141–7; discussion 155–6.
206. **Low-Beer, S.** et al. (2000). Depressive symptoms decline among persons on HIV protease inhibitors. *Journal of Acquired Immune Deficiency Syndrome* **23**, 295–301.
207. **Judd, F.K.** et al. (2000). Depressive symptoms reduced in individuals with HIV/AIDS treated with highly active antiretroviral therapy: a longitudinal study. *Australian and New Zealand Journal of Psychiatry* **34**, 1015–21.
208. **Chochinov, H.M.** et al. (1999). Will to live in the terminally ill. *Lancet* **354**, 816–19.
209. **Kissane, D.W.** (2001). Demoralisation: its impact on informed consent and medical care. *Medical Journal of Australia* **175**, 537–9.
210. **Sewell, M.C.** et al. (2000). Anxiety syndromes and symptoms among men with AIDS: a longitudinal controlled study. *Psychosomatics* **41**, 294–300.
211. **Antoni, M.H.** et al. (2000). Cognitive-behavioral stress management intervention effects on anxiety, 24-hr urinary norepinephrine output, and T-cytotoxic/suppressor cells over time among symptomatic HIV-infected gay men. *Journal of Consulting and Clinical Psychology* **68**, 31–45.
212. **Ellen, S.R.** et al. (1999). Secondary mania in patients with HIV infection. *Australian and New Zealand Journal of Psychiatry* **33**, 353–60.
213. **de Ronchi, D.** et al. (2000). Development of acute psychotic disorders and HIV-1 infection. *International Journal of Psychiatry in Medicine* **30**, 173–83.
214. **Mijch, A.M.** et al. (1999). Secondary mania in patients with HIV infection: are antiretrovirals protective? *Journal of Neuropsychiatry and Clinical Neurosciences* **11**, 475–80.
215. **Afessa, B. and Green, B.** (2000). Bacterial pneumonia in hospitalized patients with HIV infection: the Pulmonary Complications, ICU Support, and Prognostic Factors of Hospitalized Patients with HIV (PIP) Study. *Chest* **117**, 1017–22.
216. **Jacobson, J.M.** et al. (1997). Thalidomide for the treatment of oral aphthous ulcers in patients with human immunodeficiency virus infection. National Institute of Allergy and Infectious Diseases AIDS Clinical Trials Group. *New England Journal of Medicine* **336**, 1487–93.
217. **Jacobson, J.M.** et al. (2001). Thalidomide in low intermittent doses does not prevent recurrence of human immunodeficiency virus-associated aphthous ulcers. *Journal of Infectious Diseases* **183**, 343–6.
218. **Herranz, P.** et al. (2000). Successful treatment of aphthous ulcerations in AIDS patients using topical granulocyte-macrophage colony-stimulating factor. *British Journal of Dermatology* **142**, 171–6.
219. **Jacobson, J.M.** et al. (1999). Thalidomide for the treatment of esophageal aphthous ulcers in patients with human immunodeficiency virus infection. National Institute of Allergy and Infectious Disease AIDS Clinical Trials Group. *Journal of Infectious Diseases* **180**, 61–7.

220. **Knox, T.A.** et al. (2000). Diarrhea and abnormalities of gastrointestinal function in a cohort of men and women with HIV infection. *American Journal of Gastroenterology* **95**, 3482–9.

221. **Lamberts, S.W.** et al. (1996). Octreotide. *New England Journal of Medicine* **334**, 246–54.

222. **Beaugerie, L.** et al. (1996). Treatment of refractory diarrhoea in AIDS with acetorphan and octreotide: a randomized crossover study. *European Journal of Gastroenterology and Hepatology* **8**, 485–9.

223. **Holodniy, M.** et al. (1999). A double blind, randomized, placebo-controlled phase II study to assess the safety and efficacy of orally administered SP-303 for the symptomatic treatment of diarrhea in patients with AIDS. *American Journal of Gastroenterology* **94**, 3267–73.

224. **Goldstone, S.E.** et al. (2001). High prevalence of anal squamous intraepithelial lesions and squamous-cell carcinoma in men who have sex with men as seen in a surgical practice. *Diseases of the Colon and Rectum* **44**, 690–8.

225. **Bessesen, M.** et al. (1999). Chronic active hepatitis B exacerbations in human immunodeficiency virus-infected patients following development of resistance to or withdrawal of lamivudine. *Clinical Infectious Diseases* **28**, 1032–5.

226. **Lesens, O.** et al. (1999). Hepatitis C virus is related to progressive liver disease in human immunodeficiency virus-positive hemophiliacs and should be treated as an opportunistic infection. *Journal of Infectious Diseases* **179**, 1254–8.

227. **Garcia-Samaniego, J.** et al. (2001). Hepatocellular carcinoma in HIV-infected patients with chronic hepatitis C. *American Journal of Gastroenterology* **96**, 179–83.

228. **Piroth, L.** et al. (2000). Hepatitis C virus co-infection is a negative prognostic factor for clinical evolution in human immunodeficiency virus-positive patients. *Journal of Viral Hepatitis* **7**, 302–8.

229. **Daar, E.S.** et al. (2001). Hepatitis C virus load is associated with human immunodeficiency virus type 1 disease progression in hemophiliacs. *Journal of Infectious Diseases* **183**, 589–95.

230. **Staples, C.T. Jr., Rimland, D., and Dudas, D.** (1999). Hepatitis C in the HIV (human immunodeficiency virus) Atlanta V.A. (Veterans Affairs Medical Center) Cohort Study (HAVACS): the effect of coinfection on survival. *Clinical Infectious Diseases* **29**, 150–4.

231. **Saves, M.** et al. (2000). Hepatitis B or hepatitis C virus infection is a risk factor for severe hepatic cytolysis after initiation of a protease inhibitor-containing antiretroviral regimen in human immunodeficiency virus-infected patients. The APROCO Study Group. *Antimicrobian Agents and Chemotherapy* **44**, 3451–5.

232. **Greub, G.** et al. (2000). Clinical progression, survival, and immune recovery during antiretroviral therapy in patients with HIV-1 and hepatitis C virus coinfection: the Swiss HIV Cohort Study. *Lancet* **356**, 1800–5.

233. **Dieterich, D.T.** (1999). Hepatitis C virus and human immunodeficiency virus: clinical issues in coinfection. *American Journal of Medicine* **107**, 79S–84S.

234. **Volberding, P.** (2000). Consensus statement: anemia in HIV infection—current trends, treatment options, and practice strategies. Anemia in HIV Working Group. *Clinical Therapeutics* **22**, 1004–20; discussion 1003.

235. **Mocroft, A.** et al. (1999). Anaemia is an independent predictive marker for clinical prognosis in HIV-infected patients from across Europe. EuroSIDA study group. *AIDS* **13**, 943–50.

236. **Koduri, P.R.** et al. (1999). Chronic pure red cell aplasia caused by parvovirus B19 in AIDS: use of intravenous immunoglobulin—a report of eight patients. *American Journal of Hematology* **61**, 16–20.

237. **Collier, A.C.** et al. (2001). Leukocyte-reduced red blood cell transfusions in patients with anemia and human immunodeficiency virus infection: the Viral Activation Transfusion Study: a randomized controlled trial. *Journal of the American Medical Association* **285**, 1592–601.

238. **Abrams, D.I., Steinhart, C., and Frascino, R.** (2000). Epoetin alfa therapy for anaemia in HIV-infected patients: impact on quality of life. *International Journal of STD and AIDS* **11**, 659–65.

239. **Dubreuil-Lemaire, M.L.** et al. (2000). Lenograstim for the treatment of neutropenia in patients receiving ganciclovir for cytomegalovirus infection: a randomised, placebo-controlled trial in AIDS patients. *European Journal of Haematology* **65**, 337–43.

240. **Angel, J.B.** et al. (2000). Phase III study of granulocyte-macrophage colony-stimulating factor in advanced HIV disease: effect on infections, CD4 cell counts and HIV suppression. Leukine/HIV Study Group. *AIDS* **14**, 387–95.

241. **Brites, C.** et al. (2000). A randomized, placebo-controlled trial of granulocyte-macrophage colony-stimulating factor and nucleoside analogue therapy in AIDS. *Journal of Infectious Diseases* **182**, 1531–5.

242. **Oksenhendler, E.** et al. (1993). Splenectomy is safe and effective in human immunodeficiency virus-related immune thrombocytopenia. *Blood* **82**, 29–32.

243. **Sutor, G.C., Schmidt, R.E., and Albrecht, H.** (1999). Thrombotic microangiopathies and HIV infection: report of two typical cases, features of HUS and TTP, and review of the literature. *Infection* **27**, 12–15.

244. **Alberici, F.** et al. (2000). Ivermectin alone or in combination with benzyl benzoate in the treatment of human immunodeficiency virus-associated scabies. *British Journal of Dermatology* **142**, 969–72.

245. **Obasanjo, O.O.** et al. (2001). An outbreak of scabies in a teaching hospital: lessons learned. *Infection Control and Hospital Epidemiology* **22**, 13–18.

246. **Stern, R.S.** et al. (1998). HIV-positive patients differ from HIV-negative patients in indications for and type of UV therapy used. *Journal of the American Academy of Dermatology* **39**, 48–55.

247. **Breuer-McHam, J.** et al. (1999). Alterations in HIV expression in AIDS patients with psoriasis or pruritus treated with phototherapy. *Journal of the American Academy of Dermatology* **40**, 48–60.

248. **Pechere, M.** et al. (1997). Impact of PUVA therapy on HIV viremia: a pilot study. *Dermatology* **195**, 84–5.

249. **Eustace, J.A.** et al. (2000). Cohort study of the treatment of severe HIV-associated nephropathy with corticosteroids. *Kidney International* **58**, 1253–60.

250. **John, G.C.** et al. (2001). Correlates of mother-to-child human immunodeficiency virus type 1 (HIV-1) transmission: association with maternal plasma HIV-1 RNA load, genital HIV-1 DNA shedding, and breast infections. *Journal of Infectious Diseases* **183**, 206–12.

251. **McDonald, A.M.** et al. (2001). Use of interventions for reducing mother-to-child transmission of HIV in Australia. *Medical Journal of Australia* **174**, 449–52.

252. **Nduati, R.** et al. (2000). Effect of breastfeeding and formula feeding on transmission of HIV-1: a randomized clinical trial. *Journal of the American Medical Association* **283**, 1167–74.

253. **Peckham, C. and Newell, M.L.** (2000). Preventing vertical transmission of HIV infection. *New England Journal of Medicine* **343**, 1036–7.

254. **Guay, L.A.** et al. (1999). Intrapartum and neonatal single-dose nevirapine compared with zidovudine for prevention of mother-to-child transmission of HIV-1 in Kampala, Uganda: HIVNET 012 randomised trial. *Lancet* **354**, 795–802.

255. **Glare, P.A. and Virik, K.** (2001). Can we do better in end-of-life care? The mixed management model and palliative care. *Medical Journal of Australia* **175**, 530–3.

256. **Easterbrook, P. and Meadway, J.** (2001). The changing epidemiology of HIV infection: new challenges for HIV palliative care. *Journal of the Royal Society of Medicine* **94**, 442–8.

257. **Matheny, S.C.** (2001). Clinical dilemmas in palliative care for HIV infection. *Journal of the Royal Society of Medicine* **94**, 449–51.

258. **Grant, A.D. and De Cock, K.M.** (2001). ABC of AIDS. HIV infection and AIDS in the developing world. *British Medical Journal* **322**, 1475–8.

259. **Deschamps, M.M.** et al. (2000). HIV infection in Haiti: natural history and disease progression. *AIDS* **14**, 2515–21.

260. **Mwaba, P.** et al. (2001). Clinical presentation, natural history, and cumulative death rates of 230 adults with primary cryptococcal meningitis in Zambian AIDS patients treated under local conditions. *Postgraduate Medicine Journal* **77**, 769–73.

261. **Rankin, W. and Wilson, C.** (2000). African women with HIV. *British Medical Journal* **321**, 1543–4.

262. **Moore, A.** et al. (2001). Estimated risk of HIV transmission by blood transfusion in Kenya. *Lancet* **358**, 657–60.

263. **Ainsworth, M. and Teokul, W.** (2000). Breaking the silence: setting realistic priorities for AIDS control in less-developed countries. *Lancet* **356**, 55–60.

264. **Gilks, C.F.** (2001). HIV care in non-industrialised countries. *British Medical Bulletin* **58**, 171–86.
265. **Sweat, M.** et al. (2000). Cost-effectiveness of voluntary HIV-1 counselling and testing in reducing sexual transmission of HIV-1 in Kenya and Tanzania. *Lancet* **356**, 113–21.
266. **Harries, A.D.** et al. (2001). Preventing antiretroviral anarchy in sub-Saharan Africa. *Lancet* **358**, 410–14.
267. **Farmer, P.** et al. (2001). Community-based approaches to HIV treatment in resource-poor settings. *Lancet* **358**, 404–9.
268. **Merriman, A.** (1999). Hospice Uganda: 1993–1998. *Journal of Palliative Care* **15**, 50–2.
269. **Steinhauser, K.E.** et al. (2000). Factors considered important at the end of life by patients, family, physicians, and other care providers. *Journal of the American Medical Association* **284**, 2476–82.
270. **Singer, P.A., Martin, D.K., and Kelner, M.** (1999). Quality end-of-life care: patients' perspectives. *Journal of the American Medical Association* **281**, 163–8.
271. **Manfredi, P.L.** et al. (2000). Palliative care consultations: how do they impact the care of hospitalized patients? *Journal of Pain and Symptom Management* **20**, 166–73.
272. **Armes, P.J. and Higginson, I.J.** (1999). What constitutes high-quality HIV/AIDS palliative care? *Journal of Palliative Care* **15**, 5–12.
273. **James, J.H.** (2001). Healthcare financing for the under-served: UK. *Journal of the Royal Society of Medicine* **94**, 462–5; discussion 466–7.
274. **Bozzette, S.A.** et al. (1998). The care of HIV-infected adults in the United States. HIV Cost and Services Utilization Study Consortium. *New England Journal of Medicine* **339**, 1897–904.
275. **Higginson, I.J. and O'Neill, J.** (2001). Palliative care in the age of HIV/AIDS. Conclusions from the meeting. *Journal of the Royal Society of Medicine* **94**, 496–8.
276. **Martin, D.K., Emanuel, L.L., and Singer, P.A.** (2000). Planning for the end of life. *Lancet* **356**, 1672–6.
277. **Wenger, N.S.** et al. (2001). End-of-life discussions and preferences among persons with HIV. *Journal of the American Medical Association* **285**, 2880–7.
278. **Curtis, J.R.** et al. (2000). Why don't patients and physicians talk about end-of-life care? Barriers to communication for patients with acquired immunodeficiency syndrome and their primary care clinicians. *Archives of Internal Medicine* **160**, 1690–6.
279. **Ho, V.W.** et al. (2000). The effect of advance care planning on completion of advance directives and patient satisfaction in people with HIV/AIDS. *AIDS Care* **12**, 97–108.
280. **Curtis, J.R.** et al. (2000). The attitudes of patients with advanced AIDS toward use of the medical futility rationale in decisions to forego mechanical ventilation. *Archives of Internal Medicine* **160**, 1597–601.
281. **Bernard, S.A. and Bruera, E.** (2000). Drug interactions in palliative care. *Journal of Clinical Oncology* **18**, 1780–99.
282. **Evans, B.** et al. (2001). Exposure of healthcare workers in England, Wales, and Northern Ireland to bloodborne viruses between July 1997 and June 2000: analysis of surveillance data. *British Medical Journal* **322**, 397–8.
283. **Hannan, M.M.** et al. (2000). Hospital infection control in an era of HIV infection and multidrug resistant tuberculosis. *Journal of Hospital Infection* **44**, 5–11.
284. **Hannan, M.M.** et al. (2001). Investigation and control of a large outbreak of multi-drug resistant tuberculosis at a central Lisbon hospital. *Journal of Hospital Infection* **47**, 91–7.
285. **Kelly, B.** et al. (2000). Measuring psychological adjustment to HIV infection. *International Journal of Psychiatry in Medicine* **30**, 41–59.
286. **Cox, C.** (1999). Hospice care for injection drug using AIDS patients. *Hospital Journal* **14**, 13–24.
287. **Heckman, T.G.** et al. (2001). A pilot coping improvement intervention for late middle-aged and older adults living with HIV/AIDS in the USA. *AIDS Care* **13**, 129–39.
288. **Ozsoy, M. and Ernst, E.** (1999). How effective are complementary therapies for HIV and AIDs?—a systematic review. *International Journal of STD and AIDS* **10**, 629–35.
289. **Holmes, W.C. and Shea, J.A.** (1999). Two approaches to measuring quality of life in the HIV/AIDS population: HAT-QoL and MOS-HIV. *Quality of Life Research* **8**, 515–27.
290. **Swindells, S.** et al. (1999). Quality of life in patients with human immunodeficiency virus infection: impact of social support, coping style and hopelessness. *International Journal of STD and AIDS* **10**, 383–91.
291. **McDonnell, K.A.** et al. (2000). Measuring health related quality of life among women living with HIV. *Quality of Life Research* **9**, 931–40.
292. **Kemppainen, J.K.** (2001). Predictors of quality of life in AIDS patients. *Journal of the Association of Nurses in AIDS Care* **12**, 61–70.
293. **Mallinson, R.K.** (1999). Grief work of HIV positive persons and their survivors. *Nursing Clinics of North America* **34**, 163–77.
294. **Goodkin, K.** et al. (1999). A randomized controlled clinical trial of a bereavement support group intervention in human immunodeficiency virus type 1-seropositive and -seronegative homosexual men. *Archives of General Medicine* **56**, 52–9.
295. **Breitbart, W., Rosenfeld, B.D., and Passik, S.D.** (1996). Interest in physician-assisted suicide among ambulatory HIV-infected patients. *American Journal of Psychiatry* **153**, 238–42.
296. **Starace, F. and Sherr, L.** (1998). Suicidal behaviours, euthanasia and AIDS. *AIDS* **12**, 339–47.
297. **Bindels, P.J.** et al. (1996). Euthanasia and physician-assisted suicide in homosexual men with AIDS. *Lancet* **347**, 499–504.
298. **Onwuteaka-Philipsen, B.D. and van der Wal, G.** (1998). Cases of euthanasia and physician assisted suicide among AIDS patients reported to the Public Prosecutor in North Holland. *Public Health* **112**, 53–6.
299. **Slome, L.R.** et al. (1997). Physician-assisted suicide and patients with human immunodeficiency virus disease. *New England Journal of Medicine* **336**, 417–21.
300. **Sullivan, A.D., Hedberg, K., and Fleming, D.W.** (2000). Legalized physician-assisted suicide in Oregon—the second year. *New England Journal of Medicine* **342**, 598–604.
301. **Cooke, M.** et al. (1998). Informal caregivers and the intention to hasten AIDS-related death. *Archives of Internal Medicine* **158**, 69–75.
302. **McKeogh, M.** (1997). Physician-assisted suicide and patients with AIDS. *New England Journal of Medicine* **337**, 56.
303. **Lavery, J.V.** et al. (2001). Origins of the desire for euthanasia and assisted suicide in people with HIV-1 or AIDS: a qualitative study. *Lancet* **358**, 362–7.
304. **Mishara, B.L.** (1998). Suicide, euthanasia and AIDS. *Crisis* **19**, 87–96.
305. **Rosenfeld, B.** et al. (1999). Measuring desire for death among patients with HIV/AIDS: the schedule of attitudes toward hastened death. *American Journal of Psychiatry* **156**, 94–100.

10.3 Palliative medicine for children and adolescents with HIV/AIDS

Ram Yogev and James M. Oleske

Introduction

The face of the HIV/AIDS epidemic is changing. In developed countries, the number of women with AIDS has risen steadily and, in recent years, their number has increased more rapidly than that in mean. During the first year of the millennium (2000), an estimated 41 960 adults developed AIDS in the USA, 24.9 per cent of them were women.(1) In the developing world, the HIV prevalence rate among women is even higher and is equal to that in men.(2) Most HIV-infected women are of child-bearing age, and because more than 90 per cent of HIV-infected children acquire the infection from their mother (i.e. vertical transmission), the increasing number of HIV-infected women will have a direct impact on the number of HIV-infected children. The availability of antiretroviral prophylaxis (during pregnancy, delivery, and to the newborn) dramatically decreased the rate of vertical transmission from mother to child.[3–5] Yet, in many developing countries such prophylaxis is not available and transmission continues at a significant level. Although sub-Sahara Africa is currently representing almost three-fourths of the global HIV epidemic, more populous countries (e.g. India, China) and new regions (e.g. Eastern Europe) have witnessed the greatest recent growth in the epidemic. Thus, the number of HIV-infected children will continue to grow (some predictions suggest that they will be in the tens of millions) unless effective measures to change the course of the epidemic are implemented without delay.

While the pathogenesis of HIV infection maybe similar in HIV-infected adults and children, most children acquire the infection perinatally while the immune system is immature. As a result, the immunological, virological, and clinical manifestations of the HIV infection differ from those in adults. In the first part of this chapter, we will describe the epidemiology, transmission, diagnosis, and clinical manifestations of HIV infection in children, followed by discussion on available prevention methods. The second part of the chapter will be devoted to the palliative care of HIV-infected children with advanced disease.

Epidemiology

Estimates by the World Health Organization in 2000 suggest that worldwide, 56 million people had HIV/AIDS, 36 million people are currently infected with HIV, and 20 million people have already died from this disease.[2] Sub-Sahara Africa and Southeast Asia accounts for more than 80 per cent of the total, while less than 5 per cent of the patients reside in North America and Europe. Approximately 15 000 new HIV infections occur each day, 10 per cent of them in children under 13 years of age, and 47 per cent in women of child-bearing age (15–49 years of age). In sub-Sahara Africa alone it was estimated that by the end of 2000, 1.1 million children were infected with HIV.[6] Because of the predominant exposure to HIV among women in heterosexual contact, the number of HIV cases among women will continue to increase worldwide unless effective preventive measures (e.g. modifying sexual behaviour, overcoming the stigmatization of people with HIV infection) are taken. Although most children acquired their HIV infection from their mother, the course of the paediatric epidemic is different in developed countries than in most of the developing countries. In the developed countries, a significant decline in perinatal transmission was observed due to the use of zidovudine regimens given to HIV-infected women during pregnancy and labour and to the neonate for the first 6 weeks of life.[7–10] Prior to the use of zidovudine prophylaxis, it was estimated that 1600 infants will be infected yearly in the USA.[11] Yet, a meta-analysis of 15 prospective studies has shown that the rate of HIV transmission in HIV-infected women who received zidovudine prophylaxis and had an elective caesarean delivery was very low (less than 2 per cent).[12] The same low rate of transmission was observed in women who received a potent antiretroviral therapy and achieved an undetectable viral load in their plasma.[13] In the developing countries, the paediatric epidemic is getting worse. Major contributors to the increase in HIV-infected women and children are poverty, inequality for women, no change in sexual behaviour, migration, and lack of antiretroviral prophylaxis or treatment.[2] For example, in one prenatal clinic in South Africa, the prevalence of HIV-infected, pregnant women increased from 7.9 per cent in 1993 to 34 per cent in 1999.[14] In addition, the prevalence was two and half times higher in discordant migrant couples compared to discordant non-immigrant couples (30 per cent versus 12 per cent). As a result, more than 500 000 infants are expected to be perinatally infected with HIV each year worldwide.

As of December 2000, 91 per cent ($N = 8133$) of all children with AIDS in the United States acquired the infection by vertical transmission from their mother, and 7 per cent were infected from HIV-contaminated blood, blood components, or tissue.[1] In 2 per cent, the exposure risk was not yet identified. In contrast to adults, where males represent 75 per cent of the total AIDS population, the sex distribution in the paediatric patients is even (i.e. 50 per cent are males and 50 per cent are females). Most children with AIDS are from minority groups. While fewer than 30 per cent of all US children are Black or Hispanic, children of these communities account for 77 per cent of all paediatric AIDS cases.[1]

Transmission

Early in the epidemic, the transmission rate from mother to child in developed countries ranged from 12 to 63 per cent depending on the HIV plasma levels in the pregnant women.[15,16] In 1994, the US Public Health Service recommended zidovudine prophylaxis for pregnant women following the success of protocol 076 of the Pediatric AIDS Clinical Trials Group (PACTG) to reduce transmission from mother to child by two-thirds.[3,17] The effectiveness of zidovudine in reducing transmission was confirmed both in developed[10,18–20] and developing countries.[21–23] Other prophylactic regimens that are more feasible for widespread implementation in developing countries (e.g. nevirapine,[5] zidovudine plus lamivudine[24]) also showed a significant reduction in HIV transmission from mother to child.

A dramatic decline in perinatal AIDS was found since the increase in zidovudine prophylaxis of HIV-infected pregnant women and transmission rates as low as 3 per cent have been reported.[8,9] In addition, data from Europe also confirmed the efficacy of this prophylaxis.[25] Unfortunately, the lack of prevention programmes in most of the developing countries has maintained the high rate of transmission reported from these countries. By using a classification system (developed by an international working group[26] to evaluate the probability of a child born to an HIV-infected woman, to acquire the HIV infection), the estimated transmission rate in Africa ranged from 25.4 to 42.8 per cent.[27] These results suggest that the transmission rate in the developing world is significantly higher than in the developed world and while the epidemic is contained in the developed countries its devastating effect will continue to grow in the developing world.

Transfusions of infected blood or blood products have accounted for 7 per cent of the paediatric AIDS cases in the USA.[1] However, since 1985, when HIV antibody screening was available, the transmission of HIV by this mode of transmission has been dramatically reduced to 1/60 000 transfused units.[28] Again, the limited resources for blood banking, HIV screening, adequate transfusion equipments, and screening criteria for transfusion-recipients in many developing countries, are some of the reasons why blood transfusion is still an important source of HIV transmission. This is especially true for children who, in some countries, receive more than half of the blood transfusions, mostly to combat anaemia due to malaria.[29–31]

Analysis of the risk of HIV transmission through breastfeeding showed that if the mother was known to be HIV-infected before pregnancy, the infant's risk was 14 per cent (95 per cent CI 7–22 per cent). But if the mother acquired the infection postnatally, the risk increased to 29 per cent (95 per cent CI 16–42 per cent).[32] Breastfeeding substantially increases the risk of mother to child transmission. For example, in one study the HIV transmission rate in children who were exclusively breastfed was 39 per cent, while it was only 24 per cent in children who were never breastfed.[33] Because breastfeeding is a common practice in many developing countries, the WHO recommended that in countries where diarrhoea, pneumonia, and malnutrition substantially contribute to a high infant mortality, women should be encouraged to breastfeed their infants even if they are HIV-infected.[34] Thus, transmission of HIV infection through breastfeeding continues to be a major source of infection in these countries. In contrast, in developed countries, where breastfeeding can easily and safely be substituted by infant formula, promotion of exclusive formula feeding resulted in breastfeeding being the least common route of vertical transmission.

Multiple factors have been reported to be associated with mother to child transmission,[35] but the specific contribution of each factor is difficult to assess. Few studies suggested that high[37] HIV secretion in the genital secretion,[36] advanced disease in the mother, low maternal vitamin A levels,[38] and malaria during pregnancy[39] were associated with significant increase in mother to child transmission rate.

HIV-1 subtype B is the predominant cause of infection in North America. Several HIV-1 subtypes (e.g. A, C, D, E) circulate in Europe, Africa, and Asia.[40] It seems that this diversity in HIV-1 subtypes does not change the risk of transmission from mother to child.[41] In contrast, HIV-2 (mostly identified in West Africa) has been shown to be less infectious than HIV-1 and mother to child transmission rate is less than 1 per cent.[42,43]

Diagnosis

Diagnosing HIV infection in young infants (less than 18 months of age) is not as simple as in older children and adults. While in the latter group detection of antibodies against HIV [by conventional enzyme immunoassays (EIA) confirmed by HIV-specific Western blot] is sufficient to make the diagnosis of HIV infection, a positive result in the younger infant does not differentiate between the infant or the maternal antibodies. Hundred per cent of infants born to HIV-infected women will have a positive HIV-antibody test, while only a fraction of them are also infected with the virus. Because the HIV-antibody test can remain positive in an uninfected infant for up to 18 months, a positive result should not be used to establish the diagnosis of HIV infection unless the infant is older than 18 months of age.[44] To establish the diagnosis in the younger population (as well as in older children and adults), tests that identify the presence of the virus should be used. Several tests are available, including peripheral blood mononuclear cells culture, DNA or RNA polymerase chain reaction (DNA-PCR or RNA-PCR), and demonstration of the HIV p24 antigen in the blood. The PCR methods are very specific and can detect 30–45 per cent of the HIV-infected newborns when they are 2 days old and 75–95 per cent of them by 2 weeks of age.[45] Two positive PCR tests (done on two separate blood samples) are needed to verify HIV infection. The viral culture is almost as sensitive as the PCR method, but results are delayed for 2–4 weeks.[46] Both the PCR and the viral culture are expensive and require specific equipments and considerable expertise, which may not be available in many developing countries and rural areas. In these situations, the immune-complex-dissociated (ICD) p24 antigen test should be considered because it is relatively simple, rapid, and inexpensive. While the test has a high frequency of false-positive results in HIV-exposed newborns (i.e. less than 1 month of age), it has a very good sensitivity in older infants.[47,48] Infants with positive HIV antibody (i.e. EIA or WB positive) but negative viral assay test (i.e. viral culture, PCR, or p24 antigen) should be retested. The current recommendation is to repeat the viral assay at 1–2 and at 3–6 months of age. HIV infection can be excluded if at least two viral assays are negative (at least one of them after the child is older than 4 months of age). In addition, two negative HIV-antibody tests (1 month apart) in a child without clinical evidence of HIV infection and normal gammaglobulinaemia also suggest that the child is not infected.

Other laboratory findings may be used as indicators of HIV infection. Hypergammaglobulinaemia (especially IgG_1 and IgG_3) is common in HIV-infected children and may serve as a non-specific indicator of the disease. More specific indicators are HIV-specific IgM and IgA. However, HIV-specific IgA is found in only 50–60 per cent of HIV-infected infants less than 6 months of age,[49] and the assays for HIV-specific IgM are non-specific and less sensitive.[50] Another specific test is *in vitro* production assay to detect HIV-specific antibody producing B cells. Unfortunately, the sensitivity of the test may be affected by the maturity of the infant's immune system and antiretroviral therapy given to the mother and/or the child. In addition, the test is often false-positive in infants younger than 2–3 months of age due to maternal antibodies attached to the infant's B cells.

Immunological and virological parameters

Immunological (e.g. CD_4T-cell count) and virological (e.g. plasma RNA levels) measurements are recommended to monitor progression or stabilization of the HIV infection. Both the CD_4T-cells and the HIV viral load behave differently in young children than in adults. The CD_4T-cell count in healthy uninfected infants is higher than in adults and it slowly declines to the adult level by 6 years of age.[51,52] Therefore, an immunological staging system that included age-related definitions of immune suppression by the HIV infection was developed (Table 1). Of note, while the absolute CD_4T-cell count is changing with age, their percentage does not and it may be a better marker of disease progression.

The viral burden in HIV-infected infants differs from that in adults (Fig. 1). In adults, high plasma levels are found during the acute infection, but then the plasma viremia declines within a short period of time (i.e. months).[53] In contrast, the viral load in children is lower at birth, reaching its peak during the first year of life, and slowly declines throughout infancy, reflecting the immaturity of the immune system and the availability of more CD_4T-cells.[54,55]

The course of vertically acquired HIV infection is characterized by two distinct patterns: rapid progression (occurs in one fourth of all perinatally infected infants) with development of AIDS within the first year or two of life, and a non-rapid progression with gradual development of symptoms of the disease over several years.[56–58] Several studies showed that CD_4T-cell count is an independent variable for predicting outcome and disease

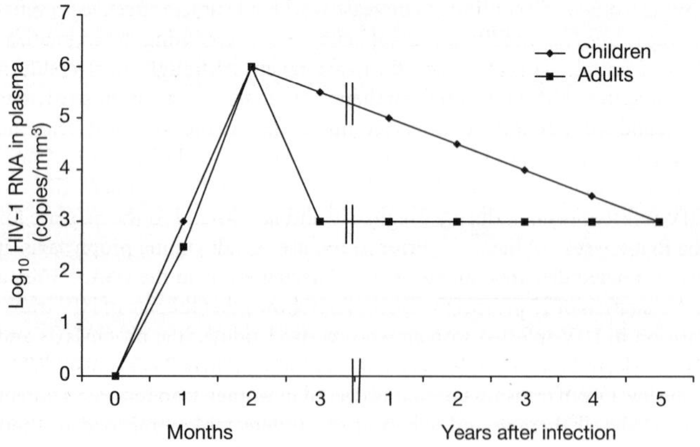

Fig. 1 Change in HIV-1 RNA level from time of infection in adults and children.

Table 1 Immune categories based on age-specific CD_4+T-cell and percentage[44]

Immune category	<12 months		1–5 years		6–12 years	
	No./mm^3	%	No./mm^3	%	No./mm^3	%
Category 1: no suppression	≥1500	≥25	≥1000	≥25	≥500	≥25
Category 2: moderate suppression	750–1499	15–24	500–999	15–24	200–499	15–24
Category 3: severe suppression	<750	<15	<500	<15	<200	<15

progression is more rapid in children with only CD_4T-cell count. In addition, infants with thymus dysfunction have even more rapid disease progression.(59) While the viral load (another independent predictor of disease progression) is not different in many infants with rapidly progressing disease compared to those who do not progress rapidly, a high viral load (>$10^{5.3}$ copies/mm^3) below 1 year of age correlated with disease progression.(54) In addition, a viral load greater than 100 000 copies/mm^3 increased by more than twice the relative risk for death.(60)

While both CD_4T-cells count and viral load can independently predict clinical outcome, the use of these two markers together increase the accuracy of the prediction.(60,61) For example, high viral load (10^5–10^6 copies/mL) was associated with 36 per cent mortality within 5 years if the CD_4T-cell percentage age was ≥15 per cent. In contrast, if the CD_4T-cell percentage was lower than 15 per cent, the mortality rate doubled (i.e. 81 per cent).(60) Similar findings have been reported for 2 years survival (i.e. lack of disease progression). Children with the highest CD_4T-cells count and lowest viral load had a slower disease progression (>89 per cent with no progression), while more than 40 per cent of the children with the highest viral load and the lowest CD_4T-cells count had progression of their disease.(61)

Clinical manifestations

The availability of potent antiretroviral treatment (HAART) for children in developed countries led to a significant change in HIV disease manifestations, progression, and morbidity.(62) In addition, side-effects specific to HAART are responsible for new clinical manifestations (e.g. lipodystrophy) that need to be recognized. The CDC developed a classification system for HIV-infected children, which reflect the stage of the disease in relation to prognosis.(44) The classification is according to clinical status and immunological status (Table 2). Children in category N have no signs or symptoms of HIV infection or only one of the symptoms listed in category A. Category A represent children who are mildly symptomatic with two or more of the following conditions but none of the conditions listed for patients in category B (Table 3(A)) or C (Table 3(B)): hyepatomegaly, splenomegaly, dermatitis, parotitis, recurrent or persistent sinusitis, otitis media or upper respiratory infection, and lymphadenopathy of more than 0.5 cm in more than two sites. All children who are classified in category C are defined as having AIDS. In addition, although lymphoid interstitial pneumonitis (LIP) is in category B it is considered to be an AIDS-defining condition.

The lack of diagnostic services in many developing countries makes the confirmation of the HIV clinical categories difficult because there is a great overlap of these manifestations in HIV-infected children and common health problems in non-HIV-infected children.(63,64) An attempt by the WHO to develop simpler clinical case definition for developing countries was not effective(63,65) because weight loss, chronic diarrhoea, acute respiratory infections, anaemia, and meningitis, the most common syndromes in HIV-infected children in developing countries, were common among HIV-uninfected children. Most HIV-infected children will have a normal physical examination at birth and the presenting symptoms of HIV such as malnutrition, hepatosplenomegaly, lymphodenopathy, oral thrush, and diarrhoea may be subtle. Only their persistence may suggest HIV infection.

In general, HIV disease progresses in children faster than in adults. Some signs and symptoms of the disease will develop in 75 per cent of the infected children by 1 year of age.(66–67) It was estimated that an infected child will remain in stage N for about 10 months and in stage A for another 4 months. Two-thirds of the children entering stage B will progress to stage C within 5 years with expected survival of 8.2 years.(65) This is in contrast to adults who remain asymptomatic for 4.4 years and progress to AIDS only after 10–15 years.(68) In addition, the paediatric population has two distinct patterns. The rapidly progressing group (about 20 per cent of the population) with a median time to reach group C of 4 months, and the more slowly progressing group with an estimated time to reach AIDS of 6.1 years.(66) In children, the spectrum of HIV infection manifestations is quite variable and the presenting illnesses vary geographically. Before the availability of antiretroviral therapy *Pneumocystis carnii*, HIV encephalopathy, recurrent bacterial infections, and lymphoid interstitial pneumonitis were the four main presentations of AIDS in HIV-infected children.(69) Other AIDS indicator conditions are shown in Table 4. Effective primary prophylaxis for *P. carinii* and increased usage of HAART continue to alter these AIDS indicators. In Africa, wasting syndrome, malnutrition, chronic diarrhoea, chronic cough, and chronic fever are the leading clinical findings, while HIV-encephalopathy and lymphoid interstitial pneumonitis are relatively uncommon.(63,64,70) In Asia, the clinical presentation is similar to that in Africa. A unique presentation in Asia is systemic infection with *Penicillium marneffei*. This disseminated infection is one of the most common opportunistic infections found in HIV-infected patients from Southeast Asia both in adults(71) and children.(72)

Skin and oral lesions

Many cutaneous and oral manifestations seen in HIV-infected children are not unique to this population, but they are usually more widely spread and slow to respond to therapy. Candidiasis is the most common manifestation of oral and cutaneous lesions with a prevalence of greater than 20 per cent. In one study, 69 per cent of the HIV-infected children had at least one episode.(73) The lesions are more common and severe in children with low CD_4+T-cells count. Persistent candidiasis has been associated with a worse prognosis,(74) and it occurred significantly less commonly in children who survived for more than 5 years.(67) Recurrent or chronic episodes of herpes simplex virus (HSV) are commonly observed.(74) Other common infections that are often difficult to control are: herpes zoster, molluscum contagiosum, and anorectal warts. An increased prevalence of atopic dermatitis and seborrhoeic dermatitis has also been noted in children infected with HIV. Allergic drug reactions (especially to trimethroprim–sulfamethoxazole and antiretroviral drugs) are relatively common and usually respond to withdrawal of the offending agent. Problems with hyperkeratotic dry skin and hair loss are seen in advanced stages of the disease. Some patients with hyperkeratotic, crusted plaques may have scabies.(75) Other more severe skin infections like pyoderma was also rarely reported.(76) Of interest, Kaposi's sarcoma is very rare in HIV-infected children.

Progression of periodontal disease and high incidence of dental caries are commonly seen in HIV-infected children and oral hygiene is very important in these children. Oral ulcers are also common and a variety of

Table 2 Paediatric human immunodeficiency virus (HIV) classification(44)

Immunological categories	Clinical categories			
	N: no signs/ symptoms	A: mild signs/ symptoms	B: moderate signs/symptoms	C: severe signs/symptoms
1: No evidence of suppression	N1	A1	B1	C1
2: Evidence of moderate suppression	N2	A2	B2	C2
3: Severe suppression	N3	A3	B3	C3

Table 3 Clinical categories of the Pediatric Classification System[44]

(A) Clinical Category B (moderately symptomatic)

Children who have symptomatic conditions other than those listed for Category A or C that are attributed to HIV infection. Examples of conditions in clinical Category B include but are not limited to:

- Anaemia (<8 gm/dL), neutropaenia (<1000/mm^3), or thrombocytopenia (<100 000/mm^3) persisting ≥ 30 days
- Bacterial meningitis, pneumonia, or sepsis (single episode)
- Candidiasis, oropharyngeal (thrush), persisting (>2 months) in children >6 months of age
- Cardiomyopathy
- Cytomegalovirus infection, with onset before 1 month of age—diarrhoea, recurrent or chronic
- Hepatitis
- Herpes simplex virus (HSV) stomatitis, recurrent (more than two episodes within 1 year)
- HSV bronchitis, pneumonitis, or oesophagitis with onset before 1 month of age
- Herpes zoster (shingles) involving at least two distinct episodes or more than one dermatome
- Leiomyosarcoma
- Lymphoid interstitial pneumonia (LIP) or pulmonary lymphoid hyperplasia complex
- Nephropathy
- Nocardiosis
- Persistent fever (lasting >1 month)
- Toxoplasmosis, onset before 1 month of age
- Varicella, disseminated (complicated chickenpox)

(B) Clinical Category C (severely symptomatic)

Serious bacterial infections, multiple or recurrent (i.e. any combination of at least two culture-confirmed infections within a 2-year period), of the following types: septicaemia, pneumonia, meningitis, bone or joint infection, or abscess of an internal organ or body cavity (excluding otitis media, superficial skin or mucosal abscesses, and indwelling catheter-related infections)

Candidiasis, oesophageal or pulmonary (bronchi, trachea, lungs)

Coccidioidomycosis, disseminated (at site other than or in addition to lungs or cervical or hilar lymph nodes)

Cryptococcosis, extrapulmonary

Cryptosporidiosis or isosporiasis with diarrhoea persisting >1 month

Cytomegalovirus disease with onset of symptoms at age >1 month (at a site other than liver, spleen, or lymph nodes)

Encephalopathy (at least one of the following progressive findings present for at least 2 months in the absence of a concurrent illness other than HIV infection that could explain the findings): (a) failure to attain or loss of developmental milestones or loss of intellectual ability, verified by standard developmental scale or neuropsychological tests; (b) impaired brain growth or acquired microcephaly demonstrated by head circumference measurements or brain atrophy demonstrated by computerized tomography or magnetic resonance imaging (serial imaging is required for children <2 years of age); (c) acquired symmetric motor deficit manifested by two or more of the following: paresis, pathologic reflexes, ataxia, or gait disturbance

Herpes simplex virus infection causing a mucocutaneous ulcer that persists for >1 month; or bronchitis, pneumonitis, or oesophagitis for any duration affecting a child >1 month of age

Histoplasmosis, disseminated (at a site other than or in addition to lungs or cervical or hilar lymph nodes)

Kaposi's sarcoma

Lymphoma, primary, in brain

Lymphoma, small, non-cleaved cell (Burkitt's), or immunoblastic or large cell lymphoma of B-cell or unknown immunological phenotype

Table 3 Continued

Mycobacterium tuberculosis, disseminated or extrapulmonary

Mycobacterium, other species or unidentified species, disseminated (at a site other than or in addition to lungs, skin, or cervical or hilar lymph nodes)

Mycobacterium avium complex or *Mycobacterium kansasii*, disseminated (at site other than or in addition to lungs, skin, or cervical or hilar lymph nodes)

Pneumocystis carinii pneumonia

Progressive multifocal leukoencephalopathy

Salmonella (non-typhoid) septicaemia, recurrent

Toxoplasmosis of the brain with onset at >1 month of age

Wasting syndrome in the absence of a concurrent illness other than HIV infection that could explain the following findings: (a) persistent weight loss >10% of baseline OR (b) downward crossing of at least two of the following percentile lines on the weight-for-age chart (e.g. 95th, 75th, 50th, 25th, 5th) in a child ≥1 year of age OR (c) <5th percentile on weight-for-height chart on two consecutive measurements, ≥30 days apart PLUS (a) chronic diarrhoea (i.e. at least two loose stools per day for >30 days) OR (b) documented fever (for ≥30 days, intermittent or constant)

Table 4 AIDS indicator conditions in 473 US children reported in 1997[69]

	Number of children[a]	%[a]
PCP	118	25
Encephalopathy	109	23
Bacterial infections	84	18
LIP	80	17
Wasting	73	15
Invasive *Candida*	61	12
CMV	39	8
MAI	32	7
Other fungi (e.g. *Histoplasma*, *Cryptococcus*, *Cryptosporidia*)	18	4
Herpes infections	15	3
Malignancy	6	<2
Toxoplasmosis—brain	3	<1

[a] The number of patient events and percentages are greater than the total number of patients and 100%, respectively, because some patients were reported with more than one event.

infections or other conditions may be the cause. Viral, fungal, and bacterial infections as well as medication and neutropenia should be investigated before the diagnosis of aphtous stomatitis is made.

Central nervous system

Neurological involvement is common in HIV-infected children. Almost half of the children have cortical atrophy and small head circumference.[77] In some children, CNS involvement is the initial manifestation of HIV disease, and deterioration in their neurological parameters indicates a poor prognosis.[78] The most common and severe presentation of encephalopathy is progressive loss or plateau of developmental milestones, cognitive deterioration, and impaired brain growth. With progression of the disease, functional and behavioural abnormalities such as flattened affect, apathy, motor dysfunction, spasticity, and weakness develop. Other language and motor skills are also lost. A less severe form of static encephalopathy also occurs in which a slower than normal development of skills and abilities is observed. These children usually score below average for their age in standardized tests. When neuroimaging studies are done, basal ganglia calcifications and leucomalacia maybe found with and without cerebral atrophy.[79]

Respiratory tract

The prevalence of acute otitis media and sinusitis in symptomatic HIV-infected children is similar to that in normal children.[80] Although the aetiological agents are usually the same as those in immunocompetent host (e.g. *S. pneumoniae, H. influenzae*), *S. aureus* is significantly more common in children with advanced HIV infection (i.e. AIDS).[81] In addition, unusual pathogens, such as *P. aeruginosa*, were found in children with chronic ear infections, which may lead to severe complications (e.g. mastoiditis) if inappropriate antibiotics are given. Bacterial pneumonia occurs more frequently in HIV-infected children, especially is those with advanced disease. *S. pneumoniae* and *H. influenzae* are the most common pathogens, but *S. pyogenes*, *S. aureus*, and gram-negative bacteria (particularly *P. aeruginosa* and *K. pneumoniae*) have received increased attention.[82] Other pathogens such as CMV, Measles, Aspergillus, and Cryptococcus were also reported. Pneumonia caused by common respiratory viruses such as adenovirus, parainfluenza, influenza, and respiratory syncytial virus (RSV) can have a protracted course and increased mortality.[83,84]

Pulmonary tuberculosis is more prevalent in HIV-infected children with an estimated rate of 20–30 times higher than the rate in immunocompetent children. It was also estimated that greater than 50 000 HIV-infected children worldwide will be co-infected with TB.[85] The diagnosis of TB in HIV-infected children may be difficult as sputum is not easily available and the PPD test is usually negative.[86] In addition, many children develop other illnesses that mimic TB and classical chest X-rays findings such as hilar adenopathy are not found. Because the presentation and progression of pulmonary TB in HIV-infected children may be atypical, children with protracted respiratory symptoms and pulmonary changes on chest X-rays of children who failed a course of antibiotics should be carefully evaluated for TB. Of note, TB cultures (e.g. gastric, bronchoalveolar lavage) are more often positive in HIV-infected children than in immunocompetent children and should be an integral part of the evaluation. In many areas of the developing world the expanding epidemics of TB and HIV will produce large number of co-infected children. Therefore, the WHO recommends to give a BCG vaccination to asymptomatic HIV-infected children (in areas where the prevalence of these infections is high), because the risk of TB in these children is greater than the BCG complications.[87]

Pneumocystis carinii pneumonia (PCP) is one of the most common AIDS-defining illnesses in children both in the developed[69,88] and developing[89,90] countries. The clinical manifestations include: fever, cough, tachypnea, dysponea, and use of accessory muscles (e.g. alae nasae, intercostal), frequently followed by an acute and rapidly progressive clinical course. Auscultation to the lung is relatively benign despite the other clinical signs and symptoms. Early in the disease, the chest X-rays may be normal, but as the disease progress bilateral pulmonary infiltrates are frequently present. While in some children a typical chest X-ray is found, in many children the chest X-ray findings cannot distinguish PCP from other causes of pneumonia. Unlike adults, the CD_4T cell count is not a good predictor for risk of PCP infection in children, especially during the first 12 months of life. Therefore, prophylaxis (mainly with trimethoprim–sulfamethoxazole) is recommended to all seropositive infants less than 1 year of age whose HIV infection status is known or indeterminate.[91] Laboratory tests are not helpful as the WBC count is usually within the normal range, but LDH levels are frequently elevated. The prognosis is relatively poor with a median survival of a year and a half.[92]

Lymphyocytic interstitial pneumonitis (LIP), a chronic interstitial process of diffuse infiltrates consisting predominantly of lymphocytes, large mononuclear cells, plasma cells, and retriculoendothelial cells, is frequently reported in HIV-infected children but rarely in adults. The median age of onset is 1 year of age with a range from 6 months to 7 years. The clinical presentation is insidious with persistent mild cough and tachypnea. The lungs are clear, with infrequent rales or wheezing. If chest X-rays are done at this stage, the bilateral diffuse retriculonodular infiltrate is surprising due to the mildness of the symptoms.[93] In some children, clubbing of the fingers or other symptoms of lymphproliferative process (e.g. lympadenopathy, hepatosplenomegaly, enlarged parotid) will be the first clues of LIP. Therefore, yearly chest X-rays should be considered in HIV-infected children to screen for LIP. As the disease progresses the child develops signs and symptoms of chronic lung disease with chronic cough, cyanosis, need for supplemental oxygen, and poor weight gain. Long standing disease may lead to development of bronchiectasis and, in rare cases, to pulmonary lymphoma.

Cardiovascular system

Cardiomyopathy is not common in older HIV-infected children as it is in short-term survivors (7 versus 21 per cent).[94] The presence of cardiac disease in an HIV infected child carries a poor prognosis. The pathogenesis is probably multifactorial and includes nutritinal deficiencies (e.g. selenium), viral infections (e.g. CMV), immunological impairment (e.g. low T-cell count), drug toxicities, and pulmonary insufficiency. The cardiovascular changes are progressive and autopsy findings ranged from abnormal cardiac growth and conduction abnormalities to myocarditis and arteriopathy.[95] Left ventricular dysfunction is probably the most common and important manifestation of the cardiac involvement.[96] Other manifestations include tachycardia, ventricular hypertrophy, arythmias, and congestive heart failure. Rarely, pericardial involvement with pericardial fluid and coronary aneurysm were reported. Because physical examination often do not correlate with the severity of the cardiac disease and electrocardiography (ECG) is of limited benefit, echocardiography (ECHO), where available, is probably the most helpful in assessing the cardiac status before the onset of clinical symptoms. Routine ECHO (every 6–12 months) should be considered in asymptomatic HIV-infected children and even more often in symptomatic children.

Renal disease

HIV-associated nephropathy seems to be increasing especially in older symptomatic children.[97] African-American and Hispanics in the USA and children in Sub-Sahara Africa are more frequently affected by this disease. Yet, North African patients or patients with North African ancestry have a lower rate of renal disease.[98,99] As with cardiac disease, the renal pathogenesis is multifactorial and include direct effect of the HIV, its immune complexes, or various cytokines on the renal parenchyma, hyperviscosity of the blood due to hyperglobulinaemia (occurring in many HIV-infected children), ischaemia, and nephrotoxic drugs.[100] The clinical manifestations may resemble nephrotic syndrome with oedema commonly seen in the lower extremities and face, or in the back if the patient is recumbent. Ascites is often present, while arthralgia is not as common. Polyuria or oliguria with or without haematuria and/or proteinuria may be present. Like most patients with nephrotic syndrome, arterial blood pressure is usually normal. If the proteinuria persists a kidney biopsy should be considered. Patients with focal glumerulonephritis usually progresses to renal failure relatively fast, while other histological patterns may remain stable for prolonged periods.[101]

Gastrointestinal and nutritional

Failure to thrive (FTT), malnutrition, and gastrointestinal symptoms are very common in HIV-infected children.[102,103] Several mechanisms contribute to the pathogenesis of FTT and malnutrition including lack of financial means to provide food, inadequate amount of food due to poor oral intake, abnormal intestinal absorption of nutrients, and increased caloric requirements. A syndrome of malabsorption with villous blunting and decreased villous surface area due to direct HIV infection has been suggested to be the cause of growth failure or weight loss. Studies in children demonstrated that carbohydrates, fats, and proteins are malabsorbed in 20–40 per cent of the patients,[104–106] while iron absorption was deficient in almost half of the investigated children.[106] Malabsorption can also be the direct result of infection with a variety of pathogens that usually cause gastrointestinal disease. Such pathogens include bacteria (e.g. *Salmonella, Campylobacter, Mycobacterium arrium-intracellulare, Shigella*), viruses (e.g. CMV, adenovirus, rotavirus), fungi (e.g. *Candida*), and protozoa (e.g. *Cryptosporidium, Micropsporidia, Isospora, Giardia*).[107] The most common symptoms are dysphagia, abdominal pain, chronic or recurrent diarrhaea and poor growth. Longitudinal studies, both in developed and developing countries, have shown that HIV-infected children are born lighter and shorter than non-infected children and they continue to grow poorly.[108–110] In addition, poor growth indicates an unfavourable outcome.[111] Micronutrients such as vitamin A, vitamin E, glutathione, β-carotene, selenium, and zinc were found to be deficient in HIV-infected children.[112]

Heptomegaly with and without splenomegaly is present in more than 75 per cent of HIV-infected children. Chronic liver involvement is evident by the abnormal serum aminotransferase levels during the course of the disease, but in most children the liver involvement is without cholestasis. In some children co-infection of HIV with Hepatitis B (HBV) or Hepatitis C (HCV) was reported. In general, co-infection with HBV does not cause a more rapid progression of the HIV infection, while HCV may cause a more rapid progression of the HIV infection.[113] Other causes of hepatitis may be infectious (e.g. *M. avium-intracellular, Candida, Cryptococcus*, CMV, EBV, *Cryptosporidium*), drug toxicity (e.g. TMP–SMX, ritonavir, nelfinavir, ddI, d4T, ZDV, pentamidine), and rarely malignancy (e.g. lymphoma) or total parenteral nutrition (TPN). The clinical presentation of liver disease is usually subtle with only elevation of liver enzymes and hepatomegagly. Liver failure is very rare and only when the bilary tract is involved (infection with CMV, *Cryptosporidium, Mycosporidia*, etc.) the child will present with abdominal pain, vomiting, and jaundice.

Acute pancreatitis usually will cause severe and diffuse abdominal pain with distention and vomiting. Opportunistic infections (e.g. CMV) can cause pancreatitis, but drug toxicity is probably the main cause. Antiretroviral medications (like ddI and ddC), anti-PCP prophylaxis (like TMP–SMZ and pentamidine) or other antimicrobial drugs are at the top of the list. Elevated serum amylase and lipase levels are found in patients with pancreatitis. Lipase levels seems to be more reliable, because in many children elevated amylase levels are from salivary origin. Recurrence of pancreatitis may occur in some patients.

Malignancy

Malignant disease in HIV-infected children are not as common as in adults. Less than 2 per cent of children with AIDS were known to have a malignancy. With the increased life expectancy of HIV-infected children in developed countries and the use of antiretroviral drugs, it is expected that the incidence of malignant diseases will increase. The most common malignancies are non-Hodgkin's lymphoma such as Burkitt lymphoma, immunoblastic lymphoma, and primary CNS lymphoma.[114] Other cancers include Kaposi's sarcoma (especially in African countries[115]) leiomysarcoma,[116] fibromyosarcoma[117] and leukaemia.[118] The clinical signs and symptoms of the malignant disease in HIV-infected children are similar to those in non-infected children.

Antiretroviral therapy

The recent developments in our understanding of the pathogenesis of HIV disease in children and the availability of more potent antiretroviral drugs profoundly changed the course of the disease in children. Yet, in general, the HAART in children is somewhat less effective than similar regimens in adults.[119,120] Although the same principles which guide HAART in adults should be used in children, the unique immunological, virological, and pharmacological parameters of this population have to be taken into account. While it is known that lower plasma viral load correlates with better outcome, the significant overlap of HIV plasma levels in infants with rapidly developing or slowly progressive disease makes the predictive value of the viral load less reliable in children. Thus, the treatment recommendation for paediatric patients (which include combinations of three antiretroviral drugs) is to start therapy in all HIV-infected children who present with clinical symptoms or evidence of immune suppression regardless of the viral load.[121] In addition, because the CD_4+T-cell count changes dramatically in the first year of life, it is recommended that antiretroviral therapy should be started in infants younger than 1 year of age as early as the diagnosis of HIV infection is made, regardless of the clinical, immunological, and virological parameters.[121] In older asymptomatic children two approaches are acceptable. Some specialists favour an early aggressive therapeutic approach for all HIV-infected children to increase the chance of preserving the immune system.[121] Others prefer to defer therapy and carefully watch for increase in viral load (three to five folds from the base- line results) or progressive decline in CD_4+T-cell count [to moderate or severe immune suppression (Table 1)] or development of clinical symptoms before initiating therapy.[121,122] In addition, many specialists start HAART if the absolute level of the HIV load is above 50 000 copies/mL.

Several factors determine the likelihood of HAART success in children. The most important is adherence to therapy, which remains a major obstacle.[121,123–126] This is especially true for regimens that include protease inhibitors because of their poor palatability, food restrictions, large number of capsules, or volume of syrup and frequent side-effects. As a result, compliance of less than 60 per cent was observed in children receiving HAART.[123] In addition, while more than half of the children with good adherence achieved suppression of viral load (<400 copies/mL) only 10 per cent of the non-adherent children had such a suppression.[123] Lack of compliance not only produces lower drug levels in the body, which are less effective in combating the virus, it also allows selection of HIV mutants with cross-resistance to other drugs which limit future treatment options.[126] Thus, major efforts are needed to ensure adherence (i.e. greater than 90 per cent of the drugs taken) if maximal suppression of HIV replication is expected.[127] Careful planning to maximize adherence such as adapting the regimen to the patient's daily routine, usage of PI-sparing regimen, or even simpler regimens (e.g. two nucleosides analogues only) should be considered.[121] Another approach to improve adherence is placement of a gastrostomy tube.[128] The lack of appropriate paediatric formulations for some of the antiretroviral drugs (especially protease inhibitors) also limits the therapeutic options available to children.

Pharmacokinetic parameters, another important factor to HAART success, are frequently different in children than in adults and dose extrapolation from adult studies may lead to sub-therapeutic levels and loss of viral suppression.[129–132] In addition, children show a greater inter-patient variability than adults partly because hepatic glucuronidation and renal excretion reaches adult levels only after 6 months of age. It is important to note that HAART side-effects and toxicity may be different in children than in adults. Thus, appropriate dosing of antiretroviral drugs in children should be derived only from specifically designed paediatric studies.

Development of drug resistance is another major barrier for HAART success. The higher viral load in HIV-infected children (compared to adults) favours a more rapid selection of HIV quasi-species with resistance mutations. In addition, if viral replication continues due to sub-therapeutic drug levels (e.g. lack of compliance or inappropriate pharmacodynamic parameters), selection of drug-resistant variants will increase leading to treatment failure. Although both genotypic and phenotypic assays are available, no specific recommendations on how to use them for antiretroviral therapy choices in children was made.[121] Although knowledge of the virus genotype may be helpful in determining which drugs to use, it only modestly improved the outcome.[133–135] Specific recommendations for initial therapy and when to change therapy are continuing to evolve over time. Thus, the reader should refer to the 'Guidelines for the use of antiretroviral agents in pediatric HIV infection', which is regularly updated and is available at http://www.hivatis.org.[121]

Prevention

Transmission of HIV from mother to child can occur during pregnancy, delivery, and from breastfeeding. The likelihood of perinatal transmission increases if the mother has an advanced HIV disease, high viral load, and low CD4T-cell count.(136) Thus, the best prevention of perinatal transmission is to prevent HIV infection in the pregnant woman through education or to identify the HIV infection before pregnancy or early during pregnancy. Early diagnosis will allow treatment with antiretroviral drugs, which will reduce the viral load and improve the mother's clinical and immunological status. A reduction in transmission rate to less than 2 per cent has been reported in HIV-infected women who received combination therapy.(137)

During labour, the transmission risk increases if delivery occurs >4 h after rupture of membranes, if maternal HIV disease is not under control, and if the mother has chorioamnionitis or another sexually transmitted disease.(138,139) Several obstetric procedures can also increase the risk.(140) Thus, reducing exposure of the newborn to the mother's blood during delivery can reduce transmission. Caesarean delivery before onset of labour (at 38 weeks gestation) in untreated HIV-infected women or those who were receiving only monotherapy (e.g. ZDV) reduced transmission by 50 per cent.(12) However, the benefit of caesarean delivery in women who received combination therapy is unknown, and the greater morbidity of this procedure compared to vaginal delivery should be considered before Caesarean section is offered to these women. Vaginal disinfection and cleansing of the newborn immediately after delivery seems to be ineffective in reducing transmission.(141)

The best strategy available today to reduce transmission from an HIV-infected woman to her newborn is to use antiretroviral prophylaxis. The most effective regimen is the three-component ZDV prophylaxis (PACTG 076 study) in which the pregnant woman receives oral ZDV during the second and third trimesters of pregnancy and intravenous ZDV during labour and delivery. The third component is administration of oral ZDV to the newborn for the first 6 weeks of life.(3) Several abbreviated prophylactic regimens were tested in developing countries and proved to be effective. Data from Thailand indicated that administration of ZDV only to the pregnant women (oral ZDV started at 36 weeks gestation and during labour and delivery) but not to the newborn reduced transmission by 51 per cent.(4) In breastfeeding mothers, the efficacy of this regimen was lower.(142,143) Other antiretrovirals were also evaluated. The combination of ZDV and 3TC given orally during labour and delivery and to the newborn and the mother for 1 week postpartum was also effective in reducing transmission.(144) In addition, a simpler regimen of only two doses of nevirapine (one dose to the mother at the onset of labour and every 3 h until delivery and a single dose to the newborn at 48–72 h of life) was more effective than the short course of ZDV.(5) A retrospective analysis of ZDV prophylaxis in pregnant women and their newborns suggests that prophylaxis of the newborn alone (started within 48–72 h of life) also offer some protection.(7) This observation is supported by studies in animals.(145)

In breastfeeding populations, breastfeeding is believed to contribute to more than one-third of all mother to child transmission. Increased transmission during breastfeeding was found if the mother had a subclinical or clinical mastitis or breast abscess or if the mother seroconverts (i.e acquired HIV infection) during lactation. Thus, in developed countries cessation of breastfeeding is recommended to reduce transmission. In contrast, in developing countries where the risk of not breastfeeding (i.e. increasing infant morbidity and mortality) may outweigh the benefit (i.e. reducing HIV transmission), the WHO recommended that in settings where common causes of death are prevalent (e.g. malnutrition, infectious diseases) HIV-infected women should be told of the risks and benefits of breastfeeding so they can make a choice.(146) Some strategies to prevent transmission during breastfeeding such as exclusive breastfeeding or early weaning at 3–6 months have been proposed.(147)

Because some studies suggested that sexually transmitted disease increase perinatal transmission, it was suggested that treatment of such diseases will reduce transmission. Unfortunately, such therapy had no effect on reducing the incidence.(148) The same occurred with nutritional supplements. While provision of supplementation had an overall benefit to the mother and her newborn, such treatment did not demonstrate reduction in HIV transmission.(149,150) The effect of malaria and chorioamnionitis treatment on reduction of mother to child transmission is currently investigated in developing countries. Both diseases were associated with increased transmission due to disruption of the placenta integrity and it has been hypothesized that their cure will decrease transmission.

Palliative care for HIV-infected children

The traditional palliative care services were aimed at managing patients with 'progressive, far-advanced disease for whom the prognosis is limited and the focus of care is the quality of life'.(151) This approach may have been acceptable earlier at the onset of the HIV epidemic when most perinatally infected children died before they were 4 years of age. Yet, recent advances in our understanding of the HIV disease pathogenesis and the dramatic effect of HAART on the course of the disease coupled with better prophylaxis therapy for opportunistic infections and good supportive care slowed the progression of the HIV infection to AIDS and the mortality of children with AIDS. Many more HIV-infected children are now living longer, well into their teen years, and are in need of a palliative care that is independent of cure-directed therapy and available from diagnosis through the entire course of the disease. Because many HIV-infected children in the developed world now have a chronic life-limiting illness, the palliative care should begin at the time an HIV-infected woman becomes pregnant and continue till the eventual death of the child. The palliative care services should be more comprehensive and include physical, psychological, social, and spiritual care.(152) Ideally, pregnant women should receive comprehensive prenatal care, which is important for the well-being of the infant and mother. If the born child is diagnosed as HIV-1 infected, all care should be aggressive, and during the course of the disease some types of the restorative care (e.g. prophylactic antibiotics) are also the best palliative care. For example, the prevention of PCP with trimethoprim/sulfamethoxazole prophylaxis is compatible with a continuum of palliative care that provides 'comfort' by avoiding the substantial morbidity of this infection. Pain and other adverse symptoms need to be assessed at each patient encounter and treated vigorously. Other treatments for HIV-1 disease complications that improve quality of life include antiretroviral therapy, continuing prophylaxis, and treatment of opportunistic infections [e.g. *P. carinii*, atypical mycobacteria infection (MAC), cryptococcal meningitis, toxoplasmosis, cytomegalovirus, herpes simplex virus], and the prevention of recurrent bacterial infections. Nutrition is another important part of supportive care and a critical component in health maintenance while adding to quality of life.(153,154)

While the use of antiretroviral therapy has had a significant impact on quality of life by improving survival, prolonging the time free of opportunistic infections, and improving and maintaining immunological health, at the end-stage disease, decisions relating to the continuation of antiretroviral therapy must be made balancing the limited effect of such treatment at this point versus its side-effects. At this stage, there should be a shift from restorative care to more supportive care; the physician and the family need to recognize when end-stage disease is present and hospice care is an appropriate option.(155–158)

During the end-stage of the disease, HIV-infected children can benefit from knowing that they are dying (in an age appropriate context) and can discuss their fears with their loved ones. In many cases, the secrecy about the disease imposed by their parents and families continue even through the terminal stages preventing an atmosphere of safety and closure. In addition, families of the dying child need to be knowledgeable, supported, and active participants in decisions about end of life care for their child. Health-care providers need to recognize the multiple difficulties experienced by these children and their families during this time, including ambivalence, fear, isolation, anger, loss of control, helplessness, and sadness. Members of the health-care team also need to balance the restorative care (disease-specific management with aggressive antiretroviral therapies and treatment of opportunistic infections) and the supportive care (nutrition, pain management, and other aspects of palliative care). The family and the child should be full partners with the health-care team in management decisions. The child's best interests are paramount and care is provided in an atmosphere of kindness and access to appropriate hospice care.(155,159,160) Hospice care should incorporate the principles of palliative care used in earlier stages of the illness but increase the emphasis on easing the burden of end of life care for the patient and the family. As part of the continuum of palliative care, hospice services should maximize the patient's dignity and allow for a smoother transition for the family and the medical staff to bereavement.[152,161,162]

Providing comprehensive and individualized palliative respite and terminal-care services for children with HIV and their families is important, yet presents a significant challenge to health-care providers and social support systems. With AIDS, more rage, shame, fear, and unresolved grief are experienced, often associated with stigmatization and disenfranchisement. Often, HIV-infected parents have difficulties in disclosing the disease to their child and experience shame and sorrow for causing their child's disease. In addition, fear of social stigma, and fears of contagion can deprive children and their families of critical community and extended family support. While the palliative care needs of HIV-infected children are similar to those of children with cancer, the care for children with HIV involves multiple medical appointments, multi-systems disease, complex home medical treatments, lengthy dying process, and frequent acute illnesses requiring constant care. Providing care is often complicated by illness in other family members, multiple social and psychological issues, and inadequate financial and community services. Unfortunately, there are no guidelines for access, delivery, or eligibility of providers for paediatric HIV palliative, hospice, and respite care. Therefore, innovative models for hospice/terminal care of children with HIV are required. The needs of children with HIV differ from traditional hospice care in that prognosis is uncertain and the medical course can be variable. Thus, multidisciplinary hospice services may be required for more extended periods of time and children often require active as well as palliative treatment. Access to appropriate programmes varies greatly in different geographical areas and availability of immediate health-care support, a critical part of hospice services, is not available in some disadvantaged areas.[163] The goal to support palliative and end of life care for HIV-affected children and families is to strengthen access to these services.

Although HAART changed dramatically the outcome for many HIV-infected children in developed countries, problems with adherence to therapy and the increasing viral resistance rate to multiple antiretroviral drugs suggest that the need for respite and hospice care for HIV-infected children will increase. In addition, some patients cannot tolerate the medications or HAART was given too late to benefit from it or the treatment is ineffective requiring palliative care services including hospice now. The picture in the resource-poor areas of the world is very different. More than 90 per cent of HIV-infected children reside in these countries and most of them lack access to many therapies (e.g. HAART, PCP or MAC prophylaxis) that would prevent disease progression and are considered part of the continuum of palliative care.[164,165] In addition, the rudimentary infrastructure of the primary care system and the lack of national programmes to identify HIV-infected pregnant women and children make palliative care even more challenging.

Even prior to the epidemic of HIV, the relief of suffering, based on the principles of palliative care and the provision of hospice services, has not always been available to most children with life-limiting illnesses.[166] For example, in 1993, only 1 per cent of US hospice patients were children (less than 2000) while it is estimated that 17 000 children die each year in the US who would benefit from palliative care and hospice services.[167] With the improved survival of HIV-infected children these services will be in increased demand.

Because autonomy is one of the three ethical principles of palliative care,[168,169] HIV-infected children need to be knowledgeable about their disease, which raises the difficult issue of disclosure of the diagnosis. The paediatric literature on disclosure of diagnosis has been based on children with cancer. These studies have shown that, in general, disclosure should occur sometime after the age of 6 and it adds to the quality of life both for the child and family.[170–171] There are unique aspects of HIV infection (e.g. social stigmatization, parent also infected with HIV) that make disclosure of the diagnosis to the child more problematic than the disclosure of cancer. Nevertheless, there is a growing consensus among care providers of HIV-infected children that disclosure of the diagnosis is as important in this disease as in cancer.[172–174]

HIV-infected children can exhibit a tremendous variability in the clinical course of their disease. End-stage disease in these children is usually characterized by progression to severe clinical disease with marked immune suppression [CDC classification C-3 (Tables 2 and 3B)]. HIV encephalopathy, nephropathy, cardiomyopathy, hepatitis, and wasting syndrome that may be associated with opportunistic infections (e.g. CMV, cryptosporidiosis, atypical mycobacterial infection) frequently are part of this progression.[160] Children often have four or more of these problems.

End-stage disease can also be associated with the development of HIV-specific malignancies (e.g. leiomyosarcoma, primary CNS lymphoma, leukaemia) and in addition to the multiple organ failure, high viral load persist (despite aggressive antiretroviral therapy) with progressive loss of CD4+ lymphocyte cells. It is at this stage that the continuum of palliative care should shift from restorative care to more supportive care and the physician needs to recognize, with the family, the end stage of the disease and that hospice care becomes the appropriate option. The physician needs to maintain a physical presence that is compassionate, recognizing the need to relieve the multiple causes of pain and suffering while balancing the maintenance of function (restorative care) and comfort (supportive care). In addition, a discussion with the family of the medical status and prognosis needs to be initiated, including age appropriate discussion of death and dying with the child. The components and the meaning of a Do Not Resuscitate (DNR) order should be explained and a joint plan developed that recognizes the need for patient and family control and assures a comfortable and pain free death at home, hospital, or hospice setting. A written notification to community ambulance and emergency room services of the child's DNR status should be given to the family. It is also advisable to document the plan in the medical records and if a conflict or disagreement arises between the patient's family and the health-care provider there should be a referral to an Ethics Committee. All DNR orders should be reviewed at intervals with the family. The discussion of the dying process should include both signs and symptoms of impending death with assurances to the family of continuous support. Implementation of the end of life care plan includes withdrawal of interventions (e.g. medication and procedures) that detract from quality of life.[175] At the time of death, the health-care and case-management team need to be available to expedite funeral arrangements and completion of the death certificate. There also needs to be initiation of bereavement support for survivors and oppor-tunity for the family to discuss the cause of death with supportive professionals.[176] Other interventions such as remembrance ceremonies to celebrate the child's life, referral to community resources to replace the medical and social support provided by the health-care team, and support groups for siblings and other family members should be considered as part of the bereavement process.

It is important for the health-care team to have opportunities to grieve over the loss of the child. Health-care professionals react differently to the dying process and death. Some grieve the loss of their close relationship with the child, while others grieve the loss and pain felt by the family or grieve their professional failure to save the child. Although the reasons for grieving maybe different, a process should be in place to support the various team members to cope with the dying process and death. The process should be on a regular basis rather than crisis-oriented. To achieve this goal, physicians and nurses should continuously exchange information (among themselves and other team members) about the dying patient and his/her care and solicit help in the medical and emotional care of this patient. In addition, staff members should share their thoughts and feelings and reflect on the value of their contributions during the child's illness and death. Physicians, who usually experience grieving as a private affair, should participate in these meetings and help in creating a safe and compassionate environment, where commendation about what has been going well and resolution of difficulties will help the team to function as a cohesive unit.

Medical aspects of palliative care

Children with progressive HIV disease have more complex medical problems because they repeatedly have life-threatening events. This unpredictable course makes it difficult for the physician to know when the child is really at the end-stage of the disease. As a result, many physicians being preoccupied with managing the HIV disease and prolonging life, frequently neglect to alleviate suffering from adverse effects of the disease, treatment interventions, or procedures. One of the major limitations in preventing HIV-infected children from receiving appropriate palliative care is the lack of appreciation of both acute and chronic pain associated with this disease and the multiple painful procedures required in the management of this syndrome.(177) In addition, physicians are not well trained in pain management, in particular, for patients with chronic illnesses that result in both somatic and neuropathic pain. Clinicians often under-treat pain because of their mistaken beliefs in erroneous myths such as: children lie about pain to get attention; children who can fall asleep or who can play cannot be in pain; and children who deny pain or do not complain, are not in pain.(177–179) Although great strides have been made in the management of paediatric pain, pain in children with HIV continues to be inadequately treated. Some of the barriers specific to the management of pain in children with HIV include: (a) the difficulty of assessing pain in young children; (b) the difficulty of assessing pain in children with neurological impairment (e.g. encephalopathy, developmentally delayed); (c) parental denial of their children's disease and, consequently, their pain; (d) physicians' resistance to the use of opioids by families who have a history of drug use; (e) unfounded fears about the addiction potential and the physical dangers of opioids (including respiratory depression); and (f) subspecialists who are not trained in assessment of pain and appropriate use of analgesics.

Even when physicians are aggressive in pain management, family members or caregivers may be resistant. Parental guilt about HIV can be profound and foster parents deny the severity of the illness and its associated pain. Additionally, the use of pain medications such as opioids may be perceived as heralding disease progression and death thereby increasing resistance to pain assessment and treatment. Families and patients may also fear addiction. Because the treatment of HIV-1 infection is complex, pain management and other supportive care efforts can be overlooked during an acute crisis or hospital admission.(180) The fact that many parents are also sick (with HIV) or are foster parents add to the complexity of identifying the severity of the pain. While parents were found to rate their child's pain more accurately than any other observer,(181) neither the sick parent nor the foster parent advocate appropriately for their child's pain,(182) thus affecting the pain management. In addition, the family's perception of pain may be affected by cultural background, social experience, and, in many cases, by substance abuse. Therefore, rigid prescriptions for pain management are inappropriate. The goals of pain management in HIV-infected children include: (a) reduce the incidence and severity of acute and chronic pain while providing appropriately aggressive medical therapy; (b) provide adequate pharmacological pain control with minimal side-effects; (c) utilize non-pharmacological approaches to pain management; (d) educate children and families to communicate about pain; (e) relieve suffering; and (f) address quality of life issues, especially in terminal illness. In end-stage disease, pain management often needs to take precedence over other aspects of medical care including antiretroviral therapy.

The incidence of pain in HIV-infected children was found to be comparable to that reported in children with cancer.(182) In one study, 59 per cent of the HIV-infected children reported pain. Younger children and girls reported even higher incidence of pain (67 and 76 per cent, respectively).(182) The pain was related to complications of the disease itself and to the multiple procedures used for diagnosis and treatment. Although no guidelines are available for the management of pain in HIV-infected children, some of the principles used in developing guidelines to other chronic life-threatening diseases (e.g. cancer, sickle cell disease) should be considered when approaching an HIV-infected child in pain.

Disease-related pain

HIV-disease-related pain syndromes result from both infectious and non-infectious processes in various organ systems that can be acute or chronic. Causes of oropharyngeal pain include candidiasis, dental problems, periodontitis, gingivitis, aphthous ulcers, and herpetic stomatitis.(183) Esophageal pain (dysphagia) can result from esophageal candidiasis, CMV, or herpetic ulcerative esophagitis. A rare cause of dysphagia may be lymphoma. Common causes of abdominal pain include pancreatitis, hepatitis, cholengitis, MAC enteritis or colitis, CMV colitis, and inflammatory or infectious colitis. Chronic diarrhoea, although not classically considered a pain syndrome, is common in HIV disease and is usually associated with abdominal discomfort including cramping and spasms.(177,182)

The oropharyngeal and gastrointestinal pain syndromes frequently result in poor oral intake and reduced absorption of nutrients, which lead to malnutrition and failure to thrive and progression to wasting syndrome. Even in the early stages of the HIV disease, the recurrent difficulty with oral intake from various causes may have a significant impact on quality of life. The wasting syndrome is commonly associated with cachexia, fatigue, depression, musculoskeletal pain, abdominal pain, and neuropathy secondary to nutritional deficiencies. The chronic pain and suffering experienced by HIV-infected children with wasting syndrome is the most challenging to effectively treat and relieve.(153,182,183)

Neurological and neuromuscular pain syndromes are relatively common in HIV-infected children. These include hypertonicity, spasticity, encephalitis (e.g. Herpes, toxoplasmosis), meningitis (e.g. *Cryptococcus neoformans*), primary CNS lymphoma, Guillain–Barre syndrome, peripheral neuropathies [the possibility that the neuropathy might be a drug side-effect, e.g. antiretroviral (ddi) should be remembered] and myopathy. Skin and soft tissue complications of HIV, which are associated with both acute and chronic pain and discomfort, include Herpes simplex, Herpes zoster (shingles), and other bacterial or fungal infections as well as adenitis due to bacterial or mycobacterial agents. Malignancies such as leukaemia, lymphoma, and leimyosarcoma, which seem to be more frequent in HIV-infected children, have cancer-associated pain syndromes in addition to the HIV-associated symptoms.(177,182)

Treatment-related pain

Some chronic pain experienced by HIV-infected children is related to the side-effects and toxicities of the multiple medications used, especially antiretroviral medications. A detailed description of the specific side-effects of each antiretroviral is available in published paediatric treatment guidelines.(121) Many of the antiretroviral medications cause abdominal discomfort, nausea, and diarrhoea. This is especially true for the protease inhibitors as a class, but is also seen with nucleoside analogues such as didanosine and zidovudine. Other painful side-effects associated with antiretrovirals drugs include headache, pancreatitis, and neuropathy. Patients often need to continue on the medications causing these symptoms and are asked to 'live with' these side-effects or risk development of drug resistance and disease progression. In addition to the pain associated with antiretroviral therapy, the stress of adherence to these complex regimens has its own adverse impact on quality of life.

Procedure-related pain experienced by children with HIV disease is similar to procedure-related pain experienced by children with cancer. Published studies indicate that the pain associated with diagnostic and therapeutic procedures can be more stressful than the disease itself and need to be addressed in a comprehensive approach to pain management.(184–186) Common painful procedures, many of which are recurrent, include venipunctures, nasogastric and gastrostomy tube placement, lumbar punctures, and IV infusions.

Many children infected with HIV, including those enrolled in clinical trials, are living longer and experience more episodes of pain due to clinical syndromes and frequent procedures. Pain assessment should be part of the routine health management of children with chronic life-limiting illnesses. Successful assessment and control of pain and anxiety depends on a positive relationship between the provider and the patient. Patients should be aware of the need for repeated invasive procedures as part of their routine care and be actively involved in pain assessment and management.(187)

Table 5 Common pain assessment instruments

Instrument	Description
Faces scale	A series of cartoon faces indicating intensity of pain
Visual analog	A vertical line with numbers indicating severity of pain
Oucher scale	A series of photos of children in pain
Pain diary	Include time, activities, medications, procedures, and rating (numerical—one to ten) of pain

Signs and symptoms, which should alert the clinician that pain may be present, include listlessness, crying, wincing, change in mood, irritability, change in sleeping pattern, change in appetite, lower activity level, loss of concentration, loss of playfulness, and loss of interest in daily activities. The child's development level and parental judgement and insight about the pain are important factors to consider while evaluating the pain intensity, duration, and distribution. There are several pain assessment instruments available that are age and developmentally appropriate for children. The faces pain scale or visual analog scale (Table 5) should be used in children 4 years and older.(188) The Oucher scale can be used in younger children (3 years and older); a pain diary is probably the best tool for adolescents. These self-reporting measurements can be followed longitudinally and are very useful in determining the quality of the pain, precipitating and aggravating factors that cause the pain, and the effect of treatment regimens.

Management of pain

Many techniques are available to minimize pain from medical procedures. Adequate preparation of the child and parent for the procedure is an important first step. Age-appropriate explanation should be used and parents should be allowed to stay with their child during the procedure. If it is anticipated that the child will have repeated procedures, appropriate pain management should be given the first time the procedure is performed. By minimizing pain during the first procedure, it is possible to prevent future anticipatory distress and anxiety. Non-pharmacological, cognitive–behavioural interventions include distraction (music, counting, blowing bubbles), relaxation (slow breathing), visualization (favourite place, imaging pain as wires going to light switch that they can turn off), play therapy, and encouraging verbalization may be sufficient for minor procedures (e.g. venipuncture). If they are ineffective topical anesthetics, such as EMLA® cream, should be applied to two potential venipuncture sites and covered by an occlusive dressing for at least 30–45 minutes prior to the procedure. If possible, the caregiver should apply EMLA® at home (prior to clinic visit) because it is effective for 4 h. Pharmacological management for more invasive procedures (such as bone marrow) should include the use of conscious sedation, which is a medically controlled state of depressed consciousness obtained through the administration of medications to obtund, dull, and reduce the intensity of pain and awareness. Through conscious sedation the patient's ability to maintain a patent airway is retained, there is no loss of protective reflexes, and the patient retains the ability to respond appropriately to physical stimulation or simple verbal commands. Conscious sedation should be provided by a qualified practitioner in an appropriate environment.(189) The recent approval of the oral transmucosal fentanyl oralet® has been shown to be an effective analgesic for paediatric patients. A simple, validated, and effective, stepwise method for treating acute and chronic pain in cancer patients has been devised by the World Health Organization.(184) This is based upon incremental use of stronger pain medications in conjunction with ongoing pain assessments and treatment of side-effects with adjunctive therapies. For mild pain acetaminophen or a non-steroidal anti-inflammatory should be used. These drugs have a ceiling effect and beyond a certain point increasing doses do not increase analgesic efficacy. If pain is not relieved, a standard dose should be maintained and a weaker opioid such as codeine or tylenol with codeine should be added. Therapy should be individualized for each patient. Intramuscular and subcutaneous routes of administration should be avoided when possible in favour of oral, transdermal, or intravenous routes. Side-effects of analgesics should be monitored for and treated but should not automatically result in discontinuing pain management.

Opioids are the backbone of the pharmacological management of severe pain and can be safely used in infants and children. It is important to be aware of the common side-effects of opioids such as constipation, nausea, vomiting, pruritus, and sedation. While side-effects are not indications for discontinuing analgesics, switching from one opioid to another may alleviate side-effects. Constipation should be anticipated with chronic opioid use, although it has not been a frequent problem for children with advanced HIV disease who often suffer from chronic loose stools or diarrhoea. Nausea should be addressed aggressively with antiemetics such as prochlorperazine (compazine), trimethobenzamide (tigan), ondansetron (zofran) and ganisetron (kytril). Respiratory depression is an uncommon side-effect of opioids and is dose-dependent.(190) Commonly used opioids include morphine, methadone, or fentanyl. If methadone is used, adjustment of the antiretroviral drugs may be needed and consultation with a pharmacist familiar with HIV therapy is encouraged. The Opioid analgesic doses should be titrated to clinical effect without adherence to 'standard doses'. The 'right' dose is the dose that is sufficient to produce pain relief, without intolerable side-effects. If inadequate, increase dose as tolerated and consider adding adjunctive medications such as tricyclic antidepressants (such as amitriptyline) for neuropathic pain or anticonvulsant (such as phenytoin or gabopentin) for shooting, stabbing pain. Other adjuvants include laxative, antiemetics, steroids, anxiolytics (benzodiazepines), and barbiturates for sedation.(191,192)

Tolerance, which is a state in which an individual is less susceptible to the effects of a drug, is commonly seen with the chronic use of opioids. Children with end-stage HIV have frequently needed doses in the range of 150–200 mg morphine per hour i.v. or even higher. It is important to determine whether increasing analgesic requirements are due to tolerance or disease progression. In most cases it is the latter. Physical dependence, which is manifested by a physiological abstinence syndrome, upon withdrawal of opioids can occur with long term use. Children can be gradually weaned off of this physiological state of dependence if pain medications are no longer necessary. Tolerance and physical dependence should not be confused with addiction, which is a psychological disorder characterized by a behaviour pattern of compulsive drug use and preoccupation with drug acquisition. Children treated with opioids for chronic pain rarely become addicted.(193)

Frequently, children with HIV come from families with a history of substance abuse and this sometimes causes clinicians to fear using opioids in some families. Clinical experience has shown that with proper monitoring and systems put in place, the incidence of addicted caregivers using a child's medication is extremely low. Fear of parental misuse is not a reason to withhold opioids from a child in pain.

A multidisciplinary team, which includes a pain management expert, a psychologist and/or a psychiatrist, a chaplin, and others should be involved when the child continues to suffer and rapid escalation of antipain, dysponea, or sedative medications cause the child to become obtunded and less responsive. It is important at this stage to discuss with the parents the concept of terminal sedation. The parents (as well as the staff) need to understand that this intervention is intended for comfort without pain or distress till the child dies with dignity.(194,195)

If the family or an adolescent patient requests physician's assisted death (i.e. euthanasia), the caring team should focus on alleviating psychological and psychosocial distress and/or physical symptoms (e.g. pain, nausea). A compassionate approach with better communication and medical care (i.e. adequate analgesia and sedation) will abort most requests.(196)

Palliative care for HIV-infected children should be part of the teaching in medical centres.(197) There is a need to educate health-care providers across disciplines on how to manage the prognostic uncertainty of HIV disease, the effective management of pain and other symptoms in these patients, develop different skills needed to negotiate DNR and life-sustaining interventions in this population, and the spiritual dimensions of their condition.(198,199) Training of home care and hospice workers, non-professional caregivers, parent aids, and volunteers should be part of this education, particularly if the HIV-infected child is not connected to an HIV specialty team. The research agenda for palliative care and hospice services for HIV-infected children has been limited.[200] If such research is developed, it will stimulate educational and training programmes at all levels of the medical training to the benefit of both health-care providers and their chronically ill patients.

References

1. **Center for Disease Control and Prevention.** HIV/AIDS Surveillance Report. 2000, vol. 12, pp. 1–44.
2. **Joint United Nations Programme on HIV/AIDS and World Health Organization.** AIDS Epidemic Update: December 2000 (UNAIDS, Geneva, 2000).
3. **Connor, E.M.** et al. (1994). Reduction of maternal–infant transmission of human immunodeficiency virus type 1 with zidovudine treatment. *New England Journal of Medicine* **331**, 1173–80.
4. **Shaffer, N.** et al. (1999). Short-course zidovudine for perinatal HIV-1 transmission in Bangkok, Thailand: a randomised controlled trial. Bangkok Collaborative Perinatal HIV Transmission Study Group. *Lancet* **353**, 773–80.
5. **Guay, L.A.** et al. (1999). Intrapartum and neonatal single-dose nevirapine compared with zidovudine for prevention of mother-to-child transmission of HIV-1 in Kimpala, Uganda: HIVNET 023 randomised trial. *Lancet* **354**, 795–802.
6. **Piot, P.** et al. (2001). The global impact of HIV/AIDS. *Nature* **410**, 968–73.
7. **Wade, N.A.** et al. (1998). Abbreviated regimens of zidovudine prophylaxis and perinatal transmission of the human immunodeficiency virus. *New England Journal of Medicine* **339**, 1409–14.
8. **Stiehm, E.R.** et al. (1999). Efficacy of zidovudine and human immunodeficiency virus (HIV) hyperimmune globulin for reducing perinatal HIV transmission from HIV-infected women with advanced diseases: results of Pediatric AIDS Clinical Trials Group protocol 185. *Journal of Infectious Diseases* **179**, 567–75.
9. **Fiscus, S.A.** et al. (1999). Trends in human immunodeficiency virus (HIV) counseling, testing, and antiretroviral treatment of HIV-infected women and perinatal transmission in North Carolina. *Journal of Infectious Diseases* **180**, 99–105.
10. **Lindegren, M.L.** et al. (1999). Trends in perinatal transmission of HIV/AIDS in the United States. *Journal of the American Medical Association* **282**, 531–8.
11. **Byers, R.H.** et al. (1998). Projection of AIDS and HIV incidence among children born infected with HIV. *Statistics in Medicine* **17**, 169–81.
12. **The International Perinatal HIV Group** (1999). Mode of delivery and the risk of vertical transmission of human immunodeficiency virus type 1: a meta-analysis of 15 prospective cohort studies. *New England Journal of Medicine* **340**, 977–87.
13. **Stek, A.** et al. (1999). The safety and efficacy of protease inhibitor therapy for HIV infection during pregnancy. *American Journal of Obstetrics and Gynecology* **180**, S7 (abstract #14).
14. **Laurence, J.** (2000). HIV/Aids in South Africa: the epidemic in numbers. *AIDS Reader* **10**, 620–1.
15. **Garcia, P.M.** et al. (1999). Maternal levels of plasma human immunodeficiency virus type 1 RNA and the risk of perinatal transmission. *New England Journal of Medicine* **341**, 394–402.
16. **Mayaux, M.J.** et al. (1997). Maternal virus load during pregnancy and mother-to-child transmission of human immunodeficiency virus type 1: the French perinatal cohort studies. *Journal of Infectious Diseases* **175**, 172–5.
17. **Centers for Disease Control and Prevention** (1994). Recommendations of the US Public Health Service Task Force on the use of zidovudine to reduce perinatal transmission of human immunodeficiency virus. *Morbidity and Mortality Weekly Report* **43** (RR-11), 1–20.
18. **Cooper, E.R.** et al. (1996). After AIDS Clinical Trial 076; the changing pattern of zidovudine use during pregnancy, and the subsequent reduction in the vertical transmission of human immunodeficiency virus in a cohort of infected women and their infants. *Journal of Infectious Diseases* **174**, 1207–11.
19. **Mayaux, M.J.** et al. (1997). Acceptability and impact of Zidovudine prevention on mother to child HIV-transmission in France. *Journal of Pediatrics* **131**, 857–62.
20. **Mofenson, L.M.** (1999). Can perinatal HIV infection be eliminated in the United States? *Journal of the American Medical Association* **282**, 577–9.
21. **Wiktor, S.Z.** et al. (1999). Short-course oral zidovudine for prevention of mother-to-child transmission of HIV-1 in Abidjan, Cote d'Ivoire: a randomised trial. *Lancet* **353**, 781–5.
22. **Dabis, F.** et al. (1999). 6-Month efficacy, tolerance, and acceptability of a short regimen of oral zidovudine to reduce vertical transmission of HIV in breastfed children in Cote d'Ivoire and Burkina Faso: a double-blind placebo-controlled multicentre trial. DITRAME Study Group. *Lancet* **353**, 786–92.
23. **DITRAME ANRS Study Group** (1999). 15-month efficacy of maternal oral zidovudine to decrease vertical transmission of HIV-1 in breastfed African children. DITRAME ANRS 049 Study Group. *Lancet* **354**, 2050–1.
24. **Saba, J.** Interim analysis of early efficacy of three short ZDV/3TC combination regimens to prevent mother-to-child transmission of HIV-1: the PETRA trial. Sixth Conference on Retroviruses and Opportunistic Infections. Chicago, IL, 1999, p. 212 (abstract S7).
25. **European Collaborative Study** (1998). The use of therapeutic and other interventions to reduce the risk of mother-to-child transmission of HIV-1 in Europe. *British Journal of Obstetrics and Gynaecology* **105**, 704–9.
26. **Dabis, F.** et al. (1993). Estimating the rate of mother-to-child transmission of HIV: report of a workshop on methodological issues Ghent (Belgium). *AIDS* **7**, 1139–48.
27. **The Working Group on Mother-To-Child Transmission of HIV** (1995). Rates of mother-to-child transmission of HIV-1 in Africa, America and Europe: results from 13 perinatal studies. *Journal of Acquired Immune Deficiency Syndrome and Human Retrovirology* **8**, 506–10.
28. **Busch, M.P.** et al. (1991). Evaluation of screened blood donations for human immunodeficiency virus type 1 infection by culture and DNA amplification of pooled cells. *New England Journal of Medicine* **325**, 1–5.
29. **Lackritz, E.M.** et al. (1993). Blood transfusion practices and blood-banking services in a Kenyan hospital. *AIDS* **7**, 995–9.
30. **Gumodoka, B.** et al. (1993). Blood transfusion practices in Mwanza region, Tanzania. *AIDS* **7**, 387–92.
31. **Colebunders, R.** et al. (1991). Seroconversion rate, mortality, and clinical manifestations associated with the receipt of a human immunodeficiency virus-infected blood transfusion in Kinshasa, Zaire. *Journal of Infectious Diseases* **164**, 450–6.
32. **Dunn, D.T.** et al. (1992). Risk of human immunodeficiency virus type 1 transmission through breastfeeding. *Lancet* **340**, 585–8.
33. **Bobat, R.** et al. (1997). Breastfeeding by HIV-1-infected women and outcome in their infants: a cohort study from Durban, South Africa. *AIDS* **11**, 1627–33.
34. **World Health Organization** (1992). Concensus statement from the WHO/UNICEF consultation of HIV transmission and breastfeeding. *Weekly Epidemiological Record* **67**, 177–9.
35. **Mofenson, L.M.** (1994). Epiedemiology and determinants of vertical HIV transmission. *Seminars in Pediatric Infectious Diseases* **5**, 252–65.
36. **John, C.G.** et al. (1997). Genital shedding of HIV-1 during pregnancy: association with immuosuppresion, abnormal cervical or vaginal discharge, and severe vitamin A deficiency. *Journal of Infectious Diseases* **175**, 57–62.
37. **Lepage, P.** et al. (1993). Mother-to-child transmission of human immunodeficiency virus type 1 (HIV-1) and its determinants: a cohort study in Kigali, Rwanda. *American Journal of Epidemiology* **137**, 589–99.
38. **Semba, R.D.** et al. (1994). Maternal vitamin A deficiency and mother-to-child transmission of HIV-1. *Lancet* **343**, 1593–7.
39. **Bloland, P.B.** et al. (1995). Maternal HIV infection and infant mortality in Malawi: evidence for increased mortality due to placental malaria infection. *AIDS* **9**, 721–6.
40. **Hu, D.J.** et al. (1996). The emerging genetic diversity of HIV. The importance of global surveillance for diagnostics, research, and prevention. *Journal of the American Medical Association* **275**, 210–6.
41. **Mayaux, M.J.** et al. (1995). Maternal factors associated with perinatal HIV-1 transmission; The French cohort Study: 7 years of follow up observation. *Journal of AIDS* **8**, 188–94.
42. **Adjorlolo, G.** et al. (1994). Prospective comparison of HIV-1 and HIV-2 perinatal transmission in Abidjan, Cote d'Ivoire. *Journal of the American Medical Association* **272**, 462–6.

43. **Del Mistro, A.** et al. (1995). HIV-1 and HIV-2 seroprevalence rates in mother-child pairs living in the Gambia (West Africa). *Journal of Acquired Immune Deficiency Syndrome* **5**, 19–24.
44. **Centers for Disease Control and Prevention** (1994). Revised classification system for human immunodeficiency virus infection in children less than 13 years of age. *Morbidity and Mortality Weekly Report* **RR-12**, 1–10.
45. **Dunn, D.T.** et al. (1995). The sensitivity of HIV-1 DNA polymerase chain reaction in the neonatal period and the relative contributions of intrauterine and intrapartum transmission. *AIDS* **9**, F7–11.
46. **McIntosh, K.** et al. (1994). Blood culture in the first 6 months of life for diagnosis of vertically transmitted human immunodeficiency virus infection. *Journal of Infectious Diseases* **170**, 996–1000.
47. **Nesheim, S.** et al. (1997). Diagnosis of perinatal human immunodeficiency virus infection by polymerase chain reaction and p24 antigen detection after immune complex dissociation in an urban community hospital. *Journal of Infectious Diseases* **175**, 1333–6.
48. **Report of a Consensus Workshop**, S. Italy (1992). Early diagnosis of HIV infection in infants. *Journal of AIDS* **5**, 1169–78.
49. **Landesman, S.** et al. (1991). Clinical utility of HIV-IgA immuoblot assay in the early diagnosis of perinatal HIV infection. *Journal of the American Medical Association* **266**, 3443–6.
50. **Rakusan, T.A., Parrott R.H., and Sever, J.L.** (1991). Limitations in the laboratory diagnosis of vertically acquired HIV infection. *Journal of Acquired Immune Deficiency Syndrome* **4**, 116–21.
51. **Denny, T.** et al. (1992). Lymphocyte subsets in healthy children during the first 5 years of life [published erratum appears in *Journal of the American Medical Association* 1992; 267: 3154]. *Journal of the American Medical Association* **267**, 1484–8.
52. **European Collaborative Study** (1992). Age-related standards for T lymphocyte subsets based on uninfected children born to human immunodeficiency virus 1-infected women. *Pediatric Infectious Disease Journal* **11**, 1018–26.
53. **Henrard, D.R.** et al. (1995). Natural history of HIV-1 cell free veremia. *Journal of the American Medical Association* **274**, 554–8.
54. **Shearer, W.T.** et al. (1997). Viral load and disease progression in infants infected with human immunodeficiency virus type 1. *New England Journal of Medicine* **336**, 1337–42.
55. **McIntosh, K.** et al. (1996). Age- and time-related changes in extracellular viral load in children vertically infected by human immunodeficiency virus. *Pediatric Infectious Disease Journal* **15**, 1087–91.
56. **Blanche, S.** et al. (1990). Longitudinal study of 94 symptomatic infants with perinatally-acquired human immunodeficiency virus infection: evidence for a bimodal expression of clinical and biological symptoms. *American Journal of Diseases in Children* **144**, 1210–5.
57. **European Collaborative Study** (1994). Natural history of vertically acquired human immunodeficiency virus. *Pediatrics* **94**, 815–9.
58. **Commenges, D.** et al. (1992). Estimating the incubation period of pediatric AIDS in Rwanda. *AIDS* **6**, 1515–20.
59. **Kourtis, A.P.** et al. (1996). Early progression of disease in HIV-infected infants with thymus dysfunction. *New England Journal of Medicine* **335**, 1431–6.
60. **Mofenson, L.M.** et al. (1997). The relationship between serum human immunodeficiency virus type 1 (HIV-1) RNA level, CD4 lymphocyte percent, and long-term mortality risk in HIV-1-infected children. National Institute of Child Health and Human Development Intravenous Immunoglobulin Clinical Trial Study Group. *Journal of Infectious Diseases* **175**, 1029–38.
61. **Palumbo, P.E.** et al. (1998). Disease progression in HIV-infected infants and children: predictive value of quantitative plasma HIV RNA and CD4 lymphocyte count. *Journal of the American Medical Association* **279**, 756–61.
62. **deMartino, M.** et al. (2000). Reduction in mortality with availability of antiretroviral therapy for children with perinatal HIV-1 infection. *Journal of the American Medical Association* **284**, 190–7.
63. **Vetter, K.M.** et al. (1996). Clinical spectrum of human immunodeficiency virus disease in children in a west African city. *Pediatric Infectious Disease Journal* **15**, 438–42.
64. **Lucas, S.B.** et al. (1996). Disease in children infected with HIV in Abidjan, Cóte d'Ivoire. *British Medical Journal* **312**, 335–8.
65. **Colebunders, R.L.** et al. (1987). Evaluation of a clinical case definition of AIDS in African children. *AIDS* **1**, 151–3.
66. **Barnhart, H.X.** et al. (1996). Natural history of human immunodeficiency virus disease in perinatally infected children: an analysis from the pediatric spectrum of disease project. *Pediatrics* **97**, 710–6.
67. **Italian Register for HIV Infection in Children** (1994). Features of children perinatally infected with HIV-1 surviving longer than 5 years. *Lancet* **343**, 191–5.
68. **Longini, I.M. Jr.** et al. (1992). Estimating the stage-specific numbers of HIV infection using a Markov model and back-calculation. *Statistics in Medicine* **11**, 831–43.
69. **Centers for Disease Control and Prevention.** HIV/AIDS Surveillance Report, 1997, Vol. 9 (2), pp. 1–43.
70. **Marum, L.** et al. Three year mortality in a cohort of HIV-1 infected and uninfected Ugandan children (abstract). XIth International Conference on AIDS STD, Vancouver, July 1996.
71. **Suparatpinyo, K.** et al. (1994). Disseminated *Penicillium marneffei* infection in Southeast Asia. *Lancet* **344**, 110–3.
72. **Sirisanthana, V. and Sirisanthana, T.** (1995). Disseminated *Penicillium marneffei* infection in human immunodeficiency virus-infected children. *Pediatric Infectious Diseases* **14**, 935–40.
73. **Kline, M.W.** (1996). Oral manifestations of pediatric human immunodeficiency virus infection: a review of the literature. *Pediatrics* **97**, 380–8.
74. **Katz, M.H.** et al. (1993). Prognostic significance of oral lesions in children with perinatally acquired human immunodeficiency virus infection. *American Journal of Diseases in Children* **147**, 45–8.
75. **Funkhouser, M.E.** et al. (1993). Management of scabies in patients with human immunodeficiency virus disease. *Archives of Dermatology* **129**, 911–13.
76. **Paller, A.** et al. (1990). Pyoderma gangrenosum in pediatric acquired immune deficiency syndrome. *Journal of Pediatrics* **117**, 63–6.
77. **Englund, J.A.** et al. (1996). Clinical and laboratory characteristics of a large cohort of symptomatic, human immunodeficiency virus-infected infants and children. *Pediatric Infectious Diseases Journal* **15**, 1025–36.
78. **Blanche, S.** et al. (1990). Longitudinal study of 94 symptomatic infants with perinatally acquired human immunodeficiency virus infection. *American Journal of Diseases in Children* **144**, 1210–16.
79. **Brouwers, P.** et al. (1995). Correlation between computed tomographic brain scan abnormalities and neuropsychological function in children with symptomatic human immunodeficiency virus disease. *Archives of Neurology* **52**, 39–44.
80. **Principi, N.** et al. (1991). Acute otitis media in human immunodeficiency virus infected children. *Pediatrics* **88**, 566–71.
81. **Marchisio, P.** et al. (1996). Etiology of acute otitis media in human immunodeficiency virus-infected children. *Pediatric Infectious Diseases Journal* **15**, 58–61.
82. **Vernon, D.D.** et al. (1998). Respiratory failure in children with acquired immunodeficiency syndrome and acquired immunodeficiency-related complex. *Pediatrics* **82**, 223–8.
83. **Chandwani, S.** et al. (1990). Respiratory virus infection in human immunodeficiency virus-infected children. *Journal of Pediatrics* **117**, 251–4.
84. **Hall, C.B.** et al. (1986). Respiratory syncytial virus infection in children with compromised immune function. *New England Journal of Medicine* **315**, 77–81.
85. **Raviglione, M., Snider, D., and Kochi, A.** (1995). Global epidemiology of tuberculosis: morbidity and mortality of a worldwide epidemic. *Journal of the American Medical Association* **273**, 220–6.
86. **Moss, W.J.** et al. (1992). Tuberculosis in children infected with human immunodeficiency virus: a report of five cases. *Pediatric Infectious Diseases Journal* **11**, 114–20.
87. **Lallemant-Le Coeur, S.** et al. (1991). Bacillus Calmette-Guerin immunization in infants born to HIV-1 seropositive mothers. *AIDS* **5**, 195–9.
88. European Collaborative Study Group (1994). CD4 T cell count as predictor of *Pneumocystis carinii* penumonia in children born to mothers infected with HIV. *British Medical Journal* **308**, 437–40.
89. **Malin, A.S.** et al. (1995). *Pneumocystis carinii* pneumonia in Zimbabwe. *Lancet* **346**, 1258–61.

90. **Lucas, S.B.** et al. (1996). Disease in children infected with HIV in Abidjan, Côte d'Ivoire. *British Medical Journal* **312**, 335–8.
91. **Centers for Disease Control and Prevention** (1991). Guidelines for prophylaxis against *Pneumocystis carinii* pneumonia for children infected with the human immunodeficiency virus. *Morbidity and Mortality Weekly Report* **40**, 1–13.
92. **Simonds, R.J.** et al. (1993). *Pneumocystis carinii* pneumonia among US children with perinatally acquired HIV infection. *Journal of the American Medical Association* **270**, 470–3.
93. **Berdon, W.E.** et al. (1993). Pediatric HIV infection in its second decade – the changing pattern of lung involvement. Clinical, plain film, and computed tomographic findings. *Pediatric Chest* **31**, 453–63.
94. **Italian Register for HIV Infection in Children** (1994). Epidemilogy of HIV infection in children in Italy. *Acta Pediatrics* **400** (Suppl.), 15–18.
95. **Lipshultz, S.E.** et al. (1992). Cardiac structure and function in children with human immunodeficiency virus infection treated with zidovudine. *New England Journal of Medicine* **327**, 1260–5.
96. **Lipshultz, S.E.** Pediatric pulmonary and cardiovascular complications of vertically transmitted HIV infection study group. Progressive cardiac dysfunction in HIV-infected children-the prospective NHLBI P2C2 HIV study (abstract). Proceedings of the 9th International Conference on AIDS, 1993, vol. 9, p. 48.
97. **Winston, J.A. and Klotman, P.E.** (1996). Are we missing an epidemic of HIV-associated nephropathy? *Journal of the American Society of Nephrology* **7**, 1–7.
98. **D'Agati, V. and Appel, G.B.** (1997). HIV infection and the kidney. *Journal of the American Society of Nephrology* **8**, 138–52.
99. **Pardo, V., Strauss, J., Abitbol, C., and Zilleruelo, G.** (1995). Renal disease in children with HIV infection. In *Renal and Urologic Aspects of HIV Infection* (ed. P. Kimmel and J.S. Berns), pp. 135–53. New York: Churchill Livingstone.
100. **Inguilli, E.** et al. (1991). Nephrotic syndrome associated with acquired immunodeficiency syndrome in children. *Journal of Pediatrics* **119**, 711–16.
101. **Strauss, J.** et al. (1993). HIV nephropathy in children: importance of early detection. *Journal of American Society of Nephrology* **4**, 288A.
102. **McKinney, R.E. and Robertson, W.R. and the Duke Pediatric AIDS Clinical Trials Unit.** (1993). Effect of human immunodeficiency virus infection on the growth of young children. *Journal of Pediatrics* **123**, 579–82.
103. **Mgone, C.S.** et al. (1991). Prevalence of HIV-1 infection and symptomatology of AIDS in severely malnourished children in Dar es Salaam, Tanzania. *Journal Acquired Immune Deficiency Syndrome* **4**, 910–13.
104. **Zuin, G.** et al. (1992). Malabsorption of different lactose loads in children with human immunodeficiency virus infection. *Journal of Pediatric Gastroenterology and Nutrition* **15**, 408–12.
105. **Calle, P.F.** et al. (1993). Protein and lipid malabsorption in children; relationship to diarrhea, failure to thrive, enteric micro-organisms and immune impairment. *AIDS* **7**, 1435–40.
106. **Costaldo, A.** et al. (1996). Iron deficiency and intestinal malabsorption in HIV disease. *Journal of Pediatric Gastroenterology and Nutrition* **22**, 359–63.
107. **Lewis, J.D. and Winter, H.S.** (1995). Intestinal and hepatobiliary diseases in HIV-infected children. *Gastroenterology Clinics of North America* **24**, 119–32.
108. **Moye, J.** et al. (1996). For the Women and Infants transmission study group. Natural history of somatic growth in infants born to women infected by human immunodeficiency virus. *Journal of Pediatrics* **128**, 58–69.
109. **Henderson, R.A.** et al. (1996). Longitudinal growth during the first two years of life in children born to HIV-infected mothers in Malawi, Africa. *Pediatric AIDS HIV Infection* **7**, 91–7.
110. **Lepage, P.** et al. (1996). Growth of human immunodeficiency type 1-infected and uninfected children; a prospective cohort study in Kigali, Rwanda, 1988–1993. *Pediatric Infectious Disease Journal* **15**, 479–85.
111. **Berhane, R.** et al. (1996). Physical growth and mortality risk in children with perinatally acquired HIV. *Pediatric AIDS HIV Infection* **7**, 281.
112. **Periquet, B.A.** et al. (1995). Micronutrient levels in HIV-1 infected children. *AIDS* **9**, 887–93.
113. **Giovanni, M.** et al. (1990). Maternal–infant transmission of hepatitis C virus and HIV infections: a possible interaction. *Lancet* **I**, 1166.
114. **Arico, M.** et al. (1991). Malignancies in children with human immunodeficiency virus type 1 infection. *Cancer* **68**, 247–57.
115. **Ziegler, J.L. and Katongole-Mbidde, E.** (1996). Kaposi's sarcoma in childhood; an analysis of 100 cases form Uganda and relationship to HIV infection. *Internation Journal of Cancer* **65**, 200–3.
116. **Chadwick, E.G.** et al. (1990). Tumors of smooth muscle origin in HIV-infected children. *Journal of the American Medical Association* **263**, 3182–4.
117. **Ninane, J.** et al. (1985). AIDS in two African children—one with fibrosarcoma of the liver. *European Journal of Pediatrics* **144**, 385–90.
118. **Arico, M.** et al. (1991). Malignancies in children with human immunodeficiency virus type 1 infection. *Cancer* **68**, 2473–7.
119. **Nachman, S.A.** et al. (2000). Nucleoside analogs plus ritonavir in stable antiretroviral therapy-experienced HIV-infected children. *Journal of the American Medical Association* **283**, 492–8.
120. **Wintergerst, U.** et al. (1998). Comparison of two antiretroviral triple combinations including the protease inhibitor indinavir in children infected with human immunoideficiency virus. *Pediatric Infectious Disease Journal* **17**, 495–9.
121. **The Working Group on Antiretroviral Therapy and Medical Management of HIV-Infected Children.** Guidelines for the Use of Antiretroviral Agents in Pediatric HIV Infection. 14 December 2001: update available at www.aidsinfo.nih.gov.
122. **Gibb, D.M. and Giaquinto, C.** (2000). Children with HIV infection: special cases. *Lancet* **356**, s34.
123. **Watson, D.C. and Farley, J.J.** (1999). Efficacy of and adherence to highly active antiretroviral therapy in children infected with human immunodeficiency virus type-1. *Pediatric Infections Diseases Journal* **18**, 682–9.
124. **Yogev, R.** (1998). HIV viral load. *Pediatric Infectious Disease Journal* **17**, 247–8.
125. **Melvin, A.J.** (1999). Anti-retroviral therapy for HIV-infected children-toward maximal effectiveness. *Pediatric Infectious Disease Journal* **18**, 723–4.
126. **Friedland, G.H. and Williams, A.** (1999). Attaining higher goals in HIV treatment: the central importance of adherence. *AIDS* **13**, S61–72.
127. **Paterson, D.L.** et al. (2000). Adherence to protease inhibitor therapy and outcomes in patients with HIV infection. *Annals of Internal Medicine* **133**, 21–30.
128. **Shingadia, D.** et al. (2000). Gastrostomy tube insertion for improvement of adherence to highly active antiretroviral therapy in pediatric patients with human immunodeficiency virus. *Pediatrics* **105**, e80.
129. **Hayashi, S.** et al. Nelfinavir pharmacokinetics in stable HIV-infected children; the effect of weight and a comparison of BID and TID dosing (abstract no. 427). Proceedings of the 6th Conference on Retroviruses and Opportunistic Infections, Chicago, IL, January 31 to February 4, 1999.
130. **Johnson, G.M.** et al. (1999). Preliminary evaluation of nelfinavir pharmacodynamics in stable antiretroviral experienced HIV-infected children following initiation of HAART (PACTG 377). *Pediatrics Research* **45**, 164A.
131. **Faye, A., Compagnucci, A., and Saidi, Y.** Evaluation of toxicity, tolerability and antiviral eficacy of early d4T + ddI + nelfinavir therapy in HIV-infected infants: 24-week preliminary results from the PENTA 7 study. (abstract no. 678). Proceedings of the 8th Conference on Retroviruses and Opportunistic Infections, Chicago, IL, February 4–8, 2001.
132. **Rodman, J.** et al. Ritonavir (RTV) pharmacokinetics and dose requirements in HIV infected children less than two years of age (abstract no. 421). Proceedings of the 6th Conference on retroviruses and Opportunistic Infections. Chicago, IL, January 31 to February 4, 1999.
133. **Palumbo, P.E.** (2000). HIV/AIDS in infants, children and adolescents. *Pediatric Clinics of North America* **47**, 155–69.
134. **Erickson, J.W., Gulnick, S.V., and Markowitz, M.** (1999). Protease inhibitors: resistance, cross resistance, fitness and the choice of initial and salvage therapies. *AIDS* **13**, S189–204.
135. **Durant, J.** et al. (1999). Drug-resistance genotyping in HIV-1 therapy: the VIRADAPT randomized controlled trial. *Lancet* **353**, 2195–9.
136. **Mofenson, L.M.** et al. (1999). Risk factors for perinatal transmission of human immuodeficiency virus type 1 in women treated with zidovudine. *New England Journal of Medicine* **341**, 385–93.
137. Dorenbaum A for the PACTG 316 Study Team. Report of results of PACTG 316: an interantional phase III trial of standard antiretroviral (ARV)

prophylaxis plus nevirpine (NVP) for prevention of perinatal HIV transmission (Abstract LB7). In: Proceedings of the 8th Conference on Retroviruses and Opportunistic Infections, Chicago IL, 4–8 February 2001.

138. **Landesman, S.H.** et al. (1996). Obstetrical factors and the transmission of human immunodeficiency virus type 1 from mother to child. *New England Journal of Medicine* **334**, 1617–23.

139. **St. Louis, M.E.** et al. (1993). Risk for perinatal HIV-transmission according to maternal immunologic, virologic, and placental factors. *Journal of the American Medical Association* **269**, 2853–9.

140. **Mandelbrot, L.** et al., and the French Pediatric HIV Infection Study Group. (1996). Obstetric factors and mother-to-child transmission of human immunodeficiency virus type 1: the French perinatal cohorts. *American Journal of Obstetrics and Gynecology* **175**, 661–7.

141. **Biggar, R.J.** et al. (1996). Perinatal intervention trial in Africa: effect of a birth canal cleansing intervention to prevent HIV transmission. *Lancet* **347**, 1647–50.

142. **Wiktor, S.Z.** et al. (1999). Short-course oral zidovudine for prevention of mother-to-child transmission of HIV-1 in Abidjan, Côte d'Ivoire: a randomised trial. *Lancet* **353**, 781–5.

143. **Dabis, F.** et al., for the DITRAME Study Group (1999) 6-month efficacy, tolerance, and acceptability of a short regimen of oral zidovudine to reduce vertical transmission of HIV in breastfed children in Côte d'Ivoire and Burkina Faso: a double-blind placebo-controlled multicentre trial. *Lancet* **353**, 786–92.

144. **Gray, G.** The PETRA study: early and late efficacy of three short ZDV/3TC combination regimens to prevent mother-to-child transmission of HIV-1. In: XIII International AIDS Conference. Durban, South Africa, July 9–14, 2000.

145. **Van Rompay, K.K.A., McChesney, M.B., and Aguirre, N.L.** (2001). Two low doses of tenofovir protect newborn macaques against oral simian immunodeficiency virus infection. *Journal of Infections Diseases* **184**, 429–38.

146. WHO Technical Consultation on Behalf of the UNFPA/UNICEF/WHO/UNAIDS Inter-Agency Task Team on Mother-to-Child Transmission of HIV. New data on the prevention of mother-to-child transmission of HIV and their policy implications, 2000. Available at http://www.unaids.org/publications/documents/mtct/index.html.

147. **Coutsoudis, A.** et al. (1999). Influence of infant-feeding patterns on early mother-to-child transmission of HIV-1 in Durban, South Africa: a prospective cohort study. *Lancet* **354**, 471–6.

148. **Wawer, M.J.** et al. (1999). Control of sexually transmitted diseases for AIDS prevention in Uganda: a randomised community trial. *Lancet* **353**, 525–35.

149. **Coutsoudis, A.** et al. (1999). Randomized trial testing the effect of vitamin A supplementation on pregnancy outcomes and early mother-to-child HIV-1 transmission in Durban, South Africa. South African Vitamin A Study Group. *AIDS*, **13**, 1517–24.

150. **Fawzi, W.W.** et al. (1998). Randomized trial of effects of vitamin supplements on pregnancy outcomes and T cell counts in HIV-1-infected women in Tanzania. *Lancet* **351**, 1477–82.

151. **Doyle, D., Hanks, G. and MacDonald, N.** (1993). Introduction. In *Oxford Textbook of Palliative Medicine* (ed. D. Doyle, G. Hanks, and N. MacDonald), pp. 1–2. Oxford: Oxford University Press.

152. **American Academy of Pediatrics** (2000). Policy Statement, Palliative Care for Children. *Pediatrics* **106**, 351–7.

153. **Oleske, J.M., Rothpletz-Puglia, P.M., and Winter, H.** (1996). Historical perspectives on the evolution in understanding the importance of nutritional care in pediatric HIV infection. *Journal of Nutrition* **126**, 2616S–19S.

154. **Oleske, J.M.** Preventing disability and providing rehabilitation for infants, children and youths with HIV/AIDS. NIH publication no. 95-3850. Bethesda MD: US Department of Health and Human Services/National Institute of Child Health and Human Development, January 1995.

155. **Committee on Bioethics on the American Academy of Pediatrics** (1994). Guidelines for forgoing life-sustaining medical treatment. *Pediatrics* **93**, 532–6.

156. **Institute of Medicine.** *Approaching Death: Improving Care at the End of Life.* Washington DC: National Academy Press, 1997.

157. **McQuillan, R. and Finlay, I.** (1996). Facilitating the care of terminally ill children. *Journal of Pain and Symptom Management* **12**, 320–4.

158. **Nelson, L.J. and Nelson, R.M.** (1992). Ethics and the provision of futile, harmful or burdensome treatments to children. *Critical Care in Medicine* **20**, 427–33.

159. **Grothe, T.M. and Brody, R.V.** (1995). Palliative care for HIV disease. *Journal of Palliative Care* **11**, 48–9.

160. **Welch, K.** et al. (1998). The clinical profile of end stage AIDS. *AIDS Patient Care STD* **12**, 125–9.

161. **American Academy of Pediatrics Committee on Psychosocial Aspects of Child and Family Health** (1992). The pediatrician and childhood bereavement. *Pediatrics* **89**, 516–18.

162. **Goldman, A.** (1996). Home care of the dying child. *Journal of Palliative Care* **12**, 16–19.

163. **Koocher, G.P. and Gudas, L.J.** (1992). Terminal and life threatening illness in childhood. In *Developmental-Behavioral Pediatrics* (ed. M.D. Levine, W.B. Carey, A.C. Crocker, and R.T. Gross), pp. 327–36. Philadelphia: WB Saunders.

164. **World Health Organization.** The World Health Report 1995—Bridging the Gap. Report of the Director-General.

165. **Oleske, J.M.** (1994). The many needs of the HIV-infected child. *Hospital Practice* **29**, 81–7.

166. **Colburn, K.** (1998). Despite the continuum of care, is hospice terminal? *American Journal of Hospice and Palliative Care* **15**, 71–3.

167. **Youngblut, J.M., Brennan, P.F., and Swegart, L.A.** (1994). Families with medically fragile children: an exploratory study. *Pediatric Nursing* **20**, 463–8.

168. **Levetown, M.** (1996). Ethical aspects of pediatric palliative care. *Journal of Palliative Care* **12**, 35–9.

169. **Pellegrino, E.D.** (1998). Emerging ethical issues in palliative care. *Journal of the American Medical Association* **279**, 1521–2.

170. **DeTrill, M. and Kovalcik, R.** (1997). The child with cancer. Influence of culture on truth-telling and patient care. *Annals of the New York Academy of Sciences* **809**, 197–210.

171. **Stevens, M.M., Jones, P., and O'Riordan, E.** (1996). Family responses when a child with cancer is in palliative care. *Journal of Palliative Care* **12**, 51–5.

172. **Tasker, M.** *How Can I Tell You? Secrecy and Disclosure with Children When a Family Member has AIDS.* Bethesda MD: Association for the Care of Children's Health, 1992.

173. **Oleske, J.M. and Ruben-Hale, A.** (1995). Enhancing supportive care and promoting quality of life: Clinical practice guidelines. *Pediatric AIDS and HIV Infection: Fetus to Adolescent* **6**, 187–203.

174. **Flanagan-Klygis, E.** et al. (2001). Disclosing the diagnosis of HIV in pediatrics. *Journal of Clinical Ethics* **12**, 150–7.

175. **Freyer, D.R.** (1992). Children with cancer: special considerations in the discontinuation of life-sustaining treatment. *Medical and Pediatric Oncology* **20**, 136–42.

176. **Bromberg, M.H. and Higginson, I.** (1996). Bereavement follow-up: what do palliative support teams actually do? *Journal of Palliative Care* **12**, 12–17.

177. **Czarniecki, L., Boland, M., and Oleske, J.M.** (1993). Pain in children with HIV disease. *PAAC Notes* **5**, 492–5.

178. **Billings, J.A. and Block, S.** (1997). Palliative care in undergraduate medical education. *Journal of the American Medical Association* **278**, 733–8.

179. **Cook, L.A. and Wachko, J.F.** (1996). Decision making for the critically ill neonate near the end of life. *Journal of Perinatology* **16**, 133–6.

180. **Oleske, J. and Boland, M.** (1997). When a child with a chronic condition needs hospitalization. *Hospital Practice* **32**, 167–91.

181. **Schechter, N.L.** et al. (1991). Individual differences in children's response to pain: role of temperament and parental characteristics. *Pediatrics* **87**, 171–7.

182. **Hirschfeld, S.** et al. (1996). Pain in pediatric human immunodeficiency virus infection: incidence and characteristics in a single-institution pilot study. *Pediatrics* **98**, 449–56.

183. **Connolly, G.M.** et al. (1989). Oesophageal symptoms, their causes, treatment and prognosis in patients with acquired immunodeficiency syndrome. *Gut* **30**, 1033–9.

184. **World Health Organization (WHO).** Cancer pain relief and palliative care in children. World Health Organization, Geneva, Switzerland, 1998.

185. **Rhiner, M.** et al. (1994). The experience of pediatric cancer pain, part II: management of pain. *Journal of Pediatric Nursing* **9**, 380–7.

186. **Breitbart, W.** et al. (1996). The undertreatment of pain in ambulatory AIDS patients. *Pain* **65**, 243–8.
187. **Zelzer, L.K.** et al. (1990). Report of the subcommittee on the management of pain associated with procedures in children with cancer. *Pediatrics* **86**, 826–31.
188. **Bieri, D.** et al. (1990). The Faces Pain Scale for the self-assessment of the severity of pain experienced by children: development, initial validation, and preliminary investigation for ration scale properties. *Pain* **41**, 139–50.
189. **Committee on Drugs** (1992). Guidelines for monitoring and management of pediatric patients during and after sedation for diagnostic and therapeutic procedures. *Pediatrics* **89**, 1110–14.
190. **DeStouz, N.D., Bruera, E., and Suarez-Almazor, M.** (1995). Opioid rotation for toxicity reduction in terminal cancer patients. *Journal of Pain and Symptom Management* **10**, 378–84.
191. **Roila, F., Aapro, M., and Stewart, A.** (1998). Optimal selection of anti-emetics in children receiving cancer chemotherapy. *Supportive Care in Cancer* **6**, 215–20.
192. **Watanabe, S. and Bruera, E.** (1994). Corticosteroids as adjuvant analgesics. *Journal of Pain and Symptom Management* **9**, 442–5.
193. **McGarth, P.J. and Finley, G.A.** (1996). Attitudes and beliefs about medication and pain management in children. *Journal of Palliative Care* **12**, 46–50.
194. **Mount, B.** (1996). Morphine drips, terminal sedation, and slow euthanasia: definitions and facts, not anecdotes. *Journal of Palliative Care* **12**, 31–7.
195. **Kenny, N.P. and Frager, G.** (1996). Refractory symptoms and terminal sedation of children: ethical issues and practical management. *Journal of Palliative Care* **12**, 40–5.
196. **Orlowski, J.P., Smith, M.L., and Van Zwienen, J.** (1992). Pediatric euthanasia. *American Journal of Diseases in Children* **146**, 1440–6.
197. **Billings, J.A. and Block, S.** (1997). Palliative care in undergraduate medical education. *Journal of the American Medical Association* **278**, 733–8.
198. **Charlton, R.** (1996). Medical education—addressing the needs of the dying child. *Palliative Medicine* **10**, 240–6.
199. **Frager, G.** (1996). Pediatric palliative care: building the model, bridging the gaps. *Journal of Palliative Care* **12**, 9–12.
200. **Corner, J.** (1996). Is there a research paradigm for palliative care? *Palliative Medicine* **10**, 201–8.

10.4 Palliative medicine and non-malignant, end-stage respiratory disease

Richard M. Leach

Introduction

Non-malignant, end-stage respiratory disease is, in many ways, the 'Cinderella' of the many chronic diseases that require 'palliative' and compassionate end-of-life management. The course of chronic respiratory disease is often one of slow inexorable decline with long periods of disabling dyspnoea, reducing exercise tolerance, recurrent hospital admissions, and premature death. Loss of dignity, self-respect, social isolation, and psychological problems are often present during and well before the terminal phase of the disease. This long deterioration places enormous pressure on family members and carers. Despite the considerable efforts of specialist respiratory nurses and chest physicians to optimize survival and quality of life, these long-suffering incurable patients have not fully benefited from the holistic approach to the management of the physical, psychological, social, and spiritual needs developed and provided by specialist palliative care medicine. Recognition of these problems is not new. When John Hinton reported the needs of dying cancer patients in 1963, he recognized that cancer patients were not alone in suffering uncontrolled symptoms in the last days of life. He reported that patients with non-malignant disease often suffered the greatest physical distress.[1] Since this seminal article, the considerable success of the hospice movement in the management of cancer patients has further highlighted the plight of terminally-ill, non-cancer patients and the widening gap in their access to adequate palliative care.[2] In recent years, there has been a growing awareness of this need for palliative care in patients dying of non-malignant disease and in countries like the United States a high proportion of patients with non-malignant disease are already admitted to hospice inpatient units (30 per cent in 1994–1995).[3] In contrast, such facilities are limited in the United Kingdom accounting for less than 4 per cent of hospice inpatient admissions in 1994–1995 and are only available to small numbers of specific groups of end-stage neurological and HIV disease (Table 1).[4] Surprisingly, there is little data examining the needs of non-malignant, end-stage respiratory disease which is a substantial cause of disability and mortality in developed countries and is likely to become increasingly important in the future.

Recent studies have recognized the similarity between symptoms in patients dying with malignant and non-malignant disease.[5,6] Although pain is often reported to be a greater problem in cancer patients,[7] recent reports suggest that moderate and severe pain can occur as often in non-cancer patients.[8,9] The SUPPORT study, a major American investigation of decision-making in the last days of life, reported severe pain in 40 per cent of patients, and moderate or severe dyspnoea in 25 per cent irrespective of the disease.[10] Similar findings in end-stage patients with renal failure,[11] motor neurone disease,[12] heart disease,[13] stroke,[14] and chronic obstructive pulmonary disease (COPD)[15–17] demonstrated the considerable physical and psychological needs of the non-malignant dying patient. This deficiency has been recognized by a number of Government Committees in the United Kingdom who have recommended that all patients needing palliative care services should have access to them.[2,18,19]

The National Council for Hospice and Specialist Palliative Care Services and the Scottish Partnership Agency for Palliative Care have recently assessed the need, potential demand, and resource implications of this directive in their 1998 publication entitled 'Reaching Out: Specialist Palliative Care for Adults with Non-Malignant Diseases'.[2] There are, without doubt, considerable difficulties to be overcome if adequate palliative care facilities are to be provided to sufferers of non-malignant disease[2] and many of these are particularly applicable to the management of end-stage respiratory disease. Not least is the potential size and resource implications of this requirement and the fear, expressed by many palliative care physicians, that this demand may be detrimental to the delivery of care to cancer patients and may reduce charitable donations. Determining when chronic disease becomes terminal is another major issue. Unlike cancer many non-malignant diseases, particularly end-stage respiratory disease, have long periods of stability interrupted by major life-threatening exacerbations, which make end-of-life management decisions difficult. Finally, concern has also been raised as to whether palliative care specialists have the necessary skills to manage a wide variety of terminal disease processes.

Table 1 Adult patients who received care from hospices/palliative care services in 1994–1995[2]

	Malignancy (%)	Neurological (%)	HIV/AIDS (%)	Other (%)
New inpatients	96.7	1.3	0.5	1.6
Home care patients	96.3	0.6	0.6	2.5
Day care patients	96.3	0.2	0.2	1.2

The potential requirement for palliative care in end-stage pulmonary disease

In most developed countries, lung cancer and chronic lung diseases are a significant and increasing cause of morbidity and mortality. Respiratory diseases accounted for 153 168 of 632 062 (24.2 per cent) deaths in the United Kingdom in 1999,[20,21] more than heart disease (132 024 cases) or non-respiratory cancer (118 922 cases). Acute infectious diseases (e.g. pneumonia) accounted for 67 591 cases and respiratory cancer for 35 879 cases. Progressive, non-malignant diseases, in particular COPD (30 634 cases), but also including less common chronic lung diseases such as pneumoconiosis, pulmonary fibrosis or circulatory disease, and cystic fibrosis (~10 000 cases) account for about 25 per cent of all respiratory disease (Table 2).

Chronic obstructive pulmonary disease is recognized as a major although neglected medical and social problem. In the United Kingdom, chronic respiratory disability causes about 13 per cent of adult disability and COPD is the major cause.[22] Exact figures for the prevelance of COPD are difficult to determine due to problems of definition. In the United Kingdom, it may affect between 7–18 per cent of men and 3–7 per cent of women[20,21,23,24] and will account for 1000 inpatient admissions and 25 000 primary care consultations annually in an average health district.[24,25] However, it should be recognized that respiratory disease, especially COPD, is twice as common in the United Kingdom (age standardized death rate: 105 per 100 000 population) as other European Union countries (57 per 100 000 population).[20,26] In the United States, about two million people have emphysema and 50 per cent of these have reduced exercise tolerance.[27] Although smoking appears to be decreasing in developed countries, and eventually the incidence of COPD will fall, it is increasing in developing countries and current low levels of COPD in these countries will rise in the future.[28]

The cause of end-stage respiratory disease requiring palliative care varies geographically in relation to socioeconomic factors. HIV-related respiratory diseases and post-tuberculous bronchiectasis are common problems in developing countries. In contrast, COPD, cystic fibrosis, restrictive chest wall diseases (e.g. scoliosis, thoracoplasty), and neuro-muscular disorders (e.g. muscular dystrophies, old poliomyelitis) are more common in the United States and Europe. In developed countries, diseases affecting younger patients, including cystic fibrosis and the muscular dystrophies, are better resourced and the terminal needs of these patients are often well managed. In comparison, COPD and the less common fibrotic lung diseases have the same palliative care requirements but there is inadequate resource to meet these needs.

From the data in Table 2 it is apparent that equal numbers of patients with non-malignant, end-stage respiratory disease (mainly COPD) and lung cancer are experiencing pre-terminal disease and are likely to require similar medical and social services. Both conditions are managed by the same health care professionals and intuition and a number of recent United Kingdom studies suggest that patients with end-stage respiratory disease do not receive the care appropriate to their needs.[2,15,16] However, in comparison to malignant disease, there has been remarkably little research into the symptomatology, survival, appropriate care, and service utilization of these patients. This information is vital if appropriate and manageable solutions to the current weaknesses in care delivery are to be addressed.

Terminal symptoms, quality of life, and survival of patients with end-stage pulmonary disease

In patients with chronic lung disease, quality of life is often poor and survival statistics may be worse than for many malignant conditions. In the Medical Research Council trial of domiciliary oxygen in stable, hypoxaemia, COPD patients, survival of men and women in the control arm was only 42 and 28 per cent, respectively, at 3 years.[29] Prognosis is inversely related to age and directly to FEV_1 and hypoxaemia. Unfortunately, in the individual case, these measurements are of little help in predicting survival. The patient may struggle from one crisis to another for many years before a sudden deterioration and death over a few days. Evidence from the SUPPORT study also indicates that judging time to death is difficult in non-malignant disease. On the day before death, hospitalized lung cancer patients were predicted to have less than 20 per cent chance of living for 2 months, compared with a 60 per cent predicted chance of doing so in patients with heart failure.[9] This inability to predict disease trajectory makes end-of-life decisions difficult and has led to some concern that hospice facilities will be blocked by non-malignant cases who are gravely ill at admission but recover to their previous state of chronic ill-health.[2] However, only half of hospice admissions in cancer patients in 1994/1995 ended in death, with many patients returning home following resolution of the immediate problem.[4]

The poor quality of life experienced by end-stage COPD patients was recognized and reported in the Nocturnal Oxygen Therapy Trial in 1980 as disturbances in both emotional and social functioning and marked impairment in activities of daily living.[30] Recent studies have documented the symptoms (Table 3), quality of life, palliative care needs, and service utilization of patients dying of chronic respiratory disease during the final weeks and months of life.[15–17] Breathlessness and pain were reported as 'very distressing' in 76 and 56 per cent of patients during the final year and the overall burden of symptoms was very similar to those experienced by lung cancer patients.[16] In chronic lung disease, symptoms had been present for longer and the severity and frequency of breathlessness was greater. In contrast, constipation and anorexia were more frequent in lung cancer patients.

A recent study indicates that COPD patients have a significantly worse quality of life than unresectable, non-small cell, lung cancer patients.[15] However, assessing quality of life is complex, being both individual and multidimensional.[31] Many quantitative instruments are available to measure 'generic' health related quality of life (HRQoL). In the medical context these grade physical symptoms, psychological well-being, and limitations in physical and social activity (e.g. Medical Outcomes Study Short Form 36

Table 2 Respiratory disease deaths, 1999[20,21]

All respiratory disease	153 168 cases (100%)
Pneumonia and TB	67 591 cases (44.1%)
Cancer	35 879 cases (23.4%)
Progressive non-malignant causes	39 939 cases (25.1%)
COPD + asthma	32 155 cases (21.0%)
Pulmonary circulatory disease	6 300 cases (4.1%)
Pneumoconiosis	1 215 cases (0.8%)
Cystic fibrosis	154 cases (0.1%)
Sarcoidosis	115 cases (0.07%)
Others (congenital, foreign body, etc.)	9 759 cases (6.4%)

Table 3 Symptoms reported in the final year of life[16]

Symptom	Chronic lung disease		Lung cancer	
	All (%)	Very distressing (%)	All (%)	Very distressing (%)
Pain	77	56	85	56
Breathlessness	94	76	78	60
Cough	59	46	56	40
Anorexia	67	15	76	19
Constipation	44	25	59	55
Insomnia	65	42	60	35
Low mood	71	57	68	51

(SF-36)). They can be compared to data from normal populations but have limitations in relation to chronic disease.[32] Disease-specific instruments examine features specific to the disease studied. The St George's Respiratory Questionnaire (SGRQ) and the Chronic Respiratory Disease Questionnaire (CRDQ) are often used to measure HRQoL in respiratory patients.[33,34] In cancer patients, the European Organisation for the Research and Treatment of Cancer Core questionnaire (EORTC QLQ-C30) and the site specific module LC-17 for lung cancer is well validated as an outcome measure.[35] In the study comparing quality of life in patients with COPD and lung cancer, both 'generic' and 'disease-specific' measures demonstrated a worse quality of life in COPD patients.[15] Physical, social, and emotional functioning, as well as activities of daily living, were worse in COPD patients. Clinical depression measured with the Hospital Anxiety and Depression Scale (HADS) affected 90 per cent of COPD compared to 52 per cent of lung cancer patients. However, some care should be exercised in interpreting the results of this study,[31] as previous studies reported greater levels of depression using HADS scores in patients with inoperable cancer[35, 36] and lower EORTC scores for emotional function in lung cancer.[37]

Current service provision and utilization by patients with end-stage pulmonary disease

In the United Kingdom, few (<5 per cent) of the 75 per cent of patients who die from non-malignant disease die in a hospice or under the care of a domiciliary palliative care team (Table 1). A recent study reported that non-cancer patients accounted for between 0 and 12 per cent (median 5 per cent) of the palliative care team's workload.[2] In contrast, at least 20 per cent of cancer patients die in a hospice and a further 40 per cent die whilst under the care of a specialist domiciliary care team.[4] These figures may be an underestimate as many cancer patients receive domiciliary care from or attended a hospice day unit and die elsewhere.

The effectiveness of palliative care in non-malignant disease is poorly studied except in motor neurone disease and dementia.[2,11,14] It is recognized that the majority of patients with heart disease and stroke die in hospital or residential/nursing homes and that there are deficits in their end of life care.[5,6,38] The proposal that patients with end-stage respiratory disease in the United Kingdom are less well served than cancer patients[15] is one that most respiratory health workers would accept. However, the assumption that there are more specialist cancer nurses than respiratory outreach nurses with an interest in COPD was questioned by a British Thoracic Society survey in 1997, which reported that less than 30 per cent of lung cancer units had access to a specialist cancer nurse.[39] Nevertheless, there is little doubt that more palliative care services are available to cancer patients.[2]

There have been two recent comparisons of end-of-life care in lung cancer and chronic respiratory disease.[15,16] Patients with chronic respiratory disease were more likely to die in hospital and lung cancer patients at home or in a hospice (Table 4). Chronic lung disease patients were often admitted as emergencies, and as a result lung cancer patients were observed to spend longer in their place of death.[16] Access to primary medical care was good for both groups[15,16] although only a small percentage received treatment for anxiety and depression despite high levels of these symptoms.[15] Available financial support (e.g. mobility allowance, income support) and aids (e.g. wheelchairs, bath aids) were utilized more frequently by COPD patients due to prolonged illness and because most of these patients were house or wheelchair bound. In both studies access to palliative care services for patients with chronic respiratory disease was poor.[15,16] Thirty per cent of cancer patients received help from a Marie-Curie nurse, Macmillon nurse, or hospice centre and a further 56 per cent had been offered or were aware of the availability of these services.[15] In contrast, none of the COPD patients received or were offered access to these services or any equivalent service. However, a respiratory nurse visited about 25 per cent of COPD patients, although her primary responsibility was for tuberculosis-contact tracing. A concern in both studies was the lack of information relating to treatment, management, and prognosis. Lung cancer patients were more likely to be told that they would die of the disease by the hospital doctor than patients with COPD. Most COPD patients determined their prognosis by talking to other health personnel (e.g. district nurse) and during acute admissions.

Table 4 Place of death in a random sample in 20 UK health districts in 1990 (adapted from refs 2,16)

Place of death	Cancer (%; *n* = 2063)	Chronic lung disease (%; *n* = 87)	Heart disease (%; *n* = 683)	Stroke (%; *n* = 229)
Home	29	12	29	9
Hospital	50	72	55	67
Hospice	14	0	0	0
Other	7	16	16	24

The effectiveness and feasibility of specialist palliative care services in end-stage, non-malignant respiratory disease have not been established. The 1997 British Thoracic Society guidelines for the management of COPD conclude that there are no data to show how severe end-stage COPD should be managed to achieve the best combination of clinical and cost effectiveness.[21] As early as 1981 the Royal College of Physicians (United Kingdom) recommended the creation of respiratory health worker posts to advise on psychosocial problems and to help with the domiciliary management of patients with chronic respiratory diseases.[40,41] Currently, there are about 140 respiratory nurses in the United Kingdom.[42] Patients under the care of these nurses live longer but their quality of life may not be improved.[41,43] However, chest clinics, employing specialist respiratory nurses, recognize their role in symptom control and compliance with therapy. In addition, despite the lack of evidence of objective improvement, patients valued these visits and wanted them to continue.[41] Recent studies in acute exacerbations of COPD demonstrated that early discharge and 'care at home programmes' run by respiratory outreach nurses are both safe and cost effective.[44,45] In addition, both patients and carer's reported that home care was their preferred option.[46]

Symptom pathophysiology and assessment

Chronic end-stage lung disease is associated with the symptoms of breathlessness, cough (± sputum production), fever (± sweats), infection (± halitosis), haemoptysis, stridor, and chest wall pain. The pathophysiology and assessment of these symptoms is examined briefly as they have been extensively reviewed in the chapter relating to malignant respiratory conditions. The treatment of each symptom and therapeutic modalities will be discussed in the management of individual disease process.

Dyspnoea

Dyspnoea is derived from the Greek *dys*: meaning painful or difficult and *pneuma* meaning breath and is used to describe a variety of sensations experienced when breathing is difficult, uncomfortable, or laboured or when the subject feels a need for more air.[47,48] This sensation of breathlessness is experienced by healthy individuals under stress (e.g. exercise) and patients with a wide spectrum of diseases. It is multifactorial being influenced by many modifying factors (e.g. psychological, social) and is clearly distinct from other symptoms like tachypnoea and hyperinflation. The American Thoracic Society in its recent consensus conference defined dyspnoea as: 'a term used to characterise a subjective experience of breathing discomfort that is comprised of qualitatively distinct sensations that vary in intensity. The experience derives from interactions among multiple physiological, psychological, social and environmental factors, and may induce secondary physiological and behavioural responses'.[49]

Like pain, breathlessness has specific descriptors and refers to a number of different sensations including chest tightness, the need for deep inspiration, frequency, and depth of ventilation.[50–52] Both normal subjects and COPD patients are able to distinguish the intensity of breathlessness from the distress it causes.[54] Unfortunately, the 'language of dyspnoea' is not specific and description is dependent on physiological context, personality, social, and ethnic factors.[53] Thus, as with pain, a good history is invaluable in the assessment of dyspnoea.

Prevalence of dyspnoea

Dyspnoea is the most frequent symptom experienced by patients with end-stage respiratory disease. In the SUPPORT trial, dyspnoea was the major complaint of 416 patients dying with COPD, and was twice as common as pain or confusion throughout the entire 6 months of their dying.[10] In chronic lung disease, breathlessness was reported in 94 per cent during the last year and 91 per cent during the last week of life, compared to 78 and 69 per cent, respectively, in lung cancer patients.[16]

Mechanisms of dyspnoea (see Chapter 8.8 relating to malignant respiratory conditions)

Figure 1 is a simplified representation of the complex and poorly understood mechanism of dyspnoea. At its simplest level the process of dyspnoea may be expressed as:

1. *A central drive or 'urge to breath' that functions to satisfy the metabolic requirements of the body by maintaining blood–gas and acid–base homeostasis by modulating ventilatory activity.* This drive to breath incorporates all the sensory afferent input from chemosensors (e.g. medulla, carotid, and aortic bodies), mechanoreceptors (e.g. chest wall, lung and pulmonary vessel receptors, peripheral muscle receptors), and higher cerebral cortex activity (e.g. anxiety, personality).
2. *As the work of breathing or 'sense of respiratory effort' associated with ventilation.* When the efferent motor command to the respiratory muscles is discharged, a corollary message is sent to higher brain centres and results in a conscious awareness of the outgoing motor command. The resulting sense of effort is the ratio of the pressure actually generated by the respiratory muscles to the maximum that could be generated.[49]

Most studies demonstrate that stimulation of ventilation is necessary for breathlessness to occur[55] and that the sensation of dyspnoea depends on the degree to which the respiratory neurons in the diffuse brainstem 'respiratory complex' are stimulated by factors like hypoxia, hypercapnia, and metabolic acidosis.[55–58] However, the relationship between ventilatory response to stimuli and dyspnoea is not maintained in all circumstances and the sensation of dyspnoea may be directly affected by inputs from chemoreceptors. Thus, relief of exercise-induced hypoxaemia by administration of oxygen in COPD patients results in a reduction of dyspnoea out of proportion to the reduction in ventilation.[59] Similarly, ventilator-dependent quadriplegics with high cervical spinal cord transactions experience breathlessness when PCO_2 is increased when there should be no change in afferent feedback from the chest wall.[60,61] Afferent input from lung (e.g. mechanical, juxta-pulmonary, irritant) and peripheral (e.g. chest wall, skeletal muscle, facial skin) receptors also modulates breathlessness.[62,63] Thus, cold air blowing on the face may decrease dyspnoea.[64] In contrast, the complete absence of dyspnoea that may occur with prolonged severe hypoxia and/or hypercapnia suggests that the respiratory centre can also adapt to prolonged stimulation.

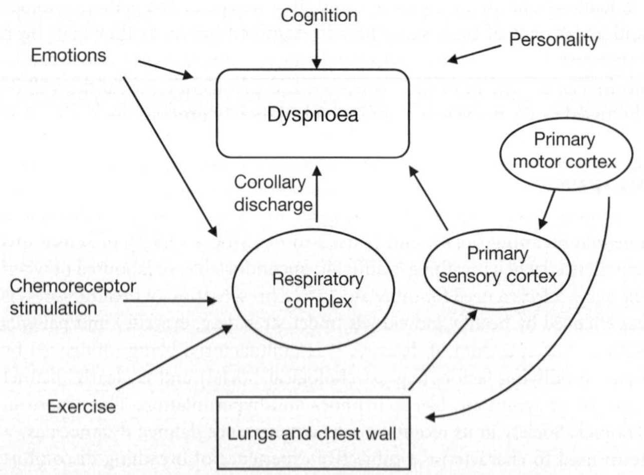

Fig. 1 Control of ventilation; involving the brainstem respiratory complex, higher cortical functions, and afferent input from the lungs, chest wall, and chemoreceptors.

The 'sense of effort' in peripheral muscles has been demonstrated to be separated from the 'urge to breath' in hyperventilating normal subjects in whom the addition of CO_2 resulted in an increased urge to breath but reduced awareness of the effort of breathing.[65] Similarly, patients with lung disease and in normal subjects with constraints to breathing (e.g. external respiratory loads) also report increased effort during breathing.[66,67] An attractive unifying theory is that dyspnoea results from a mismatch between central motor activity and incoming afferent information from chemo- and mechanoreceptors.[47,49]

An individual's emotional state, personality, experience, and cognitive function may also influence the perception of dyspnoea.[68] Dyspnoea is worse when it occurs suddenly, in inappropriate situations, or is perceived to be life threatening. The intensity of the dyspnoea is also influenced by previous experience of the sensation.[69]

Assessment of dyspnoea

A good history and examination is essential and will often establish the causal system (e.g. heart, lung, neuromuscular) and establish the underlying pathophysiology (Table 5). Diagnostic testing commonly follows to confirm the cause (Table 6). As a disease progresses, measurement of the severity of dyspnoea aids decision making and may indicate the success of a particular therapy. In general, the simpler the measurement techniques the more likely it is to be used.

1. *Verbally reported intensity:* reproducible ratings of dyspnoea intensity can be made on linear or numerical scales.[49] Simple verbal numerical scales rate dyspnoea from 0 to 10.[70] The visual analogue scale uses a 10 cm line, with 'no breathlessness' and 'maximum breathlessness' at the two ends. In response to the question 'how breathless are you', the

Table 5 The pathophysiological causes of dyspnoea

Pathophysiological mechanism	Typical causes
Increased respiratory drive	
Hypoxaemia	Many respiratory and cardiac diseases
Metabolic acidosis	Renal failure, cardiac failure
Intrapulmonary receptor stimulation	Infiltrative disease, pulmonary oedema
Mechanical impedence	
Airflow obstruction	Asthma, COPD, tumour, stenosis
Mechanical chest wall restriction	Kyphoscoliosis, obesity, pregnancy
Reduced compliance ('stiff lungs')	Interstitial fibrosis, lymphangitis carcinomatosis
Respiratory muscle failure	
Muscle disease/paralysis	Poliomyelitis, muscular dystrophy
Mechanical disadvantage	Hyperinflation, pneumothorax, pleural effusion
Wasted ventilation	
Large vessel obstruction	Pulmonary emboli, pulmonary vasculitis
Capillary damage	Interstitial lung disease, emphysema
Psychological	
Anxiety, depression	Hyperventilation syndrome

Table 6 Diagnostic tests for the evaluation of dyspnoea

Pulmonary function tests
Arterial blood gases
Exercise testing
Lung volumes and flow rates
Gas transfer/diffusing capacity (D_{LCO})
Bronchial challenge
Imaging techniques
Ventilation-perfusion scanning
High-resolution CT scanning
Angiography
Diaphragmatic fluoroscopy
Positron emission tomography (PET)
Cardiac evaluation
Echocardiography
Cardiac angiography
Myocardial perfusion scan
ECG monitoring
Other techniques
Sleep studies
Oesophageal pH monitoring
Otolaryngoscopy

Table 7 Modified Borg Dyspnoea Scale[72]

Intensity of sensation	Rating
Nothing at all	0
Very, very slight	0.5
Very slight	1
Slight	2
Moderate	3
Somewhat severe	4
Severe	5 6
Very severe	7 8
Very, very severe	9
Maximal	10

patient marks a point on the line, so that the length reflects the intensity of the dyspnoea.[71] The 12-point Borg Scale (Table 7), with extremes of 'no breathlessness' and 'maximal breathlessness', has verbal descriptors like slight and severe to assist the subject to rate the symptom.[72]

2. *Quality of life (QOL) measures:* determine the physical, emotional, and social response of a patient to their symptoms and disease.[49] Improvement may be independent of changes in the severity of the disease. Several questionnaires have been developed to assess the impact of respiratory disease on Quality of Life but are of most value in research projects rather than clinical practice. The most commonly used are the Chronic Respiratory Disease Questionnaire which evaluates dyspnoea, fatigue, emotional function, and mastery in a 20-item questionnaire,[73] the Saint Georges Respiratory Questionnaire, a 76-item questionnaire which assesses symptoms, activity, and impact of disease on daily life,[74] and the Pulmonary Functional Status Scale which measures the effect of respiratory distress on functional activity in COPD patients.[49]
3. *Physiological techniques:* including simple spirometry and oxygen saturation are relatively easy to measure even in advanced lung disease.

Table 8 Treatment of dyspnoea

Reduce work of breathing (i.e. reduce ventilatory impedence)
Bronchodilation (β_2-agonists, ipratropium bromide)
Counterbalance lung hyperinflation by
CPAP to match auto-PEEP
Breathing strategies (e.g. purse-lip breathing)
Surgical volume reduction
Rest respiratory muscles (NIPPV, cuirass)
Reduce ventilatory demand
Exercise training and oxygen therapy
Decrease central drive
Pharmacological therapy (e.g. opiates)
Altered afferent input to the medulla (e.g. facial fans)
Vagal nerve/carotid body resection
Improved CO_2 elimination by breathing therapy
Improve inspiratory muscle function
Nutrition
Rehabilitation programmes
Optimize muscle strength
Dyspnoea desensitization
Positioning (e.g. upright posture/lean forward)
Partial ventilatory support (BIPAP, CPAP, NIPPV)
Avoid oral steroids
Alter perception
Education, desensitization, coping strategies, psychotherapy
Pharmacological therapy (e.g. anxiolytics)

Table 9 Non-malignant causes of cough

Cause of cough	Typical examples
Acute infection	Viral, bronchopneumonia
Chronic infection	Bronchiectasis, cystic fibrosis
Airways disease	Asthma, COPD
Cardiovascular	Left ventricular failure
Parenchymal disease	Interstitial fibrosis
Irritant	Oesophageal reflux, foreign body
Recurrent aspiration	Motor neurone disease, stroke
Drug induced	ACE inhibitors, inhaled drugs
Pleural disease	Pneumothorax, pleural effusion
Vocal cord disease	Paralysis or nodules

Unfortunately, a patient's baseline FEV_1 has been shown to be a poor predictor of breathlessness[75,76] and improvements in dyspnoea after bronchodilators do not match changes in FEV_1.[77] Serial chest radiography is of limited value in the assessment of disease progression but may detect reversible problems (e.g. pleural effusions). Exercise tolerance (e.g. 6 min or shuttle walking) may be used to assess response to therapy even in the patient with limited mobility.[78] Many other special studies are of value in the evaluation of dyspnoea (Table 6) but these become less reliable and increasingly difficult to perform during end-stage respiratory disease.

Treatment of dyspnoea

Therapy for dyspnoea will vary depending on the underlying cause. The management of individual diseases is discussed later in this text, but a general summary of dyspnoea treatment is presented in Table 8.

Cough

Cough is not a common occurrence in normal subjects. However, in cardiothoracic disorders it may become a distressing symptom (Table 9).

Mucociliary transport is responsible for the majority of airways clearance but it is impaired in lung disease. In chronic bronchitis mucociliary, clearance is half that in healthy subjects. Cough acts as a reserve mechanism and increases clearance by 20 per cent in chronic bronchitis compared to 2.5 per cent in the healthy individual.[79] In end-stage respiratory disease, there are few data relating to the frequency, severity, and management of cough. However, in one of the few studies examining cough in the final year of life, 59 per cent of these patients complained of cough and this was very distressing in 46 per cent.[16] In the last week of life cough was reported in 52 per cent of patients. These figures were very similar to the incidence of cough in lung cancer patients.

Mechanism of cough (see Chapter 8.8 relating to malignant respiratory disease)

Involuntary cough is initiated by rapidly adapting 'irritant' receptors (RARs) that transmit through fast-velocity myelinated vagal fibres. The most sensitive sites for cough induction are the larynx, main carina, and branching points in the tracheobronchial tree. Stimulation of smaller airways and alveoli does not cause cough. RARs respond to a wide variety of chemical (e.g. smoke), inflammatory (e.g. histamine), and mechanical (e.g. foreign body) stimuli. They also cause bronchoconstriction and mucous hypersecretion.[80,81] C-fibres lying in close proximity to RARs respond to the same stimuli but do not cause cough although they may stimulate RARs to initiate cough.[82]

Cough is integrated in the medulla. Afferent fibres are relayed through the nucleus of the tractus solitarius and motor output dispatched via the nucleus ambigualis to the larynx and bronchial tree and via the nucleus retroambigualis to the respiratory muscles. The central nervous receptors for cough include serotonin, opioids, GABA, and dopamine, which may have potential therapeutic implications.[83] Voluntary cough, initiated by the cerebral cortex, can bypass these integrative centres as patients with brainstem damage and no spontaneous cough reflex can consciously induce cough to clear the airways. It is also possible for most patients to suppress involuntary cough for 5–20 min.

Cough has two functions: to prevent foreign material entering the lower respiratory tract and to clear secretions from the lungs and bronchial tree. The mechanics of cough rely on the generation of high expiratory pressures (e.g. intrapleural pressures up to 40 kPa) and rapid airflow velocity (500 miles/h). Glottic closure is not essential as the expiratory muscles are able to generate effective cough even with an endotracheal tube in place. Failure to generate an adequate airflow causes ineffective cough and subsequent atelectasis, infection, and eventually bronchiectasis. Conditions that interfere with cough and the ability to maintain a clear airway include:

- Extrapulmonary disorders—rib fractures, chostochondritis, acute abdomen, surgical procedures, respiratory muscle weakness, upper airway obstruction, and central cough depression.
- Intrathoracic conditions—COPD, pulmonary fibrosis, and bronchiectasis.

Clinical implications of cough

Excessive cough may impair quality of life by preventing sleep, interrupting communication and causing social embarrassment. In addition, the high pressures, rapid airflow, and energy associated with effective cough can cause haemodynamic changes (e.g. arrhythmias, hypotension), ruptured vessels (e.g. eyes, nasal, bronchial), urinary incontinence, hernia, neurological problems (e.g. syncope, headache), lung barotrauma (e.g. pneumothorax), and rib fractures.[84,85]

Assessment of cough and cough effectiveness

Cough assessment must determine the cause, effectiveness, and impact on quality of life. Many causes are amenable to therapy including excessive secretions, recurrent infections, bronchoconstriction, aspiration, postnasal drips, and gastric reflux. If cough is excessive or distressing (e.g. preventing sleep or communication), and a reversible component cannot be established, suppressive therapy may be indicated. Inadequate cough is a common problem and determining when there is a significant risk of atelectasis, pneumonia, or hypoventilation is important. However, the only studies assessing cough effectiveness were performed in patients with myasthenia gravis[86] and muscular dystrophy.[87] These demonstrated that maximal expiratory mouth pressures of less than 4 kPa were associated with difficulty expectorating secretions[86] and the need for enhancement of cough and secretion clearance.

Cough therapy

Cough therapy is usually successful if the cause is established[85] and includes:

Treatment of the cause

Therapy aimed at treating the underlying cause is essential.[85] Exacerbating factors should be identified and simple measures like change of posture, drainage of a pleural effusion, and oesophageal stricture dilation to prevent recurrent aspiration can be very effective. Stopping smoking abolished cough in 50 per cent of COPD cases[88] and treatment of underlying lung disease (e.g. bronchodilators, steroids) is essential. Diuretics relieve cough in heart failure, nasal anticongestants in post-nasal drip, and H_2 antagonists in gastro-oesophageal reflux.[85] Antibiotics may be required in chronic infective conditions.

Protussive therapy: makes cough more effective

Inability to clear airways secretions due to excessive production, ineffective cough, or reduced mucociliary clearance in diseases like chronic bronchitis and bronchiectasis leads to recurrent infection, dyspnoea, airways obstruction, and atelectasis. Measures to improve cough and secretion clearance are described in relation to individual diseases and include:

- Adequate hydration, steam inhalations, and nebulized saline to loosen tenacious secretions and aid expectoration.
- Physiotherapy with forced exhalation, airways vibration, postural drainage, and assisted cough techniques[85] but improvements in morbidity or mortality have not been established.[89]
- Pharyngeal suctioning.
- Mini-tracheostomy inserted through the cricothyroid membrane may occasionally be required to clear secretions that cannot be coughed past the vocal cords.
- Bronchorrhoea (watery sputum >100 mL but occasionally several litres/day) can occur in non-malignant conditions (e.g. asthma, tuberculosis) and may respond to steroids, erythromycin, and inhaled indomethacin.[90,91]
- Pharmacological therapies demonstrated to increase secretion clearance in randomized controlled trials include aerosolized hypertonic saline, which induces cough and fluid influx from the mucosa, cysteine derivatives (e.g. *N*-acetylcysteine, rhDNase), which liquefy lung secretions, and β_2-agonists (e.g. salbutamol).[85,92]

Antitussive therapy: prevents or eliminates cough

Non-specific antitussive therapy is indicated when the cause of the cough is not reversible or cannot be controlled by specific therapy. Usually, they are used for dry rather than productive coughs. Medications demonstrated to be effective in randomized, placebo controlled trials include:

- *Opioids:* are the most effective antitussive agents and act on the central cough centre. Strong opioids like morphine have the most pronounced effects. Methadone is useful at night but can accumulate because of its long half-life.[93] Hydrocodeine (5–10 mg 4–6 hourly) is preferred to codeine (15–30 mg 4–6 hourly) as it causes less constipation and neuropsychological side effects. Dextromethorphan also causes fewer gastrointestinal and neurological side effects.
- *Oral local anaesthetics:* benzonate (100–200 mg 8 hourly) is related to procaine and inhibits stretch receptors.[94] Levodroproizine modulates C-fibre activity and suppresses cough as well as dihydrocodeine but with less sedation.[95] Benzocaine and lignocaine lozenges may be useful for

laryngeal, pharyngeal, or tracheal irritation but the risk of aspiration must be considered.

- *Nebulized local anaesthetics:* lignocaine (5 mL of 2 per cent solution 6 hourly) and bupivacaine (5 mL 0.25 per cent solution 6 hourly) have been used for intractable cough but they can cause bronchospasm requiring bronchodilators. Efficacy has not been established and in view of the laryngeal anaesthesia all fluid and food intake should be stopped for at least 1–2 h after use to avoid inadvertent aspiration.[85,96]
- *Other antitussive agents:* theophyllines and β_2-agonists stimulate mucociliary clearance and may be beneficial in chronic bronchitis and bronchiectasis.[88] Sodium cromoglycate inhibits C-fibres and may reduce cough related to allergy and cancer.[85,97] Steroids are effective in many obstructive (e.g. asthma, endobronchial tumour) and pulmonary infiltrative disorders (e.g. sarcoidosis, lymphangitis carcinomatosis). A wide variety of over the counter antitussive medications including antihistamine-decongestant (e.g. pseudoephedrine, dexbrompheniramine) and expectorant (e.g. guaifenesin) preparations are available with varying and unproven efficacy.[98,99]
- *Antimuscarinics:* Antimuscarinic bronchodilators (e.g. ipratropium bromide) are useful in chronic bronchitis and may reduce secretion without increasing mucous viscosity or impairing mucociliary clearance. Hyoscine hydrobromide (0.2–0.4 mg sc prn) or glycopyrronium bromide (0.2–0.4 mg im prn) may be essential for the control of the distressing 'chest rattle' due to loose secretions in the terminal phase of chronic lung disease. Both cause sedation and dysphoria and occasionally, in the elderly, central anticholinergic syndrome with excitement, ataxia, and hallucinations.

Chest pain

Chest pain is a component of most chronic lung diseases and may exacerbate breathlessness, inhibit clearance of airways secretions, and impair quality of life. Management depends on identifying and treating the cause. Despite the proximity of various organs and the visceral nature of the pain it is usually possible to differentiate most types of pain clinically although simple investigations like chest radiography may be helpful in diagnosis.

Musculoskeletal disorders

Chest wall pain is often associated with localized tenderness. Rib fractures due to cough, tumour, or trauma, limit chest wall movement and cause hypoventilation and atelectasis. Adequate analgesia often requires oral, patient controlled opiate analgesia and local intercostals nerve blocks with subcostal bupivacaine 0.25 per cent (+adrenaline 1 : 200 000). If feasible, a thoracic epidural may be more effective.[100] Methods of external chest wall stabilization (e.g. taping, sandbagging, fixation) are ineffective and by limiting chest wall movement may encourage atelectasis. Chostochondritis (*Tietze's syndrome*), fibrositis, and subcostal pain due to diaphragmatic and intercostals muscle fatigue after prolonged difficult breathing are all recognized.[101,102] Intercostal radiculitis from osteoarthritis of the cervical and thoracic spine may cause significant chest pain in the immobile or bedridden patient with end-stage respiratory disease. Severe discomfort, anaesthesia, or hyperalgesia over the chest wall support these diagnoses. Other neuropathic pains include herpes zoster infection, which may be associated with immune suppression and brachial plexus invasion by a Pancoast's tumour.

Pleuropulmonary disorders

Inflammation of parietal pleura causes the characteristic pain of pleurisy with its unmistakable relationship to breathing movements. The character of the pain can vary but there is usually no localized tenderness. The speed of development provides a clue to the cause. Sudden onset suggests a pneumothorax, pulmonary embolism, or rib fracture. Development over days may herald pneumonia particularly if associated with fever and rigors. Slow onset with weight loss and lethargy may indicate malignancy or tuberculosis. Tracheobronchitis causes sharp, raw, or burning pain worse with coughing and is characteristically substernal. Pulmonary hypertension (PHT) is frequently associated with acute, central, crushing chest pain, which may radiate into the neck and arms and is difficult to differentiate from myocardial ischaemia. It has been reported in acute PHT (e.g. massive pulmonary embolus) and chronic PHT (e.g. primary PHT, mitral stenosis).[103]

Visceral and other disorders

A variety of cardiovascular (e.g. pericarditis), gastrointestinal (e.g oesophagitis, cholecystitis), and psychological disorders (e.g. hyperventilation syndrome) may present with chest pain. Missed diagnosis and delayed treatment may result in unnecessary discomfort.

If pain is refractory to treatment of the cause then symptomatic therapy may be necessary. The World Health Organization's guidelines for the use of analgesic drugs has been covered extensively in previous chapters and the principles of management in end-stage respiratory disease are identical.[104]

Haemoptysis

Haemoptysis is a dramatic, and occasionally life-threatening development in chronic lung disease.[105,106] The majority of episodes are mild or moderate and massive haemoptysis (defined as 500–1000 mL blood/day or any life-threatening haemoptysis in respiratory disease) accounts for less than 20 per cent of all episodes of haemoptysis.[107,108] Most cases are due to infective causes (~80 per cent) including tuberculosis, lung abscess, and bronchiectasis. Only a minority are due to malignancy (~20 per cent).[105–107] Death results from asphyxia, due to alveolar flooding, rather than circulatory collapse and mortality is directly related to the rate and volume of blood loss and underlying pathology. Haemoptysis of greater than 600 mL within a 4-, 4–16-, and 16–48-h period is associated with a mortality of 71, 45 and 5 per cent, respectively.[109]

Initial assessment

A good history and examination are essential. The characteristic clinical picture of diseases like pulmonary embolism and bronchiectasis may direct subsequent investigation and management. Examination of expectorated blood may provide clues. Food particles suggest the possibility of haematemesis whereas purulent material in the sputum may indicate bronchiectasis or a lung abscess. Microbiology may isolate tubercle bacilli and associated haematuria raises the possibility of an alveolar haemorrhage syndrome. Important diagnostic information including evidence of a mass or abscess may be detected on chest radiography, although diffuse alveolar shadowing, caused by widespread distribution of blood during coughing, may obscure the site and cause of bleeding.[108]

Management of massive haemoptysis

Active management may be inappropriate in many patients with end-stage respiratory disease. However, dying with haemoptysis is distressing for both the patient and relatives. If massive haemoptysis is a potential risk (i.e. recurrent haemoptysis) careful planning may improve management of the terminal event. Relatives should be warned and drugs immediately available. Simple measures like the use of green towels and bed linen to mask the evidence of blood, nursing the patient with the affected chest side down, and the calming influence of a controlled situation are invaluable. Palliative treatment should aim to reduce awareness and fear. Both opioid and anxiolytic therapy may be required.[93]

If resuscitation is appropriate the key aspects of management are:[105–109]

- Maintain a patent airway and ensure adequate oxygenation with supplemental oxygen as asphyxia is the immediate risk. Endotracheal intubation and mechanical ventilation may be required.
- Promote drainage and prevent alveolar 'soiling' of the unaffected lung, by positioning the patient slightly head down in the lateral decubitus position with the 'presumed' bleeding side down.
- Determine the cause, site, and severity of the bleeding (see below): haematemesis and upper airways bleeding (e.g. nose, pharynx) are often confused with haemoptysis.

- Avoid excessive chest manipulation (e.g. physiotherapy, spirometry) as this may increase or restart bleeding. Cough suppression with codeine 30–60 mg every 6 h may be helpful.
- Institute appropriate therapeutic measures depending on the underlying pathology and clinical circumstances (e.g. antibiotics in bronchiectasis, anticoagulation in pulmonary embolism).

Determining the site and cause of haemoptysis

Once the patient has been stabilized, the site and cause of bleeding must be established.

1. Early bronchoscopy is essential and is superior to other diagnostic techniques including bronchial arteriograms and computer tomography (CT) scans.[108,110]
2. If bronchoscopy is unsuccessful, CT scans with contrast may detect the bleeding site, tumours, and other structural abnormalities. Combination of bronchoscopy and CT scanning has the highest diagnostic yield.[105,106,108] Occasionally, radionucleotide scans may be useful.
3. Bronchial or pulmonary angiography are occasionally required.

Control of haemoptysis

Control of bleeding is usually required during ongoing investigation and includes immediate temporising measures or bronchial embolization. When the patient's condition has stabilized definitive surgery may be necessary.

1. *Immediate:* Control of bleeding is achieved in 95 per cent of cases with bronchoscope directed iced saline and adrenaline (10 ml; 1 : 10 000 dilution) lavage.[111] Occasionally, topical thrombin application,[112] balloon catheter tamponade,[105] or vasoconstrictors (e.g. IV terlipressin) are useful.
2. *Bronchial artery embolization:* is the established therapeutic technique for immediate control of haemoptysis. It is successful in 70–100 per cent of cases.[113,114] The best results are described in patients with dilated bronchial arteries (e.g. bronchiectasis). Early rebleeding is common but long-term control (> 3 months) has been reported in 45 per cent of cases.[115] Infarction of the anterior spinal artery and paraplegia occurs in about 5 per cent and rare complications include ischaemic necrosis of the bronchus and arterial dissection.[114]
3. *Medical versus surgical treatment:* Medical management may be mandatory due to end-stage lung disease (FEV_1 < 40 per cent predicted), poor cardiac reserve, or severe bleeding diathesis. In other patients, lesions may be multifocal or not amenable to surgical resection. However, when appropriate, surgical therapy has the best long-term outcome in patients with massive haemoptysis with success rates between 82 and99 per cent.[105,106] In conservative studies, when surgery would have been feasible, success rates were 46–68 per cent.[116]

Stridor

Obstruction of the larynx or major airways results in a hoarse inspiratory wheeze termed stridor. Airways infection (e.g. epiglottis, diphtheria), tumours, anaphylactic attacks, aspirated particulate matter, and sputum plugs can obstruct the upper airways. Immediate management requires an assessment of the cause and removal of any obstructing foreign bodies including aspirated objects (e.g. food), thick viscid sputum, blood clots, or dislodged tumour particles that have been coughed into the upper airways but are unable to pass the vocal cords. Postural manipulation and physiotherapy may relieve obstruction but occasionally laryngoscopy, bronchoscopy, or surgical intervention are required to assess the cause and direct management. Treatment with corticosteroids (dexamethasone 16 mg daily) can provide rapid relief when oedema or inflammatory changes are a significant cause of obstruction. Inhalation of helium and oxygen (ratio 4 : 1) may be beneficial in the short term by reducing airflow resistance. Endoscopically placed stents (bronchial or tracheal) or tracheostomies to bypass laryngeal obstruction may be appropriate in some cases.

Recurrent aspiration

Recurrent aspiration affects the terminal phase of many illness and may be a significant factor in the development of respiratory failure.[117,118] Bulbar involvement in neuromuscular (e.g. motor neurone disease, multiple sclerosis) and cerebrovascular disease is associated with recurrent aspiration due to impairment of the complex swallowing reflexes. Repeated micro-aspiration causes infection, bronchiectasis, and lung scarring. The right main bronchus is the most direct path for aspirated material and the right lower lobe is most commonly involved. Posture affects susceptibility to aspiration and nursing in the semi-recumbant position may reduce the risk.[118] Recurrent aspiration is not always easily recognized. Coughing after drinking or eating and crepitations in the right lower lobe are characteristic clues. Food particles or dyes (e.g. methylene blue) added to drinks may also be detected in tracheal aspirates. Recurrent pneumonia and chest radiographic changes of atelectasis or inflammation in the right lower lobe should raise suspicion of repeated micro-aspiration. Barium swallow confirms the diagnosis when barium enters the bronchial tree. It may occasionally demonstrate an oesophageal–tracheal fistula that requires stenting or surgical intervention.

If aspiration is suspected, swallowing must be assessed by a speech therapist and strategies for prevention tested, including posture manipulation and thickening of food.[117] If these fail, fine bore nasogastric feeding or gastric pegs should be considered although this will depend on the stage of the illness. The pneumonia and atelectasis associated with aspiration are treated with physiotherapy and broad spectrum antibiotics that cover nasopharyngeal organisms (e.g. anaerobes).

Management of end-stage respiratory disease

In respiratory disease there is often no clear event that signifies the onset of the end-stage after many years of gradual deterioration. Carers must be alert to the subtle change in symptoms and psychosocial status that indicate declining health and the beginning of this terminal phase including:

- persistent breathlessness despite optimization of medical therapy;
- inability to mobilize and get out of the house despite pulmonary rehabilitation;
- increasing numbers of hospital admissions;
- limited improvement following admission;
- expressions of fear or anxiety and panic attacks;
- it is not unusual for the patient to be aware of the change and to express concern about dying.

Terminal management, and particularly the last 48 h, of respiratory disease is mainly in hospital following an acute exacerbation of the chronic lung disease. About 72 per cent of patients die in hospital, 12 per cent at home, and none in hospice.[16] Recently, there has been a trend toward the management of acute exacerbations of COPD at home. This 'hospital at home' (HaH) management has been demonstrated to be safe and cost effective.[42–44] In a recent study, 95 per cent of 184 patients with acute COPD exacerbations reported satisfaction with HaH care[43] whereas, in another randomized study, COPD patient's expressed a preference for inpatient care.[119] Domicilary care is currently provided to some stable, end-stage respiratory patients by respiratory nurses and includes emotional/psychological support and assistance with oxygen and nebulizer therapy.[120]

Respiratory failure (including hypoventilation and V/Q mismatching), chronic infection (±sputum retention), pneumothorax, pleural effusions, and thromboembolic disease are all important components in the management of chronic lung disease. The emphasis of treatment will vary according to which components predominate in individual diseases. Thus, in cystic fibrosis, chronic infection and secretion clearance are paramount but the management of respiratory failure is also important. Pre-existing problems (e.g. anaemia, ascites, left ventricular failure) must also be considered.

Respiratory failure

Respiratory failure is defined as inability of the respiratory system to maintain arterial oxygenation or to clear CO_2. Most end-stage respiratory diseases are associated with respiratory failure, although the underlying mechanisms are different. The focus of treatment in neuromuscular disease is support of respiratory muscle function (e.g. with non-invasive ventilation) to prevent hypoventilation and CO_2 retention whereas in pulmonary fibrotic disease correction of hypoxaemia with oxygen therapy may be paramount. Overall, the majority of patients (~75 per cent) with end-stage respiratory disease and respiratory failure will have COPD.

Chronic obstructive pulmonary disease

End-stage management of COPD with respiratory failure[121] includes (a) *pharmacological therapies:* to reduce airways obstruction, correct hypoxaemia, and relieve dyspnoea and (b) *non-pharmacological therapies:* to improve respiratory muscle function/ventilation and enhance gas exchange.

Pharmacological therapies

Bronchodilators Inhaled β_2-agonists are well-established bronchodilators for the treatment of dyspnoea. In COPD, they reduce resting and exercise-induced dyspnoea and dynamic hyperinflation without necessarily increasing FEV_1 or FVC.[122,123] Anticholinergic agents, including ipratropium and oxitropium bromide, also reduce dyspnoea, improve exercise tolerance, and increase FEV_1.[124] Anticholinergics can aggravate prostatism and glaucoma and in patients with these conditions they should be used with care. Tiotropium bromide[125] is a newer, once daily, enhanced anticholinergic agent that has been demonstrated to relieve dyspnoea and wheeze, reduce rescue inhaler requirements, and produce a sustained improvement in vital capacity (> 10 per cent). Inhaler technique should be examined as incorrect use is a frequent cause of lack of effect. Dry powder inhalers may improve delivery in patients with poor co-ordination using metered dose aerosol inhalers.

Current evidence suggests that the clinical and bronchodilator effects of anticholinergics are greater than those of β_2-agonists in COPD. Analysis from seven trials comparing ipratropium with β_2-agonists given for at least 90 days reported a greater increase in FEV_1 with ipratropium bromide and this bronchodilation was sustained whereas the β_2-agonist effect waned with prolonged use.[126] In a randomized, controlled trial of 534 COPD patients, combining ipratropium with a β_2-agonist improved the FEV_1 beyond that with either agent alone.[127]

There is contradictory evidence for the use of nebulizer therapy in COPD,[128,129] but study comparisons are difficult because nebulizer devices differ and patient groups are small. In general, nebulizers deliver more drug to the lungs but in a less efficient manner than metered dose inhalers.[129,130] Nebulizers also cause more side effects, have increased administration times, and higher costs.[131] Comparisons between nebulizers and inhalers (±spacer) have not shown significant benefits on dyspnoea, bronchodilation, exercise tolerance, or reduced rescue therapy in patients with stable COPD.[128,132] Nevertheless, many patients prefer nebulized bronchodilators despite this lack of objective response. Benefit in acute exacerbations and in end-of-life management is reported.[128,129] It is currently recommended that metered dose inhalers be used initially, provided that patient inhaler technique is adequate. Near the end-of-life, or during acute exacerbations, patients may be too weak to use metered dose inhalers effectively and nebulized therapy both in hospital and the domiciliary situation becomes the better option.[128,133]

Inhaled and oral steroids Inhaled or oral corticosteroids are the mainstay of treatment in severe asthma, but their role in COPD is less clear. Steroids objectively benefit about 15–20 per cent of stable COPD patients but it is not possible to predict responsive patients.[134] An oral steroid trial (20–40 mg daily for ~14 d) is usually required and if FEV_1 increases by greater than 20 per cent, inhaled steroids are started as these have most of the therapeutic advantages with few of the potential side-effects.[134] Occasionally, improvement can only be maintained with oral steroids but the dose should be kept to a minimum. In acute COPD exacerbations, high-dose oral steroids are beneficial but should be stopped or replaced by inhaled steroids after 10 d as appropriate.[24]

Theophylline Theophylline, a methylxanthine, is often prescribed for COPD as an adjunct to standard bronchodilators. Recent use has declined as the pharmokinetics are unpredictable and the narrow therapeutic range risks developing toxic levels. However, theophylline therapy has been reported to reduce dyspnoea[135] and improve spirometry[136] at serum concentrations between 10 and 20 μg/mL and withdrawal of theophylline from stable COPD patients resulted in deterioration of symptoms and exercise tolerance.[137] If used judiciously, theophylline continues to have a useful role and should be prescribed once daily to achieve levels between 10 and 12 μg/mL.

Oxygen therapy Patients with severe COPD often commence oxygen therapy at home several years before the disease reaches the terminal phase. Depending on the circumstances, it will be provided from cylinders, an oxygen concentrator, or as liquid oxygen (mainly in the United States). It is commonly delivered by a face mask or nasal prongs, with or without humidification. At the onset of treatment in the hypoxaemic patient, oxygen is usually provided overnight, intermittently during the day and on exercise if a portable supply is available (i.e. liquid oxygen in the United States). As a patient becomes increasingly unwell their dependence on oxygen will increase. Continuous use is not uncommon towards the end-stage of the disease and panic may result if it is removed.[93] Oxygen saturations should be monitored. The development of headache, drowsiness, or confusion may indicate CO_2 retention and the need to check an arterial blood gas although routine blood gases are not necessary. Many patients find that the flow of air or oxygen over the face reduces breathlessness and the use of venturi masks to entrain air and increase flow may be beneficial.[64]

Long-term oxygen therapy (LTOT)

LTOT extends life expectancy in hypoxaemic COPD patients if administered for at least 12–15 h a day and benefit increases with continuous use.[29,30] In the MRC trial, mortality at 3 years was 45 per cent in patients treated with oxygen (2 L/min) for 15 h/d compared to 67 per cent in controls.[29] In the Nocturnal Oxygen Therapy Trial in the USA, mortality was 22 per cent in patients treated with continuous oxygen (~18 h/d) and 41 per cent in patients receiving nocturnal therapy.[30] Reductions in dyspnoea, haemocrit, and improved pulmonary haemodynamic performance were also reported. Quality of life was not changed significantly although there were some modest neuropsychiatric improvements.[30] In contrast, the 2001 Cochrane review identified a number of recent trials that had not shown benefit with nocturnal oxygen therapy.[138]

The criteria for LTOT prescription vary in different countries,[139] but current UK guidelines are listed in Table 10. In practice, compliance with these guidelines is poor.[140] In the United Kingdom, an oxygen concentrator is recommended for LTOT delivery as it is cheaper than cylinder oxygen. Liquid oxygen systems are preferred in the United States as they allow mobility outside the home. Nasal cannulae are a comfortable mode of administration and a flow rate of 1–3 L/min is usually adequate to achieve a saturation greater than 90 per cent. The baseline flow rate is often increased by 1 L/min at night and during exercise to prevent desaturation. The low concentrations of oxygen administered with LTOT cause only small increases in PCO_2 in patients with hypercapnea. Unfortunately, a proportion of LTOT patients continue to smoke!

Oxygen during exercise

Patients with a stable PaO_2 greater than 60 mmHg (8 kPa) on air may develop hypoxaemia during exercise. In patients with resting or exercise-induced hypoxaemia, supplemental oxygen augments exercise capacity and reduces dyspnoea.[59,141] This benefit is greater with high flow rates.[78] A diffusing capacity below 55 per cent expected, accurately predicts exercise-induced desaturation.[142] Portable cylinder or liquid oxygen systems may improve mobility and quality of life in patients who benefit in controlled exercise assessments and are widely available in the United States but less so in Europe.[78]

Palliative oxygen therapy

A significant proportion of patients with end-stage lung disease including COPD will have resting hypoxaemia, although the degree of hypoxaemia does not necessarily correlate with the level of dyspnoea.[143,144] In these

Table 10 UK Department of Health Guidelines for LTOT prescription

Indications for LTOT
COPD (+cystic fibrosis)
PaO_2 <7.3 kPa (55 mmHg) when breathing air
$PaCO_2$ may be normal or >6.0 kPa
Two measurement separated by 4 weeks when clinically stable
Clinical stability = no exacerbations or peripheral oedema for 4 weeks
FEV_1 <1.5 L and FVC <2.0 L
Non-smokers
Or
PaO_2 between 7.3 and 8.0 kPa (56–59 mmHg) together with:
Secondary polycythaemia, peripheral oedema or PHT
Nocturnal hypoxaemia (SaO_2 below 90% for > 30% of the night)
Interstitial lung disease or PHT (without parenchymal involvement)
PaO_2 <8 kPa
Other indications
Palliation of dyspnoea due to terminal disease
Obstructive sleep apnoea with persistant nocturnal hypoxaemia despite CPAP
Neuromuscular and skeletal disorders
Heart failure with PaO2 <7.3 kPa (55 mmHg) or nocturnal hypoxaemia

PHT, pulmonary hypertension.

patients, dyspnoea and exercise tolerance may be substantially improved with supplemental oxygen.[144] In patients with refractory hypoxaemia despite high flow rate oxygen, a nasal reservoir (e.g. oximizer), which stores oxygen during expiration and delivers a larger bolus at the onset of inspiration, may be useful. At high flow rates, oxygen therapy may cause CO_2 narcosis and progressive somnolence in a patient with a good saturation on oximetry should raise suspicion. A blood gas should be measured or end tidal CO_2 checked to confirm hypercapnea and the oxygen flow rate reduced whilst monitoring CO_2 and mental function.

Even in the absence of resting hypoxaemia or exercise-induced desaturation, supplemental oxygen may relieve dyspnoea in some COPD patients.[143] A 'blinded' comparison of air and oxygen may confirm this benefit. The likely mechanism for this dyspnoea relief is that oxygen reduces carotid body afferent output, altering CO_2 sensitivity, and thereby reducing minute ventilation and work of breathing. In these patients intermittent 'palliative' oxygen therapy is usually adequate, as few will require continuous therapy.[144] Oxygen is usually delivered from cylinders, although an oxygen concentrator may be supplied if life expectancy is greater than 3 months and oxygen usage high.

Drug treatment for the relief of dyspnoea

Drug treatment of dyspnoea is controversial, with differing opinions and conflicting evidence. In general, the therapeutic benefit has been small and the side-effects considerable.[145]

Anxiolytic agents and promethazine Anxiety can aggravate breathlessness and some patients experience severe panic attacks. Patients must be advised on how to stay calm by purse-lip breathing, slow expiration, and shoulder and chest wall muscle relaxation. Early work with anxiolytic therapy reported that oral diazepam reduced dyspnoea in 'pink puffer' type COPD patients,[146] but subsequent studies failed to show improvement in dyspnoea, exercise tolerance, or sense of well-being with either diazepam or alprazolam.[147,148] Indeed, diazepam caused drowsiness and decreased exercise tolerance with no change in dyspnoea.[148] The use of promethazine is equally controversial. Increased exercise tolerance and decreased dyspnoea with no notable side-effects was initially reported[148] whereas a later study found no significant changes from baseline after use for 1 month.[149] Equally conflicting reports have been published in small studies examining the use of buspirone hydrochloride, a non-sedating anxiolytic agent. Anxiety scores, exercise performance, and dyspnoea all improved on 20 mg/d for 15 d,[150] but in a second study no effect was demonstrated with at least 30 mg/d for 6 weeks.[151] Despite these inconclusive results, clinical experience suggests that low dose anxiolytics do have a beneficial role in the management of breathlessness as a consequence of their anxiolytic and muscle relaxant effects, and can result in substantial improvements in some patients (and not only those prone to anxiety or panic attacks). Concerns about respiratory depression are largely nfounded.

Antidepressant drugs A high proportion of COPD patients have psychiatric illness. Studies examining the effect of tricyclic antidepressants, serotonin reuptake inhibitors, and phenothiazines have been reported to be beneficial for anxiety but effects on dyspnoea are inconclusive.[152] However, chlorpromazine was effective for the control of dyspnoea and restlessness in advanced cancer.[153]

Oral opioids The site of action may be central (i.e. affecting brainstem opiate receptors and reducing ventilation), or on peripheral lung receptors, or by decreasing anxiety. Exogenous opiates cause a dose-dependent reduction in ventilation with increased $PaCO_2$ and a depression of ventilatory response to CO_2.[154] In contrast, dihydrocodeine reduced breathlessness in COPD without an increase in CO_2.[155,156] Oral morphine also reduced breathlessness and increased exercise tolerance but with drowsiness, a fall in PaO_2, and an increase in $PaCO_2$ as significant side-effects.[157] Sustained release morphine given for 6 weeks (mean dose of 25 mg/daily) had no effect on quality of life, exercise tolerance, or dyspnoea.[158] Studies examining diamorphine, dextromethorphan, and codeine have failed to demonstrate useful benefit and codeine elevated $PaCO_2$ significantly.[149,159] Given that opioids may cause serious side-effects including CO_2 retention, nausea, and drowsiness, and that clinical benefit is unproven, their routine prescription for COPD cannot be recommended. However, in severely dyspnoeic, end-stage COPD patients without CO_2 retention, a trial of dihydrocodeine or opiate with close monitoring is appropriate. The dose of opioid can be titrated, as for pain, but lower doses and smaller increments should be given. As little as 2.5 mg of morphine elixir every 4 h may be sufficient.[93] For patients unable to swallow, subcutaneous diamorphine is recommended. In the terminal phase, opiate therapy is justified for the relief of breathlessness and restlessness even with co-existing hypoxaemia and CO_2 retention. Excessive apprehension about respiratory depression may result in unnecessary patient suffering. Laxatives and stool softeners should be started at the onset of opioid therapy.

Nebulized opioids They act on peripheral lung receptors. Increased exercise tolerance was reported in an initial study with nebulized morphine,[160] but subsequent investigation has shown no reduction in dyspnoea in COPD or interstitial lung disease.[161,162] There is currently no good evidence to support the use of nebulized opioids in chronic lung disease.

Mucolytics Viscid or copious lung secretions due to increased mucous production and impaired mucociliary clearance often complicate chronic lung disease. Sputum expectoration varies from a few millilitres in the morning to bronchorrhea with more than 100 mL/d. Avoiding irritants, particularly cigarette smoke, may reduce secretion dramatically although cough and expectoration may increase for several weeks after stopping smoking. *N*-Acetylcysteine can be used as a mucolytic agent and improves symptoms and reduces exacerbations in COPD.[163] Recombinant human DNAse, although useful in cystic fibrosis, has not been beneficial in COPD. Thick secretions may be better expectorated after steam inhalations or nebulized normal (0.9 per cent) or hypertonic (3–7 per cent) saline, but specific expectorants like glycerol guaiacolate are of limited value.[144] Bronchorrhea may be controlled by oral steroid, inhaled atropine, or indomethacin.[164] β_2-agonists and theophyllines also aid mucociliary clearance.

Other drugs Nebulized lignocaine to anaesthetise airways receptors and reduce dyspnoea was not beneficial in interstitial lung disease.[165] No improvement in dyspnoea was reported with alcohol, caffeine, indomethacin, or carbimazole.[145]

Non-pharmacological therapies

General factors

- *Vaccinations:* Influenza and pneumococcal vaccinations should be given to severe COPD patients.
- *General nursing:* A fan to blow cool air over the face[64] or being near an open window may help relieve breathlessness. Good nursing care and regular repositioning prevent pressure sores and alleviate the musculoskeletal pain that may be associated with immobility. Relief of constipation and assistance with personal hygiene are also important.
- *Nutrition:* Patients with end-stage emphysema may loss weight and become frankly cachexic. The main consequence is reduced muscle strength with weakness of both inspiratory and expiratory muscles.[166] Weight loss is attributed to a 15–25 per cent increase in resting energy expenditure, due to increased work of breathing, increased metabolic requirement for daily activities, reduced calorie intake, and increased inflammatory cytokines.[167,168] Improved nutrition increases respiratory muscle strength but this only occurs after weight gain which can be difficult to achieve as patients tolerate nutritional supplements poorly.[169] In contrast, patients with hypercapnic COPD may be overweight and weight loss improves breathlessness and exercise tolerance.
- *Physiotherapy:* Effective cough is the best means of expelling airways mucous. The cleansing action of cough takes place during the first one or two coughs in a sequence. With controlled cough the patient takes a deep breath and coughs two to three times with the mouth open without taking another breath. The forced expiratory technique involves forced exhalation without glottic closure starting at mid lung volume ('huffing') and clears alveoli and small airways. This is followed by expectoration (or controlled cough) at full lung volume to clear central airways. In patients with large volumes of secretion, chest percussion/vibration or postural drainage in the 25° head down position for 20 min is safe and effective.[170] Patients with small quantities of secretion derive no benefit from these techniques. In the terminal phase of chronic lung disease physiotherapy may be inappropriate and the right to decline or accept physiotherapy in a modified form should be accepted.[120]
- *Psychosocial support and counselling:* The level of advice and support offered depends on the patient's level of understanding. The aim is to help them cope, provide strategies to relieve symptoms, and improve quality of life. Many patients will want to be involved with their terminal care, providing a 'living will' with instructions on levels of care and the use of mechanical ventilation. Many will simply want to 'leave their house in order' or say 'goodbye to loved ones'. Relatives as well as patients will need support and counselling. They must also be involved in discussing the issues associated with death and helped through the grieving process.[120]

Pulmonary rehabilitation Pulmonary rehabilitation attempts to return patients to their highest possible level of functional capacity and has become an essential component in the comprehensive care of patients with end-stage lung disease. Numerous studies have confirmed the value of these programmes to reduce dyspnoea, improve quality of life, increase independence, extend exercise capacity, and decrease time in hospital for COPD patients.[171–173] Exercise conditioning is the single most important aspect of rehabilitation. Patients should undertake both general exercises (e.g. stair climbing, stationary cycling) and specific muscle training, particularly the upper limbs and shoulder girdle which act as accessory muscles of respiration. Training should be continued at home, using supplemental oxygen if there is exercise-desaturation. The addition of domiciliary non-invasive positive pressure ventilation (see below) to an exercise training programme has been shown to further improve exercise tolerance and quality of life.[174]

An inspiratory resistance breathing device is the simplest, most reliable method for respiratory muscle training. The inspiratory pressure required to achieve 'training' must be 30 per cent of the maximum inspiratory pressure a patient can generate, and the training duration should be at least 30 min daily.[175] However, the value of respiratory muscle training in COPD is controversial[176,177] and recent studies have reported no benefit over general exercise reconditioning alone.[178]

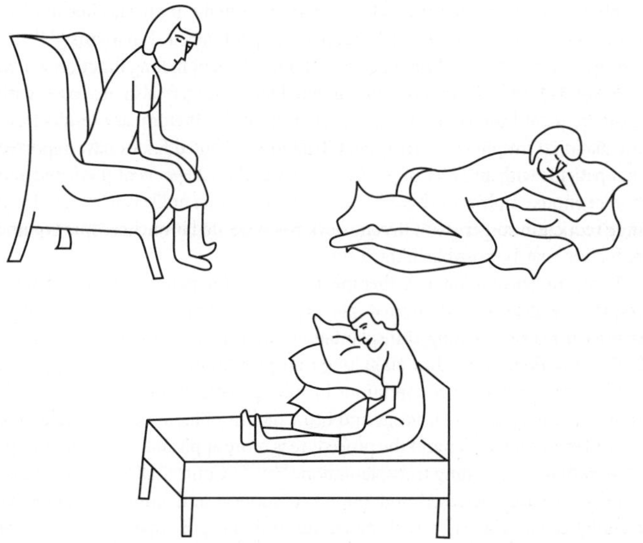

Fig. 2 Patient positioning to alleviate breathlessness.

Controlled breathing techniques These include purse lip breathing, slow expiration, manual upper abdominal compression, and the standing, bent forward position with the arms supporting the body. Purse lip breathing helps improve alveolar ventilation and gas exchange by stenting the airways, preventing dynamic airways collapse, and thus decreasing gas trapping.[179] The associated slow expiratory phase is an important component in overcoming the panic attacks that often develop in the severely breathless patient.[120] The bending forwards posture improves diaphragmatic function by increasing abdominal pressure and helps relieve dyspnoea.[180] Nursing positions that facilitate breathing and reduce respiratory distress are illustrated in Fig. 2.

Non-invasive mechanical ventilation Non-invasive ventilation, including negative and intermittent positive pressure ventilation, have been demonstrated to reduce the need for intubation, decrease the length of ICU stay, and reduce mortality in acute COPD exacerbations.[181,182] Inspiratory and expiratory (bi-level) pressure support through a nasal or full facemask is most commonly used for intermittent positive pressure ventilation. Continuous positive airways pressure (CPAP) can reduce work of breathing and hyperinflation but must be used with considerable care to avoid further gas trapping.[183] These techniques dramatically reduce respiratory distress in some patients although others are unable to tolerate the tight mask despite careful explanation and slow introduction of respiratory support. Non-invasive ventilation in acute exacerbations of end-stage COPD provides time to assess potential reversibility and to discuss whether full mechanical ventilation would be appropriate.

The value of domiciliary non-invasive ventilation to 'rest' respiratory muscles in stable COPD with chronic respiratory failure has not been established.[184,185] Failure to improve respiratory muscle function, exercise endurance, or sleep and poor tolerance has been reported.[184] A more positive view has been presented by other investigators who demonstrated reduced dyspnoea, improved ventilatory drive, reduced gas trapping, and better sleep.[185,186] Further studies are awaited.

Lung reduction surgery and lung transplantation Lung reduction surgery produces considerable improvement in both functional and quality of life measures[187–189] with increased walking distance and improvements in vitality, physical, and social functioning on quality of life questionnaires at 6 months.[190] The FEV_1 increased by 25–58 per cent (range 16–96 per cent) and FVC by 12–40 per cent, 3–6 months after bilateral surgery.[187] However, improvements were short-lived due to an increase in the annual decline in FEV_1 from ~40 mL/year to 93–163 mL/year in post-surgical patients.[191,192] Extrapolation of this decline suggests that initial benefit in lung function would only last 3–4 years. Morbidity after lung reduction surgery also increases, with more frequent hospital admissions post-surgery.[193] Preliminary results from the National Emphysema Treatment Trial in the United States have reported that patients with an FEV_1 or gas transfer lesser than 20 per cent predicted and homogenous emphysema have a high mortality and are unlikely to benefit from lung reduction surgery.[194] Recent work has suggested bronchoscopic volume reduction may be possible in the future.[195]

Lung transplantation is a therapeutic option for patients with end-stage respiratory disease and limited life expectancy. Emphysema is the most common reason for lung transplantation, often in young patients with α_1-antitrypsin deficiency. Over 6000 lung transplantations have been performed worldwide in a variety of conditions including cystic fibrosis, interstitial pulmonary fibrosis, bronchiectasis, and bronchiolitis obliterans.[196] Single lung transplantation is easier and the procedure is more applicable to an older population than double lung transplantation.[197,198] Contraindications to transplantation have decreased and improved surgical and immunosuppressive techniques are associated with better survival and post-operative quality of life. The early course of single and double lung transplantation is similar with ~70 per cent 1 year and 60 per cent 2 years survivals after which bilateral transplants tend to do better. Obliterative bronchiolitis remains a serious problem.

However, the availability of lung transplantation has greatly complicated the management of end-stage respiratory disease, especially for those with cystic fibrosis. Due to the limited organ availability only a small percentage of patients assessed will be successful recipients. Patients and their families undergo considerable stress waiting for transplants. Acknowledgement that the end-stage has been reached, and provision of appropriate palliative care is often delayed, with unnecessary pain and suffering, in the hope of a 'last minute transplant'.[120]

Interstitial/fibrotic lung disease

Table 11 lists the extensive spectrum of diseases that cause progressive fibrotic lung damage. However, these conditions are relative rare; the commonest group, the pneumoconioses account for about 1200 deaths per year and sarcoidosis for 115 deaths/year compared with over 32 000 deaths/year from COPD.[20] Idiopathic pulmonary fibrosis (also known as cryptogenic fibrosing alveolitis) has an incidence of about 3–5 per 100 000. The overall mortality is about 50 per cent at 5 years but the course is very variable and acute interstitial pneumonia (Hamman Rich Syndrome) leads to death in a few months whereas desquamative interstitial pneumonia is associated with a 28 per cent mortality at 12 years.[199] Sarcoidosis follows a relapsing course with most cases resolving spontaneously. In a small minority, pulmonary fibrosis progresses relentlessly over many years to respiratory failure. Connective tissue diseases are often associated with pulmonary fibrosis and hypertension. In systemic sclerosis, lung disease and recurrent aspiration (as a result of the oesophageal strictures) accounts for 21 per cent of all deaths.[200] Minor pulmonary fibrosis may occur in up to 60 per cent of patients with rheumatoid arthritis but severe progressive disease is rare and has a 5 year survival of less than 50 per cent. Bronchiectasis, organizing pneumonia, and obliterative bronchiolitis occasionally lead to end-stage lung disease in rheumatoid arthritis.

Table 11 Classification of interstitial lung diseases

Classification	Examples
Idiopathic fibrotic disorders	Idiopathic pulmonary fibrosis, bronchiolitis obliterans organizing pneumonia (BOOP), autoimmune pulmonary fibrosis (inflammatory bowel disease, primary biliary cirrhosis), etc.
Connective tissue diseases	Systemic lupus erythematosis, rheumatoid arthritis, scleraderma, ankylosing spondylitis, etc.
Drug-induced diseases	Antibiotics (furantoin), antiarrhythmics (amiodarone), anti-inflammatory (gold, penicillamine), chemotherapeutic agents (bleomycin), paraquat, therapeutic radiation, etc.
Occupational	*Inorganic*: silicosis, asbestosis, coal workers pneumoconiosis, beryllisosis, stanosis *Organic*: Farmer's lung, pigeon fanciers lung, etc.
Primary unclassified	Sarcoidosis, amyloidosis, pulmonary vasculitis, lymphangitis carcinomatosis, Gauchers disease, AIDS, ARDS, eosinophilic granulomatosis, etc.

AIDS, acquired immunodeficiency syndrome; ARDS, acute respiratory distress syndrome.

Immunosuppressive therapy including steroids, cyclophosphamide, azothioprine, and penicillamine are used to treat fibrotic lung diseases but success is very variable. Increasing pulmonary damage is associated with dyspnoea, decreased exercise tolerance, hypoxaemia, pulmonary hypertension, and cor pulmonale. It is rare for CO_2 retention to occur and it is safe to use high inspired concentrations of oxygen. Although benefit with oxygen therapy is poorly documented, it is widely prescribed to relieve breathlessness and improve exercise tolerance.[142] Drug therapy for relief of dyspnoea may be required as the disease progresses. The American Thoracic Society has published guidelines for the selection of patients with progressive pulmonary fibrosis for lung transplantation but shortage of organs limits the value of this therapeutic option.[201]

Neuromuscular, restrictive, and chest wall disease

Neuromuscular and chest wall disease cause restrictive defects in ventilatory function due to either respiratory muscle weakness or loss of compliance in the thoracic cage.[202] Rapid, shallow breathing, atelectasis, and aspiration due to ineffective cough result in respiratory failure and pneumonia. Neuromuscular diseases affect the respiratory muscles at multiple sites from the spinal cord (e.g. trauma, anterior horn cell disease) to the muscles themselves (e.g. myopathies, dystrophies). A number of other factors influence respiratory function:

- Ventilatory drive is increased in most of these conditions but with inadequate ventilatory response. However, patients with quadriplegia, congenital myopathies, and myotonic dystrophy may have reduced ventilatory drive.[203] These patients usually have mild respiratory muscle weakness and ventilatory response to exercise is usually good. Hypercapnia and sleep abnormalities are the main features in these patients.
- Sleep disorders commonly affect neuromuscular (~42 per cent) and quadriplegic patients (~28 per cent), with respiratory disturbance indicators greater than 15 per hour.[204]
- Unbalanced weakness of spinal and thoracic muscle leads to kyphoscoliosis in poliomyelitis and the muscular dystrophies causing loss of compliance and increased work of breathing.
- Bulbar incoordination in multiple sclerosis and amyotrophic lateral sclerosis may cause upper airways obstruction from aspirated food or foreign bodies and micro-aspiration results in recurrent pneumonia.
- Diaphragmatic paralysis is a feature of many neuromuscular diseases and may occur after trauma or thoracic surgery. Unilateral paralysis has a good outcome but bilateral paralysis is associated with severe symptoms, ventilatory failure, and pneumonia. The manifestations of bilateral paralysis are much worse in the supine position and sleep disturbances are common.
- Pulmonary embolism is a constant threat to immobilized patients but prophylactic anticoagulation reduces mortality.[205]

General supportive measures including oxygen therapy, antibiotics, and physiotherapy are required. Clearing secretions is of particular importance and techniques to improve cough capacity have been developed. Coughing can be augmented by synchronizing cough with manual abdominal compressions.[206] An insufflator/exsufflator, 'cough machine' provides a deep insufflation by mask followed by rapid decompression.[207] High cervical injury patients often learn the technique of glossopharyngeal breathing. This involves using the tongue, cheek, pharyngeal, and laryngeal muscles in a coordinated way to 'gulp/inject' small boluses of air into the trachea augmenting VC by up to 1 L. The larger inspiration is associated with better passive recoil and cough.[206,208]

Inspiratory muscle training with a daily regime of forced inspiration and expiration through resistances has been advocated in neuromuscular diseases to improve the chance of becoming independent of mechanical ventilation,[209] but not all studies have reported benefit.[210] Occasionally, phrenic or abdominal nerve stimulation may be useful[211] for those patients with failure of central drive (e.g. high cervical paralysis), but in anterior horn cell diseases, neuropathies, or myopathies the muscles are no more likely to respond to electrical stimulation than to voluntary or automatic effort. Beta-adrenergic agonists can improve mucociliary clearance in the absence of airways obstruction and mucolytics like nebulized acetylcholine may help loosen thick tenacious secretions. Nasotracheal suctioning, postural drainage, and bronchoscopy may be required to clear thick secretions.

When neuromuscular and chest wall diseases are far advanced and hypercapnic respiratory failure is developing or already established, ventilatory support is required if the patients are to survive. Advances in respiratory care and the availability of specialist respiratory facilities have made it possible for patients to live for long periods with an acceptable quality of life on mechanical ventilation with or without tracheostomy.[212] However, many patients choose not to accept either tracheostomy or ventilatory support. There are several categories of non-invasive mechanical ventilation many of which are suitable for domiciliary use:

- *Rocking beds:* utilize gravity to assist diaphragmatic movement and are useful for patients with diaphragmatic paralysis who have reasonable respiratory function when upright but not supine.
- *Abdominal pneumatic belts:* assist upward diaphragmatic movement by intermittent compression of the abdomen, with passive recoil during the non-compressive phase. It is most efficient when the patient is sitting upright.
- *Negative pressure body ventilators:* have been extensively used for many neuromuscular diseases[213] and have the advantage of allowing unimpeded speech. The early iron lungs were too cumbersome for practical use but the smaller cuirass and body wrap ventilators are more acceptable to most patients but require considerable skill for successful operation.
- *Non-invasive positive pressure ventilation:* has been used with great success in neuromuscular and chest wall diseases and may prevent the need for tracheostomy.[206,214] It is usually delivered through a nasal mask using a portable volume or pressure cycled ventilator. Full-facemasks and mouthpieces can be used. The tidal volume is adjusted for mouth and mask leaks which can be troublesome and occasionally a chin strap is required to hold the mouth closed particularly during sleep. It is generally well tolerated but skin breakdown at sites in contact with the mask and sinusitis or nasal congestion can be problems.[214]
- *Nasal continuous positive airways pressure:* prevents atelectasis, upper airways collapse, and upper airways obstruction in patients with neuromuscular and chest wall diseases. However, CPAP has the potential to worsen inspiratory muscle weakness by increasing FRC and is probably best suited to patients with upper airway obstruction due to paresis of upper airways musculature or in diaphragmatic paralysis. It should be used with caution and close monitoring in most neuromuscular diseases.

Specialist respiratory centres with domiciliary nursing facilities are needed to provide home ventilation for patients with neuromuscular and chest wall diseases. In most countries, these facilities are poorly financed and coordinated although there are exceptions as in France. Staff in these specialist facilities are skilled in the management of the terminal phase of respiratory disease and provide high-quality palliative care for patients that they may have treated and nursed for many years.

Chronic infection

Many respiratory diseases are associated with chronic or recurrent infection due to structural abnormalities, ineffective cough, or inadequate immune function. The associated parenchymal damage results in ventilation/perfusion mismatch and progressive hypoxaemic respiratory failure. Chronic infection leads to general debility, weight loss, recurrent fever, and the excessive secretions cause cough, atelectasis, and halitosis.

Bronchiectasis and cystic fibrosis

The prognosis for patients with bronchiectasis in the pre-antibiotic era was dismal with only 15 per cent of patients living for more than 20 years. Their lives were characterized by progressive decline in health punctuated by episodes of acute infection and haemoptysis.[215] This picture has been transformed by the advent of antibiotics and survival is much improved.[216] Table 12 reports conditions associated with bronchiectasis. Diagnosis was previously made with bronchography, which is now obsolete. It has been replaced by high-resolution CT scanning of the chest which has a specificity of more than 90 per cent to detect bronchiectasis at the segmental level.[217] Detection should promote a search for the underlying cause including protein electrophoresis for α_1-antitrypsin deficiency, hypogammaglobulinaemia, pilocarpine iontophoresis (sweat test) for cystic fibrosis, aspergillus precipitans for allergic bronchopulmonary aspergillosis, and electron microscopy for primary ciliary dyskinesia. Regular determination of bacterial colonization in sputum aids management.[218]

Treatment involves management of infection, secretions, haemoptysis, and obstructive airways disease and includes:

- *Antimicrobial drugs:* are the mainstay of therapy and should be directed by sputum microbiology. Combinations of broad spectrum antibiotics that have good lung penetration and cover anaerobic and gram negative organisms including *pseudomonas* are usually required and include metronidozole, augmentin, and ciprofloxcin. They often have to be administered intravenously. Most physicians only treat acute infective exacerbations but some patients may require continuous or intermittent cycles of antibiotic therapy to maintain good health. Treatment has to be given for longer periods, often 3–4 weeks and if therapy is continuous antibiotics should be cycled to minimize the risk of resistance. High doses are required to achieve therapeutic antibiotic levels in the infection filled endobronchial spaces.[219,220] Nebulized antibiotics including gentamicin and tobramycin (300 mg twice daily) have been administered successfully in cystic fibrosis to control airways inflammation and secretion.[221]
- *Bronchodilator therapy:* including β_2-agonists (metered dose and nebulized), ipratropium bromide, and oral theophyllines are all used to relieve airways bronchoconstriction (see COPD).
- *Chest physical therapy:* with postural drainage, chest clapping, humidification, and the use of mucolytics, sputum clearance increases.[222]

Table 12 Conditions associated with bronchiectasis

Cystic fibrosis
HIV infection
Rheumatoid arthritis
Infection, inflammation
Bronchopulmonary sequestration
Allergic bronchopulmonary aspergillosis
Alpha$_1$-antitrypsin deficiency
Congenital cartilage deficiency
Immunodeficiency
Yellow nail syndrome
Bronchial obstruction
Unilateral hyperlucent lung

Chest clapping can be administered by family members with considerable psychological benefit. Mucociliary clearance is increased by β_2-agonists and nebulized amiloride or hypertonic saline in cystic fibrosis.[223]

- *Nebulized recombinant human deoxyribonuclease (DNAse):* facilitates secretion clearance in cystic fibrosis[224] by hydrolysing the extracellular deoxyribonucleic acid that accumulates with other neutrophil degradation products in infected airways. It does not reduce respiratory exacerbations.[225] In bronchiectasis due to other causes it has not been so successful in reducing symptoms or sputum clearance.[226]
- *Anti-inflammatory therapy:* inhaled indomethacin improves sputum viscosity and relieves symptoms in patients with chronic bronchitis and bronchiectasis.[164] Likewise, oral ibuprofen twice daily reduces decline in lung function, radiographic deterioration, and loss of weight in patients with cystic fibrosis.[227] Oral steroids cause side-effects with little additional benefit except in allergic bronchopulmonary aspergillosis.
- *Supplemental oxygen and mechanical ventilation:* are required in hypoxaemic respiratory failure complicating bronchiectasis and cystic fibrosis[228] as for COPD.
- *Other therapies:* include immunoglobulin administration in hypogammaglobulinaemia and enzyme replacement in α_1-antitrypsin deficiency. Gene replacement therapy is currently being studied in cystic fibrosis. Good nutrition with a high caloric intake is required in bronchiectasis due to the high work of breathing and chronic infective state. Pancreatic supplements may be required in cystic fibrosis.
- *Surgery:* segmental resection may be considered in localized bronchiectasis with recurrent severe haemoptysis but otherwise the benefits of surgery are limited. Double lung and heart–lung transplantation has been most successful in the management of end-stage cystic fibrosis but is also an option in severe bronchiectasis. As previously, it is limited by donor availability.
- *Haemoptysis:* is a common problem in bronchiectasis. For the majority it is relatively minor with only flecks of blood in sputum. However, because the disease affects the high-pressure bronchial circulation it can be massive and life-threatening. Its management has been discussed above.
- *Halatosis:* is an often neglected problem in bronchiectasis. It can be severe, causing social embarrassment and difficulty managing patients both at home and in hospital. Although chronic lung infection is the most likely cause, correctable oral factors including dentistry, gum disease, and oral hygiene must be addressed. The causative anaerobic or gram negative lung infections must be managed with high dose, prolonged, broad-spectrum, antibiotic therapy (±nebulized antibiotics to sterilise airways secretions) as determined by sputum culture and sensitivity (see above). Aggressive physiotherapy and postural drainage are required to clear the foul smelling respiratory secretions. Simple measures including mouth scents, good ventilation, and air fresheners may all help particularly in the terminal phase of the disease when physiotherapy and postural drainage become more difficult.

Cystic fibrosis will affect about 1 : 2500 children and the gene responsible has been identified. The defect alters ion and water transport across epithelial cells causing recurrent pulmonary infection, bronchiectasis, lung fibrosis, and pancreatic insufficiency. Survival has improved progressively over the last 20 years and median survival is now about 30 years. Most patients with cystic fibrosis will be cared for in specialized units, with home support teams and staff trained in the principles of palliative care. Patients will have been encouraged to manage their own disease for many years and most will be familiar with the course of the disease. Psychosocial support from family and well-established carers is usually excellent. Many will have discussed their end-of-life management often at the time when a peer dies. In general, these young patients manage remarkably well although psychological problems are common. The option of lung transplantation has complicated 'end-of-life' decision making. Delay in acknowledging that the end-stage has been reached, and that lung transplantation is no longer a realistic option, should not delay effective terminal care. In comparison, terminal care support for older adults with long-standing, end-stage bronchiectasis is poor.

HIV-associated chronic infection

Pulmonary involvement in HIV disease and chronic respiratory infection is a major source of morbidity and mortality.[229,230] The Pulmonary Complications of HIV Infection Study (PCHIS) has demonstrated that the prevelance of HIV-associated pulmonary diseases depends on geographical factors and appears to be changing with time.[231,232] Although there is a wide range of pulmonary manifestations, both infectious and non-infectious (Table 13), respiratory disease is often a small component in a complex case including fever, wasting, skin disease, gastrointestinal, eye, and neurological complications. Good palliative care is a major challenge and in developed countries many patients are managed in specialized units which provide optimal medical and nursing management. The palliative management of end-stage HIV infection and its respiratory complications is extensively reviewed in a separate chapter in this textbook.

Tuberculosis

Poorly treated tuberculosis with recurrent reactivation results in severe pulmonary scarring, cavitation, and secondary aspergillus infection. In deprived populations, these patients may develop respiratory failure, recurrent bacterial and tuberculosis-related infection, and massive haemoptysis. Patients may have to be isolated in a negative pressure room particularly if multi-drug resistant tuberculosis is a factor, but otherwise treatment of the respiratory failure and chronic infection does not differ from that previously described. Considerable care must be taken by staff to avoid transmission to other patients and self-infection. The use of face masks and

Table 13 Infective and non-infective pulmonary complications of HIV disease

Pulmonary complications	Examples
Infection	
Bacterial	*Streptococcus pneumoniae, Haemophilus species, Pseudomonas aeruginosa*
Mycobacterial	*M. tuberculosis, M. avian complex, M. kanasii*
Fungi	*Pneumocystis carinii, Cryptococcus neoformans, Histoplasma capsulatum, Aspergillus species, Blastomyces dermatitidis, Penicillium marneffei*
Viruses	Cytomegalovirus
Parasites	*Toxoplasma gondii*
Malignancies	Kaposi's sarcoma, non-Hodgkin's lymphoma, bronchogenic carcinoma
Interstitial pneumonitides	Lymphocytic and non-specific interstitial pneumonitis
Other	COPD, PHT, diffuse alveolar damage, bronchiolitis obliterans organizing pneumonia, alveolar proteinosis

COPD, chronic obstructive pulmonary disease; PHT, pulmonary hypertension.

barrier nursing is essential. The tuberculosis must be actively treated with appropriate antibiotics depending on sensitivities determined from culture. Surgical and antimicrobial therapy of secondary aspergillus infection is often required.

Management of end-stage pulmonary vascular disease

Pulmonary hypertension and thromboembolic disease may be the direct cause or associated problems of end-stage respiratory disease. The breathlessness, fatigue (due to poor cardiac output), and fluid retention (cor pulmonale) that accompany these conditions are significant clinical challenges. Primary pulmonary hypertension, thromboembolic disease (e.g. antiphospholipid syndrome), and emphysema due to α_1-antitrypsin deficiency often affect young adults. In contrast, COPD and fibrotic lung disease tend to affect older age groups. Prevention of thromboembolic disease is essential in all terminally ill patients. Failure to prevent deep venous thrombosis or pulmonary embolism leads to unnecessary discomfort and may complicate care. The degree of investigation, intervention, and treatment undertaken in these conditions must be adjusted according to the needs of the individual patient and the level of terminal care.

Pulmonary hypertension and cor pulmonale

Most respiratory disease can result in pulmonary hypertension (PHT), which eventually leads to right ventricular hypertrophy, dilation, and cor pulmonale. Many mechanisms contribute to the development of PHT (Table 14), including hypoxic pulmonary vasoconstriction (HPV), multiple obstructive lesions, and primary pulmonary hypertension.

Chronic bronchitis and emphysema

They cause over 80 per cent of PHT due to progressive HPV and associated vascular remodelling.(233) Management aims to improve the underlying lung disorder. Oxygen therapy should reverse HPV and reduce right ventricular afterload, although reductions in PHT were small with LTOT.(30) In acute COPD exacerbations, non-invasive ventilation increases alveolar ventilation and CO_2 clearance which corrects acidaemia, reduces pulmonary artery vasoconstriction, and improves myocardial contractility. β_2-Agonists not only cause bronchodilation but also produce acute falls in pulmonary artery pressure and increase right ventricular ejection fraction with no significant fall in PaO_2.(234) The fluid retention in cor pulmonale is due to the effects of hypoxia on renal function and pituitary hormone release rather than right heart failure.(233) Diuretics are the mainstay of the management of fluid retention in the acute phase of cor pulmonale. With correction of hypoxaemia and improved transpulmonary blood flow, diuretic dose may be reduced or stopped. Pulmonary vasodilators (e.g. nifedipine, diltiazam) reduce pulmonary artery pressure but the effect is rarely sustained in the long term. As a consequence, function and survival are not significantly affected.(235) Futhermore, the non-specific pulmonary vasodilator action may impair ventilation/perfusion matching by enhan-cing perfusion of poorly ventilated alveoli resulting in increased hypoxaemia. Associated systemic hypotension may also be a significant problem. In severe COPD with cor pulmonale trials of the angiotensin-converting enzyme inhibitor captopril also caused systemic hypotension with no improvement in pulmonary vascular resistance, gas exchange, or ventilatory parameters.(236) In contrast, angiotensin II inhibitors reduced pulmonary vascular resistance without altering PaO_2.(237) Studies examining inhaled nitric oxide and endothelin antagonists have not produced clinically useful amelioration of PHT or cor pulmonale in chronic stable COPD to date.

Table 14 Classification of pulmonary hypertension

Idiopathic (e.g. primary pulmonary hypertension)
Hypoxic (e.g. hypoxic pulmonary vasoconstriction)
Passive (e.g. LVF/mitral stenosis/elevated LAP)
Hyperkinetic
Obliterative (e.g. chronic thromboembolic disease)
Dietary/drug induced
Vasoconstrictive

LVF, left ventricular failure; LAP, left atrial pressure.

Obstructive pulmonary hypertension

It is often caused by repetitive, silent, pulmonary emboli arising from deep vein thromboses over prolonged periods of time.(238) Other causes of obstructive PHT include vasculitis, sickle cell anaemia or infective endocarditis. World-wide schistosomiasis is one of the commonest causes of PHT due to the obstructive effect of the parasitic organism itself and the acute inflammatory response it evokes.(239) There is a high risk of chronic thromboembolic disease in many terminal conditions including chronic lung disease due to immobility and an increased tendency to coagulation.(240,241) It highlights the importance of prophylactic anticoagulation, compression stockings, and maintained mobility (see Pulmonary embolism below). Chronic thromboembolic PHT as a consequence of repeated multiple small emboli that have not previously been recognized requires careful assessment to determine whether pulmonary thromboendarterectomy is an option.(238) If accumulated clot can be successfully removed the improvement in PHT can be dramatic.(242) If surgery cannot be justified, particularly in patients with end-stage lung disease, management is focused on preventing further embolism by adequate anticoagulation, the occasional use of thrombolytic agents, and inferior vena cava filters. Pulmonary blood flow is also optimized by correcting hypoxaemia and maximizing pulmonary vasodilation.

Primary pulmonary hypertension (PPH)

PPH is a disease of unknown aetiology causing progressive PHT. The prognosis is poor with a median survival in the US registry of 2.8 years.(243) Although a rare condition, it is relatively high profile because it often cause end-stage disease in young women of child-bearing age (mean age 36, range 1–81 years). The primary clinical symptoms are progressive dyspnoea, reduced exercise tolerance, central chest pain, syncope, and occasional haemoptysis. In the terminal phase it is often associated with fluid accumulation and ankle oedema. Sudden death occurs in all forms of severe PHT due to acute right ventricular decompensation, arrhythmias, or thromboembolic events. In end-stage disease oxygen therapy provides symptomatic relief and may be beneficial in the management of the cor pulmonale. Many patients are anticoagulated because it is difficult to exclude the possibility of recurrent embolism and *in situ* thrombosis is perceived as part of the pathogenesis of the condition. Previous studies have reported improved survival in anticoagulated patients.(244,245) A wide variety of vasodilators have been used to treat PPH including hydralazine, diazoxide, nifedipine, captopril, and nitrates, and recently high-dose calcium channel blockers were shown to improve survival.(245) Sustained, beneficial haemodynamic, and clinical effects occur in about 20–40 per cent of patients,(246) but considerable care is required in their administration because of the risk of systemic hypotension. Prostacyclin, a powerful vasodilator, results in substantial haemodynamic and symptomatic improvement when given by continuous infusion or as nebulized solutions.(247) Reductions in both pulmonary artery pressure and vascular resistance are reported(248) and there is increasing evidence of improved survival. Sildenafil has recently been reported to be highly effective in PPH management but investigation is ongoing. PPH patients are often listed for heart–lung, double lung, and more recently single lung transplantation which may increase longevity(249) but lack of donor organs limits the application of this technique.

Pulmonary embolism (PE)

In the United States, approximately 5 million episodes of deep venous thrombosis (DVT) occur, 10 per cent embolize and 10 per cent of those who have an embolic event (~50 000) die.(250) The majority are not due to therapeutic failure but rather prophylactic oversight or diagnostic error. The incidence is increasing particularly in the dependent, hospitalized patient. The triad of venous stasis, alteration in coagulation, and vascular injury as primary factors in the pathogenesis of venous thromboembolism is supported by considerable scientific evidence.[251] These conditions are particularly applicable to patients in the terminal phase of chronic cardiopulmonary disease who are relatively immobile, with an increased thrombotic tendency and often longstanding peripheral vascular disease. About 90 per cent of clinically significant PE arise from the deep veins in the lower extremities. Calf vein thrombi are rarely associated with PE whereas over 50 per cent of thrombi in the popliteal or ileofemoral systems will embolize.[252] Acute cardiovascular collapse and rapid death may occur following a large embolus and this is the cause of death in many terminally ill patients who expire suddenly during an apparently unremarkable exertion.

Clinical diagnosis of PE is imprecise although acute dyspnoea is the most frequent presenting symptom in most studies.[252,253] The PIOPED study (Prospective Investigation of Pulmonary Embolism Diagnosis) examined the clinical probability of PE on the basis of history, examination, CXR, ECG, and blood gases.[254] In 90 patients estimated to have a greater than 80 per cent clinical probability of PE, 32 per cent did not have confirmatory angiographic evidence. In 228 patients estimated to have a probability of less than 19 per cent, 9 per cent had positive angiograms. In patients without prior cardiopulmonary disease in the PIOPED study, the combination of pleuritic pain and haemoptysis was the most common mode of presentation of pulmonary embolism in 65 per cent of cases, isolated dyspnoea in 22 per cent, and circulatory collapse in 8 per cent. Dyspnoea was not present in 27 per cent of patients with confirmed PE. In addition, prospective studies demonstrate that asymptomatic PE occurs in 40 per cent of high-risk patients with proximal deep vein thrombosis.[252,255] It is apparent that the 'typical' picture of PE is relatively rare and that presentation is often atypical or subtle.

The extent and type of investigations for PE in end-stage lung disease is determined by life expectancy and the level of potential discomfort that may be inflicted. Basic investigations should include blood gases, ECG, and chest radiography, but these are generally non-specific. Chest radiography was normal in 12 per cent of cases in the PIOPED study[254] and the features were often non-specific particularly in patients with concurrent respiratory disease (e.g. atelectasis, hilar enlargement, oligaemia, pleural effusion). Doppler ultrasonography and contrast venography are standard techniques for establishing the presence of DVT.[256] Investigations to establish a diagnosis of PE include ventilation/perfusion scans, angiography, and contrast spiral computed CT scans.[256] At present, V/Q scanning remains the first-line investigation.[254,257] A normal V/Q scan helps exclude, and a high probability scan confirms PE. An indeterminate scan or a low probability scan with high clinical probability suggest the need for angiography, or CT scan.[256,267] Angiography remains the 'gold' standard test but is relatively invasive.[254,256,257] CT scanning is sensitive, specific, and non-invasive and its role as the first-line investigation is currently being assessed.[256,257]

The importance of prevention in the immobile, respiratory patient cannot be overstressed. Simple factors like hydration, mobility, and prevention of venous obstruction by uncrossing legs should not be overlooked. The use of compression 'anti-embolism' stockings in end-stage disease is questionable and the associated discomfort must be balanced against likely benefit. Low molecular weight heparin offers substantial advantages over unfractionated heparin in the prevention of DVT and PE in terminally ill patients.[258] It is equally effective, has better bioavailability, predictable anticoagulant response, and less complications (e.g. bleeding, thrombocytopaenia). Once daily dosing with some preparations is feasible because of the longer duration of action. Except in renal failure and marked obesity monitoring is not required reducing the need for repeated blood tests. These properties make it a valuable hospice and domiciliary therapy if carers can be taught to provide the once daily injection. In patients with proven DVT or PE, maintenance therapy with warfarin is standard procedure after initial heparinization. The aim is to maintain the INR between 2 and 3.[259] However, the use of warfarin in patients with terminal disease can cause problems because of the need for repeated monitoring of the INR which may fluctuate according to drug therapy, liver function, and diet. As a result, continuation of low molecular weight heparin is becoming increasingly popular.[258]

The decision to use more invasive or aggressive therapies in the management of DVT and PE in end-stage chronic lung disease is difficult. In general, the use of thrombolytic therapy (e.g. recombinant tissue plasminogen activator (rt-PA)) in PE, with the associated risks of haemorrhage, should probably be reserved for those with acute, severe, haemodynamic instability and even in this situation survival benefit over heparinization alone is not proven.[260] Where risk of PE is very high but anticoagulation contraindicated, vena caval filters may be considered although lower limb oedema may be a significant problem. Catheter or surgical embolectomy must be carefully considered in patients with end-stage disease.

Pneumothorax and pleural disease

In end-stage lung disease, even a small collection of air or fluid in the pleural space may have serious implications because respiratory reserve to compensate for the loss of ventilatory capacity (due to lung compression) is reduced in these patients.[261] The incidence of 'spontaneous' pneumothorax increases with age and severity of the underlying lung disease. It is most commonly associated with COPD but may affect a wide variety of other lung diseases that damage lung architecture or the pleura. Iatrogenic damage during aspiration of a pleural effusion may also result in a pneumothorax. Early recognition and wide-bore, intercostal tube drainage with an underwater seal is necessary in most patients and is often life-saving.[261] However, in the terminally ill patient the decision may be taken to treat the patient symptomatically with oxygen, analgesics, and opioids to avoid the distress of moving them to a unit with the appropriate facilities to insert and manage a chest drain.

Pleural effusions and empyema also result in exaggerated respiratory embarrassment in chronic lung diseases due to lung compression. Intermittent aspiration or tube drainage provides valuable symptomatic relief of breathlessness in most patients. There are a wide variety of potential causes including infection, cardiac failure, hypoalbuminaemia, and renal impairment, and the underlying cause must be addressed. However, if the cause is irreversible, the possibility of chemical pleurodesis may have to be considered and these procedures have been discussed extensively in the chapter on malignant respiratory diseases. Localized pleural pain due to rib fractures, infection, or pneumothorax may respond to normal analgesic regimes. However, local anaesthetic intercostals nerve blocks or intrapleural instillation of bupivacaine may also be useful.[262]

Respiratory terminal care and palliative sedation

During the terminal phase of end-stage respiratory disease, simple nursing measures including a constant draught from an open window or fan, regular sips of water to moisten the mouth (particularly when using oxygen), and sitting upright may be very beneficial. If confined to bed, the patient may be propped up with pillows (Fig. 2) as there is a significant loss of diaphragmatic function, increased risk of pulmonary oedema associated with cardiac failure, and lower lobe atelectasis when lying flat. In addition, recurrent micro-aspiration is more likely in the recumbent position.

In the terminal stages of end-stage respiratory disease, including the neuromuscular diseases, the emphasis of management changes from active interventions to purely supportive and symptomatic measures. Non-invasive ventilatory support and active physiotherapy may be withdrawn to facilitate greater comfort for the patient. Drug treatments aimed at palliating symptoms of pain, breathlessness, constipation, and haemoptysis are often unavoidable. If possible drugs should be given orally using sustained release preparations but subcutaneous infusions or intermittent, intramuscular injections may be necessary. Often, these patients will have been on oxygen therapy for long periods and may become distressed if this is removed. Use of nasal prongs facilitates communication with relatives and carers. Similarly, nebulizers should be continued as long as practically possible to provide bronchodilators, local anaesthetic, and opioids to alleviate breathlessness and cough. The 'rattle' associated with loose respiratory secretions in the short period before death may be distressing to relatives although most patients will be unaware of the noise at this stage. Hyoscine should be administered to reduce respiratory secretions, although repositioning or gentle suctioning may be required.[263]

The use of palliative sedation for the relief of refractory dyspnoea is particularly difficult because of the perceived risk of respiratory depression. A recent multicentre study reported that the use of sedation varied considerably between different hospice units.[264] However, several studies examining the use of sedation for refractory symptoms during the terminal phase have not shown a difference in survival between sedated and non-sedated patients with respiratory distress.[264–267] As many patients approaching death with end-stage respiratory disease will have uncontrolled breathlessness, sedation and opioid use should not be withheld because of an inappropriate fear of respiratory depression. Benzodiazepines, in particular midazolam and opioids, are the sedatives most frequently used and can be titrated to achieve the desired level of sedation. When the risk of respiratory depression is considerable, the risks and benefits must be carefully considered and the justification for sedation clearly defined. Such decisions are often made by teams rather than individuals and it is appropriate that patients and families are fully involved in decision-making and should understand that the sedation is a means of relieving distressing symptoms. Before starting sedation it should be clear that other interventions to relieve refractory dyspnoea have not provided relief, or will not do so in an appropriate time period and may be associated with additional morbidity.[268]

The degree of sedation may be varied throughout the course of the terminal stage by periods of discontinuation or titrating drug effect to the desired level. However, as death approaches and if breathlessness becomes intolerable, sedation to unconsciousness may be the last resort to alleviate suffering. For those patients and their families who do not wish to accept sedation during the period of dying, it is the duty of the carer to relieve suffering as best possible and to support the patient through to death.

Summary: the future for palliative care in end-stage respiratory disease

In the United Kingdom, the number of specialist respiratory nurses is increasing but remains relatively small.[45] They are based in hospital but many make domiciliary visits. Patients cared for by these nurses live longer but quality of life is not necessarily improved.[41,46] Nevertheless, patients valued these visits and wanted them to continue. Despite the efforts of respiratory physicians and nurses, support for patients with terminal lung disease is less well developed than that available for patients with malignant disease. A number of exceptions include care for patients with cystic fibrosis and HIV-related respiratory disease. Nevertheless, there is clearly a major unmet need in the care of the patient with end-stage respiratory disease.

In response to recommendations that all patients should have access to palliative care,[2,15,16] the need, potential demand, and resource implications of this directive have been assessed.[2] There are clearly major problems that will have to be overcome if the goal of 'palliative care for all' is to be achieved.[2] These include lack of current service provision, difficulty projecting disease trajectory in chronic lung disease, the need for specialist respiratory skills, and inadequate resources. Overcoming these problems will be difficult. Education in palliative care will be essential at all levels of doctor and nurse training and it is clear that respiratory physicians and specialist nurses will need to adopt the palliative care approach. A potential solution to the current lack of palliative care provision in the management of chronic lung disease may be to expand the limited specialist respiratory nurse service following further training in the principles of palliative care. In the short-term, specialists in palliative care medicine may be able to provide consultancy services and advice on training. In addition, there may be scope for short-term involvement of the palliative care team in the management of individual patient problems.[2] In the longer term, the need for increased funding of specialist respiratory nurses with palliative skills and the possibility of specialist units for the management of end-stage respiratory disease must be explored.

References

1. **Hinton, J.M.** (1963). The physical and mental distress of the dying. *Quarterly Medical Journal* **32**, 1–21.
2. **Addington-Hall, J.** For The National Council for Hospice and Specialist Palliative Care Services and Scottish Partnership Agency for Palliative and Cancer Care. *Reaching Out: Specialist Palliative Care for Adults with Non-Malignant Diseases.* Northamptonshire UK: Land & Unwin (Data Sciences) Ltd, 1998.
3. **Lupu, D.** (1996). Hospice inpatient care: an overview of NHO's 1995 inpatient survey results. *Hospice Journal* **11**, 21–39.
4. **Eve, A., Smith, A.M., and Tebbit, P.** (1997). Hospice and palliative care in the UK 1994–5, including a summary of trends 1990–5. *Palliative Medicine* **11**, 31–43.
5. **Wilkes, E.** (1984). Dying now. *Lancet* **i**, 950–2.
6. **Mills, M., Davies, T.O., and Macrae, W.A.** (1994). Care of dying patients in hospital. *British Medical Journal* **309**, 583–6.
7. **Seale, C.** (1991). Death from cancer and death from other causes: the relevance of the hospice approach. *Palliative Medicine* **5**, 13–20.
8. **Hockley, J.M., Dunlop, R., and Davies, R.J.** (1988). Survey of distressing symptoms in dying patients and their families in hospital and the response to a symptom control team. *British Medical Journal* **296**, 1715–17.
9. **Lynn, J.** et al. (1997). Perceptions by family members of the dying experience of older and seriously ill patients. *Annals of Internal Medicine* **126**, 97–106.
10. **The SUPPORT Principal Investigators** (1995). A controlled trial to improve care for seriously ill hospitalised patients. The Study to Understand Prognoses and Preferences for Outcomes and Risks of Treatment (SUPPORT). *Journal of the American Medical Association* **274**, 1591–8.
11. **Cohen, L.M.** et al. (1995). Dialysis discontinuation. A 'good' death? *Archives of Internal Medicine* **155**, 42–7.
12. **Barby, T. and Leigh, P.N.** (1995). Palliative care in motor neurone disease. *International Journal of Palliative Nursing* **1**, 183–8.
13. **McCarthy, M., Lay, M., and Addington Hall, J.M.** (1996). Dying from heart disease. *Journal of the Royal College of Physicians* **30**, 325–8.
14. **Addington Hall, J.M.** et al. (1995). Symptom control, communication with health professionals and hospital care of stroke patients in the last year of life, as reported by surviving family, friends and carers. *Stroke* **26**, 2242–8.
15. **Gore, J.M., Brophy, C.J., and Greenstone, M.A.** (2000). How well do we care for patients with end stage chronic obstructive pulmonary disease (COPD)? A comparison of palliative care and quality of life in COPD and lung cancer. *Thorax* **55**, 1000–6.
16. **Edmonds, P.** et al. (2001). A comparison of the palliative care needs of patients dying from chronic respiratory diseases and lung cancer. *Palliative Medicine* **15**, 287–95.
17. **Skilbeck, J.** et al. (1998). Palliative care in chronic obstructive airways disease: a needs assessment. *Palliative Medicine* **12**, 245–54.
18. **Standing Medical Advisory Committee, Standing Nursing and Midwifery Advisory Committee.** *The Principles and Provision of Palliative Care.* London: Standing Medical Advisory Committee and Standing Nurse and Midwifery Advisory Committee, 1992.
19. **The Scottish Office NHS in Scotland Management Executive.** *Contracting for Specialist Palliative Care Services.*
20. **The British Thoracic Society.** *The Burden of Lung Disease.* London: Munro & Forster Communications, pp. 6–9, 2001.
21. **Office for National Statistics** (2000). *Mortality Statistics by Cause.* Series DH2 no. 26. London: The Stationary Office.
22. **Royal College of Physicians** (1986). Physical disability in 1986 and beyond. *Journal of the Royal College of Physicians London* **3**, 160–94.
23. **Cox, B.D.** (1987). Blood pressure and respiratory function. In *The Health and Lifestyle Survey.* Preliminary Report of a Nationwide Survey of the Physical and Mental Health Attitudes and Lifestyle of a Random Survey of 9003 British Adults. *London Health Promotion Research Trust*, pp. 17–33.

24. **COPD Guidelines Group of the Standards of Care Committee of the BTS** (1997). BTS guidelines for the management of chronic obstructive pulmonary disease. *Thorax* **52** (Suppl. 5), S1–28.
25. **Strachan, D.P.** (1995). Epidemiology: a British perspective. In *Chronic Obstructive Pulmonary Disease* (ed. P. Calverley and N. Pride), pp. 47–67. London: Chapman and Hall.
26. **Thorn, T.J.** (1989). International comparisons in COPD mortality. *American Review of Respiratory Disease* **140**, S27–34.
27. **Higgins, M.** (1993). Epidemiology of obstructive pulmonary disease. In *Principles and Practice of Pulmonary Rehabilitation* (ed. R. Casaburi and T.L. Pett), pp. 10–17. Philadelphia: Saunders.
28. **Gustafsson, P.M.** (2001). A world galloping into breathlessness. *Respiration* **68**, 2–3.
29. **Medical Research Council Working Party** (1981). Long term domicillary oxygen therapy in chronic hypoxic cor pulmonale complicating chronic bronchitis and emphysema. *Lancet* **i**, 681–6.
30. **Nocturnal Oxygen Therapy Trial Group** (1980). Continuous or nocturnal oxygen therapy in hypoxaemic chronic obstructive lung disease: a clinical trial. *Annals of Internal Medicine* **93**, 391–8.
31. **Hill, K.M. and Muers, M.F.** (2000). Palliative care for patients with non-malignant end stage respiratory disease. *Thorax* **55**, 978–81.
32. **McHorney, C.A., Ware, J.E. Jr, and Raczek, A.E.** (1993). The MOS 36-Item Short-Form Health Survey (SF-36). II Psychometric and clinical tests of validity in measuring physical and mental health constructs. *Medical Care* **31**, 247–63.
33. **Jones, P.W., Quirk, F.H., and Baveystock, C.M.** (1992). A self-complete measure of health status for chronic airflow limitation. *American Review of Respiratory Disease* **144**, 1321–7.
34. **Guyatt, G.H.** et al. (1987). A measure of quality of life for clinical trials in chronic lung disease. *Thorax* **42**, 773–8.
35. **Bergman, B.** et al. (1994). For the European Organisation for Research and Treatment of Cancer (EORTC) Study Group on Quality of Life. The EORTC QLQ LC-13: a modular supplement to the EORTC Core Quality of Life Questionaire (QLQ-C30) for use in lung cancer clinical trials. *European Journal of Cancer* **30**, 635–42.
36. **Aass, N.** et al. (1997). Prevalence of anxiety and depression in cancer patients seen at the Norwegian Radium Hospital. *European Journal of Cancer* **33**, 1597–604.
37. **Langendijk, J.A.** et al. (2000). Quality of life after palliative radiotherapy in non-small cell lung cancer: a prospective study. *International Journal of Radiation Oncology, Biology, Physics* **47**, 149–55.
38. **Gibbs, G.** (1995). Nurses in private nursing homes: a study of their knowledge and attitudes to pain management in palliative care. *Palliative Medicine* **9**, 245–53.
39. **British Thoracic Society (BTS) Standards of Care Committee** (1997). Survey of resources used by respiratory physicians for the diagnosis and management of lung cancer. London BTS.
40. **Royal College of Physicians** (1981). Disabling chest disease: prevention and care. *Journal of the Royal College of Physicians London* **15**, 69–87.
41. **Cockroft, A.** et al. (1987). Controlled trial of respiratory health worker visiting patients with chronic respiratory disability. *British Medical Journal* **294**, 225–8.
42. **Cotton, M.M.** et al. (2000). Early discharge for patients with exacerbations of chronic obstructive pulmonary disease: a randomised controlled trial. *Thorax* **55**, 902–6.
43. **Skwarska, E.** et al. (2000). Randomised controlled trial of supported discharge in patients with exacerbations of chronic obstructive pulmonary disease. *Thorax* **55**, 907–12.
44. **Ojoo, J.C.** et al. (2002). Patients' and carers' preferences in two models of care for acute exacerbations of COPD: results of a randomised controlled trial. *Thorax* **57**, 167–9.
45. **Heslop, A.** (1993). Role of the respiratory nurse specialist. *British Journal of Hospital Medicine* **50**, 88–90.
46. **Littlejohns, P.** et al. (1991). Randomised controlled trial of the effectiveness of a respiratory health worker in reducing impairment, disability and handicap due to chronic airflow limitation. *Thorax* **46**, 559–64.
47. **Schwartzstein, R.M.** et al. (1990). Dyspnea: a sensory experience. *Lung* **168**, 185–99.
48. **Tobin, M.J.** (1990). Dyspnea: pathophysiologic basis, clinical presentation, and management. *Archives of Internal Medicine* **150**, 1604–13.
49. **Dyspnea. Mechanisms, Assessment and Management** (1999). A consensus statement. American Thoracic Society. *American Journal of Respiratory & Critical Care Medicine* **159**, 321–40.
50. **Simons, P.M.** et al. (1990). Distinguishable types of dyspnea in patients with shortness of breath. *American Reviw of Respiratory Disease* **142**, 1009–14.
51. **Elliott, M.W.** et al. (1991). The language of breathlessness: use of verbal descriptors by patients with cardiorespiratory disease. *American Review of Respiratory Disease* **144**, 826–32.
52. **O'Donnell, D.E., Chau, L., and Webb, K.A.** (1998). Qualitative aspects of exertional dyspnea in patients with interstitial disease. *Journal of Applied Physiology* **84**, 2000–9.
53. **Mahler, D.A.** (2000). Do you speak the language of dyspnea? *Chest* **117**, 928–9.
54. **Wilson, R.C. and Jones, P.W.** (1991). Differentiation between intensity of breathlessness and the distress it evokes in normal subjects during exercise. *Clinical Science* **80**, 65–70.
55. **Freedman, S., Lane, R., and Guz, A.** (1987). Breathlessness and respiratory mechanics during reflex or voluntary hyperventilation in patients with chronic airflow limitation. *Clinical Science* **73**, 311–18.
56. **Lindsey, B.G.** et al. (2000). Respiratory neuronal assemblies. *Respiration Physiology* **122**, 183–96.
57. **Burton, M.D. and Kazemi, H.** (2000). Neurotransmitters in central respiratory control. *Respiration Physiology* **122**, 111–21.
58. **Haji, A., Takeda, R., and Okazaki, M.** (2000). Neuropharmacology of control of respiratory rhythm and pattern in mature mammals. *Pharmacology & Therapeutics* **86**, 277–304.
59. **Lane, R.** et al. (1987). Arterial oxygen saturation and breathlessness in patients with chronic obstructive airways disease. *Clinical Science* **72**, 693–8.
60. **Banzett, R.B.** et al. (1989). 'Air hunger' arising from increased P_{CO2} in mechanically ventilated quadriplegics. *Respiration Physiology* **76**, 53–67.
61. **Banzett, R.B., Lansing, R.W., and Brown, R.** (1990). 'Air hunger' from increased P_{CO2} persists after complete neuromuscular block in humans. *Respiration Physiology* **81**, 1–17.
62. **Cristiano, L.M. and Schwartzstein, R.M.** (1997). Effect of chest wall vibration on dyspnea during hypercapnia and exercise in chronic obstructive pulmonary disease. *American Journal of Respiratory & Critical Care Medicine* **155**, 1552–9.
63. **Clark, A.** et al. (1996). Leg blood flow, metabolism and exercise capacity in chronic stable heart failure. *International Journal of Cardiology* **55**, 127–35.
64. **Schwartzstein, R.M.** et al. (1987). Cold facial stimulation reduces breathlessness induced in normal subjects. *American Review of Respiratory Disease* **136**, 58–61.
65. **Demediuk, B.H.** et al. (1992). Dissociation between dyspnoea and respiratory effort. *American Review of Respiratory Disease* **146**, 1222–5.
66. **Killian, K.J.** et al. (1984). Effect of increased lung volume on perception of breathlessness, effort and tension. *Journal of Applied Physiology* **57**, 686–91.
67. **El-manshawi, A.** et al. (1986). Breathlessness during exercise with and without resistive loading. *Journal of Applied Physiology* **61**, 896–905.
68. **Chetta, A.** et al. (1998). Personality profiles and breathlessness perception in outpatients with different gradings of asthma. *American Journal of Respiratory & Critical Care Medicine* **157**, 116–22.
69. **Smoller, J.W.** et al. (1996). Panic anxiety, dyspnoea, respiratory disease: Theoretical and clinical considerations. *American Journal of Respiratory & Critical Care Medicine* **154**, 6–17.
70. **Gift, A.G. and Narsavage, G.** (1998). Validity of the numeric rating scale as a measure of dyspnoea. *American Journal Critical Care* **7**, 200–4.
71. **Muza, S.R.** et al. (1990). Comparison of scales used to quantitate the sense of effort to breath in patients with chronic obstructive pulmonary disease. *American Review of Respiratory Disease* **141**, 909–13.
72. **Borg, G.** (1978). Subjective effort and physical activities. *Scandinavian Journal of Rehabilitation Medicine* **6**, 108–13.

73. **Guyatt, G.H.** et al. (1987). A measure of quality of life for clinical trials in chronic lung disease. *Thorax* **42**, 773–8.
74. **Jones, P.W.** et al. (1992). A self-complete measure of health status for chronic airflow limitation. *American Review of Respiratory Disease* **145**, 1321–7.
75. **O'Donnell, D.E. and Webb, K.A.** (1992). Breathlessness in patients with severe chronic airflow limitation. *Chest* **102**, 824–31.
76. **Lareau, S.C.** et al. (1999). Dyspnea in patients with chronic obstructive pulmonary disease: does dyspnea worsen longitudinally in the presence of declining lung function? *Heart & Lung* **28**, 65–73.
77. **Wolkove, N., Dajczman, E., Colacone, A., and Kreisman, H.** (1989). The relationship between pulmonary function and dyspnea in obstructive lung disease. *Chest* **96**, 1247–51.
78. **Leach, R.M.** et al. (1992). Portable liquid oxygen and exercise ability in severe respiratory disability. *Thorax* **47**, 781–9.
79. **Puchelle, E.** et al. (1980). Mucociliary transport *in vivo* and *in vitro*: Relations to sputum properties in chronic bronchitis. *European Journal of Respiratory Disease* **61**, 254–64.
80. **Sant'Ambrogio, G. and Widdicombe, J.G.** (2001). Reflexes from airway rapidly adapting receptors. *Respiration Physiology* **125**, 33–45.
81. **Sant'Ambrogio, G.** (1996). Role of the larynx in cough. *Pulmonary Pharmacology* **9**, 379–82.
82. **Tatar, M., Webber, S.E., and Widdicombe, J.G.** (1988): Lung C-fibre receptor activation and defensive reflexes in anaesthetised cats. *Journal of Physiology* **402**, 411–20.
83. **Kamai, J.** (1996). Role of opioidergic and serotonergic mechanisms in cough and antitussives. *Pulmonary Pharmacology* **9**, 349–56.
84. **French, C.L. and Irwin, R.S.** (1998). The impact of cough on quality of life. *Archives of Internal Medicine* **158**, 1657–61.
85. **Irwin, R.S.** et al. (1998). Managing cough as a defence mechanism and as a symptom: a consensus panel report of the American College of Chest Physicians. Managing cough as a defence mechanism and as a symptom. *Chest* **114**, 133S–81S.
86. **Gracey, D.R., Divertie, M.B., and Howard, F.M. Jr** (1983). Mechanical ventilation for respiratory failure in myasthenia gravis: two year experience with 22 patients. *Mayo Clinic Proceedings* **58**, 597–602.
87. **Szienberg, A.** et al. (1988). Cough capacity in patients with muscular dystrophy. *Chest* **94**, 1232–5.
88. **Irwin, R.S., Curley, F.J., and French, C.L.** (1990). Chronic cough: the spectrum and frequency of causes, key components of the diagnostic evaluation, and outcome of specific therapy. *American Review of Respiratory Disease* **141**, 640–7.
89. **Jones, A.P. and Rowe, B.H.** Bronchopulmonary hygiene physical therapy for chronic obstructive pulmonary disease and bronchiectasis. *The Cochrane Library 2.*
90. **Marom, Z.M. and Goswami, S.K.** (1991). Respiratory mucous hypersecretion (bronchorrhea): a case discussion—possible mechanism(s) and treatment. *Journal of Allergy & Clinical Immunology* **87**, 1050–5.
91. **Tamaoki, J.** et al. (2000). Inhaled indomethacin in bronchorrhoea in bronchoalveolar carcinoma: role of cyclooxygenase. *Chest* **117**, 1213–14.
92. **Wills, P. and Greenstone, M.** Inhaled hyperosmolar agents for bronchiectasis. *The Cochrane Library 2.*
93. **Davies, C.L.** (1997). ABC of Palliative care: breathlessness, cough, and other respiratory problems. *British Medical Journal* **315**, 931–4.
94. **Doona, M. and Walsh, D.** (1998). Benzoate for opioid-resistant cough in advanced cancer. *Palliative Medicine* **12**, 55–8.
95. **Luporini, G.** et al. (1998). Efficacy and safety of levodropropizine and dihydrocodeine on non-productive cough in primary and metastatic lung cancer. *European Respiratory Journal* **12**, 97–101.
96. **Louie, K., Bertolino, M., and Fainsinger, R.** (1992). Management of intractable cough. *Journal of Palliative Care* **8**, 46–8.
97. **Moroni, M.** et al. (1996). Inhaled sodium cromoglycate to treat cough in advanced lung cancer patients. *British Journal of Cancer* **74**, 309–11.
98. **Morice, A. and Abdul-Manap, R.** (1998). Drug treatments for coughs and colds. *Prescriber* **9**, 74–9.
99. **Schroeder, K. and Fahey, T.** (2002). Systematic review of randomised controlled trials of over the counter cough medicines for acute cough in adults. *British Medical Journal* **324**, 1–6.
100. **Luchette, F.** et al. (1994). Prospective evaluation of epidural versus intrapleural catheters for analgesis in chest wall trauma. *Journal of Trauma* **36**, 865–70.
101. **Wise, C.M.** (1994). Chest wall syndromes. *Current Opinion in Rheumatology* **6**, 197–202.
102. **Mukerji, B.** et al. (1995). The prevalence of rheumatological disorders in patients with chest pain and angiographically normal coronary arteries. *Angiology* **46**, 425–30.
103. **Viar, W.N. and Harrison, T.R.** (1952). Chest pain in association with pulmonary hypertension: its similarity to the pain of coronary disease. *Circulation* **5**, 1–11.
104. **Adam, J.** (1997). ABC of palliative care: the last 48 hours. *British Medical Journal* **315**, 1600–3.
105. **Thompson, A.B., Teschler, H., and Rennard, S.** (1992). Pathogenesis, evaluation, and therapy for massive haemoptysis. *Clinics in Chest Medicine* **13**, 69–82.
106. **Cahill, B.C. and Ingbar, D.H.** (1994). Massive haemoptysis assessment and management. *Clinics in Chest Medicine* **15**, 147–68.
107. **Hirshberg, B., Biran, I., Glazer, M., and Kramer, M.R.** (1997). Hemoptysis; etiology, evaluation, and outcome in a tertiary referral hospital. *Chest* **112**, 440–4.
108. **Patel, U., Pattison, C.W., and Raphael, M.** (1994). Management of massive haemoptysis. *British Journal of Hospital Medicine* **74**, 76–8.
109. **Crocco, J.A.** et al. (1968). Massive haemoptysis. *Archives of Internal Medicine* **121**, 495–8.
110. **Gong, H. and Salvatierra, C.** (1981). Clinical efficacy of early and delayed fibreoptic bronchoscopy in patients with hemoptysis. *American Review of Respiratory Disease* **124**, 221–5.
111. **Conlan, A.A. and Hurwitz, S.S.** (1980). Management of massive haemoptysis with the rigid broncoscope and iced saline lavage. *Thorax* **35**, 901–7.
112. **Bense, L.** (1990). Intrabronchial selective coagulative treatment of hemoptysis. *Chest* **97**, 990–6.
113. **Saumench, J.** et al. (1989). Value of fibreoptic bronchoscopy and angiography for diagnosis of the bleeding site in haemoptysis. *Annals of Thoracic Surgery* **48**, 272–4.
114. **Tan, R.T., McGahan, J.P., Link, D.P., and Lantz, B.M.T.** (1991). Bronchial artery embolisation in management of haemoptysis. *Journal of Interventional Radiology* **6**, 67–76.
115. **Mal, H.** et al. (1999). Immediate and long-term results of bronchial artery embolisation for life-threatening hemoptysis. *Chest* **115**, 996–1001.
116. **Jones, K.D. and Davies, R.J.** (1990). Massive haemoptysis. *British Medical Journal* **300**, 889–900.
117. **Lomotan, J.R., George, S.S., and Brandsetter, R.D.** (1997). Aspiration pneumonia. Strategies for early recognition and prevention. *Postgraduate Medicine* **102**, 229–31.
118. **Drakulovic, M.B.** et al. (1999). Supine body position as a risk factor for nosocomial pneumonia in mechanically ventilated patients; a randomised trial. *Lancet* **354**, 1851–8.
119. **Shepperd, S.** et al. (1998). Randomised controlled trial comparing hospital at home care with inpatient hospital care. I; three month follow-up of health outcomes. *British Medical Journal* **316**, 1786–91.
120. **Madge, S. and Esmond, G.** (2001). End-stage management of respiratory disease. In *Respiratory Nursing* (ed. G. Esmond), pp. 229–40. London: Bailliere Tindall.
121. **Shee, C.D.** (1995). Palliation in chronic respiratory disease. *Palliative Medicine* **9**, 3–12.
122. **Belman, M.J., Botnick, W.C., and Shin, J.W.** (1996). Inhaled bronchodilators reduce dynamic hyperinflation during exercise in patients with chronic obstructive airways disease. *American Journal of Respiratory & Critical Care Medicine* **153**, 967–75.
123. **Ramirez-Venegas, A., Ward, J., Lentine, T., and Mahler, D.A.** (1997). Salmeterol reduces dyspnea and improves lung function in patients with COPD. *Chest* **112**, 336–40.
124. **Teramoto, S., Fukuchi, Y., and Orimo, H.** (1993). Effects of inhaled anticholinergic drug on dyspnea and gas exchange during exercise in patients with chronic obstructive airways disease. *Chest* **103**, 1774–82.

125. **Casaburi, R.** et al. (2000). The spirometric efficacy of once-daily dosing with tiotropium in stable COPD: a 13-week multicentre trial. *Chest* **118**, 1294–302.

126. **Rennard, S.I.** et al. (1996). Extended therapy with ipratropium is associated with improved lung function in patients with COPD: a retrospective analysis of data from seven clinical trials. *Chest* **110**, 62–70.

127. **Combivent Inhalation Aerosol Study Group** (1994). In chronic obstructive pulmonary disease, a combination of ipratropium and albuterol is more effective than either agent alone: an 85-day multicenter trial. *Chest* **105**, 1411–19.

128. **O'Driscoll, B.R.** (1997). Nebulisers for chronic obstructive airways disease. In: Current Best Practice for Nebuliser Treatment. *Thorax* **52**, S49–52.

129. **The Nebuliser Project Group of the British Thoracic Society Standards of Care Committee** (1997). Current Best Practice for Nebuliser Treatment. *Thorax* **52**, S1–106.

130. **Blake, K.V., Hoppe, M., Harman, E., and Hendeles, L.** (1992). Relative amount of albuterol delivered to lung receptors from a metered-dose inhaler and nebulizer solution: bioassay by histamine bronchoprovocation. *Chest* **101**, 309–15.

131. **Bowton, D.L., Goldsmith, W.M., and Haponik, E.F.** (1992). Substitution of metered-dose inhalers for hand held nebulizers: success and cost savings in a large, acute care hospital. *Chest* **101**, 305–8.

132. **Berry, R.B.** et al. (1989). Nebulizer vs spacer for bronchodilator delivery in patients hospitalised for acute exacerbations of COPD. *Chest* **96**, 1241–6.

133. **O'Driscoll, B.R. and Bernstein, A.** (1996). A long-term study of symptoms, spirometry and survival amongst home nebuliser users. *Respiratory Medicine* **90**, 561–6.

134. **Stokes, T.C.** et al. (1982). Assessment of steroid responsiveness in patients with chronic airflow obstruction. *Lancet* **ii**, 345–8.

135. **Mahler, D.A.** et al. (1985). Sustained release theophylline reduces dyspnea in nonreversible obstructive airways disease. *American Review of Respiratory Disease* **131**, 22–5.

136. **Eaton, M.L.** et al. (1982). Effects of theophylline on breathlessness and exercise tolerance in patients with chronic airflow obstruction. *Chest* **82**, 538–42.

137. **Kirsten, D.K., Wegner, R.E., Jorres, R.A., and Magnussen, H.** (1993). Effects of theophylline withdrawal in severe chronic obstructive pulmonary disease. *Chest* **104**, 1101–7.

138. **Crockett, A.J., Cranston, J.M., Moss, J.R., and Alpers, J.H.** (2001). Domiciliary oxygen for chronic obstructive pulmonary disease (Cochrane Review). In *The Cochrane Library* Issue 4. Oxford: Update Software.

139. **Pauwels, R.A.** et al. (2001). Global strategy for the diagnosis, management, and prevention of chronic obstructive pulmonary disease. NHLBI/WHO Global Initiative For Chronic Obstructive Lung Disease (GOLD) workshop summary. *American Journal of Respiratory & Critical Care Medicine* **163**, 1256–76.

140. **Ringbaek, T., Lange, P., and Viskum, K.** (1999). Compliance with LTOT and consumption of mobile oxygen. *Respiratory Medicine* **93**, 333–7.

141. **Woodcock, A.A., Gross, E.R., and Geddes, D.M.** (1981). Oxygen relieves breathlessness in 'pink puffers'. *Lancet* **i**, 907–9.

142. **Kelley, M.A., Panettieri, R.A., and Krupinski, A.V.** (1986). Resting single-breath diffusing capacity as a screening test for exercise-induced hypoxemia. *American Journal of Medicine* **80**, 807–12.

143. **Dean, N.C.** et al. (1992). Oxygen may improve dyspnea and endurance in patients with chronic obstructive pulmonary disease and only mild hypoxemia. *American Review of Respiratory Disease* **146**, 941–5.

144. **Luce, J.M. and Luce, J.A.** (2001). Management of dyspnea in patients with far-advanced lung disease. *Journal of the American Medical Association* **285**, 1331–7.

145. **Burdon, J.G.W., Pain, M.C.F., Rubinfeld, A.R., and Nana, A.** (1994). Chronic lung disease and the perception of breathlessness: a clinical perspective. *European Respiratory Journal* **7**, 1342–9.

146. **Mitchell-Heggs, P.** et al. (1980). Diazepam in the treatment of dyspnoea in the 'Pink Puffer' syndrome. *Quarterly Journal of Medicine* **49**, 9–20.

147. **Man, G.C., Hsu, K., and Sproule, B.J.** (1986). Effect of alprazolam on exercise and dyspnea in patients with chronic obstructive pulmonary disease. *Chest* **90**, 832–6.

148. **Woodcock, A.A., Gross, E.R., and Geddes, D.M.** (1981). Drug treatment of breathlessness: contrasting effects of diazepam and promethazine in pink puffers. *British Medical Journal* **283**, 343–5.

149. **Rice, K.L.** et al. (1987). Effects of chronic administration of codeine and promethazine on breathlessness and exercise tolerance in patients with chronic airflow obstruction. *British Journal of Diseases of the Chest* **81**, 287–91.

150. **Argyropoulou, P.** et al. (1993). Buspirone effect on breathlessness and exercise performance in patients with chronic obstructive pulmonary disease. *Respiration* **60**, 216–20.

151. **Singh, N.P.** et al. (1993). Effects of buspirone on anxiety levels and exercise tolerance in patients with chronic airflow obstruction and mild anxiety. *Chest* **103**, 800–4.

152. **Smoller, J.W.** (1996). Panic anxiety, dyspnoea and respiratory disease. Theoretical and clinical considerations. *American Journal of Respiratory & Critical Care Medicine* **154**, 6–17.

153. **McIver, B., Walsh, D., and Nelson, K.** (1994). The use of chlorpromazine for symptom control in dying cancer patients. *Journal of Pain and Symptom Management* **9**, 341–5.

154. **Zebraski, S.E., Kochenash, S.M., and Raffa, R.B.** (2000). Lung opiod receptors: pharmacology and possible target for nebulized morphine in dyspnoea. *Life Sciences* **66**, 2221–31.

155. **Woodcock, A.A.** et al. (1981). Effects of dihydrocodeine, alcohol and caffeine on breathlessness and exercise tolerance in patients with chronic obstructive lung disease and normal blood gases. *New England Journal of Medicine* **305**, 1611–16.

156. **Johnson, M.A., Woodcock, A.A., and Geddes, D.M.** (1983). Dihydrocodeine for breathlessness in 'pink puffers'. *British Medical Journal* **286**, 675–7.

157. **Light, R.W.** et al. (1989). Effects of oral morphine on breathlessness and exercise tolerance in patients with chronic obstructive pulmonary disease. *American Review of Respiratory Disease* **139**, 126–33.

158. **Poole, P.J., Veale, A.G., and Black, P.N.** (1998). The effect of sustained-release morphine on breathlessness and quality of life in severe chronic obstructive pulmonary disease. *American Journal of Respiratory & Critical Care Medicine* **157**, 1877–80.

159. **Eiser, N., Denman, W.T., West, C., and Luce, P.** (1991). Oral diamorphine: lack of effect on dyspnoea and exercise tolerance in the 'pink puffer' syndrome. *European Respiratory Journal* **4**, 926–31.

160. **Young, I.H., Daviskas, E., and Keena, V.A.** (1989). Effect of low dose nebulised morphine on exercise endurance in patients with chronic lung disease. *Thorax* **44**, 387–90.

161. **Leung, R., Hill, P., and Burdon, J.** (1996). Effect of inhaled morphine on the development of breathlessness during exercise in patients with chronic lung disease. *Thorax* **51**, 596–600.

162. **Harris-Eze, A.O.** et al. (1995). Low dose nebulized morphine does not improve exercise in interstitial lung disease. *American Journal of Respiratory & Critical Care Medicine* **152**, 1940–5.

163. **Multicentre Study Group** (1980). Long-term oral acetylcysteine in chronic bronchitis, a double blind controlled study. *European Journal Respiratory Disease* **61**, 93–108.

164. **Tamaoki, J.** et al. (1992). Effect of indomethacin on bronchorrhea in patients with chronic bronchitis, diffuse panbronchitis, or bronchiectasis. *American Review of Respiratory Disease* **145**, 548–52.

165. **Winning, A.J., Hamilton, R.D., and Guz, A.** (1988). Ventilation and breathlessness on maximal exercise in patients with interstitial lung disease after local anaesthetic aerosol inhalation. *Clinical Science* **74**, 275–81.

166. **Wilson, D.** (1986). Nutritional intervention in malnourished patients with emphysema. *American Review of Respiratory Disease* **134**, 672–7.

167. **de Godoy, I.** et al. (1996). Elevated TNF-alpha production by peripheral blood monocytes of weight-losing COPD patients. *American Journal of Respiratory & Critical Care Medicine* **153**, 633–7.

168. **Goldstein, S.** (1988). Nitrogen and energy relationships in malnourished patients with emphysema. *American Review of Respiratory Disease* **138**, 636–44.

169. **Whittaker, J.S.** et al. (1990). The effects of refeeding on peripheral and respiratory muscle function in malnourished chronic obstructive pulmonary disease patients. *American Review of Respiratory Disease* **142**, 283–8.

170. **Marini, J.J.** et al. (1984). Influence of head-dependent positions on lung volumes and oxygen saturations in chronic airflow obstruction. *American Review of Respiratory Disease* **129**, 101–5.

171. **American Association of Cardiovascular and Pulmonary Rehabilitation** (1997). Pulmonary rehabilitation: Joint ACCP/AACVPR evidence-based guidelines. ACCP/AACVPR Pulmonary Rehabilitation Guidelines Panel. American College of Chest Physicians. *Chest* **112**, 1363–96.

172. **Guell, R.** et al. (2000). Longterm effects of outpatient rehabilitation of COPD: a randomised trial. *Chest* **117**, 976–83.

173. **Lacasse, Y.** et al. (1996). Meta-analysis of respiratory rehabilitation in chronic obstructive pulmonary disease. *Lancet* **348**, 1115–19.

174. **Garrod, R., Mikelsons, C., Paul, E.A., and Wedzicha, J.A.** (2000). Randomised controlled trial of domiciliary non-invasive positive pressure ventilation and physical training in severe chronic obstructive pulmonary disease. *American Journal of Respiratory & Critical Care Medicine* **162**, 1335–41.

175. **Larson, J.L.** et al. (1988). Inspiratory muscle training with a pressure threshold device in patients with chronic obstructive pulmonary disease. *American Review of Respiratory Disease* **138**, 689–96.

176. **Weiner, P.** et al. (2000). The cumulative effect of long-acting bronchodilators, exercise, and inspiratory muscle training on the perception of dyspnea in patients with advanced COPD. *Chest* **118**, 672–8.

177. **Smith, K.** et al. (1992). Respiratory muscle training in chronic airflow limitation: a meta-analysis. *American Review of Respiratory Disease* **145**, 533–9.

178. **Berry, M.J.** et al. (1996). Inspiratory muscle training and whole body reconditioning in chronic obstructive pulmonary disease; a controlled randomised trial. *American Journal of Respiratory & Critical Care Medicine* **153**, 1812–16.

179. **Tiep, B.L.** et al. (1986). Pursed lips breathing training using ear oximetry. *Chest* **90**, 218–21.

180. **Sharp, J.T.** et al. (1980). Postural relief of dyspnea in severe chronic obstructive pulmonary disease. *American Review of Respiratory Disease* **122**, 201–11.

181. **Hillberg, R.E. and Johnson, D.C.** (1997). Noninvasive ventilation. *New England Journal of Medicine* **337**, 1746–52.

182. **Brochard, L., Isabey, D., and Piquet, J.E.A.** (1990). Reversal of acute exacerbations of chronic obstructive lung disease by inspiratory assistance with a facemask. *New England Journal of Medicine* **323**, 1523–30.

183. **Fessler, H.E., Brower, R.G., and Permutt, S.** (1995). CPAP reduces inspiratory work more than dyspnea during hyperinflation with intrinsic PEEP. *Chest* **108**, 432–40.

184. **Strumpf, D.A.** et al. (1991). Nocturnal positive-pressure ventilation via nasal mask in patients with severe chronic obstructive pulmonary disease. *American Review of Respiratory Disease* **144**, 1234–9.

185. **Elliott, M.W.** et al. (1991). Domicilliary nocturnal nasal intermittent positive pressure ventilation in COPD: mechanisms underlying changes in arterial blood gas tensions. *European Respiratory Journal* **4**, 1044–52.

186. **Krachman, S.L.** et al. (1997). Effects of non-invasive positive pressure ventilation on gas exchange and sleep in COPD patients. *Chest* **112**, 623–8.

187. **Benditt, J.O. and Albert, R.K.** (1997). Surgical options for patients with advanced emphysema. *Clinics in Chest Medicine* **18**, 577–93.

188. **Toma, T.P., Goldstraw, P., and Geddes, D.M.** (2002). Lung volume reduction surgery. *Thorax* **57**, 5–6.

189. **Geddes, D.** et al. (2000). Effect of lung volume reduction surgery in patients with severe emphysema. *New England Journal of Medicine* **343**, 239–45.

190. **Moy, M.L.** et al. (1999). Health-related quality of life improves following pulmonary rehabilitation and lung volume reduction surgery. *Chest* **115**, 383–9.

191. **Brenner, M.** et al. (1998). Rate of FEV change following lung volume reduction surgery. *Chest* **113**, 652–9.

192. **Ingenito, E.P.** et al. (1998). Relation between pre-operative inspiratory lung resistance and outcome of lung-volume-reduction surgery for emphysema. *New England Journal of Medicine* **338**, 1181–5.

193. **Fessler, H.E. and Wise, R.A.** (1999). Lung volume reduction surgery: Is less really more? *American Journal of Respiratory & Critical Care Medicine* **159**, 1031–5.

194. **National Emphysema Treatment Trial Research Group** (2001). Patients at high risk of death after lung volume reduction surgery. *New England Journal of Medicine* **345**, 1075–83.

195. **Ingenito, E.P.** et al. (2001). Bronchoscopic volume reduction. A safe and effective alternative to surgical therapy for emphysema. *American Journal of Respiratory & Critical Care Medicine* **164**, 295–301.

196. **Hosenpud, J.D.** et al. (1997). The Registry of the International Society for Heart and Lung Transplantation: Fourteenth Official Report 1997. *Journal of Heart Lung Transplantion* **16**, 691–712.

197. **Patterson, G.A.** et al. (1991). Comparison of outcomes of single and double lung transplantation for obstructive lung disease. The Toronto Lung Transplant Group. *Journal of Thoracic & Cardiovascular Surgery* **101**, 623–31.

198. **Editorial** (1991). Single lung transplantation for pulmonary emphysema. *Lancet* **339**, 216–17.

199. **Carrington, C.B.** et al. (1978). Natural history and treated course of usual and desquamative interstitial pneumonia. *New England Journal of Medicine* **298**, 801–9.

200. **Silman, A.J.** (1997). Scleroderma—demographics and survival. *Journal of Rheumatology* **48**, 58–61.

201. **International Guidelines for the Selection of Lung Transplant Candidates** (1998). *American Journal of Respiratory & Critical Care Medicine* **158**, 335–9.

202. **Frankel, H.L.** et al. (1998). Long-term survival in spinal cord injury: a fifty year investigation. *Spinal Cord* **36**, 266–74.

203. **Weng, T.R.** et al. (1985). Pulmonary function and ventilatory response to chemical stimuli in familial myopathy. *Chest* **88**, 488–95.

204. **Labanowski, J., Schmidt-Nowara, W., and Guilleminault, C.** (1996). Sleep and neuromuscular disease: frequency of sleep disordered breathing in a neuromuscular disease clinic population. *Neurology* **47**, 1173–80.

205. **Hamilton, M.G., Hull, R.D., and Pineo, G.F.** (1994). Venous thromboembolism in neurosurgery and neurology patients. A review. *Neurosurgery* **34**, 280–96.

206. **Bach, J.R. and Alba, A.S.** (1990). Noninvasive options for ventilatory support of the traumatic high level quadriplegic patient. *Chest* **98**, 613–19.

207. **Bach, J.R.** et al. (1993). Airways secretion clearance by mechanical exsufflation for post-poliomyelitis ventilator-assisted individuals. *Archives of Physical Medical Rehabilitation* **74**, 170–7.

208. **Mazza, F.G.** et al. (1984). The flow-volume loop during glossopharyngeal breathing. *Chest* **85**, 638–40.

209. **Uijl, S.G., Houtman, S., Folgering, H.T., and Hepman, M.T.** (1999). Training of the respiratory muscles in individuals with tetraplegia. *Spinal Cord* **37**, 575–9.

210. **Wanke, T.** et al. (1994). Inspiratory muscle training in patients with Duchenne muscular dystrophy. *Chest* **105**, 475–82.

211. **Lin, V.W.** et al. (1998). Functional magnetic stimulation for restoring cough in patients with tetraplegia. *Archives of Physical Medicine and Rehabilitation* **79**, 517–22.

212. **Bach, J.R.** et al. (1998). Neuromuscular ventilatory insufficiency: effect of home mechanical ventilator use v oxygen therapy on pneumonia and hospitalisation rates. *American Journal of Physical Medicine and Rehabilitation* **77**, 8–19.

213. **Braun, S.R.** et al. (1987). Intermittent negative pressure ventilation in the treatment of respiratory failure in progressive neuromuscular disease. *Neurology* **37**, 1874–5.

214. **Gay, P.C.** et al. (1991). Nocturnal nasal ventilation for treatment of patients with hypercapnic respiratory failure. *Mayo Clinics Proceedings* **66**, 695–703.

215. **Perry, K. and King, D.** (1940). Bronchiectasis: a study of prognosis based on a follow-up of 400 patients. *American Review of Tuberculosis* **41**, 531–48.

216. **Ellis, D.A.** et al. (1981). Present outlook in bronchiectasis: clinical and social study and review of factors influencing prognosis. *Thorax* **36**, 659–64.

217. **Grenier, P.** et al. (1986). Bronchiectasis: assessment by thin-section CT. *Radiology* **161**, 95–9.

218. **Angrill, J.** et al. (2002). Bacterial colonisation in patients with bronchiectasis: microbiological pattern and risk factors. *Thorax* **57**, 15–17.

219. **Ramsey, B.W.** (1996). Management of pulmonary disease in patients with cystic fibrosis. *New England Journal of Medicine* **335**, 179–88.

220. **Mendelman, P.M.** et al. (1985). Aminoglycoside penetration, inactivation, and efficacy in cystic fibrosis sputm. *American Review of Respiratory Disease* **132**, 761–5.

221. **Lin, H-C.** et al. (1997). Inhaled gentamicin reduces airway neutrophil activity and mucous secretion in bronchiectasis. *American Journal of Respiratory & Critical Care Medicine* **155**, 2024–9.

222. **Thomas, J., Cook, D.J., and Brooks, D.** (1995). Chest physical therapy management of patients with cystic fibrosis. *American Journal of Respiratory & Critical Care Medicine* **151**, 846–50.

223. **Robinson, M.** et al. (1996). Effect of hypertonic saline, amiloride, and cough on mucociliary clearance in patients with cystic fibrosis. *American Journal of Respiratory & Critical Care Medicine* **153**, 1503–9.

224. **Ramsey, B.W.** et al. (1993). Efficacy and safety of short-term administration of aerosolised recombinant human deoxyribonuclease in patients with cystic fibrosis. *American Review of Respiratory Disease* **148**, 145–51.

225. **Fuchs, H.J.** et al. (1994). Effect of aerosolised recombinant human DNAse on exacerbations of respiratory symptoms and on pulmonary function in patients with cystic fibrosis. *New England Journal of Medicine* **331**, 637–42.

226. **O'Donnell, A.E.** et al. (1998). Treatment of idiopathic bronchiectasis with aerosolized recombinant human DNAse. *Chest* **113**, 1329–34.

227. **Konstan, M.W.** et al. (1995). Effect of high-dose ibuprofen in patients with cystic fibrosis. *New England Journal of Medicine* **332**, 848–54.

228. **Benhamou, D.** et al. (1997). Long-term efficiency of home nasal mask ventilation in patients with diffuse bronchiectasis and severe respiratory failure. A case control study. *Chest* **112**, 1259–66.

229. **Murray, J.F. and Mills, J.** (1990). Pulmonary infectious complications of human immunodeficiency virus infection. Part I. *American Review of Respiratory Disease* **141**, 1356–72.

230. **Murray, J.F. and Mills, J.** (1990). Pulmonary infectious complications of human immunodeficiency virus infection. Part II. **141**, 1582–98.

231. **Wallace, J.M.** et al. (1997). Respiratory disease trends in the Pulmonary Complications of HIV Infection Study cohort. Pulmonary Complications of HIV Infection Study Group. *American Journal of Respiratory & Critical Care Medicine* **155**, 72–80.

232. **UNAIDS and WHO** (1997). Report on the Global HIV/AIDS Epidemic. Geneva: WHO, pp. 1–26.

233. **American Thoracic Society** (1995). Standards for the diagnosis and care of patients with chronic obstructive pulmonary disease. *American Journal of Respiratory & Critical Care Medicine* **152**, S77–120.

234. **MacNee, W.** et al. (1983). Effects of pirbuterol and sodium nitroprusside on pulmonary haemodynamics in hypoxic cor pulmonale. *British Medical Journal* **287**, 1169–72.

235. **Gassner, A.** et al. (1990). Differential therapy with calcium antagonists in pulmonary hypertension secondary to COPD. *Chest* **98**, 829–34.

236. **Zielinski, J.** et al. (1986). Captopril effects on pulmonary and systemic hemodynamics in chronic cor pulmonale. *Chest* **90**, 562–5.

237. **Kiely, D.G.** et al. (1997). Haemodynamic and endocrine effects of type 1 angiotensin II receptor blockade in patients with hypoxaemic cor pulmonale. *Cardiovascular Research* **33**, 201–8.

238. **Fedullo, P.F.** et al. (1995). Chronic thromboembolic pulmonary hypertension. *Clinics in Chest Medicine* **16**, 353–74.

239. **Morris, W. and Knauer, C.M.** (1997). Cardiopulmonary manifestations of schistosomiasis. *Seminars in Respiratory Infection* **12**, 159–70.

240. **Moser, K.M.** et al. (1994). Frequent asymptomatic pulmonary embolism in patients with deep venous thrombosis. *Journal of the American Medical Association* **271**, 223–35.

241. **Hyers, T.M.** (1999). Venous thromboembolism. *American Journal of Respiratory & Critical Care Medicine* **159**, 1–14.

242. **Archibald, C.J.** et al. (1999). Long-term outcome after pulmonary thromboendarterectomy. *American Journal of Respiratory & Critical Care Medicine* **160**, 523–8.

243. **Rich, S.** et al. (1987). Primary pulmonary hypertension. A national prospective study. *Annals of Internal Medicine* **107**, 216–23.

244. **Fuster, V.** (1984). Primary pulmonary hypertension: natural history and the importance of thrombosis. *Circulation* **70**, 580–7.

245. **Rich, S., Kaufmann, R.N., and Levy, P.S.** (1992). The effect of high doses of calcium channel blockers on survival in primary pulmonary hypertension. *New England Journal of Medicine* **327**, 76–81.

246. **Weir, E.K.** et al. (1989). The acute administration of vasodilators in primary pulmonary hypertension. *American Review of Respiratory Disease* **140**, 1623–30.

247. **Barst, R.J.** et al. (1996). A comparison of continuous intravenous epoprostenol (Prostacyclin) with conventional therapy for primary pulmonary hypertension. *New England Journal of Medicine* **334**, 296–301.

248. **McLaughlin, V.V.** et al. (1998). Reduction in pulmonary vascular resistance with long-term epoprostenol (prostacyclin) therapy in primary pulmonary hypertension. *New England Journal of Medicine* **338**, 273–7.

249. **Pasque, M.K.** et al. (1991). Single-lung transplantation for pulmonary hypertension. *Circulation* **84**, 2275–9.

250. **Siverstein, M.D.** et al. (1998). Trends in the incidence of deep vein thrombosis and pulmonary embolism. *Archives of Internal Medicine* **158**, 585–93.

251. **Macik, B.G. and Ortel, T.L.** (1995). Clinical and laboratory evaluation of the hypercoagulable state. *Clinics in Chest Medicine* **16**, 375–89.

252. **Ryu, J.H., Olson, E.J., and Pellikka, P.A.** (1998). Clinical recognition of pulmonary embolism: problem of unrecognised and asymptomatic cases. *Mayo Clinic Proceedings* **73**, 873–9.

253. **Wells, P.S.** et al. (1995). Accuracy of clinical assessment of deep-vein thrombosis. *Lancet* **345**, 1326–30.

254. **The PIOPED Investigators** (1990). Value of the ventilation/perfusion scan in acute pulmonary embolism. Results of the Prospective Investigation Of Pulmonary Embolism Diagnosis (PIOPED). *Journal of the American Medical Association* **263**, 2753–9.

255. **Monroel, M.** et al. (1992). Deep venous thrombosis and the risk of pulmonary embolism. A systemic study. *Chest* **102**, 677–81.

256. **Tai, N.R.M., Atwai, A.S., and Hamilton, G.** (1999). Modern management of pulmonary embolism. *British Journal of Surgery* **86**, 853–68.

257. **Miniati, M.** et al. (1996). Value of perfusion lung scan in the diagnosis of pulmonary embolism. Results of the Prospective Investigative Study of Acute Pulmonary Embolism Diagnosis (PISA-PED). *American Journal of Respiratory & Critical Care Medicine* **154**, 1387–93.

258. **Simonneau, G.** et al. (1997). A comparison of low-molecular weight heparin and unfractionated heparin for acute pulmonary embolism. *New England Journal of Medicine* **337**, 663–9.

259. **Martin, R.** (2001). Acute pulmonary embolism 2: treatment. *Heart* **85**, 351–60.

260. **Dalen, J.E., Alpert, J.S., and Hirsch, J.** (1997). Thrombolytic therapy for pulmonary embolism. Is it effective? Is it safe? When is it indicated? *Archives of Internal Medicine* **157**, 2550–6.

261. **Millar, A.C. and Harvey, J.E.** (1993). On behalf of Standards of Care Committee, British Thoracic Society. Guidelines for the management of spontaneous pneumothorax. *British Medical Journal* **307**, 114–16.

262. **Mozell, E.J.** et al. (1991). Continuous extrapleural intercostals nerve block after pleurectomy. *Thorax* **46**, 21–4.

263. **Doyle, D.** *Domiciliary Terminal Care*. Edinburgh: Churchill Livingstone, 1987.

264. **Fainsinger, R.L.** et al. (2000). A multicentre international study of sedation for uncontrolled symptoms in terminally ill patients. *Palliative Medicine* **14**, 257–65.

265. **Stone, P.** et al. (1997). A comparison of the use of sedatives in a hospital support team and in a hospice. *Palliative Medicine* **11**, 140–4.

266. **Thorns, A. and Sykes, N.** (2000). Opioid use in the last week of life and the implications for end-of-life decision-making. *Lancet* **356**, 398–9.

267. **Chater, S.** et al. (1998). Sedation for intractable distress in the dying—a survey of experts. *Palliative Medicine* **12**, 255–69.

268. **Cherny, N.I. and Portenoy, R.K.** (1994). Sedation in the management of refractory symptoms: guidelines for evaluation and treatment. *Journal of Palliative Care* **10**, 31–8.

10.5 Palliative medicine for patients with end-stage heart disease

Andrew D. McGavigan and Francis G. Dunn

Introduction

It is perhaps surprising that it has taken so long to apply the principles of palliative care to patients with end-stage cardiac disease. After all, the term cardiac cachexia has been in use now for many decades and there are some striking clinical similarities to patients with advanced cancer. It is now known that patients with end-stage cardiac disease have a greatly reduced quality of life, inadequate support in terms of counselling and communication, and an infrastructure which is not yet in place for home management. It has to be acknowledged however that there are challenges in applying palliative care principles to patients with end-stage cardiac disease as illustrated by these two short clinical scenarios.

A 72-year-old retired teacher presented initially in 1993 with progressive breathlessness and was found at that time to have severe left ventricular dysfunction. So poor was his left ventricular function that it was felt at that time that survival beyond 1 year was considered most unlikely and his family were informed of this probable outcome. He responded well to medical management and, when seen earlier this year for review, he was found to be essentially symptom free with an excellent quality of life.

A 76-year-old patient with a previous history of myocardial infarction was admitted with severe dyspnoea caused by cardiac failure. Echo assessment of left ventricular function revealed it to be substantially impaired. He made good progress with medication and was discharged 5 days later essentially symptom free. Following discharge from hospital he joined a supervised cardiac rehabilitation exercise programme which he found helpful. Two weeks later he died suddenly during the night.

The unpredictable response to therapy and the spectre of sudden cardiac death make the prediction of proximity to death particularly difficult in end-stage cardiac disease. In the vasodilator in heart failure (V-HEFT) trials, 64 per cent of cardiac deaths occurred suddenly and only 30 per cent were preceded by any reported worsening of cardiac symptoms.(1) These patients also have a lower inpatient mortality than other chronic diseases, further emphasizing the difficulty in predicting life expectancy. Furthermore, patients even within 2–3 days of death may have a life expectancy predicted by their physicians of 2–3 months.(2)

Definitions and natural history

For the purposes of this article, end-stage cardiac disease is defined as patients with heart disease who have a predicted life expectancy of no more than 6 months. Such patients usually have grade 4 breathlessness (New York Heart Association Classification—NYHA), hypotension, clinical features of cardiac failure, and an ejection fraction of less than 20 per cent.(2) In addition, the extent of the disease will also be manifest by recurrent hospital admissions. The patients who fall within this definition will usually have had a past history of cardiac failure but there are also cohorts who develop intractable heart failure or cardiogenic shock with renal failure following acute myocardial infarction and in whom palliative care is particularly appropriate. The application of palliative care to patients with end-stage cardiac disease mainly involves patients with cardiac failure. The main cause of cardiac failure in the United Kingdom is coronary artery disease.(3) Other causes include hypertension, alcohol excess, viral infections, metabolic disorders, and the cardiomyopathies.

Heart failure is an extremely common disorder affecting 1–2 per cent of the general population. There is a marked age-related increase with up to 20 per cent of elderly patients being affected.(3) With the rising number of elderly patients in the population, the burden of heart failure is likely to further increase. The incidence of heart failure ranges from one to five cases per 1000 of population per year with a dramatic increase with advancing age.(3) Coronary artery disease accounts for over 300 000 myocardial infarctions every year in the United Kingdom and over 2 million patients have angina.(4) A significant percentage of these patients will have continuing symptoms despite optimum medical management and appropriate revascularization.

The overall prognosis in patients with heart failure is equivalent to many types of advanced cancer with an estimated 1-year survival of less than 50 per cent.(5) The mortality even in the milder forms of heart failure approaches 50 per cent within 5 years, again a prognosis which is worse than many forms of cancer.(6) Heart failure has also the greatest negative effect on quality of life compared to other major chronic illnesses such as diabetes, arthritis, and hypertension.(7) The high morbidity of heart failure is reflected by the high rate of hospital admissions. Heart failure patients currently exceed 120 000 cases per year with a cost to the NHS in excess of £300 million.(8)

Clinical features

The symptoms associated with end-stage cardiac disease are diverse, ranging from the well recognized triad of breathlessness, fatigue, and ankle swelling to less specific ones of anorexia, muscle wasting, and pain. This wide range is a function of the complexity of the underlying mechanisms involved. Symptoms are often severe and have many parallels with malignancy although there are some key differences.

Mechanisms

Heart failure is a clinical syndrome characterized by the inability of the heart to maintain a cardiac output adequate for the requirements of metabolizing tissues. This is usually due to left ventricular (LV) systolic dysfunction but occasionally can be due to diastolic dysfunction.

Heart failure is associated with complex inflammatory and neurohumoral abnormalities, in addition to the mechanical problems of the failing pump. The heart responds to injury and insult by remodelling and activation of adaptive neurohumoral mechanisms that are protective in the short term.(9) With impending cardiac failure, a shift to the right along the Frank–Starling curve increases cardiac output through increased end diastolic volume. This maintenance of cardiac output is achieved through many mechanisms including activation of the Renin–Angiotensin–Aldosterone System (RAAS), which increases vascular tone through the increased circulating levels of angiotensin II. Other vasoconstrictor systems that also contribute include the endothelin system and the adrenergic nervous system, which maintain perfusion of vital organs at the expense of peripheral perfusion. Adrenergic activation also has positive inotropic effects.

These responses to the failing myocardium improve haemodynamics in the short term, but continued activation soon becomes maladaptive, and a vicious cycle ensues (Fig. 1). Increased levels of circulating adrenaline, endothelin, and effectors of the RAAS cause endothelial dysfunction, cardiac and vascular fibrosis, sodium and water retention, promote arrhythmogenesis, and facilitate ventricular and vascular remodelling. These are all improved by drugs which antagonize these systems.(10)

Heart failure is also an inflammatory syndrome with increased circulating levels of the interleukin family and tumour necrosis factor.(11) The exact role of these mediators in the pathophysiology of heart failure is an area of considerable research. They may be responsible for the reduced skeletal muscle mass and function seen in the syndrome.(12) They may also contribute to the low-grade pyrexia found in heart failure, although hyperstimulation of the adrenergic system may also play a role in this.

Overview of symptoms and signs

The diversity of symptoms found in patients with heart disease means that many of these symptoms, such as fatigue and breathlessness, are widespread

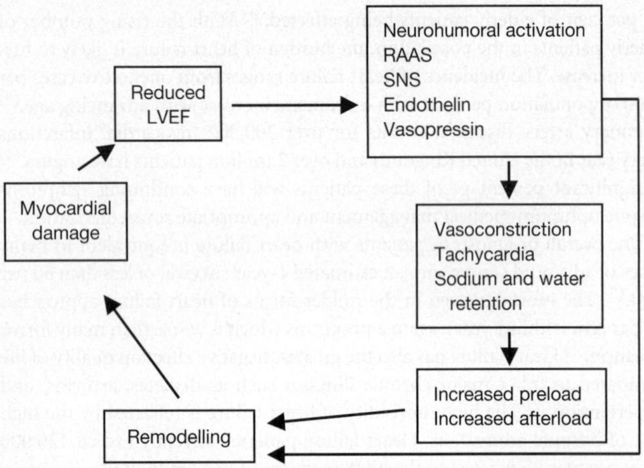

Fig. 1 Vicious cycle of neurohumoral super-activation. LVEF, left ventricular ejection fraction; RAAS, Renin–Angiotensin–Aldosterone System; SNS, sympathetic nervous system.

Table 1 Comparison of clinical characteristics between heart disease and cancer

Similarities to malignancy	Differences from malignancy
Breathlessness	Oedema more dominant in heart failure
Cachexia	Prediction of life expectancy more difficult
Weight loss (reduced muscle mass countered by fluid retention)	Mistaken belief that condition is more benign than cancer
Lethargy	Lack of local pressure effects
Poor mobility	Anaemia not as common
Pain	
Anxiety and depression	
Insomnia and confusion	
Postural hypotension	
Jaundice with abnormalities of liver function tests	
Increased infection risk	
Polypharmacy	
Fear of the future	

Adapted from O'Brien, T., Welsh, J., and Dunn, F.G. (1998). ABC of Palliative care: non-malignant conditions. *British Medical Journal* **316**, 286–9.

within the general population and are therefore not specific. However, with increasing severity of heart disease these symptoms become more specific. The patient with end-stage cardiac disease will have marked breathlessness, including orthopnoea and paroxysmal nocturnal dyspnoea. Fatigue, muscle wasting, pain, and depression are also prominent features, although not all patients will display these signs. Peripheral oedema is problematic and signs of pulmonary congestion are usually present. A resting tachycardia is characteristic of heart failure as is a gallop rhythm, displaced apex beat, and elevated jugular venous pressure.

Similarities to malignancy

The lack of specificity of symptoms and signs allows many parallels to be drawn with malignancy (Table 1). Cachexia is a frequent complication of both advanced cardiac disease and malignancy, occurring in up to 50 per cent of patients with the former, although this is sometimes masked by oedema (Fig. 2).(13) The loss of muscle mass compounds exercise

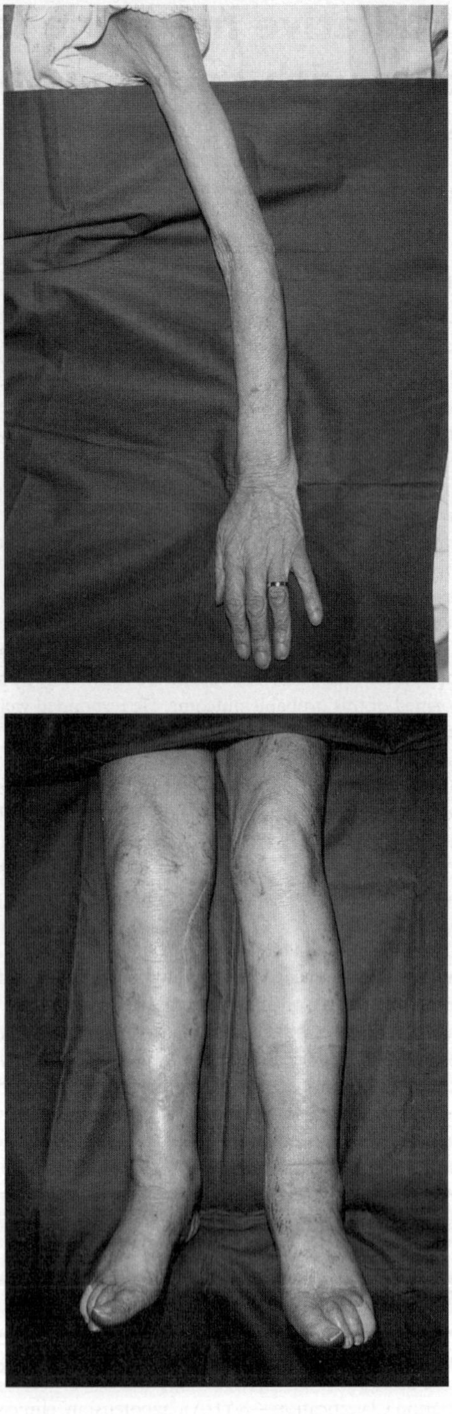

Fig. 2 Photographs of a patient with advanced cardiac failure. Note the marked oedema of the legs, but marked muscle wasting of the arms. (Adapted from ref. O'Brien, T., Welsh, J., and Dunn, F.G. (1998). ABC of palliative care: non-malignant conditions. *British Medical Journal* **316**, 286–9.)

intolerance and is an independent predictor of reduced survival.(14) Reduced energy reserve, muscle pain, and easy fatigability are also a feature due to lactic acidosis caused by poor perfusion of skeletal muscle. Increased basal metabolic rate and reduced energy intake due to anorexia contributes to the problem. Anorexia and nausea are also common symptoms in heart failure, either due to the syndrome itself or as a consequence of therapy. Reduced perfusion of intestines, activation of the sympathetic nervous system, and uraemia all play a role.

As with all patients with chronic and potentially life-threatening conditions, depression and anxiety are frequent complicating symptoms. Quality of life scores are markedly reduced in heart failure, and with advancing symptoms comes an increased incidence of depression.(7) Anxiety and fear of impending doom can be provoked by severe episodes of breathlessness and many patients report fear of attacks, especially at night. Feelings of social isolation are common.

Traditionally, pain has not been thought to be a major symptom in heart failure, although problems with concomitant angina have long been recognized. However, the recent SUPPORT study showed an incidence of pain in patients with advanced heart failure of 43 per cent, with 90 per cent of patients unhappy with the level of pain control received.(2) Perhaps increased recognition of pain as a symptom of end-stage cardiac disease may allow us to offer better analgesic regimens.

The cardinal symptoms of breathlessness and oedema are not unique to heart failure and are often found in patients with advanced malignancy. Although the mechanisms may differ, symptoms are common to the two conditions and can be very debilitating, contributing to anxiety. Other similarities are listed in Table 1.

Differences from malignancy

The key differences between advanced heart disease and malignancy are twofold. First, predicting mortality on an individual basis in heart failure is not easy and the decline in physical well-being is not uniformly progressive.(2) Heart failure patients have episodes of decompensation interspersed with periods of stability, unlike the classically progressive deteriorating course of many malignancies. Secondly, most patients and health-care professionals do not view heart failure as a terminal disease, despite the appalling mortality seen in the condition.(15) These two factors hinder the palliative care of advanced heart failure, as before palliation can be considered, one must accept that the patient's condition is terminal. This requires better identification of patients who are likely to be in the terminal stages of heart failure and a change in attitude to their treatment and prognosis, from the physician, the patient, and their families.

However, it is not only the difficulty in prediction of a terminal state or the attitudes involved which are different between severe cardiac disease and malignancy, there are several important symptomatic differences (Table 1).

Management issues

Non-pharmacological

Location of management

Many patients with end-stage cardiac disease, as with patients with advanced chronic disease, state a preference for home over hospital management.(16) This has not been achieved uniformly in the United Kingdom and the reasons for this are complex and include concerns about the patient's stability, a bias towards hospital care among health professionals, and lack of resources and suitable infrastructure. The outstanding success of Macmillan Nurses in cancer care (specialist palliative care workers) has led to an exploration of home management in patients with advanced cardiac failure using a similar set-up. In Glasgow, a programme has been developed over the past 3 years using Specialist Heart Failure Liaison Nurses who provide a link between hospital consultants and the community. Clear protocols have been drawn up identifying patients who can be managed in this shared way and when they require hospital admission. This system has already been shown to reduce hospital admission and improve the patient's quality of life.(17)

Communication

There is a well-developed support network for patients with cancer. This is not yet in place for patients with end-stage cardiac disease and there are a number of studies indicating a lack of appropriate communication between physician and patients with end-stage cardiac disease.(18) This is now recognized and there has been improvements over the past 5 years in communication between hospital staff, the GP, and patients with end-stage cardiac disease. This has been facilitated by cardiac rehabilitation programmes throughout the country. These were set up initially for patients post-myocardial infarction but have been extended in recent years to include patients with cardiac failure. Although a major plank in the rehabilitation process is exercise, it also includes education programmes with regard to drugs, diet, and psychological aspects of cardiac failure. This multi-disciplinary programme is already reaping benefits in terms of helping patients to cope with advanced cardiac failure and other forms of end stage cardiac disease.

Resuscitation issues

Discussion regarding resuscitation preferences does not come easily to either patients with end-stage cardiac disease or their doctors. Patients feel that cardiac disease is more benign than cancer and that the cardiologists have as a major part of their work keeping the heart functioning in all circumstances. Cardiologists in general remain uncomfortable about discussion of resuscitation preferences, partly because of the difficulty in predicting life expectancy and also because of their views of patients' expectations. In addition, even in end-stage cardiac disease there are many correctable causes of cardiac arrest. This is clearly a complex issue but it must be faced and approached with delicacy and understanding and in the knowledge that patients with end-stage cardiac disease may change their views from time to time regarding resuscitation preferences.

The SUPPORT study has provided important information on resuscitation preferences of patients with end-stage cardiac failure.(19) In hospital it was found that 'do not resuscitate' (DNR) orders were less common in heart failure. Such orders were written for only 5 per cent of patients admitted with cardiac failure in comparison to 47 per cent of those with malignancy and 52 per cent of patients with AIDS. In that study, only 23 per cent of patients stated that they did not wish resuscitation and 40 per cent of these patients subsequently changed their mind in favour of resuscitation.

Many hospitals have or are currently in the process of setting up DNR policies. The importance of such policies cannot be over emphasized.(20) There are three key situations in which a DNR order is appropriate. First, when cardiopulmonary resuscitation is unlikely to be effective; secondly, when it is known that the patient does not wish to receive CPR; and thirdly, where successful CPR would not increase length or, more importantly, improve quality of life.

It is always important to underscore that the DNR order only applies to cardiopulmonary resuscitation and does not in any way limit other medical or nursing care the patient is receiving. The patient will not always be able to participate in the decision-making regarding DNR. In this situation, a previous request by the patient should be adhered to and discussion with the family is also helpful. Such discussions however must be approached with sensitivity and understanding and a full explanation is extremely important so that other members of staff know the background to the decision and what the patient's resuscitation status is. This should always be recorded in the case sheet. There are situations when the DNR order may have to be reversed and the situation usually arises because of an unforeseen improvement in the patient's clinical condition but there should be no hesitation in changing this order if appropriate.

There has been some debate in the past about whether all patients presenting to hospital should be asked about their resuscitation preferences. At the moment this is done on a more selective basis but in the future advance directives may well become the norm either from the patient or after discussion with the medical team, the patient, and their family.

Diet, bed rest, and exercise

Diet has an important role in the management of end-stage cardiac disease in a number of ways. The principal goal of diet is that it should be palatable and tailored to the patient's individual needs. Restriction of sodium intake and fluid may be employed if the patient is symptomatic from fluid accumulation. With the introduction of powerful diuretics in recent years, sodium can be restricted simply to 'no added salt' and fluid intake may be restricted to 1.5–2 L. Frequent light meals are often better tolerated than heavy meals. Increased levels of tumour necrosis factor and interleukin in the circulation both contribute to cardiac cachexia and fish oils may reduce the levels of these substances.(21) In addition, fat and water soluble vitamins should be given since the absorption of these are reduced in patients with cardiac failure. It is also worth considering the use of thiamine, both because it may be a contributing factor in patients with alcohol related cardiomyopathy and also because the use of diuretics may lead to a reduction in thiamine levels.(22)

Until the last 10 years, exercise was actively discouraged in patients with end-stage cardiac disease because of concern about metabolic abnormalities and hypoperfusion of skeletal muscles giving rise to fatigue with exercise. However, inactivity can contribute to muscle atrophy and deconditioning. Furthermore, controlled trials in recent years have revealed an improvement in exercise capacity and symptomatic well-being with tailored exercise programmes.(23) There is also some evidence that the likelihood of arrhythmias will be reduced and that cardiac function will improve.

These patients therefore should all be considered for an exercise programme which will vary greatly from patient to patient. These programmes will, of course, in the final stages of disease become less appropriate, but, if possible, activity should still be encouraged with appropriate physiotherapy even in these stages.

Pharmacological

The pharmacological treatment of heart failure is a rapidly developing area, partly due to our increasing understanding of the pathophysiology of the heart failure syndrome.

The last decade or so has brought a clear evidence base for drug prescribing in heart failure of all classes to reduce mortality and hospital admissions, improve symptoms and functional status, and to delay progression of adverse remodelling. Although all these aspects are important, the severity of heart failure determines the relative importance of each one. For example, it is clear that improvement in well-being and a reduction in symptoms is the key in the palliation of end-stage heart disease and less emphasis should be placed on mortality reduction and modulation of the remodelling process.

Heart failure is characterized by symptoms of congestion and diuretics are the mainstay of treatment. They are more effective at reducing breathlessness and oedema and improving exercise tolerance than any other treatment.(24) Loop diuretics, such as frusemide, act at the loop of Henle causing a natriuresis with accompanying water loss. Close monitoring of renal function and electrolytes is required and patients will often require potassium supplementation. Diuretic requirements change and the dose of diuretic should be tailored to the patient's symptoms, fluctuation in weight, and renal function. Episodes of decompensation should be treated with intravenous diuretics to circumvent problems of poor oral absorption caused by intestinal mucosal oedema. Some patients require a continuous infusion. It may be necessary for the addition of a thiazide diuretic, such as bendrofluazide or metolazone, which works synergistically with loop diuretics through its actions on the proximal convoluted tubule. This is the principle of sequential nephron blockade and is very effective at causing a marked diuresis. Often, only a few days of treatment are required in the acute setting but a thiazide may also be given in the stable phase to patients who appear to be resistant to loop diuretics alone. Continuing with this principle, the addition of a potassium sparing diuretic (spironolactone), acting on the distal convoluted tubule and collecting duct, also increases diuresis. The need for monitoring blood chemistry is increased when using two or more different types of diuretic in combination.

Current drug therapy: the evidence base

There is now a strong evidence base for mortality reduction with a number of agents in all classes of heart failure. Importantly, there is also a good evidence base for the use of these agents in the reduction of hospital admissions and improvement in NYHA class and functional status (Table 2). Tolerability is generally good and side-effect profiles are at an acceptable level. However, this evidence is population based and, again, therapy should be tailored to the individual.

Neurohumoral modulation is a popular concept in modern heart failure management and the first agents studied were ACE inhibitors which inhibit the production of angiotensin II and, as a by-product, increase concentrations of bradykinin. In addition to their vasodilating properties, inhibition of the RAAS by ACE inhibitors causes improvements in the remodelling process, improving LV geometry and function.(25) They improve survival and symptoms in all classes of heart failure and are well tolerated with hypotension, hyperkalaemia, and cough being the common dose-limiting factors.(3) However, two points are important to remember. The first is that cough is a common symptom of heart failure itself, occurring in up to 31 per cent of patients. The incidence of cough is only 6 per cent higher with ACE inhibitors.(26) The second is that it is a common misconception that ACE inhibitors are highly nephrotoxic and are contraindicated in patients with renal impairment. ACE inhibitors cause a reduced glomerular blood flow with an associated rise in serum creatinine. This reflects a functional change and is reversible on discontinuation of the drug.(5) Creatinine values up to 200 μg/L should not be regarded as a contraindication to starting an ACE inhibitor. However, dehydration, non-steroidal anti-inflammatory drugs, and sepsis can all potentiate renal dysfunction and regular monitoring of renal function is therefore mandatory. There are many ongoing clinical trials with angiotensin II receptor antagonists, both alone and in combination with ACE inhibitors. The results of these are awaited with interest.

Inhibition of the RAAS can also be achieved by spironolactone. In addition to its diuretic effects, there seems to be improvements in fibrosis and myocyte function with antagonism of aldosterone. Clinically, it improves NYHA class and reduces hospital admissions and mortality.(27) Small doses are used and the risk of hyperkalaemia seems small although close monitoring of blood chemistry is important.

Inhibition of the sympathetic nervous system by beta-blockers is an effective form of treatment for the heart failure syndrome. Traditionally, it was thought that beta-blockade was contraindicated in heart failure. However, in the last few years, trials with carvedilol, metoprolol, and bisoprolol have all demonstrated improved symptoms and reduction in NYHA class in addition to mortality benefit, although only carvedilol to date has demonstrated safety, tolerability, and efficacy at the more severe end of the spectrum—class IV heart failure.(28) Beta-blockade should be initiated when the patient is stable, that is, not during an episode of acute

Table 2 Drugs, their use in the four classes of heart failure and their effects on survival, hospital admission, and functional status. NYHA, New York Heart Association class

Drug	NYHA I	NYHA II	NYHA III	NYHA IV	Survival	Hospital admissions	Functional status
Diuretic	X	√	√	√	→	↓	↑
ACEI	√	√	√	√	↑	↓	↑
Spironolactone	X	X	√	√	↑	↓	↑
Beta-blocker	X	√	√	√	↑	↓	↑
Digoxin	X	√	√	√	→	↓	↑

decompensation. The dose should be up-titrated as symptomatic status, heart rate, and blood pressure will allow.

Although digoxin is the archetypal treatment for heart failure, it is only recently that the question over its use in the syndrome has been answered. Digoxin does not confer a survival benefit in heart failure, but does reduce hospital admissions and improve symptoms.[29] It is therefore a useful adjunct in the treatment of severe heart failure.

Initiation of all these therapies should be attempted and continued only if well tolerated. Doses should be optimized and regular review of drugs is necessary, especially in the light of the marked polypharmacy often found in this patient group.

Risk factor management

As mentioned previously, the aetiology of heart failure in the Western world is predominantly ischaemic heart disease and hypertension. Early treatment of these conditions and adequate management of risk factors would decrease the prevalence of heart failure. However, as mortality increases dramatically with worsening classes of heart failure, risk factor management becomes less important and the emphasis lies in the palliation of symptoms. Nonetheless, risk factors should not be ignored.

In addition to the obvious adverse actions of smoking on the cardiovascular system, smoking causes changes to blood rheology and a reduction in lung function, increasing the risk of thrombo-embolism and impairing functional capacity. Cessation should be encouraged.

Thrombo-embolism is a common problem with severe LV systolic dysfunction increasing the risk of stroke by up to five times, even in patients with normal sinus rhythm. The use of anticoagulation in this setting is a topic of considerable debate, but there is agreement that anticoagulation is warranted for those with LV dysfunction coupled with atrial fibrillation or LV thrombus.[30] However, the decision to anticoagulate should not be made lightly as it brings its own attendant risks and monitoring can be a time consuming process for both the patient and the physician. There is probably only a limited role for warfarin in a truly palliative care arena.

Blood pressure control is also important. Hypertension can be an aetiological cause of heart failure, but the two can co-exist, although hypotension is much more of a problem when heart disease becomes end-stage. In hypertension, increased demand is placed on the myocardium and the associated reduction in diastolic filling may exacerbate ischaemia. A return to normotension may improve symptoms. However, the goals of treatment may be modified with a higher pressure being accepted to try and avoid symptomatic postural hypotension.

Treatment of traditional risk factors for cardiovascular disease such as hyperlipidaemia is probably less important in the severe heart failure population due to the very high mortality. However, the risk of death on an individual basis is difficult to predict and standard therapy should be maintained provided it is well tolerated.

Advanced treatment options

The variation in symptoms of patients with end-stage cardiac disease necessitates that treatment is tailored to the individual. This is true of the different treatment strategies outlined previously, but is also important in our approach to the more advanced treatment modalities such as device therapy and transplantation. This is an area within cardiology that is attracting increasing attention, but as with all treatments, the appropriate patient selection is paramount to ensure that these expensive and technically demanding management options are offered to those most likely to benefit.

Arrhythmia control

Increased understanding of the pathophysiology of arrhythmogenesis and improvements in electrophysiological techniques has widened the therapeutic options for the treatment of arrhythmias. Some of these are suitable in patients with advanced heart failure if symptoms cannot be effectively controlled by pharmacological means or side-effects of antiarrhythmic therapy occur. These include catheter-based ablative therapies, pacemakers, and implantable defibrillators. Clearly, these devices only have a limited and highly selective role in the palliation of end-stage cardiac disease.

Radiofrequency ablation is a trans-catheter means of arrhythmia control. If a discrete focus for arrhythmia can be identified, such as an area of scarring causing a ventricular re-entrant circuit, the stimulus for the tachycardia can be removed by the application of radiofrequency energy. This is performed percutaneously and is curative in some arrhythmias. However, in the heart failure patient, a discrete arrhythmogenic focus is seldom found and this approach has limited use in this setting.

Although the same may be said of attempted rhythm control with pacemaker therapy, this technique may be useful in selected patients with frequent paroxysms of atrial tachycardia or fibrillation resistant to standard anti-arrhythmic therapy. The devices used include dual site atrial pacing (utilizing two atrial wires to pace at two sites) and single wires programmed with an anti-tachycardia algorithm. The pacemakers cause alterations in atrial myocyte electrophysiology and reduce the stimulus for atrial fibrillation. Clinically they reduce the frequency of paroxysms. There are a number of ongoing clinical trials in this area and the overall efficacy and best pacing approach should become clearer. With regard to palliation of symptoms, patients could be considered for these devices if their symptoms are severe and a pacemaker is required for another, more routine indication, such as symptomatic heart block.

The most studied non-pharmocological treatment of arrhythmias in the heart failure population is the implantable defibrillator. These devices are advanced pacemaker systems with a capacitor which allow the recognition of broad complex tachycardias and ventricular fibrillation and is then able to terminate the arrythmia with anti-tachycardia pacing or the delivery of a small internal electrical shock. Up to 60 per cent of deaths in patients with severe heart failure are due to sudden cardiac death.[1] Several large trials have demonstrated a reduction in sudden cardiac death in particular groups of heart failure patients—those who have survived an episode of sudden cardiac death and those who have symptomatic sustained ventricular tachycardia.[31] Improvements in device technology have meant that these devices are now not much bigger than a standard pacemaker and can be inserted percutaneously, obviating the need for major surgery. However, it is important to remember that although they improve mortality, they do not treat the underlying arrhythmic process and control of symptoms is still required. In the palliative care setting, symptom control is more important than potential longevity and full discussion with the patient is mandatory before considering this option.

Pacemakers

Pacemakers have long been used for the treatment of bradyarrhythmias, but pacing to improve haemodynamics and symptoms in advanced heart failure is a relatively new area of interest. Many patients with severe LV systolic dysfunction will have interventricular conduction delay manifested by widening of the QRS complex on the ECG. This causes asynchronous activation and contraction of the left ventricle, resulting in reduced cardiac output. Three pacemaker leads are inserted, one to the right atrium, one to the right ventricular apex, and one in the coronary sinus, which lies over the posterior wall of the left ventricle. Synchronous pacing of both ventricles simultaneously, unlike traditional single RV pacing, improves haemodynamics including an increase in ejection fraction and cardiac index, and reducing wall stress in the short term. More importantly, it improves functional status and exercise capacity.[32] Whether this improvement in symptoms and haemodynamics will be apparent in the longer term remains to be shown and clinical trials are underway.

Pain control

Pain is obviously a distressing and limiting symptom. In addition to standard anti-ischaemic therapy and use of opioids, several additional strategies can be considered. These include coronary artery bypass grafting, transmyocardial laser revascularization techniques, and device therapy such as implantable spinal cord stimulators and external pneumatic counterpulsation.

Up to 40 per cent of patients referred for cardiac transplantation may be suitable for surgical revascularization with reasonable survival rates.(33) Traditional coronary artery bypass may be a viable option in the treatment of severe symptoms but again careful patient selection is vital. A significant area of ischaemia must be identified through non-invasive assessment and there must be suitable surgical targets apparent at angiography. An alternative strategy if full revascularization cannot be offered surgically is partial revascularization by high-risk angioplasty. This approach lacks the longer term experience supporting the use of bypass but may be useful as a bridge to transplantation and may improve symptoms.

Often, surgery or angioplasty is not an option. Interest has grown in other forms of revascularization. Transmyocardial laser revascularization aims to provide functional connections between the left ventricular cavity and the ischaemic myocardium through channels furrowed by laser therapy allowing oxygenated blood to the ischaemic area. Early studies have been conflicting, but many have reported a reduction in anginal symptoms and improved exercise capacity.(34) However, no studies have shown a reduction in ischaemic burden or improvement in ventricular function and alternative explanations for the apparent efficacy have included denervation by the therapy, stimulated angiogenesis, and a placebo effect. The technique is not widely available and its role as a treatment of severe intractable angina its own right or as an adjunct to other revascularization therapies remains unclear.

Other novel therapies for the treatment of refractory angina are external pneumatic counterpulsation devices and implantable spinal cord stimulators. External pneumatic counterpulsation consists of inflatable bands for the limbs that inflate in diastole improving diastolic blood flow to the coronary arteries and improving haemodynamics. Although this approach remains experimental, recent evidence suggests that it may be useful in the palliation of severe anginal symptoms.(35) Implantable spinal cord stimulators may also be useful in the palliation of symptoms. Their use is based on the gate theory of pain and the device is inserted into the epidural space and provides paraesthetic stimuli over the area in which anginal symptoms are present (typically T2 to T5 dermatomes). The patient controls how much stimulus is given. This is truly a palliative, symptom-orientated approach, as it does not attempt to reduce the ischaemic burden.

Transplantation

The place of orthoptic cardiac transplantation in the treatment of end-stage heart disease is constantly changing. Improved survival post-transplant has become a reality with advances in immunosuppressive therapy. Five-year survival rates post-transplant are around 60–70 per cent;(36) however improvements in medical treatments and other surgical techniques and device therapies have made the role of transplantation less clear.

The key again lies in careful patient selection. Transplantation requires great commitment from the patient and their families, starting as soon as they are placed on the registry. Psychological evaluation and continued support are essential. Patients should be considered only if they have severe symptoms from cardiac disease refractory to all other forms of conventional treatment including other surgical options. Numerous predictors of benefit have been cited in the past, but the most robust seems to be peak oxygen consumption of less than 15 mL/kg/min on a progressive exercise test.(37) However, transplantation may be considered at levels greater than this if symptoms due to refractory ischaemia or arrhythmia are causing great disability and no other treatment options are available.

A major problem lies with the shortage of donor organs. This has prompted interest in mechanical ventricular assist devices either as a bridge to, or even an alternative to, transplantation. These devices have recently been shown to improve both symptoms and survival in patients who are not candidates for transplantation and clearly represents an area of considerable promise.(38)

Integrated strategy for end-stage cardiac disease

Once a patient has been identified as having end-stage cardiac disease, management focuses on the palliation of symptoms.(39) Treatment strategies often combine many of the pharmacological, non-pharmacological, and advanced options outlined previously. However, not all these options will be appropriate and it is vital that treatment is tailored to the individual. Figure 3 gives an overview on the treatment of symptoms.

Management should be reviewed on a regular basis. Dedicated heart failure clinics and community nurse specialists have a key role in the continual assessment of the appropriateness, efficacy, and potential detrimental effects of treatment and to institute change where required. Monitoring of

Breathlessness

- Oxygen
- Drugs—diuretics, digoxin, ACE inhibitors, beta-blockers, vasodilators, sublingual GTN for acute breathlessness
- Opioids—regular quick release oral morphine, nebulized diamorphine, intravenous diamorphine if acutely distressed
- Non-drug measures—fan, positioning in bed and chair, easier access to toilet, etc.
- Assess need for admission to hospital

Oedema

- Early detection important
- Monitor weight regularly
- Aim for weight loss 0.5–1 kg/d
- Diuretics—frusemide remains first line, consider addition of metolazone 2.5 mg/d or bendrofluazide 5 mg/d in resistant oedema
- Fluid restriction—1.5–2 l/d, educate patient
- Mild salt restriction—no adding salt at table
- Decrease lower limb dependency—bed-rest in early stages, raise lower limbs by footstool or recliner when sitting
- Assess need for admission to hospital

Lightheadedness

- Check for postural hypotension
- Reassess need for drugs—vasodilator, beta-blocker, diuretic
- Exclude arrhythmia as cause of lightheadedness
- Reassure and educate patient

Muscle wasting and fatigue

- Physiotherapy
- Exercise—if possible
- Assess diet and energy intake—consider supplements
- Consider anti-cytokine therapy
- Review medications—consider stopping beta-blocker

Nausea, disturbance of taste, anorexia

- Check biochemistry—uraemia and abnormal liver function tests
- Review medications
- Assess diet and energy intake—encourage frequent small meals, consider supplements
- Consider supplementation of fat soluble vitamins
- Consider appetite stimulants—small amounts of alcohol, megesterol acetate
- Consider pro-motility agents—metoclopramide

Continued

Depression and anxiety

- Regularly assess mental state
- Morphine or temazepam at night may help reduce nocturnal anxiety
- Exercise programme
- Relaxation exercises
- Anti-depressant therapy—avoid tricyclic agents
- Reassure and educate the patient

Pain

- Analgesics—avoid NSAIDs, consider opioids
- Consider increasing anti-ischaemic medication
- Non-drug measures—relaxation exercises, TENS, hot packs, device therapy
- Review need for admission to hospital
- Reassure and educate the patient

Fig. 3 Symptomatic management of end-stage heart disease. (Adapted from O'Brien, T., Welsh, J., and Dunn, F.G. (1998). ABC of palliative care: non-malignant conditions. *British Medical Journal* **316**, 286–9.)

weight at home allows diuretic therapy to be titrated appropriately and community nurse specialists can facilitate this. They also act as a focus for patient education.

Symptoms of breathlessness, anorexia, fatigue, depression, and light-headedness should be sought from the patient on a regular basis, as should signs of oedema, muscle wasting, and postural hypotension. Drug therapy needs to be reviewed frequently and modified appropriately. Side-effects must be enquired about and therapy should be simplified if possible. Over-diuresis can cause lethargy and nausea due to uraemia. Beta-blockers often cause cold peripheries, erectile dysfunction, and fatigue. However, many of these symptoms can be due to heart failure itself and if symptoms persist after cessation of the drug, then the patient should be rechallenged if appropriate.

Consider withdrawing drugs which have been prescribed to improve prognosis but have no symptomatic benefit. Signs of depression need to be quickly identified and appropriate measures taken, keeping in mind the adverse cardiac effects of some of the well-known anti-depressant agents.

Adequate pain control is important and the need for short- and long-acting opioids should be assessed regularly. Although the intravenous route is commonly employed, perhaps a lesson can be learned from palliative care. These drugs can also be given orally, transdermally or through a nebulizer and often reduce breathlessness in addition to their analgesic properties. Non-steroidal anti-inflammatory drugs should be avoided due to their adverse effect on renal function and their propensity to increase fluid retention. In addition, it is important to control symptoms arising from myocardial ischaemia. Standard anti-anginal therapy can be used with perhaps caution with calcium antagonists, which may worsen peripheral oedema. It is important to remember that breathlessness may be an ischaemic equivalent and may be more responsive to an escalation of anti-ischaemic medication rather than increasing drug treatment for heart failure.

Arrhythmias are common in end-stage heart disease and patients who develop dizziness, syncope, or palpitations should be investigated. Most anti-arrhythmic drugs have a cardio-depressant effect and the use of some agents is associated with an increase in mortality. The drugs of choice are digoxin or beta-blockers for atrial arrhythmias and amiodarone for life-threatening ventricular arrhythmias. Restoration to sinus rhythm may improve symptoms in those who develop atrial fibrillation. Device therapy has been discussed previously.

The treatment of the patient with end-stage heart disease requires a holistic approach and is probably best served by a mutli-disciplinary team. This often allows the patient to be managed at home. Inevitably, however,

- Need for intravenous therapy—diuretics, inotropes, vasodilators
- Persistent paroxysmal nocturnal breathlessness or orthopnoea
- Refractory dependent oedema despite high dose oral therapy—120 mg of frusemide twice daily
- Fluid leakage from lower limbs
- Symptomatic postural hypotension
- Development of arrhythmias
- Refractory pain—ischaemic pain or otherwise

Fig. 4 Guide for the need for hospital admission.

- Ischaemia/myocardial infarction
- Arrhythmia
- Bacterial endocarditis
- Other sepsis, e.g. chest infection
- Pulmonary thromboembolism
- Anaemia
- Sequelae of drug treatment, e.g. digitoxicity, uraemia
- Non-compliance
- Alcohol abuse
- Thyroid disease
- Other unrelated condition, e.g. lung cancer

Fig. 5 Causes of episodes of decompensation of heart failure.

periods of hospitalization will be required to allow more intensive therapy. It is often difficult to judge when hospital admission is necessary as one has to balance the risks in inappropriately delaying hospitalisation against the psychological and other benefits of care at home. The decision to hospitalize should be made on an individual basis and will depend on many factors. Figure 4 offers a guide to those who should be considered for admission.

It is important that a cause of deterioration is sought and reversed if possible (Fig. 5). In hospital, intravenous loop diuretics are usually given, and inotropic agents such as dobutamine and low-dose dopamine may be required. Therapies to reduce afterload, such as intravenous nitrates, can also be used. Some centres advocate the use of phosphodiesterase inhibitors such as milrinone as a positive inotropic agent, but there is little evidence to support this and it should not be regarded as routine practice. Invasive haemodynamic monitoring may be useful in this situation. Although episodes of decompensation often require hospital admission, some centres adopt a 'hospital at home' approach allowing intermittent or continuous infusions of diuretics, and even inotropes, to be given at home. This is discussed in more detail below.

Future developments

The momentum, which is undoubtedly gathering in regard to palliative care for end-stage cardiac disease, must be maintained. Cardiac disease is a national priority for health in the United Kingdom but adequate financial support in the area of end-stage cardiac disease has not been forthcoming. This necessary financial commitment has to be matched by recognition within the medical profession and allied professions of the increased commitment that end-stage cardiac disease is going to require in the years ahead. There are four areas where future developments are needed.

Home management

Most of the studies of nurse-led home management of cardiac failure apply to patients before they have reached the end-stage of their life. Considerable further changes are needed to take this aspect of the care to a level where management equivalent to that in hospital can be provided right up until the time of death. Therefore, the infrastructure has to be in place to meet the patient's needs if they choose to remain at home. The provision of the Heart Failure Liaison Service is patchy at the present time. It is important that this service is deployed evenly and completely throughout the country. Thereafter, the service has to be taken to a level where in addition to all necessary appliances in the home there are facilities for intravenous infusions of opioids and other agents and round the clock nursing and medical support if required.

Hospital management

Many patients will opt for hospital management. What often appears to be the final admission may not be and the patient and their family should be made aware of the uncertainty in predicting the final days of life. All symptomatic measures mentioned previously should be in place. The staff should be aware of the patient's desired location. Some patients prefer the company of a two or four bedded area whereas others, particularly in the final days of life, may prefer the privacy of a single room with their family. The input of the cardiac liaison nursing staff who look after the patient at home is very important at this stage since this link with home becomes very important to the patient.

Psychological support and counselling

This is an important part of palliative care which has not been dealt with adequately in the past. Both the patient and the carers will at some stage suffer symptoms of anxiety and depression and the patient in particular will often experience emotions which they do not clearly recognize as being due to their disease. In addition, especially when such issues as resuscitation preference are discussed, considerable support from carers is required. Good psychological support and counselling skills are likely to make a significant impact on the patient's quality of life even to a greater extent than standard medical treatment.

Physician education

Cardiologists may be unfamiliar with the principles of palliative care and how they can be applied to the patients with end-stage cardiac disease. They are thoroughly competent in the specific aspects of management of heart failure but less familiar with the optimal method of control of pain or constipation or anxiety and depression, and the other clinical features that arise towards the end of life. Education can be most easily applied by establishing close links with the local hospice and by recognizing the similar problems that patients experience towards the end of their life whether the underlying disease is cancer or end-stage cardiac failure.

Conclusion

There is little doubt that the traditional view that hospice care be directed only towards the patient with advanced cancer is changing and it is now recognized that end-stage cardiac disease has many characteristics that lend themselves to the principles of palliative care. There is a sensitivity and realization in regard to this within palliative care. Much still needs to be achieved in this area. It may be regarded as a paradox that despite the considerable reduction in mortality and morbidity from cardiac failure because of new treatments, the number of patients with end-stage cardiac disease are likely to rise and in particular in the elderly who frequently have multiple other pathologies. In anticipation of this rise, it is important to establish a multi-disciplinary approach to the management of end-stage cardiac disease, which will greatly improve the quality of life for these patients in the final days and hours of their life. It will also ease the burden on the patient's family and friends in the same way that palliative care with cancer has done so impressively over the past 30 years.

References

1. **Cohn, J.** et al. (1986). Effect of vasodilator therapy on mortality in chronic congestive heart failure. Results of a Veterans Affairs Administration co-operative study. *New England Journal of Medicine* **314**, 1547–52.
2. **Levenson, J.** et al. (2000). Patients' experiences as death approaches: the last six months of life for patients with congestive heart failure. *Journal of the American Geriatrics Society* **48** (5), 212–16.
3. **Dargie, H.J. and McMurray, J.J.V.** (1992). Chronic heart failure: epidemiology, aetiology, pathophysiology and treatment. In *Recent Advances in Cardiology II* 2nd edn. (ed. D. Rowlands), pp. 73–114. Edinburgh: Churchill Livingston.
4. **Office of Population and Census Surveys Social Services Division.** *Health Survey for England.* London: HMSO 1993.
5. **CONSENSUS Trial Study Investigators** (1987). Effects of enalapril on mortality in severe congestive heart failure. Results of the cooperative north Scandinavian enalapril study. *New England Journal of Medicine* **316**, 1429–35.
6. **McKee, P.** et al. (1971). The natural history of congestive heart failure: the Framingham study. *New England Journal of Medicine* **285**, 1441–6.
7. **Stewart, A.** et al. (1989). Functional status and well-being of patients with chronic conditions: results form the Medical Outcomes Study. *Journal of the American Medical Association* **262** (7), 907–13.
8. **McMurray, J.J.V. and Hart, W.** (1993). The economic impact of heart failure on the UK National Health Service. *European Heart Journal* **14** (Suppl.), 113.
9. **Francis, G.** (2001). Pathophysiology of chronic heart failure. *American Journal of Medicine* **110** (Suppl. 7A), 37S–46S.
10. **Lombardi, W. and Gilbert, E.** (2000). The effects of neurohormonal antagonism on pathologic left ventricular remodeling in heart failure. *Current Cardiology Reports* **2** (2), 90–8.
11. **Matsumori, A. and Sasayama, S.** (2001). The role of inflammatory mediators in the failing heart: immunomodulation of cytokines in experimental models of heart failure. *Heart Failure Reviews* **6** (2), 129–36.
12. **Herrera-Garza, E.** et al. (1999). Tumour necrosis factor-alpha: a mediator of disease progression in the failing human heart. *Chest* **115** (4), 212–16.
13. **Carr, J.** et al. (1989). Prevalence and haemodynamic correlates of malnutrition in severe congestive heart failure secondary to ischaemic or idiopathic dilated cardiomyopathy. *American Journal of Cardiology* **63**, 709–13.
14. **Anker, S.** et al. (1997). Wasting as an independent risk factor for mortality in chronic heart failure. *Lancet* **349**, 1050–3.
15. **Lynn, J.** et al. (1997). Perceptions by family members of the dying experience of older and seriously ill patients. *Annals of Internal Medicine* **126**, 97–106.
16. **Fried, T.** et al. (1999). Older persons' preferences for site of terminal care. *Annals of Internal Medicine* **131** (2), 109–12.
17. **Blue, L.** et al. (2001). Randomised controlled trial of specialist nurse intervention in heart failure. *British Medical Journal* **323** (7315), 715–18.
18. **McCarthy, M., Addington-Hall, J., and Lay, M.** (1997). Communication and choice in dying from heart disease. *Journal of the Royal Society of Medicine* **90**, 128–31.
19. **Krumholz, H.** et al. (1998). Resuscitation preferences among patients with severe congestive heart failure: results form the SUPPORT project. *Circulation* **98**, 648–55.
20. **Handley, H.** (2001). Do not resuscitate. *Heart* **86**, 1–2.
21. **Blok, W.** et al. (1997). Pro- and anti-inflammatory cytokines in healthy volunteers fed various doses of fish oils for 1 year. *European Journal of Clinical Investigation* **27** (12), 1003–8.
22. **Seligmann, H.** et al. (1991). Thiamine deficiency in patients with congestive heart failure receiving long-term furosemide therapy: a pilot study. *American Journal of Medicine* **91**, 151–5.
23. **Meyer, K., Samek, L., and Schwalbold, M.** (1996). Physical responses to different modes of interval exercise in patients with chronic heart failure: application to exercise training. *European Heart Journal* **17**, 1040–7.

24. **Mujais, S., Nora, N., and Levin, M.** (1992). Principles and clinical uses of diuretic therapy. *Progress in Cardiovascular Disease* **35**, 221–45.
25. **Pfeffer, M.A.** et al. (1988). Effect of captopril on progressive ventricular dilatation after anterior myocardial infarction. *New England Journal of Medicine* **319**, 80–6.
26. **SOLVD Investigators** (1991). Effect of enalapril on survival in patients with reduced left ventricular ejection fractions and congestive heart failure. *New England Journal of Medicine* **325**, 293–302.
27. **Randomised Aldactone Evaluation Study Investigators** (1999). The effects of spironolactone on morbidity and mortality in patients with severe heart failure. *New England Journal of Medicine* **341**, 709–17.
28. **Tendera, M. and Ochala, A.** (2001). Overview of the results from the recent beta-blocker trials. *Current Opinion in Cardiology* **16** (3), 180–5.
29. **The Digitalis Investigation Group** (1997). The effect of digoxin on mortality and morbidity in patients with heart failure. *New England Journal of Medicine* **336**, 525–33.
30. **Diet, F. and Erdmann, E.** (2000). Thromboembolism in heart failure: who should be treated? *European Journal of Heart Failure* **2** (4), 355–63.
31. **Connolly, S.** et al. (2000). Meta-analysis of the implantable cardioverter defibrillator secondary prevention trials. AVID, CASH and CIDS studies. *European Heart Journal* **21** (24), 2071–8.
32. **Conti, J.** (2001). Biventricular pacing therapy for congestive heart failure: a review of the literature. *Cardiology in Review* **9** (4), 217–26.
33. **Elefteriades, J.** et al. (1993). Coronary artery bypass grafting in severe left ventricular dysfunction: excellent survival with improved ejection fraction and functional status. *Journal of the American College of Cardiology* **9** (22), 1411–17.
34. **Horvarth, K., Cohn, L. and Cooley, D.** (1997). Transmyocardial laser revascularization: results of a multicenter trial with transmyocardial laser revascularization used as a sole therapy for end-stage coronary artery disease. *Journal of Thoracic and Cardiovascular Surgery* **113**, 645.
35. **Arora, R., Chou, T., and Jain, D.** (1999). The multicentre study of enhanced external counterpulsation (MUST-EECP): effect of EECP on exercise-induced myocardial ischaemia and anginal episodes. *Journal of the American College of Cardiology* **33**, 1833–40.
36. **Hosenpud, J.** (1994). The registry of the International Society for Heart and Lung Transplantation: eleventh official report. *Journal of Heart and Lung Transplantation* **14**, 561–70.
37. **Mancini, D.** et al. (1991). Value of peak exercise oxygen consumption for optimal timing of cardiac transplantation in ambulatory patients with heart failure. *Circulation* **83**, 778–86.
38. **Rose, E. A.** et al. (2001). Long term use of a left ventricular assist device for end-stage heart failure. *New England Journal of Medicine* **345**, 1435–43.
39. **O'Brien, T., Welsh, J., and Dunn, F.G.** (1998). ABC of palliative care: non-malignant conditions. *British Medical Journal* **316**, 286–9.

10.6 Palliative medicine in non-malignant neurological disorders

Gian Domenico Borasio, Angela Rogers, and Raymond Voltz

Neurological disorders are among the leading causes of death in the Western world. Stroke alone accounts for around 60 deaths/100 000 population/year in Europe. Other disorders such as multiple sclerosis and Parkinson's disease are highly prevalent, and ultimately lead to premature death, although death is usually ascribed to terminal complications such as pneumonia. Finally, there is a large number of rare neurological disorders with a progressive course (amyotrophic lateral sclerosis, Huntington's disease, multiple system atrophy, central nervous system infections, muscle disorders, etc.), which nonetheless, when summed together, constitute an important group. Primary brain tumours and dementias are dealt with elsewhere in this textbook (see Chapters 8.15 and 10.7).

The differences in approach to palliative care between neurology and oncology stem primarily from the different time courses of neurological disorders, which are outlined in Table 1. In addition, the distribution and prevalence of symptoms is quite different from oncology. Generally speaking, pain is less prominent, while impairment in mobility as well as behavioural and cognitive changes are more prevalent The following section outlines principles of palliative care for source of the most important neurological disorders.

Amyotrophic lateral sclerosis/motor neurone disease

Amyotrophic lateral sclerosis (ALS, aka motor neurone disease in the United Kingdom and Lou Gehrig's disease in the United States) is the most common degenerative disorder of the motoneuronal system in adults. The incidence of ALS is 1.5–2/100 000/year and the prevalence is around 6–8 per 100 000. Most cases begin after age 40, with a mean age at onset of 58 years and an average disease duration of 3–4 years. Ten per cent of patients survive more than 10 years. There is no satisfactory treatment; the only approved drug (riluzole) prolongs life by about 3 months.

Patients present with fasciculations and slowly progressing pareses of voluntary muscles, coupled with hyperreflexia and spasticity due to concomitant involvement of upper and lower motor neurones. Bulbar onset with slurred speech (dysarthria) and/or difficulty in swallowing (dysphagia) occurs in 20–30 per cent of all cases, particularly in older females. Extraocular movements, sphincter control, and cognitive functions are usually spared, and sensation is normal. The main symptoms of ALS are shown in Table 2.

Palliative care in ALS starts with the communication of the diagnosis and goes all the way to bereavement counselling (Fig. 1). Despite first attempts at

Table 1 Different time courses of neurological disorders

(Sub)-acute progressive (days–weeks)	Progressive stroke, meningitis/encephalitis, Creutzfeldt–Jakob disease
Chronic progressive (months–years)	Amyotrophic lateral sclerosis, brain tumours, Huntington's disease, muscular dystrophies, multiple sclerosis (some), Alzheimer's disease
Chronic disability (± fluctuations)	Stroke, persistent vegetative state, multiple sclerosis (some), Parkinson's disease

Table 2 Symptoms due to ALS (either as a direct consequence of motoneuronal degeneration or indirectly as a consequence of the primary symptoms)

Directly	Indirectly
Weakness and atrophy	Psychological disturbances
Fasciculations and muscle cramps	Sleep disturbances
Spasticity	Constipation
Dysarthria	Drooling
Dysphagia	Thick mucous secretions
Dyspnoea	Symptoms of chronic hypoventilation
Pathological laughing/crying	Pain

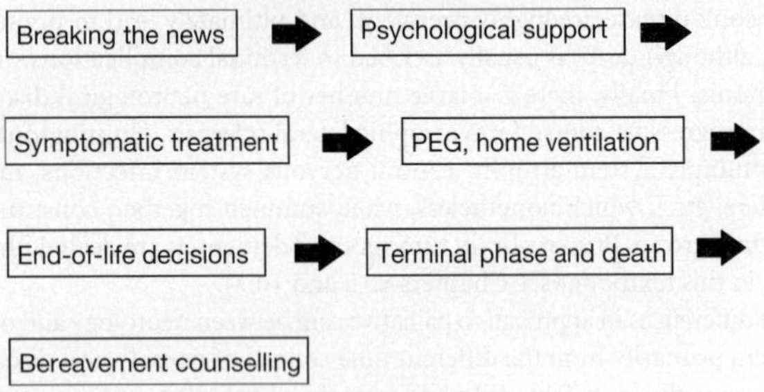

Fig. 1 The course of palliative care in ALS.

Table 3 Palliative care in ALS: who is involved?

Chaplain	Physiotherapist (physical therapist)
Counsellor	Physician
Dietitian	Psychologist
Hospice volunteers	Relatives
Lay associations	Social worker
Nurse	Speech therapist
Occupational therapist	Swallowing therapist

establishing evidence-based guidelines,[1] standards of palliative treatment in ALS are still largely based on expert opinion and differ between countries.[2]

Palliative care in ALS involves a large number of different professionals (Table 3). In the United Kingdom, at least 75 per cent of inpatient palliative care/hospice units are involved in the care of patients with ALS.[3] This figure is lower (between 25 and 50 per cent) for the rest of Europe, and no US data are currently available. In our experience, early and close cooperation between the neurologist and the local palliative care/hospice team can be of invaluable help for patients and family.[4] Ideally, all members of the palliative care team should be trained and receive ongoing support and education in this area. A comprehensive volume on this subject has been published.[5]

Breaking the news

Palliative care begins at the time of diagnosis and will influence the way it is told.[6] The patient should dictate the pace and depth of the information flow, while the doctor retains the difficult task of responding appropriately to the patient's cues.[7] Since many patients with ALS turn to alternative treatments,[8] this topic should be discussed proactively in order to protect the patient from serious financial and/or medical risks, while preserving hope and maintaining trust in the patient–physician relationship.

At the onset of symptoms of dyspnoea, symptoms of chronic nocturnal hypoventilation (see Table 4), or when the forced vital capacity (FVC) drops below 50 per cent, the patient should be offered information about the terminal phase, since most patients at this point fear that they will 'choke to death'. Describing the mechanism of terminal hypercapnic coma and the resulting peaceful death during sleep will relieve this fear in most patients.

At the same time, patients should be asked whether they would wish to be intubated and ventilated in the event of a terminal respiratory failure. Patients who have been informed about the possible subsequent clinical course, which may end up in a 'locked-in' syndrome in an intensive care unit, will usually deny permission for such a procedure. This denial must be documented in writing by the physician and should be incorporated into an advance directive.[9] The consequences of such a decision must be discussed with the patient, family, and the primary physician (e.g. concerning the use of opioids in the terminal phase). It is important to review the advance directive at 6-monthly intervals, since ALS patients' preferences for

Table 4 Symptoms of chronic hypoventilation

Daytime fatigue and sleepiness, concentration problems
Difficulty falling asleep, disturbed sleep, nightmares
Morning headache
Nervousness, tremor, increased sweating, tachycardia
Depression, anxiety
Tachypnoea, dyspnoea, phonation difficulties
Visible efforts of auxiliary respiratory muscles
Reduced appetite, weight loss, recurrent gastritis
Recurrent or chronic upper respiratory tract infections
Cyanosis, oedema
Vision disturbances, dizziness, syncope
Diffuse pain in head, neck, and extremities

life-sustaining treatments have been shown to change over this period of time.[10]

Symptom control

Muscle weakness

Should be managed by regular exercise, never to the point of fatigue, and by the use of appropriate aids (cane, ankle-foot-orthosis, wheelchair, aids for clothing and eating, etc.), in order to maintain as high as possible a degree of independence and mobility. Occasionally, a short-term (few weeks) increase of muscle strength may be achieved with pyridostigmine 40–60 mg tid. Because of its cholinergic side-effects (e.g. diarrhoea), the medication should be stopped after a week if there is no subjective benefit.

Dysphagia

Should first be treated by an adjustment in diet consistency (recipe books for ALS patients are available from several lay associations, see below). Specific swallowing techniques (such as supraglottic swallowing) can help to prevent aspiration. When the oral calorie intake is insufficient (weight loss >10 per cent) and oral food intake becomes intolerable due to choking, it is best to perform a percutaneous endoscopic gastrostomy (PEG), which is usually very well tolerated, provided the vital capacity is >50 per cent at the time of introduction.[11] Since the mortality of the procedure increases with worsening of pulmonary function, patient and family should be encouraged to make an early decision regarding PEG placement. It is important to remember that a PEG does not prevent aspiration pneumonia, which indeed is frequent if overfeeding by PEG occurs. A radiologically inserted gastrostomy may be an alternative in advanced disease.

Dysarthria

Can lead to a complete loss of oral communication abilities. Speech therapy is helpful at the beginning. In advanced cases, modern computer technology offers several options that enable even patients with almost total paresis of voluntary muscles to communicate, for example, via myoelectrically controlled switches.[12]

Dyspnoea

It is the most severe symptom in ALS. At the onset of dyspnoea, chest physiotherapy is helpful. Dyspnoeic attacks usually have a pronounced anxiety component and are best managed by short-acting benzodiazepines (lorazepam s.l. 0.5–1 mg). In acute and chronic dyspnoea, the subjective feeling of shortness of breath is reduced by the administration of morphine (2.5–5 mg po or 1–2 mg sc/iv q4h). Titration of the morphine dose against the clinical effect will almost never lead to a life-threatening respiratory depression.

Months to years before terminal respiratory failure, symptoms of chronic nocturnal hypoventilation ensue, which may considerably impair the patient's quality of life (Table 4). Non-invasive intermittent ventilation via mask (NIV) is an efficient and cost-effective means of alleviating these symptoms.[13] Patients and families should be informed about the temporary nature of the measure, which is primarily directed towards improving quality of life, rather than prolonging it (as opposed to tracheostomy). The problems with mechanical ventilation are usually not related to cost or technical difficulties, but to the increasing care needs of the ventilated patients. A slow progression, good communication skills, mild bulbar involvement, a strong motivation on the patient's part, and a supportive family environment argue in favour of the initiation of NIV. To be effective, NIV needs to be administered for at least 4 h/d, most preferably at night.[14] It is very important to reassure the patients that, whenever they may decide to stop NIV, all necessary care and appropriate medication will be available to ensure a peaceful death. The physician has a legal and ethical duty to honour a patient's request for discontinuation of such treatment.[15]

Psychological symptoms

Most if not all patients with ALS undergo a phase of reactive depression after being told the diagnosis. Counselling is of paramount importance at this stage. The reported prevalence of depression in ALS varies depending on the assessment method: although full-fledged major depression according to DSM-IV criteria is infrequent (around 10 per cent), self-reported depressive symptoms have been described in 44–75 per cent of patients.[16] Clinically significant depression should be looked for and treated at all disease stages. The most widely used drug is amitriptyline (start with 25 mg/d and slowly increase to 100–150 mg/d as tolerated), which may also exert favourable effects on other symptoms such as drooling, pseudobulbar effect (pathological laughing or crying), and sleep disturbance. If side-effects such as dry mouth or constipation are a problem, specific serotonin reuptake inhibitors (SSRIs) may be employed. Importantly, the concordance of depression and distress levels between patients and caregivers is high, thus reinforcing the notion that attention to the mental health of the caregiver may alleviate the patient's distress as well.[17]

Sleep disorders

These disorders are usually a consequence of the inability to change position during sleep. Psychological problems, muscle cramps, fasciculations, dysphagia, and dyspnoea can also impair sleep. Sedatives should be used sparingly, since they may impair residual muscle force.

Thick mucous secretions

This symptom, which results from a combination of diminished fluid intake and reduced coughing pressure, is difficult to treat. *N*-Acetylcysteine is helpful only in a small minority of cases. Suction is usually not fully effective unless performed via a tracheostomy. Physiotherapy with vibration massage may be helpful in the initial stages. Both manually assisted coughing techniques and mechanical insufflation–exsufflation can assist in extracting excess mucus from the airway.[18] Intermittent positive vibration devices are specialized inhalators, which deliver a pressurized, intermittent flow of nebulized saline with or without expectorants. They are used for 10–15 min at a time and can assist in clearing of pulmonary and bronchial secretions.[19]

Pathological laughing/crying

This symptom is also referred to as 'pseudobulbar affect' and occurs in up to 50 per cent of patients. It is not a mood disorder, but rather an abnormal display of affect, which can be very disturbing for the patients in social situations. Since this symptom is seldom volunteered, physicians should ask for it and point out that it responds well to medication (Table 5).

Other symptoms of ALS, which can be relieved by appropriate medication, include *muscle cramps, fasciculations, spasticity,* and *drooling.* Treatment options for these symptoms are shown in Table 5. For antispasticity drugs, the patient has to titrate the dose against the clinical effect, since a moderate degree of spasticity is usually better for mobility than a fully flaccid paresis.

Table 5 Symptomatic medication in ALS (in order of recommendation)

	Dosage[a]
Fasciculations and muscle cramps	
If mild	
Magnesium	5 mmol qd-tid
Vitamin E	400 IE bid
If severe	
Quinine sulphate	200 mg bid
Carbamazepine	200 mg bid
Phenytoin	100 mg qd-tid
Spasticity	
Baclofen	10–80 mg
Tizanidine	6–24 mg
Memantine	10–60 mg
Tetrazepam	100–200 mg
Drooling	
Glycopyrrolate	0.1–0.2 mg sc/im tid
Transdermal hyoscine patches	1–2 patches
Amitriptyline	10–150 mg
Atropine/benztropine	0.25–0.75 mg/1–2 mg
Clonidine	0.15–0.3 mg
Pathologic laughing/crying	
Amitriptyline	10–150 mg
Fluvoxamine	100–200 mg
Lithium carbonate	400–800 mg
L-Dopa	500–600 mg

[a] Usual range of adult daily dosage; some patients may require higher dosages, e.g., of antispastic medication.

Dantrolene should not be used as first-line medication in ALS, because it enhances weakness; however, we have witnessed a case of extreme spasticity in the terminal phase, which could only be relieved by high doses of iv dantrolene. If severe spasticity is a problem earlier in the disease, intrathecal baclofen may be an option.[20] For patients with therapy-refractory drooling, botulinum toxin injections in the salivary glands may be considered.[21]

Constipation

Lack of exercise can promote the development of constipation in patients with ALS. The first step is dietary measures (foods with high fibre content such as 'power pudding'—equal measure of prunes, prune juice, bran, and apple sauce). Care should be taken to ensure adequate fluid intake, since dysphagia-induced dehydration may worsen constipation. The next step is a review of current medication, since muscle relaxants, sedatives, and anticholinergics reduce bowel mobility. Mild laxative therapy should be prophylactically initiated in bed-ridden patients and in those receiving opioids.

Pain

Although ALS itself does not usually involve sensory fibres, musculoskeletal pain often arises in the later stages of the disease as a result of stress on the bones and joints that have lost their protective muscular ensheathment due to atrophy. In addition, muscle contractures and joint stiffness (e.g. frozen shoulder) may be painful. These symptoms are usually best treated with non-steroidal anti-inflammatory drugs (NSAIDs) and physiotherapy. Another cause of pain in ALS is skin pressure pain, due to immobility. Special attention must be given to the nursing care, which requires frequent changes in the patient's position, both at night and during daytime[22] (see Chapter 8.8.2). If NSAIDs are insufficient, opioid analgesics should be started.

Gastro-oesophageal reflux disease

It may occur in ALS due to diaphragmatic weakness involving the lower oesophageal sphincter. Particular care is needed when starting a patient on

PEG because of possible overfeeding, which may lead to gastro-oesophageal reflux and even aspiration. Treatment includes prokinetic agents (e.g. metoclopramide) and antacids.

Dependent oedema of the hands and feet

This oedema occurs in weak limbs because of reduced muscle pump activity. Limb elevation, physiotherapy, and compression hose are helpful. If pain develops or swelling persists despite prolonged elevation, a deep venous thrombosis should be ruled out.

Urinary urgency and frequency

Urinary urgency and frequency in the absence of urinary tract infections can be due to spasticity of the bladder and respond favourably to oxybutinin (2.5–5 mg qd-tid).

Jaw quivering or clenching

It may develop in patients with pseudobulbar involvement in response to noxious stimuli such as cold, anxiety, or pain, and is relieved by benzodiazepines (e.g. lorazepam sl or clonazepam).

Laryngospasm

A sudden reflex closure of the vocal chords, laryngospasm, can cause panic due to a sensation of choking. Several types of stimuli (emotions, strong flavours or smells, cold air, fluid aspiration, sinus drainage, or gastro-oesophageal reflux) may provoke this symptom, which usually resolves spontaneously within a few seconds. Repeated swallowing while breathing through the nose can accelerate resolution. Patients also benefit from reassurance and education about this distressing symptom. H_1 or H_2 blocking agents (antihistamines or antacids) may also be helpful.

Nasal congestion

Congestion in bulbar patients with a weakening of the nasopharyngeal muscles can be helped by elevating the nasal bridge with nasal tape and application of topical decongestants.

Psychosocial care

According to data from the United States, a large proportion of patients with ALS show an interest in physician-assisted suicide,[16] which in our experience is often the result of the fear of becoming a burden to their families, or the result of feeling isolated or disempowered in their relationship with the health-care team. However, suicidal actions are relatively rare in ALS.[23] When asked about the most important aspects of their quality of life (QoL), 100 per cent of the patients mentioned their family, while health-related items were nominated in about half of the cases.[24] Correspondingly, a recent study indicated that QoL in ALS depends on factors other than strength and physical function.[25] In ALS, the burden of the relatives often exceeds that of the patients and deserves particular attention. The physician must be particularly sensitive to the needs and fears of the patients' children, and the importance of helping patients in their role as parents.[26] Patients' associations* may provide invaluable help and assistance, and should be involved in patient care from the very beginning.

Spiritual care and bereavement

The role of spiritual care is often underestimated. A recent study indicated that spirituality or religiousness may affect the use of PEG and NIV in ALS, and may be a source of comfort to patients.[27] Cases of patients whose spiritual practice greatly enhanced their ability to cope with ALS have been reported.[28] Spiritual care is not limited to patients, but should encompass the whole family as a means of preventing problems during bereavement, which may be particularly severe in ALS families. It is important to acknowledge that the process of bereavement in ALS actually starts immediately after the diagnosis is communicated, in the form of the so-called 'anticipatory grief', and that callous delivery of the diagnosis may affect the psychological adjustment to bereavement.[29]

Terminal phase

A retrospective survey of 171 patients with ALS showed that around 90 per cent of the patients died peacefully, mostly in their sleep, and none of the patients choked to death.[23] If patients with ALS are not artificially ventilated, the death process usually begins with the patient slipping from sleep into coma due to increasing hypercapnia. If restlessness or signs of dyspnoea develop, morphine should be administered beginning with 2.5–5 mg po, sc, or iv every 4 h (if necessary in combination with an antiemetic). Since morphine is not an anxiolytic drug, if anxiety is present, it should be treated with lorazepam sl (beginning with 1–2.5 mg) or midazolam po/sc (beginning with 1–2 mg). The dosage of morphine and anxiolytics should be increased until satisfactory symptom control is achieved.[30] The potential of these drugs to induce respiratory depression is usually overestimated. In the terminal phase, according to the doctrine of double effect, it is legally and ethically justified to risk a shortening of the dying process if adequate symptom control cannot be achieved otherwise.[31]

Most patients with ALS wish to die at home. This can often best be achieved through enrolment of the patient in a hospice or other palliative care programme. It is advisable for the physician to initiate contact with the hospice institution, where available, well in advance of the terminal phase.

Stroke

Stroke is an heterogeneous group of diseases including brain infarction (84 per cent), intracerebral bleeding (7 per cent), subarachnoid haemorrhage (7 per cent), and various rare entities like vasculitis, dissections, and sinus thrombosis (1.4 per cent). Typical symptoms include paresis (mostly as hemiparesis), hypoesthesia, hemianopia, diplopia, visual loss, headache, acute vomiting, aphasia, and loss of consciousness. The aetiology of brain infarction includes emboli originating from the heart, aorta, or major brain supplying vessels, haemodynamic changes from severe stenosis or occlusions, *in-situ* thrombosis of intracranial arteries and microangiopathy caused by diabetes or hypertension. The long-term prognosis following a stroke is rather poor: 20 per cent of patients die within 1 month, a further 10 per cent within a year, and another 5 per cent within 2 years.[32] In addition, up to 25 per cent of patients develop poststroke dementia, and only about 25 per cent survive without disability. At least 12 per cent of stroke survivors will be admitted to institutional care within a year.

Prevalence and incidence of stroke varies between different populations and age is the major determinant. The incidence in 45–54 year olds is about 0.8/1000 rising to 9.4/1000 in the 75–84 year olds. The lowest death rates are found in USA, Canada, Australia, and Switzerland (30/100 000/year). Western European countries show rates around 60/100 000, while eastern European countries have extremely high death rates from stroke (e.g. Bulgaria with 250/100 000).[33]

About 30–50 per cent of all stroke victims present with a so-called stroke-in-evolution with progression after arrival at the hospital. In the setting of an acute stroke unit about 7–11 per cent develop a severe clinical worsening with the urgent need to transfer them to an ICU (G.F. Hamann, personal communication). In acute stroke treated with thrombolysis, clinical deterioration is often related to secondary haemorrhagic transformation or the development of brain swelling with an increase in intracranial pressure.

There are several predictors of functional recovery following stroke. These include age, previous stroke, urinary continence, consciousness at onset, disorientation in time and place, admission activities of daily living score, and level of social support.[34] Many of these factors, for example, unconsciousness and hemiplegia or incontinence are interdependent and are by themselves good indicators of death. Severe strokes appear to be more common among older patients, in which significant co-morbidity is likely to be present.

* A list of ALS patients' associations worldwide can be found at www.alsmndalliance.org; a list of ALS centres worldwide can be found at www.wfnals.org

Two different epidemiological trends exist: the growing ageing population with a rise in stroke incidence and severity, and the decline in stroke incidence and death rate caused by life style factors and healthier behaviour. On the whole, more strokes and more severe strokes are to be expected in the coming decades, which will increase the demand for palliative care in these patients. The most common types of stroke with a fatal outcome are described below.[35]

Malignant middle cerebral artery infarction

Large middle cerebral artery infarctions are likely to develop a space-occupying lesion with the danger of transtentorial herniation. The mortality in untreated patients may be as high as 80 per cent. Early clinical signs are headache, nausea with vomiting, and progressive loss of consciousness in patients with severe hemispheric syndrome (e.g. hemiplegia, aphasia, hemihypesthesia, and hemianopia). The CT scan shows a large hypodensity within the whole middle cerebral artery territory. The main space-occupying effect develops over 2–5 days. Decompressive neurosurgery may reduce mortality to about 20 per cent in patients at risk for herniation.[36] The survivors are not more severely disabled than patients with large hemispheric strokes in general. It is important to select patients early for surgery since this is when the survival rates are highest. Unresolved questions include the age limit: most centres exclude patients older than 60 or 65 from this therapeutic option. In addition, many neurologists feel uncomfortable to treat patients with complete left hemispheric syndromes including global aphasia, fearing severe long-term disability. A controlled trial is underway to attempt to answer some of these questions.

Basilar artery thrombosis/severe brain stem infarction

The most severe form of ischaemic stroke is thrombosis of the basilar artery. The blood supply to this brainstem artery is of fundamental importance since the vegetative brainstem centres for breathing, circulation control, and control of almost all basic body functions will be affected in the case of ischaemia. If untreated, about 85 per cent of all patients suffering from acute basilar thrombosis will die. The survivors often display severe brainstem dysfunction with long-term disability or even locked-in-syndrome. The state-of-the-art therapy in these patients is local intraarterial thrombolysis, which can reduce mortality to 50 per cent or less.[37] Patients with profound brainstem dysfunction (deep coma with loss of all brainstem reflexes) may not be eligible for thrombolysis if symptoms were present for longer than 5–10 h. These patients, and those where thrombolysis was unsuccessful, will usually die within a few days.

Locked-in-syndrome

This is a severe form of brainstem infarction with a decerebration state at the level of the pons cerebri. The patients are tetraplegic but fully awake. They can communicate with eye movements or closing of the eyes, they see and hear, and are fully aware of their environment. A recent essay from a locked-in patient who survived and gained substantial improvement describes this terrifying state as being 'imprisoned in your own body', being aware of everything but also being dependent for everything. The prognosis for recovery is bad, but survival after the development of a locked-in-syndrome may be as long as 2–18 years.[38] The key issues for these long-term survivors are establishing means of communication and the emotional and physical stress for the patient's caregivers. Computerized aids for communication have been developed. Most recently, very sophisticated tools have been introduced using the slow cortical potentials from the EEG to operate communicating devices. Using these devices, after training sessions with continuous feedback patients achieved 84 per cent correct communicating steps enabling them to communicate autonomously by their thoughts.[39]

Severe intracerebral haemorrhage

Supratentorial haemorrhages exceeding 50 mL of volume have a mortality of around 50 per cent. The situation is very similar to that in malignant middle cerebral artery infarction. Palliative care is required primarily for patients with large haemorrhages (>100 mL supratentorial and 50 mL infratentorial) or concomitant disorders with a poor prognosis (e.g. severe liver dysfunction with coagulopathy), as well as for patients without clinical improvement following surgery and patients with progressive transtentorial herniation or signs of severe brainstem dysfunction. These patients usually show very reduced levels of consciousness. Palliative care should include measures for acute pain relief such as opioids.

Subarachnoid haemorrhage

Patients with subarachnoid haemorrhage are usually under the age of 60. The incidence is around 6/100 000/year and most of the severe bleeds are caused either by aneurysms (85 per cent) or by arteriovenous malformations. The typical clinical pattern is of a sudden, explosive headache combined with neck stiffness and initially impaired consciousness. The prognosis is determined by the occurrence and the severity of complications, mainly re-bleeding, vasospasms with secondary brain infarction, hydrocephalus, autonomic changes, and the rise in intracranial pressure.[40] Despite advances in diagnosis and therapy (e.g. endovascular aneurysm coiling), about 50 per cent of patients suffering an acute subarachnoid haemorrhage will die, and one-third will be severely disabled.

Symptom control

A recent publication on palliative day care in the UK showed that stroke is with HIV/AIDS and motor neurone disease one of the three major diagnoses besides cancer.[41] Only very limited data are available on palliative care in stroke. In the UK, the Regional Study of Care of the Dying[42] involved 237 patients who died from stroke and showed that 65 per cent were reported to have experienced pain, 57 per cent low mood, 56 per cent urinary incontinence, and 51 per cent confusion. Pain control was judged as inadequate in 37 per cent. In 25 per cent there was a feeling of insufficient choice about treatment. A comprehensive review of symptom control and other palliative care needs in stroke has been published recently.[43]

Loss of consciousness

As outlined, a variety of stroke syndromes result in reduced levels of consciousness or alertness, which may progress to coma. This should not, however, lead to the assumption that these patients are not suffering. Non-verbal and physiological clues, such as grimacing, blushing, stiff neck, or increases in respiratory rate, blood pressure, or pulse frequency, may be indicators of distress. Adequate nursing care and analgesic medication are required, especially in situations where a cause for pain is evident, for example, large intracranial haemorrhage. It is important to always work on the assumption that the patient understands everything that is being said.

Communication

Communication is hampered by aphasia and/or dysarthria in patients who suffer strokes involving the dominant (usually the left) temporo-parietal hemisphere. The different types of speech disorders are summarised in Tables 3 and 4 of Chapter 8.15. Prolonged speech and language disorders are associated with a poorer prognosis. In addition, aphasia may significantly influence palliative care. Kehayia and co-workers[44] found that aphasic stroke patients received less pain medication than non-aphasic ones. The patients' communication abilities may be further diminished due to accompanying neuropsychological deficits such as apraxia, agnosia, neglect, and reduced visuo-spatial orientation (see Table 2, Chapter 8.15).

Stroke patients and their families are eager for information on their disease and its prognosis, but health professionals tend to avoid this subject.[45] In severe strokes, an open dialogue with the relatives is essential in establishing the patient's previous functional status and presumed wishes for the current situation. If no advance directives are present, this information will be key in any decision regarding the withdrawal or withholding of life-prolonging treatment.[46]

Incontinence and constipation

Urinary and faecal incontinence are common in stroke patients and are associated with higher mortality and morbidity.[47] Impaired communication and reduced mobility may contribute to the development of incontinence, which can reduce morale and thus influence functional recovery. The management of urinary incontinence with a catheter facilitates nursing care, but carries a risk of infection and should be restricted to severely impaired patients. Faecal incontinence is a very distressing symptom for patients and relatives. Poor management of faecal incontinence may lead to skin damage and thus to pain and discomfort. Constipation should be expected and anticipated after stroke, due to immobility and decreased oral intake. Anticholinergic and opioid medication may worsen constipation. Prophylaxis includes increased fluid intake, high fibre diet, and laxatives.

Nutrition

In the acute and subacute phases of stroke, dysphagia occurs in about 50 per cent of patients; about two-thirds of aspirations are 'silent'. Around 50 per cent of dysphagic stroke patients die or recover spontaneously within 2 weeks.[48] Predominant dysphagic symptoms after stroke are delayed pharyngeal swallow, disturbed lingual movements, and reduced tongue base retraction. In addition, stroke patients may eat less due to facial weakness, poor arm function, and fatigue. Functional swallowing therapy includes specific exercises and techniques such as supraglottic swallowing, which however require intact cognition and good co-operation from the patients. Malnutrition is present in up to 40 per cent of stroke patients and can result in reduced muscle strength, lower resistance to infection, and impaired wound healing. A naso-gastric tube (NG) for feeding is uncomfortable and often dislodges. The alternative is a PEG tube, which is inserted directly into the stomach. A controlled trial of PEG and NG feeding found greater mortality and decreased nutritional intake among NG patients.[49]

A PEG, however, does not prevent aspiration. A review of 37 patients who had a PEG tube inserted post-stroke found that only 12 patients survived for 3 months (median survival: 53 d). The question of whether to feed poor prognosis stroke patients can be a crucial issue with a strong emotional impact on the patient's family.[46] The involvement of palliative care specialists may be especially helpful when there is a disagreement between the family and the medical team. An international trial on feeding policies for stroke patients is in progress.

Pain

Pain in stroke patients may be directly due to the brain lesion, the result of pressure sores or contractures, or stem from unrelated chronic conditions such as diabetic neuropathy. Between 18 and 32 per cent of patients suffer from post-stroke headaches. The 'shoulder–hand syndrome' occurs in 20–30 per cent of patients. It begins with pain and oedema of the shoulder, wrist, and hand, and progresses to trophic skin changes, muscle atrophy, and contractures. Treatment with a rapidly tapering short course of oral steroids was effective in 86 per cent of patients in a controlled study,[50] and prevention of shoulder trauma in the acute phase reduced the frequency of shoulder–hand syndrome from 27 to 8 per cent.

Eight per cent of patients suffer from 'central post-stroke pain'; a neuropathic pain syndrome which is thought to arise from the vascular lesion and is characterized by pain in the corresponding body part. This pain is partially resistant to opioids and difficult to treat; amitriptyline and lamotrigine have shown benefit in controlled trials.[51,52]

Depression, anxiety, and confusion

A Scandinavian study in 486 stroke patients found major depression in 26 per cent and minor depression in 14 per cent. The only predictors of post-stroke depression were dependency in daily life and pre-stroke depression.[53] Post-stroke depression has both organic and psychological causes, is generally underdiagnosed, and may be relieved with appropriate psychological and medical therapies. Serotonin reuptake inhibitors are usually preferable over trycyclics in this setting.[54]

Anxiety disorders have been detected in 28 per cent of stroke patients in the acute phase. They correlate with depression and may worsen its prognosis.[55] Disorientation and confusion are common after acute stroke, and agitation may be so severe as to require sedation. The managment of confusion is discussed in Chapter 8.17.

Caregivers

Most informal care of people following a stroke is provided by spouses. The level of care needed is predicted usually by the severity of the stroke and the patients' ability to undertake activities of daily living. However, the 'burden' experienced by informal carers is also associated with the carer's personal characteristics.[56] Stroke survivors living in the community are under-served by both health and social services and have unmet personal psychosocial needs, both of which increase the load on informal carers.[42] Relatives who are involved in decision-making regarding the withdrawal or withholding of treatment may experience considerable distress and anxiety, and may benefit from counselling and bereavement support.

Care in the last days of life

Good supportive nursing care for patients dying from stroke is essential. Dysphagic patients are particularly prone to chest secretions, which can be managed with appropriate suction and medication. A timely transfer from the acute care unit to a more peaceful environment or the home setting should be considered and discussed with the family.

Multiple sclerosis

Multiple sclerosis (MS) is the most frequent inflammatory demyelinating disorder of the central nervous system. The exact cause and pathogenesis is still unknown. Several factors are discussed such as genetic influence, environmental factors—most recently human herpes virus 6 and chlamydia have been implicated—and most importantly autoimmune mechanisms. There are at least four different pathological entities with different pathomechanisms which clinically are subsumed under the term MS.[57] New diagnostic criteria proposed by an international consensus group now allow the diagnosis of MS even after a single clinical episode.[58]

The last 10 years have been dominated by the advent of effective immunomodulatory treatment options such as interferon beta, copolymer-1, or mitoxantrone.[59] The beneficial effect of these drugs, however, is still relatively modest, for example, reduction of relapse rate by one-third, or delaying the need for a wheel-chair by 6–9 months. These advances—after decades with no effective treatments—have in some respect overshadowed the need for symptomatic and palliative care for patients with MS. Although MS is not a progressive lethal disorder in the strict palliative care definition, several aspects of palliative care are important for MS and should be respected from the initial telling of the diagnosis until the patient's death.[60]

When communicating the diagnosis, the fact that MS—in general—does not reduce life expectancy, will be important to the patient. However, it should be known to the treating physician that patients with MS are at increased risk of suicide, especially within the first 5 years of diagnosis. Therefore, care must be taken to detect and treat reactive depression in the initial stages. Importantly, treatment with interferon-beta may exacerbate depressive symptoms.[61] The wish for active euthanasia is frequent in patients with MS. In the Netherlands, euthanasia is the cause of death in one out of 20 MS patients (only AIDS is higher.[62]) Risk factors for suicide or the wish for euthanasia are not so much physical symptoms, but rather loneliness, unemployment, and lack of psychosocial support or spiritual background. Therefore, from the beginning onwards, organizing or introducing any form of help—for instance via the national MS societies (visit www.ifmss.org.uk for further information)—is an essential part of palliative care.

It is a frequent experience of nurses caring for MS patients in nursing homes that many of the patients tend to overestimate their abilities, which may lead to tensions between the patient and the health-care team. On the other hand, many patients with MS perceive a reduced quality of life, which results from the effect of their disease in the physical, cognitive, and psychosocial domains (see Table 6).(60) Symptoms perceived by professionals are not necessarily the most disabling to the patients. The physician and MS sufferer Wolf(63) considers depressive symptoms to be the most disabling, spasticity to be the most frequent, bladder symptoms to be the most confusing, and bowel symptoms to be the most humiliating. For optimal symptom control, a multidisciplinary team is necessary, which includes general practitioner, neurologist, urologist, psychiatrist, pain physician, neuroradiologist, nurse, physiotherapist, social worker, occupational therapist, psychologist, speech therapist, clergy, and lay organizations.

Once advanced neurological deficits have accumulated, mortality is increased four times. Causes of death are complications of chronic illness in about half of the patients, that is, pneumonia, pulmonary embolism, renal insufficiency, or urinary tract infections. Other causes of death are tumours (16 per cent), suicide (15 per cent), heart attack (11 per cent), or stroke (5 per cent).(64) In patients with advanced disease who repeatedly develop potentially lethal complications, a shift in the goals of care may be appropriate. To this aim, DNR (do not resuscitate) orders must be discussed early with the patient and relatives. Decisions should be recorded in the medical notes, and if possible a disease-specific advance directive should be set up.(65)

Table 6 Three domains of multiple sclerosis care

Physical	Cognitive	Psychosocial
Motor function	Memory	Mood
Coordination	Thought processing	Partnership
Sensory function	Attention	Family
Vision	Judgement	Stress
Gaze	Decision making	Friendships
Speech	Concentration	Work
Swallowing	Abstract reasoning	Money
Bladder	Orientation (person, time, space, situation)	Spiritual
Bowel		
Sexual		

Table 7 Symptoms in multiple sclerosis

Primary	Secondary	Tertiary
Weakness	Disuse weakness	Psychological issues
Numbness	Bladder infections	Reactive depression
Paresthesias	Pressure sores	Social isolation
Dysbalance	Demineralization of bone	Unemployment
Visual loss	Fractures	Role changes
Incontinence	Contractures	Financial issues
Sexual problems	Falls	Divorce
Cognitive impairment	Injuries	Decreased independence
Dysarthria	Aspiration pneumonia	Denial
Dysphasia	Decreased activities of daily living	Bereavement
Dysphagia		
Epileptic seizures		
Pain		

Symptom control

Symptoms in MS may arise as a direct (primary) or indirect (secondary) consequence of the loss of myelin and axons (see Table 7).(60) Tertiary symptoms depend on the progression of the disease. A multitude of therapy options are available to MS patients, even in the later stages of their disease when immunomodulatory treatment options are no longer indicated.

Oculomotor disturbances

An acquired nystagmus may be ameliorated using either the GABA-B-agonist baclofen (orally, 5–10 mg three times daily), the GABA-A agonist clonazepam (0.5 mg three times daily), or—especially in acquired fixation pendular nystagmus—the NMDA antagonist memantine (40–60 mg/d), or alternatively gabapentin (600–1500 mg/d).(66,67)

Tremor

In some patients with MS-related tremor, wrist weights may be helpful. Despite early reports of the beneficial effect of the 5-HT_3-antagonist ondansetron, a more recent small study has found no effect in MS patients with cerebellar tremor.(68) Propranolol (10–20 mg 3/4 times/d), isoniazid (800–1200 mg/d, distributed over 3–4 doses), or clonazepam (2–4 mg/d, starting at 0.5 mg/d) may be tried. In very severe cases, tremor may be ameliorated using deep brain stimulation, which can be performed at specialized centres.

Spasticity

In a recent Cochrane review, no specific antispastic drug could be identified as being superior over the others due to insufficient data.(69) Therefore, one should use the drug one is familiar with. To avoid side-effects, it is important to start any antispastic medication at low doses, slowly titrating against the clinical effect. If overdosed, patients will complain of increasing weakness. Drug options include baclofen (orally, 3–4 × 5–25 mg; in severe cases, intrathecal application may be necessary),(70) tizanidine (3 × 2–8 mg), dantrolene (2 × 25–200 mg), memantine (2–3 × 10–20 mg), tetrazepam (1 × 50–54 × 100 mg), and other benzodiazepines. If the patient has a focal spasticity, botulinum toxin may be very helpful. Here, the effect of a single injection may last for several weeks.(71) A phase III double-blind study is underway to assess the efficacy of cannabinoids on MS-induced spasticity. Besides drugs, physiotherapy is the mainstay of management. Occasionally, orthopaedic surgery may be indicated.(72)

Urinary symptoms

Patients may develop a hyperreflexia of the detrusor muscle, if the lesion is above the sacral micturition centre. A pragmatic approach includes changes in fluid intake (more in the morning, less in afternoon) and if possible passing water every 2–4 h. Medication is based on anticholinergics such as oxybutinin (2–3 × 5 mg/d), propiverin (3 × 10 mg/d), or imipramine (3 × 10–25 mg/d). If nocturnal incontinence is still present, desmopressin (spray) at night might be very helpful.(73) If the lesion lies between the sacral and pontine micturition centre, a dyssynergia of detrusor and sphincter muscles may result. Urge incontinence and incomplete emptying of the bladder are the clinical hallmarks. In most patients—especially if the residual urine volume lies above 100 mL—intermittent catheter use will be necessary. Alpha-blockers (phenoxybenzamine, 10–20 mg bid-tid), anti-spasticity drugs (see above), or botulinum toxin injection into the external sphincter may be helpful.

Pain

Occurs in 50–60 per cent of MS patients, with increasing prevalence over time. Causes of acute pain include trigeminal neuralgia, paroxysmal dysaesthetic pain, and painful tonic spasms. Trigeminal neuralgia may be the first manifestation of MS and is clinically indistinguishable from the idiopathic form. Lhermitte's sign, the most common form of paroxysmal dysaesthetic pain, may occur spontaneously or in response to triggers such as movement (particularly neck flexion) or tactile stimuli. In painful tonic spasms (sometimes referred to as 'brainstem seizures'), paroxysmal activation of the pyramidal tract leads to sudden bursts of spasticity in the upper or lower extremities, or the whole body, without loss of consciousness but with severe pain. These paroxysmal manifestations probably arise through the loss of the insulating myelin sheath, which renders axons susceptible to uncontrolled spreading of potentials across the whole pathway ('ephaptic activation'). They respond well to anticonvulsant treatment (carbamazepine, gabapentin).[74] For painful tonic spasms, benzodiazepines and acetazolamide may also be effective.

Headache is frequent in MS and any headache type may be encountered. Optic neuritis may produce retro-orbital pain aggravated by eye movement. A case of cluster headache attributed to MS-induced demyelination has been reported.[75]

Chronic pain in MS occurs as dysaesthetic central pain, low back pain, and painful leg spasms due to spasticity. Central dysaesthetic pain arises through lesions of the spinothalamic tract and is associated with sensory abnormalities. It is usually described as a burning pain in the legs, but may affect trunk and arms as well. It may also be aching, stabbing, or squeezing, and is best treated with anticonvulsants and analgesics for neuropathic pain (see Chapter 8.2.5). For therapy-refractory cases, intrathecal analgesia (e.g. bupivacaine)[76] can be considered. Low back pain is related to degenerative changes and scoliosis of the lumbosacral spine, and is aggravated by prolonged sitting. It may overlap with spasticity-related pain. Visceral pain in MS can be due to constipation, bladder spasms, or bladder distension.

Fatigue

A very common symptom in MS, it probably is also one of the most undertreated. If the fatigue is part of a depressive syndrome, this must be treated first. For fatigue, the indirect dopaminergic agonist and NMDA antagonist amantadine (e.g. 2 × 100 mg/d) has been in use for some time with good effect. Alternatively, the potassium channel blockers 4-aminopyridine and 3,4-diaminopyridine may be tried.[77] Controlled trials are currently underway to prove their efficiency. Most recently, the antinarcoleptic drug modafinil has been shown to have some efficacy in this regard.[78]

Psychobehavioural and cognitive symptoms

Adjustment to the disease progression can be difficult and requires psychotherapeutic intervention. Denial is very frequent in late-stage MS. It is predominantly organically determined leading to reduced compliance and problems with the caregivers. Depression is frequent in MS (40–50 per cent) and is related to the amount of cerebral pathology and steroid treatment, but not to disease duration or disability. It is often under-recognized and under-treated, SSRIs are the drugs of choice because of their good tolerability. Disorders of emotional expression (pathological laughing and crying, emotional incontinence) occur in 10–25 per cent of patients and may respond to amitriptyline or SSRIs. Cognitive deficits can be detected in 40–60 per cent of patients and are severe in 21–33 per cent. Management includes education of patient and relatives, as well as cognitive retraining and learning of compensatory strategies. Personality changes may manifest as irritability, apathy, or disinhibition. They are often cause of great distress to the family and require careful psychosocial intervention.[79]

Parkinson's disease

Parkinson's disease is an example of a degenerative neurological disease with a long chronic course, which does not necessarily lie within the strict definition of palliative care.[80] However, no curative approaches are currently available, and during the course of the disease a multitude of symptoms occur that affect the quality of life of the patients and their relatives. Care requires an expert multiprofessional and interdisciplinary approach that is sometimes hard to organize. At some point, the shift of goals of care will also be relevant to patients with Parkinson's disease. This may be the case once the patient, despite optimal therapy, becomes more disabled and persistent neuropsychiatric problems arise. Whether under the current organization of care this is recognized in time and handled according to the established palliative care principles may be doubted.[81] Mortality is about twice the normal. Usually, the patients die in nursing homes or in general hospitals. There is little published information about the way these patients die. In most cases, this will probably be due to complications of the long-standing chronic disease such as bronchopneumonia or complications from falls.[82] Currently, many palliative care programmes decline to take care of these patients as it is difficult to predict prognosis. Recently, the onset of dysphagia has been shown to predict a survival time of 15–24 months in several movement disorders including Parkinson's disease, multiple system atrophy, and progressive supranuclear palsy.[83]

Table 8 Symptoms of Parkinson's disease

Parkinsonian triad	Depression	Immobility
Akinesia	Drooling	Incontinence
Rigor	Dysarthria	Orthostatic hypotension
Tremor	Dyskinesia	Pain
	Dysphagia	Postural imbalance
Other symptoms	Dystonia	Seborrhoea
Anxiety	Falls	Sleep attacks
Confusion	Freezing attacks	Weakness
Constipation	Fixed stooped posture	
Dementia	Hallucinations	

Parkinson's syndrome is a clinical diagnosis consisting of the classical triad of tremor, akinesia, and rigidity. 'Idiopathic' Parkinson's disease is highly likely if there are no obvious causes (such as drug-induced Parkinson's syndrome) and there is a good response to L-dopa therapy. L-Dopa mainly improves akinesia but does not have a positive effect on many other symptoms (Table 8). The long-term use of L-dopa therapy also leads to problems such as drug-induced fluctuations (on–off phenomenon), dyskinesias, or neuropsychological problems. Therefore, in the early stages of the disease, an L-dopa sparing approach should be taken and treatment should be started with dopaminergic agonists, especially in younger patients.

Symptom control

An essential part of palliative care for a patient with Parkinson's disease is good nursing care. Skin care (complicated by the typical seborrhoic dermatitis), positioning, constipation, and oral hygiene are only a few examples of the nursing needs of these patients.

Motor symptoms

Balance, gait and 'freezing' attacks may be ameliorated by ergonomic advice and physiotherapy (educating about cueing tricks, use of external or internal pacing). Acute episodes of hypokinesia usually respond to s.c. administration of apomorphine. Hyperkinesias, which generally are better tolerated, may still be very burdensome to some patients. In hyperkinetic crises potent neuroleptic drugs (e.g. risperidone) may be necessary. Contractures may be difficult to prevent. Recently, the use of botulinum toxin has been a very helpful addition to the therapeutic spectrum. Severe cases may require surgical tenotomies.

Pain

Although not intuitively obvious, pain is a very common problem in the end-stages of Parkinson's disease.[84] It may arise from stiffness, rigidity, or dystonic spasms. Uncomfortable posture as well as constipation may contribute to pain. If these cannot be alleviated by treating the underlying cause (e.g. with L-dopa, laxatives, nursing care), analgesics according to the WHO ladder should be used. When treating opioid-induced nausea and vomiting, the possible Parkinson-aggravating side-effects of some neuroleptics (haloperidol, prochlorperazine) should be kept in mind. Antiemetics such as domperidone, which does not block cerebral dopamine receptors, may be preferable.

Neuropsychiatric symptoms

Depression is a frequent symptom in Parkinson's disease and is often overlooked. Confusion and hallucinations may occur as part of the disease process or may be induced by dopaminergic drugs. The drugs used must be reviewed and dopaminergic or anticholinergic drugs reduced where possible. If required, atypical neuroleptics such as clozapine should be used instead of haloperidol. Development of dementia is frequent in late stages, and usually causes severe psychosocial problems. The ensuing reduction in competence should be anticipated by the early introduction of advance directives.

References

1. **Miller, R.G.** et al. (1999). Practice Parameter. The care of the patient with amyotrophic lateral sclerosis (an evidence-based review): report of the Quality Standards Subcommittee of the American Academy of Neurology: ALS Practice Parameters Task Force. *Neurology* **52**, 1311–23.
2. **Borasio, G.D., Shaw, P.J., Hardiman, O., Ludolph, A.C., Sales Luis, M.L., and Silani, V.**, for the European ALS Study Group (2001). Standards of palliative care for patients with amyotrophic lateral sclerosis: results of a European survey. *Amyotrophic Lateral Sclerosis and Other Motor Neuron Disorders* **2**, 159–64.
3. **Oliver, D. and Webb, S.** (2000). The involvement of specialist palliative care in the care of people with motor neurone disease. *Palliative Medicine* **14**, 427–8.
4. **Borasio, G.D., Voltz, R., and Miller, R.G.** (2001). Palliative care in amyotrophic lateral sclerosis. In *Palliative Care* (ed. A. Carver and K. Foley). *Neurologic Clinics* **19**, 829–47.
5. **Oliver, D., Borasio, G.D., and Walsh, D.**, ed. *Palliative Care in Amyotrophic Lateral Sclerosis (Motor Neurone Disease)*. Oxford: Oxford University Press, 2000.
6. **Doyle, D. and O'Connell, S.** (1996). Breaking bad news: starting palliative care. *Journal of the Royal Society of Medicine* **89**, 590–1.
7. **Borasio, G.D., Sloan, R., and Pongratz, D.E.** (1998). Breaking the news in amyotrophic lateral sclerosis. *Journal of the Neurological Sciences* **160**, 127–33.
8. **Wasner, M., Klier, H., and Borasio, G.D.** (2001). The use of alternative medicine by patients with amyotrophic lateral sclerosis. *Journal of the Neurological Sciences* **191**, 151–4.
9. **Borasio, G.D. and Voltz, R.** (2000). Advance directives. In *Palliative Care in Amyotrophic Lateral Sclerosis* (ed. D. Oliver, G.D. Borasio, and D. Walsh), pp. 36–41. Oxford: Oxford University Press.
10. **Silverstein, M.D.** et al. (1991). Amyotrophic lateral sclerosis and life-sustaining therapy: patients' desires for information, participation in decision making, and life-sustaining therapy. *Mayo Clinics Proceedings* **66**, 906–13.
11. **Kasarskis, E.J., Scarlata, D., Hill, R., Fuller, C., Stambler, N., and Cedarbaum, J.M.** (1999). A retrospective study of percutaneous endoscopic gastrostomy in ALS patients during the BDNF and CNTF trials. *Journal of the Neurological Sciences* **169**, 118–25.
12. **Scott, A. and Foulsum, M.** (2000). Speech and language therapy. In *Palliative Care in Amyotrophic Lateral Sclerosis* (ed. D. Oliver, G.D. Borasio, and D. Walsh), pp. 117–25. Oxford: Oxford University Press.
13. **Cazzolli, P.A. and Oppenheimer, E.A.** (1996). Home mechanical ventilation for amyotrophic lateral sclerosis: nasal compared to tracheostomy-intermittent positive pressure ventilation. *Journal of the Neurological Sciences* **139** (Suppl.), 123–8.
14. **Kleopa, K.A., Sherman, M., Neal, B., Romano, G.J., and Heiman-Patterson, T.** (1999). Bipap improves survival and rate of pulmonary function decline in patients with ALS. *Journal of the Neurological Sciences* **164**, 82–8.
15. **American Academy of Neurology** (1998). Assisted suicide, euthanasia, and the neurologist. The Ethics and Humanities Subcommittee of the American Academy of Neurology. *Neurology* **50**, 596–8.
16. **Ganzini, L.** et al. (1998). Attitudes of patients with amyotrophic lateral sclerosis and their care givers toward assisted suicide. *New England Journal of Medicine* **339**, 967–73.
17. **Rabkin, J.G., Wagner, G.J., and Del Bene, M.** (2000). Resilience and distress among amyotrophic lateral sclerosis patients and caregivers. *Psychosomatic Medicine* **62**, 271–9.
18. **Hanayama, K., Ishikawa, Y., and Bach, J.R.** (1997). Amyotrophic lateral sclerosis. Successful treatment of mucous plugging by mechanical insufflation–exsufflation. *American Journal of Physical Medicine and Rehabilitation* **76**, 338–9.
19. **Gelinas, D. and Miller, R.G.** (2000). A treatable disease: a guide to the management of amyotrophic lateral sclerosis. In *Amyotrophic Lateral Sclerosis* (ed. R.H. Broon Jr, U. Meininger, and M. Swash), pp. 405–21. London: Martin Dunitz.
20. **Marquardt, G. and Lorenz, R.** (1999). Intrathecal baclofen for intractable spasticity in amyotrophic lateral sclerosis. *Journal of Neurology* **246**, 619–20.
21. **Giess, R.** et al. (2000). Injections of botulinum toxin A into the salivary glands improve sialorrhoea in amyotrophic lateral sclerosis. *Journal of Neurology, Neurosurgery and Psychiatry* **69**, 121–3.
22. **Newrick, P.G. and Langton-Hewer, R.** (1985). Pain in motor neuron disease. *Journal of Neurology, Neurosurgery and Psychiatry* **48**, 838–40.
23. **Neudert, C., Oliver, D., Wasner, M., and Borasio, G.D.** (2001). The course of the terminal phase in patients with amyotrophic lateral sclerosis. *Journal of Neurology* **248**, 612–16.
24. **Neudert, C., Wasner, M., and Borasio, G.D.** (2001) Patients' assessment of quality of life instruments: a randomised study of SIP, SF-36 and SEIQoL-DW in patients with amyotrophic lateral sclerosis. *Journal of the Neurological Sciences* **191**, 103–9.
25. **Simmons, Z.** et al. (2000). Quality of life in ALS depends on factors other than strength and physical function. *Neurology* **55**, 388–92.
26. **Gallagher, D. and Monroe, B.** (2000). Psychosocial Care. In *Palliative Care in Amyotrophic Lateral Sclerosis* (ed. D. Oliver, G.D. Borasio, and D. Walsh), pp. 92–103. Oxford: Oxford University Press.
27. **Murphy, P.L.** et al. (2000). Impact of spirituality and religiousness on outcomes in patients with ALS. *Neurology* **55**, 1581–4.
28. **Borasio, G.D.** (2001). Meditation and ALS. In *Amyotrophic Lateral Sclerosis: a Comprehensive Guide to Management* (ed. H. Mitsumoto and T. Munsat), pp. 271–6. New York: Demos Medical Publ.
29. **McMurray, A.** (2000). Bereavement. In *Palliative Care in Amyotrophic Lateral Sclerosis* (ed. D. Oliver, G.D. Borasio, and D. Walsh), pp. 169–81. Oxford: Oxford University Press.
30. **O'Brien, T., Kelly, M., and Saunders, C.** (1992). Motor neuron disease: a hospice perspective. *British Medical Journal* **304**, 471–3.
31. **Borasio, G.D. and Voltz, R.** (1998). Discontinuation of life support in patients with amyotrophic lateral sclerosis. *Journal of Neurology* **245**, 717–22.
32. **Ebrahim, S.** *Clinical Epidemiology of Stroke*. Oxford: Oxford University Press, 1990.
33. **Wolf, P.A. and D'Agostino, R.B.** (1998). Epidemiology of stroke. In *Stroke, Pathophysiology, Diagnosis, and Management* 3rd edn. (ed. H.J.M. Barnett, J.P. Mohr, B.M. Stein, and F.M. Yatsu), pp. 3–28. New York: Churchill Livingston.
34. **Kwakkel, G.** et al. (1996). Predicting disability in stroke—a critical review of the literature. *Age and Ageing* **25**, 479–89.
35. **Hamann, G.F., Rogers, A., and Addington-Hall, J.** Palliative care in stroke. In *Palliative Care in Neurology* (ed. R. Voltz, J. Bernat, G.D. Borasio, I. Maddocks, D. Oliver, and R. Portenoy). Oxford: Oxford University Press (in press).
36. **Schwab, S.** et al. (1998). Early hemicraniectomy in patients with complete middle cerebral artery infarction. *Stroke* **29**, 1888–93.
37. **Berg-Dammer, E., Felber, S.R., Henkes, H., Nahser, H.C., and Kühne, D.** (2000). Long-term outcome after local intra-arterial fibrinolysis of basilar artery thrombosis. *Cerebrovascular Diseases* **10**, 183–8.
38. **Katz, R.T., Haig, A.J., Clark, B.B., and DiPaolo, R.J.** (1992). Long-term survival, prognosis, and life-care planning for 29 patients with chronic locked-in syndrome. *Archives of Physical Medicine and Rehabilitation* **73**, 403–8.
39. **Kaiser, J.** et al. (2001). Self-initiation of EEG-based communication in paralysed patients. *Clinical Neurophysiology* **112**, 551–4.
40. **van Gijn, J. and Rinkel, G.J.E.** (2001). Subarachnoid haemorrhage: diagnosis, causes and management. *Brain* **124**, 249–78.
41. **Higginson, I.J., Hearn, J., Myers, K., and Naysmith, A.** (2000). Palliative day care: what do services do? Palliative Day Care Project Group. *Palliative Medicine* **14**, 277–86.
42. **Addington-Hall, J.M., Lay, M., Altmann, D., and McCarthy, M.** (1995). Symptom control, and communication with health professionals, and hospital care of stroke patients in the last year of life as reported by surviving family, friends, and officials. *Stroke* **26**, 2242–8.

43. Rogers, A. (2001). Stroke. In *Palliative Care in Non-Cancer Patients* (ed. J. Addington-Hall and I.J. Higginson), pp. 11–19. Oxford: Oxford University Press.
44. Kehayia, E., Korner-Bitensky, N., Singer, F., Becker, R., Lamarche, M., Georges, P., and Retik, S. (1997). Differences in pain medication use in stroke patients with asphasia and without aphasia. *Stroke* **28**, 1867–70.
45. Becker, G. and Kaufman, S. (1995). Managing an uncertain illness trajectory in old age: patients' and physicians' views of stroke. *Medical Anthropology Quarterly* **9**, 13–18.
46. British Medical Association Discussion Document (1999). *Withholding and Withdrawing Life-Prolonging Medical Treatment: Guidance for Decision Making.* London: BMJ Books.
47. Nakayama, H., Jorgensen, H.S., Pedersen, P.M., Raaschon, H.O., and Olsen, T.S. (1997). Prevalence and risk factors of incontinence after stroke: the Copenhagen Stroke Study. *Stroke* **28**, 58–62.
48. Bath, P.M.W., Bath, F.J., and Smithard, D.G. (2002). Interventions for dysphagia in acute stroke (Cochrane Review). *The Cochrane Library* **1** Oxford: Update Software.
49. Norton, B., McLean, K.A., and Holmes, G.K. (1996). Outcome in patients who require a gastrostomy after stroke. *Age and Ageing* **25**, 493.
50. Braus, D.F., Krauss, J.K., and Strobel, J. (1994). The shoulder–hand syndrome after stroke: a prospective clinical trial. *Annals of Neurology* **36**, 728–33.
51. Leijon, G. and Boivie J. (1989). Central post—stroke pain—a controlled trial of amitriptyline and carbamazepine. *Pain* **36**, 27–36.
52. Vestergaard, K., Andersen, G., Gottrup, H., Kristensen, B.T., and Jensen, T.S. (2001). Lamotrigine for central poststroke pain. *Neurology* **56**, 184–90.
53. Pohjasvaara, T., Leppavuori, A., Siira, I., Vataja, R., Kaste, M., and Erkinjuntti, T. (1998). Frequency and clinical determinants of poststroke depression. *Stroke* **29**, 2311–17.
54. Gainotti, G. and Marra, C. (2002). Determinants and consequences of post-stroke depression. *Current Opinion in Neurology* **15**, 85–9.
55. Astrom, M. (1996). Generalized anxiety disorder in stroke patients. A 3-year longitudinal study. *Stroke* **27**, 270–5.
56. Schotte, W.J.M., deHain, R.J., Rijinders, P.T., Limburg, M., and Van der Bos, G.A.M. (1998). Burden of care after stroke. *Stroke* **29**, 1605–11.
57. Lucchinetti, C., Bruck, W., Parisi, J., Scheithauer, B., Rodriguez, M., and Lassmann, H. (2000). Heterogeneity of multiple sclerosis lesions: implications for the pathogenesis of demyelination. *Annals of Neurology* **47**, 707–17.
58. McDonald, W.I. et al. (2001). Recommended diagnostic criteria for multiple sclerosis: guidelines from the International Panel on the diagnosis of multiple sclerosis. *Annals of Neurology* **50**, 121–7.
59. Goodin, D.S., Frohman, E.M., Garmany, G.P. Jr, Halper, J., Likosky, W.H., Lublin, F.D., Silberberg, D.H., Stuart, W.H., and van Den Noort, S. (2002). Disease modifying therapies in multiple sclerosis: Subcommittee of the American Academy of Neurology and the MS Council for Clinical Practice Guidelines. *Neurology* **58**, 169–78.
60. Ben-Zacharia, A.B. and Lublin, F.D. (2001). Palliative care in patients with multiple sclerosis. In *Neurologic Clinics: Palliative Care* (ed. A.C. Carver and K.M. Foley), pp. 801–27. Philadelphia: WB Saunders.
61. Walther, E.U. and Hohlfeld, R. (1999). Multiple sclerosis: side effects of interferon beta therapy and their management. *Neurology* **53**, 1622–7.
62. van der Maas, P.J. et al. (1996). Euthanasia, physician-assisted suicide, and other medical practices involving the end of life in the Netherlands, 1990–1995. *New England Journal of Medicine* **335**, 1699–705.
63. Wolf, J.K. *Mastering MS: Handbook of Management.* Rutland, Vermont: Academy Books, 1996.
64. Sadovnick, A.D., Eisen, K., Ebers, G.C., and Paty, D.W. (1991). Cause of death in patients attending multiple sclerosis clinics. *Neurology* **41**, 1193–6.
65. Voltz, R., Akabayashi, A., Reese, C., Ohi, G., and Sass, H.M. (1998). End-of-life decisions and advance directives in palliative care: a cross-cultural survey of patients and health-care professionals. *Journal of Pain and Symptom Management* **16**, 153–62.
66. Starck, M., Albrecht, H., Pöllmann, D.M., and Straube, A. (1999). Memantine vs gabapentin in acquired pendular nystagmus: an observer-blind cross-over study. *Journal of Neurology,* **246** (Suppl. 1), 41.
67. Dieterich, M., Straube, A., Brandt, T., Paulus, W., and Buttner, U. (1991). The effects of baclofen and cholinergic drugs on upbeat and downbeat nystagmus. *Journal of Neurology, Neurosurgery and Psychiatry* **54**, 627–32.
68. Gbadamosi, J., Buhmann, C., Moench, A., and Heesen, C. (2001). Failure of ondansetron in treating cerebellar tremor in MS patients—an open label pilot study, *Acta Neurological Scandinavica* **104**, 308–11.
69. Shakespeare, D.T., Boggild, M., and Young, C. (2001). Anti-spasticity agents in multiple sclerosis (Cochrane Review). *Cochrane Library* **4**, Oxford.
70. Metz, L. (1998). Multiple sclerosis: symptomatic therapies. *Seminars in Neurology* **18**, 389–95.
71. Brashear, A. et al. (1999). Safety and efficacy of NeuroBloc (botulinum toxin type B) in type A-responsive cervical dystonia. *Neurology* **53**, 1439–46.
72. Smyth, M.D. and Peacock, W.J. (2000). The surgical treatment of spasticity. *Muscle and Nerve* **23**, 153–63.
73. Tubridy, N., Addison, R., and Schon, F. (1999). Long term use of desmopressin for urinary symptoms in multiple sclerosis. *Multiple Sclerosis* **5**, 416–17.
74. Solaro, C., Lunardi, G.L., Capello, E., Inglese, M., Messmer Uccelli, M., Uccelli, A., and Mancardi, G.L. (1998). An open-label trial of gabapentin treatment of paroxysmal symptoms in multiple sclerosis patients. *Neurology* **51**, 609–11.
75. Leandri, M., Cruccu, G., and Gottlieb, A. (1999). Cluster headache-like pain in multiple sclerosis. *Cephalalgia* **19**, 732–4.
76. Dahm, P.O., Nitescu, P.V., Appelgren, L.K., and Curelaru, I.I. (1998). Long-term intrathecal (i.t.) infusion of bupivacaine relieved intractable pain and spasticity in a patient with multiple sclerosis. *European Journal of Pain* **2**, 81–5.
77. Solari, A., Uitdehaag, B., Giuliani, G., Pucci, E., and Taus, C. (2001). Aminopyridines for symptomatic treatment in multiple sclerosis (Cochrane Review). *The Cochrane Library* **4**, Oxford.
78. Rammohan, K.W., Rosenberg, J.H., Lynn, D.J., Blumenfeld, A.M., Pollak, C.P., and Nagaraja, H.N. (2002). Efficacy and safety of modafinil (Provigil(R)) for the treatment of fatigue in multiple sclerosis: a two centre phase 2 study. *Journal of Neurology, Neurosurgery and Psychiatry* **72**, 179–83.
79. Formaglio, F., MacLeod, S., and Moiola, L. Demyelinating disease. In *Palliative Care in Neurology* (ed. R. Voltz, J. Bernat, G.D. Borasio, I. Maddocks, D. Oliver, and R. Portenoy). Oxford: Oxford University Press (in press).
80. Yahr, M.D. and Clough, C.G. (1983). Parkinson's disease. In *Houston Merritt Memorial Volume* (ed. M.D. Yahr). New York: Raven Press.
81. Clough, C.G. and Blockley, A. Parkinson's disease and related disorders. In *Palliative Care in Neurology* (ed. R. Voltz, J. Bernat, G.D. Borasio, I. Maddocks, D. Oliver, and R. Portenoy). Oxford: Oxford University Press (in press).
82. Hoehn, M.M. and Yahr, M.D. (1967). Parkinsonism: onset, progression and mortality. *Neurology* **17**, 427–42.
83. Müller, J. et al. (2001). Progression of dysarthria and dysphagia in postmortem-confirmed parkinsonian disorders. *Archives in Neurology* **58**, 259–64.
84. Quinn, N.P., Lang, A.E., Koller, W.C., and Marsden, C.D. (1986). Painful Parkinson's disease. *Lancet* **1**, 1366–9.

10.7 Palliative medicine and care of the elderly

Diane E. Meier and Anna Monias

Geriatric patients often suffer from multiple complex and chronic problems. Palliative care for the elderly needs to focus on the following: therapeutic interventions that can preserve function and help patients maintain quality of life; frank discussions on the usual course of illness so that patients and their family members can plan for the future; recognition and management of caregiver stress; and management of physical and psychological symptoms of both acute and chronic illnesses. This chapter will discuss why palliative care in the elderly is different from that needed by a younger population, provide a model for providing palliative care in the early, middle, and late stages of a chronic illness such as dementia, and discuss management and diagnostic techniques for alleviation of symptoms of distress commonly found in the elderly population.

Demographics

Improvements in sanitation and nutrition combined with advances in medicine have produced a dramatic increase in life expectancy. While a child born in 1900 could expect to live fewer than 50 years, life expectancy for a child born in 2010 is expected to increase to 86 years for a girl and 79 years for a boy.[1,2] By the year 2030, the percentage of the US population over 65 is projected to increase to 20 per cent compared with 5 per cent in 1900. Modern medicine can save a patient from a fatal myocardial infarction, cure an early malignancy, and effectively combat bacterial and parasitic diseases. Saving patients from heart attacks, early stage cancers, tragic accidents, or pneumonia, may mean that they live to develop heart failure, strokes, dementia, debilitating arthritis, emphysema, Parkinson's disease, diabetes, and other chronic diseases. In developed nations, the overwhelming majority of deaths occur in elderly patients suffering from multiple coexisting and progressive chronic illnesses.

Most research on dying has been on younger populations despite the fact that death occurs more commonly in the elderly. The largest study of adult hospital deaths in the United States had a median age of 66 while the median age of death in the United States is 77.[3] Some studies suggest that elderly patients receive fewer burdensome life-prolonging interventions irrespective of baseline functional measures.[4,5] This difference may be due to de facto rationing based on age rather than emphasis on individualizing the goals of care.

Data on treatment of pain in old age suggests that elderly patients also receive less pain medication than younger persons for chronic and acute pain. Nearly 30 per cent of elderly cancer patients living in long-term care facilities did not receive pain medication despite daily complaints of pain, and another 16 per cent received only acetaminophen/paracetamol; these percentages increased with age and minority ethnicity.[6] Age and female gender were predictors of under-treatment of pain in a study of ambulatory patients with cancer.[7] Geriatric patients with hip fracture also receive inadequate pain control, particularly if suffering from cognitive impairment.[8,9] Chronic pain syndromes such as arthritis, low back syndrome, and other musculoskeletal problems affect 25–50 per cent of the community dwelling elderly and are also typically under-treated.[10] Given the prevalence of cognitive impairment, musculoskeletal disorders, and malignant disease in the elderly, these studies indicate that pain is inadequately identified and treated in the geriatric population.

Caregiver burden

Elderly patients who require palliative treatments to control pain and discomfort are more likely than younger patients to have an increased dependence on others for basic daily activities such as dressing, meal preparation, eating, and ambulating. Typically, care needs are met by family members. Women (spouses, daughters, and daughters-in-law) provide most family (non-reimbursed) care giving. These volunteer caregivers provide labour that is worth $196 billion annually. Paid care provides the sole source of caregiver support in only 15–20 per cent of patients, particularly for elderly women who are more likely to live alone following the death of a spouse.[11]

The SUPPORT trials found that, in a younger cohort, 55 per cent of patients had persistent and intensive family caregiving needs during the course of a terminal illness, a figure that rises exponentially with increasing age.[12] Furthermore, for elderly patients with chronic illnesses, the duration of family caregiving may exceed 10 years. Caregiving has been associated with decreased immunity and is a risk factor for death, major depression, and associated co-morbidities.[13] Close to 90 per cent of caregivers say they need more help caring for their loved ones in one or more categories including transportation, homemaking, nursing, and personal care.[11]

The tremendous growth in numbers of people over 65 with chronic health problems has burdened national and personal resources. Fifty per cent of caregivers have financial difficulties. The decision to hospitalize or institutionalize is often dependent on lack of insurance reimbursement, family finances, and the availability of paid or non-paid help that would allow care at home. Growth in the elderly population in the United States has led to projections of a 73 per cent increase in Medicare and long-term expenditures over the next several decades.[14,15] Over half of all bankruptcies in people older than 65 have been attributed to medical expenses.[2] More than 25 million Americans deliver an average of 18 h of care per week to seriously ill relatives resulting in $194 billion in uncompensated care yearly based on conservative estimate of $8 hourly rate.[16]

Costs of care of Alzheimer's disease and other chronic illnesses include unpaid hours that caregivers spend with patients and lost wages due to hours missed from paid employment. The economic burden of caregiving becomes clear when the estimated 10-year cost for men with Alzheimer's disease is compared to the estimated 10-year cost for women. Expenses for a man are estimated at $67 000; however, for a woman, who frequently has less informal support, the estimated 10-year direct cost is $109 000.[17] In the United States, Medicaid and Medicare expenditures on dementia patients are significantly more than on age-matched cognitively intact patients.[18–21]

When there are no family caregivers, or care needs become too great, patients are placed in a nursing home. Twenty per cent of the population over 85 live in nursing homes.[22] Patients suffering from dementia are more likely to spend their last days in a nursing home than cognitively intact elderly patients dying from non-dementing illness.

Dementia as a model for chronic illness

While physical symptoms associated with terminal disease should be controlled throughout illness, there are unique issues to address in each stage of illness. Providing palliative care to geriatric and non-geriatric patients with chronic illness means that at different stages of illness, patients will require preventive, life-prolonging, rehabilitative, and palliative measures in varying proportions based on individual needs. In this chapter, dementia will be used as a model for a chronic illness that requires palliative care in each stage of disease (Table 1). Irreversible dementia has been chosen as the model because of its chronicity, increasing prevalence with advanced age, and the likelihood that patients with dementia will also suffer from other concurrent and chronic illnesses common amongst the elderly.

Palliative care in early stages of chronic illness

After a chronic, progressive disease such as dementia is diagnosed, medical providers should inform patients and caregivers of the diagnosis, prognosis, and treatment options. If they know what to expect, patients can think

Table 1 A checklist for palliative care throughout the course of chronic illness

Diagnosis		
Determine stage of illness		
Early	**Middle**	**Late**
Discuss diagnosis prognosis and course of disease	Assess efficacy of disease modifying therapy	Discuss goals of care with patient and family
Discuss disease modifying therapies	Review course of disease	Confirm previous advance directives
Discuss goals of care, hopes, and expectations	Reassess goals of care and expectations	Actively manage symptoms
Discuss advance care planning	Confirm advance directives and ensure a health-care proxy is appointed	Review financial resources and needs
Manage comorbidities	Recommend PT/OT therapies to preserve function and promote socialization	Review long-term care needs and discuss options
Advise financial planning/consultation with a social worker for future needs including long-term care	Behavioural and pharmacologic symptom control	Consider hospice referral/planning to ensure peaceful death
Inform patient and family about support groups	Treat mood disorders	Assess spiritual needs
Inquire about desire for spiritual support	Suggest support groups for patient and caregiver	Offer respite care
Behavioural and pharmacologic symptom control	Offer social and emotional support to caregivers	
Treat mood disorders	Review long-term care options and resource needs	

about the way in which they would like to spend their remaining functional time and discuss these wishes with their families. They will have time to make necessary financial arrangements, complete important tasks, and plan for future medical care. Patients should be advised to consult an attorney or financial advisor.

Physicians should discuss goals of care with their patients, realizing that each individual patient may have different values and belief systems. Goals may change as disease progresses. In early chronic disease, goals may include prolonging life, preserving autonomy, maintaining social activities, and forming a plan for advanced stages of disease. In later stages of disease, goals may shift to providing maximum comfort and security.

Advance directives should be discussed early in disease when the patients may still be able to make decisions for themselves. The expected decline in cognitive and functional status needs to be disclosed during discussions about advance directives because preferences for life-sustaining therapy are influenced by presumed quality of life.[23] Patients should be asked under what circumstances death would be preferable to life-sustaining treatments such as ventilator support and artificial nutrition and hydration. Health-care providers should also advise patients to appoint one or more primary decision-makers in preparation for the time that they are no longer able to make medical decisions for themselves. Discussing advance directives with the patients and their family members may reduce stress associated with surrogate decision-making later in the course of the disease.[24] Although it is important to honestly describe the course of illness, range of potential benefits, outcomes, and potential harms of therapies, these issues should be raised over the course of several visits. Otherwise, the patient and family members may become overwhelmed by the complexity and seriousness of the decisions before them.

Medical therapy should focus on preserving function and quality of life and delaying progression of the illness, if possible. For example, in dementia, this would be the period to start therapy with acetylcholinesterase inhibitors. Safe and generally well tolerated, these drugs may modestly improve cognition and functional status and have been shown to delay nursing home placement.[25,26]

Medical therapy should also treat secondary effects of the illness such as anxiety and depression. Psychiatric symptoms in patients with chronic disease are common and difficult to treat. Fifty per cent or more patients with Alzheimer's, Parkinson's, and vascular dementia suffer from depressive symptoms. Anxiety may be present in as many as 40 per cent of Alzheimer's patients. The period after diagnosis is a time of great adjustment and grief for the patient and caregivers. For many married couples, a diagnosis of dementia or another chronic illness means that the healthier spouse will need to take on chores previously done by the patient. Adult children may also have to play a caregiving role for a parent for the first time. Depressive symptoms may be confused with personality changes—indifference, limited emotional engagement, and decreased motivation—that frequently occur in Alzheimer's disease.[27] Disease-specific therapy with cholinesterase inhibitors may improve psychiatric symptoms, and should be tried before or concomitant with antidepressant therapy.

Selective serotonin reuptake inhibitors are often the first-line medication for treating depression in the elderly due to their safe side-effect profile and minimal drug interactions. In elderly patients, practitioners often use a lower starting dose to minimize side-effects; however, doses often need to be titrated to the same doses used in younger patients in order to be effective. Support groups may be helpful to both patients and caregivers at this time. Patients may suffer fear of being a burden on family members, dependency, loss of dignity, and abandonment.

Occupational and physical therapy may help the patient learn compensatory mechanisms that can help maintain their independence. Patients may derive short-term cognitive and behavioural benefits from reality orientation.[28]

Some chronic illnesses may 'skip' the early or middle stages of disease. Often, progressive dementia is not diagnosed until the middle or late stage. A patient who suffers from an acute stroke or massive myocardial infarction may transition suddenly from complete independence to total dependence. While the initial loss is sometimes partially recovered through physical and occupational therapy, the patient often remains severely debilitated. This phenomenon underscores the importance of discussing advance directives when patients are healthy. The independent patient with hypertension, hyperlipidemia, and diabetes is at risk for stroke or myocardial infarction and should be treated as having an early stage of a chronic progressive illness.

Middle stage of chronic illness

While palliative care in the early stages of chronic illness is marked by efforts to delay progression of disease and plan for the future, the middle stage of disease is defined by increased medical needs, declining function and independence, and increased dependence on caregivers for assistance with basic activities. It is important to note that each stage of a progressive chronic illness may last for years. Patients with dementia require increased supervision during this stage. Patients with Parkinson's disease, heart failure, or rheumatologic diseases may need more assistance with ambulation. Often, the home needs to be evaluated so that adaptive devices can be installed such as raised toilet seats, shower seats, and grab bars. Assistive devices can help the patient preserve independence and remain in their own homes.

The increased need for supervision results in great caregiver stress and this may lead to consideration of nursing home placement. Patients with moderate dementia but without other co-morbidities are sometimes difficult to place in nursing homes due to low reimbursement for 'custodial care'. Availability of adult day care and respite care is inadequate and costs of such services are high in the United States. Caregivers suffer increased burden during the middle stage of chronic illnesses. Many work two jobs—one at their place of employment and one at home. Demands at home may result in decreased sleep and poor job performance. Caregivers may feel unappreciated because patients, in the case of dementia, may not be able to express appreciation and in the case of other chronic illness may express resentment due to their frustration with declining functional status. Health-care providers can assist caregivers by giving them information about local resources for adult day care, respite care, homemaker services, and support groups. Physicians should encourage caregivers to attend to their own needs and to try to mobilize a regular rotating schedule of respite support from family and friends. This will help the caregiver maintain physical, financial, and emotional strength for the multi-year task before them.

Patients with moderate dementia often begin to experience weight loss, in part due to decreased acuity of taste and smell. Decreased sensitivity of thirst receptors may predispose patients to dehydration. Patients may develop apraxia for use of eating utensils. Offering frequent, nutritious snacks, preferably as finger foods, may help. Specially designed utensils such as deep dishes and large spoons may make feeding easier. Caregivers can compensate for decreased smell and taste by adding sweeteners and extra spices to food to make it more palatable. It may be helpful to relax dietary restrictions that patients are under for other concurrent illnesses.

Physical symptoms of chronic disease—pain, dyspnoea, anorexia, nausea, vomiting, changes in bowel habits, insomnia—may also become prominent during this phase of disease. These symptoms should be aggressively treated as outlined in other chapters. New symptoms that develop after diagnosis of a chronic, progressive illness should always be thoroughly evaluated in order to identify reversible aetiology and determine the most effective treatment.

Behavioural symptoms become more frequent as dementia progresses.[29] Patients often suffer from paranoia, delusions, hallucinations, sleep disorders, agitation, and combativeness; these symptoms are associated with rapid cognitive and functional decline.[27,29] Aggressive behaviours are seen in more than 50 per cent of patients with Alzheimer's disease and nearly 20 per cent assault their caregivers at some point in their illness.[30] These symptoms put an incredible burden on caregivers who may feel betrayed and unappreciated when patients cannot express gratitude and cannot realize how much they rely on their caregivers. During the middle stage, caregivers will also continue to mourn the passing of the individual they once knew. Development of aggressive behaviour and paranoia place a greater burden on caregivers than memory loss and significantly increase the likelihood of nursing home placement.[27,31]

When behavioural symptoms develop, physicians should take a careful history and examine the patient to rule out co-morbidities such as urinary tract infection, pain, constipation or faecal impaction, bladder outlet obstruction, or other source of discomfort. Patients with mild to moderate dementia may not complain of pain in the same way as cognitively intact patients.[22,32] Patients who have lost the ability to express themselves verbally can only communicate by grimacing, screaming, withdrawing, tense body posture, and expressing fear or agitation. Treating a reversible cause of discomfort relieves agitation in a significant percentage of dementia patients.

When no underlying cause for agitated behaviour is found, the caregiver should try to determine whether particular activities or settings instigate unwanted behaviours. Bathing and grooming often provoke hitting and yelling because dementia patients may perceive these activities as assaults. Encouraging patients to participate in their own grooming and bathing may decrease agitation.[33] Sponge baths and adjusting water temperature may make bathing less threatening. Playing tapes of family members telling favourite memories may also provide comfort to dementia patients.[34] Familiar music and frequent social activities may also exert calming influence. Seventy per cent of dementia patients may have insomnia or 'sundowning', a syndrome of increasing confusion during the evening. Daytime exercises, a consistent bedtime routine, and minimizing daytime napping can help improve sleep patterns.[35]

Pharmacological therapy is often needed in addition to behavioural management techniques. The primary therapy of behavioural abnormalities in dementia should be disease-specific cholinesterase inhibition such as donepezil, galantamine, or rivastigmine. Low doses of neuroleptics can ameliorate confusion, hallucinations, and delusions. Second-generation antipsychotics (risperidone, quetiapine, and olanzapine) cause less extrapyramidal toxicity than first-generation antipsychotics; however, patients still need to be monitored for parkinsonism. Electrocardiograms should be checked periodically because these medications can cause prolonged QT intervals. Successful management of agitation can prevent hospital admissions and nursing home placement.

Reassessing goals of care

Patients and family decision-makers will need to consider the goals of care in the case of superimposed acute illness in the setting of chronic illness. Do they want to continue or forego preventive health services? Would they choose medical therapy over surgical therapy for acute angina? Physicians can help weigh the risks and benefits of such procedures in light of the individual patient's current health status and their previously stated goals for medical care. Some surgeries are clearly palliative. For example, cataract surgery can make a tremendous improvement in a patient's quality of life; however, repair of an asymptomatic abdominal aortic aneurysm may not be indicated in a patient with severe disability due to chronic illness.

End-stage of chronic illness

Patients in the end-stage of a chronic disease are often bed- or chair-bound. They become completely dependent on caregivers for feeding, toileting, bathing, and dressing and are incontinent. Due to increased care demands and exhaustion of family caregivers, patients frequently require placement in a nursing home when they reach this stage of illness.

In the last few months of life, patients sometimes lose the ability to complain of pain and other symptoms. Pain is often under-treated in end-stage dementia.[9] At this stage of disease, mortality is 50 per cent at 6 months; therefore, physicians should support goals of care that promote palliation of suffering and maximum quality of life, provided that those goals are consistent with the patient's previous values and expressed wishes.[36,37]

Physicians should talk to patients and surrogate decision-makers about cessation of phlebotomy and other painful 'routine' procedures.[38] Patients who reside in a nursing home and want to remain in the comfort and security of familiar surroundings and faces may elect to have a 'do not transfer' order so that they are not routinely transferred to the hospital for intercurrent illness or for symptoms that can be managed in the nursing home.

Caring for patients in a familiar environment reduces physiological and psychosocial disturbances that occur as a result of transfer from one environment to another. These symptoms of loneliness, anxiety, depression, and agitation that occur when patients move from a familiar environment are called 'transfer anxiety' or 'relocation stress syndrome'.[39,40]

A multidisciplinary team is critical to caring for patients at the end-stage of chronic illness. In addition to the patient, the team consists of the caregiver, the physician, the nurse, the social worker, and occupational and physical therapists. For patients living at home or in a nursing home, the caregiver and nurse can alert the primary care provider to physiological and behavioural changes before hospitalization is needed. Clinical social workers can give psychotherapy, inform patients and caregivers about community resources, support groups, respite care, and home care services, and help navigate through complex insurance regulations. Physical and occupational therapists can help the patient retain their independence by teaching energy saving techniques and providing equipment that facilitates walking, using utensils, and toileting in patients with increasing levels of disability. Referral to medical specialists is often helpful in managing symptoms. For example, it may be appropriate to refer a patient to a geriatric psychiatrist for assistance with managing behavioural symptoms in end-stage dementia or Parkinson's disease. Together, the team will likely need to face issues such as development of pressure ulcers, need for supplemental nutrition, infection, and delirium. In addition to caring for the patient, the team needs to care for the caregiver.

Pressure ulcers

Patients who are bed-bound, incontinent, and poorly nourished often develop decubitus ulcers. In the end-stage of terminal disease, patients suffer cachexia secondary to poor appetite, decreased oral intake, and a catabolic state. Though ulcers are often preventable if patients are turned frequently and receive good skin care, they frequently occur in the last stages of illness because providing the level of nursing necessary for prevention is difficult. Treatment of ulcers depends on goals of care. In a patient with long life expectancy who develops an ulcer after an acute illness, the ulcer should be treated with standard management guidelines. However, in the terminal patient, care should focus on relieving pain and limiting odour. Analgesia should be provided prior to all dressing changes. Odour can be controlled with topical metronidazole gel, silver sulfadiazine, or powdered sugar. Vinegar, activated charcoal, vanilla oils, or lemon can also be used to control odours in a patient's room. Although the development of decubitus ulcers is not an independent risk factor for death, the presence of a wound is a marker of advanced stage of disease and poor prognosis.[41,42]

Artificial nutrition and hydration

Patients suffering from end-stage dementia and other chronic neurological illnesses develop dysphagia, which predisposes them to aspiration pneumonia.[43] Changing the texture of the diet to puree with liquids that are thickened with cornstarch or potato starch may support safe swallowing.[44] Caregivers should also be trained to feed the patient in an upright position, with the head forward, using small spoonfuls of a soft, puree diet. In the late stages of dementia, patients frequently refuse food, clamp their mouth shut, or hold food without swallowing. Feeding may become a frustrating battle between patient and caregiver. When patients can no longer meet their caloric needs or when recurrent aspirations have occurred, health professionals in the United States often offer artificial nutrition and hydration.

Artificial nutrition and hydration is an emotionally charged issue for many caregivers. They may believe that their loved one would suffer hunger without artificial nutrition and hydration. While many patients receive artificial nutrition in the last days of life, there is no evidence that it prolongs life or relieves suffering in patients with terminal dementia.[36,45–47] Family members should understand that loss of appetite is an integral part of the dying process. Studies of terminally ill cognitively intact patients with anorexia have shown that they do not suffer hunger and that symptoms of thirst can be relieved with good oral hygiene, artificial saliva, and sips of water.[48] Artificial nutrition has not been associated with wound healing or increased albumin levels in patients with terminal illness.[45,49] Tube feeding does not decrease the risk of aspiration pneumonia and some studies actually show an increased risk.[45,50]

Despite the lack of proven benefits from tube feeding, some caregivers will still request it for their loved ones. The decision to proceed with tube feeding should only occur after careful consideration of the patient's life goals at this stage of irreversible illness as well as the risks of operative complications and side-effects such as diarrhoea, infection, and aspiration, and need for physical restraints.[51]

Families requesting artificial nutrition and hydration should be offered a time-limited trial of therapy. If artificial nutrition does not improve the patient's quality of life after a trial of several months, it can be discontinued based on failure to achieve the desired goals. Parenteral nutrition is ill advised for patients with an intact gastrointestinal tract because placement of long-term intravenous catheters is a nidus for serious infection and loss of intraluminal nutrients may cause deterioration of the intestinal wall, leading to systemic infection from gut flora.[50]

Enteral feeding can be nasogastric or through gastrostomy or jejunostomy tube. The nasogastric tube is uncomfortable even when small-bore tubes are used. Patients often pull the tubes out even when restraints are used. This means that they have to undergo multiple nasogastric tube placements and multiple radiographic studies to check placement. Nasogastric feeding should be temporary, usually for less than 30 days. Patients who develop abrupt onset of dysphagia during an acute, concurrent illness may benefit from time-limited nasogastric feeding. Complications of nasogastric tube placement include pulmonary intubation, pneumothorax, aspiration pneumonitis, and nasal irritation. Placement of gastrostomy and jejunostomy tubes also has risks. Patients require local and in some cases general anaesthesia and sedation. Often, patients require restraints for the first 24–48 h after placement. Local wound infections are frequent and rarely perforation of viscus, necrotizing fasciitis, and colocutaneous fistula can occur. Patients can also suffer from aspiration due to supine positioning during feeding, bolus feeding, and inability to swallow oropharyngeal secretions. Diarrhoea is also common and multifactorial in origin. Causes include formula composition, rate of infusion, hypoalbuminemia, and altered bacteria flora. *Clostridium difficile* infection rate is higher in patients receiving tube feeding than in similar patients who are not receiving artificial nutrition.[52]

Infection

The late stages of many terminal illnesses are commonly complicated by life-threatening infections.[53] Immobility, malnutrition, incontinence, aspiration, and decreased immunity increase risk of pneumonia, cellulitis, decubitus ulcers, urinary tract infections, and sepsis.[54] Decreased ability to express oneself and atypical presentation may lead to delayed recognition of infections.

Palliative care should focus on reducing risk factors for infection by providing patients with good skin care, ambulation training, and aspiration precautions. Incontinent patients should have diapers changed frequently; toileting schedules may also help. Turning patients frequently will also prevent decubitus ulcers. Skin should be kept clean and dry; friction and shear should be avoided.

Comfort measures should be implemented when patients develop infection. Antipyretics can be given orally or rectally on an around the clock schedule. Analgesics for pain or dyspnoea and oxygen should also be given to alleviate symptoms. Antibiotics can be prescribed, withheld, or withdrawn in the end-stage of chronic illness depending on the goals of care.

As with all other treatments, the risks and benefits of antibiotic therapy should be weighed. For example, a patient with cellulitis may have symptomatic relief with antibiotics. A patient with *Clostridium difficile* diarrhoea will have relief of symptoms with antibiotic treatment. Antibiotics may also relieve fever, cough, dysuria, and shortness of breath. Patients with repeated aspiration pneumonia due to inability to swallow oropharyngeal secretions are less likely to have a benefit in terms of either symptom relief or survival. Antibiotics do not improve survival in advanced dementia.[55]

Disadvantages of antibiotic therapy include the risk of allergic reaction, need for repeated placement of an intravenous catheter, development of antibiotic-resistant infections, and frequent blood draws to monitor drug levels. Antibiotics can cause diarrhoea, bone marrow failure, renal failure, seizures, and vomiting. In addition, an elderly patient with end-stage dementia often will require restraints in order to tolerate placement of intravenous lines, phlebotomy, and intramuscular injections.

Delirium

More than 90 per cent of patients suffer from delirium during the last stage of their illness.(56) The risk of delirium increases with age, cognitive impairment, infection, organ failure, and fracture(57) Delirium may be agitated or apathetic. Agitated delirium is a frightening and distressing terminal symptom for both patient and family members alike. Treatment should include treating any reversibly underlying cause such as impaction, pain, urinary tract infection, electrolyte imbalance, or fever, minimizing sensory impairment by providing the patient with eyeglasses and hearing aids, and minimizing unnecessary noise and nighttime lights. Even in advanced cancer, treating the underlying cause may reverse delirium in 50 per cent of patients.(56) Antipsychotic agents provide symptomatic relief for both agitated and apathetic delirium and are preferable to benzodiazepines, which are ineffective in the treatment of delirium.(58) Sedating antipsychotic agents such as chlorpromazine may help relieve symptoms of anxiety and pain in patients with agitated delirium. In addition to providing comfort to the patient, alleviation of delirium also provides enormous comfort to family and caregivers.

Hospice

Although hospice care is appropriate for patients with end-stage dementia and other chronic illnesses, hospice is accessed less frequently for these patients than for cancer patients, probably because it is more difficult to accurately identify a 6-month survival.(36,37,59,60) In fact, hospice care with support for personal care services is critically necessary in patients suffering from long-term chronic illness who often require more help at home in the last year of life than cancer patients.(61)

Care of the caregiver

Caregivers of geriatric patients in the end-stage of chronic disease often need as much or more attention from the medical team as the patient. While family caregivers may take enormous satisfaction from their ability to provide safe and loving care for their loved one, most also feel varying degrees of exhaustion, guilt, and frustration. The patient's many-year illness typically places a significant financial burden on the caregiver. The interdisciplinary team should be called upon to help families access community resources and financial planning experts.

Simply by listening to and trying to help address the concerns of caregivers, the medical team conveys the fact that the caregiver is not alone and that her concerns are legitimate and important. Studies have shown that family caregivers' impression of having been listened to by health providers improves well-being and clinical outcomes for both patient and caregiver. Family caregivers should be reminded and helped to pay attention to their own physical and emotional needs. Community volunteers, family members, formal respite programmes in local nursing homes or through hospice programmes, or paid help may be able to stay with the patient so that the family caregiver has time off. The patient's needs can only be met if the caregiver is healthy—physically and emotionally. Caregiver stress can lead to poor care, neglect, and abuse of the patient and an increased burden of illness in both. If a caregiver appears tired, irritated, or frustrated, respite care options should be identified and recommended.

Caregiver stress does not end after placement in a nursing home. Caregivers continue to worry about the patient as well as suffer guilt over the necessity of nursing home placement. Clinicians should provide support and validation of the necessity and appropriateness of the placement decision and point out ways for family to continue to care for their loved one (e.g. regularly scheduled visits, volunteer work in the nursing home, spoon feeding, hand massage, reading aloud, bringing in favourite music or foods). Caregivers universally face difficult medical and goals of care decisions when the question of tube feeding, hospitalization for predictable infection, and use of antibiotics arise. Health professionals can facilitate both these decisions and the caregivers' confidence in the appropriateness of their ultimate choices on behalf of their loved one, by helping focus the discussion on the goals of care, the patient's values and preferences, and the benefit versus burden of the various available interventions.(62) After death, the caregiver will need to make funeral arrangements and manage financial affairs, while grieving and adjusting to a profound loss of role and purpose. Many caregivers have suspended their own lives in order to care for the deceased, often for many years. The resulting void is difficult to fill, placing these caregivers at high risk of complicated or prolonged bereavement. Bereavement support groups specific for caregivers of persons dying after years of chronic illness and decline are helpful—the caregiver feels less alone with her loss and the establishment of new social connections and relationships afforded by the group facilitates re-entry into a more interactive social existence.

Common sources of suffering and discomfort in the elderly

Patients may suffer even when they are free of pain. Practitioners need to ask about suffering as well as pain.(63) Questions should be open ended in order to help make the patient comfortable with discussing fear, anxiety, and other non-physical symptoms. A sample question to patients is 'How are you feeling inside yourself?' A sample question to family members is 'Are you concerned that your family member may be suffering or uncomfortable?' Relief of pain goes hand in hand with treatment of the emotional and spiritual components that contribute to it.(63) Patients often report pain but do not tell health-care providers about other sources of suffering. Formal assessment is crucial to management of diverse symptoms. There are many simple, validated scales to measures to assess pain and suffering. They include the Edmonton Symptom Assessment Scale (ESAS), which measures eight symptoms on visual analogue scales, and the Memorial Symptom Assessment Scale (MSAS), which delineates the intensity, frequency, and level of distress of 32 physical and psychological symptoms.(64,65) Uncomfortable physical symptoms often encountered in elderly patients with terminal and chronic disease include fatigue, pain, dyspnoea, cough, gastrointestinal complaints, anxiety, depression, dry skin, pruritis, and spiritual distress.

Pain

Treatment of pain in the elderly generally follows the same guidelines as in younger adults. In addition to the ESAS and the MSAS, pain intensity can be evaluated in frail older adults using the Simple Descriptive Pain Intensity Scale, the Numeric Pain Intensity Scale, and the Visual Analog Scale. The Functional Pain Scale has also been validated in the elderly.(66) Comprehensive pain assessment of geriatric patients should also include evaluation of mental status, functional status (ADL and IADL), and depression. Depression and functional decline can have an effect on pain perception. Studies of nursing home and community dwelling elders have shown that patients with moderate to advanced dementia can complete pain assessment scales.(67)

There is conflicting evidence on changes that occur in the nociceptive system with aging.(68) Studies on clinical pain perception indicate that pain from headache and visceral pain decrease in the elderly, but musculoskeletal, leg, and foot pain increase with aging.(69) A decrease in visceral pain perception may account for atypical presentation of myocardial infarction and acute abdomen in the elderly. Older patients also seem to experience less pain from cancer-related diagnosis.(68) However, studies also show that pain is under-treated in the elderly, and in one study, nearly 86 per cent of community dwelling patients reported some pain.(9,67) Even if nociceptive perception is decreased in the elderly, diseases likely to cause chronic pain have a higher prevalence in the elderly. These diseases include arthritis, polymyalgia rheumatica, atherosclerotic disease, temporal arteritis, cancer, zoster, and peripheral neuropathy.

When evaluating the geriatric patient, the clinician first needs to take a history and physical to determine the characteristics, precipitants, acuity, and severity of the pain. If the pain is new and acute, the characteristics of the pain and the physical exam will help the clinician determine the cause. In acute pain, treating the cause is often the best way to relieve pain. For example, a patient with acute appendicitis, bowel obstruction, or acute cholecystitis would be best served by surgery. A patient with pain secondary to cellulitis will benefit most from antibiotics, and a cancer patient with cord compression will need steroids and radiotherapy. However, the patient should be given analgesic pain relief to provide comfort in addition to treating the underlying cause. Patients suffering from moderate to severe acute pain should be started on opioids; they do not need to go through the WHO ladder in stepwise faction. The usual starting dose for opioids in the elderly is 5–10 mg of a short-acting morphine (or equivalent) every 3–4 h.

The clinician should know which, if any, analgesic medications the patient has been prescribed and whether she is taking them as prescribed. If the patient is not taking the medications, the clinician should elicit the reason. Many elderly patients avoid taking even non-opioid analgesics because of fear of dependence or addiction. They may tell you that they are not 'pill takers'. If this is the case, patients should be reassured about the safety of analgesia, and encouraged to try the pain medication. Often, patients will stop taking pain medication because of its predictable and manageable side-effects such as constipation or sleepiness. Physicians should then forewarn patients and families about common side-effects and prepare them for what to expect. For example, opioid naïve patients should be warned of the likelihood of transient sleepiness and nausea for the first several days of opioid therapy. All opioid prescriptions must be accompanied by an aggressive and comprehensive bowel regimen.

Analgesic prescribing in the elderly

Acetaminophen/paracetamol is the first-line treatment for chronic pain in the elderly due to its safety profile. Many patients with chronic pain from osteoarthritis or frequent episodes of acute, mild pain from muscle strain can control symptoms with 1 g of acetaminophen/paracetamol. The elderly should be advised not to take more than 3 g of acetaminophen/paracetamol per day. This medication also should not be prescribed in patients who abuse alcohol. Liver function tests should be monitored periodically, particularly if the patient is taking other hepatotoxic medications.

Nonsteroidal anti-inflammatory drugs (NSAIDs) are also indicated for mild pain and may be more effective than acetaminophen/ paracetamol.[70,71] These medications have a synergistic effect with acetaminophen/paracetamol and opioids. They are effective in neuropathic and musculoskeletal pain, but their use has been limited by significantly increased risk of gastrointestinal bleeding, peptic ulcer, and renal failure. Risk of serious gastrointestinal events increases with age and can be reduced with use of a cytoprotective agent or proton pump inhibitor. Patients are also at increased risk of bleeding due to decreased platelet function. The newer COX-2 inhibitors have decreased risk of gastrointestinal side-effects and have become a well-tolerated analgesic therapy in the elderly. NSAIDs are contraindicated in patients with renal failure because of direct nephrotoxicity. Patients taking NSAIDs can also develop oedema and hypertension due to increased sodium reabsorption in the loop of Henle. The elderly may be more susceptible to adverse effects from NSAIDs due to decreased hepatic and renal clearance. NSAIDs can affect warfarin metabolism and patients taking both medications should have their INR monitored more frequently. Aspirin should not be co-administered with NSAIDs.

Mild musculoskeletal and neuropathic pain can also be treated with capsaicin cream. Capsaicin, a derivative of hot peppers, inhibits substance P reuptake. Capsaicin should be used every 6–8 h; otherwise, substance P will reaccumulate. Patients should be started on the lowest strength (0.025 per cent) and warned that they may initially experience burning with application of the cream, and to avoid contact with the eyes or nasal passages. Patients will begin to feel the effects of the cream after two to three applications. Anaesthetic topical preparations may also help with neuropathic pain. Lidocaine is now available in a patch that can be placed on intact skin for up to 12 h.[72]

Both acetaminophen/paracetamol and NSAIDs have maximum doses above which there is no further therapeutic benefit but rather increased toxicity. In contrast, opioids can be titrated until pain is relieved or side-effects occur.[73] With aging, patients may require reduced doses of opioids for chronic and acute pain.[74] In addition, patients with impaired renal function should receive less frequent dosing of opioids. Choice of opioid depends on individual response and side-effect profile. Often, patients who develop side-effects with one opioid may be able to tolerate a different medication.[75] Morphine, oxycodone, and hydrocodone are the most commonly used opioids for severe pain in the elderly. Fentanyl is available in a transdermal patch and may be an excellent choice for patients who cannot tolerate oral therapy. Meperidine, a short acting mu agonist should not be used in the elderly due to the risk of accumulation of its metabolite nor-meperidine, which can cause mood irritability and seizures.

Antidepressants, anticonvulsants, and glucocorticoids have a role as adjuvant therapy, particularly for neuropathic pain. Tricyclic antidepressants have been well studied for neuropathic pain. When used for this purpose, they can be started at 1/2 to 1/3 the dose used for depression.[76] Amitriptyline is not recommended in elderly patients due to anticholinergic toxicity including constipation, dry mouth, urinary retention, and tachycardia. Nortriptyline and desipramine are better tolerated. SSRIs have not been as well studied for chronic pain, but have a better safety profile than tricyclics and are believed to be of use as an adjuvant therapy.

Carbamezapine, valproate, and gabapentin also are effective for neuropathic pain. Gabapentin has become a popular adjuvant therapy due its safety profile and it does not require monitoring of blood levels. Gabapentin dosing should be adjusted for decreased renal clearance.

Steroids can increase appetite, improve mood, and lower pain perception in patients with pain due to malignancy.[77] Steroids are effective adjuvant analgesics in pain due to bony metastases and spinal cord compression. The likely mechanism of analgesic effect is the inhibition of prostaglandin synthesis and reduction in tumour oedema.[78] Steroids are usually started at doses equivalent to 4–8 mg of dexamethasone two to three times daily. Beneficial effects are seen within a few days after beginning treatment and often wane after a few weeks. Steroids should be tapered to the lowest effective dose. Side-effects include euphoria, hypertension, osteoporosis, elevated blood glucose, oedema, and myopathy.

Non-pharmacologic treatment of pain in the elderly

Alternative therapies may also be a useful adjuvant that decreases the need for pharmacotherapy in elderly patients with chronic pain. Hypnosis in highly motivated patients can have utility in pain management.[79] Cognitive therapy, like hypnosis, encourages patients to develop a means of managing their own symptoms.[80] Modalities such as massage, heat, cold, ultrasound, and electrotherapy may play a positive role in managing musculoskeletal pain. Patients who are bed-bound secondary to stroke benefit from a range of motion exercises, which prevent development of contractures.

Nausea and vomiting

Nausea and vomiting is an extremely common source of suffering. It is a common side-effect of many medications taken by elderly patients including opioids. In addition, over 60 per cent of cancer patients have nausea and vomiting during their illness.[81] The physiology of nausea and vomiting involves the central nervous system and the gastrointestinal system. It can be caused by obstruction of the gastrointestinal tract, ulcer or irritation of the gastrointestinal lining, disturbance of the vestibular system, increased intracranial pressure, meningial irritation, and stimulation of the chemoreceptor trigger zone by medications. The neurotransmitters involved in nausea and vomiting include serotonin, dopamine, acetylcholine, and histamine; knowledge of these mediators directs drug therapy. Common causes of nausea and vomiting in the elderly are drug reactions, reaction to opioids, benign positional vertigo, gastroparesis due to diabetes, and constipation. Inferior wall myocardial infarction often presents with nausea and vomiting in the elderly. This is due to stimulation of the vagus nerve. Treatment of nausea and vomiting depends on the cause.

Nausea from opioids is usually dopamine mediated. Haloperidol is a highly effective antiemetic that works at the dopamine receptor and may cause less sedation than the phenothiazines or antihistamines. Serotonin antagonists such as ondansetron and granisetron are used in chemotherapy related nausea. Patients with a conditioned nausea and vomiting response may benefit from taking benzodiazepines prior to the noxious stimulus.

Constipation

Constipation is a nearly universal complaint of elderly patients. Over half of the community dwelling elderly report constipation.[82] Risk factors include female gender, medications, depression, and immobility.[83–86] Many chronic diseases also predispose patients to constipation—Parkinson's disease, hypothyroidism, diabetes mellitus, diverticular disease, irritable bowel syndrome, and haemorrhoids. It is also one of the few side-effects of opioids that does not decrease with time. Common medications, in addition to opioids, which predispose to constipation, include calcium, iron, calcium channel blockers, antihistamines, tricyclic antidepressants, and diuretics.

When taking a history of constipation, the clinician should ask about frequency, consistency, pain, and diet. If constipation is new or refractory, further evaluation may be necessary to exclude an obstructing mass. Usually, constipation can be managed with stool softeners, stimulants, and osmotic agents. In patients with constipation secondary to gastroparesis, prokinetic agents such as metoclopramide may be used. A patient who presents with history of constipation should always have a rectal exam to exclude impaction. If faecal impaction is present, the patient should be manually disimpacted and treated with suppositories and/or enemas prior to receiving oral laxatives. A patient who has had recent rectal or anal surgery may develop impaction due to pain causing suppression of bowel movement.

Patients receiving opioid therapy should be started on a bowel regimen at the initiation of opioid therapy. Otherwise, constipation can lead to bowel obstruction, perforation, and delirium. Initial constipation prophylaxis is a stool softener three times a day plus a mild stimulant like senna. If this does not control symptoms, then bisacodyl (suppositories or oral) can be added. The next step is addition of osmotic agents such as sorbitol or polyethylene glycol. Sodium phosphate enemas are very effective but should be avoided in renal insufficiency due to danger of elevation of serum phosphate levels. The last step in relieving constipation is giving high colonic tap water enemas. High colonic enemas are given by warming 2 l of saline or water to body temperature, hanging the bags at the ceiling level, and infusing rectally over 1 h. This should be repeated until results are obtained.

Diarrhoea

Diarrhoea can predispose elderly patients to dehydration and electrolyte disturbance. In the demented or bed-bound patient, this symptom can be particularly exhausting to caregivers who have to assist patient to the bathroom, change bed linens, and wash soiled clothes. Patients who present with diarrhoea should have a rectal exam to exclude leakage around a faecal impaction. Other common causes of diarrhoea in the elderly are antibiotics, *Clostridium difficile* enterocolitis, gastrointestinal bleeding, malabsorption, medications, and stress. After reversible causes of diarrhoea are excluded, patients can be treated symptomatically. In patients who are mobile and drink enough fluids, bulk agents/fibres may be ideal agents to control diarrhoea. If this is not efficacious, then loperamide, kaolinpectin, or tincture of opium may control symptoms. Octreotide is effective to reduce gastrointestinal secretions and fistulae.[87]

Dyspnoea

Shortness of breath can be a symptom associated with chronic disease such as emphysema and heart failure or acute bronchopulmonary pneumonia. It is a subjective symptom and patients can experience shortness of breath even if pulse oximetry and respiratory rate are normal. Seventy per cent of cancer patients and 50–70 per cent of non-cancer patients experience dyspnoea in the last 6 weeks of life.[88] Management of dyspnoea requires identification of cause, treatment of reversible causes, and therapy to relieve the symptom. Diuretics, bronchodilators, and antibiotics relieve shortness of breath due to congestive heart failure, asthma/COPD, and pneumonia, respectively. They may also be useful as a temporizing measure in patients with a pulmonary malignancy causing bronchospasm or obstructive pneumonia.

Oxygen therapy relieves symptoms, improves exercise tolerance, and is the only therapy proven to prolong life in patients with COPD. If a patient requires more than 4 l of oxygen, humidified air should be administered in order to prevent dryness. In dying patients, oxygen therapy may cause discomfort or nasal irritation without improving respiratory status. These patients may receive as much symptomatic benefit from cool air ventilation from a fan or open window as much as from oxygen. Caregivers need to monitor debilitated patients for nasal and facial irritation and decubiti from the masks and tubing.

Opioids are highly effective in reducing symptoms of dyspnoea. Often, patients require lower doses than those needed to treat pain. Although many practitioners fear respiratory depression from opioids, research shows that at doses used to control dyspnoea, there is no significant effect on respiratory rate, effort, oxygen saturation, and carbon dioxide concentration.[89] In the opioid naïve patient, 2.5–5 mg of morphine by mouth every 4 h while awake is often sufficient to relieve dyspnoea.

Opioids can also be given via nebulizer by mixing the intravenous form in 2 cc of normal saline. Clinical trials of nebulized opioids for relief of dyspnoea have yielded mixed results. The usual dose is 2.5–10 mg of morphine or 0.25–1 mg of hydromorphone. In a recent study of nebulized fentanyl, 81 per cent of patients with terminal cancer reported improvement in breathing with 25 μg of fentanyl in 2 ml of saline.[90] Patients with malignancy and chronic lung disease often derive relief from steroids. Opioids, steroids, oxygen, and bronchodilators usually are used together and have synergistic effect.

Cough

Coughing exhausts and irritates patients and presents a difficult challenge for practitioners to control. Chronic persistent cough frequently occurs in malignancies and is particularly common in pulmonary neoplasms. Non-malignant causes of chronic cough in the elderly include oesophageal reflux disease, COPD, heart failure, and post-nasal drip. It can also be a result of medications such as ACE inhibitors.

A cough, the physiologic process of clearing the airways, occurs when irritation in the upper airways stimulate sensory nerves causing deep inhalation, closure of the glottis, increased intrathoracic pressure, and forced exhalation.

Treatment of cough depends upon identifying the cause. For example, cough secondary to extension of bronchial cancer may improve with steroids and palliative radiotherapy. In a patient with malignancy and post-obstructive pneumonia, cough may improve with antibiotics. Symptomatic relief depends on quality of cough. Over the counter cough remedies including antihistamines, antitussives, expectorants, and decongestants are recommended as first-line therapy, but there is no convincing evidence that they are effective.[91]

Patients with dry cough may be given a trial of demulcents and local anaesthetics to soothe the throat. Opioids at low doses are also helpful. In severe cases of dry cough, patients can be given 2 ml of 2 per cent lidocaine in 1 ml of normal saline over 10–15 min via a nebulizer. This should not be done more than three times a day as the lidocaine can be systemically absorbed. Inhalation of lidocaine reduces cough at doses that do not affect reflex bronchoconstriction.[92] Patients given cough medicines with anesthetic properties are at higher risk for aspiration due to suppression of the cough reflex and should be advised not to eat for one hour after receiving medication.

If the cough is due to postnasal drip, then antihistamines and nasal steroids are helpful. Antihistamines should be used with caution in the elderly because they can raise blood pressure, cause delirium, sedation, and urinary retention especially in men with benign prostatic hypertrophy. Wet cough should be treated with mucolytics, expectorants, bronchodilators, and chest physiotherapy. Corticosteroids are often highly effective if other measures fail.

Terminal patients, with weak or absent cough reflex, cannot effectively clear their airways and frequently develop 'death rattle', or the sound of air passing through a thin membrane of tracheal fluid. Patients are usually moribund when this symptom develops but the sound is distressing to families and professional staff alike. Anticholinergics such as scopolamine, hycosine hydrobromide, atropine, and glycopyrrolate reduce secretions in terminal patients with death rattle. Neither glycopyrrolate nor hycosine cross the blood–brain barrier and may be preferred if sedation is a problem. However, death rattle occurs in the last days and hours of life, usually when patients are suffering from terminal delirium, and sedation is often appropriate and desired.

Dizziness

A common symptom in elderly patients with chronic disease is the sensation of dizziness. Prevalence ranges from 13 to 38 per cent.[93–97] It is multifactorial in origin and can be due to decreased propioception secondary to diabetic neuropathy, vascular disease, vestibular disorders, and cardiac arrhythmias. Dizziness has been identified as a geriatric syndrome because of its prevalence and the frequency with which no single cause is isolated.[98] The symptom is associated with falls, functional disability, syncope, nursing home placement, and death. When no concrete cause is found, treatment is difficult and relies on educating patients on avoidance of triggers and easing contributing factors such as sensory impairment. Medications such as meclizine and anxiolytics sometimes help.

Oral symptoms

Elderly patients can present with mouth pain, dryness, and halitosis. The differential diagnosis of mouth pain includes aphthous ulcers, mucositis from chemotherapy, fungal infection secondary to decreased immunity or antibiotics, dental caries, periodontal disease, and poorly fitting dentures. Infection should be treated appropriately and patients and caregivers instructed on oral hygiene. Aphthous ulcers can be treated with viscous lidocaine, topical corticosteroids, or tetracycline mouthwash. Halitosis can be due to poor oral hygiene, dental or sinus infection, medications, or dry mouth. Causes of xerostomia are multifold and the symptom is prevalent in the elderly population regardless of state of health.[99] Medications are the most common cause of dry mouth in elderly patients.[100] When symptoms are not relieved with sips of water or ice, artificial saliva or commercial preparations containing mucin may provide relief.[101,102] Some patients experience mouth pain despite a normal oropharyngeal exam. These patients often benefit from viscous lidocaine.

Spiritual suffering

Assessing patients' spiritual and existential needs is an integral part of the treatment plan.[103] The role of religion is prominent in the lives of older adults. Patients living with chronic, progressive illness frequently suffer from anxiety and fear. Regardless of their spiritual beliefs, they may question self-identity, the meaning and purpose of life, and prior decisions.[104] They may have difficulty relating to loved ones due to reluctance to discuss progressive debility and dying. By addressing spiritual and emotional needs, health-care providers can help alleviate patients' fears of abandonment.[103]

Family members and caregivers also suffer. A pending death in the family may disrupt long-time family roles. Caregivers who devote much of their lives to caring for loved ones face the thought of suddenly having a large void in their life. Guilt and a sense of abandonment are sometimes overwhelming. Patients and family members often turn to spiritual leaders and religious beliefs to assist and support them.

Physicians can help patients and caregivers address their spiritual needs by encouraging them to discuss their fears with a religious leader, counsellor, or therapist. While many patients wish to share their religious convictions with physicians, some do not; thus, physicians should be empathetic without forcing an unwanted conversation. A physician may address patients' spiritual needs by asking about membership in a formal or informal religious group and preferences for visits from a spiritual leader and other members of their faith community.[105]

Personal growth at the end of life

The end-stage of a terminal progressive illness may be a time of great suffering, but it is also a time that provides the opportunity for personal growth. Accepting death and one's self-identity in the face of and in spite of disabling illness is a sign of personal development in the last stage of life.[106] Progressive illness also affords patients and their family members the opportunity to heal old personal wounds; there is time to say goodbye.

Although in the United States and the United Kingdom there is increasing trend to discuss death openly and allow patients autonomy, this is not the case for many cultures. Native American, Asian, and many European cultures do not discuss death or terminal diagnosis openly. Physicians should do their best to respect cultural and religious attitudes towards death by asking patients and families about how much detail they wish to know about the illness and its progression—the answer to this question is a helpful guide to the clinician in terms of the desire for truth-telling.

Conclusion

Palliative care of the geriatric patient involves providing symptomatic relief for symptoms that are chronic and multi-factorial in origin. The elderly are affected by chronic, progressive illness that may persist for decades. Physicians are challenged to ameliorate symptoms, delay progression of disease, relieve caregiver stress, and assist patients with planning for the future. When treating dying patients, physicians also need to be aware of patient's psychological and spiritual suffering. Patients may not expect physicians to explore these issues with them, but they may appreciate physician acknowledgement that these concerns exist. Listening to these concerns may comfort the patient, reduce isolation, and encourage a sense of belonging in the wider human community.

References

1. **Field, M.J. and Cassel, C.K.** *Approaching Death: Improving Care at the End of Life.* In: Institute of Medicine, ed. Washington DC: National Academy Press, 1997.
2. **Future IFT.** Health and health care 2010. The forecast. The challenge. Vol. 2001, 2000.
3. **Support Principal Investigators** (1995). A controlled trial to improve care for seriously ill hospitalized patients. The study to understand prognoses and preferences for outcomes and risks of treatments (SUPPORT). The SUPPORT Principal Investigators. *Journal of the American Medical Association* **274**, 1591–8.
4. **Hamel, M.** et al. (1996). Seriously ill hospitalized adults: do we spend less on older patients? *Journal of the American Geriatrics Society* **44**, 1043–8.
5. **Perls, T. and Wood, E.** (1996). Acute care costs of the oldest old: they cost less, their care intensity is less, and they go to nonteaching hospitals. *Archives of Internal Medicine* **156**, 754–60.
6. **Bernabei, R.** et al. (1998). Management of pain in elderly patients with cancer. *Journal of the American Medical Association* **279**, 1877–82.
7. **Cleeland, C.S.** et al. (1994). Pain and its treatment in outpatients with metastatic cancer. *New England Journal of Medicine* **330**, 592–6.
8. **Feldt, K.S., Ryden, M.B., and Miles, S.** (1998). Treatment of pain in cognitively impaired compared with cognitively intact older patients with hip-fracture. *Journal of the American Geriatrics Society* **46**, 1079–85.

9. **Morrison, R.S. and Siu, A.L.** (2000). A comparison of pain and its treatment in advanced dementia and cognitively intact patients with hip fracture. *Journal of Pain and Symptom Management* **19**, 240–8.
10. **AGS Panel on Chronic Pain in Older Persons** (1998). The management of chronic pain in older persons. *Journal of the American Geriatrics Society* **46**, 635–51.
11. **Emanuel, E.J., Fairclough, D.L., Slutsman, J., Alpert, H., Baldwin, D., and Emanuel, L.** (1999). Assistance from family members, friends, paid caregivers, and volunteers in the care of terminally ill patients. *New England Journal of Medicine* **341**, 956–63.
12. **Covinsky, K.** et al. (1994). The impact of serious illness on patients' families. *Journal of the American Medical Association* **272**, 1839–44.
13. **Schulz, R. and Beach, S.** (1999). Caregiving as a risk factor for mortality: the Caregiver Health Effects Study. *Journal of the American Medical Association* **282**, 2215–19.
14. **HCFA.** HCFA Highlights—National Health Expenditures, 1998. Vol. 2001, 2000.
15. **Spillman, B. and Lubitz, J.** (2000). The effect of longevity on spending for acute and long-term care. *New England Journal of Medicine* **342**, 1409–15.
16. **Arno, P., Levine, C., and Memmott, M.** (1999). The economic value of informal caregiving. *Health Affairs* **18**, 182–8.
17. **Kinosian, B.P.** et al. (2000). Predicting 10-year care requirements for older people with suspected Alzheimer's disease. *Journal of the American Geriatrics Society* **48**, 631–8.
18. **Gutterman, E.M., Markowitz, J.S., Lewis, B., and Fillit, H.** (1999). Cost of Alzheimer's disease and related dementias in managed-medicare. *Journal of the American Geriatrics Society* **47**, 1065–71.
19. **Martin, B.C.** et al. (2000). The net cost of Alzheimer's disease and related dementia: a population based study of Georgia Medicaid recipients. *Alzheimer Disease and Associated Disorders* **14** (3), 151–9.
20. **Menzin, J.** et al. (1999). The economic cost of Alzheimer's disease and related dementias to the California Medicaid Program in 1995. *American Journal of Geriatric Psychiatry* **7**, 300–8.
21. **Taylor, D.H. and Sloan, F.A.** (2000). How much do persons with Alzheimer's disease cost Medicare? *Journal of the American Geriatrics Society* **48**, 639–46.
22. **Ferrell, B.A., Ferrell, B.R., and Rivera, L.S.O.** (1995). Pain in cognitively impaired nursing home patients. *Journal of Pain Symptom Management* **10**, 591–8.
23. **Fried, T.R., Bradley, E.H., Towle, V.R., and Allore, H.** (2002). Understanding the treatment preferences of seriously ill patients. *New England Journal of Medicine* **346** (14), 1061–6.
24. **Tilden, V.P., Tolle, S.W., Nelson, C.A., and Fields, J.** (2001). Family decision-making to withdraw life-sustaining treatments from hospitalized patients. *Nursing Research* **50**, 1–11.
25. **Birks, J.S., Melzer, D., and Beppu, H.** (2000). Donepezil for mild and moderate Alzheimer's disease (Cochrane Review). *The Cochrane Library*, Issue 4.
26. **Birks, J., Grimley Evans, J., Iakovidou, V., and Tsolaki, M.** (2000). Rivastigmine for Alzheimer's disease (Cochrane Review). *The Cochrane Library*, Issue 4.
27. **Chung, J.A. and Cummings, J.L.** (2000). Neurobehavioral and neuropsychiatric symptoms in Alzheimer's disease. *Neurologic Clinics* **18** (4), 829–46.
28. **Spector, A., Orrell, M., Davies, S., and Woods, B.** (2000). Reality orientation for dementia (Cochrane Review). *The Cochrane Library*, Issue 4.
29. **Reisberg, B.** et al. (1987). Behavioral symptoms in Alzheimer's disease: phenomenology and treatment. *Journal of Clinical Psychiatry* **48** (5), 9–15.
30. **Eastley, R. and Wilcock, G.K.** (1997). Prevalence and correlates of aggressive behaviours occurring in patients with Alzheimer's disease. *International Journal of Geriatric Psychiatry* **12**, 484–7.
31. **Donaldson, C., Tarrier, N., and Burns, A.** (1997). The impact of the symptoms of dementia on caregivers. *British Journal of Psychiatry* **170**, 62–8.
32. **Krulewitch, H.** et al. (2000). Assessment of pain in cognitively impaired older adults: a comparison of pain assessment tools and their use by nonprofessional caregivers. *Journal of the American Geriatrics Society* **48** (12), 1607–11.
33. **Wells, D.L., Dawson, P., Sidani, S., Craig, D., and Pringle, D.** (2000). Effects of an abilities-focused program of morning care on residents who have dementia and on caregivers. *Journal of American Geriatrics Society* **48** (4), 442–9.
34. **Camberg, L.** et al. (1999). Evaluation of simulated presence: a personalized approach to enhance well-being in persons with Alzheimer's disease. *Journal of the American Geriatrics Society* **47** (4), 446–52.
35. **Alessi, C.A.** et al. (1999). A randomized trial of a combined physical activity and environmental intervention in nursing home residents: do sleep and agitation improve? *Journal of the American Geriatrics Society* **47** (7), 764–91.
36. **Meier, D.E.** et al. (2001). High short-term mortality in hospitalized patients with advanced dementia: lack of benefit of tube-feeding. *Archives of Internal Medicine* **161**, 594–9.
37. **Morrison, R.S. and Siu, A.L.** (2000). Survival in end-stage dementia following acute illness. *Journal of the American Medical Association* **284**, 47–52.
38. **Morrison, R.S.** et al. (1998). Pain and discomfort associated with common hospital procedures and experiences. *Journal of Pain and Symptom Management* **15** (2), 91–101.
39. **Mallick, M.J. and Whipple, T.W.** (2000). Validity of the nursing diagnosis of relocation stress syndrome. *Nursing Research* **49** (2), 97–100.
40. **Roberts, S.L.** (1996). *Behavioral Concepts and the Critically Ill Patient.* Englewood Cliffs NJ: Prentice-Hall.
41. **Berlowitz, D.R.** et al. (1997). Effect of pressure ulcers on the survival of long-term care residents. *Journals of Gerontology. Series A, Biological Sciences and Medical Sciences* **52** (2), M106–10.
42. **Thomas, D.R., Goode, P.S., Tarquine, P.H., and Allman, R.M.** (1996). Hospital-acquired pressure ulcers and risk of death. *Journal of the American Geriatrics Society* **44** (12), 1435–40.
43. **Martin, B.J.W.** et al. (1994). The association of swallowing dysfunction and aspiration pneumonia. *Dysphagia* **9**, 1–6.
44. **Volicer, L.** et al. (1990). Discontinuation of tube feeding in patients with dementia of the Alzheimer type. *The American Journal of Alzheimer's Care and Related Disorders & Research,* July/August, 22–5.
45. **Finucane, T.E., Christmas, C., and Travis, K.** (1999). Tube feeding in patients with advanced dementia. *Journal of the American Medical Association* **282**, 1365–70.
46. **Fisman, D.N., Levy, A.R., Gifford, D.R., and Tamblyn, R.** (1999). Survival after percutaneous endoscopic gastrostomy among older residents of Quebec. *Journal of the American Geriatrics Society* **47**, 349–53.
47. **Gillick, M.R.** (2000). Rethinking the role of tube feeding in patients with advanced dementia. *New England Journal of Medicine* **342**, 206–10.
48. **McCann, R.M., Hall, W.J., and Groth-Juncker, A.** (1994). Comfort care for terminally ill patients. The appropriate use of nutrition and hydration. *Journal of the American Medical Association* **272**, 1263–6.
49. **Kaw, M. and Sekas G.** (1994). Long-term follow-up of consequences of percutaneous endoscopic gastrostomy (PEG) tubes in nursing home patients. *Digestive Diseases and Sciences* **39** (4), 738–43.
50. **Kirby, D.F., Delegse, M.H., and Fleming, C.R.** (1995). American Gastroenterological Association Technical Review on Tube Feeding for Enteral Nutrition. *Gastroenterology* **108** (4), 1282–301.
51. **Callahan, C.M., Haag, K.M., Buchanan, N.N., and Nisi, R.** (1999). Decision-making for percutaneous endoscopic gastrostomy among older adults in a community setting. *Journal of the American Geriatrics Society* **47**, 1105–9.
52. **Bliss, D.Z.** et al. (1998). Acquisition of *Costridium difficile* and *Clostridium difficile* associated diarrhea in hospitalized patients receiving tube feeding. *Annals of Internal Medicine* **129**, 1012–19.
53. **Beard, C.M.** et al. (1996). Cause of death in Alzheimer's disease. *Annals of Epidemiology* **6**, 195–200.
54. **Small, G.W.** et al. (1997). Diagnosis and treatment of Alzheimer's disease and related disorders. Consensus statement of the American Association for Geriatric Psychiatry, the Alzheimer's Association, and the American Geriatrics Society. *Journal of the American Medical Association* **278** (16), 1363–71.
55. **Fabiszewski, K.J., Volicer, B., and Volicer, L.** (1990). Effect of antibiotic treatment on outcome of fevers in institutionalized Alzheimer patients. *Journal of the American Medical Association* **263**, 3168–72.
56. **Lawlor, P.G.** et al. (2000). Occurrence, causes, and outcome of delirium in patients with advanced cancer. *Archives of Internal Medicine* **160**, 786–94.
57. **Schor, J.D.** et al. (1992). Risk factors for delirium in hospitalized elderly. *Journal of the American Medical Association* **267**, 827–31.

58. **Lawlor, P.G., Fainsinger, R.L., and Bruera, E.D.** (2000). Delirium at the end of life critical issued in clinical practice and research. *Journal of the American Medical Association* **284** (19), 2427–9.

59. **Hanrahan, P. and Luchins, D.J.** (1995). Feasible criteria for enrolling end-stage dementia patients in home hospice care. *The Hospice Journal* **10** (3), 47–53.

60. **Hanrahan, P. and Luchins, D.J.** (1993). Access to hospice programs in end-stage dementia. *Journal of the American Geriatrics Society* **41**, 25–30.

61. **McCarthy, M.** (1997). The experience of dying with dementia: a retrospective study. *International Journal of Geriatric Psychiatry* **12** (3), 404–9.

62. **Karlawish, J.H.T., Quill, T., and Meier, D.E.** (1990). A consensus-based approach to providing palliative care to patients who lack decision-making capacity. *Annals of Internal Medicine* **130**, 835–40.

63. **Chassell, E.J.** (1999). Diagnosing suffering. *Annals of Internal Medicine* **131**, 531–4.

64. **Bruera, E.** et al. (1991). Symptom Assessment system: a simple method for the assessment of palliative care patients. *Journal of Palliative Care* **7**, 6–9.

65. **Portenoy, R.K.** et al. (1994). Memorial symptom assessment scale: an instrument for the evaluation of symptom prevalence, characteristics and distress. *European Journal of Cancer* **30A**, 1326–36.

66. **Gloth, F.M.** et al. (2001). The functional pain scale: reliability, validity, and responsiveness in an elderly population. *Journal of the American Medical Directors Association* **2**, 110–14.

67. **Krulewitch, H.** et al. (2000). Assessment of pain in cognitively impaired older adults: a comparison of pain assessment tools and their use by non-professional caregivers. *Journal of the American Geriatrics Society* **48**, 1607–11.

68. **Gibson, S.J. and Helme, R.D.** (2001). Age-related differences in pain perception and report. *Clinics in Geriatric Medicine* **17** (3), 433–56.

69. **Helme, R.D. and Gibson, S.J.** (2001). The epidemiology of pain in elderly people. *Clinics in Geriatric Medicine* **17** (3), 417–31.

70. **Moskowitz, R.W.** (2001). The role of anti-inflammatory drugs in the treatment of osteoarthritis: a United States viewpoint. *Clinical and Experimental Rheumatology* **19** (6 Suppl. 25), S3–8.

71. **Pincus, T.G.** et al. (2001). A randomized, double blind, crossover clinical trial of diclofenac plus misoprostol versus acetaminophen in patients with osteoarthritis of the hip or knee. *Arthritis and Rheumatism* **44**, 1587–98.

72. **Rowbotham, M.C., Davies, P.S., Verkempinck, C., and Galer, B.S.** (1996). Lidocaine patch: double blind controlled study of a new treatment method for post-herpetic neuralgia. *Pain* **65** (1), 39–44.

73. **Mercadante, S. and Portenoy, R.K.** (2001). Opioid poorly responsive cancer pain, part 1: clinical considerations. *Journal of Pain and Symptom Management* **21**, 144–50.

74. **Cherny, N.** et al. (2001). Strategies to manage the adverse effects of oral morphine: an evidence-based report. *Journal of Clinical Oncology* **19**, 2542–54.

75. **Portenoy, R.K.** (1999). Pain: management of cancer pain. *Lancet* **353**, 1695–700.

76. **Ashburn, M.A. and Lipman, A.G.** (1993). Management of pain in the cancer patient. *Anesthesia and Analgesia* **76**, 402–16.

77. **Pereiera, J.** (1998). Management of bone pain. In *Topics in Palliative Care* Vol. 3 (ed. R.K. Portenoy and E. Bruera), pp. 79–116. New York: Oxford University Press.

78. **Twycross, R.** (1994). The risks and benefits of corticosteroids in advanced cancer. *Drug Safety* **9**, 442–5.

79. **Handel, D.L.** (2001). Complementary therapies for cancer patients: what works, what doesn't, and how to know the difference. *Texas Medicine* **97**, 68–73.

80. **Kerns, R.D., Otis, J.D., and Marcus, K.S.** (2001). Cognitive-behavioral therapy for chronic pain in the elderly. *Clinics in Geriatric Medicine* **17** (3), 503–23.

81. **Reuben, D.B. and Mor, V.** (1986). Nausea and vomiting in terminally ill cancer patients. *Archives of Internal Medicine* **146**, 2021–3.

82. **Harari, D.** et al. (1997). How do older persons define constipation? *Journal of General Internal Medicine* **12**, 63–6.

83. **Campbell, A.J., Busby, W.J., and Horwath, C.C.** (1993). Factors associated with constipation in a community based sample of people aged 70 years and over. *Journal of Epidemiology and Community Health* **47**, 23–6.

84. **Harari, D., Gurwitz, J.H., and Minaker, K.L.** (1993). Constipation in the elderly. *Journal of the American Geriatrics Society* **41**, 1130–40.

85. **Stewart, R.B., Moore, M.T., Marks, R.G., and Hale, W.E.** (1992). Correlates of constipation in an ambulatory elderly population. *American Journal of Gastroenterology* **87**, 859–64.

86. **Whitehead, W.E.** et al. (1989). Constipation in the elderly living at home: definition, prevalence and relationships to lifestyle and health status. *Journal of the American Geriatrics Society* **37**, 423–39.

87. **Muir, J.C. and von Gunten, C.F.** (2000). Antisecretory agents in gastrointestinal obstruction. *Clinics in Geriatric Medicine* **16**, 327–34.

88. **Hockely, J.M., Dunlop, R., and Davies, R.J.** (1998). Survey of distressing symptoms in dying patients and their families in hospital and their response to a symptom control team. *British Medical Journal* **296**, 1715–17.

89. **Bruera, E.** et al. (1991). Effects of morphine on the dyspnea of terminal cancer patients. *Journal of Pain and Symptom Management* **5**, 341.

90. **Coyne, P.J., Visqnathan, R., and Smith, T.** (2002). Nebulized fentanyl citrate improves patients' perception of breathing, respiratory rate, and oxygen saturation in dyspnea. *Journal of Pain and Symptom Management* **23**, 157–60.

91. **Schroeder, K. and Fahey, T.** (2002). Systematic review of randomized controlled trials of over the counter cough medicines for acute cough in adults. *British Medical Journal* **31**, 324–9.

92. **Choudry, U.B., Fuller, R.W., Anderson, N., and Larlsson, J.A.** (1990). Separation of cough and relex bronchoconstriction by inhaled local anesthetics. *European Respiratory Journal* **3** (5), 579–83.

93. **Tilvus, R.J., Hakula, S.M., Valvanne, J., and Erkinjuntti, T.** (1996). Postural hypotension and dizziness in a general aged population: a four-year follow up of the Helsinki Aging Study. *Journal of the American Geriatric Society* **44**, 809–14.

94. **Ensrud, K.E.** et al. (1992). Postural hypotension and postural dizziness in elderly women. *Archives of Internal Medicine* **152**, 1058–64.

95. **Colledge, N.R., Wilson, J.A., MacIntyre, C.C., and MacLennan, W.J.** (1994). The prevalence and characteristics of dizziness in an elderly community. *Age and Aging* **23**, 117–20.

96. **Boult, C.** et al. (1991). The relation of dizziness to functional decline. *Journal of the American Geriatrics Society* **39**, 858–61.

97. **Sloane, P., Blazer, D., and George, L.K.** (1989). Dizziness in a community elderly population. *Journal of the American Geriatrics Society* **37**, 101–8.

98. **Tinetti, M.E., Williams, C.S., and Gill, T.M.** (2000). Dizziness among older adults: a possible geriatric syndrome. *Annals of Internal Medicine* **132**, 337–44.

99. **Loesche, W.J.** et al. (1995). Xerostomia, xerogenic medications and food avoidances in selected geriatric groups. *Journal of the American Geriatrics Society* **43** (4), 401–7.

100. **Ship, J.A., Pillemer, S.R., and Baum, B.J.** (2002). Xerostomia and the geriatric patient. *Journal of the American Geriatrics Society* **50**, 535–43.

101. **Narhi, T., Meurman, J.H., and Ainamo, A.** (1999). Xerostomia and hyposalivation: causes, consequences and treatment in the elderly. *Drugs and Aging* **15** (2), 103–16.

102. **Visch, L.L.** et al. (1986). A double-blind crossover trial of CMC and mucin containing saliva substitutes. *International Journal of Oral Maxillofacial Surgery* **15** (4), 393–400.

103. **Block, S.D.** (2001). Psychological considerations, growth and transcendence at the end of life the art of the possible. *Journal of the American Medical Association* **285** (22), 2898–3014.

104. **Fainsinger, R.** et al. (1991). Symptom control during the last week of life on a palliative care unit. *Journal of Palliative Care* **7**, 5–11.

105. **Pulschaski, C.M.** (1993). Taking a spiritual history: FICA. *Spirituality and Medicine Connection* **3**, 1.

106. **Byock, I.R.** (1996). The nature of suffering and the nature of opportunity at the end of life. *Clinics in Geriatric Medicine* **12**, 237–52.

10.8 Palliative medicine in intensive care

Simon Cohen and Thomas J. Prendergast

Introduction

At first, it may seem contradictory to assert that palliative medicine has a place in intensive care. Intensive care units are hospital locations where the prime aim has been to prevent patients from dying, principally by stabilizing the pathological malfunctioning of organ systems with maximal support, often in an invasive and highly technology-dependent fashion. At the opposite end of the spectrum, palliative care directs its efforts principally towards control of suffering while emphasizing quality of life over prolonging life at all costs. These two approaches to patients meet in intensive care because, unfortunately, a significant percentage of patients entering intensive care die. Mortality figures vary between units depending on selection criteria and on the type of patients treated but, in all intensive care units, there is a realization of significant mortality.

The nature of death in the intensive care unit has evolved over the years in Europe and North America so that death now occurs most often following a planned process of withholding or withdrawing treatment modalities.(1) The high mortality rate, and the prevalence of death following considered decisions to limit therapy, together highlight the importance of integrating the rescue and palliation functions of intensive care.

There are many reasons why it is difficult to be a simultaneous advocate of rescue and palliative medicine. First, and most importantly, there is a mindset that sees acknowledgement of dying and meticulous attention to symptom control as inimical to intensive care practice. We do not agree with this mindset, and will argue that incorporating palliative care into intensive care practice improves the experience for patients and providers. There are other difficulties. Pervasive uncertainty about prognosis makes it difficult to predict which individual patient is going to die in intensive care.(2) Clinicians may feel pressure from families to persist in what appears to be futile treatment or from colleagues who may continue intrusive efforts to save patients regarded as totally hopeless by the dispassionate observer. Sometimes the switch from saving life at all costs to allowing the patient to die with a modicum of dignity may be so abrupt as to allow relatives no time to come to terms with their impending loss.

Integration of palliative and intensive care is not an easy process, but there are means to facilitate this approach, particularly through increased emphasis on communication with patients and families,(3) as well as ensuing maximal patient comfort at all times. There is clearly room for improvement in practice since many patients in intensive care die with inadequate symptom control and other unmet needs. Somogyi-Zalud et al. reported that one out of four patients in a study of 1295 adults who died during hospitalization for acute respiratory failure or multiple organ failure died with severe pain and one out of three with severe confusion.(4) Since it is rarely possible to discuss the aims and plan of treatment with the patients themselves, it is good practice to meet with the relatives of patients in intensive care, particularly of the most critically ill patients, recognizing that the decision-making role of anyone other than the patient will vary from country to country depending on the legal status of surrogates. Nonetheless, these discussions have intrinsic worth in fostering a collaborative approach to what is often a tragic situation. Active attempts to include the family also serve to enhance trust between the doctor and the family.

Communication: vital for palliative care in intensive care

Several factors contribute to the problems of communication in intensive care. Many patients come to the intensive care unit as acute emergencies, having been previously well, with no apparent reason to consider their likely imminent mortality. The sudden nature of admissions means that intensivists rarely have established relationships with their patients, and patients in intensive care usually are unable to take part in discussions on their treatment. It is difficult to predict outcomes for individuals. A further barrier to good communication in the intensive care unit may be the physician's own feelings of grief and inadequacy in dealing with dying patients.(5)

Physicians' own religious and cultural differences profoundly affect attitudes towards withdrawal of life support. In a questionnaire study by Vincent, it was found that physicians with strong religious beliefs were less likely to withdraw life support. Physicians from Southern European countries, such as Greece, Italy, and Portugal, were more reluctant to withdraw life support than their colleagues from Northern European countries.(6)

Many intensive care units, particularly in inner city areas, serve multiethnic and multicultural communities whose diverse values must be respected. Blackhall et al. in the United States have reported that African-Americans are more likely to want full and prolonged life support than European-Americans.(7)

One consistent research finding in North America is the importance that families place on communication. In a meta-analysis addressing needs of family members who have loved ones in the intensive care, eight out of 10 needs identified related to communication with clinicians.(8) Physicians usually have had little training in discussing dying in or out of the intensive care unit, so it is not surprising that the quality of such discussions is poor.(5) Effective communication depends on the clinician being able to recognize that a problematic situation exists and then to address it promptly and appropriately. If this discussion takes place too late, if it is inadequate to meet the family's needs or ends abruptly, families may feel betrayed and abandoned leading to conflict between families and physicians.(9)

Family meetings

Intensive care units contain a large team of clinicians from various medical specialities including nurses, physiotherapists, dieticians, etc. It is very important to effective communications that there is a team consensus about end-of-life decisions and planning. Thus, physicians must take the initiative to keep other members of the multi-disciplinary team aware of changing goals of care. In order to improve communication in intensive care units, particularly on end-of-life issues, the clinicians should plan and prepare the discussion.

As much preparation should be put into discussing end-of-life issues as goes into any other procedure in intensive care. This planning should include reviewing all the details of the patient's illness and any knowledge of the patient's attitudes and aspirations. It should try to examine one's own personal feelings, attitudes, biases, and grief. The clinician should plan where the discussion will take place. A quiet, private place, without disturbance from mobile telephones and beepers, is preferred. It is important to ensure that the various members of the team are represented, that is, not only the physicians but the nurses, physiotherapists, and whoever else may have been important in caring for the patient. The family should be asked as to whom they would like to be present at the discussion. It is important to ensure that the most significant, closest relatives are present, if possible.

It is important to try to put all the participants at ease, to try to find out what the patient or family understands and how much the patient or family wants to know. Most patients, when given the option, want to know the truth about their illness but some will not want to discuss end-of-life care. It is important to try to discuss the prognosis frankly and openly in a way that the family understands. Too often, families are blinded by technical jargon or misinformed by being given uninterpretable information such as 'the platelet count has risen today and the patient's five organ system failure persists'. One must not support unrealistic hopes for survival or improvement, but it is important not to discourage all hope. The crucial insight is to redirect hope towards the possible, to a focus on alleviating suffering and on healing or cementing relationships.

If withdrawal of life-sustaining treatment is suggested, it should be made abundantly clear that this does not imply withdrawal of care and that the patient is not being abandoned. It must be stressed that the emphasis of care is changing from one of cure to comfort. These discussions should not be rushed and it is useful to leave silences to give the family an opportunity to ask questions. The aim should be to achieve a common understanding of the disease and the treatment plan. One should make it clear that staff will be available for further discussions and that the patient is continuing to undergo re-assessment.

Physicians must take a leading role in this discussion. Death is often an unexpected tragedy for the family, in contrast to intensive care clinicians for whom it is part of their routine. It is commonplace for families to have feelings of guilt regarding the treatment before the patient came to the intensive care unit or hospital, and one should never leave them feeling that they are responsible for a patient's death. A decision to withdraw treatment is primarily a medical decision. A recommendation to withdraw treatment is based on the patient's clinical condition in the setting of his or her wishes for care. To the extent that the family may be involved in decisions to limit therapy, their role is to represent and support the patient rather than to initiate a change in therapy. It should be stressed that the withdrawal of treatment modalities does not hasten death so much as it stops the fruitless prolongation of dying. One should assure the family that intensive palliative care will ensure that the patient is comfortable. One should also try to inform the family as much as possible about the prognosis and mode of death expected.(5)

Some families require time to come to terms with the tragic situation. If situations of conflict do arise, it may be necessary to repeat conversations at frequent intervals. In many hospitals, ethics committees help to defuse conflict situations. Families should be encouraged to bring whomever they like including outside opinions, spiritual advisors and so on to help resolve the situation.

Symptom control in the intensive care unit

Intensive care units have a higher concentration of physicians, nurses, and professional staff than other departments of the hospital. Higher staffing ratios mean that palliation of symptoms is more readily achievable in the intensive care unit than elsewhere. Palliative care is already an essential part of intensive care nursing, and applies equally to patients who will survive as it does to those who are going to die in the intensive care unit. One of the authors (S.L.C.) is consistently impressed by the nurses in his unit who talk to the patients about every manoeuvre they are going to make, addressing them gently by name however deeply unconscious they may be. This is part of palliative care even though the nurses regard it as basic nursing care.

Many intensive care patients are unconscious on admission or rendered so shortly afterwards so that all aspects of pain—physical, psychological, emotional, and spiritual—are difficult to assess. Recent research demonstrates that many patients receiving intensive care can report their symptom burden. In this survey, hunger, thirst, and disruption of sleep were reported as moderate or severe by more than 50 per cent or intensive care unit (ICU) patients.(11) It is no surprise that disruption of sleep is very common since the difference between night and day in the ICU is usually abolished by ever present lighting and noise. In one of the author's (S.L.C.) studies, patients interviewed some months following discharge from intensive care frequently reported bad dreams during their stay in intensive care.

In those intensive care unit patients who cannot report their subjective experience, it is important to look for potential sources of pain such as pressure sores, infection, poor mouth hygiene, oesophageal candidiasis, and a host of other potential sources.(3) Many procedures regarded as routine in intensive care (such as insertion of lines, intubation, mechanical ventilation) cause pain, in addition to distress and anxiety.(3)

There is little clinical trial data about management of pain and sedation in intensive care unit patients at the end of life but there is evidence that intensivists systematically undertreat pain.(3) The SUPPORT study reported that 22 per cent of patients interviewed in the second week of the study said that they had moderate or severe pain all, most, or half the time.(11) On the other hand, excessive sedation is also a problem. Kress et al.(12) reported that daily interruption of sedative infusions in critically ill patients undergoing mechanical ventilation resulted in a shorter duration of mechanical ventilation and shorter intensive care unit stay than in a comparable group in whom sedation was not interrupted.(12) It is possible that sedation may be given excessively while analgesics are underused in intensive care units.(3)

Sometimes, one is most aware of the symptoms of intensive care patients in the recovery phase when they have come off of mechanical ventilation and are better able to communicate. A frequent request is to be moved into a darkened side room so that they may sleep. A need for privacy and an appropriate environment is another common request in recovering patients. Open visiting by family members, and on occasion by beloved pets, may be of value in this situation.

Competent symptom management depends on understanding the specific needs of different types of patient. For instance, patients with cirrhosis of the liver or renal impairment may handle drugs very differently to patients with uncomplicated respiratory failure. It is equally important to understand the pharmacology of a small number of drug families in order to achieve good symptom control. *Opioids* are of great value because of their potent analgesic properties. Opioids may improve tolerance of an endotracheal tube without coughing or fighting against a ventilator. However, they are only mildly sedative and do not have any specific anxiolytic effects apart from those consequent upon pain reduction. Occasionally, active metabolites of morphine may accumulate in patients with renal failure to contribute to excessive sedation. They may cause nausea. *Benzodiazepines* are safe and inexpensive drugs of choice for sedation in intensive care patients. They have potent anxiolytic and amnestic properties, and are mild hypnotics. They have no intrinsic analgesic effects. They may be synergistic with opioids in causing central respiratory depression. Haloperidol is the drug of choice for the management of delirium and psychosis; chlorpromazine is a more sedating agent with similar clinical effects.

When a decision to withdraw treatment has been made, it is commonplace to administer both analgesics and sedatives. The doses of opioids necessary to control acute pain or dyspnoea varies so that large doses can be necessary. It is more important to equate the dose to the patient's needs than to set rules in milligrams as to how much should be administered.(3) Sometimes, neuro-muscular blocking agents are given prior to the withdrawal of mechanical ventilation. This is not desirable because the presence of neuro-muscular blockade renders it very difficult or impossible to assess a patient's pain requirements.(13)

Many families find the experience of a family member being treated in intensive care to be distressing and even traumatic. It is part of the intensive care team's remit to try to address the problems of the family as well as the patient. Counsellors should be available for patients and relatives as part of the service.

Withholding and withdrawing intensive care treatment

An important proportion of hospital deaths occurs in the intensive care unit, usually following a considered decision to withhold or withdraw life-sustaining treatment.(1) Medical treatment is founded on beneficence and compassion for the patient. This is no different in an era when death in intensive care has become a managed process. Good communication, collaboration and consensus between doctors, patients, and families is essential, especially when treatment limitation is proposed.(14)

There are many factors involved in decisions to limit life-sustaining therapy. How this decision is made, and who is ultimately responsible, varies from institution to institution and from country to country. From the medical point of view, the first requirement is that there is at least acceptance and at best consensus agreement among all the members of the medical team, to limit therapy when hope for recovery is outweighed by burden of the treatment. This decision should be supported by the senior physician responsible for the patient. The patient's wishes for continued treatment are of paramount importance; unfortunately, in the intensive care unit, these views are usually not known directly from the patient, but may be represented by the family. It is very important that the views of the family are taken into consideration and attempts are made to avoid conflict at this sensitive time. For clinicians working in intensive care, death is a routine event. It must always be remembered that this is not the perspective of the patient or the family, for whom the passing of a loved one may be a potent source of grief and guilt, so the maximum sensitivity in handling the situation is essential.

Medical knowledge is increasingly available to the public from a variety of sources of highly variable reliability. Some very fine information is available on the internet but, at the other extreme, many popular television shows maximize recovery from critical illness and fuel families' unrealistic expectations. There is also a diminishing level of trust in the medical profession. A study by Sjokvist et al. in 1999 showed that the Swedish general public wanted the patient and family to be involved in decisions to limit treatment, with only 5 per cent of the public supporting a physician-only approach.(15) We recognize that prognosis in critical illness is often uncertain. Physicians and families may disagree about how to value a small chance of improvement or to weigh the continuing burdens of treatment.(16) This may lead to problems in communication with patients, the family and, indeed, among the doctors themselves. UK law does allow the physician to make the decision but, at the very least, this should be done with the assent of the family. The place of surrogate decision makers is unclear, and the legal position of such people is dependent on the particular country. In the United States, both the medical community and the public accuse each other of over treatment, but the evidence suggests that physicians and families are equally responsible.(17) Many physicians, unhappy with patient and family decisions that they regard as medically inappropriate, attempt to apply the concept of medical futility in order to reassert their prerogative to make the decision they favour at the end of life.(18) Such use of the concept of medical futility is seriously flawed.(18)

In the current climate, decision-making must be open and accountable to the patient, family, and all concerned. All discussions and decisions should be detailed in the patient's record.

Guidelines for limitation of intensive care treatment

Ethics (see Chapter 3.6)

Almost all ethical authorities agree that there is no moral difference between withholding and withdrawing treatments. In practice though, many doctors feel more comfortable with withholding, particularly in the first instance, rather than withdrawing treatment, although this is a point of contention.

Not only patients but also some doctors and nurses may have conscientious objection to treatment withdrawal. Their view should be respected and they should be allowed not to involve themselves with such procedures if these are against their principles. If necessary, the patient should be transferred to another physician.

Principles

Medical treatment should only be withdrawn on clinical grounds. Every withdrawal decision should be made upon its own merits and must not be made on the basis of either cost or medical convenience (e.g. to avoid the cancellation of a surgical/medical procedure or the transfer of a patient). Need for an intensive care unit bed for another patient should not be the reason for withdrawing support. Limitation of treatment should be regarded as a formal intensive care unit procedure subject to the same preparation, thought, care, and consent as for any other aspect of care.

When patients are admitted to the intensive care unit there needs to be a clear plan for their management. This should include definitions of the limits of any invasive interventions. It is good practice for the physician in charge of the patient to meet with the family shortly after the time of admission so as jointly to define the goals of treatment.

Any life-sustaining therapy may be withdrawn. This includes blood products, haemofiltration, vasopressors, parenteral nutrition, antibiotics, mechanical ventilation, and even enteral feeding and hydration; the last two may need special care and may give rise to dissent.

Training

There is a need for improved training in communications skills for all intensive care unit personnel, particularly in the breaking of bad news. Such training should emphasize the importance of good contemporaneous written records of communication with the patient and/or the family as well as with all the caring team in the widest sense. If the patient is competent, and this is rarely the case in intensive care, then the patient's wishes and preferences for treatment are of the greatest importance and must be ascertained. It is essential that all discussions and decisions be clearly recorded in the patient's notes. This may be invaluable if decisions are challenged at a later date.

It is the duty of the intensivist to recognize a dying patient and to know when palliative care should override more aggressive modalities. Families may need time to come to terms with their impending loss. Meetings with the patient and family are extremely important. One should avoid referring to the patient by his disease—'This is the case of alcoholic liver failure' is an extremely insensitive way to address the patient or his family. It is important to try to build a picture of the patient as a person in his pre-morbid state by asking about his job and his activities. This kind of approach will engender empathy between the doctors and the family. In these discussions, sufficient time must be given for the family to speak; the doctor conducting the meeting should not monopolize conversation and must allow for silences. In the case of incompetent patients without family, the physician has to determine what is in the best interest of the patient. Assistance by an Ethics Committee experienced in such matters may be invaluable.

Withdrawal of treatment

Patients and families should be given the maximum possible access and privacy at this time. If possible, the patient should be in a private room, otherwise the curtains should be drawn and all unnecessary alarms and monitors be removed from the patient. Although treatment may be withdrawn, the patient's care should continue to be compassionate and attentive at the highest level. To this end, it is important to relieve the patient's pain and distress by judicious administration of suitable drugs (such as opioids, benzodiazepines) in appropriate doses by infusion. The dosage needs to be adjusted to primarily relieve the patient's suffering but not to hasten death. At the time of withdrawal of life support, however, the comfort of the patient is paramount. If that comfort can only be achieved with doses of medications that may hasten death, such administration is appropriate.

Treatments aimed at maintaining organ function that only prolong death should be withdrawn. Examples may include vasoactive drugs, antibiotics, and intravenous fluids. The details of withdrawal of respiratory support are debated. In the sickest patients, positive end expiratory pressure is eliminated and the inspired oxygen concentration is reduced to 21 per cent. Where appropriate, the patient may be extubated. Adequate analgesia and sedation are of paramount importance. Neuromuscular blocking agents should be avoided at this time as it may make it impossible to assess the patients awareness and degree of suffering. Intensivists need to understand death and bereavement and how to support the family, in their time of despair and guilt. The place of good communication between doctors and families in the intensive care unit cannot be over emphasized.

The question sometimes arises as to whether the patient should be transferred to a different floor or facility where the purpose and atmosphere of the ward may be more conducive to dying in peace. In our experience, the nursing staff often have built up relationships with the patients and their families in intensive care so that transfer would be disruptive and may diminish the quality of care, and give rise to a feeling of abandonment.

The way forward

The intensive care unit has a role as a palliative care facility. This has been discussed in many publications. Brett[19] presents the problems of intensivists who find themselves admitting patients to the ICU who have little or no hope of survival. There are a variety of reasons for this practice, including inability to identify the dying with certainty, overwhelming pressure from the patient, family or referring physicians, the need to preserve working relationships within an institution, disagreement and uncertainty over diagnosis and prognosis among the clinicians involved. Patients who have suffered an iatrogenic injury are often preferentially admitted. It is important to transfer a very sick patient from a ward environment where they cannot be nursed properly to the intensive care unit, particularly if the atmosphere has become highly charged.

Palliative care is very important for patients and their relatives who make requests for a better death. That is not to say that patients should be deprived of curative therapy, just that the physicians in intensive care need to be sensitive to these sorts of request.[20] It is very important that physicians understand the treatment preferences of seriously ill patients. One should encourage such advance care planning at an early stage in the patients illness, preferably before they come to intensive care.[21] This may be difficult to achieve because of the reluctance of both patients and doctors to acknowledge mortality.

Key steps in implementing palliative care in the intensive care unit[3] include instituting mandatory family meetings with the physician in charge at the earliest opportunity. The purpose of such meetings is to inform the family about the patient and his illness from the perspective of the treating physicians. It also allows clinicians to orientate the family to the intensive care unit, to establish a strategy for future communication as well as reassure the family of their involvement in the process. This effort helps the clinician gain insight into the attitudes of the family. Family meetings also enable the clinician to see the patient as a person rather than a disease in a bed.

Good communication skills must be part of the training and reassessment of all intensive care clinicians. It will help them as well as families to cope with uncertainty, unstable and changing situations, intense personal relationships and emotions on both sides of the clinician/family divide. Techniques such as videotaping clinicians when they are conducting such interviews may be of great value. It is important that trainees are involved in these sorts of discussions but they should be lead by the clinician in charge.

References

1. **Luce, J.M. and Prendergast, T.J.** (2001). The changing nature of death in the ICU. In *Managing Death in the Intensive Care Unit* (ed. J.R. Curtis and G.D. Rubenfeld), pp. 19–29. New York: Oxford University Press.
2. **Teres, D. and Lemeshaw, S.** (1994). Why severity models should be used with caution. *Critical Care Clinics* **10**, 93–110; discussion pp. 111–15.
3. **Prendergast, T.J.** (2002). Palliative care in the intensive care unit setting. In *Principles and Practice of Supportive Oncology* 2nd edn., Chapter 79 (ed. A.M. Berger, R. Portenoy, and D. Weissman), pp. 1086–104. Philadelphia: Lippincott, Williams and Wilkins.
4. **Somogyi-Zalud, E., Zhong, Z., Lynn, J., Dawson, N.V., Hamel, M.B., and Desliens, N.A.** (2000). Dying with acute respiratory failure or multiple organ system failure with sepsis. *Journal of the American Geriatric Society* **48**, S140–5.
5. **Curtis, J.R. and Patrick, D.L.** (2001). How to discuss dying and death in the ICU. In *Managing Death in the Intensive Care Unit* (ed. J.R. Curtis and G.D. Rubenfeld), pp. 85–102. New York: Oxford University Press.
6. **Vincent, J.L.** (1999). Forgoing life support in Western European ICUs. The results of an ethical questionnaire. *Critical Care Medicine* **27**, 1626–33.
7. **Blackhall, I.J.** et al. (1999). Ethnicity and attitudes towards life sustaining technology. *Social Science and Medicine* **48**, 1779–89.
8. **Hickey, M.** (1990). What are the needs of families of critically ill patients? A review of the literature since 1975. *Heart & Lung* **19**, 401–15.
9. **Fins, J.J. and Solomon, M.Z.** (2001). Communication in intensive care settings: the challenge of futility disputes. *Critical Care Medicine*, **29** (2 Suppl. N), 10–15.
10. **Nelson, I.J.** et al. (2001). Self reported symptom experience of critically ill cancer patients receiving intensive care. *Critical Care Medicine* **29**, 277–82.
11. **SUPPORT** (1995). A controlled trial to improve care for seriously ill hospitalised patients. The study to understand prognosis and preferences for outcomes and types of treatments (SUPPORT). *Journal of the American Medical Association* **274**, 1591–8.
12. **Kress., J.P., Pohlman, A.S., O'Connor, M.F., and Hall, J.B.** (2000). Daily interruption of sedative infusions in critically ill patients undergoing mechanical ventilation. *New England Journal of Medicine* **342**, 1471–7.
13. **Truog, R.D.** et al. (2002). Pharmacologic paralysis and withdrawal of mechanical ventilation at the end of life. *New England Journal of Medicine* **342**, 508–11.
14. **Cohen, S.L., Ridley, S., and Goldhill, D.** (2002). *Guidelines for Limitation of Intensive Care Treatment in Adults*. UK Intensive Care Society, http://www.ics.ac.uk/downloads/LimitTreatGuidelines2003.pdf.
15. **Sjokvist, P.** et al. (1999). Withdrawal of life support—who should decide? Differences in attitudes among the general public, nurses and physicians. *Intensive Care Medicine* **25**, 949–54.
16. **Asch, D.A.** (1996). The role of critical care nurses in euthanasia and assisted suicide. *New England Journal of Medicine* **334**, 1374–9.
17. **Prendergast, T.J.** (1997). Resolving conflicts surrounding end of life care. *New Horizons* **5**, 62–71.
18. **Prendergast, T.J.** (1995). Futility and the common cold. How requests for antibiotics can illuminate care at the end of life. *Chest* **107**, 836–44.
19. **Brett, S.** Ethical questions for the new millennium. *Proceedings of the Brussels Intensive Care Symposium*, 2001, pp. 708–15.
20. **Back, A.L. and Pearlman, R.A.** (2001). Desire for physician assisted suicide requests for a better death. *Lancet* **358**, 362–3.
21. **Fried, T.R.** et al. (2002). Understanding the treatment preferences of seriously ill patients. *New England Journal of Medicine* **346**, 1061–6.

11

Cultural and spiritual aspects of palliative medicine

11 Cultural and spiritual aspects of palliative medicine

Joseph P. Cassidy and Douglas J. Davies

Pastoral care—the cure of souls

Pastoral care expresses the concern human beings show at the illness or distress of others. We perceive, understand, and react to serious illness in a variety of ways. Serious illness disrupts the regular rhythms of human life and poses a significant challenge to all personal relationships, raising questions of social integration as well as profound questions of individual destiny. In this chapter, 'pastoral care' is understood in the broadest possible sense and reflects the underlying element of depth that people sense in their relationships and in human life itself.

This sense of 'depth' is often formally expressed in religious, philosophical, or ethical ideas concerning the significance or meaning of life, with the major religious traditions speaking variously of divine love, the sanctity or value of life, or of compassion. In many societies, certain individuals are charged with particular responsibility for honouring the significance of life through their specific work of care—whether as medical personnel or as priests or ministers serving the sick. At its widest, caring and taking responsibility undergird the whole of community life, beginning in terms of family responsibilities and moving outwards into ever wider bands of responsibility.

A distinctive feature of the contemporary world involves a recognition of an increasing breadth of responsibility (often expressed in terms of universal human rights), a globalization of the ideal of care for the natural world and for the world-community, without restriction to family, region, or society. At the individual and personal level, 'human rights' is expressed more in the notion of 'dignity', especially as far as the old, sick, and, most especially, the dying are concerned. Pastoral care becomes particularly grounded in this sense of dignity.

Wounded healers—shamans old and new

More formally, especially as expressed in ritual, pastoral concern has been manifested through shamans present in many traditional societies, both of antiquity and the present. Where found, they are believed to possess power to engage with supernatural forces to bring benefit to those in need, not least to the sick.[1] Local interpretations of illness reflect both the shaman's ritual trance and the benefit claimed by the sick whose plight is taken seriously and who is afforded a cultural niche in which to find attention and hope for a positive outcome. The shaman is one widespread example of the power of personal experience of sickness when relating to others who are sick. T.S. Eliot's 'wounded surgeon' and Henri Nouwen's 'wounded healer' express this idea.[2] Shamans have often undergone some personal trauma, come close to death, and survived it. The strength of their transformed identity enables them to empathize with others who are sick and to bring them some degree of help. Ritually they were often said to have experienced 'death' and to have been reborn.

The 'wounded healer' model in contemporary society suggests the inadequacy of expert models of pastoral care, apart from those stemming from personal experience. The wounded healer model is not simply a matter of locating a source of pathos within one's experience; rather, it means that the carer reaches out to the other primarily by being wounded with the other who is wounded. This reverses ordinary expectations. In the face of a patient's fear, rather than reassure the patient with statistics about clinical outcomes, the wounded healer is more likely to share his or her own fears. The way individuals minister from their 'woundedness' will differ according to their specific roles within the palliative care team. For the surgeon to respond to a patient's fears with his or her own fears may not be appropriate, but neither is exaggerated confidence. For some in the team, however, an explicit appreciation of shared woundedness is valuable because it expresses a profound truth about shared humanity and its constraints.

Representative carers

Another aspect of pastoral care concerns the representative role, where one individual focuses the concerns of a church, community or group. Ainsworth-Smith and Speck write: 'More than most others, the minister represents a tradition which has tried over the centuries to provide some framework for integrating individuals into a larger framework of experience which attempts to make sense of fundamental issues' (ref. 3, p. 132). And these fundamental issues are quite literally issues of life and death, involving issues of faith in a providential, benevolent God; the justice or injustice of illness or issues of the seeming banality and ubiquity of suffering. The rabbi, imam, minister, or priest represents the tradition not simply in terms of ministering to co-adherents, but also, at times, in being a lightning rod for the anger or bitterness directed at the tradition, which may be perceived as having rejected them, or whose teachings may come to appear as platitudes that now ring hollow.

The representative role can, however, find itself oddly misplaced in a society consisting of persons of many diverse faiths, philosophies, and values. Even so, the deepest contribution made by official representatives often comes more from the concern reflected in their very presence than from formal doctrinal explanations of suffering. To listen and to be present offer a power of their own, as increasing numbers of ministers attest. This can be an increasingly significant component of care when related to other professional personnel whose major activity focuses on medically technical procedures, a factor that raises the issue of 'holistic' care.

Traditional pastors

In most traditional forms of major religions, ministers have shown pastoral care for individuals from birth to death. The newborn were received into family and community with its newly given name helping furnish its identity. Further care matched ongoing stages of growth and maturity, marriage, sickness, and death. In traditional Christianity, the 'cure of souls' became a developed professional field amongst priests and ministers. A major feature concerned this life as a preparation for an after-life with appropriate rituals aiding the journey through the one to the other. Not so long ago, Roman Catholic 'last rites' were known as 'extreme unction'—a solemn anointing at the time of death. Today, that rite is known as the 'sacrament of the sick', and church leaders encourage people to receive this sacrament whenever they are seriously (even if not fatally) ill, extending it to all kinds of illness. In its place, the Roman Catholic Church has re-emphasized viaticum, which is a last reception of Holy Communion as an accompaniment for the journey 'through death'. In many countries, the same shift has occurred in Anglican or Episcopalian practice. Indeed, the idea of life as a cycle or journey has, if anything, developed as an overall image of existence.

This life and afterlife

While many dedicated religious people continue to believe in traditional ideas of an afterlife, there is a growing proportion of the population who no longer believe in life after death. This is especially true in Western and Northern Europe, where the pastoral care or the 'cure of souls' has come increasingly to adopt a this-worldly emphasis, fostering self-development and self-fulfilment. Key elements include a desire for integrity of purpose, honesty with self, and as fruitful a relationship as possible with key players in a person's social world. One consequence of this self-fulfilment model of self-identity is the idea of holistic care.

Holistic care

The very notion of 'holistic' care begins with a sense of the individual viewed as an integrated self set within a distinctive community and world not as a set of 'parts'. Accordingly, holistic medicine in relation to 'scientific' medicine focuses on the wider and not narrower location of illness in relation to the 'total' person and to the overall social world that embraces both the sick and those offering care. This means that the holistic concern for 'body, mind, and spirit', for example, cannot be reducible to three or any other number of spheres of concern each with their specialist 'doctor'. Indeed, the foundation of the concept of 'total care' turns on the insight that the physical, the psychological, and the spiritual are but distinctive perspectives upon what is, in reality, a unity. Historically speaking, the background of 'holism' is complex, involving matters of philosophy, religion, and politics from ancient, traditional healing in China and India(4) to aspects of twentieth-century German medicine, some controversial branches of which have even been described in terms of 'Nazi biomedicine as holism'.(5)

This view of the individual and of sickness can also be expressed in terms of embodiment. This concept refers to the fact that, as human beings, we exist as a body, we have our being as a body. This perspective avoids any such idea as that of a separate 'soul', though even those believing in a soul, especially in Roman Catholic thought, may still see human identity as a complex outworking of the soul's capacity in and through the body. Still, embodiment is a useful way of thinking about human identity as embedded in our bodies and as something that, itself, can be profoundly affected by changes in the body brought about through illness. It is precisely the embodied identity of individuals that comes to prominence with illness.

Caring—curing and cost

While such a focus on caring may seem all too obvious, the first Director of the Kennedy Institute of Ethics, André Hellegers, noted that caring has been sidelined:

> As the caring branches of medicine were gradually pushed aside by the curing ones, there seemed to be less use for the Christian virtues. I think that shortly the need for those old Christian virtues will return and once again be at a premium. Our patients will need a helping hand and not a helping knife. This is no time to dismantle the low-technology care model of medicine. . . . We must either recapture the Christian virtues of care or we shall be screaming to be induced into death to reach the 'discomfort-free society' (ref. 6, p. 41).

Obviously, Hellegers is referring to a long-term cycle, but his identification of the shift from 'caring' to 'curing', with all the admitted blessings of curing, needs reinforcing. Issues of government funding for hospices in the UK would be but one example of this shift: when curing is no longer possible, it becomes all too obvious that caring may all too easily be devalued as real medicine. But changes in demography, with increasing numbers of people living into much older age within a broad consumerist population committed to life-style choices, may require a form of care that demands appropriate political and welfare responses.

Reverence for life

The emergence of palliative medicine has reversed the trend of cure over care in developing a branch of medicine where no external rationale is needed to commend a holistic approach to sick individuals. Here, 'healing' is not reduced to making people better, but is appreciated as helping them retain a sense of integrity even as their bodies give out. Pastoral sensitivities can help broaden the holistic approach. Still, attitudes motivating pastoral care seldom emerge from nowhere, whether derived from a theory of selfhood grounded in interpersonal relations or in some traditional religious belief. Albert Schweitzer, philosopher, theologian, and missionary doctor offered one example in his commitment to the idea of 'reverence for life', which he took to be 'the beginning and foundation of morality'.(7) More recently, the theologian Ann Loades has emphasized the term, 'the sanctity of life', arguing that 'more is affirmed by this phrase than we sometimes suppose'. She goes on to say that 'we need to keep this phrase alive, and not suppose that "quality of life" is by any means a satisfactory substitute or paraphrase for it' (ref. 8, p. 4). Loades here is emphasizing the inviolability of life, especially of the helpless, and suggests that 'sacredness' does a better job of communicating the 'preciousness' of life, which is in turn always a matter of relatedness, ultimately of our relatedness to God. Certainly, the entire issue of human 'dignity' is reflected in all these terms.

The healer

The 'status' of the healer is of paramount significance, not least in complex societies where sick people define themselves and potential helpers in different ways. Distinctions in social class, education, and varying degrees of self-knowledge all become radically important, making great demands upon medical and other personnel. Some desire the full force of scientific medicine applied by impersonal specialists, while others seek a more intimate relationship with their doctor. Alternative therapies reflect this sense of the need for interpersonal communication as a vital component of understanding one's own sickness and treatment. Given that palliative medicine is team-based, including professionals with discrete, well-honed specialisms, what is the role of pastoral care? Different emphases are possible in the task of helping people to 'live until they die' or 'live to their maximal potential'. These are issues of considerable import as evidenced in Alexander Solzhenitsyn's book *Cancer Ward*, describing what happened to someone who had cared for others for 30 years:

> During this time what she had worked out empirically for herself had become more and more indisputable, while in her mind medical theory grew increasingly coherent. . . . Then suddenly, within a few days, her own body had fallen out of this great, orderly system. It had struck the hard earth and was now like a helpless sack crammed with organs—organs which might at any moment be seized with pain and cry out . . . . The course of her disease and her new place in the system of treatment had now become equally unrecognizable to her. As from today she ceased to be a rational guiding force in the treatment; she had become an unreasoning, resistant lump of matter . . . . Her world had capsized, the entire arrangement of her existence was disrupted (Solzhenitsyn, in ref. 6, pp. 108–9).

Speech and silence

The woman described by Solzhenitsyn was not concerned about 'living to her maximal potential'. Her life was unrecognizable; she was disoriented, to the point of not knowing which way to turn. Caring, in this context, may simply mean giving a person the time to get used to this new world. Human beings inhabit complex worlds fostered by custom and convention that are generally flooded with speech. Pastoral care is alert to the changes that serious illness brings about in all these areas, not least in how people feel able to talk about their new-found situation. There is a sense in which pastoral care can help some people learn to talk, perhaps for the first time, about their present situation; about the fact that they are going to die; and about the many attaching concerns over family, friends, and life endeavours. For some, however, there is but little to say: it is not always easy to learn a new language, especially for people whose lives have not involved a great deal of self-expression. The family and friends of those who suffer and die may also stumble into a new-found form of self-expression as they give an account of their relationship with the dead.

Here, contemporary society is becoming increasingly alert to the power of story-telling, to the capacity of narrative to express relationships and emotions. This is especially true for religious people and for those who consider life to be purposeful: writing the last chapter of their lives, as it were, can give new meaning to all that preceded it. Yet, for others, life does not seem to be that kind of integrated whole, and the experience of (sometimes painful) discontinuities, of meaninglessness, will cut through any attempts to force a narrative.

Moral–somatic relationships

One significant dimension of meaning-making concerns the moral realm and the way people respond to how they are treated by others. Here, 'moral' could almost be replaced by 'social' to emphasize the widest social field of human existence and not simply a narrower sense of ethical behaviour. As social animals, humans are deeply affected by the behaviour of those with whom they live. The notion of moral–somatic relationships identifies this influence over individual well-being. Evidence shows, for example, how bereavement may affect the physical health of survivors as their world changes around them[(9)] with the idea of psycho-somatic relationships widely used to describe the complex interplay between cognitive and affective factors underlying human emotion. Similarly, there is much to be gained by also emphasizing the impact of the wider social world in 'moral–somatic' terms.[(10)]

This is significant for people in positions of authority related to the well-being of others. Doctors and other health workers are particularly important here, as are police, judges, and the clergy. Occupying prime social positions and bearing key social values, these directly affect the welfare of those they serve. They exist to 'do good' and to 'do the right thing'. However, if they behave illegally or in ways deemed improper or unjust, the outcome may have profound negative consequences upon those who see themselves as 'wronged' and whose health and sense of well-being may be deleteriously affected. People may even feel prevented from 'carrying on with life' until 'justice is done' and seen to be done. At the family level, too, some sense of injustice may trouble individuals for many years and may be amongst the issues that pastoral care can help resolve.

Death

One longstanding aspect of pastoral care has related to death both in terms of those who are dying and to their survivors. The theological beliefs of traditions are closely related to their ritual practices. In Judaism, for instance, the body is constantly attended from the moment of death; it is considered a great *mitzvah* to wash and purify the body, revering it as a sacred vessel; the body is buried either in a wooden coffin or directly into the ground, expressing the body's return to earth (Gen 3.19). This is all followed by particularly powerful expressions of grief and communal offers of comfort, which continue for at least 30 days, and then annually. The theology concerning death is perhaps most powerfully expressed in the recitation of *Kaddish*, which has little to do with the death of relatives, but everything to do with exulting God's glory. This focussing on God's glory instead of on questions of what happens in the afterlife is a forceful and characteristic expression of Jewish faith.

Christianity has involved ideas of heaven along with rites for the dying to prepare them for their journey, funeral ceremonies marking the change, and events to comfort the living. Hinduism, Buddhism, and Sikhism also prepare the dying for their next phase of existence, often through the recitation of sacred scriptures and in the belief that the capacity to hear holy words is of fundamental benefit to the dying both as comfort and to direct their life-force as it prepares for its next phase of post-mortem existence. For Muslims, belief in bodily resurrection is central, involving a test of faith after death: the recitation of the *Shahada*, by the dying or others present, is important so that the Allah will be the last thought of the dying person's mind and the first upon awakening on the day of judgement. If possible, the dying person is turned to face Mecca; and after death the head is turned to the right shoulder so that the body can be buried facing Mecca.

In the twentieth century, attitudes towards death among some Christian churches changed remarkably. Due to a theological understanding of the primordial Fall of humanity, illness, suffering, and death had been understood to be the result of sin. They were unnatural and were not willed by God. And inasmuch as they were not willed by God, they could be overcome by prayer and by God. This sense of the unnaturalness of sickness and death was exacerbated by the West's inheritance of a largely gnostic distinction between matter and spirit, between body and soul, which saw spirit and soul as timeless and superior, more God-like, and anything physical, temporal, and subject to change and decay. More recently, a number of Protestant theologians have tried to avoid the language of 'souls' and the belief that the soul 'leaves' the body and death and have preferred to use the language of resurrection to suggest that God can as easily recreate the individual person just as matter itself was created 'in the beginning'.

Roman Catholic medical ethics, with its appreciation that there is no obligation to use 'extraordinary means' to prolong human life when there is no therapeutic goal, opened the door to an appreciation that dying is perfectly natural, that death is not an evil to be avoided at all costs. The shifts in Roman Catholic practice do not stop there but have extended to funeral rites themselves, with the use of white vestments, for instance, now largely replacing the use of purple or black in many churches. Most tellingly, the funeral mass of the Roman Catholic Church is now called the 'Mass of the Resurrection'.

What is of particular interest as far as pastoral care is concerned is the fact that many of those involved in pastoral care now see funerals and post-funeral rites as directed at the survivors and not at the deceased. While the comfort of mourners has long been an aim of Christian pastoral care, this aim has grown significantly in recent decades and is, increasingly, mirrored in funeral ceremonies performed by, for example, representatives of Humanist associations. These and others often describe their work in term of 'life-centred' or 'life-directed' funerals whose stress is upon the life that has been lived and not any future life in eternity. Here, for example, in Britain and, increasingly in other European countries, family members take the cremated remains of their loved ones and hold very private and informal rites for placing these remains in places of personal significance. Along with the talks, poems, and songs used at funeral and memorial ceremonies these newly developing customs can be described in terms of the retrospective fulfilment of identity. They do not assume, with traditional Christianity, that one's identity would only be fulfilled in heaven, a kind of prospective fulfilment of identity.

Near-death experience (NDE)

Some, however, do lay great stress on what lies beyond death on the basis of what have come to be called near-death experiences, so called by Raymond Moody.[(11)] The medically resuscitated tell of having taken a journey to some other realm, often along a tunnel, where they meet deceased relatives or friends and encounter some distinctive and powerful individual who indicates that they have come to some kind of barrier beyond which they cannot currently cross. They recall seeing a powerful, welcoming light, hearing sounds, having a sense of acceptance and of being loved; and they feel charged to return to their ongoing body and life, having had an overall experience that confers a sense of calm and purpose in life and removes any fear of death.

While the media have popularized both these near-death experiences and also 'out of the body experiences' (OBEs), similar accounts are to be found in classical, historical, and anthropological texts.[(12)] The anthropologist Maurice Bloch[(13)] has described ways in which various rituals (with their attendant experiences) lead people to gain a sense of strength and power after having overcome hardship. These individuals are very like the shamans described above who seem to represent one elemental form of human response to the perils of life. Even so, Raymond Moody, the originator of the term near-death experience, now advises great caution in its use and criticizes certain types of parapsychologists, sceptical scientists, and fundamentalist Christians for using the idea for their own ends.[14] He advises a more cautious approach and hopes that such experiences will lead to a better understanding of the human mind and existence.

Spirituality, sacred and secular

Whether in religious or non-religious services for the sick or the dead, recent decades have witnessed a growth in that attitude of care towards human identity, its desires and relationships that can be described in terms of 'spirituality'. From its base within explicitly religious traditions, explicit regard for spirituality has become increasingly common among those involved in pastoral care, welfare, and well-being. While the secularization of society is related to the decrease in the explicitly religious meaning given to 'spirituality', it has, at the same time, released the word for wider use and for an expansion of meaning: it now comes to describe the depth of human life, with individuals seeking significance in their experiences and in the relationships they share with family and friends, with others who experience illness, and with those engaged in their treatment and support. To talk of the 'spiritual' is to provide the widest possible framework for an individual's experience of illness. For some this will involve an intense sense of the reality of a personal God and for some others the most general search for significance and meaning. For many, questions of ultimacy become acute.

But, at the same time, it is important not to ignore those who assume that life's ultimate meaning lies within human relationships and the numerous ventures they have pursued during their lifetime. Contemporary society allows for, and in some respects fosters, this view without labelling it as any particular kind of humanism, 'imminentism', or existentialism. The fact that most traditional religions argue that human life continues after death in some heaven or in a transmigration and reincarnation of persons has meant that the 'ultimate' meaning of life is to be sought beyond our normal life span. Fairly major changes in belief associated with life after death now leave a large number of Britons, for example, without such beliefs. This is especially true for men who tend to hold such beliefs much less frequently than do women. Pastoral care needs to be aware of such world-views and often requires of religious ministers a high degree of adaptability when relating to this worldly focused individuals.

Faith and healing

Just how individuals come to develop their world-views is an extremely complex issue, especially in contemporary societies where opinions and life-experience can vary a great deal even amongst people of a single religion, let alone amongst those of diverse backgrounds. It is precisely here that pastoral carers face a major challenge in their own approach to life and to others. This is especially true if individuals engaged in pastoral care have been nurtured in a tradition that emphasizes the importance of some ultimate meaning of life or have been deeply influenced by some particular life experience of their own.

Some pastoral carers draw from traditional religious ideas of the 'cure of souls' and seek to set their work within the ritual realm of, for example, the Christian sacraments. One contemporary feature of numerous mainline Christian churches has been in the growth of 'Healing Services'. Far removed in tone and form from popular 'faith-healing' of a more revivalistic scheme of religion, these events are often low-key and set within a Eucharist or other church occasion. The minister often prays for and may lay hands on the head of those seeking 'healing' but without any expectation of dramatic and 'miraculous' outcomes. The emphasis is upon an inward growth and acceptance of the life-situation—all within the sacramental life of the church concerned. The sense that a formal representative of that tradition as well as many group members may be praying for the sick person can be of real help to that individual. Here, the religious context of acceptance and care echoes the idea of a holistic context and many ministers involved in such work would also stress the importance of ordinary scientific medicine and of its role within holistic care.

Miracle and process

Many religious traditions speak of healing, some asserting the possibility of divine miracle to heal, with others preferring to stress the importance of healing as a transformation of the self as it accepts illness; instead of becoming resigned to the inevitable or giving up to despair, the tradition urges people to engage creatively with their circumstances.

In contrast, and this is perhaps truer among more fundamentalist Christians, the expectation of healing can be close to absolute, and a failure to be healed will be explained in terms of the lack of faith either of the person hoping to be healed or of those praying for him or her. At the same time, in every religious tradition where people pray for divine healing, there is some sort of belief that God can effect physical healing, that 'God could heal someone if God wanted to'; and so there will inevitably be challenges in coming to terms with the facts of continued illness and death.

There have been conflicting studies about links between patient health and spirituality and religion. McKee and Chappel[15] urge that spiritual issues ought to be addressed because they do make a positive impact on health. They recommend that the medical model be expanded to become a 'biopsychosocial–spiritual' one. Sloan et al.[16] are much less sanguine about an association, but they urge respect for those who have religious faith, while Larson and Koenig[17] argue for a positive association and urge medical practitioners to engage with patients' beliefs.

There is an obvious need to be cautious about any utilitarian argument for spirituality; for even though it could be argued that some people have utilitarian motives for religion (i.e. they believe in order to be saved), still this can be seen as dismissive of the way many people see their faith or spirituality as constitutive and defining of their personality. In fact, such utilitarianism could be seen as an inversion of many people's values, suggesting somehow that physical health is the highest value and the measure of all other values, including spiritual values. At the same time, if concern for spiritual issues *does* contribute to overall health, then this is a challenge to a more reductive biological medical model.

Hope and fear

Hope constitutes a major element in the dynamics of spirituality, whether religious or secular. Indeed, hope is a characteristic feature of personal identity and of interpersonal relationships, expressing their positive value and worth. Human beings not only seek meaning in the more rational areas of explaining how the world works, but also in the moral domains of the significance of life. They not only seek meaning, but they also look for the sources of meaning in different places throughout their lives.

One major feature of human cultures, especially in religious systems, lies in the fostering of hope as a form of frame for the meaning and significance of life. The early anthropologist Bronislaw Malinowski, for example, described religious practices as the 'ritualizing of human optimism'.

Fear of the unknown is a major challenge to hope. People respond differently to such fear: some try to put it out of mind; others try to learn everything they can about their illness and so try to get a purchase on hope; others become interested in religious questions: about judgement, about heaven and hell. When fear of the future-unknown is coupled with what is known of the past and present, such issues as guilt, shame, regret, trust, and anger may come to the fore. The search for meaning and hope is entangled with the search for some way to come to terms with what one has made of one's life or with what has happened in one's life. Yet, hope is not abstract. People do not have hope because they have had an insight into hopefulness. Hope is concrete; and inasmuch as people are tradition-bound, their experience of hope is likely to be expressed in their traditions, in terms of their religious stories, in terms of religious symbols, rites, and narratives that communicate the sources of life and meaningfulness.

Staged responses

Hope is one of the enduring contributions of Elisabeth Kubler-Ross's[18] original book on grief, whose developmental stage theory, along with other stage theories of grief, has otherwise experienced serious criticism and qualification. One negative feature of stage theories of grief is that, when they become popularized, they are often accepted as a 'formula' for grief that many ordinary people do not feel applies to them. In societies where many people are not often personally bereaved until they are young adults or in their early middle years, some stage theories have been almost warmly accepted in order to gain some purchase on technical knowledge in the absence of personal experience. But no amount of formal learning related to grief can replace the personal experience of individuals, a fact of considerable importance for all involved in pastoral care. One of Kubler-Ross's chief contributions was the demolishing of our expectations that grief was something akin to an illness in need of cure. It should not be forgotten just how influential her earlier stage theory was, not least in suggesting that grief was a natural process; that the denial of death, for instance, could be an entirely healthy response as part of a more complex grief process which leads to a rediscovery of hope. The initial insights into grief were applicable to those who anticipate or experience grief in terminal illness rather than to those bereaved by the death of others.

Change, control, and care

Change, whether in circumstances or in self-evaluation, typifies serious illness as it does grief in the bereaved. One major reason why such change is problematic lies in the sense of control that typifies many aspects of contemporary life. For many people with a steady job and career prospects, not to mention those who seek to plan their reproductive life and partnership relationships, life-threatening illness comes as a shock because it takes the sense of control out of their hands. As in other aspects of life there may emerge what Nicole Thoulis in her work on religious identity has called a 'crisis of presence'. In much of life individuals possess a relatively high degree of 'presence'—a term used to describe that sense of balance within one's life circumstances allowing a degree of control over one's activities and future and in relationship to other people. Developing Thoulis's perspective, one can see how a crisis of presence may be brought about by a wide variety of factors including changed employment, environment, economic circumstances, retirement, divorce, serious illness, and bereavement. One feature of the dismay that may be associated with such a crisis of presence involves the sense that other people continue to live in their ordinary and comfortable world whilst the sufferer has been thrown into a sense of unreality, into a world where the ordinary plausibility of life has fragmented. It is within that context that pastoral care comes as a kind of bridge between ordinariness-normality and the changed circumstances of the sick. One of the reasons why communication between bereaved people and others is sometimes difficult lies in the two worlds each currently inhabits.

Power

A major feature of pastoral care concerns the way individuals themselves see the world in which they are becoming sick and in which they are to die. Referring to the same Solzhenitsyn text quoted above, Richard McCormick wrote of the dual challenges of passivity and helplessness facing the terminally ill. He suggested that the difficulties are magnified by the 'asymmetrical power relationship of physician and institution to patient' (ref. 6, p. 109). Contemporary palliative medicine is, of course, based on appreciating the dignity and autonomy of patients, and it is recognized both that palliative care involves a number of decision-makers and that the patient is the primary decision-maker. But the asymmetry remains. The availability of pastoral care is but one way to address the asymmetry. This holds not just for hospitals and hospices, but also for schools, colleges, prisons, and the armed forces. One of the now-traditional roles of chaplains and other pastoral carers is that of go-between, the person who can cut through the bureaucracy and leap-frog normal chains of command, the one who can translate or relay concerns in a non-threatening manner. A team that thought it did not need such a function could be underestimating the asymmetry of power that exists and doing itself a disservice.

Controlling change

Those engaged in pastoral care have as a major feature of their life a constant passing between these two domains, a process that improves with experience but which can ever remain problematic to a degree. But, in addition to that kind of movement between realms of experience, pastoral carers also undergo their own forms of life-change, as does everyone else. These may involve many shifts in understanding and life-commitments, not least when individuals have to be mobile in their career development. For some, perhaps especially for those attracted to pastoral care, such change involves a desire to understand life in all its transitions.

Such a search may take a great variety of paths. Some, paralleling the work of such early cognitive developmental psychologists as Jean Piaget, often operate within a 'faith development' framework, emphasizing how change and development are structured by our increasing abilities to cope with new and more complex aspects of life. This approach draws heavily from biology and is based on 'an open-systems model of evolutionary biology in which the important unit of study is not the organism alone or the environment alone but the exchange of information between them' (ref. 19, p. 173). Piaget's model, for example, involved identifying invariant, sequential stages of development; and James Fowler's faith-development theory distinguishes seven levels of faith: from primal faith (a primal trust that addresses an equally primal invulnerability) to universalizing faith (movement from belief about God to a faithful abiding in God). At the same time, such faith development theorists as James Fowler and Robert Kegan subordinate the identification of actual stages to a more general appreciation of life being an 'ongoing, dynamic process of meaning-making' (ref. 19, p. 175). Faith development itself suggests a model for pastoral care, especially when the struggle with terminal illness and death is appreciated as a significant process, as a time of potential growth.

Even if one is not explicitly religious, the parallels between faith development and what one might call world-view development or life-development are apposite, and there are grounds for appreciating the complementarity of different faith and humanist perspectives.

Chaplains

Individuals representing major religious traditions are often on the staff of hospitals and other institutions, whether caring for people in a medical sense or in the ways appropriate to prisons, armies, and schools. They are an important means of allowing the complementarity of religious factors to relate to the scientific and technological dimension of medical treatment. While chaplains generally represent the distinctive group to which they belong, there is a growing trend for them to express spiritual care in a more general way. In some parts of Holland, for example, hospitals are divided into sectors each cared for by a chaplain of a distinctive tradition, including that of Humanism. Unless individuals request a chaplain of their distinctive denomination, they will meet the person appointed to their part of the hospital. This could mean that a representative of Islam, Catholicism, Protestantism, or Humanism relates to an individual of quite a different tradition.

The rationale for this approach to spiritual care is that each 'chaplain' seeks to foster the faith, spirituality, or world-view of each 'patient'. Chaplains are seen as representative human beings, as 'professional non-professionals', as having no limiting job description apart from accompanying the patient. At the same time, there should be no presumption that such a general approach suffices. Andrew Wingate[20] has written movingly of the death of a Thai woman, describing the visits he as an Anglican priest made, and how he participated in the 'loving kindness and mutual forgiveness' meditations and in the 'last rites' performed by Buddhist monks. His account of the way his friend was surrounded by the resources of both

Christianity and Buddhism underlined 'the importance of established ritual and practice.' Wingate observed:

> Rituals led by the monks seem to offer real lessons in pastoral care. They last long enough—an hour or more at a time—to give space for people to feel, reflect and move on a step. Their demeanour and the style of their chanting are sufficiently detached to be enabling of the family, and the person dying. They give a strong signal, a kind of permission, to encourage an end to the struggle. This is not resignation, however, but a sense of positive surrender to the future (ref. 20, pp. 176–7).

Rituals are, of course, expressive of traditions; and while we can enter into and be moved by rituals from other traditions, Wingate made much of the familiarity of these Buddhist traditions to the woman. One of the dangers, then, of 'expressing pastoral care in a general way' is an exaggerated emphasis on words and a reliance on more general cultural gestures. In death-denying cultures, this has obvious disadvantages.

A distinct but related role of chaplaincy is making spiritual direction available. 'Spiritual direction' is perhaps a misnomer, for spiritual directors generally do not 'direct' but help people to interpret their prayer. At crucial times of life, individual prayer can be intense, difficult, disappointing, consoling, or even overwhelming. Spiritual directors can help set the context of individual prayer within the larger context of the spiritual tradition. Even the offer of spiritual direction suggests the legitimacy of expectations of spiritual growth towards the end of life.[21]

Power of belonging

Another aspect of chaplaincy stems again from the communal representational role of chaplains: chaplains and visiting clergy often provide a link with a person's actual local church or faith community. This sense of still belonging to a community when all the normal ties are disrupted is no doubt of some therapeutic value, but it also reflects the truth of the person's continuing value to the community. In other words, fostering this sense of belonging is valuable for the community too. This aspect of chaplaincy allows people to be part of the larger rhythm of daily or weekly religious observance. For Christians, this sense of community can be expressed symbolically when a person receives communion from the same bread and wine used in the local church service or in terms simply of knowing that one is being remembered in others' prayers. But it is also expressed 'ritually' when family members bring in a piece of birthday cake from a party at home.

Training

Some chaplains, perhaps chiefly in North America (because of the existence of clinical–pastoral education or CPE), offer pastoral *counselling* as a distinct form of pastoral care. Developed in the second half of the last century, pastoral counselling grew out of Freudian psychodynamic theory and Rogerian therapy. The chief goal of pastoral counselling is to gain insight into oneself and into the conflicts one feels by engaging with one's past in some depth. Notable among those who have written on pastoral counselling are Howard Clinebell, Wayne Oates, and Seward Hiltner. Howard Stone[22] has conducted a useful study of pastoral counselling theorists, challenging their individualistic focus and questioning their over-reliance on so few and now dated theories. At the same time, he approvingly noted a growing reliance on pastoral counselling's theological roots.

Hospice

A major development in the care of the terminally ill developed in the closing decades of the twentieth century with the hospice movement. Stressing the priority of the sick individual, it exemplifies the notion of holistic care whether given at home or in a specific building. The idea of 'hospice' as an attitude of care is more important than 'hospice' as a place. It combines the centrality of the sick with a team-approach of medical, clerical, and volunteer staff to the well-being, pain-control, and the social networks of people with the opportunity for people to orientate themselves towards their forthcoming death. It is the very centrality of the dying individual that gives substance to the idea of 'dignity' that is now so often associated with death in the contemporary world. Interpreted in terms of power and control, some see the hospice movement as a corrective for the over-technological medicalization of treatment, contrasting a feminine sense of care with a masculine model of control, or even seeing it as a move on the part of clergy to regain influence over the dying (ref. 23, pp. 437–47; cf. ref. 24).

Hospice and support groups

This emergence of the hospice movement as one cultural expression of the value of human life, and of the relationships between people when life is drawing to its close, expresses four forms of care. Professional care given by paid professional staff, the care of volunteers, the care of families and friends, and the mutual care of fellow sufferers. In contemporary societies, the formation of support groups of many different kinds is one major form of response to personal trauma or to the sickness or death of family or friends. Here, 'expertise' is the expertise of those who have suffered. In some respects this contrasts with the educational expertise of medical professionals. In cultural terms, the distinction between professional and volunteer care can either be sharply maintained or dissolved depending upon a person's world-view. The very use of the term 'complementary medicine' reflects the potential divide between scientific medicine and other forms of dealing with people that are not so grounded.

Spiritual assessments

In recent years, spiritual assessments have emerged (e.g. the HOPE assessment), enabling pastoral carers and others to assess the sorts of support patients desire or need. These assessments can be very detailed, or they can be as simple as asking patients a few questions about whether they adhere to a religion, how religious they think they are, what they believe, the importance of their beliefs, and so on, including, of course, how the team can help them pastorally or spiritually. Such an assessment is undoubtedly useful to discover how best to support patients, for there will be many who will want to meet with a chaplain, to be ministered to pastorally or sacramentally.

But there are dangers in using a formal assessment tool. One danger is confusing the 'religious' with the 'spiritual', trying to manage or fit what is for many an open-ended spiritual journey into familiar religious categories. Another danger is the inappropriate use of a clinical model for the non-clinical. Do patients have 'symptoms' of spiritual needs? Do we need 'to treat' the spiritual symptoms? Do we need 'to heal' spiritual pain? While appreciating the need for some sort of 'assessment', this caution reflects the need to regard individual differences as significant, making no assumptions that religion or spirituality are strictly formulaic.

Such differences go beyond the merely individual, and include, for instance, understanding the different ways in which pastoral care is offered and received among African Americans.[25] Some feminist and womanist writers have proposed their own pastoral theology,[26] and the pastoral care of children cannot but be affected by the burgeoning interest in children's spirituality. There is a profound range of issues surrounding the care of AIDS patients, and there has been increased interest in exploring the particular spiritualities of disabled people, of the mentally handicapped, and the mentally ill. Such differences demand the broadest appreciation of spirituality and pastoral care.[27]

Conclusion

This chapter has deliberately set out to emphasize the breadth of cultural and spiritual aspects of pastoral care in palliative medicine. Without wishing to diminish the extraordinary work of chaplains, the authors are increasingly aware of the multicultural and multireligious dimensions of all caring. This may appear to make pastoral care more difficult to manage, but it also offers hope that the very real spiritual dimensions of people's lives and the unique constellation of relationships that make up those same lives will be treated as irreducibly sacred.

References

1. **Ohnuki-Tierney, E.** *Illness and Healing among the Sakhalin Ainu.* Cambridge: Cambridge University Press, 1981.
2. **Nouwen, H.J.** *The Wounded Healer.* New York: Doubleday, 1990.
3. **Ainsworth-Smith, I. and Speck, P.** *Letting Go: Care for the Dying and the Bereaved.* London: SPCK, 1999.
4. **Bowker, J.W.** (1997). Religions, society, and suffering. In *Social Suffering* (ed. A. Kleinman, V. Dons, and M. Lock), pp. 359–82. Berkeley: University of California Press.
5. **Harrington, A.** (1997). Unmasking suffering's masks: reflections on old and new memories of Nazi medicine. In *Social Suffering* (ed. A. Kleinman, V. Das, and M. Lock), pp. 181–205. Berkeley: University of California Press.
6. **McCormick, R.A.** *Health and Medicine in the Catholic Tradition.* New York: Crossroad, 1987.
7. **Schweitzer, A.** *Reverence for Life.* London: SPCK, 1975.
8. **Loades, A.** (1985). Death and disvalue: some reflections on 'sick' children'. *Hospital Chaplain* **93**, 2–7.
9. **Stroebe, W. and Stroebe, M.S.** *Bereavement and Health: The Psychological and Physical Consequences of Partner Loss.* Cambridge: Cambridge University Press, 1989.
10. **Davies, D.J.** (2000). Health, morality and sacrifice: the sociology of disasters. In *The Blackwell Companion to the Sociology of Religion* (ed. R.K. Fenn). Oxford: Blackwell.
11. **Moody, R.A.** *Life After Life: The Investigation of a Phenomenon-Survival of Bodily Death.* New York: Bantam, 1975.
12. **Davies, D.J.** *Death Ritual and Belief*, 2nd revised edn. London: Continuum, 2002.
13. **Bloch, M.** *Prey into Hunter.* Cambridge: Cambridge University Press, 1992.
14. **Moody, R.A.** *The Last Laugh.* Charlottesvile VA: Hampton Roads Pub. Co., 1999.
15. **McKee, D.D. and Chappel, J.N.** (1992). Spirituality and medical practice. *Journal of Family Practice* **35**, 201–8.
16. **Sloan, R.P., Bagiella, E., and Powell, T.** (1999). Religion, spirituality, and medicine. *Lancet* **353**, 664–7.
17. **Larson, D. and Koenig, H.G.** (2000). Is God good for your health? The role of spirituality in medical care. *Cleveland Clinical Journal of Medicine* **67**, 2.
18. **Kubler-Ross, E.** *On Death and Dying.* New York: Macmillan, 1969.
19. **Osmer, R. and Fowler, J.W.** (1993). Childhood and adolescence—a faith development perspective. In *Clinical Handbook of Pastoral Counselling* (ed. R.J. MoWicks, R.D. Parsons, and D. Capps). New York: Paulist Press.
20. **Wingate, A.** (1997). A woman of faith dies: death of a champion of Buddhism. *Theology* **795**, 170–9.
21. **Kubler-Ross, E.**, ed. *Death: The Final Stage of Growth.* Englewood Cliffs NJ: Prentice Hall, 1975.
22. **Stone, H.** (2001). The congregational setting of pastoral counseling; a study of pastoral counseling theorists from 1949–1991. *The Journal of Pastoral Care* **55** (2).
23. **Kearl, M.C.** *Endings, a Sociology of Death and Dying.* Oxford: Oxford University Press, 1989.
24. **Ariès, P.** *The Hour of Our Death.* Oxford: Oxford University Press, 1991.
25. **Wimberly, E.P.** *African-American Pastoral Care.* Nashville: Abingdon, 1991.
26. **Miller-McLemore, B. and Gill-Austern, B.L.** (ed.) *Feminist and Womanist Pastoral Theology.* Nashville: Abingdon, 1999.
27. **Pattison, S.** *Alive and Kicking: Towards a Practical Theology of Illness and Healing.* London: SPCK, 1989.

12

Emotional issues in palliative medicine

12 Emotional issues in palliative medicine

12.1 The emotional problems of the patient in palliative medicine

Mary L.S. Vachon

Emotional problems and psychosocial distress are common as individuals confront the terminal phase of illness and their impending death.(1–7) Appropriate intervention at this critical point may decrease the immediate emotional suffering for all concerned.(8) In addition, intervention can also ease the family bereavement period.(9–11)

The assessment and treatment of the psychosocial distress associated with terminal illness involve distinguishing between the normal symptoms of adjustment to a terminal illness and the symptoms of a major psychiatric disorder. The skilled practitioner must be able to identify, assess, and, when possible, treat the physical symptoms of the disease together with the increasing debility and changes in social roles and social isolation associated with the disease and the dying process. At the same time, he or she must be able to distinguish when the social isolation or change in social roles are signs of a major depression and when the pain and symptoms of the disease have a strong psychological overlay requiring psychiatric or psychological referral.

Overview of chapter

Focus of the chapter

This chapter will outline some underlying assumptions of palliative care and provide a new model of palliative care. There will then be a review of the epidemiological data on the psychosocial distress and clinical depression experienced by persons with terminal illness, identifying some of the factors associated with increased risk of psychosocial distress. Given the current interest in whether or not psychosocial factors contribute to and/or can affect the course of cancer, there will be a discussion of these variables, psychoneuroimmunology (PNI) in cancer and other illnesses and psychosocial intervention to alter the course of cancer. This will be followed by a clinical discussion of the emotional and psychosocial spiritual issues confronting dying persons.

The format of the chapter will be to discuss issues of adaptation in general, to highlight specific symptoms to alert the clinician to problems that must be addressed, and then to give some specific intervention strategies. Clinical examples as well as art and poetry from persons living with life-threatening illness and bereavement will be used to give the reader better insight into the experience of the palliative care patient and family.

Underlying assumptions of the chapter

- Illness does not occur in a vacuum.
- The illness trajectory may affect adaptation.
- Early intervention may affect later distress.
- Intervention should meet patient and family needs.
- Good palliative care involves options.
- Titrate information to patient needs.
- There is no one right way.

Illness does not occur in a vacuum

Sir William Osler has been quoted as saying, 'Ask not what disease the person has, but rather what person the disease has'.(12) The underlying premise of the chapter is that illness does not occur in a vacuum. The individual has a personal history, personality characteristics, and coping mechanisms that may prove to be helpful or unhelpful in dealing with the present situation. In addition, most individuals are members of a social network. The manner in which an individual's significant others respond to the person and his or her illness may, in part, determine the individual's response to the disease. A single mother with metastatic disease caring for young children and fighting with her husband for child support payments, knowing that he would just as soon see her dead, is in a very different position from the person who has a warm, loving supportive family structure. An individual's process of adaptation to the disease will also be determined in part by a number of other variables including:

- age and stage of family development;
- the nature of the disease;
- the trajectory or pattern of the illness;
- the individual and family's previous experience with illness and death;
- socioeconomic status;
- cultural variables.(13)

A diagnosis of AIDS in a young woman with dependent children living in rural Africa will obviously be a different disease experience requiring a different response from that of a woman of the same age living in a western society who is diagnosed with inflammatory breast cancer, carefully assesses her options, chooses to have aggressive treatment, and then relapses.

Mary Pocock[1] an artist who was diagnosed with breast cancer in her early 40s wrote (Picture 1):

> When I heard my diagnosis several years ago, my logical mind could not bend around my inevitable demise—in three to five years—treatment options—that will make you very ill—and the ravages and statistics of my two kinds of invasive cancer.

[1] The art and reflections of Mary Pocock are used with her permission.

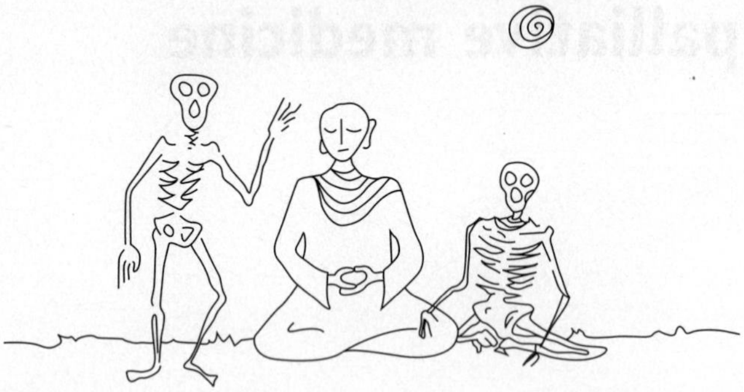

Picture 1 The very thing that we fear we carry within us right now—our corpse (milarcpa).

I sit here eight years later, wondering how and why I have survived. The cancer has spread to my bones, lungs and possibly heart sac. I have a low grade pain in my spine and my present treatment gives constant fatigue and nausea. I am happy to be alive and in the same breath contemplate how to bring contentment into an unknown future, bringing with it the probability of worsening pain and organ breakdown.

My quality of life has worsened the past few years. I am often short of breath and dog-tired, as they say. I eat not from hunger but to quell nausea. Any yet, ironically, I am much happier these days. I feel it is my meditation on this forced pilgrimage, which has allowed joy to rise in the midst of difficult circumstances.

Mary Pocock, 2001

The illness trajectory may affect adaptation

Both the person with life-threatening illness and the support network will respond differently depending on whether the illness was initially perceived as having been 'cured' and has now relapsed; whether the disease was perceived to be a chronic disease which was expected to go on 'forever' and is now at the point where treatment aimed at prolonging survival is no longer appropriate; or whether the disease has had a fairly rapid trajectory to death.[13]

Early intervention may decrease later distress

The assumption is made that if the needs of the person with a life-threatening illness and the significant others are handled reasonably well from the time of diagnosis, then even if the final outcome is death, the problems associated with this outcome will be fewer and less complicated than would be the case if there were numerous unresolved problems during the early stages of the illness.[13] Figure 1[14] shows the Square of Care developed as part of the Square of Care and Organization in the consensus document by the Canadian Hospice Palliative Care Association.[2] The preface to the document notes that people are living with illnesses for much longer. Faced with longer illness people must deal with many issues:

- How to get relief of symptoms?
- How can they carry on with life, as they have known it?
- How will the illness affect roles and relationships?
- What can be done to change the illness experience?
- How can people restore or maintain their capacity for meaningful and valuable experiences that give quality to their lives?

Each of these issues creates expectations, needs, hopes, and fears, which must be addressed in order for the ill person to carry on with life and find opportunities for growth within the illness experience. For many years, the approach used in hospice palliative care has helped patients and their families address these issues during the last stage of the illness experience: the process of dying. The same approach can now be used to enhance health-care delivery throughout the entire illness experience. All the skills developed in hospice palliative care can be applied early to help patients improve their quality of life, increase their ability to participate in therapy to fight their disease and, potentially, prolong their lives (ref. 14, p. i).

The Square of Care:

- identifies all the issues commonly faced by patients and families during an illness, respective of diagnosis;
- elaborates the norms of practice related to each element of the process of providing care during a clinical encounter.

The Square of Organization, which is not shown:

- identifies all the resources needed to run a hospice palliative care organization;
- elaborates the norms of practice related to each aspect of organizational function (see also ref. 15).

While not based directly on this model, this chapter will be dealing with many of the issues identified in the Square of Care, as this model is congruent with the author's clinical practice as a psychotherapist working with those with life-threatening illness and bereavement for over 30 years. The model is also congruent with the author's personal experience as a survivor of stage IV non-Hodgkin's lymphoma.

In September 1996, not long after completing this chapter for the second edition of the *Oxford Textbook of Palliative Medicine*,[16] the author began to experience minor abdominal pain while attending the *11th International Congress on Care of the Terminally Ill* in Montreal. The pain was 1–2 on a 10-point scale so I had no particular concerns about it, being sure that it was an ulcer. At my convenience and that of my family physician I saw her and within 2 days had an ultrasound revealing either widespread lymphoma or metastatic disease with an unknown primary. From the beginning lymphoma became the 'good news'. I immediately contacted a colleague, who I knew only peripherally, asking him to be my oncologist. I wrote him a letter informing him of my expertise in the area of palliative care and stating that if he could cure me, I would do whatever would be necessary to cooperate with him. If not, quality of life was going to be my guiding principle. I was not interested in extra days, weeks, or months (or at least at that point that was my philosophy, I know this can change with people over-time if the disease worsens). I informed him that the first bit of quality of life I wanted was to be able to participate in the *3rd Hong Kong International Congress and 7th International EBV Symposium*, in Hong Kong and Shanghai respectively. I was to present on issues such as 'Breaking Bad News' and 'Women with Cancer', but more importantly, I was to be travelling with my family—my husband, son, and daughter, and presenting papers on 'Dealing with Anger', and 'Anticipatory Loss and Grief' with my son, a former street kid and grade 9 dropout, who had just graduated with distinction from university. I figured that maybe 'my time had come'. I had fulfilled what I had been put on this earth to do, getting our son through this crisis (remember cancer does not occur in a vacuum). As I rapidly became more symptomatic while going through my workup, I began to reflect on my funeral. On a Sunday, my friend and colleague, the same Dr Frank Ferris referred to above,[14] prescribed ventalin so I could breath. On Monday I had a bone marrow biopsy, CHOP chemotherapy and on Thursday headed off to Shanghai and Hong Kong, complete with a suitcase of drugs including neuprogen and antibiotics to keep me from getting infections while abroad. Good palliative care enabled me to do what was important to me at this point in my life. People experiencing serious illness sometimes have an inner wisdom of their own that enables them to make decisions that are right for them.

Singh[17] writes of the process of transformation that may occur with serious illness—the turning point in the evolution of consciousness. 'Transformation occurs through subtraction. We begin, as we heal successive dualities, as we approach deeper and deeper levels of integration, to eliminate the nonessential. As we participate in the process, we find paradoxically, that the subtraction adds, that through the exclusion of the nonessential from our attention, we create movement and we become more inclusively essential' (pp. 90–1). Through the process of illness, I came to a deeper realization of the importance of spirituality, of my clinical work in my life, and of my lack of interest in participating in political issues in a work environment. If I was going to die of my illness, but was healthy

[2] The Square of Care is used with the permission of the Canadian Hospice and Palliative Care Association and Dr Frank Ferris.

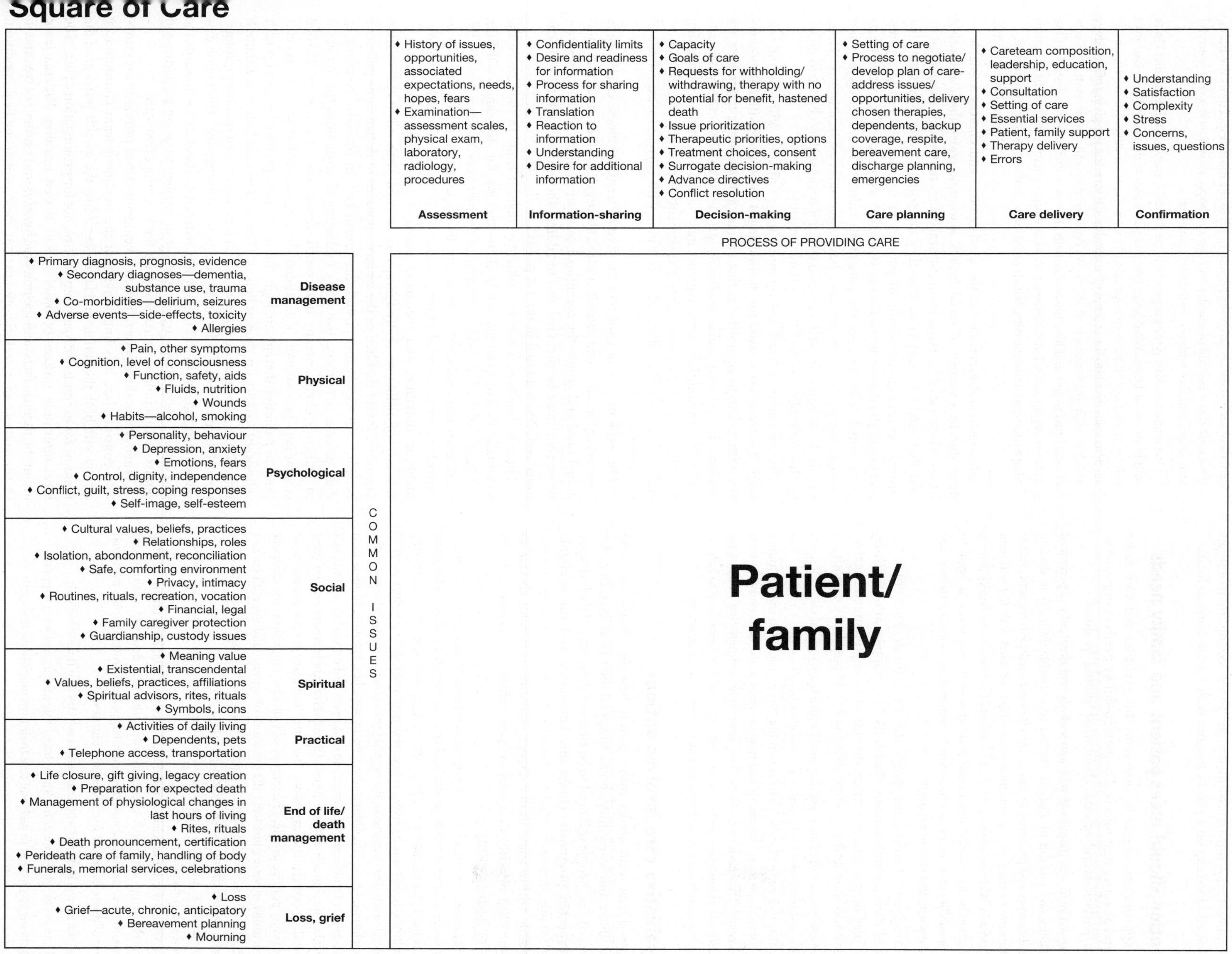

Fig. 1 Square of Care. (Used with the permission of the Canadian Hospice and Palliative Care Association and Dr Frank Ferris.[14])

enough to work, then I would just as soon use the time in a way that was valuable and helping others (while pursuing my own transforming path at the same time). Eventually, this transformation led to my leaving my role in an organization and focusing on a private practice with a more spiritual focus.

Intervention should meet patient and family needs

It is not appropriate simply to intervene. Intervention must be done carefully and at a pace best matched to patient–family needs as opposed to caregiver expectations and agendas about what 'should' be done.

A 40-year-old man was diagnosed with amyloidosis and eventually experienced kidney failure and was put on dialysis. He had considerable difficulty in dealing with the diagnosis and preferred to stay in the city near medical treatment, rather than returning to the farming community in which he lived with his wife and 14-year-old son. Although others felt that he should be closer to his family during his final months, he avoided them until such time as he was ready to begin to face the possibility of his death at which time he returned home and in his own way prepared his wife and son for his death.

While caregivers sometimes inappropriately make the decision not to tell patients and their family members what is likely to happen; at other times caregivers may inappropriately err on the side of giving too much negative information too soon and too often, allowing for no possibility of hope.

A man whose 39-year-old fiancé was diagnosed with a brain tumour said, 'I'll never forgive the residents who spoke with Sue soon after her diagnosis. They said "You might just as well go to Florida. There is nothing that we can do to change things. You are going to die soon." We barely had time to adjust to the news and they were writing her off. They gave us no hope. The surgeon let us know that things were serious, but she at least gave us some hope that they could do something to help us to have some quality time as we began to adjust to what was happening.'

Good palliative care involves options

People should have some choice with regard to how they choose to spend their final illness and where they choose to spend their final days. In order to have this choice, people will need to be aware of the extent of their disease and its expected prognosis. Given this knowledge and the available resources, people should be able to choose to continue active treatment, albeit possibly within some limits; choose palliative treatment; choose to be at home with or without a support programme or choose to be in a hospital or hospice setting.

Denise Bebenek, a mother whose 5-year-old daughter, Meagan, died of a brain tumour wrote a letter about hope during her daughter's final illness. This letter spread around the world via the Internet. Meagan died just after celebrating her fifth birthday. She was receiving active treatment until just a few days prior to her peaceful death that occurred in the hospital emergency room with her extended family including her young siblings and cousins with her. Speaking of their final journey together Denise said, 'A foundation of support and unconditional love, will help sustain one through difficult times. All palliative care journeys require great understanding and gentle compassion. Thus it is important for the patient to be surrounded by positive people. The journey of palliative care affords the caregiver the opportunity of seeing just what the dynamics of support and hopefulness can do for those afflicted. When death is a probability one has to live with hope and reality, and temper the two to keep the hope aspect alive.'

Denise spoke at a fund raising event in her daughter's honour held six months after her death and said:[3]

As we waited for a miracle for this little sweetheart, standing tall and living her own challenge with such grace, we knew that she deserved nothing but a miraculous cure. Instead we observed many happenings around us. We witnessed a number of miracles unfold from Meagan's journey:

- a very courageous little girl who embraced each day as if it were her last;
- people, many of whom we didn't know, being there for us, in loving support;
- people being challenged to seek and find their own purpose on this earth

[3] The reflections of Denise Bebenek are used with her permission.

... Yet through this particular journey with Meagan, I have come to realize the great power of hope in moving forward. Journeying with hope is not so simple. It can move mountains; it can bring an aura of joy to the most desperate of situations. If we walk just a portion of our day with greater hope, we will have a very powerful tool to face and deal with our individual challenges ...

One might ask what is the purpose of hope if a child may be destined to die? Quite simply-we never know. What keeps one going in times of despair is hope. Our lives will be much richer if we keep hope alive. What is the alternative? Not having any ay all? This spills over into the concept of unconditional love, the self-giving of ourselves, which is what this evening is all about. We don't need to wait for the most desperate of situations to live and love unconditionally. It may not change the destiny of the child, or the situation, but it bestows to those needing such love, the benefit of human compassion and understanding, which we all know is of highest value on its own.

Denise Bebenek, 2002

Obviously, not everyone has the ideal options and choices available to them due to a variety of social beliefs, economic constraints, and other issues. These variables range from cultural beliefs that people should not be told that they have cancer or that they are going to die; to settings that strongly encourage terminally ill patients to transfer to hospice settings because of the economic problems associated with expensive 'active treatment' which will not cure the patient; to cultures in which there is not enough money for even the very basic necessities of health care. Here, people die at home or even on the streets, not because they choose to do so, but because there are no other options available.

The provision of treatment options can be difficult. Within some settings, it is sometimes easier for the oncologist to proceed with chemotherapy, rather than to acknowledge that current antineoplastic treatments are inadequate and may cause morbidity greater than the underlying cancer.[6,18,19] In addition, some patients may have great difficulty accepting that there are limits to the current treatments for their particular cancer and they may push or demand to continue with current or experimental treatment.

The issue of patient choice in the face of terminal illness causes some controversy 'as clinicians cannot continue to argue for the primacy of individual need and ignore the communal cost implications of their prescriptions; they must be prepared also to address the ethics of resource allocations' (ref. 20, as quoted in ref. 18, p. 723).

There is, however, a role for palliative chemotherapy in the care of the terminally ill. For example, while chemotherapy for non-small-cell lung carcinoma of the lung and carcinoma of the pancreas may not prolong life more than minimally,[21,22] there can be documented major benefits to patients in terms of relief of pain, easing of shortness of breath, improvements in nutrition, and the maintenance of better functional status.[2] A study of palliative chemotherapy in women with advanced ovarian cancer[23] found that half of the women appeared to derive some palliative benefit from the treatment and one-fourth had an objective response in their disease. A retrospective study, evaluating all costs from the initiation of palliative chemotherapy until death, demonstrated a cost of $53 000 (Canadian) per woman. The studies demonstrated that patient expectations in palliative therapy are high and women are prepared to put up with significant toxicity for modest benefit. The authors conclude that although palliative therapy may be associated with high costs, even modest prolongation of survival can render such treatment cost-effective. The major cost saving associated with this therapy was reduced hospitalization towards the end of life. The authors suggest that future studies focus on palliative end points that include a comparison with the best supportive care.

When chemotherapy or radiation is being prescribed primarily for symptom control, then it is imperative that the treatment team communicate clearly with both the patient and family regarding the specific purpose of the therapy, for example, for symptom control, not for prolongation of life. 'The ideal informing process becomes one of shared learning. Patients learn about the medical facts, and the potential benefits and burdens of treatment, in the context of a realistic appraisal of their overall medical condition. Physicians, in turn, must learn of their patient's personal experiences and perceptions about the diagnosis, their current quality of life, and the amount of suffering they are willing to tolerate ...' (ref. 24, p. 46).

A 59-year-old widowed woman diagnosed with widespread metastatic colon cancer at presentation was at a party soon after being treated for brain metastasis, shortly before starting treatment for her lung metastasis. She said, 'I have a good understanding with my oncologist, as long as he can give me treatment that makes my life worth living then I'll take it. I've made it clear to him however that I am not interested in spending a month feeling miserable in order to get an extra week of life. I think that we understand each other quite well.'

These conversations are difficult. Caregivers must be prepared to give this information in a caring and sensitive manner, being ready to deal with the difficulty patients and families have in accepting this information. Caregivers must also be aware that patients and families may sometimes deny the reality of what is being said. Conversations to clarify the purposes of palliative therapies may have to take place periodically over the course of treatment. However, knowledgeable caregivers must also realize that they are not always correct in their prognostications.

Janet Kohut is a 46-year-old recently separated woman who was diagnosed with melanoma in 1997. The tumour was 1.22 mm in depth and was Clarks level III. In October 1998, she developed a tumour in her groin and underwent a superficial inguinal groin dissection. Six months later lesions showed up in her liver, gall bladder, abdomen, and bowel. Two noted experts in the field told her that she had 2 months to live.

At her insistence she took chemotherapy with a third physician. She completed the 3B course of the Dartmouth Protocol in June 1999. According to her notes, this protocol has a 6 per cent survival rate. Janet feels that she owes her life to her husband and daughter's help. In addition, she has used a variety of complementary approaches including: homeopathic remedies, Vitamins A, B, C; essiac tea, taheebo tea, Utilin 6, citrus pectin, cloud mushrooms, arnica, chemotherapy, steroids, zofran. She has also had spiritual healing, does reiki, qi gong, and therapeutic touch. She stopped smoking, changed her diet and takes no caffeine, steams her vegetables, eats steamed rice, fish, and chicken and takes no dairy or chocolate.

In March of 2002 she is still in remission, has left her husband, feeling that she wants more in life, and has begun a graduated return to work. She still has 'little spots' on her liver and her oncologist, with whom she has an excellent relationship, tells her that her disease will recur at some point, but in the meantime she is enjoying the life she was told that she would not have.[4]

Titrate information to patient needs

Given, that under ideal circumstances, people should have the choice of where and how to spend their final time, so too should they have the option of choosing how much information they want about their illness including the option of choosing not to know their prognosis if this is their preference. The medical practitioner must be aware that, much as there is a 'right to know', there is also a corresponding 'right not to know' provided that the patient has given the health care provider the clear message that this is his/her choice. Problems arise in this situation, however, if the patient chooses 'not-to-know' that the treatment she/he is demanding has almost no likelihood of success and the person refuses to acknowledge the possibility that death may result from this disease episode.

A young mother of two daughters, aged 6 and 8, refused to acknowledge that she might die of her colon cancer and that her children should be prepared for the possibility of her death. She kept repeating that she would search the world for treatments and would eventually manage to cure her disease, so her children did not need to be upset by discussing the possibility that she might die. She refused to speak with her children about her illness, even when their behaviour indicated that they were having considerable difficulty dealing with her obvious deterioration, while they were being reassured that all was well. When it became clear that she was dying, however, she and her husband spoke openly with their children on their own initiative, prepared them for the fact that she might die and then were open to talking as a family with the staff about what was happening. At the time of her funeral, her children read a poem describing their mother's struggle with illness and their coming to terms as a family with the need to let her go as her condition deteriorated and she slipped into unconsciousness.

[4] This anecdote is used with the permission of Janet Kohut.

The choice not to tell a person of his/her prognosis should not be a decision that the health care provider makes for the patient in order to increase the provider's comfort level. Rather, it should be an acknowledgement that the caregiver is available to 'walk with' the patient along the path that the person has chosen. When the patient chooses not to know that he or she is dying, the provider should always be open to talking with the patient about the illness and prognosis when the person is prepared to do so. The care provider should also be willing to speak with the person in 'symbolic' language as this is appropriate. If the caregiver initiates discussions in symbolic language, however, she/he must be certain that the patient understands what is being said.

One woman spoke of being told by her minister that there 'was someone inside me guiding me and telling me what to do about dying.' The woman did not understand what was meant by this comment and was afraid to ask for fear she would appear to be 'stupid.' The concept of 'letting go' and trusting in God was explained. Her face glowed as she understood what was meant. When she was asked what insights she might like to share with people reading this chapter she replied 'keep it simple. Make sure that people understand what you are saying.'

There is no one right way

Clinical examples illustrating communication with dying people will be given throughout this chapter in order to provide clarity and the understanding that there is no one 'right way' to handle the problems confronting the dying person and his/her family.

Epidemiology of psychosocial distress

Psychosocial distress

Prevalence estimates of psychological distress in terminally ill patients are higher than in a general cancer population.[(25–29)] From 61 to 79 per cent of the palliative care subgroup ($N = 69$) in a stratified, randomized, Registry-based, Canadian community cancer sample of 1319 people living with cancer[(30–32)] currently had high distress on the General Health Questionnaire (GHQ)[(33)] compared with 18–34 per cent of the general cancer population. In a replication of the original study,[(34)] 79 per cent of both terminally ill inpatients ($N = 31$) and terminally ill outpatients ($N = 14$) had high distress compared with 66 per cent of the total inpatient population ($N = 97$) and 30 per cent of the outpatient population ($N = 346$). Thirty-eight per cent of the total population ($N = 443$) had high distress.

In the original study, pain, other symptoms, and treatment side-effects, as well as cancer-related fears, were seen to have direct and indirect effects on psychological symptoms of distress. Impaired role performance was a central mediator for the indirect effects. The model explained 34 per cent of the variance in GHQ scores[(25)] and was equally applicable to all three study sites, both male and female subjects, rural and urban settings, and to all stages of illness. Pain was the single most important explaining variable, but other symptoms, including fatigue, had an impact on impaired role performance.[(25)] However, impaired role performance also had a negative effect on distress over and above the effect of pain.

Clinical depression

Wilson et al.[(28)] reported on 14 studies on the prevalence of depression in cancer patients. All studies used an interview methodology in conjunction with a criterion-based diagnostic system. The prevalence of depression ranged from 1 to 40 per cent. Five to fifteen per cent of patients with cancer will meet the criteria for major depression, even when the most stringent criteria are used.[(28)] In the North American population, the rate of 1-month prevalence of major depression has been estimated at 1.6–4.9 per cent.[(28)] In addition to major depression, another 10–15 per cent of patients with cancer present with depressive symptoms that are somewhat less severe. In some studies, these patients are classified as being 'sub-threshold' for clinical depressive disorder and are classified as not being depressed. In other studies, they may be diagnosed as having either major depression or adjustment disorder.

An Expert Working Group of the Research Steering Committee of the European Association of Palliative Care addressed the issue of depression in palliative care.[35] They concluded, as did Wilson et al.[28] that the prevalence of depression in palliative care varies depending on the type and stage of disease, setting and population characteristics. Stiefel et al.[35] reported on studies in which depression in palliative care ranged from 3.7 to 58 per cent. Among studies of patients with significant levels of physical impairment at least one-fourth of those with advanced disease experience a clinically relevant and treatable depressive illness. Only a minority of those with depression receive the necessary pharmacological treatment. Pain and depression often coexist and influence each other in palliative care settings. A close correlation between long periods of pain and depressive feelings has been demonstrated, a correlation that may be due to neurotransmitter changes, but also to psychological exhaustion.[36] On the other hand, 'pain-free periods are known to give patients new strength and to lower the incidence of mood disturbances and suicidal ideation' (ref. 37, p. 479).

In the Psychosocial Collaborative Oncology group study,[38] 39 per cent of those who received a psychiatric diagnosis experienced significant pain. In contrast, only 19 per cent of patients who did not receive a psychiatric diagnosis had significant pain. The psychiatric diagnoses of those with pain included Adjustment Disorder with Depressed or Mixed Mood (69 per cent). Fifteen per cent of patients with significant pain had symptoms of a major depression.

Spiegel and colleagues[39,40] found that major depression was significantly higher among patients with considerable pain (28 per cent) than among those without (10 per cent). However, a history of prior major depression was more prominent in the low-pain group, suggesting that pain produces major depression, since by history alone, the low-pain group should have been more likely to have current depression. The psychiatric symptoms of patients in pain must first be considered a consequence of uncontrolled pain. 'Acute anxiety, depression with despair, especially when the patient believes the pain means disease progression, agitation, irritability, uncooperative behavior, anger and inability to sleep may be the emotional or behavioural concomitants or sequele[40] of pain' (ref. 41, p. 519).

> Some days I am just too busy struggling to consider the possibility of relief from suffering, from pain, from hopelessness, from fear.
>
> Other days, when crises are but a distant memory, my mind is flooded with plans and images of walks in the park, being able to travel, getting a dog and other similar normal daily agendas.
>
> But I warn you my friend, there is nothing normal about being palliative.
>
> So I await eagerly my miracle.
>
> Mary Pocock

The prevalence of depression in those with advanced cancer is probably not significantly different from that found in patients with other major illnesses. Wells et al.[42] examined the Epidemiological Catchment Area Study data regarding psychiatric disorders and eight chronic medical conditions. Six-month and lifetime prevalence rates of psychiatric disorder were increased in the medically ill (25 and 42 per cent versus 17 and 33 per cent). In the chronically medically ill, 13 per cent had a lifetime diagnosis of affective disorder versus 8 per cent of those free from medical illness.[41] In five major neurological conditions, lifetime rates of depression have been found to range from 30 to 50 per cent.[41]

More detailed information on depression and anxiety will be found in Chapter 8.17.

The patient's experience with cancer

Psychosocial variables and the initiation and development of cancer

There has been speculation, at least since the second century, about the effect of the psyche on cancer initiation. Galen stated that 'cancer was much more frequent in melancholic than in sanguine women' (ref. 43, p. 3). During the eighteenth and nineteenth centuries, it was suggested that women who were prone to develop cancer were sedentary and melancholic and they suffered from depression and/or deep anxiety. In addition, such women were thought to have experienced numerous disasters, losses, or reversals of fortune in their lives. In the twentieth century, the focus has gradually shifted from an emphasis on the psychosocial factors that were hypothesized to be associated with the development of the disease;[44–48] to the psychosocial factors that may or may not be associated with the experience of the disease and its progression.[49–64] Numerous programmes of intervention designed either to alter the distress associated with cancer or even to alter the course of the disease have been reported.[65–73] Research on programmes that purport to alter the course of the disease may include biased samples, thus results must be viewed with caution.[70,74]

This subsection will review some of the current controversies in the field in an attempt to synthesize some of the findings on psychosocial factors that are at this point thought to be associated with the disease or its progression. The reader who wishes a more detailed overview is referred to a number of other sources.[13,64,74,75]

Do psychological factors play a role in the initiation and/or development of cancer?

The interaction between biological and psychological factors

In giving an overview of the psychosocial factors that may have a part to play in the initiation and/or development of cancer, the first point to be made is that cancer is first and foremost a biological disease that would continue to exist even if it were possible to remove stressful life events, transform personalities and create ideal social support systems.[13]

The length of time between the initiation of a tumour and its development into clinically recognized disease may take a decade or more. Therefore, if one is looking for a connection between psychosocial variables and tumour development, one must look at events and traits from at least a decade before.[13,76]

Ronson[77] suggests that in reviewing the possible impact of psychosocial variables on the initiation of cancer and its progression one should be aware that 'cellular processes that underlie malignant transformation, cancer cell behavior and response to antitumoral treatment are so complex that it will be difficult to demonstrate any direct impact of psychosocial variables. Even more elusive could be the evidence of significant correlations between psychological issues, endocrine or immunological functions, and cancer course' (p. 9). Croyle[78] suggests the need for prospective research that incorporates both biologic and psychosocial measures to begin to explore the validity of a comprehensive biopsychosocial model of cancer aetiology.

Fox[74] pointed out a number of methodological concerns in studies purporting to show the impact of some psychosocial variable on the development of cancer or its progression. He addressed the issue of bias in case–control studies and suggested that on the whole cancer patients might be expected to recall more stressful events than persons without cancer. People with negative affect report more negative events than people with average or positive affect.[79] Almost all who have cancer and know it have negative affect to varying degrees.[74] Fox used the example of the Nurses' Health Study.[80] The entire sample of 121 700 nurses who have been followed since 1976 were asked the questions 'What was the colour of your hair at 21' and 'As a child or adolescent, after repeated sun exposures, what kind of tan would you get?' Those diagnosed with melanoma between 1976 and 1982 were called the prevalent group ($n = 87$). Those diagnosed with melanoma between 1982 and 1984 were called incident cases ($n = 34$). The two groups and those who were not diagnosed with melanoma were compared in their response to a questionnaire in 1984. None changed their response with respect to hair colour at age 21, but the incident group changed their response to the tanning question. This finding suggested that the diagnosis of cancer changed their perception of hazardous events in their past life suggesting recall bias.

Psychoneuroimmunology

Psychoneuroimmunology as a scientific field attempts to demonstrate the complexities of the connections between the mind (psychology), the brain (neurology), and the immune system (immunology) and to identify the causal pathways through which the stress–health link is mediated.[81] Bovbjerg and Valdimarsdottir[82] note that the 'conventional' view of the role of PNI in psycho-oncology involves psychological influences on the immune system that provide a mechanism (mediate) the relationship between psychological factors and the development and/or progression of cancer. They argue that none of the links in the chain should be accepted as well established.

They posit that the efferent and afferent pathways in the central nervous system (CNS) and the immune system provide communication loops 'likely to be involved in the day-to-day regulation of the immune system by the central nervous system (CNS), as well as in mediating the effects of psychological factors. Consistent with this view, both feed-back and feed-forward regulation of the immune system by the CNS have been documented.[83] The possible importance of these non-psychological aspects of research into psychoneuroimmunology to cancer has received little research attention. A greater understanding of these regulatory influences may suggest novel strategies to improve immune defences against cancer' (ref. 82, p. 132). They conclude that PNI research in oncology is in its infancy. 'Only additional rigorous research will determine whether the promise of its birth is fulfilled' (p. 132).

Psychoneuroimmunology, psychosocial factors, and cancer

The argument that psychosocial factors, such as stress, could play a part in the aetiology of breast cancer is based on the observation that there is a much higher incidence of mammary neoplastic cells than ever become evident. Autopsy results have shown that between 25 and 30 per cent of all women have either in situ or invasive cancer at autopsy.[76] In men the findings are also striking. Autopsies show that 10 per cent of men at age 50 and 70 per cent at age 80 have small prostate cancers that have not spread or caused problems.[84] The release of metastatic cells does not necessarily lead to the development of metastatic disease. Presumably then, there are body conditions that may be more or less conducive to the growth of cancer. It is reasonable to assume that psychological factors could have a role to play in this situation.[76]

Bovbjerg and Valdimarsdottir[82] note that there has been little attention paid to the possibility that psychosocial factors may interact with other known risk factors for cancer.[85] They suggest that, in view of the recent explosion of information on the genetics of cancer, it would be of particular interest to consider the possibility that the impact of psychosocial variables may be more profound among individuals at familial risk than in the population as a whole. They question whether inherited deficits in immune effector mechanisms, or intercellular amplification circuits, could also contribute to poor antitumour responses.[86] Reports of lower natural killer (NK) cell activity in individuals with family histories of cancer raise the possibility that inherited deficits in putative immune defence mechanisms may contribute to familial risk.[87] On the other hand, they argued that higher levels of stress in individuals at familial risk might contribute to their immunological risk.[88]

There has been considerable interest in whether there was an increased incidence of cancer in those with depression. A meta-analytic review of evidence concerning the depression as a risk factor for cancer concluded that depression was a small and marginally statistically significant risk factor.[89] However, a more recent study provides substantial evidence of such a link, at least in the elderly.[90]

It may be that the initiation of cancer may be the result of the interaction of a number of factors, for example, the ageing process producing age-specific vulnerability to disease.

In a prospective, population-based study of 4825 persons aged 71 years and older, Penninx et al.[90] found an 88 per cent increase in cancer risk over a follow-up period that averaged 3.8 years. Depressed mood was also associated with higher cancer mortality. The authors controlled for age, sex, race, disability, hospital admissions, alcohol intake, and most importantly, smoking. Depression measured at a single point in time was not associated with cancer. The individuals in their study were chronically depressed. They were classified as being depressed only if they met the criteria for depression (a score of 20 or higher on the CES-D) at baseline and at 3 and 6 years before baseline. Jacobs and Bovasso[91] followed 1213 women from the Baltimore Epidemiological Catchment Area from 1980 through 1994–1995. Over the course of the study, 29 women were hospitalized for breast cancer and 10 women died of the disease. The factors that predicted increased risk of breast cancer were maternal death in childhood and chronic depression with severe episodes. These factors occurred at least 20 years prior to the diagnosis of cancer. Neither relatively recent life events nor other depressive and anxiety disorders were associated with increased risk. The authors suggest that the maternal deaths and chronic and severe depression may have been involved in either the causation or facilitation of the cancer and suggest meta-analysis of other prospective studies to confidently establish these variables as risk factors.

Watson et al.[92] studied 578 women with early stage breast cancer over 5 years or more. At the end of the study period 133 of the women had died. There was a significantly increased risk of death from all causes in women with a high score on the Hospital Anxiety and Depression Scale. After adjustment for known clinical prognostic factors, this association was strengthened. As the number of women scoring in the clinically depressed range was small (2 per cent), so the finding must be viewed with caution.

Holden et al.[93] hypothesized an immunological model based on dysregulation of the inflammatory cytokines to explain the pathogenesis of stress, depression, and carcinoma. They suggest that stress and depression can foster tumour progression by means of inhibiting the expression of major histocompatability complex class I and II molecules and through the reduction of NK cell activity.

The association between cancer and depression will have to be carefully assessed, particularly in view of recent findings from an epidemiological study using the data from the Saskatchewan Prescription Drug Plan[94] that was collected between 1981 and 1995. The authors reviewed the prescription records since 1970 of women 35 years of age and older with no history of cancer. They found that certain tricyclic and an SSRI (selective serotonin reuptake inhibitor) antidepressant may carry an increased risk of breast cancer. Antidepressants that are genotoxic (shown to damage DNA in laboratory experiments) were associated with a doubled breast cancer risk. Women who took non-genotoxic antidepressants did not have an increased risk of developing breast cancer. The breast cancer did not show up until 11–15 years after the initial prescription of the antidepressant. The author notes that the study needs to be replicated. Dr Alan Steingart, a psychiatrist interviewed about the findings, cautioned that the benefits of antidepressants have to be weighed against the risks. 'The benefits of antidepressants are tangible when they work. They can change lives, and save lives ... You have to weigh the risks of cancer against the risks of depression. We can't compare risk to no risk, that's a false calculus.' (ref. 95, p. A7).

Other psychosocial variables that have been implicated in the development of cancer include chronic stressors, such as loneliness, loss, and problems in living and/or an inability to cope with stressful life situations;[96] parental rejection or rejection in the early family environment.[96,97] It is hypothesized that early deprivation and loss may lead to early immunological malfunction due to abnormal neurohormonal regulation. The body's normal host resistance might then be weakened 'so as to favour the neoplastic transformation of normal cells or to lower antitumour resistance ... (and) weaken their defences against oncogenesis' (ref. 96, pp. 263–4).

In addition, 'inadequate social support, cognitively generated helplessness, and inadequate expression of negative emotion' have been associated with increased risk of developing cancer (ref. 98, p. 90). Levy and Wise suggest that in attempting to understand the role of psychosocial variables in the course of cancer, it makes sense to study cancers in which psychosocial variables might account for a fair amount of the variance, for example, those in which biological factors do not assume a primary role such as occurs in the more virulent malignancies such as pancreatic or lung cancer. In their own work, they have focused on melanoma and breast cancer, which in their intermediate stages have a more unpredictable course.[98]

Cancer relapse has been associated with severe social stress[99] while decreased survival has been found to be associated with poor coping styles[100] and low quality or quantity of social support.[100–102] Married cancer patients have been found to survive longer than unmarried persons.[102] Survivors who experienced remarkable recoveries from advanced cancer[63] spoke of 'the power of enduring marriages, devoted friendship, selfless acts, and indestructible love' (p. 210). The authors summarize studies showing that 'the link between personal relationships and immune function . . . is one of the most robust findings in psychoneuroimmunology' (p. 210) and conclude that if people without strong social support become sicker, then strengthening loving and supportive ties may be a way of stimulating the immune system. 'Love and intimacy are at a root of what makes us sick and what makes us well, what causes us sadness and what brings happiness, what makes us suffer and what leads to healing' (ref. 103, p. 3). Achterberg,[104] a noted researcher in the field of imagery and guided visualization to treat cancer and other serious diseases and herself a survivor of ocular melanoma, writes, 'We heal, and are healed, I believe by the bonds we form with one another—love, trust, hope, belief, and all those invisible qualities that have lost favor in health care' (p. 5).

Cwikel et al.[64] reviewed articles published from 1960 to 1996 on psychosocial factors that affected survival from cancer and concluded that 'the effects of psychological factors on survival are inconsistent in early stage disease and insignificant in cases of metastatic cancer, socio-demographic variables (high socio–economic status, private health insurance, and involvement in social network) are positively correlated with survival, and psychosocial factors are more apparent in patients younger than 55 years' (p. 1).

Bovbjerg and Valdimarsdottir[82] concluded from their review of many studies that while there is strong support for the hypothesis that there are relationships between stressful life events, emotional distress, and alteration in immune function; naturalistic studies do not allow one to rule out the contribution of immunomodulatory factors such as nutrition, drug use, or sleep disturbances. There are difficulties in establishing causal relations between stress and immune changes owing to the correlational nature of the research as well as difficulties in studying the underlying biologic mechanisms.

They suggest that research in immunology will prove difficult given the 'complexity of psychobiologic interactions in cancer patients. To take just one example: chemotherapy treatment can increase psychological distress in cancer patients, which ... can affect their immune system; at the same time, chemotherapy has direct suppressive effects on the immune system which can increase the risk of infection, which can (in turn) influence psychological and immune assessments' (p. 131).

Bovbjerg and Valdimarsdottir[82] suggest that whereas previous studies have focused on the psychological influences on putative immune defences against cancer, what might be studied as equally important if not more so are the 'possible effects on immune defences against infectious disease which is a major source of morbidity and mortality in cancer patients. Accumulating evidence ... supports the view that psychological stress can alter susceptibility to infectious diseases, as well as the severity and duration of the illness' (p. 131). Psychological influences on the infectious diseases of cancer patients may be particularly important because they are likely to be emotionally distressed and to receive treatments (e.g. chemotherapy) known to suppress the immune system. This 'double whammy' may leave these patients particularly vulnerable to infectious disease, which continues to be the leading cause of cancer-related death.[105] Their earlier research suggests that psychological distress on the day of the patient's first chemotherapy infusion is predictive of their subsequent risk of infection[106] (ref. 82, pp. 131–2).

Walker et al.[58] found that both the HADS depression and anxiety scores were significant independent prognostic factors for pathological response to chemotherapy—the higher the score the poorer the response. That was consistent with their previous finding that HADS scores predicted survival in patients with lymphoma treated with chemotherapy.[107] When the anxiety and depression scores were combined and the multivariate analyses repeated, the combined HADS scores emerged as the sole predictor of clinical response to chemotherapy.

Psychoneuroimmunology and psychosocial variables in the initiation, morbidity, and mortality of other illnesses

Studies in illnesses other than cancer have also linked psychosocial variables to longevity.[108] Depression has been linked to a heightened risk of heart disease,[109] especially in older persons.[110] Depression and psychological distress affect the course of cardiovascular disease.[111,112] Intimacy was found to be a protective factor in recovery from heart disease,[103] and chronic work stress and marital dissolution was associated with total and cardiovascular mortality.[113]

Depression in patients with chronic diseases has been associated with increased mortality in a number of recent studies.[114–118] In a study of 800 non-demented elderly persons with heart failure in Italy, there was an additional risk of adverse outcomes independent of physical condition in hospitalized patients even when mild to moderate depressive symptoms were considered.[118]

Personality and cancer

A Type C cancer personality,[50,55] in contrast to the Type A personality that has been associated with cardiac disease has been suggested. The Type C personality has been hypothesized to be '. . . cooperative and appeasing, unassertive, patient, unexpressive of negative emotion (particularly anger) and compliant with external authorities, in contrast to the hostile, aggressive, tense and controlling Type A individual' (ref. 50, p. 548). The Type C personality has been associated with more prognostically unfavourable lesions in cutaneous melanoma and breast cancer.[50] Watson and Greer[75] reviewed the literature on personality and coping in cancer and concluded that it is possible to conceptualize a set of behaviours frequently occurring together, which are formulated as a Type C personality. That they occur more frequently in people who have developed cancer is supported by limited evidence. There is, however, no clear evidence from well-designed prospective studies that this, or any other personality type, has a causal role in cancer. 'It would appear that the scientific community is no closer to establishing the validity of the concept of the cancer-prone personality than was Hypocrites some 2000 or more years ago' (p. 96). Furthermore, in Hirshberg and Barasch's[63] study of remarkable recoveries, they found that people with *all* types of mind/personalities can recover from life-threatening disease. Their results imply that '. . . a significant factor in recovery may be not so much what kind of individual a person is, but whether his or her behavior, beliefs and attitudes and approach to healing are congruent or resonant with his or her basic mind-style' (p. 325). The authors found that a variable these survivors had in common was that in the midst of crisis these people 'had discovered a way to be deeply true to themselves, manifesting a set of behaviors growing from the roots of their being' (p. 147).

In relating her experience with ocular melanoma, Dr Jeanne Achterberg[104] speaks of an interaction with her friend and colleague Dr Lawrence LeShan, one of the earliest pioneers in the field.[45,46] 'He reminded me of what I already knew—that the only way that you stay alive after a serious diagnosis of cancer or anything else is to find your visions. I told him that I had lost mine, at every level. But I simply could not jump into how to change my life' (p. 56).

Astin et al.[119] looked at the issue of control in women with stage I or stage II breast cancer. At 8-month follow-up, those women who were high in desire for control ('I have a strong desire for control', 'It is important for me to be in control of myself') and were low in positive yielding control (accepting, calm, letting go) showed the worst adjustment. Those who were high in desire for control and high in positive yielding made the best psychosocial adjustment. The authors suggested that the balanced use of active and yielding control efforts may lead to optimal psychosocial adjustment and quality of life in the face of terminal illness. Watson et al.[92] found that in a well-designed study that the women with early stage breast cancer ($N = 578$) that they followed for at least 5 years, those with high scores on the helplessness and hopelessness scale of the Mental Adjustment to Cancer

Scale at baseline were at significantly increased risk of relapse or death. The psychological scores 1 year after diagnosis were not statistically associated with risk of relapse or death. They suggested several possible explanations for their findings about helplessness/hopelessness and survival. 'First psychological response may influence biological response via immune function. However the link between immunosuppression and breast cancer progression remains unproven. Second, the direct effect of psychological response on stress hormones (e.g. prolactin) which might have an effect on disease processes could be investigated. Third, psychological responses may moderate important aspects of social functioning. Patients who hold a helpless attitude may be less proactive in obtaining the amount of health care needed to obtain the maximum possible survival and this effect needs to be investigated' (p. 1334). They also mention the possibility that the biology of the tumour might have caused the psychological state, but know of no evidence to support this hypothesis. There is, however, evidence that in the face of metastatic colorectal disease, tumour burden was significantly associated with pre-treatment HADS depression scores and these scores predicted survival. Allen-Mersh et al.(120) postulated that a 'toxin' released by the tumour might have caused the psychological effects.

Contrary to earlier work by members of the team,(53) Watson et al. were not able to find a survival difference when comparing one type of psychological response with another. In particular, there was no survival advantage for the category 'fighting spirit'. There was also no significant effect of scores for emotional control on survival. Specifically, they did not find evidence that the suppression of emotions suggested as a focal characteristic of the Type C personality was associated with any aspect of survival. The authors conclude that the idea that the fighting spirit improves survival has been embraced with enthusiasm by practitioners of alternative therapies, but in view of their findings such claims should be more cautious and circumspect.

Psychosocial variables and the course of disease

Hirshberg and Barasch(63) reviewed the literature to find patients who had experienced spontaneous remissions with advanced cancer. They interviewed as many of the patients and their oncologists as they could find and described the variables that these 47 survivors of metastatic cancer had in common including:

- long-standing partnerships of 20–30 years;
- a sense of 'differentness' and 'existential shift' that began many remarkable recoveries;
- a congruity between the patient and physician;
- social support;
- spirituality;
- being treated as a unique individual, not a disease category, or errant statistic in a disease protocol:
  - a sense that 'I am understood, cared for, accepted by another and seen for myself;
- changed nutrition practices;
- some artistic pursuit.

In larger studies, persons with greater depression and low self-esteem anticipated and experienced greater stress during the first few months in a nursing home.(121) In a well-designed study of 90 elderly (average age 78), advanced cancer patients, newly admitted to 10 Florida nursing homes, age, sex, marital status, and years of education did not distinguish between survivors and non-survivors.(122) In addition, none of the cancer and treatment-related variables differed significantly. However, psychosocial variables did predict early death. Those patients who died within 3 months of admission (28 per cent) more often acknowledged their condition as being terminal, anticipated greater environmental stress and adjustment problems, expected fewer visitors, and had poorer self-esteem. The authors concluded that for cancer patients undergoing the stress of nursing home placement, feelings of hopelessness and helplessness were associated with earlier death.

Ganz et al.(123) studied persons with advanced lung cancer and found that patient-rated well-being was associated with longer survival time. This finding was often, but not always, independent of initial performance status, stage of advanced disease, and type of treatment. While patient-rated quality of life was a statistically significant predictor of longevity in both married and unmarried patients, those who were married still had an increased length of survival compared with the unmarried.(123)

In a study of prognostic indicators in metastatic melanoma,(124) feeling that treatment would lead to a cure or long-term survival, minimizing the illness and anger were independent predictors of survival, controlling for demographic and disease predictors.

Psychosocial intervention to affect survival in cancer

Cwikel et al.(64) reviewed the data on psychosocial factors affecting the survival of adult cancer patients, drawing on the literature from 1960 to 1996. They concluded that psychosocial interventions to improve survival were most effective in the early stages of disease. The strongest study in this area is that of Fawzy et al.(68,69) who studied the effects of a 6-week structured group intervention on a group of 38 newly diagnosed melanoma patients and compared them with 28 control subjects. The structured psychoeducational intervention consisted of heath education, stress management, and coping skills. The intervention was done in a supportive group format consisting of six weekly sessions, lasting approximately one and one half hours each.

At the end of 6 weeks, the experimental group reported significantly lower levels of confusion, depression, fatigue, and total mood disturbance and higher levels of vigour on the Profile of Mood States (POMS). In addition, they were more likely to use active-behavioural coping techniques (defined as helping one to solve problems and/or to make one feel better in both the short and long-term) as well as active-cognitive coping methods (defined as mental thoughts and techniques that one can use that help to solve problems and/or make oneself feel better in both the short and long-term).(69) At 1-year follow-up, the experimental group continued to show significantly lower confusion and higher vigour. In immunological tests, the experimental group had an increase in their percentage of large granular lymphocytes (LGLs defined as CD57 with Leu7). 'Six months following the intervention, there continued to be an increase in the percentage of LGLs (defined as CD57 with Leu7) as well as increases in NK cells (defined as CD16 with Leu11 and CD56 with Leu19) and interferon alpha augmented NK cell cytotoxicity' (ref. 68 as quoted in ref. 69, p. 157). At the end of 6 years, there was a statistically significant greater rate of death (10/34) in the control group compared with the experimental group (3/34). Being male and having a greater Breslow depth predicted greater recurrence and poorer survival. Analysis of multiple covariants showed that only Breslow depth and the group intervention were significant. Even after adjusting for Breslow depth, the treatment effect remained significant. Higher levels of baseline distress as well as baseline coping and enhancement of active-behavioural coping over time were predictive of lower rates of recurrence and death.(69)

The most well known of the studies in metastatic cancer is that of Speigel and Bloom and their colleagues who designed a 10-year follow-up study on women with metastatic breast cancer who had participated in a 1-year programme of supportive group therapy and self-hypnosis for pain.(67) Those in the experimental group lived twice as long as those in the control group (36.6 months for the intervention group versus 18.9 months for the control group). This study has been replicated on a larger group of women with metastatic breast cancer from seven Canadian cancer centres.(73) Women were randomly assigned in a 2 : 1 ratio to weekly supportive expressive group therapy. The experimental group had a greater improvement in psychological symptoms and reported less pain than women in the control group. Women who were more distressed and women who had more pain benefited more than those with less pain and depression. The psychological intervention did not prolong survival, which was 17.9 months in the intervention group and 17.6 months in the control group.

Other randomized studies of patients with metastatic disease designed to show a survival advantage for group psychological therapy have also given null results.[72,125] More recently, however, Cunningham et al.[125] published a small, longitudinal, correlative study of 22 patients with metastatic cancer, study with an editorial comment saying that it had been rejected by two leading medical journals without review. The study was based on the assumption that underlying attempts to prolong life through psychological and spiritual self-help work is that the mind may affect rate of cancer progression via neurophysiological mechanisms. The rate of regulatory progression of cancer is influenced by regulatory mechanisms in the tissue.[126] 'To bring about the necessary neurophysiological changes by voluntary action, considerable psychological action may be required' (p. 278).

The intervention was 1 year of weekly group psychological therapy. A qualitative analysis of the extent of each patient's involvement with psychological work was conducted. Patients were classified as showing high involvement in their psychological work if they made healing their top priority and typically devoted more than 2 hours a day to practicing the techniques of relaxation, mental imaging, meditation, cognitive restructuring, and homework. Those with medium involvement demonstrated some degree of commitment to the process, but less than the high involvement group and the low involvement group showed 'relatively little involvement in psychological techniques for helping themselves, being from the start either relatively apathetic or dismissive of the idea that they could influence the course of the disease' (p. 282). At the start of the intervention, there was no difference in the expected median survival duration of the three groups as estimated by a large panel of oncologists who reviewed their medical charts at the time of entry.

The study showed a significant difference in survival times in the three groups. Those with more involvement survived significantly longer; however, it should be noted that the non-therapy group survived longer than the low involvement group. All of the low involvement patients died, while one of the medium involvement and three of the high involvement patients were still alive at follow-up. Two of the high involvement group were still in remissions of metastatic disease lasting 6 years. The advantage of this study is the prospective, longitudinal design, medical documentation, and a qualitative analysis, followed by a quantitative rating of the strength of characteristics related to the involvement of patients in psychological self-help. The main finding was that the 'data appear to show an association, not necessarily causal, between such involvement and longevity' (p. 284). The authors hypothesize that enhanced survival depends both on psychological attributes at entry (especially openness to change and motivation) and on application of the techniques taught in the therapy. Issues that do not seem to be controlled for include: social support, personality characteristics, and other activities the long-term survivors did during and after the intervention. These factors may also have contributed to long-term survival.

The patient's experience with terminal cancer

The needs of persons living with cancer studies

The framework of this section will be derived from data obtained in two Canadian studies: The Needs of Persons Living with Cancer in Three Canadian Provinces[30–32] (CCS study)[5] and The Needs of Cancer Patients and Their Families Attending Toronto–Sunnybrook Regional Cancer Centre[34] (T-SRCC study).[6] The CCS study involved a stratified, randomized Registry-based sample of 1319 people living with cancer in three Canadian provinces who were interviewed in order to assess their unmet needs. People were interviewed in the provinces of Prince Edward Island, Manitoba, and Quebec. This study represented population-based experience that provided a contrast to existing institutional or programme-based reports.

The study was replicated at Toronto–Sunnybrook Regional Cancer Centre (T-SRCC), a tertiary care cancer centre located in Toronto, Ontario.[34] T-SRCC treats 5000 new cancer patients yearly. Patients are referred from the greater Metropolitan Toronto area as well as from other cities, towns, and villages in Ontario. At the time of the study, T-SRCC consisted of an outpatient facility and an 89-bed inpatient oncology patient service unit (PSU). T-SRCC is located on the campus of Sunnybrook and Women's Health Science Centre (SWHSC), at the time of the study, a 1300-bed University of Toronto teaching hospital with 649 acute and 670 chronic care beds. An eight-bed palliative care unit was located in the continuing care wing. This has since increased in size.

The eligible sample included all outpatients who attended the T-SRCC outpatient clinic within a 3-week timeframe as well as all inpatients on the oncology PSU during a 1 month period of time. Patients in the Palliative Care Unit were interviewed over a period of a few months in order to accrue a larger sample. The T-SRCC sample consisted of 105 inpatients and 354 outpatients.

Sample

The two samples are similar, although the Manitoba sample was older and the T-SRCC sample included more younger patients. Two-thirds of those studied were females. All major cancer diagnoses were represented. Both studies were representative of persons at various stages of their cancer trajectory. The mean time since diagnosis for the Prince Edward Island and Manitoba samples was 57 months and for the Quebec and Toronto samples the mean time since diagnosis was 48 months. The median time since diagnosis for the T-SRCC sample was 25.6 months compared with 43–48 months for the three provinces. The reason for this difference is the length of time it takes for patients to be placed on the Registries from which the provincial samples were derived.

The definition of the person's stage of illness in the CCS study was a combination of self-report and author interpretation. In the T-SRCC study, the stage of illness, was from medical charts, although the same self-reported data regarding staging was obtained from subjects. The T-SRCC sample has double the percentage of terminally ill patients because of the inclusion of the inpatients on the acute and palliative care units. The T-SRCC sample also contains more patients receiving active treatment, both as inpatients and outpatients. This difference is due to the difficulty in obtaining the names of recently diagnosed persons in the CCS study and to the fact that interviews could be held with inpatients in the T-SRCC sample. Similar patients might have been screened out of the previous studies by physicians or the patients might not have had the energy to respond to the request for an interview.

One-third of the CCS sample was free of disease for 1–5 years and 16 per cent had been free of disease for 5 years or more. Over 60 per cent of the T-SRCC sample was receiving either active or palliative treatment compared with 35 per cent of the CCS sample.

The CCS cancer population was found to have a lower income and educational level than the provincial average in the CCS study.[127] The T-SRCC sample had a lower income and was less likely to have had post-secondary education than the population of Metropolitan Toronto.[128] These findings are reflective of the higher incidence, and mortality rate of certain cancers (stomach, lung, cervical, mouth, pharynx, larynx, and oesophagus) in the economically disadvantaged.[129–131] Moreover, the sample is older than the general population and, therefore, less likely to have completed secondary school while younger people with cancer were found to have their economic potential decreased.

The terminally ill subgroup

In the three provinces studied, the percentage of terminally ill persons willing to participate in the study was 5 per cent. The study was Registry-based, meaning that inpatients were eligible for inclusion, but few inpatients consented to be interviewed. The percentage of terminally ill patients in the

5 This study was initiated by the National Patients Services Committee of the Canadian Cancer Society. The study was funded by the Canadian Cancer Society (National), the Stephen Fonyo Fund and the Division of the Canadian Cancer Society in Prince Edward Island, Manitoba and Quebec.

6 This study was funded by the Toronto–Sunnybrook Regional Cancer Nursing Research Fund and Ortho Biotech.

T-SRCC study (10.5 per cent) is presumed to fairly accurately reflect the percentage of terminally ill in this setting. Because Sunnybrook and Women's College Health Science Centre is both a community hospital as well as the host hospital for the tertiary referral cancer centre, the patients interviewed included those who received chemotherapy and radiation for their disease as well as those who would not have been referred to the cancer centre. The latter group consisted of patients who might be considered to be 'surgical cures' (e.g. some breast, colon and prostate cancers, etc.) as well as patients diagnosed with cancers that would not be expected to respond to chemotherapy or radiation.

Distress in terminally ill patients

The unmet needs of terminally ill patients were correlated with level of distress as measured on the 30-item Goldberg General Health Questionnaire (GHQ).[33] The GHQ was chosen as a measure of distress because it allowed for comparison with a large 'normal' Canadian population in which 21 per cent of those surveyed were found to have high distress.[132] Not surprisingly, the terminally ill patients had much higher distress (61–79 per cent in the three provinces). Of patients who reported distressing to excruciating pain in the past week in the CCS study 90–100 per cent had high distress.[30–32] In the T-SRCC study, 69 per cent of those with distressing to excruciating pain in the past week (31 per cent of those with pain) had high distress.[34]

Box 1 shows the variables associated with high distress. These included problems with: physical functioning, physical integrity, emotional well-being, social relationships, illness adaptation, economic/occupational roles, and cognitive ability. Table 1 shows the physical and psychological symptoms of distress in the CCS[30–32] and T-SRCC[34] studies in comparison with similar studies.[4,133–135] Although there are differences in the studies, the most commonly reported problems were pain, decreased energy or weakness, fatigue, appetite disturbances, psychological disturbance, breathing problems, sleep disturbances, nausea, and constipation. Problems with

Box 1 Variables associated with high distress

Physical functioning: Difficulty with walking/climbing stairs, ability to sleep/sleeping habits, interest in food/appetite, ability to eat, ability to see/hear/speak, ability to care for personal needs, decreased energy, inability to perform normal household activities, and fatigue.

Physical integrity: Nausea, breathing problems, pain, sore mouth, physical appearance, constipation.

Emotional well-being: Thoughts and concerns regarding one's eventual death; feelings of depression, anxiety and frustration; outlook on life; ability to relax and happiness with life.

Social relationships: Time spent at social and leisure activities and inability to perform one's normal activities as a marital partner, such as going out and doing things together.

Illness adaptation: Fear of recurrence or getting worse and coming to terms with the various stages of one's disease.

Economic/occupational roles: Feeling that one will not have enough money for the future.

Cognitive ability: Difficulty with ability to concentrate or remember.

Table 1 Symptoms of distress associated with terminal cancer

Symptom (%)	Addington-Hall[a(133)]	Coyle et al.[b(134)]	Hinton[c(135)]	Vachon[(30–32)]	Vachon et al.[(34)]		Morasso et al.[d(4)]
					Inpatients	Outpatients	
	(N = 203)	(N = 90)	(N = 77)	(N = 69)	(N = 31)	(N = 14)	(N = 94)
In pain	55–56	100	92	68	53	71	91
Decreased energy/weakness		43	79	80	71	93	
Tiredness/fatigue		58		70	64	86	
Appetite disturbances	49–54		31	56	61	79	
Psychological distress	50–56 depression	21 anxiety	32	46 feelings of depression, anxiety, frustration	56 feelings of depression, anxiety, frustration	57	92 mood
	32–43 anxiety	20 suicidal ideation 4 suicidal intent	17	67 high distress 30-item GHQ	79 high 79 distress 30-item GHQ		Patients with unmet needs higher distress on Psychological Distress Inventory
Breathing problems	61	17	32	35–47	36	39	92
Nausea	19–20	12	56	44	39	57	92
Ability to walk/climb stairs		18		55	58	64	
Sleep	35–37	24		49	52	43	91
Constipation	31–36		35	36	42	50	91
Confusion/concentration		24	10	32	52	50	92

a Addington-Hall et al. reported on 203 terminally ill cancer patients in the United Kingdom who were interviewed at least twice for a study to determine the efficacy of a coordination programme. There were minimal differences between the experimental and control groups.

b Coyle et al. studied 90 consecutive terminally ill cancer patients, living at home, referred to the Supportive Care Team of the Pain Service of Memorial Sloan-Kettering Cancer Centre. The author recorded only the symptoms reported by the patients and therefore may be under-reporting them.

c Hinton studied 77 adults and their relatives in St Christopher's Hospice Home Care Service. These patients had 90% of their care at home.

d Morasso et al. studied the needs of 94 terminally ill patients randomly selected from 324 patients admitted for palliative care in 13 Italian centres.

walking and climbing stairs, and confusion were more common in the CCS and T-SRCC studies. The poem, *Time Changes* by Coni Linderoth provides a reflection on what the experience is like for the person with the illness.

Time Changes

The shape, the meaning, the passage of time
Has shifted, slipped out of my grasp
Not better or worse
Just so different
I catch myself now
Measuring time from when I was well,
Or after the fall
As if a new era began
When the tests finally came in.
A new era measured by 'on chemo' or 'off chemo',
In 'on the couch' or 'off the couch' days
Just so different.

An ordinary day used to be
Busy or relaxed, productive or wasted.
Now a normal day is hopeful or despairing
As I travel between mountain peaks and the Dead Sea.
Memories come back
Of holding my father's hand,
Trying to keep up with his business stride
On our way to work and school.
Years later, a vision of my own child's tiny hand grasping mine,
As I pull her hurriedly to our next destination.
I use to hurry to try to beat time
To fill it up to the fullest
To get the most out of it,
To win the race.
I pulled those around me along.
Fearful of leaving them behind.
Now I sit in one place for an hour or a day
Resting, contemplating, brooding, visualizing, praying, mostly drifting
With no impulse to move or shape time.
Just so different.

Coni Linderoth[7]

In Hinton's[135] study of patients on the St Christopher's Home Care program, during the final 8 weeks of life a mean of 63 per cent of patients each week reported physical symptoms and 17 per cent reported psychological symptoms. Some distress was felt by 11 per cent of the patients; this was usually due to pain, depression, weakness, dyspnoea, or anxiety. In the T-SRCC study,[34] terminally ill inpatients reported a mean of 17.6 problems in the past month (median = 15) and terminally ill outpatients had a mean of 20.92 problems (median = 19.5). Ninety-four per cent of the terminally ill group reported a current *biggest problem* compared with 73 per cent of the total sample. The most commonly reported *biggest problems* were:

- Physical side-effects of disease and treatment; 23 per cent
- Changes in lifestyle; 14 per cent
- Pain; 10 per cent
- Dealing with recurrent disease/death; 8 per cent

Pain was the *current biggest problem* most likely to be associated with high distress (88 per cent) for the total sample. This was followed by dealing with recurrent disease/death (70 per cent), physical side-effects of the disease and illness (54 per cent), and changes in lifestyle (38 per cent). In an Italian study by Morasso et al.[4], the most frequent unmet needs were symptom control (62.1 per cent) and emotional support (51.7 per cent). Low functional state was significantly associated with a high proportion of patients with unmet needs of personal care, information, communication, occupational functioning, and emotional closeness. Patients with unmet needs showed significantly higher psychological and symptom distress for most needs Picture 2.

Dr Jane Poulson was a 46-year-old blind palliative care physician who had already experienced cardiac problems before being diagnosed with inflammatory breast cancer.[136] Meeting with her oncologist 2 months after her multimodality therapy, she told him that the physician so tired that she could hardly put one foot in front of the other.

'I sure know how you feel', he said reassuringly. 'I was on call last week and I have never seen the service as busy. I didn't stop all week. I still haven't caught up yet. A day or two off would be so nice right about now, wouldn't it?' As I was that patient I wanted to shake my doctor by the collar of his lab coat and scream, 'No, that's wrong! You have no idea how I feel!' But I did not have enough energy. I could not seem to find the words or language, which would make the doctors, nurses, and other health care professionals understand just how tired I was' (p. 4180) (Picture 3).

In a group of 196 patient/caregiver dyads dealing with solid tumours or lymphomas, patients' immobility, symptom distress, and number of dependencies in activities of daily living were all moderately to highly correlated with both patients' reported levels of depression as well as with the reported depression of their caregivers[137] (Picture 4).

Kaasa et al.[26] found that patients who had impaired role performance in addition to pain were most distressed and that distress varied with

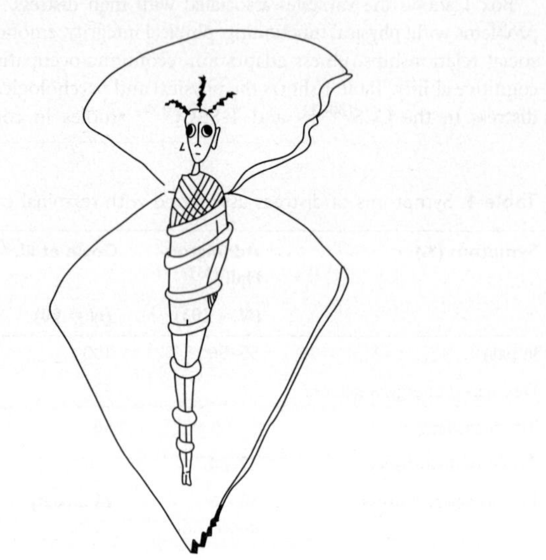

Picture 2 This is one of my prisoner series—the feeling of being trapped in a sick body, the feeling of displeasure from a husband who does not any longer have an active wife, the entrapment of pain, of fear, of not knowing when this suffering will end and how.

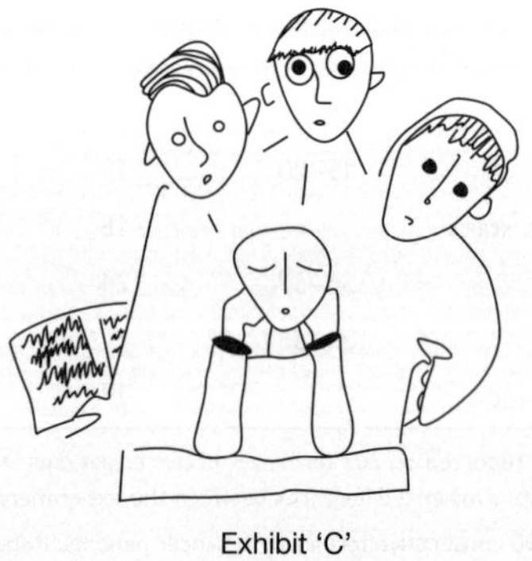

Picture 3 Cancer fatigue.

[7] This poem is used with the permission of Coni Linderoth.

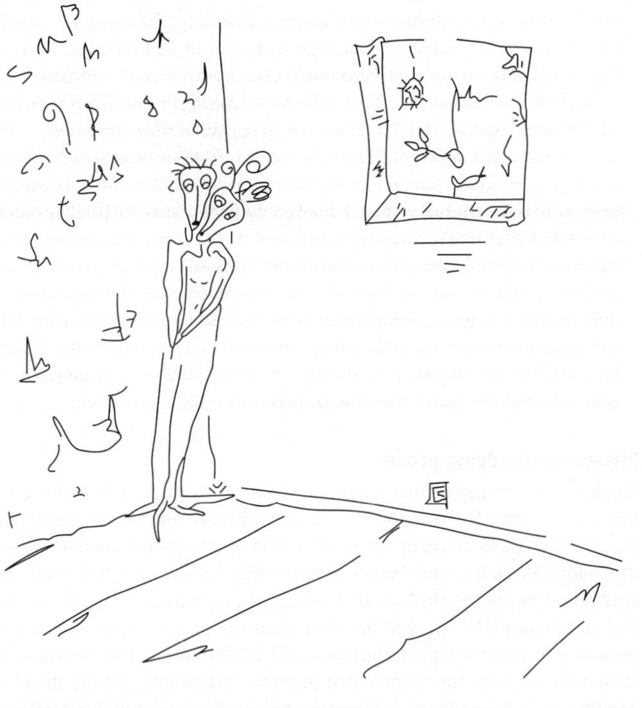

Picture 4 Wanting the intimacy so badly, yet the environment for such comfort is almost entirely removed—everything is dying untended, no furniture, and a partner with doubt and fear for himself.

severity of the pain and role impairment. In the CCS study, pain had the greatest direct impact on distress scores, followed by other symptoms and side-effects. Impaired role performance was a central mediator for the indirect effects on the level of distress.[25]

Patients from an ethnically stratified sample of oncology and HIV clinics ($N = 14$), bereaved family members who had experienced the death of a close family member 6–12 months ($N = 4$) earlier, and health care professionals and hospice volunteers ($N = 57$) participated in focus groups and individual interviews in order to determine what constituted a good death from their perspective. The participants identified six major components of a good death: pain and symptom management, clear decision-making, preparation for death, completion, contributing to others, and affirmation of the whole person. Clearly from the above information, there is still much to accomplish in this regard.

Having documented the connection between physical symptoms and impairment and psychological distress, this chapter will focus on the psychosocial issues associated with high distress.

Living with terminal illness

Having some understanding of the psychosocial problems confronting terminal patients is crucial to being able to recognize the need for, initiate, or conduct appropriate and helpful interventions for patients and/or their family members. This section will focus on the process of coping and adaptation in terminal illness and will discuss issues such as accepting or denying the disease, distress in response to terminal cancer, and factors that might alter a patient or family's response to the disease.

The meaning of the illness

The nature and extent of psychosocial vulnerability to life-threatening illness is specific to individuals and depends on the personal meaning of the disease. Meaning is defined as an 'individual's perception of the potential significance of an event, such as the occurrence of serious illness, for the self and one's plan of action' (ref. 139, p. 310). Meaning encompasses the individual's perception of the ability she/he has to accomplish future goals and to maintain the viability of interpersonal actions. The meaning of life-threatening illness comprises the set of physical, social, and intrapsychic changes that are associated with the illness. The changes associated with cancer include: (i) loss of personal control; (ii) loss of self-esteem and self-worth; (iii) changes in body image; (iv) reduced social status; (v) disruption of interpersonal relationships.

'In the head-on collision between terminal illness and the personal consciousness of the ego, hope is almost always the first powerful dynamic to come to the forefront. It arises with the first intimation of tragedy. Hope is a powerful constellation of human emotions, beliefs, and ideas, but it is a painful playground.

For the mental ego faced with a terminal prognosis, hope typically signifies one thing, the continuance of self. This is the thought: "I know that all things are impermanent, that everything must pass, and yet … and yet".' (ref. 140 in ref. 17, p. 95)

> My oncologist gave me the 'tell your friends and family speech last July. I chose not to, as I firmly believed I would have a miracle. I let them know the cancer had spread a bit, but with modern drugs, there would be no problem.
>
> Actually, I believed my spiritual practice would be at the core of my healing, the substantial cause.
>
> Medicine, chemo, nutrition stuff would be supportive causes.
>
> In September, it dawned on me that it still was a possibility that I would die, and I went on a cancer retreat where a palliative care doctor explained to me for the first time what palliative meant, and the steps I could take.
>
> I came home and registered with Trinity Home Hospice. I had found a friend in the hospice worker, Blair Henry. He and I met and we went over the present and future needs and 'travel brochures' for my eventual 'long term vacation.' At that time I had a bit of difficulty breathing and a constant cough.
>
> The next month I began to arrange my care team and think a little of my funeral. Being an organizer at heart, I have to say I enjoyed this process. My restaging in November showed a decrease in the lung mets and I could breathe freely with no cough. The pericardial effusion had also disappeared.
>
> I sheepishly e mailed Blair not to be too 'gung ho' yet, as I was showing signs of getting better. Knowing that he also had a sense of humour, I wrote, 'Please don't reject me-it appears I am not dying just yet.'
>
> I then slacked off doing anything except Xmas things and work-related activities. It is now January. I am coughing a bit and breathing goes up and down. Sometimes it seems like work to breathe.
>
> The palliative care process is really difficult and stressful from the point of view of the patient. You feel awkward when you are spiralling down and have difficulty thinking clearly enough to make decisions. There just doesn't seem to be the energy. Conversely, you feel awkward when you are spiralling up as you have to rearrange your life, priorities and tasks.
>
> Kind of like the adolescence of death (or the dying process).
>
> Mary Pocock, January 2002

Accepting the disease and prognosis

Patients in the Canadian Needs Studies[30–32,34] were asked to identify the three biggest problems they had confronted since their diagnosis. Difficulty in accepting the illness was the first or second most commonly mentioned 'biggest problem', but by the time of the interview about two-thirds of those in the CCS study and three-quarters of those in the T-SRCC study, who described it as having been one of their three biggest problems, said they had managed to resolve the problem. People said they relied upon themselves, their spouse, physicians, and family members for help in learning to accept their illness. Their primary coping methods in helping them to accept their illness were to share their concern about the problem and to confront the situation in a practical way, for example, making plans for their family in the event of their death, making a will, and taking treatment.

Terminally ill patients did not feel they were having difficulty in accepting the thought of their illness but they did acknowledge having difficulty in coming to terms with the different stages of their disease, dealing with the physical symptoms of their disease, and with thoughts of their illness coming back or getting worse.

Ben-Joshua Jaffee is a 78-year-old retired professor of social work. He was diagnosed with bulbar amyotrophic lateral sclerosis (ALS) 2 years after reconnecting with Sylvia, his college sweetheart. Ben-Joshua sent a letter to his colleagues in the International Workgroup on Death, Dying and Bereavement sharing his experience.[8] He consented to having some of his comments published.

. . . There have been some good and beautiful experiences, many, many really hard, very unpleasant, and disappointing ones, and a few dark-night-of-the-soul transformative ones. First, the positive ones. Last spring, Sylvia and I moved into a beautiful townhouse, with the fantastic help of loving friends and family . . . We have a wonderful view of Lake Washington and the Cascade Mountains, and in our east-facing bedroom, we are treated to glorious sunrises. We feel blessed to be here. Our relationship continued to deepen and be tested, honed, challenged and matured by having to face the cruel realities of ALS. This hasn't been an easy journey for either of us, but overall, for a three-year relationship, I think that we've done remarkably well in dealing with most of these realities and in meeting most of these challenges. We've also purposively scheduled concerts, dance concerts and operas into our lives so we could have some respite, pleasure and enjoyment, to counterbalance the increasing harshness of the progressive nature of this disease. And progressive it most certainly has been! Relentlessly! Even though I knew this conceptually, as is the case in most situations, it took experiencing the actuality for me to truly comprehend it. By last May, I was having such increasing difficulty eating and swallowing, that there was real danger that I could aspirate food or liquid into my lungs with resultant threat of aspiration pneumonia. So reluctantly, I followed my doctor's advice and had a PEG feeding tube inserted into my stomach . . . I take the formula by means of a pump, attached to an IV pole, which accompanies me wherever I go. I call it my Pole Star, since it plays an important role in directing where I can go and what I can do . . . I'm on the pump all night (thank goodness it's quiet!), when I take in a little more than half the formula supplement I need, leaving the remainder to be 'eaten' or 'drunk' during the day. In addition, I must also take in 700–900 cc of water each day to keep me hydrated. This I do by using a large syringe to inject the water—plus any medications—into my tube. This is another whole story: the process of tube feeding by syringe. It requires a number of different steps, each of which is essential and all of which must be done in a specified order, in order to avoid the contents of the tube and my stomach spewing all over the room. So it takes a long time to do this and requires constant attention to avoid leakage accidents. What an education in being present in the moment! I'm thinking of writing a piece on the Zen of Tube Feeding!

. . . As my swallowing became weaker, I could not eat [or even taste] progressively less and less by mouth, without danger of aspirating. For the past month or 6 weeks, I've been eating nothing orally. As you can well imagine, the losses due to this development have been manifold. Besides having to give up all my favorite foods, I miss the sensations of chewing and drinking and smelling food; the important socializing rituals around food and eating are not a pleasurable and enjoyed part of my life any more . . .

My speech, which last year was beginning to be compromised but was still intelligible, has deteriorated steadily and at what to me seems a fairly rapid pace. Up till 5–6 months ago, I could make myself at least partly understood to many people who would take the time and make the effort to listen carefully. Up to that time, Sylvia could understand close to 90%, and then 80% of what I was saying. Over the past 6 months, she has been able to understand less and less, until she can no longer understand anything, nor can anyone else. In effect, I can no longer speak at all!. Nor can I sing, or even hum! These are MAJOR, MAJOR losses for me. Throughout my life, expressing myself orally was a central aspect of my identity, and of course, even more so in my academic career. And I've always loved to sing . . .

One of my most profound losses is the loss of 'pillow talk' at night when we go to bed, and in the morning before we rise. Those deeply intimate, tender and loving exchanges, often in whispers, which were so nourishing for us, which brought us so close and which were often precursors to foreplay, are gone, no longer possible . . .

One of the principal consequences of the atrophy of the lips, palate, cheeks and swallow muscles in my type of ALS is that saliva cannot be managed well and automatically, as it is in people without the disease, and as it used to be for me. I learned that everyone generates 2 litres of saliva a day, but healthy people aren't aware of that because it is managed and swallowed unconsciously. I can no longer do that, so that saliva accumulates in my mouth, and not being fully swallowed, it leaks out. My lips are so weak that I cannot purse them at all. So I can't spit! [Nor can I swish and rinse out my mouth after brushing my teeth, nor can I really kiss!] . . .

So, right now, perhaps the MAIN difficulty I'm having to deal with is the CONSTANT drooling, ALL THE TIME, with no let up, except when I'm asleep . . . I've also concluded that at this point in my life, even if I wanted to become one, I'd make a very poor criminal; I leave my drool prints wherever I go. I've also discovered an example of true perpetual motion: I drool on the floor, and as I'm bending over to wipe it up, I drool more in roughly the same spot. As I'm wiping that spot up, I drool still more in the same place, and on and on and on. Voila! Perpetual motion [at least until I drop with exhaustion]. We've all read or heard about people who accomplish difficult tasks through the sweat of their brow. I'm destined to accomplish my difficult tasks, and indeed, any tasks, through the drool of my mouth! Really, though, my ability to joke and make puns about my drooling is really very helpful to me in getting through this aspect of the disease. In fact, it's really my salivation.

Phases in the dying process

Singh[17] is a transpersonal psychologist who has worked in hospice for many years. She has developed a Psychospiritual Journey of the Dying Process that draws on many spiritual traditions. Her model includes phases of *Chaos, Surrender*, and *Transcendence. Chaos* involves the five psychological phases enunciated by Kübler-Ross: denial, anger, bargaining, depression, and acceptance.[141] In addition, it involves the deeper experiences dying persons may pass through in the course of transformation: the experience of alienation, anxiety, the despair that leads to 'letting go', and the dread of engulfment. 'During the transformative process there are profound changes in the quality of hope. Hope in its previously known form (i.e. hope for the continuation of one's existence) is washed away like the dissolving letters of a prayer written on a beach. During the ups and downs of the ordeal of terminal illness, it is hard to say whether hope is taken away or hope is given up. Hope itself becomes difficult. The person is torn between the desire to live and the fear that allowing hope to emerge one more time would only create more misery if the treatment fails again' (ref. 17, p. 95).

Sixteen months before his death, when he had already outlived his prognosis with advanced oesophageal cancer, Graham Freeman a very successful businessman, who used both conventional and complementary forms of therapy sat at his cottage on an island and wrote a poem based on a poem that he had read.[9]

It Could Have Been Different

I rise with the morning sun
It could have been different
I sip my coffee looking out on the lake
And then sit down on my dock to feel the breeze on my cheek
It could have been different
There is no pain in my stomach and I swallow with ease
It could have been different
Every fourth wave catches a pocket under a rock
The green from the far shore is undisturbed
Its energy blends with my shore
It could have been different
The unhurried sky and earth and rock at the Island's point all come together
To encapsulate me, to take me to another presence, to fill me with awe.
It could have been different
I feel a joy and a happiness and a oneness with all
That before was an idea not a feeling at all
It could have been different
Today I can bond—be it with Susan, the earth or his light
Give praise since it definitely could have been different

Graham Freeman
Muskoka, July 2000

[8] These comments are published with the permission of Ben-Joshua Jaffee.

[9] This poem is used with permission from Graham's widow, Susan Freeman.

Singh[17] speaks of the time when hope evaporates during the process of transformation in terminal illness—the process of realizing that hope is a clinging to something other than *what is.*

'The movement into the present brings changes in identity, changes in levels of consciousness known and experienced. Arising at the same time come changes in meaning. Meaning is a powerful psychodynamic in the transformation from tragedy to grace. Meaning is the attribution of a purposeful construct to the suffering experienced. It is an important aspect of personhood and, as Viktor Frankl reveals,[142] each of us struggles for meaning in the chaos of suffering. *Our ability to intuit meaning that has value, depth, and reality is related to the ease of our transformation*' (pp. 96–7).

John was a young, very successful businessman who entered into a spiritual transformation as a result of his experience with Stage 2 lymphoma, which was unresponsive to chemotherapy. He had been hoping for a cure with chemotherapy, then to be eligible for a stem cell transplant, then to be able to have his disease kept under control for an extended time with chemotherapy. When it became clear that his disease was not responding to treatment, a physician covering for his oncologist with whom he had a very good relationship met with him and his wife. The author happened to be present for the conversation. The physician explained that his recent tests showed that his disease was progressing. John had already realized this and we had been discussing palliative care options when the physician entered the room. John pushed the physician to get information about his life expectancy. The physician reluctantly said his life would be only a very few weeks. John and his wife dealt with this information and then he said to the physician, 'there is a plan that my wife and I have had to establish a fund for others who might not have the resources to obtain some of the drugs and other things that we have been able to obtain, people who might need help with expenses such as babysitting and parking. We would like to establish a fund for such people. We would have done this if I lived, the fact that I am dying means that we should do this quickly.' The Hibiscus Fund was named for the flower the couple enjoyed on their trips to Bermuda. It is now being used to help other people dealing with lymphoma.[10]

Denial and minimization in advanced disease

Patients who do not accept the prognosis of the treating physician or who are not making appropriate life plans based on a negative prognosis are often said to be denying their illness or its negative impact. 'Denial is how one simplifies the complexity of life ... While downright denial can be harmful, denying itself is a phase of the coping process. It revises or reinterprets a portion of a painful reality avoiding what it threatens to be, and holding fast to the image of what has been' (ref. 143, p. 44).

In the St Christopher's study by Hinton,[135] on average, in each of the last 8 weeks of life, 26 per cent (SD 9 per cent) of respondents partially suppressed awareness of impending death and 8 per cent (SD 5 per cent) showed clear denial. Those rated as being more optimistic and mentally avoiding the true prognosis at the first interview more often became inpatients. 'Before admission some appeared to suffer a collapse of psychological defences and needed help; some quietly re-evaluated their situation while a few continued in denial and took inpatient treatment to be curative' (ref. 144, p. 209).

Connor[145] studied denial in terminally ill individuals and found most denial was in the service of protecting important interpersonal relationships. Interventions with significant others had positive effects by decreasing the need for use of defences and presumably facilitated the expression of anticipatory mourning. 'If denial is in the service of preserving interpersonal relationships then intervention is usually helpful and can result in growth' (ref. 146, p. 263).

In a study of prognostic indicators in metastatic melanoma,[59] feeling that treatment would lead to a cure or long-term survival, minimizing the illness and anger were independent predictors of survival, controlling for demographic and disease predictors. A review of 24 studies of survival prediction in patients admitted to hospice[147] found that clinical predictions of survival were limited. Given that clinical prediction is as yet an inexact science and that minimization may be associated with prolonged survival, how should the physician and or other health care team members respond when patients and their family members appear to be denying their prognosis? When possible, it is best to support the client's need for hope while gradually helping him/her to face the reality of current losses and the likelihood of impending death.[148]

Maguire[148] states that 'Patients use denial as a defense when the truth is too painful to bear. So, it should not be challenged unless it has created serious problems for the patient or relative. In challenging denial, it is important to be gentle so that the fragile defenses are not disrupted, but to be firm enough, that any awareness can be explored and developed.'

- Ask the patient to give an account of what has happened since the illness was first discovered. Explore how the person felt at each key point—with the first symptom, seeing a specialist, being tested, being informed about the results.
- Explore perceptions about what is wrong. This may provide glimpses of doubt ... Patients maybe ambivalent about whether they want to face reality. It is useful to confront this by saying, 'It looks as though part of you prefers to believe that it is not serious, but another part of you is willing to consider your cancer is back and not responding to treatment. Which part of you should I relate to?'
- If that strategy fails, gently challenge inconsistencies.
- If that does not work check whether there is a 'window' in it, 'I can understand that you think that it is an infection. Is there any time, even a moment, when you consider it might not be so simple?' If the person says no, accept that he or she finds it too painful to accept what is happening. If yes, explore what makes the individual think there might be something more serious.

Patient's who are single parents with dependent children, or others whose failure to acknowledge their prognosis may jeopardise their family's future may require a somewhat more directive approach. Generally, if caregivers can be respectful of patient's difficulties in facing their illness, and be willing to stick by them, gradually introducing new information as it becomes available, acceptance will come. When denial still persists it is usually reflective of a lifetime coping pattern.

Anger

'When denial cannot be maintained it is replaced in rapid succession by feelings of anger, rage, envy, and resentment ... When denial no longer has any blocking power, the scream of "NO!" turns quickly to the shout, "Why me?" ' (ref. 17, p. 185). Anger may arise from fear or feelings of impotence and is a reflection of one's response to a loss of control. A woman dying of colon cancer refused to allow her 10-year-old daughter to go to summer camp saying, 'if I have to stay in the hospital and die, there is no way you should be able to go to camp and have a good time.'

Anger can temporarily give a dying person the sense of being in control and can temporarily block off the emotion of fear. Anger can be healing and is closer to the truth than the repression of anger. Anger 'eventually, although usually painfully, works toward the experience of more and fuller life' (ref. 17, p. 186).

Anger may lead to bargaining which may also be laced with fear. In this phase one may turn to anything that might promise life. 'At this point what we want is a miracle, a reprieve from death. We plead with a Wholly other. Bargaining backtracks into older, more primitive, childlike representational thinking and the prepersonal trust that is the wellspring of the quality of earnestness. In Indian yogic terms, it is the cry of the three lower *chakras* pleading for life' (ref. 17, p. 187).

Emotional distress in response to terminal illness

The emotional response to terminal disease can range from little apparent response, through to feelings of dysphoria and some anxiety, to demoralization, through to major psychiatric disturbance. Dr Robert Shepherd, a Canadian psychiatrist, published a series of award-winning articles

[10] This anecdote is used with the permission of Nancy Poss.

chronicling his personal experience with terminal cancer. He summed up the emotional response of many people in the following: '...(E)verybody with life-threatening sickness is depressed. It is loss, you understand, catastrophic loss; you will never be the same again ... Then ... imperceptibly at first, the light starts to come back. There is less pain, less despair, longer periods of rest at night...' (ref. 149, p. 14).

Coping patterns in terminal illness

Good copers differ from poor copers in that the former seem to have a special skill that helps them to overcome many of the problems associated with cancer. Weisman[150] found that good copers were generally optimistic and self-confident, even during very difficult times. While they were aware of the possible consequences and threats implied by their disease, they were nevertheless diligent about their care and able to maintain their composure throughout adverse circumstances. Good copers were generally pragmatic about their future and seemed to exude an inner confidence that whatever happened they would be able to cope. They were generally able to confront issues directly, even if little could be done about their problems.

Poor copers were able to cope reasonably well in some situations but not at all well in others. The worst copers 'complained of having been *deserted, depressed, defeated and disappointed.* Self pity was a signal trait. Expectation of the future was usually excessive and absolute, permitting no compromise' (ref. 150, p. 81).

What determines a good or bad outcome of coping is a question of viewpoint. Patients, family members, and health care professionals may have different perspectives. '(T)he patient's subjective priority is to keep up an acceptable intrapsychic and interpersonal psychosocial equilibrium; the family wants to see the patient as a functioning member of the social network at large, whereas doctors and other healthcare providers expect optimal compliance, in view of difficult and sometimes even harmful medical procedures' (ref. 151, p. 198). In the case of terminal illness, the adaptive goals of the *patient* might be:

- overcoming insecurity and loss of control in view of self-image and orientation toward the future;
- mastering existential threat, for example, in view of terminal illness;
- preserving a meaningful quality of life under whatever circumstances.

The *family and social network* expectations might be:

- preserving or regaining an acceptable relationship with spouse;
- securing family's financial and social resources;
- sustaining social relationships with friends and acquaintances.

The *health professional's* expectations might be:

- preserving emotional stability in spite of long-term illness or progressive impairment, including terminal outcome.[151]

Prevalence of emotional distress in terminal cancer

A number of studies have shown an increased incidence of psychological distress in patients with advanced cancer.[4,26–32,34,35,41,61,152,153] In Passik et al.'s study,[153] although 36 per cent of patients had symptoms of clinical depression, only 3 per cent were seeing a mental health professional.

In the Canadian Needs studies,[30–32,34] terminally ill patients were significantly more likely to rate themselves as having difficulty with self-reported feelings of depression, anxiety, and frustration. Forty-six per cent of the terminally ill patients in the CCS study reported a problem with feelings of depression, anxiety, and frustration in the past month as did 56–57 per cent of the T-SRCC sample.

Risk assessment for emotional distress

The clinician must be able to distinguish between the psychological symptoms which are a common response to terminal cancer and are amenable to supportive interventions from staff members, and those syndromes which require a more aggressive approach from skilled mental health practitioners or psychiatrists. It is also important to identify the psychological symptoms associated with drugs such as: corticosteroids, chemotherapy agents (vincristine, vinblastine, procarbazine, asparaginase, tamoxifan, cyproterone, interferon and interleukin 2), methyldopa, reserpine, barbiturates, propanol, some antibiotics such as amphoteracin CB, cimetidine[41,154,155] metabolic alterations, such as hypercalcaemia or damage to the central nervous system by the tumour or its treatment,[154] uncontrolled pain, metabolic abnormalities, or endocrine abnormalities.[41]

Picture 5 shows the experience of pain in a woman who had experienced the death of two sons in a tragic car crash. She lived with depression and then developed excruciating pain in both hips. While her problem was not with a terminal illness, her art and comments reflect the issues involved with depression and chronic pain, and the importance of the role of the clinician in reaching out.

This chapter will focus on symptoms of depression, demoralization and anxiety, distinguishing those cases that will require intervention from those with which the primary clinician may be able to deal without the use of psychiatric professionals. Elsewhere in this text, in Chapter 8.17 much more detailed information is given about psychiatric diagnosis and pharmacological intervention in the care of people with psychiatric disturbance in response to advanced disease. Table 2 shows risk factors for depressive disorders in cancer patients.

Dying may precipitate people into psychiatric illness if they have undue vulnerability as a result of previous unresolved separation or loss experiences; a lack of support from at least one loved person or inappropriate discussions of prognosis which do not allow the natural process of adjustment and assimilation to take place.[159] A history of early parental death, loss, or strained interpersonal relationships may also leave adults susceptible to depressive episodes when confronted with later adult loss, such as a diagnosis of cancer, or the awareness that the disease is becoming worse.[160]

Depressive symptoms and depression Health care professionals are not particularly good at recognizing depression. In a study of depression[153] in

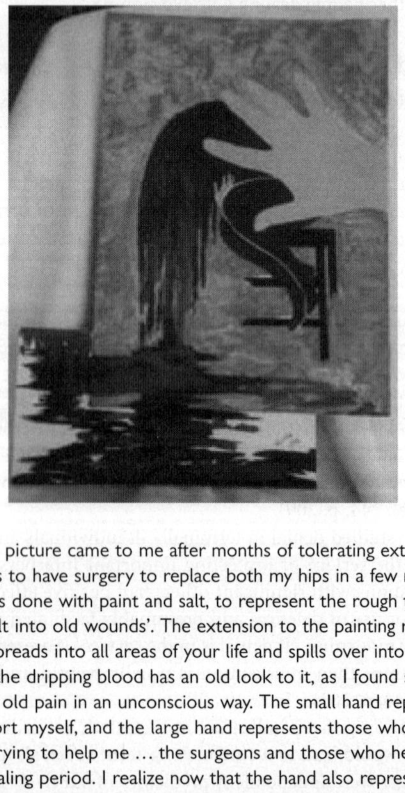

Picture 5 This picture came to me after months of tolerating extreme pain in both hips. I was to have surgery to replace both my hips in a few months. The background was done with paint and salt, to represent the rough texture of pain and 'rubbing salt into old wounds'. The extension to the painting represents the fact that pain spreads into all areas of your life and spills over into everything. The colour of the dripping blood has an old look to it, as I found severe new pain brings out old pain in an unconscious way. The small hand represents me trying to comfort myself, and the large hand represents those who comforted me and were trying to help me ... the surgeons and those who helped me through the healing period. I realize now that the hand also represents (the therapist) who helped me when my sons died. The jagged edges of the stool were meant to be jagged ... For a long time I sat only on stools or high chairs, tipped forward ... and didn't realize it until the painting was complete. (The picture and reflections are used with permission of Heather Thompson.)

Table 2 Risk factors for depressive disorders among cancer patients

Social isolation
Recent losses
Tendency to pessimism
Socio-economic pressure
History of mood disorder
Alcohol or substance abuse
Previous suicide attempt(s)
Poorly controlled pain
Depressive side-effects of medication
Advanced stage of cancer[157]
Younger age[157]
Older age[158]
Head and neck, pancreatic cancers[154]

25 ambulatory cancer centres in Indiana, 21.5 per cent of patients scored in the mild level of depression on the Zung Self-Rating Scale, 12.5 per cent had moderate depression, and 1.9 per cent severe depression. When patients were not depressed, the responses of patients and oncologists were concordant 79 per cent of the time; however, when patients had mild to moderate depression their responses were concordant only 33 per cent of the time and they were concordant only 13 per cent of the time with severe depression. Physicians' ratings of depression were most highly correlated with the patient's endorsement of more obvious symptoms such as sadness, tearfulness, and irritability. Their ratings were less strongly correlated with more subtle symptoms such as concentration difficulties, anhedonia, and somatic symptoms. The physicians' ratings were most highly associated with their own ratings of patient's anxiety and to a lesser extent pain.

Professionals do not recognize depression for a number of reasons including:

- the focus of medical visits tends to be on physiologic treatment and symptom management;
- emotional symptoms may be ignored or discounted;
- clinicians may ignore symptoms because they do not have a vocabulary to discuss them;
- patients are embarrassed to mention depressive symptoms;
- only one-fourth of patients disclose depressive symptoms because they do not want to bother staff or fear being stigmatized.[153]

A diagnosis of major depression can be made if the person has symptoms of dysphoria and/or anhedonia (loss of interest or pleasure) pervasively for at least a 2-week period. In addition, the person must have at least four of the following symptoms (at least three if the person has both dysphoria and anhedonia): sleep disorder, appetite change, fatigue, psychomotor retardation and/or agitation, low self esteem and/or guilt, poor concentration and/or indecisiveness, and thoughts of suicide and/or suicidal ideation.[161,162] Fearfulness, depressed appearance, social withdrawal, decreased talkativeness, brooding, self-pity and pessimism may also be indicative of depression.[154]

Passik et al.[153] suggest that assessment of depression could be improved by focusing on cognitive and attitudinal symptoms such as anhedonia, worthlessness, hopelessness, guilt, and the wish to die. Anhedonia is a key symptom for assessment of depression in the medically ill because it is less affected by day to day emotional changes associated with cancer than mood or neurovegetative symptoms such as weight loss, low energy, or poor sleep. While patients with terminal illness may realistically have no hope for a cure or recovery, less depressed patients may be able to hope for a painless death and good quality of life. A pervasive sense of hopelessness, accompanied by a sense of despair is a sign of depression as are feelings of being a burden, feeling useless, not needed and not wanted.[153]

Pain must always be addressed as the potential primary problem in patients with depressive symptoms. The presence of chronic pain in and of itself may be sufficient to produce depression.[163] Social support and quality of life have also been found to be associated with depression in a group of older males with cancer. Quality of life accounted for more of the variance in Beck Depression Inventory scores than did social support.[164] In another study of patients over age 55,[165] total perceived adequacy of social support and each of the three subtypes (significant other, family, and friends) were significantly associated with lower depression. The authors suggest that older cancer patients who are depressed may be good candidates for psychosocial interventions aimed at improving social support and subsequent quality of life.

It may be difficult to distinguish the withdrawal that many consider the final stage of a terminal illness from the picture of pathological depression. Attempts must be made to analyse the source of depression before treating it with medication, counselling, or psychotherapy.

Demoralization Kissane et al.[29] distinguish demoralization syndrome for depression. They propose hopelessness, loss of meaning, and existential distress as the core features for this diagnosis. The syndrome is found in palliative care settings and 'is associated with chronic medical illness, disability, bodily disfigurement, fear of loss of dignity, social isolation, and—where there is a subjective sense of incompetence—feelings of greater dependency on others or the perception of being a burden' (p. 12). Because of the sense of helplessness and impotence, those suffering from the syndrome may progress to a desire to die, or to commit suicide.

The authors distinguish demoralization syndrome from depression in that the latter is characterized by anhedonia, and the former is characterized by a sense of incompetence through loss of meaning or purpose. They further distinguish the two in that the person with demoralization syndrome can experience pleasure in the moment (consummatory pleasure), but is unable to anticipate pleasure in the future. The depressed person, on the other hand, loses both consummatory and anticipatory pleasure. This distinction is helpful clinically in that an essential characteristic of the demoralization syndrome is hopelessness, rather than happiness.

The authors propose treatment for demoralization consisting of the following:

1. 'Provide continuity of care and active symptom management.
2. Explore attitudes towards hope and meaning in life.
3. Balance support for grief with promotion of hope.
4. Foster search for renewed purpose and role in life.
5. Use cognitive therapy to reframe negative beliefs.
6. Involve pastoral counselling for spiritual support.
7. Promote supportive relationships and use of volunteers.
8. Conduct family meetings to enhance family functioning.
9. Review goals of care in multidisciplinary team meetings' (p. 17).

Suicide Chochinov et al.[166] showed that hopelessness contributed uniquely to suicidal ideation when the level of depression was controlled for. Singh[17] writes Suicidal Panic which manifests itself often in patients in the end stage of their disease: 'There seems to be a period of time for many people when, having cognitively accepted that they are going to die, but being physically and psychospiritually far from that point, they begin to say every day, sometimes several times a day, "When can I die?" "Okay, okay, I know I'm going to die. I'm tired of waiting for it. When am I going to die?"' (pp. 195–6).

Ideas of suicide in a terminally ill person might not be so much a sign of depression as of wanting to retain control over one's life to the end and of wanting to shorten the period of dying and thus relieve others of the burden of care.[161] 'Maintaining a sense of control is an important issue for the patient who expresses the wish to die. The wish for control may focus on uncontrolled pain or other symptoms; on the diminished sense of one's self and one's life; or even on family, friends, and caregivers' (ref. 167, p. 331). Not only is the patient at risk for suicide, so too are the spouse and other family members.[167]

The desire for early death in a study of 200 terminally ill inpatients was associated with ratings of pain, low family support, but most significantly with measures of depression. The prevalence of diagnosed depressive syndromes was 58.8 per cent among patients with a desire to die and 7.7 per cent in patients without such a desire. This study showed that the desire for death was closely associated with clinical depression—a potentially treatable illness.[168]

Suicide in terminal illness is discussed in detail elsewhere in this text in Chapter 8.17.

Anxiety Not surprisingly, anxiety is common in terminally ill patients.[169] Symptoms of anxiety in the latter stages of cancer may be part of a generalized response to the disease or reflective of an Adjustment Disorder with Anxious Mood (DSM IV).[162]

The clinical symptoms of anxiety including anxious mood, increased attention, fearfulness, inability to concentrate, and restlessness are easy to observe. Associated symptoms, such as dyspnoea, tremor, palpitations, or sweat, can be due to cancer or its treatment; therefore, these are less reliable for diagnosis.[170]

Anxiety has been classified[170] as follows:

Situational anxiety While some anxiety is normal in adjusting to cancer, a prolonged feeling of anxiety of an unusual intensity that interferes with the person's ability to cope with the disease or to engage in normal social activities is not normal. Imminent death is often not the most frequent source of anxiety, which may be due more to concerns regarding pain, isolation, anxiety, dependence, cachexia, and shortness of breath.

Psychiatric anxiety In addition to adjustment disorders with symptoms of anxiety, anxiety may arise as phobias about some aspect of medical care, panic, and generalized anxiety disorders. Anxiety is also a prominent symptom in up to 50 per cent of delirious patients. Withdrawal from drugs or alcohol can also cause symptoms of anxiety.

Organic anxiety It may be caused by acute pain. Organic anxiety may also be associated with asthenia; nausea; shortness of breath; metabolic disturbances, such as hypercalcaemia and hypoglycaemia; structural changes in the brain; and drugs, such as corticosteroids and morphine.

Existential anxiety It may have a spiritual dimension. This anxiety may be associated with thoughts about a wasted life, fear of the current illness situation and thoughts of the future, including the possibility of death.[170]

A more detailed review of the symptoms and treatment of anxiety are given in Chapter 8.17.

Depression and anxiety While anxiety and depression may be seen as separate and distinct symptoms, they may well occur together.[152] A high concordance between the two symptoms in cancer patients suggests that both will need to be attended to in many situations. In a Norwegian study[152] of 716 cancer patients 13 per cent had anxiety and 9 per cent had depression. The risk was greater in hospitalized patients and anxiety was higher in women than in men. Factors associated with both anxiety and depression included: impaired ability to continue professional work and/or daily life activities; impaired social life; previous psychiatric problems; significantly impaired physical functioning, fatigue, and pain. The prevalence of depression, but not anxiety, was associated with distant metastases, less than a month since diagnosis, relapse or progression of disease.

Intervention for emotional problems

There are several ways to approach an assessment of what causes most concern in a terminally ill person. One approach would be to conduct an open-minded, open-ended interview on *potential pressure points.* A second approach would be to address the issue of what the patient *wants* and is *worried about* not getting.[150]

The first approach involves inquiring into '(1) health and well being of every kind; (2) family and marital attitudes; (3) housing and money worries; (4) sexual and social activities; (5) job and daily life; (6) self image; and (7) existential issues about illness, invalidism, and death' (ref. 150, p. 84).

The second approach involves assessing what patients want and would include '(1) relief of symptoms; (2) better support; (3) firmer security; (4) sustained relationships, both personal and professional; and (5) stronger morale to face the future' (ref. 150, p. 84).

Using these approaches the interviewer can begin to assess the areas in which patients will be able to use practical assistance to help them to cope more effectively. This will also allow the clinician to decide in which areas she/he is comfortable to intervene and which will require some outside assistance. Sometimes it is possible to begin to intervene to decrease the possibility of later distress during the time of the initial interview. Simply offering the opportunity to discuss issues at the time they arise may provide a useful intervention. Caregivers may make comments such as 'it must have been very difficult to have your father die in respiratory distress. What impact do you think that has on your concerns regarding your own impending death? It must have been quite a shock finding out that you had cancer of the pancreas when you were expecting to hear that you had gallstones,' or 'It sounds like you and your wife haven't been able to talk about what your diagnosis means in your life, do you think it might be helpful to do some talking now?' Other times it might be helpful to offer the services of a social worker, mental health professional, or spiritual counsellor. Caregivers sometimes express concern that by bringing up difficult issues, they will cause patients to think about unhappy or troublesome problems. Generally, if the caregiver acts in a warm, non-judgemental, professional manner, giving the impression that such issues are a part of normal life and not particularly shocking, to the caregiver, the patient will be willing to discuss these and other difficult issues. If the caregiver avoids asking such questions, important information might be overlooked.

Intervention is indicated with an identifiable psychiatric disorder and may be indicated in situations of depression where there is poor social support and other concurrent stressors. Even those without a diagnosable psychiatric illness may have need for some type of support. Psychotherapy for the medically ill is often conducted in conjunction with appropriate psychopharmacologic treatment and consists of: emotional support, social support, cognitive restructuring, and coping skills training.

Spiegel[171] concludes that group psychotherapeutic intervention has been found to improve mood, adjustment, fatigue, and pain through helping patients cope better with their disease and live more fully. Individual and group psychotherapy have been shown to be effective in reducing depression and anxiety as well as fatigue, nausea, and pain. As already noted, such intervention may or may not also increase the quantity and generally does increase the quality of life. In addition, such interventions have been shown in numerous studies to reduce total medical costs by reducing costly and unneeded medical interventions.

Referral for psychosocial intervention When is it appropriate to refer? Although it has been estimated that 47 per cent of cancer patients suffer from psychiatric disorders, the majority of which are situational adjustment reactions,[38] and at least one-fourth of those with advanced disease experience a clinically treatable depression[35] few receive psychiatric consultations.[35,153] The reasons for the low referral rate includes the facts that staff have difficulty talking with people about emotions and a belief that depression is normal in the terminally ill.[35] Given that at least some of those not currently being referred for psychological support feel that it might be helpful, the following section will offer some guidelines regarding when the caregiver might be able to help and when outside referral might be indicated.

Intervention for depression The research data base on the treatment of depression in patients with cancer is limited. However, there is evidence that the treatment of depression improves dysphoria and other signs and symptoms of depression, improves quality of life, and may improve immune function and survival time.[157] Referral to a psychiatrist or highly skilled mental health practitioner is indicated if a difficult diagnostic problem is present, if there is evidence of a Major Depression or there is a question of suicidal ideation. Anhedonia (lack of pleasure or interest in life) is useful in distinguishing biogenic from psychogenic depression. If a person is not able to look forward to events that previously gave pleasure such as the visit of family or friends, a planned trip or if the person's sense of humour is gone then antidepressants might well be effective. Depressed patients with cancer are usually treated with a combination of supportive psychotherapy and antidepressants.[167] Depressed terminally ill patients may or may not be open to intervention that allows them to reflect on the meaning of their current situation within the context of their life, to deal with unresolved issues, and to deal with issues of loss and impending death. Chapter 8.17 contains more specific information of the treatment of depression.

Intervention for suicidal risk If there is a question of a suicidal risk, a skilled psychiatrist or mental health practitioner should be involved. Allowing cancer patients to speak about suicidal thoughts does not increase the individual's risk of committing suicide. Rather, it allows the person to feel a sense of control by allowing the person to express feelings, fears, and misconceptions. Exploring the meaning of suicidal thinking can allow the clinician to address the covert issues and tailor interventions.[167]

Despite expert care it is not always possible to prevent suicide in terminal illness.

Intervention into anxiety The following psychiatric techniques may be helpful in alleviating the anxiety and distress of cancer patients:

> 'See patients at regular intervals.
>
> Listen to what the patient is saying; avoid premature reassurance.
>
> Correct misconceptions about the disease, its treatment, and its pathophysiology.
>
> Be realistic and straightforward with both patient and family, but allow them to maintain hope.
>
> Assess the family's needs and offer preventive treatment.
>
> Allow denial and regression within reasonable bounds.
>
> Be aggressive in attempting to relieve physical discomfort.
>
> Treat anxiety, depression and insomnia pharmacologically if necessary.
>
> Keep staff conflict away from patients' (ref. 172, p. 5).

Other non-pharmacological approaches to dealing with anxiety include deep muscle relaxation, visualization and guided imagery, reiki, healing touch, or therapeutic touch. The use of non-pharmacological techniques in pain management is discussed in Section 8.2.

Acceptance of impending death

At the initial interview of patients referred to the St Christopher's Hospice Home Care Service, 78% of patients and 74% of their carers at least partly accepted the possibility of impending death but 9 per cent were clearly troubled. 'Acceptance grew more positive and, at the last interview, 50% of patients and 68% of relatives appeared fully accepting or nearly so . . . but 4% of patients and 9% of carers were troubled and unaccepting . . .' (ref. 135, p. 192).

Awareness of dying and coping attitudes of these patients at their first visit by the home care team were better predictors of which patients were likely to die at home than the symptoms they presented at that time.[144]

Singh[17] speaks of acceptance as being a cognitive stance, spiritually the transformation in consciousness begins in earnest only after the stage of acceptance begins. 'Acceptance is, in some senses, an ingathering of the attention that is the key to all transformative processes, in preparation for the arduous passage that follows' (p. 194). In Singh's psychospiritual process of dying, acceptance involves a last look backward, as well as a last look forward, in preparation for the present-centred groundedness of Surrender. She speaks of acceptance as being a moment of calm in the psychospiritual process of dying. 'There is, however, much hidden and interior movement, subterranean upheaval, and inner conversion about to take place behind this facade. This is the movement towards Surrender. The movement from Chaos to Surrender is not a straight path. It proceeds in feeling states that weave in and out of each other kaleidoscopically, chaotically, uniquely for each of us' (p. 195).

Suffering in the face of terminal illness

Singh[17] notes that as the pretence about prognosis ends, acceptance arises and opens the way to the naked experience of our alienation. 'we have cut ourselves off from our self, from others, and from Spirit. With mortality breathing down our necks, we begin to become aware of our myopic focus. Our attention shifts. This state of alienation becomes, in the dying process, painfully uncovered and revealed' (p. 198). This is an essential component of the experience of suffering in terminal illness.

Suffering has its source in challenges that threaten the intactness of the person as a complex social and psychological entity.[173] Cassel states that the relief of suffering as well as the care of disease must be seen as twin obligations of a medical profession that is truly dedicated to the care of the sick. The failure to understand the nature of suffering can result in intervention which though technically adequate not only fails to relieve suffering but becomes a source of suffering itself.

More recently, Shaver[174–176] has extended the work of Cassel. He notes that Cassel had recognized that the present concept of suffering was merely the outward expression of the injury, and not the underlying injury itself and that even less was known about the underlying injury or injuries from which human suffering arises.[175] Shaver proposes a simple paradigm 'in which the essence of suffering can be distilled into three general categories: abandonment of self, isolation and loss of significance' (ref. 175, p. 46).

First fundamental cause of suffering—abandonment of the self (ref. 174)[11]

- A sense of self develops in the first 18 months of life.
- Abandonment of the self occurs early in childhood as a result of societal influences and intolerance of negative emotions.
- The individual selectively abandons traits and emotions that society deems unacceptable.
- This removes experiential wholeness from our lives.
- What begins as a defensive posture in childhood, matures into a self-sustaining psychic structure in adulthood.
- Abandonment develops higher levels of endorphins.
- One compensates for this loss through the formation of Alternate Zones of Safety, such as the obsessive pursuit of money, power, fame, or relationships.
- This compensation does not withstand the onslaught of serious illness or impending death.
- Suffering reflects injury or removal of Alternate Zones of Safety rather than injuries to the underlying self.
- The pain of suffering occurs as a result of the unmasking of the incomplete, fractured sense of self (ref. 174, p. 9).

The clinical manifestations of abandonment of self

- Anxiety
- Inability to feel emotions
- Excessive guilt or embarrassment
- Agitation or intractable pain
- Deepening depression
- Self-deprecating or abusive behaviour

Therapeutic interventions

- Reflective listening
- Validation
- Silent presence

[11] This section is used with the permission of Dr W.A. Shaver.

- Help create a safe space
- Unconditional love

Therapeutic goals

- Reintegration of all components of self
- Restoration of experiential wholeness (ref. 174, p. 10).

Second fundamental cause of suffering

Isolation

- Occurs on a personal level through abandonment of self
- Occurs on a relational level with the breakdown of family, community, and culture

Clinical manifestations

- Personal
- Relational

Therapeutic interventions

- Relational healing
- Sharing of stories
- Emphasis on being real

Third fundamental cause of suffering

Loss of significance

- Denial of death
- Control issues

Clinical manifestations

- Death-denying culture
- Control

Therapeutic interventions

- Life review
- Re-orienting the locus of control
- Empower the patient (ref. 174, p. 11).

The value of a spiritual or religious belief system

Singh[(17)] observes that 'in the terminal phase of illness the self becomes increasingly conscious of its own disconnection from Spirit which it is beginning to intuit and encounter. Whether or not people have been religious or spiritual at other points in their lives, an experience with life-threatening illness will often lead to their exploring these issues. Those with cancer often report an increased sense of spirituality, a rise in existential concerns, and a use of religion as a coping strategy' (ref. 177, p. 121). In a study of 20 Norwegian patients with incurable cancer,[(178)] 90 per cent of patients indicated that the topic of faith was of interest to them and 75 per cent reported that they prayed.

When asked if they would welcome inquiry regarding their religious or spiritual lives if they became gravely ill, two-thirds of patients said that they would welcome such a question, 16 per cent said they would not, and, significantly, only 15 per cent reported that a physician had ever made a spiritual inquiry.[(179)] O'Connor et al.[(180)] argue that the task of 'making sense' is central to all ideas of spirituality. This 'making sense' is seen as crucial to the task of 'making the most' of the circumstances of living with dying and assist in promoting a personal sense of quality of life.[(181)]

In the Canadian study, 61 per cent of the Manitoba respondents[(31)] and 44 per cent of the Quebec respondents[(32)] turned to prayer as a way of coping with their illness. Almost everyone who used prayer (96–98 per cent) found it to be helpful. When asked how they coped with their three biggest problems since the diagnosis of cancer, turning to religion/prayer/God was specifically mentioned as a coping mechanism in Prince Edward Island.[(30)]

Of 457 cancer patients in the T-SRCC study,[(34)] 271 (59 per cent) used prayer, while in the terminally ill subgroup of 48 patients, 25 (52 per cent) used prayer. The primary reasons for using these approaches in the general cancer population and the terminally ill subgroup were similar, anxiety reduction (22 and 17 per cent, respectively) and to influence the course of disease (20 and 19 per cent, respectively). More recently, 60 patients with advanced cancer referred to the Rapid Response Radiotherapy Program at T-SRCC were interviewed with respect to the complementary approaches they were using to deal with their illness.[(182)] Spiritual approaches were the most commonly used with 69 per cent of the respondents using prayer to deal with their disease.

Singh[(17)] speaks of the period of Surrender into Transcendence as being a stage in which the individual can rest in the 'natural great peace'. In this phase, people frequently report seeing visions of spiritual figures, family members, or friends who have died. These visions may or may not be congruent with their previous belief systems. On the day before he died, a Jewish atheist with no belief in an afterlife found himself going back and forth between his hospital room and an incredibly beautiful garden. He said 'I don't believe in anything beyond this life, but it looks like I am going there.'

Singh says this period of transcendence is '*what occurs as consciousness coincides with the Ground of Being*' (p. 210). It is a time when 'dread dissipates in a profound healing and infusion' (p. 210).

Conclusions

This chapter will conclude with the story of Robert,[12] which illustrates many of the concepts discussed above:

- Illness does not occur in a vacuum.
- Intervention should meet patient–family needs.
- Good palliative care should involve options.
- There is no one right way.
- The process of illness may involve transformation—through the exclusion of the non-essential from our attention we become more inclusively essential.
- A significant percentage of patients with advanced life-threatening disease will experience periods of distress, demoralization, depression, and/or anxiety, which may respond to supportive intervention, more in depth psychosocial spiritual intervention and/ or medication.
- A variety of factors including personality and social support may or may not affect one's immune system and prolong life, and will certainly contribute to quality of life.
- Psychosocial intervention may or may not improve the length of survivorship, but can improve quality of survivorship.
- The process of terminal illness may involve periods of chaos, surrender and transcendence.

Robert was a 55-year-old married, lawyer, and father of three children aged 17–24 who was diagnosed with cancer of the colon. He did well until he recurred with liver metastases 7 years later. Robert described himself as always having been angry because of issues of feeling unloved and unworthy in his childhood. He continued to have difficulty with his parents who visited him rarely during the last 20 months of his life. He acknowledged getting into power struggles with his wife regarding issues of who was in control. Robert's life had always been a war—a battle. He saw his cancer as a battle that he had to win, for the sake of himself and his family. He suffered with thoughts of death that intruded into his consciousness and could not believe that this disease would lead to his death.

Through meditative approaches, connecting with his own non-conscious mind and his own inner healer, and through conventional psychotherapy approaches of reflective listening and support, as well as through shared stories, Robert was able to decrease his anger, come to accept that he was worthy of love, look for the lessons that he was meant to learn from cancer, and the meaning of cancer in his life.

About 3 months before his death, his oncologist let him know that his time was limited. Robert was becoming increasingly more spiritual. He awakened every

[12] The anecdote of 'Robert' is used with the permission of his widow.

morning and said good morning to the trees and God. He said that he was learning to trust his therapist, and noted that this was something that would never have happened with the person he was 10 years ago. In a meditation session he sought the answer to a question 'What do I need to learn to help others on my journey. "What cropped up is stop beefing at drivers. Calm down, be at peace, real peace, don't concern yourself with 'silly problems' don't get caught up in other people's bullshit". Having had these messages come to him, the rational part of Robert questioned, where is all this coming from?'

Through meditation he received the guidance 'Stop wasting your time on what has happened many years ago. Speak to your mother when she is on the phone; don't hang up her stupid or irrelevant remarks because they are irrelevant to survive the next 20–30 years. You have many people who want you around. Carry on with helping others, love will come from those here. Carry on; that love will be helpful in giving you what you did not get from your mother.

Having money is very important. My mother abused me over the years telling me I wasn't strong enough to get out there and achieve it. Today I helped a friend. I helped him to come up with a structure for his business. We discussed it for 10–15 minutes, which for me is a long time. We could be two men talking without problems with emotions, without feeling that I was losing my manliness.'

The lesson I have learned from my cancer is that 'there's more to life than making the almighty dollar, there are values outside of the business side of life. I can be given the time and space to take advantage of these values.'

Shortly after this conversation Robert travelled to Sedona. He returned home and noticed difficulty climbing upstairs. He had been scheduled for spinal surgery to remove metastatic disease before going to Sedona and was admitted when he experienced increasing weakness in his legs. While waiting for his surgery he spoke of his experience in Sedona saying 'I never felt God before Sedona. This was not the God of my people, or my rabbi. It was something greater than that, something so superior. I never felt an image like this before. It was all encompassing, really good.' He awakened with the sense of this 'Spirit of Sedona' with its arms outstretched to him.

While in the hospital, waiting for surgery, Robert's partners brought him a statue of an eagle to represent the inspiration he had been in their company. He was able to visualize himself soaring with the eagle.

Robert's initial surgery went well then he developed an infection and had more surgery. He had a near death experience in which he thought that he was dead and felt very calm. However, during this time he screamed for his wife who was there to comfort him. He was able to relish the love of his children and a card one of his sons gave him for his birthday telling him all the lessons he had taught him.

Robert had great difficulty recovering from his second surgery and beginning to walk. During this time we did a meditation seeking the answer to the question 'Why do I suddenly have a fear of failure? What am I meant to learn from it?'

'I learned that when you are afraid you do not accomplish anything. My big fear is what if I fall, what if I hurt my back? ... He's not to feel this fear anymore ... You have to make peace within yourself RIGHT NOW. Take your time and work it through and things will happen.'

We asked the Spirit of Sedona if there were things he could do to help the process 'Not really. Slow down and fly right would be My answer to him. Just take it a little slower. It's going to take time. Everyday you'll get a little bit stronger. Everyday you'll develop strength to get you where you need to be. Don't give up. Don't be frightened. Don't forget to soar like an eagle. Don't forget to visualize that eagles, when they start to fly many times fall out of the nest, but they keep getting up and they will do it. You will fall a few times but not physically, it will just take you a little longer to do than others.'

Robert died 2 weeks after this meditation. He recognized that the generalized oedema that affected his whole body was not going to resolve and that it was due to progressive disease. He had difficulty with his breathing and realized that it was not going to be possible to return home. Within a couple of days of coming to this recognition, Robert realized that he was going to die soon. A few days before his death he was visited by a male friend who had visited daily since his recurrence. He and Robert had not spoken of his death. The friend left the room and Robert called him back saying, 'Do you know that I am going to die?'

On the day of his death, Robert was able to have telephone contact with his sons and other family members who were not able to be there when he took a sudden downward turn. He died peacefully in the presence of several family members, his palliative care physician, and aromatherapist.[176]

References

1. **Vachon, M.L.S., Kristjanson, L., and Higginson, I.** (1995). Psychosocial issues in palliative care: the patient, the family, and the process and outcome of care. *Journal of Pain and Symptom Management* **10**, 142–50.
2. **Field, M. and Cassel, C.K.** *Approaching Death: Improving Care at the End of Life.* Washington DC: Institute of Medicine, National Academy Press, 1997.
3. **Barnard, D., Towers, A., Boston, P., and Lambrinidou, Y.** *Crossing Over: Narratives of Palliative Care.* New York: Oxford, 2000.
4. **Morasso, G., DiLeo, S., Fiore, M., Verzolatto, N., Partinico, M., Obertino, E., and Henriquet, F.** (1999). Psychosocial and symptom distress in terminal cancer patients with met and unmet needs. *Journal of Pain and Symptom Management* **17**, 402–9.
5. **The Support Principal Investigators** (1995). A controlled trial to improve care for seriously ill hospitalized patients. *Journal of the American Medical Association* **274**, 1591–8.
6. **Lynn, J. and O'Mara, A.** (2001). Reliable, high quality, efficient end-of-life care for cancer patients: Economic issues and barriers. In *Improving Palliative Care for Cancer: Summary and Recommendations* (ed. K. Foley and H. Gelband), pp. 67–95. Washington DC: National Academy Press.
7. **Ingham, J.M. and Foley, K.M.** (1998). Pain and the barriers to its relief at the end of life: a lesson for improving end of life health care. *The Hospice Journal* **1–2**, 89–100.
8. **Wilkinson, A.M., Harrold, J.K., Kopits, I., and Ayers, E.** (1998). New endeavors and innovative programs in end of life care. *The Hospice Journal* **1–2**, 165–80.
9. **Kissane, D.W., Bloch, S., McKenzie, M., McDowell, A.C., and Nitzan, R.** (1998). Family grief therapy: a preliminary account of a new model to promote healthy family functioning during palliative care and bereavement. *Psycho-Oncology* **7**, 14–25.
10. **Gilbar, O.** (1998). Length of cancer patients' stay at a hospice: does it affect psychological adjustment to the loss of the spouse. *Journal of Palliative Care* **14** (4), 16–20.
11. **Fakhoury, W.K.H., McCarthy, M., and Addington-Hall, J.** (1997). Carers' health status: is it associated with their evaluation of the quality of palliative care? *Scandinavian Journal of Social Medicine* **25**, 296–301.
12. **Sachs, O.** *An Anthropologist on Mars.* New York: Alfred A. Knopf, 1995.
13. **Vachon, M.L.S.** (1994). Psychosocial variables: cancer morbidity and mortality. In *A Challenge for Living: Death, Dying and Bereavement* (ed. I. Corless, B. Germino, and M. Pittman-Lindeman), pp. 135–55. Boston: Jones and Bartlett Publishers.
14. **Ferris, F.D., Balfour, H.M., Bowen, K., Farley, J., Hardwick, M., Lamontagne, C., Lundy, M., Syme, A., and West, P.** *A Consensus-based Model to Guide Hospice Palliative Care.* Ottawa: Canadian Hospice Palliative Care Association, March 2002.
15. http://64.85.16.230/educate/content.html
16. **Vachon, M.L.S.** (1998). The emotional problems of the patient in palliative medicine. In *Oxford Textbook of Palliative Medicine* 2nd edn. (ed. D. Doyle, G. Hanks, and N. MacDonald), pp. 882–907. Oxford: Oxford University Press.
17. **Singh, K.D.** *The Grace in Dying: How We Are Transformed Spiritually As We Die.* San Francisco: Harper San Francisco, 1998.
18. **Kearsley, J.H.** (1994). Wanted: guidelines for 'palliative' anti-cancer drug use. *The Medical Journal of Australia* **160**, 723–5.
19. **Whedon, M.B.** (2002). Revisiting the road not taken: integrating palliative care into oncology nursing. *Clinical Journal of Oncology Nursing* **6** (1), 27–33.
20. **Lowenthal, R.A.** (1992). A time of change in medical oncology. *Medical Journal of Australia* **157**, 28–30.
21. **Non-Small Cell Lung Cancer Collaborative Group** (1995). Chemotherapy in non-small cell lung cancer: a meta-analysis using updated data on individual patients from 52 randomized clinical trials. *British Medical Journal* **311**, 899–909.
22. **Chlebowski, R.T., Palomares, M.R., Lillington, L., and Grosvernor, M.** (1996). Recent implications of weight loss in lung cancer management. *Nutrition* **12**, S43–7.

23. **Patnaik, A., Doyle, C., and Oza, A.M.** (1998). Palliative therapy in advanced ovarian cancer: balancing patient expectations, quality of life and cost. *Anti-Cancer Drugs* **9**, 869–78.
24. **Quill, T.E.** *Death and Dignity: Making Choices and Taking Charge.* New York: W.W. Norton & Company, 1993.
25. **Lancee, W.J., Vachon, M.L.S., Ghadirian, P., Adair, W., Conway, B., and Dryer, D.** (1994). The impact of pain and impaired role performance on distress in persons with cancer. *Canadian Psychiatric Association Journal* **39** (10), 617–22.
26. **Kaasa, S., Malt, U., Hagen, S., Wist, E., Moum, T., and Kvikstad, A.** (1993). Psychological distress in cancer patients with advanced disease. *Radiotherapy and Oncology* **27**, 193–7.
27. **Pinder, K.L., Ramirez, A.J., Black, M.E., Richards, M.A., Gregory, W.M., and Rubens, R.D.** (1993). Psychiatric disorder in patients with advanced breast cancer: prevalence and associated factors. *European Journal of Oncology* **29A**, 524–7.
28. **Wilson, K.G., Chochinov, H.M., deFaye, B.J., and Breitbart, W.** (2000). Diagnosis and management of depression in palliative care. In *Handbook of Psychiatry in Palliative Medicine* (ed. H.M. Chochinov and W. Breitbart), pp. 25–49. New York: Oxford University Press.
29. **Kissane, D.W., Clarke, D.M., and Street, A.F.** (2001). Demoralization syndrome—a relevant psychiatric diagnosis for palliative care. *Journal of Palliative Care* **17** (1), 12–21.
30. **Vachon, M.L.S., Conway, B., Lancee, W.J., and Adair, W.K.** *Report on the Needs of Persons Living with Cancer in Prince Edward Island.* Toronto, Canada: Canadian Cancer Society, 1989.
31. **Vachon, M.L.S., Lancee, W.J., Conway, B., and Adair, W.K.** *Final Report on the Needs of Persons Living with Cancer in Manitoba.* Toronto, Canada: Canadian Cancer Society, 1990.
32. **Vachon, M.L.S., Lancee, W.J., Ghadirian, P., Adair, W.K., and Conway, B.** *Final Report on the Needs of Persons Living with Cancer in Quebec.* Toronto, Canada: Canadian Cancer Society, 1991.
33. **Goldberg, D.** *Manual of the General Health Questionnaire.* Windsor: NFER-Nelson, 1978.
34. **Vachon, M.L.S., Fitch, M., Greenberg, M., and Franssen, E.** *The Needs of Cancer Patients and Their Families Attending Toronto–Sunnybrook Regional Cancer Centre,* 1995.
35. **Stiefel, F., Die Trill, M., Berney, A., Olarte, J.M.N., and Razavi, D.** (2001). Depression in palliative care: a pragmatic report from the Expert Working Group of the European Association for Palliative care. *Supportive Care in Cancer* **9**, 477–88.
36. **Steifel, F.** (1993). Psychosocial aspects of cancer pain. *Supportive Care in Cancer* **1**, 130–4.
37. **Saltzburg, D., Breitbart, W., Fishman, B., Stiefel, F., Holland, J., and Foley, K.** (1989). The relationship of pain and depression to suicidal ideation in cancer patients (abstract). *Proceedings of the American Society of Clinical Oncology Annual Meeting* Vol. 8, p. 312.
38. **Derogatis, L.R.** et al. (1983). The prevalence of psychiatric disorders among cancer patients. *Journal of the American Medical Association* **249**, 751–7.
39. **Spiegel, D. and Sands, S.** (1988). Pain management in the cancer patient. *Journal of Psychosocial Oncology* **6**, 205–16.
40. **Spiegel, D., Sands, S., and Koopman, D.** (1994). Pain and depression in patients with cancer. *Cancer* **74**, 2570–8.
41. **Massie, M.J. and Popkin, M.K.** (1998). Depressive disorders. In *Psychooncology* (ed. J.C. Holland), pp. 518–40. New York: Oxford University Press.
42. **Wells, K.B., Golding, J.M., and Burham, M.A.** (1988). Psychiatric disorder in a sample of the general population with and without chronic medical conditions. *American Journal of Psychiatry* **145**, 976–81.
43. **Stolbach, L.L. and Brandt, U.C.** (1988). Psychosocial factors in the development and progression of breast cancer. In *Stress and Breast Cancer* (ed. C.L. Cooper), pp. 3–24. London: John Wiley & Sons.
44. **Evans, E.** *A Psychological Study of Cancer.* New York: Dodd-Mead, 1926.
45. **LeShan, L.** (1959). Psychological states as factors in the development of malignant disease: a critical review. *Journal of the National Cancer Institute* **22**, 1–18.
46. **LeShan, L.** (1966). An emotional life history pattern associated with neoplastic disease. *Annals of the New York Academy of Sciences* **125**, 780–93.
47. **Blumberg, E.M., West, P.M., and Ellis, F.W.** (1956). A possible relationship between psychological factors and human cancer. *Psychosomatic Medicine* **16**, 277–86.
48. **Greer, S. and Morris, T.** (1975). Psychological attributes of women who develop breast cancer: a controlled study. *Journal of Psychosomatic Research* **19**, 147–53.
49. **Cassileth, B.R., Lusk, E.J., Miller, D.S., Brown, L.L., and Miller, C.** (1985). Psychosocial correlates of survival in advanced malignant disease. *New England Journal of Medicine* **312**, 1551–5.
50. **Temoshok, L.** (1987). Personality, coping style, emotion and cancer: towards an integrative model. *Imperial Cancer Research Fund 1987* **6**, 545–67.
51. **Weisman, A.D. and Worden, J.W.** (1975). Psychosocial analysis of cancer deaths. *Omega* **6**, 61–75.
52. **Greer, S. and Watson, M.** (1985). Towards a psychobiological model of cancer: psychological considerations. *Social Science and Medicine* **20**, 773–7.
53. **Greer, S., Morris, T., and Pettingale, K.W.** (1979). Psychological response to breast cancer: effect on outcome. *Lancet* **2**, 785–7.
54. **Spiegel, D.** *Living Beyond Limits.* New York: Fawcett Columbine, 1993.
55. **Morris, T.A.** (1980). Type C for cancer: low trait anxiety and the pathogenesis of breast cancer. *Cancer Detection and Prevention* **3**, 102.
56. **Shekelle, R.B.** et al. (1981). Psychological depression and 17-year risk of death from cancer. *Psychosomatic Medicine* **43**, 117–25.
57. **Persky, V.W., Kempthorne-Rawson, J., and Shekelle, R.B.** (1987). Personality and risk of cancer: 20-year follow-up of the Western Electric Study. *Psychosomatic Medicine* **49**, 435–49.
58. **Walker, L.G.** et al. (1999). Psychological factors can predict the response to primary chemotherapy in patients with locally advanced breast cancer. *European Journal of Cancer* **35**, 1783–8.
59. **Butow, P.N., Coates, A.S., and Dunn, S.M.** (1999). Psychosocial predictors of survival in metastatic melanoma. *Journal of Clinical Oncology* **17**, 2256–63.
60. **Astin, J.A., Anton-Culver, H., Schwartz, C.E., Shapiro, D.H., McQuade, J., Breuer, A.M., Taylor, T.H., Lee, H., and Kurosaki, T.** (1999). Sense of control and adjustment to breast cancer: the importance of balancing control coping styles. *Behavioral Medicine* **25**, 101–9.
61. **Tross, S.** et al. (1996). Psychological symptoms and disease-free and overall survival in women with stage II breast cancer. Cancer and Leukemia Group B. *Journal of the National Cancer Institute* **88**, 661–7.
62. **Epping-Jordan, J.E., Compas, B.E., and Howell, D.C.** (1994). Predictors of cancer progression in young adult men and women: avoidance, intrusive thoughts and psychological symptoms. *Health Psychology* **13**, 539–47.
63. **Hirshberg, C. and Barasch, M.I.** *Remarkable Recovery.* New York: Riverhead Books, 1995.
64. **Cwikel, J.G., Behar, L.C., and Zabora, J.** (1997). Psychosocial factors that affect the survival of adult cancer patients: a review of research. *Journal of Psychosocial Oncology* **15** (3/4), 1–34.
65. **Siegel, B.S.** *Love, Medicine and Miracles.* New York: Harper & Row, 1988.
66. **Simonton, O.C., Simonton, S.M., and Creighton, J.L.** *Getting Well Again.* New York: Bantam Books, 1978.
67. **Spiegel, D., Bloom, J.R., Kraemer, H.C., and Gottheil, E.** (1989). Effect of psychosocial treatment on survival of patients with metastatic breast cancer. *Lancet* **2** (8668), 888–91.
68. **Fawzy, F.I.** (1993). Malignant melanoma: effects of an early structured psychiatric intervention, coping, and affective state on recurrence and survival six years later. *Archives of General Psychiatry* **50**, 681–9.
69. **Fawzy, F.I. and Fawzy, N.W.** (1994). A structured psychoeducational intervention for cancer patients. *General Hospital Psychiatry* **16**, 149–92.
70. **Morgenstern, H., Gellert, G.A., Walter, D., Ostfeld, A.M., and Siegel, B.S.** (1984). The impact of a psychosocial support program on survival with breast cancer: the importance of selection bias in program evaluation. *Journal of Chronic Diseases* **37**, 273–82.
71. **Cunningham, A.J.** et al. (1991). A group psychoeducational program to help cancer patients cope with and combat their disease. *Advances* **7**, 41–56.
72. **Cunningham, A.J.** et al. (1998). A randomized controlled trial of the effects of group psychological therapy on survival in women and metastatic breast cancer. *Psycho-oncology* **7**, 508–17.

73. **Goodwin, P.J., Leszcz, M., Ennis, M., Koopmans, J., Vincent, L., Guther, H., Drysdale, E., Hundleby, M., Chochinov, H.M., Navarro, M., Speca, M., and Hunter, J.** (2001). The effect of group psychosocial support on survival in metastatic breast cancer. *New England Journal of Medicine* **345**, 1719–26.

74. **Fox, B.H.** (1998). Psychosocial factors in cancer incidence and prognosis. In *Psycho-oncology* (ed. J.C. Holland), pp. 110–24. New York: Oxford University Press.

75. **Watson, M. and Greer, S.** (1998). Personality and coping. In *Psycho-oncology* (ed. J.C. Holland), pp. 91–109. New York: Oxford University Press.

76. **Hu, D. and Silberfarb, P.M.** Psychological factors: do they influence breast cancer? In *Stress and Breast Cancer* (ed. C.L. Cooper), pp. 27–62. London: John Wiley & Sons.

77. **Ronson, A.** (2000). Can psychosocial factors influence the prognosis of cancer? *Opinions on Topics in Supportive Care in Oncology* **35** (2), 8–9.

78. **Croyle, R.T.** (1998). Depression as a risk factor for cancer: renewing a debate on the psychobiology of disease. *Journal of the National Cancer Institute* **90**, 1856–7.

79. **Blaney, P.H.** (1986). Affect and memory: a review. *Psychological Review* **99**, 229–46.

80. **Weinstock, M.A., Colditz, G.A., Willett, W.C., Stampfer, M.J., Rosner, B., and Speizer, F.E.** (1991). Recall (report) bias and reliability in the retrospective assessment of melanoma risk. *American Journal of Epidemiology* **133**, 240–5.

81. **Bartlett, D.** *Stress Perspectives and Processes.* Buckingham: Open University Press, 1998.

82. **Bovbjerg, D.H. and Valdimarsdottir, H.B.** (1998). Psychoneuroimmunology: implications for psycho-oncology. In *Psycho-oncology* (ed. J.C. Holland), pp. 125–43. New York: Oxford University Press.

83. **Bovbjerg, D.H.** (1994). Psychoimmunology: a critical analysis of the implications for clinical oncology in the 21st century. In *The Psychoimmunology of Human Cancer* (ed. C. E. Lewis, C. O'Sullivan, and J. Barraclough), pp. 417–26. Oxford: Oxford University Press.

84. **Prostate cancer: should you get a PSA test?** *University of California Berkeley Wellness Letter*, 11:**10**, July 1995.

85. **Eysenck, H.J.** Synergistic interaction between psychosocial and physical factors in the causation of lung cancer. In *The Psychoimmunology of Human Cancer* (ed. C.E. Lewis, C. O'Sullivan, and J. Barraclough), pp. 163–78. Oxford: Oxford University Press.

86. **Schreiber, H.** (1993). Tumor immunology. In *Fundamental Immunology* 3rd edn. (ed. W.E. Paul), pp. 1143–70. New York: Raven Press.

87. **Whiteside, T.L. and Herberman, R.B.** (1994). Human natural killer cells in health and disease: biology and therapeutic potential. *Clinical Immunotherapy* **1**, 56–66.

88. **Bovbjerg, D.H. and Valdimarsdottir, H.** (1993). Familial cancer, emotional distress, and low natural cytotoxic activity in healthy women. *Annals of Oncology* **4**, 745–52.

89. **McGee, R., Williams, S., and Elwood, M.** (1994). Depression and the development of cancer: a meta-analysis. *Social Science and Medicine* **38**, 187–92.

90. **Penninx, B.W.** et al. (1998). Chronically depressed mood and cancer risk in older persons. *Journal of the National Cancer Institute* **90**, 1888–93.

91. **Jacobs, J.R. and Bovasso, G.B.** (2000). Early and chronic stress and their relation to breast cancer. *Psychological Medicine* **30**, 669–78.

92. **Watson, M., Haviland, J.S., Greer, S., Davidson, J., and Bliss, J.M.** (1999). Influence of psychological response of survival in breast cancer: a population-based cohort study. *Lancet* **354**, 1331–6.

93. **Holden, R.J., Pakula, I.S., and Mooney, P.A.** (1998). An immunological model connecting the pathogenesis of stress, depression and carcinoma. *Medical Hypotheses* **51**, 309–14.

94. **Sharpe, C.** (2002). Heavy exposure to some tricyclic antidepressants associated with elevated breast cancer risk. *British Journal of Cancer* **86**, 2–97.

95. **Picard, A.** Research finds some depression drugs raise cancer risk. *The Globe and Mail*, 14 February 2002, pp. 1–7.

96. **Baltrusch, H.F. and Waltz, M.E.** (1986). Early family attitudes and the stress process—life-span and personological model of host–tumour relationships: biopsychosocial research on cancer and stress in Central Europe. In *Cancer, Stress and Death* 2nd edn. (ed. S.B. Day), pp. 241–83. New York: Plenum.

97. **Thomas, C.B., Duszynski, K., and Schaffer, J.** (1979). Family attitudes reported in youth as potential predictors of cancer. *Psychosomatic Medicine* **41**, 287–302.

98. **Levy, S.M. and Wise, B.D.** (1988). Psychosocial risk factors and cancer progression. In *Stress and Breast Cancer* (ed. C.L. Cooper), pp. 77–96. Chichester: John Wiley.

99. **Ramirez, A.J., Craig, T.K., Watson, J.P., Fentiman, I.S., North, W.R., and Rubens, R.D.** (1989). Stress and relapse of breast cancer. *British Medical Journal* **298**, 291–3.

100. **Greer, S., Morris, T., Pettingale, K.W., and Hybittle, J.L.** (1990). Psychological response to breast cancer and 15-year outcome. *Lancet* **355**, 49–50.

101. **Marshall, J.R. and Funch, D.P.** (1983). Social environment and breast cancer: a cohort analysis of patient survival. *Cancer* **52**, 1546–50.

102. **Goodwin, J.S., Hunt, W.C., Key, C.R., and Samet, J.M.** (1987). The effect of marital status on stage, treatment, and survival of cancer patients. *Journal of the American Medical Association* **258**, 3125–30.

103. **Ornish, D.** *Love and Survival: The Scientific Basis for the Healing Power of Intimacy.* New York: HarperCollins Publishers, Inc., 1998.

104. **Achterberg, J.** *Lightening at the Gate: A Visionary Journey of Healing.* Boston: Shambhala, 2002.

105. **White, M.H.** (1993). Prevention of infection in patients with neoplastic disease: use of a historical model for developmental strategies. *Clinical Infectious Diseases* **17**, S355–8.

106. **Bovbjerg, D.H. and Valdimarsdottir, H.B.** (1996). Stress, immune modulation, and infectous agents during chemotherapy for breast cancer. *Annals of Behavioural Medicine* **18**, S63.

107. **Ratcliffe, M.A., Dawson, A.A., and Walker, L.G.** (1995). Eysenck Personality Inventory L-scores in patients with Hodgkin's disease and non-Hodgkin's lymphoma. *Psycho-Oncology* **4**, 39–45.

108. **Danner, D.D., Snowdon, D.A., and Freisen, W.V.** (2001). Positive emotions in early life and longevity: findings from the nun study. *Journal of Personality and Social Psychology* **80**, 804–13.

109. **Glassman, A.H. and Shapiro, P.A.** (1998). Depression and the course of coronary artery disease. *American Journal of Psychiatry* **155**, 4–11.

110. **Sesso, H.D., Kawachi, I., Vokonas, P.S., and Sparrow, D.** (1998). Depression and the risk of coronary disease in the Normative Aging Study. *American Journal of Cardiology* **82**, 851–6.

111. **Musselman, D.L., Evans, D.L., and Nemeroff, C.B.** (1998). The relationship of depression to cardiovascular disease: Epidemiology, biology, and treatment. *Archives of General Psychiatry* **55**, 580–92.

112. **Dwight, M.M. and Stoudemire, A.** (1997). Effects of depressive disorders on coronary artery disease: a review. *Harvard Review of Psychiatry* **5**, 115–22.

113. **Matthews, K.A. and Gump, B.B.** (2002). Chronic work stress and marital dissolution increase risk of post-trial mortality in men from the Multiple Risk Factor Intervention Trial. *Archives of Internal Medicine* **162**, 309–15.

114. **Schultz, R., Beach, S.R., Ives, D.G., Martire, L.M., Ariyo, A.A., and Kop, W.J.** (2000). Association between depression and mortality in older adults: the Cardiovascular Health Study. *Archives of Internal Medicine* **160**, 1761–8.

115. **Rozzini, R., Sabatini, S., Frisoni, G.B., and Trabucchi, M.** (2001). Association between depressive symptoms and mortality in elderly people. *Archives of Internal Medicine* **161**, 299–300.

116. **Blazer, D.G., Hybels, C.F., and Pieper, C.F.** (2001). The association of depression and mortality in elderly persons: a case for multiple independent pathways. *Journal of Gerontology, A Biol Science Medical Science* **56**, M505–9.

117. **Jiang, W.** et al. (2001). Relationship of depression to increased risk of mortality and rehospitalization in patients with congestive heart failure. *Archives of Internal Medicine* **161**, 1849–56.

118. **Rozzini, R., Sabatini, T., Frisoni, G.B., and Trabucchi, M.** (2002). Depression and major outcomes in older patients with heart failure. *Archives of Internal Medicine* **62**, 362–3.

119. **Astin, J.A., Anton-Culver, H., Schwartz, C.E., Shapiro, D.H., McQuade, J., Breuer, A.M., Taylor, T.H., Lee, H., and Kurosaki, T.** (1999). Sense of control and adjustment to breast cancer: the importance of balancing control coping styles. *Behavioral Medicine* **25**, 101–9.

120. **Allen-Mersh, T.L., Earlem, S., Fordy, C., Abrams, K., and Houghton, J.** (1994). Quality of life and survival with continuous hepatic artery infusion for colorectal metastases. *Lancet* **344**, 1255–60.

121. **Stein, S., Linn, M.W., and Stein, E.M.** (1989). Psychological correlates of survival in nursing home cancer patients. *The Gerontologist* **29**, 224–8.

122. **Stein, S., Linn, M.W., and Stein, E.M.** (1985). Patients' anticipation of stress in nursing home care. *The Gerontologist* **25**, 88–94.

123. **Ganz, P.A., Lee, J.J., and Siau, J.** (1991). Quality of life assessment: an independent prognostic variable for survival in lung cancer. *Cancer* **67**, 3131–5.

124. **Edelman, S., Lemon, J., Bell, D.R., and Kidman, A.D.** (1999). Effects of group CBT on the survival time of patients with metastatic breast cancer. *Psycho-oncology* **8**, 474–81.

125. **Cunningham, A.J., Phillips, C., Lockwood, G.A., Hedley, D., and Edmunds, C.V.I.** (2000). Association of involvement in psychological self help with longer survival in patients with metastatic cancer: an exploratory study. *Advances in Mind–Body Medicine* **16**, 276–87.

126. **Schipper, H., Goh, C.R., and Wang, T.L.** (1995). Shifting the cancer paradigm: must we kill to cure? *Journal of Clinical Oncology* **13**, 801–7.

127. *Canada Year Book 1990*. Ottawa: Minister of Regional Industrial Expansion.

128. **Statistics Canada**, *1991 Census*, Part A 93337 & 93338 and Part B 95337 & 95338. Ottawa: Statistics Canada, 1992 and 1994.

129. **Wingo, P.A., Tong, T., and Bolden, S.** (1995). Cancer statistics, 1995. *CA Cancer Journal for Clinicians* **45**, 8–30.

130. *Canadian Cancer Statistics 1990*. Ottawa: Health and Welfare Canada, 1990.

131. **Barker, D.J.P., Coggon, D., Osmond, C., and Wickham, C.** (1990). Poor housing in childhood and high rates of stomach cancer in England and Wales. *British Journal of Cancer* **61**, 575–8.

132. **D'Arcy, C.** (1982). Prevalence and correlates of nonpsychotic psychiatric symptoms in the general population. *Canadian Journal of Psychiatry* **27**, 316–24.

133. **Addington-Hall, J.M., MacDonald, L.D., Anderson, H.R., Chamberlain, J., Freeling, P., and Bland, J.M.M.** (1992). Randomized controlled trial of effects of coordinating care for terminally ill cancer patients. *British Medical Journal* **305**, 1317–22.

134. **Coyle, N., Adelhardt, J., Foley, K.M. and Portenoy, R.K.** (1990). Character of terminal illness in the advanced cancer patient: pain and other symptoms during the last four weeks of life. *Journal of Pain and Symptom Management* **5**, 83–93.

135. **Hinton, J.** (1994). Can home care maintain an acceptable quality of life for patients with terminal cancer and their relatives? *Palliative Medicine* **8**, 183–96.

136. **Poulson, M.J.** (2001). Not just tired. *Journal of Clinical Oncology* **19** (21), 4180–1.

137. **Given, C.W., Stommel, M., Given, B., Osuch, J., Kurtz, M.E., and Kurtz, J.C.** The influence of cancer patients' symptoms and functional states on patients' depression and family caregivers' reaction and depression. *Health Psychology* **12**, 277–85.

138. **Steinhauser, K.E., Clipp, E.C., McNeilly, M., Christakis, N.A., McINtyre, L.M., and Tulsky, J.A.** (2000). In search of a good death: observations of patients, families, and providers. *Annals of Internal Medicine* **132**, 825–32.

139. **Fife, B.L.** (1994). The conceptualization of meaning in illness. *Social Science and Medicine* **38**, 309–16.

140. **Kapleau, P.** *The Wheel of Life and Death: a Practical and Spiritual Guide.* New York: Anchor Books, 1989.

141. **Kübler-Ross, E.** *On Death and Dying.* New York: Macmillan, 1969.

142. **Frankl, V.** *Man's Search for Meaning.* New York: Washington Square Press, 1984.

143. **Weisman, A.** *Coping with Cancer.* New York: McGraw-Hill Book Co., 1979.

144. **Hinton, J.** (1994). Which patients terminal cancer are admitted from home care? *Palliative Medicine* **8**, 197–210.

145. **Connor, S.R.** (1992). Denial in terminal illness: to intervene or not to intervene. *Hospice* Journal **8** (4), 1–15.

146. **Connor, S.R.** (2000). Denial and the limits of anticipatory mourning. In *Clinical Dimensions of Anticipatory Mourning* (ed. T. Rando), pp. 253–65. Champaign, Ill.

147. **Viganò, A., Dorgan, M., Buckingham, J., Bruera, E., and Suarez-Almazor, M.E.** (2000). Survival prediction in terminal cancer patients: a systematic review of the medical literature. *Palliative Medicine* **14**, 363–74.

148. **Maguire, P.** (2000). Communication with terminally ill patients and their relatives. In *Handbook of Psychiatry in Palliative Medicine* (ed. H.M. Chochinov and W. Breitbart), pp. 291–301. New York: Oxford University Press.

149. **Shepherd, R.** *Living with Terminal Cancer.* Toronto: Maclean Hunter Ltd., 1991.

150. **Weisman, A.D.** (1989). Vulnerability and the psychological disturbances of cancer patients. *Psychosomatics* **30**, 80–85.

151. **Heim, E.** (1991). Coping and adaptation in cancer. In *Cancer and Stress: Psychological, Biological and Coping Studies* (ed. C.L. Cooper and M. Watson), pp. 197–235. New York: John Wiley and Sons.

152. **Aass, N., Fosså, S.D., Dahl, A.A., and Moe, T.J.** (1997). Prevalence of anxiety and depression in cancer patients seen at the Norwegian Radium Hospital. *European Journal of Cancer* **33**, 1597–604.

153. **Passik, S.D., Dugan, W., McDonald, M.V., Rosenfield, B., Theobold, D.E., and Edgerton, S.** (1998). Oncologists' recognition of depression in their patients with cancer. *Journal of Clinical Oncology* **16**, 1594–600.

154. **Razavi, D. and Stiefel, F.** (1994). Common psychiatric disorders in cancer patients. 1. Adjustment disorders and depressive disorders. *Supportive Care in Cancer* **2**, 223–32.

155. **Medical Letter** (1993). Drugs of choice for cancer chemotherapy. *Medical Letter* **35**, 43–50.

156. **Valente, S.M. and Saunders, J.M.** (1997). Diagnosis and treatment of major depression among people with cancer. *Cancer Nursing* **20**, 168–77.

157. **Harrison, J. and Maguire, P.** (1995). The influence of age on psychological adjustment to cancer, *Psycho-Oncology* **4**, 33–8.

158. **Ferrell, B.R. and Ferrell, B.** (1998). The older patient. In *Psycho-oncology* (ed. J.C. Holland), pp. 839–44. New York: Oxford University Press.

159. **Stedeford, A.** *Facing Death: Patients, Families and Professionals.* London: William Heinemann Medical Books Ltd., 1984.

160. **Vachon, M.L.S.** (1987). Unresolved grief in persons with cancer referred for psychotherapy. *The Psychiatric Clinics of North America* **10**, 467–86.

161. **McDaniel, J.S., Musselman, D.L., Porter, M.R., Reed, D.A., and Nemeroff, C.B.** (1995). Depression in patients with cancer: diagnosis, biology, and treatment. *Archives of General Psychiatry* **52**, 89–99.

162. **American Psychiatric Association.** *Quick Reference to the Diagnostic Criteria from DSM-IV.* Washington DC: American Psychiatric Association, 1994.

163. **Kathol, R.G., Mutgi, A., Williams, J., Clamon, G., and Noyes, R.** (1990). Diagnosis of major depression in cancer patients according to four sets of criteria. *American Journal of Psychiatry* **147**, 1021–4.

164. **Godding, P.R., McAnulty, R.D., Wittrock, D.A., Britt, D.M., and Khansur, T.** (1995). Predictors of depression among male cancer patients. *Journal of Nervous and Mental Disease* **183**, 95–8.

165. **Hann, D.M., Oxman, T.E., Ahles, T.A., Furstenberg, C.T., and Stukes, T.A.** (1995). Social support adequacy and depression in older patients with metastatic cancer. *Psycho-Oncology* **4**, 213–21.

166. **Chochinov, H.M., Wilson, K.G., Enns, M., and Lander, S.** (1998). Depression, hopelessness and suicidal ideation in the terminally ill. *Psychosomatics* **39**, 366–70.

167. **Massie, M.J., Gagnon, P., and Holland, J.** (1994). Depression and suicide in patients with cancer. *Journal of Pain and Symptom Management* **9**, 325–40.

168. **Chochinov, H.M., Wilson, K.G., Enns, M., Mowchun, N., Lander, S., Levitt, M., and Clinch, J.J.** (1995). Desire for death in the terminally ill. *American Journal of Psychiatry* **152**, 1185–91.

169. **Miller, R.D. and Walsh, D.** (1991). Psychosocial aspects of palliative care in advanced cancer. *Journal of Pain and Symptom Management* **6**, 24–9.

170. **Stiefel, F. and Razavi, D.** (1994). Common psychiatric disorders in cancer patients. II. Anxiety and acute confusional states. *Supportive Care in Cancer* **2**, 233–7.

171. **Spiegel, D.** (1994). Health caring: psychosocial support for patients with cancer. *Cancer Supplement* **74**, 1453–7.

172. **Silberfarb, P.M.** (1998). Psychiatric treatment of the patient during cancer treatment. In *Psychosocial Issues and Cancer,* pp.5–9. New York: American Cancer Society.

173. **Cassel, E.** (1982). The nature of suffering and the goals of medicine. *New England Journal of Medicine* **306**, 639–45.
174. **Shaver, W.A.** (2001). The origins of human suffering. *In Touch: Ohio Hospice and Palliative Care Committee Journal* **6** (4), 9–13.
175. **Shaver, W.A.** (2002). Suffering and the role of abandonment of self. *Journal of Hospice and Palliative Nursing* **4** (1), 46–53.
176. **Vachon, M.L.S. and Shaver, W.A.** (2001). Suffering in the face of terminal illness. In *Concise Oxford Textbook of Palliative Care* (ed. N. Coyle et al.). Oxford: Oxford Medical Publications (in press).
177. **Burton, L.A.** (1998). The spiritual dimension of palliative care. *Seminars in Oncology Nursing* **14** (2), 121–8.
178. **Norum, J., Risberg, T., and Solberg, E.** (2000). Faith among people with advanced cancer. A pilot study on patients offered 'no more than' palliation. *Supportive Care in Cancer* **8**, 110–14.
179. **Ehman, J.W., Ott, B.B., Short, T.H., Ciampa, R.C., and Hansen-Flaschen, J.** (1999). Do patients want physicians to inquire about their spiritual or religious beliefs if they become gravely ill? *Archives of Internal Medicine* **23**, 1803–6.
180. **O'Connor, T.S.J., Meakes, E., McCarroll-Butler, P., Gadowsky, S., and O'Neill, K.** (1997). Making the most and making sense: ethnography research on spirituality in palliative care. *Journal of Pastoral Care* **51**, 25–36.
181. **Kellehear, A.** (2000). Spirituality and palliative care: a model of needs. *Palliative Medicine* **14** (2), 149–55.
182. **Connolly, R., Vachon, M.L.S., Hollenberg, D., Librach, L., Chow, E., Danjoux, C., Franssen, E., Wong, R., Hayter, C., Szumacher, E., Loblaw, A., Andersson, L., and Pope, J.** The use of complementary and alternative therapies among patients referred to an outpatient palliative radiotherapy program (in process).

12.2 Emotional problems in the family

Joan T. Panke and Betty R. Ferrell

Introduction

Definition of the family

Advanced disease from any chronic illness impacts all of the family members surrounding the one with the diagnosis. Changing demographics of our society and an aggressive shift of health care into the living room makes the role of family caregivers in chronic and terminal illness even more significant. While the family was traditionally defined as an individual of blood relationship, a broad definition of family is most appropriate and best defined as those individuals considered as a family by the patient. Studies in oncology related to the family have generally found that approximately 70 per cent of primary family caregivers are spouses, approximately 20 per cent are children (of which daughters or daughters-in-law are most predominant), and approximately 10 per cent are friends or more distant relatives.[1,2] A review of the literature on the topic of family and palliative care reveals that most of the research has focused on pain management with the second predominant area identified as family bereavement. Family then includes biological relatives as well as persons identified by the patient as significant in their lives, intimately involved with the patient, who love the patient, and have frequent contact with the patient.[3,4]

It is important to note that opportunities for growth for both patient and family are tremendous even while they are coping with countless difficulties and sorrows as the patient's disease progresses. We may not be able to change the course of a disease or functional decline, yet professional caregivers can support and aggressively advocate for the needs of the patient and family by attending simultaneously to their physical, psychological, social, and spiritual needs and concerns. Patients and their loved ones are given the opportunity to attend to what is important to them, ultimately bringing about a more peaceful death.

Dying is recognized as a uniquely individual experience. An interdisciplinary team approach to care is necessary in order to address and respond to the many needs of the patient and family. Palliative care is appropriate at every stage of the disease regardless of whether or not the patient is seeking curative treatment. By introducing palliative care earlier in the disease trajectory, it is possible to recognize subtle shifts that take place, reassess and adapt goals as necessary, and opens the way for patients and families to begin to reframe hope, to find meaning, and to adapt as a disease progresses.

While family caregivers confront many patient symptoms, the experience of pain serves as a model for exploring the differences between the individual patient's experience as compared to that of the family caregiver. Figure 1 identifies the experience of pain from the patient's perspective beginning with nociception. Pain is influenced by many factors including prior painful experiences, meaning of pain, culture, and other factors. Pain is a subjective experience and, thus, is expressed in not only intensity, but also in the degree of distress from the pain. This perception results in the global experience of physical pain, associated symptoms and emotions, and the dimension of suffering.

Similarly, Fig. 2 describes the family caregiver's experience of pain as a model symptom of advanced illness. Family caregivers' experience of pain begins with their perceptions of the patient's suffering. However, family caregivers' perspectives of pain vary dramatically and are influenced by many factors including their own personal encounters with pain, the relationship to the patient, culture, and interpretation of cause and meaning. Observing a family member's pain and other sources of suffering can lead to severe emotional distress in the caregiver.

These models illustrate the similarities in the shared experience of pain but also the unique experience of the individual with advanced illness

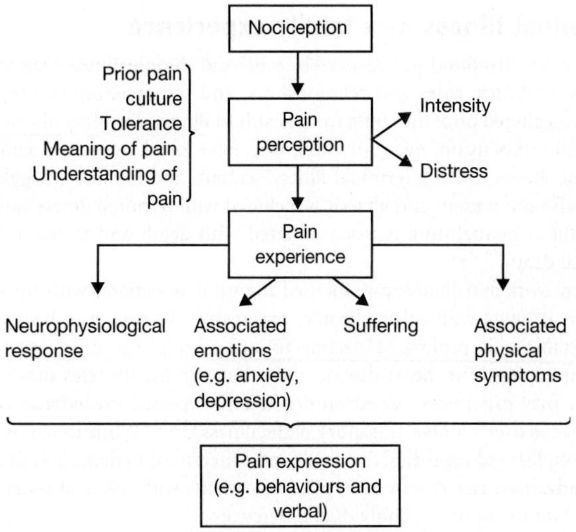

Fig. 1 Patient's experience of pain. (Adapted from Ferrel, B.R., Cohen, M.Z., Rhiner, M., and Rozek, A. (1991). Pain as a metaphor illness. Part II: family caregivers' management of pain. *Oncology Nursing Forum* **18**, 1315–21.)

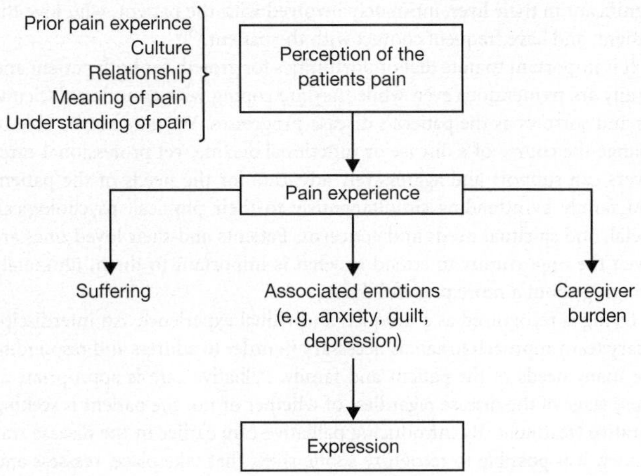

Fig. 2 Caregiver's experience of pain. [Adapted from Ferrell, B.R., Cohen, M.Z., Rhiner, M., and Rozek, A. (1991). Pain as a metaphor illness. Part II: family caregivers' management of pain. *Oncology Nursing Forum* **18**, 1315–21.]

versus those who experience it from their vision as caregivers. These same models can be applied to many other patient symptoms to illustrate the shared experiences between patient and family. It is often stated that while the patient experiences greater physical symptoms, family caregivers often experience a greater degree of suffering as they observe the patient.[5,6]

Appreciation for the caregivers' perspective is critical to the care of the patient. Decades of work in hospice and palliative care have demonstrated that support of family caregivers is an essential feature of quality care for patients with chronic advanced illness. Because family members are assuming a greater role with the shift of care to the home, quality care is dependent upon addressing family caregivers' needs.

Attention to family needs and concerns should occur throughout the trajectory of any potentially life-threatening illness. Family caregiving takes on distinct meaning in situations such as AIDS in which care is shifted to non-blood relatives and often to other individuals experiencing the same illness. Future trends in health care will also shift care from professionals to unlicensed caregivers as our society becomes increasingly dependent upon significant others such as an elderly spouse, whose ability to provide the intensive care of advanced disease is limited.[7,8]

Terminal illness as a family experience

Families are profoundly influenced by acute and chronic illness. Day-to-day family activities, roles and relationships, and the meaning of life itself becomes altered once life shifts from health to illness. Terminal illness adds an entire dimension, even for those who have faced years or decades of chronic illness. During terminal illness, patients and families struggle not only with the present and all that is included with terminal illness care but with the overwhelming issues associated with death and transcendence beyond death.[9–12]

Early work in palliative care focused attention on patients with advanced cancer. Patients with other chronic, progressive illnesses may have a less predictable and prolonged decline towards death. Family members of patients dying from heart disease and other chronic illnesses other than cancer may experience added burden due to repeated exacerbations and remissions over a longer trajectory of the illness.[13,14] While much of what has been learned regarding the needs and concerns of patients and families with advanced cancer can be applied to patients with other illnesses, it is important to appreciate individual differences.

Palliative care has the ability to prevent family crisis and create cohesion in the light of, even, a life-threatening illness. In a study of parents of children with cancer, a mother described having a child diagnosed with cancer as an experience in which the family actually came closer together. Grandparents became supportive in the care of the child. Both parents worked together to provide comfort to the child, and siblings also became co-operative and concerned about their brother with cancer. However, the mother described the experience of having the child suffering pain by saying, 'It was as if someone threw a hand grenade in our living room'.[15] Having a child with uncontrolled symptoms created an opposite environment in which the grandparents became critical of the parents' care and the parents became critical of each other. The siblings were frightened of their brother's pain and thus isolated themselves from him.

As family caregivers observe physical and emotional suffering of a loved one who is dying, they also struggle with their own losses and changing roles while dealing with their concerns about their caregiving abilities.[16] Family intervention is needed to confront the many physical and emotional issues associated with palliative care. Intervention is dependent upon assessment of family functioning and use of an interdisciplinary team to meet the diverse needs of the family.

Coping with a terminal illness can challenge both the patient and the family in terms of their spiritual beliefs. When someone is dying, hope may seem diminished, but despair is not necessarily inevitable. In fact, spiritual concerns may become more intense as death approaches. Aspects of spirituality are significant contributors to quality of life. Through assessment and intervention, family caregivers have the opportunity to find comfort and strength from their spirituality that assists in their coping.[17] The dying person may search for deeper spiritual meaning of life's work or relationship to others or God. Family members may search for the meaning in a loved one's death. Assessing what 'hope' means to an individual assists the patient and family to set realistic goals for the time that they do have remaining (see Chapter 11 for further discussion on spirituality).

Role of the family caregivers in palliative care

Whether patients are receiving aggressive treatments aimed at curing a life-threatening illness or comfort, they are likely to have multiple physical, psychological, social, and spiritual needs. Family members often have to allocate more time to caring for the patient.[18] Family caregivers furthermore may have to manage work outside the home along with caregiving roles. Many family caregivers assuming the demanding job of caring for someone they love are performing this care after completing 8 h employment outside the home each day.[19]

The role of the family caregiver involves both direct and indirect care needs. Direct care includes those aspects of care carried out directly with the patient, such as symptom management, emotional support, monitoring for changes in patient status, medication administration, and assistance with activities of daily living. Indirect care involves activities carried out on behalf of the patient, such as obtaining prescriptions and medications, transportation, scheduling and coordination of appointments, and dealing with financial issues.[18] In our research in the area of family caregivers' involvement in pain management, we have also found that family caregivers are commonly involved in 'night duty', assuming total care; making decisions at night for patients who perhaps are more independent during the day hours.[5]

Barriers to effective symptom management by family caregivers

It is notable given the extent of their involvement that there has been little attention given to family caregivers. In a study in 1998 to 1999, we analysed all end-of-life content in nursing textbooks as a part of our Robert Wood Johnson funded work on end-of-life care.[19] We reviewed 50 textbooks used in schools of nursing comprising 45 683 pages to analyse nine end-of-life topics (i.e. pain, symptom management, bereavement, quality of life, legal issues, and ethical issues). Overall only 2 per cent of content in

Table 1 Nursing textbook analysis of family caregiver content at the end of life

Roles and needs of family caregivers	0	1	11
Importance of recognizing needs of family and caregivers at EOL	57	37	6
Assessment of family needs	57	26	17
Family dynamics	83	13	4
Recognition of ethnic or cultural influences on EOL care	91	2	7
Coping strategies and support systems	70	26	4
Average	71	21	8

0 = absent; + = present; ++ = commendable; EOL = end of life.

textbooks had any relationship to any end-of-life topic, and the area most neglected was the needs and roles of family caregivers. Of the 45 683 pages, only 42 pages (or 0.1 per cent of content) were related to family. Seventy-one per cent of the texts reviewed had no content at all related to family caregivers (see Table 1). Efforts to address knowledge deficits of professionals related to care of the family are underway through initiatives such as the End of Life Nursing Education Consortium (ELNEC), which includes care of the family as a common thread throughout the curriculum (see http://www.aacn.nche.edu/ELNEC).(20)

Family caregivers frequently lack information regarding what to expect as a disease progresses, how to manage symptoms, and when to report symptoms or failure of treatments to control symptoms. Similarly, lack of adequate support has been identified as a barrier to care that negatively impacts symptom management.

Frequently cited barriers to effective pain management by family caregivers of patients with cancer include fear of respiratory depression, fear of drug tolerance, fear of drug addiction, and lack of knowledge regarding chronic pain. Investigators have documented that family members play an important role in pain management.(2,21–23) As family members assume the role of caregivers for patients, they are often required to manage complex medication regimens, parenteral infusion devices, and even parenteral and intraspinal medications in the home.(24–27) Thus, family members are assuming the responsibility for pain relief despite the need to understand basic pain management principles. Family members often deny that the patient is in pain to avoid the realization that the disease is progressing.(28–32) The family's decisions in pain management seem to range from giving pain medications aggressively (while often being quite concerned about their decisions in medicating) to restricting and withholding medications because of concern that they would be criticized for over-medicating the patient or using too much of the medications.

Caregiver burden

Caregiver burden can be described as the emotional and physical demands and responsibilities of an illness that are placed on family members, friends, or other individuals involved with the patient outside of the health care system. Families often do not know how to provide physical care, adjust to role changes, and cope with the many losses faced during the dying process and after the death. Many caregivers have physical illnesses that may impact their ability to care for the patient and themselves. Patients worry about the emotional and financial burdens placed on family members. Some families have had to drain life savings to cover costs of care.

A study by Grobe et al.(31) revealed that family members of terminally ill patients with cancer needed to learn new skills, such as assisting with ambulation, comfort care, and pain management, in order to provide effective care in the home. These family members reported that specific caregiving skills were not taught by their health care providers, and they were left with a 'trial and error' method of skill acquisition.

Tringali(33) reinforced this conclusion by observing family members of patients with cancer at three different phases of illness including initial treatment, recurrent disease, and follow-up treatment. Family caregivers were evaluated regarding their cognitive, emotional, and physical needs. Regardless of the phase of illness, informational needs were identified as most important. The results suggest that the provision of information prepares family members to support the patient, reinforces the treatment goals, and assists in managing the side-effects of therapy and disease. It is apparent from the reports of these investigators,(31,33) and others,(7,8,34–37) that the needs of family members are not being met, and that understanding needs and assisting families in meeting those needs will contribute to improved care.

Caregivers may experience severe mood disruption in the areas of depression, anxiety, and fatigue. Providing adequate pain relief is of great comfort to caregivers, who express feelings of helplessness, frustration, and sadness when unable to provide comfort. Unfortunately, caregivers often receive limited instruction in the use of pharmacologic and non-pharmacologic pain management techniques and principles, and may tend to under-medicate the patient in response to their concerns about addiction, respiratory depression, and drug tolerance.(38)

We have consistently seen a low correlation between patient and family caregivers regarding pain intensity levels and distress regarding pain. The level of concern, stress, and knowledge of the caregiver are different from the patient. Family caregivers' perception of pain may be influenced by the nature of the pain, its duration, and the patient's prognosis. An interesting finding from our recent studies is that the family caregivers' fear of addiction and tolerance were worse than the fear experienced by the patients themselves.(19)

General fears and concerns of family members

Family caregivers expect that quality care will be provided to the patient. Families also look to health care professionals to provide for information regarding the disease and dying process, physical care, symptom management needs, emotional support, and for practical guidance.(39,40)

A review of the research on the impact of cancer on the family(41) identified 11 separate issues of concern for family members. These included:

- emotional strain;
- physical demands;
- uncertainty;
- fear of the patient dying;
- altered roles and lifestyles;
- finances;
- ways to comfort the patient;
- perceived inadequacies of services;
- existential concern;
- sexuality;
- non-convergent needs among household members.

Studies of family members caring for persons with advanced cancer have shown that most experience stress in the caregiver role and significant stress in observing patient suffering. Family caregivers report distress from uncertainty about the course of the disease as well as feelings about their inability to provide care (such as effective symptom relief) or to manage the patient's psychological symptoms such as depression and anxiety.(32)

Given et al.(18) identified needs of family members of dying persons as including:

- Need for information regarding the disease
    - information about physical care and comfort measures;

- what symptoms to expect and how to manage them;
- treatment regimens;
- expectations for future care;
- patient's emotional response;
- household management procedures;
- finances;
- community resources.

◆ Need for assistance with how to structure care activities
- monitoring and reporting symptoms;
- monitoring disease status;
- transportation;
- nutritional considerations;
- co-ordination of care (scheduling);
- financial concerns.

◆ Continued guidance to alleviate stressors, overall burden, and associated depression
- escalation of care demands as patient's disease and functional status declines;
- strategies to assist with coping with disease progression and patient decline;
- detailed, specific information regarding unique psychological and social needs.

Family communication

Issues of communication frequently influence family caregiving in palliative care. Understanding family information needs is central to providing the care necessary to maintain patients in any setting. Assessing the need for information and how information is shared. The emotional and psychosocial needs of both patient and family reinforce the importance of interdisciplinary care in advanced illness.

Vachon[43] described many issues related to family communication during advanced illness. Family members, like patients, experience significant distress during the patient's illness. Three major problematic issues can be summarized from the research literature related to family communication and cancer:

1. concealing feelings;
2. acquiring information;
3. coping with helplessness.

Family communication can become restricted as family members withhold information to protect one another from difficult issues.[42–44] Patients often underreport symptoms to avoid distressing family caregivers. Three patterns of restricted communication among couples coping with the terminal phase of cancer were identified by Hinton:[36]

1. consciously avoiding any discussion of the illness as a self-protective way of preventing one's distress level from rising;
2. avoiding discussion of the illness in order to maintain the positive attitude felt to be essential to coping with the disease, thereby avoiding discussing any pessimistic feelings;
3. those who had rarely spoken openly about emotional events in the past and maintained this pattern during the terminal illness.

An important intervention by health care providers is to validate the family caregiver's contributions to the patient's comfort and reinforce their commitment. Health care providers play a central role in enhancing communication between various family members, with the patient, and with other health care professionals. In the terminal phase of illness, families often require greater support to overcome barriers to communication, which greatly affect patient care. Psychosocial services such as the care provided by a clinical psychologist or psychiatrist are important but all team members can assist in improved family communication. Encouraging expression of concerns, facilitating discussions, active listening, and providing information are all important components of this care (see Chapter 4.1).

Clinical issues in supporting family caregivers

What family caregivers need most is information and support. Family caregivers increasingly assume 24-h care that in recent years was provided in acute, inpatient settings, perhaps having received little or no education and, even more importantly, little emotional support. In many instances, family caregivers are now assuming procedures and treatments that has previously been confined to intensive care units. Health care professionals provide this care with the support of colleagues and with the assurance that the 'next shift' will relieve them soon. Family caregivers seldom have such assurance. Much can be provided in the way of home care and hospice services and yet even for those individuals with access to such services, the majority of the responsibility rests on the family members themselves.

In recent research conducted at the City of Hope National Medical Center, we evaluated a structured pain education programme in both elderly patients and family caregivers. The educational programme was successful in improving knowledge and attitudes about pain, as well as direct outcomes such as improved pain intensity and overall quality of life. However, the study also revealed the unmet emotional needs of family caregivers arising from the perceived burden of responsibility for the relief of a loved one's suffering.[27] This study, and other literature, demonstrates that providing information alone is not sufficient, but that family caregivers desperately need support for the intense roles they assume and the burdens they shoulder associated with assuming responsibility for patient comfort.

Family members often feel helpless, despite their best attempts, if symptoms persist. Family caregivers also may deny the presence of symptoms as a means of coping with the situation. Our previous decade of research has revealed the ever-present metaphor of pain as a symbol of death. In this sense, pain is unlike treatment of other symptoms, such as nausea or constipation, in that it carries with it the existential issues of suffering and death.

Realistically, professionals cannot always be present as a team to address family needs. The one-to-one encounter is significant in that it may serve to uncover important issues or concerns of both the patient and the family, which can then be shared with other team members. The value of a team meeting cannot be stressed enough as an opportunity to explore important issues and to create and reevaluate a realistic plan of care that is patient and family oriented.

Alternative therapies

Family caregivers often seek alternative therapies either as curative treatments or as palliative treatments for symptom management. Montbriand[45] reviewed alternative therapies in cancer care and categorized these as spiritual, psychological, or physical modalities. Spiritual methods include faith healing, psychic surgery, and similar modalities. Psychological therapies include visualization or other cognitive therapies. The most common alternative treatment is the use of physical methods such as herbs, vitamins, health foods, and healers.

These methods may be a valuable component of the patient's care, enhancing the effects of traditional methods. However, health providers should assess the use of these modalities to determine the potential for misuse or to identify areas of fraud or financial burden too often associated with their use. Work by Montbriand[45] and others[46–49] serves as a useful guide to direct health care providers in this important aspect of care.

Educating family caregivers to utilize alternative, non-pharmacologic approaches can enhance patient comfort. Use of gentle massage, incorporating music into daily activities, or cognitive-behavioural techniques such as distraction, relaxation, and imagery may benefit family caregivers by enhancing their sense of helpfulness and control (see Chapters 8.17 and 16).

Bereavement issues

Care provided to families during the course of a terminal illness has a profound influence on bereavement following death of the patient. All of the above-cited suggestions for family support during illness will also influence subsequent bereavement. Positive bereavement outcomes result from a sense by family caregivers of having provided optimum care and relieved symptoms. The physical and psychological burdens of caregiving may be relieved in part when family members feel that they were able to minimize the patient's distress and that the patient received appropriate professional care.[9,12] It is important that assessment of the family continue into the bereavement period, when physical symptoms can become apparent (see Chapter 19).

Ethical dilemmas encountered by family caregivers

An additional area of study is the ethical dilemmas associated with palliative care (see Section 3). The many ethical decisions and conflicts encountered by families may be in relation to the management of pain and other symptoms; initiation or withdrawing/withholding of treatments; medication management; physician relations; patient assessment; personal decisions; religious issues; balancing career and personal life; professional limitations; and nutrition and hydration.[28,29]

Studies to date have identified the important role of family caregivers and their educational needs in assuming care for the person with cancer. Research has also begun to describe conflicts and burdens faced by caregivers. The impact of cancer care on caregivers, their ethical dilemmas and resultant distress, and their knowledge of pain management principles and techniques are areas for additional study.[41,42,50,51]

Implications for future research

As care shifts into the home and family caregivers provide a greater extent of palliative care, research should also expand to understudied areas. It is important to evaluate outcomes of palliative care to include both patient and family caregivers. Outcomes should incorporate all aspects of quality of life including physical, psychological, social, and spiritual well-being (Fig. 3).

Opportunities exist in the field of pain to synthesize knowledge across studies to advance research collectively as a discipline and to strengthen clinical interventions for family caregivers in order to decrease fears and misconceptions related to pain and its treatment.[19] An example of family caregiver outcomes is the Quality of Life Questionnaire, Family Version and the Family Pain Questionnaire (questionnaires available on-line: http://prc.coh.org). The Quality of Life Questionnaire is a tool developed specifically for family caregivers, and is analogous to a questionnaire used to assess patients' quality of life.[52] This is an example of methodology which assesses the family caregiver's needs as distinct from those of the patient.

There is a need to extend family research beyond a single caregiver or beyond spouses alone. Clinical experience documents the impact of terminal care on all family members, yet the entire family unit, and particular individuals such as children, are seldom studied.[53] An effort to include family educational and supportive needs with chronic, progressive illnesses other than cancer is needed.

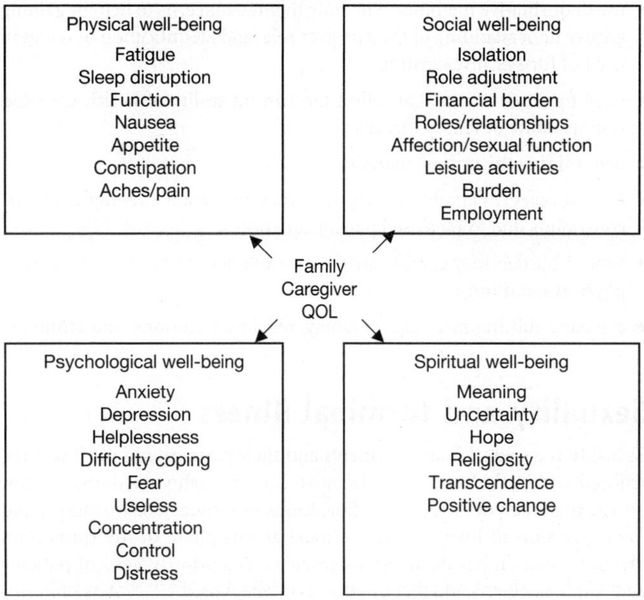

Fig. 3 Family Caregiver Quality of Life.

Future research should incorporate cost–benefit outcomes and include direct as well as indirect costs and the costs assumed by patients and families.[54,55] Cost measures are essential in the future restructuring of health care, to establish the benefits of palliative care.

We have found important methodological issues associated with conducting family research in pain management. Selection of instruments proves to be a constant challenge. A review of family literature revealed instruments frequently used in family caregiving research include (19):

- Family APGAR (adaptation, partnership, growth, affection, resolved);
- Family Pain Questionnaire;
- Quality of Life—Caregiver;
- Family communication tools;
- Social support tools;
- Family functioning tools;
- Caregiving demand assessments;
- Caregiver burden instruments;
- Barriers Questionnaire;
- Instruments applied from patient outcomes (coping, anxiety);
- Family Finances Survey;
- Interview tools.

There is a need for rigorous work to develop or adapt instruments specific to the issues of family caregiving and pain. Moreover, methodological challenges exist when including family caregivers in pain research:

- definition of family to determine who would be identified as a caregiver;
- assessing individual versus family systems outcomes to ensure individual differences are measured;
- distinguishing family caregiver response to illness versus pain since emotional responses often overlap;
- distinguishing family versus patient outcomes to identify individual needs for education, management, and support;
- assessing physical versus psychological or emotional burden and suffering;

- use of qualitative methods to identify themes/concerns to help in gaining greater understanding of the caregiver role, and identification of issues in need of further investigation;
- need for instruments that reflect the current reality of health care and responsibility of family caregivers;
- determining the unit of analysis;
- gaining access to family subjects when they are already experiencing time constraints due to increased patient care needs;
- subject burden may complicate the measurement of needs, concerns, or physical symptoms;
- assessing cultural meanings of family, religion, traditions, and ethnicity.

Sexuality and terminal illness

Sexuality is a critical issue to patients and their partners and yet it is often ignored within the context of palliative care. Sexuality encompasses not only sexual intercourse but also dimensions of intimacy, self-concept, and the expression of love, which is critical at this phase of life transition. Previous research has documented sexuality as a priority need of patients and family caregivers and that this need is often ignored.[56–58] Acts of intimacy and/or sexual intercourse have significant meaning during terminal illness, and are often important forms of communication during terminal illness. A failure to intervene with this equally important aspect of holistic care creates great distress for patients and their loved ones.

Sexuality can be addressed by first exploring with the patients their needs and assessment of physical or psychological issues associated with sexuality. Issues of sexuality are often examples of divergent needs between patients and family caregivers. Patients may have a continued or even stronger desire for sexual activity yet partners may be reluctant to reciprocate due to either fear of physical harm or avoidance of the intimacy with their loved ones given the prognosis. Tension is best addressed by allowing both partners to express their feelings or concerns associated with illness or intimacy. There are also basic considerations such as a lack of privacy within institutional settings or physical changes such as altering the hospital bed so that both patient and partner can sleep together.

The first challenge is to facilitate communication with patient or partner regarding issues of sexuality and intimacy. We have found it useful within our Quality of Life Questionnaire, Family Version (available on-line: http://prc.coh.org) to ask questions regarding distress from illness and interference with relationships as ways to begin communication and lead on to more specific aspects of intimacy. This important need is also an example of where co-ordination of the palliative care team is important, to ensure that sexuality is assessed and services are routinely offered by a member of the team and that additional services by a sexual counsellor are available as needed.

Table 2 Suggested interventions to facilitate family coping with advanced illness

Communication: Assess family communication patterns prior to and over the course of an illness
Family relationships: Acknowledge the relationship of the family member to the patient. Caregiving is significantly influenced by the distinct relationship (i.e. spouse, parent, child)
Family developmental level: Recognize the family's developmental level and its relationship to their coping with the illness. Family developmental crises (recent retirement, births, marriages, etc.), influence coping with illness. Assess whether multiple developmental crises are occurring
Family conferences: Establish mechanisms for conducting family conferences to facilitate shared communication between patient, family, and health care providers and to clarify changing goals of care
Concurrent stressors: Recognize areas of concurrent stress which may be unrelated to the patient or illness (i.e. job loss, stress in the extended family, coping with children)
Financial concerns: Provide counselling for the direct and indirect financial burdens associated with chronic illness
Education: Diminish caregiver's sense of helplessness by empowering them with knowledge and skills to enhance patient comfort (i.e. use of drug and non-drug modalities)
Pain education: Provide structured pain education to diffuse anxiety regarding issues such as addiction and tolerance
Physical aspects of care: Develop family education regarding the basic physical aspects of care giving (i.e. lifting, bathing, toileting)
Encourage expression of fears and concerns: Provide opportunities for family caregivers to express their emotions through individual or group support away from the patient
Emotional strain: Provide opportunities to verbalize the emotional strain inherent in care giving during terminal illness
Risk for dysfunctional coping: Identify families at risk for dysfunctional coping with terminal illness. Risk factors include families with poor communication patterns, prior history of family stress, and those with prior issues on non-compliance
Issues of uncertainty: Provide information regarding anticipated symptoms and discuss the distress associated with uncertainty
The actual death: Provide information regarding what to expect with the actual death event
Sources of family support: Evaluate and co-ordinate available sources of family support, i.e. social workers, spiritual support persons, clinical psychologists, psychiatrists, family counselling, peer support groups

Responding to the needs of the family

While the emotional problems facing patients and families are significant, there is much to be done to minimize the suffering of terminal illness. Palliative care programmes have demonstrated successful interventions to reduce the physical and emotional burdens of patients and families. Table 2 is a list of suggested interventions derived from the literature that serve as a guide to evaluate the adequacy of support in existing programmes as well as to guide interventions for individual families.

In order to meet the needs of the family, we must gain greater understanding and expertise in all aspects of both patient and family care covered in the other sections of this text. Enhancing clinical skills in care of the patient automatically improves assessment of family issues since attention to the physical, psychological, social, and spiritual issues related to the patient can be translated to the assessment of the family. The interdisciplinary team approach is the key to assessing and responding to both patient and family needs. The reader is referred to Table 2 for specific recommendations.

Summary

In summary, attention to family needs and concerns are an integral aspect of palliative care. Family care has been a cornerstone of the hospice philosophy and will remain so but such care demands professional support. A mother in our family research recently described having a child with cancer as 'being forced to watch your child dangled over a river'. She went on to say that having a child in pain, however, is like 'watching the child dropped into the river and drown'. Again, while experiencing terminal illness is a terrible event, and observing it perhaps even more so, the important lessons of palliative care demonstrate that much can be done to alleviate the suffering of both the patient and their family.

References

1. Ferrell, B.R., Ferrell, B.A., Rhiner, M., and Grant, M.M. (1991). Family factors influencing cancer pain management. *Post Graduate Medical Journal* **67** (Suppl. 2), S64–9.
2. Given, B. and Given, W. (1989). Cancer nursing for the elderly. *Cancer Nursing* **12**, 71–7.
3. Egan, K.A. and Labyak, M.J. (2001). Hospice care. In *Textbook of Palliative Nursing* (ed. B.R. Ferrell and N. Coyle), pp. 7–26. New York: Oxford University Press.
4. Stewart, A.L., Teno, J., Patrick, D.L., and Lynn, J. (1999). The concept of quality of life of dying persons in the context of health care. *Journal of Pain and Symptom Management* **17**, 93–108.
5. Ferrell, B.R., Cohen, M.Z., Rhiner, M., and Rozek, A. (1991). Pain as a metaphor for illness. Part II: family caregivers' management of pain. *Oncology Nursing Forum* **18**, 1315–21.
6. Ferrell, B.R., Rhiner, M., Cohen, M.Z., and Grant, M. (1991). Pain as a metaphor for illness. Part I: impact of cancer pain on family caregivers. *Oncology Nursing Forum* **18**, 1303–9.
7. Horowitz, A. (1985). Family caregiving to the frail elderly. *Annual Review of Gerontology and Geriatrics* **5**, 194–246.
8. Matthews, S.H. (1987). Provision of care to old patients: division of responsibility among adult children. *Research in Aging* **9**, 45–60.
9. Vachon, M.L.S., Freedman, K., Formo, A., Rogers, J., Lyall, W.A.L., and Freeman, S.J.J. (1977). The final illness in cancer: the widow's perspective. *Canadian Medical Association Journal* **177**, 1151–4.
10. Stedeford, A. (1984). Psychological aspects of the management of terminal cancer. *Comprehensive Therapy* **10**, 35–40.
11. Bergen, A. (1991). Nurses caring for the terminally ill in the community: a review of the literature. *International Journal of Nursing Studies* **28**, 89–101.
12. Bowen, M. (1976). Family reactions to death. In *Family Therapy* (ed. P. Guerin), pp. 335–48. New York: Gardner Press.
13. Emanuel, E.J., Fairclough, D.L., Slutsman, J., Alpert, H., Baldwin, D., and Emanuel, L. (1999). Assistance from family members, friends, paid care givers, and volunteers in the care of terminally ill patients. *The New England Journal of Medicine* **341**, 956–63.
14. Field, M.J. and Cassel, C.K. (1997). *Approaching Death: Improving Care at the End of Life* (Report of the Institute of Medicine Task Force). Washington DC: National Academy Press.
15. Ferrell, B.R., Rhiner, M., Shapiro, B., and Dierkes, M. (1994). The experience of pediatric cancer pain. Part I: impact of pain on the family. *Journal of Pediatric Nursing* **9**, 368–79.
16. Goetschius, S.K. (2001). Caring for families: the other patient in palliative care. In *Palliative Care Nursing: Quality Care to the End of Life* (ed. M.L. Matzo and D.W. Sherman), pp. 245–74. New York: Springer.
17. Johnson Taylor, E. (2001). Spiritual assessment. In *Textbook of Palliative Nursing* (ed. B.R. Ferrell and N. Coyle), pp. 397–406. New York: Oxford University Press.
18. Given, B.A., Given, C.W., and Kozachik, S. (2001). Family support in advanced cancer. *CA: A Cancer Journal for Clinicians* **51**, 213–31.
19. Ferrell, B.R. (2001). Pain observed: the experience of pain from the family caregiver's perspective. *Clinics in Geriatric Medicine* **17**, 595–609.
20. American Association of Colleges of Nursing and City of Hope National Medical Center (2000). *End of Life Nursing Education Consortium (ELNEC).* http://www.aacn.nche.edu/ELNEC (11 December 2001).
21. Cleeland, C. (1987). Barriers to the management of cancer pain. *Oncology* **1** (2 Suppl.), 19–26.
22. Ferrell, B.R. and Schneider, C. (1988). Experience and management of cancer pain at home. *Cancer Nursing* **11**, 84–90.
23. Woods, N.F., Lewis, F.M., and Ellison, E.S. (1989). Living with cancer: family experiences. *Cancer Nursing* **12**, 28–33.
24. Ferrell, B.A. and Ferrell, B.R. (1991). Pain management at home. *Clinics in Geriatric Medicine* **7**, 765–76.
25. Spross, J., McGuire, D., and Schmitt, R. (1991). Oncology Nursing Society position paper on cancer pain. *Oncology Nursing Forum* **17**, 595–614, 751–60, 943–4.
26. Whedon, M. and Ferrell, B.R. (1991). Ethical issues and high tech pain management. *Oncology Nursing Forum* **18**, 1135–43.
27. Ferrell, B.R., Ferrell, B.A., Ahn, C., and Tran, K. (1994). Pain management for elderly patients with cancer at home. *Cancer* **74**, 2139–46.
28. Ferrell, B.R., Johnson Taylor, E., Grant, M., Fowler, M., and Corbisiero, R.M. (1993). Pain management at home: struggle, comfort and mission. *Cancer Nursing* **16**, 169–78.
29. Ferrell, B.R., Johnson Taylor, E., Sattler, G.R., Fowler, M., and Cheyney, B.L. (1993). Searching for the meaning of pain: cancer patients', caregivers', and nurses' perspectives. *Cancer Practice* **1**, 185–94.
30. Dar, R., Beach, C.M., Barden, P.L., and Cleeland, C.S. (1992). Cancer pain in the marital system: a study of patients and their spouses. *Journal of Pain and Symptom Management* **7**, 87–93.
31. Grobe, M.E., Ilstrup, E.M., and Ahmann, D.L. (1990). Skills needed by family members to maintain the care of an advanced cancer patient. *Cancer Nursing* **4**, 371–5.
32. Hinds, C. (1985). The needs of families who care for patients with cancer at home: are we meeting them? *Journal of Advanced Nursing* **10**, 575–81.
33. Tringali, C.A. (1986). The needs of family members of cancer patients. *Oncology Nursing Forum* **13**, 65–9.
34. Stommel, M., Given, C.W., and Given, B.A. (1993). The cost of cancer home care to families. *Cancer* **71**, 4–11.
35. Flor, H., Turk, D.C., and Scholz, O.B. (1987). Impact of chronic pain on the spouse: marital, emotional and physical consequences. *Journal of Psychosomatic Research* **31**, 63–71.
36. Hinton, J. (1981). Sharing or withholding awareness of dying between husband and wife. *Journal of Psychosomatic Research* **25**, 337–43.
37. Hull, M.M. (1993). Coping strategies of family caregivers in hospice home care. *Caring* **12**, 78–88.
38. Juarez, G. and Ferrell, B.R. (1996). Family and caregiver involvement in pain management. *Clinics in Geriatric Medicine* **12**, 531–47.
39. Davies, B. (2001). Supporting families in palliative care. In *Textbook of Palliative Nursing* (ed. B.R. Ferrell and N. Coyle), pp. 363–73. New York: Oxford University Press.
40. Kristjanson, L.J., Leis, A., Koop, P., Carriere, K.C., and Mueller, B. (1997). Family members' care expectations, care perceptions, and satisfaction with advanced cancer care: results of a multi-site pilot study. *Journal of Palliative Care* **13**, 5–13.
41. Lewis, F.M. (1986). The impact of cancer on the family: a critical analysis of the research literature. *Patient Education and Counselling* **8**, 269–89.
42. Keitel, M.S., Zevon, M.A., Rounds, J.B., Petrelli, N.J., and Karakousis, C. (1991). Spouse adjustment to cancer surgery: distress and coping responses. *Journal of Surgical Oncology* **43**, 148–53.
43. Vachon, M.L.S. (1993). Emotional problems in palliative medicine: patient, family, and professional. In *Oxford Textbook of Palliative Medicine* (ed. D. Doyle, G.W.C. Hanks, and N. MacDonald), pp. 575–605. Oxford: Oxford University Press.
44. Oberst, M.T. and Scott, D.W. (1988). Postdischarge distress in surgically treated cancer patients and their spouses. *Research in Nursing and Health* **11**, 223–33.
45. Montbriand, M.J. (1994). An overview of alternate therapies chosen by patients with cancer. *Oncology Nursing forum* **21**, 1547–54.
46. American Cancer Society (1990). Unproven methods of cancer treatment: macrobiotic diets for the treatment of cancer. *CA: A Cancer Journal for Clinicians* **39**, 248–51.
47. American Cancer Society (1990). Unproven methods of cancer treatment: psychic surgery. *CA: A Cancer Journal for Clinicians* **40**, 184–8.
48. American Cancer Society (1990). Questionable methods of cancer management: 'nutritional' therapies. *CA: A Cancer Journal for Clinicians* **43**, 309–17.
49. Cassileth, B.R. (1986). Unorthodox cancer medicine. *Cancer Investigation* **4**, 591–8.
50. Davies, B., Reimer, J.C., and Martens, N. (1994). Family functioning and its implications for palliative care. *Journal of Palliative Care* **10**, 29–36.
51. Reimer, J.C., Davies, G., and Martens, N. (1991). Palliative care: the nurse's role in helping families through the transition of 'fading away'. *Cancer Nursing* **14**, 321–7.

52. **Ferrell, B.R., Grant, M., Chan, J., Ahn, C., and Ferrell, B.A.** (1995). The impact of cancer pain education on family caregivers of elderly patients. *Oncology Nursing Forum* **22**, 1211–18.
53. **Rhiner, M., Ferrell, B.R., Shapiro, B., and Dierkes, M.** (1994). The experience of pediatric cancer pain, Part II: management of pain. *Journal of Pediatric Nursing* **9**, 380–7.
54. **Ferrell, B.R. and Griffith, H.** (1994). Cost issues related to pain management: report from the cancer pain panel of the Agency for Health Care Policy and Research. *Journal of Pain and Symptom Management* **9**, 221–34.
55. **Ferrell, B.R.** (1995). How patients and families pay the price. *Proceedings of the Bristol Pain Symposium*, Johns Hopkins University, IASP Press.
56. **Leiber, L.** (1979). The communication of affection between cancer patients and their spouse. *Pyschomatic Medicine* **38**, 379–81.
57. **MacElveen-Hoehn, P. and McCorkle, R.** (1985). Understanding sexuality in progressive cancer. *Seminars in Oncology Nursing* **1**, 56–62.
58. **Vachon, M.L.S.** (1985). Psychotherapy and the person with cancer: one nurse's experience. *Oncology Nursing Forum* **12**, 33–40.

12.3 The stress of professional caregivers

Mary L.S. Vachon

Not only do patients and their families suffer distress when confronting terminal illness, but so do those who care for them. The professional who cares and empathizes with patients and their families can experience significant stress in response to working with dying persons as well as in response to the death of particular patients. The stress may come from a variety of sources: within the person himself/herself as a result of previous or current life experiences; because of a particular death experience with a patient/family; feelings of powerlessness or lack of control within the health care system; 'death overload' from too many patients dying too close together; frustration from not being able to give the care one would like to give to patients because of late referral; or from too much investment in patients without sufficient replenishment over too long a time. Stress may result from the work environment in which there are unrealistic expectations of the amount of work that can be accomplished or a lack of resources to carry out the work that needs to be done. In addition, there may be difficulty with communication, turf and territorial battles within the health care system.

Epidemiology of caregiver distress

A review of much of the literature of stress in palliative care over the past quarter century[1] found that many studies reported that staff working in palliative care had either less burnout and stress than other professionals or that they experienced no more stress than other health care professionals working with seriously ill and/or dying persons.

More recent studies confirm that palliative care specialists experience less stress and burnout than their oncology colleagues in the United Kingdom.[2] Palliative care nurses,[3] also experienced lower burnout than expected. When compared with oncology staff in Canada[4] and the United States,[5] the stress of the United Kingdom palliative care staff stands in marked contrast.

The fact that stress in palliative care may be less than that in other specialties does not negate the stress that does occur. The use of drugs, alcohol, and suicidal ideation of hospice medical directors and matrons was identified as an issue of concern.[6] Hospice nurses were more anxious, with associated psychosomatic complaints than hospital nurses, although the latter were more job dissatisfied. High levels of mental ill health were predicted by a lack of social support and involvement in work and high workload.[7] Hospice nurses were found to be higher on the death and dying dimension of the Nursing Stress Scale[8] and were slightly more depressed than medical/surgical or ICU nurses.

That stress may be lower in palliative care than in other specialties may be related to the fact that from the early days of the hospice movement, staff support and team development programmes were felt to be integral to effective palliative care.[1] Current educational programmes also acknowledge these as important issues of concern.[9] However, palliative care programmes developing programmes for stress management must first assess the needs and not just assume that stress will be related primarily to death and bereavement as issues may be related to organizational factors.[10] These issues have been identified previously.[1,11]

This chapter will focus on the personal and organizational variables associated with stress in palliative care in the past decade, identify the manifestations of stress and coping mechanisms, and suggest research questions for the future. The chapter will also integrate findings from caregivers, not necessarily defined as palliative care specialists, but working with dying patients and those receiving palliative treatment and end-of-life care in settings other than hospices and palliative care settings.

Models of occupational stress

Occupational stress may be viewed within the person–environment fit framework.[11,12] The underlying principle of this model is that adaptation is a function of the 'goodness of fit' between the characteristics of the person and the work environment. 'Fit' is the mesh between the needs of the individual and the supplies or resources available within the environment and/or the abilities of the individual and the demands made by the work environment. In part, fit is determined by the extent to which environmental supplies are available to meet individual needs and values; it is also determined by the ability of the person to manage the environment.[13]

In assessing one's own 'goodness of fit' within the work environment, it is important to be able to assess both one's self and the work environment. Individuals need to have an accurate understanding of their personal resources, values, and limitations. They must also be aware of the resources available within the environment to meet their needs and to facilitate their being able to perform in their professional role.[13] Other useful, complementary models of occupational stress include the demand–control[14] and the demand–control–support models of occupational stress.[15] These models state that job stress is caused by work demands and can be diminished by work control[14] and social support (ref. 15 in ref. 16).

A model of occupational stress in health care providers

The author interviewed a multidisciplinary, international sample of close to 600 caregivers caring for the critically ill, dying, and bereaved.[11] In that study, Antonovsky's[17] definition of stress was used. 'Stress is a demand made by the internal or external environment of the organism that upsets its homeostasis, restoration of which depends upon a nonautomatic and not readily available energy-expending action' (p. 72). In the model of stress developed, job stress is seen as being the result of the interaction between the person and the environment. Personal variables that affect one's perception of a situation as stressful or not include demographic variables, social support, personality, previous stressful life events, and the stressful life events one might currently be experiencing. Work stressors derive from the patients and families with whom we work, illnesses, one's occupational role, and the work environment.

A more recent study comparing burnout in two large samples of physicians in the United States and the Netherlands[16] found that background variables (sex, age, children, solo practice, academic practice, work hours) affect stress and satisfaction through mediating variables (work control, work–home interference, home support). Stress, satisfaction, and work–home interference have direct effects on burnout.

Personal variables

Demographic variables

Age

Younger caregivers have been found to report more stressors, more manifestations of stress, and fewer coping strategies.[11] In a study of Spanish physicians and nurses caring for patients dying at home,[18] professionals under age 35 reported many more problems. The chance of difficulty in relationships with patients decreased by 8 per cent for every increase in 1 year in the age of the professional. Hospital physicians under 40 years of age in Italy had less tolerance for the anxiety of terminally ill patients than did similar general practitioners.[19] As well, younger physicians reported higher degrees of burnout.[20] The later in life a respondent's first exposure to death took place, the more likely it was that he or she would avoid confronting a patient with a terminal prognosis.[21]

In the United Kingdom, being age 55 years or less was identified as an independent risk factor for burnout.[22] Increased job satisfaction was found to be associated with older age,[23] although older staff members may be more sensitive to a gap between their real and ideal work situation and, if such a gap occurs, older caregivers might be more vulnerable to stress reactions.[24]

Older physicians were less likely to believe in the need for aggressive medical interventions in advanced disease, perhaps because of the physicians' identification with the patients and their increased awareness of their own mortality. However, these older physicians had less emotional involvement with their patients allowing for an easier approach to the truth telling dilemma and potentially protecting the physicians from their patient's anxiety.[19]

Gender

At Memorial Sloan-Kettering Cancer Center (MSKCC),[5] female oncology house staff and nurses had the highest level of emotional exhaustion and psychological distress on the Maslach Burnout Scale[25] when staff physicians, house staff, and nurses were compared. Of all the groups, the female house staff showed the greatest sense of demoralization and the least sense of accomplishment within this highly stressed group. It was speculated that because of smaller numbers, females experienced less support from male colleagues.

In Italy,[19] female physicians reported somewhat more difficulty in dealing with the anxiety of a terminally ill patient, while in Spain[18] women were four times more likely to report difficulties in relationships with dying patients. When age was taken into account, the role of sex receded and the relative risk of women dropped to 2.54. The women's difficulty, in part, came from their being more inclined to disclose the diagnosis. The authors hypothesize it may be related to cultural and psychological factors, especially the fact that women show more sensitivity to the psychosocial aspects of death. In addition, women who were more fearful of death have shown a greater willingness to disclose the diagnosis.[26]

In a large study of almost 2000 British family practitioners,[27] male physicians had higher anxiety scores than the norms and had less job satisfaction and drank more alcohol than their female counterparts. Dealing with death and dying was not a major source of stress; however, it was associated with excess alcohol use, especially for female physicians.

Female physicians have been found to report greater job satisfaction and greater well-being than matched controls.[27] The latter finding was replicated in the more recent Physician Worklife Study ($N = 5704$).[28] Women were more likely than their male colleagues to report satisfaction with their specialty and with patient and colleague relationships, but less likely to be satisfied with autonomy, relationships with community, pay, and resources. Female physicians were also more likely to report less work control than their male counterparts regarding day-to-day aspects of practice, including volume of patient load. In addition, they were less well paid. There is some evidence that female physicians may be more at risk of mental health problems.[29] In The Physician Worklife study,[28] women were 1.6 times more likely to report burnout than men. The odds increased by 12–15 per cent for each additional 5 h worked per week over 40 h. Lack of workplace control predicted burnout in women, but not in men (from ref. 30).

McMurray et al.[28] hypothesize that women physicians may be more at risk of burnout because of the implicitly different gender-related work expectations that come from a variety of important sources, such as patients, physician colleagues, administrators, or non-physician co-workers. In effect, the extra stress arises from the greater time and effort being expected of them to communicate with patients and address psychosocial and health maintenance issues, rather than or in addition to the issues related to family–work conflicts.

Being married and having more children was associated with better job satisfaction in a Swedish Study.[23] Being single was an independent risk factor for burnout in the study of consultants in the United Kingdom.[22]

Dickinson and Tournier[31] surveyed male and female physicians, from five geographically distributed medical schools in the United States, about their attitude towards terminally ill patients and their families. The physicians attended a school where there was a full-term course on death and dying. They were surveyed soon after they graduated from medical school in the mid-1970s and a decade later. Over the first decade of medical practice, 'More women than men became as comfortable with dying patients as with other patients, thought of death less, found it less difficult to relate to the family of the dying patient, found it more difficult to tell a patient directly that he/she was dying, were more depressed over the death of a patient when there was nothing to be done to save him/her, and felt that dying patients were more often referred in order to avoid dealing with their terminal condition' (pp. 21–2).

Personality

Motivation

Motivation is comprised of both conscious and unconscious elements. Job stress may result when there is a discrepancy between the individual's motivation for seeking a particular job and the supplies for meeting that need existing within the job environment. Pines[32] suggests that unconscious images from childhood influence one's career decisions. People choose an occupation that enables them to replicate significant childhood experiences, gratify needs that were ungratified in their childhoods, and actualize occupational dreams and professional expectations passed on to them by their familial heritage. Given that the choice of a career involves such significant issues, caregivers enter their careers with very high hopes and expectations, high ego involvement, and passion. If one is successful in one's career, then one derives a sense of existential significance and partially heals one's childhood wounds. When one feels that one has failed to do the work the way it 'should' be done, or when work does not give one's life a sense of meaning, then individuals burn out. A lack of existential significance is the hallmark of burnout (ref. 32, from ref. 30).

Finding healthy ways of maintaining a strong sense of self is necessary for effective helping as a professional.[33] Self-psychology suggests that many helpers were sensitive and alert children who learned quickly to adapt to the needs of their parents.[34,35] 'Their own needs, programs, blueprint, or scripts were not allowed to develop. The ultimate outcome of such situations is a predisposition for diminished self-esteem and repeated attempts as adults to find the 'ideal parent' in their own children or partners' (ref. 33, pp. 620–1)—or patients. The emotionally vulnerable professional, craving admiration and appreciation may develop an ever increasing workload of patients and become dependent on the need to be needed that feeds the professional's sense of self-worth. Those who choose medicine have been found to have strong obsessive–compulsive personality traits that lead them to 'choose a career in which long hours of study, heavy responsibility and devotion to work are required. In fact, the more these traits are exaggerated the more outstanding a student may be' (ref. 36, p. 647) (from ref. 30).

Personal value systems The initial hospice movement had significant spiritual underpinning and organized religions, particularly Christianity, gave impetus to the movement.[1,37] Leaders in the British hospice movement, including Drs Cicely Saunders, Derek Doyle, and Sheila Cassidy, have written of the strong spiritual elements that underpin their work. They have a 'single-minded spiritual devotion to what they are doing' (ref. 37, p. 1366).

Spiritual and religious belief systems have been found to be helpful in oncology and palliative care. Compared with oncology nurses, hospice nurses reported a greater sense of personal spirituality, more frequent spiritual caregiving, and more positive perspectives regarding spiritual caregiving. Hospice nurses were also older and more experienced in nursing than oncology nurses. Hospice may attract nurses who have an existing sensitivity to personal spirituality, or the nature of the work might increase the nurse's spiritual sensitivity. It is also possible that more 'seasoned' nurses may have both personal and professional factors that have led to more spiritual caregiving. Hospice nurses also reported receiving stronger employer support for spiritual caregiving than did those in oncology.[38]

In the MSKCC study, nurses were more religious than other groups. Oncologists were more religious than fellows. Those quite a bit too extremely religious had significantly lower scores on diminished empathy or depersonalization and lower emotional exhaustion on the Maslach Burnout scale.[5,25,39]

Personality and coping style Hospice nurses have been found to have low death anxiety and to exhibit greater comfort in caring for the terminally ill, in contrast to hospital nurses.[40] Compared with emergency nurses, hospice nurses had lower death anxiety and were more likely to recall both good and difficult experiences related to patient care.[41] A relationship has been found between physician's fear of death and their attitudes towards informing terminally ill patients. Physicians who believe that patients 'should never be made aware that they are dying are likely to have a greater fear of their own death, to avoid references to their own death, and to express more rigid attitudes towards the problems surrounding terminal patients' (ref. 21, p. 530).

de Hennezel[42] notes that physicians have been trained to feel in control of situations through therapeutic manoeuvres to alleviate symptoms or disease. They have been taught not to get involved with patients and to keep their distance, yet palliative care requires involvement and the physicians involved with palliative care patients may be unable to control the very feelings they have been taught to control. This may engender feelings of helplessness and vulnerability. Teaching physicians will not 'help them to live with this tension; this will come only when they accept their vulnerability and are able to express and share it without fear of being judged' (ref. 43, p. 1725). David Roy, the Editor of *Journal of Palliative Care*, a mathematician, theologian, and ethicist, wrote very poignantly of his vulnerability.[44] In a final telephone call with a dying friend and colleague, who called to say goodbye, 'I spoke to her as fast as I could so that I could get the words out before I choked on them … I just barely closed with "Till soon, soon again, my dear one. Till soon, soon again." Before tears drowned my words and choked me … These last words were promises of time and words of hope. They could not possibly have had their unique source in me; certainly not in me alone. I was always too intellectually precious, too lacking in the spiritual courage and daring needed to say the great powerful words of hope that come before the first line and last long after the last line of any poetic words' (p. 228).

The Hardy Personality is effective in combating work stress.[45,46] The Hardy Personality involves a sense of commitment (as opposed to alienation) to oneself and the various areas in one's life, including work, which reflects the hardy person's curiosity about and a sense of meaningfulness of life; control (as opposed to powerlessness), reflecting the belief that one has the power to influence the course of events; and challenge (as opposed to threat), epitomizing the expectation that it is normal for life to change and for development to be stimulated. Hardiness is associated with fewer mental and physical symptoms of stress. 'Hardiness is said to lead to a perception, interpretation, and handling of stressful events that prevents excessive activation of arousal and therefore results in fewer symptoms of stress' (ref. 47, p. 652).

Hardiness has been found to be associated with decreased burnout in Greek oncology nurses[48] and was associated with less demoralization in the MSKCC study.[5] Hardy personality traits were related to a sense of accomplishment and men were found to have a greater sense of accomplishment than women. House staff and nurses had less of a sense of accomplishment than oncologists.[5]

The sense of control over things that happen in life and in the work environment was found to protect nurses from emotional exhaustion, depersonalization, and a lack of personal accomplishment on the Maslach Burnout Scale.[25,39] Nurses who experienced higher degrees of burnout reported a lack of a sense of control over external events.[48]

Although a Hardy Personality is effective in combating stress,[5,48] problems can follow if both the patient and caregiver have a strong need to control the current situation and are working at cross purposes or get into rivalry. Self-care advice for patients exhorts them to adopt a 'take-charge' attitude.[49] Caregivers may be caught in an ambiguous role-balancing their own previously unchallenged role as an authority figure with the current ethical recognition of the increased role of the patient in decision-making.[50] Barnard et al.[51] studied patients, families, and caregivers through the palliative care experience in Quebec and Pennsylvania. They give examples of power struggles between the patient and members of the palliative care team regarding treatment options. It may be helpful to caregivers in these situations to understand their own need for control and to try to work towards shared control and decision-making.

Shapiro et al.[52] wrote 'The focus of control efforts must go beyond goals of personal competence, autonomous self-identity, and positive ego development. Such control efforts should also be directed toward generativity, compassionate service for the healing of others, and interpersonal and collective well being' (refs in original) (p. 1224).

In understanding the need for control in either one's self or another, it is helpful to recognize that believing that one is in control can, in certain instances, augment feelings of threat.[53,54] Antonovsky contrasts coherence with control.[17] Coherence emphasizes the importance of predictability in both internal and external environments, coupled with the likelihood of things working out as well as can be expected. He distinguishes between a sense of coherence and control; coherence implies that one can shape one's destiny, not that one is in control.

A sense of coherence is partly personality-related and partly developed through experience. It refers in particular to personal resourcefulness. Those with a broad repertoire and good flexibility are better able to adjust to most life challenges than those with poor repertoires.[55] '(T)he sense of coherence (SOC) construct is a generalized orientation toward the world which perceives it, on a continuum, as comprehensible, manageable, and meaningful'.[56] A study of social workers[57] found that health social workers with a strong sense of coherence experienced less burnout than those with a weak sense of coherence. The manageability component of the sense of coherence was found to predict emotional exhaustion on the burnout scale.

Social support

'Although social support has many facets, a core dimension of it involves participating in a network of caring and reciprocal relationships with others and creating a sense of belonging and a reason for living that transcends one's individual self' (ref. 59, p. 22). Dr Dean Ornish found that lifestyle changes reversed coronary artery disease without drugs or surgery. He stated that the most important intervention of the study was not the finding that dietary and lifestyle changes caused significant improvements in health and well-being, but '. . . the healing power of love and intimacy, and the emotional and spiritual transformation that often result from these' (ref. 60, p. 2, from ref. 61).

Personal support systems

Female physicians with young children were 40 per cent less likely to burnout when they had the support of colleagues, spouses, or significant others for balancing work and home issues.[28]

A professional caregiver's social support system may change over time. While initially family members and friends may be useful in helping the neophyte practitioner to debrief, over time, caregivers turn more to colleagues who are better able to understand the specific stressors to which one is exposed.[61–63]

When Greek nurses working with dying children in oncology and critical care were compared[64] it was found that when the nurses were first hired they turned to family members and/or friends to discuss their work experiences and share their feelings. They learned quickly, however, that their friends and relatives found it difficult to listen to these accounts. In addition, as caregivers grow and mature, so too will the members of his/her support system. They may no longer want to play the support role.[63,65]

The role of family and friends in supporting caregivers has been found to be important but to have limits.[11] When caregivers working in HIV and oncology were compared, it was found that one-third of staff without long-term emotional relationships felt that their work kept them from being involved in such relationships. Most subjects reported spending a considerable amount of time discussing their work with partners. Thirty-nine per cent reported that their partners complained regularly about their commitment to work and one-quarter reported that their relationship had suffered as a result of their work in oncology or HIV. While friends and family of HIV staff were more supportive of their working in the field, friends and family of oncology staff were more supportive of their actual work (ref. 66, from ref. 58, 61).

Social support at work

Support from colleagues has been found to be very important for dealing with work-related stress.[11] High levels of mental ill health in hospice nurses were predicted by a lack of social support.[7] A comparison of hospice and oncology nurses showed that hospice nurses had significantly lower burnout scores than oncology nurses caring for the terminally ill on hospital-based oncology units.[24] The hospice nurses perceived a greater opportunity to express work-related feelings and to discuss problems in the workplace. A positive relationship was noted between perceived social support at work and lower burnout scores. Sixty-seven per cent of palliative care nurses used 'talking things over with a colleague' as a coping mechanism compared with 18 per cent who talked with people at home.[62]

When oncologists, house staff, and nurses were compared, nurses had the lowest scores on the Personal Accomplishment scale of the Maslach Burnout Inventory.[25,39] It was questioned whether this was because they were more overwhelmed by the enormity of the tasks of patient care or that they were less well supported by the hospital structure to meet patient needs, especially psychological needs.[5]

A lack of support and higher degrees of burnout in female physicians may well play as crucial a role as work and family issues in leading female physicians to experience difficulty with 'fit' in particular settings leading possibly to the fact that female physicians are likely to work fewer hours, retire earlier, and be inactive during part of their medical career.[28]

Stressful life events

Stressful life events may serve as a source of strength as well as a stressor. Many female physicians reported that they had chosen to enter medicine because of having had a sister with a chronic illness.[11] At other times, unresolved previous stressful life events such as the death of a parent, a history of sexual abuse, or family alcoholism might leave the caregiver vulnerable to stress reactions in one's professional practice. Selwyn[67] wrote powerfully of the burnout he experienced in his care of persons with AIDS and its relationship to his unresolved grief for his father who suicided when he was a young child.

> Once I became aware that I had never come to terms with the loss of my father, I began the work of grieving both for my father, which I had never done and for all my patients who had died. After going through this process, I found that I had become better able to be with my patients in their pain. To support them without feeling the blind compulsion to rescue them from something from which they could not be rescued, and to accompany them as they approached death without somehow feeling that I had somehow betrayed their trust (ref. 67, p. 125).

Previous experience with death may be a motivator in choosing to work in palliative care.[62] Other studies have shown a more negative impact of previous death experiences, particularly if the grief is unresolved. Recent personal bereavement and unresolved grief from deaths prior to coming into a children's hospice were associated with high distress[68] on the General Health Questionnaire.[69] Females tend to assume more of the responsibility for family life. In the MMSKC study,[5] demoralization on the burnout scale was associated with having more family, social, and residence problems; this was most common in the female house staff. It was hypothesized this was because they were assuming more responsibility for unwell family members and had greater stressors as daughters and mothers than their male counterparts.

Occupational stressors and manifestations of stress

Previous research has shown that the occupational stressors in hospice derive from the work environment (48 per cent), one's occupational role (29 per cent), patients and families (17 per cent) and illness related variables (7 per cent).[11]

More recent research has explored the interaction amongst occupational variables, personal variables and assessed the ways in which they interact, resulting in manifestations of stress, particularly burnout. In the Ramirez et al.[2] study of United Kingdom oncologists and palliative care specialists, *Job characteristics* associated with burnout included 'being overloaded and its effect on home life,' 'dealing with patients suffering,' and low levels of satisfaction from 'not having adequate resources to perform one's role.' Depersonalization was associated with 'being overloaded' and 'dealing with patients' suffering' as well as low levels of satisfaction from 'dealing well with patients and relatives.' Being a clinical oncologist, as compared with a medical oncologist or palliative care physician, and working part-time, were independent risk factors for depersonalization. 'Low Personal accomplishment was associated with stress from "being involved with treatment toxicity and errors" and low levels of satisfaction from "dealing well with patients and relatives" and from "having professional status and esteem" ' (ref. 2, p. 1268).

In a study comparing burnout in two large samples of physicians in the United States ($N = 1824$) and the Netherlands ($N = 1435$),[16] a model of burnout was tested. It was found that background variables (sex, age, children, solo practice, academic practice, work hours) affect stress and satisfaction through mediating variables (work control, work–home interference, home support). Stress, satisfaction, and work–home interference have direct effects on burnout. In that study the proportion of burnout explained is high: 50 per cent in the United States sample and 51 per cent for the Dutch. Older physicians in the Unite States felt they had more control than did younger physicians. This finding was not as marked in the Netherlands. The study found an adverse impact of academic practice on work control and work–home interference in the United States. There was a strong association between work hours and work–home interference in both countries. This was important given that work–home interference had a direct impact on burnout. There was a substantial benefit of physician work control on minimizing stress and increasing satisfaction in both countries, and there were remarkable benefits of home support on stress reduction in the United States.

> . . . (F)or both countries, work control was correlated with job stress and satisfaction, whereas work–home interference was associated with work hours, children, stress, (dis)satisfaction and burnout. Thus, the basic predictors of burnout are concordant across these two industrialized nations . . . Male U.S. physicians described significantly more work control, than female U.S. physicians, a sex difference not seen in the Netherlands (ref. 2, pp. 172–3).

In a study comparing caregivers in oncology and AIDS work, nurses reported higher levels of somatic symptoms. It was unclear whether their somatic symptoms were due to their demographic characteristics (being younger and female) or whether they were due to work characteristics. Nurses have much more direct involvement in the care of seriously ill people and cannot walk away and perform other duties as doctors can.[70]

Payne[3] surveyed 89 female nurses from nine hospices in the United Kingdom and found that while the level of burnout was generally low, in multiple regression analyses, 'death and dying', 'conflict with staff', 'accepting responsibility', and higher nursing grade contributed to emotional exhaustion. 'Conflict with staff', 'inadequate preparation', 'escape', and reduced 'planful problem-solving' contributed to depersonalization. 'Inadequate preparation', 'escape', reduced 'positive reappraisal', and fewer professional qualifications contributed to lower levels of personal accomplishment. Overall, stressors made the greatest contribution to burnout and demographic factors contributed the least (ref. 3, from ref. 30).

A study of a newly opened palliative care unit in the Netherlands[10] found most stress was attributed to organizational factors, related to management issues but also to lack of institutional support. Teamwork contributed to stress within the interdisciplinary team. Direct patient care activities also had an impact on stress through a heavy work-load of complex care, a shortage of staff, and an experienced lack of competence.

Environmental stressors

Difficulty with others in the system From the early days of hospice, caregivers have reported problems with timely referrals[11] and these issues continue with the development of the specialty of palliative care. Field[71] surveyed general practitioners in the United Kingdom working with dying patients and found that while relationships between the GPs and the district nurses with whom they work are good, the relationships with hospitals were generally 'satisfactory, but rarely more than that, and there were negative comments about the provision of information from hospitals to both patients and to GPs' (ref. 71, p. 1114). He noted that an issue of contemporary relevance was the tension over the role of hospice and specialist terminal-care services. While GPs find it helpful to be able to call on specialist care there is the concern that it might lead to the GP and team losing control of patient care. In addition, there is conflict between the district nurses and the Macmillan nurses. The GPs feel that they have the best social knowledge of the needs of the patient and family and want to be able to call on experts but not to surrender care to experts. They are not pleased with the fact that they feel that some hospices are not willing to involve the GP and team as partners but only wanted to deliver care on their terms. There are problems when there is conflict between the GPs who feel they know the patient/family unit better and the palliative care specialists who have more knowledge about symptom relief. The GPs also expressed concern that the involvement of specialist providers of palliative care can have detrimental consequences for the generalist expertise of GPs (and community nurses) by de-skilling them.

A more recent study[72] in Wales showed significant enthusiasm amongst consultant physicians, 94 per cent of whom would consider referring patients with non-malignant disease to a specialist palliative care service. The physicians thought that a system of shared care and responsibility would be most appropriate. This was seen as a means of addressing concerns regarding the lack of disease-specific expertise within the palliative care team.

In Spain, problems with the system also exist.[18] Half of physicians and 60 per cent of nurses surveyed reported that caring for terminally ill patients at home made them feel frustrated. 'Spontaneous comments pointed to the "system" as the main cause of frustration; frequently mentioned issues were bureaucracy (particularly with regard to access to narcotic analgesics), and the isolation of primary health care professionals, especially in rural areas' (ref. 18, pp. 119–20). Women, younger caregivers and those who had attended fewer patients in the past year were more likely to report feelings of frustration.

In the United States, the problem continues with difficulty with timely referral.[73] Given the documented deficiencies in end-of life care,[74] it is to be hoped that the philosophy of palliative care could be incorporated into end-of-life care for increasing numbers of people. However, Byock[75] writes of the tensions between the 'loyalists' who have generally been associated with the hospice movement and the 'progressives' who 'tend to be caring, committed clinicians and administrators, often based in hospitals, nursing homes, or home health, who have awakened to the need to improve care for the dying in their own systems and are earnestly trying to do just that' (pp. 155–6).

Rivalries are encountered as programmes try to determine with which agencies, if any, they will have preferred partner arrangements. Other settings have developed palliative care programmes in an apparent move to avoid referral to hospices, and to gain access to funding that might be made available for dying persons.[58] In addition, there are financial barriers that include reimbursement systems that provide only for the options of cure or certain death.[76,77]

Whedon, an oncology nurse whose practice changed to pain and symptom management observed, 'Patients without a care provider; unwilling to forego beneficial palliative chemotherapy, radiation, or surgery; or with a prognosis that was not absolutely certain to be six months or less, were caught in the middle. This part of the path felt treacherous; we had no trail markers, no compass, and darkness was about to fall' (ref. 77, p. 27). Some insurance companies are, however, reimbursing concurrent palliative cancer treatments and home hospice care.[78]

The Medicare Hospice Benefit limits service to patients with a life expectancy of 6 months or less, if the disease runs its normal course. Patients who elect to use this benefit must be willing to forgo further active treatment.[73] Predicting this 6-month life expectancy causes concern for physicians and hospice programme administrators who fear accusations of fraud, abuse, and payment denials.[77,79] Recent studies have also shown the limitations of physicians' ability to predict survival.[80,81]

Problems in the team In studies of caregivers to the critically ill and dying, organizational factors, such as personality issues and team conflict, were more commonly reported stressors than were problems in dealing with patients and families and issues related to death and dying.[11] This finding has recently been replicated in a new palliative care programme[10] and in a group of oncology nurses[82] in which Organizational Factors and Co-worker stress was rated as the most frequent and most intense stress cluster.

In a Finnish study[83] of the ethical dilemmas confronting patients, physicians, and nurses in the context of incurable cancer, it was found that the doctors and nurses were not communicating with each other and there was a lack of cooperation between the two groups in decision-making situations. Doctors talked primarily with one another and with patients. The nurses, as well as some of the physicians, said that it would be important to exchange views and opinions on treatments. In a group of palliative care physicians, good relationships with staff were a major source of job satisfaction; however, encountering problems in relationships with nurses was the only aspect of work in which they had more difficulties than their colleagues in other specialties.[29] Field[71] also noted communication issues amongst general practitioners, nurses, and social workers whose roles tended to be coordinated by the district nurse.

The lack of participation in planning and decision-making that may develop out of poor staff relationships has been associated with depression and increased stress in palliative care staff.[7,84,85]

Rivalry and anger often surface in team relationships. Many teams have difficulty dealing directly with anger and may use a variety of obstructive behaviours. These may involve careerism and negative rivalry—by concentrating on personal achievement and advancement, some team members' competitive instincts and energies may be channelled into rivalry among colleagues rather than on teamwork and effective patient care. Illusions of grandeur and interpersonal tugs of war occur in some teams where actual collaboration is low and mutual suspicion and antagonism is high. 'Many team members engage in tugs-of-war, have territorial disputes, and play one-upmanship, sabotage one another's programs, cut one another's throats, while all the time proclaiming what a great team they are'.[86] Lack of cooperation and discipline occurs when teams have coordination without cooperation; they will go only so far. If team members are ordered about without consultation or participation, they will not give their best effort and will fail.[58,87]

Role stressors

Role overload

When palliative care specialists were compared with clinical and radiation oncologists, problems with 'feeling overloaded and its effects on home life' were found to be significantly greater for the medical and clinical oncologists than for the palliative care specialists.[2]

Physicians in one study acknowledged that at least some of their professional work overload was self-induced. One physician said, 'Lots of us feeling overloaded and overworked create it ourselves. We start dancing to a tune that you're called to play by yourself.' Nevertheless, there is a real problem with the work overload that can occur when professionals try to juggle patient care, research, and publication while preserving some time for self and family.[11] As has been noted above, stress, satisfaction, and work–home interference have a direct effect on burnout.[16]

Role strain

Role strain involves having difficulty performing various aspects of one's professional role and may involve difficulty in decision-making.[11] Oncologists reported significantly more difficulty with two elements of role strain 'dealing with patients' suffering' and 'being involved with treatment toxicity and errors' than did palliative care specialists.[2] Seale and Cartwright[88] found 43 per cent of GP respondents needed more time to give to dying patients, around one-third had trouble coping with their own emotional responses to dying patients, and these GPs seemed most likely to have difficulty communicating with patients who were dying and their relatives.

Staff in a children's hospice were studied in the early years of the programme[89] as well as more recently.[90] Whereas initially staff felt a sense of impotence when they were unable to relieve the perceived needs or distress of patients, they now have concerns about the increasing use of life support equipment for the children, and the balance between quality of life and technical support.[58] Role strain has also been reported by nurses whose work makes them feel physically unsafe. This exposure included making visits to deserted country homes in the middle of snowstorms without access to cell phones or other ways of communicating if the nurse was in trouble; visiting in unsafe areas of the community, where the nurses do not feel safe during the day, and particularly at night; and visiting in homes where the family dynamics are such that nurses do not feel physically safe. When there are no organizational policies about how to handle these situations, staff can feel quite stressed.[58]

Role strain in palliative care can also evolve from constant exposure to the terminally ill and the need to be open to developing intimate relationships with dying persons and their families. Barnard et al.[51] state that 'palliative care is whole-person care not only in the sense that the whole person of the patient (body, mind, spirit) is the object of care, but also in that the whole person of the caregiver is involved. Palliative care is, par excellence, care that is given through the medium of a human relationship' (p. 5). He notes that the education for palliative care involves the art of building and sustaining relationships and in using the self as a primary instrument for diagnosis and treatment. This involves psychological risk taking that may be unique in the health field.

Earlier, Barnard[91] discussed the tension between the promise of intimacy and the fear of our own undoing in the care of the terminally ill. He notes the need to give full weight to both the promise and the fear of intimacy in palliative care and refers to palliative care as challenging caregivers to leap into the confrontation with the forces of chaos and disintegration. 'We live in the tension between the promise of intimacy and the fear of our own undoing. Surprised by intimacy, we are exhilarated and lifted beyond ourselves, as if we have not only made contact with another person but also with another dimension of living. At the same time we are brought face to face with forces of chaos and destructiveness, internal as well as external, and we fear that we ourselves shall be destroyed' (p. 26). These feelings can lead to significant role strain.

Issues of power and control

As has been indicated above, useful models of occupational stress involve demand–control[14] and demand–control–support.[15] Current research suggests that restructuring high-demand, low-control jobs may enhance productivity and reduce disability costs.[92] Recent practices in hospice led by fiscal constraints have raised increasing concern. Nurses are sometimes expected to perform procedures in the community for which they have not been prepared and for which no supervision is provided. When people are expected to assume responsibility with inadequate training, they have difficulty functioning.[23,62,93]

Nurses report being in situations both in the hospital and in the community where they feel responsible for alleviating the pain of a palliative care patient, yet do not have a physician willing to order the medication they feel will be sufficient to control pain. In addition, with the earlier discharge of sicker patients, nurses with limited experience may be expected to care for seriously ill palliative care patients in their home, without access to physicians skilled in effective palliative care and symptom management.[94] MacDonald[95] testified before a Senate Subcommittee on End of Life Care in Canada that in a study of Quebec oncologists and palliative care physicians, their opinion was that the big problem in managing cancer pain was the reluctance on the part of physicians to use opioids and the misunderstanding of patients about the use of pain.

Stressors versus rewards in palliative care

Although palliative care can be stressful, some authors have also tried to measure its rewards. Some of the satisfactions that may be received from working in palliative care include:

- the care of the dying is important, rewarding and satisfying; GPs saw themselves as part of a team of carers. They derived satisfaction from the fact that the patient and family were both recipients of care;[71]
- GPs see themselves as part of a team of largely equal carers;[71]
- valuing each individual; experiencing the reciprocity of giving and receiving in relationships; having a sense of interconnectedness and of mutual nurturing; being close to patients and sharing a part of one's self; having the chance to make a difference in people's lives;[96]
- helping patients achieve optimum health by enabling them to do all they are capable of doing; being able to give patients options, recognizing that patients are the directors of their own decision-making; being able to personalize the hospital environment so that patients can feel more at home;[96]
- experiencing positive feedback from patients and families; effectively relating with and communicating with patients and families;[97]
- witnessing the smooth termination of life; initiating innovative, effective intervention for the patients, involving the right decisions at the right times; and peace for the patient;[97]
- being able to provide families with good memories in the midst of difficult times;[97]
- helping patients to find meaning in suffering;[98]
- experiencing positive relationships and support from colleagues;[97,99]
- dealing well with patients and relatives;[2]
- having professional status and esteem, deriving intellectual satisfaction, and having adequate resources to perform one's role[2,99] (adapted from refs 30, 58).

Manifestations

Table 1 shows a number of the manifestations of job stress. This section will focus primarily on the psychological signs of stress. Peabody[100] stated 'the secret of the care of the patient is in caring for the patient' (ref. 43, p. 1720). Palliative care encourages such caring and resulting closeness to the patient. Some of the difficulties associated with the care of dying persons may in part be due to the close connections palliative care staff often develop with their patients. Whereas, traditionally, professionals have been taught to

Table 1 Signs of stress

Physical symptoms
Behavioural
Staff conflict
Job–home interaction
Errors in judgement
Psychological
Depression, grief, and guilt
Anger, irritability, and frustration
Feelings of helplessness and insecurity
Overinvestment and overinvolvement
Anxiety and difficulty with decision making[11,101]

maintain a boundary between themselves and their clients, in palliative care very close relationships can and do develop.[102] 'The caring person listens, responds, and relates to the patient as a unique individual, attempting to understand the other's needs and feelings (refs 103, 104 in ref. 43). Empathic communication demands good listening and may result in the palliative care worker going 'beyond the dimensions of listening to emotional realms that are neither easy nor comfortable'.[105] The closeness and exposure to repeated difficult illness experiences and deaths may lead to the experience of 'Secondary Traumatic Stress' (STS) or compassion stress. Secondary Traumatic Stress is defined as 'the natural consequent behaviours and emotions resulting from knowing about a traumatizing event experienced by a significant other—the stress resulting from helping or wanting to help a traumatized or suffering person' (ref. 106, p. 7). Secondary Traumatic Stress Disorder is a more severe manifestation of STS and 'is a syndrome of symptoms nearly identical to PTSD (Post Traumatic Stress Disorder), except that exposure to knowledge about a traumatizing event experienced by a significant other is associated with the set of STSD symptoms, and PTSD symptoms are directly connected to the sufferer, the person experiencing the primary traumatic stress' (ref. 106, p. 8). Compassion fatigue is identical to STSD and is the equivalent of PTSD[106] (from refs 30, 58). Garfield et al.[107] writes of the compassion fatigue that exists amongst AIDS/HIV caregivers. In contrast to caregivers heading for burnout who unconsciously begin to wall off more and more strong feelings associated with their work, those with compassion fatigue are able to monitor their decrease in empathy and feeling and remain emotionally accessible. However, they have greater difficulty in processing their emotions, are anxiety-ridden or distressed, have images that intrude on their days and nights and painful memories that flood their world outside the caregiving arena (from refs 30, 58).

Burnout

Over the past 20 years, many aspects of medical practice have changed: autonomy is declining, the status of physicians has diminished, and work pressures are increasing. Burnout is an unintended and adverse result of such changes. In the Netherlands, physician disability insurance premiums have risen from 20 per cent to 30 per cent owing to an increasing incidence of burnout and stress-related complaints (ref. 108 in ref. 16). Table 2 shows the signs and symptoms of burnout.

Brenninkmeyer et al.[110] differentiated burnout from depression. Given that the clinical picture of depression seems to reflect a general sense of self-defeat, they hypothesized that individuals high in burnout and low in superiority (how individuals see themselves in comparison to others) would experience depressive symptoms. Depressive symptomatology was highest among individuals high in burnout who experienced a decline in superiority. 'Depression was more strongly related to superiority than emotional exhaustion and depersonalization. In fact, emotional exhaustion, which constitutes the core symptom of burnout, did not have a significant association with superiority' (p. 879).

They concluded 'reduced sense of superiority and a perceived loss of status are more characteristic of depressed individuals than for individuals who are burnt-out. It seems that burnt-out individuals are still "in the battle" for obtaining status and consider themselves as potential winners, while depressed individuals have given up' (p. 879).

Table 2 Signs and symptoms of burnout

Fatigue
Physical and emotional exhaustion
Headaches
Gastrointestinal disturbances
Weight loss
Sleeplessness
Depression
Boredom
Frustration
Low morale
Job turnover
Impaired job performance (decreased empathy, increased absenteeism)[101]
Deterioration in the physician–patient relationship and a decrease in the quantity and quality of care[16]
Burned out physicians are less satisfied, more likely to want to reduce their time seeing patients, more likely to order tests or procedures, and more interested in early retirement than other physicians[109]
An inability to leave work (working longer hours), absenteeism, lower job satisfaction, or a decreased sense of personal accomplishment[16]

Table 3 shows a comparison of professionals with high scores on the three aspects of the Maslach Burnout Inventory[39] across a number of studies.

The generally higher rates in Ontario oncologists[4] is perhaps due to the difficulty they had been experiencing with increasing workloads and cuts to the health care system being experienced at the time of the study.

Many of the variables associated with burnout have been identified above. Sources of burnout can be seen in Table 4.

In a study of 440 nurses in the US,[112] subjects with greater hardiness[45,46] reported less burnout. The lowest burnout scores were found in the nurses with greater hardiness that used direct-active coping techniques (changing the source, confronting the source, finding positive aspects in the situation). The findings suggest that both hardiness and direct-active coping techniques can be used independently or in concert to reduce burnout.

Multiple grief and loss

Mount[113] has reflected on the losses associated with working in oncology and notes that these losses become an integrated part of one's professional life. 'Moreover, our losses do not occur in a vacuum. They interact with, modify, and often augment the other stressors in our personal and professional lives. Our reaction to loss may be repressed, only to surface later, associated perhaps with some other unrelated event' (p. 1127).

Papadatou[114] has defined the losses in oncology nursing as follows:

- loss of a close relationship with a particular patient;
- loss due to the professional's identification with the pain of family members;
- loss of one's unmet goals and expectations;
- losses related to one's personal system of beliefs and assumptions about life;
- past unresolved losses or anticipated future losses;
- the death of self.

Constant exposure to death and loss may leave caregivers with grief overload and considerable distress. However, participating in the death of some patients has been found to result in some nurses having intense positive responses that promote professional development.[115]

Table 3 Burnout

Professional group	Emotional exhaustion (%)	Depersonalization/ diminished empathy (%)	Low personal accomplishment (%)
UK Palliative Care Specialists (*N* = 126)[29]	23	13	25
UK Medical Oncologists (*N* = 60)[2]	25	15	34
UK Clinical Oncologists (*N* = 207)[2]	38	31	38
Ontario Oncologists (*N* = 122)[4]	53.3	22.1	48.4
Ontario Allied Health Professionals (*N* = 278)[4]	37.1	4.3	54
US AIDS, General medical, oncology, and ICU nurses (*N* = 237)[111]	23.8	7	34.6
UK AIDS doctors and nurses (*N* = 70)	21.7	7.7	33
UK Oncology doctors and nurses (*N* = 41)[70]	24.7	5.8	38.1

Table 4 Causes of and factors associated with burnout in health staff

Giving care to terminal patients
Continuous contact with human suffering
Demanding and difficult patients and family members
Lack of preparation for dealing with medical and spiritual problems
Working in new or unknown services
Inadequate working conditions—medical, personal, or insufficient time
Facing emergency situations and work overload in the daily routine
Tension and lack of organization in team work
Need to develop services to complement medical care
Lack of recognition of or indifference to effort from patients, superiors, and colleagues (ref. 114, p. 409, references in original)
Organizational factors, related to managerial issues and lack of institutional support
Heavy workload of complex care, shortage of staff, experienced lack of competence[10]
Being overloaded and its effect on home life, dealing with patients suffering, and low levels of satisfaction from not having adequate resources to perform one's role[2]
Emotional exhaustion predicted by: being a house officer, having more negative work events, using cigarettes, alcohol, or medication as a way of relaxing, having fewer hardiness traits[5]
Demoralization predicted by: being a woman, being a house officer, having more family, social, and residence problems, using fewer cathartic means of relaxing and using more cigarettes, alcohol, or medication, having fewer hardy personality characteristics and feeling less peer support[6]
Low personal accomplishment associated with being house staff or a nurse. Hardy personality traits were associated with a greater sense of accomplishment

Physicians can also derive a great sense of satisfaction from a death that goes well as can be seen from one of the general practitioner respondents in the Field study[71] '... (I)t's usually that you can see quite clearly that you're giving them something which nobody else can give because it's you they want and you're managing it as well. And the idea is to manage it at home, get the family all sorted out, get the person to the stage where they are quite ready to die and off they go, have a nice pain free death and nobody gets all distressed about it. And you feel like you've really completed a good job, um and if you accomplish that—release somebody's anxiety about death—it's a hell of a kick' (p. 1115).

Nurses have difficulty with grief if they had not been able to help the patient die a good death for whatever reason.[115] When the symptoms of dying patients are not controlled, the nurses feel responsible, and 'wanting' and, if training and experience are lacking, this may well be the case.[94] Staff members often experience difficulty dealing with their feelings of grief and loss at the time of death because of other responsibilities that must be attended to immediately. There is often a strong covert institutional message, as well as peer pressure not to dwell on the loss.[116]

Particularly since the AIDS epidemic, the concept of multiple loss has been increasingly recognized. The concept of multiple loss in AIDS caregivers reflected in part the reality that many caregivers were caring for dying patients, while partners, friends, and members of their social network were dying at the same time.[58]

Chronic compounded grief, defined as cumulative responses to losses over a period of time, has been found to be a powerful factor that contributes to resignations and turnover among oncology nurses and the ability of individual nurses to care for patients effectively. Feldstein and Gemma[116] suggest that what others refer to as burnout is really chronic, compounded grief (from refs 30, 58).

Coping with stress and burnout in palliative care

Coping comprises both behavioural and cognitive strategies aimed at managing the internal and external demands of stressful transactions.[54] These efforts, directed towards mastering, reducing, or tolerating demands, may be problem-focused or emotion-focused. Problem-focused mechanisms target the environment or self for direct intervention, whereas emotion-focused strategies target negative feelings arising from stressful episodes. Rarely will one coping mode be the answer, mostly it is a pattern that expresses a person–situation fit.

Coping can be either adaptive or maladaptive. Adaptive coping is task-oriented or goal-directed and deals with the problem or the affect (feeling) associated with the problem. Adaptive coping is an attempt to maintain an emotional and/or physiological balance called health. Maladaptive coping is more defence-oriented and focused on protection, and using these techniques predominantly can be harmful and can result in psychological or somatic disease. Maladaptive coping may include strategies such as use of drugs and alcohol, social isolation, or overuse of strategies that are normally adaptive.[117,118] Florio et al.[82] compared positive versus negative outcomes of coping strategies using problem-focused versus emotion-focused coping strategies. The coping strategies that were most effective in handling work stress included: *Emotion-focused/positive* (develop a growth perspective, positive reapprasal, affective regulation, and balancing work stress and *Problem-focused/positive* including positive involvement in treatment and co-worker support. Less effective strategies included *Emotion-focused/negative* (withdrawal, apathy, negative coping, catharsis/break room).

Personal coping strategies

A sense of competence, control, and pleasure in one's work

In a large study of caregivers,[11] this was the most common coping mechanism for physicians and the second most common for the group as a whole. When asked what it was that motivated them to be able to continue in their stressful jobs, caregivers would often say 'The bottom line is that I know what I am doing and I am good at it.' Field[71] notes that for most of the GPs he studied the quality of their care of people who were dying encapsulated their ideals of patient care and was seen by themselves and by their patients as a marker of their general standards of patient care.

This sense of competence developed through a series of stages in which caregivers developed their professional skills, set goals for themselves, had frequent tests of their competence, proved their competence in many situations, learned that because they were secure in their own competence that they could share their competence with others, and eventually were able to report being comfortable living with a sense that they were competent in their work situation.

MacLeod[43] interviewed 10 physicians practicing in New Zealand, but trained in other countries, about their care of the dying. The physicians had been in practice from less than 1 year to over 40 years. They felt that their most powerful learning experiences occurred when they found themselves in an intimate and caring situation. The physicians identified 'turning points' that had occurred as many as 20 years ago. Half of the physicians wept recalling these incidents. 'The doctors seemed to lower their defensive barriers, and open themselves to a personal vulnerability that remained alive, despite the passage of years. They had become intimately involved and in many situations had been taken aback by that intimacy. It appears as if, in David Barnard's words, reflecting Martin Buber's thinking 'the ordinary, goal-oriented transactions of everyday life—the world of "I and it"—were transformed into a moment of genuine mutuality and relationship—the world of "I and thou"[91]' (p. 1724–5).

Develop control over practice

Physicians were more apt to use the coping mechanism of developing control over their clinical practice than were other health professionals.[11] This often came with professional competence and allowed the professional to focus on a personal interest area of specialization or research.

The study of physician burnout in the Netherlands and the United States[16] suggests that the issue of work control needs to be explicitly addressed. Although speaking primarily of physicians, the literature reviewed above suggests that their ideas apply equally well to other professionals. Professionals need to have a say in how their work days are organized. 'Can they modulate the pace of their work, or minimize hassles, interruptions and paperwork? Second, the physician organization should commit to understanding and addressing work–home interference. Cross-coverage, child care, part-time practice, and flexible work hours[119] all may mitigate role conflicts and build physician loyalty to the organization.' (p. 173).

Personal philosophy

A personal philosophy of illness, death, and one's role in life is essential for many caregivers.[11] This often involves a spiritual or religious philosophy, centred on a commitment to serve others, which may be both helpful and key to deriving a sense of meaning in difficult times.[11] Caregivers in oncology[5] who responded that they were 'quite a bit to extremely religious' reported lower levels of both emotional exhaustion and diminished empathy for patients. It was hypothesized that this was the 'result of a more existential perception of the care of the critically ill and dying patients. These individuals may attach a different meaning to life and death, which provides them with greater satisfaction and reward from palliative care' (p. 1629). Remen[120] speaks of the power of a personal sense of meaning to change the experience of work, or relationship, and even of life. She refers to Viktor Frankl's book *Man's Search for Meaning*[121] in which he reported that survival itself may depend on seeking and finding meaning. 'Meaning may become a very practical matter for those of us who do difficult work or lead difficult lives. Meaning is strength. Physicians often seek their strength in competence. Indeed, competence and expertise are two of the most respected qualities in the medical subculture, as well as in our society. But important as they are, they are not sufficient to fully sustain us . . . Competence may bring us satisfaction. Finding meaning in a familiar task often allows us to go beyond this and find in the most routine of tasks a deep sense of joy and even gratitude' (p. 162).

For many caregivers, the concept of the Wounded Healer is an integral part of their philosophy of practice.[107,122–124] This concept derives from ancient universal shamanic stories of Paleolithic times. These stories are of tribal priests 'the original wounded healers, whose ability to heal others was seen as being directly linked to their having journeyed in depth into their own wounded selves' (ref. 123, p. 45).

Successful caregivers are often 'wounded healers', with wounds sustained either in childhood, adulthood, or both. 'In many cases, in trying to heal their respective wounds, these caregivers were drawn, consciously or not, to healing others' (ref. 122, p. 8). Sulmasy,[124] a physician, philosopher, and Franciscan friar contends, 'All health care professionals are wounded healers. They cannot escape suffering themselves. Moments of pain, loneliness, fatigue, and sacrifice are intrinsic to the human condition. The physician or nurse's own bleeding can become the source of the compassion in the healer's art. From the physician or nurse's own suffering can come the wine of fervent zeal and the oil of compassion . . . The physician's or nurse's wounds can become resources for healing . . .' (p. 48). Sulmasy warns, however, that wounded healers must not become so overwhelmed with the suffering of others that they are unable to offer effective care. 'Competence remains the first act of compassion. Wounded healers do not ask their patients for help, but recognize the unity between their own neediness and the needs of their patients. Wounded healers issue an invitation to patients to enter into the space of the healing relationship' (p. 48).

Team philosophy, team support, and team building

A sense of team philosophy, support, and team building has been identified as an important organizational coping mechanism for both palliative care and oncology professionals.[11] Improving inter-professional cooperation, team processes, and group support in nursing was found to provide the best protective or buffering approach to many health stressors, especially burnout.[23] The perception of social support at work was also correlated with lower burnout in a study comparing hospice and oncology nurses.[24]

Nason[125] notes that team development always involves tension and conflict. This may be viewed as the result of competition, lack of role definition, or poor leadership, but it can also be viewed as a reflection of contradictory institutional goals. Team members may become entrapped in conflicting relationships through the interaction of limited resources, competing demands, and unrealistic institutional priorities and, as a consequence, come to represent differing value systems within the organization. An effective team must have clarity of objectives, mission, and priorities that are shared by all team members. Role expectations should be realistic and well defined when they overlap. Effective decision-making and problem-solving processes should be in place to arrive at the 'best' possible solution; environmental norms should exist that support the tasks of problem solving. There should be a concern for each other's needs and an opportunity for individuals to enlarge their roles and optimize their chances for personal growth.[126]

One of the physicians in the Field study commented about the relationships amongst team members. 'I think that we all work together really. We boss them (nurses) around a bit and then they boss us back, and the Macmillan nurses boss everyone around! I think at the moment we're running quite well. We complement each other and we've got fairly defined roles ...' (ref. 71, p. 1114).

Regular opportunities to meet and talk together can also help teams to develop a respectful understanding of differences in respect to specific situations. For example, Redinbaugh et al.[127] note that physicians and nurses may prefer different coping strategies and may have different personality structures that may lead to differences in response to patient deaths. The authors draw on Holland's[128] theory of occupational interest to propose a model of grief that might help to understand team differences. Individuals have natural propensities and aversions for minimizing grief reactions. Emotion-focused coping would be used by those with a high Social score and low Realistic score. They would be likely to talk with others about their grief. Those with a high Artistic score with a low Social score would attempt to understand their grief through its depiction in literature and the arts. High Conventional scores paired with low Investigative scores are reflective of those who are less likely to dampen their grief with alcohol or drugs and more likely to use personal faith to resolve their grief.

Team meetings need to be developed to meet the needs of staff. A carefully designed training programme and staff-support activities were meant to enhance personal growth and to give emotional support and deal with death and bereavement issues.[10] The interventions did not involve mutual collaboration, practical problems, managerial and communication skills, and the skills needed to deliver complex palliative care. There was a cultural difference between the external consultants who embraced a relational therapeutical worldview and the hospice staff who came from a rational technical hospital environment. The former approach involves complete trust and openness in order to work. Not all staff members were convinced of the value of the non-directive approach. In addition, a therapeutic group is fundamentally different from a group that has to work together after the session. The authors suggest that future leaders should focus on content as well as process issues. They also suggest that adequate resources, a supportive management structure, an extensive educational training programme and attention to individual needs should accompany support groups. These issues have been identified earlier[1,11] so it is worth noting that they still exist.

Colleagues at work

Support from colleagues was very important for hospice caregivers.[1,62] The overall mental health of hospice nurses was in part predicted by staff support.[7] In addition, an association has been found between support from colleagues and low burnout scores for hospice nurses, showing the value of providing staff support within the work setting.[24] In the MSKCC study,[5] oncologists perceived significantly less support from colleagues than did either house staff or nurses. Peer support significantly decreased psychological distress and demoralization symptoms for the entire sample.

Life-style management

Life-style management includes having outside activities; engaging in physical activities and diversions; organizing non-job-related social interaction; taking time off; attending to one's needs for nutrition and adequate sleep; and meditation and relaxation techniques.[11] There is some evidence from AIDS caregivers that 'escapist' leisure engagements—those that involve high levels of distraction and allow little capacity for reflection—appear to be ineffective solutions for preventing burnout, particularly the aspect of 'attentional fatigue' that is associated with continued, focused caring. Such 'escapist' leisure activities actually appear to incur negative psychological effects. In contrast, 'restorative' activities—those which engage attention, but still provide 'room' for reflection, for example walking, gardening—influence functioning in a positive way and provide for restoration and renewal[79] (from ref. 110).

Future research agenda

Future research questions in palliative care might include the following:

- Which types of programs serve most effectively to buffer stress for which individuals or which types of hospice organizations?
- What is the impact of the changing hospice environment on patients and caregivers?
- Given the sensitivity of some hospice caregivers to work overload, how can these caregivers cope effectively with the changing hospice environment?
- Does extra support for staff new to palliative care influence their ability to provide effective care?
- Do support programmes developed in conjunction with staff help to effectively manage team stress?
- Is burnout decreased through training that considers practice size, emphasis on productivity, time pressure during office visits, societal pressure, colleague support, feeling poorly resourced, intellectual stimulation, job security, increased participation in decision-making, monitoring workload, increasing job fulfilment through goal setting, and feedback?[16]
- Do new programmes of education for health care professionals improve patient and family care?

References

1. **Vachon, M.L.S.** (1995). Staff stress in hospice/palliative care: a review. *Palliative Medicine* **9**, 91–122.
2. **Ramirez, A.J., Graham, J., Richards, M.A., Cull, A., Gregory, W.M., Leaning, M.S., Snashall, D.C., and Timothy, A.R.** (1995). Burnout and psychiatric disorder among cancer clinicians. *British Journal of Cancer* **71**, 1263–69.
3. **Payne, N.** (2001). Occupational stressors and coping as determinants of burnout in female hospice nurses. *Journal of Advanced Nursing* **33**, 396–405.
4. **Grunfeld, E., Whelan, T., Zitzelsberger, L., Willan, A.R., Montesanto, B., and Evans, W.K.** (2000). Cancer care workers in Ontario: prevalence of burnout, job stress and job satisfaction. *Canadian Medical Association Journal* **163**, 166–9.
5. **Kash, K.M., Holland, J.C., Breitbart, W., Berenson, S., Dougherty, J., Ouelette-Kobasa, S., and Lesko, L.** (2000). Stress and burnout in oncology. *Oncology* **14**, 1621–37.
6. **Finlay, I.G.** (1990). Sources of stress in hospice medical directors and matrons. *Palliative Medicine* **4**, 5–9.

7. **Cooper, C.L. and Mitchell, S.** (1990). Nursing the critically ill and dying. *Human Relations* **43**, 297–311.
8. **Bene', B. and Foxall, M.J.** (1991). Death anxiety and job stress in hospice and medical–surgical nurses. *The Hospice Journal* **7** (3), 25–41.
9. **Von Gunten, C.F., Ferris, F.D., and Emanuel, L.L.** (2000). Ensuring competency in end-of-life care: communication and relational skills. *Journal of the American Medical Association* **284**, 3051–7.
10. **Van Staa, A.L., Visser, A., and van der Zouwe, N.** (2000). Caring for caregivers: experiences and evaluation of interventions for a palliative care team. *Patient Education and Counseling* **41**, 93–105.
11. **Vachon, M.L.S.** *Occupational Stress in the Care of the Critically Ill, the Dying and the Bereaved.* New York: Hemisphere Press, 1987.
12. **French, J.R.P., Rodgers, W., and Cobb, S.** (1974). Adjustment as person–environment fit. In *Coping and Adaptation* (ed. G.V. Coelho, D.A. Hamburg, and E. Adams), pp. 316–33. New York: Basic Books.
13. **Harrison, R.V.** (1979). Person–environment fit and job stress. In *Stress at Work* (ed. C.L. Cooper and R. Payne), pp. 175–205. Chichester: Wiley.
14. **Karasek, R. et al.** (1981). Job decision latitude, job demands and cardiovascular disease: a prospective study of Swedish men. *American Journal of Public Health* **71**, 694–705.
15. **Johnson, J.V. and Hall, E.M.** (1988). Job strain, work place, social sup-port and cardiovascular disease: a cross-sectional study of a random sample of the Swedish working population. *American Journal of Public Health* **78**, 1336–42.
16. **Association of Professors of Medicine [Linzer, M., Visser, M.R., Oort, F.J., Smets, E.M.A., McMurray, J.E., and de Haes, H.C.J.M. for the Society of General Internal Medicine (SGIM) Career Satisfaction Study Group (CSSG)]** (2001). Predicting and preventing physician burnout: results from the United States and the Netherlands. *The American Journal of Medicine* **111**, 170–5.
17. **Antonovsky, A.** *Health, Stress and Coping.* San Francisco, Jossey-Bass, 1979.
18. **Porta, M., Busquet, X., and Jariod, M.** (1997). Attitudes and views of physicians and nurses towards cancer patients dying at home. *Palliative Medicine* **11**, 116–26.
19. **Annunziata, M.S., Talamini, R., Tumolo, S., Rossi, C., and Monfardini, S.** (1996). Physicians and death: comments and behaviour of 605 doctors in the north-east of Italy. *Supportive Care in Cancer* **4**, 334–40.
20. **Deckard, G., Meterko, M., and Field, D.** (1994). Physician burnout: an examination of personal, professional, and organizational relationships. *Medical Care* **32**, 745–54.
21. **Barroso, P., Osuna, E., and Luna, A.** (1992). Doctors' death experience and attitudes towards death, euthanasia and informing terminal patients. *Medicine and Law* **11**, 527–33.
22. **Ramirez, A.J., Graham, J., Richards, M.A., Cull, A., and Gregory, W.M.** (1996). Mental health of hospital consultants: the effect of stress and satisfaction at work. *Lancet* **347**, 724–8.
23. **Beck-Friis, B., Strang, P., and Sjödén, P.-O.** (1993). Caring for severely ill cancer patients: a comparison of working conditions in hospital-based home care and in hospital. *Support Care Cancer* **1**, 145–51.
24. **Bram, P.J. and Katz, L.F.** (1989). A study of burnout in nurses working in hospice and hospital oncology settings. *Oncol Nursing Forum* **16**, 555–60.
25. **Maslach, C. and Jackson, S.E.** *The Maslach Burnout Inventory (Manual)* 2nd edn. Palo Alto CA: Consulting Psychologists Press, 1986.
26. **Amir, M.** (1987). Considerations guiding physicians when informing cancer patients. *Social Science and Medicine* **24**, 741–8.
27. **Cooper, C.L., Rout, U., and Faragher, B.** (1989). Mental health, job satisfaction, and job stress among general practitioners. *British Medical Journal* **298**, 366–70.
28. **McMurray, J.E., Linzer, M., Konrad, T.R., Douglas, J., Shugerman, R., and Nelson, K., for the SGIM Career Satisfaction Study Group** (2000). The work lives of women physicians: results from the physician work life study. *Journal of General Internal Medicine* **15**, 372–80.
29. **Graham, J., Ramirez, A.J., Cull, A., Gregory, W.M., Finlay, I., Hoy, A., and Richards, M.A.** (1996). Job stress and satisfaction among palliative physicians: a CRC/ICRF Study. *Palliative Medicine* **10**, 185–94.
30. **Vachon, M.L.S.** (2002). Staff stress and burnout. In *Principles and Practice of Palliative Care and Supportive Oncology* 2nd edn. (ed. A.M. Berger, R.K. Portenoy, and D.E. Weissman). Philadelphia PA: Lippincott Williams & Wilkins.
31. **Dickinson, G.E. and Tournier, R.E.** (1993). A longitudinal study of sex differences in how physicians relate to dying patients. *Journal of the American Medical Women's Association* **8**, 19–22.
32. **Pines, A.M.** (2000). Treating career burnout: a psychodynamic existential perspective. *Psychotherapy in Practice* **56**, 633–42.
33. **Grosch, W.N. and Olsen, D.C.** (2000). Clergy burnout: an integrative approach. *Psychotherapy in Practice* **56**, 619–32.
34. **Maeder, T.** *Children of Psychiatrists and Other Psychotherapists.* New York: Harper and Row, 1989.
35. **Miller, A.** (1979). The drama of the gifted child and the psychoanalyst's narcissistic disturbance. *International Journal of Psychoanalysis* **60**, 47–58.
36. **Kash, K.M. and Holland, J.C.** (1989). Special problems of physicians and house staff in oncology. In *Handbook of Psycho-oncology* (ed. J.C. Holland and J.H. Rowland), pp. 647–57. New York: Oxford University Press.
37. **James, N. and Field, D.** (1992). The routinization of hospice: charisma and bureaucratization. *Social Science and Medicine* **34**, 1363–75.
38. **Taylor, E.J., Highfield, M.F., and Amenta, M.** (1999). Predictors of oncology and hospice nurses' spiritual care perspectives and practices. *Applied Nursing Research* **12** (1), 30–37.
39. **Maslach, C. and Jackson, S.E.** *The Maslach Burnout Inventory (Manual)* 2nd edn. Palo Alto CA: Consulting Psychologists Press, 1986.
40. **Carr, M. and Merriman, M.** (1996). Comparison of death attitudes among hospice workers and health care professionals in other settings. *Omega* **32**, 287–301.
41. **Payne, S.A., Dean, S.J., and Kalus, C.** (1998). A comparative study of death anxiety in hospice and emergency nurses. *Journal of Advanced Nursing* **28**, 700–6.
42. **de Hennezel, M.** (1998). Intimate distance. *European Journal of Palliative Care* **5** (2), 56–9.
43. **MacLeod, R.D.** (2001). On reflection: doctors learning to care for people who are dying. *Social Science and Medicine* **52**, 1719–27.
44. **Roy, D.J.** (2001). Last words. *Journal of Palliative Care* **17**, 227–8.
45. **Kobasa, S.C.** (1979). Stressful life events, personality and health: an inquiry into hardiness. *Journal of Personality and Social Psychology* **37**, 1–11.
46. **Kobasa, S.C., Maddi, S.R., and Courington, S.** (1982). Hardiness and health: a prospective study. *Journal of Personality and Social Psychology* **42**, 168–77.
47. **Kash, K.M. and Hollalnd, J.C.** (1989). Special problems of physicians and house staff in oncology. In *Handbook of Psycho-oncology* (ed. J.C. Holland and J.H. Roland), pp. 647–57. New York: Oxford University Press.
48. **Papadatou, D., Anagnostopoulos, F., and Monos, D.** (1994). Factors contributing to the development of burnout in oncology nursing. *British Journal of Medical Psychology* **67**, 187–99.
49. **Spiegel, D.** *Living Beyond Limits.* New York: Fawcett Columbine, 1993.
50. **Gregory, D.R. and Cotler, M.P.** (1994). The problem of futility: III. The importance of physician–patient communication and a suggested guide through the minefield. *Cambridge Quarterly of Healthcare Ethics* **3**, 257–69.
51. **Barnard, D., Towers, A., Boston, P., and Lambrinidou, Y.** *Crossing Over: Narratives of Palliative Care.* New York: Oxford, 2000.
52. **Shapiro, D.H., Schwartz, C.E., and Astin, J.A.** (1996). Controlling ourselves, controlling our world. *American Psychologist* **51**, 1213–30.
53. **Folkman, F.** (1984). Personal control and stress and coping processes: a theoretical analysis. *Journal of Personality and Social Psychology* **6**, 839–52.
54. **Lazarus, R.S. and Folkman, S.** *Stress, Appraisal and Coping.* New York: Springer Publishing, 1984.
55. **Antonovsky, A.** *Unraveling the Mystery of Health: How People Manage Stress and Stay Well.* San Francisco, Jossey-Bass, 1987.
56. **Antonovsky, A.** (1996). The salutogenic model as a theory to guide health promotion. *Health Promotion International* **11**, 11–18.
57. **Gilbar, O.** (1998). Relationship between burnout and sense of coherence in health of social workers. *Social Work in Health Care* **26** (3), 39–49.
58. **Vachon, M.L.S.** (2001). The nurse's role: the world of palliative care nursing. In *The Oxford Textbook of Palliative Nursing* (ed. B. Ferrell and N. Coyle), pp. 647–62. New York: Oxford University Press.

59. **Larson, D.G.** *The Helper's Journey.* Champaign Il: Research Press, 1993.

60 **Ornish, D.** *Love and Survival: The Scientific Basis for the Healing Power of Intimacy.* New York: HarperCollins Publishers, Inc., 1998.

61. **Vachon, M.L.S.** (2002). Social support of the health provider. In *Social Support: A Reflection on Humanity* (ed. J.D. Morgan), pp. 127–37. Amityville NY: Baywood Publishing, Inc.

62. **Alexander, D.A. and Ritchie, E.** (1990). 'Stressors' and difficulties in dealing with the terminal patient. *Journal of Palliative Care* **6** (3), 28–33.

63. **Vachon, M.L.S.** (1993). Emotional problems in palliative medicine: patient, family, and professional. In *Oxford Textbook of Palliative Medicine* (ed. D. Doyle, G.W. Hanks, and N. MacDonald), pp. 577–605. Oxford: Oxford University Press.

64 **Papadatou, D., Papazoglou, I., Petraki, D., and Bellali, T.** (1999). Mutual support among nurses who provide care to dying children. *Illness, Crisis and Loss* **7**, 37–48.

65. **Mc Cue, J.D.** (1982). The effects of stress on physicians and their medical practice. *New England Journal of Medicine* **306**, 458–63.

66. **Miller, D. and Gillies, P.** (1996). Is there life after work? Experiences of HIV and oncology health staff. *AIDS Care* **8**, 167–82.

67. **Selwyn, P.A.** *Surviving the Fall.* New Haven: Yale University Press, 1998.

68. **Woolley, H., Stein, A., Forrest, G.C., and Baum, J.D.** (1989). Staff stress and job satisfaction at a children's hospice. *Archives of Disease in Childhood* **64**, 114–18.

69. **Goldberg, D. and Williams, P.** *A User's Guide to the General Health Questionnaire.* Windsor, Berkshire: NFER-Nelson Publishing, 1988.

70. **Catalan, J.** (1996). The psychological impact on staff of caring for people with serious diseases: the case of HIV infection and oncology. *Journal of Psychosomatic Research* **40**, 425–35.

71. **Field, D.** (1998). Special not different: general practitioners' accounts of their care of dying people. *Social Science and Medicine* **46**, 1111–20.

72. **Dharmasena, H.P. and Forbes, K.** (2001). Palliative care for patients with non-malignant disease: will hospital physicians refer? *Palliative Medicine* **15**, 413–18.

73. **Boling, A. and Lynn, J.** (1998). Hospice: current practice, future possibilities. *The Hospice Journal* **13** (1/2), 29–32.

74. **Field, M. and Cassel, C.K.** *Approaching Death: Improving Care at the End of Life.* Washington DC: Institute of Medicine, National Academy Press, 1997.

75. **Byock, I.** (1998). Hospice and palliative care: a parting of the ways or a path to the future? *Journal of Palliative Medicine* **1**, 165–76.

76. **Lynn, J. and O'Mara, A.** (2001). Reliable, high quality, efficient end-of-life care for cancer patients: Economic issues and barriers. In *Improving Palliative Care for Cancer: Summary and Recommendations* (ed. K. Foley and H. Gelband), pp. 67–95. Washington DC: National Academy Press.

77. **Whedon, M.B.** (2002). Revisiting the road not taken: integrating palliative care into oncology nursing. *Clinical Journal of Oncology Nursing* **6** (1), 27–33.

78. **Montana, J. and Duffy, M.** *Blue Cross Blue Shield Report on Insurer's Redesign of the Hospice Benefit to Improve End-of-Life Care.* Paper presented at the annual grantee meeting on promoting excellence in end-of-life care of the Robert Wood Johnson Foundation, Tuczon, AZ, September 1999.

79. **Herbst, L.H. and Cetti, J.** (2001). Management strategies for palliative care: promoting quality, growth, and opportunity. *American Journal of Hospice and Palliative Care* **18**, 327–33.

80. **Viganò, A., Dorgan, M., Bruera, E., and Suarez-Almazor, M.E.** (1999). The relative accuracy of the clinical estimation of the duration of life for patients with end of life cancer. *Cancer* **86**, 172–6.

81. **Viganò, A., Dorgan, M., Buckingham, J., Bruera, E., and Suarez-Almazor, M.E.** (2000). Survival prediction in terminal cancer patients: a systematic review of the medical literature. *Palliative Medicine* **14**, 363–74.

82. **Florio, G.A., Donnelly, J.P., and Zevon, M.A.** (1998). The structure of work-related stress and coping among oncology nurses in high-stress medical settings: a transactional analysis. *Journal of Occupational Health Psychology* **3**, 227–42.

83. **Kuuppelomäki, M. and Lauri, S.** (1998). Ethical dilemmas in the care of patients with incurable cancer. *Nursing Ethics* **5**, 283–93.

84. **Alexander, D.A. and MacLeod, R.D.** (1992). Stress among palliative care matrons: a major problem for a minority group. *Palliative Medicine* **6**, 111–24.

85. **Hart, G., Yates, P., Clinton, M., and Windsor, C.** (1998). Mediating conflict and control: practice challenges for nurses working in palliative care. *International Journal of Nursing Studies* **35**, 252–8.

86. **Heming, D.** (1988). The Titanic triumvirate: teams, teamwork and teambuilding. *Canadian Journal of Occupational Therapy* **55** (1), 15–20.

87. **Vachon, M.L.S.** (1996). What makes a team? *Palliative Care Today* **5** (3), 34–5.

88. **Seale, C. and Cartwright, A.** *The Year before Death.* Aldershot: Avebury, 1994.

89. **Woolley, H., Stein, A., Forrest, G.C., and Baum, J.D.** (1989). Staff stress and job satisfaction at a children's hospice. *Archives of Diseases of Children* **64**, 114–18.

90. **Forrest, G. and Woolley, H.** 15 Years of staff support in a children's hospice. 1999 (unpublished data).

91. **Barnard, D.** (1995). The promise of intimacy and the fear of our own undoing. *Journal of Palliative Care* **11** (4), 22–6.

92. **Yandrick, R.M.** (1997). High demand low control. *Behavioral Healthcare Tomorrow* **6** (3), 41–4.

93. **Copp, G. and Dunn, V.** (1993). Frequent and difficult problems perceived by nurses caring for the dying in community, hospice and acute care settings. *Palliative Medicine* **7**, 19–25.

94. **Coyle, N.** (1997). Focus on the nurse: ethical dilemmas with highly symptomatic patients dying at home. *Hospice Journal* **12** (2), 33–41.

95. **MacDonald, N.** Testimony before The Subcommittee to Update 'Of Life and Death' of the Standing Senate Committee on Social Affairs, Science and Technology, Ottawa, Ontario: March 28, 2000.

96. **Perry, B.** *Moments in Time: Images of Exemplary Nursing Care.* Ottawa: Canadian Nurses Association, 1998.

97. **Schneider, R.** (1997). The effects on nurses of treatment-withdrawal decisions made in ICUs and SCBUs. *Nursing in Critical Care* **2**, 174–85.

98. **Kearney, M.** (1992). Palliative medicine—just another specialty? *Palliative Medicine* **6**, 41.

99. **Barni, S., Mondin, R., Nazzani, R., and Archili, C.** (1996). Oncostress: evaluation of burnout in Lombardy. *Tumori* **82**, 85–92.

100. **Peabody, F.W.** (1927). The care of the patient. *Journal of the American Medical Association* **88**, 877–82 (1984; 252: 813–18).

101. **Vachon, M.L.S.** (2000). Burnout and symptoms of stress in staff working in palliative care. In *Handbook of Psychiatry in Palliative Medicine* (ed. H.M. Chochinov and W. Breitbart), pp. 303–19. New York: Oxford University Press.

102. **Trygstad, L.** (1986). Professional friends: the inclusion of the personal into the professional. *Cancer Nursing* **9**, 326–32.

103. **Kutner, J.S., Steiner, J.F., Corbett, K.K., Jahnigen, D.W., and Barton, P.L.** (1999). Information needs in terminal illness. *Social Science and Medicine* **48**, 1341–52.

104. **Watson, J.** (1988). Human care in nursing. In *Nursing: Human Science and Human Care: A Theory of Nursing* (ed. J. Watson), pp. 27–30. New York: National League for Nursing Press.

105. **Boston, P., Towers, A., and Barnard, D.** (2002). Embracing vulnerability: risk and empathy in palliative care. *Journal of Palliative Care* **17**, 248–53.

106. **Figley, C.R.** (1995). Compassion fatigue as a secondary traumatic stress disorder: an overview. In *Compassion Fatigue* (ed. C.R. Figley), pp. 1–20. New York: Brunner/Mazel.

107. **Garfield, C., Spring, C., and Ober, D.** *Sometimes My Heart Goes Numb: Love and Caring in a Time of AIDS.* San Francisco: Jossey-Bass, 1995.

108. **Ankone, A.** (1999). Burnout bij artsen bijna verdubbeld. (Burnout among physicians almost doubled.) *Medlisch Contact* **54**, 494–7.

109. **Schmoldt, R.A., Freeborn, D.K., and Klevit, H.D.** (1994). Physician burnout: recommendations for HMO managers. *HMO Practice* **8**, 58–66.

110. **Brenninkmeyer, V., Van Yperen, N.W., and Buunk, B.P.** (2001). Burnout and depression are not identical twins: is devline of superiority a distinguishing feature? *Personality and Individual Differences* **30**, 873–80.

111. **Van Servellen, G. and Leake, B.** (1993). Burn-out in hospital nurses: a comparison of acquired immunodeficiency syndrome, oncology, general medical, and intensive care unit nurse samples. *Journal of Professional Nursing* **9**, 169–77.
112. **Simoni, P.S. and Paterson, J.J.** (1997). Hardiness, coping, and burnout in the nursing workplace. *Journal of Professional Nursing* **13**, 178–85.
113. **Mount, B.M.** (1986). Dealing with our losses. *Journal of Clinical Oncology* **4**, 1127–34.
114. **Papadatou, D.** (2000). A proposed model of health professional's grieving process. *Omega* **41**, 59–77.
115. **Saunders, J.M. and Valente, S.M.** (1994). Nurses' grief. *Cancer Nursing* **17**, 318–25.
116. **Feldstein, M.A. and Gemma, P.B.** (1995). Oncology nurses and chronic compounded grief. *Cancer Nursing* **18**, 228–36.
117. **Heim, E.** (1991). Job stressors and coping in health professions. *Psychotherapy and Psychosomatics* **55**, 90–9.
118. **Cohen, M.Z., Haberman, M.R., Steeves, R., and Deatrick, J.A.** (1994). Rewards and difficulties of oncology nursing. *Oncology Nursing Forum* **21** (8) (Suppl.), 9–17.
119. **Foster, S.W. et al.** (2000). Results of a gender climate and work environment survey at a Midwest Academic Health Center. *Academic Medicine* **75**, 653–60.
120. **Remen, R.N.** *Kitchen Table Wisdom.* New York: Riverhead Books, 1996.
121. **Frankl, V.** *Man's Search for Meaning.* New York: Washington Square Press, 1984.
122. **Nouwen, H.** *The Wounded Healer.* Garden City NJ: Doubleday, 1972.
123. **Kearney, M.** *Mortally Wounded.* New York: Scribner, 1996.
124. **Sulmasy, D.P.** *The Healer's Calling.* New York: Paulist Press, 1997.
125. **Nason, F.** (1981). Team tension as a vital sign. *General Hospital Psychiatry* **3**, 32–6.
126. **Beckhard, R.** (1974). Organizational implications of team building. In *Making Health Teams Work* (ed. H. Wise, R. Beckhard, I. Rubin, and A.L. Kyte), pp. 69–94. Cambridge UK: Ballinger.
127. **Redinbaugh, E.M., Schuerger, J.M., Weiss, L., Brufsky, A., and Arnold, R.** (2001). Health care professionals' grief: a model based on occupational style and coping. *Psycho-Oncology* **10**, 187–98.
128. **Holland, J.L.** *Making Vocational Choices: A Theory of Vocational Personalities and Work Environments.* Odesssa FL: Psychological Assessment Resources, 1985.
129. **Canin, L.H.** *Psychological Restoration among AIDS Caregivers: Maintaining Self-care.* Unpublished doctoral dissertation, University of Michigan, 1991.

13

Social work in palliative medicine

13 Social work in palliative medicine

Barbara Monroe

Introduction

Social work is a necessary and appropriate part of palliative care. Palliative care starts with specific physical symptoms but it can only be completed by consideration of the patient's feelings, family and friendship networks, and social circumstances. This requires a variety of skills and roles, including the social work skills and roles considered in this chapter. The chapter describes the forces that shape the social work role in palliative care, examines the social work task, provides a practical illustration, looks at the work that social workers do, and considers the social worker's contribution to extending the resources and values of palliative care.

Shaping the social work role

Three forces shape the social work role: the non-medical social goals that palliative care teams set themselves; the teamwork and multiprofessional skills required to meet these social goals; and the expectations of patients, carers, relatives and friends, and the various palliative care professionals, of social work and social workers.

Non-medical social goals

Relieving a patient's physical symptoms reveals their and their families' emotional, spiritual, and practical needs. Because doctors can often release patients from the horror of a physically painful and unpleasant death, palliative care teams are able to set themselves non-medical social goals aimed at these non-medical needs.

The patient's first non-medical need is to express emotional pain. Terminal illness frightens people, may make them angry, sad, or guilty, and often distances them from those to whom they are close. Helping patients to express their feelings can reduce their fear and anguish and put them back in touch with their partners, families, and friends.[1] It allows patients to say a proper good-bye and gives them the opportunity to heal rifts and complete unfinished business.

The second need is the exploration of spiritual pain.[2] Dying people want to explore 'why'; why me, why now, for what purpose? Helping them in this journey will alleviate their isolation and give them the comfort of knowing that their concerns, even if unanswered, are real, important, and valid.

The third need is for practical help. Dying people are often reduced to passive patienthood; however, they need to make decisions and exercise choice, both for practical reasons and in order to maintain their own sense of dignity and worth. For instance, they may need to make a will or to discuss and influence a child's future care. They may need the most basic assistance in order to pay a bill or get a telephone at home.

Patients' partners, families, and friends will experience the same three needs and ensuring that their needs are also met is a proper goal for palliative care. They may also feel frightened or angry. They too will ask 'why', and they too may have practical needs, such as some relief from a 24-h caring role. They will need to feel involved in the processes of dying and that they did what they could to help the patient. Research indicates that whether or not these needs are met can have a profound impact on their health in bereavement and their ability to cope with future crises. For example, Kissane et al.'s work emphasizes the importance of an assessment of family functioning during terminal illness since it influences subsequent grief outcomes.[3] They also report on the impact of time-limited focused family sessions provided to 'at risk' families by social workers and others.[4]

Teamwork

The non-medical goals permitted by good symptom control require different and extra skills beyond those traditionally accruing to the doctor and nurse. In addition, patients may want to discuss emotional, spiritual, or practical problems with someone who is not involved in their physical care, or someone wearing a different label, such as a minister of religion or a social worker. As a result, good palliative care is delivered by multiprofessional teams. Each member of the team will have a range of overlapping roles, some medical and some non-medical, each focused on a specific set of patient, family, or carer needs. Whilst medical needs will be met from the medical disciplines, no one discipline has the monopoly in fulfilling the non-medical roles. Patients' other needs do not come in neat boxes with discreet professional labels. Doctors, nurses, social workers, and ministers will all have to respond to patients' emotional, spiritual, and practical concerns. What matters is the definition and delivery of the social work task, and not the allocation of a role or task to the social worker or any other non-medical discipline. All disciplines will do some social work, and patients and those close to them will expect a consistent, careful, and effective approach to be adopted by all of them.

The social work profession does, however, bring its own perspective and approaches, and the exposition and demonstration of these is an important part of the contribution that a social worker should make within a palliative care team.[5] These perspectives come in three forms: the first reflects what social workers cannot do. They cannot cure pain, dress wounds, or offer the appropriate religious rituals. Their professional starting point has to be that defined by the patient and his or her family, not that defined by their professional role.

The second perspective is that of the patient as part of a family and friendship network with a past and a future and a social and cultural context. For the social worker, the patient is not just an individual with problems but part of a whole social network, which has a variety of strengths and resources that can be marshalled to cope with the consequences of the individual's illness and death and reflects attitudes that may impact on the possibilities available. For example, cultural expectations within the immediate circle of the family about the rights and responsibilities of individual members may affect decisions about caregiving.

Lastly, the social worker will have a perspective of how the patient and their family will be affected by the law and other social institutions. For instance, the social worker will understand the implications of family and mental health legislation in particular cases. He or she will know what community services might be applicable and what social welfare provision may be available. He or she may have to balance individual needs and wishes against a social control and protection function as in child protection work.

Expectations and attitudes

The role of the social worker is also shaped by expectations and attitudes of society, of colleagues, and of patients and families.

People in Western economies expect the welfare state to provide a safety net when things go wrong; a residential home for the elderly disabled widow whose carer has died or foster parents for the children of a dying single parent. Society sees the social worker as an agent for the welfare state, able to manipulate its institutions to the patient's advantage. For example, social workers may be expected to negotiate financial benefits from government agencies or organize child care from a statutory agency. Palliative care colleagues expect social workers to provide them with a safety net for managing difficult social work tasks. Palliative care teams will frequently meet situations that are emotionally exhausting and difficult to deal with. A young dying mother or a suicidal relative may need both extra time and specialist social work skills that are best provided by a separate resource, rather than by stretching—both physically and emotionally—the team responsible for the day-to-day care of a group of patients.

Patients and their families will also have specific expectations from organizations that provide palliative care. They increasingly expect access to professional counselling services in order to help them manage emotional difficulties. They will expect expert advice on personal family matters, such as how much should a young child know about and be involved with a parent's death and how they should be told what they need to know.[6]

The core social work task

The core social work task concerns the social and psychological health of the patient, family, friends, and carers, before and after death. It has two parts: assessment and intervention.

Assessment

The assessment of the patient at home or in an in-patient setting will often start with a medical or nursing 'clerking-in' procedure and the formulation of a care plan. This initial assessment should identify any need for further assessment, for co-ordination between disciplines, and for specialist help. Sometimes the process by which the patient has arrived in a service will have already identified problems that require a more detailed psychosocial assessment. For instance, in admitting the mother of a dependent adult with severe learning difficulties the normal in-patient admission routine might be expanded to involve the social worker as well as the doctor and the nurse. There may be immediate care needs and the patient's adult child may need particular help to become involved in and to understand his mother's impending death.[7]

In an important text on ethics in palliative care, Randall and Downie[8] question the potential intrusiveness of assessments in the psychosocial domain. They raise significant ethical concerns about the sensitive issues that may be touched upon. However, effective assessment creates a working partnership between the professional, the patient, and those close to him. Professionals should explain the reasons for their enquiries, establish consent, and check on it regularly: 'If there is something I ask that you would rather not discuss, please let me know.' The assessment process can never be a one-off event as circumstances alter and people change their minds. A failure to assess may diminish the options available to the patient and their family or mean that those at risk remain unidentified.

Assessments will vary in their formats and formality but will usually cover four perspectives: the individual, the family, physical resources, and social resources.

The individual

There is substantial evidence that psychological distress is a vital factor in the individual's experience of illness and interacts with physical distress.[9] It is influenced by perceptions of family and social support, of personal control, and attributions of meaning[10] and hope.[11] There is also evidence for links between the experiences of the dying individual and family functioning.[12]

In assessing the individual, we need to establish what changes their illness has wrought, as well as who they are. We need to know how their life has changed since the illness and who or what currently supports them. We need to understand their reaction to the illness and its implications for them. We need to identify any practical or emotional unfinished business they may have. Assessing practical issues will lead us on to values and beliefs. What are their aims now that they have entered palliative care; do they, for instance, want to die at home or in a hospital or hospice?

The family

The individual must be placed in the context of his family and friendship network. The family can be regarded as a complex system that changes over time. In order to assess the strengths and difficulties of a family and its members, we need to understand how it works.[13] We must discover the normal patterns of communication, support, and conflict in the family, and the extent to which they have been disrupted by the illness.[14]

The history of the current family and their individual experiences within their previous families will be significant factors in their ability to cope with the present crisis. For example, a wife who watched her own mother nurse her father through a protracted, exhausting, and painful terminal illness will in consequence approach her husband's death with reduced confidence and may value additional support. We need to understand the family's methods of coping with crisis and whether they are facing any additional change at the moment such as a house move, a redundancy, or a pregnancy. Lastly, we should enquire about the existence of other vulnerable individuals within the family such as children, dependent elderly, or disabled relatives. The terminal illness of a family member can be the final burden that topples a delicately balanced system of nurture and support and it may be necessary to provide additional external help.

Whatever the place of care immediately prior to death, most palliative care takes place at home and most care is provided by informal, related carers. They may also become clients in their own right. Numerous studies attest to the burden of caring with reports of increased risk of physical and psychological morbidity running alongside a recognition of the importance of the social and practical support provided to patients by those close to them.[15] The literature is clear about the needs of informal carers for information, education, and support.[16] Recent changes in the structure of families; geographical distance, divorce, split and reconstituted families, may add to carers' difficulties.

Physical resources

The assessment should cover the family's physical resources, such as money and housing.[17] We need to know about unmet physical needs because they may become the patient's biggest concern, and our expertise may be able to unlock money from charities or the state to relieve the problem. For instance, a washing machine for the exhausted carer of a patient with night sweats and incontinence may be of more value than extra counselling or nursing support. A patient's physical resources may also affect how we care for them. Adaptations to their home or the provision of domestic help may avoid or delay the need for inpatient care.

Social resources

Finally, the family themselves must be placed within the context of their community and social network. The team should attempt to understand their ethnic, cultural,[18] and religious background and the potential impact of these influences on the individual and his illness. This means enquiring about informal and formal helping systems available to the family within their community such as churches, social groups, and schools.

Field has argued that the use of the portmanteau word 'psychosocial', rather than 'psychological and social', has diminished the understanding and importance of social factors in people's lives.[19] He also points out that not all palliative care services have a social worker on the team 'and where they do these may well be part-time and marginal to decision-making processes.'

An assessment made with the individual, their family, and friends, of the emotional, spiritual, physical, and social resources available to them will lead to decisions. At one end of the spectrum the decision will be to do nothing. Assessment may reveal adequate coping mechanisms in the patient and their family and community. The result of the assessment may, however, be a decision to intervene in order to support the patient and family in managing the situation facing them.

Interventions

Interventions will be aimed at patients and families who need help in order to cope with their situation.[20] They will typically want support because: they do not have the information they need; they cannot communicate sufficiently with each other to reach a solution; they lack the confidence to act; or they do not have the resources they need. In addition, an intervention may be addressed at the needs of bereaved individuals or families after the patient has died.

Information

Sometimes patients or families cannot manage simply because they lack information, leaving them at the mercy of their fears and fantasies. For instance, many patients and their relatives will be very frightened of the moment of death because they do not know how it will happen. They need information about what normally happens and what their options are. Patients will want to know how their illness will progress to death and how difficult symptoms will be treated.[21] Parents will want to know what to expect from their child in bereavement and what options they should consider for involving their child in the death. Relatives may want information about arranging funerals and registering the death.

The way information is delivered is vital to its accurate reception. The style must be appropriate to the recipient both in terms of vocabulary and venue. Some people, for example, can discuss the implications of 'bad news' better in their own homes, others prefer the professional anonymity of a clinic. Pace is another important component. Information must be offered when requested and at a speed that allows absorption. Too much information delivered too quickly can paralyse and frighten; giving information is a two-way process that involves as much listening as talking. The person who delivers the information may also be important; one of the advantages of the multiprofessional team is the flexibility it provides. People often make their own choices about who to ask. For example, an elderly wife may be frightened to ask how her husband will die for fear of wasting the doctor's time. The social worker may be seen as less daunting.

Communication

The second objective for intervention is to help patients and their families communicate. Communication is particularly difficult at the time of a bereavement, and a family that cannot share information and feelings cannot easily resolve the problems that death brings. The immediate barrier to communication is likely to be the strong, unfamiliar, and often conflicting feelings that each family member may experience in relation to the forthcoming death. These will disrupt their normal approach to communicating with each other. In addition, death and crisis often encourage people to protect one another. Loyalty and a conventional dislike of emotional display and upset may inhibit discussion of what is going on both emotionally and practically. Many carers will also be struggling with rapid and anxiety provoking changes in the physical capacities and needs of the ill person.

More specific barriers to communication may reflect the redistribution of roles within the family; a husband may be assuming unfamiliar parenting roles and responsibilities just as his dying wife is experiencing their loss. Communicating both the practical and emotional material within this transaction will be difficult. Similarly, the different perspectives of family members will reduce their ability to communicate; the husband's experience of his wife's impending death may be very different from his father-in-law's pain in losing a much loved daughter and this new difference may not be understood by the daughter, the husband, or the father. Old relationship difficulties will be placed under even greater strain and the progression of the illness may have disrupted comforting routines of interaction at work and leisure for all involved.

Intervention will be aimed at overcoming these barriers and ensuring that the family and patient can communicate effectively. The intervention will work because a skilled outsider can often provide the security and sense of control that family members may need to release their emotions. The outsider will ensure that every member of the family hears a shared story that is as complete as possible and that all understand how each one reacts to it. Most families will manage well with just a little help. Most want to support each other, to say important things, to plan for the future, it is just that they do not know where to begin or what to say in a situation with so many uncertainties, that many will be facing for the first time.

Improving a family's communication can be a very powerful tool, releasing the existing strengths within the family, allowing them to solve their own problems and to establish new roles and relationships. For some families a bereavement may provide an opportunity for resolving historic arguments; exploiting the shared love of a dying parent to restore communication between family members who have not spoken for many years may allow the parent to see some meaning in his or her death, as well as releasing resources to deal with the immediate problems.

Intervention in a family's communication can also achieve very rapid results. The Hollywood cliché of the deathbed reconciliation is a real image. The crisis of impending bereavement can loosen the glue surrounding gummed-up communication patterns. Even in the final hours of life it is possible to reopen communication and this can have a profound effect on the survivor's future emotional health. Equally, professionals must respect people's capacity to choose. Forgiveness and reconciliation cannot be imposed, but support can always be offered.

Communicating with individuals and couples about issues of body image, sexuality, and intimacy can be particularly challenging to professionals in palliative care. However, discussion of these topics is important to quality of life. Life-threatening illness can deeply affect intimate relationships and self concepts. For example, partners may find that physical changes in the patient or their own change of role to carer alters their feelings or desires. Professional anxieties about the subject area may mean that the issues are seldom addressed in practice. In addition, there is evidence that most patients will not ask for help spontaneously. Whilst it would clearly be inappropriate to expect all professionals in palliative care to have specialist skills in psycho-sexual counselling, all should be able to offer and respond to cues about a wish to discuss sexuality and know how to refer on for specialist support where appropriate.[22] Sensitive support may involve finding questions that can be responded to at a variety of levels: 'In what ways has your illness changed how you can get close to people you particularly care about?' Generalizing can create a sense of permission: 'People often have questions they'd like to ask about the sexual side of life.'

The confidence to act

The dying patient and those close to them will often believe that they have no influence on events and may lack the confidence to take decisions for themselves. Physical disability may be reinforcing their emotional conclusion. They will have emerged from medicine's final attempt to cure them; they will not know how long they have before they die; they may have been confused by the changing series of professionals they have met.

For patients to have the confidence to act they may need to be reminded of the resources available to them and about how they have coped with crises in the past. They may need help to segment their problems and to focus on one or two difficulties that can be tackled out of a chaos that threatens to overwhelm. They may simply want the comforting presence of a concerned outsider as they think each stage through. For instance, the individual will often already know who or what can help them; the sympathetic teacher who can assist their child, the local church group who can mobilize a rota of supplementary carers. Sometimes, the patient may only need to be asked in order to provide their own answers.

The confidence to act depends on setting realistic goals. Dying patients and their families will have experienced a dramatic change in what is achievable. They may need to be encouraged to plan for what is left and to decide what is important to them; some things may not be possible, but much will be. For instance, a dying mother can attend her daughter's birthday party but may not be able to spend the whole weekend preparing party games and food.

The resource to act

Patients and families may have the information they require, the ability to discuss and resolve their problems, and the confidence to do what is needed. Ultimately, however, they may simply not have the resources to do what needs to be done. If you are threatened with eviction for rent arrears because your dying husband cannot work, it may be difficult to focus on other needs. More prosaically, patients may not have access to the resources they need; what aids to daily living or housing adaptations are available and who will supply them? A raised toilet seat may help the patient to continue using the lavatory rather than a commode, a ramp may allow access to the garden for a wheelchair user.

Families need information about financial resources and sources of social support. These services should not be imposed but must be provided in a way that allows families to obtain the kind of help that they decide they need. Effectiveness in this role requires advocacy and influence with social services departments, government agencies, and charities.

Helping patients with resources can usefully be separated from counselling work even though both carry the social work label. Knowledge of available physical resources and welfare rights may be acquired by a member of staff without a specific social work qualification. Intimate and frequent contact with local resources is as important as the theoretical knowledge of institutions and welfare legislation that should underpin it. Checklists can help any palliative care professional to screen for a potential requirement for practical assistance.

It is important to recognize that the task of the palliative care institution is to manipulate whatever is already available in society, rather than rushing to set up specialist services, expending time and energy that should be devoted to direct patient and family care. One of the most important components of the social work task is to act on behalf of the patient in order to get other agencies to do their job properly.

After the death

Further interventions may be necessary following the death of the patient. The normal process of providing palliative care should include efforts to identify those individuals at special risk in bereavement.(23) Loss and the grief that follows it are normal human experiences, but some people may need additional support with their grief either because of their previous experiences and relationships or because of the particular circumstances of their bereavement. Complicated and unresolved responses to grief may result in physical symptoms, obsessive behaviours, and can precipitate individual or family breakdown.(24)

Bereavement services aiming to respond to these needs can take many forms. A brief and possibly routine intervention following the bereavement can offer relatives, including children, the opportunity to view the body, to say a final farewell, to ask questions about the illness and death, and to begin the necessary but painful process of remembering.(25) It may be important to offer longer-term help, perhaps from a volunteer bereavement counsellor who represents the community from which the patient came and to which the relative or friend is returning. Specialist help may be required when circumstances are more extreme, such as the widower who plans to commit suicide so that he can avoid what he sees as a pointless life by joining his dead wife.

Social work methods

Interventions can provide information, increase communication, give confidence, provide resources, or help the bereaved. There are three traditional methods for making these interventions: one-to-one meetings, meetings with families or couples, or groups involving unrelated individuals with shared circumstances or problems. For all forms of intervention adolescents(26) and young children will often represent the most challenging and draining group, and palliative care teams will typically want to take extra care in these cases. Finally, all interventions will be made by listening and talking and here too there are particular skills and particular responsibilities.

One-to-one help

Any member of the team may find themselves talking to the patient or a family member with therapeutic intent. There are no solutions to the emotional anguish experienced by dying people but they can be helped by being heard. It is not necessary to approve what the patient says or does; it is important to show understanding of the feeling behind his words and actions. Staff may fear being overwhelmed by the intensity of emotion they release in the patient and more particularly that in talking about things they may have made them worse. However, it is often through tears or the expression of anger that individuals become more aware of the nature and origin of their pain and more able to decide how to cope with it.(27)

Meeting the patient or members of the family on a one-to-one basis may be an important precursor to work with the whole family. It ensures that we understand individual perspectives and problems. For example, the loving wife of a dying patient may need privacy to begin acknowledging her resentment at the exhausting task of caring. She may want to rehearse the exposure of her conflicting feelings with a sympathetic outsider before seeking a reconciliation between her resentment and grief with her husband. It should be remembered that dying people and their carers cannot act as proxies for one another's needs and feelings.(28) The dying individual and those close to them will have different needs at different times, may require different types of support and often have conflicting agendas.

Family meetings

Meeting with a family group can be a powerful tool for change and the resolution of problems.(29) It is important to prepare properly for such meetings, and to decide, usually with the patient, who should be there and which members of staff will be the most appropriate facilitators. It is often helpful for the team to work in pairs; for example, the doctor might begin with an overview of the illness and its history, to be followed by the social worker exploring the family's reaction to it. The family should do most of the talking. The aim is to help them resolve the issues that they identify as significant in a way that feels reasonably comfortable for them, not to assume responsibility for solving all the problems for them. The family may need to experience new ways of relating to one another. For example, they may need to be prompted to allow each other to talk without interruption; a child may need to be invited to speak for herself/himself. They may need help to address painful issues: 'I think everyone in this family is wondering what will happen when Mum isn't here to look after you all.'

Groups

Group work will normally involve people who share similar problems or experiences, but who are otherwise strangers to each other. For instance, bereaved fathers may meet to share the practical and emotional problems of bringing up their children alone. Patients may use a group to explore feelings about their illness. Bereaved children and adults may gain increased confidence from the normalization of grief that group work permits in contrast to their social communities where they may feel excluded or misunderstood.

Such groups have many benefits.(30) Members will hear others express the difficulties they felt too embarrassed, guilty, or frightened to share. Individuals within the group will increase their self-esteem by giving support as well as receiving it. Group work does not represent a 'cheap' alternative in terms of manpower or time. Groups are often more effectively run by two leaders who will need time for preparation before a session and time for assessment and discussion after it. Leaders themselves will need supervision, training, and support.

Working with children

Children facing bereavement have similar needs and emotions to adults. However, they may be expressed differently, for example, through behaviour rather than words.(31) Many studies make clear the cost of inadequate support and involvement for children facing the death of someone close to them.[32] Children may respond with emotional and behavioural disturbance both at the time, throughout childhood, and on into adulthood. Significant factors influencing the outcome of bereavement include the relationship of the child with the ill person before the death, the openness of family communication, the availability of peer and community support, and most importantly, the extent to which the child's parenting needs have continued and will continue to be met.[33] Palliative care professionals have a responsibility to ensure that potential difficulties for children are minimized and social workers possess specialist skills in this area. Christ's work demonstrates their role and gives clear pointers for helping based on developmental observations.[34]

It is impossible not to communicate with children. Terminal illness causes enormous changes within the family and children quickly sense when something so serious is happening. They pick up the emotions around them, read body language, overhear conversations, piece together chance remarks by neighbours and school friends, and see the evidence of physical deterioration. However, children's apparent vulnerability often evokes an impulse in both parents and professionals to protect children from the truth. The difficulties of deciding what level of information is appropriate and what words to use, added to the fear that saying the wrong thing will make matters worse, often lead to an excluding silence. Exclusion leads to isolation, leaving children unprotected from their fantasies and unsupported in their feelings. Like adults, children need appropriate involvement, an opportunity to ask questions and to receive information and reassurance, a chance to express and share their feelings in safety and help to remember.[35] This support needs to be delivered in ways that are appropriate to their age and individual level of understanding and this can only be determined by asking them about their experiences.[36]

Help for children has to start with their parents and families who will be around long after the professionals have disappeared. The task of professionals is to help parents to help their children. Parents may have good reasons for their reluctance to share information about illness and death with their children. They will be struggling to maintain some control in an uncertain situation. They themselves will be grieving and they may want to protect their children from this pain. The child may also want to protect its parents by trying to pretend that nothing is happening. It is often necessary to work with parents on their own before children's needs can be addressed. For example, a couple who cannot openly acknowledge impending death between themselves are not well placed to help their children.

We do not help parents by taking over from them—they know their children best, but we can offer them support, encouragement, and practical help. We can begin by creating environments that release parents from the expectation that children should not be involved. We can invite their presence in an in-patient unit, perhaps with a designated area with small chairs and a toy box. Equipment, such as dolls in beds, puppets, toy medical kits, and telephones, can help children to act out their concerns and to ask questions. Drawing can help them to express and control powerful emotions that they lack the vocabulary to voice. There are a number of specially designed drawing and creative workbooks available for this purpose.[37,38] Parents may appreciate advice about their child's likely understanding of death, their needs as they face bereavement, and the kinds of explanation and vocabulary appropriate to their developmental needs at different ages. Professionals must, of course, respect the family's own belief system. Lists of books and leaflets for parents to read for themselves[39] or to read with their children[40] will often be appreciated. For many parents this will be sufficient and they will then want to speak to their children alone. Others may welcome sharing the task with a professional.

Parents may be reassured by the suggestion that a professional meet them and their children to discuss changes in the family and to answer questions about the illness. Just being part of one such direct conversation can help parents to feel confident enough to continue for themselves.[41] Children facing the death of a parent need reassurance about their own continuing care and assistance in managing their inevitable separation anxieties. Whether we raise it or not they will be wondering who will look after them and perform the familiar activities such as taking them to school. It is an enormous relief to them and their parents when these painful issues are addressed. This is particularly important when a single parent is dying. Children also need explicit reassurance about the illness itself, for example, whether it is contagious, and to know that their own thoughts or behaviour could not have caused the death. Parents may need encouragement to widen their child's support network by involving other adults close to them such as teachers, clergy, or friends and relatives. Parents sometimes need assistance to anticipate and understand altered or difficult behaviour in their grieving children.

Children learn to grieve by observing others and families can be encouraged to understand that sharing feelings often helps, as does involvement in important rituals such as viewing the body, attending the funeral, or being given something that belonged to the dead person. Such activities help children to feel included and act as tangible reminders of the existence of the dead person and their importance. Professionals help parents by giving them information so that they and their children can decide together about what they feel comfortable with. Klass and Silverman's work on 'continuing bonds' emphasizes the importance of memories and shared remembering.[42]

Listening and talking

Listening and talking to patients is one of the key tasks in palliative care. Most dying patients are not looking to carers, professional or family, for solutions to their situation. They want someone to share the problems with; what helps people who are grieving is someone trustworthy who will listen to their experiences and help them explore the depths of their pain without offering false reassurance.

People facing loss awaken powerful feelings in the professionals who meet them. We cannot listen properly to the loss of others if our own losses, actual or feared, are unexplored and unresolved. Work with the dying often makes us worry about not coping or about becoming over-involved. We do not know what to say; we do not know how to 'make things better'. We have to learn how to share what we do not know as well as our knowledge, and above all, how to listen accurately.

Silence is an important part of listening. Professionals often misinterpret and feel uncomfortable with silence. They may interrupt too readily rather than allowing the patient to express his concern for himself. Silence is a necessary part of the individual's exploration of his thoughts and feelings. Prompts should be gentle and open—'You have been quiet for a long time now. I wonder if it would help you to share some of your thoughts.'

The professional must use language sensitively. Questioning should be direct but unassertive: 'What is the worst thing for you at the moment?' The use of clear, simple, feeling words such as 'sad, angry, death, guilty' helps in the expression of emotions. Body language can be both observed and used. 'You say you are feeling fine, but you look so very tense and anxious.' Appropriate touch can convey understanding and comfort when words seem inadequate.

For some people and some circumstances talking and listening may be ineffective.[43] Ritual is an alternative way of reaching feelings. Familiar rituals can offer great comfort, such as a cup of tea or the rites of prayer and religious observance.[44] New rituals can be created to meet new needs. A team member may encourage a whole family to hold hands or to spend a moment in silence remembering their love for one another. A bereaved daughter may finally be able to express her ambivalent feelings towards her dead mother and to forgive her, by writing a letter to her and burying it at the grave.

Sharing information

Personal information received from patients and families places particular responsibilities on team members. All palliative care professionals will operate within a professional framework requiring respect for the individual's privacy and autonomy and underlining the ethic of confidentiality. However, confidentiality can sometimes suffer unnecessarily in the particular atmosphere of the multiprofessional team. The need to pass on personal information must always be questioned; it is neither right nor necessary that every team member should know everything a patient or relative shares with an individual within that team. Patients choose who they talk to. Wherever possible the permission of the patient or family member should be sought explicitly: 'Thank you for telling me such an important and difficult thing. Would you mind if I tell other members of the team looking after you?' No one needs to know more than will enable them to fulfil their own role in caring for the patient. A volunteer car driver, for example, does not need to know details of the patient's diagnosis but will need to know that he uses a walking frame.

Within teams we must be clear about why we want information. Often, in the rapidly developing environment engendered by terminal illness, the emotional truth perceived and expressed by patient or family is more important than amassing painstaking details about the past. The desire for more information can represent power, confirmation of inclusion in the 'inner circle', or just plain inquisitiveness. A test of the trust necessary for teams to function well is the willingness of members to accept that another may hold confidential information and use it appropriately.

Recording of information also demands great care. What is written, particularly if it is subjective opinion, can easily assume the status of objective truth. Recording should always be undertaken with regard to the possibility of patient and family access. Good recording can assist co-ordinated care and avoid duplication of enquiry.

Case study

Introduction

This case study is intended to illustrate the most demanding form that the social work task takes. Janet Skinner (no real names are used here) and her family faced a series of difficult and interconnected medical and social problems associated with Janet's death. These concerned her attempted suicide, her marriage, her children, and the threat of breast cancer in succeeding generations. The scale and breadth of her problems are untypical but they illustrate the sequence of assessment and intervention, and the value of a competent and thoughtful professional approach.

Janet was 36 when she was admitted to St Christopher's Hospice. She had been married to her husband Rob for 12 years and they both knew she could no longer be cured. She had two children, Susan aged 7 and Paul aged 5. Her breast cancer had been diagnosed 5 years previously and was at that time treated with surgery, radiotherapy, and chemotherapy. She remained well and disease free for two and half years when evidence of metastatic disease in the lung and liver was discovered. She received further chemotherapy which she tolerated very poorly.

Three months later she presented with multiple brain metastases and an enlarged liver, and was again treated with chemotherapy and cranial irradiation, despite her previous low tolerance of the treatment and her poor prognosis. She developed a left sided weakness, walking became increasingly difficult, and she began to use a wheelchair. She was cushingoid. She became depressed and cancelled a hospital appointment. On the evening before her rescheduled appointment she took an overdose of drugs and cut her wrists whilst her husband was busy getting tea for the children. Janet was admitted to the hospice from the local hospital who had treated her following the suicide attempt.

The assessment

Individual

Janet expressed sadness and anger about the many losses she was facing; she had lost her role as mother, involvement in and a sense of security about her children's future, her physical attractiveness, a normal family life, and her faith in a caring God. She was also angry about the treatment she had endured, given its eventual futility. She felt she had been trapped into continuing with active treatment and on the day of her admission said that she 'just wanted to die'.

Janet experienced her pain as total and unendurable but she also desperately wanted to live to be a mother for her children. She described them

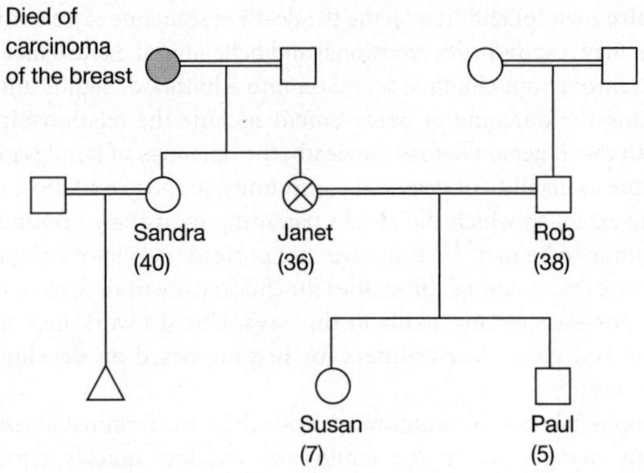

Fig. 1 Family structure.[45]

being shunted between friends and neighbours and told us that it was her son's birthday next week and that she would be useless to him. Janet felt very guilty about her suicide attempt and asked about the possibility of having further chemotherapy at the hospice. Above all, she felt completely powerless.

Family

Everyone in the family was affected by Janet's illness. It emerged that Janet's mother had also died of breast cancer when Janet was the same age as her own daughter was now (Fig. 1). Her father was reliving the loss of his wife in the loss of his daughter.

Janet's older sister, Sandra, was pregnant. She had been trying to conceive for many years. Amniocentesis the previous week had confirmed that the foetus was both healthy and female. Sandra and Janet knew what it was like to lose a mother. Sandra felt that giving birth while her sister was dying was 'obscene'.

Janet's husband, Rob, concerned the team by his noticeable reticence. He was silent throughout the procedures of his wife's admission, merely expressing concern that he might be late collecting the children from school.

The team was informed that the children had not been told about their mother's specific illness or prognosis, just that she was 'ill'. The family said that they had become clinging and difficult to get to bed at night.

Physical

Money was not a problem for this family. However, concerns were expressed about how Janet could manage at home, even on a visit, in her wheelchair with increasing weakness making transfers difficult. How would she get to the lavatory, could she negotiate the stairs, what would happen if she fell?

Social

Janet and Rob had had a wide circle of friends and an active social life. However, the stresses and upheaval of her illness and treatment had caused them to become isolated. The consequences of this isolation were that Janet and Rob were no longer getting emotional support or sufficient practical help from their friends, family, and community network. Janet was refusing visitors and had stopped attending the local church or seeing the vicar. The children's teachers were not fully informed about Janet's illness. Rob was relying on a series of temporary arrangements with neighbours to care for his children while he tried to continue with his job. Janet's and Rob's parents wanted to help but they were uncertain both about how to offer help, and what help they could best give.

Intervention

This family were perceived to be in emotional crisis, unable to cope with the problems facing them. Just as the scream of pain demands a response from the palliative care team, so does the scream of emotional anguish. The family did not appear to be able to communicate with one another. They were all stunned by Janet's suicide attempt. The team thought that if this pain and guilt was not addressed, Janet's wider family, and in particular her husband, would be unable to offer both Janet and her children the support and care they needed so badly. However, at this stage it was impossible to assess the problem fully and it was clear that there were many potentially conflicting individual needs. The team therefore decided to see the family individually, both to allow them to express their emotional pain and in order to understand what was going on.

Individual meetings

Rob and Janet both individually revealed that a major source of anguish and anger was a love affair of Rob's which had resulted in a child. The love affair had ended but Rob knew that Janet had not forgiven him for his betrayal of her, particularly whilst she was ill. Rob felt guilty and wanted to repair his relationship with Janet, yet felt trapped by his past. Janet feared that once she was dead he would create a new family for his daughters by marrying his former girlfriend.

Janet's sister was uncertain about continuing her pregnancy. Both she and Janet had lost their mother; Janet's children were now losing theirs. Sandra was wondering whether the same would happen to her unborn child. Janet and Sandra both feared that their daughters would repeat the same cycle of events.

Although the team had decided that the social worker needed to have a prominent and co-ordinating role in these meetings, the variety of team members involved allowed significant later interventions. For example, an early meeting with the chaplain paved the way for a later service in the hospice chapel focusing on peace and forgiveness with the laying on of hands. This ritual was profoundly helpful to Janet.

The data from these initial, individual meetings seemed to predict an even more hopeless future. It did, however, pinpoint some important issues for joint meetings. The team began to create a series of specific objectives against known problems.

Having met Janet and Rob individually we were aware of their conflict and the source of the distance between them. We needed to try to achieve a sufficient reconciliation between them for them at least to address their children's needs together. Sandra needed to talk to her husband about her fears and her pregnancy. The children needed information and support.

Joint meetings

Rob and Janet voiced a wish to be seen together, although neither of them was hopeful about the outcome. They expressed enormous and vociferous anger towards one another. It was necessary to confront them very directly: 'Is this really how you want things to end?' The turning point was Rob's open expression of anguish at his inadequacies as a father. He wept at his inability to iron his daughter's dress for her brother's birthday party. He and Janet began to share their pain as well as their anger, and their common purpose in loving and caring for their children.

Sandra, Janet's sister, was seen with her husband and told him for the first time of her anxieties. He had felt excluded and he had not known why. Sharing their fears enabled him to support Sandra and together they decided that the pregnancy should continue.

Family meetings and the children

Susan and Paul joined their parents in a series of meetings with the social worker and the doctor. They were encouraged to ask questions: 'What is wrong with Mummy?' 'Why hasn't Mummy got any hair?' 'Why does her breathing sound funny?' They expressed their feelings: 'I try hard not to cry because I'm scared I'll upset Daddy.' They gradually came to a realization of the gravity of their mother's illness and it was Rob who Susan finally asked: 'Is Mummy going to die?'. He was able to answer her directly and began to express more confidence in his role of father. Janet was very upset by these meetings but also reassured and moved by the children's expression of love for her: 'I love you Mummy, I want you to come home.'

These meetings and meetings with other family groupings succeeded in creating a calmer and more positive atmosphere in which Janet and her husband could set goals for the future. The couple began to request and share appropriate information and take control. During the family meetings, and subsequently, they took a number of decisions and actions.

1. Janet decided against further active treatment.
2. Janet's family and her sister's family had a meeting with a consultant who specialized in genetic cancer counselling.
3. Janet planned her own funeral and had special watches engraved for the children to keep after her death. She had not been given any proper explanation of her mother's death nor attended the funeral, and wanted things to be different for her children.
4. The family as a whole discussed the approach they would take towards the children's needs as they faced bereavement. With Janet's help they planned an advertisement for a nanny.
5. The headmaster of the children's school came to the hospice to discuss future options for their education with Janet and Rob.
6. Janet and Rob's parents and friends arranged a rota for visiting and helped Janet to get home most weekends and to go out to the theatre and restaurants.
7. With the help of a nurse escort from the hospice Janet and Rob planned and successfully completed a short holiday abroad with the children. It was important to Janet that the children had one last family memory involving her that was fun.

After death

The social worker saw Rob and the children on three occasions. Together they discussed the impact of the death, the funeral, the children's behaviour at school and home, and the family's grief. With Rob's permission the social worker again contacted the children's class teachers to discuss the help that might be offered in school. A volunteer bereavement counsellor was in touch with the parents of Janet and Rob.

Difficulties

Helping this family posed many difficulties for the team. It was difficult not to become personally involved with the intensity of their pain. We certainly neglected this area for the nurse who accompanied them on holiday. As the social worker I can remember how difficult it was to say good-bye to Janet when I went on annual leave knowing she might well be dead on my return. Janet herself solved this for me: 'I want to say good-bye. I probably won't be here when you get back.'

We had to grapple with setting boundaries for Janet and her family, boundaries that they could not be expected to set for themselves. Rob needed us to tell Janet when he and she could no longer cope with the visits home. However, we also needed to remember that we were not part of the family and that they needed to make their own decisions and to experience their own pain. Janet died peacefully 8 weeks after her admission to the hospice. Rob and her father were present.

The wider role

So far we have examined the social work task to which all members of a palliative care team will contribute, including the social worker. Next we examine the wider and more specific roles of the social worker within palliative care.

The balance of the social worker's work will depend on the circumstances of the institution in which they work and on the other skills that are available within the team. For instance, a part-time worker, whose colleagues are experienced at counselling patients, might focus on bereavement services; a social worker at a day centre might specialize in group work. However, the components of the social worker's task are likely to include internal consultancy, community liaison, user involvement, equality of access, training and the development of social work practice, and staff support and management.

Internal consultancy

The basic component of a typical social worker's role will be the support of nurses and doctors in carrying out the social work task. At one extreme the support will be simple advice; at the other it will be taking a leadership role in the management of a specific patient and their family. In effect the social worker will operate as an internal consultant and as such must understand the major concerns of the other professionals. In fulfilling this role the social worker should be involved in the day-to-day decisions about how best to manage individual patients. He or she will not be an effective resource if they are only summoned from their office when someone thinks they are needed. Social workers will also contribute to policy advice within the palliative care team: how to respond to suicide threats; what facilities should be provided for children.

Community liaison

Social workers will normally assume responsibility within the palliative care team for liaison with the community and its non-medical resources. This task requires both routine general contact and specific action on behalf of individual patients and their families. The specific action will be to create a 'package of care' for the patient in question perhaps involving both the resources of the social worker's institution and those of the wider community. For example, these might include domestic help, adaptations to the home, meals on wheels, childminders, and nightsitters. The community resources which may be available for tapping include money from government agencies or charities, or the time and attention of community social workers or local voluntary groups. Help may also be available from or through school teachers, community nurses, and family doctors.

User involvement

Any assessment of the role of social work in palliative care is incomplete without the opinions of the users of the services provided.[46] Social workers may also play an important part in developing user involvement not just in commenting on existing services but as active partners in the design and development of new ones.[47] For example, two parent users of a children's bereavement service drew attention to the particular needs of bereaved adults who had become single parents through the death of a partner rather than divorce or separation. They established and led a new service, supervised by a social worker.[48] Social workers may also be involved in providing for the training needs of both users themselves and the professional staff who work with them.

Equality of access

The training and community experience of social workers mean that they should be key resources in the important moves to examine and respond to the challenges of equal access and opportunity in palliative care. Many palliative care services operate in multicultural communities and are increasingly seeking to improve access to their services. If services are to become truly available, thought needs to be given to the different groups in any given population and the different ways in which they may use health services. This process operates at every level, from the efforts to extend primarily cancer centred palliative care services to those patients with progressive non-malignant disorders,[49] to the consideration of ways of improving knowledge of palliative care services and access to them by people from ethnic minority communities. Issues of disability, gender, race, and sexual orientation represent challenges to develop antidiscriminatory practice both for staff responding to patients and families and for institutions in their plans for training and recruitment of those staff, both paid and voluntary.[50] For example, do the volunteer counsellors in a bereavement service represent a cross-section of the communities they seek to serve? Social workers should assist their services to develop equal opportunity strategies including clear and well-publicized codes of conduct and complaints procedures. They should also be available to help with the training needs of other staff.

Culture affects us all. The crisis of death may make an individual's relationship with his or her culture and spiritual roots deeper and closer, or may reveal conflicts, with generations in transition between their family's culture and local cultural practices.[51] The dying who have experienced previous persecution as a result of political, racial, or religious differences will often have special needs as they re-experience traumatic losses. Everyone deserves respect for their individual cultural values and expectations. It is important, therefore, to clarify individual preferences about cultural and religious practices as well as improving general knowledge about the likely needs of specific groups.[52]

In 1995, the National Council for Hospice and Specialist Palliative Care Services in the United Kingdom published a report on access to services by members of black and ethnic minority communities in which the need to monitor take-up of services was emphasized.[53] We cannot assess whether our services are accessible until we are aware of how much potential users know about the services, and until we have accurate and detailed data on who is actually using our services and the reason why those who choose not to do so, decline. In 2001, in a follow-up report for the National Council, Firth commented that inadequate ethnic monitoring, an exclusive cancer focus, insensitivity, racism, and lack of cultural awareness, remained key issues.[54] However, she also noted progress in studies and fieldwork on patient and carer needs; for example, research on Bangladeshi carers[55] and Black Caribbean carers.[56] Simplified fact files about cultural practices are criticized as de-skilling by Gunaratnam.[57] Firth comments that what is 'missing in much of the culture/ethnicity discourse is an empathetic appreciation of the importance of faith to many individuals from religious communities.'

Training and the development of social work practice

Social workers should lead the development of social work practice within their institutions. This should include both the development of the service provided and the development of the skills required to support the service. Service development activities might include setting up a multiprofessional group to examine potential improvements in the care offered to relatives immediately after the death. They will also include individual activity; for example, social workers should ensure that their colleagues have access to good written material such as booklists for a bereaved child or leaflets explaining how to claim state benefits. Social workers will want to develop and write their own publications, particularly where these need to be tailored to their institutions or their local community.

Development of social work practice within the institution should extend naturally into skills training and development. Sharing and passing on skills should also flow from the internal consultancy role; all joint work with patients is an opportunity to learn new skills and understand new perspectives, both for the social worker and his or her colleagues. More formal contributions to the development of skills might include, for example, training sessions for nurses, preferably integrated into the nursing profession's own training and development programmes. Training is also a way of changing practice within the team; for example, informal training sessions for multiprofessional teams on subjects such as 'coping with anger' or 'talking about sex' can be used to improve the whole team's performance and confidence in dealing with specific problems.

In the United Kingdom and other countries, palliative care can also form a substantial part of formal social work training at both qualifying and post-graduate levels.

Staff support and management

Social workers who successfully involve themselves in service and skill development are likely to find themselves also involved in staff support. Palliative care workers can enrich their work from their experience of the death of their own friends or relatives; however, the commonality between their own experience and those for whom they care is also a potential difficulty with which they may need help. For instance, the ethics of sedation and the proper response to relatives' questions such as 'Why can't you put Dad out of his misery?' may arise both as practice issues and as personal issues for those involved. Social workers who take some leadership in the service development of their institution will, in setting policy on ethical questions, also need to take some leadership on ethical questions in training and in response to the personal concerns raised by staff. They may also become members of clinical ethics committees.

Occupational stress is increasingly seen as the result of a dynamic interaction between the person holding an individual job and the environment in which he or she is employed.[58] It is now generally recognized that an effective support system will include both personal and organizational mechanisms. Papadatou's studies begin to examine the impact of culture and inter-professional differences.[59,60] She notes that meaning making is a social as well as a personal process and that individual values and assumptions may be supported or undermined by the explicit and implicit rules and values of the working environment. Social workers and counsellors are well placed to examine the unconscious processes of projection and denial that exist in palliative care.[61,62] Social work's insistence upon the value of clinical supervision is beginning to be recognized by other professional groups. Sheldon's study of the specialist social worker in palliative care also emphasizes the value of recognizing limits and the importance of working creatively within them.[63]

Social workers should also have a role in managing the wider issues within their institution. They should be involved in setting policy on patient care, as well as decisions on individual patients. They are likely to be involved in admissions, staff recruitment, quality control, clinical governance, and education and training services, both internal and external. They will specifically manage their own responsibilities such as welfare services and volunteer bereavement services. They may be called upon to initiate and manage innovative interprofessional practice.[64] Ideally, social workers will also be able to influence and take part in the management process of the institution itself.

Extending the service

The wider values and goals of palliative care are often under-resourced and poorly acknowledged. Support is improving; for instance, in the United Kingdom specific bereavement services are now normally established after major disasters. However, the extent to which the community provides resources or acknowledges the need for such services depends on how those in the field spread their message and how they demonstrate their effectiveness and value. Social workers have a particular duty in this area as they are the professional group in palliative care that claims to have the strongest links into the community. The social worker's response to under-resourcing and poor acknowledgement should take two forms: the use of volunteers and spreading the word.

The use of volunteers

Used properly, volunteers can extend enormously the variety and scope of services offered to patients and families. Volunteers also have the advantage of representing the community from which patients come and therefore have the ability to educate and influence that community about loss, bereavement, and palliative care values. Volunteers can be used in many areas, for example, as nursing aides, hairdressers or car drivers. Social workers in palliative care will frequently want to provide counselling for bereaved relatives. One social worker can supervise a team of six volunteers, each carrying a caseload of six people, thus providing a considerable volume of service at reasonable cost. The use of volunteers should not be a reason for reduced quality; an effective volunteer bereavement service should select its volunteers rigorously and provide appropriate training.[68] It will have a programme for extending and maintaining skills through group events and supervision and will certainly aim to be a genuinely professional service and not a untutored or unfocused provision of 'tea and sympathy'.

Spreading the word

The message of palliative care is relevant in many settings within the wider community, and the resources that the community devotes to palliative care depend upon effective advocacy of both our work and our message. Social workers within palliative care should be involved in a broad spectrum of activities that serve to spread the message. At one end of the spectrum these will be an extension of the normal liaison with other local organizations concerned with the care of patients, at the other it may include political lobbying and direct attempts to influence decisions in favour of palliative care.

The direct task of liaising with other local caring organizations for the benefit of individual patients may broaden in a number of ways. For example, a social worker may become involved in lecturing to staff in a general hospital about the care of dying patients, or in helping a local health centre to develop its approach to terminal care in the community. Other contacts, such as with school teachers, funeral directors, community social workers, or welfare workers in large public or commercial organizations, may turn into opportunities to offer training or support to other professionals who have to deal with the consequences of death.[65] For instance, a social worker in palliative care may be the most experienced resource within the community to advise a school on how to cope after the murder of a pupil. The Social Work Department at St Christopher's Hospice in the United Kingdom ran a series of training sessions for the Metropolitan Police Force on breaking bad news, in particular, informing relatives of a sudden death. This involvement eventually led to the development of a new community based service offering support to children and families bereaved through sudden death.[66]

In addition to influencing attitudes locally, social workers should participate in the development of palliative care regionally, nationally, and internationally. By the nature of their work, social workers in palliative care are widely dispersed, and it is important that this fragmentation does not cause the social workers' perspective to be lost. Social workers should seek roles on advisory committees and offer their expertise and advice both to specialist groups, such as the specialist disease charities, and to government. When appropriate, social workers should be prepared to lobby actively for change. For instance, in the United Kingdom the Association of Hospice Social Workers spearheaded a successful campaign to change welfare benefit rules so that terminally ill patients could claim a special attendance allowance more quickly. They are also active in campaigning for the palliative care needs of those with severe mental health problems and those with learning disabilities.[67]

Finally, social workers must be involved in defining the future of palliative care. We have come to understand more and more about the medical aspects of palliative care, but we know little about the long-term impact of terminal illness on family members and even less about what helps them. Social workers should increasingly be involved in developing a better understanding of the psychosocial aspects of palliative care, and in the implementation of new ways of caring for patients and their families. It is vital that social work's unique perspectives remain integrated with the mainstream provision of palliative care. These perspectives offer reminders of the importance of the patient's relationship with society and its institutions and community attitudes, cultural beliefs, and values. In a health care environment in which most professionals are still only trained in one-to-one communication skills, the skills of working effectively with the relationships, groups, and systems in which most of life is lived and dying takes place, must not be ignored.

References

1. **Earnshaw-Smith, E.** (1982). Emotional pain in dying patients and their families. *Nursing Times* **78**, 865–7.
2. **Speck, P.W.** *Being There—Pastoral Care in Times of Illness.* London: SPCK, 1995.
3. **Kissane, D., Bloch, S., and McKenzie, D.** (1997). Family coping and bereavement outcome. *Palliative Medicine* **11**, 191–201.

4. **Kissane, D.** et al. (1998). Family grief therapy: a preliminary account of a new model to promote healthy family functioning during palliative care and bereavement. *Psychooncology* **7**, 14–25.
5. **Oliviere, D., Hargreaves, R., and Monroe, B.** *Good Practices in Palliative Care: A Psychosocial Perspective.* Aldershot: Ashgate, 1997.
6. **Monroe, B.** (1995). It is impossible not to communicate – helping the grieving family. In *Interventions with Bereaved Children* (ed. S.C. Smith and M. Pennells), pp. 87–106. London: Jessica Kingsley.
7. **Oswin, M.** *Am I Allowed to Cry?* London: Souvenir Press, 1991.
8. **Randall, F. and Downie, R.S.** *Palliative Care Ethics. A Companion for all Specialities* 2nd edn. Oxford: Oxford University Press, 1999.
9. **Vachon, M., Kristjanson, L., and Higginson, I.** (1995). Psychosocial issues in palliative care: The patient, the family and the process and outcome of care. *Journal of Pain and Symptom Management* **10**, 142–50.
10. **Barkwell, D.P.** (1991). Ascribed meaning: a critical factor in coping and pain attenuation in patients with cancer-related pain. *Journal of Palliative Care* **7**, 5–14.
11. **Herth, K.** (1989). The relationship between level of hope and level of coping response. *Oncology Nursing Forum* **16** (1), 67–72.
12. **Hodgson, C.** et al. (1997). Family anxiety in advanced cancer: a multicentre prospective study in Ireland. *British Journal of Cancer* **76**, 1211–14.
13. **Kirschling, J.M., ed.** *Family-Based Palliative Care.* New York: Howarth Press, 1990.
14. **Smith, N.** (1990). The impact of terminal illness on the family. *Palliative Medicine* **4**, 127–35.
15. **Payne, S., Smith, P., and Dean, S.** (1999). Identifying the concerns of informal carers in palliative care. *Palliative Medicine* **13**, 37–44.
16. **Kristjanson, L.** et al. (1997) Family members care expectations, care perceptions, and satisfaction with advanced cancer care. *Journal of Palliative Care* **1**, 5–13.
17. **Bechelet, L. and Boultwood, L.** (2001). Welfare and benefits issues affecting people with terminal illness. *Palliative Care Today* **X** (1), 10–11.
18. **Oliviere, D.** (1999). Culture and ethnicity. *European Journal of Palliative Care* **6**, 53–6.
19. **Field, D.** (2000). What do we mean by psychosocial? National Council Briefing Paper, No. 4, London.
20. **Sheldon, F.** (1997). *Psychosocial Palliative Care. Good practice in the Care of the Dying and Bereaved.* Cheltenham: Stanley Thornes, 1997.
21. **Gallagher, D. and Monroe, B.** (2000). Psychosocial care. In *Palliative Care in Amyotrophic Laterel Sclerosis* (ed. D. Oliver, B.G. Borasio, and D. Walsh), pp. 83–103. Oxford: Oxford University Press.
22. **Monroe, B.** (1998). A sexual-sensitive approach to palliative care. In *Good Practices in Palliative Care: A Psychosocial Perspective* (ed. D. Oliviere, R. Hargreaves, and B. Monroe), pp. 96–111. Aldershot: Ashgate.
23. **Sheldon, F.** (1998). ABC of palliative care. Bereavement. *British Medical Journal* **316**, 456–8.
24. **Middleton, W.** et al. (1993). Pathological grief reactions. In *Handbook of Bereavement: Theory Research and Intervention* (ed. M. Stroebe, W. Stroebe, and R. Hansson), pp. 44–61. New York: Cambridge University Press.
25. **O'Brien, T. and Monroe, B.** (1990). Twenty four hours before and after death. In *Hospice and Palliative Care: An Interdisciplinary Approach* (ed. C. Saunders), pp. 46–53. London: Edward Arnold.
26. **Bremner, I.** (2000). Working with adolescents. *Bereavement Care* **19** (1), 6–7.
27. **Stedeford, A.** *Facing Death: Patients, Families and Professionals.* Oxford: Sobell Publications, 1994.
28. **Field, D.** et al. (1995). Terminal illness: views of lay patients and their carers. *Palliative Medicine* **9**, 45–54.
29. **Monroe, B.** (1993). Psychosocial dimensions of palliation. In *The Management of Terminal Malignant Disease* 3rd edn. (ed. C. Saunders and N. Sykes), pp. 174–201. London: Edward Arnold.
30. **Oliviere, D., Hargreaves, R., and Monroe, B.** (1998). Working with groups. In *Good Practice in Palliative Care: A Psychosocial Perspective,* pp. 71–93. Aldershot: Ashgate.
31. **Jewett, C.** *Helping Children Cope with Separation and Loss.* London: Free Association Books, 1997.
32. **Silverman, P.R.** *Never Too Young to Know. Death in Children's Lives.* Oxford: Oxford University Press, 2000.
33. **Worden, W.J.** *Children and Grief. When a Parent Dies.* New York: Guilford Press, 1996.
34. **Christ, G.H.** *Healing Children's Grief. Surviving a Parent's Death from Cancer.* Oxford: Oxford University Press, 2000.
35. **Dyregov, A.** *Grief in Children.* London: Jessica Kingsley, 1991.
36. **Lansdown, R.** (1985). The development of the concept of death in childhood. *Bereavement Care* **4**, 15–17.
37. **Social Work Department.** *My Book About…* London: St Christopher's Hospice, 1989.
38. **Heegard, M.** *When Someone has a Very Serious Illness.* Minneapolis, Minnesota: Woodland Press, 1991.
39. **Couldrick, A.** *Grief and Bereavement: Understanding Children.* Oxford: Sobell Publications, 1988.
40. **Social Work Department.** *Someone Special Has Died.* London: St Christopher's Hospice, 1989.
41. **Hildebrand, J.** (1989). Working with a bereaved family. *Palliative Medicine* **3**, 105–11.
42. **Klass, D., Silverman, P., and Nickman, S.L., ed.** *Continuing Bonds.* Philadelphia: Taylor and Francis, 1996.
43. **Kearney, M.** (1992). Image work in a case of intractable pain. *Palliative Medicine* **6**, 152–7.
44. **Ainsworth-Smith, I. and Speck, P.** *Letting Go* 2nd edn. London: SPCK, 1999.
45. **McGoldrick, M. and Gerson, R.** *Genograms in Family Assessment.* New York: Norton, 1985.
46. **West, A.** (2000). What service users want from specialist palliative care social work. *Hospice Bulletin* May, 3–4.
47. **Oliviere, D.** (2001). User involvement in palliative care services. *European Journal of Palliative Care* **8** (6), 238–41.
48. **Sinclair, S., Paul, A., and Kraus, F.** (2001). A self-help group for bereaved parents and carers. *Book of Abstracts 7th Congress of EAPC, 59.* Palermo, Italy.
49. **Addington-Hall, J.M. and Higginson, I.J., ed.** (2001). *Palliative Care for Non-Cancer Patients.* Oxford: Oxford University Press.
50. **Field, D., Hockey, J., and Small, N., ed.** (1997). *Death, Gender and Ethnicity.* London: Routledge.
51. **Parkes, C.M., Laungani, P., and Young, B.** *Death and Bereavement Across Cultures.* London: Routledge, 1997.
52. **Gunaratum, Y.** *Health and Race Check List.* London: Kings Fund Centre, 1993.
53. **Hill, D. and Penso, D.** (1995). *Opening Doors: Improving Access to Hospice and Specialist Palliative Care Services by Members of the Black and Ethnic Minority Communities.* London: National Council for Hospice and Specialist Palliative Care Services, 1995.
54. **Firth, S.** *Wider Horizons: Care of the Dying in a Multicultural Society.* London: National Council for Hospice and Specialist Palliative Care Services, 2001.
55. **Spruyt, O.** (1999). Community-based palliative care for Bangladeshi patients in East London. Accounts of bereaved carers. *Palliative Medicine* **13**, 119–29.
56. **Koffman, J. and Higginson, I.J.** (2001). Accounts of carers' satisfaction with health care at the end of life: a comparison of first generation black Caribbeans and white patients with advanced disease. *Palliative Medicine* **15**, 337–45.
57. **Gunaratnam, Y.** (1997). Culture is not enough: a critique of multi culturalism in palliative care. In *Death, Gender and Ethnicity* (ed. D. Field, J. Hockey, and N. Small), pp. 166–86. London: Routledge.
58. **Vachon, M.** (1995). Staff stress in hospice/palliative care: a review. *Palliative Medicine* **9**, 91–122.
59. **Papadatou, D.** (2001). The grieving healthcare provider. Variables affecting the professional response to a child's death. *Bereavement Care* **20** (2), 26–9.
60. **Papadatou, D., Martinson, I., and Chung, B.** (2001). Caring for dying children: a comparative study of nurses' experience in Greece and Hong Kong. *Cancer Nursing* **24** (5), 402–12.
61. **Speck, P.** (1996). Unconscious communications. *Palliative Medicine* **10**, 273–4.

62. **Nimmo, S.** (1997). On being a counsellor in a hospice. *Psychodynamic Counselling* **3** (2), 133–41.
63. **Sheldon, F.** (2000). Dimensions of the role of the social worker in palliative care. *Palliative Medicine* **14**, 491–8.
64. **Monroe, B.** (1997). *The Development of a Hospice Consultancy Service.* Proceedings of the 5th Congress of the European Association of Palliative Care, London.
65. **Shipman, C., Kraus, F., and Monroe, B.** (2001). Responding to the needs of schools in supporting bereaved children: a questionnaire survey. *Bereavement Care* **20** (1), 6–7.
66. **Stokes, J.** et al. (1999). Developing services for bereaved children: a discussion of the theoretical and practical issues involved. *Mortality* **4** (3), 291–307.
67. **McEnhill, L.** *Palliative Care and People with Learning Disabilities Network.* London: Hospice Bulletin, 1998.
68. **Doyle, D.**, ed. *Volunteers in Hospice and Palliative Care: A Handbook for Volunteer Service Managers.* Oxford: Oxford University Press, 2002.

14

Rehabilitation in palliative medicine

14 Rehabilitation in palliative medicine

Adrian J. Tookman, Katherine Hopkins, and Karon Scharpen-von-Heussen

Rehabilitation—a new concept or an established approach in palliative care?

The concept of rehabilitation may seem paradoxical in palliative care, especially for patients with an advanced illness who are approaching death. However, the World Health Organization identified that palliative care offers a support system to help patients live as actively as possible until death.[1] In this context, rehabilitation becomes an essential component of palliative care rather than an additional luxury. It is an approach to care that focuses on setting goals, re-enabling patients, and in helping them to adapt to their changed circumstances so that they may live fulfilling lives.[2] Maximizing an individual's psychological and physical potential should be realistic objective for all patients at all stages of their illness.

Cancer patients are now being referred earlier to specialist palliative care in their disease trajectory and are often in receipt of concomitant active therapies. Increasing numbers of patients with non-malignant conditions are being referred for palliative care advice. Palliative care has both welcomed and embraced these changes. As palliative care continues to diversify, it is likely that specialists will care for an increasing number of patients who have disabilities as a result of either their disease process or their treatment. These specialists have developed appropriate skills in multidisciplinary teamworking and patient-centred care and are ideally placed to develop further key skills in goal-setting and in helping patients to readapt. The change in the pattern of referral to palliative care has significant implications for services that adopt a rehabilitative model. Whether the provision of rehabilitation for patients with progressive disease should be the preserve of specialist palliative care clinicians is the subject of ongoing debate. There is scant evidence that such expertise is currently being provided by specialists outside of palliative care. We suggest that Specialist Palliative Care needs to be proactive in supporting patients with both palliative and rehabilitative care needs, and the emerging picture of cancer as a chronic illness makes this provision all the more imperative. These individuals require a multiprofessional approach to their care that addresses their complex and varied needs. The rehabilitative approach acknowledges these issues and, in doing so, enhances quality of life. It enables patients to find positive meaning in situations that may previously have been perceived as hopeless and, when appropriate, enables patients to prepare for their approaching death.[2]

The aim of this chapter on rehabilitation is to describe an approach to care that is appropriate for all patients who are living with advanced illness and have palliative care needs. It aims to define the role of rehabilitation in palliative care, to discuss its component parts, and to describe how it can be provided.

What is rehabilitation?

It has been estimated that approximately 14 per cent of the population in the United Kingdom and Canada has some form of disability.[3] This estimate does not include those who have a disability that has occurred as a result of cancer. The concept of rehabilitation in orthopaedics, in acute illness, for example, cardiac disease and stroke, or in chronic neurological disease, for example, motor neurone disease (MND) or multiple sclerosis (MS), is well established. Traditionally, the term rehabilitation has engendered the vision of improving and restoring health, physical function, role, family life, and employment in patients with residual disability and a prolonged life expectancy. It is therefore unsurprising that an incongruity exists in the concept of rehabilitation in the palliative care setting, where patients experience advancing, progressive disease and a limited prognosis. However, if a more inclusive definition is considered (Box 1), it becomes clear that the rehabilitative approach can be applied to any patient with palliative care needs, wherever they are in their disease trajectory. Indeed, it can be argued that using a rehabilitative approach should be an integral component of specialist palliative care.

Box 1 A definition of rehabilitation

> (The purpose of rehabilitation is to) improve the quality of survival, so that patients' lives will be as comfortable and productive as possible and he/she can function at a minimum level of dependency regardless of life expectancy.[4]

Historically, rehabilitation services have been based on a medical model that focuses on functional assessments and defines impairment, disability, and handicap as being closely allied to disease. A growing movement amongst disabled people themselves, their representative organizations, increasing numbers of health care professionals and policy makers rejects this model in favour of a social model. The social model defines impairment as: 'the functional limitation within the individual caused by physical, mental or sensory impairment', and disability as: 'the loss or limitation of opportunities to take part in the normal life of the community on an equal level with others due to physical and social barriers'.[5] The World Health Organization International Classification of Functioning, Disability and Health (ICF), previously the International Classification of Impairments, Disabilities and Handicaps (ICIDH), reflects this changing focus,[6] but goes one step further. It integrates both medical and social models into a 'biopsychosocial approach', and uses less stereotyping terminology. 'Disability' becomes an umbrella term for 'impairments, activity limitations, or participation restrictions' and the term 'handicap' does not feature. This change in focus suggests that rehabilitation should be available for all those who experience some form of disability, not just those in whom recovery is expected. The model has huge implications for those with advanced, progressive illness whether the cause is malignant or non-malignant in nature.

Cancer rehabilitation

Patients are surviving longer with cancer.[7] Prolonged survival (Box 2) can be accompanied by complex physical and psychological problems that are the result of both treatment and disease. In certain circumstances, prolonged survival can affect the recognized natural history of the disease. New patterns of disease are being recognized, with metastatic spread to unusual sites. The effect of cancer and ongoing treatment may disrupt many aspects of the patient's lifestyle. The psychological and emotional sequelae of stoma formation, radical surgery, and amputation are well documented. The long-term effects of chemotherapy, radiation therapy, and surgery can cause specific irreversible problems in the lung, pericardium, pituitary, hypothalamus, testis, kidney, liver, thyroid, etc.

The concept that palliative care is solely reserved for end-of-life issues is outdated; it is now an integral part of cancer care actively engaged in the management of patients with complex problems. The challenge for palliative care is to acknowledge these complexities and to develop skills to support cancer survivors, helping them to adopt effective coping strategies, and to live fulfilling lives. Specialists in oncology and palliative care must work collaboratively. This partnership will ultimately lead to appropriate patterns of referral and improved management. Several authors[4,9] have described the appropriateness of rehabilitation throughout the cancer journey. Their classifications are helpful in focusing on the purpose of rehabilitation at each phase of the illness (Box 3).

Significant changes have taken place in the way in which cancer care is provided within the United Kingdom in order to ensure an equitable and nation-wide structure for the organization of cancer services. The government-commissioned report[10] that outlined this reorganization supported the concept of cancer rehabilitation, but the provision of rehabilitative cancer care has yet to feature prominently in service developments. This neglect is reflected by the paucity of published literature on cancer and palliative care rehabilitation world-wide, suggesting that limited resources are available for such provision. If individuals with a diagnosis of cancer are to reach their full potential, rehabilitation needs to be brought into sharp focus and should be routinely considered as an adjunct to cancer management in the treatment, recovery, and palliative phases.[11]

The palliative care physician should be equipped with an expanded range of skills in order to respond to the changing needs of this population of patients. We have a responsibility to address all the issues faced by patients who are living with advanced cancer. It is unacceptable to encourage early referrals to palliative care and then to be unable to respond to patients' complex needs.

Box 2 Comparison of 5-year survival figures over 20 years by year of diagnosis, primary cancer site, and sex[8]

	1971–1975		1986–1990	
	Male (%)	Female (%)	Male (%)	Female (%)
Oesophagus	3	5	5	8
Stomach	4	5	9	11
Colon	22	23	38	39
Rectum	25	27	36	39
Pancreas	2	2	2	2
Lung	4	4	5	5
Melanoma	46	65	68	82
Breast	57	52	70	66
Cervix	N/A	52	N/A	61
Uterus	N/A	61	N/A	70
Ovary	N/A	21	N/A	28
Prostate	31	N/A	41	N/A
Bladder	44	42	62	57
Kidney	28	28	38	35
Hodgkin's lymphoma	55	60	71	73
Non-Hodgkin's lymphoma	27	31	41	45
All leukaemias	12	13	24	26

Rehabilitation in non-malignant conditions

It is not only those with a cancer diagnosis who may benefit from the rehabilitative approach. In recent years, specialist palliative care has developed an increasingly important role in dealing with patients with progressive non-malignant conditions whose unmet needs for symptom management have been documented.[12,13] Specialist palliative care clinicians now provide advice on symptom management and end-of-life issues to increasing numbers of these patients.[14] Clinicians should be aware that this population of patients also have unmet rehabilitative needs that require further specialist support.

Box 3 Two established classifications of rehabilitation in cancer care—these are particularly relevant to palliative care, where they are helpful in focusing on the purpose of rehabilitation at each phase of the illness

Wells (1990)[9]	Dietz (1981)[4]
Where life expectancy is good and where no residual disfigurement or disability has occurred: rehabilitation should enable resocialization and promotion of healthy life choices	Preventative rehabilitation: designed to reduce the impact and severity of expected disabilities and designed to assist the patient and carers with coping. May include pre-operative counselling. Information and education focused
Where life expectancy is good but where physical or psychological disability or disfigurement has occurred: intensive physical, psychological, and social rehabilitation may be required in order to restore meaning	Restorative rehabilitation: restores patient to their pre-illness state. Likely to move from acute to outpatient or domiciliary setting as patient returns to valued roles
Where treatment has failed and life expectancy is short: a full range of selective rehabilitation services may be required to enable optimum restoration of function and maximize remaining quality of life	Supportive rehabilitation: goal is to limit functional changes and provide support to reduce any disability or loss of function to allow the individual to overcome handicap. Focus is on adaptation to changed circumstance rather than restoration
	Palliative rehabilitation: goal is to limit the impact of the advancing disease process. Symptom control plays an increasingly important role, promoting independence wherever possible

The precise role of palliative care rehabilitation in non-cancer conditions is evolving and will inevitably undergo refinement and definition in the future. As the speciality focuses on need rather than diagnosis, it should adopt a rehabilitative approach to care that is compatible with its underlying philosophy and should not seek to duplicate existing services or to operate outside its sphere of expertise.

The rehabilitative approach

A rehabilitative approach to care places an emphasis on the maintenance or improvement of the quality of a patient's survival in physical, psychological, social, vocational, and spiritual terms. It uses the expertise of an interdisciplinary team. The approach focuses on providing a well co-ordinated service in which a patient and their family and/or carers can be supported in learning to adapt and to cope with the changing circumstances that result in disability. In the case of palliative care it occurs within the context of a progressive illness, and one in which there can be very rapid changes in both the illness and care setting. It is therefore essential to develop a strong emphasis on speed of response and careful forward planning to take account of both predictable and unpredictable deterioration.

The key elements of a rehabilitative approach include:

- support;
- an interdisciplinary approach to care;
- enabling maximization of comfort and minimization of dependence;
- enabling adaptation to current situation, coming to terms with illness and changed circumstances;
- enabling the facing of uncertainty and loss;
- realistic approaches to patient goals;
- rapid response of the team to changing need;
- anticipation by the team of potential deterioration, allowing time to address relevant issues with the patient and/or family and carers;
- effective co-ordination and liaison across care boundaries to promote seamless care;
- education and commitment of all staff to enable consistency of approach.

This approach may seem familiar; however, its application provides the specialist palliative care team with a consistent and useful framework. It allows the team to develop skills that enable patients to deal with uncertainty, to adapt to potentially distressing situations, to feel supported through transitions of their illness, and to prepare for death.

Teamwork

The Donabedian[15] framework in Box 4[16] is helpful in determining the criteria by which rehabilitation services in both cancer and palliative care services can be developed. These criteria sit well within the philosophy of specialist palliative care with its focus on multidisciplinary teamwork.

Collaborative working and partnerships between key professionals is of fundamental importance to the rehabilitative approach. Several professional groups may be involved in joint working to design a care plan that enables a patient to adapt to disability. This may result in the blurring of professional roles, which can create difficulties.[17] It can, however, result in creative and truly patient-focused care. The value of multiprofessional working is well known, but sometimes difficult to achieve. An acceptance of the primary task/objectives and a shared sense of common purpose enable a group of professionals to work as a team. The development of an agreed operational policy or a philosophy of care will allow the team to agree and define both uniprofessional and team boundaries. Engaging in such an activity identifies a team's commitment to a rehabilitative approach.

Box 4 Definitions of rehabilitation[16]

1. *Structure*—the operational characteristics of a rehabilitation service
   A rehabilitation service comprises a multidisciplinary team of people who:
   - Work together towards common goals for each patient
   - Involve and educate the patient and family
   - Have relevant knowledge and skills
   - Can resolve most of the common problems faced by their patients
2. *Process*—how a rehabilitation service works
   Rehabilitation is a reiterative, active, educational, problem-solving process focused on a patient's behaviour (disability), with the following components:
   - Assessment—the identification of the nature and extent of the patient's problems and the factors relevant to their resolution
   - Goal-setting
   - Intervention, which may include either or both of (a) treatments, which affect the process of change; (b) support, which maintains the patient's quality of life and his or her safety
   - Evaluation—to appraise the effects of any intervention
3. *Outcome*—the aims of a rehabilitation service
   The rehabilitation process aims to:
   - Maximize the participation of the patient in his social setting
   - Minimize the pain and distress experienced by the patient
   - Minimize the distress of, and stress on, the patient's family and carers

A continuum exists between multidisciplinary teamwork, where group members practice alongside other disciplines but retain autonomy and independent decision-making within their own sphere of influence, and interdisciplinary teamwork where a further degree of integration and collaboration exists, resulting in consensus decision-making. Conflict can often be avoided by anticipating that there is the potential for blurring of roles and acknowledging that certain professional groups can be dominating. Consensus views are important but do not always result in the best outcomes and it is important to clarify which member of the team has the expertise to deal with the specific issue. A properly functioning team acknowledges the strengths and weaknesses of its constituent members. It is aware of the 'unconscious processes'[18] that can take place, such as envy, rivalry, competition, etc., and will have a structure to address these issues. If these complex issues of teamwork can be tackled then this is an indication that the team is mature and functioning well. An individual team member who works outside of the agreed stated aim or agreed programme, whether through ignorance or non-compliance, may jeopardize the success of the programme for the patient. The success of any rehabilitation programme will be dependent on commitment from all involved.

The principles of goal-setting

The essence of rehabilitation is to set goals that are realistic. Rehabilitation in palliative care differs from rehabilitation in general medicine. In palliative care, a rehabilitation programme must be seen in the context of an illness that is uncertain and will cause deterioration. Consequently, both patients and professionals need to understand the implications of a poor prognosis. Patients must be supported with strategies to cope with a life-threatening illness and, where possible, to come to terms with impeding death. In these circumstances, goals that foster insight and understanding may be more important than those that facilitate physical independence. For some individuals, the focus may be their comfort, ease, and solace.[19]

Adopting a rehabilitative approach empowers the multidisciplinary team and enables it to support the patient in attaining their chosen goals.

The process of setting achievable goals can seem daunting. Goals need to be acceptable within single disciplines, between disciplines and, most essentially, to the patient.[17] The ability to determine priorities will be influenced by prognosis, and an ability to predict the most likely course of a patient's illness within a realistic timeframe is very important.

It is fundamental to involve the patient in the process of goal-setting. Patients and carers should be given clear and unambiguous information about the purpose of adopting a rehabilitative approach ensuring, at all times, that she/he understands the importance of setting realistic goals. Acknowledging a patient's priorities and having clear rationales for treatment decisions avoids conflict, confusion, and non-compliance with management plans. Goal-setting requires open and honest communication amongst all team members.

Patients eagerly accept the concept of enabling independence and self-care wherever possible. Self-determination in some aspects of life can be welcomed as an antidote to the loss of control felt as a result of the disease and treatment. Setting regular review dates and explaining the full purpose of a review to the patient at the outset can act as a further catalyst to their full participation in the programme. Their concerns and ideas should be incorporated into active goals. For some individuals review dates will be very short, perhaps a matter of a few weeks. For others a date may be set some months hence. Both the prognosis and the goals that are to be achieved will influence this. Sensitive negotiation and counselling may be required to overcome unrealistic expectations in both patients and professionals. Where the needs of family members, or carers, conflict with those of the patient, it is necessary to make carefully balanced judgements to resolve the issues. In all cases goal-setting needs to remain flexible and sensitive, responding to the changing physical, psychological, spiritual, and social domains within which all patients live. Goal-setting offers a focused care management plan providing structure and an environment for evaluation.

Delivering the rehabilitative approach in the hospital, community, and hospice/specialist palliative setting

The rehabilitative approach in palliative care is appropriate in all health care settings. Resources will dictate the capacity of an individual service to respond to the rehabilitative needs of their patients, and these will vary according to the setting in which the care is being delivered.

Within an acute hospital setting, there are many professional groups whose expertise in rehabilitation may be called upon. These will include physiotherapists, occupational therapists, speech therapists, dietitians, social services, counsellors, etc. The inpatient specialist palliative care team can be pivotal in assessing a patient's need for rehabilitation. They can discuss the rehabilitative approach with the referring team, signposting interventions and contributions from other members of the multidisciplinary team. This collaborative, rather than prescriptive, approach is often the best way of educating professional colleagues.

In the community the locus of control is different. There may be resources for rehabilitation that are part of the palliative care team's specialist services; for example, an attached physiotherapist, occupational therapist, social worker, or dietitian. Alternatively, the rehabilitation resource may be part of the generic/primary care service. The palliative care team has an important role; first, in ensuring that the rehabilitation needs of patients are assessed and met and, secondly, in enabling other health care professionals to appreciate that a rehabilitative approach can positively enhance the patient's quality of life.

The Specialist Palliative Care Unit provides further opportunities for the development and provision of a rehabilitative approach to palliative care. Inpatient, outpatient and day care facilities can provide a supportive environment where rehabilitation can become an integral component of the broad spectrum of palliative care provision. Such developments may require a philosophical shift for staff who have historically cared for highly physically dependent and frail patients by being reactive to their multiple needs rather than adopting a proactive approach to care.[20] Careful preparation and support of staff is required if rehabilitative approaches to care are to be incorporated throughout a unit. This will potentially improve clinical management by allowing staff to take a wider view of the opportunities available for assessment and intervention. It is also our experience that this approach will affect referral patterns. It is, perhaps, to be expected that there will be increasing numbers of referrals for rehabilitation in the day care/outpatient setting. However, we have also seen a growing demand for inpatient admissions for rehabilitation. Some patients are referred after periods of intense oncological treatments in acute units. These patients have multiple physical and psychosocial needs and require intensive interventions to allow them to rehabilitate fully. Some of these patients may have relatively early disease and most have complex and ongoing problems. This, in itself, presents palliative care with new challenges and opportunities to refine our approach to symptom control. It gives us the impetus to look at new strategies to manage intractable and common symptoms such as breathlessness and fatigue. It may encourage palliative care units to take a fresh view of the appropriateness of such admissions and to reflect on the position of specialist palliative care in the wider provision of health care for patients with progressive disease.

Day care/day therapy

Day care can act as a bridge between the inpatient specialist palliative care unit and the community. There is an increasingly wide range of indications for referrals to day care (Box 5)[21] and a proactive unit will have the flexibility and vision to be able to respond to changes in health care. It is a unique environment and resource that can adopt a central role in rehabilitation. A rehabilitative approach can be appropriate in the day care/day therapy setting, whatever the patient population, and a belief in the value of rehabilitation by the unit is probably the single most important factor that will determine whether or not this approach to care is adopted.

A number of factors will dictate whether a social or a medical model of care predominates in the day care unit. These include resources, geographic locality, expertise, and enthusiasm to develop innovative approaches to care. A social model may serve a population well but will not provide the fundamental package of resources that will enable a specialist rehabilitative programme for palliative care patients to be developed. A therapeutic model can be ideally placed to be a specialist rehabilitation resource (Box 6). This model is focussed on goal-setting by a defined process of

Box 5 Referral to a day therapy unit can occur for a variety of reasons[21]

- Pain and symptom control advice
- Introduction to hospice care and preparation for death
- Support for both physical and psychological problems following definitive cancer treatment. Many patients can express feelings of abandonment at this time, perceiving that support is only available during acute treatment. Some of these patients may have early disease but significant physical and/or psychosocial morbidity
- Management of long-term physical and psychological handicaps due to their cancer treatment and/or the disease itself, for example, lymphoedema management, paraplegia following spinal cord compression, radiation plexopathies
- Management of advanced progressive non-cancer conditions, particularly exploiting expertise in symptom control and pain management

Box 6 An example of a Specialist Palliative Care Rehabilitation Service

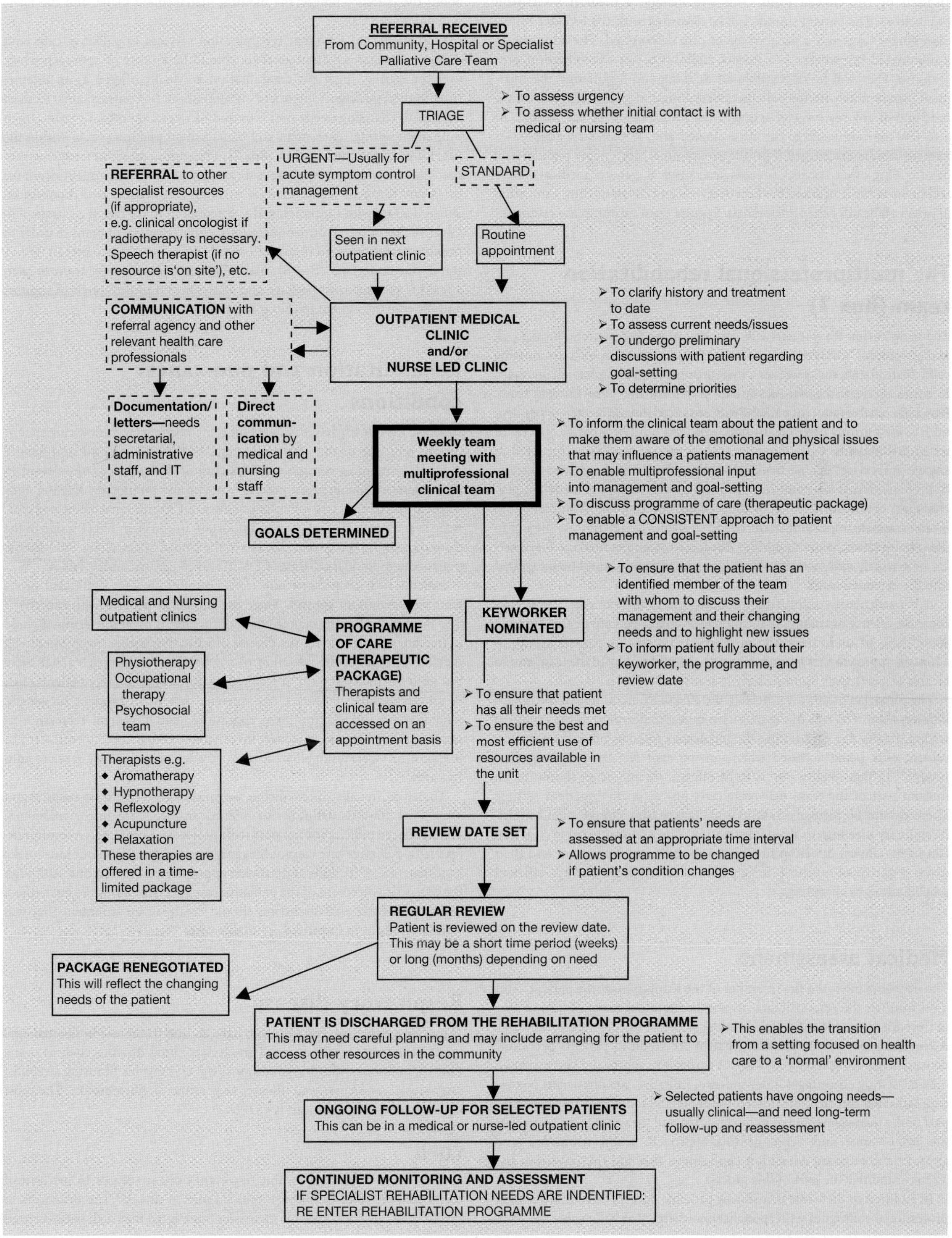

assessment and management. All patients referred to such a unit are fully assessed by the clinical team. This will include a medical assessment (see below). The patient's needs will be discussed with the broader multidisciplinary team and a programme of care determined. The adoption of a nominated key worker is a helpful addition to any rehabilitation programme. They will be responsible for defining and negotiating the treatment programme with the patient, undertaking and giving feedback on the outcome of any review, and acting as the lead contact for the patient. At a review the care package can be evaluated and, if necessary, adapted or patients can be discharged from the programme. Since many patients will be attending other services (oncological, surgical, general medical), there will be need for continued medical overview and constant communication between all health care professionals. Regular team meetings are essential.

The multiprofessional rehabilitation team (Box 7)

The team caring for patients will vary according to resources, local need, and geographic variations in skill mix. The clinical team includes nursing staff, medical staff, social worker, physiotherapist, and occupational therapist. In some services, these professionals may form the 'core' clinical team. However, rehabilitation of patients with advanced disease is often dependent on a wider group of professionals who can address specific needs of individual patients. Cross-boundary working may need to be explored to engage the services of a particular discipline. The list of the 'extended team' of professionals is long and can include a speech therapist, dietician, psychologist, counsellor, art therapist, dietician, and chaplain. Volunteers can be an extremely important resource and strategies to incorporate them into the rehabilitation team should be considered. Complementary therapists are now widely embraced into orthodox practice and should be integrated into the extended team.

It is particularly useful if the professionals in the extended team have some experience or training/education in specialist palliative care. This will allow them to understand the problems faced by this patient group, to adopt an approach that is consistent with the philosophy of the unit, and to be able to participate appropriately in teamwork.

The physician's skills are crucial to the effective functioning of the rehabilitation team. The role of the physician is best understood in the inpatient setting. In the day care setting the physician's role has often been undervalued, only being accessed when nursing staff feel there is a medical need.[23] If high-quality care is to be offered, the physician should be an integral part of the team delivering care, just as in the inpatient setting. There should be regular access to a physician, who should attend multidisciplinary meetings to share information. The result will enable clear and consistent clinical direction to be given to the team, the patient and their carers—clarity of purpose is key to delivering high-quality, efficient rehabilitation in all settings.

Medical assessment

The doctor is often the first member of the team to meet the patient. This gives him/her the responsibility of introducing the concept of goal-setting to the patient and identifying their initial priorities during the consultation. A reactive approach to symptom control can result in patients becoming dependent on clinical services whereas a proactive approach to care focused on goal-setting encourages independence. Palliative care physicians possess core skills that can facilitate this. However, rehabilitation can only become a part of the management plan if the physician and the wider team appreciate the importance and value of this approach. Good teamwork and appropriate, ongoing education can achieve this and the physician has a responsibility to be part of this process.

In addition to their role in assessing patients, doctors can empower their professional colleagues with specialist knowledge that will enable the team to plan future management effectively. The physician informs the team about the patient's illness, the medical management plans, and the likely outcomes (Box 8).

Outpatient and inpatient rehabilitation services in palliative care have different emphases. Although there should be a unity of approach whatever the setting, inpatient rehabilitation is usually offered as an intense, time-limited package. Outpatient rehabilitation, by contrast, aims to meet a patient's changing needs over a period of weeks, months, or years. In an outpatient setting, assessment and management planning occur within the timeframe of the consultation (Box 9). This contrasts with management of patients in a ward, where there is a capacity to delay non-urgent decisions in an environment where there is constant observation and supervision. When dealing with outpatients, it is essential to make rapid, accurate, and effective diagnoses, treatment decisions, and management plans in order to provide straightforward information and advice that the patient can understand and undertake (Box 8). This allows the day therapy team to plan a realistic management package and allows health professionals to support and observe the patient in the community.

Rehabilitation and non-cancer conditions

Palliative care clearly has an important role in patients with non-cancer conditions who are in the advanced stages of their illness and imminently dying.[13] The most common serious chronic diseases that are relevant to a non-cancer rehabilitation practice are chronic pulmonary disease, end-stage cardiac disease, and neurological disease. Chronic renal failure and end-stage liver disease (ESLD) are also important to consider. ESLD is one of the three most common chronic diseases in the United States, along with chronic obstructive pulmonary disease (COPD) and congestive cardiac failure.[24]

Patients with progressive non-cancer conditions have significant problems with symptom control. These are similar to patients with cancer.[13] The need for symptom management occurs not only in the terminal phase of the illness but earlier in the disease process. Our earlier involvement will inevitably result in the adoption of a rehabilitative approach. That there is a need for rehabilitation in respiratory, cardiac, neurology patients, etc., is unquestionable. However, the current lack of investment in generic rehabilitation services for these conditions, and a general reluctance of physicians to become involved in rehabilitation, could potentially put pressure on specialist palliative care services to extend its services into this area.

Therefore, in palliative medicine, we must be clear of our boundaries and must work towards defining our referral protocols, treatment guidelines, and discharge policies for patients with progressive non-cancer conditions. Specialist palliative care cannot fill gaps in service provision but must make legitimate use of its skills and provide appropriate interventions. Although the precise involvement of the palliative care specialist has yet to be defined, dialogue, debate, and discussion should create an environment that will ultimately result in improved, equitable care.

Respiratory disease

A specialist palliative care team can have an important role in the management of patients with advanced progressive lung diseases such as cystic fibrosis, pulmonary fibrotic conditions (e.g. cryptogenic fibrosing alveolitis, sarcoidosis), and chest wall diseases (e.g. scoliosis, fibrothorax). The most common of these conditions is COPD.

COPD

In the United Kingdom, chronic respiratory disease causes 13 per cent of adult disability and COPD is a major cause of this.[25] The prognosis in severe COPD is poor, and it is increasingly accepted that such patients need

Box 7 Operation of Specialist Palliative Care Team in different care settings

The specialist palliative care team operates in different care settings and has an ability to adopt a rehabilitative approach by utilizing the following resources:

Hospital

The Specialist Palliative Care Team has an important role highlighting rehabilitation aspects of clinical management. Although not directly responsible for managing the patient, the team will have a role in assessing the rehabilitation needs of patients, co-ordinating care and ensuring that referrals are made to the appropriate professional team.

Services in a hospital will include:
Site-specific clinical nurse specialists*
Physiotherapy
Occupational therapy
Social services
Speech therapy
Dietician
Chaplaincy and Psychology
Other therapists

*Site-specific nurses have an important role to play in helping the individual to adapt to the impairments caused by both disease and treatment. The preparation of patients before surgery can be seen as a key element of preventative rehabilitation for colorectal, breast, head and neck, and urology site-specific nurses. They have become an indispensable part of the cancer team. Often they are the key contact professionals and hence can be the first professional to identify new relevant symptoms. Site-specific nurse specialists may be a part of a treatment pathway or may take responsibility for specific treatment programmes. For example, the development of a nursing approach to managing breathlessness in lung cancer patients. This has, as a key aim, the identification of 'effective strategies for ameliorating the symptom of dyspnoea which can be used in addition to medical intervention'.[22] Site-specific nurses can have a focus on the preventative and restorative phases of rehabilitation. Specialist palliative care nurses can focus on the palliative phases. Both groups should have a role in supportive rehabilitation.

Community

The Specialist Palliative Care Team works with the community services and will make the primary care team aware of the rehabilitative needs of the patient.

Services in the community may include (amongst others):
Community physiotherapy
Community occupational therapy
Community dietician
Social services

Specialist Palliative Care Unit

Rehabilitation can take place on the wards and in a day therapy/day care setting. The Specialist Palliative Care Unit may also provide a resource for specialist rehabilitation.

The services may include:
Physiotherapy[a]
Occupational therapy
Complementary therapists[b]
Psychosocial support
Social support
Counselling
Spiritual resources

[a] Physiotherapy is an important part of the rehabilitation service. In addition to 'one to one' treatments, there is an important role for the physiotherapist in group work. Exercise has been shown to improve muscle strength in frail elderly populations and it is expected that similar improvements will be seen in palliative patients. In addition to physical benefits, exercise in a group setting (e.g. gym) will have emotional and social benefits. It gives patients control and is a positive approach to their treatment.

[b] Large surveys demonstrate that at least two-thirds of all cancer patients are engaged in some form of complementary and alternative practice. These treatments are often used in conjunction with standard cancer treatments. Certainly many therapies are now embraced into 'orthodox' practice and there is a public and political pressure to increase their use. Any palliative care clinician with a rehabilitation practice will have patients who are receiving complementary and/or alternative therapies. It is important to adopt a non-judgemental approach allowing opportunities for patients to discuss their use of therapies. This will also give an opportunity for the clinician to assess the therapy and give advice on its safety. The fact that orthodox practitioners now embrace many of these therapies recognizes that, although many treatments are not evidence-based, they seem to be perceived as beneficial both by patients and clinical staff. To integrate these into routine practice protects the patient from harm and exploitation. Regular medical review also protects the therapist within the rehabilitation team as it allows assessment of the patient, helping to prevent inappropriate and potentially harmful interventions from occurring. When patients wish to discuss the use of complementary therapy it presents an opportunity to forge stronger relationships. Most patients will be gratified by the chance to have a frank and honest discussion. These discussions give greater empowerment and choice in health care by encouraging patients to participate more directly in decisions about their care.

Box 8 The physician shares information with the patient and the team

Important points when sharing information with the patient:

- Aim—At all stages of illness the aim is to give patients control by assessing, then providing, a level of information that they are comfortable to receive.
- The biographic account—Many patients are keen to reiterate the details of their diagnosis and treatment to date. This allows them to express any fears or anger that they associate with those episodes or to feel reassured that the decisions enacted by their hospital teams (with or without the patient's involvement) were appropriate at the time. The doctor's role is to explain any misconceptions, to answer any questions, and to give accurate information, if available. This information can help decrease anxiety and give reassurance.
- Anticipation—The doctor has an important role in anticipating changes in a patient's condition, their future needs, deterioration, and the impact that this may have on the patient and their carers. Knowledge of oncology and general medicine is advantageous in helping to predict likely response to treatment and the course of the future illness.
- Prognosis—Some patients and/or their relatives may wish to ask about prognosis, and it is the doctor's remit to prepare the patient, family, and team for this news. The information that the doctor has gathered from the history and clinical examination and an assessment of prognostic indicators could be the key to focusing the patient, family, and team about prognosis, and this should enable realistic goals to be set. The aim is to help to prepare and to support the patient and their family to deal with uncertainty and to face loss.

Important points when sharing information with the team:

- Resource to the team—The doctor is a resource for the interdisciplinary team, and can empower the team by sharing information. It is essential to communicate the outcomes of discussions with patients, and any relevant clinical information. Reciprocity in sharing knowledge allows the whole team to consider the most effective means to support the patient and relatives, to help the patient adapt to a new level of functioning and to help the patient deal with uncertainty and loss.
- Shared learning—The clinician can endorse the value of the rehabilitative approach reinforcing the value of joint working.
- Support—Sharing information encourages a culture of openness with all members of the team. This benefits the patient; for example, new symptoms will be reported to the clinician. It also enables opportunities for relevant members of the team to be made aware of potential deterioration in a patient's condition or of anticipated death. This can be particularly important in patients who have been maintained for a long period under the care of the team where there may be a false belief that the patient is 'stable'.

Box 9 Key elements of medical care in an outpatient rehabilitation service[23]

- Initial assessment and management—Misconceptions and doubts about previous treatments can be discussed. Previous diagnoses can be confirmed or challenged. Symptom control needs are assessed.
- Contribution to initial goal-setting—This approach to management should be explored with the patient. Explanation that, even in the context of a progressive illness, management plans can achieve realistic goals.
- Contribution to development of a care package—There should be full discussion with the team, empowering the team to make realistic plans for the care package. The physician has a key role in ensuring that the team is aware of medical problems, complications, and likely future outcomes.
- Observation and monitoring—The physician needs to assess the progress of the patient continually, being aware that unpredictable changes are common.
- Co-ordination of care—With the referring team, primary care team, and the hospital. This will ensure that all relevant details about the illness are collected.
- Liaison with community and hospital services—Continuous liaison will ensure seamless care.
- Reassessment and re-evaluation—including review of symptoms and of goals.
- Rapid response to changes in patient's condition.
- Anticipation of deterioration.
- Support for patients, family, and professional carers during all phases of illness.
- Ability to discharge patients when appropriate.

good palliative care.[26] By the time advanced hypoxia is present the majority of patients, if not given long-term oxygen, will die within 3 years.

Pulmonary rehabilitation is an important part in the management of this group of patients. However, there are limited pulmonary rehabilitation programmes and patients with far advanced disease are sometimes followed-up within the specialist palliative care setting. The experience in palliative care of treating breathlessness and the value of breathlessness clinics can be exploited in this group of patients.[22,27] An active rehabilitative approach can maximize the potential in these patients whose quality of life can be extremely poor.

There are established pulmonary rehabilitation programmes in COPD that adopt a multidisciplinary programme of physiotherapy, education, exercise training, and psychotherapy to help the patient return to the highest possible functional capacity.[28] With palliative medicine having greater involvement in caring for patients with chronic pulmonary disease, there is little doubt that a rehabilitative approach can enhance the quality of life of patients. There have been few properly controlled trials looking at the benefit of pulmonary rehabilitation; however, there is increasing evidence that rehabilitation reduces symptoms and number of hospital admissions, and improves performance, exercise endurance, and quality of life.[29]

Apart from the sensory-nociceptive aspect, there are cognitive, affective, and motivational dimensions. Stress, anxiety, and isolation are all factors that can exacerbate breathlessness. Pulmonary rehabilitation aims to improve not only function, but also self-image. Psychosocial issues can be addressed and instruction in relaxation techniques can be provided. Breathlessness is a frightening symptom and, in order to avoid it, many patients become progressively less active and less fit. Exercise is an essential component of any programme and most investigators have claimed success despite wide variation in training modes, intensity, and frequency.[30] Patients often need encouragement and medical 'permission' to exercise to breathlessness. By experiencing dyspnoea in a controlled environment, they may be helped to overcome the anxiety and apprehension associated with exercise. Post-exercise dyspnoea is not harmful and, if people become fitter and more mobile, general well-being often improves.

Collaboration with the respiratory team (physicians and specialist nurses) will give a clear understanding of the management of the underlying condition and optimize palliation. In the United Kingdom, there are increasing numbers of specialist respiratory nurses whose contribution is valued by patients.[31,32]

Box 10 Adapted from text[33]

Multiple sclerosis (MS) can be identified as four different types:

1. Relapsing–remitting MS: categorized by exacerbations and remissions. Incomplete recovery leads to a stepwise progression in disability and, therefore, this category includes people with varying levels of impairment and disability. The majority of people with this form may have long periods free from new symptoms. Most eventually develop a secondary progressive course.
2. Primary progressive (or chronic progressive) MS: categorized by a relentless decline in neurological function and progressive disability following the initial attack.
3. Secondary progressive MS: occurs when relapsing–remitting MS converts to a disease pattern of a gradual accumulation of irreversible disability. This proceeds in different patterns in different people. Most commonly there is a slow deterioration, but sometimes an initial rapid progression is followed by a slow accumulation of disability. Other variations are possible.
4. Benign MS: In this group there may be a period of 10 years or more between the recognized onset of the disease and the development of a significant disability. Some of these cases convert to a secondary progressive course.

Neurological disease (see Chapter 10.6)

Specialist palliative care has an established role in the management of patients with advanced progressive neurological disease, traditionally managing patients with amyotrophic lateral sclerosis (ALS)/MND. The rehabilitation skills of a specialist palliative care team can be exploited in this group of patients who have complex symptom control needs. These are well described elsewhere in this textbook. A proactive approach to this group of patients can significantly improve their quality of life. Physiotherapy, counselling, addressing nutritional issues, and regular respite can be supportive to patients with ALS/MND. It is easy to see how this approach can be transferred into selected progressive neurological diseases, for example, new variant CJD.

The role of specialist palliative care in other progressive neurological conditions is less certain. Parkinson's disease and multiple sclerosis are two examples in which specialist palliative care has a potential role. In these conditions there is a large unmet need and if specialist palliative care takes responsibility for patients with these relatively common conditions then the services could potentially become overwhelmed. It may be more appropriate that specialists in palliative care work alongside the practitioners responsible for the care of these patients and provide advice about the most appropriate management of their palliative care and rehabilitation needs. Selected patients may benefit from the full rehabilitative resources that a specialist palliative team can provide.

Multiple sclerosis

Multiple sclerosis (MS) is an illness of progressive impairment resulting in disability. Thus, similarities can be drawn between rehabilitation in MS and rehabilitation in cancer, although the time frames differ significantly. In addition, the nature and course of disease progression in MS is variable, so that the population is heterogeneous. Expectations for outcome must be modest, and measurement should be focused on quality of life issues. The natural course of the illness is extremely variable and symptoms may appear, resolve, and reappear. This presents a challenge to workers in palliative medicine, who need to be aware of the differing presentations and patterns of disease[33] (Box 10) to allow a more accurate assessment of the likely course of the illness.

It is important to minimize the impact of disability by providing access to neurological rehabilitation. Patients with chronic progressive MS may require periodic courses of rehabilitation perhaps every 9–12 months in order to preserve the functional gains achieved at initial presentation. An extended outpatient rehabilitation programme for patients with MS appears effectively to reduce both fatigue and the severity of other symptoms associated with MS.[34]

The palliative care team may have a role working collaboratively with the neurologist and neuro-rehabilitation team in managing difficult symptoms. The patient with very advanced disease can present with multiple symptoms—spasticity, pain, urinary, or bladder dysfunction can be particularly disabling. Decisions regarding suitability for admission to an inpatient unit can be difficult because of the uncertain prognosis. However, short periods of respite or symptom control can dramatically improve the quality of life for patients with MS. Care at home can be supplemented by the effective rehabilitative approach of the community palliative care team. This approach and the responsibility of the palliative care services to manage the terminal phase of the illness give specialist palliative care services an important role in the management of patients with MS.

End-stage cardiac disease (see Chapter 10.5)

Palliative care can benefit patients with advanced heart failure.[35] Congestive cardiac failure can be considered a terminal condition, as the annual mortality in severe untreated cases approaches 60 per cent.[36] Even in mild cases, the 5-year mortality rate for patients with chronic heart disease is 50 per cent,[37] comparable with many of the common cancers. This has led some[38] to suggest that heart failure should be considered a 'malignant disease' although, at an individual level, death from heart disease may be less predictable than for cancer.

In the United Kingdom, the Regional Study of Care for the Dying[39] showed that one in six patients with end-stage cardiac disease experienced symptoms as severe as those cancer patients under the care of community or hospice palliative care services.[35]

There are well-established rehabilitation programmes for patients with cardiac disease that are primarily focused on the post-myocardial infarction phase. Palliative care rehabilitation can be important for those patients with advanced symptomatic disease who need the holistic skills that palliative care can offer. These patients often have to live with the prospect that they have an advanced illness from which they will deteriorate and ultimately die. They may have had experience of acute episodes in which they have had to face the prospect of death, and they live with the knowledge that a future acute episode may ultimately lead to their death.

Patients with cardiac disease have complex symptom control issues of which the specialist palliative care rehabilitation team needs to be aware. Lung congestion, V/Q mismatch, altered ventilatory pattern, hyperventilation, and abnormal ventilatory control all play a part in dyspnoea in cardiac failure. Fatigue, a limited exercise capacity, pain, nausea, constipation, and low mood also affect the quality of life in these patients significantly.[40]

There are many transferable skills that can enhance the quality of life of patients with heart failure and a rehabilitative approach can be particularly appropriate. A critical component of management is to enrol patients in a programme of education, counselling, physical activity, and ongoing support. The specialist palliative care physician must be aware of the available interventions and close collaboration with the referring cardiologist is critical to optimize treatment.

Box 11 Specialist palliative care skills that are transferable to a non-cancer practice

- Team approach to care
- An all-inclusive approach to symptom control, addressing physical, psychosocial and spiritual dimensions
- Specialist diagnostic and therapeutic skills in symptom control
- Decision-making appropriate to context (e.g. appropriate to stage of illness, to social situation etc.)
- Acknowledgement that patients exist in their own homes and have a family
- Specialist knowledge in the use of opioids and an awareness of alternative opioids
- Ability to recognize the dying process
- Management of the dying process

Management of chronic pain in patients who have progressive non-cancer conditions

As specialist palliative care becomes an established part of health care, referrals come from an ever-widening range of specialities. Patients with chronic severe pain can pose a specific challenge to a specialist palliative care rehabilitation practice. Peripheral vascular disease, diabetes, advanced rheumatological conditions, for example, rheumatoid arthritis and progressive systemic sclerosis are some of the progressive painful non-malignant conditions that can benefit from the skills of a palliative care physician and the experience she/he has in treating pain (Box 11). Since there is the potential for overlap between specialist palliative care and the chronic pain services, a close collaborative working relationship is crucial for best-quality care. Specialist palliative care can make a real impact in managing these patients, especially those taking opioids.

The use of opioids in chronic cancer pain is well established. Although there continues to be controversy about their use in non-cancer conditions, opioids are recommended in non-cancer pain by many experts.[41–43] Indeed, they would suggest that opioids significantly improve the function and quality of life for patients with severe intractable pain secondary to chronic advanced, progressive non-malignant conditions. The best prescribing patterns have yet to be determined and one approach is described (Box 12).

Box 12 An approach for the use of opioids in chronic non-cancer pain

- Careful patient selection is crucial.
- Pain must be opioid sensitive—a trial of opioids is a reasonable approach to assess this.
- Use controlled release preparations.
- Lay down clear ground rules about the maximum dose of opioid and the number of doses of rescue medication.
- Strictly limit the use of rescue doses of opioids—in chronic non-cancer pain it is easy for a patient to escalate both the dose of regular and rescue medication simultaneously.
- Titrate slowly, assessing effectiveness and side-effects—it can be difficult to assess effect. A functional assessment, rather than subjective reporting of pain control, is often the best guide.
- Be prepared to switch or rotate opioids—it is believed that receptor tolerance develops in very long-term use in some patients. Receptor tolerance can cause problems when assessing relative potencies of different opioids. Great caution is therefore advised when switching and rotating opioids in these situations: the new opioid may be far more potent than anticipated.
- Regular and long-term follow-up is mandatory.

Patients with advanced progressive non-cancer conditions can benefit from a rehabilitative approach. Pain impacts on all dimensions of their lives and can have significant effects on their family and friends. Current services to support these patients are limited and specialist palliative care can have a real and important part to play in these patients' management programmes. Working collaboratively with the physicians from other specialities enhances care and will ensure that patients will have their underlying pathology optimally treated.

Conclusion

Rehabilitation is an all-encompassing term, difficult to define and the responsibility of all clinicians. It is both an approach to care and a specialist area within palliative care. Rehabilitation should be an integral part of palliative and supportive care. It can bring considerable improvements in function and quality of life for seriously ill people and their families and can reduce psychological and spiritual distress. It is an approach that can give a patient the opportunity to find purpose, self-worth, and control at a time when they are experiencing a loss of independence. Rehabilitation in palliative care must be seen in the context of an illness that is often uncertain and that will inevitably progress. Therefore, the service must be able to respond rapidly, to help people adapt to their illness, to take a realistic approach to defining goals, and to help people prepare for death.

As specialist palliative care services mature and diversify it is becoming clear that they have an important role in rehabilitation for increasing numbers of patients. Referral patterns are changing for both cancer and non-cancer patients and many palliative care clinicians are responding to this by developing closer collaborative working relationships with referring teams, exploring the boundaries of their care. This evolving process is in need of evaluation (Box 13). Hopefully, it will lead to improved care resulting in meaningful and hopeful lives.

Box 13 Measurement of outcome in rehabilitation (adapted from 'Basket' of measures from The British Society of Rehabilitation medicine)

This is a list of outcome measures recommended by the British Society of Rehabilitation Medicine following a survey of rehabilitation measures in 1997.[44] These measures are now widely used. Their usefulness in the context of rehabilitation in palliative care is not yet determined. The list is a guide to available, commonly used outcome measures rather than a complete list. The scales are scientifically validated and in routine use in clinical practice in the United Kingdom by at least 10 rehabilitation units

Specific motor function tests

Generalized

Motricity Index[45]—Short measure of motor loss primarily after stroke: validity and reliability proven

Motor Assessment Scale[46]—Long test of eight hierarchical scales: good support for reliability and validity

Mobility

10 Metre Walk[47]—Simple, useful, and relevant: reliable and valid

Rivermead Mobility Index[48]—Simple to use, clinically relevant: reliable

Functional Ambulation Categories[49]—Gives detail about physical support needed by patients who are walking, particularly sensitive for transition from immobile to walking: valid and reliable

Global disability/ADL measures

Barthel Index[50]—Very widely used assessment of dependency in activities of daily living. Many different versions and modifications. Indicator of gross functional change

UK FIM ± FAM[51]—The Functional Independence Measure is a widely used measure in the United States. It assesses function globally and also addresses cognitive and psychological domains

The Functional Assessment Measure was developed specifically for use in brain injury and adds a further 12 measures to the FIM

Health Assessment Questionnaire (HAQ)[52]—Developed primarily for those with rheumatic disease

Handicap

London Handicap Scale[53]—Simple six-item assessment of handicap following stroke. Demonstrated to be equally applicable in arthritis, multiple sclerosis, and elderly care

Life Satisfaction Index[54]—Primarily designed for use with elderly people: some evidence to support its validity and reliability

Craig Handicap Assessment and Reporting Tool[55]—Developed originally for assessment of handicap in patients following spinal cord injury; recently validated for use in stroke patients

General health/mood

General Health Questionnaire (GHQ-12 or GHQ-22)[56]—Widely used, simple, and quick. It can be used to measure stress on carers. There are many versions: well-validated measure of good reliability

Hospital Anxiety and Depression Scale (HAD)[57]—Specifically designed for use with hospitalized, medically ill patients. Attempts to overcome bias caused by somatic complaints

Chronic pain rehabilitation

McGill Pain Score[58]—Widely used and translated as a standard assessment of pain in a large range of conditions: reliability, validity, and responsiveness have been tested. The value of verbal pain questionnaires over visual analogue scales is still a matter for debate,[59] much depending on whether pain itself is the focus or its effect on function

Carers

Care-givers Strain Index[60]—Short measure designed to assess strain on the carer. Used in a number of studies to assess carer strain in care of the elderly and stroke

References

1. **WHO (World Health Organization).** *Cancer Pain Relief and Palliative Care: Report of a WHO Expert Committee.* Technical Report Series, no. 804. Geneva: World Health Organization, 1990.
2. **National Council for Hospice and Specialist Palliative Care Services.** *Fulfilling Lives: Rehabilitation in Palliative Care.* London: National Council for Hospice and Specialist Palliative Care Services, 2000.
3. **Badley, E.M. and Tennant, A.** (1997). Epidemiology. In *Rehabilitation of the Physically Disabled Adult* 2nd edn. (ed. C.J. Goodwill, M.A. Chamberlain, and C. Evans), pp. 7–20. Cheltenham: Stanley Thornes.
4. **Dietz, J.H.** *Rehabilitation Oncology.* New York: John Wiley, 1981.
5. **Union of Physically Impaired against Segregation.** *Fundamental Principles of Disability.* London: Union of Physically Impaired against Segregation, 1976.
6. **World Health Organization.** *ICF: International Classification of Functioning, Disability and Health.* Geneva: World Health Organization, 2001 (www.who.int/icidh/index.htm, last accessed 1 August 2003).
7. **Capocaccia, S.M.** et al. (2001). Cancer survival increases in Europe, but international differences remain wide. *European Journal of Cancer* **37**, 1659–67.
8. **Coleman, M.P.** et al. *Cancer Survival Trends in England and Wales, 1971–1995: Deprivation and NHS Region.* Studies in Medical and Population Subjects no. 61. Cancer Research Campaign, London School of Hygiene and Tropical Medicine, Office for National Statistics. London: The Stationery Office, 1999.
9. **Wells, R.J.** (1990). Rehabilitation: making the most of time. *Oncology Nursing Forum* **17**, 503–7.
10. **Department of Health.** *A Policy Framework for Commissioning Cancer Services: A Report by the Expert Advisory Group on Cancer to the Chief Medical Officers of England and Wales (Calman-Hine Report).* London: Department of Health and Welsh Office, 1995.
11. **David, J.** (1995). Rehabilitation: adding quality to life. In *Cancer Care: Prevention, Treatment and Palliation* (ed. J. David), pp. 351–75. London: Chapman and Hall.

12. **National Council for Hospice and Specialist Palliative Care Services and Scottish Partnership Agency for Palliative and Cancer Care.** *Reaching Out: Specialist Palliative Care for Adults with Non-Malignant Diseases.* Occasional Paper 14. London: National Council for Hospice and Specialist Palliative Care Services, 1998.
13. **Addington-Hall, J., Fakhoury, W., and McCarthy, M.** (1998). Specialist palliative care in non-malignant disease. *Palliative Medicine* **12**, 417–27.
14. **Kite, S., Jones, K., and Tookman, A.** (1999). Specialist palliative care and patients with noncancer diagnoses: the experience of a service. *Palliative Medicine* **13**, 477–84.
15. **Donabedian, A.** (1966). Evaluating the quality of medical care. *Milbank Memorial Fund Quarterly* **44**, 166–206.
16. **Wade, D.T. and de Jong, B.A.** (2000). Recent advances in rehabilitation. *British Medical Journal* **320**, 1385–8.
17. **McGrath, J.R. and Davis, A.M.** (1992). Rehabilitation: where are we going and how do we get there? *Clinical Rehabilitation* **6**, 225–35.
18. **Speck, P.** (1996). Unconscious communications (editorial). *Palliative Medicine* **10**, 273–4.
19. **Watson, P.G.** (1992). The optimal functioning plan: a key element in cancer rehabilitation. *Cancer Nursing* **15**, 254–63.
20. **Flanagan, J. and Holmes, S.** (1999). Facing the issue of dependence: some implications from the literature for the hospice and hospice nurses. *Journal of Advanced Nursing* **29**, 592–9.
21. **Hopkins, K.F. and Tookman, A.J.** (2000). Rehabilitation and specialist palliative care. *International Journal of Palliative Nursing* **6**, 123–30.
22. **Corner, J., Plant, H., and Warner, L.** (1995). Developing a nursing approach to managing dyspnoea in lung cancer. *International Journal of Palliative Nursing* **1**, 5–11.
23. **Tookman, A.J. and Scharpen-von Heussen, K.S.** (2001). The role of the doctor in day care. In *Palliative Day Care in Practice* (ed. J. Hearn and K. Myers), pp. 79–93. Oxford: Oxford University Press.
24. **Fox, E.** et al. (1999). Evaluation of prognostic criteria for determining hospice eligibility in patients with advanced lung, heart or liver disease. *Journal of the American Medical Association* **282**, 1638–45.
25. **Royal College of Physicians of London** (1986). Physical disability in 1986 and beyond. A report of the Royal College of Physicians. *Journal of the Royal College of Physicians of London* **20**, 160–94.
26. **Shee, C.D.** (1995). Palliation in chronic respiratory disease. *Palliative Medicine* **9**, 3–12.
27. **Corner, J. and O'Driscoll, M.** (1999). Development of a breathlessness assessment guide for use in palliative care. *Palliative Medicine* **13**, 375–84.
28. **Petty, T.L.** (1993). Pulmonary rehabilitation in chronic respiratory insufficiency: 1. Pulmonary rehabilitation in perspective: historical roots, present status, and future projections. *Thorax* **48**, 855–62.
29. **Casuburi, R.** (1993). Exercise training in chronic obstructive lung disease. In *Principles and Practice of Pulmonary Rehabilitation* (ed. R. Casaburi and T.L. Petty), pp. 204–24. Philadelphia: WB Saunders.
30. **Belman, M.J.** (1993). Exercise in patients with chronic obstructive pulmonary disease. *Thorax* **48**, 855–62.
31. **Heslop, A.** (1993). Role of the respiratory nurse specialist. *British Journal of Hospital Medicine* **50**, 88–90.
32. **Cockcroft, A.** et al. (1987). Controlled trial of respiratory health worker visiting patients with chronic respiratory disability. *British Medical Journal Clinical Research Edition* **294**, 225–8.
33. **Ko Ko, C.** (1999). Effectiveness of rehabilitation for multiple sclerosis. *Clinical Rehabilitation* **13** (Suppl. 1), 33–41.
34. **Di Fabio, R.P.** et al. (1998). Extended outpatient rehabilitation: its influence on symptom frequency, fatigue, and functional status for persons with progressive multiple sclerosis. *Archives of Physical Medicine and Rehabilitation* **79**, 141–6.
35. **Gibbs, L.M.E., Addington-Hall, J., and Gibbs, J.S.R.** (1998). Dying from heart failure: lessons from palliative care (editorial). *British Medical Journal* **317**, 961–2.
36. **The CONSENSUS Trial Study Group** (1987). Effects of enalapril on mortality in severe congestive heart failure. Results of the Co-operative North Scandinavian Enalapril Survival Study. *New England Journal of Medicine* **316**, 1429–35.
37. **McKee, P.A.** et al. (1971). The natural history of congestive heart failure: the Framingham study. *New England Journal of Medicine* **285**, 1441–6.
38. **Dargie, H.J. and McMurray, J.J.** (1994). Diagnosis and management of heart failure. *British Medical Journal* **308**, 321–8.
39. **Addington-Hall, J. and McCarthy, M.** (1995). Regional study of care for the dying: methods and sample characteristics. *Palliative Medicine* **9**, 27–55.
40. **McCarthy, M., Hall, J.A., and Lay, M.** (1997). Communication and choice in dying from heart disease. *Journal of the Royal Society of Medicine* **90**, 128–31.
41. **Moulin, D.E.** et al. (1996). Randomised trial of oral morphine in non-cancer pain. *Lancet* **347**, 143–7.
42. **Savage, S.R.** (1999). Opioid use in the management of chronic pain. *Medical Clinics of North America* **83**, 761–86.
43. **Conigliaro, D.A.** (1996). Opioids for chronic non-malignant pain. *Journal of the Florida Medical Association* **83**, 708–11.
44. **Turner-Stokes, L. and Turner-Stokes, T.** (1997). The use of standardised outcome measures in rehabilitation centres in the UK. *Clinical Rehabilitation* **11**, 306–13.
45. **Demeurisse, G., Demol, O., and Robaye, E.** (1980). Motor evaluation in vascular hemiplegia. *European Neurology* **19**, 382–9.
46. **Carr, J.H.** et al. (1985). Investigation of a new motor assessment scale for stroke patients. *Physical Therapy* **65**, 175–80.
47. **Brandstater, M.E.** et al. (1983). Hemiplegic gait: analysis of temporal variables. *Archives of Physical Medicine and Rehabilitation* **64**, 583–7.
48. **Collen, F.M.** et al. (1991). The Rivermead Mobility Index: a further development of the Rivermead Motor Assessment. *International Disability Studies* **13**, 50–4.
49. **Holden, M.K., Gill, K.M., and Magliozzi, M.R.** (1986). Gait assessment for neurologically impaired patients. Standards for outcome assessment. *Physical Therapy* **66**, 1530–9.
50. **Mahoney, F.I. and Barthel, D.W.** (1965). Functional evaluation: the Barthel Index. *Maryland State Medical Journal* **14**, 61–5.
51. **Turner-Stokes, L.** et al. (1999). The UK FIM + FAM: development and evaluation. Functional Assessment Measure. *Clinical Rehabilitation* **13**, 277–87.
52. **Kirwan, J.R. and Reeback, J.S.** (1986). Stanford Health Assessment Questionnaire modified to assess disability in British patients with rheumatoid arthritis. *British Journal of Rheumatology* **25**, 206–9.
53. **Harwood, R.H.** et al. (1994). Measuring handicap: the London Handicap Scale, a new outcome measure for chronic disease. *Quality in Health Care* **3**, 11–16.
54. **Neugarten, B.L., Havighurst, R.J., and Tobin, S.S.** (1961). The measurement of life satisfaction. *Journal of Gerontology* **16**, 134–43.
55. **Whiteneck, G.G.** et al. (1992). Quantifying handicap: a new measure of long-term rehabilitation outcomes. *Archives of Physical Medicine and Rehabilitation* **73**, 519–26.
56. **Cooper, P.** et al. (1982). Evaluation of a modified self-report measure of social adjustment. *British Journal of Psychiatry* **141**, 68–75.
57. **Zigmond, A.S. and Snaith, R.P.** (1983). The Hospital Anxiety and Depression Scale. *Acta Psychiatrica Scandinavica* **67**, 361–70.
58. **Melzack, R.** (1975). The McGill Pain Questionnaire: major properties and scoring methods. *Pain* **1**, 277–99.
59. **Flaherty, S.A.** (1996). Pain measurement tools for clinical practice and research. *AANA Journal* **64**, 133–40.
60. **Robinson, B.C.** (1983). Validation of a Caregiver Strain Index. *Journal of Gerontology* **38**, 344–8.

15

The contribution to palliative medicine of allied health professions

15

The contribution to palliative medicine of allied health professions

15 The contribution to palliative medicine of allied health professions

15.1 The contribution of occupational therapy to palliative medicine

Jo Bray and Jill Cooper

Occupational therapy is the treatment of physical and psychiatric conditions through specific activities to help people reach their maximum level of function and independence in all aspects of daily life.

Occupational therapy practice within palliative care is underpinned by the principle that the patient sets the agenda. Time is of the essence and events are constantly changing. Patients have limited and fluctuating energy levels, numerous symptoms, and ongoing complications with which they are dealing and to which they have to adjust.

The core skills of the occupational therapist are outlined in this chapter and are applied to the individual to give meaning and quality to their life.

Traditionally, the success of occupational therapy has been measured in terms of maintaining and increasing function; hence, deterioration or death appears to be in conflict with life-enhancing goals and the aim of improving function. Within palliative care, occupational therapy is evolving to apply a rehabilitation approach in keeping with the key principles of palliative care as recognized by the World Health Organization:

- relief for the patient from pain and other distressing symptoms;
- psychological and spiritual care;
- a support system to help patients live as actively as possible in the face of impending death;
- a support system to sustain patients' friends and families during illness and bereavement.[1]

Rehabilitation in palliative care (see also Chapter 14)

Rehabilitation in palliative care differs from mainstream rehabilitation as the patients are likely to experience rapid change and deterioration. This places emphasis on the speed of response of the occupational therapist and careful forward planning to take account of present and future needs. A flexible approach is required to deal with uncertainty and respond to the changing circumstances.

Rehabilitation in palliative care aims to improve the quality of survival so that patients' lives will be as comfortable and productive as possible and they can function at a minimum level of dependency regardless of life expectancy. There are four stages within a rehabilitation programme for patients:

- *Preventative rehabilitation*—treatment in anticipation of potential disability to lessen severity.
- *Restorative rehabilitation*—to enable clients to return to their premorbid status without significant disability.
- *Supportive rehabilitation*—to support clients through their decline, the disease being progressive but stabilized, so that they can remain as functional as possible, retaining an element of choice and control.
- *Palliative rehabilitation*—to assist in symptom control, the disease being progressive and in its advanced stages, the rehabilitation preventing complications, for example, through positioning, pressure care, and preventing contractures.[2]

In identifying these four stages the occupational therapist is provided with a realistic treatment approach to facilitate patient-centred goals. The principles of occupational therapy within palliative care are underpinned, therefore, by a supportive or palliative rehabilitation approach to treatment planning.

Unique core skills of occupational therapy

The central values and beliefs of occupational therapy are that people with disabilities are valued as people with physical, emotional, intellectual, social, and spiritual needs. Occupational therapists use their core skills to enable them to empower people to make choices and achieve a personally acceptable lifestyle, with a goal of maximizing health and function.

The core skills of occupational therapy are:

- use of purposeful activity and meaningful occupation as therapeutic tools in the promotion of health and well-being;
- ability to enable people to explore, achieve, and maintain balance in the daily living tasks and roles of personal and domestic care, leisure, and productivity;
- ability to assess the effect of, and then to manipulate, physical and psychosocial environments to maximize function and social integration;
- ability to analyse, select, and apply occupations as specific therapeutic media to treat people who are experiencing dysfunction in daily living tasks, interactions, and occupational roles;
- enabling of people to maximize their physical, emotional, cognitive, social, and functional potential;
- anticipation and prevention of the effects of disability and dysfunction through education and therapeutic intervention in a functional context;
- enabling of people to achieve a meaningful lifestyle by the preparation for, or return to, work or the development of the quality use of time through leisure, education, training, and opportunities for voluntary work;
- provision of professional advocacy for people about matters such as access to premises and equal opportunity issues;
- provision of practical advice and support for the families and carers of people with disabilities;

- ability to change, adapt, and modify practices according to the needs of people with disabilities and their environment;
- ability to work in partnership with others, to facilitate the development of services for people with disabilities;
- the ability to influence social policy and legislation relating to impairment, disability, handicap, and economic self-sufficiency.[3]

Occupational therapy and dysfunction

Occupational therapy intervention is symptom-led rather than disease- or diagnosis-led and functional problems are dealt with as they arise. A proactive approach is taken to anticipate problems and prepare for patients and carers to avoid crisis intervention. Occupational therapy in palliative care encompasses all life-threatening illnesses such as advanced oncological, cardiac, and neurological illnesses and includes other problems that may already be present, for example, other chronic health conditions and mental illnesses.

Occupational therapy and function

Activity is the core element of the treatment medium used by occupational therapists, incorporating function and quality of life. Occupational therapy has always retained its links with activity as one of its central core skills on which the profession is based:

- The use of purposeful activity and meaningful occupation as therapeutic tools.
- Maintaining a balance in the daily living tasks and roles of personal and domestic care, leisure and productivity.
- Assessing the effect of and then manipulating the physical and psychological environments to maximize function and social interaction, independence, interdependence, and dependence. It is a matter of critical value in facilitating a person's sense of mastery and competence, and putting substance into quality of living.[4]

Occupational therapy in activities of daily life

The analysis of function is a core principle of occupational therapy and there are several models and frameworks of reference that underpin occupational therapy practice. Within a palliative care setting, the most applicable model to maximize quality of life assesses activities carried out on a daily basis under the headings of self-maintenance, productivity, and leisure. The focus is on 'wellness' though it is not based on a medical model but one of 'human occupation'. The theory focuses on a balance of activities being carried out in daily life, activities or occupations here meaning any activity requiring the individual's time and energy and thus using skills that have a value. This approach is essential in enabling patients to retain a sense of control in their own lives and helping them face change and loss.

Self-maintenance refers to washing, dressing, and looking after oneself. *Productivity* refers to making a productive contribution to life, either in the form of domestic activities or by earning a living. *Leisure* refers to hobbies, interests, and pursuits.

In using the model of occupational therapy shown in Fig. 1, a patient-centred, problem-oriented approach complements the palliative care philosophy in improving the individual's quality of life.

Assessment and treatment planning is based on the following core principles (see Fig. 1):

- *Motor skills*—the level, quality, and/or degree of range of motion, gross muscle strength, muscle tone, endurance, fine motor skills, and functional use of these. For many patients in palliative care, motor skills are affected by muscle wastage or weakness, resulting in loss of range of movement and mobility. The early introduction and supply of equipment, for example, bathing or toilet aids, can maintain their independence, thus giving a positive experience. Once the rapport is established with the occupational therapist, the patient and carers know whom to contact when function deteriorates and more help is needed. General advice on alternative techniques for carrying out activities can also be taught.

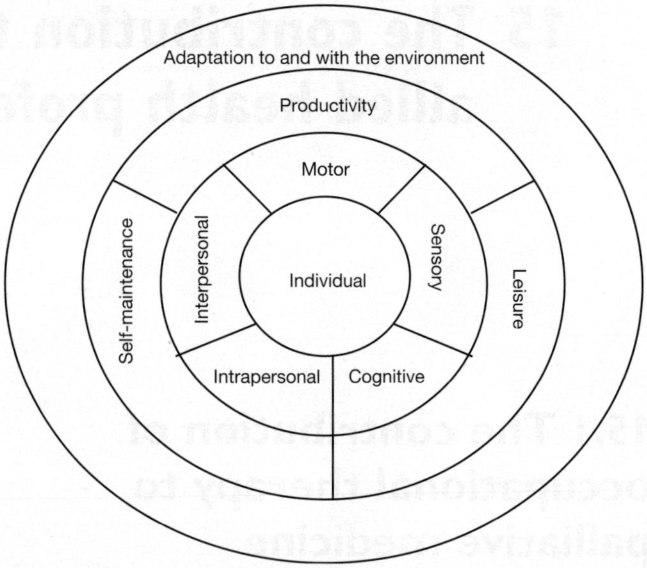

Fig. 1 Human occupations model. (Adapted from Reed, K. and Sanderson, S. *Concepts of Occupational Theraphy* 2nd edn. Baltimore: Williams & Wilkins.)

- *Sensory skills*—skills concerned with perceiving and differentiating external and internal stimuli. Patients experience many different degrees and varieties of pain. The concept of pain and its influence over the occupations and activities needs to be considered when implementing occupational therapy assessment and treatment programmes. Patients may have distortion or loss of sensation as a result of tumour growth on a nerve, fibrosing of tissue, or medically induced loss of sensation for pain control. Advice and supply of equipment may be necessary to avoid accidents, for example, when working in the kitchen.
- *Cognitive skills*—the level, quality, and/or degree of comprehension, communication, concentration, problem-solving, time management, conceptualization, integration of learning, judgement, and time/place/person orientation. All aspects of communication, comprehension, concentration, and organizational skills need to be assessed by the occupational therapist as these are vital to the performance of activities.
- *Intrapersonal skills*—the level, quality, and/or degree of self-identity, self-concept, and coping skills. Poor self-image can inhibit an individual's ability to cope with daily life. Feelings of anxiety and stress should be recognized and relaxation programmes should be taught to develop coping mechanisms to deal with such feelings. Patients whose occupational performance is affected by their intrapersonal skills may need psychological support. Goal-setting has the positive benefit of facilitating patients' involvement in, and subsequent control of, their lives.
- *Interpersonal skills*—the level, quality, and/or degree of dyadic and group interaction skills. The advanced stage of the disease often becomes the focus of patients' lives. They become disease-orientated, lose control of their lives, lose their roles and self-confidence, self-worth, and self-respect. Patients should set goals to provide an element of control and increase their motivation. The use of a structured programme of activity

can help them work towards the goals. Having addressed the performance components or skills required by the individual, the occupational therapist focuses on occupational components and the activities in routine daily life.

- *Self-maintenance occupations*—those activities or tasks that are carried out routinely to maintain the client's health and well-being in the environment such as dressing, eating, bathing, toileting, and domestic activities such as shopping, cooking, laundry, cleaning, and general household duties. The occupational therapist assesses the patient's abilities to carry out self-maintenance tasks. This assessment should not focus exclusively on performance outcomes/achievements but should also evaluate performance on those tasks that are of significance to the patient and address how the goals can be achieved. The occupational therapist corrects underlying problems, teaches alternative techniques and methods, or supplies equipment in order to maintain independence. Activities that are not a priority can be carried out by carers or health care professionals, giving patients the choice wherever possible and thus maintain control.
- *Productivity occupations*—those activities or tasks that are carried out to enable clients to provide support to themselves, their families, and society. It is important that patients feel productive throughout all stages of their decline. They may have lost employment, the role associated with this, income, role as a parent, spouse, partner and the focus becomes disease-led. This can lead to feelings of passivity and dependency. The occupational therapist can provide some structure or a new role to encourage productivity, ranging from advice on constructively filling free time by changing their role, for example, from breadwinner to housekeeper. If energy levels are severely limited, the patient could co-ordinate the shopping list for a home carer.
- *Leisure occupations*—those activities or tasks carried out for the enjoyment and renewal that the activity or task brings to the patient. They may contribute to the promotion of health and well-being. Everyone's psychological well-being requires that they gain pleasure or enjoyment for some part of every day. This is even more important for palliative care patients and, in assessing their occupational components, care must be taken to address this area, ensuring that energy levels and functional abilities still allow pleasurable experiences. As patients decline their leisure goals are often small but are of great importance to them.

Implementation of occupational therapy practice in palliative care

Occupational therapists are part of the multiprofessional team in palliative care with specialist skills in the rehabilitation of patients. Patients access palliative care in differing settings from hospital, home, and specialist units, so the rehabilitation team must establish effective means of communication in order to maximize a patient's ongoing and changing rehabilitation needs across care boundaries. The patient should receive continuity of care throughout their journey with a seamless, integrated approach of occupational therapy. Local initiatives should be in place between the voluntary sector, health, and social care providers of occupational therapy to ensure minimum disruption to the patients' lives and maximum efficiency of resources.

Occupational therapists work in all areas of health care from acute hospitals to social services, community teams as well as hospice and palliative care units. They have a tradition of working with patients suffering from chronic conditions and disabilities, where rehabilitation is a longer-term process. However, with the shift in recent health care trends to community-based care,[5] occupational therapy services have responded to focus on enabling patients as they return home from hospital, maintaining and supporting them in their own environment. Hence, there has been a growth in community and social care roles. This is in keeping with palliative care principles where services aim to help patients be at home for as long as possible.

The role of occupational therapy in palliative care

The role of occupational therapy in palliative care encompasses:

- *Assistance with psychological adjustment and goal-setting related to loss of function.* Within an undergraduate education programme, occupational therapists are trained to assess and treat physical and mental dysfunction. In palliative care, the patients' experience of and adjustment to the loss of roles within their lives are carefully considered when assessing and planning treatment to achieve realistic goals and treatment outcomes.
- *Assisting patients with activities for the treatment of physical dysfunction.* Occupational therapy has a sound working knowledge of anatomy, physiology, and normal function. When problems arise, the occupational therapist analyses the loss of function and the associated difficulties and impact on the activities within their lives. A treatment plan is prepared for each patient.
- *Retraining patients in personal and domestic activities that are necessary for daily living.* Within palliative care, it is the priorities of the patients and carers that need to be considered. The patient sets the agenda of their normal daily personal or domestic activities, which they strive to achieve independently. Conversely, if they wish to conserve their energy for other activities, arrangements can be made for assistance in these areas.
- *Assessment and prescription of wheelchairs and seating and pressure care needs.* Wheelchairs are a means of independence and the occupational therapist approaches assessment and prescription for these items of equipment with proactive planning. A patient's mobility and accessibility within a community can be greatly enhanced with early acceptance of a wheelchair. A wheelchair should not just be viewed as loss of the ability to walk but should be viewed positively as it enables family life and roles to be maintained, thus reducing the patient's isolation. Seating and pressure care needs are vital considerations in deteriorating conditions.
- *Retraining patients to help them with cognitive and perceptual dysfunction.* Cognitive and perceptual skills may be compromised by primary and/or secondary disease or treatment regimes. Depending on the underlying cause, this may be temporary or permanent dysfunction. The occupational therapist assesses and analyses the presenting problems, distinguishing cognitive, perceptual, and functional limitations. Within palliative care it may be inappropriate to use recognized, standardized, and validated screening tools to establish a baseline of dysfunction. Although they can give an indication of specific dysfunction, these are often lengthy and tiring for the patients and, with conditions that are likely to deteriorate, any re-assessment will only confirm decline for the patient.
- *Splinting to prevent deformities and control pain.* Occupational therapists assess and analyse the deformities and dysfunction of any joints, particularly those of hand and feet. Splints may be made by the occupational therapist from sheets of thermoplastic material and moulded to the individual or a commercially made one might be appropriate. These keep the joints in a comfortable resting or functional position to prevent deformity, maximize function, and control discomfort pain.
- *Home assessments and referral to community agencies for assessment and provision of equipment.* Assessment may be carried out in the patient's home environment (either as an in- or outpatient and with or without the patient present) to assess for and provide equipment and adaptations to aid daily living. This may be an essential part of complex discharge planning to enable the patient and carers to be supported and maintained at home. It provides the opportunity for carers and supportive agencies to see the patient at home with their present level of function. Goal-setting is, therefore, realistic and achievable and may also clarify whether a patient is likely to cope or not. Outcomes are dependent on the local resources.
- *Lifestyle management/investigating hobbies and leisure pursuits and roles within family life.* The occupational therapist analyses the patient's daily

routine and advises on how to manage those activities that are of importance to the patient so that they are achievable. As patients in palliative care decline, their leisure goals are often small but have immense significance to them. Incorporating hobbies and leisure into patients' daily routines can provide pleasure and enjoyment for some part of the day. This is a particularly valuable role for occupational therapists working within specialist palliative care day care settings and day therapy.

- *Relaxation techniques.* From the moment of diagnosis and throughout the disease process, patients face many potential stressors.[6] The occupational therapist teaches a range of coping mechanisms and relaxation techniques to the patient. Patients in palliative care often experience excessive fatigue and occupational therapy offers practical advice on how to negotiate daily living activities and workload to avoid exhaustion.
- *Support and education for carers.* In order to achieve goals set by and for the patient, the carers need to be involved, supported, and advised on how to help the patient and themselves. In every setting, carers and families should be consulted about what they want, and their preferences taken into account. This includes supporting and advising them on practical issues such as equipment to aid daily living as well as carer support groups.

Much has been achieved in palliative care relating to good symptom control. Patients present with numerous symptoms that have an impact on their daily lives. Whilst medical advances endeavour to address and relieve symptoms, numerous patients present with ongoing complex issues including, for example, total pain, incapacitating fatigue or breathlessness.[7]

Specific roles of occupational therapy

Occupational therapy has a specific role in the management of complex symptoms like breathlessness and fatigue.

Breathlessness

Within a multiprofessional breathlessness programme,[8] the occupational therapist assesses a patient's home environment and arranges adaptations to minimize the respiratory distress that is exacerbated by mobility within the home. 'Quick fix', short-term measures need to be realistic to address functional difficulties, for example, provision of equipment such as bathing aids or wheelchair.

Much can also be achieved by the occupational therapist analysing components of specific activities, the frequency, duration, and pacing of these in order to avoid worsening symptoms. This distressing symptom can be well managed by teaching relaxation techniques to avoid panic. These coping mechanisms need to be integral to the patient's lifestyle and activity roles, so the occupational therapist addresses these issues whilst considering equipment to aid daily living within a holistic treatment programme.

Fatigue

Fatigue has a much greater effect on patients with cancer than any other mental or physical consequence of the disease or its treatment and it has a major impact on patients' quality of life.[9]

Fatigue involves weariness, exhaustion, and lack of energy, which impacts on functional independence. It also results in increased discomfort and reduced efficiency, affecting mental and physical activities.[10] Working on the principle that fatigue is whatever the patient says it is, whenever the patient says it is,[11] the occupational therapist assesses the impact of this symptom on the whole of the patient's life, lifestyle, and roles.

The assessment addresses the patient's current activity tolerance, with peaks and troughs throughout the day and week. The occupational therapist analyses the demands and expectations of their routine, whether they are attending medical appointments or more pleasurable activities. A balance of activity is sought throughout the day and week.

The concept of pacing and scheduling is introduced in order to provide the patient with an understanding of their energy levels and tolerance of activity. A daily balance of rest and effort is the prime aim. More complex tasks can be broken down and analysed once the basic daily routine is established. Once the patient understands these principles, it is easier for them to take control, manage, and tolerate the demands on their energy levels.

The next stage goes on to establish what they want to achieve, that is, the desired outcome, and applies a clinical knowledge in order to set realistic goals. A staged and graduated treatment programme is agreed in order to work towards these goals and continuous reassessment ensures they are realistic.

The impact of these two symptoms (breathlessness and fatigue) alone has an enormous effect on all functional activities of daily living, independence, and quality of life.

Discharge home

A key role of occupational therapy within palliative care is the occupational therapist assessing the home situation in order to enable the patient and carers to cope as safely, comfortably, and confidently as possible at home. Many studies show that patients would prefer to be at home if their physical condition allowed. Returning home is not simply about assessing the physical environment as the patients and carers anxieties and concerns will determine the success or failure of discharge home.

Discharge planning is a multi-faceted complex skill. The occupational therapist works with the patient and carers to identify functional and psychological limitations, assesses the physical and environmental requirements and acts as a key worker within the palliative care team establishing communication links with the community support team.

The environmental assessment

The occupational therapist assesses the environmental requirements.

Accommodation

Assessment is made of physical limitations related to type of housing, access to property, permission for adaptations. Measurements will be taken to identify external door widths, height and number of steps, need for rails or ramps. Safety issues including personal alarms, telephone links, and preparation and coping in the event of falling over at home.

Living areas

Specific measurements will be taken of heights of furniture to ensure they are of optimum height for safe and independent transfers as furniture can be raised in a number of ways that are safe and comply with Health and Safety regulations. This is essential for patients with muscle wasting, fatigue, and breathlessness and who have difficulties or are unable to transfer on and off their furniture unassisted. The type of heating, power supply, door widths, limitations of turning space for mobility aids, wheelchair and hoist, safety of flooring, and hazardous rugs and furniture are also considered. This includes any additional furniture, equipment or adaptations required to enable the patient to cope at home. If living areas need to be rearranged, for example, the bedroom area to be moved downstairs, this is discussed and negotiated with the rest of the family or carers involved.

Bathroom/toileting

Measurements are taken of heights of bath, shower, toilet to enable specific equipment to be installed. This enables patients to transfer on and off the furniture independently or with assistance safely. Alternative washing facilities might need to be considered, a wide range of equipment is available to facilitate independence or support from a carer.

Food and meal preparation

Kitchen safety is the prime aim of assessing and practising for independence. Equipment and advice can be key for energy conservation. In cases where a patient is considered unsafe or at risk, a range of alternative options can be negotiated with carers and appropriate safety measures taken.

Involving patients and carers in discharge planning and good preparation for returning home provides significant opportunity for patients to relay any fears, anxieties, and apprehensions. Thus, attention is turned to roles and activities that will enhance meaning within their remaining life. Therefore, occupational therapy in palliative care aims to maximize quality of life regardless of the disability and life expectancy.

Equipment

Provision of equipment is not a quick fix solution to a functional problem. If assessment, supply, fitting, and evaluation of the use of equipment is not carried out and supervised by a qualified occupational therapist, it can hinder daily living and put patients at risk.

Within the commercial world, a huge range of equipment is available for purchase. However, sales and marketing techniques will not provide impartial advice. Patients and carers facing life-threatening illnesses may be particularly vulnerable to such pressures. Equipment will always be available for private purchase, but in some statutory social and health care systems, a range of simple equipment may be available free of charge or means-tested.

There is no prescriptive list of equipment that will solve every problem. The early and appropriate supply of equipment should support a patient's independence in carrying out activities of daily living. For example, the supply of bathing equipment may support a patient's independence in the early stages, and in the later stages this may assist professionals in carrying out bathing with the patient. If a patient no longer finds the equipment useful, it should be removed as it could be a potential hazard. Sensitivity needs to be applied when removing equipment after the patient's death. Many carers ask for this to be removed prior to the funeral.

The purpose of any equipment is to facilitate functional independence. However, accurate assessment of existing functional ability is essential to identify the need for, purpose of, and solution that the supply of equipment would resolve. Table 1 lists some of the equipment that ideally ought to be available to the occupational therapist, the member of the team best qualified to prescribe the equipment.

Outcome measures

No occupational therapy intervention is in isolation as the patient receives input from the interprofessional team.

Table 1 Some of the equipment and aids available to occupational therapists in the United Kingdom

Difficulties with transferring
Aim of equipment will be to:
Enable safe transfers
Facilitate ability to sit and stand independently or at least with minimal support, bearing in mind manual handling and safety implications
Optimize use of energy and strength in arms and legs
Reduce stress and avoid exacerbating shortness of breath
Ensure the patient and carers understand the use of the equipment and improve their skills to use it safely
Encourage good positioning and seating, for example, hips and knees flexed at 90°
Bed
Back rest to support patient sitting up
Leg strap to help patients lift their legs in/out of bed
Specifically designed blocks to raise the height of the bed to enable improved transfers in and out
Hydraulically operated lift which straps under the head end of the mattress and lifts the patient from lying to sitting and similar device to lift legs in and out of bed
Electrically operated height adjustable bed, particularly when nursing care is required at home as this helps both patient and carers
Chair
Wide range of blocks to raise heights of furniture and fit safely on legs of chairs
High-back, orthopaedic-type armchair with firm armrests and at least 450 mm seat height for independent transfers
Seat with riser/recliner options to enable patient to sit with legs elevated and which also brings patient into standing position from sitting down
Toilet
Range of raised toilet seats to facilitate safe and easier transfers from low toilets. These clip on to porcelain bowl of lavatory and can be removed for hygiene and if other family members do not wish to use them
Frames to fit round lavatory, adjustable height to give support for patients pushing up with arms to stand up from toilet
Grabrail strategically positioned on wall for similar support, safely fitted
Frames with raised toilet seat built in to help patients on/off toilet safely
Commode, bottle, female urinal bottle to help patients who cannot walk far from bed or gain access to toilet if it is up or down some steps or if walking frame or wheelchair does not fit through the doorway
Bathing
Range of boards and seats to fit over and/or in the bath, to fit plastic or enamel baths, standard or corner baths. Patient is instructed in how to use these safely, how to fit and clean them
Specific boards and seats designed for use in the shower, either over the bath or standing in a shower cubicle
Hydraulically operated bath seat which lifts patients in/out bath with safe back support if sitting balance is poor
Strategically placed grabrails, measured for and fitted safely to enable patients to manoeuvre in/out of bath or shower
Wheelchair
Detachable sides of wheelchair assist in safe transfers, correctly adjusted heights of footrests, and full assessment to ensure the chair suits the patient's needs as well as fitting in their own environment
Boards to facilitate sliding transfers if patient is unable to weight bear, with full assessment and training for all those concerned in using this equipment
Appropriate model of pressure relieving cushion to ensure potential pressure areas remain intact
Car
Full assessment and training is needed to ensure patients and carers can use sliding boards and turning discs to help them in/out car safely

(Continued)

Table 1 Continued

Manual handling
The risk to patients and carers has to be assessed and considered when supplying any equipment. Safety is paramount
It may be necessary to use hoists, either manually or electrically operated, and the correct sling has to be used
Sliding sheets and other transfers boards are available and the individual requires full assessment and training for safe use
Walking aids
Many patients rely on the support of a stick or frame
A kitchen trolley can enable them to walk using the trolley for support whilst carrying items. As this has wheels, the stability of the patient needs to be assessed thoroughly
Stairs
Rails. Bannister rails may assist safety on the stairs, either on one or both sides. Strategically placed grabrails at specific points on the stairs can also help
Stairlifts. Electrically operated lift with a seat on to which patients needs to transfer. These may be expensive although some companies use reconditioned ones, hire them, or buy them back when no longer required. Expense depends on whether the stairs are straight or curved. Thorough assessment is essential to ensure patient can transfer on to the seat, has sufficiently safe sitting balance, and the cognitive ability to use the controls
Through-floor lift. If the patient is dependent on a wheelchair and cannot move onto a stairlift seat, a lift might be required which has a platform on which the wheel chair and patient wheel, then it goes vertically up through the floor into the upstairs room
Assessment also depends on whether the patient will use this independently or with a carer, the time and expense of installing it with patients in advanced stage of disease is also an issue in many cases
Activities of daily living
Kitchen and meal preparation
Kitchen aids range from jar and can openers, adapted cutlery and crockery, tap turners, boards to help prepare food, large-handled and adapted plugs. All these items aim towards safety, avoiding the risk of burns and cutting, adapting to altered cognitive ability, and maximizing strength, dexterity, and energy
Washing and dressing
Long-handled equipment to help put on/take off shoes, underwear and clothes are designed to optimize independence and save energy. Some include: long-handled shoe horn, long-handled sponge for reaching feet, small frame for putting on socks or stockings, button hooks, elastic shoelaces, velcro fastenings rather than buttons. These are all used with training in techniques to overcome the functional difficulties which vary depending on the causes

In order to measure any changes that have occurred as the result of a treatment intervention, realistic goals must be set that have significance to the patient. The goals are likely to be of a practical nature such as provision and use of equipment or implementation of a treatment technique such as relaxation or energy conservation. A treatment goal is set by analysing the difficulty or task, allowing flexibility to adapt to the patient's fluctuating or deteriorating condition. Therefore, treatment goals and any outcome of the treatment intervention need to be evaluated and re-evaluated to ensure the patient's needs are being addressed.

Within this treatment planning process the occupational therapist breaks down the tasks of the overall treatment aim into smaller activities and goals. It is, therefore, these smaller goals that are evaluated and provide the evidence for reflective practice. Considering the effectiveness of the intervention and how this influences future treatment with the patient provides the outcome of the intervention. It is this outcome that can be formally measured using standardized and validated measurement tools of occupational therapy intervention. All have their strengths and weaknesses. However, elements can be applied to occupational therapy practice within palliative care as there is no one specifically acknowledged outcome measure for occupational therapy in this speciality. Standardized occupational therapy outcome measures that are applicable to palliative care include:

- *Canadian Occupational Performance Measure (COPM).* This recognizes the influence of physical, socio-cultural, mental, and spiritual domains of a patient's occupational performance.[12] It measures problems identified by the occupational therapist and patient together in terms of the patient's performance in carrying out an activity, the importance of the activity to the patient, and the patient's satisfaction with their performance.
- *The Westcotes Measure.* This uses goal-setting to measure outcomes with a scoring system that is able to identify statistically significant change. It is newly developed and needs widespread use to further test its validity and reliability.[13]
- *Goal-setting.* A system of outcome measurement that mirrors clinical practice makes measurement more acceptable, and enables assessment to be unobtrusive and low-key in the palliative care setting.[14]
- *The reintegration to Normal Living Index.* This uses a 10-point Likert scale to comment on 11 statements, for example, 'I move around in my living quarters as I feel necessary (wheelchairs, other equipment, or other resources may be used)'; 'I am able to participate in recreational activities as I want to (using adaptive equipment, supervision or assistance may be used)'; 'I assume a role in my family which meets my needs and those of other family members (with adaptive equipment, supervision or assistance)'; 'I feel that I can deal with my life events as they happen'.

Conclusion

Occupational therapy optimizes quality of life and gives patients choice in what they wish to achieve in the advanced stages of their disease. Specific occupational therapy intervention reduces anxiety, promotes self-esteem and dignity, facilitates privacy, and avoids the patient becoming dependent on others any sooner than is necessary. As the patient is not treated in isolation, the carers and family are involved in establishing goals and treatment programmes to maximize safety and comfort for all those concerned. Realistic goal-setting is reflected in outcome measures that evaluate the impact of occupational therapy intervention on the patient.

In palliative care, the occupational therapist values an individual's remaining life, helping the patient to live in the present, recognizing an individual's right to self-determination, and acknowledging and preparing for the approaching death.[15]

The unique role of the occupational therapist compliments the multiprofessional team in palliative care by its contribution towards optimizing functional independence. The problem solving approach does not provide a set answer for each individual's problems, it focuses on the individual and assessment and treatment as an ongoing process. Occupational therapy has a vital function in the delivery of palliative care.

References

1. **National Council for Hospice and Specialist Palliative Care Services.** *Fulfilling Lives. Rehabilitation in Palliative Care.* London: NCHSPCS, 2000.
2. **Bray, J.** (1997) on Dietz (1982) in: Occupational therapy in hospices and day care. In *Occupational Therapy in Oncology and Palliative Care* Chapter 10 (ed. J. Cooper). London: Whurr.

3. **College of Occupational Therapists (UK).** *Core Skills and a Conceptual Framework for Practice.* London: College of Occupational Therapists, 1992.
4 **Roberts, G.** (2000). Clinical specialisms and clinical specialist/higher/advanced level practitioner. *Occupational Therapy News* **8** (3), 12–13.
5. **Department of Health.** *National Service Framework for Older People.* London: HMSO, 2001.
6. **McVey, G.** (1997). Occupational therapy in stress and anxiety management. In *Occupational Therapy in Oncology and Palliative Care* Chapter 6 (ed. J. Cooper), London: Whurr.
7. **Kaye, P.** *A–Z of Hospice and Palliative Medicine.* Northampton: EPL Publications, 1994.
8. **Institute of Cancer of Research, Diana Princess of Wales Memorial Project, Macmillan Cancer Relief.** *A Breath of Fresh Air: An Interactive Guide to Managing Breathlessness in Patients with Lung Cancer,* CD ROM. London: ICR, 2001.
9. **Stone, P., Richardson, A., Ream, E., Smith, A.G., Kerr, D.J., and Kearney, N.** (2000). Cancer-related fatigue: inevitable, unimportant and untreatable? Results of a multi-centre patient survey. *Annals of Oncology* **11**, 971–5.
10. **Cooper, J.** *Occupational Therapy in Oncology and Palliative Care.* London: Whurr, 1997.
11. **Glaus, A.** (1993). Assessment of fatigue in cancer and non-cancer patients. *Support Cancer Care* **1**, 305–15.
12. **Law, M., Baptiste, S., Carswell, A., McColl, M.A., Polatajko, H., and Pollock, N.** *Canadian Occupational Performance Measure* 2nd edn. Toronto: CAOT Publications, 1994.
13. **Eva, G.** *Guidelines for Measuring Occupational Therapy Outcomes.* In *HIV/AIDS, Oncology & Palliative Care.* London: HOPE, 2000.
14. **Johnson, M.** (1997). Outcome measurement: towards an interdisciplinary approach. *British Journal of Therapy and Rehabilitation* **4** (9), 472–7.
15. **Bye, R.** (1998). When clients are dying: occupational therapists' perspectives. *Occupational Therapy Journal of Research* **18** (1), 3–24.

15.2 The contribution of music therapy to palliative medicine

Clare O'Callaghan

> ... watch and listen to her playing and bring it (the music) to life and me too.
> (patient with cancer)
>
> ... (memories in MT) give back life to people who no longer see the value of their lives.
> (cancer hospital staff member)
>
> ... hearing the music and people singing told me that Peter Mac (the cancer hospital) is a caring and sharing place
> (visitor)[1]

Introduction

Music therapy (MT) is the creative and professionally informed use of music in a therapeutic relationship with people identified as needing physical, psychosocial, or spiritual help, or with people aspiring to experience further self-awareness, enabling increased life satisfaction. This chapter will illustrate how MT can allow the human spirit to triumph in clinical contexts where the fragility of human life is clearly evident. Following a definition of MT in palliative care and mention of its historical origins, the contextual influences on the styles of MT palliative care practices will be discussed. The scope of MT methods used in sessions will be described alongside reports of their therapeutic benefits. MT in palliative care is increasingly being informed by both quantitative and qualitative research findings, and these are highlighted throughout the chapter.

The scope of MT and palliative care has broadened considerably since it was first described over 20 years ago by Susan Munro and Balfour Mount at Royal Victoria Hospital's Palliative Care Unit, Montreal.[(2)] Many music therapists have since discussed the palliative care components of their work with children and adults living with advanced cancer, degenerative neurological conditions, and AIDS.[(3–5)] In 1973, Lucanne Magill introduced a music programme at Memorial Sloan-Kettering Cancer Center, New York, and, alongside Munro, has inspired the continuing expansion of MT and palliative care services throughout the Western world.[(6,7)] In 2000, the Third International Symposium on MT in Palliative Care was held jointly with the 13th International Congress on Care of the Terminally Ill. An entire issue of *The Journal of Palliative Care* devoted to MT (Volume 17, Issue 3, 2001) emerged from this meeting.

While many people may offer helpful musical experiences to patients,[2] music therapists are accredited by national associations and have received extensive tertiary (university) training in a variety of MT methods, as well as music performance skills, music history and theory, psychotherapeutic theories, counselling techniques, and biopsychosocial knowledge. Music therapists attempt to work as members of multidisciplinary health-care teams, contributing to holistic patient care.

Definition

Numerous definitions of MT and palliative care exist[(5)] and include the following features. The music therapist offers patients, and occasionally their visitors and carers, opportunities to creatively experience a wide range of live and pre-recorded musical activities or 'methods' (see Table 1). Music therapists focus on the therapeutic process rather than the musical products of sessions. The musical elements (melody, harmony, rhythm, tempo, instrumentation, and volume) and evolving therapeutic relationship provide the foundation for altered thoughts, or affective, physiological, or transcendental sensations congruent with improved psychosocial adjustment and symptom alleviation.

Attention to cognitive and physical components is not always enough when attempting to address the holistic care of people with advanced, degenerative illnesses. Acknowledgement of a patient's non-discursive (nonverbal) level of awareness, accessed and expressed through creative interaction with aesthetic modalities, may be vital for improved well-being. Verbal reflection on such contemplative activities may either promote or impede the therapeutic experience. Therefore, the balance of music activity and discussion, including insight-oriented counselling, is highly variable and monitored in sessions.

For whom is music therapy appropriate?

Music therapy is suitable for patients, and those close to them, who want to explore whether varying kinds of musical experiences can help them to encounter the illness experience. Participants do not have to have 'musical backgrounds' to benefit from MT.

Historical precursors

Music has been a major factor in health maintenance and restoration among members of cultures throughout the world, both historically and geographically. Music in rituals, often led by a shaman and with tribal

[1] Anonymous, written statements from respondents in a study on the relevance of music therapy in a cancer hospital.[(1)]

[2] Including those associated with the Council for Music in Hospitals, a charity in the United Kingdom, and music thanatologists, who 'prescribe' music specifically for dying patients.[(8)]

Table 1 Music therapy methods (individual and group work)

Replaying the music of one's life
Live performance, by therapist and/or patients, visitors, staff
Word substitution in known songs
Music listening (taped or live)
Musical life review
Exploring 'new' music
Music improvization, by patient (and perhaps visitors) with or without therapist
Song writing
Unfamiliar pre-composed music (live and taped)
Musically inspired guided imagery

participation, commonly supported one's trajectory into the next life when cure did not eventuate, and helped the bereaved to adjust. Since industrialization in Western societies, however, music was increasingly viewed as irrelevant as biomedical models of health understanding and promotion became increasingly valued.[9] The limits of biomedical models of health though are especially apparent when considering the lives of people with life-threatening and incurable illnesses. Rather than being regarded as an innovation, MT in palliative care may therefore be considered as a 'reawakening' of the scope of music in aiding the community to encounter life-threatening illnesses.

Contextual influences on styles of music therapy practices

While palliative care music therapists are united by their commitment to offer music to improve quality of life, styles of practice vary according to clinical contexts and the therapists' educational backgrounds. Clinical contexts where palliative care principles are pertinent to music therapists include hospital- and home-based palliative care programmes, as well as cancer treatment settings, neurological units, and nursing homes. In clinical settings, patients' conditions and moods fluctuate, visitors often appear unpredictably, and irregularly scheduled treatments may be required. Therapists often offer sessions at flexible times, adapting MT methods to suit participants' abilities. Referrals may come via staff, the patients themselves, or others who care for them.

At Sir Michael Sobell House, a hospice/specialist palliative care unit in Oxford, an MT room with a variety of tuned and untuned musical instruments are available for patients to visit and play freely, often in an improvised manner with the therapist. Unfortunately, such facilities are unusual. Often, therapists visit patients at their bedsides in hospitals and, increasingly, homes with accompanying instruments, sheet music, or recorded music.[10] Patients may experience MT either individually or in groups with families or other patients. 'Interruptions' by overhearing patients or staff may lead to shared therapeutic group experiences.

Music therapy assessment, methods, and effects

The palliative care aims that MT could address are listed in Table 2. Upon meeting a patient, the music therapist may offer music in a general manner, for example, to increase comfort, relaxation, and enjoyment, or for more specific needs such as pain control. Assessment includes determining the patients' music preferences and the relevance of music throughout their lives. Typically, the therapist then invites patients to experience any of the methods listed in Table 1, which may be used at any stage of the illness. The following is an expanded description of some of these methods and clinical aims. Specific approaches for family and group work, seriously ill children, people with neurological impairment, ethnic minorities, bereavement, and staff support will be described later.

Table 2 Palliative care aims that music therapy can address

Supportive validation	One's feelings and thoughts A life having been lived One's relevance in meaningful relationships
Increased self-awareness	Self-discovery Reawakening or reworking of an earlier awareness Private contemplation; a time to simply 'be'
Symptom relief and relaxation	Including pain, tension, dyspnoea, nausea, insomnia, restlessness
Connection with others, reduced isolation	Those with cognitive impairment Those with language barriers and communication difficulties Expanded opportunities for interactions with other patients, visitors, and staff
Aesthetic experience	Pleasure Creative expression Transcendence

Replaying the music of one's life

Familiar live and recorded music can be offered in sessions and for patients' private use. The author often took sheet music with about 5000 songs and classical pieces that she could spontaneously play on a 6.5 octave electric piano when she visited patients in hospices, cancer wards, and a neurological unit. Therapists, patients, visitors, and staff may all actively participate in music making, singing, dancing, 'airplaying' (i.e. pretending to play) instruments, and conducting. In the author's MT practice, many seriously ill patients have been inspired to perform on musical instruments again (particularly the mouth organ, which can be sterilized) for the first time in up to 50 years, bringing considerable delight to not only themselves, but also their families, other patients, and staff. Extensive tape libraries may also be provided. For example, 3000 tapes and CDs are available for patients, families, and staff associated with Bethlehem Hospital's hospice and neurological facilities in Melbourne, Australia. This tape library is an adjunct to an extensive MT programme offering a range of MT methods in the Hospital and local community.[10]

Our lifetime songs and music often profoundly touch our entire being. Therefore, when people revisit that music in MT, they can revisit those all-encompassing experiences of their life histories that, for many, substantially underpin their current identities. Through experiencing music from one's earlier life, one has the opportunity to re-experience who one is, as well as to 'rethink' what one thought, and rediscover who one was, at both verbal and non-verbal levels of consciousness.

The following vignette illustrates the invigorating and life affirming properties of music:

> The patient suddenly started moving her bottom from side to side while sitting in bed, waving her hands like she was doing the 'Charleston', and laughed about a neighbour saying that she was doing the 'bum bum dance.' Not understanding what was going on, the music therapist begged her pardon. Her daughter was laughing and then finally recalled a neighbour who teased the patient about the way she had moved her bottom as she danced. (The patient died three days later).

Music potentially enables a transcendence of the person/patient split. It can empower patients to feel, experience, and express more of their whole, historically situated selves. In a study on the relevance of MT in a cancer hospital,[1] one anonymous female respondent (aged between 20 and 45) wrote:

> Any experience like this reminds me that I am much more than a 'cancer patient', I am a person with all sorts of needs, like everyone around me, who happens to have cancer. Music is one way I am reminded of this duplicity.

Through choosing music that they wish to hear, patients have some control over the memories of people, places, and emotions experienced. Replayed music from people's lifetimes is always experienced anew, creatively perceived and expressed.[11] In the author's study, a male (aged 70 plus) anonymously wrote after MT:[1]

> The memories were happy ones and so I felt better because it had awakened new thoughts for me, that is a different line of thinking, instead of just my problems.

The potency of MT usually results from both the patients' reactions to the music, and also their interaction with the music therapist. The therapist's supportive live and musical presence may be conceptualized as providing a musical 'human mirror' in the psychoanalytic Winnicottean sense. Winnicott suggested that in psychotherapy the therapist 'reflects back' aspects about the patient, enabling the person to exist 'as an expression of I AM, I am alive, I am myself' (ref. 12, p. 56). In MT, the patient may be 'reflected back' in a multisensorial manner, that is, musically, verbally, and non-verbally, expanding the potential for the patient's creative reintegration. Hence, while the upsurge of electronic possibilities in music provision may enable patients to have easy access to a breadth of helpful musical requests, the added therapeutic impetus encapsulated in live musical involvement with a trained music therapist cannot be underestimated.

Table 3 Themes in 64 songs written by 39 palliative care patients and the frequency that they recurred in the songs[17]

Themes	%
Messages	87
Self-reflections	66
Compliments	50
Memories	45
Reflections upon significant others, including pets	31
Self-expression of adversity	25
Imagery	17
Prayers	11

Music and life review

While patients often spontaneously reminisce in sessions, the active encouragement of patients to do a musical life review has also been described by some therapists. Patients' life stories and musical selections or performances may be placed on an audio- or video-tape, which can be left as a legacy for their loved ones.

Reported benefits of using music, which stimulates reminiscence in palliative care, include improved communication between patients and those close to them. Reminiscence also validates patients' lives, and can enable improved self-esteem, sense of worth and identity, enhanced insight, as well as ethnic and cultural affirmation.[13]

Exploring 'new' sounds and songs

Improvisation

The therapist and client can improvise together vocally and on various tuned and untuned percussion instruments, creating the development of a musical relationship. Within this relationship, the client musically expresses aspects of oneself and creatively realizes new self-understanding congruent with improved well-being.

Magee has used improvisation extensively with people with advanced neurological conditions including multiple sclerosis, Huntington's disease, Parkinson's disease, and motor neurone disease (ALS).[14] Improvisation in MT can heighten these individuals' sense of achievement, being capable, successful, and independent. It also promotes emotional expression and interaction with others.

Salmon described how music improvisation enabled a man with motor neurone disease to symbolically express anxiety and frustration about, and possibly adjustment to, his deterioration.[15] Although his verbal expression was becoming increasingly difficult, Jacques was able to play on tuned bells and percussion instruments with limited movement in one hand. At the end of an improvisation with Salmon and her student, Jacques spontaneously titled it, 'Nowhere to go but to Heaven'.

Hartley presented poignant statements made by HIV positive men who described their experience of improvisation in MT.[16] Not long before Mario's death he stated that improvising in MT allowed 'the inside of me (to be) living... it grows and expands.' During the times that Mario felt 'totally one' improvising with the music therapist he said that he felt 'completely well; in fact I never felt so alive!' (ref. 16, p. 112).

Song writing

Lyric substitution in well-known songs has provided enjoyment and a safe form of self-expression in MT sessions with people of all ages. Music therapists may also help patients to express thoughts and feelings that may be too difficult to talk about, through song writing. Patients may be invited to 'brain storm' ideas on a specific issue, assisted to transform the ideas into song lyrics, and offered a variety of musical styles, melodies, and harmonies for its accompaniment. The patient or the therapist may perform and record it, and it can then be presented as a gift to a loved one.

Patients with advanced neurological conditions such as multiple sclerosis and motor neurone disease have written many songs in group and individual sessions, ranging from the celebration of a home-brew kit arriving in their hospital, to the expression of feelings about the death of someone close to them. Thematic analysis from grounded theory, as well as content analysis, were used to examine the lyrics of 64 songs written by these patients, and others with advanced cancer (39 patients in total), in individual and group MT sessions over 7 years. The themes that emerged, and the frequency with which they recurred in the songs, are listed in Table 3.[17]

The following song lyrics were written by a mother for her two young children a few days before her death:

> The inspiration you give me.
> How sad I feel leaving you
> I don't want to leave this world
> It's been so beautiful, thanks to you
>
> We'll get through this well together
> Please carry on with the strength you've shown
> Not being afraid to cry when you need to
> To be what you are meant to be
> You are a child of the universe
> With a right to be here
> As much as the birds and the bees
>
> Don't forget you're put in this world to enjoy it and to care for it

Song writing sometimes enables people to express important thoughts and feelings, including farewell messages. Songs as parting gifts may also help the bereaved, as will be further discussed later.

Selected music for symptom alleviation

While the aforementioned MT methods may helpfully alter patients' pain sensation and alleviate other symptoms, the specific application of musical elements may also enhance patient comfort levels. Unfamiliar instrumental music with slow, regular rhythms may, for example, be used to aid in tension reduction. Therapists do not 'prescribe' music but, rather, usually help patients to explore different kinds of music that they might find helpful. Human musical response is idiosyncratic and seldom predictable. Therefore, music therapists do not advocate the indiscriminate use of 'piped' music in palliative care settings because music must be tailored to the patients' wishes. A musical work that one patient finds helpful may be aggravating for another.

Theoretical rationales for pain reduction in MT include direct physiological response to music stimuli that alter neural components of pain sensation, as well as cognitive and emotional changes aligned with increased self-awareness, thereby altering one's sense of the meaning, and thus perception, of pain.[6]

Musically inspired guided imagery

Guided imagery and music (GIM) is a specialist form of MT training directed at eliciting a client's imagery, enabling increased self-understanding and personal growth. The therapist assists a patient to listen to selected music in a relaxed state and then inquires about the patient's resultant mental imagery, which is believed to be connected to their deeper conscious selves. The patient may then discuss thoughts about their imagery with the therapist or continues to work in a symbolic manner through creative drawing, movement, or claywork. GIM has been used to help alleviate fear in terminally ill patients, as well as to help them to spiritually prepare for death. It tends to be offered in a modified form when used with patients with advanced illness and is not usually useful for people with cognitive impairment and limited attention spans.[18]

Family and groupwork

Music therapy can provide an intimate context for patients and those close to them to express supportive and validating messages about the role each has had in the others' lives. In shared MT sessions, patients and families have opportunities to choose music to enjoy and relax together, and often indirectly communicate special messages through lyrics expressed, and shared memories identified with selected songs and instrumental pieces. Thoughts may remain private, but can be indirectly expressed through 'knowing' looks and smiles, hand-holding, and embraces. Often patients and families sing and may even spontaneously dance together.

> While the therapist played 'Edelweiss' for one family the patient's son moved toward his dying mother's bedside. They wrapped their arms around each other, cried, and when the music ceased, sat back looking at each other. The son commented, 'We both needed that'. He then looked to the therapist and said, 'I suppose that's what you aim to do as well.'

Shared sessions among patients on wards also offer forums where seemingly isolated patients can discover shared interests, and offer mutual support.

Work with other therapists

Conjoint family sessions with a music therapist and social worker have been successfully used to promote supportive communication among young children and their parents when one of the parents was dying. Children have substituted lyrics in or composed new songs to express significant messages to dying parents before their deaths.[19]

While music can be used to accompany exercises in MT and physiotherapy groups, the physical benefits of MT may also occur indirectly when people sing and move in sessions. MT used to promote relaxation may also promote the successful administering of treatments by other health carers, for example, feeding a patient with dysphagia.

Specific populations

Music therapy with children and adolescents

Aims and methods in Tables 1 and 2 are often relevant in MT with children and adolescents with advanced illnesses, as well as the children of dying patients. Younger patients' developmental levels are considered as therapists tailor their interventions to their cognitive abilities and emotional states. While children and adolescents may not be able or wish to discuss the nature of their illness and associated feelings in a verbal manner, they may symbolically express aspects about their condition and experience increased self-understanding through music activities. Validating experiences of being 'heard' through the supportive medium of music may alleviate anxiety and instigate behavioural changes identified as a healthier response to the illness. For example, Daveson and Kennelly described an 8-year-old child with cystic fibrosis whom the hospital staff described as 'miserable and depressed'. She was eventually able to express her sadness and grief, as well as express a message to her best friend, through writing a song shortly before her death.[20]

Aasgaard highlighted the therapeutic importance of providing opportunities for patients and their families to 'have fun' through his description of 7-year-old Mary, who had acute myeloid leukaemia. Barely able to talk due to chemotherapy side-effects, Mary wrote a text about receiving adverse clinical treatment from 'A suspiciously cheerful lady', which was also the song title. Aasgaard used the text to compose and record a song that helped Mary to adjust to lengthy periods of treatment and isolation. The song also brought much joy to her younger brother (who added flatulence joke lyrics), other family members, patients, staff, and her school classmates.[21]

Cognitive impairment

Cerebral areas and neural systems activated during some musical activities are 'relatively independent from the areas used for verbal tasks' (ref. 22, p. 108). Furthermore, long-term memories, especially familiar lyrics and melodies, are relatively preserved in people with cognitive impairment.[23] Therefore, therapists who use both language and music therapeutically are likely to have a greater chance of activating preserved neural pathways and cerebral areas in people with cognitive impairment than therapists who use language alone. Such therapists may offer these patients expanded opportunities to encounter aesthetic experiences and to communicate meaningfully with others. Many patients who had language expression and/or comprehension difficulties due to advanced cancer or other degenerative neurological conditions have sung, shared songs with families, knowingly laughed at musically inspired reminiscences, and have even written songs in MT sessions.[17,23] Recent attention has also focused on the potential of MT to accelerate the emergence from coma and orientation of children with severe traumatic brain injury.[24]

Ethnic minorities

While it can be difficult for any music therapist to cater for the diverse musical interests of patients in multicultural contexts, music therapists usually attempt to offer a wide variety of musical styles from many cultures. Patients who have difficulties with the dominant language in the ward culture may experience reduced isolation and joy as they listen to and sing songs that are offered in their language of origin.

Bereavement

While few music therapists have the resources to actively follow-up bereaved relatives, it is likely that the memories of, and songs written in, patients' sessions can ameliorate relatives' distress following the death. The mother of a young patient who had died of a rapidly progressive form of multiple sclerosis told the author that whenever she felt sad, playing one of her son's MT song compositions, which had since been recorded by her daughter, helped her greatly. The lyrics included a story that the mother had told her son when he was child about his parents' courtship in countries separated by thousands of miles. She had not realized that her son had even remembered the story.

Skewes and Erdonmez Grocke described a qualitative research study on a MT group for six bereaved adolescents, highlighting how group improvisation and the sharing of significant songs enabled the adolescents to creatively express pent up feelings. It also helped some to feel less isolated as they discovered, in a non-confronting manner, that they were not alone.[25]

Staff support

Music therapy can indirectly support and help staff as they witness and occasionally participate in public ward sessions. This was evident in the author's study on the relevance of MT in a cancer hospital.[1] One staff member anonymously wrote:

> For me personally, seeing the patients' responses (in MT) has heightened my awareness of each person's need to be listened to, to be cared for + to have 'time out'—in an environment such as the ward, where the hectic pace + unfamiliar procedures can at times be overwhelming.

And another wrote:

> MT certainly allows me to go about my work in a more relaxed state + gives me a common point of reference between myself + patient + family.

Music therapy may also provide formal staff support in workshops enabling members to musically improvise and discuss their experiences caring for people with advanced illnesses.[26]

Further research

Music therapists have used various research methods to provide a spectrum of insights about the efficacy of MT in palliative care. Research may focus on either examining MT participants' interpretations about their experiences, or verifying whether treatment effects identified by the researcher as important have occurred. Many music therapists, however, struggle with providing evidence acceptable to hospital managers who favour findings from randomized controlled trials (RCTs) when considering resource allocation. This may explain why there are few music therapists employed in health care. The author believes that the following major methodological difficulties would exist if RCTs were used to assess the efficacy of MT:

1. *Diverse characteristics of the source population.* The range of therapies simultaneously being used with patients, their highly fluctuating physical and emotional responses to those treatments, and their diverse psychosocial and musical backgrounds, means that randomization is likely to be ineffective in distributing confounders evenly between groups.
2. *Music therapy exposure.* Music therapists tailor their approach according to patients' responses, that is, the MT process does not allow for a standardized treatment. Furthermore, the blinding of patients to the therapy is not possible.
3. *Measurement of outcome.* The use of quality of life and associated scales may measure criteria important to the researcher, but they do not necessarily capture respondents' idiosyncratic voices reflecting whether the experience was important to them.[27]

Three different studies examining the effects of MT in palliative care follow.

Patients' interpretations of their MT experiences were examined in Hogan's research on the phenomenology of MT with the terminally ill. Semi-structured interviews were conducted with nine terminally ill cancer patients who received MT sessions that included a variety of methods, mainly therapist or patient-selected live or pre-recorded music. Their reported experiences were condensed into a final statement indicating that MT was a positive, emotional experience that could elicit social interaction, inspire improved well-being and coping mechanisms, and elicit spiritual reflections and memories.[28]

An example of research examining whether MT treatment effects identified by the researchers as important have occurred is an observational study conducted by Gallagher et al.[29] An effective MT intervention was defined as when two or more positive responses were identified by the researcher (who was also the music therapist) at the end of individual patient sessions. Most frequent positive responses ascribed to 106 patients who experienced MT in this 6-month study were verbally expressed interest (74 per cent), positive verbal response (61 per cent), and relaxed/changed affect (57 per cent).

The author used the constructivist research paradigm[3] when comparing patients', visitors', staff, and her own views about the relevance of MT in a cancer hospital.[1,31] Over a 3-month period, virtually all patients who participated in sessions, patients who overheard MT sessions, and involved visitors and staff, were invited to anonymously respond to open-ended questionnaires. Feedback was received from 258 people, and the music therapist's interpretations were written in a clinical journal. The textual data was condensed into themes using thematic analysis from grounded theory, with the support of qualitative data management software.

Findings were that MT elicited a range of affective responses and altered imaginings, especially among patients who experienced MT, and the visitors. Their predominantly positive experiences were characterized by memories being revisited, as well as their 'transportation' to new places or thoughts and physical sensations. Numerous staff and visitors also reported that MT helped them while they were with the patients. The music therapist (author) also described considerably more expressions of sadness, distress, grief, and humour, and instances of 'community' interaction in sessions than the other respondents did.

This study of the relevance of a 16-hour-a-week MT position in a cancer hospital provides hospital administrators with some perspective about what a similar MT programme might offer another similar hospital context in a 3-month time frame.[31] Briefly, 207 patients experienced MT in 356 individual or group sessions. Two hundred and two people refused MT in that time. Sixty-two per cent of the patients who experienced MT provided anonymously and spontaneously written feedback. Virtually all found MT helpful. All except one of the 27 patients who overheard MT, and anonymously wrote about that experience, indicated that MT did not annoy them. Many found it helpful, as did the 61 staff members and 42 visitors who also anonymously responded.

Adverse effects

As long as MT participants have a sense of control over the music experienced in sessions, adverse effects are rare. People tend to choose music that elicits memories and affective responses that they wish to experience (consciously or unconsciously) and are usually able to shift the musical evocations by simply requesting or performing different kinds of music. For this reason, MT is often described as a non-intrusive, albeit potentially transformative, form of therapy. Music therapists attempt to ensure that neighbouring patients are consulted whenever sessions are about to commence in public ward settings and avoid conducting sessions in locations where others find them disturbing.

Contraindications for MT in palliative care are rare, except when patients do not like the available music. Occasionally, however, neural damage can result in distorted and unpleasant musical perception. Although rare, music therapists should also be wary of patients likely to experience musicogenic epilepsy (a condition in which music can directly trigger an epileptic seizure) and musically induced catastrophic reactions (heightened anxiety or distress triggered in some people with dementia when hearing specific music).[23]

Closure

Difficulties are inherent in using words to convey the multiplicity of potential messages contained within music. Music's potential to transcend cognitive forms of knowing is fundamental to its impetus as a therapeutic treatment modality. In palliative care, music therapists provide a wide range of creative musical experiences that often help patients with degenerative and terminal illnesses and those close to them. Sonic components of music can alleviate physical distress, mnemonic components reinforce feelings of a life having been and still being lived, and aesthetic components inspire transcendental experiences.

Lullabies and 'motherese' (adults' sung communication to babies) introduce babies to their culture, and an infant's repetitive use of a tune represents transitional phenomena enabling negotiation between one's inner and external reality.[12] Re-experiencing the music from one's lifetime, and improvising music and writing songs informed by that life, can help to affirm one's presence, sustain through adversity, and ease one's path from mortal reality to the reality that lies beyond.

Addis proposed that music has such 'power' in human life because it can represent a level of consciousness of which one is not aware.[32] Perhaps

[3] The constructivist research paradigm rejects the positivist view that research can uncover 'truth', that is, one acceptable reality. Constructivism acknowledges that different people can view a phenomenon in different but equally valid ways. One's view of reality is 'socially and experientially based, local and specific in nature' (ref. 30, p. 110) although some understandings may be shared among individuals and cultures. The investigator cannot be entirely objective and is inevitably linked with the object of the investigation. Knowledge is developed as multiple constructions of reality among different people are interpreted, compared, and contrasted.[30]

that explains how music can powerfully aid one's ultimate journey to the realm where one's consciousness ceases.

> Which of the two powers, love or music, is able to lift man to the sublimest heights? It is a great question, but it seems to me that one might answer it thus: love cannot express the idea of music, while music may give an idea of love. Why separate the one from the other? They are two wings of the soul.
>
> Hector Berlioz (1803–69)

References

1. **O'Callaghan, C.** (2001). Bringing music to life: music therapy and palliative care experiences in a cancer hospital. *Journal of Palliative Care* **13** (3), 155–60.
2. **Munro, S. and Mount, B.M.** (1978). Music therapy in palliative care. *Canadian Medical Association Journal* **119**, 1029–34.
3. **Lee, C.A.**, ed. *Lonely Waters: Proceedings of the International Conference, Music Therapy in Palliative Care*, Oxford, 1994. Oxford: Sobell Publications, 1995.
4. **Martin, J.A.**, ed. *The Next Step Forward: Music Therapy with the Terminally Ill*. New York: Calvary Hospital, 1989.
5. **Rykov, M. and Salmon, D.** (1998). Bibliography for music therapists in palliative care. *The American Journal of Hospice and Palliative Care* **15** (3), 174–80.
6. **Magill-Leverault, L.** (1993). Music therapy in pain and symptom management. *Journal of Palliative Care* **9** (4), 42–8.
7. **Munro, S.** *Music Therapy in Palliative/Hospice Care*. St Louis: Magnamusic-Baton, 1984.
8. **Schroeder-Sheker, T.** (1993). Music for the dying: a personal account of the new field of music thanatology—history, theories, and clinical narratives. *Advances, The Journal of Mind–Body Health* **9** (1), 36–48.
9. **Laderman, C. and Roseman, M.**, ed. *The Performance of Healing*. New York: Routledge, 1996.
10. **Hogan, B.** (1999). Searching for the rite of passage. In *Music Therapy in Palliative Care: New Voices* (ed. D. Aldridge), pp. 68–81. London: Jessica Kingsley Pub Ltd.
11. **McAdam, S.** (1984). The auditory image: a metaphor for musical and psychological research on auditory organization. In *Cognitive Processes in the Perception of Art* (ed. W.R. Crozier and A.J. Chapman), pp. 289–323. Amsterdam: North-Holland.
12. **Winnicott, D.W.** *Playing and Reality*. London: Routledge, 1971.
13. **Forrest, L.C.** (2000). Addressing issues of ethnicity and identity in palliative care through music therapy. *The Australian Journal of Music Therapy* **11**, 33–7.
14. **Magee, W.** (1999). Music therapy in chronic degenerative illness. In *Music Therapy in Palliative Care: New Voices* (ed. D. Aldridge), pp. 82–94. London: Jessica Kingsley Pub Ltd.
15. **Salmon, D.** (1995). Music and emotion in palliative care: assessing inner resources. In *Lonely Waters: Proceedings of the International Conference, Music Therapy in Palliative Care*, Oxford, 1994 (ed. C.A. Lee), pp. 71–84. Oxford: Sobell Publications.
16. **Hartley, N.** (1999). Music therapists' personal reflections on working with those who are living with HIV/AIDS. In *Music Therapy in Palliative Care: New Voices* (ed. D. Aldridge), pp. 105–25. London: Jessica Kingsley Pub Ltd.
17. **O'Callaghan, C.** (1996). Lyrical themes in songs written by palliative care patients. *Journal of Music Therapy* **33** (2), 74–92.
18. **Marr, J.** (1998–99). GIM at the end of life: case studies in palliative care. *Journal of the Association for Music and Imagery* **6**, 37–54.
19. **Slivka, H.H. and Magill, L.** (1986). The conjoint use of social work and music therapy with children of cancer patients. *Music Therapy* **6A** (1), 30–40.
20. **Daveson, B. and Kennelly, J.** (2000). Music therapy in palliative care for hospitalised children and adolescents. *Journal of Palliative Care* **16** (1), 35–8.
21. **Aasgaard, T.** (2000). A suspiciously cheerful lady: a study of a song's life in the paediatric oncology ward and beyond .... *British Journal of Music Therapy* **14** (2), 70–82.
22. **Sergent, J., Zuck, S., Tenial, S., and McDonald, B.** (1992). Distributed neural network underlying musical sightreading and keyboard performance. *Science* **257**, 106–9.
23. **O'Callaghan, C.** (1999). Recent findings about neural correlates of music pertinent to music therapy across the life span. *Music Therapy Perspectives* **17** (1), 32–6.
24. **Rosenfeld, J.V. and Dun, B.** (1999). Music therapy in children with severe traumatic brain injury. In *MusicMedicine* (ed. R. Rebollo Pratt and D. Erdonmez Grocke), pp. 35–46. Melbourne: Faculty of Music, University of Melbourne.
25. **McFerran-Skewes, K. and Erdonmez Grocke, D.** (2000). Group music therapy for young bereaved teenagers. *European Journal of Palliative Care* **7** (6), 227–9.
26. **Murrant, G.M., Rykov, M., Amonite, D., and Loynd, M.** (2000). Creativity and self-care for caregivers. *The Journal of Palliative Care* **16** (2), 44–9.
27. **McGrath, P.** *Confronting Icarus: A Psychosocial Perspective on Haematological Malignancies*. Aldershot UK: Ashgate, 2000.
28. **Hogan, B.** (1999). A phenomenological research project. In *MusicMedicine* (ed. R. Rebollo Pratt and D. Erdonmez Grocke), pp. 242–52. Melbourne: University of Melbourne.
29. **Gallagher, L.M., Huston, M.J., Nelson, K.A., Walsh, D., and Steele, A.L.** (2001). Music therapy in palliative medicine. *Supportive Care Cancer* **9**, 156–61.
30. **Guba, E.G. and Lincoln, Y.S.** (1994). Competing paradigms in qualitative research. In *Handbook of Qualitative Research* (ed. N. Denzin and Y.S. Lincoln), pp. 105–17. Newbury Park: Sage.
31. **O'Callaghan, C.** Music therapy's relevance in a cancer hospital researched through a constructivist lens. PhD thesis, University of Melbourne: University of Melbourne, 2001.
32. **Addis, L.** *Of Mind and Music*. Ithaca NY: Cornell University Press, 1999.

Further reading

Aldridge, D., ed. *Music Therapy in Palliative Care: New Voices*. London: Jessica Kingsley Pub Ltd, 1999.

Bailey, L. (1983). The effects of live versus tape recorded music in hospitalised cancer patients. *Music Therapy* **3** (1), 17–28.

Beggs, C. (1991). Life review with a palliative care patient. In *Case Studies in Music Therapy* (ed. K. Brusica), pp. 611–16. Phoenixville PA: Barcelona.

Lee, C. *Music at the Edge: The Music Therapy Experiences of a Musician with AIDS*. London: Routledge, 1996.

Magill Bailey, L. (1984). The use of songs in music therapy with cancer patients and their families. *Music Therapy* **4** (1), 5–17.

Mandel, S.E. (1991). Music therapy in the hospice: 'Musicalive'. *Journal of Palliative Care* **9** (4), 42–8.

O'Brien, E. (1999). Cancer patients' evaluation of a music therapy program. In *MusicMedicine* (ed. R. Rebollo Pratt and D. Erdonmez Grocke), pp. 285–300. Melbourne: Faculty of Music, University of Melbourne.

O'Callaghan, C. (1996). Pain, music creativity and music therapy in palliative care. *The American Journal of Hospice and Palliative Care* **13** (2), 43–9.

Porchet-Munro, S. (1995). The supportive role of music. *European Journal of Palliative Care* **2** (2), 77–80.

Porchet-Munro, S. (1998). Music therapy. In *Oxford Textbook of Palliative Medicine* (ed. D. Doyle, G. Hanks, and N. MacDonald), pp. 855–60. Oxford: Oxford University Press.

Rykov, M. (1999). Sometimes there are no reasons: Marco's song. In *Inside Music Therapy: Client Experiences* (ed. J. Hibben), pp. 202–7. Gilsum NH: Barcelona.

Salmon, D. (1993). Music and emotion in palliative care. *Journal of Palliative Care* **9** (4), 48–52.

The Journal of Palliative Care **17** (3), 2001. (Music therapy in palliative care thematic issue.)

15.3 The contribution of the dietician and nutritionist to palliative medicine

Rosemary Richardson and Isobel Davidson

How to perform a true physician's art
And show I am a perfect master of my art
I will prescribe what diet you should use
What food you ought to take and what to refuse?

Ovid 45BC

Nutritional management of patients receiving palliative care has not, until recently, been considered an explicit element of care. The features of cachexia such as anorexia are often considered by health care professionals as milestones of disease progression. Traditionally, the input from palliativists relating to nutrition is one of ethics and may centre on the withdrawal of food and fluids. Nevertheless, many patients present with and are distressed by the presence of symptoms that affects their ability to eat 'normally', that is, dysphagia, taste changes, xerostomia, dementia (see Chapter 8.4.3). The deterioration and alteration in nutritional intake results in weight loss, accompanying fatigue, and distressing alterations in body image.

The futility of approaches that merely seek to improve patients' nutritional intake, either enterally or parenterally, and replete body mass may have contributed to the lack of enthusiasm in considering the nutritional care of this vulnerable group. This is apparent in the education of the nursing profession where analysis of 46 key textbooks in palliative care have shown that 59 per cent of books make no mention of nutrition and the content of only 13 per cent was rated as commendable.[1] This study serves to confirm that nutrition is not viewed as important by experts (editors and authors) in this field and as a consequence their readership.

However, our improved understanding of the metabolic sequelae of disease and an appreciation of nutritional strategies that may be used to ameliorate or manage symptoms (see Table 1) should result in the recognition of nutrition as a component of holistic palliative care. Perhaps, what many professionals have lost sight of is that the aim of nutritional counselling and/or intervention is to improve the patient's quality of life (see Fig. 1).

Embedding nutritional care in palliative medicine must be paralleled by formal and rigorous evaluation (i.e. randomised controlled trials) of practice. To a large part, this remains to be addressed and it would be naïve not to appreciate the inherent difficulties of conducting nutritional research in the palliative care environment. For example, to avoid the distress experienced by weight-losing patients, weight is not monitored. Moreover, weighing scales are often not available in hospices or patients' homes and this poses a dichotomy for the dietitian and care team in monitoring the effectiveness of any nutritional strategies. This obstacle can be overcome by informing and involving the patient and their carer as to the value of

Table 1 Nutritional strategies to improve symptom control

Symptom	Causes of decrease in dietary intake	Management
Psychological stress/depression	Poor appetite	Antidepressant, complementary therapies (i.e. aromatherapy, reflexology), small frequent meals
Altered taste and smell	Food aversions	Dietary counselling and identification of food aversions/preferences
Oral thrush/ulceration	Blunting of taste	Pharmacological treatment of symptoms (i.e. Nystatin, lignocaine) Increase use of nutrient-dense cold fluids Optimize oral hygiene
Reduced flow and altered consistency of saliva	Induce gagging and nausea	Use of artificial saliva To encourage flow of saliva—chew gum or suck on boiled sweets Optimize oral hygiene
Nausea and vomiting	Physical obstruction Drugs, i.e. opioids Radio/chemotherapy	Pharmacological treatment that is effective at mealtimes Small frequent meals Avoidance of food aversions Consume fluids after meals
Dysphagia	Physical obstruction/construction	Altered consistency of food semi-solid → puree Use of nutrient-dense supplements Consider initiating PEG feeding
Respiratory distress	Focus on breathing rather than food intake	Medication before mealtimes Ensure patient wears loose clothing Relaxation exercises Small meals and presentation foods that do not require a list of chewing
Early satiety	Cytokine mediated	Maximize availability of food Small frequent meals Encourage food consumption when patients feel at their best/less agitated
Altered bowel function		
Constipation	Feeling bloated Abdominal discomfort	Mild laxatives Encourage fluid intake Encourage consumption of dietary fibre If possible optimize mobility
Diarrhoea	Abdominal discomfort Fear of symptom leads to food avoidance	Medication (i.e. Lomita) Temporarily avoid dairy products Increase intake soluble fibre (i.e. bananas, oranges, oatmeal)
Fatigue/lethargy	Neurological Loss of muscle mass	Maximize intake when patient feels at their best Avoid foods that require a lot of chewing

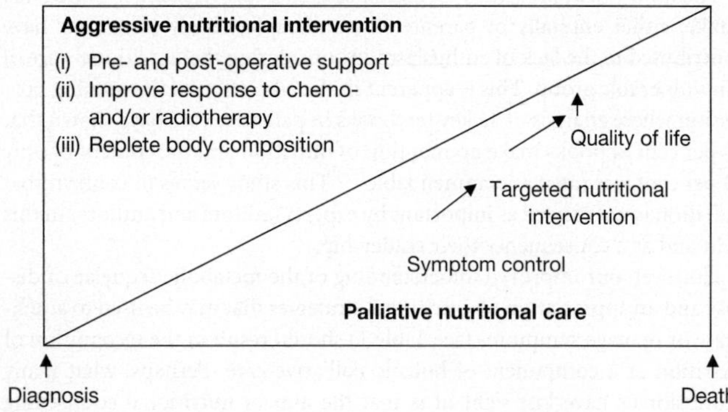

Fig. 1 The role of nutritional support in palliative care. (Adapted from ref. 2.)

monitoring weight, but as with all other elements of nutritional assessment, this procedure should only be carried out with consent.

Dietary counselling

Dietary counselling should serve to provide the dietitian with an understanding of the patients' nutritional problems, their needs, and an appreciation of limitations and barriers to complying with nutritional advice/prescriptions. Dietary counselling is a time-consuming process and an initial interview, which may or may not involve the informal carer, can last about an hour. In light of this, the atmosphere in which the interview is to be conducted should be relaxed and conducive to frank and open discussion.

Developing a relationship of trust between the dietitian, patient, and their support network is central to evaluating nutritional intervention. Patients are surprisingly good at providing information the dietitian wants to hear and whilst patients may verbally confirm their compliance to nutritional treatment on careful and sensitive questioning, adherence may be limited or non-existent. This may account for the disappointing results of one of the few randomized control trials that examined the effect of dietary counselling on food intake, body weight, and quality of life in cancer patients.[3] Patients ($n = 57$) were randomized to receive nutritional counselling (twice a month for 5 months) and offered nutritional supplemental drinks. The control group ($n = 48$) ate *ad libitum* and had no counselling. Results showed that, when compared with controls, 5 months of dietary counselling increased total energy intake by 15 kcal/day and 0.6 g protein/day and not surprisingly no differences in body weight or quality of life were observed. No details of the structure of the counselling interview were provided other than that its aim was for patients to achieve recommended intakes. Similarly, a study[4] of patients with advanced colorectal and non-small-cell lung cancer showed no differences in intake in patients receiving and not receiving dietary counselling.

There remains a paucity of studies that have examined the effect of dietary counselling in palliative care. Evaluation of counselling should be determined not only by quantitative parameters, that is, intake, change in body weight, but also by qualitative elements; for example, determining patients' and their carers' understanding of nutritional advice/prescription, patient satisfaction (i.e. is the counselling process itself too onerous), and level of symptom relief from dietary advice.

Many dietitians undertake additional training to develop their counselling skills and enlisting the expertise of an information manager can assist in formal evaluation of counselling interviews. In conducting and evaluating patient interviews, the interviewer may find it helpful to construct a template of 'probes' that forms the construct of the interview and facilitates the patient/carer taking the lead in discussion (Table 2). Prior to interview construction the dietitian should be fully cognisant of the patient's medical history.

Often, patients and their informal carers have high expectations of nutritional intervention and have themselves made a clear but inappropriate choice of treatment (i.e. TPN).[5,6] Thoughtful counselling acts to improve patient management, but by involving the patient there is scope to redefine the selection and expectations of dietary intervention. It should be remembered that the Internet is a source of dietary information accessed by many patients and their carers. This may result in alternative therapies being used, that is, macrobiotic diets, supra-dosing of vitamins and homeopathy, and should be reviewed.

Table 2 Effective dietary counselling

Suggestions for constructing patient interview
What changes in your diet had there been over the last few months?
Quantity
Food aversion/taste changes
Consistency
Diet history
Do you think nutrition is an important part of your care?
Any symptoms around mealtimes that are troublesome?
Pain
Respiratory distress
How are you managing with nutritional supplemental drinks?
Compliance
Change prescription
Taste fatigue
Is there anytime of the day when you feel at your best?
Opportunity to optimize intake
How is your informal carer? (if patient interviewed)
Pressure for patient to eat (alone)
Anxiety of carer
Identify home enteral feeding problems
Are you happy that your nutritional status is monitored?
Objectives

If the patient cannot be interviewed then the carer becomes the source of dietary information.

Innovative approaches to increase nutritional intake

Nutritional supplements

Timing of consumption

Control of ingestive behaviour in cachexia (see Chapter 8.4.3) permits re-examination of traditional approaches to nutritional intake. An extensive range of commercially produced supplements are available. These normally provide 1.5 kcal/ml and 0.6 g/ml of protein may be presented in 200–250 ml cartons. Patients are generally encouraged to consume these supplements after meals.

However, for many patients there may be amplification of the satiety cascade (neural and humoral), prolonging the inter-meal interval and negate post-prandial consumption (see Chapter 8.4.3). A more targeted approach may be to present energy and protein-dense supplements before meals (1 h) when feelings of hunger are strongest. In addition, patients should be discouraged from consuming low-nutritive fluids at the beginning of meals, that is, soups. The reason for this is to minimize the volumetric effect of fluids on satiety. In cachexia, sensitization of the afferent nerves (Chapter 8.4.3) may result in early afferent 'firing' (satiety signal) at relatively low gastric volumes. Whilst this approach is based on the translation of pathophysiology to practice, it remains to be evaluated.

Indeed, there may be some concerns that consumption of supplements before meals would result in compensation at mealtimes. Interestingly,[7] in a study that examined the effect of nutritive pre-loads (high fat, high carbohydrate) on meal consumption in elderly subjects and younger controls, the elderly subjects did not compensate for the pre-load. These results are encouraging given that the majority of patients in palliative care are elderly, but no subject in this study had metabolically active disease.

Recent work in patients with advanced pancreatic cancer[8] examined the effect of a fish-oil-enriched supplement (ecosapentanoic acid, energy and protein dense) on total dietary intake. Nutrient intake (meals and supplement) was significantly greater in those patients receiving the fish oil than in the group randomized to energy and protein supplements without fish oil. These supplements were offered after meals and future studies should evaluate supplementation before meals and include ratings of hunger and satiety.

Patient acceptance

The sensory evaluation of oral supplements is rarely carried out in patients receiving palliative care. Many patients complain of aberrant olfaction and taste,[9,10] contributing to the poor acceptance and compliance with nutritional supplements. Patients should be offered a range of flavours and this applies to 'normal' diet as well as supplements. This strategy may prevent the development of sensory specific satiety.[11]

Meal priorities

Health care professionals should appreciate that mealtimes can be a stressful event for patients and the family. For example, the food presented may be modified in consistency, too much food on the plate and coping with symptoms, that is, pain and eating, can all reduce intake. In addition, the pressure that the informal carer can put on the patient to eat often goes unrecognized.

> My husband is doing his best he cooks my favourite foods and brings it to me on a tray. It's too much, I just can't eat it so I scoop half of it into a bag
>
> Cancer patient

These issues should be explored during dietary counselling.

Attention to detail is important in encouraging dietary intake and many issues are addressed in Table 1. It is important to make sure the patient is comfortable, that is, correct positioning, toileting, and the environment is conducive to eating (catheter bag covered, table/tray attractively presented).

Home artificial nutrition

The majority of palliative care patients on home feeding are prescribed enteral nutrition (naso-gastric and percutaneous endoscopic gastrostomy). The prevalence and efficiency of artificial nutrition is considered in Chapter 8.4.3. Implementation of home artificial nutrition support requires significant education and training of patients and/or their carers. Meticulous discharge planning, communication between care team, and a structured monitoring process are key elements to making home enteral nutrition an acceptable treatment modality.

Education and training

The informal carer is most likely to take responsibility for maintaining patency of the feeding tube, feed administration, and routine mentoring. It should be remembered that the patients and their families may consider home enteral feeding to be second best when compared with parenteral feeding.[12] These apprehensions should be explored before discharging the patient.

Wherever possible, a named nurse and dietitian should be involved in training carers for home feeding. Using a stepwise approach the informal carer should become actively involved in clinical tasks relating to enteral feeding, that is, syringing tube, changing giving set, cleaning gastrostomy. By exploring one area of care at any one time allows the carers to gain confidence and demonstrate their ability and develop an understanding of the patient's needs. The use of video and written materials is helpful in reinforcing teaching sessions.

Prior to starting feeding or sending patients home on feeding, the patient's home should be visited to evaluate practical issues such as:

- What storage space is available to stock feed and related consumables, that is, giving sets.
- Can a drip stand be moved freely round the house. Steps and loose carpets may increase the patient's risk of tripping.
- Is there a phone.

Life should be made as easy as possible and a homecare company may be involved in feed delivery. Carers should also be provided with a contact number for support from health care professionals.

Nutritional assessment

Evaluation of nutritional intervention in palliative care relies on nutritional assessment. This not only involves determination of nutrient intake (dietary and/or artificial nutritional support), a procedure generally well accepted by the patient, but should also include sequential monitoring of patients' nutritional status. The latter provides information relating to the progression or attenuation of loss of body mass. Sensitivity by the individual undertaking the assessment is paramount.

Body weight

If a patient in the terminal stage of disease is immobile and/or severely demented, undertaking a nutritional assessment may be inappropriate. Furthermore, some patients might not wish their weight to be monitored and of course their wishes should be respected.

An individual's body weight can be compared with tables[13] that provide 'normal' values for individuals of the same sex, age, and height. However, consideration of recent weight loss (i.e. 3 months) allows an insight into the magnitude and progression of weight loss.

Weight loss as percentage of 'used' body weight:

$$\text{Percentage weight loss} = \frac{\text{used body weight (kg)} - \text{current weight}}{\text{usual body weight}} \times 100$$

This approach allows patients to provide their own reference value. An unintentional weight loss of 10 per cent in 3 months is indicative of significant weight loss and 20 per cent protein energy undernutrition.[14]

Body mass index

Another method of using weight as a nutritional parameter is to express height as a power index of weight:

$$\text{Body mass index (BMI) units } (\text{kg m}^2) = \frac{\text{Weight (kg)}}{\text{Height}^2\ \text{(m)}}$$

- a BMI less than 20 is indicative of mild undernutrition;
- a BMI less than 18 is indicative of moderate undernutrition;
- a BMI less than 16 is indicative of severe undernutrition.

The assessor should be aware that the presence of oedema or ascites may mask the degree of undernutrition and care in interpretation of weight data is required.

Arm anthropometry

Triceps skinfold thickness provides an indication of fat reserves. This measurement is taken using skinfold callipers at the mid-point between the acnomium process and the olecranon, and results are compared with standard values.[15]

An indication of skeletal muscle mass may be obtained by subtracting the skinfold thickness from the mid-upper arm circumference. This technique assumes the upper arm circumference is a perfect circle.

$$\text{Arm muscle circumference} = \text{mid-upper arm circumference} - (\text{triceps skinfold} \times \Pi)$$

The upper arm is easily accessible and less prone to oedema. Information on arm anthropometry should be considered with weight data.

Hand grip dynamometry

Weakness, asthenia, and fatigue are common symptoms of palliative care patients. Whilst weight and arm anthropometry provide quantitative information relating to body mass, handgrip dynamometry is a functional marker of mass. If one aim of nutritional intervention is to improve lean body mass, it is important that both the quantity and quality of this tissue increases.

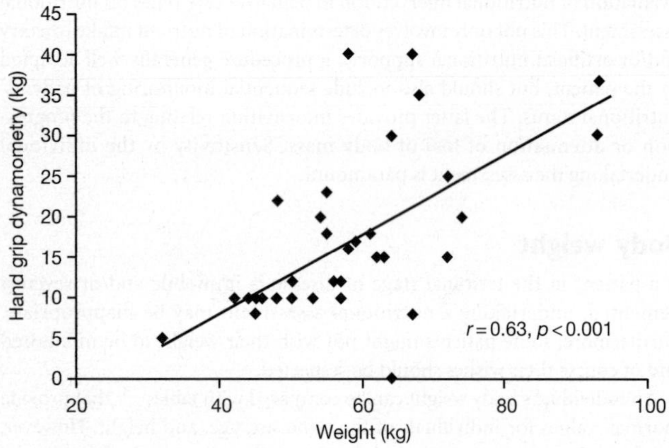

This non-invasive technique involves determination of patient's maximal grip strength.[16]

The overriding component of nutritional management in palliative care is ensuring the wishes of the patient and family are fulfilled. Today patients are more informed than ever before and actively seek information relating to their disease and management. This means that the boundaries of practice for health care professionals has shifted and will continue to do so. There is now a need for professionals to integrate their understanding of clinical science and current research to inform their practice.

References

1. **Ferell, B.** et al. (2000). Analysis of palliative care content in nursing textbooks. *Journal of Palliative Care* **16**, 39–47.
2. **Finlay, I.** (2001). UK strategies for palliative care. *Journal of the Royal Society of Medicine* **94**, 437–41.
3. **Ovensen, L.** et al. (1993). Effect of dietary counselling on food intake, body weight, response rate, survival and quality of life in cancer patients undergoing chemotherapy: a prospective, randomised study. *Journal of Clinical Oncology* **13**, 2043–9.
4. **Evans, W.K.** et al. (1987). A randomised study of oral nutritional support versus ad lib nutritional intake during chemotherapy for advanced colorectal and non-small cell lung cancer. *Journal of Clinical Oncology* **5**, 113–24.
5. **McCann, R., Hall, W., and Groth-Juncker, A.** (1994). Comfort care for terminally ill patients. The appropriate use of nutrition and hydration. *Journal of the American Medical Association* **272**, 1263–6.
6. **Plaisance, L.** (1997). The litany of the last meal. *American Journal of Nursing* **97**, 60–1.
7. **Rolls, B.J.** et al. (1991). Time course of effects of preloads high in fat or carbohydrate on food intake and hunger ratings in humans. *American Journal of Physiology* **260**, 756–63.
8. **Richardson, R.** et al. (2001). A protein and energy dense, n-3 fatty acid enriched oral nutritional supplement improves dietary intake and weight in patients with cancer cachexia. *Proceedings of the Nutrition Society* **61**, 27a.
9. **Krishnasamy, M.** (1995). Oral problems in advanced cancer. *European Journal of Cancer Care* **4**, 173–7.
10. **Davidson, H.I.M., Paltison, R.M., and Richardson, R.A.** (1998). Clinical undernutrition states and their influence on taste. *Proceedings of the Nutrition Society* **57**, 1–6.
11. **Rolls, E.T. and Rolls, J.H.** (1996). Olfactory sensory-specific satiety in humans. *Physiology and Behaviour* **61** (3), 461–73.
12. **Ireton-Jones, C., Orr, M., and Hennessy, K.** (1997). Clinical pathways in home nutrition support. *Journal of the American Dietetic Association* **97**, 1003–7.
13. **Metropolitan Height and Weight Fables.** (1983). Metropolitan Life Foundation. *Statistical Bulletin* **64** (1).
14. **Kinney, J.M.** (1988). The influence of calorie and nitrogen balance on weight loss. *British Journal of Clinical Practice* **12**, 114–20.
15. **Jelliffe, D.B.** *The Assessment of the Nutritional Status of the Community.* WHO Monograph 53, Geneva: WHO, 1996.
16. **Windsor, J.A. and Hill, G.L.** (1988). Grip strength: a measure of the proportion of protein loss in surgical patients. *British Journal of Surgery* **75**, 880–2.

15.4 The contribution of physiotherapy to palliative medicine

Luke Doyle, Jenny McClure, and Sarah Fisher

Introduction

The value of physiotherapy in palliative care has been increasingly recognized over the past few decades, with a shift in emphasis from a predominantly medical/nursing model of care, which focused primarily on symptom control, to a more inter-disciplinary, rehabilitative approach. Furthermore, with the increasing survival of patients because of advances in treatment, and the inclusion of non-cancer patients within palliative care, increasing numbers of patients are living with chronic disability, creating new challenges for physiotherapists working in this area.

Physiotherapists have much to offer this patient group with their expertise in the treatment of pain, respiratory and neurological dysfunction, and rehabilitation. The inclusion of physiotherapists in palliative care teams in hospitals, hospices, and in the community is therefore of vital importance in helping to minimize patients' discomfort and maximize functional potential. In patients with advancing disease, where functional limitations are unavoidable, the physiotherapist is the expert in helping both patients and carers cope with these changes, whilst maximizing their potential to achieve realistic goals and thereby achieve optimal quality of life.

The principal problems encountered by physiotherapists when dealing with palliative care patients are shown in Table 1.

Table 1 Key problems addressed by the physiotherapist in palliative care

Pain
Loss of mobility and function
Neurological impairment
Respiratory dysfunction
Fatigue and weakness
Orthopaedic and musculoskeletal problems
Lymphoedema

Principles of physiotherapy in palliative care

Physiotherapy in the palliative setting should aim to enhance the patient's quality of life. This may be achieved by improving function, or where this is not possible, by improving the patient's and carer's ability to cope with the patient's deterioration.

Safe, effective physiotherapy intervention involves:

- medical screening prior to referral to physiotherapy;
- thorough assessment and regular reassessment of the patient's physical status with an acute awareness of their psychological, social, and spiritual well-being;
- an awareness of the multidimensional nature of symptoms such as pain, dyspnoea, and fatigue and an holistic approach to their assessment and management;
- appropriate goal-setting according to the patient's identified problems and priorities;
- modification of goals as the patient's condition changes;
- a problem-solving approach to management;
- clear and sensitive communication with the patient, carers, and the inter-disciplinary team;
- effective communication between hospital, hospice, and community settings;
- the fostering of hope and prevention of feelings of abandonment.

Although rehabilitation is a relatively new concept in palliative care, it is a central part of physiotherapy practice, and translates well to this field. Rehabilitation is described as 'the restoration to the maximum degree possible either of function (physical or mental) or role (within the family, social network, or workforce)'.[1] This is best achieved through the combined expertise of the inter-disciplinary team.[2]

Achievable, specific, realistic goals should be negotiated between the therapist, the patient, carers, and other members of the inter-disciplinary team. This process can be an effective way of restoring a sense of hope to the palliative patient, and avoiding feelings of abandonment commonly experienced in this group.[2,3] Rehabilitation is explored in more depth in Chapter 14.

Physical disability is often a major impediment to quality of life. The range of symptoms experienced in patients with advanced disease can lead to poor mobility and reduced function, which in turn can cause limitations in social, psychological, spiritual, and sexual spheres. The danger is that the patient may become more dependent, reduce their activity levels, and become more disabled. Physiotherapy can interrupt this self-perpetuating cycle, and assist the patients to regain some independence and control of their situation (see disability diagram).

Often, the palliative care patients and their families may express a wish to return home either for a short period, or for the remainder of their life. In this situation, the physiotherapist's skill in assessing the patient's current level of mobility and ability to perform activities of daily living is important to establish the level of support needed for both patient and carers to facilitate safe discharge.

Disability cycle

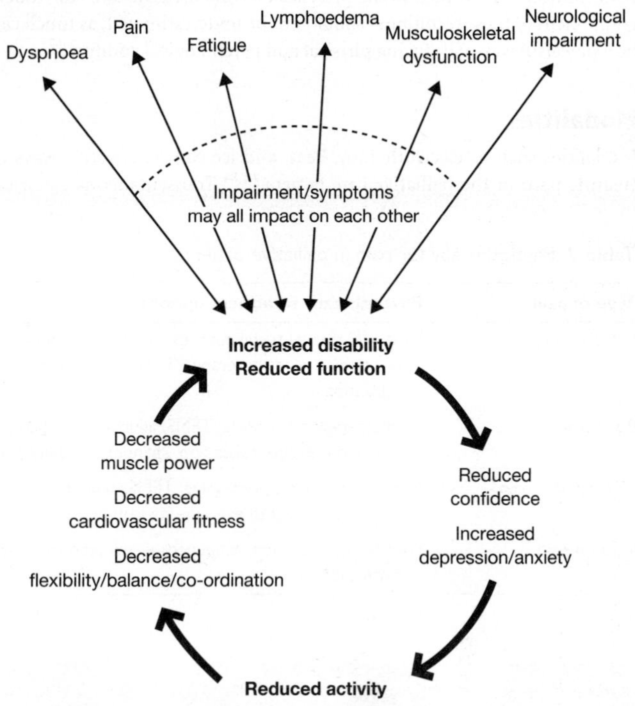

With the increasing emphasis on evidence-based practice, validated outcome measures should be used where appropriate. Physiotherapists are also increasingly becoming involved in audit and research to back up their interventions.

Pain management

Pharmacology has traditionally been the mainstay of pain management in palliative care. However, non-pharmacological treatments such as those offered by physiotherapy are increasingly being sought by patients, and combined with medication may offer improved analgesia.[4] Physiotherapists have a major role to play in the treatment of pain because of their expertise in biomechanical assessment, manual therapies, therapeutic exercise, and the use of electrotherapy and physical modalities. Physiotherapy is primarily effective in the management of bone, soft tissue, and neuropathic pain rather than visceral pain[5] (see Table 2).

Effective communication within the inter-disciplinary team is essential to optimize timing of analgesia with physiotherapy intervention, and to promptly report any significant changes in pain or movement noted by the therapist that may indicate treatable complications such as spinal cord compression. When the pain is chronic, physiotherapists can play a key role in breaking its vicious cycle by adopting the cognitive behavioural approach and other interventions used in chronic pain clinics such as coping skills, pacing, and relaxation.[6]

Physiotherapy for the treatment of pain can be divided into five main categories:

- manual therapies,
- modalities (electrotherapy, acupuncture, heat, and ice),
- exercise and movement,
- positioning,
- relaxation.

Manual therapies

The wide range of manual techniques available to the physiotherapist include soft tissue mobilization, massage, acupressure, manual lymphatic drainage (Fig. 1), and joint mobilizations (Fig. 2) (the latter should be used with caution and avoided in the presence of bone metastases). The 'touch' component of these techniques should not be underestimated, as touch can be a powerful way of inducing physical and psychological comfort.(7)

Modalities

Modalities such as electrotherapy, heat, and ice can be effective ways of treating pain in the palliative care patient.(4,8) Transcutaneous electrical nerve stimulation (TENS) is the most frequently used form of electrotherapy in the palliative setting, generally used in the treatment of neuropathic, bone, and chronic pain.(4,8) Other electrotherapy treatments are used less commonly in the palliative setting and should not be used directly over tumour sites in the absence of research to evaluate their effect on tumour growth. Physiotherapists working in palliative care are now increasingly using acupuncture to treat pain in palliative patients. Both TENS and acupuncture are explored in greater depth in Chapters 8.2.8 and 8.2.9.

Table 2 Physiotherapy for pain in palliative patients

Type of pain	Physiotherapy treatment options
Soft tissue pain	Heat, ice, manual techniques, exercise, hydrotherapy, positioning, electrotherapy, TENS, acupuncture, relaxation
Bone pain	Hydrotherapy, positioning, TENS, acupuncture, heat, selected exercise, relaxation, splinting, mobility aids
Neuropathic pain	Manual techniques, positioning, TENS, acupuncture, relaxation, selected exercise, hydrotherapy
Visceral pain	Positioning, relaxation, acupuncture, selected exercise, hydrotherapy

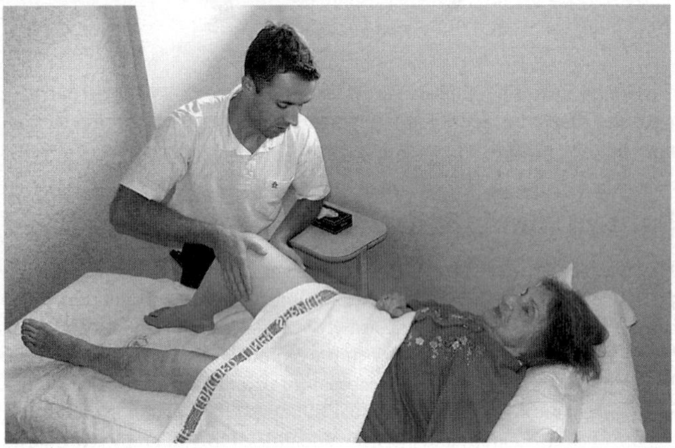

Fig. 1 Manual lymphatic drainage performed on a lymphoedema patient.

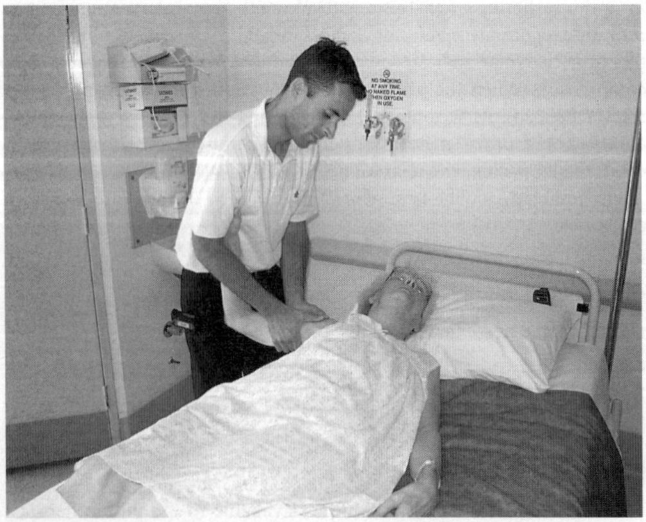

Fig. 2 Gentle shoulder mobilizations.

Exercise and movement

Encouraging the patient to mobilize with appropriate walking aids, and changing position regularly can negate pain and stiffness caused by immobility.(4) Passive, assisted, or active range of movement exercises may be given depending on the patient's level of activity, with the aim of easing joint stiffness and muscle spasm.(4,8,9) Specific exercises may be given to address postural changes and muscle imbalance with the aim of relieving pain.(10) Hydrotherapy can be another effective and enjoyable alternative in the pain management of the palliative care patient.(8)

Positioning and relaxation

Positioning the patient so as to provide support both locally to the painful body segment and generally can relieve pain and maximize function.(4) Advice with regard to positioning in bed, wheelchair, or armchair should be given to both patient and carers. Supportive measures such as the provision of collars, slings, splints, wheelchairs, and walking aids can also reduce pain whilst optimizing function and mobility.(8,9) The physiotherapist may employ general relaxation techniques to control anxiety that often augments other symptoms, including pain.(4)

Although the mechanism of analgesia for many of these therapies is not yet fully known, there are a number of possibilities. The gate control theory(11) postulates that peripheral sensory stimulation, such as that from massage or TENS, modulates the transmission of ascending pain signals at a spinal level. Another possible mechanism is the mediation of the pain response by an increase in endogenous opioids.(12) In addition, at a cognitive level, the physiotherapist may facilitate analgesia.(13) Thus, physiotherapy as part of an inter-disciplinary team can successfully target pain management from a biopsychosocial perspective.(6)

Management of the neurological patient

In the palliative care setting, patients may present with neurological impairment at a central or peripheral level, ranging from neurological tumours and complications of HIV, to neurodegenerative diseases such as multiple sclerosis (MS) and motor neurone disease (MND/AML). Impairments of muscle control, muscle tone, and sensation can lead to abnormal movements and posture, thus leading to a loss of function in everyday activities. This can be compounded by cognitive or perceptual deficits. For example, the patient with no awareness of their left side may be unable to use it.

During assessment, the physiotherapist identifies abnormal postures and movement patterns that hinder purposeful movement, and therefore function. A problem-solving approach is then used to devise an appropriate treatment programme aiming to:

- optimize function;
- re-educate movement patterns whilst taking into account any muscle tone problems;
- prevent or minimize secondary complications; for example, soft tissue contractures and pain.(14)

It is worth reiterating the importance of setting clear realistic goals, especially where perceptual problems or poor insight has been identified. In this situation, carers' and family members' involvement is imperative.

In palliative care especially, the concept of maximizing function should underpin most physiotherapy treatments. For example, whereas a patient with

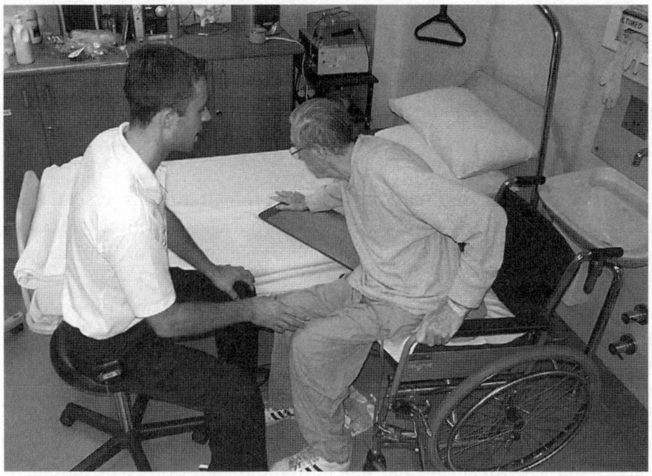

Fig. 3 Transfer practice with a spinal cord compression patient.

incomplete spinal cord injury may be rehabilitated to their highest level possible over a course of many months, this would be inappropriate for the patient with spinal cord compression in the context of advanced cancer. In this case, short-term rehabilitation goals must be set that maximize the patient's function and quality of life,[15] such as independent mobility[16] and safe transfers in and out of the wheelchair (see Fig. 3). One should not, however, assume that some palliative care patients will not tolerate or benefit from intensive rehabilitation programmes. On the whole, this will be dictated by prognosis, exercise tolerance, and fatigue.

Ideally, treatment should aim to restore normal movement patterns, and therefore function. The therapist can achieve this by using specific handling techniques. However, where this is not feasible, the physiotherapist should attempt to maximize function by encouraging appropriate compensatory movement strategies.[17]

Prevention of secondary complications such as contractures is vital, and the physiotherapist may be involved in assessing the patient's seating, splinting or educating the patient and carer about a home management programme.[17,18]

Although manual handling can be an issue in all palliative care patients, it is often a key factor in preparing for safe discharge of the neurological patient. The physiotherapist must assess the patient's ability to move safely, and their carer's ability to assist. Safe moving and handling techniques and use of equipment such as a hoist must be taught, and support from community services established.[19] It should be noted that the physiotherapist is not always the nominated manual handling representative, and may not legally be able to teach manual handling techniques. Although the patient's independence in transfers should be encouraged, this must not be at the expense of the carer's health. These issues should be explored sensitively and explained clearly and openly to avoid any misunderstanding.

Respiratory physiotherapy may also be indicated in the patient with upper spinal cord neoplasm, or progressive neurological disease. This is discussed elsewhere.

Respiratory care

Respiratory symptoms are particularly common in palliative care patients with advanced lung cancer, chronic lung disease, cardiac disease, and progressive neuromuscular disease. The role of the physiotherapist in these patients is most significant in the management of dyspnoea and retained secretions and the functional limitations that may arise from these symptoms (Table 3).

Dyspnoea

The aims of physiotherapy in the management of the breathless patient are to:

- reduce fear and anxiety;
- improve knowledge and understanding;
- maintain or improve exercise tolerance and functional ability;
- reduce breathlessness and the work of breathing;
- improve the efficiency of ventilation;
- mobilize and aid expectoration of secretions;
- reduce thoracic pain.[20]

Table 3 Physiotherapy techniques used for respiratory symptoms

Symptom	Physiotherapy techniques available
Dyspnoea	Positioning at rest and on exercise Breathing control at rest and during activity Relaxation Modified pulmonary rehabilitation (exercise) Energy conservation Mobility aids (walking frames, sticks, wheelchairs) Advice on oxygen delivery/humidification/nebulization Explanation of the mechanisms of breathlessness/ hyperventilation Non-invasive ventilation (NIV)[a]
Retained secretions and productive cough	Positioning (modified postural drainage) Mobility/exercise Active cycle of breathing techniques (ACBT) Forced expiratory technique (FET) Cough/assisted cough Autogenic drainage and other adjuncts Humidification and hydration Suction Chest percussion and vibrations[b]
Chest pain	See 'Pain Management'

[a] NIV is only set up in specialist centres by specialized health professionals.

[b] Only to be used with extreme caution in palliative patients (due to risk of osteoporosis or bone metastases in the ribs or vertebral column).

Reducing anxiety, improving understanding, and maintaining exercise tolerance

Dyspnoea can provoke intense feelings of anxiety and have a significant impact on quality of life. The physiotherapist can help to address anxiety related to dyspnoea through the use of education, relaxation techniques, breathing control (Fig. 4), and supervised exercise. The philosophy used incorporates elements of pulmonary rehabilitation with aspects of hyperventilation management. This approach aims to increase exercise tolerance, reduce the sensation of breathlessness, and reassure the patient that breathlessness need not be a frightening, abnormal experience.

Patients who are too breathless to walk unaided may benefit from a walking frame, walking stick, or wheelchair to improve mobility. Supplementary oxygen may also be used to allow patients to tolerate longer periods of activity (see Fig. 5). Energy conservation, activity pacing, and task analysis are all important aspects of care to improve function in dyspnoeic patients (see Chapter 15.1).

Reducing the work of breathing

The physiotherapist aims to improve the efficiency of breathing through education of patients and carers on positioning, breathing control, and clearance of secretions.

Positioning the patient appropriately utilizes gravity to minimize the work of breathing, maximize the efficiency of ventilation, and encourage the drainage of secretions. The efficiency of breathing is usually optimized in sitting and standing or side-lying positions and poorest in supine and slumped sitting.[21] Whilst the negative effects of the slumped position are well documented,[22] this is a common position adopted by patients. Thus, a simple measure such as changing the patients position may significantly

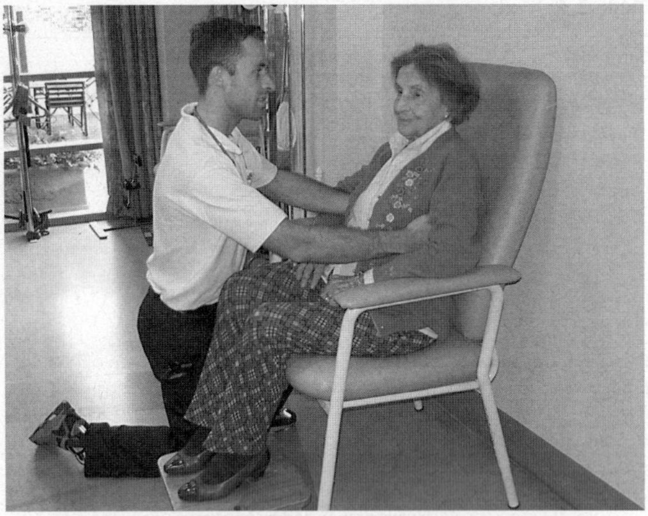

Fig. 4 Breathing control.

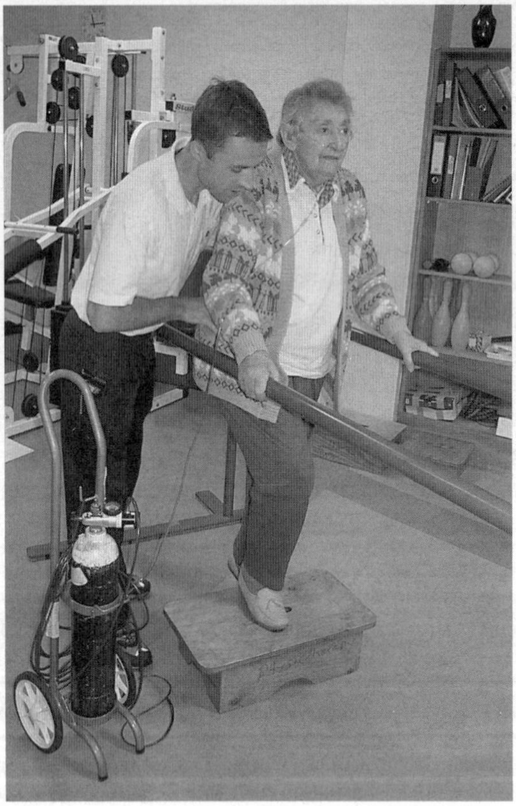

Fig. 5 Exercising to strengthen lower limbs whilst using oxygen.

reduce breathlessness, and may be the only physiotherapy intervention appropriate in the severely dyspnoeic patient.

Management of secretions

Sputum retention can be distressing for both patient and carers and can increase the risk of respiratory infection. The physiotherapist has an important role in assisting and teaching patients and carers on how to clear secretions using positioning, clearance techniques, assisted cough techniques and suction when the cough is less effective.[18,23]

Interventions such as the active cycle of breathing technique (ACBT) and the forced expiratory technique (FET) are frequently used and have been shown to be effective in the clearance of bronchial secretions.[24,25] Techniques such as chest percussion, vibrations, and shaking should only be used with caution in palliative patients and are contraindicated in patients with or at risk of osteoporosis or metastatic deposits in the ribs or vertebral column.[22,26]

Ensuring adequate humidification and hydration is essential to complement other treatments and encourage secretion clearance particularly during periods of infection, oxygen therapy, or in those with tracheotomies.[26]

The use of suction, whilst sometimes considered inappropriate in palliative care, can be useful in selected patients, particularly in those with progressive neurological disease. Even in the dying patient, when excessive upper airways secretions are usually managed pharmacologically, there may be more instances where secretions already present in the trachea may be more effectively removed using gentle suction.[27] Suction should always be carried out with great care and skill to minimize any distress or trauma. It can easily be seen as distressing by relatives sitting at the bedside.

Patients with progressive neuromuscular disease such as MND are particularly at risk of respiratory complications. The physiotherapist has an important role in assisting and teaching patients and carers on how to clear secretions using positioning, assisted cough techniques, and suction to clear secretions when the cough is no longer effective.[18] With the onset of respiratory failure, non-invasive ventilation (NIV) has been found to prolong life in these patients. Whilst there are concerns about the ethics of prolonging life in the presence of progressive disability,[28] physiotherapists working in palliative care may be increasingly involved with patients using NIV in the future.

Lymphoedema management (see Chapter 8.9.3)

Many physiotherapists are involved in the management of lymphoedema as specialist practitioners. Their unique skills in

- the diagnosis and treatment of musculoskeletal dysfunction and pain,
- postural re-education,
- exercise therapy, and
- neurological rehabilitation,

can further benefit the palliative lymphoedema patient. Complications such as brachial plexopathy, chest wall or shoulder pain, and even end-stage lymphoedema can often benefit from physiotherapy intervention, which should focus on pain relief, the amelioration of further chronic disability, and the maintenance or improvement of function. The same principles can be applied for the patient with lower limb lymphoedema.

Orthopaedic management

Skeletal metastases and pathological fractures are the most common orthopaedic conditions in patients with cancer, and can have devastating implications on the individual's quality of life. Where surgical intervention is indicated, post-operative physiotherapy is important to prevent respiratory complications, and regain mobility, function, and independence as quickly as possible.

Some palliative patients may not be appropriate candidates for surgery, resulting in pain, risk of pathological fracture, or skeletal instability. Risk of fracture may be minimized by avoiding submitting the affected limb to large forces, rotation, or full weight-bearing. Walking aids may be useful, and splints or braces may be used for bony instability. A balanced view is needed when advising the terminally ill patient with lower limb bony metastases at risk of fracture whether or not to mobilize. The risks must be discussed with the patient and weighed up against quality of life issues. Hydrotherapy is often ideal due to the water's buoyancy reducing the risk of fracture, and the warmth of the water relieving pain.

Fatigue

Fatigue is a common cause of disability and reduced quality of life in patients with cancer and HIV and has a high prevalence in both populations.[29] It can also be a major problem for other palliative patients including those with neurological or respiratory disease.

Effective management requires identification and treatment of physical causes (e.g. anaemia, infection) and a combination of:

- education about the cause and effect of fatigue;
- exercise and mobility to avoid the consequences of inactivity;
- energy conservation techniques.

Many authors advocate the inclusion of exercise in fatigue management programmes.[29,30] Exercise has been shown to be beneficial in the management of cancer-related fatigue in patients undergoing chemotherapy,[31] physically active patients receiving anti-cancer treatment,[32] and cancer survivors with extreme fatigue.[33] There is a need, however, for further research investigating the effect of exercise on fatigue in patients with more advanced disease.

This move towards using exercise as an intervention for cancer-related fatigue appears to mirror developments in the management of chronic fatigue syndrome, where researchers have found that graded exercise programmes significantly improve fatigue levels amongst other benefits.[34]

Energy conservation is another key concept when attempting to facilitate patients' adaptation to the fatigue experience, and re-establishing their role.[30] The physiotherapist may be involved in teaching principles such as activity pacing, providing equipment, and modifying the home or work environment.

Pain and dyspnoea have been demonstrated to correlate significantly with fatigue severity in patients with advanced cancer.[35] This is possibly due to inefficient function following alterations in posture, guarding, muscle weakness, and spasm.[30] The physiotherapist can address both pain and dyspnoea directly, as well as any associated changes in posture or movement that may occur.

Exercise and deconditioning

It is now widely acknowledged that symptoms such as pain,[4] dyspnoea,[36] neurological dysfunction,[18] and fatigue[29,37] can be exacerbated by inactivity. Historically, patients complaining of these symptoms in the palliative setting were advised to rest and avoid unnecessary activity. This inactivity, however, often causes:

- deconditioning in many of the body's systems (in particular the cardiorespiratory and musculoskeletal systems),
- social isolation,
- a worsening of symptoms,
- fear of movement,
- loss of independence and hence loss of role within family or relationship,

which can all contribute to a decreased quality of life. The physiotherapist can break this vicious cycle of inactivity by encouraging exercise and general mobility.

Cancer places an increased metabolic demand on the patient. Normal protein-sparing mechanisms that preserve muscle mass are reduced or absent and motor activity is reduced in response to the disease and effects of treatment. Physical and functional consequences may include low blood counts, fatigue, reduced cardiovascular and pulmonary function, muscle weakness and atrophy, weight change, sleeping disturbance, nausea, vomiting, and pain.[38] When these changes occur in addition to the effects of inactivity listed above, it is apparent how quickly the patient can lose function, independence, and quality of life. Similarly, deconditioning secondary to inactivity is thought to lead to functional losses greater than those caused directly by the disease in conditions such as HIV[29] and MND/AML.[18]

Therapeutic exercise is now an accepted part of the management of numerous chronic conditions including cardiac disease, pulmonary disease, chronic fatigue syndrome, HIV infection, renal insufficiency, intermittent claudication, and in the frail elderly. A graded exercise programme has also been recommended for MS and MND patients in stable periods of their disease.[18,39] Fatigue in these patients must be avoided by keeping exercise duration brief and allowing sufficient rest between sessions.[18] A recent systematic review investigating the effect of exercise during and following cancer treatment indicates consistent improvement in quality of life measures in addition to improvements in many physical and psychological aspects.[38]

Exercise is an effective holistic intervention as the patient may experience physical benefits such as improved endurance, muscle strength and power, flexibility, and balance in addition to psychological benefits such as improvements in body image, confidence, social interaction, and depression. It also gives the patient an opportunity to participate in what is seen as a 'normal' activity, and to initiate something positive with their body.[3]

Supervised exercise need not require expensive gym equipment and may simply involve functional exercise such as walking or stair climbing (see Fig. 6). This form of exercise is often indicated in the palliative setting as its exercise specificity means skills can be transferred directly across into daily tasks. This becomes particularly salient when planning patient discharge home.

Hydrotherapy provides an alternative medium in which to exercise, and may be more appropriate for patients with pain or bone metastases. It is

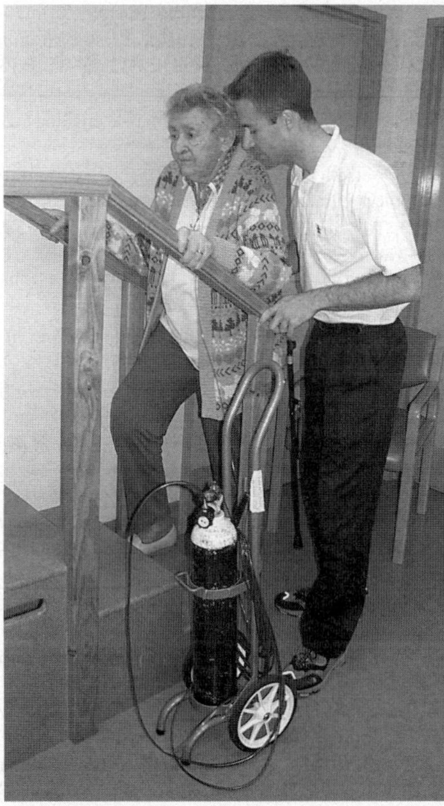

Fig. 6 Stair climbing as a functional exercise.

also recommended for MS[40] and MND[18] patients; however, the pool temperature should be kept lower than that normally maintained in hydrotherapy pools to avoid inducing fatigue.[40]

General principles of exercise such as progression must be encouraged. However, with this population, regular reassessment and goal modification are necessary. Prior to starting an exercise programme, the physiotherapist must screen for risk factors such as bone metastases, cardiomyopathy, and deep vein thromboses. It should be noted that absolute contraindications are rare; one must weigh up potential risks of exercise against the risks of immobility and hence quality of life.

Conclusions

The physiotherapist has a vital role to play in maintaining an optimal level of physical functioning in the palliative patient. This must be achieved via a process of realistic goal-setting with the patient, being aware of the patient's psychosocial needs, constant reassessment of the patient, and appropriate goal-modification. This translates to maximizing the patient's independence, and maintaining their hope in the face of progressive disability. Physiotherapy may be indicated for any of the conditions discussed above, throughout all stages of the disease process, whether for symptom control, rehabilitation, or in the terminal stages.

References

1. **Nocon, A. and Baldwin, S.** *Trends in Rehabilitation Policy: A Review of the Literature.* London: Kings Fund Publishing, 1998, cited by Hopkins, K.F. and Tookman, A.J. (2000). Rehabilitation and specialist palliative care. *International Journal of Palliative Nursing* **6** (3), 123–30.
2. **Hockley, J.** (1993). Rehabilitation in palliative care—are we asking the impossible? *Palliative Medicine* **7** (Suppl. 1), 9–15.
3. **Hopkins, K.F. and Tookman, A.J.** (2000). Rehabilitation and specialist palliative care. *International Journal of Palliative Nursing* **6** (3), 123–30.
4. **O'Gorman, B. and Elfred, A.** (2000). Physiotherapy. In *Cancer Pain Management: A Comprehensive Approach* (ed. K.H. Simpson and K. Budd), pp. 63–73. Oxford: Oxford University Press.
5. **Rashleigh, L.** (1996). Physiotherapy in palliative oncology. *Australian Journal of Physiotherapy* **42**, 307–12.
6. **Harding, V. and Watson, P.J.** (2000). Increasing activity and improving function in chronic pain management. *Physiotherapy* **86** (12), 619–30.
7. **Sims, S.** (1988). The significance of touch in palliative care. *Palliative Medicine* **2**, 58–61.
8. **Robinson, D.** (2000). The contribution of physiotherapy to palliative care. *European Journal of Palliative Care* **7** (3), 95–8.
9. **Marcant, D. and Rapin, C.** (1993). Role of the physiotherapist in palliative care. *Journal of Pain and Symptom Management* **8** (2), 68–71.
10. **Richardson, C.A. and Jull, G.A.** (1995). Muscle control–pain control. What exercises would you prescribe? *Manual Therapy* **1**, 2–10.
11. **Melzack, R. and Wall, P.D.** (1983). The gate control theory of pain. In *The Challenge of Pain* (ed. R. Melzack and P.D. Wall), pp. 222–39. New York: Basic Books.
12. **Portenoy, R.K.** (1996). Basic mechanisms. In *Pain Management: Theory and Practice* (ed. R.K. Porteroy and R.M. Kanner), pp. 19–39. Philadelphia: FA Davis Company.
13. **Rabey** (2001). Interaction between pain physiology and movement-based therapy. *Physiotherapy* **87** (7), 338–40.
14. **Kilbride, C. and McDonnell, A.** (2000). Spasticity: the role of physiotherapy. *British Journal of Therapy and Rehabilitation* **7** (2), 61–4.
15. **Hillier, R. and Wee, B.** (1997). Palliative management of spinal cord compression. *European Journal of Palliative Care* **4** (6), 189–92.
16. **Association of Chartered Physiotherapists in Oncology and Palliative Care.** *Guidelines for Good Practice.* London: Chartered Society of Physiotherapy, 1993.
17. **Edwards, S.** (1996). An analysis of normal movement as the basis for the development of treatment techniques. In *Neurological Physiotherapy: A Problem Solving Approach* (ed. S. Edwards), pp. 15–40. London: Churchill Livingstone.
18. **Dal Bello-Haas, V., Kloos, A.D., and Mitsumoto, H.** (1998). Physical therapy for a patient through six stages of amyotrophic lateral sclerosis. *Physical Therapy* **78** (12), 1312–24.
19. **Fisher, S.N.** (1998). Multidisciplinary teamwork. In *Neuro-oncology for Nurses* (ed. D. Guerrero), pp. 221–52. London: Whurr Publishers Ltd.
20. **Bott, J. and Moran, F.** (1996). *Clinical Practice Guide-lines—A.C.P.R.C. Association of Chartered Physiotherapists in Respiratory Care Standards for Respiratory Care.* London: Association of Physiotherapists in Respiratory Care.
21. **Jenkins, S.C., Soutar, S.A., and Moxham, J.** (1988). The effects of postureon lung volumes in normal subjects and inpatients pre and post coronary artery surgery. *Physiotherapy* **74**, 492–6.
22. **Webber, B. and Pryor, J.** (1998). Physiotherapy techniques. In *Physiotherapy for Respiratory and Cardiac Problems* 2nd edn. (ed. B. Webber and J. Pryor), pp. 137–209. London: Churchill Livingstone.
23. **Oppenheimer, E.A.** (1993). Decision making in the respiratory care of amyotrophic lateral sclerosis: should home mechanical ventilation be used? *Palliative Medicine* **7** (Suppl. 2), 49–64.
24. **Wilson, G.E., Baldwin, A.L., and Walshaw, M.J.** (1995). A comparison of traditional chest physiotherapy with the active cycle of breathing techniques in patients with chronic suppurative lung disease. *European Respiratory Journal* **8** (Suppl. 19), 171S.
25. **Webber, B.A., Hofmeyr, J.L., Morgan, M.D.L., and Hodson, M.E.** (1986). The effects of postural drainage incorporating the forced expiratory technique in cystic fibrosis. *British Journal of Diseases of the Chest* **80**, 353–9.
26. **Mitchie, J.** (1994). An introduction to lung cancer. *Physiotherapy* **80** (12), 844–7.
27. **Ahmedzai, A.** (1998). Palliation of respiratory symptoms. In *Oxford Textbook of Palliative Medicine* 2nd edn. (ed. D. Doyle, G. Hanks, and N. MacDonald), pp. 583–616. Oxford: Oxford University Press.
28. **Turkington, P.M. and Elliott, M.W.** (2000). Rationale for the use of non-invasive ventilation in chronic ventilatory failure. *Thorax* **55**, 417–22.
29. **Groopman, J.E.** (1998). Fatigue in cancer and HIV/AIDS. *Oncology* **12** (3), 335–44.
30. **Donovan, E.S. and the University of Texas MD Anderson Cancer Centre Rehabilitation Services Team** (2000). What the rehabilitation therapies can do. In *Fatigue in Cancer: A Multidimensional Approach* (ed. M.L. Winningham and M. Barton-Burke), pp. 301–21. Sudbury: Jones and Bartlett Publishers.
31. **Dimeo, F.C.** et al. (1999). Effects of physical activity on the fatigue physiologic status of cancer patients during chemotherapy. *Cancer* **85** (10), 2273–7.
32. **Schwartz, A.L.** (1998). Patterns of exercise and fatigue in physically active cancer survivors. *Oncology Nursing Forum* **25** (3), 485–91.
33. **Langeveld, N., Ubbink, M., and Smets, E.** (2000). 'I don't have any energy': the experience of fatigue in young adult survivors of childhood cancer. *European Journal of Oncology Nursing* **4** (1), 20–8.
34. **Powell, P., Bentall, R.P., Nye, F.J., and Edwards, R.H.T.** (2001). Randomised controlled trial of patient education to encourage graded exercise in chronic fatigue syndrome. *British Medical Journal* **322**, 387.
35. **Stone, P.** et al. (1999). Fatigue in advanced cancer: a prospective controlled cross-sectional study. *British Journal of Cancer* **79** (9/10), 1479–86.
36. **Dudgeon, D.** et al. (2001). Dyspnoea in cancer patients: prevalence and associated factors. *US Cancer Pain Relief Committee* **21**, 2.
37. **Dimeo, F., Rumberger, B.G., and Keul, J.** (1998). Aerobic exercise as therapy for cancer fatigue. *Medicine and Science in Sports and Exercise* **30**, 475–8.
38. **Courneya, K.S.** (2001). Exercise interventions during cancer treatment: biopsychosocial outcomes. *Exercise and Sports Science Review* **29** (2), 60–4.
39. **Van Sint Annaland, E. and Lord, S.** (1999). Vigorous exercise for multiple sclerosis: a case report. *New Zealand Journal of Physiotherapy* **27** (3), 42–5.
40. **Edwards, S.** (1996). Longer-term management for patients with residual or progressive disability. In *Neurological Physiotherapy: A Problem Solving Approach* (ed. S. Edwards), pp. 189–206. London: Churchill Livingstone.

15.5 The contribution of speech and language therapy to palliative medicine

Alison MacDonald and Linda Armstrong

> Carers should not underestimate how distressing a speech and language problem can be for a patient who is already suffering the loss of faculties or fearing that loss. Communication difficulties may prevent patients from understanding their treatment choices and stop them from expressing their opinions. They may avoid communicating altogether and become withdrawn and passive.[1]

Introduction

General weakness, fatigue, and the (side-)effects of drugs may cause a range of communication difficulties for many patients in palliative care through their effects on breath control, mobility of the speech musculature, and also on swallowing, memory, attention, and word recall. A reduced level of consciousness will clearly affect a person's ability to communicate effectively. Indeed, significant speech and language deviations in a study of 12 hospice patients with cancer have been recorded.[2] It is also recognized that radiation therapy to the head and neck area may lead to transient voice changes.[3]

There are, however, a significant number of terminally ill patients who, as part of their condition, will have specific speech, language, and/or swallowing difficulties. A retrospective study of hospice records identified communication disorders in 27 per cent of a group of 335 patients.[4] Several of these patients had speech production difficulties as a direct consequence of the physical symptoms of their disease, while others showed language or cognitive changes arising from their neurological deterioration. In Hunt and Burne's study, 31 per cent of the children had difficulty in swallowing their saliva and 27 per cent were tube-fed as a result of swallowing difficulty.[5] This chapter will address the problems of people with impaired communication and/or related oral and pharyngeal stage swallowing difficulties (dysphagia and saliva control), and will focus on a description of the role in their care of the speech and language therapist.

Speech and language therapists assess and treat both communication and swallowing difficulties. Palliative care would not usually be considered as a routine care-group within acute hospitals or community-based services. However, the speech and language therapist can make a valuable contribution within multi-disciplinary care of people with terminal illness, whether that is a result of, for example, head and neck cancer or progressive neurological disease.

The aims of speech and language therapy

The overall aims of such intervention in palliative care are:

- to help people with communication difficulties make the most of their abilities for as long as possible and
- to help people having difficulty eating and/or drinking to swallow as safely as possible and to inform the medical team if the swallow appears unsafe.

The Royal College of Speech and Language Therapists' (RCSLT) service delivery standards and guidelines for people with progressive neurological disorders, can be extended to include those receiving palliative care for a range of other diseases. Their aims include to:

- promote and encourage early referrals ... through education of relevant medical staff and other professionals
- provide structured management programmes, to ensure clients are able to receive therapy, advice, and/or support throughout the progression of the disorder
- maximize a client's communication potential within his/her environment and enable maintenance of communication skills for the longest possible duration
- provide ongoing assessment and management of swallowing disorders
- provide information and advice to clients, carers, and other professionals regarding the use of AAC equipment
- keep clients, carers, and other professionals informed regarding the nature of the clients' communication and/or swallowing difficulties and the ongoing goals of intervention
- maintain a close liaison with other professionals and voluntary agencies
- assist the client's carers in communicating with the client in a positive way throughout the progression of the client's illness.[6]

Communication disorders

There are many ways in which communication may be affected and it is important to recognize that difficulties in the use of language as well as in speech production may be evident within the one person, that is, there may be linguistic and/or motor elements contributing to communication problems.

Speech production and voice

Impairment in motor functioning may affect speech intelligibility by reducing control at different levels of the vocal tract, that is, respiratory, laryngeal, velo-pharyngeal, and oral mechanisms. The causes may be local, as in the case of oral or laryngeal cancer, or neurological in origin (dysarthria). The ability to articulate clearly may be affected by anatomical alterations caused by surgical excision or malignant growth, but also by the neuro-motor impairment of function of the lips, tongue, jaw, or velum. Reduced or asynchronous velo-pharyngeal closure will cause abnormalities in nasal resonance. Disturbance to the nerve supply to, or restricted movement of the vocal cords will affect the ability to produce a normal voice quality, resulting in whispery, gravelly, or overloud voice and possibly in abnormal pitch. Altered airstream pathways, as in tracheostomy or laryngectomy, will result in a complete absence of voice (aphonia). Rhythm and rate may also be affected in some conditions, particularly those of basal ganglia or cerebellar origin, for example, Parkinson's disease, Friedreich's ataxia.

Language

An impairment in the ability to use language effectively (aphasia or dysphasia) takes many forms depending on the site of the brain damage and on the level(s) of linguistic processing that has been affected. The ability to follow spoken language or to interpret written material, the ability to recall words, to formulate grammatical sentences, to pronounce words or to spell, may be affected separately or in combination and to a varying extent, producing mild to severe impairments. Aphasia is most commonly associated with cerebrovascular accident. However, it may equally arise from space occupying lesions or traumatic brain injury. A subtle decline in language use may also be evident in some deteriorating conditions, particularly in the later stages, for example, Parkinson's disease and Huntington's disease.[7] Cognitive deterioration or confusional states may also affect the effective use of language. Short-term memory deficit and disorientation can, for example, significantly reduce a person's ability to participate in conversations or to make informed choices.

Children with deteriorating conditions may have particular communication difficulties depending on the time of onset of their condition. For example, in Hunt and Burne's cohort of 127 children with neurodegenerative diseases, nearly all the children had impaired or no speech.[5] Where onset has been in infancy the child may have had difficulty in developing language. Such children may be taught some basic manual signs or picture symbols with which to communicate (see also the section on augmentative and alternative communication).

Table 1 summarizes the effects that different medical diagnoses can have on communication, cognition, access to communication aids, and swallowing. Thus, the range of patients who may benefit from speech and language therapy intervention can be delineated.

Non-verbal communication

The extent to which we rely on non-verbal signals (e.g. facial expression, body movements, or gesture) to support our spoken output is not often fully recognized. The patient who is seriously ill, weak, or in pain, may find these non-verbal signals difficult to produce; and the person with severe motor impairment, particularly if this affects the facial muscles, may unintentionally give signals that are misinterpreted. It may, therefore, be important for the speech and language therapist to discuss this with the patient and his family and to look at possible options for circumventing this potential breakdown in communication.

For others, where verbal communication is reduced through aphasia or cognitive changes, the non-verbal channel can provide an alternative and effective main mode of both message-receiving and giving. The suggestions that follow (for the person with severe dementia) can be used as a model for other patients who present with severe linguistic difficulty in terminal illness, and serve to demonstrate ways in which some degree of interpersonal communication can be preserved through non-verbal channels:

- maintain social communication (helps to maintain dignity),
- keep talking (some of the non-verbal aspects may be understood),
- use touch judiciously,
- use non-verbal communication (gestures, pictures, etc.),
- assume the person understands,
- look for signs of comfort or discomfort,
- encourage attempts to communicate, and
- provide other types of stimulation.[13]

The speech and language therapist's role in the management of communication impairment

A model of care to describe in outline the pathway of a patient (child or adult, with whatever pathology) through an episode of care with speech and language therapy is shown in Fig. 1.

Timely referral

Timely referral will allow the speech and language therapist to carry out baseline assessments and monitor changes in language use and to advise other staff and relatives on how to facilitate communication. It may be necessary to alert staff and relatives to changes in verbal comprehension and to suggest ways of simplifying language input.

In the early stages of their illness, people may have difficulty in accepting or even in being aware of their speech deterioration so that referral to a speech and language therapist may be postponed. While it is important to be sensitive to each individual's level of acceptance of their illness, delayed referral unfortunately means that, particularly where cognitive changes are taking place, the ability to adapt and learn new techniques may become progressively more difficult. If compensatory strategies can be introduced or a communication aid explained and training given while the person is still able to cope with new learning, then their ability to use this effectively may be greatly extended. In a study of the use of augmentative and alternative communication (AAC) by people with Parkinson's disease speech and language therapists, patients and carers agree that earlier referral would be beneficial.[35]

Communication impairment of sudden onset

Speech or language breakdown or voice loss may be of sudden onset following a cerebrovascular accident or surgery. Where this can be anticipated, for example, following laryngectomy, it is good clinical practice that the speech and language therapist is called in before the event takes place. This allows support to be offered to both the patient and relatives, questions to be answered, communication strategies planned, and also allows the speech and language therapist to assess the level of pre-operative communication. Those who receive instruction on the use of a communication board prior to mechanical ventilation, score higher on patient satisfaction ratings than those whose communication support was unplanned.[25]

Deteriorating communication

The speech and language therapist's contribution to the support of the patient with a progressive disease may initially be for assessment and counselling only. The patient and their relatives may wish to discuss early speech changes that they notice and to consider the implications of further deterioration (see the stages described below). It may be important for the speech and language therapist to carry out baseline assessments and to monitor change. Exercises to facilitate breath control, voice use, articulatory precision, and to reduce alterations to nasal resonance may be effective in the early stages. Compensatory speech techniques may help to maximize intelligibility as speech becomes less clear. The speech and language therapist may also be able to discuss and introduce augmentative back-up in a gradual and acceptable way as speech continues to deteriorate. Augmentative and alternative communication is described more fully later.

The rate of deterioration in speech production in diseases such as motor neurone disease, Parkinson's disease, Friedreich's ataxia, or Huntington's disease is variable and in some cases may fluctuate. The type of support given by the speech and language therapist will be influenced by the stage in the progression of speech production difficulties.[36]

Stage 1: No detectable speech disorder. No alterations in speech production are noted.

Stage 2: Obvious speech disorder with intelligible speech. Some signs of speech deterioration are evident, particularly when the person is tired or stressed. Mild slurring or alterations in voice quality, intonation, loudness and speech breathing co-ordination may be noted. Speech is intelligible but compensations may include slowing rate, careful articulation, etc. Amplifiers may be useful in cases of reduced loudness, for example, associated with Parkinson's disease.

Stage 3: Reduction in speech intelligibility. Articulation, rate, and resonance are impaired and speech may be difficult to understand. Strategies to increase intelligibility need to be developed. Some people may begin to require back up to speech, for example, pointing to key words, topic headings, or initial letters on a board, or the use of a pacing board to regulate speaking rate.

Stage 4: Natural speech supplemented with augmentative communication. Only highly predictable messages, for example, greetings or expected responses to questions are understood. Speech may be supplemented by writing/typing messages on a communication aid or spelling out words on a letter board.

Stage 5: No useful speech. Some individuals may be able to vocalize to indicate emotional expression and 'yes' or 'no' but speech cannot be understood. Support may include establishing eye-gaze systems, yes/no signals, memory aids, and more elaborate communication systems where appropriate (see the following section).

Augmentative and alternative communication (AAC)

'Because maintenance of optimum communication is critical to quality of life, AAC management is central to palliative care.'[37] This field, which offers

Table 1 Communication and swallowing problems associated with various medical diagnoses

Medical diagnosis	Communication difficulties	Communication aids/AAC	Swallowing difficulties	Sources
Degenerative neurological conditions				
MND/ALS	Spastic and/or flaccid dysarthria: first signs often early	Need to adapt rapidly to deterioration: VOCA (keyboard → switch) → eye/body movements; yes/no system	Often early, rate of deterioration linked to speech deterioration	7, 8
Parkinson's disease	Hypokinetic dysarthria: weak voice, imprecise articulation, monotone, possible language processing deficits	Pacing board → first letter cueing → VOCA (introduce before cognitive changes affect learning)	Variable onset, often in later stages, tongue pumping and inefficient peristalsis	7–10
Huntington's disease	Hyperkinetic dysarthria, onset variable, language comprehension affected by cognitive deterioration, reduced output	Cognitive deterioration may affect usefulness of AAC: large display; phrases; memory aids; yes/no system	Variable onset—oral stage co-ordination problems prominent	7
Multiple sclerosis	Mixed spastic/ataxic dysarthria, may be mild, impaired control of loudness and harsh voice quality	Less frequently required	Variable, not common, possible medication side-effects, e.g. dry mouth	7, 8
Dementias				
Alzheimer's disease	Speech production and grammar usually spared until later in the disease, meaning and interpersonal aspects of communication affected earlier	Difficult to implement because of short-term term memory deficit but improvements have been documented	Memory-related eating problems (e.g. forgetting to swallow or how to use utensils), oral and pharyngeal stage changes	11–16
Vascular dementia	Depends on location of infarcts, may include dysarthria, and dysphasia	Difficult to implement because of short-term memory deficit	Depends on location of infarcts, may have oral and pharyngeal problems at any stage of the illness	11, 17
Pick's disease	Increasing dysphasia, often with eventual mutism	May be possible in the early stage in the light of relatively intact memory and other cognitive abilities	No known literature but may have eating problems related to reduced judgement, e.g. putting too much food in at once	17, 18
(v)CJD	Often rapid deterioration in speech and language functioning	Difficult to implement because of rapid change and cognitive problems	Can present at oral and/or pharyngeal stage	12, 17, 19
Lewy body dementia	Variability with fluctuations in cognition, communication affected by hallucinations, dysarthria possible (as yet little available literature)	Fluctuating ability would affect AAC implementation	No known literature, but likely to be affected by altered consciousness, memory difficulties and concomitant Parkinsonism if present	18, 20, 21
Other neurological conditions				
Acute confusion	Dysarthria, dysgraphia and some naming errors as well as confabulation and perseveration may be present	Not strongly indicated because of fluctuating cognitive status and short time-span for training	Swallowing may be affected by reduced attention	17, 22
Brain tumour	Language impairment usually relatively mild in cerebral tumour compared to post-stroke, anomia common. Varies with tumour type and location	No known research literature	Oral and/or pharyngeal problems dependent on cranial nerves affected	8, 23
Stroke	Dysarthria, dyspraxia, and/or dysphasia	Effectiveness influenced by language comprehension and reading ability. Communication book: photographs, pictures, personal word lists/topics; VOCA	Oral and/or pharyngeal problems common especially early post-onset	24, 25
HIV and AIDS	Wide range of problems documented, either primary or secondary: voice disorder, interaction problems, dysarthria, dyspraxia, dysphasia. In children, language development can be negatively affected	May provide useful communication support—little evidence in this area as yet	Problems result from AIDS dementia complex	26–29

(Continued)

Table 1 Continued

Medical diagnosis	Communication difficulties	Communication aids/AAC	Swallowing difficulties	Sources
Head and neck surgery				
Laryngectomy	Aphonia: no voice	Electrolarynx; writing; VOCA	Occasional pharyngeal/oesophogeal stricture; aspiration following hemi-laryngectomy or supraglottal laryngectomy	30, 31
Tracheostomy; ventilator dependent patient; paralyzed vocal cords	Aphonia: no voice	Tracheostomy tube with speaking valve; talking tracheostomy tube; writing; VOCA; yes/no system	Possibility of compromise due to restricted laryngeal elevation or cuff inflation.	30, 32
Oropharyngeal tumours glossectomy	Restricted articulation	Writing or gesture supplement if necessary	Restricted tongue, jaw, lip movement; pharyngeal inefficiency, or obstruction	8, 31, 33, 34

Key: VOCA, voice output communication aid.

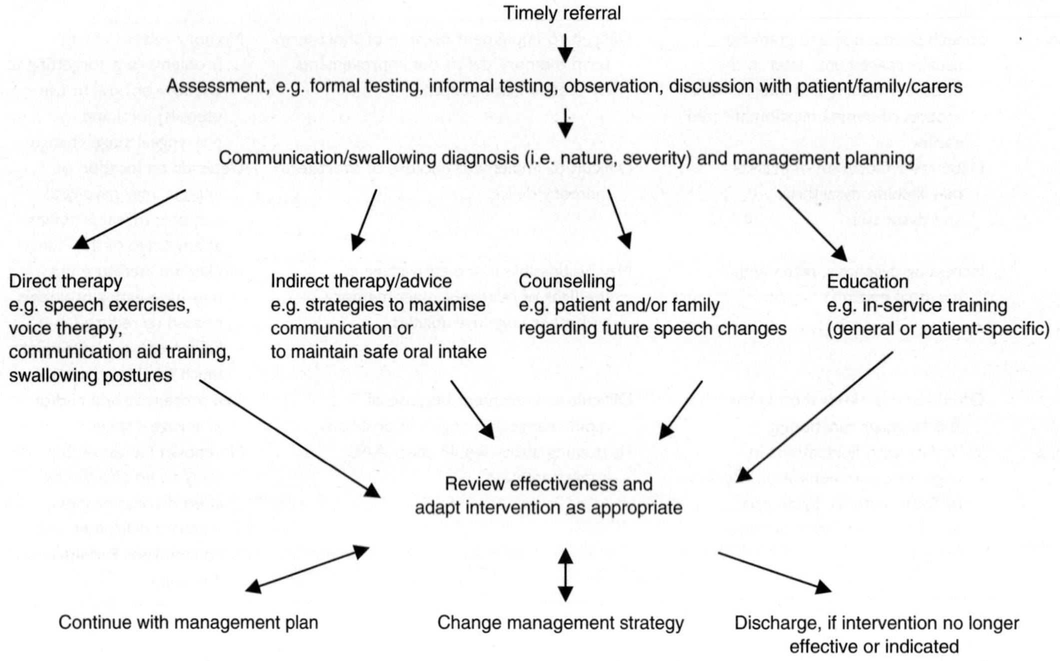

Fig. 1 A model of care for speech and language therapy.

a range of strategies and communication devices to support the person with poor intelligibility or no speech, has expanded considerably in recent years. There are now more flexible options to offer the person at different stages in their illness (see previous section on stages in the progression of speech production difficulties). Many speech and language therapists have some experience in this field,(9) and in many areas referral can be made to a communication aids centre with a team of specialist therapists and technicians.

Careful assessment by the speech and language therapist will be required in order to ensure that the most appropriate communication support is given to each individual. Visual, motor, linguistic, and cognitive impairments will influence the selection. Some may reject or fail to make much use of the communication systems offered, possibly due to increasing passivity and lack of motivation to communicate, but every person should be provided with the opportunity to try relevant aids to communication.

High-tech aids

Despite the terminal nature of their condition, some people will remain cognitively able and alert and will retain a fairly sophisticated level of communication. A range of voice output communication aids (VOCA) is available. See Fig. 2 for an example.

Many of these offer features such as banks of stored phrases, which can be triggered by one or two presses of a key or switch, or word prediction in which a choice of words appears on the screen as the individual types, predicted from the initial letters and from the grammar of the preceding words. These features greatly reduce the effort required by the user. There may also be a range of options for inputting text, from enlarged keyboards and special key guards to letter displays operated by a single switch. This allows the communication aid to be adapted to the user's abilities as motor control deteriorates.

Low-tech aids

This term refers to less technologically sophisticated support systems, for example, a chart with letters, words, or phrases, to which the individual can point. For weak or very physically disabled people, a display with a selection of messages to which the user can direct their eye gaze can be constructed. Where spelling or recognition of the written word is difficult, small pictures or symbols can be used as message signifiers. In Fig. 3, an eye-pointing frame is shown and explained.

Yes/no systems

For people who are in the very final stages of their illness, weakness, fatigue, and confusion may make even a simple system of communication difficult. It may, however, be possible to find a way for them to signal 'yes' and 'no' successfully. This may involve the use of some small body movement or eye signal, for example eye gaze up = 'yes', eye gaze down = 'no', or directing the eyes to the words 'yes' and 'no' mounted on either side of the bed. This allows the individual to continue to experience some level of control and involvement in everyday activities and decision-making.

Case study A case described in RCSLT Bulletin (October 2000, p. 4) exemplifies the significance of having a yes–no response when no other form of communication is possible. A ventilated 19-year old with motor neurone disease has been allowed through High Court agreement to have the ventilator switched off when he loses the ability to blink with his left eyelid.

Special considerations for children

Preliterate children will require specific considerations and assessment for appropriate communication support. For some children with well-maintained hand function, manual signs (usually taken from the sign language used by the deaf community) may prove the most effective means of communication. Other children may be taught to use either a high-tech communication aid or a low-tech communication chart. In either case the speech and language therapist will work in close consultation with family and educational staff in selecting and teaching a set of pictorial symbols with which the child can communicate. These will either be displayed on a chart or communication aid screen or on the overlay or keys of some communication aids. Symbol communication systems are also widely used by people of all ages with learning disabilities.

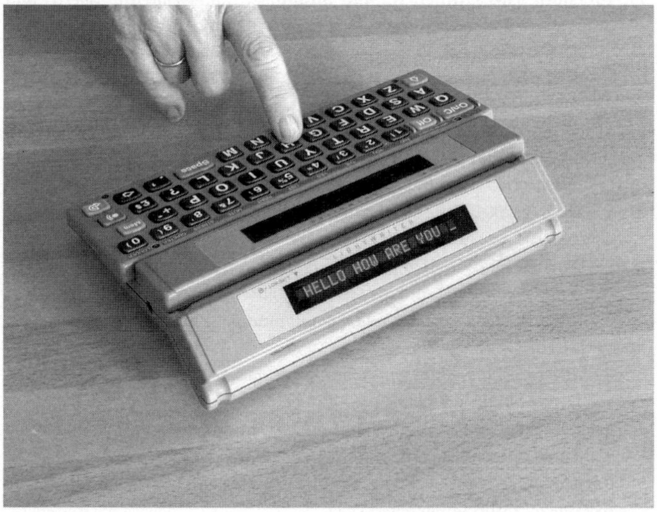

Fig. 2 A Lightwriter: an example of a high-tech communication aid.

Aids to oral communication

Patients who have undergone surgical procedures that interfere with voice production and/or speech intelligibility, may be offered a range of prostheses or mechanical aids. These include speaking tracheostomy valves, artificial larynxes and prostheses to assist velo-pharyngeal closure (palatal lift), to lower the palate in order to facilitate articulatory contact or to supply missing contact surfaces.[30] The speech and language therapist should be included in assessment for these aids, in conjunction with the medical team and possibly an orthodontist. Intensive training will probably be required once the device is available. Those with weak, low voice volume but relatively precise articulation may be helped by the use of a speech amplifier. There are several lightweight head mountable models available.

Swallowing problems

Drugs prescribed to alleviate one aspect of a patient's condition may adversely affect the ability to swallow or the amount of saliva produced. Oral tumours and glossectomy will restrict tongue movement, and tumours in the pharynx will affect the efficiency of the swallowing mechanism.[33] Radiotherapy to the head and neck may cause changes to tissue and muscle function, alterations to taste, reduced saliva flow, and possibly diminished swallow reflex both during and after radiotherapy. Dysphagia is also a symptom of many of the deteriorating neurological conditions (see Table 1).

The symptoms may vary. Chewing may be affected by the lack of graded jaw movement or by muscle weakness or rigidity. Poor control of the glossal, buccal, and labial musculature will reduce the ability to manipulate food within the oral cavity and cause delayed transit towards the pharynx or disintegration of the food bolus interfering with the co-ordination and timing of the swallow. Weak or asyncronous triggering of the pharyngeal swallow, decreased or slowed laryngeal elevation, or reduced pharyngeal peristalsis, may result in pooling in the valleculae and pyriform sinuses and risk of aspiration.[8,38,39]

Dysphagia can result in difficulty in swallowing food, fluid, saliva and medication.

The speech and language therapist's role in the management of swallowing difficulties

Many professional disciplines will be involved in supporting the person with eating and swallowing difficulties. The specialist speech and language

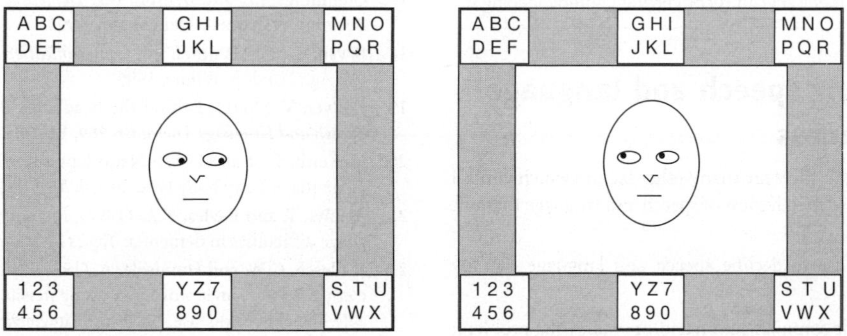

Fig. 3 Eye-pointing frame: an example of a low-tech communication aid. The user first points to the block of letters containing the target letter (in this example 'S'), then to the block corresponding to the position of that letter within the first block, i.e. top left.

therapist is trained to assess and advise on the oral control of food, liquid, and oral secretions (saliva), and the safety of the swallowing mechanism, particularly at the pharyngeal level. Problems at the oesophageal level, lie outside the remit of speech and language therapy intervention. The specialist speech and language therapist will assess the quality and safety of a patient's swallow. They may suggest head postures or alternative positioning for safer swallowing and/or different food and liquid consistencies, for example, the addition of thickener to liquids or the pureeing of solid food may be appropriate depending on the findings, as well as possible exercises to improve the swallow.[8] The speech and language therapist may request referral for videofluoroscopy (modified barium swallow)[8] or other instrumental investigations (e.g. fibreoptic endoscopic evaluation of swallowing—FEES).[40] These procedures not only help to determine whether the patient is aspirating but will also guide the therapist in appropriate management. However, in locations where radiological or instrumental evaluations are not readily accessible (e.g. in rural communities), dependence on bedside assessment may be necessary.

It is important that a person exhibiting even early signs of chewing or swallowing difficulty, for example, occasional coughing or choking when eating or drinking, chestiness, or a 'wet', gurgly voice after swallowing or poor saliva control, should be referred to the speech and language therapist as soon as possible. For people with degenerative conditions, small changes in posture and food/liquid consistency may be effective at first. If the patient appears to be at risk of aspiration then this will need to be carefully monitored and if necessary non-oral feeding considered by the medical team.

Eight factors will influence best practice in dysphagia management (particularly for people with degenerative diseases, but also more widely applicable to people with terminal illness):[10]

- cognitive/communicative and comprehension ability during interaction with caregivers for purposes of self-determination;
- cognitive/communicative and comprehension ability during execution of a plan of care;
- dependence–independence levels during execution of compensatory manoeuvres and therapeutic plans;
- matching changes in treatment plans to changes in the physiology of swallowing;
- establishing realistic expectations and goals for advancing conditions;
- determining appropriate times for surgical intervention and/or medication;
- developing sensitivity to personal, cultural, and familial wants, needs, and desires of patients/clients; and
- deciding when to terminate swallowing treatment and when to initiate palliative or supportive treatment.

Case study A paediatric example of the role of the speech and language therapist in ethical decision–making relating to dysphagia in palliative care: a child with Tay–Sachs disease was assessed and found to be a 'nonfunctional oral feeder'. From this information, the medical team recommended enteral feeding.[41]

Factors influencing speech and language therapy effectiveness

Apart from disease progression, there are many other factors which clinical experience shows will affect the effectiveness of speech and language therapy. These include:

- the patient's right to choose to decline speech and language therapy intervention;
- the patient's attitude to their communication and/or swallowing problem;
- the effect of the communication or swallowing problem in relation to other medical symptoms as perceived by the individual;
- the level of alertness (related to medication, fatigue, pain);
- family and health carer attitudes; and
- family/staff training, for example, in AAC, swallowing problems.

Conclusion

In this chapter, the role of the speech and language therapist for patients with communication and/or swallowing problems has been discussed. We stress the importance of timely referral for initial assessment so that appropriate intervention (support, counselling, advice, or therapy) can be offered.

References

1. **Salt, N., Davies, S., and Wilkinson, S.** (1999). The contribution of speech and language therapy to palliative care. *European Journal of Palliative Care* **6**, 126–9.
2. **Salt, N. and Robertson, S.** (1998). A hidden client group? Communication impairment in hospice patients. *International Journal of Language & Communication Disorders* **33** (Suppl.), 96–101.
3. **Stoicheff, M.** (1991). Post-radiotherapy voice. In *Voice Disorders and their Management* 2nd edn. (ed. M. Fawcus), pp. 333–6. London: Chapman and Hall.
4. **Jackson, P., Robbins, M., and Frankel, S.** (1996). Communication impediments in a group of hospice patients. *Palliative Medicine* **10**, 79–80.
5. **Hunt, A. and Burne, R.** (1995). Medical and nursing problems of children with neurodegenerative disease. *Palliative Medicine* **9**, 19–26.
6. **Royal College of Speech and Language Therapists**. *Communicating Quality 2.* London: Royal College of Speech and Language Therapists, 1996.
7. **Yorkston, K.M., Miller, R., and Strand, E.** *Management of Speech and Swallowing in Degenerative Diseases.* Tucson AZ: Communication Skill Builders, 1995.
8. **Logemann, J.** *Evaluation and Treatment of Swallowing Disorders* 2nd edn. Austin TX: Pro-Ed, 1998.
9. **Armstrong, L., Jans, D., and MacDonald, A.** (2000). Parkinson's disease and aided AAC: some evidence from practice. *International Journal of Language & Communication Disorders* **35**, 377–89.
10. **Sonies, B.** (2000). Patterns of care for dysphagic patients with degenerative neurological diseases. *Seminars in Speech and Language* **21**, 333–45.
11. **Bayles, K.A. and Kaszniak, A.W.** *Communication and Cognition in Normal Aging and Dementia.* London: Taylor & Francis Ltd, 1987.
12. **Lubinski, R.**, ed. *Dementia and Communication.* Philadelphia: BC Decker, 1991.
13. **Rau, M.T.** *Coping with Communication Challenges in Alzheimer's Disease.* San Diego: Singular, 1993.
14. **Priefer, B.A. and Robbins, J.** (1997). Eating changes in mild-stage Alzheimer's disease: a pilot study. *Dysphagia* **12**, 212–21.
15. **Boylston, E.W. and O'Day, C.P.** *Successful EATing: Dementia Swallowing Assessment.* Bisbee: Imaginart, 1999.
16. **Bourgeois, M.** et al. (2001). Memory aids as an augmentative and alternative communication strategy for nursing home residents with dementia. *AAC* **17**, 196–210.
17. **Cummings, J.L. and Benson, D.F.** *Dementia: A Clinical Approach* 2nd edn. Boston: Butterworth-Heinemann, 1992.
18. **Bryan, K. and Maxim, J.**, ed. *Communication Disability and the Psychiatry of Old Age.* London: Whurr, 1996.
19. **Collyer, V.** (2001). Behind the headlines. *Bulletin of the Royal College of Speech and Language Therapists* **589**, 12–14.
20. **McKeith, I.** et al. (1992). Neuroleptic sensitivity in patients with senile dementia of Lewy body type. *British Medical Journal* **305**, 673–8.
21. **Azuma, T. and Bayles, K.A.** (1997). Memory impairments underlying language difficulties in dementia. *Topics in Language Disorders* **18**, 58–71.
22. **Wallesch, C.W. and Hundsalz, A.** (1994). Language function in delirium: a comparison of single word processing in acute confusional states and probable Alzheimer's disease. *Brain and Language* **46**, 592–606.
23. **Thomson, A.-M.** *Communication Disorders in Patients with Hemispheric Intracranial Neoplasm.* PhD Thesis, University of Edinburgh, 1997.
24. **Chapey, R.**, ed. *Language Intervention Strategies in Adult Aphasia* 3rd edn. Baltimore: Williams & Wilkins, 1994.

25. **Beukelman, D., Yorkston, K. and Reichle, J.**, ed. *Augmentative and Alternative Communication for Adults with Acquired Neurologic Disorders*. Baltimore: Paul Brookes, 2000.
26. **O'Keefe, C.** et al. (1993). Developments in HIV/AIDS. *Bulletin of the Royal College of Speech and Language Therapists* **473**, 12.
27. **Vogel, D. and Carter, J.E.** *The Effects of Drugs on Communication Disorders*. San Diego: Singular, 1995.
28. **Davis-McFarland, E.** (2000). Language and oral-motor development and disorders in infants and young toddlers with Human Immunodeficiency Virus. *Seminars in Speech and Language* **21**, 19–36.
29. **McNeilly, L.G.** (2000). Communication intervention and therapeutic issues in pediatric Human Immunodeficiency Virus. *Seminars in Speech and Language* **21**, 63–78.
30. **Dikeman, K.J. and Kazandjian, M.S.** *Communication and Swallowing Management of Tracheostomized and Ventilator-dependent Adults*. San Diego: Singular, 1995.
31. **Forbes, K.** (1997). Palliative care in patients with cancer of the head and neck. *Clinical Otolaryngology* **22**, 117–22.
32. **Tippet, D.C.**, ed. *Tracheostomy and Ventilator Dependency: Management of Breathing, Speaking and Swallowing*. New York: Thieme, 2000.
33. **Saunders, C. and Sykes, N.** *The Management of Terminal Malignant Disease* 3rd edn. London: Edward Arnold, 1993.
34. **Lazarus, C.** (2000). Management of swallowing disorders in head and neck cancer patients: optimal patterns of care. *Seminars in Speech and Language* **21**, 293–309.
35. **Armstrong, L., Jans, D., and MacDonald, A.** (1999). Parkinson's disease and the use of AAC: looking for some evidence. *Communication Matters* **13/3**, 5–6.
36. **Yorkston, K.M. and Beukelman, D.R.** (2000). Decision making in AAC intervention. In *Augmentative and Alternative Communication for Adults with Acquired Neurologic Disorders* (ed. D. Beukelman, K. Yorkston, and J. Reichle), pp. 55–82. Baltimore: Paul Brookes.
37. **Klasner, E.R. and Yorkston, K.M.** (2000). AAC for Huntington disease and Parkinson's disease: planning for change. In *Augmentative and Alternative Communication for Adults with Acquired Neurologic Disorders* (ed. D.R. Beukelman, K.M. Yorkston, and J. Reichle), pp. 237–70. Baltimore: Paul Brookes.
38. **Leopold, N. and Kagel, M.** (1997). Pharyngo-esophageal dysphagia in Parkinson's disease. *Dysphagia* **12**, 11–18.
39. **Nagaya, M.** et al. (1998). Videofluorographic study of swallowing in Parkinson's disease. *Dysphagia* **13**, 95–100.
40. **Langmore, S.E. and McCulloch, T.M.** (1997). Examination of the pharynx and larynx and endoscopic examination of pharyngeal swallowing. In *Deglutition and its Disorders* (ed. A.L. Perlman and K. Schulze-Delrieu), pp. 201–26. San Diego: Singular.
41. **Sharp, H.M. and Geneson, L.B.** (1996). Ethical decision-making in dysphagia management. *American Journal of Speech-Language Pathology* **5**, 15–22.

15.6 The contribution of art therapy to palliative medicine

Michèle Wood

In Britain, Art Therapy is a state-registered profession allied to medicine and its practitioners complete a postgraduate training for 2 years full-time or equivalent. As in some other European countries, Canada, Australia, and the USA, art therapy is a recognized profession taught at the postgraduate level and practised within a wide range of settings.

In the United Kingdom, art therapy had its beginnings in the tuberculosis sanatoria of the 1940s but quickly developed within psychiatric and educational settings. Integrated with other care, it has since been widely incorporated into the fields of mental health and learning disabilities. However, there is a growing interest in art therapy with the medically and terminally ill[1–6] and, in a recent survey,[7] just over 6 per cent of all art therapists in the United Kingdom indicated that they worked in palliative care.

What is art therapy?

Art therapy provides a supportive therapeutic relationship within which a person may explore personal issues. It involves the use of art materials for this exploration so that thoughts, feelings, and other issues of personal significance can be expressed. As such it is an alternative to spoken language providing a means of communication and symbolic representation. The art therapist's task is to facilitate the patient's expressive capacities and to help him or her reflect upon what they have produced, including their chosen media and style of working. The ultimate aim of art therapy is to enable the patient to change and develop on a personal level. Art therapy does not aim to distract or divert a person from their difficulties but through encouraging an experience of creativity these difficulties can be perceived and worked with in a new way.

An important aspect of art therapy is that it provides an opportunity to express emotions that may feel unacceptable to the patient. The patient may have repressed feelings of anger, envy, and sadness for fear of upsetting the family or staff. In art therapy, pounding clay, pouring paint, and scribbling violently on paper gives the patient permission to express strong feelings, and the presence of the therapist ensures the patient is not left alone with their distress. Art therapy also allows for the development and expression of more positive feelings such as tenderness, hope, or beauty. The breadth of emotional expression possible through art therapy demands a working environment that provides confidentiality and in which the patient can feel free to be vulnerable. A separate therapy or quiet room designated for art therapy sessions is ideal.

The loss of control in many areas of patients' lives is an inevitable consequence of illness, and one that art therapy aims to address. The physicality of art therapy, where an individual must actively engage with the materials to produce a picture or object, provides an experience which reinforces the person's ability to make choices and their sense of their own vitality. The artwork represents not only something of the patient's mental state but also, by capturing in its marks and traces the movement and pressure of the patient's pencil, brush, or finger, it represents something of their physical condition too. This articulation through the artwork of the mind–body relationship is intrinsic to art therapy. Some practitioners suggest that art therapy's potency resides in this link[8] and thus art therapy is ideally placed to respond to the psychological effects of physical trauma. The developments in psycho-neuro-immunology appear to be providing exciting explanations for the links between imagery and improvements in physical health. This is an area of increasing investigation.[4]

Art therapy and creative art: similarities and differences

It is important to distinguish art therapy from creative arts activities.[9] Although there are some areas of overlap, art therapy and creative arts projects have different yet complementary functions within palliative care. Both engage the patient in actively using art media and provide a focus and sense of purpose. Both result in an increased sense of control, self-confidence, and make a positive contribution to patients' quality of life. Creative arts projects may aim to help the patient produce artwork for sale, or to bequeath to relatives. Although the artwork produced in art therapy may on occasion have a similar outcome its focus is different. As patients strive to express and explore their inner emotional landscape through their art there is no expectation that work should be aesthetically 'good' in a conventional sense, or that it will be viewed outside the therapy space. Consequently, the artwork may have a rough undeveloped quality to it. The process by which the artwork is made offers an additional level for expression and communication and contributes to the material with which the therapist and the patient engage. The need to witness the patient's process is one reason for the therapist's presence in the art therapy sessions. Although the primary aim of art therapy is to facilitate communication within the patient, the permanent nature of the artwork means that it can continue to communicate from session to session and outside of the therapeutic relationship. Patients have been known to use their pictures to communicate with friends, family,(10) other patients in similar situations,(6) and their doctors and other members of the multidisciplinary team.

Art therapists, artists in residence, and art tutors can and do work alongside each other in many establishments; their combination of skills is particularly effective where their differences are understood. While both encourage the patients' creativity and improve the overall milieu of the health care environment, art therapy works with the psychological and emotional needs of the patient, which includes their barriers to creativity and their difficulties with self-expression. It can be hard for a patient or a professional to know whether art therapy or recreational art is more appropriate. Most art therapists provide assessment sessions in which the patients' needs may be discerned. Kennett's phenomenological study of a creative arts project(11) at St Christopher's Hospice in London is a good example of a setting where both art therapy and art activities are offered alongside each other. Case 1 describes the dual functioning of art making in a palliative care setting showing the different roles played by art therapy and art activity for a woman with motor neurone disease.

Case 1: 'Rosemary' by Jackie Coote, art therapist

Whilst working in a large London hospice I was introduced to Rosemary, who had recently been diagnosed with motor neurone disease. Having become paralysed down one side of her body and rapidly losing the power of speech she had expressed a wish to 'paint her feelings'. She was, by the time I met her, using an electronic writer to communicate and only had the use of her right arm. Anything she 'said' was through the writer. Although unfamiliar with the use of art materials, she engaged in the process very quickly, allowing herself to paint freely. She began to look forward to 'the unexpected', which presented itself to her in each session, like the painting she referred to as her 'Devastated Woodland—half dead, struggling for survival' (Fig. 1). She was able to relate the image to her feelings about her own situation. Her 'fun' painting became a way to address serious issues around her encroaching illness. Through it she began to express her thoughts and feelings about the adjustments she had to make, not just physically, but psychologically. Through her images she was able to express her painful recognition of change and loss. With the loss of spontaneity and inflexion in speech Rosemary's painting became her 'voice'. Her choice of materials would often indicate her tone and mood. On one occasion she chose bright, cheerful colours, but the black paper she used reflected her underlying melancholy, and the resulting picture helped her to recognize the tendency to 'put on a cheerful front' when all behind it was not well.

In the course of using art therapy to express difficult and painful feelings, Rosemary discovered another side to her image making. She began to paint alone in her room. This work took on a 'painterly' quality. She painted gardens resembling images from 'The Arabian nights' that contained a sense of richness and fertility. Staff and other patients would come and see what she had been doing each day, and her self-esteem increased considerably. Her images enabled her to become empowered at a time of increasing powerlessness and dependency. With the increase in Rosemary's use of her newly found creative skills, it became important to differentiate between her 'public art' and her 'private art'. She needed reassurance that she still had a private and safe space in the art therapy sessions where she could pour out what she called her 'madness'. She seemed at this point to have moved into a third and what was to be the final phase of the art therapy sessions where, as her body deteriorated, the emotional floodgates opened. Fear, grief, anger, hatred, and despair appeared in the images before us. Her art therapy sessions provided the container necessary to hold the overwhelming grief she poured out in torrents. It was the coping strategy she needed in order to carry on throughout the rest of the day.

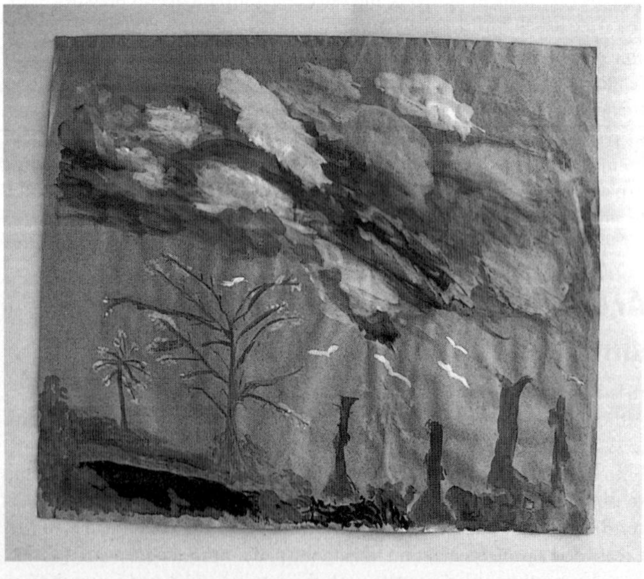

Fig. 1

Who would benefit from art therapy?

Art therapists work in a range of settings: patients' own homes,(12) prisons,(13) day centres,(14–17) specialist in-patient units,(6,18) hospices,(19–24) and private practice.(25) A brief overview is given in Table 1 of some recent literature documenting the use of art therapy with people suffering life-threatening or terminal illnesses. People with a wide range of conditions including HIV/AIDS, rheumatoid illness, multiple sclerosis, cancer, dementia, and Niemann Pick's disease have been reported as benefiting from art therapy. The range of conditions and variety of settings in which art therapy is offered indicate something of the multiple contributions art therapy can make to patients' care.

Whilst recognizing this breadth of application, is it possible to discern which conditions or types of patients would benefit most? Since art therapy is a means of facilitating communication, it is particularly useful for patients, their family, or carers, who are having difficulty with other modes of communication. Such difficulties can be physical, cognitive, emotional, or even spiritual in origin, and thus provide different starting points and ways of working for the therapist. Case 1 clearly illustrates how art therapy can extend a patient's capacity to communicate when this has been curtailed for physical reasons. Similarly, the person with AIDS dementia may no longer be able to coherently discuss their fears and anxieties but may be able to use the qualities available in art to express themselves and relieve their frustrations. In this case, the art therapist may not focus on discussion or interpretation.(24) By contrast, where there are emotional difficulties the therapist may well explore in depth the patient's associations to their image and their behaviour. Coote(21) illustrates this in her work with an attention-seeking patient where art therapy allowed an expression of bitterness and resentment, unrecognized aspects of the patient's inner self. Connell(6) gives an example of how art therapy was used to address and work through a patient's spiritual struggles. Trauger-Querry and Haghighi(22) describe an approach using art therapy and music therapy in the reduction of pain.

Young children, whose developing capacities for verbal expression limit their use of talking therapies, are an obvious group for art therapy, as art and drawing are more familiar means of self-expression.(5,10) Farrell Fenton,(25) who works with children and young people who have cystic fibrosis, suggests that art therapy works on two levels simultaneously: by providing a means of emotional catharsis while at the same time harnessing the young person's coping strategies.

Table 1 Range of conditions and settings in which art therapists work—overview of literature

Diagnosis/reason for referral to art therapy	Location of therapy	Relevant details of intervention	Evaluation/presentation of material	Reference
Acute lyphoblastic leukaemia	USA, children's hospital	Work included a strategy for dealing with family dynamics	Description of practice with 9-year-old girl	Teufel[10]
AIDS	UK, hospice	Single session where patient presents himself as the art work	Case study	Wood[23]
AIDS dementia	UK, hospice	Seven years analysed	Qualitative analysis	Wood[24]
AIDS/HIV	UK, day care	Drop-in art therapy group	Description of practice	Bartholomew[14]
AIDS/HIV	UK, prison	Closed art therapy group	Description of practice	Beaver[13]
Bone marrow transplant	USA	Individual sessions with patients in isolation	Description of practice and some qualitative analysis	Gabriel et al.[31]
Cancer	UK, patients' homes	Individual and family art therapy	Description of practice	Bell[12]
Cancer	UK, specialist cancer hospital	Art therapy—individual and group sessions; group notebook	Descriptions of a range of practices using patients' pictures	Connell[6]
Cancer	Sweden, day centre	Expressive arts and music therapy	Description of short-term practice	Olofsson[16]
Cystic fibrosis	USA, private practice	Art therapy with young people	Description of practice	Farrell Fenton[25]
Dementias	UK, day centres	Art therapy groups	A control group study	Sheppard et al.[29]
Melanoma	UK	Patient reports on art therapy and other resources used	Personal account	Morley[34]
Mixed diagnoses	UK, hospice	Art therapy group	Description of practice	Mayo[26]
	UK, hospice	Pain control mentioned as one outcome of art therapy	Description of practice. Art therapy presented alongside artist in residence	Thomas and Kennedy[20]
	UK, hospice	Individual work	Description of practice	Coote[21]
Multiple myeloma	USA	Individual work	Qualitative case study	Zammit[8]
Multiple sclerosis	UK	Individual work	Description of practice	Szespanski[18]
Niemann Pick's disease	UK, day centre	Individual work and referral to music therapy	Description of practice	Stevens and Lomas[17]
Pain control	USA, hospice with adults	Art and music therapy	Theoretical discussion illustrated by case material	Trauger-Querry and Haghighi[22]
Post-treatment cancer	USA, outpatients	Short-term structured art therapy group work	Qualitative analyses using questionnaires and follow-up interviews	Luzzatto and Gabriel[30]
Rheumatoid illness	Germany, day care	Art therapy group work	Description of practice	Dannecker[15]
Terminal cancer	UK, hospice	Short-term work in final phase of life	Case study	Gold and Ahmedzai[19]

Many factors including class, educational levels, and ethnic backgrounds influence the patient's comfort in expressing and addressing their emotional responses to illness.[5,26] In my experience of serving an ethnically diverse population, art therapy can be a welcome tool for patients who have to negotiate their experiences of illness and treatment through a language and in a cultural setting that is not their own. Art therapy can strengthen their own 'voice' and validate their own experiences. The value of art as a tool for cultural communication can be seen in the project described by Fried[27] where Aboriginal artists were commissioned to paint about end of life issues. Although this is not an example of art therapy, it illustrated the need to find more culturally relevant modes of communication for people needing palliative care services. It also indicates the value of non-verbal and symbolic levels of expression.

Any hazards of art therapy?

The hazards due to art therapy are minimal but the following pitfalls are worth mentioning. There can be a concern from some staff that the expression of feelings through image-making may unleash a flow of emotion that will overwhelm the patient and those around them. Usually, these concerns dissipate when it is realized that the processes and boundaries of art therapy provide a safe container that prevents this from happening. The patient never fully relinquishes control, but through the manipulation of the art materials their usual defences can give way to more symbolic expressions of feeling states (see Case 2). The therapist's skill in keeping the boundaries of therapy ensures that these feelings are contained and that both the patient and themselves are kept safe.

The therapeutic value of art therapy may be undermined if the position of the art therapist in relation to the interdisciplinary team is not respected or clearly understood. One example of this can be seen when art therapy sessions are interrupted for procedures or questions that can be done at another time. Another example is where the art therapist is placed at the periphery of the team working without reference to colleagues. This can lead to unnecessary replication of work, or of the art therapist's important perspective on the patient being lost to the team.

Another hazard of therapeutic work, and indeed of all work in palliative care, relates to the emotional well-being of staff. Therapists need to ensure that they themselves are adequately supported through the use of supervision, supportive teamwork, and possibly their own personal therapy. All these strategies have proved to be beneficial in guarding against staff burnout and inappropriate behaviour. Art therapy itself is often used for staff support and can facilitate a valuable level of creativity, communication, and expression in tired staff teams.[28]

On a practical level, the hazard posed to patients by the art materials does need to be considered. Most materials used in art therapy are non-toxic, but where materials could pose a risk (e.g. fixative) therapists ensure that usual precautions are taken. In cases where cross-infection between patients may be an issue it is standard practice that separate sets of equipment are used.

Outcomes of art therapy

Summarizing the literature outlined in Table 1 the following outcomes of art therapy have been identified:

- development of a creative attitude by the patient towards their circumstances;
- an increased sense of control;
- better communication;
- wider range of expressive capabilities;
- increased insight into patient's own behaviour;
- body image issues addressed;
- a cathartic release of emotive issues;
- increased self-esteem;
- increased ability to confront existential questions and relieve spiritual distress;
- development of positive coping strategies;
- reduction in experiences and reports of physical pain;
- increased quality of life.

Adjusting to multiple losses (purpose, health, and social position), and facing one's own mortality, is equally central to care of the elderly. There has been much work done by art therapists with this population who are often cared for outside of palliative settings. One UK-based study[29] evaluated art therapy with people suffering from dementia using a control group design where the control situation was a standard day centre mixed activity social group. The researchers found that there was a significant difference between the patients participating in art therapy and those in the control group.

Evaluating art therapy

The list of benefits of art therapy given above is extensive. However, as indicated in Table 1, a comprehensive evaluation of art therapy is difficult since its benefits are often based on anecdotal descriptions of case material and single group studies. Developing research methodologies that can accurately and ethically assess the complexities of the art therapy process is a considerable challenge. Some practitioners are making strides in this direction.[8,24,29–31] A recent review[32] of the art therapy literature on effectiveness suggests that art therapy can positively contribute to patients' well-being, and that in certain cases it may be more effective than other interventions. Evaluating what it is that is unique to art therapy and how best to harness its therapeutic efficacy requires an investment in art therapy research that should run alongside the current interest and development in evidence-based palliative care services.

How quickly can the benefits of art therapy be seen?

Patients are referred to art therapy for a variety of reasons and at differing stages of their journey from diagnosis to terminal care. What is clear from many practitioners' reports is that patients with life-threatening and terminal illnesses are motivated to make the most of the time they have left.[19] There is evidence[21,23] that even a single session can be of value, as Case 2 shows:

Case 2: 'Robert'[1]

Robert, a man in his early thirties, was diagnosed with AIDS and was in hospital for respite care and symptom control. He had a detached and objective approach to his diagnosis and liked to be informed of all medical facts. When we met he had announced to staff he no longer wished to discuss his condition.

Robert began the art therapy session by being somewhat surprised by the range of art materials available, and that we had a whole hour together. He said he was unsure about what to do, and I invited him to experiment with the materials to see what marks they made, and what he liked using. Robert said he was anxious about making a fool of himself and of making a mess; he wanted to do things properly. We talked about this initially in relation to his life outside the hospital, and then how he felt about making an image with me watching. Once we had acknowledged these concerns Robert began to draw.

Robert worked with some skill and concentration. As he worked he began to cry. Initially he was embarrassed, but did not stop himself. In fact he was glad to cry. He said that he had not realised he could still feel the things the drawing had brought to mind. He allowed himself to cry freely as he continued with his picture (Fig. 2). His starting point had been to draw an image of the leaves on the tree outside his bedroom window. However, despite attempts to draw autumn leaves he found himself only able to make them green. He noticed that he concentrated on the veins of the leaves, and made a link with his constant examination of his own veins, which he did to monitor his health. We talked about his green leaves being separate from the tree in the background, and his feelings of being plucked from the tree of life before his autumn years.

The tree he had drawn was beginning to blossom, and Robert felt very positive about it. The scene in the background was one that he had drawn several times

[1] Adapted from Wood (1990), with kind permission from *Inscape: British Journal of Art Therapists*.

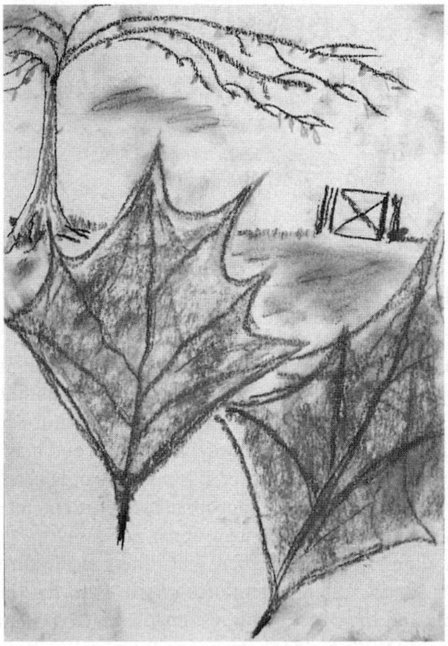

Fig. 2

before when he was a schoolboy. He remembered growing up in the countryside and talked of the dreams he had then for his adult life. Aspirations he regretted that would never now be fulfilled. Robert noticed that he had omitted a fence, which meant that the gate was useless. There seemed to be nothing separating him from the unknown place that lay beyond this field.

At the end of the session Robert reported feeling exhausted but light inside as though a burden had been lifted. This session had enabled Robert to connect with the grief he felt about having AIDS. Although we talked about some of the issues raised in the picture the main focus was allowing him to feel and to cry. His announcement to staff indicated that he had gone as far as he could with words. This one-off session prompted a positive change in Robert that was noticed by hospital staff and his partner.

Art therapy and other therapies

There is growing evidence from outside palliative circles that its fundamental principle of integrated care (based upon good interdisciplinary team work) leads to positive benefits for the patient.[33] How the different disciplines of the palliative team work together is a matter for consideration and in particular art therapy's part in this. For example, should a patient have art therapy at the same time as counselling or other emotional/psychological therapies? Art therapy works at verbal and non-verbal levels and therefore it can be possible for an art therapist to work in conjunction with a counsellor or psychologist. On these occasions good communication between staff is crucial to avoid splitting staff or confusing the patient. Art therapy has also been known to work well alongside more body-based therapies such as aromatherapy and massage. There is some evidence that art therapy may evoke issues that can be further explored in work with another discipline such as music therapy or chaplaincy.[16,17] However, the principle of patients' choice is central in this matter—the patient's own wishes must be the guide by which members of the palliative team are actively involved. After all the patients are the ones who must (together with our support) make sense of all that is happening to them. Morley describes her own journey with illness in which she used art therapy to integrated her experiences of the doctors, surgery, prayer, and her changing body.[34]

Art therapy and bereavement work

Palliative care aims to support not only the patient but also those who are close to them. Support is often provided at hospices for partners, spouses, children, and other significant family members and friends while the patient is ill and after the patient has died. Art therapy with the bereaved has been well documented over the past 20 years and in some settings has become an integral part of bereavement services.[35]

Conclusion

Art therapy is being practised in many parts of the world with adults and children living with life-threatening and terminal illnesses. There is a continuing recognition that art therapy does positively benefit patients, their carers and the professional team. The flexibility of art therapy to address a wide scope of issues ranging from pain to a patient's search for meaning makes it a valuable aspect of palliative care. To ensure that the benefits of art therapy are more clearly understood and that its efficacy is maximized there needs to be an increasing investment in research into this discipline.

References

1. **Kaye, C. and Blee, T.** *The Arts in Health Care.* London: Jessica Kingsley, 1997.
2. **Bejjani, F.** *Current Research in Arts Medicine.* Chicago: A Cappella Books, 1993.
3. **Haldane, D. and Loppert, S.**, ed. *The Arts in Health Care: Learning from Experience.* London: King's Fund Publishing, 1999.
4. **Malchiodi, C.** *Medical Art Therapy with Adults.* London: Jessica Kingsley, 1999.
5. **Pratt, M. and Wood, M.J.M.** *Art Therapy in Palliative Care: the Creative Response.* London: Routledge, 1998.
6. **Connell, C.** *Something Understood.* London: Wrexham Publications, 1998.
7. **Bint, J.** *A Report on the Exploration of Arts Therapies in Palliative Care, Cancer, AIDS and Bereavement.* The Omega Foundation, 2000.
8. **Zammit, C.** (2001). The art of healing: a journey through cancer: implications for art therapy. *Art Therapy: Journal of the American Art Therapy Association* **18** (1), 27–36.
9. **Frampton, D.** (1998). Creative therapies. In *Oxford Textbook of Palliative Medicine* 2nd edn. (ed. D. Doyle, G. Hanks, and N. Macdonald), pp. 861–4. Oxford: Oxford University Press.
10. **Teufel, E.S.** (1995). Terminal stage leukaemia: integrating art therapy and family process. *Art Therapy: Journal of the American Art Therapy Association* **12** (1), 51–5.
11. **Kennett, C.** (2000). Participation in a creative arts project can foster hope in a hospice day centre. *Palliative Medicine* **14**, 419–25.
12. **Bell, S.** (1998). Will the kitchen table do? Art therapy in the community. In *Art Therapy in Palliative Care: the Creative Response* (ed. M. Pratt and M.J.M. Wood), pp. 88–101. London: Routledge.
13. **Beaver, V.** (1998). The butterfly garden: art therapy with HIV/AIDS. In *Art Therapy in Palliative Care: the Creative Response* (ed. M. Pratt and M.J.M. Wood), pp. 127–39. London: Routledge.
14. **Bartholomew, A.** (1998). A narrow ledge: art therapy at London Lighthouse. In *Art Therapy in Palliative Care: the Creative Response* (ed. M. Pratt and M.J.M. Wood), pp. 115–26. London: Routledge.
15. **Dannecker, K.** (1991). Body and expression: art therapy with rheumatoid patients. *American Journal of Art Therapy* **29**, 110–17.
16. **Olofsson, A.** (1995). The value of integrating music therapy and expressive arts therapy in working with cancer patients. In *Lonely Waters: Proceedings of the International Conference on Music Therapy in Palliative Care UK 1994* (ed. C. Lee), pp. 147–52. Oxford: Sobell Publications.
17. **Stevens, G. and Lomas, H.** (1995). Working with the unknown: music and art therapy with a young man with Niemann Pick disease. In *Lonely Waters: Proceedings of the International Conference on Music Therapy in Palliative Care UK 1994* (ed. C. Lee), pp. 153–62. Oxford: Sobell Publications.
18. **Szepanski, M.** (1988). Art therapy and multiple sclerosis. *Inscape: Journal of the British Association of Art Therapists* Spring, 4–10.

19. **Gold, M. and Ahmedzai, S.** (1993). A transitional journey: a case study of art therapy in a hospice. In *Current Research in Arts Medicine* (ed. F. Bejjani). Chicago: A Cappella Books.
20. **Thomas, G. and Kennedy, J.** (1995). Art therapy and practice in palliative care. *European Journal in Palliative Care* **2** (3), 120–3.
21. **Coote, J.** (1998) Getting started: introducing the art therapy service. In *Art Therapy in Palliative Care: the Creative Response* (ed. M. Pratt and M.J.M. Wood), pp. 53–63. London: Routledge.
22. **Trauger-Querry, B. and Haghighi, K.R.** (1999). Balancing the focus: art and music therapy for pain control and symptom management in hospice care. *The Hospice Journal* **14** (1), 25–37.
23. **Wood, M.J.M.** (1998). The body as art: individual session with a man with AIDS. In *Art Therapy in Palliative Care: The Creative Response* (ed. M. Pratt and M.J.M. Wood), pp. 140–52. London: Routledge.
24. **Wood, M.J.M.** Making the connection: exploring art therapy practice with people who have AIDS-related dementia. MA thesis, Goldsmiths College, University of London, 1999.
25. **Farrell Fenton, J.** (2000). Cystic fibrosis and art therapy. *The Arts in Psychotherapy* **27** (1), 15–25.
26. **Mayo, S.** (1996). Symbol, metaphor and story: the function of group art therapy in palliative care. *Palliative Medicine* **10**, 209–16.
27. **Fried, O.** (1999). Many ways of caring: reaching out to aboriginal palliative care clients in Central Australia. *Progress in Palliative Care* **7** (3), 116–19.
28. **Belfiori, M.** (1994). The group takes care of itself: art therapy to prevent burnout. *The Arts in Psychotherapy* **12** (2), 119–26.
29. **Sheppard, L., MacInally, F., Rusted, J., Waller, D., and Shamash, K.** *Evaluating the Use of Art Therapy for People with Dementia: A Control Group Study.* A report commissioned by the Brighton Branch of the Alzheimer's Disease Society, 1998.
30. **Luzzatto, P. and Gabriel, B.** (2000). The creative journey: a model for short term group art therapy with post-treatment cancer patients. *Art Therapy: Journal of the American Art Therapy Association* **17**, 265–9.
31. **Gabriel, B. et al.** (2001). Art therapy with adult bone marrow transplant patients in isolation: a pilot study. *Psycho-oncology* **10** (2), 114–23.
32. **Reynolds, M.W., Nabors, L., and Quinlan, A.** (2000). The effectiveness of art therapy: does it work? *Art Therapy: Journal of the American Art Therapy Association* **17** (3), 207–13.
33. **Jackson, C. and DeJong, I.** *Achieving Effective Health Care Integration: The Essential Guide.* Brisbane: Mater University of Queensland Centre for General Practice, 2000.
34. **Morley, B.** (1998). Sunbeams and icebergs, meteorites and daisies: a cancer patient's experience of art therapy. In *Art Therapy in Palliative Care: The Creative Response* (ed. M. Pratt and M.J.M. Wood), pp. 176–85. London: Routledge.
35. **Pratt, M.** (1998). The invisible injury: adolescent griefwork group. In *Art Therapy in Palliative Care: the Creative Response* (ed. M. Pratt and M.J.M. Wood), pp. 153–68. London: Routledge.

Recommended reading

Connell, C. *Something Understood.* London: Wrexham Publications, 1998.
Malchiodi, C. *Medical Art Therapy with Adults.* London: Jessica Kingsley, 1999.
Pratt, M. and Wood, M.J.M. *Art Therapy in Palliative Care: The Creative Response* London: Routledge, 1998.

15.7 The contribution of stoma therapy to palliative medicine

Mave Salter

Introduction

Patients with stomas face multiple adjustment demands. Typically, the focus both before and after operation is on physical problems and care of the stoma. Because of limited time available, feelings about other issues may not be addressed. It is assumed that the patient will return to a normally functioning lifestyle but this is not always the case,(1) and may be especially prohibitive in palliative care. However, it is not the stoma itself, but the disease that may cause this and thus appropriate support and intervention are imperative in caring for patients with a stoma.

In chronic illness, especially when that illness is life-threatening, the body 'loses its silence' calling attention to itself. Ignoring the body is no longer possible and the person with a stoma is forced to manage physical functions in a way that would see strange to their healthy peers.(2)

Patients with stomas performed earlier on in their illness trajectory may well require help when their disease reaches the terminal stages. However, a few patients may have a stoma raised when they are in the palliative stage of their disease to relieve symptoms, such as obstruction. Whilst most patients will be able to care for their own stoma, there may well be those who require help as their health deteriorates.

The role of the stoma care nurse

More than 20 years ago, an eminent London surgeon described a stoma as 'an affront, difficult to bear, so that I marvel that our patients have put up with it for so long'.(3) The concept of the stoma care nurse was one of the first specialities in nursing. Common problems in this client population include coming to terms with the diagnosis and prognosis, and adjuvant treatment required. Issues around employment, family and other social support networks, body image, and sexuality, may also need to be addressed by the stoma care nurse.(4)

The stoma care nurse is, therefore, pivotal in ensuring the patient receives appropriate care. He/she works closely with ward staff and the multidisciplinary team in optimizing patient-focused care. This may include, for example, acting as care coordinator or patient advocate.

Definition of a stoma

The term 'stoma' derives from the Greek word for mouth or opening. A stoma is an opening on the body surface where an organ is brought to the exterior. Advances in medical treatment and surgical techniques have ensured that fewer permanent stomas are made, but temporary stomas remain a standard method of managing certain disorders that necessitate diversion of the gastrointestinal or urinary tract.(5)

Reasons for stoma formation

Surgery, which is the primary treatment for most solid tumours, plays a role in prevention, cure, and palliation. The malignancies that most commonly require construction of a stoma include colorectal, bladder, and cervical cancer.(6) Fistulae formation (e.g. rectovaginal fistula) and damage to tissue following pelvic radiotherapy may also be a reason for stoma formation.

Palliative surgery, undertaken to improve the quality of life, is primarily to relieve pain, perforation, or obstruction.(6) The primary goal is not to prolong life but to ensure a more comfortable life.[7] Examples of palliation include decompression or bypass of obstructive bowel, diversion of the faecal steam above a colonic fistula (rectovaginal, rectovesical, or entercutaneous), complications resulting from chemotherapy and radiation therapy such as skin breakdown, fistulas, radiation proctitis, and radiation cystitis. Perforation may also necessitate surgical intervention.[6]

A stoma is *permanent* when the surgical excision for trauma or disease prevents the tract or the sphincter mechanisms beyond the stoma from functioning normally again.

A *temporary* stoma is made to divert the faecal or urinary stream away from a diseased or damaged part of the tract until normal function is restored. The temporary stoma may be surgically closed later. Where the stoma may be temporary the patient may delay becoming involved in practical care in the hope of an early reversal of the stoma, while others suspend their normal living pattern and isolate themselves as they await the reversal operation. The decision not to proceed to closure may have a profound adverse effect on the patient, especially as about one-fourth to one-third of temporary stomas may become permanent. Reasons include physical factors, for example, disease advancement, and some patients simply decide to keep the stoma rather than undergo further surgery.[8]

Types of stomas (raised in patients with/at risk of cancer)

There are four main types of stoma (see Figs 1–3):

- An end (usually permanent) colostomy—this can be a simple operation where the divided bowel is brought through the abdominal wall and anastomosed to the skin. However, in an abdominoperineal excision of rectum (often done as a curative measure), the rectum and anus are removed.
- A transverse (usually temporary) colostomy.
- An ileostomy.
- A urostomy (ileal conduit).

End colostomy

A colostomy is normally formed in the left-hand quadrant of the abdomen (iliac fossa) and is used to divert faecal flow away from the anastomosis. The main portion of the colon is able to continue its normal function. If the colostomy is in the descending colon or the sigmoid colon, the faecal output from the colostomy normally results in a formed stool, with normal faecal odour.[9]

Transverse colostomy

A loop of intestine is brought out through a surgical opening.

This stoma is commonly constructed when diversion is needed but when minimal surgical intervention is required. It is not divided, but opened along the anterior surface. The opened edges are then everted and sutured to the skin. This type of stoma has two distinct openings that remain connected.[5]

A double-barrel stoma is formed when the colon is divided. The proximal and distal ends are both brought out through one opening in the abdominal wall then everted and sutured to the skin to form two stomas side by side. Complete division of the colon prevents faecal matter overflowing from the functioning into the non-functioning section. One end is a proximal, functioning stoma, the other is a distal, non-functioning one.[5] The distal stoma is generally referred to as a mucous fistula.

Ileostomy

A stoma is created from the terminal ileum and fashioned to protrude 1–2 cm from the abdominal wall at a preselected site. It may be temporary or

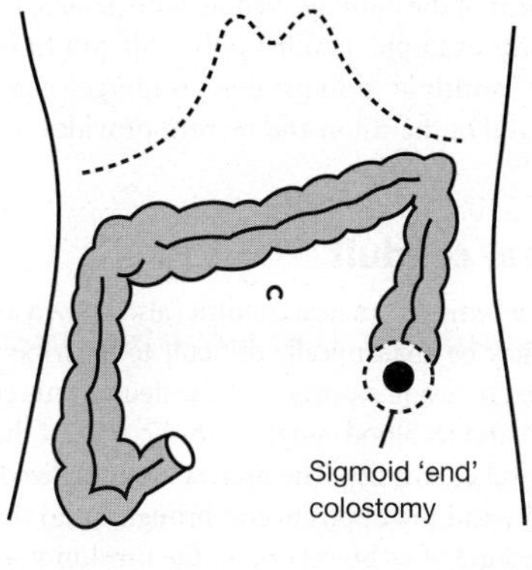

Fig. 1 Sigmoid 'end' colostomy.

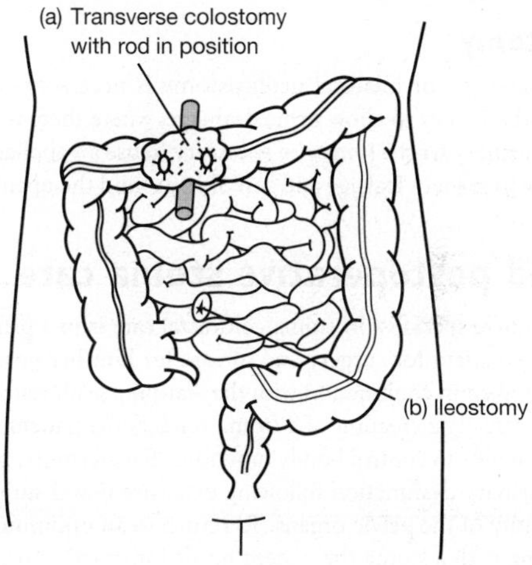

Fig. 2 (a) Transverse colostomy and (b) ileostomy.

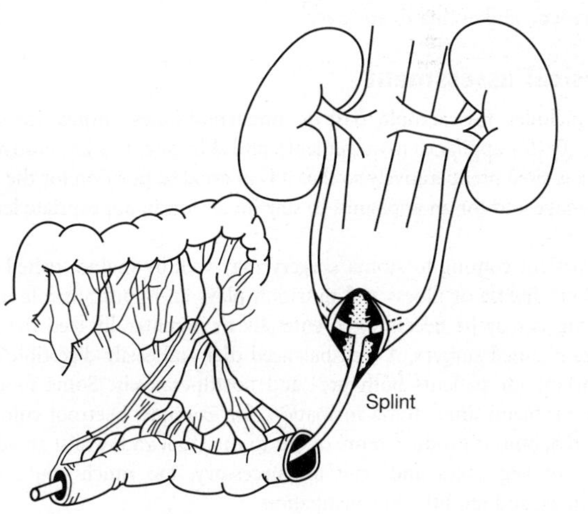

Fig. 3 Urostomy.

permanent. When an end ileostomy is raised, a mucous fistula may also be raised from any part of the small or large intestine.[10] A mucous fistula is a second non-functioning end stoma, the opening to the distal intestine may be exteriorized.

An ileostomy may be indicated if medical management is no longer appropriate in inflammatory bowel disease (ulcerative colitis and Crohn's disease). In extensive ulcerative colitis, colon cancer will develop within

25 years in one-third of the patients. People with genetic conditions may be at risk of cancer, for example, familial polyposis coli (a hereditary disease where there are multiple polyps that undergo cancerous change). Prophylactic removal of the colon and rectum provides protection for both types of patients.[6]

Urostomy/ileal conduit

When the bladder is removed an ileal conduit (also known as a urostomy) will be formed. This may be anatomically difficult to describe to the lay person because it is formed by using a portion of the ileum. This entails isolation of 10–20 cm of ileum and its blood supply with the ends of the ileum anastomosed to restore bowel continuity. The ureters are mobilized into the isolated ileum (the conduit) and the opposite end brought onto the abdominal surface as a stoma. Because of its bowel origin, the urostomy secretes mucus.

Other surgical interventions

Nephrostomy

Sometimes, a single or bilateral nephrostomy is necessary (insertion of tube(s) into the kidney to allow urine drainage, where there is obstruction of the lower urinary tract). It may be necessary to use an appliance over the nephrostomy to prevent leakage and sore skin around the opening.

Pre- and postoperative stoma care

The clinical nurse specialist in stoma/colorectal care is in a prime position to prepare the patient for surgery and to care for him/her postoperatively. This is undertaken in conjunction with the ward nurse allocated to oversee the patient's care. The creation of a stoma renders the patient incontinent and thereby unable to control bodily functions. Furthermore, patients may experience urinary dysfunction following extensive bowel surgery because of the proximity of the pelvic organs. To return to an optimum lifestyle or adapt to living with a stoma the patient needs information on a variety of issues.[1] Pre- and postoperative care includes educating the patient on what the stoma will look like, where it will be placed, how to change appliances, and the adaptation process. It is imperative to assess, plan, implement, and evaluate care given.

Physical assessment

This includes, for example, past or concurrent illness, fitness for surgery, dexterity (for appliance management), and skin care. It is imperative that a stoma is sited preoperatively so that it is in an ideal position for the patient to manage and for an appliance to stay intact for an appropriate length of time.[11]

A patient coming to stoma surgery may well be malnourished due to previous disease or illness and nutrition plays an important role in intervention. It may be necessary to enterally or parenterally feed the patient before planned surgery. A well-balanced diet and easily digestible food is important for patients both pre- and postoperatively. Some foods may cause problems after stoma formation, for example, beetroot colours the stool red, onions produce more odour to the stool and, whilst an adequate intake of vegetables and fruit are necessary, too much could lead to diarrhoea, and too little to constipation.

Patients in the palliative care stages of their disease may well have anorexia and therefore small meals interspersed with light snacks or high calorie drinks should be suggested. Taste may be altered and a patient may have a preference for savoury drinks and soups (see also Chapter 15.3).

General assessment

Age, gender, and personality/coping mechanisms should form part of the patient's overall assessment discussing with the patient their personality and coping mechanisms. Age may influence how a person responds to having a stoma, for example, a young person may respond more positively than an older one. Cultural beliefs influence lifestyle and can be associated with a religious or spiritual background. Beliefs and traditions affect an individual's attitudes towards physical and social well-being. Having a stoma can create many difficulties for ethnic groups in regard to dietary considerations, personal hygiene, social communication, religious observances, bereavement, and grief.[12]

Psychological assessment

This includes the affect of a stoma on the person's body image and sexuality.[13] Some people react with shock and disgust when told they may require a stoma, for this type of surgery has a profound effect on the mind as well as the body. It reverses the healthy body image a person may have of themselves. This reaction can occur at any age and it may not be just to the stoma itself, red, swollen, and unsightly following surgery, but also the connotations that go with it. No wonder research into techniques to do away with wearing a bag or to eliminate the need for a stoma are now a reality.[14]

Effects on sexual activity and attitudes

The implications that pelvic surgery involving a stoma has on a patient's sex life may be either physiological, for example, causing nerve damage, or psychological, due to altered body image, or both. The physical alteration that a stoma brings may result in the person with a stoma having a poor self-concept and reduced self-esteem. In Nordstrom's study,[15] patients very often perceived themselves to be less sexually attractive to their partner. It is important that the patient and their partner understand the potential impact that stoma surgery may have on sexual function and sexuality, regardless of age, marital status, illness, or sexual orientation. Postoperatively, there may be sexual difficulties to varying degrees, and for some patients impotence will occur. If, following surgery, intercourse is not possible or is difficult/painful, the patient may need help in making some adjustments in the relationship. If wide excision has been undertaken, causing a shortening or narrowing of the vagina, leading to dyspareunia, the use of lubricating jelly for a female patient can be advocated. Where the patient is impotent (either temporary or permanently), advice on alternative methods to induce erection should be made available, for example, Viagra, penile implants, etc.[13]

The experiences, concerns, and needs of gay and lesbian ostomates parallel those of anyone who has had ostomy or related surgery. However, many gay and lesbian patients are reluctant to bring up issues and concerns that in any way reveal their sexual orientation, thus making it difficult for them to receive the help they need. The stoma care nurse is ideally placed to demonstrate sensitivity and receptiveness to persons who are same-sex orientated, thus helping the patient to reveal significant personal concerns.[16]

Specific cultural issues

The Hindu patient

Hindu women are modest and may be reluctant to undress or allow a male nurse or doctor to examine them. Hindu patients believe the cow is sacred, and therefore will not eat beef. Some are vegans and will not take medication that has a gelatine capsule, or eat jelly. This can cause problems in Hindu women who need to take loperamide to slow bowel transit time down as the medication comes in capsule form.[9]

The Sikh patient

Sikhs should not have their hair cut or bodily hair removed unless it is really necessary, and then only a minimum should be removed. Many Sikh women will prefer to be examined by a female health care professional. Most Sikhs prefer not to eat beef and may refuse medication unless it is really necessary.[9]

The Muslim patient

A Muslim is expected to pray at set hours, five times a day, and before each prayer session has to perform a washing ritual. This washing signifies cleanliness of the body both inside and out. However, because this is difficult for patients with a stoma, special dispensation has been granted, although the use of a two-piece stoma appliance allows a clean pouch to be attached to the flange at each new prayer interval, thereby leaving the patient clean and pure for prayer. Muslims are very particular about cleanliness, and faeces are considered unclean. A stoma sited above the umbilicus is viewed as food content that is being put out and therefore acceptable for the patient to self-care. A further factor to be considered in Muslim patients is that the right hand is used for eating and greeting, and the left hand for cleaning oneself. Thus, careful thought is necessary to determine which appliance will be easier to use.[9]

Stoma appliances

The key to successful management of a stoma is a well-constructed, well-fitting, and skin-protective appliance (also known as a pouch). There are many different types of appliances, though all work on the same principle. The basis is a sheet of adhesive with an aperture, which can be cut by the patient to fit the stoma. Appliances are either one piece (where the faceplate is integral to the bag) or two piece (where the bag and flange clip together). Additionally, they can be clear or opaque. Most appliances come with a fibre or net backing on the body side to help absorb perspiration. Two-piece appliances consist of a flange and a bag that is clipped to this flange. Irregularities and discrepancies around the stoma can be filled in with pastes or by using convex appliances. Convexity is the outward curving of a faceplate that begins at the aperture and extends outward.[17] The bags can be drainable (for use with an ileostomy or transverse colostomy where the stool is unformed), closed (for use with an end colostomy where the stool is more formed), and with a tap (for a urostomy). This tap can also be connected to a night bag that has a capacity of up to 2 l, which means the patient will not have to get up frequently at night to drain the appliance.

Urostomy pouches come as one- or two-piece appliances and have a non-flux valve inside the bag to prevent urine washing up over the stoma and causing leakages. It is important that the peristomal skin is protected from any leaking effluent and the appliance emptied and changed regularly. Appliances should never be patched up when they leak, but the skin cleaned carefully and a new appliance fitted.[5,9]

Because the output from a left-sided colostomy can be malodorous, closed colostomy bags are manufactured with a flatus filter, which also has a charcoal centre to allow for absorption and dispersion of the odour. One-piece appliances are available for colostomy, ileostomy, and urostomy with a film that is transparent or opaque. In a two-piece appliance, the stoma aperture in the flange may need to be cut to the correct size each time it is changed.

Appliances for fistulas

Whilst a standard stoma appliance may be appropriate on some fistulas, wound management needs to consider the size of the wound. Skin surrounding a draining wound rapidly becomes macerated or denuded by biologically active substances contained in fistula efflux. Protection with hydrocolloid sheets is appropriate.[5]

Routine care of the stoma

Mild soap and water, or water only, are sufficient for skin and stoma cleaning. Detergents, disinfectants, antiseptics, and oil-based substances such as vaseline should *not* be used. The stoma is not a wound and should be regarded as a resited urethra or anus.[18]

Stoma complications

Retraction of the stoma

The stoma recedes into the abdominal opening, leading to 'pouching' problems. It may be necessary to use a convex appliance so that leakage and sore skin do not occur.

Sore skin

This is caused by leakage, or incorrect fitting of the faceplate or flange (i.e. where the opening is too large). The stoma should be measured regularly during the first few weeks following surgery and the aperture size adjusted accordingly. Leaving an appliance intact for 3–4 days (or longer) helps.

Various pastes or skin-care aids are available to help heal the area. Pastes are used to fill creases, crevices, or gullies in the skin to provide a smooth surface for the application of an appliance. However, these should not be used on broken skin as these products contain alcohol and will cause stinging.[19]

Hydrocolloid wafers are used to protect skin from proteolytic secretions. They are used to provide an even, flat surface on areas where paste has been used to fill increases, crevices, or gullies prior to application of an appliance.[19]

Prolapse

This is frequently seen in patients who have had a transverse colostomy. It can result from inefficient 'fixing' of the bowel as it emerges onto the abdominal surface. Prolapse can be corrected by surgery, but often it is held in by a belt.[5] However, if the latter method is used, the stoma will continue to prolapse from time to time and a large appliance/aperture may be required. It is often unsightly and can be distressing to the patient. Inflammation of the stoma often occurs with a prolapse and the appliance should be cut large enough to make provision for the inflammation of the stoma, but without compromising the peri-stomal skin, so that soreness develops. This is best achieved by diagonal slits around the faceplate or flange.

Herniation

This is more likely to occur in patients with colostomies than those with ileostomies and urostomies. As with all patients who have undergone abdominal and bowel surgery, patients should be advised to avoid lifting heavy weights (such as a saucepan) for 3 months following surgery. It may be necessary for the patient to undergo hernia repair.

Stenosis

This occurs when the stomal opening becomes narrower, making effluent difficult to come to the surface. Surgery may be implicated, but the use of dilators may help.[9]

Bleeding

Due to the colon's rich blood supply, occasional bleeding from the peri-stomal area is not uncommon. Causative factors include tearing an appliance off the skin, instead of removing it gently, scratching, and too rigorous cleaning around the stomal area.

Bleeding from inside the stoma, although uncommon, should be referred for a medical opinion. The writer has known this to occur in a patient with a urostomy, where a ureteric stone had formed in the ileal conduit. Bleeding episodes ceased when the stone was removed.

General effects of illness in the patient with palliative care needs

For palliative patients, who may have lost weight (due to anorexia), or gained weight (due to steroids), appliance changes may be difficult. This could be due to the body shape of the patient or because the stoma has been sited awkwardly. In such cases, a flexible one-piece appliance may be most suitable. However, for the patient who does not want to keep removing the whole appliance, a two-piece appliance is more appropriate.[5] Supportive care by a partner or family member may be necessary, and information given on stoma care.

The effect of adjuvant treatment on the person with a stoma

Radiotherapy to the pelvic area often causes diarrhoea. Increased oral intake will help with possible dehydration and increasing dietary fibre may also assist. Additionally, dietary fibre helps the constipated patient, and if the patient is unable to eat, an enema or suppositories via the colostomy may help,[9] although these are not always successful. Other gastro-intestinal symptoms such as anorexia, nausea, and vomiting could be apparent and it may be necessary for a carer to take over the management of the stoma until this resolves.

Similarly, chemotherapy could lead to nausea and vomiting, or peripheral neuritis. During such times the patient may be unable to manage their stoma/appliance as indicated above, especially if there is a change in the consistency of output from the stoma. It is important to remember that other side-effects of chemotherapy, for example, alopecia, may well have a further impact on a negative body image.

Other considerations—fistula care and abdominal wounds

A fistula is any normal tube-like passage within body tissue between two organs or an organ and the body surface. However, spontaneous intestinal fistulas can occur as a result of, for example, malignancy. Where radiation damage is the cause, the urinary bladder or vagina and rectum are common sites. Discharge from gastrointestinal fistulas can excoriate the skin.[5] A malignant tumour may invade adjacent organs and tissues causing an obstruction. Perforation may also result in an internal fistula or a cutaneous fistula.

A further complication may arise if the abdominal wound breaks down. Fistulas and large abdominal wounds, which may be associated with fistulas, are often challenging to the health care professional because of the leakage problem that damages the surrounding skin, causing excoriation, and pain. Dehiscence of a suture line can occur and patients may be very distressed on seeing the contents of their abdomen.[9] The importance of a full and comprehensive assessment of complex or chronic wounds cannot be over-emphasized. A chronic wound is one that does not heal as expected according to the 'normal' healing process. It is usually associated with an underlying disease process. A complex wound (not necessarily chronic) requires specialized assessment and management interventions.[19] Dressings and appliances may have to be changed regularly and this is demoralizing and tiring for the patient. However, appliances should never be 'patched up' as any leakage will cause more skin breakdown. Often the abdominal breakdown may be extensive, and the effluent output high, requiring a large appliance, or wound-care system. The appliance allows for easy observation of the wound, a large volume of effluent to be collected, as well as irrigating the wound, if required.[9]

Supportive/ongoing care

In palliative care, an integrated approach is required for the management of stomas and fistulas. Not only do patients have to cope with the fact that no further active treatment is appropriate, but that their body is 'letting them down'.[2]

The Hospital Palliative Care Team and the Primary Health Care and Community Palliative Care Teams have much to offer in support of the patient, who is actually the most important person in the team. Close liaison in discharge planning is essential. It may be appropriate to introduce the patient to a suitable ostomy voluntary organization/self-help group, where they may gain additional social support.

Symptoms, such as diarrhoea, should be treated with medication to slow the gut motility (loperamide or diphemoxylate) and constipation with arachis oil enemas. However, in the palliative stages of disease, invasive procedures such as a irrigation of the bowel should only be done with extreme caution and if no other resolution can be found.

The final stages of illness

It is imperative to offer the patient and all their carers sensitive care and intervention when the patient is no longer able to care for their own personal needs, such as a stoma. Frequent checks should be made on the appliance and area under the faceplate/flange to ensure there is no leakage or sore skin.

Attention to detail regarding a patient's appearance (thus deflecting from the stoma) may well be a way of demonstrating ongoing care at this difficult time in their illness and dignity in death. No patient should be left in isolation; no patient should take this journey alone.[20]

Conclusion

It is important that the stoma care nurse works with all members of the inter-disciplinary team: doctors, nurses, dietitians, occupational therapists, community nurses, etc., in giving holistic care to the patient with a stoma. Such care should be participative, collobarative, and empowering.[21]

References

1. **Walsh, B., Grunert, B., Telford, G., and Otterson, M.** (1995). Multidisciplinary management of altered body image in the patient with an ostomy. *Journal of Wound, Ostomy and Continence Nursing* **22** (5), 227–35.
2. **Bleeker, H. and Mulderij, K.** (1992). The experience of motor disability. *Phenomenology and Pedagogy* **10**, 1–18.
3. **Dudley, H.A.F.** (1978). If I had carcinoma of the middle third of the rectum. *British Medical Journal* **1**, 1035–67.
4. **Baxter, A. and Salter, M.** (2000). Stoma care nursing. *Nursing Standard* **14** (19), 59.
5. **Blackley, P.** *Practical Stoma, Wound and Continence Management.* Victoria: Research Publications Pty Ltd., 1998.
6. **Hampton, B. and Bryant, R.** *Ostomies and Continent Diversions: Nursing Management.* St Louis: Mosby Year Book, 1992.
7. **Watson, P.** (1983). The effects of short term post operative counselling on cancer/ostomy patients. *Cancer Nursing* February, 21–9.
8. **Allinson, M.** (1995). Comparing methods of stoma formation. *Nursing Standard* March, 25–8.
9. **Black, P.** (1996). Practical stoma care *Nursing Standard,* **11** (47), 49–55.
10. **Reasbrook, P., Smithers, M., and Blackley, P.** (1989). Construction and management of colostomies and ileostomies. *Digestive Diseases* **7**, 265–80.
11. **Salter, M.** *Altered Body Image: The Nurse's Role* 2nd edn. London: Bailliere Tindall, 1997.
12. **Gardner, J.** *Asians in Britain. Some Cultural Considerations in Stoma Care. Nursing 21.* London: Balliere Tindall, 1987.
13. **Garnet, E., Russell, E., and Evans, Y.** *Principle: A Framework of Nursing Designed Specifically for Meeting the Needs of Stoma Patients.* London: Royal College of Nursing, 1995.
14. **Wynreib, R., Gusavsson, J., Liljeqvist, L., Poppen, B., and Rossel, R.** (1995). A prospective study of the quality of life after pelvic pouch operation. *Journal of the American College of Surgeons* **180**, 589–95.
15. **Nordstrom, G.** (1985). Urostomy patients—a strategy for care. *Nursing Times* **85** (18), 32–4.
16. **Etnyre, W.** (1990). Meeting the needs of gay and lesbian ostomates. Proceedings of the 8th Biennial Congress, World Council of Enterostomal Nurses, Hillister, Canada.
17. **Rolstad, B. and Boarini, J.** (1996) Principles and techniques in the use of convexity. *Ostomy Wound Management* **42**, 24–32.
18. **Mallett, J. and Dougherty, L.** *The Royal Marsden Hospital, Manual of Clinical Nursing Procedures* 5th edn. London: Blackwell Science, 2000.

19. **Naylor, W., Laverty, D., and Mallett, J.** *The Royal Marsden Hospital Handbook of Wound Management in Cancer Care.* London: Blackwell Science, 2001.
20. **Slade, D.** (2000). The voice of experience. *Journal of Wound, Ostomy and Continence Nursing* **27**, 201–6.
21. **Corner, J.** (1997). Cancer nursing as a therapy: the contribution of specialist nurses. *Oncology Nurses Today* **2** (3), 11–14.

15.8 The contribution of clinical psychology to palliative medicine

Fiona Cathcart

Introduction

This chapter describes ways in which psychology can make palliative care more effective. It will describe evidence that psychological knowledge applied at the level of the individual as a patient, a group such as a family or staff team, or the wider application of psychology in the design of the treatment environment or delivery of health care can improve outcome. The chapter will focus primarily on work with patients with metastatic disease or advanced illness but will describe psychological interventions earlier in the disease process or with other types of problem if it seems likely these interventions may be relevant but have not been researched in palliative care yet.

Background

During the last two decades, clinical psychologists have extended their services to physical health care. Psychological interventions have improved outcome for patients with a range of illness from acute events such as myocardial infarction to disabling conditions such as chronic pain. People with cancer and other life-threatening disease often experience significant psychosocial distress. The psychological literature focuses predominantly on the care of patients newly diagnosed or those receiving curative treatment, but until recently there was less published literature on psychological assessment and intervention in palliative care specifically. Also, psychological studies with palliative care patients have focused on the needs of those with cancer rather than those with advanced illness caused by non-malignant conditions such as heart failure. This may reflect the methodological difficulties in assessing effective outcome in palliative care[1] as well as the lack of clinical psychologists available to undertake the work.

Psychological models

Psychologists base their interventions on the evidence base of modern psychology. These interventions are based on psychological research into how individuals learn, think, feel, and interact both with their environment and the people within it. A psychologist may suggest that a problem could be tackled more effectively by changing an aspect of the care system or the physical environment rather than working with the person directly. Clinical psychologists may direct their efforts to improve psychosocial care at the level of the individual, a group of individuals such as a family, patient, or staff group, or at an organizational level. The choice of intervention will be influenced also by the setting in which it is delivered. This may be the person's home in the community, a palliative care ward in a large general hospital, or a purpose-built specialist unit such as a hospice.

Psychological assessment

Many people enter palliative care services having had a long history of interventions with gradually deteriorating health. They will have had an opportunity to acknowledge their increasing frailty but this does not mean that they will have done so. Others will have progressed rapidly from apparent good health to a poor prognosis and may experience a sense of shock and confusion. Some carers neglect their own health to care for dependants.

One elderly man visited his sick wife daily and spent hours by her bedside, occasionally rubbing his sore back. After her death, he attended his physician and discovered the ache was caused by bone metastases from an unsuspected primary tumour. His shock was compounded by his recent bereavement.

Communicating bad news is seen as significant at the time of diagnosis but issues are revisited later as the disease progresses when other specialities no longer maintain follow-up or interventions that had been helpful are no longer effective. The person who adjusted well initially to the life-threatening diagnosis may experience great distress subsequently and require more support. Efforts have been made to reduce the sense of confusion and loss of control and facilitate informed decision-making by using leaflets, audio, and videotapes. These are helpful but it is important to address the emotional component of communication as well as the need for factual information. Innes[2] cautioned against psychologists directing too much effort in assisting draft medical information that is easily understood but does not address the concerns prioritized by the patient. Other authors suggest that patients are looking for information that acknowledges the serious nature of the problem but conveys hope and potential gains such as more valued priorities.[3]

Many studies indicate that staff caring for patients with advanced disease do not detect their distress. A variety of psychological measures is available but staff in busy clinics are more likely to use a brief screening instrument and refer to specialist help if necessary. Cull et al.[4] found that the more distressed patients attending an oncology out-patient clinic were referred to the clinical psychology service but that the psychological scores of those patients *not* referred indicated that 30 per cent warranted further assessment for anxiety and 23 per cent for depression. Asking the simple question. 'Are you depressed?' can be as effective in detecting depressed patients as more lengthy assessments.[5] This suggests that a willingness to explore patients' distress can be effective in itself but staff may need training in communication skills to ensure that the appropriate questions are asked and in a way that does not preclude answers that are uncomfortable to the questioner.

Consultations can be steered to elicit only those problems that the clinician can solve.[6] This may help the clinician maintain a sense of professional optimism that is important but it leaves the patient with unresolved problems. Clinicians may be more willing to elicit psychological problems if they believe that there are effective psychological interventions.

Psychosocial interventions are effective with cancer patients but it is unclear which are the effective components.[7,8] The methodological problems in evaluating the outcome of psychosocial interventions in patients with advanced disease are formidable. Studies face the challenge of recruitment, attrition, the selection of appropriate psychometric measures, and precise description of the intervention used. Frequently, the intervention combines several treatment strategies. A range of strategies is described below.

Interventions with the individual patient (Table 1)

Goal-setting (see also Chapter 14)

Early in the development of palliative care, it was argued that palliative care would be improved by goal-setting rather than by eliciting problem check-lists.[9] This process does not deny the limits set by the disease but keeps the focus of care on what might still be achieved. Generating a problem list can be a demoralizing exercise for both patient and carer but identifying simple goals informs the direction of care and enables short-term targets to be negotiated. Goal-setting is used extensively in rehabilitation services but it could assist palliative care patients and those caring for them maintain a sense of purpose when efforts seem futile. Goal-setting is most effective when certain conditions are met. It should be realistic, time limited, specific, and also patient centred in that the goal is valued by the patient rather than imposed by another. The goals are reviewed and modified as appropriate,

> A woman hopes to enjoy her first grandchild due in 2 months. She is no longer mobile and it is uncertain if she will live long enough but it is possible. Small steps are negotiated which would help her achieve her ultimate goal if her illness progresses slowly but which have intrinsic value if not. She may decide to perform simple daily exercises to maintain strength in the arms with which she hopes to hold the baby; she may speak into an audiocassette for a few minutes each day to record for the future bedtime stories or favourite recipes.

Patients can learn to pace themselves by identifying a goal and its component parts. Pacing reduces the sense of powerlessness when patients face many losses. The overactivity/rest cycle is a familiar concept to those working with patients with chronic pain but has relevance in palliative care. The person feels too fatigued to accomplish activities and tries to compensate by doing as much as possible when feeling a little stronger. The ensuing exhaustion confirms the belief that all energy is being drained by the disease when a more realistic explanation may be that the fatigue is a combination of the limits set by the disease *and* the way of responding to it.

Problem-solving

Patients are taught to tackle problems in a structured way over a limited number of sessions (see Table 2).

Teaching problem-solving can help reduce the sense of being overwhelmed and help regain lost confidence. A small pilot study teaching problem-solving skills to patients indicated that this approach is feasible in the palliative care setting.[10] The intervention was given to patients chosen on the basis of consecutive referrals to a palliative home-care team. They were not selected on the basis of psychological distress. The participants had an estimated prognosis of at least 3 months but only half survived to complete the 3-month assessment. This small pilot study was left with very few patients who completed all assessments. Those who completed treatment were positive about the intervention despite little or no change being reflected in the scores of the assessment measures. There was no control group so it could be possible that patients appreciated the extra individual attention rather than the nature of the intervention itself.

Table 1 Types of interventions

Goal-setting
Problem-solving
Relaxation
Hypnosis
CBT
Counselling and psychotherapy
Behavioural strategies

Table 2 Problem-solving for patients

Clarify and prioritize problems
Set realistic goals
Review available resources and options
Choose preferred solution
Decide what is needed to be achieved
Review progress

Relaxation

The use of relaxation in the management of anxiety is widely accepted. It is practised with both individuals and in groups. A frail and bed-bound patient can access this type of intervention with the use of modern lightweight audiocassette or minidisc players with earphones. Patients should be assessed on an individual basis and the rationale for using relaxation explained carefully. A small minority of patients experience an increase in anxiety or panic attacks when practising relaxation. This paradox may be caused by feelings of vulnerability and loss of control. Identifying the reasons for this and modifying the approach may be necessary.

There have been many studies indicating relaxation can reduce anticipatory and nausea associated with chemotherapy.[11] A recent meta-analysis concluded relaxation training reduced treatment-related symptoms and improved emotional adjustment in patients receiving acute non-surgical cancer treatments.[12] The SIGN Guidelines for the control of cancer pain stated there was enough evidence to recommend 'patients with cancer pain should be given an opportunity to be trained in some form of relaxation as an adjunct to pharmacological pain control.'[13]

Commercially made relaxation cassettes and CDs are readily available but specific advice tailored to the individual's needs may also be necessary.

> A woman who was anxious during radiotherapy tried to practise the deep relaxation she had learned at antenatal classes but found the noise of the treatment equipment interfered. It was suggested that incorporating the extraneous sound into her imagery would be more effective than trying to block the sound out. Her chosen imagery was relaxing in a cornfield and she successfully incorporated the sound as agricultural machinery working nearby.

Teaching patients to transform an image can be a potent intervention itself. There is evidence from the mental health setting that recurrent nightmares and intrusive imagery can be alleviated by rehearsing alternative positive endings.

> A woman with breast cancer had distressing dreams of her body being devoured by snakes. This was discussed and she created alternative images successfully herself. At the next session she recounted a dream in which the menacing snakes were being devoured by jewelled serpents and her nightmare ceased.

Walker et al. report a randomized controlled trial of 96 women with locally advanced breast cancer using relaxation and guided imagery as a psychosocial intervention and reported positive effects on mood, quality of life for the intervention group, and changes in host defences. They found no significant clinical and pathological effects and acknowledge that the significance of the biological changes is unclear. Both the intervention and control groups reported little distress and were satisfied with the emotional support given. The authors attribute this to the effect of the 'homely, drop-in' centre in which treatment including chemotherapy was administered rather than the traditional clinical environment. They suggest that it could be cost-effective to direct resources in this way and not wait for psychological casualties to emerge.[14]

Hypnosis

There is debate as to whether hypnosis is a distinct state or if it differs only in emphasis from other interventions such as relaxation with guided imagery. The terms are often used interchangeably. Imagery is a key component, but in practice the clinician may use a combination of strategies to achieve the desired effect of a sense of calm and focused attention and will be guided by the preferences of the patient. A study using the additional strategy of cognitive–behaviour therapy did not make the treatment more effective.[15] Hypnosis has been used to alleviate the distress of painful procedures in the paediatric[16] and adult setting.[17]

Hypnosis may be helpful for patients who are too frail to engage in more active ways of reducing pain or discomfort. Hypnosis has been used in palliative care but there are few large controlled studies. A retrospective study of 41 day hospice patients who had received hypnotherapy found that nearly two-thirds reported improved coping with their illness and very few (7 per cent) reported it as being unhelpful or negative. Hypnotherapy was offered to patients who appeared to be tense or have difficulties in coping or who simply requested it. The majority of those whose coping was unchanged reported hypnotherapy had been a pleasant experience. There was no formal evaluation other than the self-report.[18]

Cognitive–behaviour therapy

Cognitive therapy teaches patients to challenge habitual ways of thinking that may exacerbate emotional distress The addition of behavioural strategies has led to cognitive–behaviour therapy, which is recommended for a wide range of mental health problems.[19] Cognitive–behavioural interventions have been used successfully in oncology and palliative care.[20,21] A prospective randomized controlled trial with patients experiencing psychological morbidity favoured this type of intervention over counselling at 1-year follow-up.[22] It is not clear how feasible it may be to use this approach close to the end of life. Fatigue, poor concentration, and increasing frailty near the end of life may limit cognitive exploration. Santos and Greer[23] report a man who was able to benefit within days of his death but this intervention seems to have been successful because of the goal-setting component and the opportunity to discuss his fears rather than his gaining understanding of the way in which his cognitions influenced his mood.

Counselling and individual psychotherapy

Counselling may be part of the care given by health-service staff or it may be offered through a separate agency. A recent study of an independent cancer counselling service in London indicated that it was positively viewed by those who completed evaluations but it is not clear from this report how many of those using this service were newly diagnosed and what proportion had advanced disease.[24] As the majority of clients were young women it is probable that there were fewer in the latter category. The authors comment on the gender and social class bias of those who choose to use such a service and whether or not it would meet the needs of other sectors of the population.

A psychodynamic model of psychotherapy has been influential[25] but interest is growing in existential psychotherapy where the emphasis is on assisting the patients construct meaning from their lives and death.[26]

Behavioural strategies

As people live longer with cancer, the issues relevant in chronic disease become relevant in cancer. People learn to live with their pain and impairment but in ways that may be unhelpful to them. The approaches used to minimize disability in chronic pain can have relevance for palliative care.[27] It can be difficult to assess whether a new complaint indicates disease progression, but careful observation and recording may reveal an association with other factors such as visiting time or an adjacent patient receiving care. The social context of care is important and readily recognized by nursing staff but rarely acknowledged in the literature. A clinical unit may be busy for staff but boring for patients and staff attention may be given only for symptom complaints. Also, some individuals may have used health complaints to control relatives for many years and it is unlikely that these dynamics change at the door of the palliative care unit. Redd[28,29] describes interventions in oncology and a palliative care setting in which symptoms that were troublesome to the patient or disruptive to the care of other patients were modified successfully by changing the staff response to them. This type of approach does not appear to have been used often for a number of reasons. There are difficulties in using a behavioural programme consistently in a busy unit with many staff where few staff have training or experience in operant conditioning methods.[30] Also, staff who are attracted to palliative care may find it difficult to redirect their attention. They may obtain gratification by caring for helpless patients rather than supporting autonomy as long as possible. Even when staff have found a behavioural approach helpful, they hesitate to use it again.[31] In practice, several types of psychological intervention may be applied at once as the following two examples illustrate

A widow was diagnosed with end-stage cardiac failure. She was referred to the clinical psychologist for bereavement support and advice on managing the psychological component of her breathlessness. Additional issues emerged including the significance of past sibling dynamics which caused friction among the current carers and a tense relationship with her adult child. Intervention required anxiety management, bereavement counselling, ventilation of past and present resentments, and family therapy. Sufficient progress was made that when she died peacefully a few weeks later her family was present and there was no rivalry at the bedside.

A woman in her early forties was diagnosed with advanced cancer. She was withdrawn, angry, and complained frequently of pain that was difficult to assess and manage. She kept curtains drawn in her room and her husband fed her despite her being able to feed herself. She refused psychological intervention initially but at the third attempt she agreed and thereafter used the sessions constructively. She distrusted health professionals attributing this to her mother's unexpected death after a routine procedure some years before. She had filed a formal complaint about this. Offers of professional support were met with suspicion, for example, she expressed the belief that staff would discriminate against her when she received treatment at the local hospital where her mother had died. The hospital consultant suggested she contact him directly with any concerns and see only him. This was interpreted as confirming the basis for her fears rather than reassurance that her needs would be met. She challenged the medical and nursing staff by demanding more help while rejecting all their efforts as useless. Her way of thinking about her pain exacerbated it in that she 'catastrophized' her sensations. The psychological intervention targeted her pain cognitions and helped her develop other strategies for coping with it. The relevance of her anger at her mother's death to her own situation was explored. Modest goals were negotiated, which gave her another focus and enabled the staff to engage in a more rewarding interaction. She had been the dominant partner and was dismissive of her husband's ability to manage the household. Her husband shared her view and the couple agreed on practical ways of transferring her knowledge to him. The prepubertal daughter was a close observer who modelled on her mother. She was frequently present in the room and witnessed her mother's distress and hostility. The girl's own understanding and expectations of health care were being shaped by her interpretation of events. When efforts to engage the mother were successful, the girl interacted more positively with staff. This countered the developing family myth that health professionals are untrustworthy. Two days before her death, the patient was enjoying visitors in the hospice garden. In this case, the effective care given has not only made the daughter's memories of her mother's dying less distressing but also been an investment for the future when the girl may be on the receiving end of health care herself.

These two examples illustrate that pain and symptoms are not experienced in an interpersonal vacuum. Pharmacological and physical interventions are important but are less effective unless psychological issues are also addressed.

Interventions with groups

Groups may be viewed as a more cost-effective way of delivering the same intervention to large numbers or as having intrinsic worth because of the group dynamics.[32,33] Spiegel et al.[34] reported that weekly psychological support meetings for women with metastatic breast cancer provided psychological benefits and also increased survival time compared to those in the control group. A recent meta-analyses of psychological interventions indicated that group therapy was at least as effective as individual therapy, but advised that further research should be undertaken in other cultural contexts because many studies are with the American population.[8] A group therapy intervention was undertaken with women with metastatic breast cancer living in north-east Scotland.[35] The psychometric scores did not show significant changes but the process analysis revealed that the group was helpful to some participants. The authors concluded their results 'did not provide strong endorsement for the use of group support in this particular cultural context'. An Australian study of women with metastatic breast cancer reported that those randomized to group cognitive–behaviour therapy improved on a number of psychological measures in the short term but this was not sustained at 6 month follow-up. There was no survival advantage.[36] A Canadian study, also with women with metastatic breast cancer who were randomized to group support, found little difference in outcome over time on psychometric measures and no clear survival advantage.[37] Despite the lack of strong evidence to support the efficacy of these group interventions, all these centres reported a strong clinical impression that some participants did benefit. Cunningham et al.[38] argue that a correlative approach, which relates the survival of individuals to their psychological work as measured by qualitative data, does suggest a relationship between intervention and outcome.

In summary, studies undertaken with groups of patients with metastatic disease face problems with recruitment, retention, choice of methodology, and choice of psychometric measure. Further research is being undertaken in this area which may clarify some of these issues.

The family

Many families are able to offer emotional and practical support to the patient and work with the team. Others are distrustful of staff and both demanding and challenging of any care given. Jenkins and Bruera[39] cite the 'Daughter from California syndrome'. This describes the tensions that arise when an absent relative returns to be confronted with a deteriorating patient and decisions being made by others. One explicit way to demonstrate concern and assert one's presence is to question the care given. A high standard of care may mean more vigorous attempts to fault-find. It can help to engage the relative in practical tasks in the care process so that there is less need to prove concern. There may be other reasons.

A daughter was making increasingly frantic attempts to communicate with her unresponsive dying mother. She persistently asked if her mother could hear or understand. On interview it emerged that the daughter had been sexually abused by the father and it was her last chance to resolve this with her mother and confirm whether she had known. Support through this crisis and subsequent referral to the community psychologist was arranged.

The contribution of clinical psychology to the team

People face a psychological challenge when living with life-limiting illness but this does not mean that all patients need to see a psychologist. The skills of the clinical psychologist may be more appropriately used in developing the psychological skills of other staff. The concept of triage is familiar in medicine when there is a need to deploy limited resources effectively and the principle applies to psychological care also. If a palliative care unit has access to a weekly session of clinical psychologist time, it would be misguided to fill that time with the psychologist seeing patients individually only. More patients could benefit from psychological expertise if time were spent in staff training and supervision (Table 3).

Table 3 Helping staff formulate a problem in a psychological way

Helping staff formulate a problem in a psychological way
Teach a specific skill, e.g. relaxation
Supervise specific cases
Joint working
Support team decision-making and cohesiveness

Raise psychological awareness

General medical and nursing staff work hard to achieve pain and symptom control and may feel bewildered or angry when these attempts fail. Raising awareness of psychological issues can lead to more useful interventions and less wasted effort. A relevant analogy is the person running faster but up the wrong ladder. Given the scarcity of clinical psychologists in general medical settings, the pyramid approach in which a psychologist acts as a consultant/trainer to a staff member supervising others can be an effective way of ensuring that more patients benefit from psychological knowledge. This model has been used with carers and nurses and more recently with physiotherapists.[40]

Teach a specific skill

Relaxation is an effective way of alleviating anxiety that is widely used by mental health professionals but fewer general trained staff are confident in its use. There is a clear advantage in making psychological treatments available to more patients by teaching them to direct care staff. Doctors and nurses in oncology who were trained in behavioural treatments were as effective as clinical psychologists in reducing chemotherapy-induced nausea and vomiting.[41]

Supervision with specific cases

Supervision with specific cases can enable the regular carer to maintain the existing relationship with the patient and deliver a psychological intervention under supervision.

A team had been supporting a woman over many months during which her condition deteriorated. Her professional carers felt increasingly helpless as she became more distressed. A cognitive–behavioural intervention was used supervised by the psychologist, which enabled her existing carers to maintain their relationship and relieve some of her distress.[42] This not only helped the immediate situation but also developed their future clinical skills.

Joint working

Joint working can enable each professional to achieve desired outcomes more easily.

A man with advanced lung cancer was referred to the clinical psychologist because of low mood and anxiety. There were many issues but it emerged that the main focus of his sadness was his fear he would be forgotten by his young son who lived with his estranged wife. This fear was explored and after some discussion the man decided to make a gift for his son and future grandchildren which he could leave in safekeeping with his own parents. The feasibility of this project was discussed with the occupational therapist who enabled the patient to complete the task despite the limits of his concentration and fatigue.

An elderly woman with a disfiguring facial tumour, limited mobility, and a Parkinsonian tremor experienced anxiety and low self-esteem. A cognitive–behavioural intervention helped her leave the confines of her room and become more confident in social situations. Nurses and other staff were primed for her early ventures and praised any attempts to extend her range. Finally, she used her wheelchair expeditions to purchase items from the craft department which she used as gifts for visitors. This enabled her to regain her sense of herself as a giver rather than a passive receiver of care and helped her overcome her sense of self-worth.

Support team decision-making and cohesiveness

Some patients or families may have interacted in an aggressive or manipulative way for many years with the people and the organizational systems they encounter. They have the potential to disrupt the team, which can mirror the angry or rejecting relationships.[43] The realistic role of the mental health professional may be one of limiting damage to themselves and others.[44] Personal relationships are highly valued by palliative care staff and they can find it challenging to work with those who do not or cannot share this.

There can be barriers to organizing team support in a large system such as a general hospital. Cull[45] describes a practical way of eliciting and addressing staff problems when it is not possible for group discussion to take place. A forum for ventilating concerns can help staff feel problems have been identified and the lesson incorporated into practice. There may be no new lesson to be learned but simply a need to express sadness or anger. A reflective group is less intimidating for some team members but more intimidating for others. Support groups are not necessarily helpful and can deteriorate into a 'grouse group' but when functioning well they can be an effective resource for the team. Individual professional supervision can help junior staff manage challenging situations but having seniority does not confer emotional immunity although it helps one understand what is happening.[46]

Palliative care staff tend to criticize the efforts of those staff in other specialities who seek 'a cure' and who abandon patients when their efforts fail but they themselves pursue the goal of a 'good death' and may feel equally frustrated when they cannot alleviate distress. This can lead to criticism of oneself, the team, or the patient. There is a need to find a balance between complacency and accepting fallibility. Unrealistic goals lead to low morale and dissatisfaction. A high degree of self-criticism was found to be linked to professional stress in a study of general practitioners.[47] More training may increase professional knowledge but professional maturity can remain elusive. Bennet discusses the doctor's loss in surrendering idealistic illusions but argues they are exchanged for more rewarding realities.[48]

Caring for the patient with cognitive and sensory impairments

Cognitive impairment is prevalent in many patients receiving palliative care. Confusion may be reversible but for some patients, such as those with primary brain tumours or cerebral metastases, the impairment may be permanent. As people live longer, it is possible that some cognitive problems will be caused by ageing rather than the disease process. Some neuropsychological tests are lengthy but shorter screening measures are available and unless used routinely there is a risk cognitive problems will not be detected.[49] A formal cognitive assessment is relevant if there is conflict about whether the person is competent to give informed consent. The report should include guidance for staff caring for the person. The person may attempt to assault staff giving care. In some circumstances, this challenging behaviour can be reduced by increasing the patient's sense of control and predictability over the immediate environment, for example, the patient could have a personal box that contains prompts for routine procedures. A person with visual and auditory impairments could touch items that would help anticipate the planned interaction such as a toothbrush, a cup, a dosette tube, lavatory paper, a piece of dressing material.

The person's impaired sensory and cognitive abilities require assistance to help the person function as independently as possible. As a reaction against the impersonal white and clinical surrounding of a hospital ward, hospices create a home-like atmosphere with soft pastels and flowery prints. Unfortunately, neither environment may be helpful to the elderly person trying to reach the toilet independently but unable to find the correct door in time. Units that have been designed for the care of people with cognitive impairments address the need for a 'prosthetic environment'. The judicious use of colour and shape can facilitate orientation by attracting attention to some areas and minimizing others. One unit for people with multiple disabilities used sections of floor textured with a rippled effect to signal to anyone in a wheelchair when one area was being left and another area entered. Guidelines on corridor walls at shoulder height may help a disoriented person. A sailing ship for people with disabilities had ropes at wheelchair height leading along gangways with markers set at intervals to indicate in which direction the person was moving. If an ocean-going sailing ship can do this, is it unrealistic to expect a health unit to make efforts to maintain a person's failing abilities as long as possible? These ideas cost a fraction of a unit's drug bill and little time, yet are rarely used in palliative care. There is a danger that the lessons learned in one speciality are ignored as new ones develop. There is a wealth of relevant clinical experience in the care of people with learning disabilities and neuro-rehabilitation units but the boundaries between specialities would do credit to the strictest infection protocols and the opportunities for the transfer of skills are missed.

The vulnerable patient

Palliative care is practised in a social context and has to adapt to its changing society. The closure of large institutions for people with learning disabilities or severe mental illness and the subsequent integration of their former residents into the community has challenged mainstream services to deliver an equitable service. Palliative care staff may have had little training and experience in caring for these people and so they may share the same prejudices and fears of their community. A study of the experiences of people with learning disabilities in general hospitals revealed that basic needs for comfort and information were unrecognized.[50] The person may have had years of being told to 'behave properly' and not be a nuisance. Staff need to be proactive in their assessment of pain and symptom control, which may be made more difficult by communication difficulties. People who have lived on the edges of their community during life may die there with little understanding of their needs when facing death or bereavement.[51]

A different type of challenge is faced by the team caring for a patient who is a health professional because it is assumed that this person fully understands everything that is happening. They are familiar with the jargon, smells, and procedures *but this intellectual knowledge is not the same as psychological comfort.* The patient may adopt the familiar and comfortable role of 'expert' and present a heroic front that can make it more difficult to acknowledge fears or uncertainties. The more eminent the patient the harder it can be for the team members to give support because they feel professionally intimidated. Consultations may focus on laboratory results and natural expressions of warmth or empathy are inhibited by rank. Another danger lies in the temptation of colleagues to take short-cuts through the health care system that can have unforeseen and negative consequences.[52]

Summary

1. Psychology can make a contribution to the organization and delivery of health care provision in addition to providing care at the individual level.
2. Palliative care services are facing new challenges as people live longer with advanced disease. The psychological issues faced in chronic disease and rehabilitation services are increasingly relevant in palliative care and more lessons could be learned from other specialities.
3. The palliative care needs of people with leaning disabilities or severe mental health disorders have received little attention. There is evidence that they face obstacles in accessing care and receive inadequate care from services. Staff secondments to other services would be one way of developing skills and gaining confidence.

This chapter has not addressed bereavement, which is discussed in Chapter 19.

References

1. **Alexander, D.A.** (1998). Psychosocial research in palliative care. In *Oxford Textbook of Palliative Medicine* 2nd edn. (ed. D. Doyle, G.W.C. Hanks, and N. MacDonald), pp. 187–92. Oxford: Oxford University Press.
2. **Innes, J.** (1977). Does the professional know what the client wants? *Social Science and Medicine* **11**, 635–8.

3. **Sardell, A. and Trierweiler, S.** (1993). Disclosing the cancer diagnosis. *Cancer* **72** (11), 3355–65.
4. **Cull, A., Stewart, M., and Altman, D.G.** (1995). Assessment of and intervention for psychosocial problems in routine oncology practice. *British Journal of Cancer* **72**, 229–35.
5. **Chochinov, H.M., Wilson, K., Enns, M., and Lander, S.** (1997). Are you depressed? Screening for depression in the terminally ill. *American Journal of Psychiatry* **54**, 674–6.
6. **Rogers, M. and Todd, C.** (2000). The right kind of pain: talking about symptoms in outpatient oncology consultations. *Palliative Medicine* **14**, 299–307.
7. **Meyer, T.J. and Mark, M.M.** (1995). Effects of psychosocial interventions with advanced cancer patients; a meta-analysis of randomised experiments. *Health Psychology* **14**, 101–8.
8. **Sheard, T. and Maguire, P.** (1999). The effects of psychological interventions on anxiety and depression in cancer patients: results of two meta-analyses. *British Journal of Cancer* **80**, 1770–80.
9. **Hillier, E.R. and Lunt, B.** (1980). Goal-setting in terminal cancer. In *The Continuing Care of Terminal Cancer Patients* (ed. R.G. Twycross and Ventafridda), pp. 271–8. Oxford: Pergamon Press.
10. **Wood, B.C. and Mynors-Wallis, L.M.** (1997). Problem solving therapy in palliative care. *Palliative Medicine* **11**, 49–54.
11. **Morrow, G., Roscoe, J.A., and Hickok, J.T.** (1998). Nausea and vomiting In *Psycho-oncology* (ed. J.C. Holland), pp. 476–84. Oxford: Oxford University Press.
12. **Luebbert, K., Dahme, B., and Hasenberg, M.** (2001). The effectiveness of relaxation training in reducing treatment-related symptoms and improving emotional adjustment in acute non-surgical cancer treatment: a meta-analytical review. *Psycho-oncology* **10**, 490–502.
13. **SIGN Guidelines (Scottish Intercollegiate Guidelines Network).** *Control of Pain in Patients with Cancer.* Edinburgh: Royal College of Physicians, 2000.
14. **Walker, L. et al.** (1999). Psychological, clinical and pathological effects of relaxation training and guided imagery during primary chemotherapy. *British Journal of Cancer* **80** (1/2), 262–8.
15. **Sryjala, K. and Abrams, J.** (1996). Hypnosis and imagery in the treatment of pain. In *Psychological Approaches to Pain Management* (ed. R.J. Gatchel and D.C. Turk), pp. 231–58. London: Guilford Press.
16. **Duhamel, K., Johnson Vickberg, S.M., and Redd, W.** (1998). Behavioural interventions in paediatric oncology. In *Psycho-oncology* (ed. J.C. Holland), pp. 962–77. Oxford: Oxford University Press.
17. **Williams, D.** (1996). Acute pain management. In *Psychological Approaches to Pain Management* (ed. R.J. Gatchel and D.C. Turk), pp. 55–77. London: Guilford Press.
18. **Finlay, I. and Jones, O.L.** (1996). Hypnotherapy in palliative care. *Journal of the Royal Society of Medicine* **89**, 493–5.
19. **Department of Health.** *Treatment Choices in Psychological Therapies and Counselling.* London: Department of Health Publications, 2001.
20. **Turk, D.C. and Feldman, C.S.** (2000). A cognitive–behavioural approach to symptom management in palliative care: augmenting somatic interventions. In *Handbook of Psychiatry in Palliative Medicine* (ed. H.C. Chochinov and W. Breitbart), pp. 223–39. New York: Oxford University Press.
21. **Jacobsen, P.C. and Hann, D.** (1998). Cognitive–behavioural interventions. In *Psycho-oncology* (ed. J.C. Holland), pp. 717–29. Oxford: Oxford University Press.
22. **Moorey, S., Greer, S., Bliss, J., and Law, M.** (1998). A comparison of adjuvant psychological therapy and supportive counselling in patients with cancer. *Psycho-Oncology* **7**, 218–28.
23. **Santos, M.J.H. and Greer, S.** (1991). Adjuvant psychological therapy with a terminally ill patient; a case-report. *Behavioural Psychotherapy* **19**, 277–80.
24. **Boulton, M. et al.** (2001). Dividing the desolation: clients' views on the benefits of a cancer counselling service. *Psycho-Oncology* **10**, 124–36.
25. **Stedeford, A.** *Facing death.* Sir Michael Sobell House, Churchill Hospital, Oxford: Sobell Publications, 1994.
26. **Spira, J.** (2000). Existential psychotherapy in palliative care. In *Handbook of Psychiatry in Palliative Care* (ed. H.C. Chochinov and W. Breitbart), pp. 197–214. New York: Oxford University Press.
27. **Turk, D.C. and Fernandez, E.** (1991). Pain: a cognitive-behavioural perspective. In *Cancer Psychosocial Care; Psychosocial Treatment Methods* (ed. M. Watson), pp. 15–44. Great Britain: British Psychological Society.
28. **Redd, W.** (1982). Treatment of excessive crying in a terminal cancer patient; a time series analysis. *Journal of Behavioural Medicine* **5**, 225–35.
29. **Redd, W.** (1982). Behavioural analysis and the control of psychosomatic symptoms of patients receiving intensive cancer treatment. *British Journal of Clinical Psychology* **21**, 351–8.
30. **Zaza, C. et al.** (1999). Health care professionals familiarity with non-pharmacological strategies for managing cancer pain. *Psycho-Oncology* **8**, 99–111.
31. **Hillier, R.**, Personal communication (Countess Mountbatten House, Moorgreen Hospital, Southampton, UK).
32. **Yalom, I.D. and Grieves, C.** (1977). Group therapy with the terminally ill. *American Journal of Psychiatry* **134**, 396–400.
33. **Spiegel, D., Bloom, J.R., and Yalom, I.** (1981). Group support for patients with metastatic cancer. *Archives of General Psychiatry* **38**, 527–33.
34. **Spiegel, D., Bloom, J.R., Kraemer, H.C., and Gottheil, E.** (1989). Effects of psychological treatment on survival of patients with metastatic breast cancer. *Lancet* **334**, 888–91.
35. **Llewelyn, S.P., Murray, A.K., Johnston, M., Johnston, D.W., Preece, P.E., and Dewar, J.A.** (1999). Group therapy for metastatic cancer patients; report of an intervention. *Psychology, Health and Medicine* **4**, 229–40.
36. **Edelman, S., Lemon, B., and Kidman, A.D.** (1999). Effects of group CBT on the survival of patients with metastatic breast cancer. *Psycho-Oncology* **8**, 474–81.
37. **Edmonds, C.V.I., Lockwood, G.A., and Cunningham, A.C.** (1999). Psychological responses to long-term group therapy. *Psycho-Oncology* **8**, 74–91.
38. **Cunningham, A.C. et al.** (2000). A prospective longitudinal study of the relationship of psychological work to duration of survival in patients with metastatic cancer. *Psycho-Oncology* **9**, 323–39.
39. **Jenkins, C. and Bruera, E.** (1998). Conflict between families and staff; an approach. In *Topics in Palliative Care* Vol. 2 (ed. E. Bruera and R. Portenoy), pp. 311–25. New York: Oxford University Press.
40. **Milne, D.** (1999). Training others to train others: an illustration of the educational pyramid. *Clinical Psychology Forum* **123**, 7–12.
41. **Morrow, G.R., Asbury, R., Hammon, S., Dobkinn, P., Caruso, L., Pandya, K., and Rosenthal, S.** (1992). Comparing the effectiveness of behavioural treatment for chemotherapy-induced nausea and vomiting when administered by oncologists, oncology nurses and clinical psychologists. *Health Psychology* **11** (4), 250–6.
42. **Jones and Johnston, M.** (1989). Despair felt by the patient and the professional carer; a case-study of the use of cognitive-behaviour methods. *Palliative Medicine* **3**, 39–46.
43. **Bruera, E. and Portenoy, R.** *Topics in Palliative Care* Vol. 2. New York: Oxford University Press, 1998.
44. **Hay, J. and Passik, S.D.** (2000). The cancer patient with borderline personality disorder. *Psycho-Oncology* **9**, 91–100.
45. **Cull, A.** (1991). Staff support in medical oncology: a problem-solving approach. *Psychology and Health* **5**, 129–36.
46. **Rothenberg** (1974). Problems posed for staff who care for the child. In *Care of the Child Facing Death* (ed. L. Burton), pp. 39–45. London: Routledge and Kegan Paul.
47. **Firth-Cozens, J.** (1997). Predicting stress in GPs: 10 year follow-up postal survey. *British Medical Journal* **315**, 34–5.
48. **Bennet, G.** (1998). Coping with loss: the doctor's losses; ideals versus realities. *British Medical Journal* **316**, 1238–40.
49. **Robinson, J.** (1999). Cognitive assessment of palliative care patients. *Progress in Pallative Care* **7** (6), 291–8.
50. **Hart, S.** (1998). Learning disabled people's experience of general hospitals. *British Journal of Nursing* **7** (8), 670–7.
51. **Cathcart, F.** (1995). Death and people with learning disabilities; interventions to support clients and carers. *British Journal of Clinical Psychology* **34**, 165–75.
52. **Higgs, R.** (1991). Looking after yourself. In *Developing Communication and Counselling Skills in Medicine* (ed. R. Corney), pp. 137–45. London: Routledge.

15.9 The contribution of the clinical pharmacist to palliative medicine

Helen Fielding and Dorothy McArthur

Introduction

Pharmacy is a dynamic, evolving, patient-focused profession. In developed countries, the traditional pharmacist role of medicine procurement and dispensing is gradually being devolved to pharmacy technicians and support staff. Clinical pharmacists are emerging and clinical pharmacy services are now an established part of hospital and hospice health care in the United Kingdom.[1–3] Many clinical pharmacists will have additional qualifications in the form of a Postgraduate Diploma or Master of Science in Clinical Pharmacy.

Clinical pharmacists apply their pharmaceutical expertise to help maximize drug efficacy and minimize drug toxicity. They work with individual patients, making pharmaceutical contributions to their care. Hepler and Strand have formally defined pharmaceutical care (see Box 1).

The effective provision of clinical pharmacy services relies on the knowledge and skills of clinical pharmacists and the quality of the traditional pharmacy support services. Dedicated time is required by a pharmacist to develop and provide clinical pharmacy services.[2,5]

The involvement of pharmacists in palliative care in the United Kingdom, United States, Canada, and Australia has been reported. However, these reports have in the main been descriptive.[6–9] In one published study where the impact of a pharmacist was assessed, 13 per cent of patients' care was either improved clinically or made more cost-effective by the intervention of the pharmacist.[10] There is a need for further practice research in this area. Worldwide, the roles of clinical pharmacists vary depending on the time commitment they have to palliative care patients, as well as the extent of clinical pharmacy development in their country. In addition to clinical pharmacy and supply activities, the pharmacist's role in influencing cost containment is common.

Palliative care specialist interest groups for pharmacists are established in many countries including Scotland, United Kingdom, Canada, and New Zealand. These groups allow networking and peer review among palliative care pharmacists, which is essential as they are often professionally isolated. The groups also facilitate collaboration on research and education matters and enable pharmacists to have their voice heard within palliative care organizations at a national level, for example, Clinical Standards Board for Scotland.[2] There are no postgraduate palliative care qualifications aimed specifically for pharmacists. Options for training in palliative care for pharmacists include specifically written distance learning packages for pharmacists (e.g. The Pharmacist in Palliative Care Distance Learning Package produced by the Scottish Centre for Pharmaceutical Post Qualification Education[11]), undertaking postgraduate multidisciplinary palliative care courses, and research-based Master of Philosophy courses.

Clinical pharmacy service

There are two major components of a clinical pharmacy service: (a) the pharmaceutical care of individual patients and (b) the overall management of medicines.

Box 1 Pharmaceutical care

> Pharmaceutical care is: 'the responsible provision of drug therapy for the purpose of achieving definite outcomes which improve the patient's quality of life'[4]

Pharmaceutical care of individual patients

The aim of drug therapy in palliative care is to control symptoms and therefore improve the patient's quality of life. The drug regimen should not provoke unacceptable side-effects or become an unbearable burden for patients and carers. Patients often require many drugs to control all of their symptoms and the resulting polypharmacy increases the risk of side-effects, drug interactions, and non-compliance. Balancing the benefit and detriment of the drug regimen can be difficult to achieve. To obtain the correct balance, the clinical pharmacist becomes involved in a number of key activities in caring for individual patients.[12] (see Table 1).

Pharmaceutical care can only be achieved with good multidisciplinary communication and documentation. Drug-related problems can be detected by formulating a problem-orientated list that involves asking a number of questions: what is the indication (the need) for the drug; is the patient on the correct dose; is the drug appropriate for the disease state; is the patient experiencing an adverse reaction or problem due to drug interactions; are there contraindications to the use of the drug; and is there a medical problem untreated? Patient information required to determine drug-related problems include: characteristics (age, sex, height, and weight); current and past medical problem; history of present illness; present and past medications; allergies; relevant laboratory results; concordance/compliance with medicines and ability to take the medicine in the formulation prescribed.[3,13]

On collection of this patient-specific information, the clinical pharmacist constructs a pharmaceutical plan listing the patient's drug-related problems (care issues), treatment recommendations, and future plans for monitoring outcomes to ensure that the prescribed therapy is producing the desired effect.

The palliative care patient's condition is often labile and their response to drug therapy is variable. Drug treatment must be tailored to the patient's individual response to therapy. Accurate, repeated assessment of the patient's condition is essential to ensure successful drug treatment. Repeated assessment enables the response of treatments to be correctly assessed and encourages methodical prescribing in relation to the choice of therapy. Pharmacists need to work closely with other health care professionals to ensure that symptom assessment is carried out at appropriate intervals.

There is a need for good documentation of pharmaceutical care and systems to share this information effectively among the health care team(s). This is an essential requirement if pharmaceutical care is to be integrated into palliative care. Sharing information on the patient's response to medication can help to maintain optimized drug treatment. Improvements in symptoms that indicate a successful response to treatment and identification of therapeutic failures should be recorded as part of the patient's drug history. This information should prevent repeated trials of drugs that have previously failed to give the desired effect or have led to unacceptable side-effects. A pharmacy transfer record has been proposed for palliative care

Table 1 Key activities of a clinical pharmacist in caring for individual patients in palliative care

Maintain familiarity with patients' condition and drug-related needs
Attend multidisciplinary meetings to discuss and advise on patient care
Design, implement, and monitor therapeutic plans with specific outcomes for patients
Prevent, detect, solve, and report drug-related problems
Maintain continuity of care by sharing information with pharmacists in all care settings
Educate and counsel patients and carers
Provide drug information and advice
Provide advice on wound management
Record a medication history for all prescribed and purchased medicines
Compare drug choice against local protocols, clinical guidelines, and standards

patients (see Box 2). This record could be transferred as the patient moves between different care settings.[9]

Non-compliance with the medication regimen has been reported in up to 60 per cent of palliative care patients at home.[14] Identification of the reasons that make patients more likely to be non-compliant is essential. The most commonly occurring reasons are the presence or fear of side-effects, practical difficulties in taking medication, lack of monitoring, inadequate adjustment of therapy, old age, depression, and lack of understanding of the disease and treatments.[14–16] Identified patients require help to improve their concordance and compliance with the medication regimen.

Ignorance and fear about symptomatic drug treatment is common in advanced cancer. One-third of palliative care patients managing their own medicines are in some way unclear about the purpose of their medication or its correct use, and a small number will not take their medication because they have no instructions on how to do so. Administration of medicines is seen as a main task for caring for the patient by 78 per cent of carers, yet as many as 90 per cent may not be given any written information about the illness and use of drug treatments.[17] The pharmacist has a clear role to play in providing education for patients and carers about the role and use of drug treatments. Oral communication should be supported by written information. The drug regimen should be documented in full, providing a clear instruction for the patient and family to follow. Written information should include the name and strength of drugs, times to be taken, indication, dose (specified as number of tablets or volume of liquid). Written information is often provided in the form of a medication card. An example is shown in Figs 1 and 2.

Box 2 Palliative care pharmacy transfer record

- Patient identity and community care contact details
- Specialist palliative care team contact details (where involved)
- Primary diagnosis, symptoms present
- Full drug history including drug therapy, previous therapeutic failures, adverse effects, and their management
- Local treatment protocols being followed
- Risk factors for non-compliance, measures to address these, including patient education
- Use and availability of unlicensed or unusual medication, including stability of drugs being given by subcutaneous infusion

A pharmacist's advice is more likely to be followed if the person is satisfied with it. This can be achieved by adopting the correct manner, dedicating an appropriate amount of time, avoiding the exclusive use of closed questions (i.e. yes/no answers), and allowing the patient and carer to ask questions. Advice needs to be reinforced as failure to remember or understand what they have been told is common. Carers have identified the value of repeating information and they look for reassurance and reiteration of advice given previously. Retention of information is improved by providing information in several different formats. When providing education, it is important to know what has been said to the recipient by other members of the multidisciplinary team so that confusion or doubts are not introduced. Good liaison with the care team is therefore necessary.

The pharmacist has a major role to play in preventing and overcoming any practical difficulty with taking medicines. Many patients are unable to use oral syringes accurately. The correct use of an oral syringe should be demonstrated and the competence of the patient and carer assessed in the use of this device. Compliance aids may be appropriate for selected patients. Assessment of the patient for the compliance aid is essential to ensure appropriate use and optimal use of resources. Compliance aids range from simple measures such as large print labels, plain bottle tops, medicine charts, and diaries to commercially available aids to compliance, including inhaler spacer devices and domiciliary dosage systems (e.g. dosett).

Many medicines used in symptom control have similar or overlapping side-effect profiles that may result in the development of intolerable side-effects. For example, the use of a tricyclic antidepressant with an antiemetic such as cyclizine can cause an unbearable dry mouth. The clinical pharmacist can tailor the medication regimen to minimize toxicity. It is also essential to anticipate and ensure the prescription of prophylactic treatments to control the predictable side-effects of medicines. For example, opioid-induced constipation, nausea, sedation, and dry mouth can often be effectively managed. Medication regimens should be reviewed frequently to identify such issues. Patients taking newer drugs should be monitored for any adverse reaction

Appliances and dressings

Item	Manufacturer and code	Quantity

Equipment loaned

Date	Description

Allergies

Date	Medicine

General information about medicines

- Take your medicines as directed on your card
- Take your medicines with half a glass of water either sitting or standing
- Keep your medicines in a cool, dry place out of reach of children
- Never share your medicines
- If you have unwanted or old medicines return them to your local chemist

Name of palliative care unit

Address

Telephone number

Date of preparation

Medication card

Patient's name ____________
Address ____________
____
Telephone number ____________

GP ____________
Address ____________
____
Telephone number ____________

Community pharmacy ____________
Address ____________
Telephone number ____________

Home care sister ____________

Fig. 1 Side one of patient medication card.

Date	Medicine	Dose	Times of administration of Medicine						What is it for	Special instructions	Date stopped	Written/ checked by
			7 a.m.	11 a.m.	3 p.m.	7 p.m.	11 p.m.	3 a.m.				
1/1/02	Morphine sulphate MR 30 mg tablet (MST Continus)	30 mg twice daily		One			One		Pain relief	Take 12 hours apart Swallow whole		DM/HW
1/1/02	Diclofenac 75 mg MR tablet	75 mg twice daily		One			One		Pain relief	Take 12 hours apart Swallow whole		DM/HW
1/1/02	Co-danthramer strong capsule	One twice daily		One			One		To prevent constipation	May turn urine orange/brown		DM/HW
1/1/02	Bendrofluazide 2.5 mg tablet	One daily		One					High blood pressure			DM/HW
												/
												/
												/
												/

Medicines to be taken when required

Date	Medicine	Dose	What is it for	Special instructions	Date stopped	Written/checked by
1/1/02	Morphine solution 10 mg/5 ml (Sevredol)	5 ml	Severe breakthrough pain	Use a 5ml spoon to measure dose. Take hourly as needed		DM/HW
						/
						/

Patient's name	Medicines discontinued: any supplies remaining at home should be returned to your local pharmacy.
Date issued	

Fig. 2 Side two of patient medication card.

or unexpected event. In the United Kingdom, all unexpected events should be reported to the Committee on Safety of Medicines using the 'yellow card' system.[18] The clinical pharmacist should ensure that patients and carers are educated on predicable side-effects to avoid any misunderstandings or confusion surrounding occurrence of unwanted effects.

Advice is often needed on how to administer the required medication regimen by an alternative route when a patient develops nausea, vomiting, dysphagia, or is too weak to take drugs orally. Often, there is a rapid change in the patient's condition and the necessary drugs and equipment are required immediately. Arrangements must be in place to ensure that these demands can be met.

Over the past 10 years, networks of community pharmacies within geographical areas have been established in the United Kingdom to allow continuity of supply of medicines. In Scotland, such networks have been formalized under the model schemes initiative.[19] These networks of palliative care community pharmacists have been created to provide information and advice and access to medicines 24 h a day.

There are risks associated with the administration of subcutaneous infusions of drug combinations via portable infusion devices. The risks can be minimized by the clinical pharmacist providing specialist advice on isotonicity and stability of small-volume drug combinations. In addition, the clinical pharmacist has a key role in liaising with university pharmacy departments to undertake compatibility and stability studies.

In palliative care, many drugs are administered out with their product license. Deviations from the product license include alternative indication (e.g. amitriptyline for neuropathic pain), route of administration (e.g. subcutaneous administration of cyclizine), and dose (e.g. low-dose levomepromazine for nausea). Several care issues arise in relation to the frequent use of unlicensed medicines. The clinical pharmacist must address issues relating to product availability, advice on use, formulation and monitoring.

Overall management of medicines

The clinical pharmacist working in palliative care becomes involved in a number of key activities in the overall management of medicines (see Table 2).

The use of medicines in palliative care can be rationalized through the introduction and effective management of formularies, clinical guidelines, and treatment protocols. Formularies contain lists of medicines approved for use within a local area and are accompanied by information to assist in rational prescribing (see Appendix 1). Access to medicines utilization data, and other drug information places the clinical pharmacist in an ideal position for driving the process of formulary development and maintenance.

Clinical pharmacists can contribute to the production of clinical guidelines for symptom control in palliative care.[20] Clinical guidelines are systematically developed statements that assist in decision-making about appropriate health care for a specific clinical condition. They are developed through liaison with medical, nursing, and pharmacy staff and other health care professionals. Clinical guidelines should be reviewed at appropriate intervals to incorporate new information and changing trends in clinical practice. The clinical pharmacist should be involved in, and may have delegated responsibility for this process.

Although the supply of medicines is not a direct role of the clinical pharmacist, he/she has a responsibility to ensure the availability of medicines.

Table 2 Key activities of the clinical pharmacist in the overall management of medicines

Agree and maintain an approved list of medicines for routine use, accompanied with prescribing/drug information (formulary)
Agree clinical guidelines and treatment protocols
Agree stock lists of medicines for palliative care units and community palliative care pharmacies
Implement and review systems to assure availability of stock and non-stock medicines for palliative care in-patient units
Implement and review systems to assure the safe supply, storage, and administration of medicines for palliative care in-patient units
Implement and review systems for managing patients' own medicines in palliative care in-patient units
Review of formulary, clinical guidelines, and treatment protocols
Participate in education and training of health care professionals
Provide evaluated information on medicine expenditure and advise on the management of the medicine budget for palliative care in-patient units
Undertake and support research and audit

Table 3 Systems to assure the efficient, safe supply, and administration of medicines to patients requiring palliative care in in-patient units

Local procedures, policies, and/or guidelines should exist for the:

Supply of medicines (ordering medicines, handling of patients' own medicines, ordering medicines to take home (discharge supply) and destruction of expired medicines)

Storage of medicines (to ensure compliance with national guidelines and the law. This includes medicines for self-administration, and procedures to ensure regular checks on stock to remove expired items)

Administration of medicines (prescription of medicines, administration of medicines, assessment of patients for self-administration of medicines, training of staff in drug administration, availability of drug administration equipment and disposable sundries, use and servicing of drug administration equipment)

Specialist intervention (initiation of specialist intervention, ongoing monitoring of intervention and arrangements for on-going care following discharge)

Medicines must be available on time and in good condition. An agreed list of medicines should be stocked in palliative care units providing in-patient care. This stock list should be based on formulary choices and recommendations made within clinical guidelines. Systems also need to be in place to assure the availability of non-stock (non-formulary) medicines, as the particular clinical needs of an individual patient may take precedence over any formulary or clinical guideline. The supply of non-formulary medicines should be carried out with the knowledge and active approval of the clinical pharmacist. Liaison with the pharmacist supplying the medicines is essential.

Some medicines in palliative care require specialist intervention or equipment for drug delivery (e.g. syringe driver, enteral feeding tubes, nebulizers). To ensure safe drug administration it is essential to provide staff with education and training on the use of this equipment. Drug administration equipment must be subject to regular servicing. The clinical pharmacist has an important role in developing well-designed systems to assure the efficient, safe supply, and administration of medicines to patients requiring palliative care (see Table 3). Pharmacy technicians can take on the responsibility for a number of these tasks.[21]

A clinical pharmacist can evaluate medicines utilization information, such as the amount, cost, and patterns of prescribing. The information is evaluated in relation to workload (i.e. bed-occupancy, patient turnover, case mix) and agreed criteria for the appropriate use of medicines (i.e. formulary, clinical guidelines, and standards for the use of medicines). The clinical pharmacist may be able to highlight areas of medicine use where a change in prescribing practice may achieve a more cost-effective use of resources (e.g. oral morphine in preference to transdermal fentanyl and subcutaneous diamorphine). The resource implications of patterns of medicine use can be predicted, situations that will result in overspending can be identified and predictions made of the amount of additional resources required to fund justifiable developments.

Box 3 Education and training provided by a clinical pharmacist for the multidisciplinary team

- Education on local clinical guidelines and formulary choices
- Training in drug administration (e.g. local policies), use of equipment (e.g. syringe drivers, nebulizers)
- Pharmacology and therapeutics of palliative care medicines to doctors, undergraduate, and postgraduate nurses
- Contribute to local and national courses providing palliative care education

Clinical pharmacists can also make a valuable contribution to educational initiatives for other health care professionals (see Box 3). In addition, they have a responsibility to establish links with university departments who offer a pharmacy degree and should be willing to contribute to undergraduate, pre-registration, and postgraduate education for pharmacists on palliative care. Pharmacists can support and participate in research and development projects.

Traditional pharmacy support services

The traditional pharmacy support services are described in Table 4.

The traditional pharmacy services are essential in ensuring optimal pharmaceutical care for the patient. Dispensing for individual patients in accordance with a prescription from a practitioner is one of the key traditional activities of the pharmacist. In the United Kingdom, dispensing is governed by regulations including the Medicines (labelling) Regulations (1976) and the Misuse of Drugs Regulations (1985). The label should include the name of the product, directions for use, and precautions related to the product.

Assessment of the patient for a compliance aid such as domiciliary dosage system is done by clinical staff including the clinical pharmacist. Liaison with the dispensing pharmacist is required so that the system is filled correctly. The dispensing pharmacist must ensure that the medicines' quality is maintained following its removal from the original packaging.

Medicines are occasionally required in an alternative dosage form than that which is commercially available (e.g. levomepromazine liquid, ketamine liquid). The pharmacist may be required to produce extemporaneously prepared medicines or source unlicensed 'specials'. The pharmacist must be satisfied with the quality of extemporaneous items and assign a relevant expiry date to the finished product. Timely supply of these infrequently used medicines is essential.

For in-patient units, medicines may be supplied as stock in accordance with an agreed stock list. Liaison with the clinical pharmacist is essential in obtaining approval for the supply of non-stock medicines. The production of medicine utilization data by the dispensing pharmacist for the clinical pharmacist to analyse is useful in the review of medicine stock lists, audit of the formulary and clinical guidelines, as well as in production of medicine expenditure reports. In many hospitals in the United Kingdom, pharmacy technician management of stock medicines has been introduced, which releases nursing staff time to perform clinical activities. Such systems are advocated in palliative care in-patient units.[2]

Disposal of out of date medicines needs to be performed safely and with due consideration to the legislation, in particular, in relation to controlled drugs. The pharmacist is key to this activity.

The traditional pharmacist activities discussed are essential for the overall management of the patient. Effective liaison with the clinical pharmacist facilitates the seamless pharmaceutical care of the patient.

Table 4 Traditional pharmacy support services

Medicine procurement
Dispensing medicines for individual patients
Supply of stock and non-stock medicines for palliative care units/in-patients
Supply of aseptic preparations (e.g. intrathecal analgesics)
Dispensing medicines in compliance devices (e.g. dosett)
Dispensing clinical trial medicines
Ordering named patient medicines (e.g. ketamine)
Preparation of extemporaneous medicines (e.g. levomepromazine liquid)
Disposal of out of date medicines
Provision of medicines utilization data
Liaison with clinical pharmacist
Pharmacy technician management of stock and non-stock medicines in palliative care units/in-patients
Provision of controlled drug checks in palliative care units

Summary

The clinical pharmacist's role in palliative care is evolving. Pharmaceutical care is designed to meet the patients' medicine-related needs. The application of pharmaceutical care facilitates a systematic approach to patient care. Benefits of the clinical pharmacist in palliative care are considerable due to the complexity of medication regimens. Clinical pharmacists are able to advise on medicines used in symptom control, offer treatment choices for the management of side-effects, and ensure appropriate records are made of medicines. The development of formularies and clinical guidelines allows a standardized approach to symptom control, facilitating audit. The skills of the clinical pharmacist should be utilized alongside traditional pharmacy services to ensure the appropriate, effective, safe, and convenient use of medicines.

References

1. **Department of Health.** *Pharmacy in the Future—Implementing the NHS Plan. A Programme for Pharmacy in the National Health Service.* London: Department of Health, 2000.
2. **CSBS (Clinical Standards Board for Scotland).** *Clinical Standards. Specialist Palliative Care.* Edinburgh, June 2002.
3. **CRAG (Clinical Resource and Audit Group).** *Clinical Pharmacy in the Hospital Pharmaceutical Service: A Framework for Practice.* Edinburgh: The Scottish Office, 1996.
4. **Helper, C.D. and Stand, L.M.** (1990). Opportunities and responsibilities in pharmaceutical care. *American Journal of Hospital Pharmacy* **47**, 533–43.
5. **The Scottish Office, Department of Health.** *Commissioning Cancer Services in Scotland: Guidance on Pharmaceutical Services and Nursing Services,* NHS MEL (1997)66. Edinburgh: The Scottish Office, 1997.
6. **Hanif, N.** (1991). Role of the palliative care unit pharmacist. *Journal of Palliative Care* **7** (4), 35–6.
7. **Mitchell, K. and Clark, C.** (1996). The provision of pharmaceutical care to hospice patients. *Pharmaceutical Journal* **256**, 352–4.
8. **Arter, S. and Berry, J.** (1993). The provision of pharmaceutical care to hospice patients: Results of the National Hospice Pharmacist Survey. *Journal of Pharmaceutical Care in Pain and Symptom Control* **1**, 25–42.
9. **Urie, J.** et al. (2000). Pharmaceutical care: palliative care. *The Pharmaceutical Journal* **265**, 603–14.
10. **Lucas, C., Glare, P., and Sykes, J.** (1997). Contribution of a liaison clinical pharmacist to an inpatient palliative care unit. *Palliative Medicine* **11**, 209–16.
11. **SCPPE (Scottish Centre for Post Qualification Pharmaceutical Education).** Distance learning courses. Glasgow: SCPPE.
12. **Cipolle, R., Strand, L., and Morley, P.** *Pharmaceutical Care Practice.* New York: McGraw-Hill Health Professions Division, USA, 1998.
13. **Burch, P.L. and Hunter, K.A.** (1996). Pharmaceutical care applied to the hospice setting: a cancer pain model. *The Hospice Journal* **11**, 55–69.
14. **Zeppetella, G.** (1999). How do terminally ill patients at home take their medication? *Palliative Medicine* **13**, 469–75.
15. **Horne, R. and Weinman, J.** (1999). Patients' beliefs about prescribed medicines and their role in adherence to treatment in chronic physical illness. *Journal of Psychosomatic Research* **47**, 555–67.
16. **Spiers, M.V. and Kutzik, D.M.** (1995). Self-reported memory of medication use by the elderly. *American Journal of Health Systems Pharmacy* **52**, 985–90.
17. **Sykes, N., Pearson, S., and Chell, S.** (1992). Quality of care of the terminally ill: the carer's perspective. *Palliative Medicine* **6**, 227–36.
18. **Medicines Control Agency, Committee on Safety of Medicines,** London, UK.
19. **Scottish Executive, Health Department.** *Community Pharmacy: Model Schemes for Pharmaceutical Care NHS MEL* (1999)78. Edinburgh: Scottish Executive, 1999.
20. **SIGN (Scottish Intercollegiate Guideline Network).** Control of pain in patients with cancer SIGN publication number 44. Edinburgh: SIGN, 2000.
21. **Thomas, S. and Groves, K.** (2000). Two way drug traffic; the pharmaceutical aspects of the primary/secondary interface in palliative care. *Pharmacy Management* **16**, 50–1.

Appendix 1

Local formulary

The aim

To promote safe, effective, and economic prescribing of medicines. Formularies can apply to one care setting (e.g. hospital), but they may also extend across a range of local care settings (e.g. community, hospital, and in-patient palliative care units). They promote the use of the same commonly prescribed drugs from each major class (e.g. opioid of choice for managing a moderate to severe pain: oral morphine). The drugs listed are routinely stocked by local pharmacies and should therefore be immediately available for patients. Formularies often provide prescribers with guidance on first- and second-choice drugs.

Developing a formulary

Hospital specialists, general practitioners, senior nurses, and pharmacists agree on which drugs to include in the formulary. Working groups with representation from across the local care settings meet and consider current prescribing patterns and relative cost. They also take into account the evidence of clinical effectiveness, safety, cost-effectiveness, and patient acceptability when making their recommendations. Proposals of the working groups are often distributed to other practitioners for further consultation. Finally, the choices of medicines and content of the formulary are approved by a multidisciplinary Drug and Therapeutics Committee.

What is a formulary?

It is a selective list of medicines, but it may also contain prescribing notes that highlight key messages about the drugs and/or conditions being treated. Drugs are often listed in therapeutic categories (e.g. antidiarrhoeal agents) with separate sections providing drug choices and information on clinical conditions and specialist areas such as palliative care. Formularies should be dynamic documents and should be reviewed regularly. They are often produced in paper form (A5 pocket size) and may also be maintained in an electronic form (e.g. http://www.lothianhealth.scot.nhs.uk).

An extract from the palliative care section of a Scottish formulary is shown. This formulary provides information on managing a range of symptoms, including pain, anorexia, breathlessness, confusion, agitation, and mouth problems. Guidance on the compatibility and stability of drugs in a syringe driver is included. Details on how to access information and supplies of palliative care medicines are listed.

Extract from formulary (a sample page)

Management of anorexia in palliative care

Practical advice should be given to the patient and carer regarding nutrition:

- Nutritional value of food may be increased by adding sugar, honey, cream, and butter.
- Nutritious drinks and snacks may be of benefit.
- If taste changes, try other foods, marinate, or add strong flavours.
- Gently encourage what the patient can manage.
- Give permission to eat less, and provide smaller portions of food.
- Don't talk about food all the time; if a person has no appetite they 'fancy' nothing.
- Encourage participation in the social aspect of meal times, if possible.
- Alcohol, if previously enjoyed, may reduce the sensation of fullness, reduce stress, and provide extra calories.
- Supplementary drinks, if advised by a dietician.

First choice: dexamethasone *or* **megestrol acetate**

Dose

- **Dexamethasone** *tablets 500 μg, 2 mg:* initially 4 mg once daily before 2 p.m. reducing weekly to the lowest effective dose. Prescribe initially for 1 week and stop if no benefit. Otherwise continue for 3–4 weeks. Usually doses of up to 6 mg daily taken for less than 3 weeks may be stopped abruptly. Dexamethasone 750 μg is equivalent to prednisolone 5 mg.
- **Megestrol** *tablets 160 mg:* 160 mg daily, increased weekly to a maximum of 160 mg three times daily. Stop if no benefit.

Prescribing notes

- Dexamethasone may provide short-term improvement in appetite, energy, and general well-being in patients with advanced cancer.
- Megestrol may increase appetite and improve nutritional status. It may take a few weeks to obtain benefit but has a more prolonged effect than dexamethasone. It is more appropriate for patients with a longer prognosis, and at risk of gastro-intestinal toxicity. It should not be given to those with a history of heart failure or thrombo-embolism.
- Metoclopramide or domperidone are useful for patients with anorexia and early satiety or nausea. They are indicated in gastroparesis due to autonomic failure or tumour infiltration. Domperidone has fewer long-term side-effects than metoclopramide.

16

Complementary therapies in palliative medicine

16 Complementary therapies in palliative medicine

Barrie R. Cassileth and Glenn Schulman

Complementary therapies represent an extension and expansion of supportive care, and as such are especially beneficial to palliative care patients. With increased use and ever greater numbers of high-quality research documentation, many complementary therapies are now integrated into mainstream health care systems. Complementary modalities are available to patients at all stages of disease. However, nowhere are they of greater value and assistance than for patients in terminal phases of disease.

Complementary therapies aim to provide supportive and palliative care through the control of symptoms and the overarching goal of enhancing quality of life for both patients and family members. This is the essential meaning of palliative care as defined by the World Health Organization.(1)

Nomenclature

The language associated with complementary medicine is problematic and requires mention. Although 'complementary' is frequently applied in North America and parts of Europe to describe patient-selected modalities, the term 'complementary and alternative medicine' (CAM) has becomes increasingly popular and in many areas is now the commonly accepted terminology. 'Questionable', 'unconventional', and 'unproven' are examples of previous adjectives.

Regardless of which contemporary term is applied—conventional, alternative, or CAM—the meaning includes a vast collection of treatment modalities, from simple relaxation techniques to unproven, potentially harmful cancer treatments. Frequently, CAM is discussed in the aggregate, but it is necessary clinically and conceptually to distinguish between these two categories. The differences are essential, particularly with regard to patients with end-stage disease or those with diagnoses of cancer or other potentially fatal illnesses.

Alternative therapies are promoted as viable options to mainstream care, and sometimes as cures for cancer, AIDS, and other major diseases. Often they are promoted as literal alternatives for use instead of mainstream therapy, and too often terminally ill patients are drawn to what turn out to be useless, time-wasting remedies. Alternative therapies are unproved by definition. If backed by solid data, they would not be alternative. Rather, they would be available and used in every medical programme as viable treatments for serious illnesses.

Alternative regimens typically are invasive and biologically active. They are rarely backed by scientific data. These treatments usually are expensive and potentially harmful. A patient may be harmed directly by physiologic activity, contaminants, or toxic ingredients, or indirectly when patients postpone receipt of mainstream care, expend their family's funds on therapies of no value, or spend their remaining weeks away from their loved ones in a clinic receiving uncomfortable treatments. Late-stage patients are vulnerable to these therapies, as such regimens often promise cure even of advanced or terminal disease.

Complementary therapies are used to control symptoms and enhance quality of life. They are promoted neither as cures for disease nor to be used in lieu of mainstream therapy. Rather, complementary therapies are applied in an adjunctive fashion to reduce pain and other symptoms. They are non-invasive, comforting, effective, and inexpensive; in many respects the antithesis of alternative medicine.

In complementary medicine, therefore, we must work with both poles of the continuum. Patients need the knowledge and encouragement to forego the siren calls to receive unproven therapies; to self-treat with shark cartilage, high-dose vitamins, or other products sold over the counter or delivered intravenously in alternative-medicine clinics. They need the information and the guidance to avoid the claims of disease remission made by self-proclaimed healers as well as purveyors of the numerous useless products and regimens currently available.

Simultaneously, patients need access to the comfort of supportive complementary modalities. These therapies are becoming increasingly available not only directly to patients on a private basis, but also in hospitals, clinics, and homes as part of symptom control and the general effort to ease the physical, psychosocial, and spiritual distresses associated with terminal illness.

This chapter will address the state of CAM in the larger health care system, and review the alternative therapies, widely available to patients and families, with which physicians and other caregivers should be familiar. Helpful complementary therapies are discussed following that overview.

Acceptance of complementary and alternative medicine in the health care system

The acceptance of unconventional therapies, along with advances in biotechnology and other significant medical and societal events, marked health care in the 1990s and must be included among the significant changes of that decade throughout the developed world. The popularity of complementary and alternative medicine affected every component of the health care system and all specialties of medicine, including palliative care. It has left its mark on the thinking and practice of physicians and other health professionals, and broadened patients' influence and involvement in their own care.

No longer a collection of underground practices, unconventional cancer medicine today is highly visible, and information about it is widely available to the general public. It is a multi-billion dollar business in the United States, and of equivalent impact and importance throughout the developed world.

The use of CAM for cancer and other illnesses is widespread. An international e-mail survey of oncologists in 33 countries, including China, Australia, Zimbabwe, Brazil, United Kingdom, United States of America, Latvia, Malaysia, Israel, Tasmania, Japan, and elsewhere, revealed use of a great variety of alternative therapies, variation by country, and many local therapies. Dietary cures, shark products and other unconventional agents, vitamin therapies, botanicals, and energy healing were among those most commonly noted.(2) Other investigations substantiate these results.

Surveys involving members of the US general public, not patients, uncovered prevalence rates in 1997 to be 50 per cent of 113 family practice patients[3] and 42 per cent of 1500 members of the general public.[4] A 1998 publication reports that 42 per cent of 2055 people surveyed used CAM.[5] A large, 1999 survey of over 24 000 individuals found 8 per cent use of CAM with or without mainstream care.[6]

The US experience appears to be typical. Prevalence rates from all CAM studies conducted internationally vary from less than 10 per cent to more than 50 per cent. This broad range with its apparent discrepancies is attributable primarily to variable understandings and definitions of CAM. Often surveys do not define CAM or, more typically, define it extremely broadly, resulting in the inclusion of lifestyle activities such as weight loss efforts, exercise, church attendance, and support activities such as group counseling, thus resulting in bloated figures for CAM use. Moreover, few studies fail to distinguish between alternative therapies (used instead of mainstream care) versus adjunctive use of complementary modalities.

Although research evidence is scanty, it appears that approximately 8–10 per cent of tissue-biopsy diagnosed cancer patients decline mainstream therapy and immediately seek alternative care. The vast majority of CAM users, however, seek complementary, not alternative therapies for serious illnesses.[6]

The profound influence of 1994 legislation in the United States allowing herbal medicines and other 'food supplements' to be sold over the counter without government review is evident in the increased use of herbal remedies from 3 per cent in 1991 to 17 per cent in 1997. It is estimated that sales of dietary supplements more than doubled in the 6 years since passage of the 1994 law. However, herbal supplements sales began to decline in 1998, growing by just 12 per cent that year, and sales grew by only 1 per cent in 2000.[7] The decline probably is due to unrealistically high public expectations, media reports about safety concerns and questionable effectiveness, and public confusion about the vast and still growing array of products.

Despite the drop in sales of herbal remedies, there is indication of a growth in CAM use by cancer patients during the same time frame. A secondary analysis of close to 3000 cancer patients estimates a 64 per cent increase after 1987.[8] It is likely that this reflects expanded use and variety of over-the-counter remedies in addition to herbal products, broader availability of complementary therapies in mainstream cancer programmes and centres, and increased use of non-food supplement complementary therapies.

Virtually all studies conducted to date of cancer patients and of the general public internationally show that those who seek CAM therapies tend to be female, better educated, of higher socioeconomic status, and younger than those who do not. They tend to be more health conscious and to utilize more mainstream medical services than people who do not use CAM.

Prevalence of CAM use among paediatric patients

The use of CAM methods among late-stage paediatric patients represents a special and understudied issue.[9] Surveys in Australia, Finland, British Columbia, the Netherlands and the United States indicate substantial interest in CAM, especially in more recent years, with 40–50 per cent of paediatric oncology patients in those countries receiving complementary or alternative therapies. Imagery, hypnotherapy, prayer, and exercise account for a majority of CAM use by children.

Excluded from this sample and from studies of adults, however, are patients brought to alternative therapy clinics. Patients who receive only alternative cancer therapies do not appear in CAM surveys, because all but one such survey were conducted in mainstream clinics or hospitals.

Access to information

New technologies and expanded media coverage have made CAM a very open and public issue in today's society. Information in a variety of formats is readily accessible. The Internet allows users instantaneous access to information from around the world, and magazines, newspapers, and television specials provide the general public with details about new CAM therapies and published research.

The material presented in all media, however, varies widely in accuracy. Searches performed on the Internet for CAM-related topics reveal scores of websites that appear to be professional and objective, but actually are commercial endeavours that promote and sell unproved alternative products and devices. In 1999, the US Federal Trade Commission announced that it had identified hundreds of websites promoting and selling phony cures for cancer and other serious ailments among the estimated 15 000–17 000 existing health-related websites.

Legal action has been pursued in some cases. Examples include a company claiming that the parasitic cause of cancer and Alzheimer's disease can be eradicated with electric current, and sites promoting herbal supplements as primary alternatives to surgery, chemotherapy, and other mainstream treatments for cancer and HIV.

The US Department of Health and Human Services released a report expressing concern regarding consumers' lack of information to properly evaluate the credibility of Internet health material. Government agencies advise patients to be wary of quick cure-alls, of amazing testimonials that are not documented in the scientific literature, and of claims that the government and the scientific community are attempting to suppress the advocated treatment. Patients and practitioners must be extremely cautious when interpreting Internet and other CAM information. Misleading and false information abound. A saving grace is the proliferation of solid studies of CAM reported in scientific medical journals.

CAM in mainstream journals and physician practice

A marker of mainstream interest in CAM is the publication of research articles in major mainstream medical journals. Articles about CAM in major journals have shifted from letters and editorials in the 1970s expressing realistic concern about quackery, to surveys of patients' knowledge and prevalence of unproven methods in the 1980s, to reports of actual research results, starting primarily in the mid-1990s. The *Journal of the American Medical Association*, the *New England Journal of Medicine*, the *Lancet*, the *British Medical Journal*, and specialty journals such as *Cancer* and the *Journal of Clinical Oncology* have published reports of CAM research in recent years.

A survey of 295 family physicians in the US Maryland–Virginia region revealed that up to 90 per cent view complementary therapies such as diet and exercise, behavioural medicine, and hypnotherapy as legitimate medical practices. A majority refer patients to non-physicians for these therapies or provide the services themselves. However, homeopathy, Native American medicine, and traditional Chinese medicine were not seen as legitimate practices.

Two hundred Canadian general practitioners held a similar view and noted that chiropractic especially interested their patients. These physicians perceived chiropractic care, hypnosis, and acupuncture for chronic pain as the most effective CAM therapies. Homeopathy and reflexology were regarded as less efficacious. A meta-analysis of 12 studies in Great Britain suggests that British physicians view complementary medicine as only moderately effective,[10] although homeopathy and some other unproven methods seem to be viewed more positively in Britain than in other countries.

Therapies and practitioners

CAM therapies may be categorized in a variety of ways. The Office of Alternative Medicine (OAM), now the Center for Complementary and Alternative Medicine, originally developed the seven categories noted here: diet and nutrition; mind–body techniques; bioelectromagnetics; alternative medical systems; pharmacologic and biologic treatments; manual healing methods; and herbal medicine. Most of these approaches are unproven methods, frequently promoted as alternatives to mainstream care. Helpful complementary or adjunctive therapies are discussed separately at the end of this chapter. Currently popular therapies within each of these categories are discussed briefly below.

Diet and nutrition

Advocates of dietary treatments for cancer typically extend mainstream assumptions about the protective effects of fibre, fruits, and vegetables along with avoiding excessive dietary fat in reducing the risk of cancer, to the idea that food or vitamins can cure cancer. Proponents of this belief make their claims in books with titles such as 'The Food Pharmacy: Dramatic New Evidence that Food is your Best Medicine', 'Prescription for Nutritional Healing', and 'New Choices in Natural Healing'.

The macrobiotic diet remains a classic example of these dietary approaches. As currently constructed, it is similar to the recommendations for healthful eating, except that macrobiotic diets omit all dairy products and meat. Deriving 50–60 per cent of its calories from whole grains, 25–30 per cent from vegetables, and the remainder from beans, seaweed, and soups, this diet may be nutritionally deficient. Limited consumption of fruits, white-meat fish, and nuts may be allowed; however, all processed foods, animal meat and fat, artifical colours, preservatives, and soda are to be avoided. Inadequate caloric intake can cause weight loss, which may be especially problematic for patients with advanced disease. Despite claims in its publications and on websites, no studies have been conducted to determine whether the macrobiotic diet can cure or benefit patients with cancer. The co-founder of macrobiotics, Adelaide Kushi, died of cancer in 2001.

Some alternative practitioners preach that consumption of large doses of vitamins and minerals, consisting typically of hundreds of pills a day, or intravenous infusions of high-dose vitamin C, can cure disease. In 1968, Nobel Laureate Linus Pauling coined the term 'orthomolecular' to describe the treatment of disease with large quantities of nutrients. His claims that massive doses of vitamin C could cure cancer were disproved in clinical trials.[11,12] Despite the research, megavitamin and orthomolecular therapy, which adds minerals and other nutrients, remain popular among patients with major illnesses. There is no evidence that megavitamin or orthomolecular therapies are effective in treating any disorder.

Mind–body techniques

The potential to influence health with our minds is an extremely appealing concept in many countries because it affirms the power of individuals to heal themselves against all odds. Although some mind–body interventions such as mental imagery were promoted initially as cures or treatments for cancer, mind–body therapies today represent helpful complementary care backed by good data. Documentation exists, for example, for the effectiveness of meditation, biofeedback, and yoga in stress reduction and in the control of some physiologic reactions, such as blood pressure and heart rate.

Attending to the psychological health of patients is a fundamental component of responsible care. Support groups, good doctor–patient relationships, and the emotional and instrumental help of family and friends are vital. The argument that patients can use mental attributes or mind–body work to cure disease, however, is not tenable. The idea that patients can influence the course of their disease through mental or emotional work is not substantiated. Furthermore, as the underlying disease progresses despite patients' best spiritual or mental efforts, feelings of guilt and inadequacy can develop.[13]

Bioelectromagnetics

Bioelectromagnetics is the study of interactions between living organisms and their electromagnetic fields. According to proponents of related therapies, magnetic fields penetrate the body and heal damaged tissues, including cancers. There is no published research regarding assertions that bioelectromagnetic therapy heals illness or relieves pain. Despite the lack of data and the patent emptiness of these claims, proponents continue to sell electromagnetic therapy as a cure for cancer and other major illnesses, as well as for pain reduction.

Metabolic therapies and detoxification

Metabolic regimens are based on the importance of 'detoxification', which is thought necessary for the body to heal itself. Practitioners view cancer and other illnesses as directly related to the accumulation of toxins. This is a non-physiologic but venerable concept that originated in ancient Egyptian, Ayurvedic, and other early civilizations. Illness and death were believed caused by the putrefaction of food in the colon. Decay and purging were major themes in early cultures' view of disease and its treatment.

Metabolic therapies persist today. The contemporary version of this ancient idea is the belief that toxic products from diseased cells accumulate in the liver and lead to liver failure and death. Treatments aim to counteract liver damage with a low-salt, high-potassium diet, coffee enemas, pancreatic enzymes, and large daily amounts of fresh fruit and vegetable juice.

Modern variations on the older approach to internal cleansing are drinkable cleansing formulas, said to detoxify and rejuvenate the body. A variety of products can be purchased in health food stores, on the Internet, or ordered through catalogues. A shake of liquid clay, psyllium seed husks, and fruit juice, for example, is said to remove harmful food chemicals and air pollutants. These products tend to produce an osmotic or stimulant laxative effect and are potentially dangerous when taken daily, repeatedly over weeks, or on a regular basis as recommended by promoters. Neither the existence of gastrointestinal toxins nor the benefit of colonic cleansing has ever been documented.

There are many metabolic and 'detoxification' clinics in Tijuana, Mexico. Therapists offer treatments with practitioner-specific combinations of diet plus vitamins, minerals, enzymes, and 'detoxification'. Oral or injectable laetrile has been included as well. Between January and August 2000, approximately 20 such clinics have been ordered to cease operations by Mexican health officials. One clinic was found to be using mixtures containing chicken livers, tissue from guinea pigs, and human tissue samples from cancer patients as a therapy to be given to patients by injection.[14]

Alternative medical systems

Several popular ancient systems of healing are based on concepts of human physiology that differ from those understood by modern science. Two of the most popular healing systems are India's Ayurvedic medicine, popularized by best-selling author Deepak Chopra, MD, and traditional Chinese medicine.

'Ayurveda', is derived from the Sanskrit words 'ayur', meaning life and 'veda', pertaining to knowledge. This system classifies people into one of three predominant body types. There are specific remedies for disease and regimens to promote health for each body type. This medical system has a strong mind–body component, stressing the need to maintain balanced consciousness. Techniques such as yoga and mediation are used to focus and unite mind and body. Ayurveda also emphasizes regular detoxification and cleansing through all body openings.

Traditional Chinese medicine explains the body in terms of its relationship to the environment and the cosmos. Qi, or chi, pronounced 'chee', is the life force said to run through all of nature and flow through the human body via vertical energy channels known as meridians. The 12 primary meridians are believed dotted with acupoints. Each acupoint corresponds to a specific body organ or system, so that needling or pressing the acupoint can redirect the life-force imbalance causing the problem in that particular organ.

Traditional Chinese medicine also includes a full herbal pharmacopoeia with remedies for most ailments, including cancer. Chinese herbal teas and relaxation techniques are soothing and appealing to many patients, who use them as complementary therapies. The potential anticancer benefits of many Chinese herbal compounds and other botanicals are under investigation.

Tai chi is an effective gentle exercise technique that has gained increasing popularity in the United States. Research demonstrated that it is particularly useful in preventing falls among the frail or elderly,[15–17] and is helpful even for bedridden patients.

Pharmacologic and biologic treatments

This group of alternative treatments is invasive, biologically active, and highly controversial. The Di Bella regimen in Italy[2] and Burzynski's antineoplastons in the United States are among the most popular unproved pharmacologic therapies sought today. The Di Bella regimen utilizes a combination of medications including somatostatin, vitamins, retinoids, melatonin, bromocriptine, and occasionally subtherapeutic doses of oral cyclophosphamide or hydroxyurea to treat cancer. Burzynski's antineoplastons are peptides derived from human urine. No clinical study has demonstrated efficacy for either regimen.

Immunoaugmentive therapy (IAT) was developed by the late Lawrence Burton, PhD, and offered in his clinic in the Bahamas. Injected IAT is said to balance four protein components in the blood and to strengthen the patient's immune system. Burton claimed that IAT was particularly effective in treating mesothelioma. Documentation of IAT's efficacy remains anecdotal. The clinic has continued to operate following Burton's death, but its popularity seems to have waned.

Laetrile, an illegal and documented useless product long thought banished since the 1970s, was only dormant. It returned in the year 2000, readily available on the Internet. Also known as amygdalin, it is derived from apricot kernels. Repeated clinical trials have reported no activity and documented adverse events consistent with symptoms of cyanide poisoning.[18]

Interest in shark cartilage as a cancer therapy was activated by a 1992 book by I. William Lane, PhD, *Sharks Don't Get Cancer.* Advocates base their therapy on its putative antiangiogenic properties. Although extensive research is being conducted on small peptide extracts purified from shark cartilage,[19] over-the-counter formulations are comprised of large complex protein molecules that are too large to be absorbed by the gut. Shark cartilage actually decomposes into inert ingredients and is excreted. A recent phase I–II trial of shark cartilage found no clinical benefit;[20] the American National Cancer Institute (NCI) is recruiting patients for a phase III study to confirm this finding.[21]

Cancell, also known as Entelev, is another biologic remedy that appears to be especially popular in Florida and the Midwestern United States. Proponents claim that it returns cancer cells to a 'primitive state' from which they can be digested and rendered inert. Cancell is known to be composed of common chemicals including nitric acid, sodium sulfite, potassium hydroxide, sulfuric acid, and catechol. *In vitro* laboratory studies conducted by the Food and Drug Administration (FDA) and the American NCI found no basis for proponent claims of Cancell's effectiveness against cancer.

Manual healing methods

Osteopathic and chiropractic doctors were among the earliest groups to employ manual healing methodology. Today, there are numerous approaches that involve touch and manipulation techniques, including hands-on massage. A National Institutes of Health consensus conference in the United States supported the benefits of chiropractic treatment for low back pain, but its value is still widely disputed by mainstream physicians.

One of the most popular manual healing methods is therapeutic touch, which, despite its name, involves no direct contact. Therapeutic touch (TT), and other type of general energy healing, healers move their hands a few inches above a patient's body and sweep away 'blockages' to the patient's energy field. Although studies showed that experienced practitioners are unable to detect 'energy fields',[22] and despite mainstream scientists' unwillingness to accept its fundamental premises, TT and spiritual healing are widely practiced in North America, Britain, and other countries.

Related to therapeutic touch are several therapies that involve manipulation of a putative human energy field, or use of an individual's special gift for energy healing. Healing of this type, which has remained popular over the centuries in less-developed areas of the world, has gained increasing public interest and acceptance in Britain and the United States. Healers claim to have the ability to cure cancer and other major diseases. Although only minor difficulties may occur when healing is combined with mainstream care, some patients are so firmly convinced of their healer's abilities that they decline surgical removal of early stage tumours in favour of the healer's ministrations.

A large ad in the *New York Times* (July, 1999) claimed the ability of a Dr Yan Xin to emit healing Qi. The charge was given as US$ 5000 for stress release, weight reduction, or 'other health improvements', and US$ 3.5 million to cure a fatal disease.

Herbal treatments for cancer

Herbal remedies have a significant history of use and are a fundamental component of traditional and folk medicine. Medicinal herbs are used across all cultures of the world today and historically. Although many herbal remedies are said to have anticancer effects, these claims are either unsubstantiated or based on anecdotal studies. A handful of these therapies have gained sustained popularity as alternative cancer treatments.

Essiac, for example, has remained for decades a popular cancer treatment in North America, and more recently has been adopted by patients in Europe as well. It is thought an Ojibwa healer from Southwestern Canada created the concoction and gave it in the 1920s to a Canadian nurse, Rene Caisse (Essiac is Caisse spelled backwards). Essiac is a mixture of four botanicals: burdock root, rhubarb root, sheep sorrel root, and slippery elm bark. Researchers at the Canadian and American NCIs found that it has no anticancer effect. Essiac is illegal in Canada, but widely available elsewhere.

Iscador, a derivative of mistletoe, is a popular cancer remedy in Europe, where it is said to have been in continuous use as folk treatment since the Druids. It is used in many mainstream European cancer clinics, typically in conjunction with chemotherapy. Interest in Iscador increased in the United States after a celebrity with breast cancer acknowledged use of Iscador instead of chemotherapy. Despite many studies, data do not clearly support Iscador.

Herbal remedies

Patients use a variety of herbal supplements in addition to or instead of mainstream treatments for cancer and other diseases. Extracts from some of these herbs have been isolated to become important pharmaceutical products. Paclitaxel, an important antineoplastic agent that inhibits depolymerization of cellular microtubules, is derived from the Pacific Yew tree; digoxin was derived from foxglove (*Digitalis purpurea*); opium from the poppy (*Papaverum somniferum*); and vinca alkaloids from *Cantharanthus roseus.*

Non-prescription herbal remedies can be toxic and may interact with other medications (Table 1); others may help patients (Table 2).

Regulatory and safety issues

Dietary supplements, which include vitamins and minerals, homeopathic remedies, herbal treatments, antioxidants, and other readily available non-prescription products, appear to be the most popular unconventional remedies used today by seriously ill patients as well as by the public in general. According to the *Nutrition Business Journal* (*NBJ*), 1998 sales of supplements sold in the United States over the Internet alone reached US$ 40 million, an increase from US$ 12 million in 1997. *NBJ* estimates sales of food supplements at US$ 160 million for 1999 and US$ 500 million in 2001 in the United States alone.

Responsibility for food and drugs in the United States fall under the jurisdiction of the FDA. Botanicals and other dietary supplements, however, fall outside the categories of foods, pharmaceutical agents, and over-the-counter medications. Under the US Dietary Supplement Health and Education Act of 1994, the manufacturers of herbal products are responsible for ensuring their safety before marketing. The FDA may take action against any unsafe product after it reaches the market. Thanks to a major lobbying effort on the part of the food supplement industry in the United States, producers are not required to provide clinical data, to register manufacturing procedures, or to have labelling approved prior to marketing their products to the public. There are no legal standards for the processing or packaging of botanical products, and few food supplement companies voluntarily self-impose quality evaluation and control. Contaminated or falsely advertised products are common. The current US regulatory capability would prohibit full analysis and ongoing oversight of the estimated 20 000 food supplements now on the market.

This gap in quality-control standards and oversight requires redress. The magnitude and seriousness of the problem hopefully will result in the establishment of US government oversight programmes of some kind, despite anticipated efforts on the part of the food supplement industry to

Table 1 Herbal products with serious toxic effects

Chaparral tea, promoted as an antioxidant, pain reliever, etc.: case reports of hepatotoxicity and liver failure requiring liver transplantation
Chaste Tree Berry, used for PMS, can interfere with dopamine-receptor antagonists
Coltsfoot, used as a cough suppressant, expectorant, and demulcent, contains unsaturated pyrrolizidine alkaloids and has caused hepatotoxicity and liver failure. It is also potentially carcinogenic
Comfrey, ingested or used on bruises, contains unsaturated pyrrolizidine alkaloids associated with development of veno-occlusive disease
Feverfew (used for migraines, PMS), garlic (used for hypertension, hyperlipidemia, coronary artery disease, and other preventive and therapeutic uses), ginger (nausea), ginkgo (used for dementia and various vascular conditions from erectile dysfunction to Raynaud's), can interact with anticoagulants and increase bleeding. Anticoagulant effects occur in unusually high doses or when used in combination
Jin Bu Huan, used as a sedative and analgesic for pain-induced insomnia, has contained levo-tetrahydropalmatine, causing bradycardia, central nervous depression, and respiratory depression
Senna, cascara, and aloe, used as stimulant laxatives, overuse and abuse can cause hypokalaemia. Particularly dangerous when used with digitalis, diuretics, or patients with dehydration or electrolyte abnormalities
Licorice, used to treat peptic ulcers and as an expectorant: chronic use of licorice containing glycyrrhizin can cause hypokalaemia, hypernatraemia, decrease in male libido. May interact with cardiac glycosides, diuretics, corticosteroids, and insulin
Lobelia, used for asthma and bronchitis: at low doses may produce bronchodilation; higher doses can lead to respiratory depression, tachycardia, coma and death
Ma huang, used as a stimulant and appetite suppressant, contains ephedrine. Marketed as a herbal stimulant commonly known as speed, with names like Herbal Ecstasy, Cloud 9, and Ultimate Xphoria, has led to hypertension, palpitations, stroke, and psychosis
Plantain leaves cut or powdered found in Plantain Extract, Nature Cleanse Tablets, BotaniCleanse brands, Blessed Herbs, etc.: products found contaminated with digitalis glycosides
Siberian ginseng capsules: some contain instead a weed comprised of male hormone-like chemicals. Yohimbe, sold as a body builder and to enhance male performance has caused priapism, seizures, kidney failure and death

Table 2 Complementary therapies to help smooth the way during cancer treatment and recovery

Anxiety and stress

Acupressure: Performed by using the fingers of one hand to stimulate the acupoint inside the wrist of the other hand; can relieve nausea as well as anxiety and stress

Aromatherapy: Certain fragrances, such as rosemary, lavender, or camomile, can have a calming effect, although it may vary by individuals. Used by adding a few drops of 'essential oil' (available in health food stores and pharmacies) to the bath, or heated over a lit candle while relaxing

Meditation and other relaxation techniques: Patients can close their eyes, take slow deep breaths, and visualize themselves in a pleasant, peaceful place. An alternate technique is to lie down with eyes closed and consciously relax each body part starting from top to bottom. The body and mind relax accordingly

Music therapy: For many, music has important soothing physiologic as well as emotional benefits; type of effective music varies by individual

Therapeutic massage: Given by a licensed, certified massage therapist experienced with cancer patients, or a family member gently massaging neck, shoulders, hands, and feet. Patients with lymphatic cancers should receive only light touch massage

Table 2 Continued

Valerian: Available in tea bags, liquid extract, or capsule form. Said to reduce anxiety and bring about sleep. Can have additive effect like medications that cause CNS depression (i.e. benzodiazepines and barbiturates)

Yoga: Combination of deep breathing techniques and body postures. Instructional videotapes and books are widely available in libraries and bookstores. Even bedridden patients can utilize and benefit

For constipation

Water (6–8 glasses a day) and fibre (fruit, bran cereal, prunes) consumed regularly

Pureed rhubarb flavoured with apple juice, lemon, and honey

Plantago or psyllium seed, bulk-forming laxatives, taken with plenty of water

Extract of cascara works as stimulant laxatives; are often found in over-the-counter laxative products

For depression

Hypericum, or St John's wort, a proven antidepressant for mild to moderate symptoms, may cause photosensitivity. Induces cytochrome P450 3A4 and interacts with many prescription medications, especially chemotherapy, anticonvulsant, or antidepressant medications

Light therapy: Used specifically to reduce depression, bright-light boxes are placed at eye level on a desk or table. Especially effective in northern parts of the world where sunlight is rare or limited during winter months in the Northern Hemisphere. Recommended by psychiatrists to treat seasonal affective disorder (SAD)

Meditation and yoga

Tai Chi: Adapted from China, involves a gentle exercise programme practiced daily by millions of Chinese. May be learned through books, videos, and classes and practiced to benefit even by bedridden patients

For diarrhoea

Agrimony or peppermint tea

Applesauce or cooked carrots

Dried blackberry, blueberry, or raspberry leaves

Dried blueberry fruit

Pulverized seeds from the herb fenugreek

For 'heartburn'

Herb teas: Especially camomile, licorice, fennel, or anise

Salad items: Including lettuce, onion, garlic, and olives

Walnuts

For indigestion

Peppermint or chamomile tea

For nausea

Acupressure: Press inside of wrist with fingers of other hand (see Anxiety above)

Cinnamon or peppermint tea

Ginger: tea, capsules, or candy. Ginger ale or cookies. Must contain real ginger rather than artificial flavouring

Pain, chronic

Acupuncture

Useful herbs: External capsicum applied repeatedly, mountain mint leaf tea applied to skin; sunflower seeds, willow bark 'natural aspirin' tea (to be avoided by those who cannot take aspirin)

Hypnotherapy

Massage (see above)

For sleep problems

Warm bath scented with lavender oil

Lemon balm herb tea

Massage

Meditation

Tea made from fresh or dried passionflower herbs, valerian root, or chamomile

Please note that all herbs should be discontinued prior to receipt of chemotherapy (herb–drug interactions may occur), radiation therapy (skin may become photosensitized), or surgery (potential for pharmacokinetic interactions with analgesia and/or interference with coagulation pathways).

block efforts that could lead to regulation. In Canada, this problem was addressed by establishment of a government agency to supervise food supplements, but little activity has occurred. In Europe, botanical products are provided by prescription. The studies required to support their utility are viewed elsewhere as too brief in duration and involving inadequate sample sizes.

Adverse events and herb–drug interactions

Regulatory agencies in Europe, Asia, and North America rarely examine herbal remedies for safety and effectiveness. Few products have been formally tested to determine side-effects or quality control, but information is accumulating based on public experience with over-the-counter supplements. Health care professionals are encouraged to report adverse events related to herbal and other dietary supplements to the appropriate regulatory agency.

Recent reports in the literature describe severe liver and kidney damage from some herbal remedies (Table 1). These reports underscore the fact that 'natural' products, contrary to apparent consumer belief, are not necessarily safe or harmless. The general public apparently is not aware that herbs are not benign products, but more appropriately should be considered dilute pharmaceuticals that contain scores of different chemicals, most of which have not been documented. Effects are not always predictable due to variations in herbal composition, manufacturing procedures, and the possibility of contaminants.

Moreover, the potential for herb–drug interaction is sufficiently problematic. Many believe that patients on chemotherapy and other major medications should stop using herbal remedies. Similar cautions are necessary for patients receiving radiation therapy or about to undergo surgery. Several herbs, such as dong quai and coriander, contain psoralen, which can radiosensitize the skin and cause reactions, although interference with radiation therapy's effectiveness is not documented. Some herbs interfere with coagulation and produce dangerous blood pressure swings and other unwanted interactions with anaesthetics. Many popular herbs, such as feverfew, garlic, ginger, and ginkgo, have anticoagulant effects and should be avoided by patients on coumadin, heparin, aspirin, and related agents.

Asian patent medicines have been found to contain unsafe levels of mercury and other toxic metals in more than one-third of batches studied. Several instances of heart problems resulting from digitalis-contaminated supplements have been reported. Concerns were raised recently even about antioxidant capsules, which may interact with chemotherapeutic agents.

Complementary therapies

Complementary therapies are safe and non-toxic, non-invasive, easy to use, and inexpensive. Many may be self-managed, often rendering practitioners unnecessary, which offers patients the rare and important opportunity to maintain a measure of control over their own well-being. Complementary or supportive modalities also are soothing, comforting, and distracting, and backed by good efficacy data.

Some complementary therapies, such as relaxing in a warm bath or painting soothing mental pictures, are intuitively comforting and helpful. Major supportive therapies have been singled out of Table 2 for more detailed review and are presented below. These therapies—music therapy, therapeutic massage, acupuncture, and mind–body modalities—address some of the most pervasive and difficult problems faced by patients under palliative care. Although data are not always based on the patient population of concern to us here, research shows that these minimally invasive, non-toxic therapies effectively reduce anxiety, depression, pain, dyspnoea, nausea and fatigue, common problems among palliative care patients.

Music therapy (see also Chapter 15.2)

Music therapy integrates all aspects of music—listening, singing, playing instruments, and composing—specifically developed to meet the individual patient's needs. These services typically are provided by musicians who hold graduate degrees in music therapy. The didactic programmes combine history, theory, and practicalities of performing music with behavourial and therapeutic approaches necessary for patient care. Therapists are trained to deal with both psychosocial and clinical issues faced by patients, family members, and even caregivers.

Music therapy is referred to throughout history and can be found in both folklore and Greek mythology (Apollo was the god of both music and medicine). Only in recent years has it been studied scientifically. Music therapy has been shown to be particularly effective in the palliative care setting. Formal music therapy programmes in palliative medicine exist in several major institutions, including the Memorial Sloan-Kettering Cancer Center, the Cleveland Clinic, and many European centres.

Controlled trials indicate that music therapy produces emotional and physiologic benefits. Subjective responses include reductions in anxiety, stress, depression, and pain. Music intervention significantly reduced objective measures such as heart rate, respiratory rate, and anxiety scores among inpatients following myocardial infarction or receiving ventilatory assistance and outpatients undergoing flexible sigmoidoscopy. Live music was found to be more effective than recorded music in reducing anxiety.

In the preoperative setting, randomized trials found that music reduced anxiety as well as its physiologic correlates, including blood pressure and salivary cortisol, a biochemical marker of stress and anxiety. Music lowered blood pressure and anxiety scores during and after eye surgery and among women undergoing hysterectomies in a randomized controlled trial.

Music therapy was effective against experimental pain, among cancer outpatients, and among cancer patients with chronic pain. Music reduced intraoperative analgesic requirements compared to controls, and patients randomized to a music intervention reported significantly less pain and required less pain medication. In what may be the largest trial of its type, 500 surgical patients were randomized to recorded music, jaw relaxation, a music/jaw relaxation combination, or a control group receiving no intervention. Music led to significant decreases in both pain intensity and related distress associated with pain.[23] Music also has been found to help reduce depression.

Massage therapy

The American Massage Therapy Association defines massage therapy as a profession in which the practitioner applies manual techniques, and may apply adjunctive therapies, with the intention of positively affecting the health and well-being of the client. Many varieties of massage may be employed. The type of massage therapy selected is tailored to both patient preference and clinical status.

The benefits of massage therapy are documented for end-of-life populations.[24] In the largest study to date, a prospective, crossover trial evaluated 87 hospitalized cancer patients who were randomized to foot massage (also called reflexology) or to a control group. Pain and anxiety scores decreased following massage, with differences between groups achieving statistical significance in favour of massage.

Pain scores fell by nearly two-thirds immediately following an initial massage session for patients with post-burn itching and pain, and improvements appeared to be cumulative. No similar changes were seen in controls. Other studies found similar results for burn patients and patients with postoperative pain.

Massage often is enhanced by the addition of aroma therapy, the use of plant-based essential oils. Aroma therapy may take the form of the product used during massage, a scented candle, or some other means of infusing the room with a pleasant fragrance. The research in this area, conflicting and often methodologically inadequate, may be far less important than the observation that patients typically find light fragrances pleasant and relaxing. The use of aroma therapy as an independent complementary therapy is not often applied in the United States but is increasingly popular in the United Kingdom and Europe, and its independent application to help relieve serious symptoms or treat disease is not considered scientifically valid.

Acupuncture (see also Chapter 8.2.9)

Acupuncture has been a part of Chinese medicine for more than three millennia. Hair thin needles are placed into the body at specific points. The goal, according to the original construct, was to affect Qi and remove blockages to the smooth flow of life energy so that healing would occur. Although the modern mechanism of action is yet to be determined for acupuncture, it is apparent that response is dependent on the location stimulated. Acupuncture stimulates type II and III myelinated afferent nerves. The signal is transmitted to the spinal cord initiating the release of serotonin, enkephalin, and dynorphin and possibly reaction by higher central nervous system functions.

Several randomized controlled trials examined acupuncture for dyspnoea. A laboratory-based model of methacholine-induced bronchospasm allowed good experimental control in a blinded, placebo-controlled, randomized investigation. Significant differences in lung function emerged between needling true versus inactive ('sham') points for airway conductance, forced expiratory volume, and forced expiratory flow.[25]

Asthmatic children were evaluted in a laboratory setting in a similarly controlled study. Exercise-induced reductions in forced expiratory volume, peak expiratory flow rate, and forced vital capacity were significantly lower in real compared to sham acupuncture. A trial of acupressure for adult chronic obstructive pulmonary disorder also found significant improvements in subjective breathlessness between groups. An unncontrolled study evaluated 20 palliative care patients given a single session of acupuncture. Ten minutes of needle insertion resulted in a 43 per cent reduction in breathlessness. This benefit was maintained at 6-h follow-up.

Cancer-related fatigue often persists even after treatment of anaemia. It is a highly distressing and common complaint of cancer patients although there is no known effective treatment. Published case reports include fatigue associated with multiple sclerosis and chronic fatigue syndrome. One randomized trial of acupuncture with fatigue as an endpoint has been published. Although this was a small trial of only 13 patients and the acupuncture prescription was primarily for the treatment of pain and nausea, rather than fatigue, patients did experience a nearly 15 per cent reduction in fatigue scores; the mean change among controls was zero. Anecdotal information, obtained from the acupuncturists and patients in the MSKCC Integrative Medicine Service, provides additional insight. Several cancer patients who scored five or higher on a ten-point visual analogue scale experienced clinically important reductions in fatigue following acupuncture treatment.

Meta-analyses and systematic reviews of acupuncture support its utility for dental and back pain. A systematic review[26] as well as a pilot study indicate that acupuncture effectively reduces nausea. In a study of 183 cancer patients, almost half experienced decreased pain following acupuncture.

Certainly additional research, particularly with respect to patients receiving palliative care, will be useful and welcome. However, many complementary therapies are sufficiently well understood and appreciated by patients to include them whenever feasible. Music, touch therapies, non-invasive pain relief, and other modalities[27] enhance comfort and reduce distress. They should become readily available to help palliate the physical and psychic pain typically experienced by patients at the end of life.

References

1. **World Health Organization.** *Cancer Pain and Relief* (Technical Report Series 804). Geneva: World Health Organization, 1990.
2. **Cassileth, B.R.** et al. (2001). Alternative medicine use worldwide: The International Union Against Cancer survey. *Cancer* **91**, 1390–3.
3. **Elder, N.C., Gillcrist, A., and Minz, R.** (1997). Use of alternative health care by family practice patients. *Archives of Family Medicine* **6**, 181–4.
4. **The Landmark Report.** November 1997 (www.landmarkhealthcare. com).
5. **Eisenberg, D.M.** et al. (1998). Trends in alternative medicine use in the United States, 1990–1997: results of a follow-up national survey. *Journal of the American Medical Association* **280**, 1569–75.
6. **Druss, B.G. and Rosenheck, R.A.** (1999). Association between use of unconventional therapies and conventional medical services. *Journal of the American Medical Association* **282**, 651–6.
7. **Hellmich, N.** Bloom is off herbal-product sales. *USA Today* 05/08/2001 (www.usatoday.com/hlead.htm).
8. **Abu-Realh, M.H.** et al. (1996). The use of complementary therapies by cancer patients. *Nursing Connections* **9**, 3–12.
9. **Grootenhuis, M.A.** et al. (1998). Use of alternative treatment in pediatric oncology. *Cancer Nursing* **21**, 282–8.
10. **Ernst, E., Resch, K.-L., and White, A.R.** (1995). Complementary medicine: what physicians think of it: a meta-analysis. *Archives of Internal Medicine* **155**, 2405–8.
11. **Creagan, E.T.** et al. (1979). Failure of high-dose vitamin C (ascorbic acid) therapy to benefit patients with advanced cancer: a controlled trial. *New England Journal of Medicine* **301**, 687–90.
12. **Moertel, C.G.** et al. (1985). High-dose vitamin C versus placebo in the treatment of patients with advanced cancer who have had no prior chemotherapy. A randomized double-blind comparison. *New England Journal of Medicine* **312**, 137–41.
13. **Cassileth, B.R.** (1989). The social implications of mind–body cancer research. *Cancer Investigation* **7**, 361–4.
14. **Sanchez, E.G. and Crabtree, P.** Alternative tijuana clinic shut down by baja officials. *Union-tribune*, San Francisco, 27 July 2001.
15. **Lane, J.M. and Nydick, M.** (1999). Osteoporosis: current modes of prevention and treatment. *Journal of the American Academy of Orthopedic Surgeons* **7**, 19–31.
16. **Henderson, N.K., White, C.P., and Eisman, J.A.** (1998). The roles of exercise and fall risk reduction in the prevention of osteoporosis. *Endocrinology and Metabolism Clinics of North America* **27**, 369–71.
17. **Ross, M.C. and Presswalla, J.L.** (1998). The therapeutic effects of Tai Chi for the elderly. *Journal of Gerontologic Nursing* **24**, 45–7.
18. **Moertel, C.G.** et al. (1982). A clinical trial of amygdalin (laetrile) in the treatment of human cancer. *New England Journal of Medicine* **306**, 201–6.
19. **Sheu, J.R.** et al. (1998). Effect of U-995, a potent shark cartilage-derived angiogenesis inhibitor, on anti-angiogenesis and anti-tumor activities. *Anticancer Research* **18**, 4435–41.
20. **Miller, D.R.** et al. (1998). Phase I/II Trial of the safety and efficacy of shark cartilage in the treatment of advanced cancer. *Journal of Clinical Oncology* **16**, 3649–55.
21. **Anonymous** (1999). NCI to sponsor phase III trials of liquid shark cartilage angiogenesis inhibitor. *Oncology (Huntington)* **13**, 82.
22. **Abbot, N.C.** et al. (2001). Spiritual healing as a therapy for chronic pain: a randomized clinical trial. *Pain* **91**, 79–89.
23. **Good, M.** et al. (2001). Relaxation and music to reduce postsurgical pain. *Journal of Advanced Nursing* **33**, 208–15.
24. **Corner, J., Cawley, N., and Hildebrand, S.** (1995). An evaluation of the use of massage and essential oils on the wellbeing of cancer patients. *International Journal of Palliative Nursing* **1**, 67–73.
25. **Tashkin, D.P.** et al. (1977). Comparison of real and simulated acupuncture and isoproterenol in methacholine-induced asthma. *Annals of Allergy* **39**, 379–87.
26. **Vickers, A.J.** (1996). Can acupuncture have specific effects on health? A systematic review of acupuncture antiemesis trials. *Journal of the Royal Society of Medicine* **89**, 303–11.
27. **Cassileth, B.R.** *The Alternative Medicine Handbook: The Complete Reference Guide to Alternative and Complementary Therapies.* New York: WW Norton, 1998.

17

Palliative medicine in the home

17 Palliative medicine in the home

17.1 Palliative medicine in the home: an overview

Derek Doyle

Some years ago the National Council for Hospice and Specialist Palliative Care Services in the United Kingdom made these challenging assertions:(1)

- Every person with a life threatening illness has the right to receive appropriate palliative care.
- It is the responsibility of every clinician to provide appropriate palliative care to those who need it.
- Patients receiving palliative care should be enabled to receive it in the place of their choice.

This textbook is written with these statements in mind. This chapter, in particular, is a response to the third assertion and recognizes that, world-wide, most people say they would prefer to die in their own homes or those of their families though it must be noted that most studies looking at this have been based in Western countries.

This chapter will review the whole issue of palliative care in the home. It will look at where people say they would prefer to die and where they actually die. It will then examine the quality of palliative care available in the home, what influences where they die, and ask what they have a right to expect if they are cared for at home rather than in hospital. It will look at their pattern of suffering and, finally, examine what care can realistically be provided, looking at the scene in different countries and the place of specialist palliative home care teams. It must be noted, however, that there are many developing countries without any primary care professionals—no readily accessible family doctors, no nurses visiting homes, no local pharmacies where they can obtain medications. There are even some *developed* countries where primary care and essential drugs are not available. As will be demonstrated in this chapter, there are many countries where palliative care is unknown, and therefore where information and statistics on palliative care in the home are unobtainable.

The case for palliative care in the home

It is frequently claimed that most people want to be cared for at home, or in the home of a relative or friend, attended by a doctor who knows them—the primary health-care model, or general practice as it is known in Britain. We must ask whether such a model of care is necessarily the best for them and whether there is evidence that it is, or can be, high-quality care.

There is no doubt from many studies that 50–75 per cent of people, when still enjoying good health, express a preference for being cared for at home when they become terminally ill.(2–6) However, this is not to say they necessarily want to *die* at home. The nearer they get to death the more prepared patients are to be admitted to hospital or palliative care unit. In the same way, relatives usually express eagerness to have the patient at home but are relieved when the patient is admitted to an in-patient unit.(5) Hinton found that the longer home care continues the fewer patients and families want it until finally, in the week or so before death, only 54 per cent of patients and 45 per cent of relatives still want it. Weakness and fatigue were the principal reasons for them changing their minds,(7) but this is discussed in detail later in this chapter.

A paradox is that, in some places, the better the specialist home palliative care provision the more eager patients are to die in a palliative care unit than at home, even when there are beds available for them to be re-admitted to the general hospital or oncology service where they are well known.(8)

The percentage of home deaths is changing each year. It differs between neighbouring countries and even between different regions within a single country(2) (see Table 1).

Table 1 Percentage of deaths at home

Hong Kong	<1
Taiwan	1
USA	10
Canada	15
Denmark and UK	24
Belgium	27
Brazil	40
South Africa	41
Poland	48
South Korea	66

National differences in place of death

United Kingdom

A study of trends over 10 years in the United Kingdom revealed that deaths in hospitals and nursing homes fell from 58 to 47 per cent. Between 1985 and 1992, home deaths fell from 27 to 25.5 per cent then rose again to 26.5 per cent in 1994. Geographical differences were significant. In Thames region, around London and its densely populated suburbs, patients with carcinoma of lung, colon, rectum, bone, connective tissue, lip, and mouth were more likely to die at home. The researchers confirmed that the trend to death in hospital was changing and more were dying in hospice/palliative care units and in nursing homes. [For those unfamiliar with nursing homes in the United Kingdom and many other European countries a nursing home (often a converted mansion house) is usually staffed principally by untrained auxiliary nurses under the direction of a registered nurse (often the owner) and provides residential and nursing care for local people unable to be cared for at home. Medical cover usually remains the responsibility of the patient's family doctor.] Later in this chapter, we shall examine the quality of palliative care provided in such nursing homes. In the

Netherlands, nursing *houses* are larger institutions often with their own full-time doctors and a large complement of registered nurses. They offer a continuum of care from residential for those fit and mobile but unable to remain at home, through to advanced nursing for them when they become terminally ill.[9]

It appears that patients who die at home differ from those who die as in-patients in terms of informal carer support, age, sex, care dependency, diagnosis, and psychosocial status. Patients whose community support is started early in the terminal phase of their illness are less likely to die at home, possibly reflecting high levels of dependency.[10] Older people and women are less likely to die at home, perhaps because the widows are living alone having been pre-deceased by their husbands.[2] However, even though the men with terminal illness are cared for by their wives it has been shown that men usually remain at home for less time than women receiving palliative care.[11] Poor symptom control is a common reason for ending home care and transferring the patient to hospital or specialist palliative care unit.[3] Studies in Italy have shown that home-based patients, compared with those admitted to hospital, are generally younger, of higher education, usually married and usually have carcinoma of lung, breast, or prostate.[12] An interim report on a study still in progress has shown that those who die at home differ from those who die as in-patients in terms of informal carer support, age, sex, care dependency, diagnosis, and psychosocial status.[10] There does not seem to be any uniform picture. The pattern of where people die differs between countries and in most countries has changed considerably in recent years.

Israel

Loven and colleagues found that in Israel 29 per cent died at home, 40 per cent in general hospitals, and 31 per cent in chronic care hospitals. They concluded that when a patient has a close carer it should be possible, with the support of a home care service, to care for more people at home.[13]

Italy

A study of 401 patients found that 56 per cent died at home.[14] Toscani studied 1000 patients and found a growing self-determination amongst patients about choosing their place of death. The vast majority wanted to die at home possibly because, as he found, inadequacies of care were five times as many in hospitals as in the home.[15,16] Mercadente has studied the medications taken by people at home (most on more than four drugs and opioids more often used in the young than older patients) and also the impact of a home care service on the suffering of cancer patients.[17,18]

Belgium

Schrivers and colleagues studied 2784 deaths in Antwerp. Sixty-seven per cent occurred in hospital, 20 per cent at home, 8 per cent in nursing homes, and 4 per cent elsewhere. They confirmed what others have found, namely that a very high level of support from relatives was needed to keep people at home.[19] A longitudinal exploratory study on factors determining the place of death is in progress in Antwerp,[20] and a model for evaluating services as well as assessing unmet needs is being developed.[21]

France

A study of 6000 deaths over 11 years in Paris came to the same conclusion as the Belgium study.[22]

Sweden

A study of 56 patients in different specialist departments found that one-third of the last month was spent at home, that 10 died at home, and 46 in an in-patient unit.[23] Figures for Stockholm are available for the years 1991 and 1996 (Table 2). They show a dramatic decline in the percentage of deaths in hospital and a proportionate increase in deaths at home, in nursing homes, and in hospices. During the period 1991–1996, several changes occurred in the Swedish health-care system. There was a rapid expansion of palliative home care services, three hospice units were established and the care of the elderly was made a responsibility of local county authorities.[24] Hospital-based home care (HBHC) has existed for more than 30 years in Sweden and by 1999 there were more than 50 such teams operating. Studies have suggested that with such a HBHC team, which includes a doctor skilled in palliative medicine, deaths at home could be as high as 50 per cent for cancer patients.

Table 2 Changing pattern of deaths in Stockholm, Sweden

	1991, % of $n = 3635$	1996, % of $n = 3690$
Home	9.7	17.0
Hospitals	86.1	56.4
Nursing homes	2.9	14.5
Hospices	—	10.8
Other	1.2	1.3

Norway

In Norway, 16.6 per cent of all deaths (13.8 per cent of cancer deaths) occurred at home in 1996. Since 1964, there has been a steady decline in deaths outside hospitals (homes, nursing home, and other health-care institutions) falling from 41 per cent in 1964 to 25 per cent in 1981, and to about 20 per cent in 1996. The biggest change has been an increase in nursing home deaths from 23 to 28 per cent and a corresponding fall in hospital deaths.[25]

Denmark

Interestingly, the percentage of home cancer deaths is higher than Norway, 24 per cent. A random survey found that 86 per cent of cancer patients were being cared for at home and only 14 per cent in hospitals or nursing homes in Arhus but no figures for place of death were published in that study.[25]

Spain

The current position of palliative care in Spain is described by Centeno and colleagues.[26] The question whether or not care at home is a cost-saving alternative to hospital care has been studied in Catalonia.[27] Izquierdo-Porrera found that it was mainly medical factors that determined where men die, and functional dependency and social support were factors that determined where women die in Spain.[28]

Hong Kong

Palliative Home Care Services and family medicine are both well developed in Hong Kong, with nursing equipment available and medical specialists prepared to visit homes but still less than 1 per cent of cancer deaths occur at home.[29] This suggests that increasing the percentage of home deaths need not be a universal goal of palliative care services.

A cautionary note

Many, even of the developed countries, do not record the place of death in their national statistics and many of the figures quoted in this chapter have been obtained from studies conducted by palliative care workers. They may not be truly representative of the country as a whole. Some developing countries keep no statistics about either the place or the cause of death. In other countries, patients receive almost all their care in hospital but are taken home in the final hours of life to die with their families, further skewing the statistics. Finally, it has to be remembered that there is no consistency of definition of what constitutes a nursing home. In most countries, it describes a place of care relatively near the patient's home but the palliative care qualifications of the nurses and doctors are not defined, nor the staffing levels and patient : staff ratios.

Do patients achieve their wish to die in the place of their choice?

It is one thing for people to express a wish to die in a particular place but how often do they achieve that wish?

The first thing to note again is that both patients and their relatives, the informal carers, change their wishes as the illness progresses inexorably to its inevitable end, reflecting the increasing dependency of the patient and the strain and anxiety experienced by relatives.[30] The wishes they expressed 8 weeks before the death are often quite different from those nearer the end.

Dunlop and colleagues looked at 100 patients in London and found that 71 per cent achieved their choice, 50 per cent dying at home and 25 per cent in a hospice.[31] Thirteen per cent chose hospital because they saw that their relatives were unable to cope.

In a London-based study of 229 patients, 38 per cent had expressed a preference for place of death, 73 per cent asking for home.[4] Twenty-one per cent died at home and only 58 per cent achieved their wish. Stating a preference, nearly always for care at home, made it more likely they would achieve their wish. Using health and social services for social care made death at home less likely, a similar finding to that of Ward.[8] The percentage dying at home is marginally higher in the Scottish Highlands than the national average, 31 per cent as against 26.5 per cent, but at least all patients who asked to stay at home did so,[32] in contrast with another report from a general practice where patients did not achieve their choice.[3] Once again there is no consistency.

It is sometimes forgotten that whatever the availability of beds in hospital or hospice and whatever the quality of their care there, 90 per cent of the last year of life of cancer patients is spent at home.[30,33] This is yet further evidence of the need for high-quality palliative care to be available in the home and for family physicians and community nurses to be as highly trained in palliative care as is possible.

Just as it is wrong to assume that everyone wants to die at home so it is unwise to assume that every patient wants to leave their familiar hospital and be transferred to home or to a hospice/specialist palliative care unit as a London study demonstrated.[34]

Perhaps clinicians and researchers have for too long focused on the wish to die at home, expressed by the patient long before they entered the final phase, when they should be more flexible, prepared to take into account the patient's *changing* wishes. It should not be considered a failure when someone who previously had expressed a wish to die at home has to be admitted to hospital or hospice, provided that when they were under care at home it was of the highest standard in all respects. There are three questions to be asked when auditing this aspect of palliative care.

1. Did the patient achieve their expressed wish, whatever it was?
2. Did the patient manage to stay at home as long as possible even if not dying there?
3. Was the care offered both at home and in the hospital or hospice to which they were admitted of the highest standard?

We must now look at what influences where people die.

What influences where people die? (Table 3)

The gender of the patient

It has been shown that it is mainly medical factors that determine where men die, and functional dependency and social support are factors that determine where women die.[28] Another study showed that women can be cared for at home longer than most men can, even with the same palliative care and support services available to them.[11]

The availability of specialist palliative care services

The influence of a specialist Community Palliative Care Service (as 'Home Care Services' used to be called) on where people die has already been noted.[8] The quality of home care also affects how long they may be in hospital. A study of the effectiveness of a 'hospital-at-home' service comparing it with a hospital found them comparable but the former led to shorter stays in hospital.[35] Such papers raise interesting questions. Do some patients become aware of how good palliative care can be as a result of being under such a Community Palliative Care Service (CPCS) based in a nearby specialist palliative care in-patient unit and therefore elect to go there if possible? Do they change their minds because they are encouraged to go into the specialist palliative care unit by its CPCS nurses who are visiting them? Do they for some reason not trust the hospital to provide the best palliative care and therefore refuse to return there for terminal care? Have they seen terminally ill people suffering in hospital wards?

Table 3 Factors influencing whether people die in hospital or at home

The availability and accessibility of palliative care services
The patient's underlying pathology
The age of the patient
The quality of pain and symptom control
The stress experienced by caring relatives
The socio-economic class of the patient
The ethnic group to which the patient belongs
The attitudes and perceptions of the family physician
The availability of nursing equipment
The availability of appropriately trained community nurses
Societal and cultural attitudes of the patient and family

There seems little doubt that the quality of care at home can be enhanced if a CPCS is involved.[7,13,17,36–41] There is also evidence that such a specialist service enables patients to remain longer at home, though not necessarily to die at home, than might otherwise have been the case.[11] Even if the services of a palliative care team are not available, the involvement of a specialist nurse can make a difference. One UK study conducted over a 26-month period found that when a Marie Curie Nurse (a nurse with specialist training and experience in palliative care) was involved, more than 90 per cent of patients achieved their wish to die at home.[42,43] Though communications between them are sometimes less than ideal, there is evidence that generalist community nurses appreciate the contribution of specialist palliative care nurses working alongside them in a patient's care and feel it is beneficial for the patient.[44–47] It may improve the family physician's pain management skills that community nurses so frequently criticize.[44] Another way of improving the diagnosis and management of pain, of course, is to use Pain Assessment Scales[18] and a drug audit.[48] It must not be overlooked that in most countries of the world there are no palliative care services of any kind. As has been noted already, in many countries there are no primary care facilities, no family physicians, no community nurses. This issue will be addressed later in this chapter.

The underlying pathology

It has been claimed that the place of death for cancer patients partly depends on the malignancy site.[10,49] According to one study, the commonest cancer in men transferred from home to an in-patient facility is bronchogenic carcinoma, in women bronchogenic and breast carcinomata, not surprising because they are the commonest malignancies.[50] Another study found that the commonest tumours in patients being cared for at home were lung, breast, and prostate.[12] Yet another study, based in London, found those most likely to be managed successfully at home were those with bronchogenic carcinoma, colo-rectal tumours, bone and oropharyngeal malignancies.[2] Clearly, this is more complex than at first appears and is difficult to explain because the spectrum and intensity of suffering is not site specific.

The age of the patient

Most, but not all, studies suggest that the younger the patient, particularly if married, the greater the chance that he or she will be able to remain at home. The older the patient, particularly if she is a widow living alone, the more likely that transfer to hospital or hospice will be required, although women may be able to remain at home slightly longer than men.[3,5,10,11]

Quality of symptom control

It is sometimes claimed that good research cannot be done in the community and that quality of life tools cannot be used there. This is not so as will be seen from the number of references in this chapter.[51]

Unrelieved suffering at home is widely reported.[3,23,52–54] In both malignant and non-malignant disease patients, pain and dyspnoea are alarming for both patients and caring relatives and poorly treated.

A 2000 study by Hanratty found 96 per cent of patients having pain managed by their family physician but in only 52 per cent was it being relieved.[54] Urinary incontinence is, for some reason, seldom a reason for asking for hospital transfer but faecal incontinence is given as a reason even when a special laundry service is available to assist them.[55,56] Interestingly, most doctors describe a 'good death' as one without pain, hence patients not perceived by the doctor as having pain, are less likely to be referred to a palliative care unit, irrespective of other symptoms except anxiety, begging the question 'how well do doctors recognise pain?'[57,58]

Community care for stroke patients can be challenging. A study of 111 such patients found that 43 per cent needed more help with personal care, 27 per cent with domestic chores, 32 per cent needed financial help, and 63 per cent of their last year of life was spent in a nursing or residential home. Seventy-six per cent of carers had to restrict their own activities and only 32 per cent later reported that they had found the caring rewarding. They found the depression and anxiety of the patients the most difficult things to cope with.[59]

Stress experienced by relatives

Concern about relatives and the strain they are experiencing is certainly a reason for some patients electing to leave home.[34,39] The strain experienced by caring relatives is given as the principal reason for admission in most studies of family physicians and community nurses.[43,60–64] Experience shows that patients often agree to hospital transfer as a last mark of their love and concern for relatives, and not necessarily because they are themselves eager to leave home. Whether this is a valid and acceptable reason is another matter. It can be as big a strain and as tiring, visiting a patient in hospital as caring for them at home even with the support of social services and a community palliative care service. Particularly must this be the case if all pain and suffering are not relieved in the hospital as is sometimes the case.

It has also to be remembered that whereas most patients, certainly in the West, ask to be fully informed about their condition, many relatives are uncomfortable with this.[65]

Social class of the patient

Sims and colleagues, in a seminal paper, found that the place of death is related to social class.[66] They looked at 831 cancer deaths. Classes 1 and 2 (professional and managerial groups) with 15 per cent of all deaths contributed to 24 per cent of hospice deaths, 14 per cent hospital deaths, and 12 per cent home deaths. Class 3, with 24 per cent of all cancer deaths, contributed 58 per cent of hospice deaths, only 9 per cent of hospital deaths, and 35 per cent of home deaths. Classes 4 and 5 (semi-skilled and unskilled manual workers) with 61 per cent of all cancer deaths had only 18 per cent in hospice, 75 per cent in hospital, and 53 per cent at home. They conclude that the differences may be to do with access to services, perception by patients and family physicians, and accessibility of social support by different sections of the community. Some have suggested that the differences can be explained by how articulate and informed people are, factors that enable them to ask for the place of their well-informed choice.

Ethnic group

Though few figures were available it was brought to the attention of the National Council for Hospice and Specialist Palliative Care Services in England that no palliative care unit ever had more than 1 per cent of its patients from an ethnic minority in spite of a very high proportion of the general population in many cities being of African, Indian, Pakistani, or West Indian origin. Koffman and colleagues then studied this, looking at the black Caribbean population in London.[67] They questioned surviving relatives. Sixty-five per cent of the patients were aged over 65, 74 per cent having cancer and 65 per cent died in hospital. At home, only 61 per cent had contact with community nurses. Asked how they rated the quality of care received, 58 per cent said it had been excellent, 50 per cent fair or poor. Looking at all aspects of the care provided, only 44 per cent felt it had been excellent or good. A comparison of the views of white patients and first generation Afro-Caribbeans in London, all with advanced cancer, is reported by Koffman and Higginson.[68]

It is difficult to confirm because cancer registers do not have to give ethnic groups but one study in the United Kingdom suggests that no more than half the ethnic minority who might benefit from home palliative care receive it.[69]

No studies have yet confirmed it but one gains the impression that some cultural groups within the ethnic minorities to be found in most western countries have a strong tradition of caring for their dying at home and elect to do so rather than have them in an in-patient unit where their traditions and their culture might not be fully understood and respected.[70] In several cities in the western world there are moves to have palliative care units primarily for Moslems, Buddhists, and Hindus.

Attitudes and perceptions of family physicians

A study conducted in Glasgow, Scotland's largest city, with a population of 1.5 million, interviewed all family physicians and community nurses. It found that 93 per cent of the doctors and nurses preferred that death should occur at home, with 83 per cent of doctors and 86 per cent of nurses placing hospices second in preference for their patients. Nurses then placed nursing homes in third place whereas doctors selected the hospitals. When asked what were the obstacles to home deaths they listed, in order, lack of night support, lack of suitable home and environmental facilities, poor communications between service providers, and insufficient information to enable patients to make a choice.[43] Perhaps because of their experience when working in hospitals, 80 per cent of community nurses state that when the time comes to decide where *they* wish to die they would choose home rather than hospital.[71] Presumably this personal view influences the advice they give their patients.

Perhaps, not surprisingly, where people die is closely related to the views of their family physicians, something confirmed by a Yale study.[72] Many of the difficulties cited by the Glasgow doctors are evident in other major cities. A study of care services, not exclusively for palliative care, in a deprived district of London, found that many doctors were not contactable after 6 p.m. when they handed over to deputizing services. Other problems included language and communications ones, racial discrimination, poor information about the availability of services, and difficulty in getting any doctor to make a home visit in an emergency.[73]

A study in yet another deprived area of London with a population of 700 000 looked at the problems of providing and accessing out-of-hours medical care. There was found to be widespread dissatisfaction with current arrangements related to access, availability, demand for services, and interagency communication and co-operation. As a result of the study and its findings, it was decided to establish primary care co-operatives to provide out-of-hours emergency cover and to develop better interagency communications and collaboration. Forty-four per cent of the doctors were in favour of developing a telephone advice service and a central contact point for all health and social care agencies. Nurses reported that some patients, particularly the elderly, were reluctant to contact a doctor out-of-hours and this delay sometimes led to unnecessary hospital admissions.[74]

Medical co-operatives are a relatively recent development in the United Kingdom, but they are increasing in many countries, paralleling a fall in home visiting. The number of family physicians affiliated with a co-operative varies from 20 to 256 with 70 per cent of co-operatives having less than

100 members. All provide home visits, 98 per cent offer telephone advice, and 97 per cent base consultations. All report a marked shift away from home visiting to telephone advice and base consultations.[75] Reports by Macmillan GP Facilitators in the United Kingdom showed that 'out-of-hours' provision varies greatly and more needs to be done to achieve genuine continuity of care if more people are to be enabled to remain at home.[76,77]

Is one reason why they do not refer patients early enough to palliative care services because doctors perceive a shortage of beds for the terminally ill in hospices and hospitals? The same researchers mentioned above[43] reported that doctors found getting a hospital bed easier than nurses did, but nevertheless felt a hospital was not the best place for a terminally ill patient. Both family physicians and community nurses felt early referral to palliative care services was desirable but none felt it should be at the time of diagnosis. The researchers concluded that more palliative care beds were needed.[62] This question—when should referral to palliative care be made—is an important one. The Glasgow study of physicians and community nurses found that the nurses care for more terminally ill patients than the doctors, but both agreed that referral to palliative care should be 'when the family cannot cope'. Nurses preferred earlier referral than the doctors to reduce the suffering of relatives. Does their involvement with relatives in the home better qualify the nurses to recognize distress at an earlier stage?[63] A UK study of the work of community nurses found that the 'hands-on' aspects of it appeared to dominate, but they saw themselves as giving emotional support to both patients and families.[78]

It is well recognized that there is poor correlation between the assessment of symptoms by patients and their attending professionals.[79] In the same way, there is little relation between the reports by the patients of their symptoms and the assessment of their suffering by the relatives, the latter usually perceiving the patient to have more pain and anxiety than is the case.[80,81] When asked about the care they received and who provided it, 64 per cent of patients in one major study reported problems with washing and dressing, 78 per cent with cooking, 87 per cent with housework, 36 per cent with mobility, 32 per cent with eating and drinking, 45 per cent with taking medication, and 9 per cent with catheter care. Ninety per cent were attended by community nurses, 60 per cent by specialist palliative care nurses, 63 per cent by their doctor, and 39 per cent by a social worker. Thirty-seven per cent rated their professional carers as poor sources of emotional help and support for their relatives.[82] The question all doctors should ask when reviewing a case after a person's death is 'could the patient have been cared for at home?'[83] It is salutary to learn the views of surviving relatives after terminal care for a loved one and to review records.[84] One such review of 401 patients in Italy found that 76 per cent died at home, pain control was good and better than non-pain symptom control, that invasive procedures were carried out on 56 per cent at home (75 per cent in hospital), and 25 per cent were deliberately rendered pharmacologically unconscious in the final 12 h of life.[14] This contrasts with a Canadian report of few patients being sedated in the final weeks of life.[85]

Availability of nursing equipment

Home care usually necessitates having equipment such as commodes, back rests, special mattresses, syringe drivers, and even suction machines available.[86] If they cannot readily be obtained or borrowed, the problems involved in nursing the terminally ill patient can be considerable. Sometimes they are available but not accessed early enough.[87] Of course, there are other pieces of equipment that, while not essential, can improve the patient's comfort (see Table 4).

Availability of community nurses

In most Western countries, such nurses are available but whether or not they have been trained in, and feel confident and competent in, palliative care is another matter.[67,71] What is known is that keeping a terminally ill person at home increases their workload by well over 100 per cent, a fact that has major staffing and budgetary implications.[86] Several reports say that 24-h availability is essential.[76] A UK study of their place in home palliative care suggests that most such nurses see their main role as 'hands-on' nursing, but their contribution to emotional and social care can be considerable.[78]

Table 4 Useful (non-essential) equipment for home care

Radio, audio- and videotapes, and CDs
Head phone or pillow headpiece
Room-to-room communication aid or alarm system
Bath aids
Communication aids
Liquidizer
Commode
Wheelchair
Hoist
Hospital (adjustable height) bed
Laptop trays
Cushion/pressure-relieving mattress
Incontinence supplies
Elevated toilet seat
Sheepskin covers for bed and chair
Small bedside table
Electric fan
Deodorizer

Societal attitudes

Little research appears to have been done on this but it must be taken into account. The more the trend is towards fewer home deaths and more in hospitals, hospices, and nursing home, the less does the public expect to have anyone cared for at home. It has ceased to be 'the norm'. In the same way, family physicians and community nurses, while caring for people spending 90 per cent of their last year at home, will have less and less experience of caring for people in the *final* weeks and days of life.[88] It has been estimated that in the Western world few people under the age of 45 have suffered a bereavement or seen a dead body. They have nevertheless seen thousands of horrific, usually unnatural, deaths on film and television.

The spectrum of suffering of home-based patients

Patients with malignant disease

There is no denying that patients at home suffer from a wide spectrum of pain and other symptoms, all of which will at some time or other call for medical attention and all of which are amenable to good palliative care. Sadly, many studies have shown inadequate control of pain in patients who have subsequently been transferred for in-patient care[3,16,89,90] (see Table 5).

A 1995 study of 2074 cancer deaths in the United Kingdom showed that at some stage in the final year 88 per cent had pain, described as very distressing in 66 per cent, and 61 per cent were still in pain in their final week of life.[3] Partial pain relief was achieved in 47 per cent when treated by the family physician, but in only 35 per cent when treated in hospital. More than 50 per cent had anorexia, constipation, dry mouth, dyspnoea, low mood, or insomnia.

The same researcher in 1991 found that more than 50 per cent of patients had anorexia, dyspnoea, pain, insomnia and, depression in the final week of life.[49] Another study, this time by a family physician, found that 6 per cent of patients receiving palliative care at home had pain and 20 per cent of his patients in hospital had severe unrelieved pain before the final phase

Table 5 The spectrum of suffering in cancer and cardiac patients

Symptoms	Cancer patients (%)	Cardiac patients (%)
Pain	75	78
Breathlessness	40	61
Anorexia	75	43
Constipation	75	37
Nausea/vomiting	45	32
'Mental' symptoms	45	59
Convulsions/fits	10	—
Fungating lesions	5	—
Diarrhoea	4	—

Table 6 The suffering of cancer patients in India

Symptom	No. of patients	%
Pain	439	100
Weakness	365	83
Sleeplessness	340	79
Weight loss	314	71
Anorexia	212	48
Constipation	185	42
Nausea	160	36
Cough	152	35
Heartburn	131	30
Dysphagia	125	28
Sore mouth	116	26
Breathlessness	100	23
Vomiting	83	19

Reproduced from ref. 171.

of the illness.(89) Forty per cent of the patients at home had pain severe enough to merit admission, but once admitted *the percentage with pain remained unchanged.*

Terminally ill people are selective about what they reveal and to whom. Sixty per cent of concerns remain unreported and concerns about appearance, the future, and loss of independence are withheld for 80 per cent of the time under care.(56) One study showed that trained nurses only registered 40 per cent of concerns disclosed to them and that less than 20 per cent of concerns were identified appropriately. Perhaps surprisingly, hospice nurses are bad at identifying and reporting anxiety and depression.(91–93)

Patients with non-malignant disease

Traditionally, hospice care/palliative care in the West has been almost exclusively for those with malignant disease. Stroke patients have already been referred to in this chapter.(59) The same research team found that non-cancer patients were more likely to have symptoms extending over 6 months, but cancer patients were perceived as suffering more.(94) They also studied 3696 patients with non-malignant disease and interviewed their relatives 10 months after the deaths. By scoring the number and severity of symptoms, they estimate that 16.8 per cent of people who die of non-malignant disease may need specialist palliative care. This would amount to an increase of at least 79 per cent in the workload of specialist palliative care services.(95)

A study of 66 deaths from *heart disease* found that 54 per cent died in hospital, 30 per cent in their own homes, and 15 per cent in nursing homes or elsewhere. Half were said to have known or deduced how ill they were, most having deduced it. Thirty-nine per cent died without an informal carer present. More than one-fourth had wanted to die earlier, this wish being associated with older age and severity of symptoms. Like many malignancies, chronic heart disease has a 50 per cent 5-year life expectancy. The authors of the paper suggest that such patients should receive specialist palliative care and benefit from its communication skills just as cancer patients do,(88) a view also expressed in a Canadian study.(96)

Patients with chronic heart and pulmonary disease

McCarthy, looking at the suffering of people dying from *heart disease*, found that dyspnoea and low mood were experienced by more than half (see Table 5). Perhaps that was not surprising nor was the number distressed by anxiety, constipation, nausea and vomiting, urinary and faecal incontinence. What *was* startling in the report was how inadequately their suffering had been relieved. There had been little or no symptom control for 35 per cent with pain, 31 per cent with constipation, 2 per cent with dyspnoea, and 24 per cent with nausea and vomiting. In spite of that they reported satisfaction with the care staff.(97) Another study has shown that the concerns of palliative care patients and cardiac patients attending a cardiac clinic are simply not being met.(98) Perhaps, not surprisingly, the problems experienced by patients with chronic pulmonary disease are very similar to those of cancer patients and every bit as deserving of good palliative care.(99)

Patients with dementia

Until recently, palliative care seems to have neglected patients with *dementia.* They and their carers face many problems. A study of 170 such patients found that 83 per cent mental confusion, 72 per cent urinary incontinence, 64 per cent pain, 61 per cent low mood, 61 per cent constipation, and 57 per cent loss of appetite. They were seen less often by their family physicians than cancer patients and their relatives rated the doctor's assistance less highly. They needed more help at home than cancer patients and received more social services. Seventy-eight per cent of relatives of dementia patients and 64 per cent of relatives of cancer patients said they had come to terms with the patient's death. Once again it was concluded that such people would benefit from specialist palliative care.(95) In both Sweden and the United Kingdom, there are now specialist palliative care units exclusively for patients with dementia.

Rather than focusing almost exclusively on palliative care in Western countries, it might be interesting here to look at statistics from India, which reveal an almost identical spectrum of physical problems.(100,101) It is interesting that both dyspnoea and constipation are less of a problem in India than in the West. As everywhere pain heads the list. Not appearing on the Indian list are 'fits' or convulsions occurring in 10 per cent of patients in the West (Table 6).

Problems specific to home care

Though there are no symptoms that are only seen at home and never in hospital and vice versa, there are many problems that assume greater importance or are encountered more frequently in the home. They include:

- Anxiety because there are no professionals near at hand, as there would be in hospital, to allay fears or explain symptoms.
- Medications are given by untrained people who cannot be expected to be as reliable in this matter as hospital nurses would be. Particularly in the case when liquid medications have to be measured. Relatives can be very anxious lest they are responsible for the deterioration or even the death of the patient as a result of their administering a prescribed drug. It is easy to forget that most terminally ill patients are on several drugs, said to be on average 4, but ranging from 0–11.(48,102) Administering such complex drug regimens must be daunting for many relatives.
- In many parts of the world there still exists what has been termed *opiophobia*—fear on the part of lay carers (and even some doctors it must be admitted) that administering opioids for pain will lead to 'addiction' and even criminal behaviour to feed the 'habit'. There is much anecdotal evidence that, even when the opioids have been prescribed by a trusted doctor after careful and reassuring explanation, relatives may not administer them

to the patient because of their deep-rooted fears. Overcoming this calls for the closest collaboration between doctor and nurse or the added reassurance a specialist in palliative medicine or clinical pharmacy might bring. (See Chapter 15.9.)

- The patient can soon be fatigued by visitors whose numbers cannot be controlled as in hospital.
- Cooking smells are more evident at home than in a hospital, worsening any nausea.
- There is often subliminal pressure on patients to eat what has been prepared for them so as not to upset caring relatives whereas in hospital food can be refused.
- Patients may not report all they are suffering so as not to add to the anxiety of the relatives and, as we have seen, relatives may perceive the patient having more pain or anxiety than is actually the case.(61,80,103,104) However, other papers have suggested that the perceptions of relatives are valid and valuable.(65)
- There may be a greater 'conspiracy of silence' in the home than would be seen in hospital, with all parties trying to protect each other and seldom feeling free to express their true emotions.
- Relatives often report feeling very inadequate for the task of caring at home, not knowing how to make the patient comfortable, unsure how to lift or assist the patient, or help with bathing or feeding. Time spent teaching and demonstrating such care is never wasted(105) (discussed later in this chapter).
- Relatives are often anxious about 'emergencies', not being sure what constitutes an emergency, not knowing whether or not to inform/call in the professionals. What is 'normal' or to be expected has to be explained to them in preparation for such an eventuality.

None of these problems is insurmountable. They can be handled by members of the primary care team or, very helpfully, by specialist palliative care nurses called in for this purpose. Better still is a 'relatives group meeting' held in the palliative care unit to which carers can come to share experiences and have everything explained and demonstrated to them. As is so many situations, finding that others are experiencing the same as you can be helpful and reassuring.

The quality of care in the home

If we accept that palliative care is the relief of suffering (physical, psychosocial, and spiritual), we have to recognize that much of it is subjective and not readily amenable to objective measurement. We must, therefore, evaluate the care given in terms of both the views expressed by the patients themselves and their relatives, and by the professional assessment of their clinicians. It must be asked if we can trust the views of relatives, bearing in mind that they too are probably tired, very stressed, and not likely to be objective when commenting on the suffering of their loved ones. One writer has suggested that we should regard families as 'secondary patients', as their need for attention and support is great.(106) This has been researched.

There is strong evidence that many terminally ill patients continue to suffer pain at home even under treatment and when all the necessary drugs are available and accessible.(54) The study of 2074 patients in the final year of life, a study already quoted, found that 88 per cent had pain, described as very distressing in 66 per cent and still present even in the final week of life by 61 per cent.(107) Another researcher found 40 per cent of patients at home had pain severe enough to merit hospital admission and in 6 per cent it was totally unrelieved at home.(89) In Italy, it was found that 25 per cent still had pain in the final week of life.(90) In London, Hinton found that 11 per cent of patients at home had severe symptoms, predominantly pain and dyspnoea.(30) Another London study showed that of those for whom in-patient admission was requested by their family physicians 84 per cent had pain.(52) An interesting paper found that cancer pain management at home offered by the family physician was better than that under an oncologist.(107)

At the heart of palliative care are good communications, between the care professionals and the patient and relatives, and between the professionals themselves. These too seem to leave much to be desired.(108–113)

Are patients and relatives satisfied with home care?

Though most patients and their relatives seem reluctant to complain about the quality of the care and only mention deficiencies when invited to do so as part of research studies, their criticisms are important. Palliative care is, after all, a consumer-driven branch of medicine. Their views and comments are important.

Overall, patient satisfaction with the care received is often low.(73,114–117) One study found that 50 per cent thought hospital care had been inadequate for two reasons. Nurses were too busy, and communications about illness and treatment was also poor. Twenty per cent who had had contact with generalist community nurses were dissatisfied with their care because it lacked continuity. Twenty-seven per cent were dissatisfied with the family physician, 15 per cent who needed help at night had difficulty getting it, and 52 per cent needed equipment at home.(49) Another study found that 51 per cent of carers were unable to get all the information they wanted about the patient's condition.(118) Yet another study, this time of 1858 patients, found 52 per cent were satisfied with the community nurses, only 39 per cent with hospital doctors and 47 per cent with their family physicians.(119) The study of an ethnic minority population, already cited, found overall assessment of care rated as excellent by 58 per cent, care by the family physician fair or poor in 50 per cent, with 28 per cent finding communications easy with the doctor but 30 per cent rating him or her as unsympathetic. Only 38 per cent had been offered specialist home care but of these 83 per cent rated it as excellent.(67)

This chapter is primarily concerned with care at home, but how patients feel about their occasional hospital visits impinges on that care. A study of their views, published in 2000, reported poor transport arrangements, having to miss meals because of investigations or procedures being done, and having to give their personal details to different doctors and nurses on a single visit.(120) Cardiac patients receiving palliative care complained that their needs were not being met.(98) The satisfaction, or otherwise, with their care of first-generation black Caribbeans and white patients in London was reported by Koffman.(68)

A report on a family practice questionnaire found almost 100 per cent satisfaction with care received within a hospice. Forty per cent of those cared for in the 'community hospital' (a local hospital staffed by family physicians and general nurses) said that care could have been better in terms of communication, quality of nursing, and bereavement support though, to be fair, it has to be remembered that the nurse : patient ratio that was present was that of a general hospital and not a hospice/specialist palliative care unit.(116)

A report from an industrial city in the United Kingdom found only one-fourth of patients grateful to their family physician, 34 per cent critical of care citing poor communications, lack of resources, and not being given basic information.(115) Nurses are called in too late and necessary equipment is not always provided at home.(87) It is also reported that doctors are less prepared to visit elderly patients discharged from hospitals than younger ones.(121,122)

It must not be thought that it is only the consumers who express dissatisfaction with the provision of palliative care. Many doctors and nurses recognize deficiencies in their skills and in the care they offer.(123–128) One problem for them is that they see relatively few terminally patients whose suffering taxes their palliation skills.(89,129) A study of 87 physicians and 64 nurses working in primary care in Catalonia, Spain, expressed widespread dissatisfaction with the quality of palliative care they were giving and recognized the scope for its improvement.(130)

A study by a group of Italian doctors, looking at referrals to palliative care services, blames colleagues for too many late referrals leading to a mean survival under palliative care of only 37.5 days.[131] McWhinney, a professor of family medicine in Canada, suggests that family doctors can be classified as those who are reactive and the pro-active, those who deal with what has already happened, and those who try to anticipate what might happen. He believes that palliative care requires doctors to be pro-active.[132,133] The skills of anticipating what might happen and what care the patient might need are seldom taught in medical school. In spite of the amount of time allocated to palliative care in UK medical schools, newly qualified doctors report lack of confidence in communicating, breaking bad news, and hands-on care of the dying and many asked for changes in the curriculum.[102]

However, the picture is not all doom and gloom. A Scottish study found good management of pain with opioids without resort to specialist advice, and appropriate use of local hospices.[134] The number of patients referred to specialist palliative home care services and the number of doctors and nurses enrolling for training in palliative care bear testimony to the commitment of physicians and community nurses to improve the care they provide.

Why is palliative care in the home sometimes unsatisfactory?

Though little research has been done on this, some conclusions can be drawn from the papers already cited and the comments and observations of professionals working in this field.

Lack of professional experience and expertise

The average family physician has under his care at anyone time relatively few patients needing palliative care and even fewer who will have symptoms of such magnitude and severity as to seriously test his ability. Even the number of malignancies he diagnoses is smaller than many might think and most of them have several years prognosis. It is estimated that a family doctor in the United Kingdom or North America will diagnose one or two new cases of bronchogenic carcinoma each year, one new breast carcinoma every 2 years, one colonic carcinoma every 3 years, one gastric carcinoma every 5 years, and one childhood malignancy in a professional lifetime. Maintaining competence is difficult when so few cases are seen.

Naturally, the picture varies from country to country across the globe. Whereas naso-pharyngeal carcinoma is uncommon in the West, a doctor in Hong Kong or China will expect to encounter many. Likewise, a doctor in Southern Africa will see more with primary hepatoma than colleagues elsewhere. The final weeks and days of life can be particularly distressing for the patient and challenging to the caring relatives and the professionals. The trend towards fewer home deaths can only serve to further diminish professional confidence and competence at his time.

This relative lack of experience has to be seen in the context of changing patterns of work in family medicine/primary care. Home visiting is decreasing in the United Kingdom and Europe as has happened to a greater extent in the United States and Canada.[56,135] However, patients and their relatives often describe the quality of their doctor in terms of home visiting rather than his ability to relieve suffering.[136] In the United Kingdom, it is now becoming unusual for a family physician to do house visits at night, that responsibility having been delegated to 'emergency doctor' services of one kind or another. They are staffed by experienced doctors but not only have they had no previous contact with the patient and family, for security reasons they do not usually carry sufficient injectable opioids with them for palliative medicine emergencies. In the United States, patients are encouraged to attend local hospital Emergency Rooms when a palliation problem arises at night, raising problems of transport, heightened anxiety, unfamiliar doctors, and nurses, all at a time when everything was being done to keep the patient at home.

It must not be assumed that all doctors regard care and support of relatives as important. Some give it low priority. One study found that only 26 per cent thought it very important and 25 per cent felt it was not important at all, while others again stated that support of relatives was not their responsibility.[137]

Paucity of professional education and training (see Section 20)

Until recently, most doctors qualified without ever being taught about palliative care.[127] This is slowly improving in countries such as the United Kingdom, where a study of 450 randomly selected family physicians were asked about their training in pain and symptom control, bereavement, the use of syringe drivers, at different stages of their career—when they were clinical medical students, junior hospital doctors, family medicine registrars (trainees), and finally family physicians. In their earlier years one-fourth had been taught nothing at all. They recalled much more formal training as registrars and some training as principals in family medicine.[138] The situation is also said to be improving in the United States, some countries of Western Europe, Scandinavia, Australia, New Zealand, and Hong Kong.[139–141] A major Canadian study looking at the perceptions of family medicine residents on entering their residency and on leaving found equally high commitment to palliative care and expressions of concern about pain and dyspnoea management.[141,142] However, in spite of the time allocated to palliative medicine training in the UK curriculum, junior doctors still lack confidence in communicating and hands-on care and want many changes in their curriculum, according to a report published in 2001.[143] There is certainly no shortage of texts on palliative care and pain management written with the needs of family doctors in mind.[144–147]

Sadly there remain vast areas of the world where doctors have never been taught any of the necessary clinical skills in this field. Except in countries where specific training is given to doctors and nurses intending to work in the community, most doctors and nurses hone all their clinical skills in hospitals. They are, therefore, unfamiliar with how symptoms present in the home, the tensions which exist there, the coping ability and strategies of relatives, and the many other subtleties encountered there. Another difference between hospital and home care is that in the former medications are given by nurses who understand the importance of precise drug dosages and correct timing of administration, whereas at home it is in the hands of equally caring relatives who are usually untrained in such responsibilities and often daunted by them. The result is that often doses are not correct, some tablets are missed, and the rationale behind the treatment regimen is ill understood. Into this complex situation must be factored the anxiety and sense of inadequacy so often experienced and expressed by the relatives who in the home are the principal carers.[56] The inadequacy of nursing education resembles that of doctors and has been noted already.[71]

Changes in societal attitudes

Other changes are taking place in our society. As already noted, many people have reached middle age before they witness their first death or see a dead body, though they may have seen thousands die on film and television. Until very recently it was seen as undesirable, almost unacceptable, for someone to be cared for at home until death, even when the care given was excellent and the patient had expressed a wish to remain at home, in stark contrast to 75 years ago when 70 per cent of deaths occurred at home. Relatives report considerable pressure from neighbours and friends for them to have the patient admitted. To some extent this is now changing, largely as a result of Hospice at Home services.

However, contrary to what people expect and have every right to expect, care is not necessarily better in hospitals. There is abundant evidence that suffering there can be as bad as at home or even worse in spite of the availability of doctors, nurses, and sophisticated equipment.[14,49,67,89,90,117]

Drug and equipment availability

Drug availability, or rather non-availability, can be a factor militating against effective home caring in some communities. In many countries, the necessary opioids are only available in tertiary referral hospitals, and never obtainable locally in the community. Patients, or relatives acting on their behalf, have to travel vast distances (in one country over 1000 miles) to obtain supplies for the next 30 days. In others, there has been imposed an

Table 7 Essential equipment for home care

Firm mattress (a bed is not essential)
Anti-pressure sore pads/mattress
Feeding cup and spoons
Medicine measuring cup/syringe
Duvet or blankets
Air freshener
Supply of ice cubes
Commode
Male urinal
Back rest/triangular pillow
Bedside table or equivalent
Electric pad/hot water bottle
Night lamp/candle
Chair for carer

opioid dose ceiling when drugs are prescribed by a family physician but not when prescribed in a hospital. In yet other countries, not only are the strong opioids not available, neither are the weak opioids of the codeine group and several of the other drugs used in modern palliative care.

In many countries, an even more basic a reason for good palliative care not being possible in the patient's home is the total lack of doctors and nurses working in the community even in simple rural clinics. Government policy in some developing countries has been to build state-of-the art hospitals in major cities, usually staffed by ex-patriate professionals who often have no knowledge of palliative care.

The lack of equipment to facilitate nursing has already been noted. (See Table 7.)

What do home-based patients have a right to expect at home?

Skilled palliation

With the knowledge now available to us it is unacceptable for any patient to be left in pain or with any other treatable symptom. If a family physician or community nurse has a patient whose suffering, whatever its nature, is proving difficult or impossible to relieve they must be able to contact a specialist for advice, or even a home visit. Universal availability of skills and the necessary resources can only be achieved with improved professional education, heightened public awareness of what is possible, and political willingness to make resources available and to facilitate developments in care provision. These are all well recognized by family physicians themselves.(148)

It goes without saying that palliation of symptoms is not sufficient, important as it is. The patient has to be enabled to feel 'safe', a word often used when care is good, strange as it may sound coming from someone with a mortal illness. Making this possible will entail more than addressing psychosocial issues and spiritual problems. It will call for imaginative advice on how best to adapt the home so that the patient may have as full a life as possible with the minimum of dependency on others, remembering that terminally ill people complain more about feeling a burden on their relatives than about almost anything else.

Equipment found to be almost essential and other equipment found useful but not essential are shown in Tables 4 and 7.

Skilled management of emergencies in the home

No matter how effective palliative care has been until then, if any emergency is not handled skilfully and appropriately care in the home will soon come to an end. Doctors and nurses must be ready to cope with the following emergencies encountered in palliative care, wherever the patient is:(149)

- acute 'break through' pain, whatever its cause;
- acute paranoia, confusion, or panic attacks;
- malignant hypercalcaemia;
- pathological fractures;
- haemorrhage;
- superior vena caval obstruction;
- spinal cord compression;
- acute urinary retention;
- acute intestinal obstruction;
- chronic intestinal obstruction.

All are dealt with in this textbook but their occurrence in the home presents special challenges. Some can be managed in the home while others may call for admission. A knee-jerk response, immediately transferring the patient to hospital may sometimes be inappropriate. On the other hand, it has always to be remembered that it will be the relatives who have to do the additional caring with all its associated anxiety, uncertainty, and tiredness. The closest co-operation between doctor and nurse, giving the same explanations and reassurance, is essential.

There is no substitute for family physicians skilled in palliative medicine and the management of its emergencies, but one innovation to deal with emergencies which has been tried and found useful in some specialist palliative care services is the *Rapid Response Service*.(32) When an emergency develops the family physician, who may never have encountered such a situation before, calls for this service and as soon as possible the patient is visited at home by a palliative medicine specialist and a palliative care nurse specialist, with the necessary drugs and equipment to respond. After whatever necessary treatment that can be given in the home has been given the doctor may leave the nurse there and between them they monitor the situation with the family physician for the next day or so.

Drugs that might be needed for emergencies, and should therefore be readily available to the family physician, are shown in Table 8.

Table 8 Essential drugs needed for palliative care in the home

Injection Diamorphine 30 mg or injection Morphine 30 mg
Injection Dexamethasone 4 mg/2 ml
Injection Hyoscine butylbromide 20 mg
Injection Midazolam
Injection Haloperidol
Injection Lignocaine 2%
Injection Metoclopramide
Diazepam rectal solution or suppositaries

Appropriate support for relatives

Many times in this chapter it has been pointed out that the commonest reason for home care failing or coming to an end is the strain experienced by relatives.(150) The importance of the support and understanding given to them by doctors and nurses cannot be exaggerated.(57) Some of their fears, all very understandable, are shown in Table 9.

In hospital relatives are, for most of the time, anxious onlookers. At home they are the principal care givers, a role for which they often feel inexperienced and inept. Every symptom of the patient, every new experience he mentions can add to their anxiety. Often the relatives are elderly, possibly not enjoying good health, and the physical strain of caring for a dying relative, linked with their grief and sense of isolation, can only add to their burden. It is, therefore, imperative that the doctor and nurse, as a team pay

Table 9 Commonest fears expressed by caring relatives at home

Fear of the unknown
Fear of being unable to cope
Fear of becoming exhausted
Fear of hurting the patient
Fear of patient choking or bleeding
Fear of patient having convulsions
Fear of patient dying in the house
Fear of not recognizing signs of death
Fear of wrongly administering drugs

particular attention to the following:

- The relatives must be given every detail of the illness and the treatment and why each drug is being used. What may seem obvious and simple to the professional may not be so for relatives.
- The relatives must be helped to know what lies ahead, what symptoms may occur, what complications there may be, and how they will be managed. As has so often been said 'Fear of the unknown is infinitely worse than fear of the known'.
- The relatives will appreciate guidance and teaching on how best to care for the loved one, including how to assess their suffering, difficult as that can be for professionals and informal carers.(151) Their instruction might include basic nursing procedures, being taught how to bath and feed an ill person, how to give medication,(152) how to lift and move the patient, how to record pain(128) and other symptoms, and how to respond to crises. It is easy to forget that terminally ill people are usually on several different drugs, some given every 4 h and some once daily—understandably confusing for grieving, tired relatives.

In an unpublished study of 1000 such patients, it was found that only one was on no medication, the others taking, on average, 4–5 different drugs each day, some taking up to 11.(48,153) Relatives are conscious of their responsibility in giving potent medications to the patient and often say how they dread giving the last dose before the person dies, fearing that it might hasten the death. A medication chart can help them to remember when drugs are to be given and their indications. It is a useful tool for all home care but is essential for palliative care in the home. See chapter 15.9 for an example of a medication chart.

- The relatives must regularly be asked how they themselves are feeling and how they feel they are coping. It is easy for their health to be taken for granted and their tiredness and strain to be overlooked. Encouragement and praise are needed at all times.
- Time must be set aside for relatives to ask questions and no matter how trivial they may seem they must be answered honestly. It is often reported that relatives lost faith in the doctor because he was obviously not being totally honest. A simple thing to recommend to informal carers is to use a notebook, at one end of which they write the advice and suggestions made by the visiting doctors and nurses immediately after their visits and at the other end the questions that cross their minds that they must mention to the doctors and nurses when they next visit the home.

There are several books written exclusively for lay carers to enable them to care for terminally ill relatives at the home.(154,155)

- The value of a *Family Conference* can hardly be exaggerated. In hospital practice one is often aware of tensions between relatives and siblings and occasionally they affect the patient. In the home they can be so divisive and destructive that the possibility of good care at home can soon be brought to an unpleasant end. Some siblings feel territorial, others feel protective about the patient whilst others resent the arrival of a long-lost relative who has had no contact with the patient for years and suddenly appears and attempts to take control of the situation. Those who have done most of the caring and carried heavy responsibility during the final illness understandably resent what they see as intrusion. Often, one relative wants to challenge the doctors about the diagnosis, what the patient has been told, the treatment, and day-to-day management. In the home the doctor or nurse is met with palpable tension, sometimes open hostility from one sibling, and with different people all asking the same questions because they cannot trust each other. Something has to be done if home care is not to come to an abrupt and unhappy end. A family conference may be the answer, daunting as it may sound to anyone unfamiliar with the technique.

  If at all possible the doctor (family physician or palliative medicine specialist) and nurse should conduct the meeting *together*, demonstrating their professional collaboration and shared approach to the challenges they all face. Each family member is urged to attend 'so that together we can be sure that father/mother/John gets the best possible care'. It is explained that the session will last for, say, 1 h and no longer. When everyone has gathered the doctor chairs the session, thanks everyone for coming, emphasizing that what everyone wants is the best for the patient. He then gives a brief summary of the patient's medical problem, its treatment up till then, and the treatment he is now receiving and the rationale for it. It is all explained in a totally patient-centred way. Having told all present that only when he has finished will each in turn be asked to say what most troubles or upsets them; he then invites them in turn, offering to answer questions but urging that everyone is totally honest about how they feel, even if it means saying upsetting things about others present. This is the cathartic time of the meeting. Often, it is the first time they have realized how dysfunctional they are, how they are annoying each other and almost ignoring the patient, and how, inadvertently, they are making it harder for the doctor and nurse to help them. Finally, when they have all got everything off their chest the doctor sums up and expresses his professional view on how they can work together. He asks if they can devise a roster for helping in the house, for nursing, for shopping, for giving the medication, etc. Finally, said almost as an afterthought, he asks if they will appoint one of their number to be the 'go-between', someone who will ask the questions and convey information from the doctor or nurse back to the group 'so that everyone knows what is happening and how they can help in the most effective way'. They are then thanked, left to continue their conversations together and the doctor and nurse leave.
- Another way of assisting the family to help the home-based patient is by using a *Respite Relief Team*. This has been tried in several centres, some impressed with the benefits and continuing to offer it, others disappointed for one reason or another. It is, in effect, the provision of a comprehensive service for a few days rather than an advisory one, to keep a patient at home by giving the relatives a break from their round-the-clock hard work and responsibility. When the situation at home seems to be deteriorating because of the weariness of the carers the family physician discusses the situation with the CPCS. They then arrange for palliative care-trained nurses to be with the patient day and night for 3 or 4 days, bringing with them whatever nursing equipment might be needed and backed up by a palliative medicine specialist to offer advice and support to the nurses and the family doctor. Sometimes the decision to use this service, or to have the patient admitted for respite is often made too late for anyone to benefit. Indeed, it has been shown that 'respite admissions' carry a mortality of over 60 per cent, suggesting that by the time weary carers agree to it the patient is actually terminally ill. Carers apparently see their need for respite as a mark of their failure to cope.

Finally, the doctor and other members of the primary care team should, as a routine, check whether any modifications to the house and sick room would make caring easier and more comfortable (Table 10).

Admission to hospital/hospice must be possible

No matter how strongly the patient and/or relatives say they want care at home, the doctor and nurse must be able to promise that, should the need

Table 10 Home modifications to facilitate home care

Will any of the following facilitate care of the patient at home?	
Creating a bedroom downstairs?	Y/N
Moving the bed nearer a window to look out?	Y/N
Providing a hospital-type bed?	Y/N
Providing a handrail on the stairs?	Y/N
Building a wheelchair ramp at the door?	Y/N
Fitting a shower instead of a bath?	Y/N
Installing a stair lift?	Y/N
Providing a TV set for the bedroom?	Y/N
Is there a comfortable chair for relatives in the bedroom?	Y/N
Would a deodorizer/air freshener help?	Y/N

Table 11 Home to hospital transfer check-list

Before a patient is transferred from home to hospital/hospice the following list should be checked:	
Has the transfer been discussed with the patient?	Y/N
Have the patient's questions and any anxieties been addressed as much as they want?	Y/N
Has the transfer been discussed with the relatives?	Y/N
Have they had a chance to air anxieties?	Y/N
Has the receiving doctor been told:	
The primary diagnosis?	Y/N
The secondary diagnoses?	Y/N
The previous treatment?	Y/N
The present treatment?	Y/N
How much the patient understands?	Y/N
What anxieties he/she has expressed?	Y/N
What anxieties the relatives have expressed?	Y/N
Has the Community Nurse been told of the transfer?	Y/N
Have Social Services been informed (if relevant)?	Y/N
Has the Palliative Home Care Service been informed?	Y/N

Table 12 Hospital/hospice to home transfer check-list

Has the transfer been discussed with the patient?	Y/N
Has the patient had a chance to ask questions about it?	Y/N
Have the immediate relatives been informed about it?	Y/N
Have their anxieties about it been addressed?	Y/N
Has it been discussed with the family doctor?	Y/N
Has the Community Nurse been informed?	Y/N
Do either the doctor or the nurse have misgivings about it?	Y/N
Has a home assessment been done by Occupational Therapy?	Y/N
Are any home modifications needed?	Y/N
Has an assessment of the patient been done by the OT?	Y/N
Have any necessary aids been provided?	Y/N
Has a medication chart been prepared for the relatives?	Y/N
Have appropriate follow-up arrangements been made?	Y/N
Has a detailed report been prepared for the family doctor?	Y/N
Has transport been arranged for the patient?	Y/N

ever arise, the patient will be able to be admitted to an appropriate inpatient facility, and preferably not in the middle of the night as an emergency. Relatives often relate how reassuring it was to know that, should it be needed, their loved one would be able to go into an in-patient unit where the care would be excellent. It is the 'safety net' or, as others have called it 'the light at the end of the tunnel'. It follows that the patient's preference must be recorded, the admission procedures there be known and, if possible, the admitting unit be given a few days notice of the transfer. Specialist palliative care units, aware as they are of what a frightening experience it must be to being admitted there, often make arrangements for a doctor or nurse to visit the patient in their own home to establish a link. Better still is when the patient is placed under the care of a CPCS in the weeks prior to any possible admission before 'the family is unable to cope'.[43,63]

It is essential that the admitting unit has the fullest possible records on the patient, detailing not only diagnosis, investigations, and all treatment but also what the patient has been told, what he/she appears to know and understand, and what fears or anxieties have been expressed. A useful check-list is shown in Table 11. A so-called Ideal Referral Criteria tool has been field tested in New Zealand.[156]

It need hardly be said that equal care needs to be given to discharge planning when a palliative care patient returns home from an in-patient unit. A similar model check-list is suggested in Table 12.

Where should the patient be admitted?

Here, we assume that a conveniently close hospital or specialist palliative care unit exists. That nearness is important. Dying or going through a crisis with a terminal illness is a lonely enough experience without it having to be without the presence of family and friends because the hospital is so distant and difficult to visit. It is also preferable for the patient to be familiar with it from previous admissions. If the patient has not been in the specialist palliative care unit, perhaps for symptom management or rehabilitation, then the doctor or nurse should ensure that the patient attends the Palliative Care Day Unit both for its inherent benefits and to familiarize the patient with the place before urgent admission is necessary.

Only as a last resort should a terminally ill person be admitted to an acute facility with which they are not familiar, no matter how high its reputation. Not only are all members of staff new to the patient, they are likely as a matter of course to re-investigate, submitting the patient to a battery of expensive, intrusive, and unnecessary tests many of which are not likely to add anything to the quality of the patient's life. A study from the USA found differences between patients referred to palliative care units from academic medical centres and from a non-academic centres.[157] Those from the former were younger, had higher incomes, and were less likely to have Do Not Resuscitate Orders and needed both more medical and nursing care. A Yale study found that it was usually physician factors that determined the patients referred to palliative care and those not.[72]

However, this may not be the case when the hospital has its own *Specialist Hospital Palliative Care Team.* Such teams are now to be found in many of the major hospitals of the United Kingdom and North America and have been shown to reduce the cost of care by enabling shorter stay in acute units. The team can improve patient satisfaction, identify more patient and family needs, and also deal better with them.[158–161] When a hospital palliative care service is first established there is initially a fall in the number of deaths at home but this soon reverts[159] and such a team increases referral to community palliative care teams.[163]

The answer is for the doctor to make contact with his opposite number in the specialist palliative care unit or team and verify that admission will be possible and, at the same time, call in the local palliative care clinical nurse specialist who will, as a matter of routine, maintain contact with the in-patient bed facility.

An alternative to hospital or specialist palliative care unit in the United Kingdom is a nursing home, in essence a private hospital as might be found in many countries. They are usually small, within easy reach of the patient's home, and may be known by repute to the patient and family. They are well staffed with nurses though, unlike their opposite numbers in geriatric or long-stay hospitals, few if any of them are likely to have undertaken further training in palliative care though this situation is changing rapidly.[140,164,165] This is a serious problem and one that presents an important educational challenge.[166] However, one of the few papers published on this showed that the quality of care they offer is good.[167] Occasionally, there are junior doctors but the senior medical staff are, without exception, the local family physicians, a very acceptable thing for most patients. In some countries such as the United Kingdom, there are small community hospitals operated by the Health Service rather than being private, again staffed by family physicians.[168] A study of 12 community-based hospitals and a 12-bedded hospice found differences between patients admitted to a hospice and those admitted to a community hospital. Hospice patients had more challenging problems with pain and symptom management and remained in the hospice for shorter times than the patients admitted to community hospitals. The same study showed that record keeping in the hospital was not as adequate and acceptable as in the hospice.[169,170] Another study based on 106 interviews and 55 questionnaires found almost 100 per cent satisfaction with the hospice whilst 40 per cent felt care in the community hospital could have been better in terms of nursing, communication, and bereavement support. It has to be remembered that the staffing ratio in a community hospital is that of a hospital and not of a palliative care unit.[116] The presence of a community hospital (using that term to describe a small local hospital medically staffed exclusively by local family physicians) has an impact on home deaths, on the use made of the local hospice/palliative care unit, and on the work of the doctors. In a study of 1022 cancer deaths where there was no community hospital to which patients could be sent 29 per cent died at home. On the other hand, when beds were available in a community hospital the percentage of home deaths increased to 41 per cent with a 1 per cent increase in hospice deaths.[158] Presumably people were content to remain at home knowing that, should it be needed, they could be admitted to their neighbourhood hospital.

Ethical issues encountered in palliative care in the home

There are no ethical issues unique to palliative care in the home. However, there are several, listed below, which seem to loom larger or assume greater importance in the home.[171] Readers are referred to Section 3 for a fuller discussion of Ethics in Palliative Medicine.

Treating the patient for the sake of the relatives

This can take the form of administering a drug to the patient so as to reduce the distress of relatives or of administering a drug at the specific request of relatives, ostensibly for the patient's sake. An example of the former is giving hyoscine for the 'death rattle' because it is distressing for the relatives sitting by the bedside. This is probably unethical but is usually justified because it helps the relatives to cope better and may, though it is difficult to be sure, comfort the patient. Much more common is the second example, doing something urged by relatives such as setting up an intravenous infusion because they are sure the patient will die of dehydration, or giving total parenteral nutrition (TPN) because 'he is starving to death'. A common example is the relative who perceives the patient as having agonizing pain and requests higher doses of analgesics or heavy sedation. This can be particularly difficult because the doctor appreciates that the relative sees more of the patient than he does and does not want his patient to suffer, yet, at the same time, he is not persuaded the patient is suffering as much pain as described by the upset relative. It is here that a pain chart can be so useful. It is completed by the patient in respect of each pain and can usefully be regarded as objective evidence of what is otherwise a totally subjective phenomenon.[172] Another example is conceding to the relatives' request for admission because they are sure it is the patient's wish, though no documentary evidence of that exists. Agreeing to these is clearly unethical but the answer lies not in dogmatic refusal to do as requested but in patient explanations of what is happening to the patient (e.g. why he is cachectic or not eating) and why the requested intervention will not only not help, but may even hinder or hurt.

Confidentiality

The guidelines on this are no different from any other time in the care of the patient. No information may be passed on to third parties without the explicit consent of the patient. In the home, it is often assumed that every member of the family and all the friends who come to visit have a right to know every detail. Considerable pressure, albeit well-meaning, can be exerted on the visiting doctor or nurse to discuss information and details that need not be disclosed. Once again it is for the doctor or nurse to discuss with the patient how much can be disclosed and to whom, and thereafter, the situation patiently discussed with family members.

In the home it is often assumed that the family clergyman, rabbi, or other religious adviser has a right to know everything. With the best of intentions, they may then pass on the information to others, for example, during prayers, and so break the pledge of confidentiality given to the patient. No information should be given to them beyond that permitted by the patient.

Maintaining life at all cost

As in hospitals relatives may either plead that more be done to maintain or extend life, or they may suggest that euthanasia would be a more dignified and compassionate way out for the one they love. Both call for the same understanding but firm, informed response from the doctor or nurse. Palliative care is not about either shortening or extending life, nor is it about prolonging the dying process. When confronted by such requests, the family physician or community nurse should always consider whether it might be helpful to invoke the help of a specialist colleague who has probably faced this ethical challenge many times.

Specialist community palliative care services

It should be noted that in the literature such services are still often referred to as 'Home Care Services'. It is now more usual to refer to them as Community Palliative Care Services (CPCS).

In this chapter, reference has frequently been made to specialist CPCS, now a feature of palliative care provision not only in the United Kingdom where they originated but across Europe and North America, Australasia, and some countries of the Asian Pacific rim. They take two forms: Home Care Services where specialist doctors and nurses visit patients in their own homes and offer advice and support to patients, informal carers, and their attending professionals, and Day Care Units, often called Day Hospices. Most services care for people irrespective of their underlying pathology, some are exclusively for cancer patients; more recently, services have been developed exclusively for AIDS patients in Toronto, San Francisco, Kampala, South Africa, Edinburgh, and London.[173]

Models of CPCS

There are two models. The *comprehensive care model*, probably originating in Sweden[174–176] and now offered in the United Kingdom as 'Hospice at Home'. It is staffed by nurses and doctors accredited as specialists in palliative care, supported by physiotherapists, occupational therapists, and social workers. At the invitation of a family physician, the team visits the patient and thereafter carries out all the basic nursing not being done by the relatives, manages all the symptom control and psychosocial support, at all times maintaining close contact with the primary care team. The team is qualified and equipped to set up intravenous infusions, perform paracenteses, give blood transfusions and chemotherapy, and do simple nerve blocks in the home.

The *advisory model*, by far the commonest one used, is similarly staffed but does no practical 'hands-on' nursing, but focuses on specialist advice and support, seeing itself as an enabler to the primary care team.

Both have their proponents. The former probably guarantees the patient the highest standards of nursing and medical care as well as a link to the nearest specialist palliative care unit should admission ever become necessary. It runs the risk of marginalizing the members of the primary care team and of de-skilling them. On the other hand, it is a model that might be effective in areas where there are no primary care teams though it is expensive to run because of the highly skilled, highly paid staff.

In some isolated communities in Canada, this 'comprehensive care' model has been tried but there has been no trend to performing procedures in the homes in the cities.[177] It has been tried and well reported upon in Sweden.

The advisory model on the other hand, whilst recognizing the deficiencies often found in primary care, nevertheless also recognizes the genuine commitment of doctors and nurses to provide good palliative care in the home. It sets out to empower and enable the primary care team in what is usually accepted as one of their prime areas of responsibility. Fuller descriptions of the working, the work-load, and the effectiveness of such services have been published in refs 9, 16, 22, 30, 37, 38, 40, 45, 53, 86, 101, 110, 173, 178–187, 203. In the United Kingdom, many CPCS are operated by, or initially funded by, Macmillan Cancer Relief, a major national cancer charity. A comprehensive review of 12 of these services can be found in ref. 187 and their evaluations in refs 189, 190, 206.

Are specialist CPCS useful?

Before answering that important question, it has to be remembered that it tends to be the young, the married, those in severe pain, those with a long prognosis or who are anxious, and those whose relatives are perceived as not coping well who are referred to palliative in-patient units, the others being kept at home under CPCS.[191] From the many papers cited the following conclusions can be drawn:

- Patients and relatives enthusiastically appreciate such services.
- Family physicians greatly appreciate them when the co-operation with them is good.[47] Community nurses appreciate the improved pain control achieved but are initially suspicious of others encroaching into their 'territory'.
- Such services increase the length of time patients can be cared for at home and probably facilitate eventual admission to a specialist palliative care unit.
- When first established, they increase the percentage of deaths at home but this usually falls away again.
- Such services increase referrals to specialist palliative care units.
- What has not been studied in depth but may be the case is that the interest and palliation skills of family physicians are enhanced.

Research is on-going into how to optimize home care for cancer patients.[192]

Day hospices

Those seeking detailed information on day hospices are referred to ref. 193. They are usually based in specialist palliative care units, operate up to 5 day/week usually from 10 a.m. to 4 p.m., and are staffed by equal numbers of professional staff (nurses, physiotherapists, occupational therapists) and specially selected and trained volunteers.[32] Doctors are available to advise on clinical problems on request. The patients, usually first assessed at home after an invitation from the primary care team, are brought to the Day Hospice by volunteer transport and spend the day in creative activities in a homely social atmosphere. Such facilities can be divided, somewhat arbitrarily, into those who see themselves as 'social' and those who regard themselves as 'clinical'. Such a distinction is artificial. A paper on 40 Day Care Services in London, serving a population of 13.75 million, looked at management, staffing, organizational policies, patient numbers, reasons for referral, and special services they offered. The number of places was a mean of 57 per centre, equivalent to 1.77 per 10 000 of population. Thirty of the 40 services had no discharge policy, a few had a waiting list. The mean time for the longest attending patients was 4.5 years. Ninety per cent of the patients had cancer and of the 10 per cent with a non-malignant diagnosis the commonest conditions were AIDS, MND (ALS), and cerebro-vascular accident (stroke). Thirty-four centres were managed by nurses, two by social workers, and the remainder by people from other backgrounds. Most had doctors, nurses, chaplains, managers, aromatherapists, and hairdressers but there was much range between those with occupational therapists, dieticians, social workers, podiatrists, and art therapists.[194] Most common activities were symptom review and needs assessment, bathing, wound care, physiotherapy, hairdressing, and aromatherapy. No significant difference was found between those describing themselves as more medical than social and vice versa.[195] There are wide variations between day hospices and what they provide, often unrelated to need, according to one major study.[196] Most patients attend Day Hospices 2 day/week and appear to benefit from being with people with similar problems in such a positive relaxed environment, where the focus is on quality and value of life rather than on their diagnosis.[197] Having said that the same researchers found that Day Hospice is not fully understood by some patients. There is some evidence that their relatives benefit from having a respite from their caring role and time either to rest or do whatever else they need to do. It also appears that the patients find eventual admission to the in-patient unit less daunting than might otherwise be the case. It has been suggested that day care might be an alternative to in-patient care for some cancer patients, further developing the current practice of giving chemotherapy on an out-patient basis.[198] A review of the literature on Day Hospices can be found in ref. 199. In the United Kingdom, the National Council for Hospice and Specialist Palliative Care services has produced an invaluable occasional paper entitled *Care in the Community for People who are Terminally Ill: Guidelines for Health Authorities and Social Service Departments.*[200]

The relationship between specialists in palliative medicine and family doctors caring for people at home

It is often asked how these two groups of doctors should work together for the good of patients at home. Should the specialists 'take over'? Should the specialist be in charge, directing and co-ordinating the care team? That the two can and should work together very effectively has been demonstrated in several of the papers cited in this chapter. It is also easy to see where tensions could develop and threaten patient-care. One may resent the involvement of the other or see it as a threat, an implied criticism of his knowledge and skills. Often, palliative care is one of the few occasions when specialist and generalist meet, even socially, much of their routine communication being by e-mail or correspondence.

One reason for this chapter being included in this textbook is to demonstrate how caring for a patient at home differs in many respects from care in a hospital. Mutual respect for, and understanding of, the skills and knowledge of each other must be the bedrock of any professional relationship. The specialist brings a wealth of experience and clinical skills in the subject, based on contact with thousands of patients. The family doctor brings to the partnership his encyclopaedic knowledge of the patient and family often extending over very many years, his understanding of the many problems faced by patient and family carers at home, and his ability to mobilize community resources. Much can be achieved by developing better communications, even as simple as referral forms.[156]

Expressed simply, the family doctor should be the co-ordinator of care and leader of the care team. He should invoke the assistance of a specialist colleague when he has little if any experience of the patient's condition or the suffering to be palliated, when first-line treatment has failed to relieve suffering and newer, hopefully more effective but probably more sophisticated, treatment regimens are called for. Though he may have heard of them, it is unlikely he will have used them and for that reason their use must remain the responsibility of the specialist. Few specialists have much experience mobilizing community resources or conducting family conferences and both should remain the responsibility of the generalist. The benefits that have followed the establishment of Macmillan GP Facilitators in the United Kingdom have been considerable. They are experienced family doctors who are paid to work a few hours each week helping colleagues to practice better palliative care, running postgraduate training sessions for them, and fostering communications with specialists.[145,181,190]

Palliative care in the home in developing countries

Inevitably most of the information in this chapter is based on the experience of palliative care provision in the relatively sophisticated countries of the so-called developed world, especially the United Kingdom, Canada, United States, and Australasia. Readers in other parts of the world may have been depressed by it all, knowing that in their country there may not only be no palliative care in any form but possibly no primary care doctors, no community nurses, no access to opioids, no interest in palliative care amongst their colleagues. They may be tempted to ask if palliative care has to be as sophisticated as this chapter, indeed this textbook, would lead one to believe. The answer is an emphatic 'No'.

Those who would like information on services in developing countries such as India, Mongolia, Pakistan, Saudi Arabia, Swaziland, and South America are invited to see refs 101, 201–202. What then are the basic essentials needed if the benefits of good palliative care are to be made available for all who need them, whether in their own homes or in hospitals?

- Accessible, affordable doctors with a commitment to palliative care principles. By the time a patient needs palliative care they should never have to travel great distances to get medical help, nor should there be financial, cultural, or social barriers to receiving good care. Probably more important than the academic qualifications of the doctors is their interest in palliative care and their willingness to learn its principles.
- Access to available and affordable drugs, in particular the opioids, dispensed under strict but professionally informed legal conditions.
- Support and assistance, including simple instruction in home nursing, to enable loving relatives to care as they want to.
- A palliative care unit is desirable but not essential. Hospital doctors, with a commitment to palliative care principles, whatever their speciality, can greatly encourage and facilitate care in the home and provide support for the members of the primary care team.

References

1. *Specialist Palliative Care: A Statement of Definitions.* Occasional paper No. 8. London: National Council for Hospices and Specialist Palliative Care Services, 1995.
2. **Higginson, I.** et al. (1998). Where do cancer patients die? Ten year trends in the place of death of cancer patients in England. *Palliative Medicine* **12**, 353–65.
3. **Carrol, D.S.** (1998). An audit of place of death of cancer patients in a semi-rural Scottish practice. *Palliative Medicine* **12**, 51–5.
4. **Karlsen, S. and Addington-Hall, J.** (1998). How do cancer patients who die at home differ from those who die elsewhere? *Palliative Medicine* **12**, 279–87.
5. **Hinton, J.** (1994). Which patients with terminal cancer are admitted from home care? *Palliative Medicine* **8**, 197–210.
6. **Higginson, I.J. and Gupta, S.** (2000). Place of care in advanced cancer: a qualitative literature review of patient preferences. *Journal of Palliative Medicine.* (The majority of people prefer to be cared for at home and to die at home.)
7. **Hinton, J.** (1996). Services given and help perceived during home care for terminal cancer. *Palliative Medicine* **10**, 125–35.
8. **Ward, A.W.M.** *Home Care Services for the Terminally Ill.* Sheffield: Medical Care Research Unit, University of Sheffield, 1985.
9. **Baar, F.** (1999). Palliative care for the terminally ill in the Netherlands; the unique role of nursing homes. *European Journal of Palliative Care* **6** (5), 169–72.
10. **Grande, G.E.** et al. (2000). Factors associated with death at home. *Palliative Medicine* **14**, 244 (Interim report).
11. **Doyle, D.** (1991). A home care service for terminally ill patients in Edinburgh. *Health Bulletin (Edinburgh)* **49**, 14–23.
12. **Constantini, M.** et al. (1993). Palliative home care and place of death among cancer patients: a population-based study. *Palliative Medicine* **7**, 323–31.
13. **Loven, D.** et al. (1990). Place of death of cancer patients in Israel: the experience of a 'home care' programme. *Palliative Medicine* **4**, 299–304.
14. **Peruselli, C.** et al. (1999). Home palliative care for terminal cancer patients: A survey of the final week of life. *Palliative Medicine* **13**, 233–41.
15. **Toscani, F.** et al. (1991). Death and dying perceptions and attitudes in Italy. *Palliative Medicine* **5**, 334–43.
16. **Toscani, F. and Mancini, C.** (1989). Inadequacies of care in far-advanced cancer patients: a comparison between home and hospital in Italy. *Palliative Medicine* **4**, 31–6.
17. **Mercadente, S.** et al. (2000). The impact of home palliative care on symptoms in advanced cancer patients. *Support Cancer Care* **8**, 307–10.
18. **Kamel, H.** et al. (2001). Utilizing pain assessment scales increases the frequency of diagnosis of pain. *Journal of Pain and Symptom Management* **21** (6), 450–55. (Most symptoms improve but not weakness.)
19. **Schrijvers, D.** et al. (1998). The place of death of cancer patients in Antwerp (correspondence). *Palliative Medicine* **12**, 133–5.
20. **Van Den Eynden, B.** et al. (1999). Factors determining the place of palliative fare: a longitudinal explanatory design study. *Palliative Medicine* **13**, 515 (Interim report).
21. **Wiles, J.** et al. (1999). Improving palliative care services: a pragmatic model for evaluating services and assessing unmet need. *Palliative Medicine* **13**, 131–7.
22. **Gomas, J.M.** (1993). Palliative care at home—a reality or 'mission impossible'? *Palliative Medicine* **7** (Suppl. 2), 45–59.
23. **Sahlberg-Blom, E.** et al. (1998). The last month of life: continuity, care site and place of death. *Palliative Medicine* **12**, 287–97.
24. **Welin, L., Seiger, A.S., and Furst, C.J.** Dying of cancer in Stockholm. Place of death correlated to socio-demographic factors and diagnosis 1991 and 1996. Geneva. Poster presentation, 6th Congress of the European Association for Palliative Care, 1999.
25. **Mageroy, N.** Personal communication, 2000.
26. **Centeno, C.** et al. (2000). The reality of palliative care in Spain. *Palliative Medicine* **14**, 387–94. [An up-to-date report on the current provision of specialist palliative care in Spain, looking at in-patient units, home care services, and day care (still embryonic).]
27. **Serra-Prat, M.** et al. (2001). Home palliative care as a cost-saving alternative: evidence from Catalonia. *Palliative Medicine* **15**, 271–8.
28. **Izquierdo-Porrera, A.M.** et al. (2001). Predicting place of death of elderly cancer patients followed up by a palliative care unit. *Journal of Pain and Symptom Management* **21** (6), 481–90. (It is mainly medical factors which affect where men die and functional dependency and social support factors which affect where women die.)
29. **Chan, K.S.** Personal communications.
30. **Hinton, J.** (1994). Can home care maintain an acceptable quality of life for patients with terminal cancer and their relatives? *Palliative Medicine* **8**, 183–96.
31. **Dunlop, R.J., Davies, R.J., and Hockley, J.M.** (1989). Preferred versus actual place of death: a hospital support team experience. *Palliative Medicine* **3**, 197–201.
32. **King, M. and MacKenzie, J.** (1999). Evaluation of a hospice rapid response service. *Palliative Medicine* **13**, 509–10 (Interim report).
33. **Levy, B. and Sclare, A.B.** (1976). Fatal illness in general practice. *Journal of the Royal College of General Practitioners* **26**, 303–7. (Ninety per cent of the final year of cancer patients is spent at home.)
34. **Dunlop, R.J. Davies, R.J., and Hockley, J.M.** (1989). Preferred versus actual place of death: a hospital palliative care support team experience. *Palliative Medicine* **3**, 197–201.
35. **Wilson, A.** et al. (1999). Randomised controlled trail of effectiveness of Leicester hospital at home scheme compared with hospital care. *British Medical Journal* **319**, 1542–6.
36. **Haines, A. and Boroff, A.** (1986). Terminal care at home: perspective from general practice. *British Medical Journal* **292**, 1051–3.
37. **Maltoni, M.** et al. (1991). Description of a home care srvice for cancer patients through quantitative indexes of evaluation. *Tumori* **77**, 452–9.
38. **Morch, M.M.** et al. (1999). Thirty years experience with cancer and non-cancer patients in palliative home care. *Journal of Palliative Care* **15**, 43–8.

39. **Herd, E.B.** (1990). Terminal care in a semi-rural area. *Journal of the Royal College of General Practitioners* **40**, 248–51.

40. **McAdam, D.B.** (1985). A review of 715 terminal patients cared for at home by a hospice palliative care service. *Cancer Forum* **5**, 101–4.

41. **Grande, D.E.** et al. (2000). A randomised controlled trial of a hospice at home service for the terminally ill. *Palliative Medicine* **14**, 375–85. (HaH did not lead to more staying at home in the final 2 weeks of life at home but did lead to better care overall, different groups seeing it differently. 194 GPs, 225 community nurses, 144 informal carers of 229 patients all surveyed. CNs thought night cover was better and support for the carers. GPs thought anxiety and depression were less. Informal carers pain and nausea.)

42. **Wilkinson, S.** (2000). Fulfilling patients'wishes: palliative care at home. *International Journal of Palliative Nursing* **6** (5), 212. (Over a 26-month period of data collection, 90 per cent of patients who received care from a Marie Curie nurse achieved a home death.)

43. **Velupillai, T.** et al. (2000). The perceptions of general practitioners and district nurses of the patients' preferred place of death and obstacles preventing this happening. *Palliative Medicine* **14**, 347–8 (Interim report).

44. **Cartwright, A.** (1991). Balance of care for the dying between hospital and the community; perceptions of general practitioners, hospital consultants, community nurses and relatives. *British Journal of General Practice* **41**, 271–4.

45. **Boyd, K.J.** (1993). Palliative care in the community: views of general practitioners and district nurses in London. *Journal of Palliative Care* **9**, 33–7.

46. **Seale, C.** (1992). Community nurses and the care of the dying. *Social Science and Medicine* **34**, 375–82.

47. **McKenna, H.** et al. (1999). Perceptions of GPs and district nurses on the role of hospice home care nurses. *International Journal of Palliative Medicine* **5** (6), 288–95.

48. **Mercadente, S.** et al. (2001). Pattern of drug use by advanced cancer patients followed at home. *Journal of Palliative Care* **17** (1), 37–41. (Most patients are on >4 drugs. Opioids are more frequently used in young > old. Drug audit can be very useful.)

49. **Addington-Hall, J.** et al. (1991). Dying from cancer: the views of bereaved family and friends about the experiences of the terminally ill patients. *Palliative Medicine* **5**, 207–14.

50. **Bradshaw, P.J.** (1993). Characteristics of clients referred to home, hospice and hospital palliative care services in Western Australia. *Palliative Medicine* **7**, 101–7.

51. **Paci, E.** et al. (2000). Quality of life assessment and outcome of palliative care. *Journal of Pain and Symptom Management* **21**, 179–88. (A major study based in Italy shows that co-operative clinical research is possible in palliative care and QoL measures can be used to assess the outcome.)

52. **Kyle, S., Jones, K., and Tookman, A.** (1999). Specialist palliative care and patients with non-cancer diagnoses: the experience of a service. *Palliative Medicine* **13**, 477–84.

53. **Mercadente, S.** (1992). Home palliative care: results of 1991 versus 1988. *Journal of Pain and Symptom Management* **7**, 414–18.

54. **Hanratty, B.** (2000). Palliative care provided by GPs: the carer's viewpoint. *British Journal of General Practice* **50**, 653–4. (Ninety-six per cent of patients had their pain treated by their GP. It was controlled in only 52 per cent. Sixty-seven per cent felt that the patients' anxiety and depression had been adequately treated. Satisfaction with the GPs was high though the quality of palliation was less than optimal. The symptoms worst treated were pain, dyspnoea, anorexia, anxiety, and insomnia. Similar ratings to those given to the care of hospital doctors but much poorer than those given for hospice doctors.)

55. **Christopoulou, I.** (1993). Factors affecting the decision of cancer patients to be cared for at home or in hospital. *European Journal of Cancer Care* **2** (4), 157–60.

56. **Cartwright, A., Hockey, L., and Anderson, R.** *Life Before Death.* London: Kegan Paul, 1973.

57. **Pugh, E.M.G.** (1996). An investigation of general practitioner referrals to palliative care services. *Palliative Medicine* **10**, 251–9.

58. **Rees, W.D. and Addington-Hall, J.** (1999). How do patients who die at home differ from those those who die elsewhere? *Palliative Medicine* **13**, 169 (correspondence).

59. **Addington-Hall, J.** et al. (2000). Community care for stroke patients in the last year of life: results of a national retrospective survey of surviving family, friends and officials. *Health and Social Care in the Community* **6** (2), 112–19.

60. **Kissane, D.W.** et al. (1994). Psychologial morbidity in the families with cancer. *Psycho-Oncology* **3**, 47–56.

61. **Payne, S.** et al. (1999). Identifying the concerns of informal carers in palliative care. *Palliative Medicine* **13**, 37.

62. **Velupillai, Y.** et al. (2000). The perception of general practitioners and district nurses of bed availability in hospice and hospitals for palliative care patients. *Palliative Medicine* **14**, 348–9 (Preliminary report).

63. **Velupillai, Y.** et al. (2000). When is referral to a specialist palliative care team appropriate? *Palliative Medicine* **14**, 349–50 (Preliminary report).

64. **Robinson, I. and Stacey, R.** (1984). Palliative care in the community: setting practice guidelines for primary care teams. *British Journal of General Practice* **44**, 461–4.

65. **Field, C. and Copp, G.** (1999). Communication and awareness about dying in the 1990s. *Palliative Medicine* **13**, 459–68.

66. **Sims, A.** et al. (1997). Social class variation in place of cancer death. *Palliative Medicine* **11**, 369–73.

67. **Koffman, J.** et al. (1999). Care in the last year of life: satisfaction with health services in the Black Caribbean population in an inner London Health Authority. *Palliative Medicine* **13**, 522 (Interim report).

68. **Koffman, J. and Higginson, I.** (2001). Accounts of carers' satisfaction with health care at the end of life: a comparison of first generation black Caribbeans and white patients with advanced disease. *Palliative Medicine* **15**, 337–45.

69. **Eve, A. and Higginson, I.J.** (2000). Minimum dataset activity for hospices and hospital palliative care services in the UK 1997/98. *Palliative Medicine* **14**, 395–404. (Eighteen per cent of the people in the UK dying of cancer die in a hospice. Probably only half of ethnic minority who might benefit from hospice care access it but figures are deceiving. Cancer registers do not have to give country of origin or ethnic group and since most cancer deaths are in the elderly and there are fewer elderly ethnic minority people the picture is confusing.)

70. *Opening Doors: Improving Access to Hospice and Specialist Palliative Care Services by Members of the Black and Ethnic Minority Communities.* Occasional Paper Number 7, 1995. (National Council for Hospices and Specialist Palliative Care Services, Hospice House, 34-44 Britannia Street, London, WC1X 9JG.)

71. **Doyle, D.** (1982). Nursing education in terminal care. *Nursing Education Today* **2** (4), 4–6.

72. **Bradley, E.H.** et al.(2000). Referral of terminally ill patients for hospice; frequency and correlates. *Journal of Palliative Care* **16** (4), 20–6. (A Yale study of physicians and why they refer to hospice care. It is often physician factors which determine which patients are referred and which not.)

73. **Free, C.** et al. (1996). Out-of-hours care: identifying the needs of the community. *Primary Care Management* **6**, 10.

74. **Dale, J.** et al. (1996). Creating a shared vision of out-of-hours care: using rapid appraisal methods to create an interagency, community-oriented approach to service development. *British Medical Journal* **312**, 1206–10.

75. **Jessop, L.** et al. (1997). Changing the pattern out of hours: a survey of general practitioner co-operatives. *British Medical Journal* **314**, 199–200.

76. **Thomas, K.** (2000). Out-of-hours palliative care: bridging the gap. *European Journal of Palliative Care* **7** (1), 22–5. (Out-of-hours palliative care is a key issue in service provision. The main problems are communications and reduced access to support services, medical advice, and drugs/equipment. Things that might help are agreed protocols, 24-h nursing, carer support teams, handover forms, advice lines, and drug bags.)

77. **Holden, J. and Myles, S.** Out-of-hours care in general practice. *Palliative Care Today* 2001-06-27. (Report of an audit by Macmillan GP Facilitators. Out-of-hours arrangements vary greatly and more needs to be done to achieve continuity of care if more people are to die at home.)

78. **McIllatrick, S. and Curran, C.** (2001). The perceived role of the DN in palliative care. *Journal of Community Nursing* **15** (1), 4–6. (The 'hands-on' aspects of the work of community nurses in the United Kingdom appear to dominate but are important. They see themselves as also giving emotional support for patients and families.)

79. **Grande, G.E., Barclay, S.I.G., and Todd, C.J.** (1997). Difficulty of symptom control and general practitioners' knowledge of patients' symptoms. *Palliative Medicine* **11**, 399–406.
80. **Spiller, J. and Alexander, D.A.** (1993). Domiciliary care: a comparison of the views of patients and relatives. *Palliative Medicine* **7**, 109–15.
81. **Das, A. and Mannix, K.** (2000). Emotional needs and carers' perceptions in a hospice setting terminally ill patients and their family caregivers. *Palliative Medicine* **14**, 329 (Interim report).
82. **Gomm, S.A. and Holliday, L.** (2000). Views of patients with a terminal illness on the needs of their informal carers. *Palliative Medicine* **14**, 325 (Interim report).
83. **Lubin, S.** (1992). Palliative care—could your patient have been managed at home? *Journal of Palliative Care* **8**, 18–22.
84. **Parkes, C.M.** (1978). Home or hospital? Terminal care as seen by surviving spouses. *Journal of the Royal College of General Practitioners* **28**, 19–30.
85. **Fainsinger, R.** et al. (1991). Symptom control during the last week of life on a palliative care unit. *Journal of Palliative Care* **7** (1), 5–11.
86. **Doyle, D.** (1982). Domiciliary care—demands on statutory services. *Journal of the Royal College of General Practitioners* **32**, 285–91.
87. **Thorpe, G.** (1993). Enabling more dying people to remain at home. *British Medical Journal* **307**, 915–8.
88. **McCarthy, M.** et al. (1997). Communication and choice in dying from heart disease. *Journal of the Royal Society of Medicine* **90**, 128–31.
89. **Blyth, A.C.** (1991). Audit of terminal care in a general practice. *British Medical Journal* **330**, 983–6.
90. **De Conno, F.** et al. (1993). On the last days of life. *Journal of Palliative Care* **9** (3), 47–9.
91. **Heaven, C. and Maguire, P.** (1997). Disclosure of concerns by hospice patients and their identification by nurses. *Palliative Medicine* **11**, 283–90.
92. **Hileman, J.W. and Lackey, N.R.** (1990). Self-identified needs of patients with cancer at home: the carers' perspective. *Oncology Nursing Forum* **17**, 907–13.
93. **Hunt, R.W.** (1900). The community care of terminal ill patients. *Australian Family Physician* **19**, 1835–41.
94. **Addington-Hall, J.** (1998). Palliative disease in non-malignant disease. *Palliative Care Today.*
95. **Addington-Hall, J., Fakhoury, W., and McCarthy, M.** (1998). Specialist palliative care in non-malignant disease. *Palliative Medicine* **12**, 417–27.
96. **Davies, N. and Curtis, M.** (2000). Providing palliative care in end-stage heart failure. *Professional Nurse* **15**, 389–92. (Nurses should be trained and prepared to give as good palliative care to cardiac patients as to cancer patients.)
97. **McCarthy, M.** et al. (1996). Dying from heart disease. *Journal of the Royal College of Physicians of London* **30** (4), 325–8.
98. **Anderson, H.** et al. (2001). The concerns of patients under palliative care and a heart failure clinic are not being met. *Palliative Medicine* **15**, 279–86.
99. **Edmonds, P.** et al. (2001). A comparison of the palliative care needs of patients dying from chronic respiratory diseases and lung cancer. *Palliative Medicine* **15**, 287–95.
100. **Seamark, D.** et al. (2000). Palliative care in India. *Journal of the Royal Society of Medicine* **93**, 292–5.
101. **Dwyer, L.** (1997). Palliative medicine in India. *Palliative Medicine* **11**, 487–9.
102. **Charlton, R.** (2000). Perceived skills in palliative medicine of newly qualified doctors in the UK. *Journal of Palliative Care* **16** (4), 27–32. (In spite of the amount of time allocated to palliative care in UK medical schools this study of newly qualified junior doctors found they lacked confidence in communicating, breaking bad news, hands-on care, and many wanted changes in the curriculum.)
103. **Grossman, S.A.** et al. (1991). Correlation of patient and care ratings of pain. *Journal of Pain and Symptom Management* **6**, 53–7.
104. **Jones, R.V., Hansford, J., and Fiske, J.** (1993). Death from cancer at home: the carer's perspective. *British Medical Journal* **306**, 249–51.
105. **Grande, G.E., Todd, C.J., and Barclay, S.I.G.** (1997). Support needs in the last year of life: patient and carer dilemmas. *Palliative Medicine* **11**, 202–8.
106. **Randall, F.** (1999). Are families secondary patients? *Palliative Care Today* **8**, 27–8.
107. **Nowels, D.** et al. (1999). Cancer pain management in home settings: a comparison of primary care and oncologic physicians. *Journal of Palliative Care* **15** (3), 5–9.
108. **Beaver, K.** et al. (1999). The views of terminally ill people and lay carers on primary care services. *International Journal of Palliative Medicine* **5** (6), 268–74.
109. **Bennett, I.J. and Dandzak, A.F.** (1994). Terminal care, improving teamwork in primary care using significant event analysis (SEA). *European Journal of Cancer Care* **3**, 54–7.
110. **Boyd, K.J.** (1992). The working patterns of hospice-based home care teams. *Palliative Medicine* **6**, 131–9.
111. **Simpson, M.** (1991). Doctor–patient communication. The Toronto Consensus Statement. *British Medical Journal* **303**, 1385–7.
112. **Faulkner, A.** (1993). Helping relatives to cope with a diagnosis of cancer in a loved one. *Journal of Cancer Care* **2** (3), 132–6.
113. **Barclay, S.** (2000). Interprofessional communication. *Palliative Care Today* **9** (1), 6–7. (In modern cancer care the family physician is the one who is responsible for most general symptom control whilst the specialist deals with the anti-cancer treatment. Communication between them is critical and whilst increasingly we depend on computers we must not forget the benefits of communicating by telephone to help these patients.)
114. **Hockey, L.** (1991). St Columba's Hospice Home Care Service; an evaluation study. *Palliative Medicine* **5**, 315–22.
115. **Sykes, N.P., Pearson, S.E., and Chell, S.** (1992). Quality of care of the terminally ill: the carers' perspective. *Palliative Medicine* **6**, 227–36.
116. **Seabrook, D.** et al. (1998). Dying from cancer in community hospitals or a hospice. Closest lay carers' perception. *British Journal of General Practice* **48**, 1317–21.
117. **Wilkinson, S.** et al. (1999). Patient and carer preference for, and satisfaction with, specialist models of palliative care. *Palliative Medicine* **13**, 197–216.
118. **Addington-Hall, J. and McCarthy, M.** (1995). Dying from cancer: results of a national population-based investigation. *Palliative Medicine* **9**, 295–305.
119. **Fakhoury, W.K.H., McCarthy, M., and Addington-Hall, J.** (1997). The effects of the clinical characteristics of dying cancer patients on informal caregiver satisfaction with palliative care. *Palliative Medicine* **11**, 107–15.
120. **Raybes, N.V.** et al. (2000). Palliative care services: views of terminally ill patients. *Palliative Medicine* **14**, 159–60. (Terminally ill patients complained of the time they had to wait to be seen, of poor transport arrangements to get to the hospital, missing meals because of procedures being done, and complained that they have to give their personal details more than once at a clinic visit.)
121. **Williams, E.L. and Fitton, F.** (1990). General practitioner response to elderly patients discharged from hospital. *British Medical Journal* **300**, 159–61.
122. **Cartwright, A.** (1993). Dying when you are old. *Age and Ageing* **22**, 425–30.
123. **Roe, D.J.** (1992). Palliative care 2000—home care. *Journal of Palliative Care* **8**, 28–32.
124. **Reilly, P.M. and Patten, M.P.** (1981). Terminal care in the home. *Journal of the Royal College of General Practitioners* **31**, 531–7.
125. **Spencer, J.** (1991). Caring for a terminally ill person with pain, at home. An Australian perspective. *Cancer Nursing* **14**, 55–8.
126. **Doyle, D., Parry, K.M., and Macfarlane, R.G.** (1982). Education in terminal care. *Journal of the Royal College of General Practitioners* **32**, 335–8.
127. **Saunders, J.** (1993). Palliative care—the general practice challenge. *Journal of Cancer Care* **2** (1), 2–5.
128. **Rosser, J.E. and Maguire, P.** (1982). Dilemmas in general practice: the care of the cancer patient. *Social Science and Medicine* **16**, 315–22.
129. **Barrit, P.W.** (1984). Care of the dying in one practice. *Journal of the Royal College of General Practitioners* **34**, 446–8.
130. **Porta, M., Budquet, X., and Jariod, M.** (1997). Attitudes and views of physicians and nurses towards cancer patients dying at home. *Palliative Medicine* **11**, 116–26.
131. **Constantini, M.** et al. (1999). Terminal cancer patients and timing of referral to palliative care: a multicenter prospective cohort study. *Journal of Pain and Symptom Management* **18** (4), 243–52.
132. **McWhinney, I.R.** *Textbook of Family Medicine.* Oxford: Oxford University Press, 1989.

133. **McWhinney, I.M. and Stewart, M.A.** (1994). Home care of dying patients: family physicians' experience with a palliative care team. *Canadian Family Physician* **40**, 240–6.

134. **Lang, C.C., Beardon, P.H.G., and Ladlow, M.** (1992). Drug management of pain caused by cancer: a study of general practitioners' treatment attitudes and practices. *Palliative Medicine* **6**, 246–52.

135. **Cartwright, A.** The role of the general practitioner in caring for people in the last year of their lives. *King Edward's Hospital Fund Report* 1990, London.

136. **March, G. and Kaim-Caudle, P.** *Terminal Care in General Practice*. London: Croom Helm, 1976.

137. **Cartwright, A.** (1981). Changes in life and care in the year before death. *Journal of Public Health Medicine* **13**, 81–7.

138. **Barclay, S.** et al. (1997). How common is medical training in palliative care: a postal survey of general practitioners. *British Journal of General Practice* **47**, 800–5.

139. **Oneschuk, D.** et al. (2000). An international survey of undergraduate medical education in palliative medicine. *Journal of Pain and Symptom Management* **20** (3), 174–9.

140. **Kawagoe, H. and Kawagoe, K.** (2000). Death education in home hospice in Japan. *Journal of Palliative Care* **16** (3), 37–45.

141. **Burge, F.** et al. (2000). Family medicine residents' knowledge and attitudes about end of life care. *Journal of Palliative Care* **16** (3), 5–12. (A major Canadian study looking at the perceptions of residents entering and leaving family medicine training programmes. Commitment to good palliative care was equally high but concerns were expressed about opioid use, the relief of dyspnoea. PC is not taught in all Canadian medical schools and the paper discusses how existing residency training programmes can incorporate and train in palliative care.)

142. **MacDonald, N.** et al. (2000). The Canadian Palliative Care Education Group. *Journal of Palliative Care* **16**, 13–15.

143. **Komarony, C., Sidell, M., and Katz, J.T.** (2000). The quality of terminal care in residential and nursing homes. *International Journal of Palliative Nursing* **6**, 192–3. (A report of a major study of palliative care in a range of nursing homes finds that staff are committed to good care but discusses some of the many reasons why this is difficult to translate into practice.)

144. **Barclay, S.** (2000). The management of cancer pain in primary care. In *The Effective Management of Cancer Pain* (ed. Hiller, R. et al.), pp. 117–31. Aesculapius Medical Press.

145. **Doyle, D. and Jeffrey, D.** *Palliative Care in the Home*. Oxford: Oxford University Press, 2000.

146. **Lovell, T.W.I. and Hassan, W.U.** *Clinicians' Guide to Pain*. London: Arnold, 1999.

147. **Doyle, D.** *Caring for a Dying Relative*. Oxford: Oxford University Press, 1994.

148. **Hanratty, B.** (2000). GP Views on developments in palliative care services. *Palliative Medicine* **14**, 223–4. (Report on a questionnaire sent to 31 GPs in Yorkshire, UK. Three main theses emerged. The need to develop palliative care services for non-cancer patients, the need for better availability and access to palliative care beds, and the need for specialist services to provide education and advice for primary care teams.)

149. **Mantz, M. and Crandall, J.M.** (2000). Palliative care crises in the community: a survey. *Journal of Palliative Care* **16** (4), 33–8. (A Canadian study looking at palliative care crises in the home.)

150. **Smith, N.** (1980). The impact of terminal illness on the family. *Palliative Medicine* **4**, 127–35.

151. **Nekolaichuk, C.L.** et al. (1999). Comparison of patient and proxy symptom assessments in advanced cancer patients. *Palliative Medicine* **13**, 311–23.

152. **Zeppetella, G.** (1999). How do terminally ill patients at home take their medication? *Palliative Medicine* **13**, 469–75.

153. **Doyle, D.** Polypharmacy in palliative medicine. Unpublished paper presented in Turku, Finland, 1993.

154. **Doyle, D.** *Caring for a Dying Relative*. Oxford: Oxford University Press, 1994.

155. **Lee, E.** *In your own time—*: A Guide for Patients and their Carers Facing a Last Illness at Home, 2002.

156. **Rogers, A., Karlsen, S., and Addington-Hall, J.** (2000). Dying for care: the experience of terminally ill cancer patients in hospitals in an inner city health district. *Palliative Medicine* **14**, 53–5.

157. **Donaldson, N., Carter, H., and Green, R.** (2000). Quality of information on hospice referral. *British Journal of General Practice* **50**, 219–20. (Reports the testing of what they call an 'Ideal Referral Criteria tool'. Providing essential information that needs to be sent from primary care to receiving hospice. Worth further testing but seems promising.)

158. **Casarett, D.J.** (2001). Differences between patients referred to hospice from academic versus non-academic settings. *Journal of Pain and Symptom Management* **21** (3), 197. (A study from the USA looking to find if there were differences between patients referred to a hospice from academic medical centres and from non-academic centres. Those from academic centres were younger, had higher incomes, were less likely to have a Do Not Resuscitate Order and needed both more nursing and more medical care.)

159. **Ellershaw, J., Peat, S.J., and Boys, L.C.** (1995). Assessing the effectiveness of a hospital palliative care team. *Palliative Medicine* **9**, 145–52.

160. **Hearn, J. and Higginson, I.J.** (1998). Do specialist palliative care teams improve outcomes for cancer patients? *Palliative Medicine* **12**, 317–33.

161. **Higginson, I.J., Webb, D., and Lessof, I.** (1994). Reducing hospital beds for patients with advanced cancer. *Lancet* **344**, 409.

162. **Dessloch, A.** et al. (1992). Hospital care versus home nursing: on the quality of life of terminal tumour patients. *Psychotherapeutic and Psychosomatic Medicine and Psychology* **44** (12), 414–19.

163. **Barley, P. and Oliver, D.J.** (1995). The impact on community palliative care services of a hospital palliative care team. *Palliative Medicine* **9**, 256–8 (Correspondence).

164. **Bennett, M. and Corcoran, G.** (1994). The impact on community palliative care services of a hospital palliative care team. *Palliative Medicine* **8**, 237–44.

165. **Froggatt, K.A.** (2001). Palliative care and nursing homes: where next? *Palliative Medicine* **15**, 42–8. (Increasingly people are dying in nursing homes. The expertise that exists in such homes needs to be recognized and educational initiatives take them into account. Assumptions about nursing homes are explored.)

166. **Froggatt, K.** (2000). Evaluating palliative care education project in nursing homes. *International Journal of Palliative Nursing* **6**, 140. (A report of a 2-year education project for nursing home staff. Their care practice improved but such courses did not ensure essential organizational change.)

167. **Gibbs, G.** (1995). Nurses in private nursing homes: a study of their knowledge and attitudes to pain management in palliative care. *Palliative Medicine* **9**, 245–53.

168. **Thorn, C.P.** et al. (1994). The influence of general practitioner hospitals on the place of death of cancer patients. *Palliative Medicine* **8**, 122–8.

169. **Lethem, W.** (1999). Nursing homes deliver palliative care. *Nursing Times* **95**, 55.

170. **Seabrook, D.** et al. (1998). Palliative terminal care in community hospitals and a hospice: a comparative study. *British Journal of General Practice* **48**, 1312–36.

171. **Lyon, A. and Love, D.R.** (1984). Terminal care: the role of the general practitioner hospital. *Journal of the Royal College of General Practitioners* **34**, 331–3.

172. **Johnston, T.E.** et al. (1993). Managing cancer pain at home: the decisions and ethical conflicts of patients, family caregivers and home care nurses. *Oncology Nursing Forum* **20**, 919–27.

173. **Raiman, J.** (1986). Monitoring pain at home. *Journal of District Nursing* **4**, 4–6.

174. **Koffman, J., Higginson, I.J., and Naysmith, A.** (1996). Hospice at home—a new service for patients with advanced HIV/AIDS: a pilot evaluation of referrals and outcomes. *British Journal of General Practice* **46**, 539–40.

175. **Beck-Friis, B., Strang, P., and Eklund, G.** (1989). Physical dependence of cancer patients at home. *Palliative Medicine* **3**, 281–6.

176. **Beck-Friss, B. and Strang, P.** (1993). The organisation of a hospital based home care for terminally ill cancer patients: the Motala model. *Palliative Medicine* **7**, 103–10.

177. **Beck-Friss, B. and Strang, P.** (1993). The family in hospital-based home care with special reference to terminally ill cancer patients. *Journal of Palliative Care* **8**, 5–13.

178. **Librach, L.** Personal communication, 2000.

179. **Boyd, K.J.** (1995). The role of specialist home care teams—views of general practitioners in South London. *Palliative Medicine* **9**, 138–44.

180. **Copperman, H.** (1992). Hospice Home Care Service. *Palliative Medicine* **6**, 260 (Correspondence).

181. De Conno, F. et al. (1996). Effect of home care on the place of death of advanced cancer patients. *European Journal of Cancer* **32A**, 1142–7.
182. Doyle, D. (1980). Domiciliary terminal care. *Practitioner* **224**, 575–82.
183. Grande, G.E. et al. (1999). Does hospital at home for palliative care facilitate death at home: a randomised controlled trial. *British Medical Journal* **319**, 1472–5.
184. Kindlen, M. (1988). Hospice home care services: a Scottish perspective. *Palliative Medicine* **2**, 115–22.
185. Dans-Ortiz, J. and Gonzales, L.A. (1993). Home care in a palliative care unit. *Medicina Clinica (Barcelona)* **101**, 446–9.
186. Saunders, J. and Rosenthal, S. (1992). Improving domiciliary terminal care. *Nursing Times* **88**, 32–4.
187. Hodgson, C.S. et al. (1996). Family anxiety and palliative care. *Psycho-oncology* **5** (4), 354.
188. Clark, D. et al. (2000). Experiences, outcomes and costs of Macmillan nursing: the patient's perspective. *Palliative Medicine* **14**, 343 (Preliminary report).
189. Clark, D. et al. (2000). The structure and organisation of Macmillan nursing services: 12 case studies. *Palliative Medicine* **14**, 343–4 (Preliminary report).
190. Clark, D., Ferguson, C., and Nelson, C. (2000). Macmillan Care Schemes in England: results of a multi-centre evaluation. *Palliative Medicine* **14**, 129–39.
191. Hill, A. (2001). Community palliative care: the evolving role of Macmillan nurses. *Nursing Times* **97** (12), 38. (An examination of the work done by and challenges faced by Macmillan nurses in the United Kingdom.)
192. Dumphy, K.P. and Amesbury, B.D.W. (1980). A comparison of hospice and home care patients: patterns of referrals, patient characteristics, and predictors of place of death. *Palliative Medicine* **4**, 105–11.
193. Rosenquist, A., Bergman, K., and Strang, P. (1999). Optimizing hospital-based home care for dying cancer patients: a population-based study. *Palliative Medicine* **13**, 393–7.
194. Fisher, D.A. and McDavid, P. *Palliative Day Care.* London: Arnold, 1996.
195. Jones, G. (2000). An art therapy group in palliative cancer care. *Nursing Times* **96**, 42–3. (Art therapy is a dynamic psychotherapeutic treatment, not diversional or occupational therapy and helps anxiety and patients to express fears.)
196. Higginson, I.J. et al. (2000). Palliative day care: what do services do? *Palliative Medicine* **14**, 277–86.
197. Faulkner, A. et al. Hospice day care: a qualitative study. Sheffield *Help the Hospices* Report, 1993.
198. Goodwin, D.M. et al. (2000). Methodological issues in evaluating palliative day care: a multicentre study. *Palliative Medicine* **14**, 232 (Interim report).
199. Mor, V., Stalkewr, M.Z., and Gralla, R. (1998). Day hospital as an alternative to in-patient care for cancer patients: a random assignment trial. *Journal of Clinical Epidemiology* **41**, 771–85.
200. Spencer, D.J. and Daniels, L.E. (1998). Day hospice care—a review of the literature. *Palliative Medicine* **12**, 219–29.
201. *Care in the Community for People who are Terminally Ill: Guidelines for Health Authorities and Social Service Departments.* London: National Council for Hospices and Specialist Palliative Care Services (for address see ref. 70).
202. Ajithakumari, K., Sureshkumar, K., and Rajagopal, M.R. (1997). Palliative home care—the Calicut experience. *Palliative Medicine* **11**, 451–5. (A report of the first 3 years of a small but effective service in rural India. Helped people unable to go to hospital, reassured both relatives and villagers, and dispelled the notion that the disease was contagious.)
203. Brivio, E. and Gamba, A. (1992). Home care for advanced cancer patients, the efficacy of domiciliary assistance. *European Journal of Cancer Care* **1** (2), 24–8.
204. Almuzani, A.S. et al. (1998). The attitude of health care professionals towards the availability of hospice services for cancer patients and their carers in Saudi Arabia. *Palliative Medicine* **12**, 365–75.
205. Reports on visits of palliative care specialists invited to assist in China, Swaziland, Pakistan, India, Vietnam, Colombia, Philippines, Mongolia, and Malaysia and reports from palliative care workers in Romania, Saudi Arabia, South Korea, India, Ukraine, Poland, and Uganda. Available from the Executive Director, International Association for Hospice and Palliative Care, c/o Department of Palliative Care, MD Anderson Cancer Center, Houston, Texas, USA.
206. Thomas, K. and Millar, D. (2001). Catalysts for change. *Palliative Care Today*, 54–60. (Description of the work and benefits of Macmillan GP Facilitators in the United Kingdom.)

17.2 Palliative care in the home: North America

S. Lawrence Librach

The United States of America and Canada, two large democratic North American countries, share the longest undefended border in the world. These two countries have complex and comprehensive health care systems, although both have developed different approaches to health care and therefore to hospice/palliative care. Both countries have developed fairly sophisticated home care systems. The quantity and complexity of these home care services has increased and will continue to increase in the future.

Generally, in both countries, the purpose of home care programmes is to provide:

- a substitution function for services provided by hospitals and long-term care facilities;
- a maintenance function that allows patients to remain independent in their current environment rather than moving to a new and more costly venue; and
- a preventative function, which invests in patient service and monitoring at additional short-run but lower long-run costs.[1]

Similarities and differences between the USA and Canada impacting the provision of hospice/palliative home care

1. Both countries physically are quite large in size. Although most of the population of both countries is based in urban areas, provision of health care, particularly in Canada's more isolated northern areas, remains a major challenge. Over 80 per cent of the Canadian population lives within 100 km of the American border, the largest provinces being Ontario and Quebec. The densest populations in the USA are in the eastern seaboard area and in the west coast state of California.
2. The estimated population of the USA in 2000 (276 000 000) was almost 10 times the population of Canada (30 750 000). Both countries are built on waves of immigrant populations. The USA has had more of a 'melting pot' philosophy where immigrants maintain a little of their cultural identity but are expected to melt their traditions into American culture. The Black (35 million) and Hispanic (33 million) population groups in the USA are the largest minority groups with the Hispanic group growing rapidly. Canada, a bilingual country (English and French), has a policy of multiculturalism and so the cultural identity of continuous waves of immigrants has been reasonably maintained. In both countries, the provision of hospice/palliative care is often challenged by different cultural traditions especially in large urban areas. Both countries also have native populations not only with different spiritual and cultural traditions but also with significant social and economic problems. Serving these mostly rural and often remote populations with appropriate palliative care is an issue.

3. In any country, inner city poor populations have always provided a challenge to serve with home palliative care. This is a much more significant problem in the USA where the inner city population is most often Black or Hispanic and poor, lacking medical coverage and socio-economic resources. Both countries have social assistance providing somewhat of a safety net for these populations. Violence and drugs have been a much more prevalent problem in inner city US populations than in similar large cities in Canada.
4. The basic political systems differ. The USA is a republic with 50 states and several offshore territories. There is no national universal health care scheme. Much of health care in the USA is legislated centrally, particularly institutional accreditation and the home hospice benefit from US Medicare. Canada with 10 provinces and three territories has developed in the British system of parliamentary government. The federal government has responsibility for the overall direction of health care and exercises this control through the Canada Health Act and transfer of federal tax income. Recently, the Canadian Federal Government moved to create a federal Secretariat for Hospice/Palliative Care. The actual provision of health care is the responsibility of each province and territory, supplementing federal funds with provincial and territorial tax revenues. The relationship with both US and Canadian federal governments with provinces or states and territories over the issue of health care is a source of continuing conflict and concern.
5. Canada has a universal national health care scheme financed through taxes. All Canadians are guaranteed basic but comprehensive health care services including home care without cost within the principles of the Canada Health Act: accessibility, universality, comprehensiveness, portability, and public administration. All Canadian provinces and territories provide home care services and thus serve dying patients in the home. In only three of 10 provinces is palliative care considered a core health service. About one-third of Canadians are covered by private insurance that provides extended health benefits such as dental coverage, drugs, equipment, and some private duty nursing. The USA provides for health care through a combination of some national health care coverage for citizens over age 65 and for those who are disabled called Medicare and private insurance schemes. Part of Medicare is a hospice benefit. About 42 million people in the USA have no health care coverage.[2] Most of the hospice programmes in the USA derive income from multiple sources: Medicare, private insurance, private funds, and donations. The percentage of gross domestic product spent on health care in the USA is considerably greater and unit costs for service are also generally much more expensive than in Canada.
6. Both countries are challenged by similar demographics in planning hospice/palliative home care services: an aging population, an increasing prevalence of cancer, preference of people for care at home, the transfer of care from hospitals to community settings, and a need to control health care costs. The prevalence of HIV disease in the USA is greater than in Canada although death rates from HIV disease have dropped dramatically in both countries in the last 5 years.
7. In both countries, public polls have shown an overwhelming preference (>70 per cent in Canada and >90 per cent in the USA) for dying in the home. This has been a major stimulus for the development of home hospice/palliative care programmes.
8. In both countries, professional education in palliative care and in home care is limited. National continuing education programmes in palliative care for physicians have developed in both countries: the Educating Physicians in End of Life Care Project (the EPEC Project) in the USA and the Ian Anderson Education Program in End-of-Life Care in Canada. In both countries, there are also numerous other palliative care continuing education programmes for health care professionals.
9. Canada has a strong presence of general or family practitioners (50 per cent of all physicians) whereas the USA physician population is mostly specialist based. The ability of family physicians to participate in home palliative care is therefore much greater in Canada. Most physicians in Canada work on a fee-for-service basis although alternate salary-type arrangements are increasing. Physician fees for home care in many Canadian provinces are quite low compared to office fees and the number of physicians providing home care is decreasing. Both countries have just started to develop postgraduate physician programmes in palliative medicine. Graduate nursing programmes producing nurse specialists in home care or in palliative care are limited in both countries.
10. Standards for accreditation of hospice/palliative care services exist in the USA. Hospices who wish to receive home hospice benefits through Medicare need to be accredited. No similar system for accreditation exists in Canada, although a national consensus project has produced comprehensive standards for palliative care. Both countries have national hospice or palliative care organizations that are involved in these standards processes.

Home hospice care in the USA (Table 1)

Hospice care and programmes have increased rapidly in America. Hospice care including home care is funded mostly by the federal Medicare Hospice Benefit with further funding coming from Medicaid benefits provided by 43 of 50 states, private insurance, and other sources. To be a Medicare programme, a hospice must undergo regular accreditation and regular financial scrutiny. The Medicare Hospice Benefit was established in 1983, providing 75 per cent of hospice programme income and stimulating the rapid growth of hospice care including home hospice care.

Those persons eligible for hospice Medicare benefits have to meet the following criteria:

- They are over 65 years of age, a citizen or permanent resident in the USA or less than 65 if they have a disability or end-stage renal disease.
- They are certified by their doctor and the hospice medical director as having a prognosis less than 6 months.
- Patients must sign a statement choosing hospice care rather than curative treatment and standard Medicare benefits.
- They must enroll in a Medicare-approved programme.

The 6-month prognosis in the Medicare benefit has been a source of controversy as it expects an ability to prognosticate accurately, impedes access to patients who may require hospice care earlier in their illness, and trapped some patients without funding if they survived beyond 6 months although recently a renewel programme has been instituted. However, hospice programmes in the USA commit to providing care beyond 6 months as necessary and hospital palliative care consult teams are able to provide care at earlier phases of a patient's illness.

Table 1 Home hospice care in the USA, 1999

3139 operating or planned hospice programmes 44% independent free-standing agencies 33% hospital-based 17% home health-based 4% nursing home or others
76% of hospice programmes non-profit
61% of the 600 000 patients served by hospices were able to die at home or in a nursing home
1 in 4 people who died in the USA were looked after by a hospice
Average length of enrollment in hospice care was 48 days with a median of 29 days
64% of hospice patients had a diagnosis of cancer
Hospices cared for over 50% of the Americans dying of cancer

The hospice benefits covered by Medicare include both home and inpatient treatment by interdisciplinary teams, medical equipment and supplies, drugs, and volunteer support services. Hospice benefits do not cover expenses of care unrelated to the terminal illness. Regular home care is provided by experienced registered nurses and licensed practical nurses, home health aides and homemakers, and by visiting physicians. Counselling and spiritual support is also provided under the framework of hospice care in the home. Respite care, to give families a break in caring for a patient at home, can be provided in an appropriate facility. Co-payments may be required to pay for outpatient drugs and for respite care but the expenses are set at only 5 per cent of the costs of such services.

Hospice care and its home care component continue to grow rapidly in the USA under the expanding influence of well-organized and comprehensive hospice/palliative care programmes.

Home hospice/palliative care in Canada

All Canadians are covered by comprehensive, universal health care that includes home care as a part of the system. Home care in Canada has been defined as:[4]

> an array of services which enables clients, incapacitated in whole or in part, to live at home, often with the effect of preventing, delaying, or substituting for long-term care or acute care alternatives.
>
> Home care may be delivered under numerous organizational structures, and similarly numerous funding and client payment mechanisms. It may address needs specifically associated with a medical diagnosis (e.g. diabetes therapy), and/or may compensate for functional deficits in the activities of daily living (e.g. bathing, cleaning, food preparation). Home care is a health program, with health broadly defined; to be effective it may have to provide services which in other contexts might be defined as social or educational services (e.g. home maintenance, volunteer visits).
>
> Home care may be appropriate for people with minor health problems and disabilities, and for those who are acutely ill requiring intensive and sophisticated services and equipment. There are no upper or lower limits on the age at which home care may be required, although as in other segments of the health system, utilization tends to increase with age.

In all 13 jurisdictions (10 provinces and three territories) in Canada, ministries or departments of health are responsible for the implementation of home care policy and services. Most provinces have delegated responsibility for funding allocation and service delivery to regional or local health authorities. However, in most cases the provincial and territorial departments set overall policy guidelines and standards for regional service delivery, reporting requirements, and monitoring outcomes. All provinces and territories have single points of access for home care services.

There is considerable variation from province to province in the way home care is delivered and the services provided. In some provinces, public employees deliver all services. In others, there is combination of public and home care agency funded employees or a contracting out of all services to for-profit and not-for-profit agencies. The patient assessment and the consequent care plan determine services to be delivered and the extent of public funding in full or in part. The assessment process itself and nursing services are typically provided free of charge, while fees may apply to personal care and homemaking services. In some provinces, payment for certain equipment, supplies, and drugs may be the responsibility of the patient and family. Income or means-testing is done in some provinces to determine what the patient can contribute. In all provinces, persons over age 65 receive drugs with minimum charge or without any charge. Patients on home care under age 65 in some provinces are eligible for these drug benefits. There may also be direct charges or income tested co-payments to the patient for prescription drugs, medical supplies, and/or adaptive equipment.[5] There may be some restrictions on the amount of service that can be provided monthly but service may be provided for many months. In a number of areas, home palliative care patients may receive enhanced services over the usual services provided. All provinces through their home care agencies can provide special equipment such as continuous subcutaneous infusion pumps, oxygen tanks or concentrators, hospital beds, intravenous supplies, and other equipment. However, recent budget cuts and policy changes have forced some increase in co-payments for some of these supplies and equipment after a certain amount of time with some means-testing in some areas. If the patient wants services or equipment beyond those assessed for public coverage, the patient and family may pay for them privately out-of-pocket or with private third-party insurance.

There is no specific benefit for hospice/palliative care within the Canadian health care system. Palliative care units, nursing homes, and acute hospital beds are all part of the universal coverage. However, the lack of such a hospice benefit as exists in the USA has resulted in less comprehensive development of specific hospice/palliative care programmes in Canada. Only three provinces have made palliative care a core service and therefore the flow of government funding for palliative care programmes has been inconsistent across the country. Almost all acute care hospitals in Canada have palliative care programmes with variable interdisciplinary resources depending on the flow of funding from each individual institution. Full service interdisciplinary formal home palliative care programmes are relatively uncommon although recently there has been considerable planning in many provinces for regional home palliative care programmes. Family physicians often provide physician services for palliative care patients at home. In other areas, specialist palliative medicine physicians provide consult back-up for family physicians or may provide direct primary care in the home. There are a number of regions with home palliative care programmes integrated into the overall health system. Most areas of Canada also have community volunteer hospice services providing volunteer support but most are not part of formal interdisciplinary palliative care programmes. Cancer centres in Canada are often regional in nature and recently there has been much more presence of palliative care within those centres.

Canada has limited data on hospice/palliative care services. It is estimated that there are over 1000 palliative care programmes but the cumulative service data from those programmes are not known on a national basis. The percentage of home palliative care patients dying at home ranges from 20 to 70 per cent. Factors influencing this figure include presence or absence of specific home palliative care programmes, the availability of physicians to make home visits, the availability of inpatient palliative care unit beds, the presence of sufficient family support, and socioeconomic status. Efforts are now underway to begin to collect national data on palliative care.

Although Canada has a universal health care system, the application of home care services appropriate for palliative care patients varies across the country. The lack of specific funding for interdisciplinary home palliative care programmes in most provinces limits the number of Canadians who can access expert palliative care. The identification of palliative care and home palliative care as core services within the health care system in Canada hopefully will change this situation in the future.

References

1. **Health Canada.** *Report on Home Care* (prepared by the Federal/Provincial/Territorial Working Group on Home Care, a Working Group of the Federal/Provincial/Territorial Subcommittee on Long Term Care), 1990, p. 2.
2. Data from the United States National Centre for Health Statistics, 2001.
3. Excerpted from National Hospice and Palliative Care Organization document. *NHPCO Facts and Figures 2001.*
4. **Federal/Provincial/Territorial Working Group on Home Care, a Working Group of the Federal/Provincial/Territorial Subcommittee on Long Term Care**, *Report on Home Care*, Health Canada, 1990, p. 2.
5. **Federal-Provincial-Territorial Advisory Committee on Health Services Working Group on Continuing Care.** *Provincial and Territorial Home Care Programs: A Synthesis for Canada*, Health Canada, May 1999, p. 22.

18

The terminal phase

18 The terminal phase

Carl Johan Fürst and Derek Doyle

Life is short, the art long

Hippocrates (460–357 BC/BCE)

The challenges of the terminal phase

Why devote a chapter to a few days or even a week or so of a patient's life? Is it not safe to assume that if care has been satisfactory up to that point, it will continue to be adequate through the terminal phase until the patient dies? Is there something special, something different about those final weeks and days?

This chapter will answer those questions. It will remind us that the terminal phase is not simply a continuation of all that has gone before. There may be new causes of suffering for both the dying person and the relatives. Care plans may need to be changed to address this new suffering. Poorly relieved suffering in the days before a person dies is always remembered by relatives and can cause intense distress to them for months and years to come, often obliterating their recollections of all the good care their loved one received before that. It is little short of a tragedy if someone has high-quality palliative care over a period of many months only to die in poorly controlled suffering of body or mind, watched over by relatives who had understandably expected something better. Indeed some might argue that ensuring a comfortable and dignified terminal phase is one of the principal reasons for the patient being referred to a palliative care team.

The first challenge is to recognize the features of the terminal phase; to understand the multifaceted suffering experienced at that time, and how it may be addressed, and how best to care for and support the relatives and close friends.

The transition from the previous phase of very active, occasionally invasive treatment to the terminal phase should be a smooth, almost imperceptible one. It needs considerable clinical skill and sensitivity if the quality of life so recently achieved is not to be lost in the final days.[1]

The second challenge is the harder one. In many respects, it might be said to be the ultimate challenge of palliative medicine. It is to look beyond the clinical issues and care regimens to the human needs we all have; to be prepared to share not just our skills and our knowledge but also ourselves—our compassion and our humanity—with those we serve.

The original hospices were places of rest, healing, and safety on the great travel routes of Europe. Today we are all on our great journey of life. Some—the people we shall think about in this chapter—are on the last stage of that journey. The ultimate challenge to us is to accompany them as far as we can on that journey that one day we too must make. Caring in the terminal phase involves infinitely more than pain and symptom control, and dealing with the psychosocial and spiritual issues. It often turns out to be a humble sharing of our personal weaknesses as well as our strengths—doing for others what we would have others do for us when the time comes.

The features of dying

As the patient gets near to death he/she

- becomes increasingly weary, weak, and sleepy;
- becomes less interested in getting out of bed or receiving visitors;
- becomes less interested in things happening around him/her;
- often becomes confused, occasionally with features of agitated anguish.

Few of these features will be new ones. However, what should suggest to the clinician that the terminal phase is starting is that most of the above become evident at the same time. Important as it is, it can be difficult to know whether the patient has entered the terminal phase or is having yet another relapse from which there might be a remission as has happened in the past. They may be suffering from a recurrent illness unrelated to the malignancy or other mortal illness, one that merits further investigation and treatment providing neither will further reduce their quality of life. Diagnosing what is happening can be difficult but is important.[1]

On such occasions, the situation must be fully explained to relatives who need to know why investigations are being done, what is hoped to achieve with any treatment, and be reassured that such 'active' treatment will be withdrawn should it prove futile, and replaced with the best care possible for the terminal phase. It is important to be aware of the distress caused by raising false hopes in patients or relatives by ordering unnecessary investigations or futile treatment.

In this chapter, we shall look at suffering, for convenience of presentation arbitrarily and quite artificially classified as physical, psychosocial, and spiritual. In practice, the suffering of the terminal phase can never be simplified or compartmentalized in this way. It is never neat and orderly. No one suffers pain or breathlessness without experiencing fear. Few face death without looking back and wondering what they could have done differently. Dying is not merely another event a doctor must be skilled in handling, anymore than death is a mark of medical failure. Readers are asked to bear this in mind.

Physical suffering in the terminal phase

Do patients suffer much in this final stage of life? Some idea of their suffering can be gleaned from Table 1 compiled from refs 2–7. It will be seen that figures vary between different studies but why that might be so will not be addressed here because it might divert our attention from the central facts that, whatever the underlying pathology, patients suffer a kaleidoscope of symptoms and that much suffering is inadequately palliated.[9–18]

Pain

Three-fourths of all dying patients will have pain requiring strong opioid analgesics when they enter the terminal phase. In their final 48 h, 13 per cent will then have their dose reduced, 44 per cent will have it increased, and in 48 per cent it will remain unchanged.[2] One study showed that 60 per cent of patients were able to swallow until they died, a further 25 per cent needed suppositories, and 15 per cent needed an injection.[19] More than half will experience a new pain, hence the need for professional diligence at this time. In about 10 per cent complete pain relief is not achieved, but severe, unrelieved pain is both rare and avoidable.

Table 1 Symptoms of the last days of life assessed and described in different studies

	Lichter and Hunt[2]	Nauck et al.[3]	Conill et al.[4]	Grond et al.[5]	Ellershaw et al.[6]	Fainsinger et al.[7]
Estimated time until death	48 h	72 h	1 week	24 h	<48 h	<1 week
No. of patients	200	150	176	319	168	100
Mean age	—	—	67.7	58	67	62
Symptoms			%			
Anorexia			80			
Asthenia			82			
Confusion	9	55	68	25		39
Constipation			55	12		
Dry mouth			70			
Dyspnoea	22	26	47	17		46
Jerking, twitching	12	12				
Nausea	14	14	13	10		71
Noisy, moist breathing	56	45			45	
Pain	51	26	30	42/319	46	99
Restlessness, agitation	42	43			52	
Sweating	14			6		
Urinary dysfunction	53		7	4		

There may be a new pain problem or disease progression exacerbating a previous pain problem. For example:

- pain control was lost when changing drugs or routes of administration;
- the patient has sustained a pathological fracture with handling;
- oral candidiasis is making the mouth and swallowing painful;
- urinary retention or constipation has developed and not been noticed;
- bedsores have developed. It is sometimes forgotten that their discomfort can be relieved at this time with local anaesthetic gel.

As patients approach the end of life the use of radiotherapy or invasive analgesic approaches is often precluded because the likelihood of relief is small and there is the risk of adverse affects and the inconvenience of organizing the treatment.

If the patient already has an intravenous (IV) port, it will facilitate the use of an IV line but, like any equipment at this time infusion equipment should never become a barrier between the patient and the relatives. Syringe drivers and small electronic infusion devices, on the other hand, are small and unobtrusive, and particularly useful in the home where there are visiting nurses trained in their use, though there are sometimes problems with the site.[20] It is recognized, however, that in some parts of the world there are not sufficient doctors available in the community to supervise their use. Drugs that may be used in syringe drivers are shown in Table 2. Patient-controlled analgesia is generally inappropriate as the terminal phase progresses because the dying patient may not be able to operate it.

An analgesic given immediately before the patient is turned or moved can help reduce incident pain. In the United Kingdom, dextromoramide sublingually (5 mg being approximately equivalent to 10 mg oral morphine) has been a popular choice but normal-release morphine will work just as well and is now generally preferred (Table 3). Oral transmucosal fentanyl citrate (see Chapter 8.2.3) may be also useful particularly if the patient is already familiar with it. What must not be used for incident or 'break through' pain are sustained-release preparations.

Fentanyl patches are discussed elsewhere in this book (see Chapter 8.2.3). In the terminal phase, it is more convenient for a patient whose dose needs to be increased simply to add another patch but, when the opioid requirement is falling it is preferable to change to an alternative opioid preparation as early in the terminal phase as possible.

Table 2 Drugs which may be given SC via a syringe driver

	Percentage of units using drug	Range of mean maximum dose (mg/24 h)	Median dose (mg/24 h)
Diamorphine	99	300–10 000	2200
Haloperidol	95	5–100	12.5
Methotrimeprazine	93	25–400	150
Cyclizine	85	50–150	150
Midazolam	64	10–160	40
Metoclopramide	64	10–200	30
Dexamethasone	39	4–30	15.5
Hyoscine hydrobromide	39	0.4–4	1.2

Opioids can occasionally be reduced. If it is thought that the patient is unduly sleepy having previously been alert, and is known to be drinking less and becoming oliguric (suggesting that morphine metabolites are accumulating) then a reduced opioid dose can be tried. An alternative is to give the normal release morphine every 6 h instead of 4 hourly, particularly in the elderly.

It is mentioned elsewhere in this book that relatives have been shown to be poor judges of a patient's pain and anxiety.[21] In the terminal phase, relatives often suspect the patient is experiencing pain when, in fact, they are just grunting or muttering as most people do when asleep, or reaching out to find the hand of a loved one. However, unlike the patients in the study quoted, the dying patient cannot comment and *may* be experiencing as much pain as the relatives suspect. This must be borne in mind when kindly, confident reassurance is given to the relatives especially when they are inexperienced in sitting by the bedside of someone critically ill. However, it must never be forgotten that unconscious patients can experience pain.

Table 3 Drugs which may be used sublingually

Drug	Preparation	Strength	Comment
Analgesics			
Aspirin-glycine[a]	Tablet	500 mg	The glycine enhances the solubility of aspirin. For some patients it is too gritty
Buprenorphine	Tablet	0.2 mg, 0.4 mg	
Dextromoramide[a]	Tablet	5 mg, 10 mg	Rapid onset of action; relatively short-acting and may need to be used every 3 h
Diamorphine	Tablet	10 mg	
Morphine	Liquid	20 mg/ml	Supplied with calibrated dropper. Sublingual administration feasible because of small volume; probably absorbed mainly from stomach. Particularly useful for moribund patients at home
Phenazocine[a]	Tablet	5 mg	Bitter tasting like other opioids
Antiemetics and psychotropics			
Hyoscine	Tablet	0.3 mg	An over-the-counter preparation (Quick Kwells®)
Lorazepam[a]	Tablet	1 mg, 2.5 mg	Five times more potent than diazepam. Tablets are scored, permitting use of 0.5 mg

[a] Oral tablets that can be taken sublingually.

Dyspnoea

By this time, all treatable causes of dyspnoea will have been dealt with. In the terminal phase, the commonest causes of dyspnoea—or to be more precise the patient's perception of breathlessness—are

- extensive lung metastases or carcinomatous lymphangitis;
- anxiety or panic;
- secondary chest infection;
- pulmonary oedema;
- stridor presumably resulting from extratracheal pressure from nodes;
- large pericardial effusion with tamponade;
- metabolic acidosis associated with multisystem failure;
- an excessively dry atmosphere;
- a newly developed pleural effusion;
- anaemia.

Some of the treatments that would be applicable in palliative care at an earlier stage are no longer appropriate in the terminal phase. When death is imminent, it is rarely justified to drain either a pleural or a pericardial effusion. Similarly, unless it can be confidently expected that the patient will be much more comfortable as a result of being treated with an antibiotic, it is also rarely justified at this time. Preferable, if one is available, is the assistance of a physiotherapist to aid breathing and maybe the expectoration of sputum (see Chapter 15.4).

The symptomatic management of dyspnoea is reviewed in Chapter 8.8. Systemically administered morphine is titrated to effect, and remains the best treatment for the relief of breathlessness. This may be given orally or as a suppository or via a syringe driver when swallowing is unreliable (see Chapter 8.8). If breathlessness becomes a problem in someone already on opioids for analgesia the dose should be increased by 50 per cent.

Though nebulized opioids help in the control of cough most studies have not demonstrated benefit in dyspnoea (see Chapters 8.8 and 10.4). On the other hand, both oxygen—by mask or nasal cannulae—and cool air from a nearby fan can reduce the sensation of breathlessness whether or not there is clinical hypoxia.[21] In patient's homes, relatives tend to overheat rooms without moisturizing them, only adding to patient discomfort. Simple advice about opening windows, positioning the patient where there is a stream of air and having a bowl of water in the room to humidify it are usually sufficient and much appreciated.[23]

Panic when patients feel they are about to suffocate calls for skilled attention (see below for emergency care). It is usually associated with trying to move around, getting on or off a toilet or commode, or with a sense of claustrophobia.

Persistent or recurrent panic associated with a sense of breathlessness is an indication for a low dose of diazepam 2.5–5 mg/day or of midazolam 5–10 mg/day via a syringe driver. Chlorpromazine is also said to help.[24]

Vomiting

Rarely can the precise cause be found at this stage, with the exception of intestinal obstruction. Antiemetics must be used empirically and given either by suppository or via a syringe driver. Equally important are such measures as giving sips of fluids and small helpings of soft, easily swallowed foods such as sorbet, ice cream, custard, yoghurt, and stewed fruit. As the patient gets weaker and even less inclined to eat, the priority is to maintain fluid intake. Most enjoy crushed ice cubes of water, a favourite tipple, real fruit juice, or tea.

If antiemetics are put into a syringe driver (Table 2) it should be remembered that:

- Cyclizine (a popular drug in the United Kingdom but not available in many countries) will precipitate at concentrations above 20 mg/ml, or in saline, or if used with diamorphine, as the concentration of the opioid increases.
- Midazolam does not mix with betamethasone, dexamethasone, or methyl prednisolone.
- Cyclizine and metoclopramide should not be used together because the intestinal action of the metoclopramide is inhibited by the cyclizine. In any case the cyclizine precipitates.
- Prochlorperazine and diazepam cause skin inflammation when given subcutaneously (SC).
- Diclofenac and ketorolac are compatible with diamorphine but only when mixed with saline.
- Precipitation of dexamethasone can be prevented by warming the syringe before the drug is drawn up.

If vomiting is due to intestinal obstruction it is worth trying octreotide, SC via a syringe driver, 0.3–0.6 mg/day[25] (see Chapter 8.3.4). An alternative antisecretory drug is hyoscine butyl bromide SC, 60–120 mg/day.[26] Rarely, if ever, should it be necessary to hydrate a dying patient with

IV fluids but some patients may need a nasogastric tube for intermittent aspiration to relieve recurrent large volume vomits.

Parenteral rehydration

No one would dispute the need for the correction of dehydration in patients expected to live for weeks or months. Here, however, we are looking at patients with days rather than weeks to live. Whether or not they should have rehydration remains controversial.[27,28] In the cognitively intact, dehydration is a factor that can precipitate delirium and diminish interaction with relatives. On the other hand, parenteral rehydration can itself be associated with morbidity.[29] If the clinician believes that the potential benefits outweigh the disadvantages then a trial of SC or IV fluids is sometimes justified. It is frequently requested by relatives who see the patient's decline as being the result of inadequate fluid and food intake. They need to have it explained to them that rehydration will not reverse the process and that it is only a trial to palliate suffering. The clinician must be prepared for relatives being unhappy if he decides to discontinue the trial.

Patients rarely say they are dehydrated but they frequently say their mouth is dry, making speech and swallowing difficult, and often leading to halitosis.[30] A dry mouth from whatever cause is not an indication for SC or IV fluids but for regular and frequent sips of fluid or sucking from a lollipop sponge. The fluids might be cold water, an aerated drink, one with lemon flavouring, or a sorbet. Relatives can be taught how to give the drinks even to the dying person, and to assist with oral hygiene, and are happy to be helpful.

It is worth remembering that the nearer a patient is to death, the colder the drinks they ask for and enjoy. Hot drinks, such as clear soup or weak tea, become less acceptable as the illness progresses.

Anorexia

Appetite diminishes inexorably as death approaches but is also related to symptom control.[31] Artificial administration of nutrition by enteral and parenteral routes are medical interventions with the potential for associated morbidity. In imminently dying patients, there are no data to suggest that they contribute to symptom relief. Medications for this are not justified in the terminal phase and if the patient has been receiving steroids for anorexia, these can now be discontinued. Patients should be offered a tiny portion of whatever they fancy, when they want it, but no one should be surprised if they then refuse it. Relatives find this hard when they have gone to much trouble buying and cooking something special in the home.

The patient's unwillingness/inability to eat often upsets relatives who, until it is sensitively explained to them, believe his/her decline is because of lack of food or fluids. They have to be helped to understand that at this stage in the illness whatever food is taken, by whatever route, will not be metabolized or, as they might better understand it 'be made into energy' in the body.

Psychosocial suffering in the terminal phase

What does the patient know of his/her condition and prognosis?

Experience suggests that by this time most competent patients are aware how ill they are and that they will die. However, like their relatives and friends, they may be misled when investigations continue or doctors and nurses speak as though there was time left to them or of 'more that can be done'.

Most patients, if still able to articulate what they are feeling, speak of their fear of confusion (often assuming it is a feature of developing mental illness), their fears about asphyxia, 'fighting for breath', or bleeding to death. Most, given the chance, tell of their sadness at leaving loved ones and their anxiety about how they will cope. Particularly when they are at home, patients express anxiety about being a burden on their families. Even at this late stage in their illness, they may raise the question of being transferred to a hospital or palliative care unit 'if it will help the family' (see Chapter 17).

Hippocrates noted that 'Young men fear death, old men fear dying'.[32] To this day few people express much, if any, fear of death but rather of what has come to be called 'the dying process'—those final weeks and days leading up to death. They tell of their dread of further pain, dyspnoea, nausea, or vomiting. Many express the hope that as they get frailer they will not be subjected to enemata or over-enthusiastic bowel care or further invasive investigations. Some fear inappropriate treatment, which they suspect might be offered even though it is known to be futile at that stage. Many express the hope that they will die peacefully in their sleep but, paradoxically then try to keep themselves awake at night or decline hypnotics in case they die. (Trying to reassure a dying person that death is like a beautiful sleep can sometimes increase their resolve not to sleep.)

Almost all patients, once they feel able to speak of what lies ahead, seek reassurance that they will not be left alone, will not be allowed to suffer, and will not be a burden on those caring for them. What is easily forgotten is that the dying seem able to hear what is being said nearby. However, such an observation is only an anecdote recounted by many who have been at the bedside and has not been much researched. Relatives find it reassuring that their words of love and comfort to the patient will probably be heard, as will anything else that they had not thought the patient would hear. Naturally, the same applies to the professional carers in attendance. Though a patient may appear to be comatose they seem to be aware of the ambience of their surroundings especially if it is one of peace and compassion. Others have described the peace that has come over a dying patient when their favourite music is played (see Chapter 15.2).

Spiritual suffering in the terminal phase

For the patient, the terminal phase is a time to look back and a time to look forward. Obvious as this may be, it helps us to understand what people think about and ask about at this time—what, perhaps wrongly, we have called spiritual 'suffering'. It implies that all patients suffer spiritual doubts and endure agonies of self-recrimination and regret as they look back. Some certainly do but for most it is a time for reflection and self-appraisal, a time to look back on life and what they have achieved, a time to ponder on why things happen as they do in the world. Estimates vary but it has been suggested that close on 75 per cent of people receiving palliative care raise spiritual questions showing that they have been reviewing their lives and asking existential questions about the meaning of life, the meaning of suffering, and how one measures a 'useful' life.

Patients wonder whether or not they have achieved anything, are leaving the world a better place, and how they will be remembered, especially by their children. Particularly if they have been successful in worldly terms, with possessions, wealth and fame, they seem to look beyond such worldly signs of success to what they often describe as 'things that really matter' and speak of family, friends, love, parenting, and what will come to be seen as their legacy. Given the opportunity to talk about things on their minds they speak of family disputes and the break-up of the family; of losing touch with family and friends and their sense of guilt that they may have contributed to this. They often speak of their longing for reconciliation and forgiveness and wanting to be being remembered for the good in their past life.

As discussed in Chapter 11, though they are related, religion and spirituality are not the same thing.[34–39] A person with a religious faith will usually frame existential questions in familiar religious language and see most spiritual issues in terms of the relationship with their God. Existential questions and ponderings such as we have described may, however, be asked by patients professing no faith or life philosophy. In the terminal phase, as at any other time in palliative care, it is wrong to assume that underlying a spiritual question is a religious one, and that a religious response is what is sought.

Similarly, it is wrong to assume that a person with a long-standing faith will be immune to religious doubts or temporary loss of faith, both of which do constitute 'suffering'. Patients say it is difficult to articulate prayers, much as they want to. Others, after a lifetime of religious faith and observance, express doubts about key tenets of their faith. Others say that they have never thought much about leaving those they love, or about death and what comes after it, and now feel ill-prepared for what lies ahead.

How are these patients to be helped? Pastoral care workers can offer much. They are highly trained to deal with these issues and have encountered most of them. However, it is wise to ask the patient if they would like the pastoral care colleague to be invited. Some say they are too embarrassed or even ashamed to have spiritual or religious doubts and would prefer to discuss them with a lay person. Simply talking about them with a person of their choice—a doctor, a nurse, or a social worker—can be cathartic and helpful even when the carer has listened without commenting, without counselling, without being judgemental. However, as so often happens in palliative medicine, it must be remembered that patients usually only issue one invitation for someone to listen to them. If for some reason that person is unable to do so at that time, when they return, the patient may no longer want to share their thoughts.

People with a religious faith can and do gain great peace and comfort as a result of sacraments or practices sacred to their faith. For some it might be the anointing with oils, for others having their holy book or texts read to them. For many it is the caring companionship of their priest, teacher, holy man, or visitor from church or temple. Books are available which explain the beliefs surrounding death and the different practices and customs that must be respected by palliative care teams caring for those of different faiths and ethnic groups.[(40,41)]

Suffering of relatives and close friends

How much do relatives know?

The brief answer to this question might be that they often know less than the patient does. Relatives commonly say that they were given every detail of the patient's illness in its early days but have not been kept up-to-date more recently though they have always known it was a mortal illness. They may have experienced the hopes and disappointment of the remissions and relapses so characteristic of malignant disease, on several occasions being warned that death might be imminent only for the latest pulse of chemotherapy or course of radiotherapy to bring about a remission and a reprieve.

> Doctor, I have seen him as ill as this before and the doctors told me he was dying but every time he improved.
>
> He's a fighter so I know he'll be home soon.
>
> How can you say he is dying when only last month they gave him radiotherapy/chemotherapy/a chest tap/another CT scan/MRI and he has a date to go back and see that specialist?

When relatives find it difficult to accept or to understand that death is near, they may continue to urge that energetic measures be taken to feed or rehydrate their loved one, or seek alternative professional advice. They may be reluctant to accept that some medications can now be discontinued. As the truth dawns on them they may be embarrassed at not seeing what was obvious to others and feel themselves unprepared for what lies ahead.

Not only is this a sad time for relatives; it can be frightening. Many have never seen a dying person nor touched a dead body, their only knowledge of death being gleaned from film or television, usually of death quite unlike that seen with good palliative care. They fear that they will not know how to give essential medications if the patient is at home, will not be able to make the patient comfortable, will break down and cry, will not know what to do in an emergency or what to say if the patient asks questions, and if left alone, will not know when death has occurred.

All the time they are experiencing these fears and self-doubts, they are conscious of an unknown future which looms large and threatening, but which can seldom be spoken of in case they appear selfish or uncaring. All around them is change. They feel frightened and insecure. Some will ask questions; many will say little; a few will fight against the unknown and be a cause of worry (or irritation) to the palliative care team.

What are the responsibilities of the professional carers in the terminal phase?

Preparation for the terminal phase

Many times in this textbook is it stressed that palliative care should ideally be proactive and not reactive. Nowhere is that more important, and more feasible, than prior to the terminal phase. As stressed so often palliative care should always be team caring, whether in hospital or in the home. Preparations which the whole team or individuals in it will make will include:

- A review of all medications being taken, identifying those that must be continued and their routes of administration, and those that can be discontinued (Table 4).
- A review of medications that might be needed for problems arising in the terminal phase and ensuring their availability.
- A review of how much assistance and instruction relatives might need in giving medications if the patient is at home.
- A review of nursing aids that might be needed/useful in the home.
- A review of whether or not it seems likely that the patient can remain at home and, if not, where might be the most appropriate place for them—hospital, hospice/palliative care unit, or nursing home.
- Particularly when the patient is in hospital must it be decided whether any further investigations (even simple blood tests or chest X-rays) are likely to help or are ethical. And recording the decision in the case notes.
- What advice to give the family about calling distant relatives or friends, particularly when they must travel some distance.
- What advice and support the family will need and who is best placed to provide it.

This is the time, wherever the patient is being cared for, for a talk with the patient to ensure that their wishes are known and their fears and hopes expressed. It is also the time to talk to relatives, outlining what lies ahead, what the care plans are including what it is hoped to achieve with each item

Table 4 Reviewing drugs and their routes of administration for the terminal phase

Essential drugs—review route	Previously essential—consider stopping	No longer essential—stop
Analgesics	Steroids[a]	Antihypertensives
Antiemetics	Replacement hormones	Antidepressants
Sedatives	Hypoglycaemics	Laxatives
Anxiolytics	Diuretics Antiarrhythmics Anticonvulsants	Antiulcer drugs Anticoagulants Long-term antibiotics Iron, vitamins

[a] It is prudent to reduce steroid doses slowly, especially if the patient has been on high-dose dexamethasone for cerebral oedema.

of medication, and how everyone can create an atmosphere which is both peaceful and 'safe'—that word so frequently used by dying people. Time spent in these meetings is never wasted and often spoken of by relatives in their bereavement.

Reviewing medication and equipment

Drugs no longer considered essential

Polypharmacy is almost invariable in palliative care. One report showed that of 1000 patients only one was on no medication, a considerable number were on up to 11 different drugs and the average was 4.5 drugs, most of which were taken several times a day.[(42)] By the time the patient receiving palliative care enters the terminal phase, he/she is likely to be on one or more analgesics, laxatives, tranquilizers, oral antifungals, and possibly a hypnotic. In addition, he/she is probably still on drugs that he/she has taken for years—antihypertensives, diuretics, and potassium supplements, other cardiovascular drugs, and possibly oral hypoglycaemics, steroids, thyroid supplements, and soluble aspirin to name but a few. In the final days of life few of these will be needed. The challenge is to identify those no longer needed, explain that to the patient and family, and then discontinue them whilst keeping the patient under observation. In the case of long-term steroids or cardiac antiarrhythmics sudden withdrawal may be harmful and this should be kept in mind (Table 4).

The commonest drugs needed in the final days are analgesics, anticonvulsants and tranquilizers, and hyoscine-like drugs for 'death rattle', given by a reliable route with as little disturbance and discomfort to the patient as possible (Table 5).

In the final days, cardiac drugs are seldom needed because the heart is under less strain. Advanced malignant disease itself lowers blood pressure removing the need for antihypertensives. Food intake is so small that hypoglycaemics are not called for. Each drug and its original indication is reviewed in this way.

Explaining to relatives the rationale for discontinuing a drug is seldom easy and often misunderstood. They recall being told that certain drugs were essential for health and that discontinuing them might prove fatal. They ask why discontinuing them at this critical time is not harmful, or if it is being done for reasons of economy or non-availability of professional carers to administer them. Some even ask if it is designed to shorten the terminal phase.

There is no alternative to sitting down with relatives and explaining why a drug was needed in the past but is now no longer needed. Failure to do so may lead to profound distress for families both in the patient's final days and for a long time afterwards.

Essential drugs

The next thing to do is to review what have been identified as essential drugs, looking at not only the doses and timing but, often of more importance at this time, the routes of administration (Table 5).

Table 5 A suggested minimum set of drugs for the terminal phase

Class of drug	Drug	Routes of administration	PO dose
Opioid	Morphine	PO, PR, SC, IV	5–10 mg
	Diamorphine (UK)	SC, IV, IM	5–10 mg
	Hydromorphone	SC, IV	
Anticholinergic	Hyoscine Hbr	SC, IM	0.4 mg
	Hyoscine butyl bromide	SC, IM, IV	10–20 mg
Antiemetic/anxiolytic	Haloperidol	SC, IM, IV	0.5–1 mg SC
Tranquilizer sedative	Midazolam	SC, IV	5–15 mg SC
	Diazepam	IM, IV, PR	2.5–10 mg IM
Antifungal	Nystatin oral suspension		

The nearer a patient is to death, the less reliable is the oral route though one report showed that 60 per cent were able to continue with oral medication until a few hours before death. After that 25 per cent needed a few suppositories and only 15 per cent injections.[(19)] Which of the many alternatives to the oral route is chosen depends on whether the care is being given in the home or in hospital, who is available to give the medication, whether a drug is available in suppository, transdermal, or injectable form and what is likely to be the most acceptable route for the patient.

See Table 3 for sublingual formulations, Table 6 for essential drugs available as suppositories, and Table 2 for those that may be given SC via a syringe driver. Readers are referred to Chapter 15.9 for details of drug compatibility in a syringe driver.

In many, though by no means all, developing countries the rectal route is preferred with patients willing to have suppositories and their relatives prepared to insert them. It is essential, however, to be sure that the rectum is empty and absorption not prejudiced by blood or mucus. It has also to be remembered that moving patients into a position to insert suppositories may be uncomfortable and unacceptable to them.

In developed countries syringe drivers/pumps are increasingly available making it easy to give continuous SC infusions.[(20)] However, the temptation to mix a pharmacological cocktail in a syringe even at this time in the patient's life should be resisted. What is sometimes forgotten is that relatives can usually be taught how to give SC injections. Provided they are well taught, supervised until they are confident, and understand that though the patient may die at any time they are not the cause of it, this can be a means of enabling a person to stay at home until the end and give great satisfaction to the relative.

When the essential drugs are identified it must then be ascertained that they are available and, if possible, a small supply obtained in readiness. For

Table 6 Drugs available in suppository form

Drug	Available strengths
United Kingdom and United States	
Aspirin	120/130, 195/200, 300, 600/650, 1200 mg (USA) 300, 600 mg (UK)
Indomethacin	50 mg (USA) 100 mg (UK)
Morphine	5, 10, 20, 30 mg (USA) 15, 30 mg (UK)
Domperidone	30 mg
Paracetamol (acetaminophen)	120/125, 325, 650 mg (USA) 125, 500 mg (UK)
Prochlorperazine	2.5 mg (USA) 5, 25 mg
United Kingdom only	
Flurbiprofen	100 mg
Naproxen	500 mg
Diclofenac	100 mg
Oxycodone pectinate	30 mg[a]
Cyclizine	50 mg
Diazepam	10 mg[b]
United States only	
Opium and belladonna (15 mg) B & O supprettes no., 15A, 16A	30, 60 mg
Oxymorphone	5 mg
Hydromorphone	3 mg
Thiethylperazine	10 mg
Trimethobenzamide	100, 200 mg
Chlorpromazine	25, 100 mg

[a] Available on a named-patient basis, that is, supplied by manufacturers on receipt of a special order.

[b] Also available as a rectal solution.

Table 7 Equipment regarded as essential

Firm mattress (a bed is not essential)
Antipressure sore pads/mattress
Drinking cup and spoons
Medicine measuring cup/syringe
Duvet/blankets
Air freshener
Supply of ice cubes
Commode/toilet seat
Male urinal
Back rest/triangle pillow
Bedside table or its equivalent
Electric pad/hot-water bottle
Night lamp/candles
Chair for the carer

Table 8 Equipment regarded as useful but not essential

Suction machine
Drip stand
Room to room call system
Food liquidizer
Portable fan
Patient hoist
Reclining chair
Portable television set/radio
Remote control for television/radio

example, there have been times when both injection and transdermal hyoscine hydrobromide have not been available. Though most hospital pharmacies stock glycopyrronium, a useful alternative to hyoscine, it is not commonly stocked in community pharmacies.

Essential equipment (particularly for the home and nursing home)

Chapter 17 describes palliative care, including the terminal phase, in the home. Information about equipment that should be regarded as essential (Table 7) and other items found useful but not essential is given in some detail (Table 8).

It must be stressed again that advanced planning for the terminal phase is the key. At the same time, particularly when care is being given at home, the impression must never be given that successful care demands that the sick-room be turned into a intensive care facility full of sophisticated equipment.

Emergencies encountered in the terminal phase

Acute stridor

This may be caused by haemorrhage into a tumour pressing on the trachea or just be the final stage of progressive tracheal compression. The patient needs to be sedated as speedily as possible with IV midazolam 5–20 mg (depending on whether or not they have had it recently and in what dose), or rectal diazepam solution 10–20 mg (which relatives can be taught to use in the home), both effective within minutes.

Massive haemorrhage

The commonest sites of such haemorrhage are the carotid (externally) and major veins within the chest (internally) the exact sites only identified at subsequent autopsy. So acute and catastrophic are such events that there is rarely time to do anything other than to curtain the patient off from the view of other patients and visitors in a hospital.

However, where it is recognized that such a haemorrhage might occur it is prudent to have nearby a dark-coloured towel to make the amount of blood lost less obvious to the patient and to have a fast-acting sedative drawn up for immediate sedation. Midazolam 5–20 mg IV (the dose dependent on whether or not the patient was already on that drug) or propofol (an IV anaesthetic) for those familiar with its use. IV opioids have no place on such occasions but methotrimeprazine 50 mg IV can be useful if the others are not available. Usually, by the time the drug has been drawn up into a syringe and administered, the patient is unconscious and is within a minute or so from death.

Myoclonus

Multifocal myoclonus is not uncommon in dying patients and can distress the relatives. Patients are often so ill that they seem unaware of it. It may be caused by dopamine antagonists such as metoclopramide and the neuroleptics and by high-dose opioids, as well as by the withdrawal of such drugs as benzodiazepines, barbiturates, anticonvulsants, and alcohol. The treatment should include:

- Review of medication and doses, particularly opioids.
- Sedation with midazolam SC 5–10 mg every hour until the patient is settled and thereafter 20–30 mg/day by a syringe driver.
- Alternatives are rectal diazepam solution 10–20 mg every hour until settled and thereafter 20 mg each night, or clonazepam SC 0.5 mg hourly until settled and thereafter SC 1–4 mg/day via a syringe driver.

Convulsions

Ten per cent of patients experience grand mal convulsions in the terminal phase (see Chapters 8.14, 8.15, and 10.6). Some may have been long time epileptics, others only having had convulsions since neurosurgery and others as a result of primary or secondary cerebral malignancies. Some may result from sudden withdrawal of long-term anticonvulsants. Usually, anticonvulsants must be continued, using either rectal diazepam or SC midazolam via a syringe driver or aqueous solution of phenobarbitone. Phenobarbitone for injection is usually made up with 90 per cent propylene glycol (200 mg/1 ml). To give it SC it needs to be diluted 1 : 10 in water. It is compatible with diamorphine but with no other drug commonly used in a syringe driver.

Emergency treatment is with midazolam, diazepam, phenobarbitone, or clonazepam as outlined above for the management of myoclonus.

Pathological fracture

By this stage, the patient will usually be bed bound and highly dependent on others to lift up or turn in bed, assist to a bedside commode, and for washing.

It is remarkably easy for a carer to cause a fracture at the site of a malignant metastasis merely by firm handling or by allowing the patient to sit down too rapidly with insufficient support.

It may not be always appropriate to send the patient for emergency orthopaedic surgery. The decision will depend on how long the patient is expected to live, what level of activity and self-care they had immediately before the fracture, whether they could be expected to survive an anaesthetic and a major operation, and whether there are available alternative and effective pain-controlling measures.

Other options—all designed to palliate the pain of the fracture—include immobilizing the fractured leg between sandbags, bandaging a fractured humerus to the side of the trunk and supporting the arm in a sling, and often very effective, infusing local anaesthetic into the fracture site via a fine bore needle and cannula.

The technique is simple and can be done as easily in the home as in a hospital bed. The skin over the fracture site is anaesthetized in the usual way with 2 per cent lignocaine. A fine bore cannula (of the type and size usually used with syringe drivers) is gently inserted though a tiny cut in the skin no more than 5 mm in length until it touches the bone near the fracture. Two per cent lignocaine (10–15 ml) is then slowly injected at a rate of 1 ml/min. Alternatively, it may all be infused from a syringe driver over a period of 12 h after which the procedure may be repeated. The benefit is immediate and, because the duration of effect of lignocaine increases with each infusion less will be needed in succeeding days.

It is imperative that carers, whether family or professional, are reassured that no blame attaches to them for the patient sustaining a fracture. The danger is that if it happens in the home family members can be so distressed by it that they feel unable to continue caring there in case it happens again. They then urge that the patient be admitted to a surgical unit, without giving sufficient thought to the pros and cons of admission to hospital and surgery being put to them by the doctor. Whatever decisions are made, whether at home or in a hospital or palliative care unit, the patient (if able to understand what is being explained) and the family must have everything explained to them, slowly carefully and comprehensively. It can be disastrous if, days later, it is found that the patient is living longer than expected, is feeling stronger than was expected and it seems that surgical fixation might now be preferable. As always details of the emergency, the discussion with the family and whatever course of action is decided upon, must be recorded in the case notes.

Acute urinary retention

Urinary retention, particularly in men, is common in advanced disease often long before the terminal phase is reached. At those times it is important to identify the most likely cause. In the terminal phase, the priority is to ease the discomfort by draining the bladder as a matter of urgency. The patient should be catheterized in the usual sterile manner, the urethra being anaesthetized with lignocaine gel a few minutes before inserting the catheter. Thereafter the catheter may be clamped and released every few hours or left to drain freely into a catheter bag by the bedside. This is not the time for intermittent catheterization. Occasional or even daily bladder lavage with saline may be needed if there is any sign of debris.

It is sometimes argued that catheterization in a terminally ill person is such an unpleasant and undignified procedure that it should only be done as a last resort. In fact, it is not a painful procedure when done correctly, after explaining to the patient why it is being recommended and what is entailed. Most patients, whilst disappointed that it is needed when they are so frail, seem to understand and appreciate it. Unethical and therefore unacceptable would be catheterization without discussion with the patient or to reduce the work of nurses.

Some have suggested that a suprapubic catheter is preferable to a urethral one. This may be so before the terminal phase, and it is certainly easy to perform even on a bed-bound patient, but it can be a more difficult procedure at this late stage and needs special equipment, making it less useful especially in the home.

Table 9 Causes of confusion

Direct central nervous system causes	
	primary brain tumour
	metastatic spread to central nervous system
	seizures
Indirect causes	
	metabolic encephalopathy due to organ failure
	electrolyte imbalance
	treatment side-effects from
	chemotherapeutic agents
	steroids
	radiation
	narcotics
	anticholinergics
	antiemetics
	antivirals
	infection
	haematological abnormalities
	nutritional deficiencies
	paraneoplastic syndromes

Acute confusional state/delirium

Up to 40 per cent of terminally ill patients experience confusion for a variety of reasons (Table 9; see Chapter 8.17).

Once again, the challenge facing the doctor in the terminal phase is different from that in the weeks and months that have gone before. Provided the doctor is certain the patient is going to die within a very short time, this is not the time to be subjecting the patient to more X-rays, blood, bacteriological, and biochemical tests.

Principles of management

- Try to identify a possible cause such as a sudden increase in opioids, hypercalcaemia, uraemia, hepatic encephalopathy, cerebral metastases, sepsis, hyper- or hypoglycaemia, or even a change in surroundings (moved to a different room or furniture moved around), new care attendants, changes in medication (new drugs or discontinuing old ones).
- If the patient is dehydrated (a clinical rather than a biochemical diagnosis now) it is always worth a short trial of saline hypodermoclysis.[28,44] Benefit, in this case reduction in confusion, will be seen within 24 h. Because of the confusion, it may not be possible to explain the possible benefits to the patient. It is, however, usual for relatives to be relieved that 'something is being done' because many of them will have suspected that the patient's decline, and not only his/her confusion, was due to dehydration. This is discussed elsewhere in this chapter.
- Create as quiet and unchanging an environment as possible, explaining the importance of this to relatives and visitors.
- Explain to relatives how to converse with the confused person—not contradicting, not trying to correct them, not arguing with them. Bear in mind that there are often paranoid features deeply distressing to relatives—accusations of causing the illness, of not caring, of being unfaithful.
- Consider music therapy, even if it is as simple as playing the patient's favourite music or music they have always found restful or nostalgic (see Chapter 15.2).
- Consider a mild tranquilizer such as diazepam 5–10 mg once daily, or midazolam via a syringe driver. For agitated confusion haloperidol 2.5–5 mg is preferable for younger patients whilst for the elderly thioridazine is often more helpful.

Terminal anguish/'refractory' suffering

This, one of the greatest challenges in palliative medicine, may present as an emergency. So important is it that it is dealt with in detail later in this chapter.

Death rattle

Though not strictly an emergency, this development nevertheless calls for immediate action. It is seen in 25–92 per cent of dying patients.[2,45,46] This term describes the gurgling, bubbling noise made when a terminally ill patient has secretions at the back of the throat and is too weak either to swallow them or expectorate them. It does not refer to pulmonary oedema nor sputum that cannot be expectorated from lower down the respiratory tract.

By the time patients have a death rattle, they are usually unconscious and therefore not aware of the noise. The relatives sitting by the bedside, on the other hand, are very aware of it and usually upset believing that the patient is 'drowning' in his/her own secretions and that it must be causing them discomfort and distress. Reassurance that this is not the case is seldom effective. They want something to be done.

Aspiration of the secretions in the mouth and oropharynx using a suction machine occasionally helps but for little more than a few minutes before they re-accumulate. Furthermore, it has to be remembered that watching this aspiration can be upsetting to relatives because it looks painful and unpleasant. Asking them to leave the bedside while it is done is undesirable because they wonder what was done that they were not permitted to see.

- It is best to reduce the secretions with hyoscine hydrobromide, 0.4–0.6 mg SC every 4 h, or continuously via a syringe driver. Occasionally, this drug produces confusion in the elderly. More recently, it has become the practice to use hyoscine butyl bromide (Buscopan) 20 mg every 4 h or 120 mg/day by SC infusion. An alternative is glycopyrronium 0.2–0.4 mg SC every 4–6 h as required. It has been reported that 50 per cent of dying patients receive hyoscine in some form in the last 48 h of life.[46–48]

- In some countries, transdermal hyoscine (scopolamine) patches are available, applied over the mastoid promontory, at the first sign of secretions accumulating.

No drug is capable of drying up secretions that have already accumulated, hence the need to monitor the patient carefully to be able to give one of the above preparations as early as possible, as always explaining what is being given and why to the relatives sitting nearby.

The needs of the relatives as the patient is dying

Many of the emotional needs of relatives are dealt with elsewhere in this book (see Chapters 12.1, 12.2, and Section 17). Here we look exclusively at their needs in relation to the patient around the time of the death.

It must be remembered about relatives that:

- They may be physically tired with the nursing they have recently had to do and, if the patient is in hospital, with the travelling involved in visiting.
- They may be elderly or, for other reasons, not be fit and healthy.
- They may be angry that they were not fully informed about the diagnosis, the treatment, and help that was available for them, something mentioned many times in studies of general practice in various countries.[49–52]
- Like patients they are looking back and looking forward. Unlike the patients, they know what the future may hold for them—loneliness, financial problems, social change, new responsibilities, big decisions.
- They often feel helpless and useless, eager to help but not knowing what to do. This is particularly the case when the patient is in hospital or palliative care unit. There, unless special attention is paid to their needs, they can also feel in the way.
- They do not know what to say, either to the dying patient or, very often to each other. Often family members have not been in touch with each other for many years and feel like strangers round the bed.
- They may not know what to do when they sit by the bedside. Is it insensitive to read a book while the patient sleeps? Is it wrong to get up and walk around or go outside for a smoke? Should they touch the patient or hold her hand? If the patient wants a drink should they try to help or call a nurse? Does it look uncaring to chat with relatives and friends they have not seen for some time, all gathered round the bedside? If they go home for a few hours sleep will they be called in time?
- If the relationship has not been a happy one or the dying person has been unconscious for some time (and in that sense has 'died already') they worry in case they are not showing appropriate grief as they sit at the bedside. As one lady remarked 'I did all my crying months ago and I've no tears left. Is that wrong of me?'
- They may be embarrassed about religious matters for the patient or themselves if their faith has lapsed, and not be sure whether or not to call in a clergyman, priest, or rabbi. How do you organize a funeral? Where do you turn for help?
- They may not know what happens at the time of death, what physical changes occur in the patient, what to expect, and what to do. This is particularly the case in the home when there may be no nurse or doctor present. A common question there is 'How will I know he/she has died and what shall I have to do?'
- They may sit by the bedside and wonder how long it will be before they too are dying, perhaps of the same disease. Particularly, this is the case when one of an old couple dies or with partners each of whom has AIDS, or in countries where tuberculosis is now pandemic.

Experience suggests that it is *never* safe to assume that people know anything about death, know how to recognize it, what to say and what to do, or even how to behave at the bedside. It is always better to get them together and explain everything, giving each person an opportunity to ask questions and express any fears or misgivings. Time so spent is never wasted. Whether or not it is done by a doctor or nurse depends on who can do it best and is best known to family members.

However, some points are so important and occur so frequently they are worth separate mention. Relatives and friends sitting by a bedside need to be told:

- That patients may be able to hear them even though they give no responses.
- The features of death—colour changes, temperature changes, slowing of respiration, involuntary twitching, moans (usually thought by relatives to be caused by pain).
- The features of, and reason for, Cheyne–Stokes respiration. This can be very frightening for relatives, being seen as 'fighting for breath'. It can be helpful to remind them that they have probably heard their spouse or partner breathing like that during the night.
- That when the unconscious patient grips or tugs at the bedclothes as they roll over in bed, they are not in pain but doing what we all do in bed but are unaware of.

It is sometimes asked whether it is safe/right for children to be allowed to visit a dying relative. The answer is yes, provided certain conditions are met. They should first have it explained to them how ill the person is, what they may look like, and whether or not they will be able to speak to the young visitor(s). Children should always be accompanied by an adult who should encourage them to talk afterwards about their visit. Usually children are very 'matter-of-fact', less upset than might be expected by changes in appearance or speech, and often intrigued by the hospital. Their visit often brings considerable happiness to a patient still able to talk to them.

Home, hospital, hospice/palliative care unit?

Where should patients die? (See also Section 17.)

There is no one best place to die.[53–55] Check-lists to help make decisions about place of death are given below. Factors influencing the decisions regarding home, hospice, or palliative care unit include patients' care requirements, available resources (medical, nursing, family, and physical) primary disease and patient and family preference.[56]

Many patients and their families prefer that care be delivered in the home rather than in an institutional setting.[57,58] The availability of palliative/hospice home care and, where necessary, high-tech nursing has made this option more feasible for more patients but the provision of such services varies widely even with individual countries. Home care generally requires the availability of a family or other supports to assist in patient care.[59–64] Care resources should be evaluated before offering home care. It has to be remembered that, as a result of disease progression and increasing care needs, patients' and family attitudes regarding preferred place of death frequently change.[55] Contingency plans for inpatient respite or ongoing care are prudent.

A study to identify reasons for admitting terminally ill cancer patients to hospital found that the two major reasons were requirement of special medical and nursing care unavailable in the home (40 per cent) and to provide care for some patients with no family or friend support (27 per cent).[65] Standards for the care of dying patients have been developed and the care of such patients should be subjected to critical audit.[66–71]

Inpatient care can be delivered in a specialist hospice/palliative care setting or in an acute care hospital. There are data to suggest that there are advantages and disadvantages in each setting. A study of the quality of life of 182 terminally ill cancer patients in two specialist palliative care units with that of those in a general hospital found that the patients in a specialist palliative care unit showed less indirectly expressed anger, more positive feelings, and less anxiety about isolation but that they had more anxiety about death than those cared for in an acute care ward.[72] Since many cancer patients die in acute care hospitals, adequate provision must be made for their specific care needs.[73–75] The skills of a hospital palliative care team can be particularly helpful at this time, or in the absence of such a multiprofessional team, the help of a palliative medicine specialist.

Whenever possible, imminently dying patients should be cared for in private/single room facilities with adequate room for family members. Visiting restrictions should either be lifted completely or be flexible to meet patient and family needs.

Here we are not looking at where care might be given in the final months *but in the final days and hours.* Prior to that time it should have been agreed by everyone, including the patient, where the terminal phase is to be spent. There are exceedingly few reasons why anyone should need to be moved from home to hospital (including a palliative care unit) in this late terminal phase. In some cultures, however, patients who may have been a long time in hospital are taken home within hours of dying so important is it to them and their families that they die at home.

The advantages of care at home

- Familiar, and often much cherished, surroundings for the patient.
- An atmosphere less threatening and unfamiliar than a hospital for patient and relatives.
- Being cared for by a family doctor and community nurse known to the patient and family.
- No strain or fatigue as a result of travelling to see the patient in hospital.

The disadvantages of care at home

- A sense of isolation for relatives having to care without the reassuring presence of nurses and doctors and what might be regarded as essential equipment near at hand.
- A sense of daunting responsibility for relatives giving medication and nursing the patient.
- The possibility that if medical help is needed, the doctor who comes may not know anything about the patient, or that it might result in an emergency admission to an unfamiliar hospital.
- The problem of disturbing noise from neighbours affecting either the patient or relatives in need of sleep.
- The number of well-meaning visitors who can exhaust the patient, and phone enquirers who tire the relatives.

The advantages of care in an acute hospital ward

- If in the ward/unit where the patient has been before, the care will be given by experienced staff familiar with the patient and some of the relatives.
- Case notes, with all the essential clinical information about the patient, will be available.
- It is reassuring to relatives to know that should there be a crisis there will be trained staff and any necessary equipment on hand.
- Even though the patient knows death is inevitable, there is something reassuring about being in a place with a positive ethic.
- There may be a specialist hospital palliative care team to advise.

Disadvantages of care in an acute hospital ward

- If the patient has not previously been in that ward/unit, they will find themselves being cared for by total strangers.
- Particularly if they are admitted to a hospital they have not been in before it may be thought necessary by the doctors to subject the patient to diagnostic tests, to discontinue such essential drugs as opioids while pain is assessed, and to embark on new treatments.
- Some hospitals insist that dying patients have electrocardiogram monitoring and a few even insist on encephalogram monitoring. In the view of the authors and the editors of this book neither can be justified in the terminal phase.
- In many hospitals, there are no specialist hospital palliative care teams or palliative medicine specialists. In some hospitals, the quality of palliative care is less than optimal.[76] Even patients admitted for pain control may suffer more rather than less pain after their admission.[50]
- The distance for relatives to travel to/from the hospital may make travel expensive and tiring, adding to the worries of the relatives.
- In some countries, depending on the health care system, there may be financial burdens incurred by hospital care.

Palliative care unit

A study comparing the relative merits of a palliative care unit and a ward in an acute hospital has been cited above.[14] However desirable it may seem to admit all dying people to palliative care units, it must be asked if this is the right thing to do and if it is realistic. Should they not be reserved for patients with particularly complex or rare problems, or for patients unable to remain at home for sociofinancial reasons? Will there ever be sufficient palliative care beds to admit everyone who wants to (rather than who needs to) be admitted there? Would admitting everyone there not de-skill the countless doctors and nurses who want to care better for their patients at the end of life? Perhaps all that can be said with confidence is that if, before the patient enters the terminal phase, it is recognized that his/her care may be exceptionally challenging and complex, then admission to a specialist palliative care unit should be arranged well in advance or the help and advice of a palliative medicine specialist be invited.

Terminal anguish/terminal sedation

Occasionally, the suffering of the patient is so severe that it merits the term 'anguish'. As always in palliative medicine, it may be physical, emotional, or spiritual. It may be caused by 'refractory' symptoms or new symptoms. It may be difficult to distinguish between the different causes and components of the suffering.

The term 'refractory' is here applied to symptoms that cannot adequately be controlled despite aggressive efforts to identify a tolerable therapy that does not compromise consciousness. The diagnostic criteria for the designation of a refractory symptom include that the clinician must perceive that further invasive and non-invasive interventions are: (i) incapable of providing adequate relief; (ii) associated with excessive and intolerable acute or chronic morbidity; or (iii) unlikely to provide relief within a tolerable time frame. Terminally ill patients with such refractory symptoms may need sedation. The clinical and ethical issues involved will now be discussed.

Physical symptoms

The prevalence of refractory pain at the end of life remains controversial.[77–79] In their 1990 paper, Ventafridda et al. in Milan reported that 63 of 120 terminally ill patients developed unendurable symptoms that required deep sedation for adequate relief. In almost half the problem was pain.[8 Fainsinger et al. in Edmonton found that 16 out of 100 patients dying in a specialist palliative care unit required sedation for symptom control, six of them for pain.[7] Stone et al.[80] retrospectively comparing two such units in London found that 26 per cent of 115 patients needed sedation, the commonest reasons being delirium, mental anguish, pain, and dyspnoea.

Ethically, clinicians want neither to subject severely distressed patients to therapies that provide inadequate relief or excessive morbidity, nor to sacrifice conscious function when viable alternatives remain unexplored. The doctor has a responsibility both to distinguish between a 'refractory' symptom and a 'difficult-to-control' symptom and to identify new symptoms. This is particularly the case with pain.

Knowledge in the assessment and management of cancer pain is frequently deficient amongst physicians who lack specific training in this field.[81] A specialist consultation service can be helpful. A paper from the Pain Service at Memorial Sloan-Kettering Cancer Center, NY, reported a previously unidentified aetiology for the pain in 64 per cent of 376 referred patients, including new neurological features in 36 per cent of patients and an unsuspected infection in 4 per cent.[82] Coyle et al., working in the same hospital, reported a series of cases of crescendo pain with unsuspected delirium, treatment of which restored adequate pain control.[83] An unpublished study from Scotland of 500 consecutive admissions to a specialist palliative care unit because of severe pain found that 52 per cent were on the wrong analgesics, in the wrong dose, or by an inappropriate route.[84] Clearly, the clinician has a moral responsibility to evaluate the patient both thoroughly and repeatedly and, if needs be, to call in an expert in pain management if pain is identified as one of the causes of the anguish.

In the case of pain, questions that *must* be asked include:

- Have the different pain syndromes been identified?
- Have all the appropriate treatments for each syndrome been given?
- Have opioid doses been titrated up to the maximum tolerated dose?
- Have any side-effects been appropriately dealt with?
- Have spinal opioids been considered?
- Have anaesthetic or neurosurgical options been considered?

Reference has already been made to dyspnoea. This is known to increase in the days immediately before death and to be difficult to treat.[85] Ten to fifteen per cent of dying patients have convulsions.

Psychological and existential suffering

This can be extremely difficult to diagnose and to treat appropriately. Fear and panic may erupt in a previously settled patient. Existential/spiritual issues can suddenly overwhelm a person who has appeared serene and confident in his/her faith.[35–37,86,87] Other patients have terrifying recall of traumatic events in their past lives. To make their care more difficult there are few established strategies for the management of existential suffering. It has also to be remembered that psychological distress and the desire for death do not necessarily indicate an advanced state of psychological deterioration[88] and that psychological adaptation and coping are common.[89]

How is this complex picture of suffering to be evaluated?

Individual clinician bias can affect decision-making.[90,91] No one clinician is at the bedside observing the dying patient throughout 24 h. Many different skills are necessary to evaluate such complex problems. The answer lies in case conferences/team meetings attended by all members of the care team plus such invited specialists as oncologists, anaesthetists, psychiatrists, clinical psychologists, social workers, and pastoral care staff. Though not necessarily invited in to the meeting, relatives can often contribute significant insights and details of history previously unknown to the care team.

Before embarking on 'terminal sedation' the following steps must be followed:

- Every symptom should be evaluated by clinicians experienced in this work, if needs be calling in experts for advice, and who have established a relationship with the patient.
- Every aspect of the suffering and its management should be discussed at a specially convened team meeting as described above.[92–94]
- The ethical issues involved in terminal sedation should be discussed in the team meeting.
- If the decision is made to employ sedation ground rules must be laid down for regular, frequent assessment of its effectiveness, side-effects, the views of relatives, how long it should be maintained, and the indications for discontinuing it.

Ethical considerations in terminal sedation

The use of sedation in the management of refractory symptoms has been examined in several studies.[7,8,80,95–97]

Clinicians are committed to the ethical principles of beneficence and of non-maleficence. They want to neither subject severely distressed patients to therapies that provide inadequate relief or excessive morbidity, nor sacrifice conscious function when viable alternatives remain unexplored, hence the need for thorough ongoing patient evaluation.

Terminal sedation can have two effects. One is the desired effect—to reduce physical and psychological suffering. The other is the undesired effect—to shorten life. In this case it is the *intention* rather than the *consequence* that is important in judging whether the action is ethically acceptable or not. In other words, the principle of beneficence takes precedence over the principle of non-maleficence.

The extreme distress of these patients does not absolve the doctor from discussing the option of short-term sedation with the patient, assuring them that it will be kept under continuous review, and trying to ascertain the patient's wishes.

Sedation is something suggested by distressed relatives but in speaking to them the doctor must stress that:

- Though they may be relieved to see the patient 'at peace', it is being done primarily for the patient and not for the relatives.
- Thorough evaluation has been carried out and no reversible condition has been identified.
- Sedation may be discontinued at any time for further evaluation of the patient's suffering and needs.
- When the sedation is given they will be unable to converse with the patient.
- Cardiopulmonary resuscitation will not be carried out.
- Terminal sedation is not a form of euthanasia.
- Terminal sedation is not being used to prolong life.

Terminal sedation should not be regarded as a unique ethical issue, different from others met in clinical care. The principles underpinning its use are the same as for any clinical intervention.[94,98] It should be regarded as part of a continuum of care of which palliative care is also a part. It is not, as some have suggested, a form of euthanasia even though it has the potential to shorten life. In the landmark 1957 English case of Regina *v* Adams, Lord Justice Devlin wrote in his judgement 'If the first purpose of medicine, the restoration of health, can no longer be achieved, there is still much for a doctor to do, and he is entitled to do all that is proper and necessary to relieve pain and suffering, even if the measures he takes may coincidentally shorten life'. He went on to say 'the cause of death is the illness or the injury, and the proper medical treatment that is administered and that has an incidental effect on determining the exact moment of death is not the cause in any sensible use of the term'.[99] A judgement of the Supreme Court of the United States rejected assisted suicide but endorsed the use of terminal sedation in the management of refractory symptoms at the end of life.[100]

There is the potential for abuse of terminal sedation. Data from the Netherlands indicate that such sedation, ostensibly to relieve distress but with the manifest intent of hastening death is commonplace[101–104] and from the United States[105,106] indicate that the practice is not uncommon. Hence the term 'slow euthanasia'.[107–109]

Terminal sedation is not euthanasia for the following reasons:

- The intent is to provide symptom relief—a continuum of the palliative care which preceeded the terminal phase.

- The intervention is proportionate to the prevailing symptom, its severity, and the prevailing goals of care.
- The death of the patient is not a criterion for the success of the treatment.
- The sedation is occasionally reduced to ascertain whether or not the patient still needs it, something promised by the doctor and the care team to the patient and the relatives. There is considerable anecdotal evidence that patients can return to a state of physical and emotional peace needing minimal sedation after a day or two of heavy sedation as described below.

Methods of sedation

Only when, as discussed above, all appropriate treatment has been given for pain and other symptoms, can the following be tried. Their modes of action differ and in other respects they are not pharmacologically comparable but we start with the one most commonly used.

- Midazolam, SC via a syringe driver, 20–200 mg over 24 h, bearing in mind that tolerance develops rapidly. If it is decided to reduce the dose, it should be remembered that midazolam has an anterograde amnesic effect. The patient will have no recollection of what happened before the sedation (including explanations and reassurances).
- Methotrimeprazine, intramuscular (IM), SC, or IV for rapid effect. It may be necessary to give as much as 250 mg every 4 h.
- Chlorpromazine in similar doses but it is less sedative than methotrimeprazine and has no analgesic properties.

The use of midazolam,[96,97,110–115] lorazepam,[89] and flunitrazepam[116] is well documented.

- Thioridazine 10–75 mg given as an IV bolus followed by a continuous infusion 60–400 mg/day.
- On the rare occasions when benzodiazepines cause paradoxical agitation, barbiturates might be tried instead.[117,118] In one report on managing refractory symptoms in 17 dying patients, nine were given amobarbital and eight thiopentone with symptom relief achieved in all cases. The median survival of these patients after initiation of the infusion was 23 h (range 2 h to 4 days). All died in their sleep.
- In skilled hands propofol, a pure sedative, is a useful drug at this time in a patient's life.[119,120] It has also been reported as useful in paediatric palliative care.[121]

It is inappropriate to use escalating dose of opioids to tranquilize such patients. Opioids are analgesic agents, not primarily sedatives. Not only may they be ineffective but neuroexcitatory side-effects such as myoclonus or agitated delirium may develop only adding to the distress.[122–124]

Death itself

In the days and hours leading up to the patient's death:

- The pulse gets weaker but, unless it was previously arrhythmic, will remain regular.
- Blood pressure gradually falls (and incidentally need not be taken because it adds nothing to the care plan).
- Respiration become shallower, slower and varies in amplitude, often in a Cheyne–Stokes pattern.
- Consciousness is slowly lost except in the few patients who retain it until a few minutes before they die.
- The skin gets colder, from the periphery inwards, and feels clammy.
- The colour of the skin of the extremities and round the mouth becomes faintly cyanotic.
- Eventually, all signs of cardiorespiratory function cease and the corneal reflex is lost.

In a hospital or palliative care unit it is essential, unless the family explicitly say they do not want it, that a nurse or doctor is with the patient and family when the patient dies. It may mean sitting with them, or standing unobtrusively at the back of the room but their presence, even though they are not doing anything to the patient, can bring great comfort and reassurance to the family.

As we have seen, the family will have been told what to expect but it still helps them when the nurse confirms that death has occurred and then, in hospital, informs the doctor. Trying to sense what is best for that family and what they might want, she then offers to leave them together sharing their sorrow or to stay with them as long as they want her to. The presence of a nurse or doctor is all that is needed. Platitudes and expressions of sympathy seldom help. Letting people cry, hold each other, and behave in the traditional way for their culture is all important. For some, it is a time for silence, each relative locked in their own grief. In others, there are vocal expressions of their pain and loss. All are 'normal'. They should be enabled to remain with the body of their loved one as long as they want to and then be given the opportunity to sit together in a room set aside for such occasions as this. It is there that the doctor should join them, thank them for the privilege of caring for the patient, explain what has been written in the death certificate and, if the team feel such a request is justified, ask if they would give consent for a post mortem. When they eventually leave the hospital they should, unless they decline the offer, be accompanied to the door as a final mark of respect. Many hospices/palliative care units provide a car and volunteer driver to take them home to save them using their own cars or public transport.

Post mortems

Until a few years ago it was an anathema to suggest conducting post mortems on palliative care patients. More recently, it has come to be appreciated that autopsies to identify or confirm the aetiology of symptoms, rather than defining pathology, can be very helpful.[125] The pathologist can be told of inexplicable or difficult to control pains, of inexplicable dyspnoea or hiccups, or confirm the clinical suspicion of cerebral metastases not shown on scans. Such reasons for doing an autopsy and what might be learned that could help others must be explained to the responsible relatives, and a promise always given that not only will their general practitioner get a detailed report but the palliative medicine doctor will explain everything found to whichever members of the family want this information.

Ethical issues

Advanced directives ('living wills')

It goes without saying that in a country where advanced directives are legally binding they must be respected. In other countries, the patient may have expressed their feelings about resuscitation to a family member, doctor, or lawyer. It is the responsibility of the doctor caring for the dying patient to familiarize himself/herself with these wishes or to discuss the issue with the patient. This need not be stressful or embarrassing.

If the principles outlined in this chapter are followed, the doctor will be able to reassure the patient that everything possible will be done to ensure comfort, dignity, peace, and respect for his wishes and for the relatives. Nothing will be done to hasten death nor will futile treatment be given for any reason. When death comes, he/she will not be alone and, unless he/she so wishes, will not be kept alive artificially and will not be resuscitated.

Occasionally, a patient has signified that he/she wishes his/her organs to be donated for transplantation. If this wish is known before the death, the clinician must discuss the implications not only with the relevant transplant surgeons and organ transplant coordinator for the region but with the relatives. However, relatives need to be advised that organs can seldom be used from cancer patients with the occasional exception of patients with primary cerebral neoplasm. There may be few problems if the patient is dying in a tertiary referral hospital but if the patient is in a palliative care unit or hospice, transfer in the terminal phase to the larger centre may be necessary, something that neither the patient nor the relatives might want. It can sometimes be a comfort to relatives if the organs are not acceptable for transplantation if the body is subjected to post mortem or accepted by an anatomy department, in both instances helping to extend our knowledge.

Other ethical issues such as rehydration, total parenteral nutrition (TPN), and the use of antibiotics, are all discussed in other chapters in this book.

Further discussion of ethical issues encountered during the terminal phase will be found in refs[126–128] and in Chapters 3.3 and 3.7 of this book.

And finally…

The responsibility of the palliative care team does not stop when the patient has died and they have said good-bye to the grieving relatives. There is one last thing to do—review every aspect of the care they have given, from the time of first involvement, through the terminal phase to the death.

- Was all suffering relieved and if not, what more could have been done?
- Was the patient given every opportunity to express their feelings and fears and were they addressed appropriately?
- Was death peaceful and dignified in all respects?
- Was everything possible done to support and care for the relatives?
- Where could the care have been better?
- How does each member of the care team feel?
- What lessons have been learnt that might lead to better care for others?

Perhaps the final words of this chapter should be those of a patient, speaking to one of us only minutes before she died.

> There are times when you want your doctor to have lots of letters after his name to show how clever he is. There are other times when you want your doctor to be your friend as well as being your doctor. This is the loneliest time I have ever known in my life—a time when all I want is a friend, particularly if he is also my doctor. Please stay with me for just a few minutes more. You don't need to talk unless you want to. Just be there.

References

1. **Morita, T.** et al. (2001). Improved accuracy of physicians' survival prediction of terminally ill patients using the Palliative Prognostic Index. *Palliative Medicine* **15**, 419–24.
2. **Lichter, I. and Hunt, E.** (1990). The last 48 hours of life. *Journal of Palliative Care* **6** (4), 7–15.
3. **Nauck, F., Klachik, E., and Ostgathe, C.** (2001). Symptom control during the last three days of life. *European Journal of Palliative Care* **10**, 81–4.
4. **Conill, C.** et al. (1997). Symptom prevalence in the last week of life. *Journal of Pain and Symptom Management* **14** (6), 328–31.
5. **Grond, S.** et al. (1991). Validation of WHO guidelines for cancer pain during the last days and hours of life. *Journal of Pain and Symptom Management* **9**, 341–5.
6. **Ellershaw, J.** et al.(2001). Care of the dying: setting standards for symptom control in the last 48 hours of life. *Journal of Pain and Symptom Management* **21**, 12–17.
7. **Fainsinger, R.** et al. (1991). Symptom control during the last week of life on a palliative care unit. *Journal of Palliative Care* **7** (1), 5–11.
8. **Ventafridda, V.** et al. (1990). Symptom prevalence and control during cancer patients' last days of life. *Journal of Palliative Care* **6** (3), 7–11.
9. **Parkes, C.M.** (1978). Home or hospital? Terminal care as seen by surviving spouses. *Journal of the Royal College of General Practitioners* **28**, 19–30.
10. **McCarthy, M.** et al. (1996). Dying from heart disease. *Journal of the Royal College of Physicians of London* **30** (4), 325–8.
11. **Edmonds, P.** et al. (2001). A comparison of the palliative care needs of patients dying from chronic respiratory disease and lung cancer. *Palliative Medicine* **15**, 287–95.
12. **Davies, N. and Curtiss, M.** (2000). Providing palliative care in end-stage heart failure. *Professional Nurse* **15**, 389–92.
13. **Sykes, N.P., Pearson, S.E., and Chell, S.** (1992). Quality of care of the terminally ill: the carers' perspective. *Palliative Medicine* **6**, 227–46.
14. **Seabrook, D.** et al. (1998). Dying from cancer in community hospitals or in a hospice. Closest carers' perceptions. *British Journal of General Practice* **48**, 1317–21.
15. **Addington-Hall, J. and McCarthy, M.** (1995). Dying from cancer: results of a national population-based investigation. *Palliative Medicine* **9**, 295–305.
16. **Barritt, P.W.** (1984). Care of the dying in one practice. *Journal of the Royal College of General Practitioners* **34**, 446–8.
17. **Peruselli, C.** et al. (1999). Home palliative care for terminal cancer patients: a survey on the final week of life. *Palliative Medicine* **13** (3), 233–41.
18. **Neudert, O.** et al. (2001). The course of the terminal phase in patients with amyotrophic lateral sclerosis. *Journal of Neurology* **248**, 612–16.
19. **Twycross, R.G. and Lack, S.** *Symptom Control in Far-advanced Cancer: Pain Relief.* London: Pitman, 1983.
20. **Dickman, A., Littlewood, C., and Varga, J.** *The Syringe Driver: Continuous Subcutaneous Infusions in Palliative Care.* Oxford: Oxford University Press, 2002.
21. **Spiller, J. and Alexander, D.** (1993). Domiciliary care: a comparison of the views of terminally ill patients and their care-givers. *Palliative Medicine* **7**, 109–15.
22. **Bruera, E.** et al. (1993). Effects of oxygen on dyspnoea in hypoxaemic terminal cancer patients. *Lancet* **342**, 13–14.
23. **Schwartzstein, R.M.** et al. (1987). Cold facial stimulation reduces breathlessness in normal subjects. *American Review of Respiratory Diseases* **136**, 58–61.
24. **McIver, B., Walsh, D., and Nelson, K.** (1994). The use of chlorpromazine for symptom control in dying cancer patients. *Journal of Pain and Symptom Management* **9**, 341–5.
25. **Khoo, D.** et al. (1994). Palliation of malignant intestinal obstruction using octeotride. *European Journal of Cancer* **30**, 28–30.
26. **De Conno, F.** et al. (1991). Subcutaneous infusion of hyoscine butylbromide reduces secretions in patients with gastro-intestinal obstruction. *Journal of Pain and Symptom Management* **6**, 484–6.
27. **Fainsinger, R. and Bruera, E.** (1994). The management of dehydration in terminally ill patients. *Journal of Palliative Care* **10** (3), 55–9.
28. **Fainsinger, R.** et al. (1994). The use of hypodermoclysis for rehydration in terminally ill cancer patients. *Journal of Pain and Symptom Management* **9**, 298–302.
29. **Regnard, C. and Mannix, K.** (1991). Reduced hydration or feeling in advanced disease. *Palliative Medicine* **5**, 161–4.
30. **Musgrave, C.F., Brtal, N., and Opstad, J.** (1995). The sensation of thirst in dying patients. *Journal of Palliative Care* **11**, 17–21.
31. **Feuz, A. and Rapin, C.-H.** (1994). An observational study of the role of pain control and food adaptation of elderly patients with terminal cancer. *Journal of the American Dietetic Association* **94** (7), 767–70.
32. **Hippocrates** (460–357 BC/BCE). Aphorisms translated by Chaucer.
33. **Speck, P.W. and Ainsworth-Smith, I.** *Letting Go: Caring for the Dying and the Bereaved.* London: SPCK, 1982.
34. **Speck, P.W.** (1998). Spiritual issues in palliative care. In *Oxford Textbook of Palliative Medicine* 2nd edn. (ed. D. Doyle, G.W.C. Hanks, and N. Macdonald), pp. 805–14. Oxford: Oxford University Press.
35. **Georgesen, J. and Dungan, J.M.** (1996). Managing spiritual distress in patients with advanced cancer pain. *Cancer Nursing* **19** (5), 376–83.
36. **Speck, P.W.** *Being There—Pastoral Care at Times of Illness.* London: SPCK, 1988.
37. **Millison, M.B.** (1988). Spirituality and the care giver. Developing an underutilized facet of care. *American Journal of Hospital Care* **5** (2), 37–44.
38. **Kearney, M.** (1987). Palliative medicine—just another specialty? *Palliative Medicine* **6**, 39–46.
39. **Doyle, D.** (1992). Have we looked beyond the physical and psychosocial? *Journal of Pain and Symptom Management* **7**, 302–11.
40. **Neuberger, J.** *Caring for Dying Patients of Different Faiths.* St Louis MO: Mosby, 1994.
41. **McIllmurray, M.B.** et al. (2003). Psychosocial needs in cancer patients related to religious belief. *Palliative Medicine* **17**, 49–54.

42. **Doyle, D.** (1993). Polypharmacy in palliative medicine. Unpublished data on 1000 consecutive admissions, presented in Turku, Finland.
43. **Mercadente, S.** et al. (2001). Pattern of drug use by advanced cancer patients followed at home. *Journal of Palliative Care* **17** (1), 37–41.
44. **Bruera, E. and Fainsinger, R.** (1997). Clinical management of cachexia and anorexia. In *Oxford Textbook of Palliative Medicine* (ed. D. Doyle, G.W.C. Hanks, and N. Macdonald), pp. 948–95. Oxford: Oxford University Press.
45. **Ellershaw, J., Sutcliffe, C., and Sanders, C.M.** (1995). Dehydration and the dying patient. *Journal of Pain and Symptom Management* **10**, 192–7.
46. **Bennet, M.** (1996). Death rattle: an audit of hyoscine (scopolamine) use and review of management. *Journal of Pain and Symptom Management* **12**, 229–33.
47. **Hughes, A.** et al. (2000). Audit of three antimuscarinic drugs for managing retained secretions. *Palliative Medicine* **14**, 221–2.
48. **Dawson, H.R.** (1989). The use of transdermal scopolamine in the control of death rattle. *Journal of Palliative Care* **5**, 31–3.
49. **Carrol, D.S.** (1998). An audit of place of death of cancer patients in a semi-rural Scottish practice. *Palliative Medicine* **12**, 51–5.
50. **Toscani, F. and Mancini, C.** (1989). Inadequacies of care in far-advanced cancer patients: a comparison between home and hospital in Italy. *Palliative Medicine* **4**, 31–6.
51. **Blyth, A.C.** (1991). Audit of terminal care in a general practice. *British Medical Journal* **330**, 983–6.
52. **De Conno, F.** et al. (1993). On the last days of life. *Journal of Palliative Care* **9** (3), 47–50.
53. **Goh, C.** (1998). Preferred place of death. *Singapore Medical Journal* **39** (10), 430–1 (editorial).
54. **Hinton, J.** (1994). Can home care maintain an acceptable quality of life for patients with terminal cancer and their relatives? *Palliative Medicine* **8**, 183–96.
55. **Hinton, J.** (1994). Which patients with terminal cancer are admitted from home care? *Palliative Medicine* **8**, 197–210.
56. **Higginson, I.J.** et al.(1998). Where do cancer patients die? Ten year trends in the place of death of cancer patients in England. *Palliative Medicine* **12** (5), 353–63.
57. **Lee, A. and Pang, W.S.** (1998). Preferred place of death: a local study of cancer patients and their relatives. *Singapore Medical Journal* **39** (10), 447–60.
58. **Townsend, J.** et al. (1990). Terminal cancer care and patients' preference for place of death: a prospective study. *British Medical Journal* **301** (6749), 415–17.
59. **De Conno, F.** et al. (1996). Effect of home care on the place of death of advanced cancer patients. *European Journal of Cancer* **32A** (7), 1142–7.
60. **Hinton, J.** (1996). Services given and help perceived during home care for terminal cancer. *Palliative Medicine* **10** (2), 125–34.
61. **Sims, A.** et al. (1997). Social class variation in place of cancer death. *Palliative Medicine* **11** (5), 369–73.
62. **Smeenk, F.W.** et al. (1998). Cost analysis of transmural home care for terminal cancer patients. *Patient Education and Counselling* **35** (3), 201–11.
63. **Smeenk, F.** et al. (1998). Effectiveness of home care programmes for patients with incurable cancer on their quality of life and time spent in hospital: systematic review. *British Medical Journal* **316** (7149), 1939–44.
64. **Stajdugar, K.I. and Davies, B.** (1998). Death at home: challenges for families and directions for the future. *Journal of Palliative Care* **14** (3), 8–14.
65. **Walsh, D. and Kingston, R.D.** (1988). The use of hospital beds for terminally ill cancer patients. *European Journal of Surgical Oncology* **14** (5), 367–70.
66. **Ajemian, I.C.** (1992). Hospitals and health care facilities. *Journal of Palliative Care* **8** (1), 33–7.
67. **Joint Commission on Accreditation of Health Care Organisations** (1991). Care of the dying patient standards for the 1991 CSM. *Joint Commission Perspectives* **11** (3), B1–3.
68. **American College of Physicians** (1992). American College of Physicians Ethics Manual. Third edition. *Annals of Internal Medicine* **117** (11), 947–60.
69. **American Geriatrics Society** (1995). The care of dying patients: a position statement from the American Geriatrics Society. AGS Ethics Committee. *Journal of the American Geriatrics Society* **43** (5), 577–8.
70. **American Medical Association** (1996). Good care of the dying patient. Council on Scientific Affairs, American Medical Association. *Journal of the American Medical Association* **275** (6), 474–8.
71. **Latimer, E.** (1991). Caring for seriously ill and dying patients: the philosophy and ethics. *Canadian Medical Association Journal* **144** (7), 859–64.
72. **Viney, L.L.** et al. (1994). Dying in palliative care units and in hospital: a comparison of the quality of life of terminal cancer patients. *Journal of Consulting and Clinical Psychology* **62** (11), 157–64.
73. **Adelstein, W. and Burton, S.** (1998). Palliative care in the acute hospital setting. *Journal of Neuroscience Nursing* **30** (3), 200–4.
74. **Bircumshaw, D.** (1993). Palliative care in the acute hospital setting. *Journal of Advanced Nursing* **18** (1), 1665–6 (editorial).
75. **Constantini, M.** et al. (1993). Palliative home care and place of death among cancer patients: a population-based study. *Palliative Medicine* **7**, 323–31.
76. **Nowels, D.** et al. (1999). Cancer pain management in home settings: a comparison of primary care and oncologic physicians. *Journal of Palliative Care* **15** (3), 5–9.
77. **Mount, B.** (1990). A final crescendo of pain? *Journal of Palliative Care* **6** (3), 5–6.
78. **Roy, D.J.** (1990). Need they sleep before they die? *Journal of Palliative Care* **6** (3), 3–4 (editorial) (see comments).
79. **Enck, R.E.** (1991). Drug-induced terminal sedation for symptom control. *American Journal of Hospital and Palliative Care* **8** (5), 3–5.
80. **Stone, P.** et al. (1997). A comparison of the use of sedatives in a hospital support team and in a hospice. *Palliative Medicine* **11** (2), 140–4.
81. **Von Roenn, J.H. and Cleeland, C.S.** (1993). Physician attitudes and practice in cancer pain management. A survey from the Eastern Cooperative Oncology Group. *Annals of Internal Medicine* **119** (2), 121–6.
82. **Gonzales, G.R.** et al. (1991). The impact of a comprehensive evaluation in the management of cancer pain. *Pain* **47** (2), 141–4.
83. **Coyle, N.** et al. (1994). Delirium as a contributing factor to 'crescendo' pain: three case reports. *Journal of Pain Symptom Management* **9** (1), 44–7.
84. **Doyle, D.** (1992). Unpublished data on 500 consecutive admissions to St Columba's Hospice, Edinburgh.
85. **Heyes-Moore, L.H., Ross, V., and Mullee, M.A.** (1991). How much of a problem is dyspnoea in advanced cancer? *Palliative Medicine* **5**, 20–6.
86. **Stepnick, A. and Perry, T.** (1992). Preventing spiritual distress in the dying patient. *Journal of Psychosocial Nursing and Mental Health Services* **30** (1), 17–24.
87. **Kissane, D.W.** et al. (1997). Cognitive-existential group therapy for patients with primary breast cancer—techniques and themes. *Psychooncology* **6** (1), 25–33.
88. **Chochinov, H.M.** et al. (1995). Desire for death in the terminally ill. *American Journal of Psychiatry* **152** (8), 1185–91.
89. **Breitbart, W.** et al. (1998). Psychiatric aspects of palliative care. In *Oxford Textbook of Palliative Medicine* 2nd edn. (ed. D. Doyle, G.W.C. Hanks, and N. Macdonald), pp. 933–54. Oxford: Oxford University Press.
90. **Christakis, N.A. and Asch, D.A.** (1993). Biases in how physicians choose to withdraw life support. *Lancet* **342** (8872), 642–6.
91. **Feldman, H.A.** et al. (1997). Nonmedical influences on medical decision making: an experimental technique using videotapes, factorial design, and survey sampling. *Health Services Research* **32** (3), 343–66.
92. **Cherny, N.I.** et al. (1994). The treatment of suffering when patients request elective death. *Journal of Palliative Care* **10** (2), 71–9.
93. **Cherny, N.I. and Portenoy, R.K.** (1994). Sedation in the management of refractory symptoms: guidelines for evaluation and treatment. *Journal of Palliative Care* **10** (2), 31–8.
94. **Fins, J.J.** et al. (1997). Clinical pragmatism: a method of moral problem solving. *Kennedy Institute of Ethics Journal* **7**, 129–45.
95. **Morita, T.** et al. (1996). Sedation for symptom control in Japan: the importance of intermittent use and communication with family members. *Journal of Pain and Symptom Management* **12** (1), 32–8.
96. **Fainsinger, R.** et al. (1998). Sedation for uncontrolled symptoms in a South African Hospice. *Journal of Pain and Symptom Management* **16** (3), 145–52.
97. **Chater, S.** et al. (1998). Sedation for intractable distress in the dying—a survey of experts. *Palliative Medicine* **12** (4), 255–69.

98. **Miller, F.G.** et al. (1996). Clinical pragmatism: John Dewey and clinical ethics. *Journal of Contemporary Health Law Policy* **13** (1), 27–51.

99. **Devlin, P.** *Easing the Passing.* London: Bodley Head, 1985.

100. **Burt, R.A.** (1997). The Supreme Court speaks—not assisted suicide but a constitutional right to palliative care. *New England Journal of Medicine* **337** (17), 1234–6.

101. **van der Maas, P.J.** et al. (1992). Euthanasia and other medical decisions concerning the end of life. An investigation performed upon request of the Commission of Inquiry into the Medical Practice concerning Euthanasia. *Health Policy* **21** (1–2), vi–x, 1–262.

103. **van der Maas, P.J.** et al. (1996). Euthanasia, physician-assisted suicide, and other medical practices involving the end of life in the Netherlands, 1990–1995. *New England Journal of Medicine* **335** (22), 1699–705.

103. **Stevens, C.A. and Hassan, R.** (1994). Management of death, dying and euthanasia: attitudes and practices of medical practitioners in South Australia. *Archives of Internal Medicine* **154** (5), 575–84.

104. **Kuhse, H.** et al. (1997). End-of-life decisions in Australian medical practice. *Medical Journal of Australia* **166** (4), 191–6.

105. **Meier, D.E.** et al. (1998). A national survey of physician-assisted suicide and euthanasia in the United States. *New England Journal of Medicine* **338** (17), 1193–201 (see comments).

106. **Willems, D.L.** et al. (2000). Attitudes and practices concerning the end of life: a comparison between physicians from the United States and from The Netherlands. *Archives of Internal Medicine* **160** (1), 63–8.

107. **Brody, H.** (1993). Causing, intending, and assisting death. *Journal of Clinical Ethics* **4** (2), 112–17.

108. **Brody, H.** (1996). Commentary on Billings and Block's 'Slow euthanasia'. *Journal of Palliative Care* **12** (4), 38–41 (comment).

109. **Mount, B.** (1996). Morphine drips, terminal sedation, and slow euthanasia: definitions and facts, not anecdotes. *Journal of Palliative Care* **12** (4), 31–7 (comment).

110. **Burke, A.L.** et al. (1991). Terminal restlessness—its management and the role of midazolam. *Medical Journal of Australia* **155** (7), 485–7 (see comments).

111. **Johanson, G.A.** (1993). Midazolam in terminal care. *American Journal of Hospital and Palliative Care* **10** (1), 13–14.

112. **Power, D. and Kearney, M.** (1992). Management of the final 24 hours. *Irish Medical Journal* **85** (3), 93–5.

113. **Burke, A.L.** (1997). Palliative care: an update on 'terminal restlessness'. *Medical Journal of Australia* **166** (1), 39–42.

114. **Collins, P.** (1997). Prolonged sedation with midazolam or propofol. *Critical Care Medicine* **25** (3), 556–7 (letter; comment).

115. **Nordt, S.P. and Clark, R.F.** (1997). Midazolam: a review of therapeutic uses and toxicity. *Journal of Emergency Medicine* **15** (3), 357–65.

116. **Smales, E.A. and Sanders, H.G.** (1989). Flunitrazepam in terminal care. *Lancet* **2** (8661), 501 (letter).

117. **Greene, W.R. and Davis, W.H.** (1991). Titrated intravenous barbiturates in the control of symptoms in patients with terminal cancer. *Southern Medical Journal* **84** (3), 332–7.

118. **Truog, R.D.** et al. (1992). Barbiturates in the care of the terminally ill. *New England Journal of Medicine* **327** (23), 1678–82.

119. **Mercandte, S., De Conno, F., and Ripamonte, C.** (1995). Propofol in terminal care. *Journal of Pain and Symptom Management* **10**, 639–42.

120. **Moyle, J.** (1995). The use of propofol in palliative medicine. *Journal of Pain and Symptom Management* **10** (8), 643–6.

121. **Tobias, J.D.** (1997). Propofol sedation for terminal care in a pediatric patient. *Clinical Pediatrics* **36** (5), 291–3.

122. **Portenoy, R.K.** (1987). Continuous intravenous infusion of opioid drugs. *Medical Clinics of North America* **71** (2), 233–41.

123. **Dunlop, R.J.** (1989). Excitatory phenomena associated with high dose opioids. *Current Therapy* **30** (6), 121–3.

124. **Potter, J.M.** et al. (1989). Myoclonus associated with treatment with high doses of morphine: the role of supplemental drugs. *British Medical Journal* **299** (6692), 150–3 (see comments).

125. **Carter, R.L.** (1987). The role of limited, symptom-directed autopsies in terminal malignant disease. *Palliative Medicine* **1**, 31–6.

126. **Dickey, N.W.** (1986). Withholding or withdrawing life-prolonging treatment. *Journal of the American Medical Association* **256**, 471.

127. **Randall, F. and Downie, R.S.** *Palliative Care Ethics: A Companion for all Specialties* 2nd edn. Oxford: Oxford University Press, 1999.

128. **Hastings Center.** *Guidelines on the Termination of Life-sustaining Treatment and the Care of the Dying.* Indianapolis IN: Hastings Center, Indiana University, 1987.

19

Bereavement

19 Bereavement

David W. Kissane

Introduction

Mourning is an essential adaptive response to the inevitable experience of loss. In many ways it is the debt that has to be repaid for investment in the joys of life. Familiarity with and confidence in responding to grief is a sine qua non for all clinicians working in palliative medicine, including the capacity to differentiate healthy from maladaptive adjustment. Many losses are experienced as patients and their families move through the phases of progressive illness towards death. Related grief is thus current as well as anticipatory of future loss. Support for the grieving process in both the patients and their carers clearly begins during palliative care and places the clinician in an ideal position to sustain continuity of this care into bereavement.

Family-centred care is integral to this supportive process as the family's understanding of the illness and its treatment influences their later adjustment. Every word uttered by the treating team, the related tone, and sensitivity shown contributes to the experience for the bereaved, who generally need to understand the process of death and discuss any features of concern. Palliative care teams are ideally placed to recognize those at greater risk of poor outcome and provide care prophylactically to prevent bereavement morbidity.

Although words such as grief, mourning, and bereavement are commonly used interchangeably, the following definitions indicate their use in this chapter:

- *Bereavement* is the state of loss resulting from death.[1]
- *Grief* is the emotional response associated with loss.[2]
- *Mourning* is the process of adaptation, including the cultural and social rituals prescribed as accompaniments.[3]
- *Anticipatory grief* precedes the death and results from the expectation of that event.[3]
- *Complicated grief* represents a pathological outcome involving psychological, social, or physical morbidity.[4]
- *Disenfranchised grief* represents the hidden sorrow of the marginalized where there is less social permission to express many dimensions of loss.[5]

In this chapter, the theoretical models that have been developed to explain bereavement phenomena and the process of mourning are considered with a view to generating an understanding of the clinical features of grief. Recognition of those at risk of complicated outcome is mandatory to offer preventative interventions. Models of follow-up and management of complicated grief are fully explored, as is variation across the life-cycle and the impact of stigmatized deaths. Spiritual aspects of bereavement highlight the contributions of the world's major religions in supporting the bereaved. Bereavement research in the future will be aided by use of validated measures, which are summarized towards the chapter's end as a handy resource. Finally, to conclude, the recognition that personal growth is a common outcome despite the sadness of loss reminds us that creativity often emerges as a result of resolution of the mourning process.

Theoretical models of bereavement phenomena

Dating from Darwin's observation of monkeys 'weeping' from grief, ethology has pointed out that social birds and mammals do grieve.[6] Indeed, mourning appears to be the price paid for the evolutionary adaptiveness of social relationships. This universality of grief suggests it is imprinted into the biological processes of the species, consistent with the experience that death seems to be difficult for people everywhere. Yet, social constructionists remind us that the shape and content of grief is culturally determined. It varies markedly across places, times, and social groups, with noteworthy differences in the expression of anger, emotionality, self-mutilation, rituals, and public versus private grief.[7]

A conceptual framework that illuminates what underpins the phenomena of bereavement aids our clinical understanding of the experience of the bereaved (see Table 1). Explanatory models favoured by bereavement researchers were ranked in the following order of importance: attachment, psychodynamic, sociological, cognitive–behavioural, and ethology.[8]

Table 1 Theoretical models explaining bereavement phenomena

Name of model	Key contributors	Main features
Attachment theory	Bowlby, Ainsworth, Parkes, Weiss	The bonds of close relationships are severed by loss
Psychodynamic theory	Freud, Klein, Horowitz, Kohut	Early relationships lay down a template that guide future relationships
Interpersonal model	Sullivan, Bonnano, Horowitz, Benjamin	Relational influences are dominant in grief outcome
Psychosocial transition	Parkes, Janoff-Bulman	Changed assumptive world view
Sociological model	Rosenblatt, Klass, Walter	Cultural influences shape the form and content of grief
Family systems theory	Walsh, McGoldrick, Kissane, Shapiro	Family are the main source of support; family functioning determines outcome
Cognitive stress coping theory	Stroebe, Kavanagh	Conditioned or learnt patterns become entrenched
Traumatic model	Horowitz, Pynoos, Prigerson, Jacobs	Intrusive aspects of trauma dominate
Ethology	Darwin, Lorenz	Biological and physiological processes underpin the phenomena across species

Although limited by the available list of potential theories (for instance, continuing bonds, interpersonal, systemic, and traumatic were not offered), these models help practitioners work flexibly with pertinent issues.

Attachment theory posits that the development of close affectionate bonds to particular others generates security and survival potential.[9] From a secure base, the capacity for curiosity emerges to generate creativity in autonomous adult life. Parents, especially the mother, constitute the usual subject of primary attachments, but these behaviours become enduring throughout adult life and the spouse eventually replaces the parents as the recipient of the strongest bonds. The family thus forms the setting for the major constellation of bonds. Through studying parent–child relationships, Mary Ainsworth differentiated secure from insecure attachments, the latter appearing as either anxious, avoidant, or disorganized/hostile.[10] A trans-generational influence is evident between the parental style of attachment and that found in children, such that families can transmit insecure patterns of relating through the generations. The nature of attachments in a person's life influences the impact of loss when these bonds are changed, determining the work of mourning as this separation is dealt with.[11,12]

While related to attachment theory, the psychodynamic model places greater emphasis on the development of the person, with all of their childhood and earlier life influences, including their sense of self, confidence, and resilience that comes with a robust self-esteem, and their learnt capacity to mourn. Schematic representations of early relationships construct a template (technically termed object relations) that lays down the operating principles guiding the emotional experience of relationships. Once the infant has developed feelings of concern for its mother, Klein described the early pining evident when the mother was absent.[13] Mourning was thus recognized as a life-long mechanism of adaptation to cope with the inevitable traumas of life.

Interpersonal theories have emerged recently to throw further light on bereavement[14] and complement the psychodynamic model. Cyclical relational patterns are understood to result from current relational selections based on their resonance with the past, often confirming previous expectations. Schemas of the 'who the self is' are constructed through relational interactions to establish a role for the person pertaining to these relationships. Horowitz has made particular use of these schemas using a stress–response model for grief.[15] For instance, ambivalence towards the deceased is associated with greater distress, but restructuring the 'ambivalent' schema is possible through its observation in current relational patterns and the introduction of strategic variations to alter this habitually dysfunctional pattern. Horowitz and colleagues have tested a model of therapy based on these premises.[16]

Transition theorists highlight the adaptation to change that is inherent in any resolution of grief. Parkes suggested that alteration to an individual's set of ideas and beliefs about their environment—their assumptive world—was central to adaptation.[17] Development of acceptance of change is implicit in such a view.

In their contribution to a sociological model of bereavement, post-modern writers emphasize the various discourses that indicate a multiplicity of perspectives. The notion of the 'breaking of the bonds' of relationship, first hinted at by Freud in 1912,[18] is thus socially determined. Klass and colleagues highlighted the process of continuing bonds through reverence for the dead as both ancestors and moral guides.[19] Walter noted that conversations about and with the deceased served as one means of sustaining a relationship.[20] It becomes a personal choice whether the bereaved moves on to a new relationship or sustains the attitude of a 'broken heart'.

The sociological view also recognizes the loneliness of the bereaved and the value of groups or networks, including the family, to counter the social isolation that otherwise might prevail. Patterns of socialization of the bereaved vary with cultures, but networks of support have a vital influence on adjustment. The manner in which a family grieves and how its members continue to relate to each other is crucial to outcome. Families wreaked by conflict, reduced cohesion, and poor communication struggle to support each other—high rates of psychosocial morbidity are found in dysfunctional families.[21] Family systems theory makes particular use of intergenerational and family life-cycle perspectives.[22]

Mourning can be triggered by unexpected life events, natural disasters, and traumas that violate the person and introduce an unwelcome element to the experience that is described as 'shocking'. Traumatic grief captures something that is unique to the trauma and challenges the bereaved with the intrusion of any resultant distressing memories. Prigerson and Jacobs have argued for recognition of the specifically traumatic nature of some deaths and their impact on grief.[23]

Finally, behavioural models offer their contribution to bereavement theory through the challenge of chronic grief, in which the bereaved become stuck in an entrenched state of distress.[24] Patterns such as social withdrawal, 'memorialization' of the deceased through preserving their bedroom, clothes and possessions intact as if a shrine, or chronic weeping upon mention of the deceased's name illustrate these behaviours. Cognitive–behavioural approaches such as activity scheduling generate clinical improvement and point to an element of conditioned response in chronic grief.

The number of overlapping dimensions to these conceptual models is noteworthy, yet none by itself is a sufficient and complete explanation of bereavement phenomena. However, the intrapsychic, interpersonal, systemic, and sociological features of these models deliver an intersecting and overall coherence, which aids our eventual understanding of the complex phenomena observed in grief.

Stroebe and Schut have pointed out that while these general theories of grief explain the broad range of phenomena observed, they do not inform fully about the specific coping pathways that grieving individuals go down.[25] They have suggested a dual process model of bereavement-specific coping, in which oscillation occurs between loss-orientation, in which there is a focus on the loss itself, and restoration-orientation, in which the focus shifts to attending to ongoing life. Active 'grief work' occurs when the bereaved are loss-oriented, but excessive negative emotion could lead to a deterioration in coping, and so active confrontation of grief sits in a dynamic equilibrium with some degree of avoidance of grief. The individual needs at times to pull back and take 'time out' from the distress of the loss. They may do so through use of the restorative track in which the negative emotions are countered by some degree of positive reappraisal and of construction of meaning about the event. This promotes positive affects and eventually opens up new goals and plans for the future. Complex regulation exists in getting this balance right between grieving and restoring, with both interpersonal and cultural influences guiding this balance. Dissonance between bereaved members of a family, for instance, will challenge the balance and lead systemically to some readjustment by some or more members.

The bereaved cope therefore through adjusting the balance between expression of negative and positive emotions in emotion-based coping, and incorporating appropriate degrees of problem-solving and meaning-generation to guide their sense of purpose and control. They need to sustain the normal operation and functioning in their lives while also grieving the loss that has occurred irrevocably.

The nature of normal grief

The expression of normal grief is evident through its emotional, cognitive, physical, and behavioural features.[1] Eric Lindemann provided the first systematic study of these through his observations of people who lost a relative in Boston's *Cocoanut Grove Nightclub* fire.[26] Somatic distress with numbness, preoccupation with sad memories of the deceased, guilt, anger, loss of the regular patterns of conduct, and identification with symptoms of the deceased formed the key dimensions that Lindemann observed.

Emotional distress occurs in waves that last for minutes at a time and involves unavoidable crying, lost of concentration and purpose while preoccupied with thoughts about the deceased, and a range of associated affects including sadness, anger, despair, anxiety, and guilt. Cognitive processes become dominated by memories, reflected in story telling, reminiscences, and conversations about the deceased. Physical responses include numbness, restlessness, tension, tremors, sleep disturbance, anorexia, weight loss, fatigue, and a variety of aches and pains. Finally, behavioural aspects are variously reflected in social withdrawal, wandering, searching, and seeking company and consolation.

A number of physiological changes have been identified in neuroendocrine functioning[27] (for instance, challenge studies like the dexamethasone suppression test), immune indices[28] (e.g. natural killer cell functioning), and sleep efficiency.[29] Exploration of these physiological changes not only suggests that grief and depression lie on a biological continuum but also provides understanding for the morbidity, both somatic and psychosocial, that is associated with bereavement.

The clinical presentations of grief

As the family journey through palliative care, the clinical phases progress from anticipatory grief through to the immediate news of the death, to the stages of acute grief and, potentially for some, the complications of bereavement.

Anticipatory grief

When news of cancer recurrence or disease progression reaches the patient and family, grief is initiated as they anticipate eventual death. However, not all of this grief is about the final loss, as many changes unfold with the illness and its treatment. Loss of health can be accompanied by loss of work, leisure activities, financial security, independence, sense of certainty about life and further physical impairments, body image change, and altered perception of well-being. The clinician is challenged to understand the meaning of the loss to each person and evaluate therein their grief response.

Anticipatory grief generally draws the supportive family into a configuration of mutual comfort and greater closeness as the news of the illness and its proposed management is grappled with. For a time this perturbation advantages the care of the sick, until the pressures of daily life draw the family back towards their prior constellation. Movement back and forth is evident thereafter as news of illness progression unfolds. Periods of grief become interspersed with phases of contentment and happiness. When the family is engaged in the domiciliary care of their ill member, their cohesion potentially increases as they share their fears, hopes, joy, and distress.

In contrast, difficulties emerge for some families as they express their anticipatory grief. Impaired coping is exhibited through protective avoidance, denial of the seriousness of the threat, anger, or withdrawal from involvement. Sometimes family dysfunction is so glaring that clinicians are rapidly drawn into its snares. More commonly, however, subthreshold or mild depressive or anxiety disorders develop gradually as individuals struggle to adapt to unwelcome changes. While anticipatory grief was historically suggested to reduce post-mortem grief,[30] intense distress is now well recognized as a marker of risk for complicated grief.

During this phase of anticipatory grief, clinicians can usefully help the family that is capable of effective communication by encouraging them to openly share their feelings as they pay attention to the material needs of their dying family member or friend. Saying goodbye needs to be recognized as a process that evolves over time, with opportunities for reminiscence, celebration of the life and contribution of the dying person, expressions of gratitude and completion of any unfinished business.[31] These tasks have the potential to generate creative and positive emotional aspects of what is otherwise a sad time for all.

Grief of family and friends gathered around the death bed

When relatives or close friends gather to keep watch by the bed of a dying person, not only do they support the sick, but they also help their own subsequent adjustment. The solidarity shared through this experience cements these carers into mutually supportive relationships. As staff go about nursing the ill patient, they need to comfortably relate to the family, whether in the home, hospice, or hospital. For years to come, these poignant moments will be recalled in immense detail—the sensitivity and courteous respect of health professionals is crucial.[32] Clinicians can helpfully comment on the process of dying, explaining the breathing patterns, and commenting on any noises, secretions, patient reactions, and comfort. The experience needs to be normalized empathically and the family reassured whenever concern develops. Discussion about pain, reasons for medications, and skilled prediction of events will assuage worry and build a collaborative approach to the care of the dying.

Religious rituals warrant active facilitation, including appropriate notification of a religious minister or pastoral care worker. Respect for the body remains paramount once death has occurred and the expression of sympathy from clinicians is greatly appreciated. The family will be invariably grateful for time spent alone with the deceased, while regard for cultural approaches to the laying out of the body is essential[33] (discussed later in the section on Cross-cultural bereavement practices). The bereaved are commonly bewildered and benefit from guidance about what to do next—making contact with the undertaker is an obvious example.

When relatives have not been present at the moment of death, informing them by telephone of the fact is generally undesirable. The invitation for them to attend in person is often based on a stated deterioration in the patient's condition. On arrival, the news can be sensitively shared in an appropriate setting before accompanying them to see the deceased. To help the family to integrate an understanding of all that has occurred, clinicians should explain the sequence of medical events culminating in the death. Questions need to be sensitively answered and time taken to comfort the bereaved in their distress.

From time to time, the cause of death will remain uncertain and an autopsy may be indicated. A senior clinician should outline the pertinent issues, emphasizing the positive aspects of the information that will be gleaned and indicating that it will be subsequently shared with the family in a follow-up meeting. Unless there is a legal requirement for a coroner's post-mortem, the family's views on autopsy need to be fully respected.

Sometimes staff will have concerns about the emotional response of the bereaved. If there is uncertainty about its cultural appropriateness, consultation with an informed cultural intermediary may prove helpful. The prescription of short-acting benzodiazepines will help some, while others will prefer to manage without medication. A follow-up telephone call on the next day is worthwhile to check on coping and identify the need for continued support.

Caution is needed in settings where grief could be marginalized, well exemplified by ageism.[5] If a death is normalized because it appears in step with the life-cycle, family members can be given less support and reduced permission to express many aspects of their loss. In the process, the disenfranchised can be ignored in their sorrow.

Acute grief and time course of bereavement

The sequence or phases through which the bereaved move over time are never rigidly demarcated but merge gradually one into the other.[1,3] They assist the clinician to recognize aberration from the normal evolution. From the (i) initial numbness and sense of unreality, (ii) waves of distress begin to occur as the bereaved suffer intense pining and yearning for their lost one. Memories of the deceased trigger these acute pangs of grief. Then as the pain of separation grows, (iii) a phase of disorganization emerges as loneliness resulting from the loss sets in. Hofer described this phase aptly as a constant background disturbance of restlessness, inattention, sadness, and despair with social withdrawal that can last for several months.[34] Eventually (iv) a phase of reorganization and recovery develops as nostalgia replaces sadness, morale improves, and an altered world view is constructed. Personal growth can be recognized at this stage and new creativity is expressed.[35]

The time course of mourning is proportional to the strength of attachment to the lost person and also varies with cultural expression, there being no sharply defined end point to grief. Just as a mother's grief following sudden infant death syndrome lasts longer than grief following a neonatal death, so to with adult loss, the mourning that follows many years of marriage is generally longer than brief relationships. Older widows and widowers may continue to display their grief for several years.[36] This can correspond with a continuing relationship with the deceased, which for some is their choice and leads to chronic grief. The clinical task is then to differentiate those who remain within the spectrum of normality from those who cross the threshold of complicated grief.

Complicated grief

Normal and abnormal responses to bereavement span a spectrum in which intensity of reaction, presence of a range of related grief behaviours, and time course determine the differentiation. The common psychiatric disorders include clinical depression, anxiety disorders, alcohol abuse or other substance abuse and dependence, psychotic disorders, and post-traumatic stress disorder (PTSD). When frank psychiatric disorders complicate bereavement, their recognition and management is straightforward; subthreshold states present the greater clinical challenge as studies of the bereaved indicate groups in which clusters of intense grief symptoms are distinct from uncomplicated grief.[37–39] Their recognition calls for an experienced clinical judgement that does not normalize the distress as understandable (see Table 2). In practice, the location of these patients in high-risk groups and the application of preventive models of bereavement care eliminate some of the academic debate about their characteristics.

Inhibited or delayed grief

While use of avoidance may serve some as a temporary coping mechanism, its persistence is usually associated with relationship difficulties or the emergence of a hypomanic state in individuals with bipolar disorder. Grief may be understandably absent, however, when there has been no bond of attachment to the deceased. Cultural variation obviously influences grief expression. Empirical studies have generally identified avoidant forms of complicated grief in up to 5 per cent of the bereaved—it may not always present clinically, but reappear in later years as an unresolved issue.

Chronic grief

This common form of complicated grief is particularly associated with overly dependent relationships in which a sense of abandonment is avoided by perpetuation of the relationship through memorialization of the deceased and maintenance of continuing bonds. A stuck situation emerges in which the tearfulness is induced by any reminder of the deceased without any cognitive transition being achieved in the world view of the bereaved. Social withdrawal and depression are common. A fantasy of re-union with the deceased can cause suicide to be an increasingly attractive option. Active treatment using pharmacology for depression and cognitive–behavioural therapy to reality test the loss and promote socialization (via activity scheduling) is appropriate for chronic grief.

Traumatic grief

When death has been unexpected or its nature in some way shocking—traumatic, violent, stigmatized, or perceived as undignified—its integration and acceptance may be interfered with by the arousal and increased distress that memories can trigger. Intensive recollections including flashbacks, nightmares, and recurrent intrusive memories cause hyperarousal, disbelief, insomnia, irritability, and disturbed concentration, which distorts normal grieving.[23] The shock of the death can precipitate mistrust, anger, detachment, and an unwillingness to accept its reality. These reactions at a subthreshold level merge with the full features of PTSD, but the subthreshold state has been observed to persist for years and contribute substantial morbidity.

Table 2 Clinical presentations of complicated grief

Category	Features
Inhibited or delayed grief	Avoidance postpones expression
Chronic grief	Perpetuation of mourning long-term
Traumatic grief	Unexpected and shocking form of death
Depressive disorders	Both major and minor depressions
Anxiety disorders	Insecurity and relational problems
Alcohol and substance abuse/dependence	Excessive use of substances impairs adaptive coping
Post-traumatic stress disorder	Persistent, intrusive images with cues
Psychotic disorders	Manic, severe depressive states, and schizophrenia

Depressive disorders

Rates of major depression in the bereaved have varied between 16 and 50 per cent, peaking over the first 2 months,[40,41] and gradually decreasing to 15 per cent across the next 2 years.[42,43] The features of any major depressive episode post-bereavement resemble major depression at other points of the life-cycle.[44] There is a tendency to chronicity, considerable social morbidity, and risk of inadequate treatment.

Anxiety disorders

These take the form of adjustment disorders, generalized anxiety disorder, and phobic states and occur in up to 30 per cent of the bereaved.[45] Patients present commonly to general practitioners with a range of somatic concerns. Separation anxiety of a heightened nature can be distinguished from anxiety symptoms of a general kind.

Alcohol and substance abuse/dependence

Typically an exacerbation of pre-existing psychiatric states, individuals predisposed to alcohol abuse or dependence on other substances such as benzodiazepines relapse during bereavement.[45] Other family members often raise the alarm.

Post-traumatic stress disorder

While clearly related to unnatural deaths, deaths involving profound breakdown of bodily surfaces, gross disfigurement due to head and neck cancers, or other causes of relatives perceiving the illness to cause loss of dignity may generate traumatic memories in the bereaved. Schut and colleagues found that PTSD was often correlated with the perceived inadequacy of the good-bye, and suggested that rituals to complete this be incorporated into related grief therapies.[46]

Psychotic disorders

Bereavement is a common precipitant of relapse of psychotic illnesses such as bipolar disorder or schizophrenia in individuals so predisposed; occasionally, mania presents for the first time in such a setting.

Family grief

Family therapists have long recognized the salience of family processes to mourning and their systemic influence on outcome.[47] Exploration of the association between family functioning and bereavement morbidity highlighted the manner in which family dysfunction predicts increased rates of psychosocial morbidity in the bereaved.[21] Family-centred care that focuses on the well-being of the family during palliative care is uniquely placed to reduce rates of morbidity in those subsequently bereaved.

A typology of family functioning during both palliative care and bereavement was created using cluster analysis in the Melbourne-based family grief studies.[21,48] Dimensions of cohesiveness, expressiveness, and conflict from the Family Environment Scale[49] determined five classes of families illustrated in Table 3. While over half the families met in a palliative care setting demonstrate resilience through their family functioning, and do not need particular psychological assistance to achieve an adaptive outcome from bereavement, the remainder have identifiable characteristics predictive of a higher risk of morbid outcome and can be specifically targeted through a preventive model of family care.[50]

During early bereavement, families at risk have been shown to decompensate through deterioration in their functioning with loss of cohesiveness,

Table 3 Typology of palliative care and bereaved families[21,48]

Category	Family type	Rate of occurrence (%)	Features
Well functioning types	Supportive	32	Strongly cohesive families who grieve adaptively
	Conflict resolving	20	Cohesion and effective communication empowers tolerance of difference of opinions
Dysfunctional types	Hostile	6–12	Poorly cohesive with high conflict, ineffective communication, and fractured relationships; families resist help
	Sullen	9–18	Muted anger generates highest levels of depression; families seek help
	Intermediate	20–33	Mid-range levels of communication, cohesion, and conflict place these families at risk of deterioration when stressed by life events

communication breakdown, and increased conflict. A proportion of families with *Intermediate* characteristics of functioning changes to become *Sullen* or *Hostile* in type. Importantly, these dysfunctional families carry the bulk of the psychosocial morbidity observed to occur during bereavement, thus highlighting the potential benefits of a family form of intervention. Screening of families on their admission to palliative care through the use of a well-validated measure such as the Family Relationships Index[49] provides an ideal means to recognize those families at greater risk of morbid outcome during bereavement. Rules to interpret family functioning and thus recognize those at risk when screening (on admission to the palliative care service) are summarized in Table 4.

Recognizing those at risk of complicated bereavement outcome

Palliative care teams are ideally placed to recognize those at increased risk of complicated grief and plan preventive interventions in an endeavour to circumvent morbidity. To accomplish this, bereavement care planning does not begin post-death but at the point of entry into the palliative care service. The continuity of supportive care that flows from this builds a strong therapeutic alliance, which will be more likely to survive ambivalence about the death than if a bereavement counsellor attempts to begin post-death. Avoidance hinders many attempts to engage the bereaved after the death.

In times of resource scarceness and economic rationalism, services are under pressure to direct their clinical staff to appropriate areas of need. When relatives appear resilient and well supported, clinicians can wisely respect their capacity to cope with loss adaptively. Indeed, empirical evidence confirms that when preventive interventions are targeted to those at risk, benefits ensue,[51] whereas when they are broadly offered to a bereaved population regardless of risk, no such benefit is discernible.[52] In the latter type of study, the well functioning dilute any evidence of benefit to those at risk. In contrast with a broadly supportive bereavement follow-up programme that utilizes condolence cards and invitations to memorial services, seriously intended preventive interventions should be directed towards those at increased risk.

Risk factors to aid recognition of those at greater risk of complicated grief are summarized in Table 5. These should be assessed at entry to the service

Table 4 Screening rules to recognize families at greater risk of dysfunction and complicated grief through use of the Family Relationships Index (FRI)[a(67)]

(a) *Well-functioning families (low risk)*
Cohesiveness score of 4 (out of maximum 4) *plus* FRI > 9 (out of maximum 12)

(b) *Families considered at some risk*
Cohesiveness score <4 *or* FRI ≤9

FES[a] subscales	Typical range of scores for family types		
	Intermediate	Sullen	Hostile
Cohesiveness	3–4	2–3	0–1
Expressiveness	1–3	1–2	0–1
Conflict	0–1	1–2	2–4
FRI	8–9	5–7	0–4

[a] FRI (Family Relationships Index) is derived from the FES (Family Environment Scale).[49] FRI is the sum of the cohesiveness, expressiveness, and reversed (out of 4) conflict score; its maximum sum is 12.

Table 5 Risk factors for complicated grief

Category	Range of circumstances
Nature of the death	Untimely within the life-cycle (e.g. death of child) Sudden and unexpected (e.g. death from septic neutropaenia during chemotherapy) Traumatic (e.g. gross cachexia and debility) Stigmatized (e.g. AIDS or suicide)
Strengths and vulnerabilities of the carer/bereaved	Past history of psychiatric disorder (e.g. depression) Personality and coping style (e.g. intense worrier, low self-esteem) Cumulative experience of losses
Nature of the relationship with the deceased	Overly dependent (e.g. clinging, symbiotic) Ambivalent (e.g. angry and insecure with alcohol abuse, infidelity, gambling)
Family and support network	Dysfunctional family (e.g. poor cohesiveness and communication, high conflict) Isolated (e.g. new migrant, new residential move) Alienated (e.g. perception of poor support)

and upgraded during the phase of palliative care, including revision shortly after the death. Completion of the family genogram presents an ideal time for such assessment as relationships, prior losses, and coping are considered. Some palliative care services have developed checklists based on such risk factors to generate a numerical measure of risk. There has been insufficient validation of such scales at this stage, but the presence of any single factor in Table 5 signifies greater risk. Continued observation of the pattern of grief evolution over time is appropriate whenever such concern exists.

Health consequences of bereavement

Over 15 studies of mortality following bereavement provide evidence for an increased rate of deaths in the 45–75 age range, with these occurring over the first year post-loss, particularly the first 6 months from acute cardiovascular causes.[53] While some studies have only identified increased mortality in men, a well-controlled study of 12 522 spouse pairs in a prepaid health care plan showed increased mortality for both women and men, adjusting for age, education, and other mortality predictors.[54] Other noteworthy causes of death in addition to cardiovascular events include accidents, suicide, alcohol and substance abuse, and cirrhosis, while the association evident in large epidemiological studies of increased mortality with social isolation and alienation is also relevant.[55]

Early studies by Saunders[56] and Parkes[57] identified the increased use of health services—both greater consultations and hospitalizations—by the recently bereaved, with increased psychological distress, somatic health complaints, more days of disability, and greater reliance on medications. Some 20–25 per cent were noted to develop depressive disorders,[40] but increased rates of anxiety disorders, including PTSD in settings of traumatic loss, also occur.[45] Some of the explanations for these health consequences lie in the development of complicated grief, others in altered behaviours and life-style including diet, smoking, and alcohol consumption. Studies have also highlighted effects on the cardiovascular, neuroendocrine, and immunological systems: several studies have shown increased rates of myocardial infarction post-bereavement;[53] altered cortisol levels were seen in parents following death of their children from leukaemia;[58] altered lymphocyte response to mitogens and lowered natural killer cell activity were also seen in bereaved spouses.[59–61] Immunosuppressed patients, either chemically induced or as a result of AIDS, develop specific malignancies such as lymphomas or Kaposi's sarcomas. However, the clinical relevance of the immunological changes described in bereavement is uncertain in the light of a series of large epidemiological studies that fail to show increased rates of cancer in the bereaved.[62–64]

Bereavement follow-up by the treatment team

Once the patient has died, the palliative care team should routinely review the death and the bereavement-related risk factors in the next available multidisciplinary team meeting. Was the death perceived to impact significantly on key family members? What level of bereavement follow-up should be adopted?

Two broad levels of follow-up are possible. The first involves the expression of condolences via the telephone, sympathy card, visit by the nurse or general practitioner, staff attendance at the funeral, and subsequent family invitation to a periodic commemorative service arranged by the palliative care team. This model provides both encouragement and support while normalizing the grief that relatives express and respecting their mourning process without undue intrusion. Where greater concern does emerge, an opportunity presents to intervene appropriately. The staff who have developed the closest relationships with the family are wisely selected by the team to take up this observing model of follow-up as it provides them with a means of gradual farewell. Their formal identification and documentation is nonetheless important to ensure completion of the process over time. Final contact is often shortly after the first anniversary.

The second model of follow-up is for those individuals or families judged to be at greater risk and thought likely to benefit from a preventive intervention. Studies have shown that such prevention effectively reduces morbidity when delivered to those 20 per cent likely otherwise to develop complicated grief.[51] Teams vary in their pursuit of this depending on staff availability; in other instances, general practitioners provide active individual support. Individual, group, or family approaches are valid and selected on the basis of personal needs. Where continuity of involvement of the counsellor from palliative care into bereavement is possible, direct knowledge of the deceased is advantageous, as is the continuing relationship with the bereaved. Attempts to establish bereavement counselling only after the death meet high rates of defensive avoidance blocking this form of support. Where social isolation is noteworthy, the additional support derived from a group approach maximizes connectedness.[65,66] Others will seek the personal support of individual therapy. For many, a family approach is cost-effective in reaching several at risk when the nature of the family's functioning has been shown by screening to be dysfunctional. *Family Focused Grief Therapy* (FFGT) offers continuity from palliative care through to bereavement and, in promoting family functioning, it fosters the role of the family as a prime source of support.[67] Asian cultures including the Chinese and Japanese are especially suited to family models of care.[68]

The diverse range of clinicians in palliative care teams, including chaplains or pastoral care workers, nurses, social workers, psychologists or psychiatrists, general practitioners, volunteers, and generic bereavement counsellors ensure that there is no shortage of staff to support the bereaved. Nevertheless, staff caught up with the business of acute patient care will neglect the bereaved despite their best of intentions. Team leadership needs to actively monitor programmes of bereavement follow-up to ensure its adherence to an intended protocol and to initiate appropriate cross-referral of those at greater risk.

Grief therapies

As loss is so ubiquitous within palliative care, all clinicians need skill in the application of grief therapies. The most basic model is a supportive–expressive intervention in which the person is invited to share their feelings about the loss to a health professional who will listen and seek to understand the other's distress in a comforting manner. The key therapeutic aspects of this encounter are the sharing of distress and, through the relational understanding that is acknowledged, some shift in cognitive appraisal of the reality that has been forever altered. There are hundreds of small losses involving aspects of health and well-being as well as hopes and dreams that are experienced by the patient during their terminal illness. Support is needed from all members of the treatment team in response to these before the major loss of the patient is ultimately experienced through death.

Formal interventions that are possible for bereaved people are multiple, but the very first question is whether 'an intervention' is actually warranted. For the majority, although bereavement is painful, their personal resilience will ensure their normal adaptation. There can, therefore, be no justification for routine intervention as grief is not a disease. Those considered at risk of maladaptive outcome are the ones that should be treated preventatively and those who later develop complicated bereavement need active treatments.

The spectrum of interventions spans individual, group, and family oriented therapies, and encompasses all schools of psychotherapy as well as appropriately indicated pharmacotherapies. Adoption of any model (or parts thereof) is predicated on the clinical issues and associated predicaments that arise. Thus, variation will be influenced by age, perception of support, the nature of the death, the personal health of the bereaved, and the presence of co-morbid states. Clinicians generally plan for an intervention to proceed as six to eight sessions over several months and do well to map this out at the beginning. In this sense, grief therapy is focused and time-limited, but multi-modal therapies are commonplace. Thus, group as well as individual therapies better support the lonely so that socialization complements interpersonally any intrapersonal change.

Guided mourning as an approach to 'grief work' promotes narrative review with repetitive recollections of the deceased being actively encouraged to relive and eventually revise the relationship experienced, ultimately redefining the reality of self and situation.[69,70] In the process, Worden emphasized the accomplishment of four basic tasks of mourning: accepting the reality of loss; working through the pain of grief; adjusting to a new environment without the loved person; and establishing a collection of positive and useful memories of the deceased for future reference.[71] Reality testing and adaptation to the separation leads to what Parkes termed an altered assumptive world in which the ideas, attitudes, and beliefs about the self and the world are fundamentally altered.[17,72,73] The inherent cognitive change is vital to future equanimity. Even when culture prescribes some level of continuing bonds with one's ancestors, creativity and generativity emerge from resolution of the mourning process.[35] Raphael has tended to understand much of this guided grief therapy within the rubric of 'crisis' intervention, placing additional emphasis on the mobilization of support to assist and comfort the bereaved[51] (Table 6).

As well as the supportive–expressive model described above, interpersonal therapy places emphasis on the nature of relationships and how the bereaved functions within these.[74] The psychodynamic model overlaps considerably with these interpersonal approaches.[75] The mixed feelings underpinning ambivalent relationships warrant expression and understanding, while the past influences on insecure and overly dependent patterns of relating help to consider future needs. The nature of the continuing relationship with the

Table 6 Models of grief therapy

Name of model of therapy	Potential focus for the model's application	Clinical issues when indicated
Supportive–expressive therapy (guided grief work, crisis intervention)	Individual and/or group	Avoidance of emotional expression Inhibited or delayed grief Isolated and needing support Established psychiatric disorders including depression
Interpersonal or psychodynamic therapy	Individual and/or group	Relational issues dominate Role transition difficulties
Cognitive–behavioural therapy	Individual and/or group	Chronic grief with stuckness of behaviours Traumatic grief Post-traumatic stress disorder
Family focused grief therapy	Family	Family either at risk or clearly dysfunctional in its relating Adolescents or children at risk
Combined pharmacotherapies with any of the psychotherapeutic models	Individual	Depressive disorders Anxiety disorders Sleep disorders

Group interventions can be given in parallel with individual approaches to intervention.

deceased is explored alongside any desire to replace the lost person. The urge for reunion with the deceased merits active discussion as suicidal desire easily grows out of persistence of such ideas. Gersie highlighted the dangerous pull that reunion fantasies can have when the dependent bereaved lament their loss and search to re-establish connection.[76] Increased suicide risk also occurs among socially isolated, elderly widowers, those who abuse alcohol, and those with a current or past history of depressive disorder.

Cognitive–behavioural therapy offers a special contribution to chronic grief.[24] Here, continued connectivity with the deceased may be valued and bring benefits to the bereaved that are cherished, promoting some memorialization as 'stuckness' that prevents other progress in life. Furthermore, repeated exposure to cues that induce sadness may deepen depressive illness in these circumstances. Behavioural approaches regulate exposure to these cues, optimize socialization through activity scheduling, moderate inappropriate drug and alcohol use, and promote graduated involvement in new roles and experiences. Related cognitive reframing of negative ideas such as unfairness and hopelessness steers towards a constructive adaptation.

When an overly dependent relationship has formed the basis of a complicated grief reaction, the bereaved's self-image changes from 'being valued and cared for' to being now 'alone and useless'. Patterns of perceived abandonment may re-emerge from earlier relationships. Therapy needs to target boosting self-esteem, confidence, and sense of security. The combination of both group and individual therapy has special merit since the group process promotes socialization in an individual otherwise at risk of isolation.[77] Brief group psychotherapy[66] can be offered as a complementary programme of support for the more needy, and both variety and creativity can enhance such programmes, exemplified by one programme that combined group behaviour therapy with art therapy.[78]

A family approach to grief intervention is exemplified by FFGT.[50] Such a model aims to improve family functioning while also supporting the expression of grief and, as mentioned, can be applied preventatively to those families judged through screening to be at high risk of such morbid outcome.[50] Commencing thus during palliative care and including the ill member in the family work, FFGT continues through the early phases of bereavement until there is confidence that morbidity has been prevented or appropriately treated. This approach invites the family to identify and agree to work on aspects of family life that they recognize as a cause of concern. Through enhancing cohesion, promoting open communication of thoughts and feelings, and teaching effective problem-solving to reduce conflict and optimize tolerance of different opinions, the improved functioning of the family as a unit becomes the means to accomplish adaptive mourning. The continuity of care and the personal knowledge that the therapist achieves of the dying family member empowers considerable maturation in the family unit not only as carers but also as comforters of the bereaved.

Basic aids to any form of grief counselling include the use of evocative rather than sensitive language to assist the expression of feelings, the sharing of photo albums and special letters from the loved person, writing about any unfinished business to draw it to a close, and optimizing attendance at cultural or religious rituals to support the process of mourning. Children can be encouraged to make up a 'scrap' or memory book about a deceased parent as an aide to their adaptive mourning. Complementary forms of therapy such as art[79] and music[80] therapy can also make a valuable contribution to any programme for the bereaved. Any individual differences in the intensity and progress of mourning need to be normalized as appropriate. For instance, research has repeatedly confirmed that mothers express grief more intensely than fathers do.[47] Time must be allowed to permit the process to unfold naturally and the length of mourning is helpfully appraised as proportional to the strength of attachment to the deceased.

Where the experience of death has been in some manner 'shocking', incomplete assimilation of the event can develop, leading to intrusive recollections and numbing. Here, the bereaved need to make clear sense of the loss, understanding the mechanisms involved in the death, and attributing responsibility to appropriate factors.[81] Benzodiazepines have a particular role in reducing autonomic arousal, lessening intrusive symptoms, and allaying anxiety so that avoidant responses are minimized.[45] The treatment team helps further by bringing the bereaved back in the weeks after the death to review overall understanding of events and report on findings from any autopsy. Whenever a coroner's inquiry follows a death, the bereaved are to be encouraged to attend to increase their integration of understanding of such events.

Pharmacotherapies are widely used to support the bereaved—judicious prescribing is nonetheless important. Benzodiazepines allay anxiety and assist sleep, but words of caution should be offered about intermittent use to avoid tachyphylaxis and dependence. Antidepressants are indicated whenever bereavement is complicated by the development of depressive disorder, panic attacks, and moderate to severe adjustment disorders.[82,83] If insomnia is prominent, tricyclics (e.g. dothiepin, nortriptyline, desipramine) or tetracyclics (e.g. mianserin) are beneficial; otherwise, selective serotonergic reuptake inhibitors (e.g. sertraline, paroxetine, citalopram, fluvoxamine, fluoxetine) or combined noradrenergic and serotonergic reuptake inhibitors (e.g. venlafaxine, mirtazapine) are indicated. Occasionally, antipsychotics are needed for hypomania or other forms of psychosis.

The best predictors of an adaptive outcome include a gradually resolving trajectory of emotional distress that began from a moderate rather than excessive initial level, open communication with others, good supports, robust self-esteem, and evidence of personal competency in the daily tasks that are ordinarily pursued.[84] In contrast, pathological grief can be considered dimensionally through greater degrees of separation distress, emotional numbing and dissociation, mood symptoms, impaired social functioning, and maladaptive coping styles. Categorical approaches to pathological grief incorporate elements of avoidance or denial, distortion through excessive anger, despair, guilt, idealization or somatization, and prolongation that culminates in chronicity of distress. An integrated approach to the treatment of complicated grief incorporates balanced combinations of pharmacology (e.g. antidepressants or antianxiety agents), individual psychotherapy, and socialization through family or group work.[45]

The notion of recovery is important and recognized by the return of equanimity in discussion of the deceased. A process of social transition has been accomplished.[85] New interests or roles are adopted, with new friendships emerging. Eventually, the bereaved see their future with reprioritized and altered world views. As ultimate evidence of completed mourning, new generativity and creativity emerges in the activities and lives of the bereaved.[35]

Special types of loss

Particular needs arise for bereaved children, the very elderly, and when loss is especially stigmatized, for instance death from AIDS. The timing of such deaths within the life-cycle explains some of the special considerations that arise.

Children and bereavement

The general principle of open communication with children about cancer or serious illness, its nature and meaning, treatment, and prospect of death is important.[86,87] Concepts need to be presented in an age-appropriate manner, recognizing that the finality of death only becomes more completely understood around the age of 9–10 years.[88] Younger children believe that death is reversible; after age 5, the understanding is more in terms of separation with a gradual recognition of its irreversibility. Families can teach children a healthy understanding of the life-cycle and support the child through identification of and reassurance by available, surviving adults who commit to remaining involved with the child in the future. Such processes may help a child to mature more rapidly and grow in their appreciation of death as cessation of life. Children display a variety of bereavement symptoms including sadness, fear, guilt, insecurity, and behavioural problems.[89] A programme that guides parents in what to say and do to assist their children was found to be helpful.[90]

The death of either a parent or sibling is a significant and distressing occurrence that prompts many children to ask questions such as: 'Why? Did I cause it? Who will care for me?' Careful discussion of death causation is worthwhile to avoid prophylactically any misinterpretation by the child. In the setting of advanced cancer, when death can be anticipated, preparation of the child through involvement in care activities and open discussion of realities facilitates acceptance and adjustment. Subsequent involvement of children in funeral and anniversary rituals[91] normalizes the experience of loss and promotes the family as the continuing, supportive environment.[92]

The long-term effects of childhood bereavement are not completely clear, as studies have been hampered by being retrospective, but they have suggested that the loss of a mother prior to age 12 predicts an increased risk of adult depression. However, the quality of the relationship to subsequent careproviders may be more significant in determining outcome than the parental loss.[93] Nonetheless, should such children develop cancer themselves in adult life, their memories of their dying parent and related identifications are powerful influences on their overall adjustment.

After accidents, cancer is the second leading cause of death in childhood. The family typically focuses on the dying child with the risk of relative neglect of other children. They in turn may try to replace the dead child and experience survivor guilt. Openness of family communication about all aspects of the illness and death is the best formula to promote normal grieving and family meetings can especially model this. The grief of the parents needs support alongside the grief of the children, empowering the parents to attend to their children's grief, rather than the children being parentified as a support for their parents. Parents may become hypervigilant about their surviving children's health, unwittingly promoting hypochondriasis in later life if too much attention is placed on somatic symptoms and fear of cancer. Attention to the functioning of the family provides the most useful model for recognition of those at greater risk of poorer outcome.[94] Families that block discussion, suppress sharing of feelings, and concentrate rigidly on concrete events fare more poorly than families that comfort one another with empathy and teamwork.

The elderly and bereavement

When couples have been married for many years, the length and depth of their attachment may predispose them to profound grief, further complicated by the acute loneliness they can experience if many of their friends and sources of support have already died. Elderly bereaved men can have particular needs in these circumstances.[95] Moreover, despite apparent support from within the family, the bereaved spouse may carry an especially painful level of loneliness.[96] The social support of the elderly bereaved warrants special consideration, including use of volunteer programmes.[97]

Bereavement during adulthood

Although the loss of a spouse has received most attention in research, loss of a parent or sibling during adult life is a common event and will generate distress proportional to the degree of emotional closeness to the deceased. Increased maturity is one potential outcome of such losses.[98] Where there is a high familial incidence of cancer raising questions of genetic risk, as in familial polyposis, breast, or colon cancer, the death of a sibling increases the sense of vulnerability of family members and highlights the importance of genetic testing and counselling when relevant.

When comparisons have been made between the death of a spouse, parent, or child, the most intense bereavement reactions are found following the death of a child, an event clearly out of step with life-cycle expectations.[99,100] Parents have a strong and powerful investment in their children such that their premature death shakes the adult personality to its very roots.[101] Its impact is life-long—although the distress slowly declines with the passage of time, it plateaus eventually to a steady state of continued influence, although the meaning of this continues to change throughout the life-cycle.[102] For many it is a disruptive and life-shattering experience, necessitating a continuing life-long accommodation, but this is affected to some degree by the quality of the relationship before the child's death and the relationship that exists with other surviving children.

Aware of such inherent challenges, palliative care teams do well to involve parents in the care of terminally ill children (including adult offspring), foster open communication of feelings about the death, and seek views on their philosophy of life. Where parents can find some meaning and sense of purpose in their child's life, their acceptance of the death, despite its inherent unfairness, is likely to be greater.[103] The incorporation of parents into the model of family-centered care remains important when a middle-aged adult is dying and predeceasing elderly parents; often the focus of the palliative care team is on the nuclear family, supporting the spouse and children to the neglect of parental grief.

Hospices for dying children allow particular care to be taken of the family, including continuity of this care into bereavement. Active discussion of the choice between death at home or in the hospice is important and a family-centered model of care will consider the potential impact on usually three generations of family membership. Well-functioning families are perceived to cope better with death in the home, while respite admissions can bring relief to those families more stressed by the emotional demands of caring for the dying child. Irrespective of whether death is affecting a young child, an adolescent, or young adult, grief is intense and potentially protracted;

sustained support of family members is especially important when the functioning of the family has been stressed or is clearly dysfunctional.

Bereavement and AIDS

The stigma associated with human immunodeficiency virus (HIV) infection handicaps the adjustment of both patients and their families and adds a risk factor for complicated grief. Caregiving partners of men with AIDS experience several stressors that induce role conflict and burden.(104) Mean scores for depressive symptoms were found in one longitudinal study to remain at one standard deviation above the general community norm 3 years after the death.(105) The families also display complex dynamics related to their degree of acceptance of a homosexual relationship, any ambivalence about which potentially complicates the mourning process.(106)

Spirituality and bereavement

The existential quest to understand the meaning of life creates an endeavour to understand the uniqueness and special contribution of each and every person. This spiritual orientation influences adaptation both to dying and to bereavement. Clinicians do well to inquire about the spiritual dimensions and philosophy of life of both their patients and families.(107) For some, this will be expressed in the language of their religious beliefs; for others, cultural custom and traditions will inform their set of values and the philosophy by which they have lived. Using these values to understand the life of the deceased helps in appraising their accomplishments, the sort of person they were, and the meaning their life had. When consensus about this can be achieved with the bereaved, it assists their acceptance of the death. Moreover, when the latter has been peaceful, this will console the bereaved, but when the death was difficult, disappointing, or in some manner horrifying, there is considerable work to do in helping the bereaved to understand and come to terms with this final outcome. A spiritual understanding of the person's life may help in accepting the limitations of palliative care or coming to terms with any unfinished business that remained in the deceased's life. Philosophically this may be akin to letting go of the ideal and accepting a life lived with a goodness that is sufficient.

Ritual is an important component of religious and cultural tradition as it creates a proven pathway down which the bereaved tread.(108) The wisdom of centuries is often woven into such rituals as a means of assisting the bereaved to mourn. Respect for such ritual is important and clinicians help the bereaved by endorsing its value. Familiarity with different ethnic traditions is worthwhile in palliative care. Nonetheless, should a clinician meet an unfamiliar ethnic group, they should seek from the relatives an understanding of their tradition and strive to co-operate with them in a culturally sensitive manner.

Bereavement practices across cultures

Palliative care practitioners need at least some rudimentary knowledge of cross-cultural bereavement customs to inform sensitive clinical practice. Most cultures do sanction the expression of emotions such as crying, fear, and anger, while each of the world's major religions have developed comprehensible practices to guide their bereaved. Eastern religions sustain greater belief in a spirit world, reflecting an animism underlying Asian religious traditions. Western religions in contrast are theistic in nature. An overview of the contribution of the world's major religions to bereavement practices follows, but further information about other ethnic and religious practices can be found in the references listed in the further reading section.

Hindu bereavement practices

Hindus believe in rebirth with transmigration of the *jeevatma* or subtle personality of the person into another life until eventually the *atma* (soul) merges with God.(109) The theory of *karma* and its reciprocal reactions explains suffering that can be endured through detachment. Fear of death is reduced through belief in rebirth. It is the sacred duty (*dharma*) of the family to follow the teachings of the *shastras*, the sacred religious texts, and to perform the rituals and acts of piety and charity to ensure the peaceful repose of the departed soul, although variation occurs according to caste, regions, and finances.

Death is preferred at home and with the patient on the floor. A drop or two of water from the Ganges is sprinkled from a basil leaf onto the lips or mouth of the person just before or soon after death.(110) Loud shrieks of emotion are able to be expressed when death has happened. Then a ritual washing of the body occurs, and the widow removes her wedding mark from her forehead, while the heads of the men can be shaved and all dress in white. Condolences are shared freely. Priests read from sacred texts, recite verses from the *Bhagavad Gita*, and sing devotional songs. In India, after the body is anointed and garlanded, it would be cremated at the burning ghat, where the eldest son would ignite the pyre. Mourners chant or wail. The spirit is said to depart the body when the skull cracks. The funeral rites last for a traditional 12 days, during which all sleep on the floor and eat vegetarian food. After ablutions, the recital of prayers occurs twice daily and special gatherings of the mourners—termed *markha* or *utthama* ceremonies—ensure the open sharing of grief by all involved. The empty handed display of the palms of the hands symbolizes their sense of devastation. After 12 days, the ashes would be traditionally scattered into the waters of the Ganges and charitable acts performed to aid beggars.

Hindu death outside of India can still respect traditional customs such as ritualistic washing, preparation of the body, pall-bearing to gain virtue, and the prayer ceremonies as described. Hindu traditions are indeed the most ancient of the world religions.

Buddhist bereavement practices

Buddhist tradition also began in India during the sixth century BC and believed in repeated rebirth. Through attaining the state of a clear and calm mind undisturbed by worldly events and full of compassion, the diligent person can escape the continuous cycle of rebirth to attain enlightenment (*nirvana*). Theravada Buddhism, which concentrates on teachings found in the Four Noble Truths and the Eightfold Path, is found in Sri Lanka, Myanmar, Thailand, Cambodia, and Laos. Mahayana Buddhism in its various faith and devotional forms is practiced widely in China, Japan, Korea, Taiwan, and Vietnam. Vajrayana Buddhism places emphasis on rituals and initiation rites and is found in Tibet, Nepal, Mongolia, and parts of India.(111) While the Vietnamese prefer death at home, for instance, the vast majority of Chinese families seek admission to hospital to directly avoid death in the home.

As the Buddhist person approaches death, chanting certain *sutras* has a calming effect on the mind and helps concentrate on the Buddha or Pure Land. Ceremonial instructions can be quietly read to the dead to guide it through the *bardo* (transitional state) between life forms. The ceremony can be repeated for 49 days until rebirth is assured. The body is wrapped in a white silk cloth; incense and votive papers are burned; both cremation and below-ground burial are practiced; and a series of prayer ceremonies are conducted. Mourners wear white clothes and head bands and can walk with sticks, symbolizing that their grief has left them in need of support. An altar of commemoration for the dead is usually erected in the home; daily offerings are made and prayers recited. Family dinners are held on the 49th, 100th, and 365th days after the death; temple ceremonies are observed on the first and 15th days of each lunar month, the lunar new year, and the first anniversary. Filial duty is particularly laid down for the first son to commemorate his family's ancestors; custom requires the open display of grief as a mark of loyalty.

Confucianism and death

Confucius taught the right way of relating to others to achieve peace, harmony, and happiness.(112) Social rituals optimized the expression of mutual respect. The attitude of the living towards the dead is similarly respectful and one of continuous remembrance and affection. Family-centered rituals are at the core of such expressions of gratitude and grief, consistent with strong traditions of filial duty, and they guide members to follow the middle way, always avoiding extremes.[113] These rituals model the ultimate dignity of human relationships and bring grace and beauty to human behaviour through continuity with the past and tradition.

Confucian philosophy views the human person as part of an infinite biological chain, the value of each person lying in their part of one's family and society. Accepting one's fate and bearing sorrow in silence is part of the maintenance of human dignity.[114] Public prescribed rituals are the place to express grief. For the Chinese to be buried in China or have their ashes returned to China means reunion with their ancestors in the town their family originated from—understanding the significance of such wishes can help to reassure and comfort the dying.

Taoism and death

The second great spiritual tradition that originated in China focuses more on nature than man in providing a means of transcending the limits of one's world.[114] Everything is in a state of continuous change, necessitating acceptance of the spontaneity of things. Spiritual tranquillity is achieved by freeing oneself from worldly pursuits, even by adopting an element of playful fun.

The circle of the yin and yang is the symbol of the Supreme Reality and the cosmic forces underpinning natural change.[112] Yin is the feminine, passive, dark, cold, wet, and soft aspects of life while yang represents the masculine, active, bright, hot, dry, and hard elements. Their complementary and interactional relationship leads to ceaseless transformations in the forms of life and death. Positive admiration of such beauty in nature promotes acceptance and counters any anxiety about death.

Grief is recognized as part of the normal emotions of life, but it is moderated in intensity by acceptance of the unending change of nature and the transformation of the spirit within the cosmic world. Taoist philosophy clearly posits that the dominant perspective on death is one of acceptance.[113]

Jewish bereavement practices

Judaism splits into several denominations ranging from the Orthodox to the Reform, with further variations being culturally based on Ashkenazic (Central-Eastern European) or Sephardic (Spanish-African) origins. Basic beliefs include the concept of one God, the sanctity of the person created in the image of God, the immortality of the soul and an afterlife following judgement, and a period of purification. The Talmud states that one should not hasten death. Visitation of the sick and accompaniment of the dying are ancient traditions. The rabbi should be called at the approach of death to say a confessional prayer (the *Vidui*) and recite the fundamental affirmation of faith, the *Shema*.

The process of life review prior to death has generated one interesting tradition taking the form of writing an ethical will. In this document, the dying person records his/her legacy to his/her family. It states the hopes and dreams held for the family, the values considered important, and any thoughts or messages that the family should remember. Such ethical wills are usually warmly and lovingly written and thus are a source of great comfort to the bereaved.

After death, the body should be cleansed and prepared by the burial society (*Chevrah Kadisha*) through a religious ritual (*Taharah*). Dressed in white and robed in a prayer shawl (*tallit*), burial of the body in the ground is desirable within 24 h and fulfils the notion of 'returning to dust'. Post-mortem examinations, embalming, and cremation are prohibited. A simple funeral service honours the dead with an eulogy, psalms, and a reading of the Memorial Prayer. The family, whose garments may be torn as a symbol of grief, then accompany the coffin to the cemetery to conclude the burial.

While the period between death and burial is termed the *Aninut*, the time of intense shock, the first 3 days following the funeral are seen as the time for weeping and lamentation at home in private mourning. The period of 7 days following the burial corresponds with the tradition of *shiva*, in which the primary mourners sit on low stools and allow others to prepare their food. Their energy is focused on grief, knowing that their friends will take care of them. The community gathers at the home to make up a *minyan* (quorum of 10) so that the mourner's prayer, The *Kaddish*, may be recited. The *Kaddish* affirms faith in God and hope in an everlasting resurrection. The burning of a memorial candle is also a common tradition during this time.

The period of 30 days following the burial is termed the *sheloshim*, a time when business can be resumed but grief continues and due allowance is made for the distress of the mourners. In the 10 months after the *sheloshim*, lives are expected to gradually return to normal, but the *Kaddish* is recited at Sabbath services each week, thus supporting the bereaved's grief within their community. At the first anniversary, the commemorative tombstone is unveiled at the cemetery and the formal period of mourning is concluded. The dead are, however, remembered each year during the *Yizkor* memorial service and at the *Yahrzeit* (the family meeting on the anniversary of the day of death).

Christian bereavement practices

Many of the rituals of Christianity are derived from their Jewish origins. The basic tenets are that *Jesus* of Nazareth was the *Messiah*, the Son of God, who was crucified to redeem the sins of mankind, and rose from the dead on the third day as evidence of his divinity. Reconciliation with monotheism is achieved through the doctrine of the *Trinity* (God the Father, Son, and Holy Spirit), three persons in one God. Christ's teachings were laid down in the *Gospels* and *Acts of the Apostles* as the *New Testament*, which was then added to the Jewish Bible. There is belief in the soul, forgiveness of wrongdoing, resurrection of the body, and everlasting life in the place commonly termed heaven. The *Eastern Orthodox Churches* split from the *Roman Catholic Church* in the eleventh century, while the *Protestant Reformation* occurred during the sixteenth century.[115]

Priesthood is followed in the tradition of the rabbis, with study in preparation and ordination bringing responsibility for the conduct of the major rituals. These are perceived as a source of spiritual grace and connectedness with God and are known as the *sacraments*. *Baptism* with water is an initial cleansing ritual celebrating entry into the community, while the *Mass* is the major sacrament celebrating the life of Jesus in the form of a Jewish Passover meal with communion, the sharing of the sacred bread and wine. Christian tradition recognizes *Mary* as the mother of Jesus, introducing a female element missing from other major world religions.

For the sick, in the Roman Catholic rite both the sacrament of *Confession or Reconciliation*, in which sins are repented before a priest and forgiven, and the sacrament of *Anointing the sick*, formerly called *Extreme Unction* in keeping with the blessed oils that are used, are a means of spiritual uplifting and prayerful connectedness with God. In the Eastern rites, the priest will chant the *Office for the Sick* and the *Office for the Parting of the Soul*, while in the Anglican rite, *Prayers for the Sick* are said. Contact with a priest or minister of the appropriate church is important for Christians to access these rituals before death. The family would traditionally gather around the bed of the dying keeping prayerful watch, including recital of the *Rosary* prayer to invoke the support of Mary in the Roman Catholic tradition.

Once death has occurred, funeral directors play a dominant role in arranging services with the priest and plans for burial or cremation. Viewing of the body is common and may be accompanied by prayers. The funeral occurs when practical within a few days of the death, usually occurring in a church or chapel. Traditionally, a *Vigil* service on the night preceding the funeral involves prayers, psalms, or recitation of the *Rosary*. In Roman Catholicism, the *Requiem Mass* incorporates the regular sacrament with a commemorative service, while in Orthodox services, mourners prostrate themselves and kiss the cross. If there is a burial, a *Service of Internment* takes place at the graveside; if cremated, the ashes are placed in an urn for later internment or scattering by the family.

Within the Eastern rites, memorial services (*Panikhidi*) are held 3, 8, and 40 days after the funeral with chanting of traditional psalms and anthems (*Contakion & Trepanion*). Catholic rites include the offering of *Votive*

Masses to commemorate the dead, especially at times of the anniversary and at the calendar *Feasts of All Saints and All Souls.* Considerable variation occurs across the range of Protestant and Free Churches of Christian tradition, incorporating differing emphasis on beliefs about communion, Bible interpretation, and church rules. Members of African communities converted to Christianity retain some beliefs in Voodoo, spirit healing, and witchcraft, while fundamentalist practice has emerged in many churches to counter the drift away from religious practice. *Mormons* (*Church of the Latter-Day Saints*) wear a sacred undergarment, which should not be removed after death.

Thus, within Christian tradition, the prayers for the sick before death play a potentially spiritual healing role, while the bereavement practices orientate around church services but provide continuing support for the bereaved from their church communities.

Islamic bereavement practices

Muhammad saw himself around 610 AD as one of a succession of Semitic prophets following in the tradition of Moses, Abraham, and Jesus who preached God's judgement on each person according to their works, culminating in the resurrection of the dead. The Islamic religion has been based on the *Quran* and teachings of its prophet and quickly spread across the Arabic nations from Morocco to Egypt to Pakistan to Indonesia.[116]

As death approaches, the Imam should be called to attend the dying. They may be helped to sit up or turn their face towards Mecca and their confession of faith is prayed as their relatives gather around and provide support. Following death, ritual washing occurs to prepare the body. As a rule, only men wash a man's body and only women a woman's. A *Quran* reader chants from the holy book during this cleansing ablution. Washing proceeds in a fixed pattern and with great respect for the body, which is then wrapped in three pieces of white cloth and thus prepared for burial. Cremation is forbidden through belief in resurrection of the body. Cultural variation exists within Islamic sects with regard to the expression of grief: it ranges from extreme wailing to restrained composure. Burial is encouraged within 24 h. News of the death and invitation to pray for the deceased is announced by loudspeaker from the village minaret.

During the final ceremony, the face of the deceased is made visible for the mourners to look at and bid farewell. Recitation from the *Quran* or construction of a personal dirge is common. The Imam invites the community to forgive the deceased any wrong deeds and the *Prayer for the Dead* is recited. The body is then ready for burial. The body lying on a bier is carried in procession to the graveside and lowered into the grave, positioning the face and eyes towards Mecca and laying a board across the face to permit a little room. The *Quran* is read while the grave is filled with soil and the Imam gives a final blessing. Then, while the mourners leave in silence, Islamic belief states that two angels visit the deceased to ask the final five questions as an expression of their faith. The Imam, standing at the head of the grave acts for the angels and calls the deceased to answer these questions: Who is your God? Prophet? Book? Iman? Qibla (prayer direction)? The Imam listens for the head of the dead to bump against the wooden board in reply and continues to call the name of the deceased until the response is heard.

In North Africa, bereaved women wear white, while in the Middle East, they wear black—young women for 3 months; older women for 1 year. Special sweet food is eaten on the third, seventh, and 40th days and prayers are offered. The story of the prophet's birth is read on the 40th day as a source of consolation and a special stone is laid at the tomb on the anniversary of the burial. Traditionally, children have been excluded from Islamic burial ceremonies although these practices appear to be changing. The rituals clearly draw in community support for the bereaved as they foster hope in the belief of resurrection.

Secular bereavement practices

Many in society are non-religious, whether agnostic or atheistic, and see death as a natural process, albeit considerably medicalized. There is grief at the closure of life and mourning for those left behind. The funeral industry provides support for the bereaved and helps them celebrate the life of the deceased person with appropriate eulogy, poetry, and story, conducting a secular service in the funeral parlour while other self-help groups are available to support the bereaved. For the non-religious, such processes continue to nurture the expression of grief and affirm the normality of mourning.

Research and measurement in bereavement

Although generic measures of psychiatric symptomatology (see Chapter 5.5) are commonly used in bereavement research, a number of self-report measures of bereavement phenomena make it now possible to specifically evaluate the process and outcome of both the grief over the loss and the supportive therapies used by palliative care services to intervene. The psychometric properties and key references of these bereavement measures are summarized in Table 7 as a resource for researchers.

Qualitative studies of bereavement are ideally suited to reveal the unique meanings that inform the reactions of individuals or cultural groups to death and loss.[117] They are derived from constructivist philosophy that recognizes the socially and personally constructed realities of human experience and are helpful in generating theory, but limited in providing causal explanations for grief phenomena or demonstrating the efficacy of particular interventions. Yet mixed qualitative–quantitative methodologies continue to provide valuable insights, well exemplified by the work of Folkman's group in studying the bereavement experience of carer's of gay men dying from AIDS.[118] Here, they recognized the value of positive emotion and spirituality, leading to an enriched understanding of the contribution of meaning-based coping to the adaptive responses of the bereaved. There is a substantial need for quantitatively based observational and interventional studies in bereavement.

Positive outcome and personal growth

The adaptation that follows the wrenching loss of bereavement is associated with personal growth for a sizeable proportion. Although this personal growth manifests itself most clearly after the acute pain of grief, it is actually identifiable across all phases of the bereavement process.[119] Renewed sense of meaning, self-awareness, increased empathy, appreciation of family and relationships, independence, reprioritized goals and values, deepened spirituality, and increased altruism can all result from positive reappraisal, seeking for help and enhanced social resources.

Clinicians can helpfully reassure bereaved people about these beneficial outcomes, especially at times when the going is hard. Providing information about the longitudinal course of the mourning process including the prospect of such personal growth creates a feedback loop that nurtures adaptive recovery through cognitive appraisal and active coping.

Conclusion

Bereavement care is an integral dimension of palliative medicine as clinicians sustain continuity of care in assisting the family or carers of their deceased patient. Knowledge of and competence in assessing grief is essential to enable recognition of the 20 per cent of the bereaved who get into difficulties and need additional assistance. Routine assessment of the bereaved for risk factors for complicated grief provides a responsible method through which treatment teams can intervene preventatively or early to reduce unnecessary morbidity. Effective therapies are available to assist in the management of complicated grief and palliative care practitioners should be skilled in their application or understand the circumstances when referral for further specialist help is appropriately made. Grief is an inevitable dimension of our humanity, an adaptive adjustment process, and one that with support can be approached with courage. Grief that is shared is grief that is healed.

Table 7 Psychometric properties of grief and bereavement self-report measures

Instrument name	Item number and response style	Subscale or factor structure	Reliability	Validity	Comments on utility
Texas Revised Inventory of Grief (TRIG)[120]	21-item, 5-point response	Past behaviour at time of death Present feelings	Cronbach's α 0.77–0.87	Satisfactory predictive validity	Comparison between past and present responses invalidated by memory; subscale 2 useful as a change measure
Grief Experience Inventory (GEI)[121]	135-item, true–false response	Validity scales of denial, atypical response, and social desirability Clinical scales of despair, anger, guilt, isolation, control, rumination, depersonalization, somatization, and death anxiety	Cronbach's α 0.34–0.84; test–retest 0.53–0.87 over 9 weeks	Satisfactory concurrent and predictive validity	Long measure, some items using past tense wording in a fixed manner; true–false response style less useful as a change measure
Core Bereavement Items (CBI)[122] and Bereavement Phenomenology Questionnaire (BPQ)[95,123]	17-item, CBI and 22-item BPQ; 4-point response	CBI—1 scale BPQ—1 factor[124]	Cronbach's α 0.91 (CBI); 0.93 (BPQ)	Satisfactory concurrent and predictive validity	Sensible focus on core bereavement phenomena. CBI best measure of normal responses; BPQ better as measure to include symptoms of non-resolution. CBI derived in part from BPQ
Inventory of Complicated Grief (ICG)[38]	19-item, 5-point response	Separation distress Traumatic grief	Cronbach's α 0.94; test–retest 0.80 over 6 months	Satisfactory concurrent and predictive validity	Derived from research on bereaved elderly spouses whose loss resulted from cancer
Inventory of Traumatic Grief (ITG)[23]	30-item, 5-point response	Separation distress Traumatic grief	Cronbach's α 0.95	Concurrent validity with SF-36	Permits application of proposed diagnostic criteria for traumatic grief
Sibling Inventory of Bereavement (SIB)[125]	46-item, 5-point response	Grief factor Personal growth	Cronbach's α 0.88–0.95	Satisfactory predictive validity	Instrument only used with adolescents (13–18 years) although developed from qualitative data from children
Grief Experience Questionnaire (GEQ)[126]	55-item, 5-point response	Eight factors from principal components analysis: abandonment, stigma, searching, guilt, somatic, personal responsibility, self-destructive, and shame	Cronbach's α 0.68–0.89	Differentiates suicidally bereaved from other losses	Useful for stigmatized deaths from suicide, AIDS

References

1. **Parkes, C.** *Bereavement: Studies of Grief in Adult Life* 3rd edn. Madison: International Universities Press, 1998.
2. **Stroebe, M., Stroebe, W., and Hansson, R.**, ed. *Handbook of Bereavement*. Cambridge: Cambridge University Press, 1993.
3. **Raphael, B.** *The Anatomy of Bereavement*. London: Hutchinson, 1983.
4. **Rando, T.** *Treatment of Complicated Mourning*. Illinois: Research Press, 1993.
5. **Doka, K.** (1989). Disenfranchised grief. In *Disenfranchised Grief: Recognizing Hidden Sorrow* (ed. K. Doka), pp. 3–11. Lexington MA: Lexington Books.
6. **Darwin, C.** *The Expression of the Emotions in Man and Animals*. London: Murray, 1872.
7. **Rosenblatt, P.** (2001). A social constructionist perspective on cultural differences in grief. In *Handbook of Bereavement Research. Consequences, Coping, and Care* (ed. M. Stroebe, R. Hansson, W. Stroebe, and H. Schut), pp. 285–300. Washington DC: American Psychological Association.
8. **Middleton, W., Moylan, A., Raphael, B., Burnett, P., and Martinek, N.** (1993). An international perspective on bereavement related concepts. *Australian and New Zealand Journal of Psychiatry* **27**, 457–63.
9. **Bowlby, J.** (1977). The making and breaking of affectional bonds I & II. *British Journal of Psychiatry* **130**, 201–10 and 421–31.
10. **Ainsworth, M., Blehar, M., Waters, E., and Wall, S.** *Patterns of Attachment: A Psychological Study of the Strange Situation*. Hillsdale NJ: Erlbaum, 1978.
11. **Parkes, C.** (1985). Bereavement. *British Journal of Psychiatry* **146**, 11–17.
12. **Jacobs, S., Kosten, T., Kasl, S., Ostfeld, A., Berkman, L., and Charpentier, P.** (1987/88). Attachment theory and multiple dimensions of grief. *Omega* **18**, 41–52.
13. **Klein, M.** (1940). Mourning and its relation to manic-depressive states. *International Journal of Psycho-analysis* **21**, 125–53.
14. **Shapiro, E.** (2001). Grief in interpersonal perspective: theories and their implications. In *Handbook of Bereavement Research. Consequences, Coping, and Care* (ed. M. Stroebe, R. Hansson, W. Stroebe, and H. Schut), pp. 301–27. Washington DC: American Psychological Association.
15. **Horowitz, M.** (1989). A model of mourning: change in schemas of self and other. *Journal of the American Psychoanalytic Association* **38**, 297–324.
16. **Horowitz, M., Bonanno, G., and Holen, A.** (1993). Pathological grief: diagnosis and explanations. *Psychosomatic Medicine* **55**, 260–73.
17. **Parkes, C.** (1975). What becomes of redundant world models? A contribution to the study of adaptation to change. *British Journal of Medical Psychology* **48**, 131–7.
18. **Freud, S.** *Totem and Taboo*. London: Hogarth Press, 1912.

19. **Klass, D., Silverman, P., and Nickman, S.**, ed. *Continuing Bonds: New Understandings of Grief.* Washington DC: Taylor & Francis, 1996.
20. **Walter, T.** (1996). A new model of grief: bereavement and biography. *Mortality* **1**, 7–25.
21. **Kissane, D., Bloch, S., Dowe, D., Snyder, R., Onghena, P., McKenzie, D.** et al. (1996). The Melbourne family grief study I & II. *American Journal of Psychiatry* **153**, 650–8 and 659–66.
22. **Walsh, F. and McGoldrick, M.**, ed. *Living Beyond Loss.* New York: Norton, 1991.
23. **Prigerson, H. and Jacobs, S.** (2001). Traumatic grief as a distinct disorder: A rationale, consensus criteria, and a preliminary empirical test. In *Handbook of Bereavement Research. Consequences, Coping, and Care* (ed. M. Stroebe, R. Hansson, W. Stroebe, and H. Schut), pp. 613–37. Washington DC: American Psychological Association.
24. **Kavanagh, D.** (1990). Towards a cognitive–behavioural intervention for adult grief reactions. *British Journal of Psychiatry* **157**, 373–83.
25. **Stroebe, M. and Schut, H.** (2001). Models of coping with bereavement: a review. In *Handbook of Bereavement Research. Consequences, Coping, and Care* (ed. M. Stroebe, R. Hansson, W. Stroebe, and H. Schut), pp. 375–403. Washington DC: American Psychological Association.
26. **Lindemann, E.** (1944). Symptomatology and management of acute grief. *American Journal of Psychiatry* **101**, 141–8.
27. **Jacobs, S., Bruce, M., and Kim, K.** (1997). Adrenal function predicts demoralisation after losses. *Psychosomatics* **38**, 529–34.
28. **Esterling, B., Kiecolt-Glaser, J., and Glaser, R.** (1996). Psychosocial modulation of cytokine-induced natural killer cell activity in older adults. *Psychosomatic Medicine* **58**, 264–72.
29. **Hall, M., Baum, A., Buysse, D., Prigerson, H., Kupfer, D., and Reynolds, C.** (1998). Sleep as a mediator of the stress–immune relationship. *Psychosomatic Medicine* **60**, 48–51.
30. **Parkes, C.** (1975). Determinants of outcome following bereavement. *Omega* **6**, 303–23.
31. **Meares, R.** (1981). On saying goodbye before death. *Journal of the American Medical Association* **246**, 1227–9.
32. **Maguire, P.** (1985). Barriers to psychological care of the dying. *British Medical Journal* **291**, 1711–13.
33. **Parkes, C., Laungani, P., and Young, B.**, ed. Death and bereavement across cultures. London: Routledge, 1997.
34. **Hofer, M.** (1984). Relationships as regulators: a psychobiologic perspective on bereavement. *Psychosomatic Medicine* **46**, 183–97.
35. **Polloch, G.** *The Mourning-Liberation Process.* New Haven CT: International University Press, 1989.
36. **Zisook, S. and Schuchter, S.** (1985). The first four years of widowhood. *Psychiatric Annals* **16**, 288–94.
37. **Parkes, C. and Weiss, R.** *Recovery from Bereavement.* New York: Basic Books, 1983.
38. **Prigerson, H., Maciejewski, P., Newson, J., Reynolds, C., Bierhals, A., Miller, M.** et al. (1995). Inventory of complicated grief. *Psychiatry Research* **59**, 65–79.
39. **Prigerson, H., Frand, E., and Kasl, S.** (1995). Complicated grief and bereavement-related depression as distinct disorders: preliminary empirical validation in elderly bereaved spouses. *American Journal of Psychiatry* **152**, 22–30.
40. **Clayton, P.** (1990). Bereavement and depression. *Journal of Clinical Psychiatry* **51**, 34–8.
41. **Zisook, S. and Schuchter, S.** (1991). Depression through the first year after the death of a spouse. *American Journal of Psychiatry* **148**, 1346–52.
42. **Harlow, S., Goldberg, E., and Comstock, G.** (1991). A longitudinal study of the prevalence of depressive symptomatology in elderly widowed and married women. *Archives of General Psychiatry* **48**, 1065–8.
43. **Zisook, S., Schuchter, S., and Sledge, P.** (1994). The spectrum of depressive phenomena after spousal bereavement. *Journal of Clinical Psychiatry* **55** (Suppl. 4), 29–36.
44. **Karam, E.** (1994). The nosological status of bereavement-related depressions. *British Journal of Psychiatry* **165**, 48–52.
45. **Jacobs, S.** *Pathological Grief.* Washington DC: American Psychiatric Association Press, 1993.
46. **Schut, H., Stroebe, M., de Keijser, J., and van den Bout, J.** (1997). Intervention for the bereaved: gender differences in the efficacy of two counselling programmes. *British Journal of Clinical Psychology* **36**, 63–72.
47. **Kissane, D. and Bloch, S.** (1994). Family grief. *British Journal of Psychiatry* **164**, 728–40.
48. **Kissane, D., Bloch, S., Burns, W., Patrick, J., Wallace, C., and McKenzie, D.** (1994). Perceptions of family functioning and cancer. *Psycho-oncology* **3**, 259–69.
49. **Moos, R. and Moos, B.** *Family Environment Scale Manual.* Palo Alto CA: Consulting Psychologists' Press, 1981.
50. **Kissane, D. and Bloch, S.** *Family Focused Grief Therapy: A Model of Family-Centered Care during Palliative Care and Bereavement.* Buckingham: Open University Press, 2002.
51. **Raphael, B.** (1977). Preventive intervention with the recently bereaved. *Archives of General Psychiatry* **34**, 1450–4.
52. **Parkes, C.** (1981). Evaluation of a bereavement service. *Journal of Preventive Psychiatry* **1**, 179–88.
53. **Stroebe, M. and Stroebe, W.** (1993). The mortality of bereavement: a review. In *Handbook of Bereavement. Theory, Research, and Intervention* (ed. M. Stroebe, W. Stroebe, and R. Hansson), pp. 175–95. Cambridge: Cambridge University Press.
54. **Schaefer, C., Quesenberry, C., and Wi, S.** (1995). Mortality following conjugal bereavement and the effects of a shared environment. *American Journal of Epidemiology* **141**, 1142–52.
55. **House, J., Landi, K., and Umberson, D.** (1988). Social relationship and health. *Science* **241**, 540–5.
56. **Saunders, C.** *Grief: The Mourning After: Dealing with Adult Bereavement* 2nd edn. New York: Wiley, 1999.
57. **Parkes, C.** (1984). The effects of bereavement on physical and mental health: a study of the case records of widows. *British Medical Journal* **2**, 274–80.
58. **Hofer, M., Wolff, C., Freedman, S., and Mason, J.** (1972). A psychoendocrine study of bereavement: parts I & II. *Psychosomatic Medicine* **34**, 481–507.
59. **Bartrop, R., Lazarus, L., Luckhurst, E., Kiloh, L., and Penny, R.** (1977). Depressed lymphocyte function after bereavement. *Lancet* **1**, 834–6.
60. **Schleifer, S., Keller, M., Camerino, J., Thornton, C., and Stein, M.** (1983). Suppression of lymphocyte stimulation following bereavement. *Journal of the American Medical Association* **250**, 374–7.
61. **Irwin, M., Daniels, M., and Weiner, H.** (1987). Immune and neuroendocrine changes after bereavement. *Psychiatric Clinics of North America* **10**, 449–65.
62. **Jones, D. and Goldblatt, P.** (1986). Cancer mortality following widow(er)hood: some further results from the Office of Population Censuses and Surveys Longitudinal Study. *Stress Medicine* **2**, 129–40.
63. **Kaprio, J., Koskenvuo, M., and Rita, H.** (1987). Mortality after bereavement: a prospective study of 95,647 widowed persons. *American Journal of Public Health* **77**, 283–7.
64. **Helsing, K., Comstock, G., and Szklo, M.** (1982). Causes of death in a widowed population. *American Journal of Epidemiology* **116**, 524–32.
65. **Yalom, I. and Vinogradov, S.** (1988). Bereavement groups: techniques and themes. *International Journal of Group Psychotherapy* **38**, 419–46.
66. **Lieberman, M. and Yalom, I.** (1992). Brief group therapy for the spousally bereaved: a controlled study. *International Journal of Group Psychotherapy* **42**, 117–32.
67. **Kissane, D.** (2000). Family grief therapy: a new model of family-centered care during palliative care and bereavement. In *Cancer and the Family* 2nd edn (ed. L. Baider, G. Cooper, and Kaplan De Nour). Chichester: Wiley.
68. **Kissane, D.** (1999). Importance of family-centred care to palliative medicine. *Japanese Journal of Clinical Oncology* **29**, 1–3.
69. **Melges, F. and Demaso, D.** (1980). Grief-resolution therapy: reliving, revising and revisiting. *American Journal of Psychotherapy* **34**, 51–61.
70. **Mawson, D., Marks, I., Ramm, L., and Stern, R.** (1981). Guided mourning for morbid giref: a controlled study. *British Journal of Psychiatry* **138**, 185–93.
71. **Worden, J.** *Grief Counseling and Grief Therapy: A Handbook for the Mental Health Practitioner* 2nd edn. New York: Springer, 1991.

72. **Janoff-Bulman, R.** (1989). Assumptive worlds and the stresss of traumatic events: application of the schema concept. *Social Cognition* **7**, 113–36.
73. **Janoff-Bulman, R.** *Shattered Assumptions. Towards a New Psychology of Trauma.* New York: Free Press, 1992.
74. **Klerman, G., Weissman, M., and Rounsaville, B.** *Interpersonal Psychotherapy of Depression.* New York: Basic Books, 1984.
75. **Horowitz, M., Marmar, C., Weiss, D, Dewitt K.N., and Rosenbaum, R.** (1984). Brief psychotherapy of bereavement reactions. *Archives of General Psychiatry* **41**, 438–48.
76. **Gersie, A.** *Storymaking in Bereavement. Dragons Fight in the Meadow.* London: Jessica Kingsley Publishers, 1991.
77. **Vachon, M., Sheldon, A., Lancee, W., Lyall, W., Rogers, J., and Freeman, S.** (1980). A controlled study of self-help intervention for widows. *American Journal of Psychiatry* **137**, 1380–4.
78. **Schut, H., de Keijser, J., van den Bout, J., and Stroebe, M.** (1996). Cross modality grief therapy: description and assessment of a new program. *Journal of Clinical Psychology* **52**, 357–65.
79. **Simon, R.** (1982). Bereavement art. *American Journal of Art Therapy* **20**, 135–43.
80. **Bright, R.** *Grieving: A Handbook for Those Who Care.* St Louis MO: MMB Music Inc, 1986.
81. **Rynearson, E.** (1987). Psychotherapy of pathologic grief. *Psychiatric Clinics of North America* **10**, 487–99.
82. **Jacobs, S., Nelson, J., and Zisook, S.** (1987). Treating depressions of bereavement with antidepressants: a pilot study. *Psychiatric Clinics of North America* **10**, 501–10.
83. **Pasternak, R., Reynolds, C., and Schlernitzauer, M.** (1991). Acute open-trial nortriptyline therapy of bereavement-related depression in late life. *Journal of Clinical Psychiatry* **52**, 307–10.
84. **Lund, D., Caserta, M., and Dimond, M.** (1993). The course of spousal bereavement. In *Handbook of Bereavement: Theory, Research and Intervention* (ed. M. Stroebe, W. Stroebe, and R. Hansson), pp. 240–54. Cambridge: Cambridge University Press.
85. **Silverman, P.** *Widow to Widow.* New York: Springer, 1986.
86. **Adams-Greenly, M.** (1984). Helping children communicate about serious illness and death. *Journal of Psychosocial Oncology* **2**, 62–72.
87. **Eiser, C. and Havermans, T.** (1992). Children's understanding of cancer. *Psycho-oncology* **1**, 169–81.
88. **Rowland, J.** (1989). Developmental stage and adaptation: child and adolescent model. In *Handbook of Psycho-oncology* (ed. J. Holland and J. Rowland), pp. 519–43. Oxford: Oxford University Press.
89. **Webb, N.**, ed. *Helping Bereaved Children.* London: Guilford, 1993.
90. **Adams-Greenly, M. and Moynihan, R.** (1983). Helping the children of fatally ill parents. *American Journal of Orthopsychiatry* **53**, 219–29.
91. **Silverman, P. and Worden, J.** (1992). Children's understanding of the funeral ritual. *Omega* **25**, 319–31.
92. **Wells, R.** *Helping Children Cope with Grief.* London: Sheldon, 1988.
93. **Tennant, C., Bebbington, P., and Hurry, J.** (1980). Parental death in childhood and risk of adult depressive disorders: a review. *Psychological Medicine* **10**, 289–99.
94. **Davies, B., Spinetta, J., Martinson, I., McClowry, S., and Kulenkamp, E.** (1986). Manifestations of levels of functioning in grieving families. *Journal of Family Issues* **7**, 297–313.
95. **Byrne, G. and Raphael, B.** (1994). A longitudinal study of bereavement phenomena in recently widowed elderly men. *Psychological Medicine* **24**, 411–21.
96. **Large, T.** (1989). Some aspects of loneliness in families. *Family Process* **28**, 25–35.
97. **Lopata, H.** (1986). Becoming and being a widow: reconstruction of the self and support systems. *Geriatric Psychiatry* **19**, 203–14.
98. **Malinak, D., Hoyt, M., and Patterson, V.** (1979). Adults' reactions to the death of a parent: a preliminary study. *American Journal of Psychiatry* **136**, 1152–6.
99. **Saunders, C.** (1979). A comparison of adult bereavement in the death of spouse, child, and parent. *Omega* **10**, 303–22.
100. **Middleton, W., Raphael, B., Burnett, P., and Martinek, N.** (1998). A longitudinal study comparing bereavement phenomena in recently bereaved spouses, adult children and parents. *Australian and New Zealand Journal of Psychiatry* **32**, 235–41.
101. **Rubin, S.** (1993). The death of a child is forever: the life course impact of child loss. In *Handbook of Bereavement* (ed. M. Stroebe, W. Stroebe, and R. Hansson), pp. 285–99. Cambridge: Cambridge University Press.
102. **Neimeyer, R., Keese, B., and Fortner, M.** (2000). Loss and meaning reconstruction: propositions and procedures. In *Traumatic and Non-traumatic Loss and Bereavement: Clinical Theory and Practice* (ed. R. Malkinson, S. Rubin, and E. Witztum), pp. 197–230. Madison CT: Psychosocial Press/International Universities Press.
103. **Spinetta, J., Swarner, J., and Shepost, J.** (1981). Effective parental coping following death of a child from cancer. *Journal of Pediatric Psychology* **6**, 251–63.
104. **Folkman, S., Chesney, M., and Christopher-Richards, A.** (1994). Stress and coping in caregiving partners of men with AIDS. *Psychiatric Clinics of North America* **17**, 35–53.
105. **Moskowitz, J., Acree, M., and Folkman, S.** (1998). Depression and AIDS-related bereavement: a 3-year follow-up. New perspectives on depression in AIDS-related caregiving and bereavement. In *Annual Meeting of the American Psychological Association.* San Francisco CA. Cited by Folkman, S. Revised coping theory and the process of bereavement, In *Handbook of Bereavement Research* (ed. M.S. Stroebe, R.O. Hansson, W. Stroebe, and H. Schut), pp. 563–84, Washington DC: American Psychological Association.
106. **Wolfe, B.** (1993). AIDS and bereavement. In *Death and Spirituality* (ed. K. Doka and J. Morgan), pp. 257–78. New York: Baywood.
107. **Doka, K.** (1993). The spiritual crisis of bereavement. In *Death and Spirituality* (ed. K. Doka and J. Morgan), pp. 185–93. New York: Baywood.
108. **Imber-Black, E.** (1991). Rituals and the healing process. In *Living Beyond Loss: Death in the Family* (ed. F. Walsh and M. McGoldrick). New York: Norton.
109. **Sharma, D.** (1990). Hindu attitude toward suffering, dying and death. *Palliative Medicine* **4**, 235–8.
110. **Laungani, P.** (1997). Death in a Hindu family. In *Death and Bereavement Across Cultures* (ed. C. Parkes, P. Laungani, and B. Young), pp. 52–72. London: Routledge.
111. **Truitner, K. and Truitner, N.** (1993). Death and dying in Buddhism. In *Ethnic Variations in Dying, Death, and Grief: Diversity in Universality* (ed. D. Irish, K. Lundquist, and V. Nelsen), pp. 125–36. Washington DC: Taylor & Francis.
112. **Ryan, D.** (1993). Death: eastern perspectives. In *Death and Spirituality* (ed. K. Doka and J. Morgan), pp. 76–92. Amityville: Baywood.
113. **Joachim, C.** *Chinese Religions.* Englewood Cliffs NJ: Prentice-Hall, 1986.
114. **Overmyer, D.** *Religions of China.* New York: Harper & Row, 1987.
115. **Ter Blanche, H. and Parkes, C.** (1997). Christianity. In *Death and Bereavement Across Cultures* (ed. C. Parkes, P. Laungani, and B. Young), pp. 131–46. London: Routledge.
116. **Jonker, G.** (1997). The many facets of Islam. Death, dying and disposal between orthodox rule and historical convention. In *Death and Bereavement Across Cultures* (ed. C. Parkes, P. Laungani, and B. Young), pp. 147–65. London: Routledge.
117. **Neimeyer, R. and Hogan, N.** (2001). Quantitative or qualitative? Measurement issues in the study of grief. In *Handbook of Bereavement Research* (ed. M. Stroebe, R. Hansson, W. Stroebe, and H. Schut), pp. 89–118. Washington DC: American Psychological Association.
118. **Folkman, S.** (2001). Revised coping theory and the process of bereavement. In *Handbook of Bereavement Research. Consequences, Coping, and Care* (ed. M. Stroebe, R. Hansson, W. Stroebe, and H. Schut), pp. 563–84. Washington DC: American Psychological Association.
119. **Hogan, N., Morse, J., and Tason, M.** (1996). Toward an experiential theory of bereavement. *Omega* **33**, 43–65.
120. **Faschingbauer, T.** *Texas Revised Inventory of Grief Manual.* Houston TX: Honeycomb, 1981.
121. **Saunders, C., Mauger, P., and Strong, P.** *A Manual for the Grief Experience Inventory.* Blowing Rock NC: Center for the Study of Separation and Loss, 1985.

122. **Burnett, P., Middleton, W., Raphael, B., and Martinek, N.** (1997). Measuring core bereavement phenomenon. *Psychological Medicine* **27**, 49–57.

123. **Burnett, P., Middleton, W., Raphael, B., Dunne, M., Moylen, A., and Martinek, N.** (1993). Concepts of normal bereavement. *Journal of Traumatic Stress* **24**, 8–30.

124. **Kissane, D., Bloch, S., and McKenzie, D.P.** (1997). The bereavement phenomenology questionnaire. *Australian and New Zealand Journal of Psychiatry* **31**, 370–4.

125. **Hogan, N. and Greenfield, D.** (1991). Adolescent sibling bereavement symptomatology in a large community sample. *Journal of Adolescent Research* **6**, 97–112.

126. **Barrett, T. and Scott, T.** (1989). Development of the Grief Experience Questionnaire. *Suicide and Life-Treatening Behaviour* **19**, 201–15.

Further reading

Irish, D.P., Lundquist, K.F., and Nelsen, V.J., ed. *Ethnic Variations in Dying, Death and Grief: Diversity in Universality.* Washington DC: Taylor & Francis, 1993. A useful resource to cross-cultural bereavement.

Jacobs, S. *Pathologic Grief. Maladaptation to Loss.* Washington DC: American Psychiatric Press, 1993. A concise account of complicated mourning.

Kissane, D.W. and Bloch, S. *Family Focused Grief Therapy. A Model of Family-Centered Care during Palliative Care and Bereavement.* Buckingham: Open University Press, 2002. An innovative, integrated and preventive approach to family care.

Parkes, C.M. *Bereavement. Studies of Grief in Adult Life* 3rd edn. Madison: International Universities Press, 1998. A classic and worthwhile introduction.

Parkes, C.M., Laungani, P., and Young, B., ed. *Death and Bereavement Across Cultures.* London: Routledge, 1997. Useful reference to cross-cultural bereavement practices.

Raphael, B. *Anatomy of Bereavement.* New York: Basic Books, 1983. A classic work with excellent discussion of grief across the life cycle.

Stroebe, M.S., Hansson, R.O., Stroebe, W., and Schut, H., ed. *Handbook of Bereavement Research. Consequences, Coping, and Care.* Washington DC: American Psychological Association, 2001. An excellent, up-to-date review of recent research that comprehensively explores theory, culture, coping and intervention.

Stroebe, M.S., Stroebe, W., and Hansson, R.O., ed. *Handbook of Bereavement. Theory, Research and Intervention.* Cambridge: Cambridge University Press, 1993. Excellent compilation of phenomenology, bereavement studies and approaches.

20

Education and training in palliative medicine

20 Education and training in palliative medicine

20.1 Introduction

Kenneth Calman

We are all now part of a learning society and medicine and medical education must be part of that process. Medical education itself is a continuum, beginning at the undergraduate level progressing to specialist training and then entering the phase of continuing education. This continuum is critical for those involved in palliative medicine in that at each stage there are different levels of knowledge, skills, and attitudes required. These three factors need emphasizing, as all are important. The clinician in palliative care needs an effective and growing knowledge base, together with a widening range of skills. In addition, the attitudes adopted will be the component with which patients are likely to identify, and are the focus of much of the dissatisfaction with the care provided. However, all three are essential. There is not much point in a caring and communicative doctor if the knowledge base is not up to date and technical skills are limited. Here lies the ethical justification for continuing education. Patients expect their doctors to be fully aware of advances in diagnosis and treatment. Anything less would be doing patients a disservice.

Much of the debate on this subject relates to the purpose of medicine and of medical education. It is concerned with the attributes of the doctor and the relationship between these attributes and the curriculum and the educational process. It is also concerned about the concept of a profession, and what it means to be a professional. These are very important issues that should be considered before entering into the more detailed aspects of education and training in palliative care.

The profession of medicine

It is suggested that the purpose of medicine is to serve the community by continually improving health, health care, and quality of life, for the individual and the population by health promotion, prevention of illness, treatment and care, and the effective use of resources, all within the context of a team approach. In terms of palliative medicine, this emphasizes the issues of quality of life, care, and the team approach. It also highlights the importance of service to patients and this leads to a discussion of the concept of a profession.

It is not easy to define a profession but it has some, or all of the following characteristics. It is a vocation or calling and implies service to others. It has a distinctive knowledge base that is kept up to date and determines its own standards and sets its own examinations. It has a special relationship with those whom it serves—patients, clients. It has particular ethical principles, the ethical base, and is self-regulating and accountable to patients and to the profession itself.[1–5]

Flowing from this it is possible to list a series of attributes that might be expected of the doctor, or other health professional. These include:

1. A high standard of ethical practice. This is a key part of the role of the doctor and in a medical world that is constantly changing and developing and within which the principles are regularly challenged. There is greater scrutiny of medical practice and this is to be welcomed.
2. Continuing professional development is an issue that is broader than continuing education. It is concerned with personal growth and satisfaction with performance. Its main feature is that it emphasizes the need to keep up to date.
3. Ability to work as part of a team. As medicine and palliative care increase in complexity, it is necessary to ensure that all the skills of team members are used to the full.
4. Patient focussed. This should be an explicit part of the role of the doctor and of the palliative care service.
5. A concern with standards, outcomes effectiveness, and audit. This must be part of the practice of palliative medicine. There are considerable variations in standards across the world and it is our patients who suffer.
6. An interest in change, improvement, research, and development. Medicine cannot and should not stand still. It is continually evolving and changing. All professionals need to be involved in that quest for improvement.
7. Ability to communicate. This is a key attribute of the doctor. Arrogance and discourtesy reflect badly on a profession whose primary purpose is to care for patients.

Some of these attributes will be discussed in more detail later in this chapter and in other sections of the book. They are set out here because the purpose of medical education is to pursue these attributes and, in addition to factual knowledge, provide a basis for the wider range of skills and attitudes to be developed. The concept of personal growth alluded to above is an interesting one. It includes how we spend our time, our outside interests, and everything that makes us a broader person. It is about being a whole person with connections beyond medicine into hobbies, art, literature, and all aspects of recreation in the original sense of the word. In practical terms, the process of education should assist the doctor to answer the following questions, posed by the patient and by the professional:

1. What is wrong with me? What is the diagnosis, and while this may be difficult, patients are often seeking an explanation for their symptoms.
2. What does this mean for me? The prognosis. This may be the most difficult issue of all. In spite of considerable experience in palliative care it is easy to get this aspect wrong.
3. What can be done for me? This is the caring and management component and can and should be explained to the patient and the family.
4. What can I learn from this patient? The research dimension. How will an understanding of this patient's problems help others in the future?
5. What can I teach others from this experience? This identifies the educational opportunities for both patients and professionals.

Education and learning

This then is the justification for a section in this textbook on the subject of education. It is a complex process about which we still have much to learn and before looking at the subject in more detail a few definitions will be set out. Teaching is the process by which learning is facilitated by another person who guides, directs, and assesses progress. Learning is the outcome of a process that results in a change in knowledge, skills, attitudes, and/or behaviour. It is usually assessed in a variety of different ways to reflect acquisition of the knowledge, skills, or attitudes that have been learned. A wide variety of methods have been used for this purpose. In this chapter, the use of the term 'student' covers all levels of the continuum and not just the undergraduate level.

The process of learning in a formal sense is brought together in a curriculum that has three components. The objectives (what will the student be expected to know or do at the end of the module or course); the methods used (small group, lecture, computer based, problem based, etc.); and the methods of assessment (essay, multiple choice, clinical or practical, oral, dissertation, Objective Structured Clinical Examination (OSCE), etc.). The assessment may be formative in which the process takes place throughout the course, or summative, which takes place at the end. Both have advantages and disadvantages.

Two further definitions are important. The first is that of training. This implies the learning of specific knowledge, skills, or attitudes to tackle a particular clinical problem. For example, the doctor might be trained to manage pain, or understand pain mechanisms. Education, on the other hand, is not concerned only with task-based problems, but is broader and deeper. Education always has a value base while training does not have to have one. You can be trained to steal, pick pockets, or break into cars. You could not be educated to do these activities. Perhaps the best way of illustrating this difference is to note that 'to be trained is to have arrived, to be educated is to continue to travel'. Not surprisingly, both are necessary in the field of palliative medicine.

For those interested in further reading of the general aspects of education a short reading list is appended. Several journals are published specifically on medical education and are a most useful source of reference. It should be emphasized again that there is a strong moral imperative for the clinician in palliative care to keep up to date, and for those involved in the education of professionals to be aware of the range of methods of teaching and assessment now available. The remainder of this chapter will deal with more specific topics and which are developed further in subsequent chapters.

The process of learning

There are many different theories of how learning occurs and its molecular and psychological basis. In general, it must involve memory and the ability to solve problems using existing knowledge or by thinking out new solutions. Learning can be superficial (some facts are recalled) or deep (when the mechanism behind the facts is understood), in general deep learning is preferable. Learning may be active (the student is positively involved in searching for information or developing skills) or passive (they sit in a lecture class being 'taught'). Again there are advantages and disadvantages of both. Increasingly, medical schools are using problem-based learning where the process is student-centred and its purpose is to engage the student in the topic and to encourage critical thinking and analysis, as well as the acquisition of factual knowledge. This method of learning is self-directed and sometimes called 'learning from experience'. For the student beyond the undergraduate phase, the learning can be even more self-directed and be specifically related to deficiencies in practice or in the development of new skills.

The learning cycle is a useful way of summarizing the above discussion (Fig. 1). It begins with the assessment of the learning needs of the group, class, or individual student. This is then translated into a curriculum. The next stage is the planning of the learning experience and the choice of method and setting to be used. This is then implemented and the process, including the student learning, is evaluated. The cycle is completed by a review of the learning requirements and the progression to the next stage of the learning experience.

A phrase that occurs frequently in other chapters is that of the 'reflective practitioner', or 'reflective learning'. This refers to the process by which the

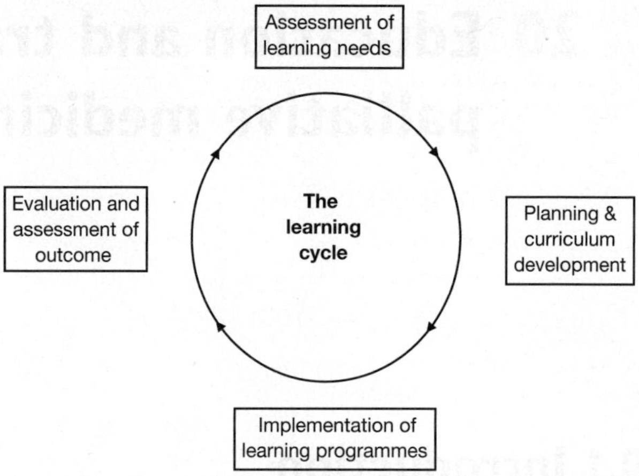

Fig. 1 The learning cycle.

student takes time to think through a particular problem or patient issue, or to think about the process of care through an audit of a particular group of patients or type of problem. In some instances, a diary of work can be helpful for this purpose and the use of creative writing[6] may be particularly useful. The process of audit is a particularly powerful one. It involves the critical analysis of outcome and compares these to those in the literature or by other colleagues. It is an educational process that should lead to changes or modifications in practice.

Increasingly then, learning is student centred, relevant to their needs, and the outcomes of the learning process defined. A key part of the process is feedback on performance, and letting the student know how they are progressing. This can be both formal and informal but is an important role of the supervisor or mentor. There is no point in allowing a young clinician from any professional background progress up the career ladder if the competencies that she or he demonstrates are inadequate. There is room for remedial work, but this should occur during the process of education when deficiencies can be remedied, not at the end. This is unfair to the student.

Learning palliative medicine

Students require support during their time in a palliative care service. It is not an easy area to work in, particularly if the placement is part of a rotational programme and the student intends practising in a different branch of medicine. They may not have been exposed to the problems in the same way before, nor as closely involved with patients who are dying. They will need help and the team as a whole needs to be alert to potential problems and to identifying those who are vulnerable. This is relevant at all levels of the continuum of medical education. Of particular interest is the development of a trusting environment in which it is easy for the student to seek help or support or to talk through their own feelings and concerns.

In many medical schools the student is encouraged to consider special study modules. These allow the student to spend time in a specialist area and increase their understanding of the subject. This is an ideal way to gain experience in palliative care and directors of services should be alert to the opportunities available.

In all of this role models are of particular importance. If a student attends a seminar on communication skills, practices their skills, and reflects on them, only to be confronted in clinical practice with a clinician, from any professional background who demonstrates exactly the opposite attributes, then confusion will arise. The student picks up attitudes and approaches to patients by such mechanisms. This is sometimes called the 'hidden curriculum'. The apprenticeship model is a very powerful one and where it works well it can enthuse and enlighten the student. Habits learned by osmosis, by watching the senior person in action, are copied and personalized. The formal curriculum may be powerless to interfere with this and it needs to be recognized by those who teach. The process of 'socialization' into a profession is part of the ritual of becoming a professional and to change attitudes in clinical practice in those working in other specialties may be an important part of the work of the palliative care unit.

Facilitating learning

A wide variety of methods may be used to facilitate learning and each has advantages and disadvantages and these are discussed in more detail in subsequent chapters. This is well illustrated by the process of learning communication skills, at the heart of palliative care practice. In educational terms there are several implications for the methods employed, which are also relevant to many other aspects of professional practice. First, should this be a short course, or should it be seen as a continuing thread throughout the curriculum? Second, should it be seen as a topic that is taught outside the clinical setting or at the bedside? Third, how can it be evaluated, and what is the role of the patient in that process? Finally, what happens when the young professional meets resistance to new thinking on communication skills in a clinical setting when his or her superior does not agree with the approach? These questions are not specific to communication skills but reflect the kinds of difficulties in converting good practice into real life situations. Similar issues are raised in the teaching of ethical issues.

In the development of the curriculum, a balance will need to be struck between the scientific basis of medicine and those aspects of clinical practice that use the social sciences or the arts. This is of particular relevance in palliative medicine where both are required. The second dichotomy is between research and practice. How much learning needs a research focus? There is certainly an agreement that practice needs to be evidence based and the role of case conferences, literature searches, the use of the Internet are all relevant to this. Patients now expect their professional carers to be up to date and aware of recent developments in their own and related fields.

Advances in clinical management come about in several ways, one of which is the curiosity of the doctor, and a wish to find out more and do things better. This curiosity leads to new methods of thinking, to observations that are built on and repeated and the hypothesis developed is then tested against the best available therapy. The methodology for such developments is part of the work of the doctor and should be a component of the curriculum. Palliative medicine needs research, and an attitude of questioning should be part of the practice of the doctor or other professional.

The assessment of learning

Part of the educational process is the assessment of the outcome of the learning. This can be done in a wide variety of ways.[7] The commonest ways include written essays, short questions, multiple choice questions, and OSCEs. Such methods are particularly good at determining the knowledge base, and in some instances clinical skills. Clinical examination of patients by students provide an additional way of assessing skills. However, attitudes are more difficult to assess and increasingly patients are used for this purpose.

However, it is also useful to consider the role of assessment in education and why it is needed. It has a clear role in the motivation of students, and in the facilitation of learning. It helps facilitate choices and options and gives feedback on the learning outcome. It is also used to satisfy accrediting bodies and determine student progression. It is a fundamental part of learning. Outside bodies use such assessments to benchmark the clinical unit or institution against known standards. Such processes are increasingly widespread and the clinician of the future will need to be sure that the standards that are in place meet the external quality requirements.

Increasingly, the end point of education is the assessment of the competence of the professional to perform tasks or to solve problems. This is more than just the assessment of factual knowledge and the ability to recall certain packets of information, important as that is. It is also about putting this information into practice. It is the component of medical education that the patient sees and experiences.

Relevant to this is the question as to who should assess the student? The most obvious answer is the relevant professional body, but it should be more than this. The role of the nurse or the dietician in the assessment of medical competence also has a place, as would the role of the patient. Increasingly, input from patients is informing the way in which professionals are assessed. The use of actors, professional patients, or simulated patients is a good way of finding out how students will cope with difficult situations and how they will communicate with patients. Communication, it should be recalled remains the major cause of concern for many patients and the object of most complaints. Anything that will improve this position should be welcome.

In recent years, the role of the humanities in the teaching of palliative care has increased, hence the chapter on this topic in this section of the textbook. The use of the arts such as literature and music can help to encourage students to think in different ways about patients and their feelings and emotions. There is now considerable experience world-wide on this topic.[8,9] The use of narrative and stories to help understand the patient perspective are also relevant. Doctors and other health professionals are privileged to listen to patient's stories (histories, narratives) and help interpret them and in doing so facilitate the healing of the patient. Writing down what has happened, sharing it with others can be a powerful therapeutic and educational experience.

In this context, Howard Brody uses an interesting phrase. He recalls a patient who said 'My story is broken, can you help me fix it'. A comment that encapsulates so many of the issues in palliative care and uses the language of narrative to describe the problem.

Traditionally, learning takes place in classes and adopts several forms including lectures, seminars, and tutorials. Newer methods are much more problem based and involve the student in finding out for himself or herself what the answers are to the problems set. In addition, especially for more experienced staff, learning sets provide an effective method of sharing and improving practice. Such sets, usually of five to seven people, meet on a regular basis and draw up an agenda for their own learning and find the people or the resource to help. They also share their own problems and experiences. Groups, for example, of newly appointed palliative care physicians would be ideal for this as a supportive and cohesive group facing many similar problems.

Increasingly, the use of electronic media will be used to assist in learning both for patients and professionals. The chapter in this section (Chapter 20.6) devoted to this topic highlights the major issues. The availability of large databases on the World Wide Web, and the access to journals and literature make the acquirement of the knowledge base much easier. This, however, needs to be placed in the context of the clinical practice of the individual doctor and the facilities available. It can lead to the development of special interest groups and bulletin boards on the web facilitating discussion and problem-solving.

Mentoring is another useful, and growing, innovation. In this process a colleague, often not in the particular clinical field, acts as a sounding board and reflects back to the person views and experience. He or she can guide or be simply a person to listen. For those working in palliative care where there are difficult clinical issues to deal with, where the stress and strain of every day work can become overwhelming, such mentors can not only be of educational value but can assist in the performance of the clinical work.

Competencies of the specialist in palliative medicine

Increasingly, there is discussion about the competencies required of the clinician and how such competencies are generally defined by the specialist body.[10] Competence should cover the three aspects of learning and reflect not only the level of knowledge, skills, and attitudes but the ability to solve problems, think critically, work as part of a team, and show an appetite to continue to learn. For most specialties such competencies are now published and against which individuals can be assessed.

Multi-disciplinary learning: learning in teams

A further theme that is developed throughout the volume is that of teamwork and that applies equally to inter-disciplinary learning. How this is carried out will vary from setting to setting but in each instance requires that the team members learn from each other and respect the skills of other professionals. Again this may best be done with specific problems and involve the use of different experience and expertise to manage the problem. The use of the humanities is another vehicle that can assist in this process.

Teaching the teachers

So far it has been assumed that all professionals are natural teachers, able to inspire and motivate students. This is clearly not always the case. Teaching is a special series of skills, many of which can be learned and improved with practice. In professional terms, most people who are involved in educational programmes will be asked to produce a portfolio of teaching activity along with evidence of student feedback as the end point of the process. External accrediting organizations will also wish to see evidence that teaching is being taken seriously and that those involved are aware of the of new developments in methods, curricular design, and assessment of learning. The reading list develops these themes further. The teacher is also an academic leader whose function as a role model is critical. In education as in other areas of clinical practice the early experiences are so important in sending messages of enthusiasm for the subject, of its excitement, its place in medicine as a whole, and its value to patients and the public. Palliative care needs such teachers and leaders if it is to continue to grow and develop as a specialty. As public scrutiny of professional practice increases so will the need for such professional leadership in setting out professional standards and values.

References

1. **Freidson, E.** *Profession of Medicine. A Study of the Sociology of Applied Knowledge.* New York: Dodd, Mead and Co, 1975.
2. **Calman, K.C.** (1994). The profession of medicine. *British Medical Journal* **309**, 1140–3.
3. **Irvine, D.** (1997). The performance of doctors. II. Maintaining good practice, protecting patients from poor performance. *British Medical Journal* **314**, 1613.
4. **Alberti, G.** (2002). Professionalism—time for a new look. *Clinical Medicine* **2**, 91.
5. **Medical Professionalism Project.** (2002). Medical professionalism in the new millennium: a physician's charter. *Lancet* **359**, 520–2.
6. **Bolton, G.** *The Therapeutic Potential of Creative Writing.* London: Jessica Kingsley Publishers, 1999.
7. **Grant, J.** (2002). Learning needs assessment: assessing the need. *British Medical Journal* **324**, 156–9.
8. **Greenhalgh, T. and Hurwitz, B.** *Narrative Based Medicine. Dialogue and Discourse in Clinical Practice.* London: British Medical Journal Publishing Group, 1998.
9. **Calman, K.C.** *Storytelling, Humour and Learning in Medicine.* London: The Stationery Office, 2000.
10. **Calman, K.C.** (2000). Postgraduate specialist training and continuing professional development. *Medical Teacher* **22**, 448–51.

Reading list

Newble, D. and Cannon, R. *A Handbook for Medical Teachers* 2nd edn. Lancaster: MTP Press Ltd, Kluwer Academic Publishing Group, 1987.

David, T., Patel, L., Burdett, K., and Rangachari, P. *Problem Based Learning in Medicine.* London: Royal Society of Medicine Press, 1999.

Cox, K.R. and Ewan, C.E. *The Medical Teacher* 2nd edn. Edinburgh: Churchill Livingstone, 1988.

Wear, D. and Bickel, J., ed. *Educating for Professionalism. Creating a Culture of Humanism in Medical Education.* Iowa City: University of Iowa Press, 2000.

Peyton, J.W.R. *Teaching and Learning in Medical Practice.* Rickmansworth: Manticore Europe Ltd, 1998.

Miller, G.E. *Educating Medical Teachers.* Harvard University Press, 1980.

Sweet, J., Huttly, S., and Taylor, I. Effective Learning and Teaching in Medical, Dental and Veterinary Education. London: Kogan Page Ltd., 2003.

Journals

The list below does not include specialist journals in palliative care, or other medical and professional journals which include regular articles on education.

Education for Primary Care. Radcliffe Medical Press, Abingdon, Oxford.

Academic Medicine. Journal of the Association of Medical Colleges. Washington. Previously the *Journal of Medical Education.*

Journal of Medical Ethics. British Medical Journal Publishing Group, UK. Medical Humanities, special edition of the *Journal of Medical Ethics.*

Medical Education. Published for the Association for the study of Medical Education. Blackwell Science, Oxford, UK.

Medical Teacher. An International Journal of Education in the Health Sciences. In collaboration with the Association for Medical Education in Europe. Taylor and Francis Ltd, Basingstoke, Hants, UK.

20.2 Training family physicians

Ilora Finlay and Simon R. Noble

Introduction

Every family physician is, at some time, involved in the care of patients with incurable disease. They present many challenges, with complex physical, social, emotional, and spiritual needs, but also can be the most rewarding aspect of clinical care when things go right. To competently address the many issues of a dying person and continue to support their loved ones through their bereavement requires wisdom, knowledge, and skill accrued from training and from many years of experience, as most of the final year of life of a dying patient is spent at home under the medical care of the family physician and the community team.[1]

Until recently, palliative care training was a postgraduate specialty with sporadic undergraduate training. However, in the United Kingdom all medical students are now taught about palliative medicine and the past 16 years have seen increases in the number of taught hours about death, dying, and bereavement,[2] with a broadening of the topics covered. This lays the foundation for ongoing postgraduate education, particularly for those entering family practice. The role of the palliative care physician is vital in the training of family physicians, empowering them to be more involved in complex issues whilst continuing to facilitate professional development and self-directed learning throughout their career.

The importance of training the family physician

Out of all the medical specialities, palliative care, better than any, embraces an interdisciplinary approach, which spans the gap between the community and acute sector. Likewise, the palliative care team has much to offer the learning process within the community. Whilst most patients would like to die at home, within the United Kingdom only 26 per cent of cancer patients and 20 per cent of non-cancer patients achieve this.[3]

Many reasons are given for this, including difficulty in controlling symptoms at home. Improving the training of the family physician and empowering the community teams in supporting patients and families at home may help to improve patient choice about place of death. It is important to recognize that many patients will have been under the care of the family physician for several years, some even from birth. The palliative care teams must be careful not to deprive community colleagues of some of the most challenging, yet rewarding parts of clinical practice. Too often, a call for assistance is misinterpreted as an invitation to take over, which undermines the family doctor's role and previous work, as well as destroying a unique leaving opportunity for both family physician and palliative care team to share.

The family physician is used to studying and learning, having been in the educational system from the beginning of their school life. Most learning will have been from didactic teaching with clear goals and standardized assessment. The process of learning is likely to have been prescriptive with self-directed study focused towards examinations. However, adults appear to learn in a way that is quite distinct from children, so the teacher's role and relationship with the learner must necessarily shift.

Areas of postgraduate learning

Assessment often focuses around knowledge, with different assessment methods tending to test knowledge more than other attributes to learning. However, there are four principal domains[4] to be considered in any learning/teaching cycle:

1. knowledge and understanding;
2. skills and competencies;
3. attitudes and professional behaviour;
4. professional development.

In planning any educational event or course, it is important that the learning outcomes that are expected have been defined in terms of these domains, to ensure that all aspect of learning and professional development have been covered. Different teaching methods will cover different domains, so a mixture of methods is required. The didactic lecture may impart facts and increase 'knowledge', but will not develop 'understanding' unless the application of the facts to the clinical scenario is explored and understood; without understanding of the application the facts have little meaning and may be dangerous if wrongly applied. Similarly, communication skills training will not correct a poor underlying attitude to clinical practice; the attitudinal difficulties of the practitioner may emerge during a teaching session and must be separately addressed if change is to occur.

It is much easier to increase knowledge and understanding, or to improve skills and competencies, than to change attitudes and professional behaviours. Change in behaviour is subject to many other influences, but will only occur when the person concerned recognizes the need to change and has begun to contemplate action to initiate change. Most work on the ways that people alter behaviour has been studied in smokers and in the need to promote illness prevention.[5] The stages of change are seen in learners who need to move from pre-contemplation of attitudinal change, when they may feel there is nothing wrong with their approach, to contemplation, when they realize their attitude may be making things harder for themselves and for others, to the initiation of change as true insight develops. Examples of areas where attitudinal change is more frequently required include: the approach to patients whose lifestyle or behaviours are unpleasant; and the management of conflict with other team members. Many problems in team working are linked to lack of insight in the practitioner of behaviours that cause difficulties or irritation.

Learning outcomes

In the past, the goals of any training were defined as the aims and objectives to be achieved. However, this concept has been largely replaced by the process of defining the desired learning outcomes from each part of the training process. Learning outcomes are the explicit statement of what the learner should be able to demonstrate at the end of training. They should be written as explicit statements and each one should be able to be assessed, although the mode of assessment will vary widely. For instance, written answers and multiple choice questions may only test factual recall, clinical problem-solving may demonstrate understanding, but the practical skills of a procedure, such as the insertion of a chest drain, will only be assessed by the practical demonstration of this skill. The evaluation of such a skill is incomplete without the process of consent being included in the assessment.

An example of some learning outcomes for communication skills teaching are given in Box 1.

It should be noted that the assessment schedule for a simulated consultation covers many of these areas, so the assessment is explicitly matched to the learning outcomes.

When learning needs are being defined, it is helpful for the student to think about the activities and skills that need to be improved proactively and then to write the learning outcomes in these terms. This will help the learner to be able to demonstrate that learning has occurred, a process that is becoming increasingly important in the current climate of revalidation of professional groups in some countries, such as the United States and the United Kingdom.

Adult learning

The principle characteristics of adult learning, as described by Knowles,[6] are summarized in Table 1. First, adult learning needs to be purposeful; adults are more likely to engage in learning when they have a specific purpose in mind. This does not preclude learning as a means of enjoyment, but adults are more likely to engage if there is a specific objective to fulfil, such as career advancement, or to gain confidence in handling difficult topics or situations. Also, adults are more likely to learn if they wish to learn. Involuntary participants on a course will do the bare minimum to get

Box 1 Communication

At the end of the module the students will be able to:

- Demonstrate non-verbal ways of:
  - facilitating a patient feeling comfortable and safe
  - opening up a communication
  - helping a patient disclose their problems
- Demonstrate the use of open questions
- Demonstrate the use of focused questions
- Demonstrate the process of checking that a patient has understood information
- Demonstrate the process of closure of a consultation
- Demonstrate a stepwise approach to breaking bad news
- Demonstrate respect of the patient and the patient's concerns
- List potential barriers to communication with patients, with patients' families, and with colleagues
- Suggest ways to overcome barriers to communication
- Reflect on their own communication style
- Analyse the processes they use in a consultation

Table 1 Principles of adult learning[4]

Adult learning must be purposeful
Adults must be voluntary participants in learning
Adults require active participation in learning
Adults require clear goals and objectives to be set
Adults need feedback
Adults need to be reflective

through, having learned very little; they are more likely to be keen to learn if they see relevance in the subject matter. Within palliative care, for example, a workshop on managing epidurals is unlikely to motivate a family physician no matter how well it is taught since he/she is unlikely to envisage needing such skills. A workshop on setting up and prescribing for syringe drivers will be viewed as far more relevant.

Adults need to be active participants in learning. The same information can be given in a lecture or a small group, but the student is likely to learn more if able to discuss and explore the topic. The two-way interaction in a small group seminar, for example, enhances the learning process. Similarly, a lecture that encourages active participation will consolidate greater understanding than a one-way talk.

Adult learners need clear goals (learning outcomes) to be set, these will specify what is to be learned and ensure that assessment is matched to the aims of the course. Within palliative care, the derived learning outcomes for the family physician are likely to vary between individuals, depending on their current circumstances and previous experience. In any learning process, it is important for the learner to have feedback and this can take many forms, be it formal or informal. Finally, adult learners need to be reflective and this will be covered later in the chapter.

Tools necessary to train the family physician

The Association for Palliative Medicine for Great Britain and Ireland published a joint statement with the Royal College of General Practitioners on the palliative medicine content of vocational training, outlining a core curriculum applicable throughout the training scheme.[7] The curriculum aims for doctors to understand and gain experience in all aspects of care. The curriculum outlines:

1. physical aspects of care including the disease process and symptom control;
2. psychosocial aspects of care including communication skills, psychological responses, grief, sexuality, and dealing with ones own feelings;
3. cultural issues;
4. ethical issues;
5. the importance of team-work;
6. practical aspects including regulations relevant to palliative care.

Within the United Kingdom, those wishing to become a family physician must complete a minimum of 3 years post-registration training within what is known as a Vocational Training Scheme. They are required to complete at least 6 months of paediatrics, accident and emergency, and obstetrics in addition to a year as a General Practice Trainee. They are encouraged to complete further speciality jobs such as psychiatry, dermatology, and genitourinary medicine but only a few get the opportunity to work in a palliative care unit. Many aspects of the Vocational Training Scheme will touch on areas of the palliative care curriculum and need not be covered in isolation. Development and demonstration of competency in communication skills, for example, is essential in all aspects of the physician's training and will not be restricted to palliative care training. However, the learner needs to be aware that particular issues within the palliative care consultation may differ from those in other aspects of training and competency in one does not necessarily imply competency in the other.

The importance of a sound knowledge base cannot be over emphasized. In addition to those skills unique to the care of the dying, palliative care physicians need a breadth of knowledge that spans almost all specialities within medicine, since almost all specialties involve diagnosis and treatment of life-limiting disease. Likewise, the palliative care physician and family physician, for that matter, will practice in environments without immediate access to various investigations and imaging. Good clinical acumen is essential as many management decisions will be made on the basis of clinical signs, a knowledge of the disease process, and understanding of treatment options available.

It is essential that the trainee family physician has access to sufficient palliative care patients as it is a speciality that one learns best through experience. In addition to providing care to patients within the community, the trainee should have the opportunity to work within a specialist palliative care unit. Some vocational training schemes now include a period of time working within such a unit and trainees may take it upon themselves to work within a palliative care setting prior to committing themselves to full time work as a family physician. Such trainees tend to be in the minority and it is important that we give them exposure to the work of a specialist palliative care team. It is not enough to arrange an afternoon's tour of a hospice, as this is unlikely to teach little more than where the local facilities are and what they look like. Prior to undertaking any training of the family physician, individual educational needs must be identified, recognizing that they differ from one individual to another. Each learner should identify their perceived educational needs and recognize that these may alter with time.

The trainer/facilitator may identify that certain topics are more important for the trainer to learn than others. It is sometimes useful to negotiate a set of educational objectives between learner and facilitator so that both views of educational need are addressed. There may be topics that the specialist deals with on a daily basis, and hence feels are vital to teach, whilst the family physician may encounter these situations only rarely. It is also possible that the corollary is also true: many issues the family physician faces in the community, are dealt with there and palliative care teams rarely become involved with them.

The perceived training need of general practitioners in the United Kingdom has been explored by questionnaire.[8] Educational needs varied between rural and inner city GPs but some topics are frequently identified (see Table 2).

Interestingly, over 50 per cent wanted training on symptom control of non-cancer patients. This may be due to the apparent imbalance of palliative care services to cancer patients, resulting in the family physician caring for non-cancer patients for a longer period of time.

The teaching and learning of palliative medicine lends itself to a wide range of educational methods. The adult learner is likely to be more comfortable with some methods rather than others and this is usually a throwback to their good or bad experiences of learning at school and university. All of the following methods of learning (see Table 3) may help in the training of the family physician and they should not be used in isolation.

It has often been a criticism of undergraduate medical training that students are expected to memorize vast amounts of information in a didactic fashion, with little apparent relevance to clinical practice. This information would often have little application other than being something that might come up in an examination. As mentioned before, adult learners need to see relevance in their learning and so the trainee will learn most effectively when encouraged to focus their learning around experiences they have had or cases they have looked after. This provides a focus for study and demonstrates relevance, which lies at the heart of experiential learning through reflective practice.

Tacit knowledge

The traditional method of learning described as 'technical–rational' mainly involved teaching clearly defined procedures with problems and

Table 2 Topics frequently identified as learning needs by general practitioners

Education in opioid prescribing
Controlling nausea and vomiting
Counselling skills
Communication skills
Using a syringe driver
Symptom control of non-cancer patients

Table 3 Different educational methods in palliative care

Lectures
Bedside teaching
Reading
Case studies
Audit
Reflective practice/experiential learning through: Portfolio learning; Small group discussions; Project work; One to one tutorials
Inter-disciplinary conferences
Computer-assisted learning
Hands-on practice

assignments. These were usually artificial academic examples, which were well defined and had identifiable correct answers. In other words, topics were taught in such a way that every problem had a clear and identifiable solution implying that logical thinking should prevail if all the facts are available. This method of teaching has its limitations within medicine, especially palliative care, since it is as much an art form as a science. Only too often the clinician is expected to deal with a situation for which there is no straightforward answer. Schon describes this zone of indeterminate practice as the *swamp*.[9] Schon believed that most of the routine work of a professional is *tacit* and situations are often dealt with, and problems solved, without deeply thinking about how the decision was reached or procedure followed. This almost conscious routine is what Schon calls *knowing-in-action*.[7]

For example, when we originally learned to drive every action was deliberate and thought out: *accelerator up, clutch down, change gear, clutch up, accelerator down*, and so on. Now these actions are so familiar to us that we can make a long journey without having given any thought to the pedal dynamics that previously challenged us. Even if we saw a car careering towards us and safely took evasive action, it is still likely that we would do this without consciously thinking about the practicalities of driving a car. Driving lessons will not have prepared us for this, nor are we likely to have had practice sessions with cars careering towards us; yet if asked to verbalize what we did to avoid the other car we may find it hard. This is because our tacit knowledge enabled us to undertake the appropriate manoeuvre by *knowing-in-action*. Since *knowing-in-action* is often employed by physicians, it is not uncommon to find they are able to perform a task themselves, but have difficulty in explaining to someone else how to do it. No doubt this is one of the reasons that the 'See one. Do one. Teach one' approach to learning skills has been used for so long. Schon recognizes that not all professional practice is governed by *knowing-in-action* and that a learner also engages in a period of reflection.

Reflective practice

The term reflective practice, within the context of learning, has been used since the early 1930s. The most celebrated description by Donald Schon has become a major adjunct to adult learning over the past 15 years. Reflection involves thinking about what we are doing, for example, when solving a problem, sometimes even while tackling it. It helps us understand what steps we have taken to solve the problem by consciously considering how we undertake a task normally done without thought. Such questions we may ask are:

- What features do I notice when I recognize this situation?
- What are the criteria by which I make this judgment?
- What procedures am I enacting when I perform this skill?
- How am I framing the problem that I am trying to solve?

To understand an approach to a problem, the learner also needs to reflect on related knowledge and experiences. This then allows him or her to criticize, restructure, and apply these principles for further learning. Schon calls this type of thinking *reflection-on-action*. In practical terms, reflective practice encourages us to review past experiences (*reflection-on-action*) or experiences as they occur (*reflection-in-action*) and critically analyse what has lead us to different actions. The learner is encouraged to do this in a non-threatening way so that the learning experience is not demoralizing. Mistakes or unsatisfactory outcomes often provide the best stimuli for learning, yet such events must be handled sensitively and appropriately. Asking the question 'What would you do differently next time?' will have a far more worthwhile effect on learning than asking 'What did you do wrong there?'. A non-threatening approach to reflective practice is even more important in palliative care because of the complexity of the clinical scenarios often encountered, the management of a patient who has died or a particularly challenging consultation will be subject to review. Many situations faced by the palliative care or family physician are likely to be upsetting, with difficult and sometimes imperfect resolutions to problems. A blameless approach to reflection is necessary to allow learning, without damaging the learner.

There are some limitations to Schon's work since it only concentrates on *reflection-in-action* and *reflection-on-action*. Greenwood in particular criticized the limitations of Schon's model since it fails to recognize the importance of *reflection-before-action*, that is, thinking through what one intends to do before doing it.[10] Within palliative care, *reflection-before-action* is vital, as it enables the learner to use previous experiences to prepare for future challenges; reflective practice loses much of its value if it is not used to prepare us for future challenges.

Reflective practice as applied to palliative care

The process

Boud et al. depict a model of the reflective process, which can be readily applied to palliative care. They define reflection as 'an important human activity in which people recapture their experience, think about it, mull it over and evaluate it'.[11] In this context, the focus of reflection in learning is the individuals' experience. The reflective process involves both cognition and feelings, as the two are closely interrelated and interactive. Feelings may be 'positive' or 'negative' but will cue the individual to the initial stage of the reflective process. The model suggests that as an individual encounters an experience, he or she responds and initiates the process of reflection. By returning to the experience, recalling what has occurred, and replaying the experience, re-evaluation takes place. There are four main components to the process of re-evaluation:

1. Association—relating new experiences to existing knowledge.
2. Integration—seeking relationships amongst new and already known data.
3. Validation—determining the validity of feelings and ideas that have resulted.
4. Appropriation—making this knowledge one's own.

The role of the tutor

Many family physicians may be new to reflective practice, so their reservations and discomfort must be acknowledged and considered. A verbal contract, setting out goals of a reflective session should be established, including assurance of confidentiality if the discussion becomes candid. The session may be as a one-to-one or within a small group. Participation by all present is important, so that larger groups (over six) are less likely to benefit those present. The supervisor should act as facilitator, encouraging someone to offer a situation, case, clinical problem they encountered and share it with those present. Often it is helpful to ask the individual to highlight particular areas they wish to concentrate on.

First, the student is encouraged to reflect on areas that they felt went well. This is important in maintaining a safe environment, supporting the individual, and it also reinforces good practice. The rest of the group may then wish to comment on any other things they could identify from the case that appeared to have gone well, facilitated as before by the supervisor. The student should then be encouraged to highlight things that they would like to do differently, were they to face a similar situation again, followed by non-threatening feedback from the rest of the group. Those familiar will recognize that this session follows Pendleton's method[14] of feedback, which is considered one of the best ways of appraising. Hopefully, once the group becomes familiar with the concept of reflective practice and feels comfortable with the proposed format, the supervisor can then encourage the sessions to become more sophisticated. Rather than just describe things that went well, the student should be encouraged to describe what they were thinking, how they felt at the time, and whether past situations had influenced their decision-making. Likewise, in identifying areas for improvement and things that did not go so well, the student could be encouraged to describe how they had felt, and what steps they would take to do things differently next time. With time, a successful group should be able to run itself. It is important always to have one person acting as facilitator and retaining a degree of outsider's objectivity, but this role can be rotated between individuals at each meeting.

Stimuli for reflection

The learner's every-day practice within the palliative care environment offers many stimuli for reflection. It is important for the individual to be open to reflection as they go about their daily work, noting interesting or stimulating situations as they occur. Major events, such as a difficult family conflict or problematic symptom, are often easy to reflect on as they have a major impact on all around but one must also be vigilant to more subtle stimuli. The perception of a colleague, a letter from a relative, or taking time to write a discharge summary may give a different slant to a situation and further opportunity to reflect. Many palliative care teams now use protected time for reflective practice in small groups. This can be successful within uni-professional and inter-professional groups, provided it is conducted in a safe non-threatening environment paying particular attention to confidentiality within the group.

One of the most useful tools to capture and record reflection and personal development is by portfolio learning.

Portfolio learning

Portfolio learning is now widely recognized as a valuable learning tool as it provides a record of learning and also acts as a stimulus to reflection. Portfolio learning is designed to provide a chronological record of the learning process of the student. The learning process is self-directed; the learner chooses the areas within a subject of particular interest. In the context of training the family physician, this enables each learner to meet their own individual learning objectives. For example, a student who identifies a need to develop skills in the controlling of nausea and vomiting can focus their portfolio on this topic, whilst another colleague may concentrate on bereavement.

Those unaccustomed to this learning style will require gentle support and supervision, as it differs greatly from their previous technical–rational learning experiences. The beauty and simplicity of a reflective portfolio, which allows the learner to determine format, learning objectives, and emphasis to the learner may be seen by some as too unstructured and challenging. Most physicians are new to the relative lack of prescribed formal structure in the portfolio. Depending upon the experience of the educational supervisor, even the method of presenting the portfolio can be relaxed if the reasons are clear. The learner should be encouraged to develop the portfolio in a similar way to an artist's portfolio, reflecting their freedom of creativity in presentation (Box 2).

Within the realms of self-directed learning, the portfolio will act both as a tool for learning and as evidence to the supervisor that learning has taken place. It is important that adult learners have feedback on their progress. This can sometimes be difficult with portfolio marking, since the scope and form of portfolios may differ greatly. Formative assessment between the supervisor and student, in an informal setting, is essential. It enables the supervisor to give constructive feedback to the student and provide support, especially to those new to the concept of portfolio learning. The supervisor will need to identify those students who require more frequent feedback sessions and extra support. Summative assessment can help the student identify areas of learning that they may wish to consider in the future. Examples of a mark schedule for a portfolio are given in Tables 4 and 5.

Box 2 The elements in a successful portfolio

Most successful portfolios consist of the following elements, which are interrelated and cross-referenced:[12]

- Factual case histories around which the learning usually occurs.
- References to items that have influenced the clinical decision-making process and have been foci of learning.
- References to diverse sources, e.g. text-book reading, literature search, lay press, conversations with colleagues.
- A record of the clinician's own decision-making processes, including details of decisions made and how the student came to them.
- Documentation of how the student felt at the time: sources of stress or doubts are as useful as the outcome, since the personal feelings of the learner will influence how they were able to approach a problem.
- Ethical considerations.
- Illustrative items such as photographs, drawings, quotations, poetry, etc. may clarify points being made.
- Some form of indexing is important, so the learner and supervisor can follow the learning process and refer to specific items at a later date.

Table 4 Summative portfolio mark schedule

Contextual description of case	5%
Biological issues of the case	5%
Individual issues of the case	5%
Team working	10%
Clarity of presentation	10%
Decision-making logic	20%
Attribution of evidence	20%
Critical analysis	15%
Index and discretionary marks	10%
Total	100%

Table 5 Student's guidance

Academic background	15%
Display appropriate use of academic literature/research, other influences in learning	
Coverage of topic	40%
Biology of cancer	10%
The natural history of cancer	
Cancer screening and diagnosis	
Staging and metastatic disease	
Impact of cancer	10%
The psychological response to cancer and the importance of honest communication	
The social impact of cancer on patients and their families/carers	
The spiritual response to a diagnosis of cancer	
Clinical management	10%
Treatment options and how decisions are made	
Symptom control	
Co-ordinated care	10%
Multi-disciplinary team working	
The response to loss and bereavement	
Approach to patient and problems	10%
Warmth	
Caring	
Empathy	
Respect	
Humanity	
Holistic assessment and management	25%
Communication and personal insight	10%
Physical, psychological, social, and spiritual assessment	
The ability to engage and talk to a patient with cancer, and their carers about their experience and develop a relationship with them	
Display insight into their own emotional reactions to difficult and sad situations	
Patient responses	5%
The identification of the patient's problems, hopes, and fears	
Critical analysis of care	10%
The process of evaluating the efficacy of care from both the medical and patient perspective	
Display evidence of clear critical analysis and synthesis of issue	
Commitment	10%
Throughout the 6 months, the student should have displayed commitment to learning about cancer in tutorials and in self-directed learning time	

When assessing a learning portfolio it often becomes apparent that some factual clinical details of the portfolio cannot be verified or crosschecked, as the patients or episodes described are not known to the reader. It is always better to base a learning portfolio around real cases and events rather than a fabricated scenario. The learner will gain more from *reflection-on-action* with which they have first-hand experience. The suggested marking schedules attribute only a small proportion of marks to the description of the case, awarding the majority of marks to evidence that learning has occurred. The biological evolution of the disease process is balanced by social and personal issues in the case history. The marking scheme reflects the importance placed upon team working within palliative care and the supervisor should actively encourage an appreciation of this if it is felt to be lacking in the portfolio.

For the family physician in training, a portfolio gives excellent opportunity to focus their experiences. It also can act as a documentation of learning objectives, since it records the clinical situations commonly faced and areas of difficulty. For the supervisor it helps identify any topics requiring further experience or teaching. Often, small group tutorials can be organized around subjects identified by several learners, all in a position to contribute in this environment with experiences to reflect upon and share.

Portfolio learning should be viewed as a dynamic, fluid learning process, which should ideally continue as long as the individual keeps learning. As all medical professionals become more accountable and are required to give evidence of continuing learning, the portfolio may become a more prominent educational tool within the whole of medicine, not just palliative care.

The portfolio provides a unique opportunity for learning to occur in the wider context of the humanities. Relevant facets are incorporated and cross-referenced, giving validity to the learned experience described by others through art or literature.

Communication skills

Communication skills are essential for all medical practitioners, but even more so for those dealing with the dying and their families. Training schemes for family physicians appear to recognize the need for communication skills training to a greater extent than general internal medicine rotations. In the United Kingdom, general practice trainees are required to submit a portfolio of videotaped consultations with patients for formative and ultimately summative assessment. Membership of the Royal College of General Practitioners cannot be obtained until the candidate has provided this evidence of proficiency in communicating with patients. However, this does not obviate the need to concentrate on communication skills in relation to palliative care when training the family physician. Such general assessment does not test the physicians' communication skill with terminally ill patients for several reasons. First, as the general practice trainee is required to submit a selection of videotaped consultations for assessment, the best ones are submitted; the worst ones will not be reviewed, even though they may have the most valuable triggers for reflection. Second, the consultations are from routine practice and contain a wide mix of cases and problems. Palliative care cases are unlikely to be included, especially as many significant palliative care consultations occur at the patient's home.

Palliative care consultations are often the most challenging, since they may involve breaking bad news and talking about dying and loss. Videotaping such sensitive consultations is extremely difficult. The trainee may feel particularly nervous about the consultation. Consent needs to be given by the patient prior to filming and a trainee may feel uncomfortable subjecting a patient to a video camera during what they anticipate will be a potentially difficult consultation. Some of the most complex consultations, such as with an angry relative, dealing with collusion or breaking bad news are unlikely, if ever, to be recorded. Since the palliative care consultation is potentially difficult and may have wide ramifications if badly handled, the trainer must create a safe learning environment where the trainee can feel comfortable making mistakes without repercussions. It necessarily follows that the use of real patients is not always appropriate.

Role-play

Role-play using either actors or colleagues as patients, has long been established as a useful tool for developing communication skills.(13) It is best done as a small group of learners with one or more trained facilitators. It is important to keep the groups small enough to ensure that everyone gets the opportunity to role-play in the time allocated. People are initially wary of role-play since, for many, it is unlike any other training they may have encountered. Maintaining a small group will help them feel more comfortable in the process.

The strength of role-play is its ability to train people for situations they may rarely encounter, but when they do, need to be ready. The skills a learner can develop for breaking bad news or dealing with anger are best learned prior to encounter in the real world. Also in the real world, one will not get a second opportunity to tackle a difficult consultation from scratch, over and over again. Role-play affords the learner this luxury.

Role-play sessions are best planned in advance so that participants can give due thought to the process. It is often helpful if learners come with specific situations in mind that they would like to explore. These can be discussed at the beginning of the session so that the agenda is fixed according to the learners' needs. Participants can share an experience or hypothetical situation, which can then be acted out. It is often helpful for the person who brought the scenario to role-play the medical role. Another member of the group or actor will play the patient.

Critics of role-play feel that it has limited benefit due to the artificial situation. At its best, role-play can be so realistic that debriefing and 'coming out of role' are often required after particularly intense scenarios. The use of professional actors has cost implications but enhances the process. They are not only able to adapt to different scenarios quickly but also learners find it more realistic since they are not interacting with familiar colleagues. Sometimes the most powerful feedback will come from the actors who, remaining in character, can share their feelings and understanding from the consultation. Many departments use a cohort of health workers who have been trained as actor patients for these sessions. Their knowledge of the medical system enables them to add authenticity to their role. However, they should play the role of someone younger than their own age, so there is no potential to foretell a feared future illness.

The role of the educator in facilitating a role-play learning session cannot be underestimated. Training sessions for this task and regular personal appraisal for the facilitator are strongly recommended. It is beyond the scope of this chapter to outline fully how one should facilitate a role-play session. Many useful books have explored this subject and the best way to learn is to attend an appropriate training course. However, there are several basic principles that should be considered in any such learning session:

- clearly established rules of role-play;
- strict adherence to confidentiality;
- safe environment;
- avoidance of role-playing situations that are potentially distressing for learners;
- option to call 'time-out' at any point;
- opportunity for all learners to participate;
- non-confrontational feedback;
- time for those involved to 'come out of role' after a session;
- review of learning points and de-brief at end of each session.

There are different ways that feedback can be given. Pendleton's method is one of the safest ways to give feedback singly or involving other participants. It involves the application of four enquiries:[14]

- asking the learner what they felt they did well or were particularly happy with;
- asking other learners what they observed to be done well;
- asking the learner what they felt could be improved;
- asking the other learners what they felt could be improved.

This approach to feedback has the merit of first highlighting what was done well, thereby reinforcing good practice and offering positive suggestions for improvement. It is useful to engage members of the group who are not role-playing to take an active part in the appraisal system. In addition to involving them in the group, it also gives them an insight and experience of peer appraisal. Recently, the Calgary–Cambridge approach to communication skills teaching has been developed as an excellent facilitation tool.[15] It differs from other methods as it encourages a far more agenda-led approach to communication skills, encouraging learners to focus on specific areas of the consultation that they otherwise avoid through lack of confidence.

The skills needed to facilitate such sessions are far more sophisticated than the ones we have described and training in this method is strongly recommended before embarking on it. Most learning of value will occur from the role-play itself and the feedback session. Some learners benefit from more summative assessment in order to focus on particular areas they need to concentrate on. It is worth noting that role-play does not need to be used in isolation. Selected videotaped consultations can be used for discussion and specific points explored further using role-play. Table 6 illustrates a suggested marking scheme for the palliative care consultation. Marks are given in each section out of 10, five being a pass mark.

Table 6 Summative marking schedule for palliative care consultation

1.	Puts patient at ease
2.	Establishes problems sufficiently to erect hypothesis
3.	Prioritizes problems/hypothesis
4.	Checks back on problem list agreement
5.	Elicits fears/concerns
6.	Elicits beliefs/concepts/attitudes
7.	Establishes physical/psychosocial relationship of complaints
8.	Explores physical issues appropriately
9.	Evolves plan acceptable to patient
10.	Checks back that plan is understood/agreed
11.	Overall—non-verbals facilitate
12.	Overall—verbals appropriate
13.	Overall—patient appears comfortable/safe
14.	Overall—respects patient's pace
15.	Overall—closes interview well

Ethics

Ethical dilemmas abound in care of patients at the end of life. Ethical decision-making is never straightforward and mastering the art of reflection will at least help the learner function better within zones of indeterminate practice or as Schon describes it as 'the swamp'. Ethical decision-making needs a sound understanding of the principles of autonomy, beneficence, non-maleficence, and justice within the patient's clinical context.[16] Gillon has also highlighted the wide issues around each decision, which require the clinician to reflect on the 'scope' of application of the decision-making process and its outcomes.[17] Although a formal lecture may appear useful to inform, the complex decision-making around each case requires ongoing reflection-in-action by both tutor and learner. Resources available include the ethical sections of the BMA and GMC websites.[18]

Support of the family physician

The training of the family physician should be a dynamic, continually developing process. It should not end once the learner has finished an attachment or completed a formal course. The concept of life-long learners means continued support and recognition of learning needs. The palliative care physician, working in a specialist palliative care unit, is surrounded by colleagues from the many disciplines involved in the care of the dying. Working in such an environment, a multidisciplinary approach becomes part of daily practice; personal support discussion with colleagues to 'bounce ideas around' is often available. The family physician, however, tends to by contrast, be more isolated and less supported.

It is important to maintain a strong working relationship with community colleagues and nurture good communication on both sides. Palliative care units may offer a telephone advice service to community teams, such advice given should be as supportive as possible, acknowledging good practice and responding in a non-judgemental way to problems. Colleagues should be encouraged to recognize the limitations of their skills and feel comfortable to request assistance at this time. Telephone advice calls and joint domiciliary visits are opportune times to anticipate further problems the patient may face and to jointly plan care.

A community palliative care service is another practical way of supporting the community teams and also gives us in the context as educators insight into the learning needs of the family physician. Where at all possible, the home visit should be done alongside the community team so that they are able to observe another person's approach to the problem and discuss the learning issues around it.

Inter-professional learning

Much of this chapter has discussed how palliative care physicians can facilitate the learning of colleagues in the community. All members of the inter-professional team should be involved in teaching, as different professionals will be experts on different topics. Inter-professional learning does not occur simply by putting people in the same setting and teaching them the same core material. It involves letting the different professions learn together where they have common core skills and responsibilities, and helping them define the competencies that exist in others. They will then be able to work better as a team through enhanced respect, as the individual members feel empowered to use their own skills and competencies, whilst also recognizing which other profession has the required competencies for the problem in hand.

Covering a topic such as bereavement will be enhanced by input from all specialties including the team chaplain and social worker. Discussions on the management of cord-compression are not complete without nurse, physiotherapist, and occupational therapist input on rehabilitation aspects. Learning as well as teaching may effectively occur as a multi-professional group. Regular community team meetings between doctors, community nurses, physiotherapists, and occupational therapists offer excellent opportunities for each other. Recent cases could be presented focusing on learning points as a team and those relevant to different professions.

Problem-based learning

Training the family physician in palliative care can also be very effectively undertaken by peer group learning, where a group of family practitioners, either only doctors or as a mixed professional group, form a self-directed learning group.

In problem-based learning, the group takes a defined problem and some or all group members research different aspects of it, presenting their findings to the rest of the group for discussion and critique.[19] The group needs to have one member acting as chair and another as evaluator, to ensure that the discussions remain focused on the topic in hand. The critique should explore positive attributes to the feedback given to the presenters as well as identifying areas for further study.

Problem-based learning does not always require an expert to facilitate a particular subject. However, facilitation requires particular skills, which should be learnt before attempting to run a problem-based learning group.

Further learning opportunities

Individual family physicians and their work partners are likely to identify their learning needs within palliative care. It is up to individual local palliative care units to provide the teaching required. Evening update meetings covering common topics such as morphine prescribing, use of syringe drivers, etc., may do little to increase the factual knowledge of attendees. Their main function is to assist the learning process, by encouraging the sharing of ideas and mutual support.

Day courses with update lectures fulfil a similar function. Workshops in communication skills or ethics are other ways of disseminating the principles of palliative care, by ensuring that new knowledge is consolidated in understanding and new skills acquired are developed to become professional competencies.

Those who develop a particular interest in the care of the dying should consider undertaking a diploma or MSc in palliative medicine. These courses are predominantly long-distance learning with residential weekends to address particular topics. Attended by hospital, hospice, and family physicians, often from all over the globe, they explore palliative care in far more depth, encourage critical appraisal and reflective practice. Many of the courses require an audit project or some form of research which learners find both interesting and challenging. It affords individuals the chance to explore palliative care with like-minded colleagues, yet each brings something unique to the experience.

The Internet has enhanced the learning of palliative care. Many distance-learning courses have developed their own web pages so that participants can share ideas from around the world and liase with their tutors. There are several excellent websites with stimulating discussion groups where learners can participate or just observe ongoing dialogue. Sites such as 'palliativedrugs.com' allow users to post difficult problems on their bulletin board for advice from other users. Participants can thus gain the benefit of other colleagues' experience and learn at the same time. Literature searches can also be done online via sites such as Med-line.

As computer technology becomes more advanced and accessible, so does its scope as a useful learning tool in medical education. CD-ROMs can store vast quantities of information and many textbooks are now produced on disc as well as on paper. International conferences are often recorded onto CD or DVD format so that delegates can watch talks again or browse through abstracts on their computer at a later date. Interactive CDs have been used for sometime in medical training. There are many applications for this technology to palliative care. Interactive CDs are a useful tool for interactive tutorials on topics with questions and extended answers. Difficult clinical problems can be simulated on a computer program with a 'virtual patient' in whom the learner is faced with questions as how best to manage a problem. Some departments are building up a library of simulated patient encounters that will fill some of the gaps in the clinical exposure that can be provided to a student.[20] As technologies develop, it will only be a matter of time before realistic communication skills programmes are developed and we will be breaking bad news to virtual patients and virtual families.

Conclusions

If palliative care teams are to have a valuable role in training the family physician, they must respect the prior learning and experiences of these physicians. Each person will come with his or her own abilities, experiences, and expectations. No one learning tool will suit all, so different teaching methods must be adopted for different situations. To teach we also need to recognize our own limitations and be open to learn from those we are supervising.

As David Henry Thoreau once wrote 'A man needs to be turned around once in this world with his eyes shut to be completely lost. Not until we are lost, do we begin to find ourselves'.[21]

References

1. **Barclay, S.** (1997). Palliative care in the community—the role of the primary health care team. *European Journal of Palliative Care* **6**, 46–7.
2. **Hillier, R. and Wee, B.** (2001). From cradle to grave: palliative medicine education in the UK. *Journal of the Royal Society of Medicine* **94**, 468–71.
3. **Office for National Statistics.** *Mortality Statistics.* London: HMSO, 1995.
4. **Beard, R.M. and Hartley, J.** *Teaching and Learning in Higher Education.* London: Paul Chapman, 1984.
5. **Prochaska, J.O. and Velicer, W.F.** (1997). The transtheoretical model of health behavior change. *American Journal of Health Promotion* **12** (1), 38–48.
6. **Knowles, M.** *Self Directed Learning.* New York: Association Press, 1988.
7. **Association for Palliative Medicine of Great Britain and Ireland.** *Palliative Medicine Curriculum.* Southampton: APMGBI, 1993.
8. **Shipman, C.** et al. (2001). Educational opportunities in palliative care: what do general practitioners want? *Palliative Medicine* **15**, 191–6.
9. **Schon, D.** *Educating the Reflective Practitioner: Towards a New Design for Teaching and Learning in the Professions.* San Francisco: Jossey-Bass, 1987.
10. **Greenwood, J.** (1998). The role of reflection in single and double loop learning. *Journal of Advanced Learning* **27**, 1048–53.
11. **Boud, D., Keogh, R., and Walker, D.** *Reflection: Turning Experience into Learning.* London: Kogan Page, 1985.
12. **Finlay, I.G., Stott, N.C.H., and Marsh, H.M.** (1993). Portfolio learning in palliative medicine. *European Journal of Cancer Care* **2**, 41–3.

13. **Mansfield, F.** (1991). Supervised role-play in the teaching of the process of consultation. *Medical Education* **25**, 485–90.
14. **Pendleton, D.** et al. *The Consultation: an Approach to Learning and Teaching*. Oxford: Oxford University Press, 1984.
15. **Kurtz, S., Silverman, J., and Draper, J.** *Teaching and Learning Communication Skills in Medicine*. Oxford: Radcliffe Medical Press, 1988.
16. **Beauchamp, T.L. and Childress, J.F.** *Principles of Biomedical Ethics*, 3rd edn. Oxford: Oxford University Press, 1989.
17. **Gillon, R.** (1994). Medical ethics: four principles plus attention to scope. *British Medical Journal* **309** (6948), 184–8.
18. www.bma.org.uk; www.gmc-uk.org
19. **David, T., Patel, L., Burdett, K., and Rangachari, P.** *Problem-Based Learning in Medicine: A Practical Guide for Students and Teachers*. London: Royal Society of Medicine, 1999.
20. **McGee, J.B., Neill, J., Goldman, L., and Casey, E.** (1998). Using multimedia virtual patients to enhance the clinical curriculum for medical students. *Medinfo* **9**, 732–5.
21. **Thoreau, D.H.** Walden, or, Life in the Woods: selections from the American Classic. In: *A Week on the Concord and Merrimack Rivers/Walden; or, Life in the Woods/The Maine Woods/Cape Cod*. New York: Library of America, 1985.

20.3 Training specialists in palliative medicine

Andrew M. Hoy

Introduction

Palliative medicine has now become a global activity. For a single author to give an accurate and balanced global perspective has become all but impossible. This is, therefore, an account of the evolution of palliative medicine and will concentrate on specific aspects of the development of education and training in terms of the specialty itself and also training for non-specialist colleagues. Clearly, each national context will develop different approaches to education, in general, and to this specialty, in particular. Inevitably this account will concentrate heavily on the experience of the United Kingdom.

Evolution of palliative medicine

The specialty of palliative medicine as a specific entity dates from the mid-1980s. However, medical activity related to terminal care, care of the dying, hospice care, and end-stage cancer is, of course, as old as medical practice itself.[1] Palliative medicine is the medical component of what has become known as palliative care.

Palliative medicine was first recognized as a medical specialty by the Royal Colleges of Physicians in the United Kingdom in 1987. For several years doctors had been recruited to work in the charitable hospices. They had been attracted to work in this field of terminal care or care of the dying from a variety of backgrounds. As most of the voluntary hospices had a strong Christian ethos, many doctors were similarly motivated. Several medical missionaries returning to the United Kingdom found scope for the development of a new vocation in the Hospice Movement. However, the fields of general practice, anaesthetics, pharmacology, and oncology also provided able recruits to the hospices.

The official recognition of the new specialty in 1987 implied that training would be formalized. Initially, a small number of training posts was recognized. These posts now had to conform to accepted criteria laid down for all specialist training. The institutions and would be educational supervisors required external inspection before such posts could gain educational approval. The trainees themselves were selected competitively to become senior registrars in palliative medicine. Previously, education in palliative medicine ideas had been by ad hoc apprenticeship arrangements and the size of the job market for physicians who had completed training was indeed limited. Aspiring specialists would seek experience at one of the few units practising palliative care. In the United Kingdom, these were the hospices. Outside the United Kingdom sphere of influence, these were palliative care units such as the Palliative Care Service at the Royal Victoria Hospital, Montreal, or specialist pain services such as at Memorial Sloane-Kettering Cancer Center, New York, and University of Washington in Seattle.

Funding for higher specialist training in the United Kingdom has for many years been provided jointly by the training hospitals and centrally from funds distributed via regional postgraduate deans. As experience and educational supervision was almost exclusively within the charitable hospice sector, which had hitherto not been recognized by the postgraduate deans, there was no budget for these new senior registrar posts. Funding, therefore, came from the charitable hospices and from the national cancer care charity Cancer Relief Macmillan Fund (now known as Macmillan Cancer Relief). As the number of trainees nationally has grown from the initial 11 to approximately 150 (2002), the funding arrangements have been accepted as the responsibility of the central government. Currently, 100 per cent of core funding is now provided from central sources via the postgraduate deanery structures throughout the United Kingdom. Funding for the on-call component of training is provided by the institution.

The history of the hospice movement during the nineteenth and twentieth centuries demonstrates the innovations of several charismatic leaders. These practitioners were enthusiasts for their own particular contribution to care of the dying, and they were also the teachers of the next generation of palliative physicians. Although they were products of their original background and training, they all shared the vision of regarding patients who happened to be dying as whole people. They naturally brought their own approaches from specific disciplines of pharmacology, oncology, surgery, anaesthetics, or general practice. This whole person attitude has been labelled as 'holistic care'. Comfort and freedom from pain and distress were of equal importance to diagnostic acumen and cure. However, rather than being a completely new philosophy of care, palliative medicine can be regarded more as a codification of existing practices from past generations.

Histories of the development of palliative medicine illustrate the thread of ideas from figures such as Snow, who developed the Brompton Cocktail in the 1890s, to Barrett who developed the regular giving of oral morphine to the dying at St Luke's, West London, to Saunders who expanded these ideas at St Joseph's and St Christopher's Hospices. Worcester, in Boston, was promoting the multiprofessional care of whole patients in lectures to medical students at a time when intense disease specialization was very much the fashion as it was yielding great therapeutic advances.[2] Winner and Amulree, in the United Kingdom in the 1960s, were promoting whole person care particularly for the elderly, first challenging and then re-establishing the ethical basis for palliative medicine.

As the previous generation of palliative medicine teachers developed their interest in the specialty from their own specialty base or from general practice, it is not surprising, therefore, that the curricula of today should represent a hybrid of the various influences that have been contributed. This is reflected in the recommendations for preparation for specialist training (General Professional Training or GPT). However, the essence of palliative medicine training will necessarily be that of clinical apprenticeship. Alfred Worcester, in the preface to his lectures, notes that '. . . the younger members of the profession, although having enormously greater knowledge of the science of medicine, have less acquaintance than many of their elders with the art of medical practice. This like every other art can of course be learned only by imitation, that is, by practice under masters of the art. Primarily, it depends upon devotion to the patient rather than to his disease'.[2]

Specialist palliative medicine

Palliative medicine is recognized as a specialty in the following countries: United Kingdom, Ireland, Australia, New Zealand, Hong Kong, Taiwan, Poland, and Romania. It will probably be recognized in Sweden during 2003. There are other countries where important educational developments have taken place, but where the specialty is not as yet officially recognized, such as Canada, the United States of America, and Singapore.

United Kingdom

The European Specialist Medical Qualifications Order 1995 came into force in the United Kingdom in 1997. This stipulated that a specialist medical register be held by all European Union states. Entry to the specialist register would be by successful completion of specialist training and acquisition of a Certificate of Completion of Specialist Training (CCST). Previously recognized specialists could obtain entry to the specialist register in the United Kingdom provided that they had been appointed by an appropriately constituted appointment procedure, or any training undertaken elsewhere had been at least as rigorous as that in the United Kingdom.[3]

Specialist registration in European Union states is covered legally by European Directives. It is the responsibility of governments to ensure that these directives are implemented. At present, in the United Kingdom, it is the Specialist Training Authority (STA) that checks and approves CCSTs. This function will be taken over in the near future by a new body to be called the Postgraduate Medical Education and Training Board (PMETB). The expanded functions of this new board will include standard setting for all postgraduate medical education and training, both specialist and generalist, and for assessment of equivalent training of foreign medical graduates.[4]

In the United Kingdom, the academic body responsible for the practicalities of standard setting and monitoring of training and educational achievement in all medical specialties, including palliative medicine, is the Joint Committee for Higher Medical Training (JCHMT). This body draws from the four Royal Colleges of Physicians (London, Edinburgh, Glasgow, and Ireland). It has represented on it all the 23 medical specialties with which it is concerned. These individual specialties all have specialty associations that are responsible for writing and updating the syllabus and curriculum for their own specialty. The Association for Palliative Medicine of Great Britain and Ireland (APM) is the specialty association that originally wrote the curriculum in 1993 and has continued to develop it subsequently.[5] The syllabus, curriculum, and competency assessment was updated in 2001 and will be discussed below.[6]

The broad sections of the current syllabus are as follows:

- Introduction to palliative care,
- Physical aspects of palliative care,
- Psychosocial care,
- Culture, language, religion, and spirituality,
- Ethics,
- Legal frameworks,
- Teamwork,
- Learning and teaching,
- Research,
- Management.

Ireland

Postgraduate medical structures in Ireland have historically been very close to those in the United Kingdom. The Royal College of Physicians of Ireland has formal representation on the UK JCHMT, and the Irish equivalent body the Irish Committee on Higher Medical Training (ICHMT) adopted the same curriculum when it came to advise on the recognition of palliative medicine. The entry requirements for higher specialist training in Ireland are similarly almost identical to those in the United Kingdom.[7]

Australia and New Zealand

The development of the specialty of palliative medicine in Australia and New Zealand has paralleled that in the United Kingdom. The 3-year training is completed after first satisfying the requirements and examinations for Fellowship of the Royal Australasian College of Physicians. The specialty training is broadly comparable to that in the United Kingdom. Indeed, it has been possible for trainees to arrange to gain assessable supervised experience on exchange visits, thus providing valuable cross-fertilization between Australia, New Zealand, and the United Kingdom. In both Australia and New Zealand, part of the training includes compulsory exposure to oncology.[8]

Hong Kong

Traditionally, medical specialist structures in Hong Kong have depended heavily on input from the UK Royal Colleges. Although, there are clear demographic and cultural differences from the United Kingdom, palliative care in Hong Kong has developed through a similar bipartite pathway of charitable and hospital-based services. The Membership examination of the UK Royal College of Physicians is held in Hong Kong, and is the entry qualification to Higher Specialist Training (HST). Furthermore, there has been demand from Hong Kong doctors to follow the Diploma in Palliative Medicine developed at the University of Wales College of Medicine in Cardiff. This diploma course has now been held and examined in Hong Kong in parallel with the main course in the United Kingdom.

Palliative medicine was recognized as a specialty under the Hong Kong College of Physicians of the Academy of Medicine in 1998. The training consists of a 4-year dual accreditation programme in conjunction with Internal Medicine.[9]

Taiwan

The Taiwan Academy of Hospice Palliative Medicine was established in 1999, and in 2000 certification procedures were instituted to recognize specialists in palliative medicine.[10,11]

Singapore

Although specialist hospice and palliative care has been practised in Singapore for several years, a recent application to recognize the specialty of palliative medicine was unsuccessful.[12]

Poland

Among all the eastern European states, it is Poland that has led the development of hospice ideas. This movement goes back to the 1970s and parallels the evolution and growth of the political *Solidarity* movement. Furthermore, there has been a close collaboration between palliative care structures in Poznan, founded by Professor Jacek Luczak, and the specialist unit of Sir Michael Sobell House in Oxford, UK. For many years, Poznan has been the centre for educational activity in palliative care. This has included advanced and basic courses attended by faculty from Poland, United Kingdom, Canada, and the United States of America. Course students have come from all over Eastern Europe.

Poland now has a sophisticated network of specialist units, including the Warsaw Children's Hospice Service. Many of these services have been supported by the Roman Catholic Church and have often depended on volunteer staffing to run them. Training for Polish doctors has been greatly facilitated by charitable funding from the Polish Hospices Fund, the Stefan Batory Foundation, and the Open Society Institute.

Palliative medicine was recognized officially as a medical specialty in 1999. Higher specialist training can only be undertaken following primary specialization in another discipline such as oncology, anaesthetics, or general internal medicine.[13]

Romania

Although Romania has had a less tranquil transition politically from communism to capitalism than Poland, it has nevertheless been able to develop its own hospice movement. The pioneering unit of Casa Sperantei at Brasov has acted as the national educational centre for palliative care. It has received both academic and financial support for this initiative from abroad, particularly from the United Kingdom. Although doctors can now demonstrate subspecialist competence following training in Romania, it would not be equivalent to full specialty recognition.

Canada

It is ironic that the term *Palliative Care* was coined in Canada in the 1970s, yet the specialty of palliative medicine has still not been formally recognized. Much of the seminal early work in the discipline was done by Mount, MacDonald, Bruera, and others in Canada. Academic departments of palliative medicine have been built up and teaching has been innovative and well received, particularly at undergraduate and generic postgraduate levels.[14] There is recognition, however, of a 1-year programme of added competence in palliative medicine. This is a jointly accredited course by the Royal College of Physicians and Surgeons of Canada and the College of Family Physicians of Canada.[15]

The specific standards are designed to train physicians to have the ability to provide secondary, consultant-level expertise to support other physicians and their patients. The course has also been designed to provide the basic clinical training needed for academic careers in palliative medicine.

United States of America

The United States of America has over 2000 separate hospice services. These include free-standing and hospital-based institutions as well as community programmes. Although there has been considerable interest in the medical support of these services, they have tended to be led by non-medical professionals and volunteers. Since 1995, it has been possible to obtain certification in Pain and Palliative Care in the United States of America. There are currently approximately 50 palliative care fellowship programmes to achieve this. Full specialization, however, is not yet possible. In 2002, there were over 1000 physicians who had achieved such certification.

General preparation for higher specialist training

Higher specialist training (HST) is the final pathway leading to specialist registration. All specialties require basic undergraduate training leading to a first medical degree or other qualification. Such basic medical education requires some form of practical apprenticeship such as pre-registration house officer posts or internship. General professional training (GPT) is the training and experience obtained immediately following full registration as a doctor. In the United Kingdom, this experience is gained in the senior house officer (SHO) grade. In the United States of America, the SHO grade is equivalent to that of a resident. GPT must clearly be of relevance to the future career aspirations of the individual. However, most authorities agree that narrow specialization at too early a point in a doctor's career is undesirable.

Historically, palliative medicine specialists brought a diversity of experience to the new specialty. General practitioners, anaesthetists, oncologists, pharmacologists, and internists represented the majority. In the United Kingdom, therefore, the specialty has argued successfully for the acceptability of experience in these disciplines as useful background preparation for HST. Consequently, postgraduate diplomas from the Royal Colleges of General Practitioners, Anaesthetists and Radiologists are accepted alongside the membership examination of the Royal College of Physicians as the entry qualification for HST in palliative medicine.[16]

Because palliative medicine is under the umbrella of the Royal College of Physicians as a medical monospecialty, some experience of acute unselected medical emergency work has been required. This is also true of other monospecialties such as dermatology, medical oncology, neurology, nephrology, rehabilitation medicine etc. Clearly, the so called 'acute' specialties, such as cardiology, endocrinology and diabetes, gastroenterology, geriatrics, respiratory medicine, and rheumatology, which are usually combined with general internal medicine (GIM), have an overriding need to experience emergency medical problem-solving.

In a specialty where there are competitive pressures to achieve appointment to a higher training post, prior experience of the discipline is not only a useful introduction to the type of work involved, but also shows commitment to the specialty. However, the rapid growth of the specialty in the United Kingdom and the majority of inpatient beds being in the charitable sector have resulted in a dearth of palliative medicine posts at junior level. Furthermore, it is at that level that palliative medicine experience may be most useful for the training of specialists in other disciplines.

Reform of the early years of postgraduate education (SHO grade) in the United Kingdom is currently under consideration. It is acknowledged that development of the grade has not kept pace with improvements in pre-registration education and HST. Young, newly qualified doctors in the SHO grade in the United Kingdom have often found that the educational content of these posts is disorganized and variable. Approximately half of all doctors in training are SHOs. Half of the posts are short-term in duration and do not form part of a coherent training rotation or programme. Half of the SHOs are female and this proportion is increasing. There are insufficient opportunities for flexible or part-time training and the workload is increasing. There is no defined end-point to SHO training other than successful competitive entry to HST.

The consultation document entitled 'Unfinished Business' has been published by the Department of Health for England.[17] This sets out detailed proposals for reform that will have a significant impact on all specialties including palliative medicine. The training would be programme-based rather than grade-based. The first 2 years would be a broadly based *foundation programme* that would include the current pre-registration year. It would 'develop and enhance core or generic clinical skills essential for all doctors (e.g. team-working, communication, ability to produce high standards of clinical governance and patient safety, expertise in accessing, appraising and using evidence as well as time management skills)'.

The second part of the new structure would be any one of eight or so broad-based, time-capped *basic specialist training programmes.* This would include training for general practice. Entry to a basic specialist training programme would be competitive and would have followed sample experience during the foundation programme. This second part of training would last 2–3 years and may enable HST in some specialties to be shortened to as little as 2 years. The eight suggested Basic Specialist Training Programmes include: medicine in general, surgery in general, general practice, child health, mental health, obstetrics and gynaecology, pathology in general, and anaesthetics. There would be scope for flexibility, career breaks, and entry for overseas graduates.

As far as palliative medicine is concerned, there could be opportunities to insert palliative experience into some or all of the clinical subjects on this list of eight. The Federation of Royal Colleges of Physicians published a Core Curriculum and Appraisal Record for SHOs in GIM and the medical specialties in 2001. This curriculum includes some aspects of palliative medicine as core skills to be acquired.[18]

Palliative medicine for specialists other than palliative physicians

Undergraduate training

During the last 10 years, there has been acceptance that most palliative care is provided by non-specialists, rather than by palliative medicine specialists. The National Council for Hospice and Specialist Palliative Care Services in the United Kingdom made a clear distinction between specialist palliative care services and what it termed general palliative care services.[19,20] The former included care provided by a full multiprofessional team including recognized specialists in the key professions of medicine and nursing. The latter was the application of palliative care principles in the context of every branch of clinical practice. This has been called the 'palliative care approach'. The education and training of generalists and specialist in other disciplines is, therefore, of great importance.

From the beginnings of the modern hospice movement, it was recognized that the inclusion of teaching about death, dying, terminal care, and palliative care should be integrated into undergraduate and postgraduate education wherever possible. Soon after St Christopher's Hospice opened in London in 1967, Cicely Saunders lectured regularly to open student meetings held in the London undergraduate medical schools. She also initiated open ward rounds at St Christopher's. This continues to this day and is replicated in all of the specialist palliative care units throughout the United Kingdom. Many of the current generation of palliative physicians (including the author) were introduced to the subject by these voluntary educational contacts.

From 1980, there has been the recommendation that palliative care should be an essential part of the undergraduate curriculum. The Wilkes Report in the United Kingdom argued for the dissemination of palliative care philosophy into mainstream medicine and that there should be integration of hospice ideas into the community.[21] In 1994, the case for increased educational effort was reinforced by a House of Lords Select Committee recommendation. This was in response to examination of the issue of legalization of euthanasia.[22]

When the original palliative medicine curriculum was written by a working party of the Association for Palliative Medicine in the early 1990s, it was published as three different syllabuses that were considered to be appropriate for medical students, general professional medical training, or HST in palliative medicine. The curriculum specifically for vocational trainees for general practice was written jointly with the Royal College of General Practitioners.[5] At much the same time, the Canadian Committee on Palliative Care Education, lead by MacDonald, published the Canadian Palliative Care Curriculum.[23] This document had been commissioned by the deans of the majority of the medical schools of Canada. The object was to facilitate specific palliative care programme development in the medical schools. The contents of the Canadian and UK curricula are broadly similar.

In the United Kingdom, Field and Wee have shown that over the last 19 years, palliative medicine teaching has become the norm in all medical schools.[24] Comparison with surveys performed in 1983 and 1994 shows that improvements in the use of integrated curricula have taken place.[25] It is now more likely for medical students to have direct involvement with dying patients. Ideas of palliative care are often covered in several different part of the undergraduate course. However, emphasis on aspects of physical treatment including symptom control seems to reflect the expansion of the specialty of palliative medicine.

Surveys of the effectiveness of this training indicate that there is still considerable room for improvement. Lloyd-Williams showed that newly qualified house officers were frustrated by their lack of skills and knowledge of palliative care, especially communication skills.[26,27]

Dickinson and Field compared the current status of teaching of end-of-life issues in UK and US medical schools.[28] They surveyed all medical schools in 2000 and found great interest and activity in both countries. All clinical schools offered some training, although teaching methods, professional background of the instructors, and content varied significantly (Tables 1–3). The mean number of teaching hours during the undergraduate course was 20 in the United Kingdom and 14 in the United States of America.

Although the traditional lecture format was still commonly used, both countries favour small group learning. There would seem to be a particular emphasis in the United Kingdom on clinical case discussions and communication skills development with role-play. Visits to hospices were commoner in the United Kingdom, perhaps reflecting the relative medicalization of the hospice model. However, US schools stated that more extensive hospice visiting was planned for the future.

Table 1 Methods used in teaching about death, dying, and bereavement[28]

	UK[a] (%)	US[b] (%)
Lecture	21 (88)	91 (81)
Role-play	22 (92)	44 (39)
Hospice visit	22 (92)	55 (49)
Video/film	19 (79)	50 (45)
Seminar/small group discussion	23 (96)	94 (84)
Simulated patients	5 (21)	37 (33)
Clinical case discussions	23 (96)	77 (69)

[a] N = 24.
[b] N = 112.

Table 2 Professional background of instructors[28]

	UK[a] (%)	US[b] (%)
Physician/general practitioner[c]	20 (83)	105 (94)
Palliative medicine specialist	24 (100)	—
Psychiatrist	10 (42)	34 (30)
Social worker	11 (46)	35 (31)
Nurse	3 (13)	40 (36)
Nurse specialist in palliative care	15 (63)	—
Psychologist	7 (29)	29 (26)
Sociologist	6 (25)	9 (8)
Philosopher	–	17 (15)
Theologian/religious minister	11 (46)	49 (44)
Ethicist	4 (17)	8 (7)

[a] N = 24.
[b] N = 112.
[c] Includes all specialists except palliative medicine (United Kingdom only) and psychiatrists.

Perhaps the most interesting feature of Table 2 is that medical student education in death, dying, and bereavement is a multiprofessional activity. The obvious differences in availability of palliative medicine and nurse specialists in the United Kingdom account for the other major differences.

The curricular topics covered are shown in Table 3 and indicate some interesting discrepancies between the United Kingdom and the United States of America. Death certification issues and euthanasia are seen to be more important in the United Kingdom, while AIDS end-of-life issues are more commonly included in the United States of America. Neither country offers much about neonatal topics or physical therapies. Symptom control, pain relief, communication, and attitudinal aspects are particularly prominent in the United Kingdom. The authors note that their findings reflect prevalent negative attitudes to pain control in the United States of America. They also comment that the culture of 'death as a medical failure' in US medical circles is responsible for the relative slowness in introducing and developing end-of-life topics in medical school curricula.[28]

Postgraduate training

The acquisition of appropriate attitudes, skills, and knowledge are extremely important prior to medical qualification; however, it is when junior doctors are required to make management decisions themselves that such training is

Table 3 End-of-life topics covered in the curriculum

	UK[a] (%)	US[b] (%)
Attitudes towards death and dying	24 (100)	90 (80)
Communication with dying patients	21 (89)	97 (87)
Communication with family members	23 (96)	85 (76)
Grief and bereavement	22 (92)	81 (72)
Social contexts of dying	21 (89)	71 (63)
Psychological aspects of dying	22 (92)	80 (71)
Religious and cultural aspects of dying	16 (67)	74 (66)
The experience of dying	19 (79)	68 (61)
Analgesics for chronic pain	23 (96)	87 (78)
Analgesics for cancer pain	23 (96)	83 (74)
Symptom relief in advanced terminal disease	24 (100)	74 (66)
End-of-life hydration	16 (67)	55 (49)
End-of-life nutrition	14 (58)	57 (51)
Other physical therapy	8 (33)	5 (4)
Neonatal issues	8 (33)	29 (26)
Relating to patients with AIDS	9 (37)	58 (52)
Euthanasia	21 (89)	51 (46)
Advance directives	18 (75)	91 (81)
Death certificates	20 (83)	29 (26)

[a] N = 12.

[b] N = 112.

crucial. Over the past 20 years, newly qualified doctors have felt ill-prepared for the palliative care role that they were required to fulfil as soon as they became house officers or interns.[29] Despite widespread acknowledgement that undergraduate palliative medical education was improving, junior doctors still feel insecure.[30]

Various approaches have been developed to improve the situation. Hospital palliative care units and teams have offered not only clinical advice but also education and training to general hospital colleagues. Early examples of hospital support teams include St Luke's Hospital Center Hospice Team in New York, the Palliative Care Service at the Royal Victoria Hospital, Montreal, the St Thomas' Hospital and St Bartholomew Hospital terminal care support teams, both in London.[31–33]

Incorporation of palliative medicine material into the curricula of specialties other than palliative medicine has taken place. Specialties that have overlapping interests, such as clinical oncology and anaesthetics, now have palliative care in their curricula.[34,35] However, the indicative content is not large or detailed in either specialties curriculum. Perhaps of more importance, however, is that candidates sitting the appropriate specialty examinations now know that palliative medicine topics may be included.

In the United Kingdom, surgical specialty training has been encouraged following the Kennedy Report[36] to emphasize communication skills, team working, leadership skills, and use of evidential base for clinical decision-making. The basic surgical training, therefore, now includes as part of the syllabus for Membership of the Royal College of Surgeons items about breaking bad news and other communication topics.[37]

In the general medical specialties in the United Kingdom, the curriculum for senior house officers (residents) now includes the acquisition of palliative medicine topics as core skills. The three examples that have been suggested are problems of pain, constipation, and breathlessness. There is a further section intitled 'additional topics for SHOs in the specialties'. These are topics that a SHO in any particular specialty would expect to cover during his/her time in the post, but are not regarded as core topics. For palliative medicine posts the following are included: organization of palliative care services, eligibility for financial support, quality of life issues in late-stage disease, cultural and religious influences on patient and family attitudes to death and dying.[18] In addition to specialty specific skills, there is particular emphasis on communication, breaking bad news, maintaining trust, and communication with colleagues. Perhaps one of the more significant changes to traditional training in general internal medicine is the use of cross-specialty clinical scenarios. These include various symptoms that patients might present with, but which they might equally well suffer from as symptom management problems. From a palliative perspective, it is refreshing that alleviation of symptoms is of equal importance to diagnosis.

The specialty association, the APM, has published a curriculum for Continuing Professional Development, called palliative medicine for other specialties. It poses three questions that are intended to provoke further learning. They are:

- Can you control at least 80 per cent of cancer pains effectively?
- Do you know why people ask for euthanasia?
- Do you worry about breaking bad news?

There follows a short curriculum concerned with symptom management, psychosocial issues, and ethical issues in advanced disease.[38]

Postgraduate trainees in general practice in the United Kingdom currently gain experience in a variety of specialties as well as a supervised year with a general practice trainer in the community. Some of the general practice vocational training schemes include supervised time in a specialist palliative care unit/hospice. This form of experience could be expanded when the new arrangements for basic specialist training programmes are implemented (see above). It has also been possible for funding to be obtained from postgraduate deans to allow additional hospice and community experience after vocational training has been completed, immediately prior to seeking a permanent partnership in general practice. Such top-up training has included joint domiciliary visiting with palliative medicine specialists.

Postgraduate courses

The last few years have seen the initiation of several postgraduate certificate, diploma, and masters programmes that have included palliative medicine. Some of these courses have been aimed at trainees who will become palliative medicine specialists, but many others have catered for non-specialists.

One example of such a course is the Diploma in Palliative Medicine offered by the University of Wales College of Medicine. This started in 1989 as a distance learning course for general practitioners, consultants of all specialties, and interested trainees. The core curriculum of the APM was used as the basis for the programme. This included specific communication skills at the residential weekends held during the year-long course. To date, over 400 doctors have been awarded the diploma. They come from diverse geographical, social, and cultural backgrounds as well as many different countries. A recent assessment of the relevance of the curriculum to the diplomates in their own practice context indicated that the large majority found the core topics covered of either 'great or very great' importance to them subsequently. The elements of the curriculum of particular importance were communication with patients and families, assessment, diagnosis and treatment of pain, multiprofessional team working, and psychological responses to illness and bereavement.[39]

Most other postgraduate courses in the United Kingdom and elsewhere have been multiprofessional. These include diplomas and masters courses at Kings College, London, Sheffield, Bristol, Glasgow, Dundee, Cape Town, Adelaide, Sydney, Australia, and Canada. Bearing in mind that good palliative care is almost always an activity performed in a multiprofessional context, it would seem logical to develop multiprofessional learning. Indeed, there is a growing literature showing examples where the multiprofessional approach has been very successful.[40–42] Students, patients, and carers are all positive about such multiprofessionalism. However, in the assessment of the educational process there is the need to find generalities that can be tested across all professions. One solution to this problem has been proposed whereby the examiners work in multiprofessional pairs. This approach is used in a course for the 'Certificate of Essential Palliative Care' at the Princess Alice Hospice in Surrey.[43] It would seem that generic, psychological, and social subjects are better learned across the professional boundaries, whereas technical issues such as specialist pharmacology may be more difficult to accommodate.

Preparation for palliative medicine practice in various contexts

Selection for higher specialist training in palliative medicine

Over the last 20 years, questions have been posed concerning what type of doctor is most suited to palliative medicine: whether 30 or more years of unrelenting palliative medicine is sustainable and whether it is incompatible with maintaining mental stability. How should we select entrants into the specialty and how should we support them? What little evidence there is suggests that palliative physicians suffer no more from psychiatric morbidity and burn-out than their oncological counterparts.[44]

Clearly, an educational process must take account of how the students will eventually be employed and what job opportunities will be available once specialist status has been achieved. In the United Kingdom, palliative medicine as a specialty has been one of the most rapidly growing on record. Over the last 8 years, consultant posts have grown at a rate of 375 per cent. Admittedly, the baseline was very low to begin with. However, national cancer plans that include access to specialist palliative medical opinion indicate that the number of consultants must double from 260 currently (2002) within the next 10 years. At present there are over 100 vacant consultant posts, so the challenge is to expand the training opportunities and ensure adequate educational supervision.[45] There will, therefore, be no shortage of employment opportunities for specialists in palliative medicine in the United Kingdom for the foreseeable future. As other countries recognize the specialty, so will the demand grow for suitably trained specialists. At present, doctors from other European Union countries have sought training posts in the United Kingdom. Eventually, there will need to be replication elsewhere in Europe of the development of training opportunities on the same scale as the United Kingdom.

Other factors will also influence the shape of palliative medicine practice in the future. In the United Kingdom, 80 per cent of trainees are female. At present, 56 per cent of consultants are female, but the figure will obviously rise over the next generation. Thirty per cent of the trainees are training flexibly, that is, part-time. Presumably, there will also be a trend for these individuals to work part-time for at least some of their consultant careers. Perhaps because female trainees may have family responsibilities as well as career aspirations, there is a tendency for them to be less mobile in the job market than their male counterparts. These factors mean that each region or geographical area will need to appoint trainees who will be likely to fill the consultant post in that same area. These regions will also need to find ways of offering more flexible work opportunities than perhaps previously. MacLeod has speculated thoughtfully about how we can provide the best environment in which to learn to care as palliative physicians.[46] There may also be clues to do with empathic, feminine, nursing values as to why such work results in such a marked gender difference. However, he does not offer suggestions as to how we can select the most appropriate trainees to fulfil this role, other than to encourage an empathic and humanistic philosophy alongside the biomedical model throughout training.

Career context of palliative physicians of the future

In the Western world, the majority of people die in an institution, usually a hospital. However, most of us would choose to die in our own home if we could. Hospitalization is almost always costly, to the individual, the family, or society. If we are to achieve a reversal of the trend of institutional death, then a palliative medicine training must have a thorough grounding in community practice and skills. There must be an understanding of the possibilities and compromises involved in domiciliary care. Adaptation of palliative medicine practice is required for the nursing home sector and for community beds in what is now termed 'intermediate care'. Not withstanding this desire for community care, death in a specialist unit such as a hospice may be preferable to death in hospital, and such units will continue to be centres of excellence and numbers will probably expand. Similarly, however effective the hospitals of the future are at maintaining their role as diagnostic and active management facilities, the majority of deaths will still take place in them. The palliative physician of the next generation will, therefore, also need to be skilled in relating to his/her specialist hospital colleagues, understanding their problems, and advocating the application of palliative principles. The changing requirements for all medical specialties can be found in a document from the Royal College of Physicians.[47]

The reality of future palliative medicine practice is that it will be demanding medically and psychologically and will require selection not only for medical and technical excellence but also for qualities of empathy, compassion, toughness, and the ability to handle raw emotions. It will inevitably be a hybrid specialty that has highly developed interprofessional work practices. The myth of the 'do-gooding pious hand-holder' could not be further from reality.[48]

Curriculum design, assessment, and appraisal during higher specialist training

There has been a trend towards ever more explicit curricula and tighter supervision and assessment during training. In the mid-1990s in the United Kingdom, much needed reforms in higher specialist training changed what had largely been an apprenticeship into a structured course of training with regular external review. This process demanded an explicit syllabus, and a detailed curriculum for all specialties. Initially, the review process was performed on an annual basis by a deanery specialty training committee and inspection of the trainee's Record of In-Training Assessment (RITA).[49] The RITA is a folder that contains individual curriculum topics, records of the trainee's educational objectives, achievements, external courses attended, research undertaken, and annual RITA review reports. This process was a great improvement on the completely unstructured approach previously, but there were criticisms that it tended to be a rather automated 'tick-box' exercise nevertheless.

The next step has been to rewrite all curricula and link the topics therein with descriptors of competencies that are to be achieved during each part of training. The APM completed this task of curriculum revision and it has been accepted by the statutory registration body.[6] The descriptors of competencies are now being piloted in selected deaneries.[50]

The syllabus consists of 10 broad topics. These are broken down as follows:

1. Introduction to palliative care
    - 1.1. History, philosophy, and definitions
    - 1.2. Personal qualities and attributes of palliative medicine physicians
    - 1.3. Communication between services
2. Physical care
    - 2.1. Disease process and management
        - 2.1.1. Management of life limiting, progressive disease
        - 2.1.2. Specific disease processes
        - 2.1.3. Management of concurrent clinical problems encountered in palliative care

- 2.2. Symptoms—understanding and management
  - 2.2.1. General principles of symptom management
  - 2.2.2. Pain
  - 2.2.3. Other symptoms and clinical problems
  - 2.2.4. Emergencies in palliative medicine
  - 2.2.5. Practical procedures
- 2.3. Pharmacology and therapeutics
  - 2.3.1. General
  - 2.3.2. Drug specific
- 2.4. Rehabilitation
- 2.5. Care of the dying patient and their family

3. Psychosocial care
   - 3.1. Social and family relationships
   - 3.2. Communication with patients and relatives
   - 3.3. Psychological responses of patients and carers to life-threatening illness and loss
   - 3.4. Attitudes and responses of doctors and other professionals
   - 3.5. Grief and bereavement
   - 3.6. Patient and family finance
4. Culture, language, religious, and spiritual issues
   - 4.1. Culture and ethnicity
   - 4.2. Religion and spirituality
5. Ethics
   - 5.1. Theoretical ethics
   - 5.2. Applied ethics in clinical practice of palliative care
6. Legal frameworks
   - 6.1. Death
   - 6.2. Treatment
   - 6.3. Doctor/patient relationship
   - 6.4. Organizational
   - 6.5. Charity and company law
7. Teamwork
8. Teaching and learning
   - 8.1. Teaching
   - 8.2. Learning
9. Research
10. Management
    - 10.1. Human resources
      - 10.1.1. Recruitment
      - 10.1.2. Staff development
      - 10.1.3. Disciplinary procedures
    - 10.2. Leadership skills
    - 10.3. Management of work
    - 10.4. Information management
    - 10.5. Structures
    - 10.6. Running a palliative care unit
    - 10.7. Financial management
    - 10.8. Clinical governance
    - 10.9. Audit

Table 4 Section 3 summary of palliative medicine curriculum: Psychosocial care

3. Psychosocial care
   - 3.1. Social and family relationships
   - 3.2. Communication with patients and relatives
   - 3.3. Psychological responses of patients and carers to life-threatening illness and loss
   - 3.4. Attitudes and responses of doctors and other professionals
   - 3.5. Grief and bereavement
   - 3.6. Patient and family finance

The format of the curriculum is that for each of these 10 sections learning outcomes are defined. The subject matter is specified, with relevant teaching/learning methods, assessment, and evidence of competence for inclusion in the record of training. An example is given in Tables 4 and 5 for part of the psychosocial care section of the curriculum. All parts of the curriculum have been developed in this way.

Competencies have been defined for each part of the curriculum in terms of knowledge, skills, and attitudes. When assessment takes place, a template is applied that categorizes the trainee's competence as: (a) satisfactory for that particular stage of training; (b) needing more or specific targeted training; (c) unsatisfactory or training need unmet. Table 6 shows the competencies using the first part of the psychosocial care section of the curriculum as an example. The purpose of 'targeted training' lying between 'satisfactory' and 'unsatisfactory' enables the current or future educational supervisor to specify a particular educational activity for the trainee that could then become their next educational objective, rather than the trainee being required to repeat the whole of that part of the course.

The activity of assessment of competence is quite distinct from appraisal. Assessment takes place infrequently and is likely to involve external assessors. Appraisal in the context of a higher specialist trainee should occur every 3–4 months between the educational supervisor and the trainee. Although structured, it can be relatively informal. It is a two-way process to maximize the learning potential of the specific placement. It may also be an early warning system that training is not proceeding as well as it could for any particular reason. Records of appraisal should be kept by both parties, but should not form part of the RITA.

Research and the development of a specific evidence base for palliative medicine

For a new specialty to grow and develop, it must have an active, questioning philosophy. To fail to develop a specific evidence base for the practice of palliative medicine runs the risk of a static, complacent discipline. It also lays the specialty wide open to criticism from outside that it is reactive rather than proactive. A specialty without research energy and ideas will soon dwindle and cannot expect to earn the respect of mainstream medicine. The new specialty must, therefore, recruit, train, and grow its academic wing. It must set its standards based on such research evidence. It must develop audit procedures that are measured against those standards. In short, research is necessary to initiate the audit cycle.

Palliative care in general, however, is concerned with the provision of care to very ill patients only some of whose problems are necessarily physical. The purely biomedical philosophy that has delivered such spectacular advances in other disciplines may be less than adequate for palliative medicine. Furthermore, many palliative physicians are by nature carers and doers, rather than experimentalists or academics. However, they are unlikely not to be philosophers and reflective thinkers.

Table 5 Psychosocial care. 3.1: Social and family relationships

Learning outcomes	Subject matter	Teaching/learning method	Assessment	Evidence of competence for inclusion in record
The trainee will demonstrate skills in assessing the ill person in relation to family, work, and social context. The trainee will undertake this assessment with tact and compassion	Application of the ill person in relation to his/her family, work, and social circumstances Impact of illness on interpersonal relationships Impact of illness on body image, sexuality, and role Construction and use of genograms Assessment of the response to illness and expectations among family members When and how to use family meetings Concept of resonance Concept of family scripts, homeostasis in families, and the impact of illness and loss on the family system Awareness of transference and counter-transference in professional relationships with patients and family members	Participation in multidisciplinary assessment and review Personal study Participation in family meetings Appropriately supervised role-play	Observed behaviour Multiprofessional feedback Portfolio of cases	Satisfactory trainer's report Satisfactory completion of portfolio
The trainee will have acquired the skills to adapt his/her approach to care to meet the patients' individual and family needs	Ways to accommodate needs of partners and families in provision of palliative care in an inpatient unit or home setting Palliative care provision in relation to the homeless and those in custody	Spent time with social workers Attend case conferences		

Table 6 Competencies for Section 3.1: Social and family relationships

3.1 Assessing patients in relation to their family, work, and social context

	Satisfactory (for year . . . of training)(2)	Needs more or specifically targeted training(3)	Unsatisfactory or training need unmet(4)
Knowledge	The trainee demonstrates a broad knowledge of the impact of illness on the patient and his/her family, and the effect of family, work, and social setting on the patient and the way in which he/she manages his/her illness	The trainee demonstrates a patchy or superficial knowledge, such that clinical care might be compromised without close supervision	Knowledge is limited to the point where patient care provided by the trainee is frequently compromised
Skills	The trainee: ◆ Routinely assesses patients in relation to family, work, and social context ◆ Consistently adapts his/her approach to meet the patient's individual and family needs ◆ Arranges and leads family meetings appropriately and effectively	The trainee: ◆ Sometimes fails to take into account the family, work, or social context sufficiently when assessing patients ◆ Adapts his/her assessment approach only partially, or with assistance, to meet individual and family needs ◆ Initiates and manages family meetings haphazardly at times	The trainee: ◆ Routinely fails to take the family, work, or social context into account when assessing patients ◆ Cannot adapt his/her assessment approach to meet individual and family needs, in spite of feedback and training ◆ Cannot or does not arrange and manage family meetings
Attitudes	The trainee: ◆ Appreciates the importance of the patient's family, work, and social setting on the way in which he/she manages his/her illness ◆ Uses tact and compassion in assessing the patient's needs ◆ Is confident in arranging and managing family meetings	The trainee: ◆ Needs prompting in recognizing the importance of assessing patients in relation to their family, work, and social context ◆ May appear lacking in tact or compassion towards patients and families at times ◆ May lack confidence in arranging or leading family meetings	The trainee: ◆ Regularly upsets patients and families ◆ Does not see the social context of the patient as important ◆ Is unwilling to arrange or lead family meetings

The practicalities of clinical research in a palliative care setting are difficult (see Chapter 5.2 'Research'). Although some research questions are amenable to conventional randomized trial methodology, attitudinal and quality of life research may require a more qualitative approach. Most hospice or palliative care units cater for patients who, by definition, are deteriorating rapidly from a disease process that will be fatal. Such an unstable population represents a moving target for randomized, cross-over trial methodology. There may also be powerful ethical and humanitarian considerations when including palliative care patients in research, which may be less pressing in different patient populations. This is not to argue that such research should not be attempted, but there must be particular education in the most appropriate techniques.

Access to academic funding varies by country, and is likely to be linked with the arrangements for health care funding in general. A predominantly state-funded system such as the UK National Health Service values care provision primarily; educational and research funding are of secondary concern. Furthermore, the administrative structures for commissioning and providing care, the primary care trusts (PCTs) and acute hospital trusts, are quite separate from the academic, educational, and research structures of the universities, medical, and nurse training schools. During HST for most medical specialties, only 1 year of pure research is accountable towards a CCST.[(49)] This is clearly inadequate time to complete a PhD, a research MD, or even a Masters degree. Furthermore, the funding of the trainee's salary must be found. This is often not covered by hospice, hospital, or deanery sources. 'Soft' money from large academic departments has been used in the past, but such resources are increasingly difficult to access. The NHS does have a large research and development (R&D) budget, but there are invariably strings attached to R&D funding, in terms of targeted topics and projects.

Canada, Australia, the United States of America, and some European countries such as Norway and Sweden have managed to create academic departments with chairs and senior lecturers. These departments have acted as very effective foci for research and educational activity. However, this does not necessarily correlate with recognition of the specialty. The United Kingdom has currently six professors, one reader, and several senior lecturers of palliative medicine throughout the country. This number is inadequate to cater for the research needs of a rapidly growing specialty, or to be able to supervise the registrars who have declared a particular research interest.

To try to improve the situation in the United Kingdom, the Association for Palliative Medicine convened a group of trainees and academics to keep a register in each region of research leads, potential supervisors, possible sources of funding, and current research activity.[(51)] It is too early to tell how successful this has been in stimulating and supporting new research activity.

Palliative medicine as a specialty

Any new field in medical practice meets with at least questions as to its relevance and often there will be initial hostility. Palliative medicine has been no exception. Medicine is an intrinsically conservative occupation. New ideas can all too easily become threats and be viewed as implied criticism. It is no coincidence that hospices in the United Kingdom placed themselves outside mainstream clinical care for many years until the justification for reintegration became self-evident. Arguments have been put forward that redefining end-of-life care as a specialty will 'de-skill' generalists. It is certainly true that a body of special knowledge that is guarded jealously without the desire to educate and train will result in restricted care for patients and hostility from colleagues. Palliative medicine, as with all palliative care, is concerned with enabling and facilitating, not preservation of a limited cartel.[(52)]

Experience in the United Kingdom suggests that it was only when palliative medicine was recognized as a distinct entity that purposive training could be organized. The development of the specialty as part of a multiprofessional activity provided recruits with a model of work that did not result in isolationism and de-skilling of colleagues.[(53)] There have been criticisms that it is illogical to lavish extra care and expertise on the minority of patients who are dying of cancer, rather than the greater numbers who die from other causes.[(54)] The challenge, therefore, as the specialty matures, is to incorporate into our educational programmes applications of hospice philosophy to progressive neurological conditions, incurable heart disease, and other progressive degenerative illnesses.

In the United States of America, it has been recognized that physician education in end-of-life issues is inadequate. The American Academy of Hospice and Palliative Medicine was founded over 10 years ago 'to promote hospice care for the terminally through medical education, research, and training'.[(55)] There has been great interest among physicians in pursuing palliative medicine fellowships, which have been organized on a 'apprenticeship' model. However, it has been suggested that only a more academic training with specialty recognition will result in rigorous enough standards to produce the desired growth of the discipline in the future.[(56)] Accordingly, the American Board of Hospice and Palliative Medicine was formed in 1995 and has created and run certification procedures.[(57)] However, specialty recognition is still awaited.

Continuing professional development (CPD)

Many countries, including the United Kingdom, have recognized that maintenance of professional standards and clinical governance demand structured continuing professional development (CPD). This is irrespective of specialty or discipline. CPD can take various forms and will differ for individuals and specialty. It is becoming an essential component of revalidation and continuing registration.

Design of CPD programmes provides opportunities for palliative physicians to influence and update colleagues. Activities usefully include hospital grand rounds, case presentations, audit sessions, and study days. These educational activities may be internal for colleagues of the institution or external for all interested parties. Local, regional, national, and international meetings will all have valuable CPD functions. A national specialty association will usually have as one of its main functions that of convening such meetings, conferences, or congresses. International organizations that provide academic congresses in palliative care include the European Association for Palliative Care, the Asia Pacific Hospice Palliative Care Network, the International Association for Hospice and Palliative Care, and the National Hospice and Palliative Care Organization (VA, USA).[(58–61)]

Courses running in the immediate future in the United Kingdom are listed by the organization *hospice information*.[(62)]

References

1. **Saunders, C.** (1993). Introduction—history and challenge. In *The Management of Terminal Malignant Disease* (ed. C. Saunders and N. Sykes), pp. 1–14. London: Edward Arnold.
2. **Worcester, A.** *The Care of the Aged, the Dying and the Dead.* Springfield IL: Charles C. Thomas, 1935.
3. **Information concerning training in the medical specialties in the United Kingdom.** London: JCHMT (available at www.jchmt.org.uk/gen_training.htm).
4. **Department of Health.** *Postgraduate Medical Education and Training—Statement on Policy.* London, 2002 (available at www.doh.gov.uk/medicaltrainingintheuk).
5. **Association for Palliative Medicine of Great Britain and Ireland.** *Palliative Medicine Curriculum.* Southampton: APM, 1993.
6. **Association for Palliative Medicine.** *Palliative Medicine Syllabus and Curriculum.* Southampton: APM, 2002 (available at www.palliative-medicine.org).
7. **The Irish Committee on Higher Medical Training.** *Curriculum for Higher Specialist Training in Palliative Medicine.* Dublin: RCPI, 1997.

8. **Royal Australasian College of Physicians.** *Requirements for Physician Training (Mango Book). Vocational Training in Palliative Medicine for 2003.* Sydney: RACP, 2002 (available at www.racp.edu.au/training/adult2003/advanced/vocational/palliative.htm).
9. **Hong Kong College of Physicians.** *Guidelines for Higher Physician Training.* Hong Kong: HKCP, 2002 (available on www.hkcp.org/protocol.htm).
10. **Hospice Foundation of Taiwan** (www.hospice.org.tw).
11. **Taiwan Academy of Hospice Palliative Medicine** (www.hospicemed.org.tw).
12. **Singapore Hospice Council** (www.singaporehospice.org.sg).
13. **Wright, M. and Clark, D.** (2003). The development of palliative care in Poznan, Poland. *European Journal of Palliative Care* **10**, 26–9.
14. **Oneschuk, D.** (1999). The evolution of palliative medicine education in Canada. *European Journal of Palliative Care* **6**, 198–202.
15. **Royal College of Physicians and Surgeons of Canada.** *Specific Standards of Accreditation for a 1-Year Program of Added Competence in Palliative Medicine.* Ottawa: RCPSC, 2002 (available at www.rcpsc.medical.org/english/residency/accreditation/ssas/palliativemed_e.html).
16. **Joint Committee on Higher Medical Training.** *Curriculum for Higher Specialist Training in Palliative Medicine.* London: RCP, 2000 (available at www.jchmt.org.uk/curricula/curr_palliative.htm).
17. *Unfinished Business. Proposals for Reform of the Senior House Officer Grade.* A Report by Sir Liam Donaldson, Chief Medical Office for England (available at www.doh.gov.uk/shoconsult).
18. **Federation of Royal Colleges of Physicians.** *Core Curriculum for Senior House Officers in General (Internal) Medicine and the Medical Specialties* 3rd edn. London: RCP, 2001.
19. **National Council for Hospice and Specialist Palliative Care Services.** *Palliative Care 2000. Commissioning Through Partnership.* London: NCHSPCS, 1999.
20. **National Council for Hospice and Specialist Palliative Care Services.** *Definitions of Supportive and Palliative Care.* Briefing number 11. London: NCHSPCS, 2002.
21. **Standing Medical Advisory Committee.** Report of the Working Group on Terminal Care (The Wilkes Report). London: SMAC, 1980.
22. **House of Lords Select Committee on Medical Ethics.** Report. London: HMSO, 1994.
23. **MacDonald, N.** *The Canadian Palliative Care Curriculum.* The Canadian Committee on Palliative Care Education, 1991.
24. **Field, D. and Wee, B.** (2002). Preparation for palliative care: teaching about death, dying and bereavement in UK medical schools 2000–2002. *Medical Education* **36**, 561–7.
25. **Field, D.** (1995). Education for palliative care: formal education about death, dying and bereavement in UK medical schools in 1983 and 1994. *Medical Education* **29**, 414–19.
26. **Lloyd-Williams, M.** (1996). Communication skills—the house officer's perception. *Journal of Cancer Care* **11**, 151–3.
27. **Lloyd-Williams, M.** (2001). Assessing training needs to extend the scope of palliative care. *European Journal of Palliative Care* **8**, 28–9.
28. **Dickinson, G.E. and Field, D.** (2002). Teaching end-of-life issues: current status in United Kingdom and United States medical schools. *American Journal of Hospice and Palliative Care* **19**, 181–6.
29. **Charlton, R. and Smith, G.** (2000). Perceived skills in palliative medicine of newly qualified doctors in the UK. *Journal of Palliative Care* **16**, 27–32.
30. **Block, S.D.** (2002). Medical education in end-of-life care: the status of reform. *Journal of Palliative Medicine* **5**, 243–8.
31. **Mount, B.M.** (1976). The problem of caring for the dying in a general hospital; the palliative care unit as a possible solution. *Canadian Medical Association Journal* **115**, 119–21.
32. **Bates, T.D., Hoy, A.M., Clarke, D.G., and Laird, P.P.** (1981). The St Thomas' Hospital terminal care support team—a new concept of hospice care. *Lancet* **1**, 1201–3.
33. **Dunlop, R. and Hockley, J.** *Terminal Care Support Teams: The Hospital–Hospice Interface.* Oxford: Oxford University Press, 1990.
34. **Royal College of Radiologists.** *Structured Training in Clinical Oncology.* Ref: EBCO (95)1, 1995 (available at www.rcr.ac.uk).
35. **Royal College of Anaesthetists.** *CCST in Anaesthesia parts I, II, III,* 2002 (available from: www.rcoa.ac.uk/publications).
36. **The Bristol Royal Infirmary Inquiry** (2001). *Kennedy Report.* London: HMSO, 2001 (available at www.bristol-inquiry.org.uk/final_report/report).
37. **Royal College of Surgeons of England.** *Manual of Basic Surgical Training,* 1998 (available at www.rcseng.ac.uk/surgical/trainees/sho_bst/bluebook.pdf).
38. **Association for Palliative Medicine of Great Britain and Ireland** (1999). *Continuing Professional Development. Palliative Medicine Curriculum for Specialists in Other Fields and General Practitioners.* Southampton: APM, 1999 (available from: 11 Westwood Road, Southampton, SO17 1DL, UK).
39. **Rawlinson, F. and Finlay, I.** (2002). Assessing education in palliative medicine: development of a tool based on the Association for Palliative Medicine core curriculum. *Palliative Medicine* **16**, 51–5.
40. **Nash, A. and Hoy, A.** (1993). Terminal care in the community—an evaluation of residential workshops for general practitioner/district nurse teams. *Palliative Medicine* **7**, 5–17.
41. **Wee, B., Hillier, R., Coles, C., Mountford, B., Sheldon, F., and Turner, P.** (2001). Palliative care: a suitable setting for undergraduate interprofessional education. *Palliative Medicine* **15**, 487–92.
42. **Koffman, J.** (2001). Multiprofessional palliative care education: past challenges, future issues. *Journal of Palliative Care* **17**, 86–92.
43. **Watson, M.** (2003). *Evaluation of Assessment Methods in a Palliative Care Education Course,* MSc Thesis. University of Wales College of Medicine
44. **Graham, J., Ramirez, A.J., Cull, A., Finlay, I., Hoy, A., and Richards, M.A.** (1996). Job stress and satisfaction among palliative physicians. *Palliative Medicine* **10**, 185–94.
45. **Federation of Medical Royal Colleges.** *Census of Consultant Physicians in the UK, 2001. Data and commentary.* London: RCP, 2002.
46. **MacLeod, R.** (2000). Learning to care: a medical perspective. *Palliative Medicine* **14**, 209–16.
47. **Royal College of Physicians of London.** *Consultants Physicians Working for Patients. The Duties, Responsibilities and Practice of Physicians* 2nd edn. London: RCP, 2001.
48. **Hoy, A.** (2001). Palliative medicine. In *So You Want to be a Brain Surgeon?* 2nd edn. (ed. C. Ward and S. Eccles), pp. 116–17. Oxford: Oxford University Press.
49. **NHS Executive** (1998). *A Guide to Specialist Registrar Training.* London: Department of Health, 1998, pp. 139–54.
50. **Association for Palliative Medicine.** *Descriptors of Competencies.* Southampton: APM, 2002 (available at www.palliative-medicine.org).
51. **Association for Palliative Medicine.** *Specialist Registrars' Research. The Way Ahead.* Southampton: APM, 2001 (available at www.palliative-medicine.org).
52. **O'Keefe, K.** (1999). Specialist palliative care needs specialists. *Palliative Medicine* **13**, 181–2.
53. **Fordham, S., Dowrick, C., and May, C.** (1998). Palliative medicine: is it really specialist territory? *Journal of the Royal Society of Medicine* **91**, 568–72.
54. **Douglas, C.** (1992). For all the saints. *British Medical Journal* **304**, 579.
55. **Holman, G.H. and Forman, W.B.** (2001). On the 10th anniversary of the organization of the American Academy of Hospice and Palliative Medicine (AAHPM): the first 10 years. *American Journal of Hospice & Palliative Care* **18**, 275–8.
56. **Casarett, D.J.** (2000). The future of the palliative medicine fellowship. *Journal of Palliative Medicine* **3**, 151–5.
57. **Von Gunten, C.F., Sloan, P.A., Portenoy, R.K., and Schonwetter, R.S.** (2000). Physician board certification in hospice and palliative medicine. *Journal of Palliative Medicine* **3**, 441–7.
58. **European Association for Palliative Care (online)** (www.eapcnet.org).
59. **Asia Pacific Hospice Palliative Care Network** (www.APHN.org).
60. **International Association for Hospice and Palliative Care** (lidelima@iahpc.com).
61. **National Hospice and Palliative Care Organization** (www.nhpco.org).
62. www.hospiceinformation.info

20.4 Learning counselling

Peter Maguire and Carolyn Pitceathly

Counselling in palliative care should have two objectives: first, to identify accurately the key concerns of patients and carers, whether they be physical, social, psychological, or spiritual in nature; second, to help patients and carers find strategies to resolve those concerns that can be resolved or adapt to those that cannot. Achieving these objectives should reduce levels of emotional distress and the likelihood of patients and/or carers developing an affective disorder (adjustment disorder, generalized anxiety disorder, or major depressive illness) for strong links have been found between concerns and psychological morbidity.

Concerns and psychological adjustment

The number and severity of concerns provoked by a diagnosis of cancer and treatments employed has been found to predict high levels of emotional distress 6 months later.[1] Similarly, Parle et al.[2] followed up over 600 cancer patients and found the number and severity of concerns patients reported within 8 weeks of diagnosis predicted the development of affective disorders over the next year. Patients were only included if they were judged by the treating clinician to have a strong chance of surviving 2 years or more. Similar relationships between concerns and psychological morbidity have been confirmed in patients receiving palliative care,[3] who report even more concerns than those with earlier stages of disease.

Unfortunately, regardless of disease stage, only 40 per cent of patients' concerns[2,4] are likely to be known to health professionals involved in their care. Consequently, there can be a considerable disparity between the known and undisclosed concerns. Heaven and Maguire[3] compared the responses of patients in audio-taped interviews with hospice nurses, with responses the same patients gave when a short checklist of concerns was administered by a research nurse. Patients talked mainly to the hospice nurses about physical symptoms. Important psychosocial concerns like worry about being a burden to the family, the impact of cachexia on their loved ones, and fears of how they might die were only disclosed to the research nurse. Yet, these patients would have welcomed an opportunity to talk about these issues had they been actively encouraged to do so.

If patients fail to disclose their main concerns, attempts to counsel them will be less effective. The problem is likely to be even greater with their carers[5,6] as carers believe the patient should be the priority and they do not voice their own concerns.

The low disclosure and identification of patients' and carers' concerns may explain, in part, why the prevalence of affective disorders remains high. In 1983, Derogatis et al.[7] found up to one-third of cancer patients were so affected. Nearly 20 years later Hoptof et al.[8] found that 29 per cent of palliative care patients were probable cases of depression.

Affective disorders seriously impair quality of life, relationships within the family, and hinder open communication and resolution of unfinished business. This can hinder the processing of grief by carers and lead to psychiatric morbidity. Yet, affective disorders are recognized in only half of those patients and carers who develop them.[9,10] As discussed later, counselling patients and carers who are too depressed or anxious to benefit can intensify their problems.

It is crucial, therefore, to understand the barriers to disclosure, learn how to overcome them, and recognize when patients are suffering from depression and/or anxiety.

Barriers to disclosure

Patients, carers, and health professionals all create barriers to full disclosure and the main reasons will be discussed.

Patient and carer barriers

Patients and carers tend to believe that problems that develop as a result of cancer progression and lack of curative treatment are inevitable. Anxious or depressed mood is viewed as an understandable reaction to their predicament for which nothing can be done.[11] Physical symptoms like pain and breathlessness are often unreported for similar reasons.[12] Patients have usually come to respect and like the doctors and nurses who are doing their best to care for them. So, they are particularly reluctant to burden them with concerns about dying or fears of how they might die for which there are no easy answers.

Patients who are struggling to cope emotionally may fear that admitting this will lead them to being viewed as 'ungrateful', 'neurotic', or 'pathetic', particularly as other patients and carers appear to be coping well. They fail to realize that many others are putting on 'a brave face' for similar reasons.

These beliefs are reinforced by health professionals who do not actively enquire about patients' key concerns, perceptions of their predicament, and the emotional and practical impact of it on them and their families. Even when patients give signals that all is not well they are likely to be met by doctors and nurses using strategies designed to block disclosure.[11,13] For example, distress may be dismissed as normal and remain unexplored. Most commonly, concerns will be responded to with premature reassurance ('there is no need to worry, we'll get your pain under control'). This reassurance was premature because the doctor had not understood the basis for the concern. This patient with advanced ovarian cancer had seen her husband suffer intractable pain before he died from lung cancer only 6 months previously.

Overcoming patient and carer barriers

Health-care professionals need to be proactive in their assessments by asking patients and carers about their perceptions of and emotional reactions to key events, such as diagnosis of cancer recurrence, cessation of active treatment, or serious deterioration in health ('when your breathing got worse again what did you think was going on? how did you feel about it? what has been the effect of this on you and your family?'). This style of questioning educates patients that they can disclose their views and feelings about key events and the impact on them and their families.

Asking the basic questions is insufficient. The responses they generate must be acknowledged and clarified so that the nature and extent of the patients' or carers' concerns are established.

> You mention you have been devastated about losing so much weight. Exactly how much weight have you lost? . . . over what period of time? . . . what was your normal weight before you became ill?

It is then important to explore the reasons for the patient's concerns about weight loss rather than assume what they are.

> You say you are devastated about losing all this weight. Can you bear to tell me why?

This may reveal that the patient is concerned about body image, the aggressiveness of the cancer, dying, exhaustion, or other issues.

The use of negotiation ('can you bear to tell me?') allows patients who find it too distressing to discuss such issues to decline to do so ('I'd prefer not to go into it. It is too painful').

Hints about how patients and carers are feeling emotionally should be pursued similarly.

> You say you feel miserable. Can you tell me just how miserable you have been? What are you like at your lowest? How much of the time do you feel so low?

Active responding like this educates patients and carers that it is legitimate to talk about their emotional reactions as well as physical problems.

Sometimes when patients or carers claim all is well their non-verbal behaviour suggests otherwise. The health professional should feed back this intuition in the form of an educated but tentative guess.

> You say you have no pain. But as we talk I get the feeling from how you are sitting and moving you might be in some pain?
>
> Yes I am. I'm getting a lot of pain in my back where the cancer is. I find it hard to get comfortable. It is very frustrating. It keeps reminding me my cancer is not going to get better.

Putting educated guesses in a tentative form allows patients or carers to elaborate, correct, or refute it. It does not matter if the guess is wrong. It educates the patient or carer that the health professional is trying to understand what they are experiencing.

The use of empathy also signals that the health professional is trying to understand the patients' or carers' reactions.

Mrs B

What really gets to me is I got my cancer three months after Sarah was born. Despite chemotherapy it is back. I know I won't make it and see her grow up.

Dr A

It must be awful for you to realise you are not going to see your child grow up?

Mrs B

It seems so unfair, so cruel.

If patients and carers are to develop sufficient trust to disclose all their key concerns they need feedback that they have been heard and understood. The frequent use of summarizing by the health professional provides this evidence. It also allows for the correction of any misunderstandings.

Can I just check what you have been saying? Your wife had high dose chemotherapy and a bone marrow transplant after her lymphoma came back. This went well initially but then she got a cytomegalovirus. She's now desperately ill and may die. You are finding it hard to cope with the strain of it all and afraid you won't be able to live without her. Have I understood?

The use of these strategies maximizes patient and carer disclosure. An increasing number of health professionals in palliative care are aware of these strategies or have acquired them through courses or workshops.[14,15] Yet, they may not use them in practice when they encounter certain difficult situations that they are not confident to deal with. These situations are described in the next section and strategies for dealing with them outlined.

Other reasons for health professional's reluctance to explore patients' and carers' concerns were discussed in Chapters 12.1 and 12.2.

Handling difficult situations

Patients whose fears seem understandable

There is a considerable risk when patients say they fear the future, are worried about dying, or do not know how they will tolerate the difficult treatments on offer, that their concerns will be dismissed as understandable and not explored. Health professionals may feel it is stupid or insensitive to ask why patients are worried when they know they have a terminal illness and there is nothing that can be done to change that reality. However, there are two reasons why health-care professionals should overcome their fears of asking a question like: 'can you bear to say what you are worried about?'

First, patients' and carers' concerns are not predictable. A patient who says he is worried about dying may be worried about how he will die, not seeing his children grow up, being cared for in hospital instead of home, or about who will look after his dog when he dies. The patient or carer is the expert on what his/her worries are and needs to be asked about them.

Second, even when patients' and carers' concerns cannot be resolved they experience great relief from sharing them with a health professional who wants to understand where they are in their cancer journey.

Patients or carers who appear to have no problems

Health professionals are more likely to be thrown when palliative patients appear cheerful and say there is nothing they wish to talk about than when they acknowledge they are distressed. It is important for health professionals to be honest about their concerns, and not avoid checking out the situation. For example, they may say 'You always seem so cheerful. I want you to know, however, that if you have any concerns we're here to help. Can I just check if there is anything at all at the moment that is worrying you about your illness or the situation in general, even though you say you are coping well?'

This approach encourages patients and carers who are putting on a brave face to talk about issues that they have not disclosed. It enables them to explain why they are untroubled by their situation. For example, a palliative care team was concerned when a young woman recently diagnosed as suffering from terminal breast cancer, and with only a few weeks to live, said that she did not have any problems she needed to discuss with the team. She explained she just wanted to talk to her husband on the ward and then be allowed to go home, so that she could die there.

The team were convinced that she must have undisclosed concerns. After her death, her husband returned to the ward and thanked the team for the care they gave his wife. He was grateful that they had allowed her to spend what little time she had left with him at home. He made it clear that his wife had come to terms with her imminent death, had talked through key issues with him and close friends, and had no need of counselling.

So it is important to acknowledge that many patients and carers cope well using their own resources and the support of friends and relatives and do not need counselling imposed upon them.

Patients and relatives who are not talking together

Health professionals may be worried when they think that the dying patient and key relative are not talking together about their shared predicament, even though they are willing to talk separately to staff about their concerns.

It is easier not to intrude and let them get on with this way of coping. However, gentle acknowledgement that they are not finding it easy to talk to each other about what is happening may allow the couple to agree that there is a problem and they need help to be more open. Alternatively, they may acknowledge that it is too painful to talk together and that they need support as separate individuals.

Patients or relatives who are angry

Health professionals in palliative care will usually have done their best to ensure that patients and relatives obtain good symptom control and as optimal a social and psychological adjustment as possible. It can be upsetting, therefore, when a patient or carer is angry about the care being given (especially if the health professional is feeling tired at the end of a demanding shift).

It is tempting for health professionals to become defensive, argue back, and suggest that the patients' and relatives' anger is unjustified. Such defensiveness will merely serve to escalate the level of anger instead of containing it and lead to complaints about the care given and litigation.

The hardest, but most effective step is to accept that their anger may have a rational basis and be related to real concerns. So, it is important for health professionals to remain calm, acknowledge that the patient or relative is angry, and invite them to explain how angry they are and the reasons they have for their anger. It is important to elicit all the possible reasons contributing to the anger before any attempt is made to respond: ('I can see you're angry, can you bear to tell me exactly how angry you are and why? Are there any other reasons why you're angry?'). This will lead patients and relatives to disclose the level of their anger, and all the concerns that are contributing to it. As they are encouraged to express feelings and concerns there should be an obvious lessening in the intensity of anger. A clear transition should occur when they volunteer other feelings like sadness or despair. These should be acknowledged and explored.

In the following example, a palliative care nurse working in the community was faced with anger from a relative who believed that her mother's care was inadequate:

Nurse M

I gather you wanted to talk to me.

Mrs S

I certainly do. What kind of care do you call this? You've been coming round to see my mother for some weeks now. You promised you'd be able to help her, but she is getting much worse. She's in constant pain. She cannot get out of her bed. She is getting increasingly upset and distressed by what's happening. I want to know what's going on.

Nurse M

I can see you're very angry about all this, would you like to say if there is anything else making you angry.

Mrs S

Isn't it obvious? You can see the state my mother's in. She is suffering all the time. She's very upset and weepy. You wouldn't allow a dog to suffer like this?

Nurse M

Are there any other reasons why you're angry?

Mrs S

She's been a wonderful mother. There's no way she should suffer like this. I can't bear the thought I'm going to lose her soon; we've been so close (begins to weep). I don't know how I'm going to live without her.

Nurse M

I can see it's hard for you to see her suffering like this, especially as you've been so close. I can also understand that you're upset about the thought that you're going to lose her soon. Before we talk more about these concerns, can I check if you have any other concerns?

Mrs S

I'm desperate that something be done to ease her suffering.

Nurse M

Is that your main concern or is there anything else you would like me to start with?

Mrs S

(Still crying) I'm just desperate about her suffering, can anything be done?

Nurse M

Let's look at what we've tried so far and what we might do differently, is that alright?

At the end of this session Mrs S felt calmer in herself. She was much less angry, but still concerned about whether adequate pain control could be achieved.

Sometimes, these strategies for defusing anger fail. This is usually because the patient has hidden reasons for being so angry. These reasons cannot be guessed at. Instead the patient or carer should be invited to consider 'Is there anything else that might be making you so angry, maybe relating to experiences you have had in the past?' This usually produces answers like 'I just can't believe this is happening again. I lost my first wife from cancer. She endured terrible pain. I can't believe it's happening to my second wife in the same way'.

Once the anger is defused and the current concerns elicited it is possible to move on to counselling.

Patients or relatives in denial

When patients or relatives are in denial, it is impossible to elicit their concerns and worries because they have none. Others will not be in true denial. The question is how far to probe to see if they are willing to consider what is going on. The key is to offer patients and carers opportunities to reflect on their predicament rather than force these realities on to those who may find them unbearable.

There are two ways this can be done safely. The first is to challenge inconsistencies in the history. 'I am puzzled. You say you are going to be alright and recover, but you also say you have been losing weight again and have been coughing up more blood?' The patient may respond by saying 'I'm sure the coughing up blood and losing weight are due to an infection' or give an opening 'I guess I'm just trying to kid myself that everything is alright'. When patients give an opening it is important to follow this up quickly by saying, 'When you stop kidding yourself what do you think about?'.

If challenging inconsistencies in the history does not overcome apparent denial, it is important to ask if there is ever a moment when they consider that things would not work out. If there is such a 'window on denial' they should be asked if they are prepared to talk more about their doubts.

If patients are willing they should be asked to explain what their doubts are and the reasons for them. They should be encouraged to talk about how they feel and to voice the associated concerns.

It is important to check if they are finding this discussion too painful and wish to put it on the 'back burner' or would be prepared to talk again on another occasion.

When patients prefer to remain in denial it is important to let them know that if a time comes when they want to talk about what is happening the team will be there for them.

The withdrawn patient

Some patients can be difficult to engage in conversation especially when their disease is advancing and they are suffering pain or other major physical symptoms like breathlessness. It is important, therefore, to establish whether they wish to remain 'cut off' from conversation, or are willing to talk.

In beginning to talk with such patients the difficulty soon becomes apparent. They may have muttered that they cannot be bothered to talk or do not want to. Acknowledge this behaviour by saying 'I can see we are having difficulty getting into a conversation. Can you give me any clues as to why that is'. They will usually respond with helpful clues like 'I'm feeling too down', 'too confused', 'too angry', or by saying 'there is no point in talking'. These clues should be followed up to establish whether the lack of conversation is due to the patient feeling depressed, angry, confused, hopeless, or whether there are other reasons. It should then be possible to negotiate with the patient whether to either have a dialogue or postpone it until an underlying problem like depression or confusion has been dealt with. Where the patient believes that talking will not help, it is important to acknowledge this and say 'You are quite right, talking won't help in the sense of curing your disease, but it might help you feel less distressed about what is going on. I can't promise talking will be of help, but, perhaps we should give it a try to see if it will'.

Dealing with distress and despair

Health professionals often feel inhibited by patients or carers who appear very distressed or in despair at the outset of the consultation. They avoid probing because they fear the distress will be overwhelming and cause psychological damage. Paradoxically, highly distressed or despairing patients and carers need to feel that the health professional is prepared to cross this barrier in order to engage with them and understand what they are feeling and why. Health professionals should, therefore, acknowledge the distress and despair they are witnessing by saying 'I can see you're extremely upset at the moment'. They should then negotiate with the patient or carer to determine whether they are prepared to take this further 'Can you bear to tell me why you're so distressed?' If the patient or carer says 'No it's too painful', this should be respected. However, most patients or carers will give permission for further exploration. It is then important to say, 'In that case can you tell me exactly why you are so distressed'. This will allow patients and carers to disclose their main concerns. They should then be helped to put these into priority order. They can then be dealt with in turn, as 'time allows'.

When a health professional uses these strategies, the patient's level of distress or despair should ease. If it does not, the possibility that he/she is suffering from a depressive illness and/or anxiety state should be considered.

Dealing with the manipulative patient or relative

It can be off-putting for health professionals to be faced with patients who appear manipulative. For example, they may claim to have consistent pain and demand painkillers frequently. When observed by other staff they appear to be comfortable within the ward and pain free. Alternatively, patients may split staff by saying one thing to one member and something else to another. The sooner manipulative behaviour is acknowledged and explored the better, if there is going to be any hope of the patient's behaviour becoming more appropriate. Health professionals should share with the patient or carer their recognition of the behaviour without being judgemental. The patient or carer should then be invited to consider why they might be behaving like that. This will usually reveal major concerns they have not disclosed. It is important to check if there has been manipulative behaviour in the past since it may be as much a product of their personality as their current predicament.

When it is a product of their current predicament they should be encouraged to disclose their true concerns and these should be discussed and dealt with. If it is a product of their personality it is important to set limits about what they can and cannot do within the consultation or ward setting.

> I am concerned that you tell some of the nurses you have no problems you need help with. Then you complain to other nurses that you are in constant pain and say you are being neglected. I know this has happened before when you have been ill. Unless you trust us all with what is going on, we will not be able to help you.

Collusion—requests for the patient or carer not to be told the truth

Some relatives insist that patients be kept ignorant of their prognosis. Similarly, patients might insist that relatives should not be told the truth. Since collusion leads to greater anxiety and depression in the short and longer term, attempts should be made to overcome it.

The patient or carer should be invited to explain their reasons for colluding. These should be acknowledged and respected. For example, a husband may say 'my wife has always said she would not want to know if she were dying'. He should be asked to consider the costs of collusion in terms of the distress it may be causing him and how it is affecting his relationship with his wife, who is the victim of the collusion. This usually reveals that collusion is being maintained at considerable emotional cost to the colluder and has resulted in a barrier forming between himself and the wife he loves.

Awareness of these costs causes most patients or carers to reconsider their strategy. The health professional can then suggest they have a joint meeting to promote openness about what is going on and discuss current concerns. At this point carers may be reassured to know that if patients signal that they do not want to know, it will not be thrust upon them.

As well as acquiring the strategies and confidence to elicit concerns and deal with difficult situations, health professionals involved in counselling should be equipped, as discussed earlier, to recognize and refer patients and carers with significant mental health problems.

Recognizing mental health problems (see Chapter 8.17)

When patients have developed major depressive illnesses and/or anxiety disorder it is unlikely they will respond to counselling alone. Being clinically depressed means that patients or carers will find it extremely hard, or impossible, to connect with positive thoughts about their predicament. Talking about it, without suitable medical help may make them more anxious or depressed and even suicidal. It is, therefore, crucial that health professionals involved in counselling in palliative care know how to identify when patients or carers are clinically anxious and depressed. It is also critical that they can identify those who may be at risk of suicide or, albeit rarely, homicide.

Unfortunately, health professionals involved in counselling patients with advanced disease or their carers often delay referring them for help. They believe the mood disturbance is understandable, that nothing can be done about it, or believe it will respond to counselling alone.

Depression

Depression should be diagnosed when a patient or carer complains of persistent low mood for more than 2 weeks or loss of ability to enjoy life, over a similar period. The change in natural mood should be substantial, quantitatively and qualitatively, even when compared with periods when the patient has been unhappy. Despite their best efforts, they cannot pull themselves or be pulled out of it. The mood change should be accompanied by at least four or more other symptoms. These could be sleep disturbance (repeated or early morning wakening, excessive sleep), irritability, impairment of attention and concentration, restlessness or retardation, social withdrawal, negative ideation (ideas of hopelessness, self-blame, guilt, worthlessness, feeling a burden, seeing no future, seeing life as pointless), suicidal ideation (where life does not seem worth living and ways of committing suicide may have been contemplated), and diurnal variation of mood where mood is obviously worse at a particular time of day.

In arriving at a diagnosis of depression it is important to base it on the presence of depressed mood plus the associated symptoms rather than any consideration of how understandable it is in the context of advancing disease. Otherwise, all depression will be dismissed as understandable and not worthy of medication. The extent to which symptoms, like sleep disturbance, can be fully explained by physical symptoms like pain, disease progression, or medication should be taken into account.

Patients and carers who are experiencing low mood should be asked 'What are you like at your lowest?', 'How do you see the future?', and 'Have you ever felt so low you have considered ending your life?' If suicide risk appears a problem a psychiatric assessment should be arranged urgently.

Anxiety

Anxious mood should be diagnosed when a patient complains of a persistent inability to relax or stop worrying and this represents a significant change both qualitatively and quantitatively. The patient cannot distract himself or herself out of it or be distracted by others. The anxious mood must be accompanied by four or more of the following symptoms before a generalized anxiety disorder can be diagnosed: difficulty getting off to sleep, irritability, sweating, tremor or nausea, impaired concentration, indecisiveness, and spontaneous panic attacks. Patients with generalized anxiety may also suffer from fear of specific situations like meeting people or leaving the house alone.

Referral

When patients with mood disturbance are encountered it is important to ensure they are assessed medically so that they can be given appropriate medication by a palliative care doctor, general practitioner, or psychiatrist to alleviate their anxiety and depression. The mood disturbance must be treated promptly since it should assist symptom control and aid counselling.

Patients who are referred to a psychiatrist or offered medication should be given an explanation about why they have become anxious or depressed. For example, it helps to explain that depression is due to changes in brain chemistry caused by the stress patients experience on hearing that their cancer had progressed or is no longer treatable. So, medication is needed to help the brain produce the necessary chemicals again and will need to be continued for 4–6 months to forestall any relapse.

It is important to emphasize that medication is only the first step in helping them. They can then be given psychological support to deal with any residual concerns as their mood begins to lift. Tablets should be taken as prescribed and not just on an 'as needed' basis.

When first-line treatment by the palliative care doctors or general practitioner has not worked, health professionals may avoid making a psychiatric referral. They fear that patients and carers will feel stigmatized. The patient may think the health professional believes that he is going mad or is pathetic in his inability to cope. It is also important that health professionals are aware when patients are becoming confused. They may complain of changes in memory and problems in orientating themselves to time, date, and place. Where there is any doubt about their capacity to cope with counselling a medical opinion should be sought to clarify their mental state and suitability.

Methods of learning counselling skills

Several components are necessary if health professionals are to improve their ability to identify patients' and carers' concerns, and help them resolve or adapt to them.[16]

The barriers to effective communication, the contribution of patients, carers, and health professionals to these and the reasons for them should be made explicit. Strategies for overcoming these barriers should be presented before giving health professionals a chance to practice them in safe conditions, for example, in role-play.

Presenting of strategies

Videotapes demonstrating how to do it and how not to do it have been used.[17] The disadvantage of video tapes is that the patient or carer is not there to validate the strategies used. Participants have to accept the word of the tutor or facilitator that strategies were positive both in terms of disclosure and emotional impact. If they disagree there is no way to resolve this. The use of interactive demonstration overcomes this problem.

Interactive demonstration

In an interactive demonstration a facilitator simulates the history of a patient or carer he or she has encountered in clinical practice. The story is adapted to fit the facilitator's own real-life situation. The simulated patient is then interviewed by a second facilitator who seeks to elicit the patient's or carer's current concerns and feelings. In doing so the facilitator follows his or her normal assessment task, whether it be as doctor, nurse, or social worker.

The facilitator asks the group of health professionals for advice about how to start the interview and elicits the reasons for their suggestions. The interview is audiotaped so that the strategies tried can be listened to again and the participants views about their effectiveness and impact on the patient can be discussed. These views are then validated or refuted by asking the patient how he or she was affected.

The interview is continued and particular attention is paid to eliciting and trying out competing strategies. For example, the patient said she was very upset by news that there was no more active treatment. The facilitator stopped the interview and asked the group how he should respond. Half the group said he should ignore the cue since it was obvious why she was upset. Enquiry would upset her even more. The remainder wanted him to acknowledge her cue and negotiate to explore it.

Both strategies were tried in turn. It was evident from the patient's feedback that ventilating and explaining the basis of her upset was beneficial to her.

Practice in role-play

Participants are asked to define the exact communication situations they find difficult and are then encouraged to practice tackling them in role-play. Role-play is used because the nature of the task and the level of complexity can be tailored to participants' needs. Since they have chosen a difficult task they are encouraged to stop the interview if they feel stuck and ask the group what they should do next. The reasons for their getting stuck are explored by the facilitator. The problem may be a fear of explaining painful feelings, or uncertainties about how to move the interview forward. Either way, the participant's difficulties are made explicit and they have an opportunity to try out different strategies. Participants also gain valuable insight from simulating patients or carers they found difficult to deal with in their recent practice.

If role-play is to result in effective learning two conditions need to be met. First, the apprehensions of participants about role-play and exposing their communication and counselling behaviours in front of others should be addressed. Explicit ground rules for making it as safe as possible and minimizing the risks of deskilling should then be introduced. These include making the task realistic and clear, checking it is personally safe for the interviewer to take on and will not trigger past adverse experiences, ensuring the agreed level of complexity is adhered to, checking the simulator feels all right to take on the role, reminding interviewers to stop if they feel stuck, and then the group will advise them on what they might do next. Positive feedback must be exhausted before constructive criticisms are offered.

Workshops using these methods help health professionals improve their ability to elicit concerns and respond to them.[14] A major question is how well they transfer these basic methods of counselling to the workplace.

Promoting transfer

Short workshops and courses help participants acquire the skills needed to elicit patients' and carers' concerns, respond to them, handle difficult situations, and learn to recognize anxiety and depression.[18,19] However, this is not sufficient to ensure the application and maintenance of skills in the workplace. Booster workshops have proved helpful in maintaining skills, but facilitators giving feedback to health professionals on audio- or videotape recordings of real consultations is likely to prove the most effective method of promoting transfer.[20] Feedback from supervisors who were present at real consultations produced definite but limited transfer.[21] Unfortunately, there are still too few facilitators capable of giving the necessary feedback.

More advanced counselling

More specialist palliative care nurses are seeking to augment their basic counselling skills by obtaining diplomas in counselling and/or attending courses that teach behavioural, cognitive–behavioural, or psycho-dynamic methods. Some of these methods are mentioned to illustrate the range available, but their exact merits in palliative care remain unclear.

Methods of counselling

Greer et al.[22] developed an adjuvant psychological therapy. It is based on cognitive behavioural principles and requires between six and eight hourly sessions. It aims to help cancer patients increase their self-esteem, overcome feelings of helplessness, and promote a fighting spirit. It has been applied successfully to patients with advanced cancer and appears more effective than non-directive counseling.[23]

Nezu et al.[24] have advocated a problem-solving therapy. Regardless of disease stage, it aims to help patients improve their problem-solving skills, to reduce their emotional distress, and increase their sense of control.

Spira[25] developed a method of existentialist psychotherapy. This encourages patients to use their predicament as an opportunity to shed habitual assumptions about life and help them engage in activities that bring the greatest meaning, purpose, and value to their lives.

Speigel and colleagues[26] have evaluated weekly support groups for patients with advanced cancer. Their methods include: encouraging mutual support, discussion of specific fears, helping patients reorder their priorities and identify areas of unfinished business, and make better use of health professionals and other support networks.

Pitceathly and Maguire[6] have developed a flexible one to six session intervention for partners of cancer patients when the patients have become clinically depressed. A substantial minority of these patients have been receiving palliative care. The parties are invited to share their experiences of the patient's illness, identify their current concerns, and explore how they might resolve these difficulties, whether by problem-solving or cognitive reappraisal.

Personal boundaries

Even at the basic concerns level, counselling can be emotionally demanding. Health professionals have a right to protect themselves from an excessive load and set limits. Thus, patients and carers need to be orientated to the goals of counselling, the duration, and likely number of sessions. Progress can be reviewed after this period. This structure protects the health professional from patients or carers becoming over-dependent and having unrealistic expectations. It also reduces the risk of health professionals becoming over-involved and devaluing the ability of patients and carers to find effective ways of coping, using their own resources.

Over-involvement is likely to occur when the patient or carer reminds the health professional, consciously or unconsciously, of someone important in their own life. When patients or carers demand more than the offered time or contact between sessions the reasons should be explored. Signs of over-involvement include giving much more time than usual, being available at any time and preoccupation with thoughts of the patient or carer. The health professional should ask himself or herself 'Why am I so involved? Do they remind me of someone in my past or present life?'.

When a health professional giving counselling is going through a personal crisis like a recent bereavement, relationship break-up, or finds that a clinical situation triggers intensely painful memories of past illness or loss, he/she should question the wisdom of counselling that patient or carer. Similarly, if the patient or carer triggers strong feelings of anger or dislike, the health professional should reflect on the origin of these feelings and consider referring on to a colleague.

Despite a realistic initial assessment and decision to counsel, health professionals can soon find themselves out of their depth. For example, a patient who seemed straightforward revealed in a subsequent session that her disease progression had reactivated strong memories of childhood abuse. The specialist nurse had the sense to refer the patient to a psychotherapist.

Continuing to counsel patients and carers when they are not making progress and are sounding 'like a gramophone record' or have become clinically depressed or anxious should cause the health professional to ask 'What are my personal reasons for holding on?'.

When health professionals in palliative care are counselling in isolation from colleagues it is hard to acknowledge and observe these boundaries. Burnout can then occur with the development of feelings of emotional detachment, emotional exhaustion, and low personal accomplishment. Burnout is less likely when support and supervision are provided.

Support and supervision

If health professionals are to relinquish the use of strategies designed to block patient or carer disclosure they need to feel they are valued as persons within the workplace and know they can obtain help if they encounter difficulties.[27] They should be able to talk to colleagues with a similar role and share successes as well as problems regularly.

Ideally, those involved in counselling should attend a supervision group. They can talk about problems they are encountering with patients, carers, and colleagues and receive advice and support. They can reflect on issues like over-involvement, dislike of clients, or problems of patient advocacy. These groups should be run by skilled facilitators with a knowledge of the counselling methods being used and of group dynamics.

One-to-one personal supervision can permit health professionals to work through relevant issues at a more personal level. It can help them become aware of 'blind spots', may be situations they are less effective with or avoid consistently. They can then explore the reasons for this which are usually rooted in their own biography or professional experience and can try to resolve their conflicts.

For example, a specialist palliative care nurse found herself unable to represent her patients' counselling needs to the medical team. They would try to minimize these and restrict discussions to medical matters. She found she became defensive, upset, and gave up trying. Then she felt guilty and pathetic. Supervision helped her trace the origins of this reaction to an overcritical authoritarian father and she found ways of successfully asserting her patients' needs.

While support and supervision are essential to effective counselling and emotional survival of the health professional they are often not provided at an adequate level. Health professionals, in particular, can then pay too high a price for their commitment to patients and carers.

References

1. **Weisman, A.D. and Worden, J.W.** (1977). The existential plight of cancer: significance of the first 100 days. *International Journal of Psychological Medicine* **7**, 1–15.
2. **Parle, M., Jones, B., and Maguire, P.** (1996). Maladaptive coping and affective disorders in cancer patients. *Psychological Medicine* **26**, 735–44.
3. **Heaven, C.M. and Maguire, P.** (1998). The relationship between patients' concerns and psychological distress in a hospice setting. *Psycho-Oncology* **7**, 502–7.
4. **Heaven, C.M. and Maguire, P.** (1997). Disclosure of concerns by hospice patients and their identification by nurses. *Palliative Medicine* **11**, 283–90.
5. **Maguire, P., Walsh, S., Jeacock, J., and Kingston, R.** (1999). Physical and psychological needs of patients dying from anorectal cancer. *Palliative Medicine* **13**, 45–50.
6. **Pitceathly, C. and Maguire, P.** (2000). Preventing affective disorders in partners of cancer patients: an intervention study. In *Cancer and the Family* (ed. L. Baider, C.L. Cooper, A. Kaplan De-Nour), pp. 137–54. New York: John Wiley.
7. **Derogatis, L.R., Morrow, G.R., Fetting, J., Penman, D., Piasetsky, S., Schmale, H.M., Henrichs, M., and Carmickel, L.M.** (1983). The prevalence of psychiatric disorders among cancer patients. *Journal of the American Medical Association* **249**, 751–7.
8. **Hoptoff, M., Chidgey, J., and Addington-Hall, J.** (2002). Depression in advanced disease: a systematic review Part 1. Prevalence and case finding. *Palliative Medicine* **16**, 181–97.
9. **Hardman, A., Maguire, P., and Crowther, D.** (1989). The recognition of psychiatric morbidity on a medical oncology ward. *Journal of Psychosomatic Research* **33**, 235–7.
10. **Fulton, C.** (1998). The prevalence and detection of psychiatric morbidity in patients with metastatic breast cancer. *European Journal of Cancer Care* **7**, 232–9.
11. **Maguire, P.** (1985). Barriers to psychological care of the dying. *British Medical Journal* **291**, 1711–13.
12. **Glajchen, M., Blum, D., and Calder, K.** (1995). Cancer pain management and the role of social work: barriers and interventions. *Health and Social Work* **20** (3), 200–6.
13. **Wilkinson, S.** (1991). Factors which influence how nurses communicate with cancer patients. *Journal of Advanced Nursing* **16**, 677–88.
14. **Maguire, P., Faulkner, A., Booth, K., Elliott, C., and Hillier, V.** (1996). Helping cancer patients disclose their concerns. *European Journal of Cancer* **32A**, 78–81.
15. **Wilkinson, S., Roberts, A., and Aldridge, J.** (1988). Nurse–patient communication in palliative care: an evaluation of a communication skills programme. *Palliative Medicine* **12**, 13–22.
16. **Parle, M., Maguire, P., and Heaven, C.** (1997). The development of a training model to improve health professionals' skills, self-efficacy and outcome expectancies when communicating with cancer patients. *Social Science and Medicine* **16**, 483–91.
17. **Maguire, P. and Faulkner, A.** (1988). Improving the counselling skills of doctors and nurses in cancer care. 1. How to do it. *British Medical Journal* **297**, 847–9.
18. **Maguire, P., Booth, K., Elliott, C., and Jones, B.** (1996). Helping health professionals involved in cancer care acquire key interviewing skills: The impact of workshops. *European Journal of Cancer* **32A**, 1486–9.
19. **Fallowfield, L., Jenkins, V., Farewell, V., Saul, J., Duffy, A., and Eves, R.** (2002). Efficacy of a Cancer Research UK communication skills training model for oncologists: a randomised controlled trial. *Lancet* **359**, 650–6.
20. **Aspegren, K., Birgegard, G., Ekeberg, O., Hietonen, P., Holm, U., Jensen, A.B., and Lindfors, O.** (1996). Improving awareness of the psychosocial needs of the patient—a training course for experienced cancer doctors. *Acta Oncologica* **35** (2), 246–8.
21. **Heaven, C.** The role of clinical supervision in communication skills training. Unpublished PhD thesis, University of Manchester, 2001.
22. **Greer, S., Moorey, S., Baruch, J.D.R., Watson, M., Robertson, B., Mason, A., Rowden, L., Law, M.G., and Bliss, J.M.** (1992). Adjuvant psychological therapy for patients with cancer: a prospective randomised trial. *British Medical Journal* **304**, 675–80.
23. **Moorey, S., Greer, S., Bliss, J., and Law, M.** (1998). A comparison of adjuvant psychological therapy and supportive counselling in patients with cancer. *Psycho-Oncology* **7**, 218–88.

24. **Nezu, A.M., Maguth Nezu, C., Houts, P.S., Friedman, S.H., and Faddis, S.** (1999). Revelance of problem solving therapy to psychosocial oncology. *Journal of Psychosocial Oncology* **5**, 26.
25. **Spira, J.L.** (2000). Existential psychotherapy in palliative care. In *Handbook of Psychiatry in Palliative Medicine* (ed. H. Chochinov and W. Breitbart), pp. 197–204. Oxford: Oxford University Press.
26. **Spiegel, D., Bloom, J.R., Kraemer, H.C., and Gottheil, E.** (1989). Effect of psychosocial treatment on survival of patients with metastatic cancer. *Lancet* **2**, 888–91.
27. **Booth, K., Maguire, P., Butterworth, T., and Hillier, V.F.** (1996). Perceived professional support and the use of blocking behaviours by hospice nurses. *Journal of Advanced Nursing* **24**, 522–7.

20.5 The role of the humanities in palliative medicine

Deborah Kirklin

> My journey has two intertwined threads, elements which mirror each other as exactly as the two chains of the double helix. One is the medical history: the physical injury, the illness, the happening, the happened, the inevitable, and the unavoidable. The parallel thread is my emotional response: the disbelief, the grief, the doubt, the flung out, the banter, the bargaining, the accepting, the clenching of teeth, the sick to the teeth, the pain, the no-gain. Why me? Why me now?
>
> Michele Petrone in 'The healing touch: the necessity for humanity in medicine and the humanities in medical education'. Chapter 3 in *Medical Humanities: A Practical Introduction.* RCP, London, 2001. Ed. Kirklin, D. and Richardson, R.

All journeys have highs and lows. Palliative medicine has come a long way in its own physical and spiritual journey. The care of those whose condition is not amenable to cure has for many been transformed by Cicely Saunders' determination to allow patients to chart their own courses. By including the humanities in the education section of this volume the editors are encouraging practitioners and educators to draw on the wealth of human experience and wisdom embodied in the arts and humanities in their important work. This chapter will examine the potential role of the humanities in the education and training of all those looking after other human beings in the final part of their life journey. Firstly, the power of words to not only reflect our conception of palliative medicine but also to shape its nature, will be examined. Secondly, an overview of the framework whereby educational initiatives are and could be delivered, will be provided. Thirdly, the educational objectives that can be specifically addressed in this way will be illustrated with extracts from poetry and prose. Finally, the special area of caring for dying children will be highlighted. Educational resources which may be of interest to practitioners and educators will be suggested.

Background

> A biomedical education cannot equip someone in their late teens or early 20s to understand the reactions of a bereaved person, the reactions of someone terrified to learn they have a life-threatening condition or the devastation of long-term disability.
>
> Ilora Finlay, p. 156, 'Portfolio learning: the humanities in medical education'. In *Medical Humanities.* BMJ Books, London, 2001. Ed. Evans M, and Finlay, I.

> (What I'm looking for is a doctor) who is a close reader of illness and a good critic of medicine . . . someone who can treat body and soul . . . I'd like my doctor to scan me, to grope for my spirit as well as my prostate.
>
> Anatole Broyard in 'The patient examines the doctor' from *Intoxicated by My Illness* quoted in Shapiro.(1)

The last few years have seen increasing enthusiasm to establish a role for the arts and humanities in both undergraduate and postgraduate medical education, and in continuing professional development. The humanities place expressing, exploring and interpreting the human condition as central to human philosophical and artistic endeavour. It is the deceptively simple imperative to healthcare practitioners, to make these pursuits integral to their daily clinical practice that is fundamental to the humane practice of medicine. There is, however, no consensus about precisely which disciplines constitute the inter-disciplinary field of medical humanities. Literature, art, medical history, anthropology, theology, and philosophy are integral to many courses. Creative writing, music, medical journalism, and drama are also widely used. Andrew Hoyd has outlined the history of the development of palliative care in his chapter and clearly an understanding of this historical context provides useful and interesting insights into current practice.

Learning how to address the complex and important needs of those requiring palliative care poses as many emotional as intellectual challenges.(2,3) Willingness to think about and be open to new and sometimes uncomfortable ideas, an ability to use metaphors of life and death to help explain feelings there are no other words for, and a capacity to engage with the person at the centre of the medical drama are all vital. Later in this chapter three educational objectives, that between them aim to facilitate this ideal of learning, will be detailed. First however the importance of the words used to describe the subjects of those doctors' concern will be examined.

The power of words

Definitions and their consequences

> Palliative medicine is 'the study and management of patients with active, progressive, far-advanced disease for whom the prognosis is limited and the focus of care is the quality of life.'
>
> . . . the active total care of patients whose disease is not responsive to curative treatment. Control of pain, of other symptoms, of psychological, social and spiritual problems is paramount. The goal of palliative care is achievement of the best quality of life for the patients and their families.
>
> WHO definition.

In attempting to mark out the area of medical practice that falls within the province of palliative care, the importance of an ability to critically evaluate and select the language used in medicine, and specifically in this field, will be illustrated. These terms have practical implications for patients and their families that are increasingly apparent as palliative medicine develops as a speciality with its own guiding principles, clinical goals and established practices. The words used to categorize the condition of patients help decide who does and does not fall under the care of palliative physicians. This in turn affects the resources that can be made available to the patient and family both in terms of medical and nursing care and social support. Use of the language of palliative care for a particular person implies changed expectations, for patients, carers and professionals, about the quality and length of life of the patient and the nature of the medical interventions they will be offered. Thinking about the words used in this field and examining what these terms imply is a practical way to initiate the learning process discussed above whereby learners must be willing to think about and be open to new and sometimes uncomfortable ideas.

Cure, care, and compassion

> Above all else, those with distressing chronic or terminal illnesses need continuity of care—that is, the attention and friendship of one doctor whom they can come to trust and with whom they can share their hopes and fears.
>
> David Weatherall in *The Inhumanity of Medicine.*(4)

He was so pathetically reduced that Pelagia felt no shame in remaining with him even when he was naked, and she did not have to resort to delivering instructions from the far side of the door. His muscle was gone, and the skin hung about his bones in flaccid sheets.

She did not feel very much like a healer when she saw those feet, however; they were unrecognisable as such. They were a necrotic, multi-hued pulp . . . The stench was inconceivably stupefying, and at last Pelagia felt herself flood with the sacred compassion whose absence had so previously appalled her.

Quote from 'Pelagia's first patient' in Louis de Bernieres' *Captain Corelli's Mandolin*, pp. 135–6.

'The surgeons
Are not going
To operate.
They've had a look
At your scan,'
He said,
'And it's too near
All the lymph glands
And all like that,
The arteries.'
He said.
It was too dangerous.
I was
Disappointed.
I think that
Was more disappointing
Than being told
I had cancer,
Because that
Was my cure.
To cut it out
And then it was
Away.

From 'I knew . . . ' BJGP, September 2001, p. 777. A patient recently diagnosed as having inoperable lung cancer speaks of their experience. Presented by S. Murray et al.

alliative medicine has of course already been defined on numerous occa-ons throughout this book. One part of those definitions inevitably focuses n the incurable nature of the conditions being addressed. Pellegrino and homasma[5] equate cure with 'the eradication of the cause of an illness or isease, to the radical interruption and reversal of the natural history of the isorder'. One danger of the cure-orientated model of healthcare[6] is that hen cure is no longer possible words and phrases such as 'untreatable' and eyond help' become all to easy to employ. In contrast to the bleak, efeatist and demoralizing assumptions implied by these terms, the palli-ive care model requires strident and proactive efforts to be directed wards the alleviation of distressing symptoms and the maximization of uality of life. Words do matter and the words used in palliative care can nd should provide hope, dignity, control and choice at a time when they e sorely needed.

The use of the word care in this context is also worthy of attention. Care is nphasized in palliative medicine and yet surely caring for patients is some-ing that all physicians should do. Care is juxtaposed to treatment and treat-ent is somehow associated with cure. Caring is a positive goal and one hich all patients would surely wish their doctors to aspire to. The implicit ade-off between care and treatment is not only erroneous given the ngoing treatment of distressing symptoms central to good palliative medi-ne and the care inherent in curative treatment, but potentially distressing to atients and their families who fear that the initiation of palliative care means e ending of the treatment of any conditions. The fostering of the inherent oility of all human beings to care for others is to be encouraged in all doctors. aring should be integral to all medical care whether curative or palliative.

Finally if care involves compassion, then the response of Louis de Bernières elagia to the diseased and pitiful form of her ex-lover, Mandras, provides an teresting paradox. Only when Pelagia gains some psychological detachment om Mandras does she finally feel a sense of compassion for him. Before then her private anxieties and physical revulsion left this emotion disturbingly absent. This apparent contradiction, that only through emotional distance was compassion made possible, is in some sense underlies the friendship that David Weatherall says a good doctor–patient relationship entails.[4] Whilst we will not always like our patients and would not perhaps choose them as friends in our private lives, nevertheless our compassion for them can enable us to value them and hopefully thereby to earn their trust and friendship.

Terminal

Of course, if incurability were the only element characterizing those conditions where care was deemed palliative, then much of medical practice would fall within the remit of palliative medicine. In chronic conditions such as arthritis and asthma, despite the clear intention to prevent premature death, we currently have no cure. A significant emphasis is placed on the alleviation of distressing symptoms. These conditions are kept under control rather than cured and often contribute to the person's death.

In order to more precisely define those areas that palliative care physicians might be responsible for the terminal nature of the condition is usually emphasized, as in the WHO definition. This, however, raises its own questions. Brief consideration of just two of those questions will serve to exemplify the sort of conundrum that might keep philosophers, linguists and physicians engaged for a considerable time. Firstly, precisely how long need the remaining (predicted) life span be to qualify as terminal, and secondly, is old age terminal? Few in this field would argue with the assertion that the answer to the first question is inevitably arbitrary depending as much on matching workload to available resources as on logic and consistency although this statement might come as more of a surprise to the lay public. The mere posing of the second question, whilst contentious is not easily dismissed.[7] Ironically, if we choose not to designate old age as incurable and terminal then the need to develop and deliver properly resourced and co-ordinated care, now considered core in palliative care, might not be adequately acknowledged. Given the physical, social, and psychological vulnerability of very old and frail people this is precisely the sort of care they would benefit from. The answers given by a society, a healthcare system or by individual practitioners to questions like these can and daily does have profound effects on the patient's experience of the last part of their life. The irony inherent in this apparently sharp demarcation between curative medicine and palliative medicine has not escaped the latter's practitioners and indeed the proper areas of concern of the palliative care team constitutes an ongoing debate.

The emphasis on the terminal nature of conditions although of value in helping define educational objectives has the potential to distract the gaze of caregivers from the life being lived as attention is paid to the act of dying. Palliative care physicians are therefore often at pains to point out that palliative care is concerned with the life lived as well as the death of the individual concerned. For individuals, there is no sharp demarcation between the life they are living before and after the designation of incurable and terminal is made and so the emphasis on caring in palliative medicine is one that we would do well to re-embrace in curative medicine. Moreover, with the growing debate in recent years about the provision of palliative care and training in the context of both critical care and long-term care, the relevance of palliative care training to all physicians is once more underlined.

An appreciation of the tendency of patients, their families and their professional carers to focus on the impending death of the patient is important in understanding a number of important educational needs that the humanities can help address. Nevertheless it behoves us all to remember that the emotional and spiritual needs of those who are ill and those who care for them do not magically appear when the patient becomes eligible for the services of the palliative care team. Thus, any lessons the humanities can offer to the palliative care physician must surely be of value to all those living through the experience of illness. Carefully facilitated discussions involving healthcare practitioners, patient representatives, managers, economists, and policy makers about these and other issues would be beneficial not only for palliative care but also for areas of patient care outside of the palliative physicians remit.

Unbearable words

> 'You know perfectly well you can do nothing to help me, so leave me alone.'
> 'We can ease your suffering,' said the doctor.
> 'You can't even do that; leave me alone.'
> ... The doctor said [to the patient's wife] his physical suffering was dreadful, and that was true; but even more dreadful was his moral agony, and it was this that tormented him most.
> ... What had induced his moral agony was that during the night ... It occurred to him that what had seemed utterly inconceivable before—that he had not lived the kind of life he should have—might be true.
> *The Death of Ivan Ilyich* by Leo Tolstoy. Bantam Classics, p. 126.

The physical, moral and spiritual agony of Ivan Ilyich stands in sharp contrast to Cicely Saunders' vision. A good education in palliative care should ensure that physicians do all that is in their power to minimize all of these agonies. Unfortunately, not all of the causes of these agonies, particularly the moral and spiritual ones, will be either apparent or amenable to physician directed intervention. Seeing this anguish at first hand can be unbearable for all concerned and can result in a protective distance being placed between the patient and carer. Leo Tolstoy feared a death like Ivan Ilyich's for himself and chose to confront his own fears in his writing. Palliative care physicians although not perceiving their patient's death as a failure may interpret suffering like Ivan Ilyich's as just that. Meeting him on paper and trying to understand the origin of his difficulties may provide some preparation for patients they meet who are struggling to find peace.

Unspeakable words

Other words have the potential to be so unbearable that they can become unspeakable. These are the words that can come from patients who are thinking about ending their own lives or seeking help to do so. In many ways, this appears to be a taboo subject within palliative medicine and Cicely Saunders sincerely felt opinion that a call for euthanasia is an indictment of the care being given is oft quoted in response. Undoubtedly, there will be cases in which more can be done to ease the many types of suffering already alluded to and as a consequence people may well change their minds and want to live out what remains of their natural life span. However, there will remain cases where despite optimal symptom control and psychosocial support the patient remains steadfast in their wish to control the manner and time of their death. A recent UK legal case involving a woman in the terminal phase of motor neurone disease wanting her right to assisted suicide to be recognized as a human right provides an example of this.

Whilst death is clearly not viewed as a sign of failure in palliative care, it would seem that a call from the patient for help in dying often is. It is not my intention to discuss the case either for or against euthanasia and for a more detailed discussion of this important issue readers are encouraged to read Randall and Downie's excellent book about palliative care ethics. It is, however, important to consider the potential consequences that could flow from the over-simplistic equation of calls for euthanasia with failure of palliative care. There is a danger that the wishes of the individual concerned would then be de-emphasized in the efforts of the team to 'get it right' and 'sort things out'. Some things cannot be sorted out and no matter how disturbing and distressing and contrary to the values of the attending physician, the wishes of the patient at this time deserve to be listened to and acknowledged. One can only assume that the public support given by her GP to the lady with motor neurone disease mentioned above has been very important to her. I do not know what that GP's personal moral views are in this case but his support of his patient's right to have her views listened to are an example to us all.

Spiritual words

> When the priest came and heard his confession, he relented, seemed to feel relieved of his doubts and therefore of his agony, and experienced a brief moment of hope.
> *The Death of Ivan Ilyich* by Leo Tolstoy. Bantam Classics, p. 128.

> The dying man was still screaming desperately and flailing his arms. One hand fell the boy's head. The boy grasped it, pressed it to his lips, and began to cry. At that ve moment Ivan Ilyich fell through and saw a light, and it was revealed to him that life had not been what it should have been but that he could still rectify the situatic

(He then feels overwhelming compassion for his son and wife, who, he nc realises, are suffering enormously. The focus of his concern is to ease the pain, not his own. Finally his life is what it should be.)

> He searched for his accustomed fear of death and could not find it. Where w death? What death? There was no fear because there was no death. Instead of dea there was light.
> ...
> 'It is all over,' said someone standing beside him.
> He heard these words and repeated them to his soul.
> 'Death is over,' he said to himself. 'There is no more death.'
> He drew in a breath, broke off in the middle of it, stretched himself out, and diec
> *The Death of Ivan Ilyich* by Leo Tolstoy. Bantam Classics, pp. 132–

> Happy the man, and happy he alone,
> He who can call today his own; he who, secure within, can say,
> Tomorrow, do they worst, for I have lived today.
> John Dryden (1631–1700).

Whilst it is clearly beyond the scope of this chapter to give even a curso overview of the many sources of spiritual comfort and distress, I offer th prose and poetry to encourage quiet contemplation about the spiritu journeys that patients make a short time before the rest of us. For some, t journey is eased by religious belief, for others the love of close frien and family allows peace. Sadly, the journey is often lonely and demandin The palliative care practitioner has both the honour and the duty to be true and steadfast travel companion.

Delivering education and training

> ... too many patients are unprepared for death, too many have symptoms l untreated and too many families are left to face this time feeling isolated and alo
> Emmanuel 1997 quoted in MacLeod.

There is and always will be more to do in the education and training of phy cians, and the humanities can only hope to contribute to that importa work. Literature can help students and practitioners to think through ma of the important issues in palliative care. By describing work currently taki place in this field, this chapter is intended to offer the reader insight in some of the approaches which the humanities can offer. By providing su gestions for further reading as well as highlighting available education resources, it is hoped that those interested in this work will feel encourag to include the humanities in their educational programmes. Like all areas education, clear learning objectives need to be identified and appropria assessment of students and evaluation of teaching effectiveness undertake

The General Medical Council (GMC)

When, in 1993, The General Medical Council's document 'Tomorrov doctors'[9] suggested that the humanities could be gainfully employed undergraduate medical education, the media suggested were already famili to those working with patients in palliative care. Art therapy and poet therapy are just two examples of widely used approaches to enable patier to contemplate their own responses to their illness. *Tomorrow's Doctc* required medical schools to develop and deliver optional undergradua courses called special study modules (SSMs) to allow students to purs areas of particular interest to them in further depth. Specifically, tho planning SSMs were encouraged to provide humanities modules such literature and medicine.[10] A number of medical schools in the Unit Kingdom have responded by doing just that.

Moreover, the GMC's plans for revalidation will require all physicians provide evidence of reflective practice, good communication skills, sens ivity to ethical concerns and a demonstration of both appropriate attitud and patient-centred practice. The humanities can offer palliative ca physicians practical and enjoyable ways to meet those expectations.

ndergraduate medical education

'he development of humanities courses in this field has been patchy but ncouraging. Many of these courses remain unreported and those developng them often work in relative isolation unaware of similar efforts lsewhere. In the United States and Canada, work began several years ago to ollate all available information about medical humanities courses on one niversally accessible on-line database. This initiative has proven both poplar and practical with a large number of courses now listed of which many re directly or indirectly relevant to palliative care. Many of these courses in Jorth America remain optional but in an increasing number of centres this vork is now core and compulsory. In the United Kingdom details of only a mall proportion of courses have been published and there has been until ecently no central database. A database of UK medical humanities courses now available at the Centre for Medical Humanities. Details of how to ccess both of these databases are provided under Further reading. So far, 83 ourses are listed of which seven are directly relevant to palliative medicine nd many others are in some way pertinent to palliative care.

ostgraduate training

ostgraduate training in palliative care should address not only the clinical nd psychosocial needs of patients and relatives but also those of the practioner. There are encouraging signs in medicine as a whole that issues eyond the clinical management of a patient are being given more weight. eginning in 2001 and for the first time since the Royal College of hysicians (RCP) began to examine doctors for membership, communicaon skills and appreciation of ethical and legal concerns are now systematcally assessed. As a result postgraduate training will now need to address nese issues. In the same year the RCP published the first UK textbook in Medical Humanities thus endorsing the educational value that such courses an offer. Despite these promising signs, a lack of familiarity with the techiques and learning opportunities afforded by the humanities as well as ariable access to expert support in this area will remain a problem for the oreseeable future. One of the important tasks facing academics in this field therefore to develop educational resources to support those wishing to ncorporate medical humanities into local training programmes and details f existing resources will be provided at this end of this chapter. In addition, aining courses need to be available to interested clinicians and educators enhance their confidence and skills base as well as guiding them to local xpertise and support. Again details will be given below.

ontinuing professional development

'he concept of continuing professional development (CPD) represents a earning ideal where the educational and support needs of the maturing ractitioner are addressed from the perspective of all those involved in the nerapeutic context of his or her work. Thus, the needs of patients, their amilies, the community, the healthcare team and those of the practitioner re all determinative of the ongoing programme of education and support nat CPD should be. Implicit in this definition of CPD are three elements nat medical humanities purports to address. The first requires the doctor appreciate the varied and often conflicting perspectives of patients, families nd professionals. The second involves reflection on the strengths and eaknesses of the individual's practice—an ability to build on the former nd address the reasons behind the latter. The third focuses on the support nat a practitioner engaged in caring for the sick needs both as a profesonal and as a person. These three educational objectives will be considered elow with examples from existing educational initiatives.

n integrated approach

Films, music, poetry, music, artworks, other visual stimuli may all be potent sources of learning and directly relevant to the problems of the patient being studied.

Ilora Finlay, p. 159 in *Medical Humanities*. BMJ Books, London, 2001. Ed. Evans, M. and Finlay, I.

Although optional courses such as SSMs are extremely valuable in allowing students to consider important areas in greater depth, there is a compelling argument for the incorporation of training in palliative care into the core curriculum. If the humanities are to contribute to this training then this too will need to be within the core curriculum and this might be either as part of the standard clinical training described earlier in this volume or as a complementary but independent component of the courses. The value of this is attested to by educators such as Ilora Finlay. The section 'Painting a roomful of bad news', provides a practical example of how this can be done.

Educational objectives

Reflecting

The first objective I will explore aims to enable practitioners to reflect on their own thoughts, feelings, inclinations, practice and experience. The process of reflection offers practitioners the opportunity to gain new insights into the strengths and weaknesses of their own practice and into the nature of their own spiritual journey. This objective acknowledges both the participation of practitioners in the lived experience of illness, and the fact that illness affects not only patients and their families but also those caring for them. The response of physicians to illness is far more than a scientific answer to biomedical challenges. Recognition of the individual needs, fears and values of physicians is essential if they are to move beyond their own feelings and concerns and be able to place those of the patient central to their endeavours. To illustrate how the humanities might help this reflection, I will describe the use of practical art in enabling both students and established practitioners to understand how fears for their own mortality can be evoked by the illness of patients. Recognizing this is an important step if practitioners are to be psychologically prepared to help another individual face their own death.

The wounded healer

The ailing physician remains a paradox to the average mind, a questionable phenomenon. May not his scientific knowledge tend to be clouded and confused by his own participation, rather than enriched and morally reinforced? He cannot face disease in clear-eyed hostility to her; he is a prejudiced party, his position is equivocal. With all due reserve it must be asked whether a man who himself belongs among the ailing can give himself to the cure or care of others as can a man who is himself entirely sound.

Magic Mountain, p. 133. Thomas Mann.

While (the doctor) inevitably feels superior to me because he is the doctor and I am the patient, I'd like him to know that I feel superior to him, too, that he is my patient, and I have my diagnosis of him.

Anatole Broyard in 'The patient examines the doctor' from *Intoxicated by My Illness* quoted in Shapiro.(1)

O body swayed to music, O brightening glance,
How can we know the dancer from the dance?

W.B. Yeats, from '*Among school children*'.

How can we know the physician from the care he gives, the doctor from the therapy? In medicine, the practitioner not only diagnoses and administers treatment, he is part of the diagnosis and part of the treatment. In the curative model of medicine, being a patient is about being sick and maybe dying and being a doctor is about making the patient better and sending death packing. As Anatole Broyard points out, diagnosing is also the domain of the patient. This may involve a conscious act as in Broyard's case. More often perhaps an unconscious recognition of the healer's own wounds, psychological and spiritual acts as an empathic bridge to the shared humanity which underpins a close doctor–patient relationship. This recognition of the wounds of the healer has led some to wonder who it is in fact that is the greatest beneficiary in the therapeutic relationship between doctor and patient.

The concept of the wounded healer underlies a psychological interpretation of the nature of the doctor–patient relationship that has resonance for many experienced practitioners. At the same time, as the healer within the doctor reaches out to the wounded within the patient, so the wounded within the doctor reaches out to the patient for healing. Moreover, the participation of the wounded part of the healer in the relationship is essential for its success. Without this part of his or herself the doctor cannot fully connect with the patient. The wounds of the healer may be overt and apparent or the doctor may not even be conscious of their existence. These wounds, which include a recognition of one's own mortality, represent the shared vulnerability that enable us to relate at an emotional and psychological level with another human being. If these wounds are unacknowledged, even at the subconscious level, then the result may be an inability to forge a fully therapeutic relationship between doctor and patient. Put simply, it will be difficult to establish rapport and trust.

Mortality

If, as Thomas Mann asserts, the ailing physician is a paradox to the average mind then the mortal physician is a paradox too. In the cartoon world of doctors doing battle with death there is indeed a paradox if the doctor's own mortality, his personal identity with death, is acknowledged. Yet, the palliative care physician, like all other practitioners, has at least one very important thing in common with his or her patient—they will both die. Uncertainty is something humans deal with poorly but this particular certainty, that we will all die, is one we seem psychologically adept at ignoring. The diagnosing of a 'terminal' condition is an unwelcome and public affirmation of this certainty for the individual concerned. The shunning experienced by dying patients or those diagnosed with conditions such as cancer (often equated in the lay mind with death), reflects in part the unwelcome reminder this gives to us all of our own mortality. The psychological slight of hand by which we maintain our immortality is found wanting. The trick is exposed as cheap and flawed. Yet, unlike the lay public, doctors cannot shun the bearers of this uncomfortable reminder of their own mortality. In bringing himself or herself, the wounded healer, to the therapeutic relationship, doctors must face not only their patient's mortality but also their own. They must face their own fears as well as those of the patient. I will describe next how practical art can be used with both students and practitioners to help them do just that.

Painting a roomful of bad news

Clinical communication skills, now formally taught as part of all undergraduate medical courses, are also beginning to be introduced into the postgraduate training of various specialities. Breaking bad news is one of the topics frequently included. Students are often daunted by the enormity of the task involved when conveying bad news. Moreover, they find it difficult to believe that anyone can be taught how to break bad news and phrases such as 'you'll only know when you actually try it' and 'each time must be different' are familiar to communications skills tutors. There is of course some truth in these assertions although there are doubtless many approaches and ideas that can be usefully worked through before the student or young doctor is faced with a real patient in genuine distress. Nevertheless, the objections raised draw our attention to the importance of responding to the individual needs of the patient or carer with whom the conversation is taking place. Implicit in this apparently obvious statement is the requirement for a good doctor–patient relationship. This in turn, hinges on a recognition by the practitioner, at some level, of his or her own vulnerability and when the news is of impending death, of his or her own mortality.

The exercise described below has been used with numerous students and experienced practitioners. The following description relates to a group of students scheduled for a communications skills class about 'breaking bad news'. They were not self-selected, had minimal warning of what the class would involve and had not been primed with any theoretical information about the psychology discussed above. Instead they had been told that we would use, amongst other things, painting to think about what bad news is.

Twenty students took part in the class. The students were asked to close their eyes and using guided visual meditation they were taken to a room with 'bad news' written on the door. In their mind's eye they were asked to walk down a long corridor to this door, to look at and decide whether to go in. Once inside, they were instructed to look around the room and wer given time to do so. They were then instructed to leave the room and wal back up the corridor. The students were then told to open their eyes anc without talking, to spend 10 minutes drawing or painting the room the had visited. Whilst initially quite nervous about the proposed paintin ('I can't paint', 'help', 'I'm no artist'), all 20 set about their tasks with focu and care. Once the work was complete, the students were asked to describ what they had drawn with one other person in the group. The discussior were lively and good humoured with anxiety broken by smiles and encou aging words between peers. Students were invited, if they wished, to te the larger group about their painting. The process became infectious as became apparent that between them they had only painted two rooms.

The first room was grey, bare, dusty and depressing, It seemed that hop joy and pleasure were not to be found in this room. Any small signs of lif indistinct and remote, were only to be glimpsed through a grimy windov The second room was, by contrast, bright and pleasant. A neat bed wit colourful cover, beautiful flowers in a vase, a painting hanging on the wa and a carefully curtained window onto a world filled with sunshine. As th students described their pictures it became clear to them what these pic tures were about. The first was what life would be like after bad news. Th second represented the future life, on which they had previously countec which would now be very different.

Using practical art, these students, and many others in similar group have used their own creativity to gain greater insight into hopes and fears c which they were often not conscious. This recognition of one's own feeling is a powerful preparation for the development of empathy.

Connecting

Fortunately, most doctors, qualifying in their mid-twenties, have littl personal experience of death although it is important to realize that a sig nificant number will. This may be the death or terminal illness of an elder relative such as a grandparent, a closer relative such as a parent or sibling c of a friend or fellow pupil at school. As a young doctor, they often exper ence death as the end result of a failed resuscitation attempt. When th death is anticipated then they may well be called after the event and require to make legal confirmation of this event and to talk to the recently bereave relatives. By the time the doctor has completed postgraduate training and responsible for training others then, depending on the speciality chosen, th doctor will be expected to guide the healthcare team as they care for thos with incurable conditions in the final part of their lives. MacLeod[10] talks c the 'turning points' described by experienced practitioners in palliative car The moment when they first began to understand what their work was a about. This invariably occurred when they found themselves in an intima and caring situation with a patient. Like Cicely Saunders caring for a relativ stranger and suddenly understanding what was needed, so these docto learnt from these close and moving experiences.

The second objective I will therefore explore aims to help practitioners t further appreciate the experience of illness for patients and their carers an what their journey entails. This process is sometimes referred to as 'improvin empathy'. One view of empathy as vicarious introspection comes close t describing the way in which the arts can connect doctors and patient Practitioners are required to step outside of their professional role and t think, feel and listen person-to-person, and not professional to patient. will now illustrate the use of literature to facilitate improved understandin of the perspective of patients, carers and professionals in palliative care wit reference to specific poetry and prose.

The patient's perspective

> As soon as you're diagnosed the medical profession sees you as being the illness wi the patient attached. Actually you are an ordinary person, with something dreadf that has happened to you, absolutely dreadful. That doesn't mean that all the rest your life isn't carrying on. Maybe you're going to have to withdraw from some of because of the physical limits, but things like relationships will still be there.
>
> Tracy quoted by Michele Petrone in 'The healing touch'
>
> *Medical Humanities: A Practical Introductio*

opened this chapter with a quote from Michele Petrone, a professional rtist who has painted and written about his experience of Hodgkin's mphoma. When Michele was in isolation following a stem cell transplant e painted square pictures to fill the glass pane on his door. These paintings eveal his emotional journey of illness in ways that even he was initially naware of. This collection of pictures has toured widely and been used in ormal and informal settings to allow all of those caring for patients with erious illness to explore the feelings that are so often generated.

Fortunately, there are many generous individuals willing to share their motional journeys with us through their writing, art, music, drama and ance. This growing body of work constitutes a rich and varied teaching esource. The authenticity of such work is appreciated by students of all ges and can provide convincing and useful guides to the agendas and priorities of patients. In his writing and through his subsequent work with atients, Michele Petrone has chosen to give a voice to others, like Tracey, truggling to cope in a world that has been turned upside down by illness. Ie reinforces Tracey's plea to all doctors to not let the person be hidden by eir illness, not to view patients as illnesses with people attached. Through eading and discussing what patients write and say we can all help ensure at those voices are heard.

he carer's perspective

Why is a scar on a man a mark of distinction,
on a woman a mark of disfigurement?
  I don't know.
Why is it funny when a man loses his hair,
And tragic when a woman loses hers?
  I don't know.
What will you tell her
when the X-Rays turn the scar
on her breast raw-
hamburger red?
  I don't know.
When she's bald, lost the hair
From her eyebrows,
And lies with closed eyes,
With a skeletal look,
Will you kiss her
and tell her
she's beautiful?
  I don't know.
What do you do
In the bedroom,
When she is thinking
of death,
and she cries?
  I hold her hand, and I breathe.

'I don't know' by Joe Milosch in *Poetic Medicine* by John Fox.

... I am relieved to leave you, relieved to be in the bus. New York is beautiful as we come in, at dusk. There is a patch of green under the flyover, and a man lives there, alone, in a shack he has made himself....

It is not until tomorrow, in Manhattan, as I am crossing the street to post a letter, that a sense of your unhappiness will come crashing down on me, it will be as though you are with me, and in the road, in the traffic, a desolation will overwhelm me, which is both yours and mine. I will hurry back to your loft and as I close the door behind me the telephone will be ringing and it will be you: you unhappy, alone and lost.

Extract from 'Flight' by James Loader, in *Cold Comfort* edited by James Loader.

don't know, is a moving poem written by a husband trying to come to erms with his wife's breast cancer and the physical and psychological nguish that followed. Aware of the many issues this man would have to eal with, the medical team asked him lots of questions, to see how he was oing to cope. These questions made him angry and this poem began as an ngry poem. Subsequently, it also became a love poem—a poem full of ain, uncertainty, anger, love. Through writing the poem, he came to accept the fact that not knowing is OK, acceptable, appropriate. All this wisdom and more can be accessed and understood by reading this poem.

Flight by James Loader is a wonderful description of the lonely and claustrophobic experience that caring for the sick and dying can be. Students reading this piece feel themselves intuitively disapprove of the narrator and his desire to run away, not to be responsible. As they read on, as he runs only to know he must return, they begin to see the fuller picture, the man behind the carer with needs, fears and hopes of his own. This story has many analogies in the world they are more familiar with. The late night admission of a dying woman who'd be better off at home but whose partner says he can't cope anymore can all too easily be interpreted by the young admitting houseman as the consequence of a selfish and heartless carer. The snap-shot of the human tragedy seen in casualty almost certainly is just that—a two-dimensional representation of a moment in time—and gives only a limited idea of what has bought patient, carer and doctor to this place at this time. And yet, the admission history will purport to do just that, to sum up the situation, when instead it can only offer a fragment of the emerging narrative of illness. Analysis of the feelings pieces such as *Flight* evokes in the reader, can provide unanticipated insights into the carer's perspective and this in turn can have direct relevance to subsequent clinical work.

The professional's perspective

The frisson you get from a fine line of poetry comes chiefly, I think, from the sheer pleasure that someone has recorded something you thought only you had felt before. More that that, it comes from the realisation that many others have shared and will share with you this moment that you had thought was unique and inexpressible. The loneliness of the individual life is dissolved briefly in the flicker of that same sensation, of coherence.

Martyn Harris, *Odd Man Out*, p. 302. Pavilion Books Ltd, 1996.

Most students have little idea of what being a doctor is really like. They will have been exposed to many and varied representations and interpretations of doctors. Examining how doctors are portrayed in popular culture provides insights into the expectations that society and patients have of doctors and doctors have of themselves. For a detailed description of how this can work the reader is referred to Glasser's paper.[11] In palliative medicine, the doctor's perspective can be all too easily ignored and the problems this can cause are discussed in the next section.

Support

The third objective is to enable those working in this field to draw on the arts and humanities for their own personal development and support. Given the demanding nature of the work and the well-documented stress felt by numerous professionals in this area, this last objective addresses a pressing need.

Crying in stairwells

I mumbled condolences to the parents and hurried from the room. Walking rapidly down the hall, looking neither right nor left, finally I reached the stairwell.... A soft wail emanated from some place deep within me. Warm tears began to flow down my cheeks as I wept quietly for Joshua. Soon, however, angry sobs racked my body as all the frustration and impotence overwhelmed me.

From 'Joshua knew' by Liana Roxanne Clark.

When this piece was published it provoked a flurry of impassioned correspondence. Why, the letters asked, was the only support available to most doctors in this position still so inadequate and why do doctors still feel a need to hide their own feelings by crying in stairwells? Fortunately, for an increasing number of health professionals writing allows creative expression of the emotions elicited by their work and there is a growing body of publicly available doctor-generated literature in this field. However, for many doctors, nurses and others working in, for example, palliative care, the burdens are great and the sources of support few. MacLeod[10] has written about the types of stress encountered by young doctors. For many the experience of becoming emotionally close to a dying patient is formative and yet this experience is seldom acknowledged or considered from the viewpoint of the professionals concerned. As Copp and Dunn have reported,[12] nurses also suffer from emotional stress when looking after dying patients. Not surprisingly, they report that patients who have not accepted their prognosis are particularly upsetting to look after. They also report that poor inter-professional communication and support can be frustrating and demoralizing. The opportunity exists therefore not only to use the humanities to support individuals but also to support teamwork and the mutual respect and understanding that are its prerequisites.

In some centres, there have been welcome attempts to address these issues either using existing resources or by inviting in outside facilitators. This is, however, far from universally available. Support of this sort could be a valuable resource for doctors in palliative care and a proactive approach to the provision of these continuing educational needs throughout the speciality would benefit not only doctors but also the patients they would feel more equipped to help.

Mutual support through listening

Another source of support, familiar to those working in medical humanities, is that which comes from listening to each other's stories. Work involving patients, carers and professionals listening to each other can be particularly powerful. Turner describes the support received by both carers and professionals when, as part of an educational exercise, carers were asked to tell their story to a student.[13] The carers were very pleased to be able to tell someone their story and felt that they were in some sense heard for the first time. The students felt that they gained far more from the storytelling than information. They felt a closeness to the teller which they found supportive and accepting. Sharing of stories, as opposed to eliciting histories, can facilitate mutual respect, greater understanding of alternative perspectives and can reduce the sense of isolation and loneliness sometimes felt by those involved in palliative care either as patient, carer or professional.

The care of dying children

He straightens, looks up, and our eyes lock. 'What happened?' he repeats softly, but more clearly.

I only have to look into those eyes for a second to know what he is asking . . . what happened to the baby he already loved more than he thought it was possible to love.

. . .

I stand in the center of the room. I don't know what to say, and very quickly I am unable to say anything. It is all I can do to suppress the ball of grief that is growing in my chest. Images of my own son fill my mind: the toothless grins and sweet breast-milk breath as a baby, the squeals of laughter of a mischievous toddler, the warmth of his sleeping body nestled in my protecting arms, the innocent questions that challenge me, make me pause, make me smile.

From 'A father's eyes' by Stephen Schultz.

As I leaned over to listen to his chest with my stethoscope, Joshua awakened. His teal blue eyes fixed on my face.

'I don't need this anymore,' he said, and pulled off the oxygen mask. 'I'm ready to die now.'

I looked at his mother trying to hide my shock. For three weeks I had struggled to make this child well enough to go home for what would inevitably be his last Christmas. Now, on December 17, Joshua was telling me that the fight was over.

. . . as I left the room, I struggled with my emotions. I had felt so helpless, standing by, watching Joshua die, unable to heal him.

From 'Joshua knew' by Liana Roxanne Clark.

The care of dying children is one that many of us find particularly difficult.[14] Few of us feel emotionally prepared to deal with the death of a child and yet faced with parental grief the professionals involved often view their own feelings as intrusive and relatively insignificant. In addition, the circumstances in which the child will die can be very different to those in which adults die. Parents, often capable of providing most it not all of the personal care, may not need or want outside help. Reading, writing and discussing literature like *A father's eyes* and *Joshua knew* enables the practitioner not only to reflect on his or her one own practice and feelings but also to share these with their peers. As in all other areas of life it can be a deep source of comfort to find out that someone else has felt just as you now feel.

Conclusion

I will not profess bravery,' said Lydgate, smiling, 'but I acknowledge a good deal of pleasure in fighting, and I should not care for my profession, if I did not believe that better methods were to be found and enforced there as well as everywhere else.'

George Eliot, *Middlemarch*, p. 152. Penguin Books, 1981.

Palliative medicine has a history of setting standards by which other specialities are subsequently measured, of continually looking for better methods. Expertise in symptom control including pain relief is to a great extent now concentrated in the palliative care team and indeed team members often provide advice in these areas to those in other specialities. One of the reasons for this success may be the rather introspective nature of the speciality. Every intervention is questioned, the patient's wishes are paramount, and every effort is made to ensure that the emotional, spiritual and physical needs of the patient and family are met. Nevertheless, addressing the complex and diverse educational needs of those who will be involved in the care of individuals with incurable conditions has not proved easy. It remains a challenge to ensure that doctors in training have direct experience of caring for the dying and where training is provided to young doctors the retention of skills and knowledge can be poor. Thanks to concerted efforts, both in the United Kingdom and in numerous other countries, an increasing number of both undergraduate and postgraduate medical programs do now incorporate some element of training in palliative care.

By emphasizing the powerful role that the humanities could play in the education, training and support of doctors, and other healthcare professionals, who care for patients who cannot be cured, the editors of this volume have shown foresight and courage. It is now up to educators and clinicians in palliative medicine to embrace this opportunity to draw on the wealth of human wisdom and understanding embodied in the arts. In doing so they will, once more, be at the forefront of constructive change in medicine.

Acknowledgements

I would like to thank all the writers—patients, carers, and professionals—who have so generously shared their deepest feelings with us all. I would also like to commend the editors of this volume for their vision in introducing the humanities into this important and influential clinical textbook.

References

1. **Shapiro, J.** (2000). Literature and the arts in medical education. *Family Medicine* **32** (3), 157–8.
2. **Field, D.** (1995). Education for palliative care: formal education about death, dying and bereavement in UK medical schools in 1983 and 1994. *Medical Education* **29**, 414–19.
3. **Oliver, D.** (1998). Training and knowledge of palliative care of jumior doctors. *Palliative Medicine* **12**, 297–9.
4. **Weatherall, D.** (1994). The inhumanity of medicine. *British Medical Journal* **309**, 24–31.
5. **Pellegrino, E. and Thomasma, D.** *The Virtues in Medical Practice.* New York: Oxford University Press, 1993.
6. **Fox, E.** (1997). Predominance of the curative model of medical care. *Journal of the American Medical Association* **278** (9), 761–3.
7. **Steel, K.** et al. (1997). Incorporating education on palliative care into the long-term care setting. *Journal of the American Geriatrics Society* **47**, 904–7.
8. **MacLeod, R.** (2001). On reflection: doctors learning to care for people who are dying. *Social Science and Medicine* **52**, 1719–27.
9. **General Medical Council.** *Tomorrow's Doctors—Recommendations on Undergraduate Medical Education.* London: General Medical Council, 1993.
10. **Calman, K.** (1999). Literature in the education of the doctor. *Lancet* **29**, 1622–5.

11. Glasser, B. (2001). From Kafka to casualty doctors and medicine in popular culture & the arts—a special studies module. *The Journal of Medical Ethics: Medical Humanities* **27**(2), 99–101.
12. Copp, G. and Dunn, V. (1993). Frequent and difficult problems perceived by nurses caring for the dying. *Palliative Medicine* **7**, 19–25.
13. Turner, P. et al. (2000). Listening to and learning from the family carer's story: an innovative approach in interprofessional education. *Journal of Interprofessional Care* **14** (4), 387–95.
14. Charlton, R. (1996). Addressing the needs of the dying child. *Palliative Medicine* **10**, 240–6.

Further reading

The arts and medicine: general works

Cassell, E.J. *The Nature of Suffering and the Goals of Medicine.* Oxford: Oxford University, Press, 1991.

Downie, R.S., ed. *The Healing Arts: An Anthology.* Oxford: Oxford University Press, 1994.

Evans, M. and Finlay, I., ed. *Medical Humanities.* London: BMJ Publishing, 2001.

Fox, J. *Poetic Medicine: The Healing Art of Poem-Making.* New York: Tarcher/Putnam, 1997.

Kirklin, D. and Richardson, R., ed. *Medical Humanities: A Practical Introduction.* London: Royal College of Physicians, 2001.

Philipp, R., Baum, M., Mawson, A., and Calman, K. *Humanities in Medicine: Beyond the Millennium.* London: Nuffield Trust, 2000.

The role of narrative in medicine

Campo, R. *The Desire to Heal—A Doctor's Education in Empathy, Identity and Poetry.* London: WW Norton, 1997.

Greenhalgh, T. and Hurwitz, B., ed. *Narrative-based Medicine.* London: BMJ Publishing, 1998.

Montgomery Hunter, K. *Doctors' Stories: The Narrative Structure of Medical Knowledge.* Princeton NJ: Princeton University Press, 1991.

Patient perspectives

Brighton, J. and Savage, A., ed. *The Patient Knows.* Cardiff: Marches Cancer Care, 1997.

Diamond, J.C. . . . *because cowards get cancer too.* London: Vermillion, 1998.

Harris, M. *Odd Man Out.* Pavilion Books Ltd, 1996.

Picardie, R. *Before I Say Goodbye.* Middlesex: Penguin Books, 1998.

Zola, I. *Ordinary Lives: Voices of Disability and Disease.* Cambridge: Applewood Books, 1982.

The doctor as patient

Vaughan, C. (1996). Teach me to hear mermaids singing. *British Medical Journal* **313**, 565.

Wyoka, J. (1995). Hospice at home. *British Medical Journal* **311**, 1687–8.

The carer's perspective

Herriot, B. (1996). The need to protect colleagues. *British Medical Journal* **313**, 369.

Jayes, A. (1996). Open letter from a carer. *British Medical Journal* **313**, 370.

Loader, J., ed. *Cold Comfort.* London: Serpents Tail, 1996.

Martz, S., ed. *If I had my Life Over I would Pick More Daisies.* Watsonville CA: Papier Mache Press, 1992.

Spark, D. *Last Things.* Boston MA: Ploughshares, 1994.

The doctor's perspective

Singh, S. (1996). Around every tumour there's a person. *British Medical Journal* **316**, 560.

Schultz, S. (1994). A father's eyes. *Journal of the American Medical Association* **271**, 1146.

Clark, L. (1993). Joshua knew. *Journal of the American Medical Association* **270**, 2902.

Seigel, B. (1994). Crying in stairwells: how should we grieve for dying patients? *Journal of the American Medical Association* **272**, 659.

Illness, patients, and doctors in fiction

De Bernières, L. *Captain Corelli's Mandolin.* London: Minerva, 1995.

Solzenitsyn, A. *Cancer Ward.* Middlesex: Penguin, 1979.

Welsh, I. *Trainspotting.* London: Secker & Warburg, 1993.

Informative texts in humanities subjects relevant to this field

Randall, F. and Downie, R. *Palliative Care Ethics. A Companion for All Specialties.* Oxford University Press, 1999.

Porter, R. *The Greatest Benefit to Mankind: A Medical History of Humanity from Antiquity to the Present.* London: Fontana Press, 1997.

Educational resources

http://www.mhrd.ucl.ac.uk, Database of UK medical humanities courses including reviews of the texts, images and films used in the courses.

http://endeavor.med.nyu.edu, Database of literature and medicine including details of courses available throughout North America.

Kirklin, D., Meakin, R., Lloyd, M., and Singh, S. Living with and dying from cancer: an educational pack incorporating teaching materials for tutors and students. London: Centre for Medical Humanities, 2001.

20.6 Internet and IT learning

Claud Regnard

Introduction

> Progress just means bad things happen faster.
>
> *Granny Weatherwax*, in *Witches Abroad* by *Terry Pratchett.* London: Corgi, 1992.

Information overload

Experienced clinicians use about 2 million pieces of information to care for their patients, but unfortunately some of that information is wrong, out of date, or inaccessible.[1] As if this was not worrying enough, the clinicians are faced with fourfold increases in biomedical knowledge during their career, and in some specialities such as AIDS there is a doubling time of 22 months.[1] This daunting task is effectively a barrier to achieving a clinical governance setting where clinicians have the knowledge and skills that are current and appropriate for safe, caring, and efficient practice.[2]

Information patchwork

It is not just the sheer volume of information that is an obstacle to learning, but also that much of this information exists in patches that are of variable quality and difficult to access or interpret. Most learning has depended on a wide variety of sources including clinical experience, observation of colleagues, reflection, protocols, standards, guidelines, workshops, lectures, textbooks, research articles, reviews, and the much vaunted meta-analysis (combining data from multiple trials). With so many sources it may seem unnecessary to develop new ones, but all of these learning sources have problems that can prevent the learners from understanding or relying on the information sufficiently to use it in their practice. For example, reading one specialist journal may mean missing a subject altogether. In a recent review the distribution of 458 selected ethics articles varied from 20 per cent in *Palliative Medicine* to none in the *European Journal of Palliative Care.*[3] In addition, published research has biases caused by negative results that remain unpublished and positive data that is published several times. This results in reviews that are based on selected evidence and meta-analyses that may be wrong in up to a third of cases.[4] Further bias is present in the way that pharmaceutical companies control the design of drug studies, the interpretation and analysis of data, and the dissemination of the results.[5] This has prompted the International Committee of Medical Journal Editors to require contributors to disclose details of the roles of sponsors.[5] Searching for so-called 'grey literature' (literature that has not been formally published in the peer-reviewed journals) is an attempt to reduce this bias when conducting systematic reviews, but recent experience suggests this is not a useful tool in palliative care.[6]

When these problems are added to the difficulty of finding relevant journal articles, it is not surprising that clinicians view learning from colleagues as more relevant to their work than journal articles (see Table 1).[1] Textbooks are viewed by clinicians as highly relevant, but in addition to the sheer physical weight and size of current multi-volume medical texts, they are out of date as soon as they are published. Despite these problems, doctors believe they can cope with the increasing flow of medical information, even though they are spending less time reading and attending courses than before.[7] This lack of insight may explain why doctors in one study reported using printed information sources two-thirds of the time, when in reality they only used them one-fourth of the time and used colleagues over half the time.[8]

Access to learning in palliative care has been further hampered by the lack of suitable education materials in palliative care, and the focus on diploma, degree, and masters courses, which are lucrative for Universities but expensive and difficult to access for learners. When materials are produced that could aid learning their aims are often missing, unclear, or misunderstood. A typical example is the repeated problem of confusing guidelines (a systematically developed statement to assist decisions), review criteria (a systematically developed statement used to assess health-care decisions), protocols (a comprehensive set of criteria for a single situation), and standards (a percentage of events that should comply with the criterion).[9] More learning might be possible from these sources if it was made clear that guidelines are the map, review criteria the compass heading, protocols the routes, and standards the destinations.

The consequence of this information patchwork is that there are few workplace or home-based learning opportunities in palliative care convenient to learners, and very little has been done at a foundation level to ensure a basic level of palliative care knowledge amongst professionals.

Table 1 Characteristics of learning resources (adapted from ref. 1)

Source	Relevance	Validity	Work needed	Usefulness
Colleagues	High	Moderate	Low	Moderate
Lectures	Moderate	Moderate	Low	Moderate
Guidelines	Moderate	Moderate	Low	Moderate
Journal articles	Low	High	High	Low
Standard textbook	High	Low	Moderate	Moderate
Updated IT textbook	High	High	Low	High
Internet now	Low	Low	High	Low
Future Internet?	High	High	Low	High

Information technology

Imagining future technology has often been 50 years or more ahead of reality. For example, videoconferencing was first described in science fiction films of the late 1920s, but had to wait until 1975 for the advent of adequately powerful computers, and it is only in the last 10 years that it has become a reality.[10,11]

Three advances have now brought us firmly into the information technology (IT) age.

Computing speed and memory capacity

The computer used for the manned landing on the moon in 1969 had less power than one of today's cheap calculators. The doubling time for increasing computing speed is currently about a year, and processors are available in the shops today that are capable of handling over 2 billion discrete operations per second (2 GHz). Memory capacity has kept pace with this increase in speed, and temporary storage routinely exceeds 128 million discrete bits of information called 'bytes' (128 MB) and permanent storage routinely exceeds 20 billion bytes (20 GB). The consequence is that complex computing tasks are now possible on home desktop computers that were inconceivable 10 years ago.

Data transmission

An essential advance has been the ability to send and receive large amounts of data, rapidly and accurately. Standard telephone lines can transmit 50 000 bytes every second (50 kB/s), although because of demand on the networks speeds can be as low as 1 kB/s. Low speeds manage text and simple graphics without problems. Higher speeds cope with still pictures but cannot cope with the smooth transmission of live video or simultaneous live video and data. These problems are resolved when transmission rates are increased up to 128 kB/s using digital Integrated Services Digital Network (ISDN) links with the advantage that these can use existing telephone lines at home. 384 kB/s ISDN links are common in commercial sectors but are becoming more common in health care. Asymmetric Digital Subscriber Line (ADSL) is an alternative means of fast data transfer, which can run up to 2 million bytes per second (2 MB/s). So far these have been used mainly on existing domestic telephone lines mainly for rapidly downloading information from the Internet (so-called 'broadband'); however, the lines can be used for videoconferencing and open up the possibility of good-quality links to patients' homes. Very high speeds of over 600 MB/s are possible, which give broadcast-television quality, but they need dedicated and expensive links not available in homes or most health settings.

The Internet

In 1973, Vinton Cerf and Robert Kahn led a project conducted by the Advanced Research Projects Agency, part of the United States Department of Defence, to link up computers over the telephone network. In 1984, the technology and the network were turned over to the private sector and in the ensuing years the network has become a global information system with rapid, easy, and cheap access to data anywhere in the world. It has rightly become known as the World Wide Web, and the initials 'www.' are the prefix to many Internet addresses.

IT learning

The massive growth in IT is all around us. Five years ago, it was unusual to attend a lecture with a digital presentation. Today, presenters using slides are in the minority, and even those using overheads will have prepared them on computers. This pace of change is unlikely to ease and we need to understand what is currently available and what is in development to make the most of this change in learning.

IT learning currently in wide use

Digital presentations

Despite the reality that an almost infinite variety of problems can ruin a computer-based presentation compared with the simplicity of using photographic slides, digital presentations are becoming widely used. Even if some presenters cannot resist the novelty and throw clarity to the wind, this new medium usually results in professional-looking presentations, allows last minute changes, rapid preparation of accompanying audience notes, simple updating, and presentations can be sent to staff and colleagues by e-mail. The presentations can also be placed (with sound if wanted) on to the Internet as a web-based lecture allowing learners to access the lecture at any time convenient to them. This level of flexibility is a key feature of IT-based learning.

Learning by e-mail

The use of e-mail is likely to become ubiquitous in the next 5 years. Already widely used for messaging within and between organizations, it is regularly used as a means to share information in mailing groups such as *Palliative Medicine Mailbase, Palliativedrugs Bulletin Board* and *Onco-Pain* (see Table 2). Some recent reports describe its use in supplementing a teaching round for junior doctors,[12] continuing medical education (CME) case discussions for physicians,[13] and evaluations for fourth-year medical students.[14] In evaluating its use in ward round teaching, although only seven out of 15 doctors attended a teaching round, most read the e-mail summary of the discussion and over half found they learnt as much or more from the e-mail.[12] In contrast, medical students were more likely to complete educational evaluations when reminded to do so by post, than when reminded by e-mail.[13] Paper still has a 'presence' and importance not shared by e-mail.

Learning by CD-ROM

Large amounts of data can be stored on compact discs (CD). Currently, this is routinely at least 600 million bytes (600 MB), but is much higher with digital video disc (DVD) technology. This means that the current three-volume, 4363-page *Oxford Textbook of Medicine* is available on a single CD where it can be rapidly searched with much greater speed and convenience.[15] The purchase cost is often less than the printed version, but for a modest additional cost it can be placed on an IT system within an organization allowing much greater access. Unfortunately, publishers have been slow at putting texts on CD, tending to do this only for texts with large numbers of sales. This seems a missed opportunity as CD readers are now standard on computers. However, a computer today is more likely to include a CD reader and writer that allows large amounts of data to be downloaded from the Internet and stored on CD for future use. This opens up the possibility of storing textbooks on the Internet, which can be regularly updated. Educational teams can now easily distribute their own educational programmes by copying them onto CDs. Using CDs to deliver learning material is well received by nurses,[16] rural doctors,[17] surgeons,[18] and allied health professionals.[19] When two 30-min multimedia tutorials were placed on a departmental computer, professionals interacted for a median of 22 min and 34 per cent of the interactions led to the tutorial being completed.[19] Although this seems a low response, in reality it is surprisingly high since they were accessing this learning at their workplace during working hours. Such CD-based learning seems as effective as face-to-face delivery of factual information,[18] and allows the use of pictures and video clips in the material.[20] Examples of educational CD-ROMs in palliative care are *Palliative Care Challenge*, teaching junior doctors about pain control, and *A Breath of Fresh Air: An Interactive Guide to Managing Breathlessness in Patients with Lung Cancer.*[21,22]

Internet information

In 2000, it was estimated that there were 15 000 medical websites covering all specialties.[23] Increasing numbers of sites are dedicated to palliative care, pain, and related areas, and a selection is shown in Table 2. Quality varies from sites that are clear, reliable, regularly updated, and informative to those that are little more than advertisements. Surveys of health information sites have shown that less than 40 per cent of sites contain information on authorship, references, writing date, and disclosure, and it is rare for a site to have all four.[24–26] As a consequence, reviewers of websites are checking these factors when assessing sites,[27] and new sites have appeared that check the quality of health information websites (see Table 2). Search sites are increasing and the percentage of professionals accessing the Internet has increased dramatically over the last 10 years. Several surveys show that over 80 per cent of health-care professionals now have access.[27–30] Access to full versions of Medline, EMBASE, and CINHAL are restricted to universities or health-care organizations, but simpler versions are available for free (see Table 2). Free sites such as PubMed Central provide free access to the full text of peer-reviewed articles, a 'decentralized' model that is challenging the traditional restrictions of publishers to information dissemination.[31]

IT learning growing in use

Online journals

Some journals such as the *British Medical Journal* provide free and unlimited access to full text articles, having learnt that, contrary to expectation, full and free access on the Internet increases sales.[32] One palliative care journal (*Innovations in End of Life Care*) is an online journal available free after registration. Sadly, no other palliative care journals are as accessible. Some provide no more than a table of contents while some web addresses seem designed to ensure that no one finds their site (see Table 2). Online journals allow rapid and thorough searches to be made, if necessary from home. Three times as many people access an online journal than read its paper copy.[33] Despite this, however, professionals still find it easier to read a full issue as a paper copy, thus ensuring the publishers receive the income they need to produce the journal.[33,34]

Online research

Publishing research in journals has many problems including long delays from writing to publication, rapidly increasing subscription costs paid to publishers (a 207 per cent increase between 1986 and 1999), variable policies about publishing competing interests, bias in selecting articles, and a reliance on researchers and clinicians to edit and peer review the articles for free.[35,36] Pre-publication electronic articles (eprints) are versions that have been placed on the Internet before publication in a peer-reviewed journal. The experience of eprints in high-energy physics over the last 10 years is that rapid and direct reader feedback helps to streamline the peer-review process in a transparent way.[35] Authors are able to revise their articles from readers comments and the resultant submission to peer-reviewed journals are of a higher quality. The *Clinical Medicine NetPrints* website is a good example and is sponsored by a UK medical publishing group and a US University libraries service (see Table 2). Such sites have not led to the demise of peer-reviewed journals and some palliative care professionals are already submitting articles to these sites.

Online textbooks

In addition to the rapid search facility with CD-textbooks, an online textbook allows the authors and publisher to continuously update the text as new information and evidence appears. This eliminates the long lag time between writing and publishing a textbook, often a year or more. An excellent example of an online palliative care textbook is the *Palliative Care Formulary* (see Table 2), which is available in full, is free after registration, can be searched, and is regularly updated. Because health professionals still prefer to have a paper copy to carry around such websites are encouraging sales. In 2002, a palliative care textbook, *A Clinical Decision Guide to Symptom Relief in Palliative Care* (5th edition), was written 'online' on the Palliative Medicine Mailbase, with each section posted as it was written, with the aim of encouraging feedback and consensus on its content.[37]

Table 2 Selection of Internet websites. Preference has been given to websites offering full and free access to all their contents. Some websites offering partial access have been included, but websites where all access is restricted by subscription or by membership of an organization have been excluded

Title and web address	Access	Description
Information		
Learn the Net (www.learnthenet.com)	Full free	A site that teaches you how to use the Internet
British Lymphology Society (www.lymphoedema.org/bls)	Full free	Information on the treatment of lymphoedema
British National Formulary (www.bnf.org.uk)	Full free	Access to full text
Cancer BACUP (www.cancerbacup.org.uk/info)	Full free	Source of patient information
Cancer Symptoms (www.cancersymptoms.org)	Full free	Information on cancer symptoms set up by the US Oncology Nursing Forum
Cancer Net (www.cancernet.nci.nih.gov)	Full free	Cancer information set up by the US National Cancer Institute
Cochrane collaboration (www.cochrane.org)	Partly free	Organization carrying out systematic reviews
Cochrane review abstracts (www.update-software.com/abstracts/mainindex.htm)	Subscription	
Edmonton Regional Palliative Care Program (www.palliative.org)	Full free	Resource site with assessment tools, palliative care tips, and nursing notes
Growth House (www.growthhouse.org)	Full free	Link site to other sites with some information
Hospice Information (www.hospiceinformation.info)	Full free	Search for UK and international palliative care services
Manual of Palliative Care (www.hospicecare.com/manual/IAHPCmanual.htm)	Full free	Full text of this symptom control book
MAPI Research Institute (www.mapi-research-inst.com/index02.htm)	Partial free	Database of 800 quality of life tools. Details only available on subscription
National Electronic Library for Health (www.nelh.nhs.uk)	Partial free	Gateway to extensive range of health-related sites, most free and full
OncoLink (www.oncolink.upenn.edu)	Full free	Comprehensive online oncology information resource
Palliative Care Drug Formulary (www.palliativedrugs.com)	Registration, full free	Thorough and continuously updated text on palliative drugs
Palliative Care Matters (www.pallmed.net)	Full free	Information site on palliative care issues, including the full text of a symptom control manual
TIME (Toolkit of Instruments to Measure End-of-Life Care) (www.chcr.brown.edu/pcoc/toolkit.htm)	Full free	Resource reviewing current outcome measures with links and references
Mail groups		
Palliative Medicine Mailbase (www.mailbase.ac.uk/lists/palliative-medicine)	Registration, full free	E-mail group of over 600 professionals discussing a range of palliative care issues
Palliative Drugs Bulletin Board (www.palliativedrugs.com)	Registration, full	E-mail group of over 6000 professionals with discussions on drugs used in palliative care
OncoPain (www.multi-med.com/oncology/oncopain)	Registration, full free	E-mail group on aspects of cancer pain. No search facility
Quality check sites		
The Health on the Net Foundation (www.hon.ch/home.html)	Full free	Quality assessment site checking reliability and credibility of sites
Clinical journals		
BioMed Central (www.biomedcentral.com)	Full free	Online journal with peer-reviewed articles
British Medical Journal (www.bmj.com)	Full free	Full text available
European Journal of Palliative Care (www.ejpc.co.uk)	Subscription	Brief summaries only
Hospice Information Bulletin (www.hospiceinformation.info)	Free to PC services	E-mailed information on organizational issues for PC
International Journal of Palliative Care Nursing (www.internationaljournalofpalliativenursing.com)	Part free	Abstracts only
Innovations at the End of Life Care (www.edc.org/lastacts)	Registration, full free	Peer-reviewed, online journal
Journal of Clinical Oncology (www.jco.org)	Part free, subscription	Abstracts free, subscription for full text
Journal of Pain and Symptom Management (www.elsevier.nl/inca/publications/store/5/0/5/7/7/5)	Subscription	Abstracts only for free
Journal of Palliative Care (www.ircm.qc.ca/bioethique/english/publications/journal_of_palliative_care.html)	Subscription	Table of contents only for free
Journal of Palliative Medicine (www.liebertpub.com/jpm)	Subscription	Subscription only
Pain (www.elsevier.nl/inca/publications/store/5/016/0/8/3)	Registration	Text available after registration
Palliative Medicine (www.arnoldpublishers.com/Journals/Journpages/02692163.htm)	Subscription	Abstracts free, subscription for full text
Progress in Palliative Care (www.leeds.ac.uk/lmi/ppc/ppcmain.html)	Subscription	Table of contents only

Table 2 Continued

Title and web address	Access	Description
Search facilities		
Biomedical Resources on the Internet (www.lib.monash.edu.au/medicine/sites.html)	Full free	Catalogues interesting websites with brief descriptions
Cancer Index (www.cancerindex.org/clinksib.htm)	Full free	Extensive source of links to cancer-related sites
Clinical Medicine and Health Research (http://clinmed.netprints.org)	Full free	Site for pre-publication or original research (sponsored by BMJ and Stanford University)
International Association for Hospice and PC (www.hospicecare.com)	Full free	Links to large number of international PC sites
Medical Journal Search (www.sciencekomm.at)	Full free	Large collection of links to medical and biomedical journals
National Electronic Library for Health Clinical Guidelines Database (www.nelh.nhs.uk/guidelinesfinder)	Part free	UK NHS site listing guidelines. Some parts only available to NHS staff
NICE (National Institute for Clinical Excellence) (www.nice.org.uk)	Full free	UK NHS site providing guidance on current 'best practice'
PubList (www.publist.com)	Full free	Links to 150 000 journals
PubMed (www.ncbi.nlm.nih.gov/PubMed)	Full free	Full access to Medline, but with limited search facilities
HSTAT (USA Health Services/Technology Assessment Texts) (http://text.nlm.nih.gov)	Full free	Access to guidelines, clinical guides, evidence reports, and assessments

All sites checked on 15th February 2002.

Palm-sized computers

Increases in speed and storage capacity have been accompanied by reductions in size. Desktop computers of the storage and speed of 10 years ago can now be made small enough to fit in a pocket and yet retain a word-processor, full diary and agenda, contact lists, spreadsheet, presentation software, and multiple other programmes. Recently, these devices have also added coloured, touch-sensitive screens, they can record sound and pictures, and most can be linked with a larger computer to share files and synchronize diaries. This means that learning programmes, updates, and patient information systems can be downloaded from the Internet.

Videoconferencing

Videoconferencing is possible over the Internet using standard desktop computers and ordinary telephone lines, but the picture quality is poor, although still images are well transmitted.(38) Installing a Coder/Decoder (CODEC) into the same computer produces better-quality live video and sound if the sites are linked by an ISDN or ADSL line. A small number of palliative care sites in the United Kingdom are now beginning to use this type of desktop videoconferencing and by the end of 2002 at least six UK hospices will have videoconferencing equipment.(5,39) In one 4 year study, the use of videoconferencing was closely evaluated.(39) The study found that:

- Twenty-two sites were linked world-wide reaching 136 professionals, and two patients in the United Kingdom were linked with their families in Australia.
- Savings on travel and time within the United Kingdom alone would have paid for the equipment in less than 1 year.
- Sites only continued with videoconferencing if they reached a point at which their organization saw the advantages of videoconferencing.
- Links were easy to establish, rarely failed regardless of distance, users rapidly adapted to the new medium, and links could be used in a variety of settings and audiences, including journal clubs and expert workshops.

In a randomized, controlled study, the Open University in the United Kingdom compared face-to-face palliative care teaching with delivering the same material over a videoconferencing link.(40) Although the learners preferred face-to-face workshops, they were shown to learn as much from a videoconferenced workshop. Videoconferencing was less suitable for discussions on psychological or emotional issues, but some features of videoconferencing suggest it could be used effectively in helping learners to discuss sensitive issues.

CME can be delivered effectively by videoconferencing. In one study of rural doctors, 77 per cent said they would not have attended the CME programme if it had not been available by videoconference, while 73 per cent said is was as effective as having the presenter in the room.(41) Videoconferencing can be used to support multicentre trials,(42) and to deliver training skills such as ultrasound use.(43) Desktop systems are low cost,(44) and produce significant savings in travel and time.(39) One oncology centre in Japan now organizes 130 videoconferences each year that reach 16 000 people.(45)

Future IT developments

IT mergers

Palm-sized computers and mobile phones

A few devices are now available that combine these technologies, but at the present time even the latest generation of mobile phone technology is too slow to allow videos or rapid still-picture transfer. However, it is possible to download text updates from the Internet without difficulty and carry out text searches. Over the next 5 years, devices will appear that combine the best of palm size and mobile phone technologies. This will allow learning materials and updates to be easily transmitted by e-mail to personal hand-held devices.

Computer and television

Already computers are available with television receivers and some televisions can access the Internet for information and shopping. Although these developments are being driven by the entertainment industry, the merger may increase Internet access in the home. The Open University in the United Kingdom has been successfully using television as a learning medium for the past 20 years, as well as the Internet. Such organizations are likely to embrace this IT merger.

Computerized documentation and information access

Health care to date has relied on paper documentation. Anyone developing patient documentation, care pathways, care plans, and outcome measures soon discovers the inflexibility of the paper format. For several years in the United Kingdom, the Hospice Information Service has been collecting a yearly dataset from all palliative care teams and many teams extract this data from their existing computerized databases. Very few teams use IT for routine documentation, although reliable and detailed electronic documentation software for palliative care has been available for more than 5 years,(46) and at least one palliative care patient information system is available for hand-held computers.[47] However, as teams develop networks and partnerships, joint databases and documentation become essential and there will be increasing use of computerized documentation. This would make it easy to include guidelines and protocols in optional menus in the documentation as well as rapid access to information sources (electronic textbooks and Internet sites) and e-mailed updates.

Web-based courses

Web-based courses in palliative care are becoming available,[48] and an online Oncology and Palliative Care Masters course is now available in the United Kingdom.[49] In planning such courses, organizers need to consider not just the content but also the speed of access of a web page onto the computer.[50] When content and access speed are good the effects are impressive as shown in an online course on bioethics, which was compared with face-to-face teaching.[51] The computer-based learning students scored higher examination scores and felt better clinically prepared than those attending lectures and small group discussions. There is an obvious attraction to such courses for students living away from University centres or unable to travel because of home commitments. In one US online course for dental hygienists, more than 86 per cent of the participants lived outside the major metropolitan centres.[52] The Open University in the United Kingdom has been successfully running distance learning courses at all levels for years, including online information and lectures.[53]

Linked web-based databases

Websites at present exist on their own, at most providing links to other websites. Linking electronic databases would allow a patient or doctor to search for one subject through a series of databases without the frustration of having to search anew in multiple databases. Creating such links, and making them freely available, would transform the usefulness of detailed searches.[54]

IT learning barriers

Access to the technology

In Norway, the number of physicians accessing the Internet has risen from 38 per cent in 1997 to 90 per cent in 2000.[30] Although access is high amongst health professionals and is increasing rapidly at home, almost all of this increase has been in developed countries and the gap has been widening.[55] Perhaps as little as 5 per cent of the world's population currently have access to the Internet, but this is likely to change as technologies merge, especially in health-care settings. For example, in 2000 India had 1 million people with Internet access, but this is expected to rise to 40 million by 2005.[56] In remote rural Australia, access to the Internet is high.[57]

There have been criticisms that videoconferencing is not appropriate in developing countries on two counts, first that it may produce a dependence on Western commercial exports, and second that it may divert funds away from the basic primary care needs.[58] In palliative care, the experience is proving very different. Regular palliative care teaching sessions are now held over a videoconferencing link between St Oswald's Hospice, Newcastle upon Tyne, UK, and St Luke's Hospice in Capetown, SA.[5,39] The Capetown service could not afford to send or receive staff, let alone buy videoconferencing equipment. This service had the use of videoconferencing facilities donated to them by telecommunications firms, a model that could be used in many developing countries with the help of large multinational firms with videoconferencing equipment. This reflects well locally on the commercial companies while providing links free to palliative care teams with no commercial ties. Initially, the UK tutors had little experience of the issues faced by the teams in South Africa but the regular links every 1–2 months are resulting in a dialogue that exposes the tutors to more issues than could be possible in a brief visit. There are no commercial pressures in setting up such links and there is no evidence that such teams develop any dependency on the distant tutors.

Technophobia

While some health professionals embrace change like a fresh set of clothes, most of us need time to learn and accept new ways of working. Having an enthusiastic technophile on an IT project does not ensure that an organization will embrace the new technology.[39] Training in the use of the technology is essential and needs to be continuous.[39,59] Websites on how to use the Internet are now available (see Table 2) and it is likely other similar sites will grow in the future. Experience with videoconferencing shows initial unease and discomfort, but also show that this rapidly disappears, often after only a few sessions.[39,60]

Adapting to change

When looking into the faces of tired, jet-lagged clinicians at meetings and conferences, it makes one wonder why so many believe travel is the only option. Similarly, organizations continue to spend a large percentage of their training budgets on travel and accommodation for staff. It takes time for individuals and organizations to think in alternative patterns, and to consider IT such as videoconferencing as an alternative.[39] Multicentre trials continue to be organized and run by face-to-face meetings when technology could link teams as often as they wished, at low cost and with large time savings.[42] Clinicians continue to prefer using paper-based books even if these are often out of date and difficult to search rapidly or effectively. Even clinicians who regularly use computers in their work have difficulty believing computer-aided learning is useful.[61] However, attitudes towards IT do not seem to be influenced by the enthusiasm for IT, which suggests that establishing IT learning does not depend on having IT enthusiasts.[62] When IT is embraced, numerous and profound organizational changes occur, which make it difficult for individuals and organizations to envision those changes and prepare for them.[63] This slowness to change habits of a lifetime is one of the greatest barriers to IT learning, although it is salutary to realize that none of us are immune!

IT usefulness

A group of public health graduate students were monitored for their use of the Internet.[64] Initially, 96 per cent of the students found it their most useful resource, but 6 months later it was no longer their most useful source. Unless information is provided in forms that are reliable, referenced, updated, concise, and relevant to the learner, the learner will soon revert to traditional information sources. There is a desperate need for learning translation services that are able to 'translate' information such as research articles, reviews, and meta-analyses into concise summaries and into learning materials.

What can a palliative care team do now?

As increasing numbers of health organizations put their laboratory results, patient databases, and policies on internal networks, it is a necessity for teams to have access to a computer and the network. Although this is happening more slowly in the community, access to the Internet should be a basic requirement of all palliative care teams. This gives them access to the online discussions through e-mail, as well as access to many useful information and search sites. They can also use CD-ROM resources such as textbooks and learning materials. New computers should have a minimum of 1 GHz speed processors, 128 MB memory, 20 GB hard disc, Internet access, and a CD reader/writer, although each year these minimal requirements will increase. Such computers can be purchased for under £750 (Euro 1160). Organizations such as hospices should at least be networked internally to enable rapid sharing of information by internal e-mail as well as using shared CD-ROM textbooks. At least one computer should have Internet access, but ideally this should be available to most on the network. It could be argued that not having access to Internet information may prevent staff from accessing current knowledge and so threaten clinical governance. At least one person should have direct responsibility for IT in an organization as part of their job description. It is also essential to have external, contracted IT support for faults and when developments are planned. The decision to use videoconferencing should be taken by an organization, rather than one enthusiast. Key people should experience its use first hand in an interactive session—conducting a meeting with someone at least 100 miles away soon brings home it cost-effectiveness in terms of time and cost. As the number of hospices using videoconferencing grows, it will be easier to have such experiences.

An information quilt?

IT alone is not the answer to information overload. The problems with current sources of learning do not rest simply with the medium used, but with the way information is collected, presented, and accessed. In seeking to change an information patchwork into a useful quilt, changes are needed in these three areas and information technology offers the means to make these changes possible.

The potential changes to the way we learn are as great as the changes in technology. The traditional conference is likely to change as important lectures are placed on the Internet and downloaded at any time convenient to the learner. This would free conferences from the constraints of back-to-back lectures into productive consensus meetings, as well as opportunities to share views and meet colleagues. Research articles in the future may well be published only online, allowing rapid feedback and modification. Clinical journals would print reviews, the deliberations of consensus conferences and, if they are sufficiently imaginative, could become the 'learning translation services', we need. Institution-based learning will become work-based and home-based learning while CME will go online for the convenience of clinicians and governing bodies.

Such views of the future are no longer science fiction, they are already happening.

Key points

- Many clinicians are unaware of the daunting task that faces them in keeping up to date.
- Despite the mass of available information, much of it is patchy in terms of access, quality, and format.
- Technology now allows rapid transfer of information and pictures into the workplace and the home.
- Learners, educators, and publishers have been slow to take advantage of this technology.
- Future learning using IT will be more accessible, concise, and interactive.

References

1. **Smith, R.** (1996). What clinical information do doctors need? *British Medical Journal* **313**, 1062–8.
2. **Department of Public Health**. *Clinical Governance in North Thames*. London: NHSE North Thames Region Office, June 1998 (www.doh.gov.uk/pub/docs/doh/cgrept.pdf; site checked 1 July 2002).
3. **Hermsen, M.A. and ten Have, H.A.M.J.** (2001). Moral problems in palliative care journals. *Palliative Medicine* **15**, 425–31.
4. **Naylor, C.D.** (1997). Meta-analysis and the meta-epidemiology of clinical research. *British Medical Journal* **315**, 617–19.
5. **Smith, R.** (2001). Maintaining the integrity of the scientific record. *British Medical Journal* **323**, 588.
6. **Cook, A.M., Finlay, I.G., Edwards, A.G.K., Hood, K., Higginson, I.J., Goodwin, D.M., Normand, C.E., and Douglas, H.-R.** (2001). Efficiency of searching the grey literature in palliative care. *Journal of Pain and Symptom Management* **22**, 797–801.
7. **Nylenna, M. and Aasland, O.G.** (2000). Primary care physicians and their information-seeking behaviour. *Scandinavian Journal of Primary Health Care* **18**, 9–13.
8. **Covell, D.G., Uman, G.C., and Manning, P.R.** (1985). Information needs in office practice: are they being met? *Annals of Internal Medicine* **103**, 596–9.
9. **Baker, R. and Fraser, R.C.** (1995). Development of review criteria: linking guidelines and assessment of quality. *British Medical Journal* **311**, 370–3.
10. **Elford, R.** (1998). Telemedicine activities at memorial University of Newfoundland: a historical review, 1975–1997. *Telemedicine Journal* **4**, 207–24.
11. **Regnard, C.** (2000). Videoconferencing and palliative care. *European Journal of Palliative Care* **7**, 168–71.
12. **Pusic, M.V. and Taylor, B.W.** (2001). E-mail amplification of a mock code teaching round. *Journal of Emergency Medicine* **20**, 307–14.
13. **Marshall, J.N., Stewart, M., and Ostbye, T.** (2001). Small-group CME using e-mail discussions. Can it work? *Canadian Family Physician* **47**, 557–63.
14. **Paolo, A.M., Bonaminio, G.A., Gibson, C., Partridge, T., and Kallail, K.** (2000). Response rate comparisons of e-mail and mail-distributed student evaluations. *Teaching and Learning in Medicine* **12**, 81–4.
15. **Wetherall, D.J., Ledingham, J.G.G., and Warrell, D.A.**, ed. *Oxford Textbook of Medicine on CD-ROM*, Version 1.10. Oxford: Oxford University Press and Electronic Publishing BV, 1996.
16. **Mangan, J.M. and van Soeren, M.H.** (2000). Development of a pathophysiology CD-ROM for nurse practioner. *Computers in Nursing* **18**, 87–92.
17. **Short, M.W.** (1999). CD-ROM use by rural physicians. *Bulletin of the Medical Library Association* **87**, 206–10.
18. **Rosser, J.C., Herman, B., Risucci, D.A., Murayama, M., Rosser, L.E., and Merrell, R.C.** (2000). Effectiveness of CD-ROM multimedia tutorial in transferring cognitive knowledge essential for laparoscopic skill training. *American Journal of Surgery* **179**, 320–4.
19. **Pusic, M., Johnson, K., and Duggan, A.** (2001). Utilization of a paediatric emergency department education. *Archives of Paediatrics and Adolescent Medicine* **155**, 129–34.
20. **Bacro, T., Gilbertson, B., and Coultas, J.** (2000). Web-delivery of anatomy video clips using a CD-ROM. *Anatomical Record* **261**, 78–82.
21. *Palliative Care Challenge (CD-ROM)*. Dundee: Macmillan Education Resource Unit, Centre for Medical Education, University of Dundee, 1998.
22. *A Breath of Fresh Air: An Interactive Guide to Managing Breathlessness in Patients with Lung Cancer (CD-ROM)*. London: Interactive Education Unit, The Institute of Cancer Research, 2001.
23. **Rolland, Y., Bousquet, C., Pouliquen, B., Le Beux, P., Fresnel, A., and Duvauferrier, R.** (2000). Radiology on Internet: advice in consulting websites and evaluating their quality. *European Radiology* **10**, 859–66.
24. **Shon, J. and Mussen, M.A.** The low availability of metadata elements for evaluating the quality of medical information available on the World Wide Web. *Proceedings/AIMA Annual Symposium*, 1999, pp. 945–9.
25. **Hoffman-Goetz, L. and Clarke, J.N.** (2000). Quality of breast cancer sites on the World Wide Web. *Canadian Journal of Public Health* **91**, 281–4.
26. **Hellawell, G.O., Turner, K.J., LeMonnier, K.J., and Brewster, S.F.** (2000). Urology and the internet: an evaluation of internet use by urology patients and of information available on urological topics. *BJU International* **86**, 191–4.
27. **Ahmedzai, H.H.** (2001). Internet reliability and credibility issues. *Progress in Palliative Care* **9**, 151–2.
28. **Pereira, J., Bruera, E., and Quan, H.** (2001). Palliative care on the net: an online survey of health care professionals. *Journal of Palliative Care* **17** (1), 41–5.
29. **Polyakov, A., Palmer, E., Devitt, P.G., and Coventry, B.J.** (2000). Clinicians and computers: friends or foes? *Teaching and Learning in Medicine* **12**, 91–5.
30. **Nylenna, M. and Aasland, O.G.** (2000). Nine out of ten Norwegian physicians have access to the Internet. *Tidsskrift for Den Norske Laegeforening* **120**, 3280–2.
31. **Delamothe, T.** (2001). Navigating across medicine's electronic landscape, stopping at places with Pub or Central in their name. *British Medical Journal* **323**, 1120–2.
32. **Dealmothe, T.** (1997). Developing www.bmj.com. *British Medical Journal* **315**, 1558.

33. **Delamothe, T. and Smith, R.** (1999). The joy of being electronic. *British Medical Journal* **319**, 465–6.
34. **Delamothe, T. and Smith, R.** (1999). Revel in electronic and paper media. *British Medical Journal* **321**, 192.
35. **Delamothe, T. and Smith, R.** (1999). Moving beyond journals: the future arrives with a crash. *British Medical Journal* **318**, 1637–9.
36. **Smith, R.** (2001). Electronic publishing in science. *British Medical Journal* **322**, 627–9.
37. **Regnard, C. and Hockley, J.** *A Clinical Decision Guide to Symptom Relief in Palliative Care* 5th edn. Abingdon: Radcliffe Medical Press, 2003.
38. **Broderick, T.J., Harnett, B.M., Merriam, N.R., Kapoor, V., Doran, C.R., and Merrell, R.C.** (2001). Impact of varying transmission bandwidth on image quality. *Telemedicine Journal and E-Health* **7**, 47–53.
39. **Regnard, C.** (2000). Using videoconferencing in palliative care. *Palliative Medicine* **14**, 519–28.
40. **van Boxel, P., Anderson, K., and Regnard, C.** (2003). The effectiveness of palliative care education delivered by videoconferencing compared with face-to-face delivery. *Palliative Medicine* **17**, 344–58.
41. **Callas, P.W., Ricci, M.A., and Caputo, M.P.** (2000). Improved rural provider access to continuing medical education through interactive videoconferencing. *Telemedicine Journal and E-Health* **6**, 393–9.
42. **Kennedy, C., Kirwan, J., Roux, P., Stulting, A., and Murdoch, I.** (2000). Telemedicine techniques can be used to facilitate the conduct of multicentre trials. *Journal of Telemedicine and Telecare* **6**, 343–9.
43. **Hussain, P., Melville, D., Mannings, R., Curry, D., Kay, D., and Ford, P.** (1999). Evaluation of a training and diagnostic ultrasound service for general practtioners using narrowband ISDN. *Journal of Telemedicine and Telecare* **5**, S95–9.
44. **Mattioli, P., Klutke, P.J., Baruffaldi, F., Villar-Guzman, A., Toni, A., and Englmeier, K.H.** (1999). Technical validation of low-cost videoconferencing systems applied in orthopaedic teleconsulting services. *Computer Methods and Programs in Biomedicine* **60**, 143–52.
45. **Mizushima, H., Uchiyama, E., Nagata, H., Matsuno, Y., Sekiguchi, R., Ohmatsu, H., Hojo, F., Shimodo, T., Wakao, F., Shinkai, T., Yamaguchi, N., Moriyama, N., Kakizoe, T., Abe, K., and Terada, M.** (2001). Japanese, experience of telemedicine in oncology. *International Journal of Medical Informatics* **61**, 207–15.
46. **Patient Management Systems.** Eider computers Ltd. (www.eider.com/products.htm; site checked 1 July 2002).
47. **Panacea Patient Information System** (www.iyb.ca/pan.html; site checked 1 July 2002).
48. **Edmonton Palliative Care Programme: Pilot Web Base Course** (www.palliative.org/pallcareednet/course_goals.html; site checked 1 July 2002).
49. **University of Newcastle upon Tyne (UK) Palliative Care Masters Course** (www.ncl.ac.uk/cancereducationonline/information.htm; site checked 1 July 2002).
50. **Sekikawa, A., Aaron, D.J., Acosta, B., Sa, E., and Laporte, R.E.** (2001). Does the perception of downloading speed influence the evaluation of web-based lectures? *Public Health* **115**, 152–6.
51. **Fleetwood, J., Vaught, W., Feldman, D., Gracely, E., Kassutto, Z., and Novack, D.** (2000). MedEthEx online: a computer-based learning program in medical ethics and communication skills. *Teaching and Learning in Medicine* **12**, 96–104.
52. **Fehrenbach, M.J., Baker-Eveleth, L., and Bell, N.** (2001). Online continuing education for dental hygienists: DH forum. *Journal of Dental Hygiene* **75**, 45–9.
53. Open University: www.open.ac.uk.
54. **Smith, R. and Chalmers, I.** (2001). Britain's gift: a 'Medline' of synthesised evidence. *British Medical Journal* **323**, 1437–8.
55. **Tan-Torres Edejer, T.** (2000). Disseminating health information to developing countries: the role of the Internet. *British Medical Journal* **321**, 797–800.
56. **Godlee, F., Horton, R., and Smith, R.** (2000). Global information flow. *British Medical Journal* **321**, 776–7.
57. **White, C., Sheedy, V., and Lawrence, N.** (2002). Patterns of computer usage among medical practitioners in rural and remote Queensland. *Austrial Journal of Rural Health* **10** (3), 137–46.
58. **Rigby, M.** (2002). Impact of telemedicine must be defined in developing countries. *British Medical Journal* **324**, 47–8.
59. **Blignault, I. and Kennedy, C.** (1999). Training for telemedicine. *Journal of Telemedicine and Telecare* **5**, S112–14.
60. **Sawada, I., Suigiyama, A., Ishikawa, A., Ohyanagi, T., Saeki, K., Izumi, H., Kawase, S., and Matsukura, K.** (2000). Upgrading rural Japanese nurses' respiratory rehabilitation skills through videoconferencing. *Journal of Telemedicine and Telecare* **6** (Suppl. 2), S69–71.
61. **Polyakov, A., Palmer, E., Devitt, P.G., and Coventry, B.J.** (2000). Clinicans and computers: friends or foes? *Teaching and Learning in Medicine* **12**, 91–5.
62. **Snowden, S., Harrison, R., and Wallace, P.** (2001). General practitioner participants in a telemedicine trial: comparison with their peers. *Journal of Telemedicine and Telecare* **7**, 32–7.
63. **Aas, I.H.** (2001). A qualitative study of the organizational consequences of telemedicine. *Journal of Telemedicine and Telecare* **7**, 18–26.
64. **Blumberg, P. and Sparks, J.** (1999). Tracing the evolution of critical skills in student's use of the Internet. *Bulletin of the Medical Library Association* **87**, 200–5.

21

Palliative medicine—a global perspective

21 Palliative medicine—a global perspective

Jan Stjernswärd and David Clark

Introduction

The great certainty of human existence is that we are all born to die. 'No death is evil, but a shameful death.'[1] Palliative care has much to offer in easing our passage at the end of life and it has the potential to do this for many millions of people around the world.

At present, 56 million people die annually, but palliative care reaches only a small fraction of those who could benefit from it. Yet, there is a moral responsibility to give those who leave life—elderly people, those terminally ill, those dying slowly of AIDS and cancer—the same care and attention that we give to those who enter life. This should be achievable. There now exist valid and simple methods, which cost little, are acceptable and maintainable at the community level, and can ensure the relief of suffering on a large scale.[2–5] The World Health Organization (WHO) has promoted clear public health policies and advice for the rational implementation of pain relief and palliative care.[6–16] By enabling the implementation of knowledge available in the field of palliative care, both the quality of life and the quality of death of terminally ill people can be improved significantly. Unfortunately, palliative care is not available in many of those countries where it is the only realistic and effective therapy/care to offer.[12] What is needed is the political will to act, to formulate clear policies for pain relief and palliative care, to educate and train health workers, and to empower family members. In particular, it is necessary to make the right inexpensive drugs, especially morphine sulfate tablets or solutions, easily available in most countries of the world.

The application of existing knowledge according to rational public health principles is paramount if we are to reach the majority of those in need of palliative care. Palliative medicine has the advantage of being a new and emerging speciality. It is relatively unencumbered by vested interests and capable of avoiding the mistakes sometimes made in other areas of medicine; in particular, the risk of achieving a lot for a few, whilst the needs of the majority remain unmet. For such an approach, it is important that we have a worldwide perspective, that we identify where the 'consumers' are and how they can be helped, and that we place the problem in a wider context.

It is clear that the problems faced are not only medical, but are often socio-economic, cultural, and ethical in character.[14–18] 'West is not always best.' Many countries with scarce medical facilities have at the same time avoided the institutionalization and professionalization of death, whilst also retaining strong cultural, ritual, community, and family support systems in end-of-life care—precisely those that have been lost, medicalized, or commercialized in the west. Accordingly, each country needs to work out the best way of looking after its dying persons in accordance with its own culture and resources.

The World Health Organization defined the term palliative care officially [6] together with the world leaders on the subject in an expert committee in 1989 as:

> Palliative care is the active total care of patients whose disease is not responsive to curative treatment. Control of pain of other symptoms, and of psychological, social and spiritual problems is paramount. The goal of palliative is the achievement of the best quality of life for patients and their families. Many aspects of palliative care are applicable earlier in the course of the illness, in conjunction with treatment

Palliative care:

- affirms life and regards dying as a normal process
- neither hastens nor postpones death
- provides relief from pain and other distressing symptoms
- integrates the psychological and spiritual aspects of patient care
- offers a support system to help patients live as actively as possible until death
- offers a support system to help the families cope during the patients' illness and in their own bereavements.

A more recent definition of palliative care as 'an approach',[19] with 'impeccable assessment' and that 'includes *those investigations* needed to better understand and manage distressing clinical complication' may be ambiguous and give the wrong impression of an over medicalized approach being compulsory for offering palliative care, unfortunate in two thirds of the world where its application is desperately needed. In this chapter the WHO Expert Committee Definition of palliative care is being used.[6]

In this chapter, we address the following issues:

- the size of the problem now and in the future;
- the development and current provision of palliative care in the world today;
- key issues, priorities, and strategies to achieve optimal coverage of patients in need of palliative care, and recommendations for the rational implementation of existing knowledge through a public health approach.

> We ought to give those who are to leave life, the elderly, the terminally ill, those dying slowly of AIDS and cancer the same care and attention that we give to those who enter life—the newborn.

The need for palliative care—demography and epidemiology

Total deaths globally

The total number of deaths in the world each year is at present 56 million (Table 1). The great majority of these deaths, 44 million, occur in the developing countries.[20,21] It can be estimated that around 60 per cent of those dying would benefit from palliative care. Thus, over 33 million would need pain relief and palliative care. Since death also affects family members and close companions, perhaps one to two persons giving care and support for every one who dies, then a conservative figure might be 100 million people who would benefit from the availability of basic palliative care. Since in

Table 1 Size of problem. Estimated number of people who would need palliative care (in millions)

Annual deaths globally	56
Annual deaths in developing countries	44
Annual deaths in developed countries	12
Estimated numbers needing palliative care[a]	33

[a] It can be estimated that approximately 60% of the dying need palliative care.

Table 2 Cancer burden: global picture. Yearly burden of new cancer cases (in millions)[a]

Population	2000	2025	2050
Total	6.0	7.8	8.9
Developed countries	1.2	1.2	1.2
Developing countries	4.7	6.6	7.8
65+	0.4	0.8	1.5
Developed countries	0.2	0.3	0.3
Developing countries	0.2	0.7	1.2

[a] WHO: *Ageing programme*. Database, 2001.

some cultures up to 10 family members may be involved in the care of a dying person, the figure able to benefit globally could be much higher.

Among those dying there are some major groups who clearly need palliative care: those with cancer, with AIDS-related diseases, and some older people affected by chronic and/or terminal illness.

The ageing of the world populations

Table 2 shows that the world population is expected to increase by one-third in the next 50 years, from 6 billion today to 9 billion.[22] This increase will occur in the developing countries, while the population will remain the same in the developed countries. There will be a fourfold increase worldwide among those aged 65 and over, from 0.4 to 1.5 billion. While the numbers will be more or less stable in the developed world, there will be a dramatic sixfold increase in older people in the developing world, from 0.2 to 1.2 billion. In 2000, 62 per cent of those aged 60 and over lived in the developing regions; by 2050, this will increase to 80 per cent.[23]

The change in the percentage of populations aged 60 or over in selected countries is given in Table 3. Over one-fifth of the population in some countries is made up of those over the age of 60; this is expected in certain cases to increase to 40 per cent over the next 50 years.[22,24]

The ageing of the populations will lead to a significant shift in the dependency ratio of those economically active to those reliant upon them (Table 4), raising major issues about health care costs, welfare, and insurance benefits.[14] The number of persons of working age per person aged 65 or older has been changing significantly around the world since at least 1950.[25]

These demographic changes will result in an increased need for social and economic support, including palliative care, and this will have to be provided by a proportionally decreased working-age population of caregivers. The ratio of tax payers/caregivers to care receivers, which is now 4 : 1, will soon change to 2 : 1 in many developed countries.

In developed countries, for example, the United Kingdom, the penalty of a long life may be high costs of residential care from admission to death, resulting in changing patterns of inheritance and intergenerational dependency.[26–28] The amount spent on residential and nursing home care could more than double in real terms over the first four decades of the twenty-first century. Other changes in family structure, such as geographical dispersion of the three-generation family, increased female participation in the workforce, and high divorce rates, raise questions about whether the amount of care now provided by the families can continue. In contrast, in the developing countries, empowerment of family members as effective caregivers at the end of life is the most realistic approach to achieving meaningful coverage. At the same time, in view of the intensive urbanization and social changes taking place in these countries, it is not certain whether it will be possible to rely on the three-generation family for the care of older people and dependent groups in the future. The devastating effect of AIDS on the family support system in Africa can already be seen. China's policy of only one child per family will mean that each member of its future generation will have to take care of six persons: four grandparents and two parents.

Table 3 Percentage of population aged 60 years or more in selected countries, years 2000 and 2050[a,b]

Country	2000	2050
Italy	24	41
Germany	23	35
Japan	23	38
Spain	22	43
Czech	18	41
USA	16	28
China	10	30
Thailand	9	30
Brazil	8	23
India	8	21
Indonesia	7	22
Mexico	7	24

[a] United Nations Population Database: *The Sex and Age Distribution of the World Populations*. New York: UN Publications, updated 1998.

[b] WHO: *Health and Ageing*. A discussion paper. WHO/NMH/HPS/0.1/2001.

Table 4 The dependency ratio: number of persons of working age (15–64), per person aged 65 or older[a]

Country	1950	2000	2050
Japan	12.06	3.99	1.75
European Union	6.97	4.06	1.89
USA	7.83	5.21	2.57

[a] United Nations Population Division, New York, 2002.

Cancers

What will be the common diseases of the twenty-first century? As a group, the non-communicable diseases (cancer, cardiovascular, diabetes) will increase from 27 to 43 per cent of the global burden of diseases up to 2020, while communicable diseases (infections and tropical and parasitic diseases) will decrease from 50 to 22 per cent.[19] For cancer, one-third of cases are preventable; one-third are curable if found early and standard therapies are available; for the remaining, freedom from pain and other symptoms is possible. However, around the world the majority of cancers when found are incurable, though pain relief and palliative care are not offered to most of those in developing countries who suffer from the disease.

Table 5 shows that the global burden of cancer will increase from 10 to 24 million over the next 50 years and that 17 million of these will be in developing countries.[29] Until early referral/diagnosis occurs and standard therapies are able to be deployed for the majority of those with cancer, pain relief and palliative care will remain the most relevant provision for large numbers affected. The inaction of the west in doing so little for cancer in developing countries is unacceptable, particularly given the double burden in these countries created by the high prevalence of both communicable and non-communicable diseases.

It is interesting to consider the similarities between lung cancer and AIDS. While neither disease was known at the beginning of the twentieth century, both are rapidly increasing worldwide. They are emerging as major health problems in many developing countries. Both are virtually preventable because the primary causes—lifestyle factors—are known. However, the health sector is finding it extremely difficult, in practical terms, to bring about the changes in human behaviour necessary for their prevention. Both lung cancer and AIDS are essentially incurable—the overall survival curves are quite similar. While considerable resources are spent on treating advanced cases, the curative effort is usually fruitless and a major role of the health care services should be to provide palliative care. In the case of tobacco-related diseases, high mortality rates are spreading from industrialized countries to the rest of the world. Lung cancer is already the most frequent cancer worldwide and 90 per cent of cases are incurable, with most patients in need of palliative care. Currently, tobacco use is estimated to account for 3 million deaths per year, with slightly more than half of these occurring in the developed world where the cumulative exposure (primarily smoking) has been higher than in the developing world. At the global level, the annual number of tobacco-related deaths is expected to rise dramatically, from 3 to about 10 million, by the year 2025. Of this estimated 10 million, about 3 million are expected to occur in China alone; almost a million of these will be exclusively from lung cancer. Moreover, with current trends, about 200 million children and teenagers living in China today will become regular smokers. Of these, about 50 million or one-fourth will die prematurely of smoking-related illnesses.

Table 5 Cancer burden: global picture. Number of new cancer cases (in millions)[a]

Where	2000	2020	2050
World	10.6	15.3	23.8
Developing countries	5.4	9.3	17.0
Developed countries	4.6	6.0	6.8

[a] Parkin, D.M., Bray, F.I., and Devesa, S.S. (2001). Cancer burden in the year 2000. The global picture. *European Journal of Cancer* **37**, 4–66.

AIDS

A global summary of the HIV/AIDS epidemic as at end of 2002 is given in Table 6. The number of people living with HIV/AIDS is 42 million, the great majority of whom (38.6 million) are adults. There are 3.2 million children living with HIV/AIDS. During 2002, a total of 5 million people were newly infected with HIV and 3.1 million died of AIDS.[30]

The regional HIV/AIDS statistics and features are given in Table 7. Sub-Saharan Africa carries the major burden of disease, with close to three-fourths of all cases—29.4 out of 42 million, worldwide. Sub-Saharan Africa also has the highest adult prevalence rate: 8.8 per cent of adults, 58 per cent of whom are women. It also has the highest number of newly infected adults and children, 3.5 million out of a global total of 5 million in 2002. Heterosexual transmission is the main cause of infection in Sub-Saharan Africa, in contrast to Western Europe and North America where the main route of transmission is between men who have sex with men, or through injecting drug misuse.

Reduced life expectancy, from 59 to 45 years, is a major consequence of the epidemic in Sub-Saharan Africa. In Zimbabwe, life expectancy is likely to go down from 61 to 33 years by 2010. In contrast, in Uganda, under wise leadership, the *prevalence* rate of the disease is going down. In some countries, up to one-fourth of the adult working population are infected.

Table 6 Global summary of the HIV/AIDS epidemic, end of 2002 (in millions)[a]

Number of people living with HIV/AIDS	
Total	42
Adults	38.6
Women	19.6
Children under 15 years	3.2
People newly infected with HIV in 2002	
Total	5
Adults	4.2
Women	2
Children under 15 years	0.8
AIDS deaths in 2002	
Total	3.1
Adults	2.5
Women	1.2
Children under 15 years	0.6

[a] UNAIDS/WHO, December 2002.

Table 7 Regional HIV/AIDS statistics and features, end of 2002 (in millions)[a]

Region	Adults and children living with HIV/AIDS	Adults and children newly infected with HIV/AIDS	Adult prevalence rate[b] (%)	% HIV positive adults who are women	Main mode(s) of transmission for those living with AIDS[c]
Sub-Saharan Africa	29.4	3.5	8.8	58	Hetero
North Africa	0.55	0.083	0.3	55	Hetero, IDU
Middle East, South and South East Asia	6.0	0.7	0.6	36	Hetero, IDU
East Asia Pacific	1.2	0.27	0.1	24	IDU, Hetero, MSM
Latin America	1.5	0.15	0.6	30	MSM, IDU, Hetero
Caribbean	0.44	0.06	2.4	50	Hetero, MSM, IDU
Eastern Europe	1.2	0.25	0.6	27	
Central Asia, Western Europe	0.57	0.03	0.3	25	MSM, IDU
North America	0.98	0.045	0.3	20	MSM, IDU, Hetero
Australia and New Zealand	0.015	0.005	0.1	7	MSM
Total	42	5	1.2	50	

[a] UNAIDS/WHO, December 2002.

[b] The proportion of adults (15–49 years of age) living with HIV/AIDS in 2002, using 2002 population numbers.

[c] Hetero, heterosexual transmission; IDU, transmission through injecting drugs; MSM, sexual transmission among men who have sex with men.

Together with the high number of orphaned children in Africa, major socio-economic and cultural changes are occurring that will have an impact on how and in what form palliative care can be delivered. Where poverty and the alleviation of hunger are major priorities for most families and governments, it is clear that medical strategies must be coordinated with these wider efforts and will be ethically, morally, and technically difficult to carry out in isolation. Furthermore, Africa is home to half of the world's refugee population—themselves the victims of war, violence, corruption, and corporate capitalism. Fortunately, there is some hope, as shown by the examples of Uganda and South Africa.

India and China, with a major part of the world population, still have low adult prevalence rates of HIV/AIDS, but the epidemic seems to have got a foothold in these countries, which now acknowledge its existence.

The estimated number of persons dying needing palliative care is just over 33 million. Death also affects family members and with one to two persons shouldering the heavy daily routine of care, this gives a conservative figure of 100 million people who would benefit by the availability of basic palliative care.

The global village

Such demographic and epidemiological trends mean that in planning palliative care developments in every part of the world, and particularly in the resource-poor regions, it is essential to consider the necessary costs and required human resources if meaningful coverage is to be achieved. The poor are the most price-sensitive users of health services and high prices are known to significantly reduce their levels of utilization. Almost half of the world's people, an estimated 2.8 billion, live on less than US$ 2 per day, and 1.2 billion people live on less than US$ 1 a day.(31) In India, with one-sixth of the world population, 89 per cent live on less than US$ 2 a day and 53 per cent on less than US$ 1. There are examples of absurdly high prices charged by pharmaceutical companies for certain pain-relieving drugs in developing countries (see below), where 1 month's medication supply for a single patient may be two or three times the salary of a nurse or doctor. This makes freedom from unacceptable, unnecessary, but controllable pain unrealistic and it has sunk many national initiatives aimed at widening the impact of cancer pain relief. Instead, as WHO recommends, generic immediate-release morphine sulfate tablets or hydrochloride solution, coupled with appropriate national policies and leadership (as in Uganda) can mean that a 1-week course of medication can cost no more than a loaf of bread, and can (again as in Uganda, from 2003) be offered free of charge for all.(14)

The developing countries have two-thirds of the global disease burden, but only around 5 per cent of the world's resources (doctor, nurses, drugs, equipments, funds) for controlling/combating disease. Around 1.2 billion do not have clean drinking water and around two-thirds of the world population have never made a telephone call. Thus, an uncritical copying of western approaches and a purely medical approach should be avoided. Major social changes are set to occur in the coming 50 years, when for the first time in our history the majority (two-thirds) of the word's population will live in cities. It seems unlikely that the old cultural support systems will survive. In many countries in Africa, over half of the population will never encounter a nurse or a doctor in an entire lifetime! For these people, unique culturally specific community systems and rituals exist, which for many generations have structured communal approaches to dying and suffering. Certainly, old cultural traditions for curbing pain, which is spiritual, existential, and physical, could be harnessed to simple modern techniques for the relief of suffering. Symptom care, bedsore prophylaxis, appropriate food, and hygiene could be enhanced through the empowerment of family members. Finding ways to empower families and communities in such ways is an urgent priority and in this socio-economic and cultural solutions will be as important as medical ones if meaningful palliative care coverage is to be achieved.

Socio-economic and cultural solutions will be as important as the medical efforts in achieving meaningful palliative care coverage.

Palliative care developments around the world

The rise of hospice and palliative care in its distinctly modern guise (combining clinical care, education, and research) is generally traced to the late 1950s and early 1960s(32) when there is evidence in many countries of a new interest in the improvement of care for dying people. In the wake of developments at the local level and as hospice and palliative care services began to establish in individual countries, there quickly emerged a range of international associations concerned to promote and develop the work of hospice-palliative care, as well as the cognate field of pain medicine. These focused on professional development, education, and training; on clinical innovation and research; on lobbying and advocacy. Table 8 contains a timeline of these international organizations and initiatives.(33–42) A 1999 listing of palliative care organizations with a global perspective(43) also includes: British Aid for Hospices Abroad; the Hospice Education Institute; and the WHO Collaborating Centre for Palliative Cancer Care, Oxford. Other groups include WHO experts and international collaborators and WHO collaborating centres in Milan, Saitama, and Wisconsin.

With a few exceptions,(44,45) the published literature contains little comparative analysis of hospice and palliative care developments in different regions of the world. There is, however, a considerable literature on individual country initiatives and this is summarized here. It is estimated(46) that hospice or palliative care services now exist, or are under development, on every continent of the world, in around 100 countries. The total number of hospice or palliative care initiatives is in excess of 8000 and these include inpatient units, hospital-based services, community-based teams, day care centres, and other modes of delivery.

North America

After the foundation of the first hospice initiative in New Haven in 1974, the United States saw striking growth in hospice services, with 516 hospices in

Table 8 International associations and initiatives in support of hospice-palliative care

1973	International Association for the Study of Pain, founded Issaquah, Washington, USA
1976	First International Congress on the Care of the Terminally Ill, Montreal, Canada
1980	International Hospice Institute, became International Hospice Institute and College (1995) and International Association for Hospice and Palliative Care (1999)
1982	World Health Organization Cancer Pain and Palliative Care Programme initiated
1988	European Association of Palliative Care founded in Milan, Italy
1990	Hospice Information Service, founded at St Christopher's Hospice, London, UK
1998	Poznan Declaration leads to the foundation of the Eastern and Central European Palliative Task Force (1999)
1999	Foundation for Hospices in Sub-Saharan Africa founded in USA
2000	Latin American Association of Palliative Care founded
2001	Asia Pacific Hospice Palliative Care Network founded
2002	UK Forum for Hospice and Palliative Care Worldwide founded by Help the Hospices

existence just 10 years later. A federal benefit was created in 1982 under *Medicare* for patients with terminal disease and a prognosis of 6 months and this legislation proved a stimulus to both not-for-profit and for-profit hospices. By the end of the twentieth century, some 3000 hospice organizations were operating in the United States. In 1989, the place of death for the majority (64.1 per cent) of Americans who died of chronic illnesses was an acute care hospital; by 1997, this had decreased to 51.8 per cent and, overall, more persons in the United States are now dying in nursing homes and at home, although this varies state by state.(47) In the richest country in the world, however, the major identified challenge is for the care of the seriously ill and dying to be recognized as a public health issue, requiring: *Medicare* to be reframed towards population needs; widespread programmes of professional education across all levels; demonstration projects to identify and experiment with new models of care delivery; public education and support for advocacy groups.(48) There has been considerable progress on these areas in recent years through the activities of the Project on Death in America, the Robert Wood Johnson Foundation's Last Acts programme, as well as the work of the National Hospice and Palliative Care Organization, and the American Academy of Hospice and Palliative Medicine. Nevertheless, research evidence from the mid-1990s shows that dying in America is unnecessarily painful and isolating, that patients' wishes are not well understood, and that the associated financial costs are also high.(49) A state-by-state review of end-of-life care indicates that: 'In most states, too few patients are accessing hospice and palliative care services, there are too few professionals trained in pain management and palliative care, and there are too many patients dying in hospitals and nursing homes—in pain—rather than at home with their families'.(50) Working with regulators is one important way in which standards of care in pain management are being improved in the United Sates, for example, through the introduction of accreditation standards for pain on the part of the Joint Commission on Accreditation of Healthcare Organizations (JCAHO), which covers more than 19 000 American health care organizations.(51)

In Canada,(52) 220 000 people die each year, around 73 per cent of them in hospital.(53) In 1997, over 600 services were listed in a palliative care directory.(54) In June 2000, the Canadian Senate commissioned a report, *Quality End of Life Care: The Right of Every Canadian*; it concluded that little progress had been made in the extension of palliative care provision since 1995. Less than 15 per cent of Canadians receive optimal palliative care; access to services is uneven; funding is inadequate. There were several responses to this situation.(55) A 'Quality End of Life Care Coalition' developed a *Blueprint for Action* in 2001 and in the same year, a special Secretariat for palliative and end-of-life care was established by Health Canada, with a one million dollar budget. In 2002, the Secretariat considered seven priority themes for end-of-life care, including: availability and access; ethical, cultural, and spiritual considerations; education for health care providers; support for families and caregivers; public education and awareness; research; and surveillance. There is considerable scope for improvement in end-of-life care in the very country where the term 'palliative care', in the modern sense that it is now used, was first coined.(56)

Latin America and the Caribbean

It is estimated that by the year 2020 close to a half million people each year will be in need of palliative care services in this region of the world; meanwhile, seven Latin American countries offer some form of palliative care and pain relief services, but public health models of service development are weakly articulated in most places.(57) There are major concerns in the region about the availability and use of opioids for medical purposes. Less than 1 per cent of the global consumption of morphine for medical and scientific purposes occurs in the Latin American countries.(58) A concerted effort to address this issue took place in 1994 when representatives of palliative care programmes in eight Latin American countries met with others from WHO and produced the Declaration of Florianopolis,(59) which made a series of recommendations covering the availability of opioid analgesics, the production of opioid preparations, and the monitoring of costs. A related initiative has been that of the Pan American Health Organization (PAHO), working with WHO, the International Association of Hospice and Palliative Care (IAHPC), and other partners, to organize a series of workshops and an associated demonstration project, on opioid availability and accessibility; and in which particular work has been done to educate narcotics regulators in issues concerning availability. In Argentina, with a population of approximately 32 million people, there are 25–30 palliative care and supportive care teams, mostly in Buenos Aires, with services mainly delivered by doctors and nurses working in a voluntary capacity.(60,61) Morphine consumption in the country increased fivefold over a 5-year period to 2000(62) and there has been a reported fall in the price of opioids.(63) Major support to the whole of Latin America is coming from the IAHPC, as well as from palliative care colleagues in Spain and elsewhere.

Asia Pacific region

One commentator,(64) on the basis of extensive palliative care teaching experience in east Asia, concludes that Hong Kong and Singapore have 'eminently recognizable' palliative care programmes; that Malaysia has begun to achieve governmental recognition for palliative care; and that Japan, South Korea, and Taiwan have established models of palliative care, but without comprehensive coverage. In North Korea, Myanmar, Vietnam, and Mongolia, hospice and palliative care development is locked into deeply rooted issues of inadequate resources for the wider health care system. Somewhere in the middle, between these extremes, are Thailand, China, and the Philippines. Table 9 presents data on palliative care services in 14 countries of the Asia-Pacific region in 2002 and highlights the wide variations in preferred organizational models across these settings.

In 1965, the Catholic Sisters of the Little Company of Mary, from Australia, created a service for dying patients in Korea at the Calvary Hospice of Kangnung;(65) by 1999, there were 60 hospice/palliative care programmes in the country.(66) Hospice services, unrecognized in Korean health care law, are mostly affiliated to general hospitals or clinics and operate on a 'fee for service basis', whereby even those with insurance must pay 20–50 per cent of the service costs. Korea lacks any national policy on palliative care and there are no government-recognized specialist courses. Short-acting oral morphine is unavailable and there are widespread concerns about the use of opioids among patients, families, and health care professionals. Nevertheless, there are two national hospice associations (one Catholic, one protestant) and the Korean Society for Hospice/Palliative Care was formed in 1998.(66) An original research study has pointed to the economic benefits of hospice home care in the country.(65) Comparing four settings, the following costs in US dollars were generated by patients being cared for in the last year of life: charity hospice hospital unit ($54.4); home hospice programme ($87.6); university hospital hospice unit ($585.1); and university hospital unit ($864.5). The authors conclude that 'home hospice services should be extended much more widely in Korea, and deserve enthusiastic support and subsidy by the government',(65) though they recognize that the frugal cost regimes of pioneering hospice services run by religious foundations could not be maintained by others in the future.

Protocols for the introduction of the WHO three-step analgesic ladder were first introduced in China in 1991, leading to increased opioid use and greater interest in pain and palliative care; since 2000, certificated training for opioid prescribing for all clinicians who care for cancer patients has been required by the government and there are said to be hundreds of hospice and palliative care units providing services in urban areas of China.(67)

In Japan, cancer is the principal cause of death, accounting for about 295 000 deaths in 2000. The country's first service for dying people was organized in the Yodogwa Christian Hospital in 1973; in 1979, the Japanese Association for Clinical Research on Death and Dying was established; and in 1981, the first hospice ward inside a hospital was created; by 1993, the Ministry of Health and Welfare had recognized palliative care units in 11 hospitals, with 231 beds in total; by 1997, there were 35 such hospitals with 623 beds;(68) by 2000, there were a total of 80 inpatient units.(69) Hospice medical care in Japan was made eligible for health insurance in 1990 and there were 86 government-approved hospices by the beginning of 2001,

Table 9 Palliative care services in the 14 sectors of the Asia Pacific Hospice Palliative Care Network[a]

Sector	Organizations providing hospice/palliative care	Population (millions)	Estimated annual cancer deaths	Estimated coverage by palliative care services (%)
Australia	230	19	34 587	56
Hong Kong	15	7	10 000	50
India	49	1000	—	—
Indonesia	6	225	60 991[b]	—
Japan	102	127	295 482	5
Korea	28		—	—
North Korea		21		
South Korea		45		
Malaysia	30	22	7825[b]	24
Myanmar	1	50	—	<1
New Zealand	42	4	7461	83
Philippines	20	72	35 000	—
Singapore	10	4	4237	66
Taiwan	28	22	32 000	5
Thailand	3	60	—	—
Vietnam	5	79	51 000[b]	<1

[a] Goh, C.R. (2002). The Asia Pacific Palliative Care Network: a network for individuals and organizations. *Journal of Pain and Symptom Management* **24** (2), 128–33.

[b] Actual statistics not available.

with one hospice bed per 80 000 people.[70] Japan is also notable for the links between hospice/palliative care developments and a wider interest in thanatology, including death education.[71,72] Japan became involved in the field testing of the WHO pain ladder from 1982, and morphine consumption has increased more than 100 times since 1979. Indeed, there is said to be 'an unlimited supply' of opioid analgesics in health care settings, but an urgent necessity to educate health professionals in their use for effective pain relief.[73] There are also reported on-going concerns among patients about the use of morphine.[74]

In Australia, the country that established the world's first academic chair in the specialty, funds for palliative care from both the commonwealth and state governments have been increasing since 1980; and in 2000, Foundation Fellowships were created in the Royal Australasian College of Physicians' new Chapter of Palliative Medicine. Since 1988, the Australian universal health insurance system, Medicare, has provided enhancement funding for palliative care services, and there were 250 services employing designated palliative care staff by 2002, caring for more than 24 000 Australians annually.[75] A study in South Australia estimates that 70 per cent of terminally ill cancer patients receive assistance from palliative care services.[76] In neighbouring New Zealand, there were 42 hospice/palliative care organizations affiliated to the national organization in 1999, but service development here is said to be patchy, with major unmet needs in the upper North Island, where the majority of New Zealand's population is based.[77]

India, with one billion inhabitants, contains one-sixth of the world's population and is a country of striking ethnic, cultural, and religious diversity. Around one million new cases of cancer occur each year; and the vast majority are incurable at diagnosis. An Indian Association of Palliative Care was formed in 1994 with the support of WHO and by 2000 there were nearly 100 palliative care initiatives across the country.[78] A detailed analysis of opioid availability problems in India shows that approximately one million people experience cancer pain in India every year. There was no official source of morphine in India in the 1980s,[11] only 'pump-priming' supplies for specific centres and projects, so levels of morphine consumption for pain relief were low. By 1997, they reached a low of just 18 kg and per capita consumption ranked 113th among 131 countries around the world.[79] There is evidence of an imbalance in policies concerning the regulation of opioids in India, in favour of control and to the detriment of making such drugs easily available. Such regulations have been shown to be highly complex, bureaucratic, and often poorly understood. In a collaborative project involving the Pain and Policy Studies Group in Wisconsin, together with palliative care leaders in India, attempts have been made to press for the simplification of state narcotic rules; there is evidence that these have had the effect of reversing the downward trend in morphine consumption up to 1997, though a great deal remains to be done at the state level to simplify rules governing opioid availability. In Kerala, one of the more progressive states and the first to adopt more streamlined procedures for the control of opioids, striking innovations in palliative care have been achieved against a background of extremely limited resources[80] and the mode of organization and presenting problems of patients at a palliative care service have been described.[81,82]

The Middle East

The first hospice initiative in Israel got underway in 1981 and by 1997 there were 20 hospices in the country, with a coverage of 1.1 hospice beds per million population; the Israel Palliative Care Association was established in 1993.[83] Nevertheless, a study from Israel reports considerable problems in the relief of cancer pain: knowledge deficits, and a disparity between physicians' perceived and actual competence.[84] In both Jordan and Saudi Arabia, pioneering attempts to found a hospice development have been described, along with the attendant difficulties of establishing an appropriate cultural model;[85,86] in Lebanon, work has been undertaken to train the first cohort of physicians to work in palliative care.[87] In 1999, the European School of Oncology sponsored a symposium on 'modern cancer management' at the King Faisal Specialist Hospital in Saudi Arabia. Within the symposium, a session took place on 'the availability and distribution of narcotics', during which several problems were identified, including: the lack of information; religious acceptance and education for patients, professionals, and government; the availability of medications; and of palliative care. A paper published 2 years after the symposium reiterates the complexity of the problems, but reports both 'openness and willingness' on the part of the Saudi government in the subsequent discussions.[88]

Africa

Slowly, attention is being given to the needs of those dying from AIDS-related disease in Africa.[89] The scale of the public health crisis caused by the epidemic of HIV/AIDS has already been described earlier in this chapter. Radical and imaginative solutions are required if effective palliative care can be delivered on the scale required. The HIV/AIDS pandemic has caused the international community, at all levels, to pay increased attention to Africa. Amongst the patchwork of responses, support has been forthcoming from governmental and non-governmental organizations; from community and faith groups; and from institutions offering informal partnership or 'twinning' arrangements. The Diana, Princess of Wales Memorial Fund has initiated palliative care initiatives in Ethiopia, Tanzania, Uganda, Zimbabwe, Kenya, Malawi, Rwanda, South Africa, and Zambia.[90] The WHO is currently involved in a joint palliative care project for cancer and HIV/AIDS patients in the five countries of Botswana, Ethiopia, Tanzania, Uganda, and Zimbabwe.[91] The Foundation for Hospices in Sub-Saharan Africa is also active in the area.[92] In addition to these developments, interest is growing in Morocco and Egypt and services appear to have been established in Congo, Ghana, Namibia, Nigeria, Sierra Leone, The Gambia, and Swaziland.

The first hospice in Africa, established in Zimbabwe in 1980, seems to have been greatly modelled on British lines; a charitable institution, relying on volunteers, initially with patients who were elderly, middle class, and mostly white.[93,94] As it developed, more black and younger patients were cared for, black nurses were employed, and the service sought ways to work alongside the Shona culture of medicine. At the policy level, the country, with WHO involvement, developed a national cancer control initiative, with a nationwide palliative care programme to be integrated within the Ministry of Health. The programme is still to be implemented. In 2000, there were no palliative care posts in the public sector and 20 years from inception, the charitable hospice continued to be the main source of palliative care.

Hospice Uganda was started in 1993 and aims to provide home palliative care services within the immediate area of Kampala; to provide palliative care across Uganda; and to encourage other initiatives elsewhere in Africa.[95,96] The service expanded to include Mobile Hospice Mbarara and Little Hospice Hoima in 1998. By 2002, it had trained over 600 health professionals in pain and symptom control. It is notable that Uganda is a country that has achieved a government policy commitment to palliative care, that oral morphine is becoming available, and that palliative care is one of the essential clinical services in the government's 5-year plan for 2000–2005.[15,95] A distance-learning Diploma in Palliative Care for Africa was developed by Hospice Uganda in conjunction with Makerere University and began in 2002.[97]

In South Africa, the first services were started by non-governmental charitable hospices in the early 1980s; the Hospice Association of South Africa was established in 1986; and in 2002 there were more than 50 hospices throughout the country, though large areas of the country have no hospice services.[98]

Eastern Europe and Central Asia

A large-scale review has been undertaken of hospice and related developments in Eastern Europe and Central Asia.[99] Here, we find that the collapse of communism has removed old certainties and created new risks. Health care systems are de-centralizing and moving to insurance-based models of reimbursement. Wider social and economic problems create chronic underfunding. These seem uncongenial conditions for the development of improved end-of-life care. Yet, it is precisely in these circumstances that hospice and palliative care activists have gained support from the public, policy makers, and fellow professionals.

Some limited hospice developments did take place in this region before the end of the communist era, in Poland (from 1976) and in Russia (from 1985); but, in general, progress only began to occur from the early 1990s. In a region of more than 400 million people, just 467 adult and paediatric hospice-palliative care services exist in 23 out of 28 countries (Table 10). Adult services total 417 and are distributed across 22 countries. There are six countries (Belarus, Georgia, Kazakhstan, Tajikistan, Turkmenistan, and Uzbekistan) that appear to have no adult services whatever. Home care is the type of service most frequently found; there are 221 home care services in 17 countries. There are 173 inpatient units in 13 countries; 80 of these services are free-standing and 92 are within hospitals. Only five hospital mobile teams exist, in four countries. Nursing home teams, five in total, exist in one country only. Day care services total 14, in four countries. Paediatric services total 50 and are found in only nine countries: 19 countries in the region have no paediatric hospice or palliative care services. There are 11 inpatient paediatric services in five countries and 37 paediatric home care services in five countries. There is one day care service. In Poland and the Russian Federation combined, there is a total of 331 adult and paediatric palliative care services, making up 71 per cent of the total for the whole region. Indeed, Poland alone (261 services), has more palliative care than all the other 27 countries in the region combined.

This study found that Poland has the most comprehensive national policy recognition for palliative care, with reimbursement through sickness funds. Hungary has also made substantial strides towards policy assimilation, with recognition from the National Health Service since 1993. Romania has secured reimbursement for palliative care through recognition from the House of Insurance. In Russia, hospices are funded through region and city health administration budgets, which are topped up by district funds. There is some recognition for palliative care by sickness funds in Estonia, Latvia, and Lithuania. In the Czech Republic, hospice and palliative care services are recognized by health authorities and the public health insurance system as types of nursing home, thereby restricting reimbursement potential. In 2000, the Slovak government named palliative care as a priority within the state health policy. The Minister of Health in Belarus has appointed a coordinator for palliative care. In Bulgaria, the Palliative Care Fund is addressing policies and standards. In Croatia, a working party on palliative care policy and legal recognition was established in 2002. In all countries in this region, palliative care services are dependent for their continued development upon charitable funds, project grants, and other subventions.

Five 'beacons' of excellence in palliative care were identified in this study, located in four countries.[100] In each of these there was evidence of: the historical significance of the service within the national scheme of development of palliative care; involvement of personnel of national/international repute; a centre for education and training; impacts upon national health policy. These 'beacons', therefore, provide good evidence of service innovation, partnership approaches, and successful use of international mechanisms of support. Palliative care 'beacons' were found in: Brasov, Romania; Budapest, Hungary; Poznan and Warsaw, Poland; and St Petersburg, Russian Federation.

Western Europe

Palliative care development in Western Europe made rapid progress from the early 1980s. Nevertheless, a comparative analysis of provision, conducted in 1999 as part of the seven-nation European *Pallium* Project,[101,102] showed striking differences in the onset of palliative care developments, country by country and massive inequities in provision when measured at the population level (see Table 11).

It was at St Christopher's Hospice, in London in 1967, that the first hospice service in these seven countries became operational. Next came the Motala-based Hospital-based Home Care Service (1977), followed by the home care programme of the Pain Therapy Division of the National Cancer Institute in Milan, Italy (1980). In Germany, a hospital inpatient unit began in Cologne in 1983 and the first service in Spain was in the Medical Oncology Department of Valdicella Hospital, Santander (1984). In Belgium, palliative care initiatives got underway in 1985, in Brussels, and the first hospice to open in Holland was in Vleuten (1991). By the late 1990s, palliative care services in these seven European countries were at various stages of development. In the United Kingdom, a phase of maturation had been reached, measured

Table 10 Hospice and palliative care services in Central and Eastern Europe (2002)[a]

Country/ territory	Adult: Inpatient Free-standing	Adult: Inpatient Hospital unit	Adult: Hospital mobile team	Adult: Nursing home	Adult: Home care	Adult: Day care	Adult: Total	Paediatric: Inpatient	Paediatric: Home care	Paediatric: Day care	Paediatric: Unspecified	Paediatric: Total	Grand total
Albania	0	0	0	0	3	0	3	0	0	0	0	0	3
Armenia	0	0	0	0	3	0	3	0	0	0	0	0	3
Azerbaijan	0	0	0	0	1	0	1	0	0	0	0	0	1
Belarus	0	0	0	0	0	0	0	0	3	0	0	3	3
Bosnia-Herzegovina	0	0	0	0	1	0	1	0	0	0	0	0	1
Bulgaria	1	0	0	0	20	0	21	0	1	0	0	1	22
Croatia	0	0	0	0	1	0	1	0	0	0	0	0	1
Czech Republic	6	0	1	0	2	0	9	0	1	0	0	1	10
Estonia	0	0	0	0	9	0	9	0	0	0	0	0	9
Georgia	0	0	0	0	0	0	0	0	0	0	0	0	0
Hungary	0	4	2	5	13	2	26	1	0	0	0	1	27
Kazakhstan													
Kyrgyzstan	1	1	0	0	0	0	2	0	0	0	0	0	2
Latvia	0	1	0	0	0	3	4	1	0	0	0	1	5
Lithuania	1	0	0	0	5	0	6	0	0	0	0	0	6
Macedonia	0	1	0	0	0	0	1	0	0	0	0	0	1
Moldova	0	0	0	0	3	0	3	0	0	0	0	0	2
Mongolia	0	1	0	0	0	0	1	0	0	0	0	0	1
Poland	23	50	1	0	149	8	231	25	5	0	0	30	261
Romania	1	5	0	0	4	1	11	6	3	1	0	10	21
Russia	45	25	0	0	0	0	70	0	0	0	0	0	70
Serbia	0	0	0	0	1	0	1	0	0	0	0	0	1
Slovakia	0	2	0	0	1	0	3	0	0	0	1	1	4
Slovenia	0	0	1	0	5	0	6	0	0	0	0	0	6
Tajikistan													
Turkmenistan													
Ukraine	2	2	0	0	1	0	5	1	1	0	0	2	7
Uzbekistan													
Total services	80	92	5	5	221	14	418	34	13	1	2	48	466
Total countries	8	10	4	1	17	4	22	5	5	1	2	9	23

Blank rows indicate no information identified; '0' indicates no existing service.

[a] Clark, D. and Wright, M. *Transitions in End of Life Care: Hospice and Related Developments in Eastern Europe and Central Asia*. Buckingham: Open University Press, 2002.

Table 11 Palliative care services in seven European countries (1999)[a] (populations are given in parentheses)

	Belgium (10.1 m)	Germany (81.9 m)	Italy (57.4 m)	The Netherlands (15.6 m)	Spain (40.0 m)	Sweden (8.8 m)	United Kingdom (57.1 m)
Inpatient hospice	1	64	3	16	1 }	69 (both rows)	219 (both rows)
Inpatient palliative care unit	49	50	0	2	23 }		
Hospital (and nursing home) teams	55	1	0	34	45	41	336
Home care	45	582	88	286	75	67	355
Day care	2	9	0	0	0	13	248

[a] ten Have, H. and Clark, D., ed. *The Ethics of Palliative Care: European Perspectives*. Buckingham: Open University Press, 2002.

Table 12 Ratio of inpatient hospice and palliative care beds to population in seven European countries (1999)[a]

Country	Beds	Ratio of beds to population
United Kingdom	3196	1:17 866
Belgium	358	1:28 212
Sweden	298	1:29 530
Spain	812	1:49 261
Germany	989	1:82 812
Netherlands	119	1:131 092
Italy	30	1:1 913 333

[a] ten Have, H. and Clark, D., ed. *The Ethics of Palliative Care: European Perspectives.* Buckingham: Open University Press, 2002.

by: recognition as a health care specialty, extensive education programmes, and a growing culture of research and academic enquiry. Only in one country (Spain) was there evidence of a strategic approach to palliative care service development using a public health model.(103–105) In all seven countries, the provision of palliative care had moved beyond isolated examples of pioneering services run by enthusiastic founders. Palliative care is being delivered in a variety of settings (domiciliary, quasi-domiciliary, and institutional) though these are not given uniform priority among countries. An example of this can be found in Table 12, which lists the provision of specialist palliative care beds to population, and in which we see the existence of one specialist palliative care bed in the United Kingdom for every 17 000 people, but only one per 1.9 million in Italy.(106)

Beyond these seven western European countries, there is little in the way of comparative information, though data does exist for individual states. In Norway, the first palliative care initiatives occurred in Oslo in 1973; the country's first university-based unit for palliative care was established in Trondheim in 1992; the 1990s saw three key strategy documents for palliative care development; and in 2001 palliative medicine was recognized as a specialty by the Norwegian Medical Association.(107) In Switzerland, only Suisse Romande has a governmental strategy for palliative care;(108) in the country as a whole in 2000 there were nine hospital units, six hospices, six home care teams, and five hospital mobile teams. In France, developments got underway in the mid-1980s, but by 1998 only 55 mobile teams and 51 fixed units (averaging 10 beds each) were in existence.(109)

In 2002, a Council of Europe expert group reporting to the European Health Committee was developing proposals on the legislative framework needed for palliative care development, including: the relevant structures for practice (including the place of the family); the necessary reforms to medical practice; innovative forms of delivery; and the improvement of training for health professionals in palliative care.

Underlying themes

Three key areas can be identified when reviewing the current development of palliative care around the world.

Cultural sensitivity

There is a welcome and growing interest in the question of developing services that are sensitive to the cultural context of those they serve. The Calicut Declaration of 1997 reflects this in its determination to devise 'Asian solutions to Asian problems'.(110) A volume from Hong Kong shows this vividly in documenting the rise of psycho-oncology and palliative care on the island.(111) A project in China highlights some of the issues that occur when western palliative care models encounter cultural systems from the east.(112) Reflecting this concern with cultural sensitivity are examples of the translation of commonly used English-language quality-of-life measures into other languages, with adaptation to the cultural setting.(113) In addition to the traditional preserve of palliative care in the context of cancer, and acknowledging the interest which is now developing in palliative care for those with conditions such as heart disease, lung disease, and stroke,(114) there is also a great need to consider the provision of palliative care to those disadvantaged in other or multiple ways. This includes homeless people, those in prisons, those in poverty, those dying of AIDS, malaria, rabies, tuberculosis, and other conditions, many of them eminently curable where the resources are available.

There is increasing sophistication in the understanding of issues of language, gender, power, and oppression when configuring the work of palliative care. Some striking examples can be found in the literature. A review of palliative care work with 'marginalized communities' in Australia describes those disadvantaged *within* palliative care, because they do not have a diagnosis of cancer, but, in particular, draws attention to those marginalized by *imprisonment*, by *geography*, and by *culture*.(115) In work with aboriginal peoples, the concept of 'cultural safety' has become a guiding principle that attends to: beliefs about illness, dying, and death; folk and popular health care practices; language and cultural practices (rituals, ceremonies, spirituality); and social organization (families, kin, communities). A project of the Central Australian Palliative Care Service involved commissioning a series of paintings by aboriginal artists about palliative care in the local context; the paintings were found to create new understandings and served as a vehicle for referral and a tool for education.(116) Such approaches merit wider exposure and can contribute to an evolving methodology whereby palliative care becomes more attuned to its cultural context. Improved understanding of the place of death and bereavement within the major religious traditions is a further aspect of this.(117)

Policy awareness

Sustainable development in palliative care is dependent on integration within the prevailing policy framework; in particular, the framework of reimbursement. In this respect, palliative care activists have had a great deal to do in lobbying and convincing policy makers. One commentator observes: 'The resources for, and legitimation of, high-quality end-of-life care will depend on broader support than that which emerges piece by piece, or institution by institution, as a result of local initiatives.'(118) Policies relating to opioids are perhaps the most obvious barrier to the development of palliative care in many countries of the world. Here, the guiding principle of 'balance' must be observed: allowing adequate availability of opioids for medical purposes, whilst controlling illegal use; 'diversion' from the former to the latter is an important inhibitor to the easier availability of opioids for medical purposes. Particularly in Asia, the long history of addiction associated with the widespread use of opium—itself the product of British nineteenth-century foreign policy—continues to cast a shadow over easier medical availability.(119) International measures to restrict illicit trade and usage first developed in the early twentieth century with the International Opium Convention, held in Shanghai in 1909. From here a direct line can be traced to the Single Convention on Narcotics of 1961, which led to the creation of the International Narcotics Control Board (INCB).(120)

In general, it is cost that restricts the availability of new drugs to the poorer regions of the world, but regulatory and educational barriers are also at work.(121) Opioids alone are not the solution to the wider availability of palliative care, but they are an important marker of progress and the current variations in levels of availability and consumption are a major outstanding concern at the policy level. Beyond the regulatory field lie the attitudinal and cultural barriers, reported from many countries, and relating to patients, families, and professional care givers, which militate against the use of strong opioids.(122)

Ethical maturity

It is increasingly apparent that the ethics of the rich western world, in which modern palliative care originated, cannot form the ethical code for all peoples and settings. Three authors from Malaysia make the important observation that '. . . decision making in palliative care in this part of the world is far removed from the ideals of autonomy, informed consent and individualism described in the classic textbooks on medical ethics'.(123)

Elsewhere in Asia, but also in Europe and in Southern Africa, there are examples in the literature of growing insight into the different ethical and cultural systems that promote or discourage 'truth telling', disclosure, and the sharing of information.[124–127]. In a post-modern world, there is a need to move beyond the four principles of bio-ethics[128] (autonomy, justice, beneficence, and non-maleficence) to a much richer ethical landscape encompassing care ethics, virtue ethics, and the ethics of authenticity.

A parallel has been drawn between human mortality and the fragile existence of planet earth itself, beset with global problems of poverty, pollution, war, and disease: 'Palliative care offers an example of what can be won from a desperate situation of impending demise; it acknowledges a hope founded in love and courage and patience rather than desperate survival, and so it proclaims a still, small message for a terminal world'.[129] To this can be added the observation that: 'it is better to have poorer and older technologies that are available to all, than more recent technologies that must be rationed. A fair and general allocation of health care resources, even with less than up-to-date technologies, is better than a system creating a massive technological gap between rich and poor'.[130]

What can be done? It is imperative that palliative care leaders in the rich world give greater attention to supporting their colleagues in the resource-poor regions of the world. There is a great 'unfinished agenda' to be tackled. Indeed, the agenda has become larger, and far more complex than could have been imagined when western palliative care began to develop in the 1970s. Over the last 30 years, there has been an extended period of international hospice and palliative care development, fuelled by charismatic leadership, individual motivation and commitment, as well as rich and spontaneous networks of support and assistance across countries and continents. These have been vital to the successes achieved so far. They have generated 'beacons' of excellence in an ocean of suffering, even in the most difficult of circumstances. They will be crucial to further development in many places. It is important to go on encouraging such networks and centres. Nevertheless, they are a *necessary*, but not *sufficient* condition for achieving the goal of palliative care for all who require it. For this to occur there must be engagement with policy makers, politicians, and the wider political and health economy. One initiative aimed specifically at this issue on a global scale and building on the work initiated by WHO is the International Observatory on End of Life Care,[131] which aims to speed up the pace of development by (i) providing clear and accessible research-based information about hospice and palliative care provision in the international context, from a public health perspective incorporating demographic, epidemiological, and health care systems analysis; (ii) complementing this information with data drawn from the social and cultural analysis of end-of-life issues, from a perspective incorporating ethno-graphic, historical, and ethical perspectives; and (iii) making such information available country by country, in ways that facilitate cross-national and regional comparison and analysis.

Key issues, priorities, and strategies

Key issues and priorities

Globally, palliative care remains a neglected area, despite the progress reported in the previous section of this chapter. Notwithstanding the scale of the problem, however, practical solutions can be identified that are affordable and make use of relatively simple methods, applicable and maintainable at the community level. For these to succeed, political commitment must be assured and combined with powerful advocacy from community groups, the professions, and the wider public. Much can be learned from the AIDS movement.

There is a need for a comprehensive approach to the development of a coherent palliative care policy for cancer, AIDS, and the care of older people with chronic illnesses that can be implemented worldwide. For palliative care, a common generic approach covering all diseases will be the most efficient, coupled with some disease-specific variations, for example, anti-retroviral prophylaxis for HIV infection.

It will be necessary to harmonize palliative care into a variety of other structures. These include the institutionalized health care system, as well as systems of family and community support. Cultural, spiritual, and socio-economic support systems in a country are also important, together with both governmental and non-governmental (NGO) efforts. Public engagement and consumer involvement are likewise vital. In particular, palliative care should be integrated with, and not separated from, the mainstream of medical practice and health care.

Research addressing health service and public health questions that affect palliative care development will be an important driver of innovation and may prove a higher priority in the developing world than studies in biomedicine.

The ethical and moral questions and the value systems of different cultures and socio-economic systems must continuously be addressed, as they will be of key importance for what type of palliative care ultimately can be delivered. Freedom from pain could become a human rights issue and care of the dying a human responsibility issue in the near future.

There is a need for a more concerted effort to deliver death-related education to young people in schools in many developed countries in the west. In these societies, religious pluralism, taboos relating to modern death, and high expectations of the capacity of biomedical technology often result in a sense of death as both an individual and collective 'failure'. Each country will be required to identify an approach to the care of dying people in accordance with its own culture and resources. Individual and social norms will have an important role in this, at least as significant as the achievements of the biomedical system.

Accountability, on the part of governments, service providers, and other stakeholders, will become an increasingly important issue, particularly in the context of rising health care costs, shortages of carers, and pressures to adopt new health care technologies. Palliative care programmes and strategies should, therefore, give attention to quality assurance, cost analysis, evaluation, standardization, and coverage.

> A medically institutionalized governmental approach will not reach all in need of palliative care in a society, nor on their own will the usual hospice approaches.

Strategies

National public health programmes for palliative care

The guiding principle of the public health approach recommended here is that, in order to achieve coverage, the methods and approaches adopted must be scientifically valid as well as acceptable, maintainable, and affordable at the community level. This is exemplified by the consensus, established in 1982 by WHO, that drugs are the mainstay of cancer pain relief and that a relatively inexpensive and easily applicable method exists.[2] This method, known as the WHO pain ladder, has become accepted worldwide. Policies and recommendations for rational public health implementation have been undertaken,[6–16] essential drug policies established,[132–141] and national policies established for pain relief, palliative care and/or end-of-life care in wide-ranging and well-documented programmes of activity.

Guidelines on policies and strategies for the effective implementation of palliative care development are extremely important. The establishment of public health programmes in palliative care has now been described extensively.[142–152] The principles have been outlined in detail in a series of WHO documents,[6–8] and good examples exist concerning the establishment of public health programmes in palliative care.

Around the world, some outstanding examples exist of demonstration projects and initiatives, supported by WHO, which have had a demonstrable impact on palliative care development and the improvement of pain management services.

The pioneering Wisconsin Pain Initiative, a WHO Demonstration Project, was one of the earliest state initiatives in the United States and has been a major stimulus to the state pain initiatives that now exist in most parts of America.[153] A federal policy has been established in the United States[154] together with excellent reference guides for clinicians covering the management of cancer pain in adults[155] and children[156] and guides for patients.[157]

Generally, the same recommendations for an effective public health approach can be applied not only for patients with cancer, but also for adults with other serious life-threatening illnesses[13,14] and for children with chronic non-communicable diseases, such as congestive heart failure, cerebrovascular insults, and neuro-degenerative diseases. A comprehensive generic approach benefiting as many as possible in the country is desirable. That this can be done effectively has been proven by the 10-year evaluation of a WHO demonstration project in Catalonia. This covered the majority of those terminally ill with cancer, elderly persons with chronic illness, and those with HIV/AIDS, and successfully provided palliative care and pain relief at the home care level, backed up by hospital provision.[104] It has been shown that a national or state programme for pain relief and palliative care offers the most rational and effective approach for improving the quality of life for the greatest number of patients and families,[148] and will work even where resources are severely limited.[15,152]

A WHO Demonstration Project in the state of Kerala, India, began in 1989 with a 10-year action plan for cancer,[152] which included pain relief and palliative care. During the 10 years, a much earlier diagnosis was observed of cancers of the mouth, breast, and cervix; in addition, one of India's largest radiotherapy centres, in Trivandrum, the capital of Kerala, established a palliative care unit with 24 beds and full-time doctors in palliative care, and equipment was purchased to produce affordable normal release morphine sulfate tablets. India is made up of over 500 districts, with between two and five million people per district. If the problem of coverage for palliative care could be solved in one or two model districts, it could then be applied elsewhere, with the chance of having a major impact. The Pain and Palliative Care Society in Calicut, northern Kerala, was designated a WHO Demonstration project for a 'bottom up approach' in the mid-1990s. By its example, by motivating medical colleges elsewhere in the district of over four million people and, by working with lay volunteers, palliative care services are available to over 50 per cent of terminally ill persons. This model of 'for, with, and through the people' has minimal governmental input, but could serve as a guide for similar districts in India and show that the two approaches ('bottom up' and 'top down') are interdependent and complementary. Both will be needed in an attempt to achieve meaningful national coverage. At the same time, foundation measures through, for example, government policies on morphine availability and handling will also be necessary, and after years of little progress, a breakthrough may occur.[158,159] While consumption of morphine has increased significantly in countries with clear policies, like the Nordic countries, the United Kingdom, United States, Canada, and Japan, the consumption of morphine in India has remained close to zero, going from just below 1 mg to zero.[160]

Uganda is the first and only country in Africa that has made palliative care for people with AIDS and cancer a priority in its National Health Plan (Fig. 1), where it is classed as 'essential clinical care'.[95–97,161–163]

Detailed specifications (outputs, indicators, verification of indicators, and activities at the operational level) concerning the implementation of palliative care into all parts of the health care system is given in Uganda's Health Sector Strategic Plan for 2000–2005 (Table 13).[162]

Uganda has established all the foundation measures as recommended by WHO.[13] A clear national policy has been established, education in palliative care is incorporated into the undergraduate curricula of doctors and nurses, health professionals at all levels are exposed to courses and workshops in pain relief and palliative care, and affordable morphine has been made easily available and is being produced generically in the country. Nurses qualified in palliative care will be able to give morphine. The Ministry of Health has published detailed guidelines for handling of class A drugs.[167] Hospice Uganda is the major resource for education and training in palliative care at all levels and is developing models for community and home-based care. TASO,[164] a pioneering AIDS support organization is providing counselling and support services and the Mildmay Centre for HIV/AIDS Care in Entebbe is extending its activities from a referral centre to rural home-based care. The various missionary hospitals play an important role for achieving coverage, complementing the government health care services, and they are also addressing pain relief and palliative care.

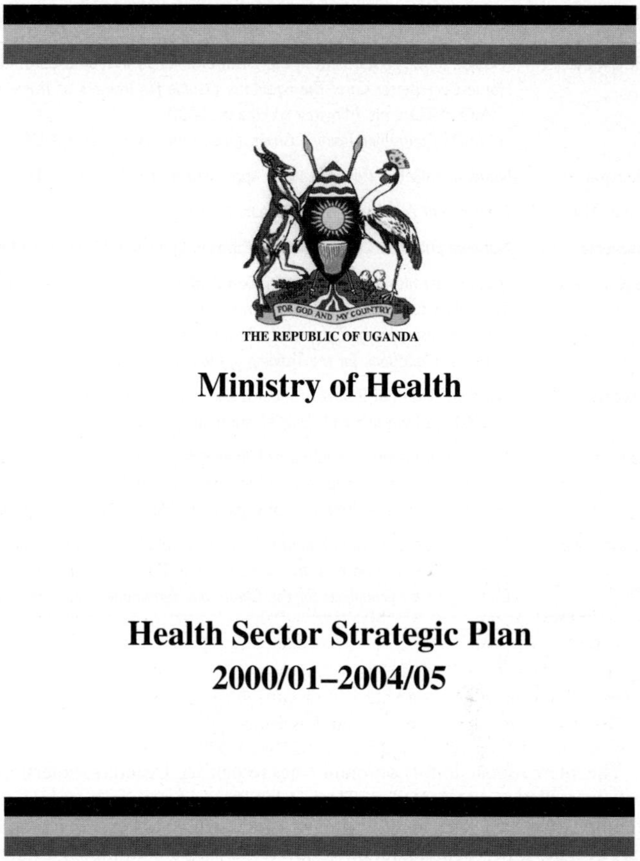

Fig. 1 Uganda establishing palliative care as part of 'essential clinical care', with specifications for output, indicators, and evaluation.

Table 13 Uganda's National Health Sector Strategic Plan: output, indicators, activities of palliative care[a]

Output	Indicators	Verification	Activities at operational level
Accessibility of palliative care for chronically ill and terminally ill increased	Proportion of patients receiving palliative care Number of health providers trained in palliative care	Field visits, feedback from communities, district and health facility reports Training reports, performance appraisal reports	Carry out training of health providers in palliative care Provide supplies for palliative care at all levels of health care Integrate palliative care into curricula of training institutions Provide technical backup to the districts

[a] Ministry of Health, Republic of Uganda: *National Sector Strategic Plan 2000/01–2004/05*[162] and *National Health Policy*.[161]

Table 14 Governmental policies for pain and palliative care (indicative), 1998–2003

Botswana	*A Guide to the Assessment of the Client and Family in Home Care*. Gaborone: WHO and AIDS/STD Unit, Ministry of Health, 2000 *Home Care Better Care: The Facilitator's Guide for Trainers of Trainers on the Use of Modules on Community Home Based Care*. Gaborone: WHO and AIDS/STD Unit, Ministry of Health, 2000 *HIV/AIDS Counsellor Training Guide*. Gaborone: WHO and AIDS/STD Unit, Ministry of Health, 2001
Croatia	*National Palliative Care Program*. Approved draft. Ministry of Health, 2002
Mongolia	*Government Act 1949*. UlaanBataar: Ministry of Health, 1999
Slovenia	*National Palliative Care Program*. Proposal. Ljubljana: Ministry of Health, 2002
South Africa	*South Coast Hospice's Community Based HIV/AIDS Home Care Model*. Pretoria: Directorate, HIV/AIDS and STD, Department of Health, 1999 *Curriculum for the Training of Community Based Home Caregivers*. Pretoria: Directorate, HIV/AIDS and STD, Department of Health, 2001 *Comprehensive Home/Community Based Care Training Manual*. Pretoria: Directorate, HIV/AIDS and STD, Department of Health, 2001 *Learners' Handbook for the Training of Home/Community Based Caregivers*. Pretoria: Directorate, HIV/AIDS and STD, Department of Health, 2001
Sweden	Swedish National Board of Health and Welfare. *Death Concerns Us All—Dignified Care at End of Life*. Expert report 2001 : 6. Stockholm: Socialstyrelsen, 2001 (in Swedish with English summary)
Uganda	Ministry of Health, Republic of Uganda. *National Health Policy*. Kampala: Ministry of Health, 1999 Ministry of Health, Republic of Uganda. *National Sector Strategic Plan 2000/01–2004/05*. Kampala: Ministry of Health, 2000 Ministry of Health, Republic of Uganda. *Guidelines for Handling Class A Drugs*. Kampala: Ministry of Health, 2001
Zimbabwe	*National Cancer Control Program*. Harare, Zimbabwe: Ministry of Health, 1994 and 1995 (approved plan, activated but aborted due to lack of resources) *Community Home Based Care Policy*. Harare, Zimbabwe: Ministry of Health and Child Welfare, 2001 *Discharge Plan Guidelines for the Chronically/Terminally Ill Patients*. Harare, Zimbabwe: Ministry of Health and Child Welfare, 2001

The international donor community has recognized Uganda's leadership role in palliative care in Africa. Thus, it has become a main recipient of funding from the Diana, Princess of Wales Memorial Fund.[165,166] Uganda has become a key demonstration country in WHO's community health approach to palliative care for HIV/AIDS and cancer patients in Africa, a joint project between Botswana, Ethiopia, Tanzania, Uganda, Zimbabwe, and South Africa. Hospice Uganda is doing important work outside Uganda too in the form of workshops in other African countries, sensitizing them to introduce foundation measures for education and drug availability and establish policies, as well as running courses in palliative care.

Uganda has demonstrated the importance and success of a harmoniously integrated government approach with clear policies and a decentralized community-based approach, linked to its HIV/AIDS programme. Uganda and Senegal are the only two African countries where the prevalence of HIV/AIDS has declined[167]—clear evidence of the value of strategic policy-making.

There is evidence that governments at many levels (national, provincial, federal, and state) have begun to recognize the importance of pain relief and palliative care through the development of officially formulated policies. Palliative care has also been incorporated into several cancer control and some HIV/AIDS programmes. Some of these policies have had real impact, others have been 'paper tigers' with little effect. Often, failure results from the lack of a *comprehensive* strategy, for example, omitting the community system. Nor will a government approach in the absence of hospice developments, or unconnected to them, be likely to achieve meaningful coverage or vice versa. Table 14 gives an indicative list of governmental policies and strategies in different countries that have appeared since the second edition of this textbook.

Governmental policy

Establishing a national policy offers the best way to ensure, in a cost-effective manner, adequate palliative care for the greatest number of patients and families. WHO recommends three foundation measures based on: governmental policy, education, and drug availability.[8,14] They cost very little, but have a large potential impact. They are important for establishing sustainable palliative care and achieving meaningful coverage (Fig. 2):

- establish a national policy of palliative care with solutions specific for the country/culture;
- establish commitments to educate and train all health professionals by including palliative care in the curricula for undergraduate doctors, nurses, pharmacists, social workers, and others;
- develop advocacy and education for the public;
- ensure availability of affordable drugs for pain control and symptom management and their use by appropriately trained professionals;
- ensure that pain and palliative care programmes are incorporated into the country's health care system;
- ensure a multidisciplinary and multidisease approach.

> Uganda serves as a brilliant model, like Wisconsin and Catalonia, for the importance of an integrated government and community non-governmental approach. Each one by themselves in isolation, will not achieve much.

Points found valuable to address when establishing a national policy for palliative care are summarized in Table 15.

Assessing the magnitude of the problem is important, as it will demonstrate the high number in need of palliative care. To come to an overall figure, either the figure for the total number of deaths in the previous year can be used, or if this is not available then the crude death rates can be utilized. Approximately 60 per cent of the figure arrived at gives the number needing palliative care. Estimating the approximate number of cancer patients does not demand a cancer registry in the country. As a rule of thumb if 50 per cent of the country's population is under the age of 20, then a cancer incidence of 100/100 000 population can be assumed: and if 50 per cent are over the age of 20 assume an estimated cancer incidence of 180/100 000. In many developing countries this method has been proved to give a realistic estimate. Developed countries usually have population-based cancer registries and also a much higher cancer incidence.

A medically institutionalized governmental approach will not reach all in need of palliative care in a society, nor will the usual hospice approaches.

By coordinating all efforts to incorporate palliative care into the national health care services and with the importance of home care and community support clearly spelt out in the policy, it should be possible to achieve adequate coverage. Appropriate hospital support and backup for the home-based care will be important for the degree of effectiveness. However, it should be recognized that a large part of the population, for example, in Africa, will not be reached by conventional health services. Thus, other existing traditional approaches and culturally specific support systems will need to be supported and incorporated.

Nothing is more stimulating to future nurses and doctors wishing to do palliative care than seeing it at work in real life. An identified clinical centre of excellence will, therefore, be an important focal point for the training of future trainers in palliative care. Hospices[168–170] have indeed played an important role in this respect as a model and source of inspiration to others.

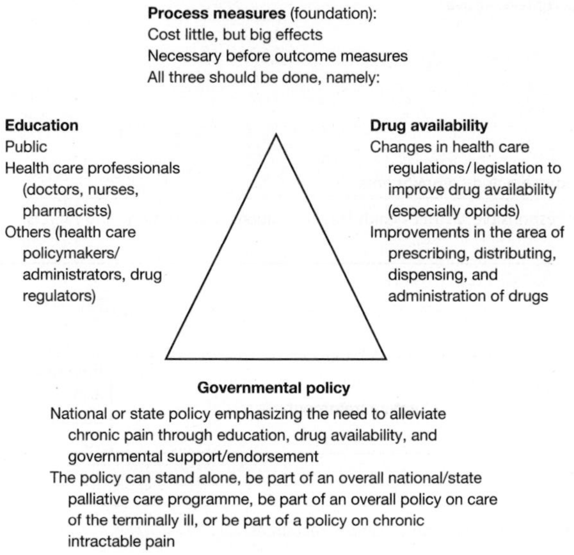

Process measures (foundation):
Cost little, but big effects
Necessary before outcome measures
All three should be done, namely:
Education
Public
Health care professionals (doctors, nurses, pharmacists)
Others (health care policymakers/ administrators, drug regulators)
Drug availability
Changes in health care regulations/legislation to improve drug availability (especially opioids)
Improvements in the area of prescribing, distributing, dispensing, and administration of drugs
Governmental policy
National or state policy emphasizing the need to alleviate chronic pain through education, drug availability, and governmental support/endorsement
The policy can stand alone, be part of an overall national/state palliative care programme, be part of an overall policy on care of the terminally ill, or be part of a policy on chronic intractable pain

Fig. 2 Foundation measures necessary for an effective national programme.

Table 16 contains a self-explanatory checklist of points that will be important to consider when establishing a national palliative care programme.[6,8,12,14] UNAIDS has developed guidelines for national responses to HIV/AIDS that address situation analysis, response analysis, strategic planning, and resource mobilization.[171] Also useful, especially for developed countries, is the Canadian Palliative Care Association's guidelines for 'Standardized Principles and Practice of Palliative Care'.[172]

The allocation of limited resources is becoming an increasingly important question to address within a country's overall national health plan. The pressures for applying costly high technology with minimal applicability in many countries, especially resource-poor settings, is also increasing. Already an uncritical application of costly diagnostic and curative approaches with rather limited effects in a situation of mainly late-stage incurable patients is ongoing in many developing countries and makes large demands on the health budget. Nothing would have a greater impact on the care of patients with advanced incurable disease than instituting and implementing the knowledge we have today to improve their quality of life. Indeed, a fraction of the costs spent on curative efforts with minimal results would, if spent on palliative care, have a major positive impact on both patients and their families. A model for allocation of resources in both developed and developing countries is given in Figs 3–5.

With limited resources worldwide for palliative care, rational approaches are essential. Even limited resources may have an impact, provided that the relevant priorities are set and strategies are implemented.

Palliative care should attract more of the available resources. Yet, in both developed and developing countries it is an option that is all too often ignored and not offered to the patient until too late in the course of the disease (Fig. 3). Palliative care should be seen as an integral part of patient care from the outset, and in many cases it should be introduced at the time of diagnosis (Figs 4 and 5). Curative care and palliative care are not mutually exclusive. The present allocation of resources should be changed in future strategies in both developed (Fig. 4) and developing countries (Fig. 5). This form of resource allocation (Fig. 4) would have a much bigger effect than present arrangements (Fig. 3).

A better allocation of resources for cancer control than presently being practised is to be encouraged strongly, requiring relevant national policies. There are yearly 10 million new cancer patient years, and the figure will soon rise to 24 million yearly; a major part of those who will need

Table 15 Establishing a national public health policy for palliative care. Points to consider

• Assess magnitude of problem • Point out solutions, e.g., simple affordable methods applicable and maintainable at community level exist
Set objectives: • To improve control of symptoms of all that would benefit from palliative care: patients with CANCER and AIDS/HIV (all ages); those terminally ill, some elderly persons; those with congestive heart failure, cerebrovascular diseases, and other incurable chronic diseases; neurodegenerative diseases • To establish WHO Foundation measures of a national policy, drug availability, and education of the health professions and public. These cost little but will have major effects • To make optimal use of limited resources so as to benefit all in need of palliative care • To ensure equity of access
Evaluate strategies and approaches: • Need for incorporating palliative care into the national health care system, at all levels by the Government • The importance of home care and community approaches for achieving coverage • The national policy to include home-based palliative care • Hospitals and specialized palliative care centres should be able to offer support to home-based care • Importance of empowering the families in palliative care, what to do and how • Importance of non-medical approaches, social cultural support systems • Importance of advocacy and public information • Importance of obtaining highest possible political commitments
Set priorities; identify indicators for monitoring and evaluation
Identify key persons, champions, and how to support them
Action plan, including time schedules, responsible persons and budget. Details for implementation, e.g., national conference for launch and follow-up workshops in the country

Table 16 Checklist for development of national palliative care programmes

Identification of the capacities of today's health care system and what needs to be added for palliative care to be delivered
Get commitments from deans and directors of nursing schools to introduce palliative care education in curricula
Identify future trainers of trainers and persons who will deliver undergraduate education of doctors and nurses in palliative care
Identify legislative changes that may be needed, for example, for easy availability of morphine and prescription. Review economic reimbursements for palliative care
Estimate new national quota of morphine to be requested from the International Narcotic Control Board (INCB), Vienna
Specify in national policy that over 80 % of new quota when tendering for it should be generic immediate-release morphine sulfate tablets. For those countries that do not ignore cost-effectiveness considerations in their abilities to cover all in need
Consultations with NGOs
Review role of existing organizations
Identify resources for and organize a national multidisciplinary workshop, including leading doctors, nurses, pharmacists, social workers, representatives of Ministry of Health, drug regulating authorities, universities, relevant NGOs, patients representatives, representatives from the country's international donor community, religious representatives, traditional healers, press and TV representatives, and the country's WHO representative
Identify legislative changes that may be necessary
Secure a budget for catalytic palliative care key activities and persons needed
Prepare a national plan
Prepare short concise positive advocacy and public information materials
Plan national conference for launching the programme, including highest possible political leadership and commitments
Plan and find budget for follow-up targeted workshops around the country, for example, for responsible district health leaders, patient organizations and NGOs, pharmacists and drug regulator, GPs, leading educational centres

palliative care are cancer patients competing for scarce resources. Table 17 summarizes the state of the art in cancer control—priorities and strategies for the eight most common cancers. It shows the importance of prevention and palliative care. Unfortunately, most resources for cancer control, usually over 90 per cent, go to therapy, with proportionally fewer going to primary prevention (in spite of the fact that six to seven out of the eight most common cancers are preventable), and often none go to palliative care. Only four of the eight most common cancers are curable, if diagnosed early. However, in developing countries most of the cancers listed as curable are incurable because of delays in diagnosis. Of the eight most common cancers worldwide, five are more prevalent in developing countries. Even if diagnosis is made at an early stage of the disease, treatment is curative in only four of these cancers but palliative care is needed in all eight.

About 70–80 per cent of total health care spending, both public and private, in developing countries is on to curative treatment. Within the curative sector, hospitals often account for more than 80 per cent of the total health care costs. Most of these hospitals are located in urban areas, whereas most of the population still lives in rural areas. Thus, considerable resources are spent on treating advanced cases when the main role of the health care services should be to provide palliative care. A better balance must be achieved: not a question of either/or but an integration of palliative care into the early stages of therapy. Curative efforts for the clearly incurable at the time of diagnosis are costly, often with additional morbidity, and doomed to fail.

The following recommendations are valid for countries that want to introduce pain relief and palliative care through the implementation of rational public health strategies:

1. Governments should establish national policies and programmes for palliative care.
2. Governments should ensure that palliative care programmes are incorporated into their existing health care systems; separate systems of care are neither necessary nor desirable.
3. Governments should ensure that health care workers (physicians, nurses, pharmacists, or other categories appropriate to local needs) are adequately trained in palliative care.

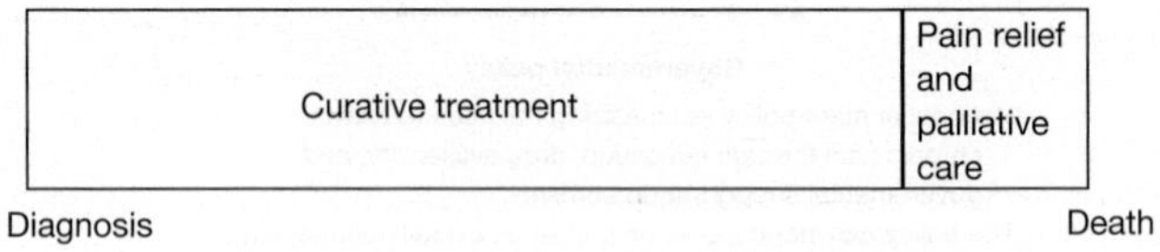

Fig. 3 Present allocation of cancer resources.

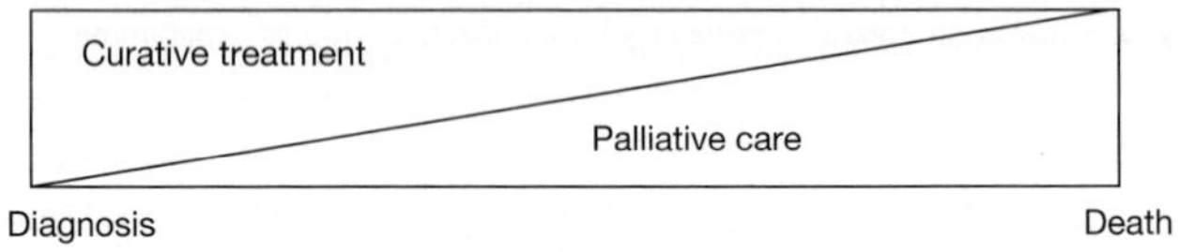

Fig. 4 Proposed allocation in developed countries.

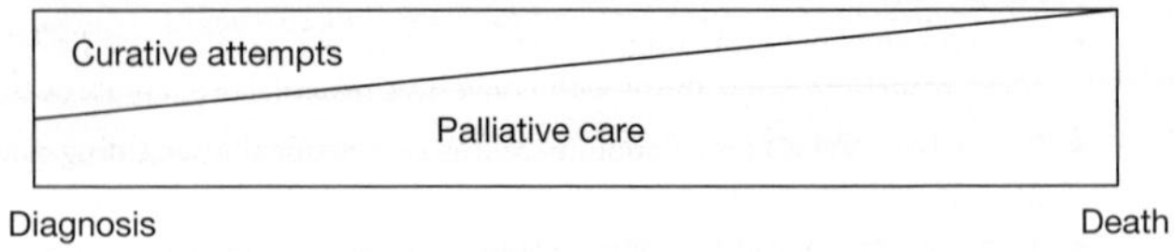

Fig. 5 Proposed allocation in developing countries.

4. Governments should review their national health policies to ensure that equitable support is provided for programmes of palliative care at all levels in the health care system and in the home.
5. In the light of the financial, emotional, physical, and social burdens carried by family members who are willing to care for chronically and terminally ill persons in the home, governments should consider establishing formal systems of recompensation for the principal family caregivers.
6. Governments should recognize the singular importance of home care for patients with advanced diseases and should ensure that hospitals are able to offer appropriate back-up and support for home care.

Table 17 Cancer control—priorities and strategies for the eight most common cancers globally

Tumour[a]	Primary prevention	Early diagnosis	Curative therapy[b]	Pain relief and palliative care
Lung	++	—	—	++
Stomach	+	—	—	++
Breast	—	++	++	++
Colon/rectum	+	+	+	++
Cervix	++	++	++	++
Mouth/pharynx	++	++	++	++
Oesophagus	—	—	—	++
Liver	++	—	—	++

++, Effective; +, partly effective; —, not effective.

[a] Listed in the order of the eight most common tumours globally.

[b] Curative for the majority of cases with a realistic opportunity of finding them early.

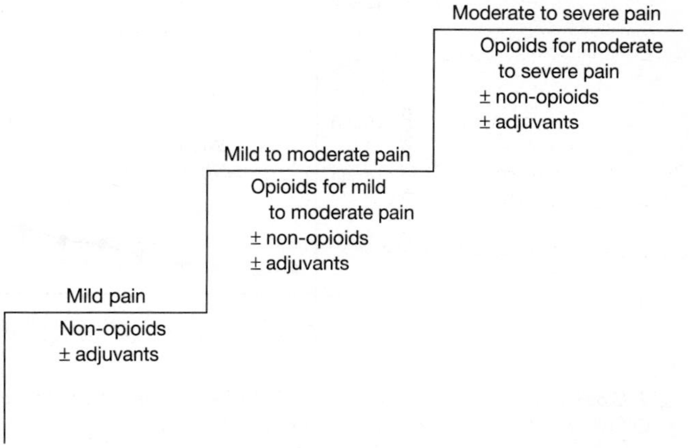

Fig. 6 WHO Pain Ladder.

7. Governments should ensure the availability of both opioid and non-opioid analgesics, particularly morphine for oral administration. Further, they should make realistic determinations of their opioid requirements and ensure that annual estimates submitted to the INCB reflect actual needs.
8. Governments should ensure that their drug legislation makes full provision for the following:
   (a) regular review, with the aim of permitting importation, manufacture, prescribing, stocking, dispensing, and administration of opioids for medical purposes;
   (b) legally empowering physicians, nurses, pharmacists, and, where necessary, other categories of health care worker to prescribe, stock, dispense, and administer opioids;
   (c) review of the controls governing opioid use, with a view to simplification, so that drugs are available in the necessary quantities for legitimate use.

Drug availability

WHO recommends that countries establish an Essential Drug List, based on the medical needs of the majority of the population.[(132)] A national palliative care strategy should address the necessary legislation, procurement, tender or generic national production and administrative process for drugs essential for palliative care of people with cancer, HIV/AIDS, and those chronically ill at the end of life. In the early 1980s, WHO used pain as the priority symptom for these patients and established technical guidelines for its control.[(2)] The WHO Pain Ladder became the accepted standard method worldwide (Fig. 6).

> The brief given to achieve consensus for the WHO Pain Ladder was that it should be a simple, effective, and scientifically valid method for pain relief, applicable, affordable, and maintainable at community level, so as to be able to reach all globally.

Only a handful of drugs (all given orally) are needed for the implementation of the WHO Pain Ladder, all generic and thus inexpensive but effective, and it has been shown that up to 90 per cent of severe pain can be controlled by its use. The approach was originally suggested by Professor V. Ventafridda to Chief Cancer, WHO, and after a first WHO meeting in 1982, draft guidelines were produced, followed by field testing, and subsequent wide dissemination, advocacy, adoption, and evaluation. The consumption of morphine worldwide, constant and low between 1972 and 1983, started to increase from 1984 onwards (see Fig. 7).[(173)] WHO policy guidelines to governments were produced at a WHO Expert Committee Meeting in 1999.

Collaboration with the International Narcotics Control Board, Vienna,[(174–176)] was established in the mid-1980s to promote the availability of morphine for pain-relieving purposes. A WHO Collaborating Centre to help with drug policies was established in Wisconsin, USA, and guidelines for governments on morphine availability were produced together with WHO[(3)] in 1992.[(177)]

Over the last 15 years, there has been increasing evidence that vague and ambiguous laws and regulations, at both state and national levels, are being revised to accommodate the legitimate use of opioids, particularly for patients with chronic pain. Methods of assessing and monitoring the medical need for opioids are being improved. This is reflected in the substantial increase in the estimated annual requirements for morphine reported by various countries to the INCB. Morphine consumption has increased rapidly. Global medical morphine consumption was relatively constant between 1972 and 1984, below 2 tons. In 1984, it started to increase and by 1992 it had reached 12 tons. Today, it is close to 25 tons. However, between 1984 and 1993, most morphine use was concentrated in the 10 industrialized countries that have consistently ranked highest in per capita consumption: Australia, Canada, Denmark, Iceland, Ireland, New Zealand, Norway, Sweden, the United Kingdom, and the United States. During this period, morphine consumption in the top 10 countries increased by 450 per cent, while in the remainder of the world it increased by 150 per cent. Although the top 10 consuming countries represent only 7 per cent of the world's population, in 1993 they accounted for approximately 77 per cent of the total morphine used. By contrast, in 1993, approximately 120 countries representing more than 80 per cent of the world's population consumed only 23 per cent of the total morphine used. These are mainly, but not exclusively, developing countries in Asia, all of South America, Africa, Eastern Europe, and the Mediterranean region. There may be small quantities of opioids in some hospitals in these countries, but most cancer patients have extremely limited access to them, if any. There are still about 50 countries where no oral morphine is available (Fig. 8). Yet in these countries most cancer patients are incurable and symptom control is at present the only pragmatic and realistic approach that can be offered.

Under the Single Convention on Narcotic Drugs, to which most governments are party, governments are responsible for assuring the availability of opioid analgesics for medical purposes in their country. Medical organizations have a parallel duty to relieve pain and suffering. Several national health ministries have initiated actions to develop policy, education, and drug availability. However, if there is no cooperative medical and government

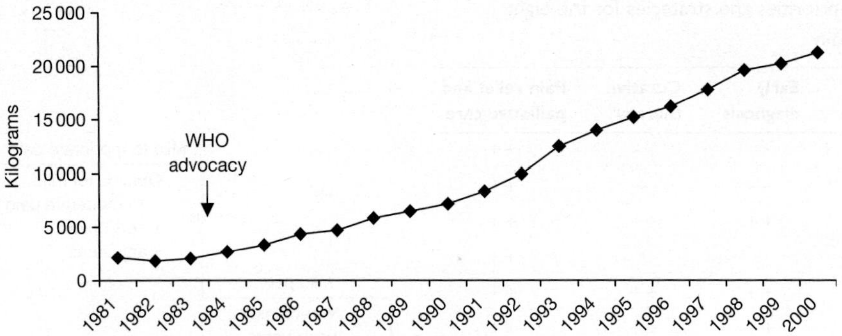

Fig. 7 Global consumption of morphine, 1981–2000. (*Source:* International Narcotics Control Board (INCB). *Demographic Yearbook*. United Nations, 1999 and WHO Collaborating Center, University of Wisconsin, WI, 2002.)

leadership, there will be little improvement in opioid availability and relief of cancer pain, one of the major symptoms in palliative care.

Importance of specifying availability of cost-effective morphine

For most of the world's countries consideration of cost-effectiveness[132–140] will be absolutely essential for achieving coverage of their populations with pain relief and palliative care, especially in resource-poor settings. Generic normal-release morphine sulfate tablets or morphine hydrochloride solution should not cost more than around US$ 0.001 or 1 cent US for 10 mg (as in Kerala or Uganda). Normal-release morphine sulfate tablets are effective, yet many times when a country has established a national programme there have been commercial pressures to adopt newly developed and more expensive pain-relieving drugs. Thus, in many countries with health expenditure of less than US$ 10 per capita per year, 1 month's supply of drugs promoted or offered by the many large multinational companies may cost between US$ 60 and 180. One month's supply of morphine sulfate tablets should only cost between US$ 1.8 and 5.4.

The recommendations on these issues are therefore:

- when establishing a national policy for pain relief and palliative care, specify that it should be normal-release generic morphine for treating moderate to severe pain, and of the new quota requested from INCB 80 per cent of the amount, when tendering for its import, should be the cost-effective normal-release generic morphine;

> Scientifically valid, effective but inexpensive methods, applicable and maintainable at community level exist for controlling pain. Provided the right visionary leadership also exist, every country should be able to offer *freedom from pain*.
>
> With the correct policies and strategies every country should be able to secure freedom from pain. Using morphine sulfate tablets, immediate release morphine or morphine hydrochloride solutions, freedom from pain can cost less than aspirin, or—as in Uganda—less than the price of a loaf of bread.

- targeted tendering from the few companies providing this may be necessary;
- many countries are able to produce their own generic medicines, and an alternative to consider would be to import the opioid base and produce the tablets/solutions in the country.

Other symptoms

Whenever introducing opioids for pain relief, it is essential that other symptoms and drugs for their control are addressed, for example: constipation, bowel obstruction, anxiety, depression, insomnia, confusional states, agitation, nausea, and vomiting. Additional drugs to cover the frequent opportunistic infections and their side-effects in HIV/AIDS patients should also be included. An example of the latest essential drug list for palliative care compiled by WHO[135] is given in Table 18.

Many countries have established their own essential drug list. Wherever there is an 'equally efficient drug', as the generic drugs are called in Sweden, this is recommended for prescription. Such drugs are included in the reimbursement policy of the government.[141] Other more expensive drugs can, of course, be prescribed, but are not included by the reimbursement policy, and have to be paid for in full by the patients. The escalating drug cost is one of the major concerns of many countries, even in developed countries, as drugs costs account for a major part of the health budget. Implementing wise policies can make great savings. Zimbabwe and Uganda have long since established their national essential drug list, and these include drugs for the relief of cancer pain,[140,164] but a comprehensive list of palliative care drugs has yet to appear in these countries.

Any essential drug list for palliative care will include opioid drugs and WHO has produced guidelines for their handling.[3,6,132] Key points include:

- *Legal issues:* doctors, nurses, and pharmacists should be empowered legally to prescribe, dispense, and administer opioids to patients in accordance with their needs.
- *Accountability:* opioids must be dispensed for medical use only, with responsibility in law.
- *Prescription:* a prescription for opioids should contain at least the following information:
  - patient's name,
  - date of prescription,
  - drug name, dosage, strength and form, quantity prescribed,
  - instructions for use,
  - the doctor's name and business address,
  - the doctor's signature.
- *Accessibility:* opioids should be available in locations that will be accessible to as many patients as possible.

In countries where a great deal of effort has been expended in the introduction of clear national policies for pain relief and palliative care, including making opioids available, educating and training the health professionals in the use of opioids, and establishing necessary guidelines is also essential if adequate coverage is to be achieved. The main concern for all involved, including the pharmaceutical companies, should be effective pain relief for all in need of it and it is hoped a constructive balance and *modus operandi* can be achieved. The ideal would be morphine sulfate tablets for starting and maintaining pain control in the majority of patients, availability of

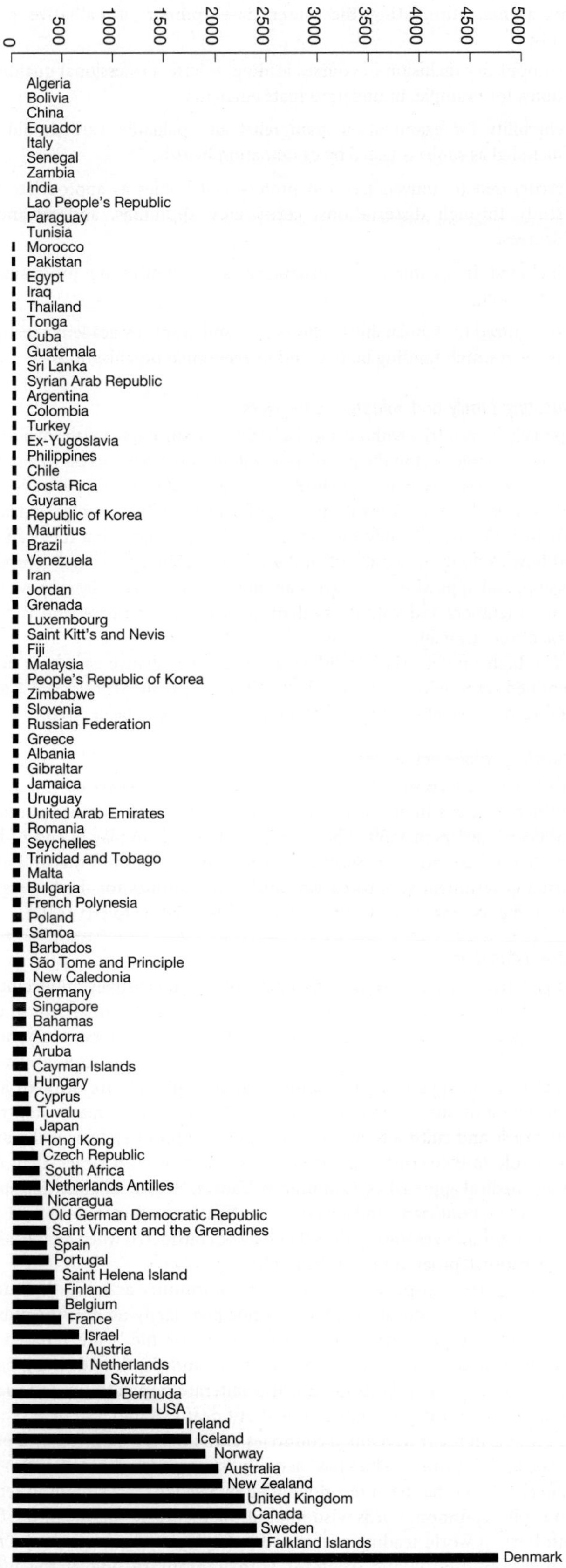

Fig. 8 Average daily consumption of defined daily doses of morphine per million inhabitants.

Table 18 Example of a suggested essential drug list for palliative care[a]

Analgesics	
Non-opioids (mild pain)	Acetylsalicylic acid
	Paracetamol
	Ibuprofen
Opioids (mild to moderate pain)	Codeine
Opioids (moderate to severe pain)	Morphine
	Methadone
Opioid antagonist	Naloxone
Corticosteroids	Dexametasone
	Prednisone
Laxatives	Senna
	Sodium ducosate
	Mineral oil
	Lactulose
	Magnesium hydroxide
Anxiety, depression, insomnia, psychosis, epileptic seizures	Amitryptiline
	Diazepam
	Lorazepam
	Chlorpromazine
	Haloperidol
	Phenytoin
	Sodium valproate
Appetite	Prednisole
Bowel obstruction (when surgery not indicated)	Dimenhydrinate
	Haloperidol
	Hyoscine butylbromide
	Metoclopramide
Diarrhoea	Codeine phosphate
	Loperamid
Gastric protection	Omeprazol
Fluid retention	Furosemide
	Spironolactone
Oral candidiasis	Cotrimoxazole
	Ketoconazole
	Nystatin
Nausea and vomiting	Dimenhydrinate
	Holoperidol
	Metoclopramide
	Prednisolone
	Prochlorperazine
Neuropathic pain	Amitriptyline
	Phenytoin
	Diazepam
Repiratory problems	Hyoscine butylbromide
	Lorazepam
	Morphine
	Prednisolone
	Salbutamol
Cough	Codeine
Excessive secretion at end of life	Hyoscine butylbromide
Skin problems (fungating tumours, decubitus ulcers)	Metronidazole
	Dressing supplies

[a] Modified from Olweney, C., Sepúlveda, C., Merriman, A., Fonn, S., Borok, M., Ngoma, T., Doh, A., and Stjernswärd, J. (2003). Guidelines for the treatment and palliative care of HIV disease patients with cancer in Africa. *Journal of Palliative Care* (in press).

slow-release morphine for those willing or able to pay the much higher price for the convenience of taking the tablets twice instead of four to six times per 24 h, and in those few countries that can afford it, fentanyl patches for transdermal delivery in selected cases.

Education

Education and training is the third foundation measure, a priority for ensuring effective implementation of palliative care in a national public health approach.

Multiprofessional education

Teamwork is at the core of palliative care and this includes professional disciplines, volunteers, family members, and persons leading culturally specific community support systems. For the professions, training programmes should be in place for nurses, doctors, pharmacists, social workers, spiritual-religious carers, and community-based home care workers. The introduction of palliative care into the curricula of the undergraduate education of all doctors and nurses is recommended as an efficient way to broaden the base of palliative care coverage at the national level. Before that it is necessary to establish a critical mass of educators and trainers of the trainers in most countries. Selected training of family doctors, radiotherapists/oncologists, geriatricians, and HIV/AIDS doctors and workshops for District Chief Medical Officers are advisable.

Training in palliative care should cover:

- symptom control;
- management of disease complications and treatments;
- decision-making;
- communication;
- psychosocial care of patient and family;
- care of the dying.

WHO recommends that education should address:[6] attitudes, beliefs, and values, as well as the appropriate knowledge base and practice skills (Table 19).

Education integrated into the system

Targeted education and training may be a necessary start in many countries, but the goal should be to maximize the impact of the educational programme, stimulating the wider development of palliative care, that is:

- compulsory inclusion in courses leading to basic professional qualifications, for example, in undergraduate curricula;
- eligibility for examination: pain relief and palliative care should be included as subjects tested by examination boards;
- recognized by universities and professional bodies as appropriate for study through dissertations, certificates, diplomas, and advanced degrees;
- included in postgraduate programmes of continuing professional education;
- recognized for scholarships, fellowships, and grants by academic institutions, research funding bodies, and international organizations.

Table 19 Education in palliative care to cover knowledge, attitude, and practice (KAP)—suggested topics

Attitudes, values, beliefs
The philosophy and ethics of palliative care
Personal attitudes towards the disease (cancer, HIV/AIDS, terminal patients) pain, dying, death, and bereavement
Illness as a state with physical, social, psychological, and spiritual dimensions
Team work multiprofessional
The family as the unit of care
Knowledge
Principles of effective communication
Pathophysiology of the common symptoms
Assessment and management of pain and other symptoms
Psychological and spiritual needs of seriously ill and dying patients and family
Treatment of emotional and spiritual distress
Availability of community resources to assist patients and families
Physiological and psychological responses to bereavement
Practice/skills
Practice of learned knowledge in the classroom, use of role play and discussion of real case-histories
Goal-setting in physical, psychological, social, and spiritual dimensions
Development of family trees and of a family care plan
Monitoring of pain and symptom management

Educating family and volunteer caregivers

Especially in countries without a social health insurance system (the majority) or where a large part of the population will not even have access to a nurse or a doctor, empowerment of family members and volunteers in palliative care will be the most realistic approach for meaningful coverage, particularly in rural areas. Family care givers should be taught what they can do and how to do it. Personal care and services, social support and companionship, and applied medical care can often be done better by empowered family members and volunteers than, for example, a nurse who is only available occasionally.

The high unmet needs of informal carers in palliative care have been identified, especially in the west[178–183] and also in Africa[184–193] and valid recommendations for how to support carers have been given.

Educating traditional healers

This has been a controversial subject. Provided the healers do not cause significant delays in access to treatment for otherwise curable diseases, traditional healers may often have an important role to play in end-of-life care. Several countries in Southern Africa have recognized this and also started government-sponsored education programmes for the healers to extend the coverage of palliative care, especially relating to HIV/AIDS.

Public education

For effective implementation of national policies, it is usually important to have the general public well informed. This is especially important in the case of pain relief and palliative care, for several reasons. First, everyone is going to die, but few are aware of what can be done for controlling severe symptoms and supporting the families. Second, opioids are involved and there are lot of misconceptions about morphine. Third, in many countries individuals and culturally specific community support systems will play a major role in delivering palliative care, equal to or even larger, than the purely medical approaches. Community leaders, NGOs, religious and spiritual leaders, politicians, and government officials also need to be informed. Table 20 summarizes some points that may be considered when establishing an educational programme for the public.

Direct person-to-person education in community activities is a most powerful form of education. Media campaigns clarifying how the public can benefit by palliative care ('what is in it for me?') are important. Videos on national TV, covering pain relief and death and dying have been very effective in both literate and illiterate populations, and radio too in the latter category. Education about death should also be given in the schools in many developed countries in the west as an integrated part of social education. This has actually started in the UK[194] and France,[195] and has been recommended in Sweden.[196] Common sense is not very common, nor is wisdom; but the memories of one of the few with both, a world leading pioneer of palliative medicine, captures the human condition giving solutions with humour to one of the most important events, death, that all have to go through, and ought to be compulsory reading not only for health professionals but also the informed public.[197]

Educational resources and material

The publications of WHO on cancer and palliative care have already been cited in this chapter. These monographs are published in several of the major world languages, are often translated into numerous other languages, and should be available at reduced prices for developing countries. They have wide application. Excellent monographs for professional education have been published,(198–213) and many are in their third or fourth editions, indicating their popularity and usefulness. Adaptation to developing countries has been done(214,215) and several governmental or professional society guidelines have been produced that also are useful.

For physicians, thorough curricula for palliative care exist in the United Kingdom and the United States. One of the most concentrated empowering didactic training courses (EPEC) deserves particular mention and takes the form of a train-the-trainers curriculum and a $2\frac{1}{5}$ day course.(216) A core curriculum for professional education in pain, developed by the International Association for the Study of Pain (IASP) was one of the earliest educational programmes(217) and a Canadian training module for palliative care for HIV/AIDS also exists.(205) For nurses, a core curriculum in palliative care has been established, which has served as a model over the years.(218) A train-the-trainer curriculum and an intensive $2\frac{1}{5}$ day course for nurses (ELNEC), similar to that for doctors (EPEC), also merits attention.(219)

For informal carers, unmet needs have been identified and recommendations for support have been produced both by the professions as well as by governments.(57,184–193)

For the public, many countries are producing their own information and advocacy materials, though most have not been evaluated. Among those that appear to have had a significant impact, however, are the Bill Moyers TV series, now available on tapes(220) and the Last Acts website,(221) both in the United States.

Table 20 Points to consider when establishing an educational programme for the public

Palliative care will improve the patient's quality of life, even if the disease is incurable
Treatment exists that can relieve pain and many other symptoms
The pain drugs ought to be inexpensive
There is no need for patients to suffer prolonged and intolerable pain or other distressing symptoms
Drugs for the relief of pain can be taken indefinitely without losing their effectiveness
'Addiction' (psychological dependence) does not occur when morphine is taken to relieve pain
The medical use of morphine does not lead to abuse
Family, volunteers, and the community support systems can do much to improve the quality of life of the patients

Table 21 Networks: some organizations, associations, and initiatives covering international and regional palliative care

Organizations		
World Health Organization	WHO	www.who.int
United Nations AIDS programme	UNAIDS	www.UNAIDS.org
Foundations		
Diana, Princes of Wales Memorial Fund	DPWMF	www.theworkcontinues.org
Robert Wood Johnson Foundation	RWJF	www.rwjf.org
Last Acts		www.lastacts.org
Open Society Institute	OSI	www.soros.org
Associations		
International Association for Hospice and Palliative Care	IAHPC	www.hospicecare.com
Foundation for Hospices in Sub-Saharan Africa	FHSSA	PHarper@hospiceny.org
International Association for the Study of Pain	IASP	www.iasp-pain.org
European Association of Palliative Care	EAPC	www.eapcnet.org
Help the Hospices, UK Forum for Hospice and Palliative Care Worldwide		www.helpthehospices.org.uk
Indian Association of Palliative Care	IAPC	
Eastern and Central European Palliative Care Task Force	ECEPT	free.med.pl/ecept/index.html
Latin American Association of Palliative Care		
Asia Pacific Hospice Palliative Care Network		www.APHN.org
International Psycho-Oncology Society	IPOS	www.ipos-aspboa.org
International Association of Physicians in AIDS Care	IAPAC	www.iapac.org
Others		
WHO Collaborating Centre, Wisconsin, USA		www.medsch.wisc.edu/painpolicy
WHO Collaborating Centre, Oxford, UK		www.palliativecourses.com
WHO Collaborating Centre, Seoul, South Korea		www.cuk.ac.kr
International Observatory on End of Life Care, UK		www.eolc-observatory.net
Newsletters		
Cancer Pain Release		www.WHOcancerpain.wisc.edu
Hospice Information		www.hospiceinformation.info
IAHPC		www.hospicecare.com
Hospice Information Bulletin		www.hospiceinformation.info
World Hospice Palliative Care Online		avril@hospiceinformation.info
Palliatif (French)		irzpalli@vtx.ch
Manuals		
Doyle, D. and Woodruff, R. *Manual for Palliative Care*		www.hospicecare.com/manual/IAHPCmanual.htm

Networks

Organizations, foundations, and associations, like countries, are not excellent per se; but excellent individuals make excellent organizations, foundations, associations, and countries. Table 21 gives a list, with some known focal points, of excellent organizations and associations who play an important role in international networking, speeding up the global development of palliative care. The WHO, with its collaborating centres and global network, like UNAIDS, is truly worldwide and tends to prioritize developing countries. The International Association of Hospice and Palliative Care is truly international, with a comprehensive website. *Last Acts* is a campaign to implement end-of-life care through a coalition of professional and consumer organizations. Its website is open to all and represents an excellent model internationally for securing political commitment and action on the ground. The International Observatory on End of Life Care is a newly developed community effort seeking to provide research-based intelligence concerning policy-making, service development, and evaluation, which will promote the development of palliative care services internationally; it actively seeks collaborators and providers of information around the world. Other networks are mainly regional or national but also have helpful and informative websites and publications. The Open Society Institute, concentrates its support on Eastern Europe and Southern Africa. The Diana, Princess of Wales Memorial Fund is supporting the development of palliative care in Eastern and Southern Africa, as well as global advocacy. The European Association for Palliative Care has wide-ranging involvement across many countries. India has its own national association for palliative care and a quarterly journal. Many of these organizations produce newsletters for wide circulation, specially the electronic ones and provide updated information. The number of scientific and professional journals in palliative care continues to increase steadily and includes: *The Journal of Palliative Care, Palliative Medicine, The Journal of Palliative Medicine, The European Journal of Palliative Care, The Journal of Pain and Symptom Management, The International Journal of Palliative Nursing, Progress in Palliative Care, and The American Journal of Hospice and Palliative Care.*

The networks and activities suggest great promise for the future. 'Nothing can stop an idea whose time has come.'

References

1. **Epictetus.** *Discourses, Book II, AD 60–138,* quoting Euripides' 'Fragments', 480–906 BC.
2. **WHO.** *Cancer Pain Relief.* Geneva: WHO, 1987.
3. **WHO.** *Cancer Pain Relief. With a Guide to Opioid Availability* 2nd edn. Geneva: WHO, 1990.
4. **WHO.** *Symptom Relief in Terminal Illness.* Geneva: WHO, 1998.
5. **WHO.** *Cancer Pain Relief and Palliative Care in Children.* Geneva: WHO, 1998.
6. **WHO.** *Cancer Pain Relief and Palliative Care.* WHO Technical Report Series 804. Geneva: WHO, 1990.
7. **WHO.** *National Cancer Control Programmes: Policies and Managerial Guidelines.* WHO/CAN/92.1. Geneva: WHO, 1992.
8. **WHO.** *National Cancer Control Programmes: Policies and Managerial Guidelines.* Geneva: WHO, 1995.
9. **Swerdlow, M. and Stjernsward, J.** (1982). Cancer pain relief—an urgent public health problem. *World Health Forum* **3**, 329.
10. **Stjernswärd, J.** (1985). Cancer pain relief: an important global public health issue. In *Advances in Pain Research and Therapy* Vol. 9 (ed. H.L. Field et al.), pp. 555–8. New York: Raven Press.
11. **Stjernswärd, J., Stanley, K., and Tsechkovski, M.** (1985). Cancer pain relief: an urgent public health problem in India. *Clinical Journal of Pain* **1**, 95–7.
12. **Stjernswärd, J.** (1988). WHO Cancer Pain Relief Programme. *Cancer Surveys* **7**, 196–208.
13. **Stjernswärd, J., Colleau, S., and Ventafridda, V.** (1996). The World Health Organization cancer pain and palliative care program: past, present and future. *Journal of Pain and Symptom Management* **12** (2), 65–72.
14. **Stjernswärd, J.** (1993). Palliative medicine—a global perspective. In *Oxford Textbook of Palliative Medicine* 1st edn. (ed. D. Doyle, G. Hanks, and N. MacDonald), pp. 805–16. Oxford: Oxford Medical Publications.
15. **Stjernswärd, J.** (2002). Uganda: establishing a government public health approach to pain relief and palliative care. *Journal of Pain and Symptom Management* **3,** 257–64.
16. **Foley, K., Aulino, F., and Stjernswärd, J.** (2003). Palliative care in resource-poor settings. In *A Guide to Supportive and Palliative Care of People with HIV/AIDS* (ed. J. O'Neil and P. Selwyn), Rockville MD: HRSA, HIV/AIDS Bureau (in press).
17. **Stjernswärd, J.** (1989–1990). Editorial. *Newsletter. European Association for Palliative Care* No. 2, Winter.
18. **Stjernswärd, J.** (1994). The case for palliative care: a global problem addressed. *European Journal of Palliative Care* **1** (1), 6–7.
19. **Sepúlveda, C., Marlin, A., Yoshida, T., and Ullrich, A.** (2002). Palliative care: the World Health Organization's global perspective. *Journal of Pain and Symptom Management* **24** (2), 91–6.
20. **Murray, C. and Lopez, A.** *The Global Burden of Disease.* Oxford: Oxford University Press, 1996.
21. **WHO.** (2001). *World Health Report.* Annex, Table 2 (www.WHO.int/whr/2001/main/en/annex 2.htm and www.WHO.int/whr/2001/archives/1999/en/pdf/statistical annex.pdf).
22. **WHO.** *Ageing Programme.* Database. Courtesy of Dr A Kalache. Geneva: WHO, 2001.
23. **United Nations.** *United Nations Population Database: The Sex and Age Distribution of the World Populations.* New York: United Nations, 1998.
24. **WHO.** *Health and Ageing.* WHO/NMH/HPS/0.1. Geneva: WHO, 2001.
25. **United Nations.** *Population Division.* New York: United Nations, 2002.
26. **Stephen, P.** (1995). The curse of long life. *Financial Times,* 4 August, p. 18.
27. **Harding, J.** (1997). Is there a responsibility to die? Review. *Hastings Center Reports* **27** (2), 34–42.
28. **Callahan, D.** *What Kind of Life: The Limits of Medical Progress.* New York: Simon and Schuster, 1990.
29. **Parkin, D.M., Bray, F.I., and Devesa, S.S.** (2001). Cancer burden in the year 2000: the global picture. *European Journal of Cancer* **37**, 4–66.
30. **UNAIDS/WHO**, December 2002, www.who.int/hiv/pub/epidemiology.
31. **World Bank.** *World Development Report 2000/2001. Attacking Poverty.* Oxford and New York: Oxford University Press, 2000.
32. **Clark, D.** (2002). Between hope and acceptance: the medicalisation of dying. *British Medical Journal* **324**, 905–7.
33. http://www.library.ucla.edu/libraries/biomed/his/painexhibit/panel10.htm.
34. **Woodruff, R., Doyle, D., de Lima, L., Bruera, E., and Farr, W.C.** (2001). The International Association for Hospice and Palliative Care (IAHPC): history, description and future direction. *Journal of Palliative Medicine* **4** (1), 5–7.
35. **Bruera, E., de Lima, L., and Woodruff, R.** (2002). The International Association for Hospice and Palliative Care. *Journal of Pain and Symptom Management* **24** (2), 102–5.
36. **Bruera, E.** (1992). Palliative care programmes in Latin America. *Palliative Medicine* **6**, 182–4.
37. **Blumhuber, H., Kaasa, S., and de Conno, F.** (2002). The European Association for Palliative Care. *Journal of Pain and Symptom Management* **24** (2), 124–7.
38. **Saunders, C.** (2000). Global developments and the Hospice Information Service. Editorial. *Palliative Medicine* **14**, 1–2.
39. **Łuczak, J. and Kluziak, M.** (2001). The formation of ECEPT (Eastern and Central Europe Palliative Task Force): a Polish initiative. *Palliative Medicine* **15**, 259–60.
40. **The Poznan Declaration** (1998). *European Journal of Palliative Care* **6**, 61–3.
41. **Goh, C.R.** (2002). The Asia Pacific Hospice Palliative Care Network: a network for individuals and organisations. *Journal of Pain and Symptom Management* **24** (2), 128–33.
42. **Richardson, H., Praill, D., and Jackson, A.** (2002). The UK Forum for Hospice and Palliative Care Overseas. *European Journal of Palliative Care* **9** (2), 72–3.
43. **Speck, P.** (1999). Palliative care organisations with a global perspective. *Palliative Medicine* **13**, 69–74.

44. **Saunders, C. and Kastenbaum, R.**, ed. *Hospice Care on the International Scene.* New York: Springer, 1997.
45. **ten Have, H. and Clark, D.** *The Ethics of Palliative Care: European Perspectives.* Buckingham: Open University Press, 2002.
46. http://www.hospiceinformation.info/hospicesworldwide.asp.
47. http://www.chcr.brown.edu/dying/usastatistics.htm.
48. **Foley, K. and Hendin, H.** (2002). Conclusion: changing the culture. In *The Case Against Assisted Suicide* (ed. K. Foley and H. Hendin), p. 332. Baltimore: Johns Hopkins University Press.
49. **SUPPORT Principal Investigators** (1995). A controlled trial to improve care for seriously ill hospitalized patients: the Study to Understand Prognoses and Preferences for Outcomes and Risks of Treatment (SUPPORT). *Journal of the American Medical Association* **274**, 1591–8.
50. **Last Acts.** *Means to a Better End: A Report in Dying in America Today.* Washington: Last Acts, 2002: 3.
51. **Dahl, J.** (2002). Working with regulators to improve the standard of care in pain management: the US experience. *Journal of Pain and Symptom Management* **24** (2), 136–47.
52. **Grantee Profile: The Canadian Hospice Palliative Care Association.** *Project on Death in America Newsletter* Summer 2002, **10**, 8–9.
53. **Heyland, D.K., Lavery, J.V., Tranmer, J.E., Shortt, S.E.D., and Taylor, S.J.** (2000). Dying in Canada: is it an institutionalized, technologically supported experience? *Journal of Palliative Care* **16** (Suppl.) S10–16.
54. **Fainsinger, R.L.** (2002). Canada: palliative care and cancer pain. *Journal of Pain and Symptom Management* **24** (2), 173–6.
55. **Carstairs, S. and Chochinov, H.M.** (2001). Politics, palliation, and Canadian progress in end-of-life care. *Journal of Palliative Medicine* **4** (3), 396–9.
56. **Mount, B.** (1997). The Royal Victoria Hospital Palliative Care Service: a Canadian experience. In *Hospice Care on the International Scene* (ed. C. Saunders and R. Kastenbaum), pp. 73–76. New York: Springer.
57. **De Lima, L.** (2001). Advances in palliative care in Latin America and the Caribbean: ongoing projects of the Pan American Health Organization (PAHO). *Journal of Palliative Medicine* **4** (2), 228–31.
58. **Moyano, J., Ruiz, F., and Vainio, A.** (2002). Cancer pain management in Colombia. *European Journal of Palliative Care* **9** (3), 98–101.
59. **Stjernswärd, J.** et al. (1995). Opioid availability in Latin America: the Declaration of Florianopolis. *Journal of Pain and Symptom Management* **10** (3), 233–6.
60. **Bertolino, M. and Heller, K.S.** (2001). Promoting quality of life near the end of life in Argentina. *Journal of Palliative Medicine* **4** (3), 423–30.
61. **Bruera, E. and Sweeney, C.** (2002). Palliative care modes: international perspective. *Journal of Palliative Medicine* **5** (2), 319–27.
62. **De Simone, G.** (2000). Palliative care in Argentina. *Palliative Medicine* **14**, 323.
63. **Wenk, R., Bertolino, M., and Pussetto, J.** (2000). High opioid costs in Argentina: an availability barrier that can be overcome. Letter. *Journal of Pain and Symptom Management* **20** (2), 81–2.
64. **Maddocks, I.** (2000). Teaching palliative care in east Asia. *Palliative Medicine* **14**, 535–7.
65. **Yeom, C.H.** et al. (2000). Medical costs and quality of life in terminal cancer patients: a comparison of four care facilities. *Progress in Palliative* Care **8** (1), 5–11.
66. **Chung, Y.** (2000). Palliative care in Korea: a nursing point of view. *Progress in Palliative Care* **8** (1), 12–16.
67. **Wang, X.S., Yu, S., Gu, W., and Xu, G.** (2002). China: status of pain and palliative care. *Journal of Pain and Symptom Management* **24** (2), 177–9.
68. **Maruyama, T.C.** *Hospice Care and Culture.* Aldershot: Ashgate, 1999.
69. **Morita, T., Chihara, S., and Kashiwagi, T.** (2002). A scale to measure satisfaction of bereaved family receiving inpatient palliative care. *Palliative Medicine* **16**, 141–50.
70. **Ida, E., Miyachi, M., Uemura, M., Osakama, M., and Tajitsu, T.** (2002). Current status of hospice cancer deaths both in-unit and at home (1995–2000), and prospects of home care services in Japan. *Palliative Medicine* **16**, 179–84.
71. **Kawagoe, H. and Kawagoe, K.** (2000). Death education in hospice home care in Japan. *Journal of Palliative Care* **16** (3), 37–45.
72. **Takeda, F.** (1986). Results of field testing of the WHO draft interim guidelines on relief of cancer pain. *Pain Clinic* **1**, 83–9.
73. **Takeda, F.** (2002). Japan: status of cancer pain and palliative care. *Journal of Pain and Symptom Management* **24** (2), 197–9.
74. **Morita, T., Tsunoda, J., Inoue, S., and Chihara, S.** (2000). Concerns of Japanese hospice inpatients about morphine therapy as a factor in pain management: a pilot study. *Journal of Palliative Care* **16** (4), 54–8.
75. **Currow, D.** (2002). Australia: state of palliative care provision 2002. *Journal of Pain and Symptom Management* **24** (2), 170–2.
76. **Hunt, R., Fazekas, B.S., Luke, C.G., Priest, K.R., and Roder, D.M.** (2002). The coverage of cancer patients by designated palliative services: a population-based study, South Australia, 1999. *Palliative Medicine* **16**, 403–9.
77. **Allan, S.** (1999). Palliative care in New Zealand. Letter. *Progress in Palliative Care* **7** (3), 120–1.
78. **Burn, G.** (2001). A personal initiative to improve palliative care in India: ten years on. *Palliative Medicine* **15**, 159–62.
79. **Joranson, D.E., Rajagopal, M.R., and Gilson, A.M.** (2002). Improving access to opioid analgesics for palliative care in India. *Journal of Pain and Symptom Management* **24** (2), 152–9.
80. **Rajagopal, M.R.** (2002). Kerala, India: status of cancer pain relief and palliative care. *Journal of Pain and Symptom Management* **24** (2), 191–3.
81. **Sureshkumar, K. and Rajagopal, M.R.** (1996). Palliative care in India. *Palliative Medicine* **10**, 293–8.
82. **Ajithakumari, K., Sureshkumar, K., and Rajagopal, M.R.** (1997). Palliative home care: the Calicut experience. *Palliative Medicine* **11**, 451–4.
83. **Waller, A.** (1997). Hospice and palliative care services in Israel. In *Hospice Care on the International Scene* (ed. C. Saunders and R. Kastenbaum), pp. 235–41. New York: Springer.
84. **Sapir, R., Catane, R., Strauss-Liviatan, N., and Cherny, N.** (1999). Cancer pain: knowledge and attitudes of physicians in Israel. *Journal of Pain and Symptom Management* **17** (4), 266–76.
85. **Hammad, R.** (1997). The hospice experience in Jordan: Al-Malath Foundation for Humanistic Care. In *Hospice Care on the International Scene* (ed. C. Saunders and R. Kastenbaum), pp. 242–54. New York: Springer.
86. **Gray, A.J., Ezzart, A., and Boyar, M.D.** (1997). Palliative care for the terminally ill in Saudi Arabia. In *Hospice Care on the International Scene* (ed. C. Saunders and R. Kastenbaum), pp. 255–63. New York: Springer.
87. **Daher, M.** et al. (2002). Lebanon: pain relief and palliative care. *Journal of Pain and Symptom Management* **24** (2), 200–4.
88. **Isbister, W.H. and Bonifant, J.** (2001). Implementation of the World Health Organisation 'analgesic ladder' in Saudi Arabia. *Palliative Medicine* **15**, 135–40.
89. **Defilippi, K.** (2000). Palliative care issues in sub-Saharan Africa. *International Journal of Palliative Nursing* **6** (3), 108.
90. **The Diana, Princess of Wales Memorial Fund.** *Palliative Care Initiative: Palliative Care in Sub-Saharan Africa.* London: The Diana, Princess of Wales Memorial Fund, 2002.
91. **World Health Organization.** *Community Health Approach to Palliative Care and Cancer Patients in Africa.* Progress Report. Geneva: World Health Organization, October 2002.
92. **Foundation for Hospices in Sub-Saharan Africa.** *Challenging Times.* Liverpool, NY, USA, 2002.
93. **Williams, S.** (2000). Zimbabwe. *Palliative Medicine* **14**, 225–6.
94. **Khambatta-Perkin, A.** (1995). Island Hospice Service—Harare. *International Journal of Palliative Nursing* **1** (4), 226–7.
95. **Jagwe, J.G.M.** (2002). The introduction of palliative care in Uganda. *Journal of Palliative Medicine* **5** (1), 160–3.
96. **Merriman, A. and Heller, K.S.** (2002). Hospice Uganda—a model palliative care initiative in Africa: an interview with Anne Merriman. *Innovations in End of Life Care* **4** (3) (www.edc.org/lastacts).
97. **Merriman, A.** (2002). Uganda: current status of palliative care. *Journal of Pain and Symptom Management* **24** (2), 252–6.
98. **Gwyther, E.** (2002). South Africa: the status of palliative care. *Journal of Pain and Symptom Management* **24** (2), 236–8.
99. **Clark, D. and Wright, M.** *Transitions in End of Life Care: Hospice and Related Developments in Eastern Europe and Central Asia.* Buckingham: Open University Press, 2002.

100. **Clark, D.** (2002). Beacons in Eastern Europe. *European Journal of Palliative Care* **9** (5), 180.
101. **ten Have, H. and Clark, D.**, ed. *The Ethics of Palliative Care: European Perspectives.* Buckingham: Open University Press, 2002.
102. **ten Have, H. and Janssens, R.** *Palliative Care in Europe.* Amsterdam: IOS Press, 2001.
103. **Gómez Batiste, X., Borrás, J.M., Fontanals, M.D., Stjernswärd, J., and Trias, X.** (1992). Palliative care in Catalonia 1990–95. *Palliative Medicine* **6**, 321–7.
104. **Gómez-Batiste, X.** et al. (1996). Catalonia WHO Demonstration Project on Palliative Care Implementation, 1990–1995: results in 1995. *Journal of Pain and Symptom Management* **12** (2), 73–8.
105. **Gómez-Batiste, X., Porta, J., Tuca, A., Carrales, E., Madrid, F., Treils, J., Fontanals, D., Borrás, J., Stjernswärd, J., Salva, A., and Rius, E.** (2002). Spain: the WHO Demonstration Project of Palliative Care Implementation in Catalonia. Results at 10 years (1991–2001). *Journal of Pain and Symptom Management* **24** (2), 239–44.
106. **Toscani, F.** (2002). Palliative care in Italy: accident or miracle? Editorial. *Palliative Medicine* **16**, 177–8.
107. **Kaasa, S., Breivik, H., and Jordhoy, M.** (2002). Norway: development of palliative care. *Journal of Pain and Symptom Management* **24** (2), 211–14.
108. **Ligue Suisse Contré le Cancer and Societé Suisse de Medicin et Soins Palliatifs.** *Les soins palliaitifs en Suisse: état des lieux, 1999–2000.* Bern: Ligue Suisse Contré le Cancer/Societé Suisse de Medicin et Soins Palliatifs, 2000.
109. **Poulain, P.** (1998). The evolution of palliative care in France. *European Journal of Palliative Care* **5** (1), 4.
110. **Kumar, S.** (1998). The Calicut Declaration, November 1997. *European Journal of Palliative Care* **5** (3), 78.
111. **Fielding, R. and Chan, C.L.-W.** *Psychosocial Oncology and Palliative Care in Hong Kong.* Hong Kong: Hong Kong University Press, 2001.
112. **Ross, M.M., Dunning, J., and Edwards, N.** (2001). Palliative care in China: facilitating the process of development. *Journal of Palliative Care* **17** (4), 281–7.
113. **Tolentino, V.R. and Sulmasy, D.P.** (2002). A Spanish version of the McGill quality of life questionnaire. *Journal of Palliative Care* **18** (2), 91–6.
114. **Addington Hall, J.M. and Higginson, I.**, ed. *Palliative Care for Non-Cancer Patients.* Oxford: Oxford University Press, 2001.
115. **Prior, D.** (1999). Palliative care in marginalised communities. *Progress in Palliative Care* **7** (3), 109–15.
116. **Fried, O.** (1999). Many ways of caring: reaching out to aboriginal palliative care clients in Central Australia. *Progress in Palliative Care* **7** (3), 116–19.
117. **Morgan, J.D. and Laungani, P.**, ed. *Death and Bereavement Around the World. Volume 1: Major Religious Traditions.* Amityville NY: Baywood, 2002.
118. **Barnard, D.** (2001). Introduction: International Policy Report. *Journal of Palliative Medicine* **4** (3), 395.
119. **Maddocks, I.** (2000). How can opioid drugs be more widely and safely available? *Progress in Palliative Care* **8** (3), 125.
120. **De Lima, L. and Bruera, E.** (2000). The role of international treaties in the opioid availability process: relationship between INCB, national governments, the pharmaceutical industry and physicians. *Progress in Palliative Care* **8** (3), 128–32.
121. **Barnard, D.** (2001). Introduction: International Policy Report. *Journal of Palliative Medicine* **4** (2), 227.
122. **Mystakidou, K., Liossi, C., Fragiadakis, K., Georgaki, S., and Papadimitriou, J.** (1998). What do Greek physicians know about managing cancer pain? *Journal of Cancer Education* **13**, 39–42. (The study showed that among 1200 physicians, 42 per cent were reluctant to prescribe opioids for cancer pain.)
123. **Ng, L.F., Shumacher, A., and Goh, C.B.** (2000). Autonomy for whom? A perspective from the Orient. *Palliative Medicine* **14**, 163–4.
124. **Lin, C.-C.** (1999). Disclosure of the cancer diagnosis as it relates to the quality of pain management among patients with cancer in Taiwan. *Journal of Pain and Symptom Management* **18** (5), 331–7.
125. **Dein, S. and Thoms, K.** (2002). To tell or not to tell. *European Journal of Palliative Care* **9** (5), 209–12.
126. **Goncalves, J.F. and Castro, S.** (2001). Diagnosis disclosure in a Portuguese oncological centre. *Palliative Medicine* **15**, 35–41.
127. **Hosking, M., Whiting, G., Brathwate, C., Fox, P., Boshoff, A., and Robbins, L.** (2000). Cultural attitudes towards death and dying: a South African perspective. *Palliative Medicine* **14**, 437–9.
128. **Beauchamp, T.L. and Childress, J.F.** *Principles of Biomedical Ethics* 5th edn. Oxford: Oxford University Press, 2000.
129. **Maddocks, I.** (1999). Connecting with a terminally-ill world. *Progress in Palliative Care* **7** (4), 169–70.
130. **Callahan, D.** (2000). Justice, biomedical progress and palliative care. *Progress in Palliative Care* **8** (1), 3–4.
131. www.eolc-observatory.net.
132. **WHO.** *The Use of Essential Drugs.* WHO TRS: 895. Geneva: WHO, 2000.
133. **WHO** (1995). Essential drugs for cancer chemotherapy. A WHO meeting. *Bulletin of WHO* **63** (6), 999–1002.
134. **Sikora, K.** et al. (1999). WHO essential drugs for cancer therapy: a World Health Organization consultation. *Annals of Oncology* **10,** 385–90.
135. **Olweney, C., Sepúlveda, C., Merriman, A., Fonn, S., Borok, M., Mgoma, T., Doh, A., and Stjernswärd, J.** (2003). Guidelines for the treatment and palliative care of HIV disease patients with cancer in Africa. *Journal of Palliative Care* (in press).
136. **Wang'ombe, J.K. and Mwabu, G.M.** (1987). Economics of essential drugs schemes: the perspectives of the developing countries. *Social Science and Medicine* **25** (6), 615–30.
137. **Reich, M.R. and Govindaraj, R.** (1998). Dilemmas in drug development for tropical diseases. Experiences with praziquantel. *Health Policy* **44** (1), 1–18.
138. **Frisk, M.** (2000). Choice of drugs—by whom, for whom and to what costs? *Lakartiidningen* **97** (39), 4343–6 (in Swedish).
139. *Standard Treatment Guidelines and Essential Drugs List.* Pretoria: Essential Drugs Programme, Primary Health Care. Directorate Pharmaceutical Programmes and Planning, 1998.
140. *Essential Drug List for Zimbabwe (EDLIZ)*, including guidelines for treatment of medical conditions common in Zimbabwe. Harare: Ministry of Health and Child Welfare, 1989.
141. **Ministry of Health and Social Affairs.** *Lag (2002: 160) om Lakemedelsformaner m.m.* Stockholm: Socialdepartementet, 2002. Also www.lagrummet.gov.se and www.mpa.se.
142. **State of Wisconsin Legislature.** *Resolution on Cancer Pain.* Madison WI: State of Wisconsin Legislature, 1987.
143. **Dahl, J., Joranson, D.E., Engber, D., and Dosch, J.** (1988). The cancer pain problem: Wisconsin's response. A report on the Wisconsin Cancer Pain Initiative. *Journal of Pain and Symptom Management* **3**, S1–5.
144. **Wisconsin Cancer Pain Initiative.** *Cancer Pain can be Relieved: A Guide for Patients and Families.* Madison WI: Wisconsin Cancer Pain Initiative, 1988.
145. **Weissman, D.E., Burchman, S.L.K., Dinndorf, P.A., and Dahl, J.L.** *Handbook for Cancer Pain Management.* Madison WI: Wisconsin Cancer Pain Initiative, 1988.
146. **Wisconsin Cancer Pain Initiative.** *Children's Cancer Pain can be Relieved: A Guide for Parents and Families.* Madison WI: Wisconsin Cancer Pain Initiative, 1989.
147. **Wisconsin Cancer Pain Initiative.** *Jeff Asks About Cancer Pain: A Booklet for Teens about Cancer Pain.* Madison WI: Wisconsin Cancer Pain Initiative, 1990.
148. **Dahl, J.** (1980). The Wisconsin Pain Initiative. *Journal of Psychosocial Oncology* **8**, 125–37.
149. **Dahl, J.L.** (1993). State cancer pain initiatives. *Journal of Pain and Symptom Management* **8** (6), 372–5.
150. **Generalitat de Catalunya, Departament de Sanitat i Seguretat Social, Direccio General d'Ordenacio i Planifacacio Sanitaria.** *Catalan Cancer Control Programme.* Barcelona: Generalitat de Catalunya, 1991.
151. **Gómez-Batiste, X.** (1994). Catalonia's five-year plan: basic principles. *European Journal of Palliative Care* **1** (1), 45–9.
152. **Nair, M.K.** *Ten year Action Plan for Cancer Control in Kerala.* State Cancer Control Advisory Board, Health and Family Welfare Department, Go(Ms) No 26/88/H&FWD. Trivandrum, Kerala: St Joseph's Press, 1988.
153. **Dahl, J.L., Bennett, M.E., Bromley, M.D., and Joranson, D.** (2002). Success of the State Pain Initiatives. *Cancer Practitioner* **10** (Suppl.1), S9–13.
154. **Jacox, A.K.** et al. *Management of Cancer Pain. Clinical Practice Guidelines No. 9.* AHCPR Publication No. 94-0592. Rockville MD: Agency for Health Care Policy and Research, 1994.

155. **Jacox, A.K.** et al. *Management of Cancer Pain. Adults. Quick Reference Guide for Clinicians No. 9.* AHCPR Publication No. 94-0593. Rockville MD: Agency for Health Care Policy and Research, 1994.

156. **Jacox, A.K.** et al. *Management of Cancer Pain. Pediatric. Quick Reference Guide for Clinicians No. 9.* AHCPR Publication No. 94-0594. Rockville MD: Agency for Health Care Policy and Research, 1994.

157. **Jacox, A.K.** et al. *Management of Cancer Pain: A Patient's Guide. Clinical Practice Guideline No. 9* (Adult version—English). AHCPR Publication No. 94-0595. Rockville MD: Agency for Health Care Policy and Research, 1994.

158. **Rajagopal, M.R., Joranson, D., and Gilson, A.M.** (2001). Medical use, misuse and diversion of opioids in India. *Lancet* **385**, 139–43.

159. **Rajagopal, M.R. and Palat, G.** (2002). Kerala, India: status of cancer pain relief and palliative care. *Journal of Pain and Symptom Management* **24** (2), 191–3.

160. **International Narcotics Control Board (INCB)**. *Demographic Yearbook.* United Nations, 1999 and WHO Collaborating Center, University of Wisconsin, WI, 2002.

161. **Ministry of Health, Republic of Uganda**. *National Health Policy.* Kampala: Ministry of Health, 1999.

162. **Ministry of Health, Republic of Uganda**. *National Sector Strategic Plan 2000/01–2004/05.* Kampala: Ministry of Health, 2000.

163. **Ministry of Health, Republic of Uganda**. *Guidelines for Handling Class A Drugs—Uganda.* Kampala: Ministry of Health, 2001.

164. **Uganda**. *TASO Uganda: The Inside Story. Participatory evaluation of HIV/AIDS counselling, medical and social services 1993–1994.* WHO/GPA/TCO/HCS/95.1. Kampala: TASO and Geneva: WHO, 1995.

165. *Diana Palliative Care Initiative.* The Diana, Princess of Wales Memorial Fund, Press Kit, 2001.

166. **Ramsay, S.** (2001). Raising the profile of palliative care in Africa. *Lancet* **358**, 734.

167. **Hunter, S.S.** *Reshaping Societies. HIV/AIDS and Social Changes: A Resource Book for Planning, Programs and Policy Making.* Glen Falls NY: Hudson Run Press, 2000.

168. **Saunders, C.** *Hospice and Palliative Care: An Interdisciplinary Approach.* London: Edward Arnold, 1990.

169. **Merriman, A.** (2002). Uganda: current status of palliative care. *Journal of Pain and Symptom Management* **24** (2), 252–6.

170. **Directorate HIV/AIDS and STD**. *South Coast Hospice's Community Based HIV/AIDS Home Care Model.* Pretoria, South Africa: Department of Health, 1999.

171. **UNAIDS**. *Guide to the Strategic Planning Process for National Response to HIV/AIDS.* New York: United Nations, 2000 (www.unaids.org/publications).

172. **Ferris, F.D. and Cummings, I.**, ed. *Palliative Care: Towards Standardized Principles of Practice.* Ottawa, Ontario: The Canadian Palliative Care Association, 1995 (www.cpca.net).

173. **Pain and Policy Studies Group/WHO collaborating Center at the University of Wisconsin**, www.medsch.wisc.edu/painpolicy/

174. **International Narcotics Control Board.** *Demand for and Supply of Opiates for Medical and Scientific Needs.* New York: United Nations, 1989.

175. **International Narcotics Control Board**. *Estimated World Requirements for 1995. Statistics for 1993.* Vienna: United Nations, 1995.

176. **International Narcotics Control Board**. Table IX: Average daily consumption of defined daily doses per million inhabitants during the years 1989 to 1993. *International Narcotics Control Board Report.* Vienna: United Nations 1995, pp. 152–6.

177. **WHO**. *Cancer Pain Relief: A Guide to Opioid Availability.* WHO/CAN/92.3. Geneva: WHO, 1992.

178. **Clark, D.** (1993). Evaluating the needs of informal care givers. *Progress in Palliative Care* **1**, 3–5.

179. **Ferrell, B.R., Grant, M., Chan, J., Ahn, C., and Ferrell, B.A.** (1995). The impact of cancer pain education on family care givers of elderly patients. *Oncology Nursing Forum* **22**, 1211–18.

180. **Vachon, M.L., Kristjanson, L., and Higginson, I.** (1995). Psychosocial issues in palliative care: the patient, the family and outcome of care. *Journal of Pain and Symptom Management* **10**, 142–50.

181. **Stajduhar, K.L. and Davies, B.** (1998). Death at home: challenges for families and direction for the future. *Journal of Palliative Care* **14** (3), 8–14.

182. **Doyle, D.** *Caring for a Dying Relative: A Guide for Families.* Oxford: Oxford University Press, 1999.

183. **Harding, R., Leam, C., Pearce, A., Taylor, E., and Higginson, I.J.** (2002). A multiprofessional short-term group intervention for informal caregivers of patients using a home palliative care service. *Journal of Palliative Care* **18** (14), 275–81.

184. **Directorate HIV/AIDS and STD.** *South Africa: Curriculum for the Training of Community Based Home Caregivers.* Pretoria: Department of Health, 2001.

185. **Directorate HIV/AIDS and STD.** *South Africa: Comprehensive Home/Community Based Care Training Manual.* Pretoria: Department of Health, 2001.

186. **Directorate HIV/AIDS and STD.** *South Africa: Learners Handbook for the Training of Home/Community Based Caregivers.* Pretoria: Department of Health, 2001.

187. *Zimbabwe: Community Home Based Care Policy.* Harare, Zimbabwe: Ministry of Health and Child Welfare, 2001.

188. *Zimbabwe: Discharge Plan Guidelines for the Chronically/Terminally Ill Patients.* Harare, Zimbabwe: Ministry of Health and Child Welfare, reprinted 2001.

189. *Botswana: A Guide to the Assessment of the Client, and Family in Home Care.* Gaborone: WHO and AIDS/STD Unit, Ministry of Health, 2000.

190. *Botswana: HIV/AIDS Counsellor Training Guide.* Gaborone: WHO and AIDS/STD Unit, Ministry of Health, 2001.

191. *Botswana: Home Care Better Care: The Facilitator's Guide for Trainers of Trainers on the Use of Modules on Community Home Based Care.* Gaborone: WHO and AIDS/STD Unit, Ministry of Health, 2000.

192. *Tanzania: Needs Assessment Report for Tanzania. Community Health Approach to Palliative Care for HIV/AIDS and Cancer Patients Joint Project: WHO/Botswana, Ethiopia, Tanzania, Uganda, Zimbabwe.* Dar es Salaam: Tanzania Palliative Care Team, Ocean Road Cancer Institute, 2002.

193. **Kikule, E.** A study to assess the palliative care needs in terminally ill persons and their caregivers in Kampala District, Uganda. Dissertation. Kampala: Makerere University, 2000.

194. **Department of Education and Skills.** *A Teacher's Guide to Personal, Social and Health Education.* London: The Stationery Office, 1999.

195. **Abras, M.A.** (2002). Teaching children to understand death and grieving. *European Journal of Palliative Care* **6** (6), 256–7.

196. **Swedish National Board of Health and Welfare.** *Death Concerns Us All—Dignified Care at End of Life.* Expert Report. Stockholm: Socialstyrelson, 2001 (in Swedish with English summary).

197. **Doyle, D.** *The Platform Ticket: Memories and Musing of a Hospice Doctor.* Edinburgh: Pentland Press, 1999.

198. **Doyle, D.** *Palliative Care: The Management of the Far Advanced Illness.* London: Croom Helm, 1984.

199. **Wilkes, E.**, ed. *A Source Book of Terminal Care.* Sheffield: University of Sheffield, 1986.

200. **Saunders, C. and Baines, M.** *Living with Dying: The Management of Terminal Disease* 2nd edn. Oxford: Oxford University Press, 1989.

201. **Foley, K.M.** (1985). The treatment of cancer pain. *New England Journal of Medicine* **313**, 84–95.

202. **Twycross, R.G. and Lack, S.A.** *Therapeutics in Terminal Cancer* 2nd edn. London: Churchill Livingstone, 1990.

203. **MacDonald, N.**, ed. *Palliative Medicine: A Case-based Manual.* Oxford: Oxford University Press, 2001.

204. **Ferris, F.D. and Cummings, I.**, ed. *Palliative Care: Towards Standardized Principles of Practice.* Ottawa, Ontario: The Canadian Palliative Care Association, 1995 (www.cpca.net).

205. **Ferris, F.D., Flannery, J. S., McNeal, H.B., Morissette, M.R., Cameron, R., and Balley, G.A.**, ed. *A Comprehensive Guide for the Care of Persons with HIV Disease, Module 4: Palliative Care.* Toronto, Ontario: Mount Sinai Hospital and Casey House Hospice, 1995.

206. **Victoria Hospice Society.** *Pocket Booklet: Medical Care of the Dying.* Victoria BC, Canada: Victoria Hospice Society, 1999.

207. **Regnard, S. and Tempest, S.** *A Guide to Symptom Relief in Advanced Cancers.* Oxford: Butterworth-Heinemann, 1993.

208. **Librach, L. and Squires, B.P.** *The Pain Manual, Principles and Issues in Pain Management.* Montreal, Canada: Pegasus International, 2000.

209. **Spross, J.A., McGuire, D.B., and Schmitt, R.M.** *Oncology Nursing Society Position Paper on Cancer Pain.* Oncology Nursing Press, 1991. (Also published as three parts in *Oncology Nursing Forum* 1991, **17**, 4–6.)

210. **Ferrell, B.R. and Coyle, N.** *Textbook of Palliative Nursing.* New York: Oxford University Press, 2001.

211. **Doyle, D. and Jeffrey, D.** *Palliative Care in the Home.* Oxford: Oxford University Press, 2000.

212. **Doyle, E.**, ed. *Domiciliary Palliative Care: A Handbook for Family Doctors and Community Nurses.* Oxford General Practice Series. Oxford: Oxford University Press, 1994.

213. **Doyle, D., Hanks, G.W.C., and MacDonald, N.**, ed. *Oxford Textbook of Palliative Medicine* 1st and 2nd edn. Oxford: Oxford University Press, 1993 and 1998.

214. **Merriman, A.** *Palliative Medicine. Pain and Symptom Control in the Cancer and/or AIDS Patients in Uganda and Other African Countries* 3rd edn. Kisubhi, Entebbe, Uganda: Marianum Press, 2002. (Adapted from D. Doyle and T.F. Benson, *Palliative Medicine: Pain and Symptom Control,* 1991.)

215. **Ministry of Health, Bostwana and WHO.** *Clinical Management of HIV Infection in Adults, Vol. 1: Botswana Guidelines for District, Referral and Primary Hospitals.* Gaborone: AIDS/STD Unit, Ministry of Health, 1998.

216. **The Robert Wood Johnson Foundation and American Medical Association.** *Education for Physician on End of Life Care, EPEC Trainers Guide.* USA: Robert Wood Johnson Foundation and American Medical Association, 1999.

217. **Fields, H.L.**, ed. *Task Force on Professional Education in Pain: Core Curriculum for Professional Education in Pain.* Seattle WA: International Association for the Study of Pain Publications, 1991.

218. **International Society of Nurses in Cancer Care (ISCNN)** (1990). A core curriculum for a post-basic course in palliative care nursing. *Palliative Medicine* **4**, 261–70.

219. **End of Life Nursing Education Consortium.** ELNEC, Training Program. USA: Robert Wood Johnson Foundation and American Association of Colleges of Nursing.

220. **Moyers, W.J.** *On Our Own Terms: Moyers on Dying.* A four-part documentary, PBS Public Television (broadcast September 2000) (www.rwj.org).

221. www.lastacts.org.

Appendix

Useful sources of information

International

European Association for Palliative Care, National Cancer Institute of Milan, Via Venezian 1, 20133 Milan, Italy
www.eapcnet.org

Hospice Information, Hospice House, 34 Britannia Street, London WC1X 9JG, UK
www.hospiceinformation.info

Help the Hospices, Hospice House, 34 Britannia Street, London WC1X 9JG, UK
www.helpthehospices.org.uk

Macmillan Cancer Relief, 89 Albert Embankment, London SE1 7UQ, UK
www.macmillan.org.uk

Marie Curie Cancer Care, 89 Albert Embankment, London SE1 7TP, UK
www.mariecurie.org.uk

National Council for Hospice and Specialist Palliative Care Services, Hospice House, 34 Britannia Street, London WC1X 9JG, UK
www.hospice-spc-council.org.uk

Sue Ryder Care, Health Care Services, PO Box 5044, Ashby de la Zouch, Leics, LE65 1ZP, UK
www.suerydercare.org

Hospice Educational Institute, 3 Unity Square, PO Box 98, Machiasport, Maine 94655-0098, USA
www.hospiceworld.org

World Health Organization, Programme on Cancer Control, 20 Avenue Appia, Geneva 1211, Switzerland

WHO/PANO Focal Point for Palliative Care, To Latin America and the Caribbean, UT MD Anderson Cancer Center, 1515 Holmcombe Bouleward #8, Houston, TX, USA
www.mdanderson.org/departments/palliative

European and Central Europe Palliative Care Task Force, (EDEPT), C/o Palliative Care Department, Ul. Lakowa, 61-878 Poznan, Poland

Palliative Care in Eastern Europe (EAPC Propect), Stockholms Sjukhem Foundation, Mariebergspatan, 22, S-112 35 Stockholm
www.eapceast.org

International Association for Hospice and Palliative Care, MD Anderson Cancer Center, 1515 Holmcombe Boulevard #8, Houston, Texas, USA.
www.hospicecare.com

National organizations

Argentina

AAMCYP, Av.Roque Saenz Pena 94433 6 to '67', Buenos Aires, Argentina

Australia

National Palliative Care Organisation, PO Box 24 Deakin West, ACT 1600, Australia
www.pallcare.org.au

Austria

Hospiz Österreich, Menschenwurde Bis Zuletzt, Lainzerstrasse 138, A-1130 Vienna, Austria
www.hospiz.at

Belgium

Societe Belge de Medicine Palliative, Centre de Douleur, CHU de Liege, Domaine Universitaire du Sart Tilman, BB-4000 Liege 1

Brazil

Associacao Brasileira de Cuidados Palliativos, Rua Bissau 88 Cep 04543-020, San Paulo, SP, Brazil

Canada

Canadian Hospice Palliative Care Association, 131c-43 Bruyere Street, Ottawa, Ontario K1N 5C8, Canada
www.chpca.net

Colombia

Assiocion Colombiana de Cuidados Palliativos, Clle 130 B No. 11-26 Apto 401, Edif Pinos del Norte, Bogota, Colombia

Costa Rica

Unidad de Cuidados Palliativos, Hospital Max Peralta de Cartago, PO Box Apartado postal 13 codigo 7100, Paraiso de Cartago, Costa Rica

China

National Hospice Society, C/o Tiajin Medical University, Qixiangtai Road, Tiannjin 3000700, PRC

Croatia

CSHPC—Croatian Society for Hospice/Palliative Care, Gunduliceva 49, Zagreb 10000, Croatia
www.mefst.hr

Czech Republic

Association of Providers of Hospice Care, Betlemska 14, 110 00 Praha 1, Czech republic

Denmark

Danish Society of Palliative Medicine, Kristianiagade 14, 4 tv, DK2100 Copenhagen, Denmark

Finland

Finnish Association of Palliative Care, Pirkanmaa Hospice, PL60, 33501 Tampere, Finland

France

SFAP, 106 avenue Emile Zola, Paris 75015, France

Germany

DGP Deutsche Gesellschaft für Palliativmedizin Malteser Krankebhaus Bonn Hardberg, Zentrum für Palliativmedizin Rheinische Fredrich-Wilhems-Universitat Bonn, Von Hompesch Str 1, 53123 Bonn, Germany
www.dgpalliativmedizin.de

Greece

Hellenic Society of Palliative–Symptomatic Care Anaesthetic Department, University of Athens, 452 Mesogeoin Str, 15342 Athens, Greece

Hong Kong

Hong Kong Society of Palliative Medicine, C/o Haven of Hope Hospice, Po Lam Road South, Tseung Kwan O, Kowloon, Hong Hong

Hungary

Magyar Hospice-Palliativ Egyesulet, 1091 Budapest Ulloi ut 47-51, Hungary

India

Indian Association of Palliative Care/Pain and Palliative Care Society, Medical College and Hospital, Calicut 673008, Kerala, India

Indonesia

Indonesia Palliative Society, C/o Palliative care Unit, Dr Soetomo Hospital, JL Mayjen Prof. Dr Moestopo 6-8, Surabaya 60286, Indonesia

Ireland

Irish Association for Palliative Care, PO Box 5593, Ballsbridge, Dublin 4, Ireland
www.iapc.ie

Israel

Israel Association for Palliative Care, PO Box 324, 36046 Kiryat Tivon, Israel

Italy

SICP, Piazza Castello 4, 20133, Milan, Italy
www.sicp.it

Japan

Japan Society for Palliative Medicine, Ayumi Corporation, 507 Tenshin-bill 1-12-14 Hori, Kyomachi Osaka-shi 5500003, Osaka, Japan

Japanese Association of Hospice and Palliative Care Units, Seirei-Mikatahara General Hospital, 3454 Mikagataha-oho Hamamatsu-shi, Shiziouka 433-8558, Japan

Korea

Korean Society for Hospice and Palliative Care, Department of Internal Medicine, The Catholic University, St Mary's Hospital, #62 Youido-Dong Youngdungpo-Gu, Seoul 150-713, South Korea

Latvia

PAAL, Latvijas Onkologijas Centrs, Hipocrata iela 4, LV 1079 Riga, Latvia

Luxembourg

OMEGA 80, 138 rue Adolphe Fischer, 1521 Luxembourg

Malaysia

Malaysian Hospice Council/The National Cancer Society, A2 27 Komtar, .0000 Penang, Malaysia

Malta

Malta Hospice Movement, 35 Good Shepherd Avenue, Balzan, BZN 16, Malta

Mexico

Unidad de Cuidados Palliativos, Instituto Nacionale de Cancerologia, San Fernando 22, Tialpan, Mexica, DF 1400

Netherlands

NPTN, PO Box 189 3980, GB Bunnik, The Netherlands
www.palliatief.nl

New Zealand

Hospice New Zealand, 6th Floor, Molesworth House, 101 Molesworth Street, PO Box 12 481, Wellington, New Zealand
www.hospice.org.nz

Nigeria

Hospice Nigeria, 14 Obanikoru Street, off Ikorodu Road, Lagos, Nigeria

Norway

Nordisk forening—omsorg ved livets slutt for Sykepleivitenskap, Hans Tanksgt 11 N 5008, Bergen, Norway

Philippines

National Hospice Coordinating Council, C/o Philippine Cancer Society, 310 San Rafael Street, San Miguel, Manila

Poland

Polish National Council for Palliative/Hospice Services, C/o Palliative Care Department, Karol Marchinkowski University of Science, ul, Lakowa 1/2 Poznan 61-878, Poland

Portugal

ANCP, Unidade de Cuidados Palliativos, Instituto Portugues de Oncologia, Rua DR, Antonio Bernardino de Almeida, 4200–070 Porto, Portugal

Romania

Asociatia Nationale de Ingrijire Palliativa, Centru de Studii Pentru Medicina Palliativa, St Piatra Mare Nr 101, Brasov 2200, Romania

Russia

Association of Russian Hospices, C/o Samara Hospice, Entyziastiov 29, Samara 443067, Russia

Saudi Arabia

Section of Palliative Care Medicine, Dept. Of Oncology MBC 64, King Faisal Specialist Hospital and Research Centre, PO Box 3354, Riyadh 11211, Saudi Arabia

Singapore

Singapore Hospice Council, C/o 10 Jalan Tan Tock Send, Singapore 308436

South Africa

Hospice and Palliative Care Association of South Africa, PO Box 38785, Pinelands 7439, Cape Town
www.hospice.co.za

Spain

www.secpal.com/directorio

Sweden

Swedish Association for Palliative Medicine, Magle Lilia Kyrkog 17, S 223 51 Lund, Sweden
www.sfpm.org

Switzerland

SSMPS, Equie mobile de Soins Palliatifs, 36 Avenue Cardinal Mermillod, 1227 Carouge, Switzerland

Taiwan

Taiwan Academy of Hospice Palliative Medicine (TAHPM), No. 45 Min Sheng Road, Tamsui, Taipei
www.hospicemed.org.tw

Hospice Foundation of Taiwan, 16F, No 92, Sec 2, Chung San North Road, Taipei 10449, Taiwan
www.hospice.org.tw

Uganda

Ugandan Palliative Care Association, C/o Hospice Uganda, PO Box 7757, Kampala
hospice-Africa.Merseyside.org

United Kingdom

Association for Palliative Medicine of Great Britain and Ireland, 11 Westwood Road, Southampton, SO17 1DL, UK
www.palliative-medicine.org

USA

National Hospice and Palliative Care Organization, 1700 Diagonal Road, Suite 625, Alexandria, VA 22314, USA
www.nhpco.org

Hospice Association of America, 228 Seventh Street, SE, Washington DC 20003–4306, USA
www.nahc.org (click on 'affiliates')

Index

Main index entries are given in **bold.**
Page numbers in *italics* refer to tables.